Clinical Immunology
Principles and Practice

Commissioning Editor: *Thu Nguyen*
Development Editor: *Martin Mellor Publishing Services Ltd, Louise Cook*
Project Manager: *Gemma Lawson*
Design Manager: *Charles Gray*
Illustration Manager: *Bruce Hogarth*
Illustrator: *Danny Pyne, Martin Woodward*
Marketing Manager (UK/USA): *Clara Toombs / William Veltre*

Clinical Immunology
Principles and Practice

THIRD EDITION

Edited by

ROBERT R. RICH MD

Senior Vice President
Dean of School of Medicine
Professor of Medicine and Microbiology
University of Alabama at Birmingham
Birmingham, AL
USA

THOMAS A. FLEISHER MD

Chief, Department of Laboratory Medicine
Chief, Immunology Service, DLM
NIH Clinical Center
National Institutes of Health
Bethesda, MD
USA

WILLIAM T. SHEARER MD, PhD

Chief, Allergy and Immunology Service
Medical Director, AIDS Center
Texas Children's Hospital
Professor of Pediatrics and Immunology
Head, Section of Allergy and Immunology
Department of Pediatrics
Baylor College of Medicine
Houston, TX
USA

HARRY W. SCHROEDER, JR MD, PhD

Professor
Departments of Medicine, Microbiology and Genetics
University of Alabama at Birmingham
Birmingham, AL
USA

ANTHONY J. FREW MD, FRCP

Professor of Allergy and Respiratory Medicine
Department of Respiratory Medicine
Brighton General Hospital
Brighton
UK

CORNELIA M. WEYAND MD, PhD

David Lowance Professor of Medicine
Director, Lowance Center for Human Immunology
and Rheumatology
Director, Division of Rheumatology
Emory University School of Medicine,
Atlanta, GA
USA

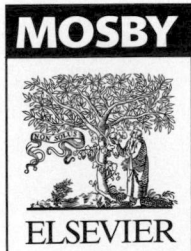

MOSBY

ELSEVIER

MOSBY
ELSEVIER

An imprint of Elsevier Limited

First edition 1996
Second edition 2001
Third edition 2008

The right of Robert R. Rich, Thomas A. Fleisher, William T. Shearer, Harry W. Schroeder Jr., Anthony J. Frew, and Cornelia M. Weyand to be identified as authors of this work has been asserted by them in accordance with the Copyright, Designs and Patents Act 1988.

Dr. Fleisher edited this book in his private capacity and no official endorsement of support by the National Institutes of Health or the Department of Health and Human Services is intended or should be inferred.

ISBN 978-0-323-04404-2

British Library Cataloguing in Publication Data
A catalogue record for this book is available from the British Library

Library of Congress Cataloging in Publication Data
A catalog record for this book is available from the Library of Congress

Notice
Medical knowledge is constantly changing. Standard safety precautions must be followed, but as new research and clinical experience broaden our knowledge, changes in treatment and drug therapy may become necessary or appropriate. Readers are advised to check the most current product information provided by the manufacturer of each drug to be administered to verify the recommended dose, the method and duration of administration, and contraindications. It is the responsibility of the practitioner, relying on experience and knowledge of the patient, to determine dosages and the best treatment for each individual patient. Neither the publisher nor the author assume any liability for any injury and/or damage to persons or property arising from this publication.

The Publisher

ELSEVIER
your source for books, journals and multimedia in the health sciences
www.elsevierhealth.com

Working together to grow libraries in developing countries
www.elsevier.com | www.bookaid.org | www.sabre.org

ELSEVIER   BOOK AID International   Sabre Foundation

The Publisher's policy is to use paper manufactured from sustainable forests

Printed in China
Last digit is the print number: 9 8 7 6 5 4 3 2 1

Contents

PART 1: FUNDAMENTAL PRINCIPLES OF THE IMMUNE RESPONSE

Contents

Contents

Contents

Contents

Contributors

SHIZUO AKIRA MD, PhD

Director, Akira Innate Immunity Project
Exploratory Research for Advanced Technology (ERATO)
Japan Science Technology Agency (JST);
Professor, Department of Host Defense
Research Institute for Micorbial Diseases
Osaka University
Osaka
Japan

JUAN ANGUITA PhD

Assistant Professor
Veterinary and Animal Sciences
University of Massachusetts
Amherst, MA
USA

GREGORY M. ANSTEAD MD, PhD

Director, Immunosuppression Clinic
South Texas Veterans Healthcare System;
Assistant Professor, Department of Medicine
Division of Infectious Diseases
University of Texas Health Science Center at San Antonio
San Antonio, TX
USA

CYNTHIA ARANOW MD

Associate Professor
Center of Autoimmune Disease
The Feinstein Institute for Medical Research
Manhasset, NY
USA

HOWARD A. AUSTIN III MD

Clinical Investigator
Clinical Research Center
National Institute of Diabetes and Digestive and Kidney Diseases
National Institutes of Health
Bethesda, MD
USA

SUBASH BABU MBS, PhD

Staff Scientist, Helminth Immunology Section
Laboratory of Parasitic Diseases
National Institute of Allergy and Infectious Diseases
National Institutes of Health
Bethesda, MD
USA

JAMES R. BAKER JR MD

Division Chief, Allergy and Clinical Immunology
Department of Internal Medicine;
Director, The MI Nanotechnology Institute for Medicine
and Biological Sciences
Ann Arbor, MI
USA

CHRISTOPHER S. BALIGA MD

Resident, Department of Medicine
University Hospitals of Cleveland
Case Western Reserve University
Cleveland, OH
USA

MARK BALLOW MD

Chief, Division of Allergy and Immunology
Department of Pediatrics SUNY Buffalo School of Medicine
Women and Children's Hospital of Buffalo
Buffalo, NY
USA

JAMES E. BALOW MD

Clinical Director
Clinical Research Center; Kidney Disease Section
National Institute of Diabetes and Digestive and Kidney Diseases
National Institutes of Health
Bethesda, MD
USA

EMIL J. BARDANA JR MD, CM

Professor of Medicine
Division of Allergy and Clinical Immunology
Oregon Health and Science University
Portland, OR
USA

MATTHIAS D. BECKER MD, PhD, FEBO

Professor of Ophthalmology
Interdisciplinary Uveitis Center
University of Heidelberg
Heidelberg
Germany

JOHN W. BELMONT MD, PhD

Professor
Department of Molecular and Human Genetics
Baylor College of Medicine
Houston, TX
USA

DINA BEN-YEHUDA MD

Head, Department of Hematology
Hadassah Hebrew University Medical Center
Jerusalem
Israel

CLAUDIA BEREK PhD

Senior Scientist
B Cell Immunology
Deutsches Rheuma-ForschungsZentrum (DRFZ)
Berlin
Germany

THOMAS BIEBER MD, PhD

Professor of Dermatology and Allergy
Chairman and Director
Department of Dermatology and Allergy
University of Bonn
Bonn
Germany

JOHANNES W.J. BIJLSMA MD, PhD

Rheumatologist
Professor and Head
Department of Rheumatology and Clinical Immunology
University Medical Center Utrecht
Utrecht
The Netherlands

JACK J.H. BLEESING MD, PhD

Attending Physician
Division of Hematology/Oncology
Cincinnati Children's Hospital Medical Center
Cincinnati, OH
USA

SARAH E. BLUTT PhD

Assistant Professor
Department of Molecular Virology and Microbiology
Baylor College of Medicine
One Baylor Plaza
Houston, TX
USA

ELENA BORZOVA MD, PhD

Clinical Research Fellow
Dermatology Centre
Norfolk and Norwich University Hospital
Norwich
UK

PROSPER N. BOYAKA PhD

Associate Professor
Department of Veterinary Biosciences
The Ohio State University
Columbus, OH
USA

KNUT BROCKOW MD

Dermatologist, Allergologist;
Senior Medical Staff; Lecturer
Department of Dermatology and Allergy Biederstein
Technical University Munich
Munich
Germany

RALPH C. BUDD MD

Director
Vermont Center for Immunology and Infectious Diseases;
Professor of Medicine
University of Vermont College of Medicine
Burlington, VT
USA

FRANK BUTTGEREIT MD

Deputy Clinical Director
Department of Rheumatology and Clinical Immunology
Charité University Hospital
CCM, Berlin
Germany

VIRGINIA L. CALDER PhD

Lecturer in Immunology
Institute of Ophthalmology
University College London
London
UK

FABIO CANDOTTI MD

Senior Investigator
Genetics and Molecular Biology Branch;
Head, Disorders of Immunity Section
National Human Genome Research Institute
National Institutes of Health
Bethesda, MD
USA

SEBASTIAN CAROTTA PhD

Erwin Schrödinger Fellow
Immunology Division
The Walter and Eliza Hall Institute of Medical Research
Parkville, Victoria
Australia

JEAN-LAURENT CASANOVA MD, PhD

Professor of Pediatrics
Laboratory of Human Genetics and Infectious Diseases
Faculty of Medicine
René Descartes University of Paris;
Department of Immunology and Paediatric Hematology
Necker Sick Children's Hospital
APHP
Paris
France

MARILIA CASCALHO MD, PhD

Assistant Professor
Departments of Surgery, Immunology and Pediatrics
Mayo Clinic
Rochester, MN
USA

EDWIN S.L. CHAN MD, FRCPC

Assistant Professor
Department of Medicine
New York University School of Medicine
New York, NY
USA

JAVIER CHINEN MD, PhD

Assistant Professor
Department of Pediatrics
Allergy and Immunology Section
Baylor College of Medicine
Houston, TX
USA

MONIQUE E. CHO MD

Clinical Investigator
Kidney Disease Branch
National Institute of Diabetes and Digestive and Kidney Diseases
National Institutes of Health
Bethesda, MD
USA

LISA CHRISTOPHER-STINE MD, MPH

Co-Director
Johns Hopkins Myositis Center;
Assistant Professor, Division of Rheumatology
Department of Medicine
Johns Hopkins University School of Medicine
Baltimore, MD
USA

Contributors

HELEN L. COLLINS PhD

Lecturer in Immunology
Division of Immunology
Infection and Inflammatory Diseases
Kings College London
London
UK

ANDREW P. COPE BSc, PhD, MBBS, FRCP, ILTM

Head of Molecular Medicine
Reader in Molecular Medicine;
Honorary Consultant in Rheumatology
The Kennedy Institute of Rheumatology
Faculty of Medicine
Imperial College London
London
UK

IRENE CORTESE MD

Clinical Fellow
Neuroimmunology Branch
National Institute of Neurological Disorders and Stroke
National Institutes of Health
Bethesda, MD
USA

BRUCE N. CRONSTEIN MD

Professor of Medicine, Pathology and Pharmacology
Department of Medicine (Clinical Pharmacology);
Department of Pathology and Pharmacology
New York University School of Medicine
New York, NY
USA

ADNAN CUSTOVIC MD, PhD

Professor of Allergy
University of Manchester
Manchester
UK

MARINOS C. DALAKAS MD

Chief, Neuromuscular Diseases Section
National Institutes of Health
Bethesda, MD
USA

BLYTHE H. DEVLIN PhD

Assistant Research Professor
Department of Pediatrics
Duke University Medical Center
Durham, NC
USA

BETTY DIAMOND MD

Chief, Center of Autoimmune Disease
The Feinstein Institute for Medical Research
Manhasset, NY
USA

ANGELA DISPENZIERI MD

Associate Professor of Medicine
Division of Hematology
Mayo Clinic
Rochester, MN
USA

JOOST P.H. DRENTH MD, PhD

Professor of Molecular Gastroenterology and Hepatology
Division of Gastroenterology and Hepatology
Department of Medicine
Radboud University Nijmegen Medical Center
Nijmegen
The Netherlands

TERRY W. DU CLOS MD, PhD

Professor, Department of Internal Medicine
University of New Mexico School of Medicine;
Chief of Rheumatology
Veteran's Administration Medical Center
Albuquerque, NM
USA

MARK S. DYKEWICZ MD, FACP, FAAAAI

Professor of Internal Medicine
Allergy and Immunology Program Director
Saint Louis University School of Medicine
St Louis, MO
USA

TODD N. EAGAR PhD

Assistant Professor
Department of Neurology and Department of Immunology
University of Texas Southwestern Medical School
Dallas, TX
USA

GEORGE S. EISENBARTH MD, PhD

Executive Director
Barbara Davis Center for Childhood Diabetes;
Professor of Pediatrics, Immunology and Medicine
University of Colorado Health Sciences Center
Aurora, CO
USA

CHARLES O. ELSON III MD

Professor of Medicine and Microbiology
University of Alabama at Birmingham
Birmingham, AL
USA

DORUK ERKAN MD

Associate Physician-Scientist
The Barbara Volcker Center for Women and Rheumatic Disease;
Assistant Attending Physician
Hospital for Special Surgery;
Assistant Professor of Medicine
Weill Medical College of Cornell University
New York, NY
USA

MARK FEINBERG MD, PhD

Vice President
Policy, Public Health and Medical Affairs
Merck Vaccines
West Point, PA
USA

EROL FIKRIG MD

Professor of Medicine, Microbial Pathogenesis
Epidemiology and Public Health
Section of Rheumatology
Department of Internal Medicine
Yale University School of Medicine
New Haven, CT
USA

ALAIN FISCHER MD, PhD

Professor of Pediatrics
Director of the Pediatric Immunology Department and INSERM
Laboratory 'Normal and Pathological Development of the Immune
System'
Feculté de medicine
René Descartes
Paris
France

THOMAS A. FLEISHER MD

Chief, Department of Laboratory Medicine
Chief, Immunology Service, DLM
NIH Clinical Center
National Institutes of Health
Bethesda, MD
USA

ANDREW P. FONTENOT MD

Henry N. Clamen Associate Professor
Department of Medicine
University of Colorado at Denver and Health Sciences Center
Denver, CO
USA

KAREN A. FORTNER PhD

Research Assistant Professor
Immunobiology Program
Department of Medicine
The University of Vermont College of Medicine
Burlington, VT
USA

ANTHONY J. FREW MD, FRCP

Professor of Allergy and Respiratory Medicine
Department of Respiratory Medicine
Brighton General Hospital
Brighton
UK

THEA M. FRIEDMAN PHD

Associate Scientist
Director, Laboratory Services
The Cancer Center
Hackensack University Medical Center
Hackensack, NJ
USA

KOHTARO FUJIHASHI DDS, PhD

Professor, School of Dentistry;
Co-Director, Immunobiology Vaccine Center
The University of Alabama
Birmingham, AL
USA

STEPHEN J. GALLI MD

Mary Hewitt Loveless Professor
Professor of Pathology and of Microbiology and Immunology;
Chair, Department of Pathology
Stanford University School of Medicine
Stanford, CA
USA

MOSHE E. GATT MD

Fellow, Lecturer
Department of Hematology
Hadassah Hebrew University Medical Center
Jerusalem
Israel

M. ERIC GERSHWIN MD

Distinguished Professor of Medicine
The Jack and Donald Chia Professor
of Medicine;
Chief, Division of Rheumatology
Allergy and Clinical Immunology
Genome and Biomedical Sciences Facility
University of California at Davis
Davis, CA
USA

JÖRG J. GORONZY MD, PhD

Mason I. Lowance MD Professor of Medicine
Director, Kathleen B. and Mason I. Lowance Center for Human
Immunology
Department of Medicine
Emory University School of Medicine
Atlanta, GA
USA

CLIVE E.H. GRATTAN MD, FRCP

Consultant Dermatologist
Dermatology Centre
Norfolk and Norwich University Hospital
Norwich
UK

NEIL S. GREENSPAN MD, PhD

Professor, Department of Pathology
Case Western Reserve University
Cleveland, OH
USA

BEATRIX GRUBECK-LOEBENSTEIN MD

Director, Institute for Biomedical Aging Research
Austrian Academy of Sciences
Austria

GABRIELLE HAEBERLI MD

Senior Resident, Division of Allergology
Bern Ziegler Hospital
Bern
Switzerland

RUSSELL P. HALL III MD

J. Lamar Callaway Professor and Chief
Division of Dermatology
Department of Medicine;
Professor, Department of Immunology
Duke University Medical Center
Durham, NC
USA

ROBERT G. HAMILTON PhD, D.ABMLI

Professor of Medicine and Pathology
Johns Hopkins Asthma and Allergy Center
Johns Hopkins University School of Medicine
Baltimore, MD
USA

GREGORY R. HARRIMAN MD

Vice President, Research and Development
Therakos, Exton, PA
USA

KHALED M. HASSAN BA

BS Pre-Doctoral Research Fellow
Division of Dermatology
Department of Medicine
Duke University Medical Center
Durham, NC
USA

ARTHUR HELBLING MD, FAAAI

Professor of Internal Medicine and Allergology
Department for Rheumatology and Clinical Immunology/
Allergology
Inselspital
University of Bern
Bern, Switzerland

DAVID B. HELLMANN MD, MACP

Vice Dean and Chairman
Department of Medicine
Johns Hopkins Bayview Medical Center;
Aliki Perroti Professor of Medicine
Johns Hopkins University School of Medicine
Baltimore, MD
USA

VIVIAN HERNANDEZ-TRUJILLO MD

Attending Physician
Division of Allergy and Clinical Immunology
Miami Children's Hospital
Miami, FL
USA

MELANIE HINGORANI MBBS, MD, FRCOphth

Consultant Ophthalmologist
Eye Department
Hinchingbrooke Hospital
Huntingdon
UK

STEVEN M. HOLLAND MD

Chief, Laboratory of Clinical Infectious Diseases
National Institute of Allergy and Infectious Diseases
National Institutes of Health
Bethesda, MD
USA

HENRY A. HOMBURGER MD

Professor of Laboratory Medicine
Mayo College of Medicine;
Consultant, Department of Laboratory Medicine and Pathology
Mayo Clinic
Rochester, MN
USA

MCDONALD HORNE MD

Senior Clinical Investigator
Hematology Service
Department of Laboratory Medicine
National Institutes of Health
Clinical Center
Bethesda, MD
USA

GABOR ILLEI MD, PhD, MHS

Chief, Sjögrens Syndrome Clinic
National Institute of Dental and Craniofacial Research
National Institutes of Health
Bethesda, MD
USA

JOHN IMBODEN MD

Professor, Department of Medicine
University of California
San Fransisco, CA
USA

KEN J. ISHII MD, PhD

Group Leader, Akira Innate Immunity Project
Exploratory Research for Advanced Technology (ERATO)
Japan Science Technology Agency (JST);
Associate Professor, Department of Protozoology
Research Institute for Micorbial Diseases
Osaka University
Osaka
Japan

SHAI IZRAELI MD

Head, Research Section on Childhood Malignancies
Cancer Research Center
Sheba Medical Center
Tel-Hashomer
Ramat Gan
Israel

ELAINE S. JAFFE MD

Chief, Hematopathology Section;
Acting Chief, Laboratory of Pathology
Center for Cancer Research, National Cancer Institute
National Institutes of Health
Bethesda, MD
USA

Contributors

SIRPA JALKANEN MD, PhD

Professor of Immunology
Director, MediCity Research Laboratory
University of Turku
Turku
Finland

CARL H. JUNE MD

Professor of Pathology Laboratory Medicine
Director of Translational Research Programs
Abramson Cancer Center
Philadelphia, PA
USA

BARRY D. KAHAN MD, PhD

Professor of Surgery
Director
Division of Immunology and Organ Transplantation
Department of Surgery
The University of Texas Medical School at Houston
Houston, TX
USA

AXEL KALLIES PhD

PhillipDesbrow Memorial Fellow
Immunology Division
The Walter and Eliza Hall Institute of Medical Research
Parkville, Victoria
Australia

STEFAN H.E. KAUFMANN PhD

Professor of Immunology and Microbiology
Director, Max-Planck-Institute for Infection Biology
Department of Immunology
Berlin
Germany

ARTHUR F. KAVANAUGH MD

Professor of Medicine
Center for Innovative Therapy
Division of Rheumatology, Allergy and Immunology
University of California at San Diego School of Medicine
La Jolla, CA
USA

GARY KORETZKY MD, PhD

Leonard Jarett Professor of Pathology Laboratory Medicine
Chief, Division of Rheumatology
Department of Medicine
University of Pennsylvania;
Investigator and Director
Signal Transduction Program
AFCRI
Philadelphia, PA
USA

ROBERT KORNGOLD PhD

Chief, Research Division
Cancer Center
Hackensack University Medical Center
Hackensack, NJ
USA

RANIA D. KOVAIOU PhD

Institute for Biomedical Aging Research
Austrian Academy of Sciences
Innsbruck
Austria

DOUGLAS B. KUHNS PhD

Head, Neutrophil Monitoring Laboratory
Clinical Services Program
SAIC-Frederick, Inc.
NCI Frederick
Frederick, MD
USA

ROGER KURLANDER MD

Medical Officer
Hematology Section
Department of Laboratory Medicine
NIH Clinical Center
National Institutes of Health
Bethesda, MD
USA

ROBERT A. KYLE MD

Professor of Medicine
Laboratory of Medicine and Pathology
Mayo Clinic College of Medicine
Rochester, MN
USA

H. CLIFFORD LANE, MD

Chief, Clinical and Molecular Retrovirology Section
Laboratory of Immunoregulation
National Insitute of Allergy and Infectious Diseases
National Institutes of Health
Bethesda, MD
USA

ARIAN LAURENCE PhD, MRCP, MRCPath

Visiting Postdoctoral Fellow
Molecular Immunology and Inflammation Branch
National Institute of Arthritis and Musculoskeletal and Skin
Diseases
National Institutes of Health
Bethesda, MD
USA

FRANÇOISE LE DEIST MD, PhD

Professor of Immunology
Department of Microbiology and Immunology
University of Montreal
Montreal, QC
Canada

SUSAN J. LEE MD

Assistant Professor
Division of Rheumatology, Allergy and Immunology
University of California at San Diego School
of Medicine
La Jolla, CA
USA

STEVEN J. LEMERY MD

Hematologist
Hematology Branch NHLBI
Department of Laboratory Medicine
National Institutes of Health
Clinical Center
Bethesda, MD
USA

MICHAEL J. LENARDO MD

Section Head
Molecular Development of the Immune System Section
Laboratory of Immunology
National Institute of Allergy and Infectious Diseases
National Institutes of Health
Bethesda, MD
USA

ARNOLD I. LEVINSON MD

Professor of Medicine and Neurology
Chief, Allergy and Immunology Section
University of Pennsylvania School of Medicine;
Director, Penn Center for Clinical Immunology
Philadelphia, PA
USA

DAVID B. LEWIS MD

Professor and Member of the Program in Immunology
Department of Pediatrics
Stanford University School of Medicine;
Attending Physician at Lucile Salter Packard Children's
Hospital
Stanford, CA
USA

DOROTHY E. LEWIS PhD

Professor,
Internal Medicine, Microbiology & Immunology, and
Pathology
University of Texas Medical Branch
Galveston, TX
USA

JAY LIEBERMAN, MD

Resident Physician
Department of Internal Medicine
Washington University
St Louis, MO
USA

PHIL LIEBERMAN MD

Clinical Professor of Medicine and Pediatrics
University of Tennessee College of Medicine
Memphis, TN
USA

SUE L. LIGHTMAN PhD, FRCP, FRCOphth, FMedSci

Professor of Clinical Ophthalmology
Consultant Ophthalmologist
Department of Clinical Ophthalmology
Moorfields Eye Hospital
London
UK

MICHAEL D. LOCKSHIN MD, MACR

Director
Barbara Volcker Center for Women and Rheumatic Disease;
Co-Director, Mary Kirkland Center for Lupus Research
Hospital for Special Surgery;
Attending Physician, Hospital for Special Surgery;
Professor of Medicine and Obstetrics-Gynecology
Joan and Sanford Weill College of Medicine of Cornell University
New York, NY
USA

MICHAEL T. LOTZE MD

Professor of Surgery and Bioengineering
Vice Chair
Research
Department of Surgery;
Director
Strategic Partnerships
University of Pittsburgh Cancer Institute
University of Pittsburgh School of Medicine
Pittsburgh, PA
USA

MEGGAN MACKAY MD

Assistant Investigator
Autoimmune Disease Center
The Feinstein Institute for Medical Research
Manhasset, NY
USA

JONATHAN S. MALTZMAN MD, PhD

Assistant Professor
Renal-Electrolyte and Hypertension Division
Department of Medicine
University of Pennsylvania
Philadelphia, PA
USA

MICHAEL P. MANNS MD

Professor and Chairman
Department of Gastroenterology
Hepatology and Endocrinology
Hannover Medical School
Hannover
Germany

MARKUS Y. MAPARA MD, PhD

Associate Professor of Medicine
Scientific Director
Hematopoietic Stem Cell Transplantation Program
Division of Hematology/Oncology
University of Pittsburgh Cancer Institute
Pittsburgh, PA
USA

SUSANA MARINHO MD

Allergist Clinical Immunologist
Research Fellow
North West Lung Centre
Wythenshawe Hospital
University of Manchester
Manchester
UK

M. LOUISE MARKERT MD, PhD

Associate Professor of Pediatrics
Department of Pediatrics
Division of Allergy and Immunology
Duke University Medical Center
Durham, NC
USA

ALBERTO MARTINI MD

Professor and Head, Department of Pediatrics
University of Genoa and Istituto G. Gaslini
Genoa
Italy

SETH L. MASTERS PhD

Visting postdoctoral Fellow
Inflammatory Biology Section
National Institute of Arthritis and Musculoskeletal and Skin Diseases
National Institutes of Health
Bethesda, MD
USA

EVELINA MAZZOLARI MD

Assistant Professor
Chief, Bone Marrow Transplantation Unit
Department of Pediatrics
University of Brescia
Italy

HENRY F. MCFARLAND MD

Chief, Neuroimmunology Branch
National Institute of Neurological Disorders and Stroke
National Institutes of Health
Bethesda, MD
USA

JERRY R. MCGHEE PhD

Adjunct Professor
Department of Microbiology
University of Alabama at Birmingham
Birmingham, AL
USA

FRANK MCKENNA BA, MD, FRCP

Consultant Physician and Rheumatologist
Rheumatic Diseases Unit
Trafford General Hospital
Manchester
UK

PETER C. MELBY MD

Professor, Department of Medicine
Division of Infectious Diseases
The University of Texas Health Science Center
San Antonio, TX
USA

DEAN D. METCALFE MD

Chief, Laboratory of Allergic Diseases
National Institute of Allergy and Infectious Diseases
National Institutes of Health
Bethesda, MD
USA

MARTIN METZ MD

Post-Doctoral Scholar
Department of Pathology
Stanford University School of Medicine
Stanford, CA
USA

JOANN M. MICAN MD

Staff Clinician
Division of Clinical Research
National Institutes of Allergy and Infectious Diseases
National Institutes of Health
Bethesda, MD
USA

STEPHEN D. MILLER, PhD

Congressman John E. Porter Professor
Director, Interdepartmental Immunobiology Center
Department of Microbiology-Immunology
Feinberg School of Medicine
Northwestern University Medical School
Chicago, IL
USA

CAROLYN MOLD PhD

Professor
Department of Molecular Genetics and Microbiology
University of New Mexico School of Medicine
Albuquerque, NM
USA

DAVID R. MOLLER MD

Associate Professor of Medicine
Department of Medicine
Johns Hopkins Bayview Medical Center
Johns Hopkins University School of Medicine
Baltimore, MD
USA

ANTHONY MONTANARO MD

Professor of Medicine
Head, Division of Allergy and Clinical Immunology
Oregon Health and Sciences University
Portland, OR
USA

SCOTT N. MUELLER PhD

Postdoctoral Fellow
Emory Vaccine Center and Department of Microbiology and Immunology
Emory University
Atlanta, GA
USA

ULRICH R. MÜLLER MD

Professor
Consultant
Spital Ziegler
Spital Netz Bern
Bern
Switzerland

Contributors

PHILIP M. MURPHY MD

Chief, Laboratory of Molecular Immunology
National Institute of Allergy and Infectious Diseases
National Institutes of Health
Bethesda, MD
USA

PIERRE NOEL MD

Chief, Hematology Service
Department of Laboratory Medicine
National Institutes of Health
Clinical Center
Bethesda, MD
USA

LUIGI D. NOTARANGELO MD

Professor of Pediatrics and Pathology
Harvard Medical School;
Director of Research and Molecular Diagnosis Program on Primary Immunodeficiencies
Division of Immunology
Children's Hospital
Boston, MA
USA

THOMAS B. NUTMAN MD

Head, Helminth Immunology Section;
Head, Clinical Parasitology Unit
Laboratory of Parasitic Diseases
National Institutes of Health
Bethesda, MD
USA

STEPHEN L. NUTT PhD

Pfizer Australia Research Fellow
Immunology Division
The Walter and Eliza Hall Institute of Medical Research
Parkville, Victoria
Australia

JOÃO BOSCO DE OLIVEIRA MD

Staff Scientist
Molecular Immunology and Genetics Section
Laboratory of Medical Investigation 56
University of São Paulo-USP
São Paulo
Brazil

STEPHEN N. OLIVER, MD

Assistant Professor
Department of Medicince
Division of Clinical Pharmacology
New York University School of Medicine
New York, NY
USA

CHRIS M. OLSON JR.

Graduate Student
Department of Veterinary and Animal Sciences
University of Massachusetts at Amherst
Amherst, MA
USA

JOHN O'SHEA MD

Chief, Molecular Immunology and Inflammation Branch;
Chief, Lymphocyte Cell Biology Section;
Scientific Director, Intramural Research Program
National Institute of Arthritis and Musculoskeletal and Skin Diseases
National Institutes of Health
Bethesda, MD
USA

MARY E. PAUL MD

Associate Professor
Pediatric Allergy and Immunology
Baylor College of Medicine
Texas Children's Hospital
Houston, TX
USA

ERIK J. PETERSON MD

Assistant Professor
Department of Medicine
Division of Rheumatic and Autoimmune Diseases
Center for Immunology
University of Minnesota
Minneapolis, MN
USA

CAPUCINE PICARD, MD, PhD

Immunologist and Paediatrician
Director of Immunodeficiencies Study Center
Necker Sick Children's Hospital
APHP;
Laboratory of Human Genetics and Infectious Diseases
Faculty of Medicine
René Descartes University of Paris
Paris
France

WERNER J. PICHLER MD

Head of Allergology
Department for Rheumatology and Clinical Immunology/
Allergology
Inselspital
University of Bern
Bern
Switzerland

STANLEY R. PILLEMER MD

Vice President
Clinical Research and Product Safety Macrogenics
Rockville, MD
USA

STEFANIA PITTALUGA MD, PhD

Staff Physician
Laboratory of Pathology
National Cancer Institute
National Institutes of Health
Hematopathology Section
Bethesda, MD
USA

JEFFREY L. PLATT MD

Director, Transplantation Biology;
Professor of Surgery
Immunology and Pediatrics
Mayo Clinic
Rochester, MN
USA

PAUL H. PLOTZ MD

Chief, Arthritis and Rheumatism Branch
National Institute of Arthritis and Musculoskeletal and Skin
Diseases
National Institutes of Health
Bethesda, MD
USA

ANDREAS RADBRUCH PhD

Scientific Director
Deutsches Rheuma-Forschungszentrum (DRFZ)
Berlin
Germany

ANGELO RAVELLI MD

Associate Professor
Department of Pediatrics
University of Genoa and Istituto G. Gaslini
Genoa
Italy

JOHN D. REVEILLE MD, FACR

Professor
Director, Division of Rheumatology
The University of Texas Health Sciences Center at Houston
Houston, TX
USA

ROBERT R. RICH MD

Senior Vice President
Dean of School of Medicine;
Professor of Medicine and Microbiology
University of Alabama at Birmingham
Birmingham, AL
USA

MARGARET E. RICK MD

Assistant Chief, Hematology Service
Department of Laboratory Medicine
National Institutes of Health
Clinical Center
Bethesda, MD
USA

KIMBERLY A. RISMA MD, PhD

Assistant Professor of Pediatrics
Division of Allergy/Immunology
Cincinnati Children's Hospital Medical Center
Cincinnati, OH
USA

JOHN R. RODGERS PhD

Assistant Professor
Department of Immunology
Baylor College of Medicine
Houston, TX
USA

Contributors

ANTONY ROSEN, MD

Mary Betty Stevens Professor of Medicine
Professor of Medicine and Pathology;
Director, Division of Rheumatology
Johns Hopkins University School of Medicine
Baltimore, MD
USA

JAMES T. ROSENBAUM MD

Edward E. Rosenbaum Professor of Inflammation Research
Departments of Ophthalmology
Medicine and Cell Biology
Oregon Health and Science University
Portland, OR
USA

MARC E. ROTHENBERG MD, PhD

Director Endowed Chair
Division of Allergy and Immunology;
Professor of Pediatrics
Cincinnati Children's Hospital Medical Center
University of Cincinnati College of Medicine
Cincinnati, OH
USA

BARRY T. ROUSE DVM, DSc

Distinguished Professor
Department of Pathobiology
College of Veterinary Medicine
University of Tennessee
Knoxville, TN
USA

SCOTT ROWLEY MD

Division Chief, Blood and Marrow Stem Cell Transplantation
The Cancer Center
Hackensack University Medical Center
Hackensack, NJ;
Clinical Associate Professor
University of Medicine and Dentistry of New Jersey
Newark, NJ
USA

MARTINA RUDELIUS MD

Postdoctoral Research Fellow
National Cancer Institute
National Institutes of Health
Bethesda, MD
USA

SHIMON SAKAGUCHI, MD, PhD

Professor and Chair
Department of Experimental Pathology
Insititute for Frontier Medical Sciences
Kyoto University
Kyoto
Japan

MARKO SALMI MD, PhD

Director of Laboratory
Department of Bacterial and Inflammatory Diseases
National Public Health Institute
MediCity Research Laboratory
University of Turku
Turku
Finland

ULRICH E. SCHAIBLE PhD

Professor of Immunology
Chair, Department of Infectious and Tropical Diseases
London School of Hygiene and Tropical Medicine
London
UK

HARRY W. SCHROEDER JR, MD, PhD

Professor, Departments of Medicine, Microbiology
and Genetics
University of Alabama at Birmingham
Birmingham, AL
USA

MARVIN I. SCHWARZ MD

James C. Campbell Professor of Medicine
University of Colorado at Denver and Health Sciences
Center
Denver, CO
USA

MARKUS J.H. SEIBEL MD, PhD, FRACP, FGABJS

Professor and Chair of Endocrinology
The University of Sydney;
Head, Bone Research Program
ANZAC Res Inst;
Director, Department of Endocrinology and Metabolism
Concord Hospital Medical Center
Concord, NSW
Australia

CARLO SELMI, MD

Assistant Professor of Medicine
Division of Rheumatology
Allergy and Clinical Immunology
University of California at Davis
Davis, CA
USA;
Division of Internal Medicine and Liver Unit
San Paolo School of Medicine
University of Milan
Milan
Italy

WILLIAM M. SHAFER PhD

Senior Research Career Scientist
VA Medical Research Service;
Professor of Microbiology and Immunology
Department of Microbiology and Immunology
Emory University School of Medicine
Atlanta, GA
USA

PREDIMAN K. SHAH MD

Director, Division of Cardiology
Cedars-Sinai Medical Center
Los Angeles, CA
USA

MARYAM SHAHBAZ-SAMAVI MD, MRCP

Specialist Registrar in Rheumatology
Rheumatology Department
North Manchester General Hospital
Manchester
UK

ALAN R. SHAW PhD

President
Chief Executive Officer
Vaxinnate
Cranbury, NJ
USA

WILLIAM T. SHEARER MD, PhD

Chief, Allergy and Immunology Service;
Medical Director, AIDS Center
Texas Children's Hospital;
Professor of Pediatrics and Immunology;
Head, Section of Allergy and Immunology
Department of Pediatrics
Baylor College of Medicine
Houston, TX
USA

SCOTT H. SICHERER MD

Associate Professor of Pediatrics
The Elliot and Roslyn Jaffe Food Allergy Institute
Division of Allergy and Immunology
Department of Pediatrics
Mount Sinai School of Medicine
New York, NY
USA

RICHARD SIEGEL MD, PhD

Investigator, Autoimmunity Branch
National Institute of Arthritis and Musculoskeletal and
Skin Diseases;
Head, Immunoregulation Unit;
Director, National NIH-MSTP partnership
National Institutes of Health
Bethesda, MD
USA

RAVINDER JIT SINGH PhD

Assistant Professor of Laboratory Medicine
Co-Director, Endocrine Laboratory
Department of Laboratory Medicine and Pathology
Mayo Clinic
Mayo Foundation
Rochester, MN
USA

JUSTINE R. SMITH MBBS, PhD, FRANZCO, FRACS

Associate Professor of Ophthalmology
Casey Eye Institute
Oregon Health and Science University
Portland, OR
USA

PHILLIP D. SMITH MD

Mary J. Bradford Professor in Gastroenterology
Professor of Medicine and Microbiology;
Director, Mucosal HIV and Immunobiology Center
Department of Medicine (Gastroenterology)
University of Alabama at Birmingham
Birmingham, AL
USA

MICHAEL C. SNELLER MD

Medical Officer
Clinical and Molecular Retrovirology Section
Laboratory of Immunoregulation
National Insitute of Allergy and Infectious Diseases
National Institutes of Health
Bethesda, MD
USA

JOHN W. STEINKE PhD

Assistant Professor of Research
CAFGC Director
Asthma and Allergic Diseases Center;
Beirne B Carter Center for Immunology Research
University of Virginia
Charlottesville, VA
USA

DAVID S. STEPHENS MD

Stephen W. Schwarzmann Distinguished Professor of Medicine
Professor of Microbiology and Immunology;
Director, Division of Infectious Diseases;
Executive Associate Dean for Research
Emory University School of Medicine
Atlanta, GA
USA

JOHN H. STONE MD, MPH

Clinical Director, Rheumatic Diseases Unit
Massachusetts General Hospital
Boston, MA;
Deputy Editor for Rheumatology
UpToDate, Inc.
Waltham, MA
USA

HELEN C. SU MD, PhD

Assistant Clinical Investigator
Molecular Development of the Immune
System Section
Laboratory of Immunology
National Institute of Allergy and Infectious Diseases
National Institutes of Health
Bethesda, MD
USA

CRISTINA M. TATO PhD

Post-Doctoral Fellow
Molecular Immunology and Inflammation Branch
National Institute of Arthritis and Musculoskeletal and Skin
Diseases
National Institutes of Health
Bethesda, MD
USA

RAUL M. TORRES PhD

Associate Professor
Department of Immunology
University of Colorado Health Sciences Center
and National Jewish Medical
and Research Center
Denver, CO
USA

GÜLBÛ UZEL MD

Clinical Investigator
Laboratory of Clinical Infectious Diseases
National Institute of Allergy and Infectious Diseases
National Institutes of Health
Bethesda, MD
USA

JEROEN C.H. VAN DER HILST MD

Internal Medicine Resident
Department of General Internal Medicine
Radboud University Nijmegen Medical Center
Nijmegen
The Netherlands

JOS W.M. VAN DER MEER MD, PhD, FRCP, FRCP (Edin)

Head, Department of General Internal Medicine
Radboud University Nijmegen Medical Center
Nijmegen
The Netherlands

JOHN VARGA MD

Hughes Professor of Medicine
Division of Rheumatology
Northwestern University Feinberg School
Chicago, IL
USA

JOSÉ A. VILLADANGOS PhD

Laboratory Head
The Leukemia and Lymphoma
Society Scholar
Immunology Division
The Walter and Eliza Hall Eliza Institute
of Medical Research
Parkville, Victoria
Australia

SU HE WANG MD, PhD

Research Assistant Professor
Department of Internal Medicine
University of Michigan Medical Center
Ann Arbor, MI
USA

BIRGIT WEINBERGER PhD

Institute for Biomedical Aging Research
Austrian Academy of Sciences
Innsbruck
Austria

PETER F. WELLER MD

Professor of Medicine
Harvard Medical School;
Co-Chief, Infectious Disease Division;
Chief, Allergy and Inflammation
Division;
Vice Chair of Research
Department of Medicine
Beth Israel Deaconess Medical Center
Boston, MA
USA

CORNELIA M. WEYAND MD, PhD

David Lowance Professor of Medicine;
Director
Lowance Center for Human Immunology
and Rheumatology;
Director, Division of Rheumatology
Emory University School
of Medicine
Atlanta, GA
USA

FREDRICK M. WIGLEY MD

Professor of Medicine;
Associate Director, Division of Rheumatology;
Director, Scleroderma Center
Johns Hopkins University School of Medicine
Baltimore, MD
USA

ROBERT J. WINCHESTER MD

Professor of Medicine
Pediatrics and Pathology;
Director, Division of Rheumatology
Department of Medicine
College of Physicians and Surgeons
Columbia University
New York, NY
USA

Contributors

KAJSA WING PhD

Research Associate
Department of Experimental Pathology
Insititute for Frontier Medical Sciences
Kyoto University
Kyoto
Japan

LOUISE J. YOUNG BSc(Hons)

Graduate Student, Immunology Division
The Walter and Eliza Hall Institute of Medical Research
Victoria
Australia

LI ZUO MD, MS

Clinical Fellow
Division of Allergy and Immunology
Cincinnati Children's Hospital Medical Center
University of Cincinnati
Cincinnati, OH
USA

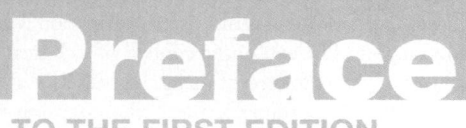

Preface
TO THE FIRST EDITION

Clinical immunology is a discipline with a distinguished history, rooted in the prevention and treatment of infectious diseases in the late nineteenth and early twentieth centuries. The conquest of historical scourges such as smallpox and (substantially) polio and relegation of several other diseases to the category of medical curiosities is often regarded as the most important achievement of medical science of the past fifty years. Nevertheless, the challenges facing immunologists in the efforts to control infectious diseases remain formidable; HIV infection, malaria and tuberculosis are but three examples of diseases of global import that elude control despite major commitments of monetary and intellectual resources.

Although firmly grounded in the study and application of defenses to microbial infection, since the 1960s clinical immunology has emerged as a far broader discipline. Dysfunction of the immune system has been increasingly recognized as a pathogenic mechanism that can lead to an array of specific diseases and failure of virtually every organ system. Pardoxically, although the importance of the immune system in disease pathogenesis is generally appreciated, the place of clinical immunology as a practice discipline has been less clear. As most of the non-infectious diseases if the human immune system lead eventually to failure of other organs, it has been organ-specific subspecialists who have usually dealt with their consequences. Recently, however, the outlook has begun to change as new diagnostic tools increasingly allow the theoretical possibility of intervention much earlier in disease processes, often before irreversible target organ destruction occurs. More importantly, this theoretical possibility is increasingly realized as clinical immunologists find themselves in the vanguard of translating molecular medicine from laboratory bench to patient bedside.

In many settings, clinical immunologists today function as primary care physicians in the management of patients with inmune-deficiency, allergic, and autoimmune diseases. Indeed many influential voices in the clinical disciplines of allergy and rheumatology support increasing coalescence of these traditional subspecialities around their intellectual core of immunology. In addition to his or her role as a primary care physician, the clinical immunologist is increasingly being looked to as a consultant, as scientific and clinical advances enhance his or her expertise. The immunologist with a 'generalist' perspective can be particularly helpful in the application of unifying principles of diagnosis and treatment across the broad spectrum of immunologic diseases.

Clinical Immunology: Principles and Practice has emerged from this concept of the clinical immunologist as both primary care physician and expert consultant in the management of patients with immunologic diseases. It opens in full appreciation of the critical role of fundamental immunology in this rapidly evolving clinical discipline. Authors of basic science chapters were asked, however, to cast their subjects in a context of clinical relevance. We believe the result is a well-balanced exposition of basic immunology for the clinician.

The initial two sections on basic principles of immunology are followed by two sections that focus in detail on the role of the immune system in defenses against infectious organisms. The approach is two-pronged. It begins first with a systematic survey of immune responses to pathogenic agents followed by a detailed treatment of immunologic deficiency syndromes. Pathogenic mechanisms of both congenital and acquired immune deficiency diseases are discussed, as are the infectious complications that characterize these diseases. Befitting its importance, the subject of HIV infection and AIDS receives particular attention, with separate chapters on the problem of infection in the immuno-compromised host, HIV infection in children, anti-retroviral therapy and current progress in the development of HIV vaccines.

The classic allergic diseases are the most common immunologic diseases in the population, ranging from atopic disease to drug allergy to organ-specific allergic disease (e.g., of the lungs, eye and skin). They constitute a foundation for the practice of clinical immunology, particularly for those physicians with a practice orientation defined by formal subspecialty training in allergy and immunology. A major section is consequently devoted to these diseases, with an emphasis on pathophysiology as the basis for rational management.

The next two sections deal separately with systemic and organ-specific immunologic diseases. The diseases considered in the first of these sections are generally regarded as the core practice of the clinical immunologist with subdisciplinary emphasis in rheumatology. The second section considers diseases of specific organ failure as consequences of immunologically mediated processes that may involve virtually any organ system. These diseases include as typical examples the demyelinating diseases, insulin-dependent diabetes mellitus, the glomerulonephritides and inflammatory bowel diseases. It is in management of such diseases that the discipline of clinical immunology will have an increasing role as efforts focus on inetervention early in the pathogenic process and involve diagnostic and therapeutic tools of ever-increasing sophistication. One of the major clinical areas in which the expertise of a clinical immunologist is most frequently sought is that of allogeneic organ transplantation. A full section is devoted to the issue of transplantation of solid organs, with an introductory chapter on general principles of transplantation and management of transplantation rejection followed by separate chapters dealing with the special problems of transplantation of specific organs or organ systems.

Appreciation of both the molecular and clinical features of lymphoid malignancies is important to the clinical immunologist regardless of subspecialty background, notwithstanding the fact that primary responsibility for management of such patients will generally fall to the haematologist/oncologist. A separate section is consequently devoted to the lymphocytic leukemias and lymphomas that constitute the majority of malignancies seen in the context of a clinical immunology practice. The separate issues of immune responses to tumors and immunological strategies to treatment of malignant diseases are subjects of additional chapters.

Another important feature is the attention to therapy of immunologic diseases. This theme is constant throughout the chapters on the allergic and immunologic diseases, and because of the importance the editors attach to clinical immunology as a therapeutic discipline, an extensive section is also devoted specifically to this subject. Subsections are devoted to issues of immunologic reconstitution, with three chapters on treatment of immunodeficiencies, malignancies and metabolic diseases by bone marrow transplantation. Also included is a series of chapters on pharmaceutical agents currently available to clinical immunologists, both as anti-allergic and anti-inflammatory drugs, as well as newer agents with greater specificity for T cell-mediated immune responses. The section concludes with a series of chapters that address established and potential applications of therapeutic agents and approaches that are largely based on the new techniques of molecular medicine. In addition to pharmaceutical agents the section deals in detail with such subjects as apheresis, cytokines, monoclonal antibodies and immunotoxins, gene therapy and new experimental approaches to the treatment of autoimmunity.

The book concludes with a section devoted to approaches and specific techniques involved in the diagnosis of immunologic diseases. Use of the diagnostic laboratory in evaluation of complex problems of immunopathogenesis has been a hallmark of the clinical immunologist since inception of the discipline and many clinical immunologists serve as directors of diagnostic immunology laboratories. Critical assessment of the utilization of techniques ranging from lymphocyte cloning to flow cytomeric phenotyping to molecular diagnostics are certain to continue as an important function of the clinical immunologist, particularly in his or her role as expert consultant.

In summary, we have intended to provide the reader with a comprehensive and authoritative treatise on the broad subject of clinical immunology, with particular emphasis on the diagnosis and treatment of immunological diseases. It is anticipated that the book will be used most frequently by the physician specialist practicing clinical immunology, both in his or her role as a primary physician and as a subsequent consultant. It is hoped, however, that the book will also be of considerable utility to the non-immunologist. Many of the diseases discussed authoritatively in the book are diseases commonly encountered by the generalist physician. Indeed, as noted, because clinical immunology involves diseases of virtually all organ systems, competence in the diagnosis and management of immunological diseases is important to virtually all clinicians. The editors would be particularly pleased to see the book among the references readily available to the practicing internist, pediatrician and family physician.

Robert R. Rich
Thomas A. Fleisher
Benjamin D. Schwartz
William T. Shearer
Warren Strober

Preface
TO THE THIRD EDITION

In the 12 years since publication of the first edition of Clinical Immunology much has changed; as we have increasingly appreciated the nature of the molecular mechanisms underlying inflammatory responses to specific antigens, the discipline has surely become more complex, more interesting and more demanding of its practitioners. Acquired immunity, the specialized development of vertebrate host defenses, was for many decades the primary focus of attention. Recently, however, we have witnessed an explosion of information relating to the phylogenetically older systems of innate immunity, which has concurrently enlarged the purview of clinical immunology. In addition to those classical diseases of the acquired immune system, clinical immunologists today are increasingly interested in a range of inflammatory diseases where rearranged antigen-specific receptors have not been demonstrated or may not be involved. Rather than specific antigen receptors, these disorders are mediated by pathogen-recognition systems such as Toll-like receptors on NK lymphocytes and phagocytic cells. These trigger inflammatory effector processes that were later adopted by the acquired immune system, such as elaboration of soluble inflammatory mediators (cytokines and chemokines), complement activation, phagolysosome-mediated pathogen elimination and programmed cell death.

The third edition reflects this improved understanding with increased attention to processes and diseases of inflammation and a broadly defined view of host defenses. We trust that this has been accomplished while retaining a principal focus on those many diseases at the core of clinical immunology arising from deficiency or aberration of functions of acquired immunity.

Two changes will be immediately apparent to readers familiar with the previous editions. The third edition is, we believe, much enhanced by production in full color throughout. Clinical case photos are increased and are presented more usefully in the context of text discussion. Similarly line drawings are not only more attractive, but utilize color effectively to enrich their information content. The second obvious change is that we have chosen to publish the book in a single (albeit large) volume rather than in the previous two-volume format. We believe that by editing to reduce redundancy, judicious referencing (with an emphasis on recent reviews) and tightening presentation, the third edition is consequently more "user friendly," eliminating the necessity to consult more than a single volume, while not compromising overall content quality or quantity. There is also a third important change that is not immediately obvious, but which will considerably enhance the long-term usefulness of the book. This third change is the intent to provide quarterly electronic updates to registered purchasers relating to key advances in clinical immunology since the publication of this edition. We are confident that such updates will help to keep the book fresh as our field advances.

The process of editing a book of this size represents the combined efforts of many individuals in addition to the editors and authors. Two persons, however, warrant special thanks for their essential roles in shepherding this work to its conclusion: Martin Mellor and Randell Baker, whose efforts on behalf of the editors, authors and, finally, the readers, is gratefully acknowledged.

We trust that the book continues to find a useful place on the desks and book shelves of clinical immunologists of many stripes—from the specialized practitioner of clinical immunology (either generalized or organ-system oriented), to the generalist or organ-based specialist who is interested in state-of-the-art approaches to management of inflammatory conditions, and to the fundamental immunologist interested in mechanisms of immunologic diseases. Finally, upon reviewing this comprehensive text on clinical immunology, which delves into the many and increasingly diverse areas of immune system related diseases, the editors hope that this recording of the expanse and depth of knowledge in our specialty will impart a sense of pride and possession to those clinicians and researchers who call themselves clinical immunologists.

Robert R. Rich
Thomas A. Fleisher
William T. Shearer
Harry W. Schroeder, Jr.
Anthony J. Frew
Cornelia M. Weyand

Dedication

To:
Cathryn and Kenneth Rich and Lynn Todorov
Mary, Jeffrey, Jeremy and Matthew Fleisher
Lynn Des Prez and Christine, Mark, Christopher, Martin, John, Jesse and Melissa Shearer
Dixie, Trey, Elena and Jenny Schroeder
Helen, Edward, Sophie, Georgina and Alex Frew
Jörg Goronzy and Dominic and Isabel Weyand Goronzy

part 1

FUNDAMENTAL PRINCIPLES OF THE IMMUNE RESPONSE

The human immune response

Robert R. Rich

Arguably, clinical immunology touches as many organs and diseases as any other subspecialty of medicine. Indeed when 'innate' and 'acquired' immune mechanisms are both considered it would likely be possible to write a textbook relating to the immunologic diseases of virtually any organ system. The challenge for clinical immunologists is to reduce a dizzying array of disease descriptions, with increasingly defined cellular and molecular mechanisms, to a far more limited and systematic approach to disease management or, ideally, prevention. For the nonimmunologist, either generalist or specialist, the immunological forest is more important than the trees to the management of a specific patient with an immune disease. The role of a consulting immunologist is to bring understanding in depth of immune pathogenesis to bear in a particular patient setting.

This chapter is directed as a consult from a clinical immunologist to the generalist physician. It is predicated on the notion that appreciation of fundamental aspects of immune responses will facilitate understanding of immunologic diseases. The chapter is structured as an introduction to the interacting elements of the human immune system and their disordered functions in diseases. The subtleties are described in detail in the chapters that follow.

■ THE HOST–MICROBE INTERACTION ■

The vertebrate immune system is a product of eons of evolutionary struggle between rapidly evolving microbial pathogens and their much less rapidly reproducing, and hence less adaptable, hosts.[1] Unable to win the battle with microbial invaders by rapid mutation and selection, the immune system employs a strategy of complexity and redundancy involving both the individual organism and its population. Microbes respond by adaptations to particular elements of the immune system that they can turn to their own advantage. Reflecting plasticity of the response, specific defenses differ substantially based upon the nature of the infecting organism and its point of entry and distribution within the body. Regardless of the defense mechanism, an intended outcome is the destruction or neutralization of the invading organism. A secondary

consequence, however, can be collateral damage to host cells. These cells can be involved in the attack either as sites of microbial residence or as 'innocent bystanders.' Depending on the site and severity of the host defense response, it may be accompanied by local and/or systemic symptoms and signs of inflammation.

ACQUIRED AND INNATE IMMUNITY

Immune responses are traditionally classified as acquired (or specific) and innate (or nonspecific) (Table 1.1). The acquired immune system, present uniquely in vertebrates, is specialized for development of an inflammatory response based on recognition of specific 'foreign' macromolecules that are predominantly, but not exclusively, proteins or peptides. Its primary actors are antibodies, T lymphocytes, B lymphocytes, and antigen-presenting cells (APCs).

Innate immune responses are far more ancient, being widely represented in multicellular phyla.[2,3] Rather than being based upon specific recognition of an exceedingly diverse array of macromolecules (i.e., antigens), it is focused on recognition of common molecular signatures of potential pathogens.[4,5] For responses of both types, effector mechanisms can be based upon elaboration of soluble products acting systemically (humoral immunity) or can require direct cell-to-cell contact or the activity of cytokines and chemokines acting in the cellular microenvironment (cell-mediated immunity).

The elements of innate immunity are diverse. They include physical barriers to pathogen invasion (such as skin, mucous membranes, cilia, and mucus), as well as an array of cellular and serum factors that can be activated by secreted or cell surface products of the pathogen. Consequent activation of these cells induces an inflammatory response that uses mechanisms which are broadly shared with those of the specific immune system. Among these are natural killer (NK) cell-mediated cytotoxicity, activation of phagocytic cells, the secretion of inflammatory cytokines and chemokines, and the actions of the many participants in the complement cascade.

There is substantial overlap and redundancy between the innate and acquired immune systems. The distinguishing feature of the latter is the direct activation by antigen of lymphocyte clones with specific antigen

Table 1.1 Features of innate and acquired immune systems

Distinguishing features	
Innate immunity	Acquired immunity
Receptors fixed and based on pathogen molecular patterns	Receptors clonally variable and based on gene rearrangement
Does not require immunization	Consequence of B- and/or T-cell activation
Little or no memory	Immunologic memory
Includes physical barriers to pathogen	Antibody and cytotoxic T cells

Common features
Cytokines and chemokines
Complement cascade
Phagocytic cells
Natural killer (NK) cells
Natural autoantibodies

receptors. In contrast, innate immune responses are independent of the function of cells expressing such clonotypic receptors. Because recognition of pathogens by the innate immune system relies on germline-encoded cellular receptors and does not require clonal expansion of cells with receptors that are products of gene rearrangements, innate immunity is more rapidly responsive. It can initiate in minutes to hours and generally precedes development of a primary acquired immune response by at least several days. However, for the same reason, it does not exhibit specific memory for previous encounter with a particular pathogen.

CELLS OF THE IMMUNE SYSTEM

The major cellular constituents of both innate and acquired immunity originate in the bone marrow where they differentiate from multipotential hematopoietic stem cells along several pathways to become granulocytes, lymphocytes, and APCs (Chapter 2).

GRANULOCYTES

Polymorphonuclear leukocytes (granulocytes) are classified by light microscopy into three types. By far the most abundant in the peripheral circulation are neutrophils, which are principal effectors of antibody and complement-mediated immune responses (Chapter 21). They are phagocytic cells that ingest, kill, and degrade phagocytosed microbes and other targets of an immune attack within specialized cytoplasmic vacuoles. Phagocytic activity of neutrophils is promoted by their surface display of receptors for antibody molecules (specifically the Fc portion of immunoglobulin G (IgG) molecules) and complement proteins (particularly the C3b component). Neutrophils are the predominant cell type in acute inflammatory infiltrates and are the primary effector cells in immune responses to pyogenic organisms (Chapter 24).

Eosinophils (Chapter 23) and basophils (Chapter 22) are the other circulating forms of granulocytes. A close relative of the basophil, but derived from distinct bone marrow precursors, is the tissue mast cell that does not circulate in the blood. Eosinophils, basophils, and mast cells are important in host defenses to multicellular pathogens, particularly

helminths (Chapter 29). Their defensive functions are based not on phagocytic capabilities, but rather on their ability to discharge potent biological mediators into the cellular microenvironment. This process of degranulation can be triggered by antigen-specific IgE molecules bound to basophils and mast cells, which express high-affinity receptors for the Fc portion of IgE (FcεR on their surfaces). In addition to providing a mechanism for helminthic host defenses, this pathologic process is also the principal mechanism involved in acute (IgE-mediated) allergic reactions.

LYMPHOCYTES

Three types of lymphocytes are identified based on display of particular surface molecules: B cells, T cells, and NK cells. All lymphocytes differentiate from common lymphoid stem cells in the bone marrow. T cells undergo further maturation and selection in the thymus for expression of antigen receptors useful in self/nonself discrimination (Chapter 9). B cells continue differentiation into antibody-producing cells in the bone marrow (Chapter 8).

T cells and B cells are the heart of specific immune recognition, a property reflecting their clonally specific cell surface receptors for antigen (Chapter 4). B-cell receptors for antigen (BCR) are membrane immunoglobulin (mIg) molecules of the same antigenic specificity that the cell and its terminally differentiated progeny, plasma cells, will secrete as soluble antibodies. The T-cell receptor for antigen (TCR) is a heterodimeric integral membrane molecule expressed exclusively by T lymphocytes.

Receptors for "antigen" on the third class of lymphocytes, NK cells, are not clonally expressed. Expressing receptors, however, for moieties that can be regarded as molecular signatures of pathogens, NK cells serve as major constituents of innate immunity. They also recognize target cells that might otherwise elude the immune system (Chapter 18). NK cell differentiation is particularly driven by interleukin (IL)-15. Recognition of NK cell targets is based largely on what their targets lack rather than on what they express. NK cells express receptors of several types for major histocompatibility complex (MHC) class I molecules via killer cell immunoglobulin-like receptors (KIR).[6] KIR can either inhibit or activate NK cell activity utilizing receptors for MHC class I molecules or other immune adaptor molecules that express a tyrosine-based inhibitory-motif (ITIM) or tyrosine-based activation motif, respectively, in their intracellular domain. NK cells will kill target cells unless they receive an inhibitory signal transmitted by an ITIM receptor. Because virus-infected cells and tumor cells may attempt to escape T-cell recognition by downregulating their expression of class I molecules, such cells can become susceptible to NK cell-mediated killing.

NK cells can also participate in antigen-specific immune responses by virtue of their surface display of the acvitating ITAM receptor CD16, which binds the constant (Fc) region of IgG molecules. This enables them to function as effectors of a cytolytic mechanism termed antibody-dependent cellular cytotoxicity (ADCC).[7]

In general, pathways leading to differentiation of T cells, B cells, and NK cells are mutually exclusive, representing a permanent lineage commitment. No lymphocytes express both mIg and TCR. Some T cells, however, also display NK cell surface markers, including MHC class I receptors, and exhibit both NK-like cytotoxicity and antigen-specific T-cell responsiveness.

Antigen-presenting cells

A morphologically and functionally diverse group of cells, all of which are derived from bone marrow precursors, is specialized for presentation of antigen to lymphocytes, particularly T cells (Chapter 7). Included among such cells are monocytes (present in the peripheral circulation); macrophages (solid tissue derivatives of monocytes); cells resident within the solid organs of the immune system such as dendritic cells; and constituents of the reticular endothelial system within other solid organs. B lymphocytes that specifically capture antigen by virtue of mIg receptors can also function efficiently in antigen presentation to T cells.

Cardinal features of APCs include their expression of both class I and class II MHC molecules (the latter can either be expressed constitutively or can be induced by cytokines) as well as requisite accessory molecules for T-cell activation (e.g., B7-1, B7-2/CD80, CD86).[8] Upon activation, APCs also elaborate cytokines that induce specific functions in cells to which they are presenting antigen.

APCs differ substantially among themselves with respect to mechanisms of antigen uptake and effector functions. Monocytes and macrophages are actively phagocytic, particularly for antibody and/or complement-coated (opsonized) antigens that bind to their surface receptors for Fcγ and C3b. These cells are also important effectors of

immune responses, especially in sites of chronic inflammation. Upon further activation by T-cell cytokines, they can kill ingested microorganisms by oxidative pathways similar to those employed by polymorphonuclear leukocytes. In addition, they can kill adjacent target cells by a cytotoxic mechanism. Mature dendritic cells, although efficient in antigen presentation and T-cell activation, have little phagocytic function and are not known to participate as effectors in immune responses. Immature dendritic cells, however, phagocytose apopototic cells and present antigenic peptides from such cells to T lymphocytes.

The interaction between B cells acting as APCs and T lymphocytes is particularly interesting as the cells are involved in a mutually amplifying circuitry of antigen presentation and response. The process is initiated by antigen capture through B-cell mIg and ingestion by receptor-mediated endocytosis. This is followed by antigen degradation and then display to T cells as oligopeptides bound to MHC molecules. In addition, like other APCs, B cells display CD80, thereby providing a requisite second signal to the antigen-responsive T cell via its accessory molecule for activation, CD28[8] (Fig. 1.1). As a result of T-cell activation, T-cell cytokines that regulate B-cell differentiation and antibody production are produced and T cells are stimulated to display the surface ligand CD40L (CD154) that can serve as the second signal for B-cell activation through its inducible surface molecule CD40.

BASIS OF ACQUIRED IMMUNITY

The essence of acquired immunity is molecular distinction between self constituents and potential pathogens (for simplicity, self/nonself discrimination). This discrimination is predominantly a responsibility of T lymphocytes. It reflects the selection of thymocytes that have generated specific antigen receptors, and that upon later encounter can bind both self MHC molecules and nonself antigenic peptides. The consequence of this selection process is that foreign proteins are recognized as antigens but self proteins are tolerated (i.e., are not perceived as antigens).

T lymphocytes generally recognize antigens as a complex of short linear peptides bound to MHC molecules on the surfaces of APCs (Chapter 7). With the exception noted below, T cells do not bind antigen in native conformation. Furthermore, they do not recognize antigen in solution. The vast majority of antigens for T cells are oligopeptides, although utilizing specialized antigen-presenting molecules, T cells can also recognize other molecular species such as glycolipids. Antigen recognition by T cells differs fundamentally, however, from that by antibodies, which are produced by B lymphocytes and their derivatives. Antibodies, unlike T cells, can bind complex macromolecules and can bind them either at cell surfaces or in solution. Moreover, antibodies show less preference for recognition of proteins; antibodies against carbohydrates, nucleic acids, lipids, and simple chemical moieties can be readily produced. Although B cells can also be rendered unresponsive by exposure to self-antigens, particularly during differentiation in the bone marrow, this process does not define foreignness within the context of self-MHC recognition.

CLONAL BASIS OF IMMUNOLOGICAL MEMORY

An essential element of self/nonself discrimination is the clonal nature of antigen recognition. Although the immune system can recognize a vast array of distinct antigens, all of the receptors of a single T cell or B cell

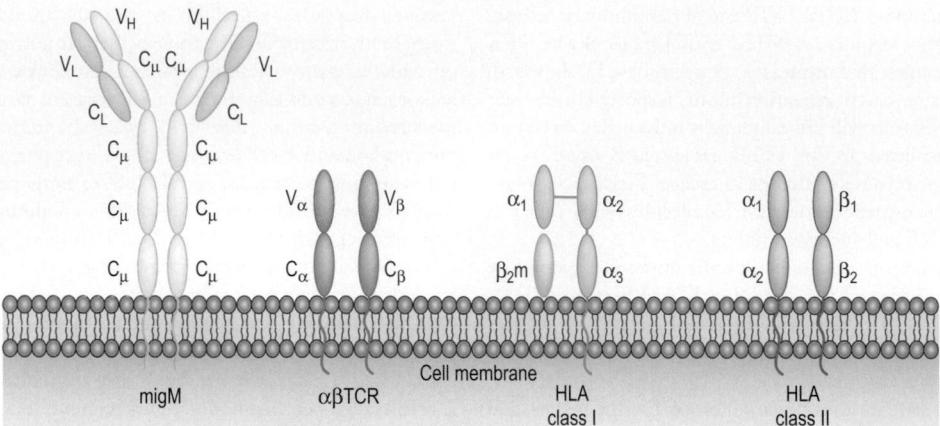

Fig. 1.1 Antigen-binding molecules. Antigen-binding pockets of immunoglobulin (Ig) and T-cell receptor (TCR) are comprised of variable segments of two chains translated from transcripts that represent random V(D)J or VJ gene segment rearrangements. Antigen-binding grooves of major histocompatibility complex (MHC) molecules are formed with contributions of α_1 and β_1 domains of class II molecules and α_1 and α_2 domains of class I molecules. In contrast to Ig and TCR, MHC binding sites do not reflect genetic rearrangements. All of these molecules are members of the immunoglobulin superfamily. HLA, human leukocyte antigen; mIgM, membrane immunoglobulin M.

(and their clonal progeny) have identical antigen-binding sites and hence a particular specificity. A direct consequence is the capacity for antigen-driven immunologic memory. This phenomenon derives from the fact that, after an initial encounter with antigen, clones of lymphocytes of appropriate specificity proliferate, resulting in a greater and more rapid response upon subsequent antigen encounter. These two hallmarks of the specific immune system, clonal specificity and immunological memory, provide a conceptual foundation for the use of vaccines in prevention of infectious diseases (Chapter 92). Immunologic memory involves not only the T cells charged with antigen recognition, but also the T cells and B cells that mediate the efferent limb of an inflammatory response. In its attack on foreign targets, the immune system may display exquisite specificity for the inducing antigen, as is seen in the lysis of virus-infected target cells by cytolytic T cells. However, an immunologic attack *in vivo* will also have important elements that are independent of antigen recognition, such as the response of phagocytes to inflammatory mediators.

■ MECHANISMS OF IMMUNOLOGIC DISEASES ■

The pathogenic pathways that lead to diseases of the immune system are based on an understanding of its physiology and its perturbations in disease states (Table 1.2). First, immunologic disease can reflect a failure or deficiency of the immune system (Chapters 30–38). This pathway is similar to that accounting for most diseases of other organ systems, i.e., a consequence of failure of physiologic function. Considering the essential role of the immune system in defenses against microbes, such failures are usually identified by increased susceptibility to infection (Chapter 31). Failure can be congenital (e.g., X-linked agammaglobulinemia) or acquired (e.g., acquired immunodeficiency syndrome (AIDS)). It can be global (e.g., severe combined immunodeficiency) or quite specific, involving only a particular component of the immune system (e.g., selective IgA deficiency).

A second mechanism, malignant transformation (Chapters 76–78), is also common to virtually all organ systems. Malignancies of the

Table 1.2 Pathways to immunologic diseases

1. Immune system deficiency or failure
   a. Congenital
   b. Acquired
2. Malignant transformation
3. Immunologic dysregulation
4. Autoimmunity
5. Untoward consequences of physiologic immune function

hematopoietic system are familiar to all physicians. Manifestations of these diseases are protean, most commonly reflecting the secondary consequences of solid-organ or bone marrow infiltration and immune system deficiency.

Dysregulation of an essentially intact immune system provides a third pathway to immune pathogenesis. Features of an optimal immune response include antigen recognition and elimination with little adverse effect on the host. Both initiation and termination of the response, however, involve regulatory interactions that can go awry when challenged by antigens of a particular structure or in a particular mode of presentation. Diseases of immune dysregulation reflect genetic and environmental factors that act together to subvert a normal immune response to some pathological end. The acute allergic diseases (Chapters 39–49) are examples of such disorders.

The fourth and fifth pathways to immunopathogenesis are more specific to the immune system. The fourth lies at the heart of specific immune system function, i.e., the molecular discrimination between self and nonself. Ambiguity in this discrimination can lead to autoimmune tissue damage (Chapters 50–75). Although such damage can be mediated by either antibodies or T cells, the frequent association of particular diseases with inheritance of specific human leukocyte antigen (HLA) alleles (Chapter 5) suggests that the pathogenesis of autoimmune diseases usually represents a failure of self/nonself discrimination by T cells. This failure to discriminate can be general, leading to development of systemic autoimmune diseases such as systemic lupus erythematosus, or local, as in the organ-specific autoimmune diseases. In the latter instance, attack is directed against specific cells and usually particular cell surface molecules. In most cases, pathology is a consequence of target tissue destruction (e.g., multiple sclerosis, rheumatoid arthritis, insulin-dependent diabetes mellitus). However, it can also reflect hormone receptor blockade (e.g., myasthenia gravis, insulin-resistant diabetes) or hormone receptor stimulation (e.g., Graves' disease). It is thought that ambiguity in self/nonself discrimination is commonly triggered by an unresolved encounter with an infectious organism or other environmental agent, although this remains a subject of controversy[9] (Chapter 50).

A fifth pathogenetic pathway to immunologic disease is disease development as a result of physiologic rather than pathologic function. Inflammatory lesions in such diseases are the result of the normal function of the immune system. A typical example is contact dermatitis to potent skin sensitizers such as urushiol, the causative agent of poison-ivy dermatitis (Chapter 44). These diseases can also have an iatrogenic etiology that can range from benign (e.g., delayed hypersensitivity skin test reactions) to life-threatening (e.g., graft-versus-host disease, organ graft rejection).

■ ANTIGEN-BINDING MOLECULES ■

Three sets of molecules are responsible for the specificity of acquired immune responses by virtue of their capacity to bind foreign antigen. These molecules are Ig, TCR, and MHC molecules (Fig. 1.1; Chapters 4 and 5). All are products of a very large family of ancestrally related genes, the immunoglobulin superfamily (IgSF).[10] Members of the IgSF, which includes many other molecules essential to induction and regulation of immune responses, exhibit characteristic structural features. The most notable of these is organization into homologous domains of approximately 110 amino acids that are usually encoded by a single exon and characteristically have an intradomain disulfide bond. Typically, each domain assumes a configuration of anti-parallel strands that form two opposing β-pleated sheets.

▌ KEY CONCEPTS

FEATURES OF THE IMMUNOGLOBULIN SUPERFAMILY

>> Large family of ancestrally related genes (probably > 100 members)

>> Most products involved in immune system function or other cell–cell interactions

>> Proteins exhibit domain structure of ~100 amino acids, usually translated from a single exon and characteristically with a single intradomain disulfide bond

>> Tertiary structure of protein typified by anti-parallel strands forming a pair of β-pleated sheets

IMMUNOGLOBULINS AND T-CELL RECEPTORS

The exquisite specificity of Ig and TCR molecules for antigen is achieved by a mechanism of genetic recombination that is unique to Ig and TCR genes (Chapter 4). The antigen-binding site of both types of molecules is comprised of a groove formed by contributions from each of two constituent polypeptides. In the case of immunoglobulins, these are a heavy (H) chain and one of two alternative types of light (L) chains, κ or λ. In the case of TCR, either of two alternative heterodimers may constitute the antigen-binding molecule, one comprised of α and β chains, and the other of γ and δ chains. The polypeptides contributing to both Ig and TCR can be divided into an antigen-binding amino-terminal variable (V) domain and one or more carboxy-terminal constant (i.e., nonvariable) domains. Ig constant region domains generally include specific sites responsible for the biological effector functions and other activities of the molecule (Chapter 15).

The most noteworthy feature of the vertebrate immune system is the process of genetic recombination that generates a virtually limitless array of specific antigen receptors from a rather limited genomic investment. This phenomenon is accomplished by the recombination of genomic segments that encode the variable portions of Ig and TCR polypeptides[11] (Chapter 4). The products of these rearranged genes provide a specific B or T cell with its unique antigen receptor. The mature receptor consists

▌ KEY CONCEPTS

COMPARISON OF T-CELL AND B-CELL RECEPTORS FOR ANTIGEN

Similarities

>> Members of the immunoglobulin (Ig) superfamily

>> Heterodimeric antigen-binding groove

>> Divided into variable and constant regions

>> Variable regions constructed by V(D)J rearrangements

>> Nongenomic N-nucleotide additions at V(D)J junctions

>> Exhibit allelic exclusion

>> Mature T cells and B cells display receptors of one and only one antigenic specificity

>> Negative selection for receptors with self-antigen specificity

>> Transmembrane signaling involving co-receptor molecules

Differences

>> Ig binds antigen in solution; T-cell receptor (TCR) binds antigen when presented by antigen-presenting cell

>> Ig can be secreted; TCR is not

>> Somatic hypermutation of Ig genes

>> Isotype switching of Ig genes

>> Inflammatory effector functions by the Ig constant domains

>> Selection of TCR for self-major histocompatibility complex (MHC) recognition

of the products of two or three such rearranged segments. These are designated V (variable) and J (joining), for IgL chains and TCR α and γ chains, and V, D (diversity) and J, for IgH and TCR β and δ chains.

DNA rearrangement involved in generating T- and B-cell receptors is controlled by recombinases that are active in early thymocytes and in pro-B cells in the bone marrow. The process is sequential and carefully regulated, leading to translation of one receptor of unique specificity for any given T or B lymphocyte. This result is achieved through a process termed *allelic exclusion*, wherein only one member of a pair of allelic genes potentially contributing to an Ig or TCR molecule is rearranged at a time.[12] If a productive rearrangement is achieved, i.e., a full-length transcript that will encode the appropriate protein product, the other member of the allelic pair is permanently inactivated. If, on the other hand, the first effort at rearrangement is not productive, resulting in a truncated transcript, two alternatives are presented. The cell can attempt a second (or more) rearrangement at the same gene, depending upon the availability of unrearranged D and/or J segments. Alternatively, the process can move to the second member of the pair on the homologous chromosome, which will similarly undergo rearrangement. This affords a cell several opportunities to construct a variable region sequence that encodes a full-length receptor transcript. The frequency of nonproductive rearrangements is high because of a secondary mechanism that contributes substantially to potential receptor diversity. This process, termed N-nucleotide addition, results in the insertion at the time of rearrangement of one or more nongenomic nucleotides at the junctions between V, D, and J segments.[11] A frequent consequence of this process is a codon frameshift and, hence, a nonproductive rearrangement.

In addition to the process of allelic exclusion, there are other control mechanisms to insure that a lymphocyte expresses a single antigen receptor. B cells exclusively rearrange Ig genes, but not TCR genes, and vice versa for T cells. Moreover, B cells sequentially rearrange L-chain genes, typically κ before γ. Thus, B cells express either κ or γ chains, but not both. Similarly, thymocytes express α and β genes or γ and δ genes, and, with the caveat that some Vδ gene segments can rearrange with some Jα and vice versa, one never finds T cells with αδ or γβ receptors. Indeed, Vα →Jα rearrangement generally deletes the DJCδ locus that is embedded within the α gene complex. Interestingly, the TCR α gene complex and IgL chain genes can occasionally rearrange independent of the constraints of allelic exclusion.[13] This allows possible expression of two different TCRα or IgL chains. However, only one of these is typically expressed by the cell – a process termed *phenotypic exclusion*.

There is one feature of V-region construction that is essentially reserved to B cells. This is *somatic hypermutation* (SHM), a process that can continue throughout the life of a mature B cell at the hypervariable sites of both the V_H and V_L genes.[11] The amino acid products of these sites, particularly at V, D, and J junctions, are the specific points of contact with antigen within the binding groove. As antigen is introduced into the system, mature B cells remain genetically responsive to the antigenic environment. As a consequence, through SHM of mIg, a few B cells increase their affinity for antigen. Such cells are preferentially activated, particularly at limiting doses of antigen. Thus, the average affinity of antibodies produced during the course of an immune response increases – a process termed affinity maturation. The process of SHM is not limited to V-region coding segments, but extends to 3′ and 5′ flanking sequences; indeed, the start of the hypermutation domain lies within the V-gene promoter. SHM is driven by an enzyme, activation-induced cytidine deaminase (AID), that catalyzes mutation of deoxycytidine to deoxyuracil in single-stranded DNA.[14] Inactivation of AID is associated with development of hyperIgM syndrome (Chapter 34). The process of SHM is also of pathogenetic importance in a variety of B-cell lymphomas and leukemias, and possibly in nonlymphoid malignancies as well.[14, 15]

The products of TCR genes generally do not show evidence of SHM. This virtual absence of hypermutation may be related to the fundamental responsibility of T cells for discrimination between self and nonself through a rigorous process of selection in the thymus that involves co-recognition of a self-MHC molecule and antigenic peptide[16] (Chapter 9). This process results in deletion by apoptosis of the vast majority of differentiating thymocytes by mechanisms that place stringent boundaries around the viability of a thymocyte with a newly expressed TCR specificity. Once a T cell is fully mature and ready for emigration from the thymus, its TCR is essentially fixed, thus reducing the likelihood of emergent autoimmune T-cell clones in the periphery.

The receptor expressed by a developing thymocyte must be capable of binding with low-level affinity to some particular MHC self-molecule, either class I or class II, expressed by a resident thymic APC. If it does not exhibit such binding affinity, the TCR can make further attempts to construct an appropriate receptor by additional Vα →Jα rearrangements. If it is not ultimately successful, the developing thymocyte dies. Because their receptors are generated by a process of random gene rearrangement, most thymocytes fail this test. They are consequently deleted as not being useful to an immune system that requires T cells to recognize self-MHC molecules. Thymocytes surviving this hurdle are said to have been "positively selected"[16] (Fig. 1.2A). Conversely, a small number of thymocytes bind with an unallowably high affinity for a combination of MHC molecule plus antigenic peptide expressed by a thymic APC. Because the peptides available for MHC binding at this site are derived almost entirely from self proteins, differentiating thymocytes with such receptors are intrinsically dangerous as potentially autoimmune. This deletion of thymocytes with high-affinity receptors for self-MHC plus (presumptively) self-peptide is termed "negative selection" (Fig. 1.2B), a process that may also involve activity of T-regulatory cells (Tregs).[17, 18]

Although not selected for recognition of foreignness in the context of self, maturing pre-B cells in the bone marrow are also subject to negative selection upon encounter with "self" soluble or particulate antigen, and B cells in peripheral tissues may be rescued by ligand engagement in a process resembling positive selection.[19, 20] Additionally, IgM-producing B cells with low-affinity specificity for autoantigens that are cross-reactive with bacterial glycoconjugates appear to be positively selected during B-cell development.[21] Conversely, studies in transgenic mice suggest that when an initial pre-B-cell mIg is cross-linked by encounter of relatively high affinity with self-antigen in the bone marrow, secondary rearrangements can occur. This process, termed receptor editing, can thus generate a new receptor lacking self reactivity[22] (Chapter 8).

Another feature that distinguishes B cells from T cells is that the cell surface antigen receptors of the former are secreted in large quantities as antibody molecules, the effector functions of which are carried out in solution or at the surfaces of other cells. Secretion is accomplished by alternative splicing of Ig transcripts to include or exclude a transmembrane segment of the Ig heavy chains.

In addition to synthesizing both membrane and secreted forms of immunoglobulins, B cells also undergo class switching. Antibody molecules are comprised of five major classes (isotypes). In order of abundance in the serum these are IgG, IgM, IgA, IgD, and IgE (Chapters 4 and 15). The IgG class is further subdivided into four

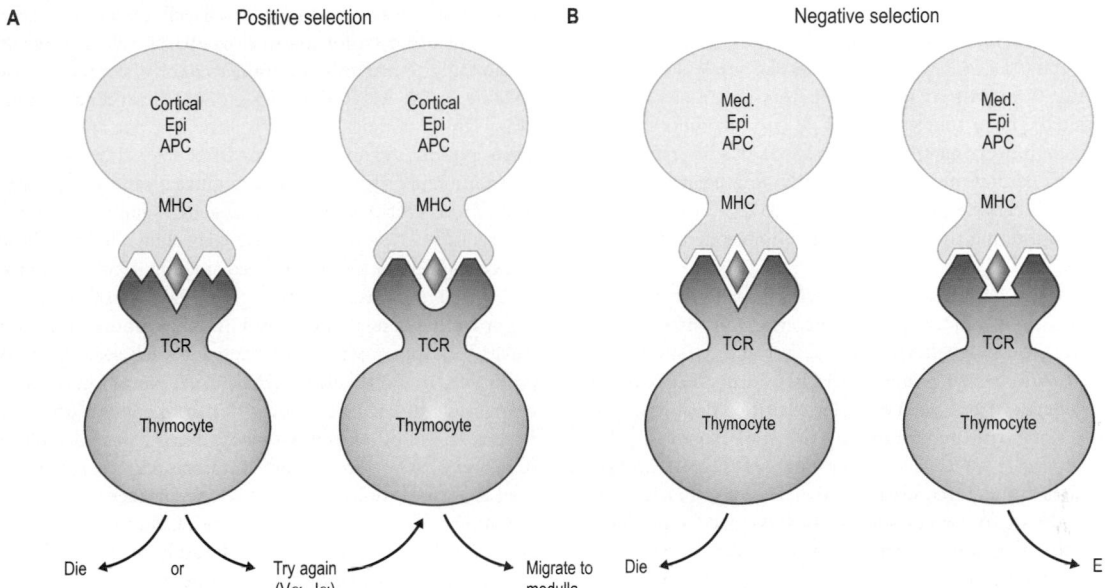

Fig. 1.2 Two-stage selection of thymocytes based on binding characteristics of randomly generated T-cell receptors (TCR). Panel A: Positive selection. "Double-positive" (CD4, CD8) thymocytes with TCR capable of low-affinity binding to some specific self-major histocompatibility complex (MHC) molecule (either class I or class II) expressed by thymic cortical epithelial cells are positively selected. This process may involve sequential attempts at a gene rearrangement in order to express an αβ TCR of appropriate self-MHC specificity. Thymocytes that are unsuccessful in achieving such a receptor die by apoptosis. The solid diamond represents a self-peptide derived from hydrolysis of an autologous protein present in the thymic microenvironment or synthesized within the thymic antigen-presenting cell (APC) itself. Panel B: Negative selection. "Single-positive" (CD4 or CD8) thymocytes, positively selected in stage one, that display TCR with *high* affinity for the combination of self-MHC plus some self (autologous) peptide present in the thymus are negatively selected (i.e., die). Those few thymocytes that have survived both positive and negative selection emigrate as mature T cells to the secondary lymphoid tissues.

subclasses and the IgA class into two subclasses. The class of immunoglobulin is determined by the sequence of the constant region of its heavy chain (C_H). The isotype-determining exons are located downstream (3′) of the heavy-chain variable (V_H) genes. Thus, an antibody-producing cell can change the class of antibody molecule that it synthesizes by utilization of different C_H genes without changing its unique antibody specificity. This process, termed class switch recombination, is regulated by cytokines and, like SHM, is accomplished through the action of activation-induced cytidine deaminase.[11, 23]

There is no process comparable to class switch recombination in T cells. The two types of TCR are products of four independent sets of V-region and C-region genes. A substantial majority of T cells express the αβ TCR. A small number express γδ TCR (usually 5% or less in peripheral blood). There is a higher representation of γδ T cells in certain tissues, particularly those lining mucous membranes, where they may be specialized for recognition of heavily glycosylated peptides or nonpeptide antigens. Thymocytes are committed to the expression of either αβ or γδ TCR and their differentiated progeny (T cells) never undergo secondary changes in the periphery.

MAJOR HISTOCOMPATIBILITY COMPLEX

MHC molecules constitute a third class of antigen-binding molecules. When an MHC class I molecule was initially crystallized, an unknown peptide was found in a binding groove formed by the first two domains

(α₁ and α₂). This binding groove has since been established as a general feature of MHC molecules.[24] It is now known that the function of MHC molecules is to present antigen to T cells in the form of oligopeptides that reside within this antigen-binding groove. The most important difference between the nature of the binding groove of MHC molecules and those of Ig and TCR is that the former does not represent a consequence of gene rearrangement. Rather, all the available MHC molecules in an individual are encoded in a linked array within the MHC, which in humans is located on chromosome 6 and designated HLA (Chapter 5).

MHC molecules are of two basic types: class I and class II. Class I molecules have a single heavy chain that is an integral membrane protein comprised of three external domains (Fig. 1.1). The heavy chain is noncovalently associated with β₂-microglobulin, a nonpolymorphic, nonmembrane-bound, single-domain molecule that is not encoded within the MHC (although it is a member of the IgSF). Class II MHC molecules, in contrast, are comprised of two polypeptide chains, α and β (or A and B), of approximately equal size, each of which consists of two external domains connected to a transmembrane region and cytoplasmic tail. Both chains of class II molecules are embedded within the cell membrane, and both are encoded within the MHC. Class I and class II molecules have a high degree of structural homology and both fold to form a peptide-binding groove on their exterior face, with contribution from the α₁ and α₂ domains for class I and from α₁ and β₁ domains for class II.[24] There are three class I loci (HLA-A, -B, and -C) and three class II subregions (HLA-DR, -DQ, and -DP) that are principally involved in antigen presentation to T cells (Chapter 5). The functions of other class I and class II genes within this complex are less clear. Some at least appear to be specialized for binding (presentation) of peptide antigens of restricted type or source (e.g., HLA-E), and others are clearly involved in antigen processing (e.g., HLA-DM). Additionally, recent studies have established that members of a family of 'nonclassical' class Ib molecules, CD1$_{a-d}$ which are encoded outside the MHC (on chromosome 1) are specialized for binding and presentation of lipid and lipid conjugate antigens to T cells.[25]

The HLA complex represents an exceedingly polymorphic set of genes. Consequently, most individuals are heterozygous at each major locus, having inherited one allele from the father and an alternative at each locus from the mother. In contrast to TCR and Ig, the genes of the MHC are codominantly expressed, i.e., allelic exclusion does not operate on MHC genes. Thus, at a minimum, an APC can express six class I molecules and six class II molecules (the products of the two alternative alleles of three class I and three class II loci). This number is, in fact, usually an underestimate for two reasons. First, there may be products of other (nonclassical) MHC genes with specialized functions. Second, the class II loci are somewhat more complex than just suggested. For example, the DRβ locus is duplicated so that most individuals express from each chromosome at least two different dimers, each comprised of a different β-chain joined to an identical nonpolymorphic α-chain. Additionally, because both the α and β loci for DQ are polymorphic and gene products can be assembled from *trans*-encoded transcripts, unique DQ αβ combinations, not represented in *cis* by either parental chromosome, are possible. Class I genes are found on almost all somatic cells, whereas class II genes are restricted in expression primarily to cells specialized for APC function.

ANTIGEN PRESENTATION

Because MHC genes do not undergo recombination, the number of distinct antigen-binding grooves that they can form is many orders of magnitude less than that for either TCR or Ig. Oligopeptides that bind to MHC molecules are the hydrolytic products of self or foreign proteins. They are derived by hydrolytic cleavage within the APC and are loaded into MHC molecules before expression at the cell surface (Chapter 6). Indeed, stability of MHC molecules at the cell surface requires the presence of a peptide in the antigen-binding groove. Since most hydrolyzed proteins are of self origin, the binding groove of most MHC molecules contains a self peptide. Class I and class II molecules differ from one another in the length of peptides that they bind, usually 8–9 amino acids for class I and 14–22 amino acids for class II. Although important exceptions are clearly demonstrable, they also generally differ with respect to the source of peptide. Those peptides binding to class I molecules usually derive from proteins synthesized intracellularly (e.g., autologous proteins, tumor antigens, viruses, and other intracellular microbes), whereas class II molecules commonly bind peptides derived from proteins synthesized extracellularly (e.g., nonreplicating vaccines, extracellular bacteria). Endogenous peptides are loaded into newly synthesized class I molecules in the endoplasmic reticulum following active transport from the cytosol. Loading of exogenous peptides into class II molecules, in contrast, occurs in acidic endosomal vacuoles.

In addition to the recognition of lipids and lipid conjugates presented by CD1 molecules, there are other exceptions to the generalization that

MHC molecules only present (and T cells only recognize) oligopeptides. It has been known for many years that T cells can recognize haptens, presumably covalently or noncovalently complexed with peptides residing in the MHC-binding groove. This phenomenon is familiar to physicians as contact dermatitis to nonpeptide antigens such as urushiol (from poison ivy) and nickel ions.

Additionally, γδ T cells can recognize a variety of nonpeptide antigens by a process that is not thought to require presentation by MHC molecules.[26] These antigens have been shown to include phosphorylated nucleotides, other phosphorylated small molecules, and alkylamines.

Another exception to the generalization of T-cell recognition of oligopeptides is represented by a group of proteins termed superantigens (SAg).[27] SAg, of which the staphylococcal enterotoxin A represents a prototype, are produced by a broad spectrum of microbes, ranging from retroviruses to bacteria. They differ from conventional peptide antigens in their mode of contact with both MHC class II molecules and TCR (Chapter 6). They do not undergo processing to oligopeptides, but rather bind to class II molecules and TCR as intact (~30 kDa) proteins outside the antigen-binding grooves. Their interaction with TCR is predominantly determined by polymorphic residues of the TCR Vβ region. Because SAg bind independently (more or less) of the TCR α-chain and the other variable segments of the β-chain, they are capable of activating much larger numbers of T cells than do conventional peptide antigens; hence the name. A secondary consequence of T-cell activation by SAg is death by apoptosis of appropriate Vβ-expressing cells. The initial response, however, is a wave of activation, proliferation, and cytokine production that can have profound clinical consequences, leading to development of such diseases as toxic shock syndrome. Interestingly, it is now apparent that certain bacterial products such as protein A of *Staphylococcus aureus* can similarly act on B cells, both to activate and then to delete, cells based on supraclonal binding to a site on products of the V$_H$3 gene family outside the conventional antigen-binding site. Such findings have led to the identification of a number of B-cell SAgs.[28]

LYMPHOCYTE ADHESION AND TRAFFICKING

The capacity to survey continuously the antigenic environment is an essential element of immune function. APCs and lymphocytes must be able to find antigen wherever it occurs in the body. Surveillance is accomplished through an elaborate interdigitated circulatory system of blood and lymphatic vessels that establish connections between the solid organs of the peripheral immune system (e.g., spleen and lymph nodes) in which the cellular interactions between immune cells predominantly occur (Chapter 2).

The trafficking and distribution of circulating cells of the immune system are largely regulated by interactions between molecules on the surfaces of such cells with ligands on vascular endothelial cells (Chapter 3). The leukocyte-specific cellular adhesion molecules can be expressed constitutively or can be induced by cytokines (e.g., as a consequence of an inflammatory process). Two families of molecules, termed selectins and integrins, regulate lymphocyte traffic and insure that mobile cells home to appropriate locations within lymphoid organs and other tissues. Selectins are proteins characterized by a distal carbohydrate-binding (lectin) domain. They bind to a family of mucin-like molecules, the endothelial vascular addressins. Integrins are heterodimers essential for the emigration of leukocytes from blood vessels into tissues. Members of the selectin and integrin families are not only involved in lymphocyte circulation and homing, but are also important in interactions between APC, T cells, and B cells in induction and expression of immune responses. A third family of adhesion molecules, distinguished as members of the IgSF, are similarly involved in promoting interactions between T cells and APCs (Chapter 12).

LYMPHOCYTE ACTIVATION

For both B cells and T cells, initial activation is a two-signal event[29, 30] (Chapters 8 and 13). This generalization is particularly true for cells that have not been previously exposed to antigen. The first signal is provided by antigen. Most commonly, antigen for B cells is a protein with distinct sites (epitopes) that bind to membrane Ig. Such epitopes can be defined by a contiguous amino acid sequence or (more commonly) can be conformationally defined by the three-dimensional structure of the antigenic molecule. Epitopes can also be simple chemical moieties (haptens) that have been attached, usually covalently, to amino acid side chains (Chapter 6). In addition to proteins, some B cells have receptors with specificity for carbohydrates, and, less commonly, lipids or nucleic acids. Antigens that stimulate B cells can be either in solution or fixed to a solid matrix (e.g., a cell membrane). As previously noted, the nature of antigens that stimulate T cells is more limited. TCRs do not bind antigen in solution, but are generally only stimulated by small molecules, primarily oligopeptides, that reside within the antigen-binding cleft of a self-MHC molecule.

The second signal requisite for lymphocyte activation is provided by an accessory molecule expressed on the surface of the APC (e.g., B7/CD80) for stimulation of T cells or on the surface of a helper T cell (e.g., CD40L/CD154) for activation of B lymphocytes. The cell surface receptor for this particular second signal on T cells is CD28 and on B cells is CD40 (Fig. 1.3). Other cell surface ligand–receptor pairs may similarly provide the second signal[29] (Chapters 8 and 13). The growth and differentiation of both T cells and B cells also require stimulation with one or more cytokines, which are peptide hormones secreted in small quantities for function in the cellular microenvironment by activated leukocytes and APC.[31]

Cells stimulated only by antigen in the absence of a second signal become unresponsive to subsequent antigen stimulation (anergic) rather than being activated (Chapter 13). T cells can also be "tolerized" by minor changes in the sequence of the stimulatory antigenic peptide that can convert an activating (agonist) signal into an inactivating (antagonist) signal.[32] This capacity to alter fundamentally the outcome of T-cell stimulation with minor changes in antigen suggests exciting opportunities for the development of future therapeutic agents.

Signal transduction through the antigen receptor is a complex process involving interactions between the specific receptor and a set of molecules co-expressed in the cell membrane. For B cells, this set of molecules is a heterodimer, Igαβ, and for T cells it is a macromolecular complex, CD3, usually comprised of γ, δ, ε, and ς chains.

Within the cell membrane, antigen receptor stimulation induces phosphorylation of CD3 subunits and hydrolysis of phosphotidylinositol 4,5-bisphosphate by phospholipase C, leading to generation of diacylglycerol (DAG) and inositol 1,4,5-trisphosphate (IP$_3$). As a consequence of signal transduction and secondarily of DAG and IP$_3$ generation, tyrosine and serine/threonine protein kinases are activated. In turn, these kinases catalyze phosphorylation of a number of signal-transducing proteins, leading to activation of cytoplasmic transcription

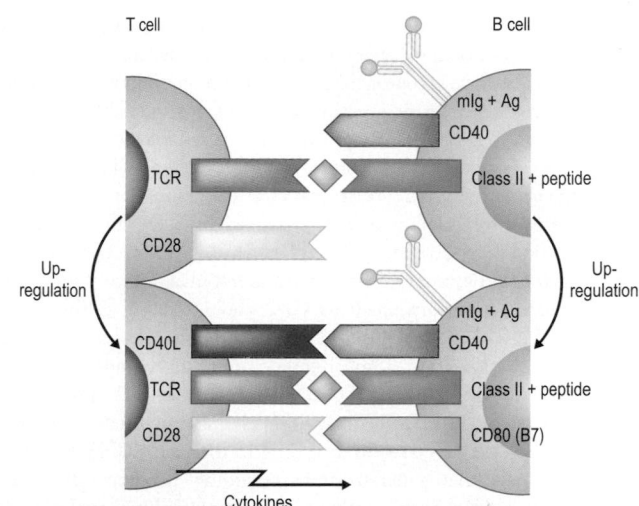

Fig. 1.3 Reciprocal activation events involved in mutual simulation of T cells and B cells. T cells constitutively express T-cell receptors (TCR) and CD28. B cells constitutively express membrane immunoglobulin (mIg) and major histocompatibility complex (MHC) class II. Activation of B cells by antigen (Ag) upregulates expression of CD80 (B7) causing activation of T cells, which upregulates CD40L (CD154) and induces cytokine synthesis. Co-stimulation of B cells by antigen, CD40L, and cytokines leads to Ig production.

factors NF-AT and NF-κB. These transcription factors then translocate to the nucleus, where they bind to 5′ regulatory regions of genes that are critical to generalized lymphocyte activation[33, 34] (Chapter 13).

CELL-MEDIATED IMMUNE RESPONSES

T-CELL SUBSETS

T lymphocytes expressing an αβ TCR can be divided into two major subpopulations based upon the class of MHC molecule that their TCR recognizes and the consequent expression of one of a pair of TCR accessory molecules, CD4 or CD8 (Chapter 4). By binding to MHC molecules on APCs, CD4 and CD8 contribute to the overall strength of intercellular molecular binding. Additionally both molecules are involved in antigen receptor-mediated signal transduction. T cells expressing CD4, commonly referred to as T helper (Th) cells, recognize antigen bound to a nonpolymorphic region of class II MHC molecules. CD8 T cells recognize antigen bound to a nonpolymorphic loop on the α$_3$ domain of class I MHC molecules. The ratio of CD4 to CD8 cells in peripheral blood is usually about 2:1, but can normally vary over a considerable range (from approximately 0.8:1 to 3:1).

CD4 T CELLS, CYTOKINES, AND CHEMOKINES

The activities of CD4 T lymphocytes (CTLs) are predominantly mediated through the secretion of cytokines[31] (Chapter 10). Cytokines are small (~12–30 kDa) protein hormones that control growth and differentiation of cells in the microenvironment. This activity may include autostimulation (autocrine function) if the cell producing the cytokine also expresses a surface receptor for it, or stimulation of other cells in the microenvironment (paracrine function) including B cells, APC, and other T cells. Although it is now recognized that their biological effects are broader than implied by their name, many of the principal cytokines active in the immune system are known as interleukins (ILs).

The specific profile of cytokines produced by CD4 T cells allows further functional subdivision[35] (Chapters 16–18). Those CD4 T cells elaborating the "inflammatory" cytokines involved in effector functions of cell-mediated immunity, such as IL-2 and interferon (IFN)-γ, are designated Th1 cells. Other CD4 T cells synthesize cytokines such as IL-4 and IL-13 that control and regulate antibody responses, and are designated Th2 cells. Differentiation of Th1 versus Th2 subsets is a process regulated by positive-feedback loops, being promoted particularly by IL-12 in the case of Th1 cells and IL-4 in the case of Th2 cells. It is important to note that generalizations regarding cytokine activity are usually oversimplifications, reflecting a remarkable overlap and multiplicity of functions (Chapter 10). For example, although IL-2 was initially identified as a T-cell growth factor, it also significantly affects B-cell differentiation. The prototypic inflammatory cytokine, IFN-γ, which promotes differentiation of effector function of CTL and macrophages, is also involved in the regulation of Ig isotype switching. And IL-4, although known primarily as a B-cell growth and differentiation factor, can also stimulate proliferation of T cells.

A distinct subset of cytokines is a large group of highly conserved cytokine-like molecules, smaller than typical cytokines (~7–12 kDa), termed *chemo*tactic cyto*kines* or chemokines. Chemokines regulate and coordinate trafficking and activation of leukocytes, functioning importantly in host defenses, and also broadly in a variety of nonimmunological processes, including organ development and angiogenesis[36, 37] (Chapter 11). They are characterized by binding to seven-transmembrane-domain G-protein-coupled receptors. The chemokines are classified based on number and spacing of cysteine residues. Of particular interest to clinical immunologists, two chemokine receptors are utilized by human immunodeficiency virus (HIV) as co-receptors (together with CD4) to gain entry into target cells.[38]

Cytokines produced by activated T cells can downregulate as well as initiate or amplify immune responses.[39] Cytokines with such activity include IL-10 (produced by both T cells and B cells) and transforming growth factor-β (TGF-β). The functions of IL-10 *in vivo* are thought to include both suppression of the production of proinflammatory cytokines and enhancement of IgM and IgA synthesis. TGF-β is produced by virtually all cells and expresses a broad array of biological activities, including the promotion of wound healing and the suppression of both humoral and cell-mediated immune responses.

In addition to their central role in initiation and regulation of immune responses, CD4 T cells are important effectors of cell-mediated immunity (Chapter 17). Through the elaboration of inflammatory cytokines, particularly IFN-γ, they are essential contributors to the generation of chronic inflammatory responses, characterized histologically by mononuclear cell infiltrates, where their principal role is thought to be the activation of macrophages. Additionally, CD4 T cells, at least in some circumstances, are capable of functioning as cytotoxic effectors, either directly as CTL (in which case the killing is "restricted" for recognition of antigen-bound self-MHC class II) or through the elaboration of cytotoxic cytokines such as lymphotoxin and tumor necrosis factor-α (TNF-α).

A third subset of Th cells, designated Th17, has been recognized more recently.[40] With differentiation driven particularly by TGF-β and IL-23 and characterized by the production of the proinflammatory cytokine IL-17, Th17 cells are important in the induction and exacerbation of autoimmunity in a variety of disease models. Recent data also suggest a role of Th17 cells in host defenses against certain bacterial, fungal, and helminthic infections.

A further subset of CD4 cells, T regulatory cells (Tregs), suppresses the functions of other lymphocytes.[41] Tregs can differentiate either in the thymus (natural Tregs) or in the periphery (induced or adaptive Tregs). They are characterized by surface expression of CD4 and CD25 and by nuclear expression of the transcription factor FOXP3. Activation of CD25+ Tregs is antigen-specific; the cells are IL-2-dependent and apparently require cell–cell contact for suppressive function. They can suppress functions of both CD4 and CD8 T cells, as well as B cells, NK cells, and NK T cells. In contrast to activation, suppressor effects are independent of the antigen specificity of the target cells. Other Tregs are noted for production of inhibitory cytokines, including TGF-β-secreting Th3 cells and IL-10-producing Tr1 cells.

CD8 T CELLS

The best understood function of CD8 T cells is that of cytotoxic effectors (CTL). Such cells are of particular importance in host defenses against virus-infected cells, where they are capable of direct killing of target cells expressing an appropriate viral peptide bound to a self-MHC class I molecule (Chapter 18). This process is highly specific and requires direct apposition of CTL and target cell membranes. Bystander cells, expressing inappropriate MHC molecules (e.g., that might be presented in an *in vitro* culture system) or different antigenic peptides are not affected. The killing is unidirectional; the CTL itself is not harmed and after transmission of a 'lethal hit' it can detach from one target to seek another. Killing occurs via two mechanisms: a death receptor-induced apoptotic mechanism, resulting in fragmentation of target cell nuclear DNA, and a mechanism requiring insertion of perforins and granzyme from the CTL into the target cell. CTL activity is enhanced by IFN-γ. As CTL function is dependent upon cell surface display of MHC class I molecules, a principal mechanism of immune evasion by viruses and tumors is elaboration of factors that downregulate class I expression (Chapter 27). As noted above, however, this increases susceptibility of such cells to cytolytic activity of NK cells.

■ ANTIBODY-MEDIATED IMMUNE RESPONSES ■

The structure of antibodies permits the possibility of a virtually limitless binding specificity of its antigen-binding groove, determined by the sequence variability of the amino-terminal segments of its light and heavy chains (Fab portion). Antigen binding can then be translated into biological effector functions based on the properties of the larger nonvariable (constant) portions of its heavy chains (Fc fragment) (Chapter 15). Moreover, in response to cytokines in the cellular microenvironment, through the mechanism of isotype switching, an antibody-producing cell can alter the biological effects of its secreted product without affecting its specificity. With functional heterogeneity determined by isotype, the antibody molecules provide an efficient

KEY CONCEPTS

BIOLOGICAL PROPERTIES OF IMMUNOGLOBULIN (IG) CLASSES

>> IgM: Principal Ig of primary immune responses

Generally restricted to vascular compartment
B-cell antigen receptor (monomer)
Fixes complement

>> IgG: Principal Ig of secondary immune responses

Binds to Fcγ receptors on neutrophils, monocytes/macrophages, NK cells
Fixes complement (except IgG$_4$ subclass)

>> IgA: Principal Ig of mucosal immunity

>> IgD: B-cell antigen receptor

>> IgE: Binds to Fcε receptors on mast cells and basophils

Antibody of immediate hypersensitivity
Important in defenses against helminths

defense system against extracellular microbes or foreign macromolecules (e.g., toxins and venoms) (Chapters 15 and 24).

Each of the antibody classes contributes differently to an integrated defense system. IgM is the predominant class formed upon initial contact with antigen (primary immune response). As a monomeric structure comprised of two light (κ or γ) and two heavy (μ) chains, it is initially expressed as an antigen receptor on the surface of B lymphocytes. It is secreted, however, as a pentamer composed of five of the monomeric subunits held together by a joining (J) chain. IgM is essentially confined to the intravascular compartment. As a multivalent antigen binder that can efficiently activate complement, it is an important contributor to an early immune response. Moreover, the synthesis of IgM is much less dependent than other isotypes upon the activity of T lymphocytes.

IgG is the most abundant immunoglobulin in serum and the principal antibody class of a secondary (anamnestic or memory) immune response. The structure of an IgG molecule is similar to an IgM monomer, i.e., two light (κ or γ) and two heavy (μ) chains joined by interchain disulfide bridges. Because of its abundance, its capacity to activate (fix) complement, and the expression on phagocytes of Fcγ receptors, IgG is the most important antibody of secondary immune responses. IgG has an additional important property of being the only isotype that is actively transported across the placenta. Thus, infants are born with a full repertoire of maternal IgG antibodies, at concentrations often greater than those found in the mother's serum. Maternal antibodies provide the neonate with an important level of antibody protection during the early months, when its own antigen-driven antibody responses are primordial.

IgA is the principal antibody in the body's secretions (Chapter 19). It is found in serum in monomeric form of two light and two heavy (α) chains or as a dimer joined by J chain. In secretions, it is usually present as a dimer also joined by J chain and is actively secreted across mucous membranes by attachment of a specialized secretory component. It is found in high concentration in tears, saliva, and the secretions of the respiratory, gastrointestinal, and genitourinary systems and is relatively resistant to enzymatic digestion. It is particularly abundant in colostrum, where its concentration may be greater than 50 times that in serum, providing passive immunity through this class of antibody to the gastrointestinal system of a nursing neonate. IgA does not fix complement by the antibody-dependent pathway. Hence, its role in host defenses is not through the promotion of phagocytosis, but rather in preventing a breech of the mucous membrane surface by microbes or their toxic products.

IgD and IgE are present in serum at concentrations much lower than that of IgG. The biological role of secreted IgD, if any, is unknown. However, IgD is important as a membrane receptor for antigen on mature B cells. Moreover, the molecular mechanisms promoting isotype switching from IgM to IgM/IgD are substantially different from those for other isotypes and can occur independent of a T-cell-regulated process.

Although IgE is the least abundant isotype in serum, it has dramatic biological effects because it is responsible for immediate-type hypersensitivity reactions, including systemic anaphylaxis (Chapter 42). Such reactions are a consequence of the expression of high-affinity receptors for Fcε on the surfaces of mast cells and basophils. Crosslinking of IgE molecules on such cells by antigen induces their degranulation, with the synthesis and/or release of the potent biological mediators of immediate hypersensitivity responses. The protective role of IgE is in host defenses against parasitic infestation, particularly helminths (Chapter 29).

COMPLEMENT AND IMMUNE COMPLEXES

As noted, the biological functions of IgG and IgM are largely reflections of their capacities to activate the complement system. Through a series of sequential substrate–enzyme interactions, the 11 principal components of the antibody-dependent complement cascade (C1q, C1r, C1s, and C2–9) effect many of the principal consequences of an antigen–antibody interaction (Chapter 20). These consequences include the establishment of pores in a target membrane by the terminal components (C5–9) leading to osmotic lysis; opsonization by C3b, promoting phagocytosis; the production of factors with chemotactic activity (C5a); and the ability to induce degranulation of mast cells (C3a, C4a, and C5a). There are three distinct pathways to complement activation.[42, 43] The pathway mediated by the binding of IgG or IgM to the first component (specifically C1q), has been termed the 'classical' pathway. The lectin pathway is similar to the classical pathway but is activated by certain carbohydrate-binding proteins, the mannose (or mannan)-binding lectin (MBL) and ficolins, which recognize certain carbohydrate repeating structures on microorganisms. MBL and ficolins are plasma proteins that are homologous to C1q and contribute to innate immunity through their capacity to induce antibody- and C1q-independent activation of the classical pathway. Finally, a large number of substances, including certain bacterial, fungal, and viral products, can directly activate the cascade through a distinct series of proteins, also leading to activation of the central C3 component. Although bypassing C1, C4, and C2, this distinct pathway results in all the biological consequences of C3–9 activation. Nonantibody-induced activation of C3 is referred to as the alternative or properdin pathway. Reflecting these separate pathways to activation, the complement system is a major contributor to the efferent limbs of both innate and acquired immune systems.

In addition to their roles in pathogen/antigen elimination, constituents of the complement system, together with antigen–antibody (immune) complexes, act at leukocyte surfaces to regulate immune functions.[44] For example, interaction of immune complexes via FcγR on B cells decreases their responsiveness to stimulation. In contrast, complement activation on B-cell surfaces co-ligates their receptors with B-cell receptors for antigen; the cells are more readily activated and become relatively resistant to apoptosis.

APOPTOSIS AND IMMUNE HOMEOSTASIS

An immune response is commonly first viewed in a 'positive' sense, i.e., lymphocytes are activated, proliferate, and carry out effector functions. It is equally important, however, that this positive response be tightly regulated by mechanisms that operate to turn off the response and eliminate cells no longer required. Under physiologic circumstances, once an immune response fades, commonly as a consequence of antigen depletion, two pathways to terminal lymphocyte differentiation become available: apoptosis or differentiation into memory cells. Memory cells are, of course, a key to the effectiveness of the adaptive immune system. Once seen effectively, a second encounter with antigen (e.g., pathogen) is both more rapid and more effective. IgG antibodies are rapidly produced and/or clones of CTL effector cells are rapidly expanded as a consequence of prior exposure and clonal expansion. But the majority of lymphocytes in an active response are not required for maintenance of immunologic memory, and for these larger populations a need for immune homeostasis leads to apoptosis.[45]

Apoptosis is a unique process of cellular death, widely conserved phylogenetically, and distinguished from death by necrosis by cellular shrinking, DNA fragmentation, and breakdown of cells into "apoptotic bodies" containing nuclear fragments and intact organelles (Chapter 14). The process depends upon the activation of cysteinyl proteases, termed caspases, that cleave proteins involved in DNA repair and cellular and organelle architecture at specific aspartyl residues. In the absence of such mechanisms, massive proliferation of lymphoid tissues is a consequence, seen clinically as the autoimmune lymphoproliferative syndrome or ALPS, which is characterized by lymphocytosis with lymphadenopathy and splenomegaly, as well as autoimmunity and hypergammaglobulinemia (Chapter 35).

HOST IMMUNE DEFENSES REVISITED

The first response upon initial contact with an invading pathogen depends upon components of the innate immune system. This response begins with expression of pathogen-associated molecular patterns (PAMPs), such as lipoproteins, lipopolysaccharide, CpG-DNA, and bacterial flagellin, among others. PAMPs bind to pattern recognition receptors (PRRs) on effector cells of the innate immune system, including dendritic cells, granulocytes, and lymphocytes. The best-characterized PRRs are the 11 Toll-like receptors (TLRs), first recognized as determinants of embryonic patterning in *Drosophila* and subsequently appreciated as components of host defenses in both insects and mammals.[46, 47] TLR subfamilies can be distinguished by expression either on the cell surface or in intracellular compartments. Binding of TLRs by a PAMP ligand triggers intracellular signaling pathways via multiple "adaptors" leading to a vigorous inflammatory response. Based on involvement of the myeloid differentiation primary response gene 88 (MyD88), two principal pathways are recognized. Most TLRs are MyD88-dependent, whereas TLR3 and -4 signal via a MyD88-independent IFN-β pathway.

As noted above, the innate immune response also includes the capacity of NK lymphocytes to identify and destroy, by direct cytotoxic mechanisms, cells lacking surface expression of MHC class I molecules, which marks them as potentially pathogenic.[7] Additionally, an innate immune response involves elements of the humoral immune system that function independently of antibody, especially the activation of the complement cascade through the lectin and alternative pathways, with consequent opsonization to promote phagocytosis and destruction.

The defenses of the specific immune system to any particular pathogenic agent are determined largely by the context in which it is encountered. Regardless, effectiveness depends upon the four principal properties of specific immunity: (1) a virtually unlimited capacity to bind macromolecules, particularly proteins, with exquisite specificity, reflecting random generation of antigen-binding receptors; (2) the capacity for self/nonself discrimination, consequences of a rigorous process involving positive and negative selection during thymocyte differentiation as well as negative selection during B-cell differentiation; (3) the property of immunological memory, reflecting antigen-driven clonal proliferation of T cells and B cells that results in increasingly rapid and effective responses upon second and subsequent encounters with a particular antigen or pathogen; and (4) mechanisms for pathogen destruction, including direct cellular cytotoxicity, release of inflammatory cytokines, opsonization with antibody and complement, and neutralization in solution by antigen precipitation or conformational alteration.

Although most specific immune responses involve a multiplicity of available defense mechanisms, several generalizations may be conceptually useful. NK-cell- and T-cell-mediated effector functions are particularly important in defenses against pathogens encountered intracellularly, such as viruses and intracellular bacteria. These responses involve the production of inflammatory cytokines by CD4 Th1 cells, as well as the direct cytolytic activity of CD8 CTL. In contrast, host defenses to most antigens encountered primarily in the extracellular milieu are largely dependent upon humoral mechanisms (antibody and complement) for antigen neutralization, precipitation, or opsonization and subsequent destruction by phagocytes. Targets of antibody-mediated immunity include extracellular bacteria and toxins (or other foreign proteins). It is worth reiterating, however, that induction of an effective antibody response (including isotype switching) and development of immunological memory (resulting from B-cell clonal expansion) require antigen activation not only of specific B cells, but also CD4 T cells, particularly of the Th2 type.

Finally, clinical 'experiments of nature' have proven particularly instructive in our efforts to understand the role of specific components of the immune system in overall host defenses[48] (Chapter 31). The importance of T-cell-mediated immunity in host defenses to intracellular parasites, fungi (Fig. 1.4), and viruses is emphasized by the remarkable susceptibility of T-cell-deficient patients to organisms such as *Pneumocystis jiroveci* and *Candida albicans,* as well as by the risks of utilizing attenuated live virus vaccines in such patients. On the other hand, patients with defects in antibody synthesis or phagocytic cell function are characteristically afflicted with recurrent infections with pyogenic bacteria, particularly Gram-positive organisms; patients with inherited defects in synthesis of terminal complement components have increased susceptibility to infection with species of *Neisseria.*

In recent years immunology has entered the lay lexicon, largely as a result of the HIV pandemic. People throughout the world are now tragically aware of the consequences of immune deficiency. The

CLINICAL RELEVANCE

CHARACTERISTIC INFECTIONS ASSOCIATED WITH IMMUNE DEFICIENCY SYNDROMES

>> Deficiencies of T-cell-mediated immunity

Mucocutaneous fungal infections, especially *Candida albicans*
Systemic (deep) fungal infections
Systemic infection with attenuated viruses (e.g., live viral vaccines)
Infection with viruses of usually low pathogenicity (e.g., cytomegalovirus)
Pneumocystis jiroveci pneumonia

>> Antibody deficiencies

Encapsulated bacterial infections (e.g., *Streptococcus* spp., *Haemophilus influenzae*)
Recurrent pneumonia, bronchitis, sinusitis, otitis media
Giardia lamblia enteritis

>> Phagocyte deficiencies

Gram-positive bacterial infection (e.g., staphylococci, streptococci)
Gram-negative sepsis
Systemic fungal infections (e.g., *Candida* spp., *Aspergillus* spp.)

>> Adhesion molecule deficiencies

Pyogenic bacterial infections (especially staphylococci)
Cutaneous and subcutaneous abscesses

>> Complement component deficiencies

C3 deficiency – infections with encapsulated bacteria
Deficiency of terminal components – Gram-negative bacteria, especially *Neisseria* spp.

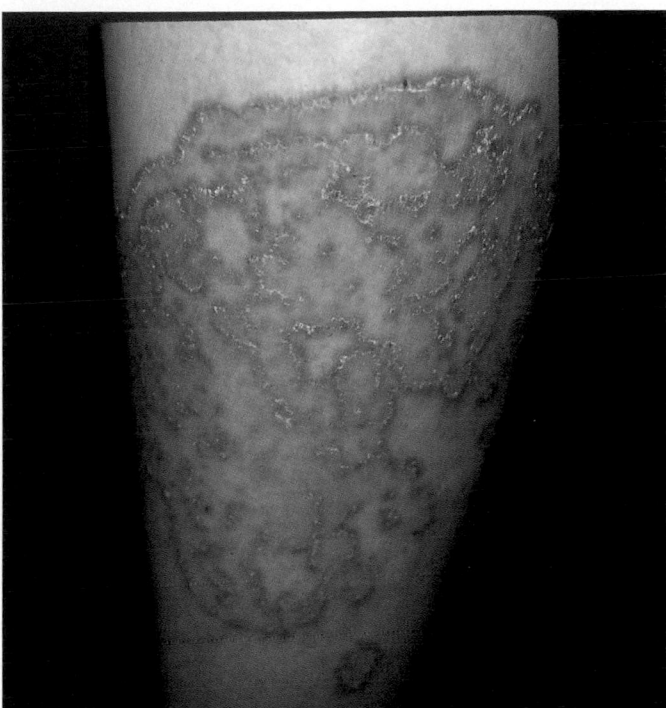

Fig. 1.4 Leg of a 16-year-old patient with chronic mucocutaneous candidiasis as a consequence of congenital T-cell deficiency associated with hypoparathyroidism.

remarkable progress in understanding of this disease, however, depended substantially upon earlier studies of relatively rare patients with primary immunodeficiency syndromes. Similarly, cure of patients with primary immunodeficiencies by cellular reconstitution, particularly bone marrow transplantation, presaged recent interest in correction of such diseases by gene replacement, which, despite formidable challenges, is likely to lead to cures of numerous other, more common, diseases in the foreseeable future. The 'present' of clinical immunology is indeed bright, but its future potential to impact prevention and treatment of many diseases that are today immense challenges is even more exciting to contemplate.[49]

Studies in experimental animal systems, especially the mouse, have been critical to our understanding of molecular aspects of immune system function and have contributed importantly to our appreciation of how aberrations of such functions are involved in the pathogenesis of disease. The new insights gained from use of transgenic mice (including murine expression of human genes) and constitutive or conditional gene knockout mice suggest that future progress will equally depend upon detailed analysis in such systems. Nevertheless, the carefully studied patient will remain the ultimate crucible for understanding human immunity and the roles of the immune system in the pathogenesis of and protection from disease.

REFERENCES

1. Kotwal GJ. Microorganisms and their interaction with the immune system. J Leukocyte Biol 1997; 62: 415.

2. Hancock RE, Brown KL, Mookherjee N. Host defence peptides from invertebrates – emerging antimicrobial strategies. Immunobiology 2006; 211: 315.

3. Kurata S, Ariki S, Kawabata S. Recognition of pathogens and activation of immune responses in *Drosophila* and horseshoe crab innate immunity. Immunobiology 2006; 211: 237.

4. Kawai T, Akira S. Pathogen recognition with Toll-like receptors. Curr Opin Immunol 2005; 17: 338.

5. Meylan E, Tschopp J, Karin M. Intracellular pattern recognition in the host response. Nature 2006; 442: 39.

6. Lanier LL. NK cell recognition. Annu Rev Immunol 2005; 23: 225.

7. Sun PD. Structure and function of natural-killer-cell receptors. Immunol Res 2003; 27: 539.

8. Wang S, Chen L. T lymphocyte co-signaling pathways of the B7-CD28 family. Cell Mol Immunol 2004; 1: 37.

9. Marks DJ, Mitchison NA, Segal AW, et al. Can unresolved infection precipitate autoimmune disease? Curr Top Microbiol Immunol 2006; 305: 105.

10. Anderson MK, Rast JP. Evolution of antigen binding receptors. Annu Rev Immunol 1999; 17: 109.

11. Dudley DD, Chaudhuri J, Bassing CH, et al. Mechanism and control of V(D)J recombination: similarities and differences. Adv Immunol 2005; 86: 43.

12. Corcoran AE. Immunoglobulin locus silencing and allelic exclusion. Semin Immunol 2005; 17: 141.

13. Malissen M, Trucy J, Jouvin-Marche E, et al. Regulation of TCR alpha and beta gene allelic exclusion during T-cell development. Immunol Today 1992; 13: 315.

14. Luo Z, Ronai D, Scharff MD. The role of activation-induced cytidine deaminase in antibody diversification, immunodeficiency, and B-cell malignancies. J Allergy Clin Immunol 2004; 114: 726.

15. Kinoshita K, Nonaka T. The dark side of activation-induced cytidine deaminase: relationship with leukemia and beyond. Int J Hematol 2006; 83: 201.

16. von Boehmer H. Selection of the T-cell repertoire: receptor controlled checkpoints in T-cell development. Adv Immunol 2004; 84: 201.

17. Coutinho A, Caramalho I, Seixas E, et al. Thymic commitment of regulatory T cells is a pathway of TCR-dependent selection that isolates repertoires undergoing positive or negative selection. Curr Top Microbiol Immunol 2005; 293: 43.

18. Hogquist KA, Balddwin TA, Jameson SC. Central tolerance: learning self control in the thymus. Nat Rev Immunol 2005; 5: 772.

19. Nemazee D, Kouskoff V, Hertz M, et al. B-cell-receptor-dependent positive and negative selection in immature B cells. Curr Top Microbiol Immunol 2000; 245: 57.

20. Cancro MP, Kearney JF. B cell positive selection: road map to the primary repertoire? J Immunol 2004; 173: 15.

21. Hayakawa K, Asono M, Shinton SA, et al. Positive selection of natural autoreactive B cells. Science 1999; 285: 113.

22. Edry E, Melamed D. Receptor editing in positive and negative selection of B lymphopoeisis. J Immunol 2004; 173: 4265.

23. Durandy A. Activation-induced cytidine deaminase: a dual role in class switch recombination and somatic hypermutation. Eur J Immunol 2003; 33: 2069.

24. Madden DR. The three-dimensional structure of peptide-MHC complexes. Annu Rev Immunol 1995; 13: 587.

25. De Libero D, Mori L. Mechanisms of lipid-antigen generation and presentation to T cells. Trends Immunol 2006; 27: 485.

26. Berkowski JF, Morita CT, Brenner MB. Human γδ T cells recognize alkylamines derived from microbes, edible plants and tea: implications for innate immunity. Immunity 1999; 11: 57.

27. Proft T, Fraser JD. Bacterial superantigens. Clin Exp Immunol 2003; 133: 299.

28. Goodyear CS, Silverman GJ. B cell superantigens: a microbe's answer to innate-like B cells and natural antibodies. Springer Semin Immunol 2005; 26: 463.

29. Janeway CA, Bottomly K. Signals and signs for lymphocyte responses. Cell 1994; 76: 275.

30. Sharpe AH, Abbas AK. T-cell costimulation – biology, therapeutic potential and challenges. N Engl J Med 2006; 355: 973.

31. Arai K, Lee T, Miyajima A, et al. Cytokines: coordinators of immune and inflammatory responses. Annu Rev Biochem 1990; 59: 783.

32. Jameson SC, Bevan MJ. T cell receptor antagonists and partial agonists. Immunity 1995; 2: 1.

33. Kehrl JH. G-protein-coupled receptor signaling, RGS proteins, and lymphocyte function. Crit Rev Immunol 2004; 24: 409.

34. Schulze-Luehrmann J, Ghosh S. Antigen-receptor signaling to nuclear factor kappa B. Immunity 2006; 25: 701.

35. Mosmann TR, Coffman RL. TH1 and TH2 cells: different patterns of lymphokine secretion lead to different functional properties. Annu Rev Immunol 1989; 7: 145.

36. Zlotnik A, Yoshie O. Chemokines: a new classification system and their role in immunity. Immunity 2000; 12: 121.

37. Viola A, Contento RL, Molon B. T cells and their partners: the chemokine dating agency. Trends Immunol 2006; 27: 421.

38. Ray N, Doms RW. HIV-1 coreceptors and their inhibitors. Curr Top Microbiol Immunol 2006; 303: 97.

39. Yoshimura A, Mori H, Ohishi M, et al. Negative regulation of cytokine signaling influences inflammation. Curr Opin Immunol 2003; 15: 704.

40. Weaver CT, Harrington LE, Mangan PR, et al. Th17: an effector CD4 T cell lineage with regulatory T cell ties. Immunity 2006; 24: 677.

41. Levings MK, Allan S, d' Hennezel E, et al. Functional dynamics of naturally occurring regulatory T cells in health and autoimmunity. Adv Immunol 2006; 92: 119.

42. Walport MJ. Complement. First of two parts. N Engl J Med 2001; 344: 1058.

43. Walport MJ. Complement. Second of two parts. N Engl J Med 2001; 344: 1140.

44. Hjelm F, Carlsson F, Getahun A, et al. Antibody-mediated regulation of the immune response. Scand J Immunol 2006; 64: 177.

45. Pinkoski MJ, Green DR. Apoptosis in the regulation of immune responses. J Rheumatol Suppl 2005; 74: 19.

46. Janssens S, Beyaert R. Role of Toll-like receptors in pathogen recognition. Clin Microbiol Rev 2003; 16: 637.

47. Uematsu S, Akira S. Toll-like receptors and innate immunity. J Mol Med 2006; 84: 712.

48. Fleisher TA. Back to basics: primary immune deficiencies: windows into the immune system. Pediatr Rev 2006; 27: 363.

49. Brent L, Cohen IR, Doherty PC, et al. Crystal-ball gazing-the future of immunological research viewed from the cutting edge. Clin Exp Immunol 2006; 147: 1.

Organization of the immune system

Dorothy E. Lewis, Gregory R. Harriman,
Sarah E. Blutt

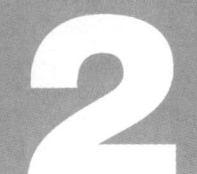

The human immune system consists of organs, including the spleen, the thymus, and the lymph nodes; and movable cells, including cells from bone marrow, blood and lymphatics. This design allows central locations for the initial production and differentiation of committed cells from naive precursors, as in the fetal liver, the bone marrow and the thymus; and more dispersed sites for the selection and further differentiation of cells into mature effector cells, as in the spleen, lymph nodes and intestinal Peyer's patches. This arrangement also allows the regulation of immune responses at locations peripheral to the primary lymphoid organs, and thus provides local control of infectious processes. The mechanisms responsible for the ability of nonspecific leukocytes and natural killer (NK) cells and antigen-specific T and B lymphocytes to respond rapidly to an assault are discussed in later chapters. This chapter is concerned with the basic features and the ontogeny of the cells involved with both specific and nonspecific immunity, and with the essential structure of the lymphoid organs.

IMMUNE CELL DEVELOPMENT

ONTOGENY OF THE CELLS OF THE IMMUNE SYSTEM

In the first month of embryogenesis in humans, stem cells capable of producing white blood cell progenitors can be found in yolk sac erythropoietic islands that are physically attached to, but not inside, the embryo.[1] A specialized endothelial cell is thought to give rise to the first progenitor cell.[2] An area adjacent to the liver, called the aorta–gonad–mesonephros (AGM), produces the progenitor cells that will subsequently develop into hematopoietic stem cells, as classically defined. The placenta has been identified as a separate possible source for fetal stem cells for both the AGM and the fetal liver.[3] The embryonic liver is the first organ β be populated by these progenitor stem cells. It begins the process of blood cell production in the sixth week of gestation, or just after the organ can first be identified histologically. By the 11th week, the liver is the major source of hematopoiesis and will remain the major organ until the sixth month of gestation.

The first progenitor cells derived from hematopoietic stem cells (HSC) are colony-forming cells that can differentiate into granulocytes, erythrocytes, monocytes, megakaryocytes, and lymphocytes. The elements of the skeleton are formed between the second and fourth months of gestation. After this process is βββ, white blood cell development shifts to the marrow of these bones. The transition from liver to bone marrow is completed in the sixth month of gestation. Cells that differentiate from early stem cells begin to populate the primary lymphoid organs, such as the thymus, by 7–8 weeks' gestation.[4] At 8 weeks' gestation, T-cell precursors that have initiated T-cell receptor (TCR) rearrangement (Chapter 9) can be detected in thymic tissue. In the fetal liver, B-cell precursors initiate immunoglobulin (Ig) rearrangements by 7–8 weeks' gestation (Chapter 8). Late in the first trimester, B-cell development spreads to the bone marrow. In the bone marrow, B-cell progenitors congregate in the areas adjacent to the endosteum and differentiate in the direction of the central sinus. The association of B cells with stromal reticular cells is thought to be essential for the eventual release of mature B cells into the central sinus. As in the case of T-cell development, a selection process causes many B-cell progenitors to die by apoptosis.

In adult humans the bone marrow is the chief source of stem cells. However, the peripheral blood contains a population of stem cells with somewhat different characteristics that are capable of limited self-renewal.[5]

TOOLS ESSENTIAL TO AN UNDERSTANDING OF IMMUNE CELL BIOLOGY

Progress beyond morphologic categorization of hematopoietic cells has been facilitated in the last 20 years by the creation of a series of monoclonal antibodies that can be used to identify stage-specific leukocyte cell surface antigens using flow cytometry. These antibodies can also be used for functional characterization. In the early 1980s, the sheer number of monoclonal antibodies raised against a multitude of human leukocyte antigens yielded a complicated nomenclature. In response, leukocyte differentiation antigen workshops were convened to provide guidance, a consistent nomenclature, and consensus regarding the reactivities of

CELLS OF THE IMMUNE SYSTEM

>> Pluripotent stem cells in the bone marrow give rise to all the lineages of immune cells.

>> The development and regulation of cells of the immune system is associated with the programmed appearance of specific cell surface molecules and responsiveness to selective cytokines.

>> The mature cells of the immune system include the antigen-presenting cells of various types; other phagocytic cells, including neutrophils, eosinophils and basophils; and lymphocytes, which are T, B or natural killer cells.

>> Each lymphocyte lineage can be divided into discrete subpopulations which subserve specialized functions. These include CD4 and CD8 T cells, T-helper (Th) subsets, CD16$^+$ and CD16$^-$ NK cells, and CD5$^+$ (B1) and CD5$^-$ (B2) B cells.

monoclonal antibody preparations. All the monoclonal antibodies that recognized a single molecule on leukocytes were grouped by the cluster pattern of cells with which they were identified, hence the term CD, or 'cluster of differentiation' antigen (Table 2.1). As of 2005, 339 CD antigens had been officially recognized, with varying levels of characterization (see Appendix 1). The identification of distinctive patterns of CD antigen expression is an important tool in understanding cellular subpopulations, the relationships between differentiating progenitor subpopulations, and the effector functions of the various cells of the immune system. Future workshops will focus on markers of functional subsets of cells. A more extensive discussion of these markers can be found at http://www.hcdm.org.

HEMATOPOIESIS AND LYMPHOPOIESIS

All mature cells of the hematopoietic and lymphoid lineages are derived from the same population of pluripotent stem cells.[6] These cells first give rise to hematopoietic and lymphoid progenitors. The hematopoietic

Table 2.1 Important cell surface antigens on hematopoietic cells

Cell type	Surface antigens	Predominant location
Hematopoietic stem cells		
Bone marrow	CD34$^-$ or	Bone marrow
HSC	CD34$^+$, Lin–, Thy1$^+$	
Peripheral blood	CD34$^+$, Lin–, CD38$^+$, CD71$^+$	Blood
HSC		
Myeloid cells		
Monocytes	CD14	Blood
	CD35 (CR1), CD64 (FcRrγ1)	
Macrophages	CD68, CD13, CD64, CD35	Tissues
Langerhans' cells	CD1a, CD207 (Langerin),	Skin
Follicular dendritic cells	CD35, CD64	B-cell areas, lymph nodes
Interdigitating	CD80, CD56, Class II,	T cell areas, lymph nodes
Dendritic cells	CD83, CD40	Mainly tissues
Dendritic cells	CD83, CD80, CD86, CD40	
Plasmacytoid dendritic cells	CD4, CCR5, CXCR4, CD40	
(IFN-α producing)		
Granulocytes	CD16 (FcγRIII), CD35 CD88 (C5aR)	Blood, tissues
Neutrophils	CD32 (FcγRII)	Blood, tissues
Eosinophils	CD23, (FcεRII), CD32	Tissues, blood
Basophils	FcεRI Alpha	Tissues, blood,
Mast cells	FcεRI Alpha	Tissues
Lymphocytes		
T cells	CD7, CD3, CD4, CD8, CD28	Thymus, spleen, lymph nodes, MALT, blood
B cells	Surface Ig, class II,	Bone marrow, spleen, lymph nodes, MALT, blood
	CD19, CD20, CD22, CD40	
NK cells	CD16, CD56, CD94	Spleen, lymph nodes, mucosal tissues, blood
NKT cells	CD3, CD56, Vα24 TCR	Blood, tissues
Tregs	CD4, CD25, Foxp3	Thymus, blood, tissues

progenitors are subsequently capable of maturing into cells of the granu-
locytic, erythroid, monocytic–dendritic, and megakaryocytic lineages
(GEMM colony-forming units, CFU-GEMM). Likewise, lymphoid
progenitors mature into B lymphocytes, T lymphocytes and NK cells
(Fig. 2.1).

In the adult, hematopoiesis and lymphopoiesis occur in two distinct
tissues. The development of hematopoietic lineage cells – that is, granulocytes, monocytes, dendritic cells, erythrocytes and platelets – occurs in
the bone marrow (Table 2.2). B-lymphocyte development, through the
stage of mature B cells, also occurs in the bone marrow (Chapter 8). On
the other hand, T-cell progenitors leave the bone marrow, migrate to the
thymus and differentiate into αβ and γδ T cells, as well as regulatory T
cells (Chapter 9). Evidence also suggests that at least some NK cells
develop from precursors in the thymus.[7] However, most NK cell development occurs extrathymically, mainly in the bone marrow.

CHARACTERISTICS OF HEMATOPOIETIC STEM CELLS

The pluripotent stem cell is thought to give rise to all the major red and
white blood cell populations. Human hematopoietic stem cells (HSC) in
the bone marrow are rare: 1 in 10 000 cells. They occupy a distant niche
in the bone marrow closest to the bone and rely on osteoblasts for this
localization.[8] Several separation methods have been used to study stem
cells and their differentiative potential in detail. Early observations
showed that the HSC had characteristic flow cytometric light-scattering
properties (low side scatter, medium forward scatter), no lineage (LIN)-
specific markers (e.g., CD2, CD3, CD5, CD7, CD14, CD15 or CD16),
and expressed CD34 on the cell surface.[9] However, hematopoietic
reconstitution can occur with CD34−, noncycling LIN− cells, suggesting
that surface expression of CD34 is not a definitive marker of the most
primitive precursors.[10]

A subpopulation of stem cells excludes nucleophilic dyes such as
Hoechst dye and is called a 'side population', which can give rise to a wide
variety of cell types. A key aspect of a long-term stem cell is its capacity
for self-renewal via asynchronous division.[11]

Hematopoietic stem cells circulate in the peripheral blood with
10–100 times less frequency. Mobilization of 'stem cells' to the
periphery can be induced with G-CSF. Of these, about 5–20% are
true stem cells.[12] Enriched peripheral blood stem cells do not express
lineage-associated antigens. A minor subpopulation expresses the
B-cell antigens, CD19 and CD20, and there is a variable level of
expression of the myeloid CD33 and CD13 antigens. Most peripheral blood stem cells express activation antigens, such as the transferrin receptor, CD71 and CD38. Peripheral blood HSC cells can
engraft 2–3 days faster than conventional bone marrow HSC.
Peripheral blood HSC are slightly more differentiated than those
obtained from the bone marrow.

REGULATION OF HEMATOPOIETIC AND LYMPHOPOIETIC CELL GROWTH AND DIFFERENTIATION

Regulation of stem cell differentiation occurs through interactions with
a variety of microenvironmental factors in the bone marrow or thymus.
Cell surface receptors recognize either soluble ligand (e.g., cytokines)
released by other cells, or surface ligands (e.g., cell interaction molecules)
expressed on adjacent cells. These receptors can facilitate differentiation.
Stem cells can be exposed to spatially and temporally regulated ligands
or factors. The differential expression of receptors on the stem cells allow
control of proliferation and differentiation along one of the hematopoietic or lymphoid lineages.[13]

Cytokines have pleiotropic effects on hematopoietic and lymphoid cell
development. They affect both the growth and maintenance of pluripotent
stem cells, as well as the development and differentiation of specific cell
lineages. The effect of the cytokine often differs, depending on whether the
cell has previously been or is concurrently being stimulated by other
cytokines. The stage of differentiation, as well as the presence or absence of
the cytokine's receptor on the cell surface, also affects the cellular response.

Stromal cells located within the bone marrow and thymus regulate
hematopoietic and lymphoid cell growth and differentiation by releasing
cytokines, such as the interleukins IL-4, IL-6, IL-7 and IL-11; leukemia
inhibitory factor (LIF); granulocyte–macrophage colony-stimulating factor (GM-CSF); granulocyte colony-stimulating factor (G-CSF); and
stem cell factor (SCF).[14] Stromal cells also participate in cell–cell interactions with progenitors by means of the engagement of cell surface molecules that provide additional regulatory stimuli. In addition, stromal
cells form the intercellular matrix (e.g., fibronectin and collagen) that
binds to selectin and integrin receptors present on hematopoietic and
lymphoid progenitors.[15]

Cytokines that affect the growth and maintenance of pluripotent and multipotent stem cells

Pluripotent stem cells are characterized by their ability to reconstitute
cells of the hematopoietic and lymphoid lineages.[16] Stem cells are resistant to 5-fluorouracil treatment, which indicates that they are nondividing. The factors that maintain these cells, as well as those that promote
their growth, are becoming better understood. Maintenance of pluripotent capacity is mediated through differentiation antagonists, termed
restrictins. Studies suggest that stromal cells maintain stem cell capacity
by the release of factors such as restrictin-D or flt-3/flk-2 ligand, which
either antagonize differentiation induced by other cytokines or facilitate
stem cell self-renewal. Because the stem cell pool is depleted as their
progeny differentiate, proliferation of the stem cells is required to avoid
exhaustion. The entry of stem cells into the cell cycle and subsequent
proliferation, as well as commitment to particular lineages, also appears
to be controlled by cytokines. Recent studies have focused on discovery
of in vitro conditions that maintain extended long-term cultures of stem
cell populations. The data suggest that flt-3 ligand, c-kit ligand and
megakaryocyte growth and development factor (MGDF) all promote
long-term stem cell expansion. The combination of c-kit ligand, IL-3
and IL-6 causes more rapid expansion, but does not allow long-term
extension of precursor cells.[16]

Several cytokines, either alone or in combination, have been
shown to promote stem cell growth (Table 2.3).[17] In general, combinations of cytokines are more effective at inducing stem cell growth
than are individual cytokines. For example, IL-1 promotes stem cell
growth by its ability to induce bone marrow stromal cells to release
additional cytokines. In addition, although IL-1 cannot stimulate
hematopoietic progenitors by itself, it can synergistically stimulate
these cells in the presence of other cytokines. One of these other
cytokines, IL-3, promotes the growth of hematopoietic progenitors.

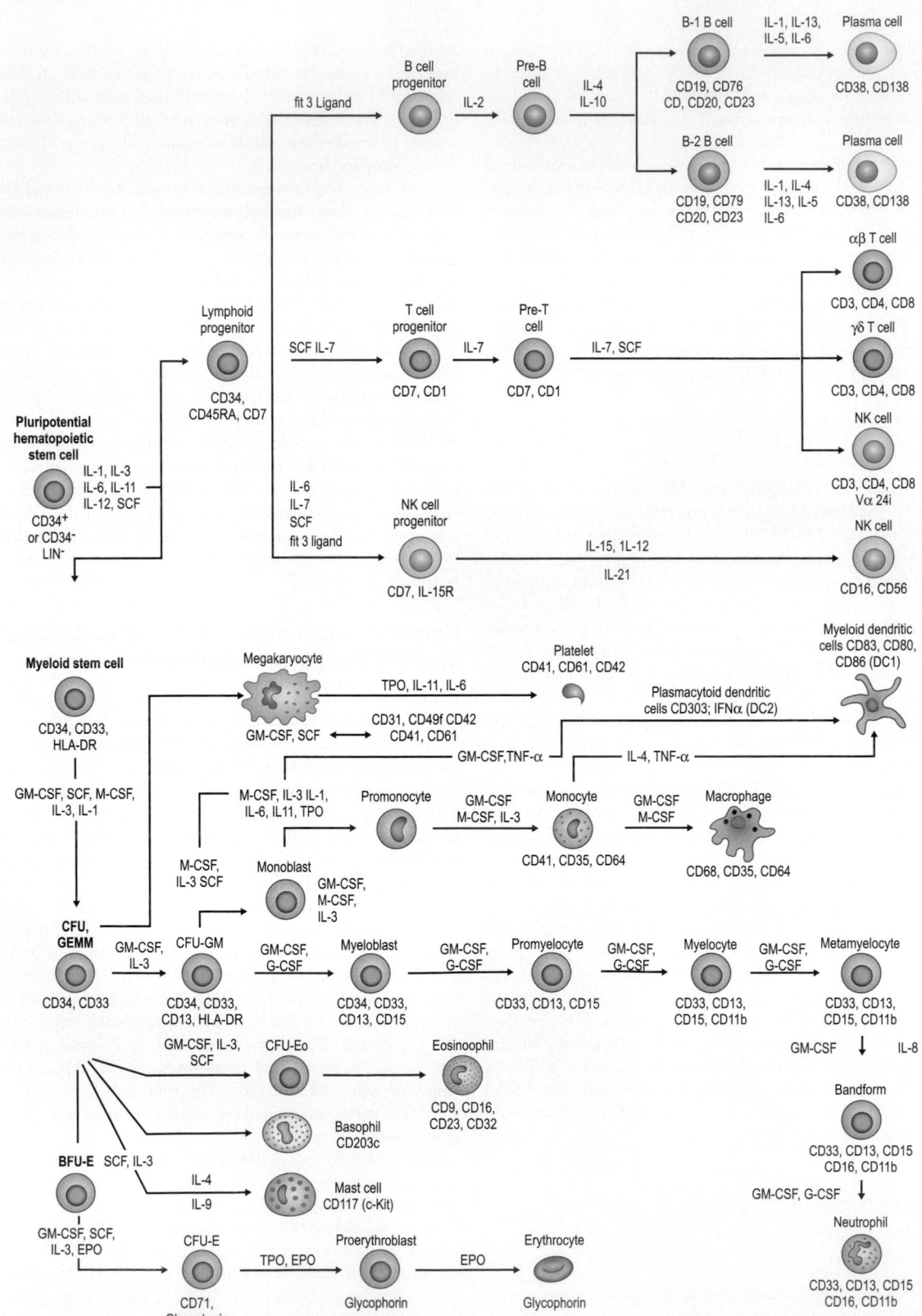

Fig. 2.1 The differentiation of hematopoietic cells.

Table 2.2 Normal distribution of hematopoietic cells in the bone marrow

Cell type	Approximate proportion (%)
Stem cells	1
Megakaryocytes	1
Monocytes	2
Dendritic cells	2
Lymphocytes	15
Plasma cells	1
Myeloid precursors	4
Granulocytes	50–70
Red blood cell precursors	2
Immature and mature red blood cells	10–20

The effect is significantly enhanced by IL-6, IL-11, G-CSF and SCF. IL-11, a stromal cell-derived cytokine, enhances IL-3-induced colony formation in 5-fluorouracil-resistant stem cells. Similarly, other cytokines secreted by stromal cells, for example IL-6, G-CSF and SCF, also exert their effects by shortening the G_0 period in stem cells. In contrast, IL-3 acts on cells after they have left G_0. IL-12 is unable to support the growth of primitive hematopoietic stem cells, either by itself or in conjunction with IL-11 or SCF. However, it does act in synergy with IL-3 and IL-11, or IL-3 and SCF, to enhance stem cell survival and growth. In some situations, cytokines can enhance the growth of hematopoietic and lymphoid cells, but under other circumstances the cytokine may inhibit cell growth or enhance differentiation. LIF is a cytokine that demonstrates such pleiotropic effects. One feature of LIF is that it enhances the growth and development of bone marrow progenitor cells along multiple lineages in media containing IL-3, IL-6 and GM-CSF. However, in the absence of cytokines or factors in serum, LIF has little effect on the growth and development of CD34+ progenitor cells. Similarly, although transforming growth factor-β (TGF-β) and IL-4 are

Table 2.3 Cytokines important for hematopoietic cell growth and differentiation

Cytokines	Stem cells	Thymocytes	B cells	NK cells
IL-1	Acts on Stromal cells	Differentiation		
IL-2		Pleomorphic	Proliferation	Proliferation
IL-3	Proliferation			
IL-4		Pleomorphic	Promotes (low) Prevents (high)	Inhibits IL-2
IL-5			Proliferation/differentiation	
IL-6	Shortens G0	Enhances stimulation	Maintains potential	Enhances IL-2
IL-7		Survival/proliferation	Proliferation of pro- and pre-B cells	Activation
IL-10			Survival	
IL-11 Oncostatin M	Shortens G_0		Maintains potential	
IL-12	Survival			Activation Proliferation
IL-13			Activation/division of mature B cells	
IL-15			Proliferation	Development/survival
Interleukin 21			Proliferation	Expansion
SCF/c-*kit*	Survival	Atrophy	Maintains potential	Expansion
G-CSF	Shortens G0		Maintains potential	
FLt3 ligand	Growth Factor		Increases proliferation	Expansion
SDF1-α		Proliferation/Regeneration	Chemoattractant	
LIF	Proliferation	Atrophy		
Thrombopoietin	Expansion			
TNF-α	Proliferation: inhibits granulocytes			
TGF-β	Inhibits growth enhanced granulocytes			
MIP-1α	Inhibits			
NGF			Proliferation/differentiation	Expansion

potent inhibitors of hematopoietic progenitor cell growth, they have been shown to enhance granulocyte development. Conversely, although tumor necrosis factor-α (TNF-α) inhibits the development of granulocytes, it can potentiate the effects of IL-3 on hematopoietic progenitor cell proliferation.

Other cytokines have effects on the proliferation and differentiation of multipotent progenitors of hematopoietic and lymphoid cells. For example, GM-CSF and IL-3 promote the development of granulocytes, macrophages, dendritic cells and erythrocytes. Similarly, IL-6 participates in the development of neutrophils, macrophages, platelets, T cells and B cells.

Cytokines that inhibit hematopoietic stem cell growth

Cytokines produced by mature cells also downregulate hematopoietic stem cell growth. For example, macrophage inflammatory protein-1α (MIP-1α) is an inhibitor of hematopoietic progenitor cell proliferation. Other factors regulate stem cell growth through a variety of mechanisms, including the promotion of terminal differentiation (e.g., interferon-γ [IFN-γ] and TGF-β) or through the induction of apoptosis (e.g., TNF-α). When pathologic conditions exist, these cytokines can have adverse effects on hematopoietic and lymphoid cell development, resulting in various deficiency states.

Cytokines affecting development and differentiation of specific cell lineages

The initial event in differentiation involves the commitment of pluripotent stem cells to a specific lineage. Cytokines are important for this process and appear to have lineage-specific effects that act specifically at late stages of differentiation. For example, erythropoietin regulates the later stages of erythrocyte differentiation, whereas G-CSF induces granulocyte differentiation and macrophage colony-stimulating factor (M-CSF) is specific for macrophage maturation.[18] Cytokines that play an important role in the growth and development of specific cell lineages are described under each cell type.

Mature cells of the immune system

The mature cells of the immune system, which arise mainly from progenitor cells in the bone marrow, include nonspecific effector cells and antigen-specific effector cells. The central player in both lines of defense is the antigen-presenting cell (Chapter 7). In addition to their nonspecific effector functions, these cells are crucial for the development of specific immune responses. With maturation, these cells enter the blood (Table 2.4), where they circulate into the tissues and organs.

Antigen-presenting cells

Cells that act as antigen-presenting cells (APC) include a diverse group of leukocytes such as monocytes, macrophages, dendritic cells and B cells. In addition, endothelial or epithelial cells can acquire antigen-presenting abilities after the upregulation of major histocompatibility complex (MHC) class II expression by various cytokines (see Chapter 5).

APC are found primarily in the solid lymphoid organs and in the skin. In most tissues the frequency of these cells varies between 0.1% and 1.0%. The specialized APC in the B-cell areas of the lymph nodes and spleen are termed follicular dendritic cells. They trap antigen–antibody complexes and thus play a key role in the generation and maintenance of memory B cells. These cells do not express class II molecules, but do have receptors for IgG and complement component C3b, FcγR (CD64) and CR1 (CD35), respectively. Antigen-presenting cells termed dendritic cells are abundant in the thymic medulla and play a role in the education (positive and negative selection) of thymocytes.

Dendritic cells residing in peripheral sites such as the skin, intestinal lamina propria, lung, genitourinary tract etc. are

Table 2.4 Normal distribution of white blood cells in the peripheral blood of adults and children.

Cell Type	Approximate percentage		Range of absolute counts (no./mm³)	
	Adults	Children (0–2 yrs)	Adults	Children (0–2 yrs)
Monocytes	4–13		400–1000	
Dendritic cells	0.5–1	ND	30–170	ND
Granulocytes	35–73		2500–7500	1000–8500
Lymphocytes	15–52	34–75	1450–3600	3400–9000
As % of lymphocytes				
T cells	75–85	53–84	900–2500	2500–6200
CD4 cells	27–53	32–64	550–1500	1300–4300
CD8 cells	13–23	12–30	300–1000	500–2000
B cells	5–15	06–41	100–600	300–3000
NK cells	5–15	03–18	200–700	170–1100

* Not determined. Child data adapted from Shearer W, Rosenblatt H, Gelman R, et al. Lymphocyte subsets in healthy children from birth through 18 years of age: The pediatric AIDS Clinical Trials Group P1009 study. J Allergy Clin Immunol 2003; 12: 973–980.

typically immature. These cells are more phagocytic and express fewer MHC class I, MHC class II and costimulatory molecules. These immature dendritic cells take up antigens in tissues for subsequent presentation to T cells. During migration to the lymph nodes, dendritic cells undergo phenotypic and functional changes characterized by increased expression of MHC class I, MHC class II and costimulatory molecules (e.g., B7–1 [CD80] and B7–2 [CD86]), which react with ligands CD28 and CTLA-4 expressed by T cells.[19]

The predominant APC of the skin are the Langerhans' cells.[20] These are found in the epidermis and are characterized by rocket-shaped granules called Birbeck's granules. Upon migration from the skin, these cells deliver antigens entering the skin to the effector cells of the lymph nodes.

The immature tissue dendritic cells in peripheral tissues also engulf and process antigens. They leave the tissues and home to T-cell areas in the draining lymph nodes or spleen.[21] At these sites they can directly present processed antigens to resting T cells to induce their proliferation and differentiation. These effector cells then home to the site of the antigenic assault. The key distinction between mature dendritic cells and macrophages in terms of antigen presentation is the ability of dendritic cells to activate resting T cells directly.

Monocytes–macrophages

Cells of the monocyte–macrophage lineage exist in blood (~10% of white blood cells) primarily as monocytes, large 10–18 μm cells with peanut-shaped, pale purple nuclei as determined by Wright's staining (Table 2.4). The cytoplasm, which is 30–40% of the cell, is light blue and has azurophilic granules that resemble ground glass. There also are numerous intracytoplasmic lysosomes. The cells have a number of characteristic cell surface molecules, including MHC class II molecules, CD14 (the receptor for lipopolysaccharide), and distinct Fc receptors (FcR) for immunoglobulin (Ig) (Chapter 21). The latter include FcγRI (or CD64), which has a high affinity for IgG, and FcγRII (or CD32), which is of medium affinity and binds to aggregated IgG. FcγRIII (or CD16) has low affinity for IgG and is associated with antibody-dependent cellular cytotoxicity (ADCC). It is expressed on macrophages, but not on blood monocytes. Monocytes and macrophages also express CD89, the Fc receptor for IgA.

Macrophages are more differentiated monocytes that reside in various tissues, including lung, liver and brain.[22] Most cells of the monocyte–macrophage lineage adhere strongly to glass or plastic surfaces, a property often used to deplete or purify them from mixed cell populations. Many cells of this lineage phagocytose organisms or tumor cells in vitro. Cell surface receptors, including CD14, Fcγ receptors and CR1 (CD35), are important in opsonization and phagocytosis. Cells of this lineage also express MHC class II molecules and some express the low-affinity receptor for IgE (CD23). Other cell surface molecules include myeloid antigens CD13 (aminopeptidase N) and CD15 (Gal (1–4) or [Fuc (1–3)] GlcNAc) and the adhesion molecules CD68 and CD29 or CD49d (VLA-4). In addition to phagocytic and cytotoxic functions, these cells have receptors for various cytokines such as IL-4 and IFN-γ that can serve to regulate their function. Activated macrophages are also a major source of cytokines, including IFN, IL-1 and TNF, as well as complement proteins and prostaglandins.

Monocytes and macrophages arise from colony-forming unit granulocyte–monocyte (CFU-GM) progenitors that differentiate first into monoblasts, then promonocytes, and finally monocytes.[23] Mature monocytes leave the bone marrow and circulate in the bloodstream until they enter tissues, where they develop into tissue macrophages (e.g., alveolar macrophages, Kupffer cells and microglial cells).

Several cytokines have been shown to participate in the development of monocytes and granulocytes. For example, SCF, IL-3, IL-6, IL-11 and GM-CSF have all been shown to promote the development of myeloid lineage cells from CD34+ stem cells, especially those in the early stages of differentiation. Another cytokine, M-CSF, acts at the later stages of development and is lineage specific, inducing maturation into macrophages.[19]

Dendritic cells

Dendritic cells are accessory cells that express high levels of MHC class II antigen and are potent inducers of primary T-cell responses. Except for the bone marrow, they are found in virtually all primary and secondary lymphoid tissues, as well as in skin, mucosa, and blood. Dendritic cells are derived from CD34+ MHC class II-negative precursors present in the bone marrow that also give rise to macrophages and granulocytes. GM-CSF and TNF-α are involved in the development of dendritic cells from their precursors in bone marrow.[24] Langerhans' cells are the immediate precursors of dendritic cells in the skin. After encountering antigen, Langerhans' cells migrate from the skin through afferent lymphatics and into draining lymph nodes, where they enter via the subcapsular sinus. Interdigitating dendritic cells, which present peptide antigens bound to MHC class II molecules to T cells in the lymph nodes and spleen, appear to derive from these Langerhans' cell immigrants. TNF-α also maintains the viability of Langerhans' cells in the skin and stimulates their migration. In Peyer's patches, immature dendritic cells occur in the dome region underneath the follicle-associated epithelium (FAE), where they actively endocytose antigens taken up by M cells in the FAE. More mature interdigitating dendritic cells are found in T-cell regions, where they appear to be the major APC type. These cells, like their counterparts in the lungs, induce T-helper type 2 immune responses. There are at least two types of dendritic cell: the DC1 type are bone marrow derived and found in lymphoid tissues. Plasmacytoid DCs or DC2 are high producers of IFN-α. Their derivation is unclear, but may be myeloid or lymphoid.[25, 26]

Polymorphonuclear granulocytes

Polymorphonuclear (PMN) granulocytes arise from progenitors that mature in the bone marrow. They are released into the blood as short-lived (2–3 days), essentially end-stage, cells. They constitute 65–75% of the white blood cells in the peripheral blood, are 10–20 μm in diameter, and have features such as a multilobed pyknotic nucleus characteristic of cells undergoing apoptosis (Table 2.4).[27] PMNs are also found in tissues and use the process of diapedesis to gain access from the blood. Granulocytes act as early soldiers in the response to stress, tissue damage or pathogen invasion. Because of their function in phagocytosis and killing, they possess granules whose unique staining characteristics are used to categorize the cells as neutrophils (Chapter 21), basophils (Chapter 22) or eosinophils (Chapter 23).

Neutrophils

Most circulating granulocytes are neutrophils (90%). Their granules are azurophilic and contain acid hydrolase, myeloperoxidase and lysozymes. These granules fuse with ingested organisms to form phagolysosomes, which eventually kill the invading organism. In some cases there is extracellular release of granules after activation via the Fc receptors. Neutrophils express a number of myeloid antigens, including CD13, CD15, CD16 (FcγRIII) and CD89 (FcαR). In response to bacterial infection there is typically an increase in the number of circulating granulocytes. This often includes the release of immature granulocytes, called band or stab cells, from the bone marrow. In a mild infection, both the number and function of neutrophils are increased. This is associated with a delay in apoptosis. With a more severe infection there may actually be impairment of function owing to the release of immature cells.

Neutrophils derive from CFU-GM progenitor cells. These give rise to myeloblasts, which in turn differentiate into promyelocytes, myelocytes, and finally mature neutrophils. The cytokines SCF, IL-3, IL-6, IL-11 and GM-CSF promote the growth and development of neutrophil precursors, whereas certain cytokines are important for differentiation of CFU-GM progenitors into mature neutrophils.[28] For example, G-CSF induces maturation of neutrophil precursors into mature neutrophils. IL-4 enhances neutrophil differentiation induced by G-CSF, while at the same time inhibiting the development of macrophages induced by IL-3 and M-CSF.

Eosinophils

Eosinophils typically comprise 2–5% of the white cells in the blood. They exhibit a unique form of diurnal variation because the peak of production occurs at night, perhaps because glucocorticoids are lower at night. Eosinophils are capable of phagocytosis followed by killing, although this is not their main function. The granules in eosinophils are much larger than in neutrophils and are actually membrane-bound organelles. The crystalloid core of the granules contains a large amount of major basic protein (MBP), which can neutralize heparin and is toxic. During degranulation, the granules fuse to the plasma membrane and their contents are released into the extracellular space. Organisms that are too large to be phagocytosed, such as parasites, can be exposed to cell toxins by this mechanism. For example, MBP can damage schistosomes *in vivo*. However, tissue damage is kept to a minimum because the MBP is confined to a small area between the eosinophil and the schistosome. Eosinophils also release products that counteract the effects of mast cell mediators.

Eosinophils derive from a progenitor (CFU-Eo) that progresses through development stages similar to those of neutrophils.[29] These stages begin with an eosinophilic myeloblast, followed by an eosinophilic promyelocyte, a myelocyte, and finally a mature eosinophil. Three cytokines are important in the development of eosinophils: GM-CSF, IL-3 and IL-5. GM-CSF and IL-3 promote eosinophil growth and differentiation; SCF also has an effect on eosinophil function (Chapter 23). IL-5 has more lineage-specific effects on eosinophil differentiation, although it also affects some subsets of T and B cells. IL-5 inhibits eosinophil differentiation, as well as apoptosis.

Basophils and mast cells

Basophils represent less than 1% of the cells in the peripheral circulation, and have characteristic large, deep-purple granules. Mast cells, found only in tissues, are much larger than peripheral blood basophils. The granules are less abundant and the nucleus is more prominent. There are two different types of mast cell, designated mucosal or connective tissue

depending on their location.[30] Mucosal mast cells require T cells for their proliferation, whereas connective tissue mast cells do not. Both types have granules that contain effector molecules. After degranulation, which is effected by cross-linkage of cell surface IgE bound to cells via the high-affinity receptor for IgE, the basophils–mast cells release heparin, histamine and other effector substances to mediate an immediate allergic attack (Chapter 22).

Basophils and mast cells share a number of phenotypic and functional features that suggest they are derived from a common precursor. They both contain basophilic-staining cytoplasmic granules; they both express the high-affinity IgE receptor (FcεRI); and they both release a number of similar chemical mediators that participate in immune and inflammatory responses, particularly anaphylaxis. However, basophils and mast cells have some distinct morphologic and functional characteristics that suggest they represent distinct lineages of cells, rather than cells at different stages within the same lineage. Basophils mature from a progenitor (CFU-BM) into basophilic myeloblasts, then basophilic promyelocytes, myelocytes, and finally mature basophils. Less is known about the stages of mast cell development, although they are probably derived from the same CFU-BM progenitor as basophils.

In human basophils and mast cells, SCF induces the most consistent effects on growth and differentiation. Recently it has been shown that IL-3, as well as SCF, is important for intestinal mast cell differentation. This probably explains why T cells are needed for their development.[31] In contrast to mouse mast cells, IL-4 and IL-9 do not appear to stimulate the development of human mast cells from progenitors. However, IL-9 does act in synergy with SCF to enhance the growth of mast cells. Additional cytokines that affect basophil growth include nerve growth factor and GM-CSF or TGF-β, and IL-5 for basophil differentiation.

Platelets and erythrocytes

Hematopoietic stem cells also give rise to platelets and erythrocytes. These cells derive from CFU-GEMM progenitors, which in turn differentiate into burst-forming units for megakaryocytes (BFU-MEG) in the case of platelets, and burst-forming units for erythrocytes (BFU-E) in the case of erythrocytes. The BFU-MEG subsequently differentiate into CFU-MEG, promegakaryoblasts, megakaryoblasts, megakaryocytes, and finally platelets.[32] Several cytokines, particularly thrombospondin, IL-1, IL-3, GM-CSF, IL-6, IL-11 and LIF, affect the growth and differentiation of platelets. In the case of erythrocytes, BFU-E differentiate into CFU-E, then pronormoblasts, basophilic normoblasts, polychromatophilic normoblasts, orthochromic normoblasts, reticulocytes, and finally erythrocytes.[33] Again, several cytokines, notably GM-CSF, SCF, IL-9, thrombospondin and erythropoietin, regulate erythrocyte development.

Lymphocytes

Lymphocytes, the central cell type of the specific immune system, represent about 25% of white cells in the blood (Table 2.4). Small lymphocytes are 7–10 μm in diameter, are characterized by a nucleus that stains dark purple with Wright's stain, and contain very little cytoplasm. Large granular lymphocytes are 10–12 μm in diameter and contain more cytoplasm and scattered granules. There are three types of lymphocyte that circulate in the peripheral blood: T, B and NK cells, representing respectively about 80%, 10% and 10% of total lymphocytes (Chapters 8, 9 and 18). In the thymus most of the lymphocytes (90%) are T cells; however, in the spleen and lymph nodes only about 30–40% are T cells. The preponderant lymphocytes in these locations are B cells (60–70%).[34, 35]

T lymphocytes

T lymphocytes arise from lymphocyte progenitors in the bone marrow which are committed to the T-cell lineage before homing to the thymus. In the early stages of embryogenesis, T-cell precursors to migrate into the thymus in waves.[36, 37] Associated with this migration is the developing ability of thymic education elements, epithelial cells, and dendritic cells to select appropriate T cells.[38] In the thymus, T cells rearrange their specific antigen receptors (TCR) and then express CD3 along with the TCR on their surface (Chapter 9). Resting T cells in the blood are typically 7–10 μm in diameter and are agranular, except for the presence of a structure termed a Gall body, not found in B cells (Table 2.4). The Gall body is a cluster of primary lysosomes associated with a lipid droplet. A minority of T cells in the blood (about 20%), are of the large granular type, meaning that they are 10–12 μm in diameter and contain primarily lysosomes, which are dispersed in the cytoplasm. Golgi apparati also are found. The preponderant form of the TCR, found on about 95% of circulating T cells, consists of α and β chains (αβTCR+).[39] Some CD3+ cells do not express either CD4 or CD8 and are characterized by having an alternative TCR of composed of γ and δ chains (γδTCR+). Further differentiation in the thymus occurs from CD3+, CD4+ and CD8+ cells to cells expressing either CD4 or CD8 but not both (Chapter 9). These mature cells then circulate in the peripheral blood at ratio of about 2:1 (CD4:CD8) and populate the lymph nodes, spleen and other secondary lymphoid tissues.

T-cell progenitors, which are CD7+, are believed to arise in the bone marrow from a multipotential lymphoid stem cell. After migration to the thymus, the CD7+ T cells give rise to a population of CD34+, CD3–, CD4–, and CD8– T-cell precursors, which undergo further differentiation into mature T cells. Cytokines produced by thymic epithelial cells, for example IL-1 and soluble CD23, promote the differentiation of these precursors into CD2+, CD3+ thymocytes (Table 2.3). IL-7 induces the proliferation of CD3+ double-negative (CD4– CD8–) thymocytes, even in the absence of comitogenic stimulation. IL-7 is absolutely required for human T-cell development.[40] IL-2 and IL-4 demonstrate complex effects on thymocyte development. Both appear capable not only of promoting the development of prothymocytes but also of antagonizing their development. IL-6 acts as a costimulator of IL-1- or IL-2-induced proliferation of double-negative (DN) thymocytes and can stimulate the proliferation of mature, cortisone-resistant thymocytes alone. Once T cells leave the thymus, a variety of cytokines affect their growth and differentiation.

Subpopulations of T cells

T cells can be divided into subsets based on their surface expression of CD4 and CD8, as well as by their function in the immune response. CD4 and CD8 T cells were originally characterized by expression of the respective antigen and association with functional ability. For example, human T cells expressing CD4 provide help for antibody synthesis, whereas cells expressing CD8 were found to develop into cytotoxic T cells. These functional distinctions are less clear today; instead, the distinction between cells expressing CD4 or CD8 involves which antigen-presenting molecule is used for TCR interaction. Thus, CD4 T cells recognize antigen in the context of MHC class II molecules, and CD8 T cells recognize antigen presented by class I molecules (Chapter 5).

T-helper (Th) cells mature in response to foreign antigens. Their function is dependent on the production of cytokine modules, which characterize them as Th type 1 (Th1), Th2 or Th17.[41] The precursor Th cell first differentiates into a Th0 cell producing interferon-γ (IFN-γ) and IL-4. The cytokine environment subsequently determines whether Th1 or Th2 cells predominate. Th1 cells produce primarily IFN-γ, IL-2 and TNF-α, and are important in cell-mediated immunity to intracellular pathogens, such as the tubercle bacillus. Th2 cells produce predominantly IL-4, IL-5, IL-6, IL-10 and IL-13, as well as IL-2, and predominate in immediate or allergic type 1 hypersensitivity. Other populations of CD4 T cells can develop and rely on IL-23 or IL-12 action upon the cells.[42] If T cells are exposed to IFN-γ, they upregulate both IL-12R and IL-23R, which then produce either conventional Th1 cells or another subset, Th17, that produces IL-17 and which has been associated with autoimmunity. Conversely, IL-17-producing CD4 cells also result from the direct action of IL-23 without IL-12 involement. It is likely that there will be other epigenetically altered T cells that allow diversity of function during an immune response.

A minor subpopulation (<5%) of CD3+ cells in the peripheral blood express γδ TCR molecules. Most of these cells do not express CD4 or CD8. However, some intraepithelial lymphocytes that express γδ TCR also express CD8 αα homodimers, rather than conventional CD8 αβ heterodimers. These cells, which are thymus independent, are thought to be involved in the initial response to bacterial antigens presented in the mucosal epithelium. Another minor subpopulation of T cells, NKT cells, can be CD4 or CD8 expressing a single Vα chain, Vα24, that recognizes glycolipids in the context of CD1a, not MHC.[43, 44] The final minor subset are regulatory T cells, which occur naturally and can be induced *in vitro*. They are CD4+ and express high levels of CD25 and the transcription factor foxp3. These cells are important in regulatory immune responses, are reduced in autommunity and increased in cancer.[45, 46]

B cells and plasma cells

B cells represent 5–10% of the lymphocytes found in the blood (Table 2.4). They are typically 7–10 μm in diameter and lack Gall bodies and granules. The cytoplasm is characterized by scattered ribosomes and isolated rough endoplasmic reticulum (RER). The Golgi is not prominent, unless B cells are activated. B cells express cell membrane immunoglobulin (mIg), the majority expressing both IgM and IgD.[47] A small minority of B cells expresses surface IgG or IgA. Plasma cells (10–15 μm) are not normally found in the blood. They display an eccentric nucleus and a basophilic cytoplasm with a well-developed Golgi. The plasma cell displays parallel arrays of expanded RER that contains Ig.

A number of other cell surface molecules are found on B cells (Chapter 8), including CD19, CD20, CD40, CD79, MHC class II, Fcγ RII receptors (CD32) and complement receptors C3b (CR1a; CD35) and C3d (CR2a; CD21). Like T cells, which surround the TCR with activation effector molecules, termed CD3, the B-cell Ig also has a B-cell receptor complex consisting of CD19, CD21 and CD81 (Chapter 4). Upon activation and cross-linking of surface Ig by specific antigen, B cells undergo proliferation and differentiation to produce plasma cells. Plasma cells are nondividing, specialized cells whose function is to secrete Ig. They lose the expression of mIg and MHC class II molecules. B-cell proliferation and differentiation processes take place in the germinal centers of the lymph nodes.

Several cytokines influence the development of B lymphocytes. *In vitro* studies of cytokines involved in the development of early B-cell progenitors have demonstrated that combinations of SCF (but not IL-3) with IL-6, IL-11 or G-CSF can maintain B-lymphoid potential.[48] Stromal cell-dependent differentiation of fetal pro-B cells occurs in conjunction with Flk-2/flt-3 ligand.

IL-4 has a variety of important effects on B-cell growth and differentiation. Low doses of IL-4 induce pre-B cells to differentiate into B cells expressing surface IgM, whereas higher doses of IL-4 inhibit differentiation into B cells. IL-4 has additional effects on mature B cells, including an increase in expression of MHC class II, CD23 and CD40 molecules; activation with progression to the G_1 stage of the cell cycle; enhancement of proliferation after stimulation through the Ig receptor; and induction of immunoglobulin class switch in human to IgG_4 and IgE (IgG_1 and IgE in mouse). IL-13, which is closely related to IL-4, has many similar effects on B cells.

Other cytokines, such as IL-2, IL-5, IL-6, IL-11 and nerve growth factor (NGF), act on mature B cells and can either enhance their proliferation or promote their differentiation into immunoglobulin-secreting cells. In addition, IL-10 enhances the viability of B cells *in vitro*, increases MHC class II expression, and augments the proliferation and differentiation of B cells after stimulation through the Ig receptor or CD40. $TGF-\beta_1$ is a major switch factor for IgA. This cytokine induces human B cells triggered with mitogen to switch to both IgA_1 and IgA_2. SDF-1 (stromal cell-derived factor) has been shown to attract early-stage B-cell precursors and is a likely mechanism whereby B cells form islands in the bone marrow.[18] There are at least two populations of B cells: those that express CD5 (B-1) and are found in the follicular mantle, and those that do not (B-2), which are primarily found in lymphoid follicles. The B-1 lineage produce natural antibodies, primarily IgM, and are the first to develop during gestation.[49, 50]

Natural killer cells

NK cells comprise the third major lymphocyte subset, i.e., 10–15% of circulating lymphocytes (Table 2.4). These cells are usually larger than typical lymphocytes (10–12 μm) and display less nuclear material and more cytoplasm than do small lymphocytes. They possess electron-dense peroxidase-negative granules and a well developed Golgi apparatus. Functional NK cells can be found in the fetal liver as early as 6 weeks' gestation. These fetal NK cells express cytoplasmic CD3 proteins, but exhibit no TCR rearrangements. Evidence suggests that an Fcγ receptor-positive cell that does not express lineage-specific markers (LIN−) exists in the fetal mouse thymus, where it normally gives rise to T cells. However, if removed from the thymus, the cells develop into CD3− NK cells. Such CD3− cells with variable CD16 expression exist in human thymocyte populations and can be induced to proliferate, to express NK-associated antigens, and to exhibit NK cell function *in vitro*. These cells also express substantial levels of CD3δ and CD3ε in the cytoplasm.[51]

Mature NK cells do not express conventional antigen receptors, such as TCR or Ig, and the genes for these receptors remain unrearranged. Some express FcγRIII (CD16) and others express CD56, an adhesion molecule. NK cells, like T cells, also express the CD2 molecule. NK cells express the β chain of the IL-2 receptor, CD122, which allows resting NK cells to respond directly to IL-2. The function of NK cells is to provide nonspecific cytotoxic activity towards virally infected cells and tumor cells (Chapter 18). NK cells also can kill specifically when they are provided an antibody. This death delivery mechanism, known as antibody-dependent cellular cytotoxicity (ADCC), occurs via binding of the antibody to the Fcγ receptor CD16. After activation, NK cells produce cytokines, such as IFN-γ, that can affect the proliferation and differentiation of other cell types. Recent evidence suggests several possible recognition molecules on human NK cells, some activating, some inhibiting, and some acting as receptors for MHC class I molecules.

The ontogeny of NK cells is now better understood. Although they express a number of membrane antigens in common with T cells and share functional properties with some T-cell subsets, suggesting a common origin, NK cells are found in fetuses before the development of T cells or the thymus. In addition, NK cells appear to develop normally in nude, athymic mice. Moreover, NK cells probably develop extrathymically, and recent data suggest that they can develop from stem cells in the lymph nodes. NK cells arise from triple-negative (CD3−CD4−CD8−) precursors that are CD56+, but do not express CD34 or CD5. T cells, on the other hand, develop from 'triple-negative' precursors that are CD34+CD5+CD56+. It is likely that T cells and NK cells arise from a common 'triple-negative' precursor with the phenotype CD7+CD34+CD5+CD56+.

Recent evidence suggests that the cytokine receptor that determines lineage specificity is the α chain of the IL-2 receptor, CD25. Once CD25 is upregulated, the cell is destined to become a T cell. The cytokines most important in the early development of NK cells are IL-15 and IL-7. Flt ligand and c-*kit* also facilitate NK cell expansion. Several cytokines have been shown to promote the growth and differentiation of mature NK cells. IL-2, the first cytokine shown to have effects on NK cells, induces the proliferation and activation of NK cells. This probably occurs via the IL-2 receptor β chain (CD122), as NK cells do not express CD25. IL-2 also induces the growth of NK cells from precursors in bone marrow cultures. Both IL-7 and IL-12, also known as NK-cell stimulatory factor, have been shown to activate NK cells. Although IL-4 inhibits the effects of IL-2 or IL-7 on NK cells, it acts synergistically with IL-12 to induce proliferation of CD56+ cells. IL-6, despite having no effect by itself, enhances NK cell activity in thymocytes cultured with IL-2. Finally, IL-15 is also involved in signalling NK cells for survival.[52]

KEY CONCEPTS

TISSUES OF THE IMMUNE SYSTEM

>> The immune system consists of central locations of immune cell production and differentiation, and dispersed organs, where encounter with and response to antigens occur.

>> B cells and T cells develop in the bone marrow and thymus, respectively.

>> The mucosal surfaces and skin provide the primary access for foreign antigens to cells of the immune system, where they first interact primarily with antigen-presenting cells.

>> The secondary lymph organs, which include the spleen, lymph nodes, tonsils and Peyer's patches, are where immune reactions occur.

■ MAJOR LYMPHOID ORGANS ■

The primary lymphoid organs are sites where lymphocytes differentiate from stem cells and proliferate and mature into effector cells. From birth to old age, these functions are carried out only in the bone marrow and the thymus.

BONE MARROW

The bone marrow provides the environment necessary for the development of most of the white blood cells of the body (Fig. 2.2). At birth, most bone cavities are filled with actively dividing blood-forming

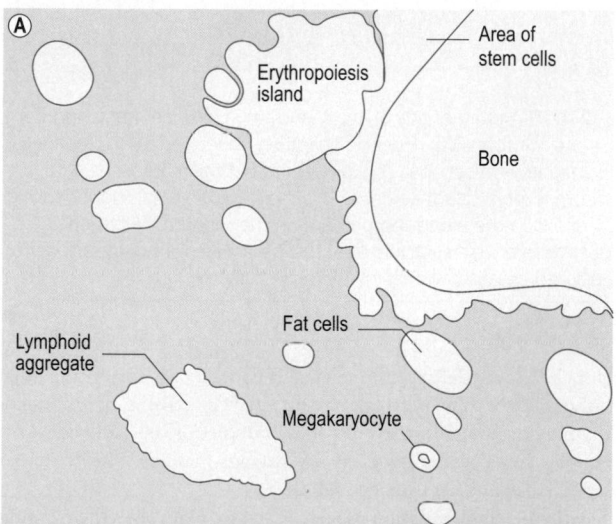

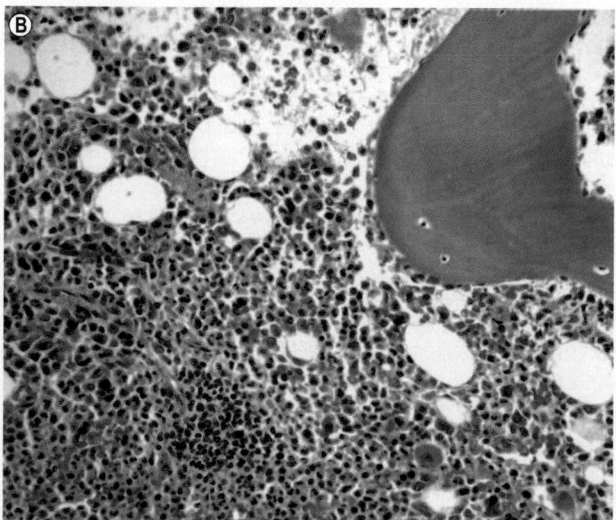

Fig. 2.2 Structure of the bone marrow, showing islands of erythropoiesis, granulopoiesis and scattered lymphocytes.

elements known as 'red' marrow. Beginning at about the age of 3–4 years, however, the tibia and femur become filled with fat cells, which limits their role in hematopoietic development. The ribs, sternum, iliac crest and vertebrae remain 30–50% cellular and continue to produce hematopoietic cells throughout life.[1] Three main components are found in the bone marrow: the blood vessels, the cells, and the extracellular matrix. The production of cells from HSC occurs in areas separated by vascular sinuses. The walls of the surrounding sinus contain a layer of endothelial cells with endocytic and adhesive properties. These specialized endothelial cells of the sinuses probably produce type IV collagen and laminin for structural support. These cells also elaborate colony-stimulating factors and IL-6. The outer wall of the sinus is irregularly covered with reticular cells, which branch into areas where cells are developing and provide anchors for those cells by producing reticular fibers. Megakaryocytes lie against this wall, touching the endothelial cells. A functional unit of marrow called a spheroid contains adipocytes, stromal cell types and macrophages. These reticular cell networks compartmentalize the developing progenitor cells into separate microenvironments called hematons.

The distribution of stem and progenitor cells across the radial axis of the bone suggests that the HSC are next to the bone surface, whereas the more mature progenitor cells are nearer the central venous sinus. This distribution serves to facilitate the eventual release of mature cells. The production of new progenitor cells from stem cells occurs as a result of interactions between stem cells and stromal cells. Given the right stimulus, most of the progeny proliferate and differentiate further, which may result in migration from the bone marrow. In migrating, the cells become detached from the stromal elements and progress toward the central sinus. Control of hematopoiesis is regulated by both positive and negative cytokines and by up- and downregulation of various adhesion molecules in committed progenitor cells. The molecules involved include the fibronectin receptor, glycoproteins IIb and IIIa, ICAM-1 (CD54), LFA-1 (CD11, CD18), LFA-3 (CD58), CD2 and CD44. Adhesion molecules on stromal cell surfaces include fibronectin, laminin, ICAM-1 (CD54), types I, III and IV collagen, and N-CAM. The most clearly established role for adhesion molecules involves fibronectin, which allows erythroid precursors to bind to stromal cells and thus facilitates progression from erythroblast to reticulocyte.

The accessory cell populations found in the bone marrow regulate many aspects of hematopoiesis, both positively and negatively. The upregulation of the growth of the earliest progenitor cells is mediated by cytokines. For example, macrophages produce IL-1, which then induces stromal cells to express growth factors such as GM-CSF, IL-6 and IL-11. However, downregulation can occur at any stage. For example, T cells can regulate hematopoiesis by producing factors that act on early erythroid progenitor cells, BFU-E. Later progenitors, CFU-E, are then more fully differentiated by erythropoietin. By contrast, activated T cells produce factors that can suppress BFU-E and CFU-E *in vitro*.

Cells in the bone marrow were originally characterized by morphology. The predominant types are those of the myeloid lineage, which account for about 50–70% of the cells (Fig. 2.3). Red blood cell precursors represent from 15% to 40% of the total cells. Other lineages exist in lower proportions (<5%). With the advent of cell surface antigen markers and flow cytometry, a more precise delineation could be made. Thus, of the mature leukocytes in the bone marrow, approximately 70% are CD3+, CD14+, CD20+ or CD11b+. These are designated as Lin+. Of the Lin− cells, about 6% are CD33+ and primarily of myeloid lineage. A Lin−CD71+ population represents about 18% of the total and is preponderantly of the red blood cell lineage.

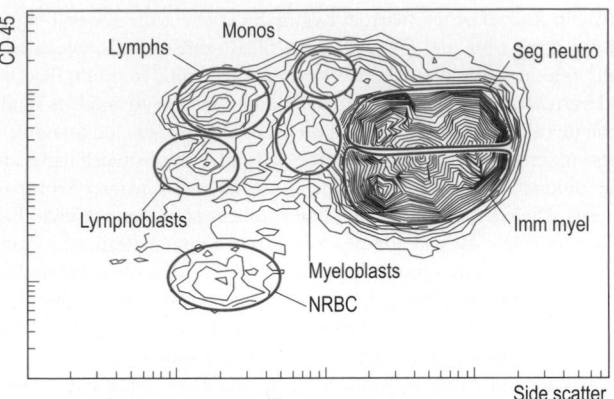

Fig. 2.3 Flow cytogram of normal human bone marrow based on CD45 expression and side scatter. Most of the major hematopoietic populations can be delineated. In this example 1.5% are red blood cell precursors (NRBC), 1.5% are lymphoblasts, 3.0% are mature lymphoytes (Lymphs), 3.0% are monocytes (Monos), 4.0% are myeloblasts, 45% are segmented neutrophils (Seg neutro) and 42% are immature myeloid cells (Imm myel).

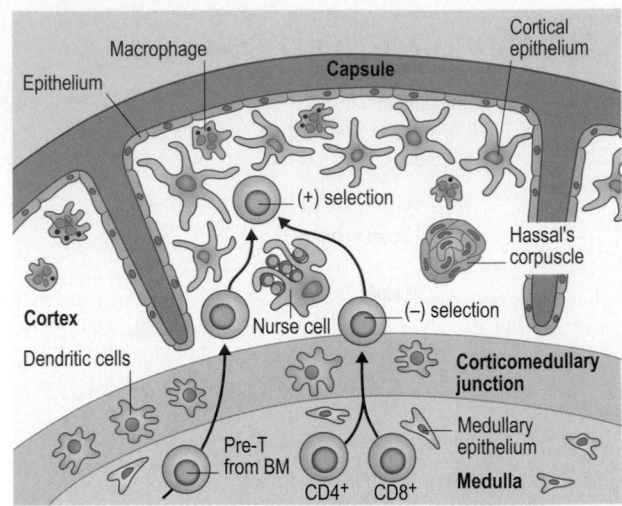

Fig. 2.4 Structure of the thymus, showing pre-T cells entering from the bone marrow (BM). Positive selection occurs on thymic epithelial cells; negative selection probably occurs during interactions with corticomedullary dendritic cells. This may explain why single-positive CD4 or CD8 cells are found primarily in the medulla. Nurse cells appear to remove negatively selected cells. Hassall's corpuscles are specialized cells producing thymic growth factors.

THYMUS

The thymus is located in the mediastinum and below the sternum. This bilobed organ develops from the third and fourth pharyngeal pouches and is endodermal in origin. It is organized into a loose lobular structure, with areas in each lobe consisting of a cortex of rapidly dividing cells and a medullary area that contains fewer, but more mature, T cells (Figs 2.4, 2.5). This arrangement has long suggested a scenario for differentiation where cells progress from the cortex to the medullary area. Nonlymphocyte cells play very important site-specific roles in the thymic development of T cells. Epithelial cells are scattered throughout the thymus. Depending on their location, they are known as nurse cells, cortical epithelial cells or medullary epithelial cells. Macrophage-type cells and interdigitating cells that are bone-marrow derived can be found at the junction between cortex and medulla. These also play an important role in T-cell selection.

It is thought that enlarged, activated T-cell precursors from the bone marrow originally colonize the subcapsular region of each lobe. These are actively proliferating and can self-renew. Selection begins when their progeny encounter MHC class II antigen-bearing cortical epithelial cells. A further education process probably occurs by interaction with macrophage-like cells found at the corticomedullary junction and in the medulla.

Thymic nurse cells, which also are found in the cortex, were originally thought to contribute to the thymic education of T cells. Because large numbers of thymic cells (50–200) can be found inside each nurse cell, it was believed that these structures provided an environment where selection and expansion could occur. However, recent evidence suggests that 'nurse' may be a misnomer because, rather than aiding in their development, the nurse cells appear to dispose of developing T cells that are selected against and which are dying by apoptosis. Nurse cells are very busy, because about 90% of cortical T cells die at this stage.

A structure known as Hassall's corpuscle, which consists of concentric whorls of epithelial cells, is found in the medulla, but its function is

unclear. These medullary epithelial cells contain secretory granules, and it is thought that this network of cells may be active in the production of thymic hormones. In the fetus these bundles of cells are widely scattered, but they become larger as the thymus matures. The center cells eventually become keratinized and die.

The thymic differentiation process (Chapter 9) involves the rearrangement of functional TCR, surface expression of CD3, and a process of positive and negative selection that allows only a small percentage of putative T cells to survive. Pre-T cells in the thymus express CD2, CD5 and CD7, as well as activation antigens such as CD38 and the transferrin receptor (CD71). Pre-T cells express intracytoplasmic CD3 and exhibit rearrangements in the TCR-β chain. Successful rearrangement of TCR-α allows the cell to progress to the next stage of development, with functional TCR and CD3 on the cell surface.[38] These later-stage cells represent most of the cells in the thymus (85%). These immature cells express both CD4 and CD8 on their surface, as well as CD1. CD69, an activation marker, is upregulated at this 'double-positive' stage. CD69 continues to be expressed until the cell reaches the single-positive stage, where it will express either CD4 or CD8, but not both. T cells are CD45RO+ at the double-positive stage and all the way to the single-positive stage. Prior to leaving the thymus, CD45RO is downregulated and CD45RA appears. The most mature thymic cells are characterized by loss of CD1 expression and loss of CD4 or CD8 expression. Most of these mature cells are also negative for activation molecules (CD38 and CD71). However, they acquire an adhesion molecule called CD44, which is necessary for homing. Upon completion of this thymic selection and education process, mature CD4 or CD8 T cells leave the thymus and enter the peripheral circulation via the postcapillary venules at the corticomedullary junction.

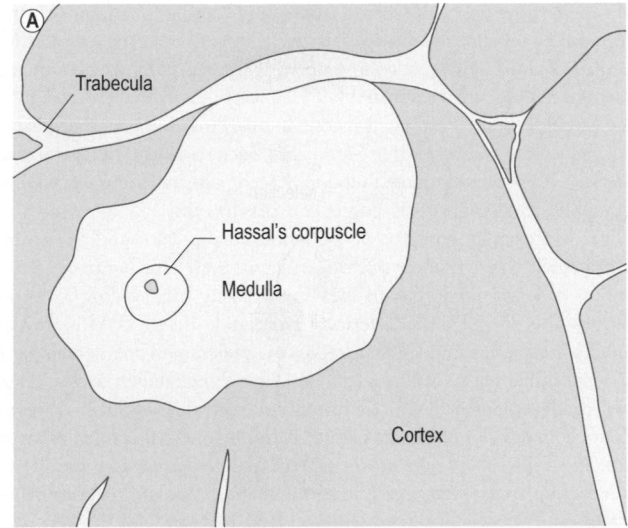

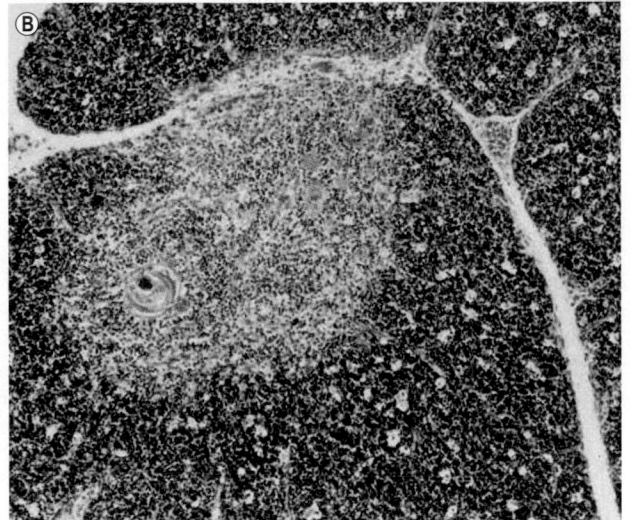

Fig. 2.5 Human thymus showing cortex and medullary areas. Cortical thymocytes are stained with an anti-CD1 antibody. Most medullary T cells do not express CD1.

After birth and during childhood the thymus continues to grow and select and educate T cells. This process is probably necessary to develop a fully normal repertoire. Prior to puberty, however, the thymus begins to involute. The rapidly dividing cortex is the first to atrophy, leaving medullary areas intact. The sensitivity of cortical thymocytes to hormone-induced death probably accounts for the involution, although there is evidence that human thymocytes are less sensitive to glucocorticosteroids than are murine thymocytes. However, an increase in steroids is known to reduce immature thymocyte numbers and enhance thymus involution. Recent evidence suggests that active TCR rearrangements, and hence T-cell development, continue to occur in the adult thymus, albeit at a lower level than during childhood.

DEVELOPMENT OF HEMATOPOIETIC AND LYMPHOID CELLS

Although most of the key steps during the growth and development of hematopoietic and lymphoid cells occur in the bone marrow and thymus, additional maturation steps occur after the cells leave those tissues. For example, monocytes and dendritic cell precursors migrate from blood vessels into tissues, where they mature into macrophages and dendritic cells, respectively. Likewise, mast cells and eosinophils undergo further differentiation in resident tissues. After leaving the bone marrow and thymus, B and T cells undergo further maturation and memory cell development in secondary lymphoid organs. Some T cells, particularly the γδ T cells residing in mucosal epithelium, may develop extrathymically.

■ SECONDARY LYMPHOID ORGANS ■

Secondary lymphoid organs are sites where mature lymphocytes reside and where immune responses are generated. Secondary lymphoid organs are part of either the systemic immune system or the mucosal immune system. The systemic immune system includes the spleen and lymph nodes and functions to protect the body from antigens present in the lymphatic drainage and circulating in the bloodstream. The mucosal immune system responds to antigens that enter through mucosal epithelium and plays an important role in the inductive phase of the immune response. Each mucosal immune system consists of organized secondary lymphoid structures, termed mucosa-associated lymphoreticular tissue (MALT), at which inductive immune responses occur, and more diffuse tissues such as the exocrine glands and lamina propria, in which effector immune responses occur. Immune responses in the mucosal immune system are initiated in the MALT, where naïve T and B cells encounter antigen, become activated, exit the tissue via efferent lymphatics, and migrate to the mesenteric lymph nodes, then into the thoracic duct and finally to the bloodstream. The cells then home to the effector sites, particularly the lamina propria of various mucosal tissues. The intraepithelial lymphocytes contained within the epithelium of mucosa and the lamina propria located immediately beneath the epithelium are the two components of the mucosal immune system responsible for carrying out effector functions (Fig. 2.6). They occur diffusely in mucosal tissues and lack the well-defined structure of the organized mucosal immune system. The ability of mucosal immune cells to circulate has led to the concept of a common mucosal immune system, so that induction of an immune response against a particular antigen leads to dissemination of lymphocytes to other mucosal tissues. Lastly, although not a systemic or mucosal lymphoid organ per se, the skin is a specialized secondary immune organ involved in the induction of immune responses.

SYSTEMIC IMMUNE SYSTEM: SPLEEN

The spleen is surrounded by a capsule of fibrous tissue with many trabeculae traversing from the capsule into the tissue of the spleen. These trabeculae branch and anastomose, forming a complex framework of lobules. Splenic blood vessels enter and exit through the hilum of the spleen and branch into smaller vessels within the trabeculae. Splenic tissue is supported by a fine network of reticular cells and fibers, called the reticulum, which connects

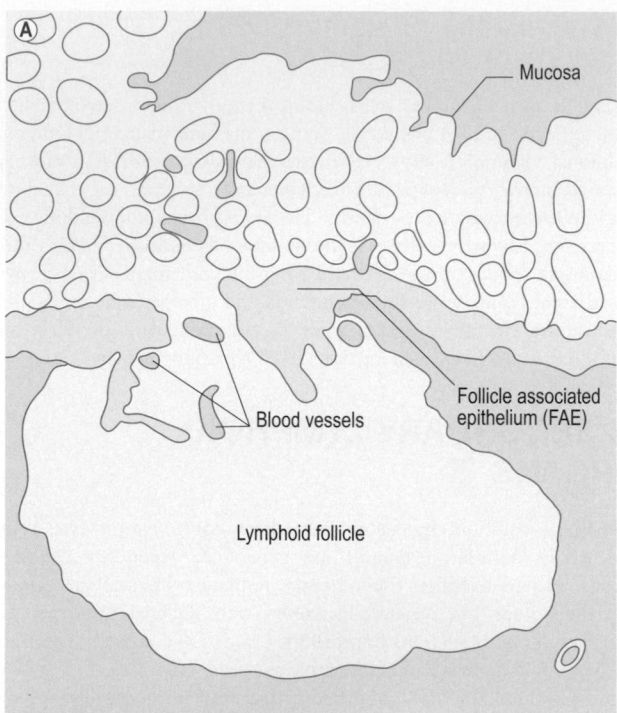

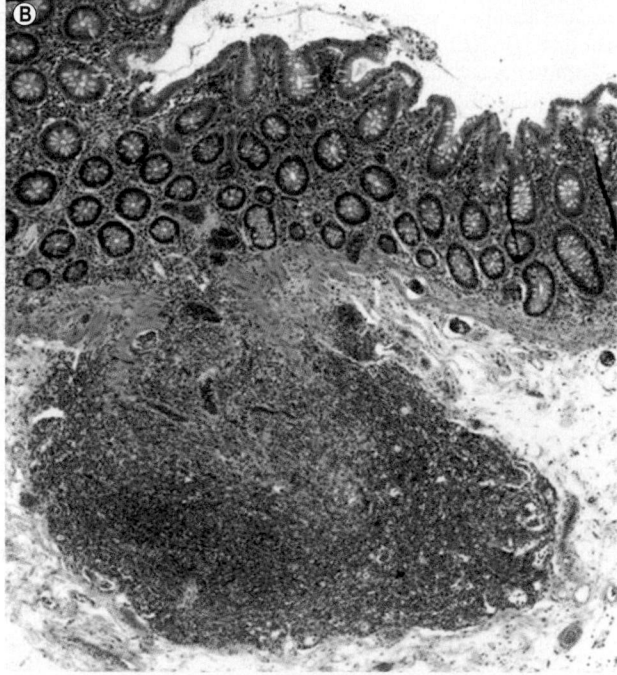

Fig. 2.6 Lymphoid follicles in the human large intestine. FAE, follicule-associated epithelium.

and supports the trabeculae, blood vessels, and capsule. The lobules of the spleen can be functionally divided into two compartments, the red pulp and the white pulp. The largest compartment is the red pulp, which contains numerous venous sinuses situated between arteries and veins. Blood is filtered through these sinuses, which contain many macrophages that phagocytose senescent red and white blood cells, bacteria, and other particulate material. Other leukocytes are found in the red pulp, including neutrophils, eosinophils, and lymphocytes, particularly plasma cells.[53]

The white pulp consists of lymphoid tissue surrounding central arterioles, which are branches of trabecular arteries. This lymphoid tissue contains a T cell-predominant area immediately surrounding a central arteriole, the so-called periarteriolar lymphoid sheath (PALS), which contains both CD4 and CD8 T cells. It is punctuated at intervals by B cell-predominant areas, follicles or so-called malpighian corpuscles. These B cell-predominant areas contain primary and secondary follicles. Primary follicles consist of only a mantle zone, without germinal centers, whereas secondary follicles contain an inner germinal center in addition to the outer mantle zone (Fig. 2.7). Within the mantle zone are predominantly resting B cells, which express surface IgM/IgD and CD23 (FcεRII). Germinal centers form in response to antigenic stimulation. It is within germinal centers that immunoglobulin class switch, affinity maturation through somatic mutation, and the development of memory B cells occur. Germinal centers are more prevalent at younger ages and diminish with aging. CD4 T cells play a key role in B-cell responses through CD40L interactions. The signaling that occurs through this interaction is central to the process of B-cell activation and the induction of class switching. In addition to activated B cells and CD4 T cells, the germinal center contains follicular dendritic cells (FDC) and macrophages.

At the interface between white pulp and red pulp is a region known as the marginal zone, that receives blood from branches of central arterioles opening into this region. It contains T cells, as well as particular subsets of macrophages and B cells. The marginal zone B cells (MZB), distinct from follicular B cells, express surface IgM but only low levels of IgD and no CD23. The function of the marginal zone involves the initial encounter of T cells and B cells with antigen from blood entering through branches of the central arteriole. Antigen presentation is enhanced by MZB cells, which are important in T cell-independent responses.

SYSTEMIC IMMUNE SYSTEM: LYMPH NODES AND LYMPHATICS

Lymph nodes occur as chains or groups located along lymphatic vessels. Lymph nodes exist in two major groups: those that drain the skin and superficial tissues (e.g., cervical, axillary, or inguinal lymph nodes), and those that drain the mucosal and deep tissues of the body (e.g., mesenteric, mediastinal, and periaortic lymph nodes). Lymph nodes are oval structures with an indentation at the region of a hilus, where blood vessels enter and leave the node (Fig. 2.8). A lymph node is surrounded by a fibrous capsule contiguous with trabeculae traversing the node. Blood vessels and nerves, which enter through the hilus, branch through these trabeculae to the various parts of the node. Immediately beneath the capsule is a subcapsular (marginal) sinus. Afferent lymph vessels enter into this sinus opposite the hilus. Dendritic cells process antigen encountered in the skin and migrate into lymph nodes from afferent lymphatics through the subcapsular sinus and into the lymph node. Lymph nodes vary in size, from barely visible in an unstimulated state to several centimeters in size when undergoing an active immune response.

2

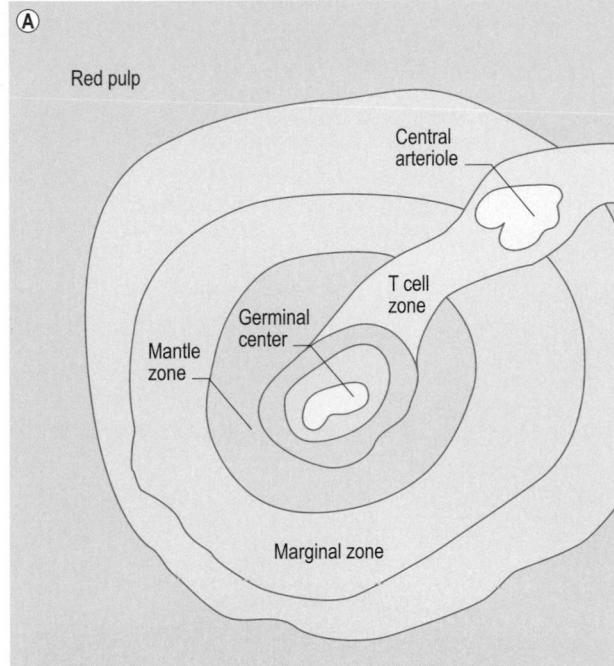

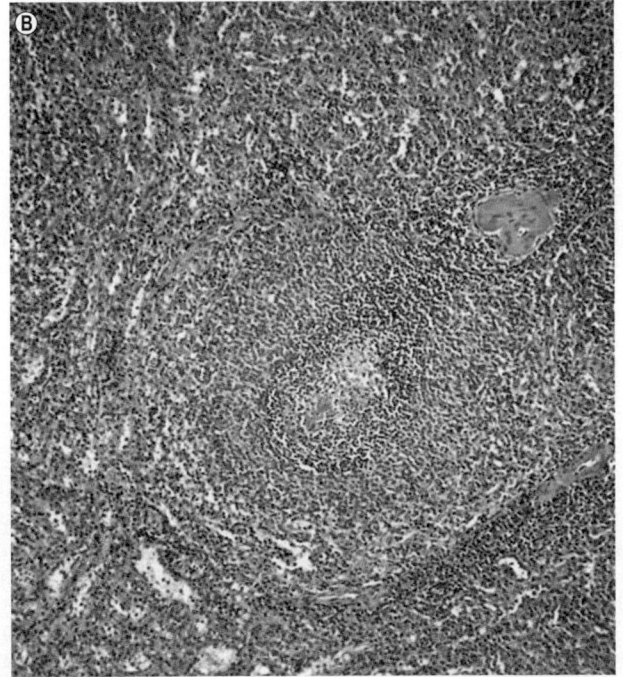

Fig. 2.7 Human spleen showing a periarteriolar lymphoid sheath and germinal center.

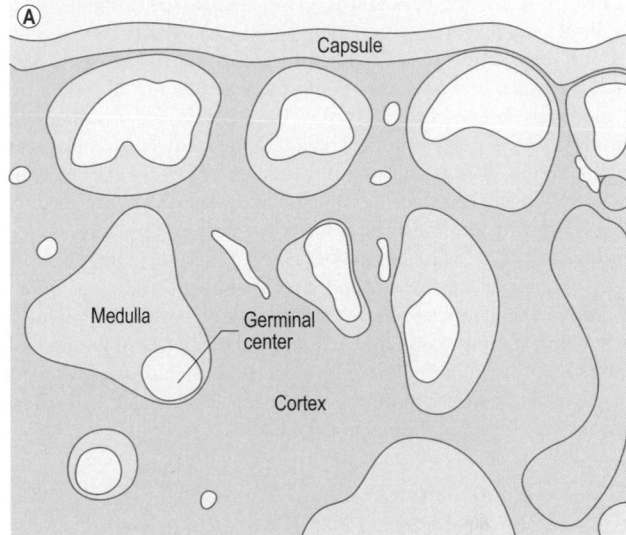

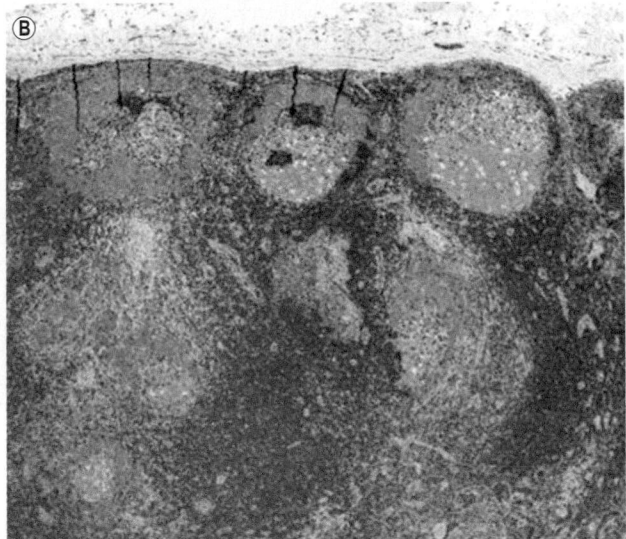

Fig. 2.8 Human lymph node showing cortex, medullary areas and germinal centers.

A lymph node is divided into two major regions, the cortex and the medulla. The cortex contains numerous primary and secondary lymphoid follicles, each approximately 0.5 mm in diameter, similar to those in the spleen. Surrounding the lymphoid follicles in the cortex is the paracortical region, which contains mostly T cells along with some macrophages and dendritic cells. Both CD4 and CD8 T cells are present in this region, as are macrophages and B cells. The accessory cells, such as interdigitating dendritic cells, present peptide antigens in association with MHC molecules to the TCR on T cells, resulting in activation of the T cells. Additional accessory molecules (e.g., B7 [CD80] or LFA-3 [CD58]) on the accessory cell and their ligands (CD28 or CD2, respectively) on the T cell provide important costimulatory signals required for activation of the T cell. Other surface antigens, particularly adhesion molecules such as LFA-1 (CD18) and ICAM-1 (CD54), are involved in stabilizing cellular interactions, as well as providing additional signals between cells.

In the center of the lymph node, beneath the cortex, lies the medulla, which is divided into medullary cords. Surrounding the medullary cords are medullary sinuses that drain into the hilus. B and T cells migrate from the follicles and paracortical region to the medulla. Medullary cords contain T cells, B cells and macrophages, as well as a large number of plasma cells, which produce immunoglobulin that drains into medullary sinuses emptying into the hilus. Efferent lymphatic vessels leave the hilus carrying antibodies, as well as mature B and T cells that migrate to other tissues and act as memory B and T cells during subsequent immune responses. The lymphatic vessel system serves to carry lymphocytes derived from various tissue spaces through the network of lymph nodes, eventually to the thoracic duct. This material is then drawn into the left subclavian vein and back into the circulation. By this mechanism, lymphocytes are circulated throughout the body.

MUCOSAL IMMUNE SYSTEM: GASTROINTESTINAL TRACT

The organized MALT of the gastrointestinal system is termed the gut-associated lymphoreticular tissue (GALT) and is comprised of Peyer's patches, cecal and rectal patches, and isolated lymphoid follicles (Chapter 19). Isolated lymphoid follicles and cecal and rectal patches are found throughout the lamina propria and are similar to an individual follicle of a Peyer's patch. Peyer's patches consist of variably sized aggregates of closely associated lymphoid follicles located in the intestinal lamina propria, occurring predominantly in the ileum[54] (Fig. 2.9). Although these structures arise during fetal life, their full development, with follicles containing germinal centers, does not occur until several weeks after birth, presumably in response to antigenic stimulation. Their number and size increase until puberty and decline thereafter. Peyer's patches and lymphoid follicles have a structural organization that belies their function of presenting antigen from the intestinal lumen to T and B cells. The epithelium overlying lymphoid follicles and Peyer's patches – that is, the follicular associated epithelium (FAE) – has a distinct structure. It lacks villi and contains very few goblet cells. Particulate antigen uptake via pinocytosis occurs in the FAE through specialized epithelial cells called M cells. The FAE expresses MHC class II antigens, with the exception of M cells; however, it does not express the polymeric immunoglobulin receptor (secretory component) required for secretion of IgA, which is expressed by crypt epithelial cells in villous epithelium.[55] A substantial number of T cells, including CD4 T cells, are found in the subepithelial region. Beneath this epithelium overlying individual follicles is a region called the dome, which contains large numbers of T cells, macrophages and dendritic cells, as well as some B cells. Antigen, which is pinocytosed by M cells, is transported to the dome region, where antigen presentation to T cells occurs. High levels of MHC class II antigens are expressed by macrophages and dendritic cells. Follicles lying beneath the dome contain mantle zones with predominantly resting B cells, most of which express IgM and IgD on their surface. Virtually all Peyer's patch follicles also have germinal centers that contain activated B cells, follicular dendritic cells (FDC), CD4 T cells, and tingible-body macrophages (so called because of their appearance after they have phagocytosed cellular debris). Many of the B cells within Peyer's patch germinal centers express surface IgA, and it is believed that this is where IgA class switch occurs. Very few CD8 T cells are located within the follicles. An interfollicular region contains

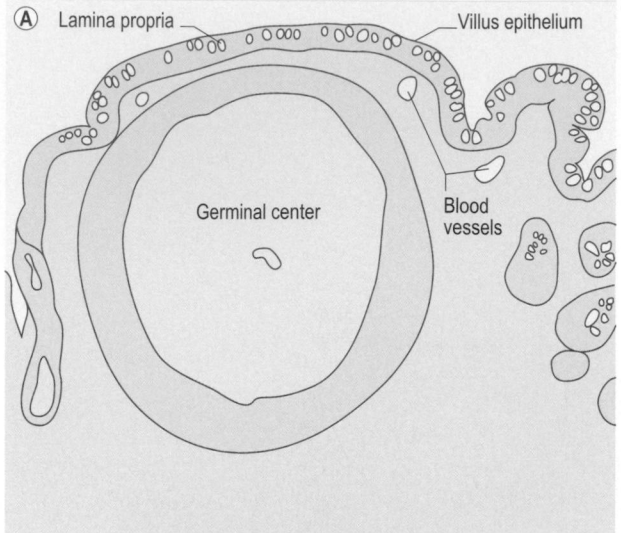

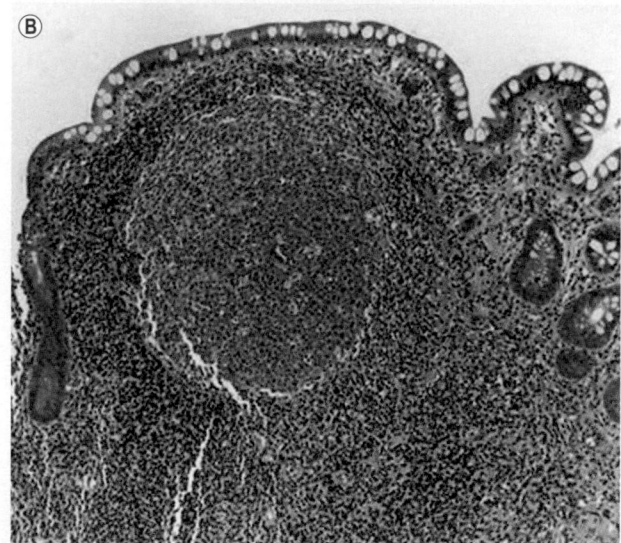

Fig. 2.9 Germinal center in terminal ilium.

predominantly CD4 and CD8 T cells, as well as dendritic cells, macrophages, and some B cells. CD4 T cells predominate over CD8 T cells in this region as well as in the dome.

The diffuse tissue of the gastrointestinal tract consists of two components: the lamina propria and intraepithelial lymphocytes (IEL). The lamina propria is located immediately beneath the epithelium. A key effector function of the lamina propria is the secretion of antibodies, primarily IgA. IgA is the major isotype produced by plasma cells in lamina propria regions; however, IgM represents 10–18% and IgG 3–5% of all Ig produced. Two IgA subclasses occur, IgA$_1$ and IgA$_2$, and the former represents >90% of IgA in the respiratory tract and >60% in the lamina propria of the small intestine.[56] Interestingly, IgA$_2$ increases in the lower ileum and becomes the predominant IgA subclass in the colon and rectum. IgA is transported from

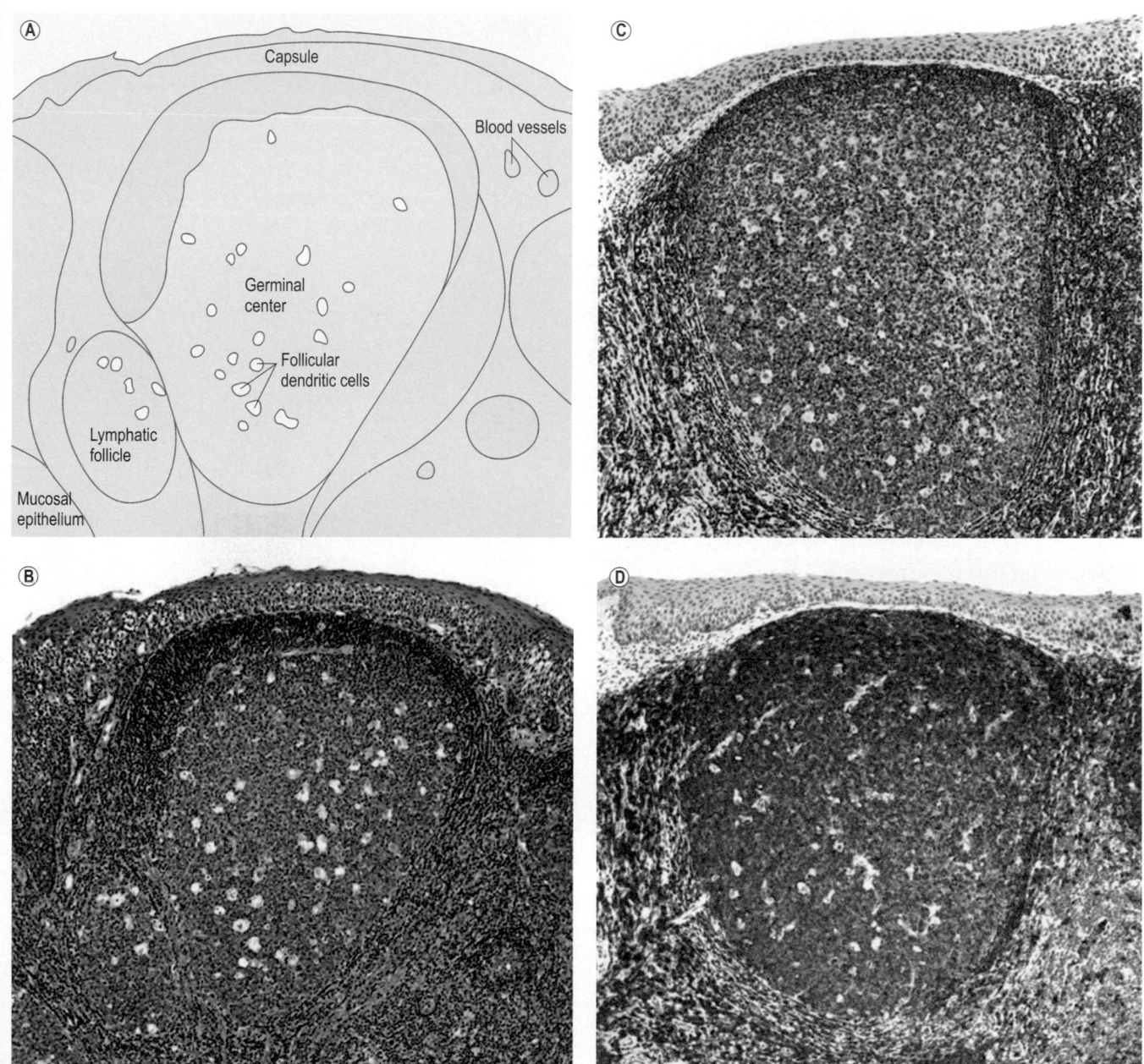

Fig. 2.10 Human tonsil. (**A**) Organization of lymphoid follicles and germinal centers. (**B**) Tonsillar tissue stained with hematoxylin and eosin. (**C**) Tonsillar tissue stained with anti-CD3 to demonstrate the distribution of T cells. (**D**) Tonsillar tissue stained with anti-CD19 to demonstrate the distribution of B cells.

the lamina propria into epithelial cells through polymeric immunoglobulin receptor-mediated uptake and subsequently secreted into the lumen. The lamina propria also contains large numbers of CD4 and CD8 T lymphocytes, CD4 T cells being about twice as prevalent as CD8 T cells. Almost all lamina propria T cells (>95%) express αβ TCR. In addition, the lamina propria contains some B lymphocytes, the majority of which express IgM. Normally, very few IgG B cells are present in the lamina propria, although in certain inflammatory conditions, such as inflammatory bowel disease, the number of IgG-producing B cells and plasma cells increases dramatically. Other cells, including macrophages, dendritic cells, eosinophils, mast cells, and a few neutrophils, are also found in the lamina propria and play a role in mediating the effector functions of this tissue. The gastrointestinal tract contains the largest number of resident macrophages in the body. These express CD68, lysozyme, ferritin, MHC II, and CD74.

Intraepithelial lymphocytes (IEL) are found at the basal surface of the epithelium as well as interdigitated with epithelial cells. The vast majority of IEL (>90%) are T cells, which are either CD8+ or CD4–CD8–.[57] Although the majority of the IEL T cells express the αβ TCR, a substantial number express the γδ TCR. The function of IEL remains incompletely understood, but they generate cytotoxic activity as well reducing oral tolerance. As part of their effector function they produce several cytokines, including IL-5 and IFNγ. Finally, epithelial cells in the small intestine express MHC class II antigens and consequently may play an important role in presenting antigen to T cells.

MUCOSAL IMMUNE SYSTEM: RESPIRATORY TRACT

Surrounding the entrance to the throat are the three tonsillar groups: palatine tonsil, lingual tonsil, and pharyngeal tonsil or adenoids.[58] They form a ring of lymphoid tissue surrounding the pharynx termed Waldeyer's ring. The tonsils reach full development in childhood and begin to involute by the time of puberty. In adults, the tonsils are usually atrophic. The palatine tonsils, one located on each side, lie at the entrance to the pharynx, each measuring approximately 2.5 × 1.25 cm. They are surrounded by a poorly organized capsule except at the pharyngeal surface, which is covered with stratified squamous epithelium. Trabeculae subdivide the tonsil into lobules. Blood vessels and nerves enter through the capsule and extend within trabeculae (Fig. 2.10). The surface of the tonsil is covered by pits, which are the openings of crypts. The crypts extend down into the tissue of the tonsil with branching, increasing the surface area exposed to contents of the pharynx. There are abundant lymphoid follicles in each lobule that contain germinal centers which are predominantly B cells. By contrast, the lymphoid tissue surrounding the follicles contains T cells, macrophages, dendritic cells, and some B cells (Fig. 2.10). The lingual tonsils consist of 35–100 separate crypts surrounded by lymphoid tissue and are located at the root of the tongue. The pharyngeal tonsils or adenoids are accumulations of lymphoid tissue, 2.5–4.0 cm long, located on the median dorsal wall of the nasopharynx. They contain a series of longitudinal folds but do not contain actual crypts. The lingual and pharyngeal tonsils also contain lymphoid nodules with germinal centers.

Inductive immune responses to inhaled antigens within the respiratory tract occur mainly in the bronchus-associated lymphoid tissue (BALT). BALT consists of lymphoid aggregates located within the bronchial wall near the bifurcations of the major bronchial branches (Fig. 2.11). These structures are analogous to the GALT present in the

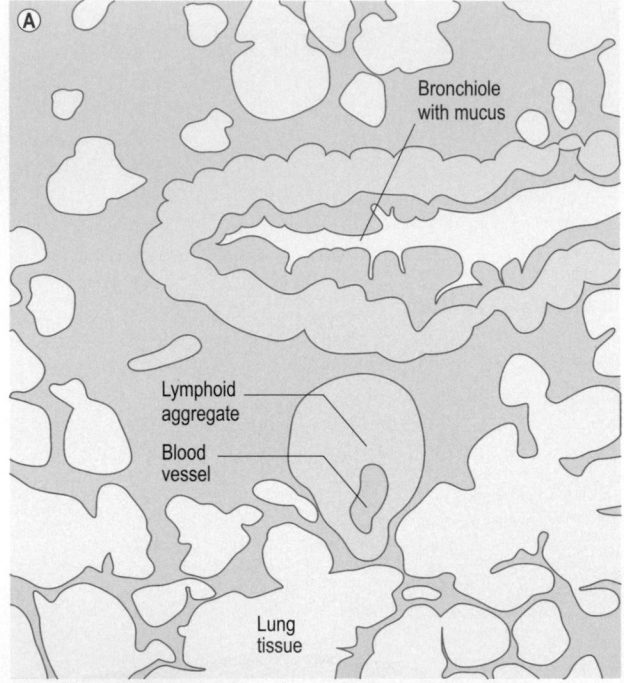

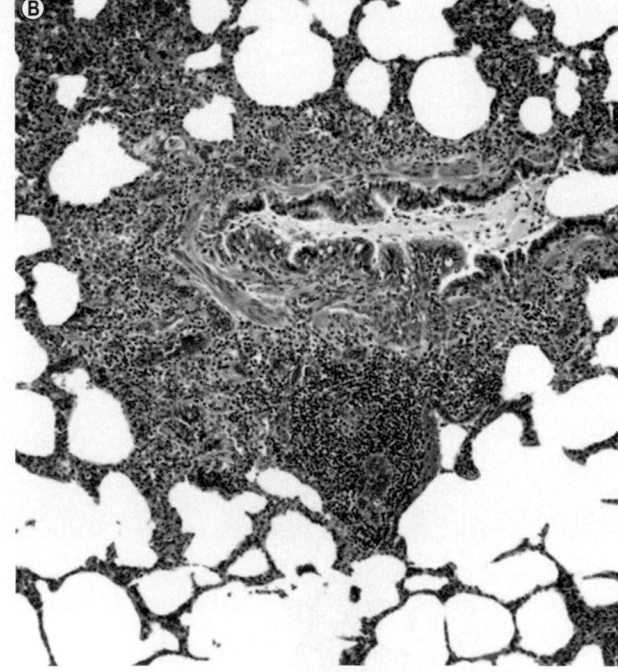

Fig. 2.11 Lymphoid regions in the human lung.

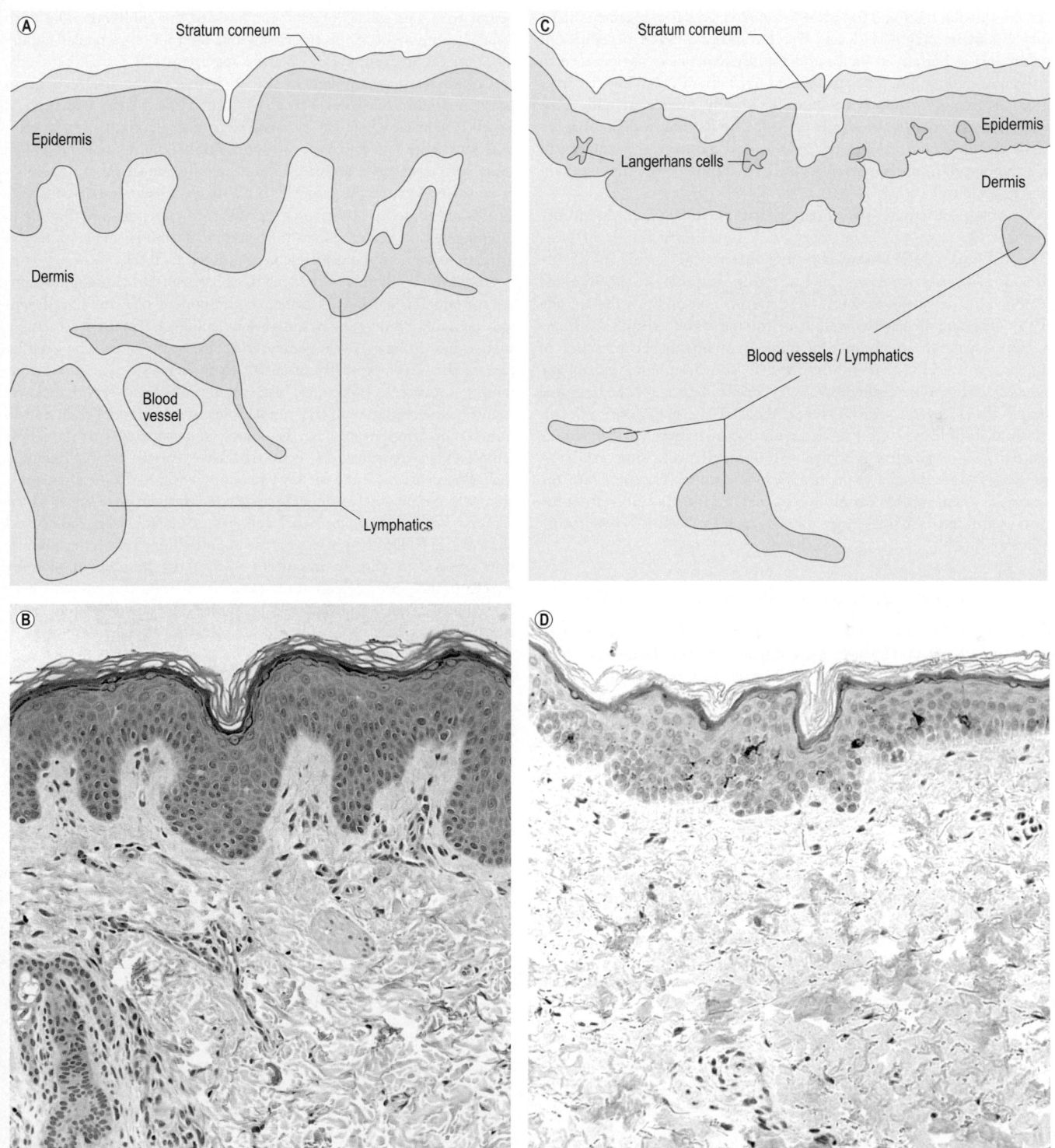

Fig. 2.12 Lymphoid regions in human skin. (**A**) Organization of the epithelial tissue. (**B**) Epithelial tissue stained with hematoxylin and eosin. (**C**) Epithelial tissue stained with anti-CD207 to demonstrate the distribution of Langerhans' cells (note brown cells).

gastrointestinal tract and function to provide a defense against inhaled microbes by induction of T- and B-cell responses. BALT development in humans is present at birth, and rapidly expands when exposed to antigenic stimulation. The specialized epithelium overlying the lymphoid aggregates consists of M cells heavily infiltrated with lymphocytes and significant dendritic cell populations present directly below the epithelium. As in the gastrointestinal tract, the main result of induction of immune responses in BALT is the production of secretory IgA.[59]

Although quite extensive in the gastrointestinal tract, the diffuse mucosal tissue of the respiratory tract is minimal. Pools of lymphocytes are present within the lung interstitium, made up of 10–20% T cells. Macrophages play a significant role in the immune response in the respiratory tract and are present on both the air side of the lung and airways as well as in the mucosa.[60] Minimal inflammation occurs in the bronchial mucosa owing to the presence of regulatory T cells that inhibit T-cell activation and expansion. Instead, antigen is carried by local macrophages to the regional lymph nodes, which are the site of most of the respiratory effector immune responses.[61] Communication occurs between the gastrointestinal and respiratory mucosae through cell trafficking. Antigen-reactive T and B cells from the Peyer's patches can populate the bronchial mucosa. This common mucosal immune system feature has been exploited to develop oral vaccines against respiratory microbes.[62]

MUCOSAL IMMUNE SYSTEM: GENITAL TRACT

The male and female reproductive tracts are also components of the common mucosal system. However, the immune system in the genital tract is unique because it must maintain a delicate balance between tolerance of germinal center cells, spermatozoa, and fetus and the recognition of microbes. Most of what is known about the mucosal response in the genital tract has been learned from the female reproductive tract. Unlike the gastrointestinal and respiratory tracts, there is a minimal amount of induction of mucosal immune responses in the genital tract.[63] Much of the population of the mucosa results from induction of immune responses at other sites, predominately in the rectum and Peyer's patches, followed by homing of IgA cell precursors to the genital tract. Although secretory IgA is the predominant antibody found in the genital tract, monomeric IgA, IgM, and IgG are also present. The production and transport of antibody produced in the genital tract is thought to depend on both hormonal and local factors, including IL-1b, IL-6, and IL-10, which all influence the maturation of B cells to plasma cells within the mucosa.[64, 65]

SKIN

The skin consists of two layers, the epidermis and the dermis. The epidermis is the outermost layer and contains three distinct cell types: keratinocytes, melanocytes, and Langerhans' cells (Fig. 2.12). Keratinocytes are squamous epithelial cells and are the principal cell type of the epidermis. Recent studies have shown that keratinocytes secrete a variety of cytokines, including IL-1, IL-6, IL-10, TGF-β, and TNF-α, that can profoundly influence immune responses. Thus, they probably play a significant role in regulation and/or modulation of immune responses in the skin. The second cellular constituent of the skin is the pigment-producing melanocyte. This cell is derived from the

neural crest and resides in the basal layer of the epidermis. The third cellular component of the epidermis, and the one of particular importance for the immune system, is the Langerhans' cell. Langerhans' cells are found scattered throughout the epidermis within the malpighian layer, or prickle cell layer. These cells play a role in the induction of T-cell responses, which can give rise to contact dermatitis, graft rejection, and other immune responses, both normal and pathologic. When these cells encounter antigen, in concert with exposure to cytokines provided by keratinocytes such as TNF-α, they migrate from the epidermis to the dermis, then enter the afferent lymphatics and migrate to draining lymph nodes. There they participate in the generation of a primary immune response, presenting antigen to T cells.[66]

Under the epidermis is the dermis, which contains abundant fibroblasts producing collagen, a principal component of skin. The dermis also contains blood vessels and various epidermal adnexal structures, such as hair follicles, sweat glands, and sebaceous glands. The vasculature of the dermis consists of an extensive network of plexuses containing arterioles, capillaries, and venules. Dermal lymphatics are found in association with the vascular plexuses. In normal skin, a small number of lymphocytes can be found in perivascular areas. These lymphocytes are mostly T cells that have certain unique features, including expression of a memory phenotype (CD45RO+) and expression of a cutaneous lymphocyte-associated antigen that binds to the vascular addressing endothelial cell leukocyte adhesion molecule-1 (ELAM-1) (CD62E) present on the endothelium. This latter interaction appears to play an important role in the homing of memory T cells to inflamed regions of the skin. The dermis also contains mast cells that play an important role in immediate hypersensitivity reactions in the skin.

ACKNOWLEDGMENTS

We would like to thank Dr Edwina Popek, Pathology Department, Texas Children's Hospital, Houston, Texas, for providing histopathological images of lymphoid tissues; Dr Gregory Stelzer and Wendy Schober for the flow cytometric display; Eleanor Chapman, Anna Wirt, Terry Saulsberry and Yvette Wyckoff for typing the manuscript; and Dr Jerry McGhee for critical review of the first edition.

REFERENCES

1. Rampon C, Huber P. Multilineage hematopoietic progenitor activity generated autonomously in the mouse yolk sac: analysis using angiogenesis-defective embryos. Int J Dev Biol 2003; 47: 273–280.

2. Dzierzak E, Medvinssky A, de Bruijn M. Qualitative and quantitative aspects of haematopoietic cell development in the mammalian embryo. Immunol Today 1998; 19: 228–236.

3. Gekas C, Dieterien-Lievre F, Orkin SH, Mikkola HK. The placenta is a niche for hematopoietic stem cells. Dev Cell 2005; 8: 297–298.

4. Haynes BF, Martin ME, Kay HH, et al. Early events in human T cell ontogeny: phenotypic characterization and immunohistological localization of T-cell precursors in early human fetal tissues. J Exp Med 1988; 168: 1061–1080.

5. Sato N, Sawada K, Koizumi K, et al. In vitro expansion of human peripheral blood CD34+ cells. Blood 1993; 82: 3600–3609.

6. Metcalf D. The molecular control of cell division, differentiation commitment and maturation in haemopoietic cells. Nature 1989; 339: 27–30.

7. Raulet D. Development and tolerance of natural killer cells. Curr Opin Immunol 1999; 11: 129.

8. Andrews RG, Singer JW, Bernstein ID. Precursors of colony-forming cells in humans can be distinguished from colony-forming cells by expression of the CD33 and CD34 antigens and light scattering properties. J Exp Med 1989; 169: 1721–1731.

9. Moore KA, Lemischka IR. Stem cells and their niches. Science 2006; 311: 1880–1885.

10. Goodell MA. CD34+ or CD34–: does it really matter?. Blood 1999; 94: 2545–2547.

11. Bunting KD. ABC transporters as phenotypic markers and functional regulators of stem cells. Stem Cells 2002; 20: 11–20.

12. Lapidot T, Petit I. Current understanding of stem cell mobilization: The roles of chemokines, proteolytic enzymes, adhesion molecules, sytokines, and stromal cells. Exp Hematol 2002; 30: 973–987.

13. Wilson A, Trumpp A. Bone-marrow haematopoietic-stem-cell niches. Nature Immunol Rev 2005; 6: 93–107.

14. Paolo Bianco, Mara Riminucci, Gronthos S, Robey PG. Bone marrow stromal stem cells: nature, biology, and potential applications. Stem Cells 2001; 19: 180–92.

15. Dorshkind K. Regulation of hemopoiesis by bone marrow stromal cells and their products. Annu Rev Immunol 1990; 8: 111–137.

16. Kondo M, Wagers MJ, Manz MG, et al. Biology of hematopoietic stem cells and progenitors: implications for clinical application. Annu Rev Immunol 2003; 21: 759–806.

17. Zandstra PW, Conneally E, Petzer AL, et al. Cytokine manipulation of primitive human hematopoietic cell self-renewal. Proc Natl Acad Sci USA 1997; 94: 4698–4703.

18. Barreda DR, Hanington PC, Belosevic M. Regulation of myeloid development and function by colony stimulating factors. Dev Comp Immunol 2004; 25: 509–554.

19. Shortman K, Liu YJ. Mouse and human dendritic cell subtypes. Nature Immunol Rev 2002; 2: 151–161.

20. Mende I, Karsunky H, Weissman IL, et al. Flk2+ myeloid progenitors are the main source of Langerhans' cells. Blood 2006; 107: 1383–1390.

21. Randolph GJ, Angeli V, Swartz MA. Dendritic-cell trafficking to lymph nodes through lymphatic vessels. Nature Immunol Rev 2005; 5: 617–628.

22. Rutherford MS, Witsell-Teutsch A, Schook LB. Mechanisms generating functionally heterogeneous macrophages. J Leukocyte Biol 1993; 53: 602–618.

23. Takahashi K, Naito M, Takeya M. Development and heterogeneity of macrophages and their related cells through their differentiation pathways. Pathol Int 1996; 46: 473–485.

24. Karsunky H, Merad M, Cozzio A, et al. Flt3 ligand regulates dendritic cell development from Flt3+ lymphoid and myeloid commited progenitors to Flt3+ dendritic cells in vivo. J Exp Med 2003; 198: 305–313.

25. Chicha L, Jarrossay D, Manz MG. Clonal type I interferon-producing and dendritic cell precursors are contained in both human lymphoid and myeloid progenitor populations. J Exp Med 2004; 200: 1519–1524.

26. Onai N, Obata-Onai A, Tussiwand R, et al. Activation of the Flt3 signal transduction cascade rescues and enhances type I interferon-producing and dendritic cell development. J Exp Med 2006; 203: 227–238.

27. Friedman AD. Transcriptional regulation of granulocyte and monocyte development. Oncogene 2002; 21: 3377–3390.

28. Lieber JG, Webb S, Suratt BT, et al. The in vitro production and characterization of neutrophils from embryonic stem cells. Blood 2004; 103: 852–859.

29. Rothenberg ME, Hogan SP. The eosinophil. Annu Rev Immunol 2006; 24: 147–174.

30. Kambe N, Hiramatsu H, Shimonaka M, et al. Development of both human connective tissue-type and mucosal-type mast cells in mice from hematopoietic stem cells with identical distribution pattern to human body. Blood 2004; 103: 860–867.

31. Matsuzawa S, Sakashita K, Kinoshita T, et al. IL-9 enhances the growth of human mast cell progenitors under stimulation with stem cell factor. Immunology 2003; 170: 3461–3467.

32. Long MW. Megakaryocyte differentiation events. Semin Hematol 1998; 35: 192–199.

33. Malik P, Fisher TC, Barsky LL, et al. An in vitro model of human red blood cell production from hematopoietic progenitor cells. Blood 1998; 91: 2664–2671.

34. Pelayo R, Welner R, Perry SS, et al. Lymphoid progenitors and primary routes to becoming cells of the immune system. Curr Opin Immunol 2005; 17: 100–107.

35. Blom B, Spits H. Development of human lymphoid cells. Annu Rev Immunol 2006; 24: 287–320.

36. Weerkamp F, Pike-Overzet K, Staal FJT. T-sing progenitors to commit. Trends Immunol 2006; 27: 125–131.

37. Haddad R, Guimiot F, Six E, et al. Dynamics of thymus colonizing cells during human development. Immunity 2006; 24: 217–230.

38. Spits H. Development of αβ T cells in the human thymus, thymic involution. Nature Immunol Rev 2002; 2: 260–772.

39. Gary DHD, Ueno T, Chidgey AP, et al. Controlling the thymic microenvironment. Curr Opin Immunol 2005; 17: 137–143.

40. Takahama Y. Journey through the thymus: stromal guides for T-cell development and selection. Nature Rev Immunol 2006; 6: 127–136.

41. Farrar JD, Asnagli H, Murphy KM. T helper subset development: roles of instruction, selection, and transcription. J Clin Invest 2002; 109: 431–435.

42. Bettelli E, Kuchroo VK. IL-12 and IL-23 induced T helper cell subsets: birds of the same feather flock together. J Exp Med 2005; 201: 169–171.

43. Kronenberg M. Towards an understanding of NKT cell biology: progress and paradoxes. Annu Rev Immunol 2005; 26: 877–900.

44. MacDonald HR. Development and selection of NKT cells. Curr Opin Immunol 2002; 14: 250–254.

45. Jonuleit H, Schmitt E. The regulatory T cell family: distinct subsets and their interrelations. J Immunol 2003; 171: 6323–6327.

46. Dejaco C, Dufner C, Grubeck-Loebenstein B, Schirmer M. Imbalance of regulatory T cells in human autoimmune diseases. Immunology 2005; 117: 289–300.

47. Nagasawa T. Microenvironmental niches in the bone marrow required for B-cell development. Nature Immunol Rev 2006; 6: 107–116.

48. LeBien TW. Fates of human B-cell precursors. Blood 2000; 96: 9–23.

49. Herzenberg LA, Tung JW. B cell lineages: documented at last!. Nature Immunol 2006; 7: 225–226.

50. Dono M, Zupo S, Colombo M, et al. The human marginal zone B cell. Ann NY Acad Sci 2003; 987: 117–124.

51. Moretta L, Moretta A. Unravelling natural killer cell function: triggering and inhibitory human NK receptors. EMBO J 2004; 23: 255–259.

52. Farag SS, Caligiuri MA. Human natural killer cell development and biology. Blood 2006; 20: 123–137.

53. Mebius RE, Kraal G. Structure and function of the spleen. Nature Immunol Rev 2005; 5: 606–616.

54. Newberry RD, Lorenz RG. Organizing a mucosal defense. Immunol Rev 2005; 206: 6–21.

55. Mac Donald TT. The mucosal immune system. Parasite Immunol 2003; 25: 235–246.

56. Woof JM, Mestecty J. Mucosal immunoglobulins. Immunol Rev 2005; 206: 64–82.

57. Yamamoto M, Vancott JL, Okahashi N, et al. The role of Th1 and Th2 cells for mucosal IgA responses. Ann NY Acad Sci 1995; 778: 64–71.

58. Bienenstock J, McDermott MRM. Bronchus- and nasal-associated lymphoid tissues. Immunol Rev 2005; 206: 22–31.

59. Lamm ME, Nedru JG, Kaetzel CS, Mazanec MB. IgA and mucosal defense. APMIS 1995; 103: 241–246.

60. Boyton RJ, Openshaw PJ. Pulmonary defences to acute respiratory infection. Br Med Bull 2002; 61: 1–12.

61. Kyd JM, Foxwell AR, Cripps AW. Mucosal immunity in the lung and upper airway. Vaccine 2001; 19: 2527–2533.

62. Boyaka PN, Tafaro A, Fischer R, et al. Therapeutic manipulation of the immune system; enhancement of innate and adaptive mucosal immunity. Curr Pharm Des 2003; 9: 1965–1972.

63. Mestecky J, Moldoveanu Z, Russell MW. Immunologic uniqueness of the genital tract: challenge for vaccine development. Am J Reprod Immunol 2005; 53: 205–214.

64. Mestecky J, Rusell MW. Induction of mucosal immune responses in the human genital tract. FEMS Immunol Med Microbiol 2000; 27: 351–355.

65. Mestecky J, Kutteh WH, Jackson S. Mucosal immunity in the female genital tract; relevance to vaccination efforts against the human immunodeficiency virus. AIDS Res Hum Retroviruses 1994; 10: S11–20.

66. Hayday A, Viney JL. The ins and outs of body surface immunology. Science 2000; 290: 97–100.

Innate immunity

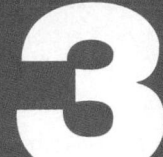

Ken J. Ishii, Shizuo Akira

All living organisms are continuously exposed to foreign entities including food, microorganisms, and unnecessary self metabolites. As a result, there is a continuing need to discriminate dangerous nonself from safe self, particularly when life-threatening microorganisms invade the body. Jawed vertebrates have evolved two arms of immune defenses against invading pathogens: innate (natural) and adaptive (acquired) immunity (Fig. 3.1). Innate immunity is the first line of host defense. It includes the physical barrier of skin and the mucosal layer, and inflammatory responses by 'innate' immune cells such as granulocytes and macrophages that can be triggered in minutes and are then followed by activation of dendritic cells and natural killer (NK) cells. Adaptive (acquired) immune responses are slower processes that are mediated by T cells and B cells, whose highly diverse antigen receptors are generated by complex DNA rearrangement events and thus have the potential to recognize novel antigens as well as conserved ones (Chapter 4).

In contrast to adaptive immunity, innate immunity had long been regarded as a relatively nonspecific system, with its main roles being to engulf and destroy pathogens, to trigger proinflammatory responses, and to help present antigen, thereby priming adaptive immune responses. However, recent studies have shown that the innate immune system has a great degree of specificity that enables it to discriminate efficiently between self and foreign entities, including microorganisms and unnecessary self molecules. This discrimination relies, to a great extent, on pattern recognition receptors (PRRs), which include the Toll-like receptors (TLRs), NOD-like receptors (NLRs), and the recently described RIG-I-like receptors (RLRs). All of these receptors can play a crucial role in early host defense against invading pathogens (Table 3.1 and Fig. 3.2). Unlike the T-cell and B-cell antigen receptors, these PRRs are entirely germline-encoded and are expressed constitutively by both immune and nonimmune cells. They recognize conserved microbial components known as pathogen-associated molecular patterns or PAMPs.[1] Following PAMP recognition, PRR activate specific signaling pathways that lead to robust but highly defined innate immune responses. These innate responses then help prime subsequent protective adaptive (antigen-specific) immune responses to the inciting pathogens.

In addition to their 'primary function' of fighting invading microbes, PRR are also involved in the pathogenesis of many diseases. In particular, PRR recognition of self-molecules derived from the host (e.g., nucleic acids) may be linked to autoimmune diseases and possibly to other immunological disorders. In humans, PRRs and their mutations (e.g., single nucleotide polymorphisms (SNPs)) have recently been linked to susceptibility, not only to infectious diseases, but also to chronic inflammatory diseases, such as atherosclerosis and asthma[2] (Chapter 40).

This potential involvement of innate immune system in a variety of human diseases has attracted the interest of a wide range of clinical fields.[3] Agonists and antagonists for TLRs, NLR and RLR, as well as inhibitors of their signaling molecules, are presently under development for a variety of therapeutic applications. Choosing highly 'effective and proper' but 'safer' PRR-agonists/antagonists is critical for the development of improved vaccine adjuvant and immunostimulatory agents. PRR antagonists or inhibitors of PRR-signaling molecules, on the other hand, may provide another opportunity for the development of drugs to prevent and/or treat diseases in which PRRs are involved in the etiology or pathogenesis. In this chapter, we discuss recent advances and understanding of the innate immunity-related research field, including the molecular and cellular mechanisms underlying PRR-mediated innate immune responses and their impact on human diseases.

KEY CONCEPTS

THE INNATE IMMUNE SYSTEM

>> The innate immune system is the first line of host defense against pathogens

>> It helps prime subsequent activation of the adaptive immune system

>> Unlike the antigen receptors of the adaptive immune system, its pattern recognition receptors (PRRs) are entirely germline-encoded

>> PRRs recognize conserved microbial components known as pathogen-associated molecular patterns or PAMPs

| KEY CONCEPTS |

THE MAJOR PATTERN RECOGNITION RECEPTORS OF THE INNATE IMMUNE SYSTEM

Toll-like receptors (TLRs)

>> Reside on the cell surface or phago/endosome membranes

>> Include 11 different type I integral membrane glycoproteins in the multigene family

>> Contain a ligand-sensing leucine-rich repeat (LRR) extracellular domain and a Toll/IL-1R homology (TIR) cytoplasmic signaling domain

Nod-like receptors (NLRs)

>> Reside in the cytoplasm

>> Include 22 different family members, most of whom remain to be fully characterized

>> Contain a ligand-sensing LRR and a domain for the initiation of signaling such as CARDs, PYRIN, or baculovirus inhibitor of apoptosis repeat (BIR) domains

RIG-I-like receptors (RLRs)

>> Reside in the cytoplasm

>> Include three different family members

>> Contain a C-terminal DExD/H box RNA helicase that can recognize RNA, with or without an N-terminal CARDs signaling domain

■ INNATE IMMUNE SENSORS AND THEIR FUNCTIONS ■

TOLL-LIKE RECEPTORS

An important role of the innate immune system in the first-line defense against pathogens and the underlying molecular and cellular mechanism(s) has recently been unveiled. The Toll pathway in *Drosophila melanogaster* was initially discovered as a receptor essential for embryonic patterning. The identification of the Toll pathway as a critical component of the host defense against fungal and Gram-positive bacterial infections in insects in 1996[4] provided the impetus for the subsequent identification of mammalian homologues, the evolutionarily conserved TLRs.[1] These mammalian TLRs form a class of PRR molecules that currently consists of 11 members that can recognize microbial components known as PAMPs.[5, 6] The TLRs are type I integral membrane glycoproteins characterized by extracellular domains that contain varying numbers of leucine-rich repeat (LRR) motifs and a cytoplasmic signaling domain homologous to that of the interleukin-1 receptor (IL-1R), termed the Toll/IL-1R (TIR) homology domain (Fig. 3.2).

Similar to the other PRRs, mammalian TLRs are widely distributed on/in the cells of the immune system. They are capable of discriminating among a variety of invading pathogens, including protozoa, fungi, bacteria, and viruses (Table 3.1). TLRs can be classified into subfamilies based on their genetic tree. The TLR1, TLR2, and TLR6 subfamily recognizes lipoproteins, whereas TLR3 and the highly related TLR7, TLR8, and TLR9 subfamily recognize nucleic acids. TLR4 recognizes lipopolysaccharide (LPS) and TLR5 is the receptor for bacterial flagellin. TLR11 recognizes a profilin-like molecule in *Toxoplasma gondii* (Table 3.1).

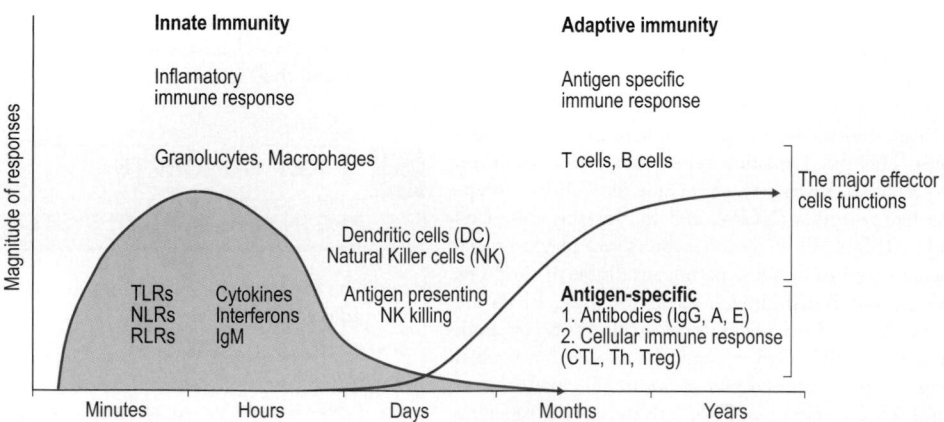

Fig. 3.1 Innate and adaptive immune responses to infection or tissue damage. When infection or tissue damage occurs, activation of innate immunity takes place within minutes and lasts for several days. Its purpose is to recognize and clear most of the microbes or damaged tissue. The adaptive immune response follows and peaks within the following weeks, resulting in an immunological memory that can last for the life of the individual.

Table 3.1 Mammalian pattern recognition receptors (PRRs)

Location	Pattern recognition receptors		Natural ligand	Species
Transmembrane	Toll-like receptors (TLRs)	TLR1 + TLR2	Triacyl lipopeptides	Bacteria
		TLR2	Zymosan	Fungi
		TLR3	dsRNA	Viruses
		TLR4	LPS	Gram-negative bacteria
		TLR5	Flagellin	Bacteria
		TLR6 + TLR2	Diacyl lipopeptides	*Mycoplasma*
		TLR7	ssRNA	Virus, host
		TLR8	ssRNA	Virus, host
		TLR9	DNA, hemozoin	Bacteria, virus, plasmodium
		TLR10	Not known	Bacteria
		TLR11	Profilin-like protein	*Toxoplasma*, bacteria
	Scavenger receptors (SR-A, CD36, and CXCL16 etc.)		Apoptotic cells, malaria-infected red blood cells, diacylglycerides	Host, plasmodium
	C-type lectin-like receptors (mannose receptors, dectin-1, DC-SIGN)		Carbohydrates on ligand	Host, bacteria, fungi, parasite
Intracellular	NOD-like receptors (NLRs)	NOD1 (CARD4)	Peptidoglycan (mDAP)	Bacteria
		NOD2 (CARD15)	Peptidoglycan (MDP)	Bacteria
		NALP1(1b)	Anthrax toxin	Host, bacteria
		NALP3	Bacterial RNA, ATP, uric acid	Bacteria, host
		IPAF	Flagellin	Bacteria
		CIITA	Not known	
		NAIP	Not known	
	RIG-like helicases (RLHs)	RIG-I	dsRNA, ssRNA	Viruses
		MDA5	dsRNA, ssRNA	Viruses

CXCL16, transmembrane CXC chemokine 16; DC-SIGN, DC-specific ICAM-3 grabbing nonintegrin; dsRNA, double-stranded RNA; LPS, lipopolysaccharide; SR-A, scavanger receptor-A; ssRNA, single-stranded RNA.

INNATE IMMUNE SENSORS AND THEIR FUNCTIONS

TLR-ligand recognition can be flexible, permitting the recognition of a diverse range of molecules. For example, although TLR4 is associated with recognition of LPS, it also recognizes the fusion protein of respiratory syncytial virus (RSV), fibronectin, and heat-shock proteins. Similarly, TLR9 recognizes hemozoin, the heme-polymeric metabolite of the malaria parasite, as well as nucleic acids.

Localization of the various subfamilies in the cell varies. While certain TLRs (TLRs 1, 2, 4, 5, and 6) are expressed on the cell surface, others (TLRs 3, 7, 8, and 9) are found almost exclusively in intracellular compartments such as the endoplasmic reticulum and endosomes (Fig. 3.2). The physiological significance of these expression patterns remains unclear, but it is the common perception that ligands easily liberated from the pathogens such as flagellin and LPS are recognized by cell surface TLRs, while ligands hidden inside the pathogens such as nucleic acids are recognized in the endosome after lysosomal degradation of microbes or cells.

TLRs are expressed on various immune cells, including macrophages, dendritic cells, B cells, granulocytes, NK cells, and T cells, as well as on nonimmune cells such as fibroblasts and epithelial cells (Fig. 3.3). TLR expression can be altered in response to pathogens, a variety of cytokines, and environmental stresses. Taken together, the ability of single TLRs to detect a unique but diverse range of ligands and their ubiquitous expression and distinct localization within and between cells may enable the

KEY CONCEPTS

TOLL-LIKE RECEPTOR (TLR) SIGNALING

>> The C-terminal Toll/IL-1R (TIR) domain can initiate differential intracellular signaling

>> Except for TLR3, most TLRs, including TLR4, signal through an adapter molecule termed myeloid differentiation primary response gene 88 (MyD88)

>> TLR3 signals through an adaptor molecule termed Toll/IL-1R domain-containing adaptor-inducing interferon-β (TRIF)

>> TLR4 can also signal through TRIF

>> Both MyD88 and TRIF can associate with tumor necrosis factor receptor-associated factor 6 (TRAF6), which leads to the activation of nuclear factor (NF)-κB and/or the mitogen-activated protein kinase (MAPK) pathway

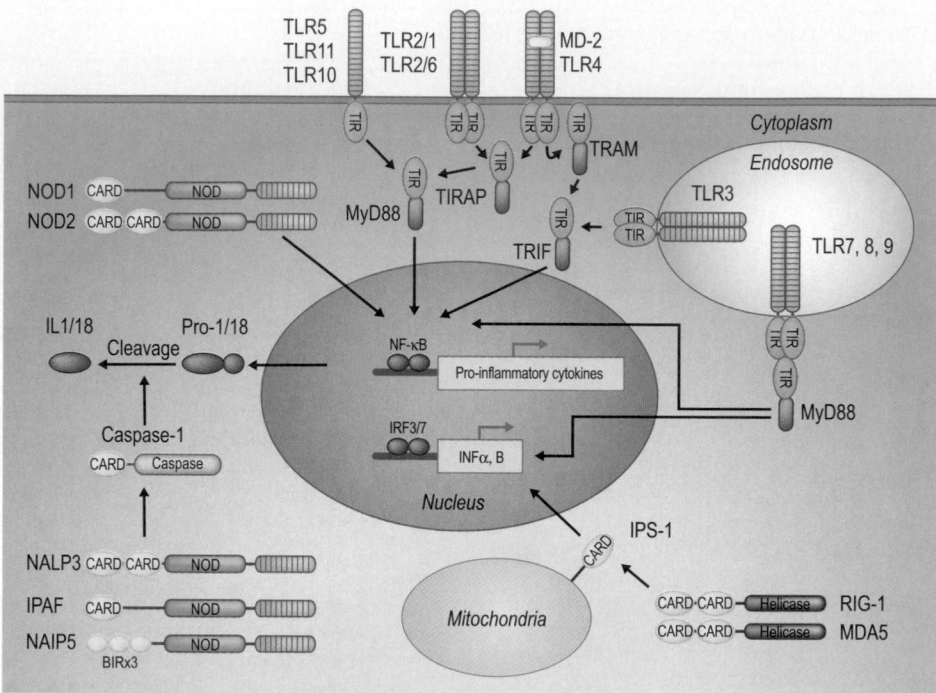

Fig. 3.2 Intracellular localization and signaling of Toll-like receptors (TLRs), NOD-like receptors (NLRs), and RIG-I-like receptors (RLRs). These pathogen recognition receptors are able to activate cells to produce proinflammatory cytokines and type I interferons. TLRs localize at the plasma membrane, such as the cell surface, and at endosomal membrane (as indicated). NLRs and RLRs are localized in the cytoplasm. Their cognate ligand (shown in Table 3.1) activates each pattern recognition receptor via distinct adaptor molecules. TLRs utilize either MyD88 and/or TRIF via their Toll/IL-1R homology (TIR) domain. RLR utilize interferon-β promoter stimulator 1 (IPS-1) via their CARD domain. NLRs activate caspase-1, leading to cleavage of pro-interleukin (IL)-1 or pro-IL-18 into the active forms.

host to sense invasion of a variety of pathogens even though the numbers of TLR genes are limited.

Direct interaction of a TLR with its cognate ligand triggers intracellular signaling pathways by means of multiple adaptors, including transduction and transcription molecules. This leads to robust immune responses that are characterized by the production of immunoglobulins, chemokines, and inflammatory cytokines with upregulation of co-stimulatory molecules (see next section), all of which are hallmarks of innate immune responses. The activation of dendritic cells via TLRs, in particular, is critically important owing to their ability to prime adaptive immune responses, thereby linking innate immunity to adaptive immune responses.

TOLL-LIKE RECEPTOR SIGNALING

Another important key to understanding TLR-mediated immune responses is the ability of the TIR domain to initiate differential intracellular signaling downstream of the TLR, with one signaling pathway that is shared with a member of the IL-1R superfamily.[7] Myeloid differentiation primary response gene 88 (MyD88) is an essential adaptor molecule for most TLRs. The exception is TLR3 (Fig. 3.2). The other adaptor molecule, Toll-IL-1R domain-containing adaptor protein (TIRAP), acts specifically as part of the MyD88-dependent TLR2 and 4 signaling process. TLR3 and 4-mediated activation signals through Toll/IL-1R domain-containing adaptor-inducing interferon-beta (IFN-β) (TRIF), the so-called MyD88-independent pathway, lead

to the induction of IFN-β and IFN-inducible genes. The TRIF-related adaptor molecule (TRAM) characterizes the TLR4 MyD88-independent, TRIF-dependent signaling pathway, and acts as a bridging adaptor between TLR4 and TRIF (Fig. 3.2).

Upon TLR stimulation, MyD88 and TRIF associate with tumor necrosis factor receptor-associated factor 6 (TRAF6), which leads to the activation of nuclear factor (NF)-κB and/or the mitogen-activated protein kinase (MAPK) pathway. This leads to the production of several proinflammatory molecules, including cytokines and chemokines (reviewed in reference 7). TRAF6 forms a complex with ubiquitin-conjugating enzymes (Ub), such as Ubc13, and activates transforming growth factor-beta-activated kinase 1 (TAK1). In turn, TAK1 activates transcription factors NF-κB and activator protein-1 (AP-1) by means of the canonical IκB kinase (IKK) complex and MAPK. The IKK complex is composed of two catalytic subunits, IKKα and IKKβ. NEMO (NF-κB essential modifier, also known as IKKκ) encodes the regulatory component of the IKK complex, which is responsible for activating the NF-κB signaling pathway. IKK phosphorylates IκB and targets it for degradation. The removal of IκB enables NF-κB to translocate into the nucleus, where it activates the transcription of various target genes.

In addition to these signaling pathways controlled by IKK complexes, TLR7/9-mediated MyD88-dependent signaling possesses a distinct signaling pathway for type I IFN production.[8] MyD88 forms a complex with IL-1R-associated kinase 4 (IRAK4) and IRAK1. Depending on the types of cells or stimuli, TLR-MyD88-dependent signaling requires

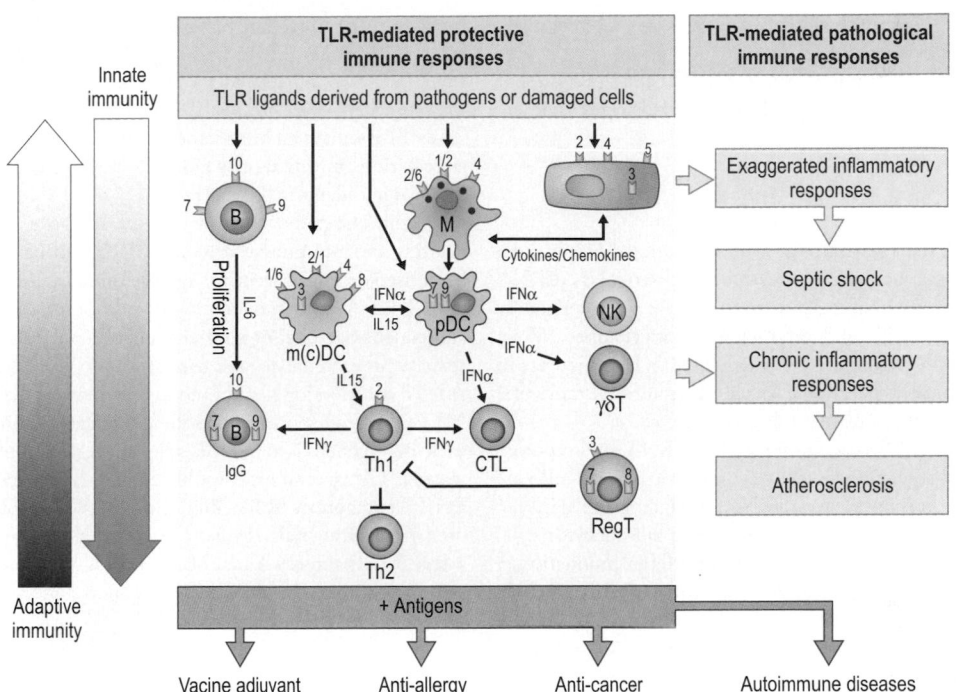

Fig. 3.3 Toll-like receptor (TLR)-mediated innate and adaptive immune responses and their roles in the immune system. Both immune and nonimmune cells can express various TLRs. Cognate ligand(s), derived from either pathogens or damaged host cells, activate the cells and trigger intercellular signaling cascades. Activation leads to the production of humoral factors such as cytokines and chemokines, as well as cell–cell interactions. These orchestrate innate immune activations, especially those derived from certain dendritic cell (DC) subsets such as myeloid (conventional) DC (m(c)DC) and plasmacytoid DC (pDC), lead to the induction of antigen-specific adaptive immune responses. These responses are characterized by B-cell production of immunoglobulin (Ig)G, CD4 Th1 (or Th2) cell production of IFNγ, and CD8 T-cell-mediated cytotoxicity. Other types of immune cells that can be involved in this process are indicated. These TLR-mediated innate and adaptive immune responses can lead to protective immune responses to antigens of vaccines, allergens, or cancer antigens. They can also result in exaggerated innate and/or adaptive immune responses, which, in turn, may have detrimental effects, including the development of septic shock, atherosclerosis, or autoimmune diseases.

IRAK4 or IRAK1. While IRAK4 is necessary for most TLR-mediated proinflammatory cytokine production by macrophages and dendritic cells, IRAK1 is only essential for TLR7- and TLR9-mediated type I IFN production by plasmacytoid dendritic cells. TLR3 and TLR4 also mediate type I IFN production via another major adaptor molecule, TRIF, and the TRAF-family-member-associated NF-κB activator (TANK)-binding kinase 1 (TBK1). TBK1 comprises a family with inducible IκB kinase (IKK-i, also known as IKK-e). Together these kinases directly phosphorylate interferon regulatory factor 3 (IRF3) and IRF7. TBK1/KK-i-mediated type I IFN induction is not restricted to TLR3 and 4, but is also involved in TLR-independent virus-, RNA- and DNA-induced type I IFN production.[8]

Transcription factors such as IRF5 and IRF7 are important mediators for TLR-dependent and -independent signaling pathways.[9] In particular, IRF5 is involved in the production of most TLR-mediated proinflammatory cytokines, excluding IFN-α. This occurs independently of NF-κB or the MAPK signaling pathway. In contrast, the IRF7 transcription factor plays a critical role in TLR7- and TLR9-mediated IFN-α production by both direct interaction with MyD88 and by TLR-independent type I IFN production that is induced by viruses.

TLR1, 2, 6, AND 10

TLR2 is a major mammalian TLR that can recognize lipoproteins derived from bacteria, viruses, fungi, and parasites. It acts by forming heterodimers with either TLR1 or TLR6.[10–12] The molecular tree of the TLR family indicates that specific recognition of lipopeptide PAMPs involves TLR1, TLR2, TLR6, and TLR10.[13] Thus, some structurally related TLRs can easily form heterodimers for the recognition of different ligands, as is the case for TLR2 together with TLR1 and TLR6. For example, *Mycoplasma* macrophage-activating lipopeptide 2 (MALP-2) is recognized by TLR2/TLR6 heterodimers, while the synthetic bacterial lipopeptide PAM_3CSK_4 is recognized by TLR2/TLR1 heterodimers. Altered ligand recognition has been attributed to the presence of a diacylated cysteine residue at the N-terminus of MALP-2. PAM_3CSK_4 contains a triacylated cysteine residue instead. Highly purified lipoteichoic acid from *Staphylococcus aureus* and *Streptococcus pneumoniae* was found to trigger innate immune responses thorough both TLR2/TLR6 and TLR2/TLR1 heterodimers. Similarly, glycophosphatidylinositols with three fatty acids derived from *Plasmodium falciparum* are preferentially recognized by TLR2/TLR1 heterodimers, whereas glycophosphatidylinositols with two fatty acids are recognized with TLR2/TLR6 heterodimers.

Human TLR10 is an orphan member of the TLR family. It is present in a locus that also contains TLR1 and TLR6, and can also heterodimerize with TLR1 and TLR2.

TLR3

Double-stranded (ds) RNA is generated in host cells during the replication of most viruses. The host innate immune system thus recognizes dsRNA as a PAMP, inducing robust immune responses that are characterized by the production of type I IFNs and proinflammatory cytokines. While poly(I:C) synthetic dsRNA analogues are widely used as IFN inducers in many research and clinical applications, specific receptor-like molecules that recognize poly(I:C) have not been fully characterized.

It has been shown that TLR3 can confer strong dsRNA-induced NF-κB activation in 293 cells when ectopically expressed and that TLR3–/– mice display reduced responses to dsRNA, including poly(I:C).[14] Accordingly, TLR3-deficient mice are susceptible to murine cytomegalovirus (MCMV) infection owing to reduced interferon production.[15] In contrast, TLR3-deficient mice survive otherwise lethal West Nile virus infection owing to reduced virus entry into the brain and fewer TLR3-induced inflammatory responses, which contribute to pathogenesis rather than to protection.[16]

Poly-I:C was one of the first therapeutic agents used to treat human immunodeficiency virus (HIV) and leukemia patients, but was abandoned due to its toxicity.[17] Several studies have been undertaken to reduce the toxicity of poly-I:C, with ongoing clinical trials against breast cancer and ovarian cancer. The dsRNA-induced, TLR3-mediated maturation of CD8 dendritic cells was shown to play an important role in the induction of antigen-specific CD4 and CD8 T-cell responses via type I interferon-mediated cross-priming.[18] Yet dsRNA still stimulates dendritic cells from TLR3–/– mice, especially when administered directly into the cytosol by transfection. This observation led to the discovery of an intracellular detection system that is independent of TLR3. This detection system is described in a later section.

TLR4

LPS is a major causative agent of sepsis. It triggers strong proinflammatory responses. The endotoxin shock that results is associated with high mortality. Although CD14 and LPS-binding protein were known to bind LPS, a sole receptor that recognize LPS to initiate proinflammatory response had been sought for decades before human Toll, homologous to fly Toll, was found. Most strikingly, it was shown that mice lacking TLR4 function were hyporesponsive to LPS.[19–21] Thus TLR4 proved to be the "long-sought" receptor for LPS. The other TLRs were also found to recognize specific microbial products, many of which are also known to cause a robust inflammatory response.

TLR4 recognizes LPS via a homodimeric form that cooperates with MD2. Unlike the other TLRs, TLR4 utilizes as many as four adaptor molecules, as described above, which creates complex signaling pathways.[7]

In a mouse model, TLR4-deficient mice were found to be resistant to experimental septic shock induced by LPS. A similar phenomenon was observed in humans, in that some people with the TLR4 polymorphisms Asp299Gly and Thr399Ile were hyporesponsive to inhaled LPS. Further studies sought to link these SNPs and susceptibility to several infections,

including RSV infection, brucellosis, severe malaria, and candidal bloodstream infections. TLR4 and several other TLR polymorphisms were then found to be related to chronic inflammatory diseases, such as *inflammatory bowel disease* (Chapter 74) and *sarcoidosis* (Chapter 72). Thus TLR4 plays an important role in both protective immune responses to various infectious diseases and in pathological responses that occur in chronic inflammatory diseases.

Despite the pathogenic roles described above, due to their potency in eliciting innate immune responses, LPS and its purified products have been used as pharmaceutical agents. Initially, purified LPS (which contains lipid A) was thought to provide prophylactic protection against subsequent bacterial or viral challenge in animals; however, its extreme toxicity prevented extensive use. Efforts to eliminate the toxicity of lipid A led to the development of monophosphoryl lipid A (MLA or MPL).[22] MLA has been shown to be safe and effective in human clinical studies as a new-generation vaccine adjuvant against infectious diseases and seasonal allergic rhinitis. Lipid A analogs have been demonstrated to act as LPS antagonists by blocking the effects of endotoxin. They have been used in clinical trials against sepsis and the complications of coronary artery bypass surgery. Thus, TLR4 ligands are apparently a double-edged sword, requiring attention to address safety concerns in order to make use of their potency for therapeutic applications.

TLR5

TLR5 recognizes flagellin, a protein that is found in the flagellar structure of many bacteria.[23] TLR5 is expressed in epithelial cells in the lung and gut, as well as residual dendritic cells, such as those located in the lamina propria of the intestine.[24] TLR5 may act as both an immune sensor and as a receptor to capture flagellated bacteria. Flagellin is a potent immune activator, stimulating diverse biologic effects that mediate both innate inflammatory responses and the development of adaptive immunity. Signaling of flagellin via TLR5 enhances the diversity of the response by engaging the MyD88-dependent pathway to activate the proinflammatory responses. Due mainly to its ease of manipulation, the protein nature of flagellin is considered an advantage for many immunotherapeutic applications, for example as a vaccine adjuvant.

TLR7 AND TLR8

Single-stranded RNA genome oligonucleotides derived from HIV or influenza virus, some ds short interference (si) RNAs developed for RNA interference (RNAi), and small synthetic compounds known as imidazoquinolins are recognized by TLR7 in mice and by TLR7 and TLR8 in humans. TLR7 and TLR8 subsequently activate various immune cells that elicit type I IFNs as well as cellular immune responses.[25–27] The immunostimulatory effect of these RNAs is abrogated by various types of methylation. In humans, TLR7, but not TLR8, is highly expressed in plasmacytoid dendritic cell to produce type I IFNs, while TLR8, but not TLR7, is highly expressed in monocytes to produce proinflammatory cytokines, especially IL-12. TLR7 and possibly TLR8 utilize MyD88 as an essential adaptor for downstream signaling pathways. Owing to its ability to stimulate type I IFN production, several TLR7 agonists have been approved for clinical use in various viral infections. The TLR7 agonist imiquimod has been shown to be effective for external genital warts, basal cell carcinoma, and actinic keratosis and is in phase I clinical trials against human papillomavirus.[3] Several other synthetic TLR7 agonist compounds have been in phase I or phase II trials against hepatitis B virus, hepatitis C virus, and cancer.

Recent evidence suggests that TLR7 also recognizes autoantigens complexed with RNA, such as U1snRNP (nuclear self-antigen) in mice. Thus TLR7 may also play an important role in the pathogenesis of systemic lupus erythematosus (SLE), functioning as a double-edged sword similar to the other TLRs.

TLR9

TLR9 recognizes unmethylated CpG (cytosine phosphate guanosine) motifs found in bacterial and viral DNA.[28] Synthetic oligo deoxy nucleotides (ODNs) that contain these CpG motifs trigger TLR-mediated, MyD88-dependent signaling of macrophages, dendritic cells, and B cells to produce proinflammatory cytokines, chemokines, and immunoglobulins.[29] Some types of CpG DNA can activate plasmacytoid dendritic cells to produce a large amount of IFN-α. The robust innate immune response to CpG ODNs enables the host to be resistant to various intracellular infectious organisms. It skews the host's immune milieu in favor of Th1 cell responses and proinflammatory cytokine production.

CpG ODNs are being developed as immunoprotective agents, vaccine adjuvants, and anti-allergens.[30] Preclinical studies provide evidence that CpG ODNs are effective for each of these uses and can modulate the immune response to co-administered allergens and vaccines. CpG ODNs have had promising results in human use and have entered phase III clinical trials against several types of cancer, including melanoma, lymphoma, and nonsmall-cell lung cancer, either alone or in combination with chemotherapy.[31] The other promising application of CpG ODN under clinical development is a vaccine composed of allergen antigen conjugated with CpG ODN to treat or prevent allergic diseases. CpG ODN skews the Th2 allergic immune milieu to a protective Th1 immune milieu, whereby allergic symptoms are diminished or reduced.

Recent evidence suggests that TLR9 can also recognize DNAs that do not contain CpG motifs. Moreover, TLR9 also recognizes molecules other than DNA, such as heme metabolites derived from malaria-infected red blood cells and self-DNA-chromatin complexes often observed in autoimmune diseases, including SLE. The physiological roles of TLR9 in the etiology and pathogenesis of malaria infection or autoimmune diseases such as SLE, however, are still unclear. As CpG ODN has become a promising compound for many immunotherapeutic applications including vaccine adjuvant, allergy, and cancer, the potential role of TLR9 in the pathogenesis of various diseases needs to be clarified in the future.

NOD-LIKE RECEPTORS AND THEIR FUNCTIONS

TLRs reside either on the cell surface or on phago/endosome membranes, suggesting that the TLR system is not optimal for the detection of pathogens that have invaded or escaped into the cytoplasm. Recent evidence suggests that such pathogens are detected by cytoplasmic PRRs, which can also activate the innate immune system.[32, 33]

A number of cytoplasmic PRRs have now been identified. Currently they are subclassified into NOD-like receptors and RIG-helicase-like receptors. These protein families are implicated in the recognition of bacterial and viral components, respectively, while both are also implicated in the intracellular recognition of endogenous components, including uric acids and nucleic acids that may become dangerous to host cells

(danger signal). Proteins in NOD families possess LRRs that mediate ligand sensing; a nucleotide-binding oligomerization domain (NOD) and a domain for the initiation of signaling, such as CARDs, PYRIN, or baculovirus inhibitor of apoptosis repeat (BIR) domains. Counting the IPAF, NAIP, and CIITA group of proteins, 22 NLR members have been identified to date. However, the biological significance of most of the NLRs remains to be determined (Table 3.1 and Fig. 3.2).

NOD1 AND NOD2

NOD1 and NOD2, initially identified and characterized as NLR, contain N-terminal CARD domains. NOD1 and NOD2 detect κ-D-glutamyl-meso-diaminopimelic acid (iE-DAP) and muramyl dipeptide (MDP), found in bacterial peptidoglycan, respectively. Although direct binding between NOD protein and their cognate ligands has not been demonstrated, consequent activation of NOD1 and NOD2 causes their oligomerization and the recruitment of RIP2/RICK, a serine/threonine kinase, to the NODs via their respective CARD domains. These homophilic interactions result in NF-κB activation. In mice, macrophages lacking either NOD1 or NOD2 fail to produce cytokines in response to the corresponding ligand. In humans, a missense point mutation in the human *NOD2* gene is correlated with susceptibility to Crohn's disease.

THE NALP INFLAMMASOME AND OTHER NLRS

It has been shown that bacterial infections often induce activation of caspase-1, which catalyzes the processing of pro-IL-1β to produce the mature cytokines. A complex of proteins responsible for these catalytic processes has been purified and designated the inflammasome.

The inflammasome consists of caspase-1; caspase-5; ASC (apoptosis-associated speck-like protein containing a CARD); and members of the NALP family, which are PYRIN-domain-containing proteins that also contain NOD-LRR. ASC is an adaptor protein that contains a PYRIN domain and a CARD. NALPs recruit ASC through a homotypic interaction between the PYRIN domains. In turn, ASC recruits caspase-1 via its CARD, leading to the activation of IL-1β and IL-18 processing. Although the ligands for many members of the NALP family are currently unknown, NALP3 has recently been shown to recognize bacterial RNA (which is also known as TLR7/8 ligand), adenosine triphosphate (ATP), and uric-acid crystals. As these compounds are not unique to bacteria or other pathogens, it seems that not only PAMPs but also the presence of host danger signals (danger-associated molecular patterns, or DAMPs)[34] can be sensed by NALP3 in inflammasomes. Despite the existence of 14 NALP families, most of the known danger signals seem to activate caspase 1 through the NALP3 inflammasome, suggesting that NALP3 may represent one of the long-sought host danger receptors.

Interestingly, mutations in the NALP3 gene have been identified and found to be associated with three autoinflammatory disorders: Muckle–Wells syndrome, familial cold autoinflammatory syndrome, and neonatal-onset multisystemic inflammatory disease.[35] These disorders are associated with constitutive release of IL-1β from monocytes of patients, suggesting that the mutations trigger spontaneous NALP3 oligomerization without the need for a ligand. Importantly, patients with NALP3 mutations are now being treated with the IL-1R antagonist, which has been shown to relieve all symptoms, including rashes, periodic fever, and arthritis.

Another NOD-LRR protein, NAIP5, is involved in caspase-1-dependent susceptibility of macrophages to *Legionella pneumophila*. It detects flagellin in cytoplasm. IPAF, another CARD-containing NOD-LRR protein, has been shown to recognize *Salmonella typhimurium*, which also results in caspase-1 activation. Interestingly, IPAF is also required for *L. pneumophila* growth restriction. Although the mechanism for how these two proteins intracellularly recognize the same ligand is not yet clear, NAIP5 and IPAF may cooperate for recognition of such bacterial components, since they can physically interact with each other. Importantly, *Legionella*-induced IL-1β release, but not bacterial growth, is restricted in ASC-deficient macrophages. This suggests that NAIP has an antibacterial role that is independent of the NALP inflammasome.

RIG-LIKE RECEPTORS

Innate immune responses against invading viruses also rely on detection of viral PAMPs and subsequent production of antiviral cytokines such as type-I IFNs. dsRNA is one of the most frequently used viral PAMP. It does not normally exist in host cells but is generated intracellularly during viral replication. While dsRNA activates macrophages and dendritic cells via TLR3 to secrete proinflammatory cytokines and type I IFNs, most virus-infected cells such as fibroblasts produce type I IFNs in a TLR3-independent manner.

Recently, three homologous DExD/H box RNA helicases were identified as cytoplasmic sensors of viral infection by means of RNA detection. These helicases are designated RLRs. Two family members, retinoic acid-inducible gene I (RIG-I; also called DDX58) and melanoma differentiation-associated gene 5 (MDA5; also called Helicard), share two N-terminal CARDs followed by an RNA helicase domain.[36] RIG-I, but not MDA5, can mount antiviral responses against the positive-strand single-stranded (ss) RNA virus Japanese encephalitis virus, and against negative-strand ssRNA viruses such as Newcastle disease virus, vesicular stomatitis virus, Sendai virus, and influenza virus. MDA5 senses the presence of the positive-strand ssRNA picornavirus encephalomyocarditis virus.[37] The protein LGP2 shares homology with RIG-I in its helicase domain, but lacks a CARD. It has been suggested that LGP2 acts as a negative regulator of RIG-I/MDA-5 signaling (Table 3.1 and Fig. 3.2).

IPS-1 (interferon-β promoter stimulator 1, also named as MAVS, VISA, or CARDIF), serves as a critical signaling adaptor for RIG-I/MDA5. IPS-1 is composed of an N-terminal CARD domain that resembles that of MDA-5 or RIG-I.[8, 32, 33] When expressed in cells, this protein has the ability to induce activation of the type I IFN promoter as well as NF-κB. This protein is present in the outer mitochondrial membrane, suggesting that mitochondria might be important for IFN responses. Downstream of RIG-I-IPS-1, noncanonical IKKs, including TBK1 and IKK-I, are activated to phosphorylate IRF-3 and IRF-7. Thus signaling pathways triggered by TLR stimulation and RIG-I converge at the level of TBK1/IKK-i.

C-TYPE LECTINS

Among the other PRRs, the mannose receptor is among the best-characterized C type lectin. It binds mannosyl/fucosyl or GlcNAc-glycoconjugate ligands on many bacteria, fungi, and protozoan parasites to mediate subsequent inflammatory responses. This mannose receptor also functions to clear glycosylated endogenous ligands. Thus it can act both to detect foreign pathogens and to help in the clearance of injurious self molecules.

Dectin-1, another C-type lectin, is the major receptor for β-1,3-glucans; ligand binding induces phagocytosis, and reactive oxygen species production in macrophages. Dectin-1 can cooperate with TLR2 to recognize ligands, thereby enhancing immune activation.

Other C-type-like receptors, including DC-SIGN, DEC-205, and BDCA-2, are known to be expressed in dendritic cells. These receptors play a role in intertissue trafficking, as well as endocytic antigen (ligand) uptake. Both help dendritic cells in their role as professional antigen-presenting cells.

THE SCAVENGER RECEPTORS

The scavenger receptors (SR) are another example of innate immune receptors that can act as a PRR with additional functions. SR-A contributes not only to the endocytosis of modified low-density lipoprotein, but also to resistance to Gram-positive bacterial infections. These dual functions of SR-A result on the one hand in resistance to septic shock induced by LPS *in vivo* and on the other to susceptibility to atherogenesis.

CD36, another type of scavenger receptor, is required for binding and internalization of apoptotic cells as well as for pathogens such as malaria-infected red blood cells. CD36 can detect diacylglycerides and is thus

---

KEY CONCEPTS

CLINICAL RELEVANCE

Toll-like receptors (TLRs) can play an essential role in the initiation of human diseases and represent potential targets for therapeutic intervention. Examples include:

>> TLR ligands serve as components of common vaccine adjuvants

>> TLR9 recognition of nucleic acids may help trigger systemic lupus erythematosus and rheumatoid arthritis

>> TLR 1, 2, 4, and 5 are expressed in atherosclerotic plaques

>> TLR agonists can skew the immune response from a Th2-allergic immune phenotype to a protective Th1 immune phenotype in asthma

By extension, TLR polymorphisms can either increase or decrease susceptibility to human diseases. Examples include:

>> Increased susceptibility to Gram-negative bacterial septic shock, respiratory syncytial virus, malaria, *Brucella*, and *Candida* in polymorphisms of TLR4, which recognize lipopolysaccharide

>> Increased susceptibility to *Legionella pneumophila* (legionnaire's disease), Crohn's disease, and ulcerative colitis in polymorphisms of TLR5, which recognize flagellin

>> Decreased susceptibility to atherosclerosis in polymorphisms of TLR4

>> Decreased susceptibility to systemic lupus erythematosus in polymorphisms of TLR5

Table 3.2 Single nucleotide polymorphisms (SNPs) of Toll-like receptors (TLRs) in human diseases

TLR	SNP(s) or genes	Effect on the disease
TLR2	Arg753Gln	Susceptibility to *Mycobacterium tuberculosis* or *Staphylococcus* infection. Increased risk for coronary restenosis. Resistance to Lyme disease. Associated with severe atopic dermatitis
	Arg677Trp	Susceptibility to leprosy. Susceptibility to *M. tuberculosis*
	GT-repeat polymorphism in intron II -16934	Susceptibility to *M. tuberculosis*. Reduced risk for asthma
TLR1, 2, 6	Nonsynonymous variants	Extension of inflammatory bowel diseases
TLR4	Asp299Gly	Hyporesponsiveness to LPS. Susceptibility to meningococcal diseases in infancy. Susceptibility to brucellosis. Susceptibility to osteomyelitis by Gram-negative bacteria. Hyporesponsive to *Porphyromonas gingivalis*. Increased risk for bacterial vaginosis. Association with Crohn's disease. Risk factor for Crohn's disease. Association with ulcerative colitis. Lower incidence of carotid artery stenosis. Lower incidence of acute coronary events. Lower incidence of myocardial infarction. Resistance to chronic obstructive pulmonary disease. Associated with the severity of asthma. Reduces the risk of developing late-onset Alzheimer's disease. Associated with gastric MALT lymphoma
	Asp299Gly and Thr399Ile	Susceptibility to septic shock. Susceptibility to severe RSV infection. Resistance to legionnaire's disease. Susceptibility to *Candida* bloodstream infections. Association with chronic sarcoidosis. Decreased susceptibility to rheumatoid arthritis. Lower incidence of allograft rejection
	Thr399Ile	Susceptibility to severe malaria. Association with ulcerative colitis. Increased risk of severe acute graft-versus-host disease
	C119A	Risk for ischemic stroke
	11381G/CVariant alleles	Increased risk of prostate cancer. Lower risk of prostate cancer
	Rare coding variants	Susceptibility to meningococcal diseases
TLR5	392STOP	Susceptibility to legionnaire's disease. Association to Crohn's disease. Resistance to systemic lupus erythematosus
TLR6	Ser249Pro	Decreased risk for asthma
TLR9	T-1237C	Association with Crohn's disease. Increased risk of pouchitis
TLR10	c.+1031G>A and c.+2322A>G; Haplotype GCGTGGC variant	Association with asthma. Association with risk for nasopharyngeal carcinoma

MALT, mucosa-associated lymphoid tissues; RSV, respiratory syncytial virus.

nonredundant for most, but not all, TLR2/6-mediated innate immune activations. *Drosophila* RNAi screening has shown that a CD36 family member is required for mycobacterial infection, indicating its important role in innate immune recognition of diverse molecules, including pathogens and damaged host cells.

THE INNATE IMMUNE SYSTEM AND HUMAN DISEASE: PATHOGENESIS, PREVENTION, AND THERAPY ■

TOLL-LIKE RECEPTORS AND HUMAN DISEASE

A number of studies have now linked SNPs in TLRs and a variety of human diseases, including infectious diseases, asthma, atherosclerosis, and autoimmune diseases.[38] Identification and functional characterization of such polymorphisms in TLRs as well as the other PRRs have the potential to provide new insights to the role played by genetic susceptibility to these diseases, to improve understanding of the natural history of the disease, and to evaluate better diagnostic and therapeutic strategies. For example, knowing the TLR SNP genotype of patients suffering from severe infectious disease may allow clinicians to individualize treatment and better predict the outcome.

TLR agonists or antagonists provide new means to treat immune disorders. For example, TLR antagonists may be useful when TLR-mediated innate immune activation in response to either infection or tissue damage is likely to result in deleterious outcomes, such as sepsis, autoimmune disease, or atherosclerosis. Conversely, agonists might be beneficial in situations where inhibition of TLR signaling leads to innate and/or adaptive immune deficiency (immunological tolerance or impaired Th1 responses).

TOLL-LIKE RECEPTORS AND INFECTIOUS DISEASES

The development of antibiotic resistance and bacterial product-related complications such as septic shock are major concerns in the treatment of Gram-negative and Gram-positive infections. Elucidation of the role of the TLRs in innate immunity has provided a number of new insights to the pathophysiology of infection and new avenues for treatment. For example, TLR4 recognizes LPS, a major component of Gram-negative bacterial cell walls that causes septic shock. Two well-known TLR4 polymorphisms, Asp299Gly and Thr399Ile, have been found to be linked not only to susceptibility to Gram-negative bacterial septic shock but also to susceptibility to a variety of other microbial infections, including RSV, malaria, *Brucella,* and *Candida* (Table 3.2).

As a result of TLR ligand diversity, individual polymorphisms can lead to either susceptibility or increased resistance to different microbial agents. For example, TLR2 recognizes a variety of bacterial, viral, fungal, and parasite components, such as the lipoprotein found in bacterial cell walls. TLR2 deficiency induces susceptibility to *Borrelia burgdorferi* in mice, permitting high bacterial loads. And humans with the TLR2 Arg753Gly polymorphism demonstrate a reduced response to *Staphylococcus* infections. Conversely, individuals with the TLR2 Arg753Gly polymorphism appear to be resistant to *B. burgdorferi* Lyme disease. The TLR2 polymorphism, Arg677Trp, is similarly associated

with susceptibility to tuberculosis and leprosy, linking TLR2 genetic variants to human mycobacterial infections.

TLR5 is another case in point. TLR5 recognizes bacterial protein flagellin, which is found in the flagellar structure of many bacteria. Humans with a stop codon polymorphism in the ligand-binding domain of TLR5 (392STOP) have been shown to be highly susceptible to *Legionella pneumophila* (legionnaire's disease: Table 3.2). The same stop codon polymorphism protects people from developing SLE, parenthetically providing another potential link between infectious diseases and autoimmunity.

TLRs AND PRIMARY IMMUNODEFICIENCY

Primary immunodeficiency diseases of humans are caused by a variety of immunological defects. These deficiencies are typically marked by an increased susceptibility to infectious agents. Recent studies have suggested that TLR signaling can be abnormal in several of these syndromes.[39] For example, patients with *X-linked hypohydrotic ectodermal dysplasia with immunodeficiency (hyper-IgM syndrome)* (Chapter 34), who exhibit increased susceptibility to pyogenic and atypical mycobacterial infections, were found to have a mutation in the *IKBKG* gene, which results in defective production of IKKγ (NEMO). NEMO encodes the regulatory component of the IKK complex, which is responsible for activating the NF-κB signaling pathway. Similarly, autosomal dominant hypohydrotic ectodermal dysplasia with immunodeficiency results from defects in the phoshorylation and degradation of IkBα, which also leads to abnormal activation of NF-κB. Mice with IRAK4 deficiency, an essential signaling molecule for most TLR-mediated signaling and human patients with autosomal recessive amorphic mutations in IRAK4 both demonstrate susceptibility to bacterial infections.

TLRs, GASTROINTESTINAL DISORDERS, AND INFLAMMATORY DISEASES

TLRs also appear to play an important role in mucosal immunity. Both TLR4 and TLR2 are involved in the recognition of LPS and HSP60 derived from *Helicobacter pylori* in gastric mucosa. TLR2, TLR4, and TLR5 play critical roles in host defense against gastrointestinal infections with *Salmonella typhimurium*. TLR4 aids in the early detection of *S. typhimurium* infection. TLR5 recognizes *S. typhimurium* flagellin, but appears to play a limited role in host defense against *S. enterica*, which causes typhoid fever. These observations suggest that innate immune responses can play a crucial role during the invasive phases of bacterial infection.

Crohn's disease and *ulcerative colitis* (Chapter 74) are chronic inflammatory diseases of the bowel. Chronic mucosal inflammation appears to be the result of excessive secretion of proinflammatory cytokines in the gastrointestinal tract. TLRs appear to be involved in this process. Indeed, TLR4 has been implicated in the triggering of Crohn's disease in mice. TLR4 expression has been found to be elevated in both ulcerative colitis and Crohn's diseases and the common Asp299Gly and Thr399Ile polymorphisms of *TLR4* have been linked to the disease etiology. Strong antibody responses to flagellin of commensal bacteria have been observed in Crohn's disease but not in ulcerative colitis. The *TLR5* stop codon polymorphism has been found to be negatively associated with Crohn's disease, suggesting that immune responses to flagellin via TLR5 may promote pathogenesis. Conversely, *TLR9* (T-1237C) polymorphisms have also been associated with Crohn's disease, but not ulcerative colitis.

Sarcoidosis is another inflammatory granulomatous multisystem disorder with an unknown etiology that pursues a chronic course in many patients. In a recent study, Asp299Gly and Thr399Ile polymorphisms of *TLR4* have been found to be associated with the chronic but not acute course of sarcoidosis, implicating TLRs in the etiology of the disease.

TOLL-LIKE RECEPTORS AND AUTOIMMUNITY

TLR-mediated innate immune activations are so potent that they may be deleterious to host in certain situations. In addition, TLR recognition of self molecules of the host (e.g., nucleic acids), which are not easily distinguishable from those of no-self (infectious organisms), has the potential to provoke autoimmune diseases and other immunological disorders. Indeed, TLR9 recognition of nucleic acids has been implicated in triggering *SLE* (Chapter 51) and *rheumatoid arthritis* (RA) (Chapter 52). Several mutations in *IRF5*, whose protein product plays an important role in the trans-activation of TLR9-mediated proinflammatory gene inductions, have been associated with an increased risk for SLE. Although it is still controversial whether TLRs are critically involved, innate immune responses seem to play an important role in the etiology and/or pathogenesis of this classic autoantibody-mediated disease.

Multiple sclerosis (MS) (Chapter 65) is an inflammatory demyelinating disease of the central nervous system with complex pathological features and disease courses. Recently, LPS recognition and *Chlamydia pneumoniae* infection have both been tentatively implicated in the pathogenesis of MS. Although TLR4 Asp299Gly and Thr399Ile mutations do not appear to influence the incidence of MS, in mice both TLR9 and MyD88 can act as essential modulators of the sterile autoimmune process during the effector phase of MS. This suggests that endogenous molecules, possibly nucleic acids, may play a role in the pathogenesis of MS. Conversely, pathological changes and disease severity of experimental inflammatory arthritis, including collagen-induced arthritis, can be reduced by guanine-rich ODN (suppressive ODN or inhibitory ODN), an antagonist of TLR9. This suggests that TLR9 may be involved in the pathogenesis of inflammatory arthritis and that TLR9 antagonists could potentially block or ameliorate the development of autoimmune diseases, such as MS or rheumatoid arthritis.

TOLL-LIKE RECEPTORS AND ATHEROSCLEROSIS

As multiple microorganisms, such as *C. pneumoniae*, *H. pylori*, and cytomegalovirus, have been shown to be involved in the inflammatory etiology of *atherosclerosis* TLR-mediated innate immune activations also appear to play a role in this disease. Most TLRs, particularly TLR1, 2, 4, and 5, are expressed in atherosclerotic plaques. Expression of these TLRs could potentially trigger the activation of NF-κB and other transcription factors, resulting in upregulation of proinflammatory mediators.[40] In support of this hypothesis, it has been shown that MyD88 deficiency, with impaired TLR signaling, leads to delays in the onset of atherosclerosis.

One example of a TLR ligand is HSP60. This protein, which is expressed by *C. pneumoniae* that can be found in atherosclerotic lesions, can activate TLR4 and enhance the inflammatory process.

It is thus not surprising that people with the TLR4 Asp299Gly polymorphism have been found to have a reduced risk for coronary artery disease. In addition, the relatively common Arg753Gln polymorphism of TLR2 has been associated with coronary restenosis, further suggesting that certain pathogens containing ligand(s) for TLR2 or TLR4 (or other PRRs) could provide a link between inflammation and atherogenesis.

TOLL-LIKE RECEPTORS AND ASTHMA

The lung epithelium plays an important role in host defense against microbial colonization and infections. Numerous epidemiologic and experimental studies have suggested an inverse correlation between the incidence of infectious diseases and allergic/autoimmune disorders that may support the so-called hygiene hypothesis.[41] In fact, microbial products or TLR ligands are being developed to treat or prevent allergic diseases. TLR agonists such as CpG DNA (TLR9 ligand) can skew the immune response from one exhibiting a Th2 allergic immune phenotype to a protective Th1 immune one. This shift can diminish or reduce allergic symptoms. However, there is also opposing evidence that an increased bacterial load or viral infections of the lung can lead to severe exacerbations of *chronic obstructive pulmonary disease* or *asthma*. Thus TLRs may serve as a double-edged sword. While certain polymorphisms of TLR6, TLR9, and TLR10 are associated with an increased risk of asthma, polymorphisms of TLR2 can reduce the risk.

TOLL-LIKE RECEPTORS AND VACCINES

Although TLRs have been discovered just recently, their ligands have been used as components of vaccine adjuvants for decades. More than 15 years ago, Charles A Janeway Jr. described these adjuvants as the 'immunologist's dirty little secret,' because they have been known to be critical components in vaccine formulation, needed in order to initiate adaptive (antigen-specific) immune responses to the vaccine antigen.[42] For example, one of the most potent adjuvants, which is often used in animal models, is complete Freund's adjuvant (CFA). CFA contains mycobacterial products (possibly with TLR2, 4, or 9 ligands), whereas the less active incomplete Freund's adjuvant does not. Aluminum hydroxide gel (alum), the only clinically approved adjuvant, does not seem to contain any TLR ligand, and is quite weak in inducing cellular immune responses. On the other hand, CpG DNA, a ligand for TLR9, strongly activates dendritic cells, inducing them to produce IL-12 and type I IFNs. Expression of IL-12 and IFNs is followed by the development of strong Th1 immune responses, including antigen-specific IFNγ-producing Th1 cells and CTL. The efficacy of the TLR9 ligand as a vaccine adjuvant has been demonstrated in both primates and in humans. MPL, another well known adjuvant, contains lipid A, which is an immunostimulatory element of LPS. MPL and R848, a potent ligand for TLR7, are also being developed as vaccine adjuvants. Finally, TLR ligands have been shown to break immunological tolerance to tumor cells, and thus are under consideration for use as 'adjuvants' for antitumor vaccines.

■ SUMMARY ■

PRR-mediated innate immune recognition of a diverse range of molecules has attracted the interest of immunologists, researchers in other fields, and physicians. The physiological roles of PRRs in innate and adaptive immune responses are still being uncovered, and the precise molecular and cellular mechanisms by which PRRs recognize the cognate ligand, influence intra- and intercellular signaling pathways and contribute to protective and/or pathological immune responses in both innate and adaptive immunity remain to be further clarified. The hope, however, is that research on innate immunity will have a direct impact on the future development of PRR agonists or antagonists as immunotherapeutic agents for infectious diseases, allergies, or cancer, as well as for immunological disorders, such as autoimmune diseases, atherosclerosis, or even diabetes.

▌ REFERENCES ▌

1. Janeway CA Jr, Medzhitov R. Innate immune recognition. Annu Rev Immunol 2002; 20: 197.

2. Cook DN, Pisetsky DS, Schwartz DA. Toll-like receptors in the pathogenesis of human disease. Nat Immunol 2004; 5: 975.

3. Hoffman ES, Smith RE, Renaud RC Jr. From the analyst's couch: TLR-targeted therapeutics. Nat Rev Drug Discov 2005; 4: 879.

4. Lemaitre B. The road to Toll. Nat Rev Immunol 2004; 4: 521.

5. Takeda K, Kaisho T, Akira S. Toll-like receptors. Annu Rev Immunol 2003; 21: 335.

6. Beutler B. Inferences, questions and possibilities in Toll-like receptor signalling. Nature 2004; 430: 257.

7. Akira S, Takeda K. Toll-like receptor signalling. Nat Rev Immunol 2004; 4: 499.

8. Kawai T, Akira S. Innate immune recognition of viral infection. Nat Immunol 2006; 7: 131.

9. Honda K, Yanai H, Takaoka A, et al. Regulation of the type I IFN induction: a current view. Int Immunol 2005; 17: 1367.

10. Ozinsky A, Underhill DM, Fontenot JD, et al. The repertoire for pattern recognition of pathogens by the innate immune system is defined by cooperation between toll-like receptors. Proc Natl Acad Sci USA 2000; 97: 13766.

11. Takeuchi O, Kawai T, Muhlradt PF, et al. Discrimination of bacterial lipoproteins by Toll-like receptor 6. Int Immunol 2001; 13: 933.

12. Takeuchi O, Sato S, Horiuchi T, et al. Cutting edge: role of Toll-like receptor 1 in mediating immune response to microbial lipoproteins. J Immunol 2002; 169: 10.

13. Roach JC, Glusman G, Rowen L, et al. The evolution of vertebrate Toll-like receptors. Proc Natl Acad Sci USA 2005; 102: 9577.

14. Alexopoulou L, Holt AC, Medzhitov R, et al. Recognition of double-stranded RNA and activation of NF-kappaB by Toll-like receptor 3. Nature 2001; 413: 732.

15. Tabeta K, Georgel P, Janssen E, et al. Toll-like receptors 9 and 3 as essential components of innate immune defense against mouse cytomegalovirus infection. Proc Natl Acad Sci USA 2004; 101: 3516.

16. Wang T, Town T, Alexopoulou L, et al. Toll-like receptor 3 mediates West Nile virus entry into the brain causing lethal encephalitis. Nat Med 2004; 10: 1366.

17. Robinson RA, DeVita VT, Levy HB, et al. A phase I–II trial of multiple-dose polyriboinosic-polyribocytidylic acid in patieonts with leukemia or solid tumors. J Natl Cancer Inst 1976; 57: 599.

18. Schulz O, Diebold SS, Chen M, et al. Toll-like receptor 3 promotes cross-priming to virus-infected cells. Nature 2005; 433: 887.

19. Poltorak A, He X, Smirnova I, et al. Defective LPS signaling in C3H/HeJ and C57BL/10ScCr mice: mutations in Tlr4 gene. Science 1998; 282: 2085.

20. Qureshi ST, Lariviere L, Leveque G, et al. Endotoxin-tolerant mice have mutations in Toll-like receptor 4 (Tlr4). J Exp Med 1999; 189: 615.

21. Hoshino K, Takeuchi O, Kawai T, et al. Cutting edge: Toll-like receptor 4 (TLR4)-deficient mice are hyporesponsive to lipopolysaccharide: evidence for TLR4 as the Lps gene product. J Immunol 1999; 162: 3749.

22. Evans JT, Cluff CW, Johnson DA, et al. Enhancement of antigen-specific immunity via the TLR4 ligands MPL adjuvant and Ribi.529. Exp Rev Vaccines 2003; 2: 219.

23. Hayashi F, Smith KD, Ozinsky A, et al. The innate immune response to bacterial flagellin is mediated by Toll-like receptor 5. Nature 2001; 410: 1099.

24. Uematsu S, Jang MH, Chevrier N, et al. Detection of pathogenic intestinal bacteria by Toll-like receptor 5 on intestinal CD11c(+) lamina propria cells. Nat Immunol 2006; 7: 868–874.

25. Hemmi H, Kaisho T, Takeuchi O, et al. Small anti-viral compounds activate immune cells via the TLR7 MyD88-dependent signaling pathway. Nat Immunol 2002; 3: 196.

26. Diebold SS, Kaisho T, Hemmi H, et al. Innate antiviral responses by means of TLR7-mediated recognition of single-stranded RNA. Science 2004; 303: 1529.

27. Heil F, Hemmi H, Hochrein H, et al. Species-specific recognition of single-stranded RNA via toll-like receptor 7 and 8. Science 2004; 303: 1526.

28. Hemmi H, Takeuchi O, Kawai T, et al. A Toll-like receptor recognizes bacterial DNA. Nature 2000; 408: 740.

29. Krieg AM. CpG motifs in bacterial DNA and their immune effects. Annu Rev Immunol 2002; 20: 709.

30. Klinman DM. Immunotherapeutic uses of CpG oligodeoxynucleotides. Nat Rev Immunol 2004; 4: 249.

31. Krieg AM. Therapeutic potential of Toll-like receptor 9 activation. Nat Rev Drug Discov 2006; 5: 471.

32. Akira S, Uematsu S, Takeuchi O. Pathogen recognition and innate immunity. Cell 2006; 124: 783.

33. Meylan E, Tschopp J, Karin M. Intracellular pattern recognition receptors in the host response. Nature 2006; 442: 39.

34. Seong SY, Matzinger P. Hydrophobicity: an ancient damage-associated molecular pattern that initiates innate immune responses. Nat Rev Immunol 2004; 4: 469.

35. Creagh EM, O'Neill LA. TLRs, NLRs and RLRs: a trinity of pathogen sensors that co-operate in innate immunity. Trends Immunol 2006; 27: 352.

36. Yoneyama M, Kikuchi M, Natsukawa T, et al. The RNA helicase RIG-I has an essential function in double-stranded RNA-induced innate antiviral responses. Nat Immunol 2004; 5: 730.

37. Kato H, Takeuchi O, Sato S, et al. Differential roles of MDA5 and RIG-I helicases in the recognition of RNA viruses. Nature 2006; 441: 101.

38. Schroder NW, Schumann RR. Single nucleotide polymorphisms of Toll-like receptors and susceptibility to infectious disease. Lancet Infect Dis 2005; 5: 156.

39. Turvey SE, Hawn TR. Towards subtlety: understanding the role of Toll-like receptor signaling in susceptibility to human infections. Clin Immunol 2006; 120: 1–9.

40. Hansson GK, Libby P. The immune response in atherosclerosis: a double-edged sword. Nat Rev Immunol 2006; 6: 508.

41. Bach JF. The effect of infections on susceptibility to autoimmune and allergic diseases. N Engl J Med 2002; 347: 911.

42. Janeway CA Jr. Approaching the asymptote? Evolution and revolution in immunology. Cold Spring Harb Symp Quant Biol 1989; 54 Pt 1: 1.

Antigen receptor genes, gene products, and co-receptors

Raul M. Torres, John Imboden, Harry W. Schroeder Jr.

4

In 1890, von Behring and Kitasato reported the existence of an agent in the blood that could neutralize diphtheria toxin. The following year, glancing references were made to 'Antikörper' in studies describing the ability of the agent to discriminate between two immune substances, or bodies. The term antigen is a shortened form of '*Anti*somato*gen*+⁻ Immunkörperbildner,' or the substance that induces the production of an antibody. Thus, an antibody and its antigen represent a classic tautology.

In 1939, Tiselius and Kabat used electrophoresis to separate immunized serum into albumin, α-goblulin, β-globulin, and γ-globulin fractions. Absorption of the serum against the antigen depleted the γ-globulin fraction, yielding the terms gammaglobulin, immunoglobulin (Ig), and IgG. 'Sizing' columns were then used to separate immunoglobulins into those that were 'heavy' (IgM), 'regular' (IgA, IgE, IgD, IgG), and 'light' (light-chain dimers).

In 1949, Porter used papain to digest IgG molecules into two types of fragments, termed Fab and Fc. The constancy of the Fc fragment permitted its crystallization, and thus the elucidation of its sequence and structure. The variability of the Fab fragment precluded analysis until Bence Jones myeloma proteins were identified as clonal, isolated light chains.

In 1976, Hozumi and Tonegawa demonstrated that the variable portion of κ chains was the product of the rearrangement of a variable (V) and joining (J) gene segment. In 1982, Alt and Baltimore reported that terminal deoxynucleotidyl transferase (TdT) could be used to introduce a nongermline-encoded sequence between rearranging V, D for diversity, and J gene segments, potentially freeing the heavy-chain repertoire from germline constraints. These discoveries clarified how lymphocytes could generate an astronomically diverse antigen receptor repertoire from a finite set of genes.

In 1982 Allison and colleagues raised antisera against a cell surface molecule that could uniquely identify individual T-cell clones. A year later, Kappler and a consortium of colleagues demonstrated that these surface molecules were heterodimers composed of variable- and constant-region domains, just like immunoglobulin. Subsequently, Davis and Mak independently cloned the β-chain of the T-cell receptor (TCR). Initial confusion regarding the identity of the companion α-chain led to the realization that there were two mutually exclusive forms of TCR, αβ and γδ.

PARATOPES AND EPITOPES

Immunoglobulins and TCRs both belong to the eponymous immunoglobulin superfamily (IgSF).[1-3] The study of antibodies precedes that of TCR by decades, hence much of what we know is based on knowledge first gleaned from the study of immunoglobulins.

Immunoglobulin–antigen interactions typically take place between the *paratope*, the site on the immunoglobulin at which the antigen binds, and the *epitope*, which is the site on the antigen that is bound. Thus lymphocyte antigen receptors do not recognize antigens, they recognize epitopes borne on those antigens. This makes it possible for the cell to discriminate between two closely related antigens, each of which can be viewed as a collection of epitopes. It also permits the same receptor to bind divergent antigens that share equivalent or similar epitopes, a phenomenon referred to as *cross-reactivity*.

Although both immunoglobulins and TCRs can recognize the same antigen, they do so in markedly different ways (Chapter 6). Immunoglobulins tend to recognize intact antigens in soluble form, and thus preferentially identify surface epitopes that can represent conformational structures that are noncontiguous in the antigen's primary sequence. TCRs recognize fragments of antigens that have been processed by a separate antigen-presenting cell and then bound to a major histocompatibility complex (MHC) class I or class II molecule (Chapter 5). This permits T cells to scan the internal, as well as the external, components of the antigen. Thus recognition of the antigen by the immune system often involves recognition of multiple epitopes on that antigen.

THE BCR AND TCR ANTIGEN RECOGNITION COMPLEX

While the ability of the surface antigen receptor to recognize antigen was appreciated early on, the mechanism by which the membrane-bound receptor relayed this antigen recognition event into the cell interior was not understood, since both B-cell receptor (BCR) and TCR cytoplasmic

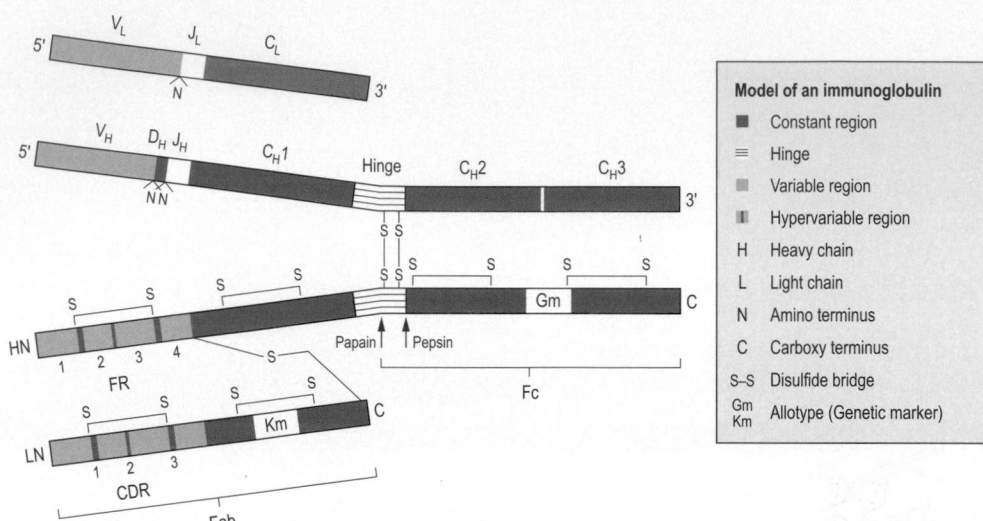

Fig. 4.1 A two-dimensional model of an immunoglobulin G (IgG) molecule. The top H and L chains illustrate the composition of these molecules at a nucleotide level. The bottom chains illustrate the nature of the protein sequence. See text for further details.

domains are exceptionally short. This conundrum was solved when it was shown that BCR and TCR each associate noncovalently with signal transduction complexes: heterodimeric Igα:Igβ for B cells and multimeric CD3 for T cells. Loss of function mutations in either of these complexes leads to cell death, which becomes clinically manifest as hypogammaglobulinemia in the case of B cells (Chapter 34), or severe combined immune deficiency (SCID) in the case of T cells (Chapter 35).

IMMUNOGLOBULINS AND TCR STRUCTURES

THE Ig DOMAIN, THE BASIC IgSF BUILDING BLOCK

Immunoglobulins consist of two heavy (H) and two light (L) chains (Fig. 4.1), where the L chain can consist of either a κ- or a λ-chain. TCRs consist of either an αβ or a γδ heterodimer. Each component chain contains two or more Immunoglobalin superfamily (IgSF) domains, each of which consists of two sandwiched β pleated sheets 'pinned' together by a disulfide bridge between two conserved cysteine residues (Fig. 4.2).[1] Considerable variability is allowed to the amino acids that populate the external surface of the IgSF domain and the loops that link the β strands. These solvent-exposed surfaces offer multiple targets for docking with other molecules.

Two types of IgSF domains, 'constant' (C) and 'variable' (V), are used in immunoglobulins and TCRs (Fig. 4.2). C-type domains, which are the most compact, have seven anti-parallel strands distributed as three strands in the first sheet and four strands in the second. Side chains positioned to lie between the two strands tend to be nonpolar in nature, creating a hydrophobic core of considerable stability. Indeed, V domains engineered to replace the conserved cysteines with serine residues retain their ability to bind antigen. V-type domains add two additional anti-parallel strands to the first sheet, creating a five-strand–four-strand

distribution. The two additional strands, which encode framework region 2 (FR2), are used to steady the interaction between heterodimeric V domains, allowing them to create a stable antigen-binding site.[4]

Each Ig and TCR chain contains only one NH2-terminal V Ig domain. Ig H chains contain three or four COOH-terminal C domains, whereas both Ig L chains and all four TCR chains contain only one C domain each. H chains with three C domains tend to include a spacer *hinge* region between the first (C_H1) and second (C_H2) domains. Each V or C domain consists of approximately 110–130 amino acids, averaging 12 000–13 000 kDa. A typical L or TCR chain will thus mass approximately 25 kDa, and a three C-domain Cγ H chain with its hinge will mass approximately 55 kDa.

IDIOTYPES AND ISOTYPES

Immunization of heterologous species with monoclonal antibodies (or a restricted set of immunoglobulins) has shown that immunoglobulins and TCRs contain both common and individual antigenic determinants. Individual determinants, termed *idiotypes*, are contained within V domains. Common determinants, termed *isotypes*, are specific for the constant portion of the antibody and allow grouping of immunoglobulins and TCRs into recognized classes, with each class defining an individual type of C domain. Determinants common to subsets of individuals within a species, yet differing between other members of that species, are termed *allotypes*, these define inherited polymorphisms that result from allelic forms of the genes.[5]

THE V DOMAIN

Early comparisons of the primary sequences of V domains identified three hypervariable intervals, termed complementarity-determining regions (CDRs), situated between four framework regions (FRs) of stable sequence (Fig. 4.1). The current definition of these regions

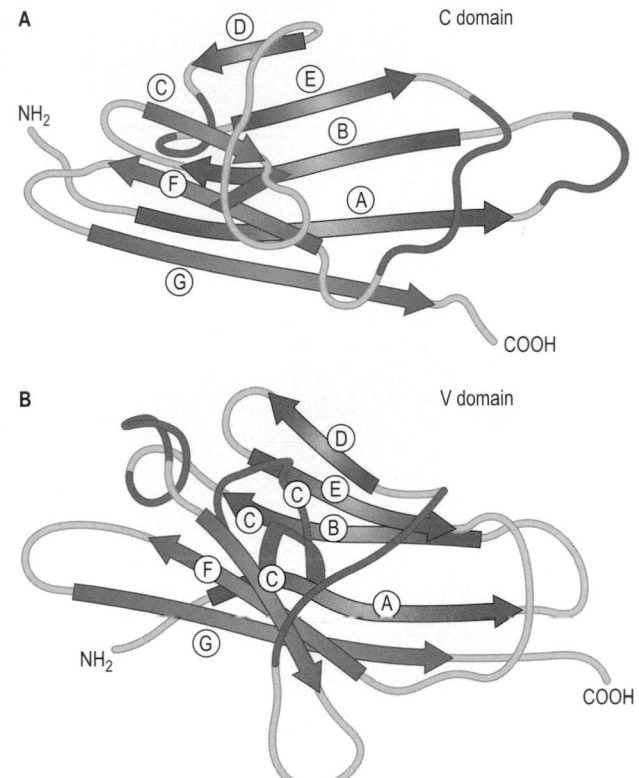

A

C domain

NH₂

COOH

B

V domain

NH₂

COOH

Fig. 4.2 Immunoglobulin superfamily (IgSF) domain structures. **(A)** A typical compact C domain structure. The β strands are labeled A through G. The sequence at the core is conserved and nonpolar. The external surface and the β-loops are available for docking and often vary in sequence. **(B)** A typical V domain structure. Two additional strands, C' and C', have been added. Note the projection of the C-C' strands and loop away from the core.

integrates sequence diversity with three-dimensional structure.[6] The international ImMunoGeneTics information system (IMGT), maintains an extremely useful website, http://imgt.cines.fr, which contains a large database of immunoglobulin and TCR sequences, as well as a multiplicity of software tools for their analysis.

ANTIGEN RECOGNITION AND THE FAB

Studies of Ig structure were facilitated by the use of papain and pepsin to fragment IgG molecules. Papain digests IgG into two Fab fragments, each of which can bind antigen, and a single Fc fragment. Pepsin splits IgG into an Fc fragment and a single dimeric F(ab)₂ that can cross-link as well as bind antigens. The Fab contains one complete L chain in its entirety and the V and C_H1 portion of one H chain (Fig. 4.1). The Fab can be further divided into a variable fragment (Fv) composed of the V_H and V_L domains, and a constant fragment (Fb) composed of the C_L and C_H1 domains. Single Fv fragments can be genetically engineered to recapitulate the monovalent antigen-binding characteristics of the original, parent antibody.[7] The extracellular domains of TCRαβ and TCRγδ correspond to Ig Fab.

EFFECTOR FUNCTION AND THE Fc

The Fc portion (Fig. 4.1) encodes the effector functions of the immunoglobulin. These functions are generally inflammatory reactions that include fixation of complement, activation of complement, and binding of antibody to Fc receptors on the surface of other cells. Each immunoglobulin class and subclass exhibits its own set of effector functions. For example, the IgG C_H2 domain plays a key role in binding to class-specific Fc receptors on the surface of effector cells.[8] Complement fixation is also focused on the C_H2 domain. Both of these interactions are important in initiating the process of phagocytosis, in allowing certain subclasses to traverse the placenta, and in influencing the biologic functions of lymphocytes, platelets, and other cells.

GM ALLOTYPE SYSTEM

A series of serologically defined genetic markers of the C domains of both H and L chains have been termed Gm for the gammaglobulin fraction of the serum in which they were first identified.[9] Different allelic forms have been defined for C domains of the γ_1, γ_2, γ_3, γ_4, α_2, and ε H chains and for the κ L chain. Associations between certain Gm allotypes and predisposition to develop certain diseases of immune function have been reported.

■ IMMUNOGLOBULIN CLASSES AND SUBCLASSES ■

The constant domains of the H chain define the class and subclass of the antibody. Table 4.1 lists the five major classes of immunoglobulins in humans and describes some of their physical and chemical features. Two

Table 4.1 Selected properties of immunoglobulin (Ig) classes

	IgG	IgA	IgM	IgD	IgE
Molecular weight	160 000	170 000 or polymer	900 000	160 000	180 000
Approximate concentration in serum (mg/dl)	1000–1500	250–300	100–150	3–30	.0015–.2
Valence	2	2 (monomer)	10 (small antigen) 5 (large antigen)	2	2
Molecular formula	$\gamma_2 L_2$	$(\alpha_2 L_2)n$	$(\mu_2 L_2)_5$	$\delta_2 L_2$	$\varepsilon_2 L_2$
Half-life (days)	23	6	5	3	2.5
Special property	Placental passage	Secretory Ig	Primary response lymphocyte surface	Lymphocyte surface	Reagin

Table 4.2 Selected biologic properties of classes and subclasses of immunoglobulins (Igs)

	IgG				IgA		IgM	IgD	IgE
	1	2	3	4	1	2			
Percentage of total (%)	65	20	10	5	90	10			
Complement fixation	++	+	++	–	–	–	++	–	–
Complement fixation (alternative)		+	+	+/–	+/–				
Placental passage	+	+	+	+	–	–	–	–	–
Fixing to mast cells or basophils	–	–	–	–	–	–	–	–	+
Binding to:									
Lymphocytes	+	+	+	+	–	–	+	–	–
Macrophages	+	+/–	+	+/–	–	–	–	–	–
Neutrophils	+	+	+	+	+	+	–	–	–
Platelets	+	+	+	+	–	–	–	–	–
Reaction with *Staphylococcus* protein A	+	+	–	+	–	–	–	–	–
Half-life (days)	23	23	8-9	23	6	6	5	3	2.5
Synthesis (mg/kg per day)	25	?	3.5	?	24	?	7	0.4	0.02

of the five major H chain classes, α and γ, have undergone duplication.[10] IgG_1, IgG_2, IgG_3, and IgG_4 all have the same basic structural design and differ only in the primary sequence of their constant regions and in the location of their interchain disulfide bonds. The H chain in each of these subclasses is referred to as γ_1, γ_2, etc. IgA consists of the two subclasses, α_1 and α_2. Table 4.2 compares the four subclasses of IgG, the two of IgA, and the classes of IgM, IgD, and IgE from the standpoint of their biologic functions. In humans, two L chain classes exist, κ and λ. No specific effector function has been identified for either L chain class.

IgM

IgM exists in monomeric, pentameric, and hexameric forms. The 8S monomeric 180 kDa IgM has the molecular formula $\mu_2 L_2$. It is a minor fraction in serum, but in its transmembrane form IgM plays a key role in B-cell development and function. The major form in serum is the 19S, 900 kDa pentameric IgM, which contains five subunits $((\mu_2 L_2)_5)$ linked together by disulfide bridges, and by one molecule of an additional polypeptide chain, the J chain, which joins two of the subunits by a disulfide bridge.[11]

IgM is the predominant immunoglobulin produced during the primary immune response. Occasionally, particularly in the case of carbohydrate Ags such as isohemagglutinins, it will remain the major or sole antibody class. IgM differs from most other immunoglobulins in having an extra C_H domain in place of a hinge.

IgM avidly fixes complement. This property is focused in $C_H 3$, the homologue of IgG $C_H 2$.[12] Although the valence of each $\mu_2 L_2$ subunit is 2, when binding to large protein antigens, five of the 10 antigen-binding sites in pentameric IgM appear blocked due to steric hindrance. As a consequence, the valence for large antigens is five.

IgG

IgG, the major immunoglobulin class, accounts for the bulk of serum antibody activity in response to most protein antigens. The four IgG subclasses are numbered in relation to their serum levels relative to each other, with IgG_1 predominant and IgG_4 the least common. IgG_1 and IgG_3 fix complement and bind phagocyte Fcγ receptors well, whereas IgG_2 fixes complement but binds Fcγ receptors more poorly. IgG_4 does not fix complement effectively in the native state, but has been reported to do so after proteolytic cleavage.[13] IgG_1 and IgG_3 are most frequently elicited by viral antigens,[14] IgG_2 by carbohydrates,[15] and IgG_4 by helminthic parasites.[16]

IgA

Although IgA generally exists in a monomeric form $(\alpha_2 L_2)$ in the serum, it can interact with J chain to form a polymer $(\alpha_2 L_2)_{2,3}$-J. Second in concentration to IgG in serum, IgA functions as the predominant form of immunoglobulin in mucosal secretions.[17]

Secretory IgA is largely synthesized by plasma cells located in, or originating from, mucosal tissues. In the secretions, the molecule usually exists in an alternative polymeric form with two subunits in association with the 70 kDa secretory component $(\alpha_2 L_2)_2$-SC. SC is synthesized by the epithelial cells that line the lumen of the gut. The complete function of SC remains uncertain, but it appears to serve as a receptor for IgA and may play a role in attracting IgA-bearing lymphocytes to the gut and other organs of secretion. It also appears to render the secretory IgA complex more resistant to proteolytic digestion.

IgE

IgE is largely found in extravascular spaces. Its plasma turnover is rapid, with a half-life of about 2 days. IgE antibodies help protect the host from parasitic infections. However, in westernized, affluent societies, IgE is primarily associated with allergy. Through their interaction with Fcε receptors on mast cells and basophils, IgE antibodies, in the presence of antigens, induce the release of histamine and various other vasoactive substances. These factors are responsible for clinical manifestations of various allergic states.[18]

IgD

Although the H chain of IgD can undergo alternative splicing to a secretory form, IgD serum antibodies in human are uncommon and are absent in the serum of mice and primates. Instead, IgD is typically found in association with IgM on the surface of mature lymphocytes. The appearance of IgD is associated with the transition of a B lymphocyte from a cell that can be tolerized to antigen to a cell that will respond to antigen with the production of antibody (Chapter 8).

■ TCR αβ AND γδ ■

As members of the IgSF, TCR α-, β-, γ-, and δ-chains share a number of structural similarities with immunoglobulin. Each chain has a leader peptide, an extracellular, a transmembrane, and an intracytoplasmic interval. The extracellular interval can be divided into three domains: a polymorphic V domain encoded by VJ (α- and γ-chains) or VDJ (β- and δ-chains) gene segments, a C domain, and a hinge region.[19] The hinge

region typically contains an extra cysteine (none in γ-chains encoded by Cγ2) that forms a disulfide bond with the other partner of the heterodimer. The transmembrane domains all include a lysine and some contain an arginine residue that facilitate the association of the TCR heterodimer with components of the CD3 signal transduction complex, each of which has a matching negatively charged residue in its own transmembrane portions (see below). The intracytoplasmic domains are tiny and play a minimal role in signal transduction.

TCR αβ

The TCR α- and β-chains are glycoproteins with molecular weights that vary from 42 to 45 kDa, depending upon the primary amino acid sequence and the degree of glycosylation. Deglycosylated forms have a molecular mass of 30–32 kDa. These chains share a number of invariant residues in common with immunoglobulin heavy and light chains, in particular residues that are thought to be important for interactions between heavy and light chains. The structures of several partial or full-length TCRs have been solved by X-ray crystallography (Fig. 4.3).[20–22] In general, the structure of the TCR αβ heterodimer is similar, but not identical, to that of an Ig Fab fragment.

TCR γδ

The TCR γ- and δ-chains are glycoproteins with a more complex molecular size pattern than α- and β-chains. TCRs that use the Cγ1 gene segment, which contains a cysteine-encoding exon, are disulfide-linked (molecular weight 36–42 kDa). TCRs that use Cγ2 exist in two nondisulfide-linked forms, one of 40–44 kDa and one of 55 kDa.[23] The differences in molecular size are due to variability of both N-linked glycosylation and primary amino acid sequence. The 55 kDa form uses a Cγ2 allele that contains three (rather than two) exons encoding the connecting piece, as well as more N-linked carbohydrate. The functional implication of three different TCR γ-chain isoforms, if any, is unknown. The TCR δ-chain is more straightforward, being 40–43 kDa in size and containing two sites of N-linked glycosylation. The overall architecture of the γδ TCR closely resembles that of αβ TCRs and antibodies, although the angle between the V and C domains, known as the elbow angle, appears more acute.

LIGAND RECOGNITION

Although TCR αβ T cells primarily recognize peptide–MHC complexes (pMHC) (Fig. 4.3; Chapters 5 and 7), other types of ligands exist. For example, some αβ TCRs can bind nonpeptidic antigens (atypical antigens) that are bound to nonclassic MHC molecules. Many γδ T cells recognize atypical antigens that may or may not be associated with an antigen-presenting molecule. Finally, many αβ TCRs bind superantigens (SAg) in a predominantly Vβ-dependent fashion (Chapter 6).

BINDING TO pMHC

TCRs recognize peptide antigens bound to the binding groove of MHC-encoded glycoproteins (Fig. 4.3). TCR recognition of pMHC requires a trimolecular complex in which all the components (antigen, MHC, and TCR) contact one another.[20–22] Thus, recognition is highly influenced by polymorphisms in the MHC molecule (Chapter 5). As in the case of Ig, TCR CDR1 and CDR2 are encoded in the germline V

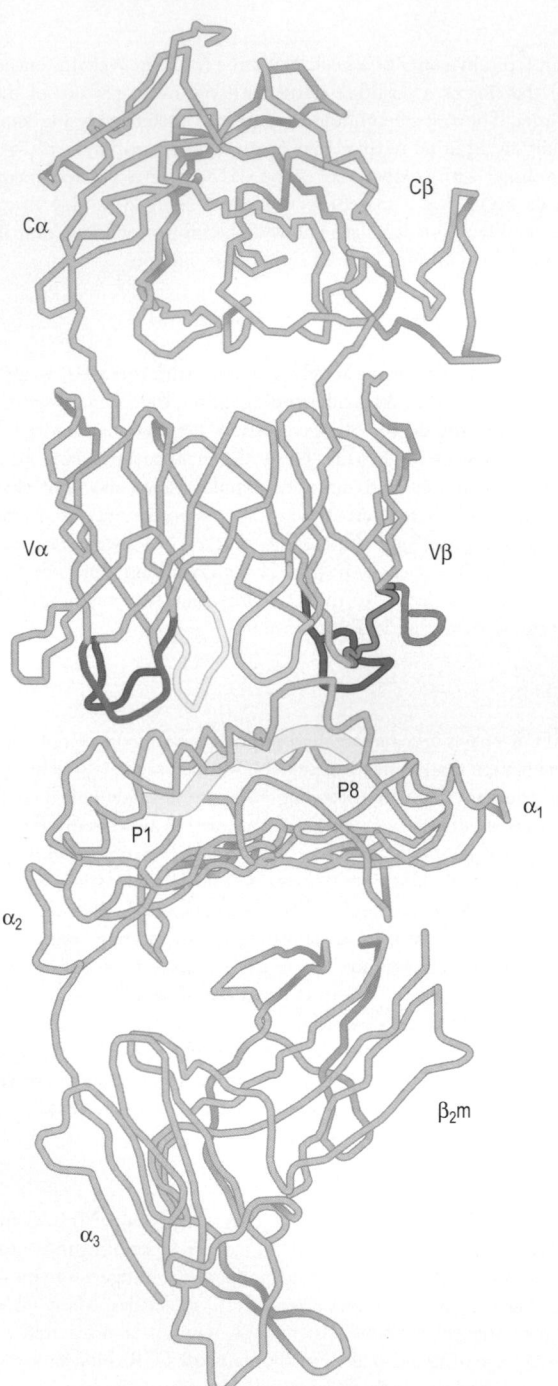

Fig. 4.3 Backbone representation of murine αβ T-cell receptor (TCR) bound to murine major histocompatibility complex (MHC) class I and an octamer peptide. The TCR is above. The Vα CDR1 and CDR2 are magenta, Vβ CDR1 and CDR2 are blue, both CDR3s are green, and the Vβ HV4 is orange. β2M refers to β2-microglobulin. The peptide is in green, and the NH2-terminal and COOH-terminal residues are designated P1 and P8. (From Garcia KC, Degano M, Stanfield RL, et al. An alphabeta T cell receptor structure at 2.5 A and its orientation in the TCR-MHC complex. Science 1996; 274: 209–219. Reprinted with permission from AAAS.)

regions, whereas CDR3 is formed at the junction of the V gene with a J gene segment (TCR α and γ) or D and J gene segments (TCR β-and δ-chains).[24] Vβ also has a fourth region of variability near the other CDRs, hypervariable region 4 (HV4) or CDR4, which can participate in SAg binding.

The co-crystallization of different combinations of soluble TCR αβ interacting with MHC class I bound to antigen peptide (pMHC) has made it possible to directly address the manner in which antigen recognition occurs (Fig. 4.3).[20–22] The TCR αβ combining site is relatively flat, allowing it to interact with a rather broad surface at the point of contact with pMHC.

The TCR footprint on the pMHC complex often occurs in a diagonal across the MHC antigen-binding groove, with TCR Vα positioned over the MHC α2 helix and TCR Vβ overlying the MHC α1 helix. This geometry would permit consistent access of the CD8 co-receptors to the MHC class I molecule. The CDR1 and CDR2 loops, which are entirely encoded by germline sequence, tend to interact more with the MHC molecule; whereas the CDR3 loops, which are composed of both germline and somatic (N-region) sequence, appear to dominate the interaction with MHC-bound peptide.

The binding of TCR to pMHC appears to be driven by enthalpy. That is, binding increases the stability of the CDR loops, especially the CDR3s. These results have led to the suggestion that initial binding focuses on the interaction between CDRs 1 and 2 and the MHC. After this initial recognition, the CDR3s change their shape to maximize the area of contact. Conformational flexibility, or 'induced fit,' would allow TCRs to sample many similar pMHC complexes rapidly, stopping only when their CDR3s are able to stabilize the interaction.

TCR-BINDING AFFINITY

The affinity with which the TCR ultimately binds its ligand is a critical determinant of T-cell activation. It is, however, only one factor in determining the overall *avidity* of the interaction, since other cell surface molecules of the T cell (e.g., CD4, CD8, CD2, and various integrins) bind to cell surface molecules on the antigen-bearing cell to stabilize cell–cell TCR–ligand interactions. Furthermore, since both the TCR and the pMHC ligand are surface membrane proteins, each T cell can provide multiple TCR in the same plane that can bind multiple pMHC molecules on the surface of the antigen-presenting cell. This makes binding of TCR to pMHC functionally multivalent, enhancing the apparent affinity of the interaction.

ATYPICAL ANTIGENS

Some αβ T cells can recognize lipid antigens when they are complexed with members of the CD1 family.[25] The interaction of TCR αβ with CD1 resembles that of TCR αβ with MHC class I. Allelic polymorphism in CD1 is limited, which theoretically would restrict the range of lipid antigens that can be bound.

Rather than binding to a single groove on the MHC, lipids attach themselves to one of several hydrophobic pockets that can be found on the surface of CD1. Pocket volume can range from 1300 Å^3 to 2200 Å^3. The number and length of the pockets differ between the various CD1 isoforms. For example, CD1b has three pockets that share a common portal of entry, as well as a fourth pocket that connects two of the three pockets to each other. This connecting pocket permits the insertion of lipids with a long alkyl chain, such as mycobacterial mycolic acid.

IMMUNOGLOBULIN GENE ORGANIZATION

Antigen recognition by γδ TCRs resembles recognition of intact antigens by antibodies more closely than recognition of pMHC by αβ TCR.[26] γδ TCRs can recognize protein antigens, such as nonclassical MHC molecules and viral glycoproteins, as well as small, phosphate- or amine-containing compounds, such as pyrophosphomonoesters from mycobacteria and alkylamines.

Binding to nonpeptide antigens plays an important role in the biology of γδ T cells. About 5% of peripheral blood T cells bear γδ TCRs, and most of these are encoded by Vγ9JγP and Vδ2[+]gene segments. (In an alternative nomenclature, Vγ9 is known as Vγ2 and JγP as Jγ1.2. See the IMGT database at http://imgt.cines.fr.) These Vγ9JγPVδ2[+]TCRs recognize nonpeptide pyrophosphate- or amine-containing antigens, such as pyrophosphomonoesters from mycobacteria or isobutylamine from various sources.[26] Other common naturally occurring small phosphorylated metabolites that stimulate γδ T cells include 2,3-diphosphoglyceric acid, glycerol-3-phosphoric acid, xylose-1-phosphate, and ribose-1-phosphate. In addition to mycobacteria, Vγ9JγPVδ2[+]T-cell populations are seen to expand in response to listeriosis, ehrlichiosis, leishmaniasis, brucellosis, salmonellosis, mumps, meningitis, malaria, and toxoplasmosis.

The atypical antigens do not require antigen processing and are not co-recognized with known antigen-presenting molecules. Although MHC presentation is not necessary, cell cell contact is required for stimulation. This suggests either that the small molecules are being presented by non-MHC molecules or that co-stimulation from neighboring cells is needed for proper γδ T-cell activation.

SUPERANTIGENS

SAgs are a special class of TCR ligands that have the ability to activate large fractions (5–20%) of the T-cell population. Activation requires simultaneous interaction between the SAg, the TCR Vβ domain, and an MHC class II molecule on the surface of an antigen-presenting cell.[27]

Unlike conventional antigens, SAgs do not require processing to allow them to bind class II molecules or activate T cells. Instead of binding to the peptide antigen-binding groove, SAgs bind to polymorphic residues on the periphery of the class II molecule. And, instead of binding to TCR β CDR3 residues, SAg bind to polymorphic residues in CDR1, CDR2, and HV4. Soluble TCR β-chains can also bind the appropriate SAg in the absence of a TCR α-chain. As a consequence, although SAg link the TCR to the MHC, the T-cell responses are not 'MHC- restricted' in the conventional sense, since a T cell with the appropriate Vβ will respond to a SAg bound to a variety of polymorphic class II molecules.

■ IMMUNOGLOBULIN AND TCR GENE ORGANIZATION ■

The component chains of immunoglobulins and TCRs are each encoded by a separate multigene family.[28, 29] The paradox of variability in the V region in conjunction with a nearly invariable constant region was resolved when it was shown that immunoglobulin V and C domains are encoded by independent elements, or gene segments, within each gene family. That is, more than one gene element is used to encode a single polypeptide chain. For example, while κ constant domains are encoded by a single Cκ exon in the κ locus on chromosome 2,[30] κ variable domains represent the joined product of Vκ and Jκ gene segments (Fig. 4.1).

KEY CONCEPTS

FEATURES COMMON TO IMMUNOGLOBULIN (IG) AND T-CELL RECEPTOR (TCR) GENES

>> Ig and TCR variable domains are created by site-specific V(D)J recombination

>> Each receptor is assembled in a stepwise fashion:

Immunoglobulins: $D_H \rightarrow J_H$; $VH \rightarrow D_H J_H$; cytoplasmic μ-chain expression; $V\kappa \rightarrow J\kappa$ and, if needed, $V\lambda \rightarrow J\lambda$; surface IgM expression

TCRαβ: $D\beta \rightarrow J\beta$; $V\beta \rightarrow D\beta J\beta$; cytoplasmic β-chain expression; $V\alpha \rightarrow J\alpha$; surface αβ TCR expression

>> In developing lymphocytes, CDRs1 and 2 contain exclusively germline sequence, whereas CDR3 is created by the (V[D]J) joining reaction and often includes nongermline sequence:

>> CDR-H3, CDR-B3, and CDR-D3 are the most variable components of IgM, TCRαβ, and TCRγδ, respectively

>> The antigen-binding site is a product of a nested gradient of diversity. Conserved framework regions flank CDR1 and CDR2, which in turn surround the paired CDR3 intervals that form the center of the antigen-binding site

>> Starting with a small set of individual gene segments, combinatorial gene segment rearrangement, combinatorial association of heavy and light chains, and mechanisms of junctional diversity generate a broad repertoire of antigen-binding structures

>> The variability of the Ig and TCR repertoires is restricted during perinatal life, limiting the immune response of the infant

KEY CONCEPTS

FEATURES SPECIFIC TO IG GENES

>> Variable-domain somatic hypermutation (SHM) permits affinity maturation

>> Class switch recombination (CSR) allows replacement of an upstream C domain by a downstream one, altering effector function while maintaining antigen specificity

V_L gene segments typically contain their own promoter, a leader exon, an intervening intron of ~100 nucleotides, an exon that encodes the first three framework regions (FR1, 2, and 3), the first two CDRs in their entirety, the amino-terminal portion of CDR 3, and a recombination signal sequence. A J_L (J for joining) gene segment begins with its own recombination signal, the remaining portion of CDR 3, and the complete FR4 (Fig. 4.1).

(Use of the same abbreviation, V, for both the complete variable domain of an immunoglobulin peptide chain and for the gene segment that encodes only a portion of that same variable domain is the result of historic precedent. It is unfortunate that one must depend on the context of the

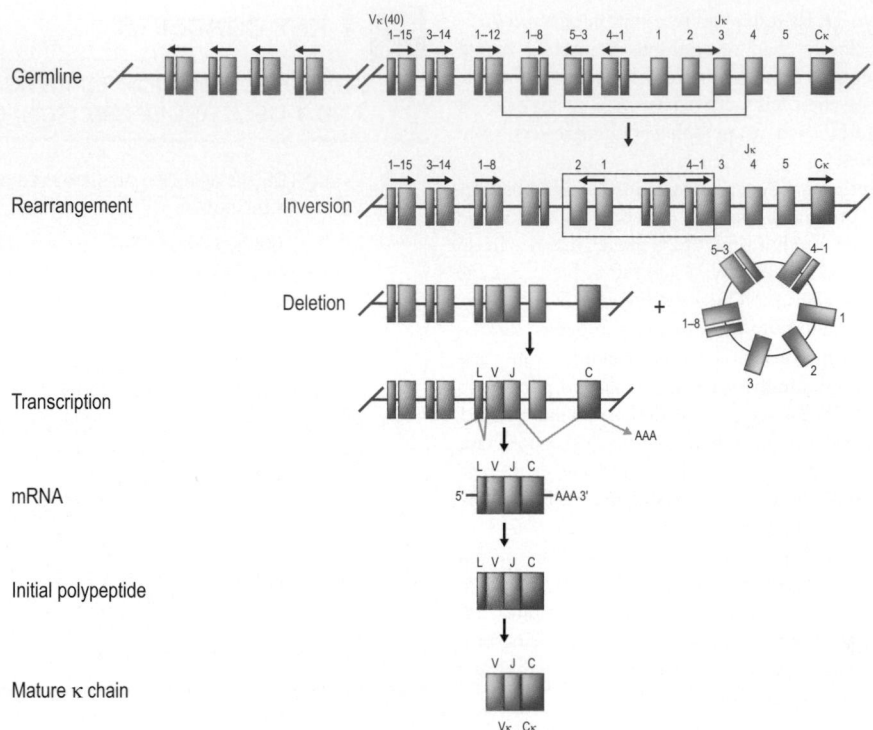

Fig. 4.4 Rearrangement events in the human κ locus. V, variable region; J, joining region; C, constant region of the κ light chain. See text for further description.

surrounding text in order to determine which V region of the antibody is being discussed. The same holds true for the use of J to represent both the J gene segment and the J joining protein.)

The creation of a V domain is directed by the recombination signal sequences (RSS) that flank the rearranging gene segments. Each RSS contains a strongly conserved 7-basepair, or heptamer, sequence (e.g., CACAGTG) that is separated from a less well-conserved 9-basepair, or nonamer, sequence (e.g., ACAAAACCC) by either a 12- or 23-basepair spacer. For example, Vκ gene segments have a 12-basepair spacer and Jκ elements have a 23-basepair spacer. These spacers place the heptamer and nonamer sequences on the same side of the DNA molecule, separated by either one or two turns of the DNA helix. A one-turn recombination signal sequence (12-basepair spacer) will preferentially recognize a two-turn signal sequence (23-basepair spacer). This helps prevent wasteful V-V or J-J rearrangements.

Initiation of the V(D)J recombination reaction requires recombination-activating genes 1 and 2 (RAG-1 and RAG-2). These genes are only expressed in developing lymphocytes.[31] RAG-1 and RAG-2 act by precisely introducing a DNA double-strand break between the terminus of the rearranging gene segment and its adjacent recombination signal sequence (Fig. 4.5). These breaks are then repaired by ubiquitously expressed components of a DNA repair process that is known as nonhomologous end-joining (NHEJ). Lack-of-function mutations in NHEJ proteins yield susceptibility to DNA damage in all cells of the body.

The NHEJ process creates precise joins between the RSS ends, and imprecise joins of the coding ends. TdT, which is only expressed in lymphocytes, adds nongermline-encoded nucleotides (N nucleotides) to the coding ends of the recombination product.

Lymphoid-specific expression of RAG-1 and RAG-2 limits V(D)J recombination to B and T lymphocytes. However, to ensure that TCR genes are rearranged to completion only in T cells and immunoglobulin genes are rearranged to completion only in B cells, V(D)J recombination is further regulated by limiting the accessibility of the appropriate gene segments to the specific lineage as well as to the specific stage of development. For example, H chain genes are assembled before L chains.

RAG-1 and RAG-2 cooperatively associate with 12- and 23-basepair RSSs and their flanking coding gene segments to form a synaptic complex. Typically, the initial event will be recognition of the nonamer sequence of a 12-basepair spacer RSS by RAG-1. RAG-1 binding to the heptamer provides specificity. RAG-2 does not bind DNA independently, but does make contact with the heptamer when in a synaptic complex with RAG-1. Binding of a second RAG-1 and RAG-2 complex to the 23-basepair, two-turn RSS permits the interaction of the two synaptic complexes to form what is known as a paired complex. Creation of this paired complex is facilitated by the actions of the DNA-bending proteins HMG1 and HMG2.

After paired complex assembly, the RAG proteins single strand cut the DNA at the heptamer sequence. The 3' OH of the coding sequence ligates to 5'phosphate and creates a hairpin loop. The clean-cut ends of the signal sequences enable formation of precise signal joints. However, the hairpin junction created at the coding ends must be resolved by renicking the DNA, usually within four to five nucleotides from the end of

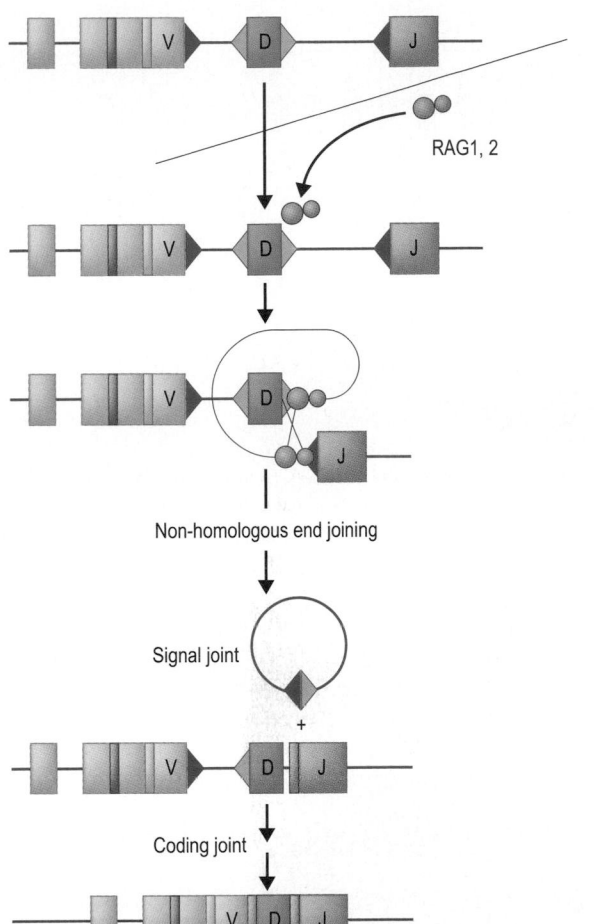

Non-homologous end joining

Signal joint

+

Coding joint

Fig. 4.5 VDJ recombination. Lymphoid-specific RAG-1 and RAG-2 bind to the recombination signal sequences (RSS) flanking V, D, or J gene segments, juxtapose the sequences, and introduce precise cuts adjacent to the RSS. Components of the nonhomologous end joining repair pathway subsequently unite the cut RSS to form a signal joint, and the coding sequences of the rearranging gene segments to form a coding joint.

the hairpin. This forms a 3' overhang that is amenable to further modification. It can be filled in via DNA polymerases, nibbled, or serve as a substrate for TdT-catalyzed N addition. DNA polymerase μ, which shares homology with TdT, appears to play a role in maintaining the integrity of the terminus of the coding sequence.

The cut ends of the coding sequence are then repaired by the nonhomologous end joining proteins. NHEJ proteins involved in V(D)J recombination include Ku70, Ku80, DNA-PKcs, Artemis, XRCC4, and ligase 4. Deficiency of any one of these proteins creates sensitivity to DNA breakage and can lead to a SCID phenotype (Chapter 35).

Ku70 and Ku80 form a heterodimer (Ku) that directly associates with DNA double-strand breaks to protect the DNA ends from degradation, permit juxtaposition of the ends to facilitate coding end ligation, and help recruit other members of the repair complex. DNA-PKcs phosphorylates Artemis, inducing an endonuclease activity that plays a role in the

opening of the coding joint hairpin. Thus absence of DNA-PKcs or Artemis inhibits proper coding joint formation. Signal joint formation is normal in Artemis deficiency, but it is impaired in the absence of DNA-PKcs. This suggests an additional, as yet undefined, role for DNA-PKcs. Finally, XRCC4 and ligase 4 help rejoin the ends of the broken DNA.

Depending on the transcriptional orientation of the rearranging gene segments, recombination may result in either inversion or deletion of the intervening DNA (Fig. 4.4). The products of inversion remain in the DNA of the cell, whereas deletion leads to the loss of the intervening DNA. The increased proximity of the V promoter to the C domain enhancers promotes the subsequent transcription of the Ig gene product.

THE κ LOCUS

The κ locus is located on chromosome 2p11.2. It contains five Jκ and 75 Vκ gene segments upstream of Cκ (Fig. 4.6). The Vκ gene segments can be grouped into six different families of varying size.[30] Each family is comprised of gene segments that share extensive sequence and structural similarity.[32, 33]

One-third of the Vκ gene segments contain frameshift mutations or stop codons that preclude them from forming functional protein, and of the remaining sequences fewer than 30 of the Vκ gene segments have actually been found in functional immunoglobulins. Each of these active Vκ gene segments has the potential to rearrange to any one of the five Jκ elements, generating a potential repertoire of more than 140 distinct VJ combinations. Even more diversity is created at the site of gene segment joining. The terminus of each rearranging gene segment can undergo a loss of 1–5 nucleotides during the recombination process. In human, but not mouse, N addition can either replace some or all of the lost nucleotides or can be inserted in addition to the original germline sequence.[34] Each codon created by N addition increases the potential diversity of the repertoire 20-fold. Thus, the initial diversification of the κ repertoire is focused at the VJ junction that defines CDR-L3.

THE λ LOCUS

The λ locus, on chromosome 22q11.2, contains four functional Cλ exons, each of which is associated with its own Jλ (Fig. 4.6). The Vλ genes are arranged in three distinct clusters, each containing members of different Vλ families.[35] Depending on the individual haplotype, there are approximately 30–36 potentially functional Vλ gene segments and an equal number of pseudogenes.

In addition to normal κ and λ peptides, H chains can also form a complex with unconventional λ light chains, known as surrogate or pseudo light chains (ΨLC). The genes encoding the ΨLC proteins, λ14.1 (λ5) and V$_{preB}$, are located within the λ light-chain locus on chromosome 22. Together, these two genes create a product with considerable homology to conventional λ light chains. The λ14.1 gene contains Jλ and Cλ-like sequences and the V$_{preB}$ gene includes a Vλ-like sequence. A critical difference between these unconventional ΨLC genes and other L chains is that λ14.1 and V$_{preB}$ gene rearrangement is not required for ΨLC expression.

THE H-CHAIN LOCUS

The H-chain locus, on chromosome 14q32.33, is considerably more complex than the κ and λ loci. There are ~80 V$_H$ gene segments near the telomere of the long arm of chromosome 14.[36] Of these, approximately 39

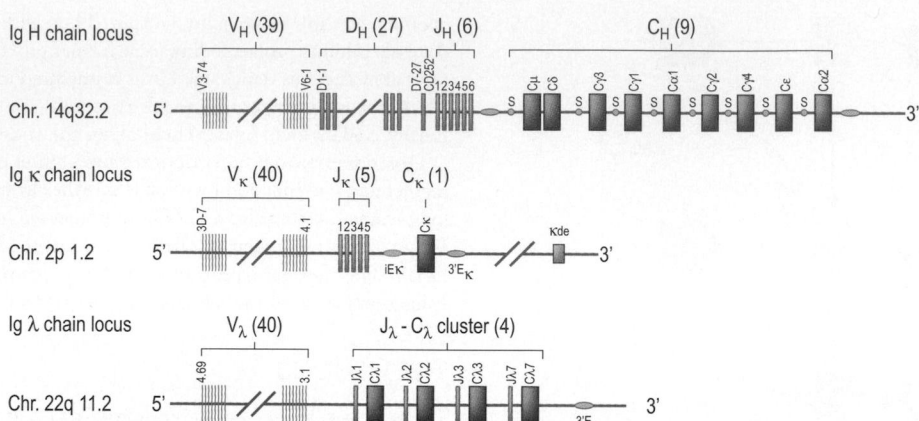

Fig. 4.6 Chromosomal organization of the immunoglobulin (Ig) H, κ, and λ gene clusters. The typical numbers of functional gene segments are shown. The κ gene cluster includes a κ-deleting element that can rearrange to sequences upstream of Ck in cells that express λ-chains, reducing the likelihood of dual κ and λ light-chain expression. These maps are not drawn to scale.

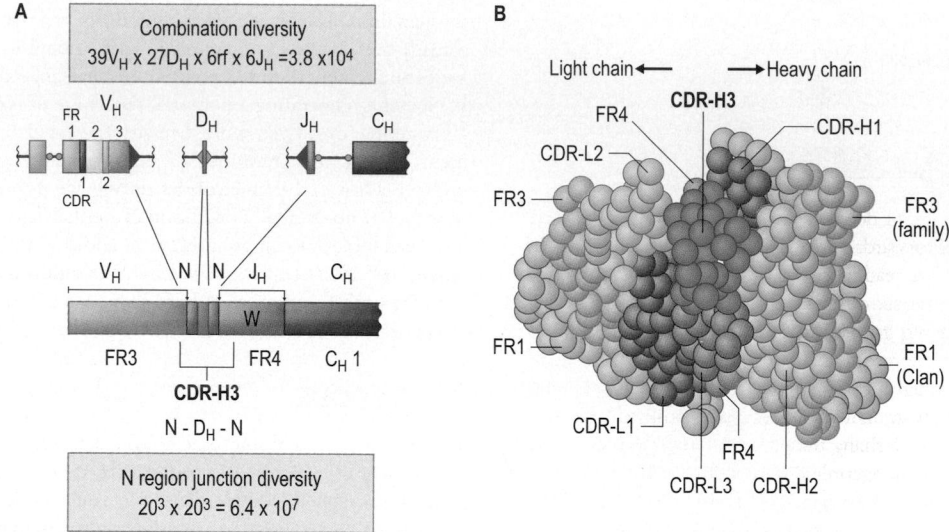

Fig. 4.7 The antigen-binding site is the product of a nested gradient of diversity. (A) VDJ rearrangement yields 3800 different combinations. The CDR-H3 sequence contains both germline V, D, and J sequence, as well as nongermline N nucleotides. The addition of nine N nucleotides on either side of the D gene segment yields 64 million different combinations. (B) The antigen-binding site is created by the juxtaposition of the three complementarity-determining regions (CDRs) of the H chain and the three CDRs of the light chain. The view is looking into the binding site as an antigen would see the CDRs. The V_h domain is on the right side. The central location of CDR-H3, which due to N addition is the focus for repertoire diversity, is readily apparent.

are functional and can be grouped into seven different families of related gene segments. Adjacent to the most centromeric V_H, V6-1, are 27 D_H (D for diversity) gene segments (Fig. 4.6)[37] and six J_H gene segments. Each V_H and J_H gene segment is associated with a two-turn recombination signal sequence, which prevents direct V→J joining. A pair of one-turn recombination signal sequences flanks each D_H. Recombination begins with the joining of a D_H to a J_H gene segment, followed by the joining of a V_H element to the amino-terminal end of the DJ intermediate. The V_H gene segment contains FR1, 2, and 3, CDR1 and 2, and

the amino-terminal portion of CDR3; the D_H gene segment forms the middle of CDR3; and the J_H element contains the carboxy-terminus of CDR3 and FR4 in its entirety (Fig. 4.1). Random assortment of one of ~50 active V_H and one of 27 D_H with one of the six J_H gene segments can generate up to 10^4 different VDJ combinations (Fig. 4.7).

Although combinatorial joining of individual V, D, and J gene segments maximizes germline-encoded diversity, the major source of variation in the pre-immune repertoire is focused on the CDR-H3 interval which is created by VDJ joining (Fig. 4.7). First, D_H gene segments can

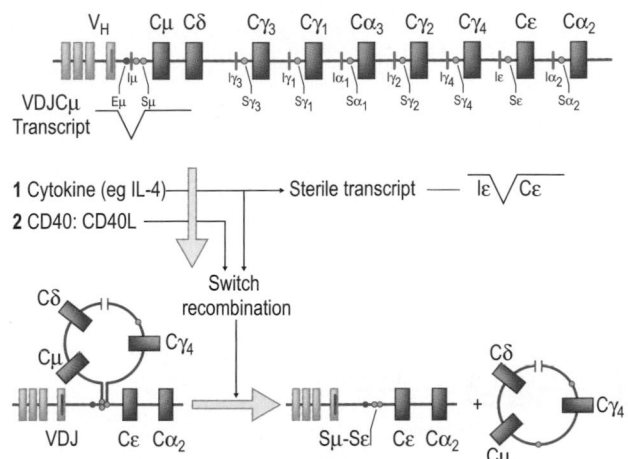

Fig. 4.8 Immunoglobulin H-chain class switching. The molecular events involved in switching from expression of one class of immunoglobulin to another are depicted. At the top is the gene organization during μ-chain synthesis. At the bottom a class switch recombination event has resulted in the deletion of the intervening DNA. Exposure to the appropriate cytokine or T-cell:B-cell interaction through the CD40:CD40L pathway results in activation of the I exon that yields a sterile epsilon transcript (Iε-Cε) (Chapter 8). The CD40:CD40L interaction is necessary for the subsequent replacement of Cμ by another constant gene (in this case, Cε). The S loci indicate switch-specific recombination signals.

rearrange by either inversion or deletion, and thus have the potential to be read backwards as well as forwards. Each D_H can be spliced and translated in each of the three potential reading frames. Thus, each D_H gene segment has the potential to encode six different peptide fragments. Second, the terminus of each rearranging gene segment can undergo a loss of one or more nucleotides during the recombination process. Third, the rearrangement process proceeds through a step that creates a hairpin ligation between the 5' and 3' termini of the rearranging gene segment. Nicking to resolve the hairpin structure leaves a 3' overhang that creates a palindromic extension, termed a P junction. Fourth, nongermline-encoded nucleotides (N regions) can be used to replace or add to the original germline sequence. Every codon that is added by N-region addition increases the potential diversity of the repertoire 20-fold. N regions can be inserted both between the V and the D, and between the D and the J. Together, the imprecision of the joining process and variation in the extent of N addition permit generation of CDR-H3s of varying length and structure. As a result, more than 10^{10} different H-chain VDJ junctions, or CDR-H3s, can be generated at the time of gene segment rearrangement. Together, somatic variation in CDR3, combinatorial rearrangement of individual gene segments, and combinatorial association between different L and H chains yields a potential preimmune antibody repertoire of greater than 10^{16} antibody repertoire of greater different immunoglobulins.

CLASS SWITCH RECOMBINATION

Located downstream of the VDJ loci are nine functional C_H gene segments (Fig. 4.8).[10] The C_H consist of a series of exons, each encoding a separate domain, hinge, or terminus. All C_H genes can undergo alternative splicing to generate two different types of carboxy termini: either a membrane

terminus that anchors immunoglobulin on the B lymphocyte surface, or a secreted terminus that occurs in the soluble form of the immunoglobulin. With the exception of $C_H1\delta$, each C_H1 constant region is preceded by both an exon that cannot be translated (an I exon) and a region of repetitive DNA termed the switch (S) region. Through recombination between the Cμ switch region and one of the switch regions of the seven other H chain constant regions (a process termed *class switching* or *CSR*), the same VDJ heavy-chain variable domain can be juxtaposed to any of the H-chain classes (Fig. 4.8).[10] Thus, the system can tailor both the receptor and the effector ends of the antibody molecule to meet a specific need.

SOMATIC HYPERMUTATION

A final mechanism of immunoglobulin diversity is engaged only after exposure to antigen. With T-cell help, the variable domain genes of germinal center lymphocytes undergo *somatic hypermutation* (SHM) at a rate of up to 10^{-3} changes per basepair per cell cycle. SHM is correlated with transcription of the locus and current studies suggest that at least two separate mechanisms are involved. The first mechanism targets mutation hot spots with the RGYW (purine/G/pyrimidine/A) motif[38] and the second mechanism incorporates an error-prone DNA synthesis that can lead to a nucleotide mismatch between the original template and the mutated DNA strand.[39] SHM allows affinity maturation of the antibody repertoire in response to repeated immunization or exposure to antigen.

ACTIVATION-INDUCED CYTIDINE DEAMINASE

Activation-induced cytidine deaminase (AID) plays a key role in both CSR and SHM.[31, 40] AID is a single-strand DNA (ssDNA) cytidine deaminase that can be expressed in activated germinal center B cells. Transcription of an immunoglobulin V domain or of the switch region upstream of the C_H1 domain opens the DNA helix to generate ssDNA that can then be deaminated by AID to form mismatched dU/dG DNA basepairs. The base excision repair protein uracil DNA glycosylase (UNG) removes the mismatched dU base, creating an abasic site. Differential repair of this lesion leads to either SHM or CSR. The mismatch repair proteins MSH2 and MSH6 can also bind and process the dU:dG mismatch. Deficiencies of AID and UNG underlie some forms of the hyper-IgM syndrome (Chapter 34).

DIVERSITY AND CONSTRAINTS ON IMMUNOGLOBULIN SEQUENCE

In theory, combinatorial rearrangement of V(D)J gene segments, combinatorial association of H and L chains, flexibility in the site of gene segment joining, N-region addition, P junctions, hypermutation, and class switching can create an antibody repertoire the diversity of which is limited only by the total number of B cells in circulation at any one time. In practice, constraints and biases on both the structure and sequence of the antibody repertoire are apparent.

The representation of individual V gene elements is nonrandom. Among Vκ and V_H elements, half of the potentially functional V gene elements contribute minimally to the expressed repertoire. Among Vλ elements these restrictions are even greater, with three gene segments contributing to half of the expressed repertoire.

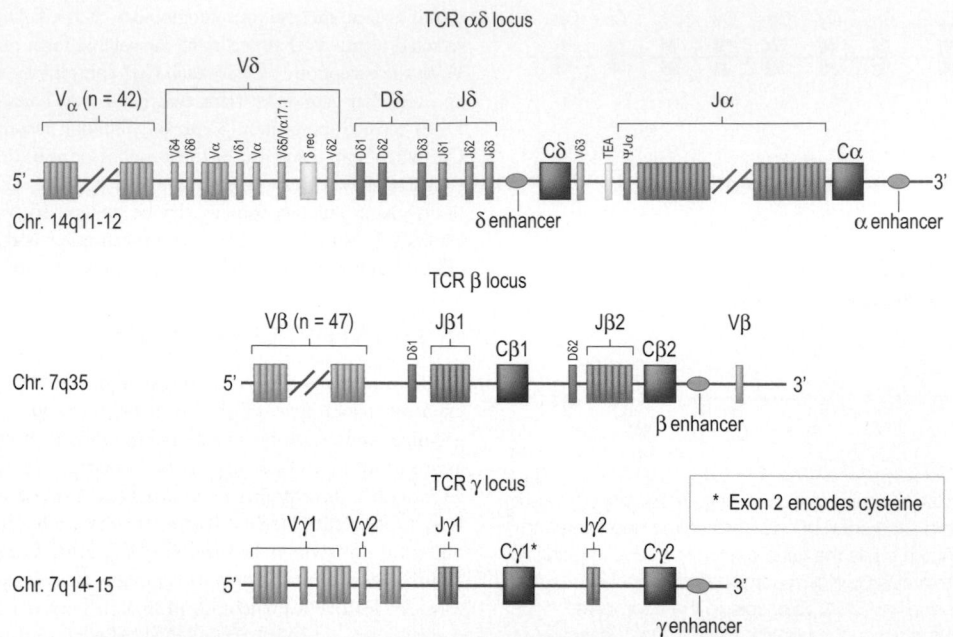

Fig. 4.9 Chromosomal organization of the T-cell receptor (TCR) αδ, β, and γ gene clusters. Typical numbers of functional gene segments are shown. These maps are not drawn to scale.

Particular patterns of amino acid composition in the sequences of the V domains create predictable canonical structures for several of the hypervariable regions. In κ chains, CDR2 is found in a single canonical structure, whereas four structures are possible for CDR1.[41] In the H chain, germline CDR1 and CDR2 elements encode one of three or one of five distinct canonical structures, respectively.[42] Preservation of these key amino acids during affinity maturation tends to maintain the canonical structure of CDR1 and CDR2 even while they are undergoing SHM.[43]

The enhanced sequence diversity of the CDR3 region is mirrored by its structural diversity. Few canonical structures have been defined for the H-chain CDR3, and even in κ chains 30% of the L chain CDR3 can be quite variable. However, at the sequence level there is a preference for tyrosine and glycine residues in the H-chain CDR3, which reflects both preferential use of only one of the six potential D_H reading frames as well as selection during development.[44]

THE TCR αδ-CHAIN LOCUS

The α and δ loci are located on chromosome 14q11-12. This region is unusual in that the gene segments encoding the two different TCR chains are actually intermixed (Fig. 4.9). There are 38–40 Vα, 5 Vα/Vδ, and 50 Jα functional gene segments, as well as one Cα gene in the locus.[45] Variation in numbers does occur between individuals. There are no Dα segments.

The δ locus lies between the Vα and Jα gene segments. There are three committed Vδ, five Vα/Vδ, three Dδ, and three Jδ gene segments, as well as one Cδ gene. Vδ3 lies 3' of Cδ, and thus must rearrange by inversion. Although V region use by α and δ chains is largely independent of one another, this unusual gene organization is accompanied by sharing of five V gene segments. For example, Vδ1 can rearrange to either Dδ/Jδ or to Jα elements, and thus can serve as the V region for both γδ and αβ TCRs.

In the large majority of αβ+ T cells analyzed, the α-chain on both chromosomes has rearranged. This occurs by the rearrangement of the 5' recombination signal sequence δRec to a pseudo-J segment, ΨJα, at the beginning of the Jα cluster (Fig. 4.9) as well as by the subsequent rearrangement of Vα to Jα on both chromosomes. Both types of rearrangement delete all of the Dδ, Jδ, and Cδ genes, preventing co-expression of αβ and γδ TCRs.

THE TCR β-CHAIN LOCUS

The β locus is positioned at chromosome 7q35.[45] It contains 40–48 functional Vβ genes, two Dβ, two Jβ clusters each containing six or seven gene segments, and two Cβ genes (Fig. 4.9). There is one Vβ immediately downstream of Cβ2, which rearranges by inversion. Each Cβ is preceded by its own Dβ–Jβ cluster. There is no apparent preference for Vβ gene rearrangement to either Dβ–Jβ cluster. Dβ1 can rearrange to the Jβ1 cluster or the Dβ2–Jβ2 cluster. Dβ2 can only rearrange to Jβ2 gene segments. The two Cβ segments differ by only six amino acids and are functionally indistinguishable from each other.

THE TCR γ-CHAIN LOCUS

The γ locus is located at chromosome 7p14-15.[45] There are four to six functional Vγ region segments intermixed with pseudogenes and two J clusters with a total of five J segments.[45] Each J cluster is 5' to its C region (Fig. 4.9). The Vγ segments have been divided into six families, although only Vγ1 (nine members, five of them functional) and Vγ2 (one member) encode functional proteins. The number of Cγ gene

KEY CONCEPTS

B-CELL RECEPTOR (BCR) AND CO-RECEPTORS

>> The BCR–antigen complex consists of a membrane-bound immunoglobulin (Ig) that is responsible for antigen recognition and an Ig-α/-β heterodimer that transduces the binding signal into the cell

>> BCR engagement leads to the phosphorylation of tyrosines in the Ig-α/-β immunoreceptor tyrosine-based activation motifs (ITAMs). This signal is then transmitted to one or more other intracellular signaling pathways

>> Recognition of antigen by B lymphocytes can also involve binding of antigen complexed with C3d and IgG to additional B-cell co-receptors

>> Binding of complexed antigen by individual co-receptors can lead to either positive or negative signals, each of which can influence the ultimate outcome of an antigen–B lymphocyte interaction

>> Deficiency of the components of the BCR–antigen complex impairs B-cell development and can produce agammaglobulinemia

exons varies: Cγ1 has three, while there are two alleles of Cγ2 that have four and five, respectively. The first Cγ exon encodes most of the extracellular portion of this region. The last Cγ exon encodes the intracytoplasmic portion of the molecule. The middle exon(s) (one for Cγ1, two or three for Cγ2) encode the connecting piece, which does (Cγ1), or does not (Cγ2), include a cysteine. Since this cysteine can form a disulfide bond with another cysteine in the δ-chain, TCRs using Cγ1 contain a covalently linked γ-δ pair, while TCRs using Cγ2 do not.

The nomenclature of the human γ locus differs between laboratories and reports, and is extensively cross-referenced on the IMGT website (http://imgt.cines.fr).

ALLELIC EXCLUSION

Because of the inherently imprecise nature of coding joints, only one in three V(D)J rearrangements will be in-frame and capable of creating a functional protein.[31, 46] Theoretically, one in nine cells might be expected to express two different Ig or TCR chains. However, almost all B cells express the functional products of only one IgH allele and one IgL allele, and mature αβ T cells express only one functional TCRβ gene. The process of limiting the number of receptors expressed by an individual cell is known as *allelic exclusion*.

Both stochastic and regulated models have been put forth to explain this process, but the precise mechanism remains unclear. The mechanism has been shown to be associated with the expression of an Ig or TCR product capable of transducing a signal. In pre-B cells, a functional μ H-chain associates with the surrogate light chain to form the pre-BCR. Similarly, in developing T-cell progenitors a productive TCR β-chain associates with pre-Tα to form the pre-TCR. These preliminary antigen receptors signal to shut down RAG expression, promote cell division, and limit the accessibility of the IgH and TCRβ loci to further

rearrangement while promoting the accessibility of the IgL and TCRα loci, respectively.

In pre-B cells, the κ locus is the first to rearrange, with λ rearrangement occurring in cells that have failed to produce a proper κ chain. Surface expression of an acceptable membrane-bound IgM BCR invokes the mechanism of allelic exclusion among the L-chain loci and promotes further maturation of the B cell.

Productive TCRα rearrangement in CD4⁺CD8⁺ T-cell progenitors allows the expression of a functional TCR αβ heterodimer. Unlike IgH and TCRβ, TCRα does not undergo allelic exclusion at the level of gene rearrangement. Instead, in cells that express two functional TCRα alleles, one of the two alleles tends to pair preferentially with the one functional TCRβ chain. This results in phenotypic allelic exclusion.

Allelic exclusion can be overcome by selection pressures. Cells that express self-reactive antigen receptors can downregulate IgH or TCR expression and reactivate gene rearrangement to replace one of the two offending chains. This process, termed *receptor editing*,[47] occurs most often in the IgL or TCRα loci, whose gene structures lend themselves to repeated rearrangement. Less commonly, the V_H in the H chain can be replaced by means of rearrangement to a cryptic RSS located at the terminus of the V_H gene segment.

■ B-CELL RECEPTOR COMPLEX: STRUCTURE AND FUNCTION ■

Although the ability of surface immunoglobulin to recognize antigen was appreciated very early, the mechanism by which membrane-bound immunoglobulin (mIg) transmitted an antigen recognition event to the cell took longer to understand. Specifically, as the predominant isotypes expressed on the surface of mature B cells, mIgM and mIgD, contain only three amino acid residues exposed to the cytoplasm, it was thought unlikely that these Ig heavy chains could function as signal transduction molecules by themselves. This presumption was eventually proved correct when it was shown that all membrane immunoglobulin isotypes associated noncovalently with a heterodimeric complex consisting of two transmembrane proteins, Ig-α and Ig-β, each of which is capable of transducing signals into the cell (Table 4.3).

MEMBRANE-BOUND IMMUNOGLOBULIN

Immunoglobulins mediate their effector functions as secreted products of plasma cells. However, as membrane-bound structures on mature B cells, immunoglobulins serve as the antigen recognition component of the BCR complex. Although all immunoglobulin classes can be expressed at the cell surface, the vast majority of circulating mature B cells coexpress membrane-bound IgM and IgD. Appropriate activation of a naïve IgM- and IgD-expressing B cell leads to plasma cell differentiation and antibody secretion. The membrane-bound forms of IgM and IgD are the product of alternative splicing of the immunoglobulin transcript at the 3′, or carboxy-terminus, of the heavy chain (Fig. 4.10). The two membrane exons encode transmembrane hydrophobic stretch of amino acids and an evolutionary conserved cytoplasmic tail encoding lysine, valine, and lysine.

Table 4.3 The B-cell receptor (BCR) and its co-receptor molecules

Molecule	M_r	Chromosome	Function
BCR			
mIgM ($\mu_2 L_2$)	180 000	14 (IgH; 14q.32)	Antigen recognition
		2 (Igκ; 2p12)	
		22 (Igλ; 22q11.2)	
Ig-α	47 000	19 (19q13.2)	Signal transducer
Ig-β	37 000	17 (17q23)	Signal transducer
Co-receptors			
CD21	140 000	1 (1q32)	Activating co-receptor
			Ligand for C3d, EBV, CD23
CD19	95 000	16 (16p11.2)	Activating co-receptor
			Signal transducer
FcγRIIB	40 000	1 (1q23-24)	Inhibitory co-receptor
			Low-affinity receptor for immunoglobulin G
CD22	140 000	19 (19q13.1)	Inhibitory co-receptor
			Adhesion molecule
			Signal transducer

mIgM, membrane-bound immunoglobulin M.

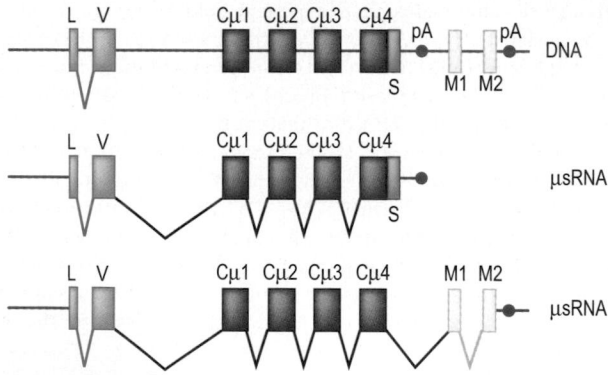

Fig. 4.10 Membrane and secretory immunoglobulin (Ig)M are created by alternative splicing. Alternative splicing of the Cm carboxy-terminal exons results in mRNA transcripts encoding either secreted IgM (μ_s RNA) or membrane-bound IgM (μ_m RNA).

SIGNAL TRANSDUCTION AND THE IG-α/β (CD79A/CD79B) HETERODIMER

The heterodimeric signal transduction component of the BCR complex that associates with mIg has been designated CD79. It is composed of Ig-α (CD79a) and Ig-β (CD79b). CD79 is responsible for transporting mIg to the cell surface and for transducing BCR signals into the cell.[48, 49]

CD79a/Ig-α is encoded by *CD79a/MB-1* (chromosome 19q13.2) as a 226-amino-acid glycoprotein of approximately 47 kDa. The exact molecular weight depends on the extent of glycosylation. *CD79b/B29*

(chromosome 17q23) encodes CD79b/Ig-β, which is a 229-amino-acid glycoprotein of approximately 37 kDa. *CD79a* and *CD79b* share an exon-intron structure, which is similar to that of the genes that encode the CD3 TCR co-receptor molecules. These similarities suggest that both BCR and TCR co-receptors are the progeny of a common ancestral gene. Ig-α and Ig-β both contain a single IgSF Ig domain (111-residue C-type for Ig-α and 129-residue V-type for Ig-β). Each also contains a highly conserved transmembrane domain and a 61 (Ig-α) or 48 (Ig-β) amino acid cytoplasmic tail that also exhibits striking amino acid evolutionary conservation.

Ig-α and Ig-β are expressed by the earliest committed B-cell progenitors and before expression of Igμ heavy chain. The CD79 heterodimer has also been observed on the surface of early B-cell progenitors in the absence of μ heavy chain, although neither protein is required for progenitors to commit to the B-cell lineage.[50] Later in development, Ig-α and Ig-β are coexpressed together with Ig of all isotypes on the surface of B cells as a mature BCR complex.[48] The CD79 proteins are specific to the B lineage and are expressed throughout B lymphopoiesis. This has led to their use as markers for the identification of B-cell neoplasms.[51, 52]

The signaling capacity of both Ig-α and Ig-β resides within an immunoreceptor tyrosine-based activation motif (ITAM) that has the consensus sequence of D/IxxYxxL(x)$_7$YxxL, where x is any amino acid. Similar ITAMs are also found within the cytoplasmic domain of the molecules that associate with, and signal for, the T-cell antigen receptor (CD3) and certain Fc receptors. The phosphorylation of both tyrosines in both Ig-α/β ITAMs is considered an obligate initial step in the propagation of an antigen receptor engagement event to the cell nucleus.[49, 53] Tyrosine-phosphorylated ITAMs serve as efficient binding sites for Src homology 2 (SH-2) domains, which are present within a large number of cytosolic signaling molecules. Whether Ig-α and Ig-β make qualitatively different

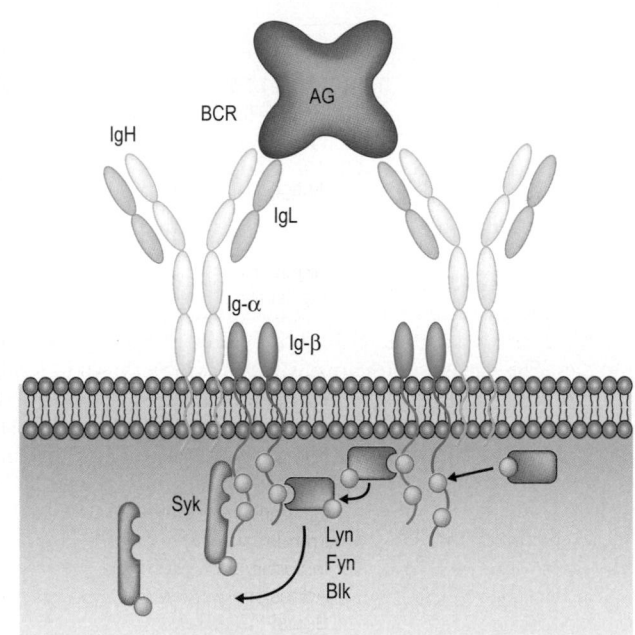

Fig. 4.11 The B-cell receptor (BCR) core complex. The BCR core complex can be divided into an antigen recognition unit fulfilled by membrane immunoglobulin M (mIgM) and a noncovalently associated signal transduction unit composed of the Ig-α/β (CD79) heterodimer. Antigen engagement of mIgM oligomerizes the BCR, allowing preassociated Src-family protein tyrosine kinases to phosphorylate neighboring Ig-α/β ITAM tyrosines. This promotes association of the SYK tyrosine kinase with the tyrosine phosphorylated immunoreceptor tyrosine-based activation motif (ITAMs), allowing SYK to become a substrate for other Syk or Src-family tyrosine kinases and leading to its activation.

contributions towards BCR signaling or are functionally redundant remains unclear, as evidence exists to support both views. Moreover, the high degree of evolutionary conservation within the non-ITAM portion of the cytoplasmic domains suggests additional, as yet uncharacterized, signaling roles for the cytoplasmic tails of these molecules over and above positive signaling via the ITAMs.

Ig-α and Ig-β are covalently associated by a disulfide bridge via cysteine residues that exist within the IgSF extracellular domains of both molecules. The association of the Ig-α/β heterodimer with mIg occurs though interaction within the transmembrane domains of these proteins.[48] The core BCR complex consists of a single Ig molecule associated with a single Ig-α/β heterodimer (H_2L_2/Ig-α/Ig-β)[54] (Fig. 4.11).

A current model for the initiation of signals originating from the BCR (Fig. 4.11) proposes that antigens induce the clustering of BCR complexes, increasing their local density. The increase in density leads to the transfer of phosphate groups to the tyrosine residues of the Ig-α/β ITAM motifs.[49, 53] Src-family tyrosine kinases, of which LYN, FYN, and BLK are most often implicated, are believed to be responsible for ITAM phosphorylation upon aggregation of Ig-α/β. They have been shown to associate physically with the heterodimer. It has been suggested that a fraction of Src-family tyrosine kinases is associated with the Ig-α/β heterodimer and, upon aggregation, transphosphorylate juxtaposed heterodimers. However, the exact mechanism by which Ig-α/β undergoes initial tyrosine phosphorylation after antigen engagement remains uncertain. Regardless of mechanism, phosphorylated ITAMs subsequently serve as high-affinity docking sites for cytosolic effector molecules that harbor SH2 domains. The recruitment of the SYK tyrosine kinase, via its tandem SH2 domains, to doubly phosphorylated Ig-α/β ITAMs is thought to be a next step in propagating a BCR-mediated signal. Association of SYK with the BCR leads to its subsequent tyrosine phosphorylation by either Src-family or other Syk tyrosine kinases, further increasing kinase activity. Together, the concerted actions of the Syk and Src-family protein tyrosine kinases activate a variety of intracellular signaling pathways that can lead to the proliferation, differentiation, or death of the cell.[55]

CLINICAL CONSEQUENCES OF DISRUPTIONS IN BCR SIGNALING

Both the development of B lymphocytes and the maintenance of the mature antigen-responsive B-cell pool demand the presence of an intact BCR and its downstream signaling pathway(s). Disruption of these pathways can present clinically with hypogammaglobulinemia and an absence of B cells.

The most common such genetic lesion is BTK deficiency, which is an X-linked trait (Chapter 34).[56] BTK plays an important role in BCR signaling both during development and in response to antigen. Loss of function mutations in *BTK* results in the arrest of human B-cell development at the pre-B-cell stage.

BTK is intact in approximately 10–15% of patients with hypogammaglobulinemia and an absence of B cells. Mouse models where BCR components or signaling pathways have been disrupted by targeted mutagenesis have provided insight into the basis of these atypical hypogammaglobulinemia disorders.[49] These studies have shown that an inability to express either a functional μ IgH chain, Ig-α, Ig-β, or the signaling adaptor molecule, BLNK, lead to an early, severe arrest in B lymphopoiesis, with subsequent agammaglobulinemia. Together, these experimental findings highlighted the central role of the BCR in the generation and function of B lymphocytes. They suggested that mutations in any component of the antigen receptor complex or immediate downstream effectors would have the potential to disrupt B-cell development and thus create an agammaglobulinemic state. These speculations were borne out when hypogammaglobulinemic individuals demonstrating an absence of B cells in the presence of normal BTK function were subsequently identified with mutations in either Igμ heavy chain, Ig-α, or BLNK.[56]

Besides its important role in the maturation, differentiation, and survival of B lymphocytes, the B-cell antigen receptor is responsible for initiating the humoral response to foreign antigen. Some of the variables that can influence the ultimate outcome of BCR–antigen interaction include the nature of the foreign antigen, the mode of activation, the developmental stage of the B cell, and the microenvironment in which antigen encounter occurs. Exactly how these variables ultimately result in the differential activation of diverse intracellular signaling pathways with fundamentally divergent outcomes is only beginning to be understood, and is an area of active investigation. Emerging from these studies is an appreciation of the role of BCR co-receptors, which have been shown to be capable of modulating antigen receptor signaling in response to antigen.

BCR CO-RECEPTORS

The initiation of a humoral immune response results from antigen interaction with the antigen receptors on mature peripheral lymphocytes. However, the manner in which mature B and T lymphocytes recognize antigen is fundamentally different (Chapter 6). Surface Ig, as a component of the BCR on B lymphocytes, recognizes antigen in its native three-dimensional configuration that, upon engagement with mIg, is capable of transmitting a signal to the cell interior. In contrast, the antigen receptor expressed by T lymphocytes recognizes an antigen-derived peptide associated with an appropriate MHC structure. Moreover, for a productive outcome of this T-cell recognition event, a CD4 or CD8 co-receptor must also bind to the MHC structure presenting the foreign antigen (Chapter 7). Similarly, antigen recognition by the BCR on B lymphocytes is also influenced by co-receptors present on mature B cells (Table 4.3). In this case the co-receptors may also recognize antigen, but only in a form that has been modified by other components of the immune system, as described below. In general, these co-receptors and co-receptor complexes can be divided into those that regulate BCR signaling in a positive manner and those that regulate in a negative manner. Thus, the ultimate outcome of signaling via the BCR depends not only on the signals transduced via the Ig-α/β heterodimer, but also how these signals are perceived by the cell in association with the signals propagated by the various co-receptors that are concomitantly engaged.

CO-RECEPTORS THAT POSITIVELY REGULATE BCR SIGNALING

CD21

Mature B lymphocytes express two receptors for complement C3 components, CD35 (CR1) and CD21 (CR2) (Chapter 20). Of these, CD21 fulfills the requirements of a BCR co-receptor, as described below. The expression of CD21 is restricted to mature B cells and follicular dendritic cells, whereas CD35 is also found on erythrocytes, monocytes, and granulocytes. CD21 is a 140-kDa surface glycoprotein encoded by the *CR2* locus on chromosome 1q32 (Table 4.3). Expression of CD21 begins at approximately the same time as IgD during B lymphopoiesis (Chapter 8). CD21 is subsequently expressed on all mature B cells until terminal differentiation. Within the mature population, marginal-zone B cells express higher levels relative to follicular B cells. The extracellular domain of CD21 is composed of 15–16 short consensus regions (SCRs), each composed of 60–70 amino acids, and a relatively short 34-amino-acid cytoplasmic tail. The two-amino-terminal SCRs constitute the region that interacts with one of the third complement component (C3) cleavage products, iC3b, C3d, g, and C3d (Chapter 20).[57]

CD21 is a known receptor for Epstein–Barr virus, which similarly binds the two N-terminal SCRs via its major envelope glycoprotein gp350/220. CD21, through its oligosaccharide chains, also binds CD23, the low-affinity IgE receptor (FcεRII). Whereas Epstein–Barr virus utilization of CD21 for cell entry has clear physiological consequences in terms of infection, B-cell immortalization, and the potential for oncogenesis, the *in vivo* relevance of a CD21–CD23 interaction remains unclear.[57]

CD19

CD19 is an IgSF surface glycoprotein of 95 kDa that is expressed from the earliest stages of B-cell development until plasma cell terminal differentiation, when its expression is lost.[58] Follicular dendritic cells also express CD19. *CD19* maps to chromosome 16p11.2, where it encodes for a 540-amino-acid protein with two extracellular C-type IgSF domains as well as a large, approximately 240-residue, cytoplasmic tail that exhibits extensive conservation between mouse and human. This relatively large cytoplasmic domain includes nine conserved tyrosine residues that, upon phosphorylation, serve as docking sites for other SH2-containing effector molecules. The signaling capacity of CD19 has been shown to result from tyrosine phosphorylation, which occurs upon engagement of the BCR, CD19 or, optimally, by co-ligation of CD19 and IgM. Known signaling effector molecules that have been identified in association with tyrosine-phosphorylated CD19 include the LYN and FYN protein tyrosine kinases, the Rho-family guanine nucleotide exchange factor, VAV, and phosphatidyl inositol 3-kinase.[58] Although specific ligands for CD19 have been proposed, the physiological relevance of CD19 engagement by putative ligands has not been demonstrated.

In vitro studies using monoclonal antibodies directed against CD21 or CD19 provided initial evidence that these B-cell surface antigens could influence mIg-mediated signaling.[57, 58] Formal demonstration that these molecules played a physiological role in regulating B-cell responses was first provided by targeted mutagenesis in mouse models. CD21- and CD19-deficient mice demonstrate impaired antibody response to T-dependent antigens.[57–59] The paucity of CD5⁺B cells in CD19-deficient mice also suggested a role for this molecule in the generation and maintenance of the B1 lineage of B cells (Chapter 8). CD19 is expressed from the earliest stages of B-cell ontogeny in both mice and humans and, accordingly, a signaling function for CD19 in B lymphopoiesis has been demonstrated.[60] CD19 deficiency has been shown to be a cause of common variable immune deficiency (Chapter 34).

CD21–CD19 co-receptor complex

A mechanism by which these molecules could augment BCR-mediated signaling was provided by the identification of a CD21/CD19 co-receptor complex on mature B cells that also includes CD81 (Fig. 4.12). CD81, also known as TAPA-1, is a 26-kDa tetraspan molecule that is widely expressed on a number of cell types, including lymphocytes. The CD21/CD19 co-receptor model predicted that, as a result of complement activation, C3d would be deposited on an antigen, thereby providing a bridge by which a CD21–CD19 receptor complex could associate with mIgM and the BCR complex.[57–59] Clustering of CD19 close to the BCR by the C3d–antigen complex would effectively recruit the signal transduction effector molecules associated with CD19 to the Ig-α/β heterodimer. As a consequence, the CD19-associated LYN and FYN tyrosine kinases, VAV, and PI3-kinase signaling effector molecules would be in a position to exert their activities on the Ig-α/β heterodimer-mediated signaling events initiated by antigen engagement of mIgM.

Strong support for CD21/CD19 co-receptor physiological function in BCR signaling was subsequently provided by experiments using a murine model of immune response. In these experiments, the immunization of mice with an antigen covalently attached to C3d dramatically

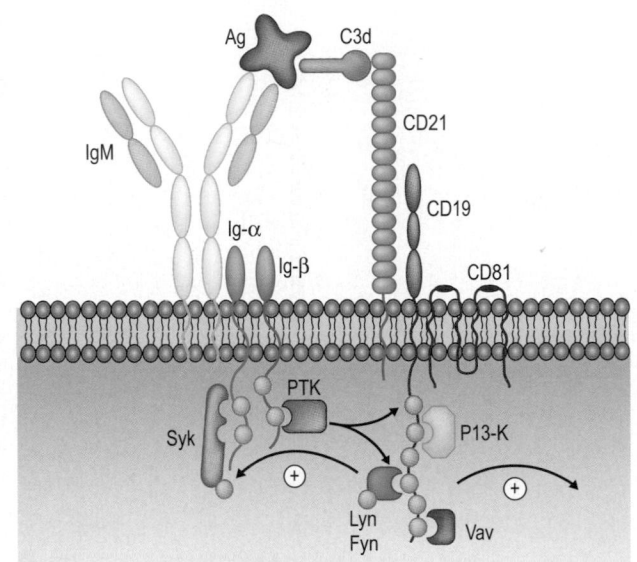

Fig. 4.12 Proposed mechanisms for the augmentation of B-cell receptor (BCR) signaling by the CD21/19 co-receptor. Co-ligation of the BCR and CD21–CD19 complex by C3d–antigen complex allows a CD79-associated Src-family tyrosine kinase to phosphorylate tyrosine residues within the CD19 cytoplasmic domain. Subsequently, tyrosine-phosphorylated CD19 effectively recruits key SH2-containing signaling molecules to the BCR complex, allowing the initial BCR-mediated signal to disseminate quickly along different intracellular signaling pathways.

reduced the signaling threshold necessary for antigen to elicit an immune response.[61] Antigen bearing either two or three copies of C3d was respectively 1000 and 10 000 times more immunogenic than antigen alone. Thus, the CD21–CD19 co-receptor complex provides a link between the innate and adaptive immune responses. *In vivo*, CD19-deficient mice appear to have more severely affected T-dependent immune responses than do CD21-deficient animals, suggesting alternative roles for CD19 in regulating BCR signals beyond the CD21/CD19 co-receptor complex.

CO-RECEPTORS THAT NEGATIVELY REGULATE BCR SIGNALING

FcγRIIB

Among the several receptors for the Fc portion of immunoglobulin expressed by B cells, the Fc receptor for IgG, FcγRIIB (a member of the CD32 cluster), has an important role in negatively regulating BCR-mediated signal transduction.[62] FcγRIIB is a 40-kDa single-chain molecule that is encoded by a single gene located on chromosome 1q23-24. Alternative splicing of different cytoplasmic exons permits expression of three isoforms. The extracellular domain of FcγRIIB is composed of two C-type IgSF domains that can bind with low affinity to IgG. All three FcγRIIB isoforms share a common cytoplasmic region that is important for negatively regulating activation signals delivered by associated surface receptors. The region within the cytoplasmic domain of FCγRIIB

responsible for the inhibitory activity of this Fc receptor towards the BCR has been identified as a sequence that contains a tyrosine residue critical for its activity.[62] In analogy to the ITAM, which provides an activation signal, this inhibitory sequence has been referred to as an immunoreceptor tyrosine-based inhibitory motif, or ITIM. The ITIM is carried by the canonical sequence of I/L/VxYxxI/V/L (where x is any amino acid).[63] ITIMs are found in a number of other transmembrane structures, all of which share the ability to regulate signaling negatively by activating receptors.

The ability of passively administered soluble antibody to inhibit humoral responses has long been appreciated and was initially thought to occur by soluble antibody, effectively masking all available antigen epitopes. The molecular mechanism accounting for this suppression is now known to be mediated by the binding of IgG to FcRγIIB and the subsequent recruitment of cytosolic phosphatases to the FcRγIIB ITIM upon tyrosine phosphorylation. Thus, the inhibitory effect of IgG on BCR-mediated B-cell activation is explained by the interaction of the FcγRIIB ITIM, and specifically associated phosphatases, with the BCR (Fig. 4.13). Co-ligation of the BCR and FcγRIIB by antigen–IgG complexes results in the tyrosine phosphorylation of the FcγRIIB ITIM, presumably by the BCR-associated tyrosine kinases. Phosphorylated FcRγIIB ITIMs then recruit two different SH2-containing phosphatases, SHIP and SHP-1, which function to remove phosphate groups from inositols or tyrosines, respectively. Although both phosphatases can negatively regulate BCR-mediated signaling events, SHIP appears to be the most relevant phosphatase in FcRγIIB inhibition of BCR signaling[64] (Fig. 4.13). Thus, once the majority of antigen exists in immune complexes together with antigen-specific IgG, attenuation of an ongoing immune response occurs by the juxtaposition of FcRγIIB with the BCR.

CD22

CD22 is a 135–140-kDa transmembrane glycoprotein that is restricted in its expression to the B lineage.[65] CD22 expression is limited to the cytoplasm of progenitor and pre-B cells in early B-cell development. Expression on the surface of the B cell occurs concomitant with the appearance of surface, or membrane, IgD. Upon B-cell activation, CD22 expression is initially transiently upregulated and subsequently down-modulated upon terminal differentiation to Ig-secreting plasma cells. Although the onset of CD22 expression follows a similar pattern during murine B lymphopoiesis, it is not restricted to the cytoplasm in early B lymphopoiesis but rather is expressed on the surface from the progenitor stage onward. The basis or function of CD22 intracellular retention in human B-cell development is not understood.

CD22 maps to chromosome 19q13.1 and encodes for alternatively spliced forms of CD22, CD22α and CD22β, of which the latter is the predominant species expressed by B cells. The CD22β isoform contains seven extracellular IgSF domains, of which all but one are of the C type. The single exception is the N-terminal domain, which is of the V type. CD22α lacks the IgSF third and fourth domains, although the significance of this minority alternatively spliced product remains unclear. The CD22 murine homolog has only been found as a full-length CD22β isoform. The extracellular domain of CD22 is homologous to the carcinoembryonic antigen subfamily of adhesion molecules, which includes the myelin-associated glycoprotein and CD33. CD22 also functions as an adhesion molecule belonging to the Siglec subfamily of the Ig superfamily, whose members function as mammalian sialic acid-binding Ig-like lectins.[65] The two amino-terminal IgSF domains have been shown

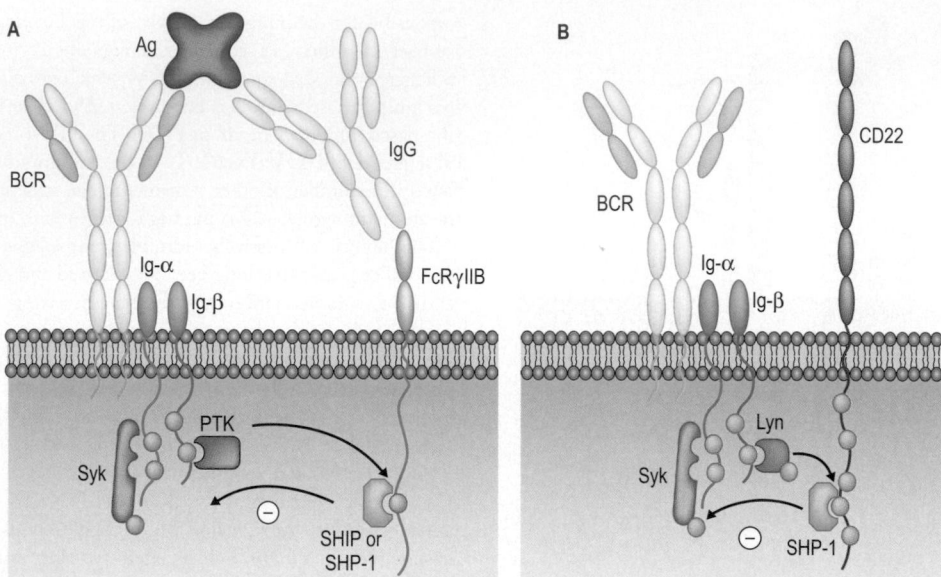

Fig. 4.13 Negative regulation of B-cell receptor (BCR) signaling by FcγRIIB and CD22. (A) Soluble immunoglobulin (Ig)G–antigen immune complexes juxtapose the BCR with FcγRIIB. The BCR-associated Lyn tyrosine kinase subsequently tyrosine phosphorylates the FcγRIIB ITIM. In turn, this leads to the recruitment of the SH2-containing inositol phosphatase SHIP and tyrosine phosphatase SHP-1 to the phosphorylated FcRγIIB ITIM. Both of these phosphatases have demonstrable inhibitory activity on BCR-mediated signaling. Although SHIP is believed to be the major effector in the FcRγIIB-mediated inhibition of BCR signaling,[64] the exact mechanism of its action in this context has not yet been fully elucidated. (B) CD22 associated with the BCR is tyrosine-phosphorylated upon antigen-BCR engagement. SH2-containing signaling molecules dock on tyrosine phosphorylated residues, including the SHP-1 tyrosine phosphatase that can subsequently dephosphorylate signaling molecules previously activated by a membrane immunoglobulin M (mIgM)-mediated signal.

KEY CONCEPTS

T-CELL RECEPTOR (TCR)–CD3 COMPLEX

>> Cell surface expression of the TCR heterodimers requires association with a complex of invariant proteins designated CD3

>> Each TCR–CD3 complex contains a single TCR heterodimer and three CD3 dimers

>> Assembly of the TCR–CD3 complex involves interactions between TCR transmembrane basic residues and transmembrane acidic residues in each of the CD3 subunits

>> Signal transduction by the TCR involves the phosphorylation of immunoreceptor tyrosine-based activation motifs (ITAMs) in the cytoplasmic domains of CD3 proteins:

>> Phosphorylated CD3 ITAMs recruit and activate the ZAP-70 protein tyrosine kinase

>> Deficiency of CD3 proteins impairs T-cell development and can produce severe combined immunodeficiency (SCID)

to mediate adhesion to both B and T lymphocytes via the binding of structures carrying α2,6 sialic acids.

In addition to acting as an adhesion molecule, CD22 is also capable of modulating BCR signaling (Fig. 4.13). A fraction of CD22 associates with the BCR, and CD22 is rapidly tyrosine-phosphorylated upon mIgM engagement. Tyrosine-phosphorylated CD22 associates with several SH2-containing signaling molecules, including the LYN and SYK tyrosine kinases, PI3-kinase, phospholipase C-γ, and SHP-1. The 140-amino-acid cytoplasmic domain of CD22 includes six conserved tyrosine residues. Three of these tyrosines are located within conserved consensus ITIM sequences and possess a demonstrable capacity to bind the SH2 domain of the SHP-1 phosphatase. The presence of the multiple ITIMs and association with SHP-1 indicated that CD22 might impinge on BCR signaling in a negative manner. Physiological evidence that CD22 could act as a co-receptor to regulate mIgM signaling negatively was provided by the generation of CD22-deficient mice by targeted mutagenesis.[65] CD22-deficient B cells exhibited hyperactive B-cell responses upon BCR triggering, and an increased incidence of serum autoantibodies. This suggests that B-cell tolerance is altered and B cells are more readily activated in the absence of this negative regulator of BCR signaling.

THE TCR–CD3 COMPLEX

The αβ and γδ TCR heterodimers, which are responsible for the recognition of specific antigen by T lymphocytes, associate with a complex of invariant proteins designated CD3. This association is necessary for

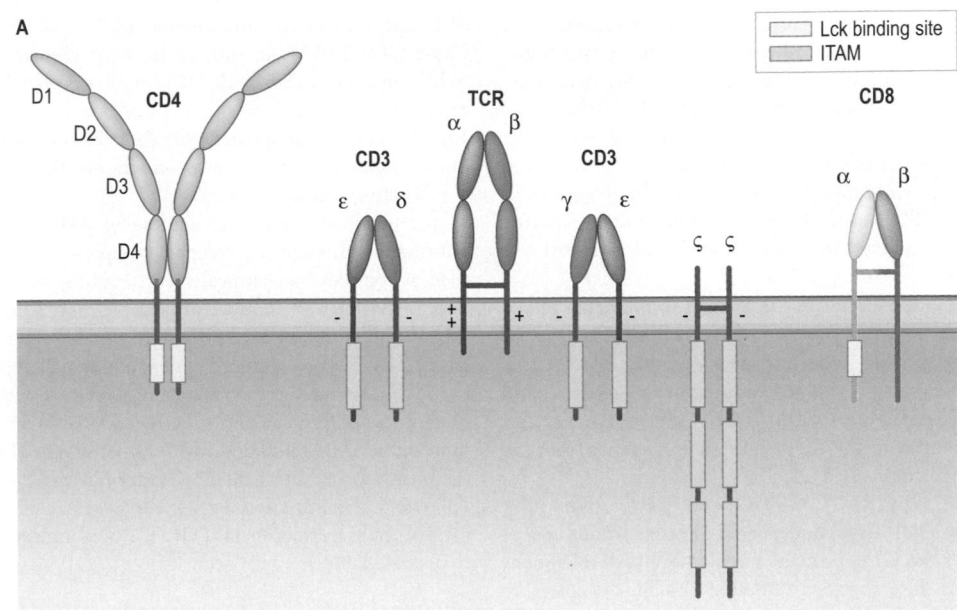

Fig. 4.14 Schematic representation of the human T-cell receptor (TCR) and CD4 and CD8 co-receptors. Immunoglobulin superfamily (IgSF) domains are represented by ovals. The four extracellular domains of CD4 are labeled D1–D4. Basic (+) and acidic (–) transmembrane charged residues are indicated, as are known and predicted sites of disulfide bonds.

TCR cell surface expression and enables the TCR heterodimers, which have only short cytoplasmic domains, to couple to the intracellular signaling events that lead to the activation of T-cell effector function. There are four CD3 proteins: γ, δ, ε, and ζ (Fig. 4.14).[66]

CD3 PROTEINS

CD3γ, CD3δ, and CD3ε are structurally similar, and the genes encoding them map to a locus in chromosome 11q23. The polypeptides range in size from 20 to 25 kDa. Each has an extracellular C-type IgSF domain, a transmembrane region that contains an acidic residue (aspartic acid in CD3δ and CD3ε, glutamic acid in CD3γ), and a cytoplasmic domain with a single ITAM. These CD3 chains are present in the TCR–CD3 complex in the form of noncovalently linked CD3εγ and CD3εδ heterodimers.[22, 66, 67]

The 16kDa CD3ζ differs substantially from the other CD3 proteins and is structurally homologous to the γ chain of the high-affinity IgE receptor (FcRγ chain). The extracellular domain of CD3ζ is very short (only nine amino acids) and is of unknown structure. Its large cytoplasmic domain has three ITAMs in tandem. As is the case with the other CD3 chains, the transmembrane region of CD3ζ contains an acidic residue (aspartic acid). CD3ζ is usually present in the TCR–CD3 complex in the form of disulfide-linked CD3ζζ homodimers.[22, 66, 67]

STOICHIOMETRY OF THE TCR–CD3 COMPLEX

The valency and stoichiometry of the TCR–CD3 complex have been the subject of considerable interest and of some past controversy. Recent data indicate that the αβTCR–CD3 complex consists of a single αβ TCR heterodimer and three CD3 dimers: CD3εγ, CD3εδ, and CD3ζζ (Fig. 4.14). The γδTCR–CD3 complex, in contrast, lacks CD3δ. On naïve T cells, this receptor complex contains two CD3εγ heterodimers and one CD3ζζ homodimer. Following activation of γδT cells, the TCR–CD3 complex incorporates the FcRγ chain, either as a homodimer or as heterodimer with CD3ζ.[22, 67]

As noted above, each of the CD3 subunits has a transmembrane acidic residue while the transmembrane domains of the αβ and γδ TCRs contain basic residues. For example, the TCR α-chain has an arginine and a lysine within its transmembrane domain while the transmembrane region of the TCR β-chain contains a lysine. Because the receptor complex consists of one TCR heterodimer and three CD3 dimers, there is an apparent 'charge imbalance' with six acidic residues but only three basic residues.[67]

ASSEMBLY AND CELL SURFACE EXPRESSION OF THE TCR–CD3 COMPLEX

Assembly begins with formation of the individual TCRαβ, CD3εδ, and CD3εγ heterodimers, processes that are driven by interactions between the extracellular domains of the pairing polypeptides. The subsequent higher-order assembly of the TCRαβ with the CD3 dimers depends upon interactions between the potentially charged residues within their transmembrane regions. Mutation of any of these transmembrane acidic or basic residues to neutral alanine impairs formation of the TCR–CD3 complex. TCRαβ appears to associate first with CD3εδ and then with CD3εγ. TCRα binds CD3εδ, and TCRβ likely interacts with CD3εγ. The incorporation of a CD3ζζ homodimer into the complex requires the prior formation of a TCRαβ-CD3γε-CD3δε hexamer.

The structure of transmembrane region of TCRα is not known. If, as seems likely, this region has an α-helical structure, then the two transmembrane basic residues would lie on opposite faces of the helix, possibly allowing TCRα to interact with CD3ζζ as well as CD3εδ.

Formation of the TCR–CD3 complex is tightly regulated. For example, when there are deficiencies of CD3γ, CD3δ, or CD3ε, TCRα and β are retained in the endoplasmic reticulum and are rapidly degraded. In the absence of CD3ζ, the TCRαβ–CD3εγ–CD3εδ hexamer is exported to the Golgi but is then targeted to a lysosomal degradation pathway rather than the cell surface.[22, 66, 67]

Because the structures of most of the individual components of the TCR–CD3 complex are known, a model of the overall structure of the receptor has been proposed. This model envisions a compact TCR–CD3, with trimeric contacts occurring within the transmembrane regions of all components (i.e., TCRα–CD3ε–CD3δ, TCRβ–CD3ε–CD3γ, and TCRα–CD3ζ–CD3ζ) and with the TCRαβ extending further from the membrane than the CD3 chains.[22, 68]

Mutations in the *CD3D*, *CD3E*, *CD3G*, and *CD3Z* have been described in human. The clinical consequences of these mutations underscore the importance of the CD3 proteins for the normal development and function of T cells. Homozygous mutations leading to complete deficiencies of either CD3δ or CD3ε protein produce a form of SCID (Chapter 35) characterized by the complete absence of T cells but the presence of phenotypically normal B cells and natural killer (NK) cells- ($T^-B^+NK^+$SCID).[69–71]

The absence of CD3ε leads to a complete block early in T-cell development, which, in CD3ε-knockout mice, occurs at the CD4$^-$CD8$^-$ "double-negative" stage (Chapter 9).

Homozygous deficiency of CD3δ produces a block at a slightly later stage in T-cell development, at the entry of thymocytes into the CD4$^+$CD8$^+$ "double-positive" stage.

Interestingly, deficiency of CD3γ produces a milder phenotype than does the absence of either CD3δ or CD3ε. Homozygous deficiency in CD3γ has been observed in two brothers but, surprisingly, manifested clinically as severe immunodeficiency and autoimmunity in only one of these.[71] The second brother survived to adulthood with only mild autoimmunity. The absence of CD3γ protein impaired, but did not abrogate, T-cell development. In peripheral blood, there were differential effects on phenotypically defined T-cell subsets, with very few CD8$^+$T cells, a 10-fold reduction in CD4$^+$CD45RA$^+$T cells ("naïve helper" subset), and normal numbers of CD4$^+$CD45RO$^+$T cells ("memory" cells). Cell surface expression of the TCR–CD3 complex on peripheral T cells was reduced by 75–80%.[71]

There have been no reports of individuals homozygous for null mutations of *CD3Z*. However, a point mutation leading to a premature stop codon within the first ITAM of CD3ζ has been identified. An individual homozygous for this *CD3Z* mutation presented with severe immunodeficiency at age 4 months. Peripheral blood CD4 and CD8 T cells were reduced in number, expressed low levels of cell surface TCR–CD3 complex, and were hyporesponsive to TCR stimulation *ex vivo*.[72]

EARLY EVENTS IN TCR–CD3 SIGNALING

Stimulation of the TCR–CD3 complex by pMHC, or by nonphysiological agonists such as anti-CD3 monoclonal antibodies, leads to the phosphorylation of tyrosine residues of the CD3 ITAMs by the SRC-like protein tyrosine kinases, LCK and FYN.[73] The phosphorylated CD3 ITAMs in turn create high-affinity binding sites for the SH2 domains of the ZAP-70 protein tyrosine kinase, leading to its recruitment to the TCR–CD3 complex and to its activation (Chapter 13).[73, 74] The consequences of ZAP-70 deficiency (selective T-cell immunodeficiency in humans) underscore the centrality of its role in T-cell activation (Chapter 35).

It is not known how the binding of pMHC to the TCR transfers information through the receptor complex, thereby triggering the cascade of complex biochemical events leading to the activation of T-cell effector function. A number of possible models have been proposed to explain the initiation of TCR–CD3 signaling by pMHC. In one set of scenarios, a pMHC-induced conformational change in the TCR causes the TCR heterodimer to change its orientation with respect to the CD3 dimers. In another, the entire TCR–CD3 complex acts as a rigid structure, and pMHC binding leads to displacement of the CD3 chains into the membrane or alters their orientation with respect to the membrane. Following the initiation of signaling, sustained signaling appears to involve multimerization of TCR–CD3 complexes and engagement of co-receptors.[66]

■ T-CELL CO-RECEPTORS: CD4 AND CD8 ■

Expression of CD4 and CD8 divides mature T cells into two distinct subsets: CD4 T cells (Chapter 17), which recognize peptides in the context of class II MHC molecules, and CD8 T cells (Chapter 18), which recognize antigens presented by class I MHC molecules. Indeed, CD4 binds directly to class II MHC molecules, and CD8 interacts directly with class I MHC molecules (Fig. 4.15); in both cases binding involves nonpolymorphic regions at the base of the MHC molecule (Chapter 5). During antigen recognition, CD4 and CD8 are thought to bind the same pMHC complex as the TCR and thus are true co-receptors for the TCR. The cytoplasmic domains of CD4 and CD8 associate with LCK, and, in current models of TCR signaling, these co-receptors bring LCK into contact with the CD3 chains of the pMHC-engaged TCR–CD3 complexes and thus play an important role in the phosphorylation of CD3 ITAMs (Chapter 13). The CD4 and CD8 co-receptors are needed for full T-cell activation.[73, 75–77]

The expression of the CD4 and CD8 co-receptors is highly regulated during T-cell development in the thymus. Thymocytes initially express neither co-receptor ('double-negative'). CD4$^-$CD8$^-$ thymocytes destined to become TCRαβ T cells progress through a CD4$^+$CD8$^+$ ('double-positive') stage to become mature CD4$^+$CD8$^-$ or CD4$^-$CD8$^+$T cells. Positive and negative selection of thymocytes on the basis of their TCR specificities and commitment to the CD4 or CD8 lineages occur during the double-positive stage (Chapter 9).

CD4: STRUCTURE AND BINDING TO MHC CLASS II MOLECULES

A member of the immunoglobulin superfamily, CD4 is a 55-kDa glycoprotein that can be expressed either as a monomer or a dimer on the cell surface. Its relatively rigid extracellular region contains four IgSF domains (designated D1–4). The cytoplasmic domain of CD4 contains two cysteine residues that mediate its noncovalent interaction with

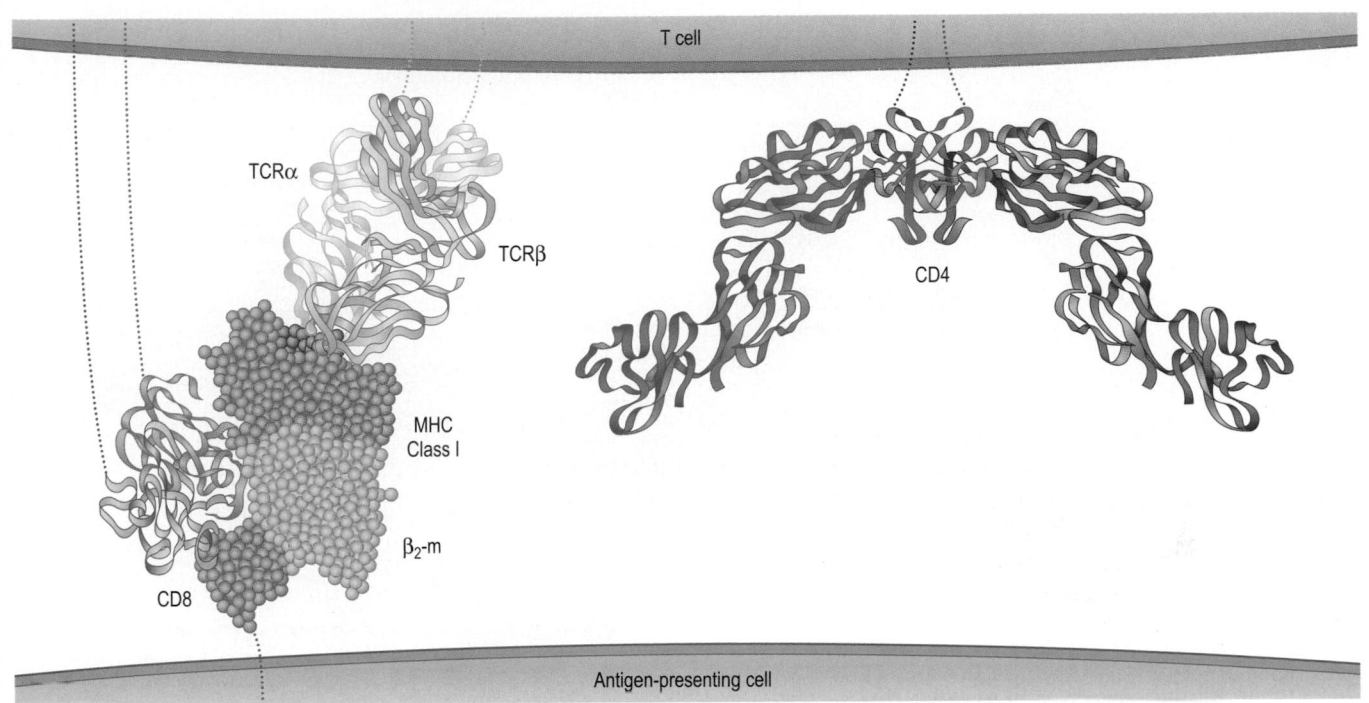

Fig. 4.15   Illustration of the interactions between the T-cell receptor (TCR), peptide–major histocompatibility complex (pMHC), and CD8. A composite illustration of the human leukocyte antigen (HLA)-A*0201 structure in complex with a Tax peptide and its cognate TCR α- and β-chains (protein databank (pdb) designation 1BD2) with the human CD8αα/HLA-A*0201 structure (pdb designation 1AKJ) was generated by superposition of the HLA moiety of the two structures. The HLA heavy chain is indicated as MHC, its light chain (β_2-microglobulin) as β_2-m, the CD8αα homodimer as CD8, the TCR α- and β-chains as TCRα and TCRβ. In addition, the CD4 homodimer (pdb file 1WIO) is shown to scale. Connecting peptides, transmembrane, and cytoplasmic domains are drawn by hand and indicated by dotted lines. Courtesy of David H. Margulies, National Institute of Allergy and Infectious Diseases, National Institutes of Health.

LCK through a 'zinc clasp'-like structure formed with a dicysteine motif in the N-terminal region of LCK.[73, 75, 76]

The crystal structure of the CD4 D1D2 fragment bound to pMHC class II demonstrates that the N-terminal domain (D1) of CD4 binds between the membrane-proximal α_2 and β_2 domains of MHC class II. Thus CD4 interacts with pMHC class II at a distance from the α-helices and peptide contacted by the TCR. This enables the TCR and CD4 to bind the same MHC class II molecule simultaneously. Models for the structure of TCRαβ–pMHC–CD4 indicate that this ternary complex assumes a V-shape with pMHC at the apex and with TCRαβ and CD4 forming the arms of the V. In this model, therefore, there is no direct interaction between the co-receptor and the TCR heterodimer, suggesting that pMHC brings the TCR and CD4 together. The model does not address the localization of the CD3 dimers, but raises the possibility that the CD3 chains lie within the open angle between TCRαβ and CD4, promoting interactions between CD3 chains and CD4-associated LCK.[73, 75, 76]

Experiments using soluble forms of CD4 and pMHC reveal that monomeric CD4 binds pMHC with very low affinity (K_d approximately 200 μM). The binding of CD4 to pMHC is of lower affinity than that TCRαβ to pMHC (K_d 1–10 μM) and displays more rapid kinetics. Because of the low affinity and the rapid off-time, it is unlikely that interactions of CD4 with MHC class II molecules initiate the interaction between a T cell and an antigen-presenting cell. Rather,

these binding characteristics are more compatible with a model in which the initial event is the interaction between the TCR and pMHC, followed by the recruitment of CD4, which then stabilizes the interaction and promotes signaling events.[73, 75–77]

CD8: STRUCTURE AND BINDING TO MHC CLASS I MOLECULES

There are two CD8 polypeptides, α and β, and these are expressed on the cell surface either as a disulfide-linked CD8αα homodimer or as a disulfide-linked CD8αβ heterodimer. On most αβ T cells, CD8αβ is the predominant form of CD8. However, NK cells (Chapter 18) and γδ T cells exclusively express CD8αα.[73, 75, 76]

CD8α, a 34–37-kDa protein, and CD8β, a 32-kDa protein, share about 20% amino acid sequence homology. Both are glycoproteins and IgSF members. Although CD8 subserves a co-receptor function similar to that CD4, in structure it differs substantially from CD4. The CD8 extracellular regions have single N-terminal IgSF V domains at the end of extended mucin-like stalk regions of 48 amino acids (CD8α) or 35–38 amino acids (CD8β). A striking difference between the two forms of CD8 lies within the cytoplasmic domain. CD8α, like CD4, contains a cysteine-based motif that enables it to interact with LCK through a 'zinc clasp'-like structure. In contrast, CD8β lacks this

Table 4.4 CD28 superfamily

Receptor	Expression	Ligand	Function on T cells
CD28	Most CD4 T cells 50% CD8 T cells	B7-1 (CD80) B7-2 (CD86)	Co-stimulation of IL-2 production and proliferation; promote T-cell survival
ICOS	Activated and memory T cells NK cells Not expressed by naïve T cells	ICOS ligand	Differentiation and effector T-cell function
CTLA-4	Upregulated after T-cell activation	B7-1 (CD80) B7-2 (CD86)	Inhibits IL-2 production and proliferation Promotes peripheral T-cell tolerance
PD-1	Upregulated after activation of T and B cells, myeloid cells	PD-L1 (B7-H1) PD-L2 (B7-DC)	Inhibits proliferations and cytokine production
BTLA	T and B cells, myeloid cells, dendritic cells	HVEM (herpes virus-entry mediator)	Inhibits T-cell proliferation

IL-2, interleukin-2; NK, natural killer.

motif and does not associate with LCK. Interestingly, CD8αβ appears to be a more effective activator of TCR signaling than CD8αα. This may reflect the palmitoylation of the cytoplasmic domain of CD8β, which allows CD8αβ to associate with lipid rafts during T-cell activation.[73, 75, 76, 78]

The structure of CD8αα–pMHC class I complexes demonstrates that CD8αα attaches primarily to the α$_3$ domain of MHC class I (i.e., a nonpolymorphic, membrane-proximal region of the molecule distinct from the peptide-binding groove engaged by the TCR) (Chapter 5). Compared to the interaction of CD4 and MHC class II, binding is more antibody-like, with a loop of the MHC α$_3$ domain locked between the CDR-like loops of the two CD8α IgSF V domains. Models of the structure of the TCRαβ–pMHC–CD8 ternary complex propose a V shape similar to that of the model for TCRαβ–pMHC–CD4, with pMHC at the apex of the V and the TCR and CD8 forming the arms of the V. CD8 binds to pMHC with lower affinity and with faster kinetics than the TCR. Thus, the binding properties of the CD8 co-receptor, like those of CD4, are consistent with a model in which the TCR initiates pMHC binding, followed by engagement of CD8 to the same pMHC.[73, 75–78]

CO-STIMULATORY AND INHIBITORY T-CELL MOLECULES: THE CD28 FAMILY

Although the T-cell response to antigen requires the binding of the TCR and its co-receptors to pMHC, additional receptor–ligand interactions can affect the outcome by delivering signals that promote activation (co-simulation) or that inhibit it (Table 4.4). Prominent among these are the interactions of members of the CD28 family with their cell surface ligands on antigen-presenting cells. This family includes CD28, inducible costimulator (ICOS), cytotoxic T-lymphocyte-associated

antigen-4 (CTLA-4), B- and T-lymphocyte attenuator (BTLA), and program death-1 (PD-1). CD28 and ICOS are co-stimulatory receptors; the major functions of CTLA-4, PD-1, and BTLA are inhibitory. CD28 and CTLA-4 are T-cell-specific whereas BTLA and PD-1 are also expressed by B cells and ICOS by NK cells.[79–81]

All members of the CD28 family have a single extracellular IgSF V domain and have, as their ligands, members of the B7 family of cell surface molecules. CD28, CTLA-4, and ICOS are expressed on the cell surface as disulfide-linked homodimers. Their cytoplasmic domains contain the SH2-binding motif YXXM. In contrast, PD-1 and BTLA are monomers whose cytoplasmic domains each contain an ITIM and an immunoreceptor tyrosine-based switch motif (ITSM).

The best-characterized members of the CD28 family are CD28 and CTLA-4. CD28 is the prototypic co-stimulatory receptor. Virtually all human CD4 T cells constitutively express CD28, as do half of the CD8 T cells. CD28 stimulation usually does not elicit a cellular response in the absence of TCR signaling. However, CD28 signals can act in concert with TCR signals to promote cytokine production, T-cell expansion, and T-cell survival. TCR signaling in the absence of CD28 co-stimulation can induce T-cell anergy (Chapter 13).

CTLA-4 inhibits the response to TCR and CD28 signals and acts to terminate T-cell responses. T-cell activation induces CTLA-4, whose cell surface expression is tightly regulated by the cytoplasmic motif YVKM. In the unphosphorylated state, this motif binds to AP-1 and AP-2 clathrin adaptor complexes that target CTLA-4 to intracellular compartments. Phosphorylation of the tyrosine releases the adaptor complexes and increases cell surface expression of CTLA-4.[79, 80]

CD28 and CTLA-4 bind to the same ligands, B7.1 (CD80) and B7.2 (CD86), and interact with these B7 ligands through a conserved hydrophobic MYPPPYY motif in their extracellular domains. Nonetheless, CD28 and CTLA-4 differ in the valency of binding. CD28 is monovalent whereas CLTA-4 binds two B7 ligands. And the affinity of CTLA-4 for B7.1 and B7.2 is substantially greater than that of CD28.[81] Thus, the inhibitory complexes formed by CTLA-4, particularly those involving B7.1, are more stable than the co-stimulatory interactions involving CD28.

Inhibition of T-cell activation by CTLA-4 appears to involve competition for B7 ligands and the generation of intracellular signals. In addition, CTLA-4 may induce 'reverse signaling' through B7.1 and B7.2 to the antigen-presenting cell, leading to the upregulation of the enzyme indoleamine 2,3-dioxygenase (IDO), which in turn breaks down tryptophan, a requirement for T-cell proliferation.[82]

The importance of CD28 co-stimulation has made it an attractive target for therapeutic intervention. Indeed, abatacept, a soluble fusion protein composed of the extracellular domain of human CTLA-4 and the constant regions of human IgG_1, is an effective therapy for the treatment of rheumatoid arthritis (Chapter 52). Abatacept is thought to inhibit CD28 co-stimulation through blockade of its B7 ligands, but some of its immunosuppressive effects may be indirect through the induction of IDO and consequent local depletion of tryptophan.[83]

■ REFERENCES ■

1. Williams AF, Barclay AN. The immunoglobulin superfamily – domains for cell surface recognition. Annu Rev Immunol 1988; 6: 381–405.

2. Harpaz Y, Chothia C. Many of the immunoglobulin superfamily domains in cell adhesion molecules and surface receptors belong to a new structural set which is close to that containing variable domains. J Mol Biol 1994; 238: 528–539.

3. Ashwell JD, Weissman AM. T cell antigen receptor genes, gene products, and co-receptors. In: Rich RR, Fleisher TA, Shearer WT, et al. (eds): Clinical Immunology: Principles and Practices, vol. 1. London: Mosby, 2001.

4. Padlan EA. Anatomy of the antibody molecule. Mol Immunol 1994; 31: 169–217.

5. Jazwinska EC, Dunckley H, Propert DN, et al. GM typing by immunoglobulin heavy chain gene RFLP analysis. Am J Hum Genet 1988; 43: 175–181.

6. Lefranc MP, Giudicelli V, Kaas Q, et al. IMGT, the international ImMunoGeneTics information system. Nucleic Acids Res 2005; 33 (database issue): issue 7.

7. Huston JS, McCartney J, Tai MS, et al. Medical applications of single-chain antibodies. Int Rev Immunol 1993; 10: 195–217.

8. Weng Z, Gulukota K, Vaughn DE, et al. Computational determination of the structure of rat Fc bound to the neonatal Fc receptor. J Mol Biol 1998; 282: 217–225.

9. Grubb R. Immunogenetic markers as probes for polymorphism, gene regulation and gene transfer in man – the Gm system in perspective. APMIS 1991; 99: 199–209.

10. Honjo T. Immunoglobulin genes. Annu Rev Immunol 1983; 1: 499–528.

11. Johansen FE, Braathen R, Brandtzaeg P. Role of J chain in secretory immunoglobulin formation. Scand J Immunol 2000; 52: 240–248.

12. Chen FH, Arya SK, Rinfret A, et al. Domain-switched mouse IgM/IgG2b hybrids indicate individual roles for C mu 2, C mu 3, and C mu 4 domains in the regulation of the interaction of IgM with complement C1q. J Immunol 1997; 159: 3354–3363.

13. Sensel MG, Kane LM, Morrison SL. Amino acid differences in the N-terminus of C(H)2 influence the relative abilities of IgG2 and IgG3 to activate complement. Mol Immunol 1997; 34: 1019–1029.

14. Skvaril F, Schilt U. Characterization of the subclass and light chain types of IgG antibodies to rubella. Clin Exp Immunol 1984; 55: 671–676.

15. Barrett DJ, Ayoub EM. IgG2 subclass restriction of antibody to pneumococcal polysaccharides. Clin Exp Immunol 1986; 63: 127–134.

16. Otteson EA, Skvaril F, Tripathy SP, et al. Prominence of IgG4 in the IgG antibody response to human filariasis. J Immunol 1985; 134: 2707–2712.

17. Suzuki K, Ha SA, Tsuji M, et al. Intestinal IgA synthesis: A primitive form of adaptive immunity that regulates microbial communities in the gut. Semin Immunol 2007; 19: 127–135.

18. Prussin C, Metcalfe DD. IgE, mast cells, basophils, and eosinophils. J Allergy Clin Immunol 2006; 117: S450–S456.

19. Davis MM, Bjorkman PJ. T-cell antigen receptor genes and T-cell recognition. Nature 1988; 334: 395–402.

20. Garcia KC, Degano M, Stanfield RL, et al. An alphabeta T cell receptor structure at 2.5 A and its orientation in the TCR–MHC complex. Science 1996; 274: 209–219.

21. Clements CS, Dunstone MA, Macdonald WA, et al. Specificity on a knife-edge: the γδ T cell receptor. Curr Opin Struct Biol 2006; 16: 787–795.

22. Rudolph MG, Stanfield RL, Wilson IA. How TCRs bind MHCs, peptides, and co-receptors. Annu Rev Immunol 2006; 24: 419–466.

23. Porcelli S, Brenner MB. Biology of the human gammadelta T-cell receptor. Immunol Rev 1991; 120: 137–183.

24. Davis MM. The evolutionary and structural 'logiC' of antigen receptor diversity. Semin Immunol 2004; 16: 239–243.

25. De Libero G, Mori L. Mechanisms of lipid-antigen generation and presentation to T cells. Trends Immunol 2006; 27: 485–492.

26. Allison TJ, Garboczi DN. Structure of gammadelta T cell receptors and their recognition of non-peptide antigens. Mol Immunol 2002; 38: 1051–1061.

27. Li H, Llera A, Malchiodi EL, et al. The structural basis of T cell activation by superantigens. Annu Rev Immunol 1999; 17: 435–466.

28. Leder P. The genetics of antibody diversity. Sci Am 1982; 246: 102–115.

29. Tonegawa S. Somatic generation of antibody diversity. Nature 1983; 302: 575–581.

30. Zachau HG. The human immunoglobulin kappa genes. In: Honjo T, Alt FW, Rabbitts PH, (eds): Immunoglobulin genes. London: Academic Press, 1995; p 173.

31. Dudley DD, Chaudhuri J, Bassing CH, et al. Mechanism and control of V(D)J recombination versus class switch recombination: similarities and differences. Adv Immunol 2005; 86: 43–112.

32. Brodeur PH, Riblet RJ. The immunoglobulin heavy chain variable region (IgH-V) locus in the mouse. I. One hundred Igh-V genes comprise seven families of homologous genes. Eur J Immunol 1984; 14: 922–930.

33. Kirkham PM, Schroeder HW Jr. Antibody structure and the evolution of immunoglobulin V gene segments. Semin Immunol 1994; 6: 347–360.

34. Lee SK, Bridges SL Jr, Koopman WJ, et al. The immunoglobulin kappa light chain repertoire expressed in the synovium of a patient with rheumatoid arthritis. Arthr Rheum 1992; 35: 905–913.

35. Kawasaki K, Minoshima S, Nakato E, et al. One-megabase sequence analysis of the human immunoglobulin lambda gene locus. PCR Methods Appl 1997; 7: 250–261.

36. Matsuda F, Ishii K, Bourvagnet P, et al. The complete nucleotide sequence of the human immunoglobulin heavy chain variable region locus. J Exp Med 1998; 188: 2151–2162.

37. Corbett SJ, Tomlinson IM, Sonnhammer EL, et al. Sequence of the human immunoglobulin diversity (D) segment locus: a systematic analysis provides no evidence for the use of DIR segments, inverted D segments, "minor" D segments or D-D recombination. J Mol Biol 1997; 270: 587–597.

38. Dorner T, Foster SJ, Farner NL, et al. Somatic hypermutation of human immunoglobulin heavy chain genes: targeting of RGYW motifs on both DNA strands. Eur J Immunol 1998; 28: 3384–3396.

39. Rada C, Ehrenstein MR, Neuberger MS, et al. Hot spot focusing of somatic hypermutation in MSH2-deficient mice suggests two stages of mutational targeting. Immunity 1998; 9: 135–141.

40. Reynaud C-A, Aoufouchi S, Faili A, et al. What role for AID: mutator, or assembler of the immunoglobulin mutasome? Nature Immunol 2003; 4: 631–638.

41. Tomlinson IM, Cox JP, Gherardi E, et al. The structural repertoire of the human V kappa domain. EMBO J 1995; 14: 4628–4638.

42. Chothia C, Lesk AM, Gherardi E, et al. Structural repertoire of the human VH segments. J Mol Biol 1992; 227: 799–817.

43. Tomlinson IM, Walter G, Jones PT, et al. The imprint of somatic hypermutation on the repertoire of human germline V genes. J Mol Biol 1996; 256: 813–817.

44. Ivanov II, Schelonka RL, Zhuang Y, et al. Development of the expressed immunoglobulin CDR-H3 repertoire is marked by focusing of constraints in length, amino acid utilization, and charge that are first established in early B cell progenitors. J Immunol 2005; 174: 7773–7780.

45. Arden B, Clark SP, Kabelitz D, et al. Human T-cell receptor variable gene segment families. Immunogenet 1995; 42: 455–500.

46. Jung D, Giallourakis C, Mostoslavsky R, et al. Mechanism and control of V(D)J recombination at the immunoglobulin heavy chain locus. Annu Rev Immunol 2006; 24: 541–570.

47. Nemazee DA, Weigert MG. Revising B cell receptors. J Exp Med 2000; 191: 1813–1818.

48. Neuberger MS, Patel KJ, Dariavach P, et al. The mouse B-cell antigen receptor: definition and assembly of the core receptor of the five immunoglobulin isotypes. Immunol Rev 1993; 132: 147–161.

49. Wang LD, Clark MR. B-cell antigen-receptor signalling in lymphocyte development. Immunol 2003; 110: 411–420.

50. Pelanda R, Braun U, Hobeika E, et al. B cell progenitors are arrested in maturation but have intact VDJ recombination in the absence of Ig-alpha and Ig-beta. J Immunol 2002; 169: 865–872.

51. Mason DY, Cordell JL, Brown MH, et al. CD79a: a novel marker for B-cell neoplasms in routinely processed tissue samples. Blood 1995; 86: 1453–1459.

52. Tsuganezawa K, Kiyokawa N, Matsuo Y, et al. Flow cytometric diagnosis of the cell lineage and developmental stage of acute lymphoblastic leukemia by novel monoclonal antibodies specific to human pre-B-cell receptor. Blood 1998; 92: 4317–4324.

53. Gauld SB, Cambier JC. Src-family kinases in B-cell development and signaling. Oncogene 2004; 23: 8001–8006.

54. Schamel WW, Reth M. Monomeric and oligomeric complexes of the B cell antigen receptor. Immunity 2000; 13: 5–14.

55. Niiro H, Clark EA. Regulation of B-cell fate by antigen-receptor signals. Nat Rev Immunol 2002; 2: 945–956.

56. Conley ME, Broides A, Hernandez-Trujillo V, et al. Genetic analysis of patients with defects in early B-cell development. Immunol Rev 2005; 203: 216–234.

57. Carroll MC. The role of complement and complement receptors in induction and regulation of immunity. Annu Rev Immunol 1998; 16: 545–568.

58. Fujimoto M, Poe JC, Inaoki M, et al. CD19 regulates B lymphocyte responses to transmembrane signals. Semin Immunol 1998; 10: 267–277.

59. Fearon DT, Carroll MC. Regulation of B lymphocyte responses to foreign and self-antigens by the CD19/CD21 complex. Annu Rev Immunol 2000; 18: 393–422.

60. Otero DC, Rickert RC. CD19 function in early and late B cell development. II. CD19 facilitates the pro-B/pre-B transition. J Immunol 2003; 171: 5921–5930.

61. Dempsey PW, Allison ME, Akkaraju S, et al. C3d of complement as a molecular adjuvant: bridging innate and acquired immunity. Science 1996; 271: 348–350.

62. Nimmerjahn F, Ravetch JV. Fcgamma receptors: old friends and new family members. Immunity 2006; 24: 19–28.

63. Coggeshall KM. Positive and negative signalling in B lymphocytes. Curr Top Microbiol Immunol 2000; 245: 213–260.

64. Ono M, Okada H, Bolland S, et al. Deletion of SHIP or SHP-1 reveals two distinct pathways for inhibitory signaling. Cell 1997; 90: 293–301.

65. Nitschke L. The role of CD22 and other inhibitory co-receptors in B-cell activation. Curr Opin Immunol 2005; 17: 290–297.

66. Kuhns MS, Davis MM, Garcia KC. Deconstructing the form and function of the TCR/CD3 complex. Immunity 2006; 24: 133–139.

67. Call ME, Wucherpfennig KW. The T cell receptor: critical role of the membrane environment in receptor assembly and function. Annu Rev Immunol 2005; 23: 101–125.

68. Arnett KL, Harrison SC, Wiley DC. Crystal structure of a human CD3-epsilon/delta dimer in complex with a UCHT1 single-chain antibody fragment. Proc Natl Acad Sci USA 2004; 101: 16268–16273.

69. Dadi HK, Simon AJ, Roifman CM. Effect of CD3delta deficiency on maturation of alpha/beta and gamma/delta T-cell lineages in severe combined immunodeficiency. N Engl J Med 2003; 349: 1821–1828.

70. de Saint-Basile G, Geissmann F, Flori E, et al. Severe combined immunodeficiency caused by deficiency in either the delta or the epsilon subunit of CD3. J Clin Invest 2004; 114: 1512–1517.

71. Fischer A, de Saint-Basile G, Le Deist F. CD3 deficiencies. Curr Opin Immunol 2005; 5: 491–495.

72. Rieux-Laucat F, Hivroz G, Lim A, et al. Inherited and somatic CD3zeta mutations in a patient with T-cell deficiency. N Engl J Med 2006; 354: 1913–1921.

73. Gao GF, Rao Z, Bell JI. Molecular coordination of alphabeta T-cell receptors and co-receptors CD8 and CD4 in their recognition of peptide-MHC ligands. Trends Immunol 2002; 23: 408–413.

74. Palacios EH, Weiss A. Function of the Src-family kinases, Lck and Fyn, in T-cell development and activation. Oncogene 2004; 23: 7990–8000.

75. Wang JH, Reinherz EL. Structural basis of T cell recognition of peptides bound to MHC molecules. Mol Immunol 2002; 38: 1039–1049.

76. van der Merwe PA, Davis SJ. Molecular interactions mediating T cell antigen recognition. Annu Rev Immunol 2003; 21: 659–684.

77. Xiong Y, Kern P, Chang H, et al. T cell receptor binding to a pMHCII ligand is kinetically distinct from and independent of CD4. J Biol Chem 2001; 276: 5659–5667.

78. Chang HC, Tan K, Ouyang J, et al. Structural and mutational analyses of a CD8alphabeta heterodimer and comparison with the CD8alphaalpha homodimer. Immunity 2005; 23: 661–671.

79. Riley JL, June CH. The CD28 family: a T-cell rheostat for therapeutic control of T-cell activation. Blood 2005; 105: 13–21.

80. Sansom DJ, Walker LS. The role of CD28 and cytotoxic T-lymphocyte antigen-4 (CTLA-4) in regulatory T-cell biology. Immunol Rev 2006; 212: 131–148.

81. Collins AV, Brodie DW, Gilbert RJ, et al. The interaction properties of costimulatory molecules revisited. Immunity 2007; 17: 201–210.

82. Grohmann U, Orabona C, Fallarino F, et al. CTLA-4-Ig regulates tryptophan catabolism in vivo. Nat Immunol 2002; 3: 1097–1101.

83. Genovese MC, Becker JC, Schiff M, et al. Abatacept for rheumatoid arthritis refractory to tumor necrosis factor alpha inhibition. N Engl J Med 2005; 353: 1114–1123.

The major histocompatibility complex

Robert J. Winchester

The term *major histocompatibility complex* (MHC) refers to the first biologic role identified for the polymorphic classical MHC molecules encoded in this region of the genome, that of governing transplant rejection. Growing appreciation of the role of MHC-encoded molecules in binding processed antigens for recognition by T cells has made it clear that MHC genes are centrally involved in regulating the adaptive immune response and determining susceptibility to many autoimmune diseases.[1] In the human the classical MHC genes are alternatively termed *human leukocyte antigen* (HLA) genes and the MHC itself is sometimes termed the *HLA region*.

Among the key aspects of the functional biology of classical MHC genes are their central function in the recognition of processed antigen by T cells, the biologic role their polymorphism plays in this recognition, and the importance of block inheritance of sets of polymorphic MHC genes encoded by different loci. In this chapter we will explore the significance of these aspects, examine the function of the various major MHC genes, and explore the implications of their polymorphisms.

■ CLASSICAL MHC MOLECULES DETERMINE HOW T CELLS RECOGNIZE PROCESSED ANTIGEN ■

T cells recognize a subset of the amino acid side chains of peptides derived from processed proteins. These peptides, which average nine amino acids in length, are anchored to pockets on the surface of classical MHC molecules by at least two of their amino acid side chains. The T cell recognizes a complex ligand composed of both the bound peptide and the presenting MHC, or *p-MHC*. Although the mode of TCR docking on MHC molecules is globally conserved, the shapes and chemical properties of the interacting surfaces found in these complexes are so diverse that no fixed pattern of contact has been recognized even between conserved TCR residues and conserved side chains of the MHC α-helices.[2]

In the adaptive immune response, the p-MHC ligand functions by presenting nonself peptide to T cells in the context of self-MHC. However, p-MHC are also the elements that select the repertoires of

T-cell clones generated during the thymic clonal selection process, as well as those that maintain the repertoire of naïve T cells (Chapter 9). Thus, in these instances self-peptide MHC complexes are surrogates for nonself peptides.[3] *Immunologic self* is the set of self-peptides and self-MHC molecules that select the TCR repertoire and which constitute the T-cell recognition component of an individual's adaptive immune system.

Basically the T-cell immune system protects the body from two major types of pathogens, viruses that commandeer the replicative machinery of a cell and bacteria that replicate autonomously and often extracellularly. The two specialized forms of MHC class I and class II molecules influence the recognition and response of the adaptive immune system to peptides derived from these two broad classes of pathogens in contrasting ways. To terminate viral infection, a cell harboring virus is killed by a cytotoxic CD8 T cell that recognizes viral peptides bound to the MHC class I molecules. In contrast a typical bacterium is eliminated by being phagocytized by a macrophage or neutrophil. The CD4 T cell recognizes the peptides of this bacterium bound to MHC class II molecules and directs the adaptive immune system either to locally activate the macrophage to a heightened state of antibacterial activity or to foster production of specific antibodies that opsonize the bacterium. The critical difference between killing or helping the antigen-presenting cell depends on whether class I or class II MHC molecules are loaded with pathogen peptide. Both the differential lineage expression of class I versus class II and the way pathogen peptides are loaded on the two classes of MHC molecules direct the recognition process.[4] The CD4 and CD8 co-receptors (Chapters 4 and 7) that interact with the class II and class I molecules respectively also appear to play an important role in this recognition process.[2]

Duplication of MHC genes involved in peptide presentation is a genetic strategy that offers additional varieties of peptide-presenting structures, which enhance the variety of presented peptides.[5] There are three types of classical MHC class I molecules, HLA-A, HLA-B, and HLA-C, and three types of MHC class II molecules, HLA-DR, HLA-DQ, and HLA-DP.[6] Each type of MHC molecule in an individual selects its own repertoire of T cells that are restricted in their ability to react only to peptides presented in the context of the same type of MHC molecule.

Virally encoded genes can decrease the expression of the class I MHC surveillance system through which they are identified.[7] This attempt to escape surveillance is countered by the extensive interaction of class I molecules with various natural killer (NK) receptors. These interactions provide a mechanism for detecting decreases in MHC class I expression, which is termed recognition of *missing self.*[8]

■ BIOLOGY OF MHC POLYMORPHISM ■

Since a given MHC molecule specifically binds particular amino acid side chains of the peptide, only a relatively few peptides from any protein are likely to bind to a given type of MHC molecule, restricting T-cell recognition. This shortcoming is compensated at the species level by the *polymorphic* nature of the MHC class I and II MHC genes. Nearly all of the polymorphic changes distinguishing individual alleles at each HLA locus encode molecules with different peptide-binding properties. This allows the individual members of a species to recognize different portions of a given protein molecule in their T-cell immune response in a manner

dependent on the binding properties of their particular HLA allotypes. This restriction constrains their T-cell repertoire to recognizing different MHC-dependent immunodominant T-cell epitopes. The three maternally and three paternally derived class I alleles of HLA-A, HLA-B, and HLA-C are codominantly expressed to create six different antigen-binding structures that are each recognized by T cells from the six separate T-cell repertoires.

A *genetic polymorphism* implies that alleles of a gene are present at a frequency greater than expected from random mutation due to selection for diversity. In the case of the HLA genes, there is no preponderant wild-type allele. Multiple MHC polymorphisms provide a major evolutionary survival benefit, since they equip the species with a large number of very specific, but alternative, MHC molecules that differ in their binding pockets and present different peptides.[1] This prevents the creation of shared antigen recognition structures that a pathogen could readily counter by means of mutation. The existence of multiple HLA alleles with no dominant wild-type allele all maintained at stable levels is an example of *balancing selection*. The most likely responsible factor driving this equilibrium is *frequency-dependent selection*, where the fitness of an individual bearing a common allele decreases because certain pathogens can adapt to the particular common structure and more efficiently infect those bearing a common MHC peptide-binding structure. The remarkably different frequency of the HLA alleles in different ethnic subsets tells the history of the successful adaptation of our ancestors' adaptive immune systems to a new environment with different pathogens, as well as bottlenecks resulting from migration and perhaps survival during periods of massive epidemics.

MHC polymorphisms have clinical consequences. The large number of different HLA alleles greatly reduces the probability that two unrelated individuals will inherit an identical set of MHC genes, making the immunologic self close to unique for each unrelated individual. The phenomenon of near-universal rejection of transplants between unrelated individuals is a reflection of this, because one person's T-cell repertoire will typically recognize another individual's self-peptide:MHC molecules as equivalent to a pathogen peptide:MHC interaction. Conversely, because the T-cell portion of the adaptive immune system is entirely selected on self-peptide presented by self-MHC allotypes in the thymus, should education of clones to respond only to nonself pathogen peptides fail, the inherent autoreactivity of the T-cell system will set the stage for the development of autoimmune diseases that are associated with the recognition of particular self-peptides which are ably presented by self MHC. This accounts for the association of certain HLA alleles with disease susceptibility.[9]

The MHC genes are organized into regions that perform different functions, but are inherited together in large blocks. The short arm of chromosome 6 (6p22.2-p21.3) contains the 3.6 million bases of the MHC. Of the 128 expressed genes in the MHC, over 50 appear likely to have an immune function. According to the distribution of the HLA genes, the MHC is subdivided into two principal regions (Fig. 5.1). The class I region is found at the telomeric end of the locus. This region, which contains the HLA-A, -B, and -C genes, as well as other class I gene family members, is principally concerned with CD8 T-cell peptide recognition and NK cell recognition. The class II region is located at the centromeric end of the locus. This region, which contains the genes encoding HLA-DR, -DQ, and -DP and other

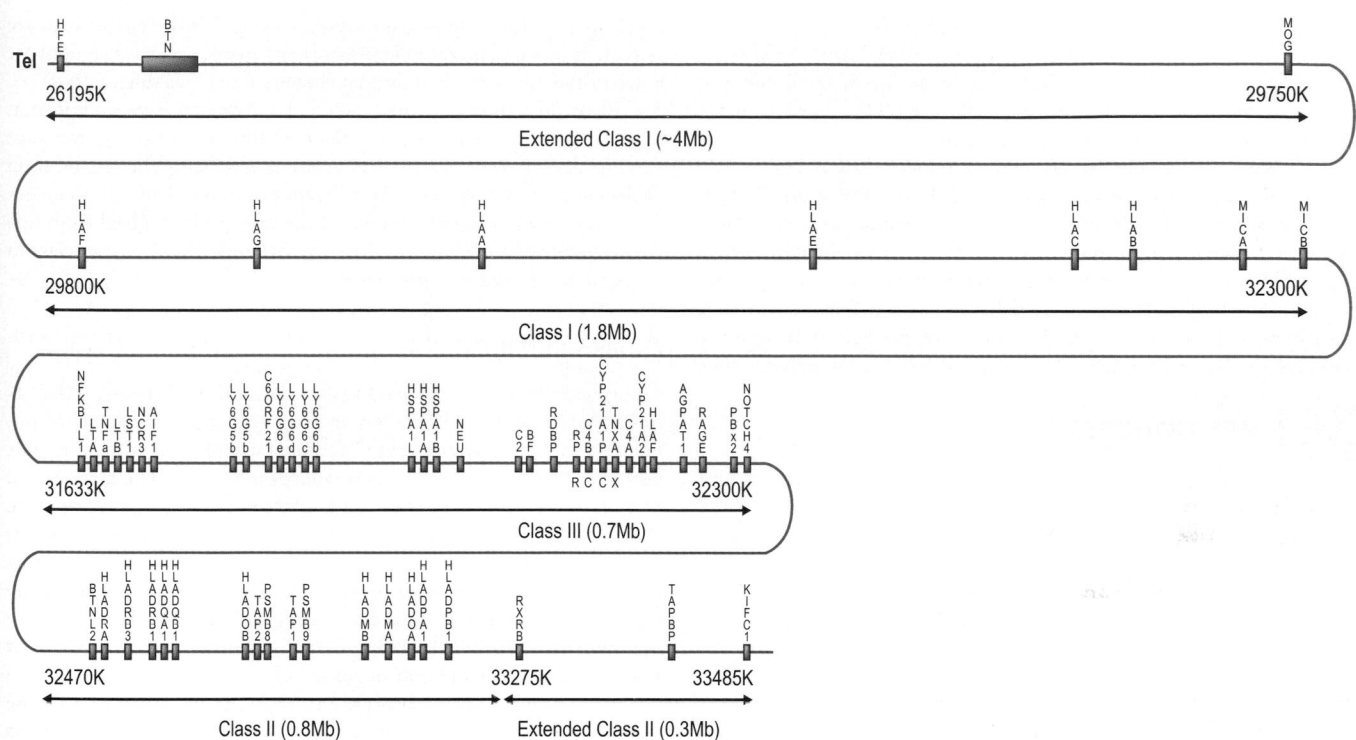

Fig. 5.1 Gene map of the extended major histocompatibility complex (MHC) depicting the immune related expressed genes, and certain reference genes. The MHC consists of five regions: extended class I, class I, class II, class II, and extended class II. Numbering of the sequence begins at the telomere. The approximate locations of genes near the start or end of the regions are indicted. The class III region is distinguished by a cluster of genes in the LY6 family that were revealed in the sequencing of the genome. The genes of the RCCX region are indicated and the order of the principal duplicated genes shown. The expressed genes in the HLA-DR haplotypes containing HLA-DRB3, e.g. HLA-DRB1*0301, are located within the class II region. (Modified from Beck S, Trowsdale J. The human major histocompatibility complex: lessons from the DNA sequence. Annu Rev Genomics Hum Genet 2000; 1: 117–137.)

members of the class II gene family, is principally concerned with CD4 T-cell peptide recognition as well as the processing of peptides for class I molecules. The identification of additional genes of immunologic importance lying on either side of the classic MHC locus has extended these class I and class II regions, enlarging the MHC locus to a span of nearly 8 million bases. Interposed between the class I and II regions is the class III region which also contains a number of genes that play a role in the immune response.

The many genes of the MHC are not inherited separately. Large regions of the MHC are virtually devoid of crossing over, with certain alleles of different gene loci inherited together far more frequently than expected from the product of their frequencies, a phenomenon termed *linkage disequilibrium*.[10] For most haplotypes, linkage disequilibrium extends over the entire extended MHC, so that large groups of genes with distinct functions are inherited together. There is an evident strong selective pressure that has apparently maintained these ancestral haplotypes over millennia and suggests that particular alleles on a haplotype function cooperatively in the adaptive immune response. This linkage of many polymorphic alleles makes it difficult to identify the genes within the MHC that determine disease susceptibility or a particular immnophenotype.[1]

■ PRINCIPAL GENES OF THE MHC AND THEIR IMMUNOLOGIC ROLE ■

THE CLASS I REGION

The class I molecule is composed of an MHC-encoded α-chain and a nonpolymorphic β₂-microglobulin chain encoded on chromosome 15. The class I region (Fig. 5.1) is distinguished by the six duplicated expressed class I α-chain genes that are subdivided into the highly polymorphic HLA-A, HLA-B, and HLA-C loci, designated class Ia genes, and the less polymorphic, nonclassical class Ib genes, HLA-E, HLA-F, and HLA-G.

The MHC class Ia and Ib molecules have different functions and tissue distributions (Table 5.1). Class Ia genes are expressed on virtually all nucleated cells. They are responsible for selecting the CD8 T-cell repertoire by engaging the clonal peptide-specific T-cell receptor (TCR). They subsequently function to present nonself peptides to the same subsets of CD8 T cells. Class Ib genes do not present nonself peptide to the TCR of CD8 T cells and contain a very limited variety of self-peptides. These self-peptides include the leader peptide of the classical class Ia MHC molecules, and their binding is an important part of the surveillance mechanism for missing self. Class Ib MHC molecules engage NK receptors (NKRs) such as heterodimeric CD94/NKG2A or CD94/NKG2C encoded by the killer cell lectin-like receptor family at 12p12-13 and expressed on NK cells, effector CD8 T cells, and the cytotoxic subset of CD4 T cells[11](Chapter 18).

The class I region also includes stress-induced MICA and MICB (MHC class I polypeptide-related sequence A and B) that are distantly related members of the class I family.[5] They are similar to MHC class I molecule α-chains, but do not associate with β_2-microglobulin or bind peptides. They encode heavily glycosylated proteins that are ligands for the activating NKG2D receptor (KLRK1), another member of the killer cell lectin-like receptor complex.[12] Binding of the MICA/B ligand to NKG2D on NK cells, CD8 αβ T cells, and γδ T cells activates their cytolytic response. These pathways involving NKR engagement are important in a number of inflammatory responses, e.g., they account for much of the injury of the intestinal epthelium in celiac disease.[13]

Half of the expressed genes in the class I region have no apparent function in the immune system, including some ancient genes that antedate the development of the adaptive immune system. The organization of the class I region is distinctly different between rodents and humans. The different class I genes in each of the two species evolved from different groups of ancestral class I genes, thus rodent and human class Ia genes are not considered *orthologues*.

CLASS I MOLECULE

The genetically polymorphic 44 kDa α-chain of the HLA-A, HLA-B, or HLA-C molecule is 362–366 amino acids long and consists of five domains. The ~30 amino acid C-terminal cytoplasmic domain is connected to a ~25-amino-acid transmembrane domain. The extracellular portion of the molecule consists of a ~90-amino-acid supporting stalk, the α_3 domain, and the similarly sized α_1 and α_2 domains that together form the peptide-binding portion of the molecule and the surface that interacts with the TCR or NKR (Fig. 5.2). The exon–intron organization of the class I gene parallels the domain organization, with exon 1 encoding the leader, exons 2–4 α1–3, exon 5 the transmembrane region, and exons 6 and 7 the cytoplasmic region.

The ends of the class I peptide-binding cleft are closed and fix the peptide's orientation to facilitate TCR recognition. The sides of the peptide-binding cleft are composed of α-helices and the floor is composed of asymmetric strands of β-pleated sheet. Typically, two amino acid side chains of the peptide bind to pockets formed into the side and base of the groove. Consistent with their surveillance role for viral infections, classical class I molecules are expressed on nearly all nucleated cells. The expression of class I molecules is upregulated by α, β, and γ-interferons, granulocyte–macrophage colony-stimulating factor, and certain other cytokines. Expression is governed by the class I regulatory element located ~160 nt upstream from the initiation site which binds a number of regulatory factors, including those induced by interferons.

During their synthesis MHC class I molecules are loaded with antigenic peptides in three steps (Chapter 6). First, following ubiquitylation,

KEY CONCEPTS

CLASS I MAJOR HISTOCOMPATIBILITY COMPLEX (MHC) GENES

>> The class I region contains the polymorphic human leukocyte antigen *(HLA)-A, -B,* and *-C* genes and the less polymorphic, nonclassical class Ib genes, *HLA-E, HLA-F, and HLA-G* genes

>> HLA-A, -B, and -C molecules are expressed on the surface of virtually all nucleated cells

>> HLA-A, -B, and -C are loaded with antigenic peptides derived from cytoplasmic proteins following their cleavage in the proteasome complex and present these peptides, both self and nonself, to clonal peptide-specific T-cell receptors (TCR) of CD8 T cells

>> Each MHC allotype selects its own T-cell repertoire. Thus there are usually six different repertoires in a person's CD8 T-cell population, each specialized for a maternally or paternally derived HLA-A, -B, and -C allotype

>> Class Ib molecules contain a very limited variety of self-peptides and engage lectin family natural killer receptors (NKR) in the recognition of *missing self*

Table 5.1 Contrast of classical and nonclassical major histocompatibility complex (MHC) class I and II molecules

MHC class	Ia	Ib	IIa	IIb
Polymorphism	High	Low	High	Low
Distribution	All nucleated cells	Restricted	Professional antigen-presenting cells	Restricted, endosome
Loci	HLA-A, B, C	HLA-E, G	HLA-DR, DQ, DP	HLA-DM, DO
Receptors	TCR αβ, γδ	CD94/NKG2A,C	TCR αβ	None, chaperone function
Presents	Many cytoplasmically self- and nonself-derived peptides	Few peptides, e.g., class Ia leader	Peptides from ingested proteins and self-peptides	HLA-DR, DQ, DP

HLA, human leukocyte antigen; TCR, T-cell receptor.

cytoplasmic proteins are targeted to the proteasome complex that cleaves them at basic and hydrophobic residues, yielding peptides suitable for binding to class I MHC.[14] Second, the peptides are actively translocated across the endoplasmic reticulum membrane by the selective TAP-1 and TAP-2 transporters that preferentially process peptides of 8–13 amino acids in length. Third, with the aid of chaperone proteins such as calnexin, calreticulin, and tapasin, the peptides are placed in the assembling MHC class I heterodimers. Some components of this system are encoded in the class II region (Fig. 5.1).

Analogous to the interaction of class Ib molecules with NKR, HLA-A, -B, or -C molecules are also ligands for a different group of NKR, the killer inhibitor receptors (KIR).[11, 15] Whether or not the molecules engage the inhibitory KIR3DL1 and thereby influence the potential for NK inhibition is determined by amino acid polymorphisms in the C-terminus of the α-helix around position 80. These polymorphisms allow subdivision of HLA-B alleles into two subclasses, designated HLA-Bw4 and HLA-Bw6.

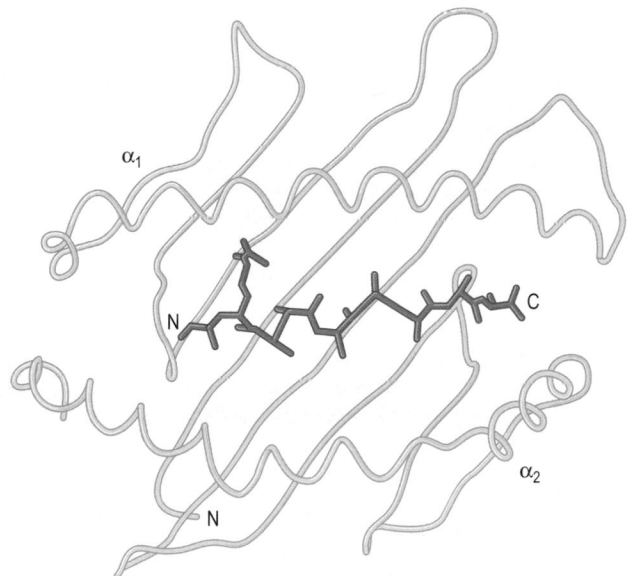

Fig. 5.2 The three-dimensional structure of human leukocyte antigen (HLA)-B27. The α-helical margins of the peptide-binding cleft contain the bound peptide RRIKAITLK, which is oriented with its amino-terminus to the left. There are extensive contacts at the ends of the cleft between peptide main-chain atoms and conserved MHC side chains, with the peptide amino and carboxyl termini tethered by H bonds and charge interactions. The peptide reciprocally stabilizes the three-dimensional fold of HLA-B27. The side chain of arginine in the P2 position of the peptide inserts into the B pocket, which contains an oppositely charged glutamic acid at its base. The resulting salt bridge is the dominant anchor for the peptide. Side chains P4, P6, and P8 make minor contributions to the interaction of the peptide with the HLA-B27 molecule. The central region of the peptide is left free to interact with a TCR. (Modified from Madden DR, Gorga JC, Strominger JL et al. The three-dimensional structure of HLA-B27 at 2.1 Å resolution suggests a general mechanism for tight peptide binding to MHC. Cell 1992; 70: 1035, with permission from Elsever.)

The HLA-C alleles are also subdivided according to the amino acid encoded at position 80 into C1, where the amino acid is asparagine, and C2, where the amino acid is lysine. The C1 subset of HLA-C molecules can serve as ligands for KIR2L2 and KIR2DL3, while the C2 subset interacts specifically and more strongly with KIR2DL1. The presence of the lysine at position 80 of HLA-C and the corresponding KIR receptors are features unique to humans and chimpanzees.[15]

The HLA-C–KIR interaction plays a major role in the tolerance of the fetal allograft. Tolerance of the paternally inherited MHC molecules of the fetus encoded by fetal allograft involves a number of mechanisms. The fetally derived trophoblast containing the paternal HLA genes does not express HLA-B and HLA-A, but expresses HLA-C along with the nonclassical MHC class Ib molecules HLA-G and HLA-E. *Pre-eclampsia* occurs in 2–10% of pregnancies. The highest risk for pre-eclampsia is in mothers who inherit two C2 HLA-C alleles and KIR haplotypes encoding KIR2DL1, a combination capable of giving the greatest inhibitory signal to the many NK cells in the placenta. This inhibition appears responsible for the underlying defect in pre-eclampsia – the failure of placental trophoblast to invade maternal arterioles sufficiently to achieve adequate fetal nourishment.[15]

The class Ib nonclassical HLA-E, HLA-F, or HLA-G molecules share a similar overall structure, but differ in their peptide-binding cleft. All have relatively few polymorphisms. HLA-E is specialized to bind the leader peptide of most HLA-A and HLA-B molecules cleaved off during synthesis. The extent of loading of HLA-E molecules becomes a reflection of the rate of class Ia molecule synthesis. Inhibitory CD94/NKG2A expressed on NK cells engages leader peptide-loaded HLA-E molecules and this holds the killing function of these cells at bay. A reduction in the level of class Ia molecule synthesis, *missing self*, as might occur during certain viral infections (Chapter 18), leads to diminished expression of HLA-E-peptide, release of NK cell inhibition, and subsequent destruction of the target cell. A complementary surveillance function monitors for cells under stress, *stressed or damaged self*. Stress induces upregulation of HLA-E, enabling engagement of activating NKR CD94/NKG2A, making the stressed target cell a target for the NK cell. This is paralleled by the MIC-A/B system. This dual regulatory mechanism plays a major role in maintaining the integrity of the intestinal epithelium.

HLA-G is highly expressed by placental trophoblast cells. It is distinguished by a series of alternative splices that result in either a membrane form lacking combinations of α2 or α3 domains or a soluble isoform that lacks the transmembrane domain. HLA-F has a small binding cleft that does not contain peptide and its functions are not well understood.

The α-chains of a separate group of class I molecules, CD1A through CD1E, are not encoded in the MHC, but on chromosome 1. These molecules also associate with β2-microglobulin, but exhibit limited genetic polymorphism. They present nonpeptide antigens, including microbial lipids and glycolipids, to γδ or NKT cells.

HFE, the hemochromatosis gene, a member of the class I family, regulates iron absorption by controlling the interaction of the transferrin receptor with transferrin. HFE has a binding cleft that is too small to contain a peptide. HFE defects can lead to hereditary hemochromatosis or porphyria.

PRINCIPAL GENES OF THE MHC AND THEIR IMMUNOLOGIC ROLE

■ HLA ALLELE DETECTION, NOMENCLATURE, AND INHERITANCE ■

The initial recognition of HLA molecules involved the use of human allosera that arose from alloimmunization during pregnancy or transplantation. The resulting nomenclature reflects the history of this discovery effort. Allotypes were designated by numbers, such as HLA-A2, HLA-B27, and HLA-Cw6; and the numbers of the HLA-A and HLA-B antigens are nonoverlapping. The letter 'w,' initially used to refer to a tentative workshop category, was retained for the HLA-C allotypes to prevent confusion with the complement components C2 and C4 that also map in the MHC. Some specificities were found not to be shared by numbers of allotypes. These are designated public specificities or epitopes. HLA-Bw4 and HLA-Bw6 are examples that are now known to define motifs recognized by the KIR receptor 3DL1.

Allosera were supplanted in order by gel analysis, DNA-based hybridization, and direct sequencing. Using these techniques, 2899 alleles of expressed class I and II HLA genes could be recognized by the end of 2007. These include 617 HLA-A, 960 HLA-B, 335 HLA-C, 9 HLA-E, 21 HLA-F, and 28 HLA-G named class I alleles, as well as 626 HLA-DRB, 34 HLA-DQA1, 87 HLA-DQB1, 23 HLA-DPA1, and 127 HLA-DPB1 alleles. The current nomenclature is a modification of the serologic classification extended to four-digit allele designations, so that HLA-A2 becomes HLA-A*0201. Currently 115 alleles differing at the nucleotide level have been identified that encode the HLA-A2 serologic specificity and belong to the same allele family. They are designated HLA-A*0202 through HLA-A*0296. The first four digits are used to distinguish alleles encoding different amino acid sequences. Alleles that have distinguishing silent nucleotide changes are assigned additional digits, so there are HLA-A*02010101, etc. Sequencing has also revealed null alleles that contain stop codons, e.g., A*0215N. Since there is no transcribed and expressed product, individuals with this null allele are not tolerized to determinants expressed by HLA-A2 molecules and may make a strong alloimmune response to tissue expressing a nonnull HLA-A2 allotype. Different alleles occur at highly different frequencies among different ethnic and racial groups (Table 5.2). Table 5.2 also illustrates the peptide-binding motifs of these allotypes.[16]

Due to the infrequency of cross-overs, combinations of genes forming haplotypes are the unit of MHC inheritance. This is measured by the Δ value of linkage disequilibrium. For example, among the Irish the haplotype frequency of HLA-A*0101 is 20.2%, of HLA-B*0801 is 16.2%, and of DRB1*0301 is 16%. If each allele occurred separately, the expected frequency of finding an HLA-A*0101-B*0801-DRB1*0301 individual would be $20.2 \times 16.2 \times 16 = 0.052\%$, but the observed frequency of the HLA-A*0101-B*0801-DRB1*0301 haplotype is 9.0%, yielding a linkage disequilibrium Δ value of $9.0 - 0.052 = 8.5$. There are two ways of counting the frequency of HLA alleles: gene or haplotype frequency. The gene frequency counts the number of alleles per haploid chromosome, totaling 100% or 1.0. The phenotype frequency, which enumerates the frequency of alleles in a population of diploid individuals, can total up to 200%.

The genetic relationships among members of a family are important for disease inheritance and transplantation. Each parent shares one haplotype with each of their children and always differs by one haplotype. Two siblings may share two, one, or no haplotypes, and thus range from being HLA-identical, through haplo-identical, to HLA-disparate.

■ PEPTIDE-BINDING FUNCTION ■

The peptide is a critical structural component of the classical class Ia and II MHC molecules. If a peptide is not loaded into a molecule or somehow escapes from the binding groove, the molecule becomes unstable and disassociates into its component chains. The purpose of this instability reflects the cell-specific surveillance function of these MHC molecules and prevents the passive acquisition of peptides from the milieu surrounding the cell that would subvert immune recognition.

Allotypes are generally distinguished by different patterns of peptide binding, as illustrated for selected HLA-B molecules in Table 5.2. In class I molecules, one or a few amino acid changes may considerably alter the functional consequences of a pocket and confer different binding properties.

In a healthy nonendocytosing cell, MHC molecules are filled with a variety of peptides from self molecules. Even during viral infection or upon pathogen phagocytosis the number of nonself peptides may not be high. Binding to MHC class I molecules follows several rules. Usually peptides are nine amino acids in length and are always oriented with their NH2 terminus to the 'left' (Fig. 5.2).

The biological consequences of the different patterns of peptide binding are significant. In the response to human immunodeficiency virus-1 (HIV-1: Chapter 37), the presence of HLA-B27 is associated with long-term nonprogression to acquired immunodeficiency syndrome (AIDS), whereas HLA-B35 denotes rapid progressors.[17] One of the striking correlates with these two HLA alleles is the number of different peptides in the HIV envelope that can bind to either type of HLA molecule. Fifteen different envelope peptides can bind to the HLA-B27 molecule, while no peptide contains motifs that preferentially bind to HLA-B35. The HIV infection is controlled by a CD8 T-cell response for a period of years, and the length of this time is proportional to the number of viral peptides recognized. The virus progressively mutates the anchor residues and the amino acids recognized by T-cell clones to evade presentation and identification.[18]

■ CONTRIBUTION OF MHC AND PEPTIDE TO THE MOLECULAR BASIS OF T-CELL RECOGNITION ■

Because the TCR repertoire is selected on self p-MHC, the molecular basis of MHC restriction of peptide recognition is affected by MHC residues that influence the peptide binding as well as by polymorphic MHC residues that contact the TCR. The specificity of recognition depends on particular amino acid differences. The dual dependency on peptide and MHC is well illustrated by a classic experiment that was performed with T-cell clones which recognize hepatitis B virus. The two T-cell clones were derived from an HLA-A*3101/A*6801 patient with hepatitis B virus hepatitis. In examining the HLA-restricted cytotoxic T-cell response to the hepatitis B nucleocapsid core antigen (HBcASg), Missale et al. identified a CTL epitope recognized by both clones that maps to a 10-residue sequence from amino acids 141–151 of HbcAg (Table 5.3).[19] HLA-A31 and HLA-Aw68 each proved to bind the same peptide, even though their amino acid sequence in domains 2 and 3 differs by 13 amino acids. The peptide-binding motif of A*3101 A*6801 and 10 of the amino acid differences influenced only the peptide-binding

Table 5.2 Different frequencies of selected human leukocyte antigen (HLA)-B alleles in various ethnic and racial populations and their peptide-binding motifs

	Ethnic groups								
Allele	Amer-indian	Guarani-Kaiowa	Han-Chinese 572	Irish	Korean	North America (Eu)	South Indian	Zulu	Peptide-binding-motifs
B*0702	0.068		0.002	0.173	0.003	0.110		0.022	.[PV]......[LA]
B*0801	0.045		0.003	0.162		0.108	0.067	0.067	.[RK].[RK]....
B*1301			0.078		0.010		0.014		
B*1302	0.021		0.019	0.017	0.045	0.014	0.014	0.025	
B*1501	0.083		0.022	0.038	0.088	0.057		0.002	.[QL]......[YV]
B*1502			0.102		0.005				.[LQ]......[YF]
B*1503	0.004	0.003		0.001				0.100	
B*1504		0.115							
B*1801	0.019		0.001	0.029		0.031	0.010	0.040	
B*2703								0.002	[RK]R......[LY]
B*2704			0.019						R[R-]......[LF]
B*2705	0.090			0.029	0.053	0.023			R[R-]F.....[-]
B*3501	0.109	0.010	0.016	0.055	0.063	0.066	0.010	0.030	.[PV]......[LY]
B*3503	0.006		0.010	0.005	0.003	0.019	0.082		
B*3505		0.139	0.010			0.003			
B*3701	0.006		0.004	0.016	0.008	0.019	0.087		.[DE].....L[I]
B*3802			0.054		0.013	0.002			
B*3901	0.041	0.049	0.014	0.009	0.018	0.005	0.010	0.002	.[HR]......[L-]
B*3903	0.004	0.003		0.001		0.003			
B*3905	0.004	0.111	0.003						
B*3906	0.015	0.090		0.009		0.007	0.005		
B*3909		0.083	0.001						.[RH]......[L-]
B*4001	0.038		0.152	0.054	0.040	0.068	0.010		.[E-]......[L-]
B*4006	0.004		0.010		0.035		0.130		.[E-]......[VA]
B*4201						0.003		0.129	.[PL]......[-]
B*4402	0.041		0.002	0.131	0.010	0.113			.[E-]......[FL]
B*4601			0.163		0.063				.[MI]......[YF]
B*5101	0.104	0.007	0.043	0.027	0.125	0.052	0.120	0.002	.[AP]......[LY]
B*5201					0.025		0.120		.[QF]......[VF]
B*5301	0.009			0.002		0.003	0.010	0.015	.[P-]......[FL]
B*5401			0.030		0.048				.[P-]......[A-]
B*5701	0.017		0.003	0.038	0.005	0.042	0.029	0.002	.[ST]......[WF]
B*5801	0.011		0.073	0.003	0.055	0.014	0.072	0.032	.[TS]......[WF]
B*5802	0.002							0.097	.[ST]......[FM]

Allele frequency data from anthropology section of IHWG. Boxes denote the three highest allele frequencies in a population.
Peptide binding motifs from Lund et al., 2004

Table 5.3 Molecular events in human leukocyte antigen (HLA)-restricted cytotoxic T-cell response to the hepatitis B nucleocapsid core peptide

Target MHC-p	T cell clone	Target killed (%)
A*3101	2D7	2
A*3101	3D11	83
A*6801	2D7	84
A*6801	3D11	1

Peptide binding motifs of HLA-A molecules

A*3101   [RK]QL......[R-]

A*6801   E[VT]......[RK]

Amino acid sequence comparison of HLA-A*3101 and HLA-A*6801

```
                    10         20         30         40         50
A*310102   GSHSMRYFTT SVSRPGRGEP RFIAVGYVDD TQFVRFDSDA ASQRMEPRAP
A*680101   --------Y- ---------- ---------- ---------- ----------

                    60         70         80         90        100
A*310102   WIEQERPEYW DQETRNVKAH SQIDRVDLGT LRGYYNQSEA GSHTIQMMYG
A*680101   -----G---- -RN------Q --T------- ---------- ----------
                 *

                   110        120        130        140        150
A*310102   CDVGSDGRFL RGYQQDAYDG KDYIALNEDL RSWTAADMAA QITQRKWEAA
A*680101   ---------- ---R------ ------K--- ---------- -T-KH-----
                                                         *

                   160        170        180
A*310102   RVAEQLRAYL EGTCVEWLRR YLENGKETLQ
A*680101   H----W---- ---------- ----------
                *
```

Peptide region of HBcAg that binds to both MHC molecules and main peptide epitope recognized by T cell clones indicated by asterisks

```
141-151 STLPETTVVRR
3D11        *
2D7          **
```

pockets. Although both MHC molecules bound the same peptide, the killing of T-cell clone 3D11 was completely restricted to HLA-A*3101 and that of 2D7 was restricted to HLA-A*6801 (Table 5.3). Subsequently it was shown that the same peptide is recognized differently, with the TCR of clone 3D11 recognizing the E at 145 (P5) while 2D7 recognized the two Ts at 146 and 147 (P6, P7). These recognition patterns reflected differences in three TCR contact amino acids on the two α-helical rims of the two HLA-A molecules, which contribute to the separate HLA-A allotype restriction of each clone.

■ AUTOIMMUNE DISEASE ■

Autoimmune diseases are generally complex diseases with indeterminate modes of inheritance that are influenced by the number and kind of susceptibility alleles that segregate at several loci throughout the genome. A monozygotic twin concordance rate on the order of 50%

suggests that stochastic events, such as TCR repertoire formation, as well as extrinsic environmental effects likely play a role in onset and progression of the disease. The primary susceptibility to develop most autoimmune diseases is associated with alleles or haplotypes of either class I or class II MHC loci.[1]

One of the more extraordinary observations in the MHC field was made in 1973 when the frequency of HLA specificity HLA-B27 was found to be 95% in those with the disease *ankylosing spondylitis* compared to 2–3% in healthy controls. The odds of being HLA-B27-positive if one has ankylosing spondylitis are 0.95/0.05 = 19, and the odds of being HLA-B27-positive if one is a control are 0.02/0.98 = 0.02. Thus, the odds of developing ankylosing spondylitis if one is HLA-B27-positive is 19/0.02 = 950:1, surely an impressive observation that implicates HLA-B27 in the pathogenesis of ankylosing spondylitis. However there are several points about this approach. First, ankylosing spondylitis is a relatively rare disease with a prevalence of ~130 per 100 000, or 0.013%. For every HLA-B27 patient with ankylosing spondylitis there are over 15

KEY CONCEPTS

CLASS II MAJOR HISTOCOMPATIBILITY COMPLEX (MHC) GENES

>> The class II region contains the genes encoding human leukocyte antigen (HLA)-DR, DQ, and DP, which are principally concerned with CD4 T-cell peptide recognition, and PSMB8, PSMB9, TAP1, and TAP2, which help process peptides for class I molecules

>> During the synthesis of MHC class II molecules, occupation of the peptide-binding groove by the N-terminus of the invariant chain prevents the binding of self-peptides

>> MHC class II molecules are constitutively expressed on professional phagocytes, thymic epithelial cells, and activated T cells

>> Interferon-γ induces the expression of MHC class II molecules on a wide variety of stromal, parenchymal, and vascular cells

healthy HLA-B27-positive persons without the disease (2.0/(0.013×0.95). Second, the impressive odds ratio, although mathematically correct, somewhat numerically overstates the impact of HLA-B27, since it is a ratio of two ratios. Third, it is quite clear that the HLA-B27 allele conferring susceptibility does not differ from the 'wild-type' allele found in the healthy population and is also positively selected in the overall population. Fourth, there are 44 alleles of HLA-B27, of which HLA-B270502 is the most common, and not all alleles are associated with susceptibility to ankylosing spondylitis. The B27 molecules associated with susceptibility are often distinguished by the presence of a cysteine in the P2 pocket that can potentially dimerize to another HLA-B27 molecule. This allele has a tendency to fold slowly and somewhat unstably, as well as a peptide-binding motif that often recognizes a large proportion of peptides. Lastly, although it has been three decades since the initial observation was made, we still do not have a precise and certain understanding of how the presence of the HLA-B27 alleles results in the autoimmune injury underlying ankylosing spondylitis, nor indeed how HLA alleles confer susceptibility for most of the many autoimmune diseases that have a large component of their susceptibility in the MHC. Nevertheless, it appears to be the particular HLA-B27 allele, rather than a gene in linkage disequilibrium with the HLA-B27 allele, because the association of the particular HLA-B27 allotypes with susceptibility appears to map to the sequence of the allele.

THE CLASS II REGION

The genes of the class II region are almost exclusively concerned either with recognition of peptide expressed by CD4 T cells or with processing of peptides for class I molecules. As with MHC class I molecule, self-peptide–MHC class II complexes expressed in the thymus positively and negatively select the CD4 TCR repertoire according to the particular MHC class II allotypes. In the course of an immune response, nonself proteins are endocytosed by 'professional' phagocytes, processed and reduced to nonself peptides, and presented by class II molecules expressed on these cells for recognition by the TCRs of CD4 T cells.

Following endocytosis, extracellular pathogens and protein antigens are digested in lysosomes to form peptides that are loaded on the MHC class II molecules that traffic to the endosome.[20] Invariant chain plays a critical role in the class II pathway, because its C-terminus contains a recognition motif that redirects the molecule to the endosome rather than to the cell membrane. The N-terminus of invariant chain occupies the peptide-binding groove during its synthesis in the endoplasmic reticulum so no endogenous peptide can load the class II molecule during its time in the endoplasmic reticulum. The acidic enzymatic environment of the endosome degrades the invariant chain to a CLIP (class II-associated invariant chain peptide) that is subsequently removed to allow peptide binding. The class II molecule is then free to travel to the cell membrane where it presents its newly acquired peptide to CD4 T cells (Chapters 6 and 7).

Of the 18 expressed genes in the class II region (Fig. 5.1), 11 encode either the α-chains, HLA-DPA, HLA-DQA, and HLA-DRA; or the β-chains, HLA-DPB, HLA-DQB, HLA-DRB1, HLA-DRB3 of the classical heterodimeric HLA-DP, HLA-DQ, HLA-DR molecules; or the analogous α- and β-chains of HLA-DM and HLA-DO molecules.[5] In some haplotypes the HLA-DRB3 gene is replaced by HLA-DRB4, HLA-DRB5, or a pseudogene. With the exception of HLA-DRA, classical class II molecules are highly polymorphic. As with class I molecules, this polymorphism determines the particular peptides they present to CD4 T cells, thus regulating their immune response. The nonpolymorphic nonclassical class II molecules HLA-DM and HLA-DO are exclusively expressed in endosomes. They regulate peptide binding to the classical MHC class II molecules. HLA-DM, a peptide editor, plays a central role in peptide loading of MHC class II molecules by helping to release the CLIP from the peptide-binding site and facilitate entry of peptides that bind with higher affinity.[21] HLA-DO interacts with HLA-DM but its expression is more restricted. Analogous with the class I region, there are a number of pseudogenes in the class II region, reflecting the number of duplication events that have shaped the number and arrangement of genes in this region.[5]

Four genes in the class II region are involved with processing and loading peptides on to class I molecules (Fig. 5.1). PSMB8 and PSMB9 are proteasome subunits and TAP1 and TAP2 transport the peptides from the cytoplasm to the endoplasmic reticulum. Of the three remaining expressed genes of the class II region, one, butyrophilin-like 2 (BTNL2), has a potential immune function. BTNL2 has been implicated in susceptibility to sarcoidosis.

CLASS II MOLECULES

Although the conformation of the classical class II molecules, HLA-DP, HLA-DQ, and HLA-DR is similar to that of class I molecules, there are several key differences (Fig. 5.3). Unlike class I, which encodes the peptide-binding pocket in a single protein chain, class II molecules are constructed from two structurally homologous α- and β-chains that each contributes half of the peptide-binding groove. Both of these molecules are encoded within the MHC. The α2 domain of the α-chain contributes the left four strands of the β-pleated sheet floor and the upper α-helix, while the β2 domain of the β-chain contributes the right four strands of the β-pleated sheet floor and the lower α-helix. The α3 and β3 domains, similar to the class I α3 domain, form a supporting stalk and are each connected to transmembrane and intracytoplasmic domains.

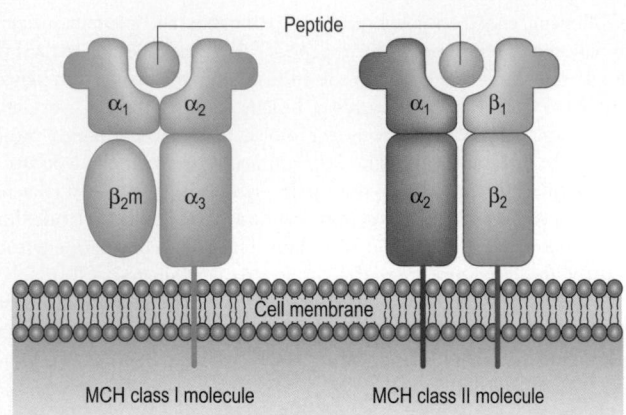

Fig. 5.3 Major histocomptability complex (MHC) class I and II molecules have a homologous domain organization, but a different chain structure.

The peptide-binding region differs from that of the class I molecule in that the antigen-binding groove is open at both ends. Thus, the MHC class II heterodimer does not interact with either the N- or C-terminus of the peptide. Accordingly, the MHC class II-binding peptides may be of varying lengths, up to about 30 amino acids, and their N- and C-termini extend outwards from the peptide-binding groove. Side chains in the middle of the peptide tether it to pockets within the groove.

The contribution of the α- and β-chains to the polymorphism in the HLA-DR molecule differs from that found in HLA-DP and HLA-DQ molecules. In the latter, both the α- and β-chains are polymorphic and each contributes to overall peptide-binding characteristics of the molecule. The α- and β-chains in HLA-DP and HLA-DQ can come either from genes on the same haplotype, *cis*, or from the α- and β-chain genes on opposite haplotypes, *trans*. This complementation between genes encoded by different parental haplotypes generates novel MHC molecules with peptide-binding characteristics not found in either parent. This is the mechanism involved in the determination of *celiac disease* susceptibility, where the inheritance of the DQA1*0501 allele and the DQB1*0201 allele confers disease risk whether or not the genes are inherited on the same paternal or maternal haplotype.

The α-chain gene of the HLA-DR molecule lacks immunologically significant polymorphisms and all of the considerable diversity in peptide-binding function arises from the more highly polymorphic DRB chain alleles. The structure of the DR region between DRA and DRB1 is a complex polymorphic region that varies across different haplotypes.[5] While all MHC haplotypes have a single DRB1 locus, additional DRB genes are found in most, but not all, haplotypes. These additional genes vary in number and position, reflecting their origin by duplication and recombination events. The DRB3 locus is present in DRB1*03 and *11, *12, *13, and *14 haplotypes and encodes the HLA-DRw52 specificity. The DRB4 locus is present in evolutionarily more ancient DRB1*04, *07, and *09 haplotypes, and encodes the DRw53 specificity. The DRB5 locus is present in DRB1*15 and 16 haplotypes and encodes the DRw51 specificity. These haplotypes also vary in intron sequences, repeat elements, and the presence of pseudogenes. Differences in genomic structure between the haplotypes prevent homologous meiotic pairing and may

contribute to linkage disequilibrium by suppressing recombination. Similar complex polymorphisms are seen in the class III region.

The expression of MHC class II molecules is much more intricately regulated than that of class I MHC.[22] In addition to professional phagocytes, class II molecules are expressed on thymic epithelial cells and activated T cells. Interferon-γ expression occurring during tissue infiltration by activated T cells or NK cells also induces MHC class II molecule expression on a wide variety of stromal, parenchymal, and vascular cells. The MHC class II molecule expression is also regulated within a lineage according to developmental stage. In the myeloid lineage committed neutrophil progenitors express class II molecules through the myeloblast stage. Expression diminishes upon maturation of monocytes to macrophages, unless it is reinduced by interferon-γ. Expression in B cells is lost upon their differentiation into plasma cells.

Expression of class II molecules is regulated by a promoter located within 150 basepairs of the transcription initiation site in exon 1. A variety of cooperative trans-acting factors bind to the promoter. MHC2TA is a critical coactivator for MHC class II expression that binds to these subunits. Genetic defects in the expression of these factors results in the *bare lymphocyte syndrome*. MHC2TA is induced in activated T cells and by interferon-γ, resulting in upregulation of class II MHC expression. This upregulation is opposed by TH2 or antiinflammatory cytokines such as transforming growth factor-β, interleukin (IL)-4, and IL-10.

CLASS II-ASSOCIATED AUTOIMMUNE DISEASES

Susceptibility to a large number of autoimmune diseases, especially those characterized by autoantibodies, is influenced by a number of MHC class II alleles. The inheritance of *rheumatoid arthritis* is an interesting instance where susceptibility maps to a set of HLA-DRB1 alleles, all of which are intriguingly characterized by similar amino acid motif involving positively charged amino acids around position 70 in the β-chain, that has been designated the *shared epitope*.[23, 24] The presence of two alleles of this group increases susceptibility and favors development of more severe disease.[25] The region around position 70 is involved in the formation of a peptide side chain binding pocket. It also interacts directly with the TCR. The apparent functional equivalence or identity by state of the DRB1*0101, *0401, *0404, *0405, *0408, *1001, and *1402 that confer susceptibility to rheumatoid arthritis explains why earlier linkage studies greatly underestimated the contribution of the MHC to disease genetics.[26]

THE CLASS III REGION

The MHC class III region is the shortest (0.7 Mb), most gene-dense (58 genes; one every ~15 kbp of DNA), and evolutionarily the most ancient and stable within the MHC since it contains highly conserved genes and the fewest pseudogenes.[5] It is delimited by the telomeric BAT1 and the centromeric NOTCH4.

The MHC class III region contains both nonimmune genes and immune-related genes involved in inflammation. However, none of these genes is involved in the presentation of peptides. Among the immune-related genes are three encoding complement components C2, fB, and C4, three members of the tumor necrosis factor (TNF) family, TNF, LTA, and LTB, members of the Ly6 superfamily, three genes encoding heat shock protein and the gene for the receptor for advanced glycation products, RAGE. Among nonimmune genes is 21-hydroxylase (CYP).

Additionally, Notch 4, PBX, and SK12 are interesting because they are ancient genes that substantially predate the adaptive immune system and form part of the fundamental framework of the MHC in many species. The region is distinguished by remarkably little recombination.

With one major exception, there is little evidence of gene duplication in the class III region. The exception is the polymorphic subregion that contains the C4 and 21-hydroxylase loci. This region is designated RCCX (Fig. 5.1) because it is composed of tandem duplications of *RP*, *C*4A/B, *CYP21*, and TN*X*B.[5] Ten different haplotypes of this subregion exist that differ markedly in terms of gene content and arrangement with one, two, or three copies of the genes, analogous to the complex haplotype organization of the DRB region. The C4 gene is duplicated, resulting in two functionally different forms C4A (acidic) and C4B (basic) (Chapter 20). Some individuals may lack either the C4A or C4B gene and the variation in copy number of the C4 gene, mainly between 2 and 6 copies, presumably contributes to the large range of stable normal C4 levels. Similarly, the 21-hydroxylase gene is duplicated, as CYP21A a pseudogene and CYP21B.[27]

EXTENDED CLASS I AND CLASS II REGIONS

The most telomeric member of the class I family, HFE marks the beginning of the extended class I region that ends with MOG. Its 4 Mb contains large clusters of histone, tRNA, zinc-finger and ribosomal protein genes that are seemingly unrelated to the regulation of the immune response.[28] It also contains two clusters of olfactory receptor genes that have been considered to play a part in mating choice. Since these olfactory receptor genes are in linkage disequilibrium with class I and class II HLA alleles, they could thus influence selection of polymorphic HLA genes.[29] The presence of linkage disequilibrium also extends centromeric from the MHC to kinesin family member C1, KIFC, that is not structurally related to the class II MHC gene family. This region contains TAPBP, TAP-binding protein (tapasin), a transmembrane glycoprotein that mediates interaction between newly assembled MHC class I molecules by binding to TAP1.

■ FUTURE LEARNING AND RESOURCES ■

This chapter provides only a limited sketch of this fascinating but complex topic. The reader is referred to *The HLA Facts Book*[6] for a more detailed and very accessible presentation of much additional information. There are also a number of websites with extremely useful information. Four stand out in terms of their utility and the curated quality of the information. The IMGT/HLA database (http://www.ebi.ac.uk/imgt/hla/index.html) contains all MHC sequences and has a variety of sequence alignments of different alleles as well as specialized sequence searches. The National Center for Biotechnology Information maintains dbMHC that includes several components of the international histocompatibility working group (IHWG) that are of interest. Among these are the anthropology database that contains HLA class I and class II allele and haplotype frequencies in various human populations: http://www.ncbi.nlm.nih.gov/projects/mhc/. Information about the genes and the genetic organization of the MHC is contained in several sites, but perhaps the most comprehensive and comprehensible is that using the Entrez search engine: http://www.ncbi.nlm.nih.gov/gquery/gquery.fcgi?itool=toolbar.

■ REFERENCES ■

1. Trowsdale J. HLA genomics in the third millennium. Curr Opin Immunol 2005; 17: 498–504.

2. Housset D, Malissen B. What do TCR-pMHC crystal structures teach us about MHC restriction and alloreactivity? Trends Immunol 2003; 24: 429–437.

3. Stefanova I, Dorfman JR, Tsukamoto M, et al. On the role of self-recognition in T cell responses to foreign antigen. Immunol Rev 2003; 191: 97–106.

4. Trowsdale J, Parham P. Mini-review: defense strategies and immunity-related genes. Eur J Immunol 2004; 34: 7–17.

5. Beck S, Trowsdale J. The human major histocompatibility complex: lessons from the DNA sequence. Annu Rev Genomics Hum Genet 2000; 1: 117–137.

6. Marsh SGE, Parham P, Barber LD. The HLA Facts Book. San Diego, California: Academic Press, 2000.

7. Lilley BN, Ploegh HL. Viral modulation of antigen presentation: manipulation of cellular targets in the ER and beyond. Immunol Rev 2005; 207: 126–144.

8. Raulet DH. Missing self recognition and self tolerance of natural killer (NK) cells. Semin Immunol 2006; 18: 145–150.

9. Winchester R. The genetics of autoimmune-mediated rheumatic diseases: clinical and biologic implications. Rheum Dis Clin North Am 2004; 30: 213–227, viii.

10. Stewart CA, Horton R, Allcock RJ, et al. Complete MHC haplotype sequencing for common disease gene mapping. Genome Res 2004; 14: 1176–1187.

11. Kelley J, Walter L, Trowsdale J. Comparative genomics of natural killer cell receptor gene clusters. PLoS Genet 2005; 1: 129–139.

12. Lanier LL. On guard – activating NK cell receptors. Nat Immunol 2001; 2: 23–27.

13. Meresse B, Curran SA, Ciszewski C, et al. Reprogramming of CTLs into natural killer-like cells in celiac disease. J Exp Med 2006; 203: 1343–1355.

14. Rivett AJ, Hearn AR. Proteasome function in antigen presentation: immunoproteasome complexes, peptide production, and interactions with viral proteins. Curr Protein Peptide Sci 2004; 5: 153–161.

15. Parham P. Immunogenetics of killer cell immunoglobulin-like receptors. Mol Immunol 2005; 42: 459–462.

16. Lund O, Nielsen M, Kesmir C, et al. Definition of supertypes for HLA molecules using clustering of specificity matrices. Immunogenetics 2004; 55: 797–810.

17. Winchester RJ, Charron D, Louie L, et al. The role of HLA in influencing the time of development of a particular outcome of HIV-1 infection. Proceedings of the Twelfth International Histocompatibility Workshop and Conference; EDK, Sevres, France; ed. Charron D. pp. 640–648, 1997.

18. McMichael AJ, Ogg G, Wilson J, et al. Memory CD8+ T cells in HIV infection. Philos Trans R Soc Lond B Biol Sci 2000; 355: 363–367.

19. Missale G, Redeker A, Person J, et al. HLA-A31- and HLA-Aw68-restricted cytotoxic T cell responses to a single hepatitis B virus nucleocapsid epitope during acute viral hepatitis. J Exp Med 1993; 177: 751–762.

20. Pieters J. MHC class II compartments: specialized organelles of the endocytic pathway in antigen presenting cells. Biol Chem 1997; 378: 751–758.

21. Karlsson L. DM and DO shape the repertoire of peptide-MHC-class-II complexes. Curr Opin Immunol 2005; 17: 65–70.

22. Ting JP, Trowsdale J. Genetic control of MHC class II expression. Cell 2002; 109(Suppl.): S21–S33.

23. Winchester R. The molecular basis of susceptibility to rheumatoid arthritis. In: Advances in Immunology, vol. 56. San Diego, CA: Academic Press, 1994; Dixon F, ed. pp 389–466.

24. Goronzy JJ, Weyand CM. Rheumatoid arthritis. Immunol Rev 2005; 204: 55–73.

25. Michou L, Croiseau P, Petit-Teixeira E, et al. Validation of the reshaped shared epitope HLA-DRB1 classification in rheumatoid arthritis. Arthritis Res Ther 2006; 8: R79.

26. Ollier W, Winchester R. The germline and genetic somatic basis for rheumatoid arthritis. Curr Dir Autoimmun 1999; 1: 166–193.

27. Gruen JR, Weissman SM. Human MHC class III and IV genes and disease associations. Front Biosci 2001; 6: D960–D972.

28. Horton R, Wilming L, Rand V, et al. Gene map of the extended human MHC. Nat Rev Genet 2004; 5: 889–899.

29. Ehlers A, Beck S, Forbes SA, et al. MHC-linked olfactory receptor loci exhibit polymorphism and contribute to extended HLA/OR-haplotypes. Genome Res 2000; 10: 1968–1978.

Antigens and antigen processing

John R. Rodgers, Robert R. Rich

A century ago the composite word 'antigen' referred to 'that which generates antibodies'. This tautology developed before the concept of a 'receptor', before the definition of macromolecular proteins, before a kinetic theory of binding specificity, and before it was known that antibodies actually bind to antigens. The antigen–antibody tautology remains central to our concepts of immunity and to the the tautology of 'self' and 'non-self'.

At a molecular level, an 'antigen' can be defined today as any molecule recognized by (i.e., binding specifically to) the antigen-binding domain of an 'antigen receptor' (antibody or T-cell receptor – TCR) (Fig. 6.1). The antigen bound by a particular antigen receptor is sometimes called its *cognate antigen*. The concept of a cognate antigen is useful when identifying the molecular rules governing antigen–antigen receptor

Fig. 6.1 Two definitions of antigen. Epitopes form the complementary molecular surfaces that engage the antigen-binding sites of clonally selected antibodies or T-cell receptors. Complete antigens or immunogens for B cells also carry T-cell epitopes. These must be released by antigen processing for presentation by major histocompatibility complex (MHC) molecules. In this model, the APC is a B cell expressing its own membrane-bound immunoglobulin. A dendritic cell would acquire antigen–antibody immune complexes through the binding of the antibody to an Fc receptor.

interactions, for predicting antigens from sequence and structural information, for designing subunit and genetic vaccines, and for understanding what the immunologist means by such terms as 'self' and 'nonself'.

Because the definition of antigen remains tautological; it requires us to know in advance what antigen receptors are, even though they must ultimately be defined as 'those structures that bind and distinguish among different antigens'. At the biologic level it is sufficient to appreciate that if an organism has already generated antibodies or TCR specific for the antigen, that antigen may be identified by means of an assay appropriate for study of the binding interaction between the two entities.

This definition begs the question of why some molecules, albeit in principle capable of binding one or more antigen receptors, do not *generate* antigens in a given organism. Three factors impinge on this functional definition. The first concerns mechanisms that affect the structure and conformation of the antigen: antigen processing (covered in this chapter) and antigen presentation (Chapter 7). The second category includes mechanisms of tolerance that delete or inactivate antigen receptors – for according to the molecular tautology mentioned above, an antigen that has no 'cognate' antigen receptor in some specific context does not function as an antigen, even if it possesses the requisite structural properties. Finally, we must consider those factors that allow the clonal expansion and functional expression of antigen receptors – that is, those permissive factors that allow an individual to express functionally an acquired immune response to the antigen.

It will require much of the rest of this book to explore these functional categories. Still, special terms make the practical distinctions required by the two kinds of definition. Thus, 'hapten', 'epitope', and 'determinant' are terms that refer to the structural definition of a cognate antigen. When a structure lacks the permissive factors required to stimulate the production of cognate antigen receptors, we call this an 'incomplete antigen'. Antigens that actually *induce* immune responses are called 'immunogens' or 'complete antigens'.

Antigens recognized by antibodies are chiefly recognized directly, in their macromolecular form, whenever the macromolecular conformation allows epitopes to be exposed on the molecular surface. In contrast, antigens recognized by T-cell receptors are acquired by an antigen-presenting cell in a macromolecular form, but are then *processed* into epitopes.

In the remainder of this chapter we discuss, first, the biochemical aspects of antigens recognized by antibodies and TCR, and second, the biochemical processing steps that convert large molecules into structures that bind antigen receptors. At a functional level, this chapter will deal with only one key aspect of complete antigens: the need for more than one epitope per antigen. For example, most antigens for antibodies are not *immunogenic* unless they also contain epitopes for helper T cells. Important exceptions to this generalization are the 'T-independent' antigens, described below, which either receive a separate signal through a conserved pattern recognition receptor or contain two or more repeating epitopes. Additionally, molecules that bind TCR are not immunogenic unless the T cell is activated. Thus, a B-cell response to a cognate antigen requires accessory or helper T antigens, which themselves are not cognate with the B-cell receptor (antibody). The equivalent cognate antigens for T cells are generated by *antigen processing*. Still, most potential immunogens for T cells will not be immunostimulatory unless accompanied by *adjuvants* that help activate *antigen-presenting cells*, such as dendritic cells.

ANTIGENS AS LIGANDS FOR ANTIBODIES

Using appropriate carriers and adjuvants, antibodies can be raised *in vivo* against almost any chemical moiety.[1] Ligands include naturally occurring proteins, lipids, steroids, sugars and nucleic acids, as well as synthetic compounds. Here the only limitation appears to be that it is difficult to raise antibodies against molecules to which the immune system has become tolerant – especially 'self' molecules expressed extracellularly. Nevertheless, it is often possible to trick the immune system into generating autoreactive antibodies, and many of these arise in autoimmune reactions. Similarly, bacteriophage libraries of recombinant antibodies (*phage display libraries*) can be screened for almost any chemical specificity without regard for self/nonself discrimination.

Haptens (from a Greek word meaning 'to hold') are the smallest molecular structures with sufficient molecular complementarity to bind antibodies, and are thus the smallest compound for which enzyme-linked immunosorbent assays (ELISA) or radioimmunoassays (RIA) can be devised. A classic example is the chemical moiety dinitrophenol (DNP), which consists of a hydrophobic aromatic ring with three polar side chains. A modern example of a hapten of great use to basic researchers is phosphotyrosine, a moiety found on many proteins subject to regulation. Haptens are too small to be complete antigens. Therefore, in order to raise hapten-specific antibodies, the moiety is chemically coupled to a

highly immunogenic carrier protein that contains a large number of epitopes for B and T cells. Immunization of animals with haptenated carriers stimulates a polyclonal antibody response that contains mostly antibodies specific for carrier epitopes not related to the hapten, as well as a useful subset with specificity for the hapten itself.

There is no obvious upper limit to the size of an antigen. For example, antibodies are routinely used to tag mammalian cells for flow cytometry in the laboratory, or to opsonize bacteria *in vivo*. Thus we can use 'antigen' loosely to refer to complex structures (virus particles, entire cells) or mixtures (tumor or mycobacterial extracts). More typically, we conceive of antigens as specific macromolecules – hence the entire cluster of differentiation (CD) nomenclature for the definition of cell-surface molecules.

Such structures or mixtures actually contain many different cognate molecular structures that bind distinct antigen receptors. Jerne[2] coined the useful term 'epitope' to refer to that part of the antigen that forms direct molecular contacts with the antigen-binding site of the antibody. We also use 'epitope' to refer to that part of an antigen peptide that engages the TCR, including those residues that primarily engage the major histocompatibility molecule (Fig. 6.1). Epitopes thus tend to be subsets of the complete antigen. In Jerne's system, 'haptens' are a subset of epitopes and thus can be even smaller than a typical epitope. The antigen-binding site of antipolysaccharide antibodies holds up to six sugar residues; antipeptide antibodies accommodate up to four amino acids; somewhat larger epitopes can be recognized on native protein antigens. The epitopes recognized by TCR are about the same size – typically peptides of a dozen or fewer amino acids.

Antibodies can bind antigens both in solution and independently of any other molecule. This property differentiates antigens for antibodies from those typically recognized by TCR, which instead recognize their epitopes bound to major histocompatibility complex (MHC) molecules (Chapter 5). The majority of protein epitopes, however, do depend on the conformation of a peptide or group of peptides within the three-dimensional structure of a folded protein.[3] These are termed *conformational* epitopes. These may vanish if a protein enters a different allosteric state or is denatured, as in most Western blot assays. A major subset of such epitopes are *discontinuous* epitopes. These are composed of noncontiguous amino acids or very short oligopeptides that are brought into close proximity in the native three-dimensional form of the protein. As a result, most epitopes of native proteins are located in exterior loops and can be predicted by a variety of structure-prediction strategies.[4] In contrast, the epitopes that are detected by Western blotting are typically neither conformational nor discontinuous: they are comprised of haptens or of a continuous or 'linear' sequence of amino acids that is not structurally disrupted by the denaturing conditions of the assay. Similarly, epitopes bound by TCR are short linear peptides within the antigen-binding cleft of an MHC molecule.

Neutralizing antibodies inactivate the activity of toxins, pathogens, enzymes or other proteins. The 'inhibitory' antibodies produced by many hemophilia patients receiving clotting factor replacement therapy are of this type. Neutralizing epitopes on virus particles may represent a transition state or otherwise altered conformation stabilized by the antibody that results in noninfectious viral particles. 'Neutralizing' antibodies in other cases refer to those that fix complement and destroy virus infectivity by physical destruction of membrane-enclosed viruses.

Not all antibodies that bind to a pathogen are strictly neutralizing. For example, most antibodies specific for the HIV gp120 envelope protein are not neutralizing, and some even facilitate the uptake of virus

---

KEY CONCEPTS

ANTIGENS FOR B CELLS

>> Immunogens contain

   Epitopes that bind to the antigen-binding sites of antibodies

   Class II epitopes for T helper cells.

>> Haptens can have almost any chemical nature.

>> Epitopes on native proteins can be discontinuous segments of amino acids at the cell surface.

into vulnerable cells such as monocytes. Nonetheless, nonneutralizing antibodies can still block function. For example, anti-insulin receptor antibodies can prevent insulin from gaining access to its receptors. Other antibodies probably block function by clearing ligands. For example, many hepatitis C patients receiving interferon therapy develop anti-interferon antibodies that clear therapeutic interferon from the bloodstream. Immunization with partially denatured proteins or with synthetic proteins may elicit antibodies recognizing epitopes that are independent of a rigid conformation. Such *nonconformation-dependent* antibodies are useful, especially in Western blot assays. This is the basis of the widely used assay for HIV infection.

ANTICARBOHYDRATE ANTIBODIES

T-independent (TI) antigens are typically polysaccharides with the ability to induce B-cell proliferation and antibody secretion *in the absence of T cells*. At relatively high doses, TI-1 antigens, typified by lipopolysaccharide (LPS or endotoxin), stimulate polyclonal proliferation of B cells, in part by activating toll-like receptor TLR-4 and its MyD88-dependent signaling pathway (Chapter 3). At lower doses TI-1 antigens stimulate the division of B cells that secrete antigen specific antibodies. This probably reflects cross-linking surface antibodies by such polyvalent antigens.

TI-2 antigens behave much as do TI-1 antigens at low doses. They include pneumococcal capsular polysaccharides and are probably effective by virtue of their repeating structure: polyvalent antigens can more easily cross-link the B-cell receptor to induce proliferative signals. Consistent with this interpretation, TI-2 antigens stimulate antigen-specific responses in athymic mice but, unlike TI-1 antigens, do not stimulate polyclonal proliferation at high doses.

A classic example of anticarbohydrate immune responses is provided by the human ABO 'blood group' system of antigens, which are expressed in many tissues of the body and by many kinds of bacteria.[5] The polymorphic *ABO* locus encodes a glycosyltransferase that functions as a haptenating enzyme in this system. The common *O* allele is functionally silent. Both active enzymes (alleles *A* and *B*) transfer a uridylate diphosphate (UDP)-charged sugar to glycoproteins and glycolipids. The *A* and *B* enzymes use UDP-*N*-acetyl-galactosamine and UDP-galactose, respectively, as sugar donors.

Individuals expressing the *A* and/or *B* alloenzymes express *A* and/or *B*-type carbohydrates as self-antigens, and are thus tolerant to them. In contrast, *O*-type individuals cannot make *A* or *B* antigens. As a result, *O individuals are intolerant to these antigens*. Thus exposure to common bacteria induces both anti-*A* and anti-*B* antibodies in *O*-type individuals. Their own blood does not contain either antigen, however, and so they are universal donors. *A* and *B* individuals may not donate blood to an *O* individual, because their donated erythrocytes are rapidly lysed by the recipient's anti-*A* or -*B* antibodies through a complement-mediated mechanism. The anti-*A* and anti-*B* antibodies of a type *O* donor could react with recipient erthrocytes but are are rapidly cleared by absorption by the other antigen-expressing cell types in the recipient.

Interestingly, the nature of antibody responses to T-independent antigens can provide an insight into important roles of T cells in conventional (T-dependent) antibody responses. For example, T-independent responses generally do not exhibit immunological memory and do not undergo isotype switching with maturation of the response (i.e., antibody responses are of the IgM class), consistent with the known requirement for T-cell help in these features of a typical T-dependent response.

With the exception of the 'T-independent antigens', antigens for antibodies are limited to those that can be coexpressed with antigens for T cells. Without T-cell help, B cells will not respond to antigen stimulation and might be tolerized. As suggested by the absence of classic immunologic memory in T independent antibody responses, strong secondary T-dependent antibody responses also require that B cells present antigen to T cells, leading to the requirement for T–B interactions. B cells capture *carrier* antigens attached by their hapten-specific antibodies, and then endocytose, process and present them to T cells. The B and T epitopes present in a vaccine do not need to derive from same targeted pathogen. For example, a 'multiantigenic peptide' vaccine might include a strong T-cell epitope for tetanus and an antibody epitope for HIV. Such a vaccine couples a primary response to the HIV epitope with a secondary response to tetanus.

■ ANTIGENS AS LIGANDS FOR T-CELL RECEPTORS[6] ■

The biochemical definition of antigen indicates that epitopes recognized by TCR should bind directly to them. This is true in some cases, but the affinity of these interactions is usually too weak. Instead, epitopes recognized by T cells are recognized in the molecular context of major histocompatibility complex (MHC) molecules (Chapter 5). This means that such epitopes have two receptors: the MHC molecule, which binds with high affinity, and the TCR, which recognizes the molecular complex of MHC and epitope. Historically, MHC class I and class II molecules were themselves viewed as antigens. 'Major histocompatibility' or 'transplantation' antigens elicit robust antibody responses as well as strong T cell-mediated alloreactions in mixed leukocyte cultures and tissue transplants. As antigens for antibodies, they behave as conventional protein antigens; it is their ability to stimulate T cells that makes them potent in transplant situations.

MHC molecules typically bind short peptides. The short length of epitopes for MHC class I molecules is enforced by a closed-ended binding cleft that binds both amino and carboxyl termini (Fig. 6.2). In contrast, both ends of the binding cleft of class II MHC molecules are open, allowing longer peptides to bind. Because the ends of these peptides are usually degraded before presentation to T cells, most epitopes for class II molecules are still short – of the order of 15–20 amino acids.

The binding cleft of both class I and class II molecules also interacts with the peptide backbone and two or three of the side chains. The latter are considered *anchor* residues of the epitope and define the *binding motif* of the MHC molecule. Amino acid side chains not used as anchors are potentially available for binding the TCR.

The need for terminal anchoring severely limits the length of epitopes for class I MHC molecules to seven to ten amino acids, though longer peptides can sometimes bind by looping out central residues. In general, the efficacy of a peptide as an epitope correlates with its binding strength. Adding or removing a single amino acid to either end of an 'optimal' peptide often effectively destroys the epitope. As a result, the proteolytic processing pathway (see below) can be very important in generating optimal epitopes from proteins. It is possible for proteins to contain peptide sequences that in their free state bind optimally to MHC molecules, but which are not converted into epitopes *in vivo*.

Antigen recognition by T cells is *MHC restricted* (Chapters 5 and 7). MHC restriction reflects molecular and genetic mechanisms and is explained by the requirement that epitopes for T cells are presented by

MHC molecules. The fact that MHC molecules are highly polymorphic, especially in the sequence positions involved in epitope and TCR contacts, means that antigen recognition by T cells is genetically restricted to only those MHC genotypes expressing the same (*syngeneic*) MHC molecules as the responder. For example, the human class I MHC molecules HLA-A31 and HLA-Aw68 are allelic forms of the same molecule. Both present the same peptide (amino acids 141–151) derived from the core antigen of hepatitis B virus. T-cell clones from an HLA-A31/Aw68 heterozygous patient that recognize this epitope bound to HLA-A31 cannot recognize the same peptide when it is presented by HLA-Aw68 (and vice versa). Such clones are described as HLA-A31 restricted and HLA-Aw68 restricted, respectively.

A given allelic form of MHC molecules recognizes two or three anchor residues with high specificity, severely limiting the 'universe' of peptides that it can present to T cells. Two different MHC alleles thus may see radically distinct antigenic universes. The high polymorphism of MHC molecules has three implications for responses to pathogens and vaccines. First, most individuals are heterozygous for each MHC locus, effectively doubling the size of their antigenic universe. Second, although some individuals may be unable to respond to certain pathogens, some are likely to be protected. This may account for the prevalence of certan MHC haplotypes in populations exposed to malaria, and for genetic vulnerabilities or resistance to HIV/AIDS. Finally, epitopes detected by one individual may be invisible to the T cells of another; subunit vaccines effective for some MHC haplotypes may be ineffective for others. For example, the hepatitis B surface antigen subunit vaccine is often ineffective in individuals homozygous for certain *HLA* haplotypes.

How can we rationalize the operation of MHC restriction? Why do T cells not recognize their antigens as do B cells, with no need for antigen presentation? Because alloreactive T cells distinguish between self and nonself MHC molecules, it is tempting to think that MHC restriction mediates self/nonself discrimination. However, it is clear that allospecific antibodies also distinguish self from nonself MHC molecules. MHC

restriction may function in two opposing ways (Fig. 6.3). First, antigen-processing increases the complexity of pathogen antigens by exposing epitopes not available on the surface of pathogens. MHC molecules are 'merely' the mechanism for presenting processed epitopes to T cells. MHC polymorphism further increases the size of the species' antigenic universe. Second, the requirement that T cells do not respond unless activated by co-stimulation from the APC is enforced by anchoring MHC molecules on the APC. This second mechanism thus minimizes autoimmunity. In this view, the experimental observations of genetic MHC restriction and alloreactivity are by-products of the polymorphism of MHC molecules.

Ligands for MHC molecules are usually oligopeptides, but there are notable exceptions. In particular, the class I-like molecule CD1 presents certain lipids, such as are found in mycobacteria. Even conventional oligopeptide epitopes may include modified amino acids such as phospho-serine or sugar residues. Chemically modified self-peptides are major determinants of allergic responses to nonprotein environmental agents, such as metals, cosmetics and antibiotics. Mediators of these responses

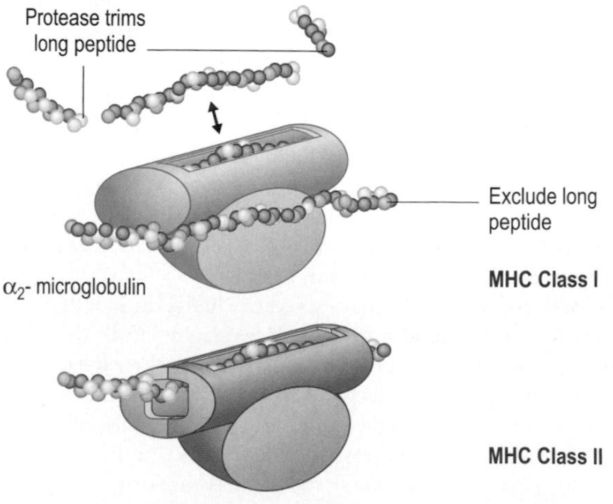

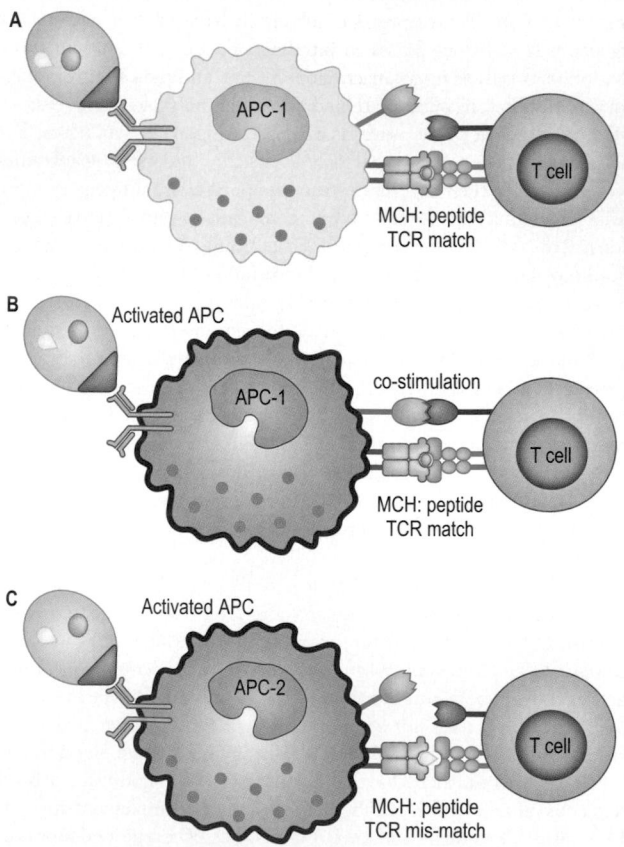

Fig. 6.3 MHC restriction carries out two critical functions. First, by presenting processed peptides derived from within proteins and pathogens, MHC molecules sample a broader antigenic landscape than antibodies, whose epitopes are surface oriented. Second, naive T cells respond to cognate epitopes only when presented by an activated APC (B) but not when the APC is resting (A). Experimentally observed MHC restriction results when an activated APC cannot present the proper MHC/peptide pair (C).

Fig. 6.2 Peptide binding by MHC class I and II molecules. Class I molecules are usually closed at both ends. The peptide termini must interact with terminal sockets. Peptides that are too long must be cleaved (arrows) prior to entry into the binding site. The clefts of class II molecules are open at the ends, permitting the binding of long peptides.

may be effector T cells, as in cell-mediated contact sensitization, or helper-T cells, as in induction of allergic antibodies.

An important clinical example is the allergic response to penicillin and other β-lactam-based antibiotics (Fig. 6.4). The β-lactam ring can cross-link itself to a patient's own proteins, thereby creating a novel set of potential epitopes. For example, human serum albumin forms adducts with β-lactams at several different lysine residues and at least one serine residue. Penicillin adducts become haptens for antibody responses, but modified peptide epitopes can be presented by MHC class I molecules to CD8 T cells and by MHC class II molecules to CD4 T cells.

SUPERANTIGENS[7,8]

'Superantigens' are protein antigen-like molecules produced by a diverse array of microbes that interact with MHC class II molecules and TCR in a manner that dramatically increases the frequency of T-cell responses compared to conventional peptide antigens. They include certain bacterial toxins (e.g., staphyloccal enterotoxin A (SEA) and toxic shock syndrome toxin (TSST)) and viral proteins (e.g., mouse mammary tumor virus superantigen). Superantigens are not processed intracellularly. Instead, they bind class II MHC molecules as intact macromolecules and bind outside the peptide–antigen-binding groove. Class II binding is independent of the specific MHC allele (albeit often with a preference for one or more of the major isotypes:

DR, DQ or DP). Each superantigen/class II complex binds TCR bearing a characteristic subset of Vβ families, thereby selectively activating T-cell clones with those TCR. By stimulating large numbers of clones of a specific Vβ family, superantigens can induce an overwhelming T-cell response with a massive release of cytokines. This can lead to such clinical conditions as staphylococcal food poisoning and toxic shock syndrome (Fig. 6.5).

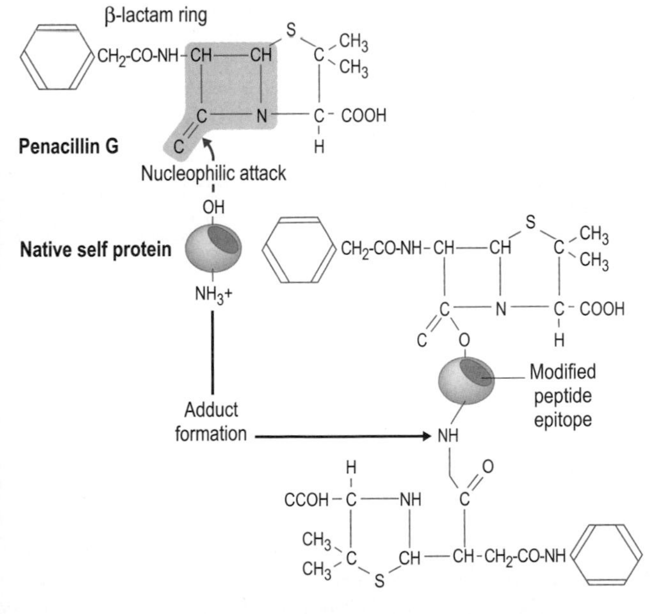

ANTIGEN PROCESSING FOR CLASS I-RESTRICTED T CELLS[9–11]

T cells recognize their cognate antigens in the form of short peptides embedded in MHC molecules. X-ray crystallography shows that roughly 90% of the molecular surface recognized by the TCR is the MHC

Fig. 6.4 Sensitizing agents create neoantigens by forming covalent adducts with self-proteins. Penicillin allergies involve both antibodies against penicillin and with T-cell responses to penicillin-modified self-proteins. The same chemical reaction that allows penicillin to inhibit peptidoglycan formation in bacteria leads to adduct formation of cellular proteins. Nucleophilic attack by penicillin G (upper left) on the β-lactam ring (shaded) opens the ring and creates an adduct (lower left) with a protein serines (shown) and lysines. The lactam adducts can be presented to B cells as modified self-proteins or processed for presentation by MHC molecules to T cells as lactam-conjugated self-peptides.

ANTIGENS AS LIGANDS FOR T-CELL RECEPTORS

95

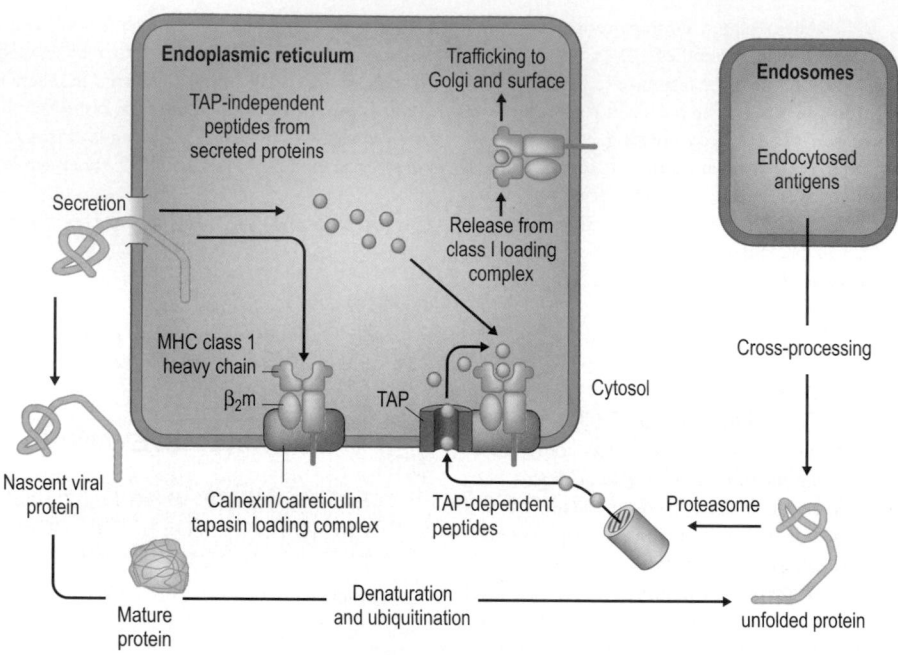

Fig. 6.5 Antigen processing for MHC class I. Two chief pathways for antigen process intersect within the cytosol. Most endogenous antigens are synthesized on cytosolic ribosomes, processed by proteasomes, and enter the ER through the TAP transporter. A minor set of antigens are processed within the ER from proteins secreted into the ER. Professional antigen-presenting cells transfer endocytosed antigens into the cytosol for processing.

molecule. *Antigen processing* excises these peptides from their parent protein antigens and loads them onto MHC molecules. It is often said that antigens presented by class I MHC molecules are necessarily endogenous, that is, synthesized by the cells that presented them, whereas class II molecules uniquely present exogenous antigens. This makes sense functionally, because CD8 cytotoxic T lymphocytes (CTL) are class I restricted and need to distinguish virus-infected cells (expressing endogenously synthesized viral antigens) from protective phagocytes such as macrophages. In contrast, CD4 T-helper cells are not usually cytolytic, but need to recognize antigens from bacteria phagocytosed by macrophages.

Although this scenario is useful in a conceptual sense, in practice it is too simplistic. For example, virus-specific CTL are primarily activated by cells – chiefly dendritic cells – that are not themselves infected. A variety of mechanisms known as cross-presentation can be used to process endocytosed antigens, including bacteria and apoptotic infected cells, for presentation on class I molecules.[12]

Endogenous peptides presented by class I molecules derive from proteins made on the cell's own ribosomes.[13] The chief mechanism for degrading large proteins into small peptides is the *proteasome*, a macromolecular tubular structure containing multiple protease activities that cleaves proteins into small fragments of eight to 14 residues.[14,15] There are at least four mechanisms that feed proteins into proteasomes. First, nascent cyoplasmic polypeptides that fail to fold properly – and most do not – are attacked by enzymes that attach chains of the protein ubiquitin to the protein targeted for destruction. Second, nascent proteins that are translocated into the endoplasmic reticulum endosome but fail to fold properly can be exported back to the cytosol by a protein transporter called Sec61.[16] Third, properly folded mature proteins are ubiquitinated in the course of normal activity – part of

ANTIGEN PROCESSING AND PRESENTATION FOR CLASS I MHC

>> Peptides presented on most cell types are synthesized endogenously.

>> Peptides acquired through endocytosis by professional APC can be cross-presented.

>> Most epitopes are processed by proteasomes and enter the ER through the TAP transporter.

>> Peptides of 8–10 amino acids are bound at both termini within the binding cleft.

the normal course of protein turnover. Finally, in cross-presentation, proteins engulfed by phagocytes are partially degraded in lysosomes before transfer – through poorly understood mechanisms – into the cytosol.

Proteasomes preferentially cleave proteins after amino acids with acidic side chains (glutamine; aspartamine). However, interferon-γ (IFN-γ) induces the expression of two additional proteasome subunits, the MHC-encoded low molecular weight proteins (LMP). Exchange of the LMP subunits into proteasomes shifts the cleavage pattern towards peptides terminating in basic or hydrophobic residues, which are favored by many class I MHC molecules.[14,15] This may be one subtle mechanism by which the immune system can distinguish between self-peptides, which are generated constitutively by proteasomes, and peptides associated with inflammation, which are generated by LMP-containing proteasomes.

Proteasomal digestion products are in turn recognized by the transporter associated with antigen processing (TAP), a member of the ATP-binding cassette (ABC) transporter family of proteins that includes the multidrug resistance protein and CFTR – the cystic fibrosis transmembrane regulator.

Heterodimers of TAP1 and TAP2 subunits form peptide pumps that burn ATP to drive peptides from the cytosol into the lumen of the endoplasmic reticulum (ER). Patients lacking either subunit of TAP cannot process most MHC class I-binding peptides. Without a ready source of peptides in the ER, class I MHC molecules are themselves unstable and are extruded into the cytosol by Sec61 for proteasomal degradation. TAP mutations are involved in many cases of type I bare lymphocyte syndrome (BLS) (Chapter 35) and many tumor cells lack class I expression owing to mutations in their TAP genes (Chapter 81).

TAP transports peptides ranging in size between six and 20 residues. Several allelic forms exist in humans. The TAP1A and 1C alleles prefer peptides with a basic residue at the carboxyl terminus (a form that is *not* preferentially generated by proteasomes), whereas the TAP1B allele shows no such preference.[17] Few of dozens of studies have found any significant associations between human diseases and TAP alleles, leaving the physiological significance of these allelic forms unresolved.[18]

A minor subset of peptides enter the ER independently of TAP through the protein secretory pathway. Nascent polypeptides bearing a signal peptide are recognized and transported into the lumen by the signal recognition particle (SRP). The signal peptide itself is cleaved by a signal peptidase. By inserting the sequence of a CTL epitope behind a signal peptide, this pathway can be used to deliver the epitope directly into the MHC class I loading compartment. Peptides that are too long to bind MHC class I molecules may be retained temporarily in the ER by additional peptide-binding proteins such as BiP, pumped back into the cytosol by an undefined non-TAP mechanism, or trimmed by aminopeptidases (also present in the cytosol) to a size that can bind MHC molecules.[19] One of these, leucine aminopeptidase (LAP), is also induced by IFN-γ.[20]

The luminal proteases appear quite efficient, apparently reducing the steady-state concentration of free antigenic peptides in the ER to very low levels. As a result of differences in protease specificities and/or kinetic effects, different epitopes may be carved out of the same protein, depending on whether it follows the proteasome/TAP or the secretory pathway into the ER. Finally, different peptides within a single protein may be degraded or protected at different rates, leading to immunodominance of a subset of potential epitopes for a given MHC molecule.

The production of an immunodominant epitope from influenza A nucleoprotein (NP) illustrates how extra-epitope residues might affect nonproteasome, nonubiquitin processing.[21] The optimal NP peptide in one mouse strain is the nonamer TYQRTRALV. The three C-terminal residues are efficiently removed from a related 12-mer peptide TYQRTRALVRTG. However, an 11-mer, TYQRTRALVTG, is impotent at producing the epitope. The terminal TG sequence represents a 'block' to epitope production. All of these complexities in antigen processing make it difficult at present to predict which potential epitopes, identified on the basis of their ability to bind to class I molecules, will be immunodominant *in vivo*.

CLASS I MHC TRAFFICKING

Nascent class I MHC molecules are inserted into the ER membrane via the protein secretory pathway. Nascent chains bind first to the membrane-bound chaperone calnexin until they begin to fold into association with β2-microglobulin light chains (β2m). Heterodimers of β2m and heavy chain are released by calnexin and bind the soluble chaperone calreticulin. This assembly engages a *class I loading complex*, which includes a 60 kDa thiol reductase, the TAP heterodimer and another MHC-encoded protein, tapasin.[22] Tapasin retains class I molecules in the complex until they bind peptide. MHC molecules failing to attract peptides misfold and are exported by Sec61 to the cytosol. Only those that bind peptide are released by tapasin from the loading complex. They migrate to the Golgi, where they undergo glycan maturation, and then traffic to the cell surface for recognition by CD8 T cells.

The noncanonical antigen processing pathway for MHC class I molecules

Noncanonical pathways for acquiring and processing exogenous antigens are very important for initiating MHC class I-restricted responses, a process mediated by 'professional' antigen-presenting cells (APC) that might not themselves synthesize viral or tumor antigens. The acquisition of such exogenous antigens leads to cross-presentation by APC and cross-priming of T cells.

Cross-presentation of class I-restricted peptides can also inhibit immune responses. For example, antigen-specific B cells endocytose their specific antigens, which they then process for presentation by their own MHC class I molecules. When this happens, antigen-specific B cells may be attacked by CTL. In this way, CTL can suppress B-cell responses to some antigens.

B cells can be extremely efficient as APC in stimulating both CD4 and CD8 T-cell 4responses to their cognate antigens, while ignoring other antigens. However, in the general case they are vastly surpassed by dendritic cells and, to a lesser extent, by macrophages. A critical difference between these cell types is that whereas B cells internalize their own surface immunoglobulins and the antigens attached to them, they endocytose their own Fc receptors inefficiently, and B cells are nonphagocytic. In contrast, DC and macrophages are phagocytic and efficiently endocytose through Fc and other surface receptors.

Receptor-mediated endocytosis probably accounts for the ability of oligopeptide-binding chaperone proteins (chaperonins) to prime class I-restricted antigen responses to antigens. Heat shock proteins gp60, hsp70, hsp90 and gp96 derived from tumors or virus-infected cells elicit peptide-specific CTL responses. These proteins have been proposed as the the basis of experimental vaccines.[23] Whether this pathway for transferring peptides from dying cells is important physiologically is controversial. An alternative mechanism focuses on the relase of whole proteins from dying cells. These released proteins can be endocytosed by APC. Other mechanisms of cross-presentation include the engulfment of apoptotic and/or 'necrotic' cells, or the endocytosis of apoptotic bodies and 'exosomes.'

All of these mechanisms lead to the uptake of antigens into the endosomes of APC. Although endosomal uptake is sufficient for MHC class II molecules, which are loaded in endosomal subcompartments themselves, antigens cross-presented by class I molecules must still enter the ER through TAP after transfer from the endosomes into the cytosol.

ANTIGEN PROCESSING FOR CLASS II-RESTRICTED T CELLS (FIG. 6.6)[24–26]

Antigens presented by MHC class II molecules come from two main sources, autophagy[27] of endogenous antigens, and endocytosis of both exogenous and cell surface (endogenous) antigens. Autophagocytosis is the engulfment by lysosomes of internal organelles, including mitochondria and endoplasmic reticulum. It is an active process in all cell types.

MHC class II molecules assemble in the ER, where they associate with *invariant* chain, a 31 Da chaperonin specific for MHC molecules. Invariant chain chaperones nascent αβ dimers of class II molecules into endosomes. A segment of this chain, called CLIP, blocks class II molecules from binding peptides in the ER. Once in the endosomes, CLIP may be removed along with the rest of invariant chain. Alternatively, a CLIP fragment may be left occupying the binding cleft. Many class II MHC molecules traffic to the cell surface with CLIP embedded.

In the absence of infection, MHC class II molecules are loaded with peptides derived from cellular self-proteins. Macrophages and dendritic cells acquire exogenous antigens through endocytosis (Fig. 6.6). Many surface molecules, such as HIV gp120 protein, are endocytosed through clathrin-coated pits. In *receptor-mediated endocytosis*, surface receptors (such as Fc receptors) drag their ligands (antigen–antibody complexes) into the cell. Very large particles, such as bacteria and opsonized viruses and apoptotic bodies, are phagocytosed. The large phagosome fuses with lysosomes, in which bacteria are killed and fragmented before antigen processing can take place.

Regardless of how they reach the endosomes, protein antigens are unfolded and partially degraded in endosomal and acidic lysosomal subcompartments by disulfide isomerase (which unlinks disulfide loops) and a variety of proteases. Most peptides presented by class II molecules are processed from parent proteins and loaded on to class II molecules within a specialized loading compartment of the endosome. Within this general scheme there at least two pathways for epitope production. These are distinguishable, in part, by their dependence on the function of DM molecules, which are heterodimers of composed of DMA and DMB subunits each of which is phylogenetically related to MHC class II proteins.[28] DM catalyze the exchange of CLIP for processed epitopes. Alternatively, in the

---

> **KEY CONCEPTS**

ANTIGEN PROCESSIN G FOR CLASS II MHC

>> Class II MHC expressed constitutively only by professional APC (dendritic cells, macrophages and B cells).

>> Epitopes presented by professional APC are acquired mostly through endocytosis and autophagocytosis.

>> Peptides (10–15 amino acids) often have terminal extensions, extending outside the antigen-binding groove.

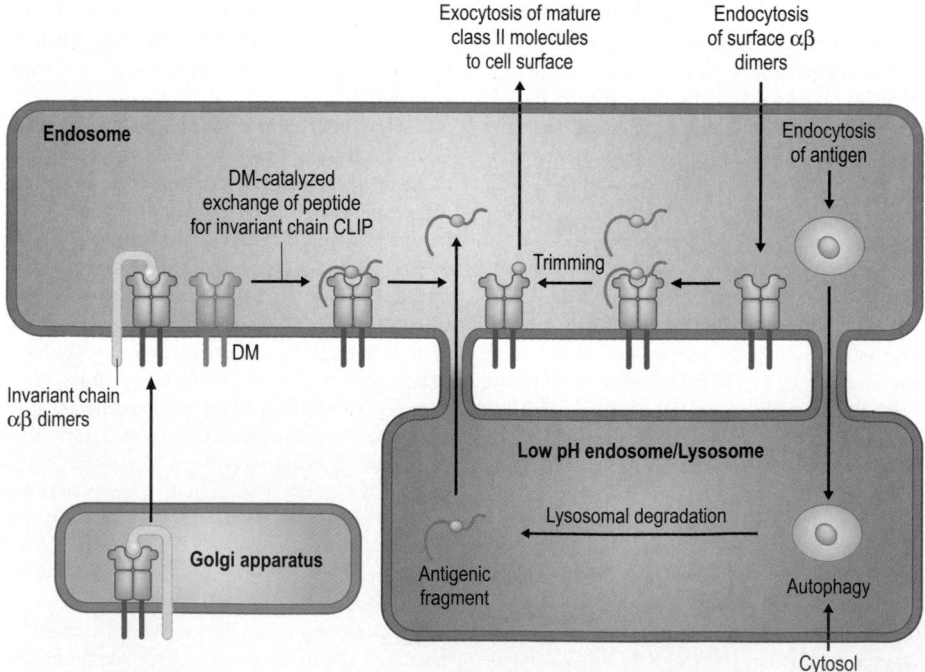

Fig. 6.6 Two pathways for loading antigens onto class II MHC molecules. Autophagy and endocytosis transfer cytosolic and external antigens, respectively, into the endosomes. Nascent class II molecules are chaperoned to the endosomes from the Golgi by the invariant chain. The DM molecules catalyze the exchange of antigenic peptides for invariant chain. Mature class II molecules recycling from the cell surface can acquire peptides in a DM-independent manner. Antigens binding initially as polypeptides are trimmed into oligopeptides in the endosomes and at the surface.

DM-independent pathway peptides are loaded on to class II molecules recycling from the cell surface in the absence of CLIP.

The initial ligand for binding class II molecules is a large unfolded protein or protein fragment, rather than the oligopeptide ultimately displayed at the cell surface. This MHC–polypeptide complex is the substrate for trimming exopeptidases. Prolines are found near the N terminus of many mature epitopes, and the endosomal aminopeptidases cannot cleave at these proline residues. Trimming of the extra-cleft residues can continue even after the MHC–peptide complex has reached the surface through the activity of the membrane-bound surface enzyme aminopeptidase N (CD13).

As in the case of epitope formation for class I molecules, the initial conformation of the antigen can affect the production of specific linear epitopes. For example, vaccinating mice with synthetic peptides elicits class II-restricted T cells specific for at least two HIV gp160 epitopes. However, only one is detected on infected cells. Similarly, prior denaturation or mutational destabilization of viral influenza hemagglutinin abolishes its ability to be processed for presentation to some T-helper cell clones.

PREDICTING EPITOPES FOR TCR

The critical role of T cell antigens in driving both T- and B-cell responses has fueled attempts to use antigen sequence information to predict T-cell epitopes.

The characterization of *binding motifs* for a large number of class I and a smaller number of class II molecules has facilitated computer-based algorithms for predicting potential epitopes from linear protein sequences. These motifs reflect the chemical affinity of the binding cleft for various amino acid side chains. In many cases it is possible to show that several alleles of class I or class II molecules recognize the same or very closely related epitopes. These groups of MHC alleles are called 'supertypes' and can permit the prediction of epitopes for a large number of alleles.[29,30] However, because of the complexity of endoprotease and exoprotease cleavage during processing of epitopes for both class I and class II MHC molecules, it is difficult to predict whether a given epitope will actually be used *in vivo*.

Because MHC-binding peptides are linear fragments, one might not expect them to coincide with discontinuous and/or surface epitopes detected by antibodies. This is often true, but one notable exception to this statement is the V3 loop of HIV gp120, which exhibits immunodominant epitopes for neutralizing antibodies overlapping with immunodominant Th epitopes. Such observations are consistent with the idea that antibodies can focus the degradative machinery on selected peptides. Following receptor-mediated endocytosis of antigen–antibody complexes on specific B cells, peptide fragments bound to the antibody might be protected from degradation or diverted into a particular degradation path that would favor the likelihood of their binding a class II molecule.

Structural features of immunodominant T-cell epitopes may reflect the probability of coinciding with a facilitating B-cell epitope and/or other factors controlling degradation rates. One such correlative feature is the aforementioned presence of proline near the N terminus of a number of class II-binding peptides and the propensity of proline to induce turns in protein structures. In this case the unique chemical structure of proline contributes independently to its propensity to induce turns, and to its resistance to proteolysis. Proximity to the protein surface may allow an epitope to unfold more readily, enabling it to bind class II molecules prior to lysosomal degradation. Earlier observations that many T-cell epitopes contained sequences prone to form helices or that were amphipathic had been interpreted as suggesting that such peptides bound as helices within the MHC cleft. X-ray crystallography showed that peptides actually bind in extended conformations, but helicity and/or amphipathicity may well affect the kinetic pathways of intracellular degradation. Such observations help establish criteria to identify likely T-cell antigens. A major criterion is that epitopes should bear sequence motifs that favor binding to self-MHC molecules. A second criterion points to the need for a kinetically favorable proteolytic pathway allowing the cell to produce the epitope in quantities sufficient to promote a T-cell response. Accurate prediction of epitope processing remains beyond current science.

TISSUE SPECIALIZATION AND REGULATION OF ANTIGEN PROCESSING

Not all cell types are equally proficient at processing antigens (Table 6.1). As should be obvious from the preceding discussions, limiting factors in different cells can include differences in endocytosis and phagocytosis rates; the presence of internalizable surface receptors; the relative efficiency of different pathways of proteolysis in different subcellular compartments; the level of expression of specialized antigen-processing molecules such as TAP, LMP, DM and invariant chain; and the level of expression of different MHC molecules.

Table 6.1 Antigen processing in representative cell types

	Feature	Endothelial cells	B cells	Dendritic cells
MHC class I	Expression Antigen acquisition	Constitutive Endogenous	Constitutive Endogenous exogenous (surface Ig-mediated)	Constitutive, Endogenous Exogenous
MHC Class II	Expression Antigen entry	Inducible Surface recycling autophagy	Constitutive, inducible Surface recycling autophagy Ig-mediated	Immature low Mature high Surface recycling autophagy Ig-mediated endocytosis phagocytosis
FcγRII	Expression/function	None	Not internalized	Internalized

Class I heavy chains, β_2-microglobulin, LMP, and TAP proteins are coordinately expressed in most cell types. Activated lymphocytes express high levels constitutively, whereas fibroblasts and liver cells express intermediate levels. Neurons are almost completely negative for expression of all four. $\alpha\beta$ and γ interferons can increase gene expression of these gene sets in most cell types.

Control of MHC class II expression and its attendant antigen-processing machinery is much more complex. Most cell types do not express MHC class II, DM or invariant chains under any circumstances. Macrophages, immature dendritic cells and B cells express these molecules constitutively at low levels. Upregulation is induced by inflammatory cytokines, especially IFN-γ, in most cells. Inflammatory cytokines, notably tumor necrosis factor-α (TNF-α), can also induce class II molecules and antigen processing in certain otherwise class II-negative cell types, including endothelial cells, dermal fibroblasts, neuronal glial cells and astrocytes. Class II molecules are induced on activated T cells in most species, including the laboratory rat, but notably not in laboratory mice. The ectopic expression of class II molecules and associated self-antigens may play a role in the induction of autoimmunity.

MICROBIAL INTERFERENCE WITH ANTIGEN PROCESSING AND PRESENTATION[31]

Considering the importance of class I-mediated immune responses in antiviral immunity, it is not surprising to find a variety of viral mechanisms for subverting antigen processing. Proteins from several serotypes of human adenovirus, as well as HIV-1 tat protein, inhibit class I MHC transcription. Other viral factors inhibit class I MHC maturation in the ER. Two proteins from human cytomegalovirus (CMV), US2 and US11, destabilize nascent class I molecules in the ER by shunting them into the Sec61 pathway for export into the cytosol before they have a chance to bind peptides.

The CMV US6 and herpes simplex virus ICP47 proteins inhibit TAP function, indirectly starving MHC molecules of peptide. In contrast, the CMV US3 proteins binds class I molecules that have already engaged peptides, but retains them in the ER. To round out these examples, the HIV-1 protein nef binds the intracellular tails of mature class I MHC molecules, targeting them for increased endocytosis and degradation.

■ A CLINICAL CODA ■

If microbes can manipulate specific mechanisms of antigen processing and presentation, it should be obvious that human genetic variation in these pathways should be able to contribute to immune competency or, through deficiency, to immune dysfunction. These may result in specific or global defects in antigen processing and recognition, such as the bare lymphocyte syndrome (BLS) (Chapter 35). Type I BLS involves general loss of class I surface expression, typically the result of mutations in the TAP peptide transporter. Type II BLS reflects loss of class II MHC expression. Defects in any of at least four different transcription factors can cause this disease. In type III BLS, defects in the RFX transcription factor depress expression of both class II MHC molecules and the β_2-microglobulin light chain shared by all class I MHC proteins.

A considerable literature indicates that allergens are unremarkable antigens. Their recognition by B- and T-cell receptors follows all the normal rules of antigen acquisition, processing and presentation. One distinguishing feature of some allergens is the formation of adducts by drugs and environmental compounds, resulting in the formation of neoantigens. Intriguing data suggest that some allergens have intrinsic protease activity that may elicit IgE-dependent allergy.[32]

As with allergens, and as expected from our chemical understanding of antigenicity, autoantigens are chemically unremarkable. The principles that govern pathological self-recognition appear to be the same as for healthy self-tolerance or recognition of foreign antigens: the availability of particular processed peptides at appropriate times for tolerance induction of T-cell activation.

Two nonexclusive models have emerged that may begin to account for why certain individuals are predisposed to autoimmunity and why certain self-antigens are likely to become autoantigens (Chapter 51). The first is the concept of *molecular mimicry*. According to this idea, exposure to sufficient doses of a pathogen-derived epitope that cross-reacts with a previously ignored or *cryptic* self-epitope can break self-tolerance to that epitope. A newer concept in autoantigenicity can explain why many autoantigens are proteins normally found intracellularly, where they are involved in nucleic acid and protein metabolism. These include small nuclear riboproteins, histones and heat-shock proteins. This involves the observation (discussed earlier with regard to cross-presentation) that apoptotic bodies are efficiently recognized by dendritic cells, and that many intranuclear and intracellular antigens are exposed on the extraverted surfaces of apoptotic bodies. Thus it is possible that, by inducing apoptosis, certain predisposing infections may elicit autoimmune reactions to cryptic self-epitopes.

Finally, tumor-specific and tumor-associated antigens are typically self-proteins.[33] In rare human cases, such as a peptide derived from papilloma virus type 16, they can be encoded by tumor viruses. Some tumor antigens, such as carcinoembryonic antigen (CEA), prostate-specific antigen (PSA), or the MAGE proteins of melanomas, are normal proteins that are merely overexpressed by tumor cells. These can serve as diagnostic

■ CLINICAL RELEVANCE

>> The tautological and complementary interactions of antigens and their antigen receptors constitute the recognitive mechanism for both acquired immunity to pathogens and tumors, and autoimmunity towards the 'self'.

>> Human genetic defects in antigen processing pathways result in three types of bare lymphocyte syndrome (BLS).

>> Structural features of certain antigens may predispose them to induction of allergic (IgE) responses by affecting antigen processing.

>> *Molecular mimicry* and exposure of cryptic self-epitopes are mechanisms leading to autoimmunity.

>> Tumor-specific neoantigens can be detected by the immune system, often leading to selection for tumor variants lacking the relevant MHC and/or antigen-processing functions.

Tumor antigens are typically self-proteins that can be:

Products of tumor viruses

Over-expressed normal proteins

Mutated products of oncogenes

Clonally expressed idiotypes of antigen receptors.

markers or as a target for tumor-selective immunity. The antigenic products of mutated tumor suppressor genes and other oncogenes, such as *HER2*, the retinoblastoma protein RB and the breast cancer-associated antigen BRAC, are also called *neoantigens* and are potentially more specific targets for immunotherapy. The neoantigens expressed by these tumors arise as chance mutations during the many steps of carcinogenesis. Finally, the immune system itself provides a unique category of neoantigens that can be targets of immunotherapy, the clonally distributed products of rearranged antigen receptor genes – idiotypes – expressed by malignancies such as myelomas.

■ REFERENCES ■

1. Landsteiner K. The specificity of serological reactions, New York: Dover Press; 1945.

2. Jerne NK. Immunological speculations. Annu Rev Microbiol 1960; 14: 341–358.

3. Laver WG, Air GM, Webster RG, Smith-Gill SJ. Epitopes on protein antigens: misconceptions and realities. Cell 1990; 61: 553–556.

4. Arnon R, Van Regenmortel MH. Structural basis of antigenic specificity and design of new vaccines. FASEB J 1992; 6: 3265–3274.

5. Yamamoto F. Review: ABO blood group system – ABH oligosaccharide antigens, anti-A and anti-B, A and B glycosyltransferases, and ABO genes. Immunohematology/American Red Cross 2004; 20: 3–22.

6. Rudolph MG, Stanfield RL, Wilson IA. How TCRs bind MHCs, peptides, and coreceptors. Annu Rev Immunol 2006; 24: 419–466.

7. Proft T, Fraser JD. Bacterial superantigens. Clin Exp Immunol 2003; 133: 299–306.

8. Silverman GJ, Goodyear CS. Confounding B-cell defences: lessons from a staphylococcal superantigen. Nature Rev Immunol 2006; 6: 465–475.

9. Cresswell P, Ackerman AL, Giodini A, et al. Mechanisms of MHC class I-restricted antigen processing and cross-presentation. Immunol Rev 2005; 207: 145–157.

10. Haque A, Blum JS. New insights in antigen processing and epitope selection: development of novel immunotherapeutic strategies for cancer, autoimmunity and infectious diseases. J Biol Regul Homeost Agents 2005; 19: 93–104.

11. Elliott T, Williams A. The optimization of peptide cargo bound to MHC class I molecules by the peptide-loading complex. Immunol Rev 2005; 207: 89–99.

12. Rock KL, Shen L. Cross-presentation: underlying mechanisms and role in immune surveillance. Immunol Rev 2005; 207: 166–183.

13. Norbury CC, Tewalt EF. Upstream toward the 'DRiP'-ing source of the MHC class I pathway. Immunity 2006; 24: 503–506.

14. Hendil KB, Hartmann-Petersen R. Proteasomes: a complex story. Curr Protein Pept Sci 2004; 5: 135–151.

15. Strehl B, Seifert U, Kruger E, et al. Interferon-gamma, the functional plasticity of the ubiquitin-proteasome system, and MHC class I antigen processing. Immunol Rev 2005; 207: 19–30.

16. Cresswell P, Hughes EA. Protein degradation: the ins and outs of the matter. Curr Biol 1997; 7: R552–555.

17. Quadri SA, Singal DP. Peptide transport in human lymphoblastoid and tumor cells: effect of transporter associated with antigen presentation (TAP) polymorphism. Immunol Lett 1998; 61: 25–31.

18. Slomov E, Loewenthal R, Korostishevsky M, et al. Pemphigus vulgaris is associated with the transporter associated with antigen processing (TAP) system. Hum Immunol 2005; 66: 1213–1222.

19. Reits E, Neijssen J, Herberts C, et al. A major role for TPPII in trimming proteasomal degradation products for MHC class I antigen presentation. Immunity 2004; 20: 495–506.

20. Kloetzel PM, Ossendorp F. Proteasome and peptidase function in MHC-class-I-mediated antigen presentation. Curr Opin Immunol 2004; 16: 76–81.

21. Yellen-Shaw AJ, Eisenlohr LC. Regulation of class I-restricted epitope processing by local or distal flanking sequence. J Immunol 1997; 158: 1727–1733.

22. Wright CA, Kozik P, Zacharias M, Springer S. Tapasin and other chaperones: models of the MHC class I loading complex. Biol Chem 2004; 385: 763–778.

23. SenGupta D, Norris PJ, Suscovich TJ, et al. Heat shock protein-mediated cross-presentation of exogenous HIV antigen on HLA class I and class II.. J Immunol 2004; 173: 1987–1993.

24. Sant AJ, Chaves FA, Jenks SA, et al. The relationship between immunodominance, DM editing, and the kinetic stability of MHC class II: peptide complexes. Immunol Rev 2005; 207: 261–278.

25. Li P, Gregg JL, Wang N, et al. Compartmentalization of class II antigen presentation: contribution of cytoplasmic and endosomal processing. Immunol Rev 2005; 207: 206–217.

26. Villadangos JA, Schnorrer P, Wilson NS. Control of MHC class II antigen presentation in dendritic cells: a balance between creative and destructive forces. Immunol Rev 2005; 207: 191–205.

27. Munz C. Autophagy and antigen presentation. Cell Microbiol 2006; 8: 891–898.

28. Karlsson L. DM and DO shape the repertoire of peptide-MHC-class-II complexes. Curr Opin Immunol 2005; 17: 65–70.

29. Doytchinova IA, Guan P, Flower DR. EpiJen: a server for multistep T cell epitope prediction. BMC Bioinformatics 2006; 7: 131.

30. Sidney J, Southwood S, Sette A. Classification of A1- and A24-supertype molecules by analysis of their MHC-peptide binding repertoires. Immunogenetics 2005; 57: 393–408.

31. Abele R, Tampe R. Modulation of the antigen transport machinery TAP by friends and enemies. FEBS Lett 2006; 580: 1156–1163.

32. Kheradmand F, Kiss A, Xu J, et al. A protease-activated pathway underlying Th cell type 2 activation and allergic lung disease. J Immunol 2002; 169: 5904–5911.

33. van der Bruggen P, Van den Eynde BJ. Processing and presentation of tumor antigens and vaccination strategies. Curr Opin Immunol 2006; 18: 98–104.

Antigen-presenting cells and antigen presentation

José A. Villadangos, Louise J. Young

7

The body is constantly being exposed to a diverse array of infectious agents. The primary function of the immune system is to alert and protect against invading pathogens. The first line of defense falls to the innate immune system, which is essential for the control of many bacterial, protozoan, fungal, and metazoan infections (Chapter 3). The effector cells and molecules of the innate immune system (e.g. macrophages, complement) react against pathogen components, such as bacterial cell wall components, that are fundamentally distinct from those normally found in our bodies. The adaptive arm of the immune system is alerted by innate mechanisms to generate a more specific and durable response that can be tailored to each particular pathogen. Adaptive immunity relies on two major devices for antigen recognition. The first are the immunoglobulins, which are expressed on the surface of B cells and secreted as antibodies during the humoral immune response. Immunoglobulins recognize (bind) antigen motifs in their native conformation, and these are accessible to the extracellular medium. Thus immunoglobulins are very effective at binding and neutralizing soluble toxins, or at attaching to the surface of pathogens to tag them for destruction by macrophages or the complement system (Chapter 20). However, immunoglobulins are ineffective against pathogens capable of living within the cells, which include viruses and some bacteria (e.g. *Mycobacterium*) and protozoans (e.g. *Plasmodium*). Detection of intracellular pathogens relies on the second major recognition device of the adaptive immune system, the eponymous T-cell receptors (TCRs).

TCRs are expressed on the surface of T cells and are structurally similar to the immunoglobulins. However, unlike immunoglobulins, TCRs are used only for antigen recognition, never as secreted effector proteins (Chapter 4). Another major difference between immunoglobulins and the TCRs is that TCRs cannot recognize antigens in their native state, nor in isolation. The structural motifs recognized by individual TCRs consist of small peptide fragments derived from proteins belonging to the intracellular pathogen. Furthermore, these peptide antigens are not recognized in isolation, but only when bound to major histocompatibility complex (MHC) molecules expressed on the surface of infected cells (Chapter 5). This constitutes the structural basis of the phenomenon of *MHC restriction* whereby the T cells of an individual are selected to recognize only peptide antigens presented by the MHC *allotypes* of that individual.[1] The process that leads to formation of MHC–peptide complexes for T-cell recognition is called *antigen presentation*.[2] This involves degradation of the antigen, which is normally referred to as *antigen processing* (Chapter 6). The term *antigen-presenting cell* (APC) is operative; it is used to refer to the cells that display MHC–peptide complexes during a particular immune response.

Some specialized cells of the immune system, termed *professional APC*, can use their MHC molecules not only to display antigens derived from pathogens that are infecting the cells themselves, but also to capture pathogens from the extracellular medium, or even other cells infected with pathogens. These professional APCs present the pathogen antigens on their own MHC molecules. Such cells can thus communicate with T cells specific for the pathogens via interactions between the MHC–peptide complexes and the TCR. This interaction plays a key role in immune protection, because a fully fledged immune response requires the

█ KEY CONCEPTS

NON-PROFESSIONAL AND PROFESSIONAL ANTIGEN-PRESENTING CELLS (APC)

>> All nucleated cells express major histocompatibility complex (MHC) class I molecules and are *nonprofesional* APCs

>> *Professional* APC constitutively express MHC class II molecules and possess one or more mechanisms for antigen capture. Within the immune system, professional APC include dendritic cells, B cells, and macrophages

>> All professional APC employ the same basic machinery for antigen processing and presentation. However, professional APC can differ in the way they capture antigens, and in the way the molecular components of the machinery are expressed and interact with each other. These sometimes subtle differences enable subsets of APCs to engage in different specific functions

NON-PROFESSIONAL AND PROFESSIONAL ANTIGEN-PRESENTING CELLS

intervention of antigen-specific T cells. This requirement acts as a safety mechanism to minimize the likelihood of self-reactivity. Self-reactivity is minimized by depleting the T-cell repertoire of autoreactive cells during negative selection in the thymus. If a T cell becomes activated, this must be because it has encountered a foreign antigen. Antigen presentation thus serves a dual purpose. On the one hand, it is used by all cells to alert the immune system about the presence of intracellular parasites; on the other hand, it allows professional APC to survey large tracts of the body and inform T cells about the presence of infections.

NON-PROFESSIONAL AND PROFESSIONAL ANTIGEN-PRESENTING CELLS ■

The term APC can be confusing, as it is sometimes used to refer to a particular cell type, and at other times to refer to the cells presenting antigen in the context of a particular immune response. For instance, in the absence of infection, all cells express MHC class I molecules and can be considered APC. However, under normal circumstances the peptides they present are derived only from normal self molecules, and as such induce little, if any, immune response. During a pathogen infection the term APC is used to refer only to those cells that are actually presenting pathogen antigens. Similarly, during an autoimmune response APC will refer to the cells that present the autoantigen. Therefore what constitutes an "APC" depends on the context in which the term is used. Because most cells of the body express MHC class I molecules, they can serve as APC for endogenous antigens derived from pathogens should they become infected with viruses or intracytosolic bacteria. This ensures that any infected cell is recognized and eliminated by cytotoxic T lymphocytes (Chapters 25 and 27).

The expression of MHC II molecules is restricted to cells that possess mechanisms to endocytose antigens and to communicate with T cells. Such cells are termed *professional* APC. Although all professional APC share the same basic machinery for antigen presentation, they differ

markedly in their mechanisms of antigen capture and in the way they handle their MHC class II molecules. In the next sections we will describe the functional specializations of the antigen presentation functions of the three major representatives of professional APC: dendritic cells (DC), macrophages, and B lymphocytes (Table 7.1).

DENDRITIC CELLS

DC are present in nearly all tissues, as well as the blood and the lymphoid organs. However, they are relatively rare; for example, they only account for 2–3% of the non-red blood cells of the spleen and lymph nodes. Yet they were one of the earliest described cell types, even though at the time they were not recognized as components of the immune system.[3] The German clinician Paul Langerhans was conducting histological studies of skin epidermis in 1868 when he described cells with long, stellate processes, which became known as *Langerhans cells*. He thought that these cells were nerve terminals, and it was not until the 1960s that Langerhans cells were recognized as components of the hematopoietic system. However, it would take another 20 years to discover that Langerhans cells are the skin representatives of a more widely distributed cell type of the immune system, namely the DC. This resulted from the convergence of studies of Langerhans cells with a different line of research initiated in 1973 by Steinman and Cohn, who used the term *dendritic cells* to describe cells with long processes ('dendrites') isolated first from the spleen and later also from the lymph nodes.[4] DC began to attract particular attention when it was found that they were the most efficient, if not the only, type of APC capable of fully stimulating ('priming') naïve T cells.[5] Indeed, naïve T cells do not become effector T cells if they only engage MHC–peptide complexes with their TCR (Chapter 13). Such interaction triggers a signaling cascade in the naïve T cell that is usually termed '*signal 1*.' To become fully activated *effector* T cells capable of fighting infection, naïve T cells also require additional signals transmitted by a combination of surface receptors and soluble cytokines that are collectively known as '*signal 2*.'[6] It turned out that DC were highly adept at providing naïve T cells with both signals 1 and 2.

When Langerhans cells were found also to be capable of priming naïve T cells, a relationship between DC and Langerhans cells was hypothesized.[7]

Table 7.1 Properties of professional antigen-presenting cells (APC)

	Dendritic cell	Macrophages	B cell
Antigen uptake	Phagocytosis, Macropinocytosis Receptor-mediated endocytosis	Phagocytosis Receptor-mediated endocytosis	Receptor-mediated endocytosis (surface immunoglobulin only)
Major histocompatibility complex (MHC) II expression	Constitutively expressed, high levels inducible upon activation	Low levels, induced by activation	Constitutively expressed, high levels inducible upon activation
Role of antigen presentation	Inititation of immune response (naïve T-cell activation)	Recruitment of helper T cells for induction of inflammation	Recruitment of helper T cells for antibody production
Location	Lymphoid tissue Connective tissue Epithelia	Lymphoid tissue Connective tissue	Lymphoid tissue

Dendritic cells, macrophages, and B cells are the three major representatives of professional APC. Although these cells share the same basic MHC class II antigen presentation machinery, they differ in their mechanisms of antigen capture, their regulation of expression of MHC class II molecules, and the role that antigen presentation plays in that cell.

This was confirmed when Langerhans cells were found to traffic from the epidermis via the lymphatic system to the local subcutaneous lymph nodes, where they appeared as DC.[8] Parallel studies that tracked the origin of DC contained in the lymph nodes draining the liver, gut, or lungs also indicated that such DC immigrated from the corresponding peripheral tissue. This led to the realization that Langerhans cells were in fact the skin epidermis representative of a wider network of DC distributed throughout the body.[5] Now we know that this network is not constituted by a single type of cell, but comprises several DC subtypes that emerge from closely related, but separate, lines of development.[9] Furthermore, the tissue localization, lifecycle and function of the DC subtypes differ, conferring on each subtype unique properties tailored to fight specific types of infection. We next describe the archetypical lifecycle of DC, commonly referred to as the 'Langerhans cell paradigm,' before delineating in more detail how the different DC subtypes fit or diverge from this paradigm.

The Langerhans cell paradigm of DC lifecycle and function

In peripheral tissues, Langerhans cells/DC form a network of interconnected cells with long, dynamic processes projecting into the extracellular spaces between the parenchymal cells (Figure 7.1). The resulting mesh provides a barrier that can easily detect any invading pathogen. DC do not passively wait to encounter pathogens in the tissues. In their so-called 'immature' state, they appear to be dedicated to sampling their surroundings. For example, immature DC are highly active at all forms of endocytosis.[10] They constitutively macropinocytose, an activity that in other highly endocytic cells such as macrophages (see below) is inducible, not constitutive. Macropinocytosis enables DC to engulf the equivalent of their own volume every hour, an impressive figure that highlights the role of DC in immunosurveillance. Immature DC are also phagocytic, an activity they use to capture bacteria, cellular fragments and even whole dying cells. Finally, they express a large array of surface receptors that they use to detect the particulate matter that has to be phagocytosed. These receptors also permit the DC to engulf soluble extracellular compounds such as immunocomplexes and glycoproteins.

A crucial feature of immature DC is their ability to detect pathogens. They express Toll-like receptors[11] and C-type lectins,[12] both of which recognize pathogen-associated molecular patterns such as components of the bacterial wall (lipopolysaccharide), or nucleic acid motifs typically found in bacteria (e.g., CpG-rich DNA) or viruses (e.g., double-stranded RNA) (Chapter 3). Detection of these molecular cues triggers activation of the DC. Activation can also occur upon recognition of so-called inflammatory or 'danger' signals released by tissues damaged by invading pathogens (Figure 7.2).[13]

Activated DC leave the tissues, enter the lymphatic system, and migrate to the T-cell areas of the lymph nodes (Chapter 2). Simultaneously, the DC undergo a series of dramatic phenotypic changes that together are known as "maturation."[7, 14] "Mature" DC are no longer endocytic. However, they become highly effective at presenting the pathogen antigens captured in the

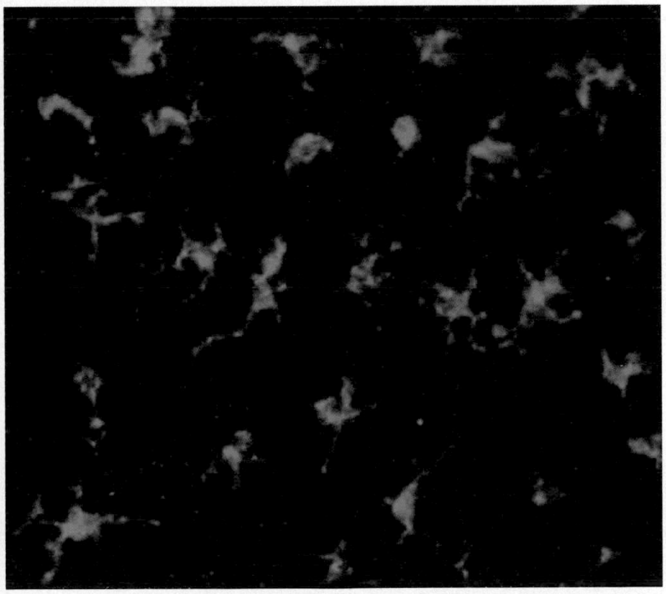

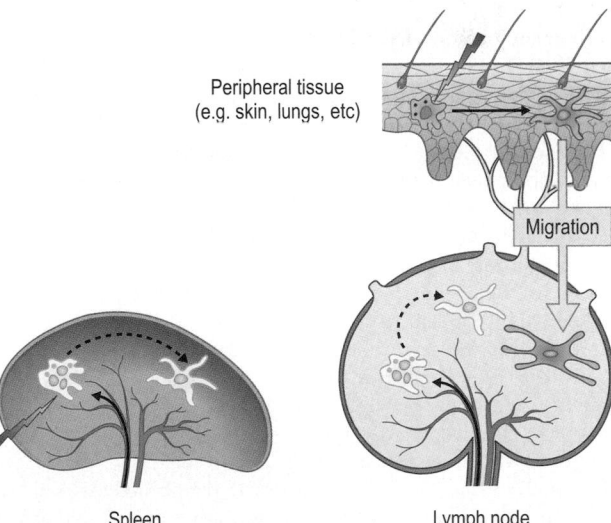

Peripheral tissue (e.g. skin, lungs, etc)

Migration

Spleen

Lymph node

Fig. 7.1 Migratory dendritic cells (DC) in the skin. This micrograph of a mouse skin explant seen from above shows Langerhans cells (one type of migratory DC) in the epidermis. The mice have been genetically altered to express a fluorescent protein only in Langerhans cells. Note the 'dendritic' shape of the cells, which form an interconnected network ready to detect the presence of invading pathogens. The dark spaces between the cells are occupied by nonfluorescent cells and connective tissue. (Courtesy of Rhys Allan and Frank Carbone, University of Melbourne.)

Fig. 7.2 Lifecycle of migratory and lymphoid organ-resident dendritic cells (DC). Migratory DC (green) and resident DC (yellow) are distributed throughout peripheral tissues and the lymphoid organs, respectively, where they are dedicated to sampling their environment in their so-called 'immature' state. Upon detection of pathogen products or inflammatory signals in the tissues (lightning bolt), migratory DC travel to the draining lymph nodes via the lymphatics where they develop into mature DC. Resident DC can detect such signals within the lymphoid organs themselves and mature *in situ*.

periphery at the time of activation. This reflects both the high expression of MHC class I and class II molecules (Chapter 5) and the ability of the DC to 'freeze' on their surface a large representation of long-lived MHC class II–peptide complexes, which are generated shortly after pathogen encounter.[15] This is an important feature found only in DC. The persistence of antigen is referred to as *antigenic memory*. This special ability allows DC to present to naïve T cells in the lymph node antigens that may have been encountered at a distant peripheral site, and gives the DC time to encounter a T cell specific for that antigen.

Another special ability found primarily in DC is the capacity to present on their MHC class I molecules peptides derived from antigens synthesized by other cells (exogenous), a mechanism known as *cross-presentation* (Chapter 6). Most cells only load their MHC class I molecules with peptides derived from antigens they have themselves synthesized (endogenous), enabling their detection by cytotoxic T lymphocytes (CTL) if they become cancer cells or are infected with viruses (Chapter 18). The problem is that CTL derive from primed naïve CD8 T cells. Since DC are the only APC that can prime naïve T cells, if they were not able to cross-present they would have to express the tumor antigens, or be infected with viruses, in order to initiate responses against these challenges. However, many viruses avoid infecting DC or inactivate the antigen-presenting machinery of infected cells, and by definition tumor antigens are only expressed (or expressed in significant amounts) by transformed cells. Cross-presentation by DC thus probably plays a major – albeit still controversial – role in immunity against viruses and cancer.[16]

Another major feature of mature DC is their acquisition of high expression levels of B7 family members and other co-stimulatory molecules that provide the 'signal 2' required to activate naïve T cells.[6] They also express high levels of CD40 which, upon engagement of CD40 ligand on activated CD4 T cells, "licenses" the DC to convert naïve CD8 T cells into effector CTL.[17] Finally, mature DC secrete cytokines that promote the differentiation of naïve CD4 T lymphocytes into Th1-, Th2-, and perhaps other types of helper T cells, each of which produces a distinct cytokine production profile. The specific mechanisms employed by DC to dictate which differentiation program will be followed by the CD4 T cells, which are often referred to as 'signal 3,' are still poorly understood.[18] DC secretion of IL-12 plays a major role in promoting Th1 differentiation, but the molecules involved in Th2 or other types of differentiation programs are less well characterized. It is believed that the type of signal 3 delivered by the mature DC may be determined by the specific compound that caused its activation when immature. In this scenario, the DC would be able to 'memorize' the type of pathogen it encountered in the periphery and promote in the lymph node the type of Th cell differentiation best suited to fight that particular pathogen.

The finding that DC migration to the lymph node is coupled to their maturation into cells capable of activating naïve T lymphocytes has had a major impact because it provides an elegant solution to a problem that had puzzled immunologists for years. Naïve T cells do not enter peripheral tissues, circulating instead amongst the secondary lymphoid organs (spleen and lymph nodes) via the circulatory and lymphatic systems (Chapter 2). How can they then detect infections restricted to a peripheral site such as the skin? DC solve this problem by acting as antigen middlemen, capturing infectious agents in peripheral tissues and transporting them into the lymph nodes for presentation to the naïve T cells. Each lymph node is therefore a communication hub where T cells can be exposed to a representation

of the antigenic material contained in the peripheral tissues in the form of MHC–peptide complexes exposed on the surface of the DC.

Departures from the paradigm: dendritic cell subtypes and their specializations

Even as the lifecycle of Langerhans cells was being characterized, studies of the development and phenotype of DC purified from lymphoid organs indicated that not all DC responded to the paradigm typified by Langerhans cells. It is now well established that DC can be subdivided into several subtypes that differ in developmental origin, anatomical localization, lifecycle, and functional properties.[19] Due to this heterogeneity, defining what constitutes a DC has become increasingly difficult. It is currently based on a combination of phenotypic and functional characteristics rather than on a single feature. These are: (1) the expression of the integrin CD11c; (2) the ability to endocytose antigens; (3) high expression of MHC class II and T-cell co-stimulatory molecules; and (4) the ability to activate naïve T cells. DC heterogeneity has been extensively characterized in mice and less so in humans. In fact, as we will point out later, the human equivalents of some of the known murine DC types have not yet been identified. Nevertheless, given the similarity between the immune systems of the two species, it is generally assumed that those equivalents do exist. We will now describe the major DC subtypes in the mouse system. Rather than providing an extensive list of the surface markers and functional features that characterize each subtype, we will focus on the major properties that distinguish them from each other.

KEY CONCEPTS

DENDRITIC CELL (DC) POPULATIONS

>> DC can be *conventional* or *plasmacytoid*

>> Among conventional DC, some subtypes first appear in peripheral tissues as *immature* DC. Upon encountering antigen, they migrate to the local lymph node, where they then acquire a *mature* phenotype. These *migratory* DCs consitute one-half of lymph node DC and are absent from spleen

>> The remaining lymph node DC, and all of the splenic and thymic DC, emerge in the lymphoid organs themselves. They spend their entire lifespan in an immature state unless they encounter pathogens. These are the *resident* DC types

>> Migratory DC can be subdivided into two major populations: *interstitial DC*, which are present in all organs, and *Langerhans cells*, which are only found in the epidermis. Resident DC can be subdivided into at least three populations. All different DC types probably play distinct, albeit still ill-defined, roles

>> In the absence of infection, DC induce tolerance. Upon pathogen detection they induce immunity. The rules governing whether DC will induce one or the other are still poorly understood

Plasmacytoid DC versus conventional DC

A major subdivision of DC can be made between *plasmacytoid DC* and *conventional DC*. The defining property of plasmacytoid DC is that upon activation they release large amounts of type I interferons, which play important roles in immunity against viruses.[20] Plasmacytoid DC were originally described as *interferon-producing cells*. They contain large amounts of endoplasmic reticulum, befitting their role as producers of a secreted cytokine. It is this ultrastructural feature, similar to that observed in antibody-producing plasma cells, that gives plasmacytoid DC their name. Although DC belonging to this subtype express MHC class II and T-cell co-stimulatory molecules, and can stimulate naïve T cells, their antigen-capturing abilities remain controversial. Moreover, their capacity to present antigens appears rather poor compared to that of conventional DC.[20] Plasmacytoid DC are found in all lymphoid organs. They are also present in the blood because they recirculate among lymphoid organs, much like lymphocytes, without entering non-inflamed peripheral tissues. This is also in contrast with conventional DC, which generally do not exit lymphoid organs and simply die there. Together, these features place plasmacytoid DC as quite separate from the conventional DC. Indeed some authors have questioned the categorization of plasmacytoid DC as part of the DC lineage.[20] In the rest of this chapter we will use the term DC to refer exclusively to the conventional ones.

Migratory versus resident DC

Analysis of DC contained in mouse lymph nodes has revealed two major groups of DC. The first can be tracked back to an origin in the peripheral tissue drained by that lymph node, for example, the skin, the airways, and the gut for the subcutaneous, mediastinal, and mesenteric lymph nodes, respectively. Thus, if a fluorescent tracker is applied to those tissues, DC labeled with the tracker accumulate in the corresponding lymph node after a few hours. These are the *migratory* DC types.[19] The migratory DC develop from earlier precursors that either multiply in the peripheral tissues themselves, or traffic from the bone marrow. The newly generated DC then stay in the tissue in an immature state until they receive the signals that trigger their migration and maturation, as described above. The migratory DC contained in most tissues appear homogeneous, so they probably represent a single population that is known as *interstitial DC*.

The DC migrating from the skin can be further subdivided into interstitial DC that migrate from the dermis (for this reason they are normally called *dermal DC*) and the classic Langerhans cells that migrate from the epidermis. The latter can be distinguished from the interstitial (dermal) DC by their expression of a unique antigen receptor called *langerin* and by their possession of *Birbeck granules*, an enigmatic racket-shaped intracellular organelle of as yet unknown function.[3] The skin appears to be the only tissue that contains two distinct types of migratory DC, suggesting that immunosurveillance of the epidermis requires a dedicated type of DC (the Langerhans cells). The reasons behind this need for a specialized cell remain unclear. Thus, although Langerhans cells are usually described as the archetypical DC, they represent a rather restricted subtype dedicated to monitor the epidermis.[19]

Approximately half of the DC contained in the lymph nodes do not become labeled with the dyes used to track the migration of DC from peripheral tissues. These are the *resident* DC types. The resident DC are the only types of DC contained in the spleen and the thymus. This would be expected since these organs are not connected with the lymphatic system and therefore cannot receive cells migrating from peripheral tissues via the lymph. Indeed, resident DC most likely develop in the lymphoid organs from earlier precursors that may continually migrate from the bone marrow or divide within the organs.[21] The lifecycle of resident DC represents a clear departure from the 'Langerhans cells paradigm.'[19] In the absence of blood infections, virtually all the resident DC display an immature phenotype analogous to that of the migratory DC contained in peripheral tissues. Most die without ever becoming mature. Their function there is probably to survey the blood. Although the blood is not usually mentioned as a 'peripheral tissue' susceptible to pathogen infection, it is the primary route of entry for the plethora of insect-borne microorganisms transmitted by blood-sucking insects. Some examples are the viruses that cause yellow fever or several forms of encephalitis, the bacterium *Borrelia burgdorferi*, which causes Lyme disease, and the malaria parasite *Plasmodium* spp. When the resident DC encounter pathogen-asociated compounds carried in the blood, they become activated, undergo maturation, and present the pathogen antigens. Thus, the lymphoid organs and the blood can be considered the 'peripheral tissue' surveyed by the resident DC of the spleen and lymph nodes.[19]

The migratory and resident DC differ not only in location and lifecycle but also in their antigen presentation capacities and the type of Th response that they promote. Resident DC can also be further subdivided into three smaller populations ($CD4^+$ DC, $CD8^+$ DC and $CD4^-CD8^-$ DC), each of which plays its own distinct role in the immune response. For example, $CD8^+$ DC are particularly efficient at capturing dead cells, cross-presenting antigens, and secreting IL-12 for the induction of Th1-type responses.[16] The resident DC of the thymus also deserve special mention because their main function is not to survey the blood but to mediate negative selection of thymocytes[22] (see below). Characterizing the functional specializations of each DC subtype and the molecular basis of their differences is an important goal of current DC research. This may allow the design of more effective immunotherapies tailored to specific outcomes.

Blood DC

Mouse blood DC have been difficult to analyze due to the obvious scarcity of starting material for cell purification. However, the blood is the preferred source for studies of human DC, so this is the tissue that has allowed the clearest comparison between the DC of the two species (see below). Mouse blood contains plasmacytoid DC and conventional DC, but conventional DC do not resemble any of the migratory or resident DC types described in the lymphoid organs. They do not appear to be their precursors either. The function and lifecycle of blood DC thus remain enigmatic.[19]

Monocyte-derived DC

Monocytes circulate through the blood and are best known as precursors of macrophages in tissues. However, they can also differentiate into DC, although it remains unclear what type of DC they generate. These do not appear to be any of the resident DC. Some reports have suggested that monocytes can differentiate into migratory DC,[23] but this may only happen in inflamed tissues. A current view holds that under normal conditions migratory DC are continually renewed by non-monocyte precursors. During inflammation, however, the monocytes represent an 'emergency' source of new migratory DC.[21] It remains unclear to what extent the newly generated monocyte-derived DC resemble the migratory DC that are normally produced in the absence of infection.

Human DC subtypes

If the preferred source for study of mouse DC has been the lymphoid organs, the blood has served as the preferred source for the study of human DC. These differences in origin have complicated efforts to establish phenotypic and functional correlations between human and murine DC subsets. However, when DC are isolated from homologous tissues, parallelisms become evident.[9] Thus, human blood, like mouse blood, contains two major subsets of DC: plasmacytoid DC (CD1d− IL3 receptor+) and conventional DC (CD1d+ IL3 receptor−). The terms *lymphoid* and *myeloid* are commonly used to refer to human plasmacytoid and conventional DC because it was once thought that each subset emerged from the lymphoid and myeloid hematopoietic lineages, respectively. Later studies have shown that this is not the case, so the two terms have become obsolete and should be avoided. Human blood is also the major source for monocytes that can be transformed into DC in culture (see below). The DC of human lymphoid organs remain poorly characterized. It is clear that both plasmacytoid and conventional DC are present, but the only human equivalent of a particular mouse lymphoid organ DC subtype described so far are the Langerhans cells. The equivalents of the interstitial and of the three resident DC subtypes described above remain unknown. This represents an important knowledge gap that limits the ability to translate to the clinic the findings of basic DC research conducted in the mouse system.

Generation of DC in culture

Studies of DC were marred for over 30 years due to their scarcity, the difficulty of the protocols required for their purification, and the lack of unique phenotypic markers to distinguish them from other hematopoietic cells. The fact that DC purified from tissues proved to be remarkably 'unstable' further compounded these technical difficulties. This is because Langerhans cells extracted from the epidermis, or resident DC purified from the spleen, undergo spontaneous maturation when put in culture, hampering the analysis of their 'immature' properties. This situation changed with the establishment of methods to generate DC *in vitro* by culturing mouse bone marrow precursors or human blood monocytes in medium supplemented with the growth factor granulocyte–macrophage colony-stimulating factor.[24, 25] Such cultures yield large numbers of DC that maintain their immature state until stimulated by the addition of pathogen-associated compounds or inflammatory mediators. This has allowed detailed studies of the mechanisms involved in DC activation and their transformation from antigen-capturing immature DC into antigen-presenting mature DC.

Human monocyte-derived DC are the most commonly used DC type in immunotherapy. However, we still do not know how to generate the migratory and resident human DC types normally found in the lymphoid organs. Only recently have protocols been established for the generation of their mouse equivalents.[26] Since these DC subtypes have functional properties that may be absent from monocyte-derived DC, it would be important to develop methods to generate them in culture because they might be more suitable for clinical applications than those derived from monocytes.

Dendritic cells and tolerance

Throughout this chapter we have described DC as initiators of immune responses. However, DC have another major role, the induction of T-cell tolerance. Elimination of autoreactive T cells occurs primarily in the thymus during the process of negative selection (Chapter 9), whereby thymocytes that react too strongly with self MHC–peptide complexes displayed on the surface of thymic APC are eliminated. The major APC of the thymus involved in this process are DC.[22]

Many autoreactive T cells escape negative selection and enter the circulation, where they can elicit autoimmune responses if they are not held in check by some mechanism of peripheral tolerance. These mechanisms can induce abortive proliferation of the autoreactive cells, their entry into an anergic state, or their regulation by suppressor or regulatory T cells (Chapters 9 and 16). The APC in charge of presenting self antigen for the induction of peripheral tolerance are also DC. This is paradoxical. How can DC promote T-cell tolerance and also be the major initiators of immune responses? The answer to this question is still unclear, but the most likely explanation is that DC that present antigens without having received activation signals associated with pathogens are tolerogenic.[27] Since peripheral tolerance occurs in the secondary lymphoid organs, such DC might be plasmacytoid DC, resident DC that have not received maturation signals, or even migratory DC that have undergone maturation in response to a constitutive differentiation program rather than to pathogen encounter. The implication of this conclusion is that tolerogenic and immunogenic DC may differ in their expression of surface molecules or cytokines that define their ability to initiate immunity or tolerance. If true, this would imply that DC could potentially be used as immunotherapeutic agents for the induction of tolerance as well as for vaccination purposes. However, the differences that distinguish tolerogenic and immunogenic DC remain poorly characterized.

▌ KEY CONCEPTS

THE ROLE OF THE B-CELL RECEPTOR (BCR) IN HUMORAL IMMUNITY

>> Each B cell expresses a unique antigen receptor, the surface immunoglobulin (Ig), whose antigen specificity is the same as the antibody (Ab) it will produce upon differentiation into Ab-secreting cells

>> Recognition of antigen by the BCR promotes B-cell activation and presentation of antigenic peptides via major histocompatibility complex (MHC) class II molecules to CD4+ helper T cells

>> The BCR keeps capturing antigen, promoting continued recruitment of T-cell help, for as long as the antigen persists in the extracellular environment. It acts as a gauge that determines when the humoral immune response should stop

B LYMPHOCYTES

B lymphocytes (B cells) constitute the major population of lymphocytes of the immune system. Generated constitutively through life, naïve B cells exit the bone marrow after negative selection and circulate the body, repopulating both the blood and the follicles of the secondary lymphoid organs (Chapter 8).

Naïve B cells become stimulated upon recognition of antigen with their specific B-cell receptor (BCR), which consists of a membrane-attached form of immunoglobulin (mIg) associated with several accessory molecules (see below). Engagement of the BCR initiates a series of events that culminate in the differentiation of B cells into plasma cells, the antibody-secreting cells responsible for eliciting the humoral arm of the adaptive immune response (Chapter 8). The capacity of B cells to capture, process, and present antigens to T cells is a requisite for the initiation of these events.[28] The reason for this is that B cells need to present antigen to helper CD4 T cells, which upon recognition of the antigen respond by providing signals back to the B cells using surface molecules and secreted cytokines. These signals further stimulate the B cells to proliferate and differentiate into antibody-producing cells.

Why don't the B cells differentiate autonomously into antibody-producing cells? The requirement for T-cell help introduces an additional layer of control to prevent formation of autoantibodies by potentially autoreactive B cells which may have escaped negative selection, as these would still need to encounter autoreactive T cells that themselves avoided being purged from the T-cell repertoire. For this "double-safe" mechanism to work, two conditions must be met. First, B cells must only present antigens recognized with their BCR; and second, B cells specific for a given antigen should be able to receive help only from previously activated T cells specific for that same antigen. The antigen-presenting function of B cells thus differs from that of DC in three important aspects. First, it is focused on presentation of antigens recognized with the BCR; second, B cells do not generally activate naïve T cells, instead they interact with helper T cells previously recruited from the naïve T-cell pool by DC; and third, B cells present antigen to T cells 'for their own benefit' rather than to stimulate T cells which will then collaborate with third-party cells.

In this section we will describe the specializations of B cells that underpin their specific antigen-presenting function, with particular emphasis on the role of the BCR in antigen endocytosis and promotion of processing and presentation of BCR-internalized antigens. We will then integrate the antigen-presenting activity of B cells in the process that culminates in the initiation of humoral immunity.

The influence of B-cell localization on their role as APC

The clonal nature of the B-cell repertoire implies the same type of problem for antigen detection that we described above for T cells. Namely, very few cells amongst the vast B-cell repertoire express the right immunoglobulin specificity capable of recognizing a given antigen. Therefore it would be impractical for B cells to circulate throughout the tissues to monitor for the presence of their antigen. Instead, B cells circulate through the secondary lymphoid organs, concentrating in the follicles. Antigens carried in the blood or seeping from tissues via the efferent lymph reach these areas and can be readily recognized by B cells. However, there must be many antigens that do not reach the follicles passively, so it has been hypothesized that DC can transport these antigens to the lymph nodes and, in addition to processing and presenting them to T cells, expose them on their surface in intact form for B-cell recognition.[29]

The role of the B-cell receptor in antigen presentation

Unlike DC and macrophages, B cells are not phagocytic or macropinocytic, and do not express multiple types of antigen receptors. Their capacity to endocytose antigen is restricted almost exclusively to those captured through their cell surface receptor, the BCR. While this makes B cells less efficient than other APC at presenting most antigens, it also makes them the most focused. The BCR consists of an mIg, which provides the antigen recognition component to the receptor, noncovalently associated to an Igα:Igβ heterodimer (Chapter 4). This dimer provides the signaling module to the receptor, as it contains an immunoreceptor tyrosine-based activation (ITAM) motif required for signal transduction that upon antigen engagement triggers internalization of the receptor–antigen complex and initiates a signaling cascade leading to B-cell activation.[28] Ig-mediated endocytosis allows B cells to concentrate in their endosomal compartments minute amounts of antigen due to the high specificity of their mIg molecules. It is easy to imagine how this process operates on soluble antigens, but less so for antigens associated with cellular membranes. However, it has recently been demonstrated that B cells can indeed endocytose antigens 'ripped' from cell surfaces,[30] so BCR-mediated endocytosis can account for presentation of even cell-associated antigens without the need to invoke a phagocytic mechanism for antigen capture.

The signaling cascade ignited by the BCR upon antigen engagement induces changes in the endocytic route that facilitate the trafficking of BCR–antigen complexes to the compartments where antigens are degraded and MHC class II molecules acquire their peptide cargo. Concurrently, BCR signaling induces increased MHC class II synthesis and delivery to the same compartments.[28] Presentation of BCR-internalized antigen is also facilitated by the expression of H-2O/human leukocyte antigen (HLA)-DO.[31] This is an MHC class II-like molecule that functions in B cells as an inhibitor of H-2DM/HLA-DM, the chaperone that facilitates the displacement of the CLIP peptide from the peptide-binding site of MHC class II molecules (Chapter 6). DO inhibits DM function, and therefore formation of peptide-receptive MHC class II molecules, in all but the most acidic late-endosomal compartments. This is advantageous because BCR-internalized antigens are difficult to degrade due their stable association with the Ig-binding site, so their processing requires their degradation in vesicles of a low pH. HLA-DO inhibition of HLA-DM in less acidic compartments preserves the peptide-binding site of the MHC class II molecules until they reach the acidic compartments, where the antigens can be processed.

B-cell activation also promotes migration towards the T-cell areas of the spleen and lymph nodes, facilitating their encounter with antigen-specific helper T cells at the margin of the lymphoid follicles.[32] T-cell-dependent activation of B cells occurs both through the interaction of CD40 on B cells and its ligand CD154 on helper T cells, and through secretion of cytokines including IL-4 by the T cell. Both signals serve to promote and sustain activation initiated by BCR engagement.

This results in the formation of primary foci, which then lead to the establishment of germinal centers – the multicellular compound where the humoral response develops.[33]

The duration of the humoral response is dictated by BCR-mediated antigen presentation.

In the germinal centers the B cells multiply, undergo isotype switching, and differentiate into antibody-producing cells.[33] The Ig-encoding regions of some of the progeny B cells undergo somatic hypermutations, resulting in generation of new Ig sequences of variable affinity for the antigen. Since the availability of helper T cells in the germinal center is limiting, these B cells compete with each other to receive proliferation and differentiation signals. Those with higher-affinity Ig are better able to capture antigen and present MHC class II–peptide complexes to the helper T cell, so they are selected for a new round of proliferation and differentiation. The efficiency of MHC class II presentation by B cells within the germinal center is thus proportional to the quality of their immunoglobulin and to the amount of antigen accessible to the BCR. This mechanism acts as a gauge for when to downregulate the humoral immune response upon the clearance of antigen. At this stage B cells can no longer present antigen to helper T cells and the humoral immune response ceases.

MACROPHAGES

Widely identified as a scavenger cell, the loose definition of a macrophage is a large mononuclear cell with a high capacity for phagocytosis. Macrophages are distributed throughout the organs and differentiate from blood monocytes upon entering the peripheral tissues (Chapter 21). Depending on their specific location within the body, macrophages are adapted to play multiple roles, resulting in their adoption of different morphologies. Consequently, they are identified by individual names, such as the Kupffer cells that line the hepatic sinusoids of the liver, the alveolar macrophage of the lung, the osteoclasts found in bones, or the marginal-zone macrophages found within the pulp of the spleen and the lining of the circular and medullary sinuses of the lymph nodes. The wide distribution and heterogeneity of macrophages reflect the multiple roles they play, many of which are unrelated to immunity. For example, they are the cells in charge of engulfing and digesting cells that have reached the end of their lifecycle, and osteoclasts play an important role in bone remodeling.

During an infection, macrophages provide the first line of defense of the innate immune response by engulfing infectious agents and destroying them (Chapters 3 and 21). Phagocytosis of these agents is triggered by recognition of carbohydrate and lipid structures on microbial surfaces by receptors such as the mannose receptor, the scavenger receptor, complement receptors, and several Toll-like receptors.[34] In addition to triggering phagocytosis, these receptors signal macrophage activation, promoting antigen presentation, expression of T-cell co-stimulatory molecules, and the secretion of chemokines that attract helper T cells to sites of infection. The antigen-presenting ability of macrophages is relatively limited because their expression of MHC II molecules is not as high as in DC or B cells. Moreover, their endosomal proteolytic machinery is geared towards the destruction of endocytosed material rather than to the production of MHC ligands.[35] Nevertheless, they do present antigens to helper T cells arriving at sites of infection. The

interaction between the two cell types induces the macrophages to express anti-microbial mediators and proinflammatory cytokines that contribute to contain pathogen spread (Chapter 3).

■ CLINICAL IMPLICATIONS ■

The events that lead to the display of MHC–peptide complexes on the surface of professional APC can be seen as the initial stages of T-cell-dependent immune responses. These events are modulated by signals delivered by innate receptors of microbial products. The characterization of the machinery involved in antigen detection, uptake, processing, and presentation, and of the functional abilities of distinct APC has practical applications for the clinical application of immunology. Considerable effort is currently being expended on finding ways to increase the efficiency of uptake, processing, and presentation of vaccine antigens (Chapter 94).

One major goal is to develop vaccine formulations that can be targeted to specific populations of APC, in particular DC, so that the dose of vaccine required to elicit a response can be kept to a minimum. For example, the antigen might be linked to antibodies specific for DC surface markers or to molecular motifs recognized by antigen receptors. Inclusion of the right pathogen products (adjuvants) or even molecular modulators of immune responses such as CD40 ligand would be predicted both to increase the efficacy of a vaccine and to promote the most effective type of T-cell response for the pathogen. A variation of this theme would be to generate vaccines against tumor antigens that might elicit immune responses against cancer cells (Chapter 94).

As we have described in this chapter, the professional APC also play key roles in the induction of tolerance. Thus, it should also be possible to design vaccines to suppress, rather than induce, immune responses. Such vaccines might be useful in the prevention or treatment of hypersensitivity (e.g. asthma: Chapter 40) or autoimmune disorders (e.g. type 1 diabetes: Chapter 70). The challenge is to understand what causes APC to initiate immunity or tolerance. Does this depend on the type of APC presenting the antigen? Or do the types of immune modulators that accompany the antigen determine the tolerogenic or immunogenic potential of a vaccine? The answers to these questions might open a future of novel vaccine formulations that exploit our knowledge of the abilities of distinct APC and their antigen-presenting functions to treat, as well as prevent, a large array of diseases.

The realization that antigen presentation is the result of complex molecular interactions has led to the development of drugs capable of enhancing or inhibiting the formation of MHC–peptide complexes. Such drugs might have immunomodulatory properties. For instance, protease inhibitors have been used in mice to impair the processing and presentation of autoantigens and model allergens and thus reduce autoimmunity and hypersensitivity, respectively.[36, 37] Developing strategies to target such drugs to particular populations of APC is another approach that may allow enhancement of the efficacy of vaccines or the prevention of autoimmunity or allergic reactions. There is still much to be learned about the functional specializations of distinct APC, but the potential benefits of such knowledge should encourage investigators to continue their studies of these fascinating components of the immune system.

REFERENCES

1. Zinkernagel RM, Doherty PC. The discovery of MHC restriction. Immunol Today 1997; 18: 14–17.

2. Germain RN. MHC-dependent antigen processing and peptide presentation: providing ligands for T lymphocyte activation. Cell 1994; 76: 287–299.

3. Romani N, Holzmann S, Tripp CH, et al. Langerhans cells – dendritic cells of the epidermis. Apmis 2003; 111: 725–740.

4. Steinman RM, Cohn ZA. Identification of a novel cell type in peripheral lymphoid organs of mice. I. Morphology, quantitation, tissue distribution. J Exp Med 1973; 137: 1142–1162.

5. Steinman RM. The dendritic cell system and its role in immunogenicity. Annu Rev Immunol 1991; 9: 271–296.

6. Sharpe AH, Freeman GJ. The B7-CD28 superfamily. Nat Rev Immunol 2002; 2: 116–126.

7. Schuler G, Steinman RM. Murine epidermal Langerhans cells mature into potent immunostimulatory dendritic cells in vitro. J Exp Med 1985; 161: 526–546.

8. Larsen CP, Steinman RM, Witmer-Pack M, et al. Migration and maturation of Langerhans cells in skin transplants and explants. J Exp Med 1990; 172: 1483–1493.

9. Shortman K, Liu YJ. Mouse and human dendritic cell subtypes. Nat Rev Immunol 2002; 2: 151–161.

10. Wilson NS, Villadangos JA. Regulation of antigen presentation and cross presentation in the dendritic cell network: facts, hypothesis, and immunological implications. Adv Immunol 2005; 86: 241–305.

11. Medzhitov R. Toll-like receptors and innate immunity. Nat Rev Immunol 2001; 1: 135–145.

12. van Kooyk Y, Geijtenbeek TB. DC-SIGN: escape mechanism for pathogens. Nat Rev Immunol 2003; 3: 697–709.

13. Matzinger P. The danger model: a renewed sense of self. Science 2002; 296: 301–305.

14. Reis e Sousa C. Dendritic cells in a mature age. Nat Rev Immunol 2006; 6: 476–483.

15. Villadangos JA, Schnorrer P, Wilson NS. Control of MHC class II antigen presentation in dendritic cells: a balance between creative and destructive forces. Immunol Rev 2005; 207: 191–205.

16. Heath WR, Belz GT, Behrens GM, et al. Cross-presentation, dendritic cell subsets, and the generation of immunity to cellular antigens. Immunol Rev 2004; 199: 9–26.

17. Lanzavecchia A. Immunology. Licence to kill. Nature 1998; 393: 413–414.

18. de Jong EC, Smits HH, Kapsenberg ML. Dendritic cell-mediated T cell polarization. Springer Semin Immunopathol 2005; 26: 289–307.

19. Villadangos JA, Heath WR. Lifecycle, migration and antigen presenting functions of spleen and lymph node dendritic cells: limitations of the Langerhans cells paradigm. Semin Immunol 2005; 17: 262–272.

20. Colonna M, Trinchieri G, Liu YJ. Plasmacytoid dendritic cells in immunity. Nat Immunol 2004; 5: 1219–1226.

21. Naik SH, Metcalf D, van Nieuwenhuijze A, et al. Intrasplenic steady-state dendritic cell precursors which are distinct from monocytes. Nat Immunol 2006; 7: 663–671.

22. Brocker T, Riedinger M, Karjalainen K. Targeted expression of major histocompatibility complex (MHC) class II molecules demonstrates that dendritic cells can induce negative but not positive selection of thymocytes in vivo. J Exp Med 1997; 185: 541–550.

23. Ginhoux F, Tacke F, Angeli V, et al. Langerhans cells arise from monocytes in vivo. Nat Immunol 2006; 7: 265–273.

24. Inaba K, Inaba M, Romani N, et al. Generation of large numbers of dendritic cells from mouse bone marrow cultures supplemented with granulocyte/macrophage colony-stimulating factor. J Exp Med 1992; 176: 1693–1702.

25. Sallusto F, Lanzavecchia A. Efficient presentation of soluble antigen by cultured human dendritic cells is maintained by granulocyte/macrophage colony-stimulating factor plus interleukin 4 and downregulated by tumor necrosis factor alpha. J Exp Med 1994; 179: 1109–1118.

26. Naik SH, Proietto AI, Wilson NS, et al. Cutting edge: generation of splenic CD8+ and CD8– dendritic cell equivalents in Fms-like tyrosine kinase 3 ligand bone marrow cultures. J Immunol 2005; 174: 6592–6597.

27. Steinman RM, Nussenzweig MC. Avoiding horror autotoxicus: the importance of dendritic cells in peripheral T cell tolerance. Proc Natl Acad Sci U S A 2002; 99: 351–358.

28. Rodriguez-Pinto D. B cells as antigen presenting cells. Cell Immunol 2005; 238: 67–75.

29. Wykes M, Pombo A, Jenkins C, et al. Dendritic cells interact directly with naïve B lymphocytes to transfer antigen and initiate class switching in a primary T-dependent response. J Immunol 1998; 161: 1313–1319.

30. Batista FD, Iber D, Neuberger MS. B cells acquire antigen from target cells after synapse formation. Nature 2001; 411: 489–494.

31. Denzin LK, Sant'Angelo DB, Hammond C, et al. Negative regulation by HLA-DO of MHC class II-restricted antigen processing. Science 1997; 278: 106–109.

32. Garside P, Ingulli E, Merica RR, et al. Visualization of specific B and T lymphocyte interactions in the lymph node. Science 1998; 281: 96–99.

33. Liu YJ, Arpin C. Germinal center development. Immunol Rev 1997; 156: 111–126.

34. Taylor PR, Martinez-Pomares L, Stacey M, et al. Macrophage receptors and immune recognition. Annu Rev Immunol 2005; 23: 901–944.

35. Trombetta ES, Mellman I. Cell biology of antigen processing in vitro and in vivo. Annu Rev Immunol 2005; 23: 975–1028.

36. Nakagawa TY, Brissette WH, Lira PD, et al. Impaired invariant chain degradation and antigen presentation and diminished collagen-induced arthritis in cathepsin S null mice. Immunity 1999; 10: 207–217.

37. Riese RJ, Mitchell RN, Villadangos JA, et al. Cathepsin S activity regulates antigen presentation and immunity. J Clin Invest 1998; 101: 2351–2363.

B-cell development and differentiation

**Claudia Berek, Andreas Radbruch,
Harry W. Schroeder Jr.**

8

B lymphocytes arise from multipotent hematopoietic stem cells that successively populate the embryonic para-aortic splanchnopleura, the fetal liver, and then the bone marrow. Stem cell daughter cells give rise to lymphoid multipotent primed progenitors (LMPPs), which in turn can give rise to either myeloid or lymphoid cells.[1, 2] LMPPs then produce common lymphoid precursors (CLPs), which can generate T cells, B cells, natural killer (NK) cells, and a special subset of dendritic cells. Final B-cell differentiation requires the exposure of CLP daughter cells to specialized microenvironments such as those found in the fetal liver and the bone marrow. These two tissues are the primary B lymphoid organs. The shift from fetal liver to bone marrow begins in the middle of fetal life and ends just prior to birth. B cells continue to be produced in the bone marrow throughout the life of the individual, although the rate of production decreases with age.

An intact and functional B-cell antigen receptor (BCR) complex, which consists of membrane-bound immunoglobulin (mIg), the Igα and Igβ co-receptors, and ancillary signal transduction components, must be present in order for the developing B cell to survive (Chapter 4). The composition of the BCR is subject to intense selection. In the primary organs, hazardous self-reactive BCRs, as well as nonfunctional ones, can be culled by altering the composition of the receptor (receptor editing), by cell anergy, or by apoptosis of the host cell. Survivors of this initial selection process are released into the blood and thence to the spleen, lymph nodes, and other secondary lymphoid tissues and organs where selection for specificity continues (Chapter 2).

B-cell differentiation (Fig. 8.1) is commonly presented as a linear process defined by the regulated expression of specific sets of transcription factors, immunoglobulin, and cell surface molecules. Given the central role of the BCR (Chapter 4), the initial developmental steps are classically defined by the status of the rearranging immunoglobulin loci. With the development of monoclonal antibody technology, analysis of cell surface markers such as CD10, CD19, CD20, CD21, CD24, CD34, and CD38 has facilitated definition of both early and late stages of development, especially in those cases where immunoglobulin cannot be used to distinguish between cell types (Table 8.1). Of these, CD19, a signal transduction molecule that is expressed throughout B-cell development up to, but not including, the

mature plasma cell stage,[3] warrants special mention as the single best clinical marker for B-cell identity.

In practice, B-cell development is a more complex process than the simple linear pathway depicted in Figure 8.1. For example, pro-B cells typically derive from a common lymphoid progenitor, but they can also develop from a bipotent B/macrophage precursor. Thus, B-lineage subsets identified by one fractionation scheme may consist of mixtures of subsets identified by others. The complexity of the process continues to yield competing nomenclatures. Therefore, it behooves the practitioner to clarify the fractionation scheme used by the reference laboratory when comparing patient findings to the literature.

KEY CONCEPTS

B-CELL DEVELOPMENT IN THE PRIMARY LYMPHOID ORGANS

>> Commitment to the B-cell lineage reflects differential activation of transcription factors that progressively lock the cell into the B-cell pathway

>> B-cell development is typically viewed as a linear, stepwise process that is focused on the assembly and testing of immunoglobulin function, first in the fetal liver and bone marrow, and then in the periphery:

Failure to assemble a functional receptor leads to cell death

Expression of a functional receptor subjects the B cell to antigen selection

B cells with inappropriate specificities tend to be eliminated

B cells responding appropriately to external antigen may develop into either immunoglobulin-secreting plasma cells or into memory cells

At the clinical level, B-cell development can be monitored by examining the pattern of expression of lymphoid-specific surface proteins

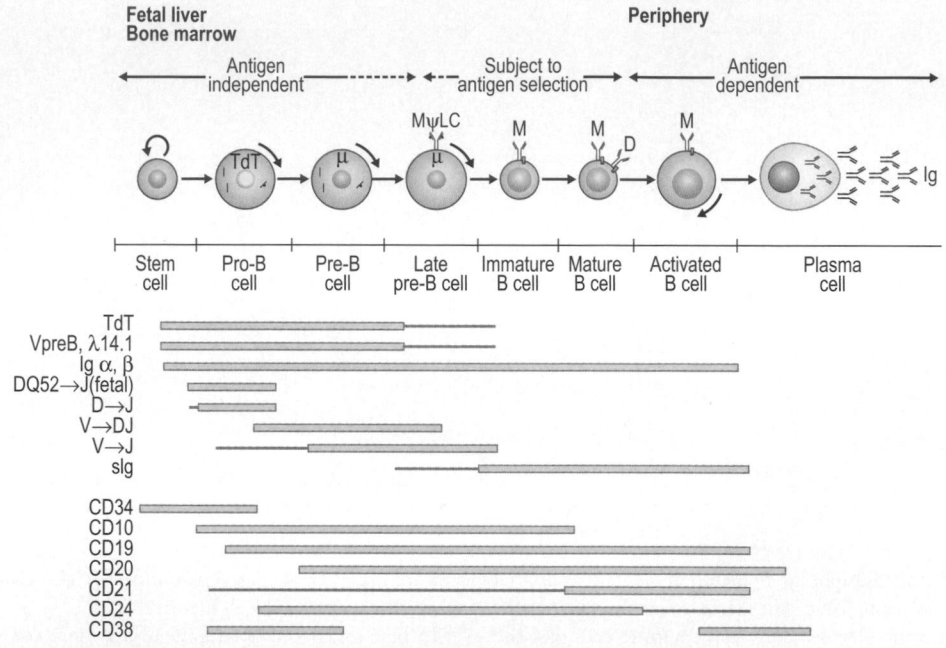

Fig. 8.1 Model of B-cell differentiation. B-cell development is typically viewed as a linear progression through different stages of differentiation: the various processes associated with the assembly of the B-cell antigen receptor complex and the expression pattern of surface molecules whose presence or absence are illustrated through use of bars. The various steps in immunoglobulin rearrangement and the pattern of expression of these surface molecules can be used to characterize stages in B-cell development.

Initial commitment to the B-cell lineage requires activation of a series of transcriptional and signal transduction pathways. At the nuclear level, the transcription factors PU.1, Ikaros, ID-1, E2A, EBF, and PAX-5 play major roles in committing progenitor cells to the B-cell lineage.[4] However, after lineage commitment has been established, it is the composition of the BCR that controls further development.

Each B-cell progenitor has the potential to produce a large number of offspring. Some will develop into plasma or memory B cells, while others – the majority – will perish.[5] Most of the defined steps in this process of development represent population bottlenecks: developmental checkpoints wherein the developing B cell is tested to make sure that its BCR will be beneficial. In the periphery, exposure to antigen is associated with class switching and hypermutation of the variable domains of the antigen receptor. A few select survivors earn long lives as part of a cadre of memory B cells. These veterans are charged with the responsibility to rapidly engage antigen to which they have been previously exposed, providing experienced protection against repeated assault.

Specialized microenvironments also play a role in peripheral B-cell development (Chapter 2), each of which enables the B cell to properly engage different types of antigens or venues of attack. In the marginal zone, mature splenic B cells lie in wait for bacterial pathogens. In the lymphoid follicles, B cells reactive with a given antigen collaborate with T cells and follicular dendritic cells (FDC) in order to maximize the immune response. In the germinal centers (GC), B cells use class switching and somatic mutation to modify and enhance the function and affinity of their immunoglobulins. And, underneath mucosal surfaces, B cells are primed to express IgA.

■ B-CELL DEVELOPMENT BEGINS IN THE PRIMARY LYMPHOID ORGANS ■

GENERATION OF A FUNCTIONING ANTIGEN RECEPTOR IS KEY TO THE VIABILITY OF A B CELL

Immunoglobulin rearrangement is hierarchical. In pro-B cells, $D_H \rightarrow J_H$ joining precedes $V_H \rightarrow DJ_H$ rearrangement (Chapter 4); and $V_L \rightarrow J_L$ joining takes place at the late pre-B-cell stage.

Production of a properly functioning B-cell receptor is essential for development beyond the pre-B-cell stage. For example, function-loss mutations in RAG-1/2 and DNA-dependent protein kinase (DNA-PKcs, Ku 70/80) preclude B-cell development. For the pro-B cell the dismal reality is that only one of three possible splices will place the V_H and J_H in the same reading frame. The opportunity to try rearrangement on the second chromosome gives failing pro-B cells a second opportunity. Together, this provides the cell with five chances out of nine for initial survival ($\frac{1}{3} + \frac{1}{3} \times \frac{2}{3}$). In-frame, functional VDJ_H rearrangement allows the pro-B cell to produce μ H chains, most of which are retained in the endoplasmic reticulum. The appearance of cytoplasmic μ H chains defines the pre-B cell. Early pre-B cells are marked by their large size.

VpreB, and $\lambda 14.1$ [$\lambda 5$], which together form the surrogate light chain (ψLC), and Igα and Igβ are constitutively expressed by pro-B cells. Pre-B cells whose μ H chains can associate with surrogate light chains form a pre-B-cell receptor. Its appearance signals the termination of further H-chain rearrangement (*allelic exclusion*), which is followed by four to

Table 8.1 Cell surface proteins active in early B-cell development

Gene	Class or alternative name	Associated or targeted genes or molecules	B-cell developmental phenotype in human or *mouse* associated with disrupted function of the indicated gene
The B-cell receptor complex			
μ-chain	Immunoglobulin superfamily	κ, λ, L chains, ΨL chain, CD79 a, b (Igα, β)	*Arrest at pre-B-cell stage*
λ14.1	Immunoglobulin superfamily	VpreB, μ H chain	*Arrest at pre-B-cell stage*
CD79a, b (Igα, β)	Immunoglobulin superfamily, cytoplasmic ITAM motifs	H chain, LYN, FYN, BLK, SYK	*Arrest at pro-B-cell stage*
Other cell surface proteins			
CD10	Type II metalloproteinase	Hydrolyzes peptide hormones, cytokines	Not expressed in murine B-cell progenitors
CD19	Immunoglobulin superfamily	mIgM, PI-3 kinase, VAV, LYN?, FYN?	Panhypogammaglobulinemia, normal numbers of CD20+ B cells in the blood
CD20	Four transmembrane domain surface molecule	B-cell Ca2+ channel subunit; indirectly interacts with LYN, FYN, LCK	*20–30% reduction in B-cell numbers*
CD21	Complement control protein	iC3b, C3dg, C3d, CD19, CD81, Leu 13, CD23	*Diminished T-cell-dependent immune responses, decreased germinal center formation, reductions in affinity maturation*
CD24	GPI-linked sialoglycoprotein	Ligand for P-selectin (CD62P)	*A57V polymorphism associated with increased risk of multiple sclerosis.* Deletion in mice leads to reductions in late pre-B and immature B-cell populations
CD34	Type I transmembrane glycoprotein	Ligand for L-selectin (CD62L) and E-selectin (CD62E)	Not expressed in murine B-cell progenitors
CD38	Type II transmembrane glycoprotein ADP-ribosyl cyclase, cyclic ADP-ribose hyroxylase	ADP ribosylates proteins	*Diminished T-cell-dependent immune responses, augmented responses to T-cell-independent type 2 polysaccharide antigens*

six cycles of cell division;[6] a process associated with a progressive decrease in cell size. Late pre-B daughter cells reactivate RAG1 and RAG2 and begin to undergo $V_L \rightarrow J_L$ rearrangement. Successful production of a complete κ or λ light chain permits expression of conventional IgM on the cell surface (sIgM), which identifies the *immature* B cell. Immature cells expressing self-reactive IgM antibodies may undergo repeated rounds of light-chain rearrangement to lessen the self-specificity of the antibody, a process termed *receptor editing*.[7]

Immature B cells that have successfully produced an acceptable IgM B-cell receptor extend transcription of the H-chain locus to include the Cδ exons downstream of Cμ. Alternative splicing permits co-production of IgM and IgD. These now newly *mature* IgM+IgD+ B cells enter the blood and migrate to the periphery where they form the majority of the B-cell pool in the spleen and the other secondary lymphoid organs. The IgM and IgD on individual cells share the same variable domains.

TYROSINE KINASES PLAY KEY ROLES IN B-CELL DEVELOPMENT

Signaling through the BCR is required for continued development. Bruton's tyrosine kinase is an important component of the phospholipase Cγ (PLCγ) pathway, which is used in BCR signaling. Deficiency of BTK function results in the arrest of human B-cell development at the pre-B-cell stage[8] and is the genetic basis of X-linked agammaglobulinemia (Chapter 34).

BLNK is a SRC homology 2 (SH2) domain-containing signal transduction adaptor. When phosphorylated by SYK, BLNK serves as a scaffold for the assembly of cell activation targets that include GRB2, VAV, NCK, and PLCγ. An agammaglobulinemic patient lacking pre-B and mature B cells has been reported with a loss-of-function mutation in BLNK.[9]

FLT3 (FLK2) is a receptor tyrosine kinase belonging to the same family as c-FMS, the receptor for colony-stimulating factor-1 (CSF-1). FLT3 ligand, which has homology to CSF-1, is a potent co-stimulator of early pro-B cells. In mice, targeted disruption of *flt3* leads to a selective deficiency of primitive B-cell progenitors.

CELL SURFACE ANTIGENS ASSOCIATED WITH B-CELL DEVELOPMENT

B-cell development is associated with the expression of a cascade of surface proteins, each of which plays a key role in the fate of the cell (Fig. 8.1 and Table 8.1). The timing of the appearance of each of these proteins can be used to analyze further the process of B-cell development.

CD34 is a highly glycosylated type I transmembrane glycoprotein that binds to CD62L (L-selectin) and CD62E (E-selectin) and thus likely aids in cell trafficking (Chapter 12). It is expressed on a small population (1–4%) of bone marrow cells that includes hematopoietic stem cells. Minimal hematopoietic defects have been documented in mice made deficient for CD34. However, such observations must be viewed with caution when extrapolated to humans, because CD34 is not expressed on hematopoietic stem cells in the mouse.

CD10, also known as neprilysin, neutroendopeptidase, and the common acute lymphocytic leukemia antigen (CALLA), is a type II membrane glycoprotein metalloprotease. CD10 has a short N-terminal cytoplasmic tail, a signal peptide transmembrane domain, and an extracellular C-terminal domain that includes six N-linked glycosylation sites. The extracellular domain contains 12 cysteines whose disulfide bonds help stabilize its zinc-binding pentapeptide motif, which is involved in its zinc-dependent metalloprotease catalytic activity. By virtue of its protease activity, it is thought to downregulate cellular responses to peptide hormones and cytokines. Inhibition of CD10 activity on bone marrow stromal cells enhances B-cell maturation. CD10 (CALLA) is used as a marker for pre-B acute lymphocytic leukemias and for certain lymphomas. Although not expressed in mouse B cells, CD10 belongs to the same family and has activity that is similar to mouse BP-1.

CD19 is a cell surface glycoprotein of the immunoglobulin superfamily that is exclusively expressed throughout B-cell development from the pro-B-cell stage up to, but not including, the mature plasma cell stage (Fig. 8.1).[3] CD19 exists in a complex with CD21 (complement receptor 2: CDR2), CD81 (TAPA-1), and Leu 13. With the help of CD21, CD19 can bind the complement C3 cleavage product C3d. The simultaneous binding of sIgM and CD19 to a C3d–antigen complex enables CD19 and the BCR to interact and thereby provides a link between innate and adaptive immune responses (Chapter 3). CD19–BCR interactions permit the cell to reduce the number of antigen receptors that need to be stimulated in order to activate the cell. Co-activation also reduces the threshold required for B-cell proliferation in response to a given antigen.

The cytoplasmic domain of CD19 contains nine conserved tyrosine residues which, when phosphorylated, allow CD19 to associate with PI-3 kinase and the tyrosine kinase VAV. Patients deficient in CD19 have normal numbers of CD20+ B cells in the blood, but are panhypogammaglobulinemic and are susceptible to sinopulmonary infections.[10]

CD20 contains four transmembrane domains and cytoplasmic C- and N-termini. It is a member of the CD20/FcεRIβ superfamily of leukocyte surface antigens. Differential phosphorylation yields three forms of CD20 (33, 35, and 37 kDa). Activated B cells have increased fractions of the 35 and 37 kDa forms of the antigen. CD20 appears to function as a B-cell Ca^{2+} channel subunit and regulates cell cycle progression. It can interact directly with major histocompatibility complex (MHC) class I and II molecules, as well as members of another family of four transmembrane domain proteins known as the TM4SF: CD43, CD81, and CD82. It also appears to interact indirectly with LYN, FYN, and LCK. In mice, loss of CD20 function leads to a 20–30% reduction in B-cell numbers. B-cell development, tissue localization, proliferation, T-cell-dependent antibody responses, and affinity maturation are otherwise normal.

CD21 (complement receptor 2: CR2) is a cell surface protein that contains a small cytoplasmic domain and an extracellular domain consisting of a series of short consensus repeats termed complement control protein domains. These extracellular domains can bind three different products of complement C3 cleavage: iC3b, C3dg, and C3d. When binding these products, CD21 acts as the ligand-binding subunit for the CD19–CD21–CD81 complex, tying the innate immune system to the adaptive immune response.[3] Mice that lack CD21 exhibit diminished T-dependent B-cell responses. However, serum IgM and IgG are in the normal range.

CD24 is a glycophosphatidylinositol-linked sialoprotein that serves as a ligand for P-selectin (CD62P). It is expressed on progenitor, immature, and mature B cells. Its expression decreases in activated B cells and is lost entirely in plasma cells. Monoclonal antibodies against CD24 inhibit human B-cell differentiation into plasma cells. In mice, CD24 is also known as HSA, or heat-stable antigen. Mice made deficient for CD24 show a leaky block in B-cell development with a reduction in late pre-B and immature B-cell populations.[11] However, peripheral B-cell numbers are normal and no impairment of immune function has been demonstrated.

CD38 is a bifunctional enzyme that can synthesize cyclic ADP-ribose (cADPR) from nicotinamide adenine dinucleotide (NAD+) and also hydrolyze cADPR to ADP-ribose. It is presumed that the enzyme exists to ADP-ribosylate target molecules. CD38 is expressed on pre-B cells, activated B cells, and early plasma cells, but not on immature or mature B cells or on mature plasma cells. Antibodies to CD38 can inhibit B lymphopoiesis, induce B-cell proliferation, and protect B cells from apoptosis. CD38 knockout mice exhibit marked deficiencies in antibody responses to T-cell-dependent protein antigens and augmented antibody responses to T-cell-independent type 2 polysaccharide antigen.[12]

TRANSCRIPTION FACTORS CONTROL EARLY B-CELL DIFFERENTIATION

Ultimately, B-cell development is a function of differential gene expression. Deficiencies in the function of the transcription factors that regulate lymphoid-specific gene expression can thus be expected to result in abnormal B-cell development (Fig. 8.2 and Table 8.2).

PU.1 is an ETS family loop-helix-loop (winged helix) transcription factor. ETS proteins contain a structure that binds purine-rich DNA sequences. PU.1 appears to regulate a number of lymphoid-specific genes, including CD79a (Igα), J chain, μ-chain, κ-chain, λ-chain, RAG1, and terminal deoxynucleotidyl transferase (TdT). ETS family members are relatively weak transcriptional activations and typically

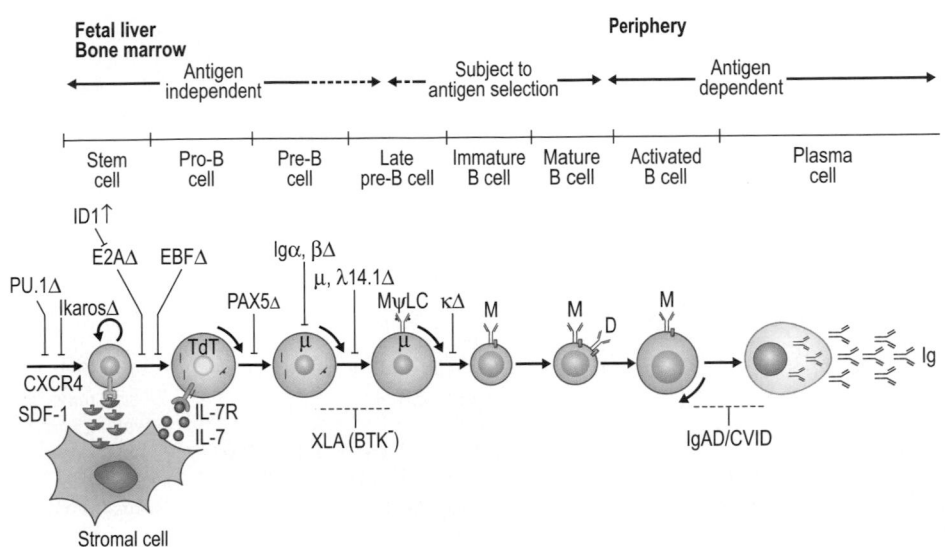

Fig. 8.2 Changes in the function of genes involved in early B-cell development can reduce or prevent the production of B cells and immunoglobulin. The stage of development at which abnormal function of selected set of transcription factors, cytokines, chemokines, and signal transduction elements can influence B-cell development is illustrated. A Greek delta (Δ) or a dash (–) indicates a loss of function of the gene in question. An upward arrow (↑) indicates an increase in the function of the gene in question.

require the presence of other factors in order to activate or repress their target genes, and PU.1 is no exception. PU.1 has been shown to cooperate with PIP (LSIRF, IRF4), c-JUN, and c-FOS. PU.1-deficient mice demonstrate defective generation of progenitors for monocytes, and granulocytes as well as B and T lymphocytes, indicating a role in the generation of MPPs as well as LMPPs. PIP-deficient mice lack GC in peripheral lymphoid organs and exhibit defects in B-cell activation.[13]

Ikaros and Aiolos belong to the same zinc finger transcription factor family. Both are expressed during lymphoid development, but Ikaros is expressed in stem cells and in mature lymphocytes, whereas Aiolos is only expressed after commitment to the B-cell lineage. Ikaros transcripts are subject to alternative splicing, generating several isoforms, each of which differs in its DNA-binding patterns, tendency to dimerize, and nuclear localization. Among the genes bound by Ikaros are TdT, λ14.1 (λ5), VpreB, and LCK. Ikaros-deficient mice lack B cells. Aiolos-deficient mice exhibit elevated levels of IgG and IgE. With age, these mice tend to develop autoantibodies and B-cell lymphomas.

The E2A locus encodes two basic helix-loop-helix transcription factors that represent two alternately spliced products, E12 and E47.[14] Targets for E2A include RAG-1 and TdT, the enzyme responsible for N addition (Chapter 4). The functions of E12 and E47 appear to overlap. However, E47 appears to play a greater role in driving TdT and RAG-1, whereas E12 is a better activator of EBF and PAX5, and thus helps commit developing cells to the B-cell lineage. In mice with disruptions in the *E2A* gene, B-cell development is arrested at an extremely early stage, prior to the first transcription of RAG-1.

ID-1 has a helix-loop-helix domain, but lacks a DNA binding domain. Thus, it can function as a dominant negative factor, inhibiting the function of helix-loop-helix transcription factors, such as E2A. ID-1 is only expressed in pro-B cells. ID-1 transgenic mice have a

phenotype that is very similar to E2A knockout mice, suggesting that Id-1 can regulate E2A function.

EBF, or early B-cell factor, is a helix-loop-helix-like transcription factor. EBF is expressed at all stages of differentiation except plasma cells and in mice has been shown to be critical in the progression of B cells past the early pro-B-cell stage. The developmental block in B-cell differentiation is similar to that seen in E2A mutants, suggesting that these transcription factors act cooperatively and regulate a common set of genes.

PAX5 is a paired-box, or domain, transcription factor that, among the progeny of hematopoietic stem cells, is expressed exclusively in cells of the B-cell lineage. PAX5 has both a positive and a negative effect on B-cell differentiation. In mice, B-cell precursors require PAX5 in order to progress beyond the pro-B-cell stage. The presence of PAX5 also prevents early B-lineage progenitors from transiting into other hematopoietic pathways, including those leading to the development of granulocytes, dendritic cells, macrophages, osteoclasts, NK cells, and T cells.

MODULATION OF B-CELL DEVELOPMENT BY CHEMOKINES, CYTOKINES, AND HORMONES

Stromal cells can influence the microenvironment surrounding B-cell precursors through cytokines and chemokines, which exert local effects on B-cell development (Fig. 8.2). For example, CXCL12, which is also known as pre-B-cell growth-stimulating factor and as stromal cell-derived factor-1 (PBSF/SCF-1), promotes pro-B-cell proliferation. Mice with a targeted disruption of this gene exhibit impaired B lymphopoiesis in fetal liver and bone marrow, and fail to undergo bone marrow myelopoiesis.[15] The mechanism by which CXCL12 regulates early B-cell development remains unclear. However, disruption of its

Table 8.2 Nuclear and cytoplasmic factors active in early B-cell development

Gene	Class or alternative name	Associated or targeted genes or molecules	B-cell developmental phenotype in human or *mouse* associated with disrupted function of the indicated gene
Transcription factors			
PU.1	Loop-helix-loop (winged helix)	CD79a (Igα), μ H chain	*Arrest prior to the pro-B cell stage*
Ikaros	Zinc finger	RAG1, TdT, IL2R, VpreB, LCK	*Arrest prior to the pro-B-cell stage*
Aiolos	Zinc finger	RAG1, TdT, IL2R	*Aging mice develop symptoms of systemic lupus erythematosus*
E2A	Basic helix-loop-helix (BHLH)	RAG1, IgH, Igκ, TdT, EBF, PAX5	*Arrest prior to the pro-B-cell stage*
EBF	EBF/Olf helix-loop-helix (HLH)-like	CD79a (Igα), λ14.1, VpreB, PAX5	*Arrest prior to the pro-B-cell stage*
PAX5	Paired-domain	CD19, λ14.1, VpreB, BLK kinase, J chain, VH promoters, Vκ promoters	Arrest at pro-B-cell stage
The recombinase complex			
RAG1, RAG2	Recombinase	Recombination signal sequences of immunoglobulin gene segments	*Arrest at pro-B-cell stage*
TdT	Nontemplated DNA polymerase	Coding ends of rearranging immunoglobulin gene segments	Absence of N nucleotides, diminished production of pathogenic anti-DNA autoantibodies in susceptible mice
DNA-PK	DNA repair complex	Multimeric complex consisting of DNA-PKcs, Ku70, Ku80 which repairs double-stranded DNA breaks	Arrest at pro-B-cell stage, original mouse SCID mutation identified as a loss of function mutation in DNA-PKcs
Protein tyrosine kinases			
FLK2/FLT3	Class III receptor tyrosine kinase	GRB2, SHC	Selective deficiency of primitive B-cell progenitors
BLNK	SH2 adapter protein	SYK, GRB2, VAV, NCK, Phospholipase Cγ (PLCγ)	*Arrest at pro-B-cell stage*
BTK	BTK/TEC protein tyrosine kinase	Phospholipase Cγ (PLCγ), SAB	*X-linked agammaglobulinemia – arrest at pre-B-cell stage*

SCID, severe combined immunoeficiency.

receptor CXCR4 leads to failure in the homing of plasma cells to the bone marrow.

Interleukin-7 (IL-7) has a minimal proliferative effect on human B-cell progenitors and, unlike in the mouse, is not essential for B-lineage differentiation. Nevertheless, IL-7 enhances CD19 expression. IL-7 treatment of human pro-B cells also leads to a reduction in the expression of RAG-1, RAG-2, and TdT and thus can modulate the process of immunoglobulin gene segment rearrangement.

Interferons-α and β (IFN-α/β) are potent inhibitors of IL-7-induced growth of B-lineage cells in mice.[16] The inhibition is mediated by apoptotic cell death. One potential source of IFN-α/β is bone marrow macrophages. Another macrophage-derived cytokine, IL-1, can also act as a dose-dependent positive or negative modulator of B lymphopoiesis.

Systemic hormones also regulate lymphopoiesis.[17] A role for sex steroids is suggested by the reduction in pre-B cells during pregnancy. Estradiol can also alter later stages of B-cell development, promoting expansion of the marginal-zone compartment. Prolactin appears to enhance production of both marginal-zone and follicular B cells. Mice with a loss of function mutation in the *Pit-1* transcription factor gene do not produce growth hormone, prolactin, or thyroid-stimulating hormone. These dwarf mice exhibit a defect in B-cell development that is correctable by the thyroid hormone thyroxine.[18]

KEY CONCEPTS

B-CELL DEVELOPMENT IN THE PERIPHERY

>> T-independent activation of naïve B cells results in terminal differentiation into short-lived plasma cells or long-lived B1 cells

>> T-dependent activation of B cells leads to germinal center formation, permitting somatic hypermutation and class switch recombination

>> T-dependent activation of naïve B cells results in differentiation into memory B cells (via CD40/CD154 interaction) or short-lived plasma cells (via OX40/OX40-ligand)

>> T-dependent activation of memory B cells results in expansion of memory B cells (via CD40/CD154) or differentiation into long-lived plasma cells (via CD27/CD70)

>> Activated T cells control late B-cell differentiation by cell-bound ligands and secreted cytokines

>> Activated B cells control T-cell development by presentation of antigen and co-stimulation

B-CELL DEVELOPMENT IN THE PERIPHERY: DIFFERENTIATION AND THE RESPONSE TO ANTIGEN

The lifespan of mature B cells expressing surface IgM and IgD appears entirely dependent on antigen selection. After leaving the bone marrow, unstimulated cells live for only a few days. Deletion of the transmembrane/intracellular domains of the B-cell antigen receptor of mature B cells disables their survival, which indicates that signaling through the BCR is essential for their survival. As originally postulated by Burnet's 'clonal selection' theory, B cells are rescued from apoptosis by their response to a cognate antigen.

The reaction to antigen leads to activation, which may then be followed by diversification. The nature of the activation process is critical. T-cell-independent stimulation of B cells induces differentiation into short-lived plasma cells with limited class switching. T-dependent stimulation adds additional layers of diversification, including somatic hypermutation (SHM) of the variable domains, which permits affinity maturation, class switching to the entire array of classes available (Chapter 4), and differentiation into the long-lived memory B-cell pool or into the long-lived plasma cell population.

BAFF AND APRIL CAN PLAY KEY ROLES IN THE DEVELOPMENT OF MATURE B CELLS

B cells leave the bone marrow while still undergoing initial maturation, demonstrating progressively higher levels of IgD expression with a commensurate lowering of IgM. They need the splenic environment in order to complete this maturation process. Immigrant splenic maturing B cells pass through two transitional stages, known as transitional stages 1 (T1) and 2 (T2). Only a minority of these cells will successfully make the transition, as this differentiation step is a crucial checkpoint for controlling self-reactivity.

Passage through this checkpoint requires the interaction of soluble B-cell-activating factor of the tumor necrosis family (BAFF), with its receptor, BAFF-R, which is primarily expressed on B cells.[19] Death signals triggered through interaction of the BCR with self antigen may be counterbalanced by stimulation of BAFF-R, which enhances expression of survival factors such as Bcl-2 and at the same time downregulates proapoptotic factors.

BAFF and a second tumor necrosis factor (TNF) family member APRIL (a proliferation-inducing ligand) can also induce isotype switching in naïve human B cells.[20] APRIL, as well as BAFF, can bind to B-cell maturation antigen (BCMA) and transmembrane activator and calcium modulator and cyclophilin ligand interactor (TACI), both of which are members of the TNF-R family. BCMA is exclusively expressed on B cells, whereas TACI is expressed on B cells and activated T cells.

T-INDEPENDENT RESPONSES

Unlike T cells, which require presentation of antigen by other cells, B cells can respond directly to an antigen as long as that antigen is able to cross-link the antibodies on the B-cell surface. Such antigens, especially those that by nature cannot be recognized by T cells (e.g., DNA or polysaccharides) can induce a B-cell response independent of T-cell help. Depending on the cytokine milieu, the B cells may even class switch, although the range of available classes appears to be restricted. B cells that are activated by antigen alone do not take part in a GC reaction (see below).

T-DEPENDENT RESPONSES

Activated B cells express both MHC class I and class II molecules (Chapter 5) on their cell surface. They can thus present both intracellular and extracellular antigens to CD4 T helper and CD8 T cytotoxic lymphocytes. Their role as antigen-presenting cells is enhanced when they present peptides from the same antigen they have taken up with their antibodies (Chapter 7). Cognate recognition of the same antigen by both a B cell and a T cell permits each of these cells to activate the other reciprocally. In particular, T-cell-activated B cells express the co-stimulatory molecules CD80 and CD86, which in turn are required for activation of T cells via CD28 as well as their inactivation by CD152 (CTLA-4). Since B cells do not express IL-12, they do not induce expression of IFN-γ in the activated T cells but rather favor the differentiation of activated T cells into IL-4, IL-5, IL-10, and IL-13-expressing Th2 cells. These cytokines can support the CD40 induced expansion of memory B cells (IL-4), OX40 or CD27-induced differentiation into short-lived and long-lived plasma cells (IL-10), and CD40-induced class switch recombination (CSR) to IgG$_4$ or IgE (IL-4). Co-stimulation also permits T-helper cells to induce SHM, permitting affinity maturation.

ORGANIZATION OF THE PERIPHERAL LYMPHOID ORGANS

Compartmentalization in the immune system facilitates efficiency and regulation of the immune response. During development, the primary and secondary lymphoid organs are built up in an organized way.[21] The process involves multiple factors that play various roles in the development, maintenance, and function of the lymphoid organs.

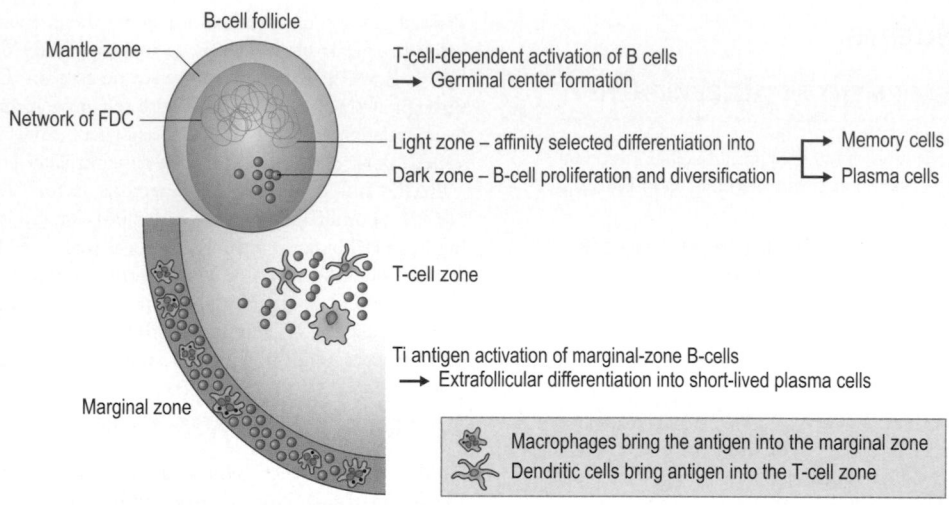

Fig. 8.3 T-cell and B-cell compartments within the white pulp of the spleen. Most splenic T cells can be found in a compartment that surrounds the central arterioles. This compartment is also referred to as the periarteriolar lymphocyte sheath (PALS). Most splenic B cells are found in two separate compartments – the marginal zone and the follicles. The marginal zone is located next to the marginal sinuses. The primary follicles are located within, but separate from, the T-cell zones. Within these primary follicles, B cells are embedded within a network of follicular dendritic cells (FDC).

B lymphocytes enter the secondary lymphoid organs through defined ways. Each organ exhibits a preferred route of entry.[22] For example, most lymphocytes enter the spleen through the bloodstream whereas lymphocytes enter lymph nodes and Peyer's patches through high endothelial venules. In general, lymphocyte migration and the tissue-specific homing are strictly controlled by chemokines (Chapter 13). Dendritic cells, macrophages, and other highly specialized cells transport antigens from peripheral sites of entry into the secondary lymphoid organs. Within these organs, circulating lymphocytes survey available antigens. Binding to a cognate antigen activates the cell. Contact between a T cell and a B cell that have been activated by the same antigen permits initiation of a T-cell-dependent immune response.

THE SPLEEN

In the secondary lymphoid organs, T cells and B cells are segregated into clearly defined areas (Chapter 2). Figure 8.3 illustrates the pattern observed in the white pulp of the spleen. It is in these areas where antigen-dependent B-cell activation occurs and where the cells subsequently undergo further differentiation. The marginal sinuses, the site of entry for lymphocytes, macrophages, and dendritic cells, separate the white pulp from the red pulp. These sinuses are lined with a mucosal addressin cell adhesion molecule-1 (MAdCAM-1) expressing endothelium (Chapter 12). In the marginal sinuses, one finds a specialized layer of metallophilic macrophages that are thought to control the entry of antigen into the white pulp.

FDC are highly specialized cells that present antigen to B cells (Chapter 7).[23] In contrast to other types of dendritic cells, FDC do not process antigen. Instead, FDC have abundant complement receptors and Ig Fc receptors that allow accumulation of antigen in the form of immune complexes within the B follicle. FDC are crucial for B-cell maintenance as well as for their activation and differentiation (see below).

Chemokines (Chapter 11) and cytokines (Chapter 10) play a major role in the organized development of the secondary lymphoid organs.[24] For example, mice deficient in the B-cell chemokine receptor CXCR5 fail to develop primary B-cell follicles in the spleen. In these mice, B cells enter the spleen through the marginal sinuses just as they do in their wild-type littermates. However, B cells in these CXCR5-deficient mice fail to move into the areas where B-cell zones would normally develop. Instead, a broad ring of B cells surrounds the T-cell zone.

The proinflammatory cytokine, TNF-α, and its receptor TNFR1 play an important role in the organogenesis of the spleen. In mice deficient for TNF-α, the marginal zones are expanded whereas the primary follicles are missing. The disruption of B-cell follicles in these mice is similar to the one observed in CXCR5-deficient mice. However, in contrast to the CXCR5-deficient mouse, no network of FDC develops.

Deficiency of lymphotoxin (LTα) has even more profound effects. This may be explained by the fact that the LTα exists in two forms, a soluble homotrimer that is released from the cell membrane after cleavage and interacts with the TNFR1 molecule and a membrane-bound heterotrimer LTα$_1$/LTβ$_2$ that interacts with the LTβ receptor (LTβR). Thus, in mice deficient for LTα, both interactions are interrupted. The expression of LTα$_1$/LTβ$_2$ on B cells is crucial for the organized development of lymphoid structures and hence the induction of memory humoral immune responses. LTα$_1$/LTβ$_2$-positive B cells by themselves are necessary and sufficient for the formation of the FDC network.

■ THE MARGINAL ZONE PROVIDES A HOME FOR B-CELL EARLY RESPONDERS ■

Mature B cells are not homogeneous. Functionally and developmentally distinct subsets exist. In the spleen, follicular B cells have a key role in the adaptive immune response, whereas marginal-zone B cells are now seen as major players at the interface between the initial innate immune response and the delayed adaptive response.[25] The ability of marginal-zone B cells to respond rapidly to encapsulated bacteria by differentiating into antigen-specific plasma cells helps keep such infections under control. Marginal-zone B cells take time to develop and are not present in young infants. The marginal zone becomes fully populated only after the age of 2. In the physiologic absence of these marginal-zone cells, a poor response to bloodborne infections is commonly observed.[26]

GERMINAL CENTERS

T-cell-dependent activation of follicular B cells can induce the formation of a GC, which is the microenvironment where affinity maturation of the humoral immune response takes place.[27] The interplay of hypermutation followed by antigen selection is the basis of affinity maturation. In the GC, B cells that express antibodies of high affinity are selected to develop into memory and long-living plasma cells.

GC develop only after T-cell-dependent activation of B cells. Their full function is dependent on the interaction between CD40 expressed on B cells and CD40L (CD154) expressed on activated T cells. Patients with loss of function mutations in CD40L have high serum levels of IgM and suffer from recurrent infections (hyper-IgM syndrome: Chapter 34).[28]

In a primary immune response, it takes about a week for the complex GC structure to develop. In the spleen, a few days after activation of antigen-specific B cells and T cells, small clusters of proliferating B cells are observed at the border of the T-cell zone and the primary B-cell follicle.[29] The rapidly expanding B-cell clone seems to push the naïve B cells towards the edge of the primary follicle. The naïve B cells form a mantle zone around the newly developing GC and the primary follicle changes into a secondary follicle. Subsequently, the network of FDC becomes filled with proliferating, antigen-activated B cells. About the second week after immunization, the GC matures into a classical structure that contains a dark zone and a light zone. At this stage of GC development, proliferation is restricted to the dark zone. In the network of FDC, the B cells differentiate into plasma cells and memory cells. In the fully developed GC, dividing cells are termed centroblasts, whereas differentiating cells within the FDC network are termed centrocytes.

In the dark zone, proliferating B cells activate a mechanism of SHM.[23, 26] This is a highly specific process that is targeted towards the gene segments that encode the antigen-binding domain of the antibody molecule. Hypermutation introduces single nucleotide changes into the rearranged variable genes of the Ig molecules. By chance a few of these mutations result in a receptor with higher affinity for antigen. B cells expressing such receptors are favored for activation, particularly late in an immune response, when availability of antigen is limiting. Thus, within the dark zone, a clone of variants expressing antigen receptors with various affinities for the antigen is generated from a single B-cell progenitor. Antigen presented by the FDC is thought to select which B cells differentiate into memory cells or plasma cells. Only the few B cells with a high-affinity receptor for the antigen ultimately survive. The rest of the B-cell variants die by apoptosis, presumably due to the lack of sufficient stimulation through the B-cell antigen receptor complex.

THE MURINE B1 AND B2 PERIPHERAL B-CELL COMPARTMENTS (CD5 B CELLS)

Differential expression of the cell surface molecules IgD, CD5, CD11b/CD18, CD23, and CD45 allows the separation of the peripheral B-cell population into two compartments, B1 and B2.[25, 26, 30] 'Conventional' B cells (B2 cells) express high levels of IgM and IgD, whereas 'CD5' B cells (B1 cells) express minimal surface IgD. B1 cells express little CD45 and virtually no CD23. They all express CD5 mRNA, although not all of them display CD5 on their cell surface. Based on the pattern of surface CD5 expression, B1 cells have been divided into B1a (CD5+) and B1b (CD5-) populations.

B1 cells seem to develop from distinct progenitors that represent a majority of B cells in fetal life.[33] Accordingly, in fetal liver all B cells are B1 cells, as are 40–60% of B cells in fetal spleen. Later in development, B1 cells comprise fewer than 10% of the splenic IgM+ B cells. In the peritoneal cavity B1 cells are abundant. In humans the subset of B1 B cells is not clearly defined.

Natural antibodies are found in every serum. These IgM antibodies are produced by B1 cells. They tend to have specificity for bacterial antigens as well as autoantigens. In general, they are both of low affinity and polyreactivity. However, these antibodies represent a second important and immediate defense against infectious organisms.

MOLECULAR MECHANISM OF SOMATIC HYPERMUTATION AND CLASS SWITCH RECOMBINATION

Immunoglobulin SHM and CSR are essential mechanisms for the generation of a high-affinity, adaptive humoral immune response. They allow the generation of effector plasma cells secreting high-affinity IgG, IgA, and IgE antibodies.

SOMATIC HYPERMUTATION

Hypermutation occurs only during a narrow window in B-cell development. The mechanism is induced during B-cell proliferation within the microenvironment of the GC.[32-35] With a high rate of about 10^{-3} to 10^{-4}/basepair per generation, single nucleotide exchanges are introduced in a stepwise manner into the rearranged V-region and its 3′ and 5′ flanking sequences. Mutations are randomly introduced, although there is a preference for transitions (cytidine → thymidine or adenosine → guanine) over transversions. Analysis of the pattern of somatic mutations has revealed that the sequence of the complementarity-determining regions (CDRs: Chapter 4), the loops that form the antigen-binding site, have been selected to form mutation hot spots.

Effective hypermutation requires the V-gene promoter and transcription enhancer sequences. Indeed, the position of the V-gene promoter defines the start of the hypermutation domain, which spans 2000 nucleotides. Any heterologous sequence that is introduced into the V-gene segment locus will become a target of the hypermutation machinery. Thus, SHM can sometimes play a role in lymphomas and leukemias where oncogenes have been linked to Ig promoters and enhancers.

CLASS SWITCH RECOMBINATION

Upon transition from the immature to the mature state and leaving the bone marrow, the B cell starts to express IgD as well as IgM. Both IgM and IgD antibodies use the same $V_H DJ_H$-exon and promoter (Fig. 8.4). The molecular basis of co-expression of IgM and IgD by the same B cell is due to differential termination of transcription and splicing of the primary transcripts. Although sequences have been identified that are required for the control of termination and splicing of the $C\mu$ and $C\delta$ transcripts, none of the proteins involved is known. The role of IgD remains unclear. In mice, targeted inactivation of IgD has shown that IgD is not critical for B-cell activation and differentiation. $IgD^{-/-}$ B cells show a slightly reduced capability for affinity maturation, but no other defect has yet been described.

Unlike IgD, the other antibody classes are not stably expressed together with IgM. B cells can switch from expression of their $V_H DJ_H$-exon with $C\mu$ to expression of the same $V_H DJ_H$-exon with any of the downstream C_H genes (e.g., $C\alpha_{1,2}$, $C\gamma_{1,2,3,4}$, or $C\varepsilon$: Chapter 4). Class switching, like SHM, is a hallmark of B-cell activation. It can be induced by T-cell-independent signals (e.g., lipopolysaccharide) or by signals derived from T cells (e.g., CD40L). CD40L-deficient humans (X-linked hyper-IgM syndrome: Chapter 34) are severely impaired in the expression of Ig classes other than IgM.

TATA-less promoters located in front of the switch regions respond to signals from cytokines and B-cell activation-inducing ligands, like CD40L binding to CD40 on the B cell. Transcription starting from these promoters is essential in targeting switch recombination to the transcribed switch region. Such transcription starts with a small I-exon located between the promoter and the switch region, continues through the switch region itself, and finishes after including the entire C_H gene sequence.

The choice of C_H gene targeted for switch recombination in a particular B cell appears to be dependent on external cytokine signals, e.g., from T cells. IFN-γ targets CSR to IgG_2 in humans and IgG_{2a} in mice, IL-4 to IgG_4 and IgE in humans and IgG_1 and IgE in mice, and transforming growth factor-β to IgA in both humans and mice. Other switch targeting cytokines have been described, although our knowledge is far from complete. It is evident, however, that those cytokines central for the organization of cellular, humoral, and mucosal immunity, respectively, recruit exactly those classes of antibodies that provide the most useful functions for their respective branches of the immune system.

BOTH SHM AND CSR REQUIRE ACTIVATION-INDUCED CYTIDINE DEAMINASE

Both molecular mechanisms, CSR and SHM, are dependent on an activation-induced cytidine deaminase (AID).[34, 35] Mice deficient for this enzyme will express only IgM antibodies without somatic mutations, and patients with homozygous AID loss-of-function mutations present with a hyper-IgM syndrome (Chapter 34). The precise mechanism of action remains controversial, with first reports implicating AID as a potential RNA editing enzyme and subsequent reports pointing to single-strand DNA modifications. In either case, in SHM AID is targeted to the rearranged V-region gene that encodes the antigen-binding portion of the antibody molecule, and in CSR AID is targeted to the switch regions located upstream (5′) of each C_H gene. Both processes, SHM and CSR, are dependent on transcription.

Hypermutation is proposed to occur in two steps.[35] The mechanism is induced by AID-catalyzed deamination of deoxycytidine (C) to deoxyuridine (U). The mispairing of U and deoxyguanosine (G) is than processed by uracil DNA glycosylase and targeted by repair pathways. As a consequence mutations at C-G pairs are observed. In the second step, mutations at A-T pairs are induced, probably during a mutagenic patch repair of U-G mismatches introduced by AID. A number of proteins, such as MSH2 and MHS6 (homologues 2 and 6 of the *Escherichia coli*

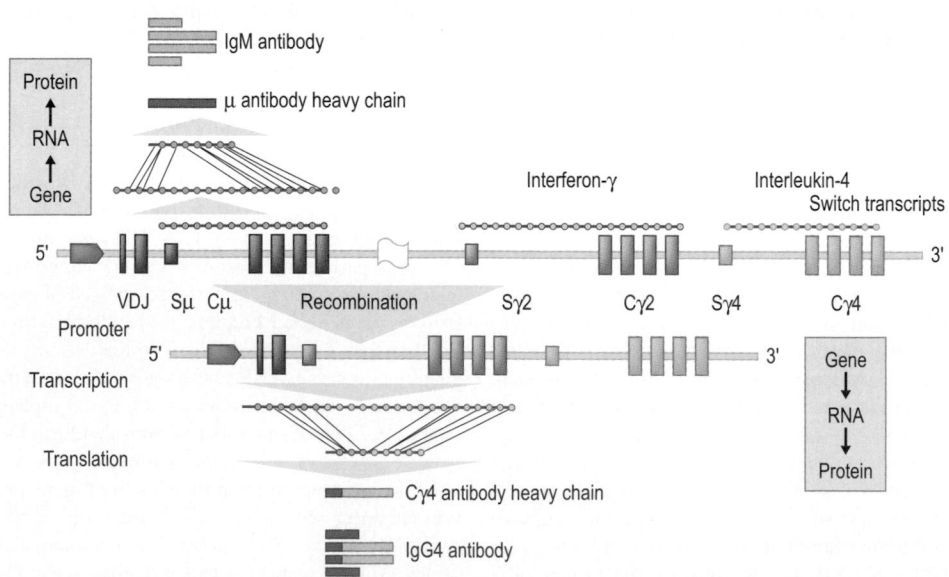

Fig. 8.4 Antibody class switch recombination. Recombination between switch regions (Sμ and Sε) is preceded by transcription of these switch regions. Transcription is targeted by cytokines to distinct switch regions.

MutS), polymerase η or exonuclease-1 seemed to be involved; however, the mechanism is not yet clear.

Switch regions are composed of 1–6 kilobase-long GC-rich repetitive sequence motifs. G-C pairs within these motifs are targeted by AID. Deamination of C and processing by uracil DNA glycosylase creates an abasic site, which facilitates the introduction of double-strand DNA breaks. Joining and repair require the presence of DNA-phosphokinases, Ku70, Ku80, and probably other members of the general double-strand repair mechanism (Chapter 4).

Both mechanisms, SHM and CSR, have to be tightly controlled, since the introduction of double-strand breaks into the DNA not only poses a risk to the longevity of the B cell, but also permits translocations involving and activating oncogenes.[36] For example, for Burkitt lymphoma cells and for plasma cell-derived myeloma cells, the translocation and ectopic expression of the c-*MYC* gene are an apparent consequence of abnormal SHM and CSR.

B-CELL MEMORY

PLASMA CELLS

One of the key features of the immune system is immunological memory for antigens encountered in the past. Immunological memory of B lymphocytes is dependent on T helper lymphocytes. While primary B-cell responses start with secreted low-affinity IgM antibodies after a lag-phase of 1–2 days and only gradually develop high-affinity antibodies of other classes, secondary responses start faster and with high-affinity antibodies of IgM and other classes. This protective humoral memory is provided by long-lived plasma cells.[37] These cells are generated in the secondary lymphoid organs and then migrate to the bone marrow or to a site affected by inflammation. In the bone marrow, they can survive for long periods without further activation and proliferating. By continuously secreting antibodies, long-lived plasma cells provide the individual with long-term humoral protection. If the original antigen recurs at higher concentrations, free antigen may activate memory B cells and induce again differentiation into high-affinity antibodies secreting effector plasma cells (Fig. 8.5).

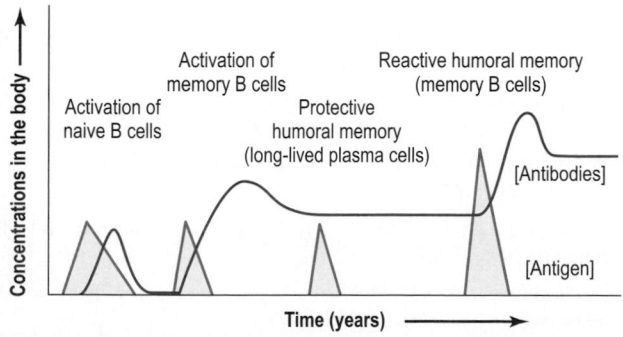

Fig. 8.5 The two types of B-cell memory: reactive memory of memory B cells and protective memory of long-lived plasma cells. The relative concentrations of antibody and antigen over time are indicated.

MEMORY B CELLS

Memory B cells are derived from naïve B cells activated by antigen and T-cell help in extrafollicular or GC reactions. The differentiation to memory B cells is critically dependent on CD40 of the B cell and CD40L expressed by T cells and FDC.[28] Inactivation of the CD40 or CD40L genes by targeted mutation in the murine germline or by accidental mutation in humans leads to a hyper-IgM syndrome and a general lack of B-cell memory (Chapter 34). Interestingly, using CD27 as a marker for B-cell memory cells, a small fraction of IgM memory B cells have been detected in the peripheral blood of some patients with hyper-IgM syndrome. The pattern of cell surface antigen expression suggested that these cells are marginal-zone B cells. In humans, hypermutation is a mechanism that occurs during a narrow window of B-cell development in the GC. However, it seems possible that under certain circumstances the mechanism of hypermutation might be induced, when B cells are activated in a T-independent response, perhaps in the gut by signals delivered through Toll-like receptors.[38]

DEVELOPMENT OF ECTOPIC LYMPHOID TISSUE IN AUTOIMMUNE DISEASE

In immune diseases such as myasthenia gravis, Sjögren's syndrome, Hashimoto's disease, or rheumatoid arthritis, ectopic lymphoid tissue may develop in the affected tissue or organ.[39, 40] The presence of proinflammatory cytokines may support the development of additional lymphoid tissue.

The growth of ectopic lymphoid tissue in rheumatoid synovium offers an excellent example of this disease-related phenomenon. In healthy individuals, the synovium is made up by a thin lining layer of synoviocytes. In contrast, in patients with rheumatoid arthritis the diseased joint is highly

---

CLINICAL RELEVANCE

ABNORMAL B-CELL DEVELOPMENT AND DISEASES OF IMMUNE FUNCTION

>> Failure to generate B cells or a normal repertoire of antibodies leads to humoral immune deficiency, which is commonly marked by recurrent sinopulmonary infections

>> Failure to prevent the formation of antibodies with high avidity or high affinity to self-antigens can lead to autoimmune diseases

>> The process of antibody repertoire diversification lends itself to the creation of mutations that can activate and modify oncogenes as well, leading to leukemia or lymphoma. Mechanisms include:

RAG1/2-catalyzed juxtaposition of an oncogene to an immunoglobulin promoter or enhancer, activating the oncogene

Activation-induced cytidine deaminase-induced somatic hypermutation of the oncogene, altering its function

infiltrated with varying numbers of T cells, B cells, plasma cells, macrophages, and dendritic cells. In the majority of patients, these mononuclear cells are loosely dispersed throughout the synovium. However, in some patients large, well-organized lymphocyte structures develop that are similar in appearance to the lymphoid follicles seen in the secondary lymphoid organs. At the center of these cell clusters one finds a network of FDC. Antigen presented by the FDC appears to activate the B cells, which induces proliferation. A layer of T cells, which may support B-cell differentiation into plasma cells, surrounds the central B cells. The analysis of the V-gene repertoire expressed in synovial B cells has demonstrated that during proliferation hypermutation is activated in a pattern similar to the one observed in normal secondary lymphoid organs. Thus, in rheumatoid arthritis a GC reaction can be induced within the synovial tissue. A central question is which antigens drive the immune response and select B cells to differentiate into memory and plasma cells. The ectopic lymphoid tissue may function as additional lymphoid tissue, in which case the immune response is no longer restricted to the peripheral lymphoid organs. Equally well, the ectopic lymphoid tissue may support a self-specific immune response. These questions remain active topics of investigation.

■ REFERENCES ■

1. Matthias P, Rolink AG. Transcriptional networks in developing and mature B cells. Nat Rev Immunol 2005; 5: 497–508.

2. Nagasawa T. Microenvironmental niches in the bone marrow required for B-cell development. Nat Rev Immunol 2006; 6: 107–16.

3. Haas KM, Tedder TF. Role of the CD19 and CD21/35 receptor complex in innate immunity, host defense and autoimmunity. Adv Exp Med Biol 2005; 560: 125–39.

4. Matthias P, Rolink AG. Transcriptional networks in developing and mature B cells. Nat Rev Immunol 2005; 5: 497–508.

5. Rajewsky K. Clonal selection and learning in the antibody system. Nature 1996; 381: 751–758.

6. Matthias P, Rolink AG. Transcriptional networks in developing and mature B cells. Nat Rev Immunol 2005; 5: 497–508.

7. Nemazee DA, Weigert MG. Revising B cell receptors. J Exp Med 2000; 191: 1813–1818.

8. Conley ME, Cooper MD. Genetic basis of abnormal B cell development. Curr Opin Immunol 1998; 10: 399–406.

9. Minegishi Y, Rohrer J, Coustan-Smith E, et al. An essential role for BLNK in human B cell development. Science 1999; 286: 1954–1957.

10. van Zelm MC, Reisli I, van der Burg M, et al. An antibody-deficiency syndrome due to mutations in the *CD19* gene. N Engl J Med 2006; 354: 1901–1912.

11. Nielsen PJ, Lorenz B, Muller AM, et al. Altered erythrocytes and a leaky block in B-cell development in CD24/HSA-deficient mice. Blood 1997; 89: 1058–1067.

12. Cockayne DA, Muchamuel T, Grimaldi JC, et al. Mice deficient for the ecto-nicotinamide adenine dinucleotide glycohydrolase CD38 exhibit altered humoral immune responses. Blood 1998; 92: 1324–1333.

13. Mittrucker HW, Matsuyama T, Grossman A, et al. Requirement for the transcription factor LSIRF/IRF4 for mature B and T lymphocyte function. Science 1997; 275: 540–543.

14. Rothenberg EV, Telfer JC, Anderson MK. Transcriptional regulation of lymphocyte lineage commitment. Bioessays 1999; 21: 726–742.

15. Nagasawa T, Hirota S, Tachibana K, et al. Defects of B-cell lymphopoiesis and bone-marrow myelopoiesis in mice lacking the CXC chemokine PBSF/SDF-1. Nature 1996; 382: 635–638.

16. Wang J, Lin Q, Langston H, et al. Resident bone marrow macrophages produce type 1 interferons that can selectively inhibit interleukin-7-driven growth of B lineage cells. Immunity 1995; 3: 475–484.

17. Grimaldi CM, Hill L, Xu X, et al. Hormonal modulation of B cell development and repertoire selection. Mol Immunol 2005; 42: 811–820.

18. Foster M, Montecino-Rodriguez E, et al. Regulation of B and T cell development by anterior pituitary hormones. Cell Mol Life Sci 1998; 54: 1076–1082.

19. Mackay F, Browning JL. BAFF: a fundamental survival factor for B cells. Nat Rev Immunol 2002; 2: 465–475.

20. Castigli E, Geha RS. Molecular basis of common variable immunodeficiency. J Allergy Clin Immunol 2006; 117: 740–747.

21. Fu YX, Chaplin DD. Development and maturation of secondary lymphoid tissues. Annu Rev Immunol 1999; 17: 399–433.

22. Butcher EC, Williams M, Youngman K, et al. Lymphocyte trafficking and regional immunity. Adv Immunol 1999; 72: 209–253.

23. Kosco-Vilbois MH. Are follicular dendritic cells really good for nothing. Nature Rev Immunol 2003; 3: 764–769.

24. Cyster JG. Chemokines and cell migration in secondary lymphoid organs. Science 1999; 286: 2098–2102.

25. Lopes-Carvalho T, Foote J, Kearney JF. Marginal zone B cells in lymphocyte activation and regulation. Curr Opin Immunol 2005; 17: 244–250.

26. Carsetti R, Rosado MM, Wardmann H. Peripheral development of B cells in mouse and man. Immunol Rev 2004; 197: 179–191.

27. MacLennan IC. Germinal centers. Annu Rev Immunol 1994; 12: 117–139.

28. Facchetti F, Appiani C, Salvi L, et al. Immunohistologic analysis of ineffective CD40–CD40 ligand interaction in lymphoid tissues from patients with X-linked immunodeficiency with hyper-IgM. Abortive germinal center cell reaction and severe depletion of follicular dendritic cells. J Immunol 1995; 154: 6624–6633.

29. Camacho SA, Kosco-Vilbois MH, Berek C. The dynamic structure of the germinal center. Immunol Today 1998; 19: 511–514.

30. Hayakawa K, Hardy RR. Development and function of B-1 cells. Curr Opin Immunol 2000; 12: 346–353.

31. Herzenberg LA, Tung JW. B cell lineages: documented at last! Nat Immunol 2006; 7: 225–226.

32. Berek C, Berger A, Apel M. Maturation of the immune response in germinal centers. Cell 1991; 67: 1121–1129.

33. Wagner SD, Neuberger MS. Somatic hypermutation of immunoglobulin genes. Annu Rev Immunol 1996; 14: 441–457.

REFERENCES

34. Honjo T, Muramatsu M, Fagarasan S. AID: how does it aid antibody diversity? Immunity 2004; 20: 659–668.

35. Neuberger MS, Harris RS, Di Noia J, et al. Immunity through DNA deamination. Trends Biochem Sci 2003; 28: 305–312.

36. Kuppers R, Dalla-Favera R. Mechanisms of chromosomal translocations in B cell lymphomas. Oncogene 2001; 20: 5580–5594.

37. Manz RA, Hauser AE, Hiepe F, et al. Maintenance of serum antibody levels. Annu Rev Immunol 2005; 23: 367–386.

38. Weller S, Reynaud CA, Weill JC. Splenic marginal zone B cells in humans: where do they mutate their Sg receptor? Eur J Immunol 2005; 35: 2789–2792.

39. Weyand CM, Klimiuk PA, Goronzy JJ. Heterogeneity of rheumatoid arthritis: from phenotypes to genotypes. Springer Semin Immunopathol 1998; 20: 5–22.

40. Kim HJ, Berek C. B cells in rheumatoid arthritis. Arthr Res 2000; 2: 126–131.

T-cell development

Ralph C. Budd, Karen A. Fortner

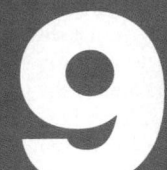

T-lymphocyte development must produce a large and diverse repertoire of functional T cells that can effectively combat a wide variety of infections without provoking a response against the host. The price for generating an increasingly varied population of antigen receptors needed to recognize a wide array of pathogens is the progressive risk of producing self-reactive lymphocytes that can manifest as an autoimmune disease, as well as other lymphocytes that make no fundamental interactions with major histocompatibility complex (MHC) molecules. The accumulation of either type of lymphocyte to critical numbers could be dangerous to the host. In order to minimize the possibility of retaining self-reactive T cells, or useless T cells that recognize no MHC–peptide complex, T lymphocytes are subjected to rigorous selection processes of positive and negative selection during development in the thymus. In addition, requiring two signals for activation prevents premature activation of T cells. Finally, the tremendous expansion of T cells that occurs during the response to an infection is resolved by the active induction of cell death. In perhaps no other organ are the processes of cell proliferation and death more dynamically displayed than by lymphocytes during an immune response. Collectively, these processes severely restrict the possibility of clonal expansion occurring without strict control. The consequences of inefficient lymphocyte removal at any one of these junctures can be devastating to the health of the organism. This is vividly displayed in both humans and mice where naturally arising mutations in death receptors such as Fas result in massive accumulation of lymphocytes and autoimmune sequelae.

THE THYMUS

Development of T cells occurs within the microenvironment provided by the thymic epithelial stroma. The thymic anlage is formed from embryonic ectoderm and endoderm. The thymic epithelium develops from the third branchial cleft and the third and fourth pharyngeal pouches.[1] Once formed, this anlage is colonized by hematopoietic cells that give rise to dendritic cells, macrophages, and developing T cells.[1] As few as 50–100 bone marrow-derived stem cells enter the thymus daily. The hematopoietic and epithelial components combine to form two histologically defined compartments: the cortex, that contains immature thymocytes and the medulla, which contains mature thymocytes.

The cortex is the earliest apparent portion of the thymus. As stem cells begin to enter the thymus, two microenvironments emerge. The subcapsular cortex is composed of epithelial cells, including the thymic nurse cells, so named because they envelop groups of immature thymocytes. In fact, however, the term "nurse cells" is misleading, since the thymocytes that are enveloped are likely those chosen for apoptotic elimination. The cortex proper is a network of epithelial cells with ubiquitous processes that are in intimate contact with densely packed immature thymocytes, most of which express both CD4 and CD8 surface proteins that bind to MHC class II and class I molecules, respectively.

The medulla is composed of epithelial cells that are packed more tightly and are associated with thymocytes that bear exclusively the mature phenotypes of expressing only CD4 or CD8. There appears to be a mutually positive benefit of thymocyte–epithelial interaction in the

KEY CONCEPTS

THE THYMUS

>> T cells develop in the thymus

>> The thymus consists of three major regions: the cortex, the medulla, and the corticomedullary junction

>> Most immature T cells, termed thymocytes, express both CD4 and CD8 and are found in the cortex

>> The corticomedullary junction contains large numbers of macrophages and dendritic cells that arise from mesodermal tissue

>> As thymocytes mature, they make their way through the corticomedullary junction to the medulla

>> Mature thymocytes express either CD4 or CD8 and are found exclusively in the medulla

medulla, as the thymic medulla remains disorganized until populated by mature T cells.

The corticomedullary junction is more than just an interphase. It contains large numbers of macrophages and dendritic cells that arise not from ectoderm or endoderm, but from mesodermal tissue (especially the bone marrow).

The diversity of cell types that make up the thymic stroma is only beginning to be appreciated. Cortical epithelial cells, for example, appear to be largely responsible for positive selection of thymocytes. Dendritic cells, predominantly at the corticomedullary junction, are potent mediators of negative selection. Medullary epithelial cells may promote the maturation of thymocytes that have successfully passed the selection requirements.

The ability of different stromal components to regulate distinct developmental events is influenced in part by the particular surface molecules expressed and their density, as well as the stage of the developing thymocytes with which they interact. As an example, although all stromal cell types appear to express both MHC class I and class II molecules, macrophages and dendritic cells express particularly high levels of class II. As a result macrophages and dendritic cells are exceptionally efficient at antigen presentation compared to epithelial cells. Macrophages and dendritic cells also differ from epithelial cells in their expression of CD80/CD86, the ligands for the co-stimulatory molecule CD28. Thymic epithelial cells have also been shown to secrete granulocyte and granulocyte–macrophage colony-stimulating factors (G-CSF, GM-CSF), as well as interleukin-6 (IL-6) and IL-7, whereas dendritic cells are unusual in their secretion of IL-10 and IL-12.[2]

■ EARLY T-CELL DEVELOPMENT ■

T-CELL DEVELOPMENT WITHIN THE THYMUS

T cells must traverse two fundamental and stringent hurdles during their development into mature cells capable of mounting an immune response. First, a T cell must successfully rearrange the pair of genes that encode a heterodimeric T-cell receptor (TCR) (Chapter 4). Second, a T cell must survive thymic selection during which self-reactive T cells are eliminated. The survival rate of these two independent selection processes is less than 3%. These processes minimize the chances of autoreactive T cells escaping to the periphery.

The most common type of T-cell receptor, TCR-αβ, is an 80–90 kDa disulfide-linked heterodimer composed of a 48–54 kDa β-chain and a 37–42 kDa α-chain. An alternate TCR is composed of γ- and δ-chains. The TCR is noncovalently associated with as many as five invariant chains belonging to its associated signal-transducing CD3 complex. The structure of a TCR gene is very similar to that first described for immunoglobulin genes in B cells (Chapter 4). The combinatorial diversity generated by gene rearrangements within the two TCR chain loci plus the additional diversity generated by the introduction of nucleotides not encoded by the genome (N-region nucleotides) yield at least 10^8 theoretical possible TCR combinations. Mutations in the genes that engage in this rearrangement process can produce an arrest in lymphocyte development. For example, a mutation in a gene encoding a DNA-dependent protein kinase required for receptor gene recombination results in a severe combined immunodeficiency, a type of disorder that is typically identified by the acronym SCID(Chapter 35) TCR gene recombination thus

▌ KEY CONCEPTS

T-CELL DEVELOPMENT IN THE THYMUS

>> In order to reach the mature T-cell stage of development, T cells must successfully rearrange a pair of genes that encode a heterodimeric T-cell receptor (TCR) (αβ or γδ) and survive thymic selection, during which self-reactive T cells are eliminated. Only 3% of thymocytes survive this process

>> For the majority of T cells, the stages of T-cell development can be defined by the status of rearrangement and expression of TCRα and β, and the expression of CD4 and CD8, which proceeds CD4⁻CD8⁻ → CD4⁺CD8⁺ → either CD4⁻CD8⁺ (cytotoxic T cells) or CD4⁺CD8⁻ (helper T cells)

>> TCRβ rearrangement begins in CD4⁻CD8⁻ cells; TCRα expression occurs in the CD4⁺CD8⁺ cells; thymocytes that are selected by class I go on to express CD8 alone; and thymocytes that are selected by class II go on to express CD4 alone

>> Two types of selection occur in the thymus: positive selection, which requires the TCR on the cell surface to recognize either a MHC class I or class II molecule that is endogenous to the individual; and negative selection, which eliminates those T cells that bind too well to the endogenous MHC molecule and are thus in danger of becoming self-reactive

presents the first of the two major hurdles for developing lymphocytes. Since the developing T cell has two copies of each chromosome, there are two chances to rearrange each of the two TCR chains successfully. As soon as successful rearrangement occurs, further β-chain rearrangements on either the same or the other chromosome are suppressed, a process known as *allelic exclusion*. This limits the chance of dual TCR expression by an individual T cell. The high percentage of T cells that contain rearrangements of both β-chain genes attests to the inefficiency of this complex event. Rearrangement of the α-chain occurs later in thymic development in a similar fashion, although without apparent allelic exclusion.

Several other mutations have been identified that regulate early T-cell development and lead to a clinical SCID phenotype (Chapter 35). These include deficiencies in IL-7Rα-chain, CD3δ, CD3ε, γ_c (X-linked SCID), CD45, JAK3, Artemis, RAG1 and RAG2, and adenosine deaminase.

The stages of thymocyte development can be defined by the status of rearrangement and expression of the two genes that encode the α- and β-chains of the TCR and the expression of CD4 and CD8. Thymocytes are divided into four main subsets based on their expression of CD4 and CD8: immature CD4⁻8⁻ and CD4⁺8⁺, and mature CD4⁺8⁻ or CD4⁻8⁺ cells (Fig. 9.1). During maturation, thymocytes proceed in an orderly fashion from CD4⁻8⁻ → CD4⁺8⁺ → CD4⁺8⁻ or CD4⁻8⁺. CD4 and CD8 define, respectively, the helper and cytolytic subsets of T cells (Chapters 17 and 18).

CD4⁻8⁻ thymocytes can be further subdivided based on their expression of CD25 (the high-affinity IL-2 receptor α-chain) and CD44 (the hyaluronate receptor). Development proceeds in the

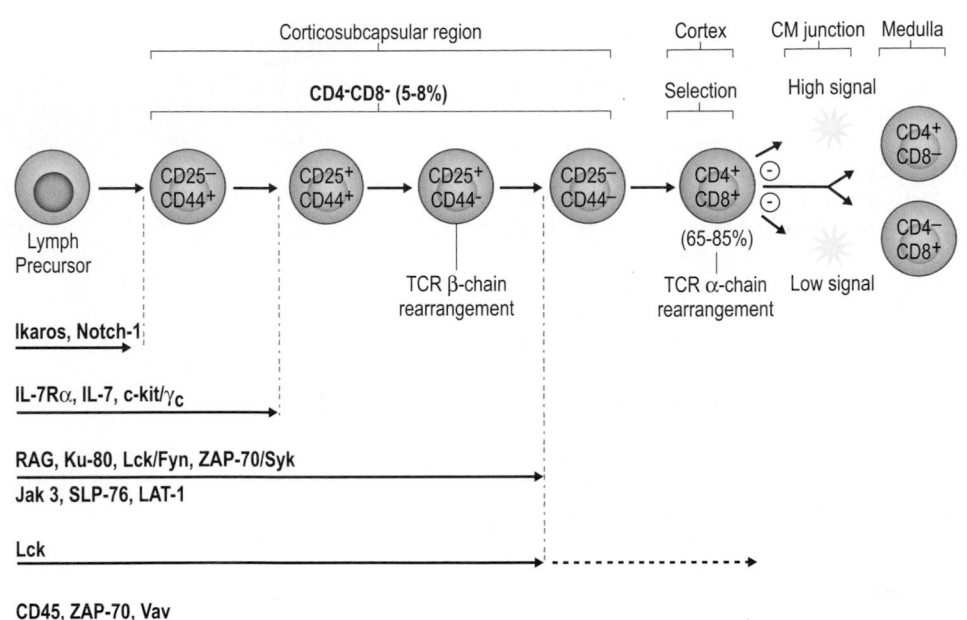

Fig. 9.1 Sequence of αβ T-cell development in the thymus. The earliest thymocyte precursors lack expression of CD4 and CD8 (CD4⁻CD8⁻). These can be further divided into four subpopulations based on the sequential expression of CD25 and CD44. At the CD25⁺CD44⁻ stage, the TCR β-chain rearranges and associates with a surrogate α-chain known as pre-Tα. Concomitant with a proliferative burst, thymocytes progress to the CD4⁺CD8⁺ stage, rearrange the TCR α-chain, and express a mature TCR complex. These cells then undergo thymic positive (+) and negative (−) selection. Thymocytes receiving a high-intensity or very low TCR signal are eliminated through apoptosis. The thymocytes that survive this rigorous selection process differentiate into mature CD4⁺ or CD8⁺ T cells. The extent of αβ T-cell development in mice deficient for certain transcription factors, cytokines, and signaling molecules required for T-cell development is shown below. Headings at top indicate the region of the thymus populated by the various thymic subsets. The percentages indicate the proportion of each subset. C-M, corticomedullary.

order: CD25⁺CD44⁺ → CD25⁺CD44⁺ → CD25⁺CD44⁻ → CD25⁻CD44⁻. These subpopulations correspond to discrete stages of thymocyte differentiation. CD25⁻44⁺ cells express low levels of CD4 and their TCR genes are in germline configuration. These cells then down-regulate CD4 and upregulate CD25 to give rise to CD25⁺CD44⁺ thymocytes, which now express surface CD2 and low levels of CD3ε. At the next stage (CD25⁺CD44⁻), there is a brief burst of proliferation followed by upregulation of the recombination-activating enzymes, RAG-1 and RAG-2, and the concomitant rearrangement of the genes of the TCR complex beginning with rearrangement of the TCR β-chain. A small subpopulation of T cells rearranges and expresses a second pair of TCR genes, known as γ and δ. Rearrangement in these cells begins with the γ-chain. These unusual γδ T cells represent only 1–3% of peripheral blood T cells and are discussed below. Productive TCR β-chain rearrangement results in downregulation of RAG and a second proliferative burst. Loss of CD25 then yields CD25⁻CD44⁻ thymocytes.

The TCR β-chain cannot be stably expressed without an α-chain. Since the TCR α-chain has not yet rearranged, a surrogate invariant TCR pre-α-chain is disulfide linked to the β-chain.[3] When associated with components of the CD3 complex, this allows a low-level surface expression of a pre-TCR and progression to the next developmental stage. Failure to rearrange the TCR β-chain successfully results in a developmental arrest at the transition from CD25⁺CD44⁻ to CD25⁻CD44⁻. This occurs in RAG-deficient mice as well as in *scid* mice and humans.

A number of molecules, including transcription factors, cytokines, and signaling molecules, are required for T-cell development (Fig. 9.1).[1] The IKAROS gene encodes a family of transcription factors required for the development of cells of lymphoid origin. NOTCH-1, a molecule known to regulate cell fate decisions, is also required at the earliest stage of T-cell lineage development. Cytokines including IL-7 promote the survival and expansion of the earliest thymocytes. In mice deficient for IL-7, its receptor components IL-7Rα or γ_c, or the receptor-associated signaling molecule JAK3, thymocyte development is inhibited at the CD25⁻CD44⁺ stage. In humans, mutations in γ_c or Jak 3 result in the most frequent form of SCID. Pre-TCR signaling is required for the CD25⁺44⁻ → CD25⁻CD44⁻ transition. Thus, loss of signaling components including Lck, SLP-76, and LAT-1 results in a block at this stage of T-cell development. TCR signals are also required for differentiation of CD4⁺8⁺ to CD4 or CD8 cells. Humans deficient in ZAP-70 have CD4 but not CD8 T cells in the thymus and periphery.

CD25⁻CD44⁻ cells upregulate expression of CD4 and CD8 to become CD4⁺8⁺. It is as a CD4⁺CD8⁺ thymocyte that the α-chain of the TCR rearranges. Rearrangement of the α-chain can occur simultaneously on both chromosomes without allelic exclusion, and if one attempt is unsuccessful, repeat rearrangements to other Vα segments are possible. Reports have been made of dual TCR expression by as many as 30% of mature T cells in which the same T cell expresses different α-chains paired with the same β-chain.

Although the structure of immunoglobulin and TCR is quite similar, they recognize fundamentally different antigens. Immunoglobulin recognizes intact antigens in isolation, either soluble or membrane-bound, and they are often sensitive to the tertiary structure. The TCR recognizes linear stretches of antigen peptide fragments bound within the grooves of either MHC class I or class II molecules (Fig. 9.2A) (Chapter 6). Thymic selection molds the repertoire of emerging TCR so that they recognize peptides within the groove of self-MHC molecules, ensuring the *self-MHC restriction* of T-cell responses. Pockets within the MHC groove bind particular residues along the peptide sequence of 7–9 amino acids for MHC class I, and 9–15 amino acids for MHC class II molecules. As a result, depending upon the particular MHC molecule, certain amino acids will make strong contact with the MHC groove while others will contact the TCR.

The contact between the TCR and antigen/MHC has been revealed by crystal structure to be remarkably flat, rather than a deep lock-and-key structure as one might imagine. The TCR axis is tipped about 30° to the long axis of the MHC class I molecule and is slightly more skewed to the MHC class II molecule.[4] The affinity of the TCR for antigen/MHC is in the micromolar range. This is less than many antibody–antigen affinities, and several logs less than many enzyme–substrate affinities. This has led to the ideas that TCR interactions with antigen/MHC are brief and successful activation of the T cell requires multiple interactions resulting in a cumulative signal.

Once the T cell has successfully rearranged and expressed a TCR in association with the CD3 complex, it encounters the second major hurdle in T-cell development: thymic selection. Selection has two phases: positive and negative. The TCR must engage antigen–MHC complexes on thymic epithelium or dendritic cells which confer a certain low-affinity signaling that permits the developing thymocyte to survive and mature beyond the CD4+CD8+ stage (Fig. 9.1). This is known as *positive selection* and is coincident with upregulation of surface TCR, the activation markers CD5 and CD69, and the survival factor Bcl-2. T cells bearing a TCR that recognizes MHC class I maintain CD8 expression, downregulate CD4, and become CD4-8+. T cells expressing a TCR that recognizes MHC class II become CD4+8-. This cell fate is also influenced by the intensity of the TCR signal, with higher-affinity interactions favoring the CD4 lineage and with lesser TCR signal intensity favoring the CD8 pathway.[5] Thymocytes bearing a TCR that does not engage any endogenous peptide–MHC complex are eliminated.

At the opposite extreme is *negative selection*, in which T cells expressing TCR complexes with too high an affinity for self-peptide–MHC complexes are eliminated by active cell death, known as apoptosis. The collective findings of several studies suggest a model in which the thymic processes of death by neglect, positive selection conferring survival, and negative selection represent a continuum of affinities from low to high of the various TCR for self-peptide–MHC complexes (Fig. 9.2B). Those at the extremes of low or high affinities are eliminated, while those with intermediate affinities survive to become mature T cells. The peptides that select the T-cell repertoire are not known. Studies in which endogenous peptides were eluted from MHC molecules found a variety of peptides, including sequences from housekeeping molecules. T cells from a transgenic mouse expressing a single MHC class II peptide complex manifest a broad repertoire and were fully functional.[6] However, the mature T cells did not respond to the selecting MHC–peptide complex. This suggested

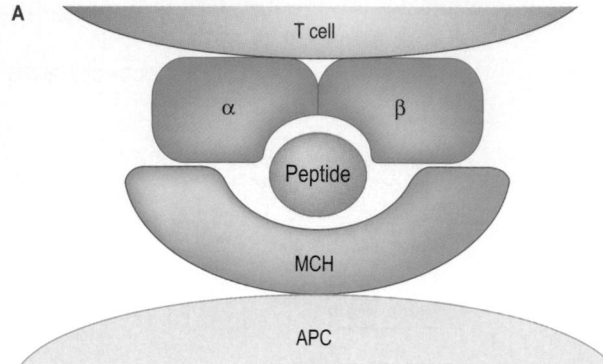

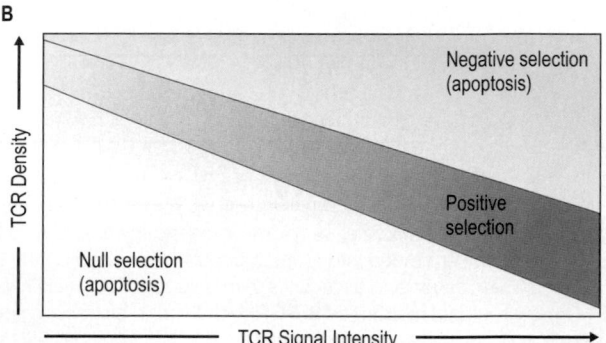

Fig. 9.2 Thymic selection. (A) Developing CD4+8+ T-cell receptor-positive (TCR+) thymocytes undergo positive selection by interaction with cortical epithelium. Those that fail to make such signals die through neglect. Surviving thymocytes then undergo negative selection primarily on medullary dendritic cells. Surviving thymocytes can then become mature CD4 or CD8 T cells. (B) TCR interaction with the major histocompatibility complex (MHC)–peptide complex. Polymorphic residues within the variable region of the α- and β-chains of the TCR make contact with determinants on the MHC molecule on an antigen-presenting cell (APC) as well as with the peptide fragment that sits in the MHC-binding groove. Schematic diagram illustrating that during thymocyte development, those TCR conferring either a very low signal intensity (null selection) or high intensity (negative selection) each lead to apoptosis. Only those thymocytes whose TCR can engage MHC/peptides and confer moderate intensity survive by positive selection.

that the threshold for triggering T cells during thymic development may be lower than that for the same T cell once it has matured.

A gene that is critical to the expression of self proteins by the thymic stromal cells is AIRE. AIRE is expressed at high levels by thymic epithelium, especially in the medulla. It is believed to promote the expression of several ectopic self proteins by the thymic epithelium, such as thyroglobulin and insulin.[7] This promotes the negative selection of T cells reacting to these self proteins. Genetic absence of AIRE results in autoimmune disease of specific organs. This is known as the autoimmune polyendocrinopathy-candidiasis-ectodermal-dystrophy syndrome (APECED or APS1: Chapter 35). Patients manifest chronic mucocutaneous candidiasis and autoimmunity most commonly of the parathyroid and adrenal glands, with lesser involvement of the skin, thyroid, and liver.[8]

Not surprisingly, a variety of signaling molecules are important to conferring positive selection. These include Lck, the Ras/Raf-1/MAP kinase cascade, the kinase ZAP-70, and the phosphatases CD45 and calcineurin, among others (Chapter 13). By contrast, although a number of molecules may promote negative selection, there appears to be sufficient redundancy so that only rarely does elimination of any one of these molecules affect deletion of thymocytes. The few exceptions include CD40, CD40L (CD154), CD30, or the Bcl-2 proapoptotic family member, Bim, where preservation of at least some thymocytes bearing self-reactive TCR could be observed in mice deficient in these molecules.

The survivors of these two stringent processes of TCR gene rearrangement and thymic selection represent fewer than 3% of total immature thymocytes. This is reflected by the presence of a high rate of cell death in developing thymocytes. This can be visualized by the measurement of DNA degradation using the TUNEL assay (Fig. 9.3) (Chapter 101). This technique labels nicked DNA using the ability of the DNA repair enzyme TdT to insert biotinylated dUTP residues at sites of double-stranded breaks. The survivors become either CD4 helper or CD8 cytolytic T cells and reside in the thymic medulla for 12–14 days before emigrating to the periphery.

EXTRATHYMIC T-CELL DEVELOPMENT

In the absence of a thymus, as in nude (*nu/nu*) mice, T-cell populations in the lymph nodes and spleen are severely reduced and oligoclonal, but they are not absent. Whereas some of this extrathymic T-cell development occurs within the liver, a significant amount also occurs in contact with the intestinal epithelium. It is less clear whether extrathymic development occurs in humans.

Intestinal intraepithelial lymphocytes (IEL) have a very different phenotype from thymus-derived T cells (Chapter 19). In contrast to the predominance of CD4 cells over CD8 T cells in normal lymph nodes, IEL contain large portions of CD8 and CD4-8- T cells.[9] Many of the CD8 IEL express only the CD8α chain as an αα homodimer. γδ T cells also comprise a significant portion of IEL. The antigens to which IEL respond are not known, although in humans some of the γδ IEL recognize the MHC class Ib molecule MICA via the stimulatory NK receptor, NKG2D.[10] IEL have a memory CD44+ T-cell phenotype (see below) and are cytolytic when freshly isolated.

■ ABNORMALITIES OF EARLY HUMAN T-CELL DEVELOPMENT ■

Given the vast number of events in T-cell development, it is not surprising that a multiplicity of causes can underlie human T-cell immunodeficiencies (Chapter 35). The influence of the thymic stroma of thymocyte ontogeny is underscored, for instance, in the DiGeorge anomaly in which development of the pharyngeal pouches is disrupted and the thymic rudiment fails to form.[11] This results, predictably, in the failure of normal T-cell development. Less severe T-cell deficiencies are associated with a failure to express MHC class I and/or class II (the "bare lymphocyte syndrome"), which are directly involved with interactions required to

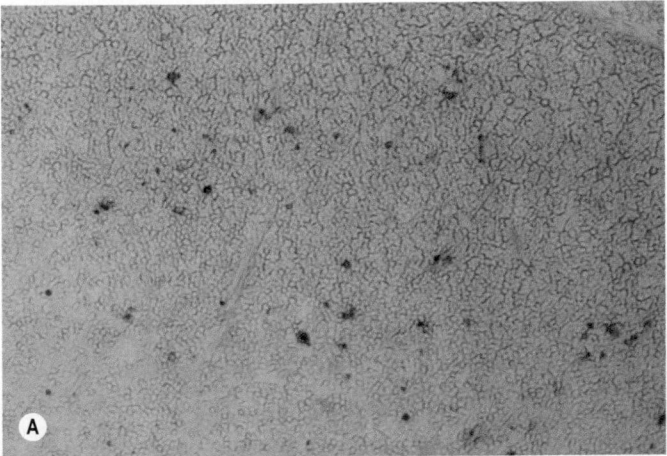
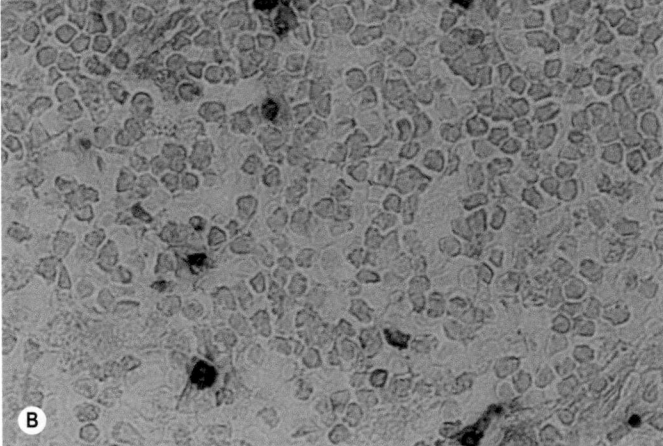

Fig. 9.3 TUNEL assay for nicked DNA in thymocytes undergoing apoptosis. Thymus sections were made from wild-type mice, fixed, and stained by the TUNEL assay. The DNA repair enzyme, TdT, inserts biotinylated dUTP residues at sites of double-stranded breaks, which is then revealed by avidin horseradish peroxidase. Shown are sections at 100× and 400×. Apoptotic thymocytes reflect those undergoing negative selection from either too intense or too weak a TCR signal.

induce the positive selection of, respectively, CD4 and CD8 single positive T cells.

Disorders can affect thymocytes more directly. The absence of functional adenosine deaminase and purine nucleoside phosphorylase results in the buildup of metabolic byproducts that are toxic to developing T and B lymphocytes, and ultimately produces forms of SCID. SCID can also result from the failure to generate lymphocyte precursors, for example due to abnormal or absent function of the RAG genes and other proteins associated with the gene rearrangement process.

The inability to express any number of surface molecules also has the potential to perturb development. The failure to express TCR-CD3 components (specifically CD3γ), CD18, and IL-2Rγ, and a defect in expression of CD3ε have all been noted among patients who exhibit varying degrees of T-cell deficiency or dysfunction.

CLINICAL RELEVANCE

ABNORMALITIES OF T-CELL DEVELOPMENT

>> The importance of the thymus is underscored by the complete absence of T cells in patients in whom a thymus has failed to develop (e.g., complete DiGeorge syndrome)

>> T-cell development can be abrogated by the accumulation of toxic metabolites, such as seen in adenosine deaminase deficiency or purine nucleoside phosphorylase

>> T-cell development requires expression of T-cell receptors (TCR), hence loss-of-function mutations in RAG and other associated genes typically results in the absence of T cells

>> T-cell survival and development require signal transduction through the TCR signaling complex and associated co-receptors, hence loss-of-function mutations in TCR-CD3 components typically result in T-cell deficiency or dysfunction

PERIPHERAL MIGRATION OF T CELLS

The migration of naïve T cells to peripheral lymphoid structures or their infiltration into other tissues requires the coordinate regulation of an array of cell adhesion molecules. T-cell recirculation is essential for host surveillance and is carefully regulated by specific homing receptors. Entry from the circulation to tissues occurs via two main anatomic sites: the flat endothelium of the blood vessels and the specialized postcapillary venules known as high endothelial venules (HEV).

HEV are distinguishable by their cuboidal shape and are found primarily in lymph nodes. Endothelium resembling HEV can occur at certain sites of inflammation such as in rheumatoid synovium. It is not clear whether this represents differentiation of normal flat endothelium to HEV or a separate lineage of endothelial cells. HEV may offer a biological advantage over flat endothelium by presentation of the optimum architecture and concentration of homing receptor ligands.

A three-step model has been proposed for lymphocyte migration: rolling, adhesion, and migration[12] (Chapter 12). The selectins (CD62) can be expressed on leukocytes (L-selectin, CD62L, and vascular endothelium E-selectin, CD62E, and P-selectin, CD62P). L-selectin expressed by naïve T cells binds via lectin domains to carbohydrate moieties of GlyCAM-1 and CD34 (collectively known as peripheral node addressin), which are expressed on endothelial cells, particularly HEV. The weak binding of CD62L to its ligand mediates a weak adhesion to the vessel wall which, combined with the force of blood flow, results in rolling of the T cell along the endothelium. The increased cell contact facilitates the interaction of a second adhesion molecule on lymphocytes, the integrin LFA-1 (CD11a/CD18) with its ligands, ICAM-1 (CD54) and ICAM-2 (CD102). This results in the arrest of rolling and firm attachment.

Migration into the extracellular matrix of tissues may involve additional lymphocyte cell surface molecules such as the hyaluronate receptor (CD44) or the integrin α4β7 (CD49d/β7) that binds the mucosal addressin cell adhesion molecule-1 (MAdCAM-1) on endothelium of Peyer's patches and other endothelial cells. Additional molecules may be involved with tissue infiltration. These include cutaneous lymphocyte-associated (CLA) antigen that is expressed by the majority

of memory T cells and binds to E-selectin on endothelium of inflamed skin, as well as other pairs such as CD49d/CD29 (α4β1/VLA-4). Expression of these receptors is regulated by inflammatory cytokines (Chapters 10 and 17). Other cytokines known as chemokines may contribute to lymphocyte homing (Chapter 11). Chemokines are structurally and functionally related to proteins bearing an affinity for heparan sulfate proteoglycan and promote migration of various cell types. The chemokines RANTES, MIP-1α, MIP-1β, MCP-1, and IL-8 are produced by a number of cell types, including endothelium, activated T cells, and monocytes, and are present at inflammatory sites such as rheumatoid synovium. A number of chemokine receptors are important for migration of developing thymocytes through the thymic stroma. These include CCR4 (ligand = CCL17 and CCL22), CCR7 (ligand = CCL19), CCR9 (ligand = CCL25), and CXCR4 (ligand = CXCL12 or SDSF1).

■ SUBSETS, FUNCTION, AND THE DEVELOPMENT OF PERIPHERAL T CELLS ■

CD4 HELPER AND CD8 CYTOLYTIC T CELLS

αβ T cells can be subdivided into two main subsets based on their recognition of peptides presented by MHC class I or class II molecules and their respective expression of CD8 or CD4. The peptides presented by MHC class I molecules are produced by the proteasome and can be derived from either self proteins or intracellular foreign proteins as might occur during viral replication. MHC class II-bound peptides are largely derived from extracellular infectious agents or self cell surface proteins that have been engulfed and degraded in the lysosomal complex.

CD4 T cells express a variety of cytokines and cell surface molecules that are important to B-cell proliferation and immunoglobulin production. Following antigen stimulation, CD4 T cells differentiate into two major classes of effector T cells called T helper 1 (Th1) and Th2 (Chapter 17). In brief, Th1 cells participate in cell-mediated inflammatory reactions, activate macrophages, and produce IL-2, LTXα, and interferon-γ. Th2 cells activate B cells and produce IL-4, IL-5, IL-6, IL-10, and IL-13. IL-4 and IL-5 are important B-cell growth factors, as are surface CD40 ligand and the recently described BAFF. In addition, IL-4 promotes B-cell secretion of IgG_1 and IgE, whereas interferon-γ drives IgG_{2a} production. Since Th1 and Th2 cells mediate different functions, the type of response generated can influence susceptibility to disease.

The CD4 molecule is structurally related to immunoglobulins and has an affinity for nonpolymorphic residues on the MHC class II molecule. In this capacity CD4 presumably increases the efficiency with which CD4 T cells recognize antigen in the context of class II molecules, which are restricted in their expression to B cells, macrophages, dendritic cells, and a few other tissues during states of inflammation. In addition, the cytoplasmic tail of CD4 binds to Lck and promotes signaling by the TCR, as described earlier. However, ligation of CD4 prior to engagement of the TCR renders the T cell susceptible to apoptosis upon subsequent engagement of the TCR. This is clinically important in human immunodeficiency virus (HIV) infections in which the gp120 molecule of HIV binds to CD4 and primes the T cell to undergo cell death when later triggered by the TCR. Accelerated apoptosis of CD4 T cells has been demonstrated in acquired immunodeficiency syndrome (AIDS) patients.[13]

CD8 T cells are very efficient killers of pathogen-infected cells. Given the ubiquitous expression of class I molecules, mature cytolytic T cells (CTL) can recognize viral infections in a wide array of cells, in distinction to the more restricted distribution of class II molecules and their recognition by CD4 T cells. CTL induce lysis of target cells through the production of perforin, which induces holes in cell membranes, and the expression of FasL and tumor necrosis factor-α (TNF-α), which induce apoptosis. In this capacity CTL kill virally infected target cells in an attempt to restrict the spread of infection. Similar to CD4, CD8 manifests an affinity for MHC class I molecules, enhances the signaling of TCR, and also binds Lck by its cytoplasmic tail.

■ T CELLS IN THE INNATE IMMUNE RESPONSE ■

In addition to the broad array of antigens recognized by αβ T cells, there is growing appreciation that the immune system also contains small subpopulations of T cells, γδ and natural killer (NK) T cells, that function as important constituents of the innate immune system. These cells may be specialized to recognize conserved structures that are either uniquely expressed by prokaryotic pathogens or on stressed host cells (Chapter 3). The receptors used to recognize these nonpolymorphic molecules may themselves be less polymorphic, such as the Toll-like receptor (TLR) family and MHC class I-like CD1 family. For example, TLR4 expressed on macrophages and dendritic cells binds lipopolysaccharide (LPS) and products of Gram-negative bacteria, whereas TLR2 binds lipopeptides from organisms such as the LPS-deficient Lyme disease spirochete, *Borrelia burgdorferi*. By focusing on such common and far less polymorphic molecules, the immune response may be able to respond quickly during the early phase of infections.

γδ T CELLS

The γδ T cell is among the oddest of immunology's distinguished oddities. Their study stems from the discovery of rearranged genes rather than a knowledge of their biological function. Transcription of rearranged γ and δ genes begins prior to αβ genes. Rearranged γ and δ genes are first expressed in the liver and primitive gut between 6 and 9 weeks' gestation. In addition to the ordered appearance of γδ TCR before αβ TCR, there is also a highly ordered expression of γ and δ V-region genes during early development. The reason for this remarkable regimentation remains unclear.

γδ T cells manifest a number of differences from αβ T cells. γδ T cells are often anatomically sequestered to epithelial barriers or sites of inflammation,[14] and frequently manifest cytotoxicity toward a broad array of targets. In contrast to αβ T cells, γδ cells can respond to antigen directly, without evidence of MHC restriction, or conversely, react to MHC molecules without peptide.

Human γδ T-cell clones, particularly those expressing the Vδ2 gene and derived from peripheral blood of normal individuals or synovial fluid of rheumatoid arthritis patients, frequently react to mycobacterial extracts.[15] While a few of these Vδ2 clones respond to a heat shock protein, the major stimulatory components have recently been identified as phosphate-containing nonpeptide molecules such as nucleotide triphosphates, prenyl pyrophosphates, and alkylamines.[16] These molecules are, respectively, subunits in DNA and RNA, substrates in lipid metabolism for the synthesis of farnesyl pyrophosphate, and products of pathogenic organisms. In mammalian cells, farnesyl addition is a critical modification for targeting certain signaling molecules, such as Ras to the cell membrane. This process appears critical to cell transformation. These phosphate-containing nonpeptides can be found in both microbial and mammalian cells. This suggests that γδ cells may recognize a class of antigens shared by a number of pathogens, as well as by damaged or transformed cells, and may provide insight into the role of γδ cells in infection and their accumulation at sites of inflammation. A subpopulation of γδ T cells typically found in the intestine and expressing the Vδ1 gene (which is also found in inflamed synovial fluid) was shown to react to MHC class I-like molecules known as MICA and MICB.[10] Unlike classical MHC class I molecules that are expressed ubiquitously and continuously, MICA and MICB expression appears to be restricted to epithelium and occurs only during times of stress, similar to that of a heat shock response. The NK receptor NKG2D on human Vδ1 T cells was determined to be a receptor for the MHC class Ib molecule MICA.[10] It remains to be determined whether Vδ1 TCR itself recognizes MICA or another as-yet undetermined structure. Some Vδ1 T cells have been suggested to respond to CD1c.

The contribution of γδ T cells to defense against infection has been examined in mice using a number of pathogens, including *Listeria*, *Leishmania*, *Mycobacterium*, *Plasmodium*, and *Salmonella*. All of these studies have shown a moderately protective role for γδ T cells. In some cases of rapid bacterial growth, γδ T cells appear to be protective early during infection by reducing bacterial growth, whereas in less virulent infections such as influenza or Sendai virus, γδ cells appear later in inflammatory lesions. In only a few instances, however, have γδ clones derived from an infected animal been shown to respond to the causative organism. In human infections, γδ T cells from cutaneous lesions of leprosy patients respond to *Mycobacterium leprae*,[17] and γδ cells from Lyme arthritis synovial fluid will respond to the causative spirochete, *Borrelia burgdorferi*.[18] This response by Lyme synovial γδ cells requires lipidated hexapeptides of the outer-surface proteins of *B. burgdorferi*, and the tripalmitate lipid moiety is as important for activation of γδ T cells as the hexapeptide portion. The same motif binds TLR2 and may thus indirectly activate γδ T cells.

γδ T cells accumulate at inflammatory sites in autoimmune disorders such as rheumatoid arthritis, celiac disease, and sarcoidosis.[19] The reason for this remains an enigma. However, there is evidence that γδ can be highly cytolytic toward a variety of tissues, including CD4 T cells, and their presence can strongly bias the cytokine profiles of the infiltrating CD4+ cells, in some instances toward Th1 profiles, and in others toward Th2.[20]

NK T CELLS

A minor subpopulation of T cells bearing the NK determinant manifest perhaps the most restricted of TCR repertoires and determinants of recognition. NK T cells are found within the CD4 and CD4−8− subsets of T cells and, in both mouse and human, express a very limited number of TCR-Vβ chains and an invariant α-chain.[21] Furthermore, NK T cells are restricted in their response to a monomorphic MHC class I-like molecule, CD1d. Crystallographic analysis of CD1 has shown that it

KEY CONCEPTS

NAÏVE VERSUS MEMORY T CELLS

CD4 and CD8 T cells emigrate from the thymus bearing a naïve phenotype

Naïve T cells:

>> Produce IL-2, but only low levels of other cytokines

>> Require continual major histocompatibility complex (MHC)/self-peptide interactions in the periphery for survival

>> Express the CD45RA isoform of CD45

Memory T cells:

>> Express a variety of surface molecules involved with cell adhesion and migration, activation, cytokine production, T-cell proliferation, and death receptors

>> Survive for long periods in the absence of MHC/peptide signaling

>> Are activated more rapidly than naïve T cells

>> Express the CD45RO isoform of CD45

---

contains a deeper groove than traditional MHC molecules and is highly hydrophobic, suggesting it may bind lipid moieties.[21] This may represent another type of innate T-cell response whereby bacterial lipids or lipopeptides may be presented to NK T cells to provoke a rapid early immune response.

The potential importance of NK T cells in autoimmune disease stems from their production of high levels of certain cytokines, particularly IL-4.[21] In this capacity, they may be important for inhibiting inflammatory responses dominated by Th1 infiltrates. This has been noted in the non-obese diabetic (NOD) mouse model of diabetes that lacks NK T cells. Adoptive transfer of NK T cells into NOD mice blocks the onset of diabetes.[22] A recent study extended this observation to human type 1 diabetes. The NK T cells of diabetic individuals produced more interferon-γ and less IL-4 than their unaffected siblings.[23] Thus, this minor population of T cells may play a pivotal role in early innate responses to certain infections and also in the regulation of inflammatory lesions.

NAÏVE VERSUS MEMORY T CELLS

CD4 and CD8 T cells emigrate from the thymus bearing a naïve phenotype. Naïve T cells produce IL-2 but only low levels of other cytokines, and as such manifest little B-cell helper activity. They express high levels of Bcl-2 and can survive for extended periods without antigen but require the presence of MHC molecules. Naïve T cells circulate from the blood to lymphoid tissues of the spleen and lymph nodes that concentrate antigen, antigen-presenting cells (APC), T cells and B cells. Particularly important in this environment as APC are dendritic cells, which are derived from both lymphoid and myeloid progenitors and are particularly adept at concentrating and presenting antigen. Dendritic cells can migrate from other areas of the body such as the skin and thus transport antigen to lymphoid tissues. These specialized cells optimize concentrations of antigen/MHC molecules, co-stimulatory molecules,

and cytokines to promote clonal expansion of antigen-specific T cells, which may be present at as low a frequency as 1 in 10^6 prior to immunization, but can increase to 1 in 1000 or more within 1 week. The development of antigen peptide/MHC tetramer technology has led to a more direct quantitation of these values using flow cytometry and suggests their frequency may be considerably higher.

During the process of clonal expansion of naïve T cells and their differentiation into effector and eventually memory T cells, as many as 100 genes are induced. These are manifest primarily as increased expression of certain surface molecules involved with cell adhesion and migration (e.g., CD44, ICAM-1, LFA-1, α4β1, and α4β7 integrins), activation (e.g., CD45 change from high-molecular-weight CD45RA to lower-molecular-weight CD45RO isotype), cytokine production (increased production of interferon-γ, IL-3, IL-4, and IL-5) and death receptors (e.g., Fas/CD95). More transiently induced are CD69, the survival factor BCL-xL, and the high-affinity IL-2 receptor α-chain (CD25), the last being necessary for T-cell proliferation.

Although the concept of immune memory has existed since the first successful vaccinations by Jenner for smallpox, the first T-cell memory marker, CD44, was not identified until 1987. Prior to the identification of this marker, memory T cells could only be identified at a functional level by demonstrating the presence of an enhanced proliferative response of peripheral blood lymphocytes from an individual previously vaccinated against an antigen such as tetanus toxoid. CD44 was absent on mature single positive T cells as they emerged from the thymus, but its expression was induced upon the first encounter with antigen stimulation in the periphery. Since then several other markers have been shown to change upon primary antigenic stimulation. Most notable for human T cells is CD45, in which an isoform known as CD45RA is expressed on naïve T cells, whereas CD45RO expression characterizes memory T cells. Using these markers it has been possible to identify a variety of differences between naïve and memory T cells. Activation of memory T cells appears to be more efficient than that of naïve T cells. The signals required for maintenance of naïve versus memory T cells also differ. Naïve T cells require continual MHC/self-peptide interactions in the periphery, while both CD4 and CD8 memory T cells can survive for long periods in the absence of MHC/peptide signaling.[24]

TH1 VERSUS TH2 T CELLS

In response to repetitive antigenic stimulation, responding CD4 cells can differentiate into effector cells expressing polarized patterns of cytokine production. Th1 cells are characterized by production of IL-2, interferon-γ, TNFα, and LTXα, whereas Th2 cells produce IL-4, IL-5, IL-6, IL-10, and IL-13[25] (Chapters 10 and 17). These patterns have been best characterized during chronic infections. In general, a Th1 response helps eradicate intracellular microorganisms, such as *Leishmania major* and *Brucella abortus*, whereas a Th2 cell response can better control extracellular pathogens, such as the helminth, *Nippostrongylus brasiliensis*. The cytokine profiles of Th1 and Th2 cells are mutually inhibitory, such that the Th1 cytokines interferon-γ and IL-12 suppress Th2 responses, whereas the Th2 cytokine IL-4 suppresses Th1 responses.

Polarization of the cytokine environment also occurs at the sites of inflammation in many autoimmune syndromes. Th2 skewing has been observed in models of systemic lupus erythematosus, where increased levels of immunoglobulins and autoantibodies are typical, as well as in chronic allergic conditions such as asthma. Frequently, however, the infiltrating lymphocytes exhibit a bias toward Th1 cytokines. This occurs with brain-infiltrating lymphocytes in multiple sclerosis and its animal model experimental allergic encephalomyelitis (EAE), β-islet lymphocytes in diabetes, and synovial lymphocytes in inflammatory arthritides.[26] Unlike the beneficial effects of Th1 responses during infections, these same cytokines can be quite deleterious in autoimmune disorders. Thus, therapies based on inhibition of certain Th1 cytokines have been of considerable interest and often are ameliorative, such as anti-TNF-α treatment of EAE and in human trials of rheumatoid arthritis.[27]

Co-stimulatory molecules and other cytokines produced by APC can also influence cytokine polarization. CD80 (B7-1) and IL-12 promote a Th1 emergence whereas CD86 (B7-2), IL-4, IL-6 can evoke a Th2 predominance. Th1 cells are also generally thought to be more easily tolerized and more susceptible to activation-induced cell death (AICD), perhaps because they express more FasL than Th2 cells. Increased expression of Fas-associating phosphatase-1 (FAP-1) by Th2 cells may also contribute to their resistance to AICD by inhibiting Fas signaling. However, other investigators have observed that Th1 and Th2 cells are equally sensitive to apoptosis upon Fas ligation.

REGULATORY T CELLS

In addition to the tolerance that results from the deletion of autoreactive T cells, a subpopulation of T cells known as regulatory T cells or Treg has been identified that suppresses the proliferation of other T cells[28] (Chapter 16). Treg have the phenotype CD4+CD25+ and arise during thymic development. Their appearance is delayed in neonatal thymectomy, and this procedure is known to lead to an autoimmune syndrome of various target organs.[28] Treg express the forkhead transcription factor Foxp3, which plays a critical role in their function, and Foxp3 expression determines the cell fate independently of any other surface marker.[28] Various autoimmune disorders have been associated with reduced levels of Treg[29] (Chapter 50).

DEATH OF T CELLS

The rapid removal of the effector T cells following clearance of the infection is as important as the clonal expansion of responding T cells for the health of the organism. Failure to clear activated lymphocytes increases the risk of cross-reactivity with self antigens and a sustained autoimmune reaction. To insure that resolution of an immune response occurs rapidly, a number of processes promote active cell death as T cells clonally expand. One means to control T-cell proliferation is through limited availability of growth factors. Upon activation, T cells express receptors for various growth cytokines for approximately 7 days, but only produce cytokines during the first 48 hours. This results in an unstable situation where T cells tend to outgrow the availability of cytokines. T cells expressing IL-2R, for example, in the absence of IL-2 will rapidly undergo programmed cell death.

The discovery of a family of death receptors expressed by T cells elucidated an additional regulatory process. These molecules are described more extensively in Chapter 14 and will only be discussed here as they relate to T-cell function. The best described of these is Fas (CD95). Ligation of Fas recruits the adaptor molecule, FADD, which in turn recruits caspase-8, the first in a series of proteases that promote cell death. Nearly all cells have some level of surface Fas, whereas expression of its ligand (FasL) is primarily restricted to activated T cells and B cells.

Consequently, regulation of Fas-mediated apoptosis is to a large extent under the governance of the immune system. FasL expression has also been reported for certain components of the eye, the Sertoli cells of the testis, and perhaps some tumors.[30]

Expression of FasL by these nonlymphoid cells is thought to prevent immune responses at sites where such inflammation might cause tissue damage. For years immunologists have been aware of these so-called "immune-privileged" sites within which immune responses are difficult to initiate.

During T-cell activation, expression of FasL is rapidly induced at the level of RNA and the ability to kill Fas-sensitive target cells is easily demonstrated. Yet expression of surface FasL protein has been difficult to demonstrate. This may be due to a sensitivity of surface FasL to certain proteinases, which results in its rapid cleavage and release from the cell in a manner similar to the release of another member of the Fas family TNF-α. Resting T cells are not sensitive to Fas-induced death, but must first enter the cell cycle for approximately 3 days. During this period, the cellular level of an endogenous inhibitor of Fas known as FLIP is downregulated, and this presumably allows Fas signaling to progress. Thus, FLIP may function to protect resting T cells from unnecessary death and restrict apoptosis to activated T cells in order to limit their expansion. The importance of FLIP as an inhibitor of cell death is reinforced by the discovery that certain herpes viruses express a homologue of mammalian FLIP called E8 that can prevent death of host cells.[31] E8 expression may alter the tumorigenic potential of herpes viruses.

Mutations of Fas have been identified in humans and these patients present with an autoimmune syndrome, often hemolytic anemia associated with hypergammaglobulinemia (both of IgG and IgA) and lymphadenopathy consisting of an unusual population of TCR-αβ+ CD4-CD8- ("double-negative") T cells. Somewhat unexpected was the finding that mutations in caspase-8 did not produce the same syndrome. Instead they result in a syndrome of immunodeficiency in which the T cells do not proliferate efficiently upon activation, have defective activation of NF-κB after TCR ligation, and produce greatly decreased levels of IL-2. A similar observation was made in mice lacking caspase-8 in T cells. These findings underscore the importance of a newly defined function of caspase-8 in T-cell activation of resting T cells, in addition to its role in cell death of actively cycling effector T cells.

The sequence of T-cell activation followed by cell death is graphically displayed following the administration to mice of bacterially or virally derived compounds called superantigens (Chapter 6). Superantigens activate T cells by directly cross-linking MHC class II molecules with particular β-chain V families of the TCR. The superantigen staphylococcal enterotoxin B (SEB) strongly activates Vβ8+ T cells.[32] This initiates a rapid expansion of Vβ8+ T cells over 2–3 days, followed by an equally rapid loss of these cells. By day 7 very few Vβ8+ T cells remain. This elimination phase is largely dependent on the pro-apoptotic Bcl-2 member, Bim.[33] A similar process occurs during homeostatic proliferation in which naïve T cells undergo spontaneous cell cycling in a lymphopenic environment[34] but are also deleted so that autoimmunity does not arise. The proliferation is regulated by IL-7 and self-MHC/peptides, whereas the deletion phase is regulated by Fas.[35] This likely explains the adenopathy that occurs in Fas-deficient lpr mice.

A similar process of superantigen-induced T-cell activation occurs in the human disease toxic shock syndrome in which a related staphylococcal superantigen/toxin, TSST, stimulates the expansion of Vβ2+ T cells.[36] The devastating illness that results from this profound activation of a large proportion of T cells underscores the need to eliminate activated T cells rapidly. At least some of the damage in toxic shock syndrome likely results from the extensive T-cell expression of FasL and TNFα, particularly in certain tissues such as the liver. Hepatocytes are exquisitely sensitive to damage by these ligands. Activation of T lymphocytes leads to homing to the liver and administration of antigen to TCR transgenic mice can yield a syndrome resembling autoimmune hepatitis. Thus, certain autoimmune disorders may result from the death or damage of 'innocent bystander' cells as a consequence of the migration of activated T cells to an organ and nonspecific damage due to the expression of FasL family members.

The life of a T cell from its infancy as a differentiating thymocyte to its death as a mature peripheral effector cell is regulated by a series of tightly coordinated genetic events linked to phases of rapid expansion of cell number followed by equally rapid programmed cell death. The expansion is paramount for combating infections while death is required to obviate the emergence of self-reactive T cells. Aberrations of either process can lead to immunodeficiency or autoimmune sequelae. The clinical consequences of each are discussed in subsequent chapters.

■ REFERENCES ■

1. Rodewald HR, Fehling HJ. Molecular and cellular events in early thymocyte development. Adv Immunol 1998; 69: 1–112.

2. Faas SJ, Rothstein JL, Kreider BL, et al. Phenotypically diverse mouse thymic stromal cell lines which induce proliferation and differentiation of hematopoietic cells. Eur J Immunol 1993; 23: 1201–1214.

3. von Boehmer H, Aifantis I, Azogui O, et al. Crucial function of the pre-T-cell receptor (TCR) in TCR beta selection, TCR beta allelic exclusion and alpha beta versus gamma delta lineage commitment. Immunol Rev 1998; 165: 111–119.

4. Reinherz EL, Tan K, Tang L, et al. The crystal structure of a T cell receptor in complex with peptide and MHC class II [see comment]. Science 1999; 286: 1913–1921.

5. Liu X, Bosselut R. Duration of TCR signaling controls CD4-CD8 lineage differentiation in vivo. Nat Immunol 2004; 5: 280–288.

6. Ignatowicz L, Kappler J, Marrack P. The repertoire of T cells shaped by a single MHC/peptide ligand. Cell 1996; 84: 521–529.

7. Gotter J, Brors B, Hergenhahn M, et al. Medullary epithelial cells of the human thymus express a highly diverse selection of tissue-specific genes colocalized in chromosomal clusters. J Exp Med 2004; 199: 155–166.

8. Su MA, Anderson MS. Aire: an update. Curr Opin Immunol 2004; 16: 746–752.

9. Lefrancois L, Puddington L. Extrathymic intestinal T-cell development: virtual reality?. Immunol Today 1995; 16: 16–21.

10. Groh V, Steinle A, Bauer S, et al. Recognition of stress-induced MHC molecules by intestinal epithelial gammadelta T cells. Science 1998; 279: 1737–1740.

11. Hong R. The DiGeorge anomaly. Immunodefic Rev 1991; 3: 1–14.

12. Butcher EC, Picker LJ. Lymphocyte homing and homeostasis. Science 1996; 272: 60–66.

13. Casella CR, Finkel TH. Mechanisms of lymphocyte killing by HIV. Curr Opin Hematol 1997; 4: 24–31.

14. Itohara S, Farr AG, Lafaille JJ, et al. Homing of a gamma delta thymocyte subset with homogeneous T-cell receptors to mucosal epithelia. Nature 1990; 343: 754–757.

15. Kabelitz D, Bender A, Schondelmaier S, et al. A large fraction of human peripheral blood gamma/delta+T cells is activated by *Mycobacterium tuberculosis* but not by its 65-kD heat shock protein. J Exp Med 1990; 171: 667–679.

16. Bukowski JF, Morita CT, Brenner MB. Human gamma delta T cells recognize alkylamines derived from microbes, edible plants, and tea: implications for innate immunity. Immunity 1999; 11: 57–65.

17. Modlin RL, Pirmez C, Hofman FM, et al. Lymphocytes bearing antigen-specific gamma delta T-cell receptors accumulate in human infectious disease lesions. Nature 1989; 339: 544–558.

18. Vincent MS, Roessner K, Sellati T, et al. Lyme arthritis synovial gamma delta T cells respond to *Borrelia burgdorferi* lipoproteins and lipidated hexapeptides. J Immunol 1998; 161: 5762–5771.

19. Brennan FM, Londei M, Jackson AM, et al. T cells expressing gamma delta chain receptors in rheumatoid arthritis. J Autoimmun 1988; 1: 319–326.

20. Zuany-Amorim C, Ruffié C, Hailé S, et al. Requirement for gammadelta T cells in allergic airway inflammation. Science 1998; 280: 1265–1267.

21. Bendelac A, Rivera MN, Park SH, et al. Mouse CD1-specific NK1 T cells: development, specificity, and function. Annu Rev Immunol 1997; 15: 535–562.

22. Baxter AG, Kinder SJ, Hammond KJ, et al. Association between alphabetaTCR+CD4–CD8– T-cell deficiency and IDDM in NOD/Lt mice. Diabetes 1997; 46: 572–582.

23. Wilson SB, Kent SC, Patton KT, et al. Extreme Th1 bias of invariant Valpha24JalphaQ T cells in type 1 diabetes [erratum appears in Nature 1999; 399: 84]. Nature 1998; 391: 177–81.

24. Swain SL, Hu H, Huston G. Class II-independent generation of CD4 memory T cells from effectors. Science 1999; 286: 1381–1383.

25. Mosmann TR. Differentiation of subsets of CD4+ and CD8+ T cells. CIBA Foundation Symposium 1995; 195: 42–50.

26. Saxne T, Palladino MA Jr., Heinegard D, et al. Detection of tumor necrosis factor alpha but not tumor necrosis factor beta in rheumatoid arthritis synovial fluid and serum. Arthritis Rheum 1988; 31: 1041–1045.

27. Elliott MJ, Maini RN, Feldmann M, et al. Repeated therapy with monoclonal antibody to tumour necrosis factor alpha (cA2) in patients with rheumatoid arthritis. Lancet 1994; 344: 1125–1127.

28. Sakaguchi S. Naturally arising Foxp3-expressing CD25+CD4+ regulatory T cells in immunological tolerance to self and non-self. Nat Immunol 2005; 6: 345–352.

29. Green EA, Choi Y, Flavell RA. Pancreatic lymph node-derived CD4(+)CD25(+) Treg cells: highly potent regulators of diabetes that require TRANCE-RANK signals. Immunity 2002; 16: 183–191.

30. Griffith TS, Brunner T, Fletcher DG, et al. Fas ligand-induced apoptosis as a mechanism of immune privilege. Science 1995; 270: 1189–1192.

31. Thome M, Schneider P, Hofmann K, et al. Viral FLICE-inhibitory proteins (FLIPs) prevent apoptosis induced by death receptors. Nature 1997; 386: 517–520.

32. Kawabe Y, Ochi A. Selective anergy of V beta 8+ CD4+ T cells in *Staphylococcus* enterotoxin B-primed mice. J Exp Med 1990; 172: 1065–1070.

33. Hildeman DA, Zhu Y, Mitchell TC, et al. Activated T cell death in vivo mediated by proapoptotic bcl-2 family member bim. Immunity 2002; 16: 759–767.

34. King C, Ilic A, Koelsch K, et al. Homeostatic expansion of T cells during immune insufficiency generates autoimmunity. Cell 2004; 117: 265–277.

35. Fortner KA, Budd RC. The death receptor Fas (CD95/APO-1) mediates the deletion of T lymphocytes undergoing homeostatic proliferation. J Immunol 2005; 175: 4374–4382.

36. Choi Y, Lafferty JA, Clements JR, et al. Selective expansion of T cells expressing Vβ2 in toxic shock syndrome. J Exp Med 1990; 172: 981–991.

REFERENCES

Cytokines and cytokine receptors

John O'Shea, Cristina M. Tato, Richard Siegel

10

Cytokines play pivotal roles in the function of a variety of cells, but are of particular interest to immunologists because of their importance in immune regulation. They are also clinically relevant in terms of both disease pathogenesis and, increasingly, treatment. However, one of the barriers to learning about cytokines is a complicated nomenclature and system of classification. In part, this reflects the nonspecificity of the term cytokine. It does not encompass a class of factors that are structurally or functionally related: rather, it includes a number of different factors produced by lymphoid and nonlymphoid cells that mediate intercellular communication. The confusion in terminology arises partly from the history of the field. The various cytokines were discovered by researchers in several disciplines, including immunology, virology and hematology, and many marked their cytokine with their original set of interests.

The term lymphokine was originally used to denote products of lymphocytes,[1] but Cohen et al.[2] coined the word cytokine to emphasize the point that these factors need not be made by one specific cell source. This was an important insight, because many immunologically relevant cytokines are made by nonlymphoid cells. Later, the term interleukin was introduced to emphasize the importance of these factors in communication between leukocytes.[3] Although this designation has remained in use, it is similarly inaccurate. Many of the polypeptides designated interleukins can also be made by or act on nonhematopoietic cells. Cytokines can be defined operationally as polypeptides secreted by leukocytes and other cells that act principally on hematopoietic cells, and whose effects include modulation of immune and inflammatory responses. However, there are clear exceptions to even this broad definition. Some definitions distinguish cytokines from hormones and growth factors, which act on nonhematopoietic cells. Thus, cytokines are typically characterized as factors made by more than one cell type and act locally, whereas hormones are secreted by specialized cells and act at a distance on a restricted set of target cells. Although many cytokines act locally in an autocrine or paracrine fashion, some do enter the bloodstream and can act in a typical endocrine fashion. Consequently, the boundary between cytokines and hormones is rather indistinct. In fact, classic hormones such as growth hormone (GH), prolactin (PRL) and erythropoietin (EPO) are clearly cytokines, as is one of the newest hormones, leptin, as evidenced by the type of receptor they bind and their modes of signaling. As we learn more, there are clear functional similarities and evolutionary relationships among these families of molecules that act on the immune, hematopoietic, endocrine and nervous systems.

A major challenge in discussing cytokines is their classification. One way is to group the factors by function, e.g., factors that regulate hematopoietic, inflammatory or immune cells. However, an important characteristic of cytokines is that they are often pleiotropic in their effects. Cytokines can have multiple target cells and consequently multiple actions. Secondly, structurally dissimilar cytokines can have overlapping but typically nonidentical actions, a given effect often being mediated by several different cytokines. This is termed cytokine redundancy. Finally, a single cytokine frequently induces or influences the action of other cytokines, and can function synergistically. Thus understanding the exact properties of a given cytokine is a challenge. However, this complexity of cytokine action has been simplified to an extent by the generation of cytokine gene targeted mice.

The complexity in terms of action provides a strong rationale for an alternative nosology, and that is to group cytokines according to the type of receptor that they bind rather than by their function. This classification is also useful because it reflects the evolutionary relatedness of cytokines, growth factors and hormones, and emphasizes similarities in modes of signal transduction. The classification used in this chapter is adapted from Vilcek[4] and includes the following receptors: the so-called type I (hematopoietin family) and type II (interferon family) cytokine

KEY CONCEPT

CYTOKINE CHARACTERISTICS

>> Cytokines have pleotropic effects: they may have more than one receptor.

>> Cytokines can be redundant – their receptors often share subunits.

>> Cytokines can have specific and unique functions – their receptors typically have ligand-specific subunits as well.

receptors, tumor necrosis factor (TNF) family receptors, interleukin (IL)-1 receptor and the related Toll-like receptors (TLRs), IL-17 receptors, receptor tyrosine kinases, and the TGF-β family receptor serine kinases (Table 10.1, Fig. 10.1). This chapter reviews in detail only a selected set of cytokines with important immunological functions.

TYPE I AND II CYTOKINE RECEPTORS (HEMATOPOIETIN FAMILY AND INTERFERON RECEPTORS) ■

LIGAND AND RECEPTOR STRUCTURE

Cytokines (Table 10.1) that bind the class of receptors termed the type I or hematopoietic cytokine receptor superfamily include hormones such as EPO, thrombopoietin (TPO), PRL, GH, and leptin; colony-stimulating factors (CSF) such as granulocyte (G)-CSF, granulocyte–macrophage (GM)-CSF; and interleukins (IL)-2–IL-7, IL-9, IL-11–IL-13, IL-15, IL-21, IL-23, IL-27, IL-31, and IL-35. Also included in this family are ciliary neurotrophic factor (CNTF), leukemia inhibitory factor (LIF), oncostatin M (OSM), and cardiotropin 1 (CT-1). Closely related are the interferons (IFN-α, -β, -τ, -ω, limitin) and IL-10-related cytokines, IL-19, IL-20, IL-22, IL-24, IL-26, and interferon-related cytokines IL-28A (IFN-γ2) IL-28B (IFN-γ3), IL-29 (IFN-γ1), which bind type II receptors. The ligands and receptors in this superfamily are structurally similar and utilize related molecules for signal transduction.[5]

A central feature of type I cytokines is a similarity in their basic structure. Each contains four anti-parallel α helices with two long and one short loop connections arranged in an up–up–down–down configuration. Because of this structure, these cytokines have also been referred to as the α-helical bundle cytokine family.

Structurally, the receptors in the type I family have conserved cysteine residues, a conserved Trp–Ser–X–Trp–Ser motif (where X indicates any amino acid), and fibronectin-like repeats in their extracellular domains. These receptors have a single transmembrane domain and divergent cytoplasmic domains. Within the cytoplasmic portion of these receptors two segments of homology can be discerned, termed the Box 1 and Box 2 motifs. The membrane proximal domain binds Janus kinases (Jaks; see below). Some of the cytokine receptors are homodimers, such as the receptors for EPO, TPO, PRL and possibly leptin; whereas other receptors for type I cytokines are heterodimers, containing two distinct receptor subunits. Based on this characteristic, the type I family of receptors can be divided into subfamilies. Each member of the subfamily uses a shared receptor subunit in conjunction with a ligand-specific subunit. For example, the receptors for IL-2, IL-4, IL-7, IL-9, IL-15 and IL-21 all use a common cytokine γ chain, $γ_c$ (Table 10.1), whereas a common β chain, $β_c$, is shared by IL-3, IL-5 and GM-CSF. Similarly, gp130 is a shared subunit for IL-6 family cytokines (IL-6, IL-11, IL-27, IL-31, CNTF, LIF, OSM and CT-1). IL-12 and IL-23 also share a receptor subunit, as do members of the IL-10 family.

Other levels of shared receptor usage also exist. For example, the receptors for LIF, CNTF, OSM, and CT-1 all share the LIF receptor subunit, whereas IL-2 and IL-15 utilize the same β and $γ_c$ chains. Conversely, IL-4 can bind two different receptor complexes. The classic IL-4 receptor is composed of the IL-4Rα chain and the $γ_c$ chain. Additionally,

IL-4 can also bind the IL-13 receptor, which comprises a heterodimer of the IL-4Rα chain and the IL-13Rα chain. IL-13 only utilizes the IL-13 receptor complex for signaling.

The utilization of common receptor subunits explains the phenomenon of shared biological activities (cytokine redundancy) between cytokines that belong to the same subfamily. Within a subfamily, actions distinct for each cytokine can be attributed, at least in part, to the ligand-specific subunits. The pleiotropic effects of a single cytokine can be accounted for by the existence of more than one receptor for that cytokine.

Family members and their actions

Homodimeric receptors

Many of the cytokines that use homodimeric receptors are classic hormones; these include the factors GH, PRL and leptin. Several hormones that regulate hematopoiesis also exist as homodimers. EPO, for example, is required for erythrocyte growth and development and is widely used to treat anemia. Similarly, TPO is required for megakaryocyte development and may have a use in the treatment of thrombocytopenia. G-CSF regulates the production of neutrophils through its action on committed progenitor cells, but also supports the survival of mature neutrophils, enhancing their functional capacity. G-CSF is widely used clinically to treat patients with granulocytopenia. As one would predict, G-CSF knockout mice have marked neutropenia. In addition, mutations of the G-CSFR result in severe congenital neutropenia in humans.

Cytokine receptors utilizing gp130

gp130 is a receptor component for IL-6, IL-11, IL-27, and IL-31, as well as for several cytokines that are important in development.[6] Targeted disruptions of the gp130 gene are lethal in early embryogenesis. The mice exhibit defects in myocardial, hematological, and placental development. LIF binds to a receptor that comprises gp130 in association with the LIF receptor (LIFR), as do the cytokines OSM, CNTF, and CT-1. Targeted disruptions of the LIFR gene are also embryonically lethal, creating defects in placental architecture and developmental abnormalities in neural tissue and bone. Targeted disruptions of LIF lead to failure of blastocyst implantation. Another critical role of LIF is the maintenance of stem cell pluripotency in culture.

Interleukin-6

The IL-6 receptor (IL-6R) consists of an 80 kDa IL-6 binding protein (α chain) and gp130. IL-6 has a wide array of biological actions on both lymphoid and nonlymphoid cells. It is important in host defense and in inflammatory responses; accordingly, IL-6-deficient mice are highly susceptible to infection by *Candida* and *Listeria*. IL-6 is an important growth and differentiation factor for B cells, inducing the production of immunoglobulin, including IgE. IL-6−/− mice have normal numbers of B cells, but have a reduced immunoglobulin response to neoantigen and a marked reduction in IgA production. IL-6 also promotes T-cell growth and differentiation. Consequently, IL-6−/− mice have reduced numbers of thymocytes and peripheral T cells. IL-6 is also important for Th17 differentiation. In addition, the cytotoxic T-cell response to viruses is impaired. IL-6 functions synergistically with IL-3 in hematopoiesis, and IL-6-deficient mice have reduced numbers of progenitor cells.

Table 10.1 Cytokines classified by receptor families

Receptor family	Subfamily	Cytokine	Signaling	Source	Target	Action	Knockout phenotype
Type 1 (hematopoietin)	Homodimeric	GH	JAK2, STAT5b	Two GH genes, pituitary, placental	Diverse tissues	Growth, adipocyte differentiation	Dwarfism
		Prl	JAK2, STAT5a	Two Prl genes pituitary, uterus	Mammary epithelium	Growth, differentiation	Infertility, lactation defects
		Epo	JAK2, STAT5	Kidney, Liver	Erythroid precursors	Erythroid differentiation	Embryonic lethal, severe anemia
		Tpo	JAK2, STAT5	Liver, Kidney	Committed stem cells and megakaryocytes	Platelet	Severe thrombocytopenia
		Leptin	JAK2/STAT3	Adipocytes	Hypothalamus, thyroid	Satiety, controls metabolic rate	Obesity
		G-CSF	JAK2, STAT3	Many tissues, macrophages, endothelium, fibroblasts	Committed progenitors	Differentiation, activates mature granulocytes	Neutropenia
	gp130-utilizing	IL-6	JAK1, STAT3	Macrophage, fibroblasts, endothelium, epithelium, T cells, other	Liver B cell, T cell, thymocytes myeloid cells, osteoclasts	Acute-phase reactants proliferation, differentiation co-stimulation	Reduced Ig, esp. IgA, T lymphopenia, impaired acute-phase response, and Th17 cells
		IL-11	JAK1, STAT3	Stromal cells	Hematopoietic stem cells	Proliferation	Female infertility
		IL-27	JAK1, STAT1, STAT3, STAT4. STAT5	DC	T and NK cells, other cells	Enhancement of Th1 responses, and IL-10; inhibition of Th1, Th2, and Th17 responses	Fatal inflammatory disease with infection
		IL-31	JAK1, STAT3, STAT5	Th2 cells	Monocytes, epithelial cells	Induces chemokines, PMN recruitment	
		CNTF	JAK1, STAT3	Schwann cells	Neuronal	Survival	Progressive atrophy and loss of motor neurons
		LIF	JAK1, STAT3	Uterus, macrophage, fibroblasts, endothelium, epithelium, T cells	Embryonic stem cells, neurons hematopoietic	Survival	Decreased hematopoietic progenitors, defective blastocyst implantation
		Osm[a]	JAK1, STAT3	Macrophage, fibroblasts, endothelium, epithelium	Myeloid cells, liver, embryonic stem cells	Differentiation, acute-phase induction	

Continued

TYPE I AND II CYTOKINE RECEPTORS (HEMATOPOIETIN FAMILY AND INTERFERON RECEPTORS)

Table 10.1 Cytokines classified by receptor families—Cont'd

Receptor family	Subfamily	Cytokine	Signaling	Source	Target	Action	Knockout phenotype
		CT-1	JAK1, STAT3	T cells, others, Myocardial	Myocardium	Growth	
	Bc-utilizing	GM-CSF	JAK1, STAT3	T cells, macrophages, endothelium, fibroblasts	Immature and committed myelomonocytic progenitors macrophages and granulocytes, DC	Growth, differentiation survival, activation	Pulmonary alveolar proteinosis
		IL-3	JAK2, STAT5	T cell	Immature hematopoietic progenitors of multiple lineages	Growth, differentiation survival	No defects in basal hematopoiesis
		IL-5	JAK2, STAT5	Th2 T cells	Eosinophil, B cells	Proliferation, activation	Decreased oesinophilla, defective CD5, B1 cell development
	γc-utilizing	IL-2	JAK1, JAK3, STAT5	T cells	T, B, NK cells, macrophages	Proliferation, cytoxicity IFN-γ secretion, antibody production	Lymphoproliferation[a]
		IL-4[c]	JAK1, JAK3, STAT6	Th2 T cells mast cells	T cell, B cell, macrophage	Proliferation, Th2 differentiation IgG[1] and IgE production Inhibition of cell-mediated immunity	Defective Th2 differentiation and IgE production, decreased allergic responses
		IL-7	JAK1, JAK3, STAT5	Bone marrow, thymic stromal cells, spleen	Thymocytes, T cells, B cells	Growth, differentiation, survival	SCID[a]
		IL-9	JAK1, JAK3, STAT5	Th2 T cells	T cells, mast cell precursors	Proliferation	Not essential for Th2 pathology
		IL-15[c]	JAK1, JAK3, STAT5	Many cells	T-cells, especially memory cells, NK cells	Proliferation, survival	Absence of NK and memory cells
		IL-21	JAK1, JAK3, STAT3	T cells, Th17 cells	T, B, and NK cells	Isotype switching, plasma cell differentiation, enhances CD8+ and NK cell responses, promotes Th17 cell differentiation	Acts in concert with IL-4 Decreased Th17 cells

Group	Cytokine	Signaling	Source cells	Target cells	Function	Phenotype/effects
Hetero-dimeric	IL-13	JAK1, TYK2, STAT6	Activated T cells	B cells, macrophage	Costimulator of proliferation, IgE increased CD23 and Class II, Inhibits cytokine secretion and cell-mediated immunity	Defective Th2 responses and IgE production, decreased allergic responses
	IL-12	JAK2, TYK2, STAT4	Macrophages, DC, B cells	T cell, NK cell	Th1 differentiation, proliferation, cytotoxicity	Defective Th1 differentiation, susceptibility to bacterial infections*
	IL-23	JAK2, TYK2, STAT3, STAT5	Macrophages, DC	T cells	IL-17 production	Reduced arthritis, inflammation,
	IL-35	?	Treg	T cells	Suppresses proliferation	Reduced Treg activity
	TSLP		Epithelial cells, keratinocytes	DC (human) B cells (mouse)	TH2 differentiation (human)	Shared receptor usage with IL-7R
Type II (interferon)	IFN-α/β	JAK1, TYK2, STAT1, STAT2	Plasmacytoid DC, Macrophages, fibroblasts, other	All, NK cell	Antiviral, antiproliferative increased MHC Class I activation	Susceptibility to viral infections[a]
	IFN-γ	JAK1, JAK2, STAT1	Th1 T cells NK cells	Macrophages, endothelium NK cells	Activation, increased MHC Class II expression, increased antigen presentation	Susceptibility to bacterial infections[a]
	IL-10	JAK1, TYK2, STAT3	Th2 T cells, other cells	Macrophages	Decreased MHC class II expression, decreased antigen presentation	Exaggerated inflammatory response and autoimmune disease
	IL-19, 20, 22, 24, 26	STAT1, STAT3	T cells, monocytes	T cells, keratinocytes	Induces production of inflammatory cytokines, Th2 responses	
	IL-28, 29, 30	STAT1, STAT2, STAT3, STAT4, STAT5	Many cells	Many cells	antiviral	
IL-1/TLR	IL-1α/β	IRAK, MyD88, TRAF6, NF-κB	Many cells, esp. macrophages	CNS, endothelial cell liver, thymocyte, macrophage	Fever, anorexia, activation acute-phase reactants co-stimulation, activation, cytokine secretion	Reduced inflammation, cooperates with TNF in host defense
	IL-1F, G					
	IL-18	IRAK, MyD88, TRAF6, NF-κB				Increased susceptibility to infection, Reduced arthritis
	IL-33			T cells	Enhanced Th2 responses	

Continued

TYPE I AND II CYTOKINE RECEPTORS (HEMATOPOIETIN FAMILY AND INTERFERON RECEPTORS)

Table 10.1 Cytokines classified by receptor families—Cont'd

Receptor family	Subfamily	Cytokine	Signaling	Source	Target	Action	Knockout phenotype
IL-17		IL-17A		Activated T cells	Endothelium, many cells	inflammation	Susceptibility to extracellular bacteria
		IL-17B,C,D		Many cells			
		IL-17E (IL-25)	TRAF2	mast cells Th2 cells	T cells	Enhanced Th2 responses	Increased susceptibility to helminths
		IL-17F		Activated T cells	Endothelium, many cells	inflammation	
TGF-β receptor serine kinase family		TGFβ 1,2,3		T cells, macrophages other	T cells, macrophages other	Inhibits growth and activation, promotes Th17	
Receptor tyrosine kinases		Stem cell factor	Ras/Raf/MAPK	Bone marrow Stromal cell	Pluripotent stem cell	Activation, growth	Defective hematopoietic stem cell proliferation, melanocyte production and development
		CSF-1 (M-CSF)	Ras/Raf/MAPK	Macrophage, endothelium, fibroblast, other	Committed myelomonocytic progenitors	Differentiation proliferation, survival	Monocytopenia, osteopetrosis, female infertility
		Flt-3 ligand	Ras/Raf/MAPK	Diverse Tissue	Myeloid cells, especially DC	Proliferation, differentiation	Reduced repopulating hematopoietic stem cells; reduced B-cell precursors
		IL-32	NF-κB, p38 MAPK	T, NK cells, monocytes, epithelia	monocytes	Induces TNF, IL-1, IL-6, IL-8	
		IL-16		T and B cells, mast cells	CD4 T cells		
		IL-34	ERK	Many cells	Monocytes	Proliferation binds CSF-1 receptors	

aHuman disease.
bLIFR is shared by these cytokines. In cases where STAT5a or STAT5b are designated, the cytokines appear to use either interchangeably.
cNote that two forms of the IL-4 and perhaps the IL-5 receptor exist.

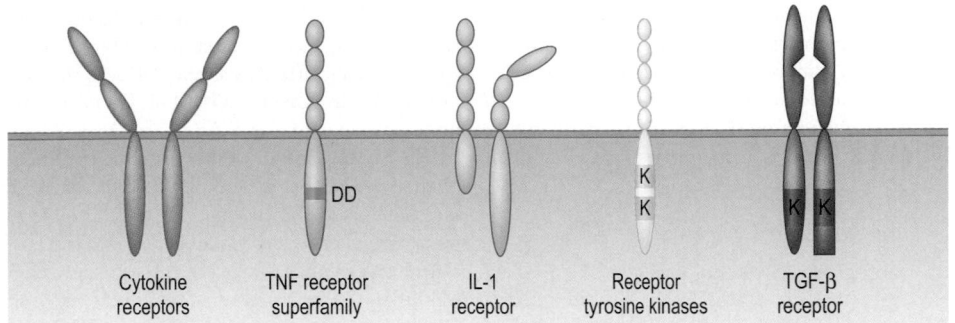

Fig. 10.1   Schematic representation of prototypical receptors from each of the five major cytokine receptor superfamilies.

CLINICAL RELEVANCE

CLINICAL RELEVANCE OF TYPES I AND II CYTOKINE RECEPTORS

>> IL-7R, γc and Jak3 mutations cause SCID

>> Tyk2 and Stat3 mutations cause Hyper IgE syndrome

>> IL-12, IL-12R, and IFNγR mutations are associated with susceptibility to intracellular infections

>> Polymorphisms of IL-2R and IL-7R are associated with multiple sclerosis

>> Polymorphism of IL-23R associated with inflammatory bowel disease

>> Polymorphism of Stat4 associated with RA and SLE

>> EPO, G-CSF, and TPO are used to treat cytopenias

>> Anti-IL-2R mAb is used to prevent transplant rejection

>> Anti-IL-12p40 is used to treat inflammatory bowel disease

IL-6 also serves as a major inducer of fever and the synthesis of acute-phase proteins (fibrinogen, serum amyloid A, haptoglobin, C-reactive protein, etc.) in the liver. The elevation of the erythrocyte sedimentation rate (ESR) in inflammatory disease largely reflects the accelerated synthesis of these proteins, and IL-6-deficient mice are defective in this response. Following exposure to IL-6, the liver reduces synthesis of albumin and transferrin and instead initiates hepatocyte regeneration. Other important functions of IL-6 include induction of adrenocorticotrophic hormone and anterior pituitary hormones such PRL, GH and luteinizing hormone. IL-6 also plays a role in osteoporosis by affecting osteoclast function. For example, IL-6-deficient mice are protected from bone loss following estrogen depletion.

Unlike many cytokines, IL-6 can be detected in the serum, although baseline levels are low in the absence of inflammation. However, IL-6 is rapidly produced in response to bacterial and viral infections, inflammation, or trauma. Patients with rheumatoid arthritis, cardiac myxoma, Castleman's disease, and other autoimmune diseases have high serum levels of IL-6. This cytokine may also contribute to malignancies such as multiple myeloma.

IL-6 is produced by a range of cell types, but its expression in mono-nuclear phagocytes has been well documented. Stimulation of monocytes with IL-1, TNF, or LPS stimulates the expression of IL-6, whereas IL-4

and IL-13 inhibit its production. The promoter of the IL-6 gene contains a number of binding sites for the following transcription factors: nuclear factor-κB (NF-κB), nuclear factor for IL-6 (NF-IL-6, or CCAAT element-binding protein), activator protein-1 (AP-1), cAMP response element-binding protein (CREB), and the glucocorticoid receptor.

Interleukin-11

IL-11 and its receptor are widely expressed. It stimulates stem cells, megakaryocytes, myeloid precursors and erythroid precursors, as well as promoting B-cell differentiation. It also acts on nonhematopoietic cells, including bone and liver. IL-11 is induced by proinflammatory cytokines (IL-1, TNF) and by TGF-β.

Interleukin-27

IL-27, like IL-12, is composed of two subunits designated EBI3 and p28. It signals through a receptor comprising gp130 and WSX-1/TCCR (T-cell cytokine receptor), which is expressed on naïve CD4 T cells. IL-27 promotes Th1 differentiation but also has essential anti-inflammatory properties.[7] It inhibits Th17 differentiation and enhances IL-10 production.

Interleukin-31

IL-31 is the most recently identified gp130-using cytokine. It is produced by Th2 cells. Overexpression of IL-31 results in atopic dermatitis.[8]

Cytokine receptors utilizing the βc chain

The cytokines IL-3, IL-5 and GM-CSF all bind to receptors that share a common β_c receptor subunit (common β subunit). Each of the individual receptors for these cytokines also has a ligand-specific α subunit. Mice, but not humans, have a second β chain, β_{IL3}. This species-specific redundancy may explain why gene targeting of β_c in the mouse did not result in loss of IL-3 responses, although β_c-null mice did have reduced GM-CSF and IL-5 responses.

Interleukin-3

IL-3 binds to a receptor composed of a unique IL-3Rα subunit and the common β_c subunit. IL-3 synergizes with other cytokines to stimulate the growth of immature progenitor cells of all lineages, and is therefore

TYPE I AND II CYTOKINE RECEPTORS (HEMATOPOIETIN FAMILY AND INTERFERON RECEPTORS)

a multilineage colony-stimulating factor (CSF). It prevents cell death and promotes the survival of macrophages, mast cells, and megakaryocytes. IL-3 is produced mainly by lymphoid cells, but also by mast cells and eosinophils. IL-3-deficient mice have no obvious defect in hematopoiesis, suggesting that the major role of IL-3 in vivo may be in the response to stress, rather than to regulate hematopoiesis under normal conditions.

Interleukin-5

IL-5 is unusual among cytokines in that it is a disulfide-linked homodimer, with each component containing three α-helical bundles. Its major action is to promote the growth, differentiation, and activation of eosinophils. As such, it is very important in pathogenesis of allergic disease. IL-5$^{-/-}$ mice fail to develop eosinophilia in response to parasitic or aeroallergen challenge. Remarkably, these mice exhibit minimal signs of inflammation and damage to the lungs. IL-5 deficiency does not affect the worm burden of infected mice, indicating that eosinophilia per se may not play an essential role in the host defense against helminths. Both IL-5 and IL-5R knockout mice have decreased numbers of CD5$^+$ B cells (B-1 cells), concomitant with low serum concentrations of IgM and IgG$_3$. IL-5 is produced by activated helper T cells of the Th2 phenotype (see below), mast cells, and eosinophils in an autocrine manner.

Granulocyte–Macrophage-CSF

GM-CSF acts on hematopoietic precursors to support myelomonocytic differentiation. It also activates mature neutrophils and macrophages, increasing their microbicidal activity and inducing the production of proinflammatory cytokines. Along with IL-4 and IL-13, GM-CSF is a major stimulatory cytokine for the in vitro production of dendritic cells (DCs). Additionally, GM-CSF induces proliferation and activation of eosinophils and upregulates adhesion molecules on fibroblasts and endothelial cells. Homozygous inactivation of the GM-CSF gene in mice, however, does not affect steady-state hematopoiesis. Instead, these animals develop alveolar proteinosis and lymphoid hyperplasia, which is not due to a detectable infectious agent. β$_c$$^{-/-}$ mice also develop alveolar proteinosis, characterized by the accumulation of surfactant in the lungs. A similar defect may be responsible for disease in a subset of humans with this abnormality.

The production of GM-CSF can be induced by proinflammatory cytokines and LPS. Unsurprisingly, GM-CSF is made by activated lymphocytes, as well as other stimulated cells. GM-CSF is not ordinarily detectable in blood except under pathologic conditions such as asthma. GM-CSF has been used clinically to treat chemotherapy-induced neutropenia, especially in the context of certain infections (e.g., fungal). It has also been tested in myelodysplastic syndrome and aplastic anemia.

Cytokine receptors utilizing the γc chain

The cytokines IL-2, IL-4, IL-7, IL-9, IL-15, and IL-21 all bind to receptors that share a common γ$_c$ receptor subunit. The γ$_c$ subunit and the ligand-specific subunits are expressed predominantly on lymphocytes, although they can be found on other hematopoietic cells as well. Accordingly, these cytokines might be expected to be important for the development and function of lymphoid cells. Proof of their importance

was provided when it was shown that mutation of the γ$_c$ gene was responsible for X-linked severe combined immunodeficiency (SCID), which is characterized by a lack of T cells and NK cells, and poorly functioning B cells (Chapter 35).[9] This disorder, which has proved to be the most common form of SCID in humans, is thus designated as a T$^-$B$^+$ SCID. Subsequently, γ$_c$ knockout mice were found to also have a SCID phenotype, but one that differed from that of the human disorder. γ$_c$ knockout mice also lack B cells, which points to species-specific functions of γ$_c$. The lack of γ$_c$ abrogates signaling by all of the cytokines that utilize this subunit (IL-2, IL-4, IL-7, IL-9, IL-15 and IL-21), but the lack of IL-7 signaling is predominantly responsible for the SCID phenotype. Thus, the lesser importance of IL-7 signaling in human B-cell development probably explains the less severe block on B-cell function seen in patients with X-linked SCID.

Interleukin-2

The IL-2 receptor consists of three subunits, α, β and γ$_c$. The latter two are members of the type I cytokine receptor family. NK cells constitutively express these latter two subunits and respond to high doses of IL-2, whereas in T cells the IL-2Rα subunit is induced upon activation, where it creates a high-affinity receptor for IL-2. IL-2Rα is also inducible in activated monocytes and B cells. IL-2Rα, however, is not a member of the type I cytokine receptor family. Rather, it resembles members of the complement family and IL-15R (see below). Thymocytes express high levels of IL-2Rα, but a role of IL-2 in thymic development is not evident. For example, IL-2 and IL-2Rα gene targeted mice exhibit normal thymocyte development.

IL-2, one of the first cytokines to be intensively studied, is produced principally by activated T cells and is a prototypical autocrine T-cell growth factor that is required for progression from the G1 to the S phase of the cell cycle in T cells activated in vitro. It is an important factor in determining the magnitude of T-cell and NK-cell responses, augmenting the cytolytic activity of T and NK cells and inducing IFN-γ secretion. IL-2 is also important in programming CD8 memory T cells, which undergo secondary expansion in viral infections.[10] IL-2 is a growth factor for B cells and induces class switching. It also activates macrophages. Targeted deletion of the genes encoding IL-2, IL-2Rα, and IL-2Rβ, however, yielded surprising phenotypes. T-cell development in these mice appears normal, but they succumb to autoimmune and lymphoproliferative disease, pointing to the existence of a separate, in vivo role of IL-2 whose function is to maintain lymphoid homeostasis and thus help prevent autoimmune disease.[11] IL-2-deficient mice develop massive enlargement of peripheral lymphoid organs, hemolytic anemia, inflammatory bowel disease, and infiltrative granulopoiesis. In addition, they have high levels of IgG$_1$ and IgE. Paradoxically, their T cells proliferate poorly in vitro in response to either polyclonal activators or antigen-specific signals. A similar phenotype is seen in humans with IL-2Rα mutations.

Whereas the T-cell hyperplasia and tissue infiltration observed in IL-2 or IL-2Rα chain-deficient individuals was originally thought to be due to a defect in the restimulation-induced cell death of activated T cells, abnormal regulatory T (Treg) cell function may provide an alternative mechanism (Chapter 16). Naturally arising Treg cells in both mice and humans express high levels of IL-2Rα, and maintenance of peripheral Treg cell numbers has been shown to be dependent on IL-2.[12] In addition, IL-2 inhibits Th17 differentiation.

IL-2 is produced almost exclusively by activated T cells. It is rapidly induced upon recognition of foreign antigen. Indeed, IL-2 production is one of the key indicators of T-cell activation. The IL-2 promoter has been extensively characterized and contains binding sites for the following transcription factors: nuclear factor of activated T-cells (NFAT), AP-1, and NF-κB. IL-2 production is also regulated by stabilization of its mRNA.

IL-2 has been used in a number of clinical circumstances both to treat malignancies and to boost CD4 T-cell counts in HIV. The clinical utility of IL-2 therapy is limited by its toxicity, two important manifestations being hepatic dysfunction and the so-called capillary or vascular leak syndrome. On the other hand, anti-IL-2Rα monoclonal antibodies, daclizumab and basiliximab, are used to prevent rejection of allotransplants. Polymorphisms of IL-2Rα are associated with multiple sclerosis.

Interleukin-4

As discussed above, two classes of IL-4R appear to exist.[13] One consists of the IL-4Rα subunit in conjunction with γ_c and is expressed on hematopoietic cells. The other, a 'type II' receptor, appears to consist of the IL-4Rα subunit in association with the α chain of IL-13R. This latter receptor appears to be widely expressed. However, two IL-13R subunits have been cloned, so the exact composition of the type II IL-4R remains uncertain. The existence of two receptors helps explain why IL-4 has diverse actions on both hematopoietic and nonhematopoietic cells. The loss of IL-4Rα would be predicted to block the actions of both IL-4 and IL-13, which could explain why gene targeting of IL-4Rα leads to a more severe phenotype than that observed in IL-4-deficient mice. Polymorphisms of IL-4Rα have been reported to be associated with a propensity towards atopy.[14]

In general, IL-4 serves to promote allergic response and to inhibit cell-mediated immune responses. Among the most important roles of IL-4 is its ability to promote differentiation of naive CD4 T cells into a subset that produces IL-4 and IL-5.[15, 16] These cells are denoted the so-called Th2 (T-helper 2) subset, as opposed to Th1 cells, which produce lymphotoxin-α and IFN-γ (Chapter 17). In conjunction with CD40 activation, IL-4 also promotes B-cell proliferation and class switching, particularly to IgG_1 and IgE in mice and to IgG_4 and IgE in humans. Mice deficient in IL-4 have normal B lymphopoiesis and marked reductions in IgG_1 and IgE production in response to parasites. Importantly, these mice have residual Th2 responses, because IL-13, which also binds IL-4Rα, can partially compensate for the defect.

IL-4 has also been shown to upregulate the expression of surface IgM, MHC class II, and CD23 on B cells. In conjunction with GM-CSF, it is also a growth factor for mast cells and basophils, as well as a potent inducer of DC differentiation. IL-4 inhibits macrophage activation and the production of proinflammatory cytokines. It antagonizes the effects of IFN-γ, blocks cytokine-induced proliferation of synoviocytes, downregulates the expression of adhesion molecules, and antagonizes the induction of some acute-phase reactants in hepatocytes by IL-6.

IL-4 is made by the Th2 subset of CD4 T cells, basophils and mast cells. A minor population of NK1.1+ CD4 T cells also produces large amounts of IL-4. Based on the tight regulation of IL-4 production, the IL-4 promoter has received considerable attention. A number of transcription factors appear to be important in regulating IL-4 production, including NFAT, NF-IL6, C/EBP, c-MAF, and GATA-3. The IL-4 promoter has a Stat6 binding site, which is consistent with the fact that IL-4 regulates its own expression. Epigenetic control and chromatin remodeling are also important aspects.[17]

Clinically, IL-4 has been tested in the treatment of malignancies and some autoimmune disorders. The ability of IL-4 to generate DCs is being exploited in the use of tumor vaccines. Conceivably, soluble IL-4R might also be useful in the treatment of allergic disease.

Interleukin-7

The IL-7 receptor consists of the IL-7Rα chain (CD127) in association with γ_c. It is expressed on both immature and mature thymocytes. Humans with mutations of IL-7Rα have T−B+ SCID, but unlike individuals with γ_c mutations, display normal NK cell development (Chapter 35).[9]

IL-7Rα expression is tightly regulated during thymocyte development (Chapter 9). It is expressed in double-negative thymocytes, downregulated in double-positive cells, and then re-expressed in single-positive thymocytes. It is also expressed in mature peripheral T cells. This suggests that IL-7 plays an important role in both developing thymocytes and mature T cells. This may be a reflection of its anti-apoptotic effects, which are attributable to the induction of Bcl-2 family members. IL-7 promotes the growth of thymocytes, as well as the expression and rearrangement of TCR genes and the expression of RAG1 and RAG2 (Chapter 4). IL-7Rα is expressed on cutaneous T-cell lymphomas, which also produce this cytokine; thus the autocrine response to IL-7 may contribute to the growth of these tumors.

IL-7- and IL-7R-deficient mice exhibit impairments in both T- and B-cell development. Postnatal B-cell development in IL-7−/− mice is blocked at the transition to pre-B cells and is arrested even earlier in IL-7Rα−/− mice. This suggests that IL-7Rα binds a cytokine other than IL-7, perhaps the thymic stroma-derived lymphopoietin. Why these abnormalities do not occur in humans with IL-7Rα mutations is not clear: presumably a factor that does not bind IL-7R regulates this step in human B-cell development.

IL-7 is produced by a wide variety of cells, including marrow and perhaps thymic stromal cells, as well as in the kidney, spleen, epithelial cells and keratinocytes. This is consistent with its role in the maintenance of function in both immature and mature lymphocytes.

Clinically, IL-7 may be useful to restore immune function in some congenital immunodeficiencies, after bone marrow transplantation, or in HIV infection. Polymorphisms of the IL-7R are associated with multiple sclerosis.

Interleukin-9

IL-9 has some of the same properties as IL-4. It strongly synergizes with stem cell factor to promote the growth and differentiation of mast cells and is a potent regulator of mast cell function. IL-9 also potentiates IgE production induced by IL-4. Although it was first identified as a T-cell growth factor, a physiologic role in T-cell development has not been established. IL-9 is produced by activated Th2 cells. Some lymphoid tumors produce IL-9, where it may serve as an autocrine growth factor.

Interleukin-15

The IL-15 receptor consists of the IL-2Rβ and γ_c subunits in association with a unique ligand-specific subunit, IL-15Rα, which is homologous to IL-2Rα.[18] These receptor proteins are not related to type I cytokine receptors. Instead, they contain protein-binding motifs termed 'sushi domains'. The relatedness of these receptors and their cognate ligands is further emphasized by the fact that in both human and mouse they are physically linked in the genome. Not surprisingly, given their shared receptor usage, there are many similarities in the actions of IL-2 and IL-15, particularly in terms of the effects on lymphoid cells. Like IL-2, IL-15 induces proliferation and cytokine production in T and NK cells. However, despite the similarities between these two ligands/receptors there are a number of important differences. IL-15Rα is more widely expressed than IL-2Rα, IL-2Rβ and γc. In addition to lymphoid cells, IL-15Rα is expressed in fibroblasts, epithelial, liver, intestine and other cells. IL-15 and IL-15Rα knockout mice are defective in NK-cell production and in the generation of memory T cells, explaining the absence of NK development in patients with γc mutations.

The production of IL-15 is also very different from that of IL-2. IL-15 mRNA is expressed broadly in hematopoietic and nonhematopoietic cells, though it is not typically produced by T cells. HTLV-I-transformed T cells are an exception in that they produce abundant IL-15. Also in contrast to IL-2, IL-15 is not controlled predominantly at the level of transcription. Instead, there are multiple upstream AUGs in the 5′ untranslated portion of the message that interfere with translation. A similar pattern of translational regulation is observed for IL-7 and IL-9, but is uncommon in other cytokine genes. IL-15 protein is also controlled at the level of secretion of the protein, but this is incompletely understood. High levels of IL-15 protein have been reported in synovial fluids from patients with rheumatoid arthritis, alveolar macrophages from patients with sarcoidosis, and peripheral blood mononuclear cells from patients with ulcerative colitis. Monoclonal anti-IL-15 antibody is being tested in rheumatoid arthritis.

Interleukin-21

IL-21 is a T cell-derived cytokine that works in concert with other γc cytokines. It synergizes with IL-7 and IL-15 to expand and activate CD8 T cells. IL-21 also augments the activity of NK cells. It further acts with IL-4 to activate B cells and induce class switching. IL-21 drives the differentiation of B cells into memory cells and terminally differentiated plasma cells.[19] IL-21 is selectively produced by Th17s cells and promotes Th17 differentiation.

Other heterodimeric receptors

Interleukin-12

IL-12 is a heterodimer composed of two disulfide-linked polypeptide chains, p35 and p40, that are the products of two distinct genes.[20, 21] IL-12 p35 shares homology with other cytokines, such as IL-6, whereas p40 resembles the IL-6 receptor. Thus, IL-12 can be viewed as being synthesized as a ligand–receptor complex. Two chains of IL-12R have been identified. Because the ligand already comprises the α subunit, the two chains of the IL-12R are denoted IL-12Rβ1 and β2. Expression of high-affinity IL-12R is very restricted, being found predominantly on T and NK cells. IL-12R expression is also notable in that it is regulated by the activation state of the cell. IL-12Rβ1 and β2 are highly inducible upon T-cell activation, and IL-4 inhibits IL-12Rβ2 expression. This is important because IL-12Rβ2 is required for IL-12 signaling and the activation

of the transcription factor Stat4. NK cells constitutively express IL-12Rβ1 and IL-12Rβ2.

IL-12 plays a pivotal role in promoting cell-mediated immune responses. Humans with IL-12R mutations, as well as mice with IL-12 and IL-12R deficiency, have very blunted immune responses and are highly susceptible to infections by intracellular pathogens.[22] An important function of IL-12 is that it promotes the differentiation of uncommitted helper T cells to the Th1 subset: i.e., T cells that produce LT-α and INF-γ. Th1 differentiation is markedly impaired in IL-12- and IL-12R-deficient mice. A major action of IL-12 is its ability to induce the production of IFN-γ, doing so synergistically in combination with IL-2 or IL-18. Consequently, many of the actions of IL-12 are blocked in IFN-γ or IFN-γR knockout mice. IL-12 also induces proliferation and cytolytic activity of T and NK cells.

Dendritic cells and macrophages are the major producers of IL-12 in response to various pathogens, occupancy of Toll-like receptors and CD40. The IL-12p40 promoter is complex and contains NF-κB sites, interferon response elements (IREs), and Ets binding sites. As with other cytokine genes, nucleosome remodeling is important in the regulation of IL-12.[23]

Because of its profound effects on cell-mediated immunity, IL-12 has been used in a number of clinical circumstances. It has been used in the treatment of malignancies and infectious diseases, but its utility has been limited due to significant toxicity. IL-12 may also have use in vaccines as an adjuvant. Conversely, antagonizing the actions of IL-12 has been found to be useful in Th1-mediated diseases, including inflammatory bowel disease (Chapter 75).

Interleukin-23

IL-23 is another heterodimeric type I cytokine. It is composed of two disulfide-linked polypeptide chains, p19 and IL-12 p40. The IL-23 receptor also shares the IL-12Rβ1 chain paired to the IL-23R.[24] The IL-23R complex is expressed on activated T cells. Its function relates to a third T lineage of differentiated helper cells, which produce high levels of the cytokine IL-17 (Th17, see below). IL-23 is thought to be important in the maintenance of Th17 cells. As such, IL-23 is thought to be important in host defense against extracellular bacteria and the pathogenesis of autoimmune and autoinflammatory disorders. It is notable in this regard that therapies that target IL-12p40 antagonize both IL-12 and IL-23. IL-23 is produced primarily by dendritic cells in response to TLR agonists. IL-23R polymorphisms are associated with inflammatory bowel disease, ankylosing spondylitis and other autoimmune diseases.

Interleukin-35

IL-35 is a newly described cytokine that is a dimer consisting of IL-12 p35 and EB13.

Interleukin-13

IL-13 has many of the same effects as IL-4 and shares a receptor subunit(s) with IL-4. IL-13-deficient mice have reduced levels of IL-4, IL-5, and IL-10. They also have lower IgE levels and eosinophilia. In mice deficient for both IL-4 and IL-13, these Th2 responses are abolished and the ability to clear parasites is severely impaired. These double-knockout mice default to Th1 responses, with concomitant production of INF-γ, IgG2a and IgG2b. Thus, it appears that IL-4 and IL-13 cooperate in promoting Th2 responses, having both overlapping and additive roles.

Thymic stromal lymphopoietin (TSLP)

TSLP is an IL-7-like cytokine expressed by epithelial cells and keratinocytes. Its receptor comprises TSLPR and IL-7Rα, which is expressed primarily on monocytes and myeloid-derived dendritic cells, as well as on B cells. Curiously, this cytokine is reported to have different effects in mouse and human cells. TSLP-treated human dendritic cells promote Th2 differentiation.[25] In the mouse, TSLP contributes to B-cell development.

INTERFERONS

Type I interferons

The type I interferons include IFN-α, IFN-ω and IFN-β. There are at least 14 separate genes that encode structurally distinct forms of IFN-α, whereas IFN-β and IFN-ω are encoded by single genes. Nonetheless, each of these molecules binds to the same receptor, termed the IFN-α/β receptor. As a result, their actions are similar. Thus, it is unclear why there are so many distinct genes. Their relative potencies do differ; hence it is possible that these genes evolved in response to various viral pathogens. The duplication of IFN genes might also simply affect the magnitude of the antiviral responses. These intronless genes are all clustered on the short arm of chromosome 9 and appear to have diverged from a common ancestor more than 100 million years ago. The receptor is a heterodimer composed of two subunits termed IFNAR1 and IFNAR2. These subunits have limited similarity to type I cytokine receptors, although they lack the WSXWS motif.

A major effect of type I interferons is their antiviral action.[26] Discovered in 1957, they act on all cells to inhibit viral replication as well as cellular proliferation. A major mechanism is the inhibition of protein translation. They also upregulate MHC class I and downregulate MHC class II expression. IFNα/β increase the cytolytic activity of NK cells. Predictably, IFNARI knockout mice are extremely susceptible to infections, even though lymphoid development is normal.

Interferons are produced ubiquitously, viral infection being a major inducer of their transcriptional regulation. Type I IFN is also induced by intracellular bacterial pathogens and LPS. Immunoregulatory effects of IFNα/β are being increasingly recognized, and it is notable that a subset of dendritic cells produces very high levels.[27, 28] The promoter for IFN-β has been intensively analyzed. It binds a variety of transcription factors, including NF-κB and interferon regulatory factor 1 (IRF-1). IRF-2 also binds to this promoter and functions as a repressor.

Type I IFN is used clinically in the treatment of certain infections, e.g., viral hepatitis. Owing to its antiproliferative action, it is also used in the treatment of certain malignancies, particularly hairy cell leukemia. IFN-β is used in the treatment of multiple sclerosis.

Newer interferon-like cytokines including IL-28A, IL-28B and IL-29 (also designated IFN-λ₁, -λ₂ and -λ₃) have been identified. They bind to a receptor designated IL-28R. However, the exact *in vivo* functions of these interferon-like cytokines are poorly understood, although they probably contribute to antiviral responses.

Interferon-γ

IFN-γ is a major activator of macrophages. It enhances their ability to kill microorganisms by augmenting their cytolytic machinery. IFN-γ exerts this effect by causing the cell to increase its production of reactive oxygen intermediates, including hydrogen peroxide, nitric oxide, and indoleamine dioxygenase. It also upregulates MHC class II expression. However, the activity of IFN-γ is by no means restricted to phagocytic cells. It has been shown to act on CD4 T cells to promote Th1 differentiation while inhibiting the generation of Th2 cells. It also promotes the maturation of CD8 T cells to cytotoxic cells. In mice, IFN-γ augments NK cytolytic activity, promotes switching to IgG$_{2a}$ and IgG$_3$, and inhibits switching to IgG$_1$ and IgE. Endothelial cells and neutrophils are also activated by IFN-γ. Like IFN-α/β, IFN-γ also contributes to antiviral defenses.

The IFN-γ receptor is a heterodimer composed of IFNγRα and IFNγRβ subunits. When one IFN-γ homodimer binds, a complex of two α and two β receptors is created.[29] Mice with a disrupted IFNγR develop normally and have normal lymphoid development, but are highly susceptible to viral and bacterial infections, especially intracellular microbes. They have diminished macrophage MHC class II expression, decreased NK function, and reduced serum IgG$_{2a}$ concentrations. Humans with mutations of IFNγR subunits are also susceptible to mycobacterial and *Salmonella* infections.

The control of IFN-γ production is tightly regulated, T cells of the Th1 subset and NK cells being the major producers. Transcription factors including STAT4, T-bet, and Eomes, play an important roles in IFN-γ gene regulation.[16] IFN-γ has been used to treat patients with immunodeficiencies (e.g., chronic granulomatous disease) and in certain patients with disseminated mycobacterial infections.[30] A monoclonal anti-IFN-γ antibody, fontolizumab, is being studied in the treatment of autoimmune disease.

Interleukin-10 and related cytokines

The major function of IL-10 is to serve as an anti-inflammatory and immunosuppressive cytokine. Unlike other cytokines in this family, it is a disulfide-linked dimer. A single IL-10R has been cloned, but the receptor may have additional components. The IL-10R is expressed on macrophages, mast cells, and most other hematopoietic cells. It is also inducible in nonhematopoietic cells by stimuli such as LPS.

IL-10 strongly inhibits the production of IL-1, IL-6, IL-8, IL-12, TNF, and other immune and inflammatory cytokines. It also inhibits macrophage antigen presentation and decreases expression of MHC class II, adhesion molecules, and the co-stimulatory molecules CD80 (B7.1) and CD86 (B7.2). The importance of IL-10 as an endogenous inhibitor of cell-mediated immunity is emphasized by the finding that IL-10-deficient mice develop autoimmune disease, which manifests with severe inflammatory bowel disease and exaggerated inflammatory responses. Delayed-type hypersensitivity and contact hypersensitivity responses are also prolonged and amplified in IL-10⁻/⁻ mice.

IL-10 is made by Th1 and Th2 cells, although a subset of T cells that preferentially produces IL-10 and TGF-β is sometimes denoted Th3. IL-10 is also produced by activated B cells, macrophages, keratinocytes, and bronchial epithelial cells. LPS and TNF are inducers of IL-10. IL-10 is readily detected in the blood of patients with septic shock and other inflammatory and immune disorders. Owing to its anti-inflammatory properties, IL-10 has been used experimentally in the treatment of some Th1-mediated autoimmune diseases. Paradoxically, IL-10 is elevated in patients with systemic lupus erythematosus, and there is a correlation between levels of IL-10 and autoantibody production.

There are viral homologs of IL-10 that may blunt the immune response to these pathogens. IL-10 also contributes to the immunosuppression

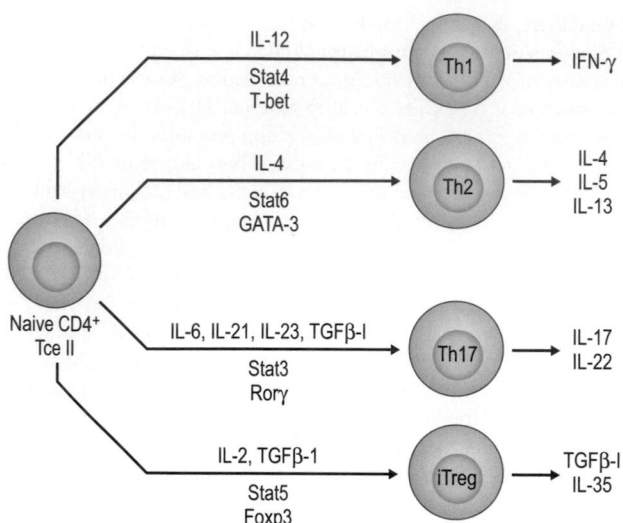

Fig. 10.2 Differentiation of T-helper cell subtypes.

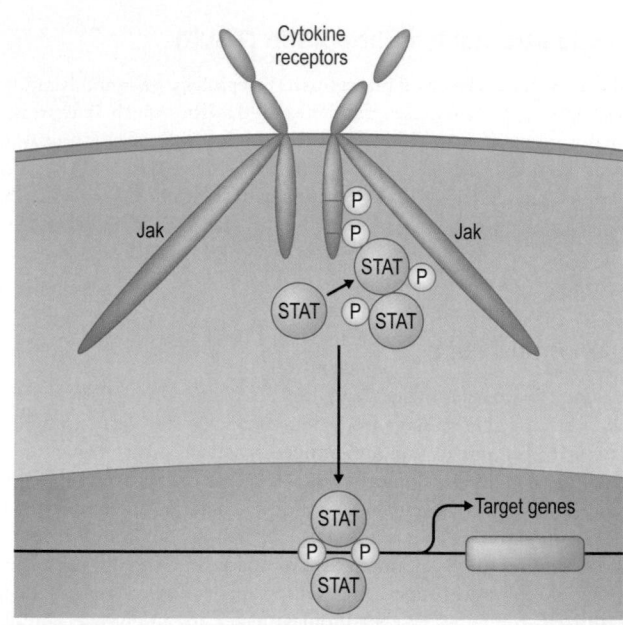

Fig. 10.3 The roles of JAKs and STATs in signal transduction by type I and II cytokine receptors.

seen in lepromatous leprosy or parasitic infestations. Other IL-10-related cytokines include IL-19, IL-20, IL-22, IL-24, and IL-26, but their biological actions are incompletely understood.[31]

Cytokines and the differentiation of T cells to helpers and effectors

Classically, precursor CD4 T-cell differentiation was viewed as polarization into one of two phenotypes: T-helper 1 (Th1) or T-helper 2 (Th2) (Fig. 10.2) (Chapter 16). More recently, other T-cell subsets have been identified, which will also be discussed. The key point is that differentiation into each of these subsets is regulated by different cytokines. Th1 cells drive the immune response towards cell-mediated immune responses, whereas Th2 cells promote a humoral or allergic response. The latter is protective against helminthic and other parasitic infestations. Th1 cells produce IL-2, LT-α and IFN-γ, whereas Th2 cells produce IL-4, IL-5 and IL-10. Both subsets produce IL-3.

The differentiation of helper T cells has important implications for host defense. In mouse models of parasitic disease, the failure of some strains to mount a Th1 response results in the majority of the animals succumbing to the infection. Conversely, in other disease models the production of a Th2 response results in enhanced survival, whereas a Th1 response causes more damage to the host. Although the mechanisms by which Th1 and Th2 development is governed are not fully understood, the cytokines themselves play important roles. Specifically, IL-4 promotes Th2 differentiation and antagonizes Th1 responses. Conversely, IL-12 and IFN-γ promote Th1 differentiation and antagonize Th2 development. A number of transcription factors have been reported to regulate this response. GATA-3, c-MAF and NFATp regulate IL-4 production and Th2 differentiation, whereas STAT4 and T-BET promote Th1 differentiation.[16, 21]

The immunopathogenesis of autoimmune disease does not fit quite so neatly into the standard Th1/Th2 dichotomy. CD4 T cells can also differentiate into cells that produce IL-10 and transforming growth factor-β (TGF-β) – so-called Th3 cells – and can become 'adaptive' Treg cells; both types appear to protect against autoimmunity.[32] As discussed above, IL-2 and TGF-β are important for Treg cell differentiation. Models of autoimmunity have pointed to the importance of yet another subset of Th cells that produces IL-17 and which are now termed Th17 cells. TGF-β and IL-6 are thought to promote Th17 differentiation from naïve progenitors, whereas IL-23 is important for the maintenance of these cells. In addition to a role in autoimmunity, IL-17 is important in host defense against extracellular bacteria.[33, 34]

SIGNALING

Neither type I nor type II receptors exhibit intrinsic enzymatic activity. However, the membrane proximal segment of each of these receptors is conserved. This segment of the molecule serves as the site at which these receptors bind Janus kinases (JAKs), which play a pivotal role in signaling via this family of cytokine receptors (Fig. 10.3).

Janus kinases

Only four mammalian Janus kinases, JAK1, JAK2, JAK3, and TYK2, have been identified so far. JAKs are structurally unique, consisting of a C-terminal catalytically active kinase domain that is preceded by a segment termed the pseudokinase domain. The latter gives JAKs their name and has regulatory functions. A key feature of the JAKs is their association with cytokine receptors, which appears to be mediated by the N terminus. The utilization of the various JAKs by different cytokine receptors is summarized in Table 10.1.

Ligand binding to type I and II receptors induces the aggregation of receptor subunits, which brings JAKs in close proximity and allows them to phosphorylate and activate each other. After activation, the JAKs phosphorylate receptor subunits on tyrosine residues, which allows the recruitment of proteins with SRC homology-2 (SH2) or phosphotyrosine-binding (PTB) domains. These proteins can also be phosphorylated by JAKs. Phosphorylation results in the activation of a number of biochemical pathways. Importantly, phosphorylation of cytokine receptors generates docking sites for a class of SH2-containing transcription factors termed the STATs (see below).

The pivotal function of the JAKs is vividly illustrated by mice or humans that are deficient in these kinases. The association of JAK3 with γ_c suggested that JAK3 mutations might also cause SCID, and indeed it was found that mutation of JAK3 results in autosomal recessive T^-B^+ SCID (Chapter 35).[35] JAK3 knockout mice were also found to exhibit SCID. Indeed, mutation of either γ_c or JAK3 leads to the same functional defects. These findings led to the notion that a JAK3 inhibitor might represent a new class of immunosuppressant drug. One such inhibitor, CP 690,550, was effective in preclinical studies.[36] This drug is currently being tested in humans. Rarely, gain-of-function mutations of JAK3 occur in leukemia.

In contrast to JAK3-deficient mice and humans, gene targeting of *jak1* and *jak2* results in more diverse abnormalities. *Jak1*$^{-/-}$ mice die perinatally from neurologic defects, but also have a SCID phenotype similar to *jak3*$^{-/-}$ mice. This is explained by the fact that γ_c-containing cytokine receptors utilize JAK1 in association with their ligand-specific receptor subunit. Other cytokines that are dependent on JAK1 include those that use gp130 cytokine receptors (IL-6, LIF, OSM, CNTF, and IL-11) and type II receptors (IL-10, IFN-γ, and IFN-α/β). Gene-targeting of *jak2* was embryonically lethal, principally because JAK2 is essential for EPO function and the mice fail to form blood. In addition, JAK2 is necessary for signaling of other cytokines, including IL-3. The importance of the JAKs has been substantiated by the identification of chromosomal translocations in various leukemias resulting in TEL (a transcription factor)/JAK fusion proteins, which have constitutive kinase activity and uncontrolled signaling. For example, a mutation in the pseudokinase domain of JAK2 underlies most cases of polycythemia vera. Mutations of Tyk2 are associated with Hyper IgE syndrome.

STATs

Members of the signal transducer and activator of transcription (STAT) family of DNA-binding proteins serve a key role in transducing signals from cytokine receptors on the cell surface to the nucleus, where they regulate gene transcription. STATs are latent, cytosolic transcription factors that have SH2 domains (phosphotyrosine-binding modules) that allow them to be recruited to phosphorylated cytokine receptors (Fig. 10.3). Different STATs bind to specific cytokine receptors (Table 10.1). STATs are themselves tyrosine phosphorylated by JAKs, and this promotes their dimerization. STATs translocate to the nucleus, bind DNA, and regulate transcription.

There are seven mammalian STATs: STAT1, STAT2, STAT3, STAT4, STAT5a, STAT5b, and STAT6. *Stat* knockout mice document the essential and specific functions of these transcription factors in transmitting cytokine signals. *Stat1*$^{-/-}$ mice develop normally, but have extreme susceptibility to viral and some bacterial infections, consistent with the defects seen in IFN$\gamma$$^{-/-}$ and IFNγR$^{-/-}$ mice, and in IFNβR-deficient humans. STAT1 also appears to be important in regulating apoptosis. Its absence is associated with tumorigenesis. Gene targeting of STAT3 leads

to early embryonic lethality, the lethality being related in part to interference with LIF function. Conditional knockouts of STAT3 in myeloid cells display exaggerated inflammatory responses, evidently due to a failure of IL-10 signaling. Stat3 is also essential for Th17 cells. Mutations of Stat3 underlie Hyper IgE syndrome. As might be expected from the fact that STAT4 is activated by IL-12; *stat4*$^{-/-}$ mice develop normally but have defective cell-mediated immune responses and Th1 differentiation combined with augmented Th2 development. This phenotype is consistent with the abnormalities seen in IL-12$^{-/-}$ mice, IL-12R$^{-/-}$ mice, and IL-12R-deficient humans.

STAT6 is activated by IL-4. *Stat6*$^{-/-}$ mice have defective Th2 development with defective IgE responses following infection with parasites. Lack of STAT6 dramatically attenuates allergic and asthmatic disease in animal models of these diseases. IL-13 also activates STAT6, and its responses are abrogated in *stat6*$^{-/-}$ mice.

STAT5a and STAT5b are highly homologous, but nonetheless have different functions. *Stat5a*$^{-/-}$ mice have impaired mammary gland development and failure of lactation, whereas *stat5b*$^{-/-}$ mice have defective sexually dimorphic growth and growth hormone-dependent regulation of liver gene expression. *Stat5a/5b* doubly-deficient mice manifest increased perinatal lethality, decreased size, female infertility, and impaired lymphocyte development. *Stat5*$^{-/-}$ mice develop lymphoproliferative disease reminiscent of IL-2- and IL-2R-deficient mice, presumably related to loss of Treg cells,

Attenuation of type-I and type-II cytokine signaling

Perhaps as important as the triggers that initiate signal transduction are the mechanisms for extinguishing the response.[37] There are several families of proteins involved in downregulating cytokine signaling. Among these are phosphatases, cytokine-inducible inhibitor molecules, and transcriptional repressors. The phosphatase SHP-1 interacts with cytokine receptors and downregulates signaling. *Motheaten* mice lack a functional SHP-1 protein and die at an early age from autoimmune disease.

Another family of proteins that attenuates cytokine signaling are the suppressors of cytokine signaling (SOCS), which are alternatively termed JAB, SSI, and CIS. These are SH2-containing proteins that bind to either cytokine receptors or to JAKs and inhibit signaling. There are at least eight members of this family. Largely due to systemic hyperresponsiveness to IFN-γ, SOCS-1$^{-/-}$ mice die within a few weeks of birth. Another family member, SOCS-3, is important in controlling Th17 differentiation.[38]

KEY CONCEPT

PROPERTIES OF THE TNF RECEPTOR SUPERFAMILY

>> Activation of a TNF receptor can lead to a wide range of effects, from proliferation to apoptosis

>> Transduction of signals through TRAFs leads to the enhancement of survival

>> Signaling through death domains leads to the induction of apoptosis

CLINICAL RELEVANCE

TNFR SUPERFAMILY CYTOKINES AND RECEPTORS AND DISEASE

>> Dominant mutations of TNFRI are associated with autosomal dominant periodic fever syndromes known as TNFR1-associated periodic syndromes (TRAPS)

>> Mutations in CD40L are associated with X-linked hyper-IgM syndrome (X-HIM)

>> Dominant mutations in FAS are associated with autoimmune lymphoproliferative syndrome (ALPS)

>> Rheumatoid arthritis often responds to therapeutic use of TNF antagonists

■ TNF RECEPTOR AND LIGAND SUPERFAMILIES ■

This large family of structurally related ligands, receptors, and inhibitory decoy receptors has various roles both within and without the immune system. The first two members of this family to be discovered were tumor necrosis factor (TNF) and lymphotoxin-α (LTα; sometimes referred to as TNF-β). These molecules are secreted principally by activated myeloid and T cells. They have similar proinflammatory functions, but are only two members of a large family of related molecules that includes CD30, CD40, Fas ligand, and TRAIL. Indeed, the TNF family now contains more than 20 members, each of which appears to exhibit marked differences in tissue expression, ligand specificity and biological function (Fig. 10.4; Tables 10.2 and 10.3). This section describes general aspects of TNF and TNFR biology, with examples from three of the best-studied TNF-family members: TNF, lymphotoxin and Fas ligand.

LIGAND AND RECEPTOR STRUCTURE

Much of our understanding of the structural and functional characteristics of the TNF ligand and receptor superfamilies has been learned from analysis of TNF (TNFSF2), LTα (TNFSF1), FasL (TNFSF6), and their receptors. TNF and LTα are closely related homotrimeric proteins (32% identity). Human TNF is synthesized as a 233 amino acid glycoprotein. It contains a long (76 residue) amino-terminal sequence that anchors it to the cell membrane as a 25 kDa type II membrane protein. A secreted 17 kDa form of TNF is generated through the enzymatic cleavage of membrane-bound TNF by a metalloproteinase termed TNF-α-converting enzyme (TACE). Both soluble and membrane forms of TNF are thought to be noncovalent homotrimers held together by a trimerization domain in the secreted molecule. When bound, both forms of TNF are biologically active. They have different affinities for the two TNF receptors and thus may exhibit different biological properties (see below).

LTα differs from TNF in that it is synthesized as a secreted glycoprotein. Human LTα is synthesized as a 205 amino acid glycoprotein that in native form exists as a 25 kDa homotrimer. It can bind both TNF receptors with affinities comparable to those of TNF, and has similar biological effects. However, a membrane-bound form of LT has been identified that consists of a heterotrimeric complex containing one LTα subunit noncovalently linked to two molecules of an LTα-related type II membrane protein termed LTβ. The $LT\alpha_1\beta_2$ heterotrimer, also known as mLT, is not cleaved by TACE and is thought to exist exclusively as a membrane-bound complex. mLT does not bind either of the two TNF receptors, but rather exerts its effects on another member of the TNF receptor superfamily, the lymphotoxin β receptor (LTβR). TNF and the two LT subunits are encoded by closely linked single-copy genes situated in the class III major histocompatibility locus, at chromosome 6p21.3 in humans (Chapter 5).

The two receptors for TNF (and LTα) are type-I transmembrane glycoproteins. They are designated TNFR1 (also termed p60 in humans, p55 in mice, official designation TNFRSF1A) and TNFR2 (also known as p80 in humans, p75 in mice, TNFRSF1B). These receptors are characterized by cysteine-rich repeats of about 40 amino acids in their amino terminal extracellular domains. Each extracellular domain consists of three or four cysteine-rich regions containing four to six cysteines involved in intrachain disulfide bonds. The cytoplasmic domains of these receptors have no obvious similarity to any known kinase and are thought to lack intrinsic enzymatic activity. Signal transduction is therefore achieved by the recruitment and activation of adaptor proteins that recognize specific sequences in the cytoplasmic domains of these receptors. Recruitment of adaptor molecules activates a number of characteristic signaling pathways that can lead to a remarkably diverse set of cellular responses, including differentiation, activation, release of inflammatory mediators and apoptosis.

FAMILY MEMBERS AND THEIR ACTIONS

Tumor necrosis factor (TNF), lymphotoxin-α (LTα) and receptors

TNF is a major physiologic mediator of inflammation.[39] It initiates the response to Gram-negative bacteria that produce lipopolysaccharide (LPS). IFN-γ also induces TNF and augments its effects. TNF has been shown to induce fever, activate the coagulation system, induce hypoglycemia, depress cardiac contractility, reduce vascular resistance, induce cachexia and activate the acute-phase response in the liver. Thus, TNF is the major mediator of septic shock. TNF also upregulates MHC class I and class II expression, activates phagocytes, and induces mononuclear phagocytes to produce cytokines such as IL-1, IL-6, chemokines and TNF itself. Activation by TNF causes increased adhesion of cells to endothelium and can be cytotoxic, particularly to tumor cells. TNF-deficient mice are resistant to septic shock induced by high doses of LPS, but have increased susceptibility to bacterial infection. The dual role of TNF in controlling bacterial replication and in septic shock emphasizes the point that although the goal of immune response is to eliminate invading microorganisms, the response itself may be injurious to normal host tissues. Septic shock is an extreme example of this. Although the primary source of TNF is the mononuclear phagocyte, it is also produced by T cells, NK cells and mast cells. LTα shares many of the same biological effects as TNF, owing mainly to its ability to bind the same receptors. However, LTβR has been shown to play a unique role in the development of secondary lymph nodes.

Table 10.2 TNF superfamily ligands

Locus link ID	Symbol	Common name	Position	Aliases	Binds to receptor(s)	OMIM ID	Key Functions	Phenotype associated with over expression	Phenotype associated with deficiency	Human Genetic Diseases
4049	TNFSF1	Lymphotoxin alpha (Ltα)	6p21.3	LT, TNFB, TNFSF1	TNFR2 (1B), TNFR1 (1A), HVEM (14)	153440	Lymphoid organ formation		Absence of LN and PP, defective GC formation	
7124	TNFSF2	Tumor necrosis factor (TNF)	6p21.3	DIF, TNFA, TNFSF2, CACHECTIN	TNFR2 (1B), TNFR1 (1A)	191160	Inflammation	Wasting syndrome, arthritis	defective GC formation, resistance to endotoxic shock and experimental arthritis	TNF2 (G-308A) promotor polymorphism associated with increased susceptability to septic shock. asthma and RA severity
405C	TNFSF3	Lymphotoxin beta (LTβ)	6p21.3	p33, TNFC, TNFSF3	As a β2α1 heterotrimer with LTα binds to LTβ receptor (3)	600978	Lymphoid organ formation	Ectopic lymphoid organ formation		
7292	TNFSF4	OX40 Ligand	1q25	GP34, OX40L, TXGP1, CD134L, OX-40L	OX40 (4)	603594	CD4 T cell expansion, survival, and Th2 development	Increased Th2 responses	Th2 deficiency, blockade improves EAE	
959	TNFSF5	CD40 Ligand	Xq26	IGM, IMD3, TRAP, gp39, CD154, CD40L, HIGM1, T-BAM,	CD40 (5)	300386	Co-stimulation and differentiation of B cells and APC	Constitutive expression in B cells or keratinocytes leads to SLE-like syndrome	Immunodeficiency due to Defective Ig class switching and germinal center formation	X-linked hyper-IGM syndrome associated with CD40L loss of function mutations

Continued

Table 10.2 TNF superfamily ligands—Cont'd

Locus link ID	Symbol	Common name	Position	Aliases	Binds to receptor(s)	OMIM ID	Key Functions	Phenotype associated with over expression	Phenotype associated with deficiency	Human Genetic Diseases
356	TNFSF6	Fas Ligand	1q23	FASL, CD178, CD95L, APT1LG1	Fas (6), DcR3 (6B)	134638	Mediator of CD4(+) T cell apoptosis due to restimulation and apoptosis in other cell types		Lymphadenopathy and Systemic Autoimmunity	Autoimmune Lymphoproliferative Syndrome (ALPS) type Ib
970	TNFSF7	CD27 Ligand	19p13	CD70, CD27L, CD27LG	CD27 (7)	602840	T cell co-stimulation	T cell hyperactivation eventually leading to immunodeficiency (HIV-like)		
944	TNFSF8	CD30 Ligand	9q33	CD153, CD30L, CD30LG	CD30 (8)	603875				
8744	TNFSF9	4-1-BB Ligand	19p13.3	4-1BB-L	4-1BB (9)	606182	T cell co-stimulation			
8743	TNFSF10	(TNF-like apoptosis inducing ligand)TRAIL	3q26	TL2, APO2L, TRAIL, Apo-2L	DR4 (10A), DR5 (10B), DcR1 (10C), DcR2 (10D)	603598	Dendritic cell apoptosis, NK-cell mediated tumor cell killing		defective NK-mediated tumor eradication	
8600	TNFSF11	RANK-L	13q14	ODF, OPGL, sOdf, RANKL, TRANCE, hRANKL2	RANK (11A)	602642	Mediates osteoclast formation and bone remodeling. Stimulation of APC			

TNF RECEPTOR AND LIGAND SUPERFAMILIES

	Symbol	Name	Location	Aliases	Receptor	OMIM	Function	Phenotype	Knockout / Disease
8742	TNFSF12	TWEAK	17p13	APO3L, DR3LG, TWEAK, MGC20669	TWEAK-R (12A)	602695	Potential role in inflammation and lymphocyte function		
8741	TNFSF13	APRIL	17p13.1	APRIL, TALL2, TWE-PRIL	TACI (13B), BCMA (17)	604472	Promotes T-independent type-2 responses through interactions with TACI	overexpression in T cells produces prolonged T cell survival and enhanced TI-2 responses	
10673	TNFSF13B	BlyS, BAFF	13q32-34	BAFF, BLYS, TALL1, THANK, ZTNF4	TACI (3B), BAFF-R (13C), BCMA(17),	603969	Promotes B cell maturation, plasmablast survival	SLE-like systemic autoimmunity and arthritis	
8740	TNFSF14	LIGHT	19p13.3	LTg, TR2, HVEML, LIGHT	HVEM (14), LT-βR (3), DcR3 (6B)	604520	CD8 T cell and APC co-stimulation,	inflammation, T cell hyperactivation Th1 bias	defective CD8 T cell costimulation
9966	TNFSF15	TL1A	9q32	TL1, TL1A, VEGI	DR3 (25)	604052	Recently identified ligand for DR3 (TNFRSF25)		Blockade impairs TCell-mediated immunopathology
8995	TNFSF18	GITR Ligand	1q23	TL6, AITRL, GITRL, hGITRL	GITR (18)	603898	T cell co-stimulation (+)CD25(+) regulatory T cells		
1896	ED1	ectodermal dysplasia 1, anhidrotic (EDA1)	X	EDA, HED, EDA1, XHED, XLHED	EDAR	305100	Tooth, hair and sweat gland formation		X-LINKED ECTODERMAL DYSPLASIA

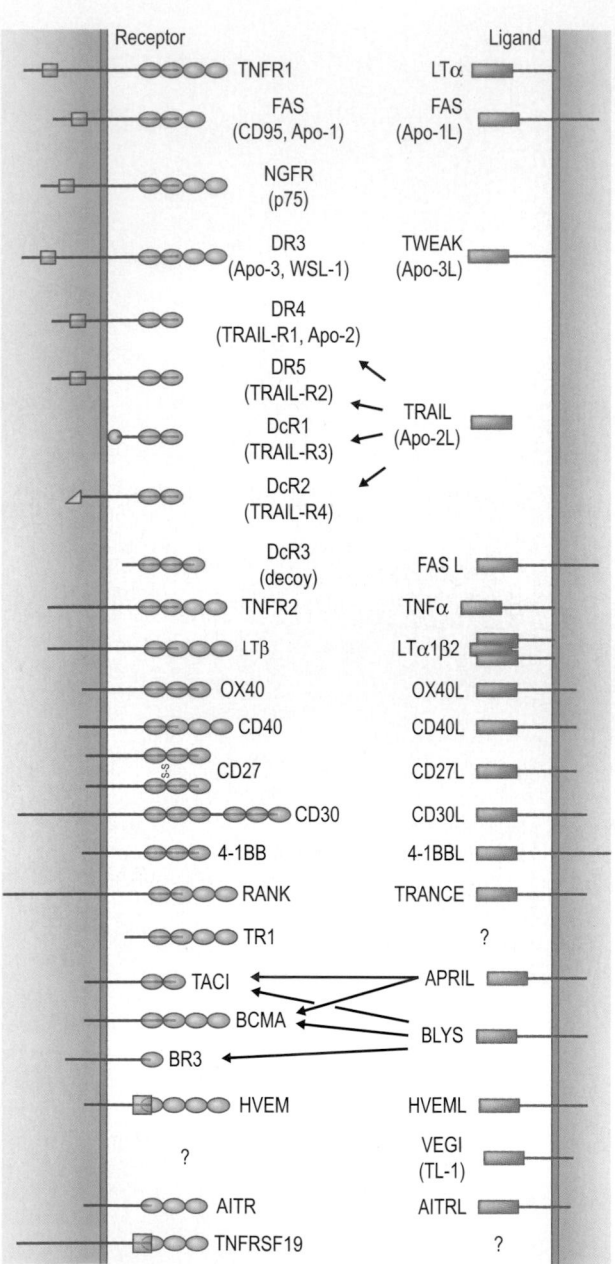

Fig. 10.4 Schematic representation of members of the TNF ligand and receptor superfamily.

T cells and NK cells. FAS-induced apoptosis is thought to play an essential role in the termination of T-cell responses, particularly in the peripheral immune system. FAS also plays a key role in the induction of cell death by cytotoxic T cells (CTLs) and natural killer (NK) cells, where it functions in conjunction with perforin.

CD40

CD40 is expressed by a variety of cell types, including B cells, dendritic cells, monocytes, macrophages and endothelial cells. It plays a major co-stimulatory role in B-cell differentiation and recombination, and promotes survival through the induction of BCL-2 family members. Studies of CD40-deficient mice reveal that its function is not restricted to the humoral immune response, and that CD40 signaling also plays a role in cell-mediated immunity. CD40 ligand (CD154) is a 39 kDa protein expressed by activated CD4 T cells that can bind to and activate CD40 by cell–cell contact.

Other members

Other members of the TNFR family play various roles in the development and function of the immune system. CD40, OX-40, CD27, CD30, and 4-1BB can mediate co-stimulation of T-cell activation, albeit through different mechanisms. CD154 on T cells triggers antigen-presenting cell (APC) activation, including upregulation of the CD28 ligands B7-1 and B7-2. This indirectly boosts co-stimulation of the T-cell response. OX-40, CD27, CD30, and 4-1BB more likely act as direct co-stimulators of T-cell activation. The TNF family ligand BAFF (BlyS/TALL1/TNFSF13B) has a special role in B-cell maturation and can bind three distinct receptors, TACI (TNFRSF13B), BADD-R (TNFRSF13C), and BCMA (TNFRSF17).

SIGNALING

The TNF receptor superfamily can be divided into three subfamilies on the basis of the types of intracellular signaling molecules recruited, e.g,. FADD, TRADD or TRAF [40] (Fig. 10.5). The cytoplasmic domains of several receptors, including TNFR1, FAS, DR3, DR4, and DR5, contain a conserved ~80 amino acid motif termed the death domain (DD). This element is required for recruitment of DD-containing adaptor molecules that are involved in the initiation of apoptotic cell death (see below). For this reason, these receptors have been termed 'death receptors.' The function of a number of death receptors may be regulated by decoy receptors, cell surface molecules that bind ligand, but lack functional intracellular domains. Other TNF receptor superfamily receptors that lack death domains (e.g., CD27, CD30, CD40, HVEM, TNFR2, LT-βR, OX-40, and 4-1BB) associate with different types of adapter molecules, most importantly members of the TRAF (TNFR-associated factor) family, as described below.

Death domains: TRADD and FADD

The primary molecule transducing signals in TNFR1 is TNF receptor-associated death domain (TRADD), which is directly recruited to TNFR1 after activation by TNF. The death domain mediates the interaction between TNFR1 and TRADD. This death domain motif is found in both adaptor molecules such as TRADD and the cytoplasmic domains

Fas ligand (FasL) and its receptor, Fas/APO-1/CD95

FAS (Apo-1/CD95/TNFRSF6) is a type I integral membrane protein that is structurally related to TNFR1. FAS is thought to trimerize and transduce proapoptotic signals upon binding of its ligand, FASL. Similar to TNF, the physiologic ligand for FAS (CD95L or FASL) is synthesized as a type II membrane protein and is expressed on activated B cells,

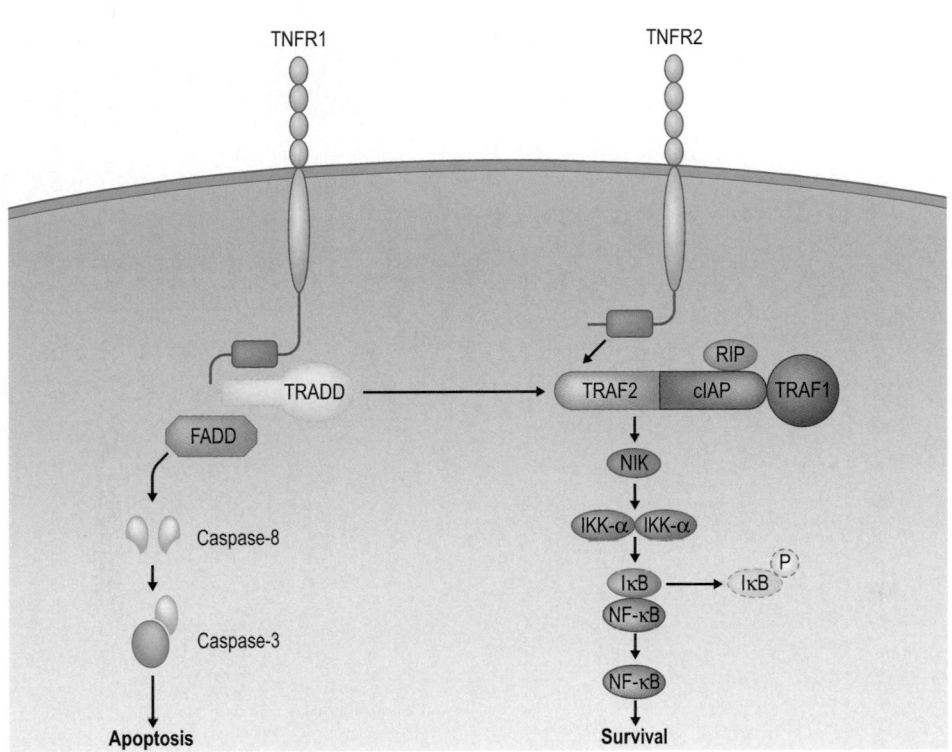

Fig. 10.5 The role of the death domain- and death effector domain-containing molecules in signaling by TNFR1 and TNFR2.

of the receptor itself (Fig. 10.5). The binding of TRADD to TNFR1 leads to the recruitment and activation of numerous associated signaling molecules. TNF-induced apoptosis is generally thought to be achieved by the interaction of TRADD with FADD (FAS-associated death domain; also known as MORT1), an ~27 kDa protein that oligomerizes with TRADD through the death domains contained in both molecules. In turn, recruitment of FADD coordinately activates several members of the caspase family.[41] Caspases are cysteine aspartate proteases that are originally synthesized as zymogens. They are typically converted to their activated form by proteolytic cleavage, often by a distinct caspase upstream in the proteolytic cascade. Caspase-8, which is generally considered to be the apical caspase in the TNF and FAS pathways, is recruited to FADD in the activated complex. It is thought to be activated by a self-cleavage reaction. Cleaved caspase-8 can subsequently activate downstream caspases, notably caspase-3, which play a more proximal role in apoptosis. In addition to FADD, TRADD also has a TRAF-binding motif that leads to the recruitment of TRAF1 and 2 and the subsequent TRAF-dependent activation of proinflammatory signaling mediated by activation of NF-κB and MAP-kinase pathways. Although cell death in tumor cells can be induced by TNF, the most common result of TNFR1 ligation in primary immune cells is inflammation and sometimes protection from TNF-induced apoptosis. Recent evidence suggests that activation of pro-apoptotic and proinflammatory signaling by TNFR1 is not simultaneous, but proceeds by sequential steps. Ligation of receptor by TNF at the plasma membrane leads to immediate recruitment of the TRAF proteins. This is followed by receptor internalization and dissociation of TRADD from the receptor, and then by a delayed recruitment of FADD and caspase-8 at later time points by TRADD .[42, 43]

Unlike TNFR1, FAS can directly recruit FADD to its cytoplasmic death domain, leading to the rapid formation of a death-inducing signaling complex (DISC), which contains FADD/MORT1 and caspase-8, thereby permitting activation of downstream caspases. The FADD death domain is recruited through interactions between charged residues in the death domains of FAS and FADD. Caspase-8 recruitment is accomplished through a structurally related domain termed the death-effector domain (DED). FADD DED contains two hydrophobic patches not present in the DD that are vital for binding to the death-effector domains in the prodomain of caspase-8 and for apoptotic activity.[44] Once bound to FADD, the proteolytic activity of caspase-8 is turned on, resulting in the cleavage of downstream substrates and the initiation of apoptotic events. How caspase-8 is maintained in a dormant state until ligation of the appropriate death receptor has been intensively studied. It has been found that oligomerization of caspase-8 is critical to activate its proteolytic activity.[45] FADD also has the ability to self-associate through separated domains in the DED. This self-association drives the formation of larger oligomers of FADD that are essential for pro-apoptotic activity.

The efficiency of apoptosis induction by death receptors is regulated at many levels. At the extracellular level, decoy receptors for FasL and TRAIL exist in the human genome. Unfortunately, their absence in mice has made it difficult to define their physiological role. The submembrane localization of FAS and TNFR1 can control signaling efficiency. The presence of receptors in lipid rafts appears to influence the efficiency of assembly of the primary signaling complex, enhancing NF-κB induction by TNFR1 and death induction by FAS.[43, 46] For FAS, the presence of receptors in lipid rafts also correlates with apoptosis that cannot be blocked by BCL-2, which has been termed 'type-I' signaling.

Table 10.3 TNF superfamily receptors (receptors in italics have a C-terminal death domain)

Locus Link ID	Symbol	Common name(s)	Position	Aliases	Binds to ligand(s)	OMIM ID	Key functions	Phenotype associated with deficiency	Human Genetic Diseases
7132	TNFRSF1A	Tumor necrosis factor receptor 1 (TNF-R1)	12p13.2	FPF, p55, p60, TBP1, TNF-R, TNFAR, TNFR1, p55-R, CD120a, TNFR55, TNFR60, TNF-R-I, TNF-R55, MGC19588	TNF-α (2), Ltα (1)	191190	Mediates TNF-induced inflammation (and apoptosis in some cells)	resistance to TNF-induced arthritis models, resistant to endotoxic shock, Increased sensitivity to bacterial pathogens	Periodic fever syndrome (TRAPS)associated with heterozygous extracellular mutaions
7133	TNFRSF1B	Tumor necrosis factor receptor 2 (TNF-R2)	1p36.3-p36.2	p75, TBPII, TNFBR, TNFR2, CD120b, TNFR80, TNF-R75, p75TNFR, TNF-R-II	TNF-α (2), Ltα (1)	191191	May enhance pro-apoptotic effect of TNFR1	still susceptible to TNF-induced arthritis models, defective CD8(+) T cell apoptosis after restimulation, Increased sensitivity to bacterial pathogens	
4055	TNFRSF3	Lymphotoxin β receptor	12p13	LTBR, CD18, TNFCR, TNFR-RP, TNFRSF3, TNFR2-RP, LT-BETA-R, TNF-R-III	LIGHT (14), LTβ (3)	600979	lymphoid organ formation	No LN, PP, defective GC formation	
7293	TNFRSF4	OX40	1p36	OX40, ACT35, CD134, TXGP1L	OX40L (4)	600315	T cell costimulation	Defective CD4 T cell responses	
958	TNFRSF5	CD40	20q12-q13.2	p50, Bp50, CD40, CDW40, MGC9013	CD40L (5)	109535	Costimulation and differentiation of B cells and APC	Defective Ig class switching and germinal center formation	Autosomal hyper-IgM syndrome associated with loss-of function mutations

355	TNFRSF6	Fas, CD95	10q24.1	FAS, APT1, CD95, APO-1	FasL (6)	134637	Apoptosis of restimulated CD4 T cells, B cells, ?others	Defective apoptosis of restimulated CD4(+) T cells	Autoimmune Lymphoproliferative Syndrome (ALPS) associated with heterozygous dominat-interfering mutations
8771	TNFRSF6B	Decoy receptor 3	20q13.3	M68, TR6, DCR3, DJ583P15.1.1	FasL (6), TL1A (15), LIGHT (14)	603361	Soluble decoy receptor for FasL, LIGHT, and TL1A. May have a role in tumor immune evason		
939	TNFRSF7	CD27	12p13	T14, CD27, S152, Tp55, MGC20393	CD27L (7)	186711	T cell co-stimulation	Defective T cell responses	
943	TNFRSF8	CD30	1p36	CD30, KI-1, D1S166E	CD30L (8)	153243	?Inhibition of CD8 T-cell effector function		
3604	TNFRSF9	4-1BB, CD137	1p36	ILA, 4-1BB, CD137 CDw137, MGC2172	4-1BBL (9;	602250	T cel co-stimulation	Defective CD8 T cell responses	
8797	TNFRSF10A	Death Receptor 4 (DR4)	8p21	DR4, APO2, MGC9365, TRAILR1, TRAILR-1	TRAIL (10)	603611	Mediator of dendritic cell and tumor cell apoptosis		
8795	TNFRFRSF10B	Death Receptor 5 (DR5)	8p22-p21	DR5, KILLER, TRICK2, TRICKB, ZTNFR9, TRAILR2, TRICK2A, TRICK2B, TRAIL-R2, KILLER/ DR5	TRAIL (10)	603612	Mediator of dendritic cell and tumor cell apoptosis		
8794	TNFRSF10C	Decoy receptor 1	8p22-p21	LIT, DCR1, TRID, TRAILR3	TRAIL (10)	603613	GPI-linked decoy receptor, interferes with TRAIL function		

Continued

TNF RECEPTOR AND LIGAND SUPERFAMILIES

Table 10.3 TNF superfamily receptors (receptors in italics have a C-terminal death domain)—Cont'd

Locus Link ID	Symbol	Common name(s)	Position	Aliases	Binds to ligand(s)	OMIM ID	Key functions	Phenotype associated with deficiency	Human Genetic Diseases
8793	TNFRSF10D	Decoy receptor 2	8p21	DCR2, TRUNDD, TRAILR4	TRAIL (10)	603614	Transmembrane decoy receptor, interferes with TRAIL function		
8792	TNFRSF11A	(Receptor activator of NF-κB) RANK	18q22.1	OFE, ODFR, PDB2, RANK, TRANCER	RANKL (11)	603499	Mediates DC co-stimulation and osteoclast maturation and activation	Osteopetrosis due to osteoclast deficiency, no lymph nodes, impaired B cell development	
4982	TNFRSF11B	Osteoprotegerin (OPG)	8q24	CPG, TR1, OCIF, MGC29565	TRAIL (10), RANKL (11)	602643	Soluble decoy receptor for RANK	osteoporosis, arterial calcification	
51330	TNFRSF12A	TWEAK-receptor	16p13.3	FN14, TWEAKR	TWEAK (12)	605914			
8791	TNFRSF12L	tumor necrosis factor receptor superfamily, member 12-like	1p36.2	DR3-Like				T-cell hyperactivation, increased susceptibility to restimulation-induced apoptosis	
23495	TNFRSF13B	TACI	17p11.2	TACI	APRIL (13), BAFF (13B)	604907	May inhibit some of the pro-survival effects of BAFF-R	Decreased TI-2 B cell responses, but B cell hyperplasia and autoimmunity	

Continued

Gene ID	Symbol	Name	Location	Other names	Ligand	OMIM	Function	Knockout phenotype
115650	TNFRSF13C	BAFF receptor (BAFF-R)	22q13.1-q13.31	BAFF/BLyS receptor 3	BAFF (13B)	606269		Impaired survival of immature transitional B cells
8764	TNFRSF14	Herpes virus entry mediator (HVEM)	1p36.3-p36.2	TR2, ATAR, HVEA, HVEM, LIGHTR	LIGHT (14), herpes viruses	602746		
4804	TNFRSF16	NGF-R	17q21-q22	TNFRSF16, p75(NTR)	NGF (not a TNF family member)	162010	NGF receptor - evolutionary outlier as NGF not classic TNF family molecule	Defective sensory neuron innervation; impaired heat sensitivity
608	TNFRSF17	B-cell maturation antigen (BCMA)	16p13.1	BCM	APRIL (13), BAFF (13B)	109545		Apparently no B cell phenotype
8784	TNFRSF18	Glucocorticoid-induced TNF receptor (GITR)	1p36.3	AITR, GITR, GITR-D	GITRL (18)	603905	T-cell co-stimulation, marker for CD4(+)CD25(+) Treg cells, modulates Treg function	T cell hyperactivation
55504	TNFRSF19	Toxicity and JNK inducer (TAJ)	13q12.11-q12.3	TROY, TRADE, TAJ-alpha		606122	Similar to EDAR, expressed in skin and brain	
84957	TNFRSF19L	RELT	11q13.3	RELT, FLJ14993			Possible T cell co-stimulator	
27242	TNFRSF21	*Death Receptor 6 (DR6)*	6p21.1-12.2	DR6, BM-018		605732	Negative regulator B- and T-cell responses	Enhanced T and B-cell activation
94098	TNFRSF22	Tumor necrosis factor receptor superfamily, member 22	11p15.5	SOBa, Tnfrh2, 2810023K06Rik				

Table 10.3 TNF superfamily receptors (receptors in italics have a C-terminal death domain)—Cont'd

Locus Link ID	Symbol	Common name(s)	Position	Aliases	Binds to ligand(s)	OMIM ID	Key functions	Phenotype associated with deficiency	Human Genetic Diseases
94099	TNFRSF23	Tumor necrosis factor receptor superfamily, member 23	11p15.5	mSOB, Tnfrh1					
8718	*TNFRSF25*	*Death Receptor 3 (DR3)*	*1p36.2*	*DR3, TR3, DDR3, LARD, APO-3, TRAMF, WSL-1, WSL-LR, TNFRSF12*	*TL1A (15)*	*603366*		*?impaired thymic negative selection*	
10913	*EDAR*	*Ectodysplasin 1, anhidrotic receptor*	2q11-q13	DL, ED3, ED5, ED1R, EDA3, EDA-A1R	E1	604095	Tooth, hair, sweat gland formation	abnormal tooth, hair, and sweat gland formation	Ectodermal Dysplasia
60401	XEDAR	XEDAR: ectodysplasin A2 isoform receptor	Xq12	EDAA2R, EDA-A2R	EDA-A2	300276			

Locuslink ID: Gene 'homepage' curated by NCBI. Go To and type the locuslink ID in the search window.
OMIM: ID in the Online Mendelian Inheritance in Man Database. Go to and type in the OMIM ID in the search window.
LN, lymph node; PP, Peyer's patch; GC, germinal center.

The recruitment and activation of caspase-8 may be another important regulatory step in FAS signaling. A cellular inhibitory protein, c-FLIP (CFLAR/FLAME/I-Flice, Usurpin/Casper/CASH). shares homology with caspase-8 but contains a functionally inactive caspase domain. c-FLIP can be recruited to the FAS signaling complex, blocking activation of caspase-8 when overexpressed. Overexpression of c-FLIP blocks B-cell apoptosis *in vivo* and leads to autoantibody production. However, endogenous levels of c-FLIP do not readily correlate with sensitivity to FAS-induced apoptosis, so the physiological role of this protein awaits mouse knockout studies. Additional molecules associating with FAS have been identified such as DAXX and FAP-1, but are not clearly present in the physiological DISC.

TRAFs

The cytoplasmic domains of many receptors in the TNFR superfamily, including TNFR2, CD30, and CD40, do not contain death domains. Instead, the cytoplasmic domains contain short peptide consensus sequences that enable recruitment of TRAF proteins, which are a different family of adaptor proteins. A separate consensus sequence has been identified for TRAF6 versus other TRAF proteins, and other mechanisms probably operate to maintain the specificity of TRAF recruitment. Structural studies have revealed a mushroom-like structure for the TRAF proteins, with a trimer of the three TRAF subunits stabilized by a stalk-like coiled-coil domain.

TRAF proteins activate NF-κB and MAP-kinase pathways through recruitment and activation of protein complexes that activate these signaling cascades. The exact mechanisms by which this occurs are not yet clear, but recent studies have called attention to the ability of TRAF proteins to catalyze ubiquitination of target signaling complexes, which can function as an activating step. TRAF6, which mediates NF-κB activation by a number of TNF-family receptors, associates with a protein complex that mediates K63-linked ubiquitination and activation of the inhibitor of κB kinase (IKK) complex, which consists of two catalytic subunits, IKKα and IKKβ and a regulatory protein IKKγ or NEMO.[47] Rather than causing degradation of IKK, K-63 linked ubiquitination activates kinase activity, leading to phosphorylation and degradation of IκB (inhibitor of NF-κB) and the release of active NF-κB subunits. Active NF-κB subunits translocate to the nucleus, where they regulate the expression of a wide variety of genes involved in the inflammatory response.

Some TNF-family receptors use other mechanisms to activate NF-κB. For example, LTβ receptor activates the IKK complex via the serine–threonine kinase NIK, which was initially identified through its ability to associate with TRAF2. A naturally occurring mouse mutation termed alymphoplasia (*aly*) is the result of a point mutation of NIK. *Aly/aly* mice lack lymph nodes and Peyer's patches, and also exhibit disorganized splenic and thymic structures. This mutation, and the phenotype of LTβR knockout mice, revealed the critical role of this receptor in normal lymph node development and the formation of 'tertiary' lymphoid tissue in inflammation.

When a single TNF-family ligand, such as TNF, binds both a death receptor (TNFR1) and a nondeath receptor (TNFR2), a number of mechanisms regulate receptor signaling and the cellular outcome. Rather than functioning in cell death, the physiological function of TNFR2 may be as a co-stimulator of lymphocyte proliferation.[48] This appears to be mediated by the direct interaction of TRAF2 with the cytoplasmic tail of

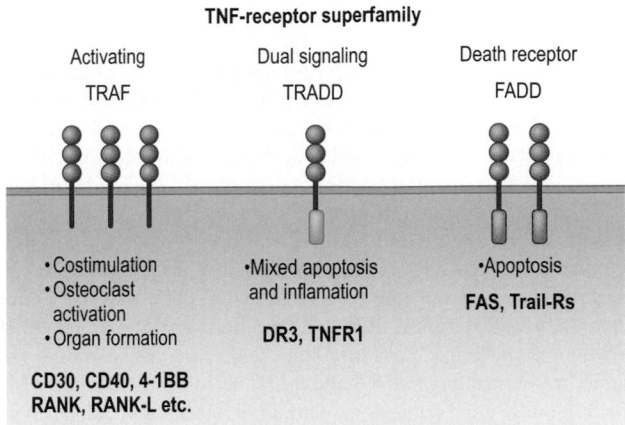

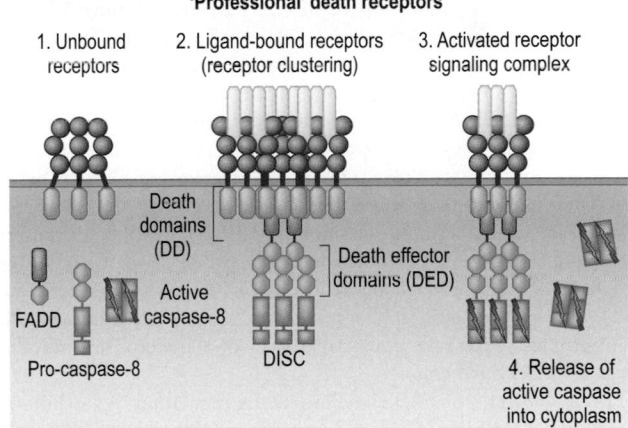

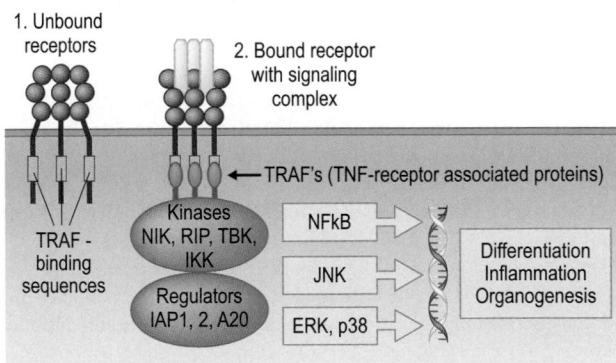

Fig. 10.6 Signaling by TNFRs

TNFR2, which leads to the activation of NF-κB and other signaling pathways (Fig. 10.6). Under some circumstances, TNFR2 can enhance apoptosis induced by TNF. This may occur through cross-talk that enhances apoptotic signaling through TNFR1, most likely by decreasing the availability of TRAF2 to bind TNFR1.

CLINICAL RELEVANCE

Many studies have implicated TNF in the pathogenesis of the chronic inflammatory diseases rheumatoid arthritis (RA) and Crohn's disease (CD). Levels of TNF are highly elevated in the synovial fluid and the serum of patients with RA, as well as in the mucosa of patients with CD. This suggests that the proinflammatory effects of TNF might underpin the severe inflammatory symptoms observed in these diseases. Of particular relevance to RA, TNF inhibits the synthesis of proteoglycan and bone formation and stimulates resorption of proteoglycan and bone. In addition, TNF-overexpressing transgenic mice develop chronic inflammatory polyarthritic disease. These findings have prompted the development of specific TNF inhibitors, which are demonstrating great promise in the treatment of RA and CD. The two best-characterized of these inhibitors are a monoclonal anti-TNF antibodies (infliximab and adalimumab) and chimeric TNFR2-Fc proteins (etanercept and lenercept). Clinical studies of these compounds have demonstrated that they can induce striking improvement in RA patients (Chapter 52). Side effects of TNF-antagonism include increased incidence of infection, particularly with *Mycobacterium tuberculosis*, and an increase incidence of cancer.[49]

Mutations of *TNFR1* are associated with autosomal dominant periodic fever syndromes[50] (Chapter 61). These patients have missense mutations in exons encoding the extracellular regions of *TNFR1* that are thought to affect normal *TNFR1* function, prompting the designation *TNFR1*-associated periodic syndromes, or TRAPS. Although the precise role of *TNFR1* has yet to be elucidated, patients with TRAPS typically have low serum levels of soluble TNF receptors that might normally serve to neutralize and control serum TNF levels. Clinical studies are in progress to test the potential efficacy of etanercept in controlling fevers in TRAPS patients.

The *in vivo* role of FAS signaling in the regulation of the immune system was confirmed when the naturally arising *lpr* and *gld* mouse strains were found to harbor homozygous mutations of Fas and Fas ligand, respectively. Both of these mouse strains are characterized by lymphadenopathy and splenomegaly due to the accumulation of unusual CD4$^-$CD8$^-$ T cells, as well as the production of autoantibodies. Subsequently, humans with heterozygous mutations in the FAS receptor were identified with similar symptoms and autoantibodies.[51] In this disease, the autoimmune lymphoproliferative syndrome or ALPS, the FAS mutations act as dominant negative inhibitors of intracellular signaling, causing defective apoptosis in all carriers of FAS mutations and overt disease in a variable percentage of family members (Chapters 14 and 35).

The gene encoding CD40 ligand is defective in X-linked hyper IgM syndrome (X-HIM), a rare inherited disorder in which affected male children generate only IgM antibodies, many of which are autoantibodies (Chapter 34). Patients with X-HIM frequently suffer opportunistic infections, usually bacterial, and have an increased susceptibility to cancer. The physiologic role of the BAFF receptor in mouse B-cell development is illustrated by BAFF-R mutations in the A/WySnJ mouse, which lacks peripheral B cells. TACI knockout mice have hyperactive B cells, but in humans, dominant negative TACI mutations have been found in patients with common variable immunodeficiency affecting B-cell numbers and function, arguing that in humans TACI serves as a positive modulator of B cells.[52, 53] Mutations of BLYS have also been found in humans with common variable immunodeficiency.[54, 55]

■ INTERLEUKIN-1/TOLL-LIKE RECEPTOR FAMILY ■

LIGAND AND RECEPTOR STRUCTURE

The IL-1/Toll-like family of receptors comprises at least 11 members, including the IL-1RI, IL-1RII, IL-1R-associated protein (IL-1RAcP), IL-18R, IL-18RAcP, IL-1Rrp2, IL-1RAPL, IL-33R(T1/ST2), TIGGIR, SIGGIR and the mammalian Toll-like receptors (TLR1–10).[56, 57] The ligands for these receptors include IL-1, IL-18 and IL-1F5–10, IL-33 (IL-1F11).[58]

FAMILY MEMBERS AND THEIR ACTIONS

Interleukin-1

There are two cell surface receptors for IL-1, type I (IL-1RI) and type II (IL-1RII). Both of these bind ligand (Fig. 10.4), but only IL-1RI transduces signals. The extracellular domain of IL-1RI has three immunoglobulin-like domains and a 200 amino acid cytoplasmic domain. Upon ligand binding IL-1RI associates with IL-1R accessory protein (IL-1RAcP), which is critical for the initiation of signaling. The IL-1RII cytoplasmic domain is extremely short and has been suggested to be a 'decoy' receptor, competing with IL-1RI for ligand binding and attenuating signaling. Both IL-1Rs are susceptible to proteolytic cleavage near the membrane surface. Therefore, they can be found as soluble proteins, functioning as another mechanism to 'buffer' IL-1 signaling. These soluble receptors are readily detectable in the circulation. Additionally, IL-1R associates with a second subunit, termed the IL-1R associated protein (IL-1Rap).

There are three members of the IL-1 gene family: two agonists, IL-1α and IL-1β, and one antagonist, IL-1 receptor antagonist (IL-1Ra). IL-1α and IL-1β are structurally similar and have similar actions, but they are regulated differently. IL-1β is regulated at the level of stabilization of the mRNA and at the level of translation. Both IL-1α and IL-1β are synthesized as precursor proteins. The pro-form of IL-1α has biological activity, whereas that of IL-1β does not. Pro-IL-1β remains in the cytoplasm until it is cleaved by caspase-1, otherwise known as IL-1β-converting enzyme (ICE). It is then transported out of the cell. IL-1α is thought to be processed by a calpain-like converting enzyme.

Principal functions of IL-1 include the induction of acute-phase protein synthesis, cachexia and fever. In fact, it was the first endogenous pyrogen to be identified. It induces the production of IL-6 and chemikines, promotes hematopoiesis, stimulates adhesion of vascular leukocytes to endothelium, and has procoagulant effects. Unlike TNF, however, it does not induce cell death. The major source of IL-1 is mononuclear phagocytes, but other cells also produce it. IL-1RI$^{-/-}$ and IL-1β$^{-/-}$ mice have blunted fever responses to some (but not all) stimuli. This indicates that despite the impressive actions of IL-1, it evidently is redundant to some extent in febrile responses.

Interleukin-18

IL-18R was first designated IL-1Rrp (IL-1R related protein) before being recognized as the receptor for IL-18. Mice lacking IL-18R fail to bind or respond to IL-18. The receptor is expressed predominantly on T cells, B cells and NK cells. It associates with an accessory protein, IL-18RAcP. A major action of IL-18 is the induction of IFN-γ, a function it typically performs synergistically with IL-12. Indeed, the ability to induce IFN-γ was the basis of its original discovery. Accordingly, IL-18-null mice have deficiencies in IFN-γ production, NK cell activity and Th1 responses. IL-18 can also induce IL-4 and IL-13 production, indicating a somewhat broader range of action. IL-18-binding protein interacts with IL-18 and prevents association with IL-18R.

Other IL-1 family members

IL-33 (IL-1F11) signals via the IL-1 receptor-related protein ST2, also known as IL-33R, and induces Th2-associated cytokines, including IL-4 and IL-5.[57] SIGIRR is a negative regulator of Toll-like receptor–IL-1 receptor signaling.[59] Other IL-1R family members have not been well studied.

SIGNALING

Ligand binding to IL-1R, IL-18R, and TLRs results in NF-κB activation (Fig. 10.7). These receptors all associate with the adapter protein MyD88. Notably, MyD88 has a C-terminal TIR domain and an N-terminal death domain. MyD88 allows the recruitment of IL-1 receptor-associated kinase (IRAK), which also has an N-terminal death domain. IRAK, in turn, permits the recruitment and activation of a member of the TNF receptor-associated factor (TRAF) family, TRAF6. This leads to the activation of the serine kinases TAB2, TAK1 and inhibitor of κB kinases, IKKα and IKKβ. With IKKγ or NEMO, these kinases phophosphorylate IκB, which leads to its degradation within proteosomes, freeing bound NF-κB for nuclear translocation. Mice deficient in MyD88, IRAK, and TRAF6 have diminished responses to IL-1R/TLR family ligands. Other adapter molecules, including Mal and TRIF, are involved in TLR signaling.

CLINICAL RELEVANCE

Because of the importance of IL-1 in the pathogenesis of fever, it would be expected that agents that inhibit IL-1 would be therapeutically useful. Indeed, IL-1Ra, the naturally produced antagonist, has been studied in a variety of settings. It has been found to be efficacious in the treatment of rheumatoid arthritis. The drug anakinra is also effective in other autoinflammatory disorders, including Muckle–Wells disease, neonatal multisystem inflammatory disease, and Still's disease.[60, 61]

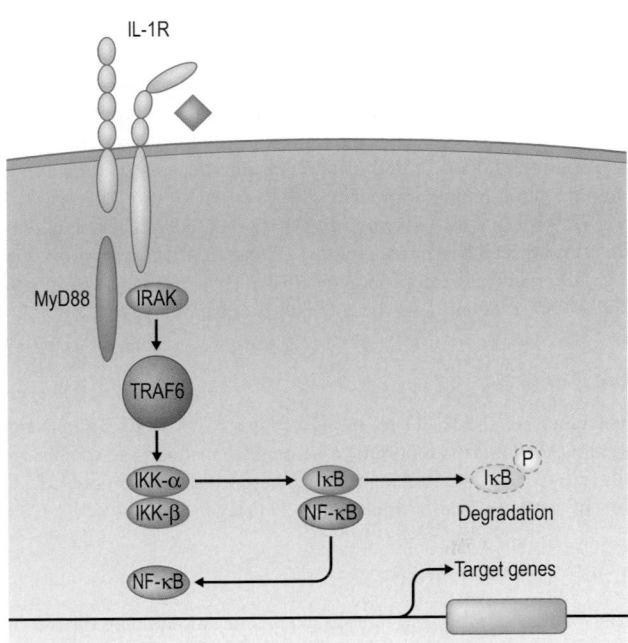

Fig. 10.7 Mechanism of signal transduction by IL-1R and related receptors.

INTERLEUKIN-17 RECEPTORS

Although their precise functions are incompletely understood, IL-17 and related cytokines are major inducers of inflammation and serve to recruit inflammatory cells.

LIGAND AND RECEPTOR STRUCTURE

The IL-17 receptor family is incompletely understood, but comprises at least five receptors, IL-17AR and IL-17BR (IL-17RH1), IL-17RL (receptor like), IL-17RD and IL-17RE, which are ubiquitously expressed.[24, 62] These receptors have a single transmembrane domain and exceptionally large cytoplasmic tails. The ligands in the IL-17 family include IL-17A-F, but the precise interactions between ligands and receptors have not been defined. A viral IL-17 homolog, designated HVS-13, is present in the herpes virus saimiri genome. Structurally, this family of cytokines forms cystine knots. In this respect, these cytokines are related to other, better-known cytokines such as nerve growth factor. IL-17 (IL-17A) is located on human chromosome 6 (mouse chromosome 1) and is produced by activated CD4 and γδ T cells. Recent findings have suggested that CD4 T cells that preferentially produce IL-17 (Th17 cells) represent a distinct lineage of effector Th cells.[63]

IL-17F is located adjacent to IL-17. Although it seems to be regulated in a similar manner, it may be more widely expressed than IL-17. Less well studied are IL-17B, IL-17C and IL-17D. All of these are thought to be expressed in a variety of nonhematopoietic tissues, although IL-17D is reported to be produced by CD4 T cells.

With respect to their biological actions, IL-17A and IL-17F are most intensively studied. These cytokines evoke inflammation largely by inducing the production of chemokines, G-CSF, and GM-CSF, with the subsequent recruitment of polymorphonuclear leukocytes. IL-17 also induces production of matrix metalloproteinase by epithelial cells, which may be an important aspect of the proinflammatory effects. IL-17 family cytokines appear to be important in host defense against *Klebsiella pneumoniae* and *Mycobacterium tuberculosis*. Abundant data also point to pathogenic roles of IL-17A in models of immune-mediated disease and in human autoimmune disorders.

IL-17E, which is also known as IL-25, is produced by Th2 cells and mast cells. It evokes an inflammatory response characterized by overproduction of Th2 cytokines, mucus production, epithelial cell hyperplasia, and eosinophilia. This cytokine is essential for the elimination of helminthic parasites.[64, 65]

SIGNALING

Engagement of the IL-17 receptor activates MAP kinases and NF-κB. Signaling via IL-25 is reported to be dependent upon the adapter molecule TRAF6. IL-17 acts synergistically with TNF.[66] The IL-17R associates with an adapter molecule called Act.

CLINICAL RELEVANCE

Many human diseases and animal models of autoimmune disease have been associated with increased levels of IL-17. The inflammatory effects of IL-23 and IL-17 also appear to be associated with malignant transformation.[67] Because of this, targeting IL-17 ligands and receptors could be a useful strategy.

■ RECEPTOR TYROSINE KINASES ■

LIGAND AND RECEPTOR STRUCTURE

Many growth factors, such as insulin and epidermal growth factor, utilize receptor tyrosine kinases (RTKs). Although most of these factors are not typically classified as cytokines, some are. These include CSF-1 (colony-stimulating factor-1 or M-CSF), stem cell factor (SCF, c-KIT ligand, or steel factor), platelet-derived growth factor (PDGF), and FLT3 ligand (FMS-like tyrosine kinase 3 ligand, FLT3-L). All of these have important hematological effects and tend to be included in discussions of cytokines. The structure of SCF and CSF-1 is similar to that of the cytokines that bind type I receptors, as they too form four α-helical bundles, even though their receptors are entirely distinct. The similarities in the three-dimensional structure points to a common evolutionary ancestor. It is therefore reasonable to define these factors as cytokines. The receptors in this subfamily typically have five immunoglobulin-like loops in their ligand-binding extracellular domains. The cytoplasmic domain contains a tyrosine kinase catalytic domain interrupted by an 'insert region' that does not share homology with other tyrosine kinases. This segment is used to recruit various signaling molecules.

FAMILY MEMBERS AND THEIR ACTIONS

Bone marrow stromal cells can synthesize stem cell factor (SCF, c-KIT ligand, or Steel factor) as either a secreted or a transmembrane protein. SCF is required to make stem cells responsive to other CSFs. SCF is widely expressed during embryogenesis and is also detectable in the circulation of normal adults. It has effects on germ cells, melanocytes, and

hematopoietic precursors, as well as important effects on the differentiation of mast cells. Naturally occurring mouse mutations of SCF (Steel) or its receptor (W) have been recognized for many years. These mice have defects in hematopoiesis and fertility, lack mast cells, and have absent coat pigmentation.

CSF-1, also known as monocyte–macrophage-CSF or macrophage-CSF (M-CSF), is a hematopoietic growth factor that supports the survival and differentiation of monocytic cells. It is produced by a wide variety of cells, including monocytes, smooth muscle cells, endothelial cells, and fibroblasts. M-CSF deficient mice manifest monocytopenia and osteopetrosis. IL-34 is a new cytokine that binds to the CSF-1 receptor. FLT3-L synergizes with other cytokines, including SCF, in inducing proliferation of hematopoietic precursors. FLT3-L is also an important regulator of dendritic cells.

SIGNALING

The first step in signaling by the RTKs is ligand-induced receptor dimerization (Fig. 10.8). Dimerization brings the two kinase domains into proximity and results in the activation of phosphotransferase activity. This leads to autophosphorylation of the receptor subunits on the tyrosine residues, which are then bound by a variety of signaling molecules, initiating signal transduction.[68] During this important step the signaling and adapter molecules recognize phosphotyrosine residues on the RTKs by virtue of either their SH2 (src homology 2) domains or their phosphotyrosine binding (PTB) domains.

A major pathway activated by RTKs is the RAS/RAF/ERK pathway. RAS is a small G protein with intrinsic low GDP/GTP exchange activity. In RTK signal transduction, two adapter proteins, GRB2 and SHC,

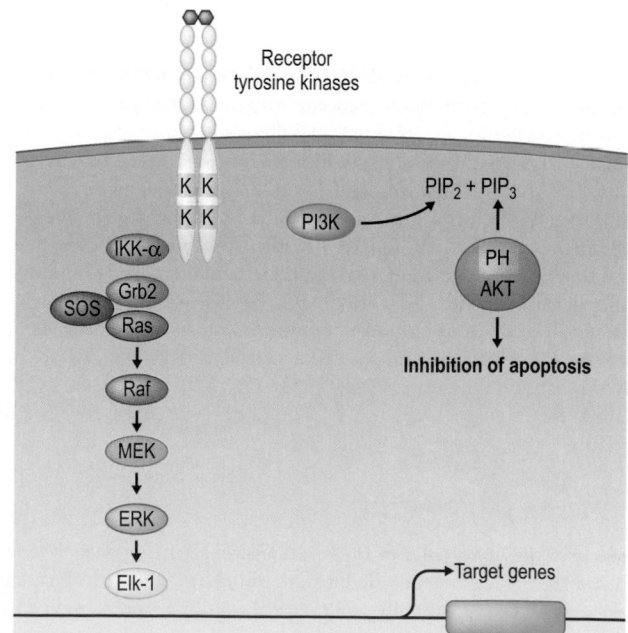

Fig. 10.8 Mechanism of signal transduction by receptor tyrosine kinases.

have important functions in RAS activation. In some cases, GRB2 binds directly to phosphotyrosine residues on the cytoplasmic tail of the receptor via its SH2 domain. Alternatively, SHC can bind first and then recruit GRB2. In addition to an SH2 domain, GRB2 has two SH3 domains that bind proline-rich segments of the guanine nucleotide exchange factor son of sevenless protein (SOS), recruiting it to the membrane and allowing it to activate RAS. Activated RAS binds and activates the serine/threonine kinase RAF, which in turn phosphorylates the dual-specificity kinase MEK. Activated MEK phosphorylates and activates ERK (extracellular signal-regulated kinase), which then translocates to the nucleus, where it phosphorylates and modulates the activity of various transcription factors, including ELK-1. Accordingly, mutations of RAS that lead to the constitutive activation of the ERK pathway have been found in a wide variety of human cancers.

Another important pathway activated by RTKs is the phosphatidylinositol 3′-OH kinase (PI3-kinase) pathway.[69] PI3-kinase catalyzes the formation of phosphatidylinositol-3,4,5-trisphosphate (PtdIns(3,4,5)P$_3$) and PtdIns(3,4)P$_2$. These phospholipids are recognized by proteins with pleckstrin homology (PH) domains. One such protein is protein kinase B (PKB or AKT), which has been implicated in the regulation of apoptosis. The PI3-kinase pathway is inhibited by the lipid phosphatase PTEN, which dephosphorylates PI3-kinase-generated phosphatidylinositides. Deletion of PTEN has been found in numerous tumor types, demonstrating a role for this protein as a tumor suppressor.

Gain-of-function mutations of c-*kit* result in a disorder termed systemic mastocytosis. Mutations resulting in a fusion between the *PDGFRA* and *FIP1L1* genes underlie hypereosinophilic syndrome.[70, 71]

TRANSFORMING GROWTH FACTOR-β LIGAND AND RECEPTOR FAMILIES

The transforming growth factor-βs (TGF-β) are a family of over 40 cytokines that inhibit cellular proliferation and can induce apoptosis of a variety of cell types. TGF-βs are involved in a number of biological processes, including tissue remodeling, wound repair, development, and hematopoiesis. Mutations of the elements in this pathway also contribute to malignant transformation. The mammalian ligands that belong to this family include TGF-β$_1$, -β$_2$, and -β$_3$, bone morphogenic proteins (BMPs), activins, inhibins, and müllerian-inhibiting substance. Despite

the name, TGF-βs inhibit the growth of many other cells, and, in combination with other cytokines and growth factors, may induce growth instead. TGF-βs also induce collagen and fibronectin production by fibroblasts, which is thought to be responsible, at least in part, for diseases characterized by fibrosis (e.g., systemic sclerosis and pulmonary fibrosis). Functionally, TGF-β inhibits many aspects of lymphocyte function, including T-cell proliferation and CTL maturation. Transgenic mouse studies have been performed using dominant negative forms of the TGF-β receptor. These mice exhibit massive expansion of lymphoid organs and develop T-cell lymphoproliferative disorders, suggesting a critical role for TGF-β in T-cell homeostasis.[32]

LIGAND AND RECEPTOR STRUCTURE

The TGF-βs are expressed as biologically inactive disulphide-linked dimers, which are cleaved to form active dimers. On translocation into the endoplasmic reticulum the N-terminal leader peptide is cleaved, and the mature protein is subsequently generated by a second cleavage event that releases an N-terminal pro-region. The pro-region can remain associated with the biologically active C-terminal region, inhibiting its activity.

The biological effects of the TGF-βs and their related ligands are mediated by two classes of receptor, designated type I (RI) and type II (RII).[72] A third group of receptors, denoted type III, also exists (e.g., TGF-βRIII in the case of TGF-β). This latter group does not actively participate in signal transduction, but is thought to function to present ligands to the functional receptors. Similar to the RTKs described previously, the cytoplasmic domains of TGF-β receptors possess intrinsic kinase activity. However, TGF-βRI and TGF-βRII encode serine/threonine kinases. The signaling cascade appears to be initiated by the binding of TGF-β to the type II receptor, inducing the assembly of a ternary complex containing TGF-β, TGF-βRII, and TGF-βRI.

FAMILY MEMBERS AND THEIR ACTIONS

The three known human TGF-βs – TGF-β$_1$, TGF-β$_2$, and TGF-β$_3$ – all have expressed molecular weights of 25 kDa. These three isoforms of TGF-β are closely related and have very similar biological functions. In humans the genes encoding TGF-β$_{1, 2}$ and $_3$ are located at 19q13, 1q41 and 14q24, respectively. TGF-β$_1$ is the most abundant form, and is the only isoform found in platelets. T cells and monocytes mainly synthesize TGF-β$_1$, a critical function of which is to antagonize lymphocyte responses.

Approximately half of TGF-β$_1^{-/-}$ mice survive until birth, and 3–4 weeks later they typically succumb to an overwhelming autoimmune state characterized by lymphoid and mononuclear infiltration of the heart, lung, and other tissues, and by autoantibody production. These studies, along with selective inhibition of TGF-β function in T cells, indicate that TGF-β plays a crucial role in T-cell homeostasis and the prevention of spontaneous T-cell differentiation. TGF-β$_1$ clearly has very complex actions, however: it induces FoxP3, promotes adaptive Treg cell differentiation, and inhibits IFN-γ production. Conversely, TGF-β$_1$ with IL-6 induces IL-17, a proinflammatory cytokine. Thus, TGF-β$_1$ has both proinflammatory and anti-inflammatory activities.

TGF-β$_2$ is the most abundant TGF-β isoform in body fluids, whereas TGF-β$_3$ is the least abundant of the three. TGF-β$_2$ and TGF-β$_3$ null mice exhibit defects distinct from those observed in TGF-β$_1$ knockouts,

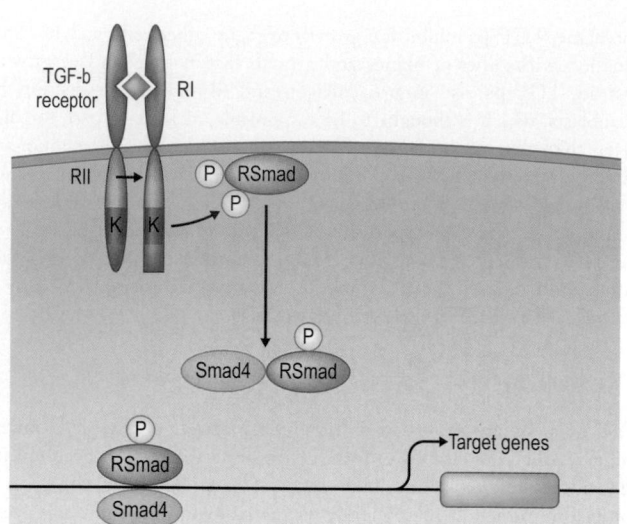

Fig. 10.9 SMADs and signaling by TGF-β superfamily receptor serine kinases.

particularly in bone and internal organ formation. Their deficiency is embryonically lethal, demonstrating that although the three isoforms functional similarly *in vitro*, they play distinct roles *in vivo*.

The human type II receptor is an 80 kDa glycoprotein which, as mentioned above, is the principal receptor for TGF-β. Upon binding of its ligand to RII, the type I receptor is recruited into the complex and activated through phosphorylation of its GS domain. The principal type I receptor in the TGF-β pathway is the ~55 kDa activin-like kinase-5 (ALK-5). ALK-1 can also be recruited into the complex and can transduce TGF-β-mediated signals.

SIGNALING

Ligand binding to the type II receptor allows the recruitment of the type I receptor (Fig. 10.9).[72] Although the receptor subunits have some affinity for one another, the complex of the receptor subunits bound to ligand is more stable. The type II receptor is thought to be a constitutively active kinase. Upon ligand binding, the type II receptor phosphorylates the type I receptor. The type I receptor is structurally distinct from the type II receptor in having a juxtamembrane domain that precedes the kinase domain, which is referred to as the GS domain. It is this site that is phosphorylated by the type II receptor. In turn, the type I receptor is responsible for phosphorylating key signaling intermediates. It is not clear whether activation of the type I receptor is due to enhancement of its kinase activity, to the appearance of substrate-binding sites, or to a combination of the two.

SMADS

The primary substrates activated by the type I receptors are SMADs, a group of related proteins that have been highly conserved throughout evolution and play a critical role in TGF-β signal transduction.[73] Eight mammalian SMADs have been identified. All exhibit a high degree of

specificity for conserved motifs in the cytoplasmic tail of type I receptors. These proteins do not contain any previously known structural or enzymatic motifs. However, they have two homology domains, termed the MH1 and MH2 domains, at the N and C termini, respectively, which are separated by a central linker domain. The extreme C terminus of some SMADs is a critical site of phosphorylation, as described below.

SMADs have been subdivided into three classes based on functional distinctions. The receptor-regulated SMADs (R-Smads) directly interact with, and are phosphorylated by, the type I receptor. These include SMAD1, -2, -3, -5, and -8. Smad2 and Smad3 are phosphorylated in response to TGF-β, whereas Smad1, -5, and -8 are primarily activated in response to BMP activation. R-SMADs bind to the GS domain of type I receptor and are phosphorylated at a conserved SSXS motif in their C terminus. The interaction of R-SMADs with TGF-β receptors may also regulated by another molecule termed SARA (SMAD anchor for receptor activation). SARA binds unphosphorylated SMAD2 and SMAD3. By virtue of its FYVE domain, SARA may bind phospholipids and localize SMADs to the plasma membrane, facilitating receptor binding. Phosphorylation of SMADs also permits dissociation from SARA.

Upon recruitment to their cognate activated type I receptor, R-SMADs are phosphorylated on C-terminal serine residues, triggering homodimerization of R-SMADs or heterodimerization with another class of SMAD, the common SMAD or C-SMAD. SMAD4 is the only known C-SMAD in vertebrates. It is thought to function as the central and essential downstream mediator of other SMADs in all TGF-β/BMP pathways. The SMAD MH2 domain is important for both receptor interaction and SMAD dimerization. However, SMAD4 lacks the SSXS element conserved in the R-SMADs and thus is not phosphorylated, rendering it unable to bind type I receptors directly.

The third subfamily of SMADs are the inhibitory SMADs or I-SMADs. In mammals, SMAD6 and SMAD7 are the I-SMADs. The I-SMADs may have different modes of function. For example, SMAD7 is induced by TGF-β and binds to TGF-β receptors inhibiting the phosphorylation of R-SMADs, thus serving as a classic feedback inhibitor. SMAD6 utilizes an alternative mechanism, and is thought to function by competing with SMAD4 for binding to an R-SMAD.

Consistent with their key functions in development, gene targeting of SMAD molecules has been shown to produce severe phenotypic abnormalities. SMAD2 null mice lack anterior/posterior specification and fail to develop mesoderm. SMAD3-deficient mice have limb malformations and defective immune function. SMAD3 null mice exhibit defective TGF-β responses. However, these mice also display accelerated wound healing compared to normal mice, which seems to contradict the role of SMAD3 as a positive regulator of TGF-β in enhancing wound healing. SMAD4-deficient mice die early in embryogenesis and exhibit severe defects in gastrulation. Of the I-SMADs, studies with SMAD6-deficient mice indicate a role in the development and homeostasis of the cardiovascular system.

Once phosphorylated, R-SMADs dissociate from the activated type I receptor and associate with SMAD4 in the cytoplasm. This is followed by nuclear translocation of the heteromeric SMAD complex, the binding to cognate DNA motifs in the promoters of TGF-β-responsive genes, and the concomitant induction of transcription. The SMAD MH1 motif mediates sequence-specific DNA binding, whereas the MH2 domain contains the transcriptional activation domain.

Other TGF-β-activated pathways

Although a canonical SMAD DNA-binding element (SBE) has been described (AGAC), comparison of the TGF-β responsiveness of synthetic promoters to natural promoters has revealed that SMADs can only partially account for the gene-regulatory effects of TGF-β signaling. SMADs also interact with a variety of other transcription factors, transcriptional co-activators, and transcriptional co-repressors to coordinately regulate transcription of a select subset of complex promoters. For example, FAST-1 (forkhead activin signal transducer), a winged helix forkhead transcription factor, associates with the SMAD2/SMAD4 complex. Moreover, SMADs also bind to c-JUN/c-FOS, and AP-1 sites frequently overlap with SBE sites in the naturally occurring promoters of TGF-β-responsive genes. SMADs can also bind ATF2, the vitamin D receptor, and other transcription factors, and can recruit the co-activators CBP/p300. Additionally, the SKI and SNON co-repressors can interact with SMADs and antagonize TGF-β signaling.

Other signaling pathways are known to mediate TGF-β signals. In particular, a number of members of the mitogen-activated protein kinase (MAPK) family are activated in response to TGF-β. TGF-β induces ERK, JNK and p38 MAPK activity. Inhibition of several of these pathways inhibits TGF-β-mediated transcriptional activation. In addition, a mitogen-activated protein kinase kinase kinase family member, TAK1 (TGF-β-associated kinase-1), has been implicated in TGF-β signaling. TAK1 is activated in response to ligand binding and has been shown to associate with another molecule, TAB1 (TAK1-asociated binding protein), which activates TAK1 kinase activity. Together, they have been reported to activate the MAPK pathway(s), leading to activation of p38/MPK2 and c-JUN N-terminal kinase (JNK), with evidence that this may take place via MKK6 and MKK4, respectively.

CLINICAL RELEVANCE

Although the relevance of TGF-β to clinical immunology remains unclear, defects in the TGF-β pathway have been identified in a range of human cancers. SMAD4 is deleted in half of all human pancreatic carcinomas. Mutations in SMAD2 have been identified in patients with colon cancer, and somatic mutations in TGF-β receptors have been identified in colon and gastric cancers. Loss of SMAD3 is associated with leukemia. In addition, oncogenic RAS has been shown to repress SMAD signaling by negatively regulating SMAD2 and SMAD3.

OTHER CYTOKINES

Several new cytokines have been identified, but their functions are less clear than those of the other cytokines discussed above. IL-16 was formerly termed lymphocyte chemoattractant factor, because of its ability to recruit CD4 T cells.[74] It is unrelated to other cytokines and its only known receptor is the CD4 molecule. It was originally identified as a product of CD8 T cells, but its message is widely expressed. CD4 T cells, eosinophils and mast cells can all secrete IL-16. It is present in bronchoalveolar lavage fluids from asthmatics and sarcoid patients. It has also been detected in blister fluid from bullous pemphigoid lesions. The physiologic function of IL-16 has yet to be clarified.

IL-32 is one of the newest cytokines and it too is structurally distinct.[75,76] It is inducible by the combination of IL-12 and IL-18. IL-32 induces the expression of various cytokines, including TNF, IL-1, IL-6 and chemokines, and can synergize with muramyl dipeptides. IL-32 signals via NF-κB and p38. IL-32 is present in rheumatoid synovium, and injection of IL-32 induces inflammation and recruitment of inflammatory cells.

IL-14 was identified as a high molecular weight B-cell growth factor produced by T cells and some B-cell tumors. The precise nature of this putative cytokine is still uncertain.

CONCLUSIONS AND SUMMARY

Cytokines encompass a wide range of molecules that are essential for communication between cells of the immune system and other nonimmune cells. Although the number of cytokines already seems vast, it is likely that more will be discovered in the future. Considerable progress has been made in defining the *in vivo* functions of various cytokines. Equally impressive have been advances in our understanding how dysregulation of cytokines and cytokine signaling contributes to human disease. Cytokine and anti-cytokine therapies are being successfully used in the clinic, and it is likely that their use will increase with advances in the understanding of the immunobiology of these cytokines.

REFERENCES

1. Dumonde DEA. 'Lymphokines': non-antibody mediators of cellular immunity generated by lymphocyte activation. Nature 1969; 224: 38.
2. Cohen S, Bigazzi PE, Yoshida T. Similarities of T cell function in cell-mediated immunity and antibody production. Cell Immunol 1974; 12: 150.
3. Thompson AW, Lotze MT. The cytokine handbook, San Diego, CA: Academic Press, 2003.
4. Vilcek J. The cytokines: an overview. In: The cytokine hand book, 4th edition. Lotte M, Thompson AW(eds), Volume I, pp.3–18. Academic Press, Amsterdam, 2003.
5. Boulay JL, O'Shea JJ, Paul WE. Molecular phylogeny within type I cytokines and their cognate receptors. Immunity 2003; 19: 159–163.
6. Taga T, Kishimoto T. Gp130 and the interleukin-6 family of cytokines. Annu Rev Immunol 1997; 15: 797–819.
7. Hunter CA. New IL-12-family members: IL-23 and IL-27, cytokines with divergent functions. Nature Rev Immunol 2005; 5: 521–531.
8. Dillon SR, Sprecher C, Hammond A, et al. Interleukin 31, a cytokine produced by activated T cells, induces dermatitis in mice. Nature Immunol 2004; 5: 752–760.
9. Kovanen PE, Leonard WJ. Cytokines and immunodeficiency diseases: critical roles of the gamma(c)-dependent cytokines interleukins 2, 4, 7, 9, 15, and 21, and their signaling pathways. Immunol Rev 2004; 202: 67–83.
10. Williams MA, Tyznik AJ, Bevan MJ. Interleukin-2 signals during priming are required for secondary expansion of CD8+ memory T cells. Nature 2006; 441: 890–893.
11. Malek TR, Bayer AL. Tolerance, not immunity, crucially depends on IL-2. Nature Rev Immunol 2004; 4: 665–674.

12. Sakaguchi S, Sakaguchi N. Regulatory T cells in immunologic self-tolerance and autoimmune disease. Int Rev Immunol 2005; 24: 211–226.

13. Nelms K, Keegan AD, Zamorano J, et al. The IL-4 receptor: signaling mechanisms and biologic functions. Annu Rev Immunol 1999; 17: 701–738.

14. Risma KA, Wang N, Andrews RP, et al. V75R576 IL-4 receptor alpha is associated with allergic asthma and enhanced IL-4 receptor function. J Immunol 2002; 169: 1604–1610.

15. Mosmann TR, Coffman RL. TH1 and TH2 cells: different patterns of lymphokine secretion lead to different functional properties. Annu Rev Immunol 1989; 7: 145–173.

16. Murphy KM, Reiner SL. The lineage decisions of helper T cells. Nature Rev Immunol 2002; 2: 933–944.

17. Lee GR, Kim ST, Spilianakis CG, et al. T helper cell differentiation: regulation by cis elements and epigenetics. Immunity 2006; 24: 369–379.

18. Tagaya Y, Bamford RN, DeFilippis AP, Waldmann TA. IL-15: a pleiotropic cytokine with diverse receptor/signaling pathways whose expression is controlled at multiple levels. Immunity 1996; 4: 329–336.

19. Leonard WJ, Spolski R. Interleukin-21: a modulator of lymphoid proliferation, apoptosis and differentiation. Nature Rev Immunol 2005; 5: 688–698.

20. Trinchieri G, Pflanz S, Kastelein RA. The IL-12 family of heterodimeric cytokines: new players in the regulation of T cell responses. Immunity 2003; 19: 641–644.

21. Watford WT, Hissong BD, Bream JH, et al. Signaling by IL-12 and IL-23 and the immunoregulatory roles of STAT4. Immunol Rev 2004; 202: 139–156.

22. Picard C, Fieschi C, Altare F, et al. Inherited interleukin-12 deficiency: IL12B genotype and clinical phenotype of 13 patients from six kindreds. Am J Hum Genet 2002; 70: 336–348.

23. Smale ST, Fisher AG. Chromatin structure and gene regulation in the immune system. Annu Rev Immunol 2002; 20: 427–462.

24. McKenzie BS, Kastelein RA, Cua DJ. Understanding the IL-23-IL-17 immune pathway. Trends Immunol 2006; 27: 17–23.

25. Watanabe N, Hanabuchi S, Soumelis V, et al. Human thymic stromal lymphopoietin promotes dendritic cell-mediated CD4+ T cell homeostatic expansion. Nature Immunol 2004; 5: 426–434.

26. Garcia-Sastre A, Biron CA. Type 1 interferons and the virus-host relationship: a lesson in detente. Science 2006; 312: 879–882.

27. Siegal FP, Kadowaki N, Shodell M, et al. The nature of the principal type 1 interferon-producing cells in human blood. Science 1999; 284: 1835–1837.

28. Asselin-Paturel C, Boonstra A, Dalod M, et al. Mouse type I IFN-producing cells are immature APCs with plasmacytoid morphology. Nature Immunol 2001; 2: 1144–1150.

29. Bach EA, Aguet M, Schreiber RD. The IFN gamma receptor: a paradigm for cytokine receptor signaling. Annu Rev Immunol 1997; 15: 563–591.

30. Rosenzweig SD, Holland SM. Defects in the interferon-gamma and interleukin-12 pathways. Immunol Rev 2005; 203: 38–47.

31. Donnelly RP, Sheikh F, Kotenko SV, Dickensheets H. The expanded family of class II cytokines that share the IL-10 receptor-2 (IL-10R2) chain. J Leukocyte Biol 2004; 76: 314–321.

32. Li MO, Wan YY, Sanjabi S, et al. Transforming growth factor-beta regulation of immune responses. Annu Rev Immunol 2006; 24: 99–146.

33. Mangan PR, Harrington LE, O'Quinn DB, et al. Transforming growth factor-beta induces development of the T(H)17 lineage. Nature 2006; 441: 231–234.

34. Bettelli E, Carrier Y, Gao W, et al. Reciprocal developmental pathways for the generation of pathogenic effector TH17 and regulatory T cells. Nature 2006; 441: 235–238.

35. Pesu M, Candotti F, Husa M, et al. Jak3, severe combined immunodeficiency, and a new class of immunosuppressive drugs. Immunol Rev 2005; 203: 127–142.

36. Changelian PS, Flanagan ME, Ball DJ, et al. Prevention of organ allograft rejection by a specific Janus kinase 3 inhibitor. Science 2003; 302: 875–878.

37. Wormald S, Hilton DJ. Inhibitors of cytokine signal transduction. J Biol Chem 2004; 279: 821–824.

38. Chen Z, Laurence A, Kanno Y, et al. Selective regulatory function of Socs3 in the formation of IL-17-secreting T cells. Proc Natl Acad Sci USA 2006; 103: 8137–8142.

39. Beutler BA. The role of tumor necrosis factor in health and disease. J Rheumatol 1999; 57: 16–21.

40. Siegel RM, Muppidi J, Roberts M, et al. Death receptor signaling and autoimmunity. Immunol Res 2003; 27: 499–512.

41. Siegel RM. Caspases at the crossroads of immune-cell life and death. Nature Rev Immunol 2006; 6: 308–317.

42. Micheau O, Tschopp J. Induction of TNF receptor I-mediated apoptosis via two sequential signaling complexes. Cell 2003; 114: 181–190.

43. Muppidi JR, Siegel RM. Ligand-independent redistribution of Fas (CD95) into lipid rafts mediates clonotypic T cell death. Nature Immunol 2004; 5: 182–189.

44. Eberstadt M, Huang B, Chen Z, et al. NMR structure and mutagenesis of the FADD (Mort1) death-effector domain. Nature 1998; 392: 941–945.

45. Boatright KM, Salvesen GS. Mechanisms of caspase activation. Curr Opin Cell Biol 2003; 15: 725–731.

46. Legler DF, Micheau O, Doucey MA, et al. Recruitment of TNF receptor 1 to lipid rafts is essential for TNFalpha-mediated NF-kappaB activation. Immunity 2003; 18: 655–664.

47. Deng L, Wang C, Spencer E, et al. Activation of the IkappaB kinase complex by TRAF6 requires a dimeric ubiquitin-conjugating enzyme complex and a unique polyubiquitin chain. Cell 2000; 103: 351–361.

48. Kim EY, Priatel JJ, Teh SJ, Teh HS. TNF receptor type 2 (p75) functions as a costimulator for antigen-driven T cell responses in vivo. J Immunol 2006; 176: 1026–1035.

49. Bongartz T, Sutton AJ, Sweeting MJ, et al. Anti-TNF antibody therapy in rheumatoid arthritis and the risk of serious infections and malignancies: systematic review and meta-analysis of rare harmful effects in randomized controlled trials. JAMA 2006; 295: 2275–2285.

50. McDermott MF, Aksentijevich I, Galon J, et al. Germline mutations in the extracellular domains of the 55 kDa TNF receptor, TNFR1, define a family of dominantly inherited autoinflammatory syndromes. Cell 1999; 97: 133–144.

51. Straus SE, Sneller M, Lenardo MJ, et al. An inherited disorder of lymphocyte apoptosis: the autoimmune lymphoproliferative syndrome. Ann Intern Med 1999; 130: 591–601.

52. Salzer U, Chapel HM, Webster AD, et al. Mutations in TNFRSF13B encoding TACI are associated with common variable immunodeficiency in humans. Nature Genet 2005; 37: 820–828.

53. Castigli E, Wilson SA, Garibyan L, et al. TACI is mutant in common variable immunodeficiency and IgA deficiency. Nature Genet 2005; 37: 829–834.

54. Losi CG, Salzer U, Gatta R, et al. Mutational analysis of human BLyS in patients with common variable immunodeficiency. J Clin Immunol. 2006; 26: 396–399.

55. Losi CG, Silini A, Fiorini C, et al. Mutational analysis of human BAFF receptor TNFRSF13C (BAFF-R) in patients with common variable immunodeficiency. J Clin Immunol 2005; 25: 496–502.

56. Dunne A, O'Neill LA. The interleukin-1 receptor/Toll-like receptor superfamily: signal transduction during inflammation and host defense. Sci STKE 2003; 25 Febuary, re3.

57. Schmitz J, Owyang A, Oldham E, et al. IL-33, an interleukin-1-like cytokine that signals via the IL-1 receptor-related protein ST2 and induces T helper type 2-associated cytokines. Immunity 2005; 23: 479–490.

58. Sims JE, Nicklin MJ, Bazan JF, et al. A new nomenclature for IL-1-family genes. Trends Immunol 2001; 22: 536–537.

59. Wald D, Qin J, Zhao Z, et al. SIGIRR, a negative regulator of Toll-like receptor-interleukin 1 receptor signaling. Nature Immunol 2003; 4: 920–927.

60. Fitzgerald AA, Leclercq SA, Yan A, et al. Rapid responses to anakinra in patients with refractory adult-onset Still's disease. Arthritis Rheum 2005; 52: 1794–1803.

61. Hawkins PN, Lachmann HJ, McDermott MF. Interleukin 1 receptor antagonist in the Muckle–Wells syndrome. N Engl J Med 2003; 348: 2583–2584.

62. Kawaguchi M, Adachi M, Oda N, et al. IL-17 cytokine family. J Allergy Clin Immunol 2004; 114: 1265–1273. quiz 1274.

63. Dong C. Diversification of T-helper-cell lineages: finding the family root of IL-17-producing cells. Nature Rev Immunol 2006; 6: 329–333.

64. Fort MM, Cheung J, Yen D, et al. IL-25 induces IL-4, IL-5, and IL-13 and Th2-associated pathologies in vivo. Immunity 2001; 15: 985–995.

65. Tato CM, Laurence A, O'Shea J. Helper T cell differentiation enters a new era: Le Roi est mort; vive le Roi!. J Exp Med 2006; 203: 809–812.

66. Maezawa Y, Nakajima H, Suzuki K, et al. Involvement of TNF receptor-associated factor 6 in IL-25 receptor signaling. J Immunol 2006; 176: 1013–1018.

67. Langowski JL, Zhang X, Wu L, et al. IL-23 promotes tumor incidence and growth. Nature 2006;442: 461–465.

68. Pawson T, Scott JD. Signaling through scaffold, anchoring, and adaptor proteins. Science 1997; 278: 2075–2080.

69. Cantley LC. The phosphoinositide 3-kinase pathway. Science 2002; 296: 1655–1657.

70. Longley BJ, Reguera MJ, Ma Y. Classes of c-KIT activating mutations: proposed mechanisms of action and implications for disease classification and therapy. Leukemia Res 2001; 25: 571–576.

71. Cools J, DeAngelo DJ, Gotlib J, et al. A tyrosine kinase created by fusion of the PDGFRA and FIP1L1 genes as a therapeutic target of imatinib in idiopathic hypereosinophilic syndrome. N Engl J Med 2003; 348: 1201–1214.

72. Heldin CH, Miyazono K, ten Dijke P. TGF-beta signalling from cell membrane to nucleus through SMAD proteins. Nature 1997; 390: 465–471.

73. Massague J, Gomis RR. The logic of TGFbeta signaling. FEBS Lett 2006; 580: 2811–2820.

74. Wilson KC, Center DM, Cruikshank WW. The effect of interleukin-16 and its precursor on T lymphocyte activation and growth. Growth Factors 2004; 22: 97–104.

75. Kim SH, Han SY, Azam T, et al. Interleukin-32: a cytokine and inducer of TNFalpha. Immunity 2005; 22: 131–142.

76. Joosten LA, Netea MG, Kim SH, et al. IL-32, a proinflammatory cytokine in rheumatoid arthritis. Proc Natl Acad Sci USA 2006; 103: 3298–3303.

Chemokines and chemokine receptors

Philip M. Murphy

11

The chemokines are a family of *chemo*tactic cyto*kines* that coordinate leukocyte trafficking and activation [in the immune system. Chemokines normally promote host defense and repair, but may also regulate non-immunological processes, such as organ development and angiogenesis. They can also be used to promote detrimental processes such as cancer and autoimmunity. Chemokines act by binding to G protein-coupled receptors, two of which, CCR5 and CXCR4, are exploited by HIV for target cell entry. This chapter describes the basic principles and clinical correlates of chemokine regulation of the immune system.

KEY CONCEPTS

Chemokine and chemokine receptor properties

>> *Definition* Chemokines, the largest subgroup of cytokines, are defined by structure, not function; chemokine receptors are defined by function not structure.

>> *Evolution* Chemokines and chemokine receptors arose in vertebrates, and have been copied or mimicked by many poxviruses, herpes viruses and retroviruses.

>> *Ligand-receptor promiscuity* Chemokines usually bind more than one receptor subtype. Chemokine receptors usually bind more than one chemokine, but from a single chemokine subclass.

>> *Cell biology* Chemokines coordinate leukocyte trafficking but may have prominent nontrafficking functions (e.g., lymphocyte proliferation/apoptosis/differentiation/activation, granulocyte degranulation/superoxide production, direct antimicrobial activity), as well as effects on other cell types in nonimmunologic contexts (e.g., development, cancer, angiogenesis).

>> *Biology* Chemokines act redundantly or nonredundantly *in vivo*, depending on the context. Host chemokine receptors mediate antimicrobial defense, but certain pathogens (e.g. HIV) can exploit chemokine receptors to infect the host. Moreover, excessive or inappropriate chemokine expression may pathologically amplify immunologically mediated disease.

■ MOLECULAR ORGANIZATION OF THE CHEMOKINE SYSTEM ■

CHEMOKINES

Chemokines are found in vertebrates from teleost fishes to humans. Copies of vertebrate chemokine genes are also found in many herpes viruses and poxviruses. Defined by structure, not by function, there are at least 45 unique human chemokines, which makes them the largest family of cytokines. Most chemokines are 66–111 amino acids long. All occupy a common sector of sequence space bounded loosely by ~20% identity for any pairwise comparison. Tertiary structure is highly conserved, partly because the disulfide-bonded cysteines are conservatively spaced (Fig. 11.1). Chemokines are subclassified according to variations in cysteine number and location. All have at least two cysteines, and all but two have at least four (Tables 11.1 and 11.2). In the four-cysteine group, the first two are either adjacent (CC motif, n = 24) or separated by either one (CXC motif, n = 16) or three (CX3C motif, n = 1) non-conserved amino acids. The C chemokines (n = 2) have only two cysteines, corresponding to C-2 and C-4 in the other subgroups. Disulfide bonds link C-1 to C-3 and C-2 to C-4. The conserved chemokine fold contains three β sheets arranged in the shape of a Greek key, overlaid by a C-terminal α-helical domain and flanked by an N-terminal domain that lacks order.[1] Sequence identity is <30% between members of different groups, but ranges from ~30% to 99% among CC and CXC chemokines considered separately. The group names are used as roots, followed by the letter 'L' and a number (e.g., CXCL1) in a systematic nomenclature that was established to resolve competing aliases.[2]

CC and CXC chemokines can be subclassified by additional motifs. The seven CXC chemokines with Glu-Leu-Arg (ELR) N-terminal to C-1 are >40% identical, attract neutrophils, bind the receptor CXCR2, and are angiogenic (Table 11.1). Among CXC chemokines lacking ELR, only CXCL12 is angiogenic and attracts neutrophils. CXCL9–11 also are >40% identical and share a receptor (CXCR3), but are angiostatic rather than angiogenic.

Class							Names	N
CX3C:		CXXXC		C		C	CX3CL1	1
Non-ELR CXC:		CX_C		C		C	CXCL#	9
ELR CXC:	ELR	CX_C		C		C	CXCL#	7
4C CC:		C_C		C		C	CCL#	19
6C CC:		C_C	C	C		C C	CCL#	5
C:		C				C	XCL#	2

Fig. 11.1 Chemokine classification and nomenclature. Chemokine classes are defined by the number and arrangement of conserved cysteines, as shown. Brackets link cysteines that form disulfide bonds. ELR refers to the amino acids glu-leu-arg. X refers to an amino acid other than cysteine. The underscore is a spacer used to optimize the alignment. The N and C termini can vary considerably in length (not illustrated). For molecules with four cysteines, there are approximately 24 amino acids between Cys-2 and Cys-3 and 15 amino acids between Cys-3 and Cys-4. At right are listed the nomenclature system and the number of human chemokines known in each class (N).

Two cysteine-defined CC subgroups exist. Both have two additional cysteines (a total of six), with one in the C-terminal domain. They are distinguished by the location of the sixth cysteine, which can be found either in the C-terminal domain or between C-2 and C-3. CXCL16 and CX3CL1 cross classes to form a unique multimodular subgroup. Each has a chemokine domain, a mucin-like stalk, a transmembrane domain, and a C-terminal cytoplasmic module. Each can exist as either a membrane-bound or a shed form, enabling either direct cell–cell adhesion or chemotaxis, respectively.

Chemokine monomer, dimer and tetramer structures may occur. Complex quaternary structures bound to glycosaminoglycans (GAGs) on the surface of cells may also be important for function *in vivo*.[1] A native heterodimer composed of CCL3 and CCL4 subunits has been purified from activated human monocytes and peripheral blood lymphocytes.

CHEMOKINE RECEPTORS

Chemokine receptors are defined as mediators that activate cellular responses upon binding chemokines. All 19 known human subtypes are members of the seven-transmembrane (7TM) domain superfamily of G protein-coupled receptors.[3] Chemokine-binding, membrane-anchoring and signaling domains come from a single polypeptide chain. Homo- and heterodimers have been reported, but the physiologic form has not been clearly delineated.

The ligand–receptor relationship is typically promiscuous, but chemokine subgroup restricted (Table 11.3). A systematic receptor nomenclature formula exploits this as follows: receptor name = ligand subgroup root + R (for 'receptor') + number in order of discovery. An exception is the C chemokine receptor XCR1, where 'X' distinguishes it from CR1, the previously assigned name for complement receptor 1. For consistency, the XCR1 ligands are named XCL1 and XCL2.

Each chemokine has a unique receptor specificity profile. Conversely, each receptor has a unique chemokine specificity profile. Almost all chemokines are chemotactic agonists, and a few are both agonists at one receptor and antagonists at another. Differential receptor usage and differential regulation of expression may account for nonredundant function *in vivo* observed for chemokines acting at the same receptor.

KEY CONCEPTS

Immunologic classification of the chemokine system

>> *Homeostatic system* Constitutively expressed ligands and receptors. Important in hematopoiesis and immune surveillance. Key receptors: CXCR4 on hematopoietic progenitors; CXCR5 on naïve B cells; CCR7 on mature dendritic cells and naïve T cells; and gut and skin-specific T-cell homing receptors CCR9 and CCR10, respectively.

>> *Inflammatory system* In innate immunity, inducible ligands and constitutively expressed receptors (e.g., neutrophil CXCR2, macrophage CCR2, eosinophil CCR3, and NK cell CX3CR1). In adaptive immunity, inducible ligands and inducible receptors (e.g., CXCR3 and CCR4 on Th1 and Th2 CD4+ T cells, respectively).

>> *Decoy receptors* Some membrane proteins that bind chemokines do not signal and act instead as scavengers/'decoy receptors' to limit chemokine action.

ATYPICAL CHEMOKINE SYSTEM COMPONENTS

Three human 7TM proteins (Duffy, D6 and CCX CKR) bind chemokines promiscuously but do not signal, and may function as scavengers.[4] Several endogenous nonchemokine ligands bind chemokine receptors, including aminoacyl tRNA synthetases and β defensin 2, possibly linking innate to adaptive immunity. In addition to chemokines, herpes viruses and pox viruses encode structurally related 7TM chemokine receptors, structurally unique chemokine-binding proteins (scavengers), and nonchemokine chemokine receptor ligands (agonists or antagonists). HIV also encodes chemokine mimics gp120 and tat. Viral chemokine elements may function to evade the immune system, to recruit new target cells, to reprogram gene expression for cell proliferation and angiogenesis, and for target cell entry.[5]

IMMUNOLOGIC CLASSIFICATION

Chemokines and chemokine receptors have differential leukocyte specificity, but together cover the full spectrum of leukocytes and populate two main subsystems, homeostatic and inflammatory (Table 11.4). Homeostatic

Table 11.1 The human CXC, CX3C and C chemokine families

ELR motif	Chemokine	Common aliases	Main source	Main immunologic roles	Chromosomal location
ELR+	CXCL1	GROα MGSA	Inducible in most hematopoietic and tissue cells Many tumors	Neutrophil trafficking	4q21.1
	CXCL2	GROβ			
	CXCL3	GROα			
ELR-	CXCL4	PF-4	Preformed in platelets	Procoagulant	
ELR+	CXCL5	ENA-78	Induced in epithelial cells of gut and lung; N, Mo, Plts, EC	Neutrophil trafficking	
	CXCL6	GCP-2	Induced in lung microvascular EC; Mo; alveolar epithelial cells, mesothelial cells, EC and Mφ		
	CXCL7	NAP-2	Preformed in platelets		
	CXCL8	IL-8	Induced in most cell types		
ELR-	CXCL9	Mig	Induced in PMN, Mφ, T cells, astrocytes, microglial cells, hepatocytes, EC, fibroblasts, keratinocytes, thymic stromal cells	Th1 response	
	CXCL10	IP-10	Induced in ECs, Mo, keratinocytes, respiratory & intestinal epithelial cells, astrocytes, microglia, mesangial cells, smooth muscle cells		
	CXCL11	I-TAC	ECs, Mo,		
	CXCL12	SDF-1, PBSF	Constitutive in bone marrow stromal cells; most tissues	Myelopoiesis HPC, neutrophil homing to BM B lymphopoiesis	10q11.21
	CXCL13	BCA-1	Constitutive in follicular HEV of secondary lymphoid tissue	Naïve B- and T-cell homing to follicles B1 cell homing to peritoneum Natural Ab production	4q21.1
	CXCL14	BRAK	Constitutive in most tissues, breast and kidney tumors	Macrophage migration	5q31.1
ELR+	(CXCL15)	(mouse only)	Constitutive in lung epithelial cells	Neutrophil trafficking	NA
ELR-	CXCL16	Sexckine	Constitutive in spleen; DCs of the T zone	T cell and DC homing to spleen	17p13
NA	CX3CL1	Fractalkine	EC, neurons, Mo, DC	NK, Monocyte, M and Th1 cell migration	16q13
	XCL1	Lymphotactin α	Epidermal T cells, NK, NK-T, activated CD8+ and Th1 CD4+ T cells	CD62L^lo T effector cell migration	1q24.2
	XCL2	Lymphotactin β			

NA, not applicable. Mo, monocyte; PMN, neutrophil; DC, dendritic cell; EC, endothelial cell; HEV, high endothelial venule; MPC, myeloid progenitor cell; plt, platelet; MΦ, macrophage; GRO, growth-related oncogene; PF-4, platelet factor-4; GCP, granulocyte chemoattractant protein; ENA-78, 78 amino acid epithelial cell-derived neutrophil activator; NAP, neutrophil activating protein; IL-8, interleukin-8; Mig, monokine induced by IFN-γ; I-TAC; interferon-inducible T-cell α chemoattractant; SDF, stromal cell-derived factor; BCA, B cell-activating chemokine; BRAK, breast and kidney associated chemokine.

MOLECULAR ORGANIZATION OF THE CHEMOKINE SYSTEM

Table 11.2 The human CC chemokine family

Chromosomal location	Chemokine	Common aliases	Sources	Main immunologic roles
17q11-12	**CCL1**	I-309	Inducible in Mo and CD4+ and CD8+ αβ and CD4-CD8- γδ T cells	Th2 response
	CCL2	MCP-1	Inducible in Mo, fibroblasts, keratinocytes, EC, PMN, synoviocytes, mesangial cells, astrocytes, lung epithelial cells and MΦ. Constitutively made in splenic arteriolar lymphatic sheath and medullary region of lymph node, many tumors, and arterial plaque EC.	Innate immunity Th2 response CD4+ T cell differentiation
	CCL3	MIP-1α LD78α MIP-1αS	Inducible in Mo/MΦ, CD8+ T cells, B cells, plts, PMN, Eo, Ba, DC, NK, mast cells, keratinocytes, fibroblasts, mesangial cells, astrocytes, microglial cells, epith cells	Innate immunity Th1 response CD4 T cell differentiation
	CCL3L1	LD78β MIP-1αP	Similar to CCL3	Probably similar to CCL3
	CCL4	MIP-1β	Similar to CCL3	Innate immunity Th1 response
	CCL5	RANTES	--Inducible in EC, T cells, epithelial cells, Mo, fibroblasts, mesangial cells, NK cells --Constitutively expressed and stored in plt and Eo granules	Innate immunity Th1 and Th2 response
NA	**(CCL6)**	Mouse only	Inducible in bone marrow and peritoneal-derived MΦ	ND
17q11-12	**CCL7**	MCP-3	Inducible in Mo, plts, fibroblasts, EC, skin, bronchial epithelial cells, astrocytes	Th2 response
	CCL8	MCP-2	Inducible in fibroblasts, PMN, astrocytes Constitutively expressed in colon, small intestine, heart, lung, thymus, pancreas, spinal cord, ovary, placenta	Th2 response
NA	**(CCL9/10)**	Mouse only	Constitutively expressed in all mouse organs except brain; highest in lung, liver and thymus Induced in heart and lung	ND
17q11	**CCL11**	Eotaxin	Epithelial cells, EC, smooth muscle, cardiac muscle, Eo, dermal fibroblasts, mast cells, MΦ, Reed–Sternberg cells	Th2 response Eosinophil trafficking Mast cell trafficking Basophil trafficking, degranulation
NA	**(CCL12)**	Mouse only	Inducible in lung alveolar MΦ and smooth muscle cells; spinal cord. Constitutive expression in lymph node and thymic stromal cells	Allergic inflammation

NA, not applicable. Mo, monocyte; PMN, neutrophil; DC, dendritic cell; EC, endothelial cell; HEV, high endothelial venule; MPC, myeloid progenitor cell; plt, platelet; MΦ, macrophage; MCP, monocyte chemoattractant protein; MIP, macrophage inflammatory protein; RANTES, regulated upon activation normal T-cell expressed and secreted; MRP, MIP-related protein; HCC, hemofiltrate CC chemokine; TARC, thymus and activation related chemokine; PARC, pulmonary and activation related chemokine; ELC, Epstein–Barr virus-induced receptor ligand chemokine; LARC, liver and activation related chemokine; SLC, secondary lymphoid tissue chemokine; MDC, macrophage-derived chemokine; MPIF, myeloid progenitor inhibitory factor; TECK, thymus expressed chemokine; CTACK, cutaneous T cell-associated chemokine; MEC, mucosa-associated epithelial cell chemokine; ND, not determined.

Continued

chemokines are differentially and constitutively expressed in specific microenvironments of primary and secondary immune organs, and recruit hematopoietic precursor cells, dendritic cells (DC) and naïve and memory lymphocyte subsets via constitutively expressed receptors. Noxious stimuli induce inflammatory chemokines in diverse tissue cells and leukocytes. Inflammatory chemokine receptors are constitutively expressed on myeloid and NK cells, but must be induced on activated effector lymphocytes. Dynamic shifts in receptor expression occur during DC and NK cell maturation and during lymphocyte maturation, activation and differentiation.[6,7]

Inflammatory CXC and CC chemokine genes are found in two main clusters on human chromosomes 4q12-q21 and 17q11-q21, respectively.

Table 11.2 The human CC chemokine family—cont'd

Chromosomal location	Chemokine	Common aliases	Sources	Main immunologic roles
17q11-12	CCL13	MCP-4	Inducible in nasal and bronchial epithelial cells; dermal fibroblasts; PBMCs; atherosclerotic plaque EC and MΦ Constitutively expressed in small intestine, colon, thymus, heart and placenta	Th2 response
	CCL14a	HCC-1	Constitutively expressed in most organs; high plasma levels	ND
	CCL14b	HCC-3	Same as CCL14b except absent from skeletal muscle and pancreas	ND
	CCL15	HCC-2; Lkn-1	Inducible in Mo and DC Constitutive RNA expression in liver, gut, heart and skeletal muscle, adrenal gland and lung leukocytes.	ND
	CCL16	HCC-4; LEC	Constitutively expressed in liver, possibly many other organs. Also, Mo, T cells and NK cells express mRNA.	ND
16q13	CCL17	TARC	Constitutive in normal DC and Reed–Sternberg cells of Hodgkin's disease	Th2 response
17q11.2	CCL18	DC-CK1, PARC	Constitutive in Mo/MΦ, germinal center DC	DC attraction of naïve T cells
9p13.3	CCL19	ELC, MIP-3β	Constitutive on interdigitating DC in secondary lymphoid tissue	Naïve and memory T cell and DC homing to lymph node
2q36.3	CCL20	LARC MIP-3α	Constitutive in lymph nodes, peripheral blood leukocytes, thymus, and appendix Inducible in PBMC, HUVEC	DC homing to Peyer's patch Humoral response
9p13.3	CCL21	SLC, 6Ckine	Constitutive in lymphatic EC, HEV and interdigitating DC in T areas of 2° lymphoid tissue, thymic medullary epithelial cells and EC	Naïve and memory T cell and DC homing to lymph node
16q13	CCL22	MDC	Constitutive in DC and MΦ Inducible in Mo, T and B cells	Th2 response
17q12	CCL23	MPIF-1	Constitutive in pancreas and skeletal muscle	ND
7q11.23	CCL24	Eotaxin-2	Inducible in Mo	Eosinophil migration
19p13.3	CCL25	TECK	Constitutive in thymic stromal cells and small intestine	Thymocyte migration Homing of memory T cells to gut
7q11.23	CCL26	Eotaxin-3	Constitutive in heart and ovary Inducible on dermal fibroblasts and EC	Th2 response
9p13.3	CCL27	CTACK, Eskine	Constitutive in placenta, keratinocytes, testis and brain	Homing of memory and effector T cells to skin
5p12	CCL28	MEC	Constitutive in epithelial cells of gut, airway	Homing of T cells to mucosal surfaces

However, homeostatic chemokine genes are on multiple chromosomes in small clusters. Thirteen of the 19 human chemokine receptor genes are clustered at 3p21–23, and *CXCR1* and *CXCR2* are adjacent at 2q34-q35. Chemokine/receptor gene repertoire may vary among closely related species. Gene copy number and sequence may also vary among individuals of a species. Such variation may affect the risk of disease.

CHEMOKINE PRESENTATION MECHANISMS

Chemokines act locally. They are probably presented tethered to matrix or to endothelial cells via glycosaminoglycans or transmembrane domains. The tethering cell may have produced the chemokine, or else imported it by transcytosis from neighbors. The ligand-binding site includes the receptor N terminus and one or more extracellular loops, which allow

MOLECULAR ORGANIZATION OF THE CHEMOKINE SYSTEM

Table 11.3 Chemokine specificities for human 7TM chemokine receptors and chemokine-binding proteins. The standard name and most commonly used alias are listed for each chemokine

	CXCR1	CXCR2 (CD128)	CXCR3 (CD183)	CXCR4 (CD184)	CXCR5	CXCR6	CXCR7	CCR1	CCR2	CCR3	CCR4	CCR5 (CD195)
CXCL1/ Groα		+++										
CXCL2/ Groβ		+++										
CXCL3/ Groγ		+++										
CXCL4/ PF-4			+++									
CXCL5/ ENA-78	+	+++										
CXCL6/ GCP-2	++	+++										
CXCL7/ NAP-2		+++										
CXCL8/ IL-8	+++	+++										
CXCL9/Mig			+++							Antag		
CXCL10/ γIP-10			+++							Antag		
CXCL11/ I-TAC			+++							Antag		
CXCL12/ SDF-1				+++			+++					
CXCL13/ BCA1			+		+++							
CXCL14/ BRAK												
*CXCL15/ lungkine												
CXCL16						+++						
CCL1/ I-309												
CCL2/ MCP-1								+	+++			
CCL3/ MIP-1α								+++				+++
CCL4/ MIP-1β								Antag				+++
CCL5/ RANTES								+++		++		+++
*CCL6/ MRP-1												

Note: For each receptor, + indicates that the corresponding chemokine is an agonist, and 'Antag' denotes an antagonist. For the 7TM chemokine-binding proteins CCX CKR, D6 and Duffy, the + signs indicate high-affinity binding without signaling.
*Mouse chemokines that may not have human counterparts.

CCR6	CCR7 (CD197)	CCR8	CCR9	CCR10	XCR1	CX$_3$CR1	CCX CKR	Duffy (CD234)	D6
								+++	
								++	
								++	
		+++							
								++	++
		+							+++
								++	+++

Continued

FUNDAMENTAL PRINCIPLES OF THE IMMUNE RESPONSE

Table 11.3 Chemokine specificities for human 7TM chemokine receptors and chemokine-binding proteins. The standard name and most commonly used alias are listed for each chemokine—cont'd

	CXCR1	CXCR2 (CD128)	CXCR3 (CD183)	CXCR4 (CD184)	CXCR5	CXCR6	CXCR7	CCR1	CCR2	CCR3	CCR4	CCR5 (CD195)
CCL7/MCP-3								+++	+++	++		Antag
CCL8/MCP-2								++	+++	++		+++
*CCL9/10/ MRP-2								++				
CCL11/ eotaxin			Antag						Antag	+++		+
*CCL12/ MCP-5									++			
CCL13/ MCP-4								+++	+++	+++		
CCL14a/ HCC-1								+++				+++
CCL14b/ HCC-3												
CCL15/ HCC-2								+++		+++		
CCL16/ HCC-4								+	+			+
CCL17/ TARC											+++	
CCL18/ PARC												
CCL19/ELC												
CCL20/ LARC												
CCL21/SLC			+									
CCL22/MDC											+++	
CCL23/ MPIF-1								+++				
CCL24/ eotaxin-2										+++		
CCL25/ TECK												
CCL26/ eotaxin-3										++		
CCL27/ CTACK												
CCL28/MEC										+		
XCL1/ Lymphotactin α												
XCL2/ lymphotactin β												
CX3CL1/ fractalkine												

11

CCR6	CCR7 (CD197)	CCR8	CCR9	CCR10	XCR1	CX$_3$CR1	CCX CKR	Duffy (CD234)	D6
									+
									+++
									+
									++
									+++
		+							
		+							
	+++						+		
+++									
	+++						+		
				+++			+		
				+++					
				+++					
					+++				
					+++				
						+++			

Table 11.4 Specificities of functional human chemokine receptors for human leukocyte subsets

	CXCR1	CXCR2	CXCR3	CXCR4	CXCR5	CXCR6	CCR1	CCR2
CD4⁻CD8⁻ thymocytes				+				
CD4⁺CD8⁺ thymocytes				+				
CD4⁺CD8⁻ thymocytes				+				
CD4⁻CD8⁺ thymocytes				+				
CD34⁺ HSC				+				
CD56^{dim} CD16⁺ NK	+	+	+	+				
CD56^{bright} CD16⁻ NK			+	+				
CD4 NK-T			+	+				+
CD8 NK-T			+	+		+	+	+
CD4⁻CD8⁻ NK-T			+	+		+	+	+
B cells			+	+	+		+	+
Plasma cells				+		+		
IgA Ab-secreting cells				+				
Naïve T cells				+				
Follicular help T cells				+	+			
Central memory T cells				+				
Effector memory T cells				+			+	
Th1 effector T cells			+	+		+		+
Th2 effector T cells				+				
Th17 effector T cells						+		
α₄β₇ + Gut-homing memory T cells			+	+				+
CLA+ skin-homing memory T cells				+				
CD4⁺ CD25⁺ regulatory T cells				+				
Immature DC	+			+			+	+
Mature DC				+				
Monocytes		+	+	+			+	+
Basophils		+		+			+	
Eosinophils			+	+			+	
Neutrophils	+	+		+			+	+
Platelets	+			+			+	

CCR3	CCR4	CCR5	CCR6	CCR7	CCR8	CCR9	CCR10	XCR1	CX₃CR1
						+			
	+			+					
+	+			+					
								+	+
		+		+					
	+	+							
		+	+						
		+	+						
			+	+					
+							+		
						+	+		
				+					
	+		+	+					
+		+							
		+		+					+
+	+			+	+				
		+				+			
	+		+	+			+		
	+				+				
	+	+	+						
				+					
		+			+				+
+		+							
+									
+	+								

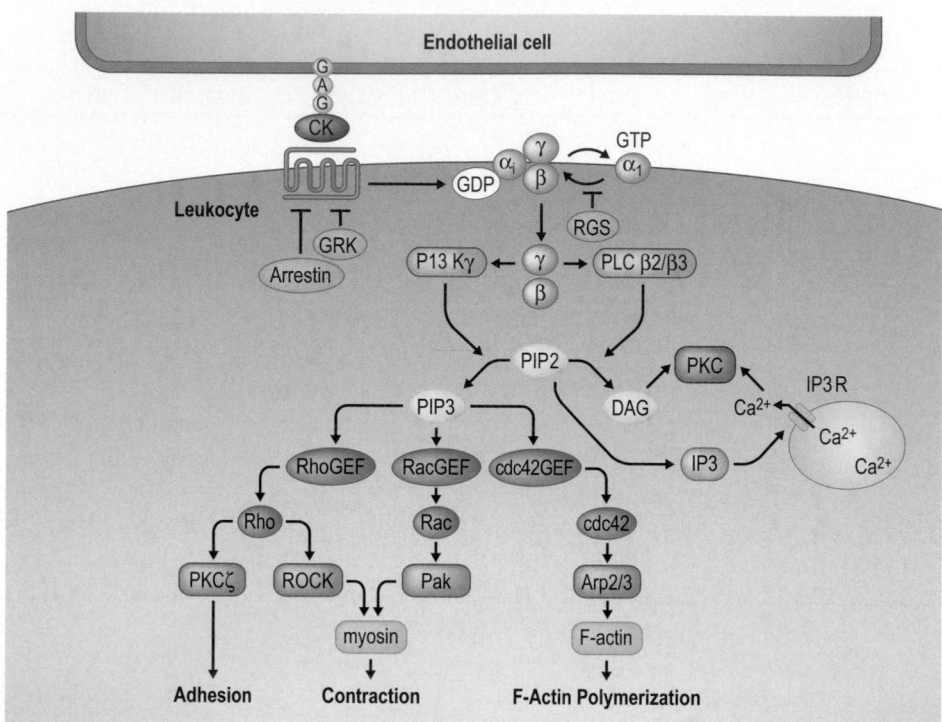

Fig. 11.2 Chemokine signal transduction in chemotaxis. Depicted are key steps in two of the main pathways induced by most chemokines. The PI3Kγ pathway is particularly important for cell migration. Chemokines are able to activate other pathways as well, including non-G$_i$-type G proteins, protein tyrosine kinases and MAP kinases. These pathways influence cell proliferation and activation. The model is modified from the Alliance for Cell Signaling (www.signaling-gateway.org). PLC, phospholipase C; PI3K, phosphatidylinositol-3-kinase; RGS, regulator of G protein signaling; DAG, diacylglycerol; IP3, inositol trisphosphate; PIP, phosphatidylinsol phosphate; GAG, glycosaminoglycan; CK, chemokine; PKC, protein kinase C; GRK, G protein-coupled receptor kinase; GEF, guanine nucleotide exchange factor.

docking of the chemokine N-loop domain and 7TM domains, which accept the chemokine's N terminus and are critical for triggering. Tyrosine sulfation on the receptor N terminus facilitates ligand binding.

LEUKOCYTE RESPONSES TO CHEMOKINES

During inflammation, leukocytes undergo transendothelial migration, a multistep process. Chemokines regulate at least two of these steps.[8] In an initial chemokine-independent step, leukocytes roll on inflamed endothelium in a selectin-dependent manner. Next, chemokines posted on endothelium stimulate rolling leukocytes to express activated β$_2$ integrins, which mediate firm adhesion via endothelial ICAMs. Leukocytes sense chemokine gradients, polarize, and become poised to crawl.[9] Motion involves shear-dependent coordinated cytoskeletal remodeling, involving expansion of the leading edge (lamellipodium), myosin-based contraction at the trailing edge (uropod), release of the uropod from substrate, and membrane lipid movement. Navigation through tissue may require relays of chemokines and adhesion molecules.

Chemokines may also modulate cell proliferation and death pathways.[10] Inflammatory chemokines may induce mediator release (e.g. defensins, proteases, perforins, histamine, eicosanoids), resulting in cytotoxic or vasomotor responses. Nevertheless, when injected systemically

chemokines are typically well tolerated. Some chemokines, e.g. CXCL9–11, have direct antibacterial activity.

■ CHEMOKINE SIGNALING PATHWAYS ■

Chemokines trigger chemokine receptors to act as guanine nucleotide exchange factors (GEF), mainly for G$_i$-type G proteins.[11,12] This results in G protein activation and dissociation into α and βγ subunits, which in turn leads to the activation of diverse G protein-dependent effectors, including phospholipases A2, C (subtypes β2 and β3) and D, phosphatidylinositol-3-kinase γ (PI3Kγ), protein tyrosine kinases (PTK) and phosphatases, low molecular weight GTPases, and mitogen-activated protein kinases (Fig. 11.2).

Cytosolic and calcium-independent PLA2 catalyze the formation of arachidonic acid from membrane phospholipids and have been shown to enhance chemokine activation of human monocyte chemotaxis. PLC hydrolyzes PI-4,5-bisphosphate (PIP$_2$) to form 1,2-diacylglycerol (DAG) and inositol-1,4,5-trisphosphate (IP$_3$). IP$_3$ induces Ca^{2+} release from intracellular stores which acts with DAG to activate protein kinase C (PKC). PI3Kγ phosphorylates PIP$_2$ to form PIP$_3$, which recruits proteins containing pleckstrin homology (PH) or PHOX (PX) domains to lamellipodium, thereby converting shallow extracellular chemokine gradients to steep intracellular effector gradients. Four PH domain-containing targets – AKT and GEFs for RAC, RHO and CDC42 – modulate distinct phases of cell movement in various model systems. RHO regulates cell adhesion and chemotaxis, and myosin contraction. RAC and CDC42 respectively control lamellipodia and filipodia formation. Downstream targets of RAC include PAK1, which also regulates myosin contraction.

G_i-INDEPENDENT EFFECTORS

Chemokines may activate effectors such as MAP kinases and nonreceptor PTKs by G_i-independent mechanisms. One proposed mechanism involves direct coupling to a scaffold/adaptor protein, such as β arrestin or a PDZ domain protein, which brings sequentially acting effectors into proximity of each other and the receptor. A second mechanism involves receptor cross-activation by inducing growth factor release. A third proposes JAK2 action upstream of G_i, e.g., for CCL2 chemotaxis of T cells. In a fourth, high concentrations of CCL5 form fibrillar aggregates that induce T-cell proliferation through a PTK-dependent mechanism.

■ REGULATION OF CHEMOKINE ACTION ■

Chemokine and chemokine receptor expression may be positively or negatively regulated at the transcriptional level by diverse factors, including proinflammatory cytokines, oxidant stress, viruses, bacterial products such as LPS and N-formyl peptides, cell adhesion, antigen uptake, T-cell co-stimulation, and diverse transcription factors including NF-κB. Proinflammatory cytokines such as IL-1, TNF and IL-15 induce expression of many of the inflammatory chemokines involved in innate immunity, such as CXCL8. Immunoregulatory cytokines such as IFN-γ and IL-4 are more tightly focused on Th1 (CXCL9–11)- and Th2 (CCL11)-selective chemokines, respectively. Interferons, glucocorticoids and anti-inflammatory cytokines (e.g., IL-10, TGF-β) may inhibit inflammatory chemokine gene expression. Chemokines may also be regulated at the level of mRNA stability.

A chemokine gene may generate families of proteins that vary in activity and potency by alternative splicing and post-translational modification, especially N- and C-terminal proteolytic trimming. Identified proteases may target many chemokines (e.g., CD26 [dipeptidyl peptidase IV] and matrix metalloproteinases [MMP]), or few or only one (e.g., TACE [the TNF-α-converting enzyme], plasmin, urokinase plasminogen activator and cathepsin G).[13] Chemokine action may be blocked by chemokine-binding proteins (e.g., Duffy), endogenous receptor antagonists, receptor decoys and autoantibodies. In addition, cytokines may convert a signaling receptor into a decoy (e.g., IL-10 inactivates CCR2 on monocytes). Also, a receptor may have different functions on different cell types. Chemokine receptor signaling can also be regulated by RGS (regulators of G protein signaling) proteins and by homologous and heterologous desensitization, which involves phosphorylation by G protein-coupled receptor kinases or PKC and PKA, respectively, and internalization by clathrin-dependent and -independent mechanisms.

■ CHEMOKINE REGULATION OF HEMATOPOIESIS ■

CXCL12 IN MYELOPOIESIS AND B LYMPHOPOIESIS

Most chemokines that modulate hematopoietic progenitor cell (HPC) proliferation *ex vivo* act early during hematopoiesis and are inhibitory.[14] CXCL12 is an important exception.[15, 16] The most abundant chemokine in bone marrow, CXCL12 was originally identified as a pre-B-cell stimulatory factor from stromal cells that also enhanced HPC colony formation *ex vivo*. Later, mice lacking CXCL12 or its receptor CXCR4 were shown to have severe defects in bone marrow myelopoiesis and B-cell lymphopoiesis (Table 11.5). CXCR4 is also critical for mobilization of human peripheral blood progenitor cells from bone marrow in humans, and for engraftment of human hematopoietic stem cells in SCID mice.

CXCR4 is also expressed on platelets, megakaryocytes, and most mature peripheral blood leukocytes. However, its precise importance in trafficking is undefined, partly because CXCL12 and CXCR4 knockout mice die in the perinatal period. These animals have multiple developmental abnormalities, including a ventricular septal defect, defective gastric vascularization, and subtle defects in neurodevelopment. Thus CXCL12 and CXCR4 comprise an essential chemokine-receptor pair with unusually pleotropic functions.

MYELOSUPPRESSIVE CHEMOKINES

When added to bone marrow culture systems *ex vivo*, many chemokines are able to suppress growth factor-dependent colony formation, apparently by acting directly on stem cells and early progenitors.[15] The *in vivo* significance of *ex vivo* myelosuppressive activity remains unclear for most chemokines and chemokine receptors. CXCR2 is a notable exception, at least in mice. CXCR2$^{-/-}$ mice develop massive neutrophilia, splenomegaly, myeloid hyperplasia, and expansion of HPCs. CXCR2-dependent myelosuppression may be important for opposing overstimulation of hematopoiesis induced by environmental flora, as this phenotype is absent in mice derived in germ-free conditions. These mice also develop lymph node B-cell hyperplasia, which may occur by an indirect mechanism.

T LYMPHOPOIESIS

During development T cells must migrate from the thymic cortex to the medulla. Chemokines and chemokine receptors are differentially expressed in the thymus and could coordinate migration. However, their precise roles remain unclear.

CCR9 and its ligand, CCL25, may be important, as competitive transplantation of CCR9$^{-/-}$ bone marrow is less efficient than normal marrow at repopulating the thymus of lethally irradiated Rag-1$^{-/-}$ mice. CCL25 is expressed by medullary dendritic cells and both cortical and medullary epithelial cells. CCR9 is expressed on the majority of immature CD4$^+$CD8$^+$ thymocytes, but is downregulated during transition to the CD4$^+$ or CD8$^+$ single-positive stage (Fig. 11.3). Just before thymic egress, thymocytes become CCR9 negative and upregulate L-selectin. Transition from CD4$^+$CD8$^+$ thymocytes in the cortex to CD4 or CD8

Table 11.5 Some phenotypes of chemokine receptor knockout mice

Receptor	Phenotype		
	Infectious disease	*Inflammation*	*Development*
CXCR2	Increased susceptibility to: *T. gondii* Brain abscess *Onchocerca volvulus* *E.coli* pyelonephritis	Reduced: Wound healing *A. fumigatus* AHR urate crystal-induced synovitis	Expansion of neutrophils and B cells in blood, marrow and lymphoid organs (not seen when derived in germ-free environment)
CXCR3	Increased susceptibility to MTb	Delayed cardiac allograft rejection	
CXCR4			Perinatal lethality Defective: Ventricular septum bone marrow myelopoiesis B-cell lymphopoiesis Gastric vascularization Cerebellar granule cell migration
CXCR5			Few Peyer's patches, no inguinal LN Defective germinal centers and B cell homing to LN
CXCR7			Defective cardiac development
CCR1	Increased susceptibility to: *T. gondii* Pneumonia virus of mice *A. fumigatus*	Increased: Th1 response and glomerular injury in nephrotoxic nephritis model Th2 response to SEA Reduced: Neutrophilic alveolitis in pancreatitis–ARDS model airway remodeling and Th2 response in *A. fumigatus* model Th1 response and resistance to EAE Th1 response to PPD Delayed cardiac allograft rejection	NR
CCR2	Increased susceptibility to: *C. neoformans* Mouse hepatitis virus *L. monocytogenes* *L. major* *M tuberculosis* Resistance to: *L. donovani* *Influenza A*	Decreased: EAE response to PPD Atherosclerosis Cardiac allograft rejection AHR to CRA Dextran sulfate-mediated colitis Thioglycollate-induced peritonitis FITC and bleomycin-induced pulmonary fibrosis recruited to injured nerve DTH monocyte extravasation Increased: AHR to OVA AHR to *A. fumigatus* glomerulonephritis in antiglomerular basement membrane antibody model	Enhanced myeloid progenitor cell cycling and apoptosis

SEA, *Schistosoma mansoni* soluble egg antigen; OVA, ovalbumin; CRA, cockroach antigen; AHR, airway hyperreactivity; LN, lymph node; DC, dendritic cell; DTH, delayed type hypersensitivity; NR, not reported.

Continued

Table 11.5 Some phenotypes of chemokine receptor knockout mice—cont'd

	Phenotype		
Receptor	Infectious disease	Inflammation	Development
CCR3		ip OVA sensitization→OVA challenge: Increased AHR and airway mast cells; decreased airway eos, trapped between elastic lamina and endothelial cells. Epicutaneous OVA sensitization→OVA challenge: Protection from allergic skin inflammation and AHR. Eos and mast cells not recruited to skin or lung	Decreased eos in gut
CCR4		Increased susceptibility to lps	
CCR5	Increased susceptibility to: L. monocytogenes C. neoformans T. gondii Influenza A L. major Resistance to: L. donovani	Decreased: Dextran sulfate-mediated colitis Lps toxicity Mouse hepatitis virus-induced demyelination due to decreased Mφ recruitment to CNS Cardiac allograft rejection Increased: DTH Humoral response to T dependent Ag	
CCR6		Defective CRA-induced allergic airway inflammation Increased contact hypersensitivity to 2,4-dinitrofluorobenzene Resistance to DTH to allogeneic splenocytes	Absent myeloid CD11b+ CD11c+ dendritic-cells in subepithelial dome of Peyer's patches. Increased T cells in intestinal mucosa Impaired humoral immune response to orally administered antigen and to rotavirus.
CCR7		Delayed humoral response Defective contact sensitivity Defective DTH	Defective lymphocyte and DC migration to LN Undeveloped T-cell zones Impaired trafficking of T cells and DC to LN
CCR8		Defective SEA-induced granuloma formation; Decreased OVA- and CRA-induced allergic airway inflammation	
CCR9			Decreased preproB cells, but nl T and B cells Decreased ratio of gut intraepithelial T-cell-to-epithelial cell ratio due to decreased γδ T cells
CX3CR1	Increased susceptibility to Salmonella infection	Resistance to cardiac allograft rejection in cyclosporine A treated animals Resistance to atherosclerosis	
Duffy		Increased or decreased neutrophil mobilization, depending on the model	
D6		Psoriasiform dermatitis	

model of *Leishmania* infection. CCR7 is also a major lymph node trafficking receptor for naïve T cells.

The CCR7 ligand CCL21 is constitutively expressed on afferent lymphatic endothelium, high endothelial venules (HEV), stromal cells and interdigitating dendritic cells in T zones of lymph nodes, Peyer's patches, mucosa-associated lymphoid tissue and spleen. It is not expressed in B-cell zones or sinuses. CCL19, another CCR7 ligand, is also restricted to the T zone and is expressed on interdigitating DCs.

CCR7$^{-/-}$ mice and the *plt* mouse, which is naturally deficient in CCL19 and a CCL21 isoform expressed in secondary lymphoid organs, have similar phenotypes: atrophic T-cell zones populated by a paucity of naïve T cells. This and the failure of activated DC to migrate to lymph node from the skin of these mice explain why contact sensitivity, delayed-type hypersensitivity and antibody production are severely impaired.

CXCR5 is expressed on all peripheral blood and tonsillar B cells, but on only a fraction of bone marrow B cells. Its ligand CXCL13 is expressed constitutively on follicular high endothelial venules (HEV) and controls trafficking of CXCR5 positive B and T cells from the blood into follicles. In CXCR5$^{-/-}$ mice B cells do not migrate to lymph node, Peyer's patches are abnormal, and inguinal lymph nodes are absent. CXCL13 is also required for B1 cell homing, natural antibody production, and body cavity immunity. CXCR5$^{-/-}$ mice still can produce antibody, perhaps partly because B cells and follicular DC are able, by an unknown mechanism, to form ectopic germinal centers within T zones of the periarteriolar lymphocyte sheath of the spleen.

CXCR5 and CCR7 are probably not the only chemokine receptors responsible for afferent trafficking of leukocytes to lymph nodes. CCL9 has been reported to mediate monocyte homing. CCR4 and CCR8 are expressed on a subset of human peripheral blood CD4^{+}CD25^{+}CTLA4^{+} T cells, which are associated with suppression of T-cell responses and may be important in the generation of tolerance.[23] Mature DCs attract these cells *in vitro* by secreting CCR4 ligands CCL17 and CCL22. In addition, inflamed peripheral tissues may exert 'remote control' over which leukocyte populations home to draining lymph nodes from the blood by 'projecting' their local chemokine profile to HEVs of the draining lymph node. Migration of T cells to splenic red pulp may involve local production of CXCL16. NK-T cells, activated CD4 T cells and activated CD8 T cells are found in this area. They express the CXCL16 receptor CXCR6. CXCL16 is also made by DCs in the T zone, and CXCR6 is also found on intraepithelial lymphocytes. Thus, CXCL16 may function in T-cell–DC interactions and in regulating movements of activated T cells in the splenic red pulp and in peripheral tissues.

Migration within lymph node microenvironments

CXCR5 is expressed on a majority of memory CD4 T cells in the follicles of inflamed tonsils. Follicular helper T cells (T$_{FH}$), a CD57^{+} subset of CXCR5^{+} T cells, lack CCR7, which licenses them to move from the T zone following activation to the follicles, where they provide help for B-cell maturation and antibody production. They do not produce Th1 or Th2 cytokines upon activation. Reciprocally, B cells activated by antigen in the follicles upregulate CCR7 and move towards the T zone. Thus B–T interaction may be facilitated by reciprocal movement of these cells, which may be influenced by the balance of chemokines made in adjacent lymphoid zones.[24] CXCR4 signaling may also be important in naïve and memory B-cell trafficking to germinal centers, and CCR5

ligands may guide naïve CD8 T cells to sites of CD4 T cell–dendritic cell interaction in lymph nodes.[25]

Efferent trafficking

Naïve lymphocytes that do not encounter antigen continue to recirculate between the blood and secondary lymphoid tissue without acquiring any tissue-specific homing properties. Most antigen-stimulated T cells die by apoptosis. The survivors may be divided into functionally distinct subsets marked by characteristic patterns of chemokine receptor expression. In general, the trafficking properties of these cells are not well understood. Within CD4 T cells, three memory subsets and two main effector subsets have been proposed. The memory subsets include T$_{FH}$ cells, described previously, effector memory (T$_{EM}$) and central memory cells (T$_{CM}$). T$_{EM}$ express L-selectin but lack CCR7. They may traffic through peripheral tissues as immune surveillance cells, rapidly releasing cytokines in response to activation by recall antigens. T$_{CM}$ express CCR7 and lymph node homing receptors. They traffic between the blood and secondary lymphoid organs, but are not polarized and lack immediate effector function. Instead, they may interact efficiently with DCs in lymph nodes and differentiate into T$_{EM}$ upon secondary stimulation. Highly heterogeneous, multifunctional human T$_{EM}$ may be produced early in differentiation and may become stable resting cells.[26] Both memory populations can be activated by APCs and antigen.

The classic effector subsets Th1 and Th2 (Chapters 17 and 18) downregulate CXCR5 and CCR7 and upregulate inflammatory chemokine receptors. This switch facilitates their exit from lymph nodes via efferent lymphatics and their homing to inflamed sites. *In vivo*, combinations of receptors rather than any single receptor appear to hold the strongest association with these functional subsets in the blood, and there is a hierarchy of chemokine receptor expression associated with the age of the cell.[26]

In vivo, Th1 cells, which by the simplest definition secrete IFN-γ but not IL-4 and control cellular and humoral immunity to intracellular pathogens, more frequently express CXCR3, CXCR6, CCR2, CCR5 and CX3CR1 than do Th2 cells. In contrast, Th2 cells, which express IL-4 but not IFN-γ and are associated with cellular and humoral immunity to extracellular pathogens and allergic inflammation, more frequently express CCR3, CCR4 and CCR8 than do Th1 cells. CXCR3 expression has been most consistently associated with Th1 immune responses and Th1-associated disease. Consistent with this, its agonists CXCL9–11 are highly induced by IFN-γ but not IL-4. Thus in Th1 immunity there is the potential for a positive feedback loop in which IFN-γ induces production of CXCL9-11, which then recruit CXCR3^{+} Th1 cells that produce IFN-γ. 'Th1 chemokines' may also help maintain Th1 dominance through their ability to block CCR3. Specific cytokines, microenvironments and inflammatory stresses may differentially regulate CXCL9-11 expression, which may account for specialized biological roles.

Similarly, in Th2 immunity IL-4 and IL-13 made at inflamed sites in the periphery may induce production of CCL7, CCL11 and other CCR3 ligands, the CCR4 ligands CCL17 and CCL22, and the CCR8 ligand CCL1. CCR3 is expressed on a subset of Th2 T lymphocytes as well as on eosinophils and basophils, the three major cell types associated with Th2 type allergic inflammation. Th2 cells are also associated with CCR4 expression. Arrival of Th2 cells amplifies a positive feedback loop through the secretion of additional IL-4. CCL7 and CCL11 may block Th1 responses by antagonizing CCR2, CXCR3 and CCR5.

Th17 cells, a recently described effector CD4 T cell subset that makes IL-17, all express CCR6.

CD4 T-cell differentiation

Some chemokines appear to also regulate the differentiation of Th1 and Th2 cells. CCL2 and its receptor CCR2 have been most extensively studied in this regard. At first glance their contribution appears contradictory, as *in vivo* CCR2 is strongly associated with Th1 immune responses and CCL2 is associated with Th2 responses. However, CCL2 appears to promote Th2 polarization directly, by inhibiting IL-12 production in monocytes and by enhancing IL-4 but not IFN-γ production in memory and activated T cells. Thus, CCL2 influences both innate immunity, through effects on monocyte trafficking, and adaptive immunity, through control of Th-cell polarization and trafficking.[27] In the case of aerosol challenge with *Mycobacterium tuberculosis* in CCR2$^{-/-}$ mice, DC migration to draining lymph nodes is markedly impaired, which preempts any direct effects of CCL2 on T cells. Why CCL2 and CCR2 have opposite effects on Th polarization is unclear, but is most likely due to ligand–receptor promiscuity.

The role of CCL3 and its receptors on T-cell polarization is also complex. In mice, CCL3 can directly enhance IFN-γ production in activated T cells, and CCL3 neutralization attenuates Th1-driven experimental autoimmune encephalomyelitis and Th1-dependent granuloma formation. Nevertheless, mice lacking the CCL3 receptor CCR1 typically have reduced Th2 responses. This suggests a role for CCR5 in mediating the Th1-polarizing effects of CCL3. This is consistent with the role of CCR5 in mediating CD8α$^+$ DC trafficking and IL-12 production in the spleen in mice injected with Stag, a soluble *Toxoplasma gondii* antigen preparation. Nevertheless, CCR5$^{-/-}$ mice have also been reported to have enhanced delayed-type hypersensitivity reactions and increased humoral responses to T cell—dependent antigenic challenge. This indicates a role for CCR5 in downmodulating certain T cell—dependent immune responses as well.

Tissue-specific lymphocyte homing

CLA$^+$ T lymphocytes, which home to skin, preferentially express CCR4 and CCR10.[28] The CCR4 ligand CCL22 is made by resident dermal macrophages and DCs, whereas the CCR10 ligand CCL27 is made by keratinocytes. Blocking both of these pathways, but not either one alone, has been reported to inhibit lymphocyte recruitment to the skin in a DTH model. This implies that these two molecules may act redundantly as well as independently of inflammatory chemokines.

Homing to the small intestine is determined in part by T-lymphocyte expression of the integrin α$_4$β$_7$ and CCR9.[28] The α$_4$β$_7$ ligand MAdCAM-1 and the CCR9 ligand CCL25 co-localize on normal and inflamed small intestinal endothelium. Most T cells in the intraepithelial and lamina propria zones of the small intestine express CCR9. These cells, which are mainly TCRγδ$^+$ or TCRαβ$^+$CD8αβ$^+$, are reduced in the small intestine of CCR9$^{-/-}$ mice.

As B cells differentiate into plasma cells, they downregulate CXCR5 and CCR7 and exit lymph nodes. B immunoblasts expressing IgG coordinately upregulate CXCR4, which promotes homing to the bone marrow, whereas B immunoblasts expressing IgA specifically migrate

to mucosal sites. Like gut-homing T cells, B immunoblasts that home to small intestine express α$_4$β$_7$ integrin and CCR9 and respond to CCL25.[29]

■ CHEMOKINES AND DISEASE ■

There is a vast literature correlating the presence of chemokines with diverse human diseases, but strong evidence that they are actually involved in pathogenesis is available for only a small subset of these.

Opposite effects of CCR5 in HIV and West Nile virus infection

HIV envelope glycoprotein gp120 mediates fusion of the viral envelope with the target cell membrane by binding to CD4 and a chemokine receptor.[30] Both CCR5 and CXCR4 physically associate with CD4 and gp120, and are therefore referred to as 'HIV co-receptors'. HIV strains are functionally classified and named according to their specificity for CXCR4 (X4 strains), CCR5 (R5 strains), or both (R5X4 strains).

▌ CLINICAL RELEVANCE

Examples of the chemokine system and disease

>> WHIM syndrome (warts, hypogammaglobulinemia, infection, myelokathexis) and truncating gain-of-function mutations in CXCR4.

>> Resistance to *Plasmodium vivax* malaria and with a nonfunctional promoter variant in Duffy.

>> Resistance to initial HIV infection and susceptibility to West Nile virus disease in patients homozygous for a loss-of-function CCR5 allele (*CCR5Δ32*).

>> Reduction of HIV viral load in AIDS patients treated with CCR5 antagonists.

>> Induction of Kaposi's sarcoma-like tumors in mice forced to express human herpes virus 8 vGPCR.

>> Atherosclerotic cardiovascular disease and CX3CR1.
Reduced risk is associated with loss-of-function CX3CR1 M280 allele.

>> Autoimmune heparin-induced thrombocytopenia and CXCL4.
Caused by autoAb production to CXCL4-heparin complexes, causing activation of platelets and microvascular endothelial cells.

>> Chronic renal allograft rejection and CCR5.
Reduced risk associated with homozygous CCR5Δ32.

>> Rheumatoid arthritis and CCR5
Reduced risk associated with CCR5Δ32.

>> Eosinophilic esophagitis and CCL26
Disease is associated with CCL26 variant.

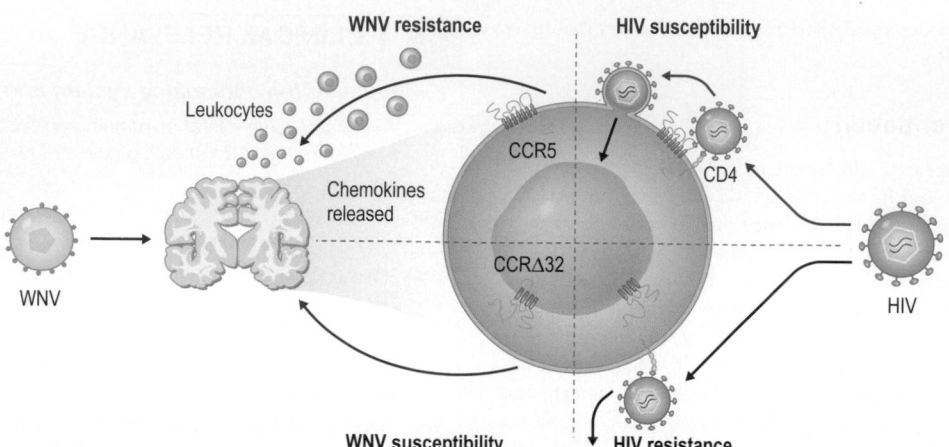

Fig. 11.4 CCR5 facilitates HIV infection, but restricts West Nile virus infection. The mutant receptor CCR5Δ32 is not expressed on the cell surface and cannot be used for cell entry by HIV or to respond to West Nile virus.

The importance of CCR5 in clinical HIV/AIDS is revealed most clearly by *CCR5Δ32*, a nonfunctional allele that occurs in ~20% of North American Caucasians. Homozygotes are highly resistant to R5 HIV, the main transmitting strain, and HIV-infected heterozygotes have slower disease progression. Homozygotes appear healthy, as do unstressed CCR5 knockout mice. This has encouraged the development of CCR5-blocking agents for application in HIV/AIDS. Recently, maravicor (Pfizer) has been approved by the FDA for this indication.

CCR5 is also important in the pathogenesis of West Nile virus (WNV) infection, but in this case it plays a protective role (Fig. 11.4).[31] In mice, WNV challenge is uniformly fatal when CCR5 has been genetically disrupted, and in humans homozygous *CCR5Δ32* is strongly associated with symptomatic WNV infection in patient cohorts. The mechanism appears to be a decrease in antiviral defense by diminishing recruitment of CCR5+ leukocytes into the brain. Thus the same receptor that appears to promote HIV infection restricts WNV infection. Theoretically, therefore, CCR5-blocking agents could increase the risk of viral infections other than HIV, particularly in the setting of HIV/AIDS, where the immune system is already compromised.

Malaria

Analogous to CCR5 and HIV, Duffy, the 7TM promiscuous chemokine-binding protein, is required for infection of erythrocytes by *Plasmodium vivax*, a major cause of malaria.[32] The parasite ligand, which is named the *Plasmodium vivax* Duffy binding protein (PvDBP), is expressed in micronemes of merozoites and binds to the N-terminal domain of Duffy via a cysteine-rich domain. This interaction is required for junction formation during invasion, but not for initial binding or parasite orientation. A deficiency of Duffy expression has been described in individuals who have inherited a single nucleotide substitution in the Duffy promoter (−46C) at an erythroid-specific GATA-1 site. This deficiency is fixed in sub-Saharan Africa, but not in other malaria-endemic regions of the world. Accordingly, *P. vivax* malaria is rare in

sub-Saharan Africa, but common in Central and South America, India and Southeast Asia. Fixation of the mutation in Africa presumably occurred because of positive selective pressure from malaria. Identification of the −46C mutation in the Melanesian Duffy allele among individuals living in a *P. vivax*-endemic region of Papua New Guinea provides an opportunity to test this hypothesis prospectively. Together with CCR5Δ32, Duffy −46C is the strongest genetic resistance factor known for any infectious disease in man. Duffy deficiency in man and knockout mice is not associated with any known health problems.

WHIM Syndrome

Truncating mutations in the C tail of CXCR4 that prolong receptor signaling by delaying desensitization and blocking internalization have been strongly linked genetically to family cohorts with WHIM syndrome (*w*arts, *h*ypogammaglobulinemia, *i*nfection and *my*elokathexis [neutropenia without maturation arrest]).[33] Myelokathexis can be explained by exaggeration of the normal bone marrow retention action of CXCR4 for myeloid cells. The exact mechanism underlying the selective predisposition to papillomavirus infection is unknown.

Atherosclerosis

Macrophages are the dominant leukocyte in atherosclerotic lesions and are associated with the presence of macrophage-targeted chemokines such as CCL2, CCL5 and CX3CL1. CCL2−/−, CCR2−/−, CX3CL1−/−, and CX3CR1−/− mice demonstrate a reduction in the accumulation of macrophages which is associated with a reduction in vessel wall lesion size. Adoptive transfer studies with bone marrow from CXCR2−/− mice have also revealed a role for that receptor in promoting atherosclerosis in mouse models, apparently by promoting monocyte adhesion to early atherosclerotic endothelium through interaction with its mouse ligand KC and activation of the VLA-4/VCAM-1 adhesion system.

KEY CONCEPTS

The viral chemokine system

Studies of the viral chemokine system can yield insight into the role of chemokines in immunoregulation. Viral chemokine elements may also have applications as therapeutic agents.

>> Structural classification

Chemokines (e.g., HHV8 vMIP-I, II and III)
7TM chemokine receptors (e.g., HCMV US28, HHV8 vGPCR)
Chemokine-binding proteins (e.g., γHV68 vCKBP-III)
Chemokine mimics (e.g., HIV gp120)

>> Functional classification

Cell entry factors (e.g., HIV gp120)
Leukocyte chemoattractants (e.g., HHV8 vMIP-II)
Immune evasion
Chemokine scavengers (e.g., γHV68 vCKBP-III)
Chemokine receptor antagonists (e.g., MCV MC148-R)
Angiogenic factors (e.g., HHV8 vGPCR)
Growth factors (e.g., HHV8 vGPCR)

The CX3CR1 genetic variant CX3CR1-M280, which lacks normal CX3CL1-dependent adhesive function under conditions of physiologic flow, has been associated with a reduced risk of atherosclerotic vascular disease in human.[34] Mechanistic studies suggest that CX3CL1 on coronary artery smooth muscle cells anchors macrophages via CX3CR1.

Kaposi's sarcoma

HHV8 provides an example of the function of virally encoded chemokines and chemokine receptors. It encodes three CC chemokines, vMIP-I, II and III, as well as a constitutively active CC/CXC chemokine receptor named vGPCR, which is encoded by ORF74. All of these factors are angiogenic and may contribute to the pathogenesis of Kaposi's sarcoma (KS), a highly vascular multicentric nonclonal tumor caused by HHV8, typically in the setting of immunosuppression such as in HIV/AIDS. Consistent with this, vGPCR induces KS-like tumors when expressed in transgenic mice.[35] The mechanism may involve activation of NF-κB and the induction of angiogenic factors and proinflammatory cytokines. This virus appears to have converted a hijacked receptor, probably CXCR2, into a regulator of gene expression.

Autoimmunity

Two human diseases have been identified in which chemokines act as autoantigens for autoantibodies. The first, heparin-induced thrombocytopenia (HIT), is the only human autoimmune disease directly linked mechanistically to chemokines. An established risk factor for thromboembolic complications of heparin therapy, HIT occurs in 1–5% of patients treated with heparin, and is the result of autoantibodies that bind specifically to CXCL4–heparin complexes in plasma. The second, autoimmune myositis, is associated with autoantibodies to histidyl tRNA synthetase, a protein synthesis factor that is also able to induce DC chemotaxis, apparently by acting as an agonist at CCR5. Its exact importance in promoting inflammation in myositis has not been established.

In general, T cell-dependent autoimmune diseases in human, such as psoriasis, multiple sclerosis (MS), rheumatoid arthritis (RA), and type I diabetes mellitus, are associated with inflammatory chemokines and tissue infiltration by T lymphocytes and monocytes expressing inflammatory chemokine receptors. The relative importance of these is not yet known. Patients homozygous for the CCR5 null allele *CCR5Δ32* have been reported who have MS, indicating that this receptor is not required for disease. An association of this allele with outcome in MS has not been firmly established. CCL2 and CCR2, and to a lesser extent CCL3 and CCR1, knockout mice have reduced disease in experimental allergic encephalomyelitis (EAE), a model of MS. Moreover, neutralization of CCL3 and CCL2 respectively markedly reduced the early and relapsing phases of EAE.

MCP-1, a dominant negative antagonist of CCL2, inhibits arthritis in the MRL-*lpr* mouse model of RA, suggesting a potential role for CCL2 and CCR2. Met-RANTES, a chemically modified variant of CCL5 that blocks CCR1, CCR3 and CCR5, was beneficial in a collagen-induced arthritis model in DBA/I mice. A meta-analysis has shown a protective effect for *CCR5Δ32* in RA. In the NOD mouse model of diabetes, insulitis and hyperglycemia were reduced in CCL3 knockout mice.

Paradoxically, in some cases blocking chemokine receptors may lead to increased inflammation, as shown for CCR1 and CCR2 in nephrotoxic nephritis and glomerulonephritis mouse models. This is associated with increased renal recruitment of CD4 and CD8 T cells, macrophages, and enhanced Th1 immune responses. The exact mechanism remains unclear.

Acute neutrophil-mediated inflammatory disorders

Many neutrophil-mediated human diseases have been associated with the presence of CXCL8, including psoriasis, gout, acute glomerulonephritis, acute respiratory disease syndrome (ARDS), rheumatoid arthritis and ischemia–reperfusion injury. Systemic administration of neutralizing anti-CXCL8 antibodies is protective in diverse models of neutrophil-mediated acute inflammation in the rabbit (skin, airway, pleura, glomeruli), providing proof of concept that CXCL8 is a nonredundant mediator of innate immunity and acute pathologic inflammation in these settings. CXCR2 knockout mice are less susceptible to acute urate crystal-induced gouty synovitis. And, SB-265610, a nonpeptide small molecule antagonist with exquisite selectivity for CXCR2, prevents neutrophil accumulation in the lungs of hyperoxia-exposed newborn rats. Together these results identify CXCL8 and its receptors as candidate drug targets for diseases mediated by acute neutrophilic inflammation. CXCR2 knockout mice also have delayed wound healing.

Transplant rejection

An advantage of transplant rejection over other animal models of human disease is that in both humans and animals the time of antigenic challenge is precisely known. The most extensive analysis of the role of chemokines in transplant rejection has been carried out in an MHC class I/II-mismatched cardiac allograft rejection model in the mouse, which is mediated by a Th1 immune response.[36] Similar sets of inflammatory chemokines are found in the mouse model as in the human disease. ELR CXC chemokines and CCL2 appear early, and are probably made by engrafted blood vessel endothelial cells. These are associated with neutrophil and mononuclear cell accumulation. On day 3 after engraftment CCL2 is still present and the three CXCR3 ligands CXCL9-11 and the CCR5 ligands

CCL4 and CCL5 appear. Of the CXCR3 ligands, CXCL10 appears earliest and in the largest amounts, probably in response to IFN-γ coming from NK cells. This phase is associated with transition to an adaptive immune response, with accumulation of trafficking of recipient T cells, macrophages and DCs to the graft, followed by acute and chronic rejection. Graft arteriosclerosis, which is distinct from the lipid-driven disease, may be driven in part by CXCL10 and IFN-γ.

Analysis of knockout mice has demonstrated that although multiple chemokine receptors contribute to rejection in this model, there is a marked rank order: CXCR3>>CCR5>CCR1 = CX3CR1 = CCR2. Most impressively, rejection and graft arteriosclerosis do not occur if the recipient mouse, treated with a brief, subtherapeutic course of cyclosporine A, is CXCR3$^{-/-}$, or if the donor heart is CXCL10$^{-/-}$. This identifies the CXCR3/CXCL10 axis as a potential drug target. Neutralization of CXCL9, a CXCR3 ligand which appears later than CXCL10, can also prolong cardiac allograft survival. It delays T-cell infiltration and acute rejection in class II MHC-disparate skin allografts. In rat, BX-471, a nonpeptide small molecule antagonist of CCR1, was reported to be effective in heart transplant rejection.

In humans, CCR5 may be important in chronic kidney allograft rejection, as in a large German kidney transplantation cohort individuals homozygous for *CCR5Δ32* were underrepresented among patients with this outcome.

Allergic airway and intestinal disease

Chemokine receptors associated with asthma include CXCR2, CCR3, CCR4 and CCR8. CCR3 is present on eosinophils, basophils, mast cells and some Th2 T cells. CCR4 and CCR8 identify airway T cells of allergen-challenged atopic asthmatics. CCR8 knockout mice have reduced allergic airway inflammation in response to three different Th2-polarizing antigens: *Schistosoma mansoni* soluble egg antigen, ovalbumin and cockroach antigen. The situation with the CCR4 axis is unsettled, as neutralization of the CCR4 ligand CCL22 was protective in a mouse model of airway hyperreactivity and eosinophilic inflammation, but CCR4 gene knockout was not. A role for the CCR3 axis in asthma has been supported by CCL11 neutralization in guinea pig, and CCR3 gene knockout in mouse.[37] Only one of three studies of CCL11 knockout mice found protection, ~40% reduction in airway eosinophils in ovalbumin sensitized/challenged mice, possibly due to compensation by other CCR3 ligands. The net effect of CCR3 knockout was expected to be more profound. However, the exact phenotype depends dramatically on the specific method of sensitization and challenge owing to complex and opposite effects on eosinophil and mast cell trafficking. Thus CCR3$^{-/-}$ mice sensitized intraperitoneally have reduced eosinophil extravasation into the lung, but an increase in mast cell homing to the trachea. The net result is a paradoxical increase in airway responsiveness to cholinergic stimulation. Mast cell mobilization is not seen after epicutaneous sensitization, and these animals have reduced airway eosinophilia on challenge and no increase in airway hyperresponsiveness. CCR6 also appears to play a role, as CCR6$^{-/-}$ mice have decreased allergic airway inflammation in response to sensitization and challenge with cockroach antigen, which is consistent with the induction of its ligand CCL20 in this model.

Eosinophilic esophagitis has been associated with a CCL26 variant.[17] Although there is no CCL26 homolog in mouse, other mouse CCR3 ligands have been implicated in a mouse model of this disease.

Cancer

Many chemokines have been detected *in situ* in tumors, and cancer cells have been shown to produce chemokines and express chemokine receptors. However, the exact role played by endogenous tumor-associated chemokines in recruiting tumor-infiltrating lymphocytes and tumor-associated macrophages and in promoting an anti-tumor immune response has not been delineated. On the contrary, there are data from mouse models suggesting that the overall effect may be to promote tumorigenesis through additional effects on cell growth, angiogenesis, apoptosis, immune evasion and metastasis.[38] Controlling the balance of angiogenic and angiostatic chemokines may be particularly important. This has been shown in several instances. The ratio of ELR to non-ELR CXC chemokine expression is high in nonsmall cell lung carcinoma (NSCLC) in humans. In a Scid mouse model, neutralization of endogenous tumor-derived CXCL8 (angiogenic) inhibited tumor growth and metastasis by about 50% through a decrease in tumor-derived vessel density, without directly affecting tumor cell proliferation. Chemokine receptors on tumor cells have been shown to directly mediate chemokine-dependent proliferation. Examples include CXCL1 in melanoma, and, CXCR4 in a mouse model of metastasis in breast cancer. It remains to be seen how general these effects are in other cancers.

■ THERAPEUTIC APPLICATIONS ■

CHEMOKINES AND CHEMOKINE RECEPTORS AS TARGETS FOR DRUG DEVELOPMENT

Although chemokine-targeted drug development is still in the early stages, there are already two accomplishments that deserve special mention. First, chemokine receptors are the first cytokine receptors for which potent, selective nonpeptide small molecule antagonists have been identified that work *in vivo*. Second, targeting host determinants, as in the case of CCR5 and CXCR4 in HIV/AIDS, is a new approach in the development of antimicrobial agents. Other reasonable disease indications are Duffy in *P. vivax* malaria; CXCR2 in acute neutrophil-mediated inflammation; CXCR3 and CCR2 in Th1-driven disease; CCR2 and CX3CR1 in atherosclerosis; and CCR3 and possibly CCR4 and CCR8 in Th2 diseases such as asthma.

Potent and selective nonpeptide small molecule antagonists of CXCR2, CXCR3, CXCR4, CCR1, CCR2, CCR3 and CCR5 have been reported.[39] These molecules share a nitrogen-rich core and appear to block ligand binding by acting at a conserved allosteric site analogous to the retinal-binding site in the transmembrane region of rhodopsin. Although small molecules taken as pills are the main goal, other blocking strategies are also under consideration, such as ribozymes, modified chemokines (e.g., amino-terminally modified versions of CCL5) and intrakines, which are modified forms of chemokines delivered by gene therapy that remain in the endoplasmic reticulum and block surface expression of newly synthesized receptors.

The fact that viral anti-chemokines typically block multiple chemokines acting at multiple receptors may hint that the most clinically effective chemokine-targeted anti-inflammatory strategy will need to provide broad-spectrum coverage. In this regard, the viral anti-chemokines themselves may have a place therapeutically, although issues of antigenicity may be limiting. There is also proof of principle from work with a distamycin analog that broad-spectrum blockade with nonpeptide small molecules is feasible.

CHEMOKINES AS BIOLOGICAL RESPONSE MODIFIERS

Both inflammatory and homeostatic chemokines are being evaluated for therapeutic potential as biological response modifiers, acting mainly as immunomodulators or as regulators of angiogenesis. Studies to date have revealed no major problems with toxicity, and efficacy has been noted in models of cancer, inflammation, and infection. So far, clinical trials in cancer and stem cell protection have been disappointing. Chemokines are also being developed as vaccine adjuvants. They can be delivered either as pure protein, as immunomodulatory plasmids, or as recombinant protein within antigen-pulsed DC. In this application, the chemokine may act at several different steps in the immune response. For example, chemokines can be used to strengthen the trafficking of specific classes of immune cell through the site of vaccination, or to enhance the uptake of antigen by APCs, or to tilt the Th1/Th2 balance to a position that is optimal for a particular disease. Impressive efficacy in infectious disease, allergy and tumor models has been observed in rodents. Chemokine gene administration has also been shown to induce neutralizing antibody against the encoded chemokine, which is able to block immune responses and to ameliorate EAE and arthritis in rodent models.

Many chemokines, when delivered pharmacologically as recombinant proteins or by plasmid DNA or in transfected tumor cells, are able to induce immunologically mediated anti-tumor effects in mouse models and could be clinically useful. Mechanisms may differ depending on the model, but can involve recruitment of monocytes, NK cells and cytotoxic CD8 T cells to the tumor. Chemokines may also function as adjuvants in tumor antigen vaccines. Chemokine–tumor antigen fusion proteins represent a novel twist on this approach that facilitates the uptake of tumor antigens by APCs via the normal process of ligand–receptor internalization. Non-ELR CXC chemokines such as CXCL4 also exert anti-tumor effects through angiostatic mechanisms. Despite impressive anti-tumor effects in animal models, efforts to translate chemokines to human therapy have been slow. In the only published study, a phase I trial of CXCL4 in colon cancer, the chemokine was well-tolerated but no efficacy was observed.

CONCLUSION

Despite the size of the chemokine and chemokine-receptor families, and the wealth of molecular and functional information from mouse models of disease available for many members,[40] with few exceptions there is as yet little known about precise roles in clinical immunology. Blocking agents targeting chemokines and chemokine receptors are beginning to enter clinical trials for numerous disease indications, driven partly by the promise of a novel class of antiretroviral agents that target CCR5 in HIV/AIDS. The next phase of chemokine research will help determine the utility of chemokine-based therapeutics and provide greater insight into the roles played by these molecules in the pathogenesis of human disease.

ACKNOWLEDGMENTS

This review was supported by funding from the Division of Intramural Research, National Institute of Allergy and Infectious Diseases, NIH.

REFERENCES

1. Handel TM, Johnson Z, Crown SE, et al. Regulation of protein function by glycosaminoglycans – as exemplified by chemokines. Annu Rev Biochem 2005; 74: 385.

2. Zlotnik A, Yoshie O. Chemokines: a new classification system and their role in immunity. Immunity 2000; 12: 121.

3. Murphy PM, Baggiolini M, Charo IF, et al. International union of pharmacology. XXII. Nomenclature for chemokine receptors. Pharmacol Rev 2000; 52: 145.

4. Locati M, Torre YM, Galliera E, et al. Silent chemoattractant receptors: D6 as a decoy and scavenger receptor for inflammatory CC chemokines. Cytokine Growth Factor Rev 2005; 16: 679.

5. Murphy PM. Viral exploitation and subversion of the immune system through chemokine mimicry. Nature Immunol 2001; 2: 116.

6. Allavena P, Sica A, Vecchi A, et al. The chemokine receptor switch paradigm and dendritic cell migration: its significance in tumor tissues. Immunol Rev 2000; 177: 141.

7. Cyster JG. Chemokines, sphingosine-1-phosphate, and cell migration in secondary lymphoid organs. Annu Rev Immunol 2005; 23: 127.

8. Campbell DJ, Kim CH, Butcher EC. Chemokines in the systemic organization of immunity. Immunol Rev 2003; 195: 58.

9. Rickert P, Weiner OD, Wang F, et al. Leukocytes navigate by compass: roles of PI3Kgamma and its lipid products. Trends Cell Biol 2000; 10: 466.

10. Luther SA, Cyster JG. Chemokines as regulators of T cell differentiation. Nature Immunol 2001; 2: 102.

11. Thelen M. Dancing to the tune of chemokines. Nature Immunol 2001; 2: 129.

12. Miller WE, Lefkowitz RJ. Expanding roles for beta-arrestins as scaffolds and adapters in GPCR signaling and trafficking. Curr Opin Cell Biol 2001; 13: 139.

13. Overall CM, McQuibban GA, Clark-Lewis I. Discovery of chemokine substrates for matrix metalloproteinases by exosite scanning: a new tool for degradomics. Biol Chem 2002; 383: 1059.

14. Youn BS, Mantel C, Broxmeyer HE. Chemokines, chemokine receptors and hematopoiesis. Immunol Rev 2000; 177: 150.

15. Murdoch C. CXCR4: chemokine receptor extraordinaire. Immunol Rev 2000; 177: 175.

16. Lapidot T, Petit I. Current understanding of stem cell mobilization: the roles of chemokines, proteolytic enzymes, adhesion molecules, cytokines, and stromal cells. Exp Hematol 2002; 30: 973.

17. Blanchard C, Wang N, Stringer KF, et al. Eotaxin-3 and a uniquely conserved gene-expression profile in eosinophilic esophagitis. J Clin Invest 2006; 116: 536.

18. Gear AR, Camerini D. Platelet chemokines and chemokine receptors: linking hemostasis, inflammation, and host defense. Microcirculation 2003; 10: 335.

19. Mukaida N. Pathophysiological roles of interleukin-8/CXCL8 in pulmonary diseases. Am J Physiol Lung Cell Mol Physiol 2003; 284. L566.

20. Morris MA, Ley K. Trafficking of natural killer cells. Curr Mol Med 2004; 4: 431.

21. Coelho AL, Hogaboam CM, Kunkel SL. Chemokines provide the sustained inflammatory bridge between innate and acquired immunity. Cytokine Growth Factor Rev 2005; 16: 553.

22. Sallusto F, Mackay CR, Lanzavecchia A. The role of chemokine receptors in primary, effector, and memory immune responses. Annu Rev Immunol 2000; 18: 593.

23. D'Ambrosio D, Sinigaglia F, Adorini L. Special attractions for suppressor T cells. Trends Immunol 2003; 24: 122.

24. Vinuesa CG, Tangye SG, Moser B, Mackay CR. Follicular B helper T cells in antibody responses and autoimmunity. Nature Rev Immunol 2005; 5: 853.

25. Castellino F, Huang AY, Altan-Bonnet G, et al. Chemokines enhance immunity by guiding naive CD8+ T cells to sites of CD4+ T cell–dendritic cell interaction. Nature 2006; 440: 890.

26. Song K, Rabin RL, Hill BJ, et al. Characterization of subsets of CD4+ memory T cells reveals early branched pathways of T cell differentiation in humans. Proc Natl Acad Sci USA 2005; 102: 7916.

27. Gerard C, Rollins BJ. Chemokines and disease. Nature Immunol 2001; 2: 108.

28. Campbell JJ, Butcher EC. Chemokines in tissue-specific and microenvironment-specific lymphocyte homing. Curr Opin Immunol 2000; 12: 336.

29. Pabst O, Ohl L, Wendland M, et al. Chemokine receptor CCR9 contributes to the localization of plasma cells to the small intestine. J Exp Med 2004; 199: 411.

30. Lusso P. HIV and the chemokine system: 10 years later. EMBO J 2006; 25: 447.

31. Lim JK, Glass WG, McDermott DH, Murphy PM. CCR5: no longer a 'good for nothing' gene – chemokine control of West Nile Virus infection. Trends Immunol 2006; 27: 308.

32. Gaur D, Mayer DC, Miller LH. Parasite ligand–host receptor interactions during invasion of erythrocytes by *Plasmodium merozoites*. Int J Parasitol 2004; 34: 1413.

33. Gulino AG. WHIM syndrome: a genetic disorder of leukocyte trafficking. Curr Opin Allergy Clin Immunol 2003; 3: 443.

34. McDermott DH, Fong AM, Yang Q, et al. Chemokine receptor mutant CX3CR1-M280 has impaired adhesive function and correlates with protection from cardiovascular disease in humans. J Clin Invest 2003; 111: 1241.

35. Jensen KK, Lira SA. Chemokines and Kaposi's sarcoma. Semin Cancer Biol 2004; 14: 187.

36. Hancock WW, Gao W, Faia KL, Csizmadia V. Chemokines and their receptors in allograft rejection. Curr Opin Immunol 2000; 12: 511.

37. Smit JJ, Lukacs NW. A closer look at chemokines and their role in asthmatic responses. Eur J Pharmacol 2006; 533: 277.

38. Strieter RM. Chemokines: not just leukocyte chemoattractants in the promotion of cancer. Nature Immunol 2001; 2: 285.

39. Wells TN, Power CA, Shaw JP, Proudfoot AE. Chemokine blockers – therapeutics in the making?. Trends Pharmacol Sci 2006; 27: 41.

40. Charo IF, Ransohoff RM. The many roles of chemokines and chemokine receptors in inflammation. N Engl J Med 2006; 354: 610.

Lymphocyte adhesion and trafficking

Sirpa Jalkanen, Marko Salmi

12

Proper control of the movement of lymphocytes through the body is a prerequisite for mounting an effective immune response. Lymphocyte trafficking provides the means by which the few lymphocytes that carry a specific antigen receptor have the opportunity to encounter their counter-antigen. Antigens can be introduced into the body via practically any surface that is exposed to the environment. Not only is the area to be protected vast (about 500 m² of epithelial surfaces in the skin, gut and lungs), but also the huge numbers of circulating lymphocytes (about 10^11), the total length of the vascular tree (>100 000 km) and the velocity of the bloodborne lymphocytes in the vessels provide formidable challenges. An elaborate process termed lymphocyte trafficking has evolved to overcome these physical constraints.[1–3] The process relies on the basic concept of compartmentalizing specific functions into discrete anatomical organs and then connecting them by means of continuous lymphocyte recirculation. Both lymphoid and nonlymphoid organs and tissues are connected by two different types of vessels. The blood vessels transport lymphocytes into the various organs, where they have a chance to leave the blood and enter the tissue stroma. Vessels of the lymphatic system then collect the extravasated lymphocytes from these various organs and return them to the circulation (Fig. 12.1).

■ EARLY LYMPHOCYTE PRECURSOR TRAFFICKING TO THE PRIMARY LYMPHOID ORGANS ■

Lymphocyte trafficking begins at an early stage of human ontogeny, when lymphocyte precursor cells first appear and migrate into the primary lymphoid organs.[4] The multipotent hematopoietic stem cells from the yolk sac and from the aorta–gonad–mesonephros migrate via the circulation to the liver, which is an important organ supporting B-lymphocyte production in the embryo (Chapter 8), and then into the bone marrow. Thereafter, the developmental maturation of B cells takes place solely in the bone marrow. T cells, on the other hand, require an additional migratory event, which involves the entry of marrow-derived T-cell progenitors into the thymus. These early T-cell progenitors enter the thymus via the vessels in the cortical region. Concomitant with their differentiation and maturation via positive and negative selection, they pass from the cortex into the medulla (Chapter 9).

■ MIGRATION OF NAIVE MATURE LYMPHOCYTES FROM THE BLOOD TO THE SECONDARY LYMPHOID ORGANS ■

After completing their initial course of development, newly arisen naive B and T cells exit the primary lymphoid organs and travel through the blood into the secondary lymphoid organs. These include the peripheral lymph nodes, the organized lymphoid tissues of the gut (e.g., Peyer's patches and the appendix) and the spleen (Chapter 2). In the lymph nodes most lymphocyte trafficking from the blood to the tissues takes place in specialized postcapillary

KEY CONCEPTS

LYMPHOCYTES RECIRCULATE

>> Lymphocytes recirculate continuously between blood and lymphoid organs.

>> 80% of lymphocytes enter the lymph nodes via specialized vessels called high endothelial venules (HEV).

>> The remaining lymphocytes enter the lymph nodes together with dendritic cells and antigens via afferent lymphatics.

>> Lymphocytes leave the lymph nodes via efferent lymphatics.

>> Lymphocyte recirculation allows the lymphocytes to meet their cognate antigens and other leukocyte subsets to evoke an efficient immune response.

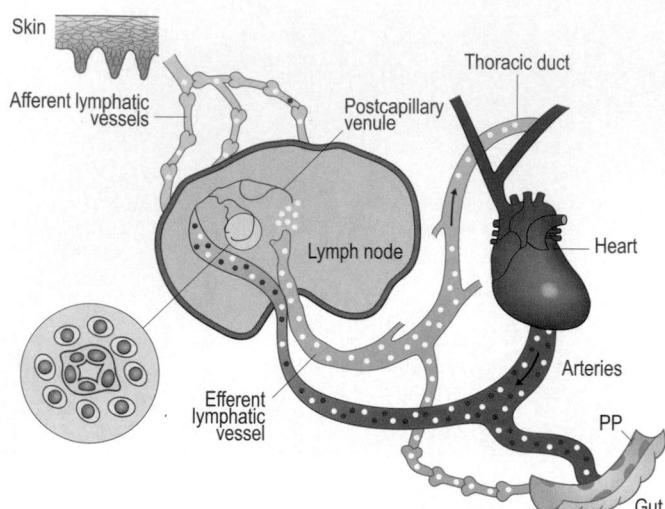

Fig. 12.1 Lymphocyte recirculation routes under physiologic conditions. A low level of continuous antigenic transport into lymphoid organs takes place via afferent lymphatics draining the skin and the epithelium of the gut. Bloodborne lymphocytes enter the organized lymphatic tissues (lymph nodes and Peyer's patches – PP) from the circulation via the arterial tree, flow through the capillary bed, and then extravasate in the postcapillary high endothelial venules (HEV). The extravasated lymphocytes percolate through the tissue parenchyma, enter the lymphatic vessels, and are then carried via the efferent lymphatics back to the systemic circulation. Most of the venous circulation has been omitted from the Figure. Inset: an HEV. (From Salmi M, Jalkanen S. How do lymphocytes know where to go: current concepts and enigmas of lymphocyte homing. Adv Immunol 1997; 64: 139, with permission from Elsevier.)

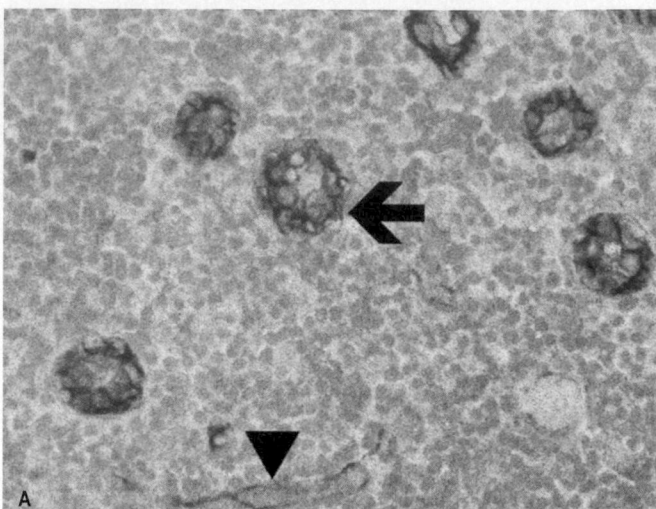

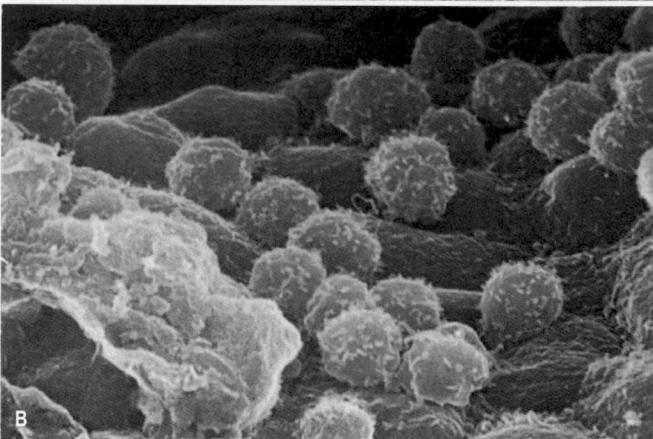

Fig. 12.2 Characteristic features of HEV. (**A**) In this immunoperoxidase staining with anti-CD31 antibody, six HEV are seen with typical plump endothelial cells. One HEV is identified by an arrow; a vessel with flat endothelium is also seen in this Figure (arrowhead). (**B**) In this scanning electron micrograph lymphocytes are adhering to HEV.

venules. The venule endothelial cells exhibit a characteristic high cuboidal morphology that has given them their name: high endothelial venules (HEV).[5] The protrusion of the surface of these endothelial cells into the vascular lumen promotes the interaction of leukocytes in the relatively low-shear venular part of the circulatory system with the endothelial surface membrane (Fig. 12.2). HEV carry many unique adhesion molecules that enable the capture of passing lymphocytes. They also have special intercellular connections that facilitate the penetration of the vessel walls by these emigrating lymphocytes. It has been estimated that more than 50% of incoming lymphocytes make transient contacts with the vascular lining in the lymph nodes, and that as many as one passing cell in four adheres to the endothelium and then extravasates into the tissue.

Antigens are gathered into these secondary lymphoid organs by a different route. Most antigens in the periphery can be taken up by dendritic cells (Chapter 7), which subsequently migrate into the secondary lymphoid organs via the afferent lymphatics.[6] These afferent lymph channels open into the subcapsular sinus of the lymph node. Individual dendritic cells subsequently penetrate the lymphatic endothelium and emigrate into the stroma. Unbound, or free, antigens that diffuse by chance into these secondary lymphoid organs can also be captured by the professional antigen-presenting cells of the lymph nodes. Lymph nodes thus serve as traps for the immune

system, collecting lymphocytes from the blood and antigens from the lymph (Fig. 12.1). In these organs, lymphocytes percolate through the tissue in search of their cognate antigens. If a given lymphocyte does not find its antigen, it will leave the organ by entering the efferent lymphatics that drain the medullary sinuses. The frustrated cell is then transported via a major lymphatic trunk, such as the thoracic duct, back into the large systemic veins. After re-entering the circulation, the cell can then randomly gain access to another lymph node, where it has another chance to extravasate into the tissue and find its cognate antigen. One round of recirculation from the blood to the lymph node stroma, to a lymphatic vessel and then back to the blood takes about 1 day. Naïve lymphocytes continue circulating in the blood until they either find their cognate antigen or die.[3, 5]

ACTIVATED LYMPHOCYTES DISPLAY SELECTIVE TISSUE HOMING PATTERNS ■

In a secondary lymphoid organ a successful encounter between a lymphocyte and its cognate antigen leads to the proliferation of the cell within the organ and the maturation of its progeny.[3, 5] Simultaneously, a process called imprinting leads to a profound change in the subsequent pattern of migration of the antigen-responsive cell. During the imprinting local dendritic cells give educational clues to the lymphocytes, which lead to changes in the chemoattractant and adhesion receptor repertoire of the lymphocytes. Although these responding cells leave the node via the lymphatics and are carried back to the systemic circulation, unlike naïve cells they no longer migrate randomly to any lymphoid tissue. Instead, imprinting primes the cells to preferentially seek the peripheral tissues in which the inciting antigen was originally ingested by the dendritic cell. In this way, selective homing of lymphocytes according to their previous history allows the organism to focus the immune response to the tissues where the effector cells can do the most good.

Among T cells, distinct pools of central and effector memory cells can be distinguished. The different profile of adhesion molecule and chemokine receptor expression allows central memory cells to continue migration through lymph nodes, whereas effector memory cells are dispersed to patrol peripheral tissues.[7]

Under normal conditions, two distinct routes of lymphocyte recirculation can be discerned.[3, 5] One targets lymphoid cells to the peripheral lymph nodes, and the second targets them to gut-associated lymphoid tissues (GALT; Chapter 19). Although the common gut-associated lymphoid system has long been considered to include both the respiratory and the genitourinary tracts, differences in the fine specificity of lymphocyte homing between these targets do exist.

DISTINCT RECIRCULATION ROUTES IN SPLEEN ■

The spleen holds a unique place in the panoply of secondary lymphoid tissues.[8] It contains more lymphocytes than all the peripheral lymph nodes put together, and the number of lymphocytes recirculating through it daily is the equivalent of the total pool of circulating lymphocytes. In the spleen, which lacks HEV, lymphocytes enter the tissue through the marginal zone sinuses, where macrophage-like cells may play an important role. Once in the splenic parenchyma, T cells accumulate in the regions surrounding the central arteriole in white pulp, a location known as the periarteriolar sheath. B cells are scattered in the corona that surrounds these T-cell areas. Most splenic lymphocytes leave the spleen via the splenic vein. The mechanisms that control the entry and exit of lymphocytes from the spleen remain incompletely understood. However, they appear to be quite distinct from those that operate in the peripheral lymph nodes and GALT.

KEY CONCEPTS

ADHESION MOLECULES IN INFLAMMATION

>> Adhesion molecules are important in directing leukocyte traffic to sites of inflammation.

>> Numerous inflammatory mediators upregulate and/or induce expression of several endothelial-cell adhesion molecules.

>> Harmful inflammation can be prevented and cured by blocking the function of adhesion molecules.

INFLAMMATION-INDUCED CHANGES IN LEUKOCYTE TRAFFICKING ■

During an acute inflammatory response to an antigenic insult, leukocytes can migrate into all nonlymphoid tissues, which are normally virtually devoid of lymphocytes. The inflammation-induced leukocyte immigration takes place in characteristic waves.[9] First, the polymorphonuclear leukocytes rapidly (typically within 1–4 hours) infiltrate into the inflammatory focus. They are followed by mononuclear cells (monocytes and lymphocytes). In a primary challenge it may take 3 days or more before antigen-specific immunoblasts are seen at the peripheral scene of inflammation. However, a secondary response by memory lymphocytes typically has a much shorter lag period. Different CD4 T-helper subpopulations (Chapters 9 and 17), CD8 T-cytotoxic cells (Chapter 18), and regulatory T cells (Chapter 16) can all enter the inflamed tissue using basically the same mechanisms, although the ratio of these populations and the individual molecules employed may vary. Successful resolution of an inflammatory reaction appears to also be dependent on a coordinated program involving lipoxins, resolvins and protectins, all of which serve to halt cell recruitment and initiate apoptosis.[10]

The normal vascular endothelium in nonlymphoid tissues has a flat, inactive morphology. With inflammation, a series of events renders postcapillary venules in these tissues capable of binding lymphocytes. The most important changes are due to the proadhesive effects of a multitude of proinflammatory cytokines that are released by a variety of cell types after being subjected to inflammatory stimuli.[9]

If inflammation becomes chronic, marked histological manifestations become apparent in affected nonlymphoid tissues.[11] Most notably, the venules in these chronically inflamed tissues acquire many of the characteristics of HEV. Also, immigrating lymphocytes can form lymphoid follicles that resemble those seen in lymph nodes. These alterations have consequences for lymphocyte recirculation pathways. For example, the inflamed skin display characteristics of lymphocyte homing that are clearly distinct from those of either mucosal or peripheral lymph node systems.[12]

■ MOLECULAR MECHANISMS INVOLVED IN LEUKOCYTE EXTRAVASATION FROM THE BLOOD INTO THE TISSUES ■

THE ADHESION CASCADE

Dynamic interactions between leukocytes and endothelial cells can be observed both *in vitro* and *in vivo*. By means of intravital microscopy, for example, leukocyte adhesion can be followed *in vivo* in experimental animals and even in human tissues (Fig. 12.3). Leukocyte–endothelial-cell interaction during the extravasation cascade can be divided into a series of phases, or steps, that all leukocyte subtypes are thought to follow (Fig. 12.4).[2, 3] First, the leukocytes marginate out of the main bloodstream and begin to tether and roll on the endothelial cell surface. This step is mediated primarily by selectin adhesion molecules and their mucin-like counter-receptors. This slow-velocity movement culminates in an activation phase, during which the leukocyte chemokine receptors transmit activation signals by recognizing their chemokine ligands presented on the endothelial-cell surface. This leads to avidity and/or affinity changes in leukocyte integrins that bind the leukocytes firmly to their immunoglobulin superfamily ligands on the endothelial cells. The lymphocytes then begin to transmigrate through the endothelium, a process that also involves leukocyte integrins and other molecules. Leukocytes diapedese between the endothelial cells through the endothelial cell junction, which opens transiently and subsequently closes.[13] This process requires proteinases, such as matrix metalloproteinase-2 (MMP-2), which is induced in T cells upon adhesion to endothelial cells, as well as other, as yet to be defined, repair mechanisms that subsequently close the path of transmigration. However, leukocytes can also migrate through the endothelial cells in a subtype-specific fashion. For example, polymorphonuclear leukocytes prefer entering via the inter-endothelial junctions, whereas nonactivated lymphocytes may choose the transcellular route.[14]

An additional complexity to the extravasation system is created by the fact that certain endothelial molecules involved in the adhesion cascade show organ-specific expression patterns. Analogously, leukocyte-associated homing molecules display subtype-specific expression profiles. Therefore, only those leukocytes that have the proper set of molecules on their surface can enter a particular tissue, because the entering leukocyte has to find a correct endothelial partner molecule at each step of the adhesion cascade. Thus, leukocyte–endothelial-cell interaction takes place in a well-coordinated multistep fashion, in which every step must be properly executed in order before the leukocyte can be guided into the tissue. The multistep nature of the leukocyte adhesion cascade is thus reminiscent of the cascades involved in blood clotting and complement-mediated killing.

KEY CONCEPTS

LEUKOCYTE-ENDOTHELIAL INTERACTIONS

>> Leukocytes interact with the vessel wall in a multistep fashion, using several leukocyte surface molecules that recognize their counter-receptors on endothelial cells.

>> The rolling and tethering of leukocytes on the vessel wall is mediated by selectins.

>> Chemokines and their receptors are needed to activate leukocyte integrins.

>> Only activated integrins are able to mediate firm adhesion between leukocytes and endothelium.

>> The transmigration of leukocytes into the tissues requires proteinases and repair mechanisms.

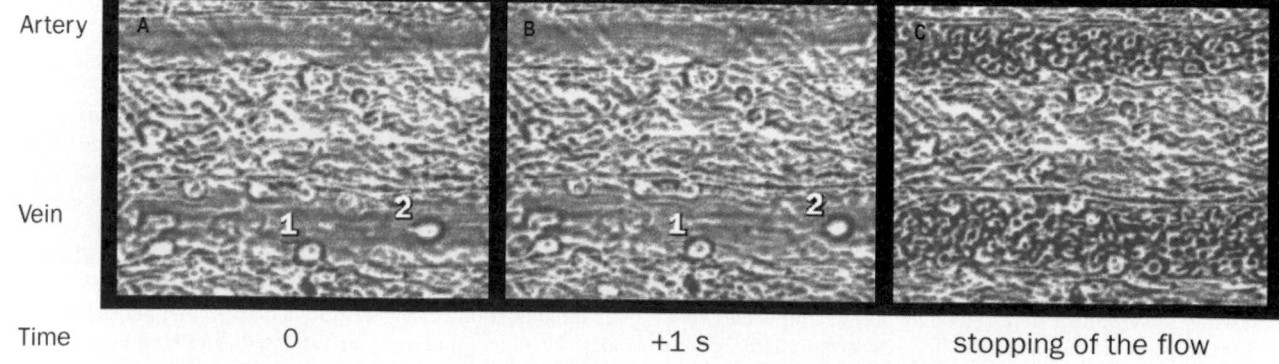

Fig. 12.3 Intravital microscopy of mesenteric vessels. In these video frames taken at indicated intervals from the same field, a vein, an artery, leukocytes and the transparent mesenteric membrane are seen. Within the vein rolling and adherent leukocytes are visible, whereas no such cells are seen in the artery. Leukocyte 1 is attached to the vessel wall and leukocyte 2 is slowly rolling. Compare the locations of these cells in A and B to stationary leukocytes outside the vessels. Leukocyte 1 is at the same location in both panels, whereas leukocyte 2 has moved a distance corresponding to roughly the length of its diameter. Under normal conditions, freely flowing cells move so fast that they cannot be visualized. However, in panel C the flow has been transiently stopped. Under this static condition, the large number of hematopoietic cells (mainly erythrocytes) traveling within the bloodstream can be seen. (Courtesy of S. Tohka, University of Turku, Finland.)

RECEPTORS AND THEIR LIGANDS IN LEUKOCYTE–ENDOTHELIAL-CELL INTERACTION

A variety of molecules belonging to several molecular families are expressed on both leukocyte and endothelial-cell surfaces and participate in the complex extravasation process.[5] Most of these molecules exert their function in successive, but overlapping, phases of the adhesion cascade. In addition, proper functioning of multiple intracellular signaling molecules is needed for execution of a successful extravasation.[15] In the following section, only the best-known surface molecules in this process are discussed (Fig. 12.5). A summary of the phenotypes exhibited by mice that are deficient for these molecules is presented in Table 12.1.

Selectins and their ligands

Three members of the selectin family mediate leukocyte trafficking. L-selectin is expressed on several leukocyte subpopulations. E-selectin is expressed on endothelium, and P-selectin is expressed on both platelets and endothelium. An important structural feature of selectins is the presence of a terminal lectin domain that is used to bind to their counter-receptors. The counter-receptor is typically decorated by a sialyl Lewis X (sLeX) carbohydrate, which is a prototype recognition domain for selectins in general.[16] The interaction between selectins and their counter-receptors is transient and weak, which allows leukocytes effectively to form and break contacts with endothelium during tethering and rolling under shear stress.

L-selectin preferentially mediates lymphocyte migration to peripheral lymph nodes. However, it also participates in the homing of lymphocytes to organized MALT, e.g., Peyer's patches (Chapter 19). L-selectin is also an important contributor to the process of leukocyte trafficking to sites of inflammation. Peripheral lymph node addressins (PNAd) are the best-characterized counter-receptors for L-selectin. This group consists of at least six different molecules that are decorated with a sulfated and fucosylated sLeX that serves as a recognition motif for L-selectin. PNAds include glycosylation-dependent cell adhesion molecule-1 (GlyCAM-1), CD34, podocalyxin, endomucin, nepmucin, and mucosal addressin cell adhesion molecule-1 (MAdCAM-1). MAdCAM-1 is decorated with recognition epitopes for L-selectin on HEV in the organized lymphoid areas of the gut, but not on the flat-walled vessels in lamina propria. The importance of post-translational carbohydrate modifications for the function of selectin ligands has been well demonstrated in knockout mice deficient for fucosyl, glucosaminyl, galactosyl, sialyl or sulfotransferases. For example, mice with a targeted disruption of fucosyltransferase VII (Fuc-TVII) are unable to glycosylate L-selectin ligands appropriately. These mice exhibit severe defects in lymphocyte homing and in the extravasation of leukocytes to sites of inflammation. In contrast, core 2 β 1,6-N-acetylglucosaminyltransferase (C2 β GlcNAcT) knockout mice that have deficient glycosylation of their P- and E-selectin ligands demonstrate normal lymphocyte homing to lymph nodes, but impaired leukocyte trafficking to sites of inflammation.[16] Interestingly, L-selectin also facilitates entry of leukocytes into the tissues by mediating leukocyte tethering and rolling of endothelium-bound leukocytes by binding to P-selectin glycoprotein ligand-1 (PSGL-1).

E-selectin and P-selectin are inflammation-inducible molecules. Within minutes, P-selectin can be translocated from intracellular storage granules onto the endothelial cell surface, where it binds to its leukocyte receptor, PSGL-1 (Fig. 12.5). P-selectin and PSGL-1 mediate rolling at early time points during inflammation. Platelet P-selectin can facilitate lymphocyte entry into the tissues, because it can simultaneously bind to PNAd on endothelium and PSGL-1 on lymphocytes. E-selectin upregulation requires new protein synthesis. It is maximally expressed about 4 hours after the induction of inflammation. E-selectin is needed for slow rolling of leukocytes. It also has an affinity towards PSGL-1, as well as a specific glycoform of PSGL-1, cutaneous lymphocyte antigen (CLA). CLA specifically directs lymphocyte trafficking to inflamed skin. In addition to PSGL-1, E-selectin has a more private leukocyte receptor called E-selectin

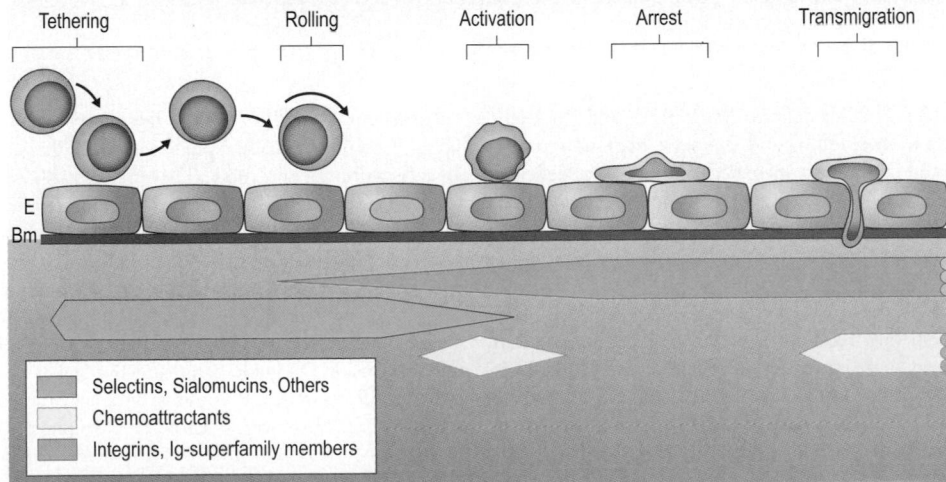

Fig. 12.4 The multistep cascade of lymphocyte extravasation. The bloodborne cell makes transient initial contacts with endothelial cells, which leads to the cell rolling along the vascular lining. If the cell becomes activated, it can subsequently adhere firmly to the endothelial cells, seek for interendothelial junctions, and then migrate through the basement membrane into the tissue. The contribution of major superfamilies of adhesion-associated molecules at each step is depicted below. E, endothelial layer; Bm, basement membrane.

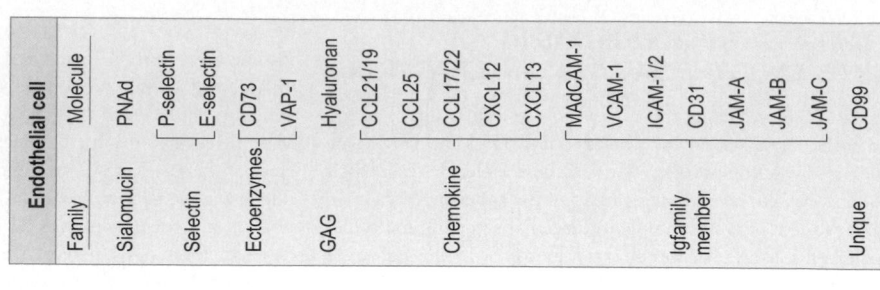
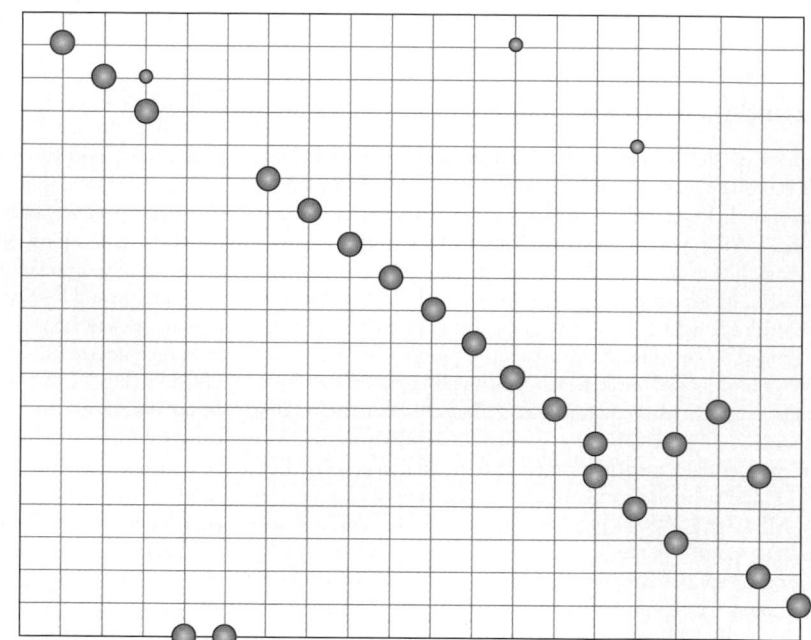

Fig. 12.5 Adhesion molecules mediating leukocyte traffic. The most relevant proteins involved in leukocyte–endothelial-cell interactions are shown as receptor–ligand pairs. GAG, glycosaminoglycan.

ligand-1 (ESL-1) (Fig. 12.5).[17] Mice deficient for both E- and P-selectin have more drastic defects in their rolling and leukocyte migration to sites of inflammation than could have been anticipated from the mice deficient in only one of the two selectins. This suggests that E- and P-selectins have overlapping functions and can compensate for each other.

Chemokines and their receptors

Chemotactic cytokines and their receptors (Chapter 11) are grouped into four different families based on their primary protein structure. The families are defined by a cysteine signature motif – CXC, CC, C and CX3C – where C is a cysteine and X any amino acid residue.[18] Most chemokines are small, soluble heparin-binding chemoattractants. The relevant chemokines for leukocyte extravasation are presented to bloodborne lymphocytes by proteoglycan molecules present on endothelial cell surfaces. During the adhesion cascade they activate integrins by signaling via serpentine receptors, which are pertussis-toxin sensitive and G-protein linked.

Different leukocyte subsets bear their own distinct sets of receptors, which enable them to respond to chemokines presented on the vascular endothelium as well as within the tissues. For example, CCL21 and CCL19 are preferentially expressed by HEV that are found in interfollicular areas within a lymph node. They preferentially attract T cells bearing the CCR7 receptor, and thus draw T lymphocytes from the blood and into these areas. Fractalkine, a CX3C chemokine, can be produced in either a soluble or a membrane-anchored form. It can be found on HEV in peripheral lymph nodes and has potent chemoattractant activity for T cells. The major attractants for B cells are CXCL12 and CXCL13. Although many chemokines are present in different organs in the body, some selectivity in their expression can guide tissue-selective leukocyte trafficking. For example, CCL25 attracts CCR9 positive lymphocytes to the small intestine, and CCL17/CCL22 attract CCR4-bearing lymphocytes to the skin.

Integrins and their immunoglobulin superfamily ligands

Integrins are a large family of heterodimeric molecules consisting of an α and a β chain.[19] Traditionally they are thought to mediate firm adhesion between leukocytes and endothelial cells, although in specific low-shear

Table 12.1 Phenotypes of the mice deficient in homing-associated molecules

Molecule	Main abnormalities in leukocyte trafficking
L-selectin	Impaired lymphocyte homing to peripheral lymph nodes
E-selectin	Increased velocity of rolling leukocytes
P-selectin	Decreased leukocyte rolling at early stages of inflammation
PSGL-1	Decreased leukocyte rolling at early stages of inflammation
ICAM-1	Impaired neutrophil migration to sites of inflammation
ICAM-2	Delayed eosinophil accumulation in the airway lumen in allergy, impaired neutrophil transmigration
VCAM-1	Embryonic lethal
CD31	Deficient migration through basement membrane
JAM-A	Increased dendritic cell homing to lymph nodes and reduced transendothelial migration
$S1P_1$	Embryonic lethal
CD11a	Reduced lymphocyte trafficking to peripheral lymph nodes and to Peyer's patches
CD11b	Decreased leukocyte trafficking to sites of inflammation
	Decreased neutrophil emigration in ischemia/reperfusion injury
β_2-integrin	No neutrophil emigration into the skin, normal emigration into inflamed peritoneum and increased migration into inflamed lung
α_4-integrin	Embryonic lethal, chimeric mice have reduced lymphocyte homing into Peyer's patches
β_7-integrin	Impaired lymphocyte migration into Peyer's patches
CD44	Decreased lymphocyte migration to peripheral lymph nodes and thymus
VAP-1	Faster rolling, decreased firm adhesion and transmigration and diminished leukocyte infiltration to sites of inflammation
CD73	Increased leukocyte traffic to sites of inflammation in ischemia
CD38	Defective chemotaxis of granulocytes and dendritic cells in severe inflammations
CCR9	Reduced number of intraepithelial T cells and IgA-positive plasma cells in lamina propria
CCR7	Defective lymphocyte entry to lymph nodes and formation of T-cell areas
CCL19/CCL21	Impaired homing of lymphocytes (especially T cells) to lymph nodes
CXCR5/CXCL13	Defect in the formation of follicles in the lymph nodes
CXCR4	Aberrant B-cell follicles
CCR4	Prolonged graft survival due to reduced T-cell trafficking

MOLECULAR MECHANISMS INVOLVED IN LEUKOCYTE EXTRAVASATION

conditions they can also participate in rolling. With regard to leukocyte trafficking, the most important integrins are $\alpha_4\beta_7$, LFA-1 and $\alpha_4\beta_1$. $\alpha_4\beta_7$ is a principal homing receptor for lymphocyte trafficking to mucosa-associated lymphatic tissues. It binds to MAdCAM-1 on HEV in organized mucosal lymphatic tissues, such as Peyer's patches and appendix, and to flat-walled venules in the lamina propria.

α_4-Integrin can also pair with a β_1 chain to form an $\alpha_4\beta_1$ dimer, which lymphocytes utilize primarily in inflammatory conditions. It binds to endothelial vascular cell adhesion molecule-1 (VCAM-1) on endothelium.

Lymphocyte function-associated antigen-1 (LFA-1/CD11a/CD18) is a member of the group of leukocyte integrins that contain a unique α chain (CD11 a, b, c and d), but share a common β chain (β2/CD18). LFA-1 is present on practically all leukocyte subsets. It interacts with its counter-receptors, intercellular adhesion molecules (ICAM-1 and ICAM-2) on the endothelial cell surface (Fig. 12.5). ICAM-1 is upregulated at sites of inflammation, whereas ICAM-2 is constitutively present on vascular endothelium. To be functional, LFA-1 needs to be activated. Activation of LFA-1 is thought to be primarily a product of chemokine signaling. However, alternative activation pathways include triggering through glycosyl-phosphatidylinositol (GPI)-linked molecules, CD44, as well as other costimulatory lymphocyte surface molecules.[15] LFA-1-dependent pathways display no significant organ specificity in their function. Mac-1 (CD11b/CD18) is also involved in leukocyte migration, although its contribution is overshadowed by LFA-1. Like LFA-1, Mac-1 uses ICAM-1 and ICAM-2 as its ligands (Fig. 12.5).

Other homing-associated molecules

Several other molecules belonging to various molecular families also participate in the adhesion cascade. CD44 is a multifunctional proteoglycan that is found on a large variety of different cell types.[20] Using endothelial hyaluronan as its ligand, it mediates lymphocyte rolling. It can form bimolecular complexes with $\alpha_4\beta_1$ that strengthens leukocyte–endothelial-cell interaction. *In vivo* inhibition studies using function-blocking antibodies indicate that CD44 plays an important role in directing lymphocyte trafficking to sites of inflammation, e.g., skin and joints.

CD31, a member of the immunoglobulin superfamily, is found on many subsets of lymphocytes and in the continuous endothelium of all vessel types. It is expressed primarily at the intercellular junctions and is involved in a stimulus-specific manner in transmigration, especially through the endothelial basement membrane. Other molecules involved in the transmigration process are CD99 and junctional adhesion molecules A and C, which are expressed both on leukocytes and endothelial cells. These molecules interact sequentially in a homotypic fashion during diapedesis. In addition, endothelial JAM-A can use LFA-1, JAM-C may utilize Mac-1, and JAM-B uses $\alpha_4\beta_1$ as leukocyte ligands.

The role of ectoenzymes in the adhesion cascade has been recently recognized.[21] Vascular adhesion protein-1 (VAP-1), CD73, and CD38 have well established roles in leukocyte trafficking. Owing to their enzymatic properties, they can rapidly modify adhesive interactions and modulate the microenvironment. VAP-1 is a homodimeric sialoglycoprotein that, under conditions of inflammation, is rapidly translocated on to the endothelial cell surface. It mediates early phases of leukocyte interaction with endothelium, as well as transmigration. Besides its adhesive

function, it also possesses an amine oxidase activity that can produce potent immunomodulators such as H_2O_2 and aldehyde as end products. CD73 is present both on a subpopulation of lymphocytes and on endothelium. It is an ectonucleotidase. The main product of its enzymatic activity in dephosphorylation of AMP is adenosine, which is highly anti-inflammatory in nature. Endothelial CD73 may also have a counter-receptor on the lymphocyte surface, because lymphocyte binding to endothelium inhibits the enzymatic activity of CD73. This facilitates the extravasation process of the lymphocyte. CD38, an ADP-ribosyl cyclase, is expressed on most lymphoid cells and can use CD31 as its endothelial cell ligand. Via its enzymatic activity it regulates calcium fluxes and the sensitivity of leukocytes to chemokine signals.

■ INTRAORGAN LYMPHOCYTE LOCALIZATION ■

Following its extravasation from the blood vessels, a lymphocyte needs to interact with several matrix molecules, such as fibronectin, laminin and collagens. Adhesive interactions between a lymphocyte and the extracellular matrix molecules are largely mediated by β_1-integrins, although

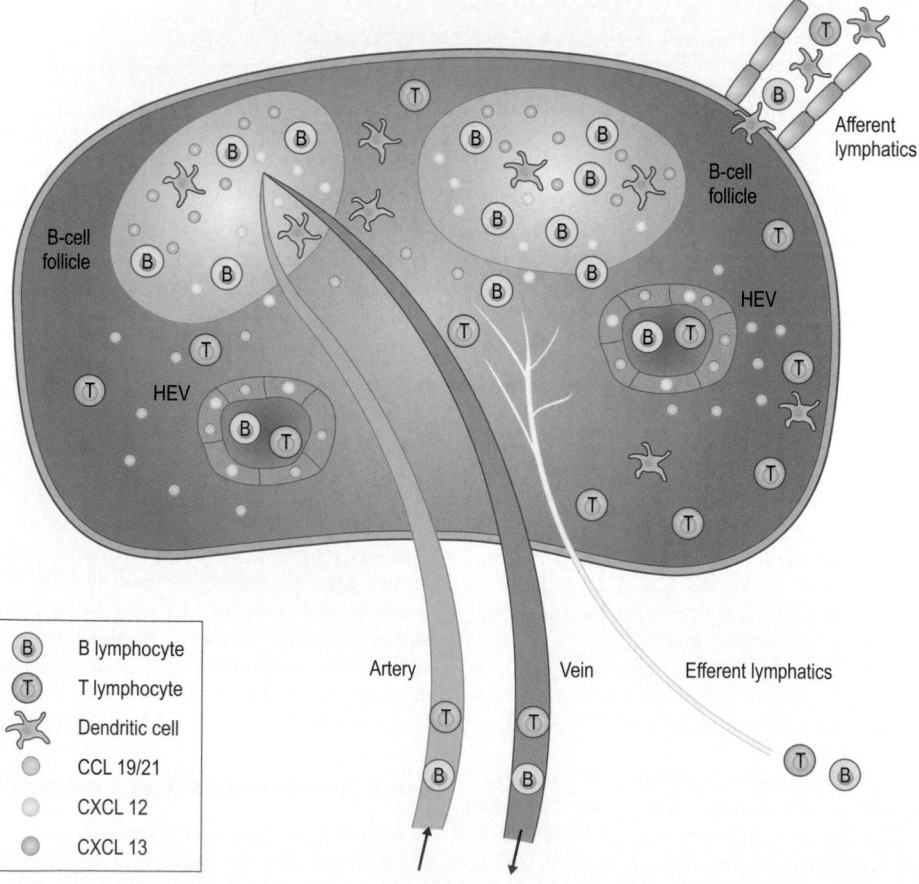

Fig. 12.6 The role of chemokines in entrance and intraorgan localization of lymphocytes. CCL19 and CCL21 are involved in T-lymphocyte entrance into the lymph node via HEV. They also guide T cells to the interfollicular areas within the node. In contrast, CXCL12 and CXCL13 attract B lymphocytes on the vessel wall and direct their localization within the follicles.

lymphocytes can also use CD44 to interact with fibronectin and collagens. The directional movement and the final localization of a lymphocyte within the tissues are controlled by chemokines.[9, 18, 22] Modern two-photon imaging has provided detailed information about the kinetics and directionality of lymphocyte movement in living tissues.[23]

Besides directing the entry of T cells into the tissues, CCL21 and CCL19 also determine the final destination of the T lymphocyte within lymph nodes, spleen and Peyer's patches. CCL19 and CCL21 produced by stromal cells in the T-cell areas within the lymphoid tissues guide the T lymphocyte into the interfollicular space. In an analogous manner, B-cell-attracting chemokine-1 CXCL13 is produced by a subset of follicular dendritic cells found in secondary lymphoid organs. It attracts B cells possessing CXCR5 to the light zone of the follicles. CXCL12, on the other hand, guides CXCR4 positive B cells to the dark zone (Fig. 12.6).

Correct localization of a lymphocyte and an antigen-presenting cell within the lymph node is a prerequisite for an optimal immune response. Dendritic cells that carry antigens from the peripheral tissues into the lymph node enter the node via afferent lymphatic vessels (Fig. 12.6). An interaction between the dendritic cell and the T cell in the T-cell area is then crucial for T-cell activation. B-cell collaboration with T cells is ensured by upregulation of CXCR5 expression on a subpopulation of T cells, and of CCR7 on certain B cells that allow the movement of these cells to the boundary of the B- and T-cell zones. The importance of CCL21 and CCL19 in lymphocyte trafficking is demonstrated by a spontaneous mutant mouse strain, *plt*, which has reduced expression of these chemokines. In these mice, both lymphocyte entry via HEV and the organization of T-cell areas within lymph nodes are defective, which is recapitulated in CCR7 knockout mice. CCL21/CCL19 and CXCL12/CXCL13 are currently the best-known determinants of lymphocyte localization within lymphoid tissues, although several other chemokines are also needed for optimal encounters between various cell populations in order to create a crisp immune response.

CELL TRAFFICKING WITHIN LYMPHATICS

Although leukocyte trafficking within the lymphatics is an essential part of the recirculation process and the immune response in general, very little is known about the molecular mechanisms that regulate this tightly controlled and cell type-selective migration. CCL21 on lymphatic endothelium attracts CCR7-positive dendritic cells and lymphocytes into the afferent lymphatics and thence to the draining lymph nodes. JAM-A may also control the traffic of dendritic cells, as dendritic cells defective for JAM-A show increased motility and enhanced trafficking via the afferent lymphatics into the draining lymph nodes. Furthermore, certain adhesion molecules, such as macrophage mannose receptor and common lymphatic endothelial and vascular endothelial receptor-1 (CLEVER-1), may mediate lymphocyte migration into the lymphatics, as lymphocytes adhere to lymphatic vessels via these molecules in *in vitro* assays.[5,14] Sphingosine 1 phosphate receptor 1 (S1P$_1$), which is expressed in many different cell types, also participates in lymphocyte exit into the lymphatics. Although its absence leads to defects in vascular development and embryonic lethality, studies of conditional knockout mice have shown that lymphocytes lacking S1P$_1$ can enter the lymph nodes normally. However, they are not able to exit from the lymph nodes into the efferent lymphatics. Additional studies indicate that S1P$_1$ may control lymphocyte trafficking by regulating endothelial permeability and/or suppressing lymphocyte chemotaxis in S1P gradients.[22, 24]

CLINICAL IMPLICATIONS

Leukocyte trafficking plays a pivotal role in the pathogenesis of all infectious and inflammatory diseases. It is essential for mounting a proper immune response against an invading microbe. However, in many other cases inappropriate leukocyte migration also causes tissue destruction. Here we have chosen a few representative examples to illustrate some of the general principles.

IMMUNODEFICIENCIES

Various defects in leukocyte trafficking have been identified during the past two decades. Leukocytes from patients with Wiskott–Aldrich syndrome, for example, show reduced migration to chemokines CCL2, CCL3 and CXCL12 owing to a mutation in the gene encoding an intracellular WAS protein responsible for proper cytoskeletal organization of the hematopoietic cells. Mutations of CXCR4 in WHIM (warts, hypogammaglobulinemia, infections and myelokathexis) patients lead to an enhanced chemotactic response to CXCL12 expressed on bone marrow endothelium and leukocyte accumulation in the bone marrow.[25] A single

Table 12.2 Clinical features of immunodeficient patients with abnormalities in homing-associated molecules

	LADI	LADII	LADIII
Clinical manifestation			
Recurrent bacterial infections	+++	+	+++
Neutrophilia	yes	yes	yes
Developmental abnormalities	no	Yes	no
Laboratory findings			
CD18 expression	Marked decrease or absence	Normal or slightly decreased	Normal
sLex expression	Normal	Absent	Normal
Neutrophil rolling	Normal	Marked decrease	Normal
Neutrophil firm adhesion	Marked decrease	Normal	Marked decrease

case of inherited dysfunction of E-selectin has also been reported. The patient had recurrent infections but did not demonstrate neutrophilia. She could not synthesize E-selectin on endothelium, although her serum level of soluble E-selectin was increased.

Three different forms of adhesion defect in integrins lead to poor or total lack of homing of certain leukocyte populations.[25, 26] Their typical features are listed in Table 12.2. These diseases are extremely rare, but they recapitulate beautifully in humans the basic principles of leukocyte trafficking first deciphered in animal models.

LAD I and LAD I variant (LAD III)

Patients with leukocyte adhesion defect-1 (LAD-1) have defects in the synthesis, pairing or expression of β_2-integrins[27] The severe form leads to the total or almost total absence of CD11a/CD18 (LFA-1), CD11b/CD18 (Mac-1), CD11c/CD18 and CD11d/CD18. Although these patients exhibit neutrophilia, they suffer from severe recurrent bacterial infections owing to defects in leukocyte extravasation into sites of inflammation. They usually die young. Patients suffering from a milder form of LAD-1 (<10% of normal β_2-integrins) demonstrate impairment in leukocyte migration and suffer from frequent infections as well, but usually survive until adulthood. In these patients lymphocyte migration to inflammatory sites is close to normal, probably because lymphocytes can utilize the VLA-4-VCAM-1 pathway to compensate for the lack of β_2-integrins.

LAD-1 variants have also been described.[26, 27] In one group, modestly reduced β_2-integrin expression has been associated with mutations which create heterodimers that do not bind ligands. A second group of LAD I variants (also known as LAD III) involves defective inside-out signaling. In these patients activation of multiple leukocyte integrins, including LFA-1 and VLA-4, by chemokine-triggered G-protein-coupled signals is genetically defective. Concurrent defects in platelet integrins lead to a bleeding diathesis. In all types of LAD I, granulocytes typically show normal rolling, but failure to arrest on endothelial cells.

LAD II

LAD II patients suffer from several abnormalities, including recurrent infections, neutrophilia, impaired pus formation, mental retardation, growth defects and deficiency in H blood group antigen.[27] The cause of the disease is impaired transport of GDP-fucose from the cytoplasm to the Golgi lumen as a result of mutations in a GDP-fucose transporter. The defect leads to impaired modification of selectin ligands, notably that of PSGL-1, with fucose. Consequently, they demonstrate a marked decrease in leukocyte rolling under flow conditions. Interestingly, some patients respond to treatment with oral fucose.

DISEASES OF AUTOIMMUNITY

Multiple sclerosis

Migration of lymphocytes through the blood–brain barrier into the central nervous system is a key pathogenetic event that occurs during the development of multiple sclerosis (MS) and its widely used animal model, experimental allergic encephalomyelitis (EAE). *In vivo* animal studies have shown that the disease course can be dramatically altered by blocking the function of leukocyte α_4-integrin.[28] This treatment is able to prevent the disease and even reverse the paralytic disease and lymphocytic infiltrations in the brain. Antibodies against $\alpha_4\beta_1$ show this remarkable efficacy even if started a month after the onset of the clinical disease. Certain EAE models can also be blocked by targeting the α_4-integrin ligand VCAM-1, or by blocking the function of CD44. In contrast, blocking of many other adhesion molecules, such as L-selectin, PSGL-1, E- and P-selectin and ICAM-1, fail to yield a consistent effect on EAE. Use of lymphocytes from MS patients in murine models has confirmed the importance of $\alpha_4\beta_1$-mediated leukocyte interaction in EAE brain, but have also revealed a role for PSGL-1. It should also be noted that although $\alpha_4\beta_1$-integrin is very important for lymphocyte homing to brain, it is not a brain-specific zip code, as it is also involved in leukocyte trafficking to other organs, such as pancreas and gut.

TRANSPLANT REJECTION

In all forms of rejection, activation of vascular endothelium of the graft with the ensuing lymphocyte infiltration is a critical parameter. In heart transplantation, for example, multiple endothelial adhesion molecules (such as P-selectin, ICAM-1 and PNAd) normally absent from the organ are rapidly induced in a rejected organ. *In vivo* studies have shown that blocking the function of these molecules prevents the unwanted binding of lymphocytes to the graft.[29] For example, in rodent allograft models rejection is significantly reduced if lymphocyte LFA-1 and endothelial ICAM-1 are rendered nonfunctional by monoclonal antibodies or by disruption of these molecules through gene deletion. The chemoattractant system has also been extensively targeted for inhibiting lymphocyte influx into transplants. For instance, FTY720, a small molecule that inhibits $S1P_1$ receptor, promotes long-term graft survival in murine models.

ISCHEMIA–REPERFUSION INJURY

When blood flow is restored to the ischemic organ a massive influx of granulocytes into the hypoxic tissue can be seen. This ischemia–reperfusion injury is due to the activation of the endothelial cells in the insulted organ. In many cases it has been shown that depletion of circulating neutrophils, or blockage of their entryinto the ischemic tissue through anti-adhesive therapy, can reduce tissue necrosis by up to 50% and prevent the death of cells in the zone of reversibly damaged tissue.[30] Myocardial ischemia–reperfusion injury, for example, is alleviated in CD18, ICAM-1, P-selectin and E-selectin-deficient mice. In many cases similar results have been obtained by using antibodies to block the function of these adhesion proteins, which are induced in the ischemic tissue.

CANCER

Lymphocyte trafficking can be harnessed to improve the outcome of cellular immunotherapy against cancer.[31] Infusion of activated or genetically modified effector T cells would benefit from a more effective targeting of the cells into the tumor. On the other hand, anti-adhesive therapies targeting inappropriate accumulation of regulatory T cells in the tumor would also enhance anti-cancer immune responses.[32]

CLINICAL IMPLICATIONS

THERAPEUTIC PRINCIPLES

>> Pro-adhesive strategies are mainly developed using gene therapy.

>> Inappropriate inflammation associated with many diseases can be dampened by anti-adhesive therapeutics.

>> Humanized, function-blocking monoclonal antibodies are effective anti-adhesive molecules.

>> Cell migration can also be blocked by ligand and receptor analogs, small molecule inhibitors and genetic means (e.g., RNA interference).

CLINICAL PEARLS

>> Efalizumab, a humanized antibody against leukocyte integrin CD11a, is efficacious in the treatment of psoriasis.

>> Blocking of α_4-integrin with natalizumab can ameliorate disease activity in multiple sclerosis.

ADHESION MOLECULES AS DIAGNOSTIC TARGETS

Immunodeficiency disorders

In classic LAD I deficiency a definitive diagnosis can be established by flow-cytometric analysis of immunofluorescent-stained CD18 integrin on blood leukocytes.[27] In normal individuals practically all peripheral blood lymphocytes are CD18 positive. In severe cases of LAD I deficiency there is a complete absence of this adhesion molecule, whereas in moderate deficiency about 1–10% of control levels is seen. Diagnosis of LAD III requires activation of the cells, the use of mAb that recognize specific activation epitopes, or functional assays.

LAD II can be diagnosed with commercially available antibodies by documenting a lack of fucosylated adhesion molecules, e.g., abnormal expression of sLeX on blood leukocytes.

Soluble adhesion molecules

Most adhesion molecules are found in soluble forms in body fluids. They can be produced by alternative splicing of the mRNA leading to the lack of transmembrane anchors, by proteolytic cleavage of cell bound proteins by various sheddases (proteases), or by cleavage of the GPI linkage. The soluble forms can either function as molecular sinks, competing for their specific ligand(s) with the membrane-bound forms, or trigger biological responses by interacting with their ligand-bearing cells.

The availability of commercial kits for measuring the levels of soluble adhesion molecules has led to numerous reports describing an increase or a decrease of certain adhesion molecules in different diseases. In most cases there appears to be little or no additional diagnostic or predictive value derived from the use of these tests compared to more traditional parameters of inflammation activity. Therefore, at present, the indications for measurements of soluble adhesion molecules, or chemokines, in inflammatory and cancerous diseases remain to be defined.

Imaging

The use of neutrophil scans or radioactively labeled nonspecific molecules to localize inflammatory foci is not satisfactory in terms of timing, expense, biohazards, specificity or sensitivity. Hence, there have been trials to radioactively or nonradioactively label monoclonal antibodies that recognize endothelial adhesion molecules, infuse them intravenously, and follow their accumulation by appropriate imaging devices.[33] Inflammation-inducible molecules such as E-selectin and MAdCAM-1 have been used as target antigens. In the case of radioactively labeled E-selectin antibodies, the utility of this approach has been verified in patients.

THERAPEUTIC APPLICATION OF ADHESION MODULATING THERAPIES

Pro- and anti-adhesive therapies have long been an obvious pharmaceutical goal in the field of leukocyte trafficking. Inflammation-promoting strategies would be beneficial in diseases such as immune deficiencies, persistent infections and cancer. Moreover, pro-adhesive control of lymphocyte traffic would benefit areas such as vaccine development and bone-marrow cell transplantation. In fact, lymphocyte recirculation routes have been already empirically exploited by choosing optimal primary and secondary vaccination regimens at different anatomical locations. Anti-adhesive therapy, on the other hand, can be seen as a form of treatment applicable to all disease categories involving an inflammatory component. In addition, it could provide novel precision drugs individually tailored for organ-specific inflammatory disorders, which would be predicted to diminish the problems of generalized immunosuppression.

FROM ANTIBODIES TO SMALL MOLECULAR DRUGS

A number of specific antagonists of adhesion molecules have been developed.[34] Function-blocking monoclonal antibodies have often been the drug candidates used for proof-of-principle experiments. These include both chimeric and fully humanized antibodies against important adhesion molecules and chemokines. In parallel, recombinant ligand or receptor analogs have been developed. Ultimately, knowledge of the structure of the adhesion molecules has allowed the design of rational, small molecular drugs such as those affecting the conformational state of leukocyte integrins.[35] Recently, the ability to modulate mRNA expression of adhesion molecules through RNAi has added another potential tool to the pharmaceutical armamentarium.

Although all these forms of therapy have been enormously successful in a panoply of different animal models, transfer to the clinic has been difficult. However, recently a small number of very potent drugs targeting adhesion molecules have been introduced.

ADHESION-MODULATING DRUGS IN CLINICAL USE

The first two selective adhesion molecule inhibitors (SAM) are efalizumab and natalizumab. Efalizumab is a humanized, function-blocking antibody directed against CD11a. It has been used in patients with plaque psoriasis. Weekly subcutaneous injections of the antibody have improved the disease score by more than 75% in 22–39% of patients, compared to a similar response in 5% of placebo-treated patients.[36] In addition, in >30% of patients other clinical endpoints, including physician-assessed disease activity, have improved significantly.

The way for natalizumab, a humanized anti-α_4-integrin antibody, was paved by the excellent results of α_4 blocking in EAE (see above). In patients with relapsing multiple sclerosis a monthly intravenous injection of natalizumab has led to >90% fewer lesions than with placebo.[37] The risk of sustained progression of disability has been reduced by >40%. Also the rate of clinical relapses has been diminished by almost 70%. Even in patients who relapsed in spite of β-interferon treatment, the addition of natalizumab to the treatment regimen reduced the formation of new or enlarging lesions by >80% and diminished the number of clinical relapses by about 50%. These data indicate that natalizumab may be more effective in the treatment of multiple sclerosis than any of the currently employed therapies. Because α_4 can also pair with β_7, natalizumab has also been tested in patients with Crohn's disease. A subpopulation of these patients have responded favorably to long-term treatment.

At the time this chapter was written, approximately 3500 patients had been treated with efalizumab and about 10 000 had received natalizumab. Compared to placebo groups, only one type of serious adverse reaction was associated with therapy. During natalizumab treatment, reactivation of a polyoma JC virus led to three cases of multifocal leukoencephalopathy, two of which were fatal. Close follow-up studies revealed that the risk of this complication is about 1 in 1000 during 1–2 years of natalizumab treatment. Reports of potentially deadly complications led to the temporary withdrawal of natalizumab from the market, but the benefits of the therapy were recently thought to outweigh the potential risks, and the drug was returned to the market. Apart from the incidence of leukoencephalopathy, only fatigue and allergic reactions have been more common in natalizumab-treated patients than in controls, and no adverse reactions specific to efalizumab have been reported. Thus, it is encouraging that targeted interference with an adhesion molecule has not been shown to lead to a generalized immunosuppression and a concomitant increase in infections. However, other potential problems with SAM therapy include rebound type of exacerbation of the disease after discontinuation of the drugs, and the induction of an immune response against the antibodies, which blunts the efficacy of the therapy. Finally, it should be emphasized that both efalizumab and natalizumab may have anti-inflammatory properties, such as an ability to block T-cell activation, that are not related to their central role in leukocyte recirculation. In any case these two antibodies are the first evidence that the understanding of lymphocyte trafficking can be successfully harnessed in clinical medicine.

■ REFERENCES ■

1. Gowans JC, Knight EJ. The route of re-circulation of lymphocytes in rat. Proc Roy Soc Lond B 1964; 159: 257.

2. Springer TA. Traffic signals for lymphocyte recirculation and leukocyte emigration: the multistep paradigm. Cell 1994; 76: 301.

3. Butcher EC, Picker LJ. Lymphocyte homing and homeostasis. Science 1996; 272: 60.

4. Moore MA. Commentary: the role of cell migration in the ontogeny of the lymphoid system. Stem Cells Dev 2004; 13: 1.

5. von Andrian UH, Mempel TR. Homing and cellular traffic in lymph nodes. Nature Rev Immunol 2003; 3: 867.

6. Randolph GJ, Angeli V, Swartz MA. Dendritic-cell trafficking to lymph nodes through lymphatic vessels. Nature Rev Immunol 2005; 5: 617.

7. Sallusto F, Geginat J, Lanzavecchia A. Central memory and effector memory T cell subsets: function, generation, and maintenance. Annu Rev Immunol 2004; 22: 745.

8. Mebius RE, Kraal G. Structure and function of the spleen. Nature Rev Immunol 2005; 5: 606.

9. Luster AD, Alon R, von Andrian UH. Immune cell migration in inflammation: present and future therapeutic targets. Nature Immunol 2005; 6: 1182.

10. Serhan CN, Savill J. Resolution of inflammation: the beginning programs the end. Nature Immunol 2005; 6: 1191.

11. Aloisi F, Pujol-Borrell R. Lymphoid neogenesis in chronic inflammatory diseases. Nature Rev Immunol 2006; 6: 205.

12. Kupper TS, Fuhlbrigge RC. Immune surveillance in the skin: mechanisms and clinical consequences. Nature Rev Immunol 2004; 4: 211.

13. Muller WA. Leukocyte–endothelial-cell interactions in leukocyte transmigration and the inflammatory response. Trends Immunol 2003; 24: 327.

14. Salmi M, Jalkanen S. Lymphocyte homing to the gut: attraction, adhesion, and commitment. Immunol Rev 2005; 206: 100.

15. Kinashi T. Intracellular signalling controlling integrin activation in lymphocytes. Nature Rev Immunol 2005; 5: 546.

16. Rosen SD. Ligands for L-selectin: homing, inflammation, and beyond. Annu Rev Immunol 2004; 22: 129.

17. Ley K, Kansas GS. Selectins in T-cell recruitment to non-lymphoid tissues and sites of inflammation. Nature Rev Immunol 2004; 4: 325.

18. Moser B, Wolf M, Walz A, et al. Chemokines: multiple levels of leukocyte migration control. Trends Immunol 2004; 25: 75.

19. Carman CV, Springer TA. Integrin avidity regulation: are changes in affinity and conformation underemphasized?. Curr Opin Cell Biol 2003; 15: 547.

20. Steeber DA, Venturi GM, Tedder TF. A new twist to the leukocyte adhesion cascade: intimate cooperation is key. Trends Immunol 2005; 26: 9.

21. Salmi M, Jalkanen S. Cell-surface enzymes in control of leukocyte trafficking. Nature Rev Immunol 2005; 5: 760.

22. Cyster JG. Chemokines, sphingosine-1-phosphate, and cell migration in secondary lymphoid organs. Annu Rev Immunol 2005; 23: 127.

23. Germain RN, Miller MJ, Dustin ML, et al. Dynamic imaging of the immune system: progress, pitfalls and promise. Nature Rev Immunol 2006; 6: 497.

24. Rosen H, Goetzl EJ. Sphingosine 1-phosphate and its receptors: an autocrine and paracrine network. Nature Rev Immunol 2005; 5: 560.

25. Badolato R. Leukocyte circulation: one-way or round-trip? Lessons from primary immunodeficiency patients. J Leukoc Biol 2004; 76: 1.

26. Etzioni A, Alon R. Leukocyte adhesion deficiency III: a group of integrin activation defects in hematopoietic lineage cells. Curr Opin Allergy Clin Immunol 2004; 4: 485.

27. Bunting M, Harris ES, McIntyre TM, et al. Leukocyte adhesion deficiency syndromes: adhesion and tethering defects involving beta 2 integrins and selectin ligands. Curr Opin Hematol 2002; 9: 30.

28. Steinman L. Blocking adhesion molecules as therapy for multiple sclerosis: natalizumab. Nature Rev Drug Discovery 2005; 4: 510.

29. Yopp AC, Krieger NR, Ochando JC, et al. Therapeutic manipulation of T cell chemotaxis in transplantation. Curr Opin Immunol 2004; 16: 571.

30. Kakkar AK, Lefer DJ. Leukocyte and endothelial adhesion molecule studies in knockout mice. Curr Opin Pharmacol 2004; 4: 154.

31. Blattman JN, Greenberg PD. Cancer immunotherapy: a treatment for the masses. Science 2004; 305: 200.

32. Zou W. Regulatory T cells, tumour immunity and immunotherapy. Nature Rev Immunol 2006; 6: 295.

33. Marshall D, Haskard DO. Clinical overview of leukocyte adhesion and migration: where are we now?. Semin Immunol 2002; 14: 133.

34. Simmons DL. Anti-adhesion therapies. Curr Opin Pharmacol 2005; 5: 398.

35. Shimaoka M, Springer TA. Therapeutic antagonists and conformational regulation of integrin function. Nature Rev Drug Discovery 2003; 2: 703.

36. Kupper TS. Immunologic targets in psoriasis. N Engl J Med 2003; 349: 1987.

37. Ropper AH. Selective treatment of multiple sclerosis. N Engl J Med 2006; 354: 965.

REFERENCES

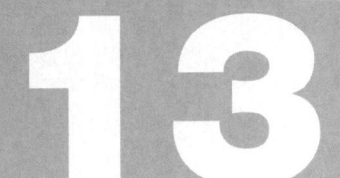

T-cell activation and tolerance

Jonathan S. Maltzman, Erik J. Peterson, Gary Koretzky

Activation of T lymphocytes during an immune response triggers a series of programmed gene regulation, proliferation, differentiation, and effector functions. These programs are designed to allow the immune system to react against foreign antigens without initiating self-reactivity or autoimmunity. Each of these functions is fully dependent on signals originating outside the cell that are recognized by cell surface receptors and then translated by means of a series of biochemical alterations within the cell. This chapter will discuss signals through one of the most studied of these receptors, the antigen-specific T-cell receptor (TCR) complex. It will address how the quality of this signal, in combination with additional co-stimulatory signals, can produce either productive activation or immune tolerance. It will also discuss how abnormal signaling can contribute to T-cell dysfunction and disease (Table 13.1).

THE T-CELL ANTIGEN RECEPTOR COMPLEX

The TCR complex consists of a ligand-binding α/β or γ/δ heterodimer in association with its CD3 complex, which provides transmembrane signal transduction capability (Chapter 4).[1] Specificity of the TCR for antigen resides exclusively within the highly polymorphic clonotypic ligand-binding α/β or γ/δ chains. Although many of the biochemical events leading to α/β and γ/δ T-cell activation are similar, it is important to note that there are differences between these cell types in regard to their development, their spectrum of antigen reactivity, and their role in specific immune responses. This chapter focuses on α/β T cells.

The α/β TCR specifically recognizes short peptide ligands bound to major histocompatibility complex (MHC) antigens (Chapter 5) on the surface of antigen-presenting cells (APCs) (Chapter 6). Co-receptor molecules expressed on subsets of α/β T cells determine whether the TCR recognizes class I or class II MHC. CD4 T cells are stimulated by processed exogenous antigen presented by class II MHC molecules on the surface of professional APCs. CD8 T cells respond to peptides synthesized by the presenting cells and presented by class I molecules. CD4 and CD8 associate with MHC class II and class I molecules, respectively, to stabilize the trimolecular interaction between the TCR, antigen, and MHC, which increases the effectiveness of TCR engagement.

Although the α/β-chains of the TCR contain all of the information necessary for antigen/MHC binding, these proteins cannot initiate the intracellular biochemical events that signal antigen recognition. Instead, signal transduction is accomplished by the noncovalently associated CD3 polypeptides, which include several pairs of transmembrane homodimers (Fig. 13.1) (Chapter 4). Each CD3 chain derives signaling capacity from the presence of a cytoplasmic region known as an immunoreceptor tyrosine-based activation motif (ITAM).[2]

CLINICAL RELEVANCE

Dysfunction or deficiency of T-cell signaling proteins (induced or spontaneous) has been causally linked to several disease states in animal or human models.

Molecules wherein mutations may lead to immune deficiency:

>> CD45
>> LCK
>> ZAP-70
>> SLP-76
>> LAT
>> IL-2R γ chain

Molecules wherein mutations may lead to lymphocyte hyperproliferation:

>> CTLA-4
>> SHP-1
>> CD95/CD95 ligand
>> SAP
>> CBL/CBL-b
>> ZAP-70

Table 13.1 Phenotypes associated with deficient function of selected T-cell signaling molecules

Molecule	Affected signaling event	Phenotype	
		Mouse	Human
TCR signaling			
CD3 γ	TCR expression	B+T+NK+ SCID	B+T+NK+ SCID
CD3 ε	TCR expression	B+T-NK+ SCID	B+T+/-NK+ SCID
CD3 δ	TCR expression	B+T-NK+ SCID	B+T-NK+ SCID
CD3 ζ	TCR expression, TCR-mediated PTK activation	B+T+NK+ SCID	B+T+NK+ SCID
ZAP-70	TCR-mediated PTK activation	B+T+/-NK+ SCID. TCRαβ T cells are absent, but TCRγδ T cells survive. Arthritis occurs in some inbred strains	B+T+/-NK+ SCID. CD8 T-cell lymphopenia. Overexpressed in some hematologic malignancies
LCK	TCR-mediated PTK activation	B+T+/-NK+ SCID. Impaired thymopoiesis and proliferation	B+T+NK+ SCID. CD4 lymphopenia, absent CD28 expression on CD8 T cells, and hypogammaglobulinemia
CD45	Maintenance of SRC family PTK in "open" conformation	B+T+/-NK+ SCID. Impaired thymopoiesis	B+T+/-NK+ SCID. Impaired thymopoiesis, decreased cytotoxic T-cell responses, progressive hypogammaglobulinemia, genetic polymorphisms may correlate with increased prevalence of autoimmune disease
SAP	SHP-2 binding to SLAM	Increased susceptibility to lymphocytic choriomeningitis virus, reduced IgE production, NKT-cell deficiency	X-linked lymphoproliferative disease (XLP) with B-cell hyper-responsiveness, NKT-cell deficiency
WASP	Actin polymerization	Decreased T-cell proliferation and IL-2 production	Wiscott–Aldrich syndrome (immunodeficiency, atopic dermatitis, thrombocytopenia, bloody diarrhea)
CBL/CBL-b[a]	E3 ubiquitin ligase. Recruitment of CrKL/C3G inhibitory complex	Hyperproliferative T cells[a]	Proto-oncogene for leukaemia
LAT	Coupling PTK activation to downstream signals	B+T-NK+ SCID. Absolute block in thymopoiesis	
SLP-76	Coupling PTK activation to downstream signals	B+T-NK+ SCID. Absolute block in thymopoiesis. Defect in vascular/lymphatic development	
Itk/Rlk	Amplification of proximal PTK signals. Activation of PLC-γ1	Defective Th2 immune responses	
CTLA-4	Inhibition of CD28-mediated co-stimulation	Fatal lymphoproliferative disease with myocarditis, pancreatitis	Allelic variants associated with autoimmunity, including Hashimoto's thyroiditis, Graves disease, and systemic lupus erythematosus
SHP-1	Downregulation of PTK activity	Autoimmunity, inflammatory lung disease. "Motheaten" mice	
IL-2R signaling			
γc	Coupling IL-2 binding to JAK activation	B+T-NK- SCID	B+T-NK- SCID, X-linked SCID
JAK3	Phosphorylation of STAT proteins	B+T-NK- SCID	B+T-NK- SCID

[a]CBL and CBL-b are closely-related; CBL-b-deficient mice develop autoimmune features and more severe lymphoproliferative disease than mice lacking CBL.
γc, common γ-chain (IL2Rγ); IgE, immunoglobulin E; NK, natural killer; SCID, severe combined immunodeficiency; TCR, T-cell receptor.

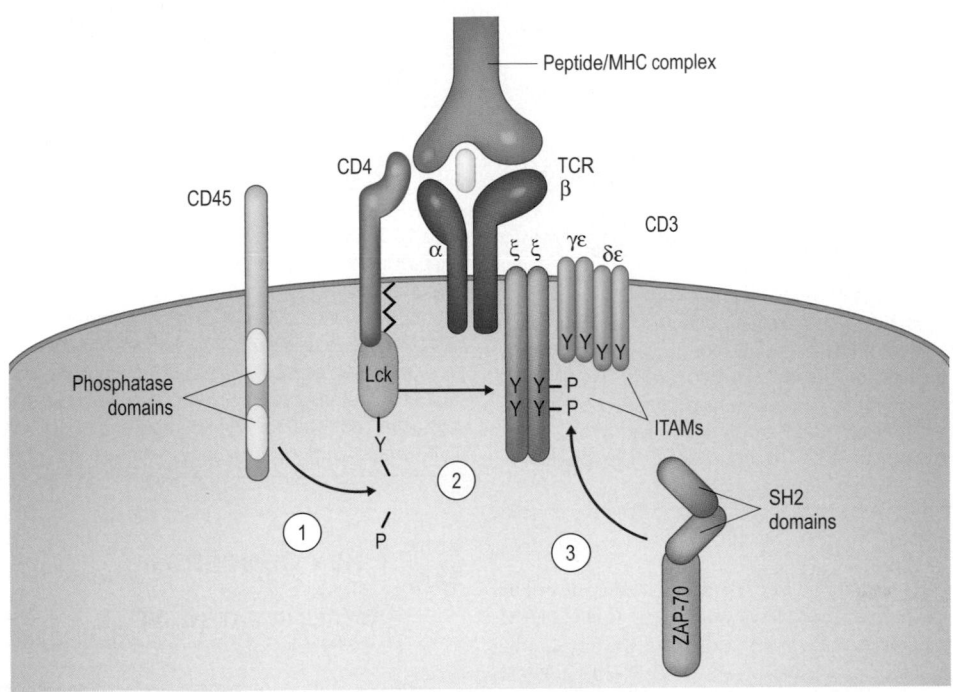

Fig. 13.1 Biochemical events in early T-cell receptor (TCR) signaling. The tyrosine phosphatase CD45 dephosphorylates the negative regulatory tyrosine residue on the CD4-associated protein tyrosine kinase (PTK) LCK, maintaining LCK in an activatable conformation (1). Engagement of the TCR α/β heterodimer and the CD4 (or CD8) co-receptors by MHC-bound peptide antigen brings activated LCK into proximity with immunoreceptor tyrosine-based activation motif (ITAM)-bearing CD3 chains. LCK phosphorylates the CD3ζ chain within ITAMs (2). The phosphorylated ζ-chain ITAMs interact with the tandem SH2 domains of the cytoplasmic PTK ZAP-70 (3), permitting activation of ZAP-70 and phosphorylation of downstream substrates.

KEY CONCEPTS

PROTEIN TYROSINE KINASE ACTIVATION

The earliest detectable biochemical event following T-cell receptor engagement is activation of protein tyrosine kinases:

>> Src family: LCK, FYN

>> Syk family: ZAP-70

>> Tec family: ITK, RLK

ACTIVATION OF PROTEIN TYROSINE KINASES BY THE TCR AND THE ROLE OF THE ITAMS

The first biochemical event known to occur following engagement of the TCR is the activation of LCK and FYN, two members of the SRC family of protein tyrosine kinases (PTKs). Similar to all SRC PTKs, LCK and FYN possess a number of features critical for their function[3] (Fig. 13.2). These include an amino-terminal myristoylation sequence that directs membrane localization; a SRC homology 3 (SH3) domain that permits associations with other proteins containing regions rich in proline residues; a SRC homology 2 (SH2) domain that dictates interactions with

proteins phosphorylated on tyrosine residues; a catalytic region, and a carboxyl-terminal tyrosine residue. The precise mechanism whereby LCK and FYN are stimulated by the TCR is not clear, but both have been shown to associate physically with TCR CD3 components and/or CD4 and CD8. SRC family PTK enzymatic function is regulated in part by the state of tyrosine phosphorylation of the kinase. When the conserved carboxyl-terminal tyrosine residue is phosphorylated, the SRC family PTKs adopt a closed conformation that is the product of an intramolecular interaction between that phosphotyrosine and the SH2 domain (Fig. 13.3). This intramolecular interaction inhibits the enzymatic activity of the PTK, limiting subsequent tyrosine phosphorylation-dependent signaling events. Phosphorylation of the carboxyl-terminal tyrosine (Y505 in LCK and Y527 in FYN) is dynamically regulated.[4] Phosphate is transferred to this residue by the cytoplasmic PTK, CSK, and removed by the transmembrane protein tyrosine phosphatase, CD45.

The phenotypes of CD45-deficient cells, mice, and humans highlight the critical regulatory importance of the carboxyl-terminal tyrosine in SRC family PTKs.[5] TCR signal transduction in cell lines lacking CD45 is blocked at the most proximal step, and mice that have been genetically modified to lack CD45 expression exhibit profound defects in thymocyte development and subsequent T-cell activation. CD45 deficiency in humans creates a T[-], B[+], NK[+] severe combined immunodeficiency (SCID) (Chapter 35). These outcomes correlate with markedly impaired LCK enzymatic activity and hyperphosphorylation on the regulatory tyrosine.

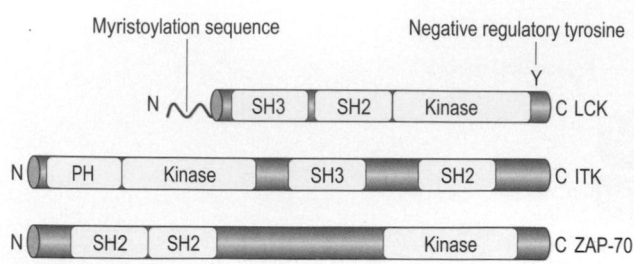

Fig. 13.2 Domain organization of T-cell receptor (TCR)-stimulated protein tyrosine kinases (PTKs). Comparative schematic representation of members of three families of PTKs required for T-cell-activating signals. In addition to catalytic domains, LCK (Src family), ITK (Tec family), and ZAP-70 (Syk family) each contain regions responsible for mediating protein–protein interactions, including SH3 and SH2 domains. SH3, Src homology 3; SH2, Src homology 2; PH, pleckstrin homology.

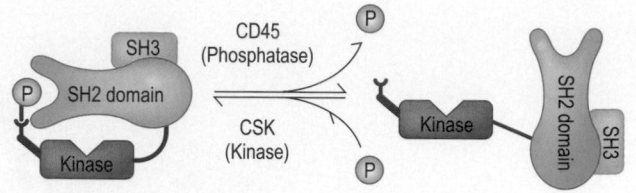

Fig. 13.3 Model for dynamic regulation of LCK by intramolecular interaction between an SH2 domain and phosphotyrosine. The transmembrane phosphatase CD45 dephosphorylates tyrosine 505 in the carboxyl-terminus of the SRC family protein tyrosine kinase (PTK) LCK. CD45 activity maintains LCK in an "open" conformation, permitting LCK kinase domain access to intracellular substrates. CSK activity opposes that of CD45; phosphorylation of tyrosine 505 results in an intramolecular interaction between the SH2 domain and phosphotyrosine. Inhibition of LCK kinase activity correlates with the "closed" conformation (left).

Following TCR engagement and PTK activation, numerous cellular substrates become tyrosine-phosphorylated, including CD3 ITAMs (Fig. 13.1). ITAM phosphorylation creates a docking site for another cytosolic PTK, zeta-associated phosphoprotein-70 (ZAP-70). ZAP-70, a member of the SYK family of PTKs, contains a catalytic domain that is located carboxyl-terminal to two tandem SH2 domains (Fig. 13.2). The ZAP-70 SH2 domains have affinity for phosphotyrosine present within ITAMs. Thus, inducible phosphorylation of CD3 γ, δ, ε, and ζ results in the recruitment of ZAP-70 to these components of the TCR. Upon TCR recruitment, ZAP-70 enzymatic activity is increased owing to phosphorylation by LCK, as well as autophosphorylation. The net result of these phosphorylations is conversion of the TCR from an enzymatically inactive complex to a potent PTK.

The critical importance of LCK, FYN, and ZAP-70 for both thymocyte development and mature T-cell activation has been established by studies in mutant cell lines, mice, and humans. Jurkat T cells (a human leukemic cell line commonly employed as a model for mature T-cell activation)[6] deficient in expression of either LCK or ZAP-70 cannot be activated via the TCR. Mice deficient in ZAP-70 or LCK, but not in FYN, exhibit a significant yet incomplete block in early T-cell development. This phenotype suggests that the pre-TCR (a complex present on immature thymocytes which includes signaling components thought similar to the TCR on mature T cells) also requires SRC and SYK family PTKs to transduce signals. ZAP-70 deficiency and abnormal LCK function in humans create a T⁻,B⁺, NK⁺ SCID (Chapter 35).[7]

Developing and mature T lymphocytes differ in their requirements for FYN and LCK.[8, 9] Fyn deficiency has no gross effect on thymocyte development, but mice deficient in both LCK and FYN have an absolute block at the pre-TCR checkpoint. Consistent with the finding that basal TCR signals are required for naïve T-cell survival, the expression of either LCK or FYN is sufficient for survival of naïve T lymphocytes. However, mice deficient in LCK and FYN exhibit defective lymphopenia-induced homeostatic proliferation of naïve T cells. LCK but not FYN expression is able to revert this phenotype and allow this type of lymphocyte expansion.

In addition to SRC and SYK family PTKs, TCR engagement also results in the activation of a third family of cytosolic PTKs, the Tec family.[10]

SIGNALING PATHWAYS

T-cell receptor engagement leads to the initiation of signaling cascades, including:

>> PLCγ1 activation
    Calcium flux
    DAG formation
>> RAS/MAPK

Members of this family in T cells include Tec, ITK, and RLK. Tec PTKs contain SH2, SH3, and catalytic domains, as well as pleckstrin homology (PH) domains that mediate interactions with membrane-localized phospholipids (Fig. 13.2). PH domains permit the recruitment of Tec family kinases to the plasma membrane, where they can phosphorylate important substrates. Studies in mutant T-cell lines suggest that the activation of Tec family members is dependent upon the prior activation of SRC and SYK family PTKs. In addition, mice made deficient in Tec PTKs display signaling defects downstream of the TCR and chemokine receptors, as evidenced by alterations in actin reorganization, adhesion, and migration.

Unlike SRC and SYK family PTKs whose loss results in an absence of TCR signaling, Tec family kinases are thought to act as modulators of TCR signal strength. Thus, deficiency results in only partial defects in thymocyte development (both positive and negative selection), and mice lacking Tec family kinases retain peripheral T cells for functional study. Rlk and Itk are differentially expressed in the Th1 and Th2 subsets. Itk, not Rlk, is expressed in Th2 cells, for example. Deficiency of Itk results in defective interleukin-4 (IL-4) secretion and *in vivo* Th2-dependent immunity.

SECOND-MESSENGER CASCADES DOWNSTREAM OF THE TCR-STIMULATED PTKS

All of the well-established signaling pathways initiated by TCR engagement are dependent upon the activation of ZAP-70 and its association with the CD3 ITAMs. The link between PTK activation and several

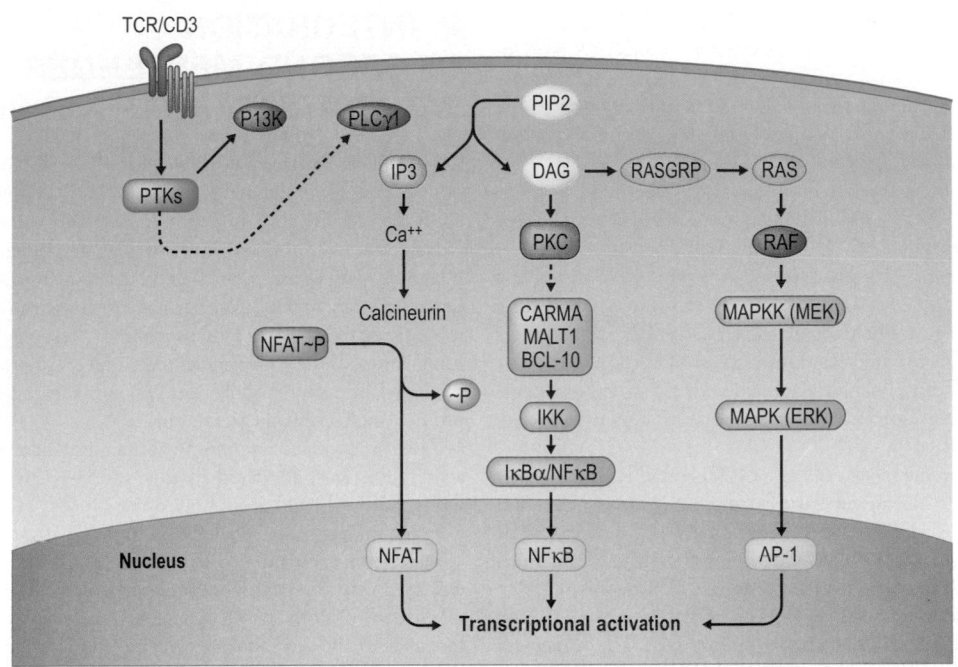

Fig. 13.4 Signaling pathways activated by T-cell receptor (TCR) engagement. TCR ligation results in activation of protein tyrosine kinases (PTKs) such as LCK and ZAP-70. Phospholipase Cγ1 (PLCγ1) becomes phosphorylated and activated by ITK and PI3K. Hydrolysis of phosphatidyl inositol bisphosphate (PIP$_2$) by PLCγ1 releases diacylglycerol (DAG) and inositol trisphosphate (IP$_3$). IP$_3$ stimulates an increase in intracellular calcium concentration, which activates the phosphatase calcineurin. Calcineurin dephosphorylates NFAT, thereby signaling NFAT translocation to the nucleus. The formation of DAG leads to activation of RAS-GRP1 GEF activity and RAS activation. Active RAS binds and stimulates the kinase RAF1, initiating a cascade of serine/threonine kinases (MAPK cascade) leading to phosphorylation and nuclear translocation of the ERK kinases. DAG formation also results in activation of the CARMA/BCL-1/MALT1 complex leading to phosphorylation of IκB kinase (IKK). Active IKK phosphorylates IκB-α, leading to IκB-α degradation and release of NF-κB to the nucleus. Transcription factors NFAT, NFκB, and those activated by the MAPK pathway cooperate to upregulate transcription of genes such as IL-2 critical for T-cell activation.

downstream second-messenger cascades is now well established. One consequence of effective TCR stimulation is activation of the membrane-associated enzyme phospholipase Cγ1 (PLCγ1) (Fig. 13.4).[11]

Phosphatidylinositol 4,5-bisphosphate (PIP$_2$), a minor phospholipid constituent of the plasma membrane, serves as a substrate for PLCγ1. PIP$_2$ hydrolysis gives rise to two biochemical second messengers, the soluble sugar inositol 1,4,5-trisphosphate (IP$_3$) and the lipid diacylglycerol (DAG). IP$_3$ binding to its cognate receptor on endoplasmic reticulum results in the release of calcium from this organelle. DAG is a physiological activator of some members of the protein kinase C (PKC) family of serine/threonine kinases. The importance of calcium mobilization and activation of PKC family members for T-cell activation was suggested by the observation that the combination of calcium ionophore and phorbol ester, pharmacologic agents which induce these biochemical events, can substitute for TCR engagement and lead to T-cell proliferation and cytokine production.[12]

Among the TCR-initiated biochemical events dependent upon calcium flux is the activation of calcineurin, a serine/threonine phosphatase. The substrates of calcineurin include members of the nuclear factor of activated T cells (NFAT) family.[13] These transcription factors are phosphorylated in the cytosol of resting T cells. Activated calcineurin dephosphorylates NFAT, allowing it to translocate to the nucleus and bind response elements in the promoters of genes important for T-cell activation.

The importance of the calcineurin pathway in T-cell activation has been exploited clinically through the use of cyclosporine A and tacrolimus, which inhibit this pathway through distinct mechanisms. These drugs are mainstays in the prevention of human solid-organ transplant rejection (Chapter 80) and are now beginning to be used to treat autoimmune diseases such as *systemic lupus erythematosus* (Chapter 51).

The mechanistic link between TCR-induced PTK activation and the PLCγ1 pathway remains incompletely understood. PLCγ1 is inducibly tyrosine-phosphorylated following TCR binding, an event that correlates with increased PLCγ1 enzymatic activity.[14] However, PLCγ1 is phosphorylated on multiple tyrosine residues, and it remains uncertain which TCR-stimulated PTK, and which tyrosine residues are most critical for PLCγ1 activation. In fact, recent work suggests that PLCγ1 is phosphorylated by multiple PTKs, including both ZAP-70 and members of the Tec family. Furthermore, TCR-stimulated tyrosine phosphorylation alone is not sufficient to activate PLCγ1; localization of the enzyme probably plays a critical role as well.

A second major signaling pathway stimulated by engagement of the TCR involves activation of the small-molecular-weight guanine nucleotide-binding protein RAS.[15] Evidence for the central importance of RAS activation for T-cell function has come from studies in cell lines and in genetically altered mice. Jurkat T cells expressing inhibitory mutant forms of RAS fail to produce IL-2 following TCR engagement. In contrast, Jurkat cells expressing an activated form of RAS produce IL-2 much more readily than do wild-type cells. Similarly, mice transgenic for activating RAS mutants show alterations in thymocyte development and demonstrate a partially stimulated state in the absence of antigen binding.

RAS is a 21-kDa protein localized to the plasma membrane owing to post-translational fatty acid modifications. In its inactive state, RAS binds guanosine diphosphate (GDP). Upon RAS activation GDP is exchanged for guanosine triphosphate (GTP), allowing RAS to interact with and activate a cascade of serine-threonine protein kinases, including RAF, MEK, and the extracellular regulated kinase (ERK). This kinase cascade culminates with the nuclear translocation of ERK. Upon entry into the nucleus, ERK can phosphorylate and activate several transcription factors that are critical for TCR-induced transactivation of cytokines and other activation genes.

In T lymphocytes, exchange of GTP for GDP-bound RAS can occur through one of two distinct molecular mechanisms involving the guanine exchange factors (GEFs) SOS or RASGRP1.[16] Following TCR activation, SOS is recruited to the plasma membrane through its interaction with the Grb2 adaptor protein. This mechanism is similar to events leading to RAS activation downstream of growth receptors with intrinsic tyrosine kinase acitivity in nonlymphoid cells. T lymphocytes express additional GEFs that are members of the Ras guanyl nucleotide-releasing protein (RasGRP) family. These proteins contain Ras exchange-, DAG binding- and EF hand-motifs. The exact mechanism of RasGRP activation remains unclear, but may involve nonclassical PKC family members such as PKC-θ or direct activation by DAG. The importance of the RasGRP pathway in TCR-mediated signaling is highlighted by the finding that deletion of RasGRP1 leads to severe defects in thymocyte development in mice. Ras activity is also regulated through the hydrolysis of RAS-bound GTP to GDP, either through the intrinsic GTPase activity of RAS or through the recruitment of GTPase-activating proteins (GAPs) to the active RAS molecule. Thus, the ability of RAS to modulate T-cell activation events is governed both by signals leading to the exchange of GTP for GDP and signals affecting the rate of GTP hydrolysis.

Stimulation of T cells also involves activation of the lipid kinase phosphatidylinositol 3'-hydroxyl kinase (PI3K) (Fig. 13.4).[17] PI3K phosphorylates phosphoinositides, which play an important role in the regulation of several downstream serine/threonine kinases. The activation of PI3K requires phosphorylation of a regulatory subunit that controls catalytic activity conferred by a 110-kDa subunit. Although TCR engagement alone can stimulate some degree of PI3K function, full activity of the lipid kinase appears to require co-stimulation of the T cell through receptors such as CD28 (see below).

Cross-linking of the TCR also leads to activation and nuclear translocation of members of the nuclear factor-κB (NFκB) family of transcription factors (Fig. 13.4).[18] Defects in immune activation result from the lack of NFκB activity. Normally, NFκB family members are sequestered in the cytoplasm through interaction with inhibitors of NFκB (IκBs). TCR stimulation results in the formation of a multimolecular complex composed of CARMA1, BCL-10, and MALT1. Formation of this complex may involve the activation of PKC-θ. Formation of the CARMA1–BCL-10–MALT1 complex leads to activation of IκB kinases (IKKs), phosphorylation and degradation of IκB, and subsequent release and translocation to the nucleus of NFκB.

INTEGRATION OF SECOND-MESSENGER PATHWAYS BY ADAPTOR PROTEINS

One of the most daunting challenges in T-cell biology is to understand how biochemical signaling pathways initiated by engagement of the TCR are coordinated to result in the appropriate biologic response. Considerable insight into how intracellular signaling pathways can be integrated has come from the recent characterization of adaptor proteins.[14,19,20] Adaptors lack enzymatic or transcriptional regulatory activity. Instead, they possess modular domains responsible for intermolecular interactions. Both constitutive and induced intermolecular interactions mediated by adaptor molecules can provide the necessary scaffold to promote signal transduction events.

Adaptor proteins commonly contain modular domains that exhibit affinity for phosphorylated tyrosine residues (Fig. 13.5A). Such regions include the SH2 and phosphotyrosine-binding (PTB) domains. Each of these domains recognizes phosphorylated tyrosine residues within a specific sequence context. For example, PTB domains obtain their specificity based on residues amino-terminal to the phosphotyrosine, whereas SH2 domains recognize particular sequence motifs carboxyl-terminal to the key phosphotyrosine. Other adaptor domains include SH3 modules, which bind proline-rich regions; WW regions responsible for interactions with proline/tyrosine or proline/leucine motifs; and PH domains that have specificity for phospholipids.

It is clear that many ubiquitously expressed adaptors, as well as others with more restricted tissue distribution, function in diverse cellular processes. Several hematopoietic-specific adaptors are now known to play essential roles in T-cell development, in coordinating the signals necessary for mature T-cell activation, and in the process of terminating T-cell responses. Two adaptors critical for T-cell activation, linker of activated T cells (LAT) and SH2 domain containing leukocyte phosphoprotein of 76 kDa (SLP-76), are described in this section.

Both LAT and SLP-76 were identified in efforts to characterize substrates of the PTKs stimulated by TCR engagement. LAT is a 36-kDa integral membrane protein that contains numerous tyrosine residues within its cytoplasmic tail (Fig. 13.5A). The tyrosines exist within the correct sequence motifs needed to bind the SH2 domains of other T-cell signaling molecules. In stimulated T cells LAT becomes associated with Grb2, GADS (another Grb2 family member), PLCγ1, and the p85 subunit of PI3K. It is likely that these induced intermolecular interactions are critical for communicating TCR engagement to downstream second-messenger cascades. The importance of LAT for T-cell activation was suggested by the signaling phenotype of LAT-deficient variants of the Jurkat T-cell leukemic line. Engagement of the TCR on these cells fails to result in signaling events downstream of ZAP-70 activation. Furthermore, examination of LAT-deficient mice revealed an essential role for LAT in T-cell development. The Lat$^{-/-}$ mice have significantly decreased numbers of thymocytes, which are arrested at an early stage during development. Arrested thymocyte development leads to the complete lack of T cells in Lat$^{-/-}$ peripheral lymphoid organs. In recent *in vivo* studies, a knockin of a PLCγ1-binding mutant of LAT partially restored thymocyte development but also resulted in a lymphoproliferative phenotype in adult animals.

Using similar approaches, it was shown that SLP-76 is absolutely required for both T-cell development and signaling via the mature TCR.

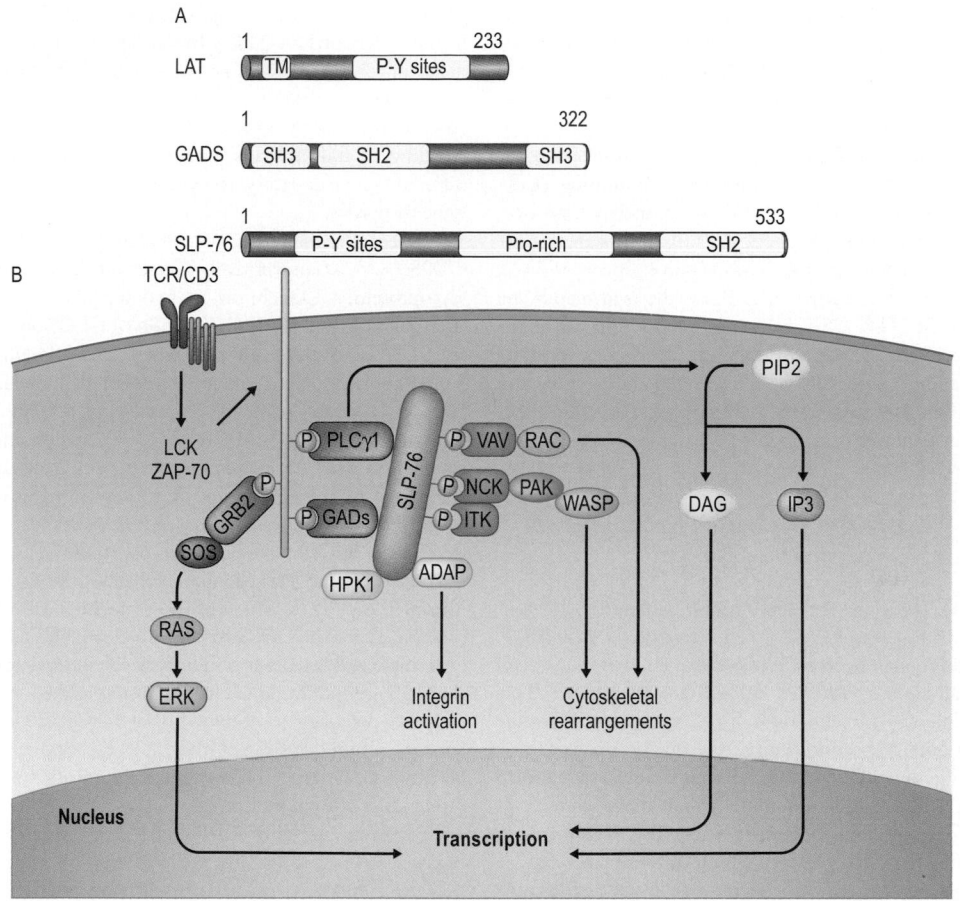

Fig. 13.5 Model for adaptor protein-mediated coupling of the T-cell receptor (TCR) to phospholipase Cγ1 (PLCγ1) activation. (A) Structural schematics of three adaptors implicated in plasma membrane proximal biochemical events. SH3 domains mediate association with proline-rich regions; SH2 domains associate with phosphorylated tyrosine residues. (B) LAT and SLP-76 are among the substrates of the TCR activated protein tyrosine kinases (PTKs). When tyrosine residues within the LAT cytoplasmic tail are phosphorylated, GADS binds to LAT through the GADS SH2 domain. Recruitment of GADS results in relocalization of SLP-76, as the proline-rich region of SLP-76 mediates constitutive association with the SH3 domain of GADS. Tyrosine-phosphorylated SLP-76, in turn, becomes associated with ITK via the ITK SH2 domain. ITK is thus brought into proximity with membrane-localized substrates, including PLCγ1. Activation of PLCγ1 leads to hydrolysis of phosphatidylinositol 4,5-bisphosphate (PIP2) and activation of transcription factors such as nuclear factor-κB (NFκB), activating protein 1 (AP-1), and nuclear factor of activated T cells (NFAT). SH2 domain containing leukocyte phosphoprotein of 76 kDa (SLP-76) also recruits several other signaling molecules, such as VAV, NCK, HPK1, and ADAP, thereby regulating changes in the actin cytoskeleton and adhesion. Phosphorylation of linker of activated T cells (LAT) also leads to recruitment of Grb2/SOS and an additional pathway for RAS activation. TM, transmembrane domain; P-Y, sites for phosphorylation of tyrosine; pro-rich, proline-rich regions.

Thus, mice deficient in SLP-76 show a complete block in thymocyte development. In mutant T-cell lines lacking SLP-76, the PLCγ1 and RAS/MAPK signaling cascades are not activated by TCR ligation, despite normal TCR-stimulated activation of ZAP-70. SLP-76 contains an amino-terminal region with tyrosine phosphorylation sites, a central proline-rich domain, and a carboxyl-terminal SH2 domain. Unlike LAT, SLP-76 does not possess a transmembrane domain. By means of its proline-rich region, SLP-76 constitutively associates with GADS and through its SH2 domain can inducibly interact with other tyrosine-phosphorylated adaptors such as HPK-1 and ADAP. Following tyrosine phosphorylation, SLP-76 inducibly binds other SH2-domain-containing proteins (e.g., VAV, an exchange factor for the RAC GTP-binding protein; NCK, an adaptor protein; and ITK, a Tec family PTK). Each of the SLP-76 domains appears critical for its function, as the overexpression of mutant variants of SLP-76 is unable to restore TCR signaling efficiency fully in either Jurkat T cells or SLP-76-deficient mice. In contrast, overexpression of wild-type SLP-76 dramatically augments TCR-stimulated second-messenger production.

One model of how SLP-76 and LAT functionally interact is as follows.[21] Following TCR engagement, the two adaptors associate with each other, bridged by GADS and perhaps PLCγ1. These interactions anchor a multimolecular "signalosome" at the plasma membrane (Fig. 13.5B). Formation of this complex brings Itk into proximity of PLCγ1, resulting in phosphorylation and activation and leading to the generation of IP₃ and DAG, as described above.

Along with LAT and SLP-76, T cells express a large number of other adaptor proteins that appear to play important roles in promoting TCR-mediated signal transduction events. Many of these are widely expressed, and some are expressed only in hematopoetic cells. Adaptors are important for the coordination of both positive and negative aspects of TCR activation. For example, in the absence of antigen, the transmembrane adaptor PAG binds to the PTK CSK, bringing it to the plasma membrane.[19] Membrane-localized CSK phosphorylates the regulatory tyrosine of LCK, thus keeping LCK inactive. Delineating the positive and negative aspects of signal transduction mediated by subcellular localization of kinases and phosphatases is an ongoing area of active research by multiple laboratories worldwide.

CO-RECEPTORS TRANSDUCE SIGNALS THAT ARE INTEGRATED WITH TCR SIGNALS

Engagement of the TCR without the concomitant stimulation of other signaling pathways does not lead to full T-cell activation. T-cell proliferation and the initiation of effector function require that the T cell must receive additional signals via other cell surface receptors.[22] This requirement for multiple signals allows the T cell to express an exquisitely sensitive TCR while protecting against the inappropriate activation of potentially dangerous effector cells. Because T cells respond to antigens presented on APCs, stimulation under physiological conditions involves the potential engagement of multiple ligand co-receptors on the T cell by various ligands on the APC. Many of these co-receptors have been characterized, and progress has been made in our understanding of how these molecules promote T-cell activation. One obvious way in which co-receptors may function is to increase the avidity of the interaction between the T cell and the APC. Interestingly, however, many co-receptors are also capable of transducing signals themselves, some independent of and others synergistic with the TCR. Additionally, co-receptors are often important as recruiters of the cytoplasmic signaling molecules and the adaptor proteins described above.

The most intensively studied co-receptors are CD4 and CD8 (Chapter 4). CD4 and CD8 expression defines subsets of T cells responding to class II or class I-bound peptide antigen, respectively (Chapter 9). In addition to increasing the affinity of the TCR–antigen interaction, both CD4 and CD8 participate in TCR-mediated signal transduction, because they each associate with LCK.[2] This constitutive interaction, which occurs via specific residues within the CD4 and CD8 cytoplasmic domains, localizes a key effector enzyme to the TCR complex.

CO-STIMULATORY MOLECULES ARE REQUIRED FOR OPTIMAL T-CELL ACTIVATION

As stated earlier, T-cell stimulation is a composite of TCR cross-linking and co-stimulatory signals. In contrast to the CD4 and CD8 co-receptors that bind to MHC molecules, other ligands on APCs interact with additional T-cell surface proteins termed co-stimulatory molecules. The importance of co-stimulatory molecules is implied by the large number of proteins expressed on the cell surface of T cells and the number of ligands expressed on APCs. Initially, it was thought that there is redundancy in co-stimulation; in other words, as long as a co-stimulatory signal is sufficient to attain an activation threshold, it does not matter which specific molecules are involved. However, recent advances in the understanding of the molecular mechanisms of co-stimulation indicate that different co-stimulatory receptor–ligand pairs confer different phenotypic responses.

The best-characterized co-stimulatory molecule present on T cells is CD28,[23, 24] a constitutively expressed homodimeric transmembrane glycoprotein. CD28 binds to two ligands expressed on APCs, B7.1 (CD80) and B7.2 (CD86). Ligation of CD28 on its own has little effect on T-cell activation; however, when CD28 is engaged along with the TCR, many TCR signals are augmented. Indeed, concomitant CD28 and TCR engagement is required for activation of naïve T cells. Co-stimulation of the TCR plus CD28 dramatically augments IL-2 production, both by increasing transcription of the IL-2 gene and by stabilizing its mRNA. If the TCR is engaged in the absence of CD28 co-stimulation, such a stimulus leads not to activation but either to T-cell death by apoptosis or to a state of unresponsiveness.

Although much has been learned about the signal transduction events mediated by CD28, which of these biochemical events is critical for the biologic effects of CD28 remains unclear.[24] CD28 contains no intrinsic enzymatic activity, but it is inducibly phosphorylated on tyrosine residues during T-cell activation. These phosphorylated tyrosines recruit several signal-transducing molecules possessing SH2 domains, including the 85-kDa subunit of PI3K, Grb2, and ITK. Several lines of evidence suggest that TCR- and CD28-dependent activation of PI3K interferes with, rather than stimulates, IL-2 gene transcription. CD28 engagement also co-stimulates activation of members of the mitogen-activated protein kinase (MAPK) family, in particular c-JUN N-terminal kinase (JNK). CD28-stimulated JNK activity plays an important role in optimizing cytokine production and protecting T cells from apoptosis. Another postulated mechanism for how CD28 promotes T-cell activation rests on the observation that stimulation of the TCR alone results in activation of RAP1, a small-molecular-weight GTP-binding protein. Activated RAP1 competes with RAS for downstream effectors and prevents the propagation of RAS-mediated signaling events. Co-stimulation of T cells via the TCR plus CD28 interferes with RAP1 activation, allowing the RAS pathways to signal effectively.

CD28 is the prototype member of a family of structurally related co-stimulatory receptors. CD28 binds to B71 (CD80) and B72 (CD86) expressed on APCs.[23] Other family members include CTLA-4 (cytotoxic lymphocyte-associated antigen 4), ICOS (inducible co-stimulator), PD-1 (programmed death 1), and BTLA (B- and T-lymphocyte attenuator). Cellular expression patterns and functional consequences vary drastically for molecules in this group. While CD28–B7 interactions are co-stimulatory, ligation of CTLA-4 by B7 is inhibitory (see T-cell anergy section below). As its name implies, ICOS is not expressed on naïve cells but is induced following stimulation. ICOS–ICOS-L interactions are important for T-cell help to B cells. Blockade of this interaction can affect the immune response in murine models of autoimmunity such as collagen-induced arthritis and experimental autoimmune encephalomyelitis (EAE), and CD28–B7 binding is thus a potential therapeutic target in solid-organ transplants. ICOS deficiency can also lead to common variable immune deficiency (CVID) (Chapter 34). PD-1 can interact with two different ligands, PDL-1 and PDL-2. PD-1–PDL-1/PDL-2 interaction can lead

KEY CONCEPTS

Mechanisms of tolerance can be divided into central and peripheral:

>> Central

   Clonal deletion/AIRE

>> Peripheral

   Immune privilege
   Anergy
   Regulation

to co-stimulation or to downregulation of the immune response depending on their cellular context and the experimental system utilized.

A second large class of co-stimulatory molecules includes members of the tumor necrosis factor receptor (TNFR) family.[25] Co-stimulatory TNFR family members include OX40 (CD134), 4-1BB (CD137), HVEM, CD30, and GITR. These are type I transmembrane proteins containing extracellular cysteine-rich domains. The cytoplasmic domains contain sequences that recruit a family of adaptor molecules known as TNF receptor-associated factors (TRAFs). For example, trimerization of OX40 leads to recruitment of TRAF2, TRAF3, and TRAF5, while GITR recruits TRAF1, TRAF2, and TRAF3. The induced downstream effector pathways also vary between the TNFRs, but NFκB induction is common among them. A substantial amount of data has been gathered regarding the cellular expression and function of each of these receptors and details of each receptor to T-cell activation, and the immune response are beyond the scope of this chapter. OX40 is preferentially expressed on activated CD4 T cells with its expression peaking approximately 48 hours after CD3/CD28 stimulation. OX40 deficiency leads to defects in CD4 T-cell proliferation and can affect survival of memory T cells. Blockade of the OX40–OX40L interaction is required for the induction of EAE and collagen-induced arthritis. *In vitro*, the engagement of OX40 enhances the proliferative response of T cells to submitogenic anti-TCR stimuli. Further, OX40 blockade partially interferes with this T-cell response. Little is yet known about the mechanism of OX40 action.

Like OX40, 4-1BB is a co-stimulatory molecule present primarily on activated T cells. Although it is expressed on both CD4 and CD8 cells, some data suggest that the engagement of 4-1BB preferentially leads to CD8 cell proliferation and protection from apoptosis. The delayed kinetics of 4-1BB expression suggest that, in contrast to the early-acting CD28, 4-1BB plays a role later in the immune response.

■ TOLERANCE ■

Tolerance is an inherent property of the immune system that governs the ability to respond against foreign antigens (nonself) without attacking the host (self). A lack of self-tolerance leads to autoimmune disease, whereas a host displaying excessive tolerance may be more susceptible to pathogens. The immune system in any individual must therefore be able to distinguish subtle differences between self and nonself. To accomplish this delicate task, multiple complementary mechanisms of immune system tolerance have developed. The remainder of this chapter will discuss tolerance in the T-cell compartment.

The concept of immune tolerance pre-dated our understanding of the cellular and molecular bases for the phenomenon. Owen's experiments in cattle showed that a shared blood supply during development led to lifelong immune tolerance. Billingham, Brent, and Medawar expanded upon the experiments in 1953 by showing that *in utero* inoculation with foreign tissue resulted in tolerance to foreign skin grafts later in life.

The process of tolerance is often divided between central and peripheral mechanisms. Central tolerance refers to tolerance that is induced during development of T cells in the thymus (Chapter 9). Central tolerance occurs in an antigen-specific fashion through the process of clonal deletion. Gene rearrangement to form the TCR is a random process that allows for the generation of T cells with an incredible repertoire of specificities (Chapter 4). Invariably, some of these receptors will react against self-protein products. It is believed that lymphocytes specific for MHC plus self-peptides will encounter most of these self-antigens during development in the thymus. In contrast to mature T cells that respond to encounter with their specific antigen with a program of proliferation and differentiation, immature lymphocytes respond by undergoing a process of activation-induced cell death. Although there are mechanisms (see below) to ensure a full repertoire of self is expressed in the thymus, it is invariable that some self-reactive cells will develop and emigrate from the thymus to the peripheral lymphoid compartment. Control of such 'escaped' autoreactive cells is achieved through peripheral tolerance mechanisms.

CENTRAL TOLERANCE/CLONAL DELETION

While the concept of T-cell tolerance is decades old, it took the development of new techniques and reagents to track the fate of clonal T-cell populations before the molecular mechanisms of clonal deletion could be elucidated.[26–28] Single-cell identification using monoclonal antibody recognizing the Vβ17 TCR variable region demonstrated clonal deletion of developing T cells that express MHC I-E. CD4⁺CD8⁺ (double-positive (DP)) thymocytes expressing Vβ17 were present, but CD4 single-positive (CD4SP) or CD8SP were not. This suggested that clonal deletion occurs at the DP to SP transition. Further studies in this model system eventually showed deletion was specific not only for the expression of I-E, but also required expression of an endogenous murine retrovirus, which appeared to serve as the dominant self-antigen.

The next significant advance in our understanding of central tolerance made use of new technologies to manipulate the mouse genome by producing transgenic mice expressing a single specificity TCR. The vast majority of developing T cells in H-Y mice, the first TCR-transgenic model of clonal deletion, are reactive against a Y-chromosome-encoded antigen, H-Y. Massive deletion of these cells results in small thymi in male mice with only a small number of DP thymocytes able to survive the antigen-induced cell death. Since these initial descriptions, significant advances have been made. Depending on the experimental system employed, deletion can occur prior to, during, or after the double-positive stage.

Deletion for self-reactivity implies that the extent of autoreactivity of the developing thymocytes is systematically calibrated. A currently favored model is one that employs strength of signal as determined by a combination of TCR affinity and co-stimulation to assess the extent of self-reactivity. Signals that go beyond a threshold of acceptability lead to clonal deletion. This model is supported by experiments in which the TCR signaling machinery has been genetically altered to increase or decrease signal intensity from each TCR. For example, an increase in the number of ITAMs (presumably leading to increases in downstream signals) enhances clonal deletion in a transgenic system.[29] Similarly, transgenic alterations of the levels of CD8, a positive regulator, or CD5, the negative regulator,[30] also affect the efficiency of clonal deletion.

An implicit assumption required for clonal deletion to be a major mechanism of tolerance is that T cells must come into contact with all self-antigens during thymocyte maturation. It is easy to recognize how deletion of cells reactive to MHC and other widely expressed protein products can occur in the thymus. However, there are also self-antigens whose expression is restricted to a specific tissue or developmental timepoint. What are the mechanisms that allow clonal deletion to antigens expressed only in the pancreas or testes, for example? One possibility is that all proteins could be transported to the thymus by APCs. Another model holds that subsets of thymus-resident APCs may "ectopically" express tissue-specific antigens. Recent work describing the function of the transcription factor AIRE supports the latter model.[31]

AIRE expression drives medullary thymic epithelial cells (mTECs) to express peptides from open reading frames ectopically. Self-reactive developing T cells are thus exposed to tissue-specific self-peptides in the thymus and are deleted. AIRE-deficient humans and mice develop autoimmune polyendocrinopathy-candidiais-ectodermal dystrophy (APS-1 or APECED in humans: Chapter 35), emphasizing the role of central tolerance in preventing T-cell-mediated autoimmune disease.

PERIPHERAL MECHANISMS OF TOLERANCE

Clonal deletion, like all biological processes, is not perfect. Given the potential for autoimmune destruction should clonal deletion fail (as typified in those individuals with an AIRE mutation), there must be backup mechanisms to control autoreactivity for those few cells that manage to escape the thymus. These mechanisms include immune privilege, anergy, and regulation.

Immune Privilege

The concept of 'immune privilege' was first described by Medawar more than 50 years ago. Typically described areas of immune privilege include the anterior chamber of the eye, the brain, and the fetus in pregnant females.[32] Both the eye and the brain have a limited capacity for regeneration, and it is believed that an immune response in these areas could have devastating effects on the individual. As a fetus expresses MHC derived from both parents, peripheral tolerance of the mother to the fetus is required for fetal survival.

Multiple mechanisms have been proposed to account for immune privilege. Medawar believed that tolerance in these areas was due to limited lymphatic drainage. In this model, lymphocytes cannot easily gain entrance to the privileged site and foreign antigens deposited there are not transported to secondary lymphoid organs, which prevents initiation of an immune response. One additional local mechanism that likely contributes to tolerance at these locations is a low level or complete absence of expression of classical MHC class Ia protein on cells of the eye and brain. Low level expression of MHC molecules may be required to protect some of these cells from CTL-mediated cell lysis (Chapters 5 and 18). In the case of the developing fetus, the cells of the villous trophoblast lack expression of class I MHC.

Cells in these areas also express cell surface and soluble factors that downregulate the immune response. For example, ocular cells express pro-apoptotic cell surface molecules such as Fas ligand (FasL) and TRAIL (Chapter 14). These TNF family members may contribute to apoptosis of infiltrating T and other inflammatory cells bearing 'death receptors.' In mice, the presence of FasL on ocular cells is critical in the acceptance of corneal allografts. Cytokines produced at sites of immune privilege are also likely to contribute to the inhibition of inflammation (Chapter 10). The presence of high levels of the anti-inflammatory cytokines TNF-β and migration inhibitory factor (MIF) leads to inhibition of NK cell-mediated cytolytic activity.

T-cell anergy

Cellular proliferation and/or potentiation of T-cell effector function are not inevitable consequences of TCR engagement. In fact, under some conditions TCR ligation results in a state of T-cell unresponsiveness to subsequent TCR engagement.[33, 34] Known as T-cell anergy, this state appears to result either when the TCR is engaged without concomitant co-stimulation, or when the ligand for the TCR is not of sufficient affinity to initiate the full spectrum of biochemical second messengers. This phenomenon was first noted by stimulating T cells in the presence of metabolically inactivated APCs. Subsequently, it was shown that CD28 co-stimulation could prevent the induction of anergy. Anergic cells are unable to proliferate or secrete cytokines upon TCR-mediated restimulation. Interestingly, supplementation of cultures with IL-2 can overcome the anergic state *in vitro*.

Several novel reagents and unique experimental systems have recently provided insights into how TCR signaling events can lead to either anergy or full T-cell activation. Mice made transgenic for specific TCR complexes have proved to be useful models for studying differential responses to TCR engagement *in vivo* and *in vitro*. TCR-transgenic mice produce T-cell repertoires largely restricted to a single specificity. T cells from such mice respond fully when presented with a specified peptide antigen, but exhibit an anergic response when that peptide is subtly altered. Opposing biologic responses of TCR-transgenic T cells isolated from these mice correlate with differences in biochemical events downstream of TCR ligation. Specifically, NFAT activity without concomitant increases in activating protein 1 (AP-1) transcription factor activity leads to anergy (Fig. 13.6A). Relatively unopposed NFAT activity can be induced experimentally either by treatment with calcium ionophore or stimulation through the TCR while blocking CD28 co-stimulation with the CLTA4-Ig recombinant protien.

Biochemical analysis of experimentally anergized T cells has shown alterations in signal transduction downstream of the TCR in the induction of anergy. For example, delivery of an anergic stimulus to T cells results in phosphorylation of the TCRζ chain at sites that differ from those phosphorylated when the TCR is stimulated with a full agonistic peptide.[35, 36] It is not yet clear how ligand binding is translated into differential ζ phosphorylation, but the downstream consequences of this alteration in proximal signaling appear to be profound.

Additional differences in TCR-mediated biochemical events have been documented in previously anergized versus fully activated T cells. One model for the generation of anergy involves the adaptor protein CBL.[37] FYN kinase activity is increased and this src family kinase can be found associated with the CBL adaptor protein in anergized cells. CBL becomes phosphorylated on tyrosines following TCR engagement, and then associates with CRKL, another adaptor protein (Fig. 13.6B). CRKL, in turn, binds to C3G, which is a guanine nucleotide exchange

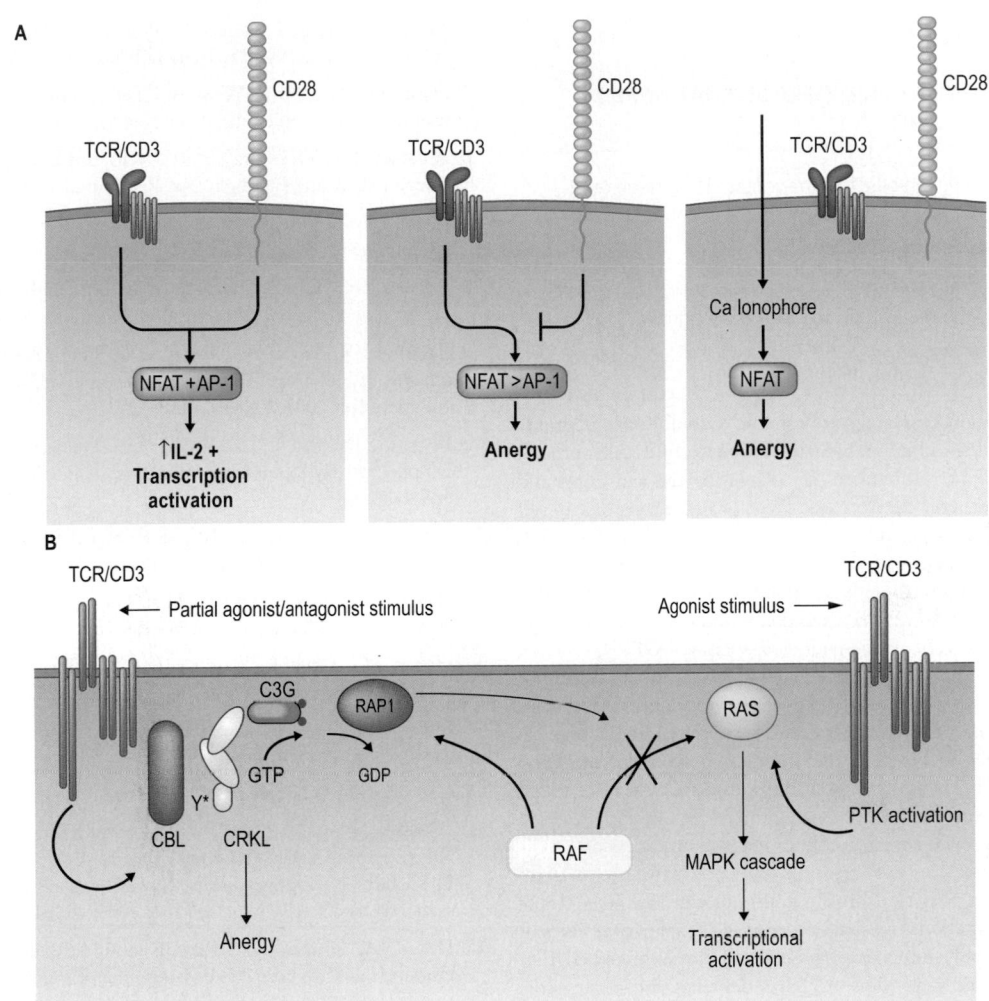

Fig. 13.6 An *in vitro* model for anergy induction. (A) Stimulation of T cells by cross-linking of both T-cell receptor (TCR)/CD3 and CD28 lead to upregulation of both the nuclear factor of activated T cells (NFAT) and activating protein 1 (AP-1) transcription factors, leading to increased transcription of the interleukin-2 (IL-2) gene and activation. An imbalance of activated NFAT and AP-1 by blockade of CD28 signals (middle) or calcium ionophore (right panel) leads to an anergic phenotype. (B) A model for anergy maintenance involving Cbl. When a partial agonist or antagonist signal is delivered to the TCR, c-CBL becomes tyrosine-phosphorylated. Phosphorylated CBL acts as a scaffold for the assembly of a complex consisting of adaptor proteins CRKL and C3G. C3G is thus positioned to perform GTP/GDP exchange for the small-molecular-weight G protein RAP1, which sequesters the RAF kinase away from the activating RAS/MAPK kinase cascade (right half of schematic).

factor for the small-molecular-weight GTP-binding protein RAP1. Formation of the ternary complex involving CBL, CRKL, and C3G results in recruitment of C3G to a position where it can activate RAP1. GTP-bound RAP1 effectively interferes with signaling molecules downstream of RAS by sequestering RAS-stimulated effector proteins. Furthermore, differential activation of members of the MAPK family has been observed. Consistent with this model, the Cbl-b, Itch, and GRAIL E3 ligases are upregulated in calcium ionophore-induced anergy and result in decreased levels of PLCγ1, PKC-θ, and RAS GRP. A complementary model centers around the LAT adaptor molecule.[38] As described above, LAT is normally palmitoylated and its membrane localization

restricted to detergent-insoluble lipid rafts. In previously anergized T cells, however, LAT palmitoylation and phosphorylation are both decreased. This defect is not due to alterations in either CD3ζ and ZAP-70 phosphorylation, nor is it directly related to Cbl-b.

Regulation

The past 10 years have seen the re-emergence of the concept of active immune regulation as a process that leads to tolerance. So-called regulatory T cells or Tregs can actively suppress the immune system (Chapter 16).[39, 40] Functional and phenotypic characterization of these

KEY CONCEPTS

IMMUNOSUPPRESSIVE DRUGS THAT AFFECT T-CELL SIGNALING

Cyclosporine/tacrolimus inhibits T-cell receptor (TCR)-generated signals

Anti-TCR antibodies block TCR signals

CTLA-4Ig blocks CD28 signals

Rapamycin inhibits interleukin-2 (IL-2)-generated signals

cells led to the revelation that Tregs are capable of inhibiting the proliferation of and cytokine production by naïve and memory T cells through a cell contact-dependent mechanism. By regulating the activation and proliferation of antigen-specific effectors, Tregs promote tolerance to self and suppress autoimmunity *in vivo*.

Identification of Treg cells was initially described based on co-expression of CD4 and CD25, but there is no single cell surface marker that is entirely specific for Tregs. CD25, for example, is found not only on Tregs, but also on activated T cells. In general, Tregs express GITR, CD103, CTLA-4, lymphocyte activation gene 3 (LAG-3), and low levels of CD45RB. More recently, expression of the transcription factor Foxp3 has been shown to correlate tightly with regulatory capacity in both humans and mice. The absence of Foxp3 either through spontaneous mutation (the scurfy mouse) or through targeted disruption of the gene leads to the absence of T cells with regulatory activity. Conversely, overexpression of Foxp3 by transgenesis or retroviral methods leads to an excess of T cells with regulatory activity.

Mice lacking Foxp3 activity exhibit autoimmune disease in multiple organs. In humans, mutations in Foxp3 account for a majority of cases of immune dysfunction/polyendocrinopathy/enteropathy/X-linked (IPEX) syndrome. The signs and symptoms of Foxp3-deficient disease are similar in mice and humans. Affected human males develop an autoimmune syndrome consisting of lymphoproliferation, thyroiditis, insulin-dependent diabetes mellitus, enteropathy, and other immune disorders.

Multiple research groups have taken advantage of using Foxp3 as a marker for regulatory T cells by generating gene-targeted mice in which a fluorescent protein has been knocked-in to the *FoxP3* locus. In these mice, cells that express FoxP3 can be identified and isolated based on fluorescence. Such reporter mice have been used to confirm that most, but not all, CD4$^+$FoxP3$^+$ cells are CD25$^+$ and that most have regulatory activity. Whether Foxp3 expression is required for maintenance of Treg function or only for commitment to the Treg lineage remains an open question.

REFERENCES

1. Weiss A, Littman DR. Signal transduction by lymphocyte antigen receptors. Cell 1994; 76: 263–274.

2. DeFranco AL. Transmembrane signaling by antigen receptors of B and T lymphocytes. Curr Opin Cell Biol 1995; 7: 163–175.

3. Sicheri F, Kuriyan J. Structures of Src-family tyrosine kinases. Curr Opin Struct Biol 1997; 7: 777–785.

4. Mustelin T, Vang T, Bottini N. Protein tyrosine phosphatases and the immune response. Nat Rev Immunol 2005; 5: 43–57.

5. Hermiston ML, Xu Z, Weiss A. CD45: a critical regulator of signaling thresholds in immune cells. Annu Rev Immunol 2003; 21: 107–137.

6. Abraham RT, Weiss A. Jurkat T cells and development of the T-cell receptor signalling paradigm. Nat Rev Immunol 2004; 4: 301–308.

7. Buckley RH. Primary immunodeficiency diseases due to defects in lymphocytes. N Engl J Med 2000; 343: 1313–1324.

8. Palacios EH, Weiss A. Function of the Src-family kinases, Lck and Fyn, in T-cell development and activation. Oncogene 2004; 23: 7990–8000.

9. Zamoyska R, Basson A, Filby A, et al. The influence of the src-family kinases, Lck and Fyn, on T cell differentiation, survival and activation. Immunol Rev 2003; 191: 107–118.

10. Berg LJ, Finkelstein LD, Lucas JA, et al. Tec family kinases in T lymphocyte development and function. Annu Rev Immunol 2005; 23: 549–600.

11. Weiss A, Irving BA, Tan LK, et al. Signal transduction by the T cell antigen receptor. Semin Immunol 1991; 3: 313–324.

12. Weiss A, Imboden J, Hardy K, et al. The role of the T3/antigen receptor complex in T-cell activation. Annu Rev Immunol 1986; 4: 593–619.

13. Hogan PG, Chen L, Nardone J, et al. Transcriptional regulation by calcium, calcineurin, and NFAT. Genes Dev 2003; 17: 2205–2232.

14. Jordan MS, Singer AL, Koretzky GA. Adaptors as central mediators of signal transduction in immune cells. Nat Immunol 2003; 4: 110–116.

15. Cantrell DA. GTPases and T cell activation. Immunol Rev 2003; 192: 122–130.

16. Roose JP, Mollenauer M, Gupta VA, et al. A diacylglycerol-protein kinase C-RasGRP1 pathway directs Ras activation upon antigen receptor stimulation of T cells. Mol Cell Biol 2005; 25: 4426–4441.

17. Deane JA, Fruman DA. Phosphoinositide 3-kinase: diverse roles in immune cell activation. Annu Rev Immunol 2004; 22: 563–598.

18. Thome M. CARMA1, BCL-10 and MALT1 in lymphocyte development and activation. Nat Rev Immunol 2004; 4: 348–359.

19. Horejsi V, Zhang W, Schraven B. Transmembrane adaptor proteins: organizers of immunoreceptor signalling. Nat Rev Immunol 2004; 4: 603–616.

20. Samelson LE. Signal transduction mediated by the T cell antigen receptor: the role of adaptor proteins. Annu Rev Immunol 2002; 20: 371–394.

21. Koretzky GA, Abtahian F, Silverman MA. SLP76 and SLP65: complex regulation of signalling in lymphocytes and beyond. Nat Rev Immunol 2006; 6: 67–78.

22. Sperling AI, Bluestone JA. The complexities of T-cell co-stimulation: CD28 and beyond. Immunol Rev 1996; 153: 155–182.

23. Greenwald RJ, Freeman GJ, Sharpe AH. The B7 family revisited. Annu Rev Immunol 2005; 23: 515–548.

24. Rudd CE, Raab M. Independent CD28 signaling via VAV and SLP-76: a model for in trans co-stimulation. Immunol Rev 2003; 192: 32–41.

25. Watts TH. TNF/TNFR family members in co-stimulation of T cell responses. Annu Rev Immunol 2005; 23: 23–68.

26. Sprent J, Kishimoto H. The thymus and negative selection. Immunol Rev 2002; 185: 126–135.

27. von Boehmer H, Kisielow P. Negative selection of the T-cell repertoire: where and when does it occur?. Immunol Rev 2006; 209: 284–289.

28. Gallegos AM, Bevan MJ. Central tolerance: good but imperfect. Immunol Rev 2006; 209: 290–296.

29. Love PE, Lee J, Shores EW. Critical relationship between TCR signaling potential and TCR affinity during thymocyte selection. J Immunol 2000; 165: 3080–3087.

30. Tarakhovsky A, Kanner SB, Hombach J, et al. A role for CD5 in TCR-mediated signal transduction and thymocyte selection. Science 1995; 269: 535–537.

31. Kyewski B, Klein L. A central role for central tolerance. Annu Rev Immunol 2006; 24: 571–606.

32. Niederkorn JY. See no evil, hear no evil, do no evil: the lessons of immune privilege. Nat Immunol 2006; 7: 354–359.

33. Schwartz RH. T cell anergy. Annu Rev Immunol 2003; 21: 305–334.

34. Schwartz RH. Models of T cell anergy: is there a common molecular mechanism?. J Exp Med 1996; 184: 1–8.

35. Sloan-Lancaster J, Shaw AS, Rothbard JB, et al. Partial T cell signaling: altered phospho-zeta and lack of zap70 recruitment in APL-induced T cell anergy. Cell 1994; 79: 913–922.

36. Kersh EN, Kersh GJ, Allen PM. Partially phosphorylated T cell receptor zeta molecules can inhibit T cell activation. J Exp Med 1999; 190: 1627–1636.

37. Macian F, Im SH, Garcia-Cozar FJ, et al. T-cell anergy. Curr Opin Immunol 2004; 16: 209–216.

38. Hundt M, Tabata H, Jeon MS, et al. Impaired activation and localization of LAT in anergic T cells as a consequence of a selective palmitoylation defect. Immunity 2006; 24: 513–522.

39. Fontenot JD, Rudensky AY. A well adapted regulatory contrivance: regulatory T cell development and the forkhead family transcription factor Foxp3. Nat Immunol 2005; 6: 331–337.

40. Sakaguchi S. Naturally arising Foxp3-expressing CD25+CD4+ regulatory T cells in immunological tolerance to self and non-self. Nat Immunol 2005; 6: 345–352.

REFERENCES

KEY CONCEPTS

APOPTOSIS

>> Programmed cell death is a normal physiologic process of mature peripheral lymphocytes:

   The best-characterized form of programmed cell death is apoptosis

>> The signaling pathway for apoptosis is conserved among worms, mice, and humans

>> Apoptosis can proceed through an extrinsic pathway involving death receptors, or an intrinsic pathway involving mitochondria (Fig. 14.2):

   Both pathways activate caspases in an intracellular enzymatic cascade that leads to the morphological features of cell death

>> Actively cycling lymphocytes are most susceptible to death:

   Excess antigen can induce apoptosis via death receptors

   Limited antigen levels can lead to cytokine withdrawal, which in turn can induce apoptosis

>> Lymphocyte and dendritic cell apoptosis serves to maintain tolerance and prevent autoimmunity

Effector caspases cleave substrates such as poly(ADP-ribose) polymerase (PARP), inhibitor of caspase-activated DNase (ICAD/DFF45), Rho-associated coil-coil-forming kinase I (ROCK I), nuclear lamins, actin, fodrin, and keratin. These proteins function to repair DNA, maintain the integrity of plasma membrane and subcellular organelle compartments, and make up nuclear and cytoskeletal architecture. Proteolysis of these substrates presumably leads to the morphologic changes seen in apoptosis, which culminates in cell death.

In mammals, two principal pathways initiate apoptosis (Fig. 14.2). The core signaling pathway elucidated in nematodes corresponds more closely to the intrinsic (mitochondrial) pathway. By contrast, the extrinsic (death receptor) pathway proceeds separately and is not found in simple invertebrates. Both intrinsic and extrinsic pathways converge at the step of caspase activation. The precisely ordered sequence of molecular events that comprise these pathways is discussed below.

INTRINSIC (MITOCHONDRIAL) PATHWAY

Many physiologically important stimuli trigger the intrinsic pathway of apoptosis. These include negative selection of T cells during thymic education, growth factor or cytokine deprivation, DNA damage, and treatment with cytotoxic drugs such as chemotherapeutic agents. Proteins of the BCL-2 family control the intrinsic pathway.[7, 11] The fine balance between the levels and activation status of the pro- and anti-apoptotic members of this family determines the cell's fate. Structurally, all members of the BCL-2 family share one or more of the four known BCL-2 homology regions (BH). The pro-survival members share three or four BH regions and include BCL-2, BCL-X$_L$, A1/BFL-1, BCL-w, BOO/DIVA/BCL-B, and MCL-1. The pro-apoptotic members, which have two or three BH regions, structurally resemble their pro-survival relatives, and include BAX, BAK, BOK/MTD, Bcl-X$_S$, and Bcl-G$_L$. Finally,

a subgroup of pro-apoptotic members, named "BH3-only" proteins, contain only one BH region. This subgroup includes BAD, BID, BIM, BIK/NBK, BLK, HRK/DP5, Bcl-G$_s$, BMF, NOXA, and PUMA/BBC3.

Although certain details of how these proteins control the intrinsic apoptosis pathway remain unclear, we summarize here the most accepted current model (Fig. 14.2). The BH-3-only proteins seem to act as sensors for different apoptotic stimuli. For example, BIM serves as a sensor for growth factor withdrawal, and PUMA for DNA damage. Activated BH-3-only proteins induce translocation of the pro-apoptotic protein BAX from the cytosol to the mitochondria, where it clusters with BAK. This leads to pore formation in the outer mitochondrial membrane, loss of inner mitochondrial transmembrane potential, and release of several apoptotic proteins such as SMAC/DIABLO, apoptosis-inducing factor (AIF), and cytochrome c. Released cytochrome c oligomerizes in the cytosol with APAF-1 and procaspase-9 to form, in the presence of Ca^{2+} and ATP, a caspase-9-activating complex called the apoptosome. Once activated within this complex, the initiator caspase-9 cleaves and activates downstream effector caspases such as caspase-3. The resulting caspase cascade leads to cell death. Anti-apoptotic BCL-2 members may promote survival by sequestering and inactivating BH-3-only proteins or other pro-apoptotic proteins, thereby preserving mitochondrial integrity and cell survival.

EXTRINSIC (DEATH RECEPTOR) PATHWAY

Apoptosis can be triggered by extracellular signals that activate cell surface death receptors of the tumor necrosis factor (TNF) receptor superfamily.[6, 12] Members of this superfamily have cysteine-rich extracellular domains and exist as pre-assembled trimers. The best-characterized death receptors are the prototypical death receptor Fas (CD95, or Apo1) and TNFR1. Others include DR3 (Apo3), DR4, and DR5 (TRAIL-R2, or Apo2). Death receptors have cytoplasmic death domains (DD) that bind to DD-containing adaptor molecules through homotypic interactions (Fig. 14.2). The adaptor molecule FADD is crucial for signal transduction because it also possesses a death effector domain (DED). This domain enables FADD to bind homotypically to the initiator caspases-8/10, which also contain DED. Upon receptor–ligand binding, recruitment of caspases-8/10 into the large death-inducing signaling complex (DISC) causes their oligomerization and enzymatic activation. Clusters of DISC form higher-order signaling protein oligomerization transduction structures (SPOTS), which promote further caspase activation. This leads to downstream caspase cascade for cell death.

The extrinsic pathway can feed into the intrinsic pathway to amplify signals for death.[13] Activated caspase-8 can cleave BID, a pro-apoptotic BH3-only BCL-2 family member analogous to the *C. elegans egl-1* gene. Truncated BID improves the binding of the pro-apoptotic multidomain BAX and BAK proteins to mitochondrial membranes, increasing mitochondrial permeability. Cells that depend upon this mitochondrial amplification for death receptor-mediated death include peripheral blood lymphocytes. By contrast, other cell types that exhibit more efficient DISC formation for caspase-8 and downstream caspase-3 activation die independently of mitochondrial involvement.

Engagement of death receptors can trigger cellular responses other than death. For example, Fas stimulation also activates the transcription factor NF-κB and mitogen-activated protein kinases (MAPK) p38 and ERK1/2. Activation of these signaling pathways can counterbalance

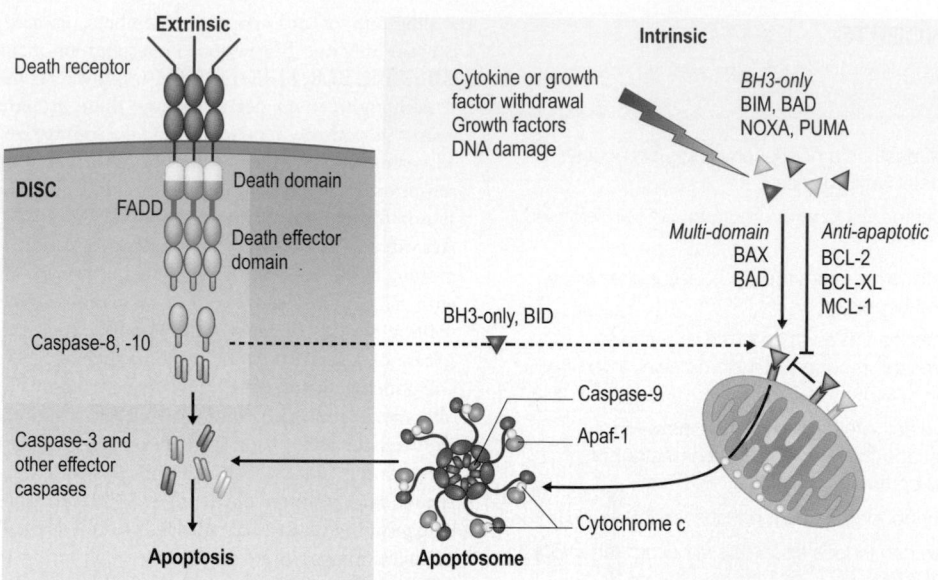

Fig. 14.2 Extrinsic and intrinsic signaling pathways for apoptosis. Two pathways exist for activating the effector caspases for lymphocyte apoptosis induction and propriocidal regulation. The extrinsic pathway activates initiator caspases-8 and -10 in death-inducing signaling complexes (DISC) anchored by death receptors. The intrinsic pathway activates initiator caspase-9 within the apoptosome. This structure is assembled when mitochondria are permeabilized. BCL-2 family members either facilitate or antagonize mitochondrial permeability and can link the intrinsic to the extrinsic pathway. See text for more details.

signals for death. However, Fas mutations generally impair death signals more readily than growth-promoting signals.

LYMPHOCYTE DEATH DURING AN IMMUNE RESPONSE

Mature peripheral lymphocytes vary in their susceptibility to apoptosis. Resting cells and cells undergoing initial activation are typically refractory to death. This property allows an effective immune response to develop against pathogens. Once cells proliferate and enter the late G1/S phase of the cell cycle, their sensitivity to death increases. The acquisition of death sensitivity occurs at the height of an ongoing immune response and at its conclusion. Thus, lymphocytes possess a built-in rheostat that can regulate cell death as a function of the rapidity by which the cells are progressing through the cell cycle.[5]

The sensitivity of lymphocytes to antigen-driven cell death during an immune response, termed propriocidal regulation, is a major negative-feedback mechanism that can be used to control the intensity of immune responses. Two events contribute to antigen receptor restimulation-induced propriocidal death (Fig. 14.3).[5] First, high levels of antigen stimulate the production of high levels of interleukin (IL)-2, which drives lymphocytes into cell cycle. Cells respond by undergoing molecular changes that render them susceptible to the extrinsic pathway or "active" apoptosis. This process is independent of new protein or mRNA synthesis, but may involve increased Fas expression and downregulation of anti-apoptotic molecules such as c-FLIP. As a consequence, T and B lymphocytes are triggered to die when their Fas receptors interact with soluble or membrane-bound FasL. CD8 cells also die when triggered through their TNF receptors. In addition, the antigen receptor

appears to connect directly to the pro-apoptotic molecule BIM. This mechanism helps limit the magnitude of the immune response, and thereby protects the host in the presence of continuous or repeated antigenic stimulation.

The second mechanism contributing to death of lymphocytes occurs when an immune response wanes (Fig. 14.3).[5] A falling level of antigen markedly decreases the amount of IL-2 produced. This in turn decreases CD25 – a component of the high-affinity IL-2 receptor complex whose expression is IL-2-dependent – and renders the cells increasingly nonresponsive to IL-2. Cytokine withdrawal drives the intrinsic pathway of apoptosis in a process that requires new protein and mRNA synthesis. Death can be blocked by the addition of common γ-chain receptor cytokines other than IL-2, such as IL-4, IL-7, and IL-15, or by overexpressing anti-apoptotic BCL-2/BCL-X_L proteins, which restrain apoptosis at the mitochondria. This mechanism facilitates contraction of the immune response following pathogen elimination.

In summary, actively cycling lymphocytes die by means of mechanisms that involve antigen receptor-induced death. These mechanisms are mediated partly by death receptors Fas and TNF, and partly by cytokine withdrawal. These complementary mechanisms limit the magnitude and duration of an immune response by eliminating activated cells.

IN VIVO IMPORTANCE OF APOPTOSIS

Studies in experimental animals and in humans have established that apoptosis is a normal physiological process that maintains immunologic tolerance and prevents development of autoimmunity.[6, 14] *Lpr* (lymphoproliferation) is a naturally arising mouse strain with a mutation in *Fas*

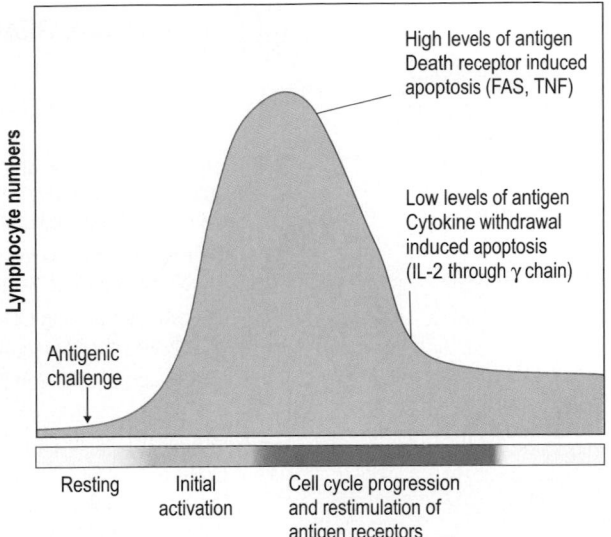

Fig. 14.3 Propriocidal regulation of actively cycling lymphocytes involves apoptosis induced (1) through death receptors at the height of the immune response, and (2) upon cytokine withdrawal at the end of the response.

resulting in its deficiency. Homozygous mutant mice develop splenomegaly and lymphadenopathy. Depending upon the genetic background, they also develop hypergammaglobulinemia, autoantibodies, glomerulonephritis, polyarteritis, sialoadenitis, arthritis, or primary biliary cirrhosis. Similar disease features are seen in another naturally arising mouse strain called *gld* (generalized lymphoproliferative disease), which has a homozygous Fas ligand (*FasL*) mutation. Recently, mice were generated in which the Fas death receptor pathway was selectively blocked in different immune cells.[15] Surprisingly, disease was more severe in the mice with Fas-blocked dendritic cells as compared to lymphocytes. Dendritic cell numbers and APC function were enhanced. The death of dendritic cells, acting in concert with propriocidal death of lymphocytes, may enforce tolerance and prevent autoimmunity *in vivo*.

■ THE AUTOIMMUNE LYMPHOPROLIFERATIVE SYNDROME ■

CLINICAL FEATURES

In 1992, Sneller and colleagues[28] described a childhood syndrome of immune cell dysregulation including autoimmunity, hypergammaglobulinemia, lymphadenopathy, and lymphocytosis. The lymphocytosis reflected expansion of an unusual T-cell population bearing rearranged T-cell receptor (TCR)-α/β but lacking CD4 or CD8 co-receptor expression (double-negative T cells; DNT). This constellation of findings resembled key phenotypic features of *lpr* and *gld* mouse strains, natural models of autoimmune disease later found to harbor *Fas* and *FasL* mutations, respectively. Like *lpr* mice, these patients had *FAS* mutations leading to the defective lymphocyte apoptosis that was critical for disease pathogenesis. The human disease was

▌ CLINICAL RELEVANCE

≫ Autoimmune lymphoproliferative syndrome (ALPS) is a genetic disorder that impairs lymphocyte apoptosis

≫ Mutations in *TNFRSF6 (FAS)* underlie most cases of ALPS:

A minority of ALPS is caused by mutations in *TNFSF6* (Fas ligand), *CASP10* (caspase 10), or somatic *FAS* mutations affecting DNT cells

These mutations all impair the Fas-mediated extrinsic pathway of apoptosis

Most are dominant interfering because they prevent formation of an effective death-inducing signaling complex (DISC)

≫ ALPS can also result from a defect in the cytokine withdrawal-induced intrinsic pathway of apoptosis:

A dominant *NRAS* gain-of-function mutation that prevents BIM induction can be responsible

≫ ALPS predisposes to autoimmunity and lymphomas:

The most typical autoimmune findings are autoantibodies, Coombs-positive hemolytic anemia, or chronic idiopathic thrombocytopenic purpura

Hodgkin and non-Hodgkin lymphomas both occur

≫ Caspase-8 deficiency state (CEDS) is characterized by combined lymphocyte immunodeficiency with susceptibility to infection, superimposed upon ALPS-like features of lymphoproliferation and apoptotic defects:

These findings stem from the participation of caspase-8 in two different signaling complexes – one for death induction, and another for NF-κB activation

KEY CONCEPTS

DIAGNOSTIC CRITERIA FOR AUTOIMMUNE LYMPHOPROLIFERATIVE SYNDROME (ALPS)

Required criteria

>> Chronic nonmalignant lymphadenopathy and/or splenomegaly

>> Increased peripheral CD4⁻CD8⁻ TCRα/β (DNT) cells

>> Lymphocyte apoptosis defect

Supporting criteria

>> Family history of ALPS

>> Characteristic histopathology

>> Autoimmune manifestations

>> Mutations in *FAS, FASLG, CASP10, NRAS*

CLINICAL PEARLS

>> Classification is based upon findings that may be present or have resolved

>> Despite its moniker, at least one-fifth of patients with autoimmune lymphoproliferative syndrome (ALPS) lack evidence of autoimmunity

>> Variable penetrance means that not all individuals with mutations manifest disease

>> TCRγ/δ cells lacking CD4 and CD8 co-receptors may falsely elevate the double-negative T-cell (DNT) count

>> Expression of B220 on DNT cells is a finding specific to ALPS

>> Elevated B_{12} levels can be used as a simple screen

>> Other helpful laboratory findings are hypergammaglobulinemia, direct Coombs test, or anti-cardiolipin antibodies

>> Patients without known mutations should be directly analyzed for somatic mutations in sorted DNT cells:

>> Apoptosis cannot be readily assessed by the usual methods, because DNT cells cannot be maintained in culture

therefore termed autoimmune lymphoproliferative syndrome (ALPS), and is likely the same clinical entity characterized in descriptive accounts by Canale and Smith[29] and others in the earlier literature.

ALPS is a rare condition with variable disease penetrance, affecting a reported 300 persons worldwide. Diagnostic criteria, discussed below, reflect deranged lymphocyte homeostasis.[6, 8, 16, 17] Patients must present with chronic nonmalignant lymphocyte accumulation, including lymphadenopathy and/or splenomegaly, elevated DNT numbers in peripheral blood, and defective *in vitro* lymphocyte apoptosis. Autoimmunity is often seen, or more rarely lymphoma, but these are not required for diagnosis.

Signs and symptoms of ALPS usually emerge in infancy or early childhood (median age of 24 months), when patients undergo medical investigation for unexplained splenomegaly, lymphadenopathy, or autoimmune destruction of blood cells. Typically there is painless enlargement of peripheral lymphoid organs, and no fever or weight loss unless complicated by lymphoma. The thymus or liver can also be enlarged. Although lymphoid hyperplasia can fluctuate, even without treatment it tends to improve gradually with age. Up to 80% of ALPS patients have circulating autoantibodies, although only half have actual autoimmune disease. Coombs-positive hemolytic anemia and chronic immune thrombocytopenic purpura are the most common autoimmune diseases. These manifestations tend to be severe, but often follow a variable course. When seen at initial presentation, ALPS can be mistaken for Evans syndrome. Neutropenia due to hypersplenism or autoimmunity can occur, but is usually mild. The high incidence of anti-cardiolipin or anti-neutrophil antibodies has no correlation with clinical manifestations of thrombosis or neutropenia. Rare autoimmune manifestations include antinuclear antibodies, rheumatoid factor, glomerulonephritis, optic neuritis or uveitis, Guillain–Barré syndrome, primary biliary cirrhosis, anti-factor VIII antibodies with coagulopathy, autoimmune hepatitis, vasculitis, and linear immunoglobulin A (IgA) dermopathy.

DNT expansion is peculiar to and required for diagnosis of ALPS. Normally, DNT comprise less than 1% of lymphocytes in the peripheral blood or in lymphoid tissues. However, they can reach up to 40% in ALPS patients. These cells are distinct from the immature DNT cells developing in the thymus that have not yet rearranged their TCR genes or expressed TCR on their cell surface. They are thought to represent aging mature

T cells that have lost CD4 or CD8 co-receptor expression, but the details of their origin are obscure. DNT express the CD45R isoform B220, a marker normally found on B cells, as well as CD27, CD57, and HLA-DR. In ALPS patients the expanded DNT produce high levels of IL-10. As elevations in IL-4 and IL-5 are also seen, the resulting T helper type 2 (Th2) cytokine profile probably contributes to the observed polyclonal hyperglobulinemia and autoantibodies. The demonstration that some ALPS patients are mosaics – with Fas mutations in DNT but not all T cells – implicates DNT in disease pathogenesis. However, understanding their exact function has been hampered by an inability to keep them alive in culture, as they do not respond well to most activating and proliferative stimuli.

Lymphoproliferation in ALPS is not limited to DNT. Patients have increased numbers of total T cells, with contributions from CD8 cells expressing CD57 as well as TCRγ/δ⁺ cells that lack CD4 and CD8 expression. Both total B cells and CD5⁺ B cells are increased. By contrast, CD4⁺CD25⁺ T cells are low, resulting in no overall change in CD4 cell numbers. Natural killer (NK) cell numbers are also unchanged. Lymph node biopsy reveals a characteristic histopathology showing follicular hyperplasia with polyclonal plasmacytosis, and paracortical expansion with infiltrating DNT.[18] Besides lymphocyte immunophenotying, high levels of circulating cobalamin (vitamin B_{12}) can be used as a simple initial screening test for ALPS. However, by itself it cannot differentiate from certain other hematologic disorders, including lymphoproliferative and myeloproliferative disorders (VK Rao, JK Dale, and SE Straus, personal communication).

A definitive diagnosis of ALPS requires the evaluation of lymphocyte apoptosis *in vitro*, a test that is typically performed only in specialized research laboratories. A key point for the appropriate interpretation of this test is that cells must be proliferating well in order to become susceptible to death-inducing stimuli. Thus, poor proliferation can be falsely interpreted as an apparent apoptosis resistance. Peripheral T cells can be activated with phytohemagglutinin and then driven into cell cycle by culturing with IL-2. Fas agonistic antibodies or TCR restimulation can then be used to induce apoptosis. A flow cytometer is subsequently used to count propidium iodide-excluding cells ('live' cells) over constant time. This number is compared to that for untreated cells, enabling calculation of the percent cell loss at any given dose of stimulus. A decrease in percent cell loss at half of normal controls is usually considered evidence of an apoptosis defect.

Although initially nonmalignant, the lymphoproliferation in ALPS predisposes to lymphoid malignancy, which develops in 10% of ALPS patients. In rare instances, ALPS patients are diagnosed when they initially present with lymphoma. Compared to the general population, ALPS patients with *FAS* mutations (type 1A) have a 51-fold and 14-fold elevated incidence of Hodgkin and non-Hodgkin lymphoma, respectively. Median age of diagnosis was 11 years for Hodgkin lymphoma and 21 for non-Hodgkin lymphoma; however, lymphomas were identified anywhere between 2 and 50 years of age. Lymphomas are of either B- or T-cell origin and of diverse histological type, thus betraying a general anti-neoplastic role for propriocidal death of lymphocytes. The lymphomas display neither loss of heterozygosity for the Fas mutation nor increased resistance to apoptosis. Most patients who develop malignancy have mutations in the DD region, with severe impairment in Fas-mediated lymphocyte apoptosis but continued Fas-mediated activation of NF-κB and MAPK for growth promotion. MAPK hyperactivation, coupled with impaired cytokine withdrawal-mediated apoptosis, was also associated with lymphoma in an individual with ALPS type IV due to *NRAS* mutation.[25]

MOLECULAR ETIOLOGY AND CLASSIFICATION

A proposed ALPS classification based on underlying genetic defects is presented in Table 14.1 and the corresponding molecular mechanisms are discussed below.[6, 8, 16]

Most ALPS patients bear heterozygous mutations in the *FAS (TNFRSF6)* gene located on chromosome 10q24.1. Mutations can be found throughout the gene, either in coding regions or in splice sites, with the majority (~2/3) affecting the intracellular DD encoded by exon 9. (A description of all mutations can be found in the ALPS database: ALPSbase: http://research.nhgri.nih.gov/ALPS/.) Autosomal dominant disease transmission occurs because most mutations exert a dominant interfering effect. This effect is explained by understanding that pre-association of three normal Fas molecules in a trimer is required for receptor death signaling function (Fig. 14.2). If 50% of Fas proteins are abnormal, as is the case for heterozygous mutations, seven out of eight Fas trimers would contain at least one mutant protein, rendering that trimer ineffective. Severity is greatest for DD mutations, which disrupt the homotypic interactions required for FADD and initiator caspase recruitment into the death-inducing signaling complex (DISC). Those that do not affect DISC formation can impair downstream higher order signaling protein oligomerization transduction structures (SPOTS) formation, which is necessary for efficient caspase activation. A few ALPS patients have compound heterozygous loss-of-function mutations that cause haploinsufficiency. Individuals with complete loss of function due to homozygous mutations have generally more severe symptoms. ALPS patients with *FAS* mutations are classified as type Ia. In some ALPS patients, *FAS* somatic mutations have been found in purified DNT cells and a fraction of peripheral lymphocytes, monocytes and hematopoietic precursors. Notably, their (non-DNT) T cells lacked

FAS mutations and apoptosis defects when expanded *in vitro*. These patients are provisionally classified as type I$_m$ (for 'mosaic').

A minority of ALPS patients harbor mutations in other components of the Fas pathway. A heterozygous mutation in Fas ligand (*FASLG, TNFSF6*) was originally reported for a patient with systemic lupus erythematosus who had lymphadenopathy, splenomegaly, and defective lymphocyte apoptosis after TCR restimulation, but no apparent DNT expansion. However, ALPS patients were also discovered who possessed either heterozygous[26] or homozygous *FASLG* mutations,[19] and these are classified as type 1b. Although caspase-10 functional polymorphisms may influence disease, at least two heterozygous caspase-10 mutations in 3 ALPS patients have been identified that cause defective apoptosis in lymphocytes and dendritic cells.[20] These patients have been classified as type II.

A subgroup of ALPS patients fulfills diagnostic criteria including increased DNT, but lacks detectable Fas-mediated apoptosis defect or known mutations in the Fas pathway. These have been termed type III. We have recently identified one such patient who demonstrated defective lymphocyte apoptosis upon cytokine withdrawal, a stimulus that triggers the intrinsic pathway. A gain-of-function mutation in the gene *NRAS* resulted in diminished downstream expression of BIM, which accounted for failure to induce apoptosis. This is the first reported defect in the intrinsic pathway of apoptosis causing ALPS.[25]

The relationship between genotype and phenotype is complex. Gene mutations are required, but are not sufficient for disease. In large kindreds, family members with the same mutation and degree of defective *in vitro* Fas-mediated apoptosis had very different clinical manifestations. In-depth analysis revealed that penetrance was greatest with intracellular DD mutations and least with extracellular mutations. This indicates that other factors, genetic and/or environmental, influence the clinical phenotype.

ALPS-LIKE DISEASE

Some patients have features overlapping with but not fulfilling diagnostic criteria for ALPS.[6] For instance, the ALPS-variant autoimmune lymphoproliferative disease (ALD) has lymphoproliferation, autoimmune disease, susceptibility to cancer, and defective lymphocyte apoptosis, but lacks DNT expansion. The responsible molecular defects are unknown. In another cohort patients display clinical features of ALPS but lack apparent apoptosis defects. Apoptotic defects are usually assessed through the Fas death receptor, which may not reveal defects that would be seen if induced by other stimuli. Apoptotic defects may also not be readily apparent due to the cells used for analyses, for example, in somatic mosaicism. Given recent evidence that dendritic cell apoptosis defects can contribute to disease pathogenesis,[15] we speculate that other diseases resembling ALPS, such as Rosai–Dorfman disease, may involve mutations within APC.[21] In sum, a proportion of ALPS-like disease likely represents variants of ALPS. However, other forms of ALPS-like disease probably reflect abnormalities in nonapoptotic pathways that also regulate lymphocyte growth and activation.

There is a growing realization that certain molecules involved in apoptosis also function integrally for lymphocyte growth and activation. One such molecule is caspase-8. Its deficiency, found in two siblings with homozygous mutations, leads to an immune regulation syndrome we term caspase-8 deficiency state (CEDS).[22] Consistent with the known role of caspase-8 as an initiator caspase in the DISC, these patients had mild lymphadenopathy and splenomegaly, as well as lymphocyte apoptotic defects. However, they had inconsistent marginally elevated

Table 14.1 Autoimmune lymphoproliferative syndrome (ALPS) classification by molecular defect

Classification	Genetic defect
Type Ia	FAS (TNFRSF6)
Type Ib	FASLG (TNFSF6)
Type Im	Somatic FAS mutations
Type II	CASP10
Type III	Unknown mutation
Type IV (provisional)	NRAS (defective intrinsic apoptosis)

THERAPEUTIC PRINCIPLES

AUTOIMMUNE LYMPHOPROLIFERATIVE SYNDROME (ALPS)

>> Disease can improve with age

>> Corticosteroids are useful for rapidly bringing autoimmune disease under control

>> If unable to discontinue medications, low-dose corticosteroids given every other day, or mycophenolate mofetil, may be useful in preventing recurrence of autoimmune disease

>> Splenectomy should only be considered when hypersplenism contributes to severe refractory cytopenias

>> The risk of post-splenectomy sepsis necessitates lifelong antibiotic prophylaxis

>> Cytotoxic agents or matched unrelated donor allogeneic bone marrow transplantation can be considered for worst-case scenarios

>> Patients should undergo periodic monitoring for development of lymphoma

>> When they develop, ALPS lymphomas tend to respond to conventional therapies

DNT, raising doubt as to whether they fulfilled ALPS criteria. More importantly, unlike classical ALPS patients, the CEDS patients had a prominent combined immunodeficiency with recurrent sinopulmonary infections and mucocutaneous herpes virus infections. They had low serum immunoglobulin levels and poor humoral responses to polysaccharide antigens, as well as impaired activation of T cells, B cells, and NK cells. Thus, they resembled patients with common variable immunodeficiency (CVID). We recently found that the impaired lymphocyte activation resulted from a defect in the kinetics of activation of the critical transcription factor NF-κB in response to stimulation through antigen receptors, TLR-4, and FcγRIII.[22] This is because caspase-8 participates in a signaling complex that includes other proteins such as BCL-10, MALT-1, and IKK in an NF-κB-activating signalosome. This complex differs from the DISC and is not affected in classical ALPS patients. It will be important to identify other patients with caspase-8 deficiency to allow further definition of the clinical spectrum of this disease.

APOPTOSIS IN OTHER IMMUNODEFICIENCIES

Although resting lymphocytes are relatively resistant to death, they appear to require antigen receptor expression with continuous low or intermittent stimulation, in addition to homeostatic cytokines such as IL-7 and IL-15 for survival.[5, 13] Mice rendered genetically deficient in anti-apoptotic BCL-2 family members (such as BCL-2, BCL-X, and MCL-1), show loss of mature or developing lymphocytes. These results suggest that inappropriately activated intrinsic pathways of apoptosis may contribute to immunodeficiency. Several studies demonstrated increased spontaneous apoptosis of lymphocytes from patients with CVID, ataxia-telangiectasia, adenosine deaminase-severe combined immunodeficiency (ADA-SCID), Omenn's syndrome, cartilage-hair hypoplasia, and DiGeorge syndrome. However, without defining biochemically how specific gene mutations affect apoptosis, it is difficult to know whether these associations are simply correlative or indeed causative.

■ THERAPIES FOR ALPS ■

Although symptoms can remit with age, some ALPS patients require continued treatment to control autoimmune disease.[17, 23] Treatment for autoimmune cytopenias is similar to that used in patients without ALPS. A high-dose pulse of corticosteroid (5–30 mg/kg methylprednisolone i.v.) is useful in bringing autoimmune cytopenias rapidly under control. This is followed by a low-dose course (1–2 mg/kg prednisone orally) that can be tapered and eventually discontinued after several weeks to months. Adjuncts to corticosteroids include intravenous immunoglobulin for autoimmune thrombocytopenia or hemolytic anemia, and granulocyte colony-stimulating factor (G-CSF, 1–2 µg/kg from three times a week to once daily) for autoimmune neutropenia. In some patients, autoimmune disease promptly recurs after discontinuing corticosteroids. These patients may need to be maintained on a minimal dose every other day. Alternatively, such patients may benefit by switching to the immunosuppressant mycophenolate mofetil (~600 mg/m2 per dose orally, twice daily) for long-term maintenance therapy. The long-term corticosteroid- and splenectomy-sparing effects of this agent are particularly advantageous in children. For patients who fail these approaches, cytotoxic agents can be tried. Success has been reported using azathioprine, vincristine, or rituxan (anti-CD20 monoclonal antibody, 375 mg/m2 per week i.v.×4), although no controlled prospective trials exist to support the widespread use of these drugs in ALPS patients. Allogeneic bone marrow transplantation has been curative when undertaken in the rare instances of severely and intractably affected patients with homozygous FAS mutations and complete absence of Fas. However, given the associated high risks of complications and death, use of matched unrelated donor allogeneic bone marrow – which is likely to be required to avoid repopulating with lymphocytes from family members having the same mutation – should be considered a therapy of last resort.

Although lymphadenopathy and splenomegaly may be unsightly, these disease manifestations are usually not treated unless medically indicated. Hypersplenism can contribute to low blood cell counts when splenic pooling exacerbates autoimmune-mediated destruction. Notably, none of the current agents used to treat ALPS improves lymph node or spleen size. Splenectomy may be required if immunosuppressant agents fail to improve cytopenias. A disproportionately increased risk for post-splenectomy pneumococcal sepsis and death in ALPS patients means that splenectomy should be undertaken only after extensive discussions with the patient and family. Patients should be immunized with vaccines against *Streptococcus pneumoniae*, *Haemophilus influenzae*, and *Neisseria meningitidis* before splenectomy. Following splenectomy, patients should be re-immunized with conjugate plus polysaccharide pneumococcal vaccines when titers wane. Lifelong antibiotic prophylaxis with penicillin or fluoroquinolones is essential. Moreover, splenectomized patients should be instructed to seek immediate medical attention to rule out bacteremia during febrile illnesses.

Given that treatment of ALPS patients aims primarily at controlling autoimmune manifestations, drugs that control lymphoproliferation or prevent lymphomagenesis are needed. Several case reports suggested that sulphadoxine-pyrimethamine (Fansidar) treatment might have utility in patients with ALPS or ALPS-like disease. Regression of lymphadenopathy and/or splenomegaly, as well as improvement in blood cell counts, were observed in 6 of 7 treated patients. Two of the treated patients sustained remission after discontinuing the drug. However, more recent studies in ALPS patients and the *lpr* mouse model failed to demonstrate any significant benefit of this agent or pyrimethamine alone on lymph node or spleen size.[27] Therefore, at present this regimen cannot be considered recommended therapy.

Finally, the predisposition to lymphoma presents a unique clinical challenge: how to distinguish a newly developing or relapsed lymphoma from benign lymphadenopathy. ALPS patients require careful periodic examinations and surveillance by serial computed tomography scans. Suspiciously enlarging lymph nodes may necessitate biopsy to assess for clonality and chromosomal abnormalities. Positron emission tomography scans, which detect areas of high cellular glucose uptake, are useful for identifying and following suspicious lesions.[24] Fortunately, lymphomas in ALPS patients tend to respond to conventional therapies.

CONCLUSION

Programmed cell death is an essential regulatory mechanism to establish equipoise with growth, differentiation, and proliferation of lymphocytes. Studies in humans with the rare genetic disorder ALPS have demonstrated that apoptosis is physiologically important for maintaining lymphocyte homeostasis, preventing autoimmunity, and suppressing lymphomagenesis. Studies in ALPS-like disorders such as CEDS have revealed that molecules responsible for death can also participate in other intracellular signaling pathways for normal lymphocyte function. Defining the genetic abnormalities responsible for ALPS and related disorders should continue to provide insights into the mechanisms that regulate immune cell homeostasis *in vivo*.

ACKNOWLEDGEMENTS

We thank Koneti Rao, Thomas Fleisher, Janet Dale, and Stephen Straus for helpful discussions. This manuscript was supported principally by the Intramural Research Program of the National Institute of Allergy and Infections Disease, NIH. H.C.S. is supported by a Cancer Research Institute Postdoctoral Fellowship and is a recipient of a Burroughs Wellcome Fund Career Award in Biomedical Science.

REFERENCES

1. Ahmed R, Gray D. Immunological memory and protective immunity: understanding their relation. Science 1996; 272: 54–60.

2. Davis MM, Bjorkman PJ. T-cell antigen receptor genes and T-cell recognition. Nature 1988; 334: 395–402.

3. Horvitz HR. Nobel lecture. Worms, life and death. Biosci Rep 2003; 23: 239–303.

4. Ranger AM, Malynn BA, Korsmeyer SJ. Mouse models of cell death. Nat Genet 2001; 28: 113–118.

5. Lenardo M, Chan KM, Hornung F, et al. Mature T lymphocyte apoptosis – immune regulation in a dynamic and unpredictable antigenic environment. Annu Rev Immunol 1999; 17: 221–253.

6. Bidere N, Su HC, Lenardo MJ. Genetic disorders of programmed cell death in the immune system (*). Annu Rev Immunol 2006; 24: 321–352.

7. Danial NN, Korsmeyer SJ. Cell death: critical control points. Cell 2004; 116: 205–219.

8. Su HC, Lenardo MJ. Lessons from autoimmune lymphoproliferative syndrome. Drug Discov Today: Dis Mechanisms 2005; 2: 495–502.

9. Kerr JF, Wyllie AH, Currie AR. Apoptosis: a basic biological phenomenon with wide-ranging implications in tissue kinetics. Br J Cancer 1972; 26: 239–257.

10. Edinger AL, Thompson CB. Death by design: apoptosis, necrosis and autophagy. Curr Opin Cell Biol 2004; 16: 663–669.

11. Marsden VS, Strasser A. Control of apoptosis in the immune system: Bcl-2, BH3-only proteins and more. Annu Rev Immunol 2003; 21: 71–105.

12. Ashkenazi A, Dixit VM. Death receptors: signaling and modulation. Science 1998; 281: 1305–1308.

13. Opferman JT, Korsmeyer SJ. Apoptosis in the development and maintenance of the immune system. Nat Immunol 2003; 4: 410–415.

14. Siegel RM, Chan FK, Chun HJ, et al. The multifaceted role of Fas signaling in immune cell homeostasis and autoimmunity. Nat Immunol 2000; 1: 469–474.

15. Chen M, Wang YH, Wang Y, et al. Dendritic cell apoptosis in the maintenance of immune tolerance. Science 2006; 311: 1160–1164.

16. Rieux-Laucat F. Inherited and acquired death receptor defects in human autoimmune lymphoproliferative syndrome. Curr Dir Autoimmun 2006; 9: 18–36.

17. Sneller MC, Dale JK, Straus SE. Autoimmune lymphoproliferative syndrome. Curr Opin Rheumatol 2003; 15: 417–421.

18. Lim MS, Straus SE, Dale JK, et al. Pathological findings in human autoimmune lymphoproliferative syndrome. Am J Pathol 1998; 153: 1541–1550.

19. Del-Rey M, Ruiz-Contreras J, Bosque A, et al. A homozygous Fas ligand gene mutation in a patient causes a new type of autoimmune lymphoproliferative syndrome. Blood 2006; 108: 1306–1312.

20. Zhu S, Hsu AP, Vacek MM, et al. Genetic alterations in caspase-10 may be causative or protective in autoimmune lymphoproliferative syndrome. Hum Genet 2006; 119: 284–294.

21. Maric I, Pittaluga S, Dale JK, et al. Histologic features of sinus histiocytosis with massive lymphadenopathy in patients with autoimmune lymphoproliferative syndrome. Am J Surg Pathol 2005; 29: 903–911.

22. Su H, Bidere N, Zheng L, et al. Requirement for caspase-8 in NF-kappaB activation by antigen receptor. Science 2005; 307: 1465–1468.

23. Rao VK, Straus SE. Causes and consequences of the autoimmune lymphoproliferative syndrome. Hematology 2006; 11: 15–23.

24. Rao VK, Carrasquillo JA, Dale JK, et al. Fluorodeoxyglucose positron emission tomography (FDG-PET) for monitoring lymphadenopathy in the autoimmune lymphoproliferative syndrome (ALPS). Am J Hematol 2006; 81: 81–85.

25. Oliveira JB, Bidere N, Niemela JE, et al. NRAS mutation causes a human lymphoproliferative syndrome. Proc Natl Acad Sci USA 2007; 104: 8953–8958.

26. Bi LL, Pan G, Atkinson TP, et al. Dominant inhibition of Fas ligand-mediated apoptosis due to a heterozygous mutation associated with autoimmune lymphoproliferative syndrome (ALPS) type 1 b. BMC Med Genet 2007; 8: 41–55.

27. Rao VK, Dowdell KC, Dale JK, et al. Pyrimethamine treatment does not ameliorate lymphoproliferation or autoimmune disease in MPL / Lpr-/-mice or in patients with autoimmune lymphoproliferative syndrome. Am J Hematol 2007; in press.

28. Snellar MC, Straus SE, Jaffe ES, et al. A novel lymphoproliferative/ autoimmune syndrome resembling murine Lpr/gld disease. J Clin Invest 1992; 90: 334–341.

29. Canale VC, Smith CH. Chronic lymphadenopathy simulating malignant lymphoma. J Pediatr 1967; 70: 891–899.

part 2

HOST DEFENSE MECHANISMS AND INFLAMMATION

Immunoglobulin function

Neil S. Greenspan

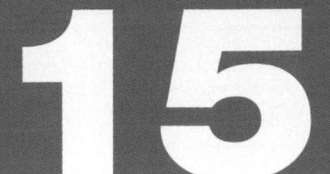

Antibody-mediated immunity generally requires noncovalent contact between antibody and antigen. The ability of an antigen to bind noncovalently to an antibody, referred to as *antigenicity*, is a physicochemical property evaluated with respect to a given antibody population. In contrast, *immunogenicity*, the ability to induce the biosynthesis and secretion of soluble antibody molecules, is a biological property, typically evaluated *in vivo* with respect to a particular immune system. Although antigenicity is necessary for immunogenicity, it is not sufficient. Moreover, the immunogenicity of a given molecule or molecular complex is influenced by host genetic variation. For example, a vaccine may be highly immunogenic in one person but be weakly immunogenic or nonimmunogenic in another.

When an antibody binds to a macromolecular antigen it directly contacts only a portion of the molecular surface of that antigen, not the entire molecule or molecular complex. Similarly, only a portion of the antibody molecule makes direct contact with the antigen. By convention, the portion of an antibody or T-cell receptor that makes physical contact with an antigen is referred to as the *paratope* or combining site. Most of the amino acids in an antibody variable domain that contact a given antigen are located in the hypervariable regions (also referred to as complementarity-determining regions or CDRs). However, X-ray crystallographic analyses of antibody–protein antigen complexes have shown that some contact residues reside in the framework regions.[1] The region of the antigen that is in physical contact with the paratope is conventionally called the *epitope* or antigenic determinant.

Although an epitope (paratope, etc.) is usually defined in terms of intermolecular contact, the region of a molecule involved in physical contact with another molecule may not correspond exactly to the structural correlates for energetics and specificity.[2]

■ ANTIGEN BINDING AND MOLECULAR IDENTITY ■

PHYSICAL ASPECTS OF BINDING

Antibody–antigen interactions are, with rare exceptions, *noncovalent*. The significance of this point is that these interactions are, in principle, spontaneously reversible under the conditions of temperature, pressure, pH, and ionic strength that generally prevail in living organisms.

Several types of noncovalent bond have been shown to contribute to antibody–antigen binding. These include van der Waals forces, hydrogen bonds, ionic bonds, and hydrophobic interactions. All of these bonds individually provide forces in the range of one to a few kcal/mol, versus 50–100 kcal/mol for covalent bonds. Because the potential to engage in these types of bond is shared by many of the components of biological macromolecules (e.g., amino acids, monosaccharides, and fatty acids), individual weak bonds do not usually confer a high degree of specificity. For example, any two atoms can interact through van der Waals forces. It is only through the simultaneous action of many such bonds that molecular specificity arises. Hence the importance of a close fit, often referred to as *complementarity* (or complementariness), between the antigen epitope and the antibody paratope.

Complementarity will be maximized when one molecule is concave and the other is convex; when one molecule is positively charged and the other is negatively charged; and where one has a hydrogen bond donor whereas the other offers a hydrogen bond acceptor, etc. It is expected that greater complementarity between receptor and ligand will in general be associated with a stronger interaction (greater affinity) between the two molecules. Specificity (see below) is also expected to be related to complementarity.[3]

In rationalizing the strength of interactions between antibodies and antigens, or other receptors and ligands, it is important to remember that the receptor competes with solvent for binding to ligand. Therefore, the thermodynamics of the interaction between two structures reflects the influence of the interaction on the solvent and other solutes, and not just the complementarity between the two molecules of special interest. Furthermore, bound water molecules may make important – even crucial – contributions to an interaction between two macromolecules or an interaction between a macromolecule and a small molecule. Apparently subtle modifications of structure can alter the thermodynamic balance (extent of binding) or the qualitative features of contact between receptor and ligand such that the agonist (e.g., a potent immunogen) becomes an antagonist or an inactive analogue (a poor immunogen).

The types of weak bond described above, and the concept of complementarity between interacting molecules, are relevant to our understanding of noncovalent interactions that can involve any biological molecules, including (but not limited to) the interactions between a T-cell receptor,

Table 15.1 Antigens and valence (Adapted from Benjamini E, Leskowitz S. Immunology: a short course, 2nd edn. New York : Wiley-Liss,1991, with permission from Wiley-Liss, Inc., a subsidiary of John Wiley & Sons, Inc.)

Number of types of epitope	Epitope copy number	Examples
Monodeterminant	Monovalent	Hapten: DNP, digoxin
Monodeterminant	Multivalent	Polysaccharide: dextran*
Multideterminant#	Monovalent	Monomeric protein: myoglobin
Multideterminant	Multivalent	Virion: influenza virus

*Even a polysaccharide composed of one type of hexasaccharide can have two or more different kinds of epitope: terminal versus internal residues, for instance. However, a given antiserum may preferentially contain antibodies specific for only one such epitope.
#Typically, multideterminance can only occur with respect to a polyclonal antibody.

its nominal antigen peptide, and an MHC class I or class II molecule; CD8 and MHC class I; CD4 and MHC class II; HIV gp120 and CD4; and LFA-1 and ICAM-1. Therefore, antibody recognition of antigen serves as a paradigm for understanding molecular recognition in the immune system in general. As will be discussed below, this fact, coupled with the inducibility of antibodies, permits antibodies to be used as surrogate ligands for almost any receptor (or vice-versa).

Affinity is the concept we use to convey how strongly two molecules bind to each other. In Table 15.1, antibody–antigen interactions are categorized with respect to the numbers of different kinds of paratope–epitope bonds and the absolute number of such bonds of each kind. Reflecting the different types of antibody–antigen interaction so identified, two categories of affinity merit consideration: *intrinsic affinity* and *functional affinity*. It should be noted that some immunologists prefer to use the term 'avidity' in place of 'functional affinity.'

Intrinsic affinity is a measure of the strength of the *monovalent* interaction between a particular paratope or antibody-combining site and a particular epitope or antigenic determinant, under defined conditions of temperature, pressure, ionic strength, and pH. By convention, the intrinsic affinity is taken to be the equilibrium association constant characterizing the paratope–epitope pair. If paratopes are represented by P, monovalent epitopes by E, paratope–epitope complexes by PE, and the equilibrium association constant by K_A, then, by the Law of Mass Action:

$$K_A = \frac{[PE]}{[P][E]}$$

The above equation says that the intrinsic affinity is the reciprocal of the concentration of monovalent antigen at which half of the paratopes will be occupied. Thus, this approach to measuring the strength of the interaction between paratope and epitope does so by determining how likely it is that epitope and paratope will be found in a complex.

Note that the intrinsic affinity, defined as above, is not an intrinsic property of either the paratope or the epitope. Instead, an intrinsic affinity characterizes the relationship between two molecules under defined conditions.

The intrinsic affinity of an antibody for a small antigenic molecule (hapten) can be determined by the technique of equilibrium dialysis (Fig. 15.1). This technique uses a semipermeable membrane to separate two compartments, one containing hapten and the other containing hapten and antibody. This membrane is referred to as semipermeable because the hapten can diffuse across it, but the antibody cannot. Free hapten will diffuse between the two compartments, and eventually the rate of diffusion between the compartments will be the same in both directions (dynamic equilibrium). At this point, the concentration of free hapten will be identical in the two compartments, but the compartment containing antibody will have more total hapten (free plus bound). By using haptens in chemical forms (e.g., radioactive) that permit quantification, one can determine the fraction of paratopes bound at known concentrations of hapten and antibody at specified temperature, pressure, ionic strength, and pH. This information permits the calculation of the intrinsic affinity.

The intrinsic affinity of an antibody for a small molecule, such as a drug (e.g., digoxin) or a hormone (e.g., insulin), can be clinically important both *in vivo* and *in* vitro.[4] For example, the *in vivo* effectiveness of antibody Fab fragments in removing toxic levels of the drug digoxin from the bodies of patients being treated for congestive heart failure is likely to be partially dependent on the intrinsic affinity of the Fab fragments for the drug. Alternatively, antibody intrinsic affinity can limit the analytical sensitivity of an *in vitro* immunoassay designed to determine the concentration of an analyte, such as a hormone (e.g., insulin, parathyroid hormone), or a drug (e.g., digoxin).

Functional affinity is defined as the equilibrium association constant characterizing the interaction between an intact antibody and an intact antigen. For a monovalent IgG antibody–antigen interaction, the intrinsic affinity and the functional affinity will be the same. However, if two paratopes interact simultaneously with two epitopes on the same antigen, which is referred to as *monogamous bivalency* (Fig. 15.2), the functional affinity of the antibody for the *multivalent* antigen may be substantially greater (as much as 10,000-fold for IgG) than the intrinsic affinity of that antibody for the relevant epitope on that same antigen.[5] Functional affinity is also influenced by the degree to which the geometric relationships among the epitopes are optimal for the paratopes, which will depend on the quaternary structure and segmental flexibility of the antibody molecule. In the presence of nonoptimal geometry, the average number of engaged sites may be less than maximal, and energy may be expended in achieving some epitope–paratope contacts. Therefore, the functional affinity for a multivalent interaction cannot necessarily be predicted precisely from the intrinsic affinity and the

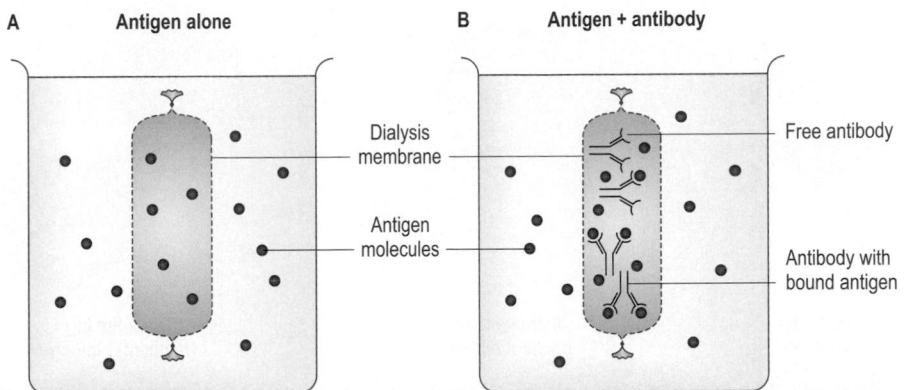

Fig. 15.1 Measurement of the intrinsic affinity characterizing an interaction between antibody and antigen (hapten) by equilibrium dialysis. At equilibrium, the amount of diffusible free hapten inside the dialysis bag will be equal to the amount of free hapten outside the bag. In the presence of antibody (B), therefore, the total hapten concentration will be greater inside of the dialysis bag (free + antibody-bound) than outside of the bag (free). The extent of this difference can be used to determine the intrinsic affinity of the antibody for the hapten. (From Abbas AK, Lichtman AH, Pober JS. Cellular and molecular immunology. WB Saunders Company, 1991 with permission from Elsevier.)

maximal number of binding sites that can be engaged simultaneously by an antibody molecule.

Intrinsic affinity provides information, with the qualifications noted above, on the degree of complementarity between epitope and paratope. Functional affinity takes account of properties influenced by structural features outside of the epitope and paratope, as normally conceived. Both concepts of affinity are valuable. Maximization of intrinsic affinity may be of prime importance for antibody-mediated inactivation of toxins or enzymes, which frequently involve monovalent interactions. In cases where antibodies bind to repetitive antigens or epitopes on the surfaces of bacteria, viruses, fungi, parasites, or mammalian cells, the functional affinity is likely to be a key factor influencing the biological consequences of the interaction.

In some instances, bivalent (IgG, IgE) or multivalent (IgA, IgM) antibodies may bind simultaneously to two or more epitopes on different antigenic particles, cross-linking them rather than engaging in monogamous bivalency or monogamous multivalency (Fig. 15.2). This phenomenon has played an important historical role in immunology. It is the basis for assays that make use of precipitation or agglutination of antigens by antibodies. Clinical methods for typing erythrocyte antigens (e.g., ABO and Rh antigens) still rely on agglutination of red cells by antibodies (or lectins).

IMMUNOLOGICAL SPECIFICITY

The concept of specificity is fundamental to an understanding of interactions between immunological receptors and antigens, but there are several senses of specificity in immunological contexts.[6] These are delineated below.

One sense of specificity is focused on the goodness of fit between paratope and epitope. Intrinsic affinity is regarded as a reasonable measure of this goodness of fit. However, substantial conformational adjustments of either paratope or epitope may be necessary for formation of the complex.[7] Such conformational changes will generally incur energetic costs. Consequently, intrinsic affinity and final complementarity may not be perfectly correlated.

A second sense of specificity corresponds to the ability of a paratope to distinguish between different epitopes. Such specificity is most readily studied when the epitope is in monovalent form. A quantitative measure of this kind of specificity is the ratio of intrinsic affinities characterizing, respectively, a paratope binding to the cognate ligand and the same paratope binding to a second ligand. This form of specificity can only be evaluated relative to a specified set of ligands. Thus, one should be cautious about extrapolating claims that one antibody is more or less specific than another with no reference to the relevant universe of ligands. However, there may be cases where it is justifiable to speak globally of more- or less-specific antibodies. Polyspecific antibodies have been described in the neonatal primary repertoire.[8] These antibodies appear to be globally less discriminating than antibodies typical of the immune repertoire (secondary or later response) when tested on large panels of antigens.

Nevertheless, it is important to note that even antibodies derived from secondary (or later) responses are not,[9] and cannot be, absolutely specific.[10,11] The impossibility of perfect recognition or discrimination can be understood in both thermodynamic and structural terms. First, perfect fit and absolute discrimination would imply infinite intrinsic affinity (negative free energy change of complex formation), which is not physically plausible.[10] Second, the convexity of atoms prevents perfect shape complementarity between antibody (receptor) and antigen (ligand).[11] Recent results also indicate that at least some antibodies can adopt two or more different unbound conformations, each of which exhibits a different ligand-binding profile. Such paratopes may undergo further structural adjustment in the process of binding to an epitope.[12]

In contrast to the epitope-centered forms of specificity just described, a third aspect relates to the ability of an antibody to discriminate among antigens that display many copies of one or more distinct epitopes. An antigen expressing many copies of one epitope is termed *multivalent*, and an antigen that expresses two or more structurally distinguishable epitopes is referred to as *multideterminant* (Table 15.1). Because two different cells, bacteria, viruses, etc., may both express multiple copies of the same or nearly the same epitope, an antibody that is highly specific (in the first sense above) for such a shared epitope may be a poor discriminator between such multivalent particles.[6] Yet an

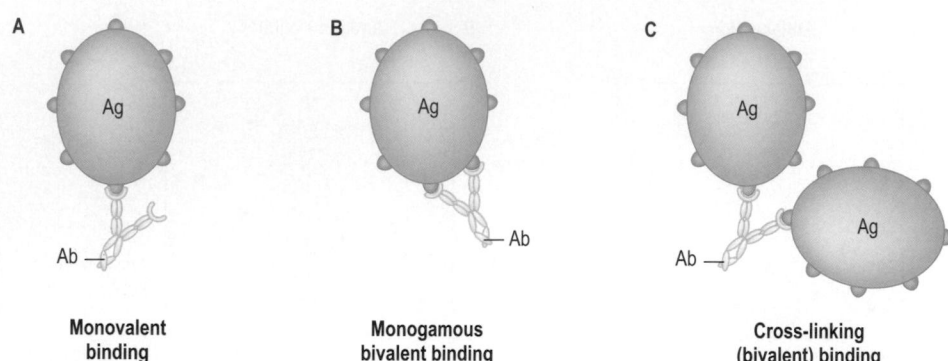

Fig. 15.2 Interaction of a bivalent antibody, such as IgG, with multivalent antigens can result in monovalent binding (**A**) monogamous bivalent binding (**B**) or cross-linking (**C**). The complexes in (**B**) are referred to as cyclic antibody–antigen complexes. (With permission from Eisen HN. General immunology. JB Lippincott, 1990.)

KEY CONCEPTS

BINDING OF ANTIBODY TO ANTIGEN

>> Paratopes interact with epitopes through multiple noncovalent (weak) bonds, each of which is reversible at room temperature.

>> Intrinsic affinity is taken to be the equilibrium association constant for a monovalent epitope-paratope interaction. It is a measure of the strength of that interaction and is influenced by the degree of complementarity between epitope and paratope and by ambient conditions: temperature, pressure, ionic strength, and pH.

>> Functional affinity is a measure of the average strength of the interaction between an intact antibody and a multivalent antigen. It can be influenced by the spatial distribution of the epitopes that are being recognized.

>> Intrinsic affinity and functional affinity can both be of biological importance, although both are not necessarily relevant in the same circumstances.

>> For the clinician, immunological specificity may sometimes need to be evaluated primarily with respect to biological as opposed to physical endpoints.

antibody with a relatively poor degree of complementarity and intrinsic affinity for an epitope found on only one of two or more multivalent targets may be superior at discriminating among these antigens. Furthermore, antibodies (or other molecules) expressing two or more binding sites of identical structure may not discriminate identically among antigens displaying the same epitope in different two- or three-dimensional distributions.[6]

Some final points regarding specificity. First, in discussing interactions between molecules such as CD4 and MHC class II, which are not clonally distributed, it is common to describe such molecules as nonspecific, meaning not specific for an antigen under consideration. The contrast being drawn is with the antigen-specific receptors, Ig or TCR. However, from the point of view of the first or second category of specificity described above (goodness of fit, discrimination between ligands), the interaction between molecules such as CD4 and MHC class II may be as biochemically specific as that between an antibody and a class II molecule. Ideally, this sense of 'nonspecific' should be modified by the term 'antigen.' If not, the meaning must be inferred from the context. Second, for many purposes immunological specificity has an ultimately biological, not a physical, definition. If the endpoint of analysis is the triggering of a complex response, such as cell activation or initiation of the complement cascade, then the presence, absence, or extent of that response, and not the extent of receptor–antigen interaction, will be the ultimate criterion for evaluating specificity. Such biological specificity is not always directly correlated with specificity as determined by the analysis of binding.[6] Third, the enormous utility of antibodies is crucially dependent on the discriminatory abilities of these molecules with respect to other molecules or molecular aggregates. However, given that the discrimination mediated by antibodies is not absolute, the usefulness of a particular antibody may depend on the context: which antigens or potential antigens in addition to the preferred target are available for binding to the antibody? Fourth, apparent antibody specificity may vary with the methods used for analysis, as these methods may differ in sensitivity and the conditions (pH, ionic strength, temperature) of application, such that the relevant intrinsic affinities may vary among the different assays.

■ PROTEIN EPITOPES ■

Several categories of epitope have been defined for protein antigens, based on the proximity of the relevant amino acids in the primary structure of the protein (Fig. 15.3). The simplest case is the *linear* epitope, where all of the relevant amino acids are derived from a contiguous stretch of the polypeptide chain. However, many – perhaps most – epitopes on globular proteins involve amino acids from two or more stretches of polypeptide that are distant from one another in the primary structure. Such an epitope is referred to as a *conformational*, or *discontinuous*, epitope. In some cases, such as with the capsids of nonenveloped viruses, it is conceivable that a conformational epitope can comprise amino acids derived from

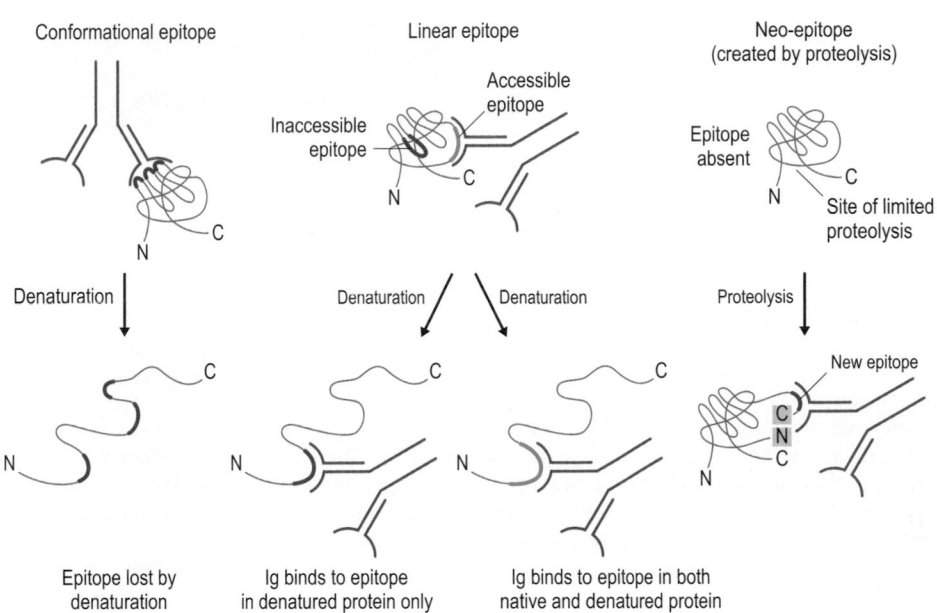

Conformational epitope   Linear epitope   Neo-epitope (created by proteolysis)

Fig. 15.3 Types of protein epitope. Some antibodies recognize structural features of proteins that arise from the folding of the polypeptide backbone (conformational epitope). Others recognize groups of amino acid residues that are contiguous, or nearly so, in the primary (covalent) structure of the protein (linear epitope). If such a linear determinant is inaccessible in the native structure of the protein, the corresponding antibodies may only be elicited by the denatured form of the protein. Neo-epitopes are created by covalent post-translational modifications, such as proteolytic cleavage. (From Abbas AK, Lichtman AH, Pober JS. Cellular and molecular immunology, 3rd edn. WB Saunders Company, 1997, with permission from Elsevier.)

separate polypeptide chains that are adjacent in the capsid. Another category of protein epitope, the *neo-epitope*, is reserved for those antigenic sites that become recognizable only after a post-translational event, such as proteolytic cleavage. For example, several neo-epitopes have been defined on cleavage products of human C1q, C3, and C9, components of the complement pathway.[13] Antibodies recognizing such neo-epitopes can be used to monitor the extent of activation of the complement pathway.[13]

Studies in the 1970s on the sizes of epitopes associated with synthetic peptide antigens yielded results suggesting that protein epitopes would maximally involve six or seven amino acids. The first structure of an antibody variable module in complex with a globular protein antigen, determined by X-ray crystallography,[1] indicated that protein epitopes, defined on the basis of intermolecular contact, could be as large as 15–20 amino acids. A similar number of amino acids in the antibody V domains constituted the paratope. Of course, it is possible that there are smaller epitopes on globular proteins, particularly for regions of proteins that protrude or have a high radius of curvature. Peptide antigen–antibody interaction can involve at least 12 peptide amino acids in contact with the antibody.

Antibodies specific for both linear and conformational epitopes have important uses. A synthetic peptide corresponding in amino acid sequence to a segment of the polypeptide chain predicted from the nucleotide sequence can be used to elicit antibodies.[14] In many cases, such antibodies will recognize a linear epitope that is available in a denatured form of the gene product. Therefore, these antibodies can be used to identify the protein following expression and blotting, or electrophoresis and blotting, under denaturing conditions. Antibodies that bind to linear epitopes may recognize a protein in denatured form, but will often not bind to or alter the function of the native protein.

Antibodies with the ability to neutralize protein function generally recognize conformations accessible to the native protein, usually at discontinuous epitopes. However, some antibodies specific for peptides (that correspond in amino acid sequence to a portion of a native protein) or denatured protein cross-react with the protein in a native (folded, functional) state. Such cross-reactivity is more likely to occur when the region being recognized is relatively unstructured in the native structure.[15]

CARBOHYDRATE EPITOPES

The classic studies of Elvin Kabat on the binding of antibodies to dextran led to the concept that epitopes on carbohydrate antigens could be as large as six or seven monosaccharide units.[16] However, minimal carbohydrate epitopes can probably be as small as one or two monosaccharides. Even in the case of larger epitopes involving three or more saccharide units, it is typical for the terminal groups to play a dominant role in determining antibody specificity for carbohydrate antigens. Recent studies suggest that, analogous to the conformational epitopes of proteins, polysaccharide epitopes can sometimes result from conformational properties of polysaccharides.

Interactions between antibodies and polysaccharides are typically characterized by relatively low intrinsic affinities compared to antibody–protein interactions.[5] Two sorts of factor may account for relatively weak antibody–carbohydrate binding: biological constraints related to protection against self-recognition and consequent tissue damage; and physicochemical constraints related to the conformational freedom and high degree of solvation of unbound carbohydrates.

Another important feature of polysaccharide antigens is that they are generally multivalent. Bacterial polysaccharide epitope densities can approach values in the millions per μm^2, which is probably one to several orders of magnitude greater than the epitope densities for protein determinants on mammalian cells. Therefore, multipoint attachment and functional affinity are likely to be critical factors in the mediation of immunity by anti-polysaccharide antibodies or other carbohydrate-specific proteins.

■ IMMUNE COMPLEXES *IN VIVO* ■

Interactions between antibodies and antigens *in vivo* can result in the formation of molecular aggregates, referred to as *immune complexes*. Deposition of immune complexes in tissues, such as blood vessels, renal glomeruli, renal tubules, the thyroid gland, and the choroid plexus, can result in pathological conditions.[17] Immune complexes can form in the circulation prior to deposition in a given tissue, or they can form directly in the affected tissue. Variables such as concentration, composition, size, charge, and antibody isotype for a given population of immune complexes will influence the magnitude and sites of tissue deposition for those complexes. The magnitude of complement activation and the extent of interaction with Fc and complement receptors, in conjunction with the sites and extent of tissue deposition, determine the biological properties of the complexes. Antigen–antibody lattice size is determined by antigen valence, epitope geometry, antibody valence, the intrinsic affinity of paratope for epitope, antibody and antigen flexibility, the ratio of antibody to antigen, and the absolute concentrations of antibody and antigen. The potential diversity of immune complex morphologies is illustrated in Figure 15.4. These complexes, between a monoclonal antibody specific for a bacterial polysaccharide and various anti-idiotypic or anti-isotypic monoclonal antibodies, are visualized by electron microscopy.

Immune complexes have also been found to have immunoregulatory effects,[18] particularly with respect to antibody responses. Immune complexes can bind simultaneously to B-cell surfaces through antigen (to B-cell surface immunoglobulin), antibody (to Fc receptors), and associated complement components (to complement receptors). The interaction with FcγRIIB, on the B-lymphocyte membrane, has the effect of diminishing the B-cell response. The molecular events underlying these immunoregulatory effects are being intensively studied and have been exploited clinically for many years. Antibody to the erythrocyte Rh antigens is used to prevent immunization of an Rh⁻ mother by an Rh⁺ fetus, thereby avoiding hemolytic disease of the newborn in a subsequent Rh⁺ fetus (Chapter 62).

■ CORRELATIONS BETWEEN C_H REGION STRUCTURE AND ANTIBODY FUNCTION ■

Antibodies are heterodimeric proteins that can be functionally divided into variable domains, which bind antigen, and constant domains, which define the effector function of the immunoglobulin. Using these domains, an antibody can physically link a specific antigen to a separate antigen-nonspecific effector molecule, such as a complement component

---

■ KEY CONCEPTS

IMMUNE COMPLEXES

>> Immune complexes are aggregates of antibody and antigen.

>> Immune complexes can form in tissues or they can form in the circulation and subsequently deposit in tissues.

>> Immune complexes can activate complement or Fc receptor-bearing cells, leading to tissue damage.

>> The composition, size, charge, and antibody isotypes characterizing a given population of immune complexes will influence the pathogenic potential of the complexes.

---

or a cell-bound Fc receptor. Many features of C_H domain structure exhibited by the immunoglobulin isotypes can be understood in the context of this requirement for linkage between antigen and effector molecules.

One property of prime significance for antibody function is intramolecular mobility, often referred to as *segmental flexibility*. Hydrodynamic methods, electron microscopy, X-ray crystallography, and fluorescence polarization have all been used to evaluate the degree of flexibility exhibited by IgG, IgM, IgA, and IgE molecules.[19] In the case of the best-studied isotype, IgG, it is clear that the structural feature most associated with relative motion of one subunit relative to another is the hinge, which connects the C_H1 domain to the C_H2 domain and is encoded by a separate exon.

Immunoglobulin flexibility has important functional consequences to the antibody. First, inter-Fab movements can play an important role in permitting antibodies to bind in monogamous bivalent (or multivalent) fashion to antigenic surfaces that display repetitive epitopes. Second, efficiency in precipitation of multivalent antigen molecules or agglutination of multivalent antigen particles can be correlated with inter-Fab flexibility. And third, optimal interactions of effector molecules with IgG antibody Fc regions has been postulated to depend on the ability of the Fc region to bend out of the plane of the Fab arms (*dislocation*) (but see discussion on complement activation below).

■ FUNCTIONS MEDIATED BY ANTIBODY ALONE ■

Although it is clear that in many *in vivo* situations antibodies mediate their effects with the aid of other molecules and, in selected cases, cells (see next section), there are circumstances where the antibody can influence antigenic targets directly. The very name 'antibody' implies the negation of some activity, and antibodies were first defined as factors that could inactivate toxins. Subsequent studies have shown inactivation of viruses, parasites, and enzymes as well.

VIRUS NEUTRALIZATION

A phenomenon of fundamental medical and biological importance is the *neutralization* of viruses by antibodies.[20] Although neutralization is defined as the elimination or reduction of the virus's ability to replicate,

KEY CONCEPTS

STRUCTURE–FUNCTION RELATIONSHIPS OF C_H DOMAINS

>> Immunoglobulin function is influenced by differences in quaternary structure and segmental flexibility.

>> The hinge region helps control segmental flexibility in IgG molecules.

>> When interacting with multivalent antigens, IgM molecules can adopt a dislocated (staple) configuration in which the Fab arms are bent out of the plane of the Fc regions.

KEY CONCEPTS

VIRUS NEUTRALIZATION

>> Antibodies can neutralize (decrease the replication of) viruses by several mechanisms, including blocking attachment to the host cell, preventing penetration of the host cell membrane, or interfering with uncoating of the virus within the cell.

>> Neutralizing antibodies typically recognize proteins or glycoproteins on the virion surface.

>> Some antibodies that bind to virion surface proteins or glycoproteins are not neutralizing. In some cases such antibodies may contribute to immunity, whereas in others they may actually enhance infection.

>> The magnitude of neutralization mediated by a given antibody may vary with the host cell used for the measurement.

>> Neutralization *in vitro* is usually related to protection *in vivo*, but these two properties are not always perfectly correlated.

it does not imply a particular mechanism of interference with the process of replication itself. Moreover, the measurement of neutralization can depend on the choice of host cell. In other words, the neutralizing activity of a given antibody for a given virus is not an intrinsic property of the antibody, but is a property of the relationship between antibody and virus, under defined conditions. Consequently, neutralization titers in serum do not always correlate perfectly with protection from infection or disease *in vivo*.

There are several mechanisms by which antibodies may inactivate viruses. Recall that the process by which a virus infects a cell involves multiple steps, including attachment to one or more membrane components, penetration of or fusion with the membrane, uncoating, and genome expression. Although the most obvious mechanism of neutralization is the prevention of viral attachment to the host cell surface, antibodies can block other steps as well. For example, some neutralizing antibodies for enveloped viruses, such as influenza virus, have been shown to prevent fusion between the virion and cell membranes, and some neutralizing antibodies for polio virus have been shown to interfere with viral uncoating in the host cell.

Different isotypes of antibodies may employ different neutralization mechanisms to varying degrees, although this statement should not be interpreted to mean that there is a one-to-one correspondence between isotypes and neutralization mechanisms. IgA, the dominant isotype in mucosal secretions, operates under conditions where complement is less plentiful than in the blood, so virus-specific IgA is more likely to utilize virus-inactivating mechanisms, such as prevention of attachment, without a requirement for complement. In the blood, IgG or IgM antibodies can mediate protection against a virus, either directly in some cases, or with the assistance of complement components in others.

Traditional thinking maintains that antibody mediates any protective effects in the extracellular environment. However, it has been reported that IgA antibodies, being transported by the polymeric immunoglobulin receptor, can mediate protection against intracellular virus.[21] In viral infections of the central nervous system there is substantial evidence for antibody-mediated clearance by incompletely understood noncytolytic mechanisms.[22]

There are several other notable features of antibody–virus interactions. Not all antibodies that bind to molecules on the virion surface will neutralize the virus. For a given virus-encoded gene product, such as the influenza virus hemagglutinin, binding of antibodies to some sites, but

not others, will effect neutralization. Some gene products on the virion surface may contain no neutralization sites, strictly defined. The neuraminidase of influenza virus may be an example of this category of virion surface protein. However, antibody to influenza neuraminidase, albeit nonneutralizing, is thought to slow the spread of infection by interfering with the escape of progeny virions from an infected cell. Nonneutralizing antibodies, or neutralizing antibodies at suboptimal concentrations, have been found in some instances to enhance the infection of host cells by virus (e.g., HIV-1 or dengue virus). Finally, some nonneutralizing antibodies can mediate protective effects *in vivo*, presumably by engaging antigen-nonspecific effector mechanisms (i.e., complement or Fc receptor-bearing cells) or perhaps through cellular signal transduction.[22]

NEUTRALIZATION OF TOXINS AND ENZYMES

In many bacterial infections the clinical consequences of infection are due more to toxic molecules liberated by the bacterial cells than to the presence of the microorganisms themselves. Antibodies to such toxins can provide life-saving protection from disease, despite not directly eliminating the bacteria producing the toxins. The classic example of this situation is infection with *Corynebacterium diphtheriae*, which secretes a potentially lethal exotoxin. Bacteria can also produce additional virulence factors, such as enzymes that facilitate spreading of the pathogen through tissues. Host antibodies that inactivate such enzymes can have a beneficial influence on the clinical course. Inactivation of toxins or enzymes is presumed to result from direct competition between antibody and the target molecule or substrate of the toxin or enzyme, or from the stabilization or induction of conformations that are to some degree incompatible with the normal function(s) of the toxin or enzyme.

In summary, antibodies can use a variety or a combination of mechanisms to play a significant role in protection against both primary infection and reinfection with a diverse array of pathogens, including viruses, bacteria, fungi, and parasites.[23]

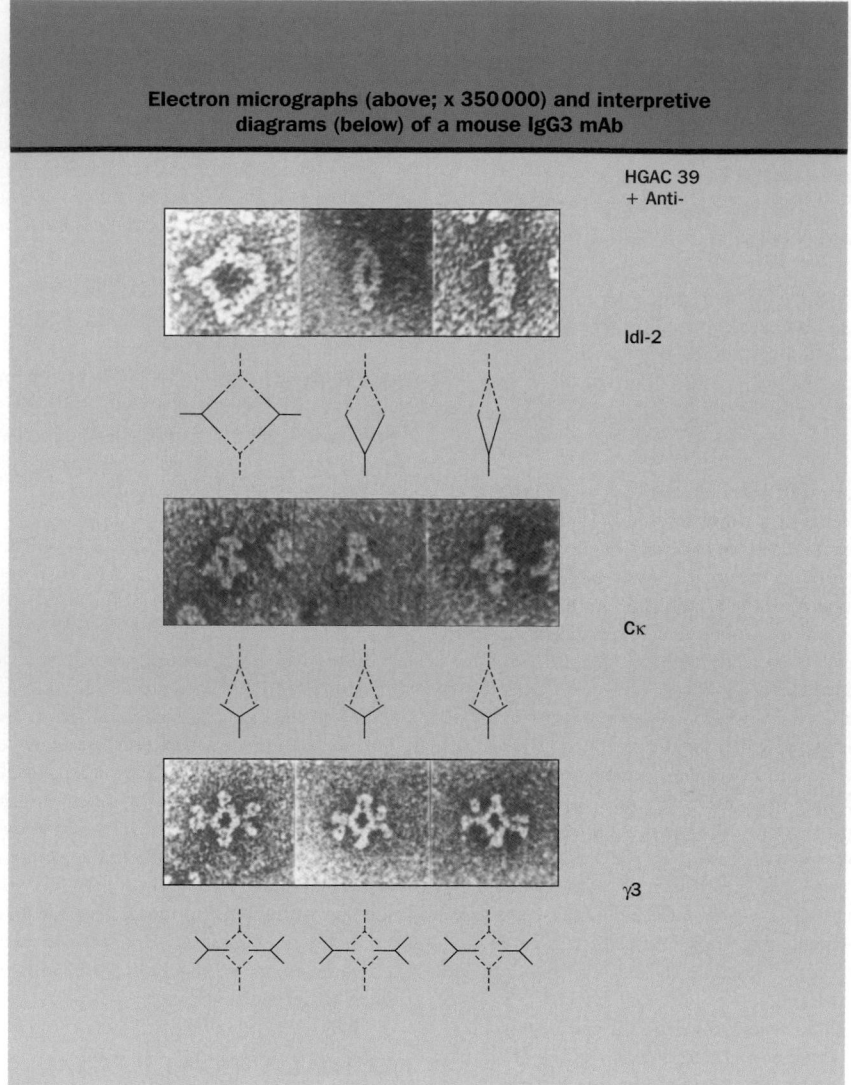

Electron micrographs (above; x 350 000) and interpretive diagrams (below) of a mouse IgG3 mAb

HGAC 39
+ Anti-

Idl-2

Cκ

γ3

Fig. 15.4 Electron micrographs (above; ×350 000) and interpretive diagrams (below) of a mouse IgG$_3$ mAb (HGAC 39; specific for a bacterial polysaccharide) in complex with mAbs specific for, respectively, an idiotope (Idl-2; top), a light chain isotypic determinant (C$_\kappa$; middle), and a heavy chain isotypic determinant (γ$_3$; bottom). The different antibodies are not intrinsically distinguishable in the electron micrographs, but the interpretations take into account information in addition to that provided directly by the electron microscopic images. In the top series of micrographs, the choice of which molecules to represent as solid or dotted figures is arbitrary. (From Greenspan NS. Analyzing immunoglobulin functional anatomy with monoclonal anti-immunoglobulin antibodies. BioTechniques 1989; 7: 1086, with permission from Eaton Publishing Company.)

■ FUNCTIONS MEDIATED BY ANTIBODY AND ADDITIONAL MOLECULES OR CELLS ■

COMPLEMENT ACTIVATION

Regardless of whether direct binding of antibody to antigen mediates protective effects, antibody bound *in vivo* will activate antigen-nonspecific effector mechanisms. The exact mechanisms will depend on the isotype of the antibody as well as on other factors. One critical set of these effector mechanisms is encompassed by the classical pathway of complement activation. The human antibody isotypes vary considerably in their intrinsic ability to activate this pathway. The consensus view is that IgM, IgG$_1$, and IgG$_3$ isotypes are effective activators. Whereas some sources state that IgG$_2$, IgG$_4$, and IgA are weak or nonactivators of the classical complement pathway, evidence suggests that when epitope density is high, IgG$_2$ can effectively activate the classical pathway.[24] Instead of attempting to decide which subclass is absolutely superior, it is probably more useful to recognize that

complement-fixing ability may not be determined solely by the sub-class of an IgG antibody.

One obvious source for the isotype-related variation in complement activating ability is variation in affinity for C1q ($IgG_3 > IgG_1 > IgG_2 > IgG_4$), the portion of the first component in the classical pathway that physically contacts the C_H2 domains of antibodies. The intrinsic affinity of the C1q globular heads for Fc regions of any isotype is relatively low, accounting for the observation that two or more IgG molecules in proximity are required for activation of the classical pathway, beginning with C1. Thus, in the activation of the classical pathway, the functional affinity of C1q for antibody Fc regions is a crucial parameter.

IgG subclass-associated differences in some measures of complement activation have been found, under some experimental conditions, to depend on quantitative differences in steps of the cascade subsequent to the binding of C1q to antibody. Although there has been speculation regarding the role of segmental flexibility in complement activation, there is probably no simple correlation between this physical property and activity in fixing the classical complement pathway.[25]

Although it is generally agreed that IgA does not activate the classical pathway, its ability to activate the alternative complement pathway has been controversial. Studies with recombinant IgA molecules have suggested that neither IgA_1 nor IgA_2 activates either complement pathway.[26]

Antibody-mediated activation of the classical complement pathway has a variety of potential consequences, including the creation of additional sites on a foreign particle to which phagocytic cells can attach and ingest the particle (opsonization), and elaboration of substances that mediate leukocyte chemotaxis, additional metabolic changes involved in the destruction of pathogens by leukocytes, and changes in vascular permeability. These inflammation-related processes are described in more detail in Chapter 20. In this scheme, it is the antibody that provides the specificity; the other molecules function similarly regardless of the epitopes involved.

RECEPTORS FOR Fc REGIONS

In addition to the complement system, the other major system with which antibodies interact in the mediation of effector functions is cellular. The specific molecules with which cells recognize antibodies are called Fc receptors (FcR).[27] In humans, there are several Fc receptors for IgG ($Fc\gamma RI$, $Fc\gamma RII$, $Fc\gamma RIII$), as well as other Fc receptors for IgA, IgE, and IgM (Fig. 15.5). We will describe selected features of Fc receptors that help to illuminate the principles by which they function.

Some receptors ($Fc\gamma RI$, $Fc\varepsilon RI$) have relatively high intrinsic affinities for antibody molecules, and can therefore bind significant fractions of monomeric Ig at physiological concentrations. For example, the high-affinity receptor for IgE ($Fc\varepsilon RI$) binds IgE with an intrinsic affinity of approximately 1×10^{10} M^{-1}. Therefore, even at relatively low concentrations, single IgE molecules can bind to mast cells or basophils through cell surface $Fc\varepsilon RI$ prior to interacting with allergen (antigen). In contrast, $Fc\gamma RII$ and $Fc\gamma RIII$ have relatively weak intrinsic affinities for IgG Fc regions. Consequently, multivalent forms of IgG, such as are found in complexes of antibody and multivalent antigens (immune complexes), are much more readily bound to these FcR. Thus, for both the complement-dependent and the FcR-dependent effector function pathways, multivalency of Fc regions (functional affinity) plays a critical role.

Several types of functional consequence can follow ligation of FcR by antibody–antigen complexes. These include activation and metabolic alteration of the FcR^+ cell, phagocytosis of antibody-coated particulate antigens, antibody-dependent cellular cytotoxicity (ADCC), and release of mediators that promote inflammation. These pathways clearly apply to IgG and IgE antibodies. Recent data suggest another possible function that depends on the interaction between antibody (IgA) and a cell surface receptor able to bind to polymeric immunoglobulins (pIgR). Transport of IgA–antigen complexes across epithelial surfaces by pIgR may represent a form of antibody-facilitated antigen excretion.[28] In mice, recent studies indicate that the effectiveness of antibodies of the various murine IgG subclasses in mediating FcR-dependent effector functions correlates with the ratio of affinities of antibodies of those subclasses for activating versus inhibiting $Fc\gamma R$.[29]

■ ANTIBODIES AS SURROGATE LIGANDS ■

The notion that one molecule can mimic a second molecule, in one respect or another, is of extraordinarily broad applicability and of profound biological significance. At least three types of mimicry can be distinguished, and each type can be regarded as a continuous (as opposed to discrete) variable.[30] First, one can conceive of limited structural mimicry of one molecule by another. By chance, two otherwise different molecules could have regions that happen to contain the same, or similar (in key respects), atoms in the same, or almost the same, three-dimensional arrangement. Second, there is mimicry at the level of noncovalent interaction. In this case, the question of interest is whether the model (object of mimicry) and the mimic bind the same receptor sites and with the same affinities. Third, there is mimicry of more complex biological functions, such as cellular or enzymatic inactivation. It is important to make these distinctions because the extent of mimicry of one type is not a perfect predictor of the extent of mimicry of another type. We have already noted that slight changes in structure sometimes have slight effects on binding affinity or specificity, yet in other cases they have dramatic effects. In other words, structural similarity (mimicry), as we perceive it, is not perfectly correlated with mimicry at the level of binding or the level of elicitation of higher biological function.

▌ KEY CONCEPTS

ANTIBODY EFFECTOR SYSTEMS

>> Multivalence of Fc regions is often important in activating antibody effector functions.

>> The occurrence and magnitude of effector function activation varies with antibody isotype.

>> Effector mechanisms are inherently nonspecific with respect to antigen.

>> Antibody Fc regions provide the mechanistic link between antigen-specific V domains and antigen-nonspecific effector mechanisms.

Receptor	FcγRI (CD64)	FcγRII-A (CD32)	FcγRII-B2 (CD32)	FcγRII-B3 (CD32)	FcγRIII (CD16)	FcεRI	FcαRI (CD89)	Fcα/μR
Structure	α 72 kDa	α 40 kDa			α 50-70 kDa or γ or ζ	α 45 kDa β 33 kDa γ 9 kDa	α 55-75 kDa γ 9 kDa	α 70 kDa
		γ~like domain	ITIM	ITIM				
Binding Order of affinity	IgG1 10^8 M^{-1} 1) IgG1=IgG3 2) IgG4 3) IgG2	IgG1 2×10^6 M^{-1} 1) IgG1 2) IgG3=IgG2* 3) IgG2	IgG1 2×10^6 M^{-1} 1) IgG1=IgG3 2) IgG4 3) IgG2	IgG1 2×10^6 M^{-1} 1) IgG1=IgG3 2) IgG4 3) IgG2	IgG1 5×10^5 M^{-1} IgG1=IgG3	IgE 10^{10} M^{-1}	IgA1, IgA2 10^7 M^{-1} IgA1=IgA2	IgA, IgM 3×10^9 M^{-1} 1) IgM 2) IgA
Cell type	Macrophages Neutrophils† Eosinophils† Dendritic cells	Macrophages Neutrophils Eosinophils Platelets Langerhans' cells	Macrophages Neutrophils Eosinophils	B cells Mast cells	NK cells Eosinophils Macrophages Neutrophils Mast cells	Mast cells Eosinophils† Basophils	Macrophages Neutrophils Eosinophils‡	Macrophages B cells
Effect of ligation	Uptake Stimulation Activation of respiratory burst Induction of killing	Uptake Granule release (eosinophils)	Uptake Inhibition of stimulation	No uptake Inhibition of stimulation	Induction of killing (NK cells)	Secretion of granules	Uptake Induction of killing	Uptake

Fig. 15.5 Domain structures, binding properties, cellular expression patterns, and functional effects of human Fc receptors. A given FcR may exhibit differences in composition depending on the cell type expressing it. For example, FcγRIII is expressed on neutrophil plasma membranes bearing a glycosylphotidylinositol anchor, without FcRγ chains, whereas it is expressed on NK cell plasma membranes as a conventional transmembrane protein in association with FcRγ chains. Similarly, FcγRII-B1 contains an additional stretch of polypeptide encoded by an exon whose product is not represented in the intracellular domain of FcγRII-B2. This additional portion of the polypeptide is believed to prevent the internalization of FcγRII-B1 subsequent to cross-linking.

*A subset of FcγRII-A allotypes bind to human IgG$_2$.

† For these cells, FcR expression is inducible, not constitutive.

‡ The molecular weight of CD89a chain is 70–100 kDa in eosinophils. (From Janeway CA Jr, Travers P, Walport M, Shlomchik M. Immunobiology: the immune system in health and disease, 6th edn. New York: Garland Science, 2004, with permission from Garland Science.)

There are two aspects of receptor–ligand interaction that antibodies can potentially mimic. First, as noted earlier, the inducibility of a vast repertoire of antibody specificities suggests the potential for identifying, through screening or selection, antibodies that can bind any given target molecule at a given site. Thus, there should be a reasonable probability of obtaining antibodies that bind to a particular receptor at a site bound by some other, perhaps physiological, ligand or co-receptor. The prediction that it should be possible to identify antibodies that can mimic the functional effects of other molecules has been supported by many investigations of anti-idiotypic antibodies and conventional anti-receptor antibodies.[31, 32]

Second, as noted earlier, the triggering event for many cellular and effector processes in the immune system is the aggregation of receptor molecules by clustered ligands. Therefore, the ability of antibodies, which naturally have a maximal valence of 2 or greater, to cross-link cell surface molecules and initiate signal transduction contributes to the abilities of antibodies to serve as surrogate co-receptors for cell surface molecules. This property of antibodies has greatly facilitated the identification and

functional characterization of many of these molecules, and is also being exploited for therapeutic use.[33]

FUNCTIONAL PROPERTIES OF ENGINEERED ANTIBODY MOLECULES

MONOCLONAL ANTIBODIES

Many modern applications of antibodies in research, medicine, veterinary medicine, and other fields rely heavily, although not exclusively, on monoclonal antibodies. By definition, a monoclonal antibody population is derived from a clonal population of B-lineage cells. Therefore, all of the molecules will express identical variable domains and identical antigen specificities. It is the homogeneity of the V domain structure associated with monoclonal antibodies that most crucially distinguishes them from polyclonal antibodies, such as those conventionally derived from the serum. Homogeneous antibodies give more reproducible and more easily interpreted results for many kinds of assay.

Monoclonal antibodies of selected specificity were first produced by cells referred to as hybridomas.[34] In contrast, a myeloma protein would be an example of a monoclonal antibody of unselected specificity. Hybridomas are hybrid transformed cells that are created by the fusion of two types of cell. Each of these parental cells endows the hybridoma with desirable properties. One parent of a hybridoma (the fusion partner) is a transformed cell, usually a myeloma cell line, which contributes a metabolism that supports unlimited growth in tissue culture and high rates of immunoglobulin synthesis and secretion. The myeloma cell lines used as hybridoma fusion partners usually have been genetically manipulated such that they no longer synthesize an immunoglobulin molecule, and they can be selected against in special culture media. The second parental cell is a B lymphocyte, usually from the spleen or lymph node of an immunized animal. This normal B cell provides the genetic information for the production of a particular antibody. Note that the choice of specificity on the part of the investigator is influenced at two stages in the process, including the choice of immunogen and the nature of the screening assay. By screening a population of hybridomas, most of which will secrete different antibodies, with an appropriately designed assay it is possible to identify the minority of cells that secrete a monoclonal antibody of desired specificity.

Monoclonal antibodies are useful for the identification and quantification of diverse molecules of biological or synthetic origin, including human immunoglobulins (e.g., paraproteins), antigens from infectious agents (e.g., HIV p24), hormones, drugs, and toxins. They have also been exploited for therapeutic purposes, such as reversing allograft rejection, killing tumor cells, or preventing cytokine activity contributing to autoimmune disease. The benefits and limitations of monoclonal antibodies for human use are discussed in Chapter 95.

RECOMBINANT ANTIBODIES

The ability to manipulate the genes that encode antibodies, and thereby manipulate the structures of antibodies, has opened a new era in the study and application of antibodies (Fig. 15.6). Progress has occurred on several fronts. This includes expression of recombinant intact IgG molecules,[35] expression of Ig fragments (Fab, Fv) in eukaryotic and

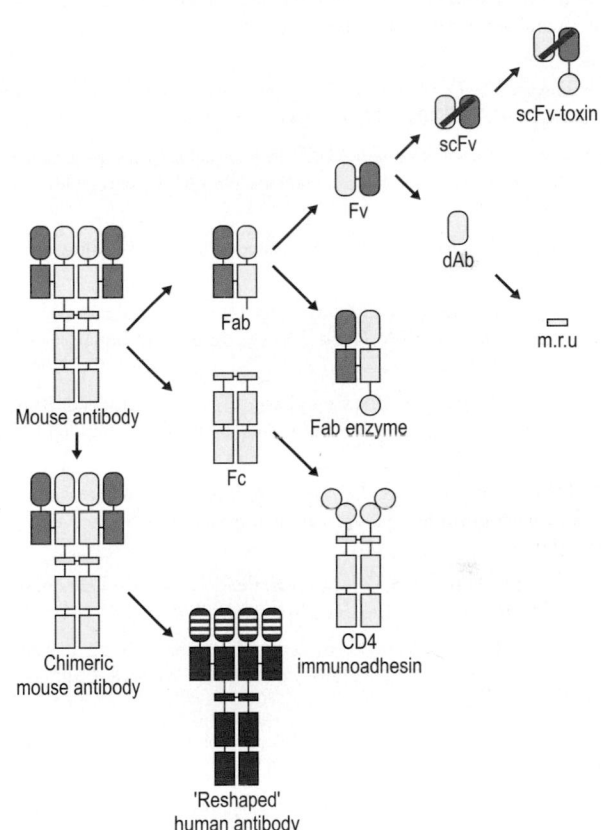

Fig. 15.6 Examples of engineered antibodies and antibody-derived fragments that can be created through the manipulation of antibody genes. Each closed rectangular (constant) or rounded (variable) box represents a domain. The molecule at the bottom of the figure represents a humanized antibody, where the constant domains and variable domain framework regions correspond to human amino acid sequences. Only the hypervariable regions, and in some cases a small number of framework residues, correspond to mouse or rat antibody amino acid sequences. Other structures depicted include an Fab fragment; an Fv fragment; a single-chain Fv fragment (scFv) in which the C terminus of the V_H domain is linked covalently by a linker peptide to the N terminus of the V_L domain; an Fab-enzyme fusion protein; an scFv-toxin fusion protein; an immunoadhesin in which extracellular domains from CD4 have been covalently attached to human heavy chain constant domains; a single V_H domain (dAb); and a peptide derived from a hypervariable region (minimal recognition unit, or mru). (From Winter G, Milstein C. Man-made antibodies. Nature 1991; 349: 293, with permission from Nature Publishing Company.)

KEY CONCEPTS

MONOCLONAL ANTIBODIES FROM HYBRIDOMAS

>> Hybridomas are created by fusing normal lymphocytes, typically from animals immunized with an antigen of choice, and transformed cells of B-lymphocyte lineage (myeloma cells).

>> Monoclonal antibodies produced by a hybridoma are homogeneous, expressing a single amino acid sequence.

>> Hybridomas can be grown indefinitely in tissue culture or in the peritoneal cavities of syngeneic mice (for murine hybridomas).

>> Hybridomas can be selected on the basis of the antigenic specificity or functional properties of the monoclonal antibody secreted by the hybridoma.

prokaryotic host cells,[36] expression of combinatorial libraries of antibody fragments displayed on the surfaces of filamentous phage particles,[36] and bispecific antibodies.[37] Details of these new forms of antibody expression, and their applications, are beyond the scope of this chapter.

■ REFERENCES ■

1. Amit AG, Mariuzza RA, Phillips SEV, et al. Three-dimensional structure of an antigen–antibody complex at 2.8 Å resolution. Science 1986; 233: 747–753.

2. Greenspan NS, Di Cera E. Defining epitopes: it's not as easy as it seems. Nature Biotechnol 1999; 17: 936–937.

3. Pauling L. Molecular structure and intermolecular forces. In: Landsteiner K. The specificity of serological reactions. New York: Dover Publications, 1962, 275–293.

4. Steward MW. The biological significance of antibody affinity. Immunol Today 1981; 2: 134–139.

5. Karush F. The affinity of antibody: range, variability, and the role of multivalence. In: Litman GW, Good RA, eds: Immunoglobulins, New York: Plenum Press, 1978; 85–116.

6. Greenspan NS, Cooper LJN. Complementarity, specificity, and the nature of epitopes and paratopes in multivalent interactions. Immunol Today 1995; 16: 226–230.

7. Rini JM, Schulze-Gahmen U, Wilson IA. Structural evidence for induced fit as a mechanism for antibody–antigen recognition. Science 1992; 255: 959–965.

8. Holmberg D, Forsgren S, Forni L, et al. Reactions among IgM antibodies derived from neonatal mice. Eur J Immunol 1984; 14: 435–441.

9. Kramer A, Keitel T, Winkler K, et al. Molecular basis for the binding promiscuity of an anti-p24 (HIV-1) monoclonal antibody. Cell 1997; 91: 799–809.

10. Alberts B, Bray D, Lewis J, et al. Molecular biology of the cell, 2nd edn. New York: Garland Publishing, 1989; 94.

11. Náray-Szabó G. Analysis of molecular recognition: steric electrostatic and hydrophobic complementarity. J Mol Recogn 1993; 6: 205–210.

12. James LC, Roversi P, Tawfik DS. Antibody multispecificity mediated by conformational diversity. Science 2003; 299: 1362–1367.

13. Mollnes TE, Harboe M. Neoepitope expression during complement activation – a model for detecting antigenic changes in proteins and activation of cascades. Immunologist 1993; 1: 43–49.

14. Walter G, Scheidtmann K-H, Carbone A, et al. Antibodies specific for the carboxy- and amino-terminal regions of simian virus 40 large tumor antigen. Proc Natl Acad Sci USA 1980; 77: 5197–5200.

15. Berzofsky JA. Intrinsic and extrinsic factors in protein antigenic structure. Science 1985; 229: 932–940.

16. Kabat EA. The upper limit for the size of the human antidextran combining site. J Immunol 1960; 84: 82–85.

17. Mannik M. Physicochemical and functional relationships of immune complexes. J Immunol 1980; 74: 333–338.

18. Heyman B. The immune complex: possible ways of regulating the antibody response. Immunol Today 1990; 11: 310–313.

19. Nezlin R. Internal movements in immunoglobulin molecules. Adv Immunol 1990; 48: 1–40.

20. Dimmock NJ. Neutralization of animal viruses. Curr Top Microbiol Immunol 1993; 183: 1–146.

21. Mazanec MB, Kaetzel CS, Lamm ME, et al. Intracellular neutralization of virus by immunoglobulin A antibodies. Proc Natl Acad Sci USA 1992; 89: 6901–6905.

22. Binder GK, Griffin DE. Immune-mediated clearance of virus from the central nervous system. Microbes Infect 2003; 5: 439–448.

23. Bachmann MF, Kopf M. The role of B cells in acute and chronic infections. Curr Opin Immunol 1999; 11: 332–339.

24. Garred P, Michaelsen TE, Aase A. The IgG subclass pattern of complement activation depends on epitope density and antibody and complement concentration. Scand J Immunol 1989; 30: 379–382.

25. Tan LK, Shopes RJ, Oi VT, et al. Influence of the hinge region on complement activation, C1q binding, and segmental flexibility in chimeric human immunoglobulins. Proc Natl Acad Sci USA 1990; 87: 162–166.

26. Chintalacharuvu KR, Morrison SL. Production and characterization of recombinant IgA. Immunotechnology. 1999; 4: 165–174.

27. Ravetch JV, Kinet J-P. Fc receptors. Annu Rev Immunol 1991; 9: 457–492.

28. Kaetzel CS, Robinson JK, Chintalacharuvu KR, et al. The polymeric immunoglobulin receptor (secretory component) mediates transport of immune complexes across epithelial cells: a local defense function for IgA. Proc Natl Acad Sci USA 1991; 88: 8796–8800.

29. Nimmerjahn F, Ravetch JV. Fcgamma receptors: old friends and new family members. Immunity 2006; 24: 19–28.

30. Greenspan NS. Relections on internal images. Nature Biotechnol 1997; 15: 123–124.

31. Sege K, Peterson PA. Use of anti-idiotypic antibodies as cell-surface receptor probes. Proc Natl Acad Sci USA 1978; 75: 2443–2447.

32. Forsayeth JR, Caro JF, Sinha MK, et al. Monoclonal antibodies to the human insulin receptor that activate glucose transport but not insulin receptor kinase activity. Proc Natl Acad Sci USA 1987; 84: 3448–3451.

33. Cragg MS, French RR, Glennie MJ. Signaling antibodies in cancer therapy. Curr Opin Immunol 1999; 11: 541–547.

34. Kohler G, Milstein C. Continuous cultures of fused cells secreting antibody of predefined specificity. Nature 1975; 256: 495–497.

35. Morrison SL. In vitro antibodies: strategies for production and application. Annu Rev Immunol 1992; 10: 239–265.

36. Hudson PJ. Recombinant antibody constructs in cancer therapy. Curr Opin Immunol 1999; 11: 548–557.

37. Fanger MW, Morganelli PM, Guyre PM. Bispecific antibodies. Crit Rev Immunol 1992; 12: 101–124.

Regulatory T cells

16

Kajsa Wing, Shimon Sakaguchi

The normal mammalian immune system protects the individual from a myriad of potentially pathogenic microorganisms while simultaneously avoiding harmful reactions against the normal constituents of the body, i.e., maintaining immunological self-tolerance. The mechanisms that balance active immunity and self tolerance are of fundamental interest to both basic and clinical immunologists, as the failure of protective immunity risks enhanced susceptibility to infectious diseases and loss of self-tolerance may trigger an autoimmune disorder. Elucidation of these mechanisms holds the promise of permitting manipulation of the immune response to enhance reactivity to self (or quasi-self) antigens, such those expressed on tumor cells, as well as to suppress the immune response to nonself antigens, such as those expressed on organ transplants.

A key feature of the adaptive immune response is that, once triggered, the effector activity against the inciting antigen, self or nonself, is the same. Its purpose is the elimination of the microbe or the destruction of self-tissue. To prevent self-destructive immune responses while permitting protective immune responses to nonself antigens, the mammalian immune system has evolved a series of regulatory mechanisms designed either to inhibit the generation of potentially harmful self-reactive T and B lymphocytes, termed *central tolerance*, or to downregulate cellular activation and expansion of lymphocytes when they encounter self-antigens, termed *peripheral tolerance*.

For T cells, central tolerance is established in the thymus. During development (Chapter 9), dangerous lymphocytes that carry T-cell receptors (TCR) with high affinity for ubiquitous self-antigens are deleted. This process of *negative selection*, which occurs at an immature stage of thymocyte development, results in the generation of a peripheral T-cell repertoire that is largely self-tolerant. Negative selection is not an absolute process, and some auto-reactive, including potentially pathogenic, T cells escape the net of thymic deletion. Nevertheless, autoimmune diseases occur infrequently, indicating that auto-reactive T cells are somehow controlled in the periphery.

Peripheral mechanisms of self-tolerance include further deletion of self-reactive T cells, the seclusion of self-antigen from T lymphocytes, low TCR affinity, lack of co-stimulation in antigen recognition (*clonal ignorance*), inactivation of auto-reactive T lymphocytes upon encounter with antigen without co-stimulation (*clonal anergy*), and active suppression of self-reactive lymphocytes by other T cells (*dominant suppression*).[1, 2]

This chapter discusses the mechanisms by which regulatory T cells (Tregs), particularly CD4 Tregs, can induce dominant suppression of self-reactive T cells. Several types of T cells with regulatory activity have been described, including subpopulations of γδ T cells, NKT cells, CD8, and CD4 T cells[3] (Table 16.1 and Fig. 16.1). Some of these Tregs are naturally produced in the immune system, while in others the phenotype is induced in naïve T cells as a product of a particular mode of antigen stimulation in a specific cytokine milieu. Although many details of how each of these populations is regulated and how each functions in the normal physiology of the organism remain to be elucidated, the abundance and apparent redundancy of Treg populations is not surprising given the essential need to maintain immune homeostasis and self-tolerance.

Naturally occurring CD4 Tregs have been the subject of the majority of recent Treg studies. which have shed new light on the mechanisms that contribute to a number of immunological disorders. For example, anomalies in natural Treg function or number can be a primary cause of autoimmune disease, allergy, and inflammatory disorders such as inflammatory bowel disease (IBD) in humans. Because of their natural presence

KEY CONCEPTS

IMMUNOLOGICAL SELF-TOLERANCE

Immunological self-tolerance is actively acquired and maintained throughout life by a series of mechanisms that cooperatively and complementarily interact to prevent the maturation and activation of potentially self reactive lymphocytes.

The mechanisms include:

>> Clonal deletion

>> Clonal anergy

>> Clonal ignorance

>> Dominant suppression

Table 16.1 Subsets of natural and induced regulatory T cells (Treg)

	CD25+Treg	Tr1/Th3	Qa-1-restricted CD8+Treg	CD8+CD28-Treg	NKT cell	γδT cell
Terminal differentiation	Thymus	Periphery/ in vitro	Periphery	Periphery/in vitro	Periphery	Periphery
Marker	Foxp3, CD25, CTLA-4, GITR	IL-10/TGF-β	Nonclassical MHC Ib Qa-1	Foxp3	Not specified TCR invariant chain Vα14 (mouse), Vα24 (human)	Various subsets Vγ5+ (mouse) Vγ1+ (human)
Specificity	Peptide plus MHC class II	Peptide plus MHC class II	Peptide plus MHC class Ib	Peptide plus MHC class I	Glycolipids plus CD1d	Glycolipids plus CD1, peptide plus MHC class Ib
Target cell	T cells, B cells, APC, NK cells NKT cells	T cell	T cell	DC/APC	T cells, APC	T cell, APC, epithelial cells
Suppressive mechanisms	Cell contact, IL-10, TGF-β	IL-10/TGF-β	CD94-NKG2	Induction of ILT3/ILT4 in DC	IL-10, Th2 cytokines	Lysis, CD95-CD95 ligand pathway, thymosin-β4
Reported suppressive function	Autoimmunity Transplantation Allergy Infection Cancer	Autoimmunity Transplantation Allergy	Autoimmunity	Autoimmunity Transplantation	Autoimmunity Transplantation Cancer	Autoimmunity Allergy (dermatitis) Infection

APC, antigen-presenting cell; DC, dendritic cell; IL-10, interleukin-10; ILT, immunoglobulin transcript; MHC, major histocompatibility complex; NK, natural killer; Th3, T helper 3 cell; TGF-β, transforming growth factor-β; Tr1, regulatory type 1 cell; Treg, regulatory T cell.

in the immune system, CD4 Tregs also provide a tempting target for the treatment and prevention of a number of diseases of immune function.[4]

CD4 REGULATORY T CELLS

CD4 Tregs can be divided into two categories: naturally occurring Tregs and induced Tregs. The so-called naturally occurring Tregs, most commonly referred to as CD25+ Tregs because of their constitutive expression of CD25, are generated in the thymus in a functionally mature form. Induced CD4 Tregs, such as interleukin-10 (IL-10)-secreting type 1 regulatory T cells (Tr1) and transforming growth factor (TGF)-β-secreting T helper 3 cells (Th3), differentiate from naïve T cells following antigen stimulation in conjunction with specific conditions in the periphery. Although both natural CD25+ Tregs and induced Tregs are suppressive in nature, differences exist in their developmental pathways, phenotype, and function. Thus, these two types of cells are considered to be of separate lineages[5] (Table 16.1 and Fig. 16.1).

THYMICALLY DERIVED CD4+CD25+ REGULATORY T CELLS

The first observation indicative of the presence of autoimmune-preventive T cells in the normal immune system and their production by the normal thymus was made more than 30 years ago when thymectomy on day 3 of life (d3Tx) was found to inflict organ-specific autoimmune diseases, such

as oophoritis, in otherwise healthy mice.[6] Subsequent studies showed that the development of autoimmune disease could be inhibited if the thymectomized animals were reconstituted with CD4+CD8- thymocytes or CD4+ splenocytes from histocompatible immune-uncompromised animals. In order to pinpoint a specific phenotype for CD4 T cells with regulatory function, surface markers with a more narrow expression pattern were explored. Among these, CD5high, CD45RBlow, CD38low, and CD62Lhigh expression was shown to characterize naturally occurring CD4 Tregs in mice.[3, 7] To date the functionally most useful and specific surface marker of natural Tregs is their high and stable expression of the IL-2 receptor α-chain, CD25. Between 5% and 10% of CD4 T cells express CD25 constitutively in the thymus and periphery of mice, and CD25 expression indeed fits the aforementioned cell surface phenotype of natural Tregs, i.e., CD25+CD4+ T cells are also largely CD45RBlow, CD38low, and CD62Lhigh.[7] Importantly, transfer of CD4 lymphocytes depleted of CD25+ cells induces autoimmunity in athymic nude mice, while co-transfer of CD4+CD25+ cells protects the mice from disease induction (Fig. 16.2).[8] Other markers shown to be associated with CD25+ Tregs are cytotoxic T-lymphocyte antigen 4 (CTLA-4, CD152) and glucocorticoid-induced tumor necrosis factor receptor protein (GITR). However, neither these nor CD25 can be appreciated as specific markers of natural Tregs since conventional T cells upregulate GITR, as well as CTLA-4 and CD25, after activation.[9] This dilemma is especially apparent when investigating naturally occurring Tregs in humans where up to 30% of CD4 T cells in peripheral blood express CD25, yet only 2–4% of CD4 T cells, enriched among cells with the highest expression level of CD25 (CD25high), have

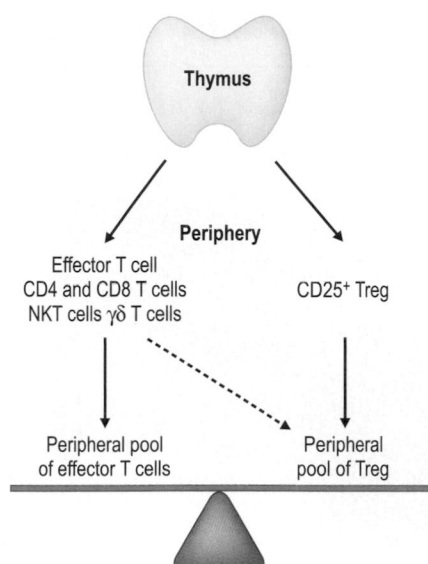

Fig. 16.1 Developmental pathways of regulatory T cells (Tregs). Tregs can develop in either the thymus or the periphery and are vital for maintaining tolerance as a counterbalance to effector T cells. Thymically generated Tregs, also known as naturally occurring Tregs or CD4+CD25+ Tregs, express Foxp3 and develop within the thymus according to a specialized combination of TCR and co-stimulatory signals. Extra thymic development of CD4+ Tregs and CD8+ Tregs can ensue from a host of different conditions, such as high concentrations of transforming growth factor-β (TGF-β), interleukin-10 (IL-10) or other particular circumstances surrounding antigen priming. The signals that control differentiation of γδ T cells and NKT cells to cells with regulatory properties are less defined.

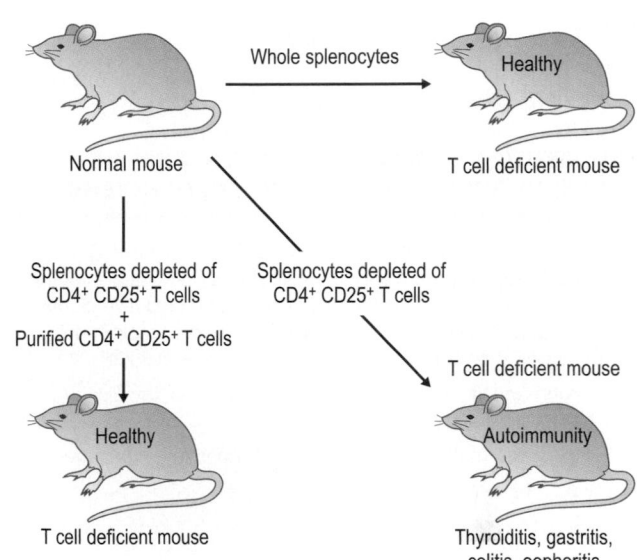

Fig. 16.2 Demonstration of Treg-mediated maintenance of self-tolerance. If a T-cell-deficient mouse receives a transfer of total spleen cells from a normal wild-type mouse of the same strain the recipient remains healthy. However, when CD4+CD25+ splenocytes are removed prior to transfer the recipient animal develops several types of organ-specific autoimmune disease, such as gastritis, thyroiditis, and type 1 diabetes. This can be prevented if a small number of purified CD4+CD25+ splenocytes are co-transferred, which shows that CD25+ Tregs are present in normal animals and protect from autoimmune disease.

suppressive properties.[10] The fact that CD25+ Tregs is not a discrete population in humans poses a problem both when obtaining cells for experimental purposes and when evaluating their role in a clinical setting. Therefore, more specific cell surface markers of CD4 natural Tregs need to be discovered. This is an active area of current research with important implications for the future clinical use of Tregs.

THYMICALLY DERIVED CD25+ TREGS EXPRESS THE TRANSCRIPTION FACTOR FOXP3

Although functional analysis of Tregs has been hampered by the lack of specific cell surface markers, a major breakthrough was achieved when the transcription factor Foxp3 was found to be specifically expressed by thymically derived natural Tregs and closely linked with their development and function.[11] The first hint as to the significance of Foxp3 was given by studies of the Scurfy mutant mouse. This mouse strain suffers from a spontaneous X-linked mutation of the *Foxp3* gene, which leads to fatal lymphoproliferative disease associated with multiorgan infiltrates and early death by 3–4 weeks of age in hemizygous males. Similarly, mutations in the human orthologue *FOXP3* is linked to IPEX (immune dysregulation, polyendocrinopathy, enteropathy, X-linked syndrome), which is an X-linked immunodeficiency syndrome associated with organ-specific autoimmune diseases such as type 1 diabetes,

IBD, allergic dermatitis, food allergy, hyperimmunoglobulinemia E, hematological disorders, and severe infections[4] (Chapter 35). Intriguingly, a common denominator for the conditions observed in mice and humans is deficient levels of CD25+ Tregs. Both CD25+CD4+ T cells and CD25+CD4+CD8- thymocytes specifically express *Foxp3* mRNA whereas other thymocytes/T cells, T helper 1 (Th), or T helper 2 (Th2) cells scarcely express *Foxp3* even after stimulation.[11] Recent analysis of intracellular staining of the Foxp3 protein has shown that, while the majority of Foxp3+ cells in mice reside in the CD4+CD25+ T-cell population, a small fraction can also be found in the CD4+CD25- population (Fig. 16.3). Most importantly, retroviral transduction of *Foxp3* in naïve CD25- T cells can convert them to regulatory cells with similar function and phenotype as natural Tregs.[11] Broadly, the same pattern of FOXP3 expression can be observed in humans, with most FOXP3+ cells among CD4+CD25bright cells and a few being CD25- or CD25low (Fig. 16.3). One difference between mice and humans is that human CD8+ T cells with suppressive function can, in some cases, express FOXP3. Another disparity is that low levels of FOXP3 seem to be transiently induced by TCR stimulation in nonregulatory T cells derived from peripheral blood; however, this expression is lower than what is seen in CD25highTregs.[9] It is likely that Foxp3 may specify the Tregs cell lineage whether Tregs are CD4+ or CD8+, class II major histocompatibility complex (MHC)- or class I MHC-restricted. Collectively, thymically derived Tregs are best recognized by their expression of Foxp3. Unfortunately, since the Foxp3 protein is present only in the cell nucleus,

CLINICAL RELEVANCE

IMMUNE DYSREGULATION, POLYENDOCRINOPATHY, ENTEROPATHY, X-LINKED SYNDROME (IPEX) IS A RESULT OF CD25+ REGULATORY T-CELL (TREG) DEFICIENCY

Loss of function mutations of *Foxp3/FOXP3. an X-linked gene,* inhibits the development and function of CD25+ Tregs in affected males. Uncontrolled activation/expansion of autoreactive clones creates a lymphoproliferative disease with severe autoimmunity with fatality at an early age. Common symptoms include:

>> Organ-specific autoimmunity (type 1 diabetes, thyroiditis, hemolytic anemia)

>> Allergy (dermatitis, hyperimmunoglobulinemia E, food allergy)

>> Inflammatory bowel disease

it is not useful for the isolation of cells. Thus at present CD25 remains the best and most commonly used marker for the isolation of Tregs.

DEVELOPMENT AND MAINTENANCE OF CD25+ TREGS

Several findings point to the thymus as central in the generation of CD25+Foxp3+ Tregs. First, the phenotype of CD25+CD4+ thymocytes is very similar to that of peripheral Tregs as they are CD25+ and Foxp3+. Second, both peripheral and thymic CD25+CD4+ T cells suppress the proliferation and cytokine production of conventional CD4+ or CD8+ T cells in a dose-dependent fashion when tested *in vitro.* Third, athymic mice transferred with CD25- T cells spontaneously develop organ-specific autoimmune diseases that can be reversed by co-transfer of either CD25+CD4+ thymocytes or CD25+CD4+ splenocytes from normal adult mice.[4] Therefore, the thymus contributes to self-tolerance by both deleting auto-reactive T cells and producing CD25+ Tregs. CD25+ Tregs are thought to arise from T-cell clones with relatively high reactivity to self-antigens that are expressed in the thymus. It is as yet unclear as to how these cells are spared from negative selection and how the Tregs developmental pathway, which apparently starts with the induction of Foxp3, is initiated.[11] It is nevertheless likely that a higher responsiveness to self-antigen is a benefit when suppressing hazardous auto-reactive T cells, since CD25+ Tregs would be more easily and strongly activated when presented with self-antigens in the case of tissue damage. In addition to TCR interaction, it seems that accessory signals, such as co-stimulation through CD28-B7 or CD40-CD40L, play an important role in the production of CD25+ Tregs in the thymus, since animals that lack CD28 or CD40 expression generate only minute numbers of Foxp3+ T cells in the thymus (Table 16.2).[4, 12]

In the periphery, the maintenance of CD25+ Tregs requires antigenic stimulation, cytokines, and signals from antigen-presenting cells (APCs). It is vital that CD25+ Tregs encounter specific antigens to remain in the Tregs pool. For example, cell transfer experiments in d3Tx models have demonstrated that Treg cells from donors of the same sex are better at

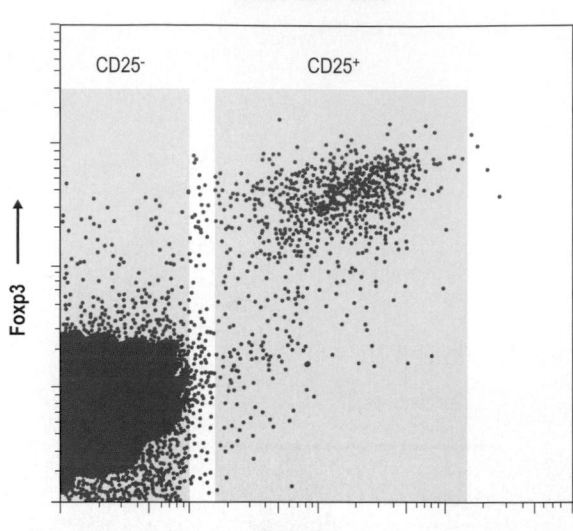

Mouse CD4 T cells

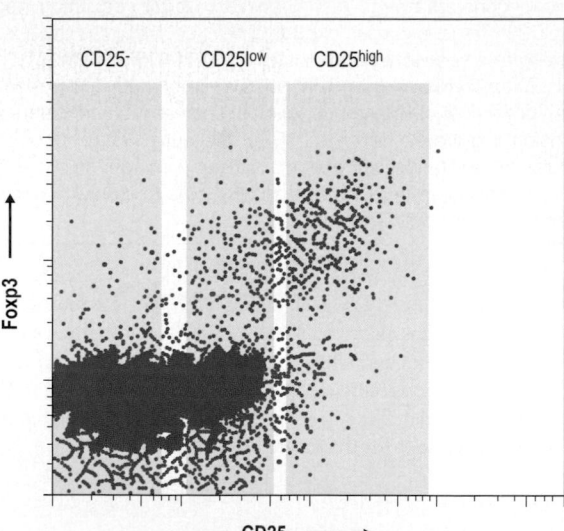

Human CD4 T cells

Fig. 16.3 Expression of CD25 and Foxp3 denotes natural regulatory T cells (Tregs) in mice and in humans. In mice, 5–10% of CD4+ T cells express CD25 and, among these, almost all are Foxp3+. In addition, a few Foxp3-expressing cells reside among CD4+CD25- T cells. In the peripheral blood of humans, approximately 30% of CD4+ T cells express CD25 but only a fraction of these cells (2–4%) express FOXP3 protein. Although some CD25- T cells are FOXP3+, generally, high expression of FOXP3 appears to correlate with high expression of CD25, which in turn represents cells with suppressive function. Foxp3 protein is localized in the nucleus and cannot be used for isolation of viable cells and therefore CD25 expression is exploited to obtain regulatory cells.

Table 16.2 Signals with impact on CD25+ regulatory T-cell (Treg) induction, maintenance, and suppression

	Differentiation	Maintenance	Suppressive function
Peptide MHC II interaction	Yes (high affinity)	Yes	Yes at least initially
CD28	Yes (crucial)	Yes (indirectly by induction of IL-2 production in effector T cells)	Not crucial for induction of suppression but high expression on APC breaks suppression
CTLA-4	No	Unclear	Yes (not crucial)
GITR	No	Modest positive effect	Breaks suppression
TLR ligands	No	Yes	TLR ligands initially break suppression but this is followed by induction of enhanced suppression
IL-2	Yes (but not crucial)	Yes (crucial)	High levels break suppression
TGF-β	Not vital for thymic differentiation but may be involved in peripheral induction	Yes	Yes (not crucial)

APC, antigen-presenting cell; CTLA-4, cytotoxic T-lymphocyte antigen 4; GITR, glucocorticoid induced tumor necrosis factor receptor protein; IL-2, interleukin 2; MHC II, major histocompatibility complex II; TGF-β, transforming growth factor-β; TLR, toll like receptor.

protecting against orchitis or oophoritis than Tregs from donors of the opposite sex, and that Tregs from ovariectomized mice are less competent in preventing oophoritis than those from normal females. Moreover, CD25+ Tregs from rats ablated of their thyroid are unable to protect rats from thyroiditis, while the capacity to protect against other organ-specific autoimmune diseases remains unchanged.[13] In general, CD25+ Tregs behave similarly to conventional T cells as they have been shown to recirculate between the blood and lymph and then home to organ-draining lymph nodes where they effectively expand in response to their specific antigen.[14]

IL-2 is vital for the maintenance of natural Tregs and CD25 is accordingly not a mere marker for natural Tregs but also a functionally indispensable molecule for them as a key component of the high-affinity IL-2 receptor. Mice genetically deficient in IL-2 or IL-2 receptor α-chain (CD25) or β-chain (CD122) develop a severe lymphoproliferative disease with lymphocyte infiltration in multiple organs, resulting in early death.[4] Genetic deficiencies of CD25 in humans generate a comparable clinical and pathological pattern. This condition was previously hypothesized to be caused by the failure of IL-2-induced cell death of self-reactive T cells. However, it is now known that IL-2-deficient animals have substantially reduced numbers of Foxp3+CD25+ T cells, and that disease can be prevented by adoptive transfer of normal CD25+ Tregs. Another cytokine that has also proven to be important for the maintenance CD25+ Tregs is TGF-β. This cytokine is shown to enhance Treg expression of *Foxp3* and render non-Treg cells susceptible to Treg-mediated suppression.[4, 15]

In addition to antigen recognition and cytokines, CD25+ Tregs require appropriate interactions with APC for their function and survival. Several molecules of cell adhesion and co-stimulation are important to CD25+ Tregs function and homeostasis, including CD18, GITR, CD28, and Toll-like receptors (TLR).[4] Although CD25+ Tregs express these markers and direct signaling takes place through these molecules, indirect effects on Tregs via effector T cells also likely exist and must be taken into account. For example, CD28 provides naïve T cells with a co-stimulatory signal for promoting IL-2 secretion and preventing cell death. Since CD25+ Tregs likely survive on the IL-2 produced by other cells, a lack of CD28 in other T cells and thus their failure to produce IL-2 results in significant reduction of CD25+Foxp3+Tregs. APCs, in particular dendritic cells (DCs), express TLRs that recognize pathogen-associated molecular patterns shared among microbes or certain self-molecules (e.g., heat shock proteins) released during inflammation. Strong activation of APCs through TLRs instigates DCs to mature and strongly activate and expand both naïve T cells and natural CD25+ Tregs. Furthermore, CD25+ Tregs express TLR 2, 5 and 8, and stimulation of Tregs through these TLRs may suppress excessive anti-microbial immune responses that could incur immunopathological tissue damage (Table 16.2).[4]

SUPPRESSIVE FUNCTION OF CD25+ TREGS

The standard assay to analyze the suppressive function of CD25+ Tregs is to co-culture purified cell fractions of T cells with Tregs and then measure the proliferative response upon antigenic stimulation in the presence of APC. Such assays show that freshly isolated CD25+ Tregs are not able to suppress T-cell responses *in vitro* unless they are first stimulated via the TCR with a specific antigen. Once activated, they suppress other CD4 and CD8 T cells irrespective of their antigen specificities.[16] CD25+ Tregs can inhibit proliferation and cytokine production of naïve T cells, which may be accomplished by downregulation of IL-2 gene transcription. CD25+ Tregs can also suppress the function of already differentiated Th1 and Th2 cells *in vitro* and have been shown to reverse ongoing immunopathology like colitis *in vivo*.[15] CD25+ Tregs are also able to suppress B cells, NK cells, and NKT cells.[13]

The mechanism behind CD25+ Treg-mediated suppression is subject to several different hypotheses that include both soluble and cell surface-bound mediators (Fig. 16.4). *In vitro* studies have shown that CD25+

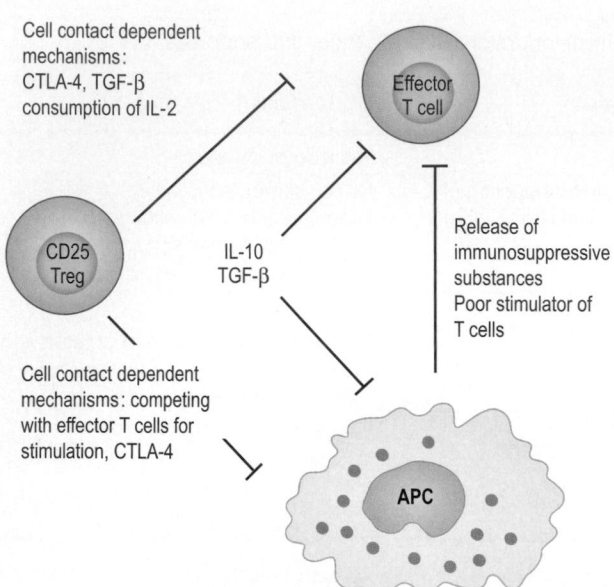

Fig. 16.4 Proposed suppressive mechanisms of CD25+ regulatory T cells (Tregs). CD25+ Tregs can inhibit many different types of effector cells and can also suppress immune responses at multiple stages, including the initial priming in the lymph node and effector actions at the site of inflammation. The precise mechanism is not known, but numerous theories have been proposed and it would not be surprising if CD25+ Tregs suppress by several different mechanisms. *In vivo* Tregs may act in a cell contact-dependent manner by competing directly for stimulatory ligands on the antigen-presenting cell (APC), by absorbing essential growth factors such as interleukin-2 (IL-2), or by directly transmitting an as-yet uncharacterized negative signal to either the T cell or APC. Alternatively, Tregs may use long-range suppressive mechanisms by means of the cytokines IL-10 and transforming growth factor-β (TGF-β).

Tregs need direct cell-to-cell contact with responder cells. Suppression does not occur if Tregs are separated from effector T cells by a semipermeable membrane, even if this allows for the passage of soluble factors.[16] Moreover, CD25+ Tregs are not prominent producers of either IL-10 or TGF-β *in vitro*. These features are quite different from Tr1 or Th3 cells, which solely rely on soluble long-range immunosuppressive cytokines, such as IL-10 and TGF-β, for their inhibitory function. Assuming that the mechanism of CD25+ Treg-mediated suppression is cell contact-dependent, one plausible theory is that CD25+ Tregs compete with effector T cells for stimulatory ligands, regardless of whether these stimulatory ligands are cell surface molecules on APC, such as CD80/CD86, or soluble growth factors, such as IL-2.[17] Other proposed mechanisms involve the transfer of downregulating signals via various molecules expressed on the cell surface of CD25+ Tregs. Candidate molecules for this theory include CTLA-4 and surface-bound TGF-β, since blocking the action of either one is shown to abolish suppression. Nevertheless, and to complicate matters further, mice deficient in either TGF-β or CTLA-4 still harbor CD25+ Tregs that are functional, at least *in vitro*. Yet another mechanism of suppression is perforin/granzyme B-mediated killing of effector cells by CD25+ Tregs, although proof of this mechanism awaits independent confirmation.[17]

Despite the fact that immunosuppressive cytokines are redundant for suppression *in vitro*, the *in vivo* situation seems somewhat different. Both TGF-β and IL-10 have been shown to take part in CD25+ Treg-mediated suppression of IBD in mice.[7] Curiously, adoptive transfer of IL-10-deficient CD25+ Tregs failed to protect against colitis, although it could inhibit the development of gastritis.[17] One important difference between gastritis and IBD is the presence of intestinal bacteria, which, together with the local cytokine environment, is likely to affect the way tolerance is mediated.

Several pieces of evidence suggest that CD25+ Tregs can interact with APC, especially DC, and through them inhibit immune responses. Current models of DC-mediated tolerance propose that T-cell antigen recognition on immature DCs is tolerizing, while recognition on mature DCs drives effector responses. In the steady state (e.g., in the absence of infection or trauma) DCs capture various auto-antigens, as well as inhaled or ingested proteins, and then migrate to the lymph node while still in an immature state. In the lymph nodes, naïve T cells will then encounter antigen and receive a suboptimal signal of activation, which is thought to drive their differentiation towards a Treg rather than an effector T-cell phenotype. On the other hand, if the same antigen is presented under different conditions in the presence of so-called "danger signals" (pro-inflammatory cytokines, microbial products), then DCs will mature fully and upregulate co-stimulatory and MHC molecules, and will initiate production of pro-inflammatory cytokines, leading to an effector T-cell response. APCs cultured with CD25+ Tregs downregulate CD80/86 and become impaired in their ability to stimulate T cells. Additionally, CD25+ Tregs can elicit the induction of the enzyme indoleamine dioxygenase (IDO) by ligation of CTLA-4 with CD80/86 on a particular class of DCs.[17] The induced IDO catalyzes the amino acid tryptophan to the metabolite kynurenine, which has negative effects on T-cell responses. Indeed, new techniques (e.g., two-photon laser-scanning microscopy) that allow for *in vivo* study antigen priming in the lymph node have shown that, while the contact between CD25+ Tregs and effector T cells is limited, stable interactions exist between CD25+ Tregs and DC during ongoing suppression.[14]

Overall, little is known about the mechanisms of suppression *in vivo* and it remains unclear whether cell contact-dependent mechanisms are involved. Nevertheless, it appears that more than one suppressive mechanism can be utilized by CD25+ Tregs, depending on the intensity of the immune response, the site of regulation, and the cytokine milieu.[17]

PERIPHERALLY INDUCED CD4+ REGULATORY T CELLS

In addition to thymus-derived natural CD25+CD4+ Tregs, there is abundant evidence supporting the peripheral development of T cells with suppressive properties and an anergic phenotype. For example, Foxp3-expressing CD25+CD4+ Tregs, functionally and phenotypically similar to natural Tregs, can be induced from naïve T cells by *in vitro* antigenic stimulation in the presence of high-dose TGF-β or by specific ways of *in vivo* antigenic stimulation, e.g., targeting of antigen to immature DC or chronic low-dose antigen administration.[9] The physiological significance of these Treg induction pathways remains to be determined. Other induced Tregs include TGF-β-secreting Th3 cells and IL-10-secreting Tr1 cells, which have been shown to be present and functional in humans following bone marrow transplantation and in response to allergens (Table 16.1).

Tr1 cells were initially generated *in vitro* from CD4 T cells rendered anergic by chronic stimulation in the presence of IL-10, which is a potent negative regulator of inflammation and lymphoproliferation.[18] T cells obtained in such a fashion produce a unique pattern of cytokines distinct from Th1 or Th2 cells, with IL-10 as the signature cytokine. Tr1 cells secrete some TGF-β, interferon-γ, and IL-5, but no IL-4 or IL-2. Tr1 cells are anergic but can proliferate in the presence of IL-2. Currently there is no specific surface marker for Tr1 cells and their identification relies on the IL-10 they produce that, together with TGF-β, forms the basis for their suppressive function. Notably, Tr1 cells do not express high constitutive levels of CD25, nor do they express Foxp3, which clearly separates them from CD25+ Tregs. Besides *in vitro* induction of Tr1 cells with IL-10 and antigen, CD4 T cells can differentiate into Tr1 cells when stimulated by APCs. This may more closely mimic what takes place *in vivo*. Antigenic stimulation with immature DCs (i.e., low levels of co-stimulatory molecules), or DCs pre-treated with IL-10/TGF-β, confers naïve CD4 T cells with an anergic and suppressive phenotype both *in vitro* and *in vivo*.[18]

Tr1 cells can participate in the induction of tolerance in humans, as well. For example, the presence of Tr1 cells can be correlated with lack of graft-versus-host disease in bone marrow transplantation. Similarly, Tr1 cells can be induced following specific immunotherapy in allergic patients. Tr1 cells specific for *Escherichia coli* proteins can be isolated from the intestinal mucosa of healthy donors. In pemphigus vulgaris, which is an autoimmune disorder with circulating autoantibodies against desmoglein-3 (Chapter 63), Tr1 cells specific for desmoglein-3 can be isolated from pemphigus vulgaris-prone but apparently healthy individuals, while pemphigus patients rarely have such cells. Collectively, Tr1 cells can be induced to auto-antigens as well as foreign antigens as a component of the mechanisms that maintain tolerance to both self and nonself.[18]

Th3 cells were identified in mice during investigations of the mechanisms of oral tolerance. Oral tolerance has presumably evolved to prevent hypersensitivity reactions to food and microbial antigens present in the mucosal flora. It was found that mice fed with myelin basic protein, a neuronal auto-antigen, developed T cells that preferentially produced TGF-β together with varying amounts of IL-4 and IL-10. These T cells had suppressive properties, mediated by TGF-β, and could prevent the induction of experimental autoimmune encephalomyelitis, the murine equivalent of multiple sclerosis (MS) (Chapter 65). There are currently no surface markers for Th3 cells but they can be generated *in vitro* when grown in the presence of TGF-β, IL-4, and IL-10. Since the intestinal mucosa has high basal levels of all these cytokines, which are upregulated after antigen administration, it is conceivable that this particular environment drives the formation of Th3 cells while a different setting may produce Tregs of another phenotype.[19]

OTHER SUBSETS OF REGULATORY T CELLS

Immunosuppressive T cells other than CD4 Tregs have been identified. They can recognize antigens that differ from those typically presented to CD4 T cells via MHC class II and thus can serve to induce tolerance in other settings. One example is CD8 T cells with TCRs that recognize

antigen presented by the MHC class Ib Qa-1 molecule (HLA-E in humans). Qa-1 has limited polymorphisms, is expressed solely by activated T cells, and can present both foreign and self-peptides. For example, Qa-1 peptide complexes on CD4 T cells can bind the inhibitory CD94–NKG2 receptor complex on CD8 T cells. This is believed to be one way that Qa-1-restricted CD8 T cells regulate T-cell responses.[20] CD8+CD28- Tregs suppress immune responses by direct interaction with APCs. These cells can be generated *in vitro* by multiple rounds of stimulation with alloantigen. They can downregulate co-stimulatory molecules or upregulate the inhibitory immunoglobulin-like transcript 3 (ILT3) and ILT4 receptors on DCs, leading to impaired activation of effector T cells.[21]

In mice, γδ T cells with a regulatory phenotype exist as a subset of epithelial γδ T cells. Mice deficient in γδ T cells do not appropriately regulate responses to various pathogens. γδ T-cell-deficient mice show accelerated autoimmune responses in models of systemic lupus erythematosus and spontaneously develop dermatitis when bred on certain genetic backgrounds. Commonly, these conditions are driven by αβ T cells and the γδ T cells function by locally inhibiting αβ T cells. Since humans lack an equivalent population of intraepithelial γδ T cells, it is plausible that this immune regulation can be provided by other types of suppressive cells.[22]

NKT cells respond to the nonclassical class I antigen-presenting molecule CD1d, which binds glycolipids rather than peptides. NKT cells can induce either pro-inflammatory (interferon-γ) or anti-inflammatory (IL-4, IL-10, IL-13) immune responses. The prerequisites for this choice remain ill defined. Nevertheless, under appropriate conditions NKT cells can clearly promote tolerance, as illustrated in studies of transplantation and oral tolerance (Table 16.1).[23]

CLINICAL RELEVANCE OF REGULATORY T CELLS

Natural Tregs are key controllers of physiological and pathological immune responses including self-tolerance. This makes them suitable targets for immunotherapy (Tables 16.1 and 16.3).

Table 16.3 Potential therapeutic approaches for regulatory T-cell (Treg)-based therapy

Increase of Treg numbers or function	Reduction of Treg numbers or function
Ex vivo expansion of natural CD25+ Treg with transplantation or known autoantigens plus growth factors such as IL-2	Transient reduction of CD25+Treg and/or perturbation of suppression *in vivo* (anti-CD25 Ab, anti-CTLA-4 Ab or anti-IL-2 Ab)
In vivo promotion of Tregs rather than effector T cells using monoclonal Ab treatment or pharmacological agents (anti-CD3 Ab, anti-CD40L Ab, etc.) *Ex vivo* induction of Treg from conventional T cells by cytokines (IL-10, TGF-β), pharmacological agents or modified DC	Render effector T cells resistant to suppression (GITR signalling)

Ab, antibody; CTLA-4, cytotoxic T-lymphocyte antigen 4; DC, dendritic cell; GITR, glucocorticoid induced tumor necrosis factor receptor protein; IL-2, interleukin-2; IL-10, interleukin-10; TGF-β, transforming growth factor β.

AUTOIMMUNITY

Natural CD25+CD4+ Tregs are engaged in active suppression of autoimmune disease. Depletion of natural Tregs leads to the development of autoimmune disease in rodents. Abnormal Treg development or function can be a direct cause of autoimmune disease in humans, as exemplified by IPEX.[4] Decreased levels of CD4+CD25high T cells in peripheral blood have been reported in systemic lupus erythematosus, psoriatic arthritis, and autoimmune liver disease. On the other hand, studies of MS and type 1 diabetes have not detected differences in Treg numbers between patients and controls and conflicting data have been reported in rheumatoid arthritis (RA) with regard to both function and numbers of CD25high Tregs. A general observation is that CD25+ Tregs increase in number at the site of inflammation.[24] In the case of RA, synovial fluid from patients with ongoing RA was found to contain increased numbers of CD25+ Tregs as compared to CD25+ Tregs levels in peripheral blood. Functional assessment of CD25+ Tregs from inflamed synovium in RA reveals increased suppressive properties of these cells, although this enhanced suppressive function of Tregs is apparently not enough to halt the inflammatory process. In contrast, CD25+ Tregs obtained from the blood of MS patients have been reported to demonstrate a decreased ability to suppress proliferation of effector T cells. Thus, reduced levels of CD25+ Tregs in peripheral blood are not a general finding in autoimmune disease, may not necessarily reflect the actual conditions at the site of inflammation, and may or may not play a causative role in common autoimmune diseases.[24]

ALLERGIC DISEASE

CD25+ natural Tregs play an important role in suppressing the development of allergic reactions to innocuous environmental substances. This is best illustrated by IPEX, which is accompanied by not only organ-specific autoimmune diseases but also severe dermatitis, high levels of serum immunoglobulin E and sometimes eosinophila.[4] Indeed, CD25+ Tregs from the blood of healthy nonallergic donors suppress both proliferation and production of Th2 cytokines when challenged with specific allergens *in vitro*. When the same experiment is performed with Tregs from allergic individuals, they fail to downregulate Th2-related responses to allergens. Since the suppressive ability for polyclonal

stimuli is retained in allergic patients, this deficiency appears to be directly related to the allergen to which the individual has been sensitized. Thus the failure of Tregs to suppress the response to the allergen probably does not reflect a general deficiency, but one specific to that allergen. The inability to suppress Th2 responses induced by birch or grass pollen is aggravated when the allergic reaction is ongoing and effector cells are fully activated, as during spring and summer compared to wintertime. Addition of IL-4 can attenuate the CD25+ Tregs-mediated suppression of Th2 clones *in vitro* in the same way as IL-2, which may provide an explanation for the insufficient control of ongoing allergic responses by Tregs.[13] It has been found that both nonallergic and allergic individuals harbor allergen-specific IL-4-producing effector T cells, IL-10-producing Tr1 cells, and CD25+ Tregs, but in different proportions. Thus, the balance between Th2 and certain Tregs populations may dictate whether clinical allergy will develop. Indeed, in the setting of curative specific allergy immunotherapy, allergen-specific, IL-10-producing T cells can be induced. Furthermore, children who grow out of their cow's-milk allergy have higher numbers of CD4+CD25+ T cells specific for β-lactoglobulin compared to children with clinically active allergy. This suggests that certain allergies can be cured by extrathymic induction/expansion of antigen-specific Tregs and that the balance of Tregs versus effector T cells is of importance to prevent allergy.[13, 25]

TRANSPLANTATION

An ultimate goal of organ transplantation is to establish tolerance to allogeneic organ grafts as effectively and stably as to self-tissues, but without the need for continuous general immunosuppression.[26] Needless to say, Tregs have sparked a lot of attention in this area of research. CD25+ Tregs were first shown to suppress graft-versus-host disease (GvHD) in murine models of allogeneic bone marrow transplantation. Similarly, nude mice transplanted with allogeneic skin rejected the graft when reconstituted with CD4+CD25- T cells alone, but retained the graft when large enough numbers of CD25+ Tregs were co-transferred. In humans, attempts have been made to prevent GvHD in bone marrow transplantation and induce graft tolerance in organ transplantation by the use of purified CD25+ Tregs.[27] Efforts have also been made to expand donor-specific Tregs *ex vivo* to enhance suppression and lower the number of Tregs needed for tolerance induction. Other means to establish tolerance to grafts are by administration of monoclonal antibodies to various cell surface molecules such as CD4, CD8, and CD40L on T cells and CD40, CD80/86 on APC or CD11a and CD54 expressed by both T cells and APC.[26] These treatments may more potently suppress the activation and expansion of effector T cells than that of CD25+ natural Tregs, and thus allow the latter to expand in a graft-specific fashion and tip the scale in favor of dominant tolerance. In addition, such monoclonal antibody treatments may induce Tregs of extrathymic origin. Indeed, several types of inducible Tregs including CD8+ Tregs and Tr1 are shown to contribute to graft tolerance.[18, 21]

A third potential way to promote the induction of Tregs in organ transplantation is to evaluate the effects of various immunosuppressants in terms of altering the balance between Tregs and effector T cells. Different immunosuppressants target different pathways in cell metabolism and can therefore have different effects on cell populations that behave in dissimilar ways, such as effector T cells and Tregs. Dosage and timing of administration, as well as specific drug combinations, seem to be a promising angle of transplantation immunotherapy with the purpose of inducing graft tolerance and preventing graft rejection. Tregs have been shown to home to, and reside within, the graft, which is stably accepted once a dominance of Tregs has become established. Treg-mediated transplantation tolerance is not a systemic phenomenon but rather localized to the graft, and as such it would not incur the dangers that accompany general immunosuppression.[26]

TUMOR IMMUNITY

It is now well known that many of the tumor-associated antigens recognized by a patient's T cells are normal self-constituents, indicating that anti-tumor immune responses are within the range of CD25+ Treg control. Therefore, the presence of natural Tregs in the normal immune system may not only prevent autoimmunity but also hamper immune surveillance of cancer.[28] In fact, CD25+ Tregs are shown to reside in the tumor mass, where they likely block any immune response targeting malignant cells. For example, the frequency of CD25+ Tregs is increased in tumors of metastatic melanoma or cancers in the pancreas and lung. Moreover, high levels of CD25+ Tregs in the tumor are correlated with a poor prognosis and survival. Whether the elevated levels are due to migration of Tregs into the tumor or to an expansion on the site is not clear, but evidence exists in support of both events. For example, ovarian tumor cells and infiltrating macrophages secrete the Treg-recruiting chemokine CCL22 and, in addition, many tumors produce TGF-β, which contributes to the maintenance of CD25+ Tregs and may also induce Foxp3 expression in non-Tregs cells within the tumor microenvironment. It is now evident that both effector T cells and Tregs have to be assessed in monitoring the efficacy of anti-cancer immunotherapy.[28]

Involvement of Tregs in tumor immunity indicates that anti-tumor immune responses can be provoked or enhanced by depleting Tregs in a host that is otherwise responding poorly. Experimental mouse models have indeed demonstrated that simple depletion of CD25+ Tregs with anti-CD25 antibody results in tumor eradication, and similar effects can be achieved with *in vivo* administration of anti-GITR or anti-CTLA-4 antibodies.[29] Depletion of CD25+ T cells also enhances the effect of vaccination with tumor antigens. Pharmacological agents are another possible way of altering the effector T cell/Tregs ratio. For example, fludarabin was shown to selectively decrease the frequency of CD25+ Tregs in patients receiving chemotherapy. Conversely, previously used

regimens, such as administration of exogenous IL-2, are now being re-evaluated, since IL-2 may expand Tregs. As expected from the role of Tregs in self-tolerance, a caveat of Treg-based therapies of cancer is the possible development of autoimmunity, which may very well depend on the degree and period of *in vivo* systemic Tregs depletion as well as the genetic makeup of the host.[28]

INFECTIOUS DISEASE

Immune responses to infectious agents, such as bacteria and viruses, often result in tissue damage, which might be more severe if it were not for the involvement of Tregs. On the downside, in many cases Tregs may contribute to the development of chronic infections. As previously discussed, CD25+ Tregs have the potential to respond directly to microbial products and are believed to suppress responses to infectious agents. A number of studies show that the outcome of an infection partly hinges on the proper balance between effector T cells and Tregs.[30] A well-documented example is the murine model of colitis, where effector T cells in the absence of Tregs are triggered by the commensal bacteria to cause intestinal inflammation in immunodeficient hosts, while co-transfer of CD25+ Tregs protects the animals through an IL-10-dependent mechanism.[7] Adoptive transfer of CD25+ Tregs prevents lethal pneumonia in T-cell-deficient mice infected with *Pneumocystis jiroveci* (formerly *P. carinii*), but at the expense of a deficient protective response and microbial clearance. Similarly, CD25+ Tregs suppress Th1 responses in mice infected with *Helicobacter pylori*, thereby limiting the mucosal inflammation, but resulting in a higher bacterial load. Human studies show that CD25+ Tregs from carriers of *H. pylori* suppress responses to *H. pylori* antigens *in vitro* and have increased frequencies of CD25high T cells in both the stomach and the duodenal mucosa compared with healthy controls. Additionally, the number of CD25+ Tregs in the circulation inversely correlates with liver damage in human hepatitis C virus infection. Taken together, modulation of the infectious response by Tregs can limit tissue damage but may enhance pathogen survival.

This sort of compromise may not always be adverse to the host. For example, in murine *Leishmania major* infection, CD25+ Tregs prevents complete eradication of the parasites, which results in the persistence of low numbers of microbes that have proved to be essential for the development of T-cell memory and prevention of re-infection. However, this delicate balance can be tipped in favor of the pathogen, which can be seen in the case of malaria and various viral infections, such as human immunodeficiency virus (HIV). For example, HIV-specific CD4 and CD8 T-cell responses are substantially suppressed by CD25+ Tregs *in vitro* in most HIV-infected individuals. Taken together, future treatments, as well as vaccines, will have to take Tregs into account and, depending on the pathogen in question, it might be necessary to reduce or enhance the activity of Tregs to achieve a favorable outcome (Table 16.3).[30]

■ REFERENCES ■

1. Palmer E. Negative selection – clearing out the bad apples from the T-cell repertoire. Nat Rev Immunol 2003; 3: 383–391.

2. Van Parijs L, Abbas AK. Homeostasis and self-tolerance in the immune system: turning lymphocytes off. Science 1998; 280: 243–248.

3. Bach JF, Francois Bach J. Regulatory T cells under scrutiny. Nat Rev Immunol 2003; 3: 189–198.

4. Sakaguchi S. Naturally arising Foxp3-expressing CD25+CD4+ regulatory T cells in immunological tolerance to self and non-self. Nat Immunol 2005; 6: 345–352.

5. Bluestone JA, Abbas AK. Natural versus adaptive regulatory T cells. Nat Rev Immunol 2003; 3: 253–257.

6. Nishizuka Y, Sakakura T. Thymus and reproduction: sex-linked dysgenesia of the gonad after neonatal thymectomy in mice. Science 1969; 166: 753–755.

7. Singh B, Read S, Asseman C, et al. Control of intestinal inflammation by regulatory T cells. Immunol Rev 2001; 182: 190–200.

8. Sakaguchi S, Sakaguchi N, Asano M, et al. Immunologic self-tolerance maintained by activated T cells expressing IL-2 receptor alpha-chains (CD25). Breakdown of a single mechanism of self-tolerance causes various autoimmune diseases. J Immunol 1995; 155: 1151–1164.

9. Wing K, Fehervari Z, Sakaguchi S. Emerging possibilities in the development and function of regulatory T cells. Int immunol 2006; 18: 991–1000.

10. Baecher-Allan C, Viglietta V, Hafler DA. Human CD4+CD25+ regulatory T cells. Semin Immunol 2004; 16: 89–98.

11. Hori S, Sakaguchi S. Foxp3: a critical regulator of the development and function of regulatory T cells. Microbes Infect 2004; 6: 745–751.

12. Fontenot JD, Rudensky AY. Molecular aspects of regulatory T cell development. Semin Immunol 2004; 16: 73–80.

13. Wing K, Suri-Payer E, Rudin A. CD4+CD25+-regulatory T cells from mouse to man. Scand J Immunol 2005; 62: 1–15.

14. Bluestone JA, Tang Q. How do CD4+CD25+ regulatory T cells control autoimmunity?. Curr Opin Immunol 2005; 17: 638–642.

15. Duchmann R, Zeitz M. T regulatory cell suppression of colitis: the role of TGF-beta. Gut 2006; 55: 604–606.

16. Piccirillo CA, Thornton AM. Cornerstone of peripheral tolerance: naturally occurring CD4+CD25+ regulatory T cells. Trends Immunol 2004; 25: 374–380.

17. von Boehmer H. Mechanisms of suppression by suppressor T cells. Nat Immunol 2005; 6: 338–344.

18. Battaglia M, Gregori S, Bacchetta R, et al. Tr1 cells: from discovery to their clinical application. Semin Immunol 2006; 18: 120–127.

19. Weiner HL. Induction and mechanism of action of transforming growth factor-beta-secreting Th3 regulatory cells. Immunol Rev 2001; 182: 207–214.

20. Sarantopoulos S, Lu L, Cantor H. Qa-1 restriction of CD8+ suppressor T cells. J Clin Invest 2004; 114: 1218–1221.

21. Filaci G, Suciu-Foca N. CD8+ T suppressor cells are back to the game: are they players in autoimmunity?. Autoimmun Rev 2002; 1: 279–283.

22. Hayday A, Tigelaar R. Immunoregulation in the tissues by gammadelta T cells. Nat Rev Immunol 2003; 3: 233–242.

23. Godfrey DI, Kronenberg M. Going both ways: immune regulation via CD1d-dependent NKT cells. J Clin Invest 2004; 114: 1379–1388.

24. Dejaco C, Duftner C, Grubeck-Loebenstein B, et al. Imbalance of regulatory T cells in human autoimmune diseases. Immunology 2006; 117: 289–300.

25. Akdis M, Blaser K, Akdis CA. T regulatory cells in allergy: novel concepts in the pathogenesis, prevention, and treatment of allergic diseases. J Allergy Clin Immunol 2005; 116: 961–968.

26. Wood KJ, Sakaguchi S. Regulatory T cells in transplantation tolerance. Nat Rev Immunol 2003; 3: 199–210.

27. Randolph DA, Fathman CG. CD4+CD25+ regulatory T cells and their therapeutic potential. Annu Rev Med 2006; 57: 381–402.

28. Baecher-Allan C, Anderson DE. Immune regulation in tumor-bearing hosts. Curr Opin Immunol 2006; 18: 214–219.

29. Yamaguchi T, Sakaguchi S. Regulatory T cells in immune surveillance and treatment of cancer. Semin Cancer Biol 2006; 16: 115–123.

30. Belkaid Y, Rouse BT. Natural regulatory T cells in infectious disease. Nat Immunol 2005; 6: 353–360.

Helper T-cell subsets and control of the inflammatory response

17

Todd N. Eagar, Stephen D. Miller

T cells play a critical role in regulating the body's defenses against pathogenic nonself. In order for T cells to participate in inflammatory processes, they must become activated, expand in number, differentiate, travel to sites of inflammation, and carry out effector functions. A substantial fraction of T cells expresses the CD4 co-receptor on the cell surface (Chapter 4), which helps stabilize the interaction between their T-cell receptors (TCR) and class II major histocompatibility complex (MHC) molecules bearing cognate antigen (Chapters 5–7). T cells expressing CD4 provide help, direction, and effector function to the immune response as well as contributing to the antigen specificity of the interaction and promoting the development of memory. This chapter focuses on the generation and function of this helper T-cell subset during inflammatory processes.

■ INITIATING IMMUNE RESPONSES ■

Inflammation is a fundamental process that the body uses in response to infection and tissue injury. Inflammation manifests with *calor* (heat), *rubor* (redness), *tumor* (swelling), and *dolor* (pain). These cardinal signs are initiated nonspecifically at the site of infection or trauma. They result from the initial release of chemical mediators that enhance vascular permeability and promote the recruitment of immune cells. Cells of the innate immune system (Chapter 3), such as granulocytes and monocytes, are rapidly recruited from the blood into the site of inflammation. Tissue-resident macrophages and dendritic cells migrate to the site from adjacent tissues. Immunosurveillance proceeds both locally and in the draining lymphoid tissues. The cells of the innate immune system use cell surface receptors, such as the Toll-like family of receptors (TLRs), to scan local tissues for the presence of infectious agents. TLRs and other innate receptors recognize conserved pathogen-associated molecular patterns (PAMPs) that are expressed by offending microbes. The detection of these molecular signals of infection leads to the rapid recruitment of additional cells and direct enhancement of the inflammatory process. Phagocytes and tissue dendritic cells act to clear damaged tissue and cell debris from the inflammatory site. Following phagocytosis, the dendritic cells traverse into the lymphatic vessels and migrate to the regional lymph nodes. In these lymph nodes, they present peptide antigens taken up at the site of tissue damage to resident T cells. Antigen presentation in the lymph nodes permits induction of an appropriate T-cell immune response against the antigens detected at the site of inflammation. These interactions between T cells and dendritic cells are critical for the activation, expansion, and differentiation of the T cell, which are required processes for the initiation of T-cell-mediated inflammation (Fig. 17.1).

CD4 T-cell activation activity can lead to self damage and even overt autoimmunity. For this reason, T-cell activation is a tightly regulated process that requires multiple stimuli. Naïve T cells exist in a quiescent state and are incapable of participating in inflammatory processes. The primary signal required for T-cell activation is an antigen-specific

■ KEY CONCEPTS ■

T-CELL-MEDIATED INFLAMMATION REQUIRES ACTIVATED OR MEMORY T CELLS

Naïve T cells

>> Traffic through spleen and lymph nodes

>> Require professional antigen-presenting cells

>> Require strong co-stimulation

>> Delayed expansion

>> Delayed cytokine production

Activated T cells

>> Traffic through most tissues

>> Respond to antigen presented by nonprofessional antigen-presenting cells

>> Require less co-stimulation

>> Rapidly expand following antigen encounter

>> Rapidly produce effector cytokines

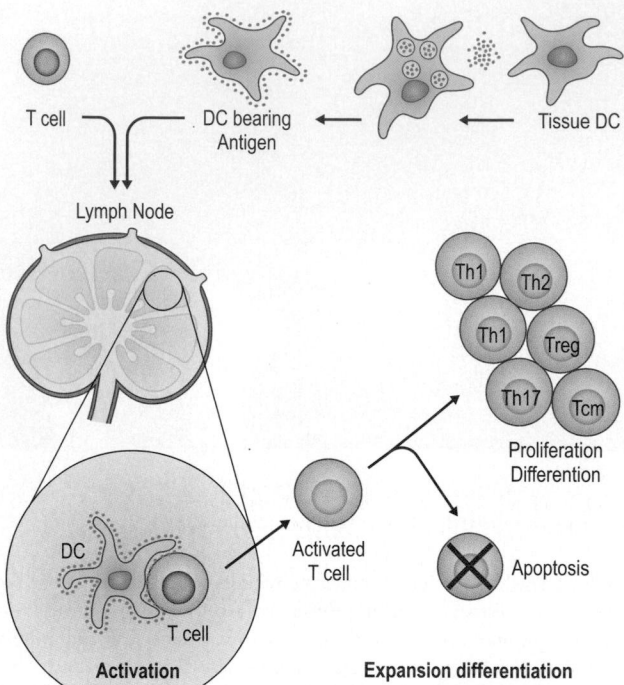

Fig. 17.1 T-cell expansion and differentiation. Following emigration from the thymus, CD4 T cells travel through the lymph nodes. Inflammation results in the recruitment of tissue dendritic cells (DCs) into the draining lymph nodes. In the lymph nodes, DCs present antigen to naïve T cells. Effective antigen presentation stimulates the activation, proliferation, and differentiation of T cells into Th1, Th2, Th17, or uncommitted T central memory (Tcm) cells.

interaction between the TCR and a self MHC molecule bearing a cognate peptide (Chapters 5, 6, and 13).

Each T cell possesses a TCR created by DNA recombination in the thymus (Chapter 4) that bears specificity for peptide epitopes presented in the context of peptide bound to self MHC. This requirement that the T cell interact with self MHC on the surface of an antigen-presenting cell (APC), such as a mature dendritic cell, provides a level of control beyond that experienced by B lymphocytes, which can interact directly with cell-free antigens in solution. The trimolecular TCR–peptide–MHC interaction permits the APC to help shape the T-cell response by providing additional information to the T cell. This information is the product of two types of interaction provided by the APC – adhesion and co-stimulation. Both types of interactions are necessary for optimal T-cell activation.

The affinity and avidity of TCR and MHC/peptide are insufficient for the T cell to maintain stable contact with an APC. However, engagement of the TCR promotes signals that activate tight adhesion between the T cell and APC by means of molecules such as the integrin LFA-1 (CD11a) binding to ICAM (CD54). Firm adhesion promoted by integrin–ICAM interactions permits a T cell to interact with an APC for up to 20 hours. These long-term interactions are necessary[1] for full activation of naïve T cells because they permit formation of the structured signaling complex known as an immunological synapse.

The immunological synapse consists of the TCR, its signaling components, and accessory or co-stimulatory molecules.[2] These co-stimulatory molecules provide an additional level of control of T-cell activation by allowing the APC to provide information about the source of the antigen. For example, dendritic cell expression of the B7 molecules, CD80 and CD86, which are ligands for the co-stimulatory receptor CD28, increases following TLR signaling. This provides the T cell with the information that the peptide it has recognized is likely to be the product of a microbial infection. Ligation of co-stimulatory molecules such as CD28 provides additional activating stimuli to the T cell and thus lowers the threshold for full activation.

Co-stimulatory molecules possess structured intracellular domains that interact with components of several intracellular signaling pathways. When properly engaged, the combination of TCR-MHC/peptide, integrin/ICAM adhesion, and co-stimulatory receptor signals triggers a series of intracellular biochemical signaling pathways whose combined effect leads to the activation of the T cell. In the presence of incomplete stimulation, i.e., if co-stimulation is lacking, T cells are prevented from participating in inflammation and may become unresponsive to further stimulation (anergy) or undergo a process of programmed cell death (apoptosis). This important safety mechanism is used to prevent inappropriate activation of T cells and helps maintain T-cell peripheral self-tolerance (Chapter 13).

Due to the critical role played by the APC in this process, T-cell activation is critically tied to the activation state of the dendritic cell. Immature dendritic cells are incapable of stimulating functional T-cell responses. Immature dendritic cells may become mature through TLR stimulation. TLR stimulation leads to increased expression of MHC class II, B7-1, B7-2, CD40 and inflammatory cytokines, all of which play a key role in permitting the mature dendritic cells to stimulate T-cell activation. This is exemplified by the result of the interaction between CD40 on the APC and its ligand CD154, whose expression by the T cell is induced following TCR signaling. Signals transduced through CD40 internally in the APC lead to the upregulation of MHC class II–peptide complexes and the ligands for co-stimulatory molecules such as B7-1 (CD80) and B7-2 (CD86). Together the enhanced expression of MHC/peptide and B7 family molecules increases the ability of the APC to stimulate other T cells. This process is known as *licensing* and is one of the methods by which CD4 T cells can act through APCs to help CD8 T-cell responses.[3]

■ T-CELL EXPANSION ■

Although T-cell activation can be detected within 8 hours of exposure to antigen, days will pass before T-cell immune responses can be detected from a naïve host. This delay is partially due to the need to generate sufficient numbers of T cells to produce a detectable and effective response. It has been estimated that the frequency of T cells specific for any given antigen is approximately one per 1×10^6 total CD4 T cells.[4] By this measure, the total number of T cells recognizing a single peptide epitope can be estimated at around 100 cells per mouse or 10^5 per human. These estimates are corroborated by experimental evidence in CD8 T cells, demonstrating that a naïve mouse possesses 100–200 CD4 T lymphocytes (CTLs) reactive against a single epitope.[5] Given this low initial frequency of T cells specific for a given epitope, T cells must go through several rounds of division to achieve sufficient numbers to mount an effective response.

Cellular proliferation following antigen exposure begins slowly, taking up to 2 days for the first divisions to occur in the lymph nodes and spleen. Peak expansion occurs around 7 days after antigen exposure. Many of the activated T cells will have undergone six or more rounds of cell division, a process known as clonal expansion. With six rounds of cell division, the original T cell can yield up to 64 daughter cells, each of which possesses the same TCR and thus the same specificity for antigen. Clonal expansion thus permits a rapid net increase in antigen-reactive T cells in the draining lymph node. To appreciate the full scope of the T-cell response against an infectious agent, it is important to realize that T-cell responses can be generated against multiple epitopes derived from multiple antigens present in that agent. Expansion of T cells specific for each epitope of each antigen permits generation of a very large number of T cells specific for the inciting pathogen. This expanded population of T cells does not persist. Following expansion, there is a period of T-cell loss from the lymph nodes. This loss of T-cell numbers is due to a combination of cell death and migration from the lymph nodes to tissues.

■ TRAFFICKING ■

Several key differences exist between naïve (resting) and activated T cells that influence their ability to participate in inflammatory processes. Among these differences is the ability of activated T cells to migrate to tissue sites and carry out effector functions. As discussed in greater detail in Chapter 12, T-cell migration relies upon three basic types of interactions between the T cell and the vascular endothelium. The first step is a rolling process mediated by the interaction of selectin molecules (L, E, or P) with their ligands. Selectins slow the T cell and allow close contact with the endothelial cell glycocalyx. The second step is mediated by chemokines (Chapter 11). Binding of chemokines to their receptors on the T cell leads to rapid G protein-coupled signaling, calcium flux, and activation of integrins. The integrins arrest T-cell movement on the luminal side of the blood vessel by stimulating strong adhesion to the endothelial cell. This sets the stage for subsequent transmigration of the T cell across the vessel wall and into the surrounding tissues.[6]

Naïve T cells and effector T cells traffic through different sets of tissues. This differential trafficking is due to varied expression of selectins, chemokine receptors, and integrins by the T cells and endothelial cells. Naïve T cells circulate almost exclusively through the lymphatic system. Following thymic maturation and export from the thymus to peripheral lymphoid tissue, naïve T cells recirculate from the blood into lymph nodes and then travel through the lymphatic ducts back into the circulation. This pattern of movement relies upon the expression of L-selectin or CD62L. L-selectin expression allows adherence to the high endothelial venules (HEV) found in the cortex of lymph nodes. Within hours of being activated by antigen, T cells downregulate expression of L-selectin and upregulate expression of ligands for E and P selectin. The change in selectin/ligand expression allows the activated T cells to interact with endothelium at sites distal from the lymph node in a tissue-specific manner. For example, while entry into the lymph nodes is mediated by L-selectin, entry into skin requires ligands for E-selectin and entry into the lung requires ligands for P-selectin.[6]

Naïve and activated T cells express different patterns of chemokine receptors and therefore follow different gradients. For example, naïve T cells expressing CCR7 follow gradients of CCL21 (SLC) as they migrate through the HEV and into T-cell-rich areas of the lymph nodes, Peyer's patches, and spleen. This promotes the retention of naïve T cells in lymphoid tissues, where they undergo initial activation. Upon activation, T cells express a new set of chemokine receptors that allow them to traffic in the periphery, but they now respond poorly to SLC. In contrast, activated T cells respond to chemokines such as CCL3 (MIP-1α).

Recent studies have shown that damage within specific tissues can influence the attraction of T cells by means of different chemokine gradients. For example, expression of CCR4 appears to assist in the homing of T cells to the skin, while other chemokine receptors are used by activated T cells trafficking to other areas. There also appears to be a temporal regulation of chemokine expression during ongoing inflammation. In a murine model of central nervous system autoimmunity, relapsing experimental autoimmune encephalomyelitis, different chemokines are expressed in the spinal cord at different stages of the immune response. This suggests a model for recruitment of T cells of different specificities, as well as monocytes, which are intimately involved in the tissue damage.[7]

Another level of control of tissue-specific migration is exerted by the integrins. Naïve T cells express predominantly LFA-1 ($\alpha_L\beta_2$, CD11a, CD18). LFA-1 interacts with ICAM-1 (CD54) and ICAM-2 (CD102). Interactions between LFA-1 and ICAM-1 are essential for extravasation into the lymph nodes of naïve T cells, as well as memory T cells and B cells. Migration to the Peyer's patches requires $\alpha_4\beta_7$ integrin in addition to LFA-1. Following activation, LFA-1 expression is markedly increased, as is the expression of other integrins. The importance of differential integrin expression is manifest as more is learned about their role in migration into specific tissues. VLA-4 ($\alpha_4\beta_1$, CD49d) is important for migration into a variety of sites, including the central nervous system and the lungs. Additional molecules other than the integrins are important in migration into the tissue. One of these, CD44, is expressed rapidly following T-cell activation. CD44 has been shown to play a role in T-cell rolling and is also important for extravasation of T cells from the vessels.

Activated T cells can traffic through many tissues. Selectivity is provided at the level of the tissue by expressing narrow subsets of selectin ligands, integrin ligands, and chemokines. The exact role of this specificity is not fully understood. Taken together, the differences in receptors and ligands expressed in naïve versus activated T cells can account for the differences in T-cell trafficking observed between these populations.[6, 8]

■ DIFFERENTIATION OF CD4 TH SUBSETS ■

Following activation, CD4 T cells have the potential to differentiate into three general categories of cell types based on function: those possessing pro-inflammatory effector characteristics, those possessing regulatory/anti-inflammatory activities, and those functioning as memory cells (Fig. 17.1). The end result of this differentiation process ultimately dictates what type of immune response will be produced.

CD4 T cells function by producing cytokines. The idea that T helper cells could be divided into subpopulations that produced a distinct set of cytokines and a specific set of effector functions was discovered through study of long-term murine CD4 T-helper cell clones and cell lines.[9] It was observed that, after repeated, long-term stimulation, CD4 T cell clones would produce two distinct patterns of cytokines. Based on the cytokine expression phenotype of the cells, the

KEY CONCEPTS

CD4 EFFECTOR PHENOTYPES

Th1

>> Produce interferon (IFN)-γ, interleukin (IL)-2, tumor necrosis factor (TNF)-α and TNF-β (LT-α)

>> Stimulate immunoglobuin (Ig)G₂ and IgG₃ class switching

>> Responses mediated by macrophage activity

>> Promote phagocytic activity via:

   Antibody-mediated FcγRIII cross-linking

   Antibody-mediated complement deposition

   Antibody-mediated opsonization

   IFN-γ-mediated macrophage activation

Th2

>> Produce IL-4, IL-5, IL-6, and IL-10

>> Stimulate IgG4 and IgE class switching

>> Responses mediated by mast cells and eosinophils

>> Increase degranulation through:

   FcεRI cross-linking

   IL-5-mediated eosinophil activation

Th17

>> Produce IL-6, IL-17, and TNF-α

>> Activate local endothelium

>> Induce cytokine and chemokine production

>> Increase infiltration by neutrophils

>> Activate cell-mediated inflammation

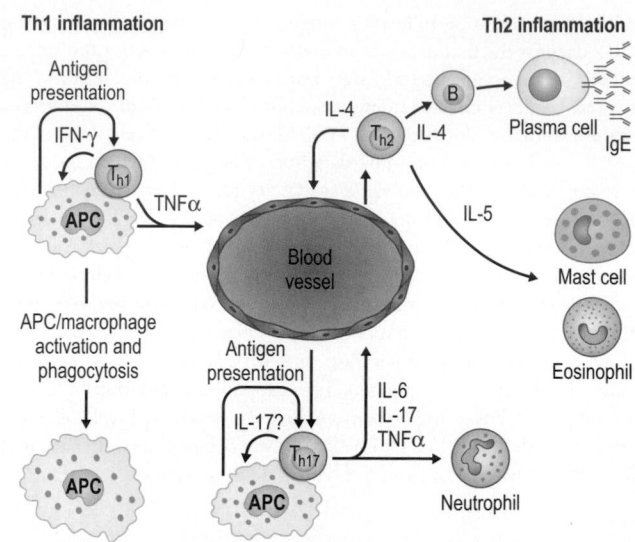

Fig. 17.2 Generalized model for Th₁ and TH₂ mediated inflammation. Top left: introduction of an infectious agent stimulates the release of chemokines and tumor necrosis factor (TNF)-α from tissue macrophages stimulating the recruitment (upward arrows) of T cells and monocytes through the local vasculature. Antigen recognition by Th₁ cells stimulates the local production of Th₁ cytokines. Interferon (IFN)-γ activates macrophages, enhancing the clearance of infectious agents. Top right: trafficking to sites of Th₂ responses is stimulated by local chemokine expression leading to T-cell recruitment. Antigen recognition leads to interleukin (IL)-4 production by Th₂ cells which stimulates B-cell immunoglobulin E (IgE) class switching. Production of IL-5 activates eosinophils. Cross-linking of FcεR1 molecules bound to IgE leads to the degranulation of mast cells (Ma) and eosinophils (E). Bottom: recruitment of Th17 cells and restimulation by antigen result in the release of IL-6, IL-17, and TNF-α, which promote the recruitment, activation, and function of many cells, particularly neutrophils.

two subsets were given the designation T helper 1 (Th1) and T helper 2 (Th2). Further study demonstrated additional CD4 T-cell phenotypes, each of which possesses its own distinct set of effector and regulatory capacities. In addition to Th1 and Th2, Th17, Tr1, adaptive regulatory T cells (Treg), central memory, and effector memory cell phenotypes have been identified.

CD4 EFFECTOR CELL PHENOTYPES

CD4 T effector cells are those that promote inflammatory processes through the release of cytokines. These cells function by modifying or promoting the activity of accessory cells, which ultimately mediate the inflammatory processes required for clearance of the antigen. Effector CD4 T cells are divided into three basic groups: Th1, Th2, and Th17. Cells belonging to these subsets are recruited and activated at sites of inflammation (Fig. 17.2) where they can be distinguished by their cytokine production profiles (Table 17.1).

Th1 cells are classically defined by the production of granulocyte–macrophage colony-stimulating factor (GM-CSF), interferon (IFN)-γ, interleukin (IL)-2 and LT (tumor necrosis factor (TNF)-β). The Th1

phenotype is elicited by the innate immune response to infection by intracellular bacteria, fungi, and viruses. Infection with these pathogens activates TLR signaling and the subsequent production by dendritic cells and NK cells of cytokines critical for Th1 development.

Th1 differentiation is promoted by IL-12, IL-18, IL-27, IFN-γ, and type 1 interferons. It is inhibited by IL-4 and IL-10. IL-12 production is critically associated with dendritic cell activation and is thought to be the critical factor associated with Th1 commitment. IL-18 plays a dual role in Th1 function by promoting Th1 commitment and eliciting IFN-γ production by fully differentiated Th1 cells. IL-27 is also produced by dendritic cells and is associated with Th1 commitment. Th1 differentiation is further enhanced by exposure to IFN-γ. A variety of cells such as NK cells and previously committed Th1 cells are thought to be important early sources of IFN-γ. The binding of IFN-γ to the IFN-γ receptor activates Stat1 signaling, which in turn stimulates the production of the Th1-restricted transcription factor Tbet. Tbet serves to reinforce the Th1 phenotype by promoting IFN-γ and IL-12Rβ₂ expression.[10]

Th1 cells help activate macrophages, natural killer (NK) cells, B cells, and CD8 T cells, thereby function in promoting cell-mediated

Table 17.1 T-helper cell effector function through cytokine secretion

Th1	
IL-2	T-cell growth and potentiation of Fas-mediated apoptosis
	NK cell growth and cytolytic activity
	B-cell growth and antibody production
IFN-γ	Increases MHC class I and class II expression on numerous cell types
	Promotes Th1 differentiation
	Macrophage activation, stimulates phagocytic killing and oxidative bursts
	Induces IgG$_2$α and IgG$_3$ class switching
	Inhibits IgG$_1$ and IgE class switching
	Inhibits Th2 proliferation
	Activates neutrophils
	Activates endothelium to promote CD4 T-cell adhesion
	Stimulates NK cell cytolytic activity
	Required for the activation of CD8 CTLs
TNF-α	Activates vascular endothelial cells, enhancing leukocyte recruitment
	Activates neutrophils, eosinophils, and macrophages
	Stimulates IL-1, IL-6, TNF, and chemokine expression by macrophages
	Protects against viral infections, similar to IFNs
	Increases MHC class I expression
	Induces fever
	Activates coagulation
LT (TNF-β)	Activates neutrophils and osteoclasts
	Activates vascular endothelial cells, enhancing leukocyte recruitment
	Cytotoxic activity against tumor cells
	Stimulates adhesion molecule expression
	Increases MHC class I expression
Th2	
IL-4	Growth and differentiation of Th2 cells
	B-cell growth and MHC class II upregulation
	Induces IgG$_1$ class switching (IgG$_4$ in humans) and IgE
	Inhibits IgG$_{2a}$ and IgG$_3$ class switching
	Mast cell growth
	Inhibits macrophage activation
	Induces VCAM expression on endothelium – recruits eosinophils/monocytes
IL-5	B-cell growth and activation
	Eosinophil differentiation
	Eosinophil activation and survival
IL-10	Inhibits cytokine and chemokine production in monocytes, especially TNF, IL-1, and IL-12
	Inhibits macrophage activation and function
	Inhibits T-cell-mediated inflammation
	Induces IgG$_1$ class switching (IgG$_4$ in humans)
IL-13	Upregulates MHC class II on monocytes and B cells
	Inhibits proinflammatory cytokine production by monocytes
	B-cell co-stimulation
	Induces IgG$_1$ class switching (IgG$_4$ in humans) and IgE
	Increases MHC class I expression
Th17	
IL-6	Activation of acute phase response inducing fever and antibacterial responses
	Stimulation of CRA and SAA production in liver
	Promotes Th2 and Th17 differentiation
	Activation and elicitation of NK responses
	Promotes plasma cell differentiation and Ig production
IL-17	Increase T-cell proliferation
	Promote neutrophil recruitment and activity
	Promote cytokine production, including IL-6 and TNF-α
	Induce chemokine production
TNF-α	See above

IFN, interferon; Ig, immunoglobulin; IL, interleukin; MHC, major histocompatibility complex; NK, natural killer; TNF, tumor necrosis factor

inflammatory responses. Macrophage function is regulated at several levels. GM-CSF promotes the production of monocyte lineage cells from the bone marrow, thereby increasing the pool of macrophage precursors. IFN-γ enhances macrophage microbiocidal activity by initiating nitric oxide (NO) production via iNOS, upregulating production of oxygen radicals, and increasing phagocytic function. IFN-γ also promotes antigen presentation by upregulating macrophage MHC class I, MHC class II, and co-stimulatory molecule expression. In mice, IFN-γ can activate NK cells and also mediate humoral responses by acting on B cells to mediate antibody class switching to an IgG$_{2a}$ isotype.[11] IgG$_{2a}$ activates the classical complement pathway and can bind Fcγ receptors expressed on phagocytic cells, thereby promoting opsonization. Lastly, IFN-γ acts in conjunction with another Th1 cytokine, IL-2, to promote the differentiation of CD8 T cells into cytotoxic effector cells. Macrophage-dependent Th1-mediated inflammatory responses are known as *delayed-type hypersensitivity* (DTH) responses. *In vivo*, DTH responses are critical for protection from intracellular pathogens, including bacteria, fungi, and viruses. Th1 cells have also been implicated in the pathogenesis of many autoimmune diseases, such as multiple sclerosis, type1 diabetes mellitus, rheumatoid arthritis, and Crohn's disease.

Th2 cells are defined by their production of IL-4, IL-5, IL-9, IL-10, and IL-13. Naïve T cells express the IL-4 receptor (IL-4R). *In vitro*, the critical step in Th2 cell differentiation is the presence of exogenous IL-4 and the absence of IFN-γ during T-cell activation. *In vivo* Th2 differentiation is thought to require IL-4 produced by basophils, eosinophils, mast cells, NKT cells, or even previously differentiated Th2 cells. The combination of TCR (NFAT), co-stimulatory (CD28 and ICOS), and IL-4R/STAT6 signaling promotes IL-4 transcription and the production of the transcription factors c-Maf and GATA3. c-Maf functions to promote IL-4 production and suppress IFN-γ, thereby helping to establish Th2 polarity. GATA3 appears to contribute to Th2 differentiation by inhibiting IFN-γ while promoting IL-5 and IL-13 production (Fig. 17.3).[10]

Th2 cells release IL-4 and IL-5, which then attract and activate eosinophils and mast cells. Th2-type cytokines promote class switching to IgG$_1$, IgE, and sIgA in mice, or IgG$_4$ and IgE in humans. Antigen triggering of IgE bound to FcεR1 receptors on eosinophils or mast cells leads to the release of inflammatory factors such as histamine, platelet-activating factor, prostaglandins, and leukotrienes (Fig. 17.2). These factors act on the local environment, producing vascular dilation and leakage, bronchial constriction, and intestinal hypermotility. Anaphylaxis can be produced on a systemic level. These eosinophil and mast cell-dependent reactions are known as *immediate-type hypersensitivity* (ITH). ITH responses are important for ridding the body of intestinal helminthes (Chapter 29). In fact, components of helminth eggs strongly promote Th2 differentiation. Th2 responses are also associated with atopy and hyper-responsive airway conditions, such as asthma (Chapter 40) and allergies (Chapters 42–44).

Recently, a third type of CD4 helper T cell has been identified. Th17 CD4 T cells are characterized by the production of IL-17, TNF-α, and IL-6. Differentiation towards the Th17 phenotype appears to require the presence of IL-6, IL-23, and TGF-β, and the absence of type 1 interferons, IFN-γ and IL-4 (Fig. 17.3). Much of the Th17 cell potency can be attributed to the production of IL-17. Other sources of IL-17 are neutrophils, CD8 T cells, and γδ T cells. IL-17 is a potent promoter of inflammation, particularly with regard to cellular recruitment. IL-17 induces the expression of adhesion molecules and the production of the pro-inflammatory mediators IL-6, G-CSF, several chemokines,

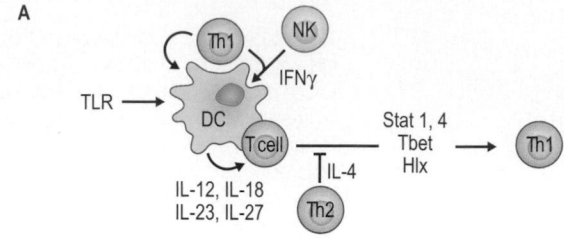

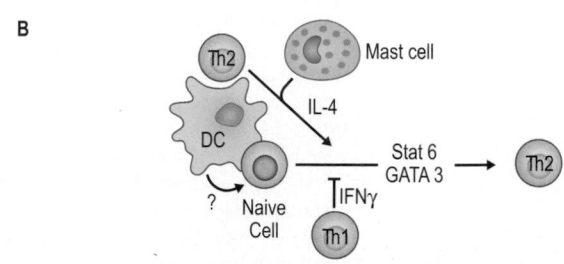

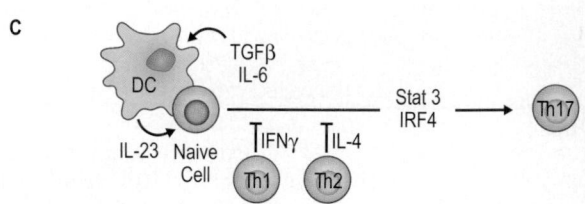

Fig. 17.3 Factors influencing T-effector differentiation. Cytokine exposure during the activation stage of naïve T cells strongly influences T-effector differentiation. Depicted here are the factors promoting and inhibiting Th1. (Top) Th2, (middle) and Th17 (bottom) differentiation following functional activation of undifferentiated T cells.

prostaglandin E$_2$, and matrix metalloproteinases (Fig. 17.2). The effect of Th17 cells on recruitment is further enhanced by the production of TNF-α. Evidence from experimental models suggest that IL-17 plays a critical role in host defense against *Klebsiella pneumoniae* and in models of autoimmune diseases, including collagen-induced arthritis and experimental autoimmune encephalomyelitis.[12] In many ways, Th17 cells appear to be potent cell-mediated effectors with similarities to Th1 cells.

■ REGULATORY T CELLS ■

The idea that T cells may possess the ability to suppress or regulate the function of others is not a new one. Our understanding of regulatory function by T cells was greatly enhanced by the discovery of CD25 as a marker for a regulatory subpopulation of CD4 T cells. This has led to a deeper understanding of Treg cells (Chapter 16) and their function in the immune system.

The majority of CD4+, CD25+, FoxP3+ Treg cells (natural Treg) are thought to develop regulatory ability in the thymus. A separate population, known as adaptive Treg cells, has been found to develop in the periphery. Once differentiated, adaptive Treg cells are similar in phenotype to natural Tregs in that they express CD4, CD25, CD38, CD62L, CD103, and FoxP3. Although not fully characterized, adaptive Tregs are thought to be generated in the periphery in response to a widely expressed antigen, through prolonged exposure to antigen, or as a result of polyclonal stimuli. Differentiation to become an adaptive Treg may therefore result from antigen presentation by poor APCs such as immature dendritic cells or other nonprofessional APCs. Stimulation in the presence of inhibitory cytokines such as IL-10 and TGF-β also appears to favor adaptive Treg differentiation. Similar to natural Tregs, adaptive Treg cells are capable of suppressing CD4 and CD8 T-cell responses both *in vitro* and *in vivo*. Unlike natural Tregs which function in a cell contact-dependent manner, adaptive Tregs appear to act at least in part through the secretion of IL-10 and TGF-β. These cytokines may regulate effector T cells directly or indirectly by inhibiting dendritic cell activity. The generation of adaptive Tregs is of great interest as a cell-based therapy for inflammatory diseases, including autoimmunity.[13]

Tr1 cells have been defined as a population of CD4 T cells that produce IL-10 in response to stimulation. Unlike adaptive Tregs, Tr1 cells do not express FoxP3, nor do they necessarily express CD25. Tr1 cells are produced *in vivo* following antigen delivery to or infection of the respiratory system. It is thought that antigen exposure in the presence of IL-10 and TGF-β, which are normally found in the lungs, is important for Tr1 differentiation. Experimentally, Tr1 cells can be induced by repeated intranasal antigen delivery.[14] In fact, it has also been found that Tr1 cells are induced during the course of infection by *Bordetella pertussis*.[15] Tr1 cells produce IL-10, which blocks proliferation of naïve T cells, prevents Th1 differentiation by blocking IL-12 production, and enhances differentiation of T cells toward a Tr1 phenotype.

■ MEMORY T CELLS ■

A critical contribution of adaptive immune cells to host defenses is the generation of immunological memory. Following an immune response, small numbers of T cells persist long-term and are called memory T cells. Memory T cells function to protect the host from re-infection by the same microorganisms. The level of protection correlates with the number of specific memory cells present in the host. Creation of a memory T-cell population is a critical component of T-cell-dependent vaccination strategies.

There are several reasons why memory cells are uniquely capable of accelerating responses against repeat antigen. First, memory cells are maintained at higher frequencies than naïve cells. Second, memory T cells proliferate and produce cytokines in response to stimulation with lower doses of antigen, less co-stimulation, and much faster kinetics than do naïve cells. Third, memory cells enhance and promote APC function and secrete polarizing cytokines, such as IFN-γ or IL-4. Finally, they accelerate the activity of naïve T cells.

Memory T cells can be divided into two general subgroups based on their patterns of migration. Central memory cells are T cells that have re-expressed the secondary lymphoid homing receptors CCR7 and L-selectin following activation. Expression of CCR7 and L-selectin allows the central memory T cells to recirculate through the secondary lymphatic organs similar to naïve T cells. Lymph node circulation is benefi-

cial because dendritic cells from diverse tissue sites continuously bring antigen to the draining lymph nodes, thereby increasing the effective area of memory cell surveillance.

Effector memory T cells express homing receptors similar to activated T cells. This not only prevents effector memory cells from trafficking through the lymph nodes, but allows the effector memory T cells to migrate through the peripheral tissues, either through uninflamed tissues or in response to localized inflammatory stimuli. Memory cell responses are thus bolstered through the process of immune surveillance at distinct sites. Differentiation to become central or effector memory cells might be through distinct mechanisms. Central memory cells develop from T cells that have failed to proliferate fully or differentiate to a specific Th phenotype.[16] These central memory cells can differentiate during subsequent antigen encounters. On the other hand, effector memory cells are thought to differentiate from previously committed T cells and retain their effector characteristics.

■ GENERAL CONSIDERATIONS IN EFFECTOR T-CELL DIFFERENTIATION ■

Several key concepts of T helper differentiation are important with regard to the cellular differentiation of CD4 T cells. First and foremost, all effector, regulatory, and memory T cells are thought to arise from naïve thymic emigrant precursors. This supposition was confirmed when it was shown that T cells from TCR transgenic mice differentiate into effector, regulatory, and memory phenotypes even though they possess the same TCR. Second, differentiation to a specific phenotype is self-promoting on the one hand and inhibitory to other phenotypes on the other (Fig. 17.3). Both promotion and inhibition result from the production of subset-specific effector cytokines. For example, IFN-γ production early in Th1 differentiation promotes signaling through the IFN-γR, triggering STAT1 signals which then promote IL-12R expression and inhibit IL-4R expression. Similarly, IL-4 expression promotes Th2 differentiation while also inhibiting responsiveness to IL-12 and IFN-γ. By regulating gene expression and chromatin remodeling, critical transcription factors such as Tbet (Th1) or Gata3 (Th2) reinforce commitment of one T-helper phenotype in lieu of the others. Third, commitment to a given Th phenotype has proven irreversible under normal conditions. That is, a fully committed Th cell cannot redifferentiate towards an alternative phenotype (Fig. 17.4). For example, Th1 cells cannot express Th2 cytokines even when they are cultured for extended periods in Th2-skewing conditions. Only by forced expression of Gata3 or Tbet can Th1 or Th2 clones change their Th phenotype.[10] Fourth, *in vitro* or *in vivo*, differentiation can be incomplete. The presence of undifferentiated precursor cells or central memory cells can adopt different Th phenotypes upon subsequent antigen stimulation (Fig. 17.4).

■ CLINICAL EXAMPLES OF EFFECTOR CD4 T-CELL FUNCTION ■

Human Th1 and Th2 populations were first described in T-helper cell clones stimulated by purified protein derivative (PPD) of *Mycobacterium tuberculosis* and *Toxocara canis* antigens, respectively. The majority of

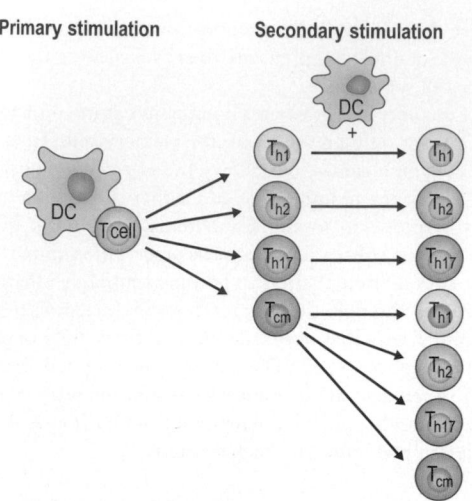

Fig. 17.4 Mechanism of Th phenotype shift. Under appropriate conditions, T-cell activation may result in daughter cells adopting one of several T-effector phenotypes. Within a polarized population of Th cells, a subset of undifferentiated T lymphocytes may exist (here referred to in the general category as Tcm). Upon restimulation, fully committed Th1, Th2, or Th17 cells will produce Th1, Th2, or Th17 phenotypes, respectively. Tcm or other uncommitted cell types retain the potential to differentiate into T effectors of any phenotype, depending on the context of the secondary stimulation.

M. tuberculosis-specific T-cell clones produced IL-2, IFN-γ, and TNF-β, while the helminth-specific Th2-type cells made IL-4 and IL-5.[17] Th1 and Th2 responses have subsequently been described in human infections and diseases. Th17 cells have been detected in humans but their function has not been well characterized. IL-17 has been isolated from human CD4 T cells and has been associated with inflammatory responses in asthma, multiple sclerosis, psoriasis, rheumatoid arthritis, and transplant rejection.[18] Table 17.2 summarizes responses to selected pathogens in which Th1 and Th2 effector responses have been indicated.

The Th1 and Th2 paradigm is not limited to infectious agents. Th1-type T cells can be isolated from the cerebrospinal fluid and peripheral blood of patients with multiple sclerosis, a T-cell-mediated autoimmune demyelinating disorder.[19, 20] These findings have been supported by results from experimental autoimmune encephalomyelitis (EAE), a rodent model of multiple sclerosis. Mouse and rat models of EAE show that Th1 cells play an important role in EAE. In these models, myelin-reactive CD4 T cells isolated from diseased animals produce primarily Th1 cytokines. Th1 cells play an important role in the initiation and continuation of disease. There is also evidence that recovery from EAE is associated with an increase in the presence of IL-10[21] and IL-4-producing cells.[22]

■ TERMINATION OF T-CELL RESPONSES ■

Termination of inflammatory immune responses and return to homeostasis requires a sharp decrease in both T-cell numbers and T-cell activity. Failure to return to pre-inflammation T-cell numbers

and activity would be predicted to have several adverse consequences. First, with each succeeding infection, the body would be increasingly burdened by the energy requirements of maintaining larger T-cell numbers. Second, there would be a loss of TCR diversity resulting from the overrepresentation of clonally expanded T cells. Third, there is an increased risk of damage to self by the presence of large numbers of activated effector T cells, which are easily retriggered. The termination of T-cell responses and restoration of homeostasis result not only from the loss of the original stimulus, but from several active control processes, including the induction of cell death, activation of inhibitory signaling pathways, and cytokine production. These processes lead to the elimination of large numbers of effector T cells and to modulation of the function of the other surviving clones.

■ CELL DEATH PATHWAYS ACTIVE IN T-CELL HOMEOSTASIS ■

Several cell death pathways are important in the restoration of homeostasis. Deletion of peripheral T cells following an immune response has been attributed primarily to the interactions of Fas (CD95) and Fas ligand (FasL), which promotes apoptosis. Following activation, T cells upregulate the surface expression of Fas and FasL. T cells are sensitized to Fas-mediated apoptosis by either exogenous stimulation from another cell (death signal) or by stimulation from endogenous molecules (suicide signal). This process is known as *activation–induced cell death* (AICD). Mutations in Fas and FasL lead to the accumulation of activated lymphocytes in the periphery, a human condition known as ALPS (Chapter 14). Another TNF-family member, TRAIL, has also been associated with AICD. Mice genetically deficient in TRAIL show enhanced susceptibility to autoimmune disease. The evidence suggests that TRAIL primarily regulates AICD in Th2 cells.[23]

Table 17.2 T-cell effector responses to selected pathogens.

Organism	Nature of the immune response
Bacteria	
Borrelia burgdorferi	Th1 responses associated with protection and joint pathology
Chlamydia trachomatis	Th1 responses protective and source of pathology
Helicobacter pylori	Th1 responses involved in ulcer formation
Legionella pneumophila	Th1 responses associated with immunity
Listeria monocytogenes	Th1 responses are protective: interferon-γ from γδ and CD8 T cells is important
Mycobacterium leprae	Severity and phenotype of disease depends on Th1 and Th2 predominance
Mycobacterium tuberculosis	Th1 responses control infection
Treponema pallidum	Th1 resolves infection, Th2 chronic
Yersinia pestis	Th1 responses associated with immunity
Fungi	
Aspergillus fumigatus	Th2 production predominates: does Th1 offer protection?
Blastomyces dermatitidis	Th1 protects: Th2 switch in progressive disease
Candida albicans	Th1 responses are protective
Cryptococcus neoformans	Susceptibility associated with Th2 response Th1 response associated with protection
Paracoccidiodes brasiliensis	Infection stimulates Th2 response, but Th1 response protects
Parasites	
Leishmania spp.	Th1 responses are protective Th2 responses allow chronic infection
Filaria	Initiates Th2 production
Schistosoma mansoni	Th1 response appears protective Th1 and humoral responses protect
Trypanisoma cruzi	Th2 responses are typically directed against eggs Th1 responses inhibit parasite replication, but protection is not completely CD4-dependent
Giardia lamblia	Th1 and Th2 responses protect
Viruses	
Measles	Th1 responses are protective
Hepatitis B	Th1 responses seen in spontaneous recovering patients
Human immunodeficiency virus	Shift from Th1 to a Th0 (Th2?) response late in disease correlates with susceptibility to pathogens
Respiratory syncytial virus	Th1 response protects, Th2 response kills

ACTION OF INHIBITORY RECEPTORS ■

T cells express several Ig-family transmembrane proteins containing immune tyrosine inhibitory motifs (ITIMs). Two of these, CTLA-4 and PD-1, are expressed on peripheral T cells following activation and play an important role in terminating T-cell responses *in vivo*. CTLA-4 binds to CD80 and CD86, thereby sharing ligands with the positive co-stimulatory molecule CD28. CTLA-4 engagement inhibits T-cell function by competing with CD28 for available ligand and inhibiting proximal TCR signaling through its association with the phosphatases SHP-2 and PP2A. Underscoring the importance of CTLA-4 in T-cell homeostasis, mice that are genetically deficient in CTLA-4 develop a severe CD28-dependent lymphoproliferative disease, tissue infiltration, and early death.[24] PD-1 interacts with two ligands, PDL1 and PDL2, which have different expression patterns throughout the immune system and peripheral tissues. Like CTLA-4, engagement of PD-1 limits T-cell cytokine production and proliferation. PD1 signals may also enhance T-cell apoptosis. Loss of PD-1 has been associated with autoimmune cardiomyopathy, arthritis, and a lupus-like glomerulonephritis disease.[25]

CYTOKINE-MEDIATED INHIBITION ■

Another method of controlling T-cell activity is through cytokine signaling. Cytokines (Chapter 10) terminate immune responses by loss or withdrawal of growth factors, by direct anti-inflammatory properties, and by promoting apoptosis, or programmed cell death (Chapter 14). In the early stages of an immune response, IL-2 functions as a growth factor by promoting T-cell survival and expansion. IL-2 and its receptors are rapidly expressed by CD4 T cells upon activation. Loss of IL-2 signals through decreased production or loss of receptor expression deprives the cell of survival signals and leads to AICD. IL-7 is another growth factor important for the survival of activated and memory T cells. Loss of IL-7 or IL-7 receptor results in increased apoptosis among activated and memory T-cell populations.[26]

Cytokines can also limit T-cell responses directly. Apart from its role in Th1 inflammation and macrophage activation, IFN-γ downregulates CD4 T-cell responses. Mice deficient in IFN-γ or IFN-γR show heightened T-cell responses. IL-10 inhibits macrophage activation, downregulating chemokine production and thus diminishing T-cell responses by suppressing co-stimulatory molecule expression by APCs. IL-10 is produced by Th2, adaptive Tregs, and Tr1 cells as well as by monocytes and macrophages. IL-10-deficient mice develop inflammatory bowel disease due to dysregulated Th1 responses. A role for IL-27 in downregulating T-cell responses has recently been described. Mice genetically deficient for the IL-27 receptor develop exaggerated CD4 T-cell responses and inflammatory diseases. These effects of IL-27 can be attributed to its role in suppressing Th1 responses and CD4 T-cell proliferation.[27] TGF-β_1 is an anti-inflammatory cytokine that is produced by subsets of regulatory T cells as well as by a variety of other cell types throughout the body. Unlike IL-10, which targets APCs, TGF-β1 directly inhibits T-cell proliferation. Mice deficient in TGF-β1 have multitissue infiltration of activated lymphocytes and macrophages. Interestingly, IL-2 signaling has also been identified to play a positive role in the termination of T-cell responses by promoting the activity of regulatory T cells. Tregs

express high levels of IL-2R and require constant IL-2 signals for survival.

Cytokines can also quell T-cell responses by promoting apoptosis. TNF-α is well characterized as possessing pro-apoptotic function. TNFR1 possesses a death domain and binding of TNF-α results in the activation of the caspase pathway and apoptosis. In addition to its role as a growth factor, IL-2 can enhance FAS-dependent apoptosis.[28]

■ THERAPEUTIC REGULATION OF IMMUNE RESPONSES ■

Inflammation is the method used to respond to foreign antigen and rid the body of unwanted microorganisms. Uncontrolled inflammation, however, is the source of tissue damage in a variety of diseases. Allergies and asthma as well as hyper-reactivity following infection are all immune system-mediated. Inflammatory responses against self antigens result in autoimmunity. Therefore, clinically it is important to be able to control inflammation. Some of the most effective techniques to control inflammation are aimed directly at T cells, especially at the various steps involved in T-cell activation and/or differentiation (Fig. 17.5).

One of the most attractive methods used to control inflammatory responses is to prevent T-cell activation. T-cell activation requires at least two signals. Signal one is antigen-specific and signal two is co-stimulatory. In the absence of signal two, T cells are rendered unresponsive (or anergic) to further stimulation. Blocking co-stimulation is an important method of controlling T-cell participation in inflammatory responses. In experimental systems, administration of antagonists of the B7/CD28 pathway have been shown to be effective at blocking the onset of T-cell responses to specific antigens, and at controlling ongoing autoimmune responses.[29] Targeting other pathways such as the CD40/CD154 co-stimulatory interaction that is involved in APC/T activation/differentiation has also been used experimentally to control ongoing Th1-mediated autoimmune diseases.[30] The CD40/CD154 pathway is required for B-cell differentiation, dendritic cell function, and production of effector cytokines, and plays an important role in Th1 differentiation via IL-12.

Regulation of inflammation by inhibiting recruitment of T cells and other effector cells is another method employed to control destructive immunopathologic responses. Because various selectins and integrins are required for efficiently targeting leukocytes to inflammatory sites, therapies directed at blocking the binding of these molecules to their ligands and at their blocking downstream signaling pathways are currently being employed to regulate inflammation. For example, the migration of T cells into the central nervous system in EAE, a Th1-mediated central nervous system-mediated autoimmune disease, can be blocked using antibodies to either the VLA-4 integrin or to CD44, which are required for T cells to cross the blood–brain barrier.[31] Knowledge of chemokine secretion profiles during various inflammatory processes has resulted in the ability to control migration to inflammatory sites more specifically. Two methods of controlling chemokine-mediated trafficking are being evaluated: interruption of the chemokine gradient by systemic injection of purified chemokines and blocking chemokine/chemokine receptor interactions by the injection of specific antibodies. For example, accumulation of Th1 cells in the central nervous system in the SJL mouse EAE model can be inhibited by using antibodies specific for the MIP-1α, a chemokine essential for migration of Th1 cells into the central nervous

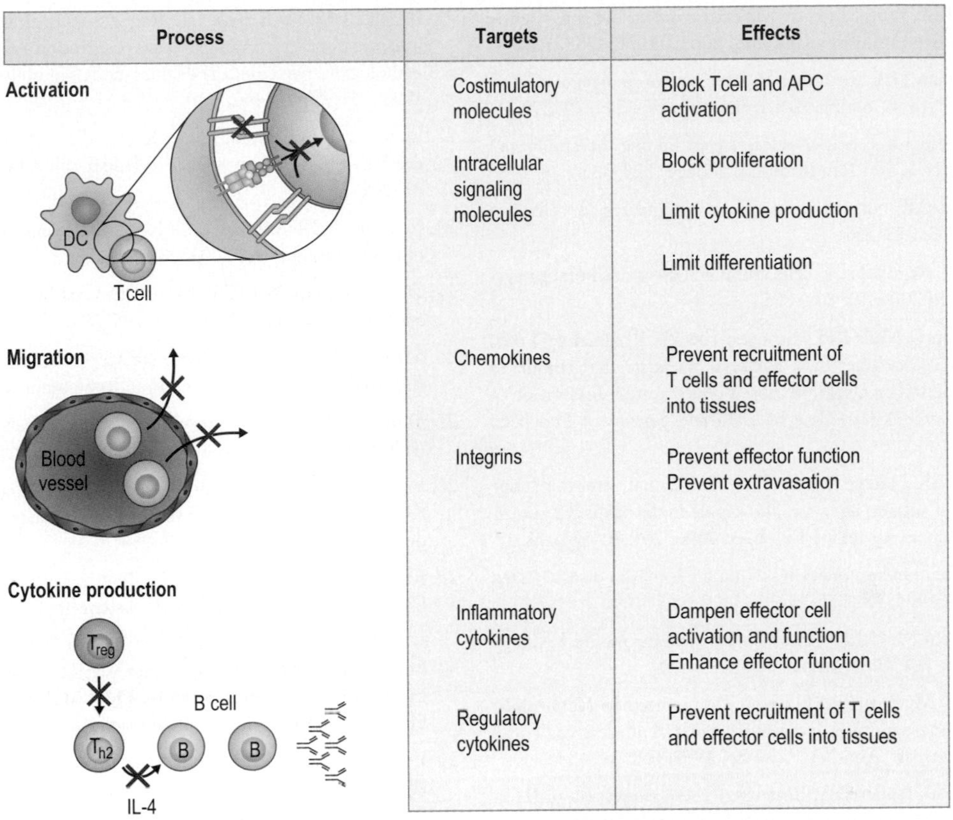

Process	Targets	Effects
Activation	Costimulatory molecules	Block Tcell and APC activation
	Intracellular signaling molecules	Block proliferation
		Limit cytokine production
		Limit differentiation
Migration	Chemokines	Prevent recruitment of T cells and effector cells into tissues
	Integrins	Prevent effector function Prevent extravasation
Cytokine production	Inflammatory cytokines	Dampen effector cell activation and function Enhance effector function
	Regulatory cytokines	Prevent recruitment of T cells and effector cells into tissues

Fig. 17.5 Therapeutic regulation of inflammation. Several techniques have been employed to reduce T-cell responses in cases of inflammation. Among these are inhibiting T-cell activation and differentiation by blocking interactions with antigen-presenting cell (APC)-expressed co-stimulatory molecules (top) inhibiting naïve and effector T-cell trafficking by blocking molecules required for chemotaxis (middle), and limiting the effect of T-helper responses by decreasing the availability of inflammatory cytokines (bottom).

system parenchyma.[7] Controlling T-cell trafficking by modulating chemokines is somewhat problematic because one must know the temporal expression pattern of the chemokines and chemokine receptors that are involved in the inflammatory process and compensate for the redundancy in chemokine/chemokine receptor binding.

Lastly, inflammatory processes can be regulated by neutralizing the pro-inflammatory cytokines (e.g., IFN-γ or TNF-α) and other effector molecules (e.g., iNOS, reactive oxygen intermediates, etc.) involved in the effector limb of the destructive processes. For example, neutralization of TNF-α using soluble TNF-receptor has proven to be an effective means of controlling inflammatory responses in an experimental autoimmune inflammatory model of multiple sclerosis[32] and is an accepted clinical treatment for rheumatoid arthritis.

■ REFERENCES ■

1. Lanzavecchia A, Sallusto F. Dynamics of T lymphocyte responses: intermediates, effectors, and memory cells. Science 2000; 290: 92–97.

2. Friedl P, den Boer AT, Gunzer M. Tuning immune responses: diversity and adaptation of the immunological synapse. Nat Rev Immunol 2005; 5: 532–545.

3. Quezada SA, Jarvinen LZ, Lind EF, et al. CD40/CD154 interactions at the interface of tolerance and immunity. Annu Rev Immunol 2004; 22: 307–328.

4. Van Parijs L, Abbas AK. Homeostasis and self-tolerance in the immune system: turning lymphocytes off. Science 1998; 280: 243–248.

5. Blattman JN, Antia R, Sourdive DJ, et al. Estimating the precursor frequency of naive antigen-specific CD8 T cells. J Exp Med 2002; 195: 657–664.

6. Ley K, Kansas GS. Selectins in T-cell recruitment to non-lymphoid tissues and sites of inflammation. Nat Rev Immunol 2004; 4: 325–335.

7. Karpus WJ, Lukacs NW, McRae BL, et al. An important role for the chemokine macrophage inflammatory protein-1 alpha in the pathogenesis of the T cell-mediated autoimmune disease, experimental autoimmune encephalomyelitis. J Immunol 1995; 155: 5003–5010.

8. Butcher EC. Leukocyte-endothelial cell adhesion as an active, multi-step process: a combinatorial mechanism for specificity and diversity in leukocyte targeting. Adv Exp Med Biol 1992; 323: 181–194.

9. Mosmann TR, Cherwinski H, Bond MW, et al. Two types of murine helper T cell clone. I., Definition according to profiles of lymphokine activities and secreted proteins.. J Immunol 1986; 136: 2348–2357.

10. Szabo SJ, Sullivan BM, Peng SL, et al. Molecular mechanisms regulating Th1 immune responses. Annu Rev Immunol 2003; 21: 713–758.

11. Coffman RL, Lebman DA, Rothman P. Mechanism and regulation of immunoglobulin isotype switching. Adv Immunol 1993; 54: 229–270.

12. Dong C. Diversification of T-helper-cell lineages: finding the family root of IL-17-producing cells. Nat Rev Immunol 2006; 6: 329–333.

13. Bluestone JA, Abbas AK. Natural versus adaptive regulatory T cells. Nat Rev Immunol 2003; 3: 253–257.

14. O'Garra A, Vieira P. Regulatory T cells and mechanisms of immune system control. Nat Med 2004; 10: 801–805.

15. McGuirk P, McCann C, Mills KH. Pathogen-specific T regulatory 1 cells induced in the respiratory tract by a bacterial molecule that stimulates interleukin 10 production by dendritic cells: a novel strategy for evasion of protective T helper type 1 responses by *Bordetella pertussis*. J Exp Med 2002; 195: 221–231.

16. Catron DM, Rusch LK, Hataye J, et al. CD4+ T cells that enter the draining lymph nodes after antigen injection participate in the primary response and become central-memory cells. J Exp Med 2006; 203: 1045–1054.

17. Romagnani S. Lymphokine production by human T cells in disease states. Annu Rev Immunol 1994; 12: 227–257.

18. Kawaguchi M, Adachi M, Oda N, et al. IL-17 cytokine family. J Allergy Clin Immunol 2004; 114: 1265–1273.

19. Benvenuto R, Paroli M, Buttinelli C, et al. Tumor necrosis factor-alpha and interferon-gamma synthesis by cerebrospinal fluid-derived T cell clones in multiple sclerosis. Ann NY Acad Sci 1992; 650: 341–346.

20. Brod SA, Benjamin D, Hafler DA. Restricted T cell expression of IL-2/IFN-gamma mRNA in human inflammatory disease. J Immunol 1991; 147: 810–815.

21. Bettelli E, Das MP, Howard ED, et al. IL-10 is critical in the regulation of autoimmune encephalomyelitis as demonstrated by studies of IL-10- and IL-4-deficient and transgenic mice. J Immunol 1998; 161: 3299–3306.

22. Begolka WS, Vanderlugt CL, Rahbe SM, et al. Differential expression of inflammatory cytokines parallels progression of central nervous system pathology in two clinically distinct models of multiple sclerosis. J Immunol 1998; 161: 4437–4446.

23. Roberts AI, Devadas S, Zhang X, et al. The role of activation-induced cell death in the differentiation of T-helper-cell subsets. Immunol Res 2003; 28: 285–293.

24. Chikuma S, Bluestone JA. CTLA-4 and tolerance: the biochemical point of view. Immunol Res 2003; 28: 241–253.

25. Okazaki T, Honjo T. The PD-1-PD-L pathway in immunological tolerance. Trends Immunol 2006; 27: 195–201.

26. Marsden VS, Strasser A. Control of apoptosis in the immune system: Bcl-2, BH3-only proteins and more. Annu Rev Immunol 2003; 21: 71–105.

27. Hunter CA. New IL-12-family members: IL-23 and IL-27, cytokines with divergent functions. Nat Rev Immunol 2005; 5: 521–531.

28. Van Parijs L, Refaeli Y, Lord JD, et al. Uncoupling IL-2 signals that regulate T cell proliferation, survival, and Fas-mediated activation-induced cell death. Immunity 1999; 11: 281–288.

29. Karandikar NJ, Vanderlugt CL, Bluestone JA, et al. Targeting the B7/CD28:CTLA-4 co-stimulatory system in CNS autoimmune disease. J Neuroimmunol 1998; 89: 10–18.

30. Howard LM, Miga A, Vanderlugt CL, et al. Mechanisms of immunotherapeutic intervention by anti-CD40L (CD154) antibody in an animal model of multiple sclerosis. J Clin Invest 1999; 103: 281–290.

31. Brocke S, Piercy C, Steinman L, et al. Antibodies to CD44 and integrin alpha4, but not L-selectin, prevent central nervous system inflammation and experimental encephalomyelitis by blocking secondary leukocyte recruitment. Proc Natl Acad Sci USA 1999; 96: 6896–6901.

32. Korner H, Goodsall AL, Lemckert FA, et al. Unimpaired autoreactive T-cell traffic within the central nervous system during tumor necrosis factor receptor-mediated inhibition of experimental autoimmune encephalomyelitis. Proc Natl Acad Sci USA 1995; 92: 11066–11070.

REFERENCES

Cytotoxic lymphocyte function and natural killer cells

Stephen L Nutt, Sebastian Carotta, Axel Kallies

18

GENERAL INTRODUCTION TO CTL AND NK CELLS

Cytotoxic T lymphocytes (CTL) and natural killer (NK) cells represent two distinct but related lineages that are important for the control of viral, bacterial, and parasitic infections. These cells also play a prominent and complementary role in the sensing and elimination of malignant cells. Although the approaches by which CTL and NK cells kill their target cells and produce immunomodulatory cytokines are quite similar, the mechanisms by which they recognize their targets are distinctly different. CTL are CD8 T cells (Chapter 9) that recognize targets via the interaction of a diverse repertoire of polyclonally rearranged T-cell receptors (TCR) (Chapter 4) with a peptide-MHC class I complex (Chapter 6) and are a component of the adaptive immune response. MHC class I molecules are expressed on virtually all cells in the body and allow the CTL to scan the tissues for cells expressing foreign or cancer-associated peptides (Chapter 5). In contrast, NK cells are members of the innate immune system (Chapter 3) that use an array of invariant activating and inhibitory receptors to control their activity and specificity.[1] These fundamentally distinct approaches to the recognition of antigen allow for complementary functions, with CTL being specialized in detecting cells infected with intracellular pathogens such as viruses, whereas a prominent function of NK cells is to eliminate those cells where the pathogen or oncogene has blocked display of MHC class I molecules on the surface of the affected cell. As one of the principal immune-evasion mechanisms of viruses and tumors is to suppress MHC class I expression, NK cells provide a key line of defense against this strategy.

The importance of the lytic function of CTL and NK cells has been demonstrated in animal models as well as in patients with defective cytotoxicity. A number of recessive genetic syndromes that affect cytotoxic function have been reported, including familial hemophagocytic lymphohistiocytosis (FHL) that results from mutations in the perforin gene.[2] FHL patients present with severe immunodeficiency often associated with uncontrolled viral infections, including cytomegalovirus (CMV), herpes simplex virus (HSV) and Epstein–Barr virus (EBV). Similarly, mice genetically deficient or depleted for CTL and NK cells

CLINICAL RELEVANCE

FUNCTIONS OF CTL AND/OR NK CELLS

Protective functions include

>> Host defense against:

most viruses, including HIV, EBV, and CMV

bacteria, including *Listeria monocytogenes*

parasites, including *Plasmodium falciparum and Toxoplasma gondii*

primary and metastatic tumors

>> Positive regulation of:

graft versus leukemia effect

placental vascularization by uterine NK cells

Uncontrolled cytotoxicity contributes to

some autoimmune disease, including diabetes and rheumatoid arthritis

hypersensitivity reactions

graft-versus-host disease

transplant rejection

are overtly susceptible to viral pathogens as well as displaying impaired tumor rejection capabilities.[2]

With this potent ability to control pathogen-infected and malignant cells, it is not surprising that the modulation of cytolytic activity is an aim of many immune therapies (see Section 10). These strategies involve either the dampening of CTL function in situations such as transplantation or autoimmunity, or enhancing CTL and NK cell function via vaccination or cytokine therapy. However, tight controls need to be maintained over these effector cells, as deregulated CTL activity plays a direct role in a variety of immunopathological settings, including autoimmune diseases, hypersensitivity reactions, graft-versus-host disease and transplant

KEY CONCEPTS

CTL AND NK CELL EFFECTOR FUNCTIONS

>> Cytotoxicity

  killing by the perforin/granzyme pathway

  death receptor mediated apoptosis, including Fas and TRAIL

>> Immune modulation

  inflammatory cytokine production, including IFN-γ and TNF

  chemokine secretion, including CCL3 (MIP1α), CCL4 (MIP1β) and CCL5 (RANTES)

  immunomodulatory cytokines, including IL-10 and GM-CSF

rejection. To maintain the right balance between killing unwanted or infected cells and not healthy neighboring cells, numerous layers of regulation operate to control cytotoxic functions.

■ EFFECTOR FUNCTIONS/ MECHANISMS ■

CYTOTOXICITY

Cytotoxic cells kill their targets via two major pathways, perforin/granzyme-mediated lysis and death receptor-induced apoptosis. Both require intimate contact between the lytic cell and its target[3] (Fig. 18.1). Although the processes are similar for CTL and NK cells, CTL lytic activity is acquired only after activation and differentiation, whereas NK cells have a 'natural killing' capacity that does not require pre-stimulation. In spite of this, NK cell killing is significantly increased by prior activation by cytokines or inflammatory signals. Both cell types also produce cytokines, most notably IFN-γ, that further enhance the immune response.

PERFORIN/GRANZYME PATHWAY

Perforin is a membrane-disrupting protein that, together with a family of serine proteases (granzymes), forms the bulk of lytic granules. The process of lysis has been most extensively studied in CTL, where, upon interaction between the TCR and an appropriate MHC class I peptide, a synaptic complex forms between the CTL and its target.[3] Lytic granules can then be observed moving along a microtubule network toward the microtubule-organizing center that localizes at the synapse (Fig. 18.1). This process allows the polarized secretion of lytic granules precisely at the CTL–target cell interface. Perforin functions to disrupt the target cell membrane, including either the plasma membrane or the lysosomal membrane. Once the lytic lysosome is internalized into the target cell, it is granzymes that are the initiators of cell death. Granzymes function directly by cleaving substrates, or indirectly via a protease cascade, some of which are shared with pro-apoptotic caspases. One important substrate of granzyme B is the pro-apoptotic protein BID (*B*H3-*i*nteracting *d*omain death agonist), which induces cell death via mitochondrial mediators such as

cytochrome c. Granzyme A, in contrast, kills via cleavage of nuclear proteins and facilitates double-stranded DNA breaks. Other granzymes must also play an important role in cytotoxicity, as mice deficient for both granzyme A and B are capable of tumor rejection and target cell lysis.[2]

DEATH RECEPTOR-INDUCED APOPTOSIS

Cytotoxic cells also have a receptor-based system to induce apoptosis of targets cells (Chapter 14). This pathway uses members of the tumor necrosis factor receptor (TNFR) superfamily that are expressed on the target cells. These receptors have an intracellular signaling motif, called the death domain, which recruits molecules such as FADD (*Fas-a*ssociated *d*eath *d*omain) that transduce the death signal. The two most prominent apoptosis-inducing TNFR family members are Fas (CD95)[4] and TRAIL (*T*NF-*r*elated *a*poptosis *i*nducing *l*igand).[5] Whereas Fas is expressed on a wide variety of tissues, Fas ligand (FasL) expression is restricted to activated CTL and NK cells, where it is stored in lytic granules and, upon activation, released to the effector cell membrane. The Fas/FasL pathway is important in controlling T-cell numbers through activation-induced cell death (AICD), as well as in the rejection of some tumors (Chapter 14). Cytotoxic cells also express TRAIL, which upon binding to TRAIL receptors induces apoptosis in a wider selection of targets.[5] Of particular therapeutic interest is the fact that tumor cells are often exquisitely sensitive to TRAIL.

CYTOKINES

Antigen-stimulated CTL and activated NK cells modulate the immune response by their ability to produce a variety of cytokines, most notably IFN-γ and TNF.[1] These potent inflammatory cytokines activate macrophages and lymphocytes at the site of infection. IFN-γ helps establish a Th1 response and further stimulates differentiated CTL. CTL and NK cells are capable of secreting a number of chemokines (Chapter 11), including CCL3, CCL4 and CCL5. These chemokines help recruit additional lymphocytes into the immune reaction.[1] NK cells are also a potent source of a diverse range of cytokines, including GM-CSF, IL-5, IL-10 and IL-13 (Chapter 10). The capacity to secrete a broad spectrum of cytokines provides NK cells with a wide range of regulatory capabilities.

■ CYTOTOXIC T CELLS ■

THE DEVELOPMENT AND TISSUE DISTRIBUTION OF CTL

CD8 T lymphocytes develop in the thymus, where they are selected for their ability to recognize nonself-peptides in the context of MHC class I molecules (Chapter 9). Upon thymic export these cells acquire a quiescent state and are termed 'naïve.' Naïve CD8 T cells circulate between the peripheral lymphoid organs such as the spleen and lymph nodes via the arterial and lymphatic systems. It is this circulation that allows the T cells to come in contact with antigen that has been brought to the lymphoid organs by dendritic cells (DC), and to initiate an immune response. The tissue distribution of lymphocytes is determined by

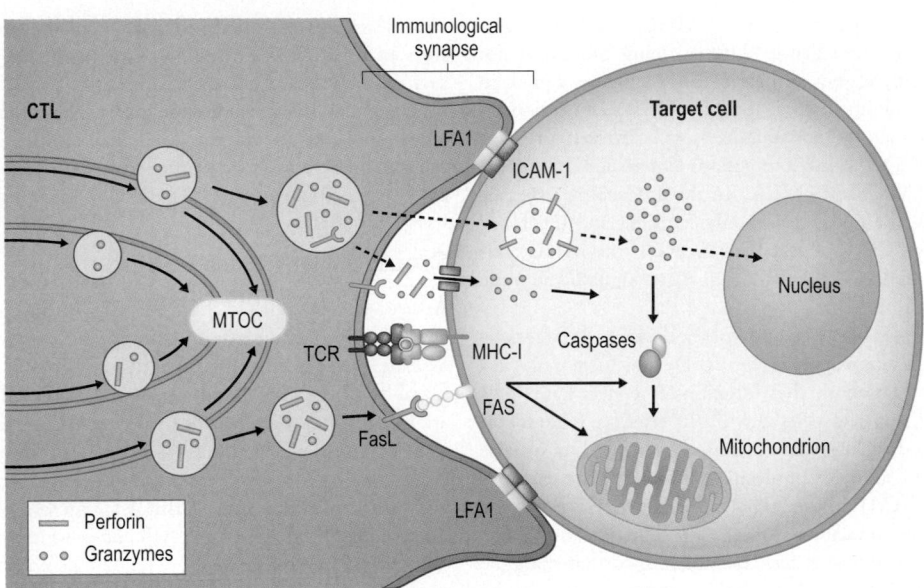

Fig. 18.1 Mechanisms of CTL-induced cell death. The CTL recognizes its target via the interaction of the TCR and the peptide-MHC class I complex on the target cell. TCR signaling induces the formation of an immunological synapse that is stabilized by the binding of LFA1 to ICAM on the target cell. Lytic granules containing perforin, granzymes and FasL are polarized along microtubules and move toward the microtubule organizing center (MTOC). Lytic granules are then either endocytosed intact into the target cell, or their contents are secreted into the synapse by a process that requires perforin. Both mechanisms permit granzymes to gain entry into the target cell and induce apoptosis by caspase-dependent and independent pathways that result in DNA cleavage and mitochondrial damage. Membrane bound FasL can bind to its receptor on target cells and induce apoptosis independently of the perforin/granzyme pathway.

targeting proteins, which can be divided into three categories: selectins, chemokine receptors, and integrins.[6, 7] Naïve and activated CD8 T cells display distinct sets of these targeting proteins, allowing for the differential homing abilities of these cells (Chapter 12). Naïve CD8 T cells express high levels of the lymph node homing receptor L-selectin (CD62L) and CCR7, a receptor which recognizes the chemokines CCL19 and CCL21 that are produced in the T-cell areas of secondary lymphoid organs[6] (Chapter 11). Here naïve T cells interact with antigen-presenting cells (APC), in particular DC (Chapter 7). If a naïve CD8 T cell does not encounter its specific peptide-MHC class I complex on the APC, it leaves the lymph node. This 'egress' is regulated by the sphingosine-1-phosphate receptor-1 (S1P$_1$).[6] If, however, a CD8 T cell encounters the correctly presented peptide–MHC-I complex, a dramatic change in its localization and homing properties ensues. These CD8 T cells upregulate the high-affinity $\alpha_L\beta_2$- integrin (LFA1) that mediates tight interaction between the CD8 T cell and the DC, shut down their egress program, and undergo multiple rounds of proliferation to become activated CTL. After the proliferative phase, the CTL then reacquire egress capacity by downregulating the molecules that recruited them to the lymph node in the first place, CD62L and CCR7.[6] Egress also requires the re-expression of S1P$_1$ and the downregulation CD69, an early activation marker of T cells.

Activated CTL travel via the circulation to nonlymphoid sites where they tether to endothelial cells and extravasate into tissue. This transmigration occurs in both inflamed and noninflamed sites, such as the skin, gut or lung. Many of the effector memory CTL are retained in nonlymphoid tissues, where they are poised to respond rapidly should the antigen be encountered again. A smaller number of memory cells reacquire CD62L and CCR7 expression and circulate through the blood and lymphoid organs and provide long-term memory.

■ THE CTL RESPONSE ■

The CTL response to an acute infection consists of three phases. First, the initial activation and proliferation of the CTL; second, the contraction of effector populations into memory cells; and third, the long-term maintenance of memory cells.

INITIAL ACTIVATION OF THE CTL RESPONSE

Naïve T cells constantly circulate through the secondary lymphoid organs, where antigen encounter occurs. For a CTL response, antigen is brought to the lymph node via the lymphatic system by APC (Fig. 18.2). These APC are typically DC that mature after antigen acquisition in the nonlymphoid tissues and migrate to the lymph node (Chapter 7). Although DC appear to be the most important 'professional' APC, macrophages and B cells are also able to present antigens in a similar manner. In the lymph node, naïve CD8 T lymphocytes scan the APC for the presence of antigenic peptides presented on the MHC class I molecules, a process termed 'immune surveillance.' The scanning process is not completely random. In the case of an infection, inflammatory signals in the lymph node induce the chemokine receptor CCR5 expression on naïve CD8 T cells, which allows individual cells to be attracted to sites of antigen-specific DC-CD4⁺ T-cell interactions as signaled by a gradient of the chemokines CCL3 and CCL4.[8] In the absence of a specific recognition by the TCR, the encounter is only transient and the T cell continues on to another APC to repeat the process. If the MHC class I–peptide complex is bound by the TCR and initiates signaling, a more lasting interaction occurs.

TCR activation promotes the polarization of the T cell and the formation of the 'immunological synapse.'[9] (Fig. 18.1) The immunological synapse is a highly structured body that functions to concentrate TCR signaling in a defined area. It is associated with the selective recruitment of signaling molecules and exclusion of negative regulators. The synapse is stabilized by a ring of adhesion molecules, including, for example, LFA1, which binds to ICAM1 on the target cell (Fig. 18.1). For a T cell to become fully active, co-stimulation through a second signaling pathway is required. Many co-stimulators have been identified that share the common characteristic of being transmembrane receptors, often of the TNFR superfamily, that bind transmembrane ligands on the APC. The most important co-stimulator, CD28, binds the ligands CD80 (B7.1) and CD86 (B7.2), both of which are expressed on activated APC. Co-stimulation results in the clonal expansion of CTL with the selected antigen specificity. The expression of CD80/86 is tightly regulated.

High-level expression occurs only after an APC receives activation signals, such as inflammatory cytokines, or components of the pathogens itself, such as lipopolysaccharide. Co-stimulation via CD28 is most critical during the initiation of the immune response, as it promotes IL-2 production which, in turn, supports the development of memory T cells.[10] Naïve T cells that receive TCR stimulation in the absence of co-stimulatory signals can become nonresponsive to antigen, a state termed 'anergy.'

Cross-presentation and priming

After it was established that only direct interaction with an APC and appropriate co-stimulation led to full CTL activity, a problem arose in explaining the mechanism by which antigens in non-APC were recognized by CTL. This dilemma was resolved by the discovery that there are two distinct mechanisms by which CTL encounter peptide–MHC class I complexes.[11] If the APC expresses the antigen, for example if it is infected by a virus, then the APC can process the antigen via the endogenous MHC class I pathway for presentation. The more intriguing situation arises when the APC does not express the antigen. In this case the APC – most notably DC, but also macrophages and B cells – are thought to acquire and process the antigen via a process termed 'cross-presentation'[11] (Chapter 7). Cross-presentation is initiated by the capture of foreign or exogenous antigens by phagosomes. The antigens are then processed by an unusual mechanism that directs the peptides to the MHC class I pathway and presentation on the cell surface. An encounter of a CTL with an antigen processed in this

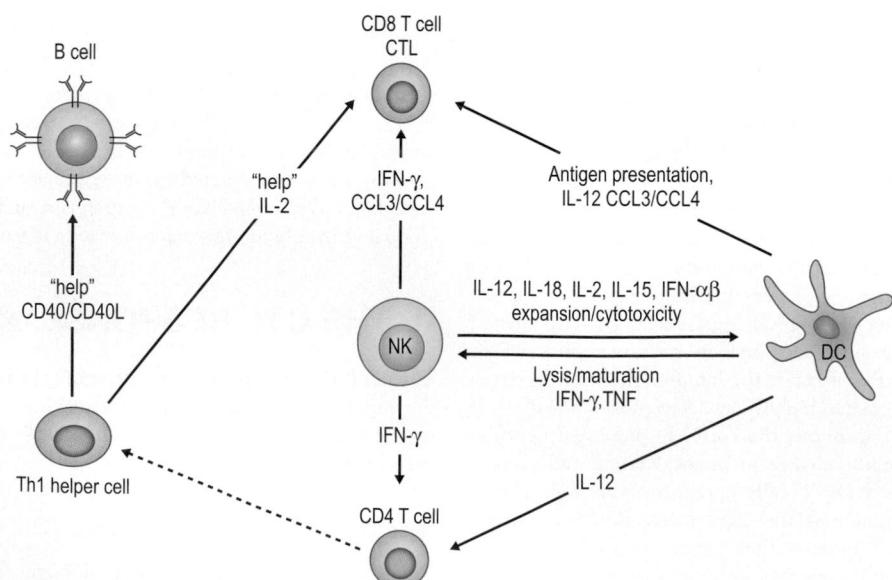

Fig. 18.2 Immune cell interactions during an immune response in the lymph node. After their encounter with antigen DC move to the draining lymph node, where they initiate an antigen-specific immune response. In the very early stages, NK cells are recruited to the lymph node and modulate various aspects of this response. NK cells provide cytokines that induce the maturation of DC, which enables these cells to efficiently present the antigen to T cells in the context of co-stimulatory signals. NK cells also have the ability to eliminate immature DC and to provide 'early' IFN-γ for the initiation of a Th1-type CD4 T-cell response. Finally, NK cells produce a range of chemokines, most notably CCL3 (MIP-1α) and CCL4 (MIP-1β), which are crucial for the recruitment of CD8 T cells into the immune response.

pathway is termed 'cross-priming.'[11] This strategy assists the CTL in viral control in two ways. First, cross-priming alleviates the need for the DC to be infected for detection, and therefore prevents viruses escaping immune detection by avoiding infecting DC. Second, viruses often attempt to evade CTL by downregulating the MHC class I pathway. Cross-priming occurs in noninfected cells that are still fully capable of MHC class I presentation, and thus remain able to stimulate CTL activity.

THE CONTRACTION OF EFFECTOR POPULATIONS INTO MEMORY CELLS

After activation of the CTL in the secondary lymphoid organs, an immune response is characterized by the rapid proliferation of antigen-specific cells and their acquisition of effector functions. CTL proliferate at one of the fastest rates known for mammalian cells, with a cell cycle time of approximately 6 hours in both humans and rodents. Infection leads to a dramatic increase in the numbers of pathogen-specific CTL, from almost undetectable initial levels to several million cells in the course of a single week. The magnitude of this response is dependent on the kind of infection and the dose of the antigen. It is controlled by the number of precursors recruited into the response.[12] The expansion phase is followed by a contraction of the CTL population that is independent of both the magnitude of the response and clearance of the antigen. This phase is essential to prevent nonspecific tissue damage through uncontrolled cytokine release and cytolytic activity. Contraction also preserves the flexibility of the T-cell response to new infections while memory of previously encountered antigens is maintained. Typically 5% of the expanded effector cell population survives in the long-lived memory pool.[13]

THE LONG-TERM MAINTENANCE OF MEMORY CELLS

The production of long-lasting antigen-independent memory cells is essential for a rapid response should re-infection occur. CTL memory provides a more vigorous response than the primary challenge for both quantitative and qualitative reasons.[14] Quantitatively, owing to the substantial clonal expansion during a primary infection, the precursor frequency of antigen-specific CTL is vastly higher in immune individuals than in naïve subjects, thus allowing for a stronger response. Qualitatively, memory CTL exhibit a striking efficiency in elaborating effector functions associated with the rapid production of IFN-γ. This enhanced response is the result of reprogramming of gene expression profiles by epigenetic changes in DNA methylation or chromatin structure. The CTL memory compartment is composed of two cell types, effector memory (T_{em}) and central memory (T_{cm}). These subsets differ in their surface molecule expression and in their ability to exhibit effector functions[12] (Table 18.1). Like their naïve counterparts, T_{cm} express high levels of CD62L and CCR7 and reside primarily in the secondary lymphoid organs. T_{cm} are capable of prolonged homeostatic self-renewal in the absence of antigen. However, upon antigen encounter they rapidly gain effector function and acquire a T_{em} phenotype. T_{em} are characterized by low expression of CD62L and CCR7 and are distributed throughout the body, including peripheral tissues such as lung and gut, where they can immediately confront invading pathogens. Both T_{em} and T_{cm} express high levels of CD44, which distinguishes them from naïve T cells (Table 18.1). The pathway(s) of development of these distinct memory cell types is not fully understood. The conventional linear model of memory formation proposes that memory cells are derived directly from the remaining effector cells after the contraction phase.[12] An alternative model proposes that pathways exist that allow the differentiation of memory cells without passing through an effector stage. CD4 T cell help and cytokines, including IL-15 and IL-7 and their receptors, have been identified as crucial for the survival and maintenance of the memory T-cell pool.[13]

■ CD4 T-CELL HELP ■

The final player in the initial activation of CTL is the 'help' provided by CD4 T cells specific for an antigen linked to the CTL epitope[10] (Chapter 17). The discovery of cross-priming by DC led to a model whereby both CD4 and CD8 T cells recognize antigen on the same APC via MHC classes II and I, respectively.[11] Subsequent studies demonstrated that the function of the CD4 T cells in the process is to activate the DC. The requirement for CD4 help to generate a CTL response in the absence of an inflammatory stimulus contrasts with the fact that CD4 T cells are not required for a strong primary CTL response to many model

Table 18.1 Properties of CTL populations

Marker	Naïve CTL	Effector memory (T_{EM})	Central memory (T_{CM})
CD62L	++	–	++
CD44	+	+++	+++
CCR7	+	–	+
IL7R (CD127)	+	–	+
IL2Rβ (CD122)	+	++	+++
Main tissue distribution	Lymph nodes, spleen, blood	Nonlymphoid tissue (lung, liver), spleen	Lymph nodes, spleen, blood
Cytotoxic function	–	++	–
IFN-γ	–	+++	+

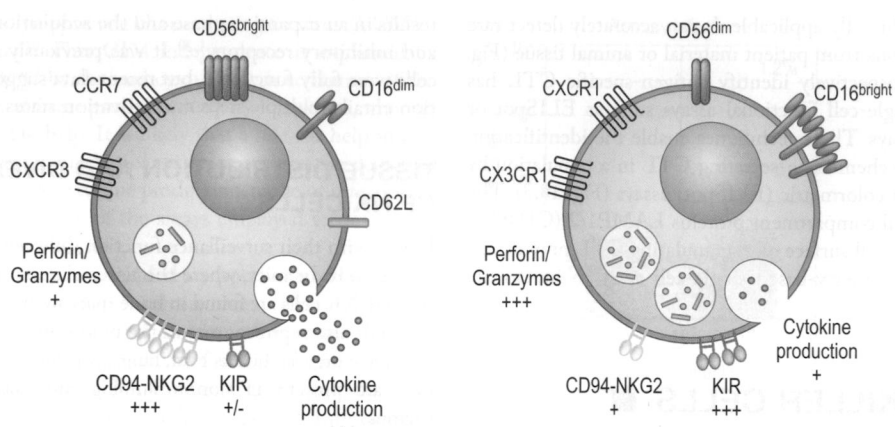

Fig. 18.4 Schematic representation of human NK cells. The human NK cell subsets show distinct receptor expression and effector functions. CD56[bright] NK cells produce high levels of cytokines and have patterns of chemokine and homing receptor expression that distinguish them from CD56[dim] NK cells. CD56[dim] NK cells express high levels of KIR and cytotoxic activity. The relative levels of receptors and effector molecules is indicated on an arbitrary scale, with +/− being weak and +++ being strong expression.

induction of NK cells that were historically called lymphokine-activated-killer or LAK cells. IL-2 activation will also induce the IL-2Rα chain to complete the high-affinity trimeric receptor. IL-4 activates human NK cells, and promotes the proliferation of a fraction of NK cells characterized by their ability to produce IL-13.

The myeloid-derived factors IL-12 and IL-18 have profound effects on NK-cell function. IL-12 and IL-18 are produced by macrophages and DC during inflammatory immune activation, such as viral infection.[26] While NK cells are present in IL-12- or IL-18-deficient mice and only marginally reduced in double mutant animals, cytotoxic activity and the ability to respond to infections such as mouse CMV (MCMV) is impaired.[26] Cultivation of NK cells in IL-12 and/or IL-18 induces short-term activation, cytotoxicity and IFN-γ production, whereas longer cultures produce more specialized cytokine-producing cells.

A recently identified NK cell-activating cytokine is IL-21.[24] IL-21 is a member of the common γ chain family of cytokines produced by CD4 T cells and, in contrast to IL-2 or IL-15, does not promote proliferation. Instead, it enhances maturation and effector function. Mouse NK cells treated with IL-21 display a broad-spectrum increase in cytotoxic function and produce cytokines including IFN-γ and IL-10.[24] Importantly, mice treated with IL-21 show a marked increase in NK cell-mediated tumor rejection, highlighting the potential for use of this cytokine in anti-cancer therapeutics.[24] Human NK cells respond similarly to IL-21, but there is also a role for IL-21 in early NK development that is not present in the mouse.

■ NK CELL RECEPTORS ■

NK cells differ from CTL in that they do not require the expression of MHC class I to recognize target cells. In fact, the re-introduction of MHC class I molecules into previously susceptible cell lines confers resistance to NK cell-mediated killing. These observations led to the missing-self hypothesis, which proposes that NK cells survey tissues

KEY CONCEPTS

NK CELL RECEPTORS

>> Inhibitory receptors:

recognize mostly MHC class I ligands with high affinity

signal via ITIM motifs

recruit phosphatases (SHP and SHIP) to prevent a cytotoxic response

required for NK cell licensing

>> Activating receptors:

do not bind MHC class I molecules with high affinity

ligands include viral molecules and stress induced proteins

signal via ITAM motifs.

use several signaling adaptors, including DAP12

for the usually ubiquitous MHC class I expression.[27] Encounter with MHC class I sends an inhibitory signal to the NK cell, which then moves on in search of other targets. However, if a cell downregulates MHC class I to avoid CTL activity, these cells are killed by NK cells. The missing-self hypothesis, although altered over time to encompass other observations, has been extremely useful in providing a predictive framework by which to investigate NK-cell receptors and the recognition of target cells (Fig. 18.5).

In the past two decades a large number of NK cell receptors have been identified,[20] the ligands for many of which are known. Although a number are the MHC class I molecules themselves, as predicted by the missing-self hypothesis, there are many other types of ligand. NK-cell receptors are classified into either activating or inhibitory types. This distinction was initially based on the *in vitro* properties of antibodies against these receptors, but is increasingly regarded as the expression of

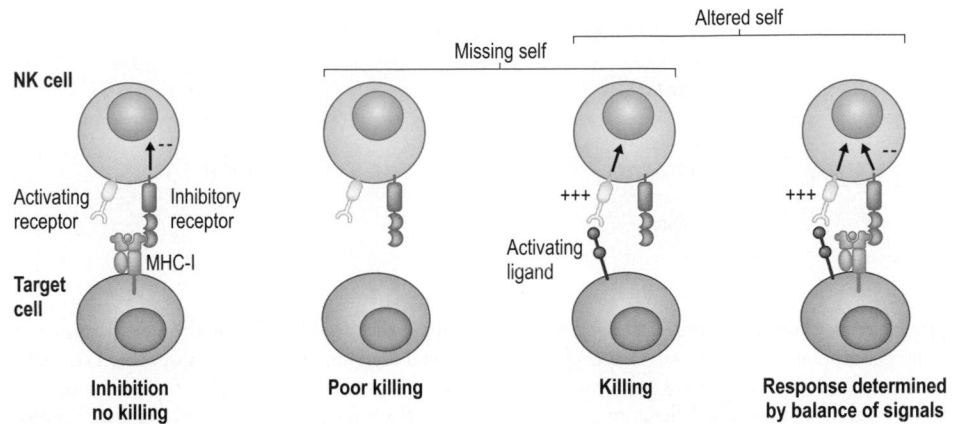

Fig. 18.5 NK cell recognition of target cells. NK cells express inhibitory receptors for MHC class I and activating receptors for a variety of cellular, viral and stress-induced ligands that alter the outcome of encounter with a target cell. The missing-self hypothesis initially predicted that NK cells would be activated to kill in the absence of MHC class I inhibition. However, an activating signal is also required. This activating signal can be provided by cellular ligands, or by viral or stress-induced proteins, termed 'altered self.' In the presence of both inhibitory and activating signals the outcome is determined by quantitative differences in signal strength between the two.

Table 18.2 Human and mouse NK cell receptors (partial list)

Gene	Function	Ligands
Human		
LILRB1	Inhibitory	HLA-A,B,C,E,F,G,CMV UL18
KIR2DL1	Inhibitory	HLA-C N77/K80
KIR2DL2, 3	Inhibitory	HLA-C S77/K80
KIR2DL4	Activating?	HLA-G?
KIR2DL5	Inhibitory	?
KIR3DL1	Inhibitory	HLA-Bw4
KIR3DL2	Inhibitory	HLA-A?
KIR3DL3	Inhibitory	?
KIR2DS1	Activating	HLA-C
KIR2DS2, 3	Activating	?
KIR2DS4	Activating	HLA-C
KIR2DS5	Activating	?
KIR3DS1, 3	Activating	?
CD94/NKG2A	Inhibitory	HLA-E
CD94/NKG2C	Activating	HLA-E
NKG2D	Activating	MICA/B, ULBP1-4
CD16 (FcγRIII)	Activating	Immune complexes
CD27	Activating	CD70
CD244 (2B4)	Activating	CD48
NKR-P1A	Activating	LLT1
Mouse		
Ly49A-C, E-G, I-O	Inhibitory	H-2 MHC-I
Ly49D	Activating	H-2 MHC-I
Ly49H	Activating	MCMV m157
CD94/NKG2A	Inhibitory	Qa-1b
CD94/NKG2C, E	Activating	Qa-1b
NKG2D	Activating	RAE-1, H60
KLRG1	Inhibitory	E-, R-, N-cadherins
CD16 (FcγRIII)	Activating	Immune complexes

Continued

Table 18.2 Human and mouse NK cell receptors (partial list)—Cont'd

Gene	Function	Ligands
CD27	Activating	CD70
CD244 (2B4)	Inhibitory	CD48
NKR-P1A,C,F	Activating	Clr-g
NKR-P1D	Inhibitory	Clr-b

the biochemical signal-transduction pathways activated by the receptor.[20] Interestingly, although this conceptual strategy of target recognition is conserved in all mammals tested, rodents and humans have evolved their receptors from two independent gene families. The killer immunoglobulin-like receptors (KIR) in humans and the Ly49 family in mice perform the same function (Table 18.2).

NK-CELL RECEPTOR SIGNALING

The signals derived from NK receptors are defined as inhibitory or activating in terms of their effect on NK-cell function. All extensively characterized inhibitory receptors carry an immunoreceptor tyrosine-based inhibitory motif (ITIM) in their intracellular domain. Ligation of ITIM-containing receptors causes tyrosine phosphorylation and the recruitment of a variety of phosphatases, including SHP and SHIP, that act to damp downstream signaling pathways and NK-cell effector functions.[20, 28] In contrast, activating receptors use immunoreceptor tyrosine-based activation motifs (ITAM) to transduce stimulatory signals. Engagement of an ITAM-containing receptor results in tyrosine phosphorylation and recruitment of adaptor molecules, including FcεR1γ, CD3ζ, or DAP12. The best-characterized activating receptor is CD16, an Fc receptor that binds IgG and is responsible for the antibody-dependent cytotoxic capacity (ADCC) of NK cells. CD16 recruits FcεR1γ and CD3ζ, which in their turn attract the tyrosine kinases syk and ZAP70.[20] These pathways then promote effector functions via multiple signal transduction pathways.

NK CELL RECEPTORS THAT RECOGNIZE MHC-I MOLECULES

NK cells recognize a wide variety of MHC class I molecules of both classic and nonclassic types. The receptors providing this recognition fit broadly into the immunoglobulin-like and lectin-like superfamilies. They show significant differences between mice and humans.

KILLER CELL IMMUNOGLOBULIN-LIKE RECEPTORS (KIR) IN HUMANS

The *KIR* genes represent a family of 15 genes that are physically linked on chromosome 19.[29] The locus shows a high degree of variation in the human population, with both the number of *KIR* genes varying between individuals and extensive allelic polymorphisms described. The KIR family was originally called killer inhibitory receptors, but subsequent studies have demonstrated that activating receptors are also encoded by the *KIR* locus. As expected, the inhibitory KIR contain ITIM, whereas all activating KIR utilize DAP12 to transduce signals from an ITAM.[20, 30] Individual *KIR* genes are expressed by only a

subset of NK cells. This expression pattern is stably maintained in a clonal manner. Similarly to most other NK-cell receptors, KIR can also be expressed by some T cells after activation.

KIR recognize the human MHC class I molecules HLA-A, B and C (Table 18.2). The specificity of the inhibitory KIR has been extensively characterized, with, for example, the different isoforms of KIR2D recognizing all known alleles of HLA-C.[20] The ligands of the activating KIR are less clear; however, they do not bind with high affinity to HLA molecules. KIR2DL4 is the most evolutionarily distinct member of the family and appears to be expressed in all activated NK cells in culture and on the CD56[bright] subset in peripheral blood. KIR2DL4 also has some distinct structural features and may act as an unconventional activating receptor binding HLA-G.[29]

There are emerging epidemiological data implicating particular KIR in a variety of autoimmune pathologies and viral responses.[29] For example, individuals with KIR2DS2 and some HLA-C alleles are predisposed to rheumatoid arthritis with vascular complications. Conversely, HIV-infected individuals who are homozygous for HLA-Bw4 progress to AIDS more slowly than those with other haplotypes, especially when they have the *KIR3DS1* gene. The mechanism by which this occurs is unknown, but the activity suggests that KIR recognize a HIV-associated peptide in the context of HLA-Bw4[31] (Chapter 37).

THE LY49 FAMILY IN RODENTS

In a remarkable example of the power of selection to shape the evolution of the immune system, a multigenic locus with functional properties almost identical to those of the *KIR* genes has evolved independently in rodents. Mice, which have only two *Kir* genes of unknown function, have an analogous cluster of type II transmembrane spanning lectin-like genes called the *Ly49* family.[20] This family consists of more than 20 members and is highly polymorphic between mouse strains. Like KIR molecules, Ly49 receptors are also highly variegated in their expression in NK cells, and they are monoallelically transcribed. *Ly49* genes encode activating and inhibitory receptors that bind to MHC class I molecules and signal via ITAM and ITIM motifs, respectively (Table 18.2). Ligand-binding studies have revealed that the inhibitory Ly49 receptors such as A, C, and I bind to MHC class I haplotypes and function to prevent autoaggression by NK cells. The function of the activating receptors has proved more difficult to elucidate. Ly49D is known to have high affinity for the MHC class I H-2D[d] allele and is involved in rejecting bone marrow allografts expressing H-2D[d], whereas the function of Ly49D in the normal immune response is unclear. For one activating receptor, Ly49H, the physiological function is known, as it recognizes the m157 molecule of MCMV and is important in viral control.[32]

CD94 AND NKG2 FAMILY

Unlike the KIR or Ly49s, the CD94/NKG2 complex is present both in rodents and humans. CD94/NKG2 receptors recognize nonclassic MHC class I ligands, such as HLA-E in humans and Qa1[b] in mice. A single *CD94* gene is physically linked to four *NKG2* (A, C, E and a truncated F) genes in humans. CD94 is found on the cell surface either alone or with the NKG2 proteins. The NKG2 family also exists in activating (C, E) and inhibitory types (A). Interestingly, both the activating and the inhibitory complexes recognize HLA-E that present predominantly the leader peptides of other HLA molecules, but not HLA-E itself. This system may provide a mechanism for the NK cells to monitor the expression of multiple MHC class I proteins using HLA-E as a surrogate.[20]

NKG2D

NKG2D, which is only distantly related to the *NKG2* family, is a single, nonpolymorphic gene that is expressed on all NK cells from an early stage. In the mouse NKG2D signals through both DAP12 and another adaptor, DAP10, whereas human NK cells use only DAP10.[20] Activation of NKG2D using a specific antibody results in enhanced cytotoxicity and cytokine secretion.[33] The ligands of NKG2D are a family of molecules with structural similarity to MHC class I proteins, including MICA/B and ULP1 4 in humans and RAE-1, H60 and MULTI in mice. These ligands represent a diverse array of sequences, yet all bind with high affinity to NKG2D.[34] Interestingly, the MIC family in human is highly polymorphic, suggesting that in this receptor–ligand interaction the diversity comes from the ligands rather than the receptors. Transfection of otherwise resistant tumor cells with NKG2D ligands restores the susceptibility of these cells to NK-cell cytotoxic function. The key to understanding NKG2D function lies in the fact that the ligands are inducible and provide a mechanism for NK cells to detect stressed tissue, such as virally infected or malignant cells,[34] a phenomenon that has been termed 'altered self' (Fig. 18.5).

■ NK RECEPTORS THAT RECOGNIZE NON-MHC-I MOLECULES ■

Beyond the multiple systems of activating and inhibitory receptors they have evolved to recognize MHC class I molecules and their structural variants, NK cells also have several other receptor families that bind nonMHC class I ligands. These include the NKR-P1 family, which is a polymorphic multigene family in rodents consisting of activating (A, C, F) and inhibitory forms (D), but consists of only a single member in humans, whose activity is inhibitory. The ligands for some family members have been recently reported and are themselves lectin family receptors, including clr-b and clr-g in mice and LLT1 in humans. The biological significance of these interactions is still unresolved.[20] Another NK receptor that is conserved between species is CD244 (2B4), a pan-NK cell-expressed molecule whose ligand is CD48. Based on antibody cross-linking studies, human CD244 is designated an activating receptor. However, recent analysis of CD244-deficient mice suggests that the mouse homolog is inhibitory.[20] A number of additional activating receptors exist, including the natural cytotoxicity receptors NKp30, NKp44 and NKp46. NKp30 and NKp46 are broadly expressed on human NK cells, and NKp46 is expressed on all mouse NK cells. NKp44 is specifically expressed on activated human NK cells. These receptors can be activated by antibody cross-linking and, although their ligands are unknown, there is evidence that heparan-sulfate proteoglycans are involved in target recognition. NKp46 binds hemagglutinin on influenza virus-infected cells, and mice deficient for NKp46 have impaired response to influenza infection.[35] Therefore, the natural cytotoxicity receptors are likely to play a critical role in some aspects of NK cell function.

■ NK CELL LICENSING AND SELF-TOLERANCE ■

The plethora of MHC class I-binding inhibitory receptors, as proposed by the missing-self hypothesis, explains the influence of MHC class I on NK-cell lytic function against tumors. However, how self-tolerance is achieved has been less clear. The initial theory to explain self-tolerance was the 'at least one receptor' model, which proposed that NK cells must express at least one self-MHC class I inhibitory receptor. A second model suggested that the receptor repertoire is shaped by selection by the specific MHC haplotype and the presence of self-ligands. The observation that NK cells are not autoreactive in the absence of any inhibitory ligands (MHC class I-deficient mice) and are actually poor killers suggests that the situation is more complex than these models would allow for.[27] A concept termed 'licensing' has been proposed to account for these observations.[36] Under this model, NK cells need to acquire functional competency through binding of at least one inhibitory receptor before they can be activated and display cytotoxic function. This model predicts that there are two types of tolerant NK cell: those that express an inhibitory receptor and are licensed, and those unlicensed NK cells that are functionally incompetent. Data to support this model come from the poor responsiveness of mouse NK cells that do not express any known inhibitory receptor. More definitive support comes from transgenic mice that express only a single MHC class I that is recognized by only a subset of NK cells expressing the inhibitory receptor Ly49C.[36] As predicted by the licensing model, only those NK cells expressing Ly49C are licensed and functionally competent to respond to stimulation. Whether unlicensed NK cells can still have a function is unclear, but inflammatory signals can, at least partially, overcome the defects in unlicensed cells, suggesting that they may play a role in some circumstances, such as viral infection. As these studies were performed in mouse models, another crucial question is whether human NK cells with their similar strategies of receptor expression and function also utilize a licensing process.

■ SPECIFIC NK-CELL FUNCTIONS ■

The increasing ability to separate NK cells from T cells both phenotypically and genetically has greatly enhanced the understanding of NK-cell functions. Although some cytotoxic and immunomodulatory capacities overlap with those of T cells, it is also apparent that some functions of NK cells are unique. Specific examples of NK-cell functions are discussed below.

CONTROL OF VIRAL INFECTIONS

NK cell activity rises early in the course of viral infection, partly driven by the release of IL-12, IL-18 and IFN- α/β, which stimulates activation[28] (Chapter 27). The evidence that NK cells are essential for host defense against viruses comes directly from patients and mice lacking NK-cell function and indirectly from viral strategies to avoid NK-cell recognition. Human patients with selective deficiencies in NK cells show a pronounced susceptibility to recurrent severe infections, especially with HSV and CMV.

A powerful example of the of role NK cell-activating receptors in viral control is NK cell-mediated resistance to MCMV. Mouse strains that lack Ly49H are highly susceptible to MCMV, leading to uncontrolled viral replication and death.[32] Importantly, this protection is mediated by the recognition of the m157 protein of MCMV by Ly49H. As a consequence, whereas in the early stages of MCMV infection the NK-cell response is nonspecific, subsequent control of the virus depends on the proliferation and effector function of the Ly49H+ NK-cell subset in the presence of the activating ligand. The rapid accumulation of Ly49H+ NK cells during MCMV infection is the first example of clonal expansion of NK cells in a manner similar to that of B and T cells.[32]

There is also emerging evidence that NK cells have direct effects on the progression of HIV infection[31] (Chapter 37). NK cells are able to lyze HIV-infected target cells either directly or by ADCC, but despite this ability, NK-cell responses are impaired in HIV-infected patients as infected T-cell blasts selectively downregulate some HLA genes to avoid CTL activity but remain resistant to NK-cell cytotoxicity. NK cells also secrete large quantities of the chemokines CCL3, CCL4 and CCL5, which are the ligands for CCR5 and inhibit CCR5-dependent entry of HIV into target cells. These findings are supported by studies that show that high-risk, but uninfected, individuals appear to have increased NK-cell activity, and that the combination of the expression of HLA-Bw4 and the KIR3DS1 gene is associated with delayed progression to AIDS.[31] Finally, HIV viraemia induces several functional abnormalities on NK cells, suggesting that this complex virus and NK cells interact at multiple levels.

CONTROL OF MALIGNANT CELLS

A function for NK cells in protective tumor immune surveillance, although hypothesized many years ago, is still uncertain. One limitation in testing this hypothesis has been the lack of a mouse model that is NK-cell deficient but has an otherwise competent immune system.[28] There is good evidence that NK cells can reject tumor cells in animal models, and that the administration of several cytokines that enhance NK-cell function, including IL-2, IL-12 and IL-21, or those that induce IFN-α production, are protective against metastasis.[37] In light of this, there have been many clinical trials to assess either cytokine treatment or the injection of *ex vivo* treated NK cells (Chapter 94). Unfortunately, the high doses of IL-2 required for efficacy are relatively toxic, and transferred NK cells have proved difficult to target to tumors.[28] Despite this, some successes have been demonstrated for melanoma, lung and hepatic cancers. Current trials are now testing combination therapies such as low dose IL-2 and IL-12 or IFN-α.

ROLE OF NK CELLS IN HEMATOPOIETIC STEM CELL TRANSPLANTATION

NK cells in an F_1 offspring of two mouse strains can reject parental bone marrow, a process termed 'hybrid resistance.' This is in contrast to organ grafts from the same mice that are tolerated by CTL owing to their expression of MHC class I molecules from each parent. This phenomenon has recently been found to be mediated by the interaction of host NKG2D and its ligands, RAE-1, on the repopulating bone marrow cells, as treatment with a neutralizing antibody to NKG2D prevented hybrid resistance.[33] These studies raise the possibility that other stem cells or tissues upregulate the expression of NKG2D ligands after transplantation, and that NKG2D may contribute to some graft rejection in immunocompetent hosts.

In humans, allogeneic bone marrow transplantation cures leukemia through the reaction of donor CTL in the graft against the residual leukemic cells. These transferred T cells also mediate graft-versus-host disease (GvHD). The need to prevent this response by strong immunosuppression is the major cause of transplantation failure, due to infection and cancer relapse (Chapter 82). It has been proposed that transplantation with a haploidentical donor (identical at one HLA haplotype and fully mismatched on the other, for example a parent) provides allogeneic NK cells with an HLA haplotype that supplies more KIR ligand than a matched recipient would provide. Hence it would yield a stronger graft-versus-leukemia effect.[38] Indeed, mice treated with alloreactive NK cells tolerate 30 times the lethal dose of mismatched bone marrow cells without developing GvHD, and alloreactive NK cells eradicated human acute myeloid leukemia (AML) transplanted into NOD/SCID mice.[38] Retrospective studies on AML patients that received haploidentical grafts revealed that transplants with alloreactive NK cells showed better engraftment and GvHD protection, and less relapse.[38] The benefit of this protocol is still controversial, as some studies have observed similar effects whereas others have found that KIR ligand mismatch was associated with reduced overall survival.[30] The discrepancy may be due to lack of functional assessment of NK-cell alloreactivity, different transplantation

---

| CLINICAL PEARLS

EXPLOITING NK CELLS IN LEUKEMIA THERAPY

>> Hematopoietic stem cell transplantation requires donor and recipient HLA matching to reduce graft-versus-host disease (GvHD) mediated by transplanted CTL.

>> Haploidentical donors and recipients (those that share only one HLA haplotype) represent 50% of unrelated transplants and undergo a stronger conditioning regimen to avoid GvHD.

>> Alloreactive NK cells are present after haploidentical transplant and provide a potent graft-versus-leukemia (GvL) effect in animal models.

>> Retrospective studies in AML patients show that haploidentical transplantation with alloreactive NK cells have enhanced long-term survival and decreased relapse rates.

>> Transplantation from NK cell-alloreactive donors controls AML relapse and improves engraftment without causing GvHD.

methods, or the genetic backgrounds of the patients and donors, and thus requires further studies.

NK CELLS AND PREGNANCY ■

During pregnancy, maternal (self) and paternal (nonself) antigens are expressed in the embryo and placenta. The reasons why the maternal immune system temporarily tolerates the fetus remain poorly understood. Interestingly, the majority of leukocytes present at the site of implantation are a distinct subset of NK cells known as uterine NK (uNK) cells. Mice deficient in uNK cells show some changes in decidual blood vessels and reduced fertility, supporting a role for these cells, but how they function is unclear.[39] uNK cells have low cytotoxic activity and, in addition to IFN-γ and TNF, secrete angiogenic factors such as vascular endothelial growth factor (VEGF-C) and angiopoietin-2.[39] This suggests that uNK cells can influence maternal arterial integrity and trophoblast invasion.

uNK cells can recognize HLA-C/E/G on paternal trophoblasts. Recently, it has been found that KIR expression on maternal uNK cells is a key factor in the development of pre-eclampsia (a serious complication of pregnancy in which the fetus receives an inadequate supply of blood due to failure of trophoblast invasion).[40] Mothers lacking most activating KIR when the fetus possessed HLA-C2 are at a greatly increased risk of pre-eclampsia. Thus, the maternal KIR and trophoblast interaction appears to play a positive physiological role related to placental development, suggesting that too great an inhibition of uNK cells is detrimental to the process.[40] This has clearly been selected against, as human populations have a reciprocal relationship between certain KIR haplotypes and HLA-C2 frequency.

INTERACTIONS OF CTL AND NK CELLS IN THE IMMUNE RESPONSE ■

Although studies of CTL and NK cells in isolation have greatly advanced our understanding of their functions, it is obvious that these immune cells function in a system that depends on numerous interactions between the various cell types at multiple levels (Chapter 2). In the case of cytotoxic cells, these immunomodulatory interactions are becoming increasingly appreciated (Fig. 18.2). In particular, it has become apparent that NK cells and DC interact specifically to promote outcomes such as the maturation of NK cells.[26] CTL activation by mature DC is influenced directly by NK cell-derived IFN-γ, and indirectly through the role of NK cells in promoting a Th1 response in CD4 T cells (Chapter 17).

Increasing evidence has emerged to implicate DC-NK cell cross-talk in various aspects of the immune response. DC produce a variety of cytokines that modulate NK-cell behavior, including IL-12, IL-15, IL-18 and IFN-α.[26] Interestingly, the outcome of these interactions for the DC depends on its maturity, with immature DC being killed by NK cells whereas mature DC are resistant to lysis. The interactions of mature DC and NK cells would be expected to occur at the site of infection, where DC provide inflammatory stimuli for NK cells. The other site of encounter is the lymph node, where, during an immune reaction, NK cells are recruited by chemokines and interact with mature DC and CD4 T cells to induce a Th1 response. This process requires IFN-γ production from NK cells[41] (Fig. 18.2).

NK-cell and CTL interactions are also important in generating an immune response to tumors that are, in general, poorly immunogenic. DC that are matured *in vitro* by NK cells show strongly enhanced ability to induce Th1 and CTL responses, including cytokine secretion. IFN-γ in particular is very important in the rejection of primary tumors and the formation of CTL memory to tumors. It is also likely that killing by NK cells and CTL provides DC with increased access to tumor antigens and promotes further adaptive immunity. Using DC to harness the helper function of NK cells as well as the cytotoxic functions of both CTL and NK cells offers therapeutic promise and is currently being tested in a variety of cancers.[26]

■ EVASION OF THE CYTOTOXIC RESPONSE ■

VIRUSES

As one principal function of CTL and NK cells is the control of viral infections, it is not surprising that viruses have evolved a number of strategies to interfere with the host response (Chapter 27). The multiplicity of these evasion strategies indicates that this is an essential step for long-term viral persistence.

These strategies include:

- *Latency*. This involves minimizing viral gene expression and thereby avoiding detection. Examples include HSV in neurons, HIV in T cells, and EBV in B cells.

- *Antigenic variation*. The virus possesses the ability to rapidly mutate its genome and produce escape variants that are no longer visible to CTL. Such mutations were shown for LCMV in mouse and HIV infection in humans.

- *Infection of immune nonaccessible sites*. Such inaccessible sites include infection of the CNS by HSV or rubella.

- *Production of viral defense molecules (immunoevasins)*. Many viruses, including adenovirus and EBV, interfere with cytotoxic activity by producing proteins that either hinder Fas or TNF-mediated killing or inhibit the function of antiviral cytokines such as IFN-α/β. A number of viruses, including EBV, produce homologs of anti-apoptotic molecules, such as Bcl2, to inhibit killing by CTL. Various members of the pox virus family have evolved homologs of the naturally occurring IL-18-binding protein that inhibits IL-18 activity and NK-cell function.[42]

- *Modulation of molecules involved in recognition*. A widely utilized viral strategy to evade the cytotoxic response is to interfere with antigen processing, presentation, or the expression of other molecules required for CTL recognition[43] (Chapters 6 and 7). Several viruses, including adenovirus, downregulate MHC class I expression on the cell surface. This can be achieved by a number of mechanisms. For example, adenovirus type 2 E3 protein forms a complex with MHC class I to prevent antigens from being processed; MCMV gpm152 protein causes retention of the MHC class I molecules in the Golgi compartment; and CMV proteins US2 and US11 promote the rapid degradation of newly synthesized MHC class I complexes. An alternative approach is to interfere with antigen presentation, either inhibiting the expression of the TAP protein, as is the case for HSV, or producing proteins that are resistant to antigen processing by

Host defenses at mucosal surfaces

19

Kohtaro Fujihashi, Prosper N. Boyaka,
Jerry R. McGhee

Mammals have evolved a sophisticated network of cells and molecules that serve to maintain homeostasis on exposed mucosal surfaces. It is noteworthy that this system, termed mucosa-associated lymphoreticular tissue (MALT), is anatomically and functionally distinct from its blood-borne counterpart and is strategically located at the portals by which most microorganisms enter the body. The development of this specific branch of the immune system alongside and separate from the peripheral immune system may have been necessitated by the size of the mucosal surfaces, which cover an area of ~400 m[2] in the adult human, as well as the large number of exogenous antigens to which these surfaces are exposed.

■ THE INNATE MUCOSAL DEFENSE SYSTEM ■

The innate defense of the mucosa includes the physical barrier provided by epithelial cells, the movement of the epithelial cilia, the production of mucus by goblet cells, the secretion of molecules with innate antibacterial activity, and the cytolytic activity of NK cells (Fig. 19.1). These innate mechanisms provide a first line of defense against exogenous antigens and invading pathogens.

PHYSICAL BARRIER PROVIDED BY EPITHELIAL CELLS

Mucosal surfaces are covered by a layer of epithelial cells that prevent the entry of exogenous antigens into the host while permitting the absorption of nutrients.[1] In the gastrointestinal (GI) tract, the barrier effect of tightly joined epithelial cells, termed enterocytes, is facilitated by the blanket of mucus that covers these cells. Mucus is secreted by goblet cells and consists of glycoproteins of various molecular sizes that tend to interfere with the attachment of microorganisms. Damaged or infected enterocytes are replaced by crypt epithelial cells, which differentiate into enterocytes as they migrate towards the desquamation zone at the villus tip. Multilayered squamous epithelial cells cover the epithelia of other mucosal surfaces, including the oral cavity, the pharynx, the tonsils, the urethra and the vagina. These epithelia lack tight junctions. They secrete a glycoprotein mucus that coats the intercellular space between the lower stratified layers. Additional barrier effects are provided by secretory IgA (SIgA), and by the renewal of exposed epithelial cell layers by cells from subjacent layers.

DEFENSINS AND OTHER MUCOSAL ANTIMICROBIAL PEPTIDES

Cells of the epithelium produce antimicrobial β-sheet proteins termed defensins, that range between 30 and 40 amino acids in length and which exhibit antimicrobial effects similar to those of antibiotics. Based upon their structure, defensins can be grouped into two distinct categories, α and β. α-defensins, which contain two contiguous cysteine residues, are smaller than β-defensins, whose cysteine residues are separated by six amino acids. In the crypt regions of villi, Paneth cells produce α-defensin granules that can be secreted into the lumen of the small intestine. α-defensins are also secreted by tracheal epithelial cells. They are homologous to peptides that function as mediators of nonoxidative microbial cell killing in neutrophils (termed human neutrophil peptides, or HNPs).[2] β-defensins, such as human β-defensin 1 (HBD-1), are expressed in the epithelial cells of the oral mucosa, trachea, bronchi, mammary glands, and salivary glands. The activity of mucosal defensins also applies to viruses. Although mechanisms that control the activation of defensins are poorly understood, inflammatory cytokines such as interleukin-1 (IL-1), tumor necrosis factor-α (TNF-α) and bacterial lipopolysaccharide (LPS) play a role in their induction.

Other potent antimicrobial products of the epithelium include lactoferrin, lysozyme, the peroxidases, secretory phospholipase A2, and cathelin-associated peptides. Some are secreted by intestinal Paneth cells, and all are produced by polymorphonuclear neutrophils (PMNs). Lactoferrin, a member of the transferrin family, is found in exocrine secretions such as milk. High concentrations of lysozyme (1209–1325 μg/mL) are found in tears and other secretions, such as saliva, colostrum, serum and urine.

Human milk contains lysozyme in concentrations ranging from 20 to 245 μg/mL, depending on the lactation period. It also contains at least two peroxidases. Milk leukocytes produce myeloperoxidase (MPO) and mammary gland cells produce human lactoperoxidase (hLPO). Both peroxidases display properties similar to those of human salivary peroxidases (hSPO). Secretory phospholipase A2 (S-PLA2) is released by Paneth cells upon exposure to cholinergic agonists, bacteria or LPS. Secretory leukocyte protease inhibitor (SLPI) is found in human saliva, nasal secretions, tears, cervical mucus and seminal fluid. It is believed to be responsible for the anti-HIV properties of external secretions.

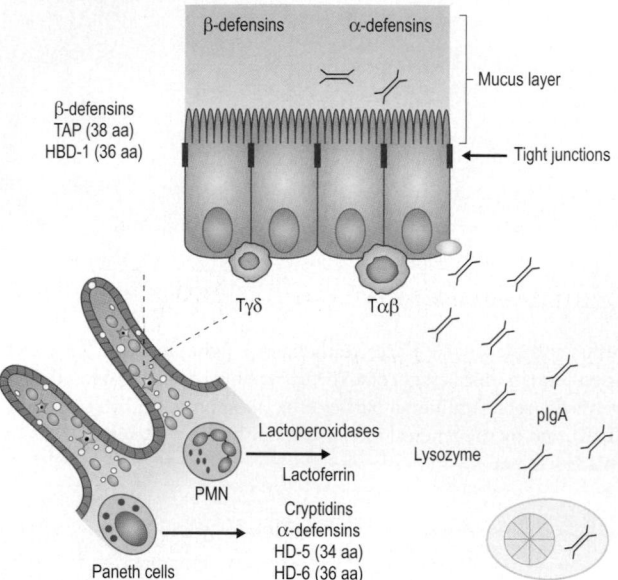

Fig. 19.1 Innate mucosal host defense factors. A thick coat of mucus prevents penetration of macromolecules and potential pathogens. The epithelial cell barrier is connected via tight junctions and contains both αβ and γδ intraepithelial lymphocytes (IELs). The crypt regions contain Paneth cells, which produce cryptins (α-defensins). The β-defensins are products of epithelial cells and form a defensin network. Other innate factors, such as lysozyme, lactoperoxidase, lactoferrin and phospholipases, also serve in antimicrobial defense.

KEY CONCEPTS

INNATE DEFENSES OF THE MUCOSAL IMMUNE SYSTEM

The innate defenses of the mucosal immune system provide a first line of defense against exogenous antigens and invading pathogens. These defenses include:

>> Physical barriers: the epithelium, the epithelial cilia, goblet cell mucus production

>> Mucosal antibacterial molecules: Paneth cell production of α-defensins in the small intestine; epithelial cell production of β-defensins in the oral mucosa, trachea, bronchi, mammary glands and salivary glands; lactoferrin, lysozyme, lactoperoxidase, and secretory leukocyte protease inhibitor (SLPI)

>> Cellular innate immunity: mucosal natural killer (NK) cells

---

MUCOSAL NATURAL KILLER CELLS

Natural killer (NK) cells are found in both the lamina propria and the intraepithelial compartment, where they appear as large granular lymphocytes. Nonspecific recruitment of cytotoxic effector cells into the intestinal mucosa occurs in either antigen-primed or virus-infected mice. As NK cells secrete IFN-γ and IL-4 after infection, they may influence the development of effector T cells as well (Chapter 18).

◼ A COMMON MUCOSAL IMMUNE SYSTEM ◼

Higher mammals have developed an organized secondary lymphoid tissue system in the GI and upper respiratory tracts. The gut-associated lymphoreticular tissues (GALT) include Peyer's patches (PPs), the appendix, and solitary lymphoid nodules in the GI tract. The tonsils and adenoids comprise the nasal-associated lymphoreticular tissues (NALT). Experimental animals such as rabbits, rats and guinea pigs exhibit organized bronchus-associated lymphoreticular tissues (BALT) that rarely occur in human airway branches.[1] Together, GALT and NALT in healthy humans, and GALT, BALT and NALT in experimental species, are termed mucosa-associated lymphoreticular tissue, or MALT.

The vast areas of the mucosal immune system characterized by diffuse collections of lymphoid cells are termed the effector tissues. These include the interstitial tissues of the mammary, lacrimal, salivary, sweat and all other exocrine glands, as well as the lamina propria and the epithelium of the GI tract. The lamina propria areas of the upper respiratory and genitourinary tracts are also lymphoid effector sites. MALT is connected with effector sites through the migratory patterns of lymphoid cells.

KEY CONCEPTS

THE COMMON MUCOSAL IMMUNE SYSTEM

The mucosa-associated lymphoreticular tissues (MALT) comprise discrete and diffuse collections of lymphoid tissues that share distinctive features, including a unique type of epithelium, a distinct architecture, a unique set of antigen-presenting cells (APCs), and B cells where switching to IgA predominates. The involved tissues include:

>> The gut-associated lymphoreticular tissues (GALT): Peyer's patches, the appendix, and solitary lymphoid nodules in the GI tract

>> The nasal-associated lymphoreticular tissues (NALT): the tonsils and adenoids

>> The effector tissues: the interstitial tissues of the mammary, lacrimal, salivary, sweat and all other exocrine glands; the lamina propria and the epithelium of the GI tract; and the lamina propria areas of the upper respiratory and genitourinary tracts

MALT AS AN INDUCTIVE SITE

MALT differs from systemic lymphoid tissues owing to the presence of a unique type of epithelium for antigen uptake. Its features include a characteristic architecture; antigen-presenting cells (APCs), such as dendritic cells that differ from APCs in spleen; and B-cell areas with germinal centers where switches of IgM to IgA bearing B cells predominate. The columnar epithelium that covers MALT is infiltrated with lymphocytes and APCs, leading to the term follicle-associated epithelium (FAE). Lacking goblet cells, the FAE is covered with far less mucus than normal enterocytes. Soluble and particulate luminal antigens are taken up by microfold (M) cells and are delivered to adjacent APCs. M cells have been described in PPs, the appendix and tonsils, and represent 10–15% of cells within the FAE.[3] M cells are also found in isolated lymphoid follicles (ILFs) and at the tips of the villus, where they are termed villous M cells.[4] The microvilli of these cells, which are less dense than those of adjacent enterocytes (Fig. 19.2), offer a portal of entry into the MALT. The M cell is often identified by an invagination of the basolateral membrane into a 'pocket' normally occupied by lymphocytes and APCs (Fig. 19.3).

M cells appear ideal for antigen uptake owing to a well developed microvesicle system that contains endosomes. However, it remains unclear whether M cells act as classic APCs. M cells also provide a portal of entry for some invasive pathogens, such as invasive strains of *Salmonella typhimurium*, but not for noninvasive strains of *S. typhimurium* and reoviruses.

GUT-ASSOCIATED LYMPHORETICULAR TISSUES (GALT)

Each PP contains a dome region that is positioned under the FAE. This dome region is populated by T cells, B cells, macrophages (Mφ) and dendritic cells (DC), and include follicles that contain germinal centers. The presence of all three major APC types in the dome, i.e., memory B cells, Mφ and DCs, makes it likely that antigen uptake occurs immediately after release from M cells (Fig. 19.4A). M cell pockets in Peyer's patches contain approximately equal numbers of T and B cells, but fewer macrophages. Approximately 75% of the T cells are T helper (Th) cells.

GALT B cell follicles differ from those in peripheral lymph nodes and spleen in that they are enriched for IgA-bearing B cells.[1] Thus, germinal centers in MALT are thought to be the major sites for B cell μ to α switching (Chapters 4 and 8). The interfollicular regions of PPs contain the high endothelial venules (HEVs), which represent the major point of entry for T and B cells, as well as an interdigitating network of dendritic cells and mature T cells. Both CD4 and CD8 TCRαβ T cells are found in these interfollicular regions, with CD4 cells representing the predominant phenotype. Both naïve and memory T cells are present in PPs, with one-third in cell cycle (Fig. 19.4, Table 19.1).

The structurally and functionally related cytokines, lymphotoxin-α (LT-α), lymphotoxin-β (LT-β), and TNF-α (Chapter 10), are critical for lymphoid organogenesis. LT-α-/- mice are markedly deficient in secondary lymph nodes,[5] whereas LT-β-/- mice have mesenteric and cervical lymph nodes, but lack peripheral lymph nodes and PPs. TNF-RI-/- mice are characterized by an absent or abnormal PP structure, whereas TNF-α-/- mice exhibit normal patches.[5] In humans, PPs develop during prenatal life, a situation also seen in sheep, pigs, dogs, and horses. ILF formation occurs postnatally in response to luminal stimuli, including the normal bacterial flora.[6] Mature ILFs contain mostly conventional B cells and small numbers of CD4 T cells.[6]

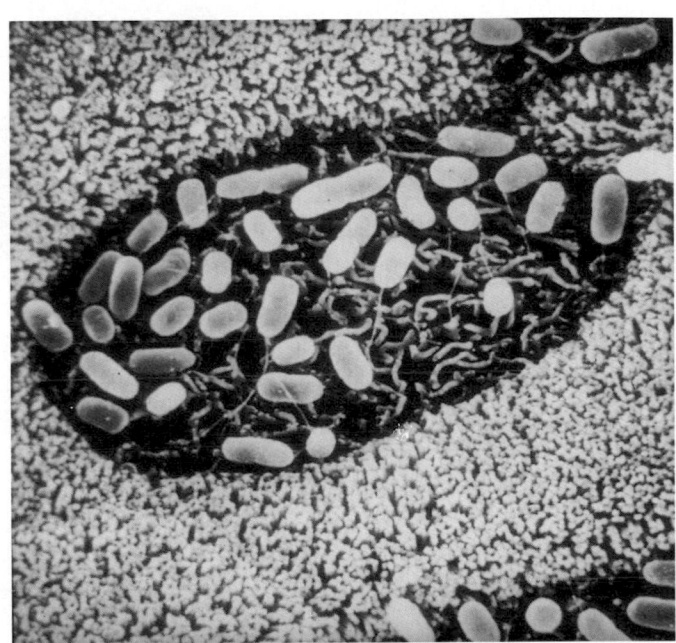

Fig. 19.2 The microfold (M) cell. A scanning electron micrograph of an M cell with adjacent enterocytes. The M cell has selectively bound *E. coli* 0157. Note that a thick brush border is lacking, facilitating the binding and uptake of microparticles. (Courtesy of Dr Tatsuo Yamamoto, Niigata University.)

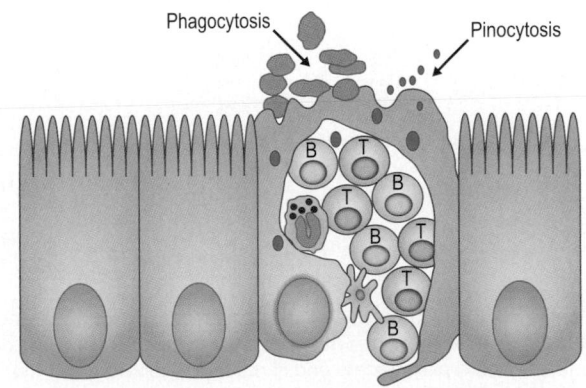

Fig. 19.3 Microanatomical features of M cells. The M cell forms a 'pocket' containing memory lymphocytes. It actively pinocytoses soluble antigens and phagocytoses particulates such as viruses, bacteria and microspheres. (Courtesy of Dr Svein Steinsvoll, University of Oslo.)

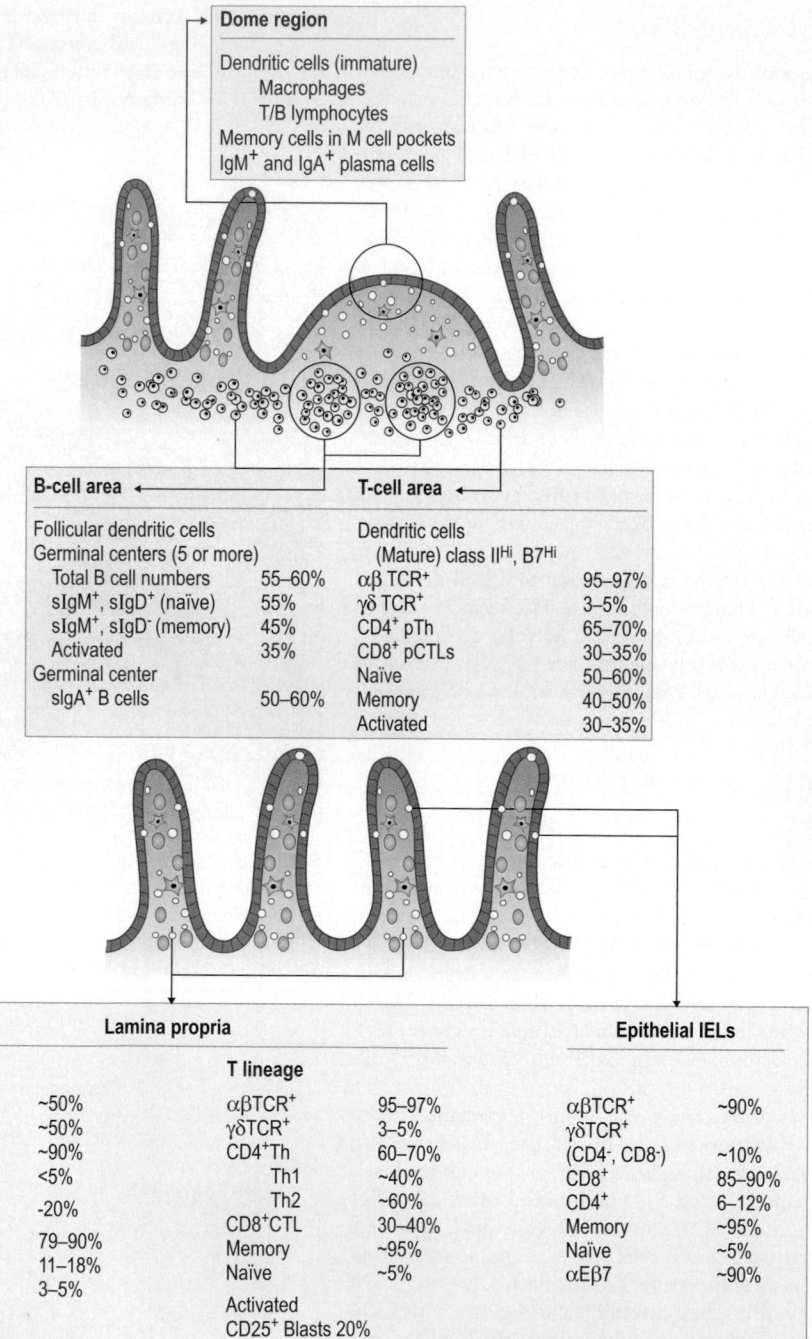

Dome region

Dendritic cells (immature)
Macrophages
T/B lymphocytes
Memory cells in M cell pockets
IgM⁺ and IgA⁺ plasma cells

B-cell area		T-cell area	
Follicular dendritic cells		Dendritic cells	
Germinal centers (5 or more)		(Mature) class II^Hi, B7^Hi	
Total B cell numbers	55–60%	αβ TCR⁺	95–97%
sIgM⁺, sIgD⁺ (naïve)	55%	γδ TCR⁺	3–5%
sIgM⁺, sIgD⁻ (memory)	45%	CD4⁺ pTh	65–70%
Activated	35%	CD8⁺ pCTLs	30–35%
Germinal center		Naïve	50–60%
sIgA⁺ B cells	50–60%	Memory	40–50%
		Activated	30–35%

Lamina propria				Epithelial IELs	
B lineage		**T lineage**			
CD5⁺	~50%	αβTCR⁺	95–97%	αβTCR⁺	~90%
CD5⁻	~50%	γδTCR⁺	3–5%	γδTCR⁺	
Memory	~90%	CD4⁺Th	60–70%	(CD4⁻, CD8⁻)	~10%
Naïve	<5%	Th1	~40%	CD8⁺	85–90%
		Th2	~60%	CD4⁺	6–12%
Plasma cells	-20%	CD8⁺CTL	30–40%	Memory	~95%
IgA⁺	79–90%	Memory	~95%	Naïve	~5%
IgM⁺	11–18%	Naïve	~5%	αEβ7	~90%
IgG⁺	3–5%	Activated			
		CD25⁺ Blasts	20%		

Fig. 19.4 Structural features and cellular components of gut-associated lymphoreticular tissues (GALT). (**A**) The dome region is covered by the follicle-associated epithelium (FAE) with its characteristic microfold or M cells. Major features of the dome include M cells with lymphocyte pockets, scattered plasma cells and immature dendritic cells (DCs). The B-cell area contains five or more germinal centers with high frequencies of surface IgA⁺ B cells. The adjacent T-cell area contains mature interdigitating DCs and precursors of CD4 Th and CD8 CTLs. (**B**) Structural features and cellular characteristics of mucosal effector sites. The lamina propria is equally populated by B1 and B2 cells, both of which differentiate into IgA⁺ plasma cells. Note that memory B and T lymphocytes are also both present in this compartment. Although intraepithelial lymphocytes (IELs) in human are mainly TCRαβ⁺, significant numbers of TCRγδ⁺ T cells are also found in this compartment.

Table 19.1 Major T-cell subpopulations associated with Peyer's patches

T-cell phenotype	Percentage of total T cells
CD3 $\alpha\beta$ TCR	95–97
CD3+ $\gamma\delta$ TCR+	3–5
CD3+, CD4+ (precursors of Th)	65–70
CD3+, CD8+ (precursors of CTLs)	30–35
Naïve (CD45RBHi)	50–60
Memory (RBLo, ROHi)	40–50
Blasts (in cell cycle)	30–35

NASAL-ASSOCIATED LYMPHORETICULAR TISSUES (NALT)

Strategically positioned at the entry of the respiratory as well as the digestive tracts are the accumulations of lymphoid tissues that comprise the palatine, lingual and nasopharyngeal tonsils, which collectively form Waldeyer's ring. These tissues resemble both lymph nodes and PPs, including an FAE with M cells in the tonsillar crypts that is essential for selective antigen uptake (Fig. 19.3). Germinal centers containing B and T cells, plasma cells and professional APCs are also present. Tonsillar tissues may serve as a source of IgA plasma cell precursors found in the upper aerodigestive tracts, as well as an inductive site for more generalized mucosal and systemic immune responses.[7] Induction through the nasal cavity may well exceed that induced by oral immunization. When viral and bacterial antigens are introduced into the nasal cavity, usually along with mucosal adjuvants such as cholera toxin (CT) and/or its B subunit (CT-B), optimal immune responses are induced in external secretions, such as saliva and, surprisingly, in secretions of the female genital tract.[1]

The $LT\alpha_1\beta_2$ signaling pathway appears to be essential for the maintenance, but not the initiation, of NALT organogenesis.[4] Thus, despite reductions in the size and the numbers of DCs and FDCs present, the NALT was still detected in LT-$\alpha^{-/-}$ and LT-$\beta^{-/-}$ mice, although the size of this tissue was reduced. Newborn mice did not contain any NALT structure in the nasal cavity, demonstrating that NALT develops postnatally. Signaling via the IL-7/IL-7R and the L-selectin/PNAd adhesion molecules plays an important part in the organization of NALT.[4] Thus cytokine signaling cascades, and in particular the $LT\alpha_1\beta_2$-LTβR signaling pathway, are essential for the maintenance of NALT architecture.

OTHER POTENTIAL SITES FOR MUCOSAL INDUCTION OF AN IMMUNE RESPONSE

The follicular structures analogous to PPs found in the large intestine and especially in the rectum, which are known as rectal-associated lymphoreticular tissues (RALT), are another IgA-inductive site and a source of IgA plasma cell precursors. Unlike most other mucosal tissues, the lamina propria of the large intestine is characterized by a predominance of IgA2- versus IgA1- producing cells.[1] This preference for IgA2 also occurs in the female genital mucosal tissues (e.g., uterus, cervix, fallopian tubes and vagina), suggesting lymphoid trafficking between these tissues. Indeed, intrarectal immunization of Rhesus macaques with simian immunodeficiency virus (SIV) induced both T- and B-cell-mediated immune responses, including

the induction of anti-SIV Abs in rectal washes and in genital secretions.[8] Rectal immunization with a bacterial vaccine (*Salmonella typhi* Ty21a) was shown to induce specific Abs not only at the site of immunization, but also in saliva, suggesting even more extensive trafficking.[9]

LYMPHOCYTE HOMING INTO MUCOSAL COMPARTMENTS

There is a direct route for B-cell migration between PPs and GI lamina propria (Fig. 19.4B). Indeed, the mesenteric lymph nodes of orally immunized animals can repopulate the lamina propria of gut, mammary glands, lacrimal glands, and salivary glands with antigen-specific IgA plasma cells (Fig. 19.4B),[1] pointing to the existence of a 'common' mucosal immune system. This concept has undergone further refinement, as studies now show that the migration of cells into and from NALT adheres to rules different from those for cell migration into and from GALT and the GI tract.

LYMPHOCYTE HOMING IN THE GI TRACT

Naïve lymphocytes enter mucosal or systemic lymphoid tissues from the blood through specialized high endothelial venules (HEV), which consist of cuboidal endothelial cells (Fig. 19.5A). In GALT, HEV are present in the interfollicular zones, which are rich in T cells.[10] In effector sites such as the lamina propria of the GI tract, the endothelial venules are less pronounced and tend to occur near villus crypt regions (Fig. 19.5B). Mucosal addressin cell adhesion molecule-1 (MAdCAM-1) is the most important addressin expressed by PP HEV or lamina propria venules (LPV) (Chapter 12). Peripheral lymph node addressin (PNAd) and vascular cell adhesion molecule (VCAM-1) are the principal addressins expressed by peripheral lymph node and skin HEV, respectively.

The major homing receptors expressed by lymphocytes are the integrins, a large class of molecules characterized by a heterodimeric structure of α and β chains (Chapter 12). In general, the type of homing receptor is determined by the integrin expressed with the α_4 chain; the β_1-integrin characterizes the homing receptor for the skin, whereas the β_7-integrin characterizes the receptor for the gut. The pairing of α_4 with β_7 is thus responsible for lymphocyte binding to the MAdCAM-1 that is expressed on HEVs in PPs and GI tract LPVs (Fig. 19.5).[11]

The C-type lectins L-, E- and P-selectin (Chapter 12) also serve as homing receptors. L-selectin has a high affinity for carbohydrate-decorated

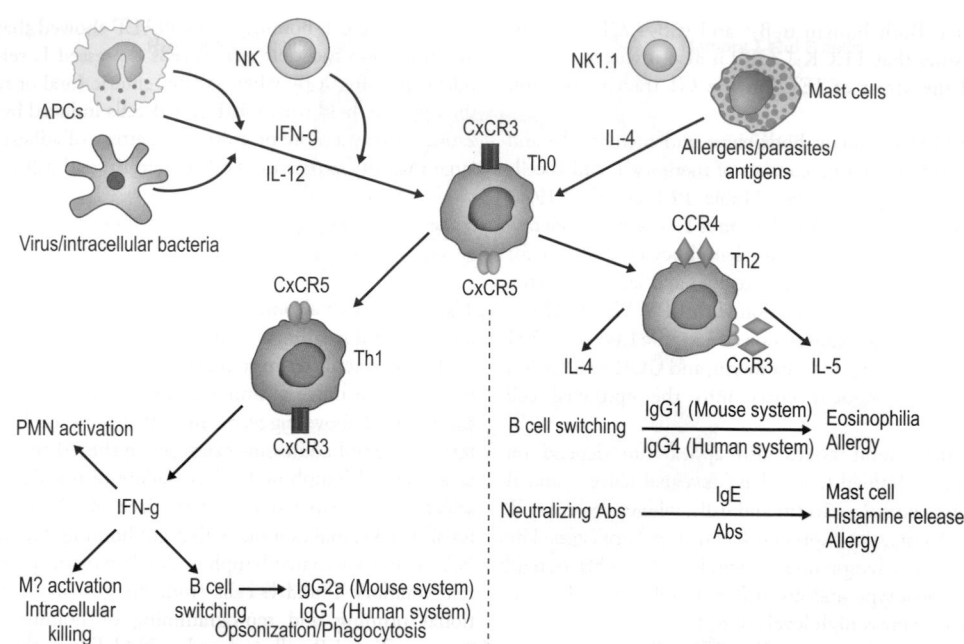

Fig. 19.6 T-helper cell subset development. The cellular and cytokine environment induces Th0 cells to develop into either Th1 or Th2 subsets. APCs produce IL-12 in response to microbial assault and, together with IFN-γ produced by NK cells, induce mature Th1 cells. Th1 cells express select chemokine receptors and, through IFN-γ synthesis, activate Mφ and induce B cells to produce opsonizing Abs. Other cells, such as NK1.1 and mast cells, respond to antigen/allergen with IL-4, which induces Th0 to Th2 switching. Th2 cells produce IL-4, IL-5, IL-6, IL-10, IL-9 and IL-13, which help regulate mucosal S-IgA Ab responses.

T-cell interfollicular areas where maturation occurs (Fig. 19.4A). DCs are also found in NALT such as human tonsils and lung, where they play the same role as in the GALT.

Intestinal epithelial cells (IECs) express MHC class II molecules and present peptides to primed CD4 and CD8 T cells. However, it is still unclear whether IECs can process antigen or if the MHC class II molecules on these cells only serve as receptors for predigested peptides that result from enzymatic lysis in the stomach. Human and murine IECs also express CD1d, a nonclassic MHC class I molecule that is also found on DCs and Mφ and which appears to be involved in the presentation of lipid and glycolipid antigens.

CD4 TH CELL SUBSETS IN MUCOSAL IMMUNITY

Th cell subsets are classified as either Th1 or Th2 according to the pattern of cytokines produced (Chapter 17). Th1 cells selectively produce IL-2, IFN-γ, LT-α, LT-β and TNF-α, whereas Th2 cells produce IL-4, IL-5, IL-6, IL-9, IL-10 and IL-13 (Fig. 19.6). The recently described Th17 produce IL-17, both Th1 and Th2 cells develop from naïve CD4 T cells through the same T-cell precursor (Th0) phase (Chapter 9). IL-2 is produced by Th0 cells upon antigen exposure and serves as an important growth factor. IL-12 induces NK cells to produce IFN-γ which, together with IL-12, triggers Th0 cells to differentiate along the Th1 pathway. Murine Th1-type responses are associated with the development of cell-mediated immunity, as manifested by delayed-type hypersensitivity (DTH) and by B-cell responses with a characteristic IgG Ab subclass (IgG2a) pattern. The Th2 cell subset is an effective

helper phenotype for supporting the production of the IgA isotype, in addition to IgG1, IgG2b and IgE responses in the mouse system. IFN-γ produced by Th1 cells inhibits both Th2 cell proliferation and B-cell isotype switching stimulated by IL-4. Likewise, Th2 cells regulate Th1 cell effects by secreting IL-10, which inhibits IFN-γ secretion by Th1 cells. This decreased IFN-γ production allows the development of Th2-type cells.

It is now accepted that polarized T-cell responses occur in humans as well. Thus, human Th1 and Th2 cells reciprocally regulate the development of the opposite subset through IFN-γ and IL-4 secretion, respectively (Fig. 19.6). Antigen-specific IgG subclass responses in patients with Lyme borreliosis, a pathology known to induce Th1 cells and strong IFN-γ responses, consisted of IgG1 and IgG3 C-fixing Abs with low IgG2 and undetectable IgG4 Ab levels.[18] Despite the differences between murine and human systems, these observations suggest that IL-4 and IFN-γ control respectively IgG1 and IgG2a in the mouse, and IgG4 and IgG1 subclasses in humans in an analogous manner (Fig. 19.6).

Adhesion molecules and chemokines also provide distinct address codes for the migration of Th1 and Th2 cells to different sites. Th1 cells express functional ligands for E- and P-selectins that allow these cells to migrate to sites of inflammation.[19] *In vitro*, Th1 and Th2 cells also express distinct patterns of chemokine receptors (Chapter 11). CCR5 and the CXC chemokine receptors CXCR3 and CXCR5 are preferentially expressed by Th1 cell clones, whereas CCR4, and to a lesser extent CCR3, are expressed by Th2 clones (Fig. 19.6).

CYTOKINES IN MUCOSAL IMMUNITY

B-cell isotype switching

Isotype switching is preceded by transcriptional activation of the isotype in question (Chapter 4). Two major cytokines, IL-4 and TGF-β, induce surface IgM-positive (sIgM[+]) B cells to switch to downstream isotypes, including IgE and IgA (Fig. 19.7). The addition of TGF-β1 to LPS-triggered mouse B-cell cultures can lead to increased IgA synthesis, an effect that can be enhanced by IL-2 or IL-5. TGF-β1 can also induce sIgM[+] to sIgA[+] B-cell switches. Anti-CD40 stimulation of tonsillar B cells, together with TGF-β1 in the presence of IL-10, further stimulates IgA synthesis.[1] Cα1 transcripts can also be induced by B-cell mitogen plus TGF-β, and Cα2 transcripts can be induced by TGF-β together with IL-10, perhaps implying that switches to IgA2 are more T cell- and Th2-cytokine dependent. TGF-β1 gene knockout (TGF-β1−/−) mice exhibit low levels of IgA plasma cells in effector sites and of S-IgA in external secretions,[1] providing further evidence that TGF-β1 can be an important factor in μ to α switching (Fig. 19.7).

IgA plasma cell differentiation

Two Th2 cytokines, IL-5 and IL-6, are of particular importance for inducing sIgA[+] B cells to differentiate into IgA-producing plasma cells.[20] In this regard, IL-6 induced strikingly high IgA responses in vitro in both murine and human systems.

■ VACCINE DEVELOPMENT AND MUCOSAL IMMUNE RESPONSES ■

Mucosal immune responses include a major B-cell component that is characterized by secretory IgA (S-IgA) Ab, as well as Th cell and CTL responses. These responses can be induced by pathogens triggering the organized mucosal inductive sites. Effective protection against strong mucosal pathogens requires prophylactic immune responses that can be achieved by mucosal vaccines. In contrast to systemic vaccines, those administered via mucosal routes can trigger both mucosal immune responses as a first line of defense at the portal of pathogen entry, and systemic immune responses that neutralize pathogens that have penetrated that barrier. Because it is now well accepted that Th1-type responses result in B- and T-cell responses distinct from those induced by Th2-type cells, mucosal adjuvants, vectors and delivery systems are being developed for vaccines that can specifically induce Th1- or Th2-type responses.

HELPER T-CELL SUBSETS IN MUCOSAL IMMUNE RESPONSES TO VACCINES

Two classes of mucosal vaccine delivery system have helped to define the role of mucosal adjuvants and recombinant vectors for the induction of Th cell subsets that support mucosal S-IgA and serum Ab responses. In mouse, the mucosal adjuvant cholera toxin (CT) has been shown to promote mucosal S-IgA as well as serum anti-vaccine and anti-CT-B subunit

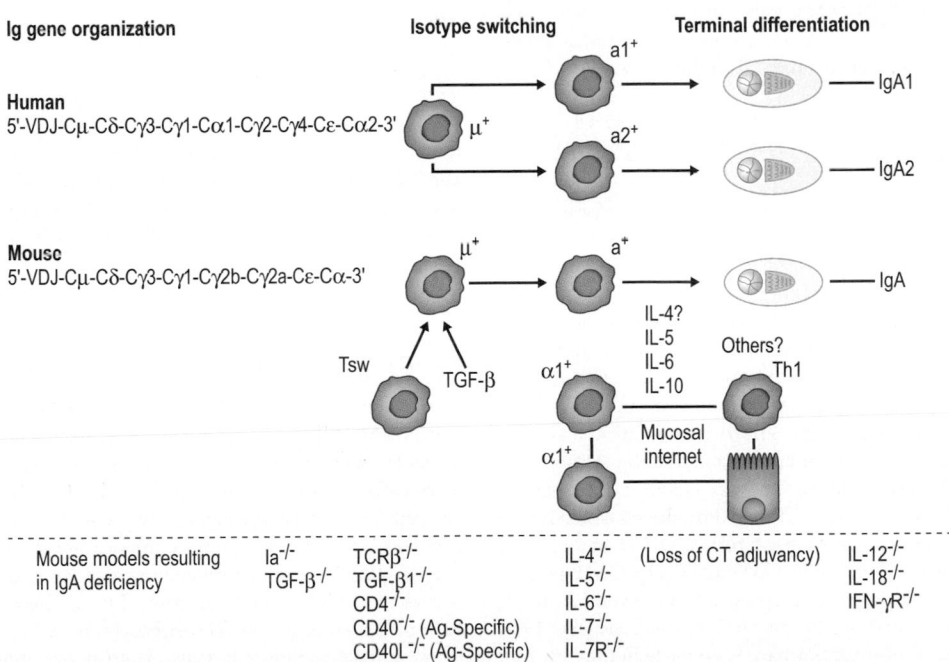

Fig. 19.7 The gene organization, switching to IgA and IgA plasma cell formation in mice and humans. Production of IgA is regulated at several steps that may become dysfunctional and result in IgA deficiency. These steps include T switch (Tsw) cells, switch cytokines (e.g. TGF-β), as well as Th cell subsets and cytokines that promote IgA synthesis. In the lower panel various mouse gene knockouts are shown which display either impaired or blocked mucosal IgA responses. Individual knockout mouse studies are described in the text. From McGhee JR, Kiyono H. The mucosal immune system. In: Paul WE, ed. Fundamental immunology. Philadelphia, Lippincott-Raven, 1999; 909.

CLINICAL RELEVANCE

MUCOSAL ADJUVANTS AND DELIVERY SYSTEMS FOR THE INDUCTION OF TARGETED IMMUNITY

A variety of adjuvants and delivery systems are being developed with the aim of targeting immunity to the mucosal immune system. These include:

>> Genetically engineered bacterial enterotoxins: e.g., cholera toxin (CT) and heat-labile (LT) toxin from *Escherichia coli*

>> Immunostimulatory DNA sequences: These sequences typically contain a transcription unit designed to express the antigen in question that is coupled to an adjuvant/mitogen unit, such as CpG motifs

>> Mucosal cytokines and innate factors as adjuvants: Mucosal delivery of specific cytokines or innate factors can reduce the risk of adverse systemic effects while targeting the immune response to the mucosa

>> Transgenic plants: Plants, such as bananas or rice, can be engineered to express both B- and T-cell antigen epitopes, providing a simple delivery system for oral vaccination or oral tolerance induction.

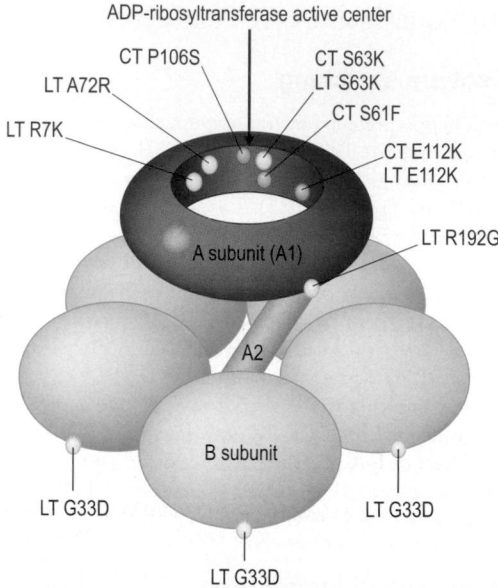

Fig. 19.8 Structure of CT/LT showing the pentameric B and the toxic A subunits. Mutants of both CT and LT have been produced through single amino acid substitutions in the A subunit. Generally, mutants of CT or LT lack residual enterotoxicity but retain mucosal adjuvant properties. (From McGhee JR, Kiyono H. The mucosal immune system. In: Paul WE, ed Fundamental immunology. 1999, 909, with permission from Lippincott, Williams and Wilkins.)

(CT-B) Ab (IgG1 and IgE) responses associated with CD4 Th2 cells.[21] Conversely, recombinant *Salmonella typhimurium* BRD 847 (*aroA-, aroD-*) expressing the C fragment of tetanus toxin has been shown to be an excellent oral vaccine vector for the induction of Th1-type responses with brisk mucosal S-IgA as well as serum Ab (IgG2a) responses.[21]

NEW MUCOSAL ADJUVANTS AND DELIVERY SYSTEMS FOR THE INDUCTION OF TARGETED IMMUNITY

Bacterial enterotoxins and their nontoxic derivatives

Two bacterial enterotoxins (i.e., cholera toxin (CT) and heat-labile toxin (LT) from *Escherichia coli*) are now established as effective for the induction of both mucosal and systemic immunity to co-administered protein antigens. Cholera toxin consists of two structurally and functionally separate A and B subunits (Fig. 19.8). The B subunit of CT (CT-B) binds to GM1 gangliosides, which on epithelia allows the A subunit to reach the cytosol of target cells, where it acts to elevate cAMP, thereby promoting secretion of water and chloride ions into the intestinal lumen. The labile toxin (LT) from *E. coli* is closely related to CT and binds to GM1 gangliosides as well. LT also binds GM2 and asialo-GM1 gangliosides. In order to circumvent toxicity, mutant CT (mCT) and LT (mLT) molecules have been generated by site-directed mutagenesis (Fig. 19.8), wherein single amino acid substitutions have been made in the active site of the A subunit of CT or LT, or in the protease-sensitive loop of LT. The levels of antigen-specific serum IgG and S-IgA Abs induced by these mutants are comparable to those induced by wild-type CT, and significantly higher than those induced by recombinant CT-B.[22] One of the mutants also induces Th2-type responses through a preferential inhibition of Th1-type CD4 T cells.

Mutant LT molecules, whether possessing a residual ADP-ribosyltransferase activity (e.g., LT-A72R) or totally devoid of it (e.g., LT-RK and LT-S63K), can also function as mucosal adjuvants when administered intranasally to mice together with unrelated antigens.[23] As LT induces a mixed CD4 Th1- (i.e., IFN-γ) and Th2-type (i.e., IL-4, IL-5, IL-6 and IL-10) response,[21] one might envisage the use of LT mutants when both Th1- and Th2-type responses are desired.

Safety of mucosal adjuvants and delivery systems

The olfactory neuroepithelium in the nasopharynx constitutes approximately 50% of the nasal surface and has direct neuronal connection to the olfactory bulbs (OBs) in the central nervous system (CNS). Although diarrhea is the primary limiting factor for the use of oral enterotoxin as an adjuvant in humans, major safety concerns with mucosal adjuvants and delivery systems for nasal vaccination are also important, as they may enter and/or target olfactory neurons and hence gain access to OBs and deeper structures in the brain parenchyma. These adverse effects appear to be mediated largely by ADP-ribosyl transferase activity and the nature of the cellular receptors targeted. Both native cholera toxin (nCT) and native labile toxin for humans (nLth-1) mutants bind to GM1 on epithelial cells and require endocytosis followed by transport across the epithelial cell to reach the basolateral membrane. GM1 gangliosides are also abundantly expressed by cells of the CNS, and their concentration on neuronal and microglial cells varies during the development of various cell types and different regions of the brain.[24]

When given nasally to mice, nCT and CT-B enter the olfactory nerves and epithelium (ON/E) and OBs by mechanisms that are selectively dependent on GM1.[25] nCT as adjuvant also promotes the uptake of nasally co-administered, unrelated proteins into the ON/E. The targeting of CNS tissues by nasally administered bacterial enterotoxins is clearly related to a higher incidence of Bell's palsy (facial paresis) among volunteers of a nasal vaccination trial given nLTh-1 as mucosal adjuvant. Bell's palsy in study subjects who in 2000 received nonliving nasal influenza vaccine (Nasalflu® led to its withdrawal from the market (www.niaid.nih.gov/dmid/enteric/intranasal.htm).

The use of GM1-receptor binding holotoxins as nasal mucosal adjuvants is currently inadvisable because of the risk of accumulation in the CNS. However, the development of nontoxic mCTs could overcome these potential problems.[26] To this end, a model adjuvant was developed by combining the ADP-ribosylating ability of nCT with a dimer of an Ig-binding fragment, D, of *Staphylococcus aureus* protein A.[27] This CTA1-DD molecule directly binds to B cells of all isotypes, but not to Mφ or DCs. Despite the lack of a mucosal binding element, the B cell-targeted CTA1-DD molecule was as strong an adjuvant as nCT. Notably, CTA1-DD promoted a balanced Th1/Th2 response with little effect on IgE Ab production. CTA1-DD did not induce inflammatory changes in the nasal mucosa, and most importantly did not bind to or accumulate in the OBs or the CNS.[28] CTA1-DD is an example of the use of nonganglioside targeting adjuvants and delivery systems as new tools for the development of safe and effective nasal vaccines.

Immunostimulatory DNA sequences

Plasmid DNA for gene vaccination can be functionally divided into two distinct units: a transcription unit and an adjuvant/mitogen unit.[29] The latter contains immunostimulatory sequences consisting of short palindromic nucleotides centered around a CpG dinucleotide core, as for example 5′-purine–purine–CG–pyrimidine–pyrimidine-3′. The adjuvant effect of these sequences is mediated by bacterial but not by eukaryotic DNA, owing to its high frequency of CpG motifs and to the absence of cytosine methylation. CpG motifs can induce B-cell proliferation and Ig synthesis as well as cytokine secretion (i.e., IL-6, IFN-α, IFN-β, IFN-γ, IL-12 and IL-18) by a variety of immune cells.

Because CpG motifs create a cytokine microenvironment favoring Th1-type responses, they can be used as adjuvants to stimulate antigen-specific Th1-type responses or to redirect harmful allergic or Th2-dominated autoimmune responses. Indeed, co-injection of bacterial DNA or CpG motifs with a DNA vaccine or with a protein antigen promotes Th1-type responses even in mice with a pre-existing Th2-type immunity. CpG motifs can enhance both systemic and mucosal immune responses when given intranasally to mice.[30]

Mucosal cytokines and innate factors as adjuvants

Mucosal delivery of cytokines offers a means to prevent the adverse effects associated with the large and repeated parenteral doses often required for the effective targeting of tissues and organs. For example, nasal delivery permits the acquisition of significant serum levels of IL-12 at one-tenth the dose required for parenteral administration, complete with inhibition of serum IFN-γ.[1] A nasal vaccine of tetanus toxoid (TT), given with either IL-6 or IL-12, induced serum TT-specific IgG

Ab responses that protected mice against a lethal challenge with tetanus toxin.[31] Also, nasal administration of TT with IL-12 as adjuvant induced high titers of S-IgA Ab responses in the GI tract, vaginal washes and saliva.[31] Similar results were reported when mice were immunized nasally with soluble influenza H1 and N1 proteins and IL-12. In related studies, IL-12 given by the oral or intranasal routes was shown to redirect CT-induced antigen-specific Th2-type responses toward the Th1 type.[1] IL-12 was also shown to promote both Th1- and Th2-type responses when administered by a separate mucosal route.[1] These observations document the power of IL-12 for the induction of targeted immunity.

Innate molecules secreted in the epithelium provide another mechanism by which the adaptive mucosal immune system may be activated. To test this concept, protein antigens were given with either IL-1, α-defensins (i.e., HNPs) or lymphotactin.[1] Lymphotactin, a C chemokine (Chapter 11) produced by NK and CD8 T cells such as TCRγδ IELs, is chemotactic for T and NK cells and induces the migration of memory T cells across endothelial cells. IL-1 is produced by a number of cells, including macrophages and epithelial cells, whereas α-defensins are produced by Paneth cells. Nasal administration of protein antigens with these innate molecules enhanced systemic immune responses to co-administered antigens. However, whereas both IL-1 and lymphotactin produced mucosal S-IgA Ab responses, the defensins failed to do so.[1] Thus, some, but not all, inflammatory cytokines and molecules of the innate immune system can be effectively administered by mucosal routes to regulate both systemic and mucosal immune responses.

Flt3 ligand (FL) binds to the *fms*-like tyrosine kinase receptor Flt3/Flk2. FL mobilizes and stimulates myeloid and lymphoid progenitor cells, dendritic cells (DCs), and natural killer (NK) cells. Although FL dramatically augments numbers of DCs *in vivo*, it fails to induce their activation. Treatment of mice by systemic injection of FL can induce a marked increase in the numbers of DCs in both systemic (i.e., spleen) and mucosal lymphoid tissues (i.e., iLP, PPs and mesenteric lymph nodes [MLNs]). Other than leading to the increase in mucosal DCs can, in some cases, initially enhance the induction of oral tolerance;[32] in many others it can favor the induction of an immune response by mucosal, systemic or cutaneous routes. In recent studies, plasmid encoding FL cDNA (pFL) has been co-administered with plasmids encoding protein Ags or linked to the Ag itself. These studies confirm the adjuvant activity of FL for both Ab and CMI responses and suggest that the costly treatment using FL protein may now be replaced by use of FL cDNA.[33]

Transgenic plants

Plants can be engineered to synthesize and assemble one or more Ags that retain both T- and B-cell epitopes and can induce systemic and mucosal immune responses in both mice and humans.[34, 35] In order to circumvent potential denaturation of antigen during cooking, recombinant bananas have been developed that can accumulate up to 1 mg of vaccine Ag per 10 g of banana. Most recently, T-cell epitope peptides of allergens of Japanese cedar pollen have been expressed under the control of the rice seed storage protein glutelin (GluB-1) promoter. Oral feeding of GluB-1 to mice resulted in the induction of oral tolerance to pollen allergens.[36] Furthermore, transgenic rice expressing CT-B using GluB-1 promoter successfully induced CT-B- specific immunity when orally immunized.[36a]

KEY CONCEPTS

SECRETORY IgA

>> Unlike serum IgA, mucosal secretion of IgA reaches adult levels early in life (1 month to 2 years).

>> The polymeric Ig receptor (pIgR) is expressed on the basolateral surface of epithelial cells and facilitates the active transport of secretory IgA, as well as pentameric IgM, into the mucosal secretions.

>> Secretory IgA protects the host by inhibiting microbial adherence; neutralizing viruses, enzymes, and toxins; and engaging in anti-inflammatory activities by means of inhibiting IgM and IgG complement activation.

>> Clinically, selective IgA deficiency, which is the most common primary immune deficiency, is characterized by recurrent mucosal infections, including sinusitis, otitis media, bronchitis, and pneumonias of viral or bacterial origin, as well as acute diarrhea caused by viruses, bacteria or parasites such as *Giardia lamblia*.

■ SYNTHESIS AND FUNCTIONS OF SECRETORY ANTIBODIES ■

In terms of both specific Ab activity and molecular size, mucosal S-IgA differs from bone marrow-derived serum IgA. In external secretions, adult levels of S-IgA are reached considerably earlier (1 month to 2 years) than in the serum (adolescence) (Chapters 32 and 34). Approximately 98% of S-IgA antibodies (Abs) are produced locally in mucosal tissues, with only a minor fraction deriving from the circulation.

Humans possess two Cα gene segments, Cα1 and Cα2 (Chapter 4), whose use defines the two IgA subclasses, IgA1 and IgA2.[37] (Fig.19.7) These IgA subtypes differ primarily in their hinge regions. IgA1 Abs contain an additional set of 13 amino acid residues in the hinge region that renders them more flexible and susceptible to IgA1-specific proteases produced by bacteria. IgA1-secreting plasma cells are prevalent in most human mucosal tissues, especially the small intestine and the respiratory tract, whereas the human colon and genital tract are enriched for IgA2-secreting cells. Although S-IgA at mucosal surfaces has often been viewed as a barrier to prevent adhesion and colonization of pathogens, as well as an effective means to neutralize viruses and toxins, these antibodies confer the additional advantage of providing anti-inflammatory properties.[8]

POLYMERIC Ig RECEPTOR AND pIgA TRANSPORT

The polymeric Ig receptor (pIgR) is synthesized as a transmembrane protein by epithelial cells and is found on the basolateral surface of epithelial cells. It acts as a receptor for the endocytosis of polymeric IgA (pIgA) and pentameric IgM, both of which typically contain a J chain. pIgR is produced by bronchial epithelial cells, renal tubules, glands, and the epithelium of the small and large intestines.[1] pIgR is not expressed by the FAE (including M cells) of PPs, but only by the adjacent columnar epithelial cells. It is expressed mainly in the upper respiratory tract (nasal cavity, tonsils, trachea, bronchi and tracheobronchial glands), expression in the lower tract being restricted to the pulmonary alveolar cells. In the female reproductive tissues the expression of pIgR is influenced by sex hormones and is low in the vagina, absent in the ovary and myometrium, and very high in the fallopian tubes and uterus. Normal kidneys do not express pIgR, whereas epithelial cells in the lower urinary tract may normally express pIgR and transport pIgA into urine. The expression of pIgR can be upregulated by cytokines such as IFN-γ, TNF-α, IL-1α, IL-1β and TGF-β.

IgA-MEDIATED INHIBITION OF MICROBIAL ADHERENCE

The inhibition of microbial adherence plays a critical initial role in the protection of the host and is mediated by both specific and nonspecific mechanisms. For example, S-IgA and pIgA are more effective at agglutinating microorganisms than is mIgA, and the agglutinating ability of S-IgA specific for capsular polysaccharides of *Haemophilus influenzae* appears to be crucial in order to prevent colonization by *H. influenzae*.[38] When a microorganism interacts with S-IgA molecules its surface becomes less hydrophobic and thus less likely to interact with the mucosal epithelium, but at the same time more likely to be entrapped in the mucus. Carbohydrate chains on the S-IgA molecule bind to bacteria and other antigens, and so represent another nonspecific mechanism that inhibits microbial adherence.

NEUTRALIZATION BY S-IgA OF VIRUSES, ENZYMES AND TOXINS

S-IgA Abs have been shown to be effective at neutralizing viruses in several experimental systems (e.g. influenza, Epstein–Barr virus, HIV, etc.) and at different steps in the infectious process. S-IgA specific to influenza hemagglutinin can interfere with the initial binding of influenza virus to target cells or with the internalization and the intracellular replication of the virus. Indeed, *in vitro* experiments using polarized murine epithelial cells have demonstrated that Abs specific to rotavirus and hepatitis virus can neutralize the viruses inside epithelial cells. Finally, S-IgA can neutralize the catalytic activity of many enzymes of microbial origin.

ANTI-INFLAMMATORY ACTIONS MEDIATED BY S-IgA Abs

IgA Abs are unable to activate complement by either the classic or the alternative pathway (Chapter 20). Nevertheless, they can interfere with IgM- and IgG-mediated complement activation.[37] S-IgA can inhibit phagocytosis, bactericidal activity and chemotaxis by neutrophils, monocytes and macrophages. IgA can downregulate the synthesis of TNF-α and IL-6, as well as enhancing the production of IL-1R antagonists by LPS-activated human monocytes. Thus, the antiflogistic properties of IgA are of significant importance for the integrity of the mucosa, in that IgA can limit bystander tissue damage that may result from the continuous interactions of the mucosa with myriad dietary and environmental antigens. Systemically, circulating IgA also appears to help limit inflammatory reactions that result from complement fixation and phagocyte activation, and contributes to the inhibition of IgE-dependent anaphylactic responses.

KEY CONCEPTS

MUCOSAL CYTOTOXIC T CELLS

>> After enteric infection or immunization, antigen-stimulated CTLs are disseminated from Peyer's patches into mesenteric lymph nodes via the lymphatic drainage.

>> Oral immunization with live virus can induce antigen-specific CTLs in both mucosal inductive and effector tissues for mucosal responses, as well as in systemic lymphoid tissues.

IgA DEFICIENCY

After AIDS, selective IgA deficiency (IgAD) is the most primary immune deficiency in individuals of European descent (Chapter 34). The clinical diagnosis of IgA deficiency depends on the relative absence of IgA in the serum. However, the most important manifestations of the disorder reflect primarily the absence of both S-IgA1 and S-IgA2 in the external secretions. Thus, IgA deficiency affects both the mucosal and systemic immune compartments, with only rare individuals exhibiting a superselective loss of either IgA1 or IgA2 alone.[39]

Approximately one-third of individuals with IgAD suffer recurrent mucosal infections, including sinusitis, otitis media, bronchitis and pneumonias of viral or bacterial origin,[39] as well as acute diarrhea caused by viruses, bacteria or parasites such as *Giardia lamblia*. Other respiratory problems seen in IgA-deficient subjects include allergies, sinusitis, asthma and eczema. It has been suggested that loss of normally protective S-IgA Abs facilitates the development of IgE-type responses.

MUCOSAL CYTOTOXIC T LYMPHOCYTES

M cells have specific receptors for mucosal virus that allow certain viruses, such as the reovirus, to enter the cells in both NALT and GALT. It is likely that enteric viruses such as rotavirus, and respiratory pathogens such as influenza and respiratory syncytial virus (RSV), also enter the mucosal inductive pathway via M cells.[40] After enteric infection or immunization, antigen-stimulated CTLs are disseminated from PPs into MLNs via the lymphatic drainage. Oral immunization with live virus can thus induce antigen-specific CTLs in both mucosal and systemic lymphoid tissues.

ENTERIC VIRUSES AND MUCOSAL CTLS

CD8 CTLs (Chapter 18) play a central role in rotavirus and reovirus immunity.[41,42] Reovirus-induced CTL precursors (pCTLs) in GALT migrate to the systemic compartment. Reovirus-specific CD8 CTLs associated with the αβ T-cell population are also observed in the IELs. Oral delivery of rotavirus increases pCTLs in GALT and results in their dissemination throughout the murine lymphoid system within 3 weeks. Moreover, adoptively transferred CD8 T cells mediate the clearance of rotavirus infection in SCID mice.

RESPIRATORY VIRUSES AND MUCOSAL CTLS

Studies of immune responses after intranasal infection with influenza virus in CD4 knockouts or other mice in which this subset had been depleted have shown that CD4 T cells do not affect the induction of pCTLs or significantly alter the clearance of infection.[43] Clearance of influenza is unaltered by the use of β2-microglobulin knockout mice, which lack CD8 T cells, or of mice that have been treated with monoclonal anti-CD8. γδ T cells with several Vδ chain specificities increase in the infected site as clearance occurs, which suggests a regulatory role for γδ T cells in antiviral immunity.[44]

Effector CTLs protect mice from respiratory syncytial virus (RSV) infection. The RSV F determinant, a 22 kDa glycoprotein, is a major target of pCTLs and CTL induction by RSV or recombinant vaccinia virus-expressing F glycoprotein-induced protective CTLs. IFN-γ-producing CD4 Th1 cells, as well as CD8 T cells, are associated with recovery, whereas CD4 Th2-type pathways are not.[45]

MUCOSAL AIDS MODELS FOR CTL RESPONSES

Approximately 80% of new HIV-1 infections result from sexual transmission (Chapter 38). Thus, significant efforts have been focused on the development of mucosal immunity in the genital tract. Studies using the Rhesus macaque and the simian immunodeficiency virus (SIV) vaginal infection model have provided direct evidence that pCTLs occur in female macaque reproductive tissues, and that infection with SIV induces CTL responses. This important finding was recently extended to vaginal infection with an SIV/HIV-1 chimeric virus (SHIV) containing HIV-1 89.6 *env* gene.[46] Recent work has shown that intranasal immunization with SIV/HIV components induces Ab responses in vaginal secretions. Intranasal immunization of mice with HIV-1 T-cell epitopes and the mucosal adjuvant CT has been shown to induce functional CTLs.

OTHER MUCOSAL CTL SYSTEMS

Salmonella can elicit CD8 T-cell responses, including CTLs, to expressed proteins, and CD8 T cells induced to the parasite *Toxoplasma gondii* have been shown to be protective. Thus, mucosal CD8 CTLs can also be induced in nonviral situations. Significant questions remain about the mechanism by which naïve CD8 T cells can be triggered to expand into pCTLs, and the rules for expression of effector CTLs and memory in the actual mucosal compartment that manifests the infection. It has been shown that pCTLs accumulate in immunologically privileged sites but do not develop a cytotoxic function until they encounter infected class I MHC-presenting target cells. It is possible that this mechanism protects the common mucosal immune system network from inadvertent cytotoxic inflammatory events.

CELLS IN THE EPITHELIUM FORM A REGULATORY INTRANET

A major hallmark of the mucosal immune system is the presence of a mucosal intranet consisting of epithelial cells, TCRαβ Th1 and Th2 T cells, TCRγδ T cells, and IgA-committed B cells for the induction and regulation of Ag-specific S-IgA Abs in external secretions. Epithelial

6. Lorenz RG, Chaplin DD, McDonald KG, et al. Isolated lymphoid follicle formation is inducible and dependent upon lymphotoxin-sufficient B lymphocytes, lymphotoxin beta receptor, and TNF receptor I function. J Immunol 2003; 170: 5475.

7. Quiding-Jarbrink M, Granstrom G, Nordstrom I, et al. Induction of compartmentalized B-cell responses in human tonsils. Infect Immun 1995; 63: 853.

8. Lehner T, Brookes R, Panagiotidi C, et al. T- and B-cell functions and epitope expression in nonhuman primates immunized with simian immunodeficiency virus antigen by the rectal route. Proc Natl Acad Sci USA 1993; 90: 8638.

9. Forrest BD, Shearman DJ, LaBrooy JT. Specific immune response in humans following rectal delivery of live typhoid vaccine. Vaccine 1990; 8: 209.

10. Youngman KR, Lazarus NH, Butcher E. Lymphocyte homing: Chemokines and adhesion molecules in T cell and IgA plasma cell localization in the mucosal immune system. In: Mestecky J, Lamm ME, Strober W, et al., eds. Mucosal immunology, 3rd ed. Vol. 1. Elsevier Academic Press, 2005: 667.

11. Holzmann B, McIntyre BW, Weissman IL. Identification of a murine Peyer's patch-specific lymphocyte homing receptor as an integrin molecule with an a chain homologous to human VLA-4 alpha. Cell 1989; 56: 37.

12. Quiding M, Nordstrom I, Kilander A, et al. Intestinal immune responses in humans. Oral cholera vaccination induces strong intestinal antibody responses and interferon-gamma production and evokes local immunological memory. J Clin Invest 1991; 88: 143.

13. Quiding-Jarbrink M, Lakew M, Nordstrom I, et al. Human circulating specific antibody-forming cells after systemic and mucosal immunizations: differential homing commitments and cell surface differentiation markers. Eur J Immunol 1995; 25: 322.

14. Csencsits KL, Jutila MA, Pascual DW. Nasal-associated lymphoid tissue: phenotypic and functional evidence for the primary role of peripheral node addressin in naive lymphocyte adhesion to high endothelial venules in a mucosal site. J Immunol 1999; 163: 1382.

15. Wolber FM, Curtis JL, Milik AM, et al. Lymphocyte recruitment and the kinetics of adhesion receptor expression during the pulmonary immune response to particulate antigen. Am J Pathol 1997; 151: 1715.

16. Quiding-Jarbrink M, Nordstrom I, Granstrom G, et al. Differential expression of tissue-specific adhesion molecules on human circulating antibody-forming cells after systemic, enteric, and nasal immunizations. A molecular basis for the compartmentalization of effector B cell responses. J Clin Invest 1997; 99: 1281.

17. Kelsall BL, Strober W. Distinct populations of dendritic cells are present in the subepithelial dome and T cell regions of the murine Peyer's patch. J Exp Med 1996; 183: 237.

18. Widhe M, Ekerfelt C, Forsberg P, et al. IgG subclasses in Lyme borreliosis: a study of specific IgG subclass distribution in an interferon-gamma-predominated disease. Scand J Immunol 1998; 47: 575.

19. Austrup F, Vestweber D, Borges E, et al. P- and E-selectin mediate recruitment of T-helper-1 but not T-helper-2 cells into inflamed tissues. Nature 1997; 385: 81.

20. Fujihashi K, McGhee JR, Lue C, et al. Human appendix B cells naturally express receptors for and respond to interleukin 6 with selective IgA1 and IgA2 synthesis. J Clin Invest 1991; 88: 248.

21. Fujihashi K, McGhee JR. Th1/Th2/Th3 cells for regulation of mucosal immunity, tolerance and inflammation. In: Mestecky J, Lamm ME, Strober W, et al, eds. Mucosal Immunology, 3rd ed. vol.1., Burlington, MA. Elsevier, Academic Press, 2005: 539.

22. Yamamoto S, Kiyono H, Yamamoto M, et al. A nontoxic mutant of cholera toxin elicits Th2-type responses for enhanced mucosal immunity. Proc Natl Acad Sci USA 1997; 94: 5267.

23. Rappuoli R, Pizza M, Douce G, Dougan G. Structure and mucosal adjuvanticity of cholera and Escherichia coli heat-labile enterotoxins. Immunol Today 1999; 20: 493.

24. Mancini P, Santi PA. Localization of the GM1 ganglioside in the vestibular system using cholera toxin. Hear Res 1993; 64: 151.

25. van Ginkel FW, Jackson RJ, Yuki Y, McGhee JR. The mucosal adjuvant cholera toxin redirects vaccine proteins into olfactory tissues. J Immunol 2000; 165: 4778.

26. Yoshino N, Lu FX, Fujihashi K, et al. A novel adjuvant for mucosal immunity to HIV-1 gp120 in nonhuman primates. J Immunol 2004; 173: 6850.

27. Agren L, Lowenadler B, Lycke N. A novel concept in mucosal adjuvanticity: the CTA1-DD adjuvant is a B cell-targeted fusion protein that incorporates the enzymatically active cholera toxin A1 subunit. Immunol Cell Biol 1998; 76: 280.

28. Eriksson AM, Schon KM, Lycke NY. The cholera toxin-derived CTA1-DD vaccine adjuvant administered intranasally does not cause inflammation or accumulate in the nervous tissues. J Immunol 2004; 173: 3310.

29. Tighe H, Corr M, Roman M, Raz E. Gene vaccination: plasmid DNA is more than just a blueprint. Immunol Today 1998; 19: 89.

30. Moldoveanu Z, Love-Homan L, Huang WQ, Krieg AM. CpG DNA, a novel immune enhancer for systemic and mucosal immunization with influenza virus. Vaccine 1998; 16: 1216.

31. Boyaka PN, Marinaro M, Jackson RJ, et al. IL-12 is an effective adjuvant for induction of mucosal immunity. J Immunol 1999; 162: 122.

32. Williamson E, Westrich GM, Viney JL. Modulating dendritic cells to optimize mucosal immunization protocols. J Immunol 1999; 163: 3668.

33. Kataoka K, McGhee JR, Kobayashi R, et al. Nasal Flt3 ligand cDNA elicits CD11c+ CD8+ dendritic cells for enhanced mucosal immunity. J Immunol 2004; 172: 3612.

34. Haq TA, Mason HS, Clements JD, Arntzen CJ. Oral immunization with a recombinant bacterial antigen produced in transgenic plants. Science 1995; 268: 714.

35. Tacket CO, Mason HS, Losonsky G, et al. Immunogenicity in humans of a recombinant bacterial antigen delivered in a transgenic potato. Nature Med 1998; 4: 607.

36. Takagi H, Hiroi T, Yang L, et al. A rice-based edible vaccine expressing multiple T cell epitopes induces oral tolerance for inhibition of Th2-mediated IgE responses. Proc Natl Acad Sci USA 2005; 102: 17525.

37. Mestecky J, Moro I, Kerr MA, Woof JM. Mucosal immunoglobulins. In: Mestecky J, Lamm ME, Bienenstock J, et al, eds. Mucosal Immunology, 3rd ed. Vol. 1. Burlington, Elsevier Academic Press, 2005: 153.

38. Kauppi-Korkeila M, van Alphen L, Madore D, et al. Mechanism of antibody-mediated reduction of nasopharyngeal colonization by *Haemophilus influenzae* type b studied in an infant rat model. J Infect Dis 1996; 174: 1337.

39. Burrows PD, Cooper MD. IgA deficiency. Adv Immunol 1997; 65: 245.

40. Neutra MR, Kreahenbuhl JP. Cellular and molecular basis for antigen transport accross epithelial barriers. In: Mestecky J, Lamm ME, Bienenstock J, et al, eds. Mucosal Immunology, 3rd ed, Vol. 1. Burlington, Elsevier Academic Press, 2005: 111.

41. Burns JW, Siadat-Pajouh M, Krishnaney AA, Greenberg HB. Protective effect of rotavirus VP6-specific IgA monoclonal antibodies that lack neutralizing activity. Science 1996; 272: 104

42. Cuff CF, Cebra CK, Rubin DH, Cebra JJ. Developmental relationship between cytotoxic α/β T cell receptor-positive intraepithelial lymphocytes and Peyer's patch lymphocytes. Eur J Immunol 1993; 23: 1333.

43. Allan W, Tabi Z, Cleary A, Doherty PC. Cellular events in the lymph node and lung of mice with influenza. Consequences of depleting CD4+ T cells. J Immunol 1990; 144: 3980.

44. Carding SR, Allan W, Kyes S, et al. Late dominance of the inflammatory process in murine influenza by γδ+ T cells. J Exp Med 1990; 172: 1225.

45. Graham BS, Henderson GS, Tang YW, et al. Priming immunization determines T helper cytokine mRNA expression patterns in lungs of mice challenged with respiratory syncytial virus. J Immunol 1993; 151: 2032.

46. Miller CJ, McChesney MB, Lu X, et al. Rhesus macaques previously infected with simian/human immunodeficiency virus are protected from vaginal challenge with pathogenic SIVmac239. J Virol 1911; 1997: 71.

47. Kiyono H, McGhee JR. Mucosal immunology: intraepithelial lymphocytes, New York: Raven Press, 1994.

48. Fujihashi K, Ernst PB. A mucosal internet: Epithelial cell–immune cell interactions. In: Ogra PL, Mestecky J, Lamm ME, Strober W, Bienenstock J, McGhee JR, eds. Mucosal Immunology, 2nd ed San Diego, CA. Academic Press, 1998, 619.

49. Challacombe SJ, Tomasi TB Jr. Systemic tolerance and secretory immunity after oral immunization. J Exp Med 1980; 152: 1459.

50. Mowat AM, Faria AMC, Weiner HL. Oral tolerance: physiological basis and clinical applications. In: Mestecky J, Lamm ME, Strober W, et al, eds: Mucosal Immunology, 3rd ed. Vol.1. Burlington, MA. Elsevier Academic press, 2005, 487.

51. Cottrez F, Groux H. Specialization in tolerance: innate CD4+ CD25+ versus acquired Tr1 and Th3 regulatory T cells. Transplantation 2004; 77: S12.

52. Miller RA. The aging immune system: primer and prospectus. Science 1996; 273: 70.

53. Fujihashi K, McGhee JR. Mucosal immunity and tolerance in the elderly. Mech Aging Dev 2004; 125: 889.

Complement and complement deficiencies

20

Terry W. Du Clos, Carolyn Mold

The complement system is an important part of the innate immune system and a major effector mechanism of humoral immunity.[1, 2] It is comprised of a group of serum proteins that are activated through sequential protease-based steps similar to the coagulation, fibrinolytic, and contact pathways. The complement activation pathways include potent amplification steps as well as critically important fluid-phase and cell membrane regulatory proteins. Complement activation is linked to cellular responses by the recognition of cleaved complement proteins by receptors on leukocytes and vascular cells. The components of the complement system, including complement regulatory proteins and receptors, are shown in Table 20.1. The three primary roles of complement in host defense against infection are: (1) to activate an inflammatory response; (2) to opsonize microbial pathogens for phagocytosis and killing; and (3) to lyse susceptible organisms. The complement system also provides a bridge between the innate and adaptive immune responses through receptors on B lymphocytes and antigen-presenting cells (APC). Three pathways have been described that share these functions. These pathways differ in their initiation steps and thus are activated in response to different threats. Activation of the complement cascade is amplified at several key steps so that it has the potential to induce a rapid, massive inflammatory response. Complement activation is normally targeted and highly regulated to focus this response. However, complement activation also contributes to tissue injury in infectious, autoimmune, and inflammatory diseases where it may amplify the response to immune complex deposition or tissue damage.

COMPLEMENT PATHWAYS

Three pathways of complement activation have been described: the classical, alternative, and lectin pathways (Fig. 20.1). The classical pathway is the complement pathway that is initiated by immunoglobulin M (IgM) and IgG antibody binding to antigen. It participates with natural IgM in early host defense,[3] and provides a mechanism for immune complex and apoptotic cell clearance.[1] The classical pathway may also be activated by innate pattern recognition molecules such as the pentraxins, C-reactive protein (CRP) and serum amyloid P (SAP) component,[4, 5]

KEY CONCEPTS

COMPLEMENT PATHWAY ACTIVATORS

Classical pathway

>> IgM-containing immune complexes

>> IgG-containing immune complexes

>> C-reactive protein and serum amyloid P–ligand complexes

>> Phospholipids on ischemic and apoptotic cells

>> C4 nephritic factor (C4NeF)

>> Myelin

Alternative pathway

>> Bacterial cell wall components: lipopolysaccharide, teichoic acids

>> Amplification from classical pathway C3b

>> Fungal cell wall polysaccharides: zymosan

>> Virus-infected cells (measles, influenza, Epstein–Barr virus)

>> Immunoglobulin A (IgA)-containing immune complexes

>> C3 nephritic factor (C3NeF)

>> Cobra venom factor

>> Some tumor cell lines

>> Deoxygenated sickle cells

Lectin pathway

>> Repeating simple sugars

>> IgA bound to antigen

>> IgM bound to antigen

>> Apoptotic cells

305

Table 20.1 Proteins of the complement system

Component	Concentration (µg/ml)	Molecular weight
Classical pathway		
C1q	66	410 000
C1r	48	170 000
C1s	34	85 000
C4	400	206 000
C2	30	117 000
Lectin pathway		
MBL	2 (wide range)	600 000
MASP-1	5	83 000
MASP-2	5	52 000
Alternative pathway		
C3	1200	195 000
Factor B	200	95 000
Factor D	3	24 000
Properdin	20	220 000
Membrane attack complex (MAC)		
C5	50	180 000
C6	60	128 000
C7	60	120 000
C8	48	150 000
C9	43	79 000
Soluble regulatory proteins		
C1-INH	190	105 000
C4bp	250	550 000
Factor H	560	150 000
Factor I	40	90 000
S protein (vitronectin)	500	80 000
Clusterin (SP-40,40, ApoJ)	60	80 000
Membrane regulatory proteins		
CD55 (DAF)		70 000
CD46 (MCP)		45 000–70 000
CD59		20 000
Receptors		
CD35 (CR1)		190 000–250 000
CD21 (CR2)		145 000
CD11b/CD18 (CR3)		170 000 α-chain
CD11c/CD18 (CR4)		150 000 α-chain
Common β-chain		95 000
CRIg		45 000–50 000
C1qRp		126 000
C5aR (CD88)		50 000
C3aR		60 000

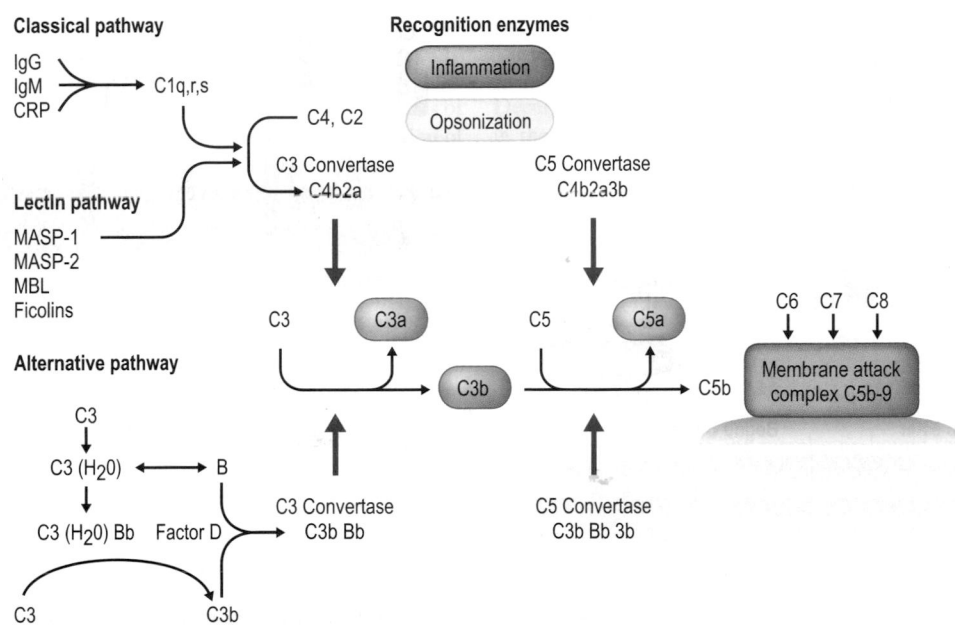

Fig. 20.1 Overview of the complement pathways indicating components required for recognition, enzymatically active components and complexes, major opsonic, inflammatory and membranolytic products.

and the membrane-bound lectin, SIGN-R1.[6] The lectin pathway uses most of the classical pathway components, but is activated by mannose (or mannan)-binding lectin (MBL) and the ficolins, which are lectins that recognize repeating carbohydrate patterns on microorganisms.[7] The alternative pathway is believed to be the most ancient pathway in an evolutionary sense, and also has the broadest recognition ability.[8] The alternative pathway is activated by surface components of all types of microorganisms, including bacteria, fungi, parasites, viruses, and virus-infected cells. The alternative pathway differs from the classical and lectin pathways in its ability to autoactivate when tightly regulated inhibitory signals are absent.[9] This mechanism promotes its function as an innate and rapid response to infection. The alternative pathway also provides an important amplification mechanism for classical or lectin pathway activation, resulting in greater opsonization and generation of the terminal pathway.[10]

CLASSICAL PATHWAY

The classical pathway is usually focused by antibody binding to a target antigen. In general, the ability of antibodies to activate complement is: $IgM > IgG_3 > IgG_1 > IgG_2 >> IgG_4$. Binding of these antibodies exposes sites in the Fc region for attachment of the first subcomponent of complement, C1q. C1 is a large calcium-dependent complex composed of C1q, and two molecules each of the proenzymes, C1r and C1s. C1q is a 410-kDa protein with six globular heads connected by a collagen-like tail. For IgM, which is pentameric, binding to antigen creates a conformational change that exposes the C1q binding site in the $C\mu3$ domain. For IgG, at least two closely bound molecules are required to provide multiple attachment points for C1q binding to the $C\gamma2$ domain. Similarly, CRP or SAP molecules bound to ligand provide multiple C1q

binding sites resulting in classical pathway activation. IgM, IgG, and CRP bind C1q through its globular head groups.[11] Membrane lipids exposed on apoptotic cells or mitochondrial membranes, polyanions, nucleic acids, and endotoxins activate the classical pathway differently through charge-based interactions with the collagen-like region of C1q.[12]

Once C1q binds to an activator through several globular heads, C1r is cleaved and activated by an autocatalytic process.[11] Activated C1r then cleaves and activates C1s, which cleaves circulating C4. C4 and C3 are highly homologous proteins that share an unusual internal thioester bond[13] (Fig. 20.2). Cleavage of C4 releases the C4a fragment, and exposes the reactive thioester bond in the larger C4b fragment. This allows C4b to attach covalently to nearby target structures, through either amide or ester bonds, to amino or carboxyl groups on proteins, glycoproteins, or polysaccharides on cell surfaces, antibodies, and antigens. The exposed thioester bond is reactive, but unstable, and only about 5% of the C4 typically becomes attached to the target prior to inactivation of the thioester site by hydrolysis. Bound C4b provides an anchor site for C2 attachment, which is then cleaved by C1s, releasing C2b.

The complex of C4b2a is termed the classical pathway C3 convertase, because it has the capacity to cleave C3, releasing C3a. The C2a component of the complex contains the active enzymatic site. C3 cleavage is similar to C4 cleavage in that the larger fragment, C3b, contains a thioester site (Fig. 20.2) that can mediate covalent attachment to nearby surface structures, including the antigen, antibody, and the attached C4b. C3 is found at higher concentration in serum than C4, and its cleavage is amplified by the alternative pathway. Thus, efficient complement activation will result in a cluster of multiple bound C3b molecules that can be recognized by cellular receptors. C3b that attaches to C4b within the C3 convertase produces the trimolecular complex C4b2a3b, which is a

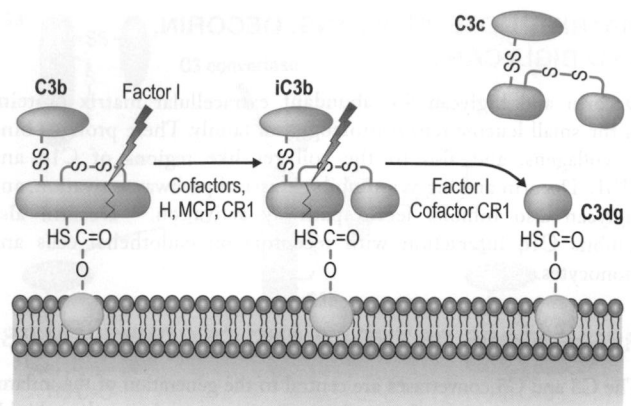

Fig. 20.4 Factor I-dependent cleavage of C3 showing the structures of the products and the required cofactors.

Membrane regulatory proteins, CD55 (DAF), CD46 (MCP), CD35 (CR1), CRIT, and CSMD1

The RCA family also includes the membrane regulatory proteins decay-accelerating factor (CD55, DAF), membrane cofactor protein (CD46, MCP), and complement receptors CR1 (CD35) and CR2 (CD21). CD55 (DAF) and CD46 (MCP), as their names imply, have decay-accelerating and cofactor activities that prevent complement activation on cell membranes. Each has an extracellular domain composed exclusively of four CCPs. CD55, a glycophosphatidylinositol (GPI)-anchored protein, and CD46, a transmembrane protein, are widely distributed on cells in contact with the blood, with the exception that erythrocytes lack CD46. Soluble CD55 is also found in most biological fluids. Both protect cells from complement-mediated lysis. CD35 (CR1) has decay-accelerating and cofactor activity as well as receptor activity for immune complexes with bound C3b. The complement receptors are discussed later in the chapter.

Two new membrane regulatory proteins have recently been described that block the classical pathway C3 convertase. The first, named complement C2 receptor inhibitor trispanning (CRIT), was originally identified on *Schistosoma* and *Trypanasoma* parasites and later found to be widely expressed on human tissues and blood cells, except for neutrophils and erythrocytes.[23] CRIT competes with C4b for C2 binding, preventing its cleavage by C1s and blocking the formation of the classical pathway C3 convertase.

The second protein, CUB and sushi multiple domains 1 protein (CSMD1), was identified by the presence of 15 CCPs homologous to those of the RCA proteins. A recombinant form of the rat homologue of human CSMD1 blocks classical-pathway, but not alternative-pathway, activation and is expressed as a membrane protein in the central nervous system, particularly during development.[24]

Properdin

In contrast to the regulatory proteins discussed above, properdin (factor P) stabilizes C3 and C5 convertases of the alternative pathway, increasing their activity.[18] Properdin is found as noncovalently linked dimers, trimers, tetramers, and larger species composed of identical 56-kDa chains.

The majority of the protein consists of a series of six thrombospondin type 1 modules. Properdin binds to C3b and to Bb, preventing the spontaneous or induced decay of the alternative-pathway C3 and C5 convertases. Its multimeric structure promotes interaction with clustered C3b. The relative affinity of properdin binding is highest for C3bBb > C3bB > C3b.

REGULATORS OF THE MAC

The MAC is also regulated by both fluid-phase and membrane regulatory proteins.

Soluble MAC inhibitors, S protein, and clusterin

Soluble hydrophobic proteins can block the incorporation of MAC into membranes. Two well-characterized proteins with this activity are S protein (vitronectin), and clusterin (SP-40,40, apolipoproteins J). S protein[25] is found in the serum and extracellular matrix and binds to C5b-7. C8 and C9 can still bind to the complex, but membrane insertion and C9 polymerization are prevented. Soluble complexes of S protein and C5b-9 are found in the serum during complement activation and an SC5b-9-specific enzyme-linked immunosorbent assay (ELISA) has been used to monitor activation of the MAC. Clusterin[26] is found in the serum, in the male reproductive tract, and on endothelial cells of normal arteries. It is also associated with amyloid deposits, including β amyloid in Alzheimer's disease. Clusterin forms an inactive complex with C5b-9, preventing membrane insertion.

Membrane MAC inhibitor, CD59

The primary membrane-bound inhibitor of MAC is CD59 (MIRL, MACIF, HRF20, P18, protectin).[27] CD59 is a GPI-anchored protein found on most cells, and may also be found in a soluble form in biological fluids. CD59 binds to C8 in the C5b-8 complex, preventing the incorporation of C9. CD59 also blocks polymerization of C9 already in the MAC.

■ COMPLEMENT RECEPTORS ■

Many of the biological effects of complement activation are mediated by cellular receptors for fragments of complement proteins. These include receptors for the small soluble complement fragments, C5a and C3a, and receptors for bound complement fragments, C1q and cleaved forms of C4b and C3b. Receptors for bound C3 are specific for not only C3b, but further breakdown products generated by the enzymatic processing by factor I in conjunction with the cofactor proteins mentioned above. The breakdown of C3 and intermediate products are shown in Figure 20.4 and the receptors for these components in Figure 20.5.

C1Q RECEPTORS

C1q shares the same general structure with a family of proteins termed 'soluble defense collagens' that includes the 'collectins' (MBL, surfactant proteins A and D, conglutinin), and the ficolins. These proteins have collagen-like regions associated with globular recognition domains. The collectins have C-type lectin carbohydrate recognition domains. Ficolins also recognize acetyl groups on carbohydrates and other molecules using fibrinogen-like recognition domains. The globular head groups of C1q bind to amino acid motifs on IgG, IgM, and pentraxins. In general, this group of proteins has broad recognition ability for both pathogen-associated carbohydrate patterns and for damaged or apoptotic cells. C1q and the soluble defense collagens share a receptor, C1qRp, to which they bind through their collagen-like regions.[28] C1qRp is expressed on phagocytic cells, endothelial cells, and platelets. On monocytes and neutrophils, binding of C1q, MBL, or SP-D to C1qRp does not directly induce phagocytosis, but can enhance Fc receptor and CR1-mediated phagocytosis of suboptimally opsonized targets. On endothelial cells C1qRp may contribute to the endothelial response to immune complexes.

CD35 (CR1), discussed further below, has separate binding sites for C3b, C4b, and C1q, facilitating binding to immune complexes or microorganisms with multiple complement components attached. CR1 also binds to MBL.

The $\alpha_2\beta_1$ integrin on mast cells, which binds to collagen and other matrix ligands, was recently reported to bind to C1q, MBL, and SP-A. The interaction of mast cells expressing $\alpha_2\beta_1$ integrin with opsonized *Listeria* resulted in C1q-dependent adhesion and secretion of interleukin (IL)-6.[29] Furthermore, mice deficient in the α_2 integrin subunit exhibited diminished neutrophil and IL-6 responses during peritonitis induced by *Listeria* or zymosan.

Other C1q binding proteins have been identified, notably calreticulin and gC1qbp. Neither of these are receptors in the classical sense, since they are not membrane proteins.[28] Calreticulin (CRT, cC1qR, collectin receptor) binds to the collagen-like regions of C1q, MBL, SP-A, and SP-D. Calreticulin is found in the endoplasmic reticulum, but is also found on the surface of macrophages and may be translocated to the cell surface during cell stress. Calreticulin lacks a transmembrane domain, but has been shown to contribute to the uptake of opsonized apoptotic cells opsonized with C1q, MBL, or SP-D by association with the α_2-macroglobulin receptor, CD91.[30]

Another intracellular protein, gC1qbp, is widely expressed and binds to the globular head groups of C1q. Secreted gC1qbp can inhibit C1 activation, suggesting a role as a regulatory protein.

COMPLEMENT RECEPTOR 1 (CD35, CR1)

There are five identified receptors for bound fragments of C3 and/or C4. CD35 (CR1) is a large protein composed of a linear string of CCPs, a transmembrane region, and a short intracytoplasmic domain. Different allelic forms of CD35 are found, the most common being composed of 30 CCPs with a molecular weight of 190 kDa. These CCPs are organized into groups of seven, creating structures termed long homologous repeats (LHRs), each of which contains a single binding site. The predominant allele of CD35 contains two binding sites for C3b, one for C4b and one for C1q. CR1 is found on human erythrocytes, monocytes and macrophages, neutrophils, B lymphocytes, a small percentage of T lymphocytes, eosinophils, follicular dendritic cells (FDC), and glomerular podocytes.

CD35 on primate erythrocytes provides a noninflammatory mechanism for clearing soluble immune complexes from the circulation. Although the number of receptors on each erythrocyte is low, the large number of erythrocytes provides the major pool of CR1 in the circulation. Soluble immune complexes that fix complement attach quickly to erythrocytes in the circulation, bypassing monocytes and neutrophils.

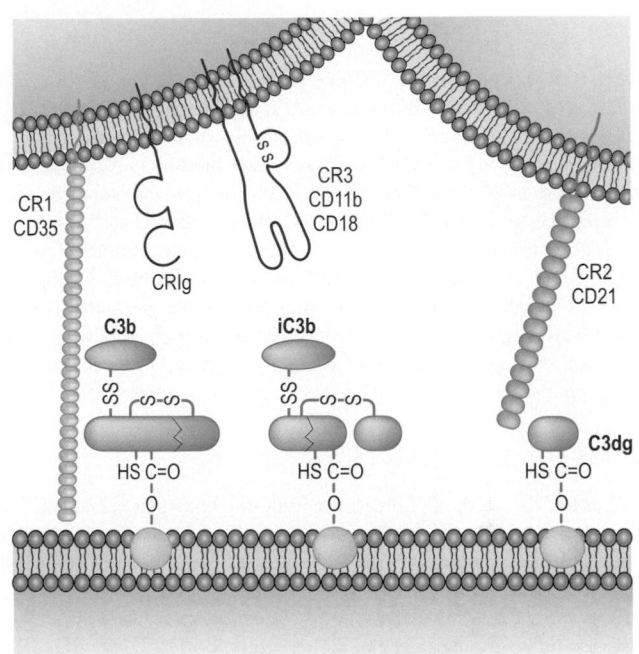

Fig. 20.5 Receptors for bound C3b and its cleavage products. Receptors shown are CD35 and CD21 composed of CCP (SCR) subunits, CD11b/CD18 (CR3), a β_2 integrin, and CRIg with 1 or 2 Ig domains. The specificities of the receptors are: CD35 for C3b, C4b > iC3b; CRIg for iC3b > C3b; CD11b/CD18 for iC3b; CD21 for C3dg, C3d > iC3b. CD11c/CD18 (CR4) is similar to CD11b/CD18 and is not shown. Receptors are not drawn to scale. Their molecular weights are listed in Table 20.1.

These erythrocyte-bound complexes are taken to the liver where they are transferred to Kupffer cells expressing Fc and complement receptors and destroyed. The erythrocytes exit into the circulation to pick up more immune complexes. This clearance pathway is impaired in patients with systemic lupus erythematosus (SLE) due to decreased complement in the circulation, decreased CD35 on erythrocytes, and saturated Fc receptors in the liver and spleen.

CD35 on monocytes and neutrophils promotes binding of microbes with bound C3b and C4b, facilitating their phagocytosis through Fc receptors. CD35 can directly mediate uptake of microbes when phagocytic cells have been activated by chemokines or integrin interactions with matrix proteins.

CD35 is a member of the RCA family and has decay-accelerating and cofactor activity in addition to its function as a receptor. It differs from the membrane regulatory proteins DAF (CD55) and MCP (CD46) in its ability to bind to C3b and C4b extrinsically (on targets other than the cell expressing it), and in its cofactor activity for C3b processing. CD35 is the most effective cofactor for factor I cleavage of C3b and iC3b to the smallest covalently bound fragment, C3dg. C3dg is the major ligand for CR2 on B lymphocytes, described below. The cofactor activity of CD35 on B lymphocytes is believed to process bound C3b to C3dg, which lowers the threshold for B-cell activation through antigen-specific receptors.

COMPLEMENT RECEPTOR 2 (CD21, CR2)

CD21 (CR2) is also an RCA family protein composed of 15–16 CCPs. CD21 has a limited range of expression that includes B lymphocytes, FDC, and some epithelial cells. CD21 is specific for the smallest covalently bound C3 fragments, C3dg and C3d, and has weaker binding to iC3b. CD21 is also the Epstein–Barr virus receptor on B lymphocytes and nasopharyngeal epithelial cells and binds to CD23, a low-affinity IgE receptor.

CD21 on B lymphocytes serves a co-stimulatory role.[31] It is expressed on mature B cells as a complex with CD19 and CD81 (TAPA-1). Co-ligation of CD21 and the B-cell antigen receptor induces the phosphorylation of CD19, activating several signaling pathways and strongly amplifying B-cell responses to antigen. This role of CD21 is believed to contribute to the strong adjuvant effect produced by attaching C3d to antigen.[32]

COMPLEMENT RECEPTORS 3 AND 4

CR3 and CR4 are the β_2-integrins commonly known as CD11b/CD18 (Mac-1) and CD11c/CD18. β_2-integrins are large heterodimers found on neutrophils and monocytes with multiple roles in adhesion to endothelium and matrix molecules as well as direct recognition of microbial pathogens. The binding activities of β_2-integrins are regulated by cellular activation often through chemokine receptors. Both CD11b/CD18 and CD11c/CD18 are expressed primarily on neutrophils, monocytes, and natural killer cells and bind to iC3b and, to a lesser extent, C3b.

CD11b/CD18 has been studied more extensively than CD11c/CD18. CD11b/CD18 expression, clustering, and conformation are all rapidly upregulated by chemokine activation of neutrophils, leading to increased responses to ligand.[33] CR3 plays an essential role in neutrophil attachment to and migration through activated endothelium to sites in inflammation and in the regulation of neutrophil apoptosis. Deficiency of the β_2-chain (CD18) results in leukocyte adhesion deficiency, characterized by recurrent pyogenic infections and defects in inflammatory and phagocytic responses. Complement receptors CD11b/CD18 and CD11c/CD18 provide an essential function for the removal of microbial pathogens following complement activation, since C3b processing often occurs rapidly following deposition.

COMPLEMENT RECEPTOR OF THE IMMUNOGLOBULIN SUPERFAMILY (CRIg)

CRIg[34] is a newly identified receptor for iC3b and C3b found on Kupffer cells in the liver as well as other tissue macrophages, but absent from splenic macrophages, peripheral blood cells, bone marrow-derived macrophages, and monocyte/macrophage cell lines. Two alternative-spliced forms of human CRIg were identified with one and two Ig domains. The mouse receptor has a single Ig domain. CRIg is thought to function in the removal of C3b or iC3b-opsonized particles from the circulation by the liver.

C5A AND C3A RECEPTORS

During complement activation, the homologous proteins C4, C3, and C5 are each cleaved near the amino-terminus of the α–chains to release a soluble peptide fragment of approximately 8 kDa. These fragments are designated C4a, C3a, and C5a. C5a may also be generated locally by direct leukocyte protease cleavage of C5. These peptides are termed anaphylatoxins because of their ability to increase vascular permeability,

contract smooth muscle, and trigger the release of vasoactive amines from mast cells and basophils. C5a is 10–100-fold more active than C3a, which is much more (1000-fold) active than C4a. These peptides are also chemotactic: C5a is specific for neutrophils, monocytes, and macrophages, whereas C3a is specific for mast cells and eosinophils. Other biological activities of complement anaphylatoxins are summarized in Table 20.2.

Structurally the anaphylatoxins are compact structures consisting of multiple helices cross-linked by disulfide bonds with more flexible carboxy-terminal regions. The C-terminal peptide of C3a interacts with the C3aR and can reproduce C3a agonist activity. In contrast, C5a interacts with the C5aR at multiple sites. Serum carboxypeptidases cleave the C-terminal arginine from C5a, C3a, and C4a producing the *des Arg* forms. This inactivates C3a and C4a; however, C5a *des Arg* retains much of its biological activity.

The C5aR (CD88 and C5L2) and the C3aR are rhodopsin-type receptors with seven transmembrane-spanning domains.[35] The C4aR has not been cloned. The C5aR and C3aR are coupled to G-protein signaling. C5L2 is not G-protein-coupled and may serve as a regulatory decoy receptor limiting the inflammatory response to C5a. The C5aR is expressed at high levels on neutrophils and is also found on macrophages, mast cells, basophils, smooth-muscle cells, and endothelial cells. When C5a is generated locally, for example in an extravascular site of infection, it helps induce an acute local inflammatory response including vasodilation, edema, neutrophil chemotaxis, and activation of neutrophils and macrophages for enhanced phagocytosis and killing.[35] The inflammatory activities of C5a may also contribute to complement-mediated pathology in conditions such as sepsis, acute respiratory distress syndrome, and ischemia–reperfusion injury, making the C5a–C5aR interaction an attractive therapeutic target.

COMPLEMENT IN HOST DEFENSE AND IMMUNITY

COMPLEMENT IN HOST DEFENSE

Complement activation provides a coordinated response to infection that results in the opsonization of microbial pathogens and the attraction and activation of phagocytic cells to kill them. Complement-dependent opsonization is of greatest importance in infections with encapsulated extracellular bacteria, and individuals with deficiencies in antibody production, neutrophil function, or C3 share increased susceptibility to these organisms, including *Streptococcus pneumoniae* and *Haemophilus influenzae*. MBL deficiency is also associated with recurrent pyogenic infections in young children. In general, activation of complement by natural antibody or MBL results in C3b and iC3b deposition on these pathogens, overcoming the anti-phagocytic effects of the capsule. Phagocytic cells ingest and kill the organisms using CD35, CD11b/CD18, and CD11c/CD18 receptors in conjunction with other innate and Fc receptors. C5a signaling activates these receptors, leading to increased phagocytosis. Gram-negative bacteria are susceptible to complement-dependent lysis. This is evident in the increased incidence of disseminated neisserial infection in individuals deficient in C3, any of the MAC components, or properdin, as discussed below.

Table 20.2 Cellular targets and effects of complement anaphylatoxins

	Target	Effects
C3a, C5a	Mast cells, basophils	Degranulation, release of vasoactive amines: contraction of smooth muscle, increased vascular permeability
C3a	Eosinophils	Chemotaxis, degranulation
C5a	Endothelium	Increased adhesion of leukocytes, chemokine and cytokine synthesis
C5a	Neutrophils, monocytes/macrophages, eosinophils, basophils, astrocytes	Chemotaxis
C5a	Neutrophils, monocytes/macrophages	Priming: activation of receptors, assembly of NADPH oxidase; activation: degranulation, respiratory burst
C5a	Resident macrophages	Regulation of FcγR expression (↑ activating, ↓ inhibitory)
C5a	Hepatocyte	Acute-phase protein synthesis
C3a, C5a	Lymphocytes, antigen-presenting cells	Regulation of T-cell responses to antigen

COMPLEMENT IN INFLAMMATION

An essential function of complement in host defense is the coordination of the local inflammatory response. C5a is the most potent complement product in this activity.[35] Sublytic deposition of MAC on endothelial cells and platelets and C3a interaction with the C3aR also contribute to the proinflammatory effects of complement activation. As discussed below, these potent inflammatory fragments of complement, when generated in high amounts or targeted inappropriately, result in many of the disease-related deleterious effects of complement. Local production of C5a at a site of infection occurs either through local complement activation or through direct cleavage of C5 by tissue macrophages. This C5a is released and sets up a chemotactic gradient for neutrophils and macrophages. In addition C5a activates endothelial cells to express P-selectin and synthesize chemokines, including IL-8. Interaction of C5a with mast cells releases vasoactive amines, increasing endothelial permeability. Neutrophils and macrophages are "primed" by interaction of C5a with its receptor. Priming includes enhancement of chemotaxis, activation of phagocytosis through complement receptors, and assembly of the NADPH-oxidase that is required for effective killing of microbes after phagocytosis. C5a also prevents neutrophil apoptosis, prolonging survival and contributing to local accumulation. Together these actions result in the attraction and activation of potent anti-microbial cells and resolution of infection (Fig. 20.6).

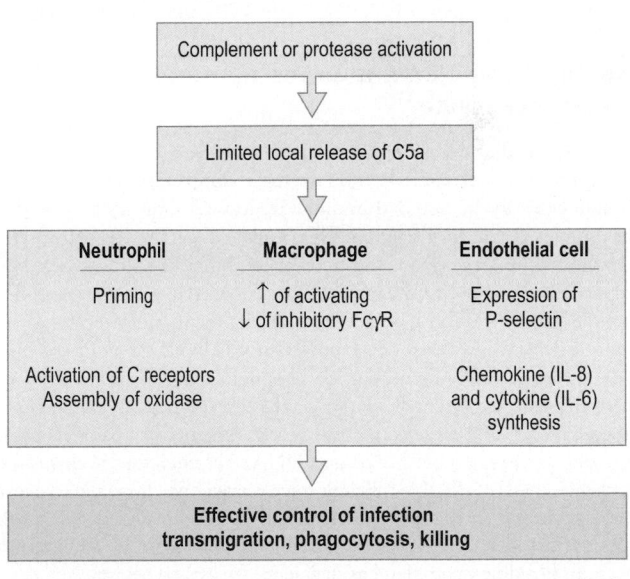

Fig. 20.6 C5a in local host defense.

PATHOGEN EVASION OF COMPLEMENT

Further evidence of the host defense function of complement is the association of complement evasion strategies with virulence. Pathogenic Gram-negative bacteria, such as *Salmonella*, have lipopolysaccharides with long O-polysaccharide side chains that promote rapid shedding of the MAC and prevent its insertion into the cell membrane. *Neisseria* species have several factor H-binding components that help restrict alternative-pathway activation and protect against lysis. Group A and B streptococci and *Streptococcus pneumoniae* have cell surface components (M protein, Bac or beta, PspC, Hic) that bind to factor H and/or C4bp, restricting complement activation. Other organisms, including type 3 group B streptococci, elaborate sialic acid-containing capsules or cell walls to limit alternative-pathway activation.

Although complement deficiencies are not generally associated with viral infections, the importance of complement in host defense against viruses is suggested by the multiple strategies used by viruses to evade complement. Several viruses produce complement regulatory proteins, including vaccinia virus complement control protein, and herpes virus glycoprotein C, which facilitate breakdown of C3b and C4b. Some viruses, such as human immunodeficiency virus (HIV), incorporate complement regulatory proteins into the viral envelope, a strategy that is also used by other pathogens, such as *Schistosoma*.

There are also many examples of complement receptors and membrane regulatory proteins being exploited as receptors for pathogens to invade cells. Examples of these are summarized in reference 1, and include strategies of direct pathogen binding to receptors as well as deposition of C3 fragments followed by invasion through host C3 receptors.

ROLE OF COMPLEMENT IN ADAPTIVE IMMUNITY

Over the past 10 years there has been renewed interest in the role of the innate immune system in adaptive immune responses. The importance of complement in humoral immunity has been recognized since the observation by Pepys in 1972[36] that complement depletion of mice prior to immunization decreased antibody responses to thymus-dependent antigens. Further studies have shown that complement receptors CR1 (CD35) and CR2 (CD21) are also required. In humans these receptors are found together on B lymphocytes and FDC. CD35 is also expressed on a number of other cell types (described above), including erythrocytes and phagocytic cells.

Effects of complement on the humoral immune response

Results obtained by experimental manipulation of C3, C4 and their receptors in mouse models indicate roles for these complement components at multiple levels in the humoral immune response.[37] One caveat regarding these studies is that in the mouse CD35 and CD21 are alternative splice products of the same gene, and genetically deficient animals lack both receptors. In humans CD35 and CD21 are encoded by separate genes. The first role of CD35/CD21 is in B-cell development, indicated by a pronounced defect in B-1 cell development in CD35/CD21-deficient mice. B-1 cells are generally found outside lymphoid follicles, have a restricted repertoire, and are essential in the production of natural antibodies to pathogens, such as *S. pneumoniae*, and to self antigens exposed on damaged cells, such as phosphatidylcholine and DNA. Although the mechanism of this defect in CD35/CD21-deficient mice is unknown, these mice have an altered repertoire of natural antibody and B-1 cells. Decreased natural antibody may contribute to susceptibility to infection and autoimmune disease in hereditary complement deficiency (discussed below).

A second role for complement in the antibody response is the well-described function of CD21 as a co-receptor for the mature B-cell response to antigen.[31] As described above, CD21 is associated with the signaling complex of CD19 and CD81 (TAPA-1) in the B-cell membrane. Co-ligation of CD21 with the B-cell antigen receptor occurs naturally when the antigen activates complement and covalently binds C3dg. This co-ligation of the B-cell receptor with CD21 greatly decreases the threshold for B-cell activation and blocks Fas-initiated apoptosis of B cells. B cells activated by complement-opsonized antigen have increased ability to present antigen as well as survival and proliferation during encounters with T dependent antigens.

The expression of CD35 and CD21 on FDC is also important in the antibody response. FDC trap antigen in the germinal centers and provide selection of somatically mutated high-affinity B-cell clones. Antigen trapped on FDC also provides a source of long-term stimulation for maintenance of memory B cells. FDC use complement receptors (CD35 and CD21) and FcγR to trap and retain antigen for these functions. Expression of CD21 on both FDC and B cells is required for effective affinity maturation of the antibody response and for the development and maintenance of memory B cells.

Complement and T-cell activation

Recent studies in primary pulmonary infection with influenza indicate that C3-deficient mice have a defect in influenza-specific CD4 and CD8 T-cell priming.[38] CR1/2 deficiency had no effect. The mechanism is unknown, but may be more efficient uptake and presentation of C3-opsonized virus by APC through CR3 and CR4 or stimulation of T-cell responses through the C3aR.

Co-stimulation of human T cells *in vitro* through CD3 and CD46 leads to the development of T cells with a regulatory phenotype characterized by synthesis of IL-10 in the absence of other Th2 cytokines (IL-2, IL-4).[39] The induction of regulatory T cells was seen in response to both anti-CD46 cross-linking and natural ligands (C3b dimers, streptococcal M protein).

CD55-deficient mice showed enhanced T-cell responses to immunization and increased T-cell-dependent autoimmune disease. These effects were complement-dependent and apparently involve the loss of CD55 regulation of local complement synthesis by APC during cognate interactions with T cells. One postulated mechanism is that CD55 inhibits the generation of C3a and C5a by APC, preventing their interactions with C3aR and C5aR on T cells.[40] Complement anaphylatoxins C3a and C5a have many important effects in inflammatory diseases that include attraction and activation of inflammatory cells, as well as regulation of APC and T-cell responses. Examples of these will be discussed in the sections below on complement in disease.

ROLE OF COMPLEMENT IN CLEARANCE OF APOPTOTIC CELLS

Damaged tissue and dead and dying cells activate complement through several pathways. This may increase local inflammation and injury, as in ischemia/reperfusion injury and hemolytic–uremic syndrome (HUS) (discussed below). Complement activation by apoptotic cells contributes to their opsonization and clearance, and may prevent the development of autoimmunity. The deleterious consequences of complement activation following tissue damage are mainly attributable to alternative-pathway-dependent generation of C5a and the MAC,[41] whereas the beneficial effects are dependent on early classical pathway components and innate recognition molecules.[42]

Necrosis as occurs following ischemic tissue injury exposes phospholipids and mitochondrial proteins that activate complement directly or indirectly. The pathways are different depending on the tissue involved.[41] For example, renal reperfusion injury appears to be initiated by the alternative pathway, possibly secondary to the loss of regulatory proteins on tubular epithelial cells. Intestinal ischemia–reperfusion injury is initiated by natural IgM antibodies and requires both the classical pathway for initiation, and the alternative pathway for injury. MBL and CRP-initiated

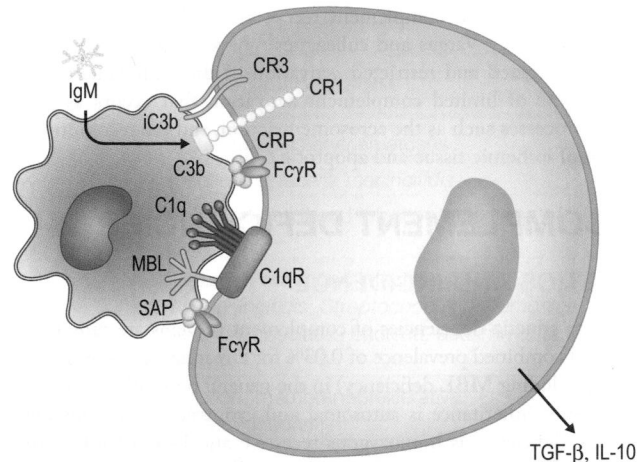

Fig. 20.7 Pathways of opsonization of apoptotic cells by complement. Innate recognition of apoptotic cells by natural immunoglobulin M (IgM), C-reactive protein (CRP), serum amyloid P (SAP), C1q, and mannose-binding lectin (MBL) is shown. Each reaction activates complement leading to opsonization by C3b and iC3b. In addition, C1q and MBL bind to collectin receptors, and CRP and SAP bind to FcγR on macrophages. Cytokine responses to apoptotic cells opsonized by complement include the anti-inflammatory cytokines, transforming growth factor-β (TGF-β) and interleukin-10 (IL-10).

complement activation have been proposed to contribute to myocardial reperfusion injury after coronary artery ligation.[43]

Apoptotic cells are recognized by multiple receptors and opsonins.[42, 44] The association between early classical pathway deficiencies and SLE (see below) has been attributed to a failure of complement-dependent opsonization, resulting in accumulation of apoptotic cells and released autoantigens.[2, 45] Support for this hypothesis is provided by studies of mice deficient in C1q, IgM, or SAP, all of which develop autoantibodies against phospholipid and nuclear antigens characteristic of SLE, and by the therapeutic effect of CRP in mouse models of SLE.[4] The role of complement in apoptotic cell recognition and uptake by macrophages is depicted in Figure 20.7. MBL, C1q, and SP-D bind to apoptotic cells and facilitate clearance through direct binding to collectin receptors as well as complement activation.[30, 42] Natural IgM antibodies, CRP, and SAP bind to phospholipids exposed on late apoptotic cells. All three proteins can also activate the classical pathway generating C1q, C4b, C3b, and iC3b ligands for complement receptors. CRP and SAP also directly opsonize apoptotic cells for uptake through Fcγ receptors.[4] Phagocytosis of apoptotic cells generally induces anti-inflammatory cytokines, transforming growth factor-β (TGF-β) and IL-10.[42, 44]

Targeted activation of complement for opsonization

Interestingly, CRP and SAP also bind complement regulatory proteins, factor H and C4bp, which helps to limit complement activation to the deposition of opsonic components with little or no lysis or generation of C5a.[46, 47] This type of complement activation was also observed on acrosome-activated spermatozoa. In this case the classical pathway was activated by CRP from follicular fluid, resulting in bound C3b and iC3b that

normal Swedish population).[50] In addition to the association of MBL deficiency in children with recurrent infections, there is a two- to three-fold increased frequency of MBL deficiency in SLE and these individuals have more frequent and more severe infections during the course of their disease. Serious infectious complications are also more frequent in the subgroups of cystic fibrosis and rheumatoid arthritis (RA) patients that have MBL deficiency.[48]

A single homozygous MASP-2 deficiency has been reported.[7] The patient was asymptomatic until the age of 13, when he was diagnosed with ulcerative colitis. Additional autoimmune manifestations developed along with recurrent severe infections with *S. pneumoniae*.

ALTERNATIVE-PATHWAY DEFICIENCIES

Individuals with complete deficiencies of factor D or properdin have been reported. Factor D-deficient patients have presented with recurrent infections due to *Neisseria* and other organisms. Properdin deficiency is X-linked and patients most commonly have severe childhood infections with *N. meningitidis*.

C3 DEFICIENCIES

C3 is central to all three complement activation pathways. Nineteen families have been reported with primary inherited deficiency of C3.[51] The most common presentation is with recurrent life-threatening infections in early childhood (before the age of 2), sometimes followed by immune complex disease. The infections observed are primarily respiratory tract infections (48%) and meningitis (34%) with a variety of pathogens, especially encapsulated bacteria. The organisms most often involved are *Neisseria meningitidis* and *Streptococcus pneumoniae*, but other encapsulated Gram-negative and Gram-positive bacteria have also been observed. Recurrent infections are seen in more than half of C3-deficient patients. This clinical presentation is similar to that seen in hypogammaglobulinemia. C3-deficient individuals may develop renal disease (26%), including membranoproliferative and mesangiocapillary glomerulonephritis and autoimmune disease (26%), most commonly SLE.

Acquired C3 deficiency: genetic deficiencies of factor H and I, C3 and C4 nephritic factors

Factors H and I are required to control the fluid-phase alternative-pathway C3 convertase. Complete deficiency of either protein results in C3 cleavage and depletion to very low levels. C5, factor B, and properdin levels may also be reduced. The clinical presentation of patients with factor H or factor I deficiency resembles that of primary C3 deficiency.[51] The highest disease association is recurrent infection with *N. meningitidis* and *S. pneumoniae*, and there is also an increased incidence of SLE. Factor H deficiency is more commonly associated with renal disease than C3 or factor I deficiency (73% of factor H-deficient individuals compared to 13% of factor I-deficient and 26% of C3-deficient individuals).

Nephritic factors (NeF) are autoantibodies specific to classical and alternative-pathway C3 convertases (C4b2a or C3bBb) or the alternative-pathway C5 convertase that stabilize these enzyme complexes and prevent normal regulatory control. The alternative-pathway C3Nef induces

unregulated complement activation, resulting in acquired C3 deficiency. NeF are most associated with membranoproliferative glomerulonephritis (MPGN) type II. C3NeF is also associated with partial lipodystrophy, a condition in which fat is lost from the waist upward.

DEFICIENCIES OF COMPLEMENT RECEPTORS

Deficiencies of CR1 (CD35) and CR2 (CD21)

Complete genetic deficiencies of CR1 or CR2 have not been reported. However, partial deficiencies of CR1 on erythrocytes, B lymphocytes, and polymorphonuclear leukocytes and of CR2 on B lymphocytes have been reported in SLE patients. Decreased CR1 on erythrocytes may be acquired as a result of immune complex clearance. CR2 has been identified as a lupus susceptibility gene in a lupus-prone strain of mice.[37]

Leukocyte adhesion deficiency (LAD): CR3 and CR4 deficiency

Leukocyte adhesion deficiency (LAD: Chapter 21) is a syndrome caused by mutations of the common β_2-integrin chain, CD18, found in LFA-1, CR3, and CR4. Defects are related to adhesion and activation of phagocytic cells and the clinical presentation includes childhood infections with pyogenic bacteria.

DEFICIENCIES OF REGULATORY PROTEINS

Hereditary angioedema: C1 INH deficiency

Hereditary angioedema (HAE) is found in individuals with heterozygous deficiency of C1-INH. Complete genetic deficiency of C1-INH has never been reported, and HAE is the only complement deficiency with an autosomal dominant pattern of inheritance. C1-INH is a serine protease inhibitor (serpin) with regulatory activity for C1r, C1s, MASP-1, and MASP-2 of the complement system, factor XII (Hageman factor), and kallikrein of the contact system, factor XI and thrombin of the coagulation system, and plasmin and tissue plasminogen activator (tPA) of the fibrinolytic system. Although previous studies implicated a C2 product (C2 kinin) as a mediator, more recent information, including studies in a C1-INH-deficient mouse model, indicate that bradykinin is the primary biological mediator of angioedema in HAE.[52, 53] In the more common form of HAE (type I, 85% of patients), reduced synthesis of C1-INH is found (5–30% of normal), along with decreased serum C4 and C2. In type II HAE, an abnormal C1-INH is synthesized, making antigenic levels normal or elevated with reduced functional activity and decreased C4 and C2. Clinically, type I and type II HAE are indistinguishable.

HAE presents in childhood or adolescence as recurrent episodes of swelling that are subcutaneous and/or submucosal, nonpainful, nonpruritic, and nonpitting.[54] Urticaria is not present. Episodes are self-limited, usually peaking at 24 hours and resolving over 2–5 days. Attacks are variable in frequency, severity, duration, and location, and initiating factors are poorly understood. The most common areas involved are the extremities, face, genitals, respiratory tract, and gastrointestinal tract. Intestinal attacks are often associated with vomiting and diarrhea and are extremely painful. Laryngeal attacks may result in life-threatening respiratory obstruction. Laryngeal attacks are 50-fold less frequent than abdominal attacks and 70-fold less frequent than skin attacks, but the overall lifetime incidence of laryngeal edema is 70%. Recurrent attacks continue throughout the life of the patient and may involve multiple sites or progress from one site to another.

Diagnosis of HAE is suggested by family history and clinical findings.[54] Confirmation is based on decreased C1-INH functional activity (< 10–35% of normal). It is important to note that, although C1-INH protein is decreased in type I HAE, it can be normal or even elevated in type II HAE. C4 levels are below normal in 95% of HAE patients. Acquired forms of C1-INH deficiency have been described, usually in elderly patients with lymphoproliferative diseases. These may be caused by autoantibodies to C1-INH and are distinguished from HAE by a lack of family history and decreased C1q, as well as C4. A small percentage (0.1–0.5%) of hypertensive patients treated with angiotensin-converting enzyme (ACE) inhibitors will experience angioedema as a result of elevated bradykinin levels, and ACE inhibitors should not be given to patients with HAE.

Management of HAE patients includes long-term prophylaxis, short-term prophylaxis, and treatment of acute attacks.[53] International consensus guidelines for diagnosis and management are given in Bowen et al.[54] Long-term therapy should be considered in patients with frequent attacks or a history of serious upper-airway episodes. Long-term therapy may be provided by attenuated androgens, such as danazol and stanozolol, which increase serum concentrations of normal C1-INH in both type I and type II HAE. The lowest dose of androgen that is clinically effective is used because of undesirable side effects. Symptomatic benefit is usually achieved at doses that are not sufficient to restore C1-INH levels. Treatment with attenuated androgens generally increases C4 protein levels and markedly reduces both the frequency of spontaneous attacks and the incidence of oral surgery-induced laryngeal edema. Anti-fibrinolytic therapy with epsilon aminocaproic acid (EACA) or tranexamic acid may be used to control HAE in patients who do not tolerate anabolic androgen therapy.

Treatment with higher doses of danazol or tranexamic acid is also useful for short-term prophylaxis 5–10 days prior to dental procedures or surgery. Infusion of fresh frozen plasma several hours before the procedure may also be effective. Although currently not licensed in the USA, C1-INH concentrates have proven effective in several case series studies for short-term prophylaxis.

Treatment of acute attacks with epinephrine, antihistamines, corticosteroids, or androgens is not effective. Anti-fibrinolytic therapy with high-dose EACA or tranexamic acid has been used, as has infusion with C1-INH concentrate or fresh frozen plasma. The efficacy of EACA therapy is currently supported only by anecdotal evidence and neither tranexamic acid nor C1-INH concentrate is licensed in the USA. Infusion of fresh frozen plasma carries a demonstrated risk of worsening the attack. In the absence of effective therapeutics, management of acute attacks is focused on symptomatic control.[53] Abdominal episodes may require fluid replacement and control of pain and nausea. Pharyngeal attacks are the most life-threatening and require hospitalization with careful airway monitoring and intubation if needed. Several new therapeutic agents are in development for acute episodes of HAE. These include recombinant human C1-INH, recombinant kallikrein inhibitor, and a bradykinin receptor antagonist.[53, 55]

Paroxysmal nocturnal hemoglobinuria: DAF and CD59 deficiency

Paroxysmal nocturnal hemoglobinuria (PNH) is a rare acquired disorder in which a somatic mutation in the *Pig*-A gene in a clone of bone marrow stem cell results in defective synthesis of GPI-anchored proteins.[56]

PNH is characterized clinically by intravascular hemolysis with periodic hemoglobinuria and venous thrombosis. DAF and CD59 are GPI-anchored complement regulatory proteins expressed on erythrocytes, and PNH erythrocytes are highly susceptible to lysis. Studies of individuals with isolated DAF and CD59 deficiencies indicate that hemolysis is more highly associated with CD59 deficiency. The basis for thrombosis in PNH is poorly understood.

Control of localized complement activation: atypical hemolytic–uremic syndrome, age-related macular degeneration

HUS is a rare disease characterized by microangiopathic hemolytic anemia, thrombocytopenia, and acute renal failure. 'Typical' HUS is found in children and is caused by *Escherichia coli*, mainly 0157:H7, producing a shigalike toxin. Atypical HUS affects older children and adults and is not associated with infection. Recently, mutations in complement regulatory proteins, factor H, factor I, or CD46 have been identified in approximately 50% of patients with atypical HUS.[57] The factor H mutations associated with HUS are clustered in the C-terminal end of the molecule in CCP20, a region that is required for factor H binding to polyanions and endothelial cells. The ability of factor H to regulate fluid-phase alternative-pathway activation is not affected and C3 levels are normal. These findings have led to the hypothesis that local complement regulation is essential for preventing renal disease following endothelial cell injury, and that factor H acts locally after binding to exposed matrix or damaged endothelium. Factor H and the membrane protein CD46 are both cofactors for factor I-mediated cleavage of C3b.

An additional factor H polymorphism (Tyr/His[402]) identified by genetic screening has been shown to be associated with the development of age-related macular degeneration (AMD), a major cause of blindness in the elderly.[58] This polymorphism is located in CCP7 in a region of factor H that binds heparin and CRP.[47] As is the case for the mutations associated with HUS, this region of factor H is not required for regulation of the fluid-phase alternative-pathway convertase. AMD develops when abnormal deposits of protein, termed drusen, form in the retina. Recent findings support the view that the local inflammatory response, including complement activation with MAC deposition, damages the retina leading to vision loss. Additional genetic analyses identified protective factor H variants as well as protective and high-risk polymorphisms in the factor B gene. Although complement factors are not the only genes linked to AMD, they are estimated to account for more than 50% of cases. These findings may lead to the development of new therapeutics that could provide protection from a very common form of age-related visual loss.

■ COMPLEMENT IN DISEASE ■

MEASUREMENT OF COMPLEMENT IN A CLINICAL SETTING

Laboratory tests for complement include functional assays for the classical pathway (CH_{50}), the alternative pathway (AH_{50}), and the lectin pathway.[48, 49] Functional and antigenic assays for each of the individual components are available in specialty laboratories. The CH_{50} is a hemolytic assay in which sheep erythrocytes sensitized with rabbit antibody are incubated with dilutions of the patient's serum. The titer is the dilution at which 50% of the sheep erythrocytes are lysed. The CH_{50} requires all of the classical pathway and terminal components (C1–C9). A comparable assay for the alternative pathway uses a buffer that blocks classical pathway activation and rabbit erythrocytes in place of sensitized sheep erythrocytes. Rabbit erythrocytes spontaneously activate the human alternative pathway and are lysed in the assay. The AH_{50} requires all of the alternative pathway and terminal components (factor B, D, P, C3–C9). The combined use of the CH_{50} and AH_{50} is the most effective screening method for genetic deficiencies of complement components. Complete deficiency will generally result in titers of < 5% in one or both assays. Because C3–C9 are common to both pathways, the combined results of the two assays can rapidly determine whether the deficiency is one of these shared components, one of the unique classical pathway components (C1, C2, C4) or one of the alternative-pathway components (factor B, D, properdin) (Fig. 20.8). Properdin deficiency results in low, but not absent, lysis in the AH_{50}, and C9-deficient patients may have values up to 30% of normal in the CH_{50}. Deficiencies of factor H and I and nephritic factors often result in very low C3 levels leading to reduced titers in both assays.

Lectin pathway function (and MBL deficiency) is determined using an ELISA in which the patient's serum is placed into wells coated with mannan. Binding MBL and activation of the lectin pathway results in the deposition of C4b and C4d that are detected with monoclonal antibodies. MBL levels may also be determined antigenically.

Heterozygous C1-INH deficiency as described above is associated with the clinical syndrome HAE.[49] The diagnosis may be made based on clinical findings and family history. C1 INH activity is reduced in these patients and C4 protein is also low in 95% of patients, especially during attacks of edema. In type I HAE (85% of cases), C1 INH protein levels are low, but in type II HAE (15% of cases), an abnormal C1 INH protein is made and antigenic levels are normal or elevated. There is an acquired form of C1 INH deficiency associated with lymphoma in which low C1 INH is accompanied by decreased C1q as well as C4 and C2.

Complement levels may also be decreased in diseases or conditions in which complement is activated, leading to consumption.[48] In contrast to genetic deficiencies, complement consumption characteristically results in low, but not absent, functional activity. In addition, multiple components of one or more pathways are expected to be low, and these decreased levels of complement are often correlated with disease activity. The most commonly used and most readily available complement tests are C3 and C4 protein and the CH_{50}. Diseases accompanied by classical pathway activation result in decreased CH_{50}, C4, and C3 levels. The alternative pathway is spared. These are primarily immune complex-associated diseases, both autoimmune and infectious, and are listed in Table 20.4. In addition 20% of cases of acute renal allograft rejection are associated with decreased CH_{50} and C2. Another cause of selective classical pathway activation is essentially a laboratory artifact in which clotting of the blood sample is associated with consumption of the early classical pathway. Plasma CH_{50}, C3, and C4 levels are all normal, but serum CH_{50} values are markedly decreased.

The alternative pathway is activated in gram-negative sepsis, poststreptococcal glomerulonephritis, MPGN, IgA nephropathy, factor H or factor I deficiency, and PNH. Laboratory values may show decreased C3 with decreased or normal CH_{50}, and normal C4 levels (Table 20.4). Alternative-pathway activation is not always reflected in decreased C3,

CLINICAL RELEVANCE

COMPLEMENT TESTS FOR DIAGNOSIS AND MONITORING OF SYSTEMIC LUPUS ERYTHEMATOSUS (SLE)

>> Decreased C3 and C4 are associated with increased severity of disease, and especially with lupus nephritis

>> On serial observation decreased C3 and C4 levels may predict flare

   Note: C4 reductions can precede C3 reductions

>> Remission after treatment of lupus often shows return to normal levels of C4, followed by increases in C3

   Note: SLE patients with partial C4 deficiency may have persistently low C4 levels

>> CH_{50} levels also decrease with flares of lupus

>> Decreased CH_{50} levels are associated with partial complement deficiencies

>> Complete absence of CH_{50} implies the existence of a hereditary deficiency of one of the classical complement pathway components (C1–C9)

because C3 is found at the highest concentration of all complement components and is an acute-phase reactant with elevated synthesis during disease states.

In clinical practice evaluation of complement levels may be useful in a variety of circumstances. Initial consideration of complement deficiency may be appropriate in patients presenting with autoimmune or infectious diseases (Table 20.3). The complement profile may also be helpful in differential diagnoses (Table 20.4). Monitoring complement levels is used to follow disease activity in SLE patients. Low complement levels are a strong predictor of renal involvement and also an indicator of response to therapy in SLE.

ROLE OF COMPLEMENT IN SPECIFIC IMMUNOLOGICAL DISEASES

The following sections briefly describe contributions of complement activation to the pathogenesis of immunological diseases. Emphasis is given to conditions in which animal models have helped to define the relative roles of different pathways and activities of complement. A general concept emerging from current research in this area is that most of the pathogenic effects of complement depend on generation of C5a and MAC. Further, it is becoming recognized that, regardless of the initial activation mechanism, alternative-pathway amplification is needed to produce sufficient quantities of these mediators to cause disease.

Systemic lupus erythematosus (Chapter 51)

Complement plays a dual role in SLE. There is a strong association of genetic deficiencies of C1, C4, C2, and C3 with SLE, indicating a protective role. Three complement-dependent mechanisms have been proposed: (1) complement-dependent clearance of immune

Table 20.4 Complement test interpretation

Pathway	CH$_{50}$	C4	C3	Related diseases
Classical	↓	↓	↓	SLE, IC disease, cryoglobulinemia, SBE
Alternative	↓	N	↓	Post-streptococcal GN, MPGN, IC disease
Fluid-phase activation of classical pathway	↓	↓	N	HAE, cryoglobulinemia, hypergammaglobulinemia
Fluid-phase activation of alternative pathway	↓	N	↓	Factor H or I deficiency
Acute-phase response	↑	↑	↑	Chronic inflammation in the absence of IC
Sample processing errors, coagulation-associated activation	↓	N	N	
Biosynthetic defects in complement proteins	↓	N	↓	Severe liver disease, decreased C3, C6, C9

GN, glomerulonephritis; HAE, hereditary angioedema; IC, immune complex; MPGN, membranoproliferative glomerulonephritis; SBE, subacute bacterial endocarditis; SLE, systemic lupus erythematosus.

complexes; (2) an essential role for complement in the development and maintenance of self-tolerance in B lymphocytes; and (3) a requirement for complement in the clearance of apoptotic cells and potential autoantigens released from such cells. On the other hand, complement activation is believed to play a pathogenic role in tissue damage induced by autoantibodies in SLE. There is evidence for complement activation in SLE skin and renal lesions as well as in autoantibody-mediated hemolytic anemia and thrombocytopenia. In mouse models of SLE genetic deficiency or blockade of alternative-pathway activation is protective, whereas deficiency of C4 exacerbates autoimmunity and disease.[41]

The pathogenesis of SLE is due in large part to the inflammatory response to immune complexes formed by autoantibody binding to antigens from dead and dying cells. The Arthus reaction is often used to study the inflammatory response to passively administered IgG antibody and antigen (usually ovalbumin) independent of autoimmune disease. The response is FcγR-dependent and includes increased vascular permeability with edema and rapid influx of neutrophils into the site. Depending on the route of injection, the Arthus reaction can be elicited in the skin, lungs, or peritoneum, with some differences in cells and effector pathways. Recent findings have shed new light on a long-standing controversy regarding the roles of complement and FcγR in the Arthus reaction. In the current model C5a has an essential role, not as a neutrophil chemoattractant, but as a modulator of FcγR expression on resident macrophages.[59] C5a may be generated through immune complex-initiated complement activation or directly from C5 by proteolytic cleavage. C5a binding to the C5aR makes resident macrophages responsive to immune complexes by increasing expression of stimulatory FcγR and decreasing expression of inhibitory FcγRIIb. This pathway is likely to apply to lupus nephritis where pathogenesis requires stimulatory FcγR, is increased in the absence of FcγRIIb, and can be treated by blocking C5 cleavage.

Anti-phospholipid syndrome (Chapter 61)

Anti-phospholipid syndrome is characterized by anti-phospholipid antibodies, recurrent fetal loss, vascular thrombosis, and thrombocytopenia. Anti-phospholipid antibodies are found in 50% of lupus patients and thrombotic events occur in about half of these patients. Anti-phospholipid antibodies found in patients without SLE have similar clinical consequences. Disease pathogenesis has been attributed to procoagulant effects of anti-phospholipid antibodies. A mouse model was recently described in which injection of pregnant mice with human IgG anti-phospholipid antibodies resulted in fetal loss and wasting.[41] In this model complement is required for pathogenesis and treatment with complement inhibitors is protective. Studies in the mouse model are consistent with initial complement activation by anti-phospholipid antibodies bound to the decidua, followed by C5a generation and recruitment of neutrophils. The alternative as well as the classical pathway was required for pathology. Interestingly, C3 deposition in the decidua was decreased if neutrophils were depleted, suggesting an amplification pathway mediated either by tissue damage or by neutrophil release of complement components.

Rheumatoid arthritis (Chapter 52)

Patients with RA generally have normal or elevated complement values systemically. There is, however, evidence for local complement activation in joint fluid, in synovium, and in rheumatoid nodules. Complement activation products in the joint are not specific to RA, but are also found in patients with osteoarthritis, SLE, Reiter's syndrome, and gout. Concentrations of C3a and C5a in joint fluid are higher in RA than in other types of arthritis. An important role for complement activation in the pathogenesis of RA is suggested by studies in two animal models – collagen-induced arthritis and the K/BxN-derived antibody transfer model. In the first model, inflammatory joint disease was ameliorated by treatment with an antibody to C5 that blocks its cleavage, preventing generation of C5a and the MAC. In the second model, disease was prevented by genetic deficiency of factor B, but not C4, indicating an essential involvement of the alternative pathway.[41]

Vasculitis (Chapter 59)

Human vasculitides encompass a spectrum of disease mechanisms and clinical manifestations. Some, such as giant-cell arteritis and the anti-neutrophil cytoplasmic antibody (ANCA)-associated vasculitides, Wegener's granulomatosis, microscopic polyangiitis, and Churg–Strauss syndrome, are not associated with local complement deposition or evidence of systemic complement depletion. In others, particularly those with circulating immune complexes, C3b, MAC and/or alternative-pathway components are deposited in lesions and complement profiles consistent with activation are found (Table 20.4). Classical pathway activation is found in polyarteritis nodosa, hypersensitivity vasculitis, rheumatoid vasculitis, SLE vasculitis, and mixed cryoglobulinemia. The vasculitis of Henoch–Schönlein purpura has features of alternative-pathway activation.

Glomerulonephritis (Chapter 67)

Complement activation is evident in most types of glomerulonephritis, with the site and pathway of activation dependent on the site of immune complex or autoantibody deposition.[60] Alternative-pathway activation is associated with IgA nephropathy, post-streptococcal glomerulonephritis, and MPGN type II. In IgA nephropathy, C3, properdin and the MAC co-localize with IgA in glomerular mesangium. Earlier studies demonstrated activation of the alternative pathway by aggregated IgA. More recent results have implicated activation of the lectin pathway in IgA nephropathy.[61] In a recent analysis of 60 renal biopsies from patients with IgA nephropathy, 25% showed deposition of MBL, along with L-ficolin, MASP, and C4d, indicating activation of the lectin pathway.[62] Glomerular deposition of MBL was associated with greater histological damage and higher proteinuria.

MPGN is a chronic progressive form of glomerulonephritis characterized by endocapillary proliferation and thickening of glomerular capillaries producing enlarged glomerular tufts. MPGN is divided into three histological groups, designated type I, II, and III based on electron microscopy of the glomerular lesion. Complement activation is present in all forms of MPGN with decreases in circulating levels and the presence of C3 on biopsy. MPGN type II differs from the other two forms in that serum levels of C4 are not decreased and renal biopsies do not usually demonstrate IgG or C4 deposition. MPGN type II is associated with three conditions that lead to unregulated alternative-pathway activation, factor H deficiency, inhibitory antibodies to factor H, and C3NeF.[51, 60] Complete factor H deficiency is rare, but strongly associated with renal disease (73% of cases), suggesting that unregulated alternative-pathway activation can damage the kidney. Factor H-deficient pigs and mice also develop MPGN that in mice could be alleviated by combined deletion of factor B.[51] C3NeF is an autoantibody that binds to the alternative-pathway C3 convertase (C3bBb), preventing its decay and regulation by factor H and I. C3NeF is found in as many as 80% of patients with MPGN type II.

In glomerulonephritis secondary to immune complex disease, such as SLE and MPGN type I, complement activation is primarily by the classical pathway and C4 is found deposited along with C3 and IgG in glomerular deposits. Complement activation contributes to disease by attracting and activating inflammatory cells through C5a and by direct damage to cells through MAC. Pathology due to inflammatory cell infiltration is predominant when subendothelial immune complex deposition and complement activation occur. Subepithelial deposits are associated with membranous disease, characterized by minimal inflammation, but direct damage to podocytes by MAC. In the Heymann nephritis model of human membranous nephropathy, there is strong experiment evidence that MAC insertion into glomerular epithelial cells is responsible for proteinuria and beneficial effects can be seen with complement activation antagonists and anti-C5 antibody.

Asthma (Chapter 39)

Asthma is a chronic inflammatory disease of the lung in which Th2 responses to environmental allergens frequently play a critical role. The development of mice deficient in receptors for C3a and C5a has led to a new understanding of the roles of the complement anaphylatoxins in asthma.[63] Several studies demonstrated a correlation between C3a and C5a release in asthmatic lungs and the influx of eosinophils and neutrophils. C3-deficient and C3aR-deficient mice were protected from development of acute bronchoconstriction, airway inflammation, and airway hyperresponsiveness. C5a inhibition had similar effects on the response to challenge in an established allergic environment. However, in contradiction to these findings, C5 deficiency was genetically linked to susceptibility to experimental allergic asthma. Further studies found that C5a signaling (most likely through the C5aR on pulmonary dendritic cells) during initial pulmonary exposure to allergen decreased Th2 cytokine and IgE production, thereby preventing the initiating of the allergic response.[63]

Ischemia/reperfusion injury

Ischemia/reperfusion (I/R) injury refers to injury induced by inflammatory mediators, such as reactive oxygen intermediates produced by activated neutrophils, following the reperfusion of hypoxic tissue. Different pathways of complement activation may be important in different sites of injury, possibly due to differences in expression of complement regulatory proteins.[41] The complement mediators of tissue injury are C5a and MAC acting locally, and in some cases C5a acting systemically. In experimental renal I/R injury and in human tubular necrosis, the alternative pathway appears to be directly activated and neither antibody nor the classical pathway are required. However, in intestinal I/R injury, the classical pathway as well as the alternative pathway is required and a natural IgM antibody to a newly exposed antigen on damaged endothelium initiates complement activation. In coronary artery ligation/reperfusion models, innate recognition of epitopes on ischemic tissue by MBL and CRP leads to classical pathway activation.

Neurological disease

Complement is found in the central and peripheral nervous system. In the central nervous system complement enters from the blood when the blood–brain barrier is impaired. Low levels of hemolytic complement (0.25% of serum levels) can be measured in the cerebrospinal fluid if care is taken to stabilize it with gelatin during storage. Complement proteins

REFERENCES

and regulatory proteins are synthesized by glial cells and astrocytes and synthesis is enhanced by inflammatory cytokines. There is evidence both from human multiple sclerosis (Chapter 65) and the animal model, experimental allergic encephalitis (EAE), that complement activation with the generation of the MAC contributes to the demyelination in these diseases. Generation of the MAC can lead to oligodendrocyte death, generation of inflammatory mediators, or a repair process in which myelin synthesis is decreased. Complement activation on myelin and oligodendrocytes is initiated by anti-myelin antibodies or directly by myelin through the classical pathway. There is evidence of MAC formation in the cerebrospinal fluid of patients with multiple sclerosis, and complement depletion, inhibition, and genetic deficiency are protective in rat and mouse models of EAE.

There is evidence of complement activation in degenerative neurological conditions such as Alzheimer's disease.[64] In Alzheimer's disease neurofibrillary tangles and senile plaques composed of β-amyloid and other proteins develop, resulting in neuronal loss and dementia with progressive loss of cognitive function. Complement activation products C1q, C4, C3, and MAC components, as well as clusterin and vironectin, are found deposited in areas of amyloid, suggesting classical pathway activation. Peptides derived from β-amyloid were shown to activate C1 directly by binding to the collagen-like domain. SAP, a component of all types of amyloid, including β-amyloid, activates the classical pathway as well. There are limited data on the role of complement in Alzheimer's disease pathogenesis, with some studies reporting enhanced disease following complement inhibition and another finding decreased inflammatory changes and neuronal degeneration C1q deficiency.

COMPLEMENT-BASED THERAPEUTICS

The multiple roles of complement in inflammatory and autoimmune diseases make it an attractive target for therapeutic intervention. Recombinant complement inhibitors, inhibitory monoclonal antibodies and peptide-based receptor inhibitors have been developed to block complement effects.[65] As described above, complement has many beneficial effects in host defense and the adaptive immune response. The detrimental effects of complement activation are for the most part

CLINICAL RELEVANCE

COMPLEMENT INHIBITORS AS THERAPEUTIC AGENTS

>> Soluble regulatory proteins: sCD35 (CR1), sCD46 (MCP), sCD55/CD46 chimera, sCD59

>> Inhibitory monoclonal antibodies to: mannose-binding lectin, properdin, factor B, factor D, C5a

>> Monoclonal antibody to C5 (eculizumab) in clinical trials was effective in paroxysmal nocturnal hemoglobinuria

>> Peptide inhibitors: C5aRa, C1q inhibitor

>> Tissue-targeted inhibitors: CD59, CD35 targeted to tissue (L-selectin, CR2)

associated with C5a and the MAC.[41] Thus targeting either the generation of C5a or the C5aR might be expected to control inflammation while maintaining other important functions such as opsonization. An anti-C5 monoclonal antibody (eculizumab) that prevents its cleavage was effective in murine lupus and Heymann nephritis.[66] In human trials, eculizumab was of benefit in patients with PNH, but had no effect on urinary protein excretion in human membranous nephropathy. C5a inhibitory peptides (C5aRa) are effective in a number of inflammatory models in animals and have potential in the treatment of sepsis, reperfusion injury, and asthma.[35] Other approaches that are being developed will target complement regulatory proteins to specific cell or tissue targets.[65] This chapter covers our current concepts of the role of complement in disease. As complement has been the object of increasing importance in a variety of inflammatory diseases, it is likely that further research will establish new complement-based therapeutic agents for additional applications.

REFERENCES

1. Walport MJ. Complement. First of two parts. N Engl J Med 2001; 344: 1058–1066.

2. Walport MJ. Complement. Second of two parts. N Engl J Med 2001; 344: 1140–1144.

3. Wessels MR, Butko P, Ma M, et al. Studies of group B streptococcal infection in mice deficient in complement component C3 or C4 demonstrate an essential role for complement in both innate and acquired immunity. Proc Natl Acad Sci (USA) 1995; 92: 11490–11494.

4. Marnell L, Mold C, Du Clos TW. C-reactive protein: ligands, receptors and role in inflammation. Clin Immunol 2005; 117: 104–111.

5. Volanakis JE. Human C-reactive protein: expression, structure, and function. Mol Immunol 2001; 38: 189–197.

6. Kang YS, Do Y, Lee HK, et al. A dominant complement fixation pathway for pneumococcal polysaccharides initiated by SIGN-R1 interacting with C1q. Cell 2006; 125: 47–58.

7. Sorensen R, Thiel S, Jensenius JC. Mannan-binding-lectin-associated serine proteases, characteristics and disease associations. Springer Semin Immunopathol 2005; 27: 299–319.

8. Farries TC, Atkinson JP. Evolution of the complement system. Immunol Today 1991; 12: 295–300.

9. Pangburn MK, Schreiber RD, Muller-Eberhard HJ. Formation of the initial C3 convertase of the alternative complement pathway. Acquisition of C3b-like activities by spontaneous hydrolysis of the putative thioester in native C3. J Exp Med 1981; 154: 856–867.

10. Harboe M, Ulvund G, Vien L, et al. The quantitative role of alternative pathway amplification in classical pathway induced terminal complement activation. Clin Exp Immunol 2004; 138: 439–446.

11. Gaboriaud C, Thielens NM, Gregory LA, et al. Structure and activation of the C1 complex of complement: unraveling the puzzle. Trends Immunol 2004; 25: 368–373.

12. Gewurz H, Ying SC, Jiang H, et al. Nonimmune activation of the classical complement pathway. Behring Inst Mitt 1993; 93: 138–147.

13. Dodds AW, Ren XD, Willis AC, et al. The reaction mechanism of the internal thioester in the human complement component C4. Nature 1996; 379: 177–179.

Phagocyte deficiencies

Gülbû Uzel, Steven M. Holland

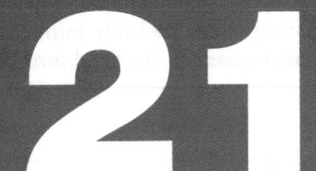

We have learned a great deal about phagocytes since their discovery by Metchnikoff in 1905. Phagocytes (neutrophils, monocytes, macrophages and eosinophils) traffic to the site of infection or inflammation and engulf microorganisms and apoptotic cells as the lead players in the innate immune response. Within the last four decades, many defects of the phagocytic system have been described and molecular genetic lesions for many have been defined. Recently, promising steps have been taken towards correcting these immunologically disabling disorders. This chapter reviews disorders of phagocytes and how they affect the immune system.

■ PHAGOCYTE DIFFERENTIATION ■

Myeloid cell differentiation has been studied at many levels and a hierarchy of maturation steps has been established. The pluripotent stem cell, residing in the bone marrow or the circulation, is the precursor for all the elements of the hematopoietic system. Precursors eventually commit to a single lineage, which terminally results in functionally distinct cells. This complex process of lineage commitment is under strict regulation by stage-specific signals derived from cytokines and growth factors (Chapter 2) that interact with their cognate receptors on cells. In response to these regulatory factors, cells change size and nuclear shape while stage-specific organelles containing critical proteins for neutrophil phagocytosis, bactericidal activity and inflammatory properties are formed.

■ PRODUCTION OF MACROPHAGES AND GRANULOCYTES ■

The pluripotent stem cell gives rise to the myeloid stem cell, from which the colony-forming unit granulocyte–erythrocyte–macrophage–megakaryocyte (CFU-GEMM) is derived. Among the growth factors that are influential at this step are stem cell factor (SCF), interleukin-3 (IL-3), and granulocyte–macrophage colony-stimulating factor (GM-CSF). The CFU-GEMM further differentiates into the colony-forming

unit–granulocyte–macrophage (CFU-GM) under the continuing influence of these growth factors. The colony-forming unit–granulocyte (CFU-G), a neutrophil lineage committed precursor, is derived from CFU-GM under the control of IL-3, GM-CSF and granulocyte colony-stimulating factor (G-CSF). Further downstream in the myeloid maturation process the myeloblast is formed from the CFU-G under the influence of GM-CSF and G-CSF. This is the first morphologically distinct cell of the neutrophil lineage. Promyelocyte, myelocyte, metamyelocyte, band form and mature neutrophil formation follow consecutively under the ongoing control of G- and GM-CSF. The maturation process from stem cell to the myelocyte stage takes 4–6 days and an additional 5–7 days for the myelocyte to form the mature neutrophil. The half-life of neutrophils in the circulation is only 7 hours, but an astounding 10^{11} neutrophils are generated daily, a number that can be further expanded in the setting of infection. The circulating and marginated granulocyte pools comprise only a small percentage of the total granulocyte pool: 3% and 4%, respectively.

Macrophage differentiation is similar to granulocyte differentiation in many respects. The CFU-GM differentiates into the colony-forming unit–macrophage (CFU-M) followed by the formation of the monoblast, promonocyte and monocyte under the influence of macrophage colony-stimulating factor (M-CSF). After monocytes are released into blood, they circulate for 1–4 days before entering tissues, where they further differentiate into macrophages. Macrophages can be found in many tissues, including pleura, alveolae, peritoneum, liver (Küpffer cells), bone marrow, bone (osteoclasts), lymph nodes and the central nervous system (microglia). They are active participants in inflammation, granuloma formation, and the appearance of multinucleated giant cells.

■ EVOLUTION OF NEUTROPHIL GRANULES ■

During myelopoiesis in the bone marrow, the first granules form at about the promyelocyte stage, stain blue with a Wright or Romanowsky stain, and are called primary or azurophilic granules

Treatment with daily subcutaneous G-CSF (1–120 µg/kg/day) results in an increase in ANC above 1000/µL, with a decrease in the frequency of infections and significant clinical improvement overall.

SHWACHMAN–DIAMOND SYNDROME (SDS)

Shwachman–Diamond syndrome was first described by Shwachman et al. in 1964 as a disorder with pancreatic exocrine insufficiency and bone marrow dysfunction.[4] Today it is recognized as the second most common cause of inherited exocrine pancreatic insufficiency after cystic fibrosis. The estimated incidence of SDS is 0.5–1:100 000 live births. It is inherited as an autosomal recessive trait.

Disease-associated mutations were identified in the gene *SBDS*, located at 7q11.[5] Recurring mutations were reported to result from gene conversion due to recombination with a pseudogene in 89% of unrelated patients; 60% carried two converted alleles. These gene conversion mutations in *SBDS* are common to different ethnic groups. The SDBS protein belongs to a highly conserved protein family involved in RNA metabolism. Mutations cause defects in the development of the exocrine pancreas, hematopoiesis and chondrogenesis.

Patients present with recurrent infections and failure to thrive in infancy. Features of SDS are hematopoietic dysfunction, metaphyseal dysostosis and growth retardation, and fatty replacement of the pancreas. Anemia and thrombocytopenia are associated with neutropenia. The majority of the patients have mild neutropenia, but a minority have neutrophil counts <500/µL Neutropenia may be intermittent or persistent. Congenital aplastic anemia is an unusual presentation of SDS.[6] Upper and lower respiratory tract pyogenic infections are the most common cause of morbidity and mortality and are related to neutropenia. An elevation in hemoglobin F is also reported in some cases. Leukemia has been observed in some SDS patients, although the exact frequency remains unknown.

Skeletal abnormalities are universal in patients with SDS. Short ribs with broadened anterior ends are the most common radiologic findings. Metaphyseal dyschondroplasia of the femoral head is frequent. Delayed bone age also may be a component of this multisystem disorder. The diagnosis can be made with the typical radiological findings, detection of abnormal pancreatic exocrine function (abnormal serum pancreatic α-amylase and total lipase activities, serum immunoreactive trypsinogen, fecal chymotrypsin and 3-day fat balance analysis) and serial hematologic evaluations. CT scans of the abdomen show typical fatty replacement of the pancreas.

Early replacement with pancreatic enzymes facilitates nutrition and growth. Subcutaneous administration of rG-CSF corrects neutropenia.

CYCLIC NEUTROPENIA

Human cyclic hematopoiesis or cyclic neutropenia (CN) is an autosomal dominant disease in which patients have approximately 21-day oscillations of blood-cell production. The neutrophils fluctuate between the lower limit of normal and zero. Platelets, monocytes and reticulocytes follow the same interval of oscillation but are out of phase with the neutrophils, hence the more appropriate title cyclic hematopoiesis. The frequency of this blood-cell disorder is estimated to be 0.5–1/1 000 000 population.

During the periods of neutropenia patients are prone to infections with pyogenic bacteria. The clinical presentation may be fever of unknown origin, gingivitis, stomatitis, oral ulcers, cellulitis, perirectal abscess, or more severe systemic pyogenic infections. Death from overwhelming infection is rare. Otherwise, it has a relatively benign course without

known predisposition to malignant disorders. Some patients may experience improvement in clinical symptoms, with the cycles being less noticeable as they grow older.

The genetic lesion has been mapped to chromosome 19p13.3 using genome-wide screening and positional cloning. Seven different single-base mutations in the gene encoding neutrophil elastase (*ELA2*) have been identified in affected families. The mutations are thought to lead to a gain of function in neutrophil elastase. Neutrophil elastase is synthesized during the promyelocyte and promonocyte stages and plays an important role in tissue destruction when released at the sites of inflammation. Various protease inhibitors, such as α_1-antitrypsin, inhibit neutrophil elastase. The reason for the disordered cycling of hematopoiesis in CN is thought to be perturbed interaction between neutrophil elastase and its substrates, but the precise mechanism remains unknown.

CN should be suspected in the setting of recurrent infections at regular intervals and cyclic hematopoiesis. To be able to document these intervals and diagnose cyclic neutropenia, a full blood count with differential should be performed 2–3 times weekly for at least 6 weeks (through two cycles).

Treatment with subcutaneous rG-CSF improves the quality of life in affected patients by increasing the ANC during both the peaks and valleys of myelopoiesis. However, this treatment does not eliminate the cyclic oscillations of other blood elements. The subcutaneous dose of rG-CSF required for the maintenance of an ANC above 1000/µL in cyclic neutropenia is typically less than that required for the same effect in SCN.

AUTOIMMUNE NEUTROPENIA

Autoimmune neutropenia (AIN) is caused by peripheral destruction of neutrophils by granulocyte-specific autoantibodies present in a patient's serum.

Primary autoimmune neutropenia

Primary AIN is seen predominantly in infancy and is not associated with other systemic immune-mediated disorders such as systemic lupus erythematosus (SLE). It is the most common form of neutropenia seen in young children and affects both genders equally. In a recently published cohort of primary AIN the average age at diagnosis was 8 months. The majority of patients present with mild skin and upper respiratory tract infections. A small minority may suffer from severe infections such as pneumonia, meningitis or sepsis. The diagnosis of primary AIN may be coincidental, as some patients remain asymptomatic despite low neutrophil counts. Neutrophil counts usually vary between 0 and 1500/µL during the neutropenic phase, the majority of patients having a count >500/µL at the time of diagnosis. The ANC may transiently increase two-to threefold during a severe infection and return to neutropenic levels following resolution. Bone marrow examination is normal or shows increased cellularity. In some cases maturation arrest may occur, but myeloid precursors reach at least to the myelocyte/metamyelocyte stage. Phagocytosed granulocytes may be seen in the bone marrow, indicating that the removal of sensitized granulocytes begins there.

Detection of granulocyte-specific antibodies is the gold standard for diagnosing primary AIN. In some patients detection may require repeated testing. Direct granulocyte immunofluorescence testing (D-GIFT) is one of the most sensitive methods available for detection of anti-granulocyte antibodies.[7] The vast majority of these are IgG; IgM antibodies are rare.

These antibodies are most commonly directed at the isolated glycoproteins of the granulocyte membrane and are designated neutrophil antigens (NA). These NA are located on the IgG receptor IIA or IIIB (FcγRIIa and FcγRIIIb). In more than 70% of primary AIN, one of the NA isoforms is recognized specifically. The etiology of this disease remains unknown unless there is a clear association with parvovirus infection.

The prognosis of primary AIN is very good, as it is self-limited. Neutropenia usually disappears within 1–2 years. Disappearance of the autoantibodies from the circulation precedes normalization of neutrophil counts. Symptomatic treatment of infections with antibiotics is usually sufficient. Prophylactic antibiotic treatment should be reserved for those with recurrent infections. Cotrimoxazole, ampicillin, or first-generation oral cephalosporins are the most commonly used prophylactic antibiotics. Alternative treatment strategies for severe infections and in the setting of emergency surgical interventions include high-dose intravenous immunoglobulin (IVIG), corticosteroids, and rG-CSF, with the latter being the most effective at increasing the ANC.

Secondary autoimmune neutropenia

Secondary AIN can be seen at any age and has a more variable clinical course, in contrast to the early onset and relatively benign, short-lived course of primary AIN. Other systemic or autoimmune diseases, such as hepatitis, SLE or Hodgkin's disease, often accompany the neutropenia. Even if it is not evident at the time of diagnosis, patients are at risk for developing other autoimmune problems. The antineutrophil antibodies have pan-FcγRIII specificity and are not specific for the NA. CD18/CD11b antibodies have been detected in a subset of patients with secondary AIN. This neutropenia responds poorly to most therapies.

ALLOIMMUNE NEONATAL NEUTROPENIA (ANN)

ANN is caused by the transplacental transfer of maternal antibodies against the fetal neutrophil antigens NA1, NA2 and NB1,[8] leading to immune destruction of neonatal neutrophils. These complement-activating antineutrophil IgG antibodies can be detected in about 1 in 500 live births. An NA-null phenotype in the mother with absence of expression of FcγRIII (CD16) has also been reported to be associated with immune neutropenia in the neonate. Antibody-coated neutrophils in ANN are phagocytosed in the reticuloendothelial system and removed from the circulation, leaving the neutropenic neonate at risk for infections. Omphalitis, cellulitis and pneumonia presenting within the first 2 weeks of life in the setting of neutropenia form the clinical picture. The diagnosis can be made by detection of neutrophil-specific alloantibodies in the maternal serum. ANN responds to G-CSF or high-dose IVIG, but most patients improve without specific treatment in a few weeks to 6 months.

■ DEFECTS OF LEUKOCYTE ADHESION ■

Migration of circulating leukocytes from the bloodstream into the tissues depends on complex bidirectional interactions between leukocytes and endothelial cells. The initial steps involve the activation of circulating leukocytes by inflammatory signals released from inflamed

tissues or by bacteria. After activation by chemotactic factors such as the complement fragment C5a, IL-8, leukotriene B_4 (LTB_4) or the bacterial product formyl-methionyl-leucyl-phenylalanine (fMLP), leukocytes rapidly become adhesive to the endothelium, other leukocytes, or laboratory surfaces. The activation process involves translocation of subcellular granules containing adhesion molecules (CD18/CD11b) to the surface of polymorphonuclear leukocytes (PMN), and qualitative alterations in the adhesion molecules constitutively expressed on the plasma membrane. Endothelial cells are similarly activated, resulting in enhanced expression of adhesion molecules. Adhesion and transmigration of leukocytes occur as a result of interactions between three groups of molecules: leukocyte integrins, endothelial intercellular adhesion molecules (ICAMs, members of the immunoglobulin supergene family), and glycosaminoglycans or selectins (Fig. 21.1).[9] The first step in targeting PMNs to inflamed tissues is the rolling or tethering of PMNs on the endothelium of postcapillary venules. This is due to the interactions between CD15s (sialyl Lewis^X or SLe^X) expressed on the leukocyte surface and P-selectin or E-selectin – members of the selectin family of adhesion molecules–expressed on the vascular endothelium. In addition, L-selectin on the leukocyte surface interacts with its counter-ligands P-selectin, CD34, glyCAM-1 and other glycoproteins located on the endothelial surface. Rolling, a relatively low-affinity interaction

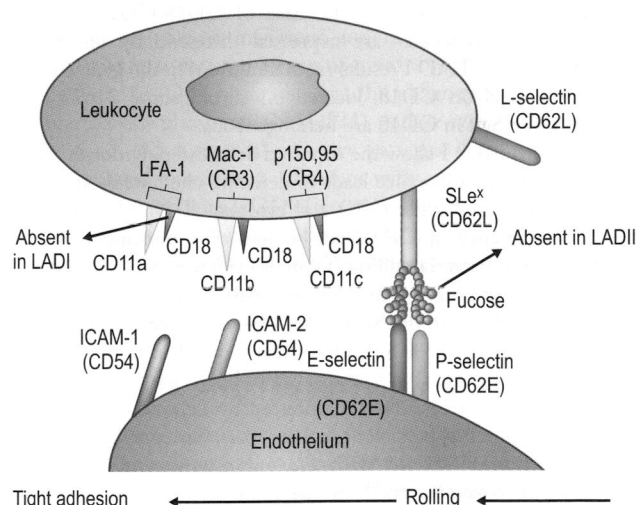

Fig. 21.1 Leukocyte adhesion to nonlymphoid endothelium. *Selectins* (L-selectin/CD62L, P-selectin/CD62P and E-selectin/CD62E), *integrins* (CD18/CD11a or LFA-1, CD18/CD11b or Mac-1 and CD18/CD11c or p150,95) and *intercellular adhesion molecules* (ICAMs) are involved in leukocyte adhesion to the nonlymphoid endothelium. Rolling, the initial step of leukocyte adhesion, is mediated by the interactions of E-selectin and P-selectin on endothelial surfaces with the sialyl Lewis^x (SLe^x or CD15s) of leukocytes as well as L-selectin on the leukocyte surfaces with its counter-ligands CD34 or glyCAM-1. This low-affinity tethering or rolling facilitates tight adhesion as a result of the interactions of LFA-1 with ICAM-1 or ICAM-2 and Mac-1 with ICAM-2. CD18 is the molecule that is missing or dysfunctional in LAD I, SLe^x is the missing molecule in LAD II.

Table 21.3 Notation used to describe different phenotypes of X-linked CGD

	X91⁰	X91⁻	X91⁺
gp91phox protein as determined by immunoblot or spectral analysis	Undetectable	Diminished	Normal
Cytochrome b558 spectrum	Absent	Low	Absent or normal
Type of mutations in CYBB	Deletions, insertions, splice site mutations, missense mutations, nonsense mutations	Missense mutation	Missense mutations

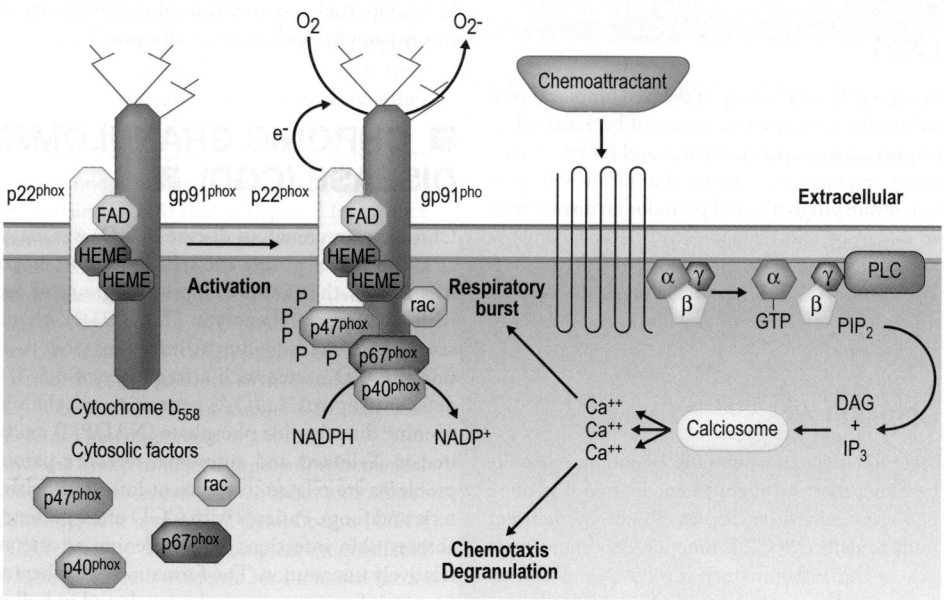

Fig. 21.4 Schematic representation of the NADPH oxidase system. Chemoattractants interact with their receptors on the neutrophil surface, leading to an increase in intracellular calcium concentration. This activation results in the assembly of the NADPH oxidase complex following phosphorylation of cytosolic factors. This is turn leads to superoxide production. DAG, diacylglycerol; PIP₂, phosphatidylinositol bisphosphate; IP₃, inositol triphosphate; α, β, γ, subunits of the GTP-coupled receptors.

proteins, p47phox, p67phox, p40phox and the small GTP binding proteins p21rac1/p21rac2. p47phox, p67phox and p40phox bind to one another via interaction of SH3 domains and proline-rich regions. This trimolecular complex docks with the cytochrome at the membrane via association of the phosphorylated p47phox and the proline-rich region of the carboxy-terminus of p22phox. The interaction between p67phox and the α helix overlying the nucleotide-binding domain of NADPH is also important. p21rac, the small GTP-binding protein of the NADPH oxidase activation complex, is involved in the regulation of oxidase activity. When stimulated, p21rac dissociates from the GDP-dissociation inhibitor protein GDI and binds to p67phox in the activation complex, leading to the translocation of the p67phox complex to the membrane. Activation of the complex results in phosphorylation of p47phox as well as p67phox, gp91phox, and p22phox.

MUTATIONS LEADING TO CGD

X-linked CGD

The most common form of CGD is caused by mutations in the gene encoding gp91phox (*CYBB*) at Xp21.1 (Table 21.3). The largest series studied to date, of 131 kindreds, found large and small deletions (11%), frame shifts (24%), nonsense mutations (23%), missense mutations (23%), splice region mutations (17%), and regulatory region mutations (2%).[16] Carrier detection revealed a functionally abnormal phagocyte population in 89% of mothers, making for a spontaneous mutation rate of approximately 11%. In several patients with large interstitial deletions, adjacent genes are affected, causing McLeod syndrome, Duchenne muscular dystrophy, or X-linked retinitis pigmentosa in addition to

CGD. The clinical phenotype of McLeod syndrome includes compensated hemolysis, acanthosis, and progressive neurodegenerative symptoms such as areflexia, dystonia and choreiform movements. McLeod syndrome is characterized by absent erythrocyte Kx protein and diminished levels of Kell blood group antigens. These patients may form anti-Kx and anti-Km antibodies when transfused, making future transfusions extremely difficult. Therefore, all X-linked CGD patients should be carefully screened for Kell blood groups.

Autosomal recessive CGD

Mutations in the genes encoding the NADPH oxidase components p47phox, p67phox and p22phox cause autosomal recessive forms of CGD, accounting for approximately 35% of all cases. Mutations in the gene encoding p22phox (*CYBA*), located at 16q24, are responsible for 6% of all CGD cases. Mutations in the gene for p67phox (*NCF2*, located at 1q25) and p47phox (*NCF1*, located at 7q11.23) cause respectively <5% and 25% of all CGD mutations. The great majority of patients with p47phox deficiency are homozygous for a GT deletion at the start of exon 2.[17] A few patients have been reported who are heterozygous for the GT deletion, with the second allele carrying a G deletion at position 502. p67phox and p22phox deficiencies are caused by deletions, insertions, missense and splice site mutations. All these genetic lesions lead to either the absence or the diminished production of the affected protein. Some CGD patients have normal amounts of nonfunctional protein due to missense mutations. So far no autosomal dominant cases have been confirmed.

CLINICAL MANIFESTATIONS OF CGD

The first severe infection is usually in infancy or childhood, although adults have been diagnosed with CGD as well. Late diagnoses usually occur in patients with some residual superoxide production. Patients with the p47phox-deficient genotype have a better prognosis and a less severe clinical phenotype overall.

The keys to diagnosis are severe infections with catalase-positive pathogens in an otherwise healthy host. Recurrent pyogenic infections with *Staphylococcus aureus*, *Burkholderia cepacia*, *B. gladioli*, *Serratia marcescens*, *Chromobacterium violaceum*, *Aspergillus* sp. and *Nocardia* sp. are highly suggestive of CGD, whereas streptococcal infections are not. Infections may be widely disseminated and fatal, but are most commonly pneumonia, lymphadenitis, liver abscess, skin abscess, perianal abscess, and osteomyelitis. As in other neutrophil defects, the most common pathogen is *S. aureus*. Staphylococcal liver abscesses, which are dense and caseous, are common in CGD and cause significant morbidity. Their fibrocaseous consistency means that percutaneous drainage is rarely successful and open surgery is required. Invasive pulmonary aspergillosis is the primary cause of death in North American CGD. *A. fumigatus* and *A. flavus* are commonly isolated, but *A. niger* and *A. nidulans*, species with low pathogenicity in the normal host, have been frequently reported in CGD. *Aspergillus* pneumonia is usually detected via computed tomography (CT) as a well-circumscribed consolidation in the peripheral lung parenchyma (Fig. 21.5). Thoracic wall invasion may occur, leading to osteomyelitis of the ribs, perforation of the diaphragm, or cutaneous abscesses. In this setting surgical resection of the infected tissue is often required, in addition to treatment with specific antifungal antibiotics. *Aspergillus* infections in CGD are often unaccompanied by systemic symptoms or signs of infection (e.g. fever,

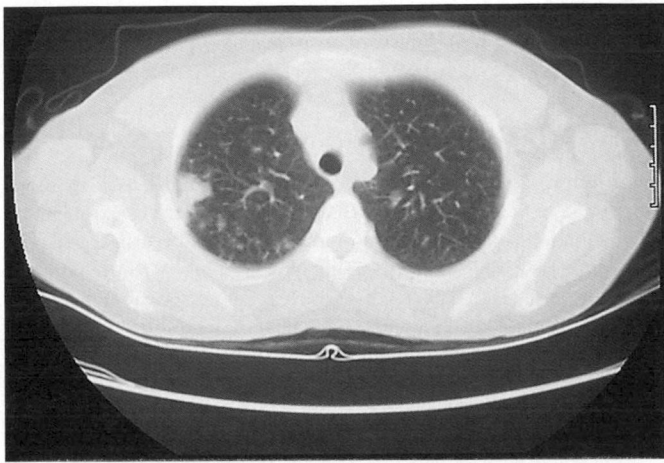

Fig. 21.5 CT scan of the lungs of a patient with chronic granulomatous disease (CGD) and *Aspergillus* pneumonia. *Aspergillus* pneumonia is detected as a peripheral consolidation in the lung parenchyma.

leukocytosis) and should therefore be suspected in any case of an asymptomatic pulmonary infiltrate. *Aspergillus nidulans* is especially likely to invade bone and be complicated. Septicemia is uncommon, but can occur with *B. cepacia*, often associated with pneumonia, *C. violaceum* following skin inoculation in brackish waters, or *S. aureus* in the setting of osteomyelitis.

Recently, a novel Gram-negative rod was identified from necrotic lymph nodes in several patients with CGD.[18] It was identified as a member of the family Acetobacteraceae and named *Granulobacter bethesdensis*.

Inflammatory granuloma formation is one of the hallmarks of CGD. The association with infection is not clear. Pyloric outlet obstruction, bladder outlet obstruction and ureteral obstruction are commonly encountered problems due to granuloma formation. A Crohn's-like inflammatory bowel disease is part of this inflammatory spectrum and may involve the esophagus (Fig. 21.6), jejunum, ileum, cecum, rectum and perirectal area in over 40% of X-linked patients. Gastrointestinal manifestations include diarrhea and malabsorption. Lipid-laden pigmented histiocytes are often seen in biopsies. GI involvement is common in CGD patients, with abdominal pain, growth delay, or hypoalbuminemia. In a large series of CGD patients evaluated for GI involvement, 43% of X-linked CGD patients and 11% of p47-deficient CGD patients had inflammatory bowel disease. The median age of initial GI manifestations was 5 years. Abdominal pain was the most frequent symptom (100%), and hypoalbuminemia was the most frequent sign (70%). GI involvement had no effect on mortality and was unaffected by the use of IFN-γ.[19]

Granulomata respond very well to steroids with a slow taper over several weeks to months. Exuberant formation of granulation tissue and dysregulated cutaneous inflammatory responses lead to wound dehiscence and impaired wound healing in CGD (Fig. 21.7). Autoimmune or rheumatologic problems, such as discoid lupus erythematosus, systemic lupus erythematosus and polyarthritis resembling juvenile rheumatoid arthritis, have been reported at higher than normal levels in CGD.

Polymorphisms in Fcγ receptors and myeloperoxidase, key molecules in host defense, have been linked to an increased risk of developing gastrointestinal or autoimmune and rheumatologic complications in CGD.

DIAGNOSIS OF CGD

In the setting of severe, recurrent infections with catalase-positive organisms involving the lung, liver or granuloma formation in the gastrointestinal or genitourinary tract, a diagnosis of CGD should be considered. The diagnosis is established by the inability of neutrophils to reduce nitroblue tetrazolium dye (Fig. 21.8), to produce chemiluminescence, or to oxidize dihydrorhodamine on appropriate stimulation. The dihydrorhodamine (DHR) assay is the most sensitive and enables quantification of the oxidative capacity of neutrophils. This flow-cytometric assay of oxidative burst can also help suggest the genotype of CGD involved.[20]

TREATMENT OF CGD

Prophylactic trimethoprim-sulfamethoxazole (TMP-SMX) significantly reduces the frequency of bacterial infections in CGD, especially those caused by *S. aureus*. TMP-SMX prophylaxis is ineffective against fungal infections but does not encourage them. Prophylactic itraconazole prevents fungal infections, as proven prospectively.[21] Leukocyte transfusions are sometimes used during severe infections in addition to antibiotics, although the benefits are unproven. Bone marrow transplants can cure CGD even in the setting of active infection However, transplant-related morbidity and mortality remains a significant problem.

IFN-γ is beneficial as a prophylactic treatment in CGD. In a multicenter placebo-controlled trial of IFN-γ the number and severity of infections were significantly reduced in the IFN-γ arm.[22] The exact

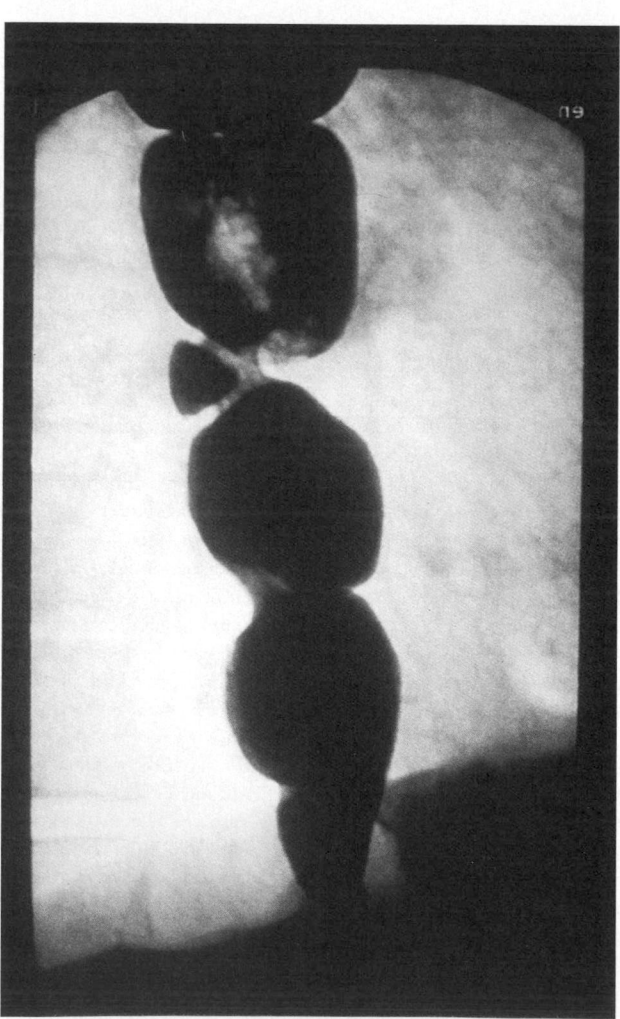

Fig. 21.6 Esophageal involvement in chronic granulomatous disease (CGD). Esophageal strictures caused by granuloma formation as seen on barium swallow.

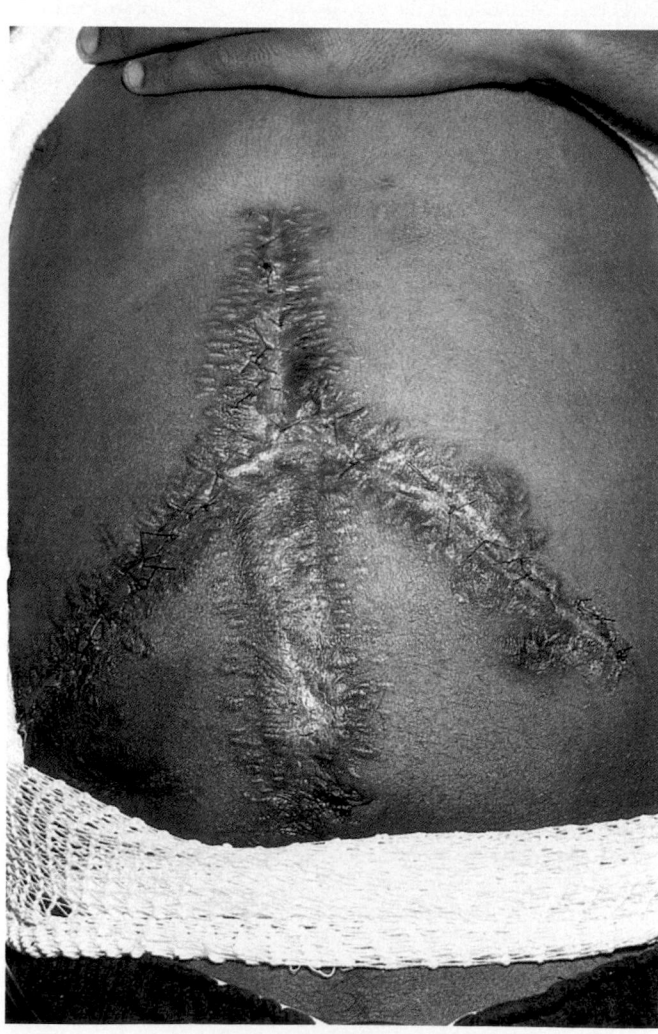

Fig. 21.7 Exuberant granuloma formation in chronic granulomatous disease (CGD). Wound dehiscence and impaired wound healing at surgical incision sites due to dysregulated inflammatory responses in an X-linked CGD patient.

CLINICAL PEARLS

CHRONIC GRANULOMATOUS DISEASE (CGD)

>> CGD comprises a group of four inherited disorders with a common phenotype.

>> Infections with catalase-positive bacteria and fungi, and granuloma formation in the gastrointestinal and urinary tract are the major problems in CGD.

>> Oral prophylactic antibiotics and subcutaneous IFN-γ injections three times a week are currently recommended for CGD.

>> Diagnosis can be made via NBT test or DHR assay, the latter being a more sensitive diagnostic tool.

mechanism of action of IFN-γ is not known, but it has a multifaceted effect, probably including stimulation of components of NADPH oxidase in partial deficiencies, increased bactericidal activity through neutrophil granule components, and Fc receptor expression. Increased nitric oxide production in CGD neutrophils with IFN-γ treatment suggests an alternative mechanism in augmenting host defense. Subcutaneous administration of recombinant IFN-γ three times a week at a dose of 50 μg/m^2 (for those with body surface area >0.5 m^2) is recommended. The adverse effects of recombinant IFN-γ in patients with CGD have been limited to fever, chills, headache, flu-like illness and diarrhea.

Gene therapy aims to provide CGD patients with genetically corrected autologous progenitor stem cells. Retrovirus-mediated gene transfer has been successful in p47^{phox} and gp91^{phox} knockout mouse models. Oxidase-positive granulocytes in patients with p47^{phox}-deficient CGD have been achieved transiently via gene therapy. Recently, two adults received gene therapy after nonmyeloablative bone marrow conditioning.[23] In these patients, gene transfer led to functionally corrected phagocytes and clinical improvement.

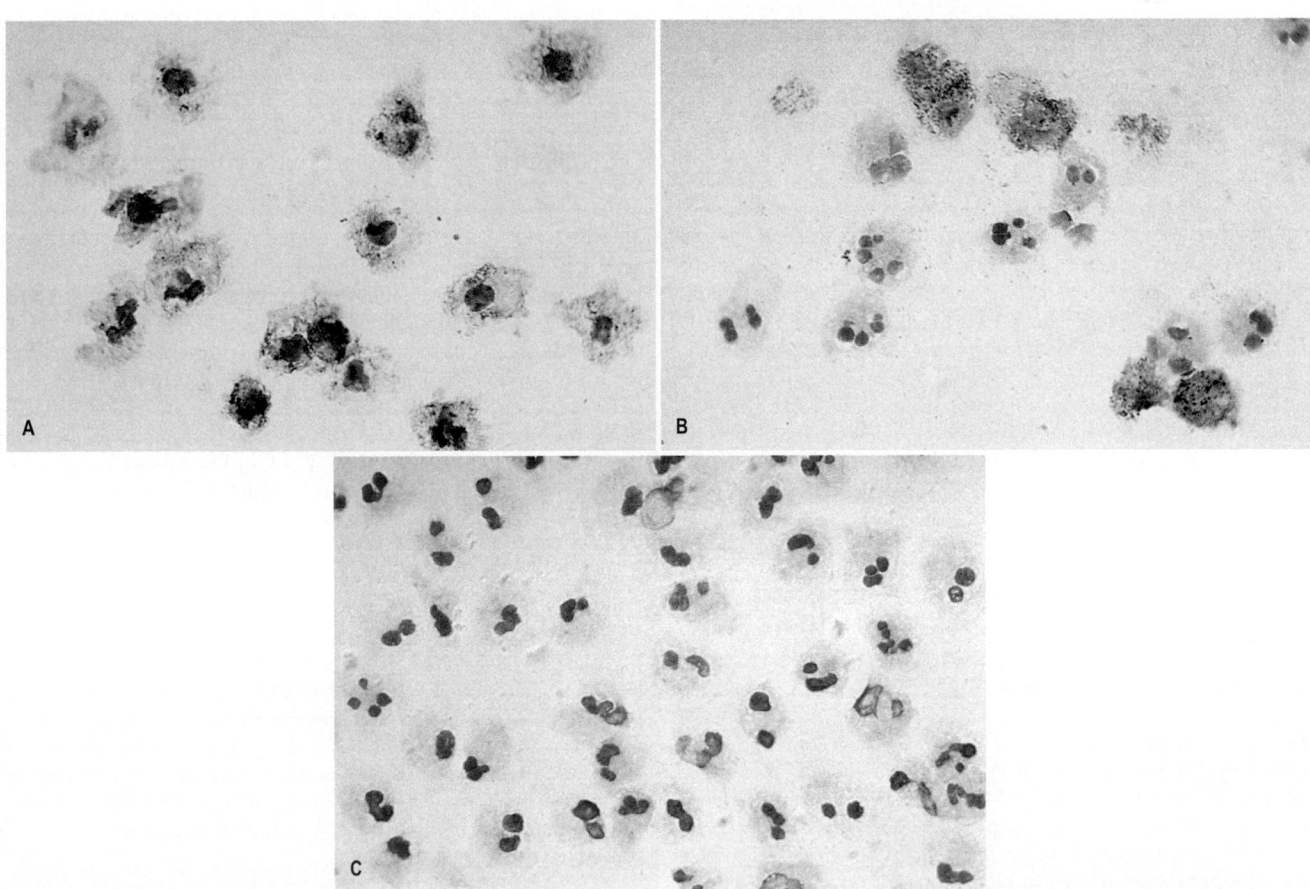

Fig. 21.8 Laboratory diagnosis of chronic granulomatous disease (CGD) with the nitroblue tetrazolium test (NBT). (**A**) NBT reduction by purified normal neutrophils following stimulation with phorbol esters and calcium ionophore. NBT is reduced by all neutrophils, showing a blue/purple deposit. (**B**) NBT reduction by purified neutrophils from an X-linked CGD carrier; two different populations of cells are seen. Normal (unaffected cells) reduce the NBT dye and stain blue/purple, whereas affected cells fail to reduce the NBT dye and appear clear. (**C**) Neutrophils from a patient with CGD fail to reduce the NBT dye and appear clear. (Courtesy of Dr Douglas B. Kuhns, SAIC, Frederick, MD.)

■ HEREDITARY MYELOPEROXIDASE DEFICIENCY ■

Hereditary myeloperoxidase deficiency (MPO) is characterized by a lack of myeloperoxidase activity. Myeloperoxidase is a heme-containing enzyme necessary for the conversion of H_2O_2 to HOCl and the subsequent killing of phagocytosed bacteria, fungi and viruses. MPO is expressed early in myeloid differentiation and resides in the azurophilic granules of neutrophils and the lysosomes of monocytes. The resulting mature protein is a symmetric molecule of four peptides, with each half consisting of a heavy-light chain heterodimer.

Neutrophils of MPO-deficient individuals fail to produce HOCl upon stimulation, but the NADPH oxidase system remains unaffected. Prolonged and higher levels of superoxide and H_2O_2 production following stimulation have been observed in MPO-deficient neutrophils. This is thought to be due to the lack of negative feedback regulation of HOCl on the NADPH oxidase, although the exact mechanism for this is unknown. MPO deficiency can be seen in two forms: primary (congenital) and secondary (acquired).

PRIMARY MPO DEFICIENCY

The primary form of MPO deficiency is the most common phagocyte defect, with a frequency of 1:4000, and is caused by germline mutations. There is heterogeneity among patients in the degree of MPO deficiency: both total and partial deficiencies have been described. Patients with primary MPO deficiency do not usually have an increased incidence of infections, probably because MPO-independent mechanisms compensate for the lack of MPO-dependent microbicidal activity. Most individuals have been diagnosed incidentally when MPO activity was used for specific neutrophil staining, for example in some automated differential readers. In some patients visceral candidiasis has occurred in the setting of concurrent diabetes. However, the frequency of such cases is very low. Affected patients may develop nonfungal infections, malignancies and certain skin disorders. In several cohorts of complete MPO-deficient patients an increased incidence of solid or hematologic tumors has been observed. Neutrophils have no apparent defect in phagocytosis of bacteria or fungi. However, microbicidal activity is slower than normal. These MPO-deficient neutrophils are unable to kill *Candida* or *Aspergillus* by *in vitro* assays, but patients do not develop *Aspergillus* infections. The association of malignancy and MPO deficiency remains uncertain, but may be related to the depressed cytotoxic activity against tumor cells.

The most common mutation is a missense change resulting in the replacement of arginine at position 569 with tryptophan (R569W). This causes a maturational arrest of the MPO precursor and prevents heme incorporation. Most patients are compound heterozygotes. The diagnosis of MPO deficiency can be made using anti-MPO monoclonal antibodies for flow-cytometric analysis of the neutrophil population. No MPO expression is seen in the congenital deficiency, whereas near-normal antigenic reactivity is seen with the acquired form.

Maintenance antibiotic or antifungal therapy is not routinely recommended. In patients with diabetes mellitus and congenital MPO deficiency, who may develop localized or systemic infections, prompt and prolonged therapy is advised.

SECONDARY OR ACQUIRED MPO DEFICIENCY

In the majority of patients MPO deficiency is partial and transient. Secondary MPO deficiency occurs under certain clinical conditions, such as some hematologic malignancies or disseminated cancers, exposure to cytotoxic agents or anti-inflammatory medications, iron deficiency, lead intoxication, thrombotic diseases, renal transplants and pregnancy. MPO activity in the bone marrow myeloid precursors as well as peripheral blood cells shows variation from cell to cell. Treatment of the underlying condition typically corrects the defect. This deficiency is most likely linked to somatic mutations in the case of malignancy or toxic–metabolic effects on MPO activity.

SPECIFIC GRANULE DEFICIENCY

Neutrophil-specific granule deficiency (SGD) is a rare disorder of leukocyte maturation in which neutrophil secondary granules are absent. SGD is characterized by frequent, severe bacterial infections. The several patients reported shared the common features of frequent, severe pyogenic infections, a paucity or absence of neutrophil-specific granule proteins and defensins, and atypical neutrophil nuclear structure with mostly bilobed nuclei. *In vitro*, these patients' cells showed diminished neutrophil migration, reduced staphylococcal killing, reduced phagocytosis and an increased cell surface/volume ratio. Eosinophils and platelets are also affected in SGD. Platelets lack high molecular weight von Willebrand factor multimers, and have reduced platelet fibrinogen and fibronectin due to diminished platelet α granules. Bleeding diatheses and neutrophil phagocytosis of platelets are seen in SGD. In addition, SGD eosinophils are deficient in the eosinophil-specific granule proteins eosinophil cationic protein (ECP), eosinophil-derived neurotoxin (EDN) and major basic protein (MBP), despite the presence of mRNA transcripts for these proteins. Early reports of normal levels of lactoferrin in saliva and mucus, but absent lactoferrin in neutrophils, indicated that the lactoferrin deficiency in SGD was tissue specific and therefore probably involved myeloid-specific transcriptional regulation. The knockout mouse model for the CCAAT/enhancer binding protein (C/EBP)ε, a member of the leucine zipper family of transcription factors expressed in myeloid cells, showed absent secondary and tertiary neutrophil-specific granule proteins, bilobed nuclei, defective chemotaxis, and a predilection to infections early in life. Based on the close similarity between the C/EBPε KO mouse and SGD, the C/EBPε locus has been identified in an SGD patient as having a 5 bp deletion leading to a frameshift and a loss of transcriptional activity of C/EBPε. This homozygous defect resulted in a promyelocyte–myelocyte transition block, absence of secondary granules and proteins, and a selective loss of the primary granule defensins, which are important elements in oxygen-independent microbicidal host defense. Few patients have been reported to have survived beyond adolescence. Bone marrow transplantation should be considered early in the disease.

■ CHEDIAK–HIGASHI SYNDROME ■

Chediak–Higashi syndrome (CHS) is a rare, autosomal recessive disorder characterized by partial oculocutaneous albinism, increased susceptibility to infections, deficient NK cell activity, and abnormal giant

SPECIFIC GRANULE DEFICIENCY (SGD)

>> SGD is caused by promyelocyte–myelocyte transition block due to a mutation in the C/EBPε gene.

>> Absence of secondary granule proteins, and a selective loss of the primary granule defensins are the pathologic findings in SGD granulocytes.

>> The prognosis is very poor in SGD.

primary granules in neutrophils. This immunodeficiency was first reported by Beguez-Cesar in 1943 and then further described by Chediak and Higashi a decade later. The hallmark of CHS is giant abnormal granules in all granule-containing cells, including melanocytes (melanosomes are members of the lysosomal lineage of organelles), neutrophils, central and peripheral nerve tissue, fibroblasts and hair. The problem is the inability to form appropriate lysosomes and cytoplasmic granules. Compared to specific granule deficiency, CHS granulocytes lack cathepsin G and elastase. On the other hand, SGD PMNs are almost completely deficient in defensins, whereas the defensin content in CHS PMNs is normal. These findings indicate that the giant granules of CHS are derived predominantly from the azurophilic granules.

CHS is classically described as a biphasic immunodeficiency, in which susceptibility to infection marks the first phase and an accelerated lymphoproliferative syndrome with histiocytic infiltration of various tissues marks the second. Disorders similar to CHS occur in many species. Rarely, the accelerated phase may be the initial presentation.[24] The giant organelles are derived from the late compartments of the endocytic pathway, affecting specifically late endosomes and lysosomes and having minimal or no effect on early endosomes. The *beige* mouse is an animal model of CHS that helped locate the *chs1* gene to chromosome 13 in the mouse and pointed out the homologous region 1q43 in humans. *CHS1* encodes a 3801 amino acid peptide (*Lyst*, lysosomal transporter) that has a vital role in lysosomal trafficking. Lysosomal exocytosis triggered by membrane wounding is impaired in both human Chediak–Higashi and beige mouse fibroblasts.[25] The reduced survival of fibroblasts after wounding indicates that impaired lysosomal exocytosis inhibits membrane resealing. Lysosomal exocytosis was increased when the normal lysosomes were restored by expression of the LYST protein. Inability of cells to repair plasma membrane lesions may contribute to the pathology of CHS. The exact mechanism by which LYST regulates lysosomal functions is yet to be identified.

The dermatologic manifestations of CHS are striking. The degree of albinism may vary from a slightly diluted skin pigment to hypopigmented skin and hair, photophobia, nystagmus, strabismus, macular hypoplasia and reduced visual acuity. Skin biopsies show large irregular melanin granules in melanocytes. Microscopic analysis of hair also shows poor distribution of melanin. Pancytopenia, neutropenia and lack of NK-cell activity result in frequent pyogenic infections, usually due to staphylococci or streptococci. Hepatosplenomegaly and lymphadenopathy are common. A mild bleeding diathesis is due to platelet storage pool deficiency. Neurologic dysfunction has been noted in CHS, including mental retardation, seizures, cranial nerve palsies and progressive peripheral neuropathy.

The lymphoma-like lymphohistiocytic accelerated phase is characterized by increased hepatosplenomegaly, lymphadenopathy and worsened pancytopenia, which may resemble the virus-associated hemophagocytic syndromes or familial erythrophagocytic lymphohistiocytosis. Although chemotherapy can induce transient remissions, relapses are common. HLA-identical bone marrow transplantation has been successful in prevention of the accelerated phase and restoration of NK-cell function, but it does not resolve the central or peripheral nervous abnormalities.

Demonstration of giant azurophilic cytoplasmic inclusions on peripheral blood smears in the setting of the clinical findings provides a diagnosis of CHS; mutation analysis can confirm the diagnosis.

■ HYPER-IGE RECURRENT INFECTION (HIES OR JOB) SYNDROME ■

HIES is now recognized to be a multisystem autosomal dominant disorder characterized by recurrent infections of the lower respiratory system and skin, chronic eczema, extremely elevated IgE levels and eosinophilia (Table 21.4). HIES occurs in all racial and ethnic groups.

FACIAL, SKELETAL AND DENTAL ABNORMALITIES

Facial abnormalities seen in the majority of patients are a protruding, prominent mandible and forehead, apparent ocular hypertelorism, a broad nasal bridge and a wide, fleshy nasal tip with increased interalar distance (Fig. 21.9). Midline anomalies common in this disorder are a high-arched palate and midline sagittal clefts of the tongue. A single patient with HIES was reported to have a cleft lip and palate.

Skeletal abnormalities are common in this disorder, with a high incidence of fractures (57%) and scoliosis (76%) (Fig. 21.10). In addition, low bone density and cortical bone loss have been observed. Other infrequent skeletal abnormalities reported in HIES are craniosynostosis, spina bifida, bifid rib, wedge-shaped lumbar vertebrae, hemivertebrae and pseudoarthritis of the hip. Hyperextensibility of joints is common. A unique dental abnormality seen in this syndrome is retained primary teeth causing delayed eruption of the permanent teeth. This may be due to reduced resorption of primary tooth roots.

INFECTIONS AND IMMUNOLOGIC CHARACTERISTICS

Moderate to severe eczema presenting within the first hours to weeks of life is almost universal in HIES. Mucocutaneous candidiasis involving finger and toenails, mouth, vagina and intertriginous areas is seen in most patients. Lung abscesses requiring surgical drainage are almost always staphylococcal. Primary pulmonary infections are predominantly due to *S. aureus* and *Haemophilus influenzae*. These pneumonias are often associated with abscess formation and usually lead to the development of pneumatoceles (Fig. 21.10). Once lung cavities are formed, they provide an attractive environment for superinfection with *Pseudomonas* or *Aspergillus* sp. Thoracotomy is frequently required for removal of pneumatoceles or drainage of infected cavities. For reasons unknown, the unresected lobes of HIES patients often do not expand appropriately to

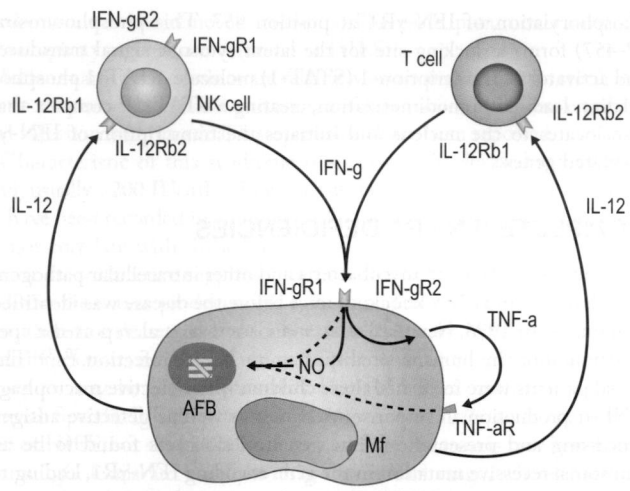

Fig. 21.11 Critical pathways in mycobacterial control. Mycobacterial infection induces IL-12 production by monocytes, which stimulates T cells and NK cells to produce IFN-γ. After binding to its cognate receptor, IFN-γ activates macrophages to produce TNF-α and to kill mycobacteria intracellularly by mechanisms not yet defined. IFN-γ also drives IL-12 production forward. AFB, acid-fast bacilli; NO, nitric oxide; IFN-γR1, interferon-γ receptor 1; IFN-γR2, interferon-γ receptor 2; IL-12Rβ1 and IL-12Rβ2, interleukin-12 receptor chains; TNF-α, tumor necrosis factor-α; TNF-αR, tumor necrosis factor-α receptors.

PARTIAL IFN-γR1 DEFICIENCY

Jouanguy et al.[35] reported two siblings with autosomal recessive IFN-γR1 deficiency due to an amino-acid substitution (I87T) in the extracellular domain of the receptor. In contrast to patients with complete IFN-γR1 deficiency, the partial IFN-γR1 defect was expressed normally on the cell surface, but only responded to IFN-γ at concentrations 100 times higher than normal. At the cellular level, the defect caused an intermediate phenotype between normal and complete IFN-γR1 deficiency. The patients were infected with BCG and *Salmonella enteritidis*; one had probable primary tuberculosis. The outcome was favorable compared to that in complete IFN-γR1 deficiency. These patients formed well-circumscribed and well-differentiated granulomas.

DOMINANT NEGATIVE IFN-γ RECEPTOR 1 DEFICIENCY (AD IFN-γR1)

A small deletion hot spot in the intracellular domain of IFN-γR1 causes autosomal dominant susceptibility to mycobacterial infection.[36] Patients with this genotype came from diverse ethnic backgrounds and presented with disseminated BCG or NTM infections, histoplasmosis, or salmonellosis. Subsequently, almost all patients with this genotype have developed multifocal NTM osteomyelitis, a manifestation that is rare in the complete IFN-γR deficiencies. The clinical presentation is usually evident later in childhood than complete IFN-γR1 deficiency. In addition, AD IFN-γR1 responds well to antimycobacterials and adjunctive IFN-γ therapy, whereas those with complete defects are often refractory to antibiotics and are unresponsive to IFN-γ.

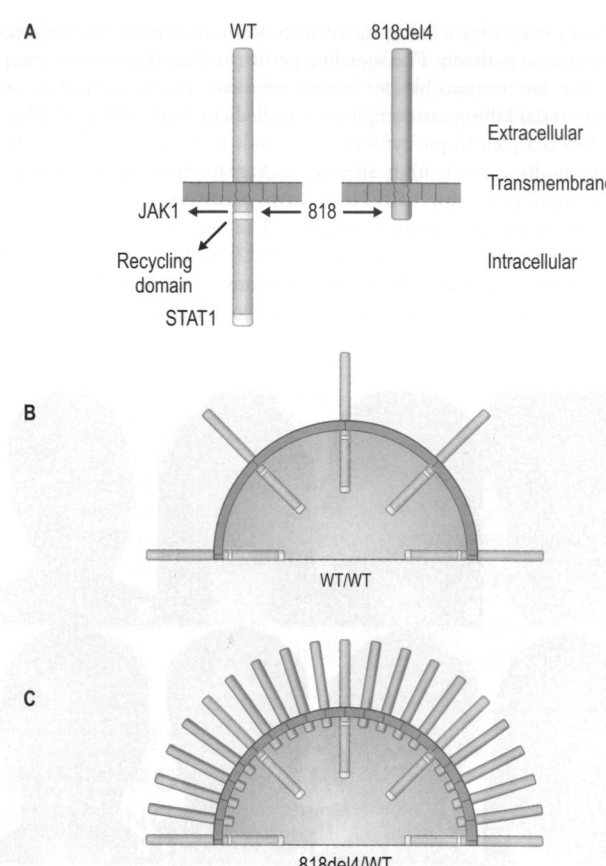

Fig. 21.12 IFN-γR proteins in wild-type and autosomal dominant conditions. (**A**) Wild-type IFN-γ receptor with intact intracellular JAK1 and STAT-1 binding sites and recycling domain (left). Truncated IFN-γR1 molecule due to 818del4/818del. The JAK1 and STAT-1 binding sites and the recycling domain are missing (right). (**B**) IFN-γR1 molecules on the surface of cells homozygous for wild type. (**C**) Mutant IFN-γR1 molecules on the surface of cells heterozygous for 818del4 and wild-type IFN-γR1 alleles. Excess truncated receptors are found on the surface of 818del4/WT cells compared to normal receptors at WT/ WT cell surface due to the lack of the recycling motif. Signaling is impaired due to the lack of intracellular signaling domains. (Modified from Jouanguy E, Lamhamedi-Cherradi S, Lammas D, et al. IFNGR1 small deletion hotspot associated with dominant susceptibility to mycobacterial infection. Nature Genet 1999; 21: 370.)

The genetic lesion can be one of four independent mutation events at a single mutation site: 816del4, 817del4, 818del4 (designated 818del4, as they cannot be distinguished from each other), or 818delT or 819delT (designated 818delT). These deletions result in frameshifts leading to a premature stop and early termination of the protein. The defect is localized to exon 6 in the IFN-γR1 open reading frame, within the intracytoplasmic segment of the receptor. Because the JAK1 and STAT-1 binding motifs are deleted, mutant chains are unable to transduce the IFN-γ signal. Mutant proteins are overexpressed at the cell surface due to a lack of the receptor-recycling domain, which is adjacent to the

low-risk patients have led to the identification of several genetic defects in this critical pathway. The signaling pathways, ligands and their receptors that are responsible for monocyte–macrophage activation and mycobacterial killing are complex but well characterized (Fig. 21.11).

IFN-γ is a pleiotropic cytokine that binds to its receptor (IFN-γR1) as a homodimer with high affinity, leading to receptor dimerization. Following dimerization of IFN-γR1, two accessory chains (IFN-γR2) aggregate with the receptor complex. The two IFN-γR2 molecules bring two Janus-associated kinase-2 (JAK2) molecules to the vicinity of the JAK1 molecules, which are constitutively associated with IFN-γR1. The trans-phosphorylation of JAK1 and JAK2 leads to tyrosine phosphorylation of IFN-γR1 at position 457. This phosphotyrosine (P-457) forms a docking site for the latent cytosolic signal transducer and activator of transcription-1 (STAT-1) molecule. STAT-1 phosphorylation leads to homodimerization, creating a STAT-1P complex that translocates to the nucleus and initiates the transcription of IFN-γ-regulated genes.

COMPLETE IFN-γR1 DEFICIENCIES

Genetic susceptibility to mycobacteria and other intracellular pathogens was identified in IFN-γ knockout mice before the disease was identified in humans. In 1996, Newport et al. and Casanova et al. reported a specific mutation in humans predisposing to NTM infection.[30, 31] The initial patients were related Maltese children with defective macrophage TNF-α production in response to IFN-γ as well as defective antigen processing and presentation. The genetic lesion was found to be an autosomal recessive mutation in the gene encoding IFN-γR1, leading to a complete absence of IFN-γR1 on the cell surface. Subsequently, a number of patients with other recessive mutations have been identified.[32, 33] Common to all patients with autosomal recessive mutations of IFN-γR1 is that the function of the mutated receptor protein and IFN-γ signaling are severely impaired. Although we think of IFN-γR1 deficiency as primarily affecting macrophages, the cells with the central role in the pathogenesis of mycobacterial infections, almost all nucleated cells display IFN-γR. Therefore, subtle aspects of the phenotype probably remain to be defined.

Patients with IFN-γR1 deficiency usually come to attention because of infections with bacille Calmette–Guérin (BCG) or nontuberculous mycobacteria (NTM) including *M. avium*, *M. fortuitum*, *M. chelonae* and *M. smegmatis*. *Salmonella* spp. infect up to 50% of patients in some series. Mycobacterial disease tends to be diagnosed in infancy or early childhood and leads to death or severe disease. A striking histopathologic finding is the failure to form well-circumscribed tuberculoid granulomas. Although this genetic defect has been predominantly associated with mycobacteria and salmonella, the recognized phenotype has been expanded to include increased susceptibility to cytomegalovirus, respiratory syncytial virus, varicella and parainfluenza virus as well as *Listeria monocytogenes*.[34]

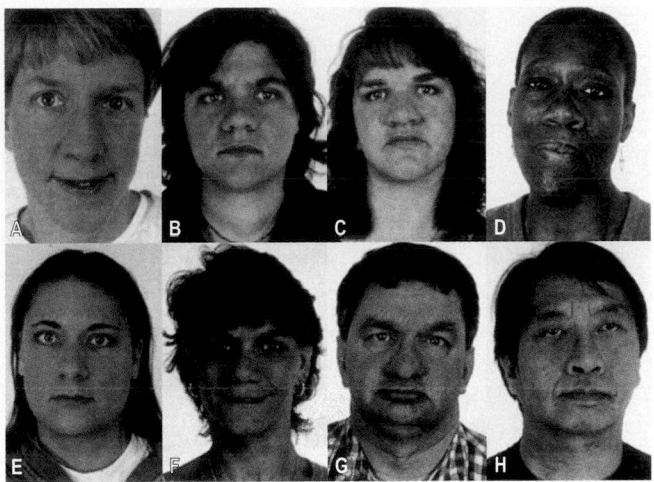

Fig. 21.9 Facial abnormalities seen in patients with hyper-IgE recurrent infection syndrome (HIES). Protruding prominent mandible and forehead, hypertelorism, broad nasal bridge with a wide nasal tip and increased interalar distance are commonly seen facial features of HIES. (Reproduced with permission from Grimbacher B, Holland SM, Gallin JI, et al. Hyper-IgE syndrome with recurrent infections – an autosomal dominant multisystem disorder. N Engl J Med 1999; 340: 692.)

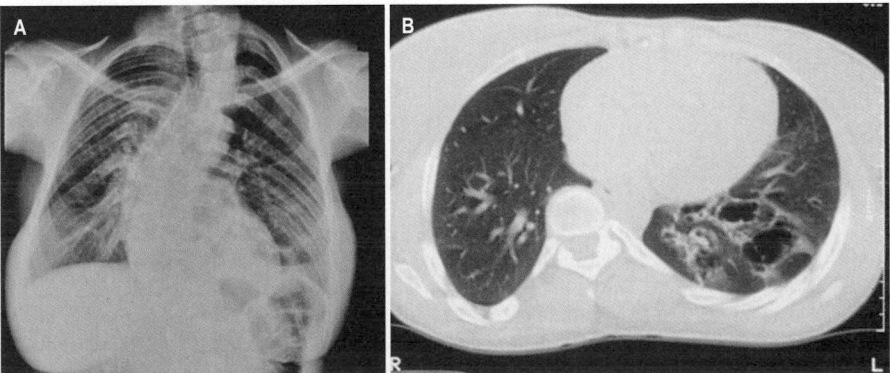

Fig. 21.10 Thoracic pathology in hyper-IgE recurrent infection syndrome (HIES). (**A**) Chest X-ray of a patient with scoliosis. (**B**) CT scan of the lungs in the same patient demonstrates multiple pneumatoceles due to prior infections.

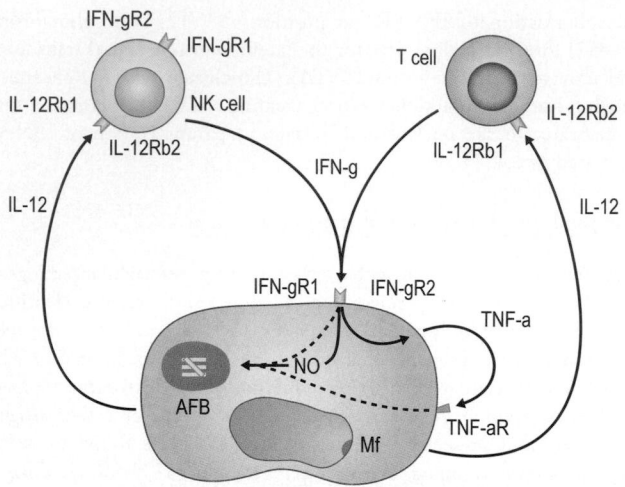

Fig. 21.11 Critical pathways in mycobacterial control. Mycobacterial infection induces IL-12 production by monocytes, which stimulates T cells and NK cells to produce IFN-γ. After binding to its cognate receptor, IFN-γ activates macrophages to produce TNF-α and to kill mycobacteria intracellularly by mechanisms not yet defined. IFN-γ also drives IL-12 production forward. AFB, acid-fast bacilli; NO, nitric oxide; IFN-γR1, interferon-γ receptor 1; IFN-γR2, interferon-γ receptor 2; IL-12Rβ1 and IL-12Rβ2, interleukin-12 receptor chains; TNF-α, tumor necrosis factor-α; TNF-αR, tumor necrosis factor-α receptors.

PARTIAL IFN-γR1 DEFICIENCY

Jouanguy et al.[35] reported two siblings with autosomal recessive IFN-γR1 deficiency due to an amino-acid substitution (I87T) in the extracellular domain of the receptor. In contrast to patients with complete IFN-γR1 deficiency, the partial IFN-γR1 defect was expressed normally on the cell surface, but only responded to IFN-γ at concentrations 100 times higher than normal. At the cellular level, the defect caused an intermediate phenotype between normal and complete IFN-γR1 deficiency. The patients were infected with BCG and *Salmonella enteritidis*; one had probable primary tuberculosis. The outcome was favorable compared to that in complete IFN-γR1 deficiency. These patients formed well-circumscribed and well-differentiated granulomas.

DOMINANT NEGATIVE IFN-γ RECEPTOR 1 DEFICIENCY (AD IFN-γR1)

A small deletion hot spot in the intracellular domain of IFN-γR1 causes autosomal dominant susceptibility to mycobacterial infection.[36] Patients with this genotype came from diverse ethnic backgrounds and presented with disseminated BCG or NTM infections, histoplasmosis, or salmonellosis. Subsequently, almost all patients with this genotype have developed multifocal NTM osteomyelitis, a manifestation that is rare in the complete IFN-γR deficiencies. The clinical presentation is usually evident later in childhood than complete IFN-γR1 deficiency. In addition, AD IFN-γR1 responds well to antimycobacterials and adjunctive IFN-γ therapy, whereas those with complete defects are often refractory to antibiotics and are unresponsive to IFN-γ.

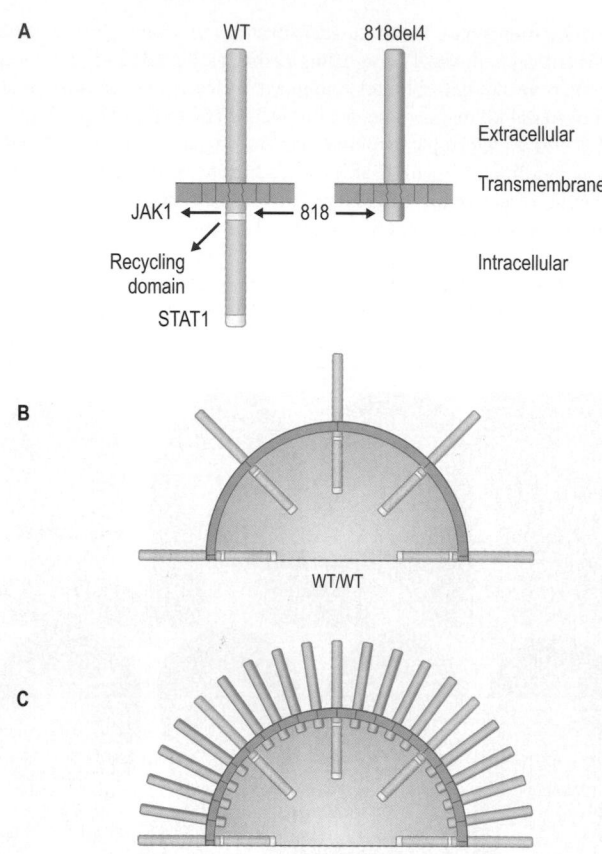

Fig. 21.12 IFN-γR proteins in wild-type and autosomal dominant conditions. (**A**) Wild-type IFN-γ receptor with intact intracellular JAK1 and STAT-1 binding sites and recycling domain (left). Truncated IFN-γR1 molecule due to 818del4/818del. The JAK1 and STAT-1 binding sites and the recycling domain are missing (right). (**B**) IFN-γR1 molecules on the surface of cells homozygous for wild type. (**C**) Mutant IFN-γR1 molecules on the surface of cells heterozygous for 818del4 and wild-type IFN-γR1 alleles. Excess truncated receptors are found on the surface of 818del4/WT cells compared to normal receptors at WT/WT cell surface due to the lack of the recycling motif. Signaling is impaired due to the lack of intracellular signaling domains. (Modified from Jouanguy E, Lamhamedi-Cherradi S, Lammas D, et al. IFNGR1 small deletion hotspot associated with dominant susceptibility to mycobacterial infection. Nature Genet 1999; 21: 370.)

The genetic lesion can be one of four independent mutation events at a single mutation site: 816del4, 817del4, 818del4 (designated 818del4, as they cannot be distinguished from each other), or 818delT or 819delT (designated 818delT). These deletions result in frameshifts leading to a premature stop and early termination of the protein. The defect is localized to exon 6 in the IFN-γR1 open reading frame, within the intracytoplasmic segment of the receptor. Because the JAK1 and STAT-1 binding motifs are deleted, mutant chains are unable to transduce the IFN-γ signal. Mutant proteins are overexpressed at the cell surface due to a lack of the receptor-recycling domain, which is adjacent to the

JAK1-binding domain (Fig. 21.12). These overabundant mutant receptors compete with wild-type receptors for binding IFN-γ. Near normal binding affinity to its ligand, defective signaling and impaired recycling combine to exert the dominant negative effect.

Flow-cytometric analysis of mononuclear cells from affected patients demonstrates a three- to fivefold increase in IFN-γR1 density compared to normal individuals. This laboratory finding supports the fact that recycling of the mutant receptor is defective. At the histologic level, patients with AD IFN-γR1 form paucibacillary and mature-looking granulomas in response to BCG, similar to those with partial recessive deficiency. At the cellular level, the response to IFN-γ as evaluated by HLA-DR expression and phosphorylation of STAT-1 requires 100–1000-fold higher concentrations of IFN-γ than do normal cells. Intracellular detection of STAT-1 phosphorylation via flow cytometry in response to IFN-γ stimulation allows cell-specific determination of IFN-γR integrity.[37]

These patients respond well to antimycobacterial agents. Administration of IFN-γ at doses of 50 μg/m2 subcutaneously, 3 days weekly, accentuates the effects of antimycobacterial agents. There have been anecdotal reports of the need to use much higher doses of IFN-γ *in vivo* to achieve a therapeutic effect.

COMPLETE IFN-γR2 DEFICIENCY

The clinical presentation of complete IFN-γR2 deficiency is similar to that of complete IFN-γR1 deficiency, with early onset of severe systemic mycobacterial infections and impaired granuloma formation.[38] Mutational analysis has shown homozygous mutations resulting in premature stop codons and missense mutations. As in complete IFN-γR1 deficiency, complete IFN-γR2 deficiency causes a lack of cellular response to IFN-γ.[39]

IL-12p40 DEFICIENCY

IL-12p40 deficiency is associated with disseminated BCG infection and *S. enteritidis* sepsis.[40] Patients have homozygous autosomal recessive deletions in the gene encoding IL-12p40. Neither IL-12p40 nor IL-12p70 subunits are detectable. Patient's lymphocytes secrete less IFN-γ, which can be corrected with recombinant IL-12 *in vitro*.

This is a milder disease than complete IFN-γR1 or IFN-γR2 deficiencies, as residual, IL-12-independent IFN-γ secretion persists, as reflected in the capacity to form organized granulomas.[41]

IL-12 RECEPTOR β1 MUTATIONS

Following the identification of patients with IFN-γR1 and IFN-γR2 mutations, several patients with disseminated mycobacterial and *Salmonella* infections and defective IL-12 receptor β1 (IL-12Rβ1)[42] chains were reported. The clinical phenotype includes severe, recurrent, disseminated *Salmonella* and NTM infections or progressive BCG infection following vaccination. Granulomatous infiltrates tend to be contained and well organized. Patients usually respond to antibiotic therapy with recovery. Most patients with IL-12R mutation lack cell surface expression of the receptor. As a result of defective IL-12R signaling, IFN-γ is produced at low levels by T cells and NK cells, thereby predisposing to infections with *Salmonella* and NTM.

Genetic lesions have been detected in the extracellular domains of the IL-12Rβ1 leading to premature stop codons and early termination of the protein. All reported patients with IL-12Rβ1 mutations show an autosomal recessive inheritance pattern, whereas heterozygous carriers are clinically healthy with normal IL-12 signaling and IFN-γ production.

Patients usually respond well to antimicrobials. Those that are not cured of infections with antimicrobials alone may benefit from exogenous IFN-γ therapy.[43, 44]

■ REFERENCES ■

1. Welte K, Dale D. Pathophysiology and treatment of severe chronic neutropenia. Ann Hematol 1996; 72: 158–165.

2. Mermel CH, McLemore ML, Liu F, et al. Src-family kinases are important negative regulators of G-CSF dependent granulopoiesis. Blood 2006; 108: 2562–2568.

3. Person RE, Li FQ, Duan Z, et al. Mutations in proto-oncogene GFI1 cause human neutropenia and target ELA2. Nature Genet 2003; 34: 308–312.

4. Scwachman H, Diamond L, Oski F, Knaw K. The syndrome of pancreatic insufficiency and bone marrow dysfunction. J Pediatr 1964; 65: 645–663.

5. Boocock GR, Marit MR, Rommens JM. Phylogeny, sequence conservation, and functional complementation of the SBDS protein family. Genomics 2006; 87: 758–771.

6. Kuijpers TW, Nannenberg E, Alders M, et al. Congenital aplastic anemia caused by mutations in the SBDS gene: a rare presentation of Shwachman–Diamond syndrome. Pediatrics 2004; 114: e387–391.

7. Bux J, Behrens G, Jaeger G, Welte K. Diagnosis and clinical course of autoimmune neutropenia in infancy: analysis of 240 cases. Blood 1998; 91: 181–186.

8. Dale DC. Immune and idiopathic neutropenia. Curr Opin Hematol 1998; 5: 33–36.

9. Etzioni A, Alon R. Leukocyte adhesion deficiency III: a group of integrin activation defects in hematopoietic lineage cells. Curr Opin Allergy Clin Immunol 2004; 4: 485–490.

10. Anderson DC, Springer TA. Leukocyte adhesion deficiency: an inherited defect in the Mac-1, LFA-1, and p150,95 glycoproteins. Annu Rev Med 1987; 38: 175–194.

11. Anderson DC, Schmalsteig FC, Finegold MJ, et al. The severe and moderate phenotypes of heritable Mac-1, LFA-1 deficiency: their quantitative definition and relation to leukocyte dysfunction and clinical features. J Infect Dis 1985; 152: 668–689.

12. Sligh JE Jr, Hurwitz MY, Zhu CM, et al. An initiation codon mutation in CD18 in association with the moderate phenotype of leukocyte adhesion deficiency. J Biol Chem 1992; 267: 714–718.

13. Bauer TR Jr, Hickstein DD. Gene therapy for leukocyte adhesion deficiency. Curr Opin Mol Ther 2000; 2: 383–388.

14. Marquardt T, Brune T, Luhn K, et al. Leukocyte adhesion deficiency II syndrome, a generalized defect in fucose metabolism. J Pediatr 1999; 134: 681–688.

15. Segal BH, DeCarlo ES, Kwon-Chung KJ, et al. *Aspergillus nidulans* infection in chronic granulomatous disease. Medicine (Baltimore) 1998; 77: 345–354.

16. Heyworth PG, Curnutte JT, Noack D, Cross AR. Hematologically important mutations: X-linked chronic granulomatous disease–an update. Blood Cells Mol Dis 1997; 23: 443–450.

17. Cross AR, Curnutte JT, Heyworth PG. Hematologically important mutations: the autosomal recessive forms of chronic granulomatous disease. Blood Cells Mol Dis 1996; 22: 268–270.

18. Greenberg DE, Ding L, Zelazny AM, et al. A novel bacterium associated with lymphadenitis in a patient with chronic granulomatous disease. Public Library of Science Pathogens 2006; 2: e28.

19. Marciano BE, Rosenzweig SD, Kleiner DE, et al. Gastrointestinal involvement in chronic granulomatous disease. Pediatrics 2004; 114: 462–468.

20. Vowells SJ, Sekhsaria S, Malech HL, et al. Flow cytometric analysis of the granulocyte respiratory burst: a comparison study of fluorescent probes. J Immunol Meth 1995; 178: 89–97.

21. Gallin JI, Alling DW, Malech HL, et al. Itraconazole to prevent fungal infections in chronic granulomatous disease. N Engl J Med 2003; 348: 2416–2422.

22. Group TICGDCS. A controlled trial of interferon gamma to prevent infection in chronic granulomatous disease. The International Chronic Granulomatous Disease Cooperative Study Group [see comments]. N Engl J Med 1991; 324: 509–516.

23. Ott MG, Schmidt M, Schwarzwaelder K, et al. Correction of X-linked chronic granulomatous disease by gene therapy, augmented by insertional activation of MDS1-EVI1, PRDM16 or SETBP1. Nature Med 2006 Apr; 12: 401–9.

24. Ahluwalia J, Pattari S, Trehan A, Marwaha RK, Garewal G. Accelerated phase at initial presentation: an uncommon occurrence in Chediak-Higashi syndrome. Pediatr Hematol Oncol 2003 Oct-Nov; 20: 563–7.

25. Huynh C, Roth D, Ward DM, Kaplan J, Andrews NW. Defective lysosomal exocytosis and plasma membrane repair in Chediak–Higashi/beige cells. Proc Natl Acad Sci USA 2004; 101: 16795–16800.

26. Grimbacher B, Schaffer AA, Holland SM, et al. Genetic linkage of hyper-IgE syndrome to chromosome 4. Am J Hum Genet 1999; 65: 735–744.

27. Grimbacher B, Holland SM, Puck JM. The interleukin-4 receptor variant Q576R in hyper-IgE syndrome [letter; comment]. N Engl J Med 1998; 338: 1073–1074.

28. Borges WG, Augustine NH, Hill HR. Defective interleukin-12/interferon-gamma pathway in patients with hyperimmunoglobulinemia E syndrome. J Pediatr 2000; 136: 176–180.

29. Renner ED, Puck JM, Holland SM, et al. Autosomal recessive hyperimmunoglobulin E syndrome: a distinct disease entity. J Pediatr 2004; 144: 93–99.

30. Newport MJ, Huxley CM, Huston S, et al. A mutation in the interferon-gamma-receptor gene and susceptibility to mycobacterial infection. N Engl J Med 1996; 335: 1941–1949.

31. Jouanguy E, Altare F, Lamhamedi S, et al. Interferon-gamma-receptor deficiency in an infant with fatal bacille Calmette–Guerin infection. N Engl J Med 1996; 335: 1956–1961.

32. Lamhamedi S, Jouanguy E, Altare F, et al. Interferon-gamma receptor deficiency: relationship between genotype, environment, and phenotype. [Review] Int J Mol Med 1998; 1: 415–418.

33. Holland SM, Dorman SE, Kwon A, et al. Abnormal regulation of interferon-gamma, interleukin-12, and tumor necrosis factor-alpha in human interferon-gamma receptor 1 deficiency. J Infect Dis 1998; 178: 1095–1104.

34. Dorman SE, Picard C, Lammas D, et al. Clinical features of dominant and recessive interferon gamma receptor 1 deficiencies. Lancet 2004; 364: 2113–2121.

35. Jouanguy E, Lamhamedi-Cherradi S, Altare F, et al. Partial interferon-gamma receptor 1 deficiency in a child with tuberculoid bacillus Calmette–Guerin infection and a sibling with clinical tuberculosis. J Clin Invest 1997; 100: 2658–2664.

36. Jouanguy E, Lamhamedi-Cherradi S, Lammas D, et al. A human IFNGR1 small deletion hotspot associated with dominant susceptibility to mycobacterial infection [see comments]. Nature Genet 1999; 21: 370–378.

37. Fleisher TA, Dorman SE, Anderson JA, et al. Detection of intracellular phosphorylated STAT-1 by flow cytometry. Clin Immunol 1999; 90: 425–430.

38. Dorman SE, Holland SM. Mutation in the signal-transducing chain of the interferon-gamma receptor and susceptibility to mycobacterial infection. J Clin Invest 1998; 101: 2364–2369.

39. Rosenzweig SD, Dorman SE, Uzel G, et al. A novel mutation in IFN-gamma receptor 2 with dominant negative activity: biological consequences of homozygous and heterozygous states. J Immunol 2004; 173: 4000–4008.

40. Altare F, Lammas D, Revy P, et al. Inherited interleukin 12 deficiency in a child with bacille Calmette–Guerin and Salmonella enteritidis disseminated infection. J Clin Invest 1998; 102: 2035–2040.

41. Picard C, Fieschi C, Altare F, et al. Inherited interleukin-12 deficiency: IL12B genotype and clinical phenotype of 13 patients from six kindreds. Am J Hum Genet 2002; 70: 336–348.

42. Altare F, Durandy A, Lammas D, et al. Impairment of mycobacterial immunity in human interleukin-12 receptor deficiency. Science 1998; 280: 1432–1435.

43. van de Vosse E, de Paus RA, van Dissel JT, Ottenhoff TH. Molecular complementation of IL-12Rbeta1 deficiency reveals functional differences between IL-12Rbeta1 alleles including partial IL-12Rbeta1 deficiency. Hum Mol Genet 2005; 14: 3847–3855.

44. Fieschi C, Dupuis S, Catherinot E, et al. Low penetrance, broad resistance, and favorable outcome of interleukin 12 receptor beta1 deficiency: medical and immunological implications. J Exp Med 2003; 197: 527–535.

Mast cells, basophils and mastocytosis

Martin Metz, Knut Brockow, Dean D. Metcalfe,
Stephen J. Galli

22

Mast cells and basophils are critical effector cells in IgE-associated allergic diseases and in host responses to parasites, as well as in a variety of other processes.[1–3] Mast cells and basophils share several features in addition to the metachromatic staining properties of their prominent cytoplasmic granules (Table 22.1). Both are derived from bone marrow progenitors, express high-affinity IgE Fc receptors (FcεRI) on their surface, are major sources of histamine and other potent inflammatory mediators, and can be activated to release a wide array of mediators after sensitization with IgE and subsequent exposure to specific multivalent antigen.[1–4] However, mast cells and basophils differ in their responsiveness to other potential activators of secretion and in the specific pattern of mediators released by the activated cells.[1–3] Moreover, basophils and mast cells exhibit several differences in morphology, particularly by transmission electron microscopy (Table 22.2 and Fig. 22.1).

different phenotypes have different roles in health and disease, and may respond differently to drugs used in clinical settings. In mice and rats, connective tissue mast cells (CTMCs) and mucosal mast cells (MMCs) exhibit significant differences in multiple aspects of phenotype.[1–3] In humans, some mast cells express immunoreactivity for both tryptase and chymase (MC_{TC}), whereas others are immunoreactive for tryptase (MC_T) but lack detectable chymase (<0.04 pg/cell).[1, 3] MC_T predominate in lung and small intestinal mucosa and MC_{TC} predominate in skin and small intestinal submucosa. A few mast cells that apparently express chymase (MC_C) but no detectable tryptase have also been reported.

Mast cell phenotypic variation could reflect any one or more of the following mechanisms: distinct mast cell lineages; the process of cellular maturation and differentiation; the functional status of the cell; and the influence of microenvironmental factors.[3]

DEVELOPMENT AND DISTRIBUTION OF MAST CELLS

DISTRIBUTION AND HETEROGENEITY

Unlike mature basophils, mature mast cells do not normally circulate in the blood but are ordinarily distributed throughout the connective tissues, where they often lie adjacent to blood and lymphatic vessels, near or within nerves, and beneath epithelial surfaces that are exposed to the external environment (e.g., lung, gut and skin).[1–3]

The numbers of mast cells in normal tissues vary considerably by anatomic site, and their distribution can change during perturbations of homeostasis.[1–3] For example, in certain inflammatory or immunologic reactions mast cells can appear within the respiratory or gastrointestinal epithelium and in their associated secretions.[1–3] Mast cell numbers at sites of chronic inflammation may be many times higher than in the corresponding normal tissues.[1–3] The extent to which such changes reflect proliferation of resident mast cell populations, as opposed to the recruitment and differentiation of mast cell precursors, remains unclear.

The phenotype of different populations of mast cells, including morphology, histochemistry, mediator content and response to drugs and stimuli of activation, can also vary.[1–3] It is possible that mast cells of

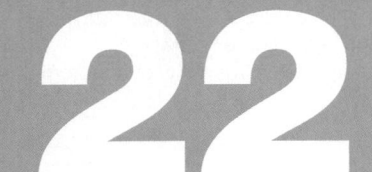

KEY CONCEPTS

ORIGINS OF BASOPHILS AND MAST CELLS

>> Mast cells and basophils represent distinct hematopoietic lineages.

>> Basophils are granulocytes that mature in the bone marrow, circulate in the blood, and can be recruited into peripheral tissues at sites of immunologic or pathologic responses.

>> Mast cell progenitors also arise in the bone marrow, but mast cells mature in peripheral tissues.

>> Mast cells are present throughout virtually all normal connective tissues, and are particularly abundant near epithelial surfaces exposed to the environment.

>> The KIT ligand stem cell factor (SCF) is critical for mast cell development and survival and can influence mast cell function.

>> IL-3 is not required for normal basophil development in mice, but is critical for the basophilia associated with Th2 responses.

Table 22.1 Natural history, major mediators and surface membrane structures of human mast cells and basophils

Characteristic	Basophils	Mast cells
Natural history		
Origin of precursor cells	Bone marrow	Bone marrow
Site of maturation	Bone marrow	Connective tissues (a few in the bone marrow)
Mature cells in the circulation	Yes (usually <1% of blood leukocytes)	No
Mature cells recruited into tissues from circulation	Yes (during immunologic, inflammatory responses)	No
Mature cells normally residing in connective tissues	No (not detectable by microscopy)	Yes
Proliferative ability of morphologically mature cells	None reported	Yes (under certain circumstances)
Life span	Days (like other granulocytes)	Weeks to months (based on studies in rodents)
Mediators		
Major mediators stored preformed in cytoplasm	Histamine, chondroitin sulfates, neutral protease with bradykinin-generating activity, β-glucuronidase, elastase, cathepsin G-like enzyme, major basic protein, Charcot–Leyden crystal protein, tryptase[a], chymase[a], carboxypeptidase A[a]	Histamine, heparin and/or chondroitin sulfates, neutral proteases (chymase and/or tryptase), many acid hydrolases, cathepsin G, carboxypeptidase
Major lipid mediators produced upon appropriate activation	Leukotriene C_4 (LTC_4)	Prostaglandin D_2, LTC_4, platelet-activating factor
Cytokines, chemokines and growth factors released upon appropriate activation	IL-4, IL-13	Tumor necrosis factor, IL-3, IL-4, IL-5, IL-6, IL-10, IL-13, IL-16, VPF/VEGF, GM-CSF, MIP-1α, MCP-1
Surface structures[b]		
Ig receptors	FcεRI, FcγRII (CDw32)	FcεRI, FcγRI, FcγRII
Cytokine/growth factor receptors	IL-1RIIb (CD121b), IL-2R (CD25), IL-3Rα, IL-4Rα, IL-5Rα, GM-CSFRα, TrK-A, CCR-2, CCR-3, CXCR1, CXCR4, KIT (some basophils express low numbers of KIT receptors)	KIT (SCF receptor), CCR-3, CCR-5, CXCR1, CXCR2, CXCR3, CXCR4, IL-4Rα, IL5Rα, IL-6R, IFN-γRα, TrkA
Cell adhesion structures	LFA-1 α chain (CD11a), C3bi receptor (CD11b), CR4 (CD11c), sLe^x(CD15s), LFA-1 β chain (CD18), β₁integrin (CD29), leukosialin (CD43), PECAM-1 (CD31), CD44, ICAM-2 (CD50), ICAM-1 (CD54), LFA-3 (CD58), L-selectin (CD62L), CD102, β₇-integrin, neurothelin (CD147), PETA-3 (CD151), BST-1 (CD157), PSGL-1 (CD162)	CD11a, CD11b, CD11c, CD18, CD29, CD43, CD44, CD49a, CD49b, CD49c, CD49d, CD49e, CD50, CD51, CD54, CD58, CD61, CD81, CD102, CD147, CD151, CD157

IL, interleukin; SCF, stem cell factor; LFA, lymphocyte function-associated antigen; CR, complement receptor; ICAM, intercellular adhesion molecule; sLe^x sialyl Lewis^x, PECAM-1, platelet-endothelial cell adhesion molecule-1; PETA-3, platelet-endothelial cell tetra-span antigen; BST-1, bone marrow stromal cell antigen-1; PSGL-1, P-selectin glycoprotein ligand-1.

[a]Expressed in peripheral blood basophils of asthma, allergy, and drug-reactive patients (Li L, Li y, Reddel SW, et al. Identification of basophilic cells that express mast cell granule proteases in the peripheral blood of asthma, allergy, and drug-reactive patients. J Immunol 1998; 161: 5079–5086).
[b]Some mast cell surface structures have been detected in either mast cells cultured from human umblilical cord blood (expression varies during differentiation), skin mast cells or lung mast cells (Valent P. Immunophentypic characterization of human basophils and mast cells. Chem Immunol 1995; 61: 34–48). Basophils and various populations of mast cells also can express several TLRs.[7,14]

MAST CELL DEVELOPMENT IN MICE AND RATS

An essentially homogeneous population of growth factor-dependent immature mast cells develops when mouse hematopoietic cells are cultured in media containing interleukin (IL)-3.[3] Although such IL-3-induced bone marrow-derived cultured mast cells (BMCMCs) share some phenotypic characteristics with mouse MMCs, both *in vivo* and *in vitro* studies indicate that these cells acquire phenotypic features more similar to those of CTMCs when placed in an appropriate environment.[1–3] *In vitro*, fibroblasts provide factors, particularly stem cell factor (SCF), that promote IL-3-induced BMCMCs to develop features of CTMCs.[1–3] Indeed, studies in both mice and humans indicate that many aspects of mast cell development

Table 22.2 Morphologic features of mature basophils and mast cells (From Galli SJ, Lichtenstein LM. In: Middleton E Jr, Reed CE, Ellis EF, et al., eds. Allergy: principles and practice, 3rd edn. St Louis: Mosby, 1988; with permission from Elsevier.)

Characteristic	Basophils	Mast cells
Size	5–7 μm	6–12 μm
Surface	Irregular, short, thick processes	Numerous, uniformly distributed, elongated thin processes
Nucleus	Segmented (usually; occasionally nonsegmented)	Nonsegmented (usually round to oval in electron micrographs)[a]
Nuclear chromatin condensation	Marked	Moderate
Cytoplasmic granules	Fewer and larger than in mast cells; contain predominantly electron-dense particulate material with occasional membranous whorls	Smaller, more numerous, and generally more variable than in basophils; contain scroll-like structures, particles, or crystals, alone or in combination
Aggregates of cytoplasmic glycogen	Present	Absent
Cytoplasmic lipid bodies	Rare	Common but not present in all cells
Granule–granule fusion during anaphylactic degranulation	Rare (granule membranes usually fuse individually with plasma membrane)	Common

[a]Human mast cells generated *in vitro* can exhibit multilobulated nuclei.

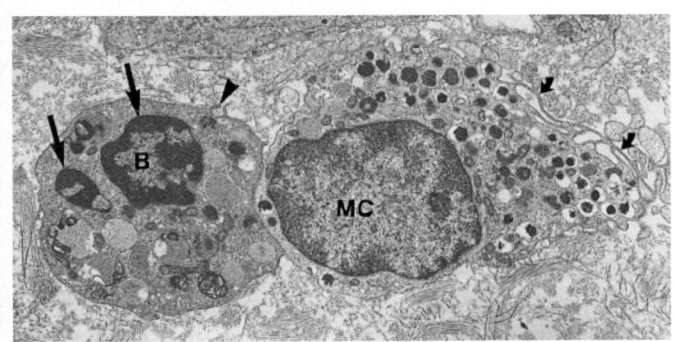

Fig. 22.1 Mast cell and basophil ultrastructure. A basophil (B) adjacent to a mast cell (MC) in the ileal submucosa of a patient with Crohn disease. The basophil exhibits a bilobed nucleus (solid arrows) whose chromatin is strikingly condensed beneath the nuclear membrane. The basophil surface is relatively smooth with a few blunt processes (arrowhead). The mast cell nucleus is larger and its chromatin less condensed than that of the basophil. The mast cell's granules are smaller, more numerous and more variable in shape and content than those of the basophil. The mast cell surface has numerous elongated, thin folds (curved arrows). (Original magnification ~×9000). (From Dvorak AM, Monahan RA, Osage JE, Dickersin GR. Crohn's disease: transmission electron microscopic studies. Hum Pathol 1980; 11: 606–619, with permission from Ann M. Dvorak.)

and survival are critically regulated by SCF, the ligand for the KIT tyrosine growth factor receptor, which is expressed on the mast cell surface.[1–3]

Several other cytokines also promote mast cell development and/or proliferation *in vitro*, including IL-4, IL-9 and IL-10.[1–3] In contrast, granulocyte–macrophage colony-stimulating factor (GM-CSF) and transforming growth factor (TGF)-β_1 can inhibit mouse BMCMC proliferation in response to IL-3.[1–3]

MAST CELL DEVELOPMENT IN HUMANS

Human mast cell progenitors are present in umbilical cord blood, as well as in the bone marrow and the peripheral blood, and highly enriched populations of mast cells develop from these and other sources of human hematopoietic cells when they are maintained *in vitro* in media containing recombinant human SCF (rhSCF).[1–3, 5] rhSCF also promotes the development of human mast cells *in vivo*.[6]

■ DEVELOPMENT AND DISTRIBUTION OF BASOPHILS ■

Basophils differentiate and mature in the bone marrow and then circulate in the blood. In the blood, the basophil is the least common blood granulocyte, with a prevalence of approximately 0.5% of total leukocytes and approximately 0.3% of nucleated marrow cells.[3] Basophils are not ordinarily found in connective tissues. Because the normal frequency of blood and bone marrow basophils is so low, accurate determinations ordinarily require absolute counting methods. The basophil's prominent metachromatic cytoplasmic granules permit it to be identified easily in Wright–Giemsa-stained preparations of peripheral blood or bone marrow cells. Both cytogenetic evidence and *in vitro* studies indicate that basophils share a precursor with other granulocytes and monocytes.[3] The ultrastructural features of human basophils are summarized in Table 22.2 and illustrated in Fig. 22.1. The extent of the biochemical similarities between basophils and mast cells continues to be explored.[7]

Under physiological conditions basophils have a lifespan measured in days. IL-3 promotes the production and survival of basophils *in vitro* and can induce basophilia *in vivo*. Findings in IL-3$^{-/-}$ mice indicate that IL-3 is not necessary for the development of normal numbers of bone marrow or blood basophils, but is essential for the bone marrow and blood basophilia associated with certain Th2 cell-associated immunologic responses.[2, 8]

BIOLOGIC MEDIATORS PRODUCED BY MAST CELLS AND BASOPHILS

Basophils and mast cells contain, or elaborate on appropriate stimulation, a diverse array of potent biologically active mediators.[1–3, 7] These agents mediate a wide array of effects in inflammation, immunity and tissue remodeling, and can also influence the clotting, fibrinolytic, complement and kinin systems. Some of these products are stored pre-formed in cytoplasmic granules (e.g. proteoglycans, proteases, histamine, certain cytokines), and others are synthesized upon activation of the cell by IgE and antigen or other stimuli (e.g., products of arachidonic acid oxidation through the cyclo-oxygenase or lipoxygenase pathways and, in some cells, platelet-activating factor [PAF], cytokines, chemokines, and growth factors).[1–3, 7]

MEDIATORS THAT ARE PRE-FORMED

Mediators stored pre-formed in the cytoplasmic granules include histamine, proteoglycans, serine proteases, carboxypeptidase A, and small amounts of sulfatases and exoglycosidases. Studies in mice indicate that

KEY CONCEPTS

MAST CELL AND BASOPHIL MEDIATORS

>> Mast cells and basophils are sources of distinct, but overlapping, panels of mediators with diverse biologic effects.

>> Some mast cell and basophil mediators are preformed and stored in cytoplasmic granules (e.g., histamine, heparin and other proteoglycans, proteases). They can be released rapidly upon degranulation induced by cellular activation.

>> Mast cells and basophils also produce lipid mediators (e.g., PGD_2, LTC_4), which are derived from arachadonic acid and are newly synthesized upon appropriate activation of the cell.

>> Mast cells can transcribe and secrete many cytokines/chemokines/growth factors, including (in mouse and/or human mast cells) IL-1, IL-2, IL-3, IL-4, IL-5, IL-6, IL-8, IL-10, IL-13, IL-16, GM-CSF, TNF, IFN-γ, TGF-β, bFGF, VPF/VEGF, NGF and many C-C chemokines.

>> In response to cellular activation (e.g., through the FcεRI), mast cells can release at least two cytokines, TNF and VPF/VEGF, from both stored and newly synthesized pools.

>> Induction of cytokine mRNA in mast cells is not always accompanied by the release of detectable cytokine bioactivity.

>> Under some circumstances, induction and/or release of mast cell cytokines can occur in response to stimuli that do not induce a detectable release of histamine.

>> Release of some cytokines (e.g., TNF) can continue for hours after initial FcεRI-dependent mast cell activation.

>> Mast cell cytokine mRNA expression and/or cytokine release can be inhibited by cyclosporine A or dexamethasone.

>> Basophils appear to produce a more restricted spectrum of cytokines than do mast cells, but these include IL-4 and IL-13.

mast cells account for nearly all of the histamine stored in normal tissues, with the exception of the glandular stomach and the CNS.[3] Basophils are the source of most of the histamine in normal human blood.[3] Mouse and rat mast cells, but not human mast cells or basophils, contain significant quantities of serotonin.[1, 3]

Human mast cells contain variable mixtures of heparin (about 60 kDa) and chondroitin sulfate proteoglycans.[1, 3] Although the sulfated glycosaminoglycans of normal human blood basophils have not been characterized, chondroitin sulfates account for the majority of the proteoglycans in the basophils of patients with myelogenous leukemia.[3]

Neutral proteases are the major protein component of mast cell secretory granules. The three major families of proteases found in mast cell granules are represented by the serine proteases chymase and tryptase and the metalloprotease carboxypeptidase A. In mice, five different chymases (mouse mast cell protease [mMCP]-1, -2, -4, -5 and -9) and four different tryptases (mMCP-6, -7 and -11 and mouse transmembrane tryptase [mTMT]) have been described;[9, 10] in humans, it appears that there is only one chymase and four different tryptases (α, β, γ and δ, encoded by several genes and alleles).[9–11] Mast cell protease content varies depending on the microenvironment, and can therefore contribute significantly to mast cell heterogeneity. Several potential functions have been associated with various mast cell proteases (e.g., effects that promote bronchomotor tone and degradation of fibrinogen, extracellular matrix proteins and endogeneous or exogenous peptides),[9, 10, 12] and it is likely that additional biological roles will be identified.

MEDIATORS THAT ARE NEWLY SYNTHESIZED

Activated mast cells initiate the de novo synthesis of several lipid-derived substances. Of particular importance are the cyclo-oxygenase and lipoxygenase metabolites of arachidonic acid, which have potent inflammatory activities and which may also play a role in modulating the release process itself. The major cyclo-oxygenase product of mast cells is prostaglandin D_2 (PGD_2), and the major lipoxygenase products derived from mast cells and basophils are the sulfidopeptide leukotriene LTC_4 and its peptidolytic derivatives LTD_4 and LTE_4.[1–3, 7, 13] Mast cells isolated from a variety of tissues release both LTC_4 and PGD_2, whereas peripheral blood basophils release LTC_4 but not PGD_2. Mast cells also produce LTB_4, although in much smaller quantities than PGD_2 or LTC_4, and some mast cell populations represent a potential source of PAF.[1–3, 7, 13]

CYTOKINES, CHEMOKINES AND GROWTH FACTORS

The ability of mast cells and basophils to produce cytokines, chemokines and growth factors greatly expands the list of possible mechanisms by which these cells may contribute to the pathophysiology of allergic and immunologic diseases, host defense or homeostasis.[1–3, 7] Mast cells are a source for IL-1, -2, -3, -4, -5, -6, -8, -10, -13, -16, GM-CSF, TNF, NGF, bFGF and VPF/VEGF, as well as several C-C chemokines (Chapters 10 and 11). These products are released when the cells are activated via IgE-dependent mechanisms, and are also produced under other circumstances (e.g., in response to stimulation by bacterial products).[1–3, 7, 14]

The first cytokine bioactivity to be clearly associated with normal mast cells was TNF.[2, 3] Some of the TNF released from mouse mast cells upon appropriate stimulation (e.g., via IgE-dependent activation) reflects cytokine that is rapidly released from pre-formed stores, and even larger amounts of newly synthesized TNF are released over a period of hours after cell activation.

The first cytokine bioactivity to be associated with normal basophils was IL-4, and mature human basophils isolated from peripheral blood can release IL-4 (and IL-13) in response to FcεRI-dependent activation.[2, 3, 15] It is possible that IL-4 derived from mast cells or basophils at sites of allergic inflammation can promote T-cell differentiation toward a Th2 phenotype. Basophils and mast cells express CD40 ligand (CD40L, CD154), and thus may also contribute to IgE production by promoting immunoglobulin class switching.[2, 7, 16]

■ MECHANISMS OF ACTIVATION OF MAST CELLS AND BASOPHILS ■

FcεRI-MEDIATED ACTIVATION

Mast cells and basophils express FcεRI, the high-affinity receptor for IgE.[1–4] Whereas high 'constitutive' levels of FcεRI expression apparently are restricted to mast cells and basophils, in humans low levels of expression are detected in Langerhans' cells, peripheral blood dendritic cells and monocytes.[1–4] In mast cells and basophils, FcεRI has a tetrameric structure composed of a single IgE-binding α chain, a single β chain and two identical disulfide-linked γ chains. All three subunits must be present for efficient cell surface expression in rodents, but human cells can express FcεRI in the absence of the β chain. In humans, the FcεRI expressed by hematopoietic cells other than mast cells and basophils consists of only the αγ form.[4] The aggregation of FcεRI that is occupied by IgE is sufficient for initiating downstream signal transduction events that activate the mast cells or basophils to degranulate and to secrete lipid mediators and cytokines.[1–4] The FcεRI β chain functions as an amplifier of signaling through FcεRI, which can markedly upregulate the magnitude of the mediator release response to FcεRI aggregation.[4] Certain mutations that result in amino acid substitutions in the human β chain may be linked to atopic disease.[4]

At the ultrastructural level, stimulation of appropriately sensitized human basophils with specific antigen provokes fusion of the membranes enveloping individual cytoplasmic granules with the plasma membrane[3] (Fig. 22.2). As a result, the granules' contents, including stored mediators, are released via multiple narrow communications between single granules and the cell surface. IgE-dependent degranulation of human lung mast cells also results in the fusion of granule membranes with the plasma membrane[3] (Fig. 22.3). However, in this cell type the first ultrastructural changes detectable in the stimulated cells are granule swelling, followed by fusion of individual granule membranes forming interconnecting chains of swollen granules; histamine release is initiated by the opening of these channels to the exterior through multiple narrow points of fusion with the plasma membrane.[3]

Both in vitro and in vivo, levels of FcεRI surface expression on mast cells and basophils correlates positively with the concentration of IgE.[2, 16] IgE-dependent upregulation of FcεRI expression in vitro, which reflects stabilization of expression of FcεRI on the cell surface, permits mast cells to secrete strikingly increased amounts of mediators after anti-IgE challenge, and to exhibit IgE-dependent mediator release at lower concentrations of specific antigen. Furthermore, mast cells that have undergone IgE-dependent upregulation of surface FcεRI expression may,

upon subsequent FcεRI-dependent activation, secrete cytokines and growth factors that are released at very low levels (or not at all) by mast cells with low levels of FcεRI expression.[2, 16] These findings strongly suggest that basophils and mast cells in subjects with high levels of IgE (as typically characterizes patients with allergic disorders or parasitic infections) may be significantly enhanced in their ability to express IgE-dependent effector functions or, via cytokine production, potential immunoregulatory functions.[2, 16] Recent in vitro data from studies with mouse or human mast cells indicates that, under some circumstances, the binding of certain IgE antibodies to FcεRI can promote mast cell survival and/or mediator secretion, even in the absence of known specific antigen.[2, 16] The clinical significance of these findings is not yet clear.

In addition to the high-affinity IgE receptor, mouse mast cells and human basophils express the low-affinity IgG receptor FcγRIIB. Co-aggregation of FcγRIIB and FcεRI has been shown to diminish IgE-dependent activation of mouse mast cells, RBL cells and human basophils in vitro and to diminish the expression of IgE- and mast cell-dependent allergic reactions in vivo.[17]

ACTIVATION BY NONIMMUNOLOGIC MEANS

In addition to IgE and specific antigen, a variety of biologic substances, including products of complement activation and neuropeptides, as well as certain bacterial products, cytokines, animal venom components, chemical agents and physical stimuli, elicit the release of basophil or mast cell mediators.[1–3, 11, 14] Morphine and other narcotics are among the pharmacological agents that can induce the release of mast cell mediators, especially from skin mast cells, and intravenous infusion of large

---

■ KEY CONCEPTS

MECHANISMS OF MAST CELL AND BASOPHIL ACTIVATION

>> Mast cells and basophils have cell-surface high-affinity IgE receptors (FcεRI) that confer on these cells the ability to express specific immunological functions.

>> Mast cells and basophils can be activated in vivo either by signaling through the FcεRI or by a variety of nonimmunologic signals (e.g., certain neuropeptides, anaphylatoxins, f-Met-Leu-Phe, bacterial products/TLR ligands, animal venom components).

>> The responses of basophils and/or different subpopulations of mast cells to stimuli other than IgE and antigen vary: some populations respond weakly or not at all to some stimuli.

>> Some stimuli activate cells to release a panel of mediators quantitatively or qualitatively more limited than that induced by IgE and antigen.

>> The susceptibility of mast cells or basophils to activation by IgE and specific antigen or other stimuli can be regulated by cytokines (e.g., SCF, IL-3), as well as other by microenvironmental factors.

>> Certain mast cell populations can exhibit down-regulation of FcεRI-dependent activation via signaling by FcγRIIb or other receptors (such as members of the KIR family).

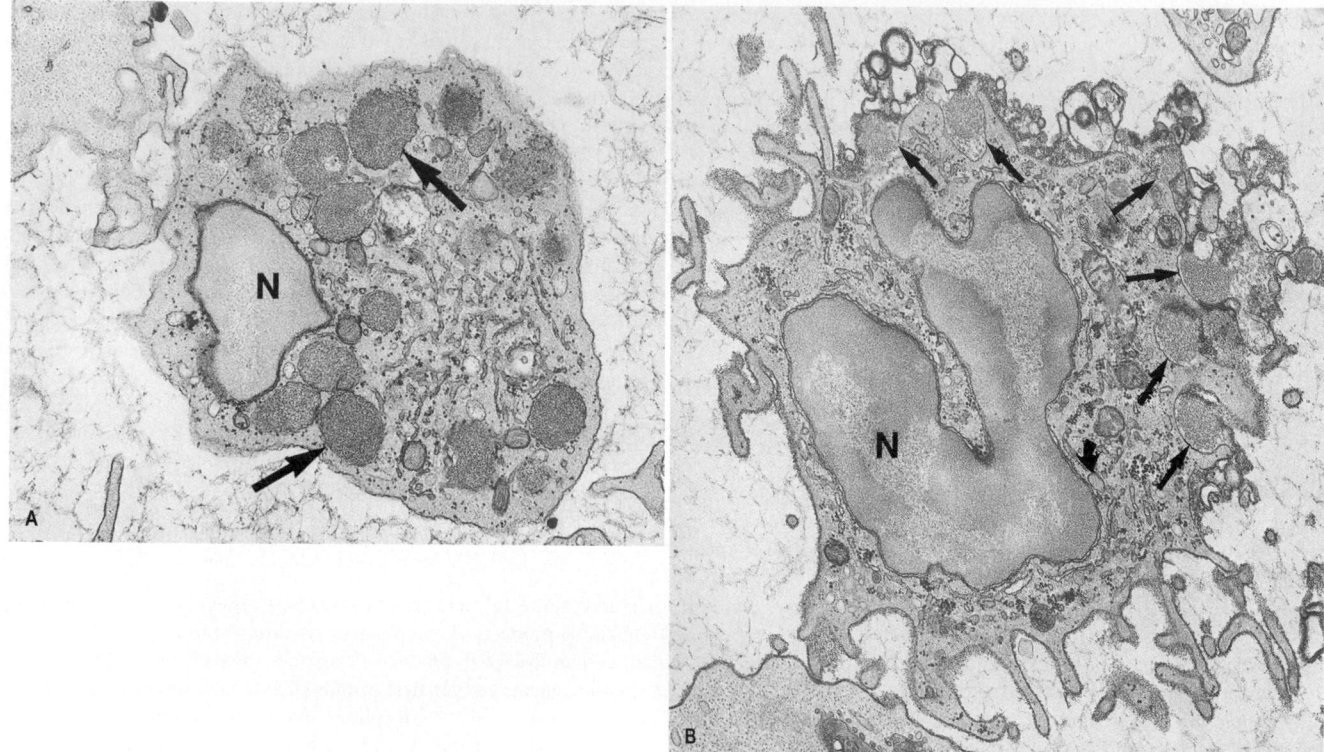

Fig. 22.2 (**A**) Transmission electron micrograph of a human basophil in a preparation of peripheral blood leukocytes obtained by separation over Ficoll-Hypaque. All of the cytoplasmic granules (some indicated by solid arrows) contain particulate electron-dense material. N, nucleus. (Original magnification ~×19800). (**B**) A human basophil 2 minutes after exposure to antigen *in vitro*. The cell exhibits extrusion of granules from six separate sites on the plasma membrane (small arrows). At this time after cell stimulation, particle-filled granules retain their shape and characteristic structure even after exposure to extracellular milieu. Cationized ferritin coats the cell surface and enters culs de sac that contain exteriorized granules. The cell exhibits no fully intracytoplasmic typical basophilic granules, but one of the smaller kind of granules (curved arrow) can be observed in perinuclear region. N, nucleus. (Original magnification ~×19 200). (From Dvorak AM, Newball HH, Dvorak HF, Lichtenstein LM. Antigen-induced IgE-mediated degranulation of human basophils. Lab Invest 1980; 43: 126-139, with permission from Nature Publishing Group Ltd.)

doses of morphine regularly causes an increase in plasma histamine levels and often results in shock.[1,3]

HIV glycoprotein 120, as well as protein Fv (pFv), which is released into the intestinal tract in patients with viral hepatitis, can interact with the heavy-chain variable domain of IgE antibodies that use V_H3 gene segments (Chapter 4) and thereby induce the release of histamine, IL-4 and IL-13 from human basophils and mast cells.[7] Basophils also respond to stimulation with immobilized secretory IgA (sIgA) by releasing both histamine and LTC_4, but only if the cells have first been primed by pretreatment with IL-3, IL-5 or GM-CSF.[18] Furthermore, certain bacterial products – including lipopolysaccharide (LPS) and other ligands of TLRs – directly induce the release of some mast cell products; pathogens can also activate mast cells indirectly via activation of the complement system.[2,3,14]

It should be emphasized that the responsiveness of basophils and different populations of mast cells to individual stimuli varies, e.g., cutaneous mast cells appear to be much more sensitive to stimulation by neuropeptides than are pulmonary mast cells.[1-3] Moreover, some stimuli induce a pattern of mediator release that differs from the one associated with IgE-dependent mast cell activation. For example, LPS induces mast cells to release certain cytokines preferentially over preformed meditors.[14]

■ MAST CELLS, BASOPHILS AND ALLERGIC INFLAMMATION ■

The immediate hypersensitivity reaction is the pathophysiologic hallmark of allergic rhinitis, allergic asthma and anaphylaxis, and the central role of the mast cell in the pathogenesis of the acute manifestations of these disorders is widely accepted. To avoid confusion between immunologic mechanisms and clinical syndromes in the discussion of these disorders, it is essential to begin by defining some key terms.

TYPE I HYPERSENSITIVITY REACTION

Also known as the allergic or immediate hypersensitivity reaction, a type I hypersensitivity reaction, as originally described by Gell and Coombs, is now understood to be a pathologic immune response initiated in

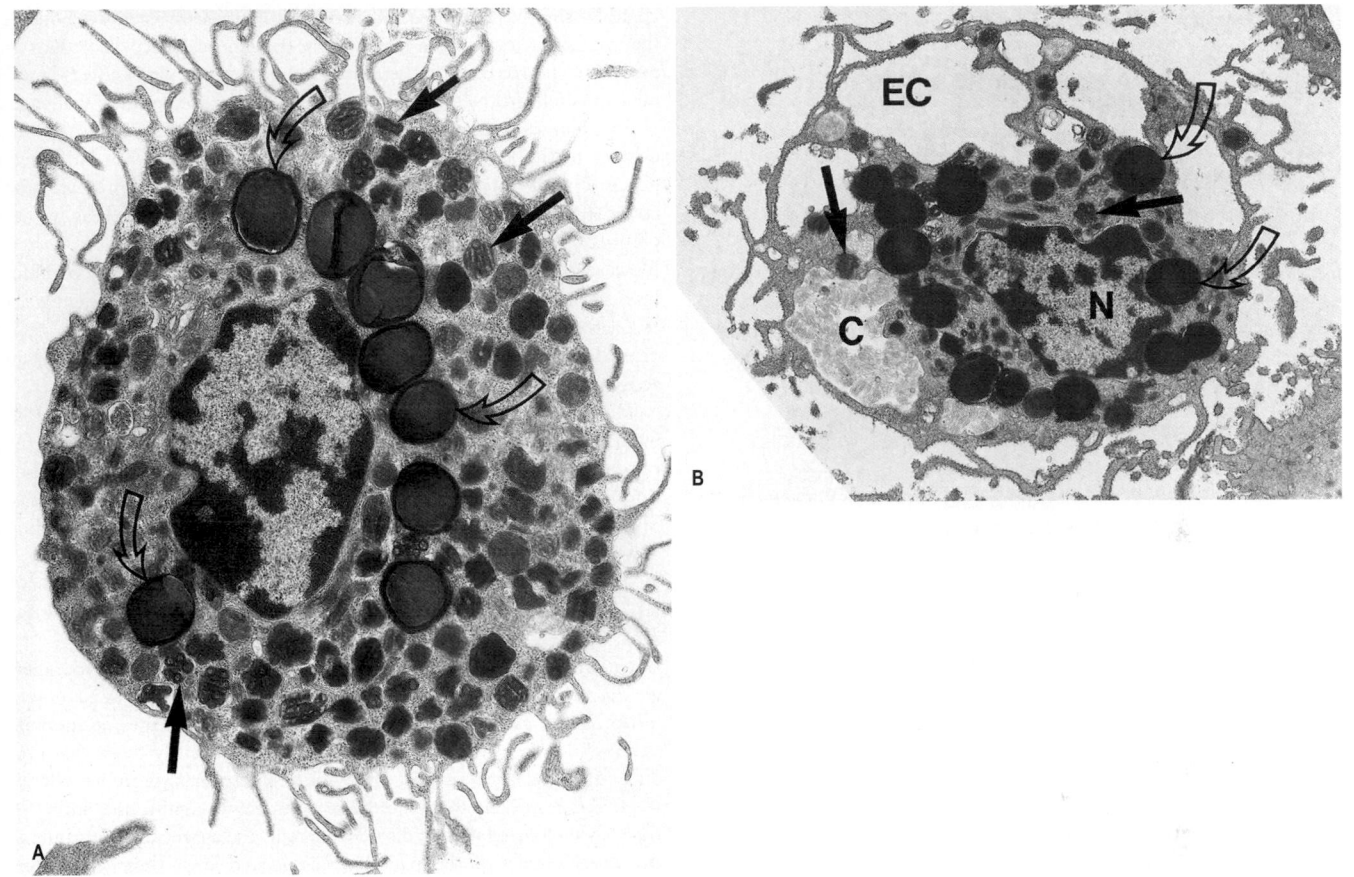

Fig. 22.3 (**A**) Mast cell purified from human lung. The cell contains many cytoplasmic granules with scroll-like substructural elements (solid arrows) and eight large nonmembrane-bound lipid bodies (open arrows). The plasma membrane has prominent folds. N, nucleus. (Original magnification ~×12 900). (**B**) An isolated human lung mast cell 10 minutes after exposure to anti-IgE *in vitro*. Some degranulation channels (C), formed by fusion of membranes surrounding individual cytoplasmic granules, contain altered granule matrix; others (EC) are empty. Cationized ferritin stains the plasma membrane and the membranes of some empty degranulation channels (EC). The membranes lining other channels (C) are unstained. A few unaltered scroll-containing granules (solid arrows) remain. Numerous lipid bodies are also present (open arrows). The cytoplasm contains prominent filaments. N, nucleus. (Original magnification ~×9100). (From Galli SJ, Dvorak AM, Dvorak HF. Prog Allergy 1984; 34: 1, with permission from Ann M. Dvorak.)

appropriately sensitized subjects by the interaction of antigen-specific IgE molecules on the surface of mast cells and/or basophils with the relevant multivalent antigen.[1–3, 16] The physiologic effects are due to the biologic responses of target cells (vascular endothelial cells, smooth muscle, glands, leukocytes, etc.) to mediators released by activated mast cells and/or basophils. The term refers to an immunopathologic mechanism: it conveys no information about the severity or distribution of the reaction.

IMMEDIATE- OR EARLY-PHASE RESPONSES

The signs and symptoms that develop at the site of antigen exposure within the first few minutes of a type I reaction reflect the biologic activities of the mast cell- and/or (especially in systemic reactions) basophil-derived mediators that are released immediately after the activation of these cells. In

sites that do not contain basophils, such as normal skin, these mediators are derived largely – perhaps exclusively – from mast cells. Thus, in most allergic patients intradermal challenge with specific antigen or anti-IgE induces an immediate wheal and flare reaction, accompanied by intense pruritus, which reaches a maximum 15–30 minutes later.[1–3, 16] Such immediate allergic reactions are usually accompanied by an increase in local levels of LTC_4 and PGD_2, and by the liberation of histamine and tryptase.

Studies in wild-type and c-*kit* mutant genetically mast cell-deficient mice, and c-*kit* mutant mice that have been selectively engrafted with mast cell populations (i.e., mast cell knock-in mice), have shown that essentially all of the augmented vascular permeability, tissue swelling and deposition of cross-linked fibrin associated with IgE-dependent passive cutaneous anaphylaxis reactions or with IgE-dependent reactions in the stomach wall were mast cell dependent.[2, 16] In humans, studies of nasal secretions or skin blister fluids induced by exposure to

CLINICAL RELEVANCE

MAST CELLS AND BASOPHILS IN HEALTH AND DISEASE

>> Mast cells and basophils are primary effector cells in atopic disorders (allergic rhinitis, allergic asthma, anaphylaxis).

>> Antigen-specific mast cell activation results in an immediate reaction, and in many cases contributes to a late-phase response in the involved tissues.

>> The late consequences of mast cell activation reflect the actions of cytokines, chemokines, growth factors and other mediators derived from mast cells and from other cells resident at or recruited to these sites whose recruitment, phenotype or function can be influenced by mast cell-derived products.

>> Mast cells and basophils may also contribute to host defense against certain parasites and have been implicated in a wide variety of other diseases and host responses, including innate immunity to microbial infection.

allergen demonstrate the release of both histamine and tryptase, with a strong correlation between levels of these two mediators, implicating mast cells in these reactions.[16]

ANAPHYLAXIS

Traditionally, this term has been used to describe an antigen-specific IgE-mediated reaction that is both life-threatening and systemic, with several organ systems involved[19] (Chapter 42). In this context anaphylaxis can be considered a severe, systemic type I immediate hypersensitivity reaction. However, because degranulation of mast cells and/or basophils can occur via non-IgE-dependent mechanisms, and because the biologic effects of the liberated mast cell and/or basophil mediators are the same regardless of the mechanism by which they are released, the term anaphylaxis sometimes also is used to describe a clinical syndrome that is severe, abrupt, and manifested by cutaneous (urticaria, angioedema), respiratory (asthma, laryngeal edema), cardiovascular (hypotension, cardiovascular collapse) and/or gastrointestinal (nausea, vomiting, diarrhea, cramping) signs and symptoms that occur either singly or in combination, whether or not the underlying mechanism is dependent on IgE.[19] When used in this fashion, the term does not imply any particular pathologic mechanism. Several lines of evidence indicate that systemic anaphylaxis in humans is associated with extensive mast cell activation. Increased levels of mast cell tryptase have been detected in the serum after the onset of anaphylactic symptoms, but little or no tryptase can be detected in serum from normal controls.[11] The histamine detected in the plasma of patients with anaphylaxis can be derived from both mast cells and basophils.[1-3]

LATE-PHASE RESPONSES

In many allergic patients the immediate reaction to cutaneous antigenic challenge is followed 4–8 hours later by persistent swelling and leukocyte infiltration, which is termed the late-phase response (LPR).[1-3, 16] LPRs can develop following IgE-dependent reactions in the respiratory tract, the nose and the skin, and in other anatomic locations. Many of the

clinically significant consequences of IgE-dependent reactions, both in the respiratory tract and in the skin, are thought to reflect the actions of the leukocytes recruited to these sites, rather than the direct effects of the mediators released by mast cells at early intervals after antigen challenge.

Both clinical and animal studies suggest that mast cell activation contributes to the leukocyte infiltration that is associated with LPRs, via effects of mast cell products on adhesion molecule expression by vascular endothelial cells and other cells at the reaction site, as well as by the production of chemokines and other chemoattractants.[1-3, 7, 11, 16] However, in actively sensitized hosts, LPRs can be induced by peptides that can activate T cells but which cannot induce IgE-dependent mast cell activation.[20] Such evidence indicates that both IgE- and T cell-dependent mechanisms can contribute to the elicitation of LPRs in actively immunized subjects.

The leukocytes recruited to sites of experimentally induced LPRs include basophils, eosinophils, neutrophils, lymphocytes and macrophages. Thus, the expression of features of LPRs reflects the contributions of mast cells, T cells and many other cell types, the relative importance of these potential effector cells probably varying depending on the individual circumstances.

CHRONIC ALLERGIC INFLAMMATION

In patients with chronic atopic diseases, including allergic asthma, allergic rhinitis and atopic dermatitis, the sites of pathology contain complex inflammatory infiltrates, including monocytes, macrophages, eosinophils, neutrophils, mast cells, basophils and T cells, especially those that produce the Th2-type pattern of cytokines that can promote allergic responses. It is likely that all of these participants significantly influence the course of these allergic disorders and, in the aggregate, contribute to the development of the pathology associated with these conditions. Although the recruitment and function of some of these leukocytes can be regulated by mechanisms that are largely independent of the activity of mast cells and basophils, recent findings suggest that mast cell and basophil products may play a larger role in the chronic manifestations of allergic inflammation than was previously supposed.

IgE-dependent activation induces mast cells to release TNF and a broad panel of other cytokines, chemokines and growth factors.[1-3] Upon appropriate activation, basophils produce IL-4 and IL-13.[1-3, 15] Such cytokines have the potential to influence many aspects of the pathophysiology at sites of allergic diseases, including some of the chronic changes (e.g., fibrosis, enhanced mucus production) associated with these disorders.[1-3, 7, 13, 16] Given that mast cell degranulation results in the local release of proteoglycans that are able to bind a variety of growth factors, FcεRI-mediated mast cell activation may also regulate the function, concentration and spatial distribution of cytokines and growth factors, whether derived from mast cells or other sources, within the tissue microenvironment. In other words, the traditional concept of the self-limited allergic reaction, which was thought to reflect the release of mast cell mediators whose biologic half-lives were measured in minutes or hours, must now be recognized as incomplete. Indeed, the complex and prolonged consequences of cytokine expression, together with the potential long-term effects of some of the cells' other mediators, suggest that mast cell activation can contribute importantly to many of the chronic features of allergic diseases and other disorders associated with mast cell activation.[1-3, 7, 13, 16] Many other factors probably also contribute to the chronicity of allergic inflammation. These include prolonged or repeated exposure to relevant allergens, and perhaps the diminished threshold for mast cell activation observed *in vivo* after even a single antigenic challenge.

■ MAST CELLS IN DISEASE AND HOST DEFENSE ■

ASTHMA

Approximately 80–90% of individuals who develop asthma before the age of 30 have an allergic component to the disease. Several lines of evidence indicate that mast cells contribute significantly to the initiation and maintenance of the pathology of allergic asthma (Chapters 39 and 40).[1–3, 7, 13, 16] In patients with allergic asthma, evidence of mast cell degranulation is provided by elevated levels of histamine and tryptase in the bronchoalveolar lavage fluid of those with moderately symptomatic asthma, and in bronchoalveolar lavage fluids after endobronchial allergen challenge.[7, 13]

There is growing agreement that the local elaboration of multiple cytokines, chemokines and growth factors, by mast cells and many other cell types, contributes importantly to the pathophysiology of asthma. Evidence includes the extended time course of release observed for some of these mast cell-derived products, the potent biological activities of such molecules, and the amplification and prolongation of the response achieved by the recruitment of additional effector cell types, each capable of contributing additional mediators to the inflammatory response. Mast cells have been proved to contribute to multiple features of asthma in certain mouse 'models' of the disorder, including allergen-induced bronchial constriction and hyperreactivity to metacholine, eosinophil and T-cell infiltration, lung collagen deposition, and increased numbers of epithelial goblet cells and proliferating cells in the airway epithelium.[2, 16] TNF may be especially important in these reactions, as this cytokine can be produced by both mast cells and eosinophils and can augment T-cell proliferation and cytokine production and enhance nonspecific bronchial hyperresponsiveness, as well as mediating many other proinflammatory effects.[2, 16] However, many cells other than mast cells, such as eosinophils and lymphocytes, as well as structural cells in the lungs such as epithelial cells, fibroblasts and smooth muscle cells, also represent a potentially important source of cytokines, chemokines and growth factors in the chronic allergic inflammation of allergic asthma.[2, 7, 13, 16] Moreover, mast cell and basophil mediators other than cytokines can also significantly influence disease pathophysiology. Clinical and *in vitro* studies indicate that LTC_4 and its peptidolytic derivatives LTD_4 and LTE_4, derived from mast cells, basophils and other sources, can contribute importantly to disease manifestations in many subjects with atopic asthma.[7, 13]

PARASITIC DISEASES

IgE-associated allergic disorders are not thought to confer any benefit to the host, and may cause significant pathology or death. What then is the selective advantage of IgE-associated immune responses? Several lines of evidence suggest that mast cells and basophils represent important components of host defense against parasites (Chapters 29 and 46).

Parasitic infections often induce strong primary and secondary IgE responses, with some of the IgE being specific for parasite antigens. Parasite infections are also associated with increased levels of circulating basophils and eosinophils, and markedly increased serum levels of IgE. This leads to enhanced expression of FcεRI on basophils and mast cells. There are also increased numbers of mast cells at sites of parasitic infection. However, it has been difficult to prove that individual components of this IgE-associated immune response to helminths are truly essential for the expression of protective host immunity to the parasite.

Studies in $Kit^{W/W-v}$ and congenic normal mice have documented increased numbers of mast cells at sites of parasite entry in the wild-type mice, and a delayed clearance of the parasite in $Kit^{W/W-v}$ mice that lack mast cells. However, expulsion of the parasite did eventually occur even in the absence of mast cells. $Kit^{W/W-v}$ mast cell-deficient mice which are also devoid of IL-3 exhibit a striking impairment in their ability to expel a primary infection with the nematode *Strongyloides venezuelensis* (*Sv*).[2, 3] In the guinea pig, basophils appear to be required for the expression of immune resistance to cutaneous feeding by larval *Amblyomma americanum* ticks, whereas the expression of IgE-dependent immune resistance to the cutaneous feeding by larval *Haemaphysalis longicornis* ticks in mice is dependent on mast cells.[3] These data, as well as many other lines of evidence, suggest that mast cells and basophils may provide similar or overlapping effector functions in parasite immunity, with the relative contributions of one or the other cell type varying according to such factors as the species of the parasite, the specific host and the site of infection. Given the importance of maintaining effective immune resistance to helminth parasites, it is perhaps not surprising that the responses remain largely intact despite the loss of a single effector component, such as IgE or mast cells.

MAST CELLS IN INNATE IMMUNITY

Mast cells may contribute significantly to several aspects of host defense during innate immune responses to bacterial infection. Mast cell knock-in mice were used to show that mast cells can represent a central component of host defense against certain bacterial infections, and that the recruitment of circulating leukocytes with bactericidal properties is dependent on mast cells.[2, 3, 14, 16] TNF is one important element of this response.[2, 3, 14, 16] Certain bacterial products – including LPS and other ligands of TLRs – also directly induce the release of some mast cell products.[7, 14]

Pathogens can also activate mast cells indirectly via activation of the complement system.[3, 14] Mast cell function in such settings can reflect the interaction between products of complement activation and complement receptors on mast cells and/or the response of mast cells to products of other cells that have been activated by complement-dependent mechanisms.[3] Clearly, a lack of mast cells can impair the effectiveness of some innate immune responses, at least in mice.

OTHER DISEASES

Mast cells or basophils or their products have been implicated in a bewildering variety of diseases not thought to be associated with an IgE response (e.g., scleroderma, pulmonary fibrosis of diverse origins, inflammatory bowel disease and peptic ulcer disease), as well as in angiogenesis, adaptive immune responses, protective responses to toxic agents, and reparative responses such as wound healing.[1–3, 7, 16] Recent data implicate mast cells in the pathogenesis of experimental allergic encephalomyelitis (an animal model of multiple sclerosis) and rheumatoid arthritis.[3] However, many of the roles proposed for mast cells or basophils in nonimmunological diseases, adaptive responses or tissue remodeling have not been evaluated using mast cell knock-in mice or other genetic approaches. Accordingly, the actual importance of the mast cell or the basophil in many of these settings remains to be determined.

MASTOCYTOSIS

Mastocytosis is a heterogeneous disorder associated with the accumulation of mast cells in the skin, bone marrow, gastrointestinal tract, liver, spleen, and lymph nodes. Its true prevalence is unknown. The incidence has been estimated between three and seven new patients per million.[21] Mastocytosis can present at any age. The onset of two-thirds of all cases is during childhood, mostly during the first 2 years of life.[22] A second peak of onset occurs in the late third to early fourth decades. Although most cases are sporadic, approximately 50 cases of familial mastocytosis have been described.

DESCRIPTION AND NATURAL HISTORY

The clinical signs and symptoms of disease observed in patients with mastocytosis are largely explained by tissue mast cell hyperplasia and an excess production of mast cell mediators (Fig. 22.4). The skin is involved in most cases, but mastocytosis does occur without visible skin manifestations. Internal organs can also be affected and constitutional symptoms can be present. The term 'systemic mastocytosis' has been used to categorize patients in whom increased numbers of mast cells are found in organ systems other than the skin.

Adults and children exhibit important differences in clinical presentation, pathogenesis, and prognosis. Whereas mastocytosis in childhood tends to be self-limited and to involve only the skin, the course in patients with adult-onset disease is usually prolonged and includes systemic involvement. Associated hematologic disorders exist or develop in up to 20–30% of adult patients.[23]

CUTANEOUS LESIONS

More than 90% of all patients with mastocytosis initially present with hyperpigmented skin lesions (maculopapular cutaneous mastocytosis [MPCM] or urticaria pigmentosa [UP]). These lesions are disseminated

brownish-red macules or slightly elevated papules that may urticate spontaneously or after trauma. This reaction elicited in lesional skin after stroking or rubbing is referred to as Darier's sign. In children, the lesions tend to be well demarcated, whereas in adults they become confluent and may form raised nodules or plaques (Fig. 22.5 A, B).[24] Although lesions may involve all sites of the integument, including mucous membranes, the trunk and proximal extremities typically have the highest density of lesions.

Mastocytosis has two additional cutaneous manifestations: solitary mastocytoma, a flat or mildly elevated, and well demarcated, solitary

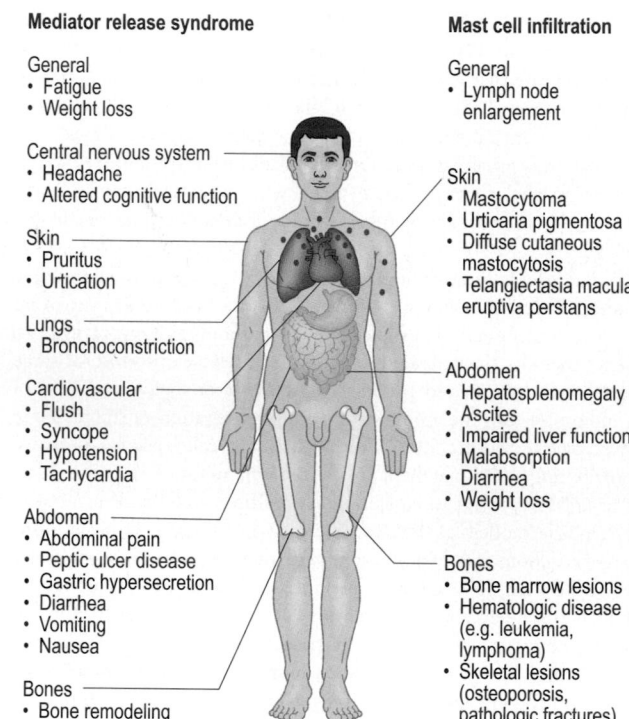

Mediator release syndrome

General
• Fatigue
• Weight loss

Central nervous system
• Headache
• Altered cognitive function

Skin
• Pruritus
• Urtication

Lungs
• Bronchoconstriction

Cardiovascular
• Flush
• Syncope
• Hypotension
• Tachycardia

Abdomen
• Abdominal pain
• Peptic ulcer disease
• Gastric hypersecretion
• Diarrhea
• Vomiting
• Nausea

Bones
• Bone remodeling

Mast cell infiltration

General
• Lymph node enlargement

Skin
• Mastocytoma
• Urticaria pigmentosa
• Diffuse cutaneous mastocytosis
• Telangiectasia macularis eruptiva perstans

Abdomen
• Hepatosplenomegaly
• Ascites
• Impaired liver function
• Malabsorption
• Diarrhea
• Weight loss

Bones
• Bone marrow lesions
• Hematologic disease (e.g. leukemia, lymphoma)
• Skeletal lesions (osteoporosis, pathologic fractures)

Fig. 22.4 Clinical manifestations of mastocytosis.

CLINICAL PEARLS

COMPARISON OF CHILDHOOD AND ADULT MASTOCYTOSIS

	Childhood	Adult
>> Etiology	Some with activating c-*kit* mutations Others unknown	Activating c-*kit* mutations SCF overproduction (?)
>> Skin involvement	Usually	Variable
>> Cutaneous patterns	Urticaria pigmentosa Mastocytoma Diffuse cutaneous mastocytosis	Urticaria pigmentosa
>> Systemic involvement	Unusual	Common
>> Course	≥50% resolution in adolescence	No resolution
>> Prognosis	Good in most cases	Depends on category

yellowish red-brown lesion, typically 2–5 cm in diameter, that occurs in infants and children, and diffuse cutaneous mastocytosis (DCM). Diffuse cutaneous mastocytosis is a rare disorder that presents in infants in the first year of life. It may involve the entire integument (erythrodermic mastocytosis). DCM presents with edema and doughy thickening of the skin. Serious systemic complications may occur, including hypotension and gastrointestinal hemorrhage, and are in part attributed to high levels of circulating mast cell-derived mediators, including histamine.

Infants and young children with mastocytosis in the skin sometimes exhibit blister formation. Blisters can form spontaneously, or in response to infection or immunization. A biopsy from a mastocytosis skin lesion typically shows increased numbers of normal-looking mast cells in the papillary dermis (Fig. 22.5C).

BONE MARROW AND HEMATOLOGIC INVOLVEMENT

Eighty percent or more of adults with systemic mastocytosis show focal to diffuse collections of spindle-shaped mast cells in the bone marrow (Fig. 22.5D). Fibrotic lesions may develop. Patients also may have a definable hematologic disorder such as a myelodysplastic syndrome, myeloproliferative disorder, acute leukemia, or a malignant lymphoma.[23] Anemia may occur in approximately one-third, and thrombocytopenia and eosinophilia in up to 25%, of all adult patients with mastocytosis.[25]

Up to 70% of patients with mastocytosis have radiologic abnormalities of bone, partially attributed to the mast cell infiltrates within the bone marrow. Approximately one in three to one in four mastocytosis patients have associated musculoskeletal to fibromyalgia-like pain. Osteoporosis, osteopenia, sclerosis, cystic lesions and, in severe disease, pathologic fractures may occur. The long bones, pelvis, ribs, skull, and vertebrae are the most common sites of skeletal involvement.

MAST CELL MEDIATOR-INDUCED SYMPTOMS

Flushing, shortness of breath, palpitations, nausea and diarrhea, hypotension and occasionally syncope are sometimes experienced by patients with mastocytosis and are believed to result from an excess release of mast cell mediators.[26] Patients may describe recurrent episodes with a combination of these symptoms. Such episodes typically last for 30 minutes. Lethargy and fatigue lasting several hours may follow. The frequency and severity of symptoms cannot be predicted by the degree of organ involvement, although such symptoms are considerably more frequent with systemic disease. Systemic episodes occur spontaneously, or they can be provoked in some individuals by stimuli such as hymenoptera insect stings, aspirin and other NSAIDs, opiates (including morphine and its derivatives), muscle relaxants, ethanol, allergies to inhalants or foods, contrast media, surgery or endoscopy, infection (bacteria, viruses, others), and certain physical stimuli such as friction, heat or exercise.

Severe or protracted anaphylaxis may occur in patients with extensive disease, and even fatal reactions have been described. Patients with mastocytosis, however, are not more likely to suffer from allergic diseases. Nevertheless, reactions may be more severe in allergic patients with mastocytosis because of an expanded effector cell population. For example, patients with mastocytosis may develop life-threatening anaphylaxis after hymenoptera stings, during the course of insect venom hyposensitization, or after being administered iodinated contrast materials.[27]

Involvement of the gastrointestinal (GI) tract is common in patients with systemic mastocytosis. Abdominal pain is the most common symptom, followed by nausea, diarrhea, and vomiting. 56% of the patients characterized their pain as dyspeptic in nature, 44% as nondyspeptic; 25% of these patients indicated that both types of pain were present.[28] Diarrhea and malabsorption occurred in 63% and 31% of patients with systemic mastocytosis, respectively. Diarrhea is not generally related to gastric hypersecretion and was attributed to altered intestinal secretion, structural mucosal abnormalities, and hypermotility. Associated malabsorption is usually mild and not clinically important.

OTHER MANIFESTATIONS

Liver disease is common in patients with mastocytosis.[28] Hepatomegaly was reported in 24%, and elevated levels of liver enzymes in 54% in one series of 41 patients. Mast cell infiltrates were frequently found in liver biopsies. However, severe liver disease was uncommon, except in those with aggressive disease. In these patients, fibrosis, cirrhosis, ascites, and portal hypertension were reported to be more frequent.

The spleen appears to be involved in 40–50% of patients with systemic disease. Splenomegaly is more pronounced in those with aggressive disease. Mast cell infiltrates are observed in biopsy specimens. Peripheral lymphadenopathy has been reported in 26–56% of patients with mastocytosis. Adenopathy is more common in patients with associated hematologic disorders and more aggressive disease.

Patients with mastocytosis sometimes report neuropsychiatric problems. Altered neurological function such as poor attention, irritability, impaired memory, personality change and depression have been observed.

PROGNOSIS AND CLASSIFICATION

The clinical course varies from asymptomatic with normal life expectancy to highly aggressive, and depends on the variant of disease. The WHO classification defines seven variants (Table 22.3).[29] The term 'systemic mastocytosis' (SM) has been used to categorize patients in whom increased numbers of mast cells are found in organ systems other than the skin. It is defined in the WHO classification by a major criterion of multifocal mast cell infiltrates in the bone marrow or in other extracutaneous organ(s) (>15 mast cells per aggregate detected by tryptase immunohistochemistry) and four minor criteria: 25% or more of mast cells in biopsy sections of bone marrow or other extracutaneous organs show a spindle-shaped or abnormal morphology, or more than 25% of all mast cells in bone marrow aspirate smears are immature or atypical mast cells; detection of a c-*kit* mutation at codon 816 in bone marrow, blood or other extracutaneous organ(s); mast cells in the bone

Table 22.3 WHO classification of mastocytosis

Cutaneous mastocytosis
Indolent systemic mastocytosis
Systemic mastocytosis with an associated clonal hematologic non-mast-cell lineage disease
Aggressive systemic mastocytosis
Mast cell leukemia
Mast cell sarcoma
Extracutaneous mastocytoma

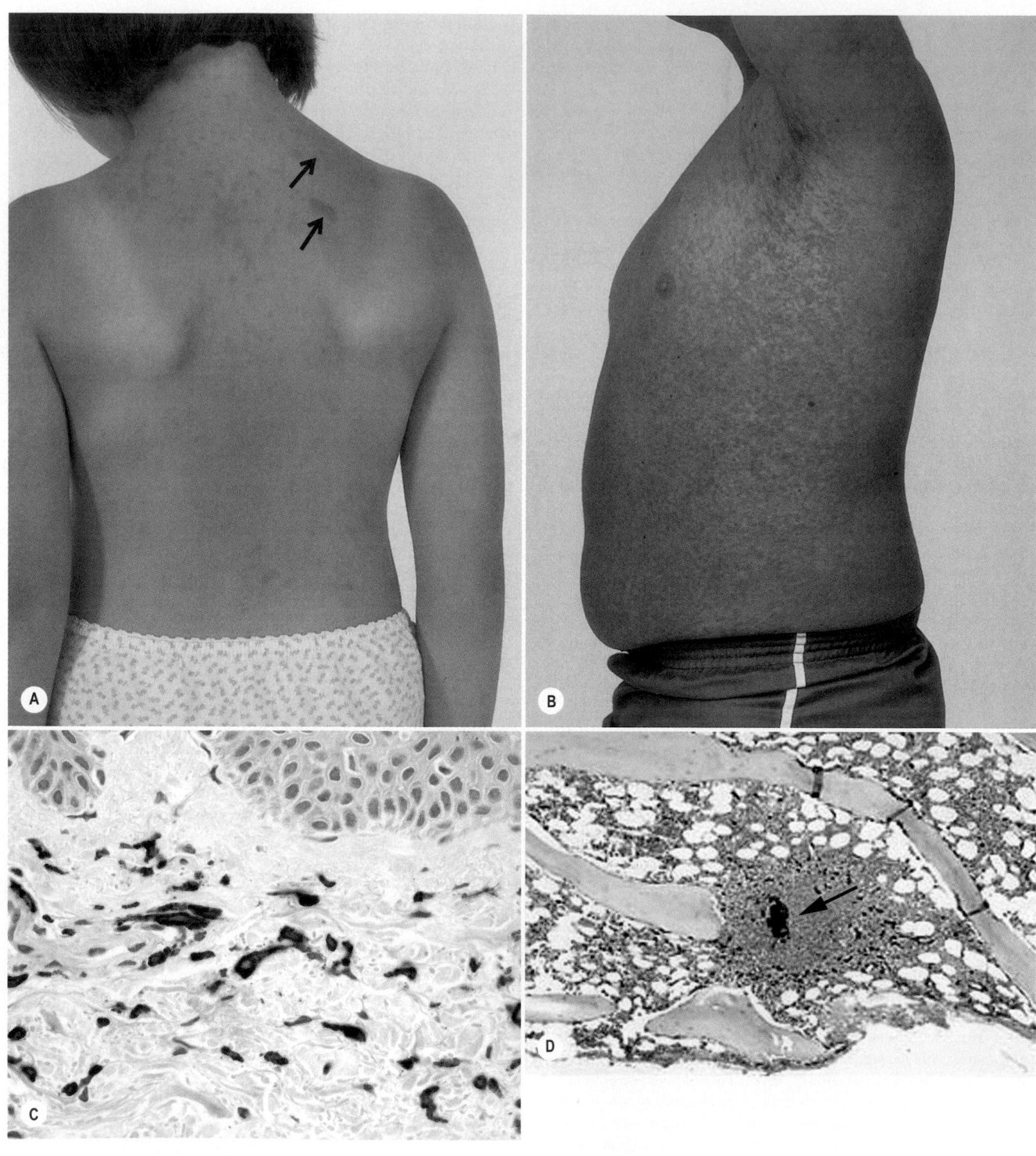

Fig. 22.5 Cutaneous mastocytosis and histopathology. Urticaria pigmentosa is the most common form of cutaneous mastocytosis. In childhood, lesions are disseminated and consist of well-demarcated hyperpigmented macules (e.g. arrows) (**A**). In adults, lesions may be numerous with less well-demarcated brownish-red macules and papules (**B**). Histopathology of cutaneous mastocytosis shows a slight perivascular mononuclear cell infiltrate with mast cells containing abundant tryptase immunoreactive cytoplasmic granules is seen in the papillary dermis (antitryptase, AA1 clone, Dako; orignal magnification ~×400) (**C**). Bone marrow pathology of indolent mastocytosis is characterized by paratrabecular lymphoid nodule containing small, well-differentiated lymphoid cells around substantial numbers of fusiform cells with prominent granules in the tryptase stain (arrow) (antitryptase, AA1 clone, Dako; original magnification ~×250) (**D**). (Courtesy of Dr Cem Akin.)

marrow or in another extracutaneous organ co-express CD117 (KIT) with CD2 and/or CD25; and serum total tryptase that is persistently greater than 20 ng/mL. If at least one major and one minor, or at least three minor criteria for SM are fulfilled, the diagnosis is SM. Criteria defining the mast cell burden, involvement of non-mast cell lineages and aggressiveness of disease are applied to subclassify SM in sub-variants.[29]

Particularly in children, mastocytosis of the skin (cutaneous mastocytosis) may be the only manifestation, and about 50% of such cases resolve during puberty.[30] Most adults fall into the indolent systemic mastocytosis category and the disease tends to remain stable over many years.[31] Progression of the skin involvement may occur, but evolution of disease into more severe forms is uncommon.

Patients in the other categories may have a less favorable prognosis and some may experience a rapid progression.[23] Patients in these categories are less likely to exhibit involvement of the skin. Factors influencing the clinical course are the associated hematologic abnormalities and the rapidity of the increase in mast cell numbers (especially in aggressive mastocytosis and mast cell leukemia).

Mast cell leukemia is the rarest form and has the most fulminant behavior. Mast cell leukemia is diagnosed when bone marrow aspirate smears show 20% or more mast cells and 10% or more of the peripheral blood nucleated cells are mast cells. Survival of those with mast cell leukemia is generally less than 1 year.

ETIOLOGY AND PATHOGENESIS

The most important survival/growth factor for mast cells is the KIT ligand SCF. At least in adults, it is thought that one initial event that can result in mastocytosis is an activating mutation in c-*kit*, the gene for KIT.[32] KIT, a transmembrane thyrosine kinase receptor encoded by the pro-oncogene c-*kit*, is expressed on mast cells, melanocytes, hematopoietic stem cells, interstitial cells of Cajal and germ cell lineages. Ligation of KIT by SCF promotes dimerization of the receptor and subsequently induces intrinsic tyrosine kinase activation. The resulting phosphorylated tyrosine residues serve as docking sites for intracellular downstream signaling pathways leading to cell proliferation and activation.

In more than 90% of adult patients with SM neoplastic mast cells exhibit a somatic 'autoactivating' mutation at codon 816 of c-*kit*. The most commonly detected mutant is Asp816Val, which has been identified not only in the bone marrow, but also in the skin and spleen in some patients. Most mutations are somatic: only rare germline mutations have been reported in cases of familial mastocytosis. These findings support the conclusion that the disease is clonal, and suggest that mastocytosis could be regarded as a clonal rather than a hyperproliferative disorder. The reason(s) for the different behavior of indolent versus aggressive variants of mastocytosis, however, remain(s) unknown. Patients with hypereosinophilia and high numbers of mast cells on the basis of a FIP1L1-PDGFRA fusion have been described.[33]

The Asp816Val c-*kit* mutation has also been described in biopsies of lesional skin of children with more severe forms of mastocytosis. However, it appears overall to be unusual in lesional biopsies of children with typical MPCM. Several additional c-*kit* mutations have been detected in some children and adults, but their clinical relevance is less clear. These findings raise the possibility that in many children mastocytosis has a different basis from that in most adults, and this could provide an explanation for the generally more benign course of some cases of childhood UP.

DIAGNOSIS

Most patients with mastocytosis present with characteristic cutaneous lesions that support the diagnosis. Histological examination of the skin should be performed at initial presentation. Mast cells within skin biopsies are identified using toluidine blue or Giemsa stains, or by immunohistochemistry using antibodies to mast cell tryptase. A 15–20-fold increase in mast cell numbers has been reported in lesions of UP, but the increase may be less pronounced.[26] However, a two- to fourfold increase in mast cell numbers has been observed in unrelated conditions, including idiopathic anaphylaxis, flushing, chronic urticaria, and eczema.

Biochemical demonstration of elevated serum levels of total mast cell tryptase (>20 ng/mL) supports the diagnosis of SM, whereas in cutaneous mastocytosis tryptase levels may be normal.[34] In addition, elevation in urinary histamine and its metabolites may be observed in SM. However, mast cell tryptase and histamine can also be elevated in association with acute exacerbations of allergic diseases, including anaphylaxis, and, in the case of tryptase, clonal myeloid disorders. Therefore such elevations in total tryptase, in isolation, are not diagnostic of mastocytosis.

In patients with elevated serum total tryptase, bone marrow biopsy and aspiration should be considered, particularly in adults. A bone marrow biopsy is also useful for staging the disease by excluding associated hematologic abnormalities. In patients with an associated hematologic disorder, identification of mast cells in the bone marrow may be difficult if the mast cells are dysplastic and when mast cell granules are more coarse than normal, or are even absent.[35] The most accurate stain for the detection of mast cells in mastocytosis is an immunohistochemical stain with antibody to mast cell tryptase. Identifying, by flow cytometry of bone marrow aspirates or by immunohistochemical analysis of bone marrow biopsies, the co-expression of CD2 and/or CD25 in CD117 (KIT)-positive mast cells has been considered the most sensitive and specific method to support the diagnosis of SM in the bone marrow.[36]

Although it can be performed on blood or peripheral tissues, c-*kit* mutation analysis is best performed on bone marrow, and particularly on sorted malignant mast cells to increase sensitivity. Inability to identify the presence of a point mutation at codon 817 in c-*kit* does not eliminate the possibility that cells bearing this mutation are present, in that the malignant clone may not have expanded to sufficient cell numbers to allow the detection of a mutation.

In patients with SM, the size of the liver and spleen should be measured by ultrasound or CT, and bone density should be measured by the DXA method to evaluate for osteoporosis. SM is classified into one of the more aggressive variants of disease when there is bone marrow involvement of non-mast cell lineages, organ dysfunction and/or a high mast cell burden.

Further studies, such as gastrointestinal endoscopy or biopsy to obtain tissue specimens from the liver, spleen, gastrointestinal tract or lymph nodes, are usually considered only when these organs are suspected to be involved and a biopsy would yield clinically useful information. A physical examination, serum tryptase determination and a complete blood count should be performed at yearly intervals in patients with indolent stable SM.

■ THERAPY ■

There currently is no cure for cutaneous or systemic mastocytosis.[37] Treatment is symptomatic and is tailored to the individual. Prominent mast cell mediator-induced symptoms include hypotension, gastric hypersecretion, abdominal pain, and pruritus. Aggressive forms of therapy are not indicated in patients with indolent mastocytosis, as this disorder has a favorable prognosis. In patients with aggressive disease or associated hematologic disorders, treatment is a therapeutic challenge.

THERAPY OF CUTANEOUS AND INDOLENT DISEASE

In patients with indolent disease, management includes reassurance, avoidance of exacerbating factors, and treatment that offers symptomatic relief. Information about the nature of the disease, an explanation

THERAPEUTIC PRINCIPLES

Avoidance of exacerbating factors

Therapy of cutaneous and indolent disease

>> H_1 antihistamines
>> H_2 antihistamines
>> Cromolyn sodium
>> Anticholinergics
>> Systemic glucocorticoids (malabsorption)
>> Epinephrine (hypotension)
>> Ultraviolet radiation (PUVA, UVA$_1$)
>> Topical glucocorticosteroids (mastocytoma)

Therapy of aggressive disease and associated hematologic disorders

>> Interferon-α_{2b}
>> Cladribine
>> Chemotherapy
>> Imatinib (in mutations other than in codon 816)
>> Experimental: new tyrosine kinase inhibitors, bone marrow transplantation

of expected symptoms, and discussion of prognosis will address the most common concerns of patients with mastocytosis. Factors known to provoke episodes of flushing and hypotension should be reviewed with the patient and avoided. Patients with mastocytosis and hymenoptera venom exposure are at risk for severe anaphylaxis. Epinephrine is the drug of choice for anaphylaxis and should be kept available by patients at risk at all times. Immediate self-administration during anaphylaxis may be life-saving. Insect venom immunotherapy, as well as premedication with antihistamines and corticosteroids prior to general anesthesia, should be seriously considered.

Nonsedating H_1 antihistamines are the agents of choice for pruritus and urtication. For prophylaxis of recurrent episodes of anaphylaxis, antihistamines should be administered daily. For some patients, classic sedating H_1 blockers, such as hydroxyzine or diphenhydramine, seem to be more effective. The addition of an H_2-receptor antagonist is also an option. Gastric acid hypersecretion, peptic ulcer disease, and reflux esophagitis are managed with H_2-receptor blockers and proton pump inhibitors. Cromolyn sodium may be used, particularly for gastrointestinal symptoms. Anticholinergics are an option for control of diarrhea. Systemic corticosteroids are used in cases of malabsorption or ascites. Calcium, vitamin D and bisphosphonates are the drugs of choice for osteoporosis.

Application of topical corticosteroids under occlusion or topical PUVA (psoralen plus UVA radiation) treatment may be considered in patients with cutaneous mastocytosis. Both are effective in reducing pruritus and urtication, but relapse typically occurs a few months after therapy is discontinued. Patients also report a diminution or decrease in intensity of skin lesions in the summer and after repeated exposure to natural sunlight. The benefits of these forms of therapy have to be weighed against the potential for inducing cutaneous malignancies associated with long-term UV radiation.

THERAPY OF AGGRESSIVE DISEASE AND ASSOCIATED HEMATOLOGIC DISORDERS

Patients with mastocytosis and an associated hematologic disorder should be managed using therapy appropriate for the associated disorder. Chemotherapy has not been shown to produce remission, or to prolong survival, in mast cell leukemia, and is not indicated in indolent mastocytosis, as it may lead to bone marrow suppression without improving the symptoms of mastocytosis. A partial response to interferon-α_{2b} has been reported in patients with aggressive mast cell disease. However, other reports of its value have been mixed.[38] Cladribine (2-cholorodeoxyadenosin) has been reported to reduce the mast cell burden and may be considered in aggressive mastocytosis.[39]

New therapeutic approaches should target neoplastic mast cells. The tyrosine kinase inhibitor imatinib is not generally considered to be indicated in patients with typical Asp 816Val mutations in KIT, as steric conformations of the receptor interfere with the action of the drug in this setting.[40] However, the drug has been reported to reduce mast cell load and symptoms in patients with mutations in other c-*KIT* exons. Other tyrosine kinase inhibitors have been developed which may also inhibit mutations in codon 816, and some of these are currently in clinical trials. Therapies that target markers such as CD25 expressed on mast cells are also currently under investigation. Bone marrow transplantation may evolve as an option, although results to date have been disappointing.

ACKNOWLEDGMENTS

We thank Dr Ann M. Dvorak for providing the electron micrographs and Drs. John J. Costa and Jochen Wedemeyer for their contributions to the first edition of this chapter. Some of the work reviewed in this chapter was supported by United States Public Health Service grants AI 23990, CA72074 and HL67674 (Project 2), by Deutsche Forschungsgemeinschaft grant ME2668/1–1, by the Intramural Research Program of NIAID and/or by AMGEN Inc.; Dr Galli consults for AMGEN Inc. under terms that are in accord with Stanford University conflict-of-interest guidelines.

REFERENCES

1. Metcalfe DD, Baram D, Mekori YA. Mast cells. Physiol Rev 1997; 77: 1033–1079.

2. Galli SJ, Kalesnikoff J, Grimbaldeston MA, et al. Mast cells as 'tunable' effector and immunoregulatory cells: recent advances. Annu Rev Immunol 2005; 23: 749–786.

3. Galli SJ, Metcalfe DD, Arber D, et al. Basophils and mast cells and their disorders. In Lichtman MA, Beutler E, Kipps TJ, eds: Williams hematology, . 7th edn, New York: McGraw-Hill Medical; 2005, p 879–897.

4. Kinet JP. The high-affinity IgE receptor (Fc epsilon RI): from physiology to pathology. Annu Rev Immunol 1999; 17: 931–972.

5. Inomata N, Tomita H, Ikezawa Z, et al. Differential gene expression profile between cord blood progenitor-derived and adult progenitor-derived human mast cells. Immunol Lett 2005; 98: 265–271.

6. Costa JJ, Demetri GD, Harrist TJ, et al. Recombinant human stem cell factor (kit ligand) promotes human mast cell and melanocyte hyperplasia and functional activation in vivo. J Exp Med 1996; 183: 2681–2686.

7. Marone G, Triggiani M, Genovese A, et al. Role of human mast cells and basophils in bronchial asthma. Adv Immunol 2005; 88: 97–160.

8. Lantz CS, Boesiger J, Song CH, et al. Role for interleukin-3 in mast-cell and basophil development and in immunity to parasites. Nature 1998; 392: 90–93.

9. Caughey GH. New developments in the genetics and activation of mast cell proteases. Mol Immunol 2002; 38: 1353–1357.

10. Hallgren J, Pejler G. Biology of mast cell tryptase. An inflammatory mediator. FEBS J 2006; 273: 1871–1895.

11. Schwartz LB. Effector cells of anaphylaxis: mast cells and basophils. Novartis Foundation Symp 2004; 2004: 276–285.

12. Metz M, Piliponsky AM, Chen C-C, et al. Mast cells can enhance resistance to snake and honeybee venoms. Science 2006; 313: 526–530.

13. Boyce JA. The role of mast cells in asthma. Prostaglandins Leukoc Essent Fatty Acids 2003; 69: 195–205.

14. Marshall JS. Mast-cell responses to pathogens. Nature Rev Immunol 2004; 4: 787–799.

15. Paul WE, Seder RA, Plaut M. Lymphokine and cytokine production by Fc epsilon RI+ cells. Adv Immunol 1993; 53: 1–29.

16. Grimbaldeston MA, Metz M, Yu M, et al. Effector and potential immunoregulatory roles of mast cells in IgE-associated acquired immune responses. Curr Opin Immunol 2006; 18: 751–760.

17. Zhu D, Kepley CL, Zhang K, et al. A chimeric human–cat fusion protein blocks cat-induced allergy. Nature Med 2005; 11: 446–449.

18. Iikura M, Yamaguchi M, Fujisawa T, et al. Secretory IgA induces degranulation of IL-3-primed basophils. J Immunol 1998; 161: 1510–1515.

19. Sampson HA, Munoz-Furlong A, Campbell RL, et al. Second symposium on the definition and management of anaphylaxis: summary report–Second National Institute of Allergy and Infectious Disease/Food Allergy and Anaphylaxis Network symposium. J Allergy Clin Immunol 2006; 117: 391–397.

20. Ali FR, Oldfield WL, Higashi N, et al. Late asthmatic reactions induced by inhalation of allergen-derived T cell peptides. Am J Respir Crit Care Med 2004; 169: 20–26.

21. Rosbotham JL, Malik NM, Syrris P, et al. Lack of c-kit mutation in familial urticaria pigmentosa. Br J Dermatol 1999; 140: 849–852.

22. Kettelhut BV, Metcalfe DD. Pediatric mastocytosis. J Invest Dermatol 1991; 96: 15S–18S.

23. Valent P, Sperr WR, Schwartz LB, et al. Diagnosis and classification of mast cell proliferative disorders: delineation from immunologic diseases and non-mast cell hematopoietic neoplasms. J Allergy Clin Immunol 2004; 114: 3–11.

24. Brockow K, Akin C, Huber M, et al. Assessment of the extent of cutaneous involvement in children and adults with mastocytosis: relationship to symptomatology, tryptase levels, and bone marrow pathology. J Am Acad Dermatol 2003; 48: 508–516.

25. Parker RI. Hematologic aspects of systemic mastocytosis. Hematol Oncol Clin North Am 2000; 14: 557–568.

26. Garriga MM, Friedman MM, Metcalfe DD. A survey of the number and distribution of mast cells in the skin of patients with mast cell disorders. J Allergy Clin Immunol 1988; 82: 425–432.

27. Oude Elberink JN, de Monchy JG, Kors JW, et al. Fatal anaphylaxis after a yellow jacket sting, despite venom immunotherapy, in two patients with mastocytosis. J Allergy Clin Immunol 1997; 99: 153–154.

28. Jensen RT. Gastrointestinal abnormalities and involvement in systemic mastocytosis. Hematol Oncol Clin North Am 2000; 14: 579–623.

29. Valent P, Horny HP, Li CY, et al. Pathology and genetics of tumors of hematopoietic and lymphoid tissue. In Jaffe E, Harris N, Stein H, Vardiman J, eds: World Health Organization classification of tumors, Lyon: IARC Press; 2001, p 293–302.

30. Caplan RM. The natural course of urticaria pigmentosa. Analysis and follow-up of 112 cases. Arch Dermatol 1963; 87: 146–157.

31. Brockow K, Scott LM, Worobec AS, et al. Regression of urticaria pigmentosa in adult patients with systemic mastocytosis: correlation with clinical patterns of disease. Arch Dermatol 2002; 138: 785–90.

32. Akin C, Metcalfe DD. The biology of Kit in disease and the application of pharmacogenetics. J Allergy Clin Immunol 2004; 114: 13–19.

33. Pardanani A, Ketterling RP, Brockman SR, et al. CHIC2 deletion, a surrogate for FIP1L1-PDGFRA fusion, occurs in systemic mastocytosis associated with eosinophilia and predicts response to imatinib mesylate therapy. Blood 2003; 102: 3093–3096.

REFERENCES

34. Schwartz LB, Irani AM. Serum tryptase and the laboratory diagnosis of systemic mastocytosis. Hematol Oncol Clin North Am 2000; 14: 641–657.

35. Horny HP, Valent P. Histopathological and immunohistochemical aspects of mastocytosis. Int Arch Allergy Immunol 2002; 127: 115–117.

36. Escribano L, Orfao A, Diaz-Agustin B, et al. Indolent systemic mast cell disease in adults: immunophenotypic characterization of bone marrow mast cells and its diagnostic implications. Blood 1998; 91: 2731–2736.

37. Worobec AS. Treatment of systemic mast cell disorders. Hematol Oncol Clin North Am 2000; 14: 659–687.

38. Worobec AS, Kirshenbaum AS, Schwartz LB, et al. Treatment of three patients with systemic mastocytosis with interferon alpha-2b. Leuk Lymphoma 1996; 22: 501–508.

39. Kluin-Nelemans HC, Oldhoff JM, Van Doormaal JJ, et al. Cladribine therapy for systemic mastocytosis. Blood 2003; 102: 4270–4276.

40. Akin C, Brockow K, D'Ambrosio C, et al. Effects of tyrosine kinase inhibitor STI571 on human mast cells bearing wild-type or mutated c-kit. Exp Hematol 2003; 31: 686–692.

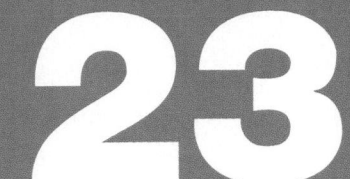

Eosinophils and eosinophilia

Peter F. Weller

Eosinophils are terminally differentiated, bone marrow-derived granulocytes that normally circulate in the blood in low numbers and tend to localize in those tissues with mucosal epithelial surfaces. Increased blood or tissue eosinophils occur with helminth parasite infections as well as with allergic diseases and a variety of other, often idiopathic conditions. Conventionally the major focus on eosinophils has been delineating the 'effector' functions of these end-stage granulocytes, including what roles these cells play as helminthotoxic effector cells and the contribution they make to the immunopathogenesis of allergic diseases. More recent findings indicate that eosinophil functions are considerably more extensive.[1–4] Eosinophils contain stores of multiple pre-formed cytokines, engage in cognate cell–cell interactions with other cell types, including lymphocytes, and have a role in varied host immune and inflammatory responses not conventionally marked by quantitatively extensive eosinophil infiltration.

■ PRODUCTION AND DISTRIBUTION OF EOSINOPHILS ■

EOSINOPHILOPOIESIS

The development of eosinophils in the bone marrow can be elicited by three cytokines. Granulocyte–macrophage colony-stimulating factor (GM-CSF), interleukin (IL)-3 and IL-5 each promote eosinophilopoiesis. In contrast to IL-3 and GM-CSF, which also promote the development of other lineages, IL-5 uniquely promotes the development and terminal differentiation of eosinophils. Although IL-5 is produced by CD8 T cells, NK cells, and other leukocytes, including eosinophils themselves, IL-5 is a defining cytokine product of Th2 CD4 T cells. The production of IL-5 by Th2 lymphocytes accounts for the eosinophilia accompanying Th2 cell-mediated immune responses characteristic of helminth infections and allergic diseases. Increases in blood IL-5 have been detectable in some, but not all, patients with eosinophilias of varying causes, including some with hypereosinophilic syndromes and parasitic infections.

Eosinophilopoiesis develops over about a week. Retained in the marrow is a pool of mature eosinophils. IL-5, alone and in concert with the chemokine eotaxin, rapidly releases this pool of mature eosinophils into the circulation to acutely increase blood eosinophilia and facilitate recruitment of eosinophils to sites of inflammation.[2] Blood eosinophils circulate with a half-life of about 8–18 hours. Eosinophils leave the circulation and localize in tissues, especially those with mucosal interfaces with the outside world, such as the respiratory, gastrointestinal and lower genitourinary tracts. Although the mechanisms governing this homing of eosinophils to mucosal tissues are not fully known, the chemokine eotaxin is involved in the homing of eosinophils to the gastrointestinal, but not the respiratory, tract.[2] Eosinophils live longer than neutrophils and probably persist in tissues for several weeks. They are principally tissue-dwelling cells: as demonstrated in rodents, for every eosinophil present in the circulation there are 300–500 in the tissues.

EOSINOPHIL ADHERENCE MECHANISMS

The transit of eosinophils from the marrow, through the circulation and into tissues is governed in part by multiple adherence molecules expressed on eosinophils (Fig. 23.1).[5] As for other leukocytes, recruitment of eosinophils into tissue sites of inflammation utilizes combinatorial interactions involving specific adhesion molecules (via their expression and altered affinity states) that mediate cellular interactions with the

---

❙ KEY CONCEPTS

ACTIONS OF EOSINOPHILOPOIETIC CYTOKINES IL-3, GM-CSF, IL-5

>> Promote eosinophil development and maturation in the marrow.

>> Release a pool of matured eosinophils from the marrow.

>> Sustain the viability and antagonize apoptosis of mature eosinophils, enhance multiple effector responses of mature eosinophils

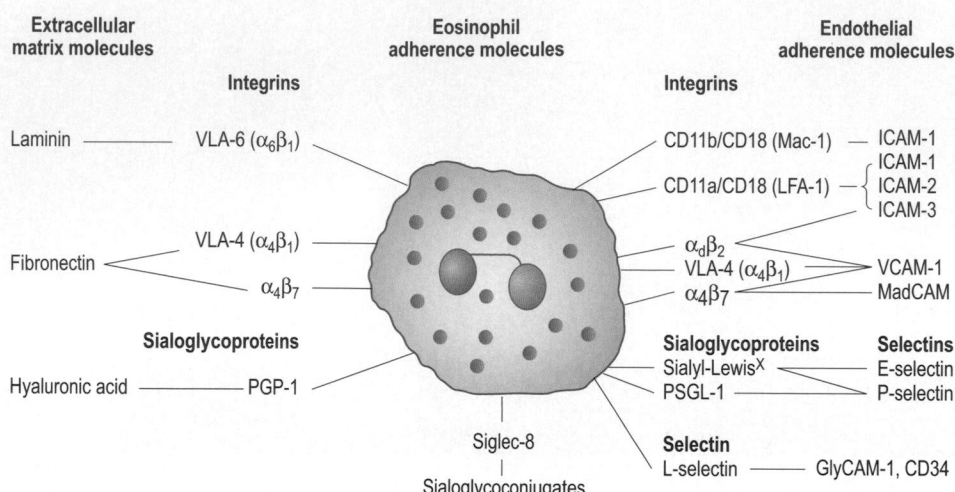

Fig. 23.1 Adherence mechanisms utilized by human eosinophils to bind to vascular endothelial cells and the extracellular matrix molecules. ICAM, intracellular adhesion molecule; VCAM, vascular cell adhesion molecule; MadCAM, mucosal addressin cell adhesion molecule; VLA, very late activation antigen.

vascular endothelium and actions of chemoattractant molecules. Eosinophils express several adhesion molecules broadly shared with other leukocytes that mediate their initial rolling and subsequent adherence to endothelial cells. Similar to neutrophils, eosinophils can adhere via CD11/CD18 heterodimeric β_2-integrins to the intercellular adhesion molecules ICAM-1 and ICAM-2. Likewise, specific sialoglycoproteins mediate adherence between eosinophils and endothelial E- and P-selectins. Unlike neutrophils, but similar to lymphocytes, eosinophils are able to bind to vascular cell adhesion molecule-1 (VCAM-1). Eosinophils express two α_4-integrins, very late activation antigen-4 (VLA-4, $\alpha_4\beta_1$) and $\alpha_4\beta_7$, that bind to VCAM-1. Moreover, $\alpha_4\beta_7$ binds to the mucosal addressin, mucosal addressin cell adherence molecule (MadCAM). The β_2-integrin, $\alpha d\beta_2$, which binds ICAM-3 and is expressed on other leukocytes, is an additional integrin that mediates eosinophil adhesion to VCAM-1. Enhanced expression of VCAM-1 on the vascular endothelium, as elicitable by IL-4 or IL-13 stimulation, may contribute to the localization of eosinophils in some tissue sites of inflammation.

In addition to mediating interactions with the endothelium, eosinophil adhesion molecules, by their interactions with extracellular matrix components, modulate the activity of eosinophils that have exited the bloodstream. Eosinophil VLA-6, $\alpha_6\beta_1$, binds laminin. Both $\alpha_4\beta_1$ and $\alpha_4\beta_7$ interact with specific domains of tissue fibronectin, and these interactions can enhance eosinophil functional responses. Eosinophils express CD44 (PGP-1), which binds hyaluronic acid. Siglec-8, a sialic acid-binding immunoglobulin-like lectin, is expressed on eosinophils and binds sialoglycoconjugates.

EOSINOPHIL CHEMOATTRACTANTS

Mobilization of eosinophils into tissues is governed by receptor-mediated chemoattractant stimuli. Chemoattractants promote the directed migration of eosinophils and may enhance the adhesion of eosinophils to vascular endothelium and their subsequent migration through the endothelium. Many compounds have been identified as eosinophil chemoattractants, including humoral immune mediators, such as platelet-activating factor (PAF) and the complement anaphylatoxins C5a and C3a; certain cytokines; and several chemokines, most notably the eotaxins. None of these is specific solely for eosinophils, but eotaxin, eotaxin-2 and eotaxin-3 exhibit the most restricted specificity.[2] Eotaxins signal through CCR3 chemokine receptors that are expressed on eosinophils as well as basophils, some Th2 cells and some mast cells. Thus, recruitment of eosinophils to sites of immunologic reactions is governed by their response to chemoattractants that facilitate intravascular emigration and direct migration of extravascular eosinophils, as well as by the functional states of eosinophil adherence molecules and the differential expression of endothelial cell adherence ligands.

STRUCTURE OF EOSINOPHILS

Human eosinophils, unlike neutrophils, usually have a bilobed nucleus (Fig. 23.2). Defining attributes of eosinophils are their large, cytoplasmic 'specific' granules that are morphologically distinct because of their unique content of crystalloid cores. Crystalloid cores are recognizable by transmission electron microscopy and usually appear electron dense (Fig. 23.2). The cores and surrounding matrices of specific granules contain cationic proteins that account for the tinctorial staining of granules with eosin. Eosinophils at sites of inflammation can exhibit morphologic changes in their specific granules, including loss of either matrix or core components from within intact granules, compatible with the extracellular release of granule constituents.

Lipid bodies, cytoplasmic structures distinct from granules (Fig. 23.2), are roughly globular in shape and range in size from minute to the size of specific granules. Lipid bodies are dissolved by common alcohol-based hematologic stains, but with osmium fixation are preserved and stain darkly. Lipid bodies lack a delimiting membrane, but contain internal membranes that are often obscured by overlying lipid. Lipid bodies are

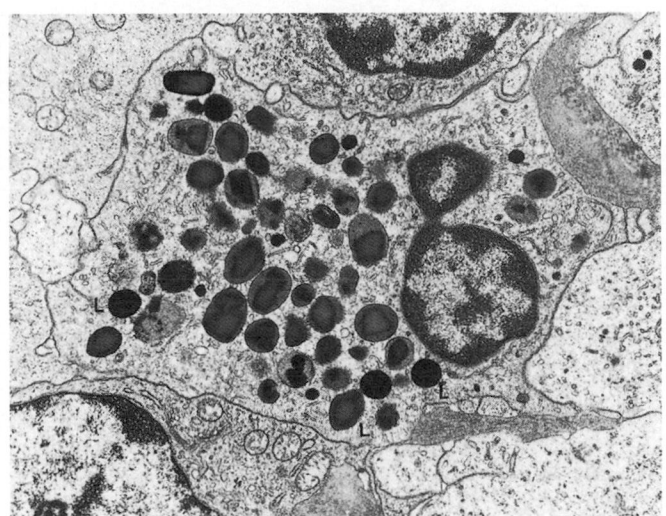

Fig. 23.2 Transmission electron micrograph of a human eosinophil. The numerous cytoplasmic specific granules (arrow heads) contain the electron-dense crystalline cores that are unique to eosinophils. In addition, lipid bodies (arrows) are visible as globular, uniformly dark structures. (Original magnification × 11,180.) (Courtesy of Dr Ann M. Dvorak, Israel Deaconess Medical Center, Harvard Medical School, Boston.)

found in neutrophils and other cells, especially in association with inflammation; but eosinophils typically contain more lipid bodies than neutrophils. Lipid body formation in eosinophils is rapidly inducible within minutes. In eosinophils, key enzymes involved in eicosanoid formation, including prostaglandin H synthase, the 5- and 15-lipoxygenases and leukotriene (LT) C_4 synthase, localize at lipid bodies; and lipid bodies are sites of eicosanoid synthesis.[6]

CELL SURFACE RECEPTORS AND PROTEINS

Eosinophil receptors for immunoglobulins include those for IgG, IgE, and IgA. The receptor for IgG on eosinophils is principally the low-affinity FcγRII (CD32), whereas neutrophils have FcγRII and FcγRIII (CD16). Exposure of eosinophils to interferon (IFN)-γ elicits expression of a phosphatidylinositol-linked form of CD16 on eosinophils, and CD16 may be expressed on eosinophils from some patients with eosinophilic disorders.

Eosinophil IgE receptors include the high-affinity IgE receptor FcεRI, typically found on basophils and mast cells, as well as FcεRII, the low-affinity IgE receptor, like CD23 found on lymphocytes, monocytes, and antigen-presenting cells. Although FcεRI α chain protein is present within eosinophils, its surface expression can be low or undetectable. Engagement of eosinophil FcεRI does not elicit exocytotic degranulation, as it does on basophils and mast cells. FcεRI may participate in IgE-mediated antigen uptake by antigen-presenting eosinophils, but the functional roles of eosinophil FcεRI remain to be delineated. Eosinophil expression of IgE receptors is notable because IgE levels and eosinophil

numbers frequently increase concomitantly in helminth parasitic infections as well as allergic diseases.

Eosinophils express FcαRI (CD89), which binds secretory IgA more potently than do other forms of IgA. Engagement of FcαRI triggers eosinophil release of granule proteins. With the characteristic localization of eosinophils to mucosal surfaces of the respiratory, gastrointestinal, and genitourinary tracts, this IgA receptor enables eosinophils to engage secretory IgA present at these mucosal sites.

Eosinophils have receptors for complement components including C1q (CR1), C3b/C4b (CR1), iC3b (CR3), C3a and C5a. Both C3a and C5a are eosinophil chemoattractants and stimulate the production of oxygen radicals by eosinophils. Eosinophils express several receptors for chemokines. CCR1 is a receptor for MIP-1α, MCP-3 and RANTES, whereas CCR3 is a receptor for eotaxin, eotaxin-2, eotaxin-3, MCP-3 and RANTES. Eosinophils express CXCR4 and respond to the ligand for this receptor, stromal cell-derived factor-1α.

Mature eosinophils, like their immature precursors, express receptors for the three cytokines, GM-CSF, IL-3, and IL-5, that promote eosinophilopoiesis and stimulate the functioning of mature eosinophils. In addition, eosinophils have receptors for a broad range of other cytokines, including IL-1α, IL-2, IL-4, IFN-α and IFN-γ, TNF-α, stem cell factor (c-*kit*) and IL-16 (which signals via CD4 on eosinophils). Thus, eosinophils are subject to stimulation by many cytokines, although little is understood about how many of them affect eosinophil functioning *in vivo*.

Of pertinence to interactions between eosinophils and B and T lymphocytes, eosinophils may express several relevant plasma membrane proteins. Class II MHC proteins, generally absent on blood eosinophils, are induced for expression on eosinophils in sites of inflammation. In addition, eosinophils can express CD40, CD154 (CD40 ligand), CD153 (CD30 ligand), CD28 (B7-2) and CD86.[7]

Eosinophils express receptors for several lipid mediators, including platelet-activating factor (PAF) and leukotriene B_4 (LTB_4), which are chemoattractants for eosinophils and stimulate eosinophil degranulation and respiratory burst activity. Eosinophils also have receptors for prostaglandin E_2 and for cysteinyl leukotrienes.

CONSTITUENTS OF EOSINOPHILS

Eosinophil specific granules contain pre-formed proteins that include both specific cationic proteins and stores of diverse cytokines and chemokines.

CATIONIC GRANULE PROTEINS

Eosinophil granule cationic proteins have been extensively studied because of their abundance in the granules and their capacity to exert multiple effects on host cells and microbial targets.[8] Major basic protein (MBP), named for its quantitative predominance within the granule and its markedly cationic (basic) isoelectric point of about 11, is a 13.8–14 kDa protein. A homolog of MBP that is somewhat smaller (13.4 kDa) and less basic (pI 8.7) has been identified. MBP lacks enzymatic activity and probably exerts its varied effects via its markedly cationic nature.

A second granule protein is eosinophil peroxidase (EPO), an enzyme distinct from neutrophil myeloperoxidase. Cationic EPO (pI 10.8) uses hydrogen peroxide and halide ions to form hypohalous acids, which are toxic for parasites, bacteria, and tumor and host cells. EPO utilizes bromide in preference to chloride and is even more active with a pseudohalide, thiocyanate, to generate oxidant products, including hypobromous and hypothiocyanous acids.

Two additional granule proteins are eosinophil cationic protein (ECP) (18 kDa, pI 10.8) and eosinophil-derived neurotoxin (EDN) (18–19 kDa, pI 8.9). EDN, never demonstrated to be neurotoxic for humans, is so named because, after it is injected intracerebrally into test rabbits, it elicits a characteristic neuropathologic response. Both ECP and EDN are ribonucleases (RNases). EDN expresses 100 times more RNase activity than does ECP, although their toxic effects on bacterial, parasitic and mammalian target cells are apparently unlikely to be due to their RNase catalytic activities.

Within the specific granule, MBP is localized to the crystalloid core, whereas ECP, EDN and EPO are localized in the matrix of the granule around the core (see Fig. 23.1). MBP is also found in low amounts (~3% of eosinophil levels) in basophils, but whether this reflects endocytosis tor endogenous synthesis is not known. Uptake of MBP and EPO into mast cells is known to occur via endocytosis. Small amounts of EDN and ECP are present in neutrophils, and as neutrophils contain mRNA transcripts for these, EDN and ECP are likely synthesized by neutrophils. Nevertheless, eosinophils are the dominant source of these four cationic proteins. The properties of these proteins and their numerous biologic effects have been reviewed,[8] as these proteins have major effects not only in the potential role of eosinophils in host defense against helminthic parasites, but also in contributing to tissue dysfunction and damage in eosinophil-related allergic and other diseases.

CYTOKINES AND CHEMOKINES

Eosinophils are capable of elaborating at least 31 diverse cytokines and chemokines, and studies continue to identify more cytokines released by eosinophils. The potential activities of eosinophil-derived cytokines are extensive. Eosinophil-derived cytokines include those with autocrine growth factor activities for eosinophils and those with a potential role in acute and chronic inflammatory responses. A notable feature of eosinophils as a source of cytokines is that they contain stores of these cytokines pre-formed within eosinophil granules and secretory vesicles.[9] Thus, in contrast to most lymphocytes, which must be induced to synthesize de novo cytokines destined for release, eosinophils can immediately release pre-formed cytokine and chemokine proteins into the surrounding milieu. Although levels of pre-formed cytokines in eosinophils may be lower than those of specifically stimulated lymphocytes, local and rapid release of eosinophil-derived cytokines in tissues could readily induce a response in various adjoining cell types.

Eosinophils synthesize the three growth factor cytokines GM-CSF, IL-3 and IL-5, which promote eosinophil survival, antagonize eosinophil apoptosis, and enhance eosinophil effector responses. Other cytokines elaborated by human eosinophils that may have activities in acute and chronic inflammatory responses include IL-1α, IL-6, IL-8, IFN-γ, TNF-α and MIP-1α. Human eosinophils can elaborate other various 'growth' factors, including transforming growth factor (TGF)-α, TGF-β1, vascular endothelial growth factor, platelet-derived growth factor (PDGF)-β, and heparin-binding epidermal growth factor. These cytokines may have a role in contributing to epithelial hyperplasia and fibrosis, as well as other activities. In addition, eosinophils are recognized as sources of specific cytokines and chemokines capable of stimulating or

inhibiting lymphocyte responses, including IL-2, IL-4, IL-10, IL-12, IL-16, RANTES and TGF-β_1. Of note, eosinophil cytokines include those associated with Th2 (IL-4, IL-5, IL-13), Th1 (IL-12, IFN-γ) and T-regulatory (IL-10, TGF-β) responses, emphasizing the diverse immunoregulatory potentials for eosinophil-secreted cytokines.

ACTIVATED EOSINOPHILS

A well recognized attribute of eosinophils is that, in conjunction with eosinophilic diseases, some blood and tissue eosinophils may exhibit various alterations indicative that these cells have been 'activated.' These changes include increased metabolic activity, diminished density ('hypodense'), enhanced LTC$_4$ formation, and morphologic alterations, including cytoplasmic vacuolization, alterations in granule numbers and size, and losses within specific granules of MBP-containing cores or matrices. Activated eosinophils may exhibit enhanced plasma membrane expression of some proteins, including CD69, HLA-DR and CD25.

Features associated with in vivo 'activated' eosinophils can be elicited in part by exposing eosinophils to specific stimuli, including GM-CSF, IL-3 and IL-5. In addition, interactions with extracellular matrix components can further contribute to eosinophil activation. Eosinophil 'activation,' however, is not a singularly binary process, and some attributes of activation can be elicited without other attributes by mediators and mechanisms that remain to be delineated.

MECHANISMS OF EOSINOPHIL DEGRANULATION

As eosinophil granules contain four major cationic proteins and a multitude of pre-formed cytokines and chemokines, the processes by which eosinophils mobilize these granule constituents for their extracellular release are important in understanding the regulated functioning of eosinophils. Unlike mast cells or basophils that undergo acute exocytotic degranulation in response to cross-linking of their high-affinity Fcε receptors, an analogous mechanism to elicit comparable exocytotic degranulation of fluid-phase eosinophils has not been identified. Cross-linking of eosinophil IgG or IgA Fc receptors can stimulate release of eosinophil cationic proteins, but this rapid FcR-mediated acute 'degranulation' process is cytolytic for eosinophils. In contrast, observations of eosinophils on the surfaces of large non-phagocytosable multicellular helminth parasites do provide evidence that eosinophils can degranulate by exocytosis to release granule contents on the surfaces of target parasites.

An alternative means of mobilizing granule contents for secretion that eosinophils utilize is a process of vesicular transport-mediated 'piecemeal' degranulation. Electron microscopic observations of lesional eosinophils provided evidence that eosinophil granule contents were mobilized in vivo by selective incorporation into small vesicles that traffic to the cell surface and release these granule contents. By this process, there may be agonist-elicited selective secretion of certain eosinophil-derived cytokines.[9, 10] Ultrastructural studies have demonstrated that secretory vesicles arise from granules and transport cytokines, such as IL-4.[11, 12] Insights into the selectivity and mechanisms of differential cytokine secretion have been indicated by finding, at least for IL-4, that a receptor for IL-4 mediates the transport of

IL-4 from granules and within secretory vesicles.[13] How this process of vesicular transport is regulated and functions to selectively mobilize specific eosinophil granule-derived cytokines or cationic proteins remains under investigation.

In addition to regulated release of granule contents from viable eosinophils, a common, but often overlooked and enigmatic, occurrence is the apparent lysis of eosinophils. Both cutaneous and pulmonary biopsies of eosinophil-associated diseases contain free, extracellular, but still membrane-bound eosinophil granules. The mechanism of cytolysis in such reactions is undefined, but may represent eosinophil apoptosis and occur more commonly than heretofore recognized. Whether this process releases granule-bound proteins is uncertain.

FUNCTIONS OF EOSINOPHILS

Conventional considerations of the roles that eosinophils may play have been guided by quantitative considerations, so that those diseases characteristically marked by more prominent eosinophilia have occasioned the most interest. Thus, studies have focused on the 'effector' roles eosinophils play in host defense against helminth infections and in the immunopathogenesis of allergic and other eosinophilic diseases. Additional roles for eosinophils must be considered in immune or inflammatory responses not conventionally recognized to contain abundant eosinophils.

ROLES IN HOST DEFENSE

Because the host response to infections with multicellular helminth parasites is characteristically associated with eosinophilia, it is often believed that eosinophils evolved to have a role in killing helminths, especially during their larval stages. Indeed, *in vitro* eosinophils can kill numerous helminths, organisms too large to be phagocytosed. Eosinophils adhere to the parasite and deposit eosinophil granule contents onto its surface. Cell products that can contribute to parasite death include MBP, ECP, EDN, and EPO.

As reviewed,[14] the helminthotoxic roles of eosinophils *in vivo* are less certain in humans and experimental rodents. In eosinophil-depleted mice (given neutralizing antibody to IL-5, or with the IL-5 gene deleted), the intensities of primary and secondary infections with some helminths have not been greater than in eosinophilic mice, nor have IL-5 transgenic mice exhibited increased resistance to infection with some helminth species. Moreover, schistosome infections in two lines of eosinophil-ablated mice have shown no differences in measures of infection compared to normal mice.[15] Nevertheless, murine studies need to be interpreted with caution. Some helminth infections elicit Th1-biased responses in mice, which differ from Th2-biased responses in humans or rats. Many experimental infections involve introducing helminth infections that are often host species-restricted into unnatural host mice, in which innate immune responses may be prominent. Natural human infections are usually a consequence of repeated exposures, during which acquired, rather than innate, immunity becomes prominent. Thus, eosinophil functions as helminthotoxic cells *in vivo* remain unclear. Eosinophils might have an alternative function in the host response to helminths, including functioning as antigen-presenting cells.[15, 16]

ROLES IN DISEASE PATHOGENESIS

The ability of eosinophils to release biologically active lipids as paracrine mediators of inflammation and to release pre-formed cationic and cytokine granule constituents enables them to contribute to the immunopathogenesis of various diseases, including asthma.[3, 17] Eosinophils form several classes of biologically active lipid. Eosinophils, like other cells, may liberate PAF. The potent, diverse activities of PAF can be mediated either directly or by stimulating other cells to release leukotrienes, prostaglandins, and complement peptides. Stimulated eosinophils also release LTC_4. LTD_4 and LTE_4 are formed from LTC_4 by the sequential enzymatic removal of glutamic acid and glycine from its tripeptide glutathione side chain. LTC_4, and especially LTD_4, has bronchoconstrictor activity, constricts terminal arterioles, dilates venules, and stimulates airway mucus secretion. Thus, eosinophils are a potential source of two major types of mediator lipids, the sulfidopeptide leukotrienes and PAF.

Oxidants released by eosinophils, including superoxide anion, hydroxyl radical, and singlet oxygen, and EPO-catalyzed hypothiocyanous acid and other hypohalous acids, have the potential to damage host tissues.

Released eosinophil granule proteins are immunochemically detectable in fluids, including blood, sputum and synovial fluids, and in tissues, including the respiratory and gastrointestinal tracts, skin, and heart, in association with various eosinophil-related diseases. The eosinophil cationic proteins, including MBP, ECP, and EPO, can damage various cell types. Thus, extracellular release of eosinophil granule proteins, by degranulation or cytolysis of eosinophils, could contribute to local tissue damage by causing dysfunction and damage to adjacent cells.

OTHER EOSINOPHIL FUNCTIONS

Other potential functions for the eosinophil are not fully defined. In addition to the acute release of lipid, peptide and cytokine mediators of inflammation, eosinophils probably contribute to chronic inflammation, including the development of fibrosis. Eosinophils are a major source of the fibrosis-promoting cytokine TGF-β in nodular sclerosing Hodgkin's disease and idiopathic pulmonary fibrosis. Additional roles of eosinophils in modulating extracellular matrix deposition and remodeling are suggested by studies of normal wound healing. During dermal wound healing eosinophils infiltrate into the wound sites and sequentially express TGF-α early and TGF-$β_1$ later during wound healing. Of note, whereas experimental administration of neutralizing anti-IL-5 monoclonal antibodies to subjects with asthma had no apparent benefit on some clinical measures of asthma,[17] anti-IL-5 monoclonal antibody has been shown to decrease TGF-β and some extracellular matrix components in the airways of asthmatics.[18] These findings suggest that eosinophils may contribute to the more chronic subepithelial airway fibrosis characteristic of chronic asthma.

Additional functions for eosinophils are suggested by the findings that they may be induced to express class II MHC proteins and can function as antigen-presenting cells. Blood eosinophils lack HLA-DR expression, but eosinophils recovered from the airways 48 hours after segmental antigen challenge have been shown to express HLA-DR. Cytokines, including GM-CSF, IL-3, IL-4 and IFN-γ, induce eosinophil HLA-DR expression. Both murine and human eosinophils can function as HLA-DR-dependent MHC-restricted antigen-presenting cells in stimulating proliferation of T cells. *In vivo*, murine eosinophils can process exogenous antigens in the airways, traffic to regional lymph nodes, and function as antigen-specific antigen-presenting cells to stimulate responses of CD4 T cells.[19]

Because eosinophils normally become resident in submucosal tissues, they undoubtedly participate in ongoing homeostatic immune responses at these sites. Eosinophils are even found in the thymus. Further investigations will help delineate their functional roles and interactions with other cells, including lymphocytes, so that the scope of eosinophil function will probably extend beyond its currently more defined role as an effector cell contributing to allergic inflammation.

■ EOSINOPHILIA AND EOSINOPHILIC DISORDERS ■

Diverse infectious, allergic, neoplastic and idiopathic disease processes can be associated with increased blood and/or tissue eosinophil numbers. Blood eosinophilia, present when eosinophil numbers are in excess of their usual level of less than 450/μL of blood, may be intermittently, modestly or less frequently markedly increased. Blood eosinophil numbers are not necessarily indicative of the extent of eosinophil involvement in affected tissues.

Some patients with sustained blood eosinophilia can develop organ damage, especially cardiac. This cardiac involvement can include the formation of intraventricular thrombi and endomyocardial fibrosis with secondary mitral or tricuspid regurgitation (Fig. 23.3). Such damage can complicate the sustained eosinophilia of hypereosinophilic syndromes and has been noted with eosinophilias accompanying other diseases, including eosinophilia with carcinomas or Hodgkin's or non-Hodgkin's lymphomas, and eosinophilia from GM-CSF or IL-2 administration, drug-reactions, and parasitic infections. Most patients with eosinophilia, however, develop no evidence of endomyocardial damage. Conversely, cardiac disease can rarely present in patients without known eosinophilia. The pathogenesis of eosinophil-mediated cardiac damage involves both usually heightened numbers of eosinophils and some activating events, as yet ill-defined, that promote eosinophil-mediated tissue damage.

Cardiac damage progresses through three stages. In the first, there is damage to the endocardium and infiltration of the myocardium with eosinophils and lymphocytes, with eosinophil degranulation and myocardial necrosis. A similar acute eosinophilic myocarditis can develop with drug hypersensitivity reactions and may be more fulminant. The first stage is frequently clinically occult, although splinter hemorrhages may be prominent. Elevations of serum troponins as a measure of myocardial injury should be evaluated. Echocardiography usually detects no abnormalities at this stage. Uncommonly, death due to acute progressive cardiac disease can occur. Corticosteroid therapy during the acute stage may help control and prevent the evolution of myocardial fibrosis.

The second stage of heart disease, the formation of thrombi along the damaged endocardium, affects either or both ventricles and occasionally the atrium. Outflow tracts near the aortic and pulmonic valves are usually spared. These thrombi can embolize to the brain and elsewhere. Finally, in the fibrotic stage, progressive scarring leads to entrapment of chordae tendineae with the development of mitral and/or tricuspid valve regurgitation and to endomyocardial fibrosis, producing a restrictive

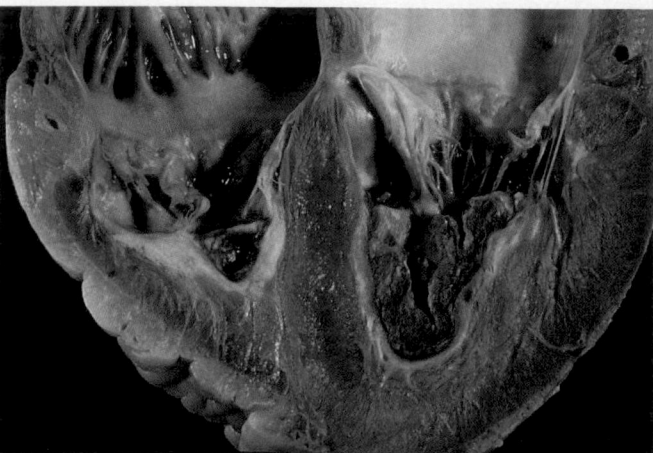

Fig. 23.3 Eosinophil endomyocardial disease. A large thrombus is present in the apex of the left ventricle and the chordae tendineae are entrapped, leading to severe mitral valve regurgitation.

cardiomyopathy. Echocardiography and magnetic resonance imaging (MRI) are valuable in detecting intracardiac thrombi and the manifestations of fibrosis. Patients with sustained eosinophilia should be monitored by echocardiography and serum troponin assays for evidence of cardiac disease. In an older series of patients referred to the NIH, much of the mortality in these patients with hypereosinophilia was attributable to end-stage congestive heart failure. In contemporary times, mitral valve replacement with bioprostheses[20] and additional therapeutic options for hypereosinophilic syndromes (see below) have largely minimized the morbidity and mortality attributable to end-stage eosinophilic endomyocardial disease.

■ INFECTIOUS DISEASES ASSOCIATED WITH EOSINOPHILIA ■

Eosinophilia is encountered only with specific infectious diseases. With active bacterial or viral infections, eosinopenia is characteristic. This suppression of blood eosinophils is due in part to heightened endogenous corticosteroid production as well as to inflammatory mediators released during these infections. This suppression of eosinophilia, with either serious bacterial infections or marked inflammation, accounts for the absence of otherwise expected eosinophilia in some patients with helminth infections, including those with hyperinfection strongyloidiasis.[21] As a general clinical guideline, patients with a febrile illness and an increased or even normal blood eosinophilia are not likely to have common bacterial or viral infections, unless they have adrenal insufficiency or a confounding medication-elicited eosinophilia.

HELMINTH PARASITES

Helminth parasites are multicellular metazoan organisms – the 'worm' parasites. Infections with diverse helminths elicit eosinophilia.[21] Although eosinophilia may provide a hematologic clue to the presence

Table 23.1 Parasitic diseases capable of causing marked (>3000/μL) or long-standing eosinophilia (Adapted from Wilson ME, Weller PF. Eosinophilia. In: Guerrant RL, Walker DH, Weller PF, eds. Tropical infectious diseases: principles, pathogens and practice, 2nd edn. Philadelphia: Churchill Livingstone, 2006; 1482)

Helminth infection	Hypereosinophilia	Chronic eosinophilia
Angiostrongyliasis costaricensis	+	
Ascariasis	+ during early lung migration	
Hookworm infection	+ during early lung migration	+ common cause of low-grade eosinophilia
Strongyloidiasis	+	+ self-perpetuating, may last >50 years
Trichinosis	+ with heavy infections	
Visceral larva migrans	+ principally in children	
Gnathostomiasis	+	+
Cysticercosis		+
Echinococcosis		+ may be episodic with cyst fluid leakage
Filariases:		
Tropical pulmonary eosinophilia	+	+
Loiasis	+ especially in expatriates	+
Onchocerciasis	+	+
Flukes:		
Schistosomiasis	+ during early infection in nonimmunes	+
Fascioliasis	+ during early infection	+
Clonorchiasis	+ during early infection	+
Paragonimiasis	+ during early infection	+
Fasciolopsiasis	+ during early infection	+

of helminth infection, the absence of blood eosinophilia does not exclude such infections. The eosinophilic response to helminths is determined both by the host's immune response and by the parasite, including its distribution, migration and development within the infected host. The level of eosinophilia tends to parallel the magnitude and extent of tissue invasion by helminth larvae or adults. For several helminth infections the migration of infecting larvae or subsequent developmental stages through tissues is greatest early in infection, and hence the magnitude of the elicited eosinophilia will be the greatest in these early phases. For established infections, local eosinophil infiltration will often be present around helminths within tissues, without a significant blood eosinophilia. Eosinophilia may be absent in those helminth infections that are well contained within tissues (e.g., intact echinococcal cysts) or are solely intraluminal within the intestinal tract (e.g., *Ascaris*, tapeworms). For some established infections, increases in blood eosinophilia may be episodic. Intermittent leakage of cyst fluids from echinococcal cysts can transiently stimulate increases in blood eosinophilia and also cause symptoms attributable to allergic or anaphylactic reactions (urticaria, bronchospasm). For tissue-dwelling helminths, increases in eosinophilia may occur principally in association with migration of adult parasites, as in loiasis and gnathostomiasis.

Helminth infections more likely to elicit prolonged hypereosinophilia in adults include filarial and hookworm infections and strongyloidiasis (Table 23.1).[21] Trichinellosis can elicit an acute hypereosinophilia. *Strongyloides stercoralis*, difficult to diagnose solely by stool examinations, is especially important to exclude, not only because it elicits modest to even marked eosinophilia, but also because, unlike other helminths, it

can develop into a disseminated, often fatal, disease (hyperinfection syndrome) in patients given immunosuppressive corticosteroids.[21] An ELISA serology has proved valuable in detecting strongyloidiasis and should be considered for eosinophilic patients likely to receive corticosteroids. Some tissue- or blood-dwelling helminths that are not diagnosable by stool examinations but which can cause marked eosinophilia require diagnostic examination of blood or biopsied tissues or specific serologic tests.[21] Infections with these include filarial infections, trichinellosis and visceral larva migrans. In children, owing to their propensity for geophagous pica and ingestion of dirt contaminated by dog ascarid eggs, visceral larva migrans due to *Toxocara canis* is a potential etiology for sustained eosinophilia. ELISA serologic testing can evaluate this possibility.

OTHER INFECTIONS: PROTOZOA AND FUNGI

Infections with single-celled protozoan parasites do not characteristically elicit eosinophilia. This is true of all intestinal, blood- and tissue-infecting protozoa, with two exceptions. Two intestinal protozoans, *Dientamoeba fragilis* and *Isospora belli*, can at times be associated with low-grade eosinophilia. Hence, in patients with symptoms of enteric infection and eosinophilia, diagnostic trophozoites of *D. fragilis* or oocysts of *I. belli* should be sought in stool examinations. Fecal examinations for *I. belli* oocysts must be specifically requested, as they are not usually detected in routine stool ova and parasite examinations. Other enteric protozoa do not elicit eosinophilia and, if detected in stool examinations, should not be accepted as causes of eosinophilia.

Two fungal diseases may be associated with eosinophilia. Aspergillosis is accompanied by eosinophilia only in the form of allergic bronchopulmonary aspergillosis, not when it is an invasive pathogen. Coccidioidomycosis, following primary infection, especially in conjunction with erythema nodosum, and at times with progressive disseminated disease, may elicit blood eosinophilia and may cause an eosinophilic meningitis.[21]

HIV AND RETROVIRAL INFECTIONS

Eosinophilia may uncommonly accompany HIV infections for several reasons. First, leukopenia may increase eosinophil percentages without reflecting true eosinophilia. Second, adverse reactions to medications may elicit eosinophilia. Third, patients with AIDS who develop adrenal insufficiency due to cytomegalovirus and other infections may exhibit eosinophilia as a consequence. In addition, usually modest, and uncommonly marked eosinophilia, is observed in some HIV-infected patients.[21] Eosinophilia also develops with HTLV-1 infections.[21]

■ ALLERGIC DISEASES ASSOCIATED WITH EOSINOPHILIA ■

Among the noninfectious diseases associated with eosinophilia (Table 23.2) are allergic diseases, notably those mediated by IgE-dependent mechanisms. In these diseases, including allergic rhinitis, conjunctivitis and asthma, eosinophils are present in involved tissues as well as often being increased in the blood.

■ MYELOPROLIFERATIVE AND NEOPLASTIC DISEASE ■

Eosinophilia may occur with specific neoplastic diseases, as well as in some disorders of uncertain etiology, including some hypereosinophilic syndromes.

HYPEREOSINOPHILIC SYNDROMES

A syndrome previously termed the idiopathic hypereosinophilic syndrome (HES) is not a single entity but rather a constellation of leukoproliferative disorders characterized by sustained overproduction of eosinophils. The three original diagnostic criteria for this syndrome are: eosinophilia in excess of 1500/μL of blood persisting for longer than 6 months; lack of an identifiable parasitic, allergic or other etiology for

---

KEY CONCEPTS
HYPEREOSINOPHILIC SYNDROMES
>> Eosinophilia sustained in excess of 1500/μL.
>> Absence of allergic, parasitic, or other etiologies for eosinophilia and distinction from other eosinophilic, organ-limited diseases.
>> Evidence of organ involvement.

---

eosinophilia and an absence of other eosinophilic syndromes clinically distinct from the hypereosinophilic syndrome; and signs and symptoms of organ involvement. In contemporary practice, one can no longer wait for 6 months before diagnostic and therapeutic interventions are needed for a hypereosinophilic patient with organ involvement. Moreover, in recent years there has been increasing recognition that hypereosinophilic syndromes (HESs) encompass a spectrum of disorders, and notable progress has been made in identifying the underlying defects in some of these (Fig. 23.4).[22–25]

It has been known that some patients with HESs exhibit features common to myeloproliferative disorders, including elevated vitamin B_{12} levels, splenomegaly, cytogenetic abnormalities, myelofibrosis, anemia, and myeloid dysplasia. In some of these with myeloproliferative HESs, the molecular defect has been identified as a chromosome 4 deletion that yields a fusion gene encoding a FIP1LI/PDGFRA (platelet-derived growth factor-α receptor) (F/P) protein that constitutively expresses receptor kinase activity.[26] This fusion gene can be diagnostically evaluated by RT-PCR or FISH (fluorescence *in situ* hybridization) (Chapter 101). Importantly, many of these patients respond to therapy with imatinib.[26, 27] Other eosinophilic patients without F/P mutations have also responded to imatinib, suggesting that other receptor tyrosine kinase mutations may underlie some of these myeloproliferative forms of HES. In addition, clonal abnormalities in the eosinophil lineage have been reported in few patients, and others may exhibit myeloproliferative features without detected F/P mutations (Fig. 23.4).

Another variant form of HES is a lymphoproliferative form due to clonal expansions of lymphocytes, often CD4+CD3- Th2-like, that elaborate IL-5.[23] These aberrant T cells can be sought by flow cytometry or T-cell receptor analysis. These patients, who may have elevated IgE levels, usually do not develop eosinophilic cardiac disease, but are at risk for developing T-cell lymphomas.[23]

In addition to these recognized variants, there are yet a substantial number of HES patients for whom the etiology of the eosinophilia remains unknown. Some such patients develop no signs or symptoms of disease and can be followed without therapy. For those who require therapy, including those with lymphoproliferative variants, glucocorticosteroids are the mainstay of treatment.[22] Second-line agents include hydroxyurea and IFN-α,[22, 28] although IFN-α is not advised for monotherapy of lymphoproliferative variants.[23] A neutralizing anti-IL-5 monoclonal antibody (mepolizumab) is being studied as a potential therapy of F/P-negative HES patients.

EOSINOPHILIA WITH TUMORS OR LEUKEMIAS

The F/P-positive myeloproliferative variant of HES can be considered a form of chronic eosinophilic leukemia.[26] Eosinophilia is a characteristic of the M4Eo subtype of acute myeloid leukemia, having the common M4 characteristic of chromosomal 16 abnormalities. Other forms of eosinophilic leukemia, often with specific cytogenetic and molecular genetic abnormalities, have been recognized.[29] Eosinophilia may accompany chronic myelogenous leukemia (often with basophilia), but is uncommon with acute lymphoblastic leukemia. Eosinophilia may accompany some lymphomas, including Hodgkin's disease, especially the nodular sclerosing form, T-cell lymphoblastic lymphoma, and adult T-cell leukemia/lymphoma. A small proportion of patients with carcinomas, especially of mucin-producing epithelial cell origin, have associated blood and tissue eosinophilia. Eosinophilia may accompany

Table 23.2 Eosinophil-associated diseases and disorders (Adapted from Weller PF. Eosinophilia and eosinophil-related disorders. In: Adkinson NF Jr, Yunginger JW, Busse WW, et al., eds. Allergy: principles and practice, 6th edn. Philadelphia: Mosby, 2003; 1105)

Allergic or atopic diseases
Myeloproliferative and neoplastic disorders
   Hypereosinophilic syndromes: myeloproliferative, lymphoproliferative and others
   Leukemia
   Lymphoma- and tumor-associated
   Mastocytosis

Pulmonary syndromes
   Parasite-induced eosinophilic lung diseases:
      Loeffler syndrome: patchy migratory infiltrates, resolving over weeks, seen with transpulmonary migration of helminth parasites, especially *Ascaris*
      Tropical pulmonary eosinophilia: miliary lesions and fibrosis; heightened immune response causing one form of lymphatic filariasis; increased IgE and antifilarial antibodies
      Pulmonary parenchymal invasion: paragonimiasis
      Heavy hematogenous seeding with helminths: trichinellosis, schistosomiasis, larva migrans
   Allergic bronchopulmonary aspergillosis
   Chronic eosinophilic pneumonia: dense peripheral infiltrates, fever; progressive, blood eosinophilia may be absent; steroid responsive
   Acute eosinophilic pneumonia: acute presentation diagnosed by bronchoalveolar lavage or biopsy
   Churg–Strauss vasculitis: small and medium sized arteries; granulomas, necrosis; asthma often antecedent; extrapulmonary (e.g., neurologic, cutaneous, cardiac, or gastrointestinal) involvement likely
   Drug- and toxin-induced eosinophilic lung diseases
   Other: hypereosinophilic syndromes, neoplasia, bronchocentric granulomatosis

Skin and subcutaneous diseases
   Skin diseases: atopic dermatitis, blistering diseases, including bullous pemphigoid, urticarias, drug reactions
   Diseases of pregnancy: pruritic urticarial papules and plaques syndrome, herpes gestationis
   Eosinophilic pustular folliculitis
   Eosinophilic cellulitis (Wells syndrome)
   Kimura's disease and angiolymphoid hyperplasia with eosinophilia
   Shulman syndrome (eosinophilic fasciitis)
   Episodic angioedema with eosinophilia: recurrent periodic episodes with fever, angioedema, and secondary weight gain; may be long-standing without untoward cardiac dysfunction

Gastrointestinal disorders
   Eosinophilic gastroenteritides
   Inflammatory bowel disease: eosinophils in lesions; occasionally blood eosinophilia with ulcerative colitis

Rheumatologic diseases
   Vasculitis: Churg–Strauss and cutaneous necrotizing eosinophilic vasculitis

Immunologic reactions
   Medication-related eosinophilias
   Immunodeficiency diseases: Job syndrome and Omenn's syndrome
   Transplant rejections

Endocrine
   Hypoadrenalism: Addison's disease, adrenal hemorrhage, hypopituitarism

Other causes of eosinophilia
   Atheromatous cholesterol embolization
   Hereditary
   Serosal surface irritation, including peritoneal dialysis and pleural eosinophilia

MYELOPROLIFERATIVE AND NEOPLASTIC DISEASE

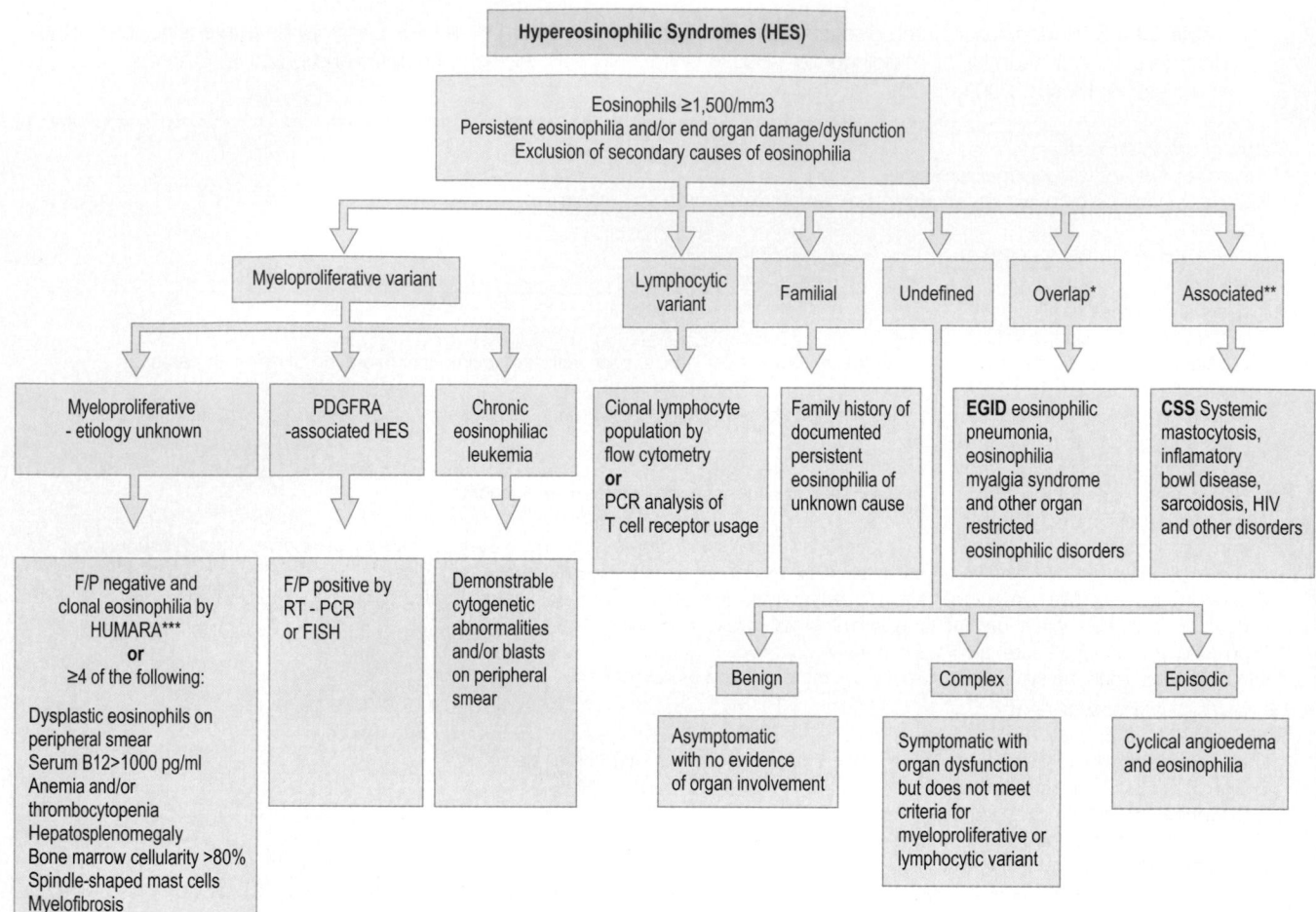

Fig. 23.4 Classification of hypereosinophilic syndromes based on a Workshop Summary report. Specific syndromes discussed at the workshop are indicated in bold. *Incomplete criteria, apparent restriction to specific tissues/organs. **Peripheral eosinophilia, 1500/mm³ in association with a defined diagnosis. †Presence of the *FLPL1/PDGFRA* mutation. *** Clonality analysis based on the digestion of genomic DNA with methylation-sensitive restriction enzymes followed by PCR amplification of the CAG repeat at the human androgen receptor gene (HUMARA) locus at the X chromosome. FISH, fluorescence *in situ* hybridization. (From Klion AD et al. Approaches to the treatment of hypereosinophilic syndromes: A workshop summary report. J Allergy Clin Immunol 2006; 117: 1294, with permission from the American Academy of Allergy, Asthma and Immunology.)

angioimmunoblastic lymphadenopathy, mycosis fungoides, Sézary syndrome and lymphomatoid papulosis. Eosinophilia occurs in about 20% of those with systemic mastocytosis and may be the presenting finding in the absence of cutaneous manifestations.

■ ORGAN SYSTEM INVOLVEMENT AND EOSINOPHILIA ■

Eosinophilic syndromes limited to specific organs, such as eosinophilic pneumonias[30] or eosinophilic gastroenteritides (Chapter 46), characteristically do not extend beyond their own target organ, and hence lack the multiplicity of organ involvement often found with nonorgan-specific hypereosinophilic syndromes. They also do not have the predilection to develop secondary eosinophil-mediated cardiac damage, for reasons that are not known.

PULMONARY EOSINOPHILIAS

Blood eosinophilia can infrequently accompany pleural fluid eosinophilia, which is a nonspecific response seen with various disorders, including trauma and repeated thoracenteses. In addition, several pulmonary parenchymal disorders may be associated with eosinophilia (Table 23.2).

Helminth parasites are responsible for four forms of eosinophilic lung disease.[21] The first of these is Loeffler's syndrome, which is marked by blood eosinophilia, eosinophilic patchy pulmonary infiltrates that appear and resolve over weeks and, at times, bronchospasm. This syndrome is typically caused by those helminth parasites (*Ascaris lumbricoides*, and less commonly hookworm and *Strongyloides*) that migrate through the lungs early in their developmental lifecycle.[21] Stool examinations are not helpful, as the pulmonary response is elicited by infecting larval forms months before productive egg-laying from later adult stages begins in the intestines. Diagnosis is made on epidemiologic grounds.[21]

The second form of helminth-induced lung disease is the syndrome of tropical pulmonary eosinophilia, which develops in a minority of patients infected with lymphatic-dwelling filarial species.[21] This syndrome is characterized by marked blood eosinophilia, a paroxysmal nonproductive cough, wheezing, and occasional weight loss, lymphadenopathy and low-grade fevers. On chest X-rays increased bronchovesicular markings, diffuse interstitial lesions 1–3 mm in diameter or mottled opacities, usually more prominent in lower lung fields, are common. Patients have markedly increased numbers of blood and alveolar eosinophils, and elevations in both total serum IgE and anti-filarial antibodies.

A third form of helminth-induced lung disease is caused by helminths that invade the pulmonary parenchyma, notably lung flukes that cause paragonimiasis. The fourth form of lung disease is caused by larger than usual numbers of helminth organisms that are carried hematogenously into the lungs. Examples include schistosomiasis, trichinellosis and larva migrans.

Bronchopulmonary aspergillosis constitutes another type of eosinophil-associated pulmonary disease. Two forms of idiopathic eosinophilic pneumonia are recognized. In chronic eosinophilic pneumonia patients may exhibit peripheral pulmonary infiltrates that may extend across lobar fissures.[30] Uncommonly, chronic eosinophilic pneumonia is antecedent to Churg–Strauss syndrome vasculitis.[30] Blood eosinophilia is present in most patients, but not all. This disease of unknown etiology is responsive to corticosteroids, but prone to relapse.[30] An acute form of eosinophilic pneumonia, manifest by fever, pulmonary infiltrates and respiratory insufficiency, is diagnosable by finding eosinophils in bronchoalveolar lavage fluids or on lung biopsy.[30] Acute eosinophilic pneumonia, which often follows new exposures to smoke or dusts, responds to corticosteroid treatment and does not relapse.[30, 31]

The major vasculitis associated with eosinophilia is the Churg–Strauss syndrome (Chapter 58). Late-onset asthma, eosinophilia, and at times transient pulmonary infiltrates, antedate the development of systemic vasculitis in about half of cases. Pulmonary involvement is seen in almost all patients, and pulmonary infiltrates occur in three-quarters. Nasal and sinus involvement is common. Corticosteroids or anti-cysteinyl leukotriene agent therapies for asthma may mask the evolution of Churg–Strauss syndrome. Neurologic, cutaneous, cardiac and gastrointestinal organ involvement is common (Chapter 58).[32] Cardiac involvement includes pericarditis and small vessel cardiac vasculitis, and much less commonly endomyocardial thrombosis and fibrosis.

Diverse medications and other drugs are capable of eliciting pulmonary eosinophilia.[33] More commonly implicated medications include nonsteroidal anti-inflammatory drugs (NSAIDs) and antimicrobial medications. Likewise, toxic agents, including from occupational exposure, can be responsible for pulmonary eosinophilia. Each of these reactions has a defined etiologic stimulus and hence differs from idiopathic and other eosinophilic diseases, but the clinical presentation of drug-and toxin-elicited pulmonary eosinophilias can resemble other forms of pulmonary eosinophilia, including acute or chronic eosinophilic pneumonia.

SKIN AND SUBCUTANEOUS DISEASES

A number of cutaneous diseases can be associated with heightened blood eosinophils, including atopic dermatitis, blistering disorders including bullous pemphigoid, drug reactions, and two diseases associated with

pregnancy, herpes gestationis and the syndrome of pruritic urticarial papules and plaques of pregnancy. Eosinophilic pustular folliculitis is seen mostly in patients with HIV infections and in those treated for hematologic malignancies or after bone marrow transplantation. For patients with cutaneous involvement and eosinophilia, angiolymphoid hyperplasia with eosinophilia and Kimura's disease, eosinophilic cellulitis (Wells syndrome), eosinophilic fasciitis, and eosinophilic pustular folliculitis can be differentiated based on the histopathology of biopsied lesions. Another syndrome, episodic angioedema with eosinophilia, is characterized by recurring episodes of angioedema, urticaria, fever, and marked blood eosinophilia. The clinical course of this disease, with its prominent periodic occurrences of angioedema and eosinophilia and its lack of association with cardiac damage, distinguishes it among hypereosinophilic syndromes. This syndrome of unknown etiology responds to glucocorticosteroid therapy.

GASTROINTESTINAL DISEASES

Eosinophilic gastroenteritis represents a heterogeneous collection of disorders in which there may be eosinophilic infiltration of the mucosa, the muscle layer or the serosa, the last of which can lead to eosinophilic ascites (Chapter 24).[34] Eosinophils are present in the lesions of collagenous colitis and ulcerative colitis, but blood eosinophilia is usually absent. Gastrointestinal eosinophilia elicited by intestinal helminths and eosinophilic enterocolitis due to hypersensitivity reactions to medications must be excluded in patients with these diseases who have tissue eosinophilia.

RHEUMATOLOGIC DISORDERS

Of the various forms of vasculitis, only two are commonly associated with eosinophilia. The principal eosinophil-related vasculitis is the Churg–Strauss syndrome (as discussed above; Chapter 58). Cutaneous necrotizing eosinophilic vasculitis with hypocomplementemia and eosinophilia is a distinct vasculitis of small dermal vessels that are extensively infiltrated with eosinophils. This form of vasculitis may occur in patients with connective tissue diseases. In addition, eosinophilia may uncommonly accompany rheumatoid arthritis itself, but is more commonly due to adverse reactions to treatment medications (including NSAIDs, gold and tetracyclines) or due to concomitant vasculitis. An uncommon disorder, characterized by the association of nodules, eosinophilia, rheumatism, dermatitis and swelling (NERDS), includes prominent para-articular nodules, recurrent urticaria with angioedema, and tissue and blood eosinophilia.

IMMUNOLOGIC DISORDERS

Adverse reactions to medications are a common cause of eosinophilia (Chapter 48). Although often considered as hypersensitivity reactions, in most instances of drug-associated eosinophilia the mechanism leading to eosinophilia is not understood. Eosinophilia may develop without other manifestations of adverse drug reactions, such as rashes or drug fevers. In addition, drug-induced eosinophilia may be associated with distinct clinicopathologic patterns in which eosinophilia accompanies drug-induced diseases that are characteristically limited to specific organs with or without associated blood eosinophilia. When organ dysfunction develops, cessation of drug administration is necessary. Drug-induced interstitial nephritis may be accompanied by blood eosinophilia, and eosinophils may be detectable in urine.[35] Unlike G-CSF therapy, therapy with GM-CSF

CLINICAL PEARLS

EOSINOPHILIA AND DRUG REACTIONS

Drug reactions	Examples
Interstitial nephritis	Semisynthetic penicillins, cephalosporins
Pulmonary infiltrates	Nitrofurantoin, sulfas, NSAIDs
Pleuropulmonary	Dantrolene
Hepatitis	Semisynthetic penicillins, tetracyclines
Hypersensitivity vasculitis	Allopurinol, phenytoin
Asthma, nasal polyps	Aspirin
Eosinophilia–myalgia	L-Tryptophan contaminant syndrome
Asymptomatic	Ampicillin, penicillins, cephalosporins
Cytokine-mediated	GM-CSF, IL-2
DRESS (drug reaction with eosinophilia and systemic symptoms)	Minocycline, allopurinol, anticonvulsants

Adapted from Weller PF. Eosinophilia and eosinophil-related disorders. In: Adkinson NF Jr, Yuninger JW, Busse WW, et al., eds. Allergy: principles and practice, 6th edn. Philadelphia: Mosby, 2003; 1105.

can lead to prominent blood and tissue eosinophilia. Administration of IL-2 or of IL-2-stimulated lymphocytes is also frequently followed by the development of eosinophilia, most likely due to stimulated production of IL-5. Reactions to medications, often anticonvulsants, minocycline and Allopurinol, can elicit DRESS, *drug reaction with eosinophilia and systemic symptoms*.[36] In addition to cutaneous eruptions, fever, lymphadenopathy, hepatitis, nephritis, eosinophilia are common but variable elements of this dug-induced syndrome, which can be fatal. The triggering medication must be stopped, and corticosteroids are often administered.

Some primary immunodeficiency syndromes are associated with eosinophilia. The hyper-IgE syndrome is characterized by recurrent staphylococcal abscesses of the skin, lungs and other sites, pruritic dermatitis, hyperimmunoglobulinemia E, and eosinophilia of the blood, sputum and tissues. Eosinophilia is characteristic of Omenn's syndrome, combined immunodeficiency with hypereosinophilia (Chapter 35).

Infiltration of eosinophils accompanies rejection of lung, kidney, and liver allografts. Tissue and blood eosinophilia occur early in the rejection process, and eosinophil counts and granule protein levels (in urine, bronchoalveolar lavage fluids and in involved allograft tissues) have correlated with prognosis, severity, and response to rejection therapy.

ENDOCRINE DISEASES

The loss of endogenous adrenoglucocorticosteroid production in Addison's disease, adrenal hemorrhage or hypopituitarism can cause increased blood eosinophilia.

OTHER CAUSES OF EOSINOPHILIA

The syndrome of atheromatous cholesterol embolization is at times associated with hypocomplementemia, eosinophilia and eosinophiluria. Uncommonly, kindreds with hereditary eosinophilia have been recognized. Irritation of serosal surfaces can be associated with eosinophilia, and related diseases can include Dressler's syndrome; eosinophilic pleural effusions; peritoneal, and at times blood, eosinophilia developing during chronic peritoneal dialysis; and perhaps the eosinophilia that follows abdominal irradiation.

■ EVALUATION OF EOSINOPHILIA ■

Because a diversity of disorders may be accompanied by eosinophilia, evaluation of the patient with eosinophilia requires a consideration of features based on the patient's history, physical examination, and other laboratory, radiographic or diagnostic testing.[37] An initial approach can focus on identifying eosinophilic diseases that have a defined treatable etiology. These include infections with helminth parasites, and for these the approach should be guided by information obtained from the history regarding potential exposures;[38] from the history and physical examinations regarding signs and symptoms of any clinically apparent associated illness; from standard biochemical and radiographic testing for evidence of organ involvement; and from specific parasitologic tests, including potentially stool, urine, blood, sputum or tissue examinations, as well as serologic tests.[21] The duration and magnitude of the eosinophilia may help suggest some entities, especially if it is prolonged or markedly elevated (see Table 23.1). Other causes of eosinophilia that are amenable to treatment include eosinophilia secondary to medications, for which cessation of the offending drug may be indicated if the eosinophilia is accompanied by organ damage. Likewise, if eosinophilia is secondary to glucocorticosteroid deficiency, diagnostic testing can corroborate this deficiency and lead to the administration of replacement corticosteroids and consequent resolution of the eosinophilia.

Because allergic diseases usually are associated with at least some degree of eosinophilia, clinical and laboratory evidence of such disease should be sought. If the eosinophilia is not attributable to allergic diseases, parasitic infections, medications or steroid deficiency, further evaluation will be guided by whether the patient has evidence of organ disease and which organs are involved (see Table 23.2). This is germane, for instance, in defining whether the patient has a distinct eosinophilic pulmonary, gastrointestinal or cutaneous syndrome. Bone marrow examinations in most patients with eosinophilia are not usually informative, revealing only evidence of enhanced eosinophilopoiesis; but marrow should be examined if there is concern for a hematologic malignancy or myeloproliferative

THERAPEUTIC PRINCIPLES

THERAPY OF SPECIFIC EOSINOPHILIC DISEASES

Eosinophil-associated diseases with identifiable etiologies

Parasitic infections	Treat causative parasite
Drug-reaction related eosinophilias	Terminate eliciting medication
Adrenal insufficiency	Corticosteroid replacement therapy
Allergic/atopic diseases	Varied, may include topical or inhaled corticosteroids

Distinct idiopathic eosinophilic syndromes involving specific organs

Eosinophilic pulmonary diseases	
Acute eosinophilic pneumonia	Corticosteroids
Chronic eosinophilic pneumonia	Corticosteroids, interferon-α
Churg–Strauss vasculitis	Corticosteroids, interferon-α

Hypereosinophilic syndromes

F/P-positive myeloproliferative	Imatinib
Lymphoproliferative and other	Corticosteroids, interferon-α, hydroxyurea, anti-IL-5 monoclonal antibody, other

disorder. For patients with sustained eosinophilia who meet the criteria for HES (see Box 23.2), diagnostic testing should aim to identify which variant form of HES the patient may have (see Fig. 23.4).

■ REFERENCES ■

1. Adamko DJ, Odemuyiwa SO, Vethanayagam D, et al. The rise of the phoenix: the expanding role of the eosinophil in health and disease. Allergy 2005; 60: 13–22.

2. Rothenberg ME, Hogan SP. The eosinophil. Annu Rev Immunol 2006; 24: 147–174.

3. Kariyawasam HH, Robinson DS. The eosinophil: the cell and its weapons, the cytokines, its locations. Semin Respir Crit Care Med 2006; 27: 117–127.

4. Munitz A, Levi-Schaffer F. Eosinophils: 'new' roles for 'old' cells. Allergy 2004; 59: 268–275.

5. Gonlugur U, Efeoglu T. Vascular adhesion and transendothelial migration of eosinophil leukocytes. Cell Tissue Res 2004; 318: 473–482.

6. Bandeira-Melo C, Bozza PT, Weller PF. The cellular biology of eosinophil eicosanoid formation and function. J. Allergy Clin Immunol. 2002; 109: 393–400.

7. Shi HZ. Eosinophils function as antigen-presenting cells. J Leukoc Biol 2004; 76: 520–527.

8. Gleich GJ. Mechanisms of eosinophil-associated inflammation. J Allergy Clin Immunol 2000; 105: 651–663.

9. Moqbel R, Coughlin JJ. Differential secretion of cytokines. Sci STKE 2006: 26.

10. Bandeira-Melo C, Weller PF. Mechanisms of eosinophil cytokine release. Mem Inst Oswaldo Cruz 2005; 100: 73–81.

11. Melo RCN, Spencer LA, Perez SAC, et al. Human eosinophils secrete preformed, granule-stored interleukin-4 through distinct vesicular compartments. Traffic 2005; 6: 1047–1057.

12. Melo RCN, Perez SAC, Spencer LA, et al. Intragranular vesiculotubular compartments are involved in piecemeal degranulation by activated human eosinophils. Traffic 2005; 6: 866–879.

13. Spencer LA, Melo RCN, Perez SAC, et al. Cytokine receptor-mediated trafficking of preformed IL-4 in eosinophils identifies an innate immune mechanism of cytokine secretion. Proc Natl Acad Sci USA 2006; 103: 3333–3338.

14. Klion AD, Nutman TB. The role of eosinophils in host defense against helminth parasites. J Allergy Clin Immunol 2004; 113: 30–37.

15. Swartz JM, Dyer KD, Cheever AW, et al. *Schistosoma mansoni* infection in eosinophil lineage-ablated mice. Blood 2006; 108: 2420–2427.

16. Padigel UM, Lee JJ, Nolan TJ, et al. Eosinophils can function as antigen presenting cells in primary and secondary immune responses to *Strongyloides stercoralis* infection in mice. Infect Immun 2006; 74: 3232–3238.

17. Kay AB. The role of eosinophils in the pathogenesis of asthma. Trends Mol Med 2005; 11: 148–152.

18. Kay AB, Klion AD. Anti-interleukin-5 therapy for asthma and hyper-eosinophilic syndrome. Immunol Allergy Clin North Am 2004; 24: 645–666, vii.

19. Shi H, Humbles A, Gerard C, et al. Lymph node trafficking and antigen presentation by endobronchial eosinophils. J Clin Invest 2000; 105: 945–953.

20. Fuzellier JF, Chapoutot L, Torossian PF. Mitral valve repair in idiopathic hypereosinophilic syndrome. J Heart Valve Dis 2004; 13: 529–531.

21. Wilson ME, Weller PF. Eosinophilia. In: Guerrant RL, Walker DH, Weller PF, eds. Tropical infectious diseases: principles, pathogens and practice, 2nd edn. Philadelphia: Churchill Livingstone, 2006 : 1478–1495.

22. Klion AD, Bochner BS, Gleich GJ, et al. Approaches to the treatment of hypereosinophilic syndromes: a workshop summary report. J Allergy Clin Immunol 2006; 117: 1292–1302.

23. Roufosse F, Cogan E, Goldman M. Recent advances in pathogenesis and management of hypereosinophilic syndromes. Allergy 2004; 59: 673–689.

24. Klion AD. Recent advances in the diagnosis and treatment of hypereosinophilic syndromes. Hematology (Am Soc Hematol Educ Program) 2005: 209–214.

25. Gleich GJ, Leiferman KM. The hypereosinophilic syndromes: still more heterogeneity. Curr Opin Immunol 2005; 17: 679–684.

26. Gotlib J, Cools J, Malone JM 3rd, et al. The FIP1L1-PDGFRalpha fusion tyrosine kinase in hypereosinophilic syndrome and chronic eosinophilic leukemia: implications for diagnosis, classification, and management. Blood 2004; 103: 2879–2891.

27. Muller AM, Martens UM, Hofmann SC, et al. Imatinib mesylate as a novel treatment option for hypereosinophilic syndrome: two case reports and a comprehensive review of the literature. Ann Hematol 2006; 85: 1–16.

28. Butterfield JH. Interferon treatment for hypereosinophilic syndromes and systemic mastocytosis. Acta Haematol 2005; 114: 26–40.

29. Bain B. The idiopathic hypereosinophilic syndrome and eosinophilic leukemias. Haematologica 2004; 89: 133–137.

30. Cottin V, Cordier JF. Eosinophilic pneumonias. Allergy 2005; 60: 841–857.

31. Shorr AF, Scoville SL, Cersovsky SB, et al. Acute eosinophilic pneumonia among US Military personnel deployed in or near Iraq. JAMA 2004; 292: 2997–3005.

32. Guillevin L, Pagnoux C, Mouthon L. Churg–Strauss syndrome. Semin Respir Crit Care Med 2004; 25: 535–545.

33. Foucher P, Camus P. Pneumotox on line: the drug-induced lung diseases. www.pneumotox.com.8/18/2006.

34. Rothenberg ME. Eosinophilic gastrointestinal disorders (EGID). J Allergy Clin Immunol 2004; 113: 11–28.

35. Kodner CM, Kudrimoti A. Diagnosis and management of acute interstitial nephritis. Am Fam Phys 2003; 67: 2527–2534.

36. Peyriere H, Dereure O, Breton H, et al. Variability in the clinical pattern of cutaneous side-effects of drugs with systemic symptoms: does a DRESS syndrome really exist? Br J Dermatol 2006; 155: 422–428.

37. Tefferi A. Modern diagnosis and treatment of primary eosinophilia. Acta Haematol 2005; 114: 52–60.

38. Hochberg N, Ryan ET. Medical problems in the returning expatriate. Clin Occup Environ Med 2004; 4: 205–219.

part 3

INFECTION AND IMMUNITY

Immune response to extracellular bacteria

David S. Stephens, William M. Shafer

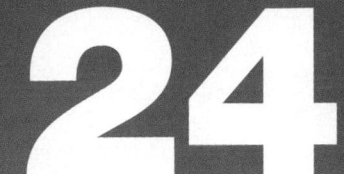

The human host has evolved protective mechanisms to deal with the multitude of bacterial species encountered in nature. These host defenses include nonspecific mechanisms of clearance, and innate as well as specific adaptive immune responses. Partly because of these mechanisms, the vast majority of bacterial species (e.g., ~10 000 different species of bacteria per gram of soil) do not cause human disease. A smaller number of bacterial species (~10^3) have established symbiotic or commensal relationships with the human host and colonize skin and mucosal surfaces.[1] These commensals are generally of low virulence except in individuals whose host defenses are compromised. A few (~10^2) pathogenic bacterial species or subpopulations of those species have evolved virulence factors or strategies that can overcome or circumvent human host defense mechanisms and cause local or invasive clinical disease. In fact, defects in host defenses are often suggested by the infecting bacteria (Table 24.1). Many of these bacterial pathogens reside mostly extracellularly. Examples are pathogens such as *Neisseria meningitidis*, *Neisseria gonorrhoeae*, *Haemophilus influenzae*, group A streptococci, *Bordetella pertussis*, and *Streptococcus pneumoniae*, which are transmitted from one individual to another by close contact. Other 'extracellular' bacterial pathogens, such as *Vibrio cholerae*, *Shigella dysenteriae*, enteropathogenic *Escherichia coli*, *Bacillus anthracis* and *Clostridium tetani*, are acquired through food, water, animal or other environmental contact. *Staphylococcus aureus* is an important extracellular pathogen for humans and can be acquired from other humans, animals, or through environmental contacts.

'Extracellular' bacterial pathogens usually produce acute inflammatory and purulent infectious diseases such as meningitis, septicemia, pneumonia, urethritis, pharyngitis, inflammatory diarrhea, cellulitis and abscesses, and/or produce disease by the release of toxins. Disease associated with some extracellular bacteria (e.g., *Helicobacter pylori*) results from chronic colonization. Susceptibility to extracellular bacterial pathogens is enhanced by hereditary, acquired or age-related defects in epithelial, humoral and phagocytic host defenses. Enhanced resistance to extracellular bacterial pathogens or their toxins can be accentuated by chemoprophylaxis, by vaccines, and by other immune modulation processes (passive immune globulin). Caution is urged in the interpretation of the term 'extracellular', as some of these pathogenic bacterial species invade host cells as a part of their normal lifecycle and during steps in the disease process.

HOST DEFENSES AND IMMUNE RESPONSES AT EPITHELIAL SURFACES

CLEARANCE AND NONSPECIFIC HOST DEFENSES AT EPITHELIAL SURFACES

Intact skin and mucosal surfaces provide a formidable barrier to most bacterial species.[2] Damage to epithelial barriers by trauma, co-infections, drugs such as those used in chemotherapy, environmental factors such as smoking, allergies or low humidity, catheterization and intubation circumvent these barriers and allow bacteria access to subcutaneous tissues, blood vessels and other normally sterile sites (Table 24.2). Skin is a relatively dry, acidic (pH 5–6) barrier that contains growth-inhibiting fatty acids and antimicrobial peptides (see below),[2] characteristics that are detrimental to many bacteria. The stratified desquamatory epithelial surface of the skin also helps in the removal of microorganisms. Repeated trauma to skin (e.g., dialysis and IV drug use) enhances skin colonization with pathogens such as *S. aureus* .

Mucosal surfaces have additional nonspecific antibacterial defenses. Lysozyme is found in most mucosal secretions and lyzes bacterial cell walls by splitting muramic acid β(1–4)- *N* -acetyl-glucosamine linkages. The mucociliary blanket of the respiratory tract (Fig. 24.1) and the female urogenital tract (fallopian tube) moves bacteria away from epithelial surfaces, as does the flushing of the urinary tract with urine and the bathing of the conjunctiva with tears. Phospholipase A_2, particularly in tears, has received attention as an antibacterial agent. The acid pH of the stomach, intestinal peristalsis and the antibacterial effect of proteolytic enzymes present in intestinal secretions are important gastrointestinal tract host defenses against bacteria.

The normal flora of the skin, upper respiratory and gastrointestinal tracts, and the genital tract of females, is also a major barrier to colonization by newly acquired pathogens.[1,3] Altering normal flora or protective barriers, for example by creating pharmacologic or surgical gastric achlorhydria or by the use of broad-spectrum antibiotics, can lead to the acquisition and overgrowth of pathogenic bacteria such as *Salmonella*

Table 24.1 Host defense defects suggested by infecting bacteria

Bacteria	Defective system
Staphylococci, aerobic Gram-negative bacilli	Skin and mucous membrane barriers, phagocyte dysfunction
Haemophilus influenzae, pneumococci	Antibody, mucous membrane barriers
Neisseria meningitidis and *Neisseria gonorrhoeae*	Complement pathways, antibody
Mycobacterium, Salmonella	Cell-mediated immunity

Table 24.2 Bacterial infections associated with impaired skin and mucous membrane barriers

Compromised physical barriers
Cystic fibrosis (mucoid *Ps. aeruginosa*)
Immotile cilia syndromes (recurrent sinopulmonary infections with pyogenic bacteria)
Tracheostomy and tracheal intubation (aerobic Gram-negative bacteria)
Urinary tract obstructive lesions and bladder catheters (Gram-negative bacilli)
IV catheters, other mucosal disruption (tumor, ulceration etc.) (*S. aureus* and Gram-negative bacilli, mixed aerobic and anaerobic infections in diabetics)
Surgical procedures and skin trauma (*S. aureus*)
Burns (aerobic Gram-negative bacilli, *S. aureus*)
Smoking (*H. influenzae,* pneumococci, meningococci)
Achlorhydria (*Salmonella,* tuberculosis)
Slowing peris talsis with opium alkaloids (prolongs symptomatic shigellosis)

Alteration of normal flora
Antibiotics: *Candida* overgrowth, *C. difficile* colitis
Alcoholism: *Klebsiella* pharyngeal colonization, tuberculosis
Severe illness: colonization of oropharynx by Gram-negative bacilli and nosocomial pneumonias
Alteration of the normal microbial flora by antibiotics, alcoholism and severe illness may lead to colonization or production of disease by extracellular bacteria. For example, colonization of the respiratory tract with aerobic Gram-negative bacilli may follow treatment with broad-spectrum antibiotics that eradicate the normal upper respiratory tract flora. Serious Gram-negative bacilli pneumonia may occur, especially if other host abnormalities are also present

typhimurium, Clostridium difficile or antibiotic-resistant Gram-negative bacilli. Normal flora also facilitate a high level of priming of the immune system by maintaining high levels of MHC class II molecule expression on macrophages and other antigen-presenting cells.[2]

Bacterial attachment and colonization of mucosal surfaces can be inhibited by bacterial binding to human cellular antigens present in secretions, such as ABO blood group antigens. Cell adhesion and extracellular matrix molecules such as fibronectin and proteoglycans can also inhibit or enhance bacterial binding to epithelial surfaces. The Tamm–Horsfall glycoprotein, found in the urine, can bind avidly to a variety of bacteria and facilitate clearance. Proteins such as lactoferrin (LF), present at mucosal surfaces, bind iron, an important requirement for bacterial growth. This action may reduce microbial proliferation, but some mucosal pathogens bind LF and remove iron for growth.

INNATE AND ACQUIRED IMMUNE DEFENSES AT MUCOSAL SURFACES

Immune pattern recognition molecules (Table 24.3) are a major arm of the innate immune system and are released or expressed by a range of host cells, including lymphocytes, macrophages or tissue histiocytes,

dendritic cells, polymorphonuclear leukocytes (PMNs) and epithelial cells (Chapter 3). These cells also protect mucosal surfaces from microbial invasion. In acquired immunity, mucosal immunoglobulins are a major protection against extracellular bacteria.

PATTERN RECOGNITION MOLECULES

The discovery and characterization of specific pattern recognition molecules has revolutionized our understanding of the initial specific events occurring between microbes and human cells. The identification and function of these molecules is rapidly expanding and include Toll-like receptors, NOD and caterpillar proteins, RNA helicases, complement proteins, antimicrobial peptides, collectin and surfactants, C- and S-lectins such as mannose-binding lectin and L-ficolin.[4–7] A family of major importance are the Toll-like receptors[4–6] (TLR1–10) (Table 24.4) found on macrophages, neutrophils and other host cells. These receptors recognize a variety of microbial ligands or pathogen-associated molecular patterns (PAMPs), including liproteins, LPS, flagellin and nucleic acids produced by Gram-negative and/or Gram-positive bacteria. Alterations (polymorphisms) in TLRs (e.g., TLR4) and other pattern recognition molecules is associated with susceptibility or severity of specific infections (e.g., sepsis).[6]

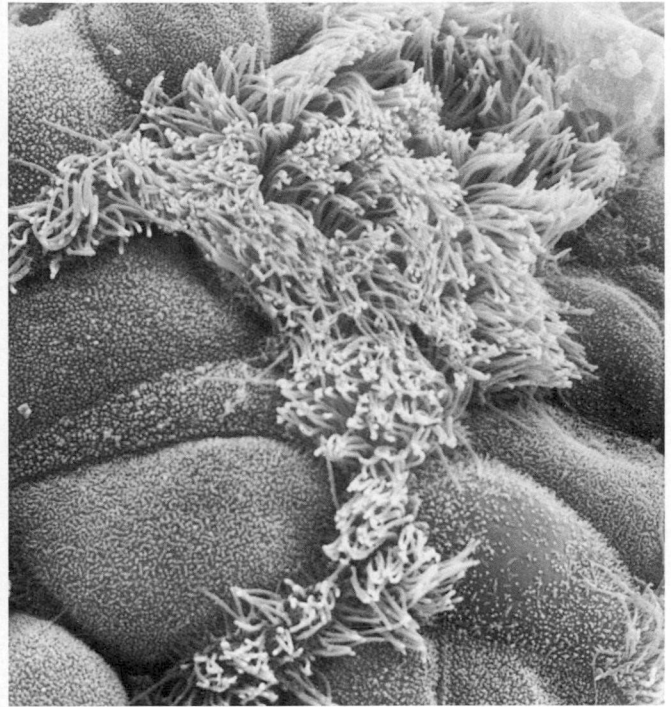

Fig. 24.1 Mucociliary host defense. Scanning electron micrograph of human upper respiratory mucosa showing the ciliated and nonciliated epithelial surface (□16 000).[35]

Table 24.3 Immune microbial pattern recognition molecules

Toll-like receptors (TLR)
NOD, Caterpillar proteins, PGRPs
RNA helicases/PkR
Complement proteins: C1q, C1 inhibitor
Antimicrobial peptides
Collectins and surfactants
C- and S-lectins: mannose-binding lectin, L-ficolin

| KEY CONCEPTS

HOST DEFENSES AND IMMUNE RESPONSE AT EPITHELIAL SURFACES TO EXTRACELLULAR BACTERIA

>> Clearance and nonspecific host defenses at skin and mucosal surfaces
>> Epithelial barriers
>> Antibacterial factors (fatty acids, antibactericidal peptides, lysozyme, phospholipase A$_2$)
>> Mucociliary activity
>> Normal flora
>> Adherence blocking molecules
>> Specific immune defenses at mucosal surfaces
>> Innate immune mechanism
>> Immunoglobulins
>> Phagocytosis at mucosal surfaces
>> Mucosal-associated lymphoid tissue (MALT, GALT, BALT)

Table 24.4 Human Toll-like receptors and microbial ligands

TLR1-lipopeptide PAMPs (pathogen-associated molecular patterns)
TLR2-lipopeptiode PAMPs
TLR3-dsRNA
TLR4-LPS
TLR5-flagellin
TLR6-lipopeptide PAMPs
TLR7-nucleic acid PAMPs
TLR8-nucleic acid PAMPs
TLR9-nucleic acid PAMPs, CpG DNA
TLR10-lipopeptide PAMPs

DENDRITIC CELLS

Discovered in the early 1970s by Steinman and Cohen,[8] dendritic cells (DCs) are now recognized as important and potent antigen-processing and -presenting cells that are crucial for the induction of T- and B-cell responses (Chapter 7). They present peptides and proteins to both T and B cells. DCs have been thought of as the pacemaker of the immune response[9] and are widely distributed in tissues, especially those that interface with the environment. They are a heterogeneous group of antigen-processing cells that arise from three pathways that are lymphoid or myeloid related in their origin. They employ pattern recognition receptors (e.g., TLRs) to detect pathogens (viruses and bacteria) in their environment. In most tissues, DCs are at low levels and are immature, but upon activation

they take up and process antigen. DC activation has a number of important consequences in immunity, including activation of naïve T cells. They perform a key role in host defense against viral and bacterial pathogens. Skin contains a major supply of tissue DCs (Langerhans' cells) and their involvement in combating skin and soft tissue infection must be considered along with their function and contribution to stimulating immunity during vaccination. Limited information is available regarding their role in host resistance to extracellular bacteria, but studies have been performed that examine the interaction of bacteria with DCs. For instance, Kolb-Maurer et al.[10] and Unkmeir et al.[11] have studied the interaction of serogroup B meningococci with DCs. Infection of DCs by meningococci resulted in a significant and rapid production of proinflammatory cytokines and chemokines, including TNF-α, IL-6 and IL-8 through a lipo-oligosaccharide (LOS)-dependent mechanism.

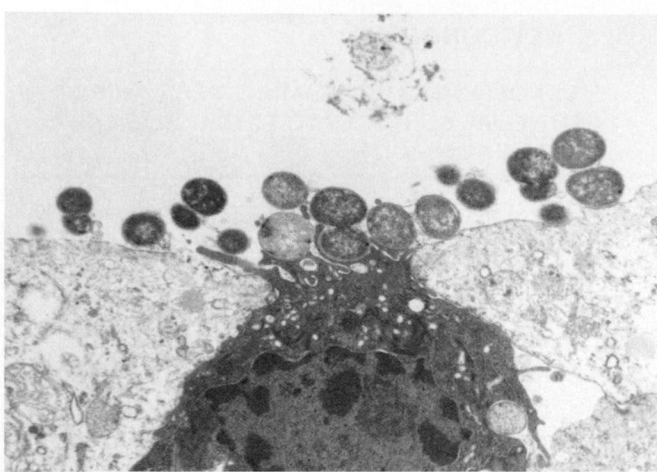

Fig. 24.2 Bacterial phagocytosis at mucosal surfaces. Transmission electron micrograph of phagocyte engulfing *N. meningitidis* at a human respiratory epithelial mucosal surface (□19 000).[35]

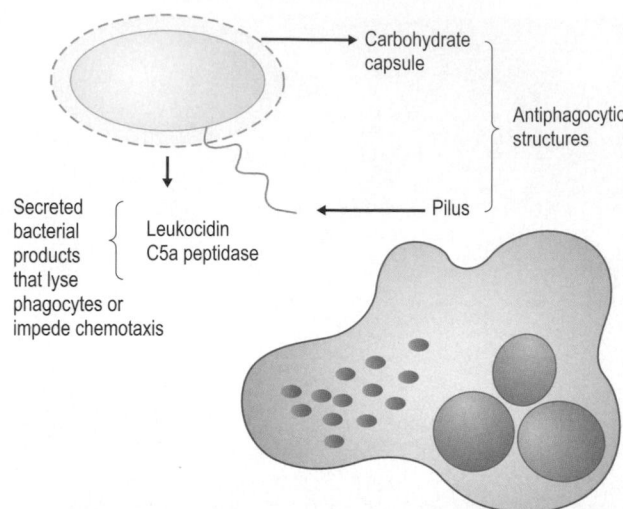

Fig. 24.3 Bacterial resistance to PMNs in the extracellular environment. The two principal mechanisms of bacterial resistance to PMN killing. These consist of resistance to phagocytosis as a result of bacterial surface components (e.g., capsule or pili) and the action of extracellular proteins that can lyse PMNs (e.g., leukocidins) or decrease chemotaxis (e.g., C5a peptidase). Bacteria growing in biofilms may be more protected from PMNs than bacteria growing in the planktonic state.

LYMPHOCYTES

Mucosa-associated lymphocyte tissue (MALT) is comprised of intraepithelial lymphocytes (IELs), lamina propria lymphocytes and lymphoid follicles (e.g., Peyer's patches), and is sometimes divided into the gut-associated (GALT), bronchial-associated (respiratory tract) (BALT) and genitourinary tract lymphocyte populations[12] (Chapter 19). These cells are important for homeostatic regulation and the maintenance of immune response against microbes at mucosal surfaces, including 'extracellular' bacteria. One in five cells in the intestinal epithelium is a lymphocyte. These cells express pattern recognition receptors (e.g., TLRs), have constitutive cytotoxic activity, secrete chemokines and cytokines important in regulation and host defense, and act in concert with mucosal epithelial cells and exocrine glands. For example, depression of IEL response (e.g., the production of IL-2/IFN-γ), is observed in experimental sepsis and following IEL exposure to lysates of enteropathogenic *E. coli* and other intestinal pathogens. *Helicobacter pylori*-associated gastritis is characterized by cytokine release and increased IEL infiltration, and can result in gastric mucosal lymphoid tissue (MALT) lymphomas. Eradication of *H. pylori* causes a reduction in IEL infiltrates.

MACROPHAGES

Phagocytic cells, macrophages and PMNs are also present at mucosal surfaces (Fig. 24.2). These cells express pattern recognition receptors and migrate to mucosal surfaces by chemotaxis and diapedesis between epithelial cells. Macrophages are also encountered after crossing the epithelial barrier. Specialized epithelial M cells of mucosal surfaces are key sites for antigen sampling, including viruses, and bacteria and macrophages surround these sites.[13] However, enteroinvasive pathogens such as *Shigella* can resist macrophages. *Shigella* induce macrophage apoptotic death by direct interaction of the bacterial protein IpaB with interleukin-1β-converting enzyme.[13] Viral co-infections may prime macrophages for LPS-induced apoptosis.[14]

POLYMORPHONUCLEAR LEUKOCYTES

In areas of epithelial inflammation, polymorphonuclear leukocytes (PMNs) or neutrophils can be recruited to mucosal and skin surfaces. PMNs are more effective in the presence of specific immune defenses, such as antibody and complement components. PMNs express pattern recognition receptors and have both oxygen-dependent and -independent mechanisms of killing (Chapter 21). Extracellular bacteria typically evade these bactericidal processes by resisting phagocytosis (Fig. 24.3). Resistance to phagocytosis can be due to the action of carbohydrate capsules, which impede the engulfment of phagocyte-associated bacteria. Other microbial surface structures, such as the pili of the gonococcus, can 'stiff-arm' neutrophils, keeping them at a distance.[15] A number of pyogenic bacteria (e.g., *S. aureus*) secrete leukocidins, which lyse phagocytes. Other pathogens (e.g., group A streptococci) inhibit chemotaxis of neutrophils through the elaboration of enzymes (e.g., C5a peptidase) that proteolytically cleave chemotactic signals. Regardless of the mechanism by which bacteria resist phagocytes, opsonic antibody can often overcome these forces and promote killing. The importance of PMNs in host defense against extracellular pathogens can best be highlighted by the increased frequency of bacteremias and other life-threatening infections in neutropenic patients or those individuals with neutrophil deficits (e.g., chronic granulomatous disease, Chediak–Higashi syndrome or specific granule deficiency, to name but a few) (Chapter 21).

ANTIMICROBIAL PEPTIDES (AMPs)

Extracellular pathogens are likely to be confronted with both myeloid-derived AMPs (e.g., the α-defensins stored within neutrophil granules) and nonmyeloid antibacterial peptides.[16] These (and similar) peptides,

THERAPEUTIC PRINCIPLES

MANAGING DEFECTS IN HOST DEFENSES

>> Impaired skin and mucous membrane barriers – protect skin from maceration and injury, frequent change of IV catheters. Antibiotic prophylaxis, such as use of trimethoprim-sulfamethoxazole remains controversial.

>> Defects or polymorphisms in innate immune mechanisms – may lead to select cytokine use or other adjuvant therapy such as activated protein C in sepsis.

>> Abnormal humoral immunity – intravenous immune serum globulin.

>> Complement system abnormalities – fresh plasma or, if available, individual complement components to replace deficient factor.

>> Defective cell-mediated immunity reversal of malnutrition – reduction in dosage of immunosuppressive drugs (corticosteroids); other therapy in selected patients (transfer factor, bone marrow transplantation, replacement of missing enzymes).

>> Phagocyte dysfunction – GM-CSF or G-CSF to increase neutrophil numbers.

>> Immunization with pneumococcal, meningococcal, *H. influenzae* and influenza vaccines in selected patients.

which are typically cationic, amphipathic molecules, represent an integral part of the innate host defense system for humans and other vertebrates, invertebrates and plants.[17] Many of these peptides from evolutionary diverse sources share structural similarities, suggesting their importance in host defense throughout evolution. In general terms, these antimicrobial peptides (often effective at micromolar concentrations *in vitro*) can either be constitutively synthesized (e.g., the α-defensins of neutrophils) or their production can be induced in a variety of epithelial cells (e.g., Paneth cells of the small intestine) by a variety of stimuli, including infection.[18] Humans produce two main classes of AMP: defensins[18] and cathelicidins.[19] Defensins (3–4 kDa) are cysteine-rich peptides and are classified as α- and β-defensins. α-Defensins are major components of neutrophil granules capable of reaching mg/mL concentrations in phagolysosomes and small intestinal Paneth cells. β-Defensins are produced by a large variety of epithelial cells, mucosal surfaces, skin and organs. The circular θ-defensins of rhesus macaques are produced by a unique ligation reaction of two peptides, but owing to a premature stop mutation are not produced by humans; θ-defensins can have potent antiviral effects. Unlike many other vertebrates, humans produce only one cathelicidin (LL-37),[19] which is synthesized by both PMNs and epithelial cells. The 'cathelin' domain of the precursor protein resembles inhibitors of cysteine proteases and is removed by proteolytic cleavage to liberate the LL-37 AMP, an α-helical, linear peptide of 37 amino acids.

AMPs probably exert their lethal effect at the bacterial inner membrane, causing rapid depolarization and loss of membrane potential,[20] although some evidence exists that certain peptides have cytosolic targets. Bacteria can avoid these peptides to some extent by reducing the electronegativity of their microbial cell surface, which reduces electrostatic interactions with

cationic regions of the peptide.[21] The importance of surface binding is further illustrated by the salt-sensitivity of a number of antibacterial peptides. This property has been advanced as one possibility to explain the antimicrobial deficit in lung airway fluid obtained from patients with cystic fibrosis.[22] Other mechanisms used by bacteria to subvert the lethal action of AMPs include energy-dependent efflux, proteolytic degradation, modification of membrane phospholipids, production of AMP-binding proteins, reduction of cytoplasmic membrane potential, and biofilm production. The regulation of genes encoding products involved in such resistance has been extensively studied and certain two-component regulatory systems[23] (e.g., *pmrAB* and *phoPQ* in *Salmonella*) or transcriptional regulators can be involved in determining levels of bacterial susceptibility to AMPs.[24]

AMPs probably contribute to host defense through their antibiotic-like action and by virtue of their immunomodulatory properties. In this respect, they should be viewed more broadly as host defense peptides.[25] They can effectively bind and neutralize endotoxin, act as chemokines, and induce chemokine synthesis that results in recruitment and accumulation of phagocytes at sites of infection. AMPs can also promote wound healing, and have been proposed to link innate and adaptive immune responses.[25, 26] Mice expressing human defensin-5 are more resistant to lethal *Salmonella* infection, providing evidence that human AMPs are important in host defense.[27] AMPs present at the human vaginal and cervical mucosal surfaces may also be important in host defense against sexually transmitted infections or in reducing the incidence of vaginosis.[28] LL-37 and β-defensins are probably important in the antimicrobial defense of human skin. Mice deficient in the murine version of LL-37 (CRAMP) are more susceptible to group A streptococcal skin and soft tissue infections and invasive disease.[24] Patients with psoriasis or atopic dermatitis provide an example of where AMP levels are altered. Thus, keratinocytes of inflamed psoriatic lesions produce increased levels of certain AMPs, and such patients rarely have secondary bacterial infections.[26] In contrast, keratinocytes from patients with atopic dermatitis do not overproduce AMPs and often have skin infections caused by *S. aureus*. Human synthesis of β-defensin 2 is significantly decreased in patients with acute burns, which may partly explain their increased susceptibility to *Pseudomonas aeruginosa* infections. The rare patient population with PMN-specific granule deficiency are deficient in defensins and other neutrophil components, and these individuals have life-threatening infections.[29] The severe congenital neutrophil deficiency termed morbus Kostmann disease can be treated with G-CSF to restore neutrophil levels, but such phagocytes fail to produce LL-37 and such patients often have frequent and life-threatening infections as well as periodontal disease.[30] Thus, taken together, there is increasing evidence that AMPs are important in the overall integrity of the human host defense scheme, and a combination of their antimicrobial and immunomodulatory activities is involved in protection against extracellular pathogens.

IMMUNOGLOBULINS

Immunoglobulins, principally secretory IgA and IgG, are present at mucosal surfaces and in mucosal secretions. Important in the generation of these immunoglobulins at mucosal surfaces is the dissemination of IgA and IgG class-committed B- and T-helper cells with specificity to an antigen encountered and processed at one mucosal site to local and distant mucosal sites. Protective mucosal antibodies against bacteria may be derived from prior colonization, vaccines, or shared cross-reactive antigens on normal flora. Mucosal immunoglobulins may neutralize bacterial toxins, facilitate phagocytosis or bactericidal activity, inhibit

Table 24.5 Bacterial and other infections associated with abnormal humoral immunity

Primary deficiency

Congenital or X-linked agammaglobulinemia (Bruton's agammaglobulinemia) is manifested by recurrent bacterial infections of the middle ear and sinopulmonary tract, often with complicating bacteremias. Infections with enteroviruses also occur

Selective immunoglobulin deficiency: IgA – variable course, often free of infection; IgG, IgG subclass deficiency, IgM – recurrent pyogenic bacterial infections

Common variable immunodeficiency ('acquired' hypogammaglobulinemia) is associated with various bacterial sinopulmonary infections, giardiasis, increased risk of lymphomas and gastric carcinomas

Secondary deficiency

Multiple myeloma and chronic lymphocytic leukemia (CLL) are associated with infections caused by encapsulated bacteria, Gram-negative bacilli, S. *aureus,* and giardiasis

Splenectomy – severe infections with pneumococci, other streptococci, H. *influenzae* and meningococci

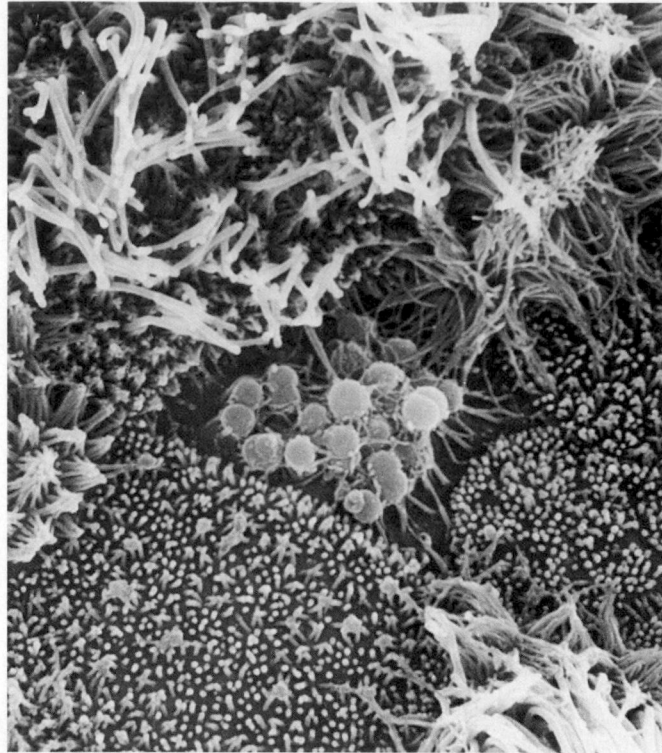

Fig. 24.4 Colonization and adherence of extracellular bacteria at mucosal surfaces. Scanning electron micrograph of *N. meningitidis* adherence and microcolony formation of a human upper respiratory mucosa (□16 250).[35]

bacterial adherence ligands, or sterically hinder other events necessary for bacterial colonization and invasion. Many extracellular bacterial pathogens (*N. meningitidis N. gonorrhoeae H. influenzae* certain streptococci) colonize and/or infect mucosal surfaces where protective IgA_1 antibodies could become available.[31] These pathogens secrete an IgA_1 protease that cleaves IgA_1, thereby inactivating it. IgA_1 protease can also recognize other substrates, notably LAMP-1, that are important in host defense. Bacterial infections associated with abnormal immunoglobulin function are summarized in Table 24.5 and Chapter 34.

BACTERIAL PATHOGENS AT EPITHELIAL SURFACES

'Extracellular' bacteria that cause disease in humans are transferred from person to person by direct contact, contact with feces, respiratory droplets or other secretions, or from contaminated food or water. Acquisition of these pathogenic bacteria may be transient, or lead to colonization or local and invasive disease. To colonize human epithelial barriers and mucosal surfaces, bacteria overcome the nonspecific clearance (e.g., mucus, ciliary activity) and other local immune defense mechanisms (e.g., mucosal cellular defenses, immunoglobulins, fatty acids, lactoferrin). For example, bacteria can transverse mucus by expressing motility factors (e.g., pili, flagella), and induce ciliostasis or decrease motility by direct contact or by the release of toxins.

Initial attachment of bacteria to human epithelial cells is, in part, mediated by pili, fimbriae or other bacteria ligands, and close adherence involves the cell wall, outer membrane proteins, lipopolysaccharide and other bacterial surface structures. The attachment of bacteria to human epithelial cells prevents loss from the host. Attachment can also induce cytoskeletal rearrangements, such as elongation and branching of the microvilli, the accumulation of actin, and calcium efflux, which facilitates close adherence and invasion of epithelial cells by normally 'extracellular' bacteria, especially at sites with rapidly moving fluid. The entry of bacteria into epithelial cells

provides access to nutrients and protection from host defenses, allows protected multiplication, and leads to shedding of organisms back to the mucosal surface, to facilitate transmission and further spread of the infection on the epithelium. Attachment can also initiate epithelial cell apoptosis or toxin-mediated cell death and lead to the breakdown of the epithelial barrier.

N. meningitidis (the meningococcus), for example, is transmitted from person to person by large respiratory droplets or close contact with secretions. During the process of colonization of human upper respiratory mucosal surfaces (e.g., the nasopharynx) meningococci utilize phase-variable meningococcal surface ligands and multiple human epithelial cell surface receptors.[32, 33] Meningococci that are acapsulate, piliated, express high levels of the outer membrane protein, Opc (formerly class 5C protein) and the nonsialylated LOS structure containing a terminal Galβ1–4Glu group (L8 immunotype) attach to and interact with human epithelial cells most effectively (Fig. 24.4). These characteristics correspond to the predominant phenotype of meningococci retrieved from the nasopharynx of human carriers. Pili facilitate twitching motility and microcolony formation, which allows the penetration of mucus and provides initial attachment. The outer membrane adhesin, Opc, mediates meningococcal attachment and invasion by binding vitronectin, which attaches to and is internalized by the vitronectin receptor $\alpha_v\beta_3$ found on epithelial cell surfaces.[32] Class V (opacity) meningococcal proteins interact directly with members of the carcinoembryonic (CD66) antigen family.[32] The expression of a sialic acid capsule and sialylatable LOS structures, such as the L3,7,9 immunotype, interfere with Opc-mediated attachment and invasion and facilitate spread and transmission.[34] Meningococci at mucosal surfaces bind and utilize lactoferrin as an iron source and secrete a protease that cleaves IgA$_1$. Meningococcal colonization of the human upper respiratory (nasopharyngeal) epithelium is also associated with ciliostasis and sloughing of ciliated cells, which occurs at a distance from the sites of bacterial attachment.[33, 35] Ciliostasis may be caused by a diffusible toxin, such as LPS, which may directly or indirectly cause cytotoxicity by the induction of inflammatory cytokines. Other cofactors, such as smoking or viral infections, facilitate meningococcal invasion at nasopharyngeal mucosal surfaces.

IMMUNE RESPONSES DURING LOCAL AND SYSTEMIC INVASION BY EXTRACELLULAR BACTERIAL PATHOGENS

Bacteria that breach mucosal and skin barriers and reach submucosal tissues and/or the bloodstream induce immune responses, including cytokine release, phagocytosis, complement activation, antibody release or production, and other local or systemic induction of the inflammatory cascade. The survival of bacteria following colonization of the epithelium and access to the bloodstream depends on the integrity of the host immune response (including variability due to genetic polymorphism) and on the ability of the bacteria to resist this response. Host factors that increase the risk for the development of systemic disease due to extracellular bacteria include polymorphisms in innate immune mechanisms, the absence of bactericidal or opsonizing antibodies, deficiencies in the complement pathways,[36] and an absence of or reduction in neutrophil function or levels.

As noted above, immune pattern recognition molecules[4] expressed or released by a variety of host cells, especially PMNs, monocytes, macrophages and dendritic cells, are important initiators of the immune response to extracellular bacteria. Interaction with microbial ligands (LPS, lipoproteins) leads to chemokine and cytokine release, including TNF-α, IL-1β, MCP-1, MIP-3a, IL-6, IL-8, 1P-10, MCP-5 and RANTES) mediate the local and systemic inflammatory response to extracellular bacteria.

Phagocytes can ingest bacteria by opsonin-independent (less efficient) or dependent mechanisms. Mononuclear phagocytes in the blood, liver, spleen and lung remove particles, including bacteria. Complement components, fibronectin or other extracellular matrix proteins that bind to bacteria facilitate recognition. Bacteria ingested by phagocytes are killed by toxic O_2 radicals and/or H_2O_2 through myeloperoxidase-dependent or -independent mechanisms. The elaboration of superoxide dismutase and catalase can reduce the efficacy of O_2-dependent killing of bacteria, but the high levels of O_2 radicals that accumulate in PMNs probably overcomes these bacterial enzymes, as evidenced by the susceptibility of *S. aureus* to intraleukocytic killing. Oxygen-independent systems caused by the action of proteins BPI, CAP 37, cathepsin G, elastase and AMPs (α-defensins and LL-37), also contribute significantly to phagocytic killing. Bacterial infections associated with phagocytic dysfunction are described in Chapters 21 and 31.

Complement, a series of more than 20 proteins, is activated by microbial surfaces (alternative complement cascade) or via antibody or by the mannose-binding lectin system (Chapter 20). Complement activation leads to microbial lysis and the release of opsonins and chemoattractant molecules for phagocytic cells. Complement activity is mediated by the

classic complement pathway, which can be initiated either by antibody binding to cell surface epitopes or by antibody-independent autocatalytic activation of C1 to form C1q. Initiation of the alternative pathways by bacterial products or mannose-binding protein leads to the direct deposition of the C3b complex on the bacterial surface. Complement activation results in the activation of the late components of the complement pathway, which results in the formation of a membrane attack complex (MAC), insertion in the bacterial cell, and bactericidal activity. Gram-positive extracellular pathogens resist the bacteriolytic action of MAC as a result of their thick peptidoglycan layer, which impedes the insertion of MAC C5b-9 complex. Gram-negative bacteria can resist MAC through structural alterations in their LPS (the possession of O antigen keeps MAC at a distance from the bacterial surface) or by masking or deleting the epitope(s) responsible for binding bactericidal antibody. The initiation of the complement cascade is also an essential step in opsonization and the eventual phagocytosis and ingestion of invading bacteria.

In infants, antibacterial activity wanes as levels of passively transferred maternal antibody fall. This waning of antibody is correlated with the highest incidence of several 'extracellular' pyogenic bacterial diseases (*S. pneumoniae, N. meningitidis, H. influenzae* type b) in young children. During childhood and adolescence, levels of bactericidal antibodies rise and rates of these diseases decline. Specific antibodies are acquired through carriage and through cross-reacting epitopes on other commensal species. For example, cross-reactive antibodies to *N. meningitidis* are acquired by colonization with commensal *Neisseria* spp. (e.g., *Neisseria lactamica*) and unrelated bacteria (e.g., *Enterococcus faecium, Bacillus pumilus* and *E. coli*). The lack of bactericidal antibodies against a strain acquired in the upper respiratory tract is an important risk factor for invasive meningococcal disease.

Complement deficiencies, either congenital or acquired, also increase the risk for invasive bacterial diseases (Chapter 20). Because C3 plays a critical role in the complement cascade, congenital C3 deficiency or conditions that reduce C3 (e.g., systemic lupus erythematosus, cirrhosis, nephritis, C3 nephritic factor) increase the risk for invasive disease due to pyogenic bacteria such as *S. pneumoniae* and *N. meningitidis*. Mannose-binding lectin (MBL) is a plasma opsonin that initiates complement activation. MBL gene polymorphisms are found in children with meningococcal and pneumococcal sepsis. Properdin deficiency, leading to defective alternative pathway killing, is also associated with severe and recurrent meningococcal infections. Terminal complement deficiencies (C5–C8) are also associated with recurrent invasive bloodstream meningococcal and gonococcal infections, indicating an important role for insertion of the complement membrane attack complex in the bactericidal activity of human serum against pathogenic *Neisseria*.[36] In adults 10–20% of invasive meningococcal disease is associated with a defect in the complement system.[36] Enteric colonization by bacteria that have similar antigenic epitopes has been proposed to induce these blocking antibodies. Screening tests useful for the evaluation of humoral, complement and other immune defects are discussed in Chapter 30.

In addition to defects in innate immunity, immunoglobulins and complement deficiencies, human genetic polymorphisms are associated with an increased risk or severity of bacterial diseases. For example, FcγIIa (CD32) receptor polymorphisms, Fcγ-receptor III (CD16), MBL, TLR4, TNF promoter region polymorphisms, plasminogen activator and inhibitor expression, and hereditary differences in cytokine induction influence susceptibility to meningococcemia.[37,38] Each of these may influence the course of invasive bacterial infection by influencing the response of the inflammatory cascade.

Table 24.6 Major agents of septicemia

Staphylococcus aureus
Enterococci
Streptococcus pneumoniae
Haemophilus influenzae
Streptococcus pyogenes
Streptococcus agalactiae
Gram-negative aerobic bacilli

E. coli	*Enterobacter* spp.
Pseudomonas aeruginosa	*Morganella morganii*
Serratia marcescens	*Proteus mirabilis*
Klebsiella pneumoniae	*Providencia stuartii*
Citrobacter spp.	*Acinetobacter* spp.
Neisseria meningitidis	*Pasteurella* spp.

KEY CONCEPTS

DEFINITIONS OF SEPTICEMIA AND SEPSIS SYNDROME

>> *Septicemia* Life-threatening bacterial infection of the bloodstream caused by Gram-positive or Gram-negative bacteria.

>> *Sepsis syndrome* Clinical evidence of infection, plus evidence of systemic response to infection and altered organ perfusion, but may not have documented bacterial infection in bloodstream. May be due to toxin, microbial product release into bloodstream.

>> *SIRS (systemic inflammatory response syndrome) or MODS (multiple organ dysfunction syndrome)* Response to a wide variety of clinical insults, both infectious and noninfectious (pancreatitis, burns); similar pathophysiology to septicemia and sepsis syndrome.

Induction of the inflammatory cascade, acute-phase reaction or response, augments humoral defense components, increases the number and function of phagocytic cells and facilitates the delivery of humoral cellular molecules to sites of bacterial invasion.[2] Components of this reaction include cytokines, mannose-binding protein, fibronectin, haptoglobin, transferrin, C-reactive protein, platelet-activating factor, prostaglandins, lipopolysaccharide-binding protein (LBP), α_1-antitrypsin and α_2-macroglobulin. Acute-phase reaction components induce fever, the catabolism of muscle protein, decrease available iron, increase phagocyte activity, increase vascular permeability, and induce the release of hormones and neurotransmitters.

Pyogenic extracellular bacteria have evolved strategies to avoid or overcome immune responses. For example, meningococci isolated from the bloodstream or cerebrospinal fluid are characteristically encapsulated and express the sialylatable lacto-*N*-neotetraose-containing L3,7,9 LPS immunotype. The co-expression of both of these structures is necessary for meningococcal systemic disease in the infant rat model, influences neutrophil activation and endothelial injury in cell monolayer models, and is required for resistance to complement-mediated killing. The similarity of capsules such as the serogroup B ($\alpha2\rightarrow8$)-linked polysialic acid and of lacto-*N*-neotetraose and other α-chain LPS structures with complex human sugars, glycosphingolipids, makes these structures infrequent targets for bactericidal antibody recognition.[39] Encapsulation of *N. meningitidis* downregulates the activation of the alternative pathway and is protective against phagocytosis by human macrophages and monocytes. Sialylation of LOS in meningococci has been shown to increase resistance to classic and alternative complement-mediated killing by decreasing the deposition of C3b and IgM on the cell surface, irrespective of capsular phenotype. Phase-variable expression of the length of the gonococcal LOS or the presence of certain forms of the major outer membrane protein (Por1A) can alter levels of gonococcal susceptibility to complement killing.

SEPSIS

Septicemia remains a leading cause of death in the United States.[40] It also accounts for several billion dollars of the US's annual healthcare expenditure. Both Gram-negative and Gram-positive bacteria can trigger sepsis and septic shock (Table 24.6). Septic shock is a result of initial and widespread overstimulation of the proinflammatory response in the systemic vasculature followed by anti-inflammatory cytokine activation, and may be characterized by a number of clinical findings, including hypotension, organ failure

and death. The severity of sepsis can also be influenced by polymorphic alleles of genes involved in the inflammatory cascade.[36–38] A related syndrome (systemic immune response syndrome, or SIRS) may be seen with the release of bacterial toxins or products from sites of colonization or local infections.

Peptidoglycan, DNA CpG motifs or LPS released by bacterial lysis or growth and toxins or superantigens are major initiators of the hypotension and shock of septicemia or SIRS, either directly through interaction with host cell membranes or indirectly through the release of host inflammatory mediators or T-cell proliferation (Fig. 24.5). The morbidity and mortality of bacteremia have been directly correlated with increased levels of proinflammatory cytokines and the amount of circulating bacterial components. Indeed, the severity of Gram-negative sepsis has been equated with high levels of endotoxin, increased levels of cytokines, and excessive activation of the alternative complement pathway. Disseminated intravascular coagulation, which often accompanies Gram-negative sepsis, is due to excessive activation of the coagulation cascade and downregulation of the fibrinolytic system associated with high levels of LPS. Levels of natural anticoagulants in the vasculature, such as antithrombin and protein C, are often low in Gram-negative sepsis. The onset and severity of DIC may be influenced by genetic polymorphisms in plasminogen activation or inhibition. The altered vascular endothelial lining facilitates thrombosis and thrombocytosis. Although much remains to be learned about the mechanisms by which Gram-negative and -positive bacteria and their products trigger sepsis, significant advances have been recently made, particularly with LPS. Advances during the past decade include the identification of certain LPS–host protein interactions that result in delivery of LPS to host cell receptors and gene activation events that result in elevated expression of a diverse array of proinflammatory mediators.

A general scheme (summarized in Fig. 24.6) for the development of endotoxic shock is as follows:

1. LPS becomes available in host fluids through rapid bacterial multiplication, release of outer membrane vesicles or the bacteriolytic action of antibiotics or antimicrobial systems (e.g., complement) in the host.

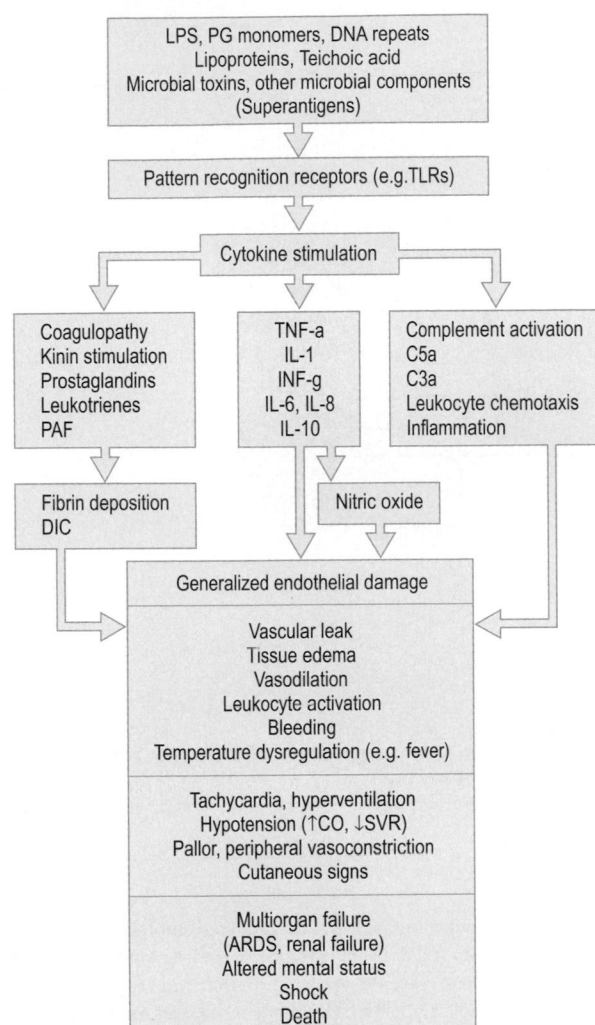

TLR4 belongs to a family of transmembrane receptors originally identified in *Drosophila* as being important in controlling dorsoventral patterning and antifungal responses. TLR4 signaling requires an accessory protein, myeloid differentiation protein-2 (MD-2)[44] that binds directly to endotoxin. The key point, however, is that the LPS engagement of MD-2/TLR4 on host cells, particularly macrophages, triggers intracellular signaling events that ultimately through NF-κB and other pathways result in cytokine gene activation and the overproduction of proinflammatory cytokines (TNF-α, IL-1, IL-6, IL-8, interferons). Different TLRs (e.g., TLR2) play a critical role in the recognition of lipoproteins and the recognition of these components is a likely key determinant in the development of septic shock seen with Gram-positive infections. TLR5 recognizes bacterial flagellae, and such recognition is of likely importance in the host response to motile bacteria; some human pathogens (e.g., *H. pylori*) produce flagellin molecules that do not engage TLR5.[45] Another TLR (TLR9) has been shown to recognize bacterial DNA CpG dinucleotides.[46] Taken together, the clinical syndrome of septic shock represents a series of interactions of bacterial products with pattern recognition molecules on serum proteins (LBP and soluble CD14), and with host cell receptors (MD-2/TLR4 and TLR2, other TLR receptors) that recognize and bind bacterial products, leading to signaling events and transcriptional factors that modulate cytokine gene expression. These events trigger further events in the inflammatory cascade, leading to massive activation of the coagulation, complement and kinin pathways.

Early and effective antimicrobial therapy is the primary goal in the treatment of sepsis. Adjuvant therapy is reviewed elsewhere.[47] For example, recombinant protein C is approved for use in patients with sepsis, but is associated with an increased risk of cerebral hemorrhage.[47] In contrast to the initial phase of sepsis characterized by the release of TNF-α, IL-1, IL-6 and interferon-γ, during the latter phase an anti-inflammatory

Fig. 24.5 Inflammatory cascade initiated during sepsis.

2. During the acute-phase response the production of a serum glycoprotein of 60 kDa, termed lipopolysaccharide-binding protein (LBP), is increased; although structurally similar to BPI, LBP lacks bactericidal activity. LBP binds lipid A, the toxic domain of LPS, with high affinity.

3. The LBP–LPS complex is then transferred to CD14, which exists in both soluble and membrane states. The primary role of LBP is to accelerate this transfer reaction.[41] CD14 is clearly important in the development of endotoxic shock, as CD14-deficient mice are resistant to lethal challenge with LPS.[42] However, membrane CD14 does not have 'signaling' ability. Soluble CD14 can accept LPS from the LBP complex and transfer it to an LPS receptor on the macrophage surface, which does have signaling ability.

4. The nature of this LPS receptor has been defined. Poltorak et al.[43] ascribed the relevant genetic defect in endotoxin-resistant C3H/HeJ mice to a missense mutation in the Toll-like receptor-4 gene (*tlr4*).

CLINICAL RELEVANCE

SIGNS OF SEPTICEMIA

➤➤ Shaking chills, spiking fevers or hypothermia (<36°C)

➤➤ Tachycardia, hyperventilation

➤➤ Pallor (peripheral vasoconstriction) and acrocyanosis, but 10–20% are flushed 'warm shock'

➤➤ Nausea/vomiting, diarrhea

➤➤ Hypotension <90 mmHg or >40 mmHg decrease from baseline, in 20–35% of cases

➤➤ Cardiac output, decreased systemic vascular resistance (SVR)

➤➤ Cutaneous signs: purpura fulminans, petechiae, palpable purpura, echthyma gangrenosum

➤➤ Change in mental status

➤➤ Signs may be more subtle in elderly and uremic (renal failure) patients

➤➤ WBC count >12 000/mm³ or <4000 cells/mm³ with >10% immature (band) forms

➤➤ Oliguria (<20 mL/h of urine)

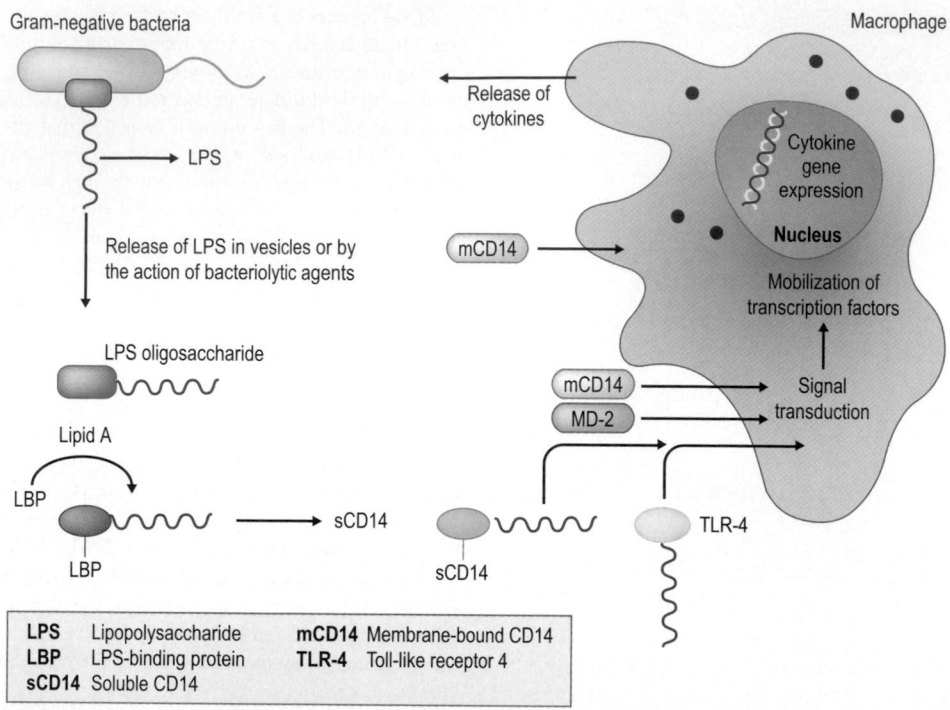

Fig. 24.6 LPS triggering of cytokine production by macrophages. Steps known or presumed to be necessary for LPS triggering of proinflammatory cytokines.

response may predominate. The failure of anti-inflammatory therapeutic mediators (anti-endotoxin antibodies, TNF-α, antagonists of IL-1 or platelet-activating factor) in sepsis may suggest that this hypoinflammatory state encountered in many patients at presentation could be an additional target of immune modulation.

ENHANCEMENT OF IMMUNE RESPONSES TO 'EXTRACELLULAR' BACTERIA (VACCINES AND IMMUNOMODULATION)

Vaccines are the most affordable and cost-effective health intervention for enhancing the immune response to extracellular bacterial and other microbial pathogens (Chapter 92).[48] The use of vaccines to prevent diphtheria, pertussis, tetanus, certain serogroups of *N. meningitidis*, *H. influenzae* b (Hib) and *S. pneumoniae* is a major public health success. The efficacy of vaccines to extracellular bacteria is most often correlated with enhanced bactericidal antibodies, opsonic antibodies and/or neutralizing antibodies, both systemically and at mucosal surfaces. Enhancement of these immune mechanisms can provide protection even in immunocompromised individuals. For example, vaccination with meningococcal capsular polysaccharide vaccines protects patients with hereditary complement deficiencies by enhancing of opsonophagocytic activity. However, some older vaccines had limitations in terms of long-lived immune responses, safety issues, and poor responses in certain populations (extremes of age) when infections with extracellular bacteria are most common.

Advances in genetic engineering, immunology, molecular pathogenesis, vaccine adjuvants and delivery systems are leading to the development of new vaccines and vaccine approaches that enhance the immune response to extracellular bacterial pathogens. The introduction of acellular pertussis vaccines, and pneumococcal and meningococcal conjugate vaccines are recent examples.

The conjugation of bacterial polysaccharides to carrier proteins such as diphtheria or tetanus toxins has been a major advance in stimulating immune responses to saccharide bacterial antigens. Polysaccharide capsules, for example, when used alone, are 'T-independent' antigens, do not require the presence of T cells to induce an immune response, and generate IgM as the dominant antibody produced (Chapter 6). There is also a failure to induce memory and failure of affinity maturation following polysaccharide immunization. Thus, polysaccharides are poorly immunogenic in infants, the elderly, and those with impaired antibody production – groups most susceptible to encapsulated bacterial pathogens. Covalent linkage of the polysaccharide to a carrier protein converts the polysaccharide to a thymus-dependent antigen generating IgG anticapsular antibodies and memory B cells. Because these vaccines induce vigorous mucosal immune responses they also protect by herd immunity. A major (and unanticipated) result of vaccination with the *H. influenzae* (Hib), meningococcal and pneumococcal conjugate vaccines was the interruption of mucosal carriage, decreased transmission[49] and herd immunity. They are now used as part of the routine childhood and adolescent immunization series.

The presentation to CD4 T cells of an antigen by MHC class II molecules is critical for an immune response and influences the amount of antibody, the affinity of that antibody and the duration of response. The two major subsets of CD4 T cells (i.e., Th1 and Th2) influence the qualitative and quantitative features of an immune response to vaccines and bacterial antigens (Chapters 16–18). Th1 responses are characterized by complement-fixing antibody and are associated with the release of IFN-γ, IL-2 and IL-12. Th2 responses result in high circulating and secreting antibody levels and the induction of cytokines IL-4, IL-5 and IL-10.

Considerable progress is being made in the development of new vaccine adjuvants and immune modulators[50–53] (Chapter 92). Aluminum salts, used since the 1930s in many vaccines against bacteria, induce a >90% Th2 response. As noted above, bacterial toxins as conjugates can be used to enhance immunogenicity. In addition, saponin adjuvants, liposomes, CpG DNA repeats and immunostimulating complexes are under development as adjuvants. Cytokines such as IL-1, IL-2, IL-12, IL-18 and GM-CSF also modify and enhance immune responses to vaccines.[53] IL-12, for example, induces strong Th1 shifts, and GM-CSF is a co-migrating signal for dendritic cells and stimulates antigen processing and presentation. Antigen recognition and processing in macrophages is critical to determining Th1 and Th2 responses and can be manipulated by selected adjuvants. Immune modulation is being evaluated not only for the enhancement of bacterial vaccines, but also as adjunct therapy for serious bacterial infections such as sepsis. Vaccines and specific immunotherapeutic approaches such as cytokines may also find use against chronic tissue-damaging inflammatory reactions created by persistent extracellular bacteria (e.g., *Helicobacter*) and autoimmune reactions that may be induced by cross-reactive bacterial antigens (e.g., *Campylobacter jejuni* and Guillain–Barré syndrome).[54]

■ REFERENCES ■

1. Gill SR, Pop M, Deboy RT, et al. Metagenomic analysis of the human distal gut microbiome. Science 2006; 312: 1355–1359.

2. Dieffenbach CW, Tramont EC. Innate (general or nonspecific) host defense mechanisms. In: Mandell GL, Bennett JE, Dolin R, eds. Principles and practice of infectious diseases, 6th edn. Vol. 1. Philadelphia: Elsevier, 2005; 34.

3. Mackowiak PA. The normal microbial flora. N Engl J Med 1982; 307: 83.

4. Pasare C, Medzhitov R. Toll-like receptors: linking innate and adaptive immunity. Adv Exp Med Biol 2005; 560: 11–18.

5. Akira S, Uematsu S, Takeuchi O. Pathogen recognition and innate immunity. Cell 2006; 124: 783.

6. Beutler B, Jiang Z, Georgel P, et al. Genetic analysis of host resistance: Toll-like receptor signaling and immunity at large. Annu Rev Immunol 2006; 24: 353–389.

7. Wright JR. Immunoregulatory functions of surfactant proteins. Nature Rev Immunol 2005; 5: 58–68.

8. Steinman R, Cohn Z. Identification of a novel cell type in peripheral lymphoid organs of mice. J Exp Med 1973; 137: 1142–1162.

9. Banchereau J, Steinman RM. Dendritic cells and the control of immunity. Nature 1998; 392: 245–252.

10. Kolb-Maurer A, Unkmeir A, Kammerer U, et al. Interaction of *Neisseria meningitidis* with human dendritic cells. Infect Immun 2001; 69: 6912.

11. Unkmeir A, Kammerer U, Stade A, et al. Lipopolysaccharide and polysaccharide capsule: virulence factors of *Neisseria meningitidis* that determine meningococcal interaction with human dendritic cells. Infect Immun 2002; 70: 2454.

12. Yoshikai Y. The interaction of intestinal epithelial cells and intraepithelial lymphocytes in host defense. Immunol Res 1999; 20: 219.

13. Sansonetti PJ, Phalipon A. M cells as ports of entry for enteroinvasive pathogens: mechanisms of interaction, consequences for the disease process. Semin Immunol 1999; 11: 193.

14. Jungi TW, Schweizer M, Perler L, Peterhans E. Supernatants of virus-infected macrophages prime uninfected macrophages for lipopolysaccharide-induced apoptosis by both an interferon-dependent and an independent mechanism. Pathobiology 1999; 67: 294.

15. Shafer WM, Rest RF. Interactions of gonococci with phagocytic cells. Annu Rev Microbiol 1989; 43: 121.

16. Ganz T, Lehrer RI. Defensins. Curr Opin Immunol 1994; 6: 584.

17. Boman HG. Antibacterial peptides: key components needed in immunity. Cell 1991; 65: 205.

18. Ganz T. Denfensins: antimicrobial peptides of innate immunity. Nature Rev Immunol 2003; 3: 710.

19. Zanetti M, Gennaro R, Scocchi M, Skerlavaj B. Structure and biology of cathelicidins. Adv Exp Med Biol 2000; 479: 203.

20. Brogden KA. Antimcrobial peptides: pore formers or metabolic inhibitors in bacteria. Nature Rev Microbiol 2005; 3: 238.

21. Peschel A, Sahl H-G. The co-evolution of host cationic antimicrobial peptides and microbial resistance. Nature Microbiol Rev 2006; 4: 529.

22. Goldman MJ, Anderson GM, Stolzenberg ED, et al. Human β-defensin-1 is a salt-sensitive antibiotic in lung that is inactivated in cystic fibrosis. Cell 1997; 88: 553–560.

23. Groisman EA. How bacteria resist killing by host defense peptides. Trends Microbiol Sci 1994; 2: 444.

24. Nizet V, Ohtake T, Lauth X, et al. Innate antimicrobial peptide protects the skin from invasive bacterial infection. Nature 2001; 4144: 454.

25. Bowdish OME, Davidson DJ, Hancock REW. Immunomodulatory properties of defensins and cathelicidins. In: Shafer WM, ed. Antimicrobial peptides and human disease, Heidelberg: Springer Verlag, 2006. : 27.

26. Braff MH, Gallo RL. Antimicrobial peptides: an essential component of the skin defensive barrier. In: Shafer WM, ed. Antimicrobial peptides and human disease. Heidelberg: Springer Verlag, 2006; 91.

27. Salzman NH, Ghosh D, Huttner KM, et al. Protection against enteric salmonellosis in transgenic mice expressing a human intestinal defensin. Nature 2003; 422: 522.

28. Cole AM. Innate host defense of human vaginal and cervical mucosae. In: Shafer WM, ed. Antimicrobial peptides and human disease. Heidelberg: Springer Verlag, 2006; 199.

29. Ganz T, Metcalf JA, Gallin JJ, et al. Microbicidal/cytotoxic proteins of neutrophils are deficient in two disorders: Chediak–Higashi syndrome and 'specific' granule deficiency. J Clin Invest 1988; 82: 552.

bacteria. Low toxicity to the host on the one hand, and dormant persistence on the other, frequently result in symptom-free infection. Hence, disease is contingent upon, but not an inevitable result of, infection with intracellular bacteria. Moreover, diseases caused by intracellular bacteria often take a chronic course and neither pathogen nor immune response succeeds. As a final characteristic corollary of this ongoing struggle, pathology is determined by the immune response and less so by the microbe directly.

Intracellular bacteria segregate into two groups. The so-called facultative intracellular bacteria, although well adapted for living inside host cells, are also found in the extracellular space (with the probable exception of *Mycobacterium leprae*). Mononuclear phagocytes (MP) provide the preferred habitat for these bacteria, yet they are not restricted to macrophages and may infect various other host cells. This group (Table 25.1) includes the pathogenic mycobacteria *M. tuberculosis*/*M. bovis* and *M. leprae*, which are responsible for tuberculosis and leprosy, respectively,[2] *M. avium-intracellulare* complex and atypical mycobacteria (mycobacterial infections in the immunocompromised host),[3] *Salmonella* spp. (typhoid and other salmonelloses),[4] *Listeria monocytogenes* (listeriosis),[5] *Legionella pneumophila* (legionnaire's disease),[6] *Francisella tularensis* (tularemia),[7] and pathogenic species of *Brucella* (brucellosis).[8]

The second group, the obligate intracellular bacteria, depends exclusively on the intracellular milieu and fails to grow outside cells. Although some of these bacteria may well survive in MP, they prefer other cells – the so-called nonprofessional phagocytes – particularly epithelial and endothelial cells. This group comprises the pathogenic *Rickettsia* and *Chlamydia*: *Rickettsia prowazekii* (louse-borne typhus), *R. tsutsugamushi* (scrub typhus), *R. rickettsii* (Rocky Mountain spotted fever), *Ehrlichia* sp. (ehrlichiosis), and *Coxiella burnetii* (Q fever).[9] Different serovars of *Chlamydia trachomatis* cause urogenital and eye infections as well as trachoma and lymphogranuloma venerum, and both *C. psittaci* and *C. pneumoniae* are responsible for atypical pneumoniae (Table 25.1).[10]

The pathogenic mycobacteria are acid-fast bacilli that grow extremely slowly, with replication times of 12 hours and 12 days for *M. tuberculosis*/*M. bovis* and *M. leprae*, respectively.[3, 11] During chronic stages of infection and disease *M. tuberculosis* seems to be exclusively restricted to MP (Fig. 25.1), although bacteria may occasionally be found in lung parenchymal cells. In contrast, during active pulmonary tuberculosis the pathogen also multiplies in the cellular detritus of liquefied lesions. *M. leprae* is found in both MP and in various nonprofessional phagocytes, notably Schwann cells.

Salmonella typhi/*S. paratyphi*, as well as *Brucella* spp., are Gram-negative rods that not only live in macrophages of various internal organs but also in nonprofessional phagocytes such as epithelial cells. They also exist in extracellular niches, and the gallbladder provides the major source of bacterial dissemination during chronic carriage following recovery from typhoid fever. *Listeria monocytogenes*, a Gram-positive rod, is localized not only to resident tissue macrophages in spleen and liver, but also to hepatocytes.[5] *Listeria* seem also to persist within the gallbladder of mice. Alveolar macrophages are the major habitat for *L. pneumophila*, which may occasionally disseminate to other tissue sites via MP. The pathogenic mycobacteria, *Salmonella*, *Brucella*, and *Legionella* primarily survive killing inside the phagosome by deviating from their intracellular fate, thereby interfering with macrophage effector functions (Figs 25.1 and 25.2). In contrast, *Listeria* primarily evade macrophage killing by leaving the phagosome and entering the cytoplasm.

Chlamydia undergo a distinct lifecycle: they infect host cells as elementary bodies and then develop into reticulate bodies that multiply in phagosomes and evade killing by inhibiting phagosome–lysosome fusion (Figs 25.1 and 25.2).[10, 12] Once sufficiently high numbers have been reached, they transmutate to elementary bodies ready to infect additional host cells. Columnar epithelial cells provide the preferential habitat for the different serovars of *C. trachomatis*. The lymphogranuloma venerum-causing serovars, however, do not remain in the epithelial layers and spread to lymphatic organs, where they infect endothelial and lymphatic cells. The pneumonia-causing *Chlamydia*, *C. psittaci* and *C. pneumoniae*, are typically located in lung epithelial cells.

Rickettsia are 'energy parasites,' that is, they depend on a supply of coenzyme A, NAD, and ATP from their host cells.[9] *Rickettsia* species, preferentially inhabit vascular endothelial cells. Their virulence in entering the host cell cytoplasm to scavenge ATP also supports their escape from being killed due to phagocytosis by macrophages (Fig. 25.2). *Ehrlichia* species are zoonotic pathogens transmitted by ticks, which cause a rare disease in humans.[13] They survive in endothelial cells and macrophages by inhibiting phagolysosome fusion. *Coxiella burnetii* preferentially parasitizes lung macrophages and parenchymal cells.[14] It resists macrophage attack within acidified phagolysosomes by interfering with macrophage effector functions.

▌ KEY CONCEPTS

CHARACTERISTIC FEATURES OF INTRACELLULAR BACTERIAL INFECTIONS

Pathogen

>> Intracellular living

>> Survival in phagocytes

>> Low toxicity for the host

Immune response

>> T-cell-dependent

>> Antibodies less important

>> Activated macrophages are prime effector cells

>> Interleukin-12/-18 and interferon-γ are key cytokines

>> Granulomatous tissue reaction (host immune-mediated)

>> Delayed-type hypersensitivity

■ DISEASES CAUSED BY INTRACELLULAR BACTERIA ■

GENERAL FEATURES

Only a few intracellular bacteria, such as *L. monocytogenes*, are sterilely eradicated once the immune response has reached its height. More often, the intracellular habitat provides a protective niche that promotes persistent infection in the face of an ongoing immune response. In this case the bacteria can persist for long periods of time without causing clinical signs

Table 25.1 Major infectious diseases caused by intracellular bacteria

Disease	Pathogen	Transmission	Distribution	Incubation time	Preferred port of entry	Preferred target cell	Intracellular location and/or evasion mechanism	Therapy
Facultative intracellular bacteria								
Tuberculosis	*Mycobacterium tuberculosis*	Inhalation of microdroplets containing pathogen	Worldwide	Years (primary infection) Weeks (reactivation)	Lung	Macrophage Dendritic cells	Early phagosome, arrest of phagosome maturation, interference with ROI, resistance against lysosomal enzymes	Multidrug therapy including isoniazid and rifampin for 6 months
Leprosy	*Mycobacterium leprae*	Intimate contact with infected persons, nasal droplets	Southeast Asia, Africa, South and Middle America	Years	Nasopharyngeal mucosa	Primarily macrophages and Schwann cells	Phagosome, cytoplasm (?) interference with ROI, resistance against lysosomal enzymes	Multidrug therapy including dapsone, rifampin
Typhoid fever	*Salmonella typhi/ S.paratyphi*	Contaminated food, fecal/oral	Worldwide	7–10 days	Gut	Macrophage	Phagosome, resistance to host defensins, inhibition of phagosome–lysosome fusion, interference with ROI	Chloramphenicol, trimethoprim plus sulfamethoxazole
Brucellosis	*Brucella sp.*	Zoonosis	Worldwide	Weeks to months	Respiratory tract, gut, broken skin	Macrophage	ER-associated phagolysosome, resistance to lysosomal enzymes	Tetracyclines
Legionnaire's disease	*Legionella pneumophila*	Aerosol transmission from aerosol-producing systems	Worldwide	2–10 days	Lung	Alveolar macrophage	ER-associated phagosome inhibition of phagosome–lysosome fusion, interference with ROI	Erythromycin and rifampin,
Listeriosis	*Listeria monocytogenes*	Contaminated food	Worldwide	Days to months	Gut	Macrophage, hepatocyte	Cytoplasm	Penicillin, ampicillin, co-trimoxazole

Continued

Table 25.1 Major infectious diseases caused by intracellular bacteria—Cont'd

Disease	Pathogen	Transmission	Distribution	Incubation time	Preferred port of entry	Preferred target cell	Intracellular location and/or evasion mechanism	Therapy
Obligate intracellular bacteria								
Rocky Mountain spotted fever	Rickettsia rickettsii	Tick bite	Western hemisphere	1 week	Blood	Vascular endothelial cell, smooth-muscle cell	Cytoplasm	Tetracycline
Epidemic (louse-borne) typhus, Brill–Zinsser disease	Rickettsia prowazekii	Louse feces	South America, Africa, Asia	1 week	Lung, broken skin, mucosa	Vascular endothelial cell	Cytoplasm	Tetracycline
Endemic (murine) typhus	Rickettsia typhi	Flea bite	Worldwide	1 week	Blood	Vascular endothelial cell	Cytoplasm	Tetracycline
Scrub typhus	Rickettsia tsutsugamushi	Mite bite	Pacific	1 week	Blood	Vascular endothelial cell	Cytoplasm	Tetracycline
Q fever	Coxiella burnetii	Inhalation of aerosols, tick bite (zoonosis)	Worldwide	2–4 weeks	Lung, respiratory tract	Macrophage, lung parenchyma cell	Phagolysosome	Tetracycline
Urogenital infection	Chlamydia trachomatis (serovars D–K)	Sexual intercourse	Worldwide	1–3 weeks	Urogenital tract	Columnar epithelial cell	Phagosome (as reticulate body), inhibition of phagosome–lysosome fusion	Tetracycline, doxycycline, quinolone
Conjunctivitis, trachoma	Chlamydia trachomatis (serovars A–C)	Smear infection congenital infection	Africa	1–3 weeks (conjunctivitis), years (trachoma)	Eye	Columnar epithelial cell	Phagosome (as reticulate body), inhibition of phagosome–lysosome fusion	Tetracycline, doxycycline quinolone
Lymphogranuloma venereum	Chlamydia trachomatis (serovars L1–L3)	Sexual intercourse	Asia, Africa, South America	1–3 weeks	Urogenital tract	Columnar epithelial cells, endothelia, lymphatic cell	Phagosome (as reticulate body), inhibition of phagosome–lysosome fusion	Tetracycline, doxycycline, quinolone
Pneumonia, psittacosis	Chlamydia psittaci	Aerosol (zoonosis), contact with infected birds	Worldwide	1–4 weeks	Lung	Macrophage, lung parenchyma cell	Phagosome (as reticulate body), inhibition of phagosome–lysosome fusion	Tetracycline
Pneumonia	Chlamydia pneumoniae	Aerosol (human to human)	Worldwide	1–4 weeks	Lung	Lung epithelial cells endothelial cells	Phagosome (as reticulate body), inhibition of phagosome–lysosome fusion	Erythromycin

ROI, reactive oxygen intermediates.

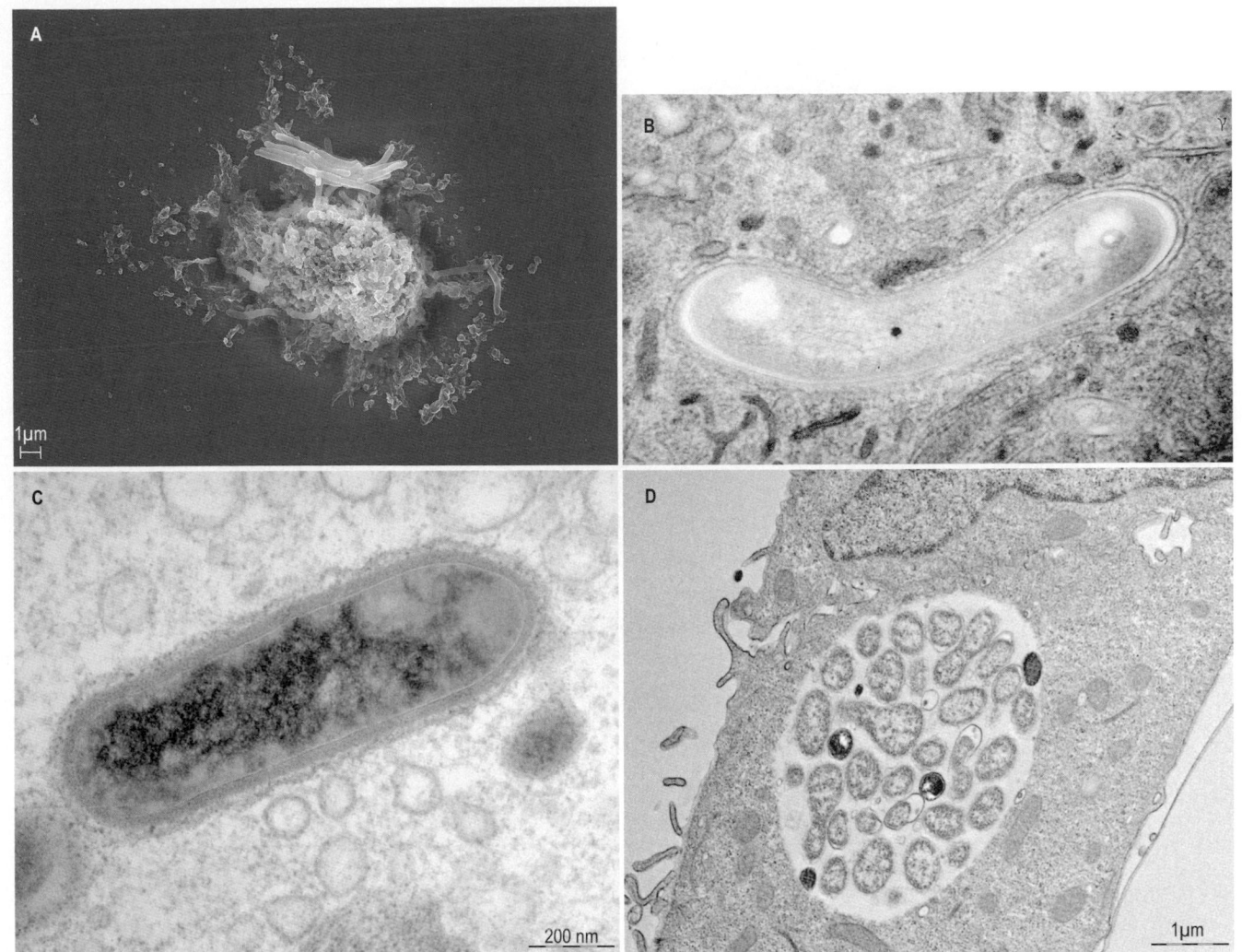

Fig. 25.1 Phagocytosis and intracellular location of bacteria. **(A)** Uptake of *Mycobacterium tuberculosis* by a macrophage (scanning electron microscopy). **(B)** *M. tuberculosis* inside phagosomes of a macrophage. **(C)** Intracytoplasmic location of *Listeria monocytogenes*. **(D)** Inclusion body containing *Chlamydia pneumoniae* reticulocytes inside a fibroblast. (Courtesy of V. Brinkmann, Max Planck Institute for Infection Biology.)

of illness, and are reactivated to cause disease only after the immune response has become compromised. This occurs in *M. tuberculosis* infection, resulting in disease years or decades after primary contact. In fact, disease need not arise from infection at all: in many regions, for example, the majority of adults harbor *M. tuberculosis* without suffering from clinical disease. Alternatively, disease can develop directly after primary infection, during maturation of the immune response, or with regression once the immune response is sufficiently strong. Yet sterile eradication of the pathogen is rarely achieved: bacteria persist latently and illness may re-emerge at a later time. For example, *R. prowazekii* may persist for decades after convalescence from typhus, to cause Brill–Zinsser disease later.

In contrast to most intracellular bacteria, some possess components that profoundly influence the course of disease, e.g., the lipopolysaccharides (LPS) of *Brucella* and *Salmonella*. Chronic persistence inside host cells, however, depends on the target cell remaining intact and physiologically

active. Accordingly, many intracellular bacteria are of low toxicity and do not have dramatic direct effects on their host. Instead, pathogenesis is largely determined by the immune response. Classic examples of this concept include granuloma liquefaction in acute tuberculosis, which severely affects lung function, and eye scarring as a consequence of chronic or recurring *C. trachomatis* infection that ultimately leads to trachoma.

The survival of intracellular bacteria in MP has major consequences for pathology. Although many intracellular bacteria show some organ tropism, dissemination to other organs frequently occurs, resulting in different disease forms. For example, tuberculosis is generally manifested in the lung, yet any other organ can be affected. In contrast to other salmonella, *S. typhi/S. paratyphi* are not restricted to the gastrointestinal tract but are disseminated to internal organs, primarily the liver and spleen. In these cases the type of clinical disease depends markedly on the infected tissue type.

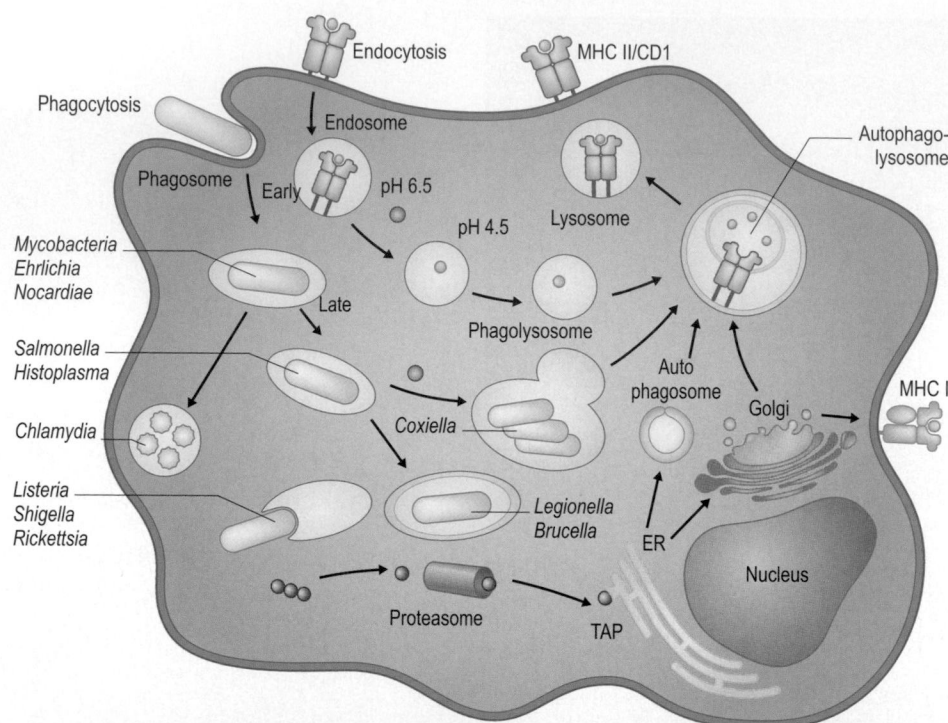

Fig. 25.2 Intracellular niches occupied by facultative and obligate intracellular bacteria. After particle uptake, the fate of the maturing phagosome parallels that of endosomes. After phagosome formation the vesicular membrane acquires the proton ATPase and acidifies towards pH 4–5, thereby maturing to the late endosomal and finally the lysosomal stage. *Mycobacterium* spp. and *Ehrlichia* spp. block maturation of their phagosomes early on, *Salmonella* allow slightly more maturation and *Coxiella* is delivered to the phagolysosome. On the way there, *Listeria* spp. and *Rickettsia* spp. escape into the cytoplasm, and *Legionella* spp. and *Brucella* spp. associate with membranes of the endoplasmic reticulum. *Chlamydia* spp. finally induce inclusion bodies associating with mitochondria.

SPECIFIC FEATURES

Tuberculosis

Tubercle bacilli are typically inhaled in microdroplets and then engulfed by alveolar macrophages, which transport the pathogens to the lung interstitia. There, as well as in the draining lymph nodes, primary lesions develop that rarely cause disease directly. The combination of both types of lesions is called a Ghon complex. Instead, the infection remains dormant under the control of the immune system. Once the immune response becomes debilitated, however, dormant bacteria are reactivated and pulmonary tuberculosis develops. Bacteria disseminate to other sites in the lung and occasionally to other organs, including the kidneys, liver, and central nervous system. Infection of immunocompromised patients, especially those with acquired immunodeficiency syndrome (AIDS), or newborns results in the rapid development of disease (miliary tuberculosis). Tuberculosis represents a major health problem worldwide, including an increasing incidence in many industrialized countries. In 2004, 3.9 million active tuberculosis cases were notified worldwide, and 1.7 million people died of the disease. However, as the incidence of reporting is much lower in countries where the estimated infection rate is greatest, the World Health Organization (WHO) estimates that there are in fact more than 9 million new cases globally. Yet, the much larger estimated number of 2 billion individuals infected with *M. tuberculosis* illustrates well the dissociation of infection from disease. The emergence of multidrug-resistant strains has further complicated the situation, and a recent study has conclusively demonstrated that, following successful treatment, reinfection can occur later in life.[15] The currently available vaccine bacille Calmette-Guérin (BCG), an attenuated strain derived from the agent of bovine tuberculosis, *M. bovis*, shows only low and variable protection against pulmonary tuberculosis in adults.

Leprosy

M. leprae is most likely transmitted by contact with patients who shed organisms in nasal secretions and lesion exudates. Leprosy primarily affects the nerves and the skin, frequently leading to stigmatizing deformities.[16] It is a spectral disease. At the more benign tuberculoid pole, strong T-cell responses succeed in restricting microbial growth in well-defined lesions containing few bacilli. In contrast, at the lepromatous pole bacterial growth is unrestricted and lesions contain abundant bacilli within macrophages lacking signs of activation. Regulatory T cells (Treg) and other types of immunosuppression have been implicated in this latter type of disease.[17] Throughout the spectrum Schwann cells are affected, promoting nerve damage and anesthesia. This results in injuries and secondary infections that significantly exaggerate the disease.

Following successful therapeutic regimens the incidence of leprosy has declined dramatically over the past decade, and in 1996 WHO estimated a global case load of 1 million with decreasing tendency.

Atypical mycobacterial infections

These environmental microbes are unable to persist within activated macrophages and thus rarely cause disease in individuals with competent immune status.[3] *Mycobacterium scrofulaceum* occasionally causes lymphadenitis in children, and *M. kansasii* primarily causes infections in elderly men with pre-existing lung disease. As a consequence of human immunodeficiency virus (HIV) infection, however, nontubercle mycobacteria (NTM), primarily *M. avium/M. intracellulare*, have gained clinical importance, and this infection is recognized as one of the most common complications of AIDS[6] (Chapter 37).

Typhoid or enteric fever

Typhoid is a foodborne disease caused by *S. typhi/S. paratyphi* in humans. The pathogens are disseminated within MP from the gastrointestinal tract to macrophage-rich organs, particularly the liver, spleen, and lymph nodes. Accordingly, typhoid is characterized by systemic symptoms such as prolonged fever and malaise with sustained bacteremia, although diarrhea or constipation may also be present. In some cases an asymptomatic carrier state can persist as a result of chronic infection of the gallbladder, which maintains the environmental reservoir of infection in endemic areas. Typhoid fever remains a major cause of morbidity and mortality, with 16 million cases and 600 000 deaths annually worldwide.

Gastroenteritis

S. typhimurium and *S. enteritidis* are the major causes of salmonella gastroenteritis in humans, which occurs mainly as a result of the ingestion of contaminated food or water. The bacteria rapidly cross the intestinal epithelia and replicate in the lamina propria, inducing an influx of polymorphonuclear granulocytes (PMN), which is generally sufficient to resolve the infection within 7 days. In rare cases the bacteria enter the bloodstream and cause systemic bacteremia, most notably in AIDS patients, where death can occur as a result of septic shock.

Brucellosis

This globally distributed zoonosis afflicts various domestic animals but is rare in humans. It is caused by *Brucella abortus, B. melitensis,* or *B. suis,* which primarily infect cows, goats, and pigs, respectively.[8] The bacteria are transmitted to humans aerogenically, through abraded skin or the gastrointestinal tract. Lesions are primarily found within macrophage-rich tissues, especially the spleen and bone marrow. Human brucellosis is characterized by systemic symptoms, particularly undulent fever. Although the disease often remains subclinical, in some patients it becomes chronic, and relapses and remissions may develop.

Listeriosis

Although epidemic outbreaks of this foodborne disease have been observed, disease manifestations are most severe in patients with a compromised immune system where the central nervous system becomes involved and fatal bacteremia can result.[5] Additionally, as these bacteria are able to cross the placenta, listeriosis is a major cause of perinatal and neonatal disease, typically resulting in abortion. The disease is increasingly recognized, with about 2000 cases in the USA in 1992, and an incidence rate of 5 cases per million population.

Legionnaire's disease or legionellosis

Legionnaire's disease is caused by *Legionella pneumophila*, an environmental bacterium that persists within ameba living in water reservoirs (e.g., air-cooling systems), from where it is spread aerogenically.[6] Infection is exacerbated by a compromised immune status. Characteristically, legionnaire's disease presents as atypical pneumonia associated with general symptoms and complicated by extrapulmonary infection, renal failure, and lung abscesses.

Lymphogranuloma venerum

Lymphogranuloma venerum, a sexually transmitted disease, is highly prevalent in Africa, Southeast Asia, and South America. It is caused by the L1, L2, and L3 serotypes of *Chlamydia trachomatis*, which are disseminated from the urogenital tract to local lymph nodes and then to the skin. Accordingly, lymphogranuloma venerum is characterized by lymph node swelling and skin lesions that are accompanied by systemic complications.

Chlamydial urethritis, cervicitis, and conjunctivitis

C. trachomatis serovars D–K remain in epithelial cells of the urogenital tract, causing cervicitis and urethritis. In women, infertility may develop as a result of chronic or recurrent infection. In neonates, congenital infection during birth may result in conjunctivitis and pneumonia. Urogenital infections by *Chlamydia* occur worldwide and are now considered to be the most common bacterial sexually transmitted disease, with an estimated 90 million new infections occurring annually.[12]

Trachoma

Smear infections of the eye with *C. trachomatis* serovars A, B, and C cause inclusion conjunctivitis.[10] As a consequence of multiple chronic infections and of the resulting immune response, scars develop that eventually injure the cornea, leading to trachoma. It is estimated that 400–600 million people suffer from *C. trachomatis* infection, and 6 million of these suffer visual impairment worldwide.

Chlamydia pneumoniae

C. pneumoniae (formerly known as *C. trachomatis* TWAR strain) is the cause of mild respiratory disease in young adults and may cause serious infections in older, more debilitated patients. Atypical pneumonia may also be caused as a result of infection with *C. psittaci*, although this zoonosis is relatively rare.

Typhus

Rickettsia prowazekii, R. typhi, and *R. tsutsugamushi* cause diseases of varying severity.[9] They are transmitted by arthropods and infect vascular endothelial cells at the site of an insect bite or scratch, causing skin reactions.

Subsequently, pathogens are disseminated to the central organs and more general symptoms develop. Globally, typhus is of minor importance.

Rocky Mountain spotted fever, ehrlichiosis

Rocky Mountain spotted fever is caused by *R. rickettsii*. Infection of the vascular endothelium leads to systemic symptoms and skin manifestations that may be followed by shock and neurological complications.[9] Worldwide, this disease, as well as Mediterranean spotted fever caused by *R. conorii*, is of minor importance, as is probably ehrlichiosis, a newly emerging zoonosis transmitted by ticks and caused by various *Ehrlichia* species, mainly *E. chaffeensis*.[13] Disease manifestations include generalized symptoms such as fever and muscle pain.

Tularemia

This rare zoonosis in humans, caused by *Francisella tularensis*, is mainly found in rabbits and has recently gained wider recognition due to its potential for dual use.[7] This Gram-negative bacterium survives in macrophages and primarily causes acute pneumonia as well as sores of the skin, with subsequent involvement of the lymph nodes.

■ THE IMMUNE RESPONSE AGAINST INTRACELLULAR BACTERIA ■

INNATE IMMUNITY

The innate immune response is a rapid and largely nonspecific reaction that coordinates the initial response to pathogens (Chapter 3). It depends critically on the ability of cells – primarily MP and dendritic cells (DC) – to recognize a broad variety of pathogens. This is accomplished by their ability to discriminate between molecules synthesized exclusively by bacteria such as LPS, bacterial lipoproteins and lipoteichoic acids, and self molecules. Phagocytic cells possess a set of germline-encoded pattern recognition receptors (PRR) that recognize invariant molecular patterns shared by a variety of microbes, the so-called pathogen, or better, microbe-associated molecular patterns (PAMP or MAMP). These receptors include the macrophage mannose receptor (MMR), DC-specific ICAM-3-grabbing nonintegrin (DC-SIGN) both of which bind mannose residues, dectin 1 (binds β-glucans), CD14 (binds LPS, lipoarabinomannan (LAM)), scavenger receptors (SR-A, SR-B), CD36 (binds microbial diacyl glycerides), and the Toll-like receptors (TLR).[18, 19] It has been suggested that, whereas PRR are required to bind and internalize the pathogen, it is the TLR that discriminate between the pathogens and provide the necessary intracellular signaling events. It should, however, be noted that intracellular signaling events can also be triggered by ligand binding to MMR, dectin 1, or DC-SIGN. Intracellular PRR include NOD-1 and -2-recognizing bacteria-derived muramyl dipeptides or diaminopimelic acid, respectively.[20] The TLR system appears as an innate scanning mechanism for microbial patterns to recognize and distinguish between a wide array of microbes, i.e., bacteria, viruses, parasites, and fungi. TLR are present as homo- or heterodimers on the plasma membrane or within endosomes/phagosomes (Fig. 25.3).[18, 21] TLR ligands of bacterial origin comprise di- and tri-acylic lipoproteins, LPS, and flagellin, which are recognized

by TLR-2/6, TLR2/1, TLR-4/4, or TLR-5/5, respectively. The vast array of mycobacterial cell wall lipids such as LAM, trehalose dimycolate (TDM), and phosphatidyl inositol mannosides (PIM) bind either TLR-2 or TLR-4. Lipoteichoic acid (LTA) of Gram-positive bacteria is recognized by TLR-2. TLR-9 binds low methylated bacterial DNA containing CpG motifs within endosomes (Fig. 25.3). Ligand binding to TLR initiates an inflammatory response, including release of proinflammatory mediators.[21]

Binding of a bacterium to certain host receptors leads to the active internalization of the organism, a prerequisite for an intracellular pathogen. Only professional phagocytes such as MP and PMN perform this host-directed process. Direct binding to a receptor is frequently supported indirectly by complement components and immunoglobulin, which bind to complement receptors and Fc receptors, respectively. Uptake via specific receptors is called the 'zipper mechanism,' which distinguishes it from internalization resulting from nonspecific adhesion, known as the 'trigger mechanism.' In some cases intracellular bacteria can exploit nonprofessional phagocytes, which provide a less hostile environment owing to their inability to mobilize antibacterial effector mechanisms. Vascular endothelial cells, epithelial cells, Schwann cells, and hepatocytes are the preferred habitats for *Rickettsia* spp., *C. trachomatis*, *M. leprae*, and *L. monocytogenes*, respectively. These host cells express minimal phagocytic activity, thereby necessitating that the bacteria induce their own internalization. This invasion process requires tight adhesion to specific cellular receptors that are capable of mediating the uptake process, including members of the integrin and growth factor receptor families. The tight binding of bacteria to these receptors activates the intracellular cytoskeleton to cause macropinocytosis, i.e., membrane ruffling, invagination, and finally phagosome formation.[4]

NATURAL KILLER CELLS

Natural killer (NK) cells were originally characterized by their capacity to lyse susceptible tumor cells in an MHC-independent fashion. They are large granular lymphocytes identified by the CD56 marker. Several lines of evidence indicate a contribution of NK cells to antibacterial resistance.[22] As NK cells express functions also performed by T lymphocytes, they contribute to early host defense before the appearance of activated T cells in normal individuals (Chapter 18). They may also fulfill an important compensatory role in T-cell-deficient patients.

Incubation of peripheral blood leukocytes from healthy individuals with a variety of intracellular bacteria induces potent NK-cell activity *in vitro*. Furthermore, infection of mice with various intracellular bacteria causes strong NK-cell activation *in vivo*. NK cells have been shown to lyse host cells infected with various intracellular bacteria, including *Legionella*, *Mycobacteria*, *Salmonella*, *Chlamydia*, and rickettsiae.[22] Moreover, NK cells are potent interferon-γ (IFN-γ) producers, thus contributing to macrophage activation (Fig. 25.4). Severe combined immunodeficiency disease (SCID) mice, which are virtually free of functionally active T and B cells, are able to control experimental listeriosis due to enhanced NK-cell activity as a compensatory mechanism. However, they are unable to eradicate the bacteria completely, and ultimately succumb to disease. To date, the exact mechanism as to how NK cells distinguish infected from uninfected cells has not been elucidated. NK cells possess two types of surface receptors. One group comprises "activating" receptors such as NKp30, NKp46, and NKG2D, which trigger killing by NK cells, whereas others inhibit cytotoxicity.[23] Of the

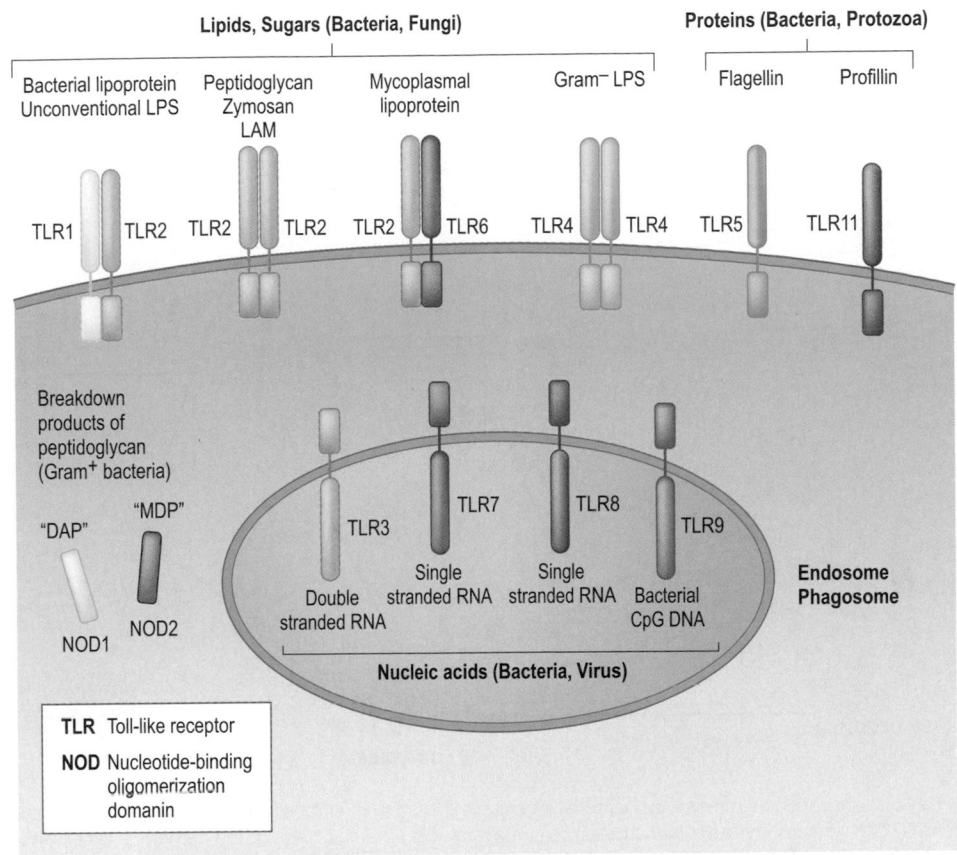

Lipids, Sugars (Bacteria, Fungi)

Proteins (Bacteria, Protozoa)

Bacterial lipoprotein
Unconventional LPS

Peptidoglycan
Zymosan
LAM

Mycoplasmal
lipoprotein

Gram⁻ LPS

Flagellin

Profillin

TLR1 TLR2 TLR2 TLR2 TLR2 TLR6 TLR4 TLR4 TLR5 TLR11

Breakdown
products of
peptidoglycan
(Gram⁺ bacteria)

"DAP" "MDP"

NOD1 NOD2

TLR3 TLR7 TLR8 TLR9

Double
stranded RNA

Single
stranded RNA

Single
stranded RNA

Bacterial
CpG DNA

Endosome
Phagosome

Nucleic acids (Bacteria, Virus)

TLR Toll-like receptor

NOD Nucleotide-binding
oligomerization
domanin

Fig. 25.3 Toll-like receptors (TLR) and nucleotide-binding oligomerization domain (NOD) are innate pattern recognition receptors (PRR) for microbe-associated molecular patterns (MAMP). As distinct homo- or heterodimers at the plasma membrane or within endosomes they recognize bacterial glycolipids, polysaccharides, lipopeptides, flagellins, and low methylated DNA (CpG). NODs are cytoplasmic receptors for the bacterial degradation products muramyl dipeptide (MDP) derived from peptidoglycan and diaminopimelic acid (DAP).

activating receptors NKp30, NKp46, and NKG2D, the latter two are induced by macrophages infected with *M. tuberculosis* and mediate NK-cell-mediated killing of infected target cells. Some of the inhibitory receptors recognize MHC class I molecules. Thus, NK cells specifically lyse target cells expressing low levels of MHC class I molecules, and therefore a possible recognition mechanism would be alteration in MHC class I expression. Notably, surface expression of MHC molecules on macrophages is often reduced as a consequence of bacterial infection.

MACROPHAGE ACTIVATION AND EFFECTOR MECHANISMS

Both MP and PMN represent major effector cells in the defense against bacterial infections. PMN are within the first line of defense and efficiently kill microbial invaders, thus contributing to limiting the size of inoculum. Lack of PMN strongly enhances susceptibility to fast-growing *Listeria* and *Salmonella*. However, because of their short lifespan, PMN are an inappropriate habitat for intracellular bacteria, particularly for slow-growing ones.[24] Against such bacteria, the highly antimicrobial potential of PMN also appears to be of low effect. In general, intracel-

lular bacteria are often less accessible to PMN because of their location inside cells. PMN, however, due to succumbing to apoptosis within less than 1 day of their lifespan, may be exploited by intracellular pathogens as 'Trojan horses' in order to enter macrophages unrecognized enwrapped within apoptotic bodies from dying PMN.[25] In contrast, tissue macrophages have a long lifespan and, in their resting stage, possess only medium antimicrobial potential. Resting tissue macrophages therefore serve as a suitable habitat for numerous intracellular bacteria (Fig. 25.2). Activation by cytokines leads to the mobilization of various antibacterial effector mechanisms, thus transforming MP from residence to effector cell (Table 25.2). Yet intracellular bacteria are able to counteract assaults by activated macrophages, at least partially, by evading, interfering with, or resisting their effector mechanisms.

The transition from resting to activated macrophage is a multifactorial and highly regulated process involving the induction of interleukin-12 (IL-12), IL-18, and related cytokines (IL-23, IL-27) by TLR ligands (Fig. 25.4). This in turn stimulates the production of IFN-γ from NK cells, which subsequently promotes development of Th1 T cells. Thereby, production of IFN-γ, the central macrophage-activating cytokine, is perpetuated, ultimately leading to tumor necrosis factor-α (TNF-α)

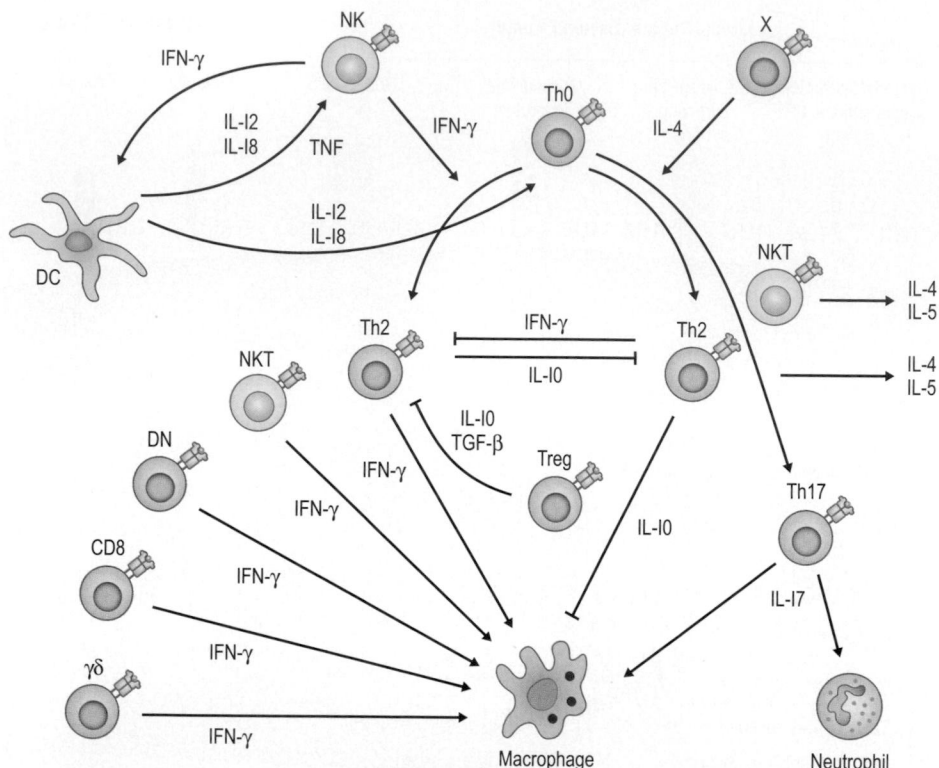

Fig. 25.4 Preferential Th1-cell activation in intracellular bacterial infections. Although in intracellular bacterial infections the activation of macrophages by interferon-γ (IFN-γ) from Th1 cells is the predominant event, this step is influenced by numerous other cytokines. Natural killer (NK) cells are the first cells upon microbial encounter to secrete IFN-γ. In terms of Th1-cell stimulation, interleukin-12 (IL-12), IL-18, and IFN-γ provide activating signals, whereas the Th2-derived cytokines IL-4 and IL-10 are inhibitory. At the level of macrophages (MP), IFN-γ, produced first by NK cells and NKT cells and later on by antigen-specific T-cell subsets, promotes the development of Th1 cells and MP activation. Th17 cells promote inflammation through IL-17 secretion and neutrophil activation. Regulatory T cells (Treg) dampen inflammation through IL-10 and/or transforming growth factor-β (TGF-β) secretion in order to minimize immunopathology. IL-10 also counteracts macrophage activation. DN represents double-negative (CD4– CD8–) T cell.

secretion (Fig. 25.4 and Table 25.2). However, IFN-γ production and macrophage activation are inhibited by microbial components such as phenolic glycolipid from *M. leprae*, as well as by anti-inflammatory cytokines such as IL-4, IL-10, and TGF-β.[17] Although these cytokines can be produced by various cell types, including DC, macrophages, B cells, NK T, and Th2 cells, Treg (CD25+/FOXP3+) have been identified as the prime players in controlling IFN-γ-mediated responses (see below). Mechanisms to counter-regulate IFN-γ function can limit exacerbated inflammation and immunopathology.

Once fully activated, MP are capable of killing most microbial pathogens, including certain intracellular bacteria. Only the most resistant bacteria, such as *M. tuberculosis*, are not fully eliminated, in which case persistent organisms may emerge. Activated macrophages not only express antimicrobial activities, they also secrete biologically active components that significantly influence the outcome of disease (Table 25.2). First, they release proteolytic enzymes that contribute to local tissue destruction; second, they secrete cytokines that regulate phagocyte attraction, granuloma formation, and macrophage activation.

Bacterial killing by toxic reactive nitrogen intermediates (RNI) and reactive oxygen intermediates (ROI)

Activation of a membrane-bound NADPH oxidase by stimulation with IFN-γ or IgG initiates an oxidative burst that generates the toxic ROI, O_2^-, H_2O_2, OH^-, $^1O_2$, and 'OH radical (Table 25.2).[26] In human PMN and blood monocytes that possess myeloperoxidase, the ROI activity is further supported by the formation of hypochlorous acid. Oxidation and/or chlorination of bacterial lipids and proteins result in the death of many bacteria. The importance of ROI in antibacterial defense is underlined by the recurrent infections in patients whose phagocytes fail to generate an oxidative burst (Chapter 21). Production of RNI from activated murine macrophages generated by inducible nitric oxide synthase (NOS-2 or iNOS) is well established (Table 25.2).[27] Expression of NOS-2 has also been detected in monocytes of patients suffering from a variety of infectious diseases. The 'NO radical is generated exclusively from L-arginine and then further oxidized to NO_2^- and NO_3^-. The formation of 'NO is catalyzed by

Table 25.2 Antibacterial effector mechanisms of activated macrophages and microbial evasion strategies

Macrophage effector mechanism	Microbial evasion strategy
Production of reactive oxygen intermediates (ROI)	Uptake via complement receptors Production of ROI detoxifying molecules (superoxide dismutase, catalase) Bacterial ROI scavengers (e.g., phenolic glycolipids, sulfatides, lipoarabinomannans)
Production of reactive nitrogen intermediates (RNI)	Inhibition of phagosome maturation Most ROI detoxifiers also affect RNI
Other types of intraphagolysosomal killing	Evasion into the cytoplasm Robust cell wall resistant to low pH / lysosomal hydrolases
Phagosome acidification Phagosome–lysosome fusion	Prevention of phagosome maturation by bacterial components, e.g., glycolipids
Defensins	Modification of cell wall lipid A
Reduced iron supply (transferrin receptor downregulation, lipocalins)	Microbial siderophores
Tryptophan degradation	Affects *Chlamydia* sp., other bacteria upregulate endogenous tryptophan synthesis

NOS-2, which is stimulated by both immunological stimuli such as IFN-γ and TNF, and microbial products such as LPS, LTA, and mycobacterial lipids. The RNI exert their bactericidal activity by destroying iron-/sulfur-containing reactive centers of bacterial enzymes, and by synergizing with ROI to form highly reactive peroxynitrite (ONOO⁻).

Tryptophan degradation

Deprivation of required nutrients appears to be an obvious strategy for microbial killing, yet it seems to be employed rarely, with restricted tryptophan supply being the best-known example. Tryptophan degradation is achieved by the enzyme indolamine 2,3-deoxygenase, which degrades tryptophan to kynurenine (Table 25.2). This reaction is induced by IFN-γ in both MP and IFN-γ-responsive nonprofessional phagocytes and inhibits the growth of *C. psittaci* and *C. trachomatis* inside human macrophages and epithelial cells.[28]

Antimicrobial peptides

Defensins and basic proteins are small lysosomal polypeptides that are microbicidal at basic pH and are particularly abundant in phagocytes.[29] Many of these compounds have been shown to have microbicidal activity against intracellular bacteria, particularly granulysin, which is present in the granules of human NK and cytolytic T cells. This molecule kills a number of pathogens *in vitro*, including *L. monocytogenes* and *S. typhimurium*, as well as intracellular *M. tuberculosis*.[30] Another antimicrobial peptide, cathelicidin, is modulated by vitamin D in a TLR-2 dependent manner to kill *M. tuberculosis*.[31]

Intracellular iron

Iron is required for many biochemical processes in both prokaryotes and eukaryotes. In light of this, competition between host cell and pathogen is established for the intracellular iron pool. Both cell types,

therefore, possess specific iron-binding proteins that promote the uptake and intracellular distribution of iron.[32] Extracellular iron is bound to transferrin and lactoferrin and is internalized by the transferrin receptor into an early recycling compartment, whose mildly acidic pH permits the uncoupling of iron from its receptor. Within the host cell most of the iron is bound to ferritin. Intracellular bacteria such as mycobacteria, *Brucella*, and *Chlamydia* have evolved a number of iron-binding proteins or siderophores which are upregulated in the intracellular environment. As countermeasures, activated macrophages downregulate surface expression of the transferrin receptor to limit intracellular iron (Table 25.2). Moreover, PMN-derived lipocalins bind bacterial siderophores, including those from mycobacteria to seclude iron from microbial usage.

MICROBIAL EVASION FROM, INTERFERENCE WITH, AND RESISTANCE TO MACROPHAGE KILLING

Strategies against toxic effector molecules

Many intracellular bacteria have exploited successful strategies against macrophage effector molecules (Table 26.2). One mechanism is determined by the receptor that is used for pathogen entry into the host cell. Internalization via complement receptors inhibits the production of IL-12, a cytokine critical in facilitating macrophage activation.[33] Engulfment by this receptor also bypasses activation of the oxidative burst, thereby avoiding ROI production. Similarly, engaging MMR and DC-SIGN for uptake triggers IL-10 and TGF-β secretion. Several intracellular bacteria also produce ROI detoxifiers, including superoxide dismutase and catalase, which nullify O_2 and H_2O_2, respectively. Finally, a number of small bacterial products, such as the phenolic glycolipid and LAM of mycobacteria, scavenge ROI. Many of the strategies used to counteract the effects of ROI also overlap in their effects on RNI. A modification of lipid A renders Gram-negative bacteria, including *Salmonella*, resistant to the effects of host antimicrobial peptides.[29]

Intraphagosomal survival

Inhibition of phagolysosome fusion represents a major intracellular survival strategy for a number of intracellular bacteria, including *M. tuberculosis*/*M. bovis*, *S. typhi*/*S. paratyphi*, *L. pneumophila*, and *C. trachomatis* (Fig. 25.2). The inclusion body formed following phagocytosis of *Chlamydia* is excluded from the classic pathway of phagosome maturation and forms tight associations with mitochondria that provide a rich source of ATP.[10] In contrast, mycobacteria arrest maturation of this compartment at an early endosomal stage. This compartment does not acidify owing to a paucity of vacuolar $H^+ATPase$; at the same time, it exchanges molecules with the plasma membrane such as the transferrin receptor to access iron.[34] The exact mechanism as to how mycobacteria influence phagosome maturation remains unclear and various suggestions have been made, such as the production of ammonia or cell wall glycolipids and their physicochemical properties. What is clear is that activation of MP with IFN-γ restores maturation of the mycobacterial phagosome, resulting in a drop in mycobacterial viability. *Salmonella* species express two secretion apparatus in order to inject effector molecules into the host cell cytoplasm to achieve invasion and intracellular survival. These effectors induce cytoskeleton rearrangements in the host cell to macropinocytose the bacteria and promote phagosome arrest at an early to late endosomal stage (Fig. 25.2). Finally, *Legionella* and *Brucella* after a transient phagosomal stage enter compartments enclosed by endoplasmic reticulum (ER) membranes, suggested to resemble autophagosomes, to escape delivery to phagolysosomes.[35]

Escape into cytoplasm

A successful strategy for survival inside activated macrophages is the egression from the phagosome into the cytoplasm, which has been exploited by *L. monocytogenes* and the various pathogenic *Rickettsia* species (Fig. 25.2 and Table 25.2). This has the advantage of both avoiding the cellular defense mechanisms within the phagosome and providing the bacteria with a nutrient-rich environment. *Listeria monocytogenes* possesses several virulence factors to facilitate its escape from the phagolysosome, a pore-forming hemolysin (listeriolysin, LLO) which acts together with a metalloproteinase, a lecithinase, and two phospholipases to promote the rupture of the phagosomal membrane efficiently, as well as spreading to other cells.[36]

Cell-to-cell spreading

For a bacterial pathogen that is very well adapted to the intracellular milieu and vulnerable to extracellular defense mechanisms, it is highly desirable to remain within host cells. Yet once a sufficiently high number of bacteria has been reached, the original cell dies and bacteria are released into the extracellular space. To avoid this fate, however, some intracellular bacteria have developed mechanisms that allow their direct spreading to other cells. *L. monocytogenes* induces polar actin polymerization by means of a surface protein, ActA. A polymerized actin tail is formed which pushes the bacteria through the cell, forcing the host cell membrane to protrude into a neighboring cell. This cell engulfs this protrusion, and eventually

both the new membrane and the host membrane are dissolved by phospholipases.[36]

ACQUIRED IMMUNITY

The adaptive immune response critically depends on the recognition of foreign antigens that are degraded to peptides and then presented to T cells in the context of MHC molecules on the surface of antigen-presenting cells (APC), including macrophages and DC.

T LYMPHOCYTES AS SPECIFIC MEDIATORS OF ACQUIRED RESISTANCE

Whereas activated macrophages act as the nonspecific executors, T lymphocytes are the specific mediators of acquired resistance against intracellular bacteria. The dramatic increase in the incidence of tuberculosis and other intracellular bacterial infections in AIDS patients well illustrates the central role of T lymphocytes. For instance, at least 0.5 million individuals are coinfected with HIV and *M. tuberculosis*. HIV increases the risk of developing tuberculosis by several orders of magnitude. At the site of microbial growth, T lymphocytes not only initiate the most potent defense mechanisms available, they also focus this response to the site of encounter, thus minimizing detriment to the host. Although protective T-cell responses are multifactorial, they can be reduced to a few principal mechanisms (Fig. 25.4).

T cells inevitably also produce pathology, and the pathogenesis of infections with intracellular bacteria is significantly determined by T cells. It is therefore important that the T-cell response be tightly controlled and can be downregulated when necessary. Regulatory mechanisms, which are executed by a number of cells, including Treg cells, are in place to limit immunopathology.

Protective immunity involves conventionally defined T-cell sets, CD4 αβ T cells, and CD8 αβ T cells, as well as unconventional T cells such as γδ, CD1-restricted αβ T cells, and nonclassical MHC class I-restricted αβ T cells (Fig. 25.4). Although these T-cell sets perform different tasks, substantial redundancy exists. Furthermore, these T-cell populations act not independently, but in a coordinated way and in close interaction with other leukocytes, such as NK cells.[22]

KEY CONCEPTS

T-CELL-MEDIATED MECHANISMS UNDERLYING PROTECTION

>> Activation of macrophages via cytokine secretion (especially interferon-γ)

>> Lysis of infected target cells

>> Bacterial killing

>> Attraction of effector cells from blood to tissue sites

>> Formation and maintenance of granulomatous lesions

>> No sterile eradication

MHC class II presentation

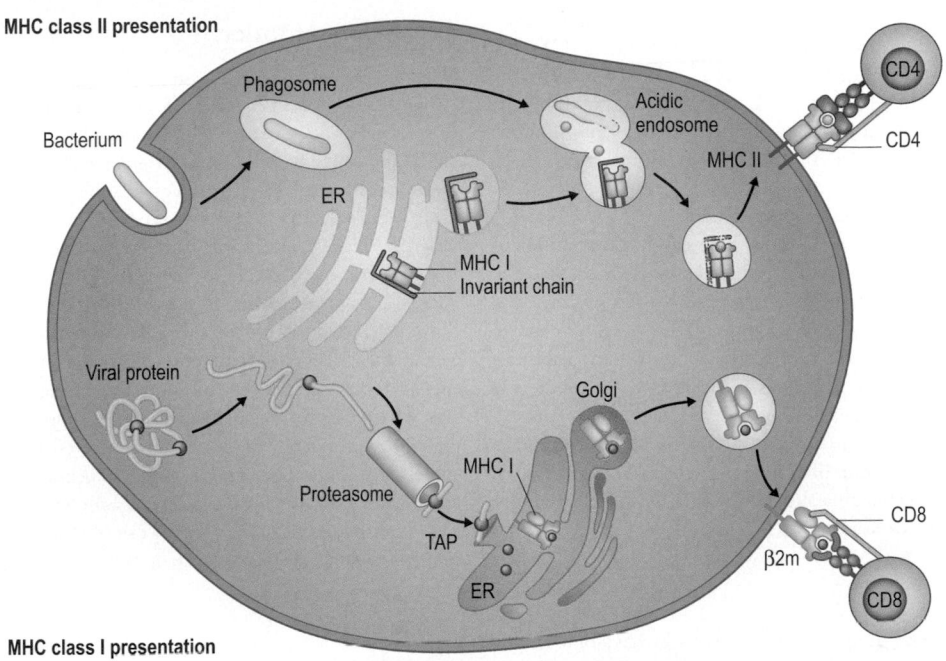

MHC class I presentation

Fig. 25.5 Pathways of antigen processing and T-cell activation. Antigens from phagosomal bacteria and their proteins secreted into the phagosome are presented by major histocompatibility (MHC) class II molecules to CD4 T cells. MHC class II molecules pick up antigenic peptides within late endosomes, termed lysosomes. Somatic and secreted proteins from bacteria within the cytoplasm are presented by MHC class I molecules to CD8 T cells. MHC class I molecules pick up antigenic peptides in the endoplasmic reticulum (ER) imported from the cytoplasm through TAP transporters and processes by proteasomes and other cytoplasmic and ER/Golgi-resident proteases. As a third pathway, cross-presentation through apoptotic blebs from infected cells going into programmed cell death facilitates presentation of antigens from phagosomal bacteria by MHC class I and MHC II to activate both CD4 and CD8 T cells.

Depending on the etiologic agent and the stage of disease, the relative contribution of the different T-cell subsets to acquired resistance may vary. The conventional αβ T cells make up more than 90% and γδ T cells make up less than 10% of all lymphocytes in the blood and peripheral organs of humans and mice. However, γδ T cells represent a significant proportion of the intraepithelial lymphocytes in mucosal tissues, suggesting a particular role at this important port of microbial entry (Chapter 19). Implication of all T-cell populations is primarily derived from studies with experimental animals and immunohistological *in-situ* hybridization studies of lesions.

CD4 T cells

The central role of CD4 T cells in immunity to intracellular bacteria is unquestioned (Fig. 25.4). Overwhelming evidence from experimental animal studies, their abundance in "protective" granulomas of patients suffering from bacterial infections, and the high prevalence of disease caused by intracellular bacteria in CD4 T-cell-deficient AIDS patients all support the salient role of CD4 T cells. Such T cells recognize antigenic peptides in the context of MHC class II molecules. MHC II molecules pick up antigenic peptides within the endosomal system (Fig. 25.5). Thus, antigens from all intracellular bacteria, even those that evade the phagosome at later stages, are accessible to processing and presentation through the MHC class II pathway. A potential drawback of CD4 T cells is related to their failure to recognize infected cells that

are constitutively MHC class II-negative. These include endothelial cells, epithelial cells, hepatocytes, and Schwann cells, the potential targets of *Rickettsia* spp., *C. trachomatis*, *L. monocytogenes*, and *M. leprae*, respectively.

The CD4 T-cell population can be further subdivided into two distinct subsets, according to their pattern of cytokine production: Th1 cells, which produce IFN-γ and TNF-β, and Th2 cells which produce IL-4, IL-5, IL-6, and IL-13 (Chapter 17). In light of this, there are differences in the host immune system induced by these T-cell sets. IFN-γ from Th1 cells promotes cell-mediated immunity, characterized by macrophage activation, stimulation of cytolytic CD8 T cells, and the production of opsonizing IgG antibodies. In contrast, Th2 cells control the differentiation of B cells and promote Ig class switching to IgE and IgA, and are subsequently responsible for protection against helminth infections as well as promoting allergic responses. The development of both T-cell subsets from a common precursor Th0 cell is under the regulation of distinct cytokines. IL-12 and IL-18, secreted by macrophages and DC, in addition to NK-cell-produced IFN-γ, promote the development of Th1 cells, whereas IL-4 is responsible for the development of Th2 cells, although the cell type responsible for the initial production of this cytokine is still under debate. NK T cells, a T-cell subpopulation expressing an evolutionary conserved TCR, which arises rapidly after infection to secrete both IFN-γ and IL-4, could be involved here (Fig. 25.4).[37, 38]

A distinct Th-cell population secretes vast amounts of IL-17, a characteristic which gave this population the term Th17 cells. Cytokines of the IL-17 family are strong inducers of granulopoiesis, of proinflammatory mediators such as IL-6, and of the chemokines CXCL1, CXCL8, and CXCL6 to attract neutrophilic and eosinophilic PMN and prolong their survival.[39] Although Th17 cells are primarily suggested to be responsible for uncontrolled inflammation in allergic and autoimmune reactions, a function in antibacterial immunity both in protection as well as in immunopathology is likely. These cells seem to be particularly important for infection control in the lung.

In general, experimental infections with intracellular pathogens induce a Th1 response that is protective. There is now evidence that the Th1/Th2 dichotomy also exists in humans, and this is best exemplified by the host response to *M. leprae* infection. Here, the tuberculoid form of the disease is characterized by a Th1-type reaction resulting in activated macrophages and effective granuloma formation with few detectable bacilli. In contrast, towards the lepromatous end of the disease spectrum, an abundance of organisms and poor granuloma formation are associated with the production of IL-4, IL-10, and IL-13 (although it should be noted here that in this situation it is CD8 T cells that are the predominant cytokine producers).

CD8 T cells

Infection of mice deficient in specific T-cell subsets has conclusively demonstrated a role for CD8 T cells in *Listeria* infections. More recently, these observations have been extended to include tuberculosis.[40] Furthermore, CD8 effector T cells have been identified in "protective" granulomas of tuberculoid leprosy patients. The cytolytic potential of these T cells can serve two roles in infection, namely target cell killing, which results directly in the inhibition of the growth of bacteria; or the lysis of cells that are unable to control the infection, thus releasing the bacteria for phagocytosis by more activated cells. Recently it has been demonstrated that populations of CD8 T cells can indeed lyse cells, resulting in a reduction in growth of *M. tuberculosis*. This microbicidal mechanism is mediated by granulysin, which is introduced into the target cell via a perforin-generated pore.[30] CD8 T cells are also a potent source of IFN-γ, and thus contribute to protective mechanisms (Fig. 25.4).

CD8 T cells recognize antigenic peptides in the context of MHC class I gene products. Initially, therefore, it was mysterious how these CD8 T cells were stimulated by intracellular bacteria, which were thought to have a uniquely restricted phagosomal residence. However, with the knowledge that many intracellular bacteria such as *L. monocytogenes* invade the cytoplasm, one major mechanism for MHC class I processing became obvious: proteins secreted by bacteria in the cytoplasm undergo antigen processing and presentation similarly to newly synthesized host proteins (Fig. 25.5).[36] However, even antigens from intracellular bacteria such as *S. typhimurium* and *M. tuberculosis*, which remain in the phagosome, are presented to CD8 T cells.[41] Hence, alternative contact points for MHC class I molecules and bacterial peptides need to be assumed. Cross-presentation by noninfected APC of antigens engulfed together with apoptotic blebs from infected cells represents a critical pathway to induce CD8 T cells by phagosomal bacteria (see below). One major advantage of CD8 T cells over CD4 T cells is their recognition of antigen bound by MHC class I gene products, which are expressed by almost all host cells. Thus, CD8 T cells recognize professional and nonprofessional phagocytes equally well.

Cross-presentation

Many intracellular bacteria such as *Chlamydia* and *Rickettsia* dwell within nonprofessional APC, which do not expose MHC II in appreciable amounts and lack expression of co-stimulatory molecules.[42] Those living inside professional APC, such as *Salmonella* and mycobacteria, interfere with expression of antigen-presenting molecules in general, thereby inhibiting T-cell activation. Mycobacteria are secluded from the classical cytoplasmic MHC I processing pathway within tight phagosomes. Despite these hindrances, basically all intracellular bacteria induce CD4 and CD8 T cells. Cross-presentation by noninfected APC is probably responsible for this phenomenon, at least in tuberculosis and salmonellosis.[43] Noninfected cells engulf bacterial antigens enwrapped within apoptotic bodies and blebs thereof, when infected cells succumb to programmed cell death. Apoptosis as a prerequisite for this pathway is induced by many intracellular bacteria, including *Salmonella*, mycobacteria, and even those escaping the phagosome, i.e., *Listeria*. For example, only *Salmonella* strains, which also induce apoptosis, elicit CD8 T cells. This cross-presentation pathway in infections with intracellular bacteria adds an essential function to the physiological role of apoptosis in maintenance of tissue integrity and growth.

γδ T CELLS

The relevance of the γδ T-cell set to bacterial immunity is less well understood. γδ T cells produce cytokines and are cytolytic; hence they cover a functional spectrum similar to that of their αβ T-cell counterparts (Fig. 25.4).[44] Although the genetic restriction of antigen recognition by γδ T cells is incompletely understood, it is clear that they are less fastidious than αβ T cells in this respect. Hence, in principle, all infected host cells are potential targets for γδ T cells. Experimental mouse studies revealed the early accumulation of γδ T cells at sites of bacterial deposition. γδ T cells have also been identified in certain forms of disease, including tuberculous lymphadenitis and leprosy lesions during reactional stages. Because of their less demanding activation and antigen recognition requirements, γδ T cells may fill a gap between nonspecific resistance and the more specific αβ T-cell response. Furthermore, transient participation of γδ T cells in protection and a unique requirement for γδ T cells in granuloma formation have been described for experimental listeriosis and tuberculosis infection in mice. In mice, antigens recognized by γδ T cells appear to comprise heat shock protein-derived peptides presented by nonpolymorphic MHC class I molecules. In contrast, human γδ T cells respond to small nonproteinaceous phosphate-containing compounds of bacterial origin.

T cells controlled by CD1 molecules

CD1 comprises a group of nonpolymorphic MHC-related molecules that can present glycolipid antigens to unconventional T cells (Fig. 25.4). They are divided into two groups. In humans, T cells that respond to group I CD1 molecules, i.e. CD1a, b, and c, are either CD4/CD8, CD4 or CD8 and express the αβ TCR. These cells can respond to a variety of microbial glycolipids, including LAM, PIM, mycolic acids, sulfatides, sulfoglycolipids, lipopeptides, and isoprenoids derived from mycobacteria.[45] Upon antigen stimulation these T cells can proliferate and secrete IFN-γ, as well as lyse macrophages infected with mycobacteria. The group II CD1 molecule CD1d, the only CD1 molecule found in mouse and rat, controls development of NKT cells that express both the

NK-cell marker NK1.1 and an invariant evolutionary conserved TCR. Upon antigen activation these T cells rapidly produce cytokines and are capable of producing both IL-4 and IFN-γ. As bacterial antigens recognized by NKT cells, PIM from mycobacteria and glycosphingolipids from *Ehrlichia* and *Sphingomonas* species have been identified so far.

Memory T cells

Similar to other infectious agents, protective immunity against intracellular bacteria relies on immune memory. In fact, memory induction forms the basis of the success of all vaccines. Protective immunity in humans can last for more than 10 years or even lifelong, as shown for infections with or vaccinations against various viruses or bacterial toxins. Immune protection in these infections, however, also depends at least partially on memory B cells (Chapter 27). For vaccine development, it is essential to identify conditions leading to long-lasting T-cell immunity.

It is thought that during an ongoing immune response, most T cells, which receive an antigen-specific signal through the TCR together with a co-stimulatory signal, and are concomitantly propagated by cytokines, become effector T cells and eventually die of exhaustion. A small proportion that receives stimulation signals of intermediate strengths change their phenotype and become long-lived memory T cells. To become a memory T cell, anti-apoptotic molecules are produced and responsiveness to the homeostatic cytokines IL-7 and IL-15 is increased through expression of the respective cytokine receptors.[46] The current concept of T-cell memory distinguishes between two types of cells, central memory T cells (T_{CM}) and effector memory T cells (T_{EM}) on the basis of differential surface molecules and functions.[46] T_{EM} lose their lymph node homing properties (CCR7, CD62L) but rather migrate to peripheral tissues where they express effector functions, i.e., cytokine secretion and cytotoxicity. Their daily proliferation rate in humans has been estimated at 4.7% compared to 1.5% for T_{CM}. T_{CM} persist in lymph nodes and express the IL-2 receptor, which enables them to propagate quickly upon IL-2 stimulation probably from NK cells during secondary infection. T_{CM} are the source of long-term immunity in *L. major* infection. Although it is generally accepted that memory T cells can survive in the absence of antigen and MHC molecules, the situation may be different in infections with intracellular bacteria, often leading to persistent and latent infections. As of today, little is known on the induction and maintenance of long-lasting cellular immunity in infections with intracellular bacteria. Infection with *M. tuberculosis* may not cause lasting immunity, at least in susceptible individuals, as it has been reported that successfully treated patients in high transmission areas can have recurrent tuberculosis often caused by distinct strains. Similarly, protection against *L. major* is provided by short-lived effector T cells constantly stimulated by persistent parasites with regulatory T cells dampening T-effector functions (see below). Long-lived memory T cells, however, maintain immunity in the absence of parasites.[47] In experimental listeriosis of mice, induction of T-memory cells depends on the duration of infection. Further studies on this issue are required to design novel vaccination strategies in a rational way to achieve long-lasting cellular immunity against intracellular bacteria.

Regulatory T cells

Similar to most infectious agents, intracellular bacteria can cause detrimental inflammation and tissue damage due to IFN-γ-mediated Th1 responses and ultimately exacerbated pathology by TNF-α. Under normal circumstances, control mechanisms are in place to limit immunopathology. Such countermeasures are elicited as part of the ongoing immune response during infection. The main cytokines that limit inflammation and control IFN-γ production are IL-10 and TGF-β. Although these cytokines are produced by macrophages and DC, their main producers are natural (Treg) and adaptive regulatory T cells, which are the prime cells involved in immune regulation. Natural Treg cells are responsive to IL-2 due to constitutive CD25 expression and are characterized by expression of the transcription factor FOXP3.[48] Expansion of Treg cells appears antigen-independent but they can be antigen-specific. However, Treg selectively express TLR and can be activated by LPS and possibly other TLR ligands. This makes their immediate activation during bacterial infection a most probable scenario. Although Treg cells limit CD8 T-cell responses in experimental listeriosis, their general role in infections by intracellular bacteria has not yet been fully elucidated. However, their regulatory function in other infections is better established. Gastrointestinal inflammation caused by *Helicobacter* species is limited by Treg cells. In murine leishmaniosis, Treg cells inhibit sterile elimination of the parasites by controlling Th1-cell responses but at the same time promote development of memory T cells, which protect against reinfection. Due to similar lifestyles of *Leishmania* parasites and intracellular bacteria, a comparable role in tuberculosis or leprosy can be envisaged. Antigen-dependent adaptive T cells with regulatory functions include CD8 Treg cells, CD4 T_R1 cells, both secreting IL-10, and Th3 cells, which produce TGF-β. Recently, T_R1 cells have been isolated from tuberculosis patients. Suppression of T-cell responses and anergy has frequently been documented for chronic infections such as tuberculosis and leprosy. Therefore, a function of Treg cells in infections with intracellular bacteria can be postulated as follows: limiting detrimental Th1-cell responses and immunopathology, prevention of total elimination of bacteria, and promotion of persistent infection and memory T cells.

B CELLS

Although B cells and antibodies appear to have a minor biological role in infections with intracellular bacteria due to their lifestyle, IgG and IgA probably play a role at the epithelial port of entry. Furthermore, facultative intracellular bacteria spend some time outside their host cells where they are accessible by antibodies. Therefore it is not surprising that antibodies are protective against *Salmonella* and *Listeria*. Finally, B cells are potent APC for soluble antigens including lipids presented by CD1c, and secrete many cytokines otherwise associated with T cells, DC, and macrophages.

ANTIGENS FOR T CELLS

Definition of the precise nature of antigens recognized by protective T cells is required for the rational design of improved vaccines and diagnostic skin test reagents. Although we understand quite well the characteristics of antigens from extracellular bacteria that are recognized by protective antibodies, virtually nothing is known about the general characteristics defining protective T-cell antigens. Three major features seem worth particular consideration.

First, it is becoming increasingly clear that bacteria capable of surviving inside host cells are a poor source of somatic antigens, and that the T-cell response against such persistent pathogens needs to focus on secreted proteins. Secreted antigens are particularly relevant to vaccine-induced immunity, which needs to be activated as soon as possible after primary infection with the natural pathogen. Much later, when MPs are activated, intracellular bacteria will be destroyed, giving rise to somatic antigens.[49] The second major concern for rational vaccine design is the appropriate distribution of antigens between the MHC class I and II processing pathways. Soluble proteins are processed through the MHC class II pathway. Consequently, CD4 T-cell activation does not pose major obstacles to subunit vaccines. In contrast, activation of CD8 T cells depends on the efficient introduction of proteins into the MHC class I pathway (Fig. 25.5). This can be achieved either by appropriate membrane translocation systems or by promoting cross-presentation through apoptosis induction. An efficient method of achieving this is the use of recombinant bacteria. This has been demonstrated using a recombinant BCG strain expressing the listerial hemolysin protein which induces apoptosis and subsequently cross-presentation.

Third, recent studies in experimental listeriosis of mice indicate that CD8 T cells not only recognize conventional peptides, but can recognize unconventional peptides containing the N-formylmethionine (N-fMet) sequence.[5] The N-fMet serves as a signal sequence for protein secretion in prokaryotes and does not exist in mammalian proteins (apart from approximately 30 proteins of mitochondrial origin). Importantly, N-fMet-containing peptides are recognized in the context of the MHC class Ib molecule H2-M3, which is far less polymorphic than classical MHC class I molecules. If preferential recognition of such peptides holds true for humans and for bacteria other than *Listeria*, this finding has far-reaching implications for vaccine development. It would promote the design of peptide vaccines applicable to a wide variety of individuals, independent of conventional MHC polymorphisms. In a similar way, lipid antigens presented by nonpolymorphic CD1 molecules can be envisaged as MHC-independent vaccines.

CYTOKINES

Cytokines serve as crucial signal transmitters between the cells participating in antibacterial immunity (Fig. 25.4). A characterization of cytokine mRNA levels in lesions of leprosy patients has provided important information about the cytokines operative in granulomas. The "protective" tuberculoid lesions express abundant mRNA levels of multiple cytokines, including IL-1, IL-2, IL-6, TNF, and IFN-γ, suggesting their relevance to granuloma formation and maintenance.[50] In contrast, IL-4, IL-5, and IL-10 mRNA levels are almost absent from this type of lesion, although they are highly increased in lepromatous lesions, suggesting inhibitory functions of these cytokines.

IL-12, IL-18, IFN-γ, and macrophage activation

Extensive studies on the activation of antibacterial effector functions in macrophages have revealed a central role for IFN-γ. Accordingly, IFN-γ neutralization with antibodies, or deletion of the IFN-γ gene by homologous recombination, markedly exacerbates infectious diseases such as listeriosis, tuberculosis, or typhoid in experimental animals (Fig. 25.4 and Table 25.2). IFN-γ is produced early in infection by NK cells, and later by Th1 cells. It is now clear that the production of IFN-γ by NK cells depends on prior activation by IL-12 and/or IL-18. This cytokine can be induced by components of intracellular pathogens, such as LPS, mycobacterial LAM, and lipoteichoic acid from *Listeria*. IL-12 in

concert with TNF-α induces a cytokine loop resulting in the production of IFN-γ, which in turn acts on macrophages both to activate bactericidal mechanisms and to sustain the production of IL-12 and IL-18. The importance of these cytokines in host defense against intracellular pathogens has been clearly demonstrated using gene knockout mice. These mice exhibit overwhelming susceptibility to infections with mycobacteria, *Salmonella*, and *Listeria*, which was demonstrated to occur as a direct result of the lack of macrophage activation mediated by IFN-γ. Recently these observations have been extended to humans, where patients with mutations in genes for the IFN-γ receptor or IL-12 and its receptor are highly susceptible to infections with *Salmonella*, atypical mycobacteria, and BCG.

Many nonprofessional phagocytes also respond to IFN-γ. Although in these cells the full antibacterial armamentarium operative in activated macrophages cannot be mobilized, IFN-γ stimulation causes some microbial growth inhibition. Important mechanisms represent trytophan and iron deprivation, which are both responsible for inhibition of chlamydial growth in epithelial cells. IFN-γ also induces an array of small GTPases such as LRG-47 and IGTP. Although functional data are very limited, these cytoplasmic enzymes are putatively involved in vesicle trafficking. Mice deficient in LRG-47 are highly susceptible to *M. tuberculosis*.[51] LRG-47 seems to control autophagy, a waste and recycling system functional in all eukaryotic cells.[52] This system is enhanced in IFN-γ-activated cells and has been suggested to contribute to elimination of mycobacteria and *Listeria*.

Proinflammatory cytokines and phagocyte attraction

The recruitment of more phagocytes to the site of infection represents a vital process in the resolution of infection. This is achieved via the secretion by macrophages and endothelial cells of cytokines such as IL-1, TNF, IL-6, and chemokines. TNF and IL-1 activate the vascular endothelium to increase the expression of adhesion molecules, which promote the extravasation of lymphocytes into the infected tissue. Chemokines are a family of structurally related proteins that can be divided into three subfamilies: C-C chemokines (MIP-1β, MCP-1, 2, 3), CXC chemokines (MIP-2, IL-8), and C chemokines (lymphotactin) (Chapter 11). These molecules are critical in controlling the migration of neutrophils (IL-8) and monocytes (MCP-1) from the bloodstream to the infected tissue.[53] Recently the role of chemokines in intracellular infections has been increasingly appreciated, with mice lacking the receptor for MCP-1 being deficient in their ability to clear *Listeria* infection. CCR7 binds CCL19 and CCL21 and is expressed by T cells but also by DC. Homing of DC from infected tissues to draining lymph nodes, in order to induce T cells by means of cross-presentation, depends on this chemokine receptor. It has been realized that distinct repertoires of chemokine receptors are expressed on Th1 and Th2 cells. Human Th2 cells selectively express CCR3, which is the receptor for eotaxin, RANTES, MCP-2, 3 and 4; and Th1 cells express CXCR3, which binds IFN-γ-inducible protein 10 (IP10), and monokine induced by IFN-γ (MIG), both of which are induced by IFN-γ. A similar selective expression of chemokine receptors has been noted in the murine system. The differential response to chemokines may influence the type of T cell that is recruited into a specific site during the course of disease, and thus influence the immune response elicited.

LYSIS, TISSUE DAMAGE, AND BACTERIAL KILLING

Cytolytic phenomena generally accompany infections with intracellular bacteria. Cells with cytolytic potential that are activated during such infections include PMN, blood monocytes, NK cells, and T cells.[22, 24, 30] PMN and blood monocytes that are attracted to foci of bacterial growth nonspecifically destroy the surrounding tissue, primarily by secreting proteolytic enzymes, including elastase, collagenase, and gelatinase. These enzymes affect the integrity of both cells and extracellular matrix. They are at least partially responsible for the exudative character of early lesions. NK cells and T cells express nonspecific or specific cytolytic activity, respectively, further contributing to tissue damage. Tissue damage is generally localized to the site of microbial implantation or persistence. Cytolytic T cells probably act at advanced stages of infection and contribute to the liquefaction that follows the reactivation of dormant bacteria. Without doubt, the tissue damage caused by cytolytic mechanisms significantly determines the pathology of infectious disease. Furthermore, the release of bacteria contained within distinct foci may promote the dissemination of pathogens to distant sites. However, cytolytic mechanisms are required for protection against microbes living in protective niches, such as deactivated macrophages or nonprofessional phagocytes. Transmission of bacteria from an incapacitated cell to a highly activated professional phagocyte significantly improves bacterial elimination. Finally, cytolytic T cells may also attack intracellular microbes. Once the target cells have been lysed, bacteria can be killed by means of a specific molecule, granulysin, that is contained within the granules of the cytotoxic T cell.[31]

GRANULOMA FORMATION

The formation of a tissue granuloma is a characteristic feature of many infections caused by intracellular bacteria. The longevity of the granuloma depends directly on the continuous presence of the microbial pathogen, and the lesion generally disappears after its sterile eradication. Granulomas form the focus of the coordinated cross-talk between different types of T cells, B cells, and MP. Even if the immune system fails to eliminate bacteria completely inside the granuloma, the latter performs a protective function by containing microbes within distinct foci and preventing their dissemination. At the same time, the granuloma can be detrimental to the host because it can interfere with physiologic organ functions.

Granulomatous lesions are generally initiated by nonspecific inflammatory signals mediated by bacterial products, chemokines, TNF-α, and IL-1, which are produced by endothelial cells and MP at the site of infection (Fig. 25.6). Inflammatory phagocytes are attracted to the site of microbial replication and an infiltrative, sometimes exudative, lesion develops. Following the accumulation and activation of increasing numbers of MPs, this lesion takes a more granulomatous form. A significant number of B cells is also found, which seem to influence granuloma morphology. Once specific T and B cells have been attracted to the lesion, it transforms into a productive granuloma that provides the most appropriate tissue site for antibacterial protection. Here, activation of macrophages by IFN-γ and TNF-α causes significant microbial growth inhibition. Bacterial transmission from inefficient host cells to more potent effector cells through lysis of infected cells by cytolytic T cells further contributes to protection. At the same time, regulatory events involving IL-10 and TGF-β by Treg, T_R1, and Th3

cells are probably in place to prevent exacerbated immunopathology. Eventually, the granuloma is encapsulated by a fibrotic wall and its center becomes necrotic.[54] Both tissue reactions are primarily protective, the former by promoting bacterial containment and the latter by reducing the nutrient and oxygen supply to the pathogen.

Frequently, such a granuloma is the result of a long-lasting standoff between microbe and host defense that may last for long periods of time. As a consequence of microbial reactivation and/or weakening of the immune response, however, this tie may break down. Exaggerated macrophage activation leads to the uncontrolled expansion of necrotic lesions, affecting the physiologic functioning of the affected organ. Moreover, extensive cytolysis by MP, T lymphocytes, and newly attracted PMN and monocytes causes liquefaction of the granuloma and its rupture.[54] This event is not only responsible for extensive organ damage: it may also favor the local replication of facultative intracellular bacteria in the cellular detritus, as well as microbial dissemination to distant tissue sites and to the environment to transmit infection.

DTH REACTION

Intradermal injection of soluble proteins from an intracellular bacterium causes local infiltration of specific T lymphocytes and MP in individuals immune to the same pathogen. The reaction generally reaches its maximum between 40 and 70 hours after antigen application. This DTH reaction has been used successfully for the diagnosis of infections with various intracellular bacteria, particularly *M. tuberculosis/M. bovis* and *M. leprae*, because of the difficulty in isolating such microbes from internal organs, where they persist without causing clinical disease: It should be emphasized that a positive DTH response directly reflects the existence of a specific T-cell response and only indirectly indicates microbial existence in the host, and is by far no conclusive indication of a protective immune status. The DTH response is mediated by CD4 αβ T cells, with recent evidence suggesting a vital role for TNF-α in the induction of chemokines. Because soluble antigens are processed inefficiently, if at all, through the MHC class I pathway, CD8 T cells, which are important elements of protective immunity, are not challenged by DTH antigens. Thus, the DTH response reflects an important arm, but not the full armamentarium, of protective immunity against intracellular bacteria. As a further complication, the DTH antigen mixture may miss antigens relevant to protection. According to the stage of disease, different ratios of secreted versus somatic antigens may be required. Whereas secreted antigens may be particularly important during persistent infection, somatic antigens may become more important once bacteria are efficiently destroyed by activated macrophages.

Although DTH responses are generally positive in immune but nondiseased individuals, they are frequently absent during full-blown disease, such as miliary tuberculosis and lepromatous leprosy. The reasons for this anergy are incompletely understood but appear to involve immunosuppression, the absence of appropriate antigens in the DTH reagent, the accumulation of specific T cells at the site of disease manifestation, and their concomitant absence from the periphery.

LOCAL IMMUNITY AT THE PORT OF ENTRY

Intracellular bacteria enter the host through two major ports. Pathogenic *Rickettsia* and *Ehrlichia* species and often *Coxiella burnetii* are introduced directly into the vascular bed by arthropod bites or through abraded skin;

A   Bacterial phagocytosis by macrophages

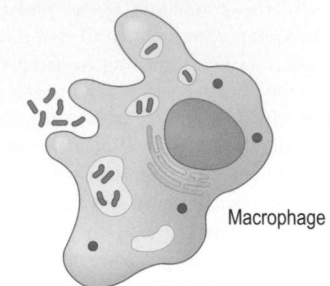

Macrophage

B   Granuloma formation at site of bacterial replication

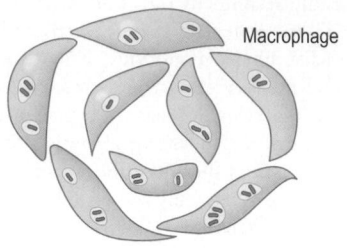

Macrophage

C   Bacterial containment in granuloma

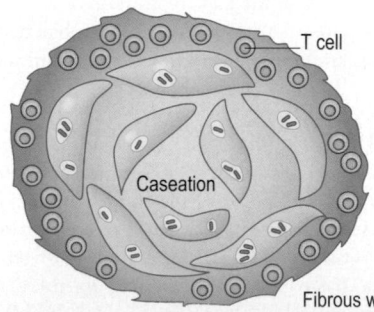

T cell

Caseation

Fibrous wall

D   Granuloma liquifaction, rupture and bacterial dissemination

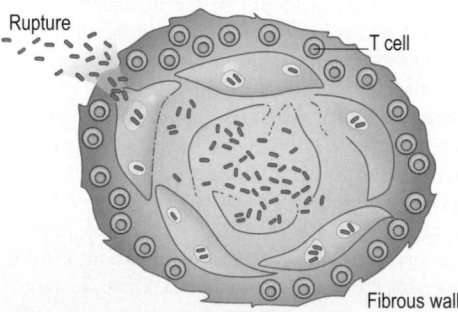

Rupture

T cell

Fibrous wall

Fig. 25.6   Cells involved in granuloma formation and rupture. This figure uses tuberculosis to illustrate the major events in granuloma formation. **(A)** Bacteria that have entered the alveolus are engulfed by alveolar macrophages, which translocate bacteria into the lung interstitium. **(B)** Inflammation develops, which causes extravasation of blood monocytes. Proinflammatory cytokines and chemokines are produced by macrophages and endothelial cells surrounding this focus. **(C)** Specific T cells are attracted to the site of microbial deposition and granuloma formation is initiated. The protective granuloma is maintained by the influence of the various T-cell subsets and cytokines. The center becomes necrotic and a fibrous wall encloses the lesion, promoting microbial containment. **(D)** Cytolytic mechanisms cause microbial release from deactivated macrophages and their inhibition by more efficacious effector cells. A preponderance of cytolytic mechanisms causes rupture of the granuloma. As a consequence, exaggerated tissue destruction and microbial dissemination occur.

all the other intracellular bacteria invade the host through mucosal tissues. *Mycobacterium tuberculosis/M. bovis, L. pneumophilia, C. burnetii, Chlamydia psittaci, C. pneumoniae,* and *Brucella* sp. preferentially intrude the lung; *S. typhi/S. paratyphi, L. monocytogenes* and sometimes *M. bovis, M. avium,* and *Brucella* sp. gain entrance through the gut; *C. trachomatis* invades the urogenital tract and eventually the ocular system; and *M. leprae* penetrates the oropharynx. The local immune response in the mucosa therefore represents an important barrier to infection (Chapter 19). The immune armamentarium at this strategically important point includes specific IgA and IgG antibodies, the intraepithelial lymphocytes, the lamina propria lymphocytes, and the cells in the local lymphoid follicles. Frequently, the immune response initiated in these follicles is directed toward the Th2 cell arm. The relatively high proportion of γδ and NKT cells among intraepithelial lymphocytes, as well as their broad antigen specificity, suggests a particular role for these cells in early immune surveillance against intruding pathogens. Many foodborne pathogens initiate infection by adherence to the microfold (M) cells distributed among intestinal epithelial cells.[55] Because these cells are specialized for the uptake of nutrients from the intestine, microbial adhesion induces transcytosis, which opens passage to the Peyer's patches beneath. Bacterial invasins are central to this step. In the Peyer's patches,

MP and DC engulf microbial invaders but fail to eradicate the majority of them. As a corollary, these cells serve as a local niche and/or transit system to deeper tissue sites. To achieve successful entrance through the lung, microbes must be inhaled within minute droplets that reach the alveolar compartment. There, alveolar macrophages and DC engulf the bacteria, yet these MP again fail to kill intracellular bacteria, and serve as a transport system to the lung interstitium as well as to the draining lymph nodes.

■ GENETICS OF HOST RESISTANCE TO INTRACELLULAR BACTERIA ■

It has been appreciated for many years that the genetic makeup of the host can influence both resistance to and the outcome of infection. Over 20 years ago, studies in the murine system revealed that a genetic factor controlled resistance to the antigenically unrelated intracellular pathogens *S. typhimurium, Leishmania major,* and *M. bovis* BCG. Subsequently this gene has been identified and termed *Nramp1* for natural resistance-associated macrophage protein. This gene encodes for a protein of phagocytic cells and a single-point mutation at amino acid 169 (glycine for aspartic acid) converts mice from a resistant to a susceptible phenotype. Functional studies using congenic mouse strains have demonstrated that *Nramp 1* plays a critical role in early macrophage activation events via pleiotropic effects such as the regulation of iNOS, TNF-α, the chemokine KC, and MHC class II expression, and ultimately biases towards Th1-cell development.[56] Nramp1 is most probably a transporter for divalent metal ions such as iron or manganese on late endosomal membranes. Despite the conflicting evidence for the role of Nramp1 in resistance of mice to *M. tuberculosis*, a large case-control study in Africans strongly associated an *NRAMP1* polymorphism with tuberculosis.[57] Polymorphisms of the genes for IFN-γ receptor, vitamin D receptor, and TLR-2 have also recently been associated with enhanced susceptibility to tuberculosis.[58–61] The latter two polymorphisms may influence production of the bactericidal peptide cathelicidin.[31] TLR-2 polymorphisms have also been associated with disease outcome in leprosy.[59] Analysis within a region of chemokine genes revealed a functional promoter polymorphism (*GG* versus *AG*) in the gene for MCP-1, a chemoattractant for monocytes and T cells, associated with increased susceptibility to pulmonary tuberculosis. Carriers of the *GG* genotype produce more MCP-1 but less IL-12, which is taken as the basis for higher susceptibility to tuberculosis of these carriers.[62]

The influence of genes of the MHC has also been examined in relation to infections caused by intracellular bacteria. Human leukocyte antigen (HLA) segregation has been described in *C. trachomatis* infections where HLA-DR53 correlated with resistance and HLA-DR16 associated with blindness. Additionally, in a large trial in Venezuela, HLA-DR genotypes were associated with responses to the mycobacterial purified protein derivative (PPD). Positive cell-mediated immune responses to PPD were associated with DR3 and DR4 and negatively associated with DR2 and DR5. The converse was observed for antibody responses, suggesting that HLA-DR alleles differentially direct Th1 and Th2 responses. In terms of HLA association in clinical mycobacterial diseases, family studies have proved an allelic association in leprosy, but the results for tuberculosis have been more conflicting, both clinically and experimentally.[63]

CONCLUSION

It is being increasingly recognized that the interaction between intracellular bacteria and the immune system is not of the 'all or nothing' type but is instead a 'continuous struggle.' This realization has far-reaching implications for preventive and therapeutic strategies against intracellular bacterial infections. First, vaccination against intracellular bacteria has not yet been effected satisfactorily because of the involvement of several distinct T-cell subsets with different modes of stimulation and activity profiles. Second, chemotherapy has frequently proved suboptimal for the sterile eradication of bacteria hidden in cellular niches. A better understanding of the complex cross-talk between cytokines, T lymphocytes, macrophages, and infected host cells will no doubt directly promote the development of improved control measures. It is interesting in conclusion to recall that the discovery of several fundamental principles of immunology was stimulated by early attempts to treat and prevent infections with intracellular bacteria. These include the characterization of macrophages and their contribution to antibacterial defense by Elias Metchnikoff, and the description of granulomatous lesions and DTH responses in tuberculosis by Robert Koch.

KEY CONCEPTS

HOST EFFECTOR MECHANISMS OPERATIVE IN GRANULOMAS

>> Macrophage activation by interferon-γ, tumor necrosis factor (TNF), and other cytokines

Microbial growth inhibition (protective)

>> Lysis of incapacitated macrophages by cytolytic T cells

Microbial release facilitating uptake by more efficient effector cells and direct killing of the bacteria (protective), or

Microbial dissemination (pathogenic)

>> Central necrosis mediated by TNF

Microbial growth inhibition (protective)

>> Fibrotic encapsulation by TNF

Microbial containment (protective)

>> Exaggerated necrosis and fibrosis

Tissue damage (pathogenic)

>> Central liquefaction by cytolytic T cells, activated macrophages, polymorphonuclear leukocytes (PMN)

Tissue damage and promotion of microbial growth (pathogenic)

>> Rupture of granuloma by cytolytic T cells, activated macrophages, PMN

Tissue damage and microbial dissemination (pathogenic)

>> Counter-regulation by regulatory T cells via interleukin-10 and transforming growth factor-β

Minimizing inflammation and tissue damage (protective)

Impairing protective immune response (pathogenic)

KEY CONCEPTS

WHAT IS REQUIRED FROM A VACCINE AGAINST INTRACELLULAR BACTERIA?

>> Activation of innate immunity (Toll-like receptor, natural killer cells)

>> Induction of interleukin-12 (IL-12) and IL-18

>> Activation of a broad array of T-cell populations

>> Promoting interferon-γ-secreting and cytotoxic T cells

>> Inhibition of regulatory T cells and induction of long-lasting T-cell memory

>> Ideal goal: induction of sterile pathogen eradication

>> Second-best goal: sustaining latent infection and prevention of disease reactivation

◼ ACKNOWLEDGMENTS ◼

This work received financial support from Fonds der Chemischen Industrie. We are grateful to Caitlin McCoull and Mary Louise Grossman for excellent secretarial assistance and Diane Schad for the figures.

◼ REFERENCES ◼

1. Kaufmann SH. Immunity to intracellular bacteria. In: Paul WE (ed:) Fundamental Immunology, 5th ed. Philadelphia, PA: Lippincott-Raven, 2003; pp1229–1261.

2. Cole ST, Eisenach KD, McMurray DN, Jacobs Jr WR , (eds): Tuberculosis and the Tubercle Bacillus Washington, DC: ASM Press, 2005.

3. Cosma CL, Sherman DR, Ramakrishnan L. The secret lives of the pathogenic mycobacteria. Annu Rev Microbiol 2003; 57: 641–676.

4. Abrahams GL, Hensel M. Manipulating cellular transport and immune responses: dynamic interactions between intracellular *Salmonella enterica* and its host cells. Cell Microbiol 2006; 8: 728–737.

5. Pamer EG. Immune responses to *Listeria monocytogenes*. Nat Rev Immunol 2004; 4: 812–823.

6. Neild AL, Roy CR. Immunity to vacuolar pathogens: what can we learn from *Legionella*? Cell Microbiol 2004; 6: 1011–1018.

7. Sjostedt A. Intracellular survival mechanisms of *Francisella tularensis*, a stealth pathogen. Microbes Infect 2006; 8: 561–567.

8. Roop RM 2nd, Bellaire BH, Valderas MW, et al. Adaptation of the Brucellae to their intracellular niche. Mol Microbiol 2004; 52: 621–630.

9. Parola P, Paddock CD, Raoult D. Tick-borne rickettsioses around the world: emerging diseases challenging old concepts. Clin Microbiol Rev 2005; 18: 719–756.

10. Dautry-Varsat A, Subtil A, Hackstadt T. Recent insights into the mechanisms of *Chlamydia* entry. Cell Microbiol 2005; 7: 1714–1722.

11. Munoz-Elias EJ, Timm J, Botha T, et al. Replication dynamics of *Mycobacterium tuberculosis* in chronically infected mice. Infect Immun 2005; 73: 546–551.

12. Fields KA, Hackstadt T. The chlamydial inclusion: escape from the endocytic pathway. Annu Rev Cell Dev Biol 2002; 18: 221–245.

13. Winslow GM, Bitsaktsis C. Immunity to the ehrlichiae: new tools and recent developments. Curr Opin Infect Dis 2005; 18: 217–221.

14. Raoult D, Marrie T, Mege J. Natural history and pathophysiology of Q fever. Lancet Infect Dis 2005; 5: 219–226.

15. van Rie A, Warren R, Richardson M, et al. Exogenous reinfection as a cause of recurrent tuberculosis after curative treatment. N Engl J Med 1999; 341: 1174–1179.

16. Scollard DM, Adams LB, Gillis TP, et al. The continuing challenges of leprosy. Clin Microbiol Rev 2006; 19: 338–381.

17. Bloom BR, Modlin RL, Salgame P. Stigma variations: observations on suppressor T cells and leprosy. Annu Rev Immunol 1992; 10: 453–488.

18. O'Neill LA. How Toll-like receptors signal: what we know and what we don't know. Curr Opin Immunol 2006; 18: 3–9.

19. Cambi A, Figdor CG. Levels of complexity in pathogen recognition by C-type lectins. Curr Opin Immunol 2005; 17: 345–351.

20. Strober W, Murray PJ, Kitani A, et al. Signalling pathways and molecular interactions of NOD1 and NOD2. Nat Rev Immunol 2006; 6: 9–20.

21. Pasare C, Medzhitov R. Toll-like receptors: linking innate and adaptive immunity. Adv Exp Med Biol 2005; 560: 11–18.

22. Orange JS, Ballas ZK. Natural killer cells in human health and disease. Clin Immunol 2006; 118: 1–10.

23. Stewart CA, Vivier E, Colonna M. Strategies of natural killer cell recognition and signaling. Curr Top Microbiol Immunol 2006; 298: 1–21.

24. Segal AW. How neutrophils kill microbes. Annu Rev Immunol 2005; 23: 197–223.

25. Laskay T, van Zandbergen G, Solbach W. Neutrophil granulocytes – Trojan horses for *Leishmania major* and other intracellular microbes? Trends Microbiol 2003; 11: 210–214.

26. Werner E. GTPases and reactive oxygen species: switches for killing and signaling. J Cell Sci 2004; 117: 143–153.

27. Bogdan C. Nitric oxide and the immune response. Nat Immunol 2001; 2: 907–916.

28. Rottenberg ME, Gigliotti-Rothfuchs A, Wigzell H. The role of IFN-gamma in the outcome of chlamydial infection. Curr Opin Immunol 2002; 14: 444–451.

29. Lehrer RI. Primate defensins. Nat Rev Microbiol 2004; 2: 727–738.

30. Stenger S, Rosat JP, Bloom BR, et al. Granulysin: a lethal weapon of cytolytic T cells. Immunol Today 1999; 20: 390–394.

31. Liu PT, Stenger S, Li H, et al. Toll-like receptor triggering of a vitamin D-mediated human antimicrobial response. Science 2006; 311: 1770–1773.

32. Schaible UE, Kaufmann SH. Iron and microbial infection. Nat Rev Microbiol 2004; 2: 946–953.

33. Stuart LM, Ezekowitz RA. Phagocytosis: elegant complexity. Immunity 2005; 22: 539–550.

34. Russell DG. *Mycobacterium tuberculosis*: here today, and here tomorrow. Nat Rev Mol Cell Biol 2001; 2: 569–577.

35. Salcedo SP, Holden DW. Bacterial interactions with the eukaryotic secretory pathway. Curr Opin Microbiol 2005; 8: 92–98.

36. Dussurget O, Pizarro-Cerda J, Cossart P. Molecular determinants of *Listeria monocytogenes* virulence. Annu Rev Microbiol 2004; 58: 587–610.

37. Salgame P. Host innate and Th1 responses and the bacterial factors that control *Mycobacterium tuberculosis* infection. Curr Opin Immunol 2005; 17: 374–380.

38. Hunter CA. New IL-12-family members: IL-23 and IL-27, cytokines with divergent functions. Nat Rev Immunol 2005; 5: 521–531.

39. Kelly MN, Kolls JK, Happel K, et al. Interleukin-17/interleukin-17 receptor-mediated signaling is important for generation of an optimal polymorphonuclear response against *Toxoplasma gondii* infection. Infect Immun 2005; 73: 617–621.

40. Harty JT, Bevan MJ. Responses of CD8(+) T cells to intracellular bacteria. Curr Opin Immunol 1999; 11: 89–93.

41. Yrlid U, Svensson M, Kirby A, et al. Antigen-presenting cells and anti-*Salmonella* immunity. Microbes Infect 2001; 3: 1239–1248.

42. den Haan JM, Bevan MJ. Antigen presentation to CD8+ T cells: cross-priming in infectious diseases. Curr Opin Immunol 2001; 13: 437–441.

43. Winau F, Hegasy G, Kaufmann SH, et al. No life without death – apoptosis as prerequisite for T cell activation. Apoptosis 2005; 10: 707–715.

44. Ziegler HK. The role of gamma/delta T cells in immunity to infection and regulation of inflammation. Immunol Res 2004; 29: 293–302.

45. Brigl M, Brenner MB. CD1: antigen presentation and T cell function. Annu Rev Immunol 2004; 22: 817–890.

46. Lanzavecchia A, Sallusto F. Understanding the generation and function of memory T cell subsets. Curr Opin Immunol 2005; 17: 326–332.

47. Scott P. Immunologic memory in cutaneous leishmaniasis. Cell Microbiol 2005; 7: 1707–1713.

48. Belkaid Y, Rouse BT. Natural regulatory T cells in infectious disease. Nat Immunol 2005; 6: 353–360.

49. Kaufmann SH, Schaible UE. Antigen presentation and recognition in bacterial infections. Curr Opin Immunol 2005; 17: 79–87.

50. Bleharski JR, Li H, Meinken C, et al. Use of genetic profiling in leprosy to discriminate clinical forms of the disease. Science 2003; 301: 1527–1530.

51. MacMicking JD, Taylor GA, McKinney JD. Immune control of tuberculosis by IFN-gamma-inducible LRG-47. Science 2003; 302: 654–659.

52. Gutierrez MG, Master SS, Singh SB, et al. Autophagy is a defense mechanism inhibiting BCG and *Mycobacterium tuberculosis* survival in infected macrophages. Cell 2004; 119: 753–766.

53. Le Y, Zhou Y, Iribarren P, et al. Chemokines and chemokine receptors: their manifold roles in homeostasis and disease. Cell Mol Immunol 2004; 1: 95–104.

54. Ulrichs T, Kaufmann SH. New insights into the function of granulomas in human tuberculosis. J Pathol 2006; 208: 261–269.

55. Niedergang F, Kweon MN. New trends in antigen uptake in the gut mucosa. Trends Microbiol 2005; 13: 485–490.

56. Forbes JR, Gros P. Divalent-metal transport by NRAMP proteins at the interface of host–pathogen interactions. Trends Microbiol 2001; 9: 397–403.

57. Hoal EG, Lewis LA, Jamieson SE, et al. SLC11A1 (NRAMP1) but not SLC11A2 (NRAMP2) polymorphisms are associated with susceptibility to tuberculosis in a high-incidence community in South Africa. Int J Tuberc Lung Dis 2004; 8: 1464–1471.

58. Roth DE, Soto G, Arenas F, et al. Association between vitamin D receptor gene polymorphisms and response to treatment of pulmonary tuberculosis. J Infect Dis 2004; 190: 920–927.

59. Texereau J, Chiche JD, Taylor W, et al. The importance of Toll-like receptor 2 polymorphisms in severe infections. Clin Infect Dis 2005; 41 (suppl 7): S408–S415.

60. Cooke GS, Campbell SJ, Sillah J, et al. Polymorphism within the interferon gamma/receptor complex is associated with pulmonary tuberculosis. Am J Respir Crit Care Med 2006; 174: 339–343.

61. Bornman L, Campbell SJ, Fielding K, et al. Vitamin D receptor polymorphisms and susceptibility to tuberculosis in West Africa: a case-control and family study. J Infect Dis 2004; 190: 1631–1641.

62. Flores-Villanueva PO, Ruiz-Morales JA, Song CH, et al. A functional promoter polymorphism in monocyte chemoattractant protein-1 is associated with increased susceptibility to pulmonary tuberculosis. J Exp Med 2005; 202: 1649–1658.

63. Nikolich-Zugich J, Fremont DH, Miley MJ, et al. The role of mhc polymorphism in anti-microbial resistance. Microbes Infect 2004; 6: 501–512.

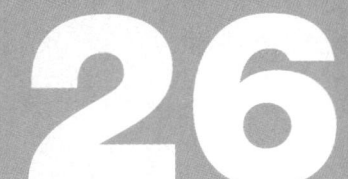

Immune responses
to spirochetes

Juan Anguita, Chris M. Olson Jr, Erol Fikrig

26

■ CHARACTERISTICS OF SPIROCHETES ■

GENERAL FEATURES

Spirochetes constitute a unique and diverse group of bacteria that inhabit many different environments such as soil, deep marine sediments, arthropods, and mammals. Spirochetes are the causative agents of numerous human illnesses, including syphilis and Lyme disease.

Spirochetes are characterized by a typical spiral shape with a distinctive flat-wave morphology. Cellular dimensions vary over a wide range among spirochetes, with a diameter of 0.09–0.75 µM, and lengths that range from 3 to 500 µm. They are motile organisms with a multilayered outer membrane that encapsulates a peptidoglycan layer surrounding their inner membrane. Motility is due to the presence of endoflagella located in the periplasmic space. These axial filaments are arranged in a bipolar fashion and extend toward the opposite end of the cell (Fig. 26.1). The viability of the organism is dependent on an intact outer membrane, which can be damaged by variations in osmolarity, antibodies, or complement, resulting in the loss of intracellular components and ultimately death of the bacterium.

Several spirochetal species are able to induce disease in mammals (Table 26.1). Lyme disease was first discovered in 1975 as an illness affecting a cluster of children in Lyme, Connecticut. In 1981 the agent of Lyme disease was identified as *Borrelia burgdorferi*.[1] In contrast, *Treponema pallidum* subspecies *pallidum* is the causative agent of venereal syphilis, a disease that has been recognized for over 500 years, although its agent was not determined until 1905.[2]

The genomes of *B. burgdorferi* and *T. pallidum* have recently been sequenced.[3,4] Despite similar ancestry and morphological features, these spirochetes have striking differences at the genetic level that may account for the differences in their lifecycles, environmental adaptations, and the diseases caused by them. Both *B. burgdorferi* and *T. pallidum* have relatively small genomes, when compared to other microorganisms. *B. burgdorferi*, however, has one of the most complex genomes known

among prokaryotes. This spirochete has a single linear chromosome and 21 plasmids, the largest number of plasmids of any characterized prokaryote. Of the 21 plasmids, nine are circular and 12 are linear. Furthermore, less than 10% of *B. burgdorferi* plasmid coding regions are found in other microorganisms, including spirochetes, which underscores the uniqueness of this spirochete amongst all bacterial microorganisms. Unlike *B. burgdorferi*, *T. pallidum* contains a single circular chromosome with no plasmids. Yet, 476 open reading frames (ORFs) in *T. pallidum* have orthologous genes in *B. burgdorferi*. Almost 60 of these orthologous genes encode proteins of unknown biological functions that are specific to spirochetes, which may be involved in the pathology associated with infection.

Typically, Gram-negative microorganisms have lipopolysaccharide (LPS)-encoding genes; however, *B. burgdorferi* and *T. pallidum* do not. Lipoproteins are the major immunogens of *B. burgdorferi* and most likely *T. pallidum*, and thus they are the dominant proinflammatory agonists of spirochetal infection. Some 5% of the chromosomal ORFs of *B. burgdorferi* encode putative lipoproteins, whereas 14.5–17% of the functionally complete ORFs contained in these plasmids encode lipoproteins. Interestingly, only 2.1% of the *T. pallidum* ORFs encode putative lipoproteins. The abundant lipoprotein-coding potential of *B. burgdorferi* suggests that lipoproteins may be important for the survival of the spirochete. In fact, as a result of increased temperature and nutrient availability, as well as reduced pH, expression of several *B. burgdorferi* lipoproteins is augmented upon tick feeding and transmission into the mammalian host.[5] For instance, the lipoprotein outer-surface protein (Osp) A is expressed at high levels in the gut of the unfed tick, but upon feeding OspA expression is downregulated, and the expression of OspC increases 90-fold.[5] It is thought that many Osps have adhesive functions, and it has been shown that OspA is involved in the attachment of *B. burgdorferi* to the gut of the tick through an interaction with the tick receptor TROSPA.[6] Furthermore, OspC may be necessary for the migration of *B. burgdorferi* from the gut of the tick to the salivary glands, where it is transmitted into the mammalian host during tick engorgement, and also for survival in the mammalian host.

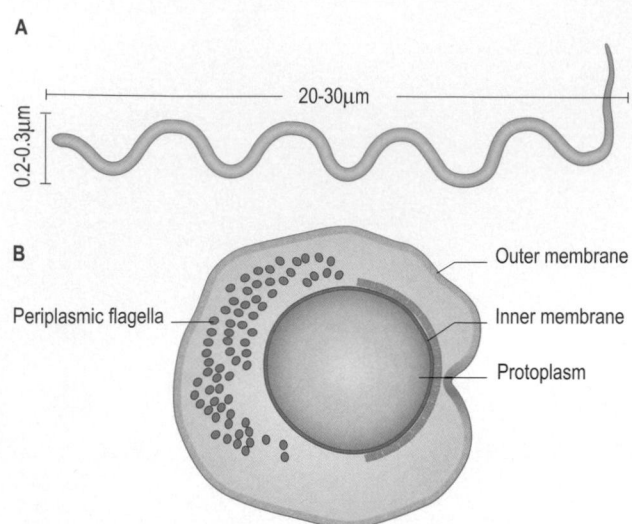

Fig. 26.1 (**A**) *Borrelia burgdorferi* structure is characterized by a distinctive flat-wave morphology consisting of approximately 18 bends and a length of 20–30 µm. (**B**) A cross-section of this spirochete reveals the endoflagella, which are responsible for the unique morphology and motility of this organism.

▮ CLINICAL RELEVANCE

>> Pathology arising from infection with Borrelia burgdorferi and Treponema pallidum in untreated individuals includes:

>> Early localized disease

>> Early disseminated disease

>> Persistent infection

▮ PATHOLOGY ARISING FROM INFECTION WITH B. BURGDORFERI OR T. PALLIDUM ▮

LYME DISEASE

B. burgdorferi sensu stricto (*B. burgdorferi*) is the etiologic agent of Lyme disease in the USA and other parts of the world, while *B. afzelii* and *B. garinii* are agents of Lyme disease that are restricted to Europe and Asia.[1] Infection with Lyme disease-causing spirochetes has also been observed in Japan, Russia, and China. In the USA, transmission of the spirochete is by hard-bodied ticks of the *Ixodes* complex, mainly *I. scapularis* and *I. pacificus*. According to the Centers for Disease Control, Lyme disease is the most common tickborne disease in the USA.[7]

An early hallmark of infection is the appearance of a skin rash known as erythema migrans (Fig. 26.2), which often appears during the first week of infection (stage I, Lyme disease). Other symptoms occurring at this time may include fever, headache, malaise, myalgia, and/or arthralgia. The spirochete then disseminates (stage II, Lyme disease) and

symptoms can include conduction system abnormalities, meningitis, and acute arthritis, which appear in 60% of untreated individuals in the USA. Some untreated individuals develop stage III Lyme disease, which is generally characterized by prolonged infection with the spirochete. Late-stage symptoms may include chronic arthritis, neuroborreliosis, or cutaneous lesions such as *acrodermatitis chronica atrophicans*.

Diagnosis

A detailed clinical history and comprehensive physical examination are critical for the accurate diagnosis of Lyme disease. Appropriate laboratory testing, however, can be a valuable diagnostic aid.

In the USA, more than 70 Food and Drug Administration (FDA)-approved serologic assays for the diagnosis of Lyme disease exist. In 1995 the Association of Public Health Laboratories and the Centers for Disease Control implemented a two-tiered approach for the serodiagnosis of Lyme disease in the USA, and this remains the gold standard today. Using this approach, serum is first tested for the presence of *B. burgdorferi*-specific antibodies by a sensitive method, such as enzyme-linked immunosorbent assay (ELISA) or an immunofluorescent assay (IFA) – an ELISA is most commonly used. Serum testing negative for antibodies generally need not be tested further; however, those found to be positive or equivocal are further evaluated by the more specific immunoblotting for immunoglobulin M (IgM) and IgG antibodies. The detection of at least two of three specific bands in IgM or five of 10 specific bands in IgG is considered positive. It should be noted that patients with early Lyme disease often report to a physician during the first few days of infection, at which time a detectable humoral response may not have developed. If these individuals are rapidly and effectively treated, then significant *B. burgdorferi*-specific antibody responses may not develop. Consequently, the two-tiered approach is considered highly sensitive during the later stages of Lyme disease (> 90%) and less sensitive during very early infection. It should be noted that a positive serologic test, particularly IgG, is evidence of exposure to *B. burgdorferi*, but does not necessarily indicate active infection. All serologic tests must be evaluated in conjunction with the clinical assessment of the attending physician.

Culture and polymerase chain reaction (PCR) detection of *B. burgdorferi* may be very useful to detect active infection, particularly of the skin, joints, and central nervous system. Culture, however, is generally limited to research labs, and the sensitivity and specificity of PCR can vary greatly among testing centers.

Treatment

During early stages of Lyme disease, such as that during which erythema migrans is present, oral administration of doxycycline (100 mg twice daily) or amoxicillin (500 mg 3 times a day) for approximately 2 weeks is recommended.[8] Doxycycline has the advantage of being effective against *Anaplasma phagocytophilum*, which may also be transmitted by ticks. In areas where *B. burgdorferi* infection is prevalent, some experts recommend antibiotic therapy for individuals who served as hosts to *I. scapularis* ticks that were attached longer than 48 hours – the time required for transmission of the spirochete. It is extremely difficult, however, to make consistently accurate determinations of the species of tick and the degree of engorgement. Furthermore, randomized double-blind clinical trials involving individuals who were bitten by *I. scapularis* ticks led to the conclusion that treating all individuals who remove vector ticks with antibiotics is probably not warranted.[8]

Table 26.1 Spirochetes are the causative agents of many diseases, which can have social as well as lasting health-related consequences

Major diseases caused by spirochetal infection				
Disease	Agents	Distribution	Transmission	Symptoms
Lyme disease	*Borrelia burgdorferi* *B. garinii* *B. afzelii* *B. andersoni* *B. japonica* *B. lusitaniae* *B. valaisiana*	North America, Europe Asia, Europe Asia, Europe North America Japan Southern Europe Europe, Ireland, UK	Tick engorgement	Development of a skin rash known as *erythema migrans,* accompanied by other symptoms such as malaise, myalgia, and/or arthralgia. Symptoms can progress to include carditis and arthritis. Persistent infection can result in chronic arthritis, neuroborreliosis, or cutaneous symptoms (acrodermatitis chronica atrophicans)
Relapsing fever	*B. hermsii* *B. turicatae* *B. parkeri* *B. mazzotti* *B. venezuelensis* *B. duttoni* *B. crocidurae* *B. persica* *B. hispanica* *B. latyschewii* *B. caucasia*	Western USA Southwestern USA, Mexico Western USA Central America Central America Sub-Saharan Africa North Africa, Middle East Middle East, Central Asia Iberian peninsula, North Africa Iran, Iraq, Eastern Europe Iraq, Eastern Europe	Tick engorgement	Clinical manifestations of infection include high-density spirochetemia, high fever, myalgias, and arthralgias, and can even include cerebral hemorrhage and fatality
Venereal syphilis	*Treponema pallidum pallidum*	Worldwide	Sexual contact	Disease progresses from a primary lesion (chancre) to a secondary eruption and then a latent period, and if left untreated tertiary symptoms may appear
Endemic syphilis or Bejel syphilis	*T. pallidum endemicum*	Eastern Mediterranean region, West Africa	Nonsexual skin contact	Symptoms begin with a slimy patch on the inside of the mouth followed by blisters on the trunk and limbs. Bone infection in the legs soon develops, and, in the later stages, lumps may appear in the nose and on the soft palate of the mouth
Yaws	*T. pertenue*	Humid equatorial countries	Nonsexual skin contact	Destructive lesions of the skin and bones, which is rarely fatal but can be debilitating

Continued

PATHOLOGY ARISING FROM INFECTION WITH B. BURGDORFERI OR T. PALLIDUM

Table 26.1 Spirochetes are the causative agents of many diseases, which can have social as well as lasting health-related consequences—Cont'd

Major diseases caused by spirochetal infection				
Disease	Agents	Distribution	Transmission	Symptoms
Pinta	T. carateum	Mexico, Central America, South America	Nonsexual skin contact	Dark skin lesions found on those areas of the body that are exposed to sunlight. Eventually, the skin lesions become discolored
Leptospirosis	L. interrogans	Worldwide	Urine from an infected animal	Symptoms include fever, headache, chills, nausea, and vomiting, eye inflammation, and muscle aches. In more severe cases, the illness can result in liver damage and kidney failure

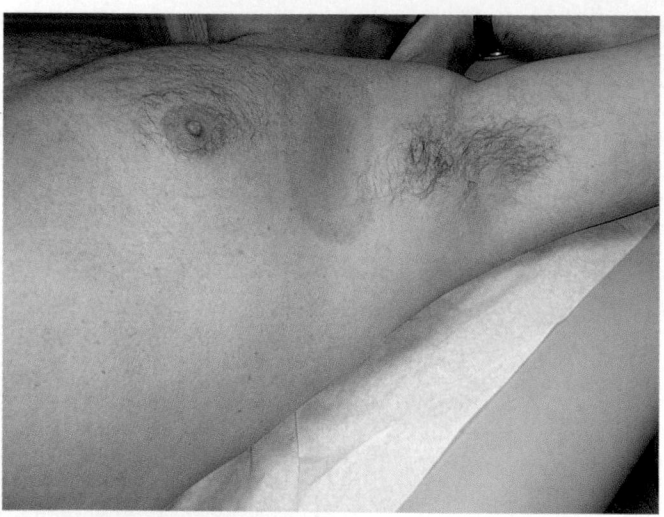

Fig. 26.2 Erythema migrans due to infection with *Borrelia burgdorferi*, the Lyme disease agent. (Courtesy of Gary Wormser, MD.)

VENEREAL SYPHILIS

Infection with the agent of syphilis, *T. pallidum* subspecies *pallidum*, occurs worldwide. *T. pallidum* is an obligate human parasite that is almost exclusively transmitted when contact with infectious exudates from lesions of the skin and mucous membranes of infected individuals occurs.

Clinically, this treponemal infection is first characterized by the formation of a hardened and painless ulcer at the initial site of infection. This primary lesion, called a chancre, forms after invasion of the bloodstream by the spirochete. Four to 6 weeks following infection, the edges of the chancre roll inwards and upwards and, in most cases, a secondary eruption appears, often accompanied by a rash on the palms of the hands and the soles of the feet. The secondary manifestations spontaneously resolve within weeks to a year. Long periods of latency, and late lesions of the skin, bone, viscera, cardiovascular and central nervous systems, can follow.

Diagnosis

Much like Lyme disease, the diagnosis for syphilis is based on the clinical presentations of the disease and serologic tests. In addition, dark-field microscopy may be used for the identification of *T. pallidum* in the serous exudates of the chancre. This approach, however, is limited by the number of live treponemes in the exudates and by the presence of nonpathologic treponemes in oral and anal lesions; as such, negative examinations on three independent days are required before a lesion is considered negative for *T. pallidum*.

Infection with *T. pallidum* leads to the production of nonspecific antibodies, which is the basis for other diagnostic tests, such as the traditional nontreponemal serologic tests, including the Venereal Disease Research Laboratory (VDRL) and rapid plasma reagin (RPR) tests. Because these tests are nonspecific, false-positive reactions may occur as a result of pregnancy, autoimmune disorders, or infections. Therefore, treponemal-specific tests, which detect antibodies to various antigens of *T. pallidum*, are often used to confirm the results of a non-specific test. Interestingly, treponemal-specific tests are just as sensitive as nontreponemal tests; however, they are much more difficult and expensive to perform, which limits their use. These tests include, but are not limited to, the enzyme immunoassay test for *T. pallidum*-specific IgG (EIA), *T. pallidum* hemagglutination test (TPHA), fluorescent treponemal antibody-absorption test (FTA-abs), and ELISA.

Treatment

Susceptibility to infection with *T. pallidum* is universal, although only 30% of exposures with lesions teeming with the spirochete result in infection. Infection results in gradual development of immunity against *T. pallidum* and often against heterologous treponemes as well. However, treatment with long-acting penicillin subverts the development of immunity against *T. pallidum*. A single intramuscular dose of 2.4 million units the day that the primary, secondary, or latent syphilis is diagnosed is effective at killing the spirochetes. For people who are allergic to penicillin, there are alternative treatments such as doxycycline.

IMMUNE RESPONSES TO B. BURGDORFERI

The Lyme disease spirochete has been the subject of intensive investigation in order to elucidate the mechanisms that contribute to its ability to cause persistent infection and multisystemic disease, despite the development of strong immune responses. The control of the number of bacteria in the mammalian host is likely to depend on several immune effector mechanisms, such as the development of antibody responses and the capacity of phagocytic cells to clear spirochetes.

INNATE IMMUNITY

The initial encounter of a pathogen with cells of the host initiates a cascade of responses that lead to the upregulation of chemokines and cytokines, adhesion molecules, and a vast array of other effector molecules (Chapter 3). These events are aimed at the recruitment of phagocytic cells, their activation, and the eventual development of the adaptive immune response. The initial recognition of pathogens by cells of the innate immune system and others, like endothelial and epithelial cells, depends on the rapid detection of the microorganism. This depends on the presence of germline-encoded pattern recognition receptors (PRRs) that distinguish infectious agents from host factors. These pattern recognition molecules are being extensively studied because they not only mediate these initial responses to microorganisms, but also modulate the extent and quality of acquired immune responses. Toll-like receptors (TLRs), identified as the mammalian counterparts of the Toll protein in *Drosophila* that mediate immune responses to fungi, are the most studied, but do not constitute the only mechanism by which innate immune cells recognize infecting microorganisms. Each PRR recognizes a specific structure that is present in a group or groups of microorganisms and that distinguishes them from the more specific recognition of spirochetal

antigens by the T- and B-cell receptors. Thus, TLR4 recognizes LPS, which is present in Gram-negative bacteria. The recognition of patterns instead of specific antigens provides the innate immune system with a rapid way to respond to infecting organisms until the more specific response mediated by T and B cells develops.

B. burgdorferi does not contain LPS, in contrast with other members of the spirochete group, and therefore does not engage TLR4. The most important pattern recognized by innate immune receptors is constituted by the surface lipoproteins of the spirochete and this seems to be true for whole spirochetes and lysates. It is not clear what the specific interaction between whole spirochetes and antigens exposed by bacterial lysis with immune cells is *in vivo*. However, it is conceivable that both elicit immune responses, since *B. burdorgferi* is likely to die *in vivo*, for example in the presence of antibody in a process that does not require complement or phagocytosis.

The interaction of *B. burgdorferi* lipoproteins with complexes formed by TLRs 1 and 2 on the surface of innate immune and other cell types initiates a series of signaling cascades that results in the production of proinflammatory cytokines (interleukin (IL)-1β, tumor necrosis factor (TNF)-α, IL-12, and IL-18, among others), chemokines (IL-8, MCP-1, KC), metalloproteinases and adhesion molecules (E-selectin, VCAM-1, and ICAM-1).[9] These proteins mediate both the inflammatory response to the spirochete through the production of proinflammatory cytokines and chemotactic factors that further induce the recruitment of inflammatory cells. These products also modulate adaptive immune responses, through increased antigen presentation, induction of co-stimulatory signals on antigen-presenting cells and the production of cytokines that influence CD4 T-cell differentiation and effector function (Fig. 26.3).

Phagocytic cell responses to the spirochete mediate a major previously unrecognized role in the control of bacterial numbers, presumably by their capacity to engulf the bacteria. Even though phagocytic cells are able to engulf bacteria in the absence of antibody through a potential interaction with the mannose receptor,[10] experiments in TLR1- or TLR2-deficient mice have shown significant increases in their bacterial burden, underscoring the importance of TLR-mediated activation of phagocytic cells. These observations emphasize the necessity to maintain an active phagocytic cell compartment in spite of the inflammatory response that it generates in response to infection.

This conclusion has been further confirmed with the infection of mice that are deficient in MyD88, an early signaling component that mediates TLR-induced signals. It is clear that TLR signaling is involved in many of the early innate immune responses to *B. burgdorferi*; however, the engagement of TLR 2/1 complexes by spirochetal lipoproteins has a role in the manifestation of pathology associated with *B. burgdorferi* infection, which exposes a puzzling dichotomy. What is the role of this interaction in the manifestation of disease versus its role in resolution of spirochetal infection? This question remains to be answered, especially because of contradicting reports of arthritis development upon infection of TLR1-, TLR2-, or MyD88-deficient mice. The development of arthritis in the absence of TLRs, CD14, or MyD88 suggests that alternative pathways exist that trigger the inflammatory response to the spirochete. It is conceivable that the interaction of *B. burgdorferi* with resident cells of the invaded tissues through the specific interaction of bacterial proteins (Bbk32, DbpA and B, P66) with host factors (fibronectin, decorin, integrins) allows their homing and the initiation of signals for the production of chemokines that attract infiltrating phagocytic cells. These basally activated infiltrating cells may still be able to induce

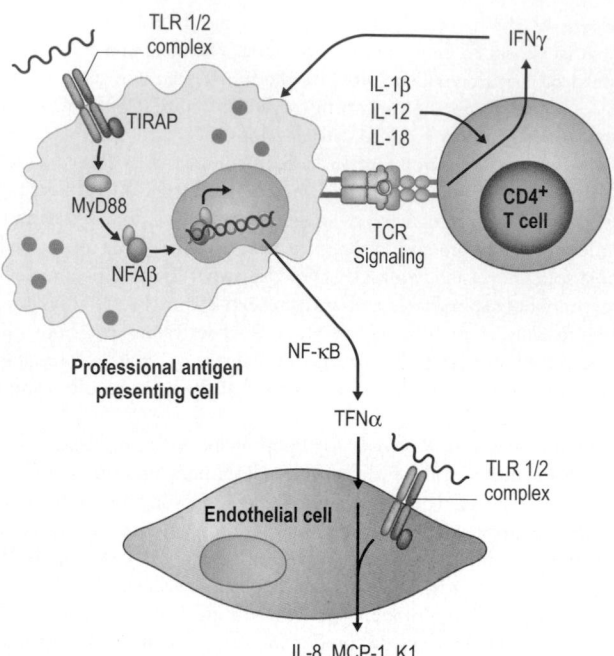

Fig. 26.3 The interaction of *Borrelia burgdorferi* with Toll-like receptor (TLR) 1/2 complexes on the surface of innate immune and endothelial cells mediates the inflammatory response to the spirochete. TLR-driven proinflammatory cytokine production as well as antigen presentation by professional antigen-presenting cells (APCs) leads to the activation of CD4 effector T cells, which is marked by the production of interferon-γ. Likewise, TLR- and tumor necrosis factor-α receptor signaling lead to the upregulation of chemokines by endothelial cells. Overall, these responses lead to increased activation and recruitment of innate immune cells in sites of infection.

low levels of inflammation that nevertheless may be compensated with the increased insult resulting from the higher number of bacteria, independent of their interaction with the spirochete with TLRs that signal through MyD88. The inability of these phagocytic cells to eliminate *B. burgdorferi* effectively even in the presence of a strong antibody response leads to increased bacterial burdens and an overall inflammatory response that is equivalent to or superior than the one produced in the presence of functional TLRs. In any case, these results highlight the complexity of the innate immune response to the spirochete. It is likely that the early control of infection through innate immune defenses is important for controlling bacterial burden until the more powerful and specific adaptive immune response can completely resolve the infection.

Phagocytic cell recruitment

The recruitment of phagocytic cells into sites of infection is mediated by the production of chemokines, increased vascular permeability, and upregulated expression of cell adhesion molecules in endothelial cells. *B. bugdorferi* induces the upregulation of these factors in different cell types. Chemokine production at sites of pathology in disease-susceptible C3H/HeJ mice and -resistant C57BL/6 mice show that

inflammation is related to increased production of neutrophil and monocyte–macrophage chemokines, KC and MCP-1, respectively.[11] In patients, the production of chemokines, especially IL-8, during the initial response to *B. burgdorferi* correlates well with the onset of symptoms known to occur during the early stages of infection, suggesting that their production is increased during the beginning of the infection to recruit phagocytic cells, which are involved in the initial clearance of the spirochete. Overall, these results also suggest that the chemokine response is modulated once the infection progresses, and that progression of the disease may be dependent on the regulation of these chemoattractants whose production might be altered by the presence of the infiltrating cells.

Complement

The complement system is a key component of the innate immune system (Chapters 3 and 20). It comprises a collection of serum proteins and cell surface receptors that are involved in the early response to pathogens, including *B. burgdorferi*.[12] Destruction of microorganisms via complement involves the formation of a pore in the microbial cell membrane by the membrane attack complex (MAC), which results in the lysis of the organism. Three different pathways elicit complement activation: the classical (antigen antibody-mediated), lectin, and alternative (pathogen surface) pathway. These pathways converge at the level of C3 convertase, a protease that cleaves complement component C3 into C3a and C3b. As a result, C3b can either bind to the surface of the bacteria and facilitate internalization of the spirochete via opsonization or bind C3 convertase and facilitate the deposition of downstream components on to the surface of the spirochete resulting in the formation of MAC and lysis of the cell.

B. burgdorferi activates the classical and alternative pathways of the complement cascade.[13] Moreover, the activation of complement has been associated with dramatic decreases in spirochetal numbers in different tissues of infected mice, indicating the importance of the complement system early in *B. burgdorferi* infection. However, complement-independent, antibody-mediated killing of spirochetes has been extensively reported, although the relative contribution of both mechanisms is not completely clear *in vivo*.

The members of the *B. burgdorferi sensu lato* group, which includes *B. burgdorferi sensu stricto*, *B. garinii*, and *B. afzelii*, have evolved a variety of mechanisms enabling them to escape complement-mediated lysis, including the expression of complement regulator-acquiring surface proteins (CRASPs). Of these CRASPs, the ERP (OspEF-related protein) family of outer-membrane proteins serves as binding sites for the complement inhibitor factor H and factor H-like protein 1 (FHL-1).[9] The interaction of factor H with these proteins recruits a protease (factor I) that cleaves and inactivates the complement serum proteins C3b and C4b. Cleavage of these two complement proteins prevents the deposition of downstream components on to the surface of the spirochete, thereby halting the formation of the MAC. *B. burgdorferi* also express a CD59-like molecule on the outer membrane, which can inactivate MAC and prevent complement-mediated lysis.[14] It has been speculated that most *Borrelia* are able to evade complement-mediated lysis, and recently a novel protein expressed by *B. hermsii* (a relapsing-fever spirochete) has been discovered that affords protection to spirochete by inactivating C3b.[15] Because of the ability for many infectious strains to avoid complement-mediated lysis, the activation of complement is not required for the resolution of many infections with *Borrelia* species.

KEY CONCEPTS

PROTECTIVE VERSUS PATHOLOGICAL RESPONSES TO *BORRELIA BURGDORFERI*

>> The early immune response to *B. burgdorferi* is necessary to control spirochetal burden; however, alone it is not sufficient to resolve infection

>> The T-cell-mediated response appears to be involved in pathology arising from infection

>> The T-cell-independent B-cell responses are critical for resolving infection with *B. burgdorferi*

ADAPTIVE IMMUNE RESPONSES

It is well established that after presentation of antigen by macrophages, dendritic cells, or B cells, to naïve CD4 T cells, these naïve cells differentiate into either Th1 or Th2 effector T cells (Chapter 17). Through their production of interferon-γ and TNF-β, Th1 cells are regulators of the cell-mediated inflammatory reaction, which is characterized by macrophage activation, stimulation of CD8 T cells, and production of opsonizing IgG antibodies. Th2 cells produce IL-4, IL-5, IL-6, IL-10 and IL-13 and regulate the antibody response to pathogens by controlling the differentiating B cells and promoting Ig class switching. Generally, infections with intracellular pathogens induce a Th1 response that is protective, while extracellular pathogens induce an antibody-mediated Th2 response. The most powerful inducer of differentiation of naïve CD4 T cells into Th1 or Th2 effector cells is the local cytokine environment. IL-12 directs the differentiation of naïve effector T cells towards the Th1 phenotype, while IL-6 (through an IL-4-dependent mechanism) and IL-4 drive differentiation towards the Th2 phenotype. Interaction of *B. burgdorferi* antigen with TLRs drives the production of IL-12 and the differentiation of naïve CD4 T cells into Th1 effector cells. Thus, TLRs are important to bridge the innate and adaptive immune responses.

The development of an imbalanced immune response can have pathological consequences. Therefore, it has been speculated that the pathology following infection with *B. burgdorferi* is often the result of a shift in the immune response towards the Th1 phenotype, resulting in more inflammation and less antibody production. In fact, it has been shown that Th1 cells dominate the immune response in the synovial fluid of patients with Lyme disease, and that the severity of arthritis correlates directly with the ratio of Th1 to Th2 cells in the synovium, such that the higher the ratio the more severe the inflammation, indicating that Th1 cells are directly involved in the pathogenesis associated with Lyme disease.[16]

The role of T-cell-mediated immunity during infection with *B. burgdorferi* and other members of the *Borrelia* genus appears to contribute to pathology associated with infection, while the resolution of spirochetal infection with *B. burgdorferi* does not require functional T cells. Furthermore, nude mice and T-cell-depleted mice resolve *B. turicatae* infection, thereby preventing the onset of symptomatology associated with relapsing fever.[17] However, carditis, which is a *B. burgdorferi*-induced inflammatory phenomenon with a higher incidence in the murine model of Lyme borreliosis than human disease, seems to require a Th1 response for resolution.

The specific contribution of Th1 effector cells in the progression of disease mediated by infection with *B. burgdorferi* is not yet known. It has been hypothesized, however, that Th1 responses sustained by presentation of autoantigens is involved in the development of an unusual form of antibiotic-resistant chronic Lyme arthritis.[18] Certain individuals possessing specific alleles of class II major histocompatibility complex (MHC) molecules (HLA-DR4) are purportedly genetically predisposed to developing treatment-resistant Lyme arthritis. One of these alleles, identified as DRB1-0401, may bind to a molecular mimic of OspA (hLFA-1), and the presentation of this molecule to OspA-reactive, Th1 effector cells in the proper context is postulated to lead to activation of T cells, long after *B. burgdorferi* infection has been resolved.[19]

Interferon-γ, which is produced by these Th1 effector cells, has been shown to be dispensable for the genesis of acute murine arthritis. These results arose from the infection of mice that lack either the cytokine or the alpha subunit of its receptor. However, the modulation of the Th1 response by alteration of the cytokines that mediate their differentiation, such as IL-12 and IL-6, suggest the opposite. Interferon-γ has also been shown to help the persistence of the spirochete in the murine host by inducing an increased rearrangement at the Vls locus.[20] It should be noted that the route of infection greatly affects the inflammatory response in both the joints and the heart of mice infected with the spirochete, and may partially account for differences in experimental results. Infection by syringe in the footpad of mice results in increased arthritis while carditis is reduced compared to mice that are infected by subcutaneous infection in the midline of the back.[21]

ANTIBODY RESPONSES

Prior to the development of an antibody-specific immune response, the degree of clearance by circulating phagocytes is very limited, indicating that the humoral response to *B. burgdorferi* might be necessary for resolution of spirochetal infection. In addition to usual T-cell-dependent antibody responses to *B. burgdorferi*, T-cell-independent humoral responses also confer protection to the host. Furthermore, T-cell-independent humoral immune responses are critical for resolving symptoms associated with *B. burgdorferi* infection. T-cell-deficient mice infected with *B. burgdorferi* mount a protective antibody response, which upon passive serum transfer affords protection to severe combined immune deficiency (SCID) mice from homologous challenge. However, mice that lack both B and T cells developed severe arthritis and carditis in response to infection with *B. burgdorferi*.

Stimulation of CD40L, which interacts with CD40 on T cells, is crucial for T-cell-dependent activation of B cells and subsequent antibody production. Mice deficient for CD40L are also able to generate protective antibody responses against *B. burgdorferi* and therefore resolve infection.[22] Additionally, class II MHC-deficient mice are able to resolve symptoms associated with *B. burgdorferi* infection.[23] Thus, it is implied that *B. burgdorferi* antigens have the ability to stimulate B cells to expand clonally and differentiate into antibody-producing plasma cells, and that T-cell-independent humoral responses are extremely important for the protective immunity against *B. burgdorferi*.

The importance of antibodies in controlling *B. burgdorferi* infection was underscored by the discovery of complement-independent bactericidal antibodies, which have the capacity to control an infection. An IgG1κ monoclonal antibody termed CB2 binds to *B. burgdorferi*-OspB via a single lysine residue, causing an alteration in the structure of OspB, thereby, increasing its susceptibility to protease degradation, and ultimately leading to the lysis of the spirochete.[24] Another bactericidal antibody, H6831, with identical specificity to OspB was reported. Both CB2 and H6831 are so effective at killing *B. burgdorferi* that their selective pressure on the growth of *B. burgdorferi* was used to generate escape mutants of *B. burgdorferi* that lacked the lysine necessary for antibody binding to OspB, which made the escape mutants less infectious.

MECHANISMS OF IMMUNE EVASION

B. burgdorferi has evolved sophisticated mechanisms for immune evasion, which is not surprising considering that this pathogen is able to establish chronic infection in the midst of a very strong immune response. Just as *B. burgdorferi* has evolved mechanisms to evade the host innate immune system, this organism has also evolved the ability to escape killing by the acquired immune system. It has long been speculated that microbes can acquire host antigens and avoid immune recognition. In addition to evading the effector mechanisms of the innate immune response, *B. burgdorferi* is able to evade the humoral response by interacting with the extracellular matrix of the mammalian host via attachment to decorin, a major component of the extracellular matrix. *B. burgdorferi* attaches to decorin with a ligand-binding lipoprotein known as decorin-binding protein A (DbpA). A deficiency in decorin reduces the incidence of Lyme arthritis in mice, suggesting that the interaction of DbpA with the extracellular matrix provides a protective niche for *B. burgdorferi*, and thus prevents humoral-mediated bacterial killing.

Another method used by members of the *Borrelia* genus to avoid clearance by the host immune system is antigenic diversity. The recurrent spirochetemia characteristic of relapsing fever is attributed to the antigenic diversity of relapsing-fever spirochetes, with each wave of spirochetemia resulting from the generation of new outer-membrane antigens not yet recognized by the host immune system. Spirochetes of a different serotype are generated by genetic rearrangement of silent variable major protein (VMP) encoding regions into an expression locus. *B. burgdorferi* differentially expresses outer-membrane antigens under pressure from the immune response, which might contribute to the spirochetes' ability to persist in the host. A mechanism that is potentially essential for spirochetal immune escape is the recombination that takes place at the *vls* locus,[20] which consists on a *vls* expression site (*vlsE*) located near the right telomere of the linear plasmid lp28-1 and 15 silent cassettes upstream. *vlsE* encodes a surface-exposed, immunogenic protein of 34 kDa.

Ticks of the *Ixodes* complex secrete a 15-kDa salivary protein known as Salp15 during engorgement. This protein binds to CD4 and inhibits the activation CD4 effector T cells. Presumably this immunosuppressive effect is beneficial for the tick as it enables the tick to engorge on the host long enough to receive an adequate blood meal. Interestingly, *B. burgdorferi* usurps Salp15 to facilitate its own transmission from the arthropod vector to the mammalian host. *In vivo* and *in vitro* adherence of Salp15 to *B. burgdorferi* through an interaction with OspC protects the spirochete from antibody-mediated killing,[25] increasing the pathogens' capacity to infect and colonize the mammalian host upon tick feeding.

IMMUNE RESPONSE AGAINST *TREPONEMA PALLIDUM*

The agent of syphilis is an extremely elusive microbe both to our immune system and to the researchers attempting to grasp the pathogenic mechanisms of this organism. For more than 500 years, syphilis

has been a recognized disease; however, due to the inability to culture these organisms *in vitro*, we have yet to elucidate many of the mechanisms by which this treponeme causes disease. Moreover, the inability to infect mice reproducibly, for which many specific immunological reagents are available, with the pathogen has limited our ability to examine specific immune responses *in vivo*. Coupled with that is the fact that our immune system is unable to recognize and successfully eliminate infection with this spirochete, resulting in persistent infections that have lasting health and social consequences. Our understanding of the immune responses to this pathogen is not nearly as detailed as our knowledge of those elicited in response to infection with *B. burgdorferi*.

Early studies showed that cell-mediated immunity had a protective role in response to infection with *T. pallidum*, which led researchers to believe that pathogenesis was a consequence of diminished cell-mediated immunity. However, more recent studies have cast doubt on this hypothesis. In genital ulcers (chancres) the immune cell population consists mostly of CD4 T cells and macrophages, and Th1 cytokines predominate in lesions of both primary and secondary syphilis.[26, 27] Furthermore, the cell-mediated immune response to *T. pallidum* correlates well with the resolution of primary and secondary syphilis.

Currently, the role of CD4 T cells in pathology resulting from infection with *T. pallidum* is still not fully understood. It is likely that the cell-mediated immune response to *T. pallidum* has a role in the manifestation of disease during infection with this spirochete, as indicated by the propensity of this organism to cause inflammatory disease. However, a dichotomy exists between the roles of the cell-mediated immune response to *T. pallidum*, in that development of pathology versus the resolution of infection are not mutually exclusive. For instance, it has been shown that an exaggerated cell-mediated immune response is involved in the manifestation of gummatous disease, which is a characteristic of tertiary syphilis.[28] Therefore, although the importance of a strong cell-mediated immune response to *T. pallidum* has been shown, the role that this specific immune response plays in the pathogenicity of the spirochete remains unclear.

Infection with *T. pallidum* invokes a humoral immune response early in the course of infection, which strengthens as the number of recognizable antigens increases during the progression of infection. A polymorphic gene family of *T. pallidum*, called *T. pallidum* repeat (*tp*r), has recently been identified and shown to be related to the major surface protein (Msp) genes of *T. denticola*.[29] It has been shown that a single member of the *tpr* family, *tpr*K, serves as an antigen for opsonizing antibodies, which suggests that this protein is a surface antigen of *T. pallidum*. However, there are only indications that surface antigens of *T. pallidum* exist. So, although candidate *T. pallidum* surface proteins have been advanced on the basis of porin activity or homology with a surface protein of *T. denticola*, there is no real evidence identifying specific surface antigens on *T. pallidum*. Furthermore, like most pathogenic organisms, *T. pallidum* has evolved various mechanisms to escape host killing. *T. pallidum* repeat protein K (TprK) is an immunogen with seven discrete variable regions differing among different isolates of the spirochete.[29] In fact, the antibody response to *T. pallidum* is directed against these variable regions, leading to the hypothesis that the antigenic diversity of TprK is involved in the reinfection of hosts despite robust immune responses.[29]

Molecular, biochemical, and ultrastructural data have indicated that this spirochete possesses a molecular architecture responsible for its remarkable ability to evade the immune response,[28, 30] and, because of this, *T. pallidum* has been termed a stealth pathogen. The outer membrane of *T. pallidum* is comprised of mostly nonimmunogenic transmembrane proteins, and the highly immunogenic lipoproteins are contained within the periplasmic space.[31] Therefore, this rare molecular architecture is thought to explain the poor antigenicity of living treponemes and its unique ability to evade killing by the host immune system.

CONCLUSION

Spirochetes are a phylogenetically ancient and distinct group of microorganisms. Because of their propensity to cause diseases in humans, *B. burgdorferi* and *T. pallidum* are the two best-studied spirochetes. However, the inability to culture *T. pallidum in vitro* has made researching this spirochete very difficult, and as a consequence our understanding of the immune response following infection with this spirochete is more limited.

The etiologic agents of Lyme disease and syphilis are similar in having relatively small genomes, surviving only in association with a host and eliciting inflammatory disease, but genomic comparison clearly shows that *T. pallidum* and *B. burgdorferi* are not closely related. It seems likely that these spirochetes evolved independently from a more complex ancestor, resulting in differences in their lifecycles, environmental adaptations, and the pathology associated with their infection, despite some similarities. Therefore, it is not surprising to learn of differences in the host immune response to *B. burgdorferi* and *T. pallidum*. Both the host response to these spirochetes and the infectivity of the bacterium determine the extent of pathology following infection.

REFERENCES

1. Burgdorfer W, Barbour AG, Hayes SF, et al. Lyme disease – a tick-borne spirochetosis?. Science 1982; 216: 1317–1319.

2. Krause RM. Metchnikoff and syphilis research during a decade of discovery, 1900–1910. Development of an animal model and a preventive treatment set the stage for progress. ASM News 1996; 62: 307–310.

3. Fraser CM, Norris SJ, Weinstock GM, et al. Complete genome sequence of *Treponema pallidum*, the syphilis spirochete. Science 1998; 281: 375–388.

4. Fraser CM, Cas jens S, Huang WM, et al. Genomic sequence of a Lyme disease spirochaete, *Borrelia burgdorferi*. Nature 1997; 390: 580–586.

5. Anguita J, Hedrick MN, Fikrig E. Adaptation of *Borrelia burgdorferi* in the tick and the mammalian host. FEMS Microbiol Rev 2003; 27: 493–504.

6. Pal U, Li X, Wang T, et al. TROSPA, an *Ixodes scapularis* receptor for *Borrelia burgdorferi*. Cell 2004; 119: 457–468.

7. Lyme disease – United States, 2001–2002. MMWR 2004; 53: 365–369.

8. Wormser GP, Nadelman RB, Dattwyler RJ, et al. Practice guidelines for the treatment of Lyme disease. The Infectious Diseases Society of America. Clin Infect Dis 2000; 31(Suppl 1): 1–14.

9. Guerau-de-Arellano M, Huber BT. Chemokines and Toll-like receptors in Lyme disease pathogenesis. Trends Mol Med 2005; 11: 114–120.

10. Cinco M, Lini B, Murgia R, et al. Evidence of involvement of the mannose receptor in adhesion of *Borrelia burgdorferi* to monocyte/macrophages. Infect Immun 2001; 69: 2743–2747.

11. Brown CR, Blaho VA, Loiacono CM. Susceptibility to experimental Lyme arthritis correlates with KC and monocyte chemoattractant protein-1 production in joints and requires neutrophil recruitment via CXCR2. J Immunol 2003; 171: 893–901.

12. Lawrenz MB, Wooten RM, Zachary JF, et al. Effect of complement component C3 deficiency on experimental Lyme borreliosis in mice. Infect Immun 2003; 71: 4432–4440.

13. Kochi SK, Johnson RC. Role of immunoglobulin G in killing of *Borrelia burgdorferi* by the classical complement pathway. Infect Immun 1988; 56: 314–321.

14. Pausa M, Pellis V, Cinco M, et al. Serum-resistant strains of *Borrelia burgdorferi* evade complement-mediated killing by expressing a CD59-like complement inhibitory molecule. J Immunol 2003; 170: 3214–3222.

15. Hovis KM, McDowell JV, Griffin L, et al. Identification and characterization of a linear-plasmid-encoded factor H-binding protein (FhbA) of the relapsing fever spirochete *Borrelia hermsii*. J Bacteriol 2004; 186: 2612–2618.

16. Gross DM, Steere AC, Huber BT. T helper 1 response is dominant and localized to the synovial fluid in patients with Lyme arthritis. J Immunol 1998; 160: 1022–1028.

17. Newman K Jr., Johnson RC. T-cell-independent elimination of *Borrelia turicatae*. Infect Immun 1984; 45: 572–576.

18. Steere AC, Gross D, Meyer AL, et al. Autoimmune mechanisms in antibiotic treatment-resistant Lyme arthritis. J Autoimmun 2001; 16: 263–268.

19. Gross DM, Forsthuber T, Tary-Lehmann M, et al. Identification of LFA-1 as a candidate autoantigen in treatment-resistant Lyme arthritis. Science 1998; 281: 703–706.

20. Zhang JR, Hardham JM, Barbour AG, et al. Antigenic variation in Lyme disease borreliae by promiscuous recombination of VMP-like sequence cassettes. Cell 1997; 89: 275–285.

21. Motameni AR, Bates TC, Juncadella IJ, et al. Distinct bacterial dissemination and disease outcome in mice subcutaneously infected with *Borrelia burgdorferi* in the midline of the back and the footpad. FEMS Immunol Med Microbiol 2005; 45: 279–284.

22. Fikrig E, Barthold SW, Chen M, et al. Protective antibodies in murine Lyme disease arise independently of CD40 ligand. J Immunol 1996; 157: 1–3.

23. Fikrig E, Barthold SW, Chen M, et al. Protective antibodies develop, and murine Lyme arthritis regresses, in the absence of MHC class II and CD4+ T cells. J Immunol 1997; 159: 5682–5686.

24. Escudero R, Halluska ML, Backenson PB, et al. Characterization of the physiological requirements for the bactericidal effects of a monoclonal antibody to OspB of *Borrelia burgdorferi* by confocal microscopy. Infect Immun 1997; 65: 1908–1915.

25. Ramamoorthi N, Narasimhan S, Pal U, et al. The Lyme disease agent exploits a tick protein to infect the mammalian host. Nature 2005; 436: 573–577.

26. McBroom RL, Syles AR, Chiu MJ, et al. Secondary syphilis in persons infected with and not infected with HIV-1: a comparative immunohistologic study. Am J Dermatopathol 1999; 21: 432–441.

27. Van Voorhis WC, Barrett LK, Koelle DM, et al. Primary and secondary syphilis lesions contain mRNA for Th1 cytokines. J Infect Dis 1996; 173: 491–495.

28. Salazar JC, Hazlett KR, Radolf JD. The immune response to infection with *Treponema pallidum*, the stealth pathogen. Microbes Infect 2002; 4: 1133–1140.

29. Centurion-Lara A, Castro C, Barrett LK, et al. *Treponema pallidum* major sheath protein homologue Tpr K is a target of opsonic antibody and the protective immune response. J Exp Med 1999; 189: 647–656.

30. Sellati TJ, Bouis DA, Caimano MJ, et al. Activation of human monocytic cells by *Borrelia burgdorferi* and *Treponema pallidum* is facilitated by CD14 and correlates with surface exposure of spirochetal lipoproteins. J Immunol 1999; 163: 2049–2056.

31. Cox DL, Chang P, McDowall AW, et al. The outer membrane, not a coat of host proteins, limits antigenicity of virulent *Treponema pallidum*. Infect Immun 1992; 60: 1076–1083.

Immune responses to viruses

Scott N. Mueller, Barry T. Rouse

27

Viruses as obligate intracellular parasites require their host to replicate them and to facilitate their spread to others. In humans, viral infections are rarely lethal, even if they are highly cytolytic to individual cells. Mortality commonly occurs when viruses jump species (such as Ebola or human immunodeficiency virus (HIV)), when the virus undergoes a major antigenic change (i.e., influenza viruses), or when host immunity is compromised. HIV represents one of the most dramatic human examples of an exotic virus that kills its host. However, HIV kills slowly, providing ample time to spread to new hosts and an effective strategy for persistence in the species. Death or dire consequences following virus infection in mammals with inadequate immunity are well illustrated by observations that fetuses or neonates, especially if deprived of passive immunity, succumb to many agents well tolerated by normal adults. The increasing wealth of immunological tools, such as transgenic animal models and major histocompatibility complex (MHC) tetramers, have provided sensitive methods for defining the relevance of immune mechanisms for antiviral defense. In most situations, defense against viruses involves multiple immune components, and the impact of a single mechanism varies greatly according to the method by which individual viruses enter, replicate, and spread within the host. In this chapter, we highlight the principal means by which the host achieves immunity following infection by viruses. Table 27.1 presents an overview.

■ VIRAL ENTRY AND INFECTION ■

Access to target tissues presents numerous obstacles for entry and infection by most human viruses. Most effective of these are the mechanical barriers provided by the skin and mucosal surfaces, as well as the chemically hostile environment of the gut (Fig. 27.1). A number of common human viral pathogens enter through the gastrointestinal tract, including rotavirus, enteric adenoviruses, and hepatitis A virus (HAV). These are usually spread via person-to-person contact or contaminated food and water. Respiratory infections caused by influenza viruses, rhinoviruses, coronaviruses, measles virus, varicella-zoster virus (VZV), and respiratory syncytial virus (RSV) are often spread by aerosol transmission, as well as person-to-person contact. Many of the herpes viruses target the skin or the mucosae, such as herpes simplex virus (HSV) and VZV. HSV in particular can infect oral and genital mucosa, the eye, and the skin through small cuts and abrasions. Other herpes viruses, such as Epstein–Barr virus (EBV) and cytomegalovirus (CMV), target the mucosa. CMV can also spread vertically from mother to baby or rarely via blood transfusions. Human papillomavirus (HPV) targets skin and mucosa and causes warts and may transform cells, inducing cancers such as cervical cancer. Viruses such as West Nile virus and Semliki forest virus may also enter through the skin via insect vectors. HIV and hepatitis B virus (HBV) are commonly spread via sexual contact. HIV, HBV, and hepatitis C virus (HCV) can also infect humans via direct entry into the bloodstream via transfusions or contaminated needles.

Most human viruses replicate only in certain target tissues, this being mainly the consequence of viral receptor distribution. Many viruses use two receptors, such as the use of the CD4 co-receptor and CCR5 by HIV. After attachment to a cellular receptor, viruses may fuse with the cell membrane or be endocytosed and then gain entry into the cytoplasm or nucleus by fusing with the vesicular membrane (enveloped viruses such as HSV and HIV), or translocate across the cell membrane or induce lysis of the endocytic vesicle once in the cytoplasm (nonenveloped viruses such as Norwalk virus and poliovirus).[1] Viruses then utilize host cell machinery and specialized virally encoded proteins to replicate rapidly within the cell. Once they have multiplied within the cell, many viruses induce cytolysis in order to facilitate release of new infectious virions (the poxviruses, poliovirus, and herpes viruses, for example). Other viruses are released from infected cells by budding through the cell membrane in the absence of cell death (i.e., HIV and influenza virus). Having entered the body, however, viruses encounter numerous innate defenses and activate the components of adaptive immunity. The latter usually assures that clinical disease, if not infection, will not become evident. Successful exploitation of these defenses through the use of vaccines remains a central challenge for many human viruses, particularly those that cause chronic infections such as HIV and HCV.[2]

Table 27.1 Viral infections and immunity

Viral event	Obstacles	Time course
Transmission	Mechanical and chemical barriers	0
Infection and replication	Innate immunity	0 →
Infection stopped or spreads	Viral antigens transported to lymphoid tissues	Within 24 hours
Infection controlled	Specific antibodies and cell-mediated immunity	4–10 days
Sterile immunity	Immune memory	14 days to years
Viral persistence if infection not controlled	Immune disruption or evasion	Weeks to years

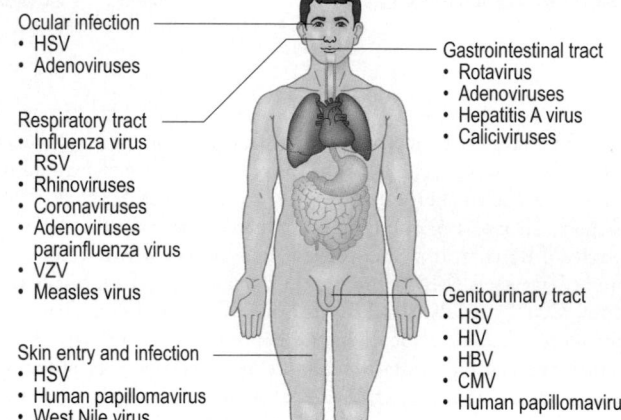

Ocular infection
- HSV
- Adenoviruses

Respiratory tract
- Influenza virus
- RSV
- Rhinoviruses
- Coronaviruses
- Adenoviruses parainfluenza virus
- VZV
- Measles virus

Skin entry and infection
- HSV
- Human papillomavirus
- West Nile virus

Gastrointestinal tract
- Rotavirus
- Adenoviruses
- Hepatitis A virus
- Caliciviruses

Genitourinary tract
- HSV
- HIV
- HBV
- CMV
- Human papillomavirus

Fig. 27.1 Common routes of entry and infection for human viral pathogens. CMV, cytomegalovirus; HBV, hepatitis B virus; HIV, human immunodeficiency virus; HSV, herpes simplex virus; RSV, respiratory syncytial virus; VZV, varicella-zoster virus.

INNATE IMMUNITY TO VIRUSES

Viral infection induces an extensive array of defense mechanisms in the host. Innate defenses come into play to block or inhibit initial infection, to protect cells from infection, or to eliminate virus-infected cells, and occur well before the onset of adaptive immunity (Chapter 3). The innate immune defenses are initiated via pathogen recognition receptors of the Toll-like receptor (TLR) family or a family of DExD/H box RNA helicases (Table 27.2).[3] These cellular sensors promote the expression of type I (α/β) interferons (IFN) and a variety of IFN-stimulated genes and inflammatory cytokines.[4] TLRs are cell surface or endosomal membrane-bound proteins expressed by numerous cells including dendritic cells (DC), macrophages, lymphocytes, and parenchymal cells.[5] Expression of TLRs is largely inducible in most cell types, though some (TLR7/8/9) are constitutively expressed at high levels by specialized plasmacytoid DC for rapid IFN production. Different TLR molecules recognize specific viral products such as single- and double-stranded RNA (TLR 3 and TLR7/8, respectively) or double-stranded DNA (TLR9). The more recently described non-TLR RNA helicases, retinoic acid-inducible gene

I (RIG-I) and melanoma differentiation-associated gene (MDA-5), mediate cytoplasmic recognition of viruses.[6] It is thought that other cytoplasmic sensors of viruses are also likely to exist such as the recently discovered cytosolic dsDNA sensor DAI (DNA-dependent activator of IFN).

The innate defense system consists of multiple cellular components and many specialized proteins. The longest-known and best-studied antiviral proteins are the α/β IFNs, which act by binding to the type I IFN receptor and result in the transcription of more than 100 IFN-stimulated genes. One consequence of this 'antiviral state' is the inhibition of cell protein synthesis and the prevention of viral replication. Type I IFNs also activate natural killer (NK) cells and induce other cytokines such as interleukin (IL)-12 that promote NK responses. NK cells produce proinflammatory

KEY CONCEPTS

MAJOR ANTIVIRAL INNATE DEFENSE MECHANISMS

>> Acting to block infection:
>> >> Natural antibodies
>> >> Complement components
>> >> Some chemokines
>> Acting to protect cells from infection
>> >> Interferon-α/β
>> >> Interferon-γ
>> Acting to destroy or inhibit virus-infected cells
>> >> Natural killer cells
>> >> NKT cells
>> >> Macrophages
>> >> Neutrophils
>> >> γδ T cells
>> >> Nitric oxide
>> Involved in regulating antiviral inflammatory response
>> >> Interleukins-1, 6, 10, 12, 18, 23
>> >> Transforming growth factor-β
>> >> Chemokines

Table 27.2 Sensors of viral infection

Toll-like receptors	
TLR3	dsRNA
	MCMV
	VSV
	LCMV
TLR7 and TLR8	ssRNA
	Influenza virus
	HIV
	VSV
TLR9	dsDNA
	HSV1/2
	MCMV
TLR2	MV hemagglutinin protein
	HSV-1
	HCMV
TLR4	MMTV envelope protein
	RSV

DExD/H box RNA helicases	
RIG-I	Influenza virus
	Paramyxoviruses
	JEV
	HCV
MDA-5	Poly(I:C)
	Measles virus
	Picornaviruses
DAI	Cytosolic dsDNA

dsRNA, double-strand RNA; HCMV, HCV, hepatitis C virus; HIV, human immunodeficiency virus; HSV1/2, herpes simplex virus 1/2; JEV, Japanese encephalitis virus; LCMV, lymphocytic choriomeningitis virus; MCMV, murine cytomegalovirus; MDA-5, melanoma differentiation-associated gene; MMTV, mouse mammary tumor virus; MV, measles virus; RSV, respiratory syncytial virus; ssRNA, single-strand RNA; TLR, Toll-like receptor; VSV, vesicular stomatis virus.

PRINCIPLES OF ANTIVIRAL IMMUNITY

>> Many human viral infections are successfully controlled by the immune system

>> Certain emerging viruses may overwhelm the immune system and cause severe morbidity and mortality

>> Other viruses have developed mechanisms to overwhelm or evade the immune system and persist

>> Individuals with defects in innate or adaptive immunity demonstrate more severe viral infections

>> T-cell immunity is more important for control than antibody with many viral infections

>> Antibody is important to minimize reinfection, particularly at mucosal sites

>> Immune memory is often sufficient to prevent secondary disease, though not in all viral infections

In addition to IFN-α/β, several other host proteins function in antiviral defense. These include natural antibody, which may play a role in defense against some virus infections, as well as the complement proteins (Chapter 20). Some viruses may be directly inactivated by complement activation or be destroyed by phagocytic cells that bind and ingest complement-bound virions. Several cytokines and chemokines induced by virus infection also play a role in defense. These include the cytokines TNF-α, IFN-γ, IL-12, IL-6, and chemokines such as MIP-1α. In particular, IL-12 is a potent inducer of IFN-γ from NK cells (Chapter 10). Inflammatory chemokines may also play an important role in innate antiviral defense by orchestrating macrophage, neutrophil, DC, and NK responses at the site of infection[9] (Chapter 11). Not only are these components of innate immunity involved in mediating initial protection against viruses, several components (such as the TLRs and type I IFN and IL-12) serve to shape the nature and effectiveness of the subsequent adaptive response to viral antigens.

ADAPTIVE IMMUNITY TO VIRUSES

Innate immunity generally serves to slow, rather than stop, viral infection, allowing time for the adaptive immune response to begin. The two major divisions of adaptive immunity, antibody and T-cell-mediated, are mainly directed at different targets. Antibodies usually function by binding to free viral particles, and in so doing block infection of the host cell. In contrast, T cells act principally by recognizing and destroying virus-infected cells. As all viruses replicate within cells and many of them spread directly between cells without re-entering the extracellular environment, resolution of infection is reliant more on T-cell function than on antibody. Antiviral antibody, however, does assume considerably more importance as an additional immunoprotective barrier against

cytokines, they can kill infected cells and interact with DC, and are an important component of innate defense against viruses (Chapter 18). NK cells are regulated by an array of activating and inhibitory receptors whose expression and function are just beginning to be understood.[7] Uninfected cells are usually protected from NK cell cytolysis as they deliver negative signals such as high expression of MHC molecules. In contrast, virus-infected cells are killed either because they deliver positive signals or because they lack adequate MHC-negative signals. The NK defense system appears important against some herpes viruses, which downregulate MHC expression in the cells they infect. NK cells are also important in resistence to mouse and human cytomegalovirus, and possibly to HIV, influenza virus, and Ebola viruses.[8] A distinct NK cell population, NKT cells, may provide some antigen-specific innate immune protection against certain viruses. Many other leukocytes are involved in innate defense, including macrophages, DC, neutrophils and perhaps T cells expressing γδ T-cell receptors for antigen (Chapter 3).

reinfection. It is the presence of antibody at portals of entry – most often mucosal surfaces – that is of particular relevance to influenza and HIV infections. Accordingly, vaccinologists try to design vaccines that optimally induce mucosal antibody.

Initiation of adaptive immunity is closely dependent upon early innate mechanisms that activate antigen-presenting cells (APC). APC and lymphocytes are drawn into lymphoid tissues by chemokine and cytokine signals and retained there for a few days in order to facilitate effective interactions between these cells. The architecture of the secondary lymphoid tissues supports the coordinated interactions between cells of the adaptive immune system through a network of supportive stromal cells and local chemokine gradients.[10] The induction events occur in lymph nodes draining the infection site, or in the spleen if virus enters the bloodstream. The passage of viral antigens to lymph nodes usually occurs in DCs. Some viruses are able to compromise the function of APC, such as HSV and measles virus, which can inhibit DC maturation.

B-cell activation occurs following antigen encounter in the B-cell follicles, and possibly the T-cell zones, in the spleen or lymph nodes[11] (Chapter 2). Some activated B cells become short-lived plasma cells while others move the edges of the B-cell follicles and interact with antigen-specific helper CD4 T cells via presentation of antigenic peptides on B-cell MHC class II molecules. These activated B cells initiate germinal center (GC) reactions, which ensure somatic hypermutation and affinity maturation for the selection of high-affinity, antibody-producing long-lived plasma cells as well as memory B cells[12] (Chapter 8). Recent advances have greatly improved our understanding of the signals that control the generation of these important B-cell subsets, particularly at the molecular level.[13] We now know that upregulation of the transcription factors Blimp-1, XBP-1, and IRF-4 dictates plasma cell formation, whereas Pax-5 expression delineates B cells destined for GC reactions and the memory B-cell lineage.

Antibody binding to epitopes expressed by native proteins at the surface of free virions usually blocks viral attachment or penetration of target cells. Sometimes the consequence is viral lysis (with complement proteins also involved), opsonization, or sensitization for destruction by Fc receptor-bearing cells that mediate antibody-dependent cellular cytotoxicity (ADCC). Occasionally, however, Fc receptor binding of antibody-bound virus may facilitate infection and result in more severe tissue damage. This occurs in dengue fever and may happen in some instances in HIV infection.[14]

As indicated previously, antibody may function most effectively to prevent reinfection, especially at mucosal surfaces. The antibody involved in humans is predominantly secretory immunoglobulin A (IgA), but serum-derived IgG may also be protective, particularly in sites such as the vaginal mucosa.[15] Both antibody isotypes act mainly to block infection of epithelial cells, although in some instances the antibody may transport antigen from within the body across epithelial cells to the outside. Mucosal antibody persists for a much shorter period than does serum antibody, which explains in part why immunity to mucosal pathogens is usually of much shorter duration than is immunity to systemic virus infections.

Like B-cell responses, T-cell responses to viral infections also begin within the lymphoid tissues. Specific CD8 cytotoxic T lymphocyte (CTL) precursors recognize antigen in the context of MHC class I–peptide antigen complexes on professional APC, such as DC. The CD8 T cells become activated, proliferate, and differentiate into effectors. Expansion of these naïve antigen-specific precursors is considerable, often exceeding 10 000-fold, and results in an effector population that

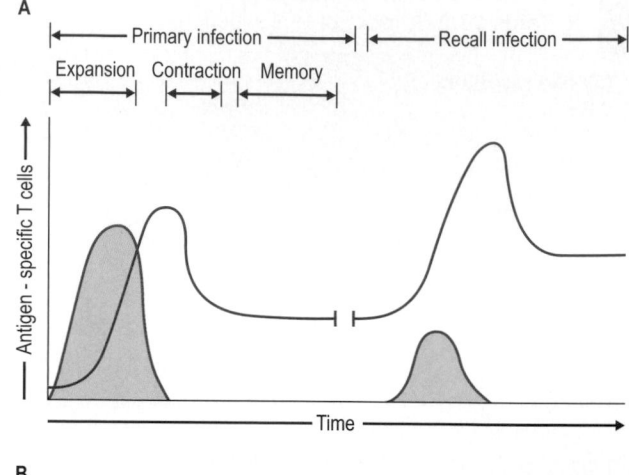

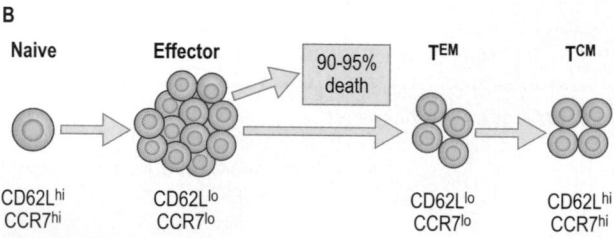

Fig. 27.2 Expansion/contraction/memory phases of adaptive immunity and memory cell subsets. (A) Dynamics of primary and secondary (recall) T-cell responses to viral infection. Both primary and recall T-cell responses undergo expansion and contraction phases, followed by stable immune memory. Recall responses induce a larger effector pool and reduced contraction further boosting the memory pool. (B) Effector and memory T-cell differentiation. Antigen stimulation expands effector cells, most of which die during the contraction phase. T_{EM} cells that are formed gradually convert to T_{CM} cells over time, with corresponding changes in surface marker expression.

can account for 40% or more of a host's total CD8 T-cell population (Fig. 27.2). Various factors, including antigen and APC, co-stimulatory molecules (such as CD28 and 4-1BB) and inflammatory cytokines (such as IFN-α/β and IL-12) are required to program the development of functional effector lymphocytes.[16] The CTL effectors enter the efferent lymph and bloodstream and access almost all body locations, including both primary and subsequent sites of infection. However, effectors do not stay activated for long once the virus is cleared, and approximately 95% die by a process termed activation-induced cell death. Following this contraction phase, the remaining cells differentiate into memory cells, which remain as a more or less stable population in the host for many years. They represent an expanded pool of CTL precursors that can be activated upon secondary encounter with antigen, and provide enhanced protection upon reinfection with the same virus. The topic of memory and homeostasis as it relates to antiviral immunity is further discussed later in this chapter.

T-cell immunity against a particular virus commonly involves both CD4 and CD8 T-cell subsets. Both CD4 and CD8 T cells recognize peptides derived from viral antigens bound to surface MHC proteins

KEY CONCEPTS

ANTIVIRAL T- AND B-CELL IMMUNITY

Effector systems	Recognized molecules	Control mechanisms
Antibody	Surface proteins or virions	Neutralization of virus, opsonization, or destruction of infected cells by ADCC
Antibody + complement	Surface proteins expressed on infected cells	Infected cell destruction by ADCC or complement-mediated lysis
Mucosal antibody (IgA)	Surface proteins or virions	Viral neutralization, opsonization, and transcytosis
CD4 T cells	Viral peptides (10–20 mers) presented on MHC class II – surface, internal or nonstructural proteins presented by APC	Antiviral cytokine and chemokine production; help for CD8 T-cell and B-cell responses; killing infected cells; regulatory functions to reduce immunopathology
CD8 T cells	Viral peptides (8–10 mers) presented on MHC class I – surface, internal or nonstructural proteins presented on infected cells or by cross-presentation	Killing infected cells or purging virus without cell death; antiviral cytokine and chemokine production

ADCC, antibody-dependent cellular cytotoxicity; APC, antigen-presenting cell; IgA, immunoglobulin A; MHC, major histocompatibility complex.

(class II and class I, respectively). Complexes of viral peptides bound to MHC class II proteins are generated by APC from scavenged and processed virus-infected cells or viral particles. Antigen–MHC class I complexes are expressed on the surface of infected cells, and antigen can also be transferred to APC from infected cells by a process known as cross-priming.[17] Recent experiments in mice have also demonstrated a role for transfer of antigen between DC[18] as they migrate from infected tissues to the lymphoid tissues. Curiously, although many peptides derived from viral proteins have an appropriate motif that permits MHC binding, the majority of CD8 T cells, and possibly CD4 T cells, are often specific for a few immunodominant epitopes.[19]

During the past few years there have been major advances in the techniques to quantify antigen-specific T-cell responses. The most revolutionary of these has been the use of MHC class I and class II tetramers to directly visualize antigen-specific CD8 and CD4 T-cell responses, respectively.[20] Many recent studies have used MHC class I tetramers to analyze virus-specific CD8 T-cell responses both in animal models and in humans. These studies demonstrated the significant size of CD8 T-cell responses to viruses and that the majority of the activated CD8 T cells seen at the peak of the response are virus-specific.

CTL function by recognizing virus-infected cells and killing them (Chapter 18). This often involves perforins and cytotoxic granules containing granzymes. Effector CTL can also induce death in target cells following engagement of Fas ligand on the CTL with Fas on target cells. Both pathways lead to apoptosis of the target cell, involving the degradation of nucleic acids, including those of the virus. Alternatively, CD8 T cells also mediate defense through the release of various cytokines following antigen recognition. Some of the cytokines and chemokines most highly produced by CTL include IFN-γ, TNF-α, lymphotoxin-α, and RANTES (Chapters 10 and 11). These cytokines can have multiple antiviral effects on infected cells and the cells around them, including purging of virus from infected cells without killing the

cell. This is particularly important for viruses like HSV which infects nonrejuvenating cells such as nerve cells.

CD4 T cells are also involved in antiviral defense. They are important, though not always essential, for controlling infections such as HSV, influenza virus, HIV, and many others. CD4 T cells participate in antiviral immunity in several ways. First, the subset acts as helper cells for the induction of both antiviral antibodies and CD8 T-cell responses to most virus antigens.[11, 21] CD4 T cells also function as antiviral effector cells, and generate stable memory cell populations similar to those of CD8 T cells.[22] The differentiation of CD4 T cells into effectors occurs in a manner very similar to that with CD8 T cells. At present less is known about the size and specificity of CD4 T-cell responses, but reports indicate that CD4 T cells undergo less expansion during virus infections, resulting in an effector pool smaller than that observed with CD8 T cells. CD4 T cells are activated by recognizing viral peptides. However, these are larger than those involved in CD8 T-cell recognition and are associated with class II MHC molecules present on more specialized cells such as APC (Chapter 6). Thus, CD4 T cells rarely recognize viral epitopes present on cells as a consequence of viral gene expression within that cell, dictating their function as helper cells for B cells and CD8 T cells, and as producers of cytokines for help and viral clearance.

In some instances CD4 T cells can perform cytotoxic functions, though not as effectively as CD8 CTL. More commonly, however, effector CD4 T cells act by synthesizing and releasing numerous cytokines following their reaction with antigen (Chapter 17). Subsets of CD4 T effectors produce different groups of cytokines. The type most often involved in antiviral defense are designated T-helper 1 (Th1) cells, and primarily produce IFN-γ, LTα, TNF-α, and IL-2 to help orchestrate the inflammatory response and act directly or indirectly in antiviral defense. Conversely, Th2 effectors produce an array of cytokines that may downregulate the protective function of Th1 cells, such as IL-4, IL-5, and two anti-inflammatory cytokines, IL-10 and transforming growth factor-β (TGF-β). Th2 T cells play a protective function against some parasite infections (Chapter 29), though in some virus infections an exuberant Th2 response may be associated with immunopathology or impaired immunity. Indeed, blocking the Th2 cytokine IL-10 was recently shown to assist in the clearance of chronic viral infection. Additionally, an IL-17-producing subset of effector CD4 T cells has also been described (Th17), with potential roles in immune pathogenesis.[23]

■ IMMUNOLOGICAL MEMORY ■

Immunological memory is a cardinal feature of adaptive immunity. The goal of vaccinology is to induce long-lived immunological memory to protect against reinfection. Following infection with certain viruses, memory can be exceptionally long-lived, potentially for the life of the host (i.e., measles and smallpox viruses).[24, 25] It is now understood that memory is defined by the persistence of specific lymphocytes and antibody-producing plasma cells, rather than persisting antigen inducing continuous lymphocyte activation. Humoral memory to viruses involves long-lived plasma cells in the bone marrow that provide a continuous low-level source of serum antibody.[26] This maintenance of humoral immunity also involves a population of homeostatically maintained memory B cells. However, the precise relationship between memory B cells and long-lived plasma cells in maintaining humoral immunity is uncertain. The pool of memory T cells is regulated by low-level homeostatic division controlled by the cytokines IL-7 and IL-15. For memory CD8 T cells, IL-7 is primarily important for survival while IL-15 is crucial for low-level proliferation to maintain the size of the memory T-cell pool.[27]

Immunological memory is defined by a pool of antigen-specific cells whose increased frequency enables rapid control of viral reinfection (Fig. 27.2).[28] Recent studies identified a population of IL-7 receptor-alpha-expressing effector cells as the precursors of this memory pool.[29] This population of cells, which constitutes ~5–10% of the effector pool, preferentially survives the contraction phase, and gradually differentiates into a stable memory population. Upon reinfection, these memory cells can be rapidly activated, and by virtue of their increased frequency mediate more rapid clearance of the viral pathogen. Moreover, repeated stimulation of memory cells via multiple infections with the same virus, or prime-boost vaccine regimes, further increases the size of the antigen-specific memory T-cell pool.[30] Re-stimulation also affects the activation status and tissue distribution of memory T cells, which may enhance protection from viral infection in mucosal, and other, tissues.

Experiments in humans and mice have demonstrated that memory T cells are heterogeneous. Memory T cells have been divided into effector memory (T_{EM}) and central memory (T_{CM}) subsets, defined by expression of two surface molecules involved in T-cell migration: CD62L and CCR7.[31] The CD62L^{lo}CCR7^{lo} T_{EM} subset is found primarily in nonlymphoid tissues and spleen, whereas the CD62L^{hi}CCR7^{hi} T_{CM} subset are largely present in the lymph nodes and spleen. The current model predicts that effector T cells form the T_{EM} subset; these cells gradually convert to a T_{CM} phenotype over time. Though the conditions that control the rate of this conversion are unknown, it is likely that the amount of antigen and inflammatory signals received during the effector phase greatly influences this. It has also been shown that CD4 T-cell help is required for the generation of long-lived memory CD8 T cells; however, exactly when this help is required during the differentiation of effector and memory T cells is uncertain.[21]

Recent studies have suggested that T_{CM} are capable of mounting stronger proliferative responses following reinfection. However, the tissue-specific homing of T_{EM} cells permits them to reside in sites of potential viral infection, such as the skin and mucosae. These differences may define the physiological raison d'être for these two memory T-cell subsets. Indeed, protection from localized viral infections such as HSV-1, influenza, and vaccinia virus in mice is more dependent upon T_{EM} cells.[32-34] However, studies suggest that memory in peripheral tissues may be less effective, or wane over time. This appears to be the case in the respiratory tract,[32] explaining in part why vaccines against respiratory viruses have a poor record.

■ IMMUNE EVASION AND IMMUNITY TO CHRONIC VIRAL INFECTIONS ■

Many, if not all, viruses employ evasion strategies to circumvent aspects of the immune system, allowing them time to replicate further or escape detection[35] (Table 27.3). One such mechanism may involve killing or infecting APC. Viruses may also delay or prevent apoptosis induced by CTL within infected cells. Other viral evasion measures aimed at the CD8 T-cell-mediated antiviral defense system serve to inhibit antigen processing, thereby minimizing effector CTL induction. Many viruses also downregulate MHC molecules on the surface of infected cells to escape CTL killing. In addition, viruses may produce various mimics or modulators/inhibitors of cytokines, chemokines, or other components of the immune system or their receptors. Viruses also resort to antigenic hypervariability to escape antibody or T-cell recognition. This can occur during transmission from host to host (i.e., influenza virus), or within hosts during chronic infection through the generation of viral escape mutants (i.e., HIV).

The success of many viral pathogens rests in their ability to subvert the host immune response. The most successful human viruses can escape the immune system and persist for the life of the host.[36] Two well-studied examples of this are CMV and EBV. T-cell responses to these viruses are prominent and readily detectable in people, yet the immune system is unable to clear either pathogen completely. However, these viruses generally remain undetectable in immunocompetent individuals. Other viral infections, such as those caused by the herpes viruses HSV and VZV, are marked by periods of latency, where no virus can be detected. Yet periods of viral reactivation, often triggered by stress, can lead to episodes of disease. These are controlled by the immune response which plays a central role in controlling herpes virus latency.[37]

Many of the most medically important human viruses are associated with persistent viremia. These include chronic infections such as HIV, HCV, HBV, and human T-lymphotropic virus (HTLV), among others.[38] Such viral infections are marked by high levels of persisting antigen and can result in skewed T-cell immunodominance hierarchies, altered tissue localization of immune cells, and severely impaired T-cell function. This altered T-cell function is hierarchical and appears to correlate directly with antigen levels, resulting in functional T-cell defects ranging from reduced cytokine production and altered proliferative capacity (exhaustion) to death (deletion) of the responding T cells[38] (Fig. 27.3). This is in stark contrast to normal memory T-cell development which occurs in the

Table 27.3 Mechanisms and examples of viral immune evasion

Mechanism	Example
Interference with viral antigen processing and presentation	HSV (ICP47), EBV (EBNA-1), HIV (Nef, Tat), HPV (E5), CMV (UL6)
Evasion of NK cell function	HIV (Nef), EBV (EBNA-1), CMV (UL40, UL18)
Inhibition of cell apoptosis	Adenovirus (RID complex and E1B), HIV (Nef), EBV (BHRF-1)
Destruction of T cells	HIV
Interference with antiviral cytokines and chemokines	EBV (IL-10 homologue), CMV (US28 chemokine receptor homologue), vaccinia virus (IL-18-binding protein), HIV (Tat chemokine activity)
Inhibition of complement action	HSV, pox viruses
Inhibition of DC maturation	HSV, vaccinia virus
Frequent antigenic variation	Influenza virus, HIV
Infection of immune privileged site	Measles virus, VZV and HSV (neurons)
Immune exhaustion	HIV, HCV, HBV

CMV, cytomegalovirus; DC, dendritic cell; EBV, Epstein–Barr virus; HBV, hepatitis B virus; HCV, hepatitis C virus; HIV, human immunodeficiency virus; HPV, human papillomavirus; HSV, herpes simplex virus; IL-18, interleukin-18; NK, natural killer; RID, receptor internalization and degradation; VZV, varicella-zoster virus.

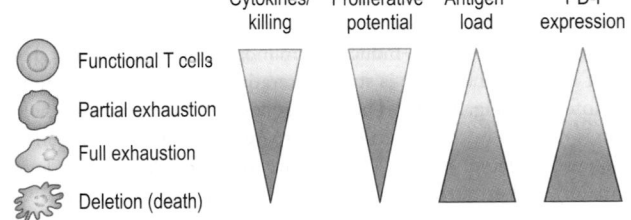

Fig. 27.3 Hierarchical model of T-cell exhaustion during persistent viral infection. T-cell function (cytokine production, killing, and proliferative potential) is negatively influenced by increasing levels of antigen. Low levels of persistent antigen may lead to partial loss of function and intermediate levels of programmed death (PD)-1 expression. High, sustained levels of antigen over time can lead to full loss of function, high levels of PD-1, and eventually cell death (deletion).

absence of persisting antigen (see previous section). Recent studies have demonstrated that signaling through programmed death (PD)-1 on effector CTL causes exhaustion during chronic infections.[39] This pathway may be essential for preventing excessive immunopathology by effector T cells, yet appears to contribute directly to failed immunity to HIV infection,[40] and other chronic human viral infections.[39] These studies implicate this pathway as a potential therapeutic target.

■ IMMUNOPATHOLOGY AND AUTOIMMUNITY ■

Immune responses against virus-infected cells often result in tissue damage, especially if cell killing is involved. If this effect is brief and without long-term consequences, it is usually judged as an immunoprotective event. A prolonged tissue-damaging effect resulting from an immune reaction against viruses is considered immunopathology.[41] Such situations most commonly involve persistent viruses, themselves at best modestly cytodestructive in the absence of an immune reaction. Chronic tissue damage initiated by viruses may also result in the response becoming autoreactive. Accordingly, some autoimmune diseases may be initiated or exacerbated by virus infections, although this notion has yet to be proved in the case of any human autoimmune disease.[42] Circumstantial evidence exists for a virus link in multiple sclerosis (MS), insulin-dependent diabetes, and possibly systemic lupus erythematosus (SLE). In MS, many viruses have been isolated from patients, though no specific one tied to the disease. The current hypothesis is that viral infections set up an inflammatory environment that may exacerbate or tip the balance towards disease in genetically susceptible individuals.[42]

Immunopathological reactions involving viruses have several mechanisms, but T cells are usually involved as orchestrators of the inflammatory events (Table 27.4). The clearest example of immunopathology involving a virus is lymphocytic choriomeningitis virus (LCMV) in the mouse. This model has dominated ideas and has set several paradigms in viral immunology in general. The first virus-induced immunopathology lesion recognized was glomerulonephritis and arteritis, noted in mice persistently infected with LCMV. The lesions were assumed to represent inflammatory reactions to tissue-entrapped immune complexes that activate complement. Similar immune complex-mediated lesions occur in other infections, but rarely have viral antigens been shown to contribute to the antigen component of the complex. An example where the inclusion of viral antigen in immune complexes has been demonstrated is chronic hepatitis B virus infection of humans. Autoimmune diseases such as SLE and rheumatoid arthritis also result from immune complex-mediated tissue damage. However, evidence linking viruses to the etiology or pathogenesis of SLE is scarce, since the immune complexes in SLE do not appear at any stage to include viral antigens.

Thanks largely to the LCMV model, it is clear that CD8 T-cell recognition of viral antigens can result in tissue damage. In LCMV, damage

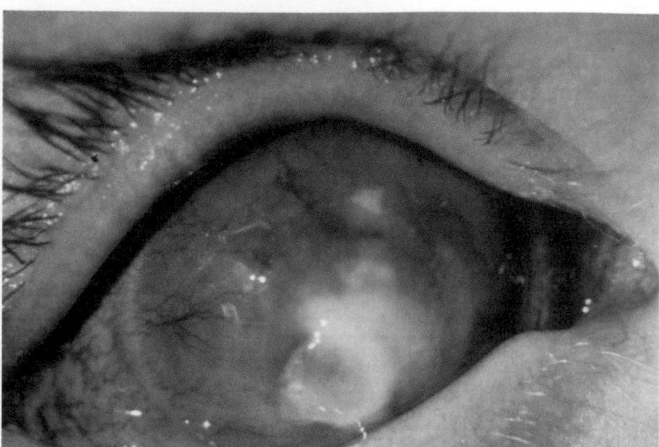

Fig. 27.5 Example of herpetic stromal keratitis (HSK) in the human eye after herpes simplex virus-1 (HSV-1) infection. Inflammation of the eye and eyelid can be observed, as well as neovascularization, and substantial necrosis, ulceration, and opacity of the cornea.

KEY CONCEPTS

PHASES OF IMMUNITY AFFECTED BY REGULATORY T CELLS

>> Interference with antigen presentation by dendritic cells

>> Inhibition T-cell responses

>> Inhibition of molecules involved in tissue-specific migration of effector cells

>> Inhibition of T-cell effector functions in lymphoid and nonlymphoid tissues

with cancer treatment, transplantation, or acquired immunodeficiency syndrome (AIDS) caused by HIV display complications. This is true for many common bacterial and viral agents, such as HSV, whose infections become far more frequent and severe in AIDS patients.

As our understanding of the mechanisms underlying innate immune defenses, antigen presentation, T- and B-cell responses and Tregs continues to improve, so too does the ability to design better vaccines and therapies to boost the immune control of viral infections. Although this remains a challenging goal, particularly for many human viruses such as HIV, HCV, and HSV, these rapid advances continue to provide many avenues for further investigation.

■ ACKNOWLEDGMENTS ■

Thanks to Bob Fujinami for Figure 27.4 and to NIH for financial support.

■ REFERENCES ■

1. Marsh M, Helenius A. Virus entry: open sesame. Cell 2006; 124: 729–740.

2. Berzofsky JA, Ahlers JD, Belyakov IM. Strategies for designing and optimizing new generation vaccines. Nat Rev Immunol 2001; 1: 209–219.

3. Kawai T, Akira S. TLR signaling. Cell Death Differentiation 2006; 13: 816–825.

4. Garcia-Sastre A, Biron CA. Type 1 interferons and the virus–host relationship: a lesson in detente. Science 2006; 312: 879–882.

5. Kopp E, Medzhitov R. Recognition of microbial infection by Toll-like receptors. Curr Opin Immunol 2003; 15: 396–401.

6. Kawai T, Akira S. Innate immune recognition of viral infection. Nat Immunol 2006; 7: 131–137.

7. Kirwan SE, Burshtyn DN. Regulation of natural killer cell activity. Curr Opin Immunol 2007; 19: 46–54.

8. Lodoen MB, Lanier LL. Natural killer cells as an initial defense against pathogens. Curr Opin Immunol 2006; 18: 391–398.

9. Esche C, Stellato C, Beck LA. Chemokines: key players in innate and adaptive immunity. J Invest Dermatol 2005; 125: 615–628.

10. von Andrian UH, Mempel TR. Homing and cellular traffic in lymph nodes. Nat Rev Immunol 2003; 3: 867–878.

11. Okada T, Cyster JG. B cell migration and interactions in the early phase of antibody responses. Curr Opin Immunol 2006; 18: 278–285.

12. McHeyzer-Williams LJ, Malherbe LP, McHeyzer-Williams MG. Checkpoints in memory B-cell evolution. Immunol Rev 2006; 211: 255–268.

13. Calame K. Transcription factors that regulate memory in humoral responses. Immunol Rev 2006; 211: 269–279.

14. Takada A, Kawaoka Y. Antibody-dependent enhancement of viral infection: molecular mechanisms and in vivo implications. Rev Med Virol 2003; 13: 387–398.

15. Mestecky J, Moldoveanu Z, Russell MW. Immunologic uniqueness of the genital tract: challenge for vaccine development. Am J Reprod Immunol 2005; 53: 208–214.

16. Mescher MF, Curtsinger JM, Agarwai P, et al. Signals required for programming effector and memory development by CD8+ T cells. Immunol Rev 2006; 211: 81–92.

17. Heath WR, Belz GT, Behrens GM, et al. Cross-presentation, dendritic cell subsets, and the generation of immunity to cellular antigens. Immunol Rev 2004; 199: 9–26.

18. Allan RS, Waithman J, Bedoui S, et al. Migratory dendritic cells transfer antigen to a lymph node-resident dendritic cell population for efficient CTL priming. Immunity 2006; 25: 153–162.

19. Yewdell JW, Bennink JR. Immunodominance in major histocompatibility complex class I-restricted T lymphocyte responses. Annu Rev Immunol 1999; 17: 51–88.

20. Altman JD, et al. Phenotypic analysis of antigen-specific T lymphocytes. Science 1996; 274: 94–96.

21. Castellino F, Germain RN. Cooperation between CD4+ and CD8+ T cells: when, where, and how. Annu Rev Immunol 2006; 24: 519–540.

22. Swain SL, Agrewaia JN, Brown DM, et al. CMD4+ T-cell memory: generation and multi-faceted roles for CD4+ T cells in protective immunity to influenza. Immunol Rev 2006; 211: 8–22.

23. Weaver CT, Harrington LE, Mangan PR, et al. Th17: an effector CD4 T cell lineage with regulatory T cell ties. Immunity 2006; 24: 677–688.

24. Ahmed R, Gray D. Immunological memory and protective immunity: understanding their relation. Science 1996; 272: 54–60.

25. Amanna IJ, Slifka MK, Crotty S. Immunity and immunological memory following smallpox vaccination. Immunol Rev 2006; 211: 320–337.

26. Manz RA, Hauser AE, Hiepe F, et al. Maintenance of serum antibody levels. Annu Rev Immunol 2005; 23: 367–386.

27. Surh CD, Boyman O, Purton JF, et al. Homeostasis of memory T cells. Immunol Rev 2006; 211: 154–163.

28. Williams MA, Bevan MJ. Effector and memory CTL differentiation. Annu Rev Immunol 2006.

29. Kaech SM, Tan JT, Wherry EJ, et al. Selective expression of the interleukin 7 receptor identifies effector CD8 T cells that give rise to long-lived memory cells. Nat Immunol 2003; 4: 1191–1198.

30. Masopust D, Ha SJ, Vezys V, et al. Stimulation history dictates memory CD8 T cell phenotype: implications for prime-boost vaccination. J Immunol 2006; 177: 831–839.

31. Sallusto F, Lenig D, Forster R, et al. Two subsets of memory T lymphocytes with distinct homing potentials and effector functions. Nature 1999; 401: 708–712.

32. Hikono H, Kohlmeier JE, Ely KH, et al. T-cell memory and recall responses to respiratory virus infections. Immunol Rev 2006; 211: 119–132.

33. Stock AT, Jones CM, Heath WR, et al. Cutting edge: central memory T cells do not show accelerated proliferation or tissue infiltration in response to localized herpes simplex virus-1 infection. J Immunol 2006; 177: 1411–1415.

34. Bachmann MF, Wolint P, Schwarz K, et al. Functional properties and lineage relationship of CD8+ T cell subsets identified by expression of IL-7 receptor alpha and CD62L. J Immunol 2005; 175: 4686–4696.

35. Finlay BB, McFadden G. Anti-immunology: evasion of the host immune system by bacterial and viral pathogens. Cell 2006; 124: 767–782.

36. Klenerman P, Hill A. T cells and viral persistence: lessons from diverse infections. Nat Immunol 2005; 6: 873–879.

37. Rouse BT, Kaistha SD. A tale of 2 alpha-herpesviruses: lessons for vaccinologists. Clin Infect Dis 2006; 42: 810–817.

38. Wherry EJ, Ahmed R. Memory CD8 T-cell differentiation during viral infection. J Virol 2004; 78: 5535–5545.

39. Sharpe AH, Wherry EJ, Ahmed R, et al. The function of programmed cell death 1 and its ligands in regulating autoimmunity and infection. Nat Immunol 2007; 8: 239–245.

40. Day CL, Kauffman DE, Kiepiela P, et al. PD-1 expression on HIV-specific T cells is associated with T-cell exhaustion and disease progression. Nature 2006; 443: 350–354.

41. Rouse BT. Virus-induced immunopathology. Adv Virus Res 1996; 47: 353–376.

42. Fujinami RS, von Herrath MG, Christen U., et al. Molecular mimicry, bystander activation, or viral persistence: infections and autoimmune disease. Clin Microbiol Rev 2006; 19: 80–94.

43. Chisari F.V, Ferrari C. Hepatitis B virus immunopathogenesis. Annu Rev Immunol 1995; 13: 29–60.

44. Radziewicz H, Ibegbu CC, Fernandez ML, et al. Liver infiltrating lymphocytes in chronic human HCV infection display an exhausted phenotype with high PD-1 and low CD127 expression. J Virol 2006; 81: 2545–2553.

45. Miller SD, Vanderlugt CL, Begolka WS, et al. Persistent infection with Theiler's virus leads to CNS autoimmunity via epitope spreading. Nat Med 1997; 3: 1133–1136.

46. Biswas PS, Rouse BT. Early events in HSV keratitis – setting the stage for a blinding disease. Microbes Infect 2005; 7: 799–810.

47. Oldstone MB. Molecular mimicry and immune-mediated diseases. Faseb J 1998; 12: 1255–1265.

48. Rouse BT, Sarangi PP, Suvas S. Regulatory T cells in virus infections. Immunol Rev 2006; 212: 272–286.

REFERENCES

Immune responses to protozoans

28

Peter C. Melby, Gregory M. Anstead

Protozoal infections are an important cause of morbidity and mortality worldwide (Table 28.1). Protozoan pathogens exact their major toll in the tropics, but infection with these parasites remains a significant problem in developed countries, owing to travel to and emigration from developing countries, the susceptibility of AIDS patients to opportunistic protozoans, and episodic transmission within communities.

Protozoan pathogens make up a group of highly diverse organisms that use a wide array of mechanisms of pathogenesis to evade the host immune response (Table 28.2). There are numerous targets for the intracellular protozoan parasites, including erythrocytes (*Babesia* and *Plasmodium*), macrophages (*Leishmania* and *Toxoplasma gondii*), or multiple cell types (*Trypanosoma cruzi*). The luminal parasitic protozoan may be extracellular, such as the amebae and the flagellates (*Giardia* and *Trichomonas*), or primarily intracellular, such as the coccidian parasite *Cryptosporidium*.

The innate and acquired immune responses to the protozoan pathogens are summarized in Table 28.3. Neutrophils and macrophages are the effector cells that mediate the innate response against the extracellular protozoan parasites. The natural killer (NK)-cell-activated macrophage system is central to the innate response to the intracellular parasites (Fig. 28.1) (Chapters 3 and 18). The innate cytokine response also plays a critical role in the generation of the adaptive immune response. For the intracellular pathogens (e.g., *Leishmania* spp., *T. cruzi*, *T. gondii*), the early production of IL-12 and IFN-γ drives the differentiation of T cells to a protective Th1 phenotype. In most cases CD4 T cells play a primary role in acquired cellular immunity, but CD8 T cells may play a critical role through cytokine production (e.g., *Plasmodium* spp., *T. cruzi*, *T. gondii*) or direct cytotoxic activity (e.g., *Cryptosporidium*). For the parasites that have an extracellular stage (e.g., *Plasmodium* spp., the trypanosomes, *Giardia* and *Trichomonas*), specific antibodies play a role in the acquired immune response.

Intensive effort has been dedicated to the development of effective vaccines for protozoal diseases, but despite their significance none has so far reached the stage of clinical use. A review of all the potential vaccine candidates is beyond the scope of this chapter and the reader is referred to a number of excellent reviews.[1-4] A discussion of the immune responses to some of the individual protozoal pathogens follows.

KEY CONCEPTS

HOST DEFENSE AGAINST PROTOZOA

>> Interaction of the parasite with host cells induces an array of cytokines which stimulate the innate and adaptive immune responses to eliminate the pathogen, and/or cytokines that inhibit or downregulate the antiparasitic responses to enable the initiation of tissue parasitism.

>> The outcome of infection is determined by the balance between the infection-promoting and the host-protective cytokines and effector cells. Often there is a mixed response, resulting in a persistent subclinical infection.

>> A persistently infected host may develop clinical disease if there is a waning of the immune mechanisms (e.g., in AIDS) that are critical to the control of infection.

PLASMODIUM SPP.

PATHOGENESIS

Soon after sporozoites of the *Plasmodium* spp. are injected into the bloodstream by the *Anopheles* mosquito they invade hepatocytes and undergo schizogony (asexual reproduction). A dormant form of *P. vivax* and *P. ovale* (hypnozoites) can reside within hepatocytes for months before causing a clinical bloodstream infection. Following schizogony, merozoites are released from ruptured hepatocytes into the bloodstream, where they invade red blood cells to produce ring-stage parasites. These parasites mature into trophozoites, which again undergo schizogony, leading to rupture of the erythrocyte and the release of merozoites. The merozoites then invade fresh red blood cells (RBC), or develop into male or female gametocytes that can then be picked up by another feeding mosquito to continue the transmission cycle.

Table 28.1 Worldwide significance of the major protozoal infections (Summarized from Markell E, John D, Krotoski W. Medical parasitology. Philadelphia: WB Saunders, 1999[44])

Parasite	Estimated worldwide cases (annual mortality)	Clinical manifestations
Trypanosoma brucei complex	100 000 new cases/year (5000 deaths)	Intermittent fever, lymphadenopathy, meningoencephalitis
Trypanosoma cruzi	24 million (60 000 deaths)	Asymptomatic infection; dysrhythmias or chronic heart failure; hypertrophy and dilation of the esophagus, colon
Entamoeba histolytica	50 million (100 000 deaths)	Asymptomatic infection, diarrhea, dysentery, or liver abscess
Cryptosporidium parvum	Prevalence 3–10% in patients with diarrhea in developing countries	Self-limited diarrhea in immunocompetent persons, severe intestinal and biliary disease in AIDS patients
Cyclospora spp.	Prevalence of ~10% in developing countries	Relapsing watery diarrhea
Giardia lamblia	200 million (most common in young children and immunocompromised)	Asymptomatic infection, chronic diarrhea
Isospora belli	Incidence unknown, rare in immunocompetent persons	Self-limited diarrhea in immunocompetent persons, chronic diarrhea in AIDS patients
Leishmania spp.	10–50 million people infected, 1.2 million new cases per year	Asymptomatic infection; skin ulcers or nodules; destructive oropharyngeal lesions; visceral disease with fever, hepatosplenomegaly, cachexia, pancytopenia
Plasmodium spp.	400–490 million (*P. falciparum:* >2 million deaths/year, primarily children)	Fever with potential complications of severe hemolysis, renal failure, pulmonary edema, cerebral involvement
Toxoplasma gondii	Several hundred million people infected worldwide. 5–70% of healthy US adults are seropositive	Self-limited fever, hepatosplenomegaly; lymphadenopathy and encephalitis (reactivation in AIDS patients); congenital infection, with fetal death, chorioretinitis, meningoencephalitis
Trichomonas vaginalis	170 million/year	Asymptomatic infection, vaginal discharge, urethritis

The clinicopathological features of malaria are caused by the intraerythrocytic stage. Schizogony and rupture of RBCs is associated with fever. Much of the tissue damage is mediated by the adherence of *P. falciparum*-infected RBCs to endothelial cells through multiple ligand–receptor interactions and plugging of microcapillary beds. Several *P. falciparum* trophozoite proteins, most notably belonging to the erythrocyte membrane protein-1 (EMP-1) family, interact either directly or indirectly with the RBC membrane, resulting in abnormalities that promote cytoadherence.[5,6] A number of endothelial adhesion molecules, including intercellular adhesion molecule-1, vascular cell adhesion molecule-1, thrombospondin, E-selectin, CD31, CD36, hyaluronic acid, and chondroitin sulphate A, mediate cytoadherence. Sequestration of parasitized RBCs in the capillary beds offers a survival advantage to the parasites by removing them from circulation through the spleen. Along with the sequestered RBCs there is accumulation of intravascular macrophages, neutrophils and platelets.

The induction of a proinflammatory cytokine cascade and counter-regulatory responses plays a central role in the pathogenesis of *P. falciparum* malaria and its complications. Parasite antigens, particularly those having glycophosphatidyl inositol membrane anchors, released during the rupture and reinvasion of RBCs, activate the innate immune response through interaction with receptors on host cells. The production of proinflammatory cytokines (IL-1, TNF-α, IL-12, and IFN-γ), which leads to fever, expression of endothelial adhesion molecules, and cytoadherence, is mediated in part by TLR-2 and is MyD88 dependent.[5,6] The induction of nitric oxide (NO) synthesis by endothelial cells may also contribute to inflammatory lesions in the brain. Cerebral malaria in the mouse model can be prevented by neutralization of TNF-α, and the risk of cerebral malaria in children is increased when the child has an allele containing a TNF-α promoter polymorphism that is associated with increased TNF-α transcription.

Table 28.2 Principal mechanisms of immune evasion by protozoal pathogens

Mechanism of immune evasion	Pathogen
Antigenic variation	*Plasmodium spp., Trypanosoma brucei, Giardia lamblia, Trichomonas vaginalis*
Entry into red blood cells	*Plasmodium spp., Babesia microti*
Resistance to complement-mediated lysis	*Leishmania spp., Trypanosoma cruzi, Trypanosoma brucei, Entamoeba histolytica*
Impaired macrophage microbicidal function	*Leishmania spp., Trypanosoma cruzi, Trypanosoma brucei, Toxoplasma gondii, Entamoeba histolytica*
Impaired antigen presentation to T cells	*Leishmania spp., Trypanosoma cruzi, Toxoplasma gondii*
Synthesis of immunosuppressive mediators (e.g. IL-10, TGF-β, PGE$_2$)	*Leishmania spp., Trypanosoma cruzi, Toxoplasma gondii, Entamoeba histolytica*
Generalized depression of T-cell responses	*Leishmania spp., Trypanosoma cruzi, Trypanosoma brucei*
Expansion of regulatory T-cell population	*Plasmodium spp., Leishmania spp., Trypanosoma cruzi*
Inhibition of phagolysosomal fusion	*Toxoplasma gondii*
Direct cytolysis of host inflammatory cells	*Entamoeba histolytica*
Degradation of host antibodies	*Entamoeba histolytica, Giardia lamblia, Trichomonas vaginalis*

PLASMODIUM SPP.

Table 28.3 Principal mechanisms of innate and acquired immunity to protozoal pathogens

Immune mechanism	Pathogen
Innate immune response	
Complement-mediated lysis	*Plasmodium spp., Leishmania spp.*
IL-12-dependent NK-cell production of IFN-γ, leading to macrophage activation	*Plasmodium spp. (pre-erythrocytic stage), Leishmania spp., Trypanosoma cruzi, Trypanosoma brucei, Toxoplasma gondii*
Cross-reactive class II-restricted CD4 T cells	*Plasmodium spp., Toxoplasma gondii*
IFN-γ production by γδ T cells	*Plasmodium spp., Toxoplasma gondii*
Activated polymorphonuclear leukocytes	*Leishmania spp., Entamoeba histolytica, Giardia lamblia, Trichomnas vaginalis, Cryptosporidium parvum*
Interferon-α/β activation of macrophages	*Leishmania spp.*
Antimicrobial peptides (defensins)	*Giardia lamblia, Cryptosporidium parvum*
Toll-like receptor signaling	*Plasmodium spp., Trypanosoma cruzi, Leishmania spp.*
Acquired immune response	
Parasite-specific IgG antibody response	*Plasmodium spp., Trypanosoma cruzi, Trypanosoma brucei, Giardia lamblia, Cryptosporidium parvum*
Class I-restricted, IFN-γ-producing CD8 T cells, which activate macrophage microbicidal mechanisms	*Plasmodium spp., Leishmania spp., Trypanosoma cruzi Trypanosoma cruzi, Cryptosporidium parvum*
Class I-restricted cytotoxic CD8 T cells	*Plasmodium spp., Leishmania spp., Trypanosoma cruzi, Trypanosoma brucei, Toxoplasma gondii, Entamoeba histolytica, Cryptosporidium parvum*
Class II-restricted, IFN-γ-producing CD4 T cells, which activate macrophage microbicidal mechanisms	*Toxoplasma gondii (cyst stage), Entamoeba histolytica, Giardia lamblia, Cryptosporidium parvum*
Mucosal IgA antibody response	

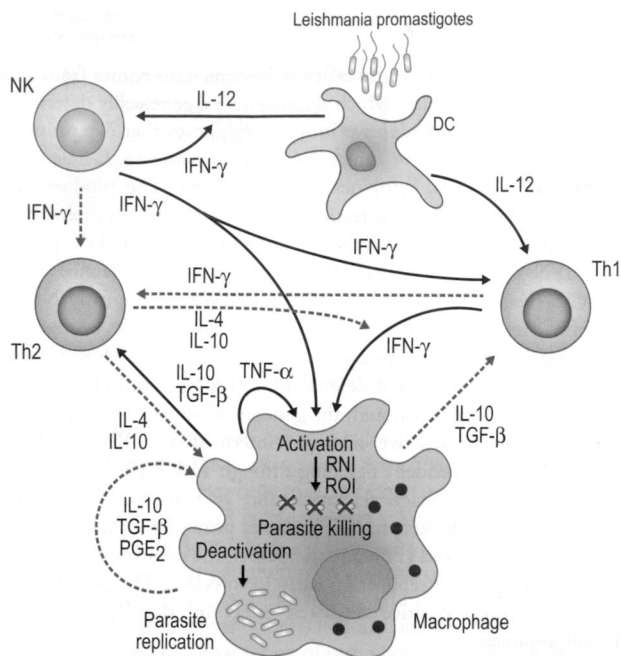

Leishmania promastigotes

Fig. 28.2 Immunity in leishmaniasis. Exposure of dendritic cells to parasites or parasite antigens leads to the release of IL-12, which induces NK cells to produce IFN-γ and drives the acquired immune response toward a protective Th1 phenotype. IL-12 production by dendritic cells and IFN-γ production by NK and Th1 cells negatively regulates the Th2 response. IFN-γ activates macrophages to kill the intracellular pathogen. In genetically susceptible individuals a counter-regulatory Th2 cytokine response can suppress the Th1 response and deactivate infected macrophages, leading to parasite replication and uncontrolled infection. Counterprotective macrophage-derived cytokines can also inhibit the Th1 response, stimulate the Th2 response, and deactivate the macrophage through an autocrine loop. Activating stimuli are shown by solid arrows, and deactivating stimuli are shown by dashed arrows.

IL-12 gene, IL-18 gene or STAT4 gene (critical to IL-12 signaling), subverts Th1 cell development and renders resistant mice susceptible. Tumor necrosis factor-α (TNF-α) contributes to protective immunity by synergizing with IFN-γ to activate macrophages. Recently, NF-κB family members have been shown to regulate T-cell responses and immunity to *L. major* infection in mice.

The generation of RNI by activated macrophages is the primary mechanism of parasite killing in the murine model.[15] The Fas/Fas ligand pathway of CD4 T cell-induced apoptosis is also involved in the elimination of parasites. Although IFN-γ-induced production of NO may not be detectable in human macrophages, inhibition of nitric oxide synthase 2 (NOS2) was shown to impair killing of intracellular *Leishmania*.

Studies in the murine model of *L. major* infection have led to the idea that two populations of CD4 T cells mediate immunity induced by primary infection.[16] Effector memory cells, which are short-lived and dependent on the persistence of antigen, respond rapidly to secondary infection by migrating to the infected tissue and generating effector cytokines. Central memory T cells, which can be maintained in the

absence of persistent antigen, circulate throughout the lymphatic system and upon secondary challenge migrate to and proliferate in the draining lymph node, gain the capacity to produce IFN-γ, and then migrate to the site of infection. Thus, central memory T cells act as a reserve of antigen-reactive T cells that can expand and become effector T cells in response to secondary antigenic challenge. There are a number of adaptive immune mechanisms that promote parasite replication and disease.[17] The progression of murine *L. major* infection has been correlated with the expansion of Th2 cells and the production of IL-4, IL-5 and IL-10. In susceptible mice, IL-4 production within the first day of infection was shown to downregulate IL-12 receptor β-chain expression and drive the response to a Th2 phenotype. However, other nonsusceptible mouse strains appear to be able to overcome an early IL-4 response and develop a resistant phenotype, and susceptibility to some *L. major* strains is not strictly mediated by IL-4 (IL-13 may contribute). Additional factors, such as IL-10, TGF-β, or PGE$_2$, are required to maintain the Th2 response and the susceptible phenotype.[16] Recent evidence indicates that susceptibility in the BALB/c mouse model of *L. major* infection is as much a result of an inherent defect in the Th1 development pathway and IL-10 production as it is related to the effects of IL-4[17]. Besides inhibition of IFN-γ production, these factors suppress macrophage activation. The antigen-specific unresponsiveness of CD4 T cells during active VL is mediated in part by the engagement of the negative co-stimulatory receptor CTLA-4.

Peripheral blood mononuclear cells (PBMCs) isolated from patients with localized or subclinical leishmaniasis demonstrate a Th1 response to *Leishmania* antigens, and in general the intralesional cytokine profile is one of a dominant Th1 response. Patients with ML exhibit vigorous T-cell responses; it is postulated that this hyperresponsive state contributes to the prominent tissue destruction of ML. Patients with DCL resemble the progressive infection caused by *L. major* in BALB/c mice. Such patients demonstrate minimal or absent *Leishmania*-specific lymphoproliferative responses, and the Th2 cytokine mRNAs were prominently expressed in DCL lesions. During active VL in humans there is a marked depression of *Leishmania*-specific lymphoproliferative and IFN-γ responses, as well as an absence of DTH response to parasite antigens. This anergy appears to be mediated, at least in part, by a suppressive effect of IL-10 and low levels of IL-12. Successful treatment of active disease restores an antigen-specific Th1 response.

EVASION OF HOST IMMUNITY

The *Leishmania* parasite has numerous ways in which it adapts to and survives within the vertebrate host.[15, 17] In the skin the promastigotes are preferentially phagocytosed by macrophages that, unlike dendritic cells, do not actively participate in T-cell priming. The parasite's surface LPG (and to a lesser extent the surface protein gp63) plays an important role in the entry and survival of *Leishmania* in the mammalian host by conferring complement resistance, and by facilitating the entry of complement-opsonized parasites into the macrophage without triggering a respiratory burst. Macrophage phagosome–endosome fusion and phagolysosomal biogenesis are also inhibited by the parasite LPG.

Leishmania-infected macrophages have a diminished capacity to initiate and respond to a T-cell response, and the impaired antimicrobial effector activity provides a safe haven for the intracellular parasite.[15] Infected macrophages have decreased synthesis of cytokines (IL-1, IL-12) and blunted IFN-γ-mediated activation (reduced MHC class II and co-stimulatory molecule expression, and reduced production of ROI and RNI) through the disruption of signal transduction pathways involving JAK/STAT, protein kinase C, p38 MAPK, ERK, AP-1, and NF-κB. Signaling mediated by tyrosine phosphorylation is reduced by the rapid induction of the host phosphotyrosine phosphatase SHP-1. Conversely, there is increased synthesis of the immunosuppressive molecules IL-10, TGF-β and prostaglandin E$_2$. Together these contribute to impaired antigen presentation to T cells. The IL-4/IL-13-enhanced expression of arginase by infected macrophages (termed alternatively activated macrophages) contributes to depletion of L-arginine and reduced NO production. Recently, IL-10-producing CD4+CD25+ T-regulatory cells at the site of chronic infection have been shown to play a role in the maintenance or progression of infection.[18] IL-10 has an essential role in parasite persistence, as mice with IL-10 deletion or IL-10R blockade are able to eliminate the parasite.[19]

■ *TRYPANOSOMA CRUZI* ■

PATHOGENESIS

Trypanosoma cruzi is transmitted to the mammalian host when the infectious metacyclic trypomastigote, which is deposited on the skin in the feces of the reduvid insect vector while it takes a blood meal, is scratched into the wound or transferred to a mucous membrane (e.g., the eyes). The trypomastigotes can infect almost any cell type, and replicate as amastigotes in the cytoplasm. Eventually the amastigotes transform back into trypomastigotes and rupture the cell to enter the bloodstream, whence they invade other cells or are picked up by another insect vector.

Following primary infection the parasites replicate locally and then disseminate through the bloodstream to a variety of tissues. Muscle and glial cells are the most frequently infected, and acute myocarditis or meningoencephalitis can develop. In most cases, however, primary infection occurs without clinical symptoms and the infected individual may enter an indeterminate phase of asymptomatic seropositivity. Only 10–30% of chronically infected individuals will ultimately develop symptomatic Chagas' disease, usually involving the heart or gastrointestinal tract. Pathologically there are few parasites observed in cardiac tissue, but an intense chronic inflammatory infiltrate with fibrosis and loss of muscle fibers is evident. In the digestive tract there is lymphohistiocytic infiltration of the myenteric plexuses, with a dramatic reduction in the number of ganglion cells.

The tissue damage of acute *T. cruzi* infection is the result of a direct effect of the parasite and the acute host inflammatory response. In chronic infection the balance between immune-mediated parasite containment and host-damaging inflammation determines the course of disease. The pathological mechanisms related to chronic Chagas' disease are controversial, but whether tissue damage is caused directly by parasites or indirectly through parasite-directed inflammatory or autoimmune mechanisms, it is clear that parasite persistence is required for disease.[20, 21] Autoimmunity could arise from molecular self-mimicry by parasite antigens, or by the release of self-molecules from damaged or dying host cells within the environment of an activated innate immune response. The production of IL-10 by *T. cruzi*-infected cells may downregulate the pathologic cellular immune response.[22]

INNATE IMMUNITY

The early innate immune response to *T. cruzi* infection is mediated primarily by NK cells and macrophages.[20] Macrophages and DCs exposed to *T. cruzi* trypomastigote antigens produce proinflammatory cytokines, including IL-12 and TNF-α, through a MyD88-dependent mechanism. MyD88-deficient mice had impaired inflammatory responses and host defense against *T. cruzi*. IL-12 activates NK cells to secrete IFN-γ, which synergizes with TNF-α to activate macrophages to control parasite replication. The generation of NO is the primary trypanocidal mechanism in murine macrophages. A number of trypomastigote antigens, including free GPI anchors, glycoinositol phospholipids (GIPLs), GPI-linked glycoproteins, and GPI-mucins activate the innate immune response, at least partly through TLR-2.

ACQUIRED IMMUNITY

In infected mice the parasitemia (trypomastigotes) increases until 3–4 weeks after infection, when either the mice die or the infection is controlled by the acquired immune response. Antibodies contribute to immunity through opsonization, complement activation and antibody-dependent cellular cytotoxicity.

Several lines of evidence establish the importance of T cells in acquired immunity to *T. cruzi* infection. Parasite-specific CD4 and CD8 T cells are activated in response to infection, and mice lacking CD4 or CD8 T cells have impaired ability to control the infection. CD8 T cells with cytotoxic activity against *T. cruzi*-infected cells have been identified in infected mice, and these cells confer protection against challenge when passively transferred to naive mice. In the early stage of infection CD4 T cells are the predominant subset recruited to the myocardium, but activated CD8 T cells soon dominate the inflammatory process in cardiac tissue. Cytokine production (IFN-γ and TNF-α) by parasite-specific CD8 T cells is more important than cytolytic activity in the control of infection.[23]

T. cruzi infection leads to a mixed Th1/Th2 cytokine response, and in general the Th1/Th2 balance determines resistance or susceptibility. As noted earlier, IFN-γ, produced in early infection by NK cells and later by T cells, clearly has an important protective function. Its protective effect is dependent on IL-12, as neutralization of IL-12 or deletion of STAT4 leads to increased parasitemia and earlier death, and the protection afforded to mice by the administration of IL-12 was abrogated by neutralization of IFN-γ and TNF-α. IL-4 does not appear to play a major role in susceptibility to *T. cruzi* infection, but IL-10 promotes parasite replication by inhibiting macrophage trypanocidal activity. IL-10 also plays a critical role in minimizing inflammation-mediated tissue pathology by regulating the Th1 and proinflammatory cytokine (predominantly TNF) responses.[22] Similarly, TGF-β has been shown to inhibit macrophage trypanocidal activity and increase parasitemia and mortality. In addition to the production of these regulatory cytokines, the secretion of prostaglandins and NO, the induction of apoptosis of T and B cells, and the expansion of a myeloid suppressor cell population serve to control the intensity of the immune response.

EVASION OF HOST IMMUNITY

A significant part of the pathogenesis following *T. cruzi* infection is its dissemination through the bloodstream to many tissues. *T. cruzi* bloodstream trypomastigotes resist complement-mediated lysis because the parasite has

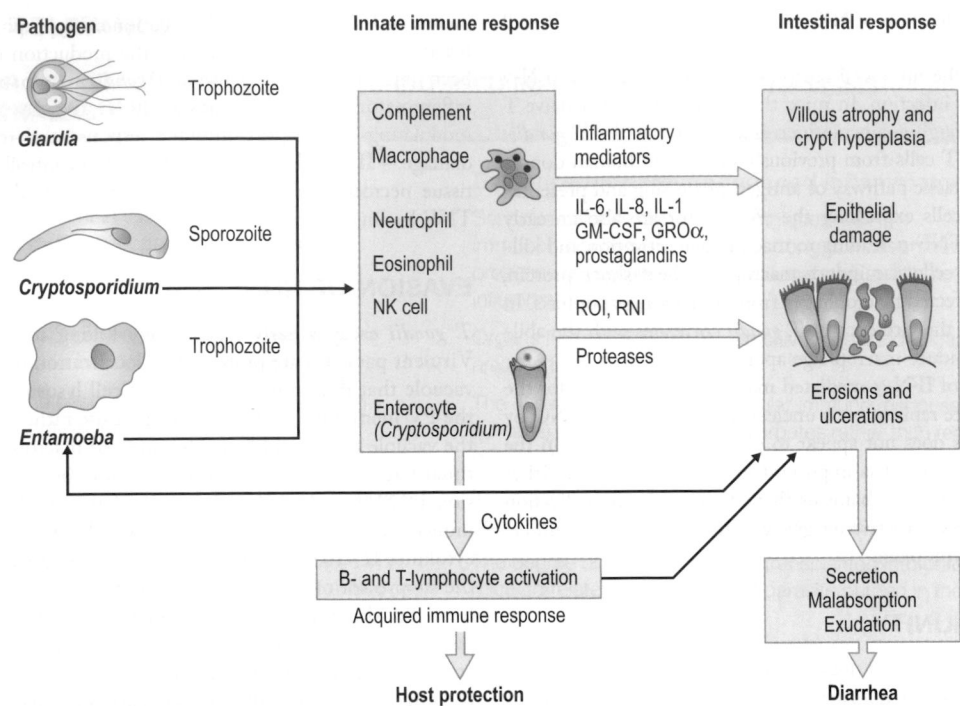

Pathogen

Giardia — Trophozoite

Cryptosporidium — Sporozoite

Entamoeba — Trophozoite

Innate immune response

Complement
Macrophage
Neutrophil
Eosinophil
NK cell
Enterocyte (*Cryptosporidium*)

Inflammatory mediators

IL-6, IL-8, IL-1 GM-CSF, GROα, prostaglandins

ROI, RNI

Proteases

Cytokines

B- and T-lymphocyte activation

Acquired immune response

Host protection

Intestinal response

Villous atrophy and crypt hyperplasia

Epithelial damage

Erosions and ulcerations

Secretion
Malabsorption
Exudation

Diarrhea

Fig. 28.3 Immunopathogenesis of intestinal protozoal pathogens. After adherence (*Giardia* and *Entamoeba*) or epithelial invasion (*Entamoeba* and *Cryptosporidium*), there is release of various inflammatory mediators from macrophages and neutrophils. This causes the activation of resident phagocytes and recruitment of phagocytes into the lamina propria. Enterocyte death may be due to direct action of the parasites or to immune-mediated damage from complement, cytotoxic lymphocytes, proteases, and reactive oxygen and nitrogen intermediates (ROI and RNI, respectively). The inflammatory mediators also act on enterocytes and the enteric nervous system, inducing the secretion of water and chloride. Under the influence of activated T lymphocytes the response to enterocyte damage is that the crypts undergo hyperplasia and the villi become shorter (villous atrophy). The immature hyperplastic cells have poor absorptive ability, but retain secretory ability. Damage to the epithelium can cause leakage (exudation) from lymphatics and capillaries. Similar mechanisms are probably responsible for the diarrhea that occurs in infection with *Cyclospora* and *Isospora*. *Isospora* is unique in causing an eosinophilic infiltrate.

which attract leukocytes to the site of invasion.[32] Neutrophils are the most important effector cells in clearing *E. histolytica* infection.[31] Studies in IFN-γ receptor gene knockout mice suggest a role for IFN-γ in innate immunity against *E. histolytica*.[30]

ACQUIRED IMMUNITY

Invasive amebiasis produces a humoral immune response in most patients, but the protection afforded is incomplete, i.e., an amebic liver abscess may progress despite an exuberant host antibody response. Nevertheless, antibodies protect against intestinal colonization and reinfection.[4] The exact role of IgA in host defense against amebiasis is unclear; IgA deficiency does not cause more frequent or severe disease.[33]

The role of cell-mediated immunity in the control of amebiasis is also not fully defined. Dissemination of infection occurs in some conditions where cell-mediated immunity is impaired,[4, 33] but the AIDS epidemic has not resulted in an increase in cases of severe amebiasis. In rodents immunized with the Gal/GalNac lectin, or in humans who have antilectin antibodies, T lymphocytes produce IL-2 and IFN-γ when stimulated with one of the lectin's subunits. The Gal/GalNac lectin also triggers IFN-γ-primed macrophages to produce the

amebicidal molecule NO. Early amebic liver abscess in gerbils is associated with a mixed Th1/Th2 response, but with chronic infection the gerbils mount a Th1-like response. Gerbils cured of amebic liver abscess by antibiotic therapy likewise have a Th1 immune response and are resistant to reinfection.

EVASION OF HOST IMMUNITY

E. histolytica utilizes a number of strategies to circumvent the immune defenses of the host. It resists complement-mediated lysis during hematogenous spread by proteolytic degradation of C3 and C5. In addition, the Gal/GalNac lectin binds to C8 and C9, preventing assembly of the C5b-9 membrane attack complex [4] (Chapter 20).

The cytolytic capability of *E. histolytica* affords protection from neutrophils, macrophages and eosinophils unless these cells are activated.[33] Cytolysis by *E. histolytica* may occur via necrosis and apoptosis; the use of the host's apoptotic machinery abrogates the local inflammatory response. Trophozoites also inhibit the macrophage respiratory burst and the production of IL-1 and TNF-α. A protective antibody response is subverted by the degradation of IgA and IgG by amebic cysteine proteases, and by capping, ingesting or shedding ameba-specific antibodies.[33]

Amebic antigens may cause selective activation of Th2-type T cells, causing macrophage deactivation and anergy.[4] Macrophages exposed to amebic lysates secrete prostaglandin E_2, which interferes with MHC II expression and TNF-α production. Patients with amebic liver abscesses have decreased CD4/CD8 T-cell ratios and decreased T-cell proliferation, which may be related to reduced IL-2 production.

GIARDIA LAMBLIA

PATHOGENESIS

After ingestion of the *Giardia* cyst in fecally contaminated food or water, excystation occurs, with the release of trophozoites. The trophozoites multiply in the small bowel. As they transit through the lower intestine they encyst, allowing the organism to survive in the environment and to be transferred to another host. The *Giardia* trophozoite initially adheres to intestinal epithelium via a surface mannose-binding lectin. Histopathologic changes in symptomatic giardiasis range from a normal appearance to villous atrophy, crypt hyperplasia, epithelial damage, and chronic inflammatory infiltrate in the lamina propria (Fig. 28.3). The factors responsible for the structural changes in the small bowel are not well defined, but may include injury from adherence, and the release of cytotoxins, including proteases. Furthermore, epithelial damage may be mediated by the host cellular immune response.[34]

INNATE IMMUNITY

Giardia has a limited capacity to neutralize reactive oxygen species, which are produced by intestinal epithelial cells. The antimicrobial peptide defensin is produced by Paneth cells and thus may also participate in host defense against *Giardia*. Few macrophages are found in the intestinal mucosa during giardiasis, which suggests they do not play an important role in the innate immune response.[35] The infection is rare in breastfed infants because breast milk contains free fatty acids lethal to *Giardia* cysts and, in endemic areas, anti-*Giardia* antibodies.[34]

ACQUIRED IMMUNITY

Several lines of evidence suggest the importance of the humoral immune response in the control of giardiasis.[35] Infection with *Giardia* results in the production of anti-*Giardia* antibodies in the serum and mucosal secretions. Human immunodeficiency syndromes that affect antibody production are associated with chronic giardiasis.

There is evidence for a role of T cell-dependent immunity in the control of giardiasis, but the mechanisms of immunity have not been fully defined.[35] T cell-deficient mice and mice treated with anti-CD4 antibody are unable to control *Giardia* infection. CD8 T lymphocytes are not important in protective immunity.

EVASION OF HOST IMMUNITY

Giardia undergoes surface antigenic variation by altering a group of variant-specific surface proteins (VSPs). Selection occurs by an immune-mediated process, because switching occurs when intestinal anti-VSP IgA responses are first detected.[36] *Giardia lamblia* also produces a protease that cleaves IgA.

CRYPTOSPORIDIUM PARVUM

There are three intestinal coccidian parasites of humans that are intracellular parasites of enterocytes: *Cryptosporidium parvum*, *Isospora belli* and *Cyclospora cayetanensis*. *Cryptosporidium* has the greatest epidemiologic significance: in 1993 a huge outbreak involving 403 000 persons occurred in Milwaukee, Wisconsin.[37] Because of their similarity, only the immunology of cryptosporidiosis will be discussed in detail.

PATHOGENESIS

Infection with *Cryptosporidium* occurs when sporulated oocysts are ingested and excyst in the proximal small bowel, invade the intestinal epithelial cells (facilitated by a cysteine protease), develop into trophozoites and undergo schizogony, with a resultant merozoite-containing schizont. The merozoites are extruded and invade other epithelial cells. The merozoites may continue an asexual cycle or develop into macro- or microgametes that fuse to form oocysts.

Histologically, in the infected small bowel there is villous atrophy and blunting, and crypt hyperplasia with increased infiltration of lymphocytes, macrophages and plasma cells. Intraepithelial lymphocytes are uncommon; neutrophils and occasional eosinophils are present between the epithelium and the lamina propria. Disorganized cells undergoing necrosis replace normal enterocyte architecture (Fig. 28.3). There is an association between the degree of intestinal injury and malabsorption and the intensity of infection, as measured by oocyst excretion.[37]

INNATE IMMUNITY

Knowledge of the immune response to cryptosporidiosis has been hampered owing to the lack of experimental models of infection. Acute infection in an immunocompetent mouse older than 3 weeks is difficult to establish, so the neonatal mouse model has been most commonly studied. The increased susceptibility of neonates (including humans) may be related to an undeveloped IL-12-dependent IFN-γ pathway.

Because of the parasite's intracellular location near the luminal surface of the enterocyte, the macrophages of the lamina propria are spatially isolated from the parasite. Thus, the intestinal epithelium mounts its own assault on the invading microbe by the activation of NF-κB and the release of TNF-α and the chemokines IL-8, RANTES, and GRO-α, which act as chemoattractants and activators of neutrophils.[38] TNF-α also inhibits parasite replication. Infected epithelial cells may attempt to eliminate the parasite through apoptosis;[38] however, NF-κB activation protects the infected epithelial cells from apoptosis, thereby facilitating parasite survival and replication.[39]

Infected intestinal cells also release TGF-β, which decreases necrosis and stimulates the synthesis of extracellular matrix proteins, which limit epithelial damage.[38] Antimicrobial peptides (the defensins) released by intestinal cells also have anti-cryptosporidial activity. There are contradictory data on the role of NO in the control of cryptosporidosis.[38]

ACQUIRED IMMUNITY

The relative contribution of antibody responses to the control of cryptosporidosis is uncertain.[39] The enterocyte membrane enveloping the parasitophorous vacuole contains *C. parvum* antigens that are recognized

Immune responses to helminths

Subash Babu, Thomas B. Nutman

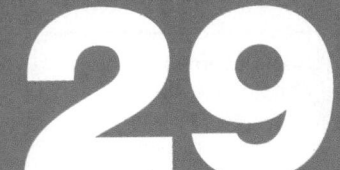

Parasitic helminths are complex eukaryotic organisms characterized by their ability to maintain long-standing chronic infections in human hosts, sometimes lasting decades. Hence, parasitic helminths are a major health care problem worldwide, infecting more than 2 billion people, mostly in developing countries (Table 29.1). Common helminth infections, such as intestinal helminths, filarial and schistosome infections, are a major medical, social, and economic burden to the countries in which these infections are endemic. Chemotherapy, while highly successful in some areas, still suffers from the disadvantages of the length of treatment, the logistics involved in the distribution of drugs and, in some cases, the emergence of drug resistance. Vector control measures are at best an adjunct measure in the control of helminth infections but also suffer from the same social, logistic, and economic obstacles as mass chemotherapy. Therefore, the study of the immune responses to helminth infections attains great importance both in terms of understanding the parasite strategies involved in establishing chronic infection and in the delineation of a successful host immune response to develop protective vaccines against infection.

■ SPECTRUM OF HOST–PARASITE INTERACTIONS ■

While both protozoa and helminths can cause parasitic infections, the biology and the host response to each are extremely different. Protozoa are small unicellular organisms that multiply intracellularly and pose an extreme immediate hazard to the host immune system. Helminths, in contrast, are large (often centimeters to meters in length), extracellular (the exception being *Trichinella spiralis*), and typically do not multiply in their vertebrate host and therefore do not present an immediate threat during initial infection.

Helminths have characteristically complex lifecycles with many developmental stages. Thus, the host is exposed during the course of a single infection to multiple lifecycle stages of the parasites, each stage with both a shared and a unique antigenic repertoire. Thus, in *Schistosoma mansoni*, infection begins with penetration of the skin of humans exposed to infested waters by the free-swimming cercariae, which then develop

into tissue-dwelling schistosomula. In the liver and mesenteric veins, schistosomula differentiate into sexually dimorphic adult worms which mate and the resultant eggs migrate through tissues into the lumen of the intestine or bladder for environmental release. Similarly, in lymphatic filarial infection, the host is exposed to the infective-stage larvae in the skin, lymph nodes, and lymphatics, to the adult worms in the lymph nodes and lymphatics, and finally to the microfilariae in the peripheral circulation. Hence, the host–helminth interaction is complex not only due to the multiple lifecycle stages of the parasite but also because of the tissue tropism of the different stages.

Antigenic differences among the lifecycle stages can lead to distinct immune responses that evolve differentially over the course of a helminth infection. In addition, depending on the location of the parasite, the responses are compartmentalized (intestinal mucosa and draining lymph nodes in intestinal nematode infection or skin/subcutaneous tissue and draining lymph nodes in onchocerciasis) or systemic (lymphatic filariasis or schistosomiasis). Moreover, the migration patterns of the parasite might elicit varied cutaneous, pulmonary, and intestinal inflammatory pathologies, as seen, for example, in *Ascaris* or *Stronglyoides* infection during their migratory phase. This is further complicated by the fact that human hosts are often exposed to multiple lifecycle stages of the parasite at the same time. Thus, a chronically infected patient with lymphatic filariasis harboring adult worms and microfilariae might be exposed to insect bites transmitting the infective-stage parasite. The immune response that ensues will not only be a reaction to the invading organism but will also bear an imprint of the previous exposures and the concurrent infection.

Helminth infections can elicit a spectrum of clinical manifestations mirroring diversity in host immune responses. For example, in lymphatic filariasis, most infected individuals remain clinically asymptomatic despite harboring significant worm burdens felt to reflect the induction of parasite-specific tolerance in the immune system. Others exhibit acute manifestations including fever and lymphadenopathy that are felt to reflect inflammatory processes induced by incoming larvae, dying worms, or superadded infections. Individuals who mount a strong but inappropriate immune response end up with lymphatic damage and subsequent immune-mediated pathology – hydrocele and elephantiasis. Finally, a group of infected individuals mount exuberant immune responses, often demonstrated to include tumor necrosis factor-β (TNF-β) and Th2 responses – IL-9 and IL-13. This polarization is driven by the cytokine environment in which CD4 T cells differentiate, thus IL-12 and, to a lesser extent, IL-23 are known inducers of Th1 responses while IL-4 is a potent inducer of Th2 responses.[2] Dendritic cells (DC) and macrophages, both professional antigen-presenting cells, are the major sources of IL-12, while differentiated T cells, natural killer (NK) T cells, eosinophils, basophils, and mast cells are sources of IL-4. More recently, the transcriptional mechanism that governs Th1/Th2 differentiation has been elucidated. The transcription factor T-bet is essential for Th1 differentiation, whereas the transcription factor GATA-3 is crucial for Th2 differentiation. These transcription factors and polarizing cytokines are known to cross-regulate each other; thus both T-bet and GATA-3 suppress the induction of the other and IFN-γ and IL-4 are mutually antagonistic.

The immunological hallmark of helminth infections is their ability to induce Th2 responses characterized by the presence of IL-4, IL-5, IL-9, IL-10, and IL-13, generalized eosinophilia, goblet and mucosal mast-cell hyperplasia, and production of immunoglobulin E (IgE) and IgG$_1$ (in mice) and IgE and IgG$_4$ (in humans).[3] While the Th2 response induced by helminth parasites is a stereotypical response of the host, the initiation, progression, and culmination of this response require interaction with many different cell types, most notably: (1) antigen-presenting cells – DC and macrophages; (2) T cells; (3) B cells; (4) eosinophils; and (5) mast cells and basophils. In addition, the host–helminth interactions lead to a variety of modulated immune responses such as the induction of regulatory T cells and alternatively activated macrophages (Fig. 29.2).

HELMINTHS AND DENDRITIC CELLS

DC are professional antigen-presenting cells that play an essential role in presenting antigen to T cells to initiate immune responses. For Th1 responses, DC present bacterial or protozoan antigens in the context of upregulated co-stimulatory molecules – CD80 and CD86; Th1 biasing pattern recognition receptors such as Toll-like receptors (TLRs: most notably); and of the presence of IL-12.[4] However, very little is known about the role of DC in the initiation of Th2 responses, as occurs in helminth infections. It has been shown that differentiation and maturation of DC in the presence of helminth antigens can lead to robust Th2 responses with inhibition of IL-12 production.[4] This has been demonstrated using: (1) excretory-secretory products from *Acanthocheilonema viteae* and *Nippostrongylus brasiliensis*, both rodent filarial parasites; (2) *Schistosoma mansoni* soluble egg antigen or the schistosomal glycan lacto-N-fucopentose III or double-stranded RNA; and (3) live microfilariae from *Brugia malayi*.[5] Although NF-κB1 activation has been found to be required for DC-mediated Th2 differentiation in helminth infections, the nature of the receptors and other signaling molecules involved is not yet known. Finally, it has been shown that helminth parasites can interact directly with TLRs on DC, either through TLR2 (for schistosomes and filariae) or TLR4 (for the filarial parasites). The modulation of DC function by helminth antigens appears to be generalizable and has been

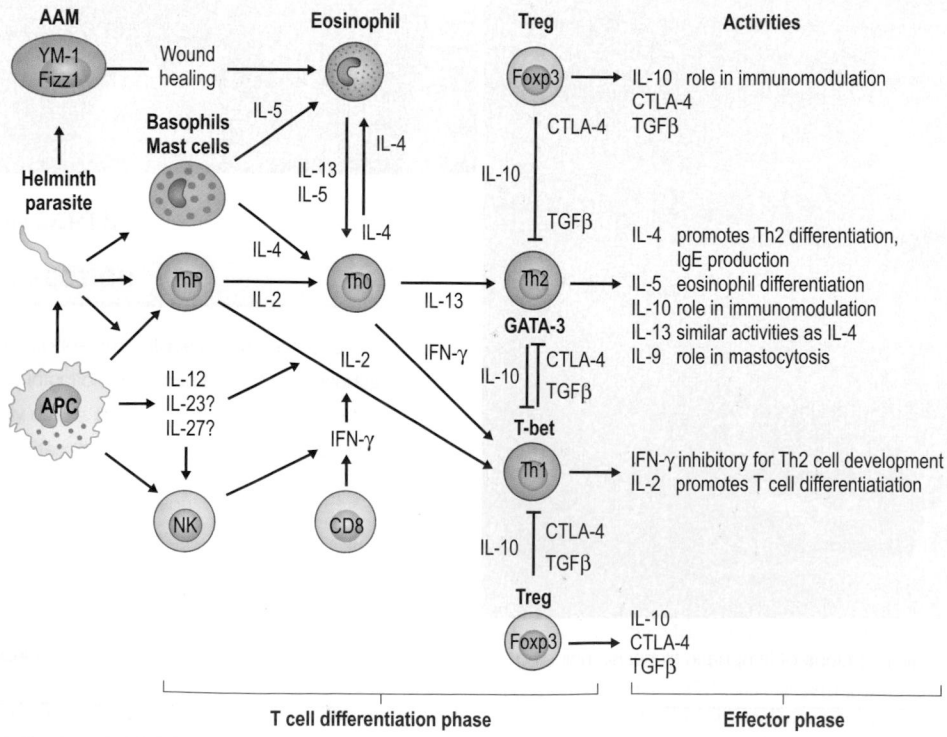

Fig. 29.2 Regulation of the T-cell response in helminth infection. AAM, alternately activated macrophages; APC, antigen-presenting cell; IFN, interferon; IL, interleukin; Th, T helper; Thp, precursor T cell; Treg, regulatory T cells.

shown to impair their ability to respond to other infectious stimuli (e.g., *Mycobacterium tuberculosis*).[6]

HELMINTHS AND MACROPHAGES

Macrophages are the other important class of antigen-presenting cells that can serve as protective effector cells in bacterial and protozoan infections by their production of nitric oxide and other mediators. Helminth interaction with macrophages induces a population of macrophages preferentially expressing arginase instead of nitric oxide due to increased activation of arginase-1 by IL-4 and IL-13. These macrophages, termed alternatively activated macrophages, are characterized by their ability to upregulate YM-1 and Fizz-1, two gene products whose function remains unknown.[7] These alternatively activated macrophages are known to be important in wound healing and have been postulated to play a potential role in repairing wound damage that occurs during tissue migration of helminth parasites. In addition, these macrophages mediate a hyporesponsiveness in cognate T cells and play an additional role in the modulation of the immune responses. While helminth infection does induce expression of these cells in humans, early interaction of parasites or parasite antigens leads to a predominantly proinflammatory response with expression of TNF-α, IL-6, IL-1β, MIP-1β, MIP-3β, IL-8 as well as CD44 and ICAM-1, genes involved in inflammation and adhesion.[8] Chronic infection then results in macrophages with downregulatory activity, as evidenced by the production of IL-10 and transforming growth factor-β (TGF-β), both potent depressants of T-cell activity.[5]

HELMINTHS AND T CELLS

Typically, acute infections with tissue-invasive helminths induce a robust Th2 response manifested by enhanced expression of IL-4, IL-5, and IL-13 in response to live parasites, parasite antigens, or mitogens.[5] The Th2 bias is often antigen-specific but in some cases bystander spillover can lead to Th2 responses to nonparasite antigens.[5] There are however exceptions to this canonical Th2 response to helminth infections. Immune responses to schistosoma cercariae are Th1 in nature and only upon egg-laying does a Th2 response emerge. Early immune responses of unexposed individuals to live filarial parasites are markedly Th1-like and in murine infections microfilariae of *B. malayi* promote Th1 responses. Finally, immune responses to the gut nematode *Trichuris muris* can be Th1 or Th2 depending on the mouse strain used for infection. Since the establishment of Th2 responses requires early induction of IL-4, one of the major research topics in helminth immunology has been on the identification of the source of this early IL-4. Depending on the model system used, it has been determined that basophils, NKT cells, and eosinophils can all serve as the early sources of IL-4 for Th2 differentiation in helminth infection. In addition to the early expression of IL-4, other factors, including expression of co-stimulatory molecules on naïve T cells, have been shown to play an important role in Th2 differentiation.[9] Thus, CD80, CD86 interaction with CD28 and ICOS–ICOS ligand as well as OX40–OX40 ligand interaction have been shown to be useful in the initiation or maintenance of the Th2 response. In addition, interaction of the Notch receptor with its ligand, Jagged, is known to induce Th2 differentiation. Finally, induction of GATA-3 and downregulation of T-bet has been shown to be an important step in T-cell differentiation to the Th2 phenotype in helminth infections.[10]

Interestingly, chronic helminth infections are associated with a downmodulation of parasite antigen-specific proliferative responses as well as IFN-γ and IL-2 production but with intact IL-4 responses to parasite antigens and global downregulation of both Th1 and Th2 responses to live parasites.[11]

HELMINTHS AND B CELLS

Helminth interactions with B cells occur both at the B-cell cytokine level and at the level of antibody production. Interactions at the cellular level primarily result in B-cell activation and cytokine production, most notably IL-10. Also, B-cell production of IL-4 has been demonstrated in mouse models of helminth infection. However, it is at the level of antibody production that B cells play a profound role in helminth infections. One of the most consistent findings in helminth infections, both in mice and humans, is the elevated level of IgE that is observed following exposure to helminths. Most of the IgE produced is not antigen-specific, perhaps representing nonspecific potentiation of IgE-producing B cells or deregulation of a normally well-controlled immune response. This potentiating effect seems to be selective for IgE (and possible IgG$_4$). Elevated levels of total serum IgE have been documented in many studies. Characteristically, individuals with invasive helminth infections have serum IgE levels approaching 100 times normal value. In addition, the IgE antibodies have specificity against a very broad range of parasite antigens. Interestingly, these IgE antibodies persist many years after the infection has been treated, indicating the presence of long-lived memory B cells or plasma cells in helminth infections.[12] IgE production in both mice and humans is absolutely dependent on IL-4 or IL-13. Other isotypes that are commonly elevated in chronically helminth-infected humans are IgG$_4$ and IgG$_1$, the former being most dependent on both IL-4 and IL-10.[13]

HELMINTHS AND EOSINOPHILS

Blood and tissue eosinophilia is characteristic of helminth infection and is mediated by IL-5 (typically in concert with IL-3 and granulocyte–macrophage colony-stimulating factor). Recruitment of eosinophils to the site of infection occurs very early in experimental helminth infection – as early as 24 hours following exposure. Kinetics in humans is harder to determine but is postulated to occur as early as 2–3 weeks following infections, as demonstrated in experimental infections of volunteers. Apart from the rapid kinetics of recruitment, eosinophils in the blood and tissue also exhibit morphological and functional changes attributable to eosinophil activation. These include decreased density, upregulation of surface activation molecules such as CD25, CD69, CD44, and HLA-DR, enhanced cellular cytotoxicity, and release of granular proteins, cytokines, leukotrienes and other mediators of inflammation.[14] Activation of eosinophils requires T cells since, in the absence of T cells, eosinophils accumulate at the site of infection but do not degranulate or become cytotoxic.

HELMINTHS AND BASOPHILS/MAST CELLS

Basophils are an important component of the immune response to helminth infections. Basophilia occurs in several animal models of helminth infections (not however in humans) and basophils can release IL-4 and histamine in response to parasite antigen stimulation. Moreover,

---

CLINICAL RELEVANCE

APPROACHES TO HELMINTH VACCINE DEVELOPMENT

>> Radiation-attenuated larval parasites have been efficacious in veterinary practice, but not feasible for wide-scale application

>> Few helminth vaccine candidates are in human clinical trials

>> Recent emphasis has been on DNA vaccines, subunit vaccines, "rational" vaccine design, parasite genome analysis, and the development of novel vectors

---

expedited the search for rational vaccine targets. Advances in proteomics and high-throughput biochemical analysis have improved and facilitated the methods to determine the structure and function of the proteins encoded by this genetic information.[46]

DNA AND RECOMBINANT PROTEIN VACCINES

DNA vaccines are made of DNA coding sequences that specify the candidate antigen protein inserted into a bacterial plasmid under the regulation of a eukaryotic promoter. DNA vaccines can be administered by multiple routes and can induce virtually all types of immune response: CD8 T-cell cytotoxicity, CD4 T-cell help and antibodies. In addition, DNA vaccines contain unmethylated DNA motifs that can stimulate the innate immune response through TLR9 and act as a self-adjuvant. DNA and protein vaccines can be administered as a prime-boost regiment with DNA used for priming and protein vaccines used for boosting. DNA and protein vaccines have been used in experimental models of schistosomiasis, filariasis, *Strongyloides* and hookworm infection. These include the candidate antigens irV5, paramyosin, Sm14, glutathione-*S*-transferase, triose phosphate isomerase and Sm23 for schistosomiasis, paramyosin, heart shock proteins, ALT-1 and ALT-2 for filariasis, chitinase and ALT-1 for onchocerciasis, Asp-1, Asp-2, metalloprotease-1 for hookworm infection and SS-eat-6 for *Strongyloides* infection.[48]

HUMAN CLINICAL TRIALS

Very few helminth vaccine candidates have reached human clinical trials. One is the 28-kDa glutathione-*S*-transferase protein from *Schistosoma mansoni*. This vaccine (in alum) has been shown to elicit antibody responses characteristic of Th2 immunity in human trials. This vaccine is primarily aimed at reducing morbidity by affecting female worm fecundity and to improve the efficacy of chemotherapy.[49] Similarly, *ASP-2* a secreted protein from *N. americanus* has been selected for evaluation as a recombinant vaccine candidate based on human epidemiological and experimental animal model studies. The vaccine is currently undergoing phase II studies.[50]

With rapid advances in the parasite genomics and proteomics as well as the newer, better vaccine delivery systems offering better and more rapid assessment development, prospects for newer anti-helminth vaccines are excellent, although the potential lack of commercial markets imposes a significant impediment to their development.

REFERENCES

1. Mosmann TR, Cherwinski H, Bond MW, et al. Two types of murine helper T cell clone. I. Definition according to profiles of lymphokine activities and secreted proteins. J Immunol 1986; 136: 2348.
2. Seder RA, Paul WE. Acquisition of lymphokine-producing phenotype by CD4+ T cells. Annu Rev Immunol 1994; 12: 635.
3. Finkelman FD, Pearce EJ, Urban JF Jr., et al. Regulation and biological function of helminth-induced cytokine responses. Immunol Today 1991; 12: A62.
4. Sher A, Pearce E, Kaye P. Shaping the immune response to parasites: role of dendritic cells. Curr Opin Immunol 2003; 15: 421.
5. Maizels RM, Yazdanbakhsh M. Immune regulation by helminth parasites: cellular and molecular mechanisms. Nat Rev Immunol 2003; 3: 733.
6. Talaat KR, Bonawitz RE, Domenech P, et al. Preexposure to live *Brugia malayi* microfilariae alters the innate response of human dendritic cells to *Mycobacterium tuberculosis*. J Infect Dis 2006; 193: 196.
7. Nair MG, Gallagher IJ, Taylor MD, et al. Chitinase and Fizz family members are a generalized feature of nematode infection with selective upregulation of Ym1 and Fizz1 by antigen-presenting cells. Infect Immun 2005; 73: 385.
8. Semnani RT, Nutman TB. Toward an understanding of the interaction between filarial parasites and host antigen-presenting cells. Immunol Rev 2004; 201: 127.
9. Jankovic D, Steinfelder S, Kullberg MC, et al. Mechanisms underlying helminth-induced Th2 polarization: default, negative or positive pathways? Chem Immunol Allergy 2006; 90: 65.
10. Babu S, Kumaraswami V, Nutman TB. Transcriptional control of impaired Th1 responses in patent lymphatic filariasis by T-box expressed in T cells and suppressor of cytokine signaling genes. Infect Immun 2005; 73: 3394.
11. Babu S, Blauvelt CP, Kumaraswami V, et al. Regulatory networks induced by live parasites impair both Th1 and Th2 pathways in patent lymphatic filariasis: implications for parasite persistence. J Immunol 2006; 176: 3248.
12. Mitre E, Nutman TB. IgE memory: persistence of antigen-specific IgE responses years after treatment of human filarial infections. J Allergy Clin Immunol 2006; 117: 939.
13. Maizels RM, Balic A, Gomez-Escobar N, et al. Helminth parasites – masters of regulation. Immunol Rev 2004; 201: 89.
14. Klion AD, Nutman TB. The role of eosinophils in host defense against helminth parasites. J Allergy Clin Immunol 2004; 113: 30.
15. Pennock JL, Grencis RK. The mast cell and gut nematodes: damage and defence. Chem Immunol Allergy 2006; 90: 128.
16. Quinnell RJ. Genetics of susceptibility to human helminth infection. Int J Parasitol 2003; 33: 1219.
17. Finkelman FD, Shea-Donohue T, Goldhill J, et al. Cytokine regulation of host defense against parasitic gastrointestinal nematodes: lessons from studies with rodent models. Annu Rev Immunol 1997; 15: 505.
18. Lawrence RA. Lymphatic filariasis: what mice can tell us. Parasitol Today 1996; 12: 267.
19. Finkelman FD, Shea-Donohue T, Morris SC, et al. Interleukin-4- and interleukin-13-mediated host protection against intestinal nematode parasites. Immunol Rev 2004; 201: 139.

20. Dombrowicz D, Capron M. Eosinophils, allergy and parasites. Curr Opin Immunol 2001; 13: 716.

21. Wynn TA, Thompson RW, Cheever AW, et al. Immunopathogenesis of schistosomiasis. Immunol Rev 2004; 201: 156.

22. Mentink-Kane MM, Wynn TA. Opposing roles for IL-13 and IL-13 receptor alpha 2 in health and disease. Immunol Rev 2004; 202: 191.

23. Amiri P, Locksley RM, Parslow TG, et al. Tumour necrosis factor alpha restores granulomas and induces parasite egg-laying in schistosome-infected SCID mice. Nature 1992; 356: 604.

24. Figueredo-Silva J, Noroes J, Cedenho A, et al. The histopathology of bancroftian filariasis revisited: the role of the adult worm in the lymphatic-vessel disease. Ann Trop Med Parasitol 2002; 96: 531.

25. Taylor MJ, Bandi C, Hoerauf A. *Wolbachia* bacterial endosymbionts of filarial nematodes. Adv Parasitol 2005; 60: 245.

26. Pearce EJ, Sher A. Mechanisms of immune evasion in schistosomiasis. Contrib Microbiol Immunol 1987; 8: 219.

27. Maizels RM, Bundy DA, Selkirk ME, et al. Immunological modulation and evasion by helminth parasites in human populations. Nature 1993; 365: 797.

28. Hartmann S, Lucius R. Modulation of host immune responses by nematode cystatins. Int J Parasitol 2003; 33: 1291.

29. Else KJ. Have gastrointestinal nematodes outwitted the immune system? Parasite Immunol 2005; 27: 407.

30. Thomas PG, Harn DA Jr.. Immune biasing by helminth glycans. Cell Microbiol 2004; 6: 13.

31. Maizels RM, Gomez-Escobar N, Gregory WF, et al. Immune evasion genes from filarial nematodes. Int J Parasitol 2001; 31: 889.

32. Loukas A, Constant SL, Bethony JM. Immunobiology of hookworm infection. FEMS Immunol Med Microbiol 2005; 43: 115.

33. King CL, Mahanty S, Kumaraswami V, et al. Cytokine control of parasite-specific anergy in human lymphatic filariasis. Preferential induction of a regulatory T helper type 2 lymphocyte subset. J Clin Invest 1993; 92: 1667.

34. Satoguina J, Mempel M, Larbi J, et al. Antigen-specific T regulatory-1 cells are associated with immunosuppression in a chronic helminth infection (onchocerciasis). Microbes Infect 2002; 4: 1291.

35. Taylor MD, LeGoff L, Harris A, et al. Removal of regulatory T cell activity reverses hyporesponsiveness and leads to filarial parasite clearance in vivo. J Immunol 2005; 174: 4924.

36. Gillan V, Devaney E. Regulatory T cells modulate Th2 responses induced by *Brugia pahangi* third-stage larvae. Infect Immun 2005; 73: 4034.

37. Steel C, Nutman TB. CTLA-4 in filarial infections: implications for a role in diminished T cell reactivity. J Immunol 2003; 170: 1930.

38. Pearce EJ, Kane CM, Sun J. Regulation of dendritic cell function by pathogen-derived molecules plays a key role in dictating the outcome of the adaptive immune response. Chem Immunol Allergy 2006; 90: 82.

39. Yazdanbakhsh M, Kremsner PG, van Ree R. Allergy, parasites, and the hygiene hypothesis. Science 2002; 296: 490.

40. Wilson MS, Maizels RM. Regulation of allergy and autoimmunity in helminth infection. Clin Rev Allergy Immunol 2004; 26: 35.

41. McKay DM. The beneficial helminth parasite? Parasitology 2006; 132: 1.

42. Summers RW, Elliott DE, Urban JF Jr, et al. *Trichuris suis* therapy in Crohn's disease. Gut 2005; 54: 87.

43. Summers RW, Elliott DE, Urban JF Jr, et al. *Trichuris suis* therapy for active ulcerative colitis: a randomized controlled trial. Gastroenterology 2005; 128: 825.

44. McCarthy JS, Nutman TB. Perspective: prospects for development of vaccines against human helminth infections. J Infect Dis 1996; 174: 1384.

45. Lightowlers MW. Vaccines against cysticercosis and hydatidosis: foundations in taeniid cestode immunology. Parasitol Int 2006; 55(Suppl): S39.

46. Tarleton RL. New approaches in vaccine development for parasitic infections. Cell Microbiol 2005; 7: 1379.

47. Dalton JP, Brindley PJ, Knox DP, et al. Helminth vaccines: from mining genomic information for vaccine targets to systems used for protein expression. Int J Parasitol 2003; 33: 621.

48. Da'dara AA, Harn DA. DNA vaccines against tropical parasitic diseases. Exp Rev Vaccines 2005; 4: 575.

49. Capron A, Riveau G, Capron M, et al. Schistosomes: the road from host–parasite interactions to vaccines in clinical trials. Trends Parasitol 2005; 21: 143.

50. Hotez PJ, Zhan B, Bethony JM, et al. Progress in the development of a recombinant vaccine for human hookworm disease: the Human Hookworm Vaccine Initiative. Int J Parasitol 2003; 33: 1245.

REFERENCES

Evaluation of the immunodeficient patient

Mary E. Paul, William T. Shearer

30

Immunodeficiency diseases can present with symptoms of susceptibility to infection but may also involve allergy, autoimmune disease or lympho-proliferation. There are over 120 primary immunodeficiency diseases (PIDs) and they can affect any aspect of the immune response. PIDS are generally hereditary and congenital deficiencies of the immune system. In contrast, secondary immunodeficiencies, discussed in detail in Chapter 38, can present at any time, in that they are acquired disruptions in immune function that increase susceptibility to infection. Examples include severe combined immune deficiencies, DiGeorge syndrome, and chronic granulomatous disease, which are usually diagnosed in infants and young children. However, common variable immunodeficiency (CVID), an immunodeficiency of impaired antibody production that has an incidence between 1:10 000 and 1:50 000, typically does not cause symptoms until the third decade of life.[1] This chapter introduces the PIDS and presents an approach to the evaluation of the immunodeficient patient.

■ FREQUENCY AND DIFFERENTIAL DIAGNOSIS ■

Nonimmune causes for recurrent infections have to be considered in the differential diagnosis of the immunodeficiency disorders. These include disorders that disrupt the usual clearance mechanisms, such as posterior urethral valves or urethral stenosis in a patient with recurrent urinary tract infection; cystic fibrosis in individuals who have recurrent sinusitis or pneumonia; and allergic rhinitis in patients who have recurrent sinusitis or otitis media. Disruption of barrier protection can lead to infection, for example in patients with skin disruption due to eczema or burns, or individuals with cerebrospinal fluid leaks following bony injury to the cranium. Patients with low antibody levels may be able to produce antibody normally, and instead have loss of antibody due to a protein-losing enteropathy, neph-ropathy, or massive protein loss through the skin, such as is found in severe eczema or burns. Secondary immunodeficiency can result from, for example, malnutrition, diabetes mellitus, and sickle cell anemia.

The incidence of congenital immunodeficiencies varies from the common selective IgA deficiency (1:300–1:700) to the rare X-linked severe combined immunodeficiency (1:50 000–1:100 000).[2] Chronic granulo-matous disease (CGD) occurs with an incidence of 1:200 000.[3]

The hallmark of immunodeficiency is recurrent serious infection with frequent treatment failures. These disorders present in a male:female ratio of 5:1 in children and infants and 1:1.4 in adults. More than 120 primary immunodeficiency disorders were recognized at the Budapest 2005 meeting of a committee of experts convened under the aegis of the International Union of Immunological Societies.[4] Examples and the typical presentation for various primary immunodeficiency disorders are listed in Table 30.1.

■ ETIOLOGY ■

Although the etiology of many immunodeficiencies has not been eluci-dated, defective genes and gene products have been identified in certain PIDs. Examples of secondary immunodeficiencies include those condi-tions that occur as a consequence of the exposure of the patient to immunosuppressive agents, infectious diseases, infiltrative diseases, and metabolic diseases as discussed throughout this book. Disruptions in the function of the immune system can occur due to problems in develop-ment, in cell-to-cell communication, and in cell function or structure. Examples of abnormalities in the immune system that result in disease are listed below. Each of these disorders is discussed fully in subsequent chapters.

> ### KEY CONCEPTS
>
> **FEATURES OF CONGENITAL ANTIBODY DEFICIENCY**
>
> >> Free of infections until 7–9 months of age, when antibodies that passed through the placenta from mother to infant are below protective levels.
>
> >> Severe infections with bacterial organisms, especially with encapsulated bacteria such as *Streptococcus pneumoniae*.
>
> >> Growth failure is generally not seen, except in the patient who has been chronically ill with severe infection.

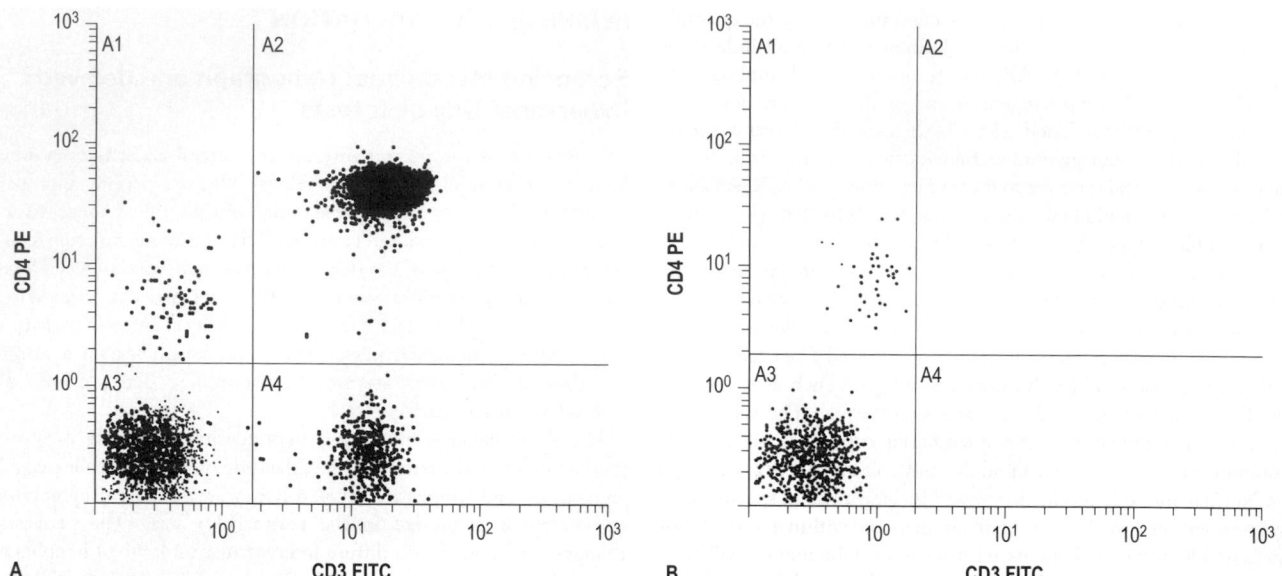

Fig. 30.5 Histograms of fluorescently stained lymphocytes. The quadrant of interest, A2, shows lymphocytes that are positive for labeling with both fluorescein isothiocyanate (FITC)-tagged monoclonal antibodies specific for CD3 and phycoerythrin (PE)-tagged monoclonal antibodies specific for CD4. The histogram on the left shows normal fluorescence due to CD4 T lymphocytes in quadrant A2. The histogram on the right shows absence of CD4 T lymphocytes in an infant with SCID.

cells can be identified and labeled using flow cytometry and fluorescent monoclonal antibodies. T-cell enumeration involves the use of a pan-T-cell monoclonal antibody specific for CD3. The CD4 marker serves as identification for T-helper (Th) cells. B cells can be identified by using monoclonal antibodies against the cell surface markers CD19 or CD20. Natural killer (NK) cells can be identified using monoclonal antibodies against CD16.[23] A histogram of fluorescence intensity is obtained (Fig. 30.5) from which the percentage of the specific lymphocyte subset can be obtained. A reference range is established for each subset by arranging values from the control population in order of magnitude and defining normals as those whose values fall between the fifth and 95th percentages for this population. Separate ranges should be used for children because infants and children generally have higher absolute numbers of T-cell subsets and higher percentages of CD4 cells (Fig. 30.6). Other factors, such as age, gender, and adrenocorticoid levels, can influence lymphocyte subset populations.

Lymphocyte functional analysis

To test lymphocyte function in the laboratory, lymphocyte proliferation or transformation studies are performed (Chapter 98). For these studies, lymphocytes are stimulated to proliferate involving new DNA synthesis and cell division. Lymphocytes from immunized or previously exposed individuals will proliferate in response to antigens to which they are sensitized. This response *in vitro* correlates with the *in vivo* delayed-type hypersensitivity response. Mitogens such as concanavalin A, phytohemagglutinin, and pokeweed mitogen can stimulate proliferation of normal cells, as can allogeneic histocompatibility antigens when leukocytes from two donors are mixed in culture. Proliferation of lymphocytes can be evaluated by the demonstration of transformed

lymphocytes, which resemble blasts, or by increased DNA synthesis. Increased DNA synthesis is monitored by the use of radiolabeled nucleic acid, usually tritiated thymidine, in culture media. A measure of the amount of radiolabeled material in the cells correlates with DNA synthesis.

SPECIAL TESTING

If autosomal recessive SCID is suspected, the ADA and PNP enzyme activities in the red blood cells should be determined. Recently transfused red blood cells will elevate the enzyme activity in deficient patients. White blood cells can be used to measure enzyme activity in recently transfused individuals. Ataxia–telangiectasia (AT) has the consistent laboratory finding of elevated α-fetoprotein levels along with variable abnormalities in B- and T-cell function. Molecular testing for many disorders, for example AT, X-linked SCID, Jak3 deficiency, X-linked agammaglobulinemia, LAD, and CGD, is available through commercial and research laboratories. Specialized functional tests for immune deficiency, for instance testing of lymphocyte apoptosis in a patient who may have ALPS, is available through research laboratories.

COMPLEMENT

Laboratory tests for complement components include tests for functional activity of the classic pathway with a CH_{50} assay and the alternative pathway with an AH_{50} assay, and immunochemical methods to measure complement component levels.[24] The CH_{50} evaluation tests the ability of fresh serum from the patient to lyse antibody-coated sheep erythrocytes. This reflects the activity of all numbered components of the classic complement pathway, C1–C9, and terminal components of the alternative

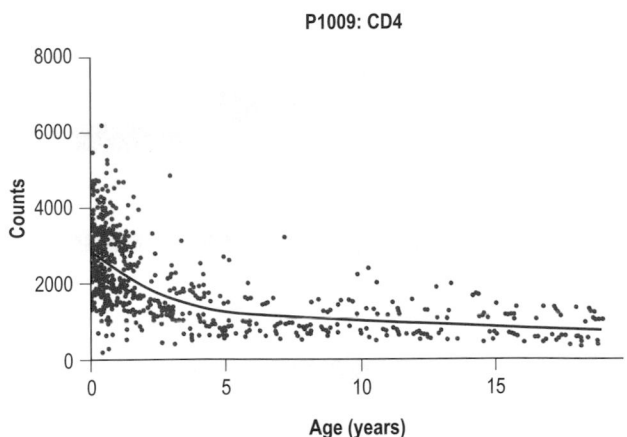

Fig. 30.6 Change in distribution of peripheral blood CD4 T-cell subsets with age in healthy children. Scatter plot indicates peripheral blood CD4 T-cell counts (cells/μL) by age, with lowest curves in healthy children from birth to 18 years of age. (From Shearer et al. Lymphocyte subsets in healthy children from birth through 18 years of age: The Pediatric AIDS Clinical Trials Group P1009 study. J Allergy Clin Immunol 2003; 112: 973, with permission from the American Academy of Allergy, Asthma and Immunology.)

complement pathway. A total deficiency of one of the classic complement pathway components will result in a CH_{50} approaching zero (Chapter 20). Nephelometry, radial immunodiffusion, RIA, and ELISA are used to measure complement components. Quantitative tests for components C3 and C4 are utilized in testing for complement deficiencies and for evaluation of complement activation (Chapter 20).

PHAGOCYTES

The evaluation of a patient with a suspected phagocyte deficiency should always begin with a complete blood count. Granulocytopenia is the most frequently encountered disorder of the phagocyte system. With granulocytopenia, a qualitative neutrophil defect is unlikely and subsequent evaluation should investigate the etiology of the granulocytopenia. Neutrophilia, although most commonly associated with acute infection, is a common finding in LAD I.

Abnormalities of white blood cell function involve difficulty with adherence, locomotion, deformability, recognition, attachment, engulfment, phagosome formation, phagocytosis, degranulation, microbial killing, and elimination of engulfed material (Chapter 21). Chronic granulomatous disease is diagnosed by demonstrating absent or markedly reduced oxidase activity in neutrophils after stimulation. Flow cytometry with the conversion of dihydrorhodamine (DHR) 123 to rhodamine 123 is a sensitive assay of oxidase activity used in the diagnosis of CGD.[25] The nitroblue tetrazolium test (NBT) measures oxidative burst activity as well, but is more subjective and can miss the diagnosis of CGD.[26] For patients with suspected LAD I deficiency, purified neutrophils or monocytes are labeled with monoclonal antibody directed against a portion of the CD11/CD18 heterodimer. The sample is then further labeled with a fluorescently tagged second antibody; fluorescence is quantified by flow cytometry.[27]

Other techniques used to identify phagocytic defects include assays for chemotaxis and bactericidal activity.

■ ILLUSTRATIVE CASES ■

CASE 1

The patient was a 6-month-old Caucasian female who presented for immunologic evaluation at 3 months of age with a history of rash and otitis media that had been recurrent since 2 weeks of age. Since birth she had had poor weight gain, frequent spitting up, coughing spells, and persistent diarrhea. There were no parental risk factors for HIV.

The physical examination showed an emaciated infant who had no palpable lymphoid tissue. The oral examination revealed white plaques consistent with thrush.

Evaluation included a radiological examination of the upper gastrointestinal tract without barium to investigate for gastroesophageal reflux, and *CFTR* gene analysis for mutations found in cystic fibrosis. Both of these were normal. Stool viral cultures were persistently positive for rotavirus.

Immunodeficiency was suspected because of the failure to thrive, persistent chronic diarrhea, and recurrent infection. An evaluation of the immune system was performed (Table 30.2). Humoral immunity was first tested with immunoglobulin levels. All were below or just above the lower limit of normal. Isohemagglutinins were not tested as the patient was less than 1 year old. As she had not been immunized, specific antibody titers to vaccines were not tested. Stool α_1-antitrypsin levels were normal, suggesting that protein was not being lost in the stool, and urinalysis did not show protein loss. The complete blood count revealed profound lymphopenia and absolute neutropenia. The neutropenia resolved on subsequent evaluations but the lymphopenia persisted. The thymic shadow was not present on chest radiograph (this finding is not unusual in children with chronic illness, in whom the thymus may involute). Delayed hypersensitivity skin tests were not placed as the patient would not have been expected to have a reliable response at this age. Evaluation of lymphocytes subsets by flow cytometry revealed that the CD4 and CD8 T- and B-lymphocyte numbers were all markedly low.

The patient receives monthly immunoglobulin replacement therapy. Subsequent infections have included recurrent otitis media, conjunctivitis, and sinusitis.

CASE 4

The patient presented at 3 years of age following hospitalization for pneumonia. The past medical history was significant for recurrent otitis media and bronchitis. The family history was negative for diagnosed immunodeficiency, although two siblings had had a history of recurrent otitis media and bronchitis. The patient had had normal growth and development.

The physical examination revealed normal tonsillar tissue in the posterior pharynx and the presence of small lymph nodes in the cervical region.

Laboratory values (Table 30.2) included a normal white blood cell count with normal numbers of granulocytes and lymphocytes. The chest radiograph showed the presence of a thymic shadow. Cellular immune function was tested with delayed hypersensitivity skin testing which was positive for *C. albicans* antigen and tetanus toxoid, and negative for purified protein derivative. Serum immunoglobulin levels were normal. The patient had been previously immunized and had adequate antibody titers to tetanus toxoid, diphtheria, and pneumococcus, suggesting the ability to form antibody when challenged. Isohemagglutinins were also positive.

The CH_{50} level was below the lowest measurable level. C3 and C4 levels were normal, but the level of C2 was 0. The patient's father, mother, and brother had levels of C2 which were half of the normal value, indicating that they were heterozygotes for the abnormal C2 allele.

C2 deficiency was diagnosed. The patient is now 7 years old and has chronically had sinusitis and bronchitis. C2 deficiency is frequently associated with autoimmune disease; this patient has no current autoimmune disease but receives yearly surveillance examinations.

■ REFERENCES ■

1. Simonte SJ, Cunningham-Rundles C. Update on primary immunodeficiency: defects of lymphocytes. Clin Immunol 2003; 109: 109–118.

2. Buckley RH. Molecular defects in human severe combined immunodeficiency and approaches to immune reconstitution. Annu Rev Immunol 2004; 22: 625–655.

3. Winkelstein JA, Marino MC, Johnston RB Jr, et al. Chronic granulomatous disease. Report on a national registry of 368 patients. Medicine (Baltimore) 2000; 79: 155.

4. Notarangelo L, Casanova JL, Conley ME, et al. Primary immunodeficiency diseases: An update from the International Union of Immunological Societies Primary Immunodeficiency Diseases Classification Committee Meeting in Budapest, 2005. J Allergy Clin Immunol 2006; 117: 883–896.

5. Cunningham-Rundles C, Ponda PP. Molecular defects in T- and B-cell primary immunodeficiency diseases. Nature Rev Immunol 2005; 5: 880–892.

6. Myers LA, Patel DD, Puck JM, Buckley RH. Hematopoietic stem cell transplantation for severe combined immunodeficiency in the neonatal period leads to superior thymic output and improved survival. Blood 2002; 99: 872–878.

7. Sayos J, Wu C, Morra M, et al. The X-linked lymphoproliferative disease gene product SAP regulates signals induced through the co-receptor SLAM. Nature 1998; 395: 462.

8. Castigli E, Geha RS. Molecular basis of common variable immunodeficiency. J Allergy Clin Immunol 2006; 117: 740–746.

9. Segal BH, Leto TL, Gallin JI, et al. Genetic biochemical and clinical features of chronic granulomatous Disease. Medicine (Baltimore) 2005; 79: 170–200.

10. Chatila TA. Role of regulatory T cells in human diseases. J Allergy Clin Immunol 2005; 116: 949–959.

11. Etzioni A, Gershoni-Baruch R, Pollack S, Shehadeh N. Leukocyte adhesion deficiency type II: long term follow-up. J Allergy Clin Immunol 1998; 102: 323–324.

12. Johnson CA, Densen P, Hurford RK Jr, et al. Type I human complement C2 deficiency. A 28-base pair gene deletion causes skipping of exon 6 during RNA splicing. J Biol Chem 1992; 267: 9347.

13. Chandra RK. Nutrition and the immune system: an introduction. Am J Clin Nutr 1997; 66: 460S–463S.

14. Villamor E, Fawzi WW. Effects of vitamin A supplementation on immune responses and correlation with clinical outcomes. Clin Microbiol Rev 2005; 18: 446–464.

15. Fraker PJ, King LE, Laakko T, et al. The dynamic link between the integrity of the immune system and zinc status. J Nutr 2000; 130: 1399S.

16. Von Bernuth H, Puel A, Ku CL, et al. Septicemia without sepsis: inherited disorders of nuclear factor-kappa B-mediated inflammation. Clin Infect Dis 2005; 41: S436–S439.

17. Folds JD, Schmitz JL. Clinical and laboratory assessment of immunity. J Allergy Clin Immunol 2003; 111: s702–s711.

18. Butler JC, Breiman RF, Lipman HB, et al. Serotype distribution of *Streptococcus pneumoniae* among preschool children in the United States, 1978–1994: implications for development of a conjugate vaccine. J Infect Dis 1995; 171: 885.

19. Breukels MA, Rijkers GT, Voorhoorst-Ogink MM, et al. Pneumococcal conjugate vaccine primes for polysaccharide-inducible IgG_2 antibody response in children with recurrent otitis media acuta. J Infect Dis 1999; 179: 1152.

20. Shearer WT, Lugg DJ, Rosenblatt HM, et al. Antibody responses to bacteriophage FX-174 in human subjects exposed to the Antarctic winter-over model of spaceflight. J Allergy Clin Immunol 2001; 107: 160–164.

21. Stites DP, Folds JD, Schmitz JL. Clinical laboratory methods for detection of cellular immunity. In: Stites DP, Terr AI, Parslow TG, eds. Medical immunology, 9th edn. Stanford: Appleton & Lange, 1997; 254–274.

22. Bothamley GH. Immunologic tests in tuberculosis and leprosy. In: Rose NR, Hamilton RG, Detrick B, eds. Manual of clinical laboratory immunology, 6th edn. Washington, DC: ASM Press, 2002; 502–510.

23. Nicholson JKA. Immunophenotyping of lymphocytes by flow cytometry. In: Rose NR, Hamilton RG, Detrick B, eds. Manual of clinical laboratory immunology, 6th edn. Washington, DC: ASM Press, 2002; 137–147.

24. Wen L, Atkinson JP, Giclas PC. Clinical and laboratory evaluation of complement deficiency. J Allergy Clin Immunol 2004; 113: 585–593.

25. Jirapongsananuruk O, Malech HL, Kuhns DB, et al. Diagnostic paradigm for evaluation of male patients with chronic granulomatous disease, based on the dyhydrorhodamine 123 assay. J Allergy Clin Immunol 2003; 111: 374–379.

26. Vowells SJ, Fleisher TA, Malech HL. Testing for chronic granulomatous disease. Lancet 1996; 347: 1048–1049.

27. Shaw JM, Al-Shamhhani A, Boxer LA, et al. Characterization of four CD18 mutants in leukocyte adhesion deficient (LAD) patients with differential capacities to support expression and function of the CD11/CD18 integrins LFA-1, Mac-1, and p150,95. Clin Exp Immunol 2001; 126: 311–318.

28. Seeborg FO, Paul ME, Abramson SL, et al. A 5-week-old HIV-1-exposed girl with failure to thrive and diffuse nodular pulmonary infiltrates. J Allergy Clin Immunol 2004; 113: 627–634.

IMMUNOLOGIC DEFICIENCIES

Table 31.1 Predominant pathogens associated with selected immunological defects[a]

Abnormality	Bacterial	Fungal	Viral	Protozoal
Neutropenia or qualitative defects of phagocytes	Gram-positive Staphylocci (coagulase-positive and negative) Streptococci (enterococcus, α-hemolytic) Nocardia spp. Gram-negative Escherichia coli, Klebsiella pneumoniae, Pseudomonas aeruginosa, other Enterobacteriaceae	Candida spp. Aspergillus spp.		
Defective cell-mediated immunity	Legionella spp. Salmonella spp. Mycobacteria Listeria spp.	Histoplasma capsulatum Coccidioides immitis Cryptococcus neoformans Candida species Pneumocystis jiroveci	Cytomegalovirus Varicella-zoster virus Herpes simplex virus Epstein–Barr virus Live viral vaccines (measles, mumps, rubella, polio)	Toxoplasma gondii Strongyloides stercoralis Cryptosporidia Microsporidia Isopora spp.
Immunoglobulin deficiency	Streptococcus pneumoniae Haemophilus influenzae		Enteroviruses	Giardia
Complement deficiency	Streptococcus pneumoniae H. influenzae Neisseria spp.			
Splenectomy	S. pneumoniae H. influenzae Neisseria spp.			Babesia spp.

[a]See text for details and exceptions.

disruption of the integrity of mucosal barriers by cytotoxic chemotherapy (e.g., oral mucositis); concurrent abnormalities of cellular or humoral immunity (related to the underlying disease or its therapy); and the presence of indwelling intravenous catheters. Thus, patients who have received cytotoxic chemotherapy for the treatment of malignant disease may have a higher frequency of infections than patients with equivalent degrees of neutropenia secondary to idiosyncratic drug reactions or aplastic anemia.

The microbiology of bacterial infections in the neutropenic host has changed significantly over the past 20–25 years. In the 1970s Gram-negative bacilli (e.g., Escherichia coli, Pseudomonas aeruginosa, Klebsiella pneumonia) were the most frequently identified bacterial pathogens in patients with chemotherapy-induced neutropenia.[2] By the 1980s, the routine use of empiric antibiotic therapy targeted primarily at Gram-negative pathogens led to the emergence of Gram-positive organisms as the predominant bacterial pathogens isolated from neutropenic cancer patients.[3]

Although virtually any bacterial organism is a potential pathogen in the neutropenic host, the Gram-negative organisms most frequently

isolated from blood cultures of febrile neutropenic cancer patients are E. coli, K. pneumonia, and P. aeruginosa. Other Gram-negative pathogens, such as Enterobacter and Citrobacter species, are less commonly isolated from these patients.[3] A clinically apparent source for Gram-negative bacteria is not usually identified, and it is presumed that these infections originate from occult sites in the gastrointestinal tract, respiratory tract, urinary tract, or soft tissues.

The Gram-positive organisms most often isolated include coagulase-negative staphylococci, Staphylococcus aureus, enterococci, and alpha-hemolytic streptococci. S. aureus and coagulase-negative staphylococci are most often isolated from the bloodstream in patients with indwelling central venous catheters. Bacteremia with S. aureus or alpha-hemolytic streptococci tends to be clinically aggressive in neutropenic patients and is frequently associated with cardiovascular collapse and shock while infections with coagulase-negative staphylococci tend to be more indolent. Other Gram-positive bacteria that are occasionally isolated include Bacillus species and Corynebacterium jeikeium. Infections with both of these organisms are associated with indwelling vascular catheters.

Pure infections with anaerobic bacteria are unusual in neutropenic patients and are invariably associated with breaches of the gastrointestinal mucosa. Mixed aerobic–anaerobic infections are usually seen in patients with intra-abdominal processes or perirectal soft-tissue infections.

Invasive fungal infections are a major cause of morbidity and mortality in the neutropenic host. Systemic fungal infections are rarely the cause of primary infections in neutropenic patients not receiving antibiotics and seen less frequently in patients with 'short-term' (< 14 days) neutropenia. Risk factors for the development of invasive fungal infections include prolonged (> 14 days) neutropenia, broad-spectrum antibiotic therapy, and concurrent glucocorticosteroid use. Of these factors, severe and prolonged neutropenia is the most important.[4] Although a wide variety of fungi can cause invasive infection in the neutropenic host, *Candida* and *Aspergillus* species are the most common pathogens encountered. The predominance of *Candida* and *Aspergillus* infections in this clinical setting attests to the importance of the neutrophil in controlling infections due to these two organisms.

The most frequent *Candida* species causing disseminated infection is *C. albicans*. Other potential *Candida* pathogens include *C. tropicalis*, *C. parapsilosis*, *C. glabrata*, and *C. krusi*. In neutropenic patients *Candida* may cause local infection of the oral cavity, esophagus, vagina, or lower gastrointestinal tract; catheter-related candidemia; or disseminated infection with involvement of the liver and spleen (hepatosplenic candidiasis), skin, or eye (endophthalmitis). The *Aspergillus* species that most frequently infect neutropenic patients are *A. fumigatus* and *A. flavus*. Aspergilli are ubiquitous in nature and infection is acquired primarily through the respiratory tract. The upper airways (nasal cavity and sinuses) and lung are the primary sites of invasive infection in neutropenic patients. *Aspergillus* usually spreads by direct invasion to contiguous tissue (Fig. 31.1), although widespread (presumably hematogenous) dissemination to the skin, kidneys, and brain can occur. Blood cultures are virtually never positive for *Aspergillus* and the diagnosis is made by biopsy and culture of the affected tissue. Other fungal pathogens that can cause invasive infection in neutropenic hosts include members of the order Mucorales (*Mucor, Rhizopus, Cunninghamella*), *Trichosporon beigelii*, *Fusarium* species, *Drechslera* species, *Pseudoallescheria boydii*, and *Malassezia furfur*.

Because neutropenia impairs the local inflammatory response to infection, fever is often the initial and only manifestation of serious infection. Approximately 20% of febrile episodes in patients with neutrophil counts below 100 cells/mm³ will be associated with bacteremia[1] which, if left untreated, can be rapidly progressive and lethal. These considerations serve as the basis for the expeditious use of empiric broad-spectrum antibiotic therapy in patients with fever and neutropenia. The initial evaluation of the febrile neutropenic patient should begin with a thorough physical examination paying particular attention to the oral cavity, perianal region, and the site of any indwelling intravenous catheter. Blood and urine cultures should be obtained and other sites of potential infection should be evaluated by biopsy or aspiration as clinically indicated. Once the initial evaluation is complete, empiric broad-spectrum antibiotic therapy should be initiated. A number of single- or multiple-agent regimens have been successfully used. The initial selection of antibiotics should be based on the institutional antimicrobial sensitivity patterns of the most likely pathogens and the clinical findings. Modification of the initial antibiotic regimen is often necessary and should be based on culture results and frequent monitoring of the patient by physical examination. Detailed guidelines for antimicrobial therapy in neutropenic hosts have been published by the

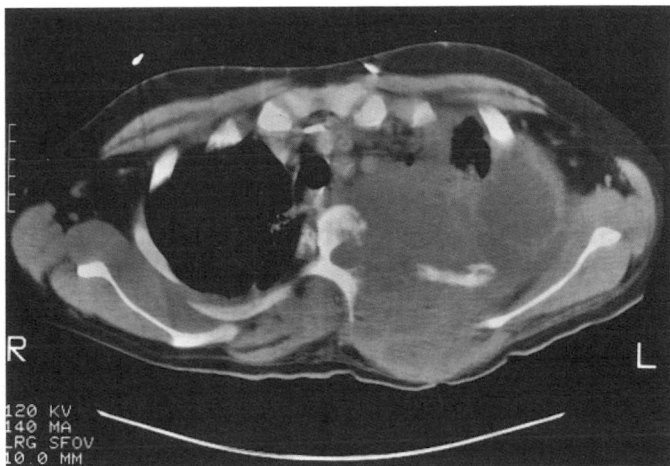

Fig. 31.1 Chest computed tomography scan of a patient with chronic granulomatous disease and pulmonary infection with *Aspergillus fumigatus*. The infection has spread by direct extension to involve the adjacent thoracic vertebral body and rib, and has partially destroyed these structures.

Infectious Diseases Society of America.[5] Results from several randomized trials suggest that selected low-risk hospitalized patients with fever and neutropenia that is expected to last less than 10 days can be safely treated with an oral antibiotic regimen.[5]

The diagnosis of invasive fungal disease in the neutropenic host is difficult. The neutropenic patient with persistent or recurrent fever after 5–7 days of antibiotic therapy is at particular risk for invasive fungal superinfection. By the time an invasive fungal infection becomes clinically apparent it is usually far advanced and difficult to treat. These considerations, along with the results of two controlled trials,[6] initially led to the routine use of empiric antifungal therapy with amphotericin B in patients with persistent or recurrent fever after 5–7 days of antibiotic therapy. In subsequent studies, liposomal amphotericin B, voriconazole, and caspofungin all appear to be as effective as conventional amphotericin B for empirical antifungal therapy in these patients, and are associated with less toxicity.[7]

A recent advance in therapy for quantitative phagocytic defects has been the use of recombinant hematopoietic growth factors to shorten the duration of neutropenia in patients treated with cytotoxic chemotherapy. Of these factors, the most widely studied are granulocyte and granulocyte–macrophage colony-stimulating factors (G-CSF and GM-CSF respectively). These glycoproteins stimulate the growth and maturation of hematopoietic progenitor cells and increase the number and function of committed phagocytic cells Both G-CSF and GM-CSF have been shown to accelerate granulocyte recovery following cytotoxic chemotherapy.[8]

QUALITATIVE ABNORMALITIES OF PHAGOCYTES

The ability of phagocytic cells to ingest and kill microorganisms involves a complex series of biochemical events. At the cellular level, these events involve the migration of phagocytic cells to the inflammatory site (chemotaxis), cell activation, phagocytosis, and the killing of organisms by oxidative-dependent and independent pathways. Primary defects in

are markedly decreased, as are *in vitro* responses to T-cell mitogens. Infectious diseases associated with this syndrome include chronic mucocutaneous candidiasis, and recurrent pneumonia (*P. jiroveci*).

The Wiskott–Aldrich syndrome (WAS) is an X-linked syndrome characterized by eczema, thrombocytopenic purpura, and increased susceptibility to infections[18] (Chapter 35). The immunologic defect most consistently found in these patients is a profound inability to mount a normal antibody response to polysaccharide antigens. Serum immunoglobulin levels are variable, but most patients exhibit low IgM, elevated IgA and IgE, and normal levels of IgG subclasses. T lymphocytes in the peripheral blood of WAS patients exhibit a progressive decline in number and function such that, by 6 years of age, profound lymphopenia is usually present. This pattern of immunologic abnormalities correlates with the types of infections seen in WAS. In younger patients, infections are predominantly due to encapsulated bacteria such as *S. pneumoniae, H. influenzae*, and other bacteria having polysaccharide capsules. Otitis media, pneumonia, meningitis, and sepsis are the most frequent types of infections caused by these organisms. Later in life, children with WAS develop opportunistic infections with agents such as *P. jiroveci* and Herpesviridae.

Ataxia-telangiectasia is a rare multisystem disease that generally presents in the first 3 years of life and culminates in death by the second decade[12] (Chapter 35). The most prominent clinical manifestations of this syndrome are cerebellar ataxia, oculocutaneous telangiectasias, chronic sinopulmonary infections, a high incidence of malignancy, and variable defects in humoral and cell-mediated immunity. Patients with ataxia-telangiectasia exhibit variably decreased levels of total IgG, IgG$_2$, IgA, and IgE. *In vitro* there is a decrease in mitogen-induced immunoglobulin synthesis that can be corrected by the addition of normal T cells. Clinically, this defect in humoral immunity is manifested by recurrent sinopulmonary infections with encapsulated bacteria. Cellular immunity is only mildly depressed at birth, but progressive impairment of delayed-hypersensitivity skin reactions and *in vitro* T-cell proliferative responses is noted in older children. Despite these defects in cellular immunity opportunistic viral, fungal, and parasitic infections are uncommon.

HIV INFECTION AND AIDS

Human immunodeficiency virus (HIV) infection leads to the progressive destruction of CD4 lymphocytes, resulting in immunodeficiency.[19] This occurs in a setting of immunosuppression due to immune system activation characterized by increased T-cell turnover and polyclonal B-cell activation. Patients with HIV infection become increasingly at risk for opportunistic infections as the CD4 T-cell count declines and/or as the levels of HIV in the blood increase. While the majority of these infections are reflective of decreased T-cell function, patients with HIV infection are also at risk for a variety of other infections as a consequence of either aberrant antibody production or drug-induced neutropenia. Recent advances in anti-retroviral therapy have led to a precipitous drop in the incidence of acquired immunodeficiency syndrome (AIDS)-defining opportunistic infections in the more developed parts of the world (Fig. 31.2).[19] Unfortunately these advances are not available to all patients with HIV infection and despite these advances, secondary infections remain a leading cause of death for patients with HIV infection and AIDS.

HIV infection can be classified into different stages depending upon the CD4 T-cell count and the clinical stage of disease (Table 31.2)

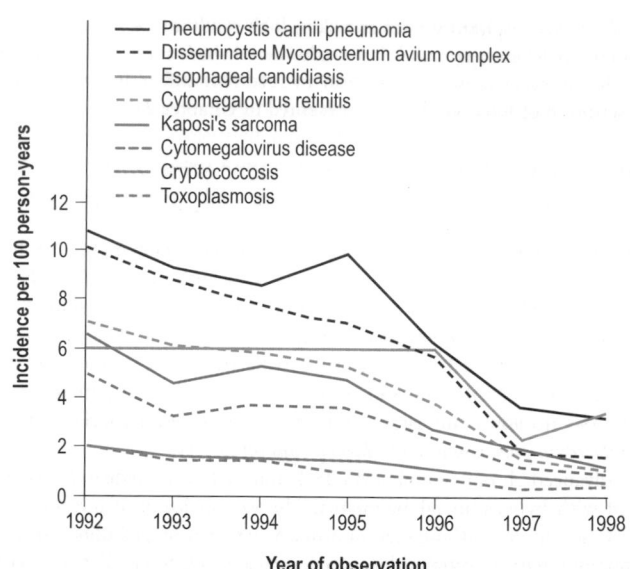

Fig. 31.2 Rates of opportunistic illness among human immunodeficiency virus (HIV)-infected patients with fewer than 100 CD4 T cells per cubic millimeter, from 1992 through 1998. (Adapted and updated from Palella FJ, et al, *New England Journal of Medicine* 1998; 338: 853–860 and Kaplan et al, *Clinical Infectious Diseases* 2000; Suppl. 1 Vol. 30: S5–S14.

(Chapter 37). This staging system utilizes the CD4 T-cell count for categories 1, 2, and 3 and the clinical stage for categories A, B, and C. Acute HIV infection (category A) may present with a clinical syndrome characterized by fever, lymphadenopathy, pharyngitis, arthralgias/myalgias, and rash.[19] In some patients this is associated with a precipitous drop in CD4 T-cell count, and opportunistic infections such as esophageal candidiasis can be seen during this time. Generally, however, patients with HIV infection remain free of secondary infections until the CD4 T-cell count falls below 500 cells per cubic millimeter (categories 2 and 3). The asymptomatic period of HIV disease following primary infection is referred to as stage B. The development of secondary diseases denotes progression to stage C.

Once the CD4 T-cell count falls below 500 cells/mm³, but remains above 200 cells/mm³, a variety of minor secondary infections can be seen (Table 31.3). These infections appear more common in patients with higher viral loads and include mucosal candidiasis, condyloma acuminata, oral hairy leukoplakia, and localized reactivation of herpes zoster (shingles) and herpes simplex. Patients with CD4 T-cell counts below 200 cells/mm³ are at risk for a wide variety of opportunistic infections (Table 31.3).

PROTOZOAL INFECTIONS

Protozoal infections are among the most common life-threatening secondary infections in patients with HIV infection. Toxoplasmosis is the most common secondary infection of the nervous system in patients with AIDS. Other protozoal infections of the CNS include focal CNS lesions due to *Trypanosoma cruzi* and meningoencephalitis due to *Acanthamoeba* spp. or *Naegleria* spp. Toxoplasmosis is generally a late complication of HIV infection and is more common in patients from the Caribbean or from France. CNS toxoplasmosis is thought to represent a reactivation

Table 31.2 1993 revised classification system for human immunodeficiency virus (HIV) infection and expanded acquired immunodeficiency syndrome (AIDS) surveillance case definition for adolescents and adults

	Clinical categories		
CD4 T-cell category	A Asymptomatic, acute (primary) HIV or PGL	B Symptomatic, not A or C conditions	C AIDS indicator conditions
> 500/µl	A1	B1	C1
200–499/µl	A2	B2	C2
< 200/µl	A3	B3	C3

PGL, progressive generalized lymphadenopathy.
(From: Morb Mort Week Rep 42, No. RR-17, December 18, 1992.)

syndrome and is 10 times more common in patients seropositive for antibodies to the etiologic agent, *Toxoplasma gondii*. In patients with AIDS, toxoplasmosis generally presents as a seizure or focal neurologic defect in association with fever. The presumptive diagnosis is based upon a magnetic resonance imaging, or double-dose contrast computed tomographic finding of multiple contrast-enhancing lesions in multiple locations (Fig. 31.3). Both *T. gondii* and trypanosomiasis can also involve the myocardium.

Protozoal infections, particularly *Cryptosporidium* and *Microsporidium* spp., can also cause diseases of the gastrointestinal tract in patients with HIV infection.[20] These organisms are responsible for clinical syndromes ranging from mild diarrhea to severe diarrhea with dehydration, nausea, and vomiting. *Cryptosporidium* can also involve the biliary tree. In addition to these two organisms one may also see diarrheal illness due to *Isospora belli*. This is an important diagnosis to make, given the fact that infection with *Isospora*, in contrast to infection with *Microsporidium* or *Cryptosporidium*, is relatively easy to treat and responds well to the combination of trimethoprim/sulfamethoxazole or ciprofloxacin.

Visceral leishmaniasis is recognized with increasing frequency in patients with HIV infection who live or travel to endemic areas. The clinical presentation is usually one of hepatosplenomegaly, fever, lymphadenopathy, and hematologic abnormalities. This disease is transmitted by sandflies. Patients usually respond well to standard therapy with pentavalent antimony compounds.

BACTERIAL INFECTIONS

Secondary bacterial infections with standard pathogens, *Mycobacterium tuberculosis*, atypical mycobacteria, and unusual organisms such as *Rhodococcus* and *Bartonella* spp. are a significant cause of morbidity in patients with HIV infection. Patients with HIV infection are particularly prone to infection with encapsulated bacteria. This similarity to patients with immunoglobulin deficiencies may reflect the defects in antigen-specific B-cell activation that have been reported in patients with HIV infection.[21] The majority of bacterial pneumonias seen in this setting are due to *Streptococcus pneumoniae* and *H. influenzae*. Patients with AIDS have a sixfold increase in the incidence of *S. pneumoniae* bacteremia. These observations emphasize the importance of pneumococcal

vaccination as a prophylaxis strategy in this group.[22] In addition, patients with AIDS have a high incidence of bacterial sinusitis, catheter-related sepsis, and pyomyositis. The standard enteric pathogens *Salmonella* spp., *Shigella* spp., and *Campylobacter* spp. are a common cause of dysenteric illness in patients with AIDS and, unlike the non-AIDS population, they are frequently associated with bacteremia.

The re-emergence of *Mycobacterium tuberculosis* as a significant public health problem and the identification of cases of tuberculosis in which the organism is resistant to two or more first-line drugs (multidrug-resistant tuberculosis) have both been a result of the HIV epidemic. In the USA, approximately 5% of patients with HIV infection have active tuberculosis. Worldwide, approximately one-third of all AIDS-related deaths are associated with tuberculosis. Given the inherent pathogenic potential of *M. tuberculosis*, active tuberculosis may be a relatively early manifestation of HIV infection and occur at CD4 T-cell counts >200 cells/mm[3].[23] Untreated tuberculosis can accelerate the course of HIV infection and treatment of tuberculosis can lead to decreases in plasma levels of HIV. In patients with early HIV infection, the clinical picture will be similar to that of classic pulmonary reactivation. In more advanced patients, the clinical picture is more likely to be that of disseminated disease. Overall 60–80% of patients will present with pulmonary disease and 30–40% will have extrapulmonary disease. Given the high probability of reactivation, it is recommended that all patients with HIV infection and a positive purified protein derivative (defined as > 5 mm at 48–72 hours) or close contact with active tuberculosis receive antimicrobial therapy. This generally consists of 9 months of isoniazid.

Infections with atypical mycobacteria are seen with an increased frequency in patients with HIV infection.[24] Infections with at least 12 different mycobacteria have been reported. The most common of these are *M. avium* and *M. intracellulare*, referred to together as the *Mycobacterium avium* complex (MAC). Infections with MAC are predominantly seen in the USA. They are rare in developing countries. One reason for this may by the observation that infection with MAC is less common in patients with prior tuberculosis. MAC infection is a late complication of HIV infection and typically occurs in patients with CD4 T-cell counts less than 50 cells/mm[3]. The average CD4 T-cell count at diagnosis is 10 cells/mm[3]. The most common clinical presentation is disseminated disease with fever, weight loss, and night sweats.

Table 31.3 Secondary infections seen in patients with human immunodeficiency virus (HIV) infection

CD4 count	Etiologic agents	Clinical manifestations
Any CD4 count	Human papillomavirus	Condyloma acuminata
	Herpes simplex	Recurrent ulcers
	Herpes zoster	Shingles
	Hepatitis B	Persistent antigenemia
	Hepatitis C	Chronic hepatitis
	Hepatitis D	Chronic hepatitis
	Rochalimaea henselae	Bacillary angiomatosis
	Encapsulated bacteria	Sinusitis
	Candida spp.	Oral thrush; vaginitis
	Coccidioides immitis	Pneumonia
≤500	Epstein–Barr virus	Oral hairy leukoplakia; lymphoma
	Human herpesvirus 8	Kaposi sarcoma; lymphoma
	Human papillomavirus	Cervical or anorectal dysplasia
	Mycobacterium tuberculosis	Pneumonia
≤200	*Pneumocystis jiroveci*	Pneumonia, disseminated infection
	Toxoplasma gondii	Encephalitis; choroiditis
	Cryptosporidia/microsporidia	Gastroenteritis; diarrhea
	Isospora	Diarrhea
	Encapsulated bacteria	Pneumonia; sinusitis
	Shigella, Salmonella, Campylobacter	Dysentery; bacteremia
	Treponema pallidum	Secondary and neurosyphilis
	Mycobacterium tuberculosis	Pneumonia; disseminated disease
≤100	Herpes simplex	Esophagitis
	Herpes zoster	Cutaneous dissemination
	Cytomegalovirus	Retinitis; colitis; neuropathy
	JC virus	Progressive multifocal leukoencephalopathy
	Candida spp.	Esophagitis
	Cryptococcus neoformans	Meningitis; pneumonia; dissemination
	Histoplasma capsulatum	Disseminated disease
	Penicillium marneffei	Disseminated disease
	Mycobacterium avium-intracellulare	Disseminated disease

Eighty-five percent of patients are mycobacteremic and liver and bone marrow involvement are common. Approximately 25% of patients with MAC infection will have an abnormal chest X-ray. The median survival following a diagnosis of MAC is in the range of 6–10 months. This may be more reflective of the late stage of underlying illness rather than the pathogenic contributions of MAC. Primary prophylaxis for MAC infection with azithromycin or clarithromycin is recommended for all patients with HIV infection and fewer than 50 CD4 T cells/mm³.[22]

The problem of syphilis has several unique features in patients with AIDS. While the majority of infections with *Treponema pallidum* are typical, there is an increased incidence of neurosyphilis, lues maligna, and nephrotic syndrome. In addition, due to the abnormalities of B-cell activation and regulation in patients with AIDS, serologic testing for syphilis may be challenging. Some patients may exhibit a false-positive rapid plasma reagin due to polyclonal B-cell activation, while others may exhibit a false-negative fluorescent treponemal antigen test due to defects in antigen-specific B-cell activation. Despite these problems, one is usually able to make a diagnosis. Syphilis is a treatable infection and should be high on the differential diagnosis when dealing with patients with HIV infection.

Two additional bacterial pathogens worthy of note in the setting of HIV infection are *Rhodococcus equi* and *Bartonella* spp. *R. equi* is a Gram-positive, pleomorphic acid-fast nonspore-forming bacillus that can cause pulmonary and/or disseminated disease in patients with HIV infection. *Bartonella* spp are fastidious, Gram-negative, *Rickettsia*-like organisms that can cause a variety of clinical syndromes. These infections are usually seen in patients with fewer than 100 CD4 T cells/mm³. The clinical manifestations of *Bartonella* infections include bacillary angiomatosis, peliosis hepatitis, cat-scratch disease, and trench fever. Bacillary angiomatosis and peliosis hepatitis are usually due to *B. henselae*. It is characterized by vascular proliferation that leads to a variety of skin lesions that often resemble the skin lesions of Kaposi's sarcoma. Peliosis hepatis is a condition in which the liver contains multiple, cystic, blood-filled spaces. Cat-scratch disease usually begins with a papule at the site of inoculation followed in several weeks by regional adenopathy and malaise. Trench fever is due to *B. quintana*, an organism typically transmitted by lice. Diagnosis of *Bartonella* infection can be made through modified conventional bacteriologic culture methods, coculture with endothelial cells, serologic

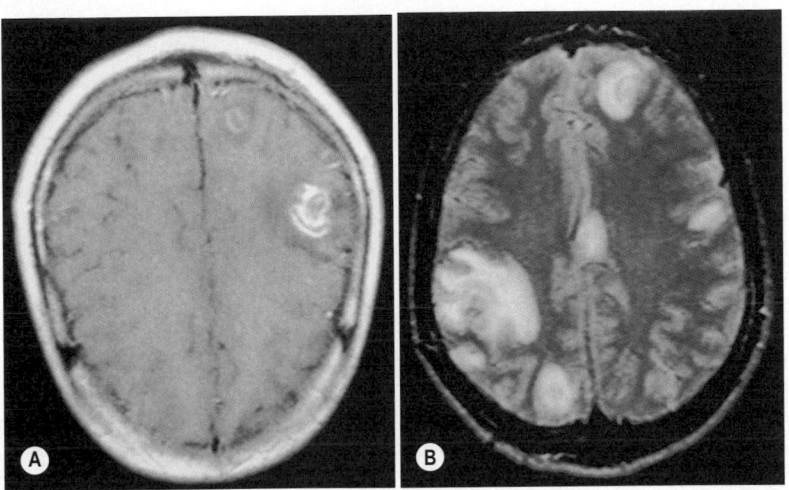

Fig. 31.3 Magnetic resonance imaging scan of a human immunodeficiency virus (HIV)-infected patient with cerebral toxoplasmosis. **(A)** T_1-weighted image showing contrast-enhancing lesions in the parietal and occipital lobes. **(B)** T_2-weighted image showing edema surrounding the two lesions seen on T_1, as well as additional areas of edema in the contralateral frontal and parietal lobes.

or immunocytochemical means, or DNA amplification, or all of these methods. Prolonged treatment with erythromycin or doxycycline is usually effective.

FUNGAL INFECTIONS

Fungal infections account for a significant degree of morbidity and mortality in patients with AIDS. *Pneumocystis jiroveci* (previously *carinii*) pneumonia (PCP) was once the hallmark of AIDS. Its incidence has decreased dramatically with the widespread use of combination antiretroviral therapy and primary prophylaxis with sulfamethoxazole/trimethoprim in patients with CD4 T-cell counts under 200 cells/mm³. Overall, 95% of patients with PCP have CD4 T-cell counts under 200 cells/mm³ and 79% of patients have CD4 T-cell counts under 100 cells/mm³. The risk of PCP is highest in patients with a prior bout of PCP. In contrast to other immunocompromised hosts, patients with AIDS-associated PCP generally present with a protracted indolent illness characterized by fever, shortness of breath, scant cough, and minimal changes on chest X-ray. Extrapulmonary disease with *P. jiroveci* may present as choroiditis, vasculitis, lymphadenopathy, and/or visceral disease

Mucocutaneous infections with *Candida* spp. can be seen prior to a diagnosis of AIDS and in that setting are associated with an increased risk of progressing to AIDS. In contrast to other immunocompromised conditions, patients with AIDS rarely develop invasive disease with *Candida*. Exceptions to this are the patient with an indwelling catheter receiving broad-spectrum antibiotics and the patient with drug-induced neutropenia. While the majority of cases of *Candida* infection involve the mucosal surfaces of the oropharynx and/or the vagina, in patients with advanced HIV infection one may also see involvement of the tracheo-bronchial tree and/or the esophagus. These latter two conditions are sufficiently indicative of advanced immunodeficiency to be included in the list of AIDS-defining illnesses.

Cryptococcus neoformans is the leading cause of meningitis in patients with HIV infection.[25] This is usually a late manifestation of HIV infection

and generally occurs in patients with fewer than 100 CD4 T cells/mm³. Cryptococcal meningitis can be indolent in onset with patients complaining of fever, headache, and nausea for weeks to months prior to diagnosis. In addition to meningitis, patients with AIDS and cryptococcal disease may present with CNS mass lesions due to cryptococcomas, pulmonary disease with focal or diffuse interstitial infiltrates on chest X-ray, or unexplained fever with positive blood cultures. Overall 50% of patients with cryptococcal disease have fungemia and over 90% have detectable levels of cryptococcal antigen in their serum.

Histoplasmosis and coccidioidomycosis are also seen with an increased frequency in patients with AIDS. Histoplasmosis is almost exclusively seen in patients from the Mississippi or Ohio river valleys, Puerto Rico, Dominican Republic, or South America. It commonly presents as disseminated disease with fever, weight loss, and hepatosplenomegaly.[26] An interstitial pattern is present on chest X-ray in about half of the patients. The bone marrow is involved in one-third of cases and one may see mucocutaneous lesions. Disseminated histoplasmosis is generally a late manifestation of HIV infection, occurring in patients with under 100 CD4 T cells/mm³. In contrast, coccidioidomycosis may occur in patients with relatively intact immune systems, although the majority of cases have been in patients with CD4 T-cell counts under 250 cells/mm³. It is also seen in a geographically limited distribution, with the highest incidence in patients who have been in the southwest USA. The most common manifestations of coccidioidomycosis are fever, weight loss, and cough with diffuse reticulonodular infiltrates on chest X-ray. As in other settings with HIV-infected individuals, serologic testing may be unreliable. Up to 25% of patients with coccidioidomycosis and HIV infection may not have a positive serology.

Penicillium marneffei is a common opportunistic infection in Southeast Asia. It is the third most common opportunistic infection in Thailand, behind tuberculosis and cryptococcosis.[27] It is most common during the rainy season. Clinical features include fever, generalized lymphadenopathy, hepatosplenomegaly, anemia, thrombocytopenia, and papular skin lesions with central umbilication. Invasive aspergillosis is not an AIDS-defining illness and is rarely seen in patients with HIV infection outside the setting of neutropenia or corticosteroid treatment. An unusual feature of respiratory tract involvement with aspergillosis in patients with AIDS is that of a pseudomembranous tracheobronchitis.

VIRAL INFECTIONS

Reactivation syndromes of human herpes viruses are among the most common problems in patients with HIV infection and AIDS. Nearly all patients with untreated AIDS actively shed CMV. Once the CD4 count drops below 100 cells/mm3, patients begin to develop clinical problems as a result of CMV reactivation.[28] The most common serious problem is CMV retinitis, which can lead to permanent blindness. In addition, CMV can cause esophagitis, colitis, pneumonia, ascending myelitis, and peripheral polyneuropathy. Herpes simplex reactivation can result in painful orolabial, genital, digital, and/or perianal ulceration that increases in severity as immunologic function declines. It can also cause an erosive esophagitis. Reactivation of varicella-zoster virus commonly results in dermatomal zoster (shingles); however, patients with advanced HIV infection may develop a form of cutaneous dissemination resembling a mild case of chickenpox. This can be a recurrent problem and patients with HIV infection who experience about of shingles may have one or more relapses.[29] Despite extensive cutaneous involvement, visceral dissemination of varicella-zoster virus is almost never seen. Epstein–Barr virus (EBV), the etiologic agent of one form of infectious mononucleosis, is also shed by the majority of patients with untreated HIV infection. It is associated with the development of oral hairy leukoplakia, a white frond-like lesion seen on the lateral aspect of the tongue. This condition is generally benign and rarely needs treatment. In addition up to 50% of the lymphomas seen in AIDS patients have been found to be contain EBV genome.[30] Human herpesvirus 8 (HHV-8) is one of the newest members of this family. It has been associated with the development of Kaposi's sarcoma, multicentric Castleman's disease, and primary effusion lymphomas in the setting of HIV infection.[31] The prevalence of HHV-8 in HIV-infected men is 30–35%, while its prevalence in HIV-infected women is approximately 4%.[32]

Approximately one-third of the deaths of patients with HIV infection are related in some way to liver disease. This is predominantly a reflection of the problems encountered in the setting of co-infection with HIV and hepatitis virus(es) coupled with drug-induced hepatic injury in association with antiretroviral therapy. Over 95% of HIV-infected individuals have evidence of infection with hepatitis B and, in the USA, > 20% of patients are chronically infected with hepatitis C. Co-infection with hepatitis D, E, and/or G viruses is also common. Patients with AIDS do not appear to have an increased risk of inflammatory liver disease in association with hepatitis B infection. This is presumably due to their underlying immunodeficiency. In contrast, hepatitis C infection is more severe in patients with HIV infection, with approximately 10-fold higher levels of hepatitis C virus in the blood and a higher incidence of liver failure.

Among the other viruses that cause problems in patients with HIV infection and AIDS are molluscum contagiosum virus, human papillomavirus (HPV), and JC virus. Diffuse, flesh-colored, umbilicated skin lesions due to molluscum contagiosum may be seen in patients with advanced HIV infection. They frequently regress with effective antiretroviral therapy. Human papillomavirus is approximately twice as common in patients with HIV infection (81%) as in the general population.[33]

This virus has been associated with epidermal dysplasia. Compared to the general population, women with HIV infection have a 10-fold increase in the incidence of abnormal Papanicolaou smears and an increased incidence of intraepithelial neoplasia. Given the potential of these lesions to progress to invasive cancer, women with HIV infection should undergo periodic Papanicolaou smear examinations. Another manifestation of HPV infection, condyloma acuminata, may present with more severe and widely distributed lesions in patients with advanced HIV infection.

JC virus is a human papova virus. It is the etiologic agent of progressive multifocal leukoencephalopathy (PML). This demyelinating disease of the nervous system is seen in 4% of HIV-infected individuals and is a late manifestation of HIV infection and AIDS. Patients typically present with multiple neurologic deficits with or without a change in mental status. Although marked recoveries have been reported following the initiation of antiretroviral therapy,[34] PML remains one of the few opportunistic infections continuing to occur with some frequency in patients with HIV infection.

■ INFECTIONS IN PATIENTS RECEIVING IMMUNOSUPPRESSIVE DRUGS ■

At pharmacologic doses, glucocorticosteroids have both anti-inflammatory and immunosuppressive properties, which result from the effects these agents have on the distribution and function of lymphocytes, monocytes, and neutrophils.[35] The major anti-inflammatory actions of glucocorticosteroids are in large part due to their suppressive effects on neutrophil function. Glucocorticosteroids inhibit neutrophil migration to inflammatory sites, reduce neutrophil adherence to vascular endothelium, reduce the bactericidal activity of neutrophils, and stabilize lysosomal membranes (Chapter 87). The latter two effects are only observed at high glucocorticosteroid concentrations and may not be of clinical importance. Glucocorticosteroid therapy produces a neutrophilic leukocytosis by accelerating release of mature neutrophils from the bone marrow, and by reducing the egress of neutrophils from the circulation into inflammatory sites.[36] The total white blood cell count may exceed 20 000/mm3, but band forms and metamyelocytes almost never increase beyond 6% of the total white blood cell count. An excess of these immature neutrophil forms is suggestive of a superimposed infectious process.

The mononuclear phagocytic system is also affected by glucocorticosteroid therapy. In contrast to the effect on neutrophils, glucocorticosteroid administration produces a peripheral blood monocytopenia. Glucocorticosteroids impair a number of monocyte functions important to host defense, including chemotaxis, bactericidal activity, clearance of antibody-coated red blood cells, and production of proinflammatory cytokines.

Glucocorticosteroids cause profound changes in lymphocyte function and induce a redistribution of lymphocytes out of the circulation. This redistribution predominantly involves T lymphocytes, with CD4 cells affected more than CD8 T cells. Glucocorticosteroids also inhibit T-lymphocyte activation, leading to decreased proliferation and lymphokine production.[37] At high doses, glucocorticosteroids are able to inhibit immunoglobulin production by B cells.[38]

In view of the broad immunosuppressive and anti-inflammatory effects of glucocorticosteroids, it is not surprising that treatment with these agents is associated with an increased frequency of infections. The infections that occur in glucocorticosteroid-treated patients are those associated with impaired phagocyte function (i.e., infections caused by staphylococci, enteric Gram-negative bacteria, *Aspergillus* spp., *Nocardia* spp.) and, to a lesser extent, those associated with suppressed cell-mediated immunity (viral, fungal, *P. jiroveci*, *Listeria* spp., and mycobacterial infections). Although there is no doubt that glucocorticoid therapy results in an increased susceptibility to infection, the exact magnitude of this problem is difficult to quantify. Experience in patients with rheumatoid arthritis, systemic lupus erythematosus, and other autoimmune diseases suggests that the incidence of infectious complications increases with doses equivalent to 20–40 mg/day of prednisone administered for longer than 4–6 weeks.[39] It is important to note that serious infections rarely occur in patients treated with alternate-day glucocorticosteroid therapy and this form of therapy should be employed whenever possible.[37]

Cytotoxic drugs such as cyclophosphamide and methotrexate disrupt host defense through their inhibitory effects on cell proliferation (Chapter 90). Cyclophosphamide is a potent immunosuppressant that interferes with B- and T-cell responses. In the treatment of rheumatic diseases, cyclophosphamide is usually given in combination with glucocorticosteroids. This combination is associated with the same types of bacterial and opportunistic infections that occur with high-dose glucocorticosteroid therapy.[40] Pneumonia due to *P. jiroveci* is the most common opportunistic infection seen in patients receiving cyclophosphamide plus daily glucocorticosteroid therapy. When cyclophosphamide is given alone or with alternate-day glucocorticosteroid therapy, the incidence of infectious complications is markedly reduced.

Low-dose methotrexate (10–20 mg once a week) is increasingly being used as a treatment for rheumatoid arthritis. Initial studies suggested that this methotrexate regimen was not associated with the occurrence of opportunistic infections. However, with widespread use of this regimen, opportunistic infections due to *P. jiroveci* and *Cryptococcus neoformans* have been reported in patients receiving low-dose weekly methotrexate therapy in the absence of concomitant glucocorticosteroid therapy or neutropenia.[41]

Cyclosporine A and azathioprine are potent immunosuppressive agents that are predominantly used to suppress rejection of transplanted organs. Treatment with these agents is associated with a variety of opportunistic infections that are described below.

In recent years, specific inhibitors of the proinflammatory cytokine, tumor necrosis factor (TNF), have become a part of treatment regimens for certain autoimmune diseases such as rheumatoid arthritis and inflammatory bowel disease. In pre-marketing trials, the use of these agents was not associated with a discernible increase in infections. However, post-marketing reporting has provided increasing evidence that treatment with TNF inhibitors (especially infliximab) may be associated with an increased incidence of tuberculosis and other infections.[42]

INFECTIONS IN SOLID-ORGAN TRANSPLANT RECIPIENTS

During the past two decades the transplantation of solid organs has gone from being an experimental procedure to an accepted therapeutic modality. Advances in surgical techniques and improved immunosuppressive

regimens have led to 1-year survival rates in excess of 70% for recipients of kidney, liver, and heart transplants (Chapter 80). Despite these advances, infection continues to be a major cause of morbidity and mortality in patients undergoing solid-organ transplantation. The types of infections along with their clinical manifestations and severity are determined by the interaction of several factors, including the specific organ transplanted, exposure to potential pathogens, and the level of immunosuppression.

TIME COURSE OF INFECTIONS AFTER TRANSPLANTATION

The majority of infectious complications occur in the first 6 months following transplantation. In the early post-transplant period (first 4 weeks), most clinically overt infections are due to nosocomial bacterial or fungal pathogens and are directly related to the surgical procedure, invasive monitoring with intravascular devices, postoperative pulmonary complications, or pre-existing infection in the organ donor or recipient.[43]

From 1 to 6 months post-transplant, infections related to the use of immunosuppressive agents predominate. A number of opportunistic infections can occur during this period (Table 31.4). Because the diversity of possible pathogens is so great, identifying the specific causative agent is essential to select appropriate and effective therapy. CMV is the dominant pathogen causing disease during this period. The majority of patients undergoing solid-organ transplantation will show evidence of CMV infection, as determined by serological rise in titer or virus isolation from the blood, urine, or throat.[43] However, not all patients with infection will develop clinical disease. There are two major determinants of whether CMV infection will progress to clinical disease. The first is the prior experience of the donor and recipient with CMV, which determines whether the infection is primary or due to reactivation of latent virus. The transplantation of an organ from a CMV-seropositive donor into a seronegative recipient will result in primary CMV infection. Primary infection is more likely to be associated with clinical disease than is CMV reactivation.[43] The second determinant of whether CMV infection will result in clinical disease is the type and intensity of immunosuppression.

Table 31.4 Time course for opportunistic infections after solid-organ transplantation

Months after transplantation	Major risk factors	Major pathogens
1	Surgical procedure, intravascular catheters; pre-existing infection in donor or recipient	Conventional nosocomial bacterial and fungal pathogens
2–6	Immunosuppressive therapy	Cytomegalovirus, *Cryptococcus neoformans*, *Listeria monocytogenes*, *Pneumocystis jiroveci*, *Toxoplasma gondii*, *Aspergillus* spp., *Candida*, *M. tuberculosis*, *Nocardia* spp., hepatitis B or C virus, Epstein–Barr virus
>6	Immunosuppressive therapy Chronic viral infection	*Cryptococcus neoformans*, *Listeria monocytogenes*, *Nocardia* spp., *Aspergillus* and non-*Aspergillus* molds Late complications of chronic hepatitis, Epstein–Barr virus Cytomegalovirus retinitis

Treatment with glucocorticosteroids alone is associated with a very low incidence of CMV disease. In fact, CMV disease was essentially unknown in transplant patients prior the introduction of agents such as cyclophosphamide, azathioprine, and cyclosporine A into anti-rejection regimens.[43] Of all the immunosuppressive agents used, polyclonal or monoclonal anti-T-cell antibodies are the most potent inducers of CMV disease.[44]

The most common type of CMV disease in the transplant recipient is a mononucleosis-like syndrome characterized by prolonged fever, leukopenia, arthralgias, and abnormal liver function tests. Splenomegaly and lymphadenopathy are usually not present. A more serious manifestation of CMV infection is interstitial pneumonitis, which can be severe and life-threatening. The clinical manifestations of CMV pneumonitis are nonspecific, and diagnosis by bronchoalveolar lavage or lung biopsy is required. Infection of the gastrointestinal tract with CMV can lead to an ulcerative disease with associated bleeding and perforation. Although chemical hepatitis is frequently seen in patients with the mononucleosis syndrome, severe CMV hepatitis is unusual. The exception is in recipients of liver transplants where CMV hepatitis may be severe and occasionally lead to hepatic failure.[45] It is important to note that CMV disease may be complicated by co-infection with other opportunistic pathogens, most notably *P. jiroveci*. The potentially severe sequelae from CMV disease in recipients of solid organ transplants have led to the widespread use of antiviral prophylaxis or pre-emptive therapy to prevent CMV disease.

Infectious complications that occur more than 6 months post-transplant are usually due to one of two possibly interrelated factors: (1) the effects of chronic viral infection acquired earlier and (2) chronic allograft dysfunction which necessitates repeated courses of high-dose immunosuppressive therapy. Examples of chronic viral infections that can become clinically manifest during this period include CMV chorioretinitis, chronic hepatitis with or without cirrhosis due to hepatitis B or C viruses, and EBV-associated lymphoproliferative disease. Patients who experience chronic allograft rejections and require high doses of immunosuppressive agents are at risk for infections with opportunistic pathogens

such as *P. jiroveci*, *C. neoformans*, *Listeria monocytogenes*, *Nocardia* species, *Aspergillus* and non-*Aspergillus* molds.

INFECTIONS IN BONE MARROW TRANSPLANT RECIPIENTS

Allogeneic bone marrow transplantation has become an accepted mode of therapy for hematological malignancies, immunodeficiency disorders, and aplastic anemia (Chapters 82 and 83). Marrow graft recipients undergo treatment with chemoradiotherapy which virtually ablates the existing hematological and immunologic marrow elements and provides a state of immunodeficiency that permits engraftment of the donor marrow. This state of profound immunosuppression places the recipient at high risk for a variety of infectious diseases. Significant abnormalities of T- and B-lymphocyte function that persist following recovery of neutrophil counts place the patient at continued risk for infection with viral and fungal pathogens.

CLINICAL PEARLS

INFECTIONS IN BONE MARROW TRANSPLANT RECIPIENTS

>> Infections 2–4 weeks post-transplantation are usually due to profound neutropenia and damage to mucosal surfaces

>> Between the period of engraftment and weeks 15–20 post-transplant, opportunistic infections predominate and are commonly associated with the development of acute graft-versus-host disease and its treatment

>> Serious infections occurring 4–6 months following transplantation are seen predominantly in patients with chronic graft-versus-host disease

TIME COURSE OF INFECTIONS AFTER TRANSPLANTATION

From an infectious diseases viewpoint, the post-transplant period can be divided into three phases that correlate with the initial ablation and ensuing recovery of hematopoietic and immunologic function. During the first weeks post-transplantation the predominant risk factors for infection are profound neutropenia and damage to mucosal surfaces that results from pre-transplant ablative radiation and chemotherapy. These host defense defects predispose the patient to the same types of bacterial and fungal infections seen in cancer patients undergoing induction chemotherapy. As would be expected, the prevalence of invasive fungal infections increases with the duration of neutropenia. Viral infections, other than herpes simplex virus, are uncommon during this period. Herpes simplex viral infections occur at a time of maximal mucosal damage by radiation and chemotherapy and may cause severe stomatitis and esophagitis. Aciclovir is effective for treatment and prophylaxis of this infection.

Between the period of engraftment and weeks 15–20 post-transplant, infections with opportunistic viral, fungal, and protozoal pathogens (i.e., CMV and *P. jiroveci*) predominate. The major predisposing factors for these infections are the immunosuppressive effect of acute graft-versus-host disease (GvHD) and its treatment. CMV is a major pathogen during this period. CMV infection occurs in 30–40% of seronegative transplant patients who receive unscreened blood products post-transplant and CMV reactivation occurs in the majority of patients who were CMV-seropositive prior to transplantation.[46] The risk of CMV infection and disease is increased in patients with acute GvHD. Manifestations of CMV infection are similar to those seen in solid-organ transplant patients, but tend to be more severe. Pneumonia is the most serious manifestation of CMV infection and, prior to the use of pre-emptive therapy, occurred in approximately one-third of marrow transplant patients. Risk factors for the development of CMV pneumonia include older age and acute GvHD.[46] In the marrow transplant recipient, the technique of centrifugation culture of bronchoalveolar lavage fluid for CMV has been shown to be both sensitive and specific for diagnosing CMV pneumonia, making open-lung biopsy unnecessary in most cases.[47] In the past, the fatality rate for CMV pneumonia was in excess of 80%. Even with the use of ganciclovir and intravenous immunoglobulin, mortality rates from CMV pneumonia are 20–50%. Thus, current strategies focus on preventing CMV disease by using pre-emptive treatment with ganciclovir or foscarnet.[48] Nonbacterial, nonfungal interstitial pneumonia that is not due to CMV infection can also occur in marrow transplant recipients. Most cases occur between days 30 and 100 post-transplant. Reported infectious causes of this syndrome include *P. jiroveci*, adenovirus, parainfluenza virus, and respiratory syncytial virus. Approximately one-third of interstitial pneumonia cases are idiopathic and may be due to toxic effects of radiation and chemotherapy.

Invasive *Aspergillus* infections are also seen during this post-transplant period. The main risk factors for the occurrence of invasive aspergillosis after day 40 of transplant are severe GvHD and glucocorticosteroid use.[49]

Serious infections occurring 4–6 months after transplantation occur predominantly in patients with chronic GvHD.[50] Following immune reconstitution, marrow transplant recipients exhibit deficient humoral immune responses to both protein and polysaccharide antigens and these abnormalities are more pronounced in patients with chronic GvHD.[51]

Clinically, the most common infections are bacterial and involve the respiratory tract and skin, or present as sepsis without apparent source. The most common organisms isolated are Gram-positive bacteria, particularly *Streptococcus pneumoniae*.[50] Thus, patients with chronic GvHD exhibit a humoral immune defect similar to that seen in patients with Hodgkin's disease who have received combined radiation and chemotherapy (see above). In patients receiving immunosuppressive therapy for chronic GvHD, invasive infections with *Aspergillus* and non-*Aspergillus* molds can also occur during this period.[49]

Herpes virus infections are also seen during the late post-transplant period. Approximately 40% of marrow transplant recipients will develop varicella-zoster virus infections, usually in the form of herpes zoster.[52] The median time to onset is 5 months after transplantation, with most cases occurring in the first year. Infections with EBV can also occur during this period and EBV-associated lymphoproliferative disease has been observed after marrow transplantation.[30]

IMPROVING HOST DEFENSE

In the patient who exhibits a defect in host defense, prevention of infection is a desirable goal, albeit difficult to attain. One of the most effective means of partially achieving this goal is through the use of prophylactic antibiotics in those settings where patients are at increased risk for a specific type of infection. An example of this is the use of trimethoprim/sulfamethoxazole for prophylaxis against PCP in patients with HIV infection and CD4 counts less than 200 cells/mm^3. Immunization against bacterial and viral pathogens has also played a major role in the prevention of certain infectious diseases. Unfortunately, active immunization is often unsuccessful in immunocompromised hosts, as they are unable to generate a protective cellular or humoral response to vaccination. On the other hand, passive immunization through the administration of pooled immune globulin may be effective in preventing certain infections in the immunocompromised host. Examples include the use of varicella-zoster immune globulin in immunocompromised children exposed to varicella and the administration of CMV hyperimmune globulin to CMV-seronegative renal allograft recipients.[53] In both of these situations the use of hyperimmune globulin is associated with a decrease in the severity of disease.

In the near future our increasing understanding of cytokines and their immunologic effects will likely lead to improved forms of immunotherapy for a variety of immunodeficiency diseases. Over the next decade, these powerful biological agents will play an important role in restoring immunologic function in the compromised host and decreasing the incidence of infectious diseases.

■ REFERENCES ■

1. Bodey G, Buckley M, Sathe Y, et al. Quantitative relationships between circulating leukocytes and infection in patients with acute leukemia. Ann Intern Med 1966; 64: 328–340.

2. Bodey GP, Rodriguez V, Chang HY, et al. Fever and infection in leukemic patients: a study of 494 consecutive patients. Cancer 1978; 41: 1610–1622.

3. Pizzo P. Management of fever in patients with cancer and treatment-induced neutropenia. N Engl J Med 1993; 328: 1323–1331.

4. Gerson SL, Talbot GH, Hurwitz S, et al. Prolonged granulocytopenia: the major risk factor for invasive pulmonary aspergillosis in patients with acute leukemia. Ann Intern Med 1984; 100: 345–351.

5. Hughes WT, Armstrong D, Bodey GP, et al. 2002 guidelines for the use of antimicrobial agents in neutropenic patients with cancer. Clin Infect Dis 2002; 34: 730–751.

6. Group EIATC. Empiric antifungal therapy in febrile granulocytopenic patients. Am J Med 1989; 86: 668–672.

7. Klastersky J. Antifungal therapy in patients with fever and neutropenia – more rational and less empirical?. N Engl J Med 2004; 351: 1445–1447.

8. Brandt SJ, Peters WP, Atwater SK, et al. Effect of recombinant human granulocyte–macrophage colony-stimulating factor on hematopoietic reconstitution after high-dose chemotherapy and autologous bone marrow transplantation. N Engl J Med 1988; 318: 869–876.

9. Cunningham-Rundles C. Clinical and immunological analyses of 103 patients with common variable immunodeficiency. J Clin Immunol 1989; 9: 22–33.

10. Winkelstein JA, Marino MC, Ochs H, et al. The X-linked hyper-IgM syndrome: clinical immunologic features of 79 patients. Medicine (Baltimore) 2003; 82: 373–384.

11. McKinney R, Katz S, Wilfert C. Chronic enteroviral meningoencephalitis in agammaglobulinemic patients. Rev Infect Dis 1987; 9: 334–356.

12. Bonilla FA, Geha RS. Primary immunodeficiency diseases. J Allergy Clin Immunol 2003; 111: S571–S581.

13. Notter D, Grossman P, Rosenberg S, et al. Infections in patients with Hodgkin's disease: a clinical study of 300 consecutive patients. Rev Infect Dis 1980; 2: 761–800.

14. Siber GR, Gorham C, Martin P, et al. Antibody response to pretreatment immunization and post-treatment boosting with bacterial polysaccharide vaccines in patients with Hodgkin's disease. Ann Intern Med 1986; 104: 467–475.

15. Ross SC, Densen P. Complement deficiency states and infection: epidemiology, pathogenesis and consequences of neisserial and other infections in an immune deficiency. Medicine (Baltimore) 1984; 63: 243–273.

16. Lynch A, Kapila R. Overwhelming postsplenectomy infection. Infect Dis Clin North Am 1996; 10: 696–707.

17. Benach J, Habicht G. Clinical characteristics of human babesiosis. J Infect Dis 1981; 144: 481.

18. Ochs HD, Thrasher AJ. The Wiskott–Aldrich syndrome. J Allergy Clin Immunol 2006; 117: 725–738.

19. Sleasman JW, Goodenow MM. HIV-1 infection. J Allergy Clin Immuno 2003; 111: S582–S592.

20. Mannheimer SB, Soave R. Protozoal infections in patients with AIDS. Cryptosporidiosis, isosporiasis, cyclosporiasis, and microsporidiosis. Infect Dis Clin North Am 1994; 8: 483–498.

21. Lane HC, Masur H, Rook A, et al. Abnormalities of B cell activation and immunoregulation in patients with the acquired immunodeficiency syndrome. N Engl J Med 1983; 309: 453–458.

22. Centers for Disease Control and Prevention. 2002 Guidelines for preventing opportunistic infections among HIV-infected persons. MMWR. 51 (RRu8); 1–46.

23. Barnes P, Bloch A, Davidson P, et al. Tuberculosis in patients with human immunodeficiency virus infection. N Engl J Med 1991; 324: 1644–1650.

24. Horsburgh C. *Mycobacterium avium* complex infection in the acquired immunodeficiency syndrome. N Engl J Med 1991; 324: 1332–1338.

25. Kovacs JA, Kovacs AA, Polis M, et al. Crytococcosis in the acquired immunodeficiency syndrome. Ann Intern Med 1985; 199: 533–538.

26. Wheat LJ, Slama TG, Zeckel ML. Histoplasmosis in the acquired immune deficiency syndrome. Am J Med 1985; 78. 203–107.

27. Duong TA. Infection due to *Penicillium marneffei*, an emerging pathogen: review of 155 reported cases. Clin Infect Dis 1996; 23: 125–130.

28. Zurlo JJ, O'Neill D, Polis MA, et al. Lack of clinical utility of cytomegalovirus blood and urine cultures in patients with HIV infection. Ann Intern Med 1993; 118: 12–17.

29. Friedman KA, Lafleur FL, Gendler E, et al. Herpes zoster: a possible early clinical sign for development of acquired immunodeficiency syndrome in high-risk individuals. J Am Acad Dermatol 1986; 14: 1023–1028.

30. Cohen JI. Epstein–Barr virus lymphoproliferative disease associated with acquired immunodeficiency. Medicine (Baltimore) 1991; 70: 137–160.

31. Aoki Y, Tosato G. Pathogenesis and manifestations of human herpesvirus-8-associated disorders. Semin Hematol 2003; 40: 143–153.

32. Kedes DH, Operskalski E, Busch M, et al. The seroepidemiology of human herpesvirus 8 (Kaposi's sarcoma-associated herpesvirus): distribution of infection in KS risk groups and evidence for sexual transmission. Nat Med 1996; 2: 918 –924.

33. Frazer IH, Medley G, Crapper RM, et al. Association between anorectal dysplasia, human papillomavirus, and human immunodeficiency virus infection in homosexual men. Lancet 1986; 2: 657–660.

34. Clifford DB, Yiannoutsos C, Glicksman M, et al. HAART improves prognosis in HIV-associated progressive multifocal leukoencephalopathy. Neurology 1999; 52: 623–625.

35. Rhen T, Cidlowski JA. Antiinflammatory action of glucocorticoids – new mechanisms for old drugs. N Engl J Med 2005; 353: 1711–1723.

36. Dale DC, Fauci AS, Guerry DI, et al. Comparison of agents producing a neutrophilic leukocytosis in man. Hydrocortisone, prednisone, endotoxin, and etiocholanolone. J Clin Invest 1975; 56: 808–813.

37. Fauci A, Dale D, Balow J. Clucocorticosteroid therapy: mechanisms of action and clinical considerations. Ann Intern Med 1976; 84: 304–315.

38. Butler WT, Rossen RD. Effects of corticosteroids on immunity in man. I. Decreased serum IgG concentration caused by 3 to 5 days of high doses of methylprednisolone. J Clin Invest 1973; 52: 2629–2640.

39. Stuck AE, Minder CE, Frey FJ. Risk of infectious complications in patients taking glucocorticosteroids. Rev Infect Dis 1989; 11: 954–963.

40. Segal BH, Sneller MC. Infectious complications of immunosuppressive therapy in patients with rheumatic diseases. Rheum Dis Clin North Am 1997; 23: 219–237.

41. LeMense GP, Sahn SA. Opportunistic infection during treatment with low dose methotrexate. Am J Respir Crit Care Med 1994; 150: 258–260.

42. Ellerin T, Rubin RH, Weinblatt ME. Infections and anti-tumor necrosis factor alpha therapy. Arthritis Rheum 2003; 48: 3013–3022.

43. Rubin R. Infection in the organ transplant recipient. In: Rubin R, Young L eds Clinical Approach to Infection in the Compromised Host, 3rd edn. New York: Plenumi 1994 : 629–705.

44. Singh N, Dummer JS, Kusne S, et al. Infections with cytomegalovirus and other herpesviruses in 121 liver transplant recipients: transmission by donated organ and the effect of OKT3 antibodies. J Infect Dis 1988; 158: 124–131.

45. Singh N. Infectious diseases in the liver transplant recipient. Semin Gastrointest Dis 1998; 9: 136–146.

46. Meyers JD, Flournoy N, Thomas ED. Risk factors for cytomegalovirus infection after human marrow transplantation. J Infect Dis 1986; 153: 478–883.

47. Crawford SW, Bowden RA, Hackman RC, et al. Rapid detection of cytomegalovirus pulmonary infection by bronchoalveolar lavage and centrifugation culture. Ann Intern Med 1988; 108. 180–185.

48. Meijer E, Boland GJ, Verdonck LF. Prevention of cytomegalovirus disease in recipients of allogeneic stem cell transplants. Clin Microbiol Rev 2003; 16: 647–657.

49. Wald A, Leisenring W, van Burik JA, et al. Epidemiology of *Aspergillus* infections in a large cohort of patients undergoing bone marrow transplantation [see comments]. J Infect Dis 1997; 175: 1459–1466.

50. Atkinson K, Farewell V, Storb R, et al. Analysis of late infections after human bone marrow transplantation: role of genotypic nonidentity between marrow donor and recipient and of nonspecific suppressor cells in patients with chronic graft-versus-host disease. Blood 1982; 60: 714–720.

51. Ambrosino DM. Impaired polysaccharide responses in immunodeficient patients: relevance to bone marrow transplant patients. Bone Marrow Transplant 1991; 3: 48–51.

52. Atkinson K, Meyers JD, Storb R, et al. Varicella-zoster virus infection after marrow transplantation for aplastic anemia or leukemia. Transplantation 1980; 29: 47–50.

53. Snydman DR, Werner BG, Heinze LB, et al. Use of cytomegalovirus immune globulin to prevent cytomegalovirus disease in renal-transplant recipients. N Engl J Med 1987; 317: 1049–1054.

Development of the fetal and neonatal immune system

David B. Lewis

32

The fetus and neonate are more vulnerable than older children and adults to severe infection with a variety of pathogens, including pyogenic bacteria, fungi, viruses, and intracellular protozoa.[1] This indicates that there are substantial limitations in innate and adaptive immunity in prenatal and early postnatal life. The results of hematopoietic stem-cell transplantation also provide compelling evidence for impairment of neonatal T-cell immunity. For example, allogeneic hematopoietic cell transplantation with cord blood results in a significantly lower risk of acute graft-versus-host disease – a disease that is mainly mediated by donor-derived naïve T cells – compared to bone marrow and peripheral blood transplants containing adult T cells.[2] These clinical observations have made defining the physiologic immaturity of the human fetal and neonatal immune system of great interest.

DENDRITIC CELLS AND ANTIGEN PRESENTATION

Activated conventional dendritic cells (cDCs) participate in antigen presentation to T cells and B cells and produce critical cytokines, e.g., interleukin (IL)-12p70 and IL-15, that provide early innate immune protection and also influence the outcome of the later adaptive immune response (Fig. 32.1). Plasmacytoid dendritic cells (pDCs) are a distinct DC population that is mainly found in lymphoid tissue and the circulation and that interacts with and enhances the activation of cDCs. Activated pDCs are an important source of interferon (IFN)-α and IFN-β, which provide early innate antiviral immunity, and also enhance the later adaptive immune response, including differentiation of Th1 lymphocytes. DCs are activated by a variety of stimuli, including the recognition of conserved structures of microbial pathogens by Toll-like receptors (TLRs) (Chapter 3).

DCS IN TISSUES

The colonization of cDCs in extra-lymphoid tissues appears to be developmentally regulated, and independent of exposure to inflammatory mediators. Immature cDC lineage cells have been identified in the interstitium of solid

CLINICAL RELEVANCE

EXAMPLES OF INFECTIONS MORE FREQUENT OR SEVERE IN THE FETUS AND NEONATE THAN IN OLDER CHILDREN AND ADULTS

>> Bacteremia and meningitis due to pyogenic bacteria, e.g., group B streptococcus – higher rate in neonatal period than any other age group

>> Primary herpes simplex virus infection – approximately 25–30% mortality in the neonate even with current antiviral therapy, e.g., aciclovir

>> Enteroviral infection – severe infection, e.g., hepatic necrosis with disseminated intravascular coagulation, which is unusual outside the neonatal period except in cases of severe T-cell immunodeficiency such as severe combined immunodeficiency (SCID)

>> Toxoplasmosis – congenital infection typically disseminates to the retina; disseminated infection is unusual in postnatally acquired infection

>> *Mycobacterium tuberculosis* acquired congenitally or perinatally has a high risk of progressing to miliary disease and meningitis

>> Mucocutaneous candidiasis in the otherwise healthy neonate is more frequent compared to older children and adults

organs, including the kidney, heart, pancreas, and lung, but not the brain, by 12 weeks of gestation, and the numbers of these cells increase progressively by 21 weeks.[3] Epidermal Langerhans cells, a cDC population unique to the dermis, are found in the skin even earlier, at 7 weeks' gestation.

CIRCULATING AND MONOCYTE-DERIVED DCs

Most studies of the developmental immunology of human DCs have analyzed circulating DCs, the main caveat being whether these results also apply to the phenotype and function of tissue DCs. Circulating

493

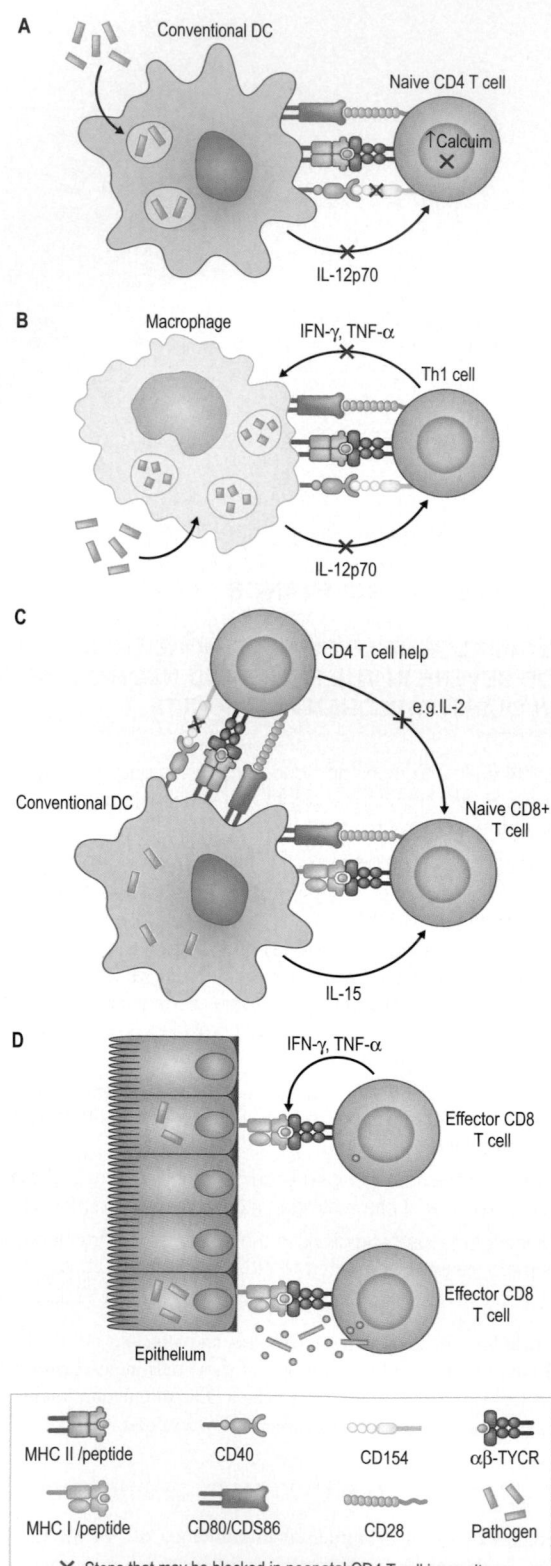

Fig. 32.1 T-cell activation and differentiation in response to antigen. Steps that may be blocked in neonatal CD4 T cells are indicated as red Xs. **(A)** Th1 generation from naïve CD4 T cells requires that conventional dendritic cells (cDCs) present antigenic peptides bound to major histocompatibility complex (MHC) class II and co-stimulatory molecules, such as CD80 and CD86. T-cell activation results in calcium-dependent increases in CD154 on the CD4 T-cell surface. The CD154–CD40 interaction enhances cDC production of interleukin (IL)-12p70, which promotes Th1 differentiation. **(B)** Differentiated Th1 cells help kill intracellular pathogens, such as *Mycobacterium tuberculosis*, that hide in the intracellular microvesicular compartments of macrophages. Pathogen-derived peptides bound to MHC class II displayed on the infected cell surface engage the αβ-T-cell receptor (TCR) of the Th1 cell, triggering its secretion of interferon (IFN)-γ and tumor necrosis factor (TNF)-α. These cytokines bind to specific surface receptors on the infected cell and increase its microbicidal activity. **(C)** The generation of CD8 T-cell effectors from naïve CD8 T cells requires αβ-TCR engagement by cognate peptide/ MHC class I complexes on the cDC, CD80/CD86-CD28 co-stimulation, cDC-derived IL-15, and, possibly, cytokines from CD4 T cells. **(D)** CD8 T-cell effectors secrete perforin and granzymes, which kill target cells displaying viral peptide/MHC class I, and IFN-γ and TNF-α, which have antiviral activity and enhance antigen presentation.

cDCs are typically CD11c^high and major histocompatibility complex (MHC) class II^high but lineage-negative (Lin–), i.e., lacking markers for other cell lineages, such as T cells, monocytes, B cells, natural killer (NK) cells, granulocytes, and erythroid cells. Human pDCs are CD11c^low Lin– and express high levels of CD123 (IL-3 receptor α-chain) and BDCA-4, a pDC-specific cell marker of unknown function. The concentrations of cDCs in cord blood and adult peripheral blood are similar.[3] Cord blood cDCs also have a surface phenotype similar to that of adult cDCs. An exception is CD86, which binds to CD28 on T cells, providing a co-stimulatory signal, and which is lower on cord blood cDCs than those of the adult. The concentration of pDCs in cord blood is significantly higher than in adult peripheral blood, and the number of these cells gradually declines after birth.[3] The relative predominance of pDCs in the neonatal circulation may reflect the relatively high rate of pDCs colonizing lymphoid tissue, which undergoes rapid expansion at this age.

Circulating neonatal DCs have selective limitations in the TLR-mediated upregulation of expression of molecules involved in T-cell co-stimulation by engagement of CD28 (CD80 and CD86) and other DC–T-cell interactions (MHC class II and CD40) compared to those of the adult.[3] For example, cord blood cDCs have reduced expression of CD40 in response to ligands for TLR-2/6 (*Mycoplasma fermentans*), TLR-3 (poly I:C), TLR-4 (lipopolysaccharide (LPS)), and TLR-7 (imiquimod), and reduced CD80 in response to TLR-3 and TLR-4 ligands. In contrast, cDC upregulation of CD40 in response to GU-rich single-stranded RNA, a TLR-8 ligand, is similar,[4] as is MHC class II and CD86 upregulation after stimulation with TLR3 and TLR-4 ligands. Cord blood and adult peripheral blood pDCs also have similar upregulation of HLA-DR, CD80, and CD86 after stimulation with TLR-9 ligands, i.e., DNA lacking methylated CpG residues (unmethylated CpG DNA).[3]

Th1 immunity may be particularly limited in the neonate and young infant compared to older individuals because of decreased IL-12p70 production by cDCs, e.g., in response to LPS plus IFN-γ.[5] However, this limitation may be pathogen-dependent, as decreased IL-12 production by cord blood cDCs is probably comparable to adult cDCs after stimulation with certain Gram-positive and Gram-negative bacteria or meningococcal outer-membrane proteins.[1] Circulating DCs from cord blood can also allogeneically stimulate cord blood T cells *in vitro*,[1] but it is unclear if they are as effective as adult DCs in promoting Th1 differentiation in an allogeneic context.

The production of type I IFNs (IFN-α and IFN-β) by circulating cDCs and pDCs is also reduced in cord blood, and could contribute to the limited ability of the neonate to control pathogens such as herpes simplex virus (HSV) (see below). For example, IFN-α production by cord blood cDCs in response to a TLR-3 ligand and by cord blood pDCs in response to TLR-9 ligands – such as live or inactivated HSV, which has a genome containing unmethylated CpG DNA sequences, or to synthetic unmethylated CpG DNA oligonucleotides – is reduced compared to adult DCs.[3] The levels of TLR-9 within the endosomes of adult and cord blood pDCs are similar, suggesting that these decreased responses are due to events downstream of TLR ligand binding.[3, 6]

Several studies have compared the function and phenotype of monocyte-derived dendritic cells (MDDCs) produced by culturing cord blood or adult peripheral blood monocytes *in vitro* with cytokines, such as granulocyte–macrophage colony-stimulating factor (GM-CSF), IL-4, and tumor necrosis factor (TNF)-α. In general, cord blood MDDCs have reduced levels of IL-12p70 expression after stimulation, but it remains unclear if these and other functional and phenotypic differences apply to neonatal and adult DCs of the tissues.

POSTNATAL DC MATURATION

Defining the role of exposure to commensal bacteria in the postnatal maturation of DC function is important, as it provides insight as to how the immune system transitions between interacting with a sterile environment to one in which pathogens versus harmless commensals must be distinguished. Impaired TLR-4 signaling in young (6-week-old) mice results in their cDCs having reduced expression of CD86 and a decreased capacity to produce IL-12 after engagement of the cDC CD40 molecule.[7] This suggests that cDCs from neonates are functionally immature until their postnatal exposure to bacterial products, such as LPS, and that a lack of such maturation could impair Th1 responses. This idea is consistent with gradual increase during the first 4–6 weeks after birth of the capacity of murine cDCs to produce IL-12p70 and to express adult levels of various surface markers.[3]

■ T CELLS ■

ONTOGENY OF THYMIC DEVELOPMENT

Initial colonization of the fetal thymus by prothymocytes occurs at 8.5 weeks of gestation, with dramatic increases in thymic cellularity during the second and third trimesters. Transient thymic involution, particularly the loss of cortical double-positive (CD4^{hi}CD8^{hi}) thymocytes, may occur at the end of the third trimester due to a prenatal surge in the circulating levels of glucocorticoids;[8] this is followed by thymic recovery at 1 month of age.

REPERTOIRE OF αβ-T-CELL RECEPTORS

The usage of T-cell receptor (TCR) D and J gene segments in the thymus is initially less diverse than subsequently. The complementarity determinant region 3 (CDR3) region of the TCR chain transcripts is also reduced in length and sequence diversity between 8 and 15 weeks of gestation. This is most likely due to decreased activity of terminal deoxytransferase (TdT), which performs N-nucleotide addition during V(D)J recombination. The impact, if any, of these limitations in αβ-TCR diversity on the ability of the fetus to respond to congenital infection is likely to be subtle and brief, as intrathymic TdT activity, CDR3 length, and V segment diversity during the second trimester are similar to that of postnatal thymic tissue.[1] The TCR repertoire expressed on cord blood T cells has a diversity of TCR usage and CDR3 length similar to that of antigenically naïve T cells in adults and infants, indicating that the functional pre-immune repertoire is fully formed by birth.[9]

TCR excision circles (TREC) are generated during TCR gene rearrangement of thymocytes, and may persist for long periods in T-lineage cells that do not proliferate. TREC levels in cord blood are relatively high compared to adult peripheral blood, as would be expected given the predominance of naïve (CD45RA^{high}CD45R0^{low}) T cells in cord blood. In addition, the cord blood CD8 T-cell compartment is enriched in recent thymic emigrants (RTEs),[10] which also have a higher TREC content than more mature circulating naïve T cells.

FETAL T-CELL DEVELOPMENT AND PHENOTYPE

By 14 weeks of gestation, CD4 and CD8 T cells are found in the fetal circulation, liver, and spleen, and CD4 T cells are detectable in lymph nodes. The percentage of circulating T cells gradually increases during the second and third trimesters of pregnancy through about 6 months of age, followed by a gradual decline to adult levels. The ratio of CD4 to CD8 T cells in the circulation is relatively high during fetal life (about 3.5) and gradually declines with age.

Circulating T cells in the term and preterm neonate and in the second and third trimester fetus predominantly express a CD45RA^{high}CD45R0^{low} surface phenotype that is characteristic of antigenically naïve T cells found in adults. About 30% of circulating T cells of the full-term neonate are CD45RA^{low}CD45R0^{low}; the cells appear to be immature thymocyte-like cells that are destined to lose expression of the CD45R0 isoform and become naïve T cells. Most neonatal CD45RA^{high} T cells express CD31 (PECAM-1), which is involved in cell adhesion, but about 10–20% are CD31$^-$. These CD31$^-$ CD4 T cells may have undergone homeostatic proliferation, which is triggered in response to unfilled niches in the periphery.[11] Cord blood T cells may be more prone than adult naïve T cells to undergo homeostatic proliferation because of a greater sensitivity to the mitogenic effects of IL-7.[1] CD38, an ectoenzyme involved in intracellular calcium mobilization, is expressed on virtually all peripheral fetal and neonatal T cells as well as fetal and postnatal thymocytes. In contrast, CD38 is absent on adult naïve T cells, suggesting that peripheral T cells in the fetus and neonate may represent a thymocyte-like immature transitional population.

CD4 T-CELL RESPONSES

Herpes virus infections

One of the most striking limitations in neonatal T-cell immunity is the reduced and delayed HSV-specific CD4 T-cell proliferation and cytokine (IL-2, IFN-γ, and TNF-α) production in neonates compared to adults after primary HSV infection.[12, 13] Older infants and young children also have reduced CD4 T-cell immunity (IL-2, IFN-γ, and CD40-ligand (CD154) expression) after primary infection with cytomegalovirus (CMV), another herpes virus, compared to adults.[14] This reduced CD4 T-cell response is associated with persistent CMV shedding in the urine and saliva of young children following primary infection. This reduced CMV-specific CD4 T-cell response also likely applies to the neonate and young infant with congenital, perinatal, or postnatally acquired CMV infection, all of whom persistently shed CMV for years following its acquisition.

Vaccines

CD4 T-cell responses to inactivated vaccines may be reduced in young infants and, likely, neonates. Vaccinated infants between 6 and 12 months of age have lower IL-2 production by CD4 T cells in response to tetanus toxoid than older children and adults,[1] suggesting that antigen-specific memory CD4 T-cell generation or function is decreased during infancy.

The robustness of the CD4 T-cell response of the neonate and young infant to live vaccines may vary with the particular agent. Vaccination with bacille Calmette-Guérin (BCG) at birth versus 2 months or 4 months of age is equally effective in inducing CD4 T-cell proliferative and IFN-γ responses to mycobacterial antigens,[15] and does not result in Th2 skewing, i.e., increased production of IL-4, IL-5, and IL-13 and reduced levels of IFN-γ. However, the Th1 responses of infant vaccinees have not been directly compared with those of older children and adult vaccinees. In contrast, the CD4 T-cell response to oral poliovirus vaccine (OPV) may be reduced in the neonate and young infant: Newborns given OPV at birth, 1, 2, and 3 months of age, have lower OPV-specific CD4 T-cell proliferation and IFN-γ production compared to adults immunized in childhood.[16] In contrast, the neonate's and infant's antibody titers are higher than those of adults, suggesting that CD4 T-cell help for B cells is not impaired. It is plausible that OPV may be less effective at inducing a Th1 response than BCG in neonates and young infants because of its limited replication (BCG vaccination results in permanent infection), its site of inoculation, or a more limited ability to stimulate antigen-presenting cells (APCs) in a manner conducive to Th1 immunity.

Mechanisms for reduced immunity

Normal CD4 T-cell activation generates a series of signals following engagement of the αβ-TCR and CD28 by MHC/peptide and CD80 and CD86 proteins respectively (Fig. 32.1). These include increases in the intracellular level of calcium and others, which activate NFAT-, AP-1-, and NF-κB-dependent transcription of genes such as IL-2 and CD154. IL-2 promotes CD4 T-cell proliferation in an autocrine and paracrine fashion, and CD154 engages CD40 on the cDC to increase its expression of CD80, CD86, and IL-12p70. In addition to limitations in DC function discussed above, there are multiple potential mechanisms intrinsic to the neonatal CD4 T cell that may limit its ability to expand into memory/

effector Th1 cells that have been revealed by *in vitro* studies using purified naïve CD4 T-cell populations (Fig. 32.1).[1, 17] These impairments include reductions in the neonatal CD4 T cell of fluxes of intracellular calcium,[18] NFAT proteins,[19] IL-2 and CD154 expression, and IL-12-induced STAT4 activation,[17] and decreased Th1 differentiation, as indicated by reduced IFN-γ mRNA and protein expression. The molecular basis for reduced calcium fluxes remains unclear, but a low level of certain NFAT proteins may contribute to reduced IL-2, CD154, and IFN-γ gene transcription. The IFN-γ gene locus may also be more highly methylated in neonatal compared to adult naïve CD4 T cells,[20] limiting its accessibility to transcription factors. Reduced CD154 expression may decrease CD40 engagement of cDCs and their production of IL-12p70.[17] Finally, decreased STAT4 signaling, which normally enhances IFN-γ gene transcription, may also impair Th1 differentiation.

CD8 T-CELL RESPONSES

The limited data available suggest that CD8 T-cell responses to herpes viruses, such as CMV, acquired congenitally are similar to those of adults[21] or the responses to infection acquired in infancy or early childhood.[22] Neonates with congenital Chagas disease also have readily detectable CD8 T-cell responses to this pathogen. These apparently robust responses do not rule out a brief, but potentially important, lag in the onset of CD8 T-cell immunity that might compromise the early control of these pathogens.

CD8 T-cell responses to human immunodeficiency virus type 1 (HIV-1) in perinatally infected infants suggest that CD8 T cells capable of mediating cytotoxicity have undergone clonal expansion *in vivo* as early as 4 months of age. However, their cytotoxicity may be reduced and delayed in appearance compared to adults. There is also decreased HIV-1specific CD8 T-cell production of IFN-γ by young infants after perinatal HIV 1 infection and a limited ability to generate HIV-1 specific cytotoxic T cells following highly active anti-retroviral therapy.[23] The role of HIV-1 itself in impairing these responses is plausible given the multiple mechanisms by which HIV-1 can suppress adaptive immunity. In general, the maintenance of

---

| **KEY CONCEPTS** |

MECHANISMS THAT MAY ACCOUNT FOR DELAYED CD4 T-CELL IMMUNITY TO INFECTION AND VACCINATION IN THE FETUS AND NEONATE

>> Decreased calcium flux and CD154 (CD40-ligand) expression by naïve CD4 T cells after activation by antigen

>> Decreased production by conventional dendritic cells of IL-12p70, a key cytokine for Th1 differentiation

>> Increased methylation of the interferon-γ gene resulting in decreased gene transcription in response to T-cell activation

>> Decreased expression of STAT4 protein and IL-12-induced STAT4 tyrosine phosphorylation in neonatal CD4 T cells

>> Reduced expression by neonatal CD4 T cells of NFAT family transcription factors required for CD154 and cytokine gene transcription

HIV-1 specific CD8 T cells with effector function depends on HIV-1 specific CD4 T cells, which tend to be selectively depleted by the virus. Interestingly, the suppressive effects of HIV-1 on CD8 T-cell responses appear to be relatively specific, as HIV-1 infected infants with poor HIV-1 specific CD8 T-cell responses maintain CD8 T cells to herpes viruses.[23]

B CELLS

ONTOGENY OF B CELLS

Pre-B cells are first detected in the human fetal liver and omentum by 8 weeks of gestation and in the fetal bone marrow by 13 weeks of gestation. By mid-gestation the bone marrow is the predominant site of pre-B-cell development, and by 30 weeks of gestation it is the sole site. The concentration of B cells in the circulation is higher during the second and third trimesters than at birth and further declines by adulthood. B cells expressing surface immunoglobulin M (IgM) but not IgD are present by 10 weeks of gestation. Such IgM+IgD B cells may be a transitory stage between pre-B cells and mature IgM+IgD+ B cells. Antigen exposure of IgM+IgD B cells may result in clonal anergy rather than activation, which may be important in maintaining B-cell tolerance to soluble self antigens present at a high concentration. This mechanism may also account for the observation that early-gestation congenital infection sometimes results in pathogen-specific defects in immunoglobulin production.

By 16 weeks of gestation, all heavy-chain isotypes are detectable in fetal bone marrow B cells. The stimulus for this fetal isotype switching remains unclear. The frequency of B cells in tissues rapidly increases so that by 22 weeks' gestation the proportion of B cells in the spleen, blood, and bone marrow is similar to that in the adult. Cord blood B cells expressing surface IgG or IgA are typically very rare (i.e., < 1% of circulating B cells). True germinal centers in the spleen and lymph nodes are absent during fetal life, but appear during the first months after postnatal antigenic stimulation.

IMMUNOGLOBULIN REPERTOIRE

The preimmune immunoglobulin repertoire consists of antibodies that can be expressed prior to encounter with antigen and is determined by the number of different B-cell clones with distinct antigen specificity. During early to mid-gestation this repertoire is limited by less diverse usage of V segments, but by the third trimester is as diverse as that of the adult. There may be over- or under-representation of a few V(D)J segments in the neonate, but these are unlikely to limit the quantity or quality of the neonatal humoral immune response significantly. The length of the CDR3 region of the immunoglobulin heavy chain, which is located at the center of the antigen-combining site, is shorter in the mid-gestation fetus than at birth or in adulthood; this is most likely due to decreased TdT activity. The length of the CDR3 region of the heavy-chain gene gradually increases from the beginning of the third trimester and birth and remains constant thereafter. As the CDR3 region is the most hypervariable portion of immunoglobulins, a short CDR3 region significantly reduces the diversity of the fetal immunoglobulin repertoire and theoretically could compromise the fetal antibody response. However, experiments with mice lacking TdT suggest this would likely be subtle. Instead, a lack of TdT may be important for the fetal development of "natural" immunoglobulin specificities that provide intrinsic protection against pathogens, such as bacteria. Somatic hypermutation appears to occur normally by birth in the B-cell compartment.[1]

B1 B CELLS

A distinct feature of fetal and neonatal B cells is their high frequency of CD5 expression, e.g., more than 40% of B cells in the fetal spleen, omentum, and circulation at mid-gestation are CD5high.[1] These CD5high B cells belong to the B-1a subset, which accounts for most production of natural IgM antibodies and also tends to produce antibodies with greater autoreactivity than do conventional B2 cells. These natural IgM antibodies can be considered a part of the innate immune system in providing protection against pathogens, such as certain encapsulated bacteria.

ONTOGENY OF RESPONSIVENESS TO T-DEPENDENT AND T-INDEPENDENT ANTIGENS

The chronology of the antibody response to different antigens differs depending on the need for cognate CD4 T-cell help (Table 32.1). Antigens that depend on cognate help (direct CD4 T-cell–B-cell interactions) include most proteins and polysaccharide–protein conjugates (T-dependent (TD) antigens). The response to TD antigens is characterized by the generation of memory B cells with somatically mutated, high-affinity immunoglobulin and the potential for isotype switching. Antigens that are partially or completely independent of CD4 T-cell help (T-independent antigens) can be divided into T-independent type 1 (TI-1) and type 2 (TI-2) antigens (Chapter 6).

Table 32.1 Postnatal ontogeny of competence for antibody responses to T-cell-dependent (TD) and T-cell independent type 1 (TI-1) and type 2 (TI-2) antigens

Antigen type	Nature of antigen	Age for competent response
TD	Proteins and protein-conjugated polysaccharides	Birth
TI-1	Certain microbial-derived products that directly activate B cells, e.g., *Brucella abortus*	Birth
TI-2	Unconjugated polysaccharides, such as those from bacterial capsules	Delayed (6–24 months of age)

Table 32.2 Postnatal antibody responses of infants 6 month of age or younger to selected vaccines

Vaccine	Antigen type	Antibody response in neonate and young infant
Diphtheria toxoid	TD	Immunogenic at birth, but response superior when vaccination series delayed until 1 month of age
Haemophilus influenzae type b polysaccharide-conjugate vaccine	TD	Immunogenic at birth, but response superior when vaccination series delayed until 2 months of age
Haemophilus influenzae type b polysaccharide unconjugated vaccine	TI-2	Not reliably immunogenic until 18–24 months of age
Hepatitis B surface antigen	TD	Moderately decreased with vaccination at birth compared to 1 month of age; decreased response in premature compared to term neonate; delay of vaccination series recommended for premature infants of HbsAg- mothers
Meningococcal polysaccharide-conjugated vaccine (types A, C, Y, W-135)	TD	Increased antibody titers in response to vaccination beginning at 2 months of age, with evidence of priming – efficacy?
Meningococcal polysaccharide vaccine – unconjugated (types A, C, Y, W-135)	TI-2	Serotype A immunogenic as early as 3 months of age; other serotypes not reliably immunogenic until 24 months of age; vaccination with type C induces tolerance to subsequent immunization in adults and presumably all age groups
Pertussis vaccine – acellular	TD	Immunogenic when series begun at 2 months of age
Pertussis vaccine – whole cellular	TD	Tolerance to pertussis toxin after vaccination at birth but not at 1 month of age; mechanism?
Pneumococcal polysaccharide-conjugate vaccine – 7 or 11 valent	TD	Protective to majority of serotypes after three doses when series is begun at 2 months of age.
Pneumococcal polysaccharide unconjugated vaccine – 23 valent	TI-2	Not reliably immunogenic until 18–24 months of age for most serotypes
Tetanus toxoid	TD	Protective in vaccinated neonates but relatively delayed response compared to 2-month-old infants

TI-1 antigens directly bind to B cells and fully activate them to produce antibodies, e.g., fixed *Brucella abortus* bacteria. TI-2 antigens include bacterial capsular polysaccharides and require additional signals for optimal antibody production, such as TLR ligands (e.g., unmethylated CpG DNA) that are directly recognized by B cells, or cytokines produced by non-B cells (e.g., NK cells, NK T cells, T cells, or DCs). The response to TI-2 antigens is characterized by a lack of B-cell memory or somatic hypermutation and isotype expression that is largely restricted to IgM and IgG_2.

The capacity of the neonate and young infant to respond to TD antigens is well established at birth, as reflected in the immune response to most protein and polysaccharide conjugate vaccines (Table 32.2). Nevertheless, there are clear differences between neonates and older infants in the magnitude of the antibody response to protein neoantigens. For example, in the case of hepatitis B surface antigen (HBsAg), the initial antibody response in term neonates immunized shortly after birth is substantially lower than if primary immunization is begun at 1 month of age. The neonate's ultimate anti-HBsAg titers achieved after secondary and tertiary immunizations are similar to those of older children, indicating that neonatal immunization does not result in tolerance. Together, these results indicate that the developmental limitations

responsible for reduced antibody responses are transient, although the precise mechanisms remain undefined.

Antibody production by human neonatal B cells to a TI-1 *in vitro* (*Brucella abortus*) is only modestly reduced (Table 32.1) and may reflect a decreased ability of antigen-activated B cells to proliferate rather than a decreased precursor frequency of antigen-specific clones.

The response to TI-2 antigen is the last to appear chronologically, and accounts for the neonate's poor antibody response to infection with encapsulated bacteria, e.g., group B streptococci (GBS) and/or vaccination with unconjugated polysaccharide antigens, such as for *Haemophilus influenzae* and *Streptococcus pneumoniae* (Table 32.2). The response to some unconjugated polysaccharide antigens can be demonstrated by 6 months of age, but the response to vaccination with *H. influenzae* type b capsule, *Neisseriae meningitidis* type C, or to most pneumococcal polysaccharides is poor until approximately 18–24 months. This poor response in children less than 2 years of age is associated with a lack of circulating memory (CD27[high]) B cells that express IgM and have not undergone isotype switching. These IgM memory B cells are also absent in adults after splenectomy, suggesting they depend on the spleen microenvironment for their generation and/or long-term survival. It is unclear whether decreased TI-2

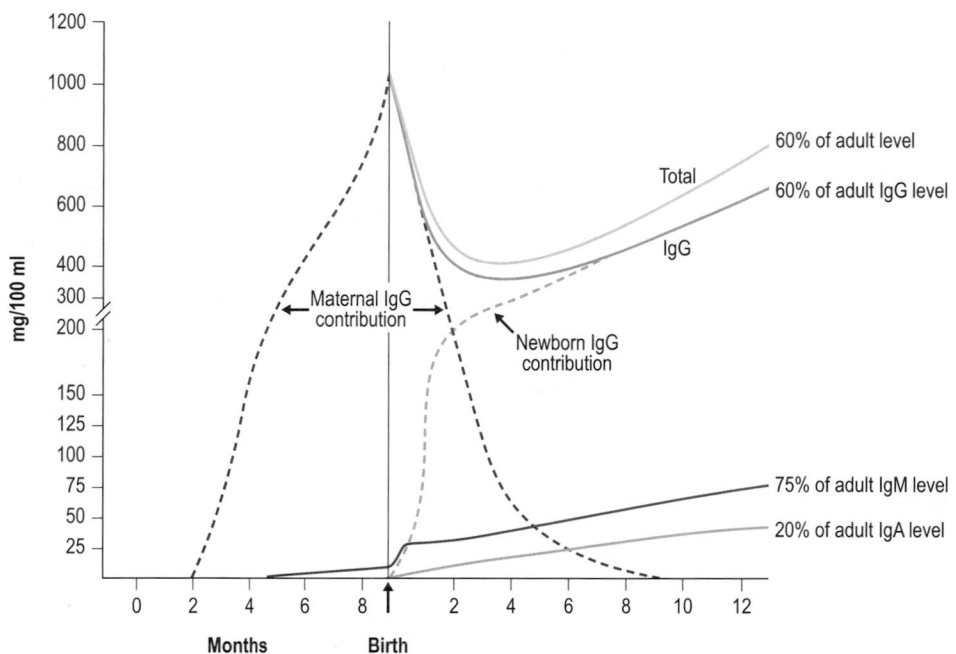

Fig. 32.2 Immunoglobulin G (IgG), IgM, and IgA levels in the fetus and in the infant in the first year of life. IgG of the fetus and newborn are solely of maternal origin. Maternal IgG disappears by 9 months of age, by which time endogenous synthesis is well established. IgM and IgA of the neonate are due solely to endogenous synthesis because these immunoglobulin isotypes do not cross the placenta. (From Remington JS, Klein JO, Wilson CB, et al. (eds) Infectious Diseases of the Fetus and Newborn Infant, 6th edn. Philadelphia: Elsevier; 2006: Fig. 4-10)

antigen responses in early childhood are due to an intrinsic immaturity in B cells or APCs of the spleen or to other limitations in the spleen microenvironment.

ANTIBODY RESPONSES OF THE PREMATURE INFANT

There is a limited antibody response of premature infants to immunization with protein antigens during the first month of life but not by 2 months of age (Table 32.2). Thus, postnatal age is more of a determinant of antibody responses to TD antigens than is gestational age. This may be of particular clinical relevance for HBsAg vaccine, which in term neonates is effective when given immediately after birth. As in term infants, the antibody responses to TI-2 antigens in premature infants are delayed until 6–24 months of age, depending on the particular antigen.

MATERNAL–FETAL TRANSFER OF IgG

IgG is transported from the mother to the fetus by transcytosis and is detectable in the fetus by 17 weeks of gestation. Circulating concentrations of IgG in the fetus rise steadily and may exceed those of the mother after 34 weeks of gestation, consistent with the transfer being an active transport mechanism. The fetus synthesizes little IgG so that the concentration *in utero* is almost entirely maternally derived (Fig. 32.2). Accordingly, the degree of prematurity is reflected in proportionately lower neonatal IgG concentrations.

FETAL AND POSTNATAL IMMUNOGLOBULIN SYNTHESIS

IgG is the predominant immunoglobulin isotype at all ages (Fig. 32.2). The IgG plasma half-life is about 21 days, and maternally derived IgG levels fall rapidly after birth. IgG synthesized by the neonate and that passively derived from the mother are approximately equal when the neonate reaches 2 months of age; by 10–12 months of age the IgG is nearly all infant-derived. Values reach a nadir of ~400 mg/dl in term infants at 3–4 months of age and rise thereafter (Fig. 32.2). The premature infant has a lower IgG concentration at birth, and reaches a nadir at 3 months of age. The slow onset of IgG synthesis in the neonate is predominantly an intrinsic limitation of the neonate rather than inhibitory effect of maternal antibody, as a similar pattern of IgG development is observed in neonates born to mothers with untreated agammaglobulinemia.

IgM, IgA, and IgE do not cross the placenta. IgM increases from a mean of 6 mg/dl in premature infants less than 28 weeks of gestation to 11 mg/dl at term, which is approximately 8% of the maternal IgM level. This IgM, which is likely to be pre-immune or "natural," is enriched for polyreactive antibodies produced by B1 cells, and may play a role in the innate defense against infection. Postnatal IgM concentrations rise rapidly in premature and term infants in the first month and then more gradually thereafter, presumably in response to antigenic stimulation (Fig. 32.2). Elevated (> 20 mg/dl) IgM concentrations in cord blood suggest possible intrauterine infections, but this is not a sensitive screen for congenital infections.

IMMUNOLOGIC DEFICIENCIES

IgA has a concentration in cord blood of about 0.1–5.0 mg/dl, approximately 0.5% of the levels in maternal sera. Concentrations are similar in term and premature neonates, and increase to 20% of those in adults by 1 year of age (Fig. 32.2). Increased cord blood IgA concentrations are observed in some infants with congenital infection, and elevated IgA is common in young infants infected by vertical transmission with HIV. IgA has a relatively short half-life in plasma of approximately 5 days. Secretory IgA is present in substantial amounts in the saliva by 10 days after birth.

The concentration of IgE in cord blood is typically only about 0.5% of those of maternal levels. The rate of postnatal increase varies, and is greater in infants predisposed to allergic disease or greater environmental exposure to allergens. The concentration of IgE at birth has limited predictive value for whether an individual will later develop atopic disease.

NK CELLS

The human fetal liver produces NK cells as early as 6 weeks of gestation, but the bone marrow is the major site for NK-cell production from late gestation onward. NK cells are present in greatest numbers in the circulation during the second trimester of fetal development, and comprise ~15% of total lymphocytes in the neonatal circulation, which is typically equal to or greater than in adults. IL-15 appears to play a central role in NK-cell development, suggesting that NK lineage cells in fetus and neonate have normal IL-15 responsiveness. Most surface receptors and markers are expressed at similar levels in neonatal and adult NK cells. An exception is CD56, which is only expressed by about 30–50% of neonatal NK cells compared to > 95% of adult NK cells.[1]

The cytolytic function of NK cells increases progressively during fetal life to reach values approximately 50% of those in adult cells at term, as determined in assays using tumor cell targets such as the K562 erythroleukemia cells. Full function is not achieved until at least 9–12 months of age. NK cells from the premature infant also have more pronounced reductions in cytotoxic function than those of the term neonate. The reduced cytolytic activity of neonatal NK cells appears to reflect primarily diminished post-binding cytotoxic activity and diminished recycling to kill multiple targets. These functional defects appear to be limited to CD56⁻ neonatal NK cells, and cytolytic activity mediated by neonatal CD56⁺ NK cells is similar to those of adult NK cells. Neonatal NK-cell cytotoxicity can be markedly increased by incubating these cells with a variety of cytokines, e.g., IL-2 or IFN-α, suggesting a potential immunotherapeutic strategy. Limited studies suggest that neonatal NK cells produce IFN-α as effectively as adult NK cells in response to exogenous IL-2 and HSV or to pharmacological stimulation, but the production of other cytokines, such as TNF-α, may be reduced.[1]

PHAGOCYTES

NEUTROPHILS

Mature neutrophils are first detected by 14–16 weeks of gestation. At midgestation, postmitotic neutrophils constitute only 10% of circulating leukocytes and are also in markedly lower numbers in the bone marrow compared to term newborns and adults. Sepsis and other perinatal complications can cause neutropenia, and severe or fatal sepsis is often associated with persistent neutropenia, particularly in preterm neonates. Neutropenia may be associated with increased margination of circulating neutrophils, which occurs early in response to infection. Sustained neutropenia often reflects depletion of the neonate's limited postmitotic neutrophil storage pool. Importantly, septic neutropenic neonates in whom the neutrophil storage pool is depleted are more likely to die than are those with normal neutrophil storage pools. Reduced G-CSF production may also be a factor in neutropenia, although this does not appear to be a major mechanism in most cases of neutropenia associated with sepsis.

Neonatal phagocytic function is also limited by reduction or delays in neutrophil migration from the blood to sites of infection and inflammation.[24] This may explain why the early inflammatory response in neonatal skin often contains a larger number of eosinophils than in adult skin and why the transition from a neutrophilic to a mononuclear cell-dominated response is delayed in the newborn. The combination of a deficiency in the abundance of L-selectin and ability to shed this protein from the surface of neonatal neutrophils, and decreased binding of these cells to P-selectin may contribute to defective cell adhesion to activated endothelium. Neonatal neutrophil chemotaxis may also be impaired based on in vitro studies using leukotrienes, IL-8, and other stimuli. In contrast, phagocytosis and killing by neonatal neutrophils, including by oxidative and nonoxidative mechanisms, are largely intact, but can be compromised when opsonins are limiting or the bacterial density is high. These deficits in uptake and killing are greater in preterm neonates.

MONONUCLEAR PHAGOCYTES

Blood monocytes from neonates are normal in number and similar to adult monocytes in phagocytic and microbicidal activity. By contrast, migration of neonatal monocytes into sites of inflammation, such as delayed-type hypersensitivity reactions, is reduced.[1] Tissue macrophages in neonatal animal models have reduced phagocytic and microbicidal activity and this may also apply to humans. The capacity of mononuclear phagocytes to produce both pro- and anti-inflammatory cytokines may be modestly reduced in term neonates and further reduced in premature neonates. These modest limitations in mononuclear cell function may be compounded by a concomitant deficiency in production of IFN-γ by neonatal T cells and NK cells, and by impaired responsiveness of neonatal mononuclear phagocytes to IFN-γ.[1]

HUMORAL MEDIATORS OF INFLAMMATION AND OPSONIZATION

Humoral factors that participate in the response to infection and inflammation include complement components, mannan-binding lectin, fibronectin, and surfactant apoproteins. Compared with adults, neonates have moderately diminished alternative complement pathway activity and slightly diminished classic complement pathway activity. Fibronectin and mannan-binding lectin concentrations are also slightly lower. Consistent with these findings, neonatal sera are less effective than adult sera in opsonization either in the absence of antibody or at low titers of antibody. Generation of complement-derived chemotactic activity is also moderately diminished.

These differences are greater in preterm than in term neonates. Preterm neonates may also have compromised lung defenses as a result of reduced abundance of surfactant apoprotein A. These deficiencies, in concert with phagocyte deficits described above, may contribute to delayed inflammatory responses and impaired bacterial and fungal clearance in neonates.

HOST DEFENSE MECHANISMS AGAINST SPECIFIC PATHOGENS

HERPES SIMPLEX VIRUS

HSV infection is severe in term infants infected at the time of parturition or postnatally up to 4 weeks of age. Characteristically, neonatal HSV infection spreads rapidly to produce disseminated or central nervous system disease in approximately 60–65% of cases. Deficiencies in the function of neonatal NK cells, cDCs, and pDCs are probably important contributors to the poor early control of infection by the mechanisms of innate immunity. Reduced type I IFN production by neonatal pDCs may be particularly relevant to infection severity, as murine studies suggest that an obligatory interaction between pDCs and cDCs is necessary to generate effective HSV-specific CD8 T-cell responses.[3] Fetal and neonatal NK cells have reduced natural and antibody-dependent cytotoxicity against HSV-infected target cells. These decreased NK-cell responses are likely to be relevant, as rare patients with selective NK-cell deficiency are also highly susceptible to severe and early disseminated infection with HSV and other herpes viruses.

As discussed above, HSV-specific CD4 T-cell responses by neonates are diminished and delayed compared to adults following primary HSV infection. Neonates do not achieve adult levels of these responses for 3–6 weeks after clinical presentation, whereas adults develop robust responses within 1 week. Since CD4 T cells provide multiple effector functions that may be critical for the resolution of HSV infection – including direct antiviral cytokine production and help for CD8 T cells and B cells – this marked lag could be an important contributor to the tendency for dissemination and severe organ damage. The basis for the delayed development of HSV antigen-specific CD4 T cells in neonates is not known and could reflect limitations in DC function or intrinsic limitations in the ability of neonatal naïve CD4 T cells to be activated and differentiate into effector cells. The age at which primary infection with HSV in children results in a similar CD4 T-cell response to that of adults is unknown, but severe or disseminated infection in otherwise healthy infants is extremely rare after 6 weeks of age.

The postinfection kinetics of HSV-specific CD8 T-cell responses in the fetus, neonate, or young infant is unknown, and it is unclear if there is a lag compared to the adult, as has been observed for the CD4 T-cell response. Whether neonates have a reduced HSV-specific antibody response following infection compared to adults with primary infection is also unknown. Passively acquired maternal antibody could play a role in decreasing transmission or ameliorating disease severity in neonatal HSV.

GROUP B STREPTOCOCCI

In the absence of maternally derived type-specific antibodies, the neonate is at risk for GBS infection. There are subtle but cumulative limitations in a number of other host defense mechanisms that account for the marked susceptibility of the neonate to GBS infection.[24] For example, neonates lack secretory IgA and have reduced amounts of fibronectin in their secretions compared to older individuals. Reduced amounts of surfactant apoprotein A in the lungs of preterm neonates, a paucity of alveolar macrophages in the lungs, particularly in preterm infants, and diminished phagocytosis and killing of GBS by these cells may facilitate invasion through the respiratory tract. Limitations in the generation of chemotactic factors and/or deficits in the chemotactic responses of neonatal neutrophils may delay recruitment of neutrophils to sites of infection. Neonatal neutrophils that reach sites of infection may kill bacteria less efficiently because of limited amounts of opsonins available for a high local density of GBS, or because the microbicidal activity of neutrophils from certain neonates is decreased. Rapidly progressive infection can deplete the limited marrow neutrophil reserve compounding this problem.

Once GBS infection is established the adequacy of neutrophil production may be critical for preventing morbidity and mortality. Severe or fatal sepsis from GBS is often associated with persistent neutropenia,

> ### KEY CONCEPTS
>
> **POTENTIAL MECHANISMS CONTRIBUTING TO THE SEVERITY OF PRIMARY HERPES SIMPLEX VIRUS (HSV) INFECTION OF THE NEONATE**
>
> » Reduced type I interferon production by plasmacytoid dendritic cells
>
> » Decreased production of IL-12p70 by conventional dendritic cells
>
> » Decreased natural killer cell-mediated cytotoxicity against HSV-infected target cells
>
> » Diminished and delayed HSV-specific CD4 T-cell responses, including Th1 cells

> ### KEY CONCEPTS
>
> **POTENTIAL MECHANISMS THAT MAY CONTRIBUTE TO THE HIGH FREQUENCY AND SEVERITY OF GROUP B STREPTOCOCCAL (GBS) INFECTIONS IN THE NEONATE**
>
> » Reduced surfactant apoprotein A in the lungs of preterm neonates
>
> » Decreased numbers of alveolar lung macrophages, particularly in the preterm neonate, that can effectively phagocytose and kill GBS in the lung
>
> » Limitations in the local generation of chemotactic factors and/or deficits in the chemotactic responses of neonatal neutrophils
>
> » Decreased neutrophil killing at sites of infection because of limited amounts of opsonins and, in some individuals, neutrophil microbicidal activity
>
> » Limited neutrophil storage pool in bone marrow compartment – important cause of neutropenia in overwhelming infection

particularly in preterm neonates, and most likely reflects the depletion of the postmitotic neutrophil storage pool in the bone marrow.

The use of intravenous immunoglobulin or subcutaneously administered colony-stimulating factors in the prevention or treatment of neonatal GBS and other pyogenic infections is theoretically attractive. However, an analysis of the outcome of multiple clinical trials suggests that this approach or the use of white blood cell transfusions in cases of established sepsis do not consistently reduce mortality.[1, 25]

SUMMARY

Careful evaluation of components of the innate and acquired immune systems of the human fetus and neonate reveals both quantitative and qualitative deficiencies. Increased bacterial infections of the neonate, as seen in neonatal nurseries and intensive care units in major medical centers, result from impaired production or function of soluble factors such as secretory IgA, opsonins, pulmonary surfactant, and defective mobility and chemotaxis. Increased viral infections in neonates obtains from functional deficiencies of NK cells, cDCs, and pDCs as well as diminished and delayed CD4 T-cell responses that stimulate cytolytic CD8 T cells. Thus, the very beginning of life is marked by a period of high risk for infection. Better countermeasures are needed for the protection of infants during this time.

REFERENCES

1. Lewis DB, Wilson CB. Developmental immunology and role of host defenses in the fetal and neonatal susceptibility to infection. In: Remington JS, Klein JO, Wilson CB, et al. (eds): Infectious Diseases of the Fetus and Newborn Infant, 6th edn. Philadelphia: Elsevier 2006, : 87–210.

2. Rocha V, Gluckman E. Clinical use of umbilical cord blood hematopoietic stem cells. Biol Blood Marrow Transplant 2006; 12: 34–41.

3. Lewis DB. Neonatal T-cell immunity and its regulation by innate immunity and dendritic cells. In: Ohls R, Yoder MC, (eds): Hematology, Immunology, and Infectious Diseases: Neonatology, Questions and Controversies; Philadelphia: Elsevier. 2008; 208–230.

4. Levy O, Suter EE, Miller RL, et al. Unique efficacy of Toll-like receptor 8 agonists in activating human neonatal antigen-presenting cells. Blood 2006; 108: 1284–1290.

5. Upham JW, Lee PT, Holt BJ, et al. Development of interleukin-12-producing capacity throughout childhood. Infect Immun 2002; 70: 6583–6588.

6. Gold MC, Donnelly E, Cook MS, et al. Purified neonatal plasmacytoid dendritic cells overcome intrinsic maturation defect with TLR agonist stimulation. Pediatr Res 2006; 60: 34–37.

7. Dabbagh K, Dahl ME, Stepick-Biek P, et al. Toll-like receptor 4 is required for optimal development of Th2 immune responses: role of dendritic cells. J Immunol 2002; 168: 4524–4530.

8. Varas A, Jimenez E, Sacedon R, et al. Analysis of the human neonatal thymus: evidence for a transient thymic involution. J Immunol 2000; 164: 6260–6267.

9. Garderet L, Dulphy N, Douay C, et al. The umbilical cord blood alpha-beta T-cell repertoire: characteristics of a polyclonal and naïve but completely formed repertoire. Blood 1998; 91: 340–346.

10. McFarland RD, Douek DC, Koup RA, et al. Identification of a human recent thymic emigrant phenotype. Proc Natl Acad Sci USA 2000; 97: 4215–4220.

11. Schonland SO, Zimmer JK, Lopez-Benitez CM, et al. Homeostatic control of T-cell generation in neonates. Blood 2003; 102: 1428–1434.

12. Sullender WM, Miller JL, Yasukawa LL, et al. Humoral and cell-mediated immunity in neonates with herpes simplex virus infection. J Infect Dis 1987; 155: 28–37.

13. Burchett SK, Corey L, Mohan KM, et al. Diminished interferon-gamma and lymphocyte proliferation in neonatal and postpartum primary herpes simplex virus infection. J Infect Dis 1992; 165: 813–818.

14. Tu W, Chen S, Sharp M, et al. Persistent and selective deficiency of CD4+ T cell immunity to cytomegalovirus in immunocompetent young children. J Immunol 2004; 172: 3260–3267.

15. Marchant A, Goetghebuer T, Ota MO, et al. Newborns develop a Th1-type immune response to Mycobacterium bovis bacillus Calmette-Guérin vaccination. J Immunol 1999; 163: 2249–2255.

16. Vekemans J, Ota MO, Wang EC, et al. T cell responses to vaccines in infants: defective IFN-gamma production after oral polio vaccination. Clin Exp Immunol 2002; 127: 495–498.

17. Chen L, Cohen AC, Lewis DB. Impaired allogeneic activation and T-helper 1 differentiation of human cord blood naïve CD4 T cells. Biol Blood Marrow Transplant 2006; 12: 160–171.

18. Jullien P, Cron RQ, Dabbagh K, et al. Decreased CD154 expression by neonatal CD4+ T cells is due to limitations in both proximal and distal events of T cell activation. Int Immunol 2003; 15: 1461–1472.

19. Kadereit S, Mohammad SF, Miller RE, et al. Reduced NFAT1 protein expression in human umbilical cord blood T lymphocytes. Blood 1999; 94: 3101–3107.

20. White GP, Watt PM, Holt BJ, et al. Differential patterns of methylation of the IFN-gamma promoter at CpG and non-CpG sites underlie differences in IFN-gamma gene expression between human neonatal and adult CD45RO- T cells. J Immunol 2002; 168: 2820–2827.

21. Marchant A, Appay V, Van Der Sande M, et al. Mature CD8(+) T lymphocyte response to viral infection during fetal life. J Clin Invest 2003; 111: 1747–1755.

22. Gibson L, Piccinini G, Lilleri D, et al. Human cytomegalovirus proteins pp65 and immediate early protein 1 are common targets for CD8(+) T cell responses in children with congenital or postnatal human cytomegalovirus infection. J Immunol 2004; 172: 2256–2264.

23. Luzuriaga K, McManus M, Catalina M, et al. Early therapy of vertical human immunodeficiency virus type 1 (HIV-1) infection: control of viral replication and absence of persistent HIV-1-specific immune responses. J Virol 2000; 74: 6984–6991.

24. Koenig JM, Yoder MC. Neonatal neutrophils: the good, the bad, and the ugly. Clin Perinatol 2004; 31: 39–51.

25. Ohlsson A, Lacy JB. Intravenous immunoglobulin for preventing infection in preterm and/or low-birth-weight infants. Cochrane Database Syst Rev. CD000361.

Aging and the immune system

Rania D. Kovaiou, Birgit Weinberger, Beatrix Grubeck-Loebenstein

33

Worldwide, the segment of the population aged 60 or over is increasing rapidly. This demographic change represents one of the most challenging problems in many countries, as it puts pressure not only on individuals and their families but also on the social security system, which has to deal with the tremendous costs of medical care for the elderly. It is therefore of great interest to society that measures are taken which contribute to healthy aging and prolong the period of life that is not compromised by age-associated deficits.

The immune system undergoes profound age-related changes, collectively termed immunosenescence. Aging affects a wide range of cell types, including hematopoietic stem cells (HSCs), lymphoid progenitors in the bone marrow and thymus, thymic stroma, mature lymphocytes in secondary lymphoid organs, and elements of the innate immune response. At the functional level, these changes are translated into an increased susceptibility to infections and suboptimal vaccine-induced protection. Furthermore, infections in the elderly are characterized by more severe symptoms, prolonged duration, and poorer prognosis. Well-known examples of infections that specifically affect the elderly are the reactivation of the varicella-zoster virus leading to herpes zoster in individuals over 50 years of age, and infection with influenza virus associated with an increased risk of severe complications. Additionally, risks for

bacterial pneumonia, urinary tract infection, pneumococcal and *Listeria* meningitis, infection with *Mycobacterium tuberculosis* and viral gastroenteritis are increased in the elderly.[1]

Although intensive research over past decades has attempted to clarify the basic mechanisms of age-related immune dysfunction, the exact nature of the underlying defects is not yet fully understood, but owing to coordinated efforts by laboratories worldwide focusing on immunosenescence and our increasing knowledge of the biology of the immune system, a convincing and clear-cut picture has started to emerge. It is the goal of this chapter to summarize recent reliable data on the cellular and molecular mechanisms of immunosenescence, and to try to interpret how basic dysfunctions may eventually lead to disability and disease in the elderly.

■ THE EFFECT OF AGING ON HEMATOPOIETIC STEM CELLS AND LYMPHOID PROGENITOR CELLS ■

It is well understood that the amount of hematopoietic tissue in the human bone marrow decreases with age.[2] Studies on humans and various animal models have indicated that HSCs are severely affected: the ability of human HSCs to proliferate correlates inversely with age, and HSCs have shortened telomeres, which may affect their proliferative and developmental potential. Age-related perturbations in the hematopoietic microenvironment combined with changes in hormones, such as the anterior pituitary-derived growth hormone, also disturb HSC self-renewal and lineage commitment.

Age-related changes to HSCs seem to affect lymphoid, but not erythroid and myeloid, progeny cells. Fewer pro-B cells are generated and fewer of these cells transit into the pre-B and B-cell pools. As a result, the total number of pre-B cells is reduced and fewer new mature B cells leave the bone marrow.[3] Bone marrow-derived T-lymphocyte precursors continuously migrate into the thymus, where they mature. The frequency and absolute numbers of intrathymic T-cell progenitors decrease with age.[4] This is partly due to age-related changes in the bone

■ KEY CONCEPTS

GENERAL INFORMATION ON AGING

- ➤➤ Aging is usually defined as the progressive loss of function accompanied by decreasing fertility and increasing mortality with advancing age.

- ➤➤ Aging begins at the moment an organism is born and is inevitable throughout life.

- ➤➤ Aging influences various systems of the organism (nervous system, endocrine system, immune system).

- ➤➤ Aging represents one of the most challenging problems of the developed countries owing to prolongation of lifespan.

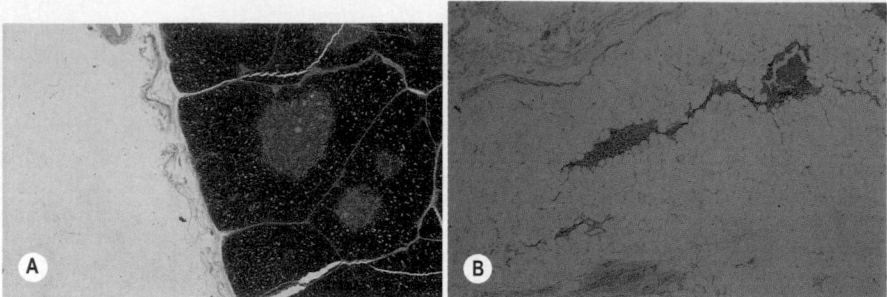

Fig. 33.1 (**A**) Pediatric thymus showing division into cortical (outer darker staining) and medullary (inner lighter-staining) areas, with lobules separated by thin septa. (**B**) Chronic involution with aging. Thymus from an 82-year-old individual showing dramatic reduction of lymphoepithelial elements (true thymus), and invasion of adipose tissue into the septa and intrathymic region immediately under the capsule. (Hematoxylin staining. Magnification × 250.) (From George AJ, Ritter MA. Thymic involution with ageing: obsolescence or good housekeeping? Immunol Today 1996; 17: 267, with permission from Elsevier.)

marrow, but is predominantly the result of thymic involution. Thymic function is at its most active during the fetal and perinatal periods, but output declines with age, resulting in a dramatic loss in the number of naïve T cells being produced. This decline in de novo T-cell production correlates with the atrophy of the thymic stroma. After puberty there is a gradual loss of thymic tissue, but the thymus can respond to T-cell lymphopenia in adulthood with renewed output of antigenically naïve T cells, such as happens with HIV infection, most likely due to the increased production of interleukin (IL)-7.[5] Elderly persons retain a very limited thymic function, with thymocytes being produced by a small thymic rudiment composed of epithelium (Fig. 33.1). TCR excision circle (TREC) analysis has been successfully used to study the age-related decline of thymic T-cell output by quantifying the amount of episomal DNA circles that are produced during the rearrangement of αβ TCR genes.[5, 6]

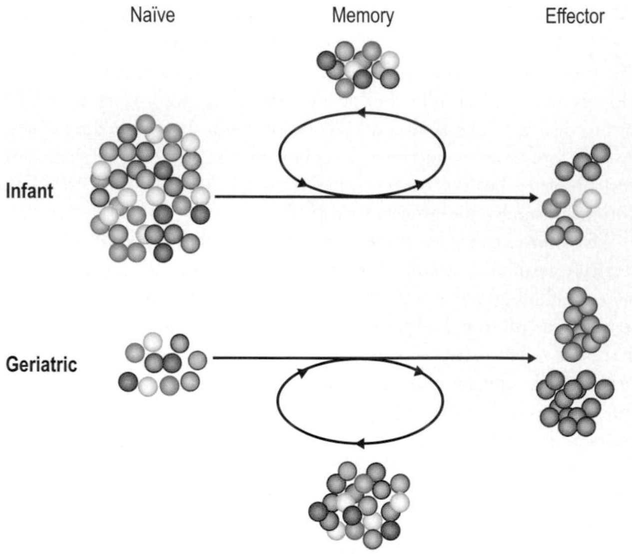

■ ADAPTIVE IMMUNITY AND AGING ■

T LYMPHOCYTES

Although the size of the mature T cell pool remains stable over the lifetime of an individual, the proportionate representation of different subsets and T cell function is greatly affected by aging.

One of the most profound age-related changes in the T-cell population is a decrease in the number of antigen-inexperienced naïve T lymphocytes combined with an increase in antigen-experienced memory and effector cells (Fig. 33.2). Although a diverse naïve CD4 T-cell compartment is maintained for decades in spite of minimal thymic function, a dramatic and sudden collapse of diversity occurs after the age of 70, which results in a severely contracted repertoire.[7] Similar changes in the CD8 T-cell pool occur even earlier in life.[8] As a result, the host's ability to respond to new antigens decreases. At the same time a progressive increase in antigen-experienced T cells occurs. Many of these cells do not express the co-stimulatory molecule CD28. Loss of CD28 expression in T cells is one of the most consistent biological indicators of aging in the human immune system.[9] CD28− T cells are long-lived lymphocytes with a

Fig. 33.2 T-cell subpopulations in youth and old age. Naïve, memory and effector T cells of different specificities are represented by different colors. All three populations are found in young and elderly persons, but their relative proportions change. With age the number and diversity of naïve cells decline as thymic output decreases. Repeated antigenic stimulation eventually leads to an increase in memory T cells and gives rise to highly differentiated, expanded effector clones, resulting in an increase in the size of the effector population that has, however, a very restricted repertoire.

limited proliferative capacity. CD28−CD8+ T cells may be CD27+ (another co-stimulatory molecule) or CD27−. In contrast, CD28−CD4+ T cells are strictly CD27−. The loss of CD28 in CD4 T cells is accompanied by a concomitant defect in CD154 (CD40L) expression, hence the capacity of CD4 T cells to provide help for B-cell proliferation and antibody production is reduced. CD28⁻CD8⁺ as well as CD28⁻CD4⁺ T cells produce large amounts of interferon (IFN)-γ and perforin, and express a variety of killer cell immunoglobulin-like receptors (KIRs). CD28⁻ T cells frequently exhibit specificity for persistent viruses, mainly for cytomegalovirus (CMV), but also for Epstein–Barr virus (EBV) and hepatitis C virus (HCV). A high frequency of these cells has been correlated with a low humoral immune response to influenza vaccination in elderly persons.[10] CD28⁻ T cells characteristically occur as large expanded clones. Expanded clones of CD8 T cells are common in old age and mostly large enough to distort the αβ T-cell repertoire. The outgrowth of CD4 T cell clonotypes is much less common and occurs mainly in diseases such as rheumatoid arthritis.[7]

At the cellular level, the activation potential of T cells is altered in old age, leading to hyporesponsiveness. This has been well documented in CD4 T cells from mice and humans, and has been attributed to alterations in the formation of the immunological synapses between T cells and antigen-presenting cells, as well as to signaling defects.[11] Age-related changes in lipid raft polarization have recently been suggested to represent an important cause of age-related changes in CD4 T-cell signaling.[12] Lipid rafts are dynamic structures, and the time-dependent recruitment or exclusion of signaling proteins in lipid rafts controls T-cell activation and immune responses. Changes in lipid raft properties in the elderly are due to an age-related increase in the cholesterol content of the CD4 T cell plasma membrane. Corresponding changes in the composition of the CD8 T-cell membrane have less effect on T-cell activation.

Cytokines are a key component in the regulatory communication process among immune cells in general, and T cells in particular. Age-related changes in cytokine production have been studied for over 20 years.[13] The long-standing notion that IL-2 production decreases while IL-4 production increases with advancing age, has recently been challenged by reports indicating an increase in proinflammatory activity in all organs, which seems at least partly due to an increase in the whole-body load of IFN-γ. The increase in the production of IFN-γ is presumably the result of the pronounced accumulation of terminally differentiated CD28⁻ T cells with a high proinflammatory activity, which is found in large subgroups of elderly persons. In contrast, high IL-4 production, which is observed in other elderly cohorts, correlates with a high number of central memory but a low number of effector T cells.[14]

Thymic involution can also lead to a decreased output of regulatory T cells (Tregs). Tregs mostly express high levels of the IL-2 receptor α chain (CD25) and the forkhead and winged-helix family transcription factor forkhead box P3 (FOXP3). Treg homeostasis may still be sustained by alternative pathways such as peripheral generation. Treg-mediated suppression has been reported to decline after the age of 50, and may contribute to age-related phenomena such as increased inflammation and autoimmunity.[15]

B LYMPHOCYTES

Like the T-cell pool, the peripheral blood B-cell pool fills up with memory cells owing to a concurrent displacement of naïve cells. The percentage of naïve B cells, which are defined by the absence of CD27, is significantly lower in the elderly than in the young, whereas the opposite is true for memory cells.[16] The production of peripheral blood B cells is similar in elderly and young persons, although there is a trend towards a

slower rate of proliferation in the elderly. Similar to the T-cell pool, aging is associated with the appearance of B-cell clonal expansions. This limits the diversity of the B-cell repertoire and may induce monoclonal serum immunoglobulins and B-cell neoplasms.[17] Additionally, there is a shift from B2 to B1 lymphocytes. Most foreign protein antigens stimulate B2 cells in the presence of T-cell help, whereas carbohydrate and autoantigens do not depend on T-cell help and stimulate B1 cells.

Age-related changes in the B-cell pool result in impaired humoral immunity in the elderly. Primary antibody responses in aged humans are often weak and short-lived, and the antibodies produced bind with lower affinity. Antibody production by elderly persons in response to vaccination has been extensively studied, and it has been suggested that the protective effect of vaccinations against *Streptococcus pneumoniae*, influenza, hepatitis B and tetanus is reduced with age. Old age is also associated with an increased occurrence of autoantibodies. However, these autoantibodies lack specificity for organs and rarely contribute to autoimmune disease.[18]

Although age-related changes in humoral immunity may be the result of intrinsic defects in B cells and change in the B-cell repertoire, the lack of the regulatory control of T cells on B cells also contributes to the low-level and brief production period of specific antibodies to foreign antigens in the elderly. CD4 T-cell help is crucial for germinal center (GC) formation. Cognate help from CD4 T cells drives the formation of GCs and enables isotype switching and affinity maturation of antibodies. A defective T-helper function at a higher age thus leads to diminished high-affinity responses in germinal centers.[19] A severe reduction in germinal center reactions has been reported in mice >22 months of age.[20] This reduction occurs gradually, and both the number and the volume of germinal centers diminish progressively (Fig. 33.3). The most important age-related changes in the adaptive immune system are summarized in Table 33.1.

■ INNATE IMMUNITY AND AGING ■

Innate immunity provides the basis for an adequate response to pathogens. It has to be tightly controlled, as excessive responses can be detrimental. However, with increasing age inflammatory processes occur ubiquitously in a variety of species and characteristically lead to a progressive proinflammatory status referred to as 'inflamm-aging.'[21] It is by now well understood that chronic inflammation supports the development and progression of age-related diseases, such as osteoporosis, atherosclerosis and neurodegeneration.[22]

At first sight, reports on enhanced inflammatory activity in old age seem to be contradicting studies demonstrating functional defects within cells of the innate immune system (Table 33.2). The accumulation of functional defects at the cellular level can, however, lead to an inability to eliminate pathogens and to a chronic ineffective activation of nonspecific responses as a consequence. The severity of inflammatory processes in old age may also depend on genetic factors, for example polymorphisms within the genes encoding for cytokines such as IL-6, IL-10 and IFN-γ, which have also been shown to be associated with changes in lifespan.[23]

Age-related changes in the function of neutrophilic granulocytes are well documented. Although their number remains constant, the production of superoxide anion in response to GM-CSF and Gram-positive bacteria is reduced in old age. Additionally, changes in membrane fluidity, chemotaxis to selected chemoattractants and various signal transduction

INNATE IMMUNITY AND AGING

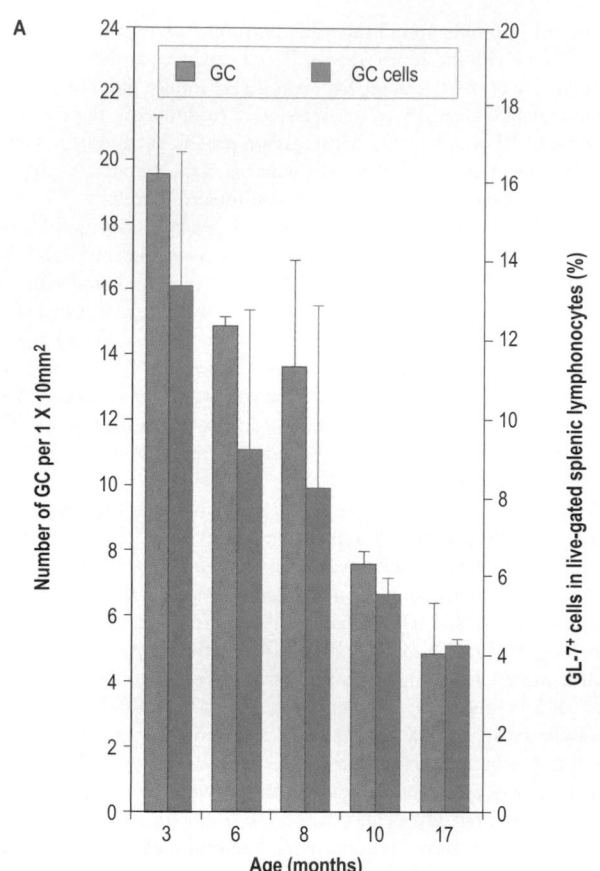

Fig. 33.3 Progressive decline in germinal center formation during aging. Spleens of C57BL/6 mice immunized 14 days earlier with NP-CGG precipitated in alum were prepared for immunohistologic or flow-cytometric analysis. For enumeration of GC (purple bars), splenic sections were stained with PNA-HRP and GCs were counted under a light microscope. For enumeration of GC cells (green bars), a single-cell suspension of splenocytes was stained with anti-B220 and GL-I7 antibodies and analyzed by flow cytometry. (From Zheng B, Han S, Takahashi Y, et al. Immunosenescence and germinal center reaction. Immunol Rev 1997; 160: 63, with permission from Blackwell Publishing Ltd.)

pathways have been observed.[24] These defects lead to a reduced bactericidal activity of neutrophilic granulocytes in old age.

Monocytes and macrophages are also affected by the aging process. An increasing number of studies shows that, similar to granulocytes, aging macrophages have an impaired respiratory burst and a reduced capacity to produce superoxide anion and nitric oxide. They have defective Toll-like receptor (TLR) expression and are unable to upregulate the expression of MHC class II genes, thus impairing their capacity to present antigen and to trigger CD4 T-cell responses. Owing to functional defects, macrophages from elderly persons may fail to eliminate pathogens. This dysfunction results in chronic activation and the prolonged production of TNF-α and IL-6, but may at the same time

increase the susceptibility to and severity of bacterial, mycotic and viral infections.[25]

The number of natural killer (NK) cells increases with age. However, NK-cell cytotoxicity and the production of cytokines and chemokines in response to activation are impaired on a per-cell basis. Probably owing to a partial loss of the high-affinity IL-2 α-chain receptor, proliferation of NK cells from healthy elderly donors in response to IL-2 is reduced.[26]

Whether dendritic cells (DC) are affected by aging is still unclear. Experiments in mice suggest that the density of DC in the skin, the expression of MHC class II and other cell surface molecules, and the capacity of DC to present antigen can all be altered with increasing age. However, only a few studies have been carried out to analyze these effects in humans.

THE ROLE OF CYTOMEGALOVIRUS (CMV) IN IMMUNOSENESCENCE

Aging is not only a major risk factor for infection, but infection itself may also contribute to the aging of the immune system, as repeated exposure to antigens directly influences immunological aging. Cytomegalovirus (CMV), a herpes virus that establishes lifelong persistence after primary infection, leads to characteristic changes in the CD4 and CD8 T-cell compartments. Comparative studies of CMV-seropositive and -seronegative aged individuals show that the age-related decrease of naïve T cells and the accumulation of CD28⁻ effector cells is strongly increased in CMV-seropositive persons (Fig. 33.4A).

The potential role of CMV and immunosenescence in healthy aging is emphasized by longitudinal studies. These studies, which enrolled individuals over the age of 86 years with a follow-up of up to 8 years, showed that a 2-year mortality can be predicted using immunological parameters summarized as 'immune risk phenotype' (IRP). The IRP is characterized by high numbers of CD8 and low numbers of CD4 T cells, leading to a CD4:CD8 ratio of <1 and a poor response of T cells after stimulation with mitogens. IRP is also associated with CMV seropositivity.[27]

In addition to the changes in the total T-cell pool, the phenotype and functional properties of CMV-specific T cells have been of particular interest. Most studies focus on CD8 T cells that are specific for the

Table 33.1 Age-related changes within the adaptive immune system

Cell type	Age-related changes
T cells	↓ Naïve T-cell counts due to involution of the thymus ↑ Memory and effector T-cell counts ↓ Diversity of the T-cell repertoire due to the accumulation of expanded clones of effector cells ↓ Expression of co-stimulatory molecules (CD28, CD27, CD40L) ↑ Expression of senescence-associated molecules (CD57, KLRG-1) ↓ Proliferative capacity ↓ T-cell signaling ↓ Activation of naïve T cells
B cells	↓ Generation of B-cell precursors ↑ Number of B1 cells ↓ Diversity of the B-cell repertoire ↓ Size and number of germinal centers ↓ Expression of co-stimulatory molecules (CD27, CD40L) ↓ Antibody affinity ↓ Isotype switch ↓ Serum antibodies specific for foreign antigens ↑ Serum antibodies specific for self-antigens ↓ Stimulation of B cells by follicular dendritic cells

Table 33.2 Age-related changes within the innate immune system

Cell type	Age-related changes
Neutrophils	↓ Oxidative burst ↓ Bactericidal activity ↓ Chemotaxis
Macrophages	↓ Phagocytic capacity ↓ Oxidative burst ↓ MHC class II expression
NK cells	↑ Number of cells ↓ Cytotoxicity ↓ Production of proinflammatory cytokines and chemokines ↓ Proliferative response to IL-2

immunodominant HLA-A2 restricted epitope NLVPMVATV, derived from the viral surface protein pp65 (aa 495-503). CMV-specific CD8 T cells of elderly donors derive from only a few clones after extensive expansion *in vivo*: representing up to several percent of the total CD8 population, they frequently dominate the repertoire (Fig. 33.4B). These cells are characterized by an effector CD28⁻CCR7⁻CD57⁺ phenotype. In contrast, a significant proportion of CMV-specific T cells from young donors exhibit a naïve (CCR7⁺CD45RA⁺) phenotype. These findings indicate that CMV infection drives CD8 T-cell differentiation and induces premature immunosenescence, with a loss of functional

CMV-specific naïve and, in the case of CD8 cells, also of memory T cells in the elderly.

It has been reasoned that the immune system is chronically fighting CMV at the expense of the capacity to respond to other pathogens. Responsiveness to new as well as to recall antigens can be impaired because the expanded CMV-specific clones fill up the immunological space, and this leads to a shrunken repertoire of other specificities. In accordance with this hypothesis, an age-related increase in Epstein–Barr virus (EBV)-specific T cells has been observed in CMV-negative donors but not in CMV-seropositive individuals.[28] Additionally, lower success rates for influenza vaccination[29] and a faster progression of AIDS[30] are associated with CMV seropositivity.

The fact that persistent infection with CMV substantially influences immunological aging raises questions about the role of other persistent pathogens, especially other herpes viruses, in immunosenescence. It has been shown that in contrast to CMV-specific T cells, EBV-specific CD8 T cells are mainly CD28⁺, indicating a lesser degree of differentiation. However, the influence of EBV on the aging immune system is not well studied, as nearly 100% of the elderly population are infected with EBV, making comparative studies of EBV-positive and -negative individuals virtually impossible. It should be taken into consideration that other persistent or recurrent pathogens might also play a role in the complex process of immunological aging.

■ VACCINATION IN THE ELDERLY ■

Vaccination is highly effective for preventing morbidity and mortality and is therefore especially required in old age. However, the protective effect of vaccination is partially lost in the elderly.[31] This holds true for

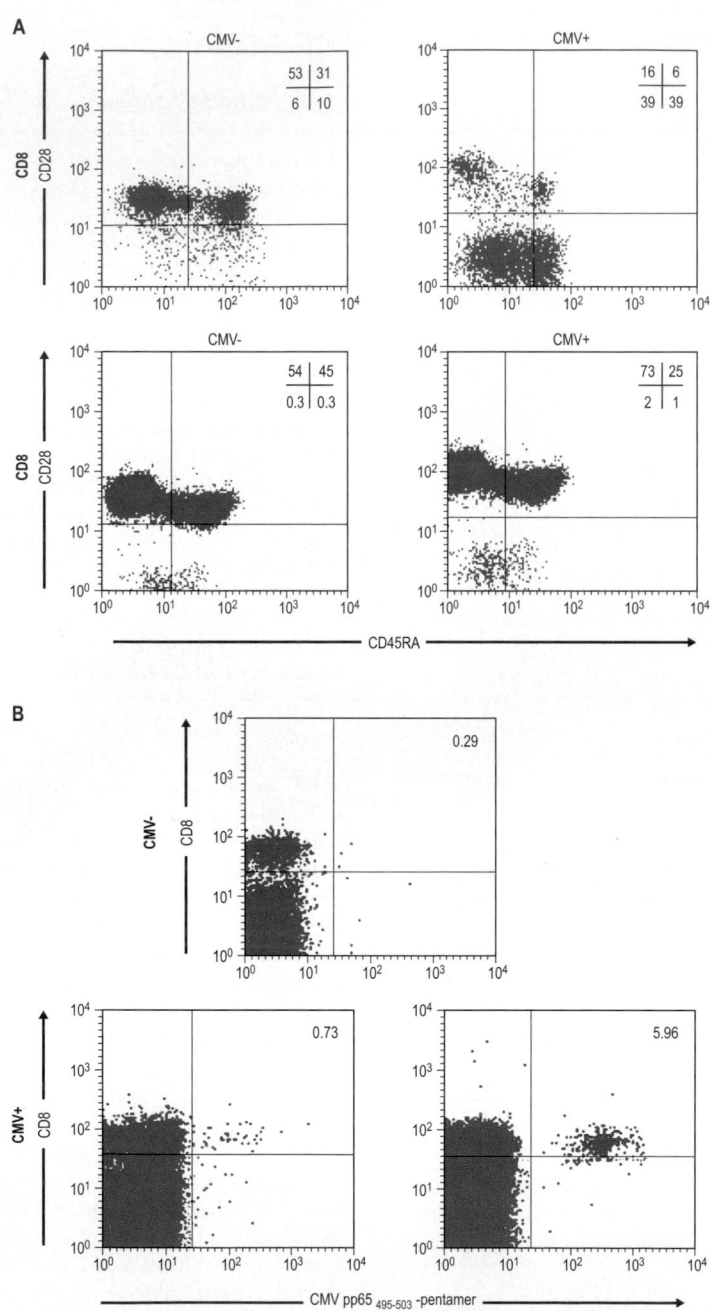

Fig. 33.4 (A) T-cell subpopulations from a CMV-seronegative and a CMV-seropositive elderly person. FACS analysis after staining with CD45RA-FITC and CD28-PE antibodies. The percentages of the respective CD8 (top panel) and CD4+ cell subsets (bottom panel) are shown in the quadrants. CD8/CD4 T cells respectively are considered as 100%. For the CD8+ population the size of the C28+CD45RA+ (naïve) and the CD28+CD45RA− (memory) T-cell populations is characteristically decreased, whereas the percentage of CD28− (effector) T cells is increased during latent CMV infection. Within the CD4+ population the percentage of naïve T cells also decreases, whereas that of memory cells increases. The percentage of CD28− effector cells is low, but still higher than in persons with a negative CMV serology. **(B)** Age-related changes in the frequency of CMV-specific CD8 T cells. FACS analysis of unstimulated CMVpp65$_{495-503}$ pentamer binding T cells in a CMV antibody-negative elderly donor and in one young and one elderly person with a positive CMV serology. In the upper right corner percentages of CMV-specific cells are shown. CD8 T cells are considered as 100%.

vaccinations against new antigens (e.g., yellow fever, rabies, new influenza strains) as well as for regularly administered vaccines (e.g., recurrent influenza strains, *Streptococcus pneumoniae*, tetanus, diphtheria, tick-borne encephalitis or hepatitis A). For instance, a meta-analysis of influenza vaccinations revealed a protection rate of only 56% in elderly persons after vaccination,[32] despite the fact that influenza is ranked among the 10 major causes of deaths in people over 65. Similarly, polysaccharide vaccines offer protection against invasive pneumococcal disease in only 65% of the elderly population.

There is thus a tremendous need to develop more immunogenic vaccines that specifically address the requirements of the aged immune system. Antigen delivery systems that convert soluble protein antigens into particulate material, which is more readily ingested by antigen-presenting cells, and immunomodulatory adjuvants can be used to overcome the age-related functional impairment of the innate immune response and to enhance the immunogenicity of subunit vaccines. In general, live-attenuated vaccines (e.g., against varicella, measles or yellow fever) are highly immunogenic by inducing long-lasting antibody production and high numbers of memory T and B cells. However, because immune function is impaired in the elderly there is an increased risk of systemic side effects when such viruses are used. For vaccination against polio it has been shown that a primary dose of live-attenuated vaccine early in life enables efficient booster with subunit vaccines in the elderly. Thus, immunization with live-attenuated virus in earlier life followed by inactivated booster vaccination in old age may be a reasonable strategy for efficient protection without the risk of complications. Shortened intervals between booster vaccinations may also be recommended for the elderly in order to sustain protective antibody titers.[33] Vaccination with peptide-loaded dendritic cells, which accelerates the generation of memory T cells, may be another possible approach for inducing a better immune response in the elderly.

STRATEGIES TO REVERSE OR DELAY IMMUNOSENESCENCE ■

THYMUS RECONSTITUTION

Thymic involution is a key event for the age-associated deterioration of immune function. For this reason, interventionist therapies aiming to rejuvenate the thymus and restore thymic output are a major challenge. Current attempts are based on the administration of IL-7[34] or growth hormone (GH) and IGF-1.[35] Administration into aged animals has shown that each of these mediators promotes thymopoiesis and stimulates thymic regrowth, but none of them alone managed to fully restore the thymic mass. Combinations of hormones (e.g. GH and IGF-1) and cytokines (e.g. IL-7) may yield greater effects on cellularity and thymic output.[36]

REDUCTION OF ANTIGENIC STIMULATION

The prevention of lifelong stimulation of the immune system with certain immunodominant antigens could reduce the accumulation of highly differentiated proinflammatory T cells that occupy immunological space and represent a basis of ubiquitous subclinical inflammatory processes. This could be achieved by eradicating chronic bacterial (e.g., in the oral cavity, the gastrointestinal tract and the urogenital tract) or viral (e.g., herpes viruses) infections. CMV is a driving force of immunosenescence, and early childhood vaccination against CMV might be one option to prevent CMV infection and CMV-associated accelerated immunosenescence. Treatment of CMV with antiviral therapies (e.g. valaciclovir) has also been discussed, but as it is unclear whether this medication leads to full eradication of the virus, long-term treatment would be needed to keep the viral load low; side-effects must also be taken into consideration.

DEPLETION OF SENESCENT T CELLS

Clonally expanded senescent T cells with specificity for antigens such as CMV compete for immunological space with T cells having specificity for other pathogens. Thus, the idea of depleting those T cells in the elderly in order to improve immune function and rejuvenate the immune system seems intriguing. However, it must be emphasized that for this approach it would be necessary to target only senescent T cells, not functionally intact T cells in earlier differentiation stages. KLRG-1 and CD57 have been suggested as surface markers for senescent T cells and could be used for sorting procedures.

CALORIC RESTRICTION

Experiments over the last few decades have shown that a 30% reduction of caloric intake supplemented with vitamins and essential elements to avoid malnutrition leads to longer life in invertebrates (*Caenorhabditis elegans*, *Drosophila melanogaster*), rodents (mice, rats, hamsters) and other vertebrates (zebra fish, birds). Caloric restriction appears to slow down many aspects of the aging process via various postulated mechanisms, including the delay of immunosenescence. In order to elucidate the possible effects of long-term caloric restriction on the human immune system, studies using rhesus macaques as a nonhuman primate model are now being conducted. Although it is still too early to determine whether caloric restriction also leads to longevity in primates, prevention of typical age-related immunological changes has been shown. Thus, dietary restriction prevents the age-related loss of naïve cells, the accumulation of memory and effector T cells, and the decrease in the proliferative capacity after antigenic stimulation.[37]

■ ACKNOWLEDGMENTS ■

We are grateful to members of the Immunology Unit, Institute for Biomedical Aging Research, who also made considerable contributions to this chapter.

■ REFERENCES ■

1. Gavazzi G, Krause KH. Ageing and infection. Lancet Infect Dis 2002; 2: 659.

2. Hartsock R, Smith E, Petty C. Normal variations with aging of the amount of hematopoietic tissue in bone marrow from the anterior iliac crest. A study made from 177 cases of sudden death examined by necropsy. Am J Clin Pathol 1965; 43: 326.

3. Allman D, Miller JP. B cell development and receptor diversity during aging. Curr Opin Immunol 2005; 17: 463.

4. Linton PJ, Dorshkind K. Age-related changes in lymphocyte development and function. Nature Immunol 2004; 5: 133.

5. Douek DC, McFarland RD, Keiser PH, et al. Changes in thymic function with age and during the treatment of HIV infection. Nature 1998; 396: 690.

6. George AJ, Ritter MA. Thymic involution with ageing: obsolescence or good housekeeping? Immunol Today 1996; 17: 267.

7. Goronzy JJ, Weyand CM. T cell development and receptor diversity during aging. Curr Opin Immunol 2005; 17: 468.

8. Effros RB, Cai Z, Linton PJ. CD8 T cells and aging. Crit Rev Immunol 2003; 23: 45.

9. Vallejo AN. CD28 extinction in human T cells: altered functions and the program of T-cell senescence. Immunol Rev 2005; 205: 158.

10. Saurwein-Teissl M, Lung TL, Marx F, et al. Lack of antibody production following immunization in old age: Association with CD8(+)CD28(-) T cell clonal expansions and an imbalance in the production of Th1 and Th2 cytokines. J Immunol 2002; 168: 5893–5899.

11. Sadighi Akha AA, Miller RA. Signal transduction in the aging immune system. Curr Opin Immunol 2005; 17: 486.

12. Larbi A, Dupuis G, Khalil A, et al. Differential role of lipid rafts in the functions of CD4+ and CD8+ human T lymphocytes with aging. Cell Signal 2006; 18: 1017.

13. Gardner EM, Murasko DM. Age-related changes in type 1 and type 2 cytokine production in humans. Biogerontology 2002; 3: 271.

14. Schwaiger S, Wolf AM, Robatscher P, et al. IL-4 producing CD8+ T cells with a CD62L++(bright) phenotype accumulate in a subgroup of older adults and are associated with the maintenance of intact humoral immunity in old age. J Immunol 2003; 170: 613–619.

15. Tsaknaridis L, Spencer L, Culbertson N, et al. Functional assay for human CD4+CD25+ Treg cells reveals an age-dependent loss of suppressive activity. J Neurosci Res 2003; 74: 296–308.

16. Johnson SA, Cambier JC. Ageing, autoimmunity and arthritis: senescence of the B cell compartment – implications for humoral immunity. Arthritis Res Ther 2004; 6: 131.

17. Weksler ME, Szabo P. The effect of age on the B-cell repertoire. J Clin Immunol 2000; 20: 240.

18. Grubeck-Loebenstein B, Wick G. The aging of the immune system. Adv Immunol 2002; 80: 243.

19. Haynes L. The effect of aging on cognate function and development of immune memory. Curr Opin Immunol 2005; 17: 476.

20. Zheng B, Han S, Takahashi Y, et al. Immunosenescence and germinal center reaction. Immunol Rev 1997; 160: 63.

21. Franceschi C, Bonafe M, Valensin S, et al. Inflamm-aging. An evolutionary perspective on immunosenescence. Ann NY Acad Sci 2000; 908: 244.

22. Blasko I, Stampfer-Kountchev M, Robatscher P, et al. How chronic inflammation can affect the brain and support the development of Alzheimer's disease in old age: the role of microglia and astrocytes. Aging Cell 2004; 3: 169.

23. Pes GM, Lio D, Carru C, et al. Association between longevity and cytokine gene polymorphisms. A study in Sardinian centenarians. Aging Clin Exp Res 2004; 16: 244.

24. Fulop T, Larbi A, Douziech N, et al. Signal transduction and functional changes in neutrophils with aging. Aging Cell 2004; 3: 217.

25. Plowden J, Renshaw-Hoelscher M, Engleman C, et al. Innate immunity in aging: impact on macrophage function. Aging Cell 2004; 3: 161.

26. Solana R, Mariani E. NK and NK/T cells in human senescence. Vaccine 2000; 18: 1613.

27. Hadrup SR, Strindhall J, Kollgaard T, et al. Longitudinal studies of clonally expanded CD8 T cells reveal a repertoire shrinkage predicting mortality and an increased number of dysfunctional cytomegalovirus-specific T cells in the very elderly. J Immunol 2006; 176: 2645.

28. Khan N, Hislop A, Gudgeon N, et al. Herpesvirus-specific CD8 T cell immunity in old age: cytomegalovirus impairs the response to a coresident EBV infection. J Immunol 2004; 173: 7481.

29. Trzonkowski P, Mysliwska J, Szmit E, et al. Association between cytomegalovirus infection, enhanced proinflammatory response and low level of anti-hemagglutinins during the anti-influenza vaccination – an impact of immunosenescence. Vaccine 2003; 21: 3826.

30. Sinicco A, Raiteri R, Sciandra M, et al. The influence of cytomegalovirus on the natural history of HIV infection: evidence of rapid course of HIV infection in HIV-positive patients infected with cytomegalovirus. Scand J Infect Dis 1997; 29: 543.

31. Grubeck-Loebenstein B, Berger P, Saurwein-Teissl M, et al. No immunity for the elderly. Nature Med 1998; 4: 870.

32. Gross PA, Hermogenes AW, Sacks HS, et al. The efficacy of influenza vaccine in elderly persons. A meta-analysis and review of the literature. Ann Intern Med 1995; 123: 518.

33. Hainz U, Jenewein B, Asch E, et al. Insufficient protection for healthy elderly adults by tetanus and TBE vaccines. Vaccine 2005; 23: 3232.

34. Aspinall R. T cell development, ageing and Interleukin-7. Mech Ageing Dev 2006; 127: 572.

35. Gray DH, Ueno T, Chidgey AP, et al. Controlling the thymic microenvironment. Curr Opin Immunol 2005; 17: 137.

36. Taub DD, Longo DL. Insights into thymic aging and regeneration. Immunol Rev 2005; 205: 72.

37. Messaoudi I, Warner J, Fischer M, et al. Delay of T cell senescence by caloric restriction in aged long-lived nonhuman primates. Proc Natl Acad Sci USA 2006; 103: 19448.

REFERENCES

Primary antibody deficiencies

Harry W. Schroeder Jr.

Primary antibody deficiency diseases are characterized by an impairment in the ability of the host to produce protective antibodies in response to hazardous antigens.[1] The impairment can be present from birth or it may be acquired at a later age. In some cases, the deficiency may either resolve or worsen with time.[2] Many of these diseases are caused by loss-of-function or altered-function mutations in genes involved in the regulation of B-cell differentiation. Others reflect mutations in the immunoglobulin genes themselves. In some of the most common conditions, a genetic predisposition has been well documented, but the underlying defect remains unclear. The typical patient presents with a history of recurrent upper respiratory or pulmonary infections and exhibits reduced serum concentrations of one or more classes of immunoglobulin (IgM, IgG, or IgA). However, patients with normal serum immunoglobulin levels may exhibit specific deficits in their ability to mount a protective response against certain antigens, and some virtually agammaglobulinemic patients can be remarkably asymptomatic. The classification of primary antibody deficiency diseases is listed in Table 34.1.

These disorders of humoral immunity can best be understood as the products of specific defects in B-cell differentiation (Chapter 8). Differentiation begins in the fetal liver, and shifts to the bone marrow in the latter stages of fetal life (Fig. 34.1). Maturing B cells are released from these primary lymphoid organs and migrate via the blood into the secondary lymphoid organs, primarily the spleen but also the lymph nodes. Contact with a polymeric cognate antigen, such as a polysaccharide, activates the B cell and allows it to differentiate into an antibody-producing plasma cell. The response to protein antigens, including toxins and viral proteins, requires T-cell help. In the germinal centers, B cells can replace the heavy (H)-chain constant domain with a downstream one, e.g., IgM to IgG_1, and they can induce a high level of mutations in the variable domains, which helps form-fit the antibody to the antigen, a process termed affinity maturation.

■ CLINICAL MANIFESTATIONS ■

Patients with antibody deficiencies most commonly present with a history of recurrent sinusitis, otitis media, bronchitis, and pneumonia. These infections typically involve encapsulated bacterial pathogens such as

---

CLINICAL PEARLS

CLINICAL MANIFESTATIONS OF ANTIBODY DEFICIENCY

>> **Recurrent bacterial infections**

>> Early in untreated disease, infections are primarily due to encapsulated pyogenic bacteria (e.g,. *Streptococcus pneumoniae* and *Haemophilus influenzae* type b)

>> Later in untreated disease, damage to mucosal surfaces engenders susceptibility to staphylococci, nontypable *H. influenzae*, and Gram-negative rods, as well

>> **Recurrent viral infections**

>> In most cases, viral infections are cleared normally, but protective immunity does not develop. For example, recurrent shingles can be a common symptom in untreated patients

>> In some cases, patients may continue to excrete virus after resolution of their clinical symptoms

>> **Increased prevalence of other immunologic disorders**

>> Paradoxic increased risk of antibody-mediated autoimmune disorders, such as idiopathic thrombocytopenia, autoimmune thyroiditis, systemic lupus erythematosus, and celiac disease

>> **Lymphoid hypertrophy**

>> **Increased risk of allergic disorders**

>> Especially among patients with immunoglobulin A deficiency

---

Streptococcus pneumoniae and *Haemophilus influenzae*. Protection against these bacteria requires production of anti-polysaccharide antibodies, which does not require T-cell help. A similar susceptibility for infection is seen among patients who are deficient in neutrophil function or in the pivotal third component of complement (C3). Thus, all three of these

Table 34.1 Primary antibody deficiencies

Disorder	Gene or locus	Chromosome
IgA deficiency (IgAD)/common variable immunodeficiency (CVID)		
IgAD/CVID (cause unknown)	MHC	6p21.3
TACI deficiency	TNFRSF 13B	17p11.2
ICOS deficiency	ICOS	2q33
BAFF-R	TNFRSF13C	22q13.1-q13.31
CD19 deficiency	CD19	16p11.2
Transient hypogammaglobulinemia of infancy (THI)		
X-linked agammaglobulinemia	BTK	Xq21.3-q22
X-linked agammaglobulinemia with growth hormone deficiency	BTK	Xq21.3-q22
Hyper-IgM syndrome		
X-linked hyper-IgM syndrome (XHIGM)	HIGM1	Xq26
Activation-induced cytidine deaminase (AID) deficiency	HIGM2	12p13
CD40 deficiency	HIGM3	20q12-q13.2
Uracil-DNA glycosylase (UNG) deficiency	HIGM5	12q23-q24.1
XHM with ectodermal dysplasia (XHM-ED)	IKBKG, NEMO	Xq28
Autosomal agammaglobulinemia		
Immunoglobulin-associated beta (Igβ) deficiency	CD79B	17q23
Immunoglobulin μ H-chain deficiencies	IGHG1	14q32.33
BLNK deficiency	BLNK	10q23.2
Surrogate light-chain deficiency	IGLL1	22q11.21
LRRC8 truncation	LRRC8	9q34.13
Selective immunoglobulin G subclass deficiencies		
Immunoglobulin γ H-chain deficiencies	IGHG1	14q32.33
Selective κ light-chain deficiency	IGKC	2p11.2
Selective λ light-chain deficiency		
Antibody deficiency with normal serum immunoglobulin levels		
Vκ A2 deficiency	IGKV2D-29	2p11.2

arms of the host defense system should be evaluated in patients who suffer with recurrent bacterial infections.

The clinical course of uncomplicated primary infections with viruses such as varicella-zoster or mumps does not differ significantly from that of the normal host. However, antibody-deficient patients have difficulty generating long-lasting immunity, thus chickenpox may repeatedly recur as shingles. This suggests that, while T cells are sufficient to control established viral infections, antibodies function best to limit the initial dissemination of virus and prevent re-infection. There are exceptions to this general rule. Hypogammaglobulinemic patients can have difficulty clearing hepatitis B virus from the circulation, poliovirus from the gut, and enterovirus from the brain, leading to progressive and sometimes fatal outcomes.

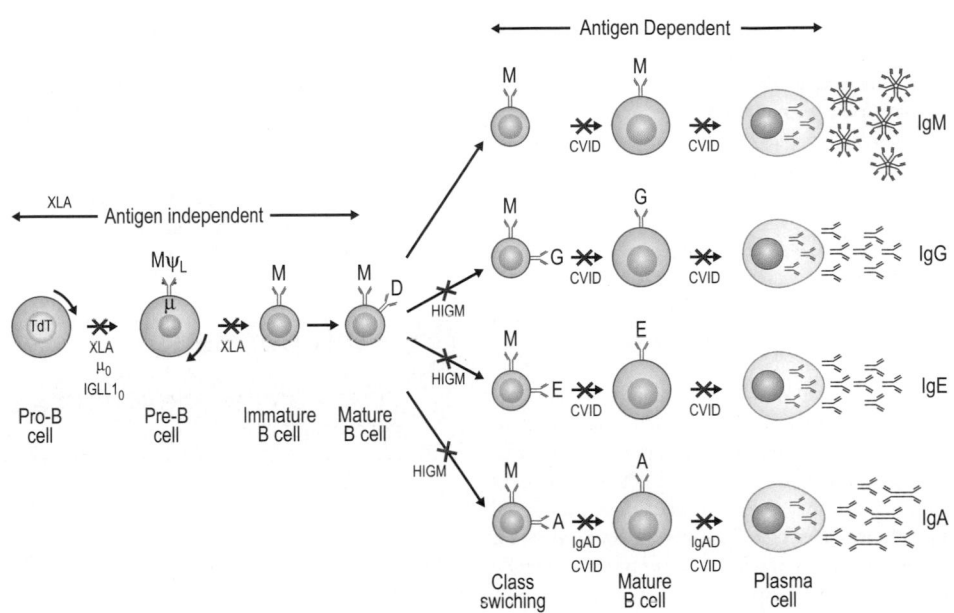

Fig. 34.1 Defects in B-cell development can lead to humoral immune deficiency. Failure to generate a functional antibody receptor (μ_0, mu heavy-chain deficiency; $\lambda 5_0$ surrogate light-chain $\lambda 5$, $\lambda 14.1$ deficiency) or to transmit signals through Bruton's tyrosine kinase (X-linked agammaglobulinemia (XLA)) can prevent or limit B-cell production. Failure to engage in proper cognate interactions with T cells (X-linked hyper-IgM syndrome (X-HIGM), CD40 deficiency) or disruptions in the genes that permit class switch recombination (activation-induced cytidine deaminase (AID), uracil-DNA glycosylase (UNG)) can prevent class switching and production of immunoglobulin G (IgG), IgA or IgE. A selective or generalized failure to progress from the immature B-cell stage to the plasma cell stage can lead to IgA deficiency (IgAD) or common variable immunodeficiency (CVID).

Because sinopulmonary infections are also commonly seen in normal infants and children, in allergic individuals, in smokers, and in patients with other diseases such as cystic fibrosis, the threshold for an extensive evaluation for immunodeficiency can be a matter of clinical judgment. However, two or more episodes of bacterial pneumonia within a 5-year period, unexplained bronchiectasis, *Haemophilus influenzae* meningitis in an older child or adult, chronic otitis media in an adult, recurrent intestinal infections and diarrhea due to *Giardia lamblia*, or a family history of immunodeficiency all warrant evaluation.

The purest forms of antibody deficiency result from mutations that allow VDJ rearrangement but prevent the expression or function of the pre-B-cell receptor. For example, a function-loss mutation of the μ heavy chain or components of the surrogate light chain (VpreB, $\lambda 14.1(\lambda 5)$) will affect only the B-cell lineage. However, these rare immune deficiencies are the exception, because most of the diseases associated with primary antibody deficiency involve more than one cell lineage. For example, *X-linked agammaglobulinemia* (XLA) is the product of loss-of-function mutations in Bruton's tyrosine kinase (*BTK)*, a key component of the BCR signal transduction pathway. BTK is also expressed in neutrophils, and under stressful conditions XLA patients have developed recurrent neutropenia. Patients with *X-linked hyper-IgM syndrome* (HIGM1) may also exhibit T-cell dysfunction, placing them at risk for infection with *Pneumocystis jiroveci*. Immune deficiency also appears to place patients at risk for autoimmunity, which is increased among patients with *IgA deficiency* (IgAD), *common variable immunodeficiency* (CVID), and hyper-IgM syndrome.

KEY CONCEPTS

HYPOGAMMAGLOBULINEMIA AND ANTIBODY DEFICIENCY

>> The genetic mutations that underlie most primary antibody deficiencies tend to affect genes that play key roles in the regulation of lymphocyte differentiation, or in the generation of the antibody repertoire

>> Clinically significant antibody deficiency is not synonymous with laboratory hypogammaglobulinemia

>> Serum immunoglobulin concentrations vary widely with age

>> Serum immunoglobulin levels vary with exposure to drugs (e.g., steroids), infectious agents, and other environmental stressors

>> A complete absence of immunoglobulin G subclasses resulting from homozygous deletions of heavy-chain genes has been observed in healthy individuals

>> Absence of a specific Vκ gene segment has been associated with an increased risk of *Haemophilus influenzae* infection in spite of normal serum immunoglobulin levels

Clinical manifestations of the primary immunodeficiency will also be heavily influenced by the patient's medical history. Patients with a delayed diagnosis or in situations wherein their infections have not been treated aggressively may suffer permanent damage to the respiratory or gastrointestinal mucosa, creating susceptibility to nontypable *H. influenzae*, staphylococci, and enteric bacteria as well.

PRINCIPLES OF DIAGNOSIS AND TREATMENT

DIAGNOSTIC TESTS AND THEIR INTERPRETATION

Laboratory testing for the diagnosis of immunodeficiency can be a time-intensive and expensive proposition. Table 34.2 illustrates four levels of testing complexity and when such testing might commonly be undertaken. In general, testing should be performed when the patient has a history of repeated infections that exceeds expectations for normal individuals, when an opportunistic pathogen or one of a low virulence is responsible for an infection, when a diagnosis of a disorder frequently associated with immunodeficiency has been made, or when a family history of immunodeficiency has been obtained.

Determination of serum immunoglobulin concentrations (IgM, IgG, and IgA), testing complement (50% hemolytic power of serum (CH_{50}) and complement components C3, and C4), a complete blood count (CBC), and an erythrocyte sedimentation rate (ESR) are among the most cost-effective screening tests available. Lymphopenia is found most often in disorders that affect the production or function of T cells (Chapter 35), but can also occur in patients with CVID. Congenital absence of an individual complement component will result in total absence of measurable complement-mediated hemolysis (Chapter 20). The ESR is often, although not always, elevated in individuals with inflammatory disorders and can be useful in the evaluation of patients with a questionable or unclear history of recurrent or chronic infection.

KEY CONCEPTS

TEST FOR IMMUNE FUNCTION SHOULD BE PERFORMED

>> When the patient's history suggests a rate or severity of infection that exceeds normal expectations

>> When the organism responsible for infection is of low virulence or is considered to be an opportunistic pathogen

>> When there is a diagnosis of a genetic syndrome or disorder associated with immune deficiency either in the patient or in the patient's family

Table 34.2 Laboratory diagnosis of primary antibody deficiency

Level	Test	Application (s)
I	Complete blood count with differential Complement (CH_{50}, C3, C4) Erythrocyte sedimentation rate Quantitative serum IgM, IgG, and IgA levels	Primary screening tests
II	B-cell functional evaluation Quantitative IgG subclasses Natural or commonly acquired antibodies (isohemagglutinins, rubella, rubeola, tetanus) Response to immunization T-cell-dependent antigens (tetanus) T-cell-independent antigens (unconjugated pneumococcal vaccine, unconjugated *Haemophilus influenzae* B vaccine)	Level I normal but history suggests antibody deficiency Better definition of a level I defect
III	Quantification of blood T- and B-cell subpopulations by immunofluoresence assays using monoclonal antibody markers T cells: CD3, CD4, CD8 B cells: CD19, CD20, CD21, Ig (μ, δ, κ, λ),	Panhypogammaglobulinemia or severely low IgM and IgA
IV	Disease-specific analysis Gene expression Gene sequencing	Gene-specific diagnosis Genetic counseling

Interpretation of the significance of the quantitative immunoglobulin determinations requires appreciation of age-related changes in immunoglobulin concentrations (Fig. 34.2).[3–6] At the end of the second trimester of pregnancy, there is active transport of IgG across the placental barrier. At birth the infant's serum IgG concentration is typically 20–25% higher than that of the mother. Catabolism of maternal IgG coupled with the slow development of endogenous antibody function leads to a physiologic nadir of serum IgG in infants 4–6 months of age. In normal infants, this loss of maternal protection is often associated with the first appearance of otitis media or bronchitis. Thus, the onset of sinopulmonary infections within the first 3 months of age should also raise the index of suspicion for immunodeficiency in the mother. After age 6 months, maternally derived IgG has largely been lost, and IgG antibodies specific for diphtheria or tetanus become useful functional measures.

IgM is the first isotype to reach young adult levels, followed by total IgG and then IgA. This physiologic delay in the production of serum IgA can complicate the diagnosis of IgA deficiency in infants and young children. Serum immunoglobulin concentrations in healthy adults tend to remain remarkably constant, but can increase dramatically in response to infection and can decline in response to immunosuppressive agents, such as corticosteroid administration. With increasing age, serum immunoglobulin concentration may continue to rise.[5] The physiologic significance of this increase in the elderly is unclear, although in some cases it reflects an accumulation of expanded B-cell clones or monoclonal gammopathies (Chapter 78).

The common laboratory practice of defining the lower range of normal for serum immunoglobulin levels as two standard deviations below the age-adjusted mean carries with it the risk of falsely labeling otherwise normal patients immunodeficient. Immunoglobulin levels vary widely with environmental exposure and normal biologic variation is much broader than that defined by the mean of the population. Symptomatic patients with IgA deficiency may demonstrate normal total IgG levels, but have sufficient IgG_1 levels that mask deficiencies of IgG_2 and IgG_4. Patients with this compound immune deficiency may benefit from more aggressive therapy; thus quantitative measurements of all four IgG subclasses IgG_1, IgG_2, IgG_3, and IgG_4 can be useful in fully defining the extent of humoral immune deficiency. Among patients with borderline serum IgG levels, tests to evaluate the host's ability to produce functional specific antibody should be performed prior to making a decision to institute replacement therapy with human immunoglobulin, especially among patients receiving corticosteroids which can lower total IgG levels while preserving function.

The most commonly employed tests include measurement of isohemagglutinins (naturally occurring IgM antibodies to the polysaccharide antigens that define the ABO blood-type system on red blood cells), antibodies to polysaccharide antigens after immunization (e.g., Pneumovax) or unconjugated *H. influenzae* B vaccine, and antibody responses to protein antigens after immunization (e.g., tetanus or diphtheria toxoids). IgM is made by the newborn, and most infants can generate isohemagglutinins, making determination of anti-A and anti-B titers a useful measurement of B-cell function even in infants. In older children and adults, isohemagglutinin titers of less than 1:8 are considered significant.[7] Serum for specific antibody titers should be obtained before and 3–4 weeks after immunization. The paired sera should be assayed simultaneously to avoid confusion that may result from

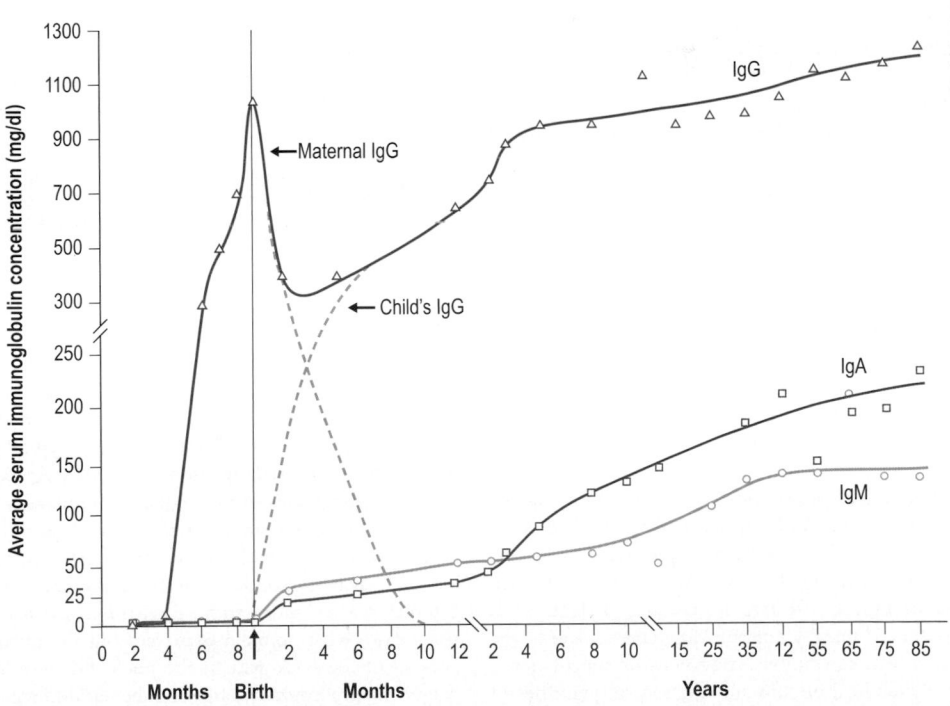

Fig. 34.2 Age-related changes in the serum concentration of immunoglobulins. Shown are average serum immunoglobulin concentrations of the major isotypes as a function of age.[5, 6]

PRINCIPLES OF DIAGNOSIS AND TREATMENT

single-tube dilution differences at the time the assay is performed. As a general rule, a high baseline titer or a fourfold or greater rise in a specific titer in individuals with a low baseline titer confirms that a specific humoral response is intact. One caveat: responses to immunization with unconjugated pneumococcal polysaccharide vaccines are not reliable measures of age-appropriate B-cell function until after the age of 2 years. The development of conjugated polysaccharide vaccines complicates analysis for children who have received such a vaccine, but information can still be gleaned from study of responses to polysaccharide antigens present only in multivalent unconjugated vaccines.

Disorders of the gastrointestinal tract or kidneys that result in protein loss through the stool or urine precipitate the selective loss of IgG because of its relatively low molecular weight and slow turnover compared with other isotypes.

An elevated IgE level may support a suspicion of allergy as an underlying explanation of sinopulmonary symptoms. Serum IgE concentrations are often elevated in patients with IgA deficiency. Extreme elevations of IgE suggest the *hyper-IgE syndrome*.

Enumeration of B cells and of T cells should be performed for any individual who has severe panhypogammaglobulinemia. The most widely used method of demonstrating B cells relies on immunofluorescent labeling of surface CD19, which is restricted in expression to mature B cells. Because an infant may have serum IgG of maternal origin for the first several months of life, the determination of the number of circulating B cells is the single most useful test in making the presumptive diagnosis of XLA, a disorder in which pre-B cells in the bone marrow fail to develop to cells of mature phenotype. Absence of circulating B cells also characterizes the *immunodeficiency associated with thymoma* in adults, whereas adults with *chronic lymphocytic leukemia* may have hypogammaglobulinemia with an overabundance of circulating B cells that typically express CD5, a common T-cell antigen.

HIGM1 represents the product of a loss-of-function mutation of the *CD154 (CD40L)* gene. CD154, a surface antigen found on activated T cells, binds CD40 on B cells to facilitate class switching, survival, and proliferation (Chapter 9). A fluorescent labeled CD40 fusion protein can be used to evaluate the expression of functional CD154 on T cells by flow cytometry. XLA reflects a loss-of-function mutation of *BTK*. As typical for previously lethal X-linked disorders, a high percentage of cases represent new mutations. Confirmation of the diagnosis, carrier detection, and prenatal diagnosis often depend on a molecular or sequence analysis of the gene in question.

REPLACEMENT THERAPY WITH HUMAN IMMUNOGLOBULIN

There are a number of commercial preparations of human immunoglobulin that are approved by the Food and Drug Administration and available in the USA (Chapter 85). No commercial preparations in this country are available to supplement IgM or IgA. All commercial human immunoglobulin preparations are effective in treating patients with immunodeficiency disorders. Clinically relevant differences relate to the route of administration, which can be by intravenous or subcutaneous means, to the method of stabilization and storage, and to quantities of contaminating serum IgA in the preparations. Low IgA content is important for those rare individuals with immunodeficiency and absent IgA who can manufacture IgG or IgE antibodies directed against IgA

and are thus at risk for anaphylactic reactions upon infusion of IgA-containing blood products.[8]

Immunoglobulin replacement therapy is not indicated for patients whose immune deficiency is limited to the selective absence of IgA. Indeed, selective IgA deficiency has long been viewed as a relative contraindication for immunoglobulin replacement because of the risk of anaphylaxis upon receipt of IgA-containing products, even though such reactions are extremely rare. Immunoglobulin replacement therapy has been found to be beneficial in patients with a combined deficit of IgA and IgG subclasses who exhibit impaired antibody responses to carbohydrate antigens.

The goal of immunoglobulin replacement is to provide sufficient concentrations of functional antibodies to prevent disease, not to achieve a target IgG level in the serum. Specific approaches to and protocols for immunoglobulin replacement therapy have been extensively evaluated by the American Academy of Allergy, Asthma, and Immunology[9] and are described in detail in Chapter 85. The only indication for immunoglobulin replacement in a patient with immunodeficiency is severe impairment of the ability to produce functional antibody. Such impairment exists in primary immunodeficiency diseases associated with low levels of all five isotypes of immunoglobulin, such as XLA, CVID, HIGM, and *severe combined immunodeficiency* (Chapter 35). Patients with normal or near-normal levels of IgG but a documented inability to produce specific antibodies after immunization are also candidates for intravenous immunoglobulin therapy if they suffer with significant infections. This is true for certain cases of IgG subclass deficiency such as those associated with compound IgA, IgG$_2$, and IgG$_4$ deficiency, for boys with Wiskott–Aldrich syndrome, and for patients with ataxia-telangiectasia. Since most patients with transient hypogammaglobulinemia of infancy can produce normal amounts of specific antibodies after immunization despite having a low total serum IgG, they are not usually candidates for immunoglobulin replacement. Intravenous immunoglobulin is unlikely to be beneficial in selective IgA deficiency or selective IgG$_4$ deficiency.[9]

■ X-LINKED AGAMMAGLOBULINEMIA ■

DIAGNOSIS

XLA, also known as Bruton agammaglobulinemia, is the prototypic humoral immunodeficiency.[10] Function-loss mutations in *BTK* lead to a block in B-cell maturation, a near-total absence of B cells in the periphery, and panhypogammaglobulinemia. Due to the transplacental transfer of maternal immunoglobulin, affected boys typically do not begin to suffer recurrent pyogenic infections until after age 6 months. The normal delay in endogenous immunoglobulin production and the presence of maternal IgG require that testing of infants known or suspected to have XLA should begin with examination of the number of B cells in the blood. Deficient expression of BTK protein can be detected by flow cytometry, a technique that can also be used for carrier detection. For those cases where protein is present but the phenotype suggests XLA, analysis of the *BTK* gene at the nucleotide level remains the definitive diagnostic procedure. A large number of different mutations have been found and collected into a disease-specific database known as BTKbase (http://bioinf.uta.fi/BTKbase). As with most X-linked lethal diseases, approximately one-third of sporadic cases are due to *de novo* mutations and diagnosis may require individual mutation analysis. There can be significant variation in the manifestations of the disease in any given family member, thus a paucity of symptoms should not prevent diagnostic evaluation.

CLINICAL MANIFESTATIONS

Although patients begin to suffer recurrent infections by age 1 year, with antibiotics and good hygiene it is not uncommon to delay suspicion of the diagnosis well into mid-childhood. Indeed, diagnoses have been made in older adults, including aged male relatives of affected probands. Recurrent upper and lower respiratory tract infections are common, including otitis media, sinusitis, bronchitis, and pneumonia. Untreated, these infections may lead to bronchiectasis (Fig. 34.3), pulmonary failure, and death at an early age. The infections are typically due to pyogenic encapsulated bacteria, including *Streptococcus pneumoniae*, *Haemophilus influenzae*, *Staphylococcus aureus*, and *Pseudomonas* species. Diarrhea due to *Giardia lamblia* is also common, although less so than in CVID. Systemic infections include bacterial sepsis, meningitis, osteomyelitis, and septic arthritis. *Mycoplasma* and *Chlamydia* infections of the urogenital tract may lead to epididymitis, prostatitis, and urethral strictures. Skin infections include cellulitis, boils, and impetigo.

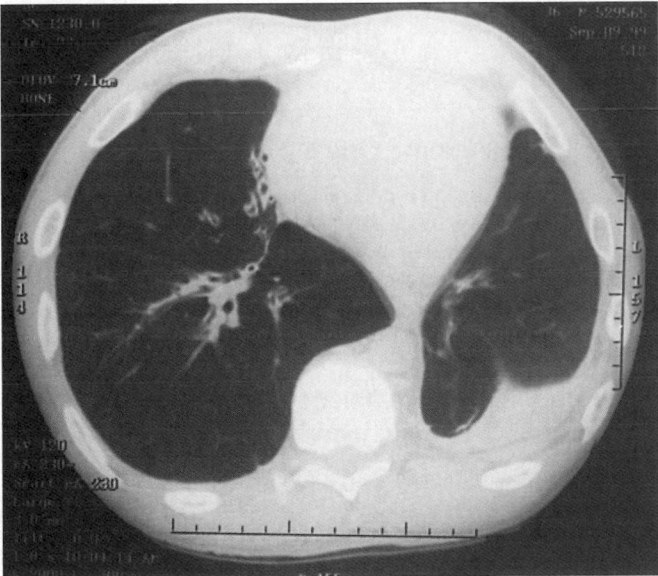

Fig. 34.3 A computed tomographic scan with contrast demonstrates bronchiectasis, bronchitis, and emphysema in the lungs of a 36-year-old man with X-linked agammaglobulinemia (XLA). Due to a left lower-lobe lobectomy, the mediastinum has shifted to the left. As a result of bronchiectatic scarring, the diameter of the bronchi in the right lung is greater than the diameter of the corresponding blood vessels, and the bronchi remain dilated in the periphery. Bronchial plugs can be seen filling some of the bronchi on the right. Finally, due to emphysema, the right upper lobe demonstrates greater radiolucency. In addition to suffering from XLA, this patient has a 30-pack-year history of smoking, which has exacerbated his clinical condition.

Although patients with XLA can resolve most viral infections, they are unusually sensitive to infections with enteroviruses, including echovirus, coxsackievirus, and poliovirus. Patients with XLA can develop paralytic poliomyelitis after vaccination with live virus. Echovirus and coxsackievirus infections may involve multiple organs, with the patients going on to develop chronic meningoencephalitis, dermatomyositis, and/or hepatitis.

Untreated patients often complain of arthritis affecting the large joints. This appears to have an infectious etiology, because the arthritis typically resolves with immunoglobulin replacement therapy. Enterovirus and *Mycoplasma* have been identified in the affected joints of these patients.

Infections with opportunistic organisms, such as tuberculosis, histoplasmosis and *Pneumocystis jiroveci*, and malignancies are rare, likely reflecting intact cell-mediated immunity.

ORIGIN AND PATHOGENESIS

BTK belongs to a subfamily of the Src cytoplasmic protein-tyrosine kinases. It includes five distinct domains: a pleckstrin homology domain (PH), a Tec homology (TH) domain, a Src homology 3 (SH3) domain, a SH2 domain, and a SH1 domain. The latter is also referred to as the catalytic, or kinase, domain. BTK is phosphorylated following activation of the B-cell receptor (BCR). Its precise role in the BCR activation pathway remains elusive; however it is now clear that BTK plays a critical role in the proliferation, development, differentiation, survival, and apoptosis of B-lineage cells. Individuals with XLA begin with normal numbers of early B-lineage progenitors in their bone marrow. These B-cell progenitors express the expected markers of B differentiation, including terminal deoxyribonucleotide transferase (TdT), CD19, and CD10. There is, however, a relative deficiency of cells containing cytoplasmic μ heavy chains in the bone marrow. Development of cells beyond the pre-B stage is even more severely impaired. Those cells that make it through the gauntlet can produce antigen-specific antibodies. Although in low numbers, the presence of these B cells in lymphoid tissues enables XLA patients to express endogenous immunoglobulin, class switch, and even suffer allergic reactions. Hypogammaglobulinemia thus appears to result from inadequate rather than absent B-cell numbers.

Patients have been described with an X-linked recessive form of agammaglobulinemia that is associated with growth hormone deficiency. Genetic analysis of the *BTK* gene in one such patient identified a frameshift mutation leading to a premature stop codon and the loss of carboxy-terminal amino acids.[11]

TREATMENT AND PROGNOSIS

The primary goal of therapy is to prevent damage to the lungs. Human immunoglobulin replacement therapy should be started as soon as the diagnosis is made. Patients treated with quantities (0.4–0.6 g/kg every 3–4 weeks) of intravenous immunoglobulin sufficient to achieve trough levels of > 500 mg/dl suffer few lower respiratory tract infections. However, these patients remain at risk for viral infections, including enteroviral meningoencephalitis. Since mucosal immunoglobulin cannot be replaced, the patients also remain at risk for recurrent upper respiratory infections, which may require prophylactic antibiotic therapy. Immunoglobulin-treated patients may lead normal lives without concern about exposure to infectious agents in childcare settings or classrooms. Immunizations of any type are unnecessary because the monthly replacement therapy will provide passive specific antibody. Since patients are unable to mount antibody responses and vaccines carry some risk of untoward side effects, they are relatively contraindicated.

An XLA patient who develops symptoms of enteroviral central nervous system or neuromuscular infection should have appropriate culture of the involved organ system. Cerebrospinal fluid culture and analysis for cells and protein should be performed and a muscle biopsy for culture should be considered if virus is not recoverable from stool or cerebrospinal fluid. Although there are no clear guidelines for managing patients with chronic enteroviral infections, immunoglobulin therapy should be accelerated for at least several weeks and higher doses maintained until symptoms cease and the virus can no longer be detected.

AUTOSOMAL AGAMMAGLOBULINEMIA

Mutations in genes whose products are required for B-cell differentiation can produce a selective block in B-cell development nearly indistinguishable from XLA.[12] Expression of the pre-B-cell receptor is a key step in the maturation of the pre-B cell. Function-loss mutations in any one of the genes that code for components of the pre-BCR can inhibit pre-B-cell development, blocking B-cell production. An absence of B cells has been reported for patients with function-loss mutations in both alleles of the the mu heavy chain region (μ_0), λ-like surrogate light chain (IGLL1), or immunoglobulin-associated beta chain (Igβ). Patients with homozygous mutations in the adaptor B-cell linker protein (BLNK), a key component of the signaling pathway for the pre-BCR, exhibit an absence of B cells and agammaglobulinemia. An absence of B cells has also been reported in a patient with a truncation of LRRC8, a gene of unknown function that is expressed in progenitor B-cell patients. In this case, the patient was heterozygous for the molecular defect. Diagnosis in each of these cases requires gene mutation analysis. Treatment follows the same guidelines given for XLA.

HYPER-IGM SYNDROME

DIAGNOSIS

Patients with the hyper-IgM syndrome exhibit markedly reduced serum concentrations of IgG, IgA, and IgE with normal to elevated levels of IgM and normal numbers of circulating B cells.[13] The altered distribution of immunoglobulin isotypes reflects a block in the ability of B lymphocytes to switch from IgM to the other isotypes. Increased IgM reflects polyclonal expansion of IgM synthesis in response to infection. HIGM patients suffer the same infections with encapsulated bacteria common to all patients with antibody deficiency. The HIGM phenotype can be either inherited or acquired. Both X-linked and autosomal recessive forms of the disease have been identified. HIGM can also develop in association with neoplasia[14] or congenital rubella.

Hyper-IgM syndrome type 1

Class switch recombination is a multistep process that requires exquisite coordination between the B cell and its cognate helper T cell. A key step in the initiation of the process is the binding of constitutively expressed CD40 on the B cell to its ligand, CD40L (CD154), which is expressed on activated T cells. The most common X form of the disease, HIGM1, results from loss-of-function mutations in *CD154*.

Hyper-IgM syndrome type 2 (HIGM2)

Activation-induced cytidine deaminase (AID), a member of the cytidine deaminase family, is required for class switch recombination between immunoglobulin H-chain constant domains and for somatic hypermutation of the immunoglobulin V domains (Chapter 4). AID is expressed only in activated B cells. Function-loss mutations on both *AID* alleles yield a hyper-IgM syndrome.

Hyper-IgM syndrome type 3 (HIGM3)

The cognate partner for CD40L (CD154) is the CD40 gene, which is located on an autosome (20q12-q13.2). HIGM3 patients with function-loss mutations on both alleles of the *CD40* gene present with a phenotype indistinguishable from HIGM1, with the exception that, as an autosomal recessive condition, females and males are equivalently affected.

Hyper-IgM syndrome type 4 (HIGM4)

Patients presenting with an HIGM-like phenotype, but lacking demonstrable mutations in genes previously associated with HIGM, such as *CD40*, *CD154*, *NEMO*, *AID*, and *UNG*, have been grouped by some immunologists into a category termed HIGM4.[15]

Hyper-IgM syndrome type 5 (HIGM5)

AID acts by deaminating cytidine nucleotides in DNA, leaving a uracil nucleotide in its place. Uracil-DNA glycosylase (UNG) can remove the uracil, permitting normal or error-prone repair. Patients with function-loss mutations on both alleles of the *UNG* gene have presented with a history of bacterial infections, hyperplasia, increased serum IgM levels, and low IgG and IgA.

Hyper-IgM immunodeficiency, X-linked, with ectodermal dysplasia, hypohidrotic (XHM-ED)

The nuclear factor kappaB (NF-κB) essential modulator (NEMO) plays a key role in the CD40 signal transduction pathway. *NEMO* is located on the X-chromosome and its protein product also influences ectodermal development. In addition to hypogammaglobulinemia, XHM-ED patients with mutations in *NEMO* may also present with conical teeth, an absence of eccrine sweat glands, and a paucity of hair follicles.

CLINICAL MANIFESTATIONS

CD40–CD154 axis (HIGM1, HIGM3, and XHM-ED)

The majority of patients with HIGM have inherited disruptions in the CD40–CD154 axis. The spectrum of disease in these patients has been well characterized. Recurrent upper and lower respiratory tract infections are the most common clinical complaint. Patients may also exhibit recurrent neutropenia with oral ulcers and perirectal abscesses and opportunistic infections with *Pneumocystis jiroveci, Toxoplasma gondii,* or *Cryptosporidium* cholangitis. Autoimmunity is observed in approximately 20% of patients, and lymph nodes and spleen are deprived of germinal centers. These features signal a compromise in cell-mediated immunity as well as the characteristic flaw in antibody production.

Without prophylaxis, one-third of patients develop *P. jiroveci* (previously *carinii*) pneumonia (PCP), which can be the presenting complaint in affected infants. These patients are also at risk for serious infections with cytomegalovirus (CMV), adenovirus, *Cryptococcus neoformans,* or mycobacteria.

Chronic diarrhea occurs in more than half of the patients. Organisms include *Cryptosporidium, Giardia lamblia, Salmonella,* and *Entamoeba histolytica.* One-quarter may require total parenteral nutrition due to diarrhea or to perirectal abscesses. Oral ulcers, gingivitis, and perirectal ulcers are associated with neutropenia, which may occur chronically or intermittently in up to two-thirds of the patients. One-fifth of the patients develop sclerosing cholangitis that can lead to hepatic failure. Cryptosporidiosis is present in half of these patients. Infections with hepatitis B and C are associated with exposure to blood products.

Although originally distinguished by the high level of serum IgM, IgM levels are often normal in affected individuals. IgG is low in all patients. IgA and IgE are usually low, but can be normal or even elevated in one-tenth of the population. B- and T-cell counts are within the normal range in more than 90% of the patients, and depressed in the rest.

Lymphoid hyperplasia is a common finding in CD40–CD154 axis patients with active infections. Individual nodes may become extremely large and some patients develop splenomegaly. Hilar adenopathy causes a diagnostic dilemma, as the risk of lymphoma is increased in HIGM. Although the lymphoid tissue is usually histologically abnormal, reactive processes are far more common than malignancy. Plasma cells may be abundant or sparse. Primary follicles are poorly developed. The most characteristic abnormality is the absence of germinal centers. Nodular lymphoid hyperplasia of the intestine is frequent and may be accompanied by malabsorption and protein-losing enteropathy. Diffuse lymphoid infiltration of various organs and tissues may also occur.

AID–UNG axis (HIGM2 and HIGM5)

Infected AID–UNG-deficient patients may present with giant germinal centers filled with highly proliferating B cells, presumably due to intense antigen stimulation. Approximately 25% of patients present with evidence of autoimmunity, which may manifest as hemolytic anemia, thrombocytopenia, or autoimmune hepatitis. Autoantibodies in these patients are of the IgM isotype. Unlike deficiencies of the CD40–CD154 axis, cell-mediated immunity is unaffected.

ORIGIN AND PATHOGENESIS

CD40–CD154 axis (HIGM1, HIGM3, and XHM-ED)

CD154 is a type II transmembrane protein belonging to the tumor necrosis factor (TNF) family that is predominantly expressed on mature, activated CD4 T cells. Its expression peaks at 6–8 hours post-activation and then falls to resting levels by 24–48 hours. CD154 is also expressed

on CD4 thymocytes, activated CD8 T cells, natural killer cells, monocytes, basophils, mast cells, activated eosinophils, and activated platelets. Newborn T cells are deficient in CD154 expression, although they can be induced to express the antigen if strongly stimulated.

CD40 is a member of the TNF receptor superfamily. It is constitutively expressed on pro-B, pre-B, and mature B cells. CD40 is also expressed on interdigitating cells, follicular dendritic cells, thymic epithelial cells, monocytes, platelets, and some carcinomas.

Engagement of CD40 on the B-cell surface with activated T cells that express CD154 and Fas ligand (CD95L or FasL) leads to the upregulation of Fas (CD95) on the B cell. If the B cell has concomitantly bound its cognate antigen and engaged the B-cell receptor signaling pathway, it becomes resistant to Fas-mediated apoptosis and expresses CD80/CD86 on the cell surface. The activated B cell can then engage CD28 on the T-cell surface and trigger the T cell to secrete its cytokines. If the B cell fails to engage its BCR, the Fas pathway predominates and the B cell is eliminated. With proper activation of the CD40–CD154 pathway, exposure to interleukin-2 (IL-2) and IL-10 induces production of IgM, IgG_1, and IgA; exposure to IL-4 induces production of IgG_4 and IgE. This change in immunoglobulin isotype reflects both induction of switching and the enhanced survival and proliferation of the B cell. In the absence of CD154, B cells can express IgM, but have difficulty switching and are likely to undergo apoptosis rather than proliferate in response to antigen.

CD40–CD154 interactions between CD154+ T cells and CD40+ macrophages lead to enhanced production of IL-12, which then stimulates T cells to release interferon-γ. Activation of this pathway appears necessary for the defense against *Pneumocystis jiroveci* and other opportunistic organisms. Its absence likely contributes to cell-mediated immune deficiency.

TREATMENT AND PROGNOSIS

The availability of human immunoglobulin replacement therapy has greatly improved the quality of life in HIGM. Adequate replacement can result in the reduction of serum IgM concentrations, prevention of infections with encapsulated bacteria, resumption of growth, and the gradual resolution of splenomegaly and lymphoid hyperplasia. Neutropenia persists but may be clinically silent.

However, in spite of the improvement granted by immunoglobulin replacement, the prognosis of patients with defects in the CD40–CD154 axis remains guarded. Among the patients in the European Registry,[16] one-quarter of HIGM1 patients died before the age of 25. These deaths were primarily the result of opportunistic infections, including PCP, cholangitis, CMV, mycobacterial infections, and cirrhosis secondary to hepatitis. Prophylaxis with trimethoprim-sulfamethoxazole can significantly reduce the risk of PCP. There is also an increased incidence of carcinomas of the liver, pancreas, and biliary tree, and perirectal abscesses can prove difficult to manage. Regular monitoring of gastrointestinal manifestations and management of neutropenia are mandatory. Bone marrow transplantation is a viable option for patients who fail to respond to supportive therapy.

■ IGA DEFICIENCY ■

Selective IgAD, selective IgG subclass deficiencies, CVID, and a syndrome of recurrent sinopulmonary infections (RESPI) with normal serum immunoglobulin levels appear to share an overlapping set of gene defects.[1, 17–20] Clinically, these disorders are marked by an increased susceptibility to sinopulmonary infections with encapsulated bacteria. IgAD and CVID feature similar B-cell differentiation arrests, but differ in the extent of immunoglobulin deficits. The correlation between serum immunoglobulin levels and severity of infection is not absolute. Virtually agammaglobulinemic patients may suffer with only occasional sinusitis, whereas patients with near-normal serum immunoglobulin levels may present with recurrent pneumonia and bronchiectasis.

DIAGNOSIS

Approximately 1 in 600 individuals of European ancestry are unable to produce detectable quantities of IgA1 and IgA2, making selective IgAD the most frequently recognized primary immunodeficiency in the Americas, Australia, and Europe. The diagnosis is dependent on the sensitivity of the laboratory measurement. The clinical laboratory typically reports serum IgA levels of less than 7 mg/dl, the concentration below which nephelometry becomes unreliable.

Uncomplicated patients with IgAD have normal serum levels of IgM and normal or elevated levels of IgG, and demonstrate normal cell-mediated immunity. A minority of patients may demonstrate additional evidence of immune dysfunction, with inability to generate appropriate IgG$_2$ anti-carbohydrate antibodies, frank IgG subclass deficiencies, or evidence of impairment of T-cell function. Patients with IgA serum levels that fall more than two standard deviations below the mean serum level for their age are considered to have partial IgA deficiency. These patients can also suffer from recurrent infections.

CLINICAL MANIFESTATIONS

The likelihood that an IgA-deficient individual who was identified serendipitously will require medical attention is difficult to assess because most studies in the literature reflect patients who were ascertained as a result of clinical symptoms. Among IgAD patients referred to immunology clinics, more than 85% present with recurrent infections, typically with encapsulated bacteria such as *Haemophilus influenzae* and *Streptococcus pneumoniae*. Among affected children, symptoms may begin in the first year of life, although the physiologic lag in serum IgA may delay the diagnosis until after the age of 2. In some patients, respiratory infections disappear with maturity. In others, infections may persist throughout adult life. Rarely IgAD patients experience recurrent bronchitis, pneumonia, and even bronchiectasis. These more severely afflicted patients often exhibit IgG$_2$ and IgG$_4$ subclass deficiencies, as well. Chronic intermittent diarrhea due to *Giardia lamblia* is a common complaint, although there are indications that this may track more closely with related deficits in IgG function. Systemic infections such as viral hepatitis, meningoencephalitis, and septicemia may also occur. Some symptomatic patients have elevated IgE levels, which can introduce an allergic or asthmatic component to respiratory dysfunction. The rise in IgE has been explained as a compensatory response to the absence of IgA. This appears to be a double-edged sword, because up to 20% of patients complain of allergic rhinitis, conjunctivitis, urticaria, and atopic eczema. Allergic reactions may be enhanced due to the lack of IgA blocking antibodies in the serum, and unusually severe asthma has also been associated with IgAD.

IgA-deficient patients rarely produce IgG or IgE anti-IgA antibodies. These uncommon patients are at risk for adverse reactions following transfusion with blood products, as mentioned previously, plasma from normal donors, or from some preparations for immunoglobulin replacement therapy which, of course, contain IgA. Patients with high anti-IgA levels (greater than 1:1000) typically have potent antibodies directed against all IgAs. These patients are at risk for severe anaphylaxis. Patients with low anti-IgA antibody titers (less than 1:256) are often multiparous or multi-transfused patients. These patients rarely demonstrate severe anaphylaxis after infusion with plasma or blood products, but do present with hives and rashes. Serum complement typically falls as a result of this type of reaction.

IgAD patients often develop autoimmune diseases. These include juvenile rheumatoid arthritis, systemic lupus erythematosus, Addison's disease, chronic nephritis, dermatomyositis, Evans syndrome, isolated hemolytic anemia, isolated idiopathic thrombocytopenic purpura, insulin-dependent diabetes mellitus, pulmonary hemosiderosis, sarcoidosis, Sjögren's syndrome, Henoch–Schönlein syndrome or hemorrhagic purpura, and thyroiditis. Gastrointestinal disorders include celiac disease, inflammatory bowel disease, intestinal disaccharidase deficiency, lactase deficiency, pancreatic insufficiency, and pernicious anemia. Hepatobiliary disorders include chronic active hepatitis, cholelithiasis, lupoid hepatitis, and primary biliary cirrhosis. Skin disorders include pyoderma gangrenosum, perinychia, and vitiligo. It is unclear whether this autoimmune diathesis is the end result of recurrent infections, the product of recurrent insult by antigens that would otherwise be cleared by IgA, or whether the underlying deficit that leads to IgAD also increases the risk of developing an autoimmune disorder. For example, autoimmune disorders such as insulin-dependent diabetes mellitus and celiac disease are associated with the same major histocompatibility complex (MHC) haplotypes (Chapter 5) as IgAD and CVID.

IgAD is associated with an increased risk for the development of malignancies,[21] including gastric and colonic adenocarcinoma and acute lymphoblastic leukemia. Hepatoma, lymphosarcoma, melanoma, multiple myeloma, ovarian carcinoma, squamous cell carcinoma, and malignant thymoma have also been reported. Cervical and bronchial lymphadenopathy can be found in IgAD patients who suffer from recurrent sinopulmonary infections. Patients with chronic gastrointestinal infections may demonstrate a nodular lymphoid hyperplasia of the small intestine that can lead to intestinal obstruction. Histologic evaluation reveals active B-lymphocyte proliferation in the germinal centers of the Peyer's patches. These "constipated" lymph nodes have been mistaken for lymphoma. In some cases, it is possible to attribute the increased risk of malignancy to the lack of protection against ingested carcinogens. In others, the simultaneous presence of IgAD and malignancy may simply reflect the high prevalence of IgAD in the Caucasian population.

ORIGIN AND PATHOGENESIS

IgAD, selective IgG subclass deficiencies, and CVID are diseases that are defined by a quantitative phenotype, a paucity of serum immunoglobulins of a given isotype in spite of the presence in the blood of B lymphocytes bearing the missing isotypes. By definition, the fundamental defect involves the failure of B lymphocytes bearing a given isotype to differentiate into plasma cells. These diseases appear to represent a common endpoint for multiple pathogenic processes. All three phenotypes may be acquired and many of the recognized precipitating causes, such as phenytoin, are the same (Table 34.3).

IgA deficiency is associated with MHC haplotypes that are more common in European populations than in the peoples of sub-Saharan

Table 34.3 Other conditions associated with humoral immunodeficiency

Genetic disorders	
Monogenic diseases	Ataxia-telangiectasia Autosomal forms of SCID Transcobalamin II deficiency and hypogammaglobulinemia Wiskott–Aldrich syndrome X-linked lymphoproliferative disorder (Epstein–Barr virus-associated) X-linked SCID
Chromosomal anomalies	Chromosome 18q-syndrome Monosomy 22 Trisomy 8 Trisomy 21
Systemic disorders Malignancy Metabolic or physical loss	Chronic lymphocytic leukemia Immunodeficiency with thymoma T-cell lymphoma Immunodeficiency caused by hypercatabolism of immunoglobulin Immunodeficiency caused by excessive loss of immunoglobulins and lymphocytes
Environmental exposures Drug-induced Infectious diseases	Antimalarial agents Captopril Carbamazepine Glucocorticoids Fenclofenac Gold salts Penicillamine Phenytoin Sulphasalazine Congenital rubella Congenital infection with CMV Congenital infection with *Toxoplasma gondii* Epstein–Barr virus Human immunodeficiency virus

CMV, cytomegalovirus; SCID, severe combined immunodeficiency virus.

African and East Asia. In the USA, the prevalence of IgAD among African-Americans is one-twentieth of that observed among Americans of European descent and in Japan the incidence is approximately 1 in 18 500. Function-loss mutations in a variety of non-MHC genes have now been defined in families with IgA-deficient/CVID members. These include the genes for ICOS, an immune co-stimulator molecule used by T cells to activate B cells in germinal centers, BAFFR and transmembrane activator and calcium modulator and cyclophilin ligand interactor (TACI), the receptors for B-cell-activating factor (BAFF), and CD19, the B-cell co-stimulatory receptor. Remarkably, several individuals with TACI mutations had also inherited MHC haplotypes associated with the disease, suggesting a complex etiology for the disorder.[22]

TREATMENT AND PROGNOSIS

Most individuals with IgAD suffer respiratory infections no more frequently than the average individual and thus require no special treatment. All individuals with IgA deficiency should be warned of the risk of serious transfusion reactions caused by antibodies to IgA. Wearing a medical alert bracelet is recommended. Should transfusion be necessary, the ideal donors are other individuals with IgAD. Washed erythrocytes are safer than whole blood.

Patients with selective IgA deficiency who suffer from clinically significant, recurrent upper respiratory infections often respond to prophylactic antibiotics. Treatment of allergy in those patients with a compensatory increase in IgE is helpful. Patients who present with combined IgA and IgG subclass deficiencies may require immunoglobulin replacement.

COMMON VARIABLE IMMUNODEFICIENCY ■

DIAGNOSIS

The diagnostic category of CVID includes a heterogeneous group of patients, mostly adults, who exhibit deficient production of all the different classes of antibodies. These patients typically have normal numbers of B lymphocytes in their blood that are clonally diverse, but phenotypically immature. B lymphocytes in CVID patients are able to recognize antigens and respond with proliferation, but they are impaired in their ability to become memory B cells and mature plasma cells. In infected patients, abortive differentiation can lead to massive B-lymphocyte hyperplasia, splenomegaly and intestinal lymphoid hyperplasia.

With an estimated prevalence of 1 in 25 000, CVID is the most prevalent human primary immunodeficiency requiring medical attention.[23] Men and women are equally affected. As with IgAD, the prevalence among African-Americans is one-twentieth that of Americans of European descent. Some patients present during childhood, but most are diagnosed in the third decade of life. The typical patient reports a normal pattern of recurrent otitis media as an infant and toddler that resolved in childhood. During adolescence, respiratory infections recur and steadily increase in frequency. Recurrent pneumonia as a young or middle-aged adult is often the precipitating complaint that brings the patient to the attention of the clinical immunologist. Although CVID thus appears to be an acquired disorder, family studies have clearly documented that susceptibility for the disease can be inherited and the manifestations of the disorder may change with time. Transitions within the spectrum of normal serum immunoglobulin concentrations to IgA deficiency to IgA deficiency with IgG subclass deficits to frank CVID have been documented in both sporadic and familial cases.[2]

Common variable immunodeficiency is a diagnostic category of primary immunodeficiencies that includes a number of immune disorders. Most CVID patients of northern European descent exhibit a distinctive phenotype characterized by a broad deficiency of immunoglobulin isotypes in spite of the presence of normal numbers of surface immunoglobulin-bearing B-cell precursors in the peripheral blood. Almost all of these patients are IgA-deficient and by definition demonstrate total serum IgG levels of less than 500 mg/dl. Some IgG subclasses are more affected than others, with the sequential order of involvement being $IgG_4 > IgG_2 > IgG_1 > IgG_3$. Most patients are also deficient in IgM and IgE. This pattern is common to patients with specific MHC susceptibility haplotypes as well as to those who have inherited function-loss mutations in the genes for ICOS, BAFFR, and TACI.

Uncomplicated patients demonstrate normal cell-mediated immunity, but a minority of patients may have evidence of T-cell dysfunction as well as other hematopoietic cell types. In some cases, B-cell numbers are reduced, although not to the extent exhibited by disorders of pre-BCR formation or signaling, as discussed in the sections on XLA and autosomal agammaglobulinemia or in the agammaglobulinemia associated with thymoma with pure red cell aplasia.

IgAD and CVID have been associated with congenital infection with rubella virus, cytomegalovirus, and *Toxoplasma gondii*. The administration of certain drugs has also been linked to a depression in serum immunoglobulin levels. Up to 20% of patients treated with phenytoin for idiopathic epilepsy suffer a mild decrease in serum IgA levels, and a minority may progress to a CVID-like phenotype. Medications used for the treatment of rheumatoid arthritis and inflammatory bowel disease can also decrease production of antibody. Persistence of antibody deficiency usually requires continued administration of the drug or continued infection with the virus or parasite. Recovery of immunoglobulin production may take months or years.

CLINICAL MANIFESTATIONS

The clinical manifestations of CVID are similar but more severe than the ones seen in IgAD. Respiratory symptoms often begin with recurrent sinusitis, otitis media, and mild bronchitis, which are typically due to encapsulated bacteria such as *Haemophilus influenzae* and *Streptococcus pneumoniae*. The frequency and severity of the upper respiratory infections worsen in the young adult and lower respiratory infections such as pneumonia become common. Apparently asymptomatic, untreated patients may suffer recurrent subclinical pulmonary infections that can lead to irreversible chronic lung damage with bronchiectasis, unilateral hyperlucent lung, emphysema, and cor pulmonale. With damage to pulmonary mucosa, the spectrum of bacterial pathogens broadens to include *Pseudomonas aeruginosa* and *Staphylococcus aureus*. Recurrent skin infections or erythroderma can be presenting complaints. The pathogenesis of these dermatologic manifestations remains unclear.

Intermittent or chronic diarrhea due to *Giardia lamblia* is a common complaint. Some unfortunate patients develop a malabsorption syndrome that resembles celiac sprue but is unresponsive to the avoidance of gluten (Fig. 34.4). Although allergic disorders are rare in CVID, antigen-specific IgE can be produced in sufficient quantities to enable anaphylactic reactions. Untreated patients often complain of an asymmetrical, oligoarticular arthritis which in some cases reflects infections with encapsulated organisms or with *Mycoplasma* species and thus requires antibiotic therapy. The arthritis typically responds to immunoglobulin replacement therapy.

CVID patients are often anergic, but only a minority suffer infections characteristic of cell-mediated immune dysfunction, such as mycobacteria, *Pneumocystis jiroveci*, and fungi. CD8 T-cell numbers may be depressed in such patients. Most viral infections are cleared normally. Exceptions include enteroviral infections, including meningoencephalitis, as well as hepatitis B and C, which can progress to a fatal chronic active hepatitis. Lack of humoral immunity enhances susceptibility to viral reactivation. Untreated patients often complain of recurrent herpes zoster infections (shingles).

Autoimmune diseases are common in CVID and include pernicious anemia, autoimmune neutropenia, Graves disease, hypothyroidism, rheumatoid arthritis, systemic lupus erythematosus, and Sjögren syndrome. Coombs-positive hemolytic anemia with idiopathic thrombocytopenic purpura, a combination known as Evans syndrome, may predate the diagnosis of CVID.

A sarcoidosis-like syndrome, characterized by noncaseating granulomas in the lung, lymph nodes, skin, bone marrow, and liver, is more common in African-Americans.[24] Occasionally the granulomas result from mycobacterial and fungal infections. In the majority of cases, the cause remains unclear and the granulomas resolve spontaneously.

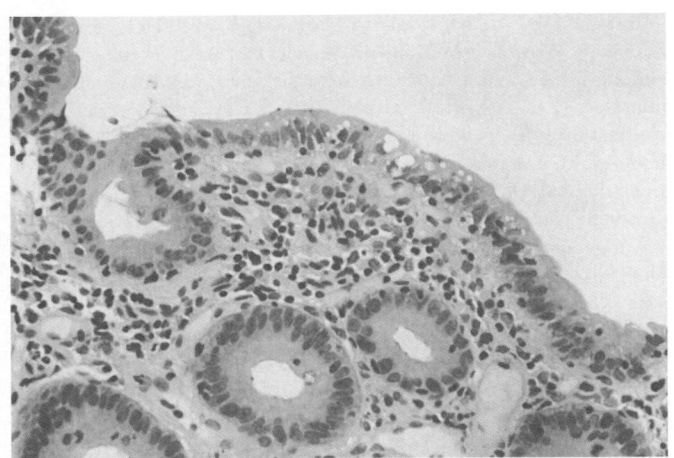

Fig. 34.4 Hypogammaglobulinemic sprue in a 41-year-old white male with common variable immunodeficiency (CVID) and insulin-dependent diabetes mellitus. The patient suffered from intractable diarrhea. Shown is a hematoxylin and eosin stain of a duodenal biopsy obtained by endoscopy. The villi are blunted and there is a marked increase in intraepithelial lymphocytes. However, unlike typical celiac disease, the villi are not completely blunted and few plasma cells are seen. The patient is homozygous for the human leukocyte antigen (HLA)-B8,-DR3 haplotype. Although the patient failed to respond to a gluten-free diet, the diarrhea resolved with corticosteroid therapy.

The development of a constellation of pulmonary abnormalities that includes granulomatous and lymphoproliferative (lymphocytic interstitial pneumonia, follicular bronchiolitis, and lymphoid hyperplasia) histopathologic patterns, termed granulomatous-lymphocytic interstitial lung disease (GLILD),[25] can be an ominous sign. These patients appear more likely to develop granulomatous liver disease, autoimmune hemolytic anemia, lymphoproliferative disease, and progressive pulmonary disease. In one study,[25] median survival was reduced by more than 50%.

There is an increased risk for the development of gastrointestinal and lymphoid malignancies, especially non-Hodgkin's lymphomas. Confounding the diagnosis of malignancy is the patient's propensity to develop benign lymphoproliferative disorders. Lymphadenopathy, splenomegaly, or both are common in untreated patients. The lymph node architecture is usually preserved, but in some patients the lymph node architecture is disrupted by a polymorphic lymphocytic infiltrate. Lymphoid aggregates with an abnormal architecture may also develop in the skin, bone marrow, or other tissues. This atypical lymphoid hyperplasia may be difficult to differentiate from a malignant lymphoma.

ORIGIN AND PATHOGENESIS

Although some CVID patients have minimal numbers of circulating B cells, the majority have normal quantities of IgA, IgG, and IgM-bearing B-cell precursors in the blood. Defects in B-cell survival, number of circulating CD27+ memory B cells (including IgM+CD27+ B cells), B-cell activation after antigen receptor cross-linking, T-cell signaling, and cytokine expression have been observed. A decrease in the relative numbers of CD4 to CD8 T cells is common. Cutaneous anergy is a frequent finding. Alteration of the CD4/CD8 ratio can reflect expansion of the

CD8 natural killer cell population or an increase in the subset of CD8+, CD57+ T cells and natural killer cells. In some patients inversion of the ratio reflects a true decline in the absolute number of CD4 helper T cells.

The TNF family members B-cell activating factor of the TNF family (BAFF) and a proliferation-inducing ligand (APRIL) can induce isotype switching in naïve human B cells.[23] APRIL and BAFF bind to two receptors, B-cell maturation antigen (BCMA) and TACI, both of which are members of the TNF-R family. BCMA is exclusively expressed on B cells, whereas TACI is expressed on B cells and activated T cells. A third receptor, BAFF-R, which is unique for BAFF, is mainly expressed on B cells but also on resting T cells. In two seminal studies,[22, 26] TACI mutations were found in 18 (10%) of 182 CVID patients, and in one of 16 IgAD patients. As is typical for CVID, symptoms in family members with TACI mutations ranged from severe to mild to nonexistent.

Function-loss mutations in the genes for ICOS, an immune co-stimulator molecule used by T cells to activate B cells in germinal centers, BAFFR, and CD19, the B-cell co-stimulatory receptor, have also been reported in isolated CVID patients. All of these genes play key roles in the maturation, proliferation, and longevity of mature B cells.

A large array of genes that play important roles in the control of the immune response are located in the MHC on chromosome 6 (Chapter 5). Studies at the University of Alabama at Birmingham have shown that in the southeastern USA the majority of IgAD and CVID patients share parts or all of one of two extended MHC haplotypes marked by either HLA-DR3,-B8 or HLA-DR7,-B44. The combined results of three studies of patients from Alabama, New England, and Australia indicate a 13% prevalence of immunodeficiency in individuals homozygous for HLA-DR3,-B8. Remarkably, several individuals with TACI mutations had also inherited MHC haplotypes associated with the disease,[22] suggesting the possibility of epistatic interactions between the MHC and TACI alleles. A deficiency of IgG subclasses and IgA may also develop in complement C2-deficient patients.[27] The typical presenting manifestation of CVID is hypogammaglobulinemia, not agammaglobulinemia, suggesting a partial or varying block in B-cell maturation. Careful analysis of B cells in patients has also revealed a spectrum of immune deficiency ranging from the nearly complete absence of memory B cells to a less severe disorder. All of these findings serve to underline the complex etiology for the disorder, and many details remain to be elucidated.

TREATMENT AND PROGNOSIS

Therapy in CVID begins with the aggressive treatment of ongoing infections and the institution of prophylactic measures to prevent or ameliorate future infection. Patients suffering from moderate upper respiratory tract infections and bronchitis will likely benefit from empiric therapy with agents effective against encapsulated organisms such as *Haemophilus influenzae* and *Streptococcus pneumoniae*. Patients with recurrent pneumonia and evidence of bronchiectasis may be infected with *Pseudomonas*, *Staphylococcus aureus*, or other aggressive organisms, thus every effort should be made to identify the inciting agent. The course of treatment for immunodeficient patients is often prolonged and intravenous administration of antibiotics may be required.

The most effective therapy for hypogammaglobulinemic patients is replacement therapy with human immunoglobulin. A number of studies have demonstrated a steadily decreasing incidence of infection with increasing frequency of immunoglobulin administration. At higher doses, even patients with bronchiectasis may experience improvement in pulmonary function. Each patient may demonstrate his or her own individual response to therapy, exhibiting dramatic differences in the frequency and severity of infections with moderate changes in the replacement dose. Patients suffering from a serious acute infection often benefit from one-time booster doses of immunoglobulin. Ultimately, replacement dosage must be individualized based upon the response of the patient. Adverse reactions occur most frequently at the time of the first administration of immunoglobulin, likely because of concurrent infection increasing the potential for generation of immune complexes. If the patient demonstrates no evidence of adverse reactions, administration of intravenous or subcutaneous immunoglobulin can be performed at home.

Some patients with CVID can sustain severe anaphylaxis when given intravenous immunoglobulin or other blood products that contain serum or plasma. These patients may possess anti-IgA antibodies, including IgE anti-A antibodies.[28] For patients with a history of severe adverse reactions, it is advisable to try lots of intravenous immunoglobulin with the lowest IgA possible and to test the patient with the different lots in an intensive care unit. Once having identified a lot that can be tolerated, the patient may receive therapy under more relaxed conditions.

Serum immunoglobulin concentrations in patients with CVID may change over time,[2] with rare patients regaining normal serum IgG levels and no longer requiring immunoglobulin therapy. Careful review of the clinical history of these patients may reveal evidence of exposure to pharmacologic agents associated with the development of hypogammaglobulinemia (e.g., phenytoin). However, the overwhelming majority of patients require replacement therapy for life.

Although IgG may be replaced, at present IgM and IgA cannot be provided to the patient. The absence of these multimeric proteins may help explain why even patients on high-dose replacement therapy may continue to suffer from chronic sinusitis or diarrhea. In such cases, patients often benefit from continued prophylactic therapy with antibiotics effective against encapsulated bacteria. Patients with CVID are also at risk from *Giardia lamblia*, as well as other enteric pathogens. Patients with chronic diarrhea often respond to treatment with empiric antibiotic therapy. Some patients develop gluten-sensitive enteropathy or lactose intolerance. These conditions often improve with avoidance of the inciting agent.[29] Others develop a malabsorption syndrome that can lead to hypoalbuminemia and hypocalcemia (due to malabsorption of vitamin D), and decreased levels of vitamin A and carotene.[30] The cause of diarrhea and malabsorption in this latter patient subset remains unclear, and treatment is limited to supportive measures, with vitamin and mineral replacement as indicated.

Patients with bronchiectasis should be treated aggressively with replacement therapy. In severe cases, aggressive pulmonary toilet will benefit the patient, including bronchodilator therapy, position and postural drainage, or other physical therapies. The use of corticosteroids should be avoided.

Splenomegaly is common in untreated patients. Hypersplenism in most patients responds to aggressive therapy with antibiotics and intravenous immunoglobulin. The presumption is that the hypersplenism is secondary to reactive hyperplasia of lymphoid follicles within the spleen attempting to respond to infection. Development of esophageal varices or other hematologic manifestations of hypersplenism (refractory thrombocytopenia, anemia, neutropenia, and lymphopenia) may require splenectomy as a therapy of last resort. The outcome for most such patients has been good, with resolution of symptoms. However, the risk of infection from encapsulated organisms increases in such patients, and they should be placed on penicillin prophylaxis (or an equivalent).

IgA-deficient mothers fail to secrete IgA in their colostrum.[31] Although colostral IgM levels may be elevated in an attempt to compensate for the lack of maternal IgA, the newborn remains relatively unprotected against intestinal pathogens. Of greater concern are the children of mothers with untreated CVID who are born in a state of humoral immunodeficiency and are at great risk for life-threatening sinopulmonary infection. In order to compensate for the loss of IgG across the placenta and to provide the infant with the passive immunity it will require, the level of intravenous immunoglobulin infusion should be increased to 600 mg/kg during the third trimester of pregnancy.

■ SELECTIVE IGG SUBCLASS DEFICIENCIES ■

DIAGNOSIS

A diagnosis of clinical immunodeficiency should be supported by clear evidence of functional impairment. Most individuals with modest reductions in serum IgG subclass levels are functionally normal. Indeed, individuals with deletions of the heavy-chain immunoglobulin gene locus, some of whom completely lack IgG_1, IgG_2, IgG_4, and IgA_1,[32] have been reported to be asymptomatic. This experiment of nature is a further reminder of the fact that absence of serum immunoglobulin is not necessarily synonymous with clinical immune deficiency.

The diagnosis of a functional IgG subclass deficiency can thus be made with confidence only when the concentration of a specific isotype is significantly depressed and there is clear evidence of abnormal specific antibody production. Among patients with deficiency of IgG_1 or IgG_3, protective titers of antibodies in response to standard tetanus toxoid and diphtheria immunizations indicate the production of adequate anti-protein antibodies and make associated immunodeficiency unlikely. Among patients with clinically significant IgG_2 deficiency, specific antibody production in response to a carbohydrate vaccine is decreased. IgG_2 levels normally begin to rise in childhood later than other subclasses, and a low value in a child may be a temporary finding. Up to 10% of normal males and 1% of normal females are IgG_4-deficient, which makes a diagnosis of immunodeficiency as a result of an isolated IgG_4 subclass deficiency problematic.

CLINICAL MANIFESTATIONS

The clinical spectrum of isolated IgG subclass deficiency is quite variable and deficiencies of each of the four IgG subclasses have been described. Some individuals are referred to the clinical immunologist with only a mild reduction of total IgG, but most symptomatic patients have marked deficiencies of one or more IgG subclass despite normal total IgG concentrations. Typically patients with IgG_1 deficiency exhibit depressed total serum immunoglobulin levels, as well.

Determination of IgG subclasses is rarely performed on asymptomatic individuals, thus most patients with an isolated IgG_2 deficiency come to medical attention as a result of recurrent sinusitis, otitis media, or pulmonary infections. Individuals may have few residual symptoms between infections, but some have severe chronic inflammation with refractory sinusitis, pulmonary fibrosis, or bronchiectasis. Because protective antibodies directed against carbohydrate antigens are usually of the IgG_2 subclass, many affected patients exhibit an impairment of their ability to mount specific protective responses to encapsulated pathogens. However, normal responses have also been described.[33] The response to polysaccharides is typically tested by challenge with a pneumococcal polysaccharide vaccine. Diagnosis is complicated by the fact that interpretation of pneumococcal polysaccharide vaccine responses remains controversial. Many clinicians would agree, however, that IgG$_2$-deficient patients who suffer with recurrent sinopulmonary infections and who respond to less than half of the polysaccharide antigens with which they have been challenged meet the standard for functional immune deficiency. Such patients warrant aggressive prophylactic therapy up to and including immunoglobulin replacement should the infections be severe.

IgG$_3$ deficiency may occur alone or in association with IgG$_1$ deficiency. Recurrent infection of the respiratory tract with chronic lung disease has been reported. With a serum half-life of only 2 weeks, IgG$_3$ levels may be consumed rapidly during the course of an active infection in an otherwise normal individual.[34] Before making the diagnosis of IgG$_3$ deficiency, serum levels of IgG$_3$ should be rechecked when the individual is asymptomatic.

When compared with the serum, IgG$_4$ is over-represented in secretions, and IgG$_4$-committed B cells are present at mucosal sites, suggesting a role in mucosal immunity. Since IgG$_4$ is normally present in the serum in very low concentrations, the significance of a low serum level in a patient with recurrent infection remains unclear.

ORIGIN AND PATHOGENESIS

The origin of IgG subclass deficiency is unknown. Homozygous deletions of portions of the immunoglobulin heavy-chain constant locus associated with total absence of IgG$_2$, IgG$_3$, and IgG$_4$ or combinations of these isotypes have been described in healthy individuals. IgG$_2$ deficiency is often found in association with selective IgA deficiency with or without IgG$_4$ deficiency, and patients with selective IgG subclass deficiencies have been shown to have inherited the same MHC haplotypes as those who suffer with IgAD and CVID.[18] These observations suggest that patients with recurrent infections have a more complex defect than the mere elimination of one or more IgG isotype. In some instances, subclass deficiency is associated with a T-cell defect, as in chronic mucocutaneous candidiasis and ataxia-telangiectasia. IgG subclass deficiency may also be acquired. Acute infections, medications, chemotherapy, irradiation, surgery, and HIV infection have all been temporally linked to the development of a deficiency in one or more IgG subclass.[35]

TREATMENT AND PROGNOSIS

The natural history of IgG subclass deficiency, especially in children, is not constant. Some children improve, whereas for others subclass deficiency may progress into frank CVID. Associated allergic rhinosinusitis and asthma must be aggressively treated with conventional therapy for these disorders, as these conditions increase the risk of purulent sinusitis and pneumonia. Causes of anatomic obstruction should be sought when persistent infection of a sinus or pulmonary segment is the presenting complaint; the role of surgical therapy for anatomic obstruction should not be overlooked. Most patients with IgG subclass deficiency do well on prophylactic antibiotics and will never need immunoglobulin supplementation.

Immunoglobulin replacement therapy should only be considered in patients with severe, recurrent infections. Patients who begin therapy should improve within the first 2 months, but to avoid the placebo effect, a full 6-month trial is recommended. A reduction in frequency of viral respiratory infections is likely to occur in any individual receiving intravenous immunoglobulin because of the broad spectrum of antibodies present, thus relative freedom from trivial infections should not be taken as evidence of need for permanent replacement therapy.

ANTIBODY DEFICIENCY WITH NORMAL SERUM IMMUNOGLOBULIN LEVELS

Occasional patients may present with normal serum immunoglobulin concentrations and a selective inability to respond to infections with pyogenic organisms. Diagnosis requires documentation of an inability to respond to antigenic challenge. These patients may respond to replacement immunoglobulin therapy. The antibody response to specific polysaccharide antigens can be very selective. In humans, most protective anti-*Haemophilus influenzae* type b (anti-Hib) antibodies utilize the rare Vκ A2 gene.[36] The Navajo population in the southwestern USA suffers a 5–10-fold increased incidence of Hib disease. This population also exhibits a high prevalence of an A2 allele with a defective recombination signal sequence, preventing use of germline-encoded antibodies that can generate protective antigen-binding sites. It is likely that many more such subtle defects that underlie susceptibility to infectious diseases will be identified in the coming years.

A recent analysis of a group of well-characterized patients, mostly female, with a history of RESPI and normal serum immunoglobulin levels revealed a high prevalence of the same MHC haplotypes observed in IgAD, selective IgG subclass deficits, and CVID.[20] This is further evidence that the presence of serum immunoglobulin is not necessarily synonymous with clinical immune sufficiency. These patients tend to respond to aggressive antibiotic therapy, including prophylaxis.

SELECTIVE LIGHT-CHAIN DEFICIENCY

A selective deficiency of κ light chains has been reported in 3 patients, and a selective deficiency of λ light chains has been reported in a fourth.[37,38] In one case, the patient was the offspring of a consanguineous (uncle–niece) union;[39] and in the second, a molecular analysis demonstrated different loss-of-function mutations in the patient's Cκ alleles.[40] The parents of these children had no health difficulties, but each of the patients required medical attention for recurrent sinopulmonary infections and diarrhea. Two of the κ-deficient patients exhibited IgA deficiency and the remaining κ-deficient and the λ-deficient patients were panhypogammaglobulinemic.

TRANSIENT HYPOGAMMAGLOBULINEMIA OF INFANCY

DIAGNOSIS

As infants make the transition from dependence on maternal immunoglobulin to reliance on endogenously produced antibodies, they experience a physiologic nadir of serum immunoglobulin at 4–6 months of

Primary T-cell immunodeficiencies

Françoise Le Deist, Alain Fischer

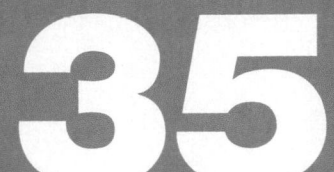

35

INTRODUCTION

Primary deficiencies of the acquired immune system are studied according to the type of lymphocyte most affected, and broadly categorized into T- and B-cell immunodeficiencies. This chapter describes primary T-cell immunodeficiencies; Chapter 34 is devoted to primary B-cell immunodeficiencies. Hematopoietic stem cell transplantation (HSCT) and gene therapy, the only available curative treatments for primary immunodeficiencies, are reviewed in detail in Chapters 83 and 86.

Primary T-cell immunodeficiency diseases originate from inherited defects of the components of the immune system involved in T-cell differentiation and function, i.e., T cells, their precursors, the thymic environment, and antigen-presenting cells. Because of the central place of T cells in immune responses, T-cell deficiencies not only affect T-cell effectors of the immune response, such as cytotoxic T cells, but also other effector cells that are activated by T cells, such as monocytes/macrophages and B cells. Profound T-cell deficiencies thus usually present as 'combined' immunodeficiencies of the different arms of the immune response. They generally present with clinical manifestations within the first year of life, although moderate deficiencies can manifest much later (up to adulthood). Statistical data from national primary immunodeficiency registries suggest that primary T-cell immunodeficiencies represent 20% of all symptomatic primary immunodeficiencies.

T-cell immunodeficiencies increase susceptibility to infections, particularly those caused by intracellular microorganisms, which may persist inside cell niches protected from immune mechanisms. Recurrent infections, chronic diarrhea and malabsorption are frequently associated with failure to thrive. Allergy, autoimmunity and lymphomas are other important characteristics of T-cell immunodeficiency, occurring with a higher frequency than in healthy individuals.

Primary T-cell immunodeficiencies can be classified into four groups according to their severity and associated features: severe combined immune deficiencies (SCIDs); T-cell immunodeficiencies with detectable T cells; T-cell immunodeficiencies with associated nonimmune defects; and miscellaneous immunodeficiencies in which the T-cell defect is less apparent than the resulting immune dysfunction.

SEVERE COMBINED IMMUNODEFICIENCIES (SCIDs)

This group of genetic disorders is characterized by profoundly defective T-cell differentiation, with or without abnormal B- and NK-cell differentiation, that leads to early death in the absence of hematopoietic stem cell transplantation (Table 35.1).[1] The overall frequency of SCID has been estimated at 1:50 000–1:100 000 live births. Various forms of SCID have been defined, based on enzymatic, genetic and immunologic criteria (Table 35.1).

CLINICAL PRESENTATION

Patients with SCID are characterized by early onset of infections, mainly of the respiratory tract and gut. The frequency of infections and the diagnosis in 117 patients with SCID who were referred to our center are shown in Table 35.2.[2] Oral candidiasis, persistent diarrhea with growth impairment, and/or interstitial pneumonitis were the most frequent infectious manifestations leading to diagnosis. There were no clinical differences between the various SCIDs, except for an earlier onset of infections in patients with adenosine deaminase (ADA) deficiency. The persistence and recurrence of infections led rapidly to growth impairment and malnutrition. Similar findings have been reported independently in another cohort of SCID patients.[3]

Common opportunistic organisms such as *Pneumocystis jiroveci* and *Aspergillus* species frequently cause infection in SCID patients. Intracellular organisms such as *Listeria* and *Legionella* can cause devastating disease, as can viruses, especially those of the herpes group and adenoviruses. Epstein–Barr virus (EBV) infection, although rare in this age group, can lead to uncontrolled B-lymphocyte proliferative disorders (BLPD) in B(+) SCID patients, as seen in immunosuppressed transplant recipients. Live vaccines can also cause life-threatening infections. We have observed BCG disease in 10 of 28 vaccinated patients, including two with local infection and eight with involvement of the liver, spleen and lungs, which was fatal in three cases.[2] Based on this experience and similar reports from other

Table 35.1 Classification of SCID

Disease	Relative frequency	Inheritance	Cells affected	Gene product	Other
Reticular dysgenesis	<1	AR	Haematopoietic cells	?	
T⁻B⁻NK⁺ SCID	15	AR	T,B	rag1/2	
	15	AR	T,B	Artemis	
Absence of T lymphocytes	45	X-L	T, NK	γc	
	10	AR	T, NK	JAK3	
	5	AR	T	Il7-Rα,	
	< 5	AR	T	CD3ε	
		AR	T	CD3δ	
		AR	T	CD45	
		AR	T	?	
ADA	12	AR	T, B, NK	ADA	Chondrodysplasia in 50% of cases

specialized centers, children with SCID or suspected to have SCID should not receive live vaccines.

Noninfectious clinical manifestations in SCID patient consist mainly of graft-versus-host disease (GVHD) caused by the patients' inability to reject allogeneic cells. The two possible sources of allogeneic cells are maternal lymphocytes and blood product transfusions. Circulating maternal T cells are detected in approximately 50% of cases. Maternal T-cell numbers range from 10 to several thousand/mm^3 of blood, and usually have a normal phenotype with poor lymphoproliferative response to mitogens, and circulate with some degree of *in vivo* activation, as shown by the expression of MHC class II molecules and/or the IL-2 receptor. The most intriguing observation regarding maternal T-cell engraftment in SCID patients is the paucity of clinical manifestations. In the majority of cases the presence of maternal T cells is entirely asymptomatic, but approximately 30–40% of patients have mild symptoms and signs, such as erythema and scaly skin with skin T-cell infiltration, eosinophilia, and elevated liver enzymes with periportal T-cell infiltration.[2] The presence of maternal T cells should not delay the diagnosis of SCID because of detection of some T cells in the periphery. It may be an obstacle to T-cell engraftment following T cell-depleted haploidentical bone marrow transplantation (BMT), especially if the donor is not the mother and if the patient is not treated with myeloablative and immunosuppressive drugs. In case of HLA-identical BMT, there is usually a dramatic expansion of donor T cells cytotoxic for maternal cells 10–12 days post BMT, which results in their rapid elimination. This 'graft-versus-graft' reaction may cause transient GVHD symptoms. In contrast, postnatal inoculation with allogeneic lymphocytes by transfusion of plasma, red cells, platelets or white cells usually causes a fatal acute GVHD syndrome, marked by diffuse necrotizing erythroderma, gut mucosa abrasion and destruction of the biliary epithelium, and is sometimes associated with stromal cell lesions in the marrow. This GVHD syndrome can occur within 2–4 weeks and is usually resistant to the most powerful immunosuppressive drugs. GVHD does not develop in a small number of cases, although allogeneic anti-host T cells can be detected and cause resistance to BM engraftment.[4] Prevention of this complication relies on T-cell depletion and irradiation of all blood products given to patients in whom SCID is suspected or cannot be excluded.

SCID patients present with profound hypoplasia of secondary lymphoid organs. The thymus is also hypotrophic, with an absence of the lymphoid component and defective differentiation of epithelial cells. There are no Hassall's corpuscles. This absence does not reflect a primary abnormality of the epithelial component of the thymus, as it becomes functional after BMT. It also indicates that the influx of hematopoietic lymphoid precursors is necessary for the differentiation of the thymic epithelium.

DIAGNOSIS

The diagnosis of SCID is suggested when there is a family history (especially in the mother's pedigree) of early death from infections and the symptoms described above. However, most SCID cases are sporadic and are diagnosed after immunologic studies are performed in an infant with unusually severe or frequent infections. In most cases, clinical examination together with very simple tests can confirm a suspicion, i.e., lack of palpable lymph nodes, especially in the inguinal area, with absence of visible tonsils, absence of a thymic shadow on the chest X-ray, and lymphocytopenia. The latter is of great value in young children, as normal absolute lymphocyte counts are high (around 6000/μL; Fig. 35.1). For example, only six out of 59 SCID patients studied in one case series had normal (or increased) lymphocyte counts.[5] Enumeration of blood T, NK and B cells, mitogen-induced lymphocyte proliferation assays, and determinations of adenosine deaminase activity are important diagnostic tests to diagnose the form of SCID. Costochondral dysplasia and, in some cases, unusual neurological manifestations (blindness, dystonia) are additional specific signs of ADA deficiency. Detection of gene mutations is important to confirm the clinical diagnosis, and for the appropriate choice of BMT treatment protocol and genetic counseling.

The differential diagnosis of SCID includes other diseases with reduced T-cell numbers, including HIV infection with severe immunodeficiency, rare cases of late-onset rubella with transient T-cell lymphocytopenia, and DiGeorge syndrome.

Given the importance of an early diagnosis in order to reach a better prognosis for BMT,[6] neonatal screening for severe T-cell immunodeficiency has been sought. One approach proposes the use of a Guthrie card

Table 35.2 Clinical features according to diagnosis (From Stephen JL, Vlekova V, Le Deist F, et al. Severe combined immunodeficiency: a retrospective single-center study of clinical presentation and outcome in 117 patients. J Pediatr 1993; 123: 564, with permission From Elsevier.)

	ADA⁻	T⁻B⁺	T⁻B⁺	Omenn syndrome	Total
Number of patients[a]	16	51	36	13	116
First hospitalization (days after birth)	45 0–100	111 0–583	93 0–402	68 0–127	91 0–583
Age at diagnosis (days after birth)	88 22–241	167 0–812	141 1–429	118 0–345	142 0–812
Growth impairment[b]	1.5mo	3.5mo	3mo	1.8mo	2.8mo
Persistent diarrhea (%)	68	57	64	66	61
Candidiasis (%)	18	40	48	16	34
Fever (%)	6	28	35	16	25
Sepsis (%)	0	4	6	16	5.4
Lung infections (%)	93	53	58	41	58
Meningitis (%)	6	6	3	0	4.4
Upper airway infections (%)	32	14	12	0	14.2
Opportunistic infections (%)	31	24	28	23	26

[a]Excluding the single case of reticular dysgenesis.
[b]Age where growth was below −2 SD.

KEY CONCEPTS

THERAPEUTIC PRINCIPLES: SEVERE COMBINED IMMUNE DEFICIENCIES (SCID)

>> Children at risk for SCID must not be given live viral vaccines.

>> All blood products administered to patients at risk for SCID must be irradiated before transfusion.

KEY CONCEPTS

SEVERE COMBINED IMMUNODEFICIENCY

>> Common element among various types of SCID is extremely low number of mature T cells.

>> B cells, present in several types of SCID, are nonfunctional, presumably because of lack of T-cell interaction.

>> Frequent opportunistic infections and unusual infections with routine pathogens lead to early demise by 1–2 years of life unless T-cell pool is reconstituted by BMT.

>> Molecular lesions in chromosomes, genes, and gene products now being discovered may lead to more selective approaches to therapy.

to detect the presence (or the absence) of T-cell receptor excision circles (TREC) in neonate blood samples, as a demonstration of functional thymopoiesis, using PCR technology.[7]

MANAGEMENT

Primary immunodeficiency patients require specialized care for diagnosis, treatment and follow-up. When a patient is suspected to have SCID, prompt immunologic evaluation is urgent in order to provide treatment before new severe and debilitating infections occur. In addition, the patient should not receive live vaccines, and if required, blood product transfusion should be irradiated, T cell-depleted, and tested negative for CMV antigen. Antibiotic prophylaxis is also indicated. Isolation measures are relative to the risk of infection with human pathogens, taking into consideration the patient's psychosocial needs.

Curative treatment for SCID is hematopoietic stem cell transplantation, which has been performed under protocols that differ regarding the donor source, the processing of the graft and the myeloablative conditioning employed. Success rates for each form of SCID treatment may not be similar (Chapter 83), emphasizing the importance of molecular diagnosis.

SCID DISEASES

Over 96% of SCID cases can be explained by four mechanisms of disease: defective VDJ recombination, defective cytokine receptor signaling, defective adenosine deaminase causing accumulation of toxic metabolites, and defective TCR signaling.

KEY CONCEPTS

CLINICAL PEARLS: FEATURES OF T-CELL DEFECTS

>> Functional deficiencies yield to discovery of molecular defects, e.g. hyper-IgM syndrome is now known as a T-cell defect (CD40 ligand deficiency on T cell).

>> Many T-cell deficiencies are due to defects in signal transduction proteins.

>> Severity of SCID is due to common γ-chain defects in IL-2R, IL-4R, IL-7R, IL-9R, IL-15R and IL-21R.

>> Defects in nonlymphocyte specific genes affect T-cell development, e.g. ADA deficiency, AT.

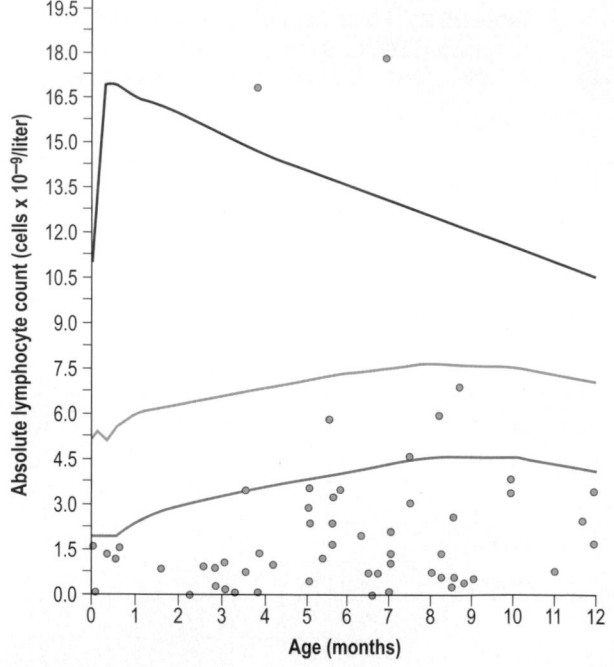

Fig. 35.1 Absolute lymphocyte counts in 59 infants with SCID at time of diagnosis. Top and bottom lines ±2 SD limits, middle line mean of normal value. (From Gossage DL, Buckley RH. Prevalence of lymphocytopenia in severe combined immunodeficiency. N Engl J Med 1990; 323: 1422, with permission From the Massachusetts Medical Society.)

Defective VDJ recombination

Autosomal recessive SCID – alymphocytosis (T-, B-, NK+ SCID)

About 20% of patients with SCID have a phenotype characterized by the absence of T and B cells; however, functional natural killer (NK) cells can be detected. These findings are similar to those found in murine SCID, which is manifested by defective V(D)J recombination of T-cell receptor (TCR) and immunoglobulin (Ig) genes (Fig. 35.2) (Chapter 4). Signal joints are formed normally but the coding segments fail to join. The murine SCID defect is caused by mutations of the gene encoding the DNA-dependent protein kinase (DNA-PK).[8] In the absence of this enzymatic activity, coding joints cannot be formed and the hairpin extremities of the V(D)J coding sequences are left apart. DNA-PK is involved in a DNA repair mechanism, i.e., nonhomologous end joining (NHEJ), utilized in the V(D)J recombination process, as all cell types of SCID mice exhibit a double-strand DNA break repair.[9] Despite phenotypic similarity, including defective V(D)J recombination as shown in marrow B-cell precursors, no SCID patients lacking T and B cells exhibit DNA-PK mutations.

Two forms of T- B- SCID can be recognized according to cell radiosensitivity. In approximately half of the patients marrow progenitor cells or fibroblasts exhibit increased cell radiosensitivity. In the other half, there is no detectable radiosensitivity anomaly. The latter phenotype results from mutations in the *RAG-1* or *RAG-2* genes.[10] RAG-1 and RAG-2 proteins are located in the nucleus of lymphoid progenitors cells undergoing the V(D)J recombination process[10] (Fig. 35.2). These proteins initiate the recombination process by interacting with the DNA recognition signal sequences that flank the coding regions, inducing a precisely targeted double-strand DNA break between the coding sequence of a V, D or J element and the signal sequence. These DNA breaks form hairpins by a transesterification reaction. These hairpins are then further resolved and joined in a second step of the V(D)J recombination process (see above). A number of *RAG-1* and *RAG-2* gene mutations have been characterized to result in preventing DNA/*RAG-1/2* complex interaction and DNA cleavage. As discussed below, mutations of these same genes allowing partial activity cause Omenn's syndrome, a condition characterized by oligoclonal T-cell expansion and immunodeficiency with γδ T-cell expansion.[11]

In those cases in which the block of T-/B-cell development and V(D)J recombination deficiency is associated with increased cell radiosensitivity, the SCID phenotype is caused by mutations of the Artemis gene.[12] This phenotype is observed with a high frequency (1:2000 live births) in North American Indians speaking the Athabascan language. Research in this ethnic group assigned the disease gene locus to the short arm of chromosome 10, which was subsequently confirmed in other ethnic backgrounds.[13] The Artemis protein has a hydrolytic endonuclease activity that is able to cleave the hairpins formed by coding ends upon *RAG-1/-2* action. Although Artemis deficiency impairs the nonhomologous end-joining (NHEJ) DNA repair pathway, no other clinical consequences of the SCID phenotype have been associated with Artemis deficiency. Hypomorphic mutations of Artemis have since been described associated either with Omenn's syndrome[14] or a severe but partial T- and B-cell immunodeficiency with a risk of EBV-associated B lymphomas.

Defective cytokine receptor signaling

X-linked SCID (SCIDX1) (T-, B+, NK- SCID)

SCIDX1 is characterized by defective T- and NK-cell differentiation, although B-cell maturation is preserved. Patients usually lack mature T cells but have a normal or increased number of B cells. Like autosomal recessive SCID, SCIDX1 can be treated by hematopoietic stem cell

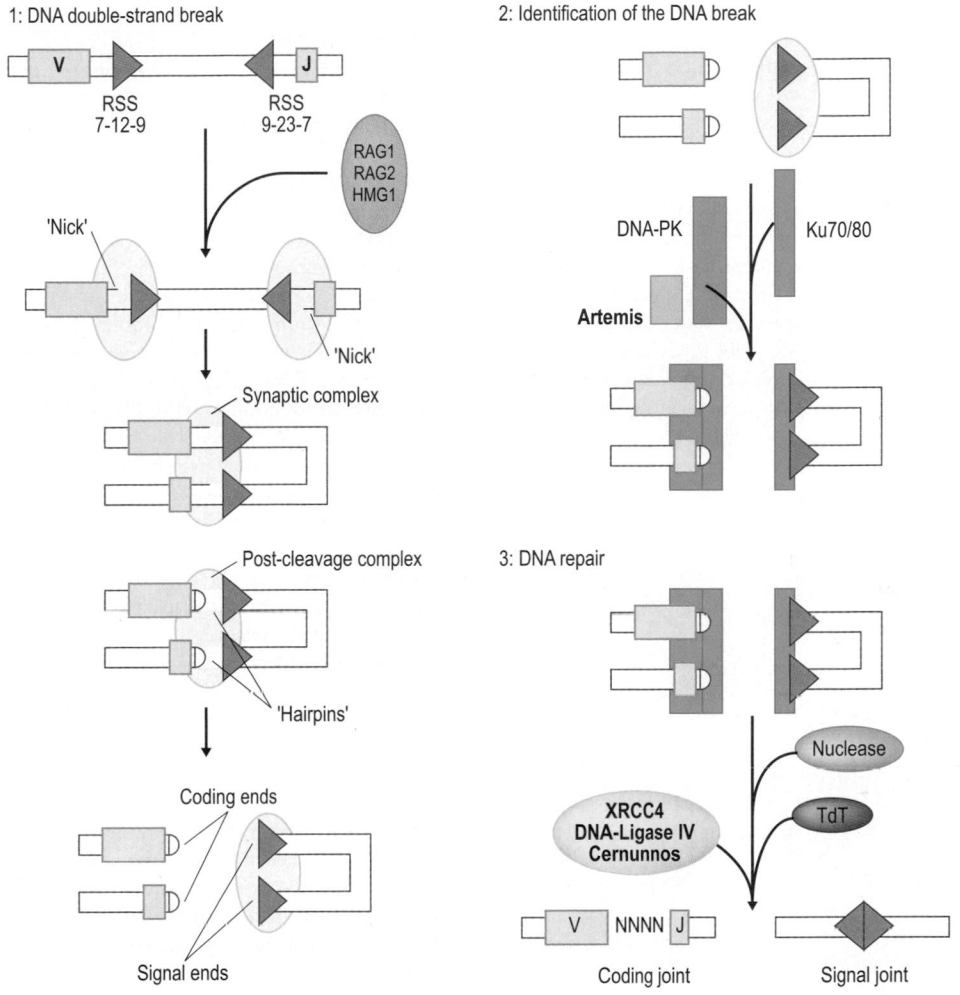

Fig. 35.2 Scheme of V(D)J gene rearrangement. The rearrangement process is divided into three steps: 1) RAG1 and RAG2 bind the RSS (recombination specific sequence), and perform single-DNA strand breaks (nick). They then form the synaptic complex in association with the architectural protein HMG1. The DNA double-strand break is performed within this complex, and the coding ends are in the form of hairpins. 2) The complex Ku70/80-DNA-PK recognizes the DNA breaks. The hairpins are opened by Artemis. 3) The recruitment of the protein XRCC4 and Cernunnos lead to the ligation action of ligases such as ligase IV. During this step, the terminal deoxynucleotidyl transferase (TdT) adds random nucleotides (N), thus increasing the diversity of the Variable chain.

transplantation (HSCT). This is the most frequent form of SCID, accounting for about 50% of cases.[2]

Precursor thymocytes are not detected in the thymus of patients with SCIDX1, indicating an early block in T-cell differentiation. Studies of X-chromosome inactivation patterns in obligate carriers have shown a skewed pattern not only in T cells but also in B cells and NK cells, whereas in the other hematopoietic cell lineages there is usually a random pattern.[15] The involvement of the product of the mutant SCIDX1 gene in B-cell maturation is also suggested by the observation that patients' B cells exhibit moderate phenotypic and functional anomalies. Following HSCT[16] the B-cell immunodeficiency is usually not functionally restored, thus requiring immunoglobulin substitution.[17, 18] This gene defect also results in faulty NK-cell differentiation.

Studies examining restriction fragment length polymorphisms (RFLP) in families localized the gene encoding SCIDX1 to Xq12-13.1, and subsequent gene mapping efforts determined that mutations in the gene encoding the IL-2 receptor γ chain were responsible for the SCIDX1 phenotype. Following binding of IL-2, the association of the IL-2 receptor γ chain (71 kDa) with the IL-2 receptor β chain is necessary for expression and signal transduction. The high-affinity IL-2 receptor comprises IL-2 receptor α, β and γ chains. Like the β chain, the γ chain is constitutively expressed by T cells. The IL-2 receptor γ chain gene (*IL2RG*) has been cloned and shown to map to Xq12–13, as does the SCIDX1 locus. These results were somewhat surprising, as in IL-2-defective mice T-cell differentiation occurs (although an immunodeficiency ensues) and IL-2 deficiency in humans (see below) is also associated with T-cell differentiation. This difference suggested that the IL-2 receptor γ chain may be part of another critical receptor for T-cell differentiation, leading to the subsequent demonstration that IL-2 receptor γ chain was also a member of one form of the IL-4 receptor, as well as the IL-7R, the IL-9R the IL-15R, and the IL-21R (Fig. 35.3)[19] (Chapter 10). The IL-2 receptor γ chain has thus been named γc (c for common). Comparison of phenotypes of γc⁻ mice and IL-7 or IL-7 Rα⁻ mice has shown that this faulty interaction of IL-7 with its receptor results in the block in T-cell development.[20] The IL-7 receptor is expressed very early in hematopoietic cell development. IL-7–IL-7R interaction delivers three different signals to thymocytes, i.e., for survival, for proliferation, and for differentiation.[21] Defective IL-15–IL-15R interaction similarly causes the block in NK-cell development, explaining the absence of NK cells in SCIDX1 patients.[22] IL-4 and IL-21 receptor deficiencies account for dysfunctional B cells. Multiple mutations of the γc gene have now been reported.[23] Most affect the extracellular region of the molecule.

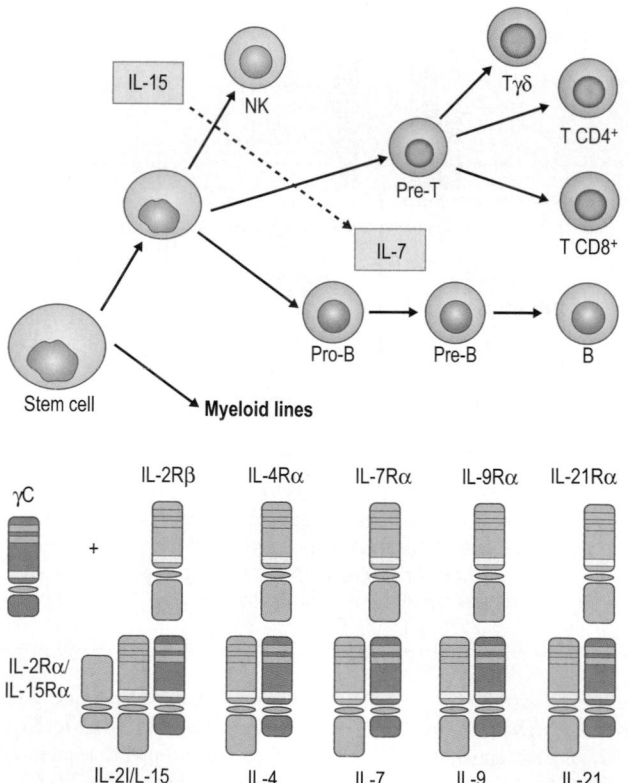

Fig. 35.3 γc-Dependent cytokines in early lymphoid development. The hematopoietic and lymphoid lines derived from a pluripotent stem cell. The NK and T-lymphocyte lineages differentiate under IL-15 and IL-7 effects, respectively. The γc chain is shared by IL-2R, IL-4R, IL-7R, IL-9R IL-15R and IL21R. Conserved cysteines are shown as orange; WS (tryptophan-serine) motif shown as yellow. (From Di Santo J, Muller W, Guy-Grand D, et al. Lymphoid development in mice with a targeted deletion of the interleukin 2γ chain. Proc Natl Acad Sci USA 1995; 92: 377, with permission From the National Academy of Sciences, USA.)

Atypical X-linked SCID

A combined X-linked immunodeficiency characterized by progressive loss of T- and B-cell function leading to death during childhood has been described in several families. In two families, T cells were found to be oligoclonal,[24] and in one family the X-chromosome inactivation pattern in obligate carriers, together with gene mapping by RFLP studies, suggested a form of SCIDX1. Analysis of the γc gene in one of these cases demonstrated two transcripts, one truncated and one of normal size, which accounted respectively for 80% and 20% of total γc mRNA.[25] A single base-pair substitution in the last position of exon 1 was found to probably disturb splicing of intron 1 (resulting in the abnormal mRNA product), whereas a less frequent normal splicing generated the normal-sized mRNA. This transcription abnormality resulted in a reduced number of normal, high-affinity IL-2-binding sites. In another case, presenting with normal numbers of T and B cells, T cells were shown to proliferate in the presence of mitogens, but IL-2 binding to T cells was reduced.[26] A mutation of γc (R222C) caused the reduced binding to IL-2. This case might thus be the consequence of defective IL-2–IL-2R interaction, although interaction of the γc receptor with other cytokines important in T-cell development, such as IL-7, is preserved. This is in contrast with the converse observation of a SCIDX1 phenotype caused by a γc mutation (A156V) affecting IL-7 (and IL-4)-mediated responses, but less so IL-2 and IL-15-mediated responses.[27]

Other atypical X-linked SCID cases included two examples of phenotype reversion. In one patient, despite a γc gene deletion encompassing most of the intracellular domain of γc, the child developed partially functional T cells that were of host origin following an unsuccessful attempt at BMT. Such T cells were detected over an 8-year period following BMT, albeit in declining numbers. Another atypical SCIDX1 patient developed an unusual phenotype characterized by the presence of host T cells (800–2000 T cells/mm³) that were able to respond (albeit not normally) to mitogens and antigens.[28] Although γc expression could not be detected on the patient's B cells, monocytes and granulocytes, T cells did express γc. The γc gene was found to be mutated in B cells (Cys→Arg substitution at position 115) but not in T cells. These results could be explained by a reverse mutation that occurs in a T-cell progenitor, differentiating into a somewhat diverse pool. By immunoscope combined with sequencing analysis, it was determined that the T-cell repertoire of this child accounted for at least 1% of the repertoire of memory T cells of a normal individual. This indicates that T-cell precursors can divide at least 10–11 times prior to the stage of *TCRB* gene rearrangement. The selective advantage conferred to this cell lineage appears very high, giving support for the feasibility of gene transfer as a treatment of SCIDX1,[29] even if conditions of hematopoietic stem cell transduction are very inefficient with currently available vectors.

SCID: JAK 3 deficiency (T⁻, B⁺, NK⁻ SCID)

A SCID phenotype similar to that of SCIDX1 is observed with an autosomal recessive pattern of inheritance in approximately 10% of cases.[30] This observation led to the hypothesis that a molecular block downstream of the γc gene could cause this condition. The immediate downstream molecule, JAK3 (Janus-associated kinase) is associated with the intracellular part of γc, is phosphorylated upon ligand binding to the receptor, and phosphorylates the Stat5 molecules.[30] Patients were indeed found to exhibit mutations in the *JAK 3* gene. The majority of described mutations affect protein expression or stability, or less commonly, result in a nonfunctional JAK3 protein. Missense mutations and small in-frame deletions may permit protein expression but interfere with kinase activity and/or γc binding. Some of these hypomorphic mutations were found in late-diagnosed patients with an atypical form of SCID characterized by oligoclonality of their T cells.[31]

SCID: IL-7R-α deficiency (T⁻, B⁺, NK⁺ SCID)

Some SCID patients present with a phenotype characterized by a selective absence of mature T lymphocytes, although maturation of NK and B cells is not affected. In most of these cases the molecular defect has now been elucidated to be mutations in the gene encoding the α chain of the IL-7 receptor.[32] All the mutations reported are clustered in the first five exons of the gene encoding the extracellular part of the protein, regardless of the type of mutation (splice-site alterations, nonsense, missense, nucleotide deletion).[33] The severe phenotype associated with these mutations indicates that integrity of IL-7 receptor-mediated signal transduction is required to promote T-cell development.

Defective adenosine deaminase causing accumulation of toxic metabolites

Adenosine deaminase deficiency (T⁻ B⁻, NK⁻ SCID)

About 20% of SCIDs are caused by adenosine deaminase deficiency. Adenosine deaminase (ADA) is a ubiquitous enzyme that reversibly transforms adenosine to inosine and 2′-deoxyadenosine (dAdo) to 2′-deoxyinosine (Fig. 35.4). The mechanism by which ADA deficiency leads to severe T, NK and B lymphocytopenia without seriously affecting other tissues is explained by the accumulation of adenosine and dAdo substrates that are preferentially toxic to lymphocytes, and especially to immature lymphocytes (thymocytes). dAdo, which diffuses freely, is phosphorylated into deoxyATP. Unlike other cell lineages, immature lymphocytes and, to a lesser extent, mature lymphocytes are poorly able to reversibly degrade dATP into dAdo.[34]

The ADA gene localizes to chromosome 20q13.11 and consists of 1089 nucleotides divided into 12 exons. Different deletions, missense mutations and splice mutations of the ADA gene that induce ADA-deficiency SCID have been characterized. Some missense mutations have been associated with partial ADA deficiency. Somatic reversions of gene mutations have been described in patients with ADA deficiency leading to the development of functional T cells.[35]

In most cases (estimated at about 85%), ADA deficiency results in a typical SCID with very low T- and B-cell counts.[2] In addition to severe infections and failure to thrive, approximately 50% of patients with ADA deficiency can develop skeletal abnormalities consisting of cupping and flaring of the costochondral junction and mild pelvic dysplasia. Some patients have neurological problems, including cortical blindness, hearing disorders and dystonia. It is difficult to exclude a diagnosis of viral encephalitis, but resolution of neurological abnormalities following specific treatment of ADA deficiency suggests that they are a direct metabolic consequence of the enzyme deficiency. Mesangial sclerosis and abnormal renal function have been noted in some patients, as well as cortical adrenal fibrosis. It is not proven that the latter lesions are specific to ADA deficiency.[34]

The typical, early-onset type of ADA deficiency is associated with barely detectable enzymatic activity in red cells and lymphocytes when erythrocyte dATP levels exceed 1000 ng/mL packed red cells. ADA

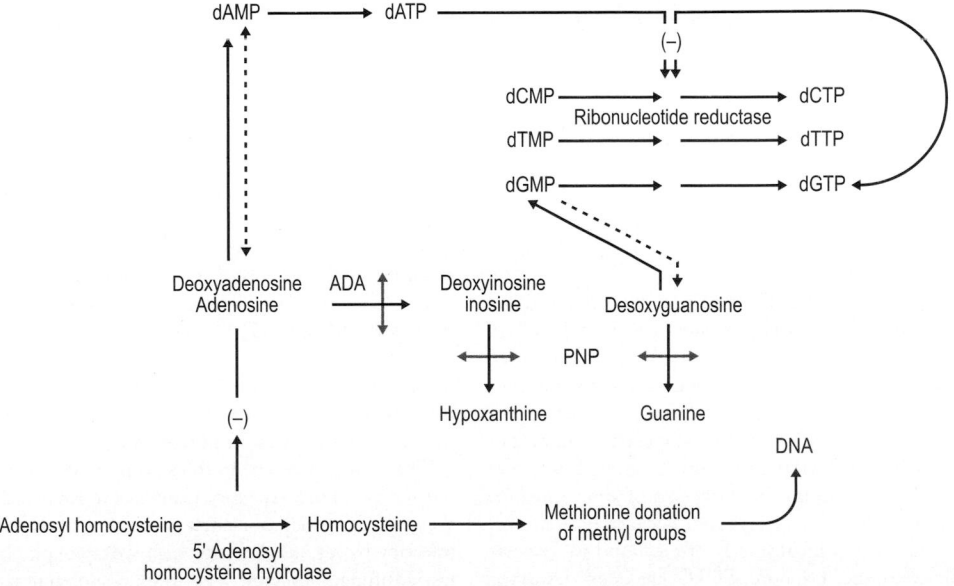

Fig. 35.4 Purine metabolism in lymphocytes. Pathway inhibition block in ADA or PNP deficiency.

gene mutations often affect the active site of the molecule or represent a deletion within the ADA gene. In some other patients, clinical onset is delayed by several months. T-cell lymphocytopenia may not be complete and there is often eosinophilia. In these patients, residual ADA activity may be found in lymphocytes. Late-onset ADA deficiency has also been described, with the first clinical manifestations occurring after 2, 3 or even 4 years. In these patients with a mild T-cell immunodeficiency, lymphocytopenia develops gradually. Autoimmune manifestations are not uncommon, as in other incomplete T-cell immunodeficiencies. For instance, refractory thrombocytopenic purpura at the age of 17 years has been described as the first manifestation of ADA deficiency.[34] In patients with late-onset ADA deficiency, dATP erythrocyte levels are usually less elevated than in the early-onset type (<1000 ng/mL packed red cells).

ADA deficiency is the only form of SCID that has a specific treatment to improve immune function, other than HSCT. Polyethylenglycol-adenosine deaminase (PEG-ADA) is a bovine-derived enzyme that replaces the deficient enzyme to eliminate toxic metabolites, which leads to increased lymphocyte survival. PEG-ADA is administered subcutaneously at least once a week and may result in normalization of cellular and humoral immunity within 8–12 weeks.[34]

Defective TCR signaling

CD3 δ, ε deficiency and CD45 deficiency

Lack of T-cell development may result from abnormal intracellular signaling after TCR binding. The CD3 complex, associated with the TCR, is composed of an assembly of four transmembrane proteins named CD3δ, ε, ζ and γ. Mutations in the genes encoding CD3 δ and ε have been shown to cause SCID in eight patients from four unrelated families and in two patients from one consanguineous family.[36] Mutations in CD3ζ and γ, and hypomorphic mutations in CD3ε, cause milder forms of immunodeficiency. These mutations, including nonsense mutations and splice site alteration, interfere with membrane receptor protein expression. The phenotypic consequences of these CD3 deficiencies are a decrease in mature CD3 T cells in the periphery, including both TCR αβ and TCRγδ T cells.[36]

Deficiency in CD45 signaling due to mutations in the CD45 gene have been described to be the cause of SCID in two patients.[37, 38]

Other SCIDs

Reticular dysgenesis

Reticular dysgenesis is a very rare SCID condition characterized not only by defective lymphoid differentiation but also by a block of myeloid differentiation. Autosomal recessive inheritance is presumed but not strictly proven, owing to the rarity of patients with this syndrome. It is not clear whether some forms of SCID with neutropenia truly represent a different syndrome or whether blocked hemopoiesis could be secondary to persistent viral infection in some cases. Not much is known about the pathogenic mechanisms of the syndrome but that its hematopoietic origin was suggested because it is curable by bone marrow transplantation. Deafness is often found in association with the SCID phenotype. Of note, SCID has been described with cyclic hematopoiesis, which resolves following bone marrow transplantation.

■ T-CELL IMMUNODEFICIENCIES WITH DETECTABLE T CELLS (COMBINED IMMUNODEFICIENCIES) (TABLE 35.3) ■

Many immunodeficient patients present with repeated infections in childhood, and occasionally autoimmunity. Immunological tests in these patients may reveal blood T cells in reduced numbers and with poor function. Antibody responses and immunoglobulin levels may also be abnormal. This clinical presentation is at least as frequent as that of typical SCID, and is associated with a large array of distinct syndromes that are far from being fully recognized and understood. This section will therefore cover the known aspects of T-cell immunodeficiencies characterized by the presence of detectable but usually abnormal T cells. This group of disorders is more commonly known as combined immunodeficiencies (CID).

CLINICAL PRESENTATION

Patients with these forms of CID do not usually develop life-threatening infections during the first years of life, but experience a variety of complications that are directly or indirectly caused by immunodeficiency: infections, autoimmunity, allergy and cancer.

In a survey of 25 patients with functional CID, infections occurred in all and were the first clinical manifestation in 22 cases.[39] Respiratory tract infections, frequently leading to bronchiectasis and recurrent or protracted diarrhea, are the most frequent complications. Cutaneous and/or mucosal candidiasis, and central nervous system infection of bacterial or viral origin, are not uncommon. Repetition of infections usually leads to failure to thrive, often necessitating parenteral nutrition. About two-thirds of patients develop repeated and/or severe viral infections, especially caused by the herpes group. Autoimmunity is a very frequent complication of CID. It occurs in at least 50% of patients, regardless of the precise diagnosis, at any time during childhood or early adulthood. The autoimmunity is caused mostly by autoantibodies against blood cells (anemia, thrombocytopenia, and neutropenia), although hepatitis, and vasculitis involving the brain and kidney have been observed. Autoimmunity is often severe and tends to relapse, requiring aggressive immunosuppression, which can worsen the immunodeficiency.

The mechanisms of autoimmunity in this setting remain unclear. It is also possible that the processes of negative selection of developing T and B cells and peripheral tolerance are impaired by the immune deficiency, resulting in the expansion of autoimmune clones. In addition, a deficiency in T-regulatory cells producing immunosuppressive cytokines such as IL-10 and TGF-β, can participate in this phenomenon.

Allergic manifestations (eczema, asthma, urticaria, etc.) are also frequent (48% in our series). Elevated serum IgE is a frequent finding in patients with CID. Cancer, and especially lymphomas, are not uncommon as a cause of death in these patients.

The natural outcome in this group of patients is generally poor, with a mean survival of 5–10 years. Causes of death usually include organ failure that is progressively worsened by poor nutritional status and uncontrolled infection by various microorganisms, despite prophylactic use of antibiotics, antifungal therapy and immunoglobulin supplementation. Early BMT is often proposed as the definite treatment, given the almost universal development of organ failure in older patients.

Table 35.3 T-cell deficiencies (combined immunodeficiencies)

Defect	Inheritance	Phenotype	Molecular defect
MHC class II deficiency (Bare lymphocyte syndrome)			
A	AR	Defective exp of MHC class II	Transactivator CIITA
B	AR	"	RFXANK
C	AR	"	RFX5
D	AR	"	RFXAP
CD3 deficiencies			
γ	AR	Mild T cell ID	CD3γ
ε (hypomorphic)	AR	"	CD3ε
Activation deficiencies			
Low CD8/abnormal CD4	AR		ZAP70
defective Ca2+ flux	AR	Functional T cell ID	ORAI1
CD25 deficiency	AR	Functional T cell ID	CD25
PNP deficiency		Progressive T cell ID	PNP
ADA deficiency (late onset)	AR	Neurological manifestations	
	AR	Progressive T cell ID	ADA
Omenn's syndrome	AR	Activated T cells in skin and gut	RAG1, RAG2
		Oligoclonality	Artemis, IL7-Rα
XL T-cell immunodeficiency	XL	Progressive T cell ID	Mild type IL2Rγ of XL SCID

XL, X-linked recessive.

DIAGNOSIS OF CID

The clinical diagnosis of CID is suggested by repeated infections, often associated with allergy and autoimmunity disease. Findings of mild T-cell lymphocytopenia and disturbances in functional T-cell assays (*in vivo* skin tests and *in vitro* proliferative tests in the presence of immunizing antigens) leads to the diagnosis in the absence of an acquired cause, such as HIV infection or malnutrition. An extended phenotype analysis, including enumeration of naïve and memory subpopulations of T cells, CD45RA+ and CD45RO+, respectively, may be useful for the diagnosis of unclear immunodeficiencies if a cell subset is absent or markedly decreased. Patients with CID may present with hyperimmunoglobulinemia of all isotypes, due to nonspecific polyclonal activation. However, partial hypogammaglobulinemia and a defective antibody response to immunizations are more commonly found.

CID DISEASES

Major histocompatibility complex (MHC) class II deficiency ('bare lymphocyte syndrome')

This is a relatively rare autosomal recessive primary immunodeficiency characterized by a profound defect in the expression of HLA class II molecules. The disease was first described in 1979, since when more than 100 cases have been identified, mostly in patients originating from the

Mediterranean area.[40] Clinical onset occurs in the first year of life, usually with recurrent bronchopulmonary infections and chronic diarrhea. The clinical course is marked by unremitting diarrhea, hepatitis and cholangitis, viral meningoencephalitis and various autoimmune manifestations. The mean age at the time of death is 4 years, often caused by overwhelming viral infections due to either enteroviruses, adenoviruses or herpes viruses. It has recently been recognized, however, that some patients can survive into adulthood with little symptomatology. Diagnosis relies on the absence of HLA DR, DQ, DP and DM molecules at the surface of all cells constitutively expressing HLA class II molecules

(B cells, monocytes, dendritic cells) and at the surface of interferon (IFN)-γ-activated cells (T cells, fibroblasts, etc.). Antigen-specific responses *in vivo* and *in vitro* are absent, whereas allogeneic responses and T-cell numbers are preserved (although CD4 T-cell counts are decreased). There is variable hypogammaglobulinemia, mainly affecting IgA and IgG$_2$. Antibody production is profoundly defective.[41]

Some MHC class II expression has been detected post mortem on medullary cells of children's thymuses and, more importantly, from aborted fetuses. This finding suggests leakiness of the defect (although leakiness in the periphery is uncommon) or the presence of an alternative regulation pattern of MHC class II gene transcription in thymic cells. In any case, this can account for partially preserved T-cell differentiation as well as a capacity for self-/nonself-discrimination. Vβ element usage by TCRs of residual CD4 T cells was found to be normal, indicating that Vβ element usage frequency is independent of selection events.

The disease genetically segregates independently of the MHC, which implies that the responsible gene(s) lie(s) outside the MHC and exert(s) a pleiotropic transregulation of MHC class II expression. Fusion experiments between MHC class II− B-cell lines from patients with this immunodeficiency have defined four complementation groups (A, B, C, D) (Table 35.4). The identification of the genetic causes of these four complementation groups has led to a better understanding of MHC class II expression regulation. MHC class II expression is regulated by a proximal promoter region that contains four *cis*-acting DNA elements called the S, X, X2 and Y boxes. RFX, X2BP and NF-Y bind respectively X, X2 and Y boxes (Fig. 35.5).[41] RFX, is expressed ubiquitously and is an heteromeric protein consisting of three elements, RFXAP (p36),[42] RFX5 (p75)[43] and RFXANK (p33)[44] or RFX-B. In MHC class II deficiency a mutation in either one of the genes has been found. Mutations affecting RFXANK/RFX-B were found in the complementation group B,[43, 44] with a common deletion observed in patients of north African origin,[44] of RFX5 in group C,[42] and of RFXAP in group D.[42] A defect in any of these proteins leads to the absence of the RFX complex. This situation is associated with nonoccupancy of the MHC class II promoter, as shown by DNAse protection assay and *in vivo* footprint experiments (Table 35.4). This indicates that binding of NF-Y and X2BP to box Y and X2 is dependent on the RFX complex showing cooperativity of these transcription factors. The MHC class II tissue specific and inducible expression is under the control of the CIITA *trans*-activator. The *CIITA* gene is transcribed constitutively in B cells, dendritic cells and activated T cells, and in other cells upon stimulation with IFN-γ.[41] Mutation in the *CIITA* encoding gene is responsible for group A of MHC class II deficiency. *CIITA* interacts with the RFX proteins to stabilize the complex and enable class II gene transcription.

TAP-1 and TAP-2 deficiencies

In 1994, de La Salle et al.[45] reported on two siblings presenting with chronic pneumonia in whom expression of HLA class I molecules was reduced and who exhibited a CD8 lymphopenia. This immunodeficiency phenotype was caused by mutation in the *TAP-2* gene. TAP-1 and TAP-2 proteins compose the HLA class I-associated peptide transporter. The TAP complex transports peptides from the cytosol to the endoplasmic reticulum, where the loading of HLA class I molecule by the peptide occurs. In the absence of the TAP complex, the HLA class I molecules are peptide free and thus unstable. The *Tap-1* and *2* encoding genes are localized on chromosome 6 within the HLA class II gene region.[46]

Table 35.4 Class II deficiency/bare lymphocyte syndrome

Complementation group		Molecular defect
A	Promoters occupied by DNA-binding proteins	Transactivator CIITA
B	Promoters unoccupied *in vivo*	RFXANK/ RFX-B
C	Promoters unoccupied *in vivo*	RFX5
D	Promoters unoccupied *in vivo*	RFXAP

The main clinical manifestations of TAP-1/TAP-2 deficiency are characteristic of an immunodeficiency. They consist of chronic lung infections, often leading in late childhood to bilateral bronchiectasis. Sinusitis and nasal polyposis are also often reported.[46] The lung manifestations can be a consequence of chronic infection, but necrotizing granulomatous lesions are also present in some cases. In none of the cases was a susceptibility to viral infections such as herpes virus noted.

The diagnosis is based on the reduced (30–100-fold) expression of HLA class I molecules on blood mononuclear cell surfaces. Expression of these molecules is not increased by PHA or IFN-γ stimulation. TcR α/β CD8 lymphopenia may be observed, but does not always occur. An excess of TcR γ/δ-bearing T cells (using more often δ$_1$ than δ$_2$) has been described in some cases: these could be autoreactive and participating in the generation of the skin lesions. The number of circulating NK cells is variable between patients, and they may be involved in the pathogenesis of vasculitis as potentially autoreactive NK cells. It has been shown that the cytotoxic activity of CD8 cells against virus-infected targets is preserved. These results suggest that a possible recognition of antigens presented by HLA class I molecules in a TAP-independent manner can occur in these patients.[47] Humoral immune responses have been found to be normal.

CD3γ and ζ deficiencies

CID due to CD3 deficiencies is extremely rare. The most prominent feature of CD3 deficiency is the defective expression (1–50% of normal expression) of the CD3/TCR complex on T cells despite normal T-cell numbers. The proportion of either CD8 or CD4 T cell could be low in these patients. In all cases, anti-CD3 monoclonal antibody-induced activation is poor, as judged by cell proliferation, CD25 expression induction and intracellular calcium increase. Antigen-induced proliferation is either low or normal, depending on the antigens tested. Antibody responses to protein antigens after vaccination are normal or only partially affected. However, antibody responses to polysaccharides could be defective.

The clinical manifestations of CD3/TCR deficiency are variable between patients. For example, in a Spanish family, one of two siblings had a severe phenotype whereas the other had no symptoms. The former developed failure to thrive, autoimmunity, protracted diarrhea and fatal pneumonia at 32 months of age. His affected brother had only infrequent respiratory tract infections and no autoimmune manifestations. Mutations in the CD3γ chain-encoding gene have been found in two patients, one

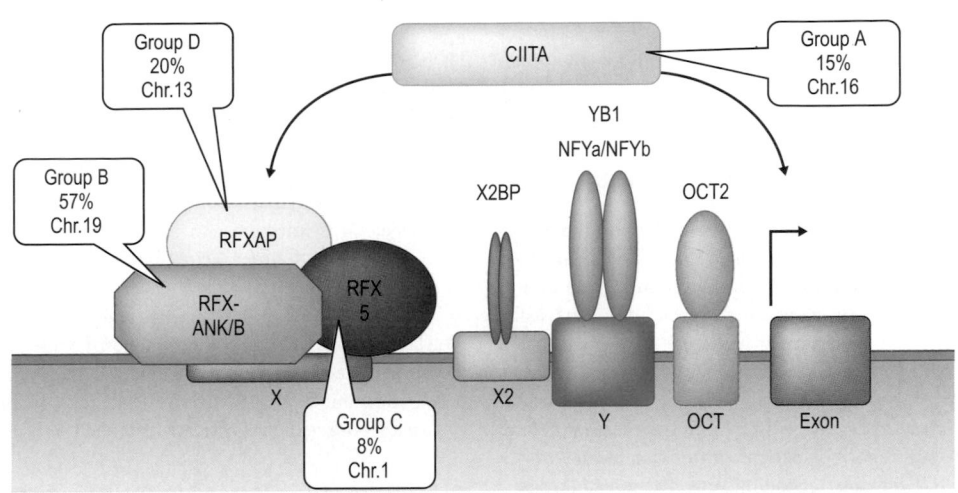

Fig. 35.5 Promoter region of HLA class II gene in HLA class II expression deficiency. The complex RFX composed of RFXAP, RFX-ANK/B, and RFX5 binds the X box and is stabilized by the transactivator CIITA. Mutations in one of these four components are involved in the four complementation groups of HLA class II deficiency. (From Masternak K, Barras E, Zufferey M, et al. A gene encoding a novel RFX-associated transactivator is mutated in the majority of MHC class II immunodeficiency patients. Nature Genet 1998; 20: 273.)

Spanish and one of Turkish origin. In the Turkish case, the parents were first cousins and the mutation was a nucleotide substitution leading to a stop codon. In the Spanish case, a point mutation affected an initiation codon on the paternal allele and a splicing site on the maternal allele. Interestingly, the absence of CD3γ protein did not completely abolish CD3/TCR expression, which was reduced to 50% of control values. CD8 T-cell counts were reduced in these patients, leading to the suggestion that CD8 interacts with CD3γ in the antigen recognition unit. More recently, a homozygous mutation of *CD3ζ* has been reported in two patients with serious infections that abolished the expression of CD3ζ chain.[48,48a] The residual expression of TCR/CD3 complex at the membrane levels was very low (1% of the normal expression) and thus T cells were incapable of activation through the antigen receptor. Surprisingly, in one patient the germline mutation of *CD3ζ* was associated with three somatic *CD3ζ* mutations in 10% of T cells. All these mutations were located at codon 70, thus restoring normal expression of the T-cell receptor–CD3 complex, which included a ζ chain presenting an amino-acid substitution. However, in spite of this normal expression, no ZAP-70 phosphorylation was detected after TCR/CD3 triggering.[48]

T-cell activation deficiencies (Fig. 35.6)

ZAP-70 deficiency

Several patients with low CD8 T-cell counts have been shown to lack expression of the lymphocyte kinase ZAP-70, resulting in defective T-cell receptor signaling and CD8 thymic selection. This disease results from mutations in the ZAP-70 encoding gene, leading to the absence of the protein.[49] The absence of peripheral blood CD8 T cells contrasts with normal or elevated counts of CD4 T cells, although they do not respond to T-cell receptor-mediated activation signals. NK cells are found in normal numbers. This immunodeficiency is associated with a low level of serum immunoglobulins and a defect in antibody responses. The phenotype of this immunodeficiency supports the key role of ZAP-70 in downstream signaling upon TCR cross-linking. ZAP-70, once

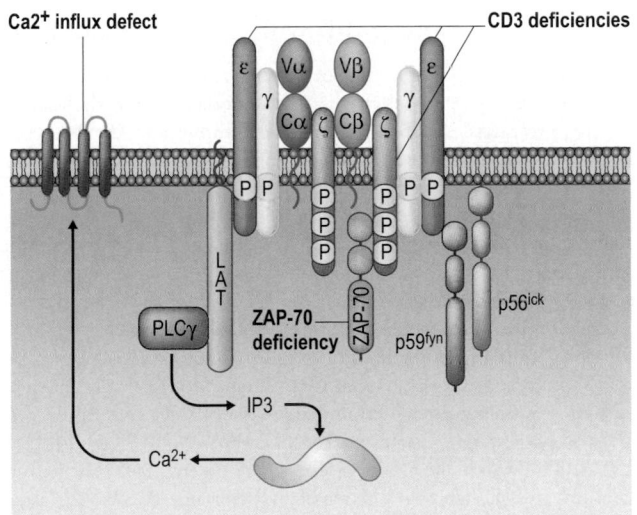

Fig. 35.6 Schema of T-cell activation deficiencies. Mutations in the CD3 component parts (γ,δ, ε, ζ) of the TCR/CD3 complex prevent cell signaling taking place from the cell surface to the cell nucleus. Likewise, mutations in cytoplasmic enzymes (e.g., ZAP-70) inhibit the transmission of cell signals to the cell nucleus via phosphorylation. Many immunodeficiencies have been described that involve this cell signaling pathway. The calcineurin pathway depends on the initial phosphorylation of phospholipase Cγ (PLCγ), which generates inositol 3P (IP3), responsible for calcium release from endoplasmic reticulum. Calcium depletion of the endoplasmic reticulum or calcium cytosolic increase leads to the opening of a membrane channel.

phosphorylated by kinases such as Lck or Fyn, binds to ITAM motifs on the CD3 complex and then phosphorylates a series of key molecules involved in T-cell activation.

Other T-cell activation immunodeficiencies: Defects in the expression of CD25 and CD8α

Patients with defective T-cell activation may present with blood lymphocyte counts and phenotypes close to normal ranges. The diagnosis is based on the observation of absent or low proliferation in response to lectins and anti-CD3 antibody. Antigen-induced proliferation is usually absent or low. In these patients, serum Ig levels are either within the normal range or elevated. Ig-restricted heterogeneity has been observed. Antibody responses have been impaired in most cases. Careful examination of T-cell activation pathways has led to finding molecular defects in some cases, such as the report of patient with a mutation in both alleles of the CD25 (IL-2Rα chain)-encoding gene. Decreased numbers of peripheral T cells that display poor proliferation capacity characterizes this immunodeficiency.[50] In a single family, a CD8 T-cell deficiency was described as a consequence of CD8α gene mutations. Clinical consequences are limited; interestingly, the presence of cytolytic CD4 T cells could be detected.[51]

Omenn's syndrome (SCID with hypereosinophilia)

This syndrome is characterized by early onset after birth of diffuse erythroderma associated with pachyderma and alopecia involving the scalp and eyebrows, protracted diarrhea with failure to thrive, and life-threatening infections. There is marked hepatosplenomegaly and lymphadenopathy. Laboratory investigations revealed frequent lymphocytosis and hypereosinophilia. Extensive T-cell infiltration involving the skin (dermis and epidermis) and gut is characteristic of this condition. In contrast, despite enlargement, lymph nodes are essentially devoid of lymphocytes, which are replaced by macrophages. As in the different SCIDs, the thymus is hypoplastic with little lymphoid differentiation.

Blood T cells express activation markers such as CD25 and HLA class II antigens. Interestingly, the T-cell phenotype is usually characterized by the presence of a predominant T-cell subset that differs from patient to patient, i.e., TCRα/β CD4+, TCRα/β CD8+ TCR α/β CD4- CD8- or TCR γ/δ. All immunoglobulins are barely detectable, with the exception of IgE, which is increased. Circulating B cells are usually undetectable. The presence of a small number of T-cell clones may be observed.[52] (Fig. 35.7)

The association of the above-mentioned phenotype with typical T-B- SCID in the same families suggested that a common gene mutation could lead either to a SCID or to an Omenn's phenotype. This hypothesis was validated by the identification of hypomorphic RAG1/RAG2 mutations in patients with Omenn's syndrome.[11] The hypomorphic mutations of RAG1/2, leading to a residual functional activity of the mutated product, could enable the generation of a low number of functional TCR gene rearrangements in the thymus. Peripheral expansion of autoreactive clones toward epithelial antigens is postulated to account for the accumulation of oligoclonal aggressive T cells, mostly in the skin and gut. Because of the low autoimmune regulator (AIRE) expression in the thymus (a possible consequence of thymopoiesis), the autoreactive nature of these clones could be the consequence of defective AIRE-dependent negative selection.[53] Omenn's T cells exhibit a Th2 phenotype, characterized by high-level production of IL-4 and IL-5. This finding explains why there is an eosinophilia and why the residual B cells make only IgE. More, recently Omenn's syndrome has been reported to occur in patients with *Artemis* mutations[14] or *IL7-Ra* mutations.[54]

Hypomorphic *RAG-1* mutations have also been found associated with expansion of oligoclonal TCR γδ T cells in a context of disseminated cytomegalovirus infection and autoimmunity.[11] In one case, γδ T cells were shown to be CMV specific. These observations emphasize the high variability of phenotypic consequences of *RAG1/2* mutations from typical SCID to milder T-cell immunodeficiency, Omenn's syndrome or only γδ T-cell expansion. It is likely that functional consequences of *RAG1/2* gene mutations, genetic background and environment (infection) interfere and define the clinical consequences. This degree of complexity is likely to be eventually observed for a number of other T-cell immunodeficiencies.

Purine nucleoside phosphorylase (PNP) deficiency

PNP deficiency is a rare cause of CID. To date, fewer than 50 cases have been reported.[55] PNP deficiency causes a progressive cellular immunodeficiency that is associated in one-third of cases with defective antibody production. Autoimmunity is also found in one-third of patients (autoimmune hemolytic anemia, thrombocytopenia, etc.). About two-thirds of patients develop neurological manifestations that appear to be specific to the disease, and consist of developmental delay, mental retardation, spasticity, or hypotonia and tremor. Diagnosis is based on PNP activity in red cells or lymphocytes in patients with immunodeficiency. Hypouricemia caused by defective transformation of inosine into hypoxanthine can also suggest the diagnosis. BMT is the sole definite therapeutic approach and has been mostly successful.

PNP deficiency is an autosomal recessive disease. So far, all the mutations of the PNP-encoding gene observed in patients – nonsense, missense or splice-site alteration – completely abolish the enzymatic activity.[55] PNP deficiency is thought to induce CID by depleting deoxynucleotides: the accumulation of dGTP inhibits ribonucleotide reductase, leading to deprivation of dCTP and dTTP and inhibition of DNA synthesis. It is likely that dGTP accumulation is toxic for resting T cells (causing lymphocytopenia) by a distinct but unknown mechanism.

▐ KEY CONCEPTS

T-CELL DEFICIENCY WITH COMBINED FEATURES

>> Variable T-cell defects are associated with some abnormality of other cell types or organ systems, as in DiGeorge syndrome, cartilage–hair hypoplasia, ataxia telangiectasia.

>> B-cell function varies according to the state of T-cell function.

>> Survival beyond infancy is common, but the quality of life may be poor because of progressive T-cell dysfunction and increasing severity of infection, autoimmunity, and premature appearance of malignancy.

>> Precise molecular defects and their effect on T-cell function are not completely understood.

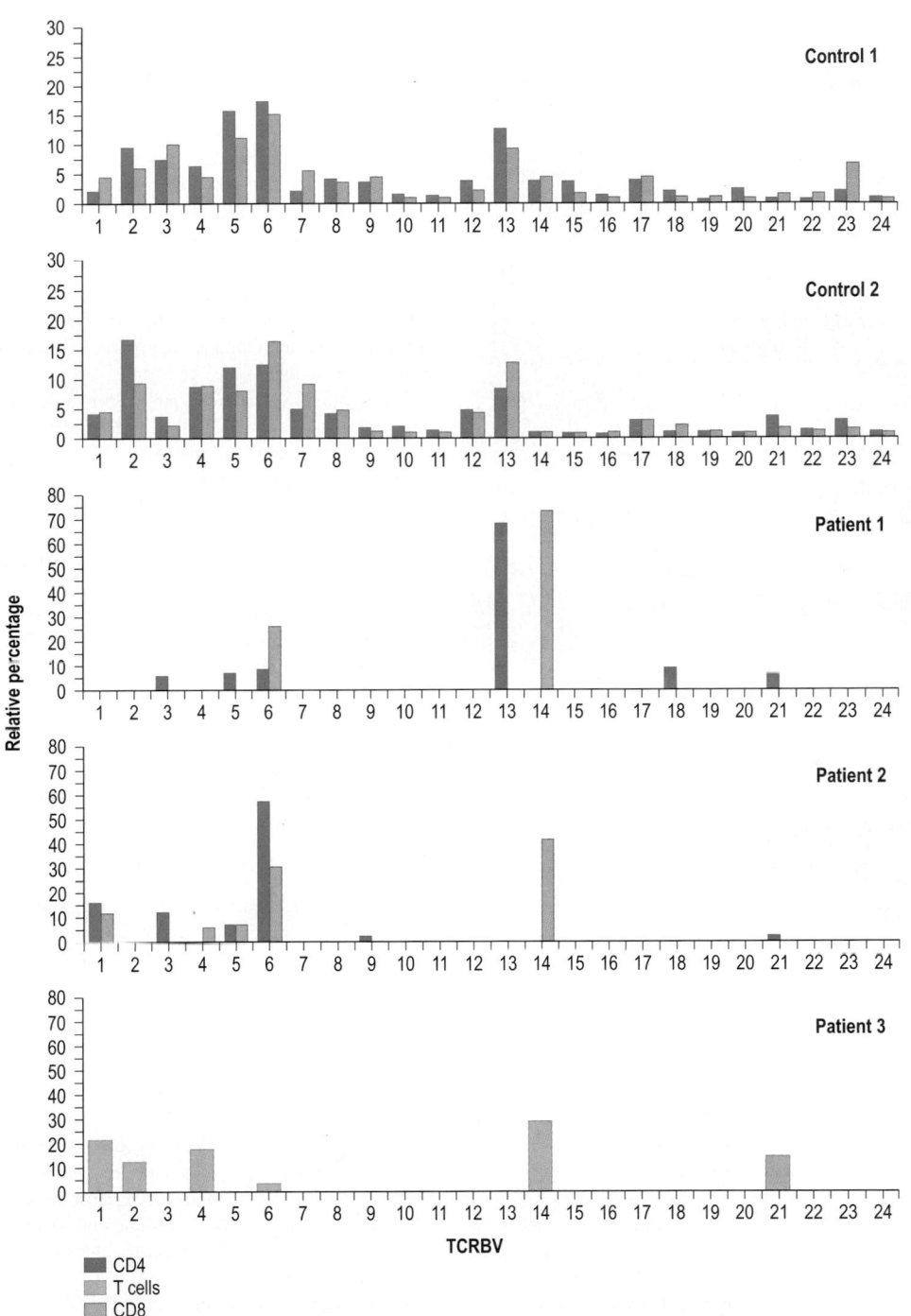

Fig. 35.7 Vβ usage by T lymphocytes for Omenn's patients. Vβ usage was analyzed by anchored PCR on either CD4, CD8 or T cells from controls and Omenn's syndrome patients.

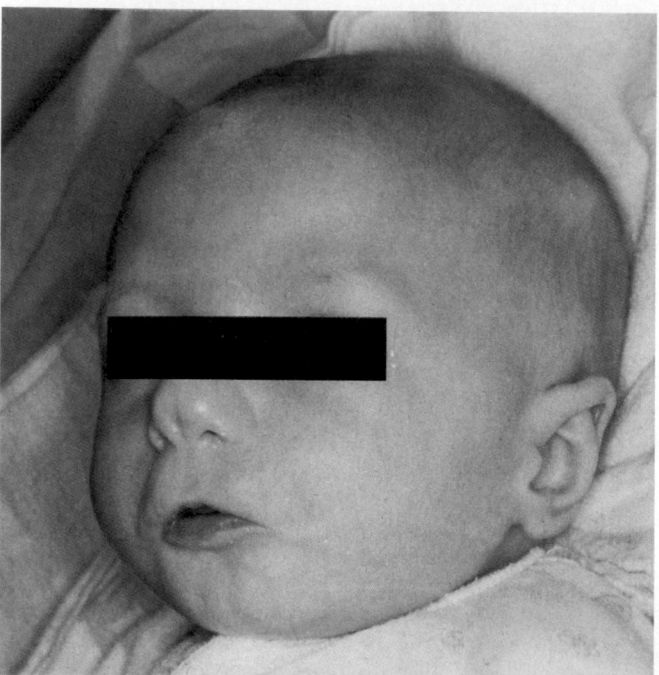

Fig. 35.8 Facies of child with DiGeorge syndrome. Note micrognathia, low-set ears and short philtrum.

■ T-CELL DEFICIENCIES WITH ASSOCIATED NON-IMMUNE FEATURES ■

DIGEORGE SYNDROME

The DiGeorge syndrome (DGS) results from faulty development of the third and fourth branchial arches, which leads to thymic, parathyroid and conotruncal cardiac defects. Facial defects are also found, and include micrognathia, low-set and posteriorly rotated ears, hypertelorism or a short philtrum (Fig. 35.8). Cardiovascular lesions usually consist of an interrupted aortic arch and truncus arteriosus. Mental retardation, suction defect and dysarthry are also common.

Depending on the degree of immunodeficiency, 'complete DGS' with thymic aplasia and very low T-cell counts is different from the more common 'partial DGS' with reduced T-cell counts and mild immunodeficiency. Parathyroid aplasia and conotruncal heart defects can be found with any degree of immunodeficiency. Heterogeneity can also be found in the clinical course, with partial resolution of the T-cell dysfunction. Thymic hypoplasia is found in most patients, but persistent immune dysfunction in only a few. Significant clinical problems secondary to T-cell lymphocytopenia are only observed in a minority of patients, in those who usually have <500 T cell/μL of blood. There is thus, a clinical spectrum of presentations, ranging from thymic aplasia with absence of T cells (<1% of DGS cases) to mild or normal T-cell counts. When T-cell counts are normal, patients may be considered in the clinically

overlapping velocardiofacial syndrome, which does not include defective development of the thymus.

DGS is a developmental field defect of the pharyngeal pouches involving neural crest derivatives. Autosomal-dominant inheritance with variable penetrance is observed. Cytogenetic abnormalities are detected in most cases, and include rare mosaic tetraploidy and 10p deletion. More than 90% of patients have a hemizygous deletion of 1.5–3 Mb interval on chromosome 22q11.2 (Fig. 35.9). This specific hemizygosity is also found in the velocardiofacial syndrome. The minimal DiGeorge gene locus has been restricted to 250 kb and includes 24–30 genes. Some of these genes are candidates to explain the complex phenotypes observed in DiGeorge patients. One candidate is *UFD1L*, an ortholog of a yeast gene involved in the degradation of ubiquinated proteins. Haploinsufficiency of *UFDIL* in a mouse model causes the same congenital heart and craniofacial defects as in DGS.[56] Of note, one DGS patient carries a monoallelic deletion of exons 1–3 of *UFD1 L* as well as of a *CDC45L*, a closely linked gene.[56] More recently mutations in *TBX1* has been found in two unrelated DGS patients without deletion at 22q11.2.[57] *TBX1* maps within the DiGeorge region and encodes a T-box transcription factor that is required for the proper development of the heart. Its complete loss in mice causes development defects similar to those seen in DGS patients. Modifier genes, such as *VEGF*, which regulates TBX1 expression, could explain the variability of the phenotype observed in patients.[58]

The most severe immunological form of DGS requires therapeutic intervention for survival. This can be accomplished either through HLA-identical bone marrow transplantation, which can provide expanding mature T cells in the absence of GVHD, or by transplantation of thymic tissue, as shown recently in a small number of patients,[59] indicating that host-derived hematopoietic cells within the thymus can govern both positive and negative steps of T-cell education.

WISKOTT–ALDRICH SYNDROME

Wiskott–Aldrich syndrome (WAS) is a complex X-linked disorder characterized by an immunodeficiency associated with thrombocytopenia, abnormal platelets and eczema. Its frequency has been estimated at one case per 250 000 live births.[60]

Patients may present with a bleeding tendency that can be apparent as early as in the first few months of life, often as bloody diarrhea. This occurs because of thrombocytopenia secondary to peripheral destruction of platelets, and in most cases splenectomy corrects it. WAS patients have abnormal megakaryocytopoiesis, resulting in a reduction of the mean platelet volume and impaired aggregation. Thrombocytopenia is of variable intensity, but can worsen during infections or because of overt autoimmune antibody production against platelets. Thrombocytopenia relapses can occur, especially in young children (less than 3 years of age). Eczema is frequent, severe, tends to be diffuse, and relapses frequently. Its association with thrombocytopenia and small platelets in young boys is strongly suggestive of WAS.

The immune deficiency in WAS is complex. It is characterized by defective production of antibodies to polysaccharides, increasing the susceptibility of infections by encapsulated organisms such as *Haemophilus influenzae* and *Streptococcus pneumoniae*, with low serum IgM but generally elevated levels of other Ig isotypes.[60] Worthy of note is that IgM serum levels are often normal or elevated during the first year of life. The T-cell deficiency consists of gradual hypoplasia with a reduction in T-cell counts, especially CD4 T cells, which correlates

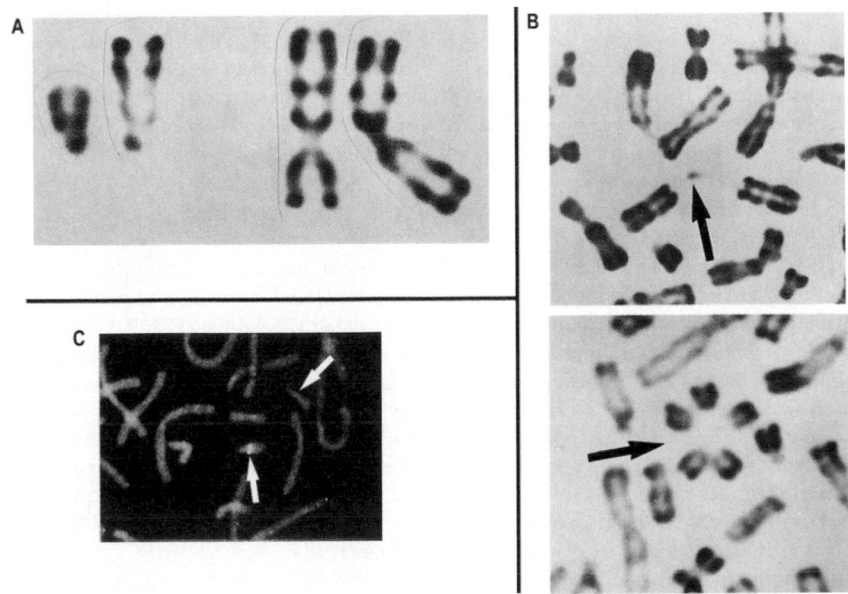

Fig. 35.9 Cytogenetic features in immunodeficiencies. (**A**) A 7.14 translocation in ataxia telangiectasia (PHA blasts). (**B**) Centromeric elongation (top) and multimeric chromosomes (bottom) in ICF syndrome. (**C**) Hemizygosity of 22q11 in DiGeorge syndrome as revealed by fluorescence in situ SC111.1 probe (arrows).

with spontaneous cell apoptosis.[61] There is no specific test that is consistently abnormal, although cytotoxic T-cell function is often defective. Nevertheless, the T-cell deficiency can be severe enough to facilitate severe viral infections and some opportunistic infections (e.g., *Pneumocystis jiroveci*).

Autoimmune manifestations are not uncommon in WAS. In addition to the production of autoantibodies to platelets, autoimmune hemolytic anemia and neutropenia can be observed, sometimes in very young children. Severe vasculitis, aneurysm and glomerulonephritis have been described, and require management by aggressive immunosuppression.[62]

The risk of cancer in WAS patients has been estimated at 2% per year. Lymphomas are the most frequent malignancies. The overall prognosis of WAS remained poor for many years, with a median survival of 5–7 years in 1980. The main cause of death was infection (59%), followed by hemorrhages (27%) and malignancies (5%). This led to the successful introduction of allogeneic BMT as a therapeutic option. BMT from an HLA-identical donor now offers a better than 90% chance of cure.[60]

Genetic segregation studies of WAS in families indicated that there was a single locus mapping to the proximal part of the short arm of the X-chromosome in Xp11-Xp1.3. The X-chromosome inactivation pattern in obligate carriers is nonrandom in all hematopoietic lineages, indicating functional expression of the WAS gene in all cell lineages. In 1994, a novel gene (*WASP*) was isolated[63] and mutations of this gene were found in WAS and in isolated X-linked thrombocytopenia (XLT).[64] The gene product, WASP, is a 53-kDa protein in which several functional domains have been identified: a pleckstrin homology domain in the N-terminal region, a GTPase-binding domain (CRIB motif) and in the C-terminal region a proline-rich domain and a Verprolin/cofilin domain. Mild forms of the disease have been observed in patients with WAS mutations, with few or no infections, mild immunodeficiency, mild

eczema and thrombocytopenia. At this end of the spectrum is XLT. XLT is more frequently associated with missense mutations and typical severe WAS with mutations leading to an absence of the WAS protein.[62]

Morphological and membrane abnormalities, as well as signal transduction defects, have been described in WAS platelets and lymphocytes. The reduced response of platelets to agonist stimulation and the poor mitogen-induced proliferation by T cells have been shown to be associated with impaired early biochemical events of activation.[65] All these data suggested a main role of WASP in the cytoskeletal arrangement and the activation pathways. The WASP protein structure is fully coherent with this hypothesis. Defective WASP expression leads to a defective formation of the immunological synapse upon TCR activation. The CRIB motif interacts with the actin-binding protein cdc42, which regulates filopodial and lamellipodal extensions. The proline-rich domain binds SH3-containing proteins such as Grb2 and Fyn, involved in activation events. In addition, a WASP-interacting protein (WIP) and the complex WASP-WIP is able to induce actin polymerization and redistribution in lymphoid cells.[62]

T-CELL DEFICIENCIES WITH DNA REPAIR DEFECTS

Ataxia–telangiectasia and AT-like disorder

Ataxia–telangiectasia (AT) is an autosomal recessive disease characterized by oculocutaneous telangiectasias and progressive cerebellar ataxia with Purkinje cell degeneration; it is usually an immunodeficiency of IgA, IgE and IgG$_2$, with a moderate reduction in T-cell counts and responses. AT patients are prone to lymphomas and epithelial cell carcinomas. A hallmark of AT is DNA fragility with abnormal chromosome translocation in lymphocytes, mainly involving TCR and Ig loci and known as illegitimate recombination. AT cells are abnormally sensitive to ionizing radiation and exhibit radioresistant DNA synthesis.

Patients have IgA and IgG$_2$ deficiency, which probably accounts for the most frequent (sinopulmonary) infections. There is, however, a T-cell deficiency, because the thymus (at autopsy) is markedly hypoplastic and peripheral T-cell counts are usually decreased. Functional *in vitro* T-cell assays usually reveal mild defects, although T-cell cytotoxicity can be more profoundly affected. Clinical consequences of the T-cell immunodeficiency appear limited: for instance, opportunistic infections are uncommon. Management includes immunoglobulin replacement and prophylaxis antibiotics to prevent and reduce the frequency of infections.

A hallmark of AT is cytogenetic abnormalities, found predominantly in T cells; these consist of chromosomal rearrangements mainly involving 7p14, 7q35, 14q12 and 14q32 (Fig. 35.9). These breakpoints correspond exactly to the respective sites of TCRγ, TCRβ, TCRα/δ and immunoglobulin heavy-chain loci. Inversions and translocations result from these chromosome rearrangements. They affect on average 10% of mitoses and form hybrid antigen-receptor genes. The site-specificity of these breaks represents abnormal 'illegitimate' lymphocyte antigen receptor rearrangements, which may explain the gradual decline in T-cell counts. About one in 10 AT patients develops T-cell clones, the proportion of which among peripheral T cells increases with time. These clones are not associated with clinical manifestations and are characterized by unique chromosomal translocations affecting chromosome 14, including a q32 breakpoint proximal to Ig heavy-chain loci. Ultimately, after several years, such clones evolve into T-cell leukemia. Many other breakpoints are also detected in leukemic T cells from AT patients.

Ubiquitous radiation hypersensitivity is another remarkable characteristic of AT. An interesting associated hallmark of the disease is the inability of AT cells to stop DNA replication following γ irradiation. This anomaly is likely to underlie the extreme susceptibility to cancer found in AT patients (200-fold increased risk) and even in AT heterozygotes (fivefold increased risk).

The AT locus has been mapped to chromosome 11q23. The ATM gene encodes a 350 kDa protein containing a functional kinase domain that is homologous to the PI-3 kinase family.[66] The ATM protein is ubiquitously expressed in all tissues and is present in both the cytosol and the nucleus. Mutations of the *ATM* gene have been found in most AT patients leading to truncated proteins, and missense mutations leading to amino acid substitutions have been reported in association with a milder phenotype.

Interestingly, clinical heterogeneity in AT has been further underlined recently with the description of patients having typical chromosomal translocations, immunodeficiency and lymphomas, but without ataxia or telangiectasia, and patients with peripheral neuropathy and spinal atrophy but without telangiectasia or immunodeficiency.

The function of ATM protein is complex and involves the control of genomic stability. The protein acts as a sensor of radiation-induced DNA damage and induces cell cycle arrest at different checkpoints through multiple steps and protein interactions.[67] It is involved in the DNA repair process by activating the double-strand break (DSB) repair protein complex hMRE-11/hRad50/Nbs1. Monitoring of DNA integrity is also mediated by radiation-induced association with a histone deacetylase (HDAC1) involved in chromatin structure modification and DNA packaging.[68] Genomic instability in AT patients probably accounts for premature cell senescence (e.g., Purkinje cells in the cerebellum) and cancer risk.

Mutations in *MRE11* have been reported in three families with AT-like disorder (ATLD), which includes progressive cerebellar degeneration and immunodeficiency, but not ocular telangiectasis. *MRE11* is part of the DSB complex, with DNA exonuclease and endonuclease activity; it senses double-strand damage and promotes the joining of noncomplementary ends.[69]

Nijmegen breakage syndrome (NBS)

Nijmegen breakage syndrome shares some of the characteristics of AT. Common features include similar chromosomal rearrangements in T cells, defective inhibition of DNA synthesis following irradiation, and an immunodeficiency. These patients have no clinical signs of ataxia or telangiectasias. They do, however, have microcephaly and developmental retardation. The immunodeficiency is more severe than in AT, with profound T-cell lymphocytopenia and depressed T-cell responses to mitogens and antigens. Panhypogammaglobulinemia is common. In addition, malignancies are very frequent and appear early in life: five of 14 patients in one series developed lymphomas between 2 and 12 years of age.[70]

The NBS gene has been identified. *NBS1* encodes the nibrine or Nbs1 protein, one member of the hMREII/Rad50/Nbs1 complex that is activated by ATM to bind and repair double-strand DNA breaks.[71] It is remarkable to observe how the study of three related diseases – AT, ATLD and NBS – has contributed to unravel a complex molecular pathway involved in the control of genomic integrity.

Immunodeficiency, centromeric instability and facial anomalies (ICF syndrome)

The ICF syndrome associates, in a heterogeneous manner, an immunodeficiency and facial anomaly to centromeric chromosome instability. About 20 cases have so far been reported in the literature.[72] A high rate of consanguinity and occurrence of the syndrome in two siblings strongly supports an autosomal recessive inheritance. Facial anomalies consist of hypertelorism, a flat nasal bridge, epicanthal folds and micrognathia. Mental retardation and malabsorption with failure to thrive have been reported in most cases. However, all these manifestations vary from one patient to another and can be absent. The immune defect is variable and most often characterized by a combined immunodeficiency with quantitative and/or functional T-cell immunodeficiency and panhypogammaglobulinemia, although B cells are normally detectable. However, in some cases only a humoral defect has been observed, and in rare cases typical cytogenetic abnormalities may be found in patients with isolated IgA deficiency.

Cytogenetic studies show typical features characterized by elongation of secondary constriction of chromosomes, which can be associated with multibranched configuration predominantly in chromosomes 1, 9, 16 and less often chromosome 2 (Fig. 35.9).[73] These features are detected in activated T cells, less often in EBV-transformed B cells, and rarely in fibroblasts. The anomaly is related to hypomethylation of classic satellites. In females, this hypomethylation also involves the inactive X without notable consequence on X-inactivation. The parent chromosomes are usually normal. Family studies allowed the mapping of the locus to the proximal long arm of chromosome 20. Mutations on both alleles of the DNA methyltransferase *DNMT3B*-encoding gene have been found in nine ICF patients from eight families.[74] These mutations include missense mutations or insertions causing an aberrant splicing.

Nonhomologous end joining DNA repair defect- DNA ligase IV (LIG4) and Cernunnos deficiencies

In a small number of patients with microcephaly, growth retardation and mild dysmorphic syndrome, a T-cell immunodeficiency of variable intensity, clinically similar to NBS, has been found to be caused by a partial DNA ligase 4 deficiency (also known as LIG4 syndrome).[75] The severity of the immunodeficiency varies from a 'quasi' SCID to no detectable immunodeficiency, the deficiency commonly detected in a setting of unusual toxicity of chemotherapy and radiation in a leukemic child. DNA ligase IV is involved in the final ligation step of the NHEJ process required for V(D)J recombination of TCR and BCR genes. It is likely that defective DNA LIG4 activity leads to a significantly reduced survival of T- and B-cell precursors, accounting for the immunodeficiency and predisposing to lymphoid malignancies because DNA LIG4 participates in the care of genome integrity.

Six patients exhibiting a similar syndrome associating microcephaly, in utero growth retardation and lymphopenia were found to carry recessive mutations of a newly identified gene called Cernunnos/XLF. Cernunnos has been shown to interact with the XRCC-DNA LIG4 complex involved in the ligation of coding end during the V(D)J recombination process.[76]

Dyskeratosis congenita

This condition is usually inherited as an X-linked recessive disease and is associated with multiple manifestations, including epithelial lesions, predisposition to cancer and progressive aplastic anemia. The most severe forms also include a combined immunodeficiency typically associating the presence of poorly functional T cells together with NK- and B-cell lymphocytopenia. This condition is known as the Hoyeraal–Hreidersson syndrome.[77] It is associated with mutations in the dyskerin-encoding gene (*DKC1*), or more rarely with the *TERC* gene in cases with autosomal dominant inheritance, but some cases the molecular basis is not yet understood.[78] Dyskerin and TERC are involved in the telomerase complex necessary for the maintenance of telomeres. When the complex is defective, it leads to premature senescence because of abnormally shortened telomeres.

SHORT-LIMB DWARFISM OR CARTILAGE–HAIR HYPOPLASIA (CHH)

CHH is an autosomal recessive form of metaphyseal chondrodysplasia characterized by short limbs, short stature, hypoplastic hair growth, a variable T-cell deficiency and an erythroid production defect. CHH is common in Finland, and among the Old Order Amish group in the United States. There is extreme variability in the expression of the features of CHH both between and within families. Short stature is, however, a constant feature. There is no clear correlation between the severity of growth failure and that of the immunodeficiency. The immunodeficiency is characterized by lymphopenia of variable magnitude with impaired mitogen-induced T-cell proliferation. The cell cycle of CHH patients' T-cell lines appears to be delayed, with both poor production of IL-2 and a poor response to IL-2. The pathophysiology remains obscure, although a ubiquitous cell-growth defect is plausible. As in other chronic T-cell deficiencies, autoimmunity (erythroblastopenia is frequent) and cancer are common. Based on a study of 14 Finnish families, the gene was mapped to chromosome 9 and encodes for *RMRP*, which is transcribed into a noncoding RNA associated with the mitochondria RNA-processing endoribonuclease.[79]

Distinct but ill-defined T-cell deficiencies have been reported in some families with other skeletal defects, such as 'Schimke immuno-osseous dysplasia,' which consists of skeletal spondyloepiphyseal dysplasia, short stature, nephropathy, pigmentary skin changes and lymphocytopenia, associated with mutations of the *SMARCAL1* gene.[80]

IMMUNODEFICIENCY AND PERIPHERAL MYOPATHY

In three cases of immunodeficiency reported to be associated with peripheral myopathy, TCR-mediated calcium influx was found to be abolished in spite of normal calcium release from intracellular stores.[81] The involvement of ubiquitous calcium release-activated calcium (CRAC) channels in this immunodeficiency was suggested and has been confirmed recently.[82] A homozygous missense mutation in exon 1 of human *ORAI1* leading to replacement of a highly conserved arginine residue by tryptophan at position 91 was found in two patients from one family. Expression of wild-type Orai1 in the patients' T cells restored calcium-ion influx triggered by TCR activation.

IMMUNODEFICIENCY ASSOCIATED WITH VENO-OCCLUSIVE DISEASE

In six patients from five families of Lebanese origin living in Australia, a combined functional cell immunodeficiency associated with veno-occlusive disease of the liver has been found to be related to recessive mutations of the *SP110* gene.[83] Sp110 is a protein associated with the PML nuclear body, probably involved in regulating gene transcription. All patients had frequent infections and hypogammaglobulinemia. Other associated features are microcephaly and left atrial endocardial fibrosis.

SCID ASSOCIATED WITH MULTIPLE GASTROINTESTINAL ATRESIA

An absence of T cells or low T-cell counts with very low B-cell counts has been associated with multiple atresias of the gastrointestinal tract. Inheritance is presumed to be autosomal recessive. It is not known whether this is a contiguous-gene syndrome, or whether a factor is involved in both the development of the 'hollow stage' of the gastrointestinal tract and lymphocyte differentiation.

■ MISCELLANEOUS T-CELL IMMUNODEFICIENCIES ■

Molecular defects in T cells may cause an immune disorder with clinical manifestations that are not traditionally attributed to cellular immunodeficiency. Two of these conditions, X-linked hyper-IgM and ICOS deficiency, present with hypogammaglobulinemia and are reviewed in detail in Chapter 34. Here we discuss T-cell defects that result in lymphoproliferative disorders and in autoimmune endocrinopathies.

MISCELLANEOUS T-CELL IMMUNODEFICIENCIES

AUTOIMMUNE LYMPHOPROLIFERATIVE SYNDROME (ALPS)

ALPS is a disorder of lymphocyte apoptosis characterized by an increased incidence of autoimmunity, nonmalignant lymphoprolifera-tion, and susceptibility to malignancy. Patients may present early in childhood with lymphadenopathy, splenomegaly and autoimmune cytopenias.[84] The disease has a wide spectrum, evidenced by the difference of clinical severity among members bearing the same gene mutation within families. Flow cytometry studies in peripheral blood may reveal increased numbers of CD3 T c ells, $\alpha\beta^+$, CD4, CD8. Lymphocyte populations show a defect to undergo induced apoptosis *in vitro*, which points to the pathogenesis of the disease. Upon binding of Fas ligand to Fas on the lymphocyte cell surface, signal transduction occur through caspases, leading to the cell and nuclear changes that are characteristic of apoptosis. Defective apoptosis leads to the accumula-tion of defective or senescent cells, which produce organomegaly and an increased risk of lymphoma, estimated to develop in 10% of patients. The differential diagnosis may include CVID if hypogammaglobuline-mia is documented; however, these patients should not present an apoptotic defect. Treatment is directed to reduce organomegaly and resolve cytopenias, and includes steroids, intravenous immunoglobu-lin and immunosuppressants.[84] ALPS is discussed in detail in Chapter 14.

X-LINKED PROLIFERATIVE SYNDROME (XLP–PURTILO SYNDROME, DUNCAN DISEASE)

EBV infection can induce uncontrolled B-cell proliferation in patients with profound T-cell deficiencies, such as SCID, or following T cell-depleted BMT. In certain otherwise healthy kindreds, EBV infection was found to have severe consequences such as hepatitis, lymphohis-tiocytic activation and bone marrow aplasia. In these cases, if not fatal, B-cell lymphoma or agammaglobulinemia may also occur. Antibodies against EBV nuclear antigen, and occasionally to the VCA (viral cap-sid antigen) and EA (early antigen), are undetectable. These patients are not prone to other severe viral infections. This abnormal X-linked lymphoproliferative-disease gene has been mapped to Xq24-q27 and identified as SH2 domain-encoding. The gene product, SLAM-associated protein (SAP/SH2 D1), was described to interact with the transmembrane receptor SLAM[85] expressed by T and B cells. SAP can act as a B-cell inhibitor by blocking the recruitment of SH2 domain-containing signal transduction molecule to SLAM, such as the phos-phatase SHP-2. The absence of the inhibitor SAP leads to inability to handle the EBV infection. However, a frequent striking feature of XLP is the uncontrolled proliferation of CD8 T cells, much more prominent that the proliferation of EBV-infected B cells. Likewise, it is possible that SAP-deficient CD8 T cells undergo proliferation because of the faulty regulatory function of SAP while being poorly able to kill EBV-infected B cells. In this way, EBV infection would act as a potent trigger of T-cell responses, which are under the control of SAP-associated proteins. NK-cell activity and the EBV-specific CTL activity of SAP-deficient cells are deficient, potentially accounting for the immunodeficiency. Another gene might also be involved in XLP syndrome, as the SAP-encoding gene has been found mutated in only 50–70% of XLP male patients. Moreover, severe EBV infection in girls has also been described.

IMMUNODYSREGULATION, POLYENDOCRINOPATHY AND ENTEROPATHY, X-LINKED (IPEX)

The IPEX syndrome was first observed in eight males of a large family comprising three generations that were related through the females, and who had some or all of the following conditions: diarrhea, eczema, hemo-lytic anemia, autoimmune diabetes mellitus and hypothyroidism. Also described was increased susceptibility to infections, and patients would usually die in infancy.[86] Subsequently, similar descriptions of other fami-lies with affected male infants were reported, including the additional observations of elevated IgE and eosinophilia, and the successful use of cyclosporine to control the disease.[87] HLA-identical BMT was shown to correct the immunological abnormalities in one patient; however, he later developed rapidly progressive hemophagocytic syndrome and died. IPEX is caused by mutations in the *FOXP3* gene, a member of a family of tran-scriptional regulators, and located in chromosome Xp11.23. FoxP3 expression confers the T-regulatory phenotype to CD4 cells. These cells play a major role in the control of autoimmunity and inflammation by decreasing the production of cytokines and other T-cell mediators using a mechanism mediated by cell–cell contact, and by secreting IL-10 to inhibit ongoing immune activation. Bacchetta et al.[88] have shown that IPEX patients present with normal numbers of regulatory T cells, but they are dysfunctional and unable to suppress autologous effector T cells.

AUTOIMMUNE POLYENDOCRINOPATHY–CANDIDIASIS–ECTODERMAL DYSTROPHY SYNDROME (APECED)

This syndrome is also known as autoimmune polyglandular syndrome I, and is diagnosed when two of the following three findings are present: Addison's disease, hypoparathyroidism and chronic mucocutaneous candi-diasis. Other associated conditions are autoimmune hepatitis, juvenile per-nicious anemia, alopecia and primary hypogonadism. Thyroid disease and diabetes mellitus are not common. Most patients present with candidiasis before 5 years of age, and almost half develop multiple endocrinopathy. The pathogenesis of the disease involves the development of autoantibodies against multiple targets, including 21-hydroxylase, liver cytochrome p450 (CYP11A), tyrosine phosphatase, tryptophan hydroxylase, and phenyla-lanine hydroxylase, all enzymes involved in hormone synthesis. The gene responsible for APECED is named 'autoimmune regulator' or *AIRE*, encoding a protein that strongly activates transcription activity, but mutated AIRE proteins found in APECED patients have lost this capacity. AIRE may induce immune tolerance by enhancing the expression of peripheral-tissue antigens in the thymus, affecting the negative selection of T-effector cells.[89, 90] This gene is located on chromosome 21q22.3 and is expressed in multiple human tissues, essentially the thymus, spleen, lymph nodes and monocytes. The disease is inherited in an autosomal dominant fashion and is most common in the Finnish, Iranian Jews and Sardinian Italians.[91]

CHRONIC MUCOCUTANEOUS CANDIDIASIS, WITH OR WITHOUT ENDOCRINOPATHY

Candidal infections can persist on the skin and mucosa in patients with a selective T-cell defect toward *Candida* antigens.[92] Such susceptibility can be inherited as an autosomal recessive or a dominant trait, and is sometimes associated with the autoimmune polyendocrinopathy caused by AIRE deficiency. *In vitro* and *in vivo*, T-cell activation by *Candida* antigens is absent as long as the infection persists. Systemic *Candida* infections are rare, and patients can be relatively free of infections if they are receiving antifungal prophylaxis. This disorder is also frequently associated with progressive hypogammaglobulinemia.

Several forms of chronic mucocutaneous candidiasis (CMC) have been described in a few families, although the genetic etiology has remained elusive. An isolated familial CMC, without endocrinopathy, has been reported in families of French-Canadian descent, showing autosomal recessive inheritance and with some predisposition to deep infection.[93] Autosomal dominant forms include the CMC restricted to nail infections and with low expression of the ICAM1 adhesion molecule in an Italian family; and a CMC form associated with nonautoimmune hypothyroidism but no other endocrinopathy, described in one family from Alabama.[94]

■ REFERENCES ■

1. Notarangelo L, Casanova JL, Conley ME, et al. Primary immunodeficiency diseases: An update from the International Union of Immunological Societies Primary Immunodeficiency Diseases Classification Committee Meeting in Budapest, 2006. J Allergy Clin Immunol 2005; (117): 883–896.

2. Stephan JL, Vlekova V, Le Deist F, et al. Severe combined immunodeficiency: a retrospective single-center study of clinical presentation and outcome in 117 patients. J Pediatr 1993; 123: 564–572.

3. Buckley RH, Schiff RI, Schiff SE, et al. Human severe combined immunodeficiency: genetic, phenotypic. functional diversity in one hundred eight infants J Pediatr 1997; 130: 378–387.

4. Hale LP, Buckley RH, Puck JM, Patel DD. Abnormal development of thymic dendritic and epithelial cells in human X-linked severe combined immunodeficiency. Clin Immunol 2004; 110: 63–70.

5. Gossage DL, Buckley RH. Prevalence of lymphocytopenia in severe combined immunodeficiency. [Letter; Comment] N Engl J Med 1990; 323: 1422–1423.

6. Myers LA, Patel DD, Puck JM, Buckley RH. Hematopoietic stem cell transplantation for severe combined immunodeficiency in the neonatal period leads to superior thymic output and improved survival. Blood 2002; 99: 872–878.

7. Chan K, Puck JM. Development of population-based newborn screening for severe combined immunodeficiency. J Allergy Clin Immunol 2005; 115: 391–398.

8. Blunt T, Finnie NJ, Taccioli GE, et al. Defective DNA-dependent protein kinase activity is linked to V(D)J recombination and DNA repair defects associated with the murine scid mutation. Cell 1995; 80: 813–823.

9. Jackson SP. DNA-dependent protein kinase. Int J Biochem Cell Biol 1997; 29: 935–938.

10. Notarangelo LD, Villa A, Schwarz K. RAG and RAG defects. Curr Opin Immunol 1999; 11: 435–442.

11. Ehl S, Schwarz K, Enders A, et al. A variant of SCID with specific immune responses and predominance of gamma delta T cells. J Clin Invest 2005; 115: 3140–3148.

12. Moshous D, Li L, de Chasseval R, et al. A new gene involved in DNA double-strand break repair and V(D)J recombination is located on human chromosome 10p. Hum Mol Genet 2000; 9: 583–588.

13. Moshous D, Callebaut R, de Chasseval R, et al. ARTEMIS, a novel DNA double-strand break repair/V(D)J recombination protein is mutated in Human Severe Combined Immune Deficiency with increased radiosensitivity (RS-SCID). Cell 2001; 105: 177–186.

14. Ege M, Ma Y, Manfras B, et al. Omenn syndrome due to ARTEMIS mutations. Blood 2005; 105: 4179–4186.

15. Conley ME, Lavoie A, Briggs C, et al. Nonrandom X chromosome inactivation in B cells from carriers of X chromosome-linked severe combined immunodeficiency. Proc Natl Acad Sci USA 1988; 85: 3090–3094.

16. Haddad E, Le Deist F, Aucouturier P, et al. Long-term chimerism and B-cell function after bone marrow transplantation in patients with severe combined immunodeficiency with B cells: A single-center study of 22 patients. Blood 1999; 94: 2923–2930.

17. Buckley RH, Fischer A. Bone marrow transplantation for primary immunodeficiency diseases in primary immunodeficiency diseases. In: Ochs HD, Smith CIE, Buck JM, cds: A molecular and genetic approach, New York: Oxford University Press, 1999; 459–476.

18. Antoine C, Muller S, Cant A, et al. Long-term survival and transplantation of haemopoietic stem cells for immunodeficiencies: report of the European experience 1968–99. Lancet 2003; 361: 553–560.

19. Sugamura K, Asao H, Kondo M, et al. The common gamma-chain for multiple cytokine receptors. Adv Immunol 1995; 59: 225–277.

20. von Freeden-Jeffry U, Vieira P, Lucian LA, et al. Lymphopenia in interleukin (IL)-7 gene-deleted mice identifies IL-7 as a nonredundant cytokine. J Exp Med 1995; 181: 1519–1526.

21. Peschon JJ, Morrissey PJ, Grabstein KH, et al. Early lymphocyte expansion is severely impaired in interleukin 7 receptor-deficient mice. J Exp Med 1994; 180: 1955–1960.

22. Cavazzana-Calvo M, Hacein-Bey S, de Saint Basile G, et al. Role of interleukin-2 (IL-2), IL-7, and IL-15 in natural killer cell differentiation from cord blood hematopoietic progenitor cells and from gamma c transduced severe combined immunodeficiency X1 bone marrow cells. Blood 1996; 88: 3901–3909.

23. Puck JM. IL2RGbase: a database of gamma c-chain defects causing human X-SCID. Immunol Today 1996; 17: 507–511.

24. Somech R, Roifman CM. Mutation analysis should be performed to rule out gamma deficiency in children with functional severe combined immune deficiency despite apparently normal immunologic tests. J Pediatr 2005; 147: 555–557.

25. DiSanto JP, Rieux-Laucat F, Dautry-Varsat A, et al. Defective human interleukin 2 receptor gamma chain in an atypical X chromosome-linked severe combined immunodeficiency with peripheral T cells. Proc Natl Acad Sci USA 1994; 91: 9466–9470.

26. Sharfe N, Shahar M, Roifman CM. An interleukin-2 receptor gamma chain mutation with normal thymus morphology. J Clin Invest 1997; 100: 3036–3043.

27. Kumaki S, Ishii N, Minegishi M, et al. Functional role of interleukin-4 (IL-4) and IL-7 in the development of X-linked severe combined immunodeficiency. Blood 1999; 93: 607–612.

28. Stephan V, Wahn V, Le Deist F, et al. Atypical X-linked severe combined immunodeficiency due to possible spontaneous reversion of the genetic defect in T cells. N Engl J Med 1996; 335: 1563–1567.

29. Cavazzana-Calvo M, Hacein-Bey S, de Saint Basile G, et al. Gene therapy of human severe combined immunodeficiency (SCID)-X1 disease. Science 2000; 288: 669–672.

30. Roberts JL, Lengi A, Brown SM, et al. Janus kinase 3 (JAK3) deficiency: clinical, immunologic, and molecular analyses of 10 patients and outcomes of stem cell transplantation. Blood 2004; 103: 2009–2018.

31. Brugnoni D, Notarangelo LD, Sottini A, et al. Development of autologous, oligoclonal, poorly functioning T lymphocytes in a patient with autosomal recessive severe combined immunodeficiency caused by defects of the Jak3 tyrosine kinase. Blood 1998; 91: 949–955.

32. Puel A, Ziegler SF, Buckley RH, Leonard WJ. Defective IL7R expression in T(-)B(+)NK(+) severe combined immunodeficiency. Nature Genet 1998; 20: 394–397.

33. Giliani S, Mori L, de Saint Basile G, et al. Interleukin-7 receptor alpha (IL-7Ralpha) deficiency: cellular and molecular bases. Analysis of clinical, immunological, and molecular features in 16 novel patients. Immunol Rev 2005; 203: 110–126.

34. Hershfield M, Mitchell B. Immunodeficiency disease caused by adenosine deaminase deficiency and purine nucleoside phosphorylase deficiency. In: Scriver C, Beaudet A, Sly W, Valle D, eds: Metabolic basis of inherited disease, 7th edn. New York: McGraw Hill, 1995; 1725–1768.

35. Ariga T, Oda N, Yamaguchi K, et al. T-cell lines from 2 patients with adenosine deaminase (ADA) deficiency showed the restoration of ADA activity resulted from the reversion of an inherited mutation. Blood 2001; 97: 2896–2899.

36. de Saint Basile G, Geissmann F, Flori E, et al. Severe combined immunodeficiency caused by deficiency in either the delta or the epsilon subunit of CD3. J Clin Invest 2004; 114: 1512–1517.

37. Kung C, Pingel JT, Heikinheimo M, et al. Mutations in the tyrosine phosphatase CD45 gene in a child with severe combined immunodeficiency disease. Nature Med 2000; 6: 343–345.

38. Tchillian EZ, Wallace DL, Well RS, et al. A deletion in the gene encoding the CD45 antigen in a patient with SCID. J Immunol 2001; 166: 1308–1313.

39. Berthet F, Le Deist F, Duliege A, et al. Clinical consequences and treatment of primary immunodeficiency syndromes characterized by functional T and B lymphocyte anomalies (combined immune deficiency). Pediatrics 1994; 93: 265–270.

40. Villard J, Masternak K, Lisowska-Grospierre B, et al. MHC class II deficiency: a disease of gene regulation. Medicine (Baltimore) 2001; 80: 405–418.

41. Reith W, Mach B. The bare lymphocyte syndrome and the regulation of MHC expression. Annu Rev Immunol 2001; 19: 331–373.

42. Steimle V, Durand B, Barras E, et al. A novel DNA-binding regulatory factor is mutated in primary MHC class II deficiency (bare lymphocyte syndrome). Genes Dev 1995; 9: 1021–1032.

43. Masternak K, Barras E, Zufferey M, et al. A gene encoding a novel RFX-associated transactivator is mutated in the majority of MHC class II deficiency patients. Nature Genet 1998; 20: 273–277.

44. Nagarajan UM, Louis-Plence P, DeSandro A, et al. RFX-B is the gene responsible for the most common cause of the bare lymphocyte syndrome, an MHC class II immunodeficiency. Immunity 1999; 10: 153–162. [Published erratum appears in Immunity 1999; 10: 399.].

45. de la Salle H, Hanau D, Fricker D, et al. Homozygous human TAP peptide transporter mutation in HLA class I deficiency Science 1994; 265: 237–241.

46. de la Salle H, Donato L, Ziummer J, et al. HLA class I deficiency. In: Ochs HD, Smith C, Puck J, eds: Primary immunodeficency disease, New York: Oxford University Press, 1998; 181–188.

47. Lee SP, Thomas WA, Blake NW, Rickinson AB. Transporter (TAP)-independent processing of a multiple membrane-spanning protein, the Epstein–Barr virus latent membrane protein 2. Eur J Immunol 1996; 26: 1875–1883.

48. Rieux-Laucat F, Hivroz C, Lim A, et al. Inherited and somatic CD3ζ mutations in a patient with T cell deficiency. N Engl J Med 2006; 354: 1913–1921.

48a. Roberts JL, Lauritsen JP, Cooney M, et al. T-B+NK+ severe combined immunodeficiency caused by complete deficiency of the CD3ζ subunit of the T-cell antigen receptor complex. Blood 2007; 109: 3198–3206.

49. Elder ME. ZAP-70 and defects of T-cell receptor signaling. Semin Hematol 1998; 35: 310–330.

50. Sharfe N, Dadi HK, Shahar M, Roifman CM. Human immune disorder arising from mutation of the alpha chain of the interleukin-2 receptor. Proc Natl Acad Sci USA 1997; 94: 3168-31.

51. de la Calle-Martin O, Hernandez M, Ordi J, et al. Familial CD8 deficiency due to a mutation in the CD8 alpha gene. J Clin Invest 2001; 108: 117–123.

52. Rieux-Laucat F, Bahadoran P, Brousse N, et al. Highly restricted human T cell repertoire in peripheral blood and tissue-infiltrating lymphocytes in Omenn's syndrome. J Clin Invest 1998; 102: 312–321.

53. Cavadini P, Vermi W, Facchetti F, et al. AIRE deficiency in thymus of 2 patients with Omenn syndrome. J Clin Invest 2005; 115: 728–732.

54. Giliani S, Bonfim C, de Saint Basile G, et al. Omenn syndrome in an infant with IL7RA gene mutation. J Pediatr 2006; 148: 272–274.

55. Grunebaum E, Zhang J, Roifman CM. Novel mutations and hot-spots in patients with purine nucleoside phosphorylase deficiency. Nucleosides Nucleotides Nucleic Acids 2004; 23: 1411–1415.

56. Yamagishi H, Garg V, Matsuoka R, et al. A molecular pathway revealing a genetic basis for human cardiac and craniofacial defects [see comments]. Science 1999; 283: 1158–1161.

57. Yagi H, Furutani Y, Hamada H, et al. Role of TBX1 in human del22q11. 2 syndrome. Lancet 2003; 362: 1366–1373.

58. Stalmans I, Lambrechts D, De Smet F, et al. VEGF: a modifier of the del22q11 (DiGeorge) syndrome?. Nature Med 2003; 9: 173–182.

59. Markert ML, Sarzotti M, Ozaki DA, et al. Thymus transplantation in complete DiGeorge syndrome: immunologic and safety evaluations in 12 patients. Blood 2003; 102: 1121–1130.

60. Ochs H. The Wiskott–Aldrich syndrome. Springer Semin Immunopathol 1998; 19: 435–458.

REFERENCES

61. Rawlings SL, Crooks GM, Bockstoce D, et al. Spontaneous apoptosis in lymphocytes from patients with Wiskott-Aldrich syndrome: correlation of accelerated cell death and attenuated Bcl-2 expression. Blood 1999; 94: 3872–3882.

62. Notarangelo LD, Notarangelo LD, Ochs HD. WASP and the phenotypic range associated with deficiency. Curr Opin Allergy Clin Immunol 2005; 5: 485–490.

63. Derry J, Ochs H, Francke U. Isolation of a novel gene mutated in Wiskott–Aldrich syndrome. Cell 1994; 78: 635–644.

64. Derry J, Kerns J, Weinberg K, et al. WASP gene mutations in Wiskott–Aldrich syndrome and X-linked thrombocytopenia. Hum Mol Genet 1995; 4: 1127–1135.

65. Remold-O'Donnell E, Rosen FS, Kenney DM. Defects in Wiskott–Aldrich syndrome blood cells. Blood 1996; 87: 2621–2631.

66. Savitsky K, Bar-Shira A, Gilad S, et al. A single ataxia telangiectasia gene with a product similar to PI-3 kinase. Science 1995; 268: 1749–1753.

67. Matsuoka S, Huang M, Elledge SJ. Linkage of ATM to cell cycle regulation by the Chk2 protein kinase. Science 1998; 282: 1893–1897.

68. Kim GD, Choi YH, Dimtchev A, et al. Sensing of ionizing radiation-induced DNA damage by ATM through interaction with histone deacetylase. J Biol Chem 1999; 274: 31127–31130.

69. Stewart GS, Maser RS, Stankovic T, et al. The DNA double strand repair gene hMRE11 is mutated in individuals with an ataxia–telangiectasia-like disorder. Cell 1999; 99: 577–587.

70. van der Burgt I, Chrzanowska KH, Smeets D, Weemaes C. Nijmegen breakage syndrome. J Med Genet 1996; 33: 153–156.

71. Varon R, Vissinga C, Platzer M, et al. Nibrin, a novel DNA double-strand break repair protein, is mutated in Nijmegen breakage syndrome. Cell 1998; 93: 467–476.

72. Brown DC, Grace E, Sumner AT, et al. ICF syndrome (immunodeficiency, centromeric instability and facial anomalies): investigation of heterochromatin abnormalities and review of clinical outcome. Hum Genet 1995; 96: 411–416.

73. Sumner AT, Mitchell AR, Ellis PM. A FISH study of chromosome fusion in the ICF syndrome: involvement of paracentric heterochromatin but not of the centromeres themselves. J Med Genet 1998; 35: 833–835.

74. Hansen RS, Wijmenga C, Luo P, et al. The DNMT3B DNA methyltransferase gene is mutated in the ICF immunodeficiency syndrome Proc Natl Acad Sci USA 1999; 96: 14412–14417.

75. Buck D, Moshous D, de Chasseval R, et al. Severe combined immunodeficiency and microcephaly in siblings with hypomorphic mutations in DNA ligase IV. Eur J Immunol 2006; 36: 224–235.

76. Buck D, Malivert L, de Chasseval R, et al. Cernunnos a novel nonhomologous end-joining factor, is mutated in human immunodeficiency with microcephaly. Cell 2006; 124: 287–299.

77. Sznajer Y, Baumann C, David A, et al. Further delineation of the congenital form of X-linked dyskeratosis congenita (Hoyeraal–Hreidarsson syndrome). Eur J Pediatr 2003; 162: 863–867.

78. Vulliamy TJ, Marrone A, Knight SW, et al. Mutations in dyskeratosis congenita: their impact on telomere length and the diversity of clinical presentation. Blood 2006; 107: 2680–2685.

79. Ridanpaa M, van Eenennaam H, Pelin K, et al. Mutations in the RNA component of RNase MRP cause a pleiotropic human disease, cartilage–hair hypoplasia. Cell 2001; 104: 195–203.

80. Boerkoel CF, Takashima H, John J, et al. Mutant chromatin remodeling protein SMARCAL1 causes Schimke immuno-osseous dysplasia. Nature Genet 2002; 30: 215–220.

81. Le Deist F, Hivroz C, Partiseti M, et al. A primary T-cell immunodeficiency associated with defective transmembrane calcium influx. Blood 1995; 85: 1053–1062.

82. Feske S, Gwack Y, Prakriya M, et al. A mutation in Orai1 causes immune deficiency by abrogating CRAC channel function. Nature 2006; 441: 179–185.

83. Roscioli T, Cliffe ST, Bloch DB, et al. Mutations in the gene encoding the PML nuclear body protein Sp110 are associated with immunodeficiency and hepatic veno-occlusive disease. Nature Genet 2006; 38: 620–622.

84. Woth A, Thrasher AJ, Gaspar HB. Autoimmune lymphoproliferative syndrome: molecular basis of disease and clinical phenotype. Br J Haematol 2006; 133: 124–140.

85. Sayos J, Wu C, Morra M, et al. The X-linked lymphoproliferative-disease gene product SAP regulates signals induced through the co-receptor SLAM Nature 1998; 395: 462–469.

86. Powell BR, Buist NRM, Stenzel P. An X-linked syndrome of diarrhea, polyendocrinopathy and fatal infection in infancy. J Pediatr 1982; 100: 731–737.

87. Seidman EG, Lacaille F, Russo P, et al. Successful treatment of autoimmune enteropathy with cyclosporine. J Pediatr 1990; 117: 929–932.

88. Bacchetta R, Passerini L, Gambineri E, et al. Defective regulatory and effector T cell functions in patients with FOXP3 mutations. J Clin Invest 2006; 116: 1713–1722.

89. Bjorses P, Halonen M, Palvimo JJ, et al. Mutations in the AIRE gene: effects on subcellular location and transactivation function of the autoimmune polyendocrinopathy-candidiasis-ectodermal dystrophy protein. Am J Hum Genet 2000; 66: 378–392.

90. Anderson MS, Venanzi ES, Chen Z, et al. The cellular mechanism of Aire control of T cell tolerance. Immunity 2005; 23: 227–239.

91. Eisenbarth GS, Gottlieb PA. Autoimmune polyendocrine syndromes. N Engl J Med 2004; 350: 2068–2079.

92. Kirkpatrick CH. Chronic mucocutaneous candidiasis. J Am Acad Dermatol 1994; 31: S14–S17.

93. Germain M, Gourdeau M, Hebert J. Familial CMC complicated with deep *Candida* infection. Am J Med Sci 1994; 307: 282–283.

94. Atkinson TP, Schaefer AA, Grimbacher B, et al. An immune defect causing dominant chronic mucocutaneous candidiasis and thyroid disease maps to chromosome 2p in a single family. Am J Hum Genet 2001; 69: 791–803.

REFERENCES

Inherited disorders of IFN-γ-, IFN-α/β-, and NF-κB-mediated immunity

Capucine Picard, Jean-Laurent Casanova

36

In the last 10 years, new primary immunodeficiencies (PIDs) affecting interferon (IFN)-γ-mediated immunity, IFN-α/β-mediated immunity, and nuclear factor (NF)-κB-mediated immunity have been identified. Some of these genetic defects are 'conventional' PIDs, associated with a broad range of infections, but others provide a molecular explanation for severe pediatric infectious diseases previously thought to be idiopathic (Table 36.1). These 'nonconventional' hereditary immunodeficiencies are associated with severe and/or recurrent infections caused by a single family of microorganisms, in contrast to what is observed in 'conventional' PIDs.[1] Standard immunologic explorations, such as leukocyte counts, lymphocyte counts, serological tests for vaccine strains, immunoglobulin levels and complement, are normal in these patients, regardless of whether they are susceptible to one or many infectious agents. Despite the lack of an evident immunological abnormality, infections in these patients are typically severe and often fatal. In this chapter, we describe these new syndromes: disorders of the interleukin (IL)-12–IFN-γ circuit (mutations in the *IFNGR1, IFNGR2, STAT1, IL12B, IL12RB1, NEMO* genes), associated with the syndrome of mendelian susceptibility to mycobacterial disease (MSMD); combined disorders of IFN-γ- and IFN-α/β-mediated immunity (other mutations in *STAT1*), associated with mycobacterial and viral diseases; and disorders of NF-κB-mediated immunity, associated with pyogenic bacterial diseases, whether isolated (mutations in *IRAK4*) or associated with mycobacterial and viral disease (other mutations in *NEMO* and mutations in *IKBA*) (Table 36.1).

KEY CONCEPTS

>> Novel primary immunodeficiencies should be sought in patients with unexplained infectious diseases.

>> Children with severe infectious diseases should be repeatedly investigated for known and unknown immunodeficiency conditions

>> The exploration of idiopathic infections leads to the discovery of new PIDs and to a better understanding of immunity against pathogens.

■ MENDELIAN SUSCEPTIBILITY TO MYCOBACTERIAL DISEASE AND INHERITED DISORDERS OF THE IL-12–IFN-γ CIRCUIT ■

Inherited disorders of the IL-12/23-IFN-γ circuit are associated with a selective susceptibility to weakly pathogenic mycobacteria and *Salmonella* (mendelian susceptibility to mycobacterial diseases, MSMD, Online Mendelian Inheritance in Man [OMIM] number 209950) (Fig. 36.1).[2] These PIDs are caused by mutations in six genes involved in IFN-γ-mediated immunity: *IFNGR1* and *IFNGR2*, encoding the two chains of the receptor for IFN-γ, a pleiotropic cytokine secreted by NK and T cells; *STAT1*, encoding a molecule essential to the IFN-γR signaling pathway; *IL12B*, encoding the p40 subunit of IL-12 and IL-23, IFN-γ-inducing cytokines secreted by macrophages and dendritic cells; *IL12RB1*, encoding the β1 chain of the receptor for IL-12 and IL-23, which is expressed on NK and T cells;[3] and *NEMO*, encoding NF-κB essential modulator (NEMO), which is involved in the CD40-dependent induction of IL-12. *NEMO* is X-linked, whereas the other five genes are autosomal. All known mutations in *IFNGR1, IFNGR2, IL12B,* and *IL12RB1* are associated with MSMD. In contrast, some mutations in *STAT1* and most mutations in *NEMO* are associated with a much broader range of infectious diseases (see below). The molecular and clinical features of MSMD have recently been reviewed.[4, 5]

COMPLETE IFN-γ RECEPTOR 1 DEFICIENCY

Complete IFN-γ receptor 1 (IFN-γR1) deficiency (OMIM 107470) is caused by recessive null *IFNGR1* mutations precluding the expression of IFN-γR1 on the cell surface[6, 7] or recognition of the ligand IFN-γ by surface-expressed receptors.[8] Affected patients therefore fail to respond to IFN-γ both *in vitro* and *in vivo* and have high serum IFN-γ concentrations after infection. So far 24 such patients have been reported.[3] All known patients suffered from disseminated infections caused by environmental mycobacteria (EM), notably rapidly growing species, and/or

Table 36.1 Novel inherited disorders

Gene	Form Mutation	Inheritance	Mycobacteria	Salmonella	Viruses	Pyogenic bacteria	Fungi	EDA	Inflammatory signs	n° P
IFNRG1	Complete	AR	+++	++	+	-	-	-	N	24
	Partial	AR	+++	++	-	-	-	-	N	3
	Partial	AD	+++	++	-	-	+/-[1]	-	N	50
IFNGR2	Complete	AR	+++	+	+	-	-	-	N	6
	Partial	AR	+++	++	-	-	-	-	N	1
IL12RB1	Complete	AR	+++	+++	-	-	+/-[2]	-	N	60
IL12B	Complete	AR	+++	+++	-	-	-	-	N	20
STAT1	Partial	AD	+++	-	-	-	-	-	N	10
	Complete	AR	+	-	+++	-	-	-	N	5
NEMO	Hypomorphic	XR	+	+	+	++	+	+/-	Weak	52
IKBA	Hypermorphic	AD	-	+	+	++	+	+	Weak	3
IRAK 4	Amorphic	AR	-	-	-	++	-	-	Weak	22

AR, autosomal recessive; AD, autosomal dominant; XR, X-recessive; EDA, ectodermal anhidrotic dysplasia; N, normal; n° p, number of patients
[1]One PD IFNGR1-deficient patient presented one episode of Histoplasma capsulatum infection.
[2]One IL12RB1-deficient patient presented one episode of Paracoccidioides brasiliensi infection.

bacille Calmette–Guérin (BCG) vaccines, with impaired granuloma formation (Fig. 36.2A).[9] Infections began early, often before the age of 3 years. A few of these patients presented nontyphoidal salmonellosis and one presented with recurrent invasive infection caused by *Listeria monocytogenes*.[9] Three patients had respiratory viral infections and one had a fatal human herpes virus-8-driven Kaposi's sarcoma.[9]

Multiple antibiotics against mycobacteria should be administered without interruption. Vaccination with live BCG is contraindicated. The prognosis is very poor, with only 25% of patients surviving to the age of 15 years without hematopoietic stem cell transplantation (HSCT).[9,10] HSCT, preferably

once mycobacterial disease is under control, is the only curative treatment for these patients, but has proved to be associated with an unusually high rate of graft rejection, making transplantation particularly difficult.

COMPLETE IFN-γ RECEPTOR 2 DEFICIENCY

Six children with complete IFN-γR2 signaling chain deficiency (OMIM 147569) have also been reported.[11–13] Mutations in the *IFNGR2* gene encoding IFN-γR2 lead to a complete loss of cellular responsiveness to IFN-γ, whether due to a lack of receptor expression[3,13] or to the surface expression of nonfunctional receptors.[13] Three of these children have the same *IFNGR2* missense mutation associated with the surface expression of nonfunctional IFN-γR2 chains.[13] This missense mutation creates a novel consensus site for *N*-glycosylation and defines a new and unexpectedly large class of human pathological mutations, designated 'gain-of-glycosylation' mutations.[13] All children with complete IFN-γR2 deficiency had severe, early-onset infections due to environmental mycobacteria and/or BCG, all requiring continuous multidrug therapy.[3,13] No mature granulomas were observed (Fig. 36.2A). Three of these patients also had cytomegalovirus infection. Two patients underwent HSCT, which was successful in one case. Two of the other four patients died of disseminated mycobacterial infection at the age of 5 years and the remaining two are currently on antibiotic therapy at the ages of 3 and 9 years, respectively.

Multiple antibiotics against mycobacteria should be administered without interruption. Vaccination with live BCG is contraindicated. These patients should therefore also be considered candidates for HSCT. Overall,

THERAPEUTIC PRINCIPLES FOR MSMD PATIENTS

>> Vaccination with live BCG is contraindicated.

>> Multiple antibiotics against mycobacteria should be administered without interruption in patients with complete IFN-γR1 or IFN-γR2 deficiency.

>> Anti-mycobacterial antibiotics may be associated with IFN-γ injections in selected patients with partial IFN-γR1 or IFN-γR2 deficiency, complete IL-12p40 and IL12Rβ1 deficiency.

>> HSCT should be considered in selected patients with complete IFN-γR1 or IFN-γR2 deficiency.

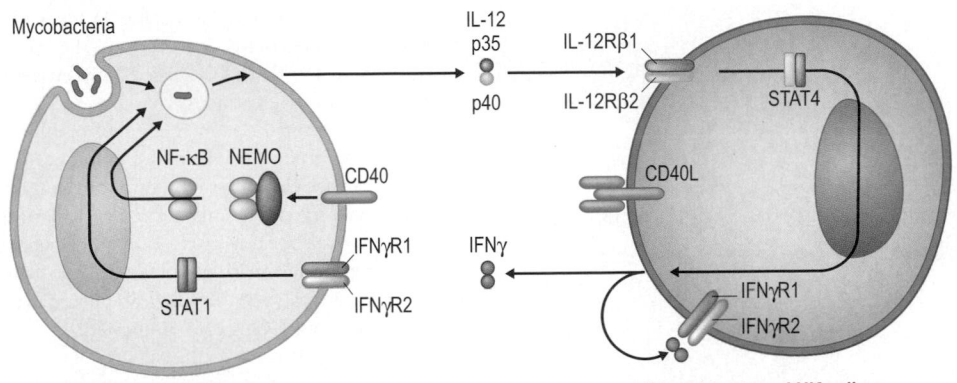

Fig. 36.1 Genetic etiologies of mendelian susceptibility to mycobacterial infection. IL-12 is secreted principally by the phagocytes and dendritic cells and binds to a heterodimeric receptor consisting of β₁ and β₂ chains, which is expressed specifically on NK and T lymphocytes. IFN-γ is secreted by NK and T lymphocytes and binds to a ubiquitous receptor made of two chains, a ligand-binding (IFN-γR1) and a signaling-associated chain (IFN-γR2). Stat-1 is phosphorylated in response to IFN-γ and is translocated to the nucleus as a homodimer. NEMO is a regulatory protein in the NF-κB pathway. The engagement of CD40 signaling via the NF-κB pathway is important for IL-12 production and for protective immunity against mycobacterial infection. The six molecules shown in red have been found to be mutated in certain patients with severe mycobacterial infection.

the immunological features of IFN-γR2-deficient patients are essentially indistinguishable from those with complete IFN-γR1 deficiency. Thus, like null recessive *IFNGR1* mutations, null recessive *IFNGR2* mutations cause susceptibility to early-onset, recurrent, multiple, and life-threatening myco-bacterial infections with impaired granuloma formation.

PARTIAL RECESSIVE IFN-γR1 AND IFN-γR2 DEFICIENCIES

Three patients from two unrelated kindreds having recessive partial IFN-γR1 deficiency (OMIM 107470) have been reported.[15] A mutation caus-ing an amino-acid substitution in the extracellular domain was identified and the encoded receptor was detected with specific antibodies at the cell surface. The cells of the patients responded only to high concentrations of IFN-γ. One of these children had disseminated BCG and *Salmonella enteritidis* infections with a favorable outcome. His sister, who had not been vaccinated with BCG, had curable symptomatic primary tuberculo-sis. The third, unrelated, patient had received BCG without complica-tions in infancy and had disseminated *Mycobacterium avium* infection with a favorable outcome at the age of 20 years. These patients had well-circumscribed and well-differentiated tuberculoid granulomas (Fig. 36.2B). These patients are currently 20, 23 and 27 years old, respectively, and have no ongoing treatment. One patient with recessive partial IFN-γR2 deficiency (OMIM 147569) has also been reported.[3] A homozygous nucleotide substitution was found in *IFNGR2*, resulting in a single amino-acid substitution in the extracellular domain. The young adult patient concerned had presented BCG and *M. abscessus* infections and is now well at 25 years of age. Thus, a diagnosis of recessive partial IFN-γR1 or IFN-γR2 deficiency should be considered in children and adults with mycobacterial and *Salmonella* infections with a mild clinical and histo-logical phenotype. For these patients, anti-mycobacterial treatment can be stopped, but not before 1 year has elapsed after the control of infection. Patients should then be closely followed.

PARTIAL DOMINANT IFN-γR1 DEFICIENCY

Patients from 28 unrelated kindreds were found to have a dominant form of partial IFN-γR1 deficiency (OMIM 107470).[3,15] These patients have a heterozygous small frameshift deletion in *IFNGR1*, downstream from the segment encoding the transmembrane domain, but upstream from the recycling motif and Jak-1 and Stat-1 docking sites. This hetero-zygous mutation is therefore loss-of-function and dominant negative and decreases (but does not abolish) cellular responses to IFN-γ in hetero-zygous cells and patients. A total of 50 patients with this condition have been identified, most bearing the same 818del4 mutation that defined the first hotspot for small deletions. The clinical phenotype is character-ized by EM and BCG infections, often affecting the bones.[9] A diagnosis of mycobacterial osteomyelitis is highly suggestive of dominant IFN-γR1 deficiency.[9] Only two patients have presented nontyphoid salmonellosis disease, and one has presented one episode of infection caused by *Histoplasma capsulatum*. Eight of these patients are asymptomatic, but two died of disseminated mycobacterial infection at the ages of 17 and 27 years, respectively. Most have had no prophylactic treatment.

Anti-mycobacterial treatment could be combined with IFN-γ injec-tion in cases of disseminated infection. Antibiotics can be stopped once the infection has been controlled. Vaccination with live BCG is contra-indicated. The clinical outcome of patients with partial dominant IFN-γR1 deficiency, like that of patients with partial recessive IFN-γR1 and IFN-γR2 deficiencies, is much better than that of children with complete IFN-γR deficiency, because there is some residual IFN-γ signaling. There is therefore a strict correlation between *IFNGR1* genotype, cellular phenotype, and clinical phenotype.[9]

IL-12 P40 DEFICIENCY

Twenty patients with complete recessive IL-12p40 deficiency (OMIM 161561) have been reported.[3,16] The mutations in *IL12B* concerned are small insertions or large deletions. Two founder mutational events have

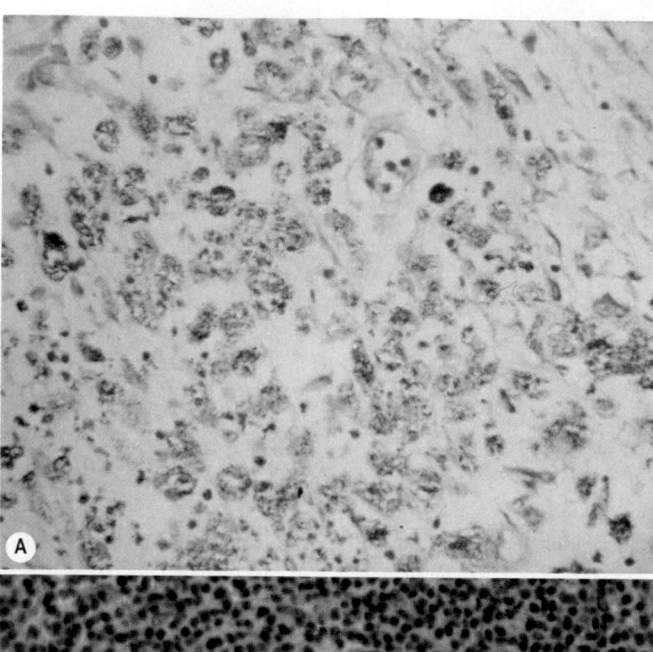

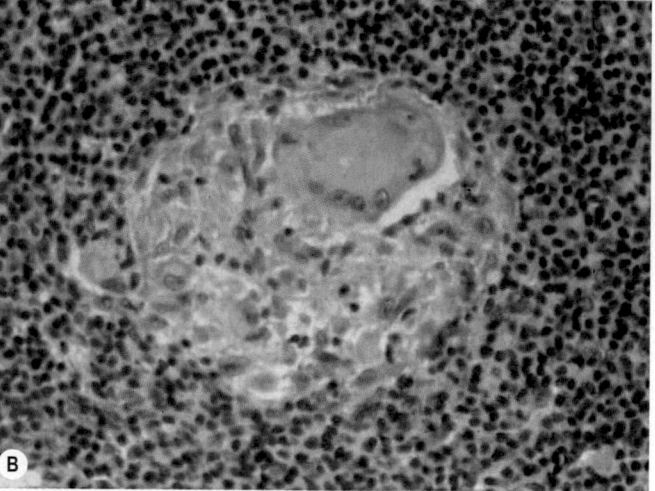

Fig. 36.2 Two types of granuloma. (**A**) The lepromatous-like type consisted of poorly defined, poorly differentiated granulomas, with few, if any giant cells and lymphocytes, but widespread macrophages loaded with acid-fast bacilli. (**B**) The tuberculoid type consisted of well-circumscribed and well-differentiated granulomas, with epithelioid and multinucleated giant cells containing very few acid-fast rods, surrounded by lymphocytes and fibrosis, occasionally with central caseous necrosis.

been identified in four kindreds from Saudi Arabia and in two kindreds from the Indian subcontinent. Children with this deficiency produce abnormally low levels of IFN-γ, due to a lack of stimulation through IL-12. This defect can be partially corrected, in a dose-dependent manner, with exogenous recombinant IL-12.[3] All children inoculated with live BCG vaccine developed clinical infection, two children had infection caused by EM, and one had an infection caused by *M. tuberculosis*. Six patients presented nontyphoid salmonellosis and one presented with a single episode of infection caused by *Nocardia asteroides*, an acid-fast

agent closely related to *Mycobacterium*.[3] One of these children is asymptomatic, but six died of infection between the ages of 2 and 11 years.[3] The survivors are currently well and aged between 6 and 29 years. Most have had no prophylactic treatment.

Anti-mycobacterial treatment can be combined with IFN-γ injection in cases of disseminated infection. Antibiotics can be stopped, but not before 1 year has elapsed after control of the infection. Granuloma formation is preserved, but may be multibacillary in these patients (Fig. 36.2B). Thus, a diagnosis of IL-12p40 deficiency should be considered in children and adults with mycobacterial and *Salmonella* infections having a mild clinical and histological phenotype. Vaccination of these patients with live BCG is contraindicated.

IL-12Rβ1 DEFICIENCY

Fifty-nine patients with recessive complete IL-12 receptor β1 (IL-12Rβ1) deficiency (OMIN 601604), with no cellular expression [3, 17] and one patient with a complete recessive form in which the affected receptor was expressed have been reported.[3] The cellular phenotype of IL-12Rβ1-deficient patients is a lack of response of NK and T lymphocytes to IL-12 and IL-23, with low levels of IFN-γ production. The clinical phenotype is characterized by EM/BCG infections, with half the patients also presenting with nontyphoid salmonellosis.[3] Twenty-nine of the 40 children inoculated with live BCG vaccine developed clinical infection, 12 children had infections caused by EM, and three had infections caused by *M. tuberculosis*.[3] The low penetrance for the case-definition phenotype of BCG/EM disease led to the discovery of tuberculosis as the sole infectious phenotype in several patients,[18] providing the first cases of mendelian predisposition to tuberculosis. Twenty-eight patients presented nontyphoid salmonellosis and one presented with a single episode of infection caused by *Paracoccidioides brasiliensis*. Five of these patients are asymptomatic, but 10 died of mycobacterial or *Salmonella* infection before the age of 8 years. The survivors are currently well and aged between 2 and 34 years. Most have had no prophylactic treatment.

Infections can be treated with antibiotics and IFN-γ. Vaccination with live BCG is contraindicated. The prognosis is good for patients with IL12-Rβ1 deficiency, partly owing to the low clinical penetrance of primary mycobacterial infection, the favorable response of infections to treatment, and the rarity of recurrent or multiple mycobacterial infections. Indeed, children with primary mycobacterial disease can mount a fully protective immune response against a secondary mycobacterial disease. However, the high incidence of recurrent salmonellosis in these patients suggests that IL-12 is required for both primary and secondary immunity against *Salmonella*.

PARTIAL STAT-1 DEFICIENCY

Four kindreds with heterozygous mutations in *STAT1* causing partial dominant Stat-1 deficiency (OMIM 600555) have been described.[19-21] Stat-1 is a critical transducer of IFN-mediated signals, either as Stat-1 homodimers – designated γ-activating factor (GAF) – or as Stat-1/Stat-2/IRF-9 trimers, known as interferon-stimulated γ factor 3 (ISGF3) (Fig. 36.3). These heterozygous *STAT1* mutations reduce the cellular response to IFN-γ, but not that to IFN-α. Indeed, the *STAT1* mutations found are loss-of-function for the IFN-γ-induced GAF activation and IFN-α/β-induced ISGF3 activation phenotypes, but are dominant for one phenotype (GAF) and recessive for the other (i.e., ISGF3) in heterozygous cells. Clinically, two patients suffered from disseminated BCG infection with tuberculoid

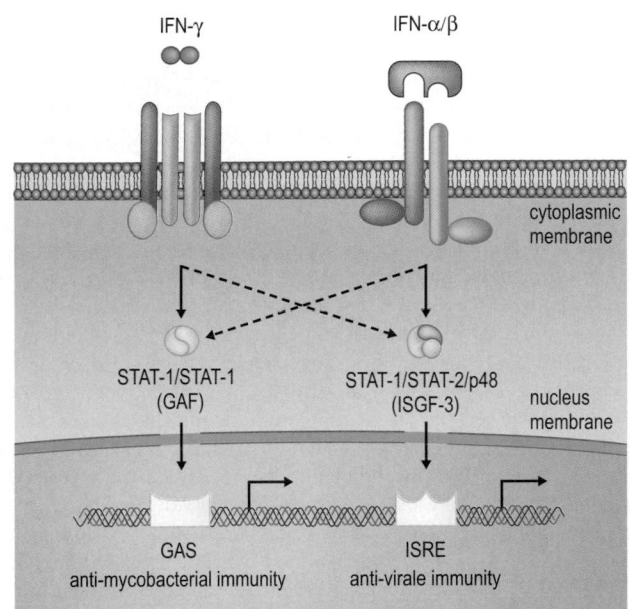

Fig. 36.3 STAT-1 pathway. The binding of homodimeric IFN-γ to its tetrameric receptor leads to the activation of constitutively associated Jak-1 and Jak-2, which then phosphorylate tyrosine residues in the intracellular part of IFN-γR1. Upon IFN-γ stimulation, unphosphorylated Stat-1 molecules are directly recruited to IFN-γR1 docking sites. They are then phosphorylated and released into the cytosol as phosphorylated Stat-1 homodimers, which form γ-activating factors (GAF), which are translocated to the nucleus. GAF binds γ-activating sequences (GAS) present in the promoters of target genes. Following monomeric IFN-α/β stimulation, Stat-2 is recruited to the phosphorylated IFN-αR1 chain of the heterodimeric IFN-αR and is itself also phosphorylated by Jak-1 and Tyk-2. This leads to the phosphorylated Stat-2-mediated recruitment of Stat-1, which is then phosphorylated. Active phosphorylated Stat-1/Stat-2 heterodimers are released into the cytosol and translocated to the nucleus with IRF-9 to form interferon-stimulated genes factor-3 (ISGF-3) heterotrimers. ISGF-3 binds IFN-α/β sequence response elements (ISRE) in the promoters of target genes via the DNA-binding domains of Stat-1 and IRF-9. In humans, recessive complete Stat-1 deficiency results in impaired responses to both IFN-γ and IFN-α/β. It is associated with a specific syndrome, different from MSMD, of susceptibility to both mycobacteria (impaired IFN-γ-mediated immunity) and viruses (impaired IFN-α/β-mediated immunity).

granulomas, one suffered from local BCG infection, and two others had disseminated *M. avium* infection. The other five patients are asymptomatic. All patients are currently well and aged between 3 and 38 years.

Anti-mycobacterial treatment can be stopped, but not before 1 year has elapsed after control of the infection. Vaccination with live BCG is contraindicated. Observations of affected patients suggest that Stat-1 and GAF are required for human IFN-γ-mediated mycobacterial immunity. In conclusion, patients with partial Stat-1 deficiency have clinical and cellular phenotypes (i.e., susceptibility to mycobacterial disease and impaired GAF activation) similar to those of patients with partial IFN-γR deficiency. These patients should be treated in a similar manner.

NEMO DEFICIENCY (XR-MSMD)

An X-linked recessive form of MSMD (XR-MSMD) was clinically described in 1996,[22] and two neighboring mutations (E315A and R319Q) in NEMO were recently discovered in three unrelated kindreds with XR-MSMD.[23] These two missense mutations, which affect two neighboring residues in the leucine zipper domain that normally form a salt bridge, are responsible only for impairing the CD40-triggered induction of IL-12 production by monocyte-derived cells upon stimulation with CD40L-expressing T cells. Four maternally related male family members in two successive generations presented *M. avium* infection and the other two, unrelated, patients suffered from mycobacterial disease. These patients had a purely infectious phenotype, with no sign of anhidrotic ectodermal dysplasia (EDA), with the exception of conical deciduous incisors in one child. The patients are currently well and aged between 8 and 57 years. It is not clear whether anti-mycobacterial treatment can be stopped once the infection has been controlled or when, as the six patients seem to have had different clinical outcomes. Vaccination with live BCG is contraindicated. These two mutations, responsible for impaired T cell-dependent IL-12 production, thus account for the observed susceptibility to mycobacteria. The MSMD-causing mutations in the NEMO leucine zipper domain define the first genetic etiology of X-linked recessive MSMD.[23]

■ INHERITED DISORDERS OF IFN-γ- AND IFN-α/β-MEDIATED IMMUNITY ■

COMPLETE STAT-1 DEFICIENCY

Three children from three unrelated kindreds with complete Stat-1 deficiency (OMIM 600555) have also been reported.[24] These patients carried homozygous mutations, which completely abolished the cellular responses to both IFN-γ and IFN-α/β. All patients had disseminated BCG disease. One patient died of recurrent encephalitis caused by herpes simplex virus, a second died of a nondocumented illness thought to be viral in origin, and the third died 3 months after HSCT, from Epstein–Barr virus lymphoproliferative disorder.[24] Recent data indicate that two other children with complete Stat-1 deficiency died of unknown viral diseases, in the course of disseminated infection with BCG (Chapgier, unpublished data). The outcome of viral illnesses in children with complete Stat-1 deficiency suggests that the Stat-1-dependent response to human IFN-α/β is necessary for viral immunity. Patients with complete Stat-1 deficiency had multiple, severe, early-onset viral infections.

Multiple antibiotics against mycobacteria, and possibly antiviral treatment directed against herpes viruses, should be administered without interruption and these patients should be considered for HSCT. Vaccination with live BCG is contraindicated.

Complete Stat-1 deficiency defines a severe innate immunodeficiency that should be considered in infants and children with severe infectious diseases, notably (but not exclusively) mycobacterial and viral diseases. Other children with viral and bacterial diseases were recently found to show an impaired cellular response to both IFN-γ and IFN-α/β, indicating that the group of disorders affecting both types of IFN-mediated immunity is likely to expand (unpublished data). Milder forms of Stat-1 deficiency should therefore be considered in children with a milder clinical course than those with complete Stat-1 deficiency.

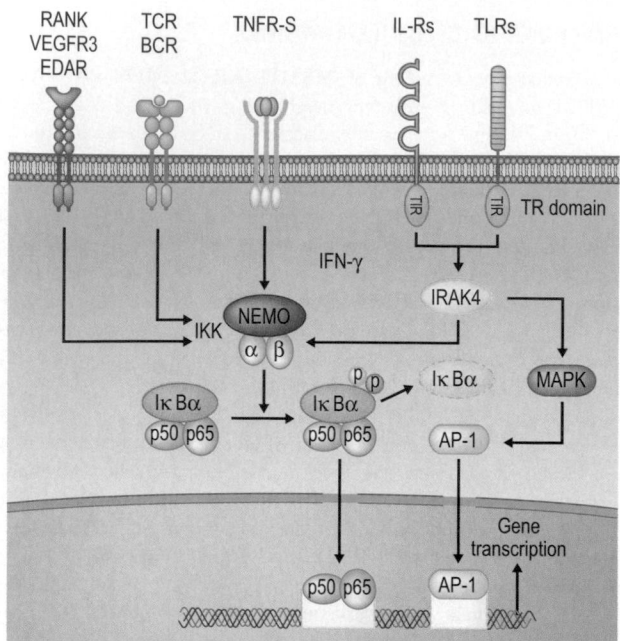

Fig. 36.4 Genetic defect of the NF-κB pathway. The NEMO-NF-κB signaling pathway is used by several groups of developmental receptors (EDAR, RANK and VEGFR) and by several groups of immune receptors (antigen receptors (TCR and BCR), members of the TNF receptor superfamily (CD40 and TFNR), and the members of the TIR superfamily). The three proteins of the NF-κB pathway (IRAK-4, NEMO, IκBα) responsible for the primary immunodeficiency are shown in red. In IRAK-4-deficient patients, TIR superfamily-induced MAPK kinase activation is also abolished.

■ INHERITED DISORDERS OF NF-ƙB-MEDIATED IMMUNITY ■

This group of inherited disorders leads to impaired NF-κB signaling and strong susceptibility to pyogenic bacteria. The affected patients bear mutations in *NEMO*, *IKBA*, or *IRAK4* (Fig. 36.4).[25] Patients with anhidrotic ectodermal dysplasia with immunodeficiency (EDA-ID) syndrome carry either X-linked recessive hypomorphic mutations in *NEMO* or autosomal dominant hypermorphic mutations in *IKBA*. Other patients with autosomal recessive amorphic mutations in *IRAK4* present a more restricted, purely immunological defect, with specific impairment of the Toll and interleukin-1 receptor (TIR)-interleukin receptor-associated kinase (IRAK) signaling pathway.[25] Diverse mutations have been found in *NEMO*, associated with a variety of cellular and clinical phenotypes (see above and below). A single type of *IKBA* mutation was found in two unrelated kindreds. All known mutations in *IRAK4* are recessive and loss-of-function, and only one cellular phenotype has been identified to date. Patients with EDA-ID and mutations in *NEMO* or *IKBA* are susceptible to multiple infectious agents, including pyogenic bacteria, mycobacteria and viruses. In contrast, patients with IRAK-4 deficiency seem to be specifically prone to pyogenic bacterial diseases, in particular pneumococcal and staphylococcal diseases.

NEMO DEFICIENCY

X-linked anhidrotic ectodermal dysplasia with immunodeficiency (XL-EDA-ID) is a rare primary immunodeficiency (OMIM 300291). To date, 52 patients with XL-EDA-ID have been reported.[25–27] Patients with XL-EDA-ID carry hypomorphic mutations in the gene encoding NEMO, a protein essential for activation of the ubiquitous transcription factor NF-κB. X-linked dominant loss-of-function mutations in NEMO are lethal in utero in males and are associated with incontinentia pigmenti in girls.[25] In the immunologic work-up of patients with EDA-ID, the only known consistent abnormality is a lack of serum antibodies against carbohydrates, which has been found in most patients reported.[25] Some patients have hyper-IgM syndrome and a few have NK-cell abnormalities.[25] Most patients bearing hemizygous *NEMO* mutations show weak blood cellular responses to TNF-α. EDA-ID is characterized by hypohidrosis, widely spaced cone- or peg-shaped teeth, and hypotrichosis (Fig. 36.5). However, the range of clinical manifestations appears to be broad, from both developmental and infectious standpoints. Two patients carrying the X420W mutation had osteopetrosis and lymphedema (defining XL-OL-EDA-ID).[25] In contrast, some children had an exclusively infectious phenotype, with no sign of EDA. The infectious phenotype is characterized mostly by infections due to encapsulated pyogenic bacteria, such as *Haemophilus influenzae* and *Streptococcus pneumoniae*. Infections caused by weakly pathogenic microorganisms, such as *M. avium* and *M. kansasii*, have also been diagnosed in patients. Other infectious diseases include salmonellosis, pneumocystosis, and viral illnesses caused by herpes simplex virus and cytomegalovirus have been reported. Infectious episodes were marked by a poor clinical and biological inflammatory response. Half the patients with EDA-ID died from invasive infection, demonstrating the severity of this disorder. Thus, NEMO deficiency is a disorder in which a PID may or may not be associated with developmental abnormalities.

All patients should receive monthly prophylactic administrations of intravenous immunoglobulins (IVIG). Prophylactic trimethoprim-sulfamethazole and/or penicillin V should also be considered, along with an intensive vaccination program, including conjugated and nonconjugated vaccines against encapsulated bacteria (pneumococcus, *H. influenzae*, meningococcus). Vaccination with live BCG is contraindicated. Patients with a severe infectious phenotype should be considered for HSCT.

┃ THERAPEUTIC PRINCIPLES FOR INHERITED DISORDERS OF NF-κB-MEDIATED IMMUNITY

➤➤ All patients should receive conjugated and nonconjugated vaccines against encapsulated bacteria (pneumococcus, *H. influenzae*, meningococcus).

➤➤ Prophylactic trimethoprim-sulfamethazole and penicillin should also be administered.

➤➤ Monthly prophylactic administrations of intravenous immunoglobulins (IVIG) should be considered in selected patients.

➤➤ HSCT should be considered in selected patients with NEMO deficiency.

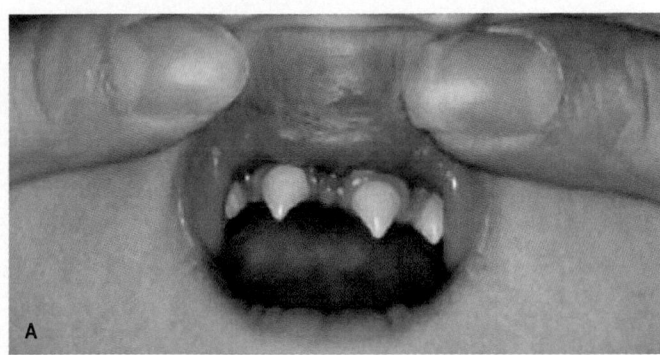
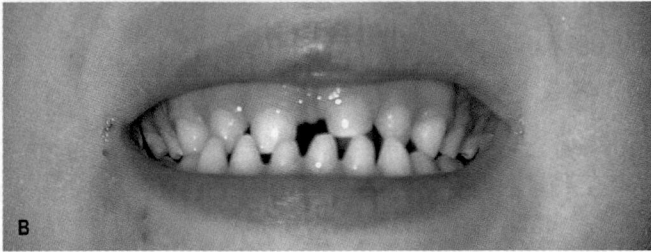

Fig. 36.5 Two patients with EDA-ID, one presented widely spaced cone- or peg-shaped teeth and the second with conical incisors.

The NEMO–NF-κB signaling pathway is used by several groups of developmental receptors (EDAR, RANK and VEGFR) and several groups of immune receptors (antigen receptors (TCR and BCR), members of the TNF receptor superfamily (CD40 and TFNR), and members of the TIR superfamily). Clinical variability results from differences in the impact of the various hypomorphic mutations in this pathway. However, the variability of the infectious phenotype seems to parallel, and may be correlated with, the variability of the immunological phenotype.

IκBα DEFICIENCY

One patient with an autosomal dominant (AD) form of EDA-ID was initially reported,[28] followed by a child and his father a year later.[29] Patients with AD-EDA-ID carried the same missense mutation (S32I) in *IKBA*, encoding an inhibitor of NF-κB (OMIM 164008). The father of the second patient has the same mutation, but displays complex mosaicism.[29] All patients were heterozygous for this mutation, which is gain-of-function/hypermorphic as it prevents the phosphorylation and degradation of IκBα, increasing the inhibitory capacity of this molecule. The mutant allele thus exerts a dominant-negative effect over the wild-type allele. Interestingly, the father of the second patient presented a milder clinical and immunological phenotype, probably owing to the complex mosaicism.[29] Both children had a lack of memory T cells and an impaired T-cell response to both antigenic and CD3 mitogenic stimulation *in vitro*. They also displayed hyper-IgM syndrome and had the EDA phenotype. From the age of 2 months onwards, they suffered from recurrent opportunistic infections and chronic diarrhea caused by pyogenic bacteria, *Pneumocystis jirovici* and virus. They also failed to thrive. The two children were treated by HSCT at the ages of 1 and 2 1/2 years, respectively. The father of the second child suffered from recurrent *Salmonella typhimurium* infection. Thus, a diagnosis of IκBα

deficiency should be considered in children with EDA and severe immunodeficiency with impaired T-cell immunity.

IL-1 RECEPTOR-ASSOCIATED KINASE-4 DEFICIENCY

Inherited interleukin-1 receptor-associated kinase-4 (IRAK-4) deficiency (OMIM 607676) is an autosomal recessive disorder first described in three unrelated patients.[30] Nineteen other patients have since been identified[3] (Casanova, unpublished data). All but one of the causal mutations concern the kinase domain of the protein (missense mutations and small insertions). The blood cells of the patients fail to produce proinflammatory cytokines upon stimulation by all known Toll-like receptor (TLR) agonists, IL-1β and IL-18. Clinically, IRAK-4-deficient patients suffer from recurrent infections caused by pyogenic bacteria, mostly Gram-positive, with little or no fever and inflammatory responses. The leading pathogen responsible for infections in these patients is *S. pneumoniae*, which was found in 21 of 22 patients with proven IRAK-4 deficiency and caused bloodborne invasive disease (septicemia, meningitis, or arthritis). The second most frequently detected infectious organism is *S. aureus*, often responsible for skin infections, but occasionally also for infection of the liver or septicemia. Invasive disease caused by Gram-negative bacteria was diagnosed in these patients on only three occasions (*Pseudomonas aeruginosa*, *Neisseria meningitidis* and *Shigella sonnei*). All sudden invasive infections occurred before the age of 10 years. IRAK-4 deficiency is a life-threatening disease, resulting in the deaths of nine of the 22 known patients, all of whom died before the age of 8 years. There is an overall trend towards improvement with age, as shown by the two adult patients doing well with no treatment at the ages of 24 and 33 years, respectively.

All IRAK-4-deficient patients should receive monthly prophylactic administrations of IVIG until the age of at least 10 years. Prophylactic trimethoprim-sulfamethazole and/or penicillin V should also be considered, along with an intensive vaccination program, including conjugated and nonconjugated vaccines against encapsulated bacteria (pneumococcus, *H. influenzae*, meningococcus). A diagnosis of IRAK-4 deficiency should be considered in children presenting with recurrent pyogenic infection with poor inflammatory responses.

■ CONCLUSION ■

An understanding of the molecular basis of these new immunodeficiencies affecting the innate immune responses mediated by IFN-γ, IFN-α/β, or NF-κB, has provided detailed insight into the pathogenesis of infections in affected patients, paving the way for genetic counseling and rational treatment design. New PIDs should be sought in patients with unexplained infectious diseases, whether caused by a single or multiple infectious agents, even if all standard immunological explorations are normal. Interestingly, even common infectious diseases, such as tuberculosis, invasive pneumococcal disease and herpes encephalitis, may be favored by mendelian immune disorders. The discovery of many new PIDs is an exciting perspective, not only increasing our understanding of immunity to pathogens, but also benefiting patients. It is thought that most children with severe infectious diseases probably suffer from an underlying PID,[31] and should be repeatedly investigated for known and unknown immunodeficiency conditions.

■ ACKNOWLEDGMENTS ■

We thank Laurent Abel and Christine Bodemer, our laboratory colleagues, our collaborators at Hospital Necker-Enfants Malades and elsewhere, and our patients and families for their assistance in making possible the studies contained in this chapter. This work was supported by the Foundation BNP-Paribas, the Foundation Schlumberger, and EU grant number QLK2-CT-2002–00846. JLC is an International Scholar of the Howard Hughes Medical Institute.

■ REFERENCES ■

1. Notarangelo L, Casanova JL, Conley ME, et al. Primary immunodeficiency diseases: an update from the International Union of Immunological Societies Primary Immunodeficiency Diseases Classification Committee Meeting in Budapest, 2005. J Allergy Clin Immunol 2006; 117: 883–896.

2. Casanova JL, Abel L. Genetic dissection of immunity to mycobacteria: the human model. Annu Rev Immunol 2002; 20: 581–620.

3. Picard C, Casanova JL. Inherited disorders of cytokines. Curr Opin Pediatr 2004; 16: 648–658.

4. Rosenzweig SD, Holland SM. Defects in the interferon-gamma and interleukin-12 pathways. Immunol Rev 2005; 203: 38–47.

5. Filipe-Santos O, Bustamante J, Chapgier A, et al. Inborn errors of IL-12/23- and IFN-γ-mediated immunity: molecular, cellular, and clinical features. Semin Immunol 2006; 18: 347–361.

6. Newport MJ, Huxley CM, Huston S, et al. A mutation in the interferon-gamma-receptor gene and susceptibility to mycobacterial infection. N Engl J Med 1996; 335: 1941–1949.

7. Jouanguy E, Altare F, Lamhamedi S, et al. Interferon-gamma-receptor deficiency in an infant with fatal bacille Calmette–Guérin infection. N Engl J Med 1996; 335: 1956–1961.

8. Jouanguy E, Dupuis S, Pallier A, et al. In a novel form of IFN-gamma receptor 1 deficiency, cell surface receptors fail to bind IFN-gamma. J Clin Invest 2000; 105: 1429–1436.

9. Dorman SE, Picard C, Lammas D, et al. Clinical features of dominant and recessive interferon gamma receptor 1 deficiencies. Lancet 2004; 364: 2113–2121.

10. Roesler J, Horwitz ME, Picard C, et al. Hematopoetic stem cell transplantation (HSCT) for complete IFNα- receptor 1 deficiency: clues for an appropriate regimen from a multi-institutional survey of eleven HSCT in eight patients. J Pediatrics 2004; 145: 806–812.

11. Dorman SE, Holland SM. Mutation in the signal-transducing chain of the interferon-gamma receptor and susceptibility to mycobacterial infection. J Clin Invest 1998; 101: 2364–2369.

12. Rosenzweig SD, Dorman SE, Uzel G, et al. A novel mutation in IFN-gamma receptor 2 with dominant negative activity: biological consequences of homozygous and heterozygous states. J Immunol 2004; 173: 4000–4008.

13. Vogt G, Chapgier A, Yang K, et al. Gains of glycosylation comprise an unexpectedly large group of pathogenic mutations. Nature Genet 2005; 37: 692–700.

14. Jouanguy E, Lamhamedi-Cherradi S, Altare F, et al. Partial interferon-gamma receptor 1 deficiency in a child with tuberculoid bacillus Calmette–Guérin infection and a sibling with clinical tuberculosis. J Clin Invest 1997; 100: 2658–2664.

15. Jouanguy E, Lamhamedi-Cherradi S, Lammas D, et al. A human IFNGR1 small deletion hotspot associated with dominant susceptibility to mycobacterial infection. Nature Genet 1999; 21: 370–378.

16. Altare F, Lammas D, Revy P, et al. Inherited interleukin 12 deficiency in a child with bacille Calmette–Guérin and Salmonella enteritidis disseminated infection. J Clin Invest 1998; 102: 2035–2040.

17. Altare F, Durandy A, Lammas D, et al. Impairment of mycobacterial immunity in human interleukin-12 receptor deficiency. Science 1998; 280: 1432–1435.

18. Alcais A, Mira M, Casanova JL, et al. Genetic dissection of immunity in leprosy. Curr Opin Immunol 2005; 17: 44–48.

19. Dupuis S, Dargemont C, Fieschi C, et al. Impairment of mycobacterial but not viral immunity by a germline human STAT1 mutation. Science 2001; 293: 300–303.

20. Chapgier A, Boisson-Dupuis S, Jouanguy E, et al. Novel STAT1 alleles in otherwise healthy patients with mycobacterial disease. PLoS Genet 2006; 2: e131.

21. Dupuis S, Dargemont C, Fieschi C, et al. Impairment of mycobacterial but not viral immunity by a germline human STAT1 mutation. Science 2001; 13: 300–303.

22. Frucht DM, Holland SM. Defective monocyte costimulation for IFN-gamma production in familial disseminated Mycobacterium avium complex infection: abnormal IL-12 regulation. J Immunol 1996; 157: 411–416.

23. Filipe Santos O, Bustamante J, Haverkamp MH, et al. X-linked susceptibility to mycobacteria is caused by mutations in the NEMO leucine zipper domain that impair CD40-dependent IL-12 production. J Exp Med 2006; 203: 1745–1759.

24. Dupuis S, Jouanguy E, Al-Hajjar S, et al. Impaired response to interferon-alpha/beta and lethal viral disease in human STAT1 deficiency. Nature Genet 2003; 33: 388–391.

25. Puel A, Picard C, Ku CL, et al. Inherited disorders of NF-kappaB-mediated immunity in man. Curr Opin Immunol 2004; 16: 34–41.

26. Doffinger R, Smahi A, Bessia C, et al. X-linked anhidrotic ectodermal dysplasia with immunodeficiency is caused by impaired NF-kappaB signaling. Nature Genet 2001; 27: 277–285.

27. Orange JS, Levy O, Brodeur SR, et al. Human nuclear factor k B essential modulator mutation can result in immunodeficiency without ectodermal dysplasia. J Allergy Clin Immunol 2004; 114: 650–656.

28. Courtois G, Smahi A, Reichenbach J, et al. A hypermorphic IkappaBalpha mutation is associated with autosomal dominant anhidrotic ectodermal dysplasia and T cell immunodeficiency. J Clin Invest 2003; 112: 1108–1115.

29. Janssen R, Van Wengen A, Hoeve MA, et al. The same I{kappa}B{alpha} mutation in two related individuals leads to completely different clinical syndromes. J Exp Med 2004; 200: 559–568.

30. Picard C, Puel A, Bonnet M, et al. Pyogenic bacterial infections in humans with IRAK-4 deficiency. Science 2003; 299: 2076–2079.

31. Casanova J.L., Abel L.. Inborn errors of immunity to infection: the rule rather than the exception. J Exp Med 2005; 202: 197–201.

HIV infection and acquired immunodeficiency syndrome

Christopher S. Baliga, Mary E. Paul, Javier Chinen,
William T. Shearer

37

The human immunodeficiency virus (HIV) has proven to be a formidable adversary for both the human immune system and medical science. After 25 years of intense research, HIV infection is still one of the most-studied infectious diseases. The clinical care for the disease caused by HIV infection, the acquired immunodeficiency syndrome (AIDS), has particular complexities due to the compromise of the immune system and the side effects of the anti-HIV drugs; consequently, it has now matured into a clinical discipline in its own right. The accumulated knowledge of this disease and its pathogenesis has led to the rapid development of effective, albeit expensive, treatment drug regimens. These anti-HIV drug therapies do not eradicate HIV infection; however, they have proven to prolong the survival of HIV-infected patients significantly. Ongoing research focuses on the discovery of new anti-HIV drugs and alternative approaches to control the spread of HIV infection, such as novel vaccines and topical microbicides.

EPIDEMIOLOGY

GLOBAL PERSPECTIVE

The face of the HIV pandemic initially varied depending on the geographic area, reflecting the different groups of people at risk in which this new infection was first described. Many of the stereotypes of the "typical" HIV-infected patient resulted from these initial reports: male homosexuals in the developed world, intravenous drug users (IDUs) in Eastern Europe, and commercial sex workers in Asia and Africa. These early descriptions do not accurately reflect today's pandemic. As of December 2006, there were about 40 million people living with HIV infection worldwide (Fig. 37.1). Of these, 43% were women and 2.3 million were children.[1] An estimated 2.9 million people died from AIDS in 2006, with more than 25 million deaths since 1981.

The developing world continues to bear the brunt of the epidemic. Sub-Saharan Africa alone is home to over two-thirds of all HIV-infected individuals and, importantly, 77% of all the HIV-infected women. Data from prenatal clinics in sub-Saharan Africa show that, in six countries – Botswana, Lesotho, Namibia, South Africa, Swaziland, and Zimbabwe – over 20% of pregnant women are infected with HIV. In Botswana and Swaziland, the incidence levels are closer to 30%. It is important to realize that the people contracting and dying from HIV infection are the young, economically productive members of society. In South Africa, the mortality rates for those aged 15 and older increased 62% between 1997 and 2002, while the rates for those aged 25–44 doubled in number.

Not all the news out of Africa is bleak. Zimbabwe is showing a decline of national HIV prevalence, apparently due to increased AIDS awareness and changes in sexual behavior. In East Africa, there is a trend of declining or stabilizing HIV prevalence. Uganda has had steadily declining adult HIV infection prevalence levels since peaking at > 15% in the early 1990s, to 6.7% in 2005. Kenya is the only other sub-Saharan country to have a declining HIV prevalence rate, from 10% in the late 1990s to 7% as of 2003, and 6% in 2005. More dramatically, the prevalence rates of HIV among attendees at urban antenatal clinics dropped from 28% in 1999 to 9% in 2003. These declines have been attributed to behavioral changes such as increased condom use with casual partners and decreased rates of multiple sexual partners, resulting from a national prevention campaign in 2000. However, the incidence of HIV infection peaked in the mid-1990s, suggesting that other factors such as the saturation of HIV infection in the population at risk may have influenced this decline.

In Asia, the prevalence data may mask the realities of the epidemic. Countries like India and China, each with a population over 1 billion, can have prevalence levels < 1%, yet still harbor millions of infected individuals. India, with 5.7 million infected patients in 2005, is one of the countries with the highest number of HIV-seropositive people in the world. India's HIV epidemic closely mirrors Africa's, being predominantly spread by heterosexual transmission. The control of HIV infection in Thailand is a qualified success. Their epidemic peaked in the mid-1990s, with HIV prevalence rates at prenatal clinics > 2.5% in some provinces. By 2004, it hovered around 1% for all provinces. The epidemic in Thailand was mainly heterosexual, being spread between commercial sex workers and their clients. Extensive education campaigns increased condom use to as high as 96%. Vigilance is required to maintain those levels, because recent surveys suggest condoms are now used only 50% of the time.

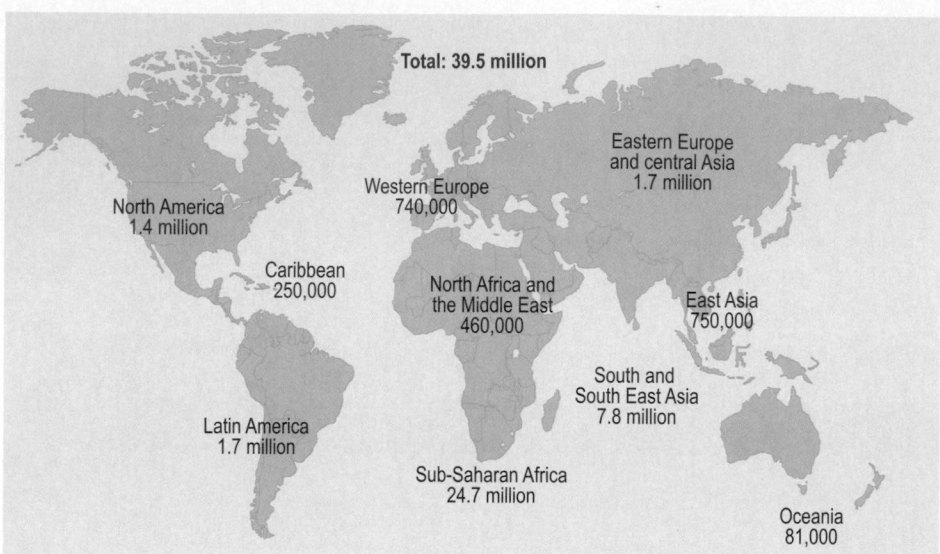

Total: 39.5 million

North America
1.4 million

Western Europe
740,000

Eastern Europe
and central Asia
1.7 million

Caribbean
250,000

North Africa and
the Middle East
460,000

East Asia
750,000

South and
South East Asia
7.8 million

Latin America
1.7 million

Sub-Saharan Africa
24.7 million

Oceania
81,000

Fig. 37.1 Global prevalence of human immunodeficiency virus (HIV) infection: 39.5 million (modified from UNAIDS, December, 2006).

Russia has the largest HIV epidemic in Europe, with approximately 350 000 cases documented since the HIV epidemic began; however it is estimated that because of the poor reporting system, the actual number of people living with HIV is 940 000. The Russian epidemic has historically been one of IDUs, with greater than 80% of all reported HIV infections belonging to IDUs. However, in time IDUs infected from sharing needles engage in sexual relations, with the potential to spread the virus. In 2001 only 6% of registered cases were due to sexual transmission; by 2004 the number was 25%. Ukraine has an HIV prevalence of 1.5% (2005), the highest in Europe. Their epidemic, like Russia, began and continues to be fueled by IDUs. In a similar pattern, commercial sex workers are beginning to change the face of the epidemic. In 1999 only 14% of new infections were related to sexual transmission, but by 2004 that number was 32%, most of whose sexual partners were infected from contaminated needles.

Although the absolute number of HIV-positive cases is relatively small, the Caribbean is the second most affected area of the world behind Africa when considering national HIV prevalences. However, the region's prevalence of 1.6% is considerably less than sub-Saharan Africa's 7.2%. The epidemic is mostly related to heterosexual transmission, with male homosexual transmission being around 10%. Latin America had 1.8 million infected individuals in 2005, mostly as a result of sexual spread. In Argentina, the epidemic began among IDUs but, as in other Latin American countries, sexual transmission is now predominant, mainly affecting men who have sex with men (MSM).

According to the UNAIDS, in North America and western and central Europe there were an estimated 2.1 million people living with HIV, 43 000 new infections, and 18 000 deaths in 2005.

KEY CONCEPTS

TRENDS IN HUMAN IMMUNODEFICIENCY VIRUS (HIV) INFECTION

>> Global rates of HIV infection continue to increase

>> The increases are mostly in heterosexual transmission

>> The age demographic most affected in the developing world, i.e., those aged 25–44 years, includes men and women who are economically productive and women of childbearing potential

>> Six African nations have prevalence rates > 20%

>> In the USA, African-American transmission in men who have sex with men is one of the key drivers of new infections

US PERSPECTIVE

The epidemic in the USA represents the changing face of the epidemic from one principally of transmission by Caucasian MSM and IDUs to a greater representation of minorities and women infected through heterosexual contact. The epidemiological data from the Centers for Disease Control and Prevention (CDC) suggest an adult and adolescent prevalence rate of 20.2/100 000 individuals, which translates into 476 095 people at the end of 2005.[2] The numbers of newly infected people in the USA decreased from 2001 to 2004, but in 2005 increased again by 1% (Fig. 37.2). The rates of new infection increased among those aged 15–29 and over 40. It decreased, however, in those aged < 13 and those aged 30–39. The incidence in those less than 13 has dropped 61% since 2000. New HIV cases increased among Caucasians, Asians, and American Indians, while decreasing by 10% in African-Americans and by 9% in Hispanics. African-Americans made up the majority of new

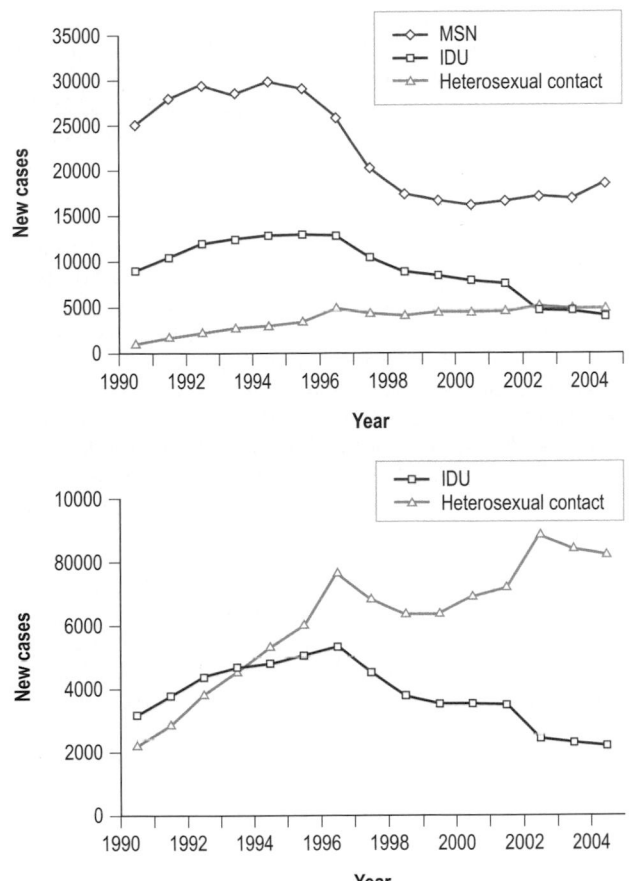

Fig. 37.2 US trends in human immunodeficiency virus (HIV) infection by sex and mode of transmission. IDU, intravenous drug users; MSM, men who have sex with men. (From Centers for Disease Control and Prevention: HIV/AIDS Surveillance Report, vol. 17, 2005, Atlanta: US Department of Health and Human Services, Centers for Disease Control and Prevention, 2006. Also available at //www/cdc/gov/hiv/topics/surveillance/resources/reports.gov.)

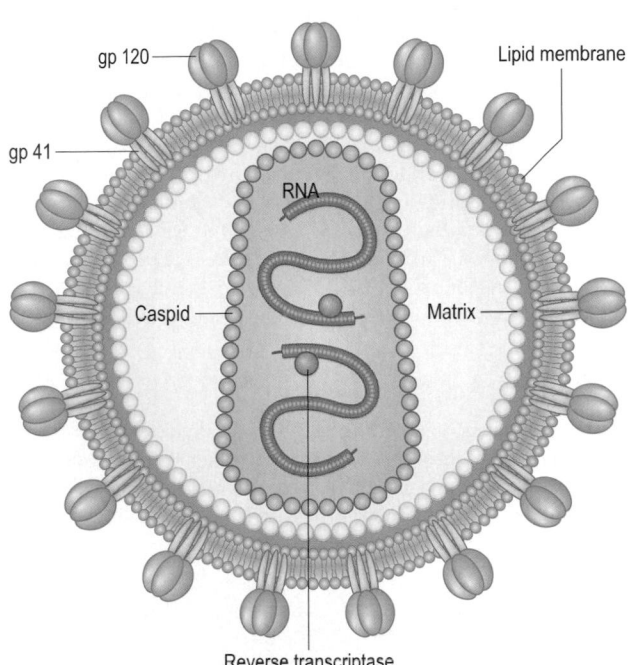

Fig. 37.3 Structure of human immunodeficiency virus (HIV) virion. (From Baliga CS, Shearer WT. HIV/AIDS. In: Fireman P (ed.) Atlas of allergy, 3rd edn. Philadelphia: Elsevier Science (USA), 2005:351–367, with permission from Elsevier.)

infections, accounting for 50% of new cases. Males represented 73% of new cases, with 64% of those being among MSM, 16% from heterosexual transmission, and 13% from IDUs. In women, heterosexual contact accounted for 78% of new cases. In children < 13 years of age, 85% of the 166 cases were from perinatal transmission. There were 44 198 newly diagnosed AIDS cases in the USA in 2005, up from 38 016 in 2001. The number of deaths among patients with AIDS declined 8% from 2000 (44%) to 2004 (36%). Since the start of the epidemic in 2004, the total US deaths due to AIDS were estimated to be 529 113.

Among adolescents (13–19 years old), there were 1268 new cases of HIV in 2005, representing a 19% increase over 2001. The total number of adolescents living with HIV/AIDS in 2005 was 5322, a 46% increase over 2001 levels. These numbers are underestimated, as it is assumed that over one-third of HIV-infected adolescents in the USA have not been tested for HIV. Half of the 40 000 new cases of HIV infection in 2004 occurred in individuals under the age of 25.[3]

VIROLOGY

CLASSIFICATION

HIV is an enveloped, positive-sense RNA virus with icosahedral symmetry and two copies of its genome. It belongs to the lentivirinae group of retroviruses (Fig. 37.3). As with all retroviruses, it contains the enzyme reverse transcriptase (RT) capable of turning its RNA genome into DNA, which is integrated into the host cell genome and can then be translated to produce viral proteins and new virions. Like other lentiviruses such as equine infectious anemia virus, visna/maedi virus, and the other immunodeficiency viruses (bovine, feline, and simian), HIV has a long latency period before causing clinical disease.

There are two distinct types of HIV, HIV-1 and HIV-2. Both cause human immunodeficiency, but HIV-2 is mostly found in West Africa, is less pathogenic than HIV-1, and may have a longer latency period. Phylogenetic studies have found that HIV-2 is more closely related to SIV_{smm} (simian immunodeficiency virus (SIV) found in sooty mangabey monkeys) and SIV_{syk} (SIV found in Skyes' monkeys) than to HIV-1. HIV-1 is more closely related to SIV_{cpz} (SIV from chimpanzees). These associations support the presumed origin theories of HIV-1 evolving from infected chimpanzees and HIV-2 from sooty mangabeys (SMs). Based on the same genetic studies and estimated mutation rates, the transmission from *Pan troglodytes* chimpanzees to humans is thought to have occurred around 1930.

HIV-1 can be further subdivided based on the genetic divergence in the *env* gene.[4] With divergences of 30–50%, HIV-1 has been divided into three groups: M (major or most), O (outlier), and N (new or non-M, non-O). The M group is further subdivided into clades (A–H, J, K, and O), each of which differs from each other by 20–30%. Clade B is most common in the industrialized world, including the USA. C is the most common clade worldwide, being present in Africa and South Asia. D is found mostly in central and East Africa. E, or rather the AE recombinant form, is the dominant strain in Southeast Asia. Clades A, D, G, H, K, and AG recombinants are found in Africa. F can be found in Africa, South America, and Eastern Europe. J can also be found in Central America.

STRUCTURAL GENES: *GAG*, *POL*, AND *ENV*

The HIV genome is 9.8 kb in length and can be divided into three groups of genes: structural, regulatory, and accessory (Fig. 37.4 and Table 37.1).

The 55-kDa Gag polyprotein (p55) is encoded by the HIV *gag* gene. After translation, the N-terminal is myristolated, causing it to localize to the cell membrane where it recruits two copies of viral RNA and other viral and cellular proteins, culminating in the budding and release of intact HIV particles. After budding, p55 is cleaved by the viral protease to give five proteins: capsid (CA, p24), matrix (MA, p17), nucleocapsid (NC, p9), p6, and p2. Gag cleavage is not required for viral particle formation, but it is necessary for the virus to be infectious. The matrix remains attached and stabilizes the viral envelope and with the capsid forms the conical core of the virus. The nucleocapsid is responsible for recognizing the "packaging signal" of the viral RNA and thus incorporating it into the developing viral particle. The p6 protein is used to recruit the HIV protein Vpr into the budding viral particle as well as being necessary for budding to occur. The last component, p2, is a spacer region between CA and NC, which is thought to be important in the stabilization of the CA core particle. Some authors consider p2 to be part of CA.

The *pol* gene encodes protease (PR, p10), integrase (IN, p50), RNAse H (p15), and RT (p31). Pol is translated in a complex with Gag (Gag–Pol, p160) by a ribosomal frame-shifting event toward the distal end of *gag*. This occurs ~5% of the time, resulting in a ratio of p55:p160 of 20:1. PR cleaves the Gag–Pol complex into Gag and Pol. It further cleaves Pol into the above components. This cleavage is often incomplete, with 50% of RT remaining complexed to RNAse H. Functional PR exists as a dimer and is an aspartyl protease. The IN protein has three functional activities: an exonuclease, endonuclease, and a ligase. It first removes the terminal two nucleotides from the linear double-stranded viral DNA through its exonuclease function. This results in the virus having "sticky ends." Then it cleaves the host DNA at integration sites, allowing the sticky ends of the viral DNA to complement the ends of the host DNA through its endonuclease function. Finally, utilizing its ligase function, it covalently joins the viral DNA with the host's. RNAse H is capable of cleaving RNA if it is part of an RNA–DNA duplex. This is important

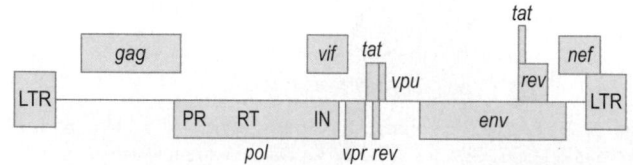

Fig. 37.4 Human immunodeficiency virus (HIV) genome: LTR, long terminal repeat; the products of *pol: IN,* integrase; PR, protease; RT, reverse transcriptase.

Table 37.1 Human immunodeficiency virus (HIV) proteins and their major functions

	Protein	Function
Structural proteins	Gag	Cleavage gives rise to capsid, matrix, nucleocapsid, and p6
	Pol	Cleavage gives rise to protease, integrase, RNAse H, reverse transcriptase
	Env	gp120 and gp41
Regulatory proteins	Tat	Stabilizes transcription complex on the LTR and increases processivity of the complex
	Rev	Allows export of the viral RNA out of the nucleus
Accessory proteins	Nef	Downregulates MHC class I expression
	Vif	Ubiquitination and subsequent degradation of APOBEC3G
	Vpr	Arrests cell in G2/M phase of cell cycle
	Vpu/Vpx	Ubiquitinates CD4 in the endoplasmic reticulum

MHC, major histocompatibility complex.

in removing the RNA template from the negative-strand DNA and allowing the positive strand of DNA to be synthesized.

The protein Env, or gp160, is the product of *env*. After translation, Env is processed in the Golgi bodies such that it is glycosylated. A cellular protease cleaves gp160 into gp120 and gp41. The transmembrane domain of Env is gp41. This is also the fusion domain involved in HIV infection. Glycoprotein 120 acts as the ligand for HIV, binding to CD4 and the chemokine receptors CXCR4 and CCR5.

REGULATORY PROTEINS: TAT AND REV

The regulatory proteins Tat and Rev are essential for HIV replication. Tat stands for trans-activating factor.[5] Without Tat the processivity is poor, although the HIV viral promoter LTR (long terminal repeat) is efficient in initiating DNA translation. This indicates that the transcription complexes easily bind on to the LTR and initiate viral RNA synthesis, but fall off the template before reaching the termination sequences. In fact, without Tat, only 10% of the RNA products are complete. Tat binds to the transactivation response element (TAR) and facilitates the binding of several accessory proteins to the transcription complex, notably the Tat-associated kinase (Tak) with cyclin T and Cdk9 (Fig. 37.5). This complex increases the processivity of the transcription complex 100-fold. Numerous other actions have been linked to Tat, especially when it is added to cultures of cells different from lymphocytes, such as neuronal cells. These include activating the target cells, inducing production of Bcl-2, a protein that inhibits apoptosis. Tat has also been implicated in neurotoxicity and in endothelial, glomerular, and myocardial cell dysfunction, using *ex vivo* or animal model systems. However, it still remains controversial whether significant effects are exerted *in vivo* where the vast majority of Tat remains confined within the nucleus and nucleolus.

HIV encodes 11 proteins from a single RNA transcript, which is then multiply spliced. To perform this task, HIV's Rev binds to the Rev responsive element (RRE) in the *env* sequence as well as to a nuclear export signal known as CRM1, which directs the RNA to an accessory pathway in the nucleus. This pathway is permissive to the passage of RNA messages containing both introns and exons into the cytoplasm. Without Rev, only Tat and Nef would be synthesized by HIV.[6]

ACCESSORY PROTEINS: NEF, VIF, VPR, AND VPU/VPX

The accessory proteins, Nef, Vif, Vpr, and Vpu (or Vpx in HIV-2) are not required for viral replication, but they help the efficiency of this process. Nef stands for negative factor, a misnomer from early studies with lab-adapted strains of HIV where mutations in *nef* led to increased viral production. Nef has numerous effects (Fig. 37.6).[7] It downregulates CD4 by promoting its endocytosis and lysosomal degradation. This helps the virus budding by removing the Env receptor from the cell surface. Nef also reduces the expression of major histocompatibility complex (MHC) class I on the cell's surface, thus limiting the ability of infected cells to be cleared by the immune system. It also activates T cells by binding to the T-cell receptor and several downstream effectors. Activated T cells translocate transcription factors NFAT and NF-κB to the nucleus where they are thought to prime the viral promoter, leading to greater HIV transcription. Recent studies have found that Nef recruits the protein Eed out of the nucleus. Eed is found to colocalize with the HIV promoter and inhibit Tat transactivation. The addition of Nef causes Eed to shift rapidly to the plasma membrane and cease acting on the viral promoter.

Vif stands for virion infectivity factor.[8] It is a 23-kDa polypeptide whose function remained unclear for many years. It was known that its

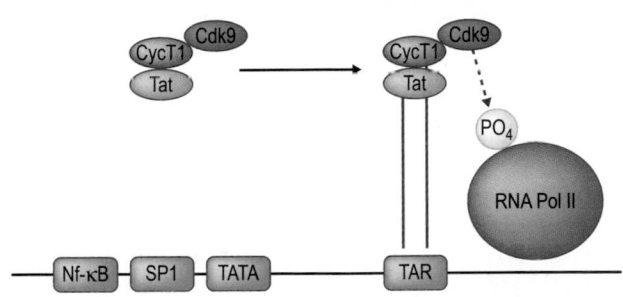

Fig. 37.5 Tat transactivation: human immunodeficiency virus (HIV) Tat forms a complex with various proteins, including cyclin T1 and Cdk9, which recognizes and binds to the TAR or transactivation response element in the nascent viral RNA. This complex then phosphorylates the carboxyl-terminal domain of RNA polymerase II (RNA Pol II), thus counteracting inhibitory factors that actively suppress transcription.

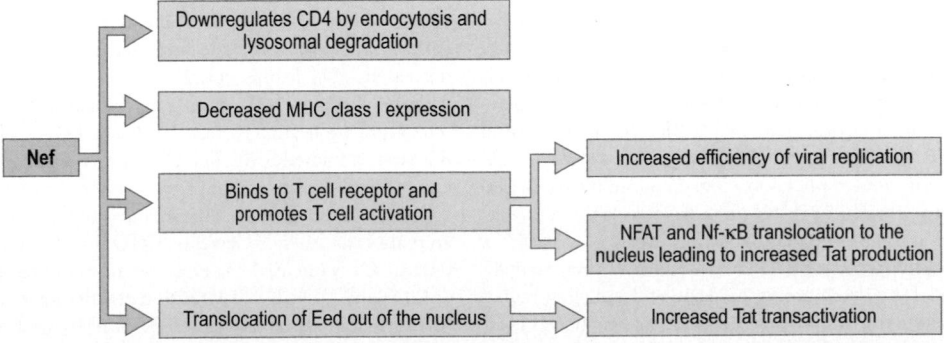

Fig. 37.6 The many functions of Nef. MHC, major histocompatibility complex.

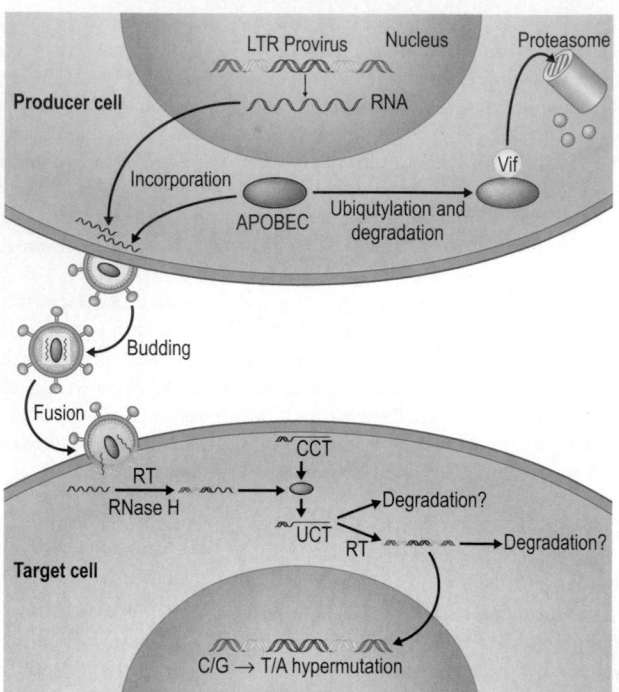

Fig. 37.7 Vif and APOBEC3G: APOBEC3G acts on the first strand of synthesized viral DNA to deaminate cytosine, thus converting it to uracil. The uracil leads to the incorporation of an adenine into the complementary DNA strand instead of a guanine, thus affecting a C/G → T/A mutation on the viral genome. The presence of uracils in single-stranded DNA can directly lead to the degradation of that DNA strand. Vif and other proteins bind to APOBEC and ubiquitinate it, leading to proteasomal degradation. (From Harris RS, Liddament NT. Retroviral restriction by APOBEC proteins. Nat Rev Immunol 2004; 4: 868–877, with permission.)

complex, which leads to the polyubiquitination of APOBEC3G and to a proteosomal degradation pathway. Interestingly, simian APOBEC3G is not affected by HIV Vif and conversely the human APOBEC3G is not affected by SIV Vif. This may help to explain the species restriction of HIV and SIV. This viral specificity is dependent on one amino acid difference in the two APOBEC3Gs (defined below). Vif does not completely negate APOBEC3G's effect, as there is still a substantial amount of G-to-A mutations occurring in HIV.

The viral protein R (Vpr) has several functions assigned to it.[10] It is best known for its ability to arrest the cell cycle in the G2/M phase through phosphorylation of Cdc2 and inhibition of the phosphorylase Cdc25C, as well as for its part in helping the pre-integration complex navigate through the cytosol into the nucleus. It recognizes various nuclear localization signals and disrupts the nuclear membrane in nondividing cells. Vpr has recently been implicated in the induction of apoptosis. While low levels of expression seem to have an anti-apoptotic effect, higher levels promote apoptosis through caspase-dependent mechanisms.

Viral protein U (Vpu) is found in HIV-1 and SIV_{CPZ}.[11] Vpx is its analogue in HIV-2 and SIV_{MAC}. Vpu has two main functions in HIV pathogenesis. The high affinity of CD4 for Env suggests that both proteins can and do interact in the ER when they cross it together. Vpu binds to CD4 in the ER and leads to the ubiquitylation of CD4 to allow free Env migration to the cell surface and into nascent HIV particles.

■ ORIGINS OF HIV ■

Phylogenetic analysis of HIV and SIV genomes has led to the hypothesis that HIV-1 originated in chimpanzees, specifically *Pan troglodytes*.[12] Recent painstaking work has identified chimpanzee communities in Cameroon that harbor endemic SIV_{cpz} infection, with prevalence rates of 29–35%. Two separate communities have been implicated as the origins of group M and group N HIV by phylogenetic analysis (Fig. 37.8).[13] Chimpanzees and SMs become infected with their equivalent of HIV, SIV_{cpz} or SIV_{smm} respectively, but they do not develop simian AIDS (SAIDS). This failure to progress to SAIDS was initially thought to be the result of effective immune control of the virus; however, research has shown that, although these animals do mount cellular and humoral immune responses against the virus, they continue to have significant levels of replicating virus. Surveys of these animals show that they have an average viral load of 171 000 copies/mL and an average CD4 T-cell count of 1076 cells/mm3. Additionally, there is no correlation between viral load and CD4 T-cell count in chimpanzees, a striking difference from human studies where increased viral load correlates directly with decreased CD4 T-cell count.

Two subsets of SMs have been described, CD4-high and CD4-low. The CD4-high animals have normal CD4 T-cell counts and compose 85–90% of studied SMs. The CD4-low animals show evidence of typical CD4 T-cell depletion, but without evidence of SAIDS. Whether these CD4-low animals represent an intermediate between the majority of animals that do not develop SAIDS and those that become sick is unclear. Only one SM has ever been documented to have SAIDS. Levels of CD4 and CD8 T-cell activation also demonstrate limited activation in SMs as defined by interferon-γ (IFN-γ) or tumor necrosis factor-α (TNF-α) secretion following exposure to pooled SIV peptides. Only 0.45% and 0.26% of CD8 and CD4 T cells were reactive, respectively.[14]

presence allowed HIV strains to replicate in peripheral blood lymphocytes and certain 'restrictive' cell lines. Even without it, Vif-deficient HIV could replicate in the majority of cell lines commonly used in labs – so-called "permissive" cell lines. This suggested the presence of a cellular factor that was inhibiting HIV replication in certain cell lines that could be counteracted by Vif. A landmark paper in 2002 by Sheehy et al.,[9] identified such a factor, APOBEC3G. This discovery also included the observation that retroviruses have genomes containing many adenines. This had also been observed in mutation studies of retroviruses in which a high frequency of guanine-to-adenine mutations was noticed, a phenomenon called retroviral hypermutation. APOBEC3G is a cytosine deaminase that mutates cytosines to uracils on the first strand of HIV DNA synthesized during viral replication (Fig. 37.7), resulting in the second strand containing an adenine instead of a guanine as the retroviral RT recognizes uracil as a thymidine. APOBEC3G is part of a family of APOBEC proteins (apolipoprotein B (APOB) mRNA-editing, catalytic polypeptide), which work by deaminating cytosine and inducing mutations, either to generate genetic diversity or inactivate viruses such as HIV or hepatitis B. Vif acts along with several other cellular cofactors like elongin B, elongin C, and cullin-5 (CUL5) to form an ubiquitin–ligase

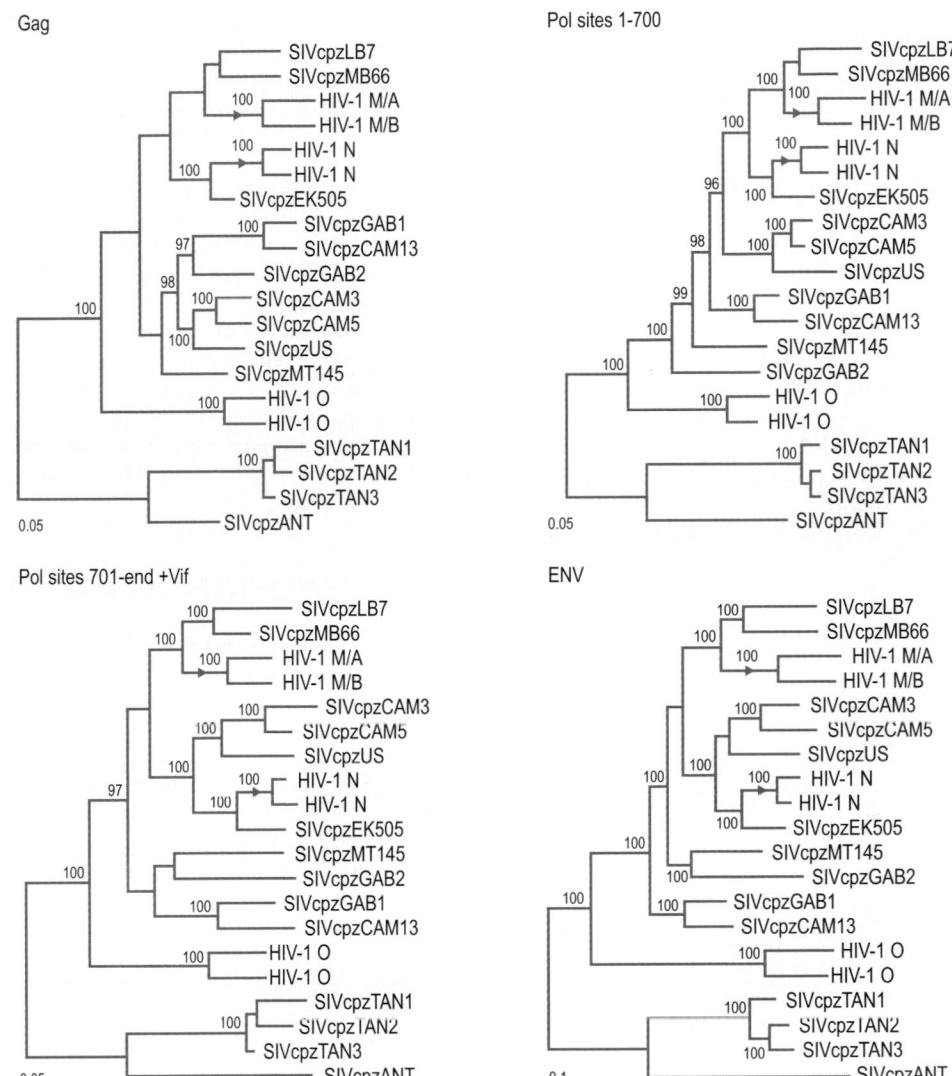

Fig. 37.8 Phylogenetic trees of the full-length human immunodeficiency virus (HIV)/SIV$_{cpz}$ genomes showing the evolutionary relationships between various chimpanzee populations and the crossover events of simian immunodeficiency virus (SIV) into the human population to give HIV groups M, N, and O. The numbers on the branches represent the posterior probability, and the arrows indicate the crossover events. (From Keele BF, Van Heuverswyn F, Li Y, et al. Chimpanzee reservoir of pandemic and nonpandemic HIV. Science 2006; 313: 523–526, with permission from AAAS.)

This again differs from human responses to HIV where 0.7% and 6.3% of CD4 and CD8 T cells, respectively, react to pooled peptides.[15]

ROUTES OF INFECTION

HIV is transmitted through three routes of infection: sexual, parenteral, and perinatal (Table 37.2). In general, higher viral loads, lower CD4 T-cell count, and viral inoculum size are all associated with a greater risk of transmission.

Sexual transmission, representing 70–80% of worldwide infections, is the most common mode of infection. Besides the factors mentioned

above, recipients of penetrative intercourse are more likely to become infected. Anal intercourse carries the greatest risk, followed by vaginal intercourse, with oral intercourse the least likely to spread the virus. The presence of other sexually transmitted diseases, especially ulcerative lesions such as those seen in herpes simplex or syphilis infection, increases the risk of transmission. In contrast, male circumcision significantly decreases transmission risk.[16]

Parenteral transmission is the second most common route of HIV infection, accounting for 8–15% of all HIV infections. Examples include contaminated needles among IDUs, accidental needlesticks among health care workers, improperly sterilized hospital equipment, and contaminated blood products. The largest component of this category is contaminated

KEY CONCEPTS

HUMAN IMMUNODEFICIENCY VIRUS (HIV) AS A ZOONOSIS

>> The natural reservoir of HIV prior to widespread human infection seems to have been chimpanzees for HIV-1, and sooty mangabeys for HIV-2

>> Each of the three groups of HIV-1 – M, N, O – is thought to represent separate transmission events from chimpanzees to humans

>> The natural hosts of the simian immunodeficiency virus (SIV) have a less robust immune response than humans, have poorer viral control, but only rarely show CD4 T-cell loss or progress to immunodeficiency

>> The ability of SIV to replicate in some nonhuman primates without causing overt disease may hold important knowledge needed for the management of the pandemic in humans

Table 37.2 Routes of human immunodeficiency virus (HIV) infection

Mode of transmission worldwide	Percentage of cases
Sexual	**70–80**
Vaginal intercourse	60–70
Anal intercourse	5–10
Perinatal	**5–10**
In utero and intrapartum	2.5–5.0
Postpartum	2.5–5.0
Parenteral	**8–15**
Injecting drug abuse	5–10
Blood transfusions	3–5

From Baliga CS, Shearer WT. HIV/AIDS. In: Fireman P (ed.) Atlas of allergy, 3rd edn. Philadelphia: Elsevier Science (USA), 2005:351–367, with permission from Elsevier.

needles by IDUs. Russia, Eastern Europe, and northeastern India all have HIV epidemics dominated by parenteral spread through contaminated needles. Epidemics of iatrogenic infections have occurred in Russia, China, and other developing countries as a result of improperly sterilized medical equipment or improper screening of blood products. Even in developed countries, prior to effective screening for HIV in 1985, many individuals were infected with blood product transfusions.

Perinatal transmission accounts for the majority of pediatric HIV cases and for 8–15% of HIV infections in all-aged patients. The virus is capable of infecting the child *in utero*, during labor, and after delivery through breastfeeding. The risk of a child contracting HIV from his or her mother during gestation or during labor is ~25%. It is thought that the majority of transmission events occur during the passage of the fetus through the birth canal, by the baby swallowing infected maternal blood, amniotic fluid, and/or cervical and vaginal secretions. An increased rate of abortions and female subfertility has been reported in HIV-infected women. This suggests an unfavorable effect of HIV on early gestation, likely reflecting transplacental passage of the virus. Breastfeeding confers an additional 15–29% increased risk of transmission of the virus from mother to child. Factors such as cracked or ulcerated nipples, mastitis, duration of breastfeeding, and prematurity of the infant may increase the risk of infection.

Recent studies suggest a role of the maternal innate immune system in modulating *in utero* and intrapartum transmission risks. Certain human leukocyte antigen (HLA)-B alleles in the mother encoding killer cell-immunoglobulin-like receptor (KIR) ligands decreases the risk of maternal transmission, suggesting that the involvement of natural killer (NK) cells in the mother is an important determinant of the risk of HIV transmission to the fetus.[17]

IMMUNOPATHOGENESIS

Following a mucosal inoculation of HIV, CD4 T cells are initially infected by CCR5-tropic virus, also called R5 or M-tropic virus. In the macaque model, it takes 3 days for HIV-infected cells to be identified. After a week, the virus becomes detectable in draining regional lymph nodes. Myeloid dendritic cells are not infected with HIV; rather HIV gp120 binds to dendritic cell-specific intercellular adhesion molecule-grabbing nonintegrin (DC-SIGN). The resulting complex is internalized as a phagosome and then presented on the cell surface. As there is no fusion of the HIV Env with the cell membrane, infection does not occur. It has been suggested that the acidic environment of the phagosome potentiates the infectivity of HIV. Plasmacytoid dendritic cells, on the other hand, express CD4 and the co-receptors CXCR4 and CCR5 and thus become infected by the virus. Infection leads to expression of CCR7, which acts as a homing signal for the lymph nodes; it is in lymph nodes where the virus infects T cells, and viral replication occurs. It is at this time that detectable viremia first occurs and the virus begins to seed lymphoid tissues.

GASTROINTESTINAL SYSTEM: EARLY TARGET

A recent advance in the understanding of HIV pathogenesis comes from the evidence of massive infection and subsequent destruction of memory T cells in the gut-associated lymphoid tissue (GALT).[18] Within days, 20% of the GALT CD4 T cells are infected and, of these, up to 80% are killed, likely by direct virus-mediated cytotoxicity or Fas-mediated apoptosis. By the time of peak viremia, 60% of the mucosal memory CD4 T cells are infected. It should be noted that the majority of the body's CD4 T cells reside in the GALT and that this massive infection and destruction of these cells occur early in the infection. Circulating CD4 T cells counts do not reflect the magnitude of CD4 T-cell death taking place in the GALT. The initial surge in viral load and its subsequent lowering to a setpoint is often attributed to the time it takes for the body's adaptive immune system to control the virus. To some extent this is true as levels of specific cellular and humoral immunity correlate with viremic control. However, given the new knowledge of the events transpiring in the GALT, one could argue that the initial rise in viral load represents the rampant proliferation and infection of cells in the GALT, and the subsequent lowering to the viral setpoint represents the depletion of most of the body's CD4 T cells. In other words, if there were fewer cells to support viral replication, levels of viremia would decline.

Following HIV infection, a massive activation of the immune system occurs. Soluble HIV proteins have long been implicated as the cause of this activation, and *in vitro* data support this theory. Lack of a memory response could lead to infection and inflammation of the entire bowel, or possibly the high level of proinflammatory cytokines released by the destruction of the memory CD4 T-cell compartment could lead to increased permeability of the mucosa and translocation of immunogenic peptides from the lumen into the tissue. In either case, the presence of these immune activators over the massive surface area of the bowel has been hypothesized to result in the profound immune activation seen in HIV.[19]

Without treatment, the viremia decreases from as high as 10 million copies of HIV RNA/ml during the acute illness to a stable level called the viral setpoint. The determinants of the setpoint remain unclear. It is known that higher setpoints, which indicate higher viral loads, are loosely predictive of shorter periods of clinical latency. On average, this plateau, or more accurately this period of gradual decline in CD4 T-cell counts and gradual rise in viral load, lasts for 7–10 years. During this time, massive immune activation persists with rapid turnover of cells and with lymph nodes becoming fibrotic. Eventually, for unclear reasons, the relative period of homeostasis between the virus and the immune system collapses and AIDS ensues.

CELLULAR IMMUNITY

The thought that cellular immunity, or specifically CD8 T cells, is important in controlling HIV is supported by several observations. Studies in macaques have shown that when CD8 T cells have been depleted, animals have experienced increased viral loads and rapid clinical progression toward SAIDS.[20] In SIV- or HIV-infected individuals, the initial control of viremia occurs with the initial expansion of HIV-specific CD8 T cells.[21, 22] HIV-exposed but uninfected individuals possess HIV-specific CD8 T-cell responses. The importance of anti-HIV cytotoxic T cells is suggested by the development of viral escape mutations.[23, 24]

HIV-infected individuals present with HIV-specific CD4 T cells, which secrete IFN-γ, even though HIV-specific CD4 T cells are severely reduced in number.[25] In other words, there is not so much a lack of CD4 T-cell response as there is a change in the quality of the response, at least early in the infection. Studies of the correlates of immunity against other chronic viral diseases like Epstein–Barr virus and cytomegalovirus (CMV) demonstrate three qualitatively different CD4 T-cell antiviral responses: (1) an IFN-γ predominant response associated with high viremia and poor immune control; (2) an IFN-γ and interleukin-2 (IL-2) response associated with low-level viremia; and (3) an IL-2 predominant response associated with clearance of viremia. Interestingly, HIV-infected patients with long-term nonprogressor disease course (LTNPs) had identifiable IL-2 and IFN-γ-secreting HIV-specific CD4 T cells. Similarly, HIV-specific CD8 T cells tend to secrete mostly IFN-γ, rather than the broader phenotype in Epstein–Barr virus and CMV infection where CD8 T cells are able to proliferate and secrete IL-2.

HUMORAL IMMUNITY

After establishment of HIV infection, neutralizing antibodies begin to be found in the circulation of patients. These antibodies are effective in neutralizing the virus; however, the virus quickly mutates to avoid them, such that the host is always chasing after the virus. The fact that antibodies can be effective in protecting hosts from HIV infection has been demonstrated in macaques and in a mouse model. Passive transfer of neutralizing antibodies to macaques was sufficient to protect them from a homologous virus challenge.[26] Similarly, in immunodeficient mice transplanted with human T cells, passive transfer of neutralizing antibodies protects against homologous HIV infection.[27] More recent studies have demonstrated protection in macaques when topical neutralizing antibodies were applied prior to challenge with homologous virus.[28] Antibodies directed against Env encounter gp120 and gp41 complexed with each other as heterodimers and homotrimers. This particular conformation has the effect that much of the surface area of Env is unavailable to the host immune system. In addition, the exposed surface of gp120 is heavily glycosylated, the so-called glycan shield. The carbohydrate moieties are provided by the host cellular machinery, and therefore are poorly immunogenic. Their locations within the gp120 molecule are driven by immune pressure. Furthermore, the external V1 and V2 loops of gp120 sterically guard the CD4 binding site, whereas the V3 loop guards the co-receptor binding site. All of the loops can vary considerably in response to host immune pressure without apparent penalty to the virus. The co-receptor binding site on gp120 is not exposed until it undergoes a conformational change caused by binding to CD4, thus limiting the time it is exposed to potential antibodies.

While many neutralizing monoclonal antibodies have been identified and studied, only five are broadly neutralizing for many different viral strains. Monoclonal antibody b12 recognizes the CD4 binding site on gp120, whereas monoclonal antibody X5 binds to the co-receptor binding site when it is exposed. Probably due to steric limitations, it is only effective as an Fab fragment. Monoclonal antibody 2G12, another neutralizing antibody, binds to mannose residues on the surface of gp120. The remaining two, monoclonal antibodies 2F5 and 4E10, bind to the membrane proximal region of gp41.

INNATE IMMUNITY

NK cells

The phenotype of NK cells is dramatically altered in HIV infection.[29] This is hypothesized to occur due to three possible mechanisms: (1) direct infection of NK cells by HIV; (2) binding of NK cell chemokine receptors by HIV; and (3) other effects of the generalized immune activation found in HIV infection. A small subset of NK cells has been found to express both CD4 and CCR5 or CXCR4. These NK cells can be infected by HIV and may serve as one of the sites of latent infection. NK cells also express chemokine receptors that can be triggered by HIV, thus altering their phenotype through downstream signaling. CCR5 levels are higher on NK cells in HIV-infected patients than in HIV-seronegative subjects. However, the increased expression of CCR5 may represent an effect of generalized immune activation rather than an HIV-specific effect. Interestingly, the expression of inhibitory NK cell receptors (for example CD94, CD85) is also increased in HIV infection,

IMMUNOLOGIC DEFICIENCIES

Table 37.3 Apoptosis by human immunodeficiency virus (HIV) products: extrinsic pathway

HIV product		Mechanism of extrinsic pathway apoptosis		
gp120	Increase CD95 and CD95L		Increase caspase-8	Increase activity of caspase-3
Nef	Increase CD95 and CD95L			Increase activity of caspase-3
Tat	Increase CD95 and CD95L	Increase TNF-related apoptosis-inducing ligand (TRAIL)	Increase caspase-8	
Protease			Increase caspase-8	

TNF, tumor necrosis factor.

but returns to normal following highly active antiretroviral therapy (HAART). Surface expression of NK cell protein 30 (NKp30), NKp44, and NKp46, receptors on NK cells that induce cytotoxic activity, is reduced in HIV infection. Antibody-dependent cell-mediated cytotoxicity (ADCC) is reduced in HIV-infected patients, as well as the NK cell responsiveness to IL-2.

NK cells detect the lower levels of MHC class I molecules on HIV-infected cell surfaces, and through ADCC or direct cytotoxic effects are able to induce death of cells infected with HIV *in vitro*. However *in vivo* studies have failed to demonstrate this effect. This is thought to be secondary to the preservation of HLA-C and -E molecules. The expression of HLA-C-specific inhibitory NK cell receptors has been found to be increased in HIV patients. Another way NK cells can inhibit HIV infection is through the production of chemokines (CCL-3, 4, and 5), which competitively inhibit HIV binding to CXCR4 or CCR5. Interestingly, studies of Vietnamese seronegative but HIV-exposed IDUs showed that their NK cells not only secreted greater quantities of chemokines than controls, but they also had greater direct cytotoxicity.

Dendritic cells: myeloid and plasmacytoid

The two subsets of dendritic cells play an important role in HIV infection, serving as antigen-presenting cells, which can prime T cells via myeloid dendritic cells, as well as stimulating innate immune responses such as the type I interferons against HIV via plasmacytoid dendritic cells. In fact, low levels of plasmacytoid dendritic cells correlate with high viral loads, low CD4 T-cell counts, opportunistic infections, and disease progression. High levels of dendritic cells are found in LTNPs. HIV infection appears to activate plasmacytoid dendritic cells by stimulation of Toll-like receptor-7.

VIRAL EFFECTS ON THE HOST

Immune activation

HIV infection induces a profound proliferation and turnover of CD4 and CD8 T cells, even though only a minority of those cells are infected with HIV. It has been thought that HIV itself, either through direct infection or through its protein products like Nef, Env, Vif, etc., induces this activation. This rampant immune activation has long been regarded as the impetus to the eventual collapse of the immune system, secondary to immune exhaustion, implying that the immune system can no longer maintain the high levels of circulating immune cells, T cells, B cells, and NK cells. Newer studies link the cause of the immune activation to an increased permeability of the gastrointestinal mucosa secondary to the heavy burden of HIV infection of mucosal immune cells.

Apoptosis

Increased apoptosis of T cells in HIV infection was established early in the epidemic. Several explanations have been offered: (1) HIV-induced apoptosis of infected cells (viral cytopathic effect); (2) a bystander effect from HIV-infected neighbor cells releasing viral proteins; (3) death of HIV-specific effectors following their migration to infected sites; (4) perturbation of pro-apoptotic signaling molecules on immune cells secondary to the chronic immune activation; and 5) destruction of HIV-infected cells by immune effectors.[30] Late HIV infection is associated with the dominance of a syncytia-inducing form of the virus. This virus induces syncytia formation (clustering of CD4 T cells and membrane fusion) through the interaction of Env and CD4/CXCR4 on neighboring cells. These cells are more prone to undergo apoptosis through a CD95-dependent pathway, likely potentiated by Vpu.

Most of the HIV proteins have been implicated at one time or another in HIV-induced apoptosis. Table 37.3 summarizes the proteins affecting the extrinsic pathway and Table 37.4 lists those affecting the intrinsic pathway.

Autophagy

Autophagy is a process by which cytoplasm and organelles are sequestered and directed toward lysosomal pathways. This process has been implicated in both preventing and inducing apoptosis, reflecting common regulating factors shared by both, e.g., TNF-related apoptosis-inducing ligand (TRAIL), FADD, DAPk, ceramide, and Bcl-2.[31] Recently, HIV Env has been proposed as a stimulus for autophagy in uninfected CD4 T cells via its interaction with CXCR4.[32] Inhibition of

Table 37.4 Apoptosis by human immunodeficiency virus (HIV) products: intrinsic pathway

HIV product			Mechanism of intrinsic pathway apoptosis	
gp120	Phosphorylation of p53	BAX insertion into mitochondrial membrane	Decreases BCL-2	
Tat		BAX insertion into mitochondrial membrane	Decreases BCL-2	
Vpr		Directly increases mitochondrial permeability		
Nef			Decreases BCL-2	Decreases BCL-XL
Protease			Cleaves BCL-2	

the autophagic pathway prevented Env-induced cell death in uninfected cells *in vitro* and demonstrates that this mechanism contributes to the loss of uninfected cells.

The effects of increased apoptosis on the immune system are obvious. The abnormal levels of apoptosis might contribute to the paucity of CD4 T cells late in the disease course. Infected cells can die by the mechanisms mentioned above. Proliferating HIV-specific T cells are also more susceptible to HIV infection and subsequent cytopathicity, depriving the host of the very cells necessary to control viremia. Noninfected cells can be killed by the above mechanisms as well.

CYTOKINES

The dysregulation of the immune system produced by HIV infection includes significant perturbation in the balance of T-cell helper 1 (Th1) and Th2 cytokine levels, which can be observed by examining infected cells *in vitro* and by measuring plasma cytokine levels in HIV-infected patients. The Th1 cytokines IL-2, TNF-α, IFN-γ, and IL-12 decrease during HIV infection, while the Th2 cytokines, IL-10 and IL-4, increase or remain normal. In addition, levels of proinflammatory cytokines such as IL-1, IL-6, and IL-8 also increase.[33] These changes are dynamic, affected by responses to infections and the deterioration of immunity. They reflect the increased state of immune activation with destruction of T cells that are known to direct antiviral responses (Th1). The increase of IL-4 correlates with the hypergammaglobulinemia observed during the early stages of HIV infection.

Viral replication in HIV-infected T cells and monocytes is induced by IL-2, IL-7, and IL-15, as well as the proinflammatory cytokines. These cytokines appear to produce this effect by activating the host cell, a requirement for HIV productive replication.[34] Some cytokines, such as IL-10, decrease HIV production, likely by inhibiting the synthesis of the activating cytokines, and by decreasing the expression of CCR5 and other chemokine receptors.[35] In addition, the HIV LTR promoter contains sequences that bind cellular factors that are activated as a response to cytokine binding, such as NF-κB and AP1. IFN-α and IFN-β have activity against HIV, although their role *in vivo* is not known. Some chemokines inhibit HIV infection by competing with their binding site.

The alpha-chemokine SDF-1 competes with the lymphotropic HIV strains for the binding of CXCR4, while the beta-chemokines MIP1α, MIP1β, and RANTES compete to bind CCR5 with the HIV macrophage-tropic strains. IL-2 and IL-7 have been tested as therapeutic adjuvants to antiretroviral therapy, in an effort to eliminate the viral reservoirs using their capacity to induce HIV replication out of latency.[36] Significant side effects and limited efficacy have decreased the enthusiasm for these strategies. The interaction of chemokines and their receptors is being investigated as a potential target for anti-HIV therapeutics.

CLINICAL FEATURES

ACUTE HIV INFECTION

The natural history of HIV involves four phases: acute retroviral syndrome, asymptomatic phase, pre-AIDS syndrome, and AIDS. There is an initial surge in viremia and loss of circulating CD4 T cells. As immune responses appear, the viremia declines to its setpoint and the CD4 T-cell counts rebound and stabilize. This balance between CD4 T-cell production and loss lasts for 7–10 years in most patients, following which the rates of CD4 T cells again begin their inexorable decline. With declining CD4 T cells, viral loads rebound (Fig. 37.9).

Acute retroviral syndrome occurs within a period of days to 6 weeks following infection with HIV. Viral loads of 10 million HIV RNA copies per ml of plasma are not uncommon. We now know that this initial burst of viremia likely represents the massive infection and subsequent destruction of the CD4 T-cell memory cells in the intestinal mucosa. Reflecting this, there is a rapid drop in circulating CD4 and CD8 T cells during the acute infection. CD8 T-cell numbers rebound, as do the CD4 T cells, albeit to a lesser extent. The symptoms of this initial illness are often described as being infectious mononucleosis-like (Table 37.5). Between 30% and 90% of patients present to the health care system at this point; however, given the nonspecific and "viral syndrome-like" nature of these complaints, they are rarely diagnosed. As the host develops cellular and humoral immunity against the virus, the viremia subsides and the symptoms abate.

Table 37.7 Opportunistic infection prophylaxis and treatment in adolescents and adults[a]

Risk factor	Agent	Prophylactic medication
CD4 cell count < 200 cells/μl	*Pneumocystis jiroveci*	Trimethoprim-sulfamethoxazole (TMP-SMX) or dapsone plus or minus pyrimethamine and leucovorin or aerosolized pentamidine or atovaquone
	Coccidioidomycosis	In endemic areas: fluconazole or itraconazole
CD4 T-cell count < 100 cells/μl	*Toxoplasma gondii*	TMP-SMX or dapsone plus pyrimethamine plus leucovorin or atovaquone plus pyrimethamine plus leucovorin
	Histoplasmosis	In endemic areas: itraconazole
CD4 T cell count < 50 cells/μl	*Mycobacterium avium complex (MAC)*	Macrolide (clarithromycin or azithromycin) or rifabutin
	Cryptococcosis	In endemic areas: fluconazole or itraconazole
PPD > 5 mm induration or recent TB contact but no active TB and no history of treatment for active or latent TB	*Mycobacterium tuberculosis*	INH + pyridoxine for 9 months; if unlikely to complete 9-month course and on HAART: rifabutin plus pyrizinamide for 2 months
Contact with chickenpox or shingles in varicella-zoster seronegative individuals	Varicella-zoster	Varicella-zoster immunoglobulins (VZIG)
HIV-infected	*Streptococcus pneumoniae*	Pneumovax
	Meningococcus – for youth attending the military or college and consider for unvaccinated adults	Menactra
Negative anti-HBc and previously unimmunized or underimmunized to hepatitis B	Hepatitis B	Recombivax-HB or Engerix-B
Negative anti-hepatitis A serology	Hepatitis A	Havrix

[a]For additional information see the current US guidelines at http://AIDSinfo.nih.gov.
HAART, highly active antiretroviral therapy; INH, ; PPD, purfiied protein derivative; TB, tuberculosis.

NONSUSCEPTIBILITY TO HIV INFECTION

Anti-CCR5 antibodies have been found in an interesting cohort of patients – those who have been repeatedly exposed to HIV but have not developed a detectable infection (i.e., HIV-exposed but seronegative patients). Many investigators have looked into this group of individuals, but have not found a good explanation for their lack of susceptibility to HIV infection. Very low levels of virus have been found in these seronegative patients, indicating that they have in fact been exposed. Other studies have implicated: (1) higher IFN-γ production by CD56+(bright) NK cells and CD3+/CD56+ cells; (2) low levels of baseline immune activation and immune responsiveness in T cell; (3) increased levels of immune responsiveness; (4) increased HIV-specific CD4 and CD8 T cells; (5) increased CD91 (low-density lipoprotein-related protein receptor) expression on monocytes; (6) mucosal CCR5-specific immunoglobulin A (IgA); and (7) mucosal HIV-neutralizing antibodies. The question is whether these immune responses are the protective factor, or rather do they result from the act of exposure, leaving an as-of-yet-undefined factor as the explanation. Because no clear or obvious correlates of immunity have been found, the immune responses that have been measured are likely reactive and not causal.

DIAGNOSIS AND MONITORING OF PATIENTS

DIAGNOSTIC TESTS

The diagnosis of HIV is conventionally a two-step process. First, a screening enzyme-linked immunoabsorbent assay (ELISA) is performed, which has a high sensitivity but low specificity. If that test is

Table 37.8 Factors affecting human immunodeficiency virus (HIV) disease progression

Inoculum size	The higher the inoculum, the faster the disease progression
Primate species	Primates infected with their native virus almost always fail to develop an immune deficiency, whereas primates infected with a nonnative strain tend to develop disease
Age	Infected infants have a higher risk of rapidly developing acquired immunodeficiency syndrome (AIDS). This is less common in adults. What makes one a rapid progressor is not known
Viral setpoint	New research is casting doubt on the long-accepted notion that the higher the setpoint, the shorter the period of clinical latency
Broad and robust cellular and humoral immune responses	These correlate with lower setpoints, but what parts of these and which one is more important are unknown
Co-receptor mutations: Δ32 CCR5, CCR2-64I, SDF 1-3' A	Homozygotes for the Δ32 CCR5 mutation fail to develop disease, heterozygotes have a much longer period of clinical latency
Th1 responses: IL-2 and interferon-γ levels Autoantibodies to CCR5 HLA-B27, -B57, -DR	Found in subsets of long-term nonprogressors
APOBEC3G levels	Higher levels are associated with slower progression
Viral fitness	Less fit viruses are associated with slower progression

positive, a second confirmatory test is done. This is usually a Western blot or a radioimmunoassay (RIA), which has a higher specificity than the ELISA, but requires a more specialized laboratory setting. The first-generation ELISAs were based on detection of HIV-1-specific IgG. They have been in widespread use for some time and are well validated. The third generation of ELISAs are designed to detect both HIV-1- and HIV-2-specific IgG and IgM. This allows one test to detect both types of HIV and also the earlier-appearing specific IgM antibodies. A fourth generation of ELISAs has the additional capacity to detect HIV antigens in patient sera, as well as antibodies. It allows the detection of viral particles in acute HIV infection when the viremia is high, but antibodies have not yet developed. An interesting additional use of the ELISAs is to record the actual antibody titers and their avidity. Studies have correlated titer and avidity to indicate duration of infection: lower titers and lower antibody avidity indicate more recent infection.

Several alternative methods of testing for HIV infection have emerged in recent years. Rapid tests can be performed in 30 minutes or less. They are simple, self-contained devices based on immunochromotography. In these tests, a sample of the patient's serum is placed on the tip of the device. As the sample diffuses through the paper substrate, it diffuses through the reagents necessary to produce a color reaction, indicating a positive or a negative result. These assays are advertised as being as sensitive and specific as ELISAs; they therefore need confirmation by a Western blot or RIA if positive. Other variants of this test are assays that use saliva or urine to diagnose HIV. Although these have been licensed by the Food and Drug Administration for use in diagnostic laboratories, none has yet been licensed for home use. However, they may offer excellent diagnostic options for clinicians in resource-poor settings.

Confirmatory testing with a Western blot is the gold standard. Interestingly, up to 15% of noninfected sera will have some reactivity on

KEY CONCEPTS

INTERPRETATION OF WESTERN BLOTS (WB)

>> Repeatedly reactive WB: patient is infected and highly active antiretroviral therapy (HAART) should be discussed, keeping in mind the likelihood of disease progression based on clinical, immunologic, and virologic criteria

>> Indeterminate: either a false positive or an early infection; repeat test in 3 and 6 months: if positive, then discuss HAART as above; if negative or still indeterminate, likely not infected

>> Unreactive: not infected

the Western blot, usually to the Gag proteins. A positive result has been defined as reactivity to two or more of the following: p24, p41, gp120/160. Reactivity to other bands is interpreted as an indeterminate result. A negative result is defined as no reactivity to any of the antigens. Indeterminate results indicate either a patient who will with time seroconvert to a full positive (i.e., an individual recently infected) or someone who will never convert to a full positive (i.e., a noninfected individual). Serial monitoring of the Western blot over the course of 6 months is recommended for indeterminate results. If after that period of time they are still indeterminate or have reverted to nonreactive, the patient can be assumed to be uninfected with HIV. Obviously, if the patient has manifestations of HIV disease, he or she was likely to have been infected at the time of the initial test. Usually, Western blots are performed on the same specimen as the positive HIV ELISA. Positive tests should be repeated on a second specimen to confirm infection in a particular patient or be confirmed with a positive viral load test.

In newborn children, maternal antibodies persist for up to 18 months of age, invalidating the use of serum ELISAs and Western blots to diagnose HIV infection in children less than 18 months of age. In infants born to HIV-infected mothers, HIV DNA polymerase chain reaction (PCR) tests should be checked within the first week of life and at 1–2 months and 4–6 months of age. Two negative tests are required to exclude infection. A positive result should be confirmed through a repeat study. There are two types of neonatal HIV infection: *in utero* infection and intrapartum infection. *In utero* infection is defined by a positive HIV PCR or viral culture within the first 48 hours of life, implying established infection by the time of birth. Intrapartum infection represents the majority of neonatal HIV infections. In these cases, confirmatory tests will document HIV infection only after 1 week of life. Infants who have negative HIV DNA PCR results should then have an HIV ELISA performed at 12–18 months of age to document loss of maternal antibody.

MONITORING TESTS

Once infection is confirmed, CDC guidelines recommend periodically checking the viral load by quantitative RNA PCR, CD4 T-cell levels, and a genotype assay. Genotype assays are based on PCR and genomic sequencing and they identify the presence or absence of key mutations that confer anti-HIV drug resistance. Other assays that can be ordered are phenotype and viral fitness assays. Phenotype assays are performed by isolating certain key regulatory genes from HIV, usually protease and RT, inserting them into a standardized viral construct containing an indicator cassette, and infecting cell lines in the presence of antiretroviral agents. The results are compared against control viral isolates and expressed as a fold-change in viral susceptibility. This provides similar information to the genotype assays, but does so in a direct way, somewhat similar to bacterial antimicrobial sensitivity results. Genotype data are used to extrapolate the resistance patterns of viruses, whereas phenotype data directly measure them. A virtual phenotype test is an extrapolated phenotype study based on comparing the genotype to known phenotypes in the test manufacturer's database. Studies have indicated that the virtual phenotype test is as good as a "real" phenotype test. While phenotyping is a useful predictor of viral susceptibilities to antiretroviral agents, large studies have failed to prove conclusively a clinical benefit of phenotypes over genotypes.

One additional test that is commercially available, but not widely used, is the viral fitness assay, which is similar to the phenotype assay in that it involves isolating viral genes of interest, incorporating them into a viral construct with an indicator cassette. However, unlike the procedure with phenotype test, the resulting viral particle is not cultured with cells in the presence of antiretroviral agents. The rate or amount of infection induced by the viral particles is compared against a wild-type virus and expressed in terms of a percent infectivity compared to the wild-type virus. Therefore, a virus that is more infectious, and presumably more pathogenic, than wild-type virus would have a value > 100% and, similarly, a virus that is less infectious and presumably less pathogenic would have a value < 100%. This assay is an attempt to quantify the loss in fitness that resistance mutations induce in HIV, with the thought that there may be an advantage in promoting the continuing presence of certain mutations in circulating viral strains.[41]

TREATMENT

INITIATION OF THERAPY

The decision to begin treatment for HIV-infected patients is currently a matter of controversy. Experimental studies showing the extent of immune destruction in the gastrointestinal mucosa early in the infection have supported those who advocate starting therapy as soon as the patient is diagnosed. However, these same studies indicate that the destruction of the mucosal CD4 T-cell compartment is not complete in the acute stages of infection. Most patients are not diagnosed during the acute infection, but rather much later in the course of the disease. Early antiretroviral drug treatment results in early development of viral resistance to drugs and medical complications secondary to the drugs' side effects. US treatment guidelines recommend starting therapy when the patient: (1) develops an AIDS-defining illness; (2) has a CD4 T-cell count of < 350 cells/mm3; (3) or has a viral load of > 100 000 copies/ml. Patients with > 350 CD4 T cells/mm3 or with viral loads < 100 000 copies/ml who are asymptomatic can be monitored without therapy.[42] In children < 12 months of age, US guidelines recommend initiating therapy in any symptomatic child or in a child with < 25% of CD4 T cells. Additionally, consider initiating treatment in any HIV-infected child < 12 months of age, since the disease tends to progress more rapidly in infants than in older children or adults.[43] For children older than 12 months, the guidelines recommend initiating therapy when children have AIDS or a CD4 T-cell percentage < 15% and to consider therapy in children with mild to moderate symptoms or 15–25% CD4 T cells or > 100 000 copies/ml of viral RNA. At any age, medication adherence issues must be addressed first. Nonadherence will lead to drug resistance and the potential loss of therapeutic options. The use of levels of viremia to initiate treatment has always been an option in the therapeutic guidelines, and not a mandate, primarily due to concerns for its predictive value in determining the rate of CD4 T-cell decline.

ANTIRETROVIRAL AGENTS

An in-depth discussion of the treatment of HIV is beyond the scope of this chapter. Generally, HIV treatment is based on antiretroviral therapy or HAART using multiple drugs, in an effort to reduce or even eliminate the chance of drug resistance and suppress HIV replication to undetectable levels. Therapy usually consists of two nucleotide RT inhibitors (NRTI) plus a protease inhibitor, or two NRTIs plus a nonnucleoside RT inhibitor (NNRTI).

There are four classes of antiretroviral agents currently available: NRTIs, NNRTIs, protease inhibitors, and a fusion inhibitor (Table 37.9). NRTIs once tri-phosphorylated *in vivo* become analogues of native nucleotides and as such are able to be incorporated into the proviral DNA by HIV RT. Once part of the proviral DNA, they induce premature chain termination as they lack the 3'-hydroxyl group on the

ribose moiety and thus inhibit successful conversion of the viral RNA to DNA (Fig. 37.10). NNRTIs act at the same step of the viral lifecycle as NRTIs; however, they act by binding to RT and inducing a conformational change such that RT is unable to bind with nucleotides. Protease inhibitors act on viral protease, preventing the cleaving of the viral polyproteins necessary for maturation and infectivity of viral particles. Fusion

THERAPEUTIC PRINCIPLE

USE OF NEWER AGENTS

>> Fusion inhibitors must be given parenterally and are poorly tolerated by patients. The approved fusion inhibitor is used primarily in salvage regimens for multidrug-resistant viruses

>> Newer agents will likely also begin as salvage regimens. However, early studies of integrase inhibitors show similar efficacy to nonnucleoside reverse transcriptase inhibitors. If well tolerated and efficacious, newer agents may advance to being first-line therapy

Table 37.9 US Food and Drug Administration-approved antiretroviral agents

Generic name	Abbreviation	Brand name	Generic name	Abbreviation	Brand name
Nucleoside reverse transcriptase inhibitors (NRTIs)			*Nonnucleoside reverse transcriptase inhibitors (NNRTIs)*		
Zidovudine	AZT, ZDV	Retrovir	Nevirapine	NVP	Viramune
Didanosine	DdI	Videx	Delavirdine	DLV	Rescriptor
Zalcitabine	DdC	Hivid	Efavirenz	EFV	Sustiva
Stavudine	d4T	Zerit	*Protease inhibitors*		
Lamivudine	3TC	Epivir	Saquinavir	SQV, hgc SQV, sgc	Invirase Fortovase
Abacavir	ABC	Ziagen	Ritonavir	RTV	Norvir
Tenofovir DF	TDF	Viread	Indinavir	IDV	Crixivan
Emtricitabine	FTC	Emtriva	Nelfinavir	NFV	Viracept
Fusion inhibitor			Amprenavir	APV	Agenerase
Enfuvirtide	T-20	*Fuzeon*	Atazanavir	ATV	Reyataz
Combination pills			Tipranavir		Aptivus
Efavirenz Tenofovir DF and emtricitabine		*Atripla*	Darunavir		Prezista
Zidovudine and lamivudine		*Combivir*	Fosamprenavir		Lexiva
Abacavir and lamivudine		*Epzicom*	Lopinavir and ritonavir		Kaletra
Zidovudine lamivudine and abacavir		*Trizivir*			
Tenofovir DF and emtricitabine		*Truvada*			

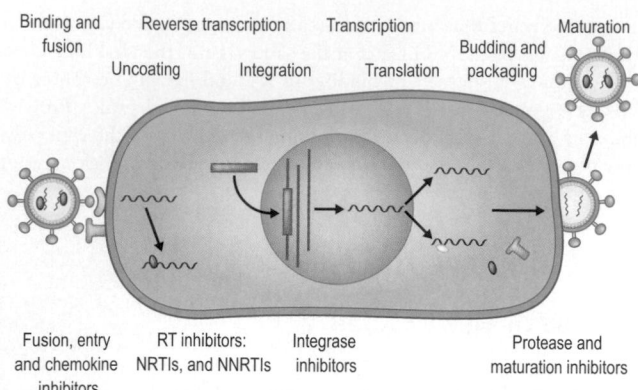

Uncoating — Integration — Translation — Budding and packaging

Fusion, entry and chemokine inhibitors — RT inhibitors: NRTIs, and NNRTIs — Integrase inhibitors — Protease and maturation inhibitors

Fig. 37.10 Lifecycle of human immunodeficiency virus (HIV) and the sites of action of antiretroviral agents: HIV binds to CD4 and its chemokine co-receptor (CCR5 and CXCR4). The viral particle is then uncoated and reverse transcription takes place. The viral DNA is then transported to the nucleus where it integrates with the host DNA. Through transcription and translation, the viral genome is copied for either packaging into new virions or for production of viral proteins. The genome and proteins are transported to the cell membrane where they are incorporated into budding viral particles. Following release, maturation occurs to create an infectious virion. Classes of antiretroviral agents are listed below the steps where they act. RT, reverse transcriptase; NRTI, nucleotide RT inhibitors; NNRTIs, nonnucleoside RT inhibitors.

inhibitors are the newest licensed class of anti-HIV medications. The currently available agent acts to block the conformational changes in gp41 necessary to induce fusion of the viral particle with the host cell. Drugs in development include various molecules acting at the steps of entry and fusion, integrase inhibitors, maturation inhibitors, and topical microbicidals (Table 37.10). New research suggests that a component of green tea, epigallocatechin gallate or EGCG, can bind to the D1 domain of CD4 and sterically prevent HIV gp120 from binding (Fig. 37.11).[44]

IMMUNORECONSTITUTION AFTER HAART THERAPY

To varying degrees, the immune system is able to recover following initiation of therapy, a process called immunoreconstitution.[45] Upon starting HAART in patients who are compliant and able to tolerate the regimen, the initial CD4 T-cell count is the best predictor of a successful outcome. Patients' viral loads are the first to respond following initiation of HAART, often rapidly becoming undetectable. This reflects the medications' ability to repress viral replication rapidly. Lagging behind the drop in viral load is the rise in CD4 T cells. An initial increase in circulating cells occurs in 3–6 months as a result of a decrease in immune activation and subsequent migration of memory T cells (CD4+CD45RO+) out of the lymphoid compartment. A more gradual rise in total CD4 T cells occurs over the course of 3–5 years with the appearance of new naïve (CD4+CD45RA+CD62L+) and memory T cells. Interestingly, a substantial minority of patients never reach a normal level of CD4 T cells,

plateauing at a lower level. Primary and some secondary drug prophylaxis for opportunistic infections can be safely discontinued in patients once the CD4 T-cell count is > 200 cells/mm3 for more than 3–6 months. Cellular and humoral responses to most pathogens also recover with rising counts. Of interest, a low CD4 T-cell count at the time of initiating HAART predicts a poor response to bacterial vaccines given after recovery of CD4 T-cell levels, suggesting a lag in the return of naïve CD4 T cells.

SCHEDULED TREATMENT INTERRUPTIONS

Scheduled treatment interruptions (STIs) were originally proposed as a way to 'auto-vaccinate' the host immune system against HIV, with the hope that stronger cellular and humoral immune responses could be elicited. It was speculated that these immune responses could result in a lower setpoint or even sustained viral suppression off HAART. While initial studies showed promise, larger studies failed to show sustained viral control and were associated with adverse events, such as a higher rate of oral candidiasis. The Staccato trial was a large randomized trial addressing STI with three arms: a 1-week-on and 1-week-off arm, an arm guided by CD4 T-cell counts in which treatment would start only when counts dropped below 350 cells/mm3, and a continuous-treatment arm.[46] The 1-week-on/1-week-off arm was discontinued prematurely as there was a high rate of failure when compared to the other arms. The remaining two arms, however, demonstrated that there was no significant difference between CD4 T-cell-guided treatment versus continuous treatment in terms of virologic response and presence of drug resistance mutations. Obviously, there was a significant difference in cost and expenses between the groups. The incidence of thrush was higher in the STI group versus the continuous-treatment arm, but the incidence of treatment-related side effects was less in the STI cohort than the other. The authors point out that the Staccato trial was not powered to detect differences in mortality or the incidence of AIDS-defining illnesses; needless to say, their data support continued studies into STI. Subsequently, a larger Strategies for Management of Antiretroviral Therapy (SMART) trial failed to demonstrate a benefit or even parity between its STI and the continuous-treatment cohorts.[47] It demonstrated an increased incidence of opportunistic illnesses and deaths in the STI group and was stopped early. One key difference is that the SMART trial withheld HAART until the CD4 T-cell count dropped below 250 cells rather than the 350 benchmark utilized in the Staccato trial.

IMMUNE RECONSTITUTION INFLAMMATORY SYNDROME

Immune reconstitution inflammatory syndrome (IRIS) is a well-known, if incompletely understood, response in AIDS patients with very low CD4 T-cell counts who begin HAART.[48] It is felt to be an inflammatory response by the rebounding host immune system to opportunistic infections, similar to the paradoxical immune response in tuberculosis or leprosy patients after starting antibiotic treatment. Other thoughts as to the etiology include a proinflammatory state secondary to "asymmetric" recovery of the immune system. In other words, there is a proinflammatory state, due to either increased secretion of proinflammatory cytokines or an imbalance between regulatory and effector cells. Risk factors

Table 37.10 Investigational agent in clinical trials[a]

Drug class	Name	Comments
Entry and fusion inhibitors	AMD070	CXCR4 inhibitor
	BMS-488043	
	GSK-873,140 (aplaviroc)	
	PRO 140	mAb
	PRO 542	CD4-IgG2
	Peptide T	
	SCH-D (vicriviroc)	CCR5 blocker
	TNX-355	
	UK-427,857 (maraviroc)	
Integrase inhibitors	GS 9137	
	MK-0518	
Microbicides	BMS-378806	Entry inhibitor
	C31G	
	Carbopol 974P (Buffer Gel)	
	Carrageenan (Caraguard)	
	Cellulose Sulfate (Ushercell)	
	Cyanovirin-N	Fusion inhibitor
	Dextran sulfate	
	Hydroxyethyl cellulose	
	PRO 2000	
	SPL 7013 (VivaGel)	
	UC-781	NNRTI
NNRTIs	Calanoldie A	
	Capravirine	
	TMC 125	
NRTIs	AVX754	
	Alovudine	
	Amdoxovir	Possible use for hepatitis B infection as well
	DPC 817 (Reverset)	
	Elvucitabine	
	KP-1461	
	Racivir	
	Foziduvine tidoxil	
Maturation inhibitor	PA-457 (bevirimat)	
Protease inhibitor	GW640385 (brecanavir)	

[a]For additional information, see the current US guidelines at http://AIDSinfo.nih.gov.

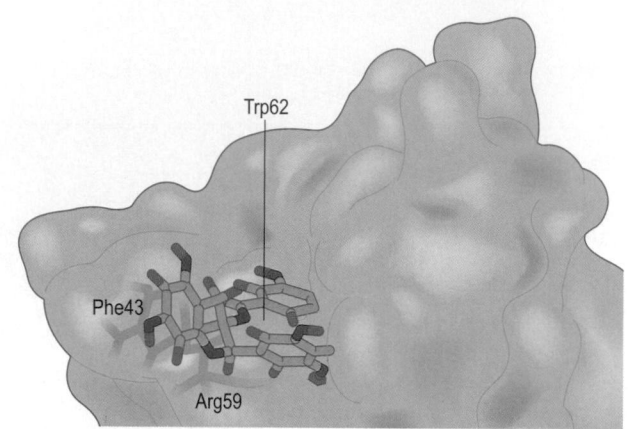

Fig. 37.11 Epigallocatechin gallate (EGCG) binding to CD4: Recent studies indicate that EGCG, a component of green tea, can bind to the human immunodeficiency virus (HIV) binding site of CD4 and potentially interfere in viral infection. (From Williamson MP, McCormick TG, Nance CL, et al. Epigallocatechin gallate, the main polyphenol in green tea, binds to the T-cell receptor, CD4: potential for HIV-1 therapy. J Allergy Clin Immunol 2006; 118: 1369–1374, with permission from the American Academy of Allergy, Asthma and Immunology.)

CLINICAL PEARL

IMMUNORECONSTITUTION INFLAMMATORY SYNDROME (IRIS)

>> IRIS is typically found 2–3 weeks after initiating highly active antiretroviral therapy (HAART)

>> Patients often become profoundly ill and require hospitalization

>> Steroids are sometimes useful in the treatment

>> Clinicians may prevent IRIS by initiating HAART only after treating opportunistic infections

---

include: (1) low CD4 T-cell counts or high viral loads at the time of initiating HAART; (2) duration of immunosuppression; (3) active opportunistic infections; and (4) rapid increase in CD4 T-cell counts. Some genetic factors implicated in IRIS include certain HLA haplotypes (HLA-B27, -Cw0202, -DR4; HLA-A2, -B44; and HLA-A1, -B8, -DR3 with TNF-α polymorphisms), and polymorphism in cytokine genes like TNF-α, IL-6, and IL-12.[49] Studies suggest that between 15% and 25% of patients started on HAART will develop IRIS within 3 months. Treatment includes steroids or other immunosupressants and treating the opportunistic infections. Clinicians try to prevent IRIS by delaying initiation of HAART in a patient with an opportunistic infection until the opportunistic infection has been treated.

An intriguing recent study in children from the Netherlands confirms a fact that many clinicians have long suspected: humoral immune responses to vaccines are abnormal in immune-reconstituted HIV-seropositive children.[50] The authors demonstrated a failure to respond to all three components of the measles, mumps, and rubella vaccine in HIV-infected children prior to initiation of HAART, in accord with prior studies. Following initiation of HAART and immune reconstitution, they demonstrated a loss of specific IgG against measles, mumps, and rubella of 40% to 11%. They also detected a loss of measurable IgG against varicella-zoster virus and herpes simplex virus. They attributed these findings to a persistent dysfunction in memory B cells in infected children. Similar studies point out failure in a substantial minority of patients to restore their CD4 T-cell compartment to normal levels in spite of undetectable HIV RNA. This result may indicate continuing levels of apoptosis or virus-induced cell death or from insufficient thymic reserve to repopulate the compartment completely. Preliminary studies show that giving IL-2 increased the survival of CD4 T cells from almost 2 weeks to almost 29 weeks.[51]

Another complication possibly associated with IRIS is the appearance of an asthma-like condition in perinatally HIV-infected children, who were given combination antiretroviral therapies since infancy. This condition may be mediated by CD4 T-cell activation, release of Th2-type cytokines, and loss of T regulatory cells and tolerance.[52] In support of this concept, Lin and Lazarus had previously observed that a CD4 T-cell count of > 200 cells/μl in the blood of HIV-infected adults was significantly associated with concurrent asthma.[53]

▪ PREVENTION ▪

As a cure to the epidemic remains elusive, prevention remains crucial to a fundamental part of the world's HIV control strategy. These methods include using condoms, providing IDUs with free sterile needles, screening blood products, administering antiretrovirals to pregnant women and their infants, and providing health care workers with antiretroviral agents after occupational exposure. From an immunologic standpoint, several areas of prevention are worth discussing, including vaccines and topical agents.

MICROBICIDES

Topical microbicidals have begun to generate increasing interest within the HIV community. They offer simple, noninvasive methods of controlling the spread of HIV that can be used on an as-needed basis. Topical microbicidals are a targeted intervention to reduce the risk of transmission during heterosexual intercourse in areas such as sub-Saharan Africa, where the risk of contracting HIV is high, but the desire to use condoms is low. Specifically, this allows women to use anti-HIV agents that reduce their risk of infection in cultures where they have little control over their sex lives and men refuse to use condoms. One class of agents is those designed to neutralize the virus.[54] These include detergents and other products that lower the intraluminal pH to < 4.5, the pH at which HIV is inactivated. Another class includes antiretrovirals, with the thought that by directly applying antiretrovirals to the mucosal surface, HIV replication can be stopped after infection occurs, but before it has a chance to spread. The third and largest class of agents includes those designed to block the receptors and co-receptors used by HIV during infection. Several different agents fall within this category. Polyanionic substances disrupt the interaction between the positively charged viral envelope and the negatively charged cell surface. Lectins and monoclonal antibodies are agents that target the glycan shield surrounding the viral particle, which hides the viral surface proteins from host defenses. However, escape mutants have been found against these agents. A monoclonal antibody directed against the CD4 binding site on gp120 has been developed, as have antibodies and agents against gp41. Monoclonal antibodies directed against CD4 that block HIV–CD4 interactions but not CD4–MHC class II are also under investigation. Antibodies and agents against DC-SIGN prevent dendritic cells from importing and presenting HIV to CD4 T cells; however, their usefulness has been limited in animal studies. Perhaps the most promising topical agents are those that target CCR5 on target cells. These agents induce the internalization of CCR5 or conformational changes, which render CCR5 unable or unavailable to bind to HIV. Without CCR5, R5 viruses are unable to infect CD4 T cells.

PREVENTIVE VACCINES

Vaccines are perhaps the greatest hope for curbing the epidemic. But to date, and despite tremendous resource allocation to study and develop them, no effective candidate vaccine has emerged. Initial attempts at vaccine development focused on the traditional methods of vaccine design: whole killed HIV, HIV protein epitopes, and live-attenuated virus.[55, 56] Whole killed virus failed to elicit a strong neutralizing antibody response and investigators remained concerned over the risk of incompletely inactivating HIV. HIV proteins are safe and well tolerated, but again failed to induce a strong neutralizing antibody response, even when coupled with adjuvants. A large phase III trial of recombinant gp120 failed to demonstrate protection from HIV infection.

Live attenuated virus vaccines

Live attenuated SIV has protected macaques from viral challenge. Concerns over the safety of attenuated HIV because of potential reversion to wild-type, however, have prevented enthusiasm for further research on live-attenuated viruses. Additional studies have demonstrated that the greater the replication capacity of the live attenuated virus, the greater its protection.[57] In other words, the more attenuated viruses, which would have greater theoretical safety, are the least protective. Several patients infected with *nef-* and LTR-deficient strains of HIV, i.e., naturally attenuated strains, eventually developed AIDS, as have several macaques infected with attenuated viruses.

DNA vaccines

Attempts at injecting naked DNA plasmids into animals, where they are taken up by cells and used as a template to make specific HIV proteins, proved promising in mice and primates. Human studies have so far been disappointing. One way to boost the immunogenicity of DNA vaccines is to follow them with a replicating viral gene vector, such as a pox virus or an adenovirus. Viral vectors are viruses engineered to express certain HIV proteins. The pox viruses in trials, principally canarypox and vaccinia, are able to elicit robust humoral immune responses, but poor or nondurable cellular immune responses. Additionally, prior immunity to smallpox would prevent the vaccine from working. The adenoviral vectors, mostly based on recombinant adenovirus serotype 5 (Ad5), are able to generate strong cellular and humoral immune responses. They have proven unable to prevent infection in primate models, but have protected animals against the development of SAIDS when challenged with a homologous virus. How well they would do against a real-world case of challenge with nonhomologous viruses in humans is still under investigation. As with the pox viral vectors, prior immunity to Ad5 determines a blunted immune response to the vaccine in some individuals. Unfortunately, many areas of the world with high pre-existing immunity to Ad5 are also some of the hardest-hit areas from the HIV epidemic. Using DNA vaccine priming followed by viral boosting probably represents the most promising vaccination strategy to date. However, even this strategy has not been able to prevent HIV infection or disease when challenged with nonhomologous viral strains.

Novel vaccines

Other potential vaccine designs include pseudovirions, or virus-like-particles. These are essentially the outer layers of HIV without enough genetic core to be infectious. They allow the immune system to encounter HIV in as realistic a manner as possible, with all the HIV surface proteins existing in the proper confirmations. The importance of this approach is demonstrated by the fact that nonnative, nontrimeric Env is unable to produce neutralizing antibodies, while trimeric Env does induce these antibodies. A final class of agents are replicons, which are similarly engineered replication-defective viruses that express HIV proteins. Ongoing vaccine clinical trials under the auspice of the HIV Vaccine Trials Network are listed in Table 37.11.

An intriguing vaccine approach reintroduced autologous monocyte-derived dendritic cells pulsed *ex vivo* with inactivated HIV in 18 patients.[58] The authors demonstrated a drop in mean viral loads of 80% within the first 112 days of follow-up. Over the course of a year, 8 patients were able to maintain a > 90% reduction in viral load. High levels of HIV-1-specific IL-2 or IFN-γ secreting CD4 T cells as well as HIV-1 gag-specific perforin-expressing CD8 T cells were associated with improved viral control.

THERAPEUTIC VACCINES

There are two possible forms for an HIV vaccine: a prophylactic vaccine and a therapeutic vaccine. The prophylactic vaccine is the traditional model, where vaccination is able to prevent or circumvent infection, usually through the induction of sterilizing immunity. A therapeutic vaccine is one in which the vaccine is used after infection occurs, aiming to induce antiviral immunity to alter the course of disease. This would be accomplished by controlling viremia or reducing the viral setpoint in infected patients. Primate models suggest that just such a result is possible, especially with cellular immunity-inducing vaccines. To date, however, data from human studies show no conclusive benefit. Using a therapeutic vaccine in combination with HAART is another approach currently under investigation.

A recent study of a therapeutic vaccine demonstrated that vaccination can induce relative sparing of the central memory T cells following challenge with SIV.[59] Macaques were immunized with a standard recombinant DNA priming vaccine, followed by a boost with a recombinant adenoviral vector vaccine and then challenged with a pathogenic SIV strain. The vaccinated animals initially demonstrated a reduced level of viremia during the acute phase of infection, but over time the viral loads of both the sham-immunized animals and the vaccinated animals' viral loads normalized. Given the similar viral setpoints, one would assume a

Table 37.11 Human immunodeficiency virus (HIV) vaccines in clinical trials[a]

Trial name (phase II)	Prime component	Boost component
HVTN 502/Merck 023	Nonreplicating adenoviral vector with clade B Gag-Pol-Nef	
HVTN 204	DNA plasmids: clade B Gag, Pol, and Nef; clade A, B, C Env	Nonreplicating adenoviral vector with clade B Gag-Pol and clade A,B,C Env
Phase I		
HVTN 042/ANRS VAC19	Canarypox vector: clade B, Env, Gag, Pro, RT, Nef	Lipopeptides: clade B Gag, Pol, Nef
HVTN 044	DNA plasmids: clade B Gag, Pol, and Nef; clade A, B, C Env	
HVTN 049	DNA plasmids: clade B Gag, Env	Protein subunit: clade B Env
HVTN 050/Merck 018	Nonreplicating adenoviral vector: clade B Gag	
HVTN 054	Nonreplicating adenoviral vectors: clade B Gag-Pol; clade A, B, C, Env	
HVTN 055	MVA vectors: clade B Env, Gag, Tat, Rev, Nef, Pol	Fowlpox vector: clade B Env, Gag, Tat, Rev, Nef, Pol
HVTN 060	DNA plasmid : clade B Gag	Peptides: clade B Env, Gag, Nef
HVTN 063	DNA plasmid : clade B Gag	Peptides: clade B Env, Gag, Nef or DNA plasmid clade B Gag
HVTN 064	Protein : T-helper epitopes from clade B Env, Gag, Pol, Vpu and DNA plasmid: Gag, Pol, Vpr, Nef	
HVTN 065	DNA plasmid: clade B Gag, Pro, RT, Env, Tat, Rev, Vpu	MVA vector: clade B Gag, Pol, Env
HVTN 068	Nonreplicating adenoviral vectors: clade B Gag-Pol, clade A,B,C Env or DNA plasmids: clade B Gag, Pol, Nef; clade A, B, C Env	

[a]For additional information see the current US guidelines at http://AIDSinfo.nih.gov.

similar outcome for the animals. Intriguingly, this was not the case: vaccinated animals fared better than sham-immunized animals. The researchers noted a significant increase in the proportion of central memory T cells in the vaccinated animals, confirming current theories that loss of memory CD4 T cells during the acute phase of infection plays an important role in the overall pathogenesis of the virus.

The recent failure of the National Institutes of Health HIV Vaccine Trials Network T-cell vaccine in a 3,000 HIV-negative subject cohort has served to emphasize again the elusive nature of designing a successful HIV vaccine and the need for more research for an HIV vaccine that works.[60]

CONCLUSION

The sudden appearance of HIV in the 1980s and subsequent pandemic reminded clinicians and scientists alike that infectious diseases have not been vanquished or relegated to developing countries. It also served as a reminder that, as the world becomes smaller with increased communication means, and as populations expand into remote areas, new and potentially deadly pathogens continue to emerge. From a basic science perspective, HIV has demonstrated how little we knew of the structure and mechanisms of the immune system and the differences in immunity between mammal species. HIV continues to impress and baffle researchers. Perhaps as a result of millions of years living and adapting in other primate species, it has developed an impressive arsenal of ways to thwart both our innate and adaptive immune systems. One could even say that it is not just a reactive virus, but one that is proactive, striking at immune cells, the very cells that are designed to control it. Our efforts at designing a vaccine have taught us much about the immunology of HIV, but have not yet developed into a successful candidate. It should be noted, however, that most current vaccines are directed against viruses or bacteria for which the body can mount an effective immune response on its own. Despite all this, immunology has made great strides in our understanding of HIV. Perhaps in no other disease has so much been learned so fast. In the developed world, HIV causes chronic infection rather than certain death, thanks in large part to the use of antiviral drugs. More novel drugs in development are due to new-found understanding of the molecular biology behind HIV. For virologists and immunologists, HIV continues to perplex and fascinate; for clinicians it continues to teach humility.

ACKNOWLEDGMENTS

Supported by National Institutes of Health grants T32 AI07456, AI27551, AI36211, AI6944I, HD41983, RR0188, HD79533, HL72705, and HD78522 and contract 202PICL05; the Pediatric Research and Education Fund, Baylor College of Medicine, and the David Fund, Pediatrics AIDS Fund, and Immunology Research Fund, Texas Children's Hospital.

Carolyn Jackson assisted with the preparation of the manuscript for publication.

Lynn Des Prez provided critical review.

REFERENCES

1. UNAIDS Joint United Nations Programme on HIV/AIDS. AIDS Epidemic Update: December 2006.

2. Centers for Disease Control and Prevention. HIV/AIDS Surveillance Report, vol. 17. Atlanta: US Department of Health and Human Services, Centers for Disease Control and Prevention; 2006.

3. CDC. Fact sheet: Young People at Risk – HIV/AIDS Among America's Youth, 2004.

4. Wainberg MA. HIV-1 subtype distribution and the problem of drug resistance. AIDS 2004; 18: S63–S68.

5. Pugliese A, Vidotti V, Beltramo T, et al. A review of HIV-1 Tat protein biological effects. Cell Biochem Funct 2005; 23: 223–227.

6. Cochrane A. Controlling HIV-1 Rev function. Curr Drug Targets Immune Endocr Metabol Disord 2004; 4: 287–295.

7. Baur A. Functions of the HIV-1 Nef protein. Curr Drug Targets Immune Endocr Metabol Disord 2004; 4: 309–313.

8. Harris RS, Liddament MT. Retroviral restriction by APOBEC proteins. Nat Rev Immunol 2004; 4: 868–877.

9. Sheehy AM, Gaddis NC, Choi JD, et al. Isolation of a human gene that inhibits HIV-1 infection and is suppressed by the viral Vif protein. Nature 2002; 418: 646–650.

10. Zhao LJ, Zhu H. Structure and function of HIV-1 auxiliary regulatory protein Vpr: novel clues to drug design. Curr Drug Targets Immune Endocr Metabol Disord 2004; 4: 265–275.

11. Binette J, Cohen EA. Recent advances in the understanding of HIV-1 Vpu accessory protein functions. Curr Drug Targets Immune Endocr Metabol Disord 2004; 4: 297–307.

12. Gao F, Bailes E, Robertson DL, et al. Origin of HIV-1 in the chimpanzee *Pan troglodytes troglodytes*. Nature 1999; 397: 436–441.

13. Keele BF, Van Heuverswyn F, Li Y, et al. Chimpanzee reservoir of pandemic and nonpandemic HIV. Science 2006; 313: 523–526.

14. Dunham R, Pagliardini P, Gordon S, et al. The AIDS-resistance of naturally SIV-infected sooty mangabeys is independent of cellular immunity to the virus. Blood 2006; 108: 209–217.

15. Betts MR, Ambrozak DR, Douek DC, et al. Analysis of total human immunodeficiency virus (HIV)-specific CD4(+) and CD8(+) T-cell responses: relationship to viral load in untreated HIV infection. J Virol 2001; 75: 11983–11991.

16. Weiss HA. Male circumcision as a preventive measure against HIV and other sexually transmitted diseases. Curr Opin Infect Dis 2007; 20: 66–72.

17. Winchester R, Pitt J, Charurat M, et al. Mother-to-child transmission of HIV-1: strong association with certain HLA-B alleles independent of viral load implicates innate immune mechanisms. J Acquir Immune Defic Syndr 2004; 36: 659–670.

18. Brenchley JM, Schacker TW, Ruff LE, et al. CD4+ T cell depletion during all stages of HIV disease occurs predominantly in the gastrointestinal tract. J Exp Med 2004; 200: 749–759.

19. Brenchley JM, Price DA, Douek DC. HIV disease: fallout from a mucosal catastrophe?. Nat Immun 2006; 7: 235–239.

20. Matano T, Shibata R, Siemon C, et al. Administration of an anti-CD8 monoclonal antibody interferes with the clearance of chimeric simian/human immunodeficiency virus during primary infections of rhesus macaques. J Virol 1998; 72: 164–169.

21. Koup RA, Safrit JT, Cao Y, et al. Temporal association of cellular immune responses with the initial control of viremia in primary human immunodeficiency virus type 1 syndrome. J Virol 1994; 68: 4650–4655.

22. Borrow P, Lewicki H, Hahn BH, et al. Virus-specific CD8+ cytotoxic T-lymphocyte activity associated with control of viremia in primary human immunodeficiency type 1 infection. J Virol 1994; 68: 6103–6110.

23. Borrow P, Lewicki H, Wei X, et al. Antiviral pressure exerted by HIV-1-specific cytotoxic T lymphocytes (CTLs) during primary infection demonstrated by rapid selection of CTL escape virus. Nat Med 1997; 3: 205–211.

24. Goulder PJ, Phillips RE, Colbert RA, et al. Late escape from an immunodominant cytotoxic T-lymphocyte response associated with progression to AIDS. Nat Med 1997; 3: 212–217.

25. Pantaleo G, Koup RA. Correlates of immune protection in HIV infection: what we know, what we don't know, what we should know. Nat Med 2004; 10: 806–810.

26. Parren PW, Marx PA, Hessell AJ, et al. Antibody protects macaques against vaginal challenge with a pathogenic R5 simian/human immunodeficiency virus at serum levels giving complete neutralization in vitro. J Virol 2001; 75: 8340–8347.

27. Gauduin MC, Parren PW, Weir R, et al. Passive immunization with a human monoclonal antibody protects hu-PBL-SCID mice against challenge by primary isolates of HIV-1. Nat Med 1997; 3: 1389–1393.

28. Veazey RS, Shattock RJ, Pope M, et al. Prevention of virus transmission to macaque monkeys by a vaginally applied monoclonal antibody to HIV-1 gp120. Nat Med 2003; 9: 343–346.

29. Fauci AS, Mavilio D, Kottilil S. NK cells in HIV infection: paradigm for protection of targets for ambush. Nat Rev Immunol 2005; 5: 835–843.

30. Gougeon ML. Apoptosis as an HIV strategy to escape immune attack. Nat Rev Immun 2003; 3: 392–404.

31. Levine B, Sodora DL. HIV and CXCR4 in a kiss of autophagic death. J Clin Invest 2006; 116: 2078–2080.

32. Espert L, Denizot M, Grimaldi M, et al. Autophagy is involved in T cell death after binding of HIV-1 envelope proteins to CXCR4. J Clin Invest 2006; 116: 2161–2172.

33. Clerici M, Galli M, Bosis S, et al. Immunoendocrinologic abnormalities in human immunodeficiency virus infection. Ann NY Acad Sci 2000; 917: 956–961.

34. Managlia EZ, Landay A, Al-Harthi L. Interleukin-7 induces HIV replication n primary naïve T cell through a nuclear factor of activated T cell (NFAT)-dependent pathway. Virology 2006; 350: 443–452.

35. Norris PJ, Pappalardo BL, Custer B, et al. Elevations in IL-10, TNF-alpha, and IFN-gamma from the earliest point of HIV type 1 infection. AIDS Res Hum Retroviruses 2006; 22: 757–762.

36. Paredes R, Lopez Benaldo de Quiros JC, et al. The potential role of interleukin-2 in patients with HIV infection. AIDS Rev 2002; 4: 36–40.

37. Rodriguez B, Sethi AK, Cheruvu VK, et al. Predictive value of plasma HIV RNA level on rate of CD4 T-cell decline in untreated HIV infection. JAMA 2006; 296: 1498–1506.

38. Martinez V, Costagliola D, Bonduelle O, et al. Combination of HIV-1-specific CD4 Th1 cell responses and IgG2 antibodies is the best predictor for persistence of long-term nonprogression. J Infect Dis 2005; 191: 2053–2063.

39. Paul ME, Mao C, Charurat M, et al. Predictors of immunologic long-term nonprogression in HIV-infected children: implications for initiating therapy. J Allergy Clin Immunol 2005; 115: 848–855.

40. Pastori C, Weiser B, Barassi C, et al. Long-lasting CCR5 internalization by antibodies in a subset of long-term nonprogressors: a possible protective effect against disease progression. Blood 2006; 107: 4825–4833.

41. Baliga CS, Sutton RE. The role of phenotyping and replication capacity in anti-HIV therapeutics. Curr Opin Mol Ther 2004; 6: 308–317.

42. DHHS Panel on Antiretroviral Guidelines for Adults and Adolescents. Guidelines for the use of antiretroviral agents in HIV-1-infected adults and adolescents. Available online at: http://AIDSinfo.nih.gov; accessed May 4, 2006.

43. Working group on antiretroviral therapy and medical management of HIV-infected children. Guideline for the use of antiretroviral agents in pediatric HIV infection. Available online at: http://AIDSinfo.nih,gov; accessed November 3, 2005.

44. Williamson MP, McCormick TG, Nance CL, et al. Epigallocatechin gallate, the main polyphenol in green tea, binds to the T-cell receptor, CD4: potential for HIV-1 therapy. J Allergy Clin Immunol 2006; 118: 1369–1374.

45. Battegay M, Nuesch R, Hirschell B, et al. Immunological recovery and antiretroviral therapy in HIV-1 infection. Lancet Infect Dis 2006; 6: 280–287.

46. Anaworanich J, Gayet-Ageron A, Le Braz M, et al. CD-4 guided scheduled treatment interruptions compared with continuous therapy for patients infected with HIV-1: results of the Staccato randomized trial. Lancet 2006; 368: 459–465.

47. Strategies for Management of Antiretroviral Therapy (SMART) Study Group. El-Sadr WM, Lundgren JD, Neaton JD, et al. CD4+ count-guided interruption of antiretroviral treatment. N Engl J Med 2006; 355: 2283–2296.

48. Shelburne SA, Montes M, Hamill R. Immune reconstitution inflammatory syndrome: more answers, more questions – authors' response. J Antimicrob Chemother 2006; 58: 1094–1095.

49. Stoll M, Schmidt RE. Adverse events of desirable gain in immunocompetence: the immune restoration inflammatory syndromes. Autoimmun Rev 2004; 3: 243–249.

50. Bekker V, Scherpbier H, Pajkrt D, et al. Persistent humoral immune defect in highly active antiretroviral therapy-treated children with HIV-1 infection: loss of specific antibodies against attenuated vaccine strains and natural viral infection. Pediatrics 2006; 118: e315–e322.

51. Kovacs JA, Lempicki RA, Sidorov IA, et al. Induction of prolonged survival of CD4+ T lymphocytes by intermittent IL-2 therapy in HIV-infected patients. J Clin Invest 2005; 115: 2139–2148.

52. Foster SB, Paul ME, Kozinetz CE, et al. Prevalence of asthma in children and young adults. J Allergy Clin Immunol 2007, In press.

53. Lin RY, Lazarus ST. Asthma and related atopic disorders in outpatients attending an urban HIV clinic. Ann Allergy Asthma Immunol 1995; 74: 510–515.

54. Lederman MM, Offord RE, Hartley O. Microbicides and other topical strategies to prevent vaginal transmission of HIV. Nat Rev Immunol 2006; 6: 371–382.

55. Duerr A, Wasserheit JN, Corey L. HIV vaccines: new frontiers in vaccine development. Clin Infect Dis 2006; 43: 500–511.

56. McMichael A. HIV vaccines. Annu Rev Immunol 2006; 24: 227–255.

57. Miller CJ, Abel K. Immune mechanisms associated with protection from vaginal SIV challenge in rhesus monkeys infected with virulence-attenuated SHIV 89.6. J Med Primatol 2005; 34: 271–281.

58. Lu W, Arraes LC, Ferreira WT, et al. Therapeutic dendritic-cell vaccine for chronic HIV-1 infection. Nat Med 2004; 10: 1359–1365.

59. Letvin NL, Mascola JR, Sun Y, et al. Preserved CD4+ central memory Tcells and survival in vaccinated SIV-challenged monkeys. Science 2006; 312: 1530–1533.

60. Cohen J. Promising AIDS vaccine's failure leaves field reeling. Science 2007; 318: 28–29.

Immunodeficiency due to congenital, metabolic, infectious, surgical and environmental factors

38

Javier Chinen, William T. Shearer

The majority of human immunodeficiencies result from factors extrinsic to the immune system, such as malnutrition, immunosuppressive agents, surgery and trauma. In addition, extremes of age (i.e., prematurity and old age), adverse environments (e.g., high altitude, space travel), and genetic conditions may also affect immune function (Table 38.1). Malnutrition, for example, is a significant factor because it affects a large percentage of the population worldwide and renders them susceptible to infection. Early and advanced ages present with increased susceptibility to infections, due in part to physiological changes corresponding to maturation and senescence of the immune response, respectively (Chapters 32 and 33). Some therapeutic agents, including chemotherapeutic drugs, may have immunosuppressive properties (Chapter 90).

In this chapter, selected clinical disorders of genetic (other than primary immune deficiencies), metabolic, and environmental etiology are discussed, conditions that are known to be associated with decreased immune function. These diseases usually cause immune defects that are heterogeneous in presentation, affecting humoral and cellular immunity with variable degrees of severity. Understanding these mechanisms of disease helps in the assessment and management of patients, because correction of the primary disorder, when it is feasible, often leads to prevention or reversal of the related immune defects.

KEY CONCEPTS

>> Immunodeficiencies commonly occur as the result of diseases or conditions extrinsic to the immune system, such as malnutrition.

>> Correction of the primary disorder leads to prevention or reversal of the related immune defects.

>> Environmental conditions, when severe, may induce immunodeficiency by acting as stressors or by suppression of the production and function of immune cells.

IMMUNOLOGICAL DEFECTS ASSOCIATED WITH GENETIC DISEASES OTHER THAN PRIMARY IMMUNODEFICIENCIES

Genetic diseases include a number of rare conditions that range from deleterious mutations in a single gene to deletions or duplications of entire chromosomes. These conditions can be inherited from the patients' parents or they can appear 'de novo' in a particular individual. There are several, albeit very rare, genetic syndromes that can be associated with mild to moderate degrees of immune compromise. The pathogenesis of the immune defects in these syndromes is hypothesized to include deficiency of proteins such as cytokines and adhesion molecules, the loss of continuity of natural epithelial barriers, and subtle defects in cell division and DNA repair. The management of increased susceptibility to infections in patients with genetic diseases relies on prevention, by promoting hygiene measures and using antibiotic prophylaxis when necessary. The most common genetic syndromes with described secondary immunodeficiency are discussed.

DOWN'S SYNDROME

Down's syndrome (DS) or trisomy of chromosome 21 is a relatively common congenital defect with an incidence of 1:600–1:800 live births. DS patients present with hypotonia, characteristic facies, heart and gastrointestinal defects and mental retardation. Infections are common but usually not severe, such as periodontitis and upper respiratory tract infections. Although the risk of frequent infections can be attributed to poor hygiene and institutionalization, immunological abnormalities have been reported, including absolute lymphopenia and a decreased number of naïve T cells,[1] possibly secondary to premature thymus involution. Also, impaired antibody response has been demonstrated, which could be associated to IgG subclass deficiency. Phagocytic cells from DS patients show decreased chemotaxis, phagocytosis and bacterial killing. Autoimmune disease occurs at a higher frequency in DS, with its most

IMMUNOLOGIC DEFICIENCIES

Table 38.1 Common conditions associated with secondary immunodeficiencies

	Cellular immunity	Humoral immunity
Congenital		
Down's syndrome	T cell cytopenia, decreased LPR to mitogens, thymus hypotrophy, decreased naïve T cells, defective NK-cell activity, decreased phagocytosis and chemotaxis	Decreased antibody response to vaccines, increased autoimmune antibodies
Turner's syndrome	T-cell cytopenia, anergy, poor LPR to mitogens	Decreased serum IgG and IgM levels
Metabolic		
Protein–calorie malnutrition	T-cell cytopenia, thymus hypotrophy, impaired cytokine secretion, decreased chemotaxis and phagocytosis	Poor antibody response to vaccines, elevated serum IgA levels, decreased serum IgG levels
Diabetes mellitus	T-cell cytopenia, decreased LPR to mitogens, decreased chemotaxis and phagocytosis.	Decreased antibody response to vaccines
Nephrotic syndrome	T-cell cytopenia, anergy, poor LPR to mitogens	Decreased serum IgG levels and response to vaccines
Uremia	Increased T-cell apoptosis, lymphopenia decreased LPR to mitogens, decreased chemotaxis and phagocytosis, decreased oxidative response.	Decreased serum IgG levels and response to vaccines
Infectious diseases		
HIV infection	CD4 T-cell cytopenia, decreased LPR to mitogens and antigens, decreased DTH, decreased naïve T cells, thymus hypotrophy. Poor NK cell and phagocytic activity	Poor antibody responses, increased serum IgG levels.
Viral infections – measles	Impaired antigen presentation, cell-mediated killing	Decreased serum IgG levels, decreased antibody responses
Stress		
Trauma	T-cell cytopenia, depressed DTH, decreased chemotaxis.	Decreased complement activity
Splenectomy	Not reported	Poor antibody responses, negligible to polysaccharides
Environmental conditions		
Radiation and UV light	T-cell anergy, poor antigen presentation, severe immunosuppression at high doses	Defective response secondary to impaired cellular immunity
High altitude	T- and NK cell cytopenia	Decreased serum IgG level
Space flight	Lymphopenia, decreased LPR to mitogens, decreased NK cell activity and cytokine secretion (IL-10, IL-1a).	Norrmal in a space flight model

LPR, lymphoproliferative response; DTH delayed-type hypersensitivity.

frequent manifestation, thyroiditis, developing before 8 years of age in about half of children with DS.[2] Recently, it has been reported that mononuclear cells from DS patients have increased expression of DSCAM (Down's syndrome cellular adhesion molecule) and SOD1 (superoxide dismutase 1), two proteins encoded in genes located in chromosome 21, which could explain impaired pathogen clearance.[3] Decreased institutionalization and better access to medical care have reduced the risk of infection and improved the life expectancy of DS patients.

TURNER'S SYNDROME

Turner's syndrome (TS) results from the presence of only one X chromosome, the other being missing or abnormally repressed. TS patients have short stature, do not develop into puberty, and are infertile. They present with frequent respiratory infections and develop bronchiectasis at an early age. However, there are no consistent immune defects in all TS patients. Low immunoglobulin levels[4] and decreased T-cell proliferative responses to mitogens[5] have been shown in some patients.

CLINICAL PEARLS

>> Sickle cell disease (SCD) patients have increased susceptibility to infections with encapsulated organisms, such as *S. pneumoniae*.

>> Autosplenectomy occurs in most SCD patients by 2 years of age, and is associated with poor antibody response to polysaccharide and inefficient complement activity.

>> Prevention of infections in SCD patients includes completion of routine immunizations and anti-pneumococcal antibiotic prophylaxis.

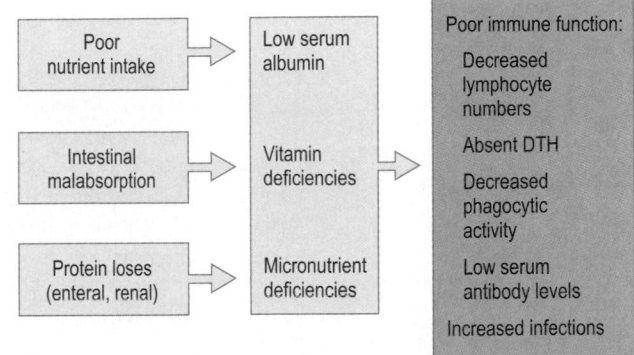

Fig. 38.1 Malnutrition results from poor access to food, decreased absorption of nutrients or loss due to inflammatory enteropathies or renal disease. Protein deficiency causes decreased production of immune cells and immunoglobulins, which increases susceptibility to infection.

SICKLE CELL DISEASE

Two genetic diseases with a significant prevalence in the general population and with increased susceptibility to infections are sickle cell disease (SCD) and cystic fibrosis (CF). SCD is an autosomal recessive disease that affects the expression of the β-hemoglobin protein and causes anemia. Its prevalence is highest in African Americans at 1:500. SCD patients have an increased susceptibility for infections from encapsulated organisms: for example, *Streptococcus pneumoniae*-related sepsis and meningitis occur 30–300 times more often than in normal children. As a result of microinfarcts, autosplenectomy occurs in most SCD patients by the second year of life, and is the major reason for the increased risk of infections, owing to the association between absence of the spleen and impaired antibody production to polysaccharides and a defective complement alternative pathway.[6] SCD patients also present with an increased frequency of osteomyelitis caused by *Salmonella* sp., although it is not well understood why susceptibility to this pathogen is increased. Prevention of infections in SCD patients should include anti-pneumococcal prophylaxis and routine immunizations to encapsulated organisms. These measures reduce the incidence of pneumococcal infections by at least 84%.[6]

CYSTIC FIBROSIS

CF is an autosomal recessive disorder caused by mutations in the cystic fibrosis transmembrane conductance regulator (CFTR) gene. It decreases the fluidity of secretions, causing blockade of secretory tubes and affecting organs such as the pancreas, salivary glands, gonads, and liver. Most significantly, the mucociliary clearance of bacteria in the lungs is impaired. CF patients often present with lungs colonized with *Pseudomonas aeruginosa*, or with pneumonia due to this pathogen and other bacteria. Several lung bactericidal factors are decreased, such as lisozymes, defensins and cathelicidins.[8] This results in poor ability to clear bacterial colonization, and eventual progression to pneumonia. The adaptive immunity is intact, demonstrated by the normal production of antibodies against *P. aeruginosa*.[7] CF patients experiencing recurrent pneumonias benefit from respiratory therapy to clear secretions and the use of antibiotic prophylaxis.

■ IMMUNOLOGICAL DEFECTS SECONDARY TO METABOLIC DISEASES: MALNUTRITION, DIABETES MELLITUS AND UREMIA ■

Severe malnutrition resulting in depletion of protein, calories and micronutrients is associated with increased morbidity and mortality from infections. Other conditions affecting the adequate absorption and metabolism of nutrients, such as diabetes mellitus and protein-losing enteropathy, impair the functioning of all organs, including the immune system.

MALNUTRITION

Malnutrition is one of the most frequent causes of secondary immunodeficiency, affecting individuals of all ages (Fig. 38.1). Protein–calorie malnutrition may result from poor intake, malabsorption or excessive loss of nutrients. Individuals with protein–calorie malnutrition progressively lose T-cell production[8] and function,[9] resulting in immunodeficiency with an increased incidence of diarrhea and respiratory infections. These conditions are complicated by a concomitant deficit of micronutrients (e.g., zinc) that augment the susceptibility of infections by inducing defects in the barrier mucosae.[10] Serum immunoglobulin levels appear to remain normal for a relative prolonged period, as does the effectiveness of vaccination to elicit antibodies.[10, 11] Nutritional replenishment in malnourished children results in reversal of deficiencies of lymphocyte proliferation and phagocytosis, and significant recovery of thymus size by ultrasonography.[12]

Micronutrient deficiencies are more prevalent in protein–calorie malnutrition but may also present alone, usually subclinically in a healthy-looking child. Feeding only half the recommended intake of iron, zinc, or vitamins B, C and E leads to oxidative damage and DNA breaks, with decreased NK-cell cytotoxicity and monocyte phagocytic activity[13, 14] (Table 38.2).

IMMUNOLOGIC DEFICIENCIES

Table 38.2 Immune defects in micronutrient deficiencies

	Cellular immunity	Humoral immunity
Vitamin A deficiency	T cell cytopenia, decreased DTH, decreased phagocytic and NK-cell function	Lower antibody response to immunization
Vitamin E deficiency	Decreased oxidative activity of phagocytes, increased PGE_2 secretion (inhibitory)	Increased IgE
Vitamin C deficiency	Decreased phagocytic activity and oxidative response to ingested organisms	Not reported
Zinc deficiency	Lymphopenia, thymus hypotrophy, decreased DTH	Decreased T cell-dependent antibody responses
Iron deficiency	T-cell cytopenia, thymus hypotrophy, decreased phagocytosis	Decreased serum IgG levels
Copper deficiency	Lymphopenia and neutropenia	Not reported
Selenium deficiency	Decreased oxidative response in phagocytes and NK cells	Not reported

DTH, delayed-type hypersensitivity; PGE_2, prostaglandin E_2.

Vitamin A deficiency is manifested by night blindness, dry and scaly skin, apathy, anemia, retarded growth, elevated intracranial pressure and increased infections. Vitamin A deficiency leads to impaired mucous membranes[15] and decreased interferon (IFN)-α production. Higher immunization rates are seen when vitamin A is given with measles vaccine in malnourished children.[16]

In contrast to protein–calorie deficiency due to other causes, malnutrition resulting from eating disorders, such as anorexia nervosa and bulimia, does not result in an increased frequency of infections.[17, 18] However, patients with these disorders show leukopenia and lymphopenia with abnormal delayed-type hypersensitivity responses. Paradoxically, infections may occur during nutritional treatment, possibly because of reactivation of latent infections.

Protein-losing enteropathy can be present in most patients with intestinal inflammatory diseases, and results in hypogammaglobulinemia; however, the ability to produce antibodies is usually preserved. Thus, the need for intravenous immunoglobulin needs to be carefully assessed, because correction of the primary defect can reduce the susceptibility to infection without requiring any other intervention. A similar disorder, intestinal lymphangiectasis, is characterized by congenital intestinal lymphatic obstruction and loss of lymph, with hypogammaglobulinemia and moderate to severe lymphopenia. A diet enriched with medium-chain triglycerides reverses the symptoms and pathological findings.[19]

DIABETES MELLITUS

Diabetes mellitus (DM) is characterized by insufficient production of insulin by the pancreas, which results in poor glucose cell metabolism. DM can result from autoimmune damage (type I, insulin dependent) or a decrease in the cell response to insulin (type II, noninsulin-dependent). Both types present with increased susceptibility to infections due to immune defects, poor glucose metabolism, poor blood supply and local denervation. Altered immune defects that have been reported include

lymphopenia, cutaneous anergy, and impaired *in vitro* lymphocyte proliferation.[20] The humoral response usually remains intact, with normal antibody responses to routine immunizations. Diabetics can exhibit abnormal phagocytic adherence, chemotaxis, phagocytosis and bactericidal activity.[21] Maintenance of blood glucose levels in the normal range results in an improvement in phagocyte function and a lower risk of infections.[22]

UREMIA

Treatment of uremia often requires either hemodialysis (HD) or peritoneal dialysis. Unfortunately, both uremia and dialysis can induce negative effects on the immune system, and can predispose patients to serious infections. Uremics have a 6–16-fold higher incidence of tuberculosis than nonuremic matched controls.[23] Sepsis secondary to vascular device or respiratory infections are common in dialysis patients. The dysregulation of their immune system is characterized by immunodeficiency with a state of cellular activation, leading to a chronic inflammatory state and increased oxidative stress.[23] Several toxins targeting phagocytes have been identified in the plasma and peritoneal fluid of uremic patients, including angiogenin, p-cresol, a form of ubiquitin, degranulatory inhibitory protein, and a protein with homology to immunoglobulin light chains. Phagocytic cell dysfunction is the most common and consistent immune defect found in uremic patients. Diminished chemotaxis, phagocytosis, intracellular killing and oxygen radical production have been documented.[24] The molecular mechanisms of these processes are not clear. It has been suggested that the increased intracellular calcium seen in end-stage renal disease could impair phagocytosis. Iron overload in HD patients is associated with decreased phagocytic bacterial killing and an increased risk of infection.[25] Improvement of such immune defects is seen after iron chelation. Decreased lymphocyte counts, depressed lymphoproliferative response to mitogens and antigens, and cutaneous anergy can also be seen in uremic patients. Impaired antigen presentation by monocytes may underlie the abnormal immune responses. Most uremic patients show an adequate response to vaccines; however, antibody titers decline rapidly within 6 months, regardless of vaccination.[23]

IMMUNOLOGICAL DEFECTS SECONDARY TO INFECTIOUS DISEASES

During the encounter between a microbial pathogen and its host a variety of complex biological processes occur, in which microbes attempt to proliferate and the host fights to eliminate them. Pathogens may interfere with a variety of immunological defenses in order to decrease their clearance and establish an infection.[26] In some cases, this action also favors infection by other pathogens. For example, during influenza infection the inflammatory response in the lung paradoxically increases the patient's susceptibility to bacterial pneumonia.[27] One infectious agent in particular, human immunodeficiency virus (HIV), targets the immune system itself by infecting CD4 T lymphocytes and causing severe immunodeficiency (Chapter 37). However, most immunological disturbances caused by microbial infections are transient and usually reflect a normal immune response rather than a weakening of the immune defenses. In some cases of chronic infection, such as tuberculosis and parasites, immune suppression may be secondary to the state of wasting induced by these diseases. The following examples describe selected individual pathogens that characteristically induce immune suppression.

VIRAL PATHOGENS

Measles virus. In the early 1900's, it was noted that the tuberculin skin response was blunted during acute measles infection. Measles infects lymphoid tissues through the CD46 molecule, a complement receptor present in monocytes and lymphocytes, affecting antigen presentation, cell-mediated killing and immunoglobin synthesis.[28] The period of immunosuppression lasts only a few weeks until the virus is cleared, but may linger in some hosts. In rare cases, persistent measles infection develops and causes subacute sclerosing panencephalitis, a progressive degeneration of the central nervous system, mediated by an inflammatory reaction triggered by persistent measles antigen, despite the presence of high levels of anti-measles antibodies.

Epstein–Barr virus (EBV)

EBV infection is present in almost 90% of the world's adult population and usually occurs subclinically. It may occasionally manifest as a self-limiting lymphoproliferative disease known as acute infectious mononucleosis. EBV targets B cells using the CD21 surface antigen and transforms them to establish a chronic infection. EBV-infected B cells fail to undergo apoptosis. Activated (also called 'atypical', because of their morphology) T cells eliminate EBV-infected B cells, developing a massive expansion of a selected oligoclonal population with limited TCR Vβ gene usage. As a result, there is a relative T-cell anergy, which can be demonstrated in *in vitro* experiments. There is also a concurrent polyclonal expansion of B cells with enhanced immunoglobulin production.[29] These changes last for only a few weeks.

The X-linked recessive lymphoproliferative syndrome (XLP) develops in individuals with mutations in the *SHD1A* gene, resulting in affected males being unable to control EBV-infected cell proliferation. Impaired immune response, splenomegaly and lymphoproliferative disease are usually fatal to the patient.[30]

Cytomegalovirus (CMV)

Infection with CMV also leads to a mononucleosis illness. CMV-infected monocytes have a decreased ability to present antigens because of reduced MHC protein expression and function, and the presence of viral molecules that resemble MHC proteins. In addition, CMV encodes a human IL-10 homolog which has been demonstrated to inhibit the activation of human lymphocytes.[31]

Influenza virus

Acute infection with influenza virus causes lymphopenia, primarily within the T-cell population. Other immunological alterations are reduced lymphocyte proliferation, increased NK-cell activity and increased generation of regulatory T cells, as well as impairment of mucus clearance that enhances bacterial adherence and increases susceptibility to secondary bacterial infections.[27, 32] Bacterial pneumonias are the most common cause of mortality during influenza epidemics.

BACTERIAL PATHOGENS

Severe bacterial infections have been associated with alterations to innate immunity, such as decreased leukocyte chemotaxis and reduced reticuloendothelial function. However, these are not seen consistently and vary with the degree of bacterial invasiveness, the production of bacterial toxic products, and the host's capacity to contain the dissemination of infection. For example, *Streptococcus* sp. and *Staphylococcus* sp. produce a family of toxins called superantigens, which bind simultaneously to the T-cell receptor β chain and to class II MHC molecules, producing nonspecific activation of T cells, massive cytokine release, and eventual cell death (Fig. 38.2). Superantigens also induce T-cell anergy. Several systemic illnesses result from the superantigens' effect, including toxic shock syndrome and scarlet fever. Over 41 bacterial superantigens have been described.[33] Early antibiotic therapy can reduce the incidence of immunological disturbances due to bacterial infections.

IMMUNOLOGICAL DEFECTS INDUCED BY SURGERY OR TRAUMA

Stress induced by surgery or trauma results in a metabolic and inflammatory response to control the injury and repair the damage. Local inflammation is necessary for wound healing and defense against microbial pathogens. The reaction to injury also initiates a systemic response, with the release of several inflammatory cytokines that can affect the ability of the host to respond to immunological challenges and also predispose the patient to infection.[34] These responses can lead to adult respiratory syndrome (ARDS) if affecting the lungs, and to multiorgan failure, or systemic inflammatory response syndrome (SIRS). The term 'sepsis' is

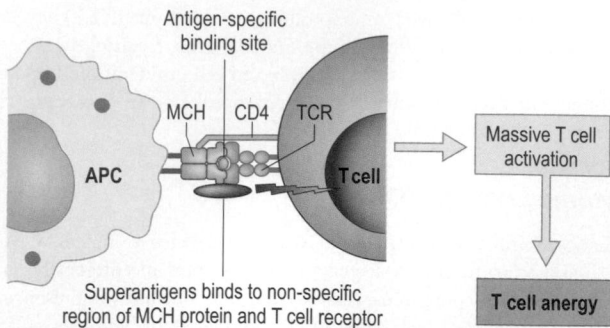

Fig. 38.2 Superantigens are microbial proteins that bind nonspecific regions of MHC molecules expressed by antigen-presenting cells, and to one of over 20 subfamilies of the Vβ chain in the T-cell receptor. This results in activation of a large number of T cells, with release of cytokines and subsequent anergy.

KEY CONCEPTS

>> Extreme environmental conditions, such as high altitude, may affect immune function.

>> Ultraviolet light induces immune tolerance and reduces inflammation.

>> Ionizing radiation impairs cell-mediated immunity by affecting the replication of lymphocytes.

>> Long space flights may induce immune defects because of microgravity and space radiation, in addition to psychological stressors such as sleep cycle alterations, confinement and isolation.

CLINICAL PEARLS

>> Surgery and severe trauma cause increased susceptibility to infections.

>> In addition to mechanical lost of mucosal barriers, the inflammatory reaction after injury is followed by up to 10 days of anergy.

>> Removal of dead tissue, foreign bodies and prompt restoration of enteral feeding reduce the time of increased susceptibility to infections.

reserved for SIRS of infectious etiology. The series of events leading to the inflammatory response to trauma, whether accidental or surgical, can be summarized into five steps: loss of epithelial barriers, vasodilation and increased vascular permeability, cellular activation and adhesion, and the neuroendocrine response. (Fig. 38.3)

Mechanical or chemical injury during trauma causes epithelial damage and allows access by vast quantities of microbial pathogens to the host. In addition, postoperative changes such as decreased motility of epithelial cilia can also affect the mucosal barrier. The release of inflammatory mediators in response to tissue damage and microbial products induces the next steps of vasodilation, increased permeability and cell activation. Chemotaxis of polymorphonuclear cells is decreased following acute depletion of complement proteins and the production of other acute plasma proteins. T-cell counts decrease between the second and fourth days after injury and correlate with injury severity, although they may not correlate with clinical outcome. Delayed-type hypersensitivity responses are depressed following major injury, with up to 90% of severely injured patients being anergic, as measured both by skin testing and by *in vitro* lymphocyte proliferation to mitogens and antigens. B-cell activation and antibody production are also impaired after trauma or major burns.

Stress, due to trauma or other causes, stimulates the neuroendocrine axis to produce hormones such as vasopressin, aldosterone, catecholamines and cortisol. Elevated levels of cortisol increase the release of neutrophils to peripheral blood and produce lymphopenia. In addition, the regulated secretion of prostaglandins, thromboxanes and leukotrienes is disturbed

and may contribute to an inefficient inflammatory response in the injured patient. Prostaglandin E$_2$ inhibits lymphocyte proliferation, decreases IL-2 release and inhibits NK cells up to 7–10 days after major injury.

Control of tissue damage, pain relief, nutritional support and avoidance of ischemia decrease the release of inflammatory mediators and hence reduce the immune abnormalities induced by surgical injury. Neutrophils from a well-perfused wound have better phagocytic and bactericidal activity than neutrophils from an ischemic wound.

The management of an injured patient should include prompt removal of all dead tissue to reduce the release of tissue degradation products and nonspecific immune activation. Although required in some cases immediately after severe injury, parenteral feeding leads to mucosal atrophy and an increased risk of sepsis, and should be replaced or supplemented by enteral feeding when possible.

Splenectomy

Surgical removal of the spleen is indicated following trauma or in cytopenias induced by certain medical conditions involving the excessive removal of red blood cells or platelets by the reticuloendothelial system. However, the risks and benefits of splenectomy should be carefully assessed, because it can result in barely detectable immunological changes that, nevertheless, significantly increase the risk of bacterial sepsis. Splenectomized patients are particularly susceptible to infections with encapsulated organisms such as *S. pneumonia* and *H. influenzae*. The mortality for sepsis in splenectomized patients is between 50% and 70%, emphasizing the need to avoid splenectomy when possible. Patients who are scheduled for splenectomy are recommended to receive anti-penumococcal, anti-*H. influenzae* and anti-meningococcal immunizations at least 2 weeks prior to surgery. Revaccination after splenectomy is not efficacious. In addition, splenectomized patients should receive lifelong anti-pneumococcal antibiotic prophylaxis.

■ ENVIRONMENTAL CONDITIONS CAUSING IMMUNODEFICIENCY ■

ULTRAVIOLET (UV) LIGHT

UV light is a form of radiant energy transmitted as electromagnetic waves, with wavelengths ranging from 230 to 450 nm. It is classified as UVA if the wavelength is between 320 and 450 nm, as UVB if it is between 280 and 320 nm, and UVC if it is less than 280 nm. The most

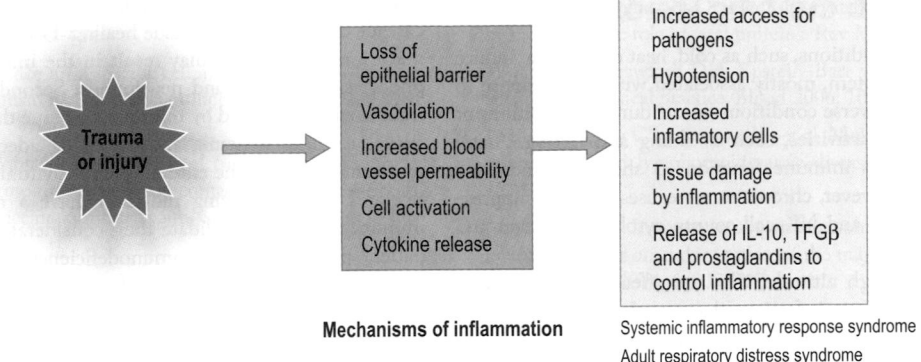

Mechanisms of inflammation

Systemic inflammatory response syndrome
Adult respiratory distress syndrome

Fig. 38.3 After trauma or injury, inflammation develops to promote healing. However, massive inflammation may result in tissue damage (e.g. systemic inflammatory response syndrome – SIRS – or adult respiratory distress syndrome, ARDS). Immune regulatory mechanisms in response to inflammation may in turn induce a transient immunosuppressive state, mediated by IL-10, TGF-β and other soluble mediators.

common source of UV light affecting humans is the sun, being most intense where the atmospheric ozone layer is thinner, such as places close to the North Pole. Immunosuppression by UV light was first suspected because the incidence of malignant skin disorders increases with increased exposure to sunlight. The effects of UVB are known to be mutagenic, by creating cross-links between thymidines in DNA. The mechanisms of UV light influence on the immune system are different, as they occur even with low doses of UVB, perhaps serving to prevent an inflammatory reaction that could damage sun-exposed skin.[35] UV light induces the activation of NF-κB, a second-signal molecule involved in T-cell activation and apoptosis (Fig. 38.4). It also affects the activation of antigen-presenting cells, the release of cytokines, and the expression of surface markers. This UV light effect may be regulated by soluble mediators released from epidermal cells, including melanocyte-stimulating hormone, which induces hapten-specific tolerance in addition to its major role of activating melanocytes to protect the skin from sunlight. This modulation of the immune system by UV light has been used to treat autoimmune skin disorders: UVB light and psoralen plus UVA light are the treatments of choice for severe psoriasis.[36] The most effective wavelength of UVB is approximately 313 nm. UVA light treatment may be combined with coal tar or an occlusive ointment for increased efficacy, and remission occurs in 80% of patients.

IONIZING RADIATION

The immunosuppressive effect of ionizing radiation has been clinically evidenced by the increased susceptibility to infections and tumors in survivors of exposure to nuclear power plant accidents and atomic bomb explosions. It has also been demonstrated when used therapeutically against neoplastic diseases in humans, and experimentally in animal models. Irradiation significantly impairs cell-mediated and humoral immunity, depending on the radiation dose, the frequency of administration, rate, and temporal relationship to antigen administration. The production of lymphocytes and neutrophils, as well as other blood cell lineages, is affected according to the radiation dose causing apoptosis of hematopoietic cells in the bone marrow. All immunological components, including total, CD4 and CD8 T cells, serum immunoglobulin levels and the proliferative response to mitogens, decrease after radiotherapy. Specific

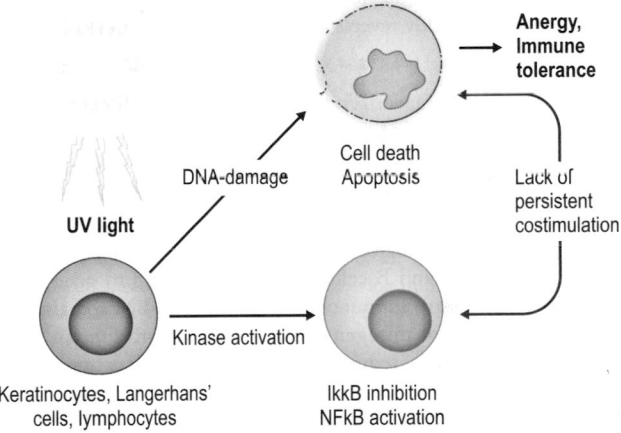

Fig. 38.4 UV light causes immunosuppression by two mechanisms: it induces apoptosis of skin lymphocytes and other immune cells by directly altering their DNA; it also activates kinases that lead to the activation of NF-κB and ultimately to cell apoptosis when other immune activation signals are missing.

immune responses are compromised primarily because of the lymphopenia. The number of macrophages can also be decreased. Phagocytosis is relatively radioresistant, whereas antigen processing by macrophages is easily impaired by low-dose radiation. Experience with the effects of ionizing radiation on the immune system demonstrates different outcomes according to applications and protocols of administration. For example, when radiation is used at therapeutic doses for myeloablation in bone marrow transplants, neutrophil counts typically recover 1 month after exposure, and lymphocyte counts recover within 3 months. Children with cancer who are treated with craniospinal irradiation have lymphopenia and impaired *in vitro* lymphoproliferative responses to mitogens for more than a year after treatment. When radiation is given in dose fractions, lymphocyte counts are reduced even more: in one experiment, when 2400 Gy were given in five fractions to children with leukemia, mean lymphocyte counts were 1840 cells/μL; when given in 12 fractions were 1120 cells/μL; and in 20 fractions were 640 cells/μL.[37]

part 5

ALLERGIC DISEASES

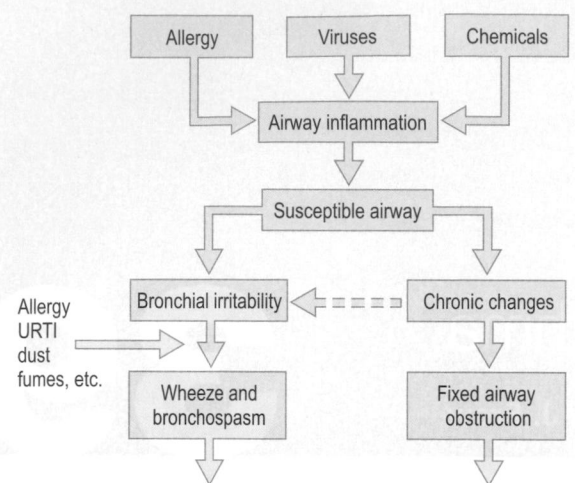

Fig. 39.1 The role of allergy and other factors in causing airways inflammation, bronchial irritability, wheeze, and fixed airways obstruction. URTI, upper respiratory tract infection.

KEY CONCEPTS

POSSIBLE ENVIRONMENTAL FACTORS RESPONSIBLE FOR THE RISE IN ASTHMA

>> Allergic sensitization

>> Factors promoting allergen exposure (especially to house dust mite)

>> Housing design
>> Increased humidity
>> Carpets/rugs
>> Bedding

>> Air pollution
>> Motor vehicles
>> Ozone
>> Particulate matter (especially diesel exhaust)

>> Diet
>> New foods
>> Food processing

>> Infections
>> Respiratory viruses
>> Environmental bacteria
>> Gut microflora

and in careful studies of birth cohorts it seems that the tendency to have eczema, rhinitis, and allergic sensitization (the so-called atopic phenotype) is inherited differently from the tendency for asthma. But in those who are atopic, asthma will show up in childhood if they also possess the genetic predisposition to asthma, whereas in those who are nonatopic, asthma is unlikely to appear in childhood, but may surface as a problem in adulthood.

Survey evidence from across the developed world has shown a clear increase in rates of asthma during the second half of the 20th century. Looking back, it seems that this rise may have started in the USA during the 1930s, while in Europe it started later – probably in the 1950s in the UK, in the 1960s in West Germany, and in the 1990s in the former socialist republics of Eastern Europe. In all cases it seems that the rise in asthma and in allergic sensitization parallels improvements in living conditions, although the precise feature of prosperity that drives these trends is not yet known. Indeed, it may well be different in different countries, due to interactions between diet, genetics, and the environment. In searching for an explanation of these secular trends, it is clear that it cannot be a simple genetic change: the timescale is too short for there to have been a sudden change in the gene pool. Equally, the risk of asthma and allergy is not evenly distributed through the population since some families are at much greater risk than others. It therefore seems likely that the change is due to one or more environmental changes operating on a genetically predisposed subset of the population.

Possible environmental factors include allergies, housing, air pollution, diet, and various aspects of infection. We sometimes forget how much our housing and daily lives have changed in the past 50 years. For example, houses are now much better heated and insulated – in the UK in the 1950s, central heating was unusual, and wall-to-wall carpeting unheard of. Partly as a result we now wear different clothes and wash them much more frequently. We also take more baths and showers, resulting in considerably more humidity inside our houses, and we have radically changed our bedding, with duvets replacing traditional blankets and quilts. Many of these changes have made our homes much

more favorable for house dust mites, and there is circumstantial evidence that exposure to house dust mite allergens is now much higher than it was in the past.

Diets have changed too – we now have year-round access to fruits and vegetables that used to be seasonal; food is picked unripe, processed, and transported halfway round the world, and all this requires new technology to make sure the fruit is ready to eat when it reaches our shelves. Artificial ripening of fruits changes their chemical composition and may alter their allergenicity. We also expect our food to be beautiful and clean, so we reject anything that is flawed or dirty. All these factors have altered what we eat and our exposure to environmental bacteria. This shows up in changes in the gut bacterial flora, which is known to be a major influence on the development of the immune system. Analysis of gut bacteria over the past 40 years in developed countries indicates that we now have a much narrower range of gut bacteria compared to 40 years ago, and that the development of allergy in childhood is associated with having a more restricted gut flora.[3]

It is clear that more people are sensitized to common airborne allergens than was the case 40 years ago. However, while allergic sensitization is a risk factor for asthma, data from Australia suggest that rates of asthma doubled during the 1980s, without any concurrent change in the rate of allergic sensitization to common allergens such as house dust mite or grass pollen.[4] This indicates that what changed in the 1980s may not have been allergy itself, but the likelihood that allergy would be translated into disease.

KEY CONCEPTS

HOW MAY POLLUTANTS AFFECT ALLERGY AND ASTHMA?

>> Promotion of immunoglobulin E (IgE) synthesis
>> Oxidative stress
>>> Direct – from redox-active metal ions on particulate matter
>>> Indirect – through recruitment and activation of inflammatory cells
>> Particulate matter acting as a vector for allergenic molecules
>> Promotion of allergic inflammation
>> Enhancement of effector cell function
>>> Releasability of basophil mediators
>> Damage to structural elements of airway
>>> Ciliary function
>>> Epithelial integrity
>>> Smooth muscle

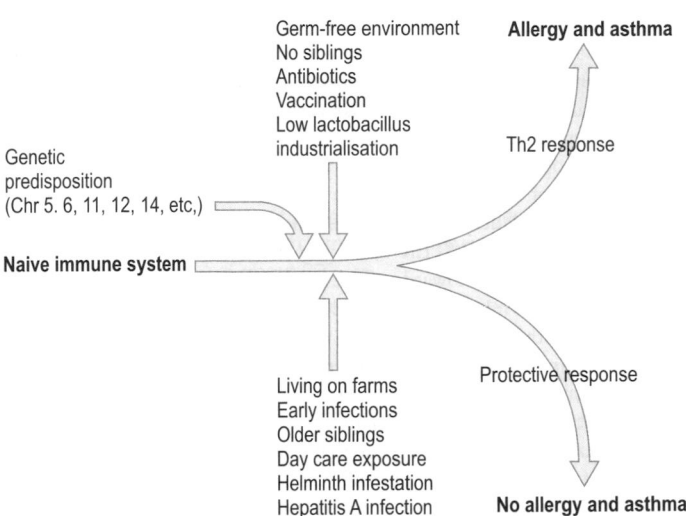

Fig. 39.2 Factors implicated in the hygiene hypothesis.

AIR POLLUTION AND ASTHMA

Air pollution has been blamed for many modern ills. It is unlikely that air pollution is good for us, but more difficult to say how bad it is. In general, air quality today is much better than in the 1950s. This reflects clean-air legislation designed to reduce the emissions from coal-burning power stations and factories. Indeed, levels of black smoke and sulfur dioxide have fallen progressively over the past 50 years, so they can hardly be blamed for the rise in allergy and asthma. The only pollutants that have increased in recent years are ozone, nitrogen oxides, and particulates, all of which are largely related to the meteoric rise in vehicular traffic during the late 20th century.

Pollutants could influence asthma in several different ways. Firstly, the organic chemicals associated with diesel exhaust particles have been shown in humans and in animal studies to enhance IgE production to newly encountered allergens.[5] Second, particulate matter (PM) can carry allergenic molecules down into the airways where they may be taken up by antigen-presenting cells and, by being presented together to immunocompetent cells, the consequent immune response may be deviated towards an allergic pattern. Moreover, in sensitized individuals, this vector function of PM allows allergen to reach sites that might otherwise have been inaccessible and trigger allergic reactions. Third, both ozone and particulate pollutants impose an oxidant stress on the airways, adding to the oxidant stress that is already present in asthma due to ongoing airways inflammation. This happens both as a direct result of oxidation by ozone and PM, and as an indirect result, through the recruitment of neutrophils to the airway. The organic chemicals on diesel exhaust particles increase the releasability of histamine and interleukin-4 (IL-4) from basophils,[6] and have adverse effects on the structural elements of the airway, including mucus release and ciliary function.[7] While some of these effects can only be shown in animal models after high-dose exposure, there is good epidemiological evidence

that small increases in ambient ozone concentrations or PM levels are associated with decrements in lung function and increased rates of admission to hospital with asthma.[8, 9]

INFECTIONS AND ASTHMA

Population surveys have shown that first-born children are more likely to develop rhinitis and asthma than those with older siblings. Interestingly, this excess risk does not apply to first-born or only children who go to day care at an early age. The general consensus is that increased exposure to respiratory viral infections is protective against the development of allergy and asthma. It is noteworthy that early use of day care does not protect against eczema. This suggests at the very least that asthma and eczema have distinct risk profiles; however they may be linked in the atopic march.

Once asthma is established, viral infections are a common trigger of symptoms.[10] This is partly because minor changes in airflow caliber may become manifest as asthmatic symptoms, and partly because viral infections appear to exacerbate the pattern of airways inflammation associated with asthma. Other forms of infection appear to protect against asthma. This concept has been entitled the "hygiene hypothesis" to explain the rise in asthma. Several strands of evidence indicate that early exposure to infection may lead to deviation of the immune response to allergens that are encountered subsequently or concurrently (Fig. 39.2). So, for example, surveys of Italian army recruits show that exposure to hepatitis A in childhood is associated with a reduced risk of asthma at age 18. This reduction in risk is not thought to be a direct effect of hepatitis A, but rather to reflect exposure to contaminated water supplies, a common problem in southern Italy. Recruits with serological evidence of other infections, not transmitted by the feco-oral route, show no protection against asthma.[11]

Other evidence of the protective effect of infections comes from studies of children raised in farming communities in the Bavarian and Swiss Alps. In these traditional communities, people live in close proximity to cows, and often take their infants to the cow barn when they are milking the cows. Children who are taken into the cow barn or who drink

asthmatic reaction in humans.[20] This suggests that tryptase may cleave and release proinflammatory chemokines from the intercellular matrix.

For many years the eosinophil has been considered a hallmark of asthma. It is certainly true that many asthmatics have eosinophils in their airways, and sometimes they may be increased in blood as well, although at any given time the vast majority of eosinophils are located in tissue rather than circulating. Eosinophils are recruited to the airways during asthma exacerbations and following allergen inhalation, when their numbers peak around the time of the LAR. Conversely, they are reduced by treatment with inhaled or systemic steroids.

In intrinsic asthma there are even more eosinophils in the airways than in allergic asthma, but their numbers are more difficult to reduce with steroid therapy. Relevant eosinophil products include the basic granule proteins (major basic protein, eosinophil cationic protein, eosinophil-derived neurotoxin, and eosinophil protein X), which can damage airways epithelium at concentrations achieved in sputum from asthmatic patients. Cysteinyl leukotrienes are also produced in large amounts by eosinophils and this seems the most likely mechanism by which they cause late-phase bronchospasm.

However there are some cautionary notes regarding the role of eosinophils in asthma. Firstly, there is no correlation between sputum eosinophilia and bronchial hyperresponsiveness (BHR). BHR is a key feature of asthma and if the eosinophil were truly critical to the pathogenesis of asthma, one might expect some degree of linkage between the degree of BHR and the number of eosinophils in sputum. Secondly, in recent studies with monoclonal anti-IL-5 antibodies it proved possible to eliminate eosinophils from the blood and sputum without materially affecting the ability of allergen to induce NSBR.[21] Moreover, treatment with anti-IL-5 monoclonal antibody seems to have no detectable effect on clinical asthma.

Alternative approaches to suppressing eosinophils include the use of chemokine antagonists, since eosinophils selectively express the CCR3 receptor, which recognizes the eotaxin family of chemokines. Eotaxin is present in increased amounts in asthma and may contribute to the increased numbers of eosinophils found in asthmatic airways. Early clinical trials with CCR3 antagonists have not yet demonstrated a clear role for CCR3 in asthma. This may be because the antagonists are inefficient, because there is biological redundancy, or of course because the eosinophil is not really important.

Interest in the neutrophil as a possible player in asthma has been rekindled lately, following the recognition of airways neutrophilia in some patients whose asthma is "difficult to control." In the absence of any specific antagonists for neutrophils and their products, it has been difficult to assess their true contribution to the clinical condition. However, asthma is definitely associated with a local oxidative stress to the airway, and neutrophils contribute to this, through their oxidative burst – the principal means by which they kill bacteria. Reactive oxygen species (ROS) cause lipid peroxidation that can be detected in BAL and serves as a direct measure of oxidative stress.[22] Low levels of ROS signal via the transcription factor Nrf2 to induce enzymes that upregulate antioxidant defenses – principally through the synthesis of glutathione. Polymorphisms in these enzymes are associated with marked variation in the risk of asthma, suggesting that failure to detoxify ROS is a permissive factor for asthma.[23] If the antioxidant defenses are overwhelmed, MAP kinase and NF-κB pathways are activated, leading to synthesis of a wide range of

KEY CONCEPTS

POSSIBLE CAUSES OF OXIDATIVE STRESS IN ASTHMA

>> Inflammation

>> Ozone

>> Particulate matter

>> Smoke (including tobacco)

>> Pollutant gases (SO_2, NO_2 etc.)

>> Chemicals (including isocyanates)

proinflammatory cytokines and chemokines, including many that have been implicated in asthma and airways inflammation. Extreme levels of oxidant stress will lead to cellular apoptosis. Although it is unclear whether this is important in clinical asthma, it is easier to induce apoptosis via oxidant stress in epithelial cells cultured from asthmatic airways as compared to epithelial cells from nonasthmatic airways.[24]

COMPARISONS WITH ALLERGIC RHINITIS

Some useful insight into the specificity of allergic inflammation in asthma can be obtained by comparing the histology of asthma with that of the lower airways of patients with allergic rhinitis who have normal bronchial reactivity and no clinical features to suggest asthma.[25] In such subjects, submucosal eosinophilic infiltration and increased numbers of epithelial mast cells are seen, at a level intermediate between that found in asthmatic subjects and healthy controls. Expression of mRNA for tumor necrosis factor-α (TNF-α) is also found in the biopsies from both asthmatic and rhinitic subjects. Eosinophil activation occurs in both groups. Taken together this adds to the doubts raised above concerning the role of eosinophils in causing asthma.

Although mast cell numbers are increased in both asthma and rhinitis, there is evidence that mast cells in asthmatics show more signs of degranulation than those in atopic controls, suggesting that it is a difference in mast cell activation status rather than in mast cell numbers that may lead to BHR.[26] IL-1β and TNF-α are both proinflammatory cytokines that can contribute to initiation and perpetuation of the inflammatory response with endothelial activation, increased adhesion molecule expression, and subsequent inflammatory cell recruitment. mRNA levels of both these cytokines were increased in both the rhinitics and asthmatics compared to normal controls, with no difference between these two atopic groups. The increased expression of these cytokines found in asthma may therefore be a feature of atopy rather than asthma. Looking for differences between rhinitis and asthma, there were increased numbers of CD8 T cells and relatively increased expression of mRNA for IFN-γ in the biopsies from the rhinitic group, suggesting that in a subject who is atopic these changes might be protective against asthma.

KEY CONCEPTS

FEATURES OF AIRWAYS REMODELING

>> Epithelial damage

>> Subbasement membrane collagen deposition

>> Mucous gland hyperplasia

>> Airways smooth muscle

>> >> Hypertrophy

>> >> Increased contractility

>> >> Decreased relaxation

>> Altered epithelial function

>> Altered intercellular matrix

REMODELING

Inflammation clearly plays an important part in the initiation of asthma, and in exacerbations of the condition, but the long-term consequence of these processes is a permanent change in the structure and function of the airway. In a broad sense, the airway is 'remodeled' so that it behaves differently when the patient is exposed to nonspecific agents such as cold air, exercise, smoke, perfume, and vehicle exhaust. The net result is that asthmatic patients have irritable airways, and that once these are constricted, the airways may remain narrowed for longer than would occur in nonasthmatic people.

There are several histological and physiological features of remodeling which occur to varying degrees in each individual with asthma. Histologically, the most obvious feature is thickening of the basement membrane, which is present in all asthmatics regardless of disease severity. When assessed by electron microscopy, the apparent thickening is due to deposition of collagen beneath the true basement membrane. Immunostaining shows that this is type III collagen, a variant associated with wound repair processes. This is produced by myofibroblasts (fibroblasts that have some ultrastructural features of smooth-muscle cells) that differentiate in the submucosa and migrate into the subbasement membrane zone. These cells are thought to be induced and regulated by growth factors released from the epithelium (see below). In addition, several regulatory cytokines produced by T cells and eosinophils have profibrotic effects. These include TGF-β, IL-10, and IL-17, all of which can be demonstrated in increased amounts in human asthmatic airways, and promote fibrosis, while at the same time downregulating T-cell and B-cell function.[27]

Asthmatic airways constrict more vigorously than normal nonasthmatic airways. There is an increased amount of muscle (hypertrophy) but the muscle is also altered in function. Muscle from asthmatic airways shortens more than normal muscle and generates more force *in vitro*. Moreover, once contracted, it is more difficult to relax than normal airways smooth muscle.[28] Pretreatment of smooth muscle with the proallergic cytokine IL-13 decreases its responsiveness to the β_2-agonist isoproterenol, demonstrating that proallergic cytokines may have pleiotropic actions, contributing both to the induction of IgE and to the remodeling process.[29]

The airways epithelium is thought to play a major role in airways remodeling. In the past, the airways epithelium was often considered as an innocent victim of the asthmatic process, becoming damaged and shed when eosinophils and other inflammatory cells released their toxic products. However, more recently it has been appreciated that growth factors and chemokines released from the epithelium play an active part in remodeling. Several chemokines, including IL-8, are present in the epithelium, where they are bound to the extracellular matrix (Chapter 11). When inflammation occurs, there is release of matrix metalloproteases which liberate and activate these chemokines, which in turn can attract neutrophils and other inflammatory cells to the area of injury. Epidermal growth factors that can induce structural alterations in the airways are also released, including many of the changes associated with airways remodeling.[30]

Recent genetic analysis has revealed a link between asthma severity and a metalloprotease (ADAM33), which is increased in patients with mild and moderately severe asthma compared to healthy controls.[31] Polymorphisms in ADAM33 have also been linked to asthma.[32] Fibronectin and collagen from the extracellular matrix may also participate in remodeling. For example, it is known that airways smooth-muscle cells from asthmatic airways produce more eotaxin than those nonasthmatic subjects. This eotaxin release is enhanced by coculture with fibronectin and type I collagen, suggesting that these extracellular matrix components are responsible for the upregulation of smooth-muscle function.[33]

Several models of airways remodeling have been developed, and there is considerable argument about how relevant these are to real-life asthma. However, both in animals and in humans, it seems that corticosteroids have little effect on the histological or physiological correlates of remodeling. This goes some way to explain why corticosteroids can damp down airways inflammation but do not abolish all symptoms. In contrast, leukotriene antagonists can reverse some features of remodeling, including airways smooth-muscle mass and subepithelial fibrosis, in animal models that are resistant to steroids.[34] Several key aspects of the remodeling process remain unclear: current research lines are attempting to work out why some exposures lead to sensitization as opposed to tolerance, why not all those who are sensitized become symptomatic, and what determines whether the responses to downstream stimuli are limited or lead on to disease progression, airway remodeling, and chronic symptomatology (Fig. 39.5).

STEROID-RESISTANT ASTHMA

A small minority of asthmatic patients are resistant to the beneficial effects of steroids. In all other respects they have asthma, i.e., their airways obstruction is variable and their failure to respond to steroids is not because they have chronic obstructive pulmonary disease (COPD) that has been misdiagnosed. Even when given large doses of oral steroids, these patients' lung function does not improve.[35] Clinically they develop the usual steroid side effects, indicating that they have receptors for steroids. The molecular and cellular basis of steroid resistance remains uncertain. Clinical investigations have shown that steroid insensitivity in these patients is associated with loss of nuclear translocation of the alpha form of the glucocorticoid receptor.[36] Some patients who have clinically severe asthma despite

25. Brown JL, Behndig A, Sekerel B, et al. Lower airways inflammation in allergic rhinitics: a comparison with asthmatics and normal controls. Clin Exp Allergy 2007; 37: 688–695.

26. Djukanovic R, Lai CK, Wilson JW, et al. Bronchial mucosal manifestations of atopy: a comparison of markers of inflammation between atopic asthmatics, atopic nonasthmatics and healthy controls. Eur Respir J 1992; 5: 538–544.

27. Molet S, Hamid Q, Davoine F, et al. IL-17 is increased in asthmatic airways and induces human bronchial fibroblasts to produce cytokines. J Allergy Clin Immunol 2001; 108: 430–438.

28. Seow CY, Schellenberg R, Pare PD. Structural and functional changes in the airway smooth muscle of asthmatic subject. Am J Respir Crit Care Med 1998; 158: S179–S186.

29. Laporte JC, Moore PE, Baraldo S, et al. Direct effects of IL-13 on signalling pathways for physiological responses in cultured human airway smooth muscle cells. Am J Respir Crit Care Med 2001; 164: 141–148.

30. Polosa R, Puddicombe SM, Krishna MT, et al. Expression of c-erbB receptors and ligands in the bronchial epithelium of asthmatic subjects. J Allergy Clin Immunol 2002; 109: 75–81.

31. Lee JY, Park SW, Chang HK, et al. A disintegrin and metalloprotease 33 protein in patients with asthma. Am J Respir Crit Care Med 2006; 173: 729–735.

32. Jongepier H, Boezen HM, Dijkstra A, et al. Polymorphisms of the ADAM33 gene are associated with accelerated lung function decline in asthma. Clin Exp Allergy 2004; 34: 757–760.

33. Chan V, Burgess JK, Ratoff JC, et al. Extracellular matrix regulates enhanced eotaxin expression in astmatic airway smooth muscle cells. Am J Respir Crit Care Med 2006; 174: 379–385.

34. Henderson WR, Chiang GKS, Tien YT, et al. Reversal of allergen-induced airways remodelling by cysLT1 receptor blockade. Am J Respir Crit Care Med 2006; 173: 718–728.

35. Heaney LG, Conway E, Kelly C, et al. Predictors of therapy resistant asthma: outcome of a systematic evaluation protocol. Thorax 2003; 58: 561–566.

36. Goleva E, Li LB, Eves PT, et al. Increased glucocorticoid receptor beta alters steroid response in glucocorticoid-insensitive asthma. Am J Respir Crit Care Med 2006; 173: 607–616.

37. Howarth PH, Babu KS, Arshad HS, et al. Tumour necrosis factor (TNFalpha) as a novel therapeutic target in symptomatic corticosteroid dependent asthma. Thorax 2005; 60: 1012–1018.

38. Berry M, Hargadon B, Shelley M. et al Evidence of a role of tumor necrosis factor alpha in refractory asthma. N Engl J Med 2006; 354: 697–708.

39. Chanez P, Springall D, Vignola AM, et al. Bronchial mucosal immunoreactivity of sensory neuropeptides in severe airway diseases. Am J Respir Crit Care Med 1998; 158: 985–990.

40. Kanazawa H, Hirata K, Yoshikawa J. Involvement of vascular endothelial growth factor in exercise induced bronchoconstriction in asthmatic patients. Thorax 2002; 57: 885–888.

41. Feltis BN, Wignarajah D, Zheng L, et al. Increased vascular endothelial growth factor and receptors: relationship to angiogenesis in asthma. Am J Respir Crit Care Med 2006; 173: 1201–1207.

Management of the asthmatic patient

40

Susana Marinho, Adnan Custovic

Asthma is a complex multifactorial disorder involving a variety of different mechanisms, in which genetic and environmental influences play intertwining roles, resulting in heterogeneous clinical phenotypes. The key role played by chronic inflammation in the pathology of asthma has implications for its diagnosis, prevention and management.

Asthma is one of the most common chronic conditions worldwide.[1] International studies have demonstrated striking geographical variations in the prevalence of asthma throughout the world, the highest being observed in English-speaking countries and Latin America, and the lowest in the Mediterranean, Eastern Europe and rural areas of Africa and China. In addition, there is considerable evidence documenting a worldwide increase in the prevalence of asthma and other allergic diseases over recent decades.[1] It remains to be seen whether this trend is ongoing, as there are recent reports suggesting that in some areas it might have reached a plateau or reversed.

◼ DIAGNOSIS ◼

Owing to the complexity and multiplicity of asthma phenotypes, there is no single measure or procedure that allows a clear-cut confirmation or exclusion of the diagnosis. Diagnosis is based on a history of episodic respiratory symptoms consistent with airflow obstruction, combined with physical findings, objective measurements of airway obstruction, and reversibility (and exclusion of other conditions with similar clinical presentation).

◼ HISTORY AND PHYSICAL EXAMINATION ◼

The medical history should focus on the type and pattern of symptoms, precipitating and/or exacerbating factors, course of the disease and response to treatment, and family and social history. The key manifestations of asthma are a variable combination of wheezing, shortness of breath, chest tightness, cough and sputum production. The pattern of symptoms and course of the illness vary between patients: it is characteristically intermittent, but ranges from mild episodic symptoms that remit spontaneously to severe and sometimes fatal exacerbations, or persistent and progressive symptoms leading to significant disability.[1] Symptoms are typically triggered/exacerbated by viral respiratory infections, exercise, indoor and outdoor pollutants and irritants, allergens, medications, food additives and preservatives, emotions and endocrine factors.[1] Asthma symptoms follow a circadian rhythm and are often worse at night, which can lead to disturbed sleep and daytime fatigue; the frequency of nocturnal episodes is one of the indicators of disease severity.[1] Because the symptoms are variable, physical examination of the chest may be normal. Wheezing is the most typical finding, but may be absent in some symptomatic patients and during severe asthma exacerbations (when other physical signs of respiratory distress are obvious). Other signs may also be observed during symptomatic periods (e.g., tachypnea, tachycardia, chest hyperinflation, use of accessory muscles with intercostal recession, hyperresonant percussion note, prolongation of expiration). Other allergic diseases (rhinitis, conjunctivitis and eczema) may also be observed.

◼ FUNCTIONAL ASSESSMENT ◼

Lung function measurements are useful in establishing the diagnosis, assessing its severity and monitoring responses to treatment. Peak expiratory flow rate (PEFR) variability is a useful test, especially in the community. Diurnal PEFR variation > 20% is considered diagnostic; it may also be used to assess asthma severity, which is broadly proportional to the magnitude of the variability. However, in mild intermittent asthma or in severe intractable disease this variability may not be present.

For patients with a history suggesting asthma but having normal lung function, measurement of airway responsiveness to methacholine, histamine or exercise may facilitate the diagnosis.[1] These methods (with the exception of exercise challenge) are sensitive but relatively nonspecific, as airway hyperresponsiveness is also found in patients with allergic rhinitis or airflow limitation due to cystic fibrosis, bronchiectasis, chronic obstructive pulmonary disease (COPD), etc.

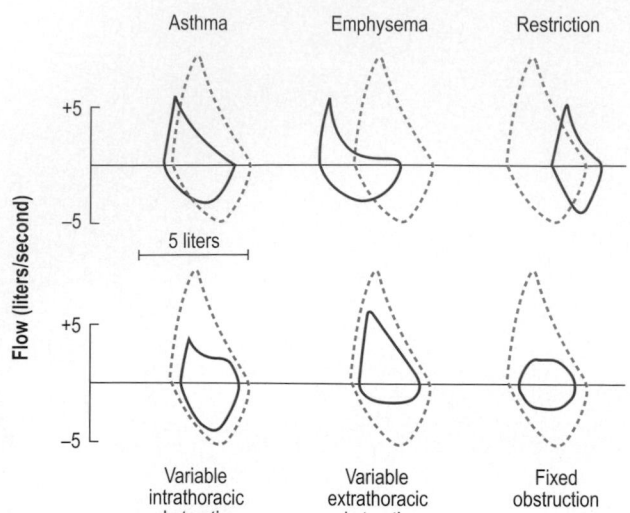

Fig. 40.1 Alteration of flow–volume loops in asthma. Six characteristic spirometric patterns of lung disease are shown. Expiratory and inspiratory flow is plotted against forced vital capacity (FVC). The expected curve is represented by the dashed line. (Adapted from Ruppel GL. Manual of pulmonary function testing, 7th edn. St Louis: Mosby, 1998, with permission from Elsevier.)

SPIROMETRY

Demonstrating reversibility of airflow limitation after bronchodilator inhalation supports a diagnosis of asthma. The forced expiratory volume in 1 second (FEV_1), forced vital capacity (FVC), and mid-expiratory flow rates obtained from flow–volume loops provide accurate and reproducible (albeit effort-dependent) information (Fig. 40.1). Characteristically, in airflow obstruction there is a decrease of both volumes and flows but FEV_1 is decreased more than FVC, resulting in a decreased FEV_1/FVC ratio (<80%).[1,2] Airflow limitation in asthma should be partially or completely reversible after inhaling a bronchodilator or after a 2-week trial of corticosteroids, with an improvement of at least 12% or 200 mL from baseline for FEV_1 or FVC considered to be clinically significant.[2] Failure to reverse should suggest other causes (especially COPD).

AIRWAY HYPERRESPONSIVENESS

Airway hyperresponsiveness (AHR) has been extensively assessed as an objective marker of asthma, as it is an important feature of the disease and is relatively easy to measure. In clinical practice, AHR is usually measured by methacholine or histamine challenges.

Most patients with symptomatic asthma show a fall in FEV_1 of > 20% after inhalation of methacholine at a concentration ≤16 mg/mL.[3] False-negative results may occur in patients who only experience symptoms at times of relevant allergen exposure and who are asymptomatic when tested.

The relevance of allergen or occupational exposures may be determined by direct airway challenge with a suspected allergen or irritant. However, this approach presents safety and practical difficulties, so its use is confined to specialist centers.

NONINVASIVE MARKERS OF AIRWAY INFLAMMATION

Airway inflammation can be indirectly assessed by measuring exhaled nitric oxide (NO)[4] or carbon monoxide (CO), which are elevated in individuals with asthma. Exhaled NO varies with disease activity and in response to anti-inflammatory therapy; it is lower in patients treated with inhaled glucocorticosteroids. However, neither measurement is specific for asthma, as both may be elevated in other conditions associated with airway inflammation. Airway inflammation can also be assessed by examining sputum for eosinophils and other inflammatory cells and mediators.[5]

ASSESSMENT OF ATOPY

Measuring allergen-specific IgE adds little to the diagnosis of asthma, but can help to identify possible triggers. Results must be interpreted in the context of the patient's history: positive results do not necessarily mean that there is a causal relationship between allergen exposure and asthma symptoms.

DIFFERENTIAL DIAGNOSIS

The differential diagnosis of asthma includes various nonasthmatic causes of wheezing, cough and shortness of breath associated with airways obstruction. These include large airway obstructions (extrathoracic), located in the lumen (primary and rarely secondary neoplasms, foreign body), in the airway wall (neoplasms, glottic webs, vascular rings, post-traumatic injury, laryngeal nerve palsy, vocal cord dysfunction, tracheomalacia) or outside the wall (extrinsic compression by a neoplastic or inflammatory mediastinal mass such as enlarged lymph nodes). Medium and small airway obstruction (intrathoracic) may be due to luminal obstruction (mucus, pus, or a fungal plug), wall obstruction (mucus, gland, and/or muscle hypertrophy, muscle spasms, or oedema), or be extrinsic (peribronchial inflammation and loss of parenchyma). Multiple conditions lead to these abnormalities and cause subsequent airway narrowing. COPD, congestive heart failure, pulmonary venous hypertension and pulmonary embolism must be considered in adults. Eosinophilic lung disease/pulmonary infiltrates with eosinophilia may be of known cause (parasitic infestations, allergic bronchopulmonary mycosis, eosinophilia-myalgia syndrome, drug-induced eosinophilic pneumonias), or unknown cause (acute or chronic eosinophilic pneumonia, Loeffler's syndrome, hypereosinophilic syndrome and Churg-Strauss syndrome). In children, CF and bronchopulmonary dysplasia should be considered. Flow–volume loops (Fig. 40.1) are useful in distinguishing the type of obstruction, which may be confirmed by direct or indirect examination.

CLASSIFICATION OF SEVERITY

Asthma severity is classified on the basis of several criteria, including symptoms, medication use and lung function: these are used to define four grades of severity (intermittent, mild persistent, moderate persistent and severe persistent) (Table 40.1).[1] If the patient is already on therapy, the classification is based on the same clinical features combined with the maintenance treatment regimen (Table 40.2).[1]

Table 40.1 Classification of asthma severity by clinical features before treatment

Asthma severity	Symptoms	Nocturnal symptoms	Lung function
Step 1 Intermittent	Symptoms < once a week Brief exacerbations (a few hours to a few days); variable severity Asymptomatic between exacerbations	≤ 2 times a month	FEV_1 or PEF≥80% predicted PEF or FEV_1 variability<20% Normal PEF between exacerbations
Step 2 Mild persistent	Once a week < symptoms < once a day Exacerbations may affect activity and sleep	> 2 times a month	FEV_1 or PEF≥80% predicted 20%<PEF or FEV_1 variability<30%
Step 3 Moderate persistent	Daily symptoms Exacerbations may affect activity and sleep; ≥ 2 times a week, may last days Daily use of inhaled short-acting β_2-agonists	> once a week	60%<FEV_1 or PEF<80% predicted PEF or FEV_1 variability > 30%
Step 4 Severe persistent	Daily/continual symptoms Frequent exacerbations Limitation of physical activity	Frequent	FEV_1 or PEF≤60% predicted PEF or FEV_1 variability >30%

The presence of one of the features of severity is sufficient to place a patient in the respective category; an individual should be assigned to the most severe grade in which any feature occurs.

(Adapted with permission from the GINA Workshop Report (2005) Global Strategy for Asthma Management and Prevention, available from http://www.ginasthma.org. Note: at the time of production of this book an updated/revised report was posted on the website, dated November 2006)

Table 40.2 Classification of asthma severity by clinical features subsequent to commencement of treatment by daily medication regimen and response to treatment

Patient symptoms and lung function on current therapy*	Current treatment step†		
	Step 1: Intermittent	Step 2: Mild persistent	Step 3: Moderate persistent
	Level of severity		
Step 1: Intermittent Normal lung function between episodes	Intermittent	Mild persistent	Moderate persistent
Step 2: Mild persistent Normal lung function between episodes	Mild persistent	Moderate persistent	Severe persistent
Step 3: Moderate persistent 60% < FEV_1 < 80% predicted OR 60% < PEF < 80% of personal best	Moderate persistent	Severe persistent	Severe persistent
Step 4: Severe persistent FEV_1 ≤ 60% predicted OR PEF ≤ 60% of personal best	Severe persistent	Severe persistent	Severe persistent

*Symptom assessment and classification based on the same classification as used for the initial assessment (see Table 40.1).
†Treatment step based on the NHLBI/WHO GINA guidelines[1] and described in Figures 40.1 and 40.2.

(Adapted with permission from the GINA Workshop Report (2005) Global Strategy for Asthma Management and Prevention, available from http://www.ginasthma.org. Note: at the time of production of this book an updated/revised report was posted on the website, dated November 2006)

CLINICAL R   ELEVANCE

RISK FACTORS FOR FATAL OR NEAR-FATAL ASTHMA AND FOR ASTHMA EXACERBATIONS

Risk factors for fatal or near fatal asthma

Indicators of asthma severity (clinical and lung function)

Previous history of life-threatening acute attacks (e.g. intubation, mechanical ventilation or respiratory acidosis)

Previous hospital admission for asthma (especially if within the previous year)

Repeated attendances to hospital emergency due to asthma exacerbations

Need for the use of three or more groups of different asthma medications

Heavy use of β_2-agonists

Recent reduction or cessation of corticosteroid therapy

Behavioral and psychosocial problems

Poor or no compliance with the medical therapy

Regular failure to attend follow up appointments (hospital and general practitioner)

Self-discharge from hospital

Alcohol or drug abuse

Psychosis, depression, other psychiatric illness

Obesity

Income or employment problems

Learning difficulties

Social isolation

Childhood abuse

Exacerbating factors for asthma

Allergen exposure
   Inhalant indoor and outdoor, food allergens

Air pollutants and irritants

Meteorological factors

Exercise and hyperventilation

Psychological/emotional factors

Drugs

Foods and food additives

Obesity

Respiratory infections

Rhinitis

Sinusitis

Gastro-esophageal reflux disease (GERD)

Vocal cord dysfunction (VCD)

KEY CONCEPTS

GOALS OF ASTHMA MANAGEMENT AND ASTHMA MANAGEMENT STRATEGIES

Goals of asthma management – Asthma control

>> Achieve and maintain control of symptoms (such as shortness of breath, cough, chest tightness)

   minimal, ideally no daytime symptoms

   minimal, ideally no nocturnal symptoms/awakenings

>> Prevent asthma exacerbations (minimal/infrequent)

   minimal 2–agonist need

   no emergency visits

>> Maintain normal activity levels, including exercise (no limitation)

>> Maintain lung function as close to normal levels as possible

   FEV_1 and PEF near normal

   PEF variability (diurnal variation) <20%

>> Avoid adverse effects from asthma medications (minimal or no)

>> Prevent progression of the disease and development of irreversible airflow limitation

>> Prevent asthma mortality

Asthma management strategies

>> Assessment and monitoring of asthma severity

   measurements of symptoms

   measurements of lung function

>> Identification and avoidance of exposure to potential risk and triggering factors

>> Pharmacological treatment

   design of individualised medication plans for long-term management in children and adults – regularly reviewed in accordance with a stepwise approach

   establishment of individualised medication plans for the management of exacerbations

>> Maintenance of regular follow up care

>> Education of patients (helping them to understand their disease and to take active part in its management, improving adherence to the management strategy)

This assessment has important implications for management, as treatment is based on a stepwise approach, adjusted according to disease severity. Asthma severity may vary over time, and patients should be assessed periodically and reclassified so that their management can be adapted to their current needs.

It is important to emphasize that any asthmatic (even those with mild persistent disease) may have a severe exacerbation, which if not recognized and treated may prove fatal.[1] Several factors increase the risk for the development of fatal or near-fatal asthma (see Clinical Relevance).[1, 6] Most patients who die from asthma have chronically severe or poorly controlled disease, with increased health service use and suboptimal self-management.[6]

MANAGEMENT GUIDELINES

Several guidelines using evidence-based methodology have been published over the last few decades, each being revised regularly to include the most up-to-date evidence.[1, 7, 8] These guidelines contain similar recommendations: the basic principles include adequate diagnosis, identification of causal/triggering/exacerbating factors, assessment of severity, achieving rapid control, and maintaining such control (Key Concepts). Although the main objective of the guidelines is to improve knowledge and standards of clinical practice in the hope of improved outcomes, it must be emphasized that guidelines are flexible recommendations.

GOALS AND PRINCIPLES OF MANAGEMENT

Although asthma cannot be cured, in most patients adequate control can be achieved and maintained. The goals of asthma management are to achieve and maintain symptom control, maintain normal activity levels and lung function, and prevent exacerbations and progression of the disease.

STEPWISE MANAGEMENT OF ASTHMA

The core principles of asthma management are to identify and avoid potential risk and triggering factors, to use appropriate pharmacotherapy, to maintain regular follow-up with continuous monitoring of severity (adjusting treatment according to response). Pharmacological treatment should be individualized and regularly reviewed. The choice of medications is dictated by the severity of the disease and directed towards suppression of airway inflammation. Once control is achieved and sustained for at least 3 months, it can be stepped down to the appropriate level until the minimum therapy required to maintain control is achieved. Failure to gain control may indicate poor compliance or an incorrect diagnosis. Regular monitoring is an essential part of this approach. Figures 40.2 and 40.3 present the stepwise approach to achieve and maintain control of asthma in adults and in children.[1]

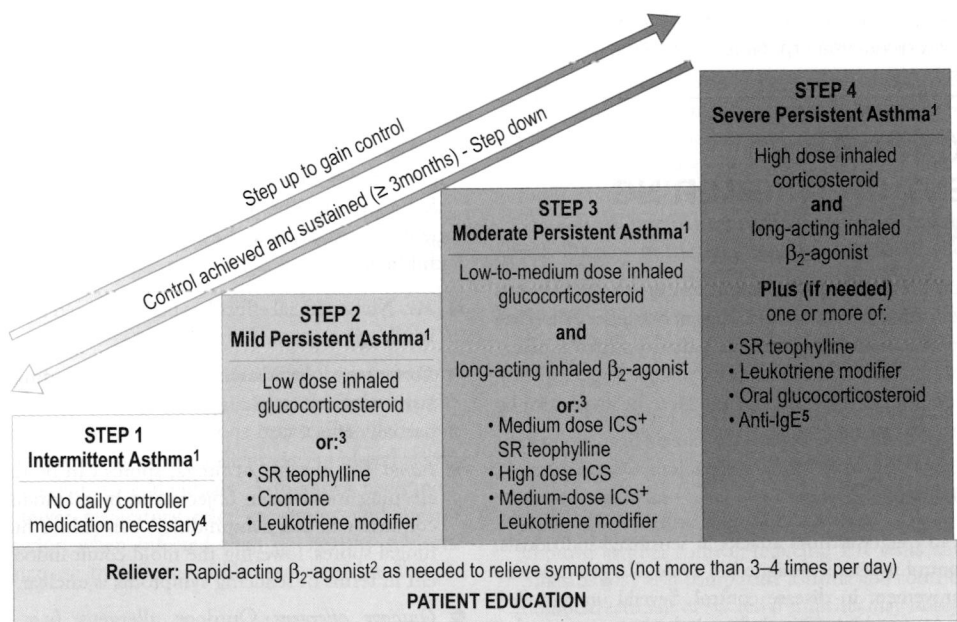

Fig. 40.2 Stepwise approach to asthma pharmacological management in adults and children older than 5 years. ICS, inhaled glucocorticosteroid; SR theophylline, slow-release theophylline. [1]See Tables 40.1 and 40.3 for classification of severity. [2]Other options for reliever medication are (in order of increasing cost) inhaled anticholinergic, short-acting oral β2-agonist, and short-acting theophylline. [3]Other treatment options listed in order of increasing cost. [4]Patients with intermittent asthma but severe exacerbations should be treated as having moderate persistent asthma – Step 3 (Evidence D[1]). [5]Current evidence supports use in adults and children ≥12 years only. Management of acute asthma exacerbations. (Adapted with permission from the GINA Workshop Report (2005) - Global Strategy for Asthma Management and Prevention, available from http://www.ginasthma.org. Note: at the time of production of this book an updated/revised report was posted on the website, dated November 2006.)

CLINICAL PEARLS

PHARMACOLOGICAL MANAGEMENT OF ASTHMA

Controllers/preventers	Relievers
Inhaled corticosteroids	Short-acting β_2-agonists
Leukotriene modifiers	Long-acting β_2-agonists
Cromones	Anticholinergics
Methylxanthines	Methylxanthines
Long-acting β_2-agonists	Systemic corticosteroids
Systemic corticosteroids	
Systemic steroid-sparing therapies	

---

systematic review of 12 trials of medical and surgical anti-reflux treatments in children and adults found no overall improvement in asthma following treatment for GERD; subgroups of patients may benefit, but it is difficult to predict responders.[18]

- *Vocal cord dysfunction (VCD)* VCD may coexist with asthma and contributes to airway obstruction in up to 40% of asthmatics.

PHARMACOLOGICAL TREATMENT

Pharmacological treatment aims to reduce airway inflammation, improve symptom control, and prevent acute exacerbations while minimizing side effects. Adequate control should be achieved as soon as possible. Treatment should start at the step most appropriate to the initial asthma severity and then be reviewed regularly, stepping up and down according to the level of control.[1, 7, 8] Anti-asthma drugs may be divided into 'controllers/preventers' (corticosteroids, leukotriene modifiers, cromones, methylxanthines and long-acting β_2-agonists) and 'relievers' (short-acting β_2-agonists, long-acting B2 agonists cholinergic antagonists). Persistent asthma is better controlled by drugs that suppress and reverse airway inflammation than by reliever drugs.[1] Clinical trials suggest heterogeneity in the individual response to asthma drugs, largely attributable to genetic background. Future developments in pharmacogenetics may allow therapy to be tailored to each patient's response to medication.

CONTROLLERS: LONG-TERM PREVENTIVE MEDICATIONS

Controllers, also called prophylactic, preventive or maintenance medications, are taken daily on a long-term basis to treat inflammation and achieve/maintain asthma control (Table 40.3).

Inhaled glucocorticosteroids

Glucocorticosteroids (Chapter 87) are the most effective anti-inflammatory asthma drugs: inhaled corticosteroids (ICS) are the first-choice controller treatment in both children and adults.[1,7,19] Glucocorticosteroids suppress airway inflammation, reduce AHR, control symptoms, improve quality of life and reduce morbidity and mortality.[20]

Role in therapy

Episodic high-dose ICS are partially effective against episodes of mild viral-induced wheeze in children, but long-term low-dose ICS cannot prevent viral-induced wheeze. In addition, early treatment of childhood wheezing with ICS does not appear to prevent subsequent asthma.[21]

Pharmacology

Glucocorticosteroids differ in their potency and bioavailability after inhalation (Table 40.4). Dose comparisons of ICS are difficult owing to their long duration of action and relatively flat dose–response curves. The delivery device has a major impact on absorption, as without the use of a spacer 70–90% of the drug is deposited in the oropharynx; dry powder inhalers (DPI) are more efficient at delivering the drug to the lungs than pressurized metered-dose inhalers (pMDI). Improvement in asthma control occurs within days of starting ICS, but several months are necessary to attain the maximum effect. Once control is achieved, the dose should be carefully reduced to the minimum needed to maintain control, reducing the potential for side effects. Because asthma sometimes remits, ICS may be withdrawn for a trial period if the patient becomes asymptomatic for a prolonged period on low-dose treatment. Because the dose–response curve for ICS is relatively flat for most outcome measures (e.g., symptoms, lung function, airway responsiveness), using higher doses rarely improves asthma control, but increases the risk of side effects.

Adverse effects

The most common adverse effects of ICS are local, including oropharyngeal candidiasis, dysphonia, and occasional coughing due to upper airway irritation. These effects are dose dependent and can be minimized by using spacer devices and rinsing the mouth or gargling after each dose.[1] Dysphonia commonly responds to vocal rest and discontinuing ICS.

All currently available ICS are absorbed from the lung, although the extent of systemic exposure varies according to their dose and potency, bioavailability, gut absorption, first-pass liver metabolism and plasma half-life.[22] The delivery system also affects the amount of systemic exposure: using a spacer reduces systemic absorption for most, but not all, ICS. Long-term treatment with high-dose ICS can cause skin thinning and easy bruising, adrenal suppression and decreased bone mineral density. Although differences exist between the various drugs and inhaler devices, treatment with doses <400 μg beclomethasone/budesonide daily is not usually associated with significant suppression of the hypothalamopituitary–adrenal (HPA) axis in children; at higher doses (≥1000 μg/day), small changes in HPA-axis function can be detected with sensitive methods. Whether these are clinically relevant remains unknown. Likewise, the question as to whether long-term ICS therapy suppresses growth in children is debatable. Dose-dependent growth retardation occurs with all ICS when sufficiently high doses are given. However, this is usually modest, transient, and unlikely to affect adult height (asthmatics treated with ICS have consistently been found to attain normal adult height).[1] However, uncontrolled or severe asthma does adversely affect final adult height.

The clinical significance of the decrease in bone formation and degradation during treatment with high doses of ICS is not yet known. Several studies have shown no effect on bone mineral density or rates of fracture.[23] Prophylactic treatment for osteoporosis is not advised for patients on ICS.[1]

Table 40.3 Glossary of asthma medications

Name	Usual doses	Side effects	Comments
CONTROLLER LONG-TERM MEDICATIONS			

Glucocorticosteroids
Inhaled
  Beclomethasone
  Budesonide
  Flunisolide
  Fluticasone
  Mometasone furoate
  Triamcinolone
	Beginning dose depending on asthma severity (see Table 40.5), then titrated down over 2–3 months to lowest effective dose once control is achieved	High daily doses may cause: skin thinning and bruises, rarely adrenal suppression.
		Local side effects: dysphonia and oropharyngeal candidiasis
			Potential but small risk of side effects is well balanced by efficacy.
			Spacer/holding chamber with pMDIs and mouth washing after inhalation with DPIs decrease local side effects and systemic absorption.
			Preparations not equivalent on per puff or μg basis

Tablets or syrups
  Hydrocortisone
  Methylprednisolone
  Prednisolone
  Prednisone
	For daily control use lowest effective dose 5–40 g of prednisone equivalent
	For acute attacks 40–60 g daily in 1 or 2 divided doses for adults or 1–2 mg/kg daily in children
		Used long-term may lead to osteoporosis, hypertension, diabetes, cataracts, adrenal suppression, growth suppression, obesity, skin thinning, muscle weakness	Long-term use: alternate day a.m. dosing produces less toxicity.
			Short-term: 3–10 day courses are effective for gaining prompt control

Cromones Sodium cromoglycate	MDI 2 mg or 5 mg/puff, 2–4 inhalations, 3–4 times/day	Minimal side effects. Cough may occur upon inhalation	May take 4–6 weeks for maximum effects to be attained. Frequent daily dosing required
Nedocromil	MDI 2 mg/puff, 2–4 inhalations, 2–4 times/day	Cough may occur upon inhalation	Some patients unable to tolerate the taste
Methylxanthines Theophylline Sustained-release tablets and capsules	Starting dose 10 mg/kg/day with 800 mg maximum in 1–2 divided doses	Nausea and vomiting are most common. Serious side effects occurring at higher serum concentrations: seizures, tachycardia, arrhythmias	Theophylline level monitoring is often required. Absorption and metabolism may be affected by many factors
Leukotriene modifiers Montelukast (M) Pranlukast (P) Zafirlukast (Z) Zileuton (Zi)	Adults M: 10 mg/day; P: 450 mg bid Z: 20 mg bid; Zi: 600 mg qid Children M: 5 mg/day (6–14 yrs); 4 mg/day (2–5 yrs) Z: 10 mg bid (7–11 yrs)	Limited data; no specific side effects at recommended doses	The position of leukotriene modifiers in asthma therapy is not fully established. Additive benefit when added to glucocorticosteroids, though not as effective as long-acting β_2-agonists.
Long-acting inhaled β_2-agonists Formoterol (F) Salmeterol (S)	DPI 1 inhalation bid (F–12 μg; S–50 μg) pMDI F or S: 2 puffs bid	May cause tachycardia, anxiety, skeletal muscle tremor, headache, hypokalemia in overdose	Always use as adjunct to anti-inflammatory therapy

Continued

PHARMACOLOGICAL TREATMENT

Table 40.3 Glossary of asthma medications—Cont'd

CONTROLLER LONG-TERM MEDICATIONS			
Name	Usual doses	Side effects	Comments
RELIEVER MEDICATIONS			
Rapid-acting inhaled β_2-agonists			
Salbutamol/Albuterol Fenoterol Metaproterenol Piributerol Terbutaline	Differences in potency exist but all products are essentially comparable on a per puff basis. For prn symptomatic use and pre-treatment before exercise: 2 puffs pMDI or 1 inhalation DPI. For asthma attacks: 4–8 puffs q1–4h, may administer q20min × 3 with medical supervision or the equivalent of 5 mg salbutamol by nebulizer.	Inhaled: tachycardia, skeletal muscle tremor, headache, and irritability. At very high dose: hyperglycemia, hypokalemia. Systemic administration as tablets or syrup increases the risk of these side effects.	Drug of choice for acute bronchospasm. Inhaled route has faster onset and is more effective than tablet or syrup. Increasing use, lack of expected effect, or use of > 1 canister a month indicate poor asthma control; adjust long-term therapy accordingly. Use of ≥ 2 canisters per month is associated with an increased risk of a severe, life-threatening asthma attack
Anticholinergics			
Ipratropium bromide (IB) Oxitropium bromide Tiotropium bromide	IB: MDI 4–6 puffs q6h or q20 min in the emergency department; Nebulizer 500 µg q20min × 3 then q2–4 hrs for adults and 250 µg for children	Minimal mouth dryness or bad taste in mouth	May provide additive effects to β_2-agonist but has slower onset of action. Alternative for patients with intolerance to β_2-agonists
Short-acting theophylline			
Aminophylline	7 mg/kg loading dose over 20 min followed by 0.4 mg/kg/h continuous infusion	Nausea, vomiting, headache. Serious side effects occurring at higher serum concentrations: seizures, tachycardia, arhythmias	Theophylline level monitoring is required. Obtain serum levels 12 and 24 hours into infusion. Maintain between 10-15 µg/ml.

(Adapted with permission from the NAEPP Guidelines–National Asthma Education and Prevention Program Expert Panel Report 2: Guidelines for the Diagnosis and Management of Asthma. Updated 1997. National Heart, Lung and Blood Institute, National Institutes of Health. NIH Publication No 97-4051. Available on http://www.nhibi.nih.gov.)

Cataracts and glaucoma have been reported in cross-sectional studies of adults using ICS, but there is no evidence of post-capsular cataracts in prospective studies.[1]

Evidence that ICS affect the central nervous system is limited to isolated case reports of hyperactive behaviour, aggressiveness, insomnia and impaired concentration, which returned to normal after discontinuing ICS.[1]

Systemic corticosteroids

Long-term systemic glucocorticosteroids may be required to control severe persistent asthma in adults, but their use is limited by the risk of significant adverse effects. If oral glucocorticosteroids (OCS) have to be administered long-term, clinicians should focus on measures that minimize their side effects: oral preparations (prednisone, prednisolone, or methylprednisolone) are preferred to parenteral preparations because of their minimal mineralo-corticoid effect, relatively short half-life and limited effects on striated muscle. OCS should normally be given as a single morning dose, either every day or on alternate days.[1] Patients with asthma on long-term OCS should receive preventive treatment for osteoporosis.[1]

Although their onset of action is 4–6 hours, systemic corticosteroids are important in the treatment of severe acute exacerbations because they prevent progression of the exacerbation, reduce the need for emergency department visits or hospitalizations, prevent early relapse after emergency treatment, and reduce morbidity.[1] Oral therapy with prednisone, prednisolone or methyprednisolone is preferred to intravenous hydrocortisone and should be continued for 3–10 days.

Table 40.4 Estimated comparative daily dosages for inhaled glucocorticosteroids

Drug	Low daily dose (µg) Adults	Children	Medium daily dose (µg) Adults	Children	High daily dose (µg) Adults	Children
Beclomethasone dipropionate – CFC	200–500	100–250	500–1000	250–500	>1000	>500
Beclomethasone dipropionate – HFA	100–250	50–200	250–500	200–400	>500	>400
Budesonide – DPI	200–600	100–200	600–1000	200–600	>1000	>600
Budesonide – nebulizer inhalation suspension		250–500		500–1000		>1000
Flunisolide	500–1000	500–750	1000–2000	750–1250	>2000	>1250
Fluticasone	100–250	100–200	250–500	200–400	>500	>400
Mometasone furoate	200–400		400–800		>800	
Triamcinolone acetonide	400–1000	400–800	1000–2000	800–1200	>2000	>1200

(Adapted with permission from the GINA Workshop Report (2005) Global Strategy for Asthma Management and Prevention, available from http://www.ginasthma. org. Note: at the time of production of this book an updated/revised report was posted on the website, dated November 2006)

In children with asthma, systemic corticosteroids are only used for acute exacerbations, where they allow earlier discharge and fewer relapses.[1]

Leukotriene modifiers

Leukotriene modifiers (LM) include cysteinyl leukotriene 1 (CysLT1) receptor antagonists (montelukast, pranlukast, zafirlukast), and 5-lipoxygenase inhibitors (zileuton).

Mechanism of action

Leukotrienes are 5-lipoxygenase products of arachidonic acid synthesized by mast cells, eosinophils and other inflammatory cells. Both LTB_4 and the cysteinyl leukotrienes (cysLTs: LTC_4, LTD_4, LTE_4) have been implicated in the pathogenesis of asthma. The cysLT are potent bronchoconstrictors and also have an effect on blood vessels, mucociliary clearance and eosinophilic inflammation. LTB_4 is a potent chemoattractant and cell activator for neutrophils and eosinophils. 5-lipoxygenase inhibitors prevent leukotriene synthesis. Leukotriene receptor antagonists block the CysLT1 receptors on airway smooth muscle and other cells. These drugs have some anti-inflammatory effects and a modest short-acting bronchodilator effect.[1, 24]

Role in therapy

The effect of LM is less than that of low-dose ICS: they should only be used as monotherapy in highly selected patients with mild persistent asthma; they have been less extensively studied as monotherapy in children, but improve lung function and asthma control in children with moderate/severe asthma, though they have advantage of oral administration.[1] LM may allow reduced doses of ICS in patients with moderate/severe asthma, and improve disease control in patients uncontrolled

on ICS.[1] However, they are less effective than long-acting inhaled β_2-agonists as add-on therapy, though they have the advantage of oral administration. LM are useful in patients with NSAID sensitivity, where there is overproduction of cysLTs (probably due to over-expression of LTC_4-synthase).[24] LM are effective in preventing exercise-induced bronchoconstriction and may reduce the symptoms of allergic rhinitis coexisting with asthma.[1, 24]

Adverse effects

LM are well tolerated and have few side effects. Zileuton has been associated with liver toxicity, and monitoring of liver function is recommended during treatment.[1, 24] There are several reports of Churg–Strauss syndrome associated with LM therapy, but in most cases this occurred when systemic glucocorticosteroids were being reduced or withdrawn,[1, 24] and a causal link is unlikely.

Cromones

Cromones (sodium cromoglycate and nedocromil sodium) are used as inhaled prophylactic treatment for mild persistent asthma, particularly in children. They have been available for over 30 years and have an excellent safety profile, but inferior efficacy to ICS.

Mechanism of action

How cromones work remains incompletely understood. There is some evidence that they partially inhibit IgE-dependent mediator release from human mast cells, and have selective suppressive effects on macrophages, eosinophils and monocytes. They also abolish or inhibit calcium channel activation triggered by cross-linking membrane-bound IgE by antigen and block chloride channels. Anti-inflammatory effects have been shown in sputum and bronchial biopsy studies. Cromones lack bronchodilator activity, but may prevent or reduce bronchoconstriction following allergen or nonspecific challenges (exercise, cold air, sulfur dioxide, aspirin); they also prevent late responses to allergens and exercise.[1]

Role in therapy

Sodium cromoglycate reduces symptoms, the frequency of exacerbations and the need for rescue medication. Lung function improves, but benefits on AHR have not been consistently demonstrated. A recent meta-analysis of 24 studies concluded that cromoglycate is not significantly effective in asthmatic children.[25] Nedocromil used before exercise reduces the severity and duration of exercise-induced bronchoconstriction. However, short-acting β_2-agonists and LMs are more effective.

Adverse effects

Cromones have minimal side effects. Occasional coughing, throat irritation and bronchoconstriction occur in a few patients; some patients find nedocromil tastes unpleasant, or report headache and nausea.

Methylxanthines

Theophylline has been available for over 50 years and remains widely prescribed for asthma. Its role has been questioned because of the frequency of side effects and relatively low efficacy; however, because it is effective, inexpensive, and widely available, several guidelines still recommend it. In richer countries it has largely been superseded by newer therapies. The most common marketed salt is aminophylline, which can also be used intravenously.

Mechanism of action

Both the mechanism and site of action remain uncertain. Several molecular mechanisms have been proposed, though many only operate at concentrations above those used clinically. These include nonselective phosphodiesterase (PDE) inhibition, adenosine receptor antagonism, stimulation of catecholamine release, mediator inhibition (prostaglandins, TNF-α), inhibition of intracellular calcium release, decreased nuclear translocation of NF-κB, and increased histone deacetylase activity. The primary effect of theophylline is assumed to be relaxation of the airway smooth muscle, which is related to PDE inhibition and seen at high concentrations (>10 mg/L); however, theophylline is a weak bronchodilator at therapeutic concentrations. Most studies show little or no effect on AHR. Theophylline may have extrapulmonary effects, including anti-inflammatory effects (demonstrable at lower concentrations [5–10 mg/L]), but whether this significantly affects chronic airway inflammation is unknown.

Role in therapy

Sustained-release theophylline and aminophylline can be used as controller medications for asthma in both adults and children.[1] Sustained-release formulations of methylxanthines are useful in controlling nocturnal symptoms and as additional bronchodilators in patients with severe asthma. They may be used as add-on therapy (adding theophylline to ICS provides better

asthma control than increasing ICS doses),[1] and although less effective than inhaled long-acting β_2-agonists,[26] theophylline is much cheaper.

Owing to the risk of adverse effects and the difficulty of monitoring therapy, theophylline is used in some countries after ICS and β_2-agonists fail to achieve therapeutic goals, but elsewhere it is recommended at an earlier stage.

Sustained-release products are preferred for maintenance therapy as they enable twice-daily dosing in most patients (particularly in children, who metabolize theophylline very rapidly and may require dosing 4–6 times/day with plain formulations). Concomitant food intake unpredictably affects the absorption of some theophylline products; preparations with reliable absorption profiles and complete bioavailability when taken with food are available.[1]

Adverse effects

One of the main limitations of theophylline is the frequency of adverse effects that are dose dependent and usually occur at concentrations exceeding 10 mg/kg body weight/day. These can generally be avoided by appropriate dosing and monitoring. Gastrointestinal symptoms (nausea and vomiting) are the most common early adverse effects, along with headaches. At higher concentrations theophylline can cause seizures and even death; these events may not be preceded by obvious central nervous system stimulation. Tachycardia, arrhythmias, and occasionally respiratory stimulation occur. Generally, serious toxic effects do not occur at serum concentrations <15 mg/L. Usual practice during long-term treatment is to aim for a steady-state serum concentration of 5–15 mg/L (28–85 μmol) for adults.[1] There is still considerable debate regarding optimal plasma levels for children; maximum bronchodilator effect is achieved at plasma levels of 10–20 mg/L (55–110 μmol),[1] but measurable effects on other outcomes may be achieved at lower concentrations (e.g. anti-inflammatory effects). So it seems reasonable to individualize the dose according to clinical effects rather than aiming for specific plasma levels. Theophylline metabolism and clearance vary with age and other factors such as multiple drug interactions, pregnancy and other conditions. Monitoring serum concentrations is advised when starting high-dose theophylline therapy (10 mg/kg/day or above) and at occasional intervals thereafter, as well as when patients develop adverse effects on their usual dose, when expected therapeutic aims are not achieved, or when situations known to alter theophylline metabolism occur.

Long-acting inhaled β_2-agonists

Long-acting inhaled β_2-agonists (LABAs) (formoterol, salmeterol) are selective β_2-agonists with an extended duration of action of more than 12 hours. They act by reversing and/or inhibiting bronchoconstriction and related symptoms of acute asthma, but do not reverse airway inflammation or reduce hyperresponsiveness.[1, 27]

Mechanism of action

Activation of β_2-adrenergic receptors induces smooth muscle relaxation, enhanced mucociliary clearance, decreased vascular permeability, inhibition of cholinergic neurotransmission and inhibition of mediator release from mast cells, basophils and other inflammatory cells.[27] Formoterol is a full β_2-agonist with a short onset of action (2–3 minutes) and a maximum effect 30–60 minutes after inhalation, whereas salmeterol is a partial agonist and has delayed onset of action (~10–20 minutes), with maximal effect attained within 1–3 hours. Owing to its rapid onset of action formoterol may be suitable for symptom relief, although this role needs further investigation.[1] LABAs protect against several bronchoconstrictive stimuli (e.g., histamine, methacholine, cold dry air and exercise).[27]

Role in therapy

LABAs should be considered in patients with moderate/severe asthma that is not controlled despite standard doses of ICS.[1] LABAs reduce asthma symptoms, frequency of nocturnal symptoms and exacerbations, decrease bronchodilator requirements, and improve lung function and asthma-specific measures of quality of life.[1, 27] As long-term treatment with LABAs does not appear to reduce the persistent airway inflammation, LABAs should *always* be combined with ICS.[1] Adding LABAs in patients whose asthma is not controlled on either low or high doses of ICS results in better control of the disease than doubling the ICS dose.[1] Fixed combination inhalers (fluticasone propionate+salmeterol, budesonide+formoterol) are convenient for patients. Although LABAs may be useful in children, there is insufficient evidence to support their general use in this age group.[1]

Adverse effects

Tremor is the major side effect, caused by stimulation of β_2 receptors in skeletal muscle. β_1-receptor stimulation may lead to increased heart rate and palpitations, prolonged QT interval, arrhythmias and myocardial ischemia. β-adrenergic relaxation of vascular smooth muscle reduces peripheral resistance, leading to reflex sympathetic cardiac stimulation. Acute metabolic responses to β_2-agonists include hyperglycemia, hypokalemia and hypomagnesemia: these diminish with regular administration.[27] Tolerance develops with regular administration of β_2-agonists, presumably due to β_2-adrenergic receptor downregulation.[27] This is found for both bronchodilator and metabolic effects; a reduced bronchodilator response develops over a few weeks, and once established it is stable with continued use of the drug (this principally affects duration of action and bronchoprotection rather than the peak effect).[27]

A recent large study comparing the safety of salmeterol or placebo added to usual asthma care in patients over 12 years of age showed a small but significant increase in asthma-related deaths in patients receiving salmeterol.[28] It was not clear whether this was directly due to the LABA or to other factors (e.g., physiologic treatment effects, genetic factors, or patient behavior). Thus far it remains uncertain whether ICS can limit or prevent the adverse outcomes (i.e., subjects underwent randomization without consideration of their corticosteroid therapy, and no records of ICS therapy were kept). A thorough analysis by the FDA concluded that the data from the SMART study are inconclusive as regards this point.[29]

RELIEVER MEDICATIONS

Relievers or rescue medications (Table 40.3) include rapid-acting bronchodilators that relieve bronchoconstriction and its associated symptoms.

Short-acting β_2-agonists

Short-acting inhaled β_2-agonists (SABAs) induce prompt bronchodilatation and provide rapid symptom relief. They include salbutamol (albuterol), terbutaline, fenoterol, reproterol and pirbuterol.

Mechanism of action

SABAs relax airways smooth muscle and have other nonbronchodilator effects related to the stimulation of β_2-adrenergic receptors[27] (see LABAs above). They can be administered via inhaled, oral, subcutaneous or intravenous routes. The inhaled route is preferred, as it allows more rapid bronchodilatation with fewer side effects. Inhaled SABAs provide significant protection against exercise-induced bronchoconstriction; their effects start within 5 minutes of administration and last 3–6 hours. Oral preparations are used in patients unable to use inhaled medication (e.g., young children).

Differential responses to SABAs have been described among asthmatic patients with different β_2-adrenergic receptor gene alleles; the clinical implications of this finding require further examination.

Role in therapy

SABAs are the medication of choice for episodic acute symptoms and for acute severe asthma in adults and children; premedication prevents exercise-induced asthma.[1] SABAs should be used as required for symptom control. Increased SABA use or decreased response to SABAs indicates the need to institute or intensify regular anti-inflammatory therapy.

Adverse effects

See section on LABAs.

Anticholinergics

Inhaled anticholinergics (ipratropium bromide, oxitropium bromide, tiotropium bromide) are short-acting bronchodilators.

Mechanism of action

These drugs block the stimulation of muscarinic cholinergic receptors (functionally selective for receptors M_1 and M_3) by acetylcholine released from autonomic nerves in the airways.[30] They also block reflex bronchoconstriction caused by inhaled irritants, but have no effect on the early- and late-phase allergic reactions or airway inflammation. In asthma, they are less potent bronchodilators than SABAs[1] and have a slower onset of action (60–90 minutes to achieve maximum effect). The duration of action of ipratropium and oxitropium is 4–8 hours, whereas tiotropium lasts for >24 hours.[30]

Role in therapy

Anticholinergics provide complete protection against bronchospasm induced by cholinergic agonists (e.g., methacholine) and β-blocking agents, but only partial protection against other bronchoconstrictors.

In acute severe asthma, nebulized ipratropium adds to the effects of nebulized SABAs with a modest improvement in lung function and reduced risk of hospital admission.[31] The benefits of ipratropium in the long-term management of asthma have not been established, although it is a useful alternative bronchodilator for patients who experience adverse effects from SABAs.[1] A subset of asthmatics may respond more favorably to anticholinergics, although it is not possible to predict response other than by therapeutic trial.[32]

Ipratropium helps in the management of acute exacerbations, as its effects are additive to those of SABAs, providing a greater and more rapid improvement in lung function and avoiding prolonged emergency treatments and hospitalization.[33] Tiotropium is a new longer-acting anticholinergic that is useful in COPD, but its role in asthma has yet to be defined.

Adverse effects

Anticholinergics have a wide therapeutic margin and are well tolerated.[30] They have few side effects, as gastrointestinal absorption is minimal, and they do not cross the blood–brain barrier. Dry mouth is the commonest side-effect, but is rarely sufficiently severe to warrant discontinuation. Other occasional complaints are a bad taste, transient cough and paradoxical bronchoconstriction.[30]

Other drugs used as relievers

Methylxanthines

Short-acting theophylline preparations may be considered for relief of symptoms (although their onset of action is slower than SABAs).[1] Although they provide no additive bronchodilator effect over adequate doses of SABAs, theophyllines may improve respiratory muscle function and prolong or sustain the response to SABAs.[1] In adults with acute asthma, intravenous aminophylline did not result in any additional bronchodilatation compared to standard care with β-agonists, and was associated with more adverse effects; no patient subgroups were identified in which aminophylline might be more effective.[34] However, in children, adding intravenous aminophylline to SABAs and glucocorticosteroids (with or without anticholinergics) improved lung function, although symptoms, treatment requirements and length of hospital stay were not reduced.[35]

OTHER PHARMACOLOGICAL AGENTS

Anti-IgE

Mechanism of action

Since IgE plays an important role in the pathophysiology of asthma, chelating IgE seems a logical therapeutic approach. Omalizumab is a recombinant humanized IgG_1 monoclonal anti-IgE antibody that binds to IgE in the region that binds IgE receptors (FcεRI and FcεRII), preventing IgE from interacting with them. Omalizumab is not anaphylactogenic, as it cannot cross-link IgE molecules bound to basophils or mast cells. Instead, it binds to circulating IgE forming small biologically inert IgE–anti-IgE complexes that do not activate complement or cause the formation of anti-omalizumab antibodies.[36] Omalizumab attenuates the early- and late-phase responses after allergen challenge, decreases eosinophil numbers in sputum and bronchial submucosa, and downregulates FcεRI expression on basophils, mast cells and dendritic cells.[36]

Role in therapy

The role of omalizumab in asthma management has yet to be precisely defined.[37] At present, the principal indication is as add-on therapy in patients with moderate to severe allergic asthma,[1] although its use is limited by its cost.[1, 37] Patients who are particularly likely to benefit include those sensitized to perennial aeroallergens who require high doses of ICS, those with frequent exacerbations, and possibly those with severe symptoms related in part to poor adherence.[36] Patients requiring daily OCS to control their asthma may be less likely to respond.[36]

Adverse effects

Anti-IgE appears safe and well tolerated.[1, 36, 37] Reported adverse effects include rash, diarrhea, nausea, vomiting, epistaxis, menorrhagia, fatigue, arthralgias, dizziness and injection-site reactions.[36] The safety profile needs further evaluation after long-term use. Potential concerns include the risk of developing malignancies and anaphylaxis. Cancer appears to develop more often in patients receiving anti-IgE than in those taking placebo, and anti-IgE is probably best avoided in patients with a personal or family history of cancer until this risk is better understood. Anaphylaxis has occurred within 2 hours of administration of omalizumab in three patients without other identifiable triggers; patients should therefore be observed in an appropriate setting after injection.[36]

Macrolide and ketolide antibacterial agents

Macrolides (azithromycin, clarithromycin, erythromycin and roxythromycin) are broad-spectrum antibiotics active against a wide range of bacteria, including *Chlamydia pneumoniae* and *Mycoplasma pneumoniae*. Ketolides are structurally related to macrolides, with a broader range of antibacterial activity; telithromycin is the first ketolide approved for clinical use. Macrolides and ketolides have anti-inflammatory and immunodulatory activity (including suppression of neutrophilic inflammation). Trials of macrolides in chronic stable asthma showed positive effects on symptoms and eosinophilic inflammation, although the small number of patients included (357 patients in five studies) limits the generalizability of these findings.

Current guidelines do not recommend antibiotics for the treatment of acute exacerbations, as viruses are usually responsible. However, continuing interest in the potential role of *Chlamydia* infection in asthma has prompted a study of telithromycin in acute exacerbations in 278 adults (TELICAST).[38] Significant improvements were reported in symptoms and lung function in patients receiving telithromycin, but there was no greater effect in patients with evidence of infection compared to those without, so the mechanisms remain unclear.[38]

Steroid-sparing agents

Several options have been tried to reduce OCS requirements in patients with severe asthma who experience significant side effects and in asthmatics who are steroid resistant defined as failure to improve FEV_1 by >15% of predicted after 7–14 days of OCS [prednisolone 20 mg twice daily]. Some steroid-resistant patients may respond to higher doses of OCS administered for longer periods, but

CLINICAL PEARLS

CHOICE OF INHALER DEVICE FOR CHILDREN

Age group	Preferred device	Alternative device
< 4 years	pMDI + dedicated spacer with face mask	Nebulizer with face mask
4–6 years	pMDI + dedicated spacer with mouthpiece	Nebulizer with face mask
> 6 years	DPI or breath-activated pMDI or pMDI + spacer with mouthpiece	Nebulizer with mouthpiece

(Adapted with permission from the GINA Workshop Report (2005) Global Strategy for Asthma Management and Prevention, available from http://www.ginasthma.org. Note: at the time of production of this book an updated/revised report was posted on the website, dated November 2006)

such courses are unacceptable owing to the adverse effects. Therapeutic options include methotrexate, cyclosporine, gold, intravenous immunoglobulin and troleandromycin. These medications should only be used in carefully selected patients under close supervision, as they have a very narrow therapeutic window and their potential steroid-sparing effect may not outweigh the risk of serious adverse effects. A meta-analysis of methotrexate studies concluded it has a small steroid-sparing effect, but the reduction in steroid dose is probably insufficient to materially alter the risk of steroid side effects and offset the adverse effects of methotrexate.[39]

Cyclosporine and gold were judged to induce small changes of questionable significance and, given the incidence of adverse effects, they are no longer recommended as steroid-sparing agents. Reviews of colchicine,[40] chloroquine[41] and dapsone[42] concluded that there is insufficient evidence to support their use as steroid-sparing drugs. Troleandomycin alters the metabolism of steroids, allowing a lower dose of methylprednisolone to be used, but may not reduce side-effects.

INHALER DEVICES

A wide range of devices is available to deliver drugs to the lung. When choosing an inhaler device, physicians should consider the efficacy of drug delivery, cost-effectiveness, safety, convenience, patient's age and ability to use the device. Pressurized metered-dose inhalers (pMDI) require training and skill to coordinate activation and inhalation. Spacers (holding chambers) improve drug delivery and reduce oropharyngeal deposition, thereby reducing systemic absorption and the risk of side effects.[1] Breath-actuated aerosols may be helpful for patients who have difficulty coordinating the pMDI. Dry powder inhalers (DPI) do not require propellants and are generally easier to use than pMDIs, but may be difficult to use during exacerbations.

Nebulizers are not preferred for maintenance treatment, as they are expensive, bulky, and require maintenance; furthermore, they deliver variable doses unless equipped with a dosimeter. It is important to emphasize that even for administration of inhaled β2-agonists during exacerbations, pMDIs with a spacer are the devices of choice, rather than nebulizers. A systematic review comparing MDI + spacer versus nebulizer delivery of SABAs in acute severe exacerbations showed equivalent clinical outcomes in adults, but the system was superior in children.[1] Simplicity of operation is especially important for treating infants and preschool children with MDI + spacer.

Whichever device is selected, patients should be instructed in its use, and their technique should be checked regularly.

FUTURE TRENDS IN ASTHMA TREATMENT

The role of specific immunotherapy in treating asthma is controversial, not least because the risk of adverse effects is much greater in patients with asthma than in those with rhinitis. Several new forms of immunotherapy are under development, which may improve the risk:benefit ratio (Chapter 93).

Various anti-cytokine strategies have been proposed and tested in asthma. TNF-α has been implicated in the pathogenesis of asthma, and in particular in the remodeling process that accompanies chronic severe asthma. A recent study in refractory asthma suggested upregulation of TNF-α, which might contribute to corticosteroid refractoriness.[43] An open study of TNF blockade with the soluble fusion protein etanercept reported improvement in asthma symptoms, lung function and quality of life, paralleled by a marked reduction in AHR.[44]

IL-4 is critical in the development of IgE but has several other actions relevant to asthma. Several approaches to IL-4 antagonism have been assessed in clinical trials, although none has yet proved very effective.[45] These include soluble humanized IL-4 receptors, a humanized anti-IL-4 monoclonal antibody, and a mutated form of IL-4 receptor that acts as a competitive antagonist of both the IL-4 and IL-13 receptors.[45] IL-4 and IL-13 signal through a shared surface receptor (IL-4 receptor α) that activates a specific transcription factor signal transducer and activator of transcription (STAT-6); this led to a search for inhibitors of STAT-6, and although peptide inhibitors that interfere with the interaction between STAT-6 and Janus kinases linked to the IL-4 receptor α have been discovered, it has proved difficult to deliver these intracellularly. Another potential target is suppressor of cytokine signaling (SOCS-1), a potent inhibitor of IL-4 signaling pathways.[45]

Intravenous infusion of anti-IL-5 antibodies (mepolizumab) markedly reduced the infiltration of eosinophils in peripheral blood and airway, but had no effect on the early or late response to allergen challenge or the baseline AHR, and proved ineffective in symptomatic asthma.[45] There is some evidence that blocking IL-13 might be more effective. Alternatively, using anti-inflammatory cytokines such as IL-10, IL-12, IL-18, IL-23 and interferon-γ might offer therapeutic potential.[45]

Several inhibitors of chemokine receptors are in development (e.g., antibodies that block IL-8; chemokine CC3 receptor antagonists). Moreover, inhibitory agents of the synthesis of multiple cytokines are also in clinical development.[45]

Another potential area for intervention is the range of adhesion molecules (selectins and their ligands, integrins, tissue matrix proteins, and members of the immunoglobulin gene superfamily) that have been identified through research into asthmatic airway inflammation. PSGL-1, ICAM-1, VCAM-1 and their ligands are all potential targets for asthma and allergy therapies because of their likely involvement in T-cell, mast cell, basophil, and eosinophil trafficking.

■ NONPHARMACOLOGICAL INTERVENTIONS ■

DIETARY MANIPULATION

Dietary interventions, such as supplementation with magnesium, sodium, antioxidants (vitamin C and selenium), omega-3 fatty acids, and calorie-controlled diets have been attempted, but in only a few controlled studies. Several Cochrane reviews have concluded that there is currently little evidence to support their use.

ALTERNATIVE/COMPLEMENTARY MEDICINE

The therapeutic efficacy of complementary/alternative treatments for asthma is not supported by currently available evidence. There is no evidence to allow any firm conclusion on the effect of herbal remedies on asthma. A Cochrane review on the role of acupuncture found no evidence of any benefit in asthma. Systematic reviews of several other unconventional approaches, such as homeopathy, manual therapy (physiotherapy, respiratory therapy, chiropractic and osteopathic techniques), psychological interventions, family therapy, relaxation therapies, and even speleotherapy, have been performed, all showing limited or no conclusive evidence of a benefit.

■ PATIENT EDUCATION AND FOLLOW-UP ■

Education is critical to ensure that patients understand the basic facts about asthma and its management, and take an active role in its control. Regular follow-up is essential to monitor symptoms and lung function, review treatment plans, inhaler technique, risk factors and methods to control them, all with the aim of ensuring that therapeutic goals are met and asthma control is achieved and maintained. The most appropriate method for follow-up will depend on the local healthcare system. A patient visit to a primary healthcare or specialist office, an outreach worker visit to patients' homes, or follow-up for asthma that is integrated with a visit for another reason can each be effective in providing ongoing care.[1]

Patient education and training should be a continual process, with the objective of providing patients and their families with adequate information so that they can successfully achieve control of the disease, adjust the medication as necessary according to a tailored plan, identify and avoid modifiable triggering factors, manage exacerbations, and maintain a satisfactory quality of life. The emphasis should be on developing an

ongoing partnership between healthcare professionals, the patient, and the patient's family. Education should focus on information regarding the disease process, its diagnosis, therapy and monitoring; patients should be taught the reasons for using the medications and the differences between 'relievers' and 'controllers,' and should receive regular training on the use of the inhaler devices. They should receive advice regarding preventive measures, detailed information on the signs and symptoms that suggest that asthma is worsening, and a contingency action plan for exacerbations, including criteria for initiating additional medicines, as well as advice on when and how to seek medical attention. Patients should be provided with written self-management plans having the most relevant information.

Table 40.5 Classification of severity of asthma exacerbations

Parameter	Mild	Moderate	Severe	Respiratory arrest imminent
Breathlessness	Walking	Talking; infant: softer, shorter cy, difficulty feeding	At rest infant stops feeding	
Speech	Sentences	Phrases	Words	Drowsy or confused
Alertness	May be agitated	Usually agitated	Usually agitated	Paradoxical
Respiratory rate	Increased	Increased	Often >30/min	Paradoxical
		Guide to rates of breathing associated with respiratory distress in awake children		
		Age	*Normal rate*	
		<2months	*<60/min*	
		2–12 months	*<50/min*	
		1–5 years	*<40/min*	
		6–8 years	*<30/min*	
Accessory muscle use	Usually not	Usually	Usually	Thoraco–abdominal movement
Wheeze	Moderate, often only end expiratory	Loud	Usually loud	Absence of wheeze
Heart rate (bpm)	<100	100–120	>120	Bradycardia
	Guide to limits of normal heart rate in children			
	Infants	*Age*	*Normal rate*	
	Preschool children	*2–12 months*	*<160/min*	
	School age children	*1–2 years*	*<120/min*	
		2–8 years	*<110/min*	
PEF After initial bronchodilator % predicted or % personal best	>80%	~60–80%	<60% 100 l/min in adults Or response lasts <2 hours	
Pao_2 (on air)	Normal (arterial blood gases not usually necessary)	>60 mmHg	<60 mmHg Possible cyanosis	
$Paco_2$	<45mmHg	<45 mmHg	>45 mmHg Possible respiratory failure	
Sat O_2% (on air)	>95%	91–95%	<90%	

*The presence of several parameters but not necessarily all indicate the severity of the attack.

(Adapted with permission from the GINA Workshop Report (2005) Global Strategy for Asthma Management and Prevention, available from http://www.ginasthma.org. Note: at the time of production of this book an updated/revised report was posted on the website, dated November 2006)

Education should be provided to patients of all ages, in a personalized fashion, over several consultations or visits. Revision and reinforcement are essential components of education provided by the healthcare professional, and a full discussion of expectations and expression of fears and concerns should be allowed.

A systematic review of 36 trials showed that compared with usual care patient education delivers significant benefits in terms of reduced morbidity and use of health services; the effects are greatest when the intervention includes written self-management action plans.[46]

COMPLIANCE

Noncompliance may be defined in a nonjudgmental way as failure to take treatment as agreed by the patient and the healthcare professional. Studies of adults and children across a broad range of diseases suggest noncompliance rates of around 50% with taking of regular preventive therapies.[1] Noncompliance may be identified by prescription monitoring, pill counting or drug assay, but at a clinical level it is best detected by asking about therapy in a way that acknowledges the likelihood of incomplete compliance.

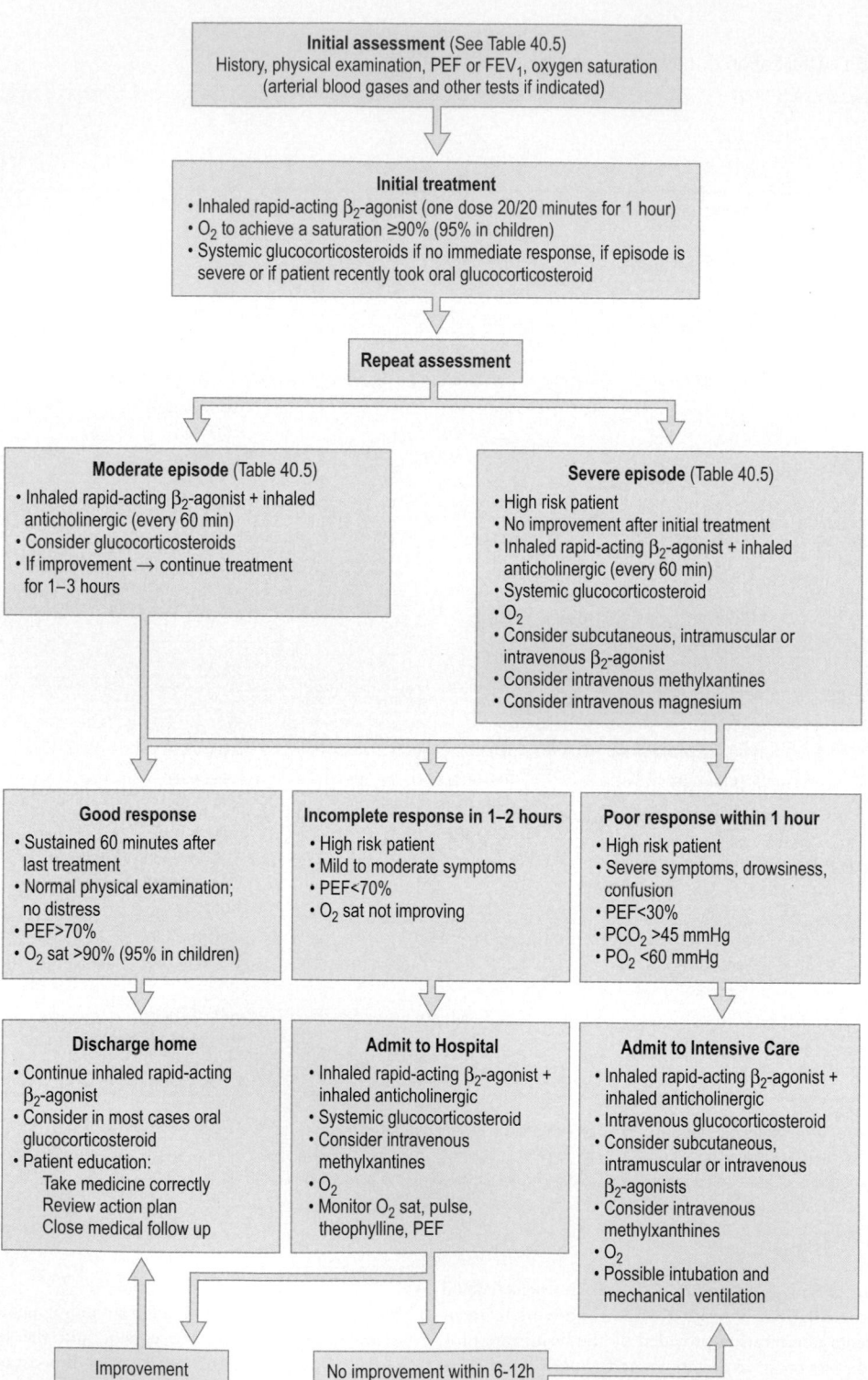

Fig. 40.4 Management of acute asthma exacerbations. (Adapted with permission from the GINA Workshop Report (2005): Global Strategy for Asthma Management and Prevention, available from http://www.ginasthma.org. Note: at the time of production of this book an updated/revised report was posted on the website, dated November 2006.)

MANAGEMENT OF ACUTE EXACERBATIONS

Acute exacerbations of asthma are what patients are most concerned about. Typically there is a progressive increase in shortness of breath, cough, wheezing, or chest tightness, or a combination of these symptoms. Exacerbations may come on gradually or over a very short timescale. The degree of exacerbation can be quantified by measuring reductions in expiratory airflow (PEF or FEV_1). Acute severe exacerbations can be life-threatening and may occur in patients at all levels of severity (see Box 40.1), and warrant prompt assessment and treatment (Table 40.5 and Fig. 40.4). In most patients deterioration progresses over hours or days, allowing action to be taken to mitigate the attack, but occasionally they can occur precipitously over a few minutes. A fatal outcome is most often associated with failure to recognize the severity of the exacerbation, inadequate action at its onset, and subsequent under-treatment.

Repeated administration of inhaled SABAs remains the mainstay of treatment, being the most effective means of relieving airflow obstruction.[1] Adding an anticholinergic drug provides more effective bronchodilatation than a $β_2$-agonist alone, resulting in a greater and more rapid improvement in lung function, avoiding prolonged emergency treatments and hospitalization.[33] Systemic glucocorticosteroids should be given early in the course of the exacerbation, even though they take some hours to become effective.[1] Oxygen should always be given, and careful attention paid to oxygen saturation. Deteriorating oxygen saturation or rising arterial CO_2 despite appropriate therapy are indications for ventilatory support. Once over the acute episode, careful review of the circumstances leading up to the exacerbation may help identify issues that could help to prevent future relapses.

CONCLUSION

Asthma management is based first on an accurate diagnosis, including the identification of specific and nonspecific triggers. Avoidance of potential risk and triggering factors is important, but unlikely to lead to resolution. As well as starting appropriate pharmacological therapy, patients should be educated on the nature and treatment of asthma, and how to recognize early signs of exacerbation. Pharmacological treatment should be individualized and tailored to the patient; it should be regularly reviewed and adjusted in a stepwise approach to achieve maximum control and minimize side effects. With appropriate management virtually all people with asthma should be able to control their condition and live full and productive lives.

REFERENCES

1. GINA Workshop Report (2005) Global Strategy for Asthma Management and Prevention. Available from http://www.ginasthma.org.

2. Pellegrino R, Viegi G, Brusasco V, et al. Interpretative strategies for lung function tests. Eur Respir J 2005; 26: 948–968.

3. Crapo RO, Casaburi R, Coates AL, et al. Guidelines for methacholine and exercise challenge testing – 1999. Am J Respir Crit Care Med 2000; 161: 309–329.

4. ATS/ERS recommendations for standardized procedures for the online and offline measurement of exhaled lower respiratory nitric oxide and nasal nitric oxide 2005. Am J Respir Crit Care Med 2005; 171: 912–930.

5. Pizzichini MM, Popov TA, Efthimiadis A, et al. Spontaneous and induced sputum to measure indices of airway inflammation in asthma. Am J Respir Crit Care Med 1996; 154: 866–869.

6. Jalaludin BB, Smith MA, Chey T, et al. Risk factors for asthma deaths: a population-based, case-control study. Aust NZ J Public Health 1999; 23: 595–600.

7. British guidelines on the management of asthma. Thorax 2003; 58: i1–94.

8. Becker A, Lemiere C, Berube D, et al. Summary of recommendations from the Canadian Asthma Consensus guidelines, 2003. Can Med Assoc J 2005; 173: S3–S11.

9. Gotzsche PC, Johansen HK, Schmidt LM, Burr ML. House dust mite control measures for asthma. Cochrane Database Syst Rev 2004; 4: CD001187.

10. Woodcock A, Forster L, Matthews E, et al. Control of exposure to mite allergen and allergen-impermeable bed covers for adults with asthma. N Engl J Med 2003; 349: 225–236.

11. Morgan WJ, Crain EF, Gruchalla RS, et al. Results of a home-based environmental intervention among urban children with asthma. N Engl J Med 2004; 351: 1068–1080.

12. Kilburn S, Lasserson TJ, McKean M. Pet allergen control measures for allergic asthma in children and adults. Cochrane Database Syst Rev 2003; 1: CD002989.

13. Johnston SL. Overview of virus-induced airway disease. Proc Am Thorac Soc 2005; 2: 150–156.

14. Johnston SL, Martin RJ. *Chlamydia pneumoniae* and *Mycoplasma pneumoniae*: a role in asthma pathogenesis?. Am J Respir Crit Care Med 2005; 172: 1078–1089.

15. Storms WW. Review of exercise-induced asthma. Med Sci Sports Exerc 2003; 35: 1464–1470.

16. Bousquet J, van Cauwenberge P, Khaltaev N. Allergic rhinitis and its impact on asthma. J Allergy Clin Immunol 2001; 108: S147–S334.

17. Harding SM. Gastroesophageal reflux: a potential asthma trigger. Immunol Allergy Clin North Am 2005; 25: 131–148.

18. Gibson PG, Henry RL, Coughlan JL. Gastro-oesophageal reflux treatment for asthma in adults and children. Cochrane Database Syst Rev 2003; 2: CD001496.

19. Barnes PJ. Corticosteroids: the drugs to beat. Eur J Pharmacol 2006; 533: 2–14.

20. Leung DY, Bloom JW. Update on glucocorticoid action and resistance. J Allergy Clin Immunol 2003; 111: 3–22.

21. Murray CS, Woodcock A, Langley SJ, et al. Secondary prevention of asthma by the use of inhaled fluticasone propionate in early childhood wheezing: double-blind, randomised, placebo-controlled study. Lancet 2006; 368: 754–672.

22. Lipworth BJ. Systemic adverse effects of inhaled corticosteroid therapy: A systematic review and meta-analysis. Arch Intern Med 1999; 159: 941–955.

23. Jones A, Fay JK, Burr M, et al. Inhaled corticosteroid effects on bone metabolism in asthma and mild chronic obstructive pulmonary disease. Cochrane Database Syst Rev 2002; 1: CD003537.

24. Lipworth BJ. Leukotriene-receptor antagonists. Lancet 1999; 353: 57–62.

25. van der Wouden JC, Tasche MJ, Bernsen RM, et al. Inhaled sodium cromoglycate for asthma in children. Cochrane Database Syst Rev 2003; 3: CD002173.

26. Shah L, Wilson AJ, Gibson PG, Coughlan J. Long acting beta-agonists versus theophylline for maintenance treatment of asthma. Cochrane Database Syst Rev 2003; 3: CD001281.

27. Nelson HS. Beta-adrenergic bronchodilators. N Engl J Med 1995; 333: 499–506.

28. Nelson HS, Weiss ST, Bleecker ER, Yancey SW, Dorinsky PM, the SMART Study Group. The Salmeterol Multicenter Asthma Research Trial: a comparison of usual pharmacotherapy for asthma or usual pharmacotherapy plus salmeterol. Chest 2006; 129: 15–26.

29. Salmeterol Postmarketing Study Review (SMART Study).Updated 2006. US Food and Drug Administration. Available on Accessed June 1, 2006, at http://www.fda.gov/ohrms/dockets/ac/05/briefing/2005–4148B1_03_02-FDA-Smart-Study.pdf

30. Gross NJ. Anticholinergic agents in asthma and COPD. Eur J Pharmacol 2006; 533: 36–39.

31. Rodrigo G, Rodrigo C, Burschtin O. A meta-analysis of the effects of ipratropium bromide in adults with acute asthma. Am J Med 1999; 107: 363–370.

32. Kanazawa H. Anticholinergic agents in asthma: chronic bronchodilator therapy, relief of acute severe asthma, reduction of chronic viral inflammation and prevention of airway remodelling. Curr Opin Pulm Med 2006; 12: 60–67.

33. Stoodley RG, Aaron SD, Dales RE. The role of ipratropium bromide in the emergency management of acute asthma exacerbation: a meta-analysis of randomized clinical trials. Ann Emerg Med 1999; 34: 8–18.

34. Parameswaran K, Belda J, Rowe BH. Addition of intravenous aminophylline to beta2-agonists in adults with acute asthma. Cochrane Database Syst Rev 2000; 4: CD002742.

35. Mitra A, Bassler D, Goodman K, et al. Intravenous aminophylline for acute severe asthma in children over two years receiving inhaled bronchodilators. Cochrane Database Syst Rev 2005; 2: CD001276.

36. Strunk RC, Bloomberg GR. Omalizumab for Asthma. N Engl J Med 2006; 354: 2689–2695.

37. Walker S, Monteil M, Phelan K, et al. Anti-IgE for chronic asthma in adults and children. Cochrane Database Syst Rev 2006; 2: CD003559.

38. Johnston SL, Blasi F, Black PN, et al. The effect of telithromycin in acute exacerbations of asthma. N Engl J Med 2006; 354: 1589–1600.

39. Davies H, Olson L, Gibson P. Methotrexate as a steroid sparing agent for asthma in adults. Cochrane Database Syst Rev 2000; 2: CD000391.

40. Dewey A, Dean T, Bara A, et al. Colchicine as an oral corticosteroid sparing agent for asthma. Cochrane Database Syst Rev 2003; 4: CD003273.

41. Dean T, Dewey A, Bara A, et al. Chloroquine as a steroid sparing agent for asthma. Cochrane Database Syst Rev 2003; 4: CD003275.

42. Dewey A, Bara A, Dean T, Walters H. Dapsone as an oral corticosteroid sparing agent for asthma. Cochrane Database Syst Rev 2002; 4: CD003268.

43. Berry MA, Hargadon B, Shelley M, et al. Evidence of a role of tumor necrosis factor alpha in refractory asthma. N Engl J Med 2006; 354: 697–708.

44. Holgate ST, Holloway J, Wilson S, et al. Understanding the pathophysiology of severe asthma to generate new therapeutic opportunities. J Allergy Clin Immunol 2006; 117: 496–506.

45. Yamagata T, Ichinose M. Agents against cytokine synthesis or receptors. Eur J Pharmacol 2006; 533: 289–301.

46. Gibson PG, Powell H, Coughlan J, et al. Self-management education and regular practitioner review for adults with asthma. Cochrane Database Syst Rev 2003; 1: CD001117.

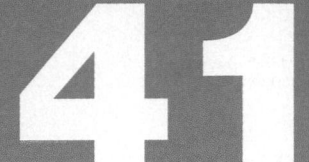

Rhinitis and sinusitus

Mark S. Dykewicz

Rhinitis and sinusitis are among the most common medical conditions, and frequently coexist.[1–6] In western societies it is estimated that 10–25% of the population suffer from allergic rhinitis.[1–3] In the US, sinusitis affects about 31 million patients annually.[6] Both rhinitis and sinusitis can have a tremendous adverse impact on individuals and society. They can significantly reduce quality of life, aggravate comorbid conditions and require significant medical expenditure. Both conditions create an even greater indirect cost to society by reducing workplace productivity and learning in school, and by causing a tremendous number of absences from work and school.

■ RHINITIS ■

Although the term 'rhinitis' connotes inflammation of the nasal mucous membranes, some rhinitis disorders are not always characterized by inflammatory cell infiltrates. Instead, rhinitis can be viewed clinically as a heterogeneous group of nasal disorders characterized by one or more of the following: nasal congestion, rhinorrhea, nasal itching and sneezing. Rhinitis can be caused by allergic, nonallergic, infectious, hormonal, occupational, and other factors.[1, 2] Although allergic rhinitis is the most

CLINICAL PEARLS

RHINITIS

>> At least one-third of perennial rhinitis patients have no allergic basis.

>> Nasal corticosteroids are the most effective drug class for allergic rhinitis.

>> Food-induced rhinitis in adults is usually a cholinergic response, and rarely involves IgE-mediated food allergy.

>> Nasal corticosteroids and oral antihistamines have similar effectiveness in relieving eye symptoms associated with allergic rhinitis.

common type of chronic rhinitis, nonallergic rhinitis has been reported to account for 30–70% of patients with chronic perennial rhinitis.[1]

NASAL ANATOMY AND PHYSIOLOGY

The nasal cavity is partitioned by the nasal septum, a structure formed from cartilage distally and bone proximally.[3] The lateral aspects of the nasal cavity contain the inferior, middle, and superior turbinates, important for humidification, temperature regulation and air filtration (Fig. 41.1). The nasal cavity is lined with mucosa composed of pseudostratified columnar ciliated epithelium that overlies a basement membrane and the submucosa (lamina propria). The submucosa contains serous and seromucous nasal glands and an extensive network of blood vessels, nerves and cellular elements. Because the nasal tissues are highly vascular, vascular changes can play a prominent role in nasal obstruction. Covering the nasal epithelium is a thin layer of mucus that is transported by ciliary action to the posterior nasopharynx. [IM1]

Sympathetic nerve stimulation causes vasoconstriction and resultant decreases in nasal airway resistance to airflow. Conversely, parasympathetic nerve stimulation can increase nasal congestion and resistance, but more importantly upregulates the secretion of mucus from nasal mucosal glands. Nonadrenergic, noncholinergic (NANC) neuropeptides (substance P, neurokinins A and K, neuropeptide tyrosine and calcitonin gene-related peptide) have a putative role in promoting vasodilatation, mucus secretion, plasma extravasation, neurogenic inflammation, and mast cell nerve interactions, but their relative clinical importance is not yet defined.[1, 3] Alterations in the autonomic tone of the nasal vasculature cause side-to-side fluctuation in nasal engorgement and airflow, called nasal cycling, with period lengths ranging from approximately 1 to 5 hours.

PATHOPHYSIOLOGY OF ALLERGIC RHINITIS

As with allergic asthma, allergic rhinitis can be caused by a variety of airborne protein and glycoprotein allergens from pollens, molds, dust mite fecal particles, cockroach residues and animal danders. After inhalation of allergenic particles, allergens are eluted in nasal mucus and subsequently

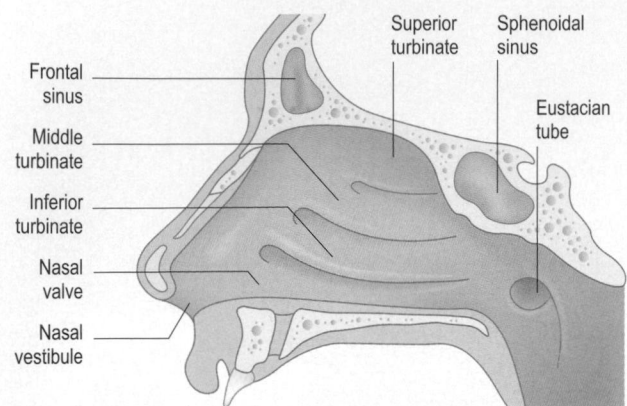

Fig. 41.1 Nasal anatomy. (Modified from: Adkinson NF Jr, Yunginger JW, Busse WW, et al. Middleton's allergy principles and practice, 6th edn. Philadelphia: Mosby, 2003; 1412.)

diffused into nasal tissues. In addition, inhaled, small molecular weight airborne chemicals (e.g., from occupational exposures or drugs) can act as haptens when they react with self proteins in the airway to form complete allergens. In nasal tissues, the sensitization process is initiated when antigen-presenting cells (dendritic cells, especially CD1+ Langerhans'-like cells, and macrophages) present allergen to CD4 T lymphocytes.[7] Next, stimulated CCR3+ CD4+ T cells, with possible contribution by CD8 Tc2 cells, release IL-3, IL-4, IL-5, IL-13, and other cytokines which produce a cascade of events that promote local and systemic IgE production by plasma cells; chemotaxis; and inflammatory cell recruitment, localization, proliferation, activation, and prolonged survival within the airway mucosa.[3,8] CD8 Tc1 cells that release IFN-γ, possibly activated by IL-15, can inhibit initiation of the process.[9]

Early/immediate allergic response

Within minutes of exposure of sensitized individuals to allergens, IgE-mediated degranulation of mast cells and basophils causes the release of pre-formed mediators such as histamine and tryptase, and de novo generation of other mediators, including cysteinyl leukotrienes and prostaglandin D_2 (PGD_2)[1,3] (Chapter 22). Mediators induce leakage of plasma from blood vessels and dilation of arteriole venule anastomoses, with resultant edema, blood pooling in the cavernous sinusoids (the predominant cause of the perceived congestion), and occlusion of nasal passages. Mediators also stimulate the secretion of mucus from goblet and glandular cells. Histamine is the principal mediator responsible for itching, rhinorrhea, and sneezing, whereas other mediators such as leukotrienes and PGD_2 probably play a greater role in the development of nasal congestion.[1] The perception of nasal itching and congestion occurs via stimulation of sensory nerves, whereas sneezing paroxysms are triggered by systemic neurogenic reflexes.[1]

Late-phase response

Mediators and cytokines released during the early phase trigger a cascade of events over the following 4–8 hours which culminate in inflammatory responses that characterize the late-phase response. Although the clinical

features of the immediate and late responses are similar, nasal congestion becomes more prominent in the late response.[1–3] Mediators and cytokines produced during the early response upregulate expression of cell adhesion molecules, such as vascular cell adhesion molecule (VCAM1) and E-selectin on post-capillary endothelial cells. As a result, circulating leukocytes adhere to the endothelium as part of the inflammatory process. Inflammation is further promoted by chemoattractant factors, including IL-5, that promote infiltration of the superficial lamina propria of the mucosa by eosinophils, neutrophils and basophils, and eventually CD4 (Th2) lymphocytes and macrophages.[1] The inflammatory cascade progresses as these cells become activated and release further mediators, which in turn activate other proinflammatory responses. Ultimately eosinophils predominate in nasal secretions, whereas CD4 (Th_2) lymphocytes predominate in nasal biopsy specimens.[10]

RELATIONSHIP BETWEEN RHINITIS AND ASTHMA

Asthma and rhinitis are comorbid conditions that are associated both epidemiologically and pathophysiologically.[1–3, 11] (Table 41.1). More than 80% of persons with allergic asthma have allergic rhinitis (AR), and AR is a risk factor for the development of asthma.[1] Guidelines recommend that patients with persistent AR should be evaluated for asthma, and patients with asthma should be evaluated for rhinitis.[1]

CLINICAL PRESENTATION OF DIFFERENT TYPES OF RHINITIS

In addition to the four classic symptoms of AR (rhinorrhea, nasal congestion, sneezing, nasal itching), patients with AR commonly experience symptoms of conjunctivitis (eye pruritus, lacrimation, chemosis) [IM4].[1] Postnasal drip occurs commonly, as do associated symptoms involving the ears, eyes, and throat. Symptoms of AR frequently overlap with symptoms associated with other forms of rhinitis and various anatomic abnormalities of the upper airway.

Nonallergic rhinitis without eosinophilia, variably termed vasomotor rhinitis (VMR) or idiopathic rhinitis,[1–3] is not caused by allergic or infectious processes, but is probably a heterogeneous group of disorders whose pathogenesis is incompletely understood. Nasal obstruction and/or rhinorrhea are prominent symptoms, with sneezing and pruritus being less common. The term VMR is sometimes used more selectively to indicate nasal symptoms that occur in response to nonallergic environmental stimuli, such as changes in temperature or relative humidity, perfumes, cleaning materials, tobacco smoke, alcohol ingestion and sexual arousal. Such hyperreactivity to nonallergic triggers may also occur in AR, a clinical picture that is sometimes termed 'mixed rhinitis.' In recent years, computerized tomography (CT) has revealed that many patients diagnosed with VMR do in fact have chronic sinusitis or other disorders.[4]

Nonallergic rhinitis with eosinophilia syndrome (NARES) is characterized by perennial nasal symptoms and typically presents with prominent nasal congestion, sneezing paroxysms, profuse watery rhinorrhea, nasal pruritus, and occasional loss of smell.[1–3] Nasal smears demonstrate eosinophils, but patients are not allergic to environmental allergens. It has been proposed that NARES may be an early stage of aspirin sensitivity.

Hormonal rhinitis can be caused by hormonal changes of pregnancy, menstrual cycle, puberty, or thyroid disorders.[1–3] During pregnancy,

Table 41.1 Comparative immunopathology and pathophysiology of allergic rhinitis and asthma (Modified from Gelfand EW. Inflammatory mediators in allergic rhinitis. J Allergy Clin Immunol 2004; 114: S135–138 with permission from Elsevier.)

Similarities	Differences
Similar immunologic processes	Nose (ectodermal) and bronchial (endodermal) airways have a different embryologic origin.
Similar pathologic findings in nasal and bronchial tissue	Genes governing repair-remodeling might be different.
Eosinophils, mast cells, Th2 lymphocytes	Smooth muscle is only present in the bronchi.
Early- and late-phase responses	Nose contains a large supply of subepithelial capillaries, arterial systems, and venous cavernous sinusoids.
Hyperresponsiveness: sensorineural in nasal passages and airways in response to allergen challenge	

congestion and other rhinitis symptoms can develop de novo during the second month of gestation and continue to term, but usually resolve shortly after delivery. However, most pregnant women with nasal symptoms have pre-existing rhinitis that may worsen, improve, or remain the same during pregnancy.[1]

Drug-induced rhinitis can be induced by either oral and topical medications.[1–3] Causal oral medications include ACE inhibitors, β-blockers, various other antihypertensive agents, aspirin and other cyclo-oxygenase-1 inhibitors, oral contraceptives or conjugated estrogens. The use of topical α-adrenergic decongestant sprays for more than 5–7 days may induce rebound nasal congestion upon withdrawal (rhinitis medicamentosa). Repeated use of intranasal cocaine and methamphetamines may also result in rebound congestion, and occasionally septal erosion and perforation.

IgE-mediated sensitivity is rarely responsible for rhinitis caused by food ingestion, in the absence of reactions involving other organ systems.[1–3] Ethanol can produce nasal symptoms via nasal vasodilation.[1] Gustatory rhinitis is a cholinergically mediated syndrome of postprandial watery rhinorrhea that may be more pronounced after eating hot and spicy foods, and becomes more common with age.

DIFFERENTIAL DIAGNOSIS OF RHINITIS

Acute viral upper respiratory infection presents with nasal symptoms and constitutional symptoms (fever, myalgias, malaise), but pruritus is typically absent and symptoms usually resolve within 7–10 days.[4–6] Acute and chronic bacterial sinusitis may be difficult to distinguish clinically from rhinitis (see Sinusitis below).

Anatomic abnormalities (e.g., septal deviation, nasal polyps) usually present with prominent obstructive symptoms but less in the way of rhinorrhea. Septal deviation, albeit often asymptomatic, may cause unilateral or bilateral congestion. Diagnosis may be made by observing external deviation of the nose or examining the anterior nasal cavity, but may require fiberoptic rhinopharyngoscopy or CT scanning.

Other differential diagnoses for nasal symptoms include nasal tumors (benign or malignant) that commonly present with obstruction.[1–3] Nasal carcinoma may present with unilateral epistaxis and nasal pain. Juvenile angiofibromas often present with bleeding in adolescent males. Young children may have intranasal foreign bodies (e.g. toy parts, or foods such as peanuts) causing a foul-smelling, purulent discharge and unilateral

nasal obstruction that predisposes to sinusitis. Adenoidal hypertrophy causes bilateral nasal obstruction in young children, with associated nocturnal mouth-breathing and snoring. Systemic diseases that cause nasal symptoms include Wegener's granulomatosis, which may present with nasal and sinus complaints, including purulent rhinorrhea and septal ulcerations and perforations; sarcoidosis, which may present with nasal congestion; and Sjögren's syndrome, which may cause nasal dryness, congestion, and crusting.

CSF rhinorrhea usually develops either immediately or within a few months of trauma, although it may occur spontaneously. Typically it presents with a unilateral, clear, watery discharge. The discharge often tests positive for glucose, although β_2-transferrin is more sensitive and specific.[12]

DIAGNOSIS

History

The history should include specific symptoms that trouble the patient (e.g., nasal congestion, pruritus, rhinorrhea, sneezing); symptom patterns (seasonal or perennial, intermittent or persistent); precipitating factors; response to previous medications; coexisting conditions (e.g., asthma, sinusitis, otitis); and a detailed environmental history, including home and occupational exposures.[1–3] In distinguishing allergic from nonallergic rhinitis, nasal itching, eye pruritus and lacrimation make allergy more likely. Because in most temperate regions trees pollinate in the spring, grasses in the late spring and early summer, and weeds in the late summer and fall, a corresponding history of seasonal symptoms suggests allergy. However, in certain regions molds and some pollens may cause perennial symptoms. Although allergens such as house dust mites, cockroaches, and animals cause perennial symptoms, approximately one-third of patients with perennial rhinitis have no underlying allergy. Family history is an important clue in making the diagnosis of AR in children.

Physical examination

Nasal examination can be performed with a handheld otoscope or nasal speculum that permits viewing of the anterior third of the nasal airway, including the anterior tip of the inferior turbinates (and occasionally the anterior tip of the middle turbinates) and portions of the nasal septum.[1-3] However, fiberoptic rhinoscopy may be required to visualize other abnormalities, such as nasal polyps, septal deviation, or masses. Typically, patients with AR have a clear discharge, swollen turbinates, and bluish or pale mucosa. Pale or erythematous mucosa can be seen in various types of nonallergic rhinitis. Both allergic and nonallergic rhinitis can cause 'allergic shiners,' infraorbital darkening attributed to chronic venous pooling, or a persistent horizontal crease across the nose in children who rub their noses upward because of nasal discomfort – the so-called 'allergic salute.' In association with rhinitis, the presence of mild bilateral conjunctivitis is suggestive of allergy. Patients with nasal disease require appropriate examination for associated diseases, such as sinusitis, otitis media and asthma.[1-3]

Diagnostic testing

Testing for specific IgE antibodies to allergens is important when avoidance measures or immunotherapy are being considered, and is of particular importance in perennial rhinitis, where it is more difficult to distinguish allergic or nonallergic rhinitis on the basis of history. Although *in vitro* tests are improving and approaching skin testing in sensitivity (Chapter 100), in a large randomized trial skin-prick tests had a better positive predictive value (48.7%) for the diagnosis of AR than did *in vitro* testing (Phadiatop) (43.5%).[13]

The presence of eosinophils in nasal cytology may aid in differentiating AR and NARES from other forms of rhinitis, such as vasomotor or infectious rhinitis, provided the correct procedure is followed and the appropriate stains are used.[1-3]

In selected cases, special techniques such as fiberoptic nasal endoscopy, inspiratory peak flow measurements, acoustic rhinometry, or rhinomanometry to assess airway function may be useful in evaluating patients presenting with rhinitis symptoms. Nasal endoscopy permits direct visualization of abnormalities of the septum, turbinates, mucosa, nasopharynx, adenoids, and eustachian tube orifice.

TREATMENT

Avoidance measures

Avoidance of inciting factors, such as allergens (house dust mites, molds, pets, pollens, cockroaches), irritants, and medications, can effectively reduce symptoms of rhinitis.[1, 2] Exposure to outdoor allergens can be reduced by keeping windows closed, using an air conditioner, and limiting the amount of time spent outdoors. Measures to reduce house dust mite exposure should focus on use of allergen-impermeable casings on the bed and pillows, including polyester pillows.[1-3]

Medications

As some medications are more effective for treating certain types of rhinitis or rhinitis symptoms, or more suitable for episodic rather than continuous use, the selection of medications should be individualized, taking into account the symptoms most troublesome to a patient, their severity, and whether they are episodic or more persistent, the likely underlying cause(s) of rhinitis, cost-effectiveness and patient preference.[1, 2] The AR guidelines published by the American Academy of Allergy, Asthma, and Immunology in conjunction with 20 other organizations, is a stepped approach that considers symptom severity, intermittent or persistent disease, and whether medications are best used on a daily or an as-needed basis (Fig. 41.2).[14] The Allergic Rhinitis in Asthma (ARIA) guidelines[1] advocate a conceptually consistent scheme for management based on the severity of rhinitis and whether symptoms are *intermittent* (defined as present <4 days per week or <4 weeks' duration) or *persistent* (present on >4 days per week or >4 weeks' duration).[1]

Oral antihistamines

Acting as competitive inhibitors for H_1 receptors, oral antihistamines act to reduce rhinorrhea, sneezing, and nasal pruritus associated with AR, but have less effect on nasal congestion.[1-3] Antihistamines are effective when taken occasionally for episodic symptoms, but work best when administered regularly. Antihistamines are a first-line therapy for milder AR,[1, 2] but have little role in treating nonallergic rhinitis syndromes. First-generation antihistamines (e.g., diphenhydramine and chlorpheniramine) can cause perceived sedation and unperceived impairment of mental functioning, and are associated with automobile accidents, decreased work performance and productivity, and impairment of children's learning and academic performance.[1-3, 15] They can also cause anticholinergic side effects, such as dry mouth and urinary retention. Second-generation antihistamines, which are associated with less risk (cetirizine) or no risk for these side effects compared to placebo (e.g., desloratadine, loratadine, fexofenadine), should usually be considered before sedating antihistamines for the treatment of AR.[1, 2]

Oral decongestants

Through their α-adrenergic vasoconstrictor effects, oral decongestants (e.g., pseudoephedrine, phenylephrine) reduce nasal congestion produced by allergic and nonallergic forms of rhinitis.[1, 2] However, they may cause insomnia, nervousness, loss of appetite, urinary retention, and may aggravate cardiac arrhythmias, hypertension, and manifestations of hyperthyroidism.

Topical decongestants

Topical decongestant nasal sprays (e.g., oxymetazoline, phenylephrine) reduce nasal congestion in both allergic and nonallergic rhinitis, but should be limited to short-term use (e.g., 3–10 days) to avoid rebound nasal congestion (rhinitis medicamentosa).[1, 2] When there is significant edema of inferior nasal mucosal structures that would impair delivery of other nasal sprays to more superior/posterior regions of the nose, guidelines advocate use of a nasal decongestant spray during the first several days of treatment with other nasal sprays in order to improve drug delivery and effectiveness.[2]

Intranasal antihistamines

Intranasal azelastine is effective in the treatment of AR and vasomotor rhinitis.[1-3] It is at least as effective as oral antihistamines, but less effective than nasal glucocorticoids.[16] It has some effect on nasal obstruction, but less than intranasal glucocorticoids. Side effects may include a bitter taste and sedation.

Severity	Daily medication	Quick-relief medication
Intermittent symptoms	None	
Persistent mild-to-moderate disease Consider referral to an allergy/immunology specialist or otolaryngologic allergy specialist for consultation or comanagement (see page 27)	Oral nonsedating H_2-antihistamine (with or without a decongestant combination). **or** Topical nasal corticosteriod (preferably start therapy 1 to 2 weeks before season and continue through season) **Consider:** Topical nasal antihistamine; nasal cromolyn sodium for children If there are prominent eye symptoms topical ocular anthistamine with or without vasoconstrictor, topical ocular mast cell stabilizer and/or topical ocular NSAID	Rapid onset oral non-sedating H_2-antihistamine **or** Topical nasal antihistamine **Consider:** Nasal cromolyn sodium as a preventive measure before anticipated allergen exposures
Severe disease Referral to an allergy/immunology specialist or otolaryngologic allergy specialist for consultation or comanagement is recomended (see page 27)	Topical nasal corticosteriod (preferably start therapy 1–2 weeks before season and continue through season) **And:** Oral nonsedating H_2-antihistamine (with or without a decongestant combination) **Consider:** Topical nasal antihistamine; nasal cromolyn sodium for children **And:** if needed A short course (3–10 days) of oral corticosteriods If there are prominent eye symptoms topical ocular anthistamine with or without vasoconstrictor, topical ocular mast cell stabilizer and/or topical ocular NSAID	

Fig. 41.2 Stepped management of allergic rhinitis. This stepped approach for treatment of seasonal allergic rhinitis considers symptom severity, intermittent or persistent disease, and whether medications are best used on a daily or as-needed basis. Although this figure depicts recommendations for seasonal allergic rhinitis, recommendations for perennial allergic rhinitis are similar. (From Rhinitis. In: The allergy report. Vol. 2. Diseases of the atopic diathesis. American Academy of Allergy, Asthma and Immunology, Milwaukee, 2000. p 20. Online. Available: http://www.aaaai.org/ar/working_vol2/020.asp 31 July 2006.)

Intranasal corticosteroids

Possessing a broad array of anti-inflammatory effects, intranasal corticosteroids are the most effective medication class for treatment of AR.[1-3, 15] Moreover, they are also useful in some forms of nonallergic rhinitis. Nasal corticosteroids and oral antihistamines have similar effectiveness in relieving eye symptoms associated with AR.[17] Modern preparations are not associated with significant systemic side effects in adults. Growth suppression in children has been associated with intranasal beclomethasone,[18] but not from several other nasal corticosteroid preparations.[19, 20] Local nasal irritation and bleeding may occur. The nasal septum should be examined periodically to assure that there are no mucosal erosions that may precede the development of perforations, which may rarely occur from intranasal corticosteroid use.[2] Although these drugs are most effective when given on a regular schedule, some agents have a demonstrated onset of effect within 24 hours or less,[1,2] and PRN use of fluticasone nasal has been demonstrated to be more effective than PRN use of oral loratadine for seasonal AR.[21]

Leukotriene receptor antagonists

In addition to their efficacy for treatment of asthma, leukotriene receptor antagonists (montekulast, zafirlukast) have been demonstrated to have benefit for all principal symptoms of AR.[22] By meta-analysis, these drugs are equivalent to oral histamine H_1 antagonists, but inferior to intranasal corticosteroids for seasonal AR. The combination of leukotriene receptor antagonists and histamine H_1 antagonists is statistically inferior to intranasal corticosteroids for relief of nasal congestion.[22] There is a low incidence of side effects with this class of drugs.

CLINICAL PEARLS

SINUSITIS

>> An acute upper respiratory illness sinusitis of less than approximately 7 days' duration is most commonly caused by viral illness, whereas bacterial sinusitis becomes more likely beyond 7–10 days.

>> Many cases of chronic sinusitis are not caused by bacterial infections, and antibiotic treatment is of unproven benefit.

>> 'Sinus headaches' are not typically caused by chronic sinusitis, but more commonly by migraines.

>> Anosmia in chronic sinusitis is suggestive of nasal polyps.

Intranasal cromolyn

Intranasal cromolyn sodium is beneficial in allergic but not nonallergic rhinitis, but is less effective than oral antihistamines or intranasal antihistamines and intranasal corticosteroids.[1, 2] Optimally administered four to six times daily, nasal cromolyn should ideally be started before major symptoms develop during a season, as it may take several weeks to be fully effective. It can also be used for acute prophylaxis before exposure to a known allergen. Cromolyn has an excellent safety profile.

Intranasal ipratropium

Intranasal ipratropium bromide is an anticholinergic agent effective in reducing rhinorrhea in AR, nonallergic rhinitis, and viral upper respiratory infections, but has no benefit for other rhinitis symptoms.[1–3] Ipratropium can provide acute prophylaxis against rhinorrhea triggered by known stimuli (e.g., food in gustatory rhinitis). It does not cause significant systemic anticholinergic effects.

Systemic corticosteroids

Short-acting oral corticosteroids (e.g., prednisone, methylprednisolone) are used in brief courses (e.g., prednisone 30 mg/day for 3–7 days for adults) for the treatment of very severe or intractable nasal symptoms.[2] The use of parenteral corticosteroids is discouraged because of their greater potential for suppression of the hypopituitary–adrenal (HPA) axis and long-term corticosteroid side effects.[2]

ALLERGEN IMMUNOTHERAPY/ALLERGY VACCINATION

Allergen immunotherapy may be highly effective in controlling the symptoms of AR, and can favorably modify the long-term course of the disease.[1–3, 23] AR patients should be considered candidates for immunotherapy on the basis of the severity of their symptoms, failure or unacceptability of other treatment modalities, presence of comorbid conditions, and possibly as a means of preventing the condition worsening or the development of comorbid conditions (e.g., asthma, sinusitis).[1, 2, 23]

■ SINUSITIS ■

Sinusitis is classically defined as inflammation of one or more of the paranasal sinuses, air-filled cavities in facial bones lined with pseudostratified ciliated columnar epithelium and mucous goblet cells. The term rhinosinusitis is increasingly used in recognition that rhinitis (whether allergic or nonallergic) typically accompanies sinusitis.[5, 6] Sinusitis without rhinitis is rare, the mucosa of the nose and sinuses are anatomically contiguous, and symptoms of nasal obstruction and discharge are prominent in sinusitis.[4] In the following discussion, the terms sinusitis and rhinosinusitis will be used interchangeably, a reflection of the varying preference for use of these terms in cited medical literature.

According to major national and international guidelines, acute sinusitis is defined as lasting less than 4 (or 12) weeks, whereas chronic sinusitis persists longer than 12 weeks.[4–6] In some guidelines, disease of 4–12 weeks' duration is termed subacute.[4] Recurrent sinusitis refers to repeated episodes of acute sinusitis, typically more than three times per year, often further defined to require the absence of intervening signs and symptoms of chronic rhinosinusitis.[4]

SINUS ANATOMY AND PHYSIOLOGY

Epithelial cilia in the sinuses normally beat in an orderly fashion to move mucus towards the ostia that communicate with the nasal cavity. Rather than draining through simple ostia, the anterior ethmoid, maxillary, and frontal sinuses drain through a comparatively convoluted and narrow drainage pathway, the ostiomeatal complex, which communicates into the middle meatus, between the inferior and middle turbinates (Fig. 41.3). Obstruction of the ostiomeatal complex is thought to be particularly important in promoting some forms of persistent sinus disease. The posterior ethmoid sinuses drain into the upper meatus, whereas the sphenoid sinuses drain into the posterior wall in the sphenoethmoidal recess. The ethmoid sinuses consist of a 'honeycomb' of cells lying medial to the orbital structures and varying between four and 17 air cells in number. Whereas the mucosa of normal paranasal sinuses has relatively few glands, inflamed sinus mucosa contains more developed and pathological mucous glands.[4]

MICROBIOLOGY

Acute viral upper respiratory infections are the most frequent cause of acute sinus inflammation.[4–6] Organisms commonly causing acute bacterial sinusitis include *Streptococcus pneumoniae*, *Hemophilus influenzae*, and *Moraxella catarrhalis*. Polysaccharide coatings typical of these bacteria impair phagocytosis. In addition, many of these bacteria secrete molecules that interfere with mucociliary clearance.[24] The most common bacterial species isolated in chronic sinusitis, in addition to those just mentioned, are *Staphylococcus aureus*, Gram-negative enteric organisms (including *Pseudomonas aeruginosa*), and anaerobes, such as *Prevotella* spp, and fusobacteria. However, the role of infection in most patients with chronic sinusitis is controversial and the microbiology results may just reflect colonization.[4] Fungal sinusitis has been traditionally divided into four primary categories: acute infectious/fulminant (invasive); chronic/indolent (invasive); fungus ball (noninvasive); and allergic. In addition, it has been proposed that noninvasive fungal colonization of the upper airway is an underlying cause of chronic sinusitis, although this is controversial.[25, 26]

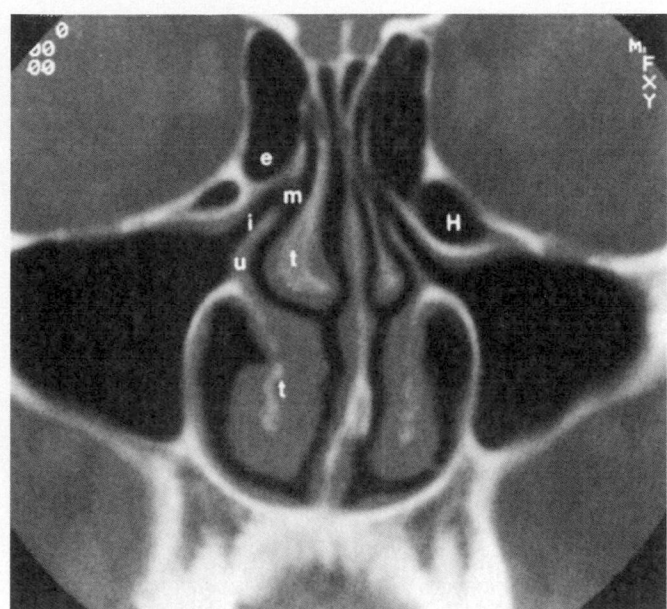

Fig. 41.3 Anatomy of sinuses with normal ostiomeatal complex. Coronal noncontrast CT scan demonstrates the ostiomeatal complex. Normal mucociliary drainage is from the maxillary sinus up through the infundibulum (i) and maxillary sinus ostium into the middle meatus (m). The ethmoid bulla (e) and uncinate process (u) form the lateral and medial walls of the infundibulum, respectively. A normal anatomic variant of a Haller air cell (H) underlying the orbit causes a mild narrowing of the left infundibulum. A smaller Haller cell is present on the right. The mild asymmetry of the mucosa of the inferior turbinates (it) and middle turbinates is part of the normal nasal cycle. (Modified from Cummings CW, Flint PW, Haughey BH, et al. Otolaryngology head and neck surgery, 4th edn. Philadelphia: Elsevier, 2005; 80.)

FACTORS INCREASING RISK FOR SINUSITIS

Many factors have been reported to predispose to sinusitis, although the level of evidence that supports such causal associations varies greatly for different factors. Reported factors include viral upper respiratory tract infections, rhinitis (allergic and non allergic), anatomical abnormalities (foreign body, nasal polyps, nasal septal deviation, enlarged tonsils and adenoids, concha bullosa and other middle turbinate abnormalities), tumors, trauma (physical, chemical, or barotrauma), cystic fibrosis, antibody deficiency, acquired immunodeficiency syndrome, ciliary dyskinesia, Kartagener's syndrome, Young's syndrome, systemic diseases (e.g., Churg–Strauss syndrome, Wegener's granulomatosis), and dental infection.[4–6] More important factors are thought to be obstruction of the sinus ostia, impaired ciliary function, and impaired host immunity (especially antibody deficiency).[4, 5] Mucosal edema, as may occur from rhinitis or anatomic abnormalities (e.g., nasal polyps, septal deviation) that obstruct drainage from or ventilation of sinuses, promotes mucus accumulation in the sinuses, serum transudation, and decreased oxygenation within the sinuses.[4] These changes result in impaired ciliary movement of mucus and promotion of bacterial growth. More recently, gastroesophageal reflux disease (GERD) has been suggested as a cause of sinusitis, and several studies report that medical treatment of GERD results in improvement in sinusitis symptoms.[4]

ACUTE SINUSITIS

Most cases of infectious rhinosinusitis of less than 7–10 days' duration are viral.[4, 5, 27, 28] Acute bacterial sinusitis in adults most often presents with 7 days of symptoms of purulent anterior rhinorrhea, nasal congestion, postnasal drip, facial or dental pain/pressure, and/or cough, often worse at night. Children with acute sinusitis most commonly have cough and rhinorrhea.[4, 28] In all age groups with acute sinusitis, less frequent symptoms may include fever, nausea, fatigue, anosmia, and halitosis. Occasionally, fungal infections can cause acute sinusitis. These are more likely to occur in diabetes mellitus and immunocompromised states.[4]

CHRONIC SINUSITIS

Historically it was thought that chronic rhinosinusitis evolved as a consequence of untreated acute bacterial sinusitis. However, linear progression from acute to chronic bacterial rhinosinusitis has not been established. In addition, the view that chronic sinusitis is primarily an infectious process is no longer held.[4–6] Instead, current data indicate that active infection may only be present in a minority of patients with chronic sinusitis, and that other patients have inflammation sustained by other processes.[4–6] Broadly, chronic sinusitis can be classified as either infectious or inflammatory (noninfectious). The following discussion reviews the principal concepts of chronic sinusitis but pertains primarily to data from adults. Because the sinus mucosa of young children with chronic sinusitis has less eosinophilic inflammation, basement membrane thickening, and mucus gland hyperplasia than in adult chronic sinusitis,[29] studies of chronic sinusitis in adults may not be fully applicable to chronic sinusitis in children.

Chronic infectious sinusitis

Bacterial chronic sinusitis can be associated with a variety of organisms, as discussed under Microbiology above. Chronic infectious sinusitis is generally associated with a significant influx of neutrophils, and is more likely to occur in patients with underlying humoral immune deficiencies, AIDS, cystic fibrosis, or Kartagener's syndrome.[4] More recently, bacterial biofilms have been proposed to be important in promoting chronic sinus infection. Biofilms are complex aggregations of interacting bacteria attached to a surface that are encased in a protective matrix of polysaccharides.[30] This encasement protects the bacterial community from antibiotic penetration and the hosts natural defenses, potentially leading to refractory infections. As with acute fungal sinusitis, chronic infectious fungal sinusitis is more common in diabetes mellitus and immunocompromised states, and in geographic areas with high humidity.

Chronic inflammatory sinusitis

Chronic hyperplastic (hypertrophic) eosinophilic sinusitis (CHES)

This noninfectious form of CS is characterized by mucosal hyperplasia with a preponderance of eosinophils and mixed mononuclear cells with relatively few neutrophils. Frequently associated with nasal polyps, asthma and aspirin sensitivity, it often responds poorly to therapy.[4, 6] Th2 lymphocytes appear to play an important role in initiating CHES.

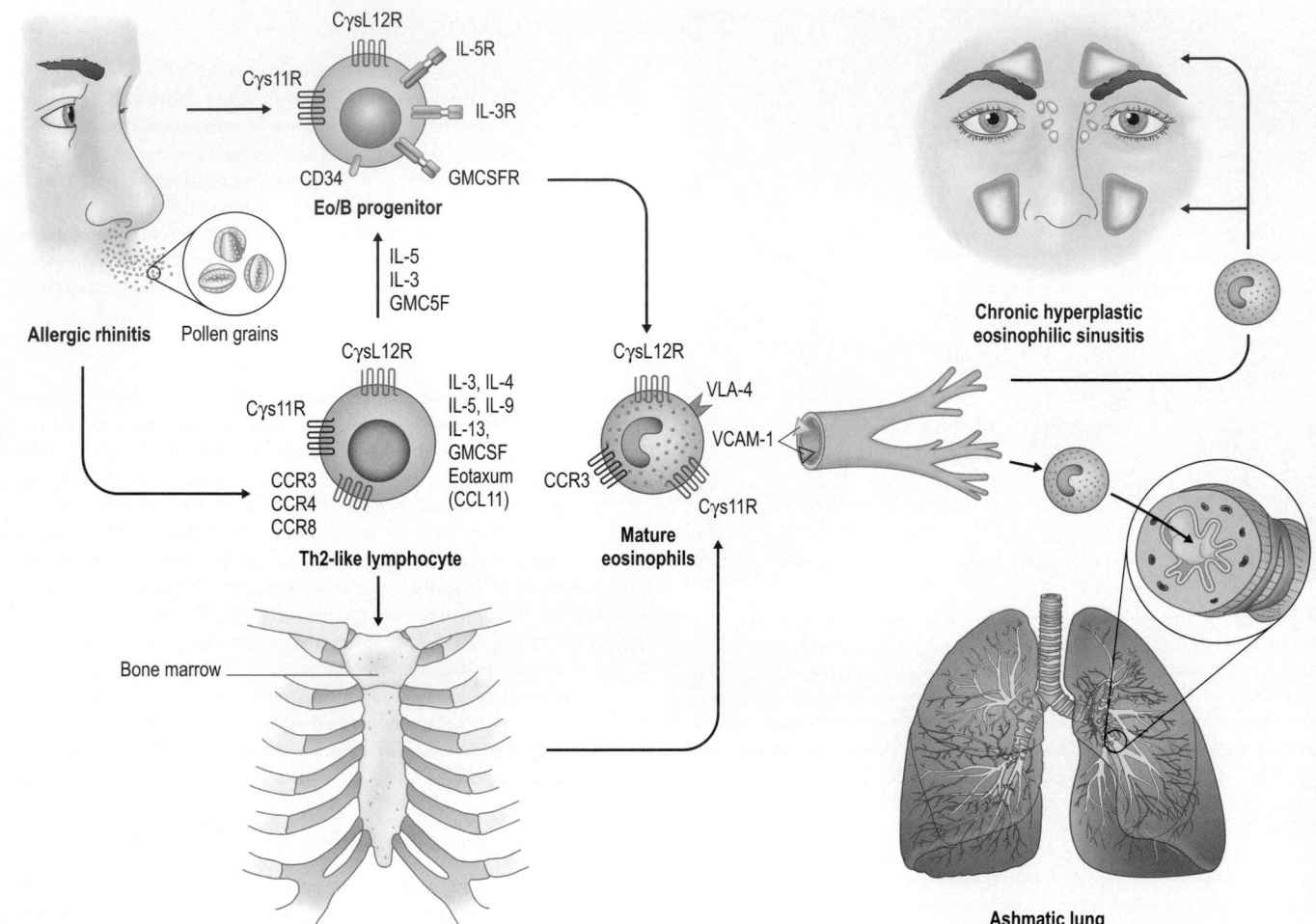

Fig. 41.4 Chronic hyperplastic eosinophilic sinusitis (CHES): part of a systemic disease of the airways. Although this figure depicts a theorized allergen-induced pathway that leads to CHES and asthma, any number of putative stimuli (see text) might initiate an analogous cascade of events driven by Th2-like lymphocytes. Here, allergen exposure activates immune cells, including Th2 lymphocytes, dendritic cells, mononuclear phagocytic cells, and mast cells within the nares and in nasal-associated lymphatic tissues. These cells might also include locally produced CD34+ IL-5Ra+ eosinophil-basophil (Eo/B) progenitors. It is presumed that the newly activated Th lymphocytes will have the phenotype of Th2-like cells characterized by their production of IL-3, IL-4, IL-5, IL-9, IL-13, eotaxin (CCL11), and GM-CSF. Such cells can migrate to the bone marrow, where they stimulate the production of inflammatory cells, including basophils, mast cells, and, most importantly, eosinophils. These newly generated inflammatory cells enter the circulatory system, from which they are selectively recruited via specific adhesion molecules (e.g., VCAM-1) and chemoattractants (e.g., eotaxin) back to the nose, but also to the lungs and sinuses, exacerbating inflammation. (From Borish L. Allergic rhinitis: Systemic inflammation and implications for management. J Allergy Clin Immunol 2003; 112: 1024 with permission from Elsevier.)

Current research is defining the role of numerous putative stimuli, including allergens, bacteria, bacteria-derived superantigens (e.g., staphylococcal enterotoxins), osteitis, biofilms, and fungal derived antigens.[4, 6, 21, 22, 26–28, 30–32] It has also been proposed that, once initiated, cellular differentiation pathways could lead to the development of an antigen-independent permanent process[27] (Fig. 41.4).

Both in the aspirin-sensitive and - tolerant patients, the disease severity of CHES and eosinophilic infiltration correlates with increased leukotriene C_4 synthase and 5-lipoxygenase activity and increased levels of cysteinyl leukotriene production.[4] The mechanism of aspirin-sensitive disease has been proposed to involve abnormal arachidonic acid metabolism, an increased absolute number of cells expressing the CysLT1 receptor, and decreased expression of certain prostanoid receptors for PGE_2, with consequent impaired braking of inflammatory cell cysteinyl leukotriene production by PGE_2.[33–35] Because there is greater expression of $cysLT_2$ than $cysLT_1$ receptors on epithelial and glandular cells, the effects of cysteinyl leukotrienes on mucosal glands and epithelium in rhinosinusitis may be mediated predominantly through $cysLT_2$.[36]

In CHES with nasal polyps (but not CHES without nasal polyps) there is a significantly increased prevalence of *Staphylococcus aureus* colonization.[37] These bacteria release enterotoxins which act as superantigens and induce topical multiclonal IgE formation, as well as a severe, possibly steroid-insensitive eosinophilic inflammation. The presence of IgE antibodies in nasal polyps is only partially related to the serum IgE and skin-prick results. Polyp specimens show follicular structures with B and T cells and diffuse lymphoid accumulations with plasma cell infiltration.[37]

Overall, studies suggest that increased production of IL-5 is likely to influence the predominance and activation of eosinophils in nasal polyps, independent of atopy.[37] However, the development of eosinophilic nasal polyps may not be simply explained as a Th2-driven process, as both Th1- and Th2-type cytokines are upregulated in eosinophilic nasal polyps, in patients with and without positive allergen skin tests.[38]

Allergic fungal sinusitis (AFS)

AFS is a distinct entity that has traditionally been viewed as the most common form of fungal sinusitis. It occurs in immunocompetent patients and results from a hypersensitivity response to saprophytic fungi such as *Aspergillus* spp. that colonize the sinuses.[39] More prevalent in certain geographic areas, AFS is often associated with nasal polyps and asthma. Typical diagnostic features include CT or MRI evidence of sinusitis, 'allergic mucin' in the sinuses (dark green or black material with the consistency of peanut butter that typically contains a few hyphae and Charcot–Leyden crystals), a positive skin test to the relevant organism, and elevated total serum IgE.[4] Treatment involves surgical exenteration and steroid therapy.

Chronic noneosinophilic sinusitis

A predominantly neutrophilic inflammatory response in chronic sinusitis is generally associated with an infectious process. In contrast to chronic sinusitis associated with eosinophilic infiltrates, nasal polyps occur less commonly, except in patients with cystic fibrosis in whom nasal polyps with predominantly neutrophilic infiltrates are frequent.[4] Other patients with chronic sinusitis can have inflammatory infiltrates characterized more by lymphocytes and mononuclear phagocytes. Although these latter patients have been thought to have chronic or recurrent sinus occlusion underlying their disease, the factors that drive differential inflammatory infiltrates in chronic sinusitis are not fully understood.

Nasal polyps

Frequently associated with sinus disease, nasal polyps are benign inflammatory growths that arise from the inflamed mucosa lining the paranasal sinuses. They may cause invariant nasal obstruction and loss of smell or rhinorrhea. The presence of nasal polyps in children is uncommon, and merits testing for cystic fibrosis.[4] Neutrophils are more characteristic of nasal polyps associated with cystic fibrosis, whereas, as discussed above, eosinophilic infiltrates are more typical of polyps associated with CHES, aspirin sensitivity and asthma. Although it had generally been assumed that allergy is a cause of nasal polyps, the prevalence of nasal polyposis in allergic patients is typically less than 5%, and the prevalence of documented allergy is not increased in patients with nasal polyps.[1, 4, 40] Corticosteroids are an effective medical treatment, although surgical polypectomy may be required.

RELATIONSHIP BETWEEN SINUSITIS AND ASTHMA

Although data relating sinus disease to asthma are far less extensive than those relating rhinitis to asthma, the relationship is conceptually analogous. In a CT study, paranasal sinus abnormalities were shown in nearly all patients with moderate to severe asthma.[41] Evidence of eosinophilia in the sinus mucosa is stronger in patients with rhinosinusitis and asthma, as opposed to rhinosinusitis alone.[1] Medical and surgical treatment of sinus disease appears to have beneficial effects on asthma outcomes, but the studies reporting such findings typically have not been randomized and the outcomes are frequently subjective.[1, 4]

DIAGNOSIS OF SINUSITIS

History

Acute bacterial sinusitis (ABS)

The principal issue in clinical practice is differentiating between an acute viral upper respiratory infection (URI) and acute bacterial sinusitis (ABS). Most viral URIs last 5–10 days, with a peak in nasal symptoms and/or cough by days 3–6 and subsequent improvement and resolution of constitutional symptoms such as fever, headache and myalgia within the first few days of illness.[4, 42] Although nasal discharge begins as clear and watery, it often becomes thicker, mucoid and even purulent for several days before reversing its appearance and then drying. ABS may have several presentations. The most common ABS presentation is onset of nasal symptoms (anterior or posterior nasal drainage, congestion) and/or cough that does not improve beyond 7–10 days. ABS may also present with severe symptoms including a fever=38.5° that persists for at least 3–4 days (longer than expected in a viral URI) with nasal discharge, and in adults, facial pain. A third presentation of ABS is a biphasic course in which a patient begins with URI-type symptoms that appears to be resolving, followed by significant worsening of nasal symptoms and/or cough with new or recurrent fever at about 1 week into the illness.

Chronic sinusitis

Chronic rhinosinusitis may cause symptoms that persist for months to years and may be less severe than those of acute rhinosinusitis. Nasal obstruction or posterior discharge are usually the chief complaints of chronic rhinosinusitis, making it difficult to distinguish this condition from rhinitis without sinusitis. Chronic cough (especially during the night, or upon waking in the morning) is also a common presenting symptom of chronic rhinosinusitis.[4-6, 43] Clinical evidence of sinusitis occasionally may be subtle, except during acute purulent episodes.

Physical examination

Typical physical signs include nasal mucosal edema, sinus tenderness (albeit neither a sensitive nor a specific finding), and purulent nasal secretions. However, purulent nasal secretions do not necessarily indicate an infectious process, let alone bacterial sinusitis.[4-6] The nose should be examined for deviated septum, nasal polyps, foreign bodies, and tumors. Maxillary sinusitis is suggested by sensitivity of the maxillary teeth. The ears and chest should be examined for signs of associated otitis media and asthma.[1]

Nasal endoscopy/rhinoscopy

Nasal endoscopy offers a significantly better visualization of the nose than a nasal speculum. The origin and extent of nasal polyps, other anatomic abnormalities and the presence of purulent ostial secretions may be identified.

Imaging studies

In routine cases of suspected acute bacterial rhinosinusitis, imaging studies are not required and may even be misleading.[3–5] Up to 40% of sinus radiographs and more than 80% of CT scans may be abnormal in viral rhinosinusitis if obtained within 7 days of the onset of illness.[42] However, imaging studies become appropriate when there is an incomplete response to initial management, or chronic sinusitis is suspected. Occipitomental view radiographs may be helpful in screening adults and children over 1 year of age, but have inadequate sensitivity.

CT scans of the sinuses can identify disease not demonstrated by standard radiographs, and are of particular value in assessing obstruction of the sinus ostia. Radiographic signs consistent with acute sinusitis include maxillary sinus findings of either mucosal thickening >6 mm in adults (>4 mm in children), or >33% loss of air space volume, or opacification or air/fluid levels in any paranasal sinus.[4, 6] A limited four- to five-image coronal sinus CT scan, with a focus on the ostiomeatal complex, may be helpful and should be considered if imaging is deemed necessary.[4] A complete series sinus CT scan fully defines sinus anatomy and is mandatory before surgery. Suspected orbital involvement is best identified by axial views. In allergic fungal sinusitis, CT scans demonstrate a characteristic heterogeneous appearance within the involved paranasal sinuses (Fig. 41.5).

MRI does not distinguish air from bone. Because examination of the air–bone interface is important in the evaluation of anatomic defects, MRI is not used for routine evaluation of suspected sinusitis. However, it may be of great value when fungal sinusitis and tumors are suspected. Fungal sinus disease is associated with a characteristic hypointense signal on T_2-weighted scans.

Transillumination is not reliable in diagnosing sinusitis.[4, 5]

Bacterial cultures and other laboratory studies

The overall presentation of history and physical findings is usually sufficient to make the diagnosis of acute, uncomplicated sinusitis. Diagnostic testing becomes important when initial therapy fails, or when symptoms are chronic or recurrent.[4, 5] Nasal cultures are not reliable for establishing the diagnosis of sinusitis, or for determining a specific causative microorganism.[4] Maxillary antrum tap with aspiration for culture is definitive in adults, but is invasive, may be uncomfortable, and is indicated only when precise microbial identification is essential.[4] Obtaining cultures of the middle meatus through endoscopically directed culture has shown promise in adults, but not in children.[4, 45]

If present, the identification of large numbers of neutrophils in nasal secretions by nasal cytology can help distinguish between infectious sinusitis and rhinitis.[4]

When patients present with recurrent or chronic sinusitis and infections of the lower respiratory tract, testing for immunodeficiency should be considered, including quantitative immunoglobulins, functional antibody tests, and HIV testing.

Quantitative sweat chloride tests and genetic testing for diagnosis of cystic fibrosis should be considered in children with nasal polyps and/or colonization of the nose and sinuses with *Pseudomonas* species and who developed chronic sinusitis at an early age.

THERAPEUTIC PRINCIPLES

ACUTE SINUSITIS

Findings in acute sinusitis that suggest complications and a possible need for immediate referral to a specialist include:

>> Facial swelling/erythema over an involved sinus

>> Visual changes; abnormal extraocular movements; proptosis; periorbital edema or erythema

>> Neurologic signs that suggest intracranial or central nervous system involvement

>> Severe headaches and high fevers

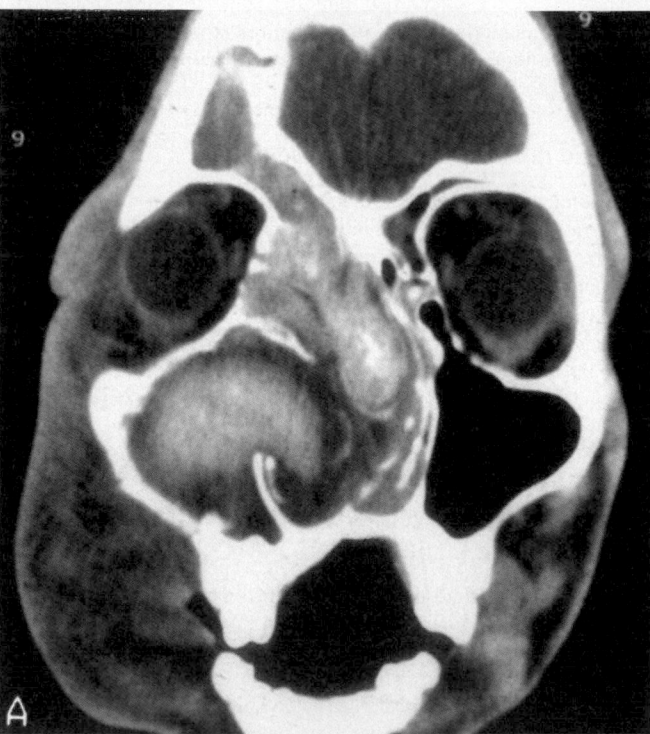

Fig. 41.5 Soft tissue algorithm CT showing findings typical of AFRS. Note heterogeneic appearance within involved paranasal sinuses. (From Meltzer EO, Hamilos DL, Hadley JA et al. Rhinosinusitis: establishing definitions for clinical research and patient care. J Allergy Clin Immunol 2004; 114: 170 with permission from Elsevier.)

Differential considerations

The differential diagnosis of sinusitis includes acute viral upper respiratory infections, various forms of rhinitis, nasal polyps, Horner's syndrome, Wegener's granulomatosis/midline granuloma, Churg–Strauss vasculitis, trauma, enlarged tonsils and adenoids, tumors, dental infections, cerebral spinal fluid (CSF) rhinorrhea, and migraine or tension headaches.[4–6] Findings on history and physical examination should direct further testing, which may include allergy testing, and other diagnostic procedures (Fig. 41.6). Although headache can be a feature, particularly in acute sinusitis, over 90% of self- and physician-diagnosed sinus headaches meet the International Headache Society criteria for migraines. Accordingly, most cases of 'sinus headache' are not in fact due to sinus disease.[46, 47]

TREATMENT

Acute sinusitis

Antibiotics

When symptoms suggestive of rhinosinusitis persist beyond approximately 7 days, bacterial rhinosinusitis becomes more likely. In an effort to promote judicious use of antibiotics, several guidelines recommend

---

Presentation Suggestive of Chronic Rhinosinusitis

⬇

Initial evaluation

- Medical history: symptoms
- Physical examination
- Anterior rhinoscopy, nasal endoscopy
- Evaluation of underlying disease and comorbidities
- Computed tomographic (CT) scan (not in an acute episode)

⬇

Based upon above, focused evaluation to address differential diagnostic considerations and underlying disease

- Allergy testing
- Microbiologic culture
- Challenge test for aspirin sensitivity
- Nasal cytology
- MRI (e.g. for fungal sinusitis, suspected tumors)
- Ciliary function studies
- Biopsy
- Blood testing (Wegener's, immunodeficiencies)
- Sweat chloride test
- Electron microscopy
- Genetic analyses
- Consultations of other specialties (e.g. ophthalmologist, neurologist)

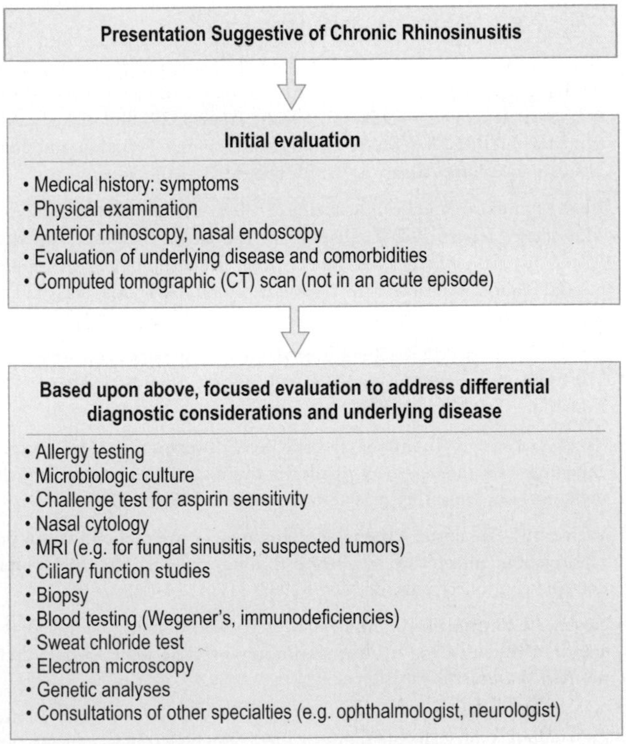

Fig. 41.6 Diagnostic approach to suspected chronic rhinosinusitis. (Adapted from Adkinson NF Jr, Yunginger JW, Busse WW, et al. Middletons allergy principles and practice, 6th edn. Philadelphia: Mosby, 2003; 78 with permission from Elsevier.)

a 7–10-day period of watchful waiting for spontaneous resolution of symptoms before prescribing antibiotics.[4, 27, 28] In such cases, antibiotic usage is appropriate when moderate to severe symptoms are present, although most cases of milder acute bacterial rhinosinusitis will resolve without the need to prescribe antibiotics. However, some guidelines also recommend that antibiotics be considered regardless of the duration of illness when severe signs or symptoms of sinusitis are present: temperature >39°C, maxillary tooth or facial pain (especially when unilateral), unilateral sinus tenderness, periorbital swelling, or worsening symptoms after 3–5 days.[4, 5] A 10–14-day antibiotic course is typically prescribed for acute sinusitis, although a shorter course may be adequate with certain newer antibiotics. The choice of antibiotic should consider cost, safety, and changing local patterns of bacterial resistance.[4] Accordingly, it is not possible to make a universally applicable recommendation for first-line agents. In many geographic areas amoxicillin is a reasonable first-line antibiotic, although surveillance studies indicate the development of significant pneumococcal resistance due to alteration of penicillin-binding proteins,[4] and there is a high frequency of β-lactamase-positive *H. influenzae* and *M. catarrhalis*.[4] In some areas, trimethoprim-sulfamethoxazole can be used as an alternative in adults, although bacterial resistance is higher in children.[4] The macrolides clarithromycin and azithromycin have extended coverage and are effective against β-lactamase-producing organisms. Other antibiotics with broader coverage include amoxicillin/clavulanate, some second- or third-generation cephalosporins (e.g., cefuroxime, cefpodoxime, cefprozil), and for adults, quinolones. First-generation cephalosporins such as cephalexin have poor *H. influenzae* coverage, whereas certain second-generation cephalosporins (e.g., cefaclor) have become less useful as *H. influenzae* and *M. catarrhalis* have become increasingly resistant to them.

When a patient fails to improve significantly after approximately 5 days' treatment, or there is a high prevalence of β-lactamase resistance, antibiotics with broader coverage should be prescribed.

Other therapies

In clinical practice, bacterial sinusitis is treated not only with antibiotics, but also with adjunctive agents and approaches such as analgesics, adequate hydration, steam inhalation, and pharmacologic measures intended to treat pathologic factors associated with sinusitis (e.g., underlying rhinitis, impaired ostial patency). Such pharmacologic measures include topical steroids, oral steroids, oral antihistamine in allergic patients, nasal saline, nasal douches/irrigation, topical and oral decongestants, and mucolytics.[4, 5] However, the use of many agents commonly prescribed for sinusitis is not based on firm evidence.[4, 5] Moreover, even when there is evidence that a pharmacologic intervention improves clinically meaningful symptoms of rhinosinusitis in controlled trials, critical analysis can question whether the improvement occurs because of effects on the rhinitis component, rather than directly improving bacterial sinus infection per se. For example, there are controlled studies in acute rhinosinusitis demonstrating that nasal steroids can decrease associated nasal symptoms, headache, facial pain, and cough after several weeks of treatment.[4, 5] However, it is argued that these endpoints may reflect the known effects of nasal steroids on rhinitis, and that other endpoints, such as greater or more rapid resolution of positive bacterial sinus cultures, would be required to demonstrate efficacy in bacterial sinusitis.[48]

When therapy fails

If the response to medical intervention is still inadequate, a sinus CT scan is indicated to confirm the presence of sinusitis and determine whether anatomic abnormalities may be predisposing to the problem. Specialist evaluation is appropriate when sinusitis is recurrent or refractory to treatment. Surgical intervention may be required in acute sinusitis to provide drainage when there is a significant risk of intracranial complications, or in patients with periorbital or intraorbital abscess or visual compromise.

Chronic sinusitis

Medical therapy

Guidelines recommend that chronic sinusitis should be treated with antibiotics for prolonged courses (at least 3 weeks; up to 3 months), although there is a relative paucity of controlled trials.[4–6] Most adjunctive agents commonly used for acute sinusitis are also commonly used for chronic sinusitis, but there is generally even less evidence in controlled trials of their efficacy. In addition, it has been proposed (but not yet convincingly proven) that other medical treatments may be useful in chronic sinusitis, including systemic and topical antimycotics, leukotriene modifiers, and proton pump inhibitors (in patients in whom gastric reflux is suspected to play a role).[4,5] Because chronic sinusitis is associated with AR in 40–80% of adults and 36–60% of children, some guidelines recommend that patients with chronic sinusitis be evaluated for allergy so that environmental control measures for allergic disease can be implemented.[4] In patients with aspirin sensitivity and hyperplastic sinus disease, aspirin desensitization has been reported to improve long-term outcomes.[49] During treatment of chronic sinusitis, but particularly if initial measures fail, there should be consideration of all factors that may be promoting chronic disease which may direct further interventions (Fig. 41.6).

Surgical therapy

Referral for surgical intervention should be considered if sinusitis does not respond to medical intervention. Functional endoscopic sinus surgery (FESS) has generally supplanted older surgical techniques.[50] FESS is typically directed at the removal of locally diseased ethmoid tissue (important in the development of frontal and maxillary sinusitis) to improve ventilation and drainage of larger, dependent sinuses.

■ REFERENCES ■

1. Bousquet J, van Cauwenberge P, Khaltaev N. Allergic rhinitis and its impact on asthma: ARIA workshop report. J Allergy Clin Immunol 2001; 108: S147–S334.

2. Dykewicz MS, Fineman S, Skoner DP, et al. Diagnosis and management of rhinitis: Complete guidelines of the Joint Task Force on Practice Parameters in Allergy, Asthma and Immunology. Ann Allergy Asthma Immunol 1998; 81: 478–518.

3. Dykewicz MS. Rhinitis and sinusitis. J Allergy Clin Immunol 2003; 111: S520–S529.

4. Slavin RG, Spector SL, Bernstein IL, et al. The diagnosis and management of sinusitis: a practice parameter update. J Allergy Clin Immunol 2005; 116: S13–S47.

5. Fokkens W, Lund V, Bachert C, et al. EAACI position paper on rhinosinusitis and nasal polyps executive summary. Allergy 2005; 60: 583–601.

6. Meltzer EO, Hamilos DL, Hadley JA, et al. Rhinosinusitis: establishing definitions for clinical research and patient care. J Allergy Clin Immunol 2004; 114: S155–S212.

7. Godthelp T, Fokkens WJ, Kleinjan A, et al. Antigen presenting cells in the nasal mucosa of patients with allergic rhinitis during allergen provocation. Clin Exp Allergy 1996; 26: 677–688.

8. Francis JN, Lloyd CM, Sabroe I, et al. T lymphocytes expressing CCR3 are increased in allergic rhinitis compared with non-allergic controls and following allergen immunotherapy. Allergy 2007; 62: 59–65.

9. Aoi N, Masuda T, Murakami D, Yajima T, et al. IL-15 prevents allergic rhinitis through reactivation of antigen-specific CD8+ cells. J Allergy Clin Immunol 2006; 117: 1359–1366.

10. Lim MC, Taylor RM, Naclerio RM. The histology of allergic rhinitis and its comparison to nasal lavage. Am J Respir Crit Care Med 1995; 151: 136–144.

11. Gelfand EW. Inflammatory mediators in allergic rhinitis. J Allergy Clin Immunol 2004; 114: S135–S138.

12. Warnecke A, Averbeck T, Wurster U, et al. Diagnostic relevance of beta2-transferrin for the detection of cerebrospinal fluid fistulas. Arch Otolaryngol Head Neck Surg 2004; 130: 1178–1184.

13. Tschopp JM, Sistek D, Schindler C, et al. Current allergic asthma and rhinitis: diagnostic efficiency of three commonly used atopic markers (IgE, skin prick tests, and Phadiatop). Results from 8329 randomized adults from the SAPALDIA Study. Swiss Study on Air Pollution and Lung Diseases in Adults. Allergy 1998; 53: 608–613.

14. 2000. Rhinitis. In: American Academy of Allergy, Asthma and Immunology. The allergy report. Vol. 2. Diseases of the atopic diathesis. American Academy of Allergy, Asthma and Immunology, Milwaukee, p 1–31. Online. Available: http://www.aaaai.org/ar/working_vol2/020.asp 31 July 2006.

15. Casale TB, Blaiss MS, Gelfand E, et al. First do no harm: managing antihistamine impairment in patients with allergic rhinitis. J Allergy Clin Immunol 2003; 111: S835–842.

16. Yanez A, Rodrigo GJ. Intranasal corticosteroids versus topical H1 receptor antagonists for the treatment of allergic rhinitis: a systematic review with meta-analysis. Ann Allergy Asthma Immunol 2002; 89: 479–484.

17. Weiner JM, Abramson MJ, Puy RM. Intranasal corticosteroids versus oral H1 receptor antagonists in allergic rhinitis: systematic review of randomised controlled trials. Br Med J 1998; 317: 1624–1629.

18. Skoner D, Rachelefsky G, Meltzer E, et al. Detection of growth suppression in children during treatment with intranasal beclomethasone dipropionate. Pediatrics 2000; 105: e23.

19. Murphy K, Uryniak T, Simpson B, O'Dowd L. Growth velocity in children with perennial allergic rhinitis treated with budesonide aqueous nasal spray. Ann Allergy Asthma Immunol 2006; 96: 723–730.

20. Schenkel E, Skoner D, Bronsky E, et al. Absence of growth retardation in children with perennial allergic rhinitis following 1 year treatment with mometasone furoate aqueous nasal spray. Pediatrics 2000; 101: e22.

21. Kaszuba SM, Baroody FM, deTineo M, et al. Superiority of an intranasal corticosteroid compared with an oral antihistamine in the as-needed treatment of seasonal allergic rhinitis. Arch Intern Med 2001; 161: 2581–2587.

22. Rodrigo GJ, Yanez A. The role of antileukotriene therapy in seasonal allergic rhinitis: a systematic review of randomized trials. Ann Allergy Asthma Immunol 2006; 96: 779–86.

23. Li JT, Lockey RF, Bernstein IL, et al. Joint Task Force on Practice Parameters. Allergen immunotherapy: a practice parameter. American Academy of Allergy, Asthma and Immunology. American College of Allergy, Asthma and Immunology. Ann Allergy Asthma Immunol 2003; 90: 1–40.

24. Scadding GK. Nonallergic rhinitis: diagnosis and management. Curr Opin Allergy Clin Immunol 2001; 1: 15–20.

25. Shin SH, Ponikau JU, Sherris DA, et al. Chronic rhinosinusitis: an enhanced immune response to ubiquitous airborne fungi. J Allergy Clin Immunol 2004; 114: 1369–1375.

26. Borish L, Lanny Rosenwasser L, Steinke JW. Fungi in chronic hyperplastic eosinophilic sinusitis: Reasonable doubt. J Allergy Clin Immunol 2006; 30: 195–204.

27. Snow V, Mottur-Pilson C, Hickner JM, et al. Principles of appropriate antibiotic use for acute sinusitis in adults. Ann Intern Med 2001; 134: 495–497.

28. Subcommittee on Management of Sinusitis. Committee on Quality Improvement, American Academy of Pediatrics. Clinical practice guideline: Management of sinusitis. Pediatrics 2001; 108: 798–808.

29. Chan KH, Abzug MJ, Coffinet L, et al. Chronic rhinosinusitis in young children differs from adults: a histopathology study. J Pediatr 2004; 144: 206–212.

30. Bendouah Z, Barbeau J, Hamad WA, Desrosiers M. Biofilm formation by *Staphylococcus aureus* and *Pseudomonas aeruginosa* is associated with an unfavorable evolution after surgery for chronic sinusitis and nasal polyposis. Otolaryngol Head Neck Surg 2006; 134: 991–996.

31. Borish L. Allergic rhinitis: Systemic inflammation and implications for management. J Allergy Clin Immunol 2003; 112: 1021–1031.

32. Zhang N, Gevaert P, van Zele T, et al. An update on the impact of *Staphylococcus aureus* enterotoxins in chronic sinusitis with nasal polyposis. Rhinology 2005; 43: 162–168.

33. Perez-Novo CA, Watelet JB, Claeys C, et al. Prostaglandin, leukotriene, and lipoxin balance in chronic rhinosinusitis with and without nasal polyposis. J Allergy Clin Immunol 2005; 115: 1189–1196.

34. Ying S, Meng Q, Scadding G, et al. Aspirin-sensitive rhinosinusitis is associated with reduced E-prostanoid 2 receptor expression on nasal mucosal inflammatory cells. J Allergy Clin Immunol 2006; 117: 312–318.

35. Sousa AR, Parikh A, Scadding G, et al. Leukotriene-receptor expression on nasal mucosal inflammatory cells in aspirin-sensitive rhinosinusitis. N Engl J Med 2002; 347: 1493–1499.

36. Corrigan C, Mallett K, Ying S, et al. Expression of the cysteinyl leukotriene receptors cysLT1 and cysLT2 in aspirin-sensitive and aspirin-tolerant chronic rhinosinusitis. J Allergy Clin Immunol 2005; 115: 316–322.

37. Gevaert P, Holtappels G, Johansson SGO, et al. Organization of secondary lymphoid issue and local IgE formation to *Staphylococcus aureus* enterotoxins in nasal polyp tissue. Allergy 2005; 60: 71–79.

38. Wagenmann M, Gärtner-Ackerboom M, Helmig P. Increased production of type-2 and type-1 cytokines in nasal polyps. J Allergy Clin Immunol 2000; 105: S210.

39. deShazo RD, Swain RE. Diagnostic criteria for allergic fungal sinusitis. J Allergy Clin Immunol 1995; 96: 24–35.

40. Settipane GA, Chafee FH. Nasal polyps in asthma and rhinitis. A review of 6,037 patients. J Allergy Clin Immunol 1977; 59: 17–21.

41. Bresciani M, Paradis L, Des Roches A, et al. Rhinosinusitis in severe asthma. J Allergy Clin Immunol 2001; 107: 73–80.

42. Wald ER. Beginning antibiotics for acute rhinosinusitis and choosing the right treatment. Clin Rev Allergy Immunol 2006; 30: 143–152.

43. Pratter MR. Chronic upper airway cough syndrome secondary to rhinosinus diseases (previously referred to as postnasal drip syndrome): ACCP evidence-based clinical practice guidelines. Chest 2006; 129: 63S–71S.

44. Gwaltney JM Jr, Philips CD, Miller RD, Riker DK. Computed tomographic study of the common cold. N Engl J Med 1994; 330: 25–30.

45. Gordts F, Abu Nasser I, Clement PA, et al. Bacteriology of the middle meatus in children. Int J Pediatr Otorhinolaryngol 1999; 48: 163–167.

46. Cady RK, Schreiber CP. Sinus headache or migraine? Considerations in making a differential diagnosis. Neurology 2002; 58: S10–14.

47. Tepper SJ. New thoughts on sinus headache. Allergy Asthma Proc 2004; 25: 95–96.

48. Starke PR, Chowdhury BA. Efficacy of intranasal corticosteroids for acute sinusitis. JAMA 2002; 287: 1261–1262.

49. Lee JY, Simon RA, Stevenson DD. Selection of aspirin dosages for aspirin desensitization treatment in patients with aspirin-exacerbated respiratory disease. J Allergy Clin Immunol 2007; 119: 157–164.

50. Senior BA, Kennedy DW, Tanabodee J, et al. Long-term results of functional endoscopic sinus surgery. Laryngoscope 1998; 108: 151–157.

REFERENCES

Urticaria, angioedema, and anaphylaxis

Elena Borzova, Clive E.H. Grattan

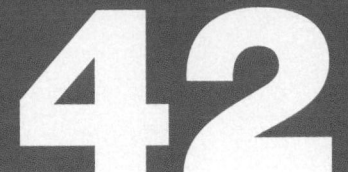

Urticaria is a common skin disorder that can lead to severe impairment of quality of life. Recently, there has been substantial progress in our knowledge and understanding of the pathophysiology of the condition, offering new diagnostic and treatment approaches for at least some patients. However, in many cases, urticaria is still a disease of unknown etiology that is difficult to manage effectively.

■ DEFINITION ■

Urticaria is a heterogeneous group of disorders that share a distinct skin reaction pattern, i.e., the development of urticarial skin lesions.[1] Urticarial lesions resulting from localized edema of the upper dermis are called wheals (Fig. 42.1), whereas pronounced swelling of deeper dermal layers, subcutis, and submucosal tissues is known as angioedema (Fig. 42.2).

■ EPIDEMIOLOGY ■

Urticaria is common: up to 25% of the general population experience some form of urticaria at least once over their lifetime, whereas the lifetime prevalence of chronic urticaria (CU) is between 0.1% and 3% of the general population.[2, 3] Acute urticaria affects mainly young adults with an obvious female preponderance,[3] whereas CU is more common in adults, affecting mainly middle-aged women, and is rare in children and adolescents.[2–4] By definition, acute urticaria resolves within 6 weeks, whereas CU lasts on average 3–5 years. Rarely, CU may last for > 10 years. However, CU is almost always a self-limiting disorder, resolving spontaneously in 50% patients within 6 months of onset.[4]

■ GENETICS ■

With the exception of hereditary angioedema and the hereditary auto-inflammatory periodic syndromes, urticaria does not show mendelian inheritance. Nevertheless, there is some evidence of genetic predisposition and human leukocyte antigen (HLA) associations in CU.[5–8]

Although earlier studies found no association between HLA class I antigens and CU, a recent study showed an increased frequency of HLA-Bw4 in CU.[5] Several associations have been reported for class II HLA antigens in CU in different ethnic populations. A link between CU and HLA DRB1*04 (DR4) and its associated allele, DQB1*0302 (DQ8), was described in British CU patients compared with a control population. This link with the HLA DR4 haplotype was also confirmed in Turkish CU patients,[7] while strong associations with HLA-DRB1*1302 and DQB1*0609 alleles were found for aspirin-induced urticaria in Korean patients.[8]

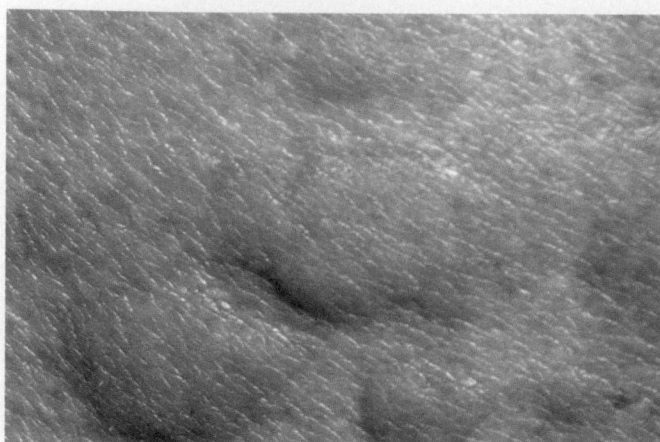

Fig. 42.1 Spontaneous wheals in severe ordinary urticaria showing superficial pink swellings with pale edematous centers.

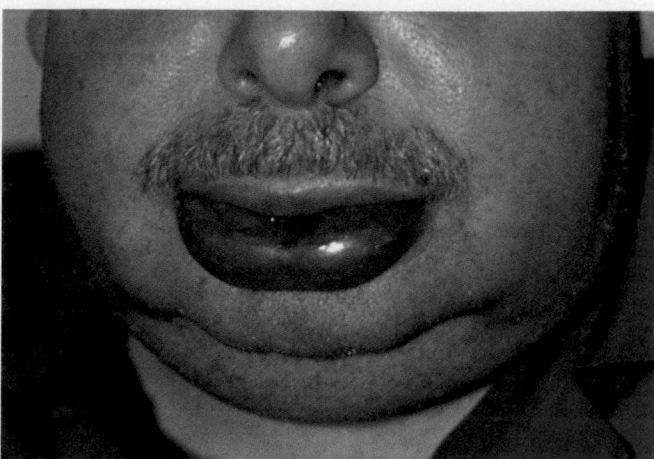

Fig. 42.2 Angioedema of the mouth in C1 esterase inhibitor deficiency.

■ CLINICAL PATTERNS ■

Urticaria is often classified by the duration of continuous activity into acute (less than 6 weeks), chronic (6 weeks of more), or episodic, where short episodes occur repeatedly over a period of time. This classification has the merit of simplicity but takes no account of etiology or clinical features that may help clinical management or research. Classification of urticaria by etiology is satisfying academically but of little value in the clinic, where the etiology is often unknown and management decisions have to be based solely on the clinical assessment.[9]

■ ETIOPATHOGENESIS AND ETIOLOGICAL CLASSIFICATION ■

Although many aspects of the pathophysiology of urticaria remain unclear, our understanding has advanced considerably over the last two decades, allowing an etiological classification (Table 42.1).

MAST CELL-DEPENDENT MECHANISMS

Skin mast cells are key players in the pathogenesis of urticaria. They are predominantly located around the small blood and lymphatic vessels as well as around or within peripheral nerves.[3] Mast cell population density is greatest at distal body areas, including the face, hands, and feet.[10] There is conflicting evidence as to whether the number of cutaneous mast cells in urticaria patients is increased but there is general agreement that they release mediators more readily than normal.

Human skin mast cells contain preformed mediators in their granules, including histamine, proteases (tryptase, chymase), and heparin. They express many membrane receptors, including high-affinity immunoglobulin E (IgE) and low-affinity IgG receptors. Unlike mast cells elsewhere (pulmonary and intestinal), skin mast cells possess complement C5a receptors and activation sites for neuropeptides and basic secretagogues.[4]

Skin mast cell activation is central to the pathophysiology of CU. Mast cells can be activated by a variety of immunological and nonimmunological triggers (Fig. 42.3).[11] Immunological and nonimmunological pathways of mast cell activation are characterized by distinct patterns of mediator release. Immunological activation of mast cells requires prior sensitization and is triggered by cross-linking of high-affinity IgE receptors (FcεRI) by antigen bound to antigen-specific IgE, by anti-FcεRIa, or by anti-IgE antibodies. Histamine release peaks at 5–10 minutes, followed by *de novo* synthesis of lipid-derived mediators (leukotriene C4 and prostaglandin D_2) and cytokines.[12] In contrast, nonimmunological stimulation of mast cells by neuropeptides, opiates, compound 48/80, or C5a leads to rapid histamine release within 15–20 seconds, without generation of eicosanoids and cytokines.[12] Moreover, prolonged and subthreshold immunological stimulation may result in a state of receptor desensitization. For example, desensitization of FcεRI may lead to basophil hyporesponsiveness to anti-IgE in autoimmune CU.[13] However, the desensitization of receptors by immunological stimulation does not affect nonimmunological release. Interestingly, enhanced responsiveness of skin mast cells to some nonimmunological stimuli has been observed in patients with CU.

Allergic urticaria

Immunological triggers of mast cell activation play an important role in different types of urticaria.[3, 11] The classical example of immunological mast cell activation via high-affinity IgE receptors is IgE-mediated urticaria (often termed allergic urticaria). In allergic urticaria, the cross-linking of receptor-bound IgE leads to the release of diverse preformed mediators and newly synthesized lipid mediators and cytokines, resulting in the early and late-phase IgE-mediated allergic inflammatory responses.

IgE-mediated mast cell activation usually presents as acute allergic urticaria in sensitized individuals and is very rarely, if ever, responsible for chronic whealing. Examples include some food- and drug-induced urticarias and latex-induced contact urticaria. Allergic urticaria to inhaled allergens (e.g., latex, animal epithelia) is often accompanied by respiratory symptoms. Generalized allergic urticaria may progress to anaphylaxis.

Table 42.1 Clinical patterns of urticaria

Ordinary urticaria
Acute
Chronic
Episodic

Physical urticaria
Mechanical: dermographism, delayed-pressure urticaria, vibratory angioedema
Thermal: cold-induced urticaria, localized heat-induced urticaria
Cholinergic urticaria and pruritus
Aquagenic urticaria and pruritus
Solar urticaria
Exercise (and food) induced anaphylaxis

Contact urticaria

Angioedema without wheals
Angioedema, due to C1 inhibitor deficiency
Angioedema with normal C1 inhibitor

Urticarial vasculitis
Normocomplementemic urticarial vasculitis
Hypocomplementemic urticarial vasculitis

Autoinflammatory syndromes (presenting with urticaria)
Hereditary (cryopyrin-associated) periodic syndromes
Familial cold autoinflammatory syndrome
Muckle–Wells syndrome
Chronic infantile neurological cutaneous and articular syndrome
Acquired
Schnitzler's syndrome

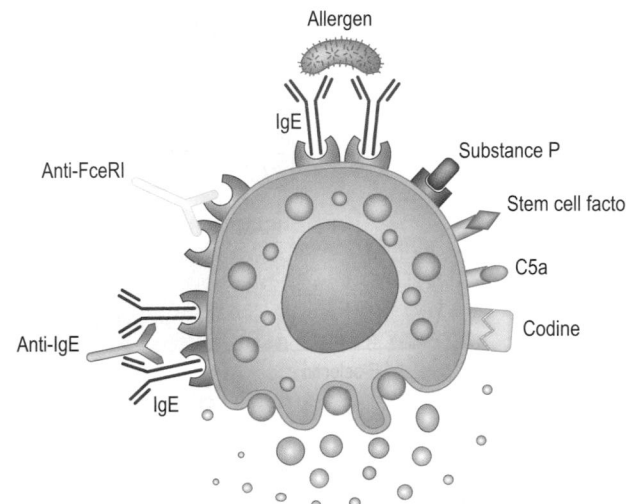

Fig. 42.3 Schematic representation of a mast cell or basophil illustrating activation of the immunoglobulin E (IgE) receptor by cross-linking with immunological stimuli (allergen/specific IgE binding, anti-IgE, or anti-FcεRI autoantibodies) or independent activation by nonimmunological stimuli (substance P, stem cell factor, codeine, or C5a) leading to degranulation.

Allergic urticaria resolves rapidly on withdrawal of allergen exposure and recurs with each re-exposure to the allergen or cross-reactive agents.

Autoimmune urticaria

Autoimmune urticaria is mediated by histamine-releasing autoantibodies directed against the extracellular α-chain of FcεRI on dermal mast cells or basophils or, less frequently, against receptor-bound IgE. These functional autoantibodies have been demonstrated by several independent research groups in 25–50% of adult and pediatric patients with the ordinary presentation of CU.[13, 14] The pathophysiology of autoimmune CU involves cross-linking of high-affinity IgE receptors by autoantibodies leading to degranulation of mast cells and basophils. There is good evidence that activation of cutaneous mast cells by IgG derived from CU sera *in vitro* is dependent on C5a but not all histamine-releasing IgG derived from CU sera are complement-dependent on basophil assays. Most functional autoantibodies are IgG_1 or IgG_3,[14] which are known to fix complement. By contrast, nonfunctional anti-FcεRI autoantibodies demonstrated by Western blot or enzyme-linked immunosorbent assay (ELISA) in other autoimmune diseases (including systemic lupus erythematosus and bullous pemphigoid) are generally from the noncomplement-fixing subclasses IgG_2 and IgG_4.[14]

Recently, anti-CD23 antibodies have also been detected in CU patients.[15] The low-affinity IgE receptor FcεRII/CD23 expressed on B lymphocytes and eosinophils may therefore be another target antigen for an autoimmune response in CU. The interaction between anti-CD23 antibodies and CD23 on eosinophils may induce release of major basic protein 1 (MBP-1), a potent IgE-independent histamine-releasing agent, resulting in activation of mast cells and basophils. The clinical relevance of anti-CD23 antibodies in CU remains to be elucidated but they may play a role in CU patients without autoantibodies against FcεRI or IgE.

Immune complex-mediated urticaria

Mast cell activation can result from binding of circulating immune complexes to FcεRIII, expressed on mast cells.[3, 11] In addition, circulating immune complexes can activate complement, leading to C3a and C5a anaphylatoxin formation. Urticaria caused by immune complexes may occur in serum sickness-like reactions, transfusion reactions, some drug-induced urticarias, and urticaria associated with infectious or autoimmune diseases. Immune complex-mediated urticaria usually develops 1–3 weeks after initial exposure to the antigen and disappears several weeks after antigen discontinuation. Chronic immune complex-mediated urticaria is known as urticarial vasculitis (UV: see below). In this condition, urticaria may be associated with systemic symptoms, such as fever, arthritis, or nephritis. Damage to postcapillary venules results from the deposition of immune complexes in the vessel wall. Immune complexes are formed on exposure to external (drug or infections) or internal (collagen-like region of C1q) antigens. Complement activation via the classical pathway leads to neutrophil chemotaxis through cytokine expression and adhesion molecule activation (Fig. 42.4). Proteolytic enzymes released from neutrophils damage vessel walls, leading to wheal formation and red blood cell extravasation.

Acute urticaria

Acute urticaria is defined as continuous disease lasting less than 6 weeks. People with an atopic predisposition are at higher risk of acute urticaria; atopic diseases are found in about half of acute urticaria patients.[3] Most acute urticaria resolves spontaneously within 3 weeks but in 10% patients may progress to CU.

Foods, drugs, and infections are the commonest identifiable causes of acute urticaria, although many cases remain unexplained. Viral upper respiratory tract infections precede the onset of acute urticaria by a few days in 40% of patients.[3] Acute urticaria can also be seen in pre-icteric viral hepatitis A, B, and C. However, a specific cause of acute urticaria will not be found in about 50% of patients. Foods are the commonest cause of acute urticaria in children but are rarely responsible for acute urticaria in adults. In infancy, cow's milk allergy is a frequent cause of acute allergic urticaria. Drug-induced urticaria is the commonest presentation of drug hypersensitivity, accounting for a quarter of all adverse drug reactions, with penicillin and NSAIDs the commonest causes of allergic and nonallergic drug-induced urticaria, respectively. Drug-induced urticaria is more likely in the elderly, perhaps reflecting polypharmacy and age-related pharmacokinetic changes, and in patients with human immunodeficiency virus (HIV) infection, renal or liver diseases. Acute NSAID-induced urticaria may be a risk factor for CU.[17]

Chronic urticaria

Some 25–50% of patients evaluated in specialist centers with continuous ordinary CU have evidence of functional autoantibodies but the majority remain idiopathic despite investigation.

Episodic urticaria

The cause of episodic urticaria often remains unknown but the possibility of an allergic or pseudoallergic cause needs to be considered.

PHYSICAL URTICARIA

Physically induced urticarias are common, accounting for 25% of all cases of CU. These include dermographism, cold contact urticaria, delayed-pressure urticaria (DPU), vibratory angioedema, localized heat urticaria, cholinergic, adrenergic, and aquagenic urticarias. Physical urticarias can coexist with chronic ordinary urticaria, and more than one physical urticaria may occur in the same patient (e.g., dermographic and cholinergic urticarias), which may lead to difficulty in diagnosis. With the exception of DPU, physical urticarias develop rapidly after exposure to the relevant trigger and fade within an hour.[2, 3]

The pathogenesis of physical urticarias is unclear. Physical stimuli lead to nonimmune activation of mast cells resulting in clinical manifestations that relate to the intensity, area, and duration of exposure. A diagnosis of physical urticaria is confirmed if the symptoms can be reproduced by challenge testing with the suspected stimulus. Challenge tests may also be used for monitoring threshold changes during treatment. In general, treatment of physical urticarias includes avoidance of known physical triggers and taking antihistamines. Sometimes tolerance may be induced for cold and solar urticarias.

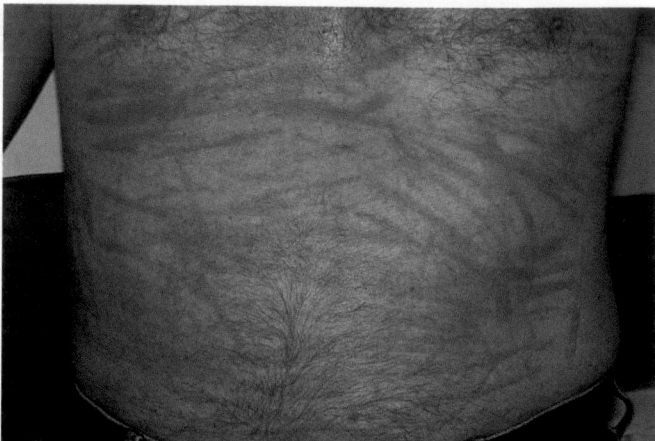

Fig. 42.6 Extensive induced dermographic whealing on the chest of a patient due to scratching.

MECHANICAL URTICARIA

Dermographism

Dermographism is the commonest physical urticaria, mainly affecting young people. Typical red, itchy, linear wheals are evoked within minutes of stroking, friction, rubbing, or scratching of skin (Fig. 42.6). Overheating, stress, and anxiety usually aggravate symptoms. Transient dermographism may occur after some bacterial and fungal infections, in scabies, parasitosis, and after treatment with penicillin. The diagnosis of dermographism is confirmed by stroking the skin with a blunt firm object, usually on the upper back. Antihistamines are the mainstay of therapy. Ultraviolet B radiation may be effective for patients unresponsive to antihistamines.

Delayed pressure urticaria (DPU)

Isolated DPU occurs in just 2% of all urticaria patients but DPU coexists with CU in up to 40% of patients. DPU is the most debilitating of the physical urticarias, and is triggered by sustained local pressure, e.g., wearing tight shoes, carrying heavy bags, long walks, sitting or leaning against firm objects, climbing ladders, jogging, driving, or hand clapping. Deep and painful swellings, clinically resembling angioedema, occur 30 minutes–12 hours after sustained pressure, and may be associated with flu-like symptoms, fever, arthralgia, and fatigue. The most frequent affected sites are hands, soles, buttocks, and shoulders, under straps and belts. DPU lesions last 12–48 hours and are usually painful rather than itchy, especially on the hands and feet. Laboratory investigation reveals transitory leukocytosis and elevated erythrocyte sedimentation rate (ESR). Hanging a heavy weight suspended on a narrow band over the forearm or thigh for 15 minutes may be used as a challenge test but more reliable results can be obtained with a dermographometer applied at 100 g/mm² for 70 seconds. The reaction should be assessed after 6 hours. DPU is difficult to treat because it responds poorly to antihistamines. High doses of steroids may be required for control in severe cases.

Vibratory angioedema

Vibratory angioedema is very rare. Familial cases have been described. Local swelling develops several minutes to 6 hours after exposure to vibrating machinery, lawn mowing, after applauding and jogging, for instance. Systemic symptoms may occur (headache, tightness in chest, diffuse flare). Placing the hand on a laboratory vortex for 5–15 minutes is a useful challenge test. Avoidance of the trigger is the only helpful treatment strategy.

THERMAL

Cold urticaria

Cold urticaria accounts for about 3% of physical urticarias.[20] It occurs in both children and adults, and is commoner in cold climates, in women, and in atopic patients. The majority of cases are primary with no identifiable cause but some cases are secondary to internal disease. Clinical manifestations can be local or generalized. Mucosal involvement may develop after drinking cold beverages. Systemic symptoms can be respiratory (laryngeal angioedema, tongue or pharyngeal swelling, wheezing), vascular (hypotension, tachycardia), gastrointestinal (hyperacidity, nausea, diarrhea), or neurological (disorientation, headache). Cold-induced urticaria can be evoked by low ambient temperature, contact with cold objects, food or beverages, and immersion in cold water. Wheals develop during the cold exposure or, more commonly, on warming up. The severity of cold urticaria depends on the intensity and duration of the cold stimulus. Cold urticaria is potentially life-threatening with a risk of anaphylaxis and death on exposure of large areas to cold, for example jumping into cold water, hypothermia in neurosurgical and cardiothoracic operations. Familial cold urticaria is due to mutations in the cold-induced autoinflammatory syndrome 1 (*CIAS1*) gene and is described below.

In 1–5% of patients, cold urticaria is secondary to cryoproteins (cryoglobulins, cryoagglutinins, cryofibrinogen, cryohaemolysin). These can be associated with infections (hepatitis C, infectious mononucleosis, syphilis, *Mycoplasma* infection), autoimmune diseases, and lymphoreticular malignancy (Waldenström's macroglobulinemia, myeloma). Cold urticaria may precede these diseases by several years. Secondary cold urticaria can also be drug-related (penicillin, oral contraceptives, angiotensin-converting enzyme (ACE) inhibitors).

The diagnosis of cold urticaria is confirmed by an ice cube challenge, although some atypical cold-induced urticarias have a negative ice cube test.

The clinical workup in cold urticaria includes measurement of cryoproteins. Patients should be cautious about bathing or swimming in cold water, and consuming cold food or drinks. Antihistamine treatment is often helpful but does not prevent anaphylaxis caused by swimming in cold water. In severe cold urticaria tolerance induction may be attempted: this involves depletion of mast cell histamine by repeated cold exposure.

Localized heat urticaria

Heat-induced urticaria is very rare. It is induced by local heating of the skin at 38–50°C. A refractory period up to 24 hours is typical. Challenge test is done by application of hot water in a tube or beaker at up to 44°C for 4–5 minutes. Symptoms develop several minutes after exposure. Management of heat-induced urticaria presents some difficulties as the clinical efficacy of antihistamines is limited.

OTHER PATTERNS

Cholinergic urticaria

Cholinergic urticaria is the second commonest physical urticaria and occurs mainly in adolescents, young adults, and atopic patients. Cholinergic urticaria usually follows a rise in core temperature due to physical exercise, fever, or external passive heat (hot bath, shower, sauna), but may also be provoked by emotional stress and spicy food. The characteristic lesions are highly pruritic pinpoint pale wheals of 1–3 mm surrounded by a red flare. They may occur anywhere except the soles and palms. Lesions usually begin on the trunk and neck, extending outwards to the face and limbs. As lesions progress, confluent areas of whealing and redness may develop. Severely affected patients may develop angioedema and even anaphylaxis. Most patients with mild disease do not seek medical help. The rash is triggered by activation of cholinergic sympathetic innervation of sweat glands but the mechanism of this remains unclear. Decreased blood protease inhibitor levels have been reported, and this is the rationale for using anabolic steroids to treat occasional severely affected individuals who are unresponsive to other measures. The prognosis is reasonably favorable, with spontaneous resolution within 8 years in most patients. However, 30% of patients are affected for >10 years.

Cholinergic urticaria can be confirmed by reproducing the rash with physical exercise or passive heating in a hot bath at up to 42°C. Treatment is primarily with antihistamines, but β-blockers, danazol, ketotifen, and montelukast have also been used. The condition is typically refractory for 24 hours and this may enable patients to prevent attacks by taking daily exercise.

Adrenergic urticaria

Adrenergic urticaria is very rare. The typical lesions are red papular wheals surrounded by a white areola, the opposite of cholinergic urticaria. It is thought that whealing is triggered by local release of norepinephrine. It is provoked by stress and may respond to β-blockers.

Solar urticaria

Solar urticaria affects > 1% of all urticaria patients with slight female predominance. It can be associated with erythropoietic porphyria. Wheals are caused by electromagnetic wavelengths ranging from 290 and 760 nm (ultraviolet B, A, and visible spectrum). It develops within minutes or hours after sun exposure and fades within 24 hours. Lesions are usually confined to sun-exposed skin, although they may also develop under clothing. Severity of solar urticaria depends on the wavelength, intensity, and duration of irradiation. Short exposures induce flare and pruritus while longer exposures cause whealing. In patients sensitive to the visible spectrum, reactions may occur through window glass.

Solar urticaria is diagnosed by monochromator phototesting. Patients are advised to use creams with a high sun protection factor (SPF), protective clothing, and protective window shields and limit time spent outdoors. Treatment of solar urticaria includes antihistamines, photochemotherapy and, occasionally, cyclosporine, or intravenous immunoglobulins.

local contact with cold water or an ice cube. Skin lesions occur after a few hours, subside in 24 hours, and are usually accompanied by fever, chills, conjunctival injection, sweating, headache, and arthralgia. During attacks there is marked leukocytosis, elevated ESR, and raised C-reactive protein.

Muckle–Wells syndrome

MWS develops in children or adolescents. It is characterized by CU, fever, aching, and malaise. Sensorineural deafness may develop in adulthood. Some MWS patients develop systemic amyloidosis (AA-type) with amyloid nephropathy. Laboratory findings in MWS include elevated ESR, C-reactive protein, IL-6, IL-1, and serum amyloid-associated protein.

Chronic infantile neurological cutaneous and articular syndrome

CINCA syndrome is more severe than FCAS or MWS, with neurological features and arthritis. Urticaria is rarely observed in infancy; other clinical features are lymphadenopathy, hepatosplenomegaly, dysmorphic features, developmental retardation, seizures, papilloedema, neurological manifestations, and overgrowth of the distal femur and patella. Affected individuals are at risk of leukemia and other malignancies, infections, and systemic amyloidosis.

Recently, it has been shown that treatment with the IL-1 receptor antagonist, anakinra, leads to complete resolution of symptoms in FCAS and MWS with normalization of inflammatory indices.

■ DIFFERENTIAL DIAGNOSIS ■

Several dermatoses may present with urticarial lesions, including erythema multiforme minor, bullous pemphigoid, and dermatitis herpetiformis.[2,3] These dermatoses can nearly always be distinguished clinically from urticaria on the basis of their polymorphic pattern, prolonged duration of individual lesions, lack of daily fluctuation, development of vesicles or blisters, and resistance to conventional therapy for urticaria. Very occasionally, skin biopsy, with or without indirect immunofluorescence, may be required to make the distinction.

Papular urticaria is an urticarial reaction to insect bites in sensitized individuals. The lesions are fixed rather than fluctuating, may take days or weeks to resolve fully, and may leave pigmentation or scars. Bites often occur asymmetrically in groups or lines. Although histamine is involved with the initial pruritic lesions, oral antihistamines are usually unhelpful and potent topical steroids may be required.

■ WORKUP IN URTICARIA PATIENTS ■

Evaluation of patients with urticaria requires a detailed history and physical examination.[1–4, 24] The history is particularly important in urticaria patients and should include a thorough search for all potential causes of the disorders, possible precipitating and aggravating factors, the timing of onset and duration of individual wheals, associated symptoms as well as travel history, recent infection, occupational exposure, food and

drug intake, and comorbidity. Patients can be asked to keep a diary of attacks, which may provide additional information about possible causes. The duration of individual lesions can be very helpful in distinguishing the different clinical patterns of urticaria.

Physical examination should focus on skin lesion morphology and careful systemic evaluation. If the patient is symptom-free at the time of evaluation, photographs may be helpful. The approximate duration of individual lesions can be assessed by outlining a particular lesion with a pen and observing it for a day. The appearance and distribution of skin lesions may suggest a diagnosis – for example, the pinpoint lesions with a large flare in cholinergic urticaria or lesions on sun-exposed areas in solar urticaria. A thorough physical examination can also offer diagnostic clues for associated comorbidities, including thyroid dysfunction.

Further evaluation of patients with urticaria is guided by the patient's history and clinical pattern of disease. However, it must be remembered that there may be more than one cause for urticaria and that different clinical subtypes of urticaria may coexist in one patient.

WORKUP IN ACUTE URTICARIA

It is well established that allergies are common causes of acute urticaria. The culprit allergens can be suspected from the clinical history, including a close temporal relationship to the time of exposure to the allergen and a history of previous exposure and prompt resolution on allergy withdrawal. Therefore, patients with acute or episodic urticaria should undergo allergy evaluation by skin testing or radioallergosorbent test (RAST) investigation if clinically indicated. In the case of food allergy, positive test results must also be verified by a trial of elimination diet followed by double-blind food challenge in supervised clinical settings.

WORKUP IN PHYSICAL URTICARIAS

When physical urticaria is suspected, appropriate challenge testing should be performed to confirm the diagnosis. Generally, there is no need for further investigations, except for cold urticaria where plasma cryoproteins (cryoglobulin, cold agglutinin, or cryofibrinogen) should be assayed.

WORKUP IN CHRONIC ORDINARY URTICARIA

No laboratory workup is recommended for patients with mild ordinary CU that is easily controlled by antihistamines, unless the history points to an underlying disease. Studies have shown that random laboratory testing very rarely yields evidence of unsuspected internal diseases as a cause of CU and this should therefore be discouraged.[25]

Screening laboratory evaluation can be considered in patients with poor response to first-line treatment. A complete blood count with differential, ESR, thyroid-stimulating hormone, liver function tests, and urinalysis will exclude most diseases associated with urticaria.

Other evaluations should be guided by abnormal findings in the history and physical examination in patients with CU. Additional tests may include stool examination for ova and parasites, antinuclear antibody titer, thyroid function and antithyroid antibodies, hepatitis viral screen, skinprick tests, or RAST for IgE-mediated reactions in episodic urticaria. Tests for immediate hypersensitivities should not be undertaken in chronic continuous urticaria unless there are compelling reasons for doing so. Rarely, CU can be caused by a specific food additive, which should be confirmed by dietary exclusion and double-blind, placebo-controlled oral challenge.

THE DIAGNOSIS OF AUTOIMMUNE CU

The diagnosis of autoimmune CU is not straightforward and involves *in vivo* and *in vitro* approaches. Autologous serum skin testing (ASST) is a simple and useful screening method for functional autoantibodies in CU patients. For skin testing, 0.05 ml of the patient's own serum should be injected intradermally into clinically uninvolved forearm skin together with an equal volume of saline and histamine (10 mg/ml) as controls at adjacent sites. The reaction is considered positive if the serum skin test forms a pink wheal at least 1.5 mm greater than the negative control at 30 minutes. The test is 80% specific and 70% sensitive for autoimmune CU as defined by a positive basophil histamine release assay.[13] A strongly positive ASST response (over 15 mm) was reported to be very specific for autoimmune CU (> 96%) when a panel of basophil and mast cell donors was used for testing.[26]

The current diagnostic gold standard in autoimmune CU is functional release assays using basophils or mast cells, but these only give indirect evidence of functional autoantibodies. Being technically difficult and time-consuming, these assays remain confined to research centers. Moreover, immunoassays (Western blotting, ELISA) based on binding of autoantibodies to relevant antigens (FcεRIα or IgE) do not correlate well with the results of functional assays.[14]

■ MANAGEMENT OF URTICARIA ■

Finding effective treatment for urticaria can be challenging for both clinician and patients. Treatment should be tailored to the clinical pattern, duration, and severity of the urticaria. Management should include nonpharmacological measures and drug therapy with a stepwise approach.[9, 26, 27]

GENERAL MEASURES

Identification and avoidance of allergens, infections, and physical triggers are of primary importance. Patients with the ordinary pattern of CU should minimize exposure to nonspecific aggravating factors, identified by a thorough history that may include overheating, stress, alcohol, dietary

THERAPEUTIC PRINCIPLES

MANAGEMENT OF URTICARIA

>> Eliminate infectious, drug, or food causes

>> Minimize nonspecific aggravators, including heat, stress, alcohol, nonsteroidal anti-inflammatories, and pressure

>> Regular oral antihistamines are the first line of therapy for all patterns of urticaria, except C1 esterase inhibitor deficiency

>> Second-line treatments, including short courses of oral corticosteroids, may be necessary for specific clinical situations

>> Immunosuppressive therapies should be reserved for patients with severe autoimmune urticaria or steroid-dependent urticaria that has not responded to other first- and second-line measures

pseudoallergens, and some drugs. NSAIDs aggravate CU in up to 30% of patients with the ordinary presentation and should generally be avoided. This probably does not apply to the physical urticarias, in particular DPU, where NSAIDs may be used as treatment. ACE inhibitors are contraindicated in angioedema without wheals and should be prescribed with caution in other patterns of urticaria. Although it is often recommended that CU patients should avoid codeine and penicillin, clinical experience suggests that this is not necessary. Cooling lotions and creams such as 1% menthol in aqueous cream may help to relieve pruritus. Some patients with ordinary but not physical CU appeared to respond to a low-pseudoallergen diet.[16] However, controlled clinical trials are lacking.

FIRST-LINE THERAPY

Antihistamines are the cornerstone of treatment in urticaria. Second-generation antihistamines offer several advantages over classical H_1 antihistamines, such as lack of sedation and impairment of performance, longer duration of action, and absence of anti-cholinergic side effects. Meta-analysis indicates that antihistamines are clinically effective in 40–90% of patients with CU. Second-generation antihistamines are inverse agonists of H_1 receptors, which stabilize H_1 receptors in the inactive conformation, and, therefore, are most effective in CU when taken regularly for prophylaxis. The timing of antihistamine intake should be adjusted to suit the diurnal pattern of urticaria. It has become common practice to increase second-generation antihistamines above their licensed doses when CU does not respond, because clinical experience shows that this achieves better control in some patients, although hard scientific evidence is still lacking. Although the evidence base for combining H_1 and H_2 antihistamines is poor, this may be helpful in some patients. Cimetidine (but not ranitidine) appears to increase the plasma concentration of H_1 antihistamines by inhibiting hepatic cytochrome P450. H_2 antihistamines also suppress the dyspepsia that often accompanies severe urticaria.

SECOND-LINE THERAPY

When urticaria does not respond to first-line measures, systemic corticosteroids are commonly used as short-term therapy for acute urticaria or severe exacerbations of CU. Long-term treatment with corticosteroids is not recommended because of safety concerns. In corticosteroid-dependent patients, an alternate-day dosing may be used and steroid-sparing drugs should also be considered. A wide variety of medications have been reported to be of benefit for antihistamine-unresponsive urticaria when oral corticosteroids might otherwise have to be considered but they are invariably used off-license and controlled trials are usually lacking. Where possible, these should be targeted at specific subgroups of urticaria patients, e.g., the leukotriene receptor antagonist montelukast has been shown to be effective in aspirin-sensitive CU patients, and thyroxine in biochemically euthyroid CU patients with evidence of thyroid autoimmunity.[28]

THIRD-LINE THERAPY

Immunosuppressive therapy is mainly considered for autoimmune CU.[3, 13] However, clinical experience suggests it may also benefit therapy-resistant CU without evidence of circulating antibodies.

The best-studied immunosuppressive therapy is cyclosporine, which has been shown in a double-blind placebo-controlled study to be effective at 4 mg/kg daily in CU patients. Patients must be monitored carefully for renal function and hypertension; treatment should normally be limited to 3 months. Cyclosporine is contraindicated for patients with previous malignant disease. Tacrolimus also appears to be effective in corticosteroid-dependent autoimmune CU.[18] There is some evidence for efficacy of plasmapheresis and immunoglobulins in chronic autoimmune urticaria, though these are expensive options and controlled clinical trials are needed. Methotrexate and azathioprine have also been used alone or with corticosteroids.

ANAPHYLAXIS

Anaphylaxis is a severe, life-threatening, systemic reaction involving difficulty with breathing, circulatory collapse or both.

Epidemiology of anaphylaxis

Estimates of the incidence of anaphylaxis in the general population vary from 3.2 cases per 100 000 inhabitants per annum in Denmark to 21 cases per 100 000 inhabitants per annum in the USA.[29] The mortality rate is estimated to be in the range of 1–2%.[30] In the UK anaphylaxis accounts for 20 deaths per year, which represents 1 death in 3 million people.[31] Anaphylaxis occurs more often in females than males[32] and in children more than adults.[33]

Hospital admissions for anaphylaxis nearly doubled in the UK in the 1990s.[34] Severe anaphylaxis was diagnosed in 1–9 per 10 000 people attending emergency departments in the UK, Australia, and the USA.[30] It is estimated that, in a 12-month period, 1 in 12 patients with previous anaphylaxis will have a recurrence, and 1 in 50 will require hospitalization or treatment with epinephrine.[33]

The pathophysiology of anaphylaxis

Although anaphylaxis is often subdivided into allergic (IgE-mediated) and nonallergic (anaphylactoid) groups, the clinical presentation is similar and some authorities do not make a distinction. In IgE-mediated anaphylaxis, allergen cross-links allergen-specific IgE antibodies on the surface of mast cells and basophils, leading to their degranulation in the

same way as in allergic urticaria. Release of mediators causes bronchoconstriction, mucus secretion, diminished cardiac contractility, increased vascular permeability, vasoconstriction of coronary and peripheral arteries, and vasodilation of venules, thereby producing clinical symptoms of anaphylaxis. IgE-mediated reactions occur in presensitized patients (e.g., penicillin-, insulin-, latex- or peanut-induced anaphylaxis). By contrast, some substances such as opioids, radiocontrast media, and some muscle relaxants are capable of direct mediator release (histamine) from basophils and mast cells without involvement of IgE. Although reactions to NSAIDs are considered to be pharmacological rather than immunological due to the downstream effects of COX inhibition, an IgE-mediated mechanism has been suspected in a few patients but is difficult to prove. Apart from IgE, other antibodies may be involved: in murine models IgG-mediated FcεRIII-dependent anaphylaxis elicited by a high dose of allergen has been described. The key participating cells in this type of anaphylaxis are macrophages, with platelet-activating factor as the main mediator.[35]

The etiology of anaphylaxis

A cause of anaphylaxis can only be identified in about 60% of patients. Anaphylaxis is most commonly caused by foods, drugs, general anesthetic agents, insect stings, and latex. Rare causes include vaccines, semen, and aeroallergen inhalation. Exercise may occasionally cause anaphylaxis either on its own (exercise-induced anaphylaxis), or after prior ingestion of a food to which the individual is sensitized (food and exercise-induced anaphylaxis). Idiopathic anaphylaxis accounts for up to 40% of all cases.[35, 36] Patients with idiopathic anaphylaxis should be investigated to exclude systemic mastocytosis.

The most common routes of allergen exposure are oral and parenteral, although inhalation of allergens (for example, fish or legume allergens after cooking, latex particles in health care settings) or percutaneous penetration after skin contact can induce anaphylaxis in highly sensitized patients. The link with atopy is not clear but anaphylaxis with predominant respiratory involvement elicited by skin and mucosal allergen contact is thought to be more often related to atopy than parenterally induced anaphylaxis (e.g., insect stings or drug-induced anaphylaxis).[35]

Food-induced anaphylaxis

Food allergy is a common cause of anaphylaxis, with an annual incidence of 7.6 cases per 100 000 person-years.[35] Anaphylactic reactions to foods have been increasing over the last two decades: a fivefold increase in food allergy was reported in France from 1980 to 1995.[30] Food-induced anaphylaxis is the most common single cause of anaphylaxis treated in emergency departments in the USA, especially in the younger population, and accounts for 29 000 estimated emergency room visits and 150–200 deaths per year.[35] Over 60% of cases of food-induced anaphylaxis occur in patients younger than 30 years.[37] Peanuts and other nuts, fish, and shellfish are the most frequent culprits in food-induced anaphylaxis but almost any food can be implicated.[37] Many cases of severe anaphylaxis are caused by unintended exposure to hidden food allergens. In addition, alcohol, NSAIDs, exercise, or concurrent infection may increase the severity of a food-induced allergic reaction.

Drug-induced anaphylaxis

Drug-induced anaphylaxis is more common in hospitalized patients than in the community. Any drug may cause anaphylaxis, though the prevalence varies: one study found 5–15 cases per 100 000 patients for most NSAIDs and antibiotics, while for penicillin and contrast agents the figure was over 30 cases per 100 000.[38] Drugs are the leading cause of fatal anaphylaxis, comprising 43.5% of such deaths.[31] The mortality rate in drug-induced anaphylaxis is about one death per 50 000–100 000 treatment courses.[38] All routes of administration can be potentially fatal, including oral, intravenous, intra-articular, intrauterine, inhalational, rectal, or topical, but the risk is greatest after parenteral administration.

Anaphylaxis during anesthesia

The incidence of anaphylaxis in general anesthesia varies between 1:3500 and 1:20 000, significantly exceeding the overall prevalence of drug-induced anaphylaxis.[36] The French registry of anaphylaxis during general anesthesia established a prevalence of one case in 13 000 episodes of general anesthesia.[39] The incidence of anaphylaxis to local anesthetics is, by contrast, extremely rare. Most cases of suspected anaphylaxis to local anesthetics are probably due to vasovagal or panic attacks; a few may follow inadvertent intravascular injection.

A network of 38 French allergo-anesthesia outpatient clinics reported that around 60% of all cases were induced by muscle relaxants (rocuronium, suxamethonium, etc.), followed by latex and antibiotics.[39] Reactions to neuromuscular blocking agents mostly occur on first exposure and were associated with a 70% rate of cross-reactivity in this group. Latex, the next most important cause of anaphylaxis, accounted for 16% of intraoperative anaphylactic reactions.[39]

Insect sting-induced anaphylaxis

Severe anaphylaxis from insect stings causes approximately 40 deaths annually in the USA and nearly 100 in Europe.[27] The intensity of reaction depends on the type of insect, amount of venom, location of sting, and the patient's sensitivity. Allergen-specific immunotherapy with venom extracts has been shown to be safe and effective in patients with hymenoptera venom allergy, providing some clinical protection within the first 8 weeks of treatment and a long-lasting effect after 3–5 years of maintenance treatment (Chapter 43). It is noteworthy that patients with systemic mastocytosis are at risk of potentially fatal anaphylaxis to insect stings even if they are not presensitized to venom: this may be due to venom components, such as phospholipase A_2, acting as mast cell liberators. Venom immunotherapy may be given to mastocytosis patients but there is quite a high risk of anaphylaxis during treatment.

Latex-induced anaphylaxis

The prevalence of latex allergy has been estimated to be as high as 1–6% in the general population, 8–17% in health care workers, and 67% in spina bifida patients.[29] Latex-induced anaphylaxis has been reported in surgery and dentistry and can be fatal. More than half of latex-allergic patients have allergies to fruits such as bananas, avocado, kiwi fruit, chestnut, pears, pineapples, grapes, and papayas.

Other rare causes of anaphylaxis

Anaphylaxis occurs during 1 in 20 000–47 000 transfusions of blood or blood products, especially in patients with IgA deficiency.[40] IgA deficiency affects 1 in 500–700 Caucasians. One-third of these patients have circulating anti-IgA antibodies, which are associated with serious life-threatening anaphylactic reactions to blood products containing IgA.

Seminal fluid allergy is extremely rare, mostly affecting atopic young women, with 20% of cases developing life-threatening anaphylaxis. These reactions can be prevented with condom usage or intravaginal desensitization with seminal fluid.

Idiopathic anaphylaxis

Idiopathic anaphylaxis is a diagnosis of exclusion. Its pathophysiology is not understood.

THE CLINICAL DIVERSITY OF ANAPHYLAXIS

In anaphylaxis, there is a remarkable range of clinical symptoms. Anaphylaxis can be preceded by prodromal symptoms such as tingling and redness of the palms and soles, anxiety, sense of doom, and disorientation. Anaphylaxis most commonly begins in the skin and mucous membranes, followed by involvement of the respiratory and gastrointestinal tracts, cardiovascular system and, finally, proceeding to cardiac and/or respiratory arrest. Generalized urticaria and angioedema are the most common manifestations of anaphylaxis observed in over 90% of cases, but may be absent. Respiratory symptoms may vary from rhinitis to laryngeal edema and airway obstruction, which are potentially life-threatening. Some patients present with only cardiovascular collapse in the absence of other signs of anaphylaxis, especially during general anesthesia.[41] The differential diagnosis of anaphylaxis includes panic attacks and vasovagal episodes.

Four clinical patterns of anaphylaxis have been described: immediate, biphasic, protracted, and delayed.[35] Anaphylaxis can occur within seconds after allergen exposure: the more rapid the onset of anaphylaxis after allergen exposure, the more severe and life-threatening the reaction. Food-induced anaphylaxis takes slightly longer to develop than drug- or insect-induced anaphylaxis. Up to 20% of patients may have biphasic anaphylaxis, with recurrence 2–12 hours after the initial attack. Recurrent episodes do not differ clinically but may require more epinephrine. The occurrence of biphasic anaphylaxis cannot be predicted from the severity of the initial attack. Some patients may develop protracted anaphylaxis, which sometimes lasts longer than 24 hours, may be extremely severe, and is often resistant to treatment. Delayed onset of anaphylaxis has been reported anecdotally but is very unusual in clinical practice.

The diversity and severity of symptoms in anaphylaxis depend on the route of allergen exposure, the extent of allergen absorption, the degree of sensitization, individual allergen threshold, target tissue sensitivity, cofactor involvement, comorbidity, and concomitant treatment. Recently, "summation anaphylaxis" has been recognized if it occurs after simultaneous exposure to various stimuli (physical exercise, infection, stress or concomitant exposure to other allergens or treatment with NSAIDs, ACE inhibitors, or β-blockers).[35] Fatal reactions to foods are usually characterized by respiratory symptoms (bronchospasm and hypoxia). In contrast, anaphylaxis induced by insect stings is more likely to lead to cardiovascular collapse. Asthma sufferers are at higher risk of fatal anaphylaxis. The risk of relapse

CLINICAL PEARLS

DIAGNOSIS OF ANAPHYLAXIS

>> Anaphylaxis is characterized by extreme difficulty with breathing due to airway obstruction from angioedema or bronchoconstriction, circulatory collapse or both

>> It is nearly always accompanied by tachycardia, usually by flushing, urticaria, and panic, and sometimes by vomiting and diarrhea

>> Panic attacks do not involve airways obstruction, hypotension, or urticaria but may be accompanied by faintness or tetany of the hands due to rapid overbreathing

>> Vasovagal attacks present with fainting, nausea, slow pulse, and pallor without respiratory difficulty, diarrhea, or urticaria

in anaphylaxis depends on the type of allergen, individual allergen threshold, success of allergen avoidance, and the availability of immunotherapy.

The most dangerous symptoms are laryngeal edema, respiratory failure, and circulatory collapse, which may lead to death. Deaths from acute asthma in anaphylaxis occur predominantly in patients with pre-existing unstable asthma. Rapidly fatal shock often occurs without other symptoms, while death from laryngeal angioedema is the least common cause of fatality. According to the UK fatal anaphylaxis registry, the earliest arrest in fatal food anaphylaxis develops within 25–35 minutes of exposure, slightly slower than for insect stings (10–15 minutes) or drugs (5 minutes or less in hospital and 10–20 minutes outside hospital).[31, 35]

THE DIAGNOSIS OF ANAPHYLAXIS

The measurement of blood tryptase level is now widely used as a marker of mast cell degranulation for *in vitro* confirmation of anaphylaxis. Beta-tryptase is released from mast cells but not from basophils and diffuses more slowly than histamine. The concentration of tryptase peaks 1–2 hours after the onset of reaction and remains elevated with a half-life of 1.5–2.5 hours. The samples for tryptase testing should be collected within 6 hours of anaphylaxis onset and again after 24 hours to check that the value has returned to normal. Tryptase can also be detected in postmortem specimens after death from suspected anaphylaxis.[31]

Normally, mature tryptase is below detection limits in the serum of healthy subjects, while it is elevated in most cases of anaphylaxis with vascular compromise, especially if it is parenterally induced. A tryptase concentration above 25 µg/l is highly suggestive of anaphylaxis.[39] However, a normal level of tryptase is quite often observed in food-induced anaphylaxis so a normal tryptase result does not exclude anaphylaxis.[35-37] The diagnostic value of other mast cell proteases in anaphylaxis is under investigation.

THE MANAGEMENT OF ANAPHYLAXIS

Early recognition of anaphylaxis facilitates removal of the cause and prompt institution of treatment. The patient with anaphylaxis should lie down with the legs elevated in order to increase venous blood return and maintain cardiac output. In drug-induced or insect-induced anaphylaxis a tourniquet may be placed proximal to the site of the injection or insect sting to slow

absorption of injected antigens. The tourniquet should be released for 3 minutes at 5-minute intervals, with the total duration of application not exceeding 30 minutes. Epinephrine should be administered at the first sign of respiratory failure or cardiovascular collapse. Milder attacks of allergy are often treated with antihistamines as a first-line measure. Epinephrine auto-injectors for self-administration are available but a single pen may be insufficient to reverse severe reactions. Their use in anaphylaxis outside hospital can be life-saving. The earlier epinephrine is administered in anaphylaxis, the better the outcome and survival rate.[42] Overall, prompt diagnosis of anaphylaxis, early administration of epinephrine, and fast transport to emergency rooms are crucial factors for successful management of anaphylaxis.

Epinephrine is both an α- and β-adrenergic agonist with cyclic adenosine monophosphate (cAMP)-mediated pharmacological effects on target organs. In patients with anaphylaxis, stimulation of α_1-adrenergic receptors increases peripheral vascular resistance, thereby improving blood pressure and coronary perfusion, reversing peripheral vasodilation, and decreasing angioedema. Activation of β_1-adrenergic receptors increases myocardial contractility (inotropy, chronotropy) while stimulation of β_2-adrenoreceptors causes bronchodilation as well as decreasing the release of inflammatory mediators from mast cells and basophils.[35, 42]

According to current recommendations, the intramuscular route for epinephrine administration is preferable to the subcutaneous route due to faster absorption and higher plasma level of epinephrine after intramuscular injection.[40] The appropriate dosage of epinephrine is 0.3–0.5 ml of a 1:1000 dilution for adults. Epinephrine has a rapid but short action, therefore the dose can be repeated every 5–15 minutes until symptoms improve. More than one dose is required in one in three patients. The intravenous administration of epinephrine (1:10 000 dilution, i.e., 100 µg/ml) should be reserved for severe anaphylaxis with profound life-threatening hypotension that is refractory to other treatment because of a risk of potentially fatal cardiac arrhythmias and myocardial infarction.

Common pharmacological adverse effects of epinephrine include anxiety, fear, headache, pallor, tremor, dizziness, and palpitation. In the event of overdose, unwanted effects may include increased QTc interval on electrocardiography, ventricular arrhythmias, angina, myocardial infarction, increased blood pressure, pulmonary edema, and intracranial hemorrhage. Patients with cardiovascular diseases and thyrotoxicosis and cocaine users are particularly prone to adverse effects of epinephrine.

The efficacy of epinephrine can be decreased by concomitant therapy with β-blockers, which is associated with unopposed stimulation of α-adrenoreceptors and reflex vagotonic effects, leading to bradycardia, hypertension, coronary artery constriction, bronchoconstriction, and augmented mediator release. Anaphylaxis in patients on β-blockers can be severe, protracted, and unresponsive to treatment. Patients treated with β-blockers may require fluid replacement and treatment with glucagon, which increases intracellular cAMP independently of β-adrenergic receptors. Glucagon can be administered in an intravenous bolus of 1 mg, followed by infusion of 1–5 mg/hour. Glucagon may improve hypotension in 1–5 minutes with maximal effect at 5–15 minutes. Side effects of glucagon include nausea and vomiting.

Corticosteroids are often administered in anaphylaxis to minimize the risk of recurrent or protracted anaphylaxis. The beneficial effects of corticosteroids develop 6–12 hours after administration. Therefore, their main role in anaphylaxis is likely to be the prevention of relapse but it is still unclear how they work.

If no response to epinephrine is observed, life support measures should be instituted. The treatment choice depends on the clinical presentation. In resistant hypotension, large volumes of fluids (crystalloids) should be given rapidly to compensate for peripheral vasodilatation and for fluid loss into the extravascular space. Other vasopressors (dopamine, glucagon) may be needed to reverse severe hypotension. Oxygen should also be administered in circulatory or respiratory failure. Bronchospasm should be treated with nebulized or inhaled β_2-agonists. If there is severe laryngeal edema, endotracheal intubation and even emergency tracheostomy may be needed to maintain the airway. All patients should be observed in a hospital setting for at least 4 hours because of the risk of biphasic anaphylaxis. In severe cases, an observation period of 24 hours is advisable.

THE PREVENTION OF ANAPHYLAXIS

The first step in prevention is to identify those at risk of anaphylaxis. Therefore, all patients with a history of anaphylaxis should be referred for assessment and undergo allergy evaluation. Patients should be instructed how to avoid culprit allergens and cross-reactive agents and should be advised on safe alternatives. The education of patients, their families and, in the case of children, caregivers and school staff about anaphylaxis and first-aid measures is of primary importance. Written treatment plans should be provided to patients at special risk. Emergency medications such as epinephrine auto-injectors should be dispensed and patients should receive training on their usage. Patients should be advised to carry an epinephrine auto-injector with them at all times. Immunotherapy is very effective for prophylaxis of bee and wasp venom-induced anaphylaxis in sensitized patients and can be life-saving. Prevention strategies for anaphylaxis should also involve public awareness and public health measures, such as appropriate food labeling, disclosure of food ingredients in restaurants, the withdrawal of peanuts from in-flight refreshments, first-aid training in anaphylaxis for school staff, and establishing national anaphylaxis registries.

■ REFERENCES ■

1. Zuberbier T, Binslev-Jensen C, Canonica W, et al. EAACI/GA2LEN/EDF guideline: definition, classification and diagnosis of urticaria. Allergy 2006; 61: 316–320.

2. Henz BM, Zuberbier T, Grabbe J, et al. (eds): Urticaria, Berlin: Springer-Verlag, 1998.

3. Greaves MW, Kaplan A (eds): Urticaria and Angioedema, New York: Marcel Dekker; 2004.

4. Beltrani VS. An overview of chronic urticaria. Clin Rev Allergy Immunol 2002; 23: 147–169.

5. Aydogan K, Karadogan SK, Akdag I, et al. HLA class I and class II antigens in Turkish patients with chronic ordinary urticaria. Clin Exp Dermatol 2006; 31: 424–429.

6. O'Donnell BF, O'Neill CM, Francis DM, et al. Human leucocyte antigen class II associations in chronic idiopathic urticaria. Br J Dermatol 1999; 140: 853–858.

7. Oztas P, Onder M, Gonen S, et al. Is there any relationship between human leucocyte antigen class II and chronic urticaria (chronic urticaria and HLA class II)? Yonsei Med J 2004; 45: 392–395.

8. Kim SH, Choi JH, Lee KW, et al. The human leucocyte antigen-DRB1*1302-DQB1*0609-DPB1*0201 haplotype may be a strong genetic marker for aspirin-induced urticaria. Clin Exp Allergy 2005; 35: 339–344.

9. Grattan CEH. The urticaria spectrum: recognition of clinical patterns can help management. Clin Exp Dermatol 2004; 29: 217–221.

10. Maurer M, Metz M. The status quo and quo vadis of mast cells. Exp Dermatol 2005; 14: 923–929.

11. Hennino A, Berard F, Guillot I, et al. Pathophysiology of urticaria. Clin Rev Allergy Immunol 2006; 30: 3–11.

12. Church MK, el-Lati S, Caulfield JP. Neuropeptide-induced secretion from human skin mast cells. Int Arch Allergy Appl Immunol 1991; 94: 310–318.

13. Sabroe RA, Greaves MW. Chronic idiopathic urticaria with functional autoantibodies: 12 years on. Br J Dermatol 2006; 154: 813–819.

14. Kaplan AP. Chronic urticaria: pathogenesis and treatment. J Allergy Clin Immunol 2004; 114: 465–474.

15. Puccetti A, Bason C, Simeoni S, et al. In chronic idiopathic urticaria autoantibodies against Fc epsilonRII/CD23 induce histamine release via eosinophil activation. Clin Exp Allergy 2005; 35: 1599–1607.

16. Zuberbier T. The role of allergens and pseudoallergens in urticaria. J Invest Dermatol Symp Proc 2001; 6: 132–134.

17. Grattan CE. Aspirin sensitivity and urticaria. Clin Exp Dermatol 2003; 28: 123–127.

18. Kozel MM, Sabroe RA. Chronic urticaria: aetiology, management and current and future treatment options. Drugs 2004; 64: 2515–2536.

19. Buhner S, Reese I, Kuehl F, et al. Pseudoallergic reactions in chronic urticaria are associated with altered gastroduodenal permeability. Allergy 2004; 59: 1118–1123.

20. Wanderer AA, Hoffman HM. The spectrum of acquired and familial cold-induced urticaria/urticaria-like syndromes. Immunol Allergy Clin North Am 2004; 24: 259–286.

21. Davis MD, Brewer JD. Urticarial vasculitis and hypocomplementemic urticarial vasculitis syndrome. Immunol Allergy Clin North Am 2004; 24: 183–213.

22. Frigas E, Nzeako UC. Angioedema. Pathogenesis, differential diagnosis, and treatment. Clin Rev Allergy Immunol 2002; 23: 217–231.

23. Almerigogna F, Giudizi MG, Capella F, et al. Schnitzler's syndrome: what's new?. J Eur Acad Dermatol Venereol 2002; 16: 214–219.

24. Kozel MM, Bossuyt PM, Mekkes JR, et al. Laboratory tests and identified diagnoses in patients with physical and chronic urticaria and angioedema: a systematic review. J Am Acad Dermatol 2003; 48: 409–416.

25. Asero R, Lorini M, Chong SU, et al. Assessment of histamine-releasing activity of sera from patients with chronic urticaria showing positive autologous skin test on human basophils and mast cells. Clin Exp Allergy 2004; 34: 1111–1114.

26. Grattan CE, Powell S, Humphreys F. British Association of Dermatologists. Management and diagnostic guidelines for urticaria and angioedema. Br J Dermatol 2001; 144: 708–714.

27. Zuberbier T, Binslev-Jensen C, Canonica W, et al. EAACI/GA2LEN/EDF guideline: management of urticaria. Allergy 2006; 61: 321–331.

28. Borzova E, Grattan C. Urticaria: current and future treatments. Expert Rev Dermatol 2007; 2: 317–334.

29. Matasar MJ, Neugut AI. Epidemiology of anaphylaxis in the United States. Curr Allergy Asthma Rep 2003; 3: 30–35.

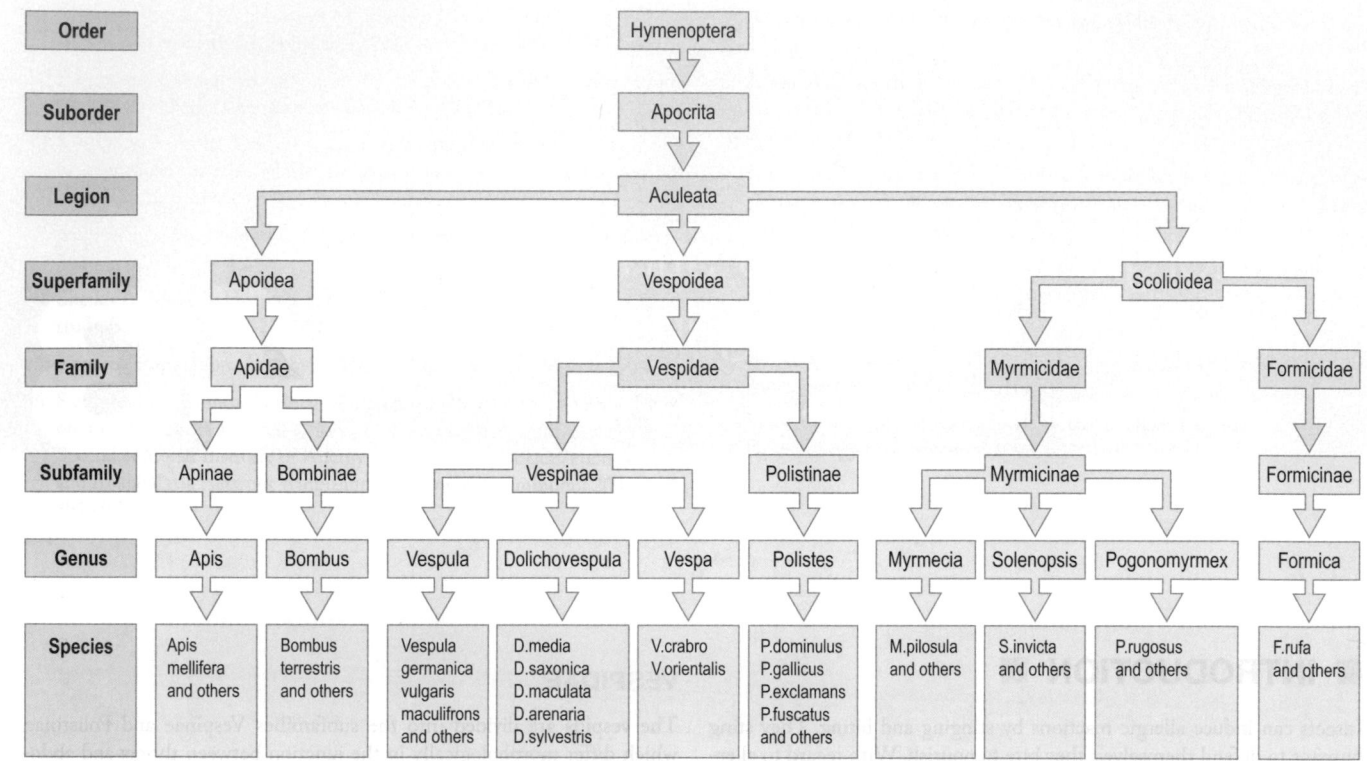

Fig. 43.1 Taxonomy of Hymenoptera.

all over Europe except for the British Isles. Their small nests consist only of one womb and are built in trees or under roofs.

ANTS (MYRMICINAE, FORMICINAE)

In south and central America, and in the southern states of the USA, the fire ants (*Solenopsis invicta, S. richteri*) are responsible for many systemic allergic sting reactions.[3] Fire ants build their mounds in yards, playgrounds and fields. Occasional allergic sting reactions have been described to *Pogonomyrmex*, the North American harvester ant, and extremely rarely to the European red ant, *Formica rufa*. In contrast, species of Myrmecinae, especially *Myrmecia pilosula*, the jack-jumper ant, are an important cause of allergic sting reactions in southern Australia.[4]

ALLERGENS IN HYMENOPTERA VENOMS

All Hymenoptera venoms contain low molecular weight substances such as biogenic amines, phospholipids, amino acids and carbohydrates, and peptides such as melittin, apamin or kinins, which contribute to the toxic effect but which – except for melittin – are probably irrelevant with regard to allergies. The allergens of the important stinging Hymenoptera are shown in Table 43.1. Most of them are glycoproteins of 10–50 kDa. The major allergens in bee venom are phospholipase A2, hyaluronidase and acid phosphatase; in vespid venoms antigen 5, phospholipase A1 and

hyaluronidase. Ant venom from *Solenopsis invicta* contains a 37 kDa and a 24 kDa allergen with some sequence homology to phospholipase A1 and to antigen 5 from vespid venom. Today the genes of many major venom allergens have been cloned, and some of them have also been expressed as recombinant proteins that are comparable in allergenic activity and enzymatic function to their natural counterparts.[5–7]

The amount of venom injected during a sting varies between and within species, especially with vespids. Bees release 50–140 µg venom per sting; vespids much less: between 2 and 17 µg.[2]

CLINICAL PICTURE

Symptoms of venom hypersensitivity are most often due to IgE-mediated, but occasionally to nonIgE-mediated immunologic mechanisms. Rarely nonimmunologic mechanisms of mediator release play a role. The clinical presentation is classified into normal, large local, systemic allergic, systemic toxic and unusual reactions.[1,2]

NORMAL LOCAL REACTIONS

The normal local reaction of a nonallergic subject to a Hymenoptera sting consists of a painful, sometimes itchy, local wheal and flare reaction, followed by a swelling of up to 5–10 cm in diameter. Usually, local symptoms resolve within a few hours, by definition within 24 hours. After stings by *Solenopsis*, the American fire ant, a vesicle remains which later develops into a pustule that only heals after 1–2 weeks.[3]

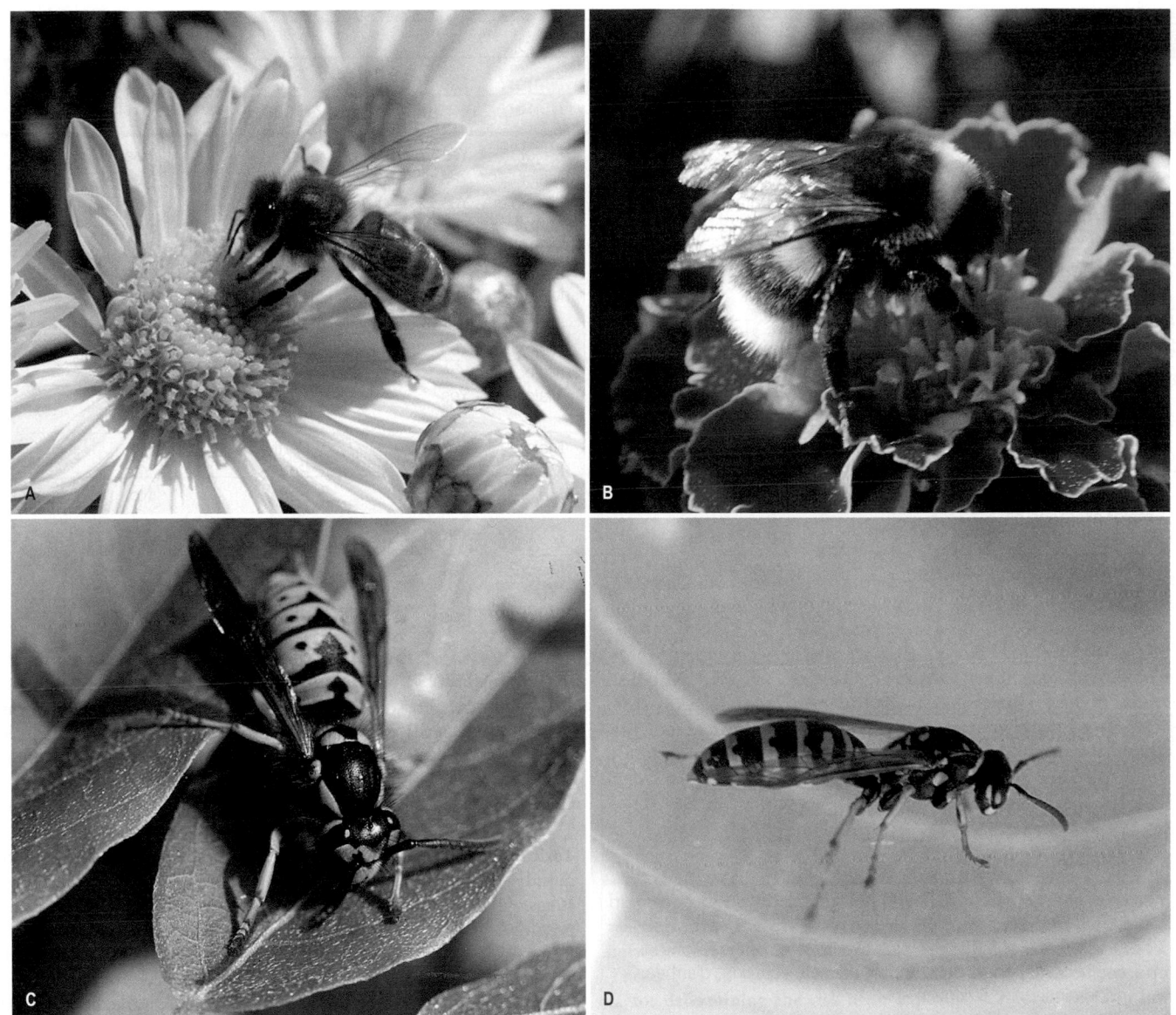

Fig. 43.2 Common Hymenoptera. (**A**) Honey bee *(Apis mellifera)*. (**B**) Bumblebee *(Bombus terrestris)*. (**C**) Wasp/yellowjacket *(Vespula* spp*)*. (**D**) Field wasp *(Polistes gallicus)*.

LARGE LOCAL REACTION (LLR)

We define an LLR as a swelling around the sting site exceeding 10 cm in diameter, developing minutes to hours after the sting and lasting over 24 hours.[1] LLR may be very disturbing, especially when they last for days or even weeks and involve a whole limb, eyelids or lips. Sometimes they are accompanied by lymphadenopathy or lymphangitis. They may also be associated with nonspecific systemic inflammatory symptoms, such as malaise, fever, shivering, or headache. However, the development of a local infection, an abscess or phlegmon at the sting site is inhibited by the bacteriostatic effect of Hymenoptera

venoms. In contrast, scratching after stings by the American fire ant *Solenopsis* or bites from blood-sucking insects such as midges, can lead to skin infection.

The pathogenesis of LLR is thought to be based on IgE- and cell-mediated immune mechanisms or a combination of both.[1,2]

SYSTEMIC ALLERGIC REACTIONS (SR)

Systemic anaphylactic reactions are usually mediated by IgE. Affected organs can include the skin (pruritus, urticaria, flush, angioedema), the gastrointestinal tract (cramps, vomiting or diarrhea, dysphagia), the

Table 43.2 Natural history of Hymenoptera venom allergy

Previous reaction	Author, year	Re-exposure by*	% with systemic reaction upon re-exposure to			
			Bee or vespid*	Bee	Vespid	Ant
Large local	Müller, 1990	FS	6			
Any systemic	Blaauw 1985, Van der Linden, 1994	CH		51	25	
Mild systemic children	Schuberth,1983	FS	16			
Mild systemic	Blaauw, 1985	CH		31	10	
Severe systemic	Blaauw, 1985	CH	44	60	33	
Severe systemic, controls of controlled studies	Hunt, 1978 Müller, 1979 Brown 2003	CH FS CH	61	75		72

*FS = field sting
CH = sting challenge.

DIAGNOSIS

HISTORY

The clinical history is the basis of the diagnosis of Hymenoptera sting allergy. This includes the date, number and circumstances of stings (e.g., environment, activities); kind and severity of symptom; sting site; retained or removed stinger; interval to onset of symptoms; emergency treatment; risk factors for a particularly severe reaction (e.g., comorbidity, drugs); tolerated stings after the first systemic reaction; and other allergies.[1,2] In individuals with only an LLR no further diagnostic tests are recommended. Basic diagnostic tests are skin tests and estimation of venom-specific serum IgE antibodies.

SKIN TESTS

Skin tests should be performed at least three weeks after an SR in order to avoid false negative results during the refractory period. They are performed by intradermal or skin-prick endpoint titration;[2] 0.02 mL of venom solution are injected intradermally in increasing concentrations – from 0.001 to 1 μg/mL – into the volar surface of the forearm. For skin-prick tests, concentrations of 0.01–300 μg/mL are used. However, even at 300 μg the sensitivity of skin prick is clearly lower than that of the intradermal test. We therefore prefer the intradermal test.

VENOM-SPECIFIC SERUM IgE ANTIBODIES (SIgE)

Several different *in vitro* immunoassays for the detection of sIgE have been derived from the original RAST (radio allergosorbent test) and are commercially available. Immediately after a sting sIgE may be low or even undetectable, but usually increases within days or weeks after an SR. If no sIgE is detectable, the test should be repeated after 2–4 weeks.[2]

SENSITIVITY AND SPECIFICITY OF SKIN TESTS AND SIgE

The sensitivity of these tests is over 90% in patients with a history of SR within the last year. As a rule the intradermal test remains positive longer than sIgE. However, so far no reliable test exists to predict the risk of future SRs in untreated or treated patients. In spite of a history of typical SRs to stings, a few patients have no detectable IgE and negative skin tests.[17] This may be due to insufficient sensitivity of the available tests, a long interval between SR and testing, with spontaneous decrease of sensitization, or nonIgE-mediated pathogenesis.

Specificity may cause problems: about 10–20% of people without a history of SR have a positive diagnostic test. Although sensitization following a previous sting is difficult to exclude, this positivity may reflect cross-reactivity (see below).

CROSS-REACTIVITY

Cross-reactivity between venom allergens is strong within a species, e.g., between *Vespula, Dolichovespula* and *Vespa*, but only limited between *Vespinae* and *Polistinae* and honeybees and bumblebees. Between bee and vespid venom there is little cross-reactivity on protein basis, mainly due to an about 50% sequence identity between hyaluronidases of the two families, but double positivity with diagnostic tests to both venoms is frequently observed. This may reflect true double sensitization or cross-reactivity. Besides partial sequence homology of hyaluronidase, carbohydrate-containing epitopes are important. Cross-reacting carbohydrate determinants (CCDs) are present in many major Hymenoptera venom allergens, such as hyaluronidase, acid phosphatase and phospholipase A2, but also in many plant proteins, e.g., in rapeseed pollen or bromelain. CCDs are certainly responsible for part of the double positivity of diagnostic tests to bee and vespid venoms. They may also explain some of the positive tests in individuals with no history of SR. The CCDs are probably of no clinical relevance.[18] The RAST-inhibition test with venoms and CCDs is helpful in distinguishing between true double sensitization and cross-reactivity, and assisting in the choice of venoms for immunotherapy, but it is not always conclusive.

For ant allergy, only whole-body extracts are commercially available. Their diagnostic sensitivity and specificity are not well documented.

CELLULAR TESTS

If routine tests in patients with a history of SR are negative, cellular tests may be helpful to demonstrate sensitization.[2]

In the *basophil histamine release test* peripheral blood leukocytes are incubated with venom allergens. The reaction with cell-bound IgE antibodies leads to histamine release from basophils. In the *cellular antigen stimulation test* (CAST) leukocytes of patients are pre-stimulated with IL-3 and exposed to venom allergens. The released sulfidoleukotrienes are determined by ELISA.

The *basophil activation test* is based on flow-cytometric demonstration of an altered membrane phenotype of basophils stimulated by IL-3 and allergen exposure. At present the most commonly used expression marker is CD63.

Cellular tests are expensive and not yet well standardized; data on sensitivity, specificity and predictive value are still scarce.

ALLERGEN-SPECIFIC IgG (sIgG)

The presence of specific IgG and IgG_4 primarily reflects exposure to the respective venom. sIgG titers increase after a sting, irrespective of the presence or absence of an allergic sting reaction. Venom immunotherapy induces a rise in sIgG. However, there is no close correlation between the concentration of sIgG or the sIgE/sIgG ratio and the clinical response to immunotherapy.[1] Routine assessment of sIgG is therefore not recommended.

BASELINE SERUM TRYPTASE

Because of the association of an elevated baseline serum tryptase level (>11.4 μg/l) with especially severe, sometimes IgE-negative, systemic sting reactions and cutaneous or systemic mastocytosis, this enzyme should be determined in all patients with a history of SR.[19] The commercially available fluorescence immunoassay measures total tryptase. α-Tryptase is secreted continuously and reflects whole-body mast-cell load. Elevated values are seen in cutaneous and systemic mastocytosis. β-Tryptase is released during mast cell activation, and is a marker of anaphylaxis.

STING CHALLENGE TESTS

Sting challenge with a live insect is not recommended as a diagnostic tool in untreated patients. A sting challenge under well supervised clinical conditions may, however, be helpful in evaluating the efficacy of venom immunotherapy.[20] A tolerated sting challenge does not, however, definitely exclude a reaction to future stings after immunotherapy, especially if these are repeated.

■ PREVENTION AND TREATMENT ■

PREVENTION

All patients with a history of SR should receive detailed instruction on the avoidance of future stings and measures to take if re-stung. Bee stings occur most often when walking barefoot on grass, wasp stings when eating outdoors, in orchards with fallen fruits and near open waste-bins. The risk of a sting is especially high near beehives or vespid nests. While gardening, long trousers, shirts with long sleeves and gloves are recommended. Strongly scented perfumes, suncreams or shampoos, as well as brightly colored garments, should be avoided.

TREATMENT OF LARGE LOCAL REACTIONS

Oral antihistamines and cooling of the sting site (e.g., with ice cubes) reduces local swelling, pain and itching. Anti-inflammatory ointments or topical corticosteroids may diminish the local inflammatory process. In cases of severe swellings oral corticosteroids together with antihistamines over several days are recommended.[21]

SYSTEMIC ALLERGIC REACTIONS

Sympathomimetics, antihistamines and corticosteroids are the most effective drugs for symptomatic treatment of SR. All patients with SR should be medically observed until the symptoms resolve and the blood pressure is stable.

Mild reactions confined to the skin may be treated with rapidly acting oral antihistamines alone. If respiratory or cardiovascular symptoms occur, intramuscular epinephrine must be given immediately, intravenous access should be established, and antihistamines and corticosteroids given IV. All patients with severe SR should be hospitalized and supervised until completely recovered. Patients with cardiovascular symptoms must be treated and transported in the supine position, and IV volume replacement is indicated.

Every patient with a systemic allergic sting reaction should be investigated by an allergist with a view to prevention measures and immunotherapy.[21]

EMERGENCY MEDICATION KIT

All patients with a history of SR should carry an emergency kit for self-administration. After a sting patients should immediately take both antihistamines and corticosteroids, whether there are symptoms or not. If systemic symptoms such as urticaria, dyspnoea, generalized weakness or dizziness occur, epinephrine should be administered IM in the lateral thigh via an auto-injector Epipen (0.3 mg of epinephrine). In children below 30 kg bodyweight the Epipen junior (0.15 mg epinephrine) and half the dose of antihistamines and corticosteroids should be used. If any SR occurs, medical care must be sought.

VENOM IMMUNOTHERAPY (VIT)[21]

Indications

VIT is indicated in children and adults with a history of severe systemic reactions (grade III/IV), if sensitization to the relevant venom is demonstrated by skin and/or blood test. LLR or unusual

THERAPEUTIC PRINCIPLES

EMERGENCY TREATMENT OF GENERALIZED ALLERGIC REACTIONS TO HYMENOPTERA STINGS

Symptoms	Medication	Other measures/comments
Mild urticaria, angioedema	Antihistamines Oral or parenteral	Check: blood pressure, peak flow or FEV_1 Observation for 1–2 hours

Severe urticaria, angioedema	Antihistamines
	   Parenteral or oral
	Corticosteroids
	   0.5–1.0 mg/kg bodyweight
	Epinephrine
	   Adults: 0.3-0.5 mg IM
	   Children: 0.01 mg/kg IM
		Check: blood pressure, peak flow or FEV_1
		Observation until symptoms disappear completely

Laryngeal edema	Epinephrine
	   inhaled
	   IM
		Oxygen supply
		In more severe cases intubation and tracheotomy may be necessary

Bronchial obstruction	β_2-agonists or epinephrine	Oxygen supply

Anaphylactic shock	Epinephrine (if necessary repeated after 10 minutes)
	   Adults: 0.3-0.5 mg IM
	   Children: 0.01mg/kg IM
	Volume replacement
	Antihistamines and corticosteroids IV
	Dopamine or norepinephrine continuous infusion
	Glucagon: 0.1 mg/kg IV
		Place in supine position, oxygen supply
		
		Hospitalization for 24 hours advisable (risk of biphasic reaction)
		
		In case of protracted hypotension or shock inpatients on β-blockers

reactions do not qualify for VIT. In patients with repeated mild, non-lifethreatening reactions who are at high risk for re-exposure, such as beekeepers or their family members, VIT is also recommended. Concomitant cardiovascular disease, mastocytosis or strongly impaired quality of life due to the venom allergy are also indications for VIT in patients with non-lifethreatening sting reactions.[22]

Contraindications for VIT are the same as for immunotherapy with other allergens. Treatment with β-blockers or ACE inhibitors is a relative contraindication: these drugs should preferably be replaced. In all patients with coronary heart disease, arrhythmias or cardiac failure, where the protective effect of these drugs is well documented, the situation should be evaluated carefully together with the family practitioner and a cardiologist.[13]

Dosage and treatment regimens

The recommended maintenance dose is 100 µg of the venom, for both children and adults. This maintenance dose is equivalent to approximately two bee stings or several vespid stings. A higher dose (e.g., 200 µg) is recommended when systemic reactions occur after re-exposure to a field sting or a sting challenge. In highly exposed subjects such as beekeepers or professional gardeners a maintenance dose of 200 µg is advised.

VIT may be initiated by a conventional or an ultra-rush protocol (Table 43.3). The injection interval for maintenance VIT is 4 weeks for the first year. Afterwards intervals may be extended to 6 weeks if VIT is well tolerated.

THERAPEUTIC PRINCIPLES

EMERGENCY MEDICATION FOR SELF-ADMINISTRATION

Prescribed emergency drugs	Epinephrine auto-injector (e.g. Epipen) Antihistamine tablets with rapid action (e.g. cetirizine 2 × 10 mg) Fexofenadine 2 x 180 mg) Corticosteroid tablets (e.g. prednisolone 2 × 50 mg)
Procedure if stung	Take the four emergency tablets as above immediately Prepare Epipen for injection If any systemic allergic symptoms arise, apply Epipen immediately in the lateral thigh; seek medical care

Adverse reactions to VIT

The overall incidence of systemic adverse reactions to VIT varies between 5% and 40%. VIT with bee venom causes more side effects than with *Vespula* venom. Ultra-rush protocols are associated with a somewhat higher rate of side effects than conventional protocols. Most systemic side effects are mild; approximately one-third will require medical treatment.

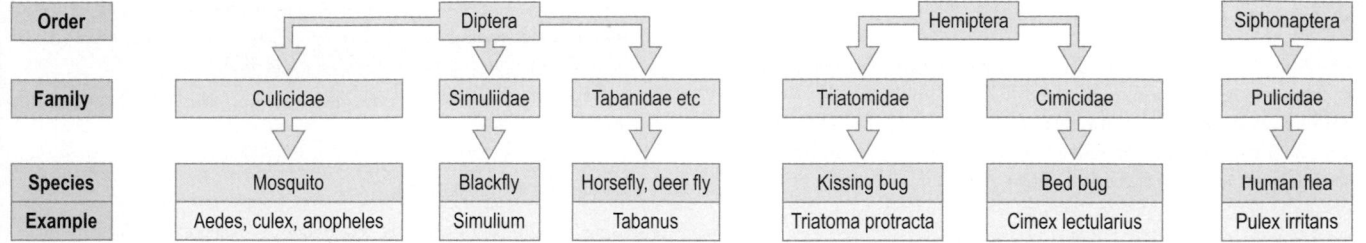

Fig. 43.4 Biting insects that may cause allergic reactions.

Premedication with antihistamines reduces large local and other cutaneous reactions such as urticaria, but severe systemic reactions may not be suppressed. Many authors recommend giving antihistamines 2 hours before injections in the up-dosing phase of VIT until the maintenance dose has been repeatedly well tolerated.

Efficacy of VIT

In addition to three prospective controlled trials, the efficacy of VIT has been confirmed by well-tolerated sting challenges during VIT in a number of uncontrolled prospective studies.[20] Treatment with bee venom results in full protection in 80–85% of patients; with *Vespula* venoms in 95–100%. The efficacy of immunotherapy with commercially available *Solenopsis* whole-body extract has not been documented in controlled studies. However, excellent results, comparable to those of VIT with *Vespula* venom, were obtained in a double-blind placebo-controlled study using *Myrmecia pilosula* venom.[4]

Duration of VIT

Lifelong treatment may be the safest recommendation, but after some years of VIT the majority of allergic individuals may lose motivation. Studies that addressed the protection rate 1–7 years after discontinuation of VIT of at least 3 years' duration showed persisting protection in over 80% of both adults and children. In most allergy centers VIT is recommended for at least 5 years. Even longer treatment should be considered in high-risk patients such as those with very severe systemic sting reactions, coexisting cardiovascular or pulmonary disease, systemic allergic reactions to VIT or stings during VIT, and for subjects with elevated basal serum tryptase levels. Lifelong VIT is advised for patients with cutaneous or systemic mastocytosis. Three of the four reported cases of fatal sting reactions after stopping VIT were in patients with mastocytosis.[21]

Risk factors for recurrence of systemic reactions after stopping VIT

A number of risk factors have been identified for relapse of Hymenoptera venom allergy after discontinuation of VIT: generally adults have a less favorable prognosis than children. Bee-venom-allergic patients have a higher relapse risk than those allergic to *Vespula* venom. The more severe the pre-treatment reactions were, the higher the risk for recurrence of systemic reactions following Hymenoptera stings. After VIT for 5 years, compared to only 3 years, the risk of relapse is reduced.

Table 43.3 Protocols for venom immunotherapy

	Conventional		Ultra-rush	
Week	Amount of venom (µg)	Day	Minutes	Amount of venom (µg)
1	0,01	1	0	0,1
2	0,1		30	1
3	1		60	10
4	2		90	20
5	4		150	30
6	8		210	50
7	10			
8	20	8	0	50
9	40		30	50
10	60			
11	80	21	0	100
12	100	49	0	100

■ ALLERGIC REACTIONS TO BITING INSECTS ■

Biting insects may cause local allergic reactions as a result of sensitization to their salivary proteins introduced during the process of blood sucking. Systemic reactions are very rare. The responsible insects belong to the orders Diptera, Hemiptera and Siphonaptera[23] (Fig. 43.4).

CLINICAL SYMPTOMS

Local reactions to insect bites may comprise immediate wheal and flare, or be delayed, with pruritic erythema and papules developing after 12–24 hours and lasting for days to weeks; combined reactions can also occur. In delayed and combined reactions, vesicular, bullous or even necrotic lesions may develop. Systemic reactions are much rarer than to Hymenoptera stings. They have, however, occasionally been described, especially following bites by horseflies (*Tabanus* spp.) and the kissing bug (*Triatoma protracta*).

ALLERGENS

The salivary proteins involved have either digestive (amylases, esterases) or hemostatic function (e.g., factor Xa inhibition). Numerous IgE-binding proteins with a molecular weight of 15–81 kDa have been described, especially in the saliva of mosquitoes, but also in horseflies and kissing bugs; some of these have been cloned.[24]

PREVENTION AND TREATMENT

The application of insect repellents and prophylactic intake of antihistamines can prevent or mitigate outdoor exposure.[25] Screens on windows and doors and mosquito nets over the beds are effective in homes. Bedbug infestation should be eliminated by appropriate pesticides; flea infestation of pet animals should be managed by a veterinarian.

Local reactions may be treated with topical steroids or oral antihistamines.

Immunotherapy for allergic reactions is controversial, because only whole-body extracts are commercially available for diagnosis and treatment.

■ FUTURE PERSPECTIVES ■

The availability of recombinant venom allergens offers several promising perspectives for both diagnosis and immunotherapy.[5,6] The specificity of these tests could be considerably improved by using recombinant cocktails with all major allergens for diagnosis instead of the whole venom. In patients with double-positive diagnostic tests using honeybee and *Vespula* venom, recombinant species-specific nonglycosylated major allergens from honeybee and *Vespula* venom should make it possible to distinguish reliably between true double sensitization and cross-reactivity, an important issue for the choice of venoms for immunotherapy.

The efficacy and safety of VIT with vespid venoms are excellent, but in bee-venom-allergic patients VIT is associated with significantly more side effects and is also less effective. With cocktails of point-mutated recombinant allergens, or of T-cell epitope peptides of bee venom allergens, it should be possible to reduce the side effects of immunotherapy with bee venom and increase the maintenance dose, and hence the efficacy of treatment.[26]

■ REFERENCES ■

1. Müller U. Insect sting allergy Stuttgart: Gustav Fischer Verlag, 1990.

2. Bilò MB, Ruëff F, Mosbech H, et al. Diagnosis of Hymenoptera venom allergy. Allergy 2005; 60: 1339–1349.

3. Reichmuth DA, Lockey RF. Clinical aspects of ant allergy. In: Levine MI, Lockey RF, eds: Monograph on insect allergy, 4th edn. Pittsburgh: Dave Lambert Associates, 2003: 133–152.

4. Brown S, Wiese M, Blackman K, Heddle R. Ant venom immunotherapy: A double blind, placebo-controlled crossover trial. Lancet 2003; 361: 1001–1006.

5. Müller U. Recombinant Hymenoptera venom allergens. Allergy 2002; 57: 570–576.

6. King TP, Lu G, Gonzales M, et al. Yellow jacket venom allergens, hyaluronidase and phospholipase. Sequence similarity and antigenic cross-reactivity with hornet and wasp homologs and possible implications for clinical allergy. J Allergy Clin Immunol 1996; 98: 588–600.

7. Grunwald T, Bockisch B, Spillner E et al. Molecular cloning and expression in insect cells of honeybee venom allergen acid phosphatase (Api m 3). J Allergy Clin Immunol 2006; 117: 848–854.

8. Mueller HL. Diagnosis and treatment of insect sensitivity. J Asthma Res 1966; 3: 331–333.

9. Reisman RE. Unusual reactions to insect stings. Curr Opin Allergy Clin Immunol 2005; 5: 355–358.

10. Graif Y, Confino-Cohen R, Goldberg A. Allergic reactions to insect stings: Results from a national survey of 10 000 junior high school children in Israel. J Allergy Clin Immunol 2006; 117: 1435–1439.

11. Müller U. Bee venom allergy in beekeepers and their family members. Curr Opin Allergy Clin Immunol 2005; 5: 343–347.

12. Antonicelli A, Bilò MB, Bonifazi F. Epidemiology of Hymenoptera allergy. Curr Opin Allergy Clin Immunol 2002; 2: 341–346.

13. Müller U, Haeberli G. Use of beta-blockers during immunotherapy for Hymenoptera venom allergy. J Allergy Clin Immunol 2005; 115: 606–610.

14. Sasvary T, Müller U. Fatalities from insect stings in Switzerland 1978 to 1987. Schweiz Med Wschr 1994; 124: 1887.94.

15. Golden DBK, Kagey-Sobotka A, Norman PS et al. Outcomes of allergy to insect stings in children, with and without venom immunotherapy. N Engl J Med 2004; 351: 668–674.

16. Brown SG. Cardiovascular aspects of anaphylaxis: implications for treatment and diagnosis. Curr Opin Allergy Clin Immunol 2005; 5: 359–364.

17. Golden DBK, Kagey-Sobotka A, Norman PS, et al. Insect sting allergy with negative venom skin test responses. J Allergy Clin Immunol 2001; 107: 897–901.

18. Hemmer W, Focke M, Kolarich D et al. Antibody binding to venom carbohydrates is a frequent cause for double positivity to honey bee and yellow jacket venom in patients with stinging insect allergy. J Allergy Clin Immunol 2001; 108: 1045–1052.

19. Ludolph-Hauser D, Ruëff F, Fries C et al. Constitutively raised serum concentration of mast cell tryptase and severe anaphylactic reactions to Hymenoptera stings. Lancet 2001; 357: 361–362.

20. Ruëff F, Przybilla B, Müller U et al. The sting challenge test in Hymenoptera venom allergy. Allergy 1996; 51: 216–225.

21. Bonifazi F, Jutel M, Bilò MB et al. Prevention and treatment of Hymenoptera venom allergy. Allergy 2005; 60: 1459–1470.

22. Oude Elberink JN, Dubois AE. Quality of life in insect venom allergic patients. Curr Opin Allergy Clin Immunol 2003; 3: 287–293.

23. Hoffman DR. Allergic reactions to biting insects. In: Levine MI, Lockey RF, eds. Monograph on insect allergy, Pittsburgh: Dave Lambert Associates, 2003; 161–174.

24. Simons FER, Zhikang Peng. Mosquito allergy. In: Levine MI, Lockey RF, eds. Monograph on insect allergy, Pittsburgh: Dave Lambert Associates, 2003; 175–203.

25. Reunala T, Lappallainen P, Brummer-Korvenkontio H, et al. Cutaneous reactivity to mosquito bites. Effect of cetirizine and development of anti- mosquito antibodies. Clin Exp Allergy 1991; 21: 617–624.

26. Blaser K, Akdis CA. Interleukin-10, T regulatory cells and specific allergy treatment. Clin Exp Allergy 2004; 34: 328–331.

Atopic and contact dermatitis

Thomas Bieber

44

Atopic dermatitis (AD) is a chronic and relapsing inflammatory skin disease affecting an increasing number of patients.[1,2] Characteristic features of AD include pruritus and chronic or chronically relapsing dermatitis, usually beginning during infancy. AD is a genetically complex disease and is often, but not always, accompanied by other atopic disorders such as allergic rhinoconjunctivitis or allergic bronchial asthma. These diseases may appear simultaneously or develop in succession during the course of disease. AD characteristically starts during early childhood, whereas allergic rhinitis and asthma predominate in adolescence. This characteristic, age-dependent sequence has been termed the *atopic march*.[3] The cutaneous manifestations of atopy often represent the beginning of this atopic career while asthma is its full expression. Therapeutic strategies should be directed towards the delay or avoidance of this development, by early intervention against skin inflammation which may prevent subsequent sensitization and progression towards rhinitis and asthma.

AD is a genetically complex disease involving gene–gene and gene–environment interactions, but much progress in understanding its pathogenesis has been achieved in recent years. Genetic linkage studies have identified several chromosomal regions linked to epidermal barrier function, and genetic variants which favor the development of AD, but several candidate genes linked to the immune system have also been detected. Stress, bacterial or viral infections, exposure to aero- or food allergens and hygienic factors have been implicated in aggravating the symptoms of AD. Although the so-called 'hygiene hypothesis' is controversial, the importance of lifestyle and environment in the mechanisms of atopic disease is well accepted. Additionally, a generalized Th2-deviated immune response is closely linked to AD, but the skin disease itself is a biphasic inflammation with an initial Th2 phase, while chronic lesions harbor Th0/Th1 cells. Both regulatory T cells (Tregs) and the innate immune system have been shown to be altered in AD. The main treatment goals for AD include the elimination of inflammation and infection, preservation and restitution of barrier function, anti-pruritic management, and control of exacerbating factors. In the longer term, the strategy in AD will likely aim to control skin inflammation in order to prevent the emergence of sensitization.

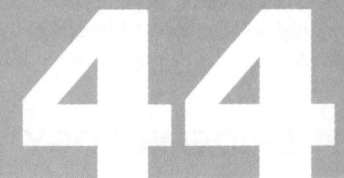

KEY CONCEPTS

PATHOPHYSIOLOGY OF ATOPIC DERMATITIS

>> Atopic dermatitis is a genetic complex disease (gene–gene and gene–environment interactions)

>> Defective epidermal barrier function and decreased epidermal innate immunity

>> Deviated immune response toward increased sensitization supported by skin inflammation

>> High microbial colonization which amplifies skin inflammation

>> Role of FcεRI/IgE-bearing dendritic cells

>> Role of IgE-mediated immune response to autoallergens

>> Decreased activity of regulatory T cells

DEFINITION

Over the last 120 years, AD has been given a multitude of different names, e.g., *Besnier's prurigo*, *disseminated neurodermitis*, or *neurodermitis constitutionalis sive atopica*, but *atopic dermatitis* and *nonatopic dermatitis* are currently the most widely used names. According to a recent consensus nomenclature by the World Allergy Organization (WAO), the term AD should be reserved for the eczematous condition with the typical clinical signs and associated with immunoglobulin E (IgE)-mediated sensitization to aeroallergens. Indeed, in 2004 a WAO consensus group proposed a revised terminology for atopy, restricting its use to conditions associated with IgE sensitization.[4] According to this classification, the term atopy should only be applied in combination with documented allergen-specific IgE antibodies in serum or with a positive skin prick test. This current terminology substitutes the former term of *extrinsic AD* and includes only patients who show IgE sensitization against inhalant and/or food allergens in skin tests or serum. A small group of approximately 20–30% of affected patients show clinical signs of AD, without

subunit may have an influence on the IL-4-receptor-related synthesis of IgE. This could be linked to the incidence of nonatopic dermatitis, which occurs without any IgE sensitization. Similarly, a dysbalance between Th1 and Th2-immune responses in AD may be explained by polymorphisms of the IL-18-gene, resulting in a Th2 predominance. At a functional level, upon stimulation with superantigens, peripheral blood mononuclear cells (PBMC) from individuals with these polymorphisms respond with upregulation of IL-18 and downregulation of IL-12 and consequently show a Th2 predominance. A particularly severe course of AD with colonization of *S. aureus* may be associated with a SNP of the Toll-like receptor (TLR)-2 gene.

DISTURBED EPIDERMAL BARRIER FUNCTION

AD is characterized by dry skin affecting lesional and nonlesional skin areas. Altered skin barrier function, resulting in increased transepidermal water loss, is typical for this condition and may be, among others, an explanation for the facilitated penetration of allergens, bacteria, and viruses. The mechanisms behind this dryness are complex and closely related to the disturbed epidermal barrier function.[14] The loss of skin ceramides, which serve as the major water-retaining molecules in the extracellular space of the cornified envelope, has been proposed to cause this modification of the skin barrier. Furthermore, variations of the stratum corneum pH may impair lipid metabolism in the skin. Overexpression of enzymes such as chymotrypsin is also likely to contribute to the breakdown of the AD epidermal barrier. Further considerations include a D-6-desaturase deficiency and a decreased conversion of ω6-linoleic acids to prostaglandin in affected patients.

Recent studies underline the importance of a primary epithelial barrier defect in the pathogenesis of AD. Mutations of filaggrin (R510X and 2282del4), a key protein in terminal differentiation of the epidermis, seem to be important risk factors for AD and for AD in combination with asthma.[15] The skin barrier may be impaired due to an alteration of keratin aggregation and hence permit the penetration of allergens, including high-molecular-weight aeroallergens.

IMMUNOLOGICAL MECHANISMS

As mentioned above, both a disturbed epidermal barrier and defects in the immune system are mandatory for the development of AD (Fig. 44.3). Having focused over the last three decades on the mechanisms directing adaptive immunity, mainly orchestrated by T and B cells for cellular and humoral immunity respectively, scientists have tended to overlook the significance of the so-called innate immunity[16] (Chapter 3).

INNATE IMMUNITY

In recent years there has been a radical transformation of our understanding of how mammalian organisms respond to microbial exposure. The innate immune system is able to react promptly to almost all kinds of microbial colonization and onslaught, while it is also involved in the initiation of the more specific but slower mechanisms of the adaptive immune response. Epithelial cells of the skin and cells residing at the interface between our environment and our organism are the first line of defense in the innate immune system.[17] They are equipped with highly conserved recognition structures, the so-called pattern recognition

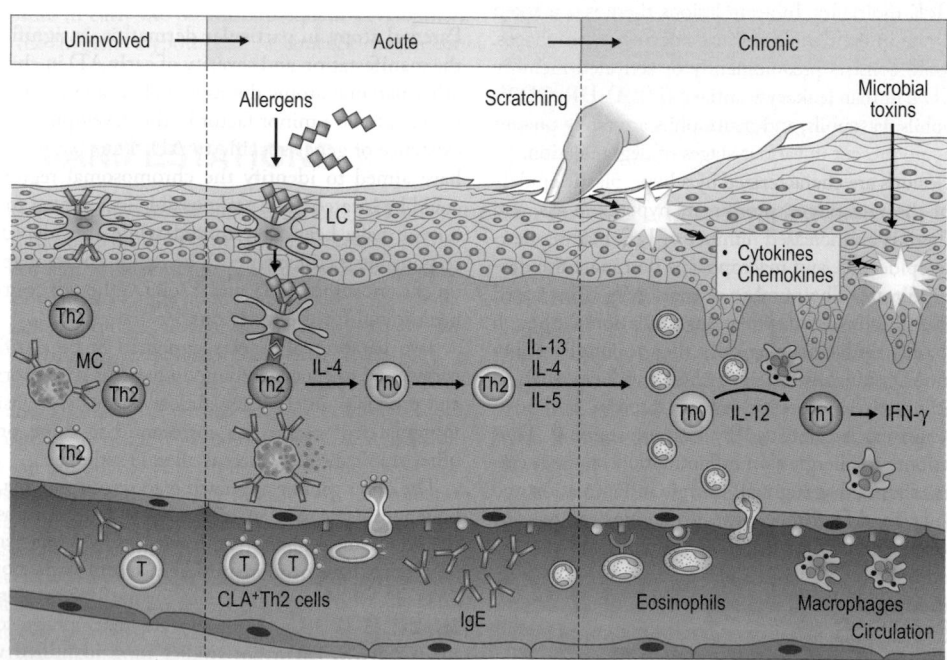

Fig. 44.3 Immunologic progression of atopic dermatitis. (Modified from Leung DYM. Atopic dermatitis: new insights and opportunities for therapeutic intervention. J Allergy Clin Immunol 2000; 105: 860.)

receptors (PRRs) such as the TLRs, which were initially described in the fruit fly. These TLRs can bind a variety of microbial structures due to highly conserved microbial surface molecules, the pathogen-associated molecular patterns (PAMP). At least 10 different TLRs have been described so far in humans and are more or less specialized in binding bacterial or fungal cell walls or viral nucleic acids (DNA or RNA with so-called CpG motifs). Hence, TLRs represent putative therapeutic targets to alter or modulate the adhesion of microbes to epithelial cells.

The binding of microbial products to the cell surface of epithelial cells leads to cellular activation, ultimately resulting in the production of molecules with anti-microbial activity: the so-called AMPs.[17] These belong to the family of defensins and cathelicidins. In human skin at least one cathelicidin (LL37) and three defensins, the human β-defensins 1, 2, and 3 (HBD1, HBD2, and HDB3) have been described.

In AD, skin is highly colonized by bacteria such as *Staphylococcus aureus*. Much attention has been focused on the putative role of the innate immune system and particularly of AMPs in the control of these bacteria as well as of viruses. Recently it has been shown that AMPs are downregulated in the skin of human atopic individuals, probably due to the particular inflammatory micromilieu created by infiltrating cells and their cytokines. These mechanisms predispose AD patients to develop extensive herpes infections such as eczema herpeticum.[18]

ACQUIRED IMMUNITY

T cells and the Th1/Th2 concept

A predominant systemic Th2 dysbalance with increased IgE levels and eosinophilia is widely accepted in the pathogenesis of atopic diseases.[19] The production of Th2 cytokines, notably IL-4, IL-5, and IL-13, can be detected in lesional and nonlesional skin during the acute phase of disease. IL-4 and IL-13 are implicated in the initial phase of tissue inflammation and in upregulating the expression of adhesion molecules on endothelial cells. IL-5 seems to increase the survival of eosinophils. A systemic eosinophilia and an increase of the eosinophilic cationic protein (ECP) are characteristic during high disease activity of AD.

However, although Th2 cytokines seem to be predominant in the acute phase of AD, they are less important during its chronic course. In chronic AD skin lesions an increase of interferon-γ (IFN-γ) and IL-12, as well as IL-5 and GM-CSF, could be detected, being characteristic for a Th1/Th0 dominance.

The maintenance of chronic AD involves the production of the Th1-like cytokines IL-12 and IL-18, as well as several remodeling-associated cytokines such as IL-11 and transforming growth factor (TGF)-β₁, expressed preferentially in chronic forms of the disease. Th-1-mediated cells seem to be responsible for apoptosis of cells, although their pathomechanisms are yet not fully understood. Clearly, a generalized Th2-deviated immune response is closely linked to the condition of AD but the skin disease itself is a biphasic inflammation with an initial Th2 phase, while the chronic phase involves Th0/Th1 cells. This biphasic pattern of T-cell activation has also been demonstrated in studies of allergen patch test skin reaction sites.[20] Twenty-four hours after allergen application to the skin, increased expression of IL-4 mRNA and protein is observed, after which IL-4 expression returns to baseline levels. In contrast, IFN-γ mRNA expression is not detected in 24-hour patch test lesions, but is strongly expressed at the 48–72-hour time points. Interestingly, the increased expression of IFN-γ mRNA in atopic patch

test lesions is preceded by a peak of IL-12 expression coinciding with the infiltration of macrophages and eosinophils.

A study using an animal model of AD examined ovalbumin-elicited allergic skin inflammation in mice with targeted deletions of the IL-4, IL-5, and IFN-γ cytokine genes to assess the role of these cytokines.[21] Allergen-sensitized skin from IL-5 knockout mice had no detectable eosinophils and exhibited decreased epidermal and dermal thickening, whereas IL-4 knockout mice displayed normal thickening of the skin layers but had decreased eosinophils. Sensitized skin from IFN-γ knockout mice was characterized by reduced dermal thickening.

Tregs are a diverse and complex family of cells with regulatory activities that became the focus of interest in the field of transplantation or tumor immunology as well as in allergy, since they have the ability to suppress T-cells (TH1 and TH2)[22] (Chapter 16). Special combinations of surface markers (CD25⁺/CD4⁺) as well as mutations of the nuclear factor Foxp3 are characteristic for these cells. It has been shown that mutations of Foxp3 result in hyper-IgE, food allergy, and dermatitis. In addition, staphylococcal superantigens can subvert the function of Tregs and may thereby augment skin inflammation (Fig. 44.4).[23]

CYTOKINES AND CHEMOKINES

The defining characteristic of the atopic immune system is the expression of proinflammatory cytokines and chemokines.[24] Cytokines from resident cells (such as keratinocytes, mast cells, or DCs) bind to receptors on the vascular endothelium and activate cellular signaling. This results in an initiation of processes leading to the characteristic extravasation of inflammatory cells.

Several different chemokines have been implicated in the pathology of AD. Large amounts of chemokines such as MIP-4/CCL18, TARC/CCL17, PARC/CCL18, MDC/CCL22, and CCL1 seem to be involved in the development of acute and chronic skin manifestations. These chemokines play an important role in the amplification of allergic reactions to bacteria or allergens. C-C chemokines (MCP-4, RANTES, and eotaxin) contribute to the infiltration of macrophages, eosinophils, and T-cells into acute and chronic AD skin lesions. An increasing number of chemokines have been shown to be up- or downregulated in patients with AD but their exact role in the pathogenesis of AD is still not resolved.

DENDRITIC CELLS

DCs are highly specialized professional antigen-presenting cells (APCs) and are essential for allergen uptake and its presentation to T cells in the context of primary and secondary immune responses (Chapter 7). The role of DC in AD has been extensively discussed elsewhere.[25] Two types of DC have been found in lesional skin of AD: myeloid (mDC) and, to a much lesser extent, plasmacytoid DCs (pDC). LC and inflammatory dendritic epidermal cells (IDEC) both belong to the group of mDC and express the high-affinity receptor for IgE (FcεRI) in lesional skin, suggesting a complex regulatory mechanism related to atopic status. While LC are present in normal skin, IDEC are mainly detected in inflamed skin.

LC and IDEC play a central role in the uptake and presentation of antigens or allergens to Th1/Th2 cells and most probably also to Tregs. Interestingly, FcεRI-expression is detected on LC from normal skin during active flare-ups of other atopic diseases such as allergic asthma or rhinitis, while FcεRI⁺ IDEC are confined to lesional skin. Although it remains to be definitely proven, there is some *in vitro* evidence that LC play a less

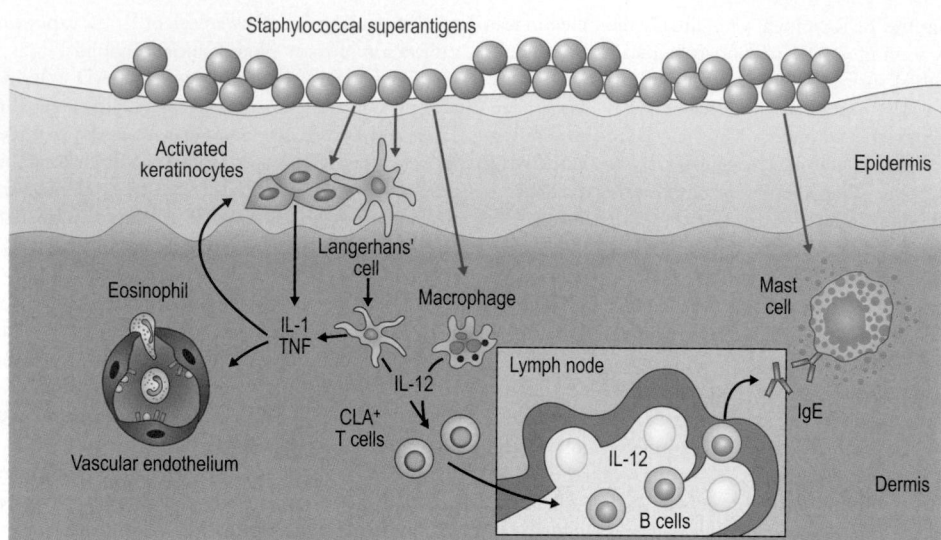

Fig. 44.4 Mechanisms of staphylococcal superantigen action in atopic dermatitis. (Modified from Leung DYM. Atopic dermatitis: new insights and opportunities for therapeutic intervention. J Allergy Clin Immunol 2000; 105: 860, with permission from Elsevier.)

dominant role than expected initially in the initiation of the allergic immune response. Nevertheless, they are active in priming naïve T cells to become T cells of Th2 type and produce distinct chemokines such as MCP-1 upon receptor ligation. In contrast, the stimulation of FcεRI on IDEC leads to a switch to Th1 response and to the release of high amounts of proinflammatory signals that amplify the allergic immune response. The atopy patch test can be used as an experimental model for AD – skin biopsies of such patch tests show that, 72 hours after allergen challenge, high numbers of IDEC invade the epidermis while alterations of the phenotype of LC and IDEC occur, including the upregulation of FcεRI.

Compared to ACD, the number of pDC is dramatically decreased in the skin of AD patients. pDC have been shown to play a major role in the defense against viral infections by producing type 1 interferons. A lower density of pDC might contribute to the susceptibility towards viral skin infections such as eczema herpeticum in these patients. In contrast to LC and IDEC, pDC seem to express FcεRI constitutively and this is upregulated in AD patients. Activation of this receptor leads to altered surface expression of major histocompatibility complex (MHC) molecules, enhanced apoptosis of pDC, and a decrease in the secretion of type I interferons.

MICROBIAL AGENTS

Staphylococcus aureus is the predominant skin microorganism in AD lesions and is found in over 90% of AD patients.[26] This high colonization rate is probably due to a defect in the production of AMP by atopic keratinocytes. Infections often provoke exacerbation or aggravation of lesional skin. *S. aureus*-derived enterotoxins have been shown to play an important role in the pathogenesis of AD.[27] Enterotoxins such as staphylococcal enterotoxin A (SEA), B (SEB), C (SEC), and D (SED) are frequently detected in patients and might provoke sensitization. Moreover, since *S. aureus* enterotoxins act as superantigens, they interact directly

with the MHC-T-cell complex on APC and provoke antigen-independent proliferation of T cells. This results in an amplification of the inflammation and may lead to typical eczematoid skin reactions of AD patients. Specific IgE antibodies directed against staphylococcal superantigens can be detected in most AD patients, correlating with their skin disease severity.

It has been shown that binding of *S. aureus* to the skin is significantly enhanced by AD skin inflammation. An altered composition of fibrin and fibrinogen of AD skin is thought to be responsible. Scratching may enhance *S. aureus* binding by disturbing the skin barrier. *S. aureus* isolated from AD patients possesses increased ceramidase activity, which may be responsible for damaging the skin barrier.

AUTOALLERGENS

The majority of sera from patients with severe AD contain IgE antibodies directed against human proteins.[28] One of these IgE-reactive autoantigens is a 55-kDa cytoplasmic protein from skin keratinocytes; it has been cloned from a human epithelial cDNA expression library and designated *Hom s 1*.[29] Although the autoallergens characterized to date have mainly been intracellular proteins, some have been detected in IgE immune complexes in sera of sensitized patients, suggesting that release of these autoallergens from damaged keratinocytes due to scratching could trigger IgE- or T-cell-mediated responses. A more recent study has shown that the emergence of IgE against self proteins can be detected as early as 1 year of age.[30] These data suggest that, while IgE immune responses are initiated by environmental allergens in combination with skin inflammation, allergic inflammation can be maintained by human endogenous antigens in patients with severe AD. Thus, if the assumed pathophysiological role of these antibodies holds true, AD should be considered as a disease at the boundary between allergy and autoimmunity.

NONATOPIC AND ATOPIC DERMATITIS IN THE CONTEXT OF THE NATURAL HISTORY OF ATOPIC DERMATITIS ■

As mentioned above, the new definition of AD requires the presence of IgE-mediated sensitization. However, this would imply that *nonatopic dermatitis* and *AD* represent two different diseases. Since dry skin is an important clinical sign of both conditions and is considered as a cardinal sign in atopic individuals as well, there is a great need for new concepts that reconcile these diverging ideas. Based on most recent genetic and immunological findings, a new picture emerges in which the natural history of AD seems to be divided into three phases: (1) an initial phase representing nonatopic dermatitis occurring in early infancy before any sensitization has taken place. This is then followed in 60–80% of cases by (2) sensitization to food and/or environmental allergens with the development of true AD (according to the new definition). In this phase, it is speculated that FcεRI+ DC play a major role in controlling the inflammation. Consequently, these AD patients will benefit from allergen avoidance measures. Finally, (3) probably due to scratching, tissue damage, and molecular mimicry, an IgE sensitization to self proteins is observed in about 25% of AD patients. Whether these specific IgE have a pathophysiological role or are just an epiphenomenon remains to be clarified. According to this concept, sensitization could be influenced by the intensity of skin inflammation, which would be in accord with the concept of the atopic march. Furthermore, attempts to control skin inflammation effectively as early as possible would putatively help to hamper the degree of subsequent sensitization.

MANAGEMENT OF ATOPIC DERMATITIS ■

The management of AD can be established on five main axes and must be adapted to the severity of the lesions: (1) skin care to restore and preserve the epidermal barrier function; (2) recognition and elimination of the provocation factors; (3) control of (even subclinical) inflammation and pruritus; (4) reduction of microbial colonization; and (5) education of patients and their parents. Throughout, topical treatment is preferred to systemic therapy, which should be reserved for the most severe forms. Successful management thus requires a multifaceted approach, and it is stressed that education of the patient is as important as pharmacological strategies.

SKIN CARE

A key feature of AD is severe dryness of the skin due to a dysfunction of the skin barrier with increased transepidermal water loss. The regular use of emollients and skin hydration is essential to improve dryness, to prevent intense pruritus, and to control subclinical inflammation during periods of remission. The choice of emollients depends on the individual skin status. Water-in-oil or oil-in-water emulsions may be substituted to support the skin barrier function. Urea allows an intensive hydration of the skin while salicylic acid can be added to an emollient for the treatment of chronic hyperkeratotic lesions.

Irritants such as soaps, clothing made from occluding or irritating, synthetic or wool material, and hot water temperature should be avoided or reduced to a minimum.

ELIMINATION OF PROVOCATION FACTORS

The patient should be educated adequately to avoid provoking factors. Specific provocation factors, such as airborne and food allergens, have to be considered and identified by serum tests for allergen-specific IgE or skin prick tests. Because of the putative role of food allergens in children, diets directed by allergological tests can be of interest but blind extensive diets, which can be nutritionally deficient, are useless. Sensitized patients should avoid house dust mites; this may include use of house dust mite-proof encasings on pillows, mattresses, and box springs. Whether patients sensitized to animal dander should be discouraged from keeping household pets is still a matter of debate.

In selected patients hospitalization may be of great benefit, especially in centers using a multidisciplinary team approach.

Food hypersensitivity affects 10–40% of children with AD. In children 90% of reactions are caused by only five allergens: eggs, milk, peanuts, soy, and wheat. Dietary restriction is only of value in patients whose allergies have been properly diagnosed, though any exclusion diets should be properly supervised by a pediatric dietician to ensure adequate nutrition. Hydrolyzed cow's-milk formula consisting of predigested peptides of whey and cytokine can be useful as its nutritional values are equivalent to normal milk, but it has a reduced capacity to induce IgE-mediated reactions.

CONTROL OF INFLAMMATION

Topical glucocorticosteroids

Topical steroids are safe and effective when used properly. Anxiety among both the general public and family physicians is often well out of proportion to the true risk. Aside from their anti-inflammatory effect, topical steroids contribute to a reduction of skin colonization with *S. aureus*. The strength and mode of application depend on disease activity and severity, the locations to be treated, and the age of the patient. Only mild to moderately potent preparations should be used on facial, genital, or intertriginous skin areas. Less potent topical steroids should be used in children less than 1 year old. The application of steroids should be limited to short courses of about 2 weeks, no more than twice a day. New steroid preparations and application protocols have reduced the risk of adverse effects and are effective when applied once daily. A number of different therapeutic schemes have been proposed: the initial treatment of acute phase can be with moderate- to high-potency steroids followed by a dose reduction or an exchange to a lower-potency preparation. However, our own experience has shown better compliance by tapering off the use of the same mid-potent topical steroid over several weeks. Intermittent use of topical steroids once or twice a week on areas prone to flare-up has been proven to reduce flares for up to 6 months, with increased compliance and better overall disease control.[31] Treatment with emollients is important both during the course of steroid treatment and as part of long-term management.

new antagonist molecules based on small-molecular-weight compounds, steroid analogues, and other treatments that are or will be in the pipeline over the next few years. Finally, beside these new pharmacological approaches, one of the most important aspects remains the strategy of very early treatment of young children by controlling skin inflammation at the earliest practical time point. This strategy may help us better control the emergence of sensitization and provide a rapid and hopefully definitive cure of the disease. If successful, physicians would be able to provide a convincing disease-modifying strategy for AD patients.

ALLERGIC CONTACT DERMATITIS

DEFINITION

Contact dermatitis is an eczematous skin eruption caused by local exposure to allergic sensitizer or irritant/toxic substances. These include immunologic, chemical, protein, or physical agents but infectious agents are excluded. Contact dermatitis is a common cause of morbidity with a life prevalence of 15% and incidence of more than 7.9 per 1000. However, the sensitization rate is higher than this – studies in Scandinavia have shown that 15–20% of the population displays at least one positive patch test reaction to contact sensitizers. In the USA, occupationally related contact dermatitis is estimated to cost $250 million per year in lost productivity, medical care, and disability payments.

PATHOPHYSIOLOGY

Genetics

ACD is a multifactorial condition in which genetic background plays an important part, as shown by twin and family studies. In case-control studies, SNPs in certain enzymes such as NAT2 (*N*-acetyltransferase) or the promoter region of IL-16 have been associated with multiple sensitization status.[41, 42]

Histology

The histological hallmark of ACD is intercellular edema or spongiosis, accompanied by a mixed inflammatory cell infiltrate around dermal vessels; eosinophils may be especially prominent in the initial acute phase. As ACD becomes chronic, the degree of spongiosis decreases while epidermal hyperplasia increases, This is seen macroscopically as lichenification.

The allergens

Most contact allergens are haptens, i.e., simple chemicals that bind to proteins (carrier) present in skin to form a complete antigen. The key to understanding the pathogenesis of contact allergy is an appreciation of the discriminate nature by which chemicals can serve as antigens (Chapter 6). Clearly, not all chemicals act as allergens. To be allergenic, the chemical must be able to penetrate the principal barrier in skin (the stratum corneum) and reach the living cells of the epidermis. Only molecules with molecular mass less than 500 Da are capable of penetrating the stratum corneum, and so most contact allergens are low-

Table 44.1 Most common contact allergens (listed in approximate order of decreasing frequency)

Allergen	Description
1. Nickel sulfate	Nickel-plated objects are omnipresent. Jewelry that looks like gold or silver has nickel in it. Gold greater than 18 carats is safe; so is aluminum; stainless steel contains nickel but it is not releasable
2. Fragrance mix	Anything that smells good has fragrance chemicals in it (e.g., cinnamates, vanillin, oak moss, eugenol, geraniol). Also used as flavorings
3. *P*-phenyldiamine	Preservative used in vaccines, antitoxins, eye and nasal medications
4. Chromate	Sensitizer in wet cement. Used as an oxidizing agent and for its anticorrosion properties. Found in glues and adhesives, leather, paints, matches, detergents, and bleaches
5. Methyldibromoglutaronitril/phenoxyethanol (MDBGN/PE)	Preservatives, antimicrobial and industrial biocides
6. Thiuram mix	Rubber accelerator and vulcanizer. Fungicide and animal repellant. Also found in lubricating oils. Cross-reacts with disulfiram
7. Methylchloroisothiazolinon/methylisothiazolinon (Kathon CG)	Preservative in paints, glues, and cosmetics
8. Formaldehyde	Preservative found in cosmetic products and topical medications. Sterilizer in cleaning agents. Fixative for tissues. Tanning agent for leather. Hardener for fabrics. Fumigant, fungicide, and insecticide
9. Parabens	Used as sunscreen agent and preservative in cosmetic products

molecular-weight compounds. Lipid solubility promotes transit through the stratum corneum. Thus, most contact allergens are small, lipophilic molecules. The most common of these chemicals are listed in Table 44.1. Once in the epidermis, the nature of the protein carrier for the hapten is very important because if the contact sensitizer is complexed to nonimmunogenic carriers, this may induce tolerance rather than sensitization.[43]

THE SENSITIZATION PHASE

The pathophysiology of ACD has been extensively reviewed elsewhere.[44] The principal event during sensitization is presentation of antigen to responder T cells by APC, culminating in activation and differentiation of T cells that proliferate in an antigen-specific clonal manner. LC are the principal APCs within the epidermis and are generally thought to be responsible for presentation of contact allergens in the primary (sensitization) phase as well as in the secondary (elicitation) phase of the immune response. However, recent studies in LC knockout animal models have seriously challenged this view.[45] Other DCs in skin, especially in the dermis, may also serve as APCs for contact allergens, including LC precursors, and dermal DCs, while macrophages may be important in the elicitation phase.

The clinical outcome of each exposure to antigen depends upon several factors. First and foremost is the integrity of the stratum corneum. An injured or diseased stratum corneum that allows greater penetration of exogenous substances will increase the chances of activating APCs in the skin. A second factor is the viability of APCs in skin, since these cells need to seek and bind appropriate responder T cells. Third is the presence or absence of extracellular factors, including cytokines produced by keratinocytes that can promote or hinder APC–T-cell engagement. The final factor is the pre-existing mix of T-cell subtypes specific for the antigen. The higher the frequency of cells of an effector subtype, the higher the likelihood that dermatitis will result, whereas a higher frequency of cells of a regulatory subtype may limit or prevent the development of dermatitis.

THE ELICITATION PHASE

The elicitation or efferent phase is characterized by invasion of the skin by antigen-specific memory T cells as well as other inflammatory cells, producing what is clinically recognized as ACD. Memory T cells and other inflammatory cells leave vessels and enter the skin through sequential activation of a number of adhesion molecules by cytokines. Memory T cells constitutively express cutaneous lymphocyte antigen (CLA). E-selectin, the ligand for CLA, is induced on vascular endothelium by inflammatory mediators such as IL-1 and tumor necrosis factor-α (TNF-α). This interaction causes memory T cells to slow down and roll along the endothelial surface as a prelude to migration to sites of inflammation. Firm adhesion and migration of leukocytes to the endothelium are mediated by T-cell VLA-4/LFA-1 and endothelial cell VCAM-1/ICAM-1, respectively. Subsequently, LFA-1⁺ T cells migrate toward ICAM-1⁺ epidermal cells.

Mast cells may also participate in the elicitation phase. In mice, mast cells can be activated by a T-cell-derived antigen-binding factor that induces release of serotonin, producing swelling 2 hours after challenge. In addition, mast cells contain preformed TNF-α, which may regulate the adhesion molecules involved in the early recruitment of helper T cells.[46]

The net result is an influx of T cells secreting IL-2 and IFN-γ into the area of allergen exposure. These cytokines enhance the immune response through activation and recruitment of more inflammatory cells, producing spongiosis and the inflammatory dermal infiltrate characteristic of ACD.

CLINICAL MANIFESTATIONS (FIG. 44.5)

As a rule, ACD takes several hours, days, or even weeks to develop, while irritant contact dermatitis may manifest within minutes to hours of contact, especially when due to strong agents. If left alone, most cases of contact dermatitis resolve completely. Unfortunately, this ideal situation is almost never realized because the accompanying itch results in scratching and attempts at topical treatment, which in turn lead to spread of the dermatitis, often with superimposed bacterial or dermatophytic infection. These and the effects of partial but incomplete treatment can produce diagnostic confusion.

The intensity of the dermatitis depends on the concentration of the inciting chemical and, in the case of ACD, on the sensitivity of the

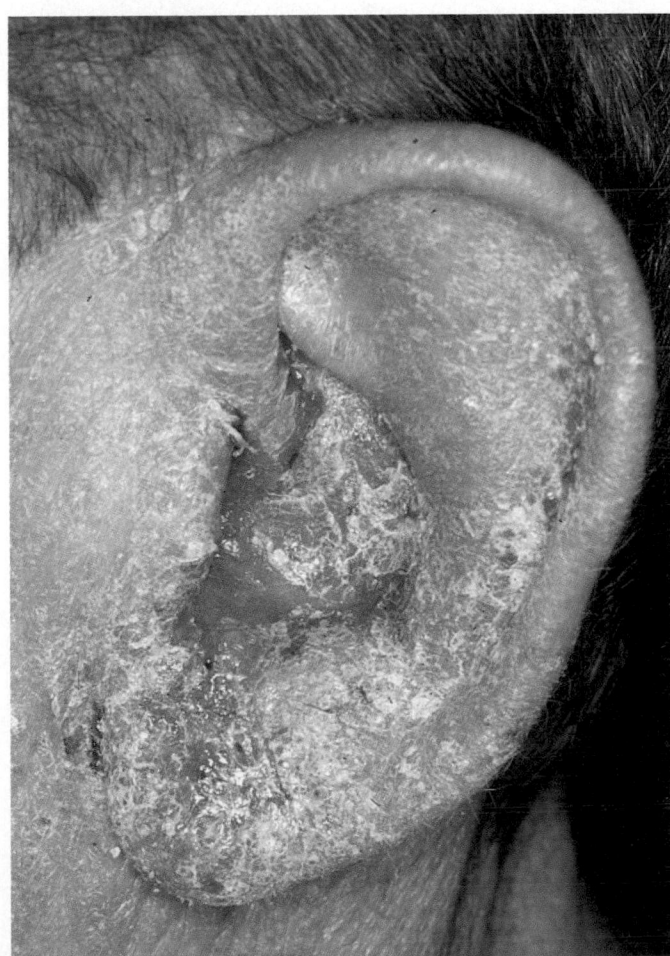

Fig. 44.5 Allergic contact dermatitis.

individual to the allergen. Acute inflammation is expressed as erythema, blistering, oozing, and crusting; rarely frank necrosis may ensue. Subacute inflammation manifests as erythema, scaling, fissuring, or a parched, scalded appearance. Chronic inflammation may have less erythema, but the skin becomes thickened with lichenification and excoriation. Itching is a cardinal feature of contact dermatitis, regardless of severity. The keys to diagnosis are recognition of the eczematous nature of the skin eruption and correlation of the pattern and distribution of the lesions to the shape of the offending substance or the nature of exposure to it.

The location of the dermatitis also serves as an important clue to the source of the offending chemical (Table 44.2). Although ACD usually affects the site of principal exposure, it can spread to other more distant sites, either by inadvertent contact or by autosensitization. Furthermore, the scalp, palms, and soles are relatively resistant to ACD and may not exhibit pathology, while surrounding areas are severely affected. A geographic approach can be very helpful in identifying the causal allergen. Although the typical presentation is eczematous, contact dermatitis may occasionally present as urticaria (contact urticaria), altered pigmentation (either hyperpigmentation or hypopigmentation), erythema multiforme, or even purpura (usually on the legs). Widespread involvement, particularly of the face and of body areas unprotected by clothing, should raise suspicions of contact dermatitis produced by airborne allergens such as plant pollen, sprays, or fumes. Photocontact dermatitis can also have a similar diffuse presentation. Rarely, contact dermatitis may become generalized, presenting as exfoliative erythroderma. In some cases ACD can be induced by body contact (e.g., to perfumes or cosmetics).

Table 44.2 Common causes of contact dermatitis by location

Scalp	Shampoos, hair dyes
Ears	Metal earrings, eyeglasses, hair care products
Eyelids	Nail polish, cosmetics, contact lens solution, airborne allergens
Face	Cosmetics, other topical preparations, including sunscreens, airborne allergens
Neck	Necklaces, perfumes, airborne allergens
Trunk	Topical preparations, clothing, including metal components and elastic in undergarments
Axillae	Deodorants, clothing
Hands	Soaps and detergents, occupational chemicals, metals, including jewelry, topical preparations, rubber gloves
Genitals	Topical preparations, condoms
Anal region	Fecal spillage, topical preparations
Legs	Topical preparations, elastic in socks
Feet	Rubber, leather, or synthetic materials in shoes.

ACD can occur at any age, but it is less frequently seen in the very old or very young. Older individuals have been shown to have various defects in the induction and/or elicitation of ACD. Children also tend to have fewer episodes of ACD but, in contrast to the elderly, this is probably due to limited exposure rather than deficient immunity. When ACD occurs in children, it is typically in older pediatric patients. The most common causes include poison ivy, nickel (jewelry), rubber (shoes), fragrance, formaldehyde (cosmetics and shampoo) and neomycin (topical antibiotics). In adults the most likely sources of ACD are allergens peculiar to the individual's occupation or hobbies.

MANAGEMENT OF ACD

Diagnosis

The clinical and histological findings of ACD are characteristic, but not diagnostic. The most widely available method for confirming the diagnosis of ACD is patch testing. Patch tests are especially indicated in cases characterized by recurrent episodes of ACD, in cases in which there is a need to identify the offending allergen, and in cases recalcitrant to conventional therapy. Patch tests document the presence of delayed-type hypersensitivity; results are usually read at 48 and 96 hours after placement of the allergens. Systemic immunosuppressive agents (e.g., systemic corticosteroids, cyclosporine, and azathioprine) or sunbathing can suppress T-cell-driven responses, and a 2–3-week washout period is advisable prior to performing patch tests in patients treated with these drugs.

The results of patch tests must be interpreted in the context of the patient's experience and exposure. A positive result does not definitively identify the cause of the ACD. False positives may be due to an irritant (rather than an allergic) effect. In these cases, patch testing in control individuals can be of great value. False negatives can occur because patch testing does not reproduce the actual environment in which the allergen is encountered. Failure to perform a second reading (between 4 and 7 days after allergen placement) may mean that late positive results are missed. Finally, only a limited number of chemicals may be tested, and although most series of allergens include the most common causes of ACD, they will not include all possible allergens. Thus a negative patch test may simply mean that the relevant allergen was not tested. Equally, some cases of contact dermatitis are due to irritants rather than to allergic sensitizers. Usually it will be clear from the history if irritant materials are being used, but if the patch tests are negative it is worth going back over the history with the patient to see whether any irritant exposures have been overlooked.

Allergen avoidance

The most important aspect of managing patients with ACD is to identify correctly the cause and provide instructions about avoiding further contact with the allergen(s). Many allergens cross-react with other compounds and thus patients should be informed of this possibility.

Symptomatic therapy

Acute forms of contact dermatitis, particularly those involving greater than 10% of the total body surface, respond well to systemic corticosteroid treatment. Topical therapy may suffice for less acute or less widespread forms of contact dermatitis.

Cold, wet compresses are highly effective during the acute blistering and oozing stage; they should be used for 15–30 minutes several times a day for 1–3 days until blistering and severe itching are controlled. Short, cool tub baths, especially with colloidal oatmeal, are soothing and help to control the acute inflammation. Antihistamine agents are not usually helpful.

Short courses of corticosteroids over 2–3 weeks are the definitive treatment. As mentioned previously, acute dermatitis and widespread involvement require systemic administration (e.g. oral prednisone, initially at a maximum dose of 1 mg/kg, tapered over at least 2 weeks). Less acute or less widespread dermatitis responds well to topical corticosteroids, the strength of which should be tailored to the age of the patient and the body part involved. For example, 1–2% hydrocortisone cream or lotions may be used in infants or on the face and mucous membranes of adults, whereas higher-potency corticosteroids like 0.1% triamcinolone cream may be used on other areas. As a rule, lotions and creams work best in the acute and subacute phases while ointments should be reserved for chronic and lichenified lesions.

CONCLUSION

ACD is a delayed-type, T-cell-mediated response following exposure to chemical sensitizers. The role of epidermal LC in the induction of ACD has recently been questioned and they may be more involved in inducing tolerance, while dermal DCs and other APC seem to play a more important role than previously believed. Irritant contact dermatitis has a similar histology, but does not involve specific sensitization.

Patch testing is the procedure of choice to confirm the diagnosis of ACD and to identify the offending contact allergens. Despite international standardization, there are still concerns about the reproducibility of patch tests and their interpretation requires both experience and judgment. The keys to management are prevention by avoiding substances containing the allergens that have been identified, and the administration of topical and/or systemic corticosteroids to get rid of any ongoing dermatitis.

REFERENCES

1. Leung DY, Bieber T. Atopic dermatitis. Lancet 2003; 361: 151–160.
2. Akdis CA, Akdis M, Bieber T, et al. Diagnosis and treatment of atopic dermatitis in children and adults: European Academy of Allergology and Clinical Immunology/American Academy of Allergy, Asthma and Immunology/PRACTALL Consensus Report. Allergy 2006; 61: 969–987.
3. Spergel JM, Paller AS. Atopic dermatitis and the atopic march. J Allergy Clin Immunol 2003; 112: S118–S127.
4. Johansson SG, Bieber T, Dahl R, et al. Revised nomenclature for allergy for global use: Report of the Nomenclature Review Committee of the World Allergy Organization, October 2003. J Allergy Clin Immunol 2004; 113: 832–836.
5. Williams H, Flohr C. How epidemiology has challenged 3 prevailing concepts about atopic dermatitis. J Allergy Clin Immunol 2006; 118: 209–213.
6. Illi S, von Mutius E, Lau S, et al. The natural course of atopic dermatitis from birth to age 7 years and the association with asthma. J Allergy Clin Immunol 2004; 113: 925–931.
7. Strachan DP. Hay fever, hygiene and household size. Br Med J 1989; 299: 1259–1260.
8. Flohr C, Pascoe D, Williams HC. Atopic dermatitis and the 'hygiene hypothesis': too clean to be true?. Br J Dermatol 2005; 152: 202–216.
9. Wollenberg A, Zoch C, Wetzel S, et al. Predisposing factors and clinical features of eczema herpeticum: a retrospective analysis of 100 cases. J Am Acad Dermatol 2003; 49: 198–205.
10. Mihm MC Jr, Soter NA, Dvorak HF, et al. The structure of normal skin and the morphology of atopic eczema. J Invest Dermatol 1976; 67: 305–312.
11. Morar N, Willis-Owen SA, Moffatt MF, et al. The genetics of atopic dermatitis. J Allergy Clin Immunol 2006; 118: 24–34. quiz 35–36.
12. Cookson W. The immunogenetics of asthma and eczema: a new focus on the epithelium. Nat Rev Immunol 2004; 4: 978–988.
13. Bowcock AM, Cookson WO. The genetics of psoriasis, psoriatic arthritis and atopic dermatitis. Hum Mol Genet 2004; 13: R43–R55.
14. Proksch E, Folster-Holst R, Jensen JM. Skin barrier function, epidermal proliferation and differentiation in eczema. J Dermatol Sci 2006; 43: 159–169.
15. Palmer CN, Irvine AD, Terron-Kwiatkowski A, et al. Common loss-of-function variants of the epidermal barrier protein filaggrin are a major predisposing factor for atopic dermatitis. Nat Genet 2006; 38: 441–446.
16. Akira S, Uematsu S, Takeuchi O. Pathogen recognition and innate immunity. Cell 2006; 124: 783–801.
17. Schroder JM, Harder J. Antimicrobial skin peptides and proteins. Cell Mol Life Sci 2006; 63: 469–486.
18. Howell MD, Gallo RL, Boguniewicz M, et al. Cytokine milieu of atopic dermatitis skin subverts the innate immune response to vaccinia virus. Immunity 2006; 24: 341–348.
19. Ong PY, Leung DY. Immune dysregulation in atopic dermatitis. Curr Allergy Asthma Rep 2006; 6: 384–389.
20. Grewe M, Walther S, Gyufko K, et al. Analysis of the cytokine pattern expressed in situ in inhalant allergen patch test reactions of atopic dermatitis patients. J Invest Dermatol 1995; 105: 407–410.
21. Spergel JM, Mizoguchi E, Brewer JP, et al. Epicutaneous sensitization with protein antigen induces localized allergic dermatitis and hyperresponsiveness to methacholine after single exposure to aerosolized antigen in mice. J Clin Invest 1998; 101: 1614–1622.
22. Beissert S, Schwarz A, Schwarz T. Regulatory T cells. J Invest Dermatol 2006; 126: 15–24.
23. Cardona ID, Goleva E, Ou LS, et al. Staphylococcal enterotoxin B inhibits regulatory T cells by inducing glucocorticoid-induced TNF receptor-related protein ligand on monocytes. J Allergy Clin Immunol 2006; 117: 688–695.
24. Homey B, Steinhoff M, Ruzicka T, et al. Cytokines and chemokines orchestrate atopic skin inflammation. J Allergy Clin Immunol 2006; 118: 178–189.
25. Novak N, Bieber T. The role of dendritic cell subtypes in the pathophysiology of atopic dermatitis. J Am Acad Dermatol 2005; 53: S171–S176.
26. Leung DY. Infection in atopic dermatitis. Curr Opin Pediatr 2003; 15: 399–404.
27. Cardona ID, Cho SH, Leung DY. Role of bacterial superantigens in atopic dermatitis: implications for future therapeutic strategies. Am J Clin Dermatol 2006; 7: 273–279.

28. Mittermann I, Aichberger KJ, Bunder R, et al. Autoimmunity and atopic dermatitis. Curr Opin Allergy Clin Immunol 2004; 4: 367–371.

29. Aichberger KJ, Mittermann I, Reininger R, et al. Hom s 4, an IgE-reactive autoantigen belonging to a new subfamily of calcium-binding proteins, can induce Th cell type 1-mediated autoreactivity. J Immunol 2005; 175: 1286–1294.

30. Mothes N, Niggemann B, Jenneck C, et al. The cradle of IgE autoreactivity in atopic eczema lies in early infancy. J Allergy Clin Immunol 2005; 116: 706–709.

31. Berth-Jones J, Damstra RJ, Golsch S, et al. Twice weekly fluticasone propionate added to emollient maintenance treatment to reduce risk of relapse in atopic dermatitis: randomised, double blind, parallel group study. Br Med J 2003; 326: 1367.

32. Wollenberg A, Sharma S, von Bubnoff D, et al. Topical tacrolimus (FK506) leads to profound phenotypic and functional alterations of epidermal antigen-presenting dendritic cells in atopic dermatitis. J Allergy Clin Immunol 2001; 107: 519–525.

33. Ashcroft DM, Dimmock P, Garside R, et al. Efficacy and tolerability of topical pimecrolimus and tacrolimus in the treatment of atopic dermatitis: meta-analysis of randomised controlled trials. Br Med J 2005; 330: 516.

34. Harper JI, Ahmed I, Barclay G, et al. Cyclosporine for severe childhood atopic dermatitis: short course versus continuous therapy. Br J Dermatol 2000; 142: 52–58.

35. Neuber K, Schwartz I, Itschert G, et al. Treatment of atopic eczema with oral mycophenolate mofetil. Br J Dermatol 2000; 143: 385–391.

36. Lear JT, English JS, Jones P, et al. Retrospective review of the use of azathioprine in severe atopic dermatitis. J Am Acad Dermatol 1996; 35: 642–643.

37. Valkova S, Velkova A. UVA/UVB phototherapy for atopic dermatitis revisited. J Dermatol Treat 2004; 15: 239–244.

38. Werfel T, Breuer K, Rueff F, et al. Usefulness of specific immunotherapy in patients with atopic dermatitis and allergic sensitization to house dust mites: a multi-centre, randomized, dose-response study. Allergy 2006; 61: 202–205.

39. Wilson DR, Lima MT, Durham SR. Sublingual immunotherapy for allergic rhinitis: systematic review and meta-analysis. Allergy 2005; 60: 4–12.

40. Wilsmann-Theis D, Martin S, Reber M, et al. Biologicals dramatic advances in the treatment of psoriasis. Curr Pharm Des 2006; 12: 989–999.

41. Schnuch A, Westphal GA, Muller MM, et al. Genotype and phenotype of N-acetyltransferase 2 (NAT2) polymorphism in patients with contact allergy. Contact Dermatitis 1998; 38: 209–211.

42. Westphal GA, Reich K, Schulz TG, et al. N-acetyltransferase 1 and 2 polymorphisms in para-substituted arylamine-induced contact allergy. Br J Dermatol 2000; 142: 1121–1127.

43. Katz DH. Carrier function in anti-hapten antibody responses. IV. Experimental conditions for the induction of hapten-specific tolerance or for the stimulation of anti-hapten anamnestic responses by 'non-immunogenic' hapten polypeptide conjugates. J Exp Med 1971; 134: 201.

44. Krasteva M, Kehren J, Ducluzeau MT, et al. Contact dermatitis I. Pathophysiology of contact sensitivity. Eur J Dermatol 1999; 9: 65–77.

45. Kissenpfennig A, Malissen B. Langerhans cells – revisiting the paradigm using genetically engineered mice. Trends Immunol 2006; 27: 132–139.

46. Groves RW. Tumour necrosis factor alpha is pro-inflammatory in normal human skin and modulates cutaneous adhesion molecule expression. Br J Dermatol 1995; 132: 345.

Food allergy

Scott H. Sicherer

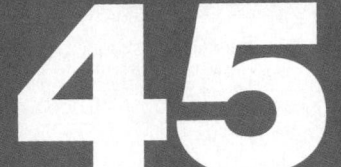

Adverse reactions to foods can result from immunologic (*food allergy*) and nonimmunologic responses.[1,2] More than one in five persons alters their diet for a presumed food allergy, but nonimmune causes can often be identified.[3] Toxins or pharmacologically active components of the diet account for a number of nonimmune adverse reactions. Recently, the term *hypersensitivity* has been applied to an exaggerated response to any food component, even a nonimmune reaction.[1] Therefore, lactose intolerance, resulting in abdominal discomfort due to a reduced ability to digest lactose, may be defined as *nonallergic hypersensitivity*. Examples of adverse reactions to foods are shown in Table 45.1. Immune responses to foods are a normal phenomenon, leading to a state of oral tolerance.[4] In contrast, aberrant immune responses to food proteins can lead to a variety of symptoms and disorders, defined together as food allergies.[5] It is conceptually and diagnostically helpful to divide food allergic disorders broadly by immunopathology, into those that are associated with detectable food-specific IgE antibodies and those that are not.[6] Disorders with an acute onset of symptoms following ingestion are typically mediated by IgE antibodies. Food-specific IgE antibodies arm tissue mast cells and blood basophils, a state termed *sensitization*. Upon re-exposure, the causal food proteins bind to the specific IgE antibodies and may trigger the release of mediators such as histamine, causing symptoms that may affect the skin, gastrointestinal tract, respiratory tract and cardiovascular system (Chapter 42). Another group of food allergic disorders, affecting primarily the gastrointestinal tract, are subacute or chronic and mediated primarily by T cells. A third group of chronic disorders that may be associated with food allergy, atopic dermatitis and eosinophilic gastrointestinal disorders, are variably associated with detectable IgE antibody (IgE associated/cell-mediated disorders).

■ PREVALENCE ■

Perceived food allergies are often not verified when standardized procedures, such as double-blind, placebo-controlled oral food challenges, are undertaken.[2] Estimated rates of food allergy, and the specific causal foods, vary by age and geographic region, and are influenced by factors such as regional diets, environmental exposures such as pollen, and the fact that many food allergies resolve in childhood.[3] It is estimated that 6% of young children and 3.7% of adults in the USA have a food allergy. In young children, the most common causal foods are cow's milk (2.5%), egg (1.3%), peanut (0.8%), wheat (~0.4%), soy (~0.4%), tree nuts such as walnut and cashew (0.2%), fish (0.1%) and shellfish (0.1%). Studies in the USA and UK have indicated at least a doubling in the rate of peanut allergy in young children during the past decade.[7,8] It is not known whether this trend is exclusive to peanuts. Studies have not implicated maternal diet as a factor, but noningestion exposures such as skin contact have been implicated as a route of sensitization.[9] Adults rarely (< 0.3%) have allergies to milk, egg, soy or wheat, and are more commonly allergic to shellfish (2%), peanut (0.6%), tree nuts (0.5%), and fish (0.4%).[3] Virtually all foods can cause an allergy in at least some individuals.[10] Reactions to fruits and vegetables are particularly common (~5%) but usually not severe, whereas reactions to seeds (e.g., sesame, poppy) are being reported with increasing frequency and can be severe. Allergy to additives and preservatives, though often suspected, are uncommon (< 1%).[11] Genetic risk factors for food allergy include a family or personal history of atopic disorders (asthma, atopic dermatitis, allergic rhinitis, food allergy).

The influence of food allergy on specific disease states varies according to the type of disease and the age group affected.[2] Anaphylaxis in the community setting is attributed to food allergy in 35–55% of episodes: common offenders are peanuts, nuts, and seafood. Food allergy is also a common cause of acute urticaria (20%) and is associated with atopic dermatitis in nearly 40% of children with mild to moderate disease, most commonly with milk and egg allergy. In contrast, food allergy is not a common cause of chronic isolated respiratory symptoms, chronic urticaria, or atopic dermatitis in adults.

■ CLINICAL MANIFESTATIONS ■

The clinical manifestations of food allergy are diverse and result from the underlying immune mechanisms and their impact on particular target organs.[3,5,12] Food allergy can present as an acute reaction following ingestion of a causal food, with a sudden onset of typical symptoms such as hives or respiratory compromise; as an increase in chronic symptoms such as exacerbation of atopic dermatitis; or as a chronic disease. Where symptoms

Table 45.1 Examples of adverse reactions to foods

Intolerance (nonallergic hypersensitivity)
Lactose intolerance (lactase deficiency)
Sucrase–isomaltase deficiency
Galactosemia
Alcohol
Caffeine (jitteriness)
Tyramine in aged cheeses (migraine)
Toxins
Bacterial food poisoning
Scombroid (in dark-meat fish, may mimic allergy)
Food allergy (immune responses)
IgE-mediated
Not IgE-associated
Mixed IgE/non-IgE (eosinophilic gastrointestinal
disease, atopic dermatitis)
Neurologic and psychological/psychiatric
Auriculotemporal syndrome (facial flush with salivation)
Gustatory rhinitis
Anorexia nervosa and food aversions

*The revised nomenclature of the World Allergy Organization uses the term 'hypersensitivity' to indicate a reproducible symptom or sign to a stimulus tolerated at the same dose by normal persons apart from an immunologic basis (e.g., lactose intolerance would be termed a nonallergic hypersensitivity).

Table 45.2 Clinical disorders

Immunopathology/disorder
IgE antibody-associated
Urticaria/angioedema
Immediate gastrointestinal reaction (GI anaphylaxis)
Oral allergy syndrome (pollen-related)
Rhinitis
Asthma
Anaphylaxis
Food-associated, exercise-induced anaphylaxis
IgE antibody associated/cell mediated, chronic
Atopic dermatitis
Eosinophilic gastroenteropathies
Non-IgE-associated
Dietary protein enterocolitis
Dietary protein proctitis
Dietary protein enteropathy
Celiac disease
Dermatitis herpetiformis
Contact dermatitis
Pulmonary hemosiderosis

are compatible with one of these patterns, a food allergy should be considered in the differential diagnosis. Specific disorders are summarized in Table 45.2. Disorders and symptoms such as behavioral problems, arthritis, and headache have not been convincingly or commonly linked to food allergy. Reflux, infantile colic and recalcitrant constipation have been attributed to food allergy in a subset of pediatric patients.

IGE-ASSOCIATED FOOD ALLERGIES

A typical feature of IgE-mediated food-allergic reactions is the timing of symptoms: reactions typically occur within minutes, and rarely more than an hour, after the ingestion of a triggering food. The organ system/systems affected and the specific symptoms additionally define these reactions. *Urticaria and/or angioedema*, pruritus and flushing are common skin manifestations of food allergy, either alone or in combination with other symptoms. The rash may occur anywhere, although the face is most commonly affected. *Contact urticaria* describes lesions that occur at the site of direct contact with the food that may or may not also induce a reaction when ingested. Chronic urticaria is not commonly associated with food allergy.

The term *gastrointestinal anaphylaxis* describes isolated, acute gastrointestinal responses such as nausea, pain, vomiting and/or diarrhea induced by IgE-mediated mechanisms. Gastrointestinal anaphylaxis is uncommon, but gastrointestinal symptoms commonly accompany other organ system manifestations of acute, IgE antibody-mediated reactions to foods. A form of contact allergy that primarily affects the oropharynx is *pollen-food syndrome (oral allergy syndrome)*.[13] Initial

KEY CONCEPTS

MANIFESTATIONS OF FOOD ALLERGY

A food allergy is likely when:

>> Typical symptoms (e.g., urticaria, pruritus, symptoms of anaphylaxis) occur minutes following ingestion of a possible causal food.

>> Certain chronic diseases are identified, such as moderate to severe atopic dermatitis in children, or eosinophilic gastroenteropathies.

>> Patterns of illness are consistent with described syndromes of food allergy, such as vomiting and lethargy about 2 hours after the ingestion of an allergen in infants (enterocolitis), or mucous, bloody stools in a breastfed infant (proctocolitis).

sensitization to pollen proteins may result in symptoms when homologous proteins in particular fruits/vegetables are ingested. For example, the birch pollen protein Bet v 1 shares homology with apple Mal d 1. Additional relationships with birch pollen proteins include other Rosaceae family fruits, such as peach and plum. It is estimated that 50% of pollen-allergic persons may be affected. Symptoms are usually limited to the oropharynx with pruritus and mild angioedema, but progression to a systemic reaction may occur. Causal proteins are presumably heat-labile, as cooking the food typically abolishes the reaction. The disorder must be distinguished from mild oral reactions

CLINICAL PEARLS

FACTORS ASSOCIATED WITH SEVERE/FATAL REACTIONS

>> Allergies to peanut, tree nuts, fish and shellfish (however other foods are potential causes)

>> Delay in treatment with epinephrine

>> Teenagers and young adults

>> Asthma

>> Lack of skin rash during a reaction

>> Reactions to trace amounts

>> Previous severe reactions

to stable proteins and oral reactions that may be a first symptom of a more progressive allergic response. The same foods that cause this oral syndrome may induce a systemic reaction in persons reactive to stable proteins they contain (e.g., lipid transfer proteins).

Chronic asthma and chronic allergic rhinitis are not typically attributable solely to food allergy. However, *respiratory symptoms* of rhinitis and wheezing may accompany systemic allergic reactions to ingested food allergens. Inhalation of airborne allergenic food proteins can also induce respiratory reactions, either in an occupational setting, e.g., baker's asthma from wheat, or when stable proteins become aerosolized during cooking or processing.

Food-induced anaphylaxis is a serious systemic allergic reaction that is rapid in onset and can cause death.[14] Symptoms can vary and may affect any of a combination of organ systems among the skin, respiratory tract, gastrointestinal tract and cardiovascular system. Symptoms may also include uterine contractions and an aura of 'impending doom.' Although a variety of mild symptoms such as urticaria and abdominal pain can occur, life-threatening symptoms include laryngeal edema, severe asthma, and cardiovascular compromise (Chapter 42). Serum tryptase elevation is often not detected during food-associated anaphylaxis. There are currently no simple tests to determine an individual's risk of severe or fatal anaphylaxis, but epidemiological factors such as age and food may define a high-risk group. Reactions can be biphasic, with initial symptoms waning and severe symptoms recurring 1–2 hours or more later. If anaphylaxis only occurs when exercise follows ingestion of the causal food, the diagnosis is *food-associated, exercise-induced anaphylaxis*. The syndrome of exercise-related food anaphylaxis is most commonly reported after eating wheat or celery, but some individuals experience anaphylaxis with exercise after any meal.

MIXED IgE/NON-IgE-ASSOCIATED (ATOPIC DERMATITIS/EOSINOPHILIC GASTROINTESTINAL DISEASE)

Studies using double-blind, placebo-controlled oral food challenges show that approximately one in three young children with moderate to severe *atopic dermatitis* has a food allergy.[15] Removal of triggering foods may improve the skin condition. Food-responsive atopic dermatitis can also

occur in adults, but appears much less common and has been less well studied. Most studies reveal that food-specific IgE antibody is detectable to the foods that cause symptoms. However, food-responsive disease has also been documented in children without detectable IgE to the causal food; therefore, cell-mediated mechanisms are also probably involved. Because of the chronic nature of the disorder, and its waxing and waning course, it is difficult to link symptoms with particular foods by history alone. More than 90% of reactions in children are attributed to milk, egg, wheat and soy. It is less common to verify a role for meats, fruits or vegetables.

Allergic eosinophilic esophagitis/gastroenteritis is a group of disorders characterized by eosinophilic inflammation in the gastrointestinal tract (Chapter 46). Symptoms overlap those of other gastrointestinal disorders and may include dysphagia, vomiting, diarrhea, obstruction, and malabsorption. Studies in children indicate that almost all patients are food responsive, although implicated foods may or may not be associated with evidence of IgE antibody.[16]

NON-IgE-ASSOCIATED DISORDERS

Similar to the IgE-associated disorders, these disorders may also affect various target organs.[2] *Contact dermatitis*, a type IV hypersensitivity response, can occur from contact with foods in occupational handling. Fixed, raised, erythematous eruptions, similar to fixed drug eruptions, have rarely been attributed to foods. *Dermatitis herpetiformis* is a papulovesicular skin rash associated with celiac disease caused by an immune response to gluten.

A rare pulmonary disorder affecting infants, *Heiner's syndrome or milk-induced pulmonary hemosiderosis*, is associated with precipitating (IgG) antibodies to cow's milk. Symptoms include anemia, pulmonary infiltrates, recurrent pneumonia, and growth failure, which resolve with milk elimination.

Several nonIgE-mediated disorders of the gastrointestinal tract have been identified in infants.[12] *Food protein-induced proctocolitis* is characterized by mucus and blood in stools. Patients are usually breastfed infants and the bleeding usually resolves with maternal exclusion of cow's milk. Rarely, foods other than milk are implicated. The infants generally appear well. Empiric dietary therapy is commonly instituted, but if rectal biopsy is performed, an eosinophilic inflammation is observed. The disorder is generally not associated with detectable IgE antibody to milk and resolves by age 1–2 years. Infants with *food protein-induced enteropathy* experience diarrhea, poor growth and edema due to hypoproteinemia caused by malabsorption. Biopsy reveals nonspecific inflammation of the jejunum with increased lymphocytes, plasma cells and eosinophils, and partial villus blunting. Enteropathy syndromes attributed to cow's milk protein usually resolve in 1–2 years. In contrast, *celiac disease*, a specific type of enteropathy, is caused by immune reactions to gluten (e.g., wheat, rye, barley) and is often associated with the HLA-DQ2 haplotype (Chapter 74). The inflammatory response remits with dietary exclusion of gluten but, unlike cow's milk enteropathy the disorder does not resolve and so lifetime exclusion of gluten is needed. A dramatic form of nonIgE mediated gastrointestinal food allergy is *food protein-induced enterocolitis*. Primarily a disorder of infants, this is characterized by a symptom complex of profuse vomiting and heme-positive diarrhea, leading to failure to thrive, and potentially to dehydration and shock during chronic ingestion of the causal protein. These infants also may develop acidemia and methemoglobinemia, and present with a sepsis-like picture including an elevated peripheral polymorphonuclear leukocyte count. Cow's milk and soy are most often responsible, but grains such as rice and oats, and poultry, are an increasingly recognized trigger. Ingestion of the causal protein may lead to a delayed (about 2 hours) recurrence of symptoms that may be severe and include shock. Resolution usually occurs in 2–3 years.

■ PATHOPHYSIOLOGY ■

IMMUNE MECHANISMS AND THE GASTROINTESTINAL BARRIER

The first line of gastrointestinal defense against microbes and allergens is the gastrointestinal surface, which poses both a physical and an immunologic barrier.[4] The mucosal surface physical barrier includes luminal contents that present enzymes, extremes of pH, and bile salts that disrupt pathogens and allergens. The mucosal surface also presents a physical barrier because glycocalyx and a thick mucous layer overlie epithelial cells joined by tight junctions. Studies in mice, and observations in humans, indicate that neutralizing gastric pH can alter the gastrointestinal barrier in a way that may promote sensitization to ingested food antigens and increase the likelihood of reactions. One theory for the disposition of infants toward allergic responses to foods is the developmental immaturity of the gut barrier: for example, enzymatic activity is suboptimal in the newborn period. Nonetheless, about 2% of ingested food antigens are absorbed and transported throughout the body in an immunologically intact form in adults; therefore, additional immune mechanisms must be active to promote tolerance.

An active immune response involving both innate immunity (e.g., NK cells, polymorphonuclear leukocytes, macrophages, epithelial cells and Toll-like receptors) and adaptive immunity (e.g., intraepithelial and lamina propria lymphocytes, Peyer's patches, sIgA and cytokines), result in a moderated immune response to food proteins and oral tolerance.[4, 17] The immunologic mechanisms involved in oral tolerance have not been fully elucidated. Central roles for antigen-presenting dendritic cells and regulatory T cells have been identified. Dendritic cells residing within the lamina propria and the noninflammatory environment of Peyer's patches produce IL-10 and IL-4, which favor the generation of tolerance. Regulatory T cells have been identified that modulate gastrointestinal inflammation and prevent adverse responses. These include Th3 cells, a population of CD4 cells that secrete TGF-β; TR1 cells, CD4 cells that secrete IL-10; CD4, CD25+ regulatory T cells; CD8 suppressor T cells; and γδ T cells. Intestinal epithelial cells may act as nonprofessional antigen-presenting cells because they present luminal antigens to T cells on an MHC class II complex, but lack a 'second signal.' The potential for allergens to transverse the gastrointestinal barrier in intact form (see below), the dose and the frequency of exposure can also influence tolerance. High dose tolerance involves deletion of effector T cells, whereas low dose tolerance is mediated by activation of regulatory T cells with suppressor functions. Commensal gut flora may also influence oral tolerance. Mice raised in a germ-free environment from birth fail to develop normal tolerance, and mice treated with antibiotics after birth are more easily sensitized to food protein.

Homing of food-responsive T cells to target organ sites of inflammation may account for organ specificity in food allergic disease. For example, when stimulated *in vitro* with milk protein, peripheral blood mononuclear cells from children with milk-responsive atopic dermatitis express the skin homing receptor cutaneous lymphocyte antigen, whereas cells from patients with isolated gastrointestinal reactions to milk do not.[18]

FOOD ALLERGENS AND ADDITIVES

Certain food allergens are relatively stable to acid and heat and typically sensitize via the oral route (traditional, or class I food allergy),[5] though they may also sensitize through ambient environmental exposures, for example in occupational asthma or skin contact with topical cosmetics. In contrast, class II food allergens are labile proteins and initial sensitization occurs primarily through respiratory exposure to homologous proteins in pollens. In accordance with the immunopathogenesis, class I food allergy typically occurs in infants or children during a presumed window of immunologic immaturity. In contrast, class II food allergy also affects adults (e.g., pollen-food related or oral allergy syndrome).

The major food allergens identified as class I allergens are water-soluble glycoproteins 10–70 kDa in size and fairly stable to heat, acid and proteases; examples include proteins in milk (caseins, β-lactoglobulin), peanut (vicillins, conglutin), egg (ovomucoid, ovalbumin), fish (parvalbumin), and nonspecific lipid transfer proteins found, for example, in apple (Mal d 3) or corn (Zea m 14). In contrast, class II allergens are generally labile, for example pathogen-related protein 10 in birch pollen (Bet v 1) that can induce sensitization through the respiratory route or can result in oral symptoms of pruritus to homologous proteins, such as in raw apple (Mal d 1) or carrot (Dau c 1). A limited number of related proteins make up the majority of food allergens (e.g., proteins in the cupin superfamily, the prolamin superfamily, and proteins in the plant defense system pathogenesis-related proteins).[19] An individual may mount an immune response to various proteins in a specific food, and towards various segments (epitopes) of a particular protein – this pattern may correlate with expression of disease. For example, major class I allergens in peanut include Ara h 1, 2 and 3, which are associated with severe peanut allergy. On the other hand, Ara h 8 is a bet v 1 homolog, class II peanut allergen, which is less likely to be associated with severe clinical reactions. The specific number of proteins or epitopes recognized may also relate to clinical outcome. Broader patterns of IgE recognition, e.g., to many proteins and epitopes of a specific food, may be associated with a higher chance of a clinical allergic reaction. It has been suggested that IgE antibodies that recognize epitopes dependent on tertiary allergen structure are associated with transient childhood allergy, whereas IgE antibodies that recognize epitopes that are not dependent on complex protein folding (i.e., linear epitopes) are associated with persistent allergy.[3] These and additional factors, such as heating a food and the matrix in which a food protein resides, can influence disease outcomes.

Whereas many botanically related proteins or animal proteins from similar species share regions of homology and may show cross-reactivity on allergy testing, clinical evidence of cross-reactivity is not as common.[20] Table 45.3 shows examples of common food allergens and describes important features and the implications for cross-reactivity. Virtually every food or derivatives (e.g., gelatin, colors or flavors) from meats, fruits, vegetables, grains, etc., has been described to cause a food allergic reaction, at least occasionally.[10] The term 'spice' is

Table 45.3 Features of selected food allergens

Food	Selected allergenic proteins	Clinical issues and cross-reactions
Cow's milk	Bos d 4 α-lactalbumin Bos d 5 β-lactoglobulin Bos d 8 casein	Allergy to most mammalian milks (goat's, sheep's) is common (>90%)
Egg	Gal d 1 ovomucoid Gal d 2 ovalbumin	
Peanut	Ara h 1 vicilin Ara h 2 conglutin Ara h 3 glycinin Ara h 8 homologue to birch Bet v 1	Uncommon to be reactive to other legumes (<5%) such as soy, pea
Codfish	Gad c 1 parvalbumin	Common to be allergic to other finned fish (~75%), but allergy to specific species possible (presumed reaction to other fish proteins)
Shrimp	Pen a 1 tropomyosin	Common to be allergic to other crustacean shellfish (~75%), but allergy to specific species possible (presumed reaction to other shellfish proteins)
Wheat	Tri a 19 ω-5-gliadin	Uncommon to be reactive to other grains
Apple	Mal d 1 homologue to birch Bet v 1 Mal d 3 lipid transfer protein Profilin actin-binding protein	Homologous protein responsible for oral allergy syndrome

often used to describe a variety of flavoring agents, such as basil, cardamom, cinnamon, fennel, garlic, parsley, pepper, peppermint, rosemary, saffron, turmeric, and many others. These 'spices' represent a huge array of types of foods having proteins that share features with other foods and pollens. Therefore, this large group could be expected to include allergens accounting for allergic reactions in a subset of patients.

A variety of substances may be added to foods to enhance flavor, preservation, color, or texture. Certain food additives are derived from natural sources and contain proteins that have been associated with allergic reactions, e.g., colors derived from turmeric, paprika, beet, seeds (annatto) and insects (carmine/cochineal). [11]

Chemical additives are not likely to cause IgE-associated allergic reactions, but some may have drug effects that cause adverse reactions, including symptoms that are allergy-like, or which may invoke an immune response. Tartrazine (Yellow #5) is a synthetic color that has been extensively investigated because of concerns that it may trigger hives, allergic reactions and asthma. However, well-conducted studies have generally not validated these concerns. Like tartrazine, many other synthetic colors (sunset yellow, erythrosine, ponceau 4R, carmoisine, quinoline yellow, patent blue and others) have not been proved to cause allergic reactions, but some have rarely been associated with illnesses such as rashes. Sulfites are added to foods as a preservative, an anti-browning agent, or for a bleaching effect. In sensitive persons, sulfites can induce asthma, and very rarely cause more significant allergic-like

KEY CONCEPTS

PATHOPHYSIOLOGIC EXPLANATIONS FOR CLINICAL MANIFESTATIONS

>> Heat- and digestion-resistant proteins are more likely to cause anaphylaxis/systemic reactions.

>> Labile food proteins are less likely to cause systemic reactions, and heating may abrogate reactions.

>> Homing of food-reactive T cells to target organs may account for particular disease manifestations, e.g., atopic dermatitis compared to isolated gastrointestinal disease.

>> Expression of IgE that binds to sequential amino acids, compared to those that bind to epitopes that depend on tertiary conformational structures, are associated with a persistent allergy.

>> The matrix in which a protein resides, and the effect of heating, may alter its presentation to the immune system, either reducing or enhancing reactions.

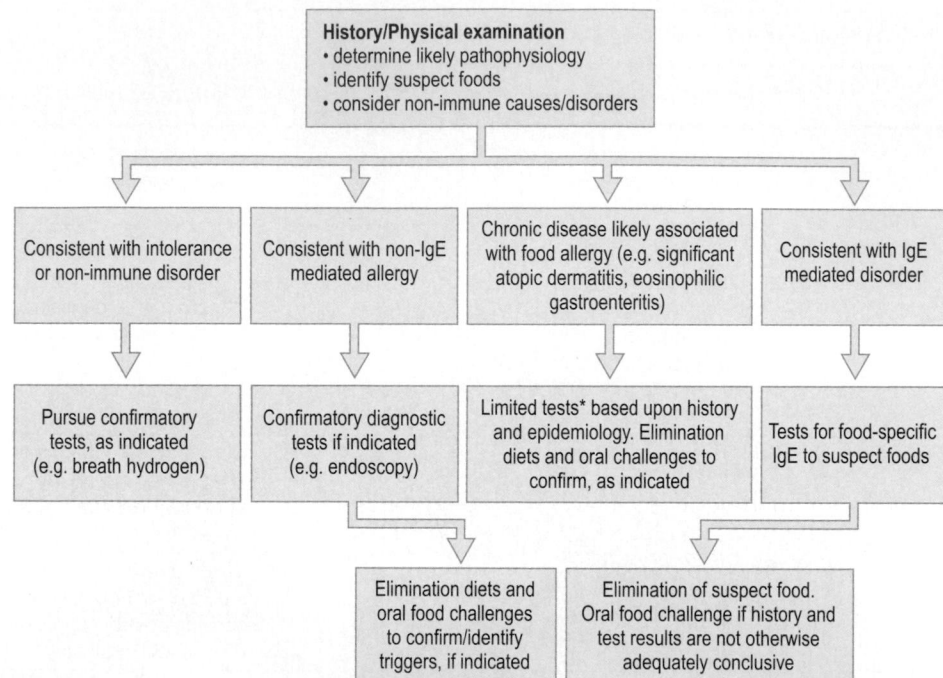

Fig. 45.1 General diagnostic scheme. The history is the key starting point toward diagnosing a food allergy, or alternative explanation for an adverse event to foods. This illustration provides a conceptual framework only, see text for additional explanations. * Certain test results may be intrinsically 'diagnostic' (see text).

responses. Sulfites are used to preserve some drugs, including epinephrine, but the low amounts used for epinephrine have never been reported to cause a reaction.

■ DIAGNOSIS ■

The clinical evaluation of an adverse reaction to food depends on a careful history and physical examination to determine the type of adverse response (as outlined in Table 45.1) and which food(s) might be responsible.[5] Important factors to consider include the types of symptoms, their chronicity, reproducibility, and possible alternative explanations. If symptoms indicate that a nonimmune response is likely, additional evaluation would follow the specific suspicion. For example, lactose intolerance can be confirmed by hydrogen breath testing. If a food allergy is likely, the pattern of illness and list of possible triggers may disclose whether an IgE- or a non-IgE-associated disorder is likely, and will establish the type of testing that might be appropriate. Figure 45.1 shows a general diagnostic scheme. For chronic disorders such as atopic dermatitis and eosinophilic gastroenteritis, the identification of suspect foods is difficult because food is ingested throughout the day and symptoms are often chronic, with a waxing and waning course. Symptom diaries are helpful, but rarely diagnostic. In addition, individuals with these disorders often test positive to multiple foods that may not be causing illness. Care in selecting and interpreting the tests is paramount.

To determine food-specific IgE antibodies, skin-prick tests (SPTs) performed using a probe to introduce food protein to the superficial skin

■ CLINICAL PEARLS

CLUES AND PITFALLS IN DIAGNOSTIC TESTING

>> The history is paramount to provide prior probability assessments to select and interpret tests.

>> In the event of a convincing reaction, a negative test should not be relied on to exclude allergy: additional testing and physician-supervised oral food challenges may be needed.

>> It is more likely that a food that is not commonly eaten is the cause of a reaction, compared to a new allergy to a routinely tolerated food.

>> Testing of large 'panels' of foods without regard to patient history or the epidemiology of allergic diseases is often misleading because sensitization (positive tests for IgE) may occur without clinical consequences.

>> The degree of positive testing may correlate positively with risk of reactions, but the exact nature of the relationship for most foods/clinical circumstances has not been determined.

layer, or serum tests, are generally sensitive (~75–95%) and specific (~30–60%).[2] SPTs are used on rash-free skin while the patient is avoiding antihistamines; intradermal skin tests should not be used. Although commercial extracts are available for performing skin-prick tests for many foods, fresh extracts may be more sensitive, particularly when testing fruits and vegetables whose proteins are prone to degradation. If IgE antibody specific for the food protein is present, a wheal and flare will occur that is compared to positive (histamine) and negative (saline–glycerine) controls. SPTs are considered positive if there is a mean wheal diameter of 3 mm or more, after subtraction of the saline control. Food-specific IgE antibodies can also be detected in serum (Chapter 100).

A positive SPT or serum IgE test merely indicates that food-specific IgE is present: it does not itself confirm an allergy. Increasingly larger wheal diameters or increasing concentrations of IgE antibodies are associated with an increasingly higher chance that the test reflects a clinical reaction. In a limited number of studies of a few foods in infants and/or children, diagnostic values associated with very high (>95%) predictive values for reactions have been determined, though not universally confirmed. A study using SPTs in young children revealed that when wheals were particularly large (> 8 mm for milk and peanut, and > 7 mm for egg) a clinical reaction was virtually certain.[21] Studies determining the concentration of specific IgE antibody measured using a particular method (CAP-RAST FEIA or UniCap reported in arbitrary units, kU_A/L) showed that a food-specific IgE concentration of >7 kU_A/L to egg, >15 to milk, and >14 to peanut was 95% predictive for a reaction among 5-year-old children.[22] For children under the age of 2 the values where most reacted were lower (e.g., > 2 kU_A/L for egg or milk). These results have not been widely confirmed.[3,5] It must be emphasized that diagnostic concentrations have not been determined for other foods, allergic disorders or age groups.

Food-specific IgE may be detected despite tolerance of a food, or may remain detectable but typically decline as a food allergy resolves. Obtaining 'panels' of food allergy tests without considering the history is not good practice because numerous irrelevant positive results can occur. The history is crucial, because tests are expected to be negative when the pathophysiology of the response is consistent with a nonIgE-mediated reaction. However, acute anaphylactic reactions may also occur despite a negative test, so caution is needed when evaluating a patient with a convincing history despite a negative test. Neither the size of the SPT nor the level of IgE in serum usefully predicts the type or severity of reaction. Additional diagnostic tests are being researched. The atopy patch test (APT), which is performed by placing the food allergen on the skin under occlusion for 48 hours and assessing for a delayed rash at 24–72 hours, shows promise for nonIgE-mediated disorders, but more studies are needed to determine their utility.[5] A host of tests have been touted for the diagnosis of food allergy, but have never been found useful in blinded studies. These include measurement of IgG_4 antibody, provocation–neutralization (drops placed under the tongue or injected to diagnose and treat various symptoms), and applied kinesiology (muscle strength testing).[5]

For evaluation of chronic disease, the amelioration of symptoms during dietary elimination of suspected foods provides presumptive evidence of causality. Elimination diets can be undertaken by removing foods suspected to be causing symptoms, removing all but a defined group of foods that are rarely allergenic (oligoantigenic diet), or by giving an elemental diet of only a hypoallergenic extensively hydrolyzed formula or a nonallergenic amino acid-based formula. The elemental diet provides the most

definitive trial. The type of elimination diet selected depends upon the clinical scenario, a priori reasoning concerning offending foods, and the results of tests for IgE antibody. The duration of the trial depends on the type of symptoms, but 1–6 weeks is usually the required range. A dietician may be needed to ensure nutritional sufficiency of trial diets. For breastfed infants, maternal dietary elimination is required. When a food to which IgE has been demonstrated is removed from the diet during a chronic disorder, it is possible for reintroduction to induce severe reactions.

When history and simple tests have not confirmed an allergy, or when tolerance is suspected, an oral food challenge (OFC) may be needed to confirm clinical allergy.[5] An oral food challenge is performed by feeding gradually increasing amounts of the suspected food over hours or days. This requires physician observation and is performed either openly or blinded by camouflaging the food in a carrier food or opaque capsules. The double-blind, placebo-controlled oral food challenge is the method least prone to bias and is considered the 'gold standard' to diagnose food allergy. The OFC can be used to evaluate any type of suspected adverse response to foods. The procedure is most often needed when several foods are under consideration, tests for specific IgE are positive, and elimination resulted in resolution of symptoms. The challenge setting also provides a safe means to introduce foods that were highly suspected to cause severe reactions but showed negative skin or IgE tests. For nonIgE-mediated reactions, OFC is usually the only means of diagnosis. These feeding tests, particularly in IgE-mediated reactions and enterocolitis syndrome, can induce severe reactions. The supervising clinician must have medications and supplies for resuscitation immediately available to manage reactions. Challenges may be optional or contraindicated in certain circumstances, and the risks of the challenge must be weighed against the social and nutritional deficits of continued avoidance. Recent, severe anaphylaxis to an isolated ingestion, with a positive test for specific IgE antibody to the causal food, is one example of a relative contraindication because this scenario represents confirmation of a convincing history. Negative challenges should always be followed by a supervised open feeding of a relevant portion of the tested food in its commonly prepared state.

■ TREATMENT ■

Various modalities to induce tolerance or reduce reaction severity, such as oral immunotherapy, injection immunotherapy using modified proteins, monoclonal antibodies to block immune responses and other strategies, are under investigation.[23] However, the mainstay of treatment is avoidance of the food and preparation for treatment in the event of an accidental ingestion leading to an allergic reaction, including anaphylaxis. Dietary management of food allergy is fraught with nutritional and other pitfalls. In most countries, manufacturing and labeling deficiencies make it very difficult to identify allergens in commercial food products. Cross-contamination and errors in packaged food and restaurants are an additional obstacle. For children, dietary management in schools can be difficult due to food sharing, school projects using foods, parties, lack of on-site medical personnel, etc.

In the event of an allergic reaction, antihistamines may be required to reduce itching/rash. However, for patients experiencing more severe symptoms of anaphylaxis, with respiratory and/or cardiovascular symptoms, additional therapies are required (Chapter 42). Self-injectable epinephrine should be prescribed for those at risk of anaphylaxis.[14] Guidelines for determining those who should have access to this

THERAPEUTIC PRINCIPLES

AVOIDANCE AND EMERGENCY CARE

Avoidance:

>> Careful reading of food ingredient labels, meal preparation to avoid cross-contact

>> Review approaches to restaurants (careful communication of allergy, avoiding higher risk cuisines based upon the allergen, caution about cross-contact in meal preparation)

>> Seek dietician support to ensure adequate nutrition when numerous restrictions are in place

Treatment:

>> Prescribe and train use of intramuscular epinephrine for self-injection

>> Medical alert bracelets

>> Alert emergency services for prompt advanced evaluation and emergency care of anaphylaxis

>> Remain under medical observation 4 or more hours following a significant reaction (biphasic reaction could occur)

>> Written/reviewed anaphylaxis action plans for schools/camps

KEY CONCEPTS

NATURAL COURSE

>> Most (85%) childhood food allergies to milk, egg, wheat, soy resolve by age 5.

>> Peanut, tree nut, fish and shellfish allergies are typically persistent.

>> 20% of young children with a food allergy to peanut become tolerant by age 5.

>> About 9% of young children with a tree nut allergy achieves tolerance.

>> Allergy to peanut can 'recur;' a risk appears to be prolonged avoidance after apparent tolerance.

>> For IgE-mediated reactions, test results may decline as tolerance develops.

>> Most infant gastrointestinal allergies resolve by early childhood, but eosinophilic gastroenteropathies appear to be more persistent.

medication are under scrutiny, but candidates include food-allergic patients with previous severe reactions, allergy to foods commonly causing severe reactions, and food-allergic patients with underlying asthma. It is essential to periodically review the indications and technique of administration of self-injectable epinephrine because mistakes are common. Patients must be instructed that following the administration of the medication they need prompt transportation to an emergency facility (by ambulance) with prolonged observation (> 4 hours), as recurrence of severe symptoms is possible. Patients should obtain medical emergency bracelets identifying their allergy, and be reminded to update expired and expended epinephrine injectors. For children, an important component of the school management of food allergy is to have a clear emergency plan in place, medications readily available, and school personnel trained in recognizing and treating reactions.

■ NATURAL HISTORY AND PREVENTION ■

Most (~85%) children lose their sensitivity to most allergenic foods (egg, milk, wheat, soy) within the first 3–5 years of life.[24] In contrast, adults with food allergy may have long-lived sensitivity. Sensitivity to peanut, tree nuts, and seafood is rarely lost. The notion that peanut and tree nut allergy is permanent derives partly from the observation that it is an allergy that affects adults; however, it has become apparent that about 20% of peanut-allergic children under age 2 years, and about 9% of those with tree nut allergy, may achieve tolerance by school age.

Evidence-based approaches to delay or prevent allergy through dietary manipulation of infants and mothers have been hampered by study design, because randomized controlled dietary trials are not possible. Studies suggest a beneficial role for exclusive breastfeeding of infants at 'high risk' for atopic disease for the first 3–6 months of life, and for avoiding supplementation with cow's milk or soy formulas in favor of hypoallergenic formulas if breastfeeding is not possible.[25] At present there are no conclusive studies indicating that the manipulation of the mother's diet during pregnancy or while breastfeeding, or the restriction of allergenic foods from the infant's diet, will prevent the development of food allergy, though such approaches have been suggested.

■ REFERENCES ■

1. Johansson SG, Bieber T, Dahl R, et al. Revised nomenclature for allergy for global use: Report of the Nomenclature Review Committee of the World Allergy Organization, October 2003. J Allergy Clin Immunol 2004; 113: 832–836.

2. Sicherer SH, Teuber S. Current approach to the diagnosis and management of adverse reactions to foods. J Allergy Clin Immunol 2004; 114: 1146–1150.

3. Sicherer SH, Sampson HA. Food allergy. J Allergy Clin Immunol 2006; 117: S470–S475.

4. Chehade M, Mayer L. Oral tolerance and its relation to food hypersensitivities. J Allergy Clin Immunol 2005; 115: 3–12.

5. Food allergy: a practice parameter. Ann Allergy Asthma Immunol 2006; 96: S1–S68.

6. Sicherer SH. Food allergy. Lancet 2002; 360: 701–710.

7. Grundy J, Matthews S, Bateman B, et al. Rising prevalence of allergy to peanut in children: Data from 2 sequential cohorts. J Allergy Clin Immunol 2002; 110: 784–789.

8. Sicherer SH, Muñoz-Furlong A, Sampson HA. Prevalence of peanut and tree nut allergy in the United States determined by means of a random digit dial telephone survey: a 5-year follow-up study. J Allergy Clin Immunol 2003; 112: 1203–1207.

9. Lack G, Fox D, Northstone K, Golding J. Factors associated with the development of peanut allergy in childhood. N Engl J Med 2003; 348: 977–985.

10. Hefle SL, Nordlee JA, Taylor SL. Allergenic foods. Crit Rev Food Sci Nutr 1996; 36: S69–S89.

11. Simon RA. Adverse reactions to food additives. Curr Allergy Asthma Rep 2003; 3: 62–66.

12. Sampson HA, Sicherer SH, Birnbaum AH. AGA Technical review on the evaluation of food allergy in gastrointestinal disorders. Gastroenterology 2001; 120: 1026–1040.

13. Ortolani C, Ispano M, Pastorello E, et al. The oral allergy syndrome. Ann Allergy 1988; 61: 47–52.

14. Sampson HA, Muñoz-Furlong A, Campbell RL, et al. Second symposium on the definition and management of anaphylaxis: Summary report – Second National Institute of Allergy and Infectious Disease/Food Allergy and Anaphylaxis Network symposium. J Allergy Clin Immunol 2006; 117: 391–397.

15. Sicherer SH, Sampson HA. Food hypersensitivity and atopic dermatitis: pathophysiology, epidemiology, diagnosis, and management. J Allergy Clin Immunol 1999; 104: S114–S122.

16. Liacouras CA, Spergel JM, Ruchelli E, et al. Eosinophilic esophagitis: a 10-year experience in 381 children. Clin Gastroenterol Hepatol 2005; 3: 1198–1206.

17. Mowat AM. Anatomical basis of tolerance and immunity to intestinal antigens. Nature Rev Immunol 2003; 3: 331–341.

18. Abernathy-Carver K, Sampson H, Picker L, Leung D. Milk-induced eczema is associated with the expansion of T cells expressing cutaneous lymphocyte antigen. J Clin Invest 1995; 95: 913–918.

19. Breiteneder H, Mills EN. Molecular properties of food allergens. J Allergy Clin Immunol 2005; 115: 14–23.

20. Sicherer SH. Clinical implications of cross-reactive food allergens. J Allergy Clin Immunol 2001; 108: 881–890.

21. Sporik R, Hill DJ, Hosking CS. Specificity of allergen skin testing in predicting positive open food challenges to milk, egg and peanut in children. Clin Exp Allergy 2000; 30: 1541–1546.

22. Sampson HA. Utility of food-specific IgE concentrations in predicting symptomatic food allergy. J Allergy Clin Immunol 2001; 107: 891–896.

23. Nowak-Wegrzyn A, Sampson HA. Food allergy therapy. Immunol Allergy Clin North Am 2004; 24: 705–725.

24. Wood RA. The natural history of food allergy. Pediatr 2003; 111: 1631–1637.

25. Muraro A, Dreborg S, Halken S, et al. Dietary prevention of allergic diseases in infants and small children. Part III: Critical review of published peer-reviewed observational and interventional studies and final recommendations. Pediatr Allergy Immunol 2004; 15: 291–307.

REFERENCES

Eosinophil-associated gastrointestinal disorders (EGID)

Li Zuo, Marc E. Rothenberg

46

Accumulation of eosinophils in the gastrointestinal tract is a common feature of numerous gastrointestinal disorders, including classic IgE-mediated food allergy, eosinophilic gastroenteritis, allergic colitis, eosinophilic esophagitis (EE),[1, 2] inflammatory bowel disease (IBD), and gastroesophageal reflux disease (GERD).[3, 4] In IBD, eosinophils are only a small percentage of the infiltrating leukocytes, but their level has been proposed to be a negative prognostic indicator. In primary eosinophilic gastrointestinal disorders (EGID), which include EE, eosinophilic gastritis, eosinophilic enteritis, eosinophilic colitis and eosinophilic gastroenteritis, the gastrointestinal tract is affected by eosinophil-rich inflammation in the absence of known causes for eosinophilia (e.g., drug reactions, parasitic infections, malignancy, etc). Patients with EGID suffer various symptoms, including failure to thrive, abdominal pain, irritability, gastric dysmotility, vomiting, diarrhea, and dysphagia. EGID appear to arise from the interplay of genetic and environmental factors. Notably, ~10% of patients suffering from EGID have an immediate family member with EGID. Several lines of evidence support an allergic etiology: ~75% of patients with EGID are atopic; some patients improve on allergen-free diets; and mast cell degranulation is seen in tissue specimens. Animal models of EGID also support a potential allergic etiology.[2] Interestingly, despite the common finding of food-specific IgE in EGID patients, food-induced anaphylactic responses occur in only a minority of patients. Thus, EGID fall between pure IgE-mediated food allergy and cellular-mediated hypersensitivity disorders (such as celiac disease) (Fig. 46.1).

Although the incidence of primary EGID has not been rigorously calculated, a mini-epidemic of these diseases (especially EE) has been noted over the last decade.[1] For example, EE has been reported in Australia,[5] Brazil,[6] England, Italy, Japan,[7] Spain, and Switzerland.[8] In a specialty clinic ~10% of pediatric patients with GERD-like symptoms who were unresponsive to acid blockade had EE.[9] Others have reported that 6% of children with esophagitis have EE.[1] Prevalence estimates vary from 1:70 000 adults in Australia to 1:2000 children in Cincinnati, USA. Collectively, these data indicate that EGID are not uncommon, and may be even more prevalent than pediatric IBD.

EGID typically occur independent of peripheral blood eosinophilia (>50% of the time), indicating the potential significance of gastrointestinal-specific mechanisms for regulating eosinophil levels. However, some patients with EGID (typically those with eosinophilic gastritis) have substantial peripheral blood eosinophilia and meet the diagnostic criteria for the idiopathic hypereosinophilic syndrome (HES). HES is defined by sustained peripheral blood eosinophilia (>1500 cells/mm²) and end-organ involvement, in the absence of known causes for eosinophilia.[10, 11] Notably, whereas HES commonly involves the gastrointestinal tract, the other organs typically affected in HES (heart and skin) are rarely involved in EGID. Some patients with HES have a microdeletion on chromosome 4 that generates an activated tyrosine kinase susceptible to imatinib mesylate therapy; the possible occurrence of this and other genetic events in EGID patients, especially those with significant peripheral eosinophilia, is currently being investigated.

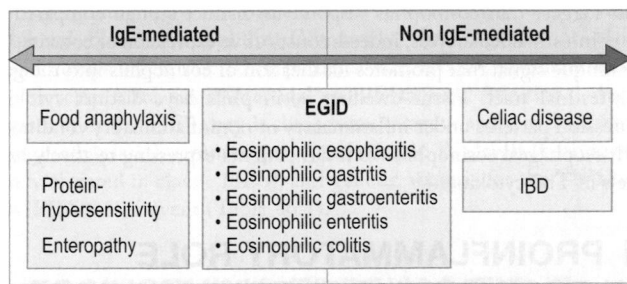

Fig. 46.1 The spectrum of gastrointestinal inflammatory disorders involving eosinophils. Gastrointestinal eosinophils accumulate in a variety of disorders with variable dependence upon IgE, ranging from predominant IgE dependence (food anaphylaxis) to nonIgE dependence (celiac disease). Primary eosinophilic gastrointestinal disorders (EGID) are in the middle of the spectrum and have some overlap with pure protein hypersensitivity disorders and inflammatory bowel disease (IBD). (Adapted From Rothenberg ME, Mishra A, Brandt EB, Hogan SP. Gastrointestinal eosinophils in health and disease. Adv Immunol 2001; 78: 291–328, with permission from American Academy of Allergy, Asthma and Immunology.)

CLINICAL PEARLS

EOSINOPHILIC ESOPHAGITIS (EE)

>> The majority of EE patients have evidence of food and aeroallergen hypersensitivity as defined by skin-prick and/or RAST testing.

>> The esophagus is normally devoid of eosinophils, so the finding of esophageal eosinophils denotes pathology. By endoscopic biopsy, up to 7 eosinophils/hpf (400×) is most indicative of GERD; 7 to 20–24 eosinophils/hpf probably represents a combination of GERD and EE; and more than 20–24 eosinophils/hpf is characteristic of EE.

>> The presence of GERD does not exclude the diagnosis of EE or food allergy, demonstrating the importance of a food allergy evaluation in these patients.

>> A trial of specific food antigen and aeroallergen avoidance is often indicated for patients with atopic EE, and if unsatisfactory or practically difficult (when patients are sensitized to many allergens), a diet consisting of an elemental formula is advocated.

>> Systemic steroids are used for acute exacerbations, while topical are used to provide long-term control. When using topical steroids we recommend the use of a metered-dose inhaler without a spacer. The patient is instructed to swallow the dose to promote deposition on the esophageal mucosa.

>> Even if GERD is not present, neutralization of gastric acidity (with proton pump inhibitors) may improve symptoms and the degree of esophageal pathology.

ETIOLOGY OF EE

The etiology of EE is poorly understood, but food allergy has been implicated. Most EE patients have evidence of specific IgE to foods and aeroallergens, but only a minority have experienced food anaphylaxis.[1] Esophageal eosinophilia may be linked to pulmonary inflammation, as repeated delivery of allergens or IL-13 to the lungs of mice induces experimental EE. In humans, patients with seasonal allergic rhinitis have increased esophageal eosinophil accumulation,[15] and patients with EE commonly report seasonal variations in symptoms. In addition to eosinophils, T cells and mast cells are elevated in esophageal mucosal biopsies, suggesting a chronic Th2-associated inflammation.[16] Consistent with this, over-expression of IL-5 induces EE, and neutralization of IL-5 completely blocks allergen- or IL-13-induced EE in mice.[17]

In a recent genome-wide microarray profile analysis of esophageal tissue[18] from patients with either EE or chronic esophagitis (typical of GERD) and normal controls, an EE genetic signature was found with dysregulated expression of ~1% of the entire human genome. Interestingly, eotaxin-3 was the most over-expressed gene in EE patients, and levels correlated with disease severity. Furthermore, a single nucleotide polymorphism (SNP) in eotaxin-3 was over-represented in EE patients. Conversely, mice lacking the eotaxin receptor (CCR3) were protected from developing experimental EE. Notably, eotaxin-3 is induced by IL-13. Taken together, these results strongly implicate eotaxin-3 in the

Table 46.2 Classification of eosinophil-associated gastrointestinal disorders (Adapted from Rothenberg ME. J Allergy Clin Immunol 2004; 113: 11–28, with permission from Elsevier).

Eosinophil-associated esophagitis
- Primary
  - Atopic
  - Nonatopic
  - Familial
- Secondary
  - Eosinophilic disorders
    - Eosinophilic gastroenteritis
    - Hypereosinophilic syndrome
  - Noneosinophilic disorders
    - Iatrogenic
    - Infection
    - Gastroesophageal reflux disease
    - Esophageal leiomyomatosis
    - Connective tissue disease (scleroderma)

Eosinophil-associated gastroenteritis
- Primary (mucosal, muscularis, and serosal forms)
  - Atopic
  - Nonatopic
  - Familial
- Secondary
  - Eosinophilic disorders
    - Hypereosinophilic syndrome
  - Noneosinophilic disorders
    - Celiac disease
    - Connective tissue disease (scleroderma)
    - Iatrogenic
    - Infection
    - Inflammatory bowel disease
    - Vasculitis (Churg–Strauss syndrome)

Eosinophil-associated colitis
- Primary eosinophilic colitis (also allergic colitis of infancy)
  - Atopic
  - Nonatopic
- Secondary
  - Eosinophilic disorders
    - Eosinophilic gastroenteritis
    - Hypereosinophilic syndrome
  - Noneosinophilic disorders
    - Celiac disease
    - Connective tissue disease (scleroderma)
    - Iatrogenic
    - Infection
    - Inflammatory bowel disease
    - Vasculitis (Churg–Strauss syndrome)

Table 46.3 Comparison of EE and GERD (Adapted from Rothenberg ME, Mishra A, Brandt EB, Hogan SP. Gastrointestinal eosinophils in health and disease. Adv Immunol 2001; 78: 291–328, with permission from Elsevier)

Characteristic features	EE	GERD
Clinical		
Prevalence of atopy	Very high	Normal
Prevalence of food sensitization	Very high	Normal
Gender preference	Male	None
Abdominal pain and vomiting	Common	Common
Food impaction	Common	Uncommon
Investigative findings		
pH probe	Normal	Abnormal
Endoscopic furrowing	Very common	Occasional
Histopathology/ pathogenesis		
Involvement of proximal esophagus	Yes	No
Involvement of distal esophagus	Yes	Yes
Epithelial hyperplasia	Severely increased	Increased
Eosinophil levels in mucosa	>24/hpf	0–7/hpf
Elevated eotaxin-3 level	Yes	No
Treatment		
H$_2$-blockers	Not helpful	Helpful
Proton pump inhibitors	Sometimes helpful	Helpful
Glucocorticoids	Helpful	Not helpful
Specific food antigen elimination	Sometimes helpful	Not helpful
Elemental diet	Helpful	Not helpful

pathoetiology of EE. Further work is needed to understand the molecular basis of the specific dysregulation of eotaxin-3 (and not other eotaxin chemokines).

CLINICAL AND DIAGNOSTIC STUDIES FOR EE

Patients with primary EE may report vomiting, epigastric or chest pain, dysphagia, and respiratory obstructive problems.[19] In a recent study of 26 adult patients, all had dysphagia and 11 had food impaction; 19 of those 26 patients responded well to EE treatment.[20] Patients are predominantly male[19] and have relatively intense esophageal eosinophilia,[2] extensive epithelial hyperplasia, and are frequently atopic compared to GERD patients (Table 46.3). The number and location of eosinophils is helpful when trying to differentiate EE from GERD. Up to 7 eosinophils/hpf (high-power field; 400×) is more indicative of GERD; 7 to 20–24 eosinophils/hpf probably represents a continuum of GERD and EE; >20–24 eosinophils/hpf suggests EE.[2] The presence of eosinophils in the proximal and distal esophagus

denotes EE, whereas eosinophil accumulation mainly in the distal esophagus suggests GERD.[1] In EE the esophageal mucosa is thickened, with basal layer hyperplasia and papillary lengthening. EE is associated with esophageal dysmotility; the etiology of the motor disturbances is unclear, but may be due to eosinophil activation and degranulation. Esophageal ultrasound shows dysfunctional muscularis mucosa in EE patients,[21] and radiographic and endoscopic studies have shown strictures, mucosal rings, furrowing, ulcerations, whitish papules and polyps.[22] Clinical assessment of EE includes analysis of food and aeroallergen sensitization and exclusion of GERD as well as other causes of eosinophils in the esophagus. Evaluation of food protein sensitization by delayed skin patch testing may increase the rate of identification of food allergy and lead to improved effectiveness of allergen avoidance.[23] Notably, the presence of GERD does not exclude the diagnosis of EE or food allergy.

TREATMENT FOR EE

A trial of specific food antigen and aeroallergen avoidance is often indicated for patients with atopic EE, and if unsatisfactory or practically difficult (when patients are sensitized to many allergens), a diet consisting of an elemental (amino acid-based) formula is advocated. Interestingly, it has been shown that an elemental diet frequently improves symptoms and reduces the number of eosinophils in the esophageal biopsies of patients with primary EE (allergic or nonallergic subtypes). Patients on elemental diets frequently require placement of a gastrostomy tube in order to achieve adequate caloric intake. Glucocorticoids have also proved effective. Systemic steroids are used for acute exacerbations, and topical steroids provide long-term control.[24] When using topical steroids we recommend metered-dose inhalers without spacers. The patient is instructed to swallow the dose to promote deposition on the esophageal mucosa. Topical fluticasone lowers the level of eosinophils, CD3+ cells, and CD8 cells in the proximal and distal esophagus,[25] and improves symptoms.[20] Side effects of inhaled glucocorticoids (e.g., adrenal suppression) are less likely with swallowed fluticasone, as this drug undergoes extensive first-pass metabolism in the liver. However, local esophageal candidiasis may occur.[25] In patients unable to use inhalers, an oral suspension of budesonide can be used.[26] Even if GERD is not present, neutralizing gastric acidity (with proton pump inhibitors) may improve symptoms and esophageal pathology. Looking to the future, anti-IgE, anti-IL5 or anti-IL13 antibodies are being assessed in clinical trials and animal models.[27,28,29]

PROGNOSIS FOR EE

It appears that EE requires prolonged treatment. Although the natural history of EE has not been extensively followed, it is not uncommon for children with EE to have a parent with long-standing esophageal strictures. In some cases, esophageal biopsies reveal long-standing EE in these parents. Typically symptoms occur sequentially, with feeding problems, vomiting, abdominal pain, dysphagia, and food impaction occurring with increasing age.[30] Thus, it seems likely that, left untreated, chronic EE can progress to esophageal scarring and dysfunction. The risk for the development of Barrett's esophagitis is unknown, but of concern. Patients with EE are at increased risk for developing other forms of EGID; thus, routine surveillance of the entire gastrointestinal tract by endoscopy is warranted.

EOSINOPHILIC ESOPHAGITIS

EOSINOPHILIC GASTRITIS AND GASTROENTERITIS

In contrast to the esophagus, the stomach and intestine have readily detectable baseline eosinophils under healthy conditions, making diagnosis of eosinophilic gastritis, enteritis, and gastroenteritis more complex than that of EE. These diseases are characterized by selective infiltration of eosinophils in the stomach and/or small intestine, with variable involvement of the esophagus and/or large intestine. Many disorders are accompanied by eosinophil infiltration in the stomach, including parasitic and bacterial infections (including *Helicobacter pylori*), IBD, HES, myeloproliferative disorders, periarteritis, allergic vasculitis, scleroderma, drug injury, and drug hypersensitivity. Similar to EE, these disorders are classified into primary and secondary (Table 46.2). Primary eosinophilic enteritis, gastritis, and gastroenteritis have also been called idiopathic or allergic gastroenteropathy. Primary eosinophilic gastroenteritis is subcategorized based on the level of histological involvement into mucosal, muscularis and serosal forms. Of note, endoscopic biopsy can be normal in patients with the muscularis and/or serosal subtypes.

ETIOLOGY OF EOSINOPHILIC GASTRITIS AND GASTROENTERITIS

Although these diseases are idiopathic, an allergic mechanism has been suggested in some patients, whereas elevated total IgE and food-specific IgE is detectable in most patients. On the other hand, no specific IgE is found in syndromes with focal erosive gastritis, enteritis, and occasionally esophagitis with prominent eosinophilia, such as the dietary (food) protein-induced enterocolitis and dietary protein enteropathy. Although most patients have positive skin tests to a variety of food antigens, they do not have typical anaphylactic reactions, suggesting a delayed form of food hypersensitivity syndrome. Indeed, eosinophilic gastroenteritis (involving the esophagus, stomach, and intestine) can be induced by feeding enteric-coated allergen beads to sensitized mice,[31] who go on to develop eosinophil-associated gastrointestinal dysfunction, including gastromegaly, delayed food transit, and weight loss.[32] Ultrastructural analysis of intestinal tissue suggested that the eosinophils were mediating axonal necrosis, as observed in patients with intestinal eosinophilia associated with IBD. Notably, mast cells are also increased in EGID and may play a critical role in the pathogenesis of allergic diarrhea.[33] In clinical studies, increased secretion of IL-4 and IL-5 by peripheral blood T cells has been reported in patients with eosinophilic gastroenteritis. Furthermore, T cells derived from the lamina propria of the duodenum of patients with EGID preferentially secrete Th2 cytokines (especially IL-13) when stimulated with milk proteins. IgA deficiency has also been associated with eosinophilic gastroenteritis and could be related to the increased rate of atopy in these patients or to occult gastrointestinal infection.

CLINICAL AND DIAGNOSTIC STUDIES FOR EOSINOPHILIC GASTRITIS AND GASTROENTERITIS

In general, these disorders present with a constellation of symptoms related to the degree and area of the gastrointestinal tract affected. The mucosal form of eosinophilic gastroenteritis (the most common variant) is characterized by vomiting, abdominal pain (which may mimic acute appendicitis), diarrhea, blood loss in stools, iron-deficiency anemia, malabsorption, protein-losing enteropathy and failure to thrive. In the muscularis form, thickening of the bowel wall may result in gastrointestinal obstructive symptoms mimicking pyloric stenosis or other causes of gastric outlet obstruction. The serosal form is characterized by exudative ascites.

There are no standards for the diagnosis of eosinophilic gastritis or gastroenteritis, but the presence of elevated eosinophils in biopsy specimens from the gastrointestinal tract wall, infiltration of eosinophils within intestinal crypts and gastric glands, lack of involvement of other organs, and exclusion of other causes of eosinophilia support a diagnosis of eosinophilic gastroenteritis. Patients with eosinophilic gastritis may have micronodules (and/or polyposis) at endoscopy, and these lesions often contain aggregates of lymphocytes and eosinophils. Food allergy and peripheral eosinophilia may be present but are not required for diagnosis.

TREATMENT OF EOSINOPHILIC GASTRITIS AND GASTROENTERITIS

Eliminating foods implicated by skin-prick or RAST testing has variable results, but complete resolution is generally achieved with amino acid-based elemental diets. Once remission has been achieved by dietary modification, specific food groups are slowly reintroduced (at ~3-week intervals for each food group) and endoscopy is performed every 3 months to identify sustained remission or disease flares. Drugs such as cromoglycate, montelukast, ketotifen, suplatast tosilate, mycophenolate mofetil (an inosine monophosphate dehydrogenase inhibitor), and 'alternative Chinese medicines' have been advocated but are not generally successful, although successful long-term remission of eosinophilic gastroenteritis has been reported following montelukast treatment. Other management includes systemic and topical steroids, noncorticosteroid therapy, management of other EGID complications (such as iron deficiency and anemia) and the management of therapeutic toxicity.[34] Anti-inflammatory drugs (systemic or topical steroids) are the main therapy where diet restriction is not feasible or has failed to improve the disease. For systemic steroid therapy, a course of 2–6 weeks of therapy with relatively low doses seems to work better than a 7-day course of burst glucocorticoids. Various topical glucocorticoid preparations are designed to deliver drugs to specific segments of the gastrointestinal tract (e.g., budesonide tablets [Entocort EC] targeted to the ileum and proximal colon). As with asthma, topical steroids have a better risk–benefit risk ratio than systemic steroids. Currently, trials are in progress with anti-IL-5 and anti-IgE.[28,29] In severe cases refractory to or dependent on glucocorticoid therapy, intravenous alimentation or immunosuppressive anti-metabolite therapy (azathioprine or 6-mercaptopurine) may help. Finally, even if GERD is not present, neutralization of gastric acidity (with proton pump inhibitors) can improve symptoms and the degree of esophageal and gastric pathology.

PROGNOSIS OF EOSINOPHILIC GASTRITIS AND GASTROENTERITIS

The natural history of eosinophilic gastritis, enteritis, and gastroenteritis is not well documented; however, they are often chronic waxing and waning disorders. Notably, the involved gastrointestinal segments often vary from time to time. In patients with clear food antigen-induced disease, abnormal levels of circulating IgE and eosinophils often serve as markers for tissue involvement. As these diseases can often be a manifestation of another primary disease process, routine surveillance of the cardiopulmonary system is recommended. When the disease presents in infancy and specific food sensitization can be identified, remission is likely by late childhood.

EOSINOPHILIC COLITIS

Eosinophils accumulate in the colon in a variety of disorders, including eosinophilic gastroenteritis, allergic colitis of infancy, infections (including pinworms and dog hookworms), drug reactions, vasculitis (e.g., Churg–Strauss syndrome), and IBD. Allergic colitis in infancy (also known as dietary protein-induced proctocolitis of infancy syndrome) is the most common cause of bloody stools in the first year of life. Similar to other EGID, these disorders are classified into primary and secondary (Table 46.2).

ETIOLOGY OF EOSINOPHILIC COLITIS

In contrast to other EGIDs, eosinophilic colitis is not usually IgE-associated. Some studies point to a T lymphocyte-mediated process, but the exact immunologic mechanisms responsible for this condition remain unclear. Allergic colitis of infancy may be an early expression of protein-induced enteropathy or protein-induced enterocolitis syndrome. Cow's milk and soy proteins are the foods most frequently implicated, but other food proteins can also provoke it. Interestingly, this condition may more commonly occur in infants who are exclusively breastfed, and can even occur in infants fed with protein hydrolysate formulas.

CLINICAL AND DIAGNOSTIC STUDIES FOR EOSINOPHILIC COLITIS

Similar to eosinophilic gastroenteritis, the symptoms of eosinophilic colitis vary depending on the degree and location of tissue involvement. Although diarrhea is a classic symptom, symptoms that can occur independent of diarrhea commonly include abdominal pain, weight loss, and anorexia. There is a bimodal age distribution, the infantile form presenting with a mean age at diagnosis of ~60 days, and the other group presenting during adolescence and early adulthood. In infants, bloody diarrhea precedes diagnosis by several weeks and anemia due to blood loss is not uncommon. Most infants affected do not have constitutional symptoms and are otherwise healthy. On endoscopic examination, patchy erythema, loss of vascularity and lymphonodular hyperplasia are seen; findings are mostly localized to the rectum, but can affect the entire colon. Histological examination often reveals preservation of mucosal architecture, with focal aggregates of eosinophils in the lamina propria, crypt epithelium and muscularis mucosa, and occasionally, multinucleated giant cells in the submucosa. There is no single gold standard diagnostic test, but peripheral blood eosinophilia or eosinophils in the stool are suggestive of eosinophilic colitis.

TREATMENT OF EOSINOPHILIC COLITIS

Treatment of eosinophilic colitis varies according to the disease subtype. For example, eosinophilic colitis of infancy is generally a benign disease. Upon withdrawal of the offending protein trigger in the diet, the gross blood in the stools usually resolves within 72 hours, but occult blood loss can persist longer. Treatment of eosinophilic colitis in older patients usually requires medical management, as IgE-associated triggers are rarely identified. Drugs such as cromoglycate, montelukast, and histamine receptor antagonists are rarely effective. Anti-inflammatory drugs, including aminosalicylates and glucocorticoids (systemic or topical steroids), are commonly used and appear to be efficacious, but careful clinical trials have not been conducted. Several forms of topical glucocorticoids are designed to deliver drugs to the distal colon and rectum, but eosinophilic colitis typically also involves the proximal colon. In severe cases, refractory or dependent upon systemic glucocorticoid therapy, intravenous alimentation or immunosuppressive antimetabolite therapy (azathioprine or 6-mercaptopurine) are alternatives.

PROGNOSIS FOR EOSINOPHILIC COLITIS

Eosinophilic colitis presenting in the first year of life has a very good prognosis, with the vast majority of patients able to tolerate the culprit food(s) by 1–3 years of age. An association between allergic colitis and the later development of IBD has been reported, but remains controversial. The prognosis for eosinophilic colitis developing in later life is more guarded. As with eosinophilic gastroenteritis the natural history has not been documented, and this disease is considered to be a chronic waxing and waning disorder. Because eosinophilic colitis can often be a manifestation of other disease processes, routine surveillance of the cardiopulmonary system and regular upper and lower gastrointestinal endoscopy are recommended.

CONCLUSION

In a variety of medical conditions, eosinophils accumulate in the gastrointestinal mucosa and cause injury. EGID are being recognized more frequently; they have strong genetic and allergic components, and share clinical and immunopathogenic features with asthma. EGID are associated with a variety of nonspecific common gastrointestinal symptoms and laboratory findings, making their diagnosis dependent on microscopic examination of gastrointestinal biopsy samples. Clinical and experimental models indicate that eosinophils have potent proinflammatory effects mediated by their cytotoxic secondary granule constituents and various lipid mediators and cytokines. In Th2-associated gastrointestinal inflammatory conditions, eosinophilia in the lamina propria is IL-5 and eotaxin dependent. Moreover, eosinophil accumulation in the esophagus can be induced experimentally by delivery to the lungs of aeroallergens or Th2 cytokine (IL-13) (Fig. 46.2). Based on these results, several new therapeutic approaches are now being developed for EGID, including humanized anti-IL-5, the tyrosine kinase inhibitor imatinib mesylate, eotaxin-3 blockers, CCR3 antagonists, and IL-4/IL-13 inhibitors. Although much progress has been made concerning gastrointestinal eosinophils and EGID, there is still a paucity of knowledge compared with other cell types and gastrointestinal diseases that may be even less common (e.g., IBD). A better understanding of the pathogenesis and treatment of EGID will emerge by combining comprehensive clinical and research approaches involving experts in the fields of allergy, gastroenterology, nutrition, and pathology.

ACKNOWLEDGEMENTS

The author would like to thank the numerous colleagues who have contributed to the body of information presented in this review, including Drs Simon Hogan, Anil Mishra, Philip Putnam, Amal Assa'ad,

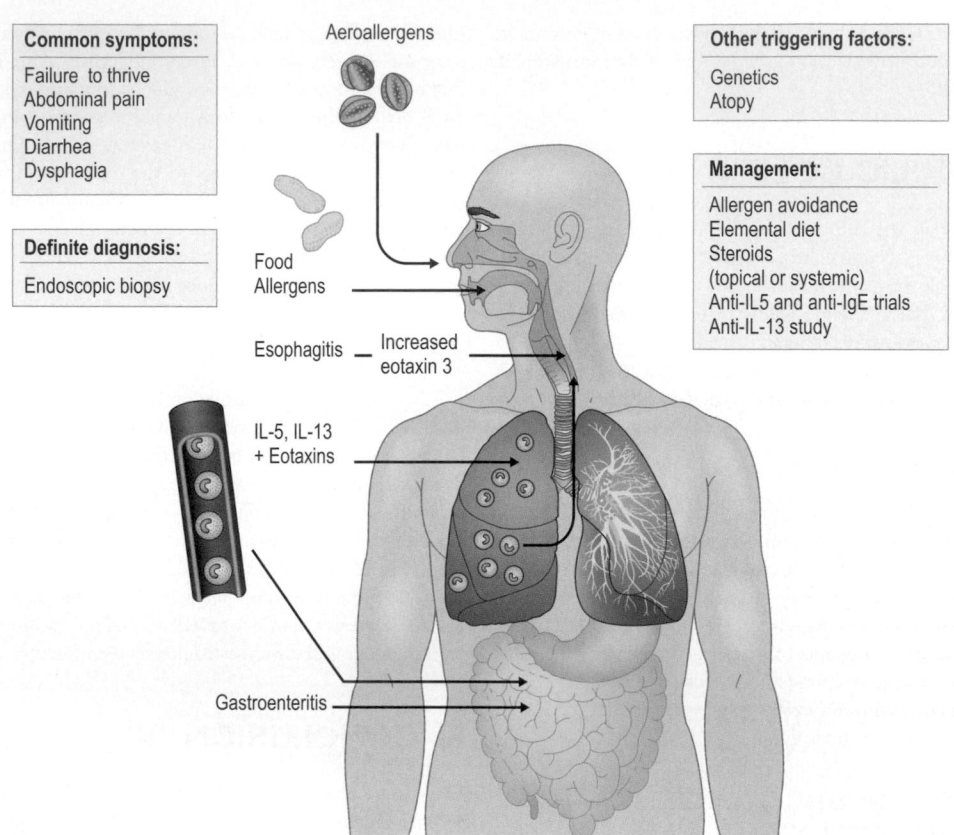

Common symptoms:

Failure to thrive
Abdominal pain
Vomiting
Diarrhea
Dysphagia

Definite diagnosis:

Endoscopic biopsy

Aeroallergens

Food
Allergens

Esophagitis — Increased
eotaxin 3

IL-5, IL-13
+ Eotaxins

Gastroenteritis

Other triggering factors:

Genetics
Atopy

Management:

Allergen avoidance
Elemental diet
Steroids
(topical or systemic)
Anti-IL5 and anti-IgE trials
Anti-IL-13 study

Fig. 46.2 Summary of pathogenesis and treatment strategies for EGID. Pathological increases in eosinophils occur in EGID, a series of disorders strongly associated with food and aeroallergen sensitization. EGID is generally a tissue-specific problem compared to HES (which has a proclivity to involve the heart, lungs, and skin); however, there can be overlap, especially when EGID is accompanied by marked blood eosinophilia. Whereas EGID may simultaneously involve multiple gastrointestinal segments (e.g., eosinophilic gastroenteritis), specific regions of the gastrointestinal tract may be selectively involved, as in eosinophilic esophagitis (EE), a disease mechanistically linked with eosinophilic airway inflammation (asthma). Recent studies have implicated an important role for the cytokines IL-5, IL-13, and eotaxins with various manifestations of EGID. Based on these collective findings, clinical intervention strategies that are currently being investigated for EGID include allergen avoidance, and therapy with anti-IL-5 and anti-IL-13 humanized antibodies, CCR3 antagonists, and imatinib mesylate. This figure also lists common symptoms of EGID, triggering factors, diagnosis and management. (Adapted from Rothenberg ME, Mishra A, Brandt EB, Hogan SP. Gastrointestinal eosinophils in health and disease. Adv Immunol 2001; 78: 291–328, with permission from American Academy of Allergy, Asthma and Immunology.)

Margaret Collins, Eric Brandt, Nives Zimmermann, Paul Foster, Carine Blanchard, Michael Konikoff, Richard Noel, Mitch Cohen, and Glenn Furuta. The authors are also grateful to Andrea Lippelman. This work was supported in part by the NIH/NIAID R01 AI42242 and AI45898, and the kind support of the CURED and Buckeye Foundations. We acknowledge that this chapter was adapted in large part from our prior publication.[35]

■ USEFUL CONTACTS ■

American Partnership for Eosinophilic Disorders: www.APFED.org.
Cincinnati Center for Eosinophilic Disorders: www.cincinnatichildrens.org/eosinophils/

■ REFERENCES ■

1. Fox VL, Nurko S, Furuta GT. Eosinophilic esophagitis: it's not just kid's stuff. Gastrointest Endosc 2002; 56: 260–270.

2. Rothenberg ME, Mishra A, Collins MH, Putnam PE. Pathogenesis and clinical features of eosinophilic esophagitis. J Allergy Clin Immunol 2001; 108: 891–894.

3. Rothenberg ME, Mishra A, Brandt EB, Hogan SP. Gastrointestinal eosinophils. Immunol Rev 2001; 179: 139–155.

4. Rothenberg ME, Mishra A, Brandt EB, Hogan SP. Gastrointestinal eosinophils in health and disease. Adv Immunol 2001; 78: 291–328.

5. Croese J, Fairley SK, Masson JW, et al. Clinical and endoscopic features of eosinophilic esophagitis in adults. Gastrointest Endosc 2003; 58: 516–522.

6. Cury EK, Schraibman V, Faintuch S. Eosinophilic infiltration of the esophagus: gastroesophageal reflux versus eosinophilic esophagitis in children – discussion on daily practice. J Pediatr Surg 2004; 39: e4–7.

7. Fujiwara H, Morita A, Kobayashi H, et al. Infiltrating eosinophils and eotaxin: their association with idiopathic eosinophilic esophagitis. Ann Allergy Asthma Immunol 2002; 89: 429–432.

8. Straumann A, Spichtin HP, Bucher KA, et al. Eosinophilic esophagitis: red on microscopy, white on endoscopy. Digestion 2004; 70: 109–116.

9. Markowitz JE, Liacouris CA. Eosinophilic esophagitis. Gastroenterol Clin North Am 2003; 32: 949–966.

10. Assa'ad AH, Spicer RL, Nelson DP, et al. Hypereosinophilic syndromes. Chem Immunol 2000; 76: 208–229.

11. Roufosse F, Cogan E, Goldman M. The hypereosinophilic syndrome revisited. Annu Rev Med 2003; 54: 169–184.

12. Straumann A, Kristl J, Conus S, et al. Cytokine expression in healthy and inflamed mucosa: probing the role of eosinophils in the digestive tract. Inflamm Bowel Dis 2005; 11: 720–726.

13. Spergel JM, Beausoleil JL, Mascarenhas M, Liacouras CA. The use of skin prick tests and patch tests to identify causative foods in eosinophilic esophagitis. J Allergy Clin Immunol 2002; 109: 363–368.

14. Ahmad M, Soetikno RM, Ahmed A. The differential diagnosis of eosinophilic esophagitis. J Clin Gastroenterol 2000; 30: 242–244.

15. Onbasi K, Sin AZ, Doganavsargil B, et al. Eosinophil infiltration of the oesophageal mucosa in patients with pollen allergy during the season. Clin Exp Allergy 2005; 35: 1423–1431.

16. Straumann A, Bauer M, Fischer B, et al. Idiopathic eosinophilic esophagitis is associated with a TH2-type allergic inflammatory response. J Allergy Clin Immunol 2001; 108: 954–961.

17. Mishra A, Rothenberg ME. Intratracheal IL-13 induces eosinophilic esophagitis by an IL-5, eotaxin-1, and STAT6-dependent mechanism. Gastroenterology 2003; 125: 1419–1427.

18. Blanchard C, Wang N, Stringer KF, et al. Eotaxin-3 and a uniquely conserved gene-expression profile in eosinophilic esophagitis. J Clin Invest 2006; 116: 536–547.

19. Orenstein SR, Shalaby TM, Di Lorenzo C, et al. The spectrum of pediatric eosinophilic esophagitis beyond infancy: a clinical series of 30 children. Am J Gastroenterol 2000; 95: 1422–1430.

20. Konikoff MR, Noel RJ, Blanchard C, et al. A randomized, double-blind, placebo-controlled trial of fluticasone propionate for pediatric eosinophilic esophagitis. Gastroenterology 2006; 131: 1381–1391.

21. Fox VL, Nurko S, Teitelbaum JE, et al. High-resolution EUS in children with eosinophilic 'allergic' esophagitis. Gastrointest Endosc 2003; 57: 30–36.

22. Fox VL. Pediatric endoscopy. Gastrointest Endosc Clin North Am 2000; 10: 175–1949

23. Spergel J, Rothenberg ME, Fogg M. Eliminating eosinophilic esophagitis. Clin Immunol 2005; 115: 131–132.

24. Liacouras CA, Spergel JM, Ruchelli E, et al. Eosinophilic Esophagitis: A 10-year experience in 381 children. Clin Gastroenterol Hepatol 2005; 3: 1198–1206.

25. Teitelbaum JE, Fox VL, Twarog FJ, et al. Eosinophilic esophagitis in children: immunopathological analysis and response to fluticasone propionate. Gastroenterology 2002; 122: 1216–1225.

26. Aceves SS, Dohil R, Newbury RO, Bastian JF. Topical viscous budesonide suspension for treatment of eosinophilic esophagitis. J Allergy Clin Immunol 2005; 116: 705–706.

27. Blanchard C, Mishra A, Saito-Akei H, et al. Inhibition of human interleukin-13-induced respiratory and oesophageal inflammation by anti-human-interleukin-13 antibody (CAT-354). Clin Exp Allergy 2005; 35: 1096–1103.

28. Stein ML, Collins MH, Villanueva JM, et al. Anti-IL-5 (mepolizumab) therapy for eosinophilic esophagitis. J Allergy Clin Immunol 2006; 118: 1312–1319.

29. Foroughi S, Foster B, Kim NY, et al. Anti-IgE treatment of eosinophil-associated gastrointestinal disorders. J Allergy Clin Immunol 2007; 120: 594–601.

30. Noel RJ, Putnam PE, Rothenberg ME. Eosinophilic esophagitis. N Engl J Med 2004; 351: 940–941.

31. Hogan S, Mishra E, Brandt E, et al. A critical role for eotaxin in experimental oral antigen-indcued eosinophilic gastrointestinal allergy. Proc Natl Acad Sci USA 2000; 97: 6681–6686.

32. Hogan SP, Mishra A, Brandt EB, et al. A pathological function for eotaxin and eosinophils in eosinophilic gastrointestinal inflammation. Nature Immunol 2001; 2: 353–360.

33. Brandt EB, Strait RT, Hershko D, et al. Mast cells are required for experimental oral allergen-induced diarrhea. J Clin Invest 2003; 112: 1666–1677.

34. Foroughi S, Prussin C. Clinical management of eosinophilic gastrointestinal disorders. Curr Allergy Asthma Rep 2005; 5: 259–261.

35. Rothenberg ME. Eosinophilic gastrointestinal disorders (EGID). J Allergy Clin Immunol 2004; 113: 11–28.

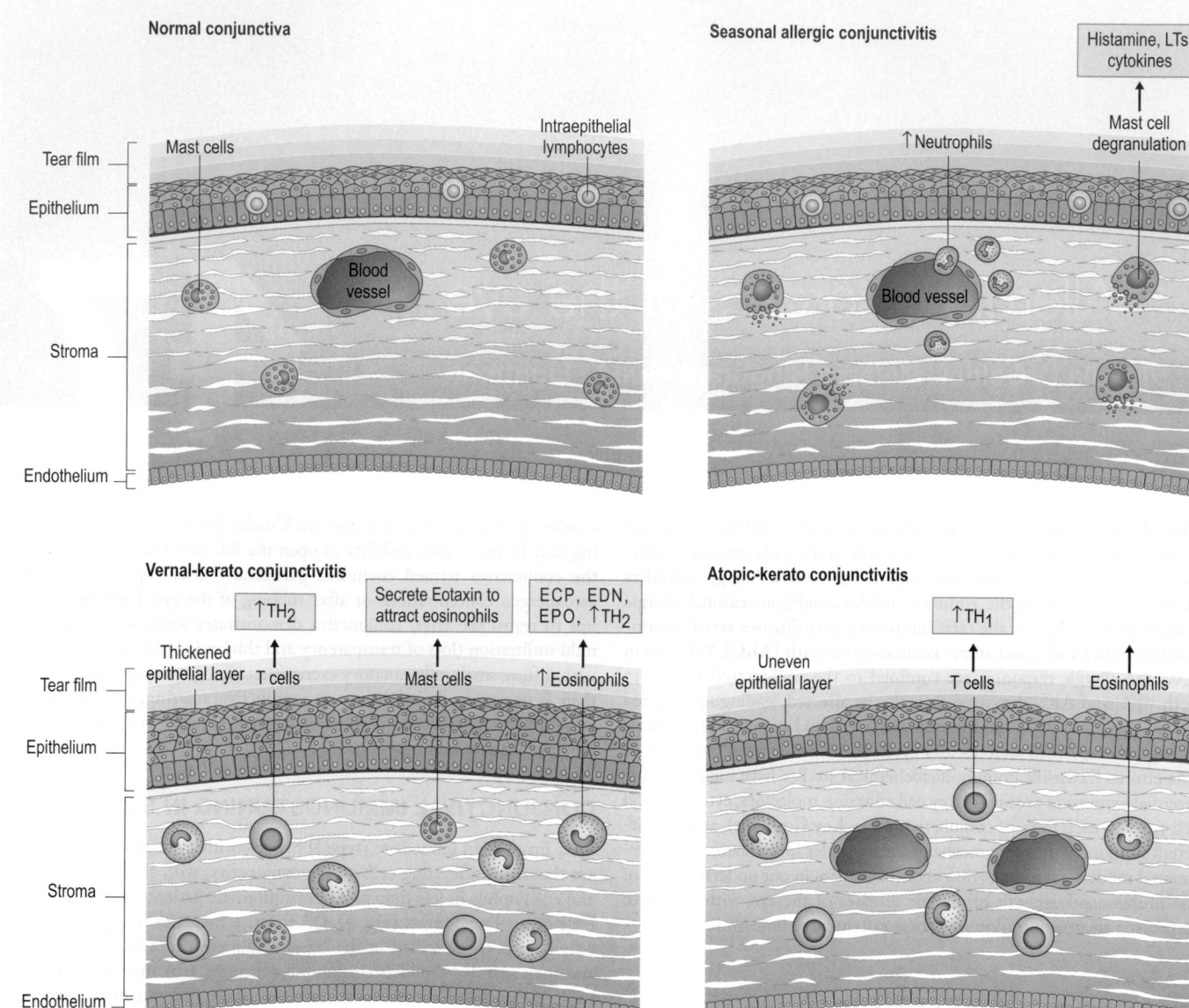

Fig. 47.1 Cross-section of conjunctival tissue biopsy, showing the cell processes involved in VKC- vs AKC-affected tissues.

count. Cold compresses and ocular lubricants (artificial tears) relieve symptoms, particularly itching.

Oral and topical H_1 antihistamines are widely used and provide rapid symptom reduction but have no preventative role and a limited potency, as they only address one arm of the inflammatory mediator response (see Clinical Pearls). Oral antihistamines also treat any concurrent rhinitis, but the onset of ocular action is slower and the local effective concentration is less than for topical therapy. Moreover, oral use exposes the patient to the risk of unwanted systemic effects. They are often used for children, where topical therapy can be difficult, and also at night when their sedative effect can be advantageous. Topical antihistamines are available in combination with a vasoconstrictor (a lower dose of antihistamine can be used as

the two components are synergistic) or as higher-potency antihistamine-only preparations (e.g., levocabastine, emedastine, azelastine). The higher-potency preparations provide a more rapid onset of symptom relief, have a more prolonged action after instillation, and avoid the worry of rebound vasodilatation and potential permanent dilatation of the conjunctival vessels associated with long-term vasoconstrictor use. Topical antihistamine drops, particularly in combination with vasoconstrictors, can cause contact allergic conjunctivitis, which may limit their use in a number of patients.

Of the several topical nonsteroidal anti-inflammatory drugs (NSAIDs) assessed in ocular allergy, ketorolac is the only one currently approved for ocular allergy. NSAIDs offer the advantage of safety, but there have been concerns that their efficacy is not well proven compared to other

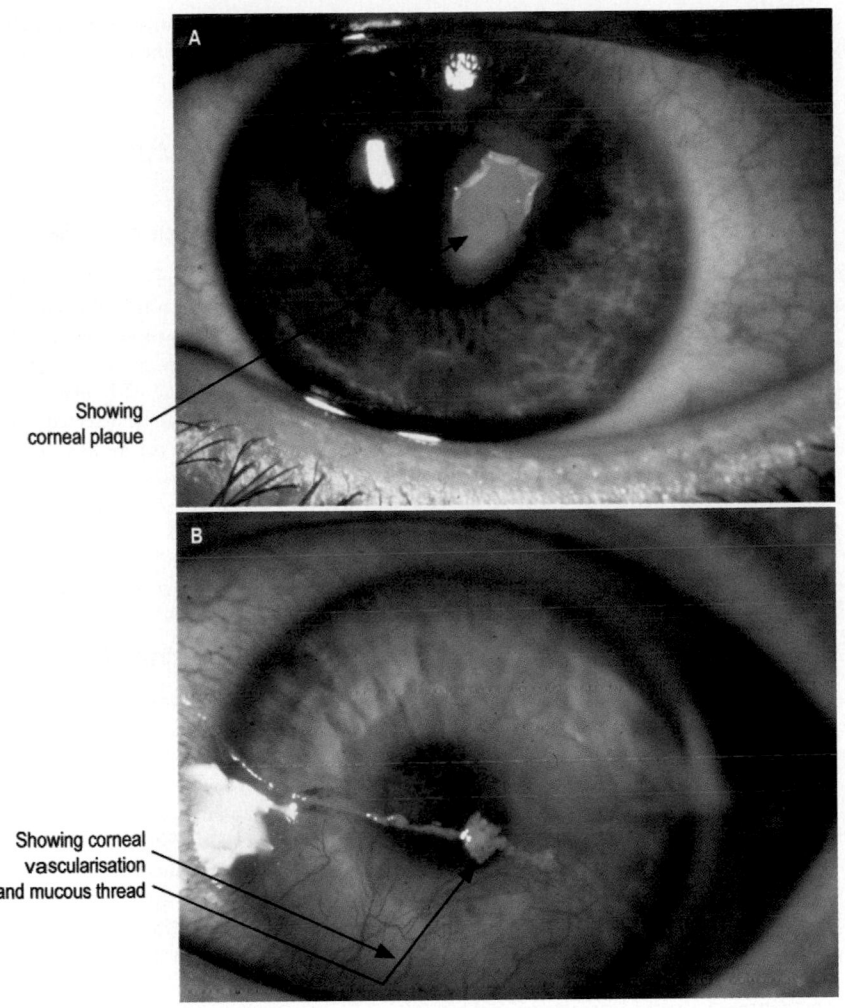

Showing
corneal plaque

Showing corneal
vascularisation
and mucous thread

Fig. 47.2   Photographs illustrating clinical features of VKC **(A)** and AKC **(B)**.

established remedies, and there are also concerns about their cost. Topical mast cell inhibitors (e.g., sodium cromoglycate) are the most useful drugs for nonsight-threatening ocular allergy. They have a number of actions that account for their ability to prevent symptoms if used early in the disease and continued throughout the allergen season, including mast cell degranulation, inhibition of leukocyte recruitment, and direct mediator antagonism. One limitation has been the slower onset of symptom relief compared to antihistamines (although this is less of an issue with the newer, high-potency preparations lodoxamide, nedocromil), and some tendency to stinging after instillation (possibly less with lodoxamide). They are almost completely safe, though very occasionally they may cause local contact allergy.

Several of the newer topical antihistamines, in particular olopatadine, epinastine and ketotifen, have additional properties, including mast cell inhibition and mediator antagonism. They offer the potential advantage of a rapid onset of action with the preventative and long-term effect of inhibiting mast cell mediator release. Olopatadine and epinastine in particular seem to offer some clinical advantage over antihistamines and

compare well with mast cell inhibitors in allergen challenge models and in clinical trials in SAC.[4]

Topical steroids have a minimal role in SAC, compared to their role in allergic rhinitis and asthma, owing to their potential for ocular adverse effects (see below). They are occasionally used in short courses for severe disease to gain control of inflammation, but their use must be supervised by an ophthalmologist.

■ PERENNIAL ALLERGIC CONJUNCTIVITIS ■

Perennial allergic conjunctivitis (PAC) is the second commonest ocular allergy.[5] It bears many similarities to SAC, but as the allergens in PAC are present for most or all of the year the disease is present all year round. PAC is most frequent and severe in children and young adults. House dust mites (*Dermatophagoides pteronyssinus*) are the commonest sensitizing allergens, but animal hair and dander, molds and other antigens may be responsible.

The symptoms comprise perennial ocular itch, discomfort, watering, redness, and some discharge. Patients may be able to correlate symptomatology with exposure to, for example, the presence of pets or a particular location. House dust mite allergy sufferers give a history of symptoms being worse in the morning. Approximately one-third have associated allergic rhinitis, and a family or personal atopic history is very common. The clinical appearance is of a mild conjunctival inflammation, and clinical signs may be very slight. The bulbar conjunctiva may be slightly red and edematous, and the tarsal conjunctiva shows mild to moderate hyperemia, infiltration and fine papillae. Lid edema is usually mild. As with SAC, there is no conjunctival scarring, corneal or serious limbal involvement, and so normal visual acuity is maintained.

IMMUNOHISTOLOGICAL STUDIES IN PAC

PAC also involves an immediate-type hypersensitivity response, but because the allergens are present continuously, unlike in SAC, the resultant inflammation is more chronic. Increased numbers of mast cells are detected in both the tarsal conjunctival epithelium and in the substantia propria, with both mucosal and connective tissue mast cell phenotypes.[2] In addition to mast cells, eosinophils, neutrophils and some T cells are present, suggesting that other cell-mediated processes are likely to be involved, although it is not yet known whether these cells contribute to the chronic inflammation in PAC. In general, little is known about the basic immunological processes occurring within the conjunctival tissues in PAC, and further research is needed.

THERAPY

In house dust mite sensitivity, advice should be provided on mite reduction. Potential manoeuvres include removal of soft furnishings in the bedroom (e.g., carpet, curtains), the use of vacuum cleaners with appropriate filters to perform intensive and regular vacuuming, including the curtains and mattress, use of mite-impermeable mattress and pillow covers, washing bedlinen and curtains at mitocidal temperatures (>55°C), and mitocidal chemicals. For patients with mold sensitivity, dehumidifying devices and mold-killing chemicals may help. For pet allergy, avoidance of the pet may be effective but is often an unpopular option.

The drug therapy of PAC is essentially as recommended for SAC (see above), but as the disease is usually prolonged, the continued use of mast cell inhibitors assumes more importance and antihistamines tend to be used episodically for flares of inflammation. Another consideration when using topical medication is the potential development of ocular

responses to the preservatives, either an allergic response, or direct damage to the ocular surface: hence preservative-free preparations should be used if at all possible.

EXPERIMENTAL MODELS OF ALLERGIC CONJUNCTIVITIS

Conjunctival allergen challenge

This model involves challenging the ocular surface to an allergen in sensitized individuals to artificially induce the ocular allergic response.[6] Symptoms are similar to those seen in SAC, and therefore the model is useful for investigating the early- and late-phase allergic responses at the ocular surface. During the early phase (20 minutes) increased levels of histamine and tryptase can be detected in tear fluid, suggesting the effector cell population to be predominantly mast cells. At 6 hours (i.e., the late phase) histamine and eosinophil cationic protein levels are elevated, but not tryptase levels, suggesting that basophils and eosinophils are recruited and contribute to the late-phase response.[7] T cells are also increased, but only in bulbar biopsy specimens. The allergen challenge model is often used to test the efficacy of eye drops.

Experimental murine allergic conjunctivitis

A model of allergic conjunctivitis has been established[8] in genetically susceptible mice, using an initial footpad sensitization with short ragweed pollen, followed 7–10 days later by conjunctival allergen challenge. An infiltration of mast cells, neutrophils and eosinophils occurs, as well as increased conjunctival chemosis and lid edema. Interestingly, although there is no significant infiltration of T cells, the model is IFN-γ dependent, as it could be inhibited by anti-IFN-γ antibody and could not be induced in IFN-γ-knockout mice.[9] Furthermore, in IL-12-deficient mice there was significantly less conjunctival inflammation, supporting a role for Th1 cytokines in this model.[8]

■ VERNAL KERATOCONJUNCTIVITIS ■

Vernal keratoconjunctivitis (VKC) is a serious ocular allergy of childhood. It constitutes 0.1–0.5% of ocular disease in the developed world but is more common and much more severe in hot dry countries, especially the Middle East, West Africa and the Mediterranean. In the UK, VKC is an unusual, self-limiting, often seasonal ocular allergy that affects children and young adults; there is a male preponderance (85%) and most sufferers have a personal or family history of atopy.

▌ KEY CONCEPTS

PREDOMINATING CELL TYPES IN THE CONJUNCTIVAL TISSUES

>> In seasonal allergic conjunctivitis, perennial allergic conjunctivitis: mast cells

>> In vernal keratoconjunctivitis: eosinophils, T cells, neutrophils, mast cells

>> In atopic keratoconjunctivitis: T cells, eosinophils, neutrophils

---

▌ CLINICAL PEARLS

SEASONAL ALLERGIC CONJUNCTIVITIS

>> Seasonal response to allergen (pollen)

>> Mast-cell mediated

>> Antihistamines, mast cell inhibitors

The link with atopy and seasonality is less clearly defined in less temperate climates.

The symptoms are worse in the spring and summer, but in severe disease can last all year. Patients complain of marked itching, discomfort or pain, photophobia, stringy discharge, blurred vision, and difficulty opening the eyes in the morning. The ocular signs may be very asymmetrical. Conjunctival signs are maximal in the superior tarsal conjunctiva and limbus, and the heavily inflamed lid may droop (ptosis). The conjunctival surfaces are hyperemic, edematous and infiltrated, and a stringy mucoid discharge is present. The tarsal conjunctiva is densely infiltrated, with papillae that are often giant (>1 mm in diameter, also known as cobblestone papillae). The limbus may show discrete swellings or, less often, diffuse hyperemia and infiltration; the presence of small white chalky deposits (Trantas' dots) is typical of vernal limbitis. In the later stages fine reticular white scarring may be seen, but this does not lead to significant shrinkage and distortion of the ocular surface, in contrast with some other cicatrizing conjunctival diseases (e.g., AKC, see below).

Visual acuity can be affected by involvement of the cornea (keratopathy), which is most marked in the upper third of the cornea owing to greater exposure to toxic inflammatory mediators, not mechanical rubbing by the papillae. At its mildest there is a punctate disturbance of the epithelium, which may coalesce to form a discrete epithelial defect (macroerosion). Deposition of mucus, fibrin and inflammatory debris can then result in the formation of a shallow oval plaque (or shield) ulcer, which repels the hydrophilic tears and the epithelial healing response (Fig. 47.2). Herpetic and bacterial corneal infection may ensue. In the later stages, scarring of the cornea may lead to a permanent reduction in vision. Steroid treatment-related complications and sensory-deprivation amblyopia (because of the young age group) also contribute to the potential for long-term visual loss (see Clinical Pearls).

IMMUNOLOGICAL STUDIES IN VKC

Several studies have identified cells of both innate and adaptive immune responses that are activated during VKC. T lymphocytes and eosinophils predominate, with mast cells, neutrophils and other activated cell types infiltrating the conjunctival epithelium and stroma. Studies of tarsal conjunctival tissue specimens have found increased numbers of activated CD4 T cells, mainly localized to the subepithelial layer of the affected tissue, and increased HLA-DR expression compared to normal subjects.[10] Increased numbers of Langerhans' cells and activated macrophages

(CD68+) were also observed. T-cell clones,[11] derived from VKC conjunctival tissues, were functionally characterized as Th2 type, and *in situ* hybridization staining demonstrated an upregulation of mRNA for IL-3, IL-4 and IL-5 in VKC in areas of maximum T-cell infiltration, supporting a Th2-cell involvement.[12] VKC tear samples were found to have increased intracellular T-cell expression of IL-4 in 67% of specimens,[13] and increased levels of IL-4, IL-10, IFN-γ, eotaxin and TNF-α compared to controls.[14] Comparison of conjunctival biopsy specimens from VKC patients against controls showed increased expression of RANTES, eotaxin, monocyte chemotactic protein (MCP)-1 and MCP-3,[15] reflecting the range of inflammatory cells present. VKC conjunctival expression of the chemokine receptor CXCR3 was found to be specifically localized to T cells,[16] and the CXC chemokine Mig was highly expressed, suggesting an important role for this ligand in recruitment of activated T cells.[17]

MANAGEMENT OF VKC

The treatment goals of VKC are to obtain adequate symptom control and to prevent both disease and iatrogenic complications that might permanently reduce visual acuity, bearing in mind that the disease is likely to remit spontaneously before adulthood. In cases where there appears to be pollen sensitivity, advice on pollen avoidance should be given, similar to that for SAC (see above). Simple measures including cold compresses, ocular lubricants and mucolytic drops may help. Antihistamines have a very limited role in the disease, and immunotherapy is not helpful.

Mast cell inhibitors are effective in VKC and should be maintained throughout the period of active inflammation, two to four times daily depending on the severity of disease and which preparation is used. Lodoxamide and nedocromil may offer some slight extra potency in clinical control. Patients with mild disease may be able to discontinue therapy during the winter months. It is important to emphasize to patients and parents that mast cell inhibitors are safe and must be continued when using steroids, in order to minimize the dose of steroids required and hence the risk of steroid complications. The role of other agents such as olopatadine in VKC is not yet established.

Steroids are highly potent controllers of allergic inflammation and are frequently required in VKC. Unfortunately, they carry a significant risk of ocular adverse effects, specifically ocular hypertension, glaucoma, and cataract, and they worsen infective keratitis. This is a particular worry in children, where examination to detect these complications may be difficult (e.g., tonometry for intraocular pressure) and also where

---

▌CLINICAL PEARLS

VERNAL KERATOCONJUNCTIVITIS

>> A chronic conjunctival inflammation with seasonal exacerbations

>> Eosinophils and T cells infiltrate the conjunctival tissues

>> Usually affects young males

>> Cornea can be affected

>> Increased expression of Th2 cytokines, adhesion molecules, eotaxin

>> Often requires steroids and topical cyclosporine

▌CLINICAL PEARLS

ATOPIC KERATOCONJUNCTIVITIS

>> The most severe form of allergic eye disease

>> Affects adults with atopic dermatitis or asthma

>> Predominant infiltration of T cells expressing IFN-γ in severe cases

>> Cornea can be affected, often by secondary infections

>> Requires steroids and cyclosporine

iatrogenic adverse effects may have long-term visual consequences well after the disease has regressed spontaneously. To minimize the risk of adverse effects, other therapies (especially mast cell inhibitors, but also cyclosporine) should be used, and steroids can be prescribed in short, sharp, rapidly tapering doses during episodes of high disease activity or significant keratopathy. In addition, it is advisable to use surface-acting preparations with a reduced intraocular effect (e.g., fluoromethalone, rimexolone), although they are not currently available in the preservative-free formulations that may be required for high-frequency use. Systemic steroids are also sometimes utilized, but expose the patient to numerous potential adverse effects. Supratarsal injections of steroids, either long-acting (triamcinolone) or short-acting (e.g., dexamethasone) may be very effective, but these are not surface-acting agents and therefore do carry a significant risk of local side effects; moreover, unlike drops, neither the treatment effect nor any adverse effects can be suddenly terminated if problems arise.

Cyclosporine is a specific T-cell inhibitor but also has a number of other inhibitory effects (e.g., on eosinophils, mast cells) that are likely to contribute to its effectiveness in ocular allergic therapy. Topical cyclosporine 2% dissolved in oil (usually maize oil) has been used to great effect in VKC[18] and is particularly effective in treating corneal complications and as a steroid-sparing agent. It has no systemic adverse effects and none of the serious ocular complications of steroids, so that generally it may be used safely long-term. It may cause temporary lid skin and corneal surface irritation, which resolves on drug cessation. However, there are difficulties with its use. It can produce intense post-instillation stinging that can prevent eye opening for some time, and the oil base can cause symptomatic visual smearing that can persist for some hours and may be enough to limit driving. In addition, drops are not commercially available at this concentration, and must be obtained from the few hospital pharmacies that manufacture on-site in a labor- and time-intensive process. The commercially available and well-tolerated 0.05% cyclosporine emulsion marketed for dry eye has unfortunately not proved efficacious in VKC. Some units have obtained the unlicensed 0.2% veterinary ointment on a named-patient basis and claim benefit.

Surgical interventions are sometimes required in VKC for the corneal manifestations; surgical or excimer laser superficial keratectomy may be used in conjunction with medical inflammation control for plaque ulcer; rarely corneal grafting may be required for scarring. Surgical removal of giant papillae or for conjunctival reconstruction is not generally recommended.

EXPERIMENTAL MODEL OF VKC

In genetically susceptible rats and mice, immune-mediated blepharoconjunctivitis is inducible by subcutaneous immunization with short ragweed pollen followed by conjunctival allergen challenge at day 10. In this model a significant eosinophilia is found 24 hours after challenge, and this has therefore been used as a model for studying eosinophil infiltration as found in VKC. It can also be induced by adoptively transferring Th2, but not Th1, T cells, demonstrating that eosinophil infiltration is Th2 mediated.[19] Similarly, transfer of antigen-specific IgE is less potent at inducing conjunctival eosinophil infiltration than transfer of antigen-primed splenocytes.[20] Modulation of co-stimulatory molecules significantly affected conjunctival eosinophil infiltration, suggesting that this may be a possible target for treating VKC.[21]

ATOPIC KERATOCONJUNCTIVITIS

Atopic keratoconjunctivitis (AKC) is the least common but most serious of the ocular allergies. It is a highly symptomatic disorder with severe itching, pain, watering, stickiness and redness of the eyelids and eye (see Clinical Pearls).[22]

AKC is a lifelong condition that affects adults with systemic atopic disease, particularly atopic dermatitis. The usual age of onset is in the late teens; occasionally the disease can begin in childhood. In contrast to VKC, the disease is persistent and may be relentlessly progressive. There is usually facial atopic dermatitis involving the eyelids. The lid margins show severe blepharitis (chronic inflammation of the lash follicles and meibomian glands) and are thickened, hyperemic, posteriorly rounded, and sometimes keratinized. The lid anatomy may be distorted with ectropion (outwardly turning eyelid), entropion (inwardly turning eyelid), trichiasis (inturning lashes), loss of lashes and notching. The whole conjunctiva is affected and shows intense infiltration, papillae (which may be giant), and sometimes scarring with linear and reticular white scar tissue, lid-to-conjunctiva adhesions (symblepharon), and shrinkage or loss of the conjunctival sac and secondary lid distortions. Marked limbal inflammation may develop and Trantas' dots may occur. The disease may spare the cornea, in which case the alternative name atopic blepharoconjunctivitis can be used; in this form of the condition the overall inflammation is generally less severe.

The cornea may be directly involved by the inflammatory process or may be damaged secondary to the extensive changes in the usually protective ocular surface by processes such as continual mechanical trauma, reduced lid protection, or severe loss of conjunctival tear production. Significant reduction in visual acuity due to corneal involvement occurs in 40–70% of cases. Keratopathy may consist of punctate and macroscopic epithelial defects, filamentary keratitis, plaque ulcer, progressive scarring, neovascularization (with or without lipid deposition), thinning and secondary corneal infections (herpetic, bacterial and fungal). Associations are recognized between AKC and eye rubbing, keratoconus, atopic cataract and retinal detachment.

IMMUNOLOGICAL STUDIES IN AKC

In AKC the predominant cell types that infiltrate the conjunctival tissues are T cells, eosinophils and neutrophils (Fig 47.1 and Key Concepts). As in VKC, increased numbers of activated CD4 T cells, HLA-DR expression, and cells of the monocyte/macrophage lineage are found in conjunctival biopsy specimens in AKC,[10] as well as mRNA expression of IL-3, IL-4 and IL-5 in the stroma. However, unlike VKC, there is a significant increase in the expression of IL-2 mRNA, and in numbers of IFN-γ-expressing T cells, suggesting a more Th1-type inflammation in this most severe of the ocular allergic diseases.[12] The production of proinflammatory cytokines by infiltrating conjunctival T cells could provide a mechanism whereby local tissue resident cells such as conjunctival fibroblasts become involved, as collagen deposition and conjunctival tissue remodeling in chronic allergic eye disease are considerable. Thus cultured human conjunctival fibroblasts have been found to respond to exogenously added IL-4, IL-13, IFN-γ and TNF-α by producing collagen and by secreting other factors, including eotaxin-1,[23] a potent chemokine for eosinophils. In severe forms of AKC, increased tear levels of eotaxin were found to correlate with increased numbers of eosinophils in tears,[24] although the cellular source of the eotaxin was not identified.

THERAPY

The therapy of AKC is not only symptomatic, but should also attempt to modify and reduce serious sight-threatening sequelae. The topical treatment of the ocular surface is similar to that for VKC, in that some general therapy may help; antihistamines are not useful; mast cell inhibitors are continued long term; and steroid and cyclosporine drops are often required. However, the disease is generally less episodic than VKC and so long-term steroid use is often needed and steroid-related complications are more problematic. In particular, herpetic keratitis, which is more common and severe in AKC, can be potentiated by topical steroids. Facial and lid dermatitis should be actively managed, if necessary in conjunction with a dermatologist, and lid margin inflammation (blepharitis) should be treated with hot compresses followed by lid hygiene, topical antibiotic and/or steroid preparations, and systemic low-dose antibiotics (especially tetracyclines), all of which will lessen the need for anti-inflammatory and immunosuppressive therapy.

Systemic therapy can be necessary in severe cases, particularly when surgical therapy is undertaken, and includes steroids, cyclosporine and sometimes other immunosuppressive agents such as mycophenolate mofetil, but all carry a risk of serious side effects and also affect atopic disease elsewhere, so consultation with physicians dealing with these other aspects is advisable.

A significant number of patients require ocular surgery, either as a consequence of the disease or because of the associated keratoconus. Surgery for AKC includes both elective procedures and emergency interventions, and may consist of corneal gluing, patch grafts, corneal transplants (partial or full thickness), conjunctival reconstruction, amniotic membrane grafts and limbal transplantation. These are generally high-risk procedures and often require support with systemic immunosuppression.

In summary, allergic disorders of the eye range in severity and duration. Studies over the past 10 years have greatly increased our understanding of the cellular mechanisms involved. Although the therapeutic options for treating mast cell-mediated forms of allergic conjunctivitis have greatly improved, there is still a need to find alternative, safer therapies for the more severe and chronic forms.

REFERENCES

1. Anderson D.F., MacLeod J.D., Baddeley S.M., et al. Seasonal allergic conjunctivitis is accompanied by increased mast cell numbers in the absence of leucocyte infiltration. Clin Exp Allergy 1997; 27: 1060.
2. Baddeley S.M., Bacon A.S., McGill J.I., et al. Mast cell distribution and neutral protease expression in acute and chronic allergic conjunctivitis. Clin Exp Allergy 1995; 25: 41.
3. Bacon A.S., McGill J.I., Anderson D.F., et al. Adhesion molecules and relationship to leukocyte levels in allergic eye disease. Invest Ophthalmol Vis Sci 1998; 39: 322.
4. Whitcup S.M., Bradford R., Lue J., et al. Efficacy and tolerability of ophthalmic epinastine: a randomized, double- , parallel-group, active- and vehicle-controlled environmental trial in patients with seasonal allergic conjunctivitis. Clin Ther 2004; 26: 29.
5. Dart J.K., Buckley R.J., Monnickendan M., Prasad J. Perennial allergic conjunctivitis: definition, clinical characteristics and prevalence. A comparison with seasonal allergic conjunctivitis. Trans Ophthalmol Soc UK 1986; 105: 513.
6. Friedlaender M.H.. Objective measurement of allergic reactions in the eye. Curr Opin Allergy Clin Immunol 2004; 4: 447.
7. Bacon A.S., Ahluwalia P., Irani A.M., et al. Tear and conjunctival changes during the allergen-induced early- and late-phase responses. J Allergy Clin Immunol 2000; 106: 948.
8. Magone M.T., Whitcup S.M., Fukushima A., et al. The role of IL-12 in the induction of late-phase cellular infiltration in a murine model of allergic conjunctivitis. J Allergy Clin Immunol 2000; 105: 299.
9. Stern M.E., Siemasko K., Gao J., et al. Role of interferon-γ in a mouse model of allergic conjunctivitis. Invest Ophthalmol Vis Sci 2005; 46: 3239.
10. Metz D.P., Bacons A.S., Holgate S., Lightman S.L.. Phenotypic characterization of T cells infiltrating the conjunctiva in chronic allergic eye disease. J Allergy Clin Immunol 1996; 98: 686.
11. Maggi E., Biswas P., Del Prete G., et al. Accumulation of Th2-like helper T cells in the conjunctiva of patients with vernal conjunctivitis. J Immunol 1991; 146: 1169.
12. Metz D.P., Hingorani M., Calder V.L., et al. T-cell cytokines in chronic allergic eye disease. J Allergy Clin Immunol 1997; 100: 817.
13. Leonardi A., DeFranchis G., Zancanaro F., et al. Identification of local Th2 and Th0 lymphocytes in vernal conjunctivitis by cytokine flow cytometry. Invest Ophthalmol Vis Sci 1999; 40: 3036.
14. Leonardi A., Curnow S.J., Zhan H., Calder V.L.. Multiple cytokines in human tear specimens in seasonal and chronic allergic eye disease and in conjunctival fibroblast cultures. Clin Exp Allergy 2006; 36: 777.
15. Abu El-Asrar A.M., Struyf S., Al-Kharashi S.A., et al. Chemokines in the limbal form of vernal keratoconjunctivitis. Br J Ophthalmol 2000; 84: 1360.
16. Abu El-Asrar A.M., Struyf S., Al-Mosallam A.A., et al. Expression of chemokine receptors in vernal keratoconjunctivitis. Br J Ophthalmol 2001; 85: 1357.
17. Abu El-Asrar A.M., Struyf S., Al-Kharashi S.A., et al. The T-lymphocyte chemoattractant Mig is highly expressed in vernal keratoconjunctivitis. Am J Ophthalmol 2003; 136: 853.
18. Secchi A.G., Tognon M.S., Leonardi A.. Topical use of cyclosporine in the treatment of vernal keratoconjunctivitis. Am J Ophthalmol 1990; 110: 641.
19. Ozaki A., Seki Y., Fukushima A., Kubo M.. The control of allergic conjunctivitis by suppressor of cytokine (SOCS)3 and SCOS5 in a murine model. J Immunol 2005; 175: 5489.
20. Fukushima A., Ozaki A., Jian Z., et al. Dissection of antigen-specific humoral and cellular immune responses for the development of experimental immune-mediated blepharoconjunctivitis in C57BL/6 mice. Curr Eye Res 2005; 30: 241.
21. Fukushima A., Yamaguchi T., Ishida W., et al. Engagement of 4-1BB inhibits the development of experimental allergic conjunctivitis in mice. J Immunol 2005; 175: 4897.
22. Foster C.S., Calonge M.D. Atopic kerato-conjunctivitis. Ophthalmology 1990; 97: 992.
23. Leonardi A., Jose P.J., Zhan H., Calder V.L. Tear and mucus eotaxin-1 and eotaxin-2 in allergic conjunctivitis. Ophthalmology 2003; 110: 487.
24. Fukugawa K., Nakajima T., Tsubota K., et al. Presence of eotaxin in tears of patients with atopic keratoconjunctivitis with severe corneal damage. J Allergy Clin Immunol 1999; 103: 1220.

Drug hypersensitivity

Werner J. Pichler

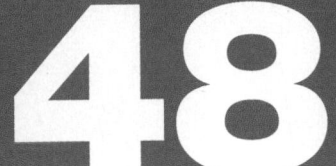

Drug-induced adverse reactions are common and may be classified into those that represent predictable side effects due to pharmacological actions of the drug and those that are not predictable, comprising idiosyncratic reactions due to some individual predisposition (e.g., an enzyme defect), and hypersensitivity reactions.[1] Drug hypersensitivity reactions account for about one sixth of all adverse drug reactions. They comprise allergic and so-called pseudoallergic reactions, the latter involving direct stimulation of immune effector cells, and thus imitating an allergic reaction, but without detectable reactions of the adaptive immune system.

Drug hypersensitivity can present in many different ways, some of which are quite severe and even fatal.[2, 3] The most common allergic reactions occur in the skin and are observed in about 2–3% of hospitalized patients.[4, 5] Any drug can elicit hypersensitivity reactions, but antibiotics and antiepileptics are the drugs most frequently responsible. The risk of sensitization and the severity of clinical symptoms depend on the state of immune activation of the individual, the dose and duration of treatment, female sex, and immunogenetic predisposition (in particular human leukocyte antigen (HLA)-B-alleles), while a pharmacogenetic predisposition has seldom been detected.

Epicutaneous application of a drug clearly increases the risk of sensitization compared to oral or parenteral treatment. Atopy – defined as the genetic predisposition to mount an immunoglobulin E (IgE) response to inhaled or ingested innocuous proteins – is not normally associated with a higher risk of drug hypersensitivity, but an atopic predisposition may prolong the detectability of drug-specific IgE in the serum.[6]

■ IMMUNE RECOGNITION OF DRUGS ■

THE HAPTEN AND PROHAPTEN CONCEPT

The recognition of small molecules like drugs by B and T cells is usually explained by the hapten concept.[1, 7] Haptens are chemically reactive small molecules (mostly < 1 kDa) that are able to undergo a stable, covalent binding to a larger protein or peptide (Chapter 6). Only by this modification of a protein or peptide does a small molecule become antigenic (Fig. 48.1). Modification can affect soluble autologous proteins (e.g., albumin), cell-bound proteins (e.g., integrins) or the peptide embedded in the major histocompatibility complex (MHC) molecule itself. Consequently, a wide array of immune responses can develop to a hapten, as many different antigens are formed, which induce different types of immune responses (Fig. 48.1A) This can lead to a great heterogeneity of clinical pictures. Indeed, drug hypersensitivity is today the great imitator of diseases, having taken over this role from syphilis, which was the great imitator a century ago.

An immune response may only arise if the hapten is also able to stimulate innate immunity. This could occur by covalent binding to cell surface structures, which might induce expression of CD40 on dendritic cells.

A typical hapten is penicillin G, which binds covalently to ε-amino groups on lysine residues within soluble or cell-bound proteins, thereby modifying them and eliciting B- and T-cell reactions. The hapten may also bind directly to the immunogenic peptide presented by the MHC-molecule. In this case no processing is required (Fig. 48.1A). Direct alteration of the MHC molecule is also possible, but evidence from mouse models suggests that this is less frequent.[8]

Many drugs are not chemically reactive but are still able to elicit immune-mediated side effects. The prohapten hypothesis tries to reconcile this phenomenon with the hapten hypothesis by stating that a chemically inert drug may become reactive upon metabolism[1, 7, 9] (Fig. 48.1B). Sulfamethoxazole is a prototype prohapten. It is not chemically reactive itself but becomes immunogenic by intracellular metabolism. Cytochrome p450-dependent metabolism leads to sulfamethoxazole-hydroxylamine, which can be found in the urine and is easily transformed to the highly reactive sulfamethoxazole-nitroso by oxidation. The latter is chemically highly reactive and binds covalently to proteins/peptides (Fig. 48.1B), forming neoantigens. The resulting clinical picture can be as variable as with haptens: sulfamethoxazole is known to cause many different diseases, affecting many organs. These side effects are mediated by antibodies and/or T cells. On the other hand,

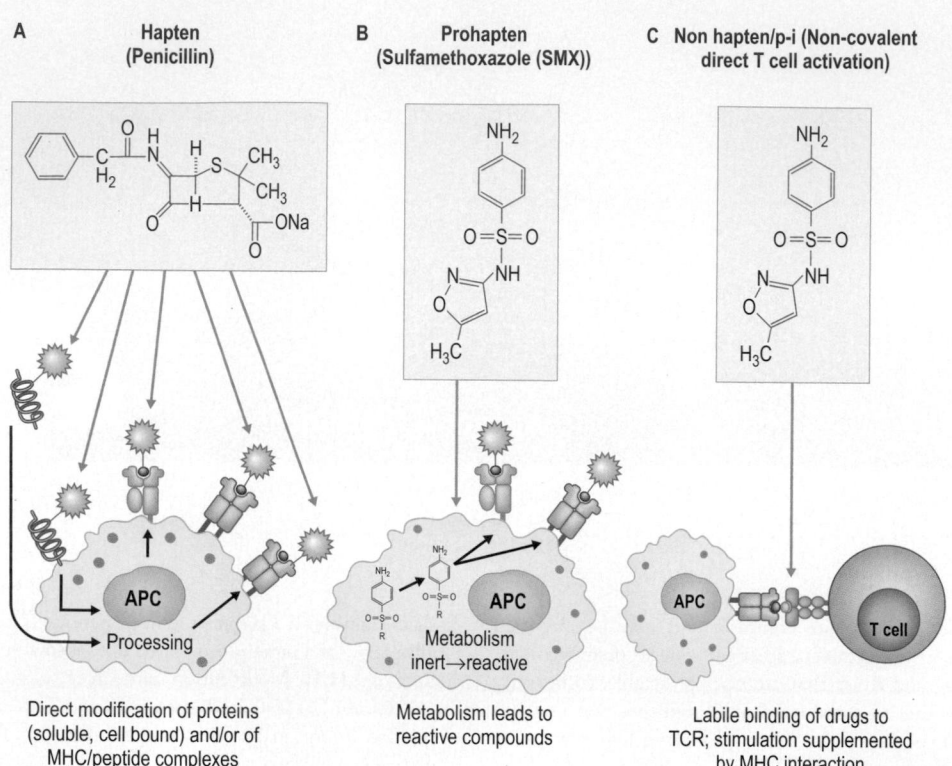

A Hapten (Penicillin) **B** Prohapten (Sulfamethoxazole (SMX)) **C** Non hapten/p-i (Non-covalent direct T cell activation)

Direct modification of proteins (soluble, cell bound) and/or of MHC/peptide complexes

Metabolism leads to reactive compounds

Labile binding of drugs to TCR; stimulation supplemented by MHC interaction

Fig. 48.1 Hapten and prohapten-concept and the noncovalent drug presentation to T cells. **(A)** Haptens: drugs are haptens if they can bind covalently to molecules, either soluble or cell-bound (e.g., penicillin G). They can even bind directly to the immunogenic major histocompatibility complex (MHC)–peptide complex on antigen-presenting cells (APC), either to the embedded peptide or to the MHC molecule itself. Thus, the chemical reactivity of haptens leads to the formation of many distinct antigenic epitopes, which can elicit both humoral and cellular immune responses. **(B)** Prohaptens: other drugs are prohaptens, requiring metabolic activation to become haptens (chemically reactive). The metabolism leads to the formation of a chemically reactive compound (e.g., from sulfamethoxazole (SMX) to the chemically reactive form SMX-NO). The resulting intake may lead to modification of cell-bound or soluble proteins by the chemically reactive metabolite, similar to a real hapten. **(C)** The p-i-concept (pharmacological interaction with immune receptors): drugs are often designed to fit into certain proteins/enzymes to block their function. Some drugs may happen also to bind into some of the available T-cell receptors. Under certain conditions (see text) this drug–T-cell receptor interaction may lead to an immune response of the T cell with a 'fitting' T-cell receptor. For a full T-cell stimulation by such an inert drug, an interaction of the T-cell receptor with the MHC molecule is required. This type of drug stimulation results in an exclusive T-cell stimulation. (Modified from Pichler WJ. Delayed drug hypersensitivity reactions. Ann Intern Med 2003; 139: 683–693, with permission from the American College of Physicians.)

transformation of a prohapten to the reactive hapten may occur exclusively in the liver or kidney and may thus cause an isolated hepatitis or interstitial nephritis.

THE P-I CONCEPT

Recently, a third possibility, namely a pharmacological interaction of drugs with immune receptors (p-i concept, Fig. 48.1C) has been elaborated.[10, 11] According to this concept, chemically inert drugs, incapable of covalently binding to peptides or proteins, can nevertheless directly activate T cells, if they happen to fit into any of the innumerable different T-cell receptors (TCRs) available. This interaction may result in selective T-cell stimulation, similar to the activation by peptide MHC. This process does not require biotransformation (to a chemically reactive compound) and thus the generation of a drug (hapten)-specific immune response to the hapten–carrier complex is not required. After drug binding to the TCR an additional MHC interaction with the TCR is required for full activation. It is assumed that the drug activates previously primed memory T cells with a certain peptide specificity and a lower threshold of reactivity than naïve T cells. This threshold might be further lowered by a massive immune stimulation of T cells such as occurs during generalized herpes or human immunodeficiency virus (HIV) infection, but also during exacerbations of autoimmune diseases. This would explain the high occurrence of drug hypersensitivity in these diseases.

The p-i concept radically changes our understanding of drug-induced hypersensitivity reactions, but may in fact explain some unusual features of drug hypersensitivity that are not explained by the hapten concept. According to the p-i concept, the symptoms are the consequence of a pharmacological reaction of immunologically competent cells, and not the result of a specific immune response. This can explain the symptoms at the first encounter with the drug, without a sensitization phase, the higher risk of drug hypersensitivity in generalized viral infections, and some peculiar *in vitro* and *in vivo* features of drug-elicited immune responses, which are reminiscent of superantigenic stimulation (Chapter 6) rather than a coordinated immune response leading to a massive over-stimulation.[11] Detailed analysis of T-cell stimulation by sulfamethoxazole, phenytoin, and carbamazepine suggests that the hapten and p-i concepts might often occur together.

■ CLASSIFICATION OF DRUG HYPERSENSITIVITY REACTIONS ■

Drug hypersensitivity reactions can cause many different diseases. To account for this heterogeneity and to explain the various clinical pictures, Gell and Coombs[43] classified drug hypersensitivity as well as other immune reactions in four categories, termed type I–IV reactions.

This classification has been revised to take into account the heterogeneity of T-cell functions[7] and the interdependence of these reactions since, for example, the maturation of B cells to IgE- or IgG-producing plasma cells depends on T-cell help. Thus, type I and type IVb reactions often occur together, as do type II or III with type IVa reactions, and the clinical picture is probably dominated by the prevalent immune reaction.

ANTIBODY-MEDIATED DRUG HYPERSENSITIVITY REACTIONS

As outlined above (Fig. 48.1), hapten-like features of a drug allow the modification of soluble and cell-bound proteins. The natural reaction of the immune system to such antigens is the development of a humoral immune response. Consequently, if a humoral immune response develops, the eliciting drug should have hapten-like features forming hapten–carrier complexes, or itself be protein-bearing "foreign" determinants (e.g., chimeric antibodies). Indeed, the majority of drugs able to elicit IgE-mediated allergies are known haptens, or contain foreign antigenic structures (Table 48.1).

TYPE I (IgE-MEDIATED) ALLERGIES

The IgE system is geared to react to small amounts of antigens. It achieves this extraordinary sensitivity by the ubiquitous presence of mast cells armed with high-affinity Fcε receptors (Fcε-RI), to which allergen/drug-specific IgE is bound. Very small amounts of a drug are apparently sufficient to interact and stimulate these receptor-bound IgE molecules, as occasionally even skin tests with drugs can elicit systemic reactions. Upon cross-linking the Fcε-RI, various mediators (histamine, tryptase, leukotrienes, prostaglandins, tumor necrosis factor-α (TNF-α)) are released, which cause the symptoms (Chapters 22 and 42).

IgE-mediated reactions to drugs are usually thought to depend on the prior development of an immune response to a hapten–carrier complex: B cells need to mature into IgE-secreting plasma cells, and T cells help in this process by interacting with B cells (i.e., CD40–CD40L interaction) and by releasing interleukin-4 (IL-4)/IL-13, which are switch factors for IgE synthesis. This sensitization phase is asymptomatic and may have occurred during a previous course of treatment. Upon renewed contact with the drug, a hapten–carrier complex is formed again, which then cross-links preformed drug-specific IgE on mast cells. The drug itself is normally too small to cross-link two adjacent IgE molecules (Fig. 48.2A).

These reactions were at one time erroneously considered to be dose-independent, as sometimes very small amounts can already cause severe reactions. But further diminishing the dose – as done in desensitization procedures – demonstrates that these reactions are *clearly dose-dependent*.

In sensitized individuals the reaction can start within seconds after parenteral administration, and minutes after oral intake (Fig. 48.2A). Anaphylactic shock can occur within 15 minutes, and asphyxia due to laryngeal edema between 15 and 60 minutes. The initial symptoms may be palmar, plantar, genital, or axillary itch, which should be seen as an alarm sign, as it often heralds a possibly severe, anaphylactic reaction, following rapidly within minutes: The skin becomes red (diffuse erythema), often first affecting the trunk, and later the whole body. In the next ~30–60 minutes an urticaria may appear, together with swelling of the periorbital, perioral, and sometimes genital areas (Fig. 48.3). Asphyxia may account for 60% of anaphylaxis-related deaths: laryngeal swelling should be suspected if the voice becomes hoarse, and the patient has difficulty speaking and swallowing due to tongue swelling. Patients may also complain of chest tightness and dyspnea – signs of acute bronchospasm. Some patients develop gastrointestinal symptoms (nausea, cramps, vomiting, and fecal incontinence). The blood pressure may collapse, either just due to a shift of volume into the extravascular space or due to cardiac arrhythmia. The full syndrome is anaphylactic shock, which is lethal in ~1% of cases. Risk factors for a severe episode are fulminant appearance, pre-existing (undertreated) asthma, and older age, as myocardial infarction or cerebral hypoxia/damage can lead to death days after the acute event. Anaphylaxis is a severe event, and survivors not infrequently have some cognitive or intellectual impairment. Table 48.1 summarizes the main drugs causing anaphylaxis.

Most IgE-mediated reactions to drugs are less severe, and often only urticaria, angioedema, or a local wheal may develop. However, *any IgE-mediated drug allergy can be potentially life threatening*, as the mild symptoms might be due to a relatively low dose, and each treatment may boost the IgE response.

PSEUDOALLERGY (NONIMMUNE-MEDIATED HYPERSENSITIVITY)

An unsolved problem are so-called *'pseudoallergic' reactions (nonimmune-mediated hypersensitivities)*, which in fact are as frequent as IgE-mediated reactions. The majority of these reactions imitate the clinical features of immediate reactions (erythema, urticaria) and are not dangerous, but some of these reactions cause anaphylaxis and can be lethal. They can appear at the first encounter with the drug and tend to arise less rapidly (often > 15 minutes) than true IgE-mediated allergies; they require higher doses, and the typical initial symptoms for anaphylaxis, namely palmar and/or plantar itch, are less common. High serum tryptase levels after some reactions underline the role of mast cell degranulation at least in some of these reactions.

'Pseudoallergic' reactions can be elicited by many drugs, but some drugs seem to elicit them more often (Table 48.1). *In vitro*, these drugs do not release mediators from basophils or mast cells. Some people seem to be more prone to react in this way, and they develop similar, mostly mild symptoms to a quite heterogeneous range of drugs, with clearly distinct chemical and pharmacological features. Neither IgE nor T-cell reactions have been demonstrated, and only very few patients have

Table 48.1 Common causes of allergic and 'pseudoallergic' drug reactions

Drugs involved in IgE-mediated allergies[a]	Drugs causing "pseudoallergic" reactions[a]
Foreign proteins (chimeric antibodies)	(Radio)contrast media
Immunoglobulin preparations (IgE anti-IgA)	Plasma expanders
β-lactam antibiotics	NSAID: acetylsalicylic acid, diclofenac, mefenamic acid, ibuprofen
Penicillin	
Cephalosporin	
Pyrazolones	Pyrazolones
Quinolones	Quinolones
Muscle relaxants	Muscle relaxants

[a]Not complete; only main groups mentioned.
IgE, immunoglobulin E; NSAID, nonsteroidal anti-inflammatory drug.

KEY CONCEPTS

THE PHARMACOLOGICAL INTERACTION OF DRUGS WITH IMMUNE RECEPTORS (P-I) CONCEPT POSTULATES DIRECT INTERACTION OF DRUGS WITH T-CELL RECEPTORS (TCR)[7,11]

>> Fixed antigen-presenting cells, unable to process antigens, can still present the drug and stimulate specific T cells

>> Many drug-specific T cells are only stimulated if the drug is constantly present. Washing the cells removes the drug, whereas covalently bound haptens are not washed away

>> Drug-reactive T-cell clones react to the drug within seconds or minutes, long before metabolism and processing can take place

>> Some T-cell reactivity to drugs can already be observed in the absence of antigen-presenting cells

>> The p-i concept has been found to be relevant for such different drugs as sulfamethoxazole, lidocaine, mepivacaine, celecoxib, lamotrigine, carbamazepine and p-phenylendiamine, causing MPE, DiHS/DRESS, AGEP, TEN, and contact dermatitis

>> AGEP, acute generalized exanthematous pustulosis; DiHS, drug-induced hypersensitivity syndrome; DRESS, drug rash with eosinophilia and systemic symptoms; MPE, maculopapular exanthem; TEN, toxic epidermal necrolysis.

constantly elevated tryptase levels as a sign of a mastocytosis. Some reactions can be suppressed by pretreatment with antihistamines.

IgG-mediated reactions (cytotoxic mechanism, type II)

Type II and type III reactions rely on the formation of complement-fixing IgG antibodies (IgG$_1$, IgG$_3$). Occasionally, IgM is involved. They are similar, as both depend on the formation of immune complexes and interaction with complement and Fcγ receptor (FcγRI, IIa and IIIa) bearing cells (on macrophages, natural killer cells, granulocytes, platelets), but the target structures and physiological consequences are different.

In type II reactions, either the antibody is directed to cell structures on the membrane (rarely) or immune complex activation occurs on the cell surface. Both events can lead to cell destruction or sequestration. Affected target cells include erythrocytes, leukocytes, platelets, and probably hematopoietic precursor cells in the bone marrow. The mechanism of type II reaction is not as clear as originally thought, since a clear hapten-specific immune reaction can often not be documented.[12, 13] One can distinguish two patterns:

1. Development of an IgG immune reaction to the hapten–carrier complex, mostly after longer duration of high-dose treatment. This is rather rare and best documented for high-dose penicillin and cephalosporin treatments. The immune reaction is due to complement-fixing antibodies (IgG$_1$, IgG$_3$, rarely IgM). Some antibody reactivity may be directed to the carrier molecule itself (i.e., autoantibodies). Onset of this autoimmune form is less abrupt, but it lasts longer (weeks instead of days) after cessation of the drug.

2. Nonspecific adherence with autoantibody induction can occur when a drug or metabolite becomes adsorbed to the erythrocyte or thrombocyte membrane, creating a new antigenic complex in combination with the cell membrane. For example, quinine-induced immune thrombocytopenia is caused by IgG and/or IgM immunoglobulins that react with selected epitopes on platelet membrane glycoproteins, usually GPIIb/IIIa (fibrinogen receptor) or GPIb/IX (von Willebrand factor receptor) only when the drug is present in its soluble form.[12] Well-documented cases are due to quinine, quinidine, or sulfonamides. The antibodies are clearly not hapten-specific, and it remains enigmatic how a soluble drug can promote binding of an otherwise innocuous antibody to a membrane glycoprotein and cause platelet destruction.

The antibody-coated cells will be sequestrated to the reticuloendothelial system in liver and spleen by Fc- or complement receptor binding. More rarely, intravascular destruction may occur by complement-mediated lysis.

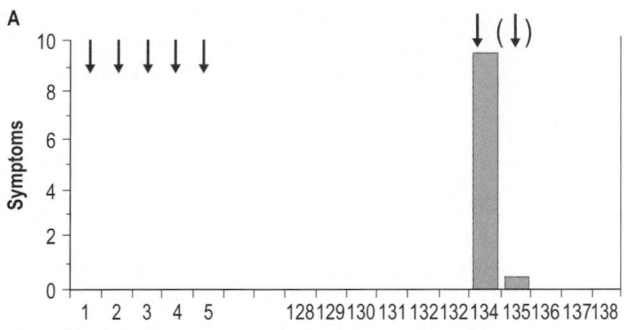

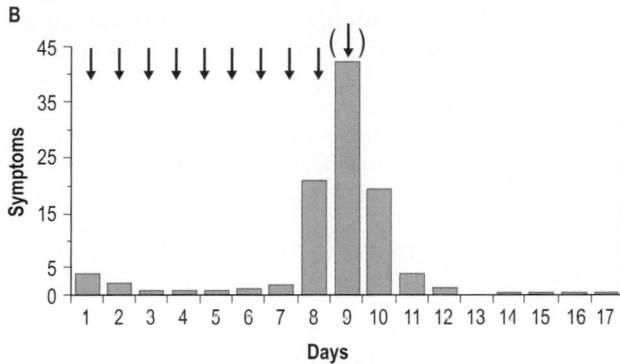

A

Possible scheme for IgE mediated, immediate reactions after a previous, silent sensitization phase

X-axis: days;
Y-axis: relative frequency of appearance

B

appearance of maculopapular exanthem in gemifloxacin treated 20–40 year old females

X-axis: Days;
Y-axis: Number of affected patients (n=270)

Fig. 48.2 Kinetic of immunoglobulin E (IgE) and T-cell-mediated reactions. (A) Schematic representation of a sensitization phase, which was symptomatic. At re-exposure at a later time point symptoms appear rapidly, mostly within 1 hour. (B) Appearance of exanthem in gemifloxacin-treated healthy volunteers. The largest study undertaken to investigate drug-induced side effects was performed with gemifloxacin, a quinolone. Initial data revealed that rashes appeared more commonly in women under 40 years of age and in those patients submitted to longer treatment (7 days). A prospective study was performed in 987 healthy women aged 18–40; 790 (80%) were treated with gemifloxacin for 10 days while the remaining 197 (20%) received ciprofloxacin for 10 days. A mostly very mild exanthem appeared in 260/790 (31.7%) gemifloxacin-treated women but only in 7/197 (4.3%) ciprofloxacin-treated women, with a clear peak on days 8–10 after treatment onset. Aminopenicillin-induced exanthems have a similar time kinetic. Data from Food and Drug Administration website: http://www.fda.gov/ohrms/dockets/ac/03/slides/3931S1_04_LFLife%20Sciences-Factive.pdf.

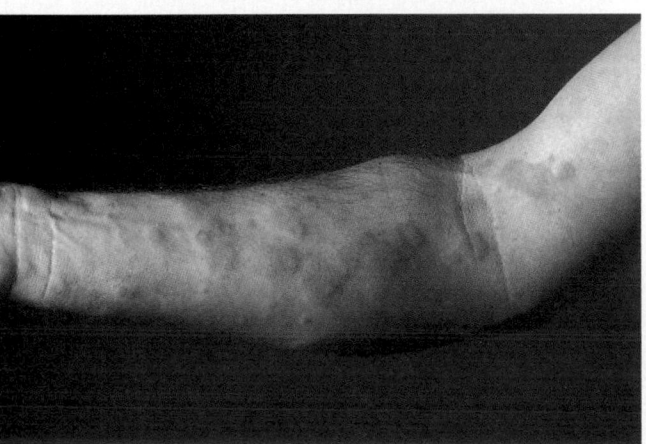

Fig. 48.3 Clinical pictures and immunohistologies of various forms of drug-induced exanthem. Urticaria with itching wheals (nonsteroidal anti-inflammatory drug intolerance reaction).

Hemolytic anemia has been attributed to penicillin and its derivatives, cephalosporins, levodopa, methyldopa, quinidine, and some anti-inflammatory drugs. Today cephalosporins are the main cause. The clinical symptoms of hemolytic anemia are insidious and may be restricted to symptoms of anemia (fatigue, paleness, shortness of breath, tachycardia) and jaundice with dark urine. Laboratory investigation may reveal reduced erythrocyte and hemoglobin levels, increased reticulocytes, and positive direct and (if the drug is present during the test) indirect Coombs tests. Unconjugated bilirubin levels are elevated and haptoglobulin is decreased. Urinary hemoglobin and hemosiderin are increased.

Thrombocytopenia is a relatively common side effect of drug treatment. Acute, sometimes severe and life-threatening thrombocytopenia is a recognized complication of treatment with quinine, quinidine, sulfonamide antibiotics, and many other medications. It can also complicate treatment with biologicals, which often contain human Fc elements themselves. Drug-induced immune thrombocytopenia usually develops after 5–8 days of exposure to the sensitizing medication or after a single exposure in a patient exposed previously to the same drug. Patients often present with widespread petechial hemorrhages in the skin and buccal mucosa, sometimes accompanied by urinary tract or gastrointestinal

> **CLINICAL PEARL**

IMMUNOGLOBULIN E (IgE)-MEDIATED DRUG ALLERGIES

>> Up to 50% of patients with IgE-induced anaphylaxis to certain drugs have no history of previous drug exposure!

>> Anaphylaxis occurs rapidly (< 20 minutes), seldom later

>> Asphyxia is probably the main cause of lethal anaphylaxis

>> Cardiac arrest can be the sole symptom of an anaphylaxis (in particular during anesthesia)

>> In certain cases desensitization procedures are possible and may allow reuse of the drug

bleeding. Intracranial hemorrhage is rare, but has been reported. After discontinuing the culprit medication, platelet counts usually return to normal within 3–5 days.

A special, intermediate form between type II and III reactions is *heparin-induced thrombocytopenia*: Platelets have low-affinity Fc-receptors (Fcγ-RIIa) that can bind immune complexes, and activate platelets.[14] Heparin is a high-molecular-weight, sulfated, linear polysaccharide that inhibits blood coagulation by activating regulatory proteins such as antithrombin III. About 50% of patients anti-coagulated with heparin for > 7 days produce antibodies that recognize complexes consisting of heparin and platelet factor 4, a CXC chemokine normally stored in platelet alpha granules. When a patient with such an antibody is given heparin, heparin–PF4 complexes are formed. These complexes react with antibodies to form immune complexes, which bind to the platelet FcIgG-RIIa receptors, leading to platelet activation, additional PF4 release and eventually, platelet destruction. Thrombocytopenia occurs in about 5% of patients given heparin and is rarely severe enough to cause bleeding. However, about 10% of affected patients experience paradoxical thrombosis that can be life-threatening.

IgG-mediated reactions (immune complex deposition, type III)

Immune complex formation is a common event during a normal immune response and does not normally cause symptoms. Immune complexes can also be formed during drug treatment, either if the drug forms a hapten–carrier complex and thus gives rise to an immune reaction or if the drug is a (partly) foreign protein that elicits an immune reaction itself (e.g., chimeric antibodies). Such immune complexes will normally be rapidly cleared, by binding to Fcγ-RI or CR1 on reticuloendothelial cells. No symptoms arise, but the efficiency of treatment decreases.

Why immune complex disease develops under certain circumstances is not clear. Very high immune complex levels, a relative deficiency of some complement components, and thus lower capacity to eliminate immune complexes or an aberrant Fcγ-R function might be responsible. Recently, a low copy number of Fcγ-RIII were found to be associated with another immune complex disease, glomerulonephritis.[15]

Type III reactions may present as small-vessel vasculitis and/or serum sickness: Serum sickness was first described with heterologous or foreign serum used for passive immunization. Antibodies are generated within

4–10 days, which react with the antigen, forming soluble circulati[ng] immune complexes. Complement (C1q)-containing immune complex[es] are deposited in the postcapillary venules and attract leukocytes by inte[r]acting with their Fcγ-RIII,[16] which then release proteolytic enzymes th[at] mediate tissue damage.

Currently, nonprotein drugs are the most common cause of seru[m] sickness. Hypersensitivity vasculitis reportedly has an incidence of 10–[3] cases per million people per year. Most reports concern cefaclor, follow[ed] by trimethoprim-sulfamethoxazole, cephalexin, amoxicillin, nonsteroi[dal] anti-inflammatory drugs (NSAIDs), and diuretics.

The main symptoms of immune complex diseases are arthralg[ia] myalgia, fever, and vasculitis. This may be localized mainly to the sk[in] as 'palpable purpura' – purplish, red spots, usually on the legs. In ch[il]dren, it is often diagnosed as Henoch–Schönlein purpura, often wi[th] arthritis. Lesions may coalesce to form plaques that occasionally ulce[r]ate. The internal organs most commonly affected are the gastrointest[i]nal tract, the kidneys, and joints. The prognosis is good when there [is] no internal involvement. Histology can reveal IgA-containing immu[ne] complexes, and the histology of kidney lesions is in fact identical to Ig[A] nephropathy.

T-CELL-MEDIATED, DELAYED DRUG HYPERSENSITIVITY REACTIONS

The original Gell and Coombs classification was established before [a] detailed analysis of T-cell subsets and functions was available. In the mean[-]time immunological research has revealed that the three antibody[-] dependent types of reactions require the involvement of helper T cell[s] Moreover, T cells can orchestrate different forms of inflammation. Therefor[e] T-cell-mediated type IV reactions have been further subclassified in[to] IVa–IVd reactions, as shown in Figure 48.4.[7] This subclassification consid[-]ers the distinct cytokine production by T cells and thus incorporates th[e] well-accepted Th1/Th2 distinction of T cells; it includes the cytotoxic activ[-]ity of both CD4 and CD8 T cells (IVc); and it emphasizes the participatio[n] of different effector cells such as monocytes (IVa), eosinophils (IVb), [or] neutrophils (IVd), which cause the inflammation and tissue damage:

Type IVa reactions correspond to Th1-type immune reactions: Th[1] type T cells activate macrophages by secreting large amounts of inter[-]feron-γ (IFN-γ), drive the production of complement-fixing antibod[y] isotypes involved in type II and III reactions (IgG$_1$, IgG$_3$), and are co[-]stimulatory for proinflammatory responses (TNF, IL-12) and CD8 T[-]cell responses. The T cells promote these reactions by secretion of IFN[-γ] and possibly other cytokines (TNF-α, IL-18). An *in vivo* correlate woul[d] be monocyte activation, e.g., in skin tests to tuberculin or even granulom[a] formation, as seen in sarcoidosis. On the other hand, these Th1 cells ar[e] known to activate CD8 cells, which might explain the common combi[-]nation of IVa and IVc reactions (e.g., in contact dermatitis).

Type IVb corresponds to the Th2-type immune response. Th2 T cell[s] secrete the cytokines IL-4, IL13, and IL-5, which promote B-cell pro[-]duction of IgE and IgG$_4$, macrophage deactivation and mast cell an[d] eosinophil responses. The high production of the Th2 cytokine IL-[5] leads to eosinophilic inflammation, which is the characteristic inflamma[-]tory cell type in many drug hypersensitivity reactions.[7] In addition, ther[e] is a link to type I reactions, as Th2 cells support IgE production by IL[-] 4/IL-13 secretion. *In vivo* correlates include eosinophil-rich maculo[-] papular exanthem (MPE), infestations with nematodes, or allergi[c] inflammation of the bronchi or nasal mucosa (asthma and rhinitis).

	Type I	Type II	Type III	Type IV a	Type IV b	Type IV c	Type IV d
Immune reactant	IgE	IgG	IgG	IFNγ, TNFα (T$_H$1 cells)	IL-5, IL-4/IL-13 (T$_H$2 cells)	Perforin/ GranzymeB (CTL)	CXCL-8. GM-CSF (T-cells)
Antigen	Soluble antigen	Cell or matrix-associated antigen	Soluble antigen	Antigen presented by cells or direct T cell stimulation	Antigen presented by cells or direct T cell stimulation	Cell-associated antigen or direct T cell stimulation	Soluble antigen presented by cells or direct T cell stimulation
Effector	Mast-cell activation	FcR$^+$ cells (phagocytes, NK cells)	FcR$^+$ cells Complement	Macrophage activation	Eosinophils	T cells	Neutrophils
Example of hypersensitivity reaction	Anaphylaxis, allergic rhinitis, asthma (with IVb)	Haemolytic anaemia, thrombocytopenia	Serum sickness, Arthus reaction	Tuberculin reaction contact dermatitis (with IVc)	Maculopapular exanthema with eosinophilia, Chronic asthma, allergic rhinitis	Contact dermatitis, maculopapular and bullous exanthem, hepatitis	AGEP Behçet disease, psoriasis

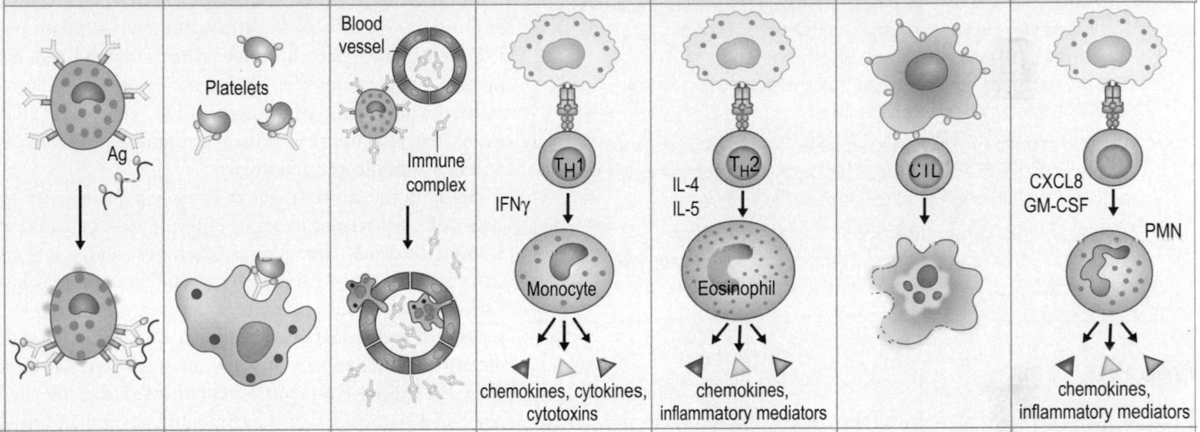

Fig. 48.4 Revised Gell and Coombs classification of drug reactions. Drugs can elicit all types of immune reactions. Although all reactions are T-cell-regulated, the effector functions are either predominantly antibody-mediated (type I–III) or rely more on T-cell/cytokine-dependent functions (type IVa–IVd). Type I reactions are IgE-mediated. Cross-linking IgE molecules on high-affinity IgE receptors (Fcε-RI) on mast cells and basophilic granulocytes leads to degranulation and release of mediators, which cause a variety of symptoms (vasodilatation, increased permeability, bronchoconstriction, itch). Type II reactions are IgG-mediated, and cause cell destruction due to complement activation or interaction with Fcγ receptor-bearing killer cells. Type III reactions are also IgG-mediated. Complement deposition and activation in small vessels and recruitment of neutrophilic granulocytes via Fcγ receptor interaction lead to a local vascular inflammation. Type IVa correspond to Th1 reactions with high IFN-γ/TNF-α secretion and involves monocyte/macrophage activation. Often, one can see also a CD8 cell recruitment (type IVc reaction). Type IVb reactions correspond to eosinophilic inflammation and to a Th2 response with high IL-4/IL-5/IL-13 secretion; they are often associated with an IgE-mediated type I reaction. Type IVc: the cytotoxic reactions rely on cytotoxic T cells (both CD4 and CD8 cells) themselves as effector cells. They seem to occur in all drug-related delayed hypersensitivity reactions. Type IVd reactions correspond to a T-cell-dependent, sterile neutrophilic inflammatory process. They are clearly distinct from the rapid influx of polymorphonuclear leukocytes in bacterial infections and seem to be related to high CXCL-8/granulocyte–macrophage colony-stimulating factor (GM-CSF) production by T cells (and tissue cells). The role of IL-17 in IVd reactions is not yet defined. (Modified from Pichler WJ. Immune mechanism of drug hypersensitivity. Immunol Allergy Clin North Am 2004; 24: 373–397, with permission from Elsevier.)

CLASSIFICATION OF DRUG HYPERSENSITIVITY REACTIONS

KEY CONCEPTS

IMMUNOLOGICAL FINDINGS IN DRUG-INDUCED EXANTHEMA

>> Drug-specific T cells are found in the blood, in affected skin, and in positive patch tests

>> Drug-specific T cells show a high frequency for many years after the reaction (1:250–1:3000 of CD4 T cells react with the drug)

>> Both drug-specific CD4 and CD8 cells can kill in a drug-dependent manner. CD4-mediated killing is perforin/granzyme B-dependent and responsible for focal, hydropic degeneration of keratinocytes in maculopapular exanthem

>> The clinical picture of the exanthem is determined by the cytokine released by the T cells infiltrating the skin. Secretion of interferon-γ → macrophage activation; secretion of interleukin-5 → eosinophil activation; secretion of CXCL-8 and granulocyte–macrophage colony-stimulating factor → neutrophil activation and recruitment

>> A high number of drug-specific CD8 T cells causes more severe, bullous skin diseases, probably because all cells are targets for CD8-mediated cytotoxicity

>> CD8-mediated severe reactions to carbamazepine, allopurinol, and abacavir show striking human leukocyte antigen (HLA)-B associations, which differ with different drugs

Type IVc

T cells can also act as effector cells: they emigrate to the tissue and can kill tissue cells like hepatocytes or keratinocytes in a perforin/granzymeB and FasL-dependent manner (Fig. 48.5).[17, 18] Such reactions occur in most drug-induced delayed hypersensitivity reactions, mostly together with other type IV reactions (monocyte, eosinophil, or polymorphonuclear leukocyte recruitment and activation). Cytotoxic T cells thus play a role in maculopapular or bullous skin diseases as well as neutrophilic inflammation, such as acute generalized exanthemtous pustulosis (AGEP), and in contact dermatitis. Type IVc reactions appear to be dominant in bullous skin reactions like Stevens–Johnson syndrome (SJS) and toxic epidermal necrolysis (TEN), where activated CD8 T cells kill keratinocytes,[7, 17, 18] but may also be dominant in drug-induced hepatitis or nephritis.

Type IVd

Another, rather neglected possibility is that T cells can coordinate sterile neutrophilic inflammation. A typical example would be AGEP. In this disease CXCL8 and granulocyte–macrophage colony-stimulating factor (GM-CSF)-producing T cells recruit neutrophilic leukocytes via CXCL8 release, and prevent their apoptosis via GM-CSF release.[19] Besides AGEP, such T-cell reactions are also found in Behçet's disease and pustular psoriasis.[20]

Tolerance mechanism

Most patients can take drugs without developing immune-mediated side effects. This could be because they lack precursor cells able to interact with the drug. But the great heterogeneity of the immune response to drugs,[7] a high precursor frequency in sensitized patients[21] and the finding that 2–4% of the normal population, but 30% to > 50% of HIV-infected patients, may react with sulfamethoxazole suggests that it is not a lack of precursor cells but other factors like the underlying immune status (preactivation of memory T cells) and "regulatory" mechanisms that may be important. Thus "regulation" may occur on different levels and may be different for drugs stimulating the immune system via hapten and the p-i concept (see above).

Maculopapular exanthem (MPE)

The most frequent manifestations of drug allergies are delayed-appearing *cutaneous reactions* – so-called 'rashes.' They comprise a broad spectrum of clinical and distinct histopathological features which appear > 6 hours to 10 days after drug intake (Fig. 48.2).

In all forms of delayed drug-induced reactions like exanthems, nephritis, and probably hepatitis, cytotoxic mechanisms seem to play an important role. The clinical picture is determined by the strength of cytotoxicity (amount of drug-specific cytotoxic T cells and tissue destruction), the generation of cytotoxic CD8 versus CD4 cells, and the type of associated effector mechanism (monocyte or activation of eosinophils and neutrophilic granulocytes).

MPE is the most frequent drug hypersensitivity reaction, affecting 2–8% of hospitalized patients, especially after treatment with β-lactams, sulfamethoxazole, quinolones, diuretics, and many more.[4, 5] In most cases it appears 8–11 days after start of treatment (Fig. 48.2), but sometimes even 1–2 days after stopping treatment (Fig. 48.6). In previously sensitized individuals it can appear on the first day of treatment. It is clearly dose-dependent. A study investigating exanthem after treatment with the quinolone gemifloxacin showed that females of childbearing age had a higher risk of exanthem, suggesting an influence of estrogens on the clinical manifestation (Fig. 48.2B) (http://www.fda.gov/ohrms/dockets/ac/03/slides/3931S1_04_LFLife%20Sciences-Factive.pdf). Most MPE, particularly if caused by β-lactams or gemifloxacin, are rather mild, and treatment with an emollient cream, and possibly topical corticosteroids, or systemic antihistamines to treat pruritus is sufficient. Some patients can continue treatment without aggravation. The exanthem often heals with desquamation within 2–10 days after stopping the incriminated drug. It is unlikely that SJS/TEN will develop from MPE, as the cells involved are different. On the other hand, some drugs may induce a mixed CD4 and CD8 cell activation (Table 48.2). In such cases prolonged treatment may lead to confluence of the papules, the patient may complain of malaise and fever, and liver function tests indicate hepatitis (more than threefold increased transaminases). Eosinophilia (> 0.5 g/l) and activated CD8 cells are found in the blood.[22] This illustrates that even "mild" drug hypersensitivity reactions are *systemic diseases*, and that cutaneous manifestations may only be the tip of the iceberg.

Immunohistology revealed drug-specific CD4. cell infiltration (CLA+, CCR6+) in perivascular areas of the dermis.[7, 22] Some T cells progress into the dermoepidermal junction zone and epidermis, where they are reactivated (MHC class II+ and CD25+) and kill keratinocytes in a contact-dependent way by releasing perforin/granzyme B. Some keratinocytes undergo hydropic degeneration, but this apoptosis is not as extensive as with CD8 T-cell-mediated killing (Fig. 48.5). In addition, the immigrating CD4 T cells exhibit a heterogeneous cytokine profile, including type 1 (IFN-γ) and type 2 (IL-4, IL-5) cytokines, suggesting

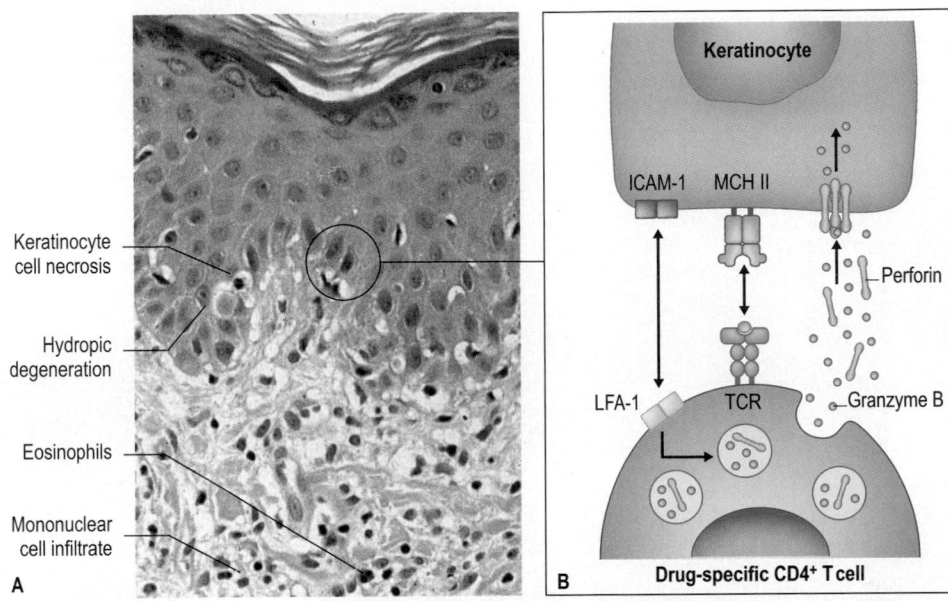

Fig. 48.5 **(A)** Typical histology of a maculopapular exanthem. Note the focal keratinocyte necrosis, often in close apposition of T cells (which have cytotoxic potential and are perforin-positive). **(B)** Schematic representation of CD4-mediated killing of activated keratinocytes, which express major histocompatibility complex (MHC) class II and ICAM1 molecules. (Modified from Pichler WJ. Delayed drug hypersensitivity reactions. Ann Intern Med 2003; 139: 683–693, with permission from the American College of Physicians.)

that both Th1 and Th2 cells infiltrate the skin. The cytokine IL-5 is also detectable in the serum. Tissue and blood eosinophilia can be found.[22–24] The recruitment of eosinophils is also enhanced by expression of the chemokines eotaxin and RANTES in MPE-lesions.

Acute generalized exanthematous pustulosis

Acute generalized exanthemtous pustulosis is a rare disease (~ 1:100 000 treatments) with an estimated incidence equal to severe bullous skin diseases (SJS and TEN combined).[19, 25] It is caused by drugs in > 90% of cases (Table 48.2). Its clinical hallmark is the rapid appearance of myriads of disseminated, *sterile* pustules in the skin (Fig. 48.7), often 3–5 days after starting treatment. Patients have fever and massive leukocytosis in the blood, sometimes with eosinophilia, but no involvement of mucous membranes. Epicutaneous patch test reactions can cause a similar pustular reaction locally (Fig. 48.7).

Immunohistology of the acute lesion reveals subcorneal or intraepidermal pustules, which are filled with neutrophilic granulocytes and surrounded by activated, HLA-DR-expressing CD4 and CD8 T cells. Keratinocytes show elevated expression of the neutrophil-attracting chemokine IL-8 (CXCL-8), and even the T cells migrating into the epidermis express CXCL-8 and GM-CSF. Analysis of sequential patch test reactions at 48–96 hours suggests that drug-specific cytotoxic T cells emigrate first, causing formation of vesicles by killing keratinocytes. Subsequently T cells and keratinocytes release CXCL8, which recruits granulocytes into the vesicles that then transform into pustules.[19] Some pustules coalesce together and can form bullae. The condition is fatal in 2–4% of cases, particularly in older people. Healing occurs within 5 days after stopping the drug. This disease and the underlying T-cell reaction

seem to be a model for sterile neutrophilic inflammations (type IVd) like pustular psoriasis and Behçet`s disease.[20]

Bullous exanthems, Stevens–Johnson syndrome, and toxic epidermal necrolysis

The most severe forms of drug-induced skin reactions involve formation of bullae. The most severe bullous skin reactions are SJS and TEN. TEN and SJS are rare (~1:1 000 000 for TEN, ~1:100 000 for SJS). They are today considered to be the milder and more severe form of the same disease (SJS < 10% skin detachment, TEN > 30% detachment). They are graded according to SCORTEN, whereby age, underlying disease and the amount of maximal skin detachment are the most important prognostic factors. According to the European study group of severe cutaneous drug reactions, SJS has a mortality of ~13%, and TEN of ~ 39%. The intermediate form with 10–30% skin detachment is called SJS/TEN overlap syndrome and has a lethality of ~ 21%.

SJS/TEN are clearly different from erythema exudativum multiforme, which is mainly caused by viral infections,[3] is often recurrent, and affects younger persons (mean age 24 years). In ~6% no drug treatment was given the week before SJS/TEN started and an infectious origin (*Mycoplasma pneumoniae, Klebsiella pneumoniae*) was suspected. It can also be due to graft-versus-host disease. Most reactions start within the first 8 weeks of treatment (mean onset of symptoms at about 17 days), with some differences according to the causing drug (e.g., it may appear later with sulfonamide antibiotics).

SJS/TEN can develop quite rapidly. Initially a macular, purple-red exanthem can often be observed, which can become painful – an ominous sign. Within 12–24 hours bullae may be seen, and the Nikolsky

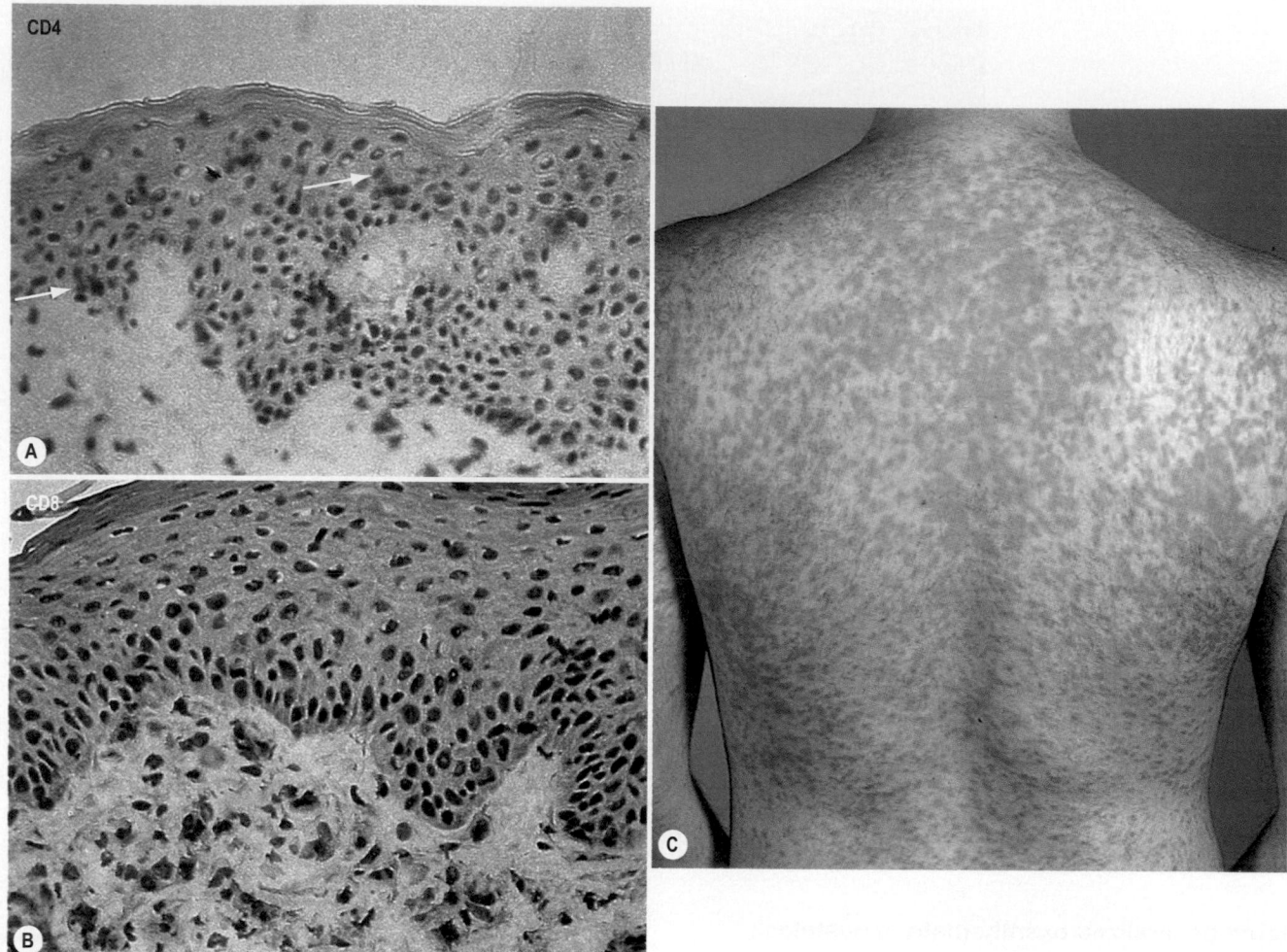

Fig. 48.6 Clinical pictures and immunohistologies of various forms of drug-induced exanthem. Maculopapular drug eruption **(C)**: the immunohistology reveals infiltration of CD4 **(A)** and only a few CD8 T cells **(B)** in the dermis and epidermis. These cells express perforin and granzyme B and, to a variable degree, FasL. (From Hari Y, Frutig-Schnyder K, Hurni M, et al. T cell involvement in cutaneous drug eruptions. Clin Exp Allergy 2001; 31: 1398–1408, with permission from Blackwell Publishing.)

sign is positive (Table 48.3). Stopping drug treatment at this stage may not prevent SJS developing, but might prevent an even more severe reaction (TEN). Mucous membranes (mouth, genitalia) are involved with blister formation, as well as a purulent keratoconjunctivitis with formation of synechiae, which may result in permanent eye damage.

The main causes for SJS/TEN are drugs (Table 48.2), which might differ in frequency in various regions due to genetic and ethnic background. Important risk factors are HIV infection (low CD4, high CD8 counts), renal diseases, and active systemic autoimmune diseases such as systemic lupus erythematosus, Still's syndrome, Sjögren's disease, and rheumatoid arthritis. In histology of toxic epidermal necrolysis, many dead keratinocytes are found, but cell infiltration is scarce. However, the bullae may be filled by cytotoxic CD8 T cells, expressing CD56 and αβ-TCRs, which kill via perforin/granzyme B but not via the Fas-mediated pathway at this stage of the disease.[17] On the other hand, the massive cell

death of keratinocytes is hard to reconcile with a cell contact-dependent killing process. It has been proposed that the apoptosis of keratinocytes is due to FasL, a soluble molecule of the TNF family, which binds to keratinocytes via Fas and functions as a so-called death receptor.[26] Since blocking anti-Fas antibodies are found in immunoglobulin preparations, it has been proposed to treat patients with TEN with immunoglobulins, but the efficacy of this therapy is unproven.[27]

Extensive research has not revealed a pharmocogenetic predisposition or low glutathione levels in affected persons. However, recent data have revealed striking HLA associations of severe, CD8-mediated drug hypersensitivity reactions.[28–30] Three factors play a role: (1) the type of drug; (2) the type of reaction, as it was found for cytotoxic CD8 reactions only; and (3) possibly race, as some reactions were mainly described in Han Chinese. The HLA-B allele, which is the most polymorphic HLA allele, seems to be involved. In carbamazepine-induced SJS/TEN it is

Table 48.2 Drugs eliciting severe cutaneous or systemic reactions[a]

Acute generalized exanthematous pustulosis (AGEP)	Stevens–Johnson syndrome (SJS) and toxic epidermal necrolysis (TEN)	Drug-induced hypersensitivity syndrome/drug rash with eosinophilia and systemic symptoms (DiHS/DRESS)
Aminopenicillins[a]	**Nevirapine**	**Carbamazepine**[b]
Cephalosporins	**Allopurinol**	Phenytoin
Pristinamycin	**Phenytoin**[b]	Lamotrigine
Celecoxib	**Carbamazepine**[b]	Minocycline
Quinolone	Lamotrigine	Allopurinol[b]
Diltiazem	Co-trimoxazole	Dapsone
Terbinafine	Barbiturate	Sulfasalazine
Macrolides	Nonsteroidal anti-inflammatory drug (oxicams)	Co-trimoxazole (abacavir)[c]

[a]List incomplete: the most frequent elicitors are given in bold.
[b]The type of reaction might be determined by the presence of a certain human leukocyte antigen (HLA)-B phenotype.
[c]Abacavir-induced systemic reactions often lack eosinophilia and preferentially affect the respiratory and gastrointestinal tract.

HLA-B*1502; for phenytoin HLA-B*5601; and for abacavir HLA-B*5701 together with hsp70. It seems that in these CD8 T-cell reactions the HLA-B alleles favor the presentation of certain peptides capable of optimally presenting the drug/hapten. Alternatively, if the stimulation occurred via the p-i concept, certain MHC molecules might supplement the T-cell stimulation better than others, while absence of the allelic product renders the T-cell unresponsive to drug binding.

The extremely high association of certain HLA-B alleles and hypersensitivity reactions to certain drugs may be used to prevent such side effects in the future, as HLA-typing may identify patients at risk. Studies to determine the benefit of such predictive testing are under way.

Systemic drug reactions – severe drug hypersensitivity syndromes

Some drugs are known to cause a severe systemic disease, with fever, lymph node swelling, massive hepatitis, and various forms of exanthems (Table 48.2). A few patients develop colitis, pancreatitis, or interstitial lung disease.[31] Over 70% have a marked eosinophilia (often > 10^12/l), and activated lymphocytes are often found in the circulation, similar to acute HIV or generalized herpes virus infections. This syndrome has many names. The most frequently used are drug (induced) hypersensitivity syndrome (DHS or DiHS) or drug rash with eosinophilia and systemic symptoms (DRESS). Importantly, the symptoms can start up to 12 weeks after starting treatment, often after increasing the dose, and may also persist and recur for many weeks, even after cessation of drug treatment. The clinical picture resembles a generalized viral infection, e.g., acute Epstein–Barr virus infection, but it is distinguished by the prominent eosinophilia. Many patients have facial swelling, and some have signs of a capillary leak syndrome, like patients having a cytokine release syndrome. Indeed, various cytokines are massively increased in the serum of these patients. As the clinical picture is quite dramatic and as the disease tends to persist in spite of stopping drug treatment, many patients *are not diagnosed correctly or in a timely manner*. However, physicians using anticonvulsants should be familiar with this syndrome, as it might occur in 1:3000 treated

patients. The mortality is ~10%, and some patients require emergency liver transplantation.

Patients with DiHS/DRESS have many activated T cells in the circulation. These drug-specific T cells are stimulated by the parent compound (p-i concept) and they secrete high amounts of IL-5 and IFN-γ.[32] A peculiar feature of this syndrome is its long-lasting clinical course despite withdrawal of the causative drug. There may also be persistent intolerance to other, chemically distinct drugs, leading to flare-up reactions to a rather innocuous drug (e.g., acetaminophen) months after stopping the initial drug therapy, further adding to the confusion. Treatment often includes high doses of corticosteroids, particularly if the hepatitis is severe.

Recently, it has been shown that in many patients with this syndrome, human herpes virus 6 DNA can be found during the 3rd or 4th week of the disease (but not before), followed by a rising antibody titer to human herpes virus 6.[33] Other reports document reactivation of cytomegalovirus infection. Thus, similar to HIV, where T-cell activation can also enhance virus production, the drug-induced massive immune stimulation may somehow reactivate these latent lymphotropic herpes viruses, which subsequently replicate and possibly contribute to the chronic course and persistent drug intolerance in affected patients.

Many drugs can induce isolated hepatitis and some (penicillins, proton pump inhibitors, quinolones, disulfiram) can cause an isolated (interstitial) nephritis. More rare are interstitial lung diseases (furadantin), pancreatitis, isolated fever, or eosinophilia as the only symptom of a drug allergy. In drug-induced interstitial nephritis eosinophils can sometimes be detected in the urine (even in the absence of blood eosinophilia).

Multiple drug hypersensitivity syndrome

The term 'multiple drug hypersensitivity' is used to describe different forms of side effects to multiple drugs. Some physicians use the term to characterize patients with multiple drug intolerance ("pseudoallergy" to NSAID), others reserve this term for well-documented repeated immune-mediated reactions to structurally unrelated drugs.[34] Cross-reactivity due to structural similarity is excluded from the definition.

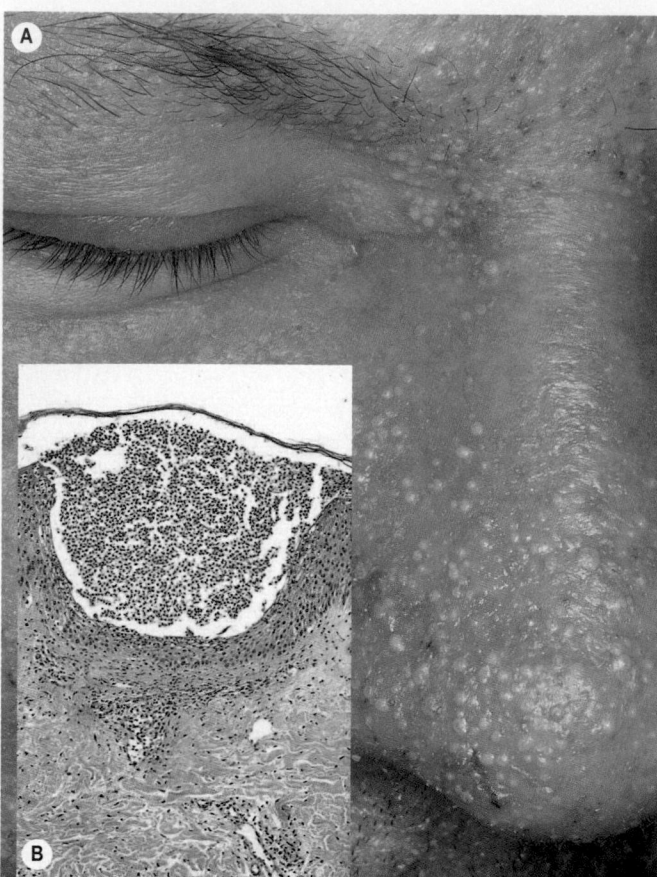

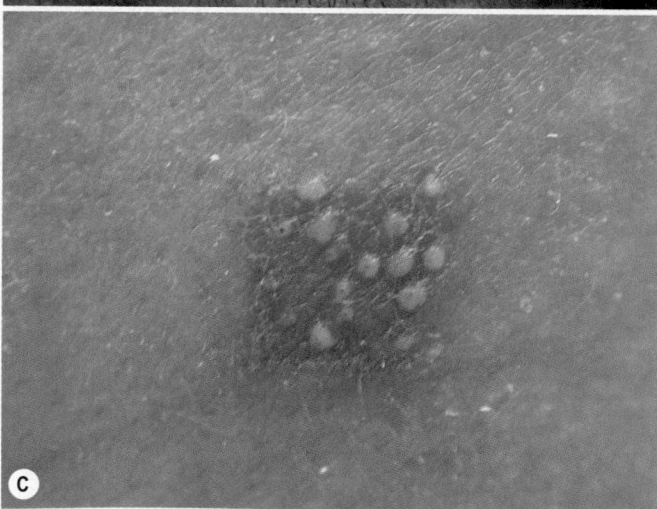

Fig. 48.7 Clinical pictures and immunohistologies of various forms of drug-induced exanthem. **(A)** Pustular drug eruption (acute generalized exanthematous pustulosis: AGEP). **(B)** Note the intraepidermal, nonfollicular pustules; **(C)** a patch test reaction leading to a pustular reaction is shown as well. (From Schaerli P, Britschgi M, Keller M, et al. Characterization of human T cells that regulate neutrophilic skin inflammation. J Immunol 2004; 173: 2151–2158. Copyright 2004, with permission from The American Association of Immunologists, Inc.)

In our experience, about 10% of patients with well-documented drug hypersensitivity (skin and/or lymphocyte transformation test positive) have multiple drug allergies.[35] For example, they may have reacted to injected lidocaine with angioedema and years later they develop contact allergy to corticosteroids. Alternatively, a patient reacts to amoxicillin, phenytoin, and sulfamethoxazole within a few months, but with different symptoms (MPE, DiHS/DRESS, erythroderma). Most of these patients have had rather severe reactions to at least one drug. An IgE-mediated reaction might be followed by a T-cell-mediated reaction. The pathophysiologic mechanism of this syndrome is unknown.

One explanation might be a deficient tolerance mechanism to small chemical compounds/xenobiotics. An immune reaction to a drug, whether via hapten or p-i mechanism, can be seen as a failure of tolerance, and the same patient might be prone to develop not only other drug allergies but also autoimmunity. Preliminary data suggest that previous drug allergy might be a risk factor for the development of delayed hypersensitivity reactions to radiocontrast media.

Multiple drug hypersensitivity should be differentiated from *flare-up reactions*. In patients with systemic drug allergies, the T-cell immune system is massively activated, similar to acute viral infections. As in the latter, these patients seem to have a higher tendency to react to a new drug and might show a flare-up of their rash to a new antibiotic, but the second drug remains negative in skin tests and is later well tolerated, if the co-stimulatory conditions are no longer present.

■ DIAGNOSIS OF DRUG HYPERSENSITIVITY ■

The diagnosis of drug hypersensitivity addresses three questions: (1) is it a drug hypersensitivity? (2) which mechanism might be involved? and (3) which drug has caused it? The symptoms can be extremely heterogeneous, and in a patient with 'bizarre' symptoms a drug hypersensitivity reaction should always be included in the differential diagnosis! On the other hand, some of the above-described skin exanthems are rather typical for drug hypersensitivity and easy to recognize.

CLINICAL DIAGNOSIS

Drug hypersensitivity is often suspected if a 'rash' appears. Differential diagnosis of this rash includes viral exanthems, occasionally other infections, food allergy, and a graft-versus-host reaction. Pruritus, blood eosinophilia, and recent administration of a new drug argue for an allergic reaction.

It is important to document the severity of the presumed drug hypersensitivity, as this may determine whether the drug can be given again. Special attention should be paid to the type and extent of skin symptoms, the involvement of mucosal areas, lymph node enlargement, fever, and subjective symptoms like malaise, as this could indicate involvement of internal organs. A painful skin and a positive Nikolsky sign might herald a severe bullous skin reaction, which can develop within hours. One should be aware of danger signs (Table 48.3) and the most important elicitors of SJS/TEN and DRESS (Table 48.2). Some patients have no skin involvement, but develop an isolated drug-allergic hepatitis or interstitial nephritis.

Different mechanisms can lead to drug hypersensitivity symptoms. They should be differentiated, as they need distinct diagnostic steps and may have a different prognosis; the combination of symptoms and time course usually helps to discriminate them. Immediate reactions start < 1

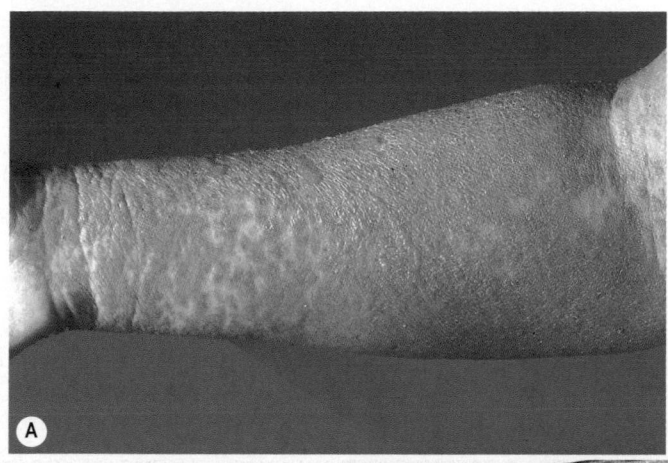

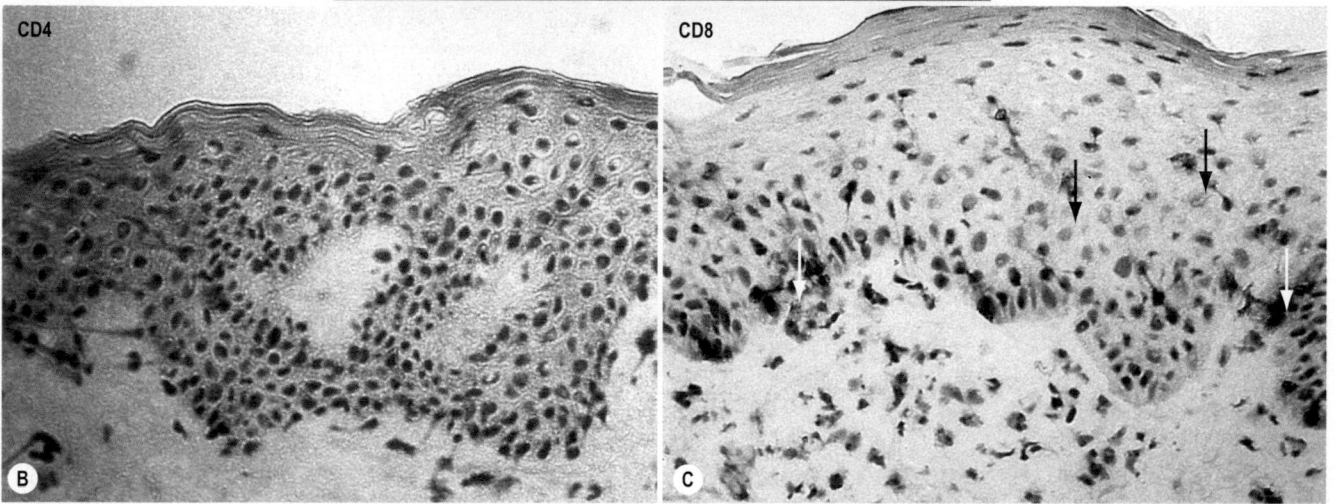

Fig. 48.8 Clinical pictures and immunohistologies of various forms of drug-induced exanthem. Maculopapular drug eruption (A) with some blisters exhibiting more CD8 T cells by immunohistology (C). (From Hari Y, Frutig-Schnyder K, Hurni M, et al. T cell involvement in cutaneous drug eruptions. Clin Exp Allergy 2001; 31: 1398–1408, with permission from Blackwell Publishing.)

Table 48.3 Clinical and laboratory investigations and *danger signs*[a] in drug-induced exanthems

Clinic	Laboratory
Extent and type of exanthem (infiltration, *bullae, pustules*) *Pain of skin, Nikolsky sign*	Eosinophilia *(> 1000–1200/μl[b]); atypical (activated) lymphocytes in the circulation (> 2%[b])*
Involvement of mucous membranes	C-reactive protein elevation
Systemic symptoms (malaise, fever) *Lymphadenopathy, hepatosplenomegaly*	Liver enzymes (ALAT, ASAT, γGT, AP) (increase >2–3×[b]) additional investigations depend on clinical signs, liver, kidney, lung, pancreas involvement (urine analysis, creatinine)

[a]Danger signs *in italics*.
[b]The cut-off values of the laboratory parameters are estimates, and are not based on prospective studies; severe reactions can also develop in the absence of these signs!

THERAPEUTIC PRINCIPLES

CROSS-REACTIVITY

>> The risk of cross-reactivity depends on the type of reaction

>> In nonsteroidal anti-inflammatory drug-induced 'pseudoallergy,' cross-reactivity seems to be due to the pharmacological action and not the structure

>> Immunoglobulin E (IgE)-mediated reactions have a higher degree of cross-reactivity than T-cell reactions, probably because antibodies can recognize small molecular components, whereas T cells tend to recognize the complete structure

>> Cross-reactivity of T cell and antibodies is common within the same class of drugs (e.g., penicillins, quinolones, pyrazolones, cephalosporins)

>> **Penicillin–cephalosporin cross-reactivity**

>> Not seen in T-cell-mediated reactions (maculopapular exanthem); in IgE-mediated reactions cross-reactivity might occur in ~4% of penicillin skin test-positive patients with first- and second-generation cephalosporins. The chance of cross-reactivity is very low if the second drug is negative in skin tests

>> **Sulfonamide cross-reactivity**

>> There is an extensive cross-reactivity between sulfonamide-containing antibacterials (sulfanilamides), which mainly induce sensitization, but not with other drugs containing a sulfonamide (e.g., furosemide, celecoxib, glibencamide)

hour after drug intake and are usually IgE-mediated (or due to drug-induced mast-cell release). Occasionally, IgE-mediated reactions occur later than 1 hour. Typical symptoms are urticaria and anaphylaxis. Delayed reactions start > 12 hours after drug intake and are mostly non-IgE-mediated, but involve T-cell orchestrated inflammation or IgG-mediated reactions. In highly sensitized individuals symptoms can arise as early as 2–4 hours after drug intake – the more drug-specific precursor T cells are present, the more rapidly symptoms may appear.

Laboratory investigations can also help to determine the severity of the reaction. In more severe acute reactions tryptase levels should be determined, optimally between 2 and 4 hours after the peak of the reaction to confirm mast cell involvement. The analysis should be repeated later (> 2 days) to rule out a constitutively elevated tryptase level (mastocytosis). Such measurements are particularly important if anaphylaxis is suspected during anesthesia, where the sole sign of anaphylaxis might be cardiac arrest, without skin symptoms.

In delayed reactions a differential blood count may reveal activated lymphocytes and eosinophilia, which is common in drug hypersensitivity (observed in up to ~40% of patients with MPE, in 30% with AGEP (together with leukocytosis, and in > 70% in DiHS/DRESS). Measurements of liver enzymes (ALAT, ASAT, ALP, and γGT) should be done in patients with malaise, in those with extensive skin involvement, or if drugs known to cause DiHS/DRESS or hepatitis/cholestasis are involved. A transient mild hepatitis is not rare and seems to occur in ~25% of patients with more severe MPE.[22] Dependent on the symptoms

other tests may also be indicated (creatinine, urinary analysis). C-reactive protein (CRP) may be elevated (e.g., in drug-induced interstitial lung or kidney diseases), but can be normal even in severe hypersensitivity reactions like DiHS/DRESS.

IDENTIFYING THE CULPRIT DRUG

The important questions are: which drugs were taken, and since when? Was the dose increased? Are there co-medications? and could they possibly interfere with drug metabolism? How were the drugs tolerated previously? Were other drugs tolerated that are known to cause similar effects? What was the underlying disease? Have similar reactions already occurred previously without or with drugs? Books listing side effects, websites (e.g., www.pneumotox.com) and pharmaceutical companies can provide information about the known side effects of a drug. In many instances, the history and these sources may allow a rather conclusive allocation of symptoms and drug intake. However, many patients have taken several drugs and the history alone may be insufficient. In these cases further tests can be justified, although these are often not well validated.

The *in vivo* (skin test) and *in vitro* tests for drug allergy diagnosis are difficult to standardize. Although drug allergy is common it only occurs rarely for each individual drug; a single drug might elicit different types of symptom, requiring different tests; provocation tests – which would prove the allergy and the sensitivity of the test – are often not performed for ethical reasons, and for some tests living cells are needed rather than serum, which requires a great logistic effort. In spite of these obstacles, many groups perform tests, but two rules are important: (1) the test can only supplement the history; and (2) the sensitivity of the tests is generally low, thus a positive test may be more meaningful than a negative test, which cannot rule out a drug allergy.

For immediate reactions both prick and intradermal tests are available. Penicillin tests are widely used. To form repetitive determinants able to cross-link two FcεRI-bound IgE molecules, the drug is coupled to polylysine, either by opening the penicillin-ring and forming penicilloyl-carriers, or by binding via the thiol structure (minor components). The pure substance (e.g., amoxicillin) can also be evaluated, since it frequently gives positive skin tests as well. The sensitivity of these tests is controversial: older studies from the USA suggested a sensitivity of > 95%; but more recent studies from Spain found only 70%.[36] Other drugs can be tested as well by prick or intradermal tests, but false-positive reactions (e.g., to quinolones) can occur and it is essential to test control individuals as well. Further information on test procedures and concentrations is available elsewhere.[37]

In vitro tests for immediate reactions include the determination of specific IgE. However, the sensitivity of commercial assays for drug-specific IgE appears to be rather low, while published "in-house" tests have been reported to help in the diagnosis and discrimination from pseudoallergic reactions.[6, 7] Various read-out systems for basophil degranulation/activation tests have been proposed to be usable for drug hypersensitivity diagnosis (e.g., Flow-Cast). Sensitivity in IgE-mediated reactions is reported to be ~40%, and in "pseudoallergic" reactions to NSAIDs up to 70%.[38]

In Europe it is common to perform patch tests for delayed reactions (e.g., for contact dermatitis).[39] The overall sensitivity is considered to be < 50%[39] and depends on the disease (often negative in macular reactions, and delayed urticarial exanthems, but more useful in severe MPE, DiHS/DRESS, AGEP: Fig. 48.7). This is a reliable test for abacavir hypersensitivity, even if only hepatitis occurs.

THERAPEUTIC PRINCIPLES

TREATMENT

>> Stop drug(s)

>> Avoid drugs, until culprit drug is identified

>> Avoid re-exposure to the drug class (cross-reactivity) in acute immunoglobulin E-mediated reactions, in acute "pseudoallergic" reactions, and in severe delayed reactions

>> Symptomatic treatment according to symptoms

>> Avoid treating through with drugs known to cause toxic epidermal necrolysis, drug-induced hypersensitivity syndrome or drug rash with eosinophilia and systemic symptoms, or if danger signs are present

The lymphocyte transformation (proliferation/activation) test (LTT) relies on the activation and proliferation of T cells cultured in the presence of the drug.[40] Reactivity can be measured by ^{3}H-thymidine incorporation after 5–6-day culture, or by ELISPOT, CSFE staining, CD69 upregulation. LTT is cumbersome, but a clearly positive value is useful. The sensitivity of LTT depends on the pathophysiologic mechanism of the drug hypersensitivity and is > 90% for DiHS/DRESS, but lower in more cytotoxic reactions like SJS/TEN. LTT is positive in drugs sensitizing via the hapten mechanism or stimulated via the p-i concept.

Provocation tests are considered to be the gold standard for the diagnosis. They are useful for immediate reactions, but less so for delayed reactions.[41] Cofactors are often important, which are absent during provocation, and the dose to elicit symptoms will often not be reached. Thus one might be able to exclude immediate reactions to the dose used in the provocation test, but treatment with higher doses might still cause symptoms.

■ THERAPEUTIC ASPECTS ■

The therapy of drug hypersensitivity diseases is dependent on the symptoms and ranges from the usual treatment of anaphylaxis to acute liver transplantation. Stopping the possible culprit drugs and avoiding them until clarity is achieved should be possible in most circumstances and might reduce the development of more severe symptoms. In some milder skin reactions, (e.g., nonbullous exanthem due to sulfamethoxazole in HIV-positive patients), experience has shown that continuation of treatment may be possible, whereas reintroducing the drug after stopping it may actually precipitate more severe symptoms.

DESENSITIZATION

Under certain circumstances a drug that causes allergic or 'pseudoallergic' side effects is essential for treatment, for example, penicillin to treat syphilis during pregnancy or certain cytostatic drugs in cancer treatments (e.g. cisplatin). Most desensitization protocols refer to hypersensitivity reactions involving mast cell degranulation, and the procedure is best established for penicillin and NSAIDs.[42]

The starting dose for desensitization is determined by the dose the patient tolerated in skin testing. This dose generally translates to 1:10 000 of the therapeutic dose. Doubling doses are administered every 15 minutes until the full dose is reached. Once desensitization is completed, the patient can receive the full therapeutic course of penicillin via the desired route. If treatment is discontinued for more than 48 hours, the patient will once more be at risk to develop anaphylaxis and the full desensitization protocol must be repeated.

In dubious, skin test-negative cases, where one actually expects *no* allergy, *graded drug challenges* under careful supervision might be used starting with ~1/100 or 1/20 of the dose, and increasing the dose stepwise (double or triple) every 30–60 minutes. The full dose may be achieved in 1 day and can be continued during the next days.

■ REFERENCES ■

1. Naisbitt DJ, Gordon SF, Pirmohamed M, et al. Immunological principles of adverse drug reactions: the initiation and propagation of immune responses elicited by drug treatment. Drug Safe 2000; 23: 483–507.

2. Lazarou J, Pomeranz BH, Corey PN. Incidence of adverse drug reactions in hospitalized patients: a meta-analysis of prospective studies. JAMA 1998; 279: 1200–1205.

3. Roujeau JC, Stern RS. Severe adverse cutaneous reactions to drugs. N Engl J Med 1994; 331: 1272–1285.

4. Bigby M, Jick S, Jick H, et al. Drug-induced cutaneous reactions. A report from the Boston Collaborative Drug Surveillance Program on 15 438 consecutive inpatients, 1975 to 1982. JAMA 1986; 256: 3358–3363.

5. Hunziker T, Kunzi UP, Braunschweig S, et al. Comprehensive hospital drug monitoring (CHDM): adverse skin reactions, a 20-year survey. Allergy 1997; 52: 388–393.

6. Manfredi M, Severino M, Testi S, et al. Detection of specific IgE to quinolones. J Allergy Clin Immunol 2004; 113: 155–160.

7. Pichler WJ. Delayed drug hypersensitivity reactions. Ann Intern Med 2003; 139: 683–693.

8. Martin S, Weltzien HU. T cell recognition of haptens, a molecular view. Int Arch Allergy Immunol 1994; 104: 10–16.

9. Griem P, Wulferink M, Sachs B, et al. Allergic and autoimmune reactions to xenobiotics: how do they arise?. Immunol Today 1998; 19: 133–141.

10. Zanni MP, von Greyerz S, Schnyder B, et al. HLA-restricted, processing- and metabolism-independent pathway of drug recognition by human alpha beta T lymphocytes. J Clin Invest 1998; 102: 1591–1598.

11. Pichler WJ. Pharmacological interaction of drugs with antigen-specific immune receptors: the p-i concept. Curr Opin Allergy Clin Immunol 2002; 2: 301–305.

12. Aster RH. Drug-induced immune thrombocytopenia: an overview of pathogenesis. Semin Hematol 1999; 36: 2–6.

13. Arndt PA, Garratty G. The changing spectrum of drug-induced immune hemolytic anemia. Semin Hematol 2005; 42: 137–144.

14. Greinacher A, Warkentin TE. Recognition, treatment, and prevention of heparin-induced thrombocytopenia: review and update. Thromb Res 2006; 118: 165–176.

15. Aitman TJ, Dong R, Vyse TJ, et al. Copy number polymorphism in Fcgr3 predisposes to glomerulonephritis in rats and humans. Nature 2006; 439: 851–855.

16. Stokol T, O'Donnell P, Xiao L, et al. C1q governs deposition of circulating immune complexes and leukocyte Fcgamma receptors mediate subsequent neutrophil recruitment. J Exp Med 2004; 200: 835–846.

17. Nassif A, Bensussan A, Dorothee G, et al. Drug specific cytotoxic T-cells in the skin lesions of a patient with toxic epidermal necrolysis. J Invest Dermatol 2002; 118: 728–733.

18. Schnyder B, Frutig K, Mauri-Hellweg D, et al. T-cell-mediated cytotoxicity against keratinocytes in sulfamethoxazol-induced skin reaction. Clin Exp Allergy 1998; 28: 1412–1417.

19. Britschgi M, Steiner UC, Schmid S, et al. T-cell involvement in drug-induced acute generalized exanthemtous pustulosis. J Clin Invest 2001; 107: 1433–1441.

20. Keller M, Spanou Z, Schaerli P, et al. T cell-regulated neutrophilic inflammation in autoinflammatory diseases. J Immunol 2005; 175: 7678–7686.

21. Beeler A, Engler O, Gerber BO, et al. Long-lasting reactivity and high frequency of drug-specific T cells after severe systemic drug hypersensitivity reactions. J Allergy Clin Immunol 2006; 117: 455–462.

22. Hari Y, Frutig-Schnyder K, Hurni M, et al. T cell involvement in cutaneous drug eruptions. Clin Exp Allergy 2001; 31: 1398–1408.

23. Pichler WJ, Zanni M, von Greyerz S, et al. High IL-5 production by human drug-specific T cell clones. Int Arch Allergy Immunol 1997; 113: 177–180.

24. Hari Y, Urwyler A, Hurni M, et al. Distinct serum cytokine levels in drug- and measles-induced exanthem. Int Arch Allergy Immunol 1999; 120: 225–229.

25. Roujeau J, Bioulac-Sage P, Bourseau C. Acute generalized exanthematous pustulosis: analysis of 63 cases. Arch Dermatol 1991; 127: 1333–1338.

26. Viard I, Wehrli P, Bullani R, et al. Inhibition of toxic epidermal necrolysis by blockade of CD95 with human intravenous immunoglobulin. Science 1998; 282: 490–493.

27. Bachot N, Roujeau JC. Intravenous immunoglobulins in the treatment of severe drug eruptions. Curr Opin Allergy Clin Immunol 2003; 3: 269–274.

28. Mallal S, Nolan D, Witt C, et al. Association between presence of HLA-B*5701, HLA-DR7, and HLA-DQ3 and hypersensitivity to HIV-1 reverse-transcriptase inhibitor abacavir. Lancet 2002; 359: 727–732.

29. Chung WH, Hung SI, Hong HS, et al. Medical genetics: a marker for Stevens–Johnson syndrome. Nature 2004; 428: 486.

30. Hung SI, Chung WH, Liou LB, et al. HLA-B*5801 allele as a genetic marker for severe cutaneous adverse reactions caused by allopurinol. Proc Natl Acad Sci USA 2005; 102: 4134–4139.

31. Knowles SR, Shapiro LE, Shear NH. Anticonvulsant hypersensitivity syndrome: incidence, prevention and management. Drug Safe 1999; 21: 489–501.

32. Naisbitt DJ, Farrell J, Wong G, et al. Characterization of drug-specific T cells in lamotrigine hypersensitivity. J Allergy Clin Immunol 2003; 111: 1393–1403.

33. Hashimoto K, Yasukawa M, Tohyama M. Human herpesvirus 6 and drug allergy. Curr Opin Allergy Clin Immunol 2003; 3: 255–260.

34. Sullivan T. Studies of the multiple drug allergy syndrome. J Allergy Clin Immunol 1989; 83: 270.

35. Gex-Collet C, Helbling A, Pichler WJ. Multiple drug hypersensitivity – proof of multiple drug hypersensitivity by patch and lymphocyte transformation tests. J Invest Allergol Clin Immunol 2005; 15: 293–296.

36. Torres MJ, Blanca M, Fernandez J, et al. Diagnosis of immediate allergic reactions to beta-lactam antibiotics. Allergy 2003; 58: 961–972.

37. Brockow K, Romano A, Blanca M, et al. General considerations for skin test procedures in the diagnosis of drug hypersensitivity. Allergy 2002; 57: 45–51.

38. Sanz ML, Gamboa P, de Weck AL. A new combined test with flowcytometric basophil activation and determination of sulfidoleukotrienes is useful for in vitro diagnosis of hypersensitivity to aspirin and other nonsteroidal anti-inflammatory drugs. Int Arch Allergy Immunol 2005; 136: 58–72.

39. Barbaud A, Goncalo M, Bruynzeel D, et al. Guidelines for performing skin tests with drugs in the investigation of cutaneous adverse drug reactions. Contact Dermatitis 2001; 45: 321–328.

40. Pichler WJ, Tilch J. The lymphocyte transformation test in the diagnosis of drug hypersensitivity. Allergy 2004; 59: 809–820.

41. Aberer W, Bircher A, Romano A, et al. Drug provocation testing in the diagnosis of drug hypersensitivity reactions: general considerations. Allergy 2003; 58: 854–863.

42. Solensky R. Drug allergy: desensitization and treatment of reactions to antibiotics and aspirin. Clin Allergy Immunol 2004; 18: 585–606.

43. Coombs RR, Gell PG. Classification of allergic reactions responsible for clinical hypersensitivity and disease. In Gell PG ed. Clinical Aspects of Immunology Oxford: Oxford University Press 1976: 575–596.

Occupational and environmental allergic disorders

Emil J. Bardana Jr., Anthony Montanaro

49

The respiratory tract is second only to the skin as the most frequently impacted organ in the workplace. The upper and lower airways are the initial point of entry for a variety of ambient dusts, gases, fumes, and vapors. When relatively low concentrations of mild irritants are encountered, transient annoyance reactions may occur in exposed workers. Increasing concentrations of soluble inhalants may irritate the mucous membranes of the upper airways. Alternatively, soluble corrosive gases may cause skin burns, ocular damage, and acute inflammation in the nasopharynx, larynx, and lower airways. Other agents may not be directly damaging, but can induce sensitization, with subsequent onset of occupational asthma (OA). To date, approximately 300 industrial agents have been implicated in the induction of OA in susceptible individuals.

■ DEFINITION ■

OA is characterized by variable airway obstruction associated with bronchial hyperresponsiveness (BHR). It is caused by inflammation of the airways secondary to inhalation of dusts, gases, fumes, or vapors that are produced at, or incidentally present at, the workplace.[1] Bronchoconstriction caused by exercise or cold air is not sufficient to diagnose OA. The definition of OA assumes variable legal importance in the context of different workers' compensation statutes.[2] Pre-existing asthma does not preclude development of a work-induced respiratory disorder. In this instance, the clinician must determine whether the suspected work exposure caused the pre-existing asthma to become transiently symptomatic, or caused a permanent worsening of the pre-existing asthma by virtue of either an intense corrosive effect on the airways, or caused the development of a unique sensitization that amplified the pre-existing disease.

There are two main variants of OA based on pathogenesis. The most common type is immunologic OA which is caused by high-molecular-weight (HMW) proteins, glycoproteins, or polysaccharides derived from natural sources (animals, plants, foods, and enzymes) via an immunoglobulin E (IgE)-mediated response after a latent period of exposure (Table 49.1). Selected low-molecular-weight (LMW) agents are also capable of acting as haptens combining with human proteins to induce OA by an immunologic mechanism. A less common nonallergic variant, reactive air-

ways dysfunction syndrome (RADS) occurs after an acute exposure to a corrosive chemical, usually soluble in water, without a latent period. Agents known to cause OA have been classified in different ways, i.e., LMW versus HMW (Table 49.1), or immunogenic versus nonimmunogenic. They have also been classified according to their biochemical nature (e.g., plastics, chemicals, wood/vegetable dusts, pharmacologic agents) (Table 49.2).

The inhalational consequences of any industrial exposure is dependent on the physicochemical properties of the dust, gas, fume, or vapor involved, its concentration and duration of exposure, as well as specific host factors (Figs 49.1 and 49.2). There is significant variability of response from person to person even when the same concentration is encountered. Some industrial irritants are capable of causing tissue damage on direct contact. The extent of acute injury induced by irritant gases and vapors is highly dependent on their water solubility. Inhalation of highly soluble gases such as ammonia, sulfur dioxide, formaldehyde, or methyl isocyanate is likely to result in

Table 49.1 Classification of selected asthmagenic agents by molecular weight

Low-molecular-weight	High-molecular-weight
Acid anhydrides	Latex constituents
Diisocyanates	Insect parts
Reactive azo-dyes	Acarid emanations
Colophony (abietic acid, pimaric acid)	Animal protein
Epoxy amine compounds	Vegetable gums
Complex salts of platinum	*Bacillus subtilis* (alcalase)
Western red cedar (plicatic acid)	Hog trypsin
Ammonium persulfate	Papain
Penicillin	Castor bean dust
Cephalosporins	Green coffee bean dust
Spiromycin	Flour
Formaldehyde	Egg powder
Freon	Tobacco leaf
Vanadium	Silkworm larva

nasopharyngeal and laryngeal inflammation associated with erythema and edema. Such exposures can also induce irritant-related contact dermatitis of the exposed skin, as well as ocular irritation. Dependent on the concentration and duration of such exposures, the most significant pathology will be observed in the upper airways, ocular tissue, and skin. On the other hand, relatively insoluble gases such as phosgene, hydrogen sulfide, and oxides of nitrogen cause little upper-airway irritation or tissue damage and are much more likely to induce pulmonary edema, bronchiolitis, or alveolitis.[3] Sustained low-level exposures to certain dusts, gases, and fumes may result in chronic fibrosing pulmonary disease such as asbestosis and silicosis. The immunologic mechanisms involved in the pathogenesis of these disorders are beyond the scope of this chapter.

PREVALENCE OF OCCUPATIONAL ASTHMA

There are few large population-based studies dealing with OA. Much of what has been published on the subject represents anecdotal case reports or descriptions of small clusters of cases. There are also a number of retrospective, observational studies dealing with specific industries. With some notable exceptions,[4–6] there are no long-term, prospective, longitudinal studies of OA. In addition, nearly all epidemiological studies have relied upon subjective data in identifying bronchial asthma. Case definition has been variable in different parts of the world and in many instances it is not possible to ascertain whether minimally symptomatic, undiagnosed nonoccupational asthma was present prior to any suspected work trigger. Equally problematic is whether pre-existing, asymptomatic BHR predisposed a worker to the development of adult-onset asthma secondary to a viral infection, exposure to a nonindustrial allergen, a pharmacologic agent, or a nonspecific environmental pollutant. There are many individuals who report having childhood asthma that completely abated, but recent studies have revealed that asymptomatic BHR in such patients may persist into adult life and cannot be modified with inhaled corticosteroids.[7] Other studies have demonstrated that a number of young adults are underdiagnosed in adolescence and are later found to have asthma.[8]

An estimated 18 million individuals in the USA are said to have asthma. The prevalence of OA has been reported to range between 9% and 15% of the asthmatic population.[9] A large population-based study of OA estimated that between 5% and 10% of cases of asthma among adults in European and other industrialized countries were due to work exposures.[10] Unfortunately, the latter study did not distinguish between new-onset OA and pre-existing asthma that was aggravated due to a subsequent work exposure. There are better prevalence data for OA within certain industries. Understandably, the highest prevalence rates are in industries where workers are exposed to HMW agents. OA has been reported in up to 30% of laboratory animal workers, 16% of snow crab processors, 10% of isocyanate workers, and up to 9% of bakers, especially in Europe.[11]

Many investigators believe the 5% prevalence for OA represents an underestimate. There are claims of some workers who develop OA but leave the industry without reporting the illness, creating a residual "healthy survivor population." Other affected workers may remain on the job with OA, neglecting to report it for fear of losing their job or their seniority. Some workers with OA are said to be misdiagnosed with nonoccupational asthma. These scenarios must be balanced against the reality that in a setting where workers are protected by unions and state workers' compensation statutes, it is highly improbable that any worker would remain silent with the possibility of an industrial injury. In addition, in the USA where some 40 million people remain uninsured, and even more underinsured, there is a tendency to implicate a work-related illness or injury as a mechanism for reimbursement in the evaluative process. Lastly, there is the occasional worker who abuses the system for personal gain.

GENETIC AND PREDISPOSING FACTORS

The development of atopy, asthma, and BHR is determined by multiple interacting genetic and environmental influences.[12] Atopy has been associated with an increased risk of sensitization and OA in workers exposed to enzymes, animal proteins, grains, flour, crab, latex, acid anhydrides,

Table 49.2 Categories of industrial agents causing occupational asthma with some representative examples and associated industries

Category of agent	Representative examples of agents	Related industry

Chemicals and plastics	Acid anhydrides
	  Phthalic
	  Trimellitic
	  Tetrachlorophthalic
		Industries using amine-based epoxy resins

	Diisocyanates
	  Toluene
	  Hexamethylene
	  Diphenylmethylene
		Polyurethane, adhesives, catalyzed paint manufacturers: textile, chemical industries; manufacturers of wire coatings

	Diamines
	  Ethylenediamine
	  Piperazine
	  Triethanolamine
		Chemical, dental, rubber industries; manufacturers of abrasives; dental, rubber, electronics industries; resin makers

	Formaldehyde
	  Formalin
	  Paraformaldehyde
		Lamination industry; adhesive manufacturing, plywood manufacturing

	Reactive azo-dyes
	  Black GR
	  Orange 3R
		Textile industry

Metallic salts and dust	Complex platinum salts	Photography, jewelry, and refinishing industries
	Cobalt, vanadium	Hard metal, smelting industries
	Nickel salts	Metal plating industry
	Chromium	Cement, tanning industries
Wood/vegetable dusts	Western red cedar (plicatic acid)	Sawmill industry, carpentry
	Flour	Food-processing industry; bakers, grain handlers, millers
	Green coffee bean	Food-processing industry; dock workers
	Castor bean	Oil, fertilizers industries

	Seeds
	  Cottonseed
	  Linseed
	  Flaxseed
		Food processing, oil product, carpet industries

	Soybean	Food-processing industry; dock workers
	Vegetable gums (karaya, acacia, gum arabic)	Printing, chewing gum industries
	Colophony (abietic acid, pimaric acid)	Electronics industry
	Cotton, hemp	Textile industry

Pharmaceuticals	Antibiotics
	  β-lactam
	  Spiramycin
	  Tetracycline
		Pharmaceutical industry; nursing

	Psyllium	Pharmaceutical industry; nursing
	Ipecac	Pharmaceutical industry; nursing
	Enflurane	Anesthesiology

Continued

Table 49.2 Categories of industrial agents causing occupational asthma with some representative examples and associated industries—Cont'd

Category of agent	Representative examples of agents	Related industry
Biologic enzymes	Bacillus subtilis (alcalase)	Detergent industry
	Trypsin	Plastic, pharmaceuticals industries
	Pancreatin	Food-processing, pharmaceuticals industries
	Papain	Laboratory, packaging industries
	Bromelin	Laboratory, pharmaceuticals industries
	Pectinase	Food-processing industries
Insecticides	Organophosphates	Farming; horticulture; chemical industry
	Carbamate	
	Pyrethrin	
Animal products, insects, birds, fish	Laboratory animals	Veterinarians; laboratories
	Fowl, poultry	Farming; breeding
	Sea squirts	Oyster processors
	Prawns	Food processing
	Insects	Grain workers, entomologists
	Grain mite	
	Grain weevil	
	Silkworm	Textile
	Crab	Food processors

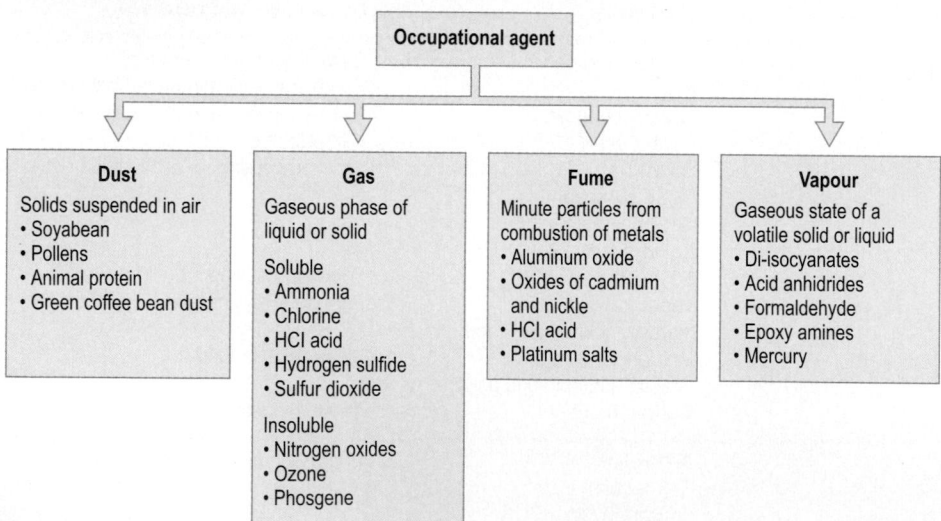

Fig. 49.1 The health effects of any industrial exposure are dependent on the physicochemical properties of the agent involved along with its concentration, duration of exposure, and specific host factors. (From Bardana EJ. Occupational asthma. In: Lieberman PL, Biaiss MS (eds) Atlas of Allergic Disease, 2nd edn. Current Medicine LLC; 2005:195–204.)

green coffee, and castor bean. When LMW agents are involved, the data are less clear. The incidence of OA secondary to exposure to toluene diisocyanates (TDI), western red cedar, or trimellitic anhydride does not appear to be influenced by atopy. However, atopy does have a role in individuals exposed to other LMW agents such as complex salts of platinum, ethylenediamine, and dimethyl ethanolamine.[13]

Genetic research related to atopic linkages has shown allelic polymorphisms associated with genes encoding the β subunit of the high-affinity IgE receptor, regulatory cytokines, the β_2 receptor and the interleukin (IL)-4α receptor.[14] There is now consistent evidence that genetic polymorphisms that code for human leukocyte antigen (HLA) class II genes may predispose to OA to a number of agents. HLA associations indicate

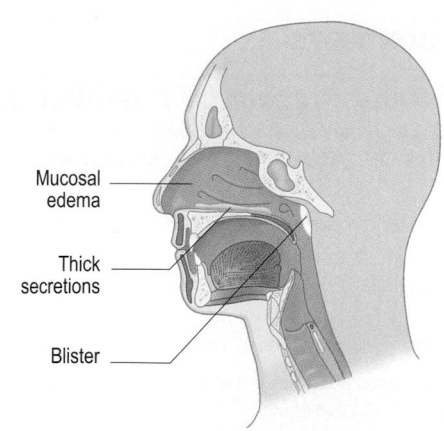

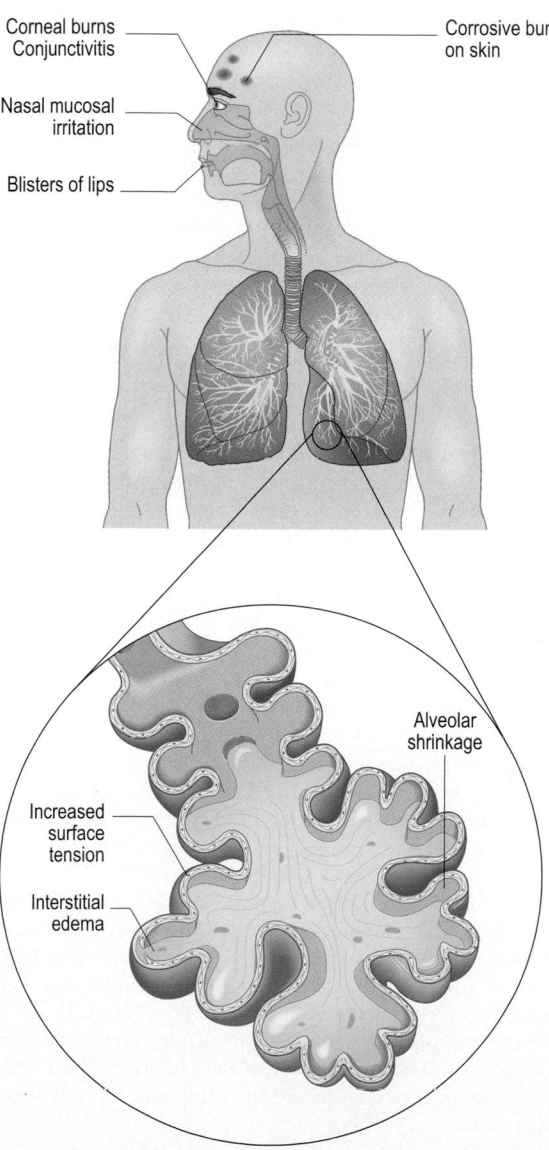

Fig. 49.2 Highly soluble gases are likely to result in nasopharyngeal and laryngeal inflammation in addition to ocular irritation. Insoluble gases cause little upper-airway irritation or tissue damage and are more likely to result in pulmonary edema, bronchiolitis, or alveolitis. (From Bardana EJ. Occupational asthma. In: Lieberman PL, Biaiss MS (eds) Atlas of Allergic Disease, 2nd edn. Current Medicine LLC; Philadelphia, PA 2005:195–204.)

a specific immunologic response in OA induced by selected LMW agents, including western red cedar, complex platinum salts, trimellitic anhydride, and TDI.[13, 15]

In addition, occupational agents may cause oxidative stress, and defects in antioxidant defenses that could contribute to the susceptibility of OA. It has been shown that absence of the MI polymorphism of glutathione-S-transferase (GST) (GSTM1-null genotype) is associated with an increased risk of isocyanate-induced asthma. It has been speculated that homozygosity for the GSTP1 valine allele could be a marker of reduced susceptibility for TDI-induced asthma.[16]

In addition to genetic factors, there are other predisposing issues related to the development of OA. A spectrum of industrial, climatic, personal, social, and other health factors have been identified as having the capacity to modulate the development of respiratory disease.

WORKPLACE FACTORS

These include the structure and inherent reactivity of the agents encountered in the workplace. Equally important are the employer's policies related to worker safety, i.e., access to material safety data sheets (MSDS), functional protective equipment, and enforcement of safety policies and appropriate industrial hygiene practices.

CLIMATIC CONDITIONS

Meteorological conditions can modify worker response to an inhaled antigen or irritant. Prevailing winds will determine the direction of an irritant stack emission. The presence of seasonal allergens or environmental pollutants (e.g., diesel exhaust particles) can augment the response to work-related antigens.[17]

TOBACCO AND RECREATIONAL DRUG ABUSE

Tobacco abuse continues to be a major problem in the USA, with an even greater prevalence in other parts of the world. The effect of smoking on the development of OA remains complex and controversial. A recent review by Siracusa et al. revealed little evidence of an increased risk of OA in workers who are smokers. However, there was evidence of an increased risk of new-onset sensitivity in smoking workers exposed to several HMW and LMW agents.[18] Clearly there is an association between chronic smoking and a higher incidence of and morbidity from respiratory tract infections. Smoking also adversely impacts asthma by enhancing inflammation, increasing airway permeability and abrogating normal healing processes.

Chronic cannabis smoking is also quite prevalent and is associated with increased symptoms of chronic bronchitis and decreased lung function. There is also an additive effect between cannabis and tobacco abuse on adversely impacting the lung.[19] Beyond these general adverse effects, nothing specific is known about the relevance of cannabis smoking to development of OA.

RESPIRATORY INFECTION

Viral infections are well recognized as important triggers of asthma exacerbations.[20] This must always be considered in the context of any worker presenting with suspected OA. Insights into the potential role of viral pathogens causing asthma have been enhanced by the employment of molecular detection techniques, i.e., polymerase chain reactions (PCR). In the 1970s viral infections were believed to be responsible for triggering 25% of asthma flares, whereas recent application of PCR detected viruses in 85% of reported episodes of cough, wheezing, and reduced peakflow.[21] A number of mechanisms have been proposed to explain the association between viral infections and asthma, including direct epithelial injury, development of viral-specific IgE, and enhanced inflammatory mediator release. Bacterial infections of the paranasal sinuses are also associated with deterioration of underlying asthma.

NONSPECIFIC BHR

BHR is the physiologic hallmark of both nonoccupational and OA. Its presence correlates with bronchoalveolar inflammatory cell infiltrate, especially eosinophils and metachromatic cells. Prior observations that occupationally induced BHR intensifies with late-phase reactions triggered by industrial agents,[22] and diminishes or normalizes after cessation of exposure,[23] suggest that BHR genetically predisposes to the development of OA. It is unclear whether the genetic tendency to nonspecific BHR is a continuous physiologic state or whether it varies over time, fluctuating according to degrees of exposure to environmental agents. Preliminary data suggest that nonspecific BHR waxes and wanes according to a variety of extrinsic factors.

Although the measurement of BHR provides quantitative insight in variable airflow obstruction, the relationship between BHR and respiratory symptoms is weak. Approximately 50% of subjects with BHR report no respiratory symptoms. BHR follows a normal distribution throughout the population, with approximately 20% of individuals without evidence of asthma or other respiratory disease having mild BHR. Although nonspecific BHR is a feature of OA, it is clearly not diagnostic of asthma. Nonspecific BHR is present in individuals with a variety of other respiratory disorders, including viral respiratory infections, current and past tobacco abuse, chronic bronchitis, atopy without asthma, and hypersensitivity pneumonitis, among others.

The relationship between nonspecific BHR and asthmatic symptoms was the subject of a large study of nearly 1400 men employed in various industries. Approximately 60% of asymptomatic workers had a PC_{20} at or below 8 mg/ml of methacholine. More importantly, approximately 35% of workers with physician-diagnosed asthma had a PC_{20} greater than 8 mg/ml. Thus, the sensitivity of a PC_{20} at or below 8 mg/ml in identifying physician-diagnosed asthma was 61% with a specificity of 85%. Ultimately, the positive predictive value of a methacholine challenge test to identify asthma was only 10%, but its negative predictive value was 99%.[24]

CLINICAL, IMMUNOLOGIC, AND PATHOLOGIC FEATURES OF OCCUPATIONAL ASTHMA

From a clinical and pathologic perspective, new-onset OA can be divided into immunologic and nonimmunologic patterns. The immunologic class can be further divided into classic IgE-mediated and polyimmunologic

SIGNIFICANCE OF NONSPECIFIC BRONCHIAL HYPERRESPONSIVENESS (NSBHR) IN THE DIAGNOSIS OF OCCUPATIONAL ASTHMA

NSBHR is regarded as a major characteristic of symptomatic asthma

NSBHR correlates with bronchoalveolar inflammatory cell infiltrates, especially eosinophils and metachromatic cells

The genetic proclivity toward NSBHR may predispose individuals to the development of occupational asthma

NSBHR probably waxes and wanes secondary to a variety of environmental and host influences

NSBHR is found in normal, asymptomatic individuals, but is also associated with viral respiratory infections, cigarette smoking, exposure to certain pollutants (e.g., ozone), and a variety of disease states (see text)

The positive predictive value of NSBHR for the presence of asthma is only about 10%, whereas the negative predictive value is about 99%

variants. The nonimmunologic category can be divided into RADS, reflex bronchoconstriction, and pharmacologic bronchoconstriction (Fig. 49.3).

ALLERGIC OR IMMUNOLOGIC OCCUPATIONAL ASTHMA

New-onset, allergic OA requires a latent period during which sensitization develops. Frequently, the exposure involves inhalation of soluble HMW proteins, glycoproteins, or other peptide-containing moieties, which in a predisposed individual result in the development of a specific IgE sensitization. There are a number of LMW agents capable of acting as haptens that cross-link with human protein to induce an IgE-mediated response. The initial step in the development of an allergic reaction is the interaction of a specific work allergen with IgE-sensitized mast cells, basophils, and other cells in airway tissue. IgE-sensitized mast cells secrete and generate bioactive mediators that facilitate development of allergic inflammation. The respiratory CD4 T cells produce predominantly type 2 helper (Th2) cytokines IL-4, IL-5, and IL-13 that play essential roles in asthma by enhancing growth, differentiation, and recruitment of eosinophils, basophils, mast cells, and IgE-producing B cells. It has recently been found that the CD4 T cells in the lungs of patients with asthma express the receptor of invariant natural killer (NK) T cells that act in concert with conventional CD4 T cells modulating inflammation in asthma.[25] The hallmark response of invariant NK T cells is their rapid and copious production of cytokines, including interferon-γ, IL-4, IL-13, IL-5, granulocyte–macrophage colony-stimulating factor, and tumor necrosis factor-α. It is not known what roles invariant NK T cells play in OA, but these recent observations offer exciting opportunities for future research.

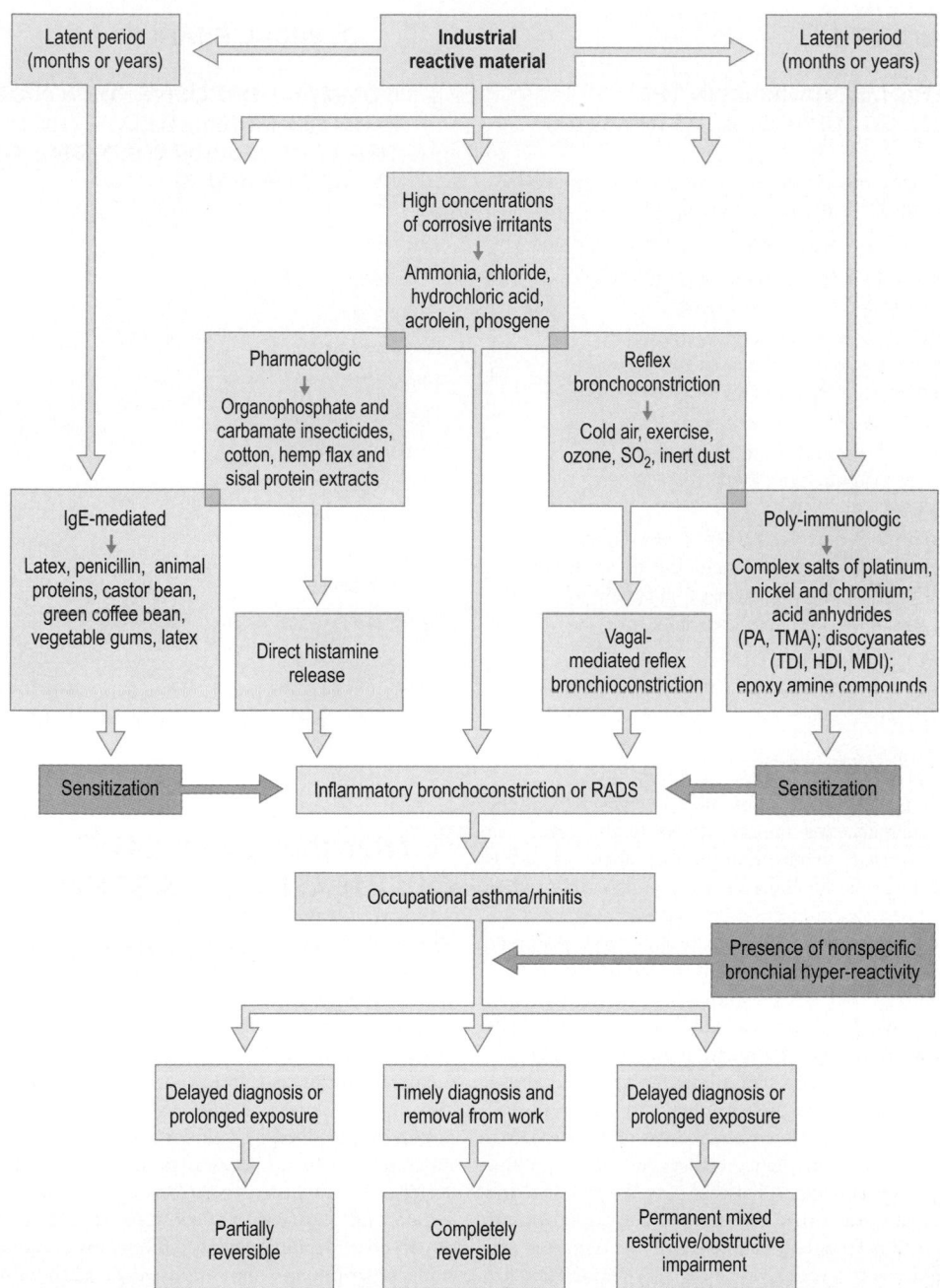

Fig. 49.3 Pathogenetic variants of occupational asthma (OA). Schematic diagram of the pathogenetic variants of OA depicting two basic mechanisms: immunologic and nonimmunologic OA. The latter has three subcategories: inflammatory, pharmacologic, and reflex bronchoconstriction. (Modified from Bardana EJ, Montanaro A. The pathogenesis and natural history of occupationally induced airway obstruction; pp 267–281. In: Bardana EJ, Montanaro A, O'Hollaren MT (eds) Occupational Asthma. Philadelphia: Hanley and Belfus; 1992, with permission.)

In addition to the classic IgE-mediated response to protein allergens, selected LMW agents are capable of inducing allergic OA by acting as copolymerizing agents producing limited immunologic responses. These include the complex salts of platinum, nickel, chromium, penicillin, and the epoxy amine compounds.

There are a group of LMW agents, including isocyanates, the acid anhydrides, and plicatic acid, that are capable of inducing immunologic OA, but the pathogenetic mechanisms are only partially elucidated.[13, 26] One critical requirement common to all chemical allergens is the requirement to form a complex with protein. It is believed that chemical

PATHOGENETIC MECHANISMS IN THE INDUCTION OF OCCUPATIONAL ASTHMA (OA)

OA is caused by two basic mechanisms: immunologically induced inflammation and several forms of irritant-induced inflammation

Most cases of OA result from exposure to work-related allergens

The majority of patients with allergic OA develop preceding or concomitant upper-airway and ocular symptoms

The allergic asthmatic response in OA is characterized by a pattern of early mast cell activation, eosinophil infiltration, fibroblast and collagen deposition, selective T-cell activation, epithelial sloughing, and mucous hypersecretion

Inflammatory bronchoconstriction and reactive airways dysfunction syndrome are similar, if not identical, disorders embodying nonimmunologic asthma

Most instances of OA are not a single, simple, or homogeneous entity, even when a single specific causal factor can be identified

Any given industrial reactant can probably induce OA by more than a single mechanism, and more than a single mechanism may be operative in any given patient

The pathogenesis of immunologic occupational asthma is similar to that of nonoccupational asthma

COMMON CORROSIVE OR NOXIOUS EXPOSURE AGENTS INCRIMINATED IN THE INDUCTION OF REACTIVE AIRWAYS DYSFUNCTION SYNDROME (RADS)

Chlorine

Phosgene

Sulfuric acid

Smoke inhalation

Phosphoric acid

Hydrochloric acid

Hydrogen sulfide

Metam sodium

Anhydrous ammonia

Toluene diisocyanate

Calcium oxide

Spray paint fumes (without isocyanates)

Asthma symptoms generally follow with work-related obstruction characterized by chest tightness, cough, and dyspnea, which may intensify during the work week.

NONIMMUNOLOGIC OCCUPATIONAL ASTHMA

The most common form of nonallergic OA is RADS, which results from a high-level exposure to a potent respiratory irritant at work. The onset is abrupt and is not associated with preceding ocular or upper-airway symptoms. Many of the incriminated agents are gases soluble in water and characteristically result in acute ocular, skin, and mucous membrane burns depending on the corrosive properties of the agent, the exposure concentration, and the duration of exposure. RADS was originally described by Gandevia in 1970[27] and referred to as "acute inflammatory bronchoconstriction." These early cases were related to accidental exposure to corrosive agents such as chlorine, hydrogen sulfide, and phosgene. Airflow obstruction followed within hours secondary to a chemically induced bronchitis or bronchopneumonia. In the initial descriptions, symptoms usually peaked within a week and usually regressed over the next several months. Some of these patients went on to manifest symptoms of chronic asthma or asymptomatic BHR. The symptom complex was redefined by Brooks and Lockey in 1981 when the term RADS was initially coined.[28] There was some initial controversy as to whether irritant-induced asthma was clearly distinguishable from allergic OA. After considerable case analysis, Alberts and doPico presented their rationale for relying on the American College of Chest Physicians (ACCP) Consensus Criteria[29] (Table 49.3). Because past and current tobacco abuse and atopy are independently associated with nonspecific BHR, and since the degree of BHR is not specified in the ACCP diagnostic criteria, five minor criteria (Table 49.4) have been

allergens are inherently protein-reactive, or must be converted at the tissue level into a protein-reactive moiety. By using the skin as a paradigm, it is assumed that chemical respiratory allergens access viable epithelium and form stable linkages with protein to become immunogenic.

Such chemical allergens must possess the innate ability to trigger type 2 immune responses resulting in sensitization of the respiratory mucosa and ultimately an allergic reaction. Recent studies have demonstrated an overexpression of matrix metalloproteinases (MMPs), including MMP-9, with resultant increase in airway inflammation and remodeling that results in the expression of asthmatic symptoms. As intimated above, there are also associations between respiratory allergy to certain chemicals and genes within the major histocompatibility complex (MHC) and, in particular, associations with genes coding for GSTs. In this respect, there is an apparent association between certain GST loci and OA to isocyanates.[13] It is possible that glutathione, a ubiquitous intracellular and extracellular transfer agent, plays a role in the transport and binding of reactive chemicals to a variety of biologically important macromolecules. Despite these recent insights, there are many chemicals for which the pathogenesis of OA remains elusive. Two large groups of chemicals in this category include certain rare wood dusts and a variety of copolymerizing compounds or hardening agents used in the manufacture of resins or plastics. The development of animal models may facilitate a better understanding of the immunopathogenesis of OA induced by these agents.

The clinical presentation of the typical patient with new-onset, allergic OA frequently parallels the symptoms of patients with classic allergic disorders. After a latent period of months or years, many develop upper-airway and ocular symptoms of occupational rhinitis or rhinoconjunctivitis.

Table 49.3 Criteria for the diagnosis of reactive airways dysfunction syndrome

American College of Chest Physicians consensus (major criteria)[29]
Documented absence of preceding respiratory complaints
Onset of symptoms after a single-exposure incident or accident
Exposure to very high concentrations of a gas, smoke, fume, or vapor with irritant properties
Onset of symptoms within 24 hours of exposure with persistence of symptoms for at least 3 months
Symptoms simulating asthma with cough, wheeze, and dyspnea
Presence of airflow obstruction on pulmonary function testing and/or presence of nonspecific bronchial hyperresponsiveness
All other pulmonary diseases excluded

Minor criteria[30]
Absence of an atopic state
Absence of peripheral or pulmonary eosinophilia
Absence of cigarette smoking for 10 years
Bronchial hyperreactivity of moderate to severe degree (i.e., positive at methacholine concentration $\leq$ 8 mg/ml)
Histopathology and/or bronchoalveolar lavage showing minimal lymphocytic inflammation

proposed which, if met, would strengthen the diagnosis considerably[30] (Table 49.3). There is growing support for the utilization of an 8 mg/ml concentration of methacholine as the upper limit for a positive test.

There are only limited pathologic studies related to RADS. Most of these studies have demonstrated a predominance of lymphocytes in bronchoalveolar lavage (BAL) with subepithelial thickening and fibrosis. The pathogenesis is postulated to be the result of extensive denudation of the bronchial epithelium with resultant airway inflammation. It is felt that nonspecific macrophage activation and mast cell degranulation result in the release of proinflammatory chemotactic and toxic mediators.

Nonallergic OA may also be secondary to agents producing a direct pharmacologic action on the respiratory mucosa (Fig. 49.3), e.g., organophosphate and carbamate insecticides. In sufficient doses, these agents inhibit acetylcholinesterase, which potentiates the effect of acetylcholine released from vagal fibers innervating bronchial smooth muscles and producing transient bronchoconstriction.

Reflex bronchoconstriction could be considered the third variant of nonallergic OA. It is distinguished from RADS by the intensity and nature of the exposure, i.e., chronic, low-to-moderate-dose, irritant-induced asthma. Certain chemicals and inert gases are felt to have the capacity to cause reflex bronchospasm by disrupting the delicate balance of adrenergic control involved in the maintenance of bronchial tone. However, it is unlikely that this mechanism induces new-onset OA. It is more likely operative in patients with pre-existent subclinical asthma, asymptomatic BHR, or atopy.[31]

PATIENT EVALUATION AND DIFFERENTIAL DIAGNOSIS OF OCCUPATIONAL ASTHMA

Though it has significant limitations, the medical history is a key element in the initial evaluation of OA. It should provide the examiner with clinical features of work-related airway disease and assist in confirming the linkage to one or more suspect work exposures. However, both the work and home environment need to be simultaneously evaluated for potential exposure to allergens, irritants, chemicals, or organic dusts. Because of time limitations, a questionnaire may be helpful as an added tool to amplify the interview process. The worker (through his or her employer) should provide Material Safety Data Sheets (MSDSs) on all relevant exposures. A complete medical record review can be rewarding for two major reasons: (1) acquisition of information of which the worker had no awareness or recollection; and (2) to corroborate other important historical benchmarks.

In reaching final conclusions related to OA, the history alone has been found to be totally unacceptable. Though the history has been found to have a high degree of sensitivity (87%), it has a low specificity (22%) for the diagnosis of OA.[32] Patient recall of past symptoms, illnesses, and medical care is often unreliable and inconsistent.

The physical examination should be carefully conducted to record the presence of ocular, nasal, oropharyngeal, and pulmonary abnormalities. It is not at all unusual for a worker with new-onset OA to have a normal examination. In those instances where the medical history is compelling, but the examination and spirometry are normal, an assessment of BHR can be useful.

LABORATORY STUDIES

The application of immunologic testing in the diagnosis of allergic OA is limited. The presence of allergen-specific IgE antibodies may be very helpful in the diagnosis and to some degree prognostication in the case of HMW allergens. However, data derived solely from cutaneous or serologic studies should not be used to conclude that a putative allergen was responsible for the OA. The presence of serum or skin-sensitizing antibody alone cannot be equated to the presence of a 'specific symptomatic state.' Antibodies of the IgG or IgE class are found in both symptomatic and unaffected workers and their value is that of a biologic marker of prior exposure. The clinician must utilize all the information assembled to differentiate between a state of asymptomatic sensitization and an active allergic symptom complex.

Table 49.4 Differential diagnostic considerations in establishing a certain diagnosis of work-related asthma

Immunologic causes of asthma
Nonoccupational allergic asthma
Allergic bronchopulmonary aspergillosis
Churg–Strauss allergic granulomatosis

Infectious causes of asthma
Viral infection (rhinovirus, Rous sarcoma virus, and para-influenza types 1, 2 and 3)
Mycoplasma pneumoniae
Chlamydia pneumoniae

Pharmaceuticals (causative or trigger)
Aspirin and related nonsteroidal anti-inflammatory drugs (NSAIDs)
β-adrenergic antagonists
Sulfiting agents

Masqueraders of asthma
Organic toxic dust syndrome
Acute tracheobronchitis
Primary vocal cord dysfunction syndrome
Secondary vocal cord dysfunction (e.g., gastroesophageal reflux)
Hypersensitivity pneumonitis
Chronic paranasal sinusitis

Conditions independently associated with asthma
Industrial bronchitis
Emphysema
Bronchiolitis obliterans

CHEST RADIOGRAPHS

Radiological observations have their principal utility in either excluding or implicating alternative conditions in the differential diagnostic process. The availability of high-resolution computed tomography has been invaluable in assessing the extent of coexisting emphysema, fibrosis, bronchiectasis, or other processes that may explain the presenting symptoms. Imaging studies may also be useful in delineating the presence of sinusitis which may be contributing to lower-airway symptoms.

PULMONARY FUNCTION STUDIES

Pulmonary function studies are essential in both the diagnosis and assessment of severity of OA. The diagnosis of OA demands as an initial premise an unequivocal demonstration of reversible airflow obstruction. The American Thoracic Society (ATS) criteria require a minimum 12% increase in forced expiratory volume in 1 second (FEV_1) with bronchodilator. When assessing spirometric data from various providers, the evaluator must consider possible inadequacies in the data. It has been shown that less than 20% of spirometry tests performed at primary care practices met ATS criteria. When spirometry is normal, methacholine provocation can be employed to demonstrate significant nonspecific

BHR. It must be carried out according to ATS criteria and positive responses at concentrations above 8 mg/ml concentration should be interpreted cautiously. In this respect, it is highly likely that exhaled nitric oxide (eNO) can be used as a safe and rapid assessment in the diagnosis of OA and eventually may replace methacholine challenge.[33]

BRONCHIAL PROVOCATION STUDIES

The suspected temporal adverse effect of a putative work agent can be initially explored by serial determination of peak expiratory flow rates during a period of work abstinence and following a return to work. The information gleaned from such a study should be interpreted cautiously because the maneuver is effort-dependent and can be relied upon only when executed under direct observation using published guidelines. A more secure pragmatic approach would be to compare the degree of nonspecific BHR after a period of continuous occupational exposure with a baseline following a 3–4-week period of total abstinence from exposure to the suspected agent. Provided there are no significant changes in medication, a change in bronchial reactivity of more than two doubling concentrations (or doses) is considered significant. Alternatively, eNO could be used as the endpoint in this process, with a 20% increase in eNO at a flow rate of 250 ml regarded as significant. There are as yet

KEY CONCEPTS

CRITERIA FOR THE DIAGNOSIS OF *DE NOVO* OCCUPATIONAL ASTHMA

Absence of pre-existing bronchial asthma

Demonstration of variable airway obstruction

Rational association of either allergic or irritant symptoms with an established work-related asthmagenic agent

Demonstration of variable airway obstruction with exposure to the putative asthmagenic agent

Controlled bronchial provocation with subirritant doses of incriminated industrial agent

Regression of symptoms with timely diagnosis and removal from the incriminated agent

THERAPEUTIC PRINCIPLES

PREVENTION AND MANAGEMENT OF OCCUPATIONAL ASTHMA

Protect at-risk workers from potentially hazardous agents

Institute regular surveillance

When diagnosis is established, remove patient from all further exposure

Treat residual symptoms in accord with usual asthma management

no studies in the occupational setting to verify the use of eNO, but these are likely to be reported in the near future. A third alternative would utilize cross-shift spirometric data, i.e., pre- and post-shift spirometry over the course of an entire work week.

The gold standard confirming the causal role of a specific work-related immunogen is a controlled bronchial challenge with subirritant concentrations of the suspected immunogen. The worker must be observed for immediate as well as delayed responses for 8–12 hours. These tests are invasive, time-consuming, pose some risk to the worker, and therefore must be performed with appropriate informed consent. A limited number of medical facilities are equipped and capable of performing this type of study.

DIFFERENTIAL DIAGNOSIS

Assuming that there has been a reliable demonstration of variable airflow obstruction by reliable physiologic testing, the clinician must consider the possibility that the asthma in question is not work-related. Pre-existent asthma should be excluded particularly in an individual with an atopic phenotype in whom asthma may have existed in a subclinical state or inappropriately labeled. Since OA is linked to causes and/or conditions at work, the examiner must exclude the possibility that the asthma is related to nonoccupational allergens or irritants. Other variants of asthma such as allergic bronchopulmonary aspergillosis, aspirin-sensitivity syndrome, and Churg–Strauss allergic granulomatosis must be excluded. Finally, unrelated disorders masquerading as asthma must be excluded. Chief among these disorders is vocal cord dysfunction (VCD). VCD is a common and frequently unrecognized masquerader and confounder of asthma. It may occur in up to 40% of patients who present with treatment-resistant asthma: one-quarter of these have isolated VCD, and the remainder have coexistent asthma. The diagnosis of VCD is dependent on a high index of suspicion related to the clinical presentation and the performance of flexible fiberoptic rhinolaryngoscopy during a symptomatic state in order to visualize the anterior portion of the vocal cords adducting during inspiration while the posterior glottis remains open (the so-called posterior chink). Other disorders that should be considered in the differential

diagnostic process include chronic bronchitis, congestive heart failure, hypersensitivity pneumonitis, and organic dust toxic syndrome, among others (Table 49.4).

PREVENTION AND MANAGEMENT

The most effective manner of preventing OA is to protect at-risk workers from potentially hazardous exposures. This requires the employer to adopt and enforce optimum industrial hygiene measures that will reduce or eliminate ambient levels of known immunogens or respiratory irritants. This can be accomplished by mandating approved respirators that have been properly fit-tested, by installation of effective exhaust systems, or by development of enclosed and automated robotic processes. Many employers conduct surveillance of their workers and their industrial hygiene practices by regular measurements of potentially harmful agents and regular medical examinations focused on airway integrity (e.g., chest radiographs, spirometry).

Management of OA is identical to that of non-OA except the patient must be removed from further exposure to the causative agent in a timely manner. Therapeutically, a combination of anti-inflammatory and bronchodilator drugs is advocated. However, the use of pharmacologic treatment is not a substitute for complete avoidance.

PROGNOSIS

The major determinants of patient outcome include the total duration of exposure, asthma severity at diagnosis, and the pathogenic mechanisms operative in the original induction of OA.[34] In addition, coexisting factors such as cigarette smoking, chronic sinusitis, and gastro esophageal reflux disorder (GERD) may also play an important role as prognostic modifiers. Prompt removal of the patient with OA from the offending immunogen or irritant should result in clinical improvement (Fig. 49.3). Recently, Ameille and Descatha[34] reviewed the literature on the outcome of OA and reported a number of conclusions: (1) nonspecific BHR in OA generally improves following cessation of exposure and occurs over several years; (2) PC_{20} or PD_{20} methacholine at the time of diagnosis is the best predictor of BHR during subsequent follow-up; (3) prognosis does not appear to be influenced by the molecular weight of the causal agent; (4) continuing airway inflammation is associated with persistence of symptoms and nonspecific BHR;

and (5) significant reduction of immunogenic exposure could represent an acceptable compromise in instances where exposure cannot be totally avoided, but can be reduced to a threshold level at which the patient is unaware of ongoing symptoms. The majority of motivated patients who are diagnosed in a timely fashion and removed from further exposure achieve good control of their asthma and are capable of resuming full employment in an alternative job. This should parallel what generally happens in nonoccupational asthma when an avoidable allergen is removed, e.g., cat.

In instances where the diagnosis of OA is delayed, or where the worker refuses to comply with warnings regarding avoidance, chronic symptoms persist with concomitant pulmonary deterioration. It should be noted that *specific* BHR to an inciting agent may persist after removal from further exposure in individuals who are asymptomatic, who no longer use medications, and who lack *nonspecific* BHR.[35]

▌ REFERENCES ▌

1. Brooks SM. Bronchial asthma of occupational origin. Scand J Work Environ Health 1977; 3: 53.

2. Rischitelli DG. A workers' compensation primer. Ann Allergy Asthma Immunol 1999; 83: 614.

3. Smith DD. Acute inhalation injury: how to assess, how to treat. J Respir Dis 1999; 20: 405.

4. Diem JE, Jones RN, Hendrick DJ, et al. Five-year longitudinal study of workers employed in a new toluene diisocyanates manufacturing plant. Am Rev Respir Dis 1982; 126: 420.

5. Chan-Yeung M, Desjardins A. Bronchial hyperresponsiveness and level of exposure in occupational asthma due to western red cedar (*Thuja plicata*). Am Rev Respir Dis 1992; 146: 1606.

6. Walusiak J, Henke W, Gorski P, et al. Respiratory allergy in apprentice bakers: do occupational allergies follow the allergic march? Allergy 2004; 59: 442.

7. Koh YY, Sun YH, Lim HS, et al. Effect of inhaled budesonide on bronchial hyperresponsiveness in adolescents with clinical remission of asthma. Chest 2001; 120: 1140.

8. Nish WA, Schwietz LA. Underdiagnosis of asthma in young adults presenting for USAF basic training. Ann Allergy 1992; 69: 239.

9. Nicholson PJ, Cullinan P, Newman-Taylor AJ, et al. Evidence based guidelines for the prevention, identification, and management of occupational asthma. Occup Environ Med 2005; 62: 290.

10. Kogevmas M, Anto JM, Sunyer J, et al. Occupational asthma in Europe and other industrialized areas: a population based study. Lancet 1999; 359: 50.

11. Piipari R, Keskinen H. Agents causing occupational asthma in Finland in 1986–2002: cow epithelium bypassed by moulds from moisture-damaged buildings. Clin Exp Allergy 2005; 35: 1632.

12. Blumenthal MN. The role of genetics in the development of asthma and atopy. Curr Opin Allergy Clin Immunol 2005; 5: 141.

13. Mapp CE. Genetics and the occupational environment. Curr Opin Allergy Clin Immunol 2005; 5: 113.

14. Cookson WOCM. Genetic aspects of atopic allergy. In: Van Hoge Hamsten M, Wichman M (eds) 30 Years with IgE. Copenhagen: Munksgaard; 1998: 13.

15. Newman-Taylor AJ. Role of human leukocyte antigen phenotype and exposure in development of occupational asthma. Curr Opin Allergy Clin Immunol 2001; 1: 157.

16. Mapp CE, Fryer AA, DeMarzo H, et al. Glutathione S-transferase G-STP1 is a susceptibility gene for occupational asthma induced by isocyanates. J Allergy Clin Immunol 2002; 99: 245.

17. Parnia S, Frew AJ. Is diesel the cause for the increase in allergic disease? Ann Allergy Asthma Immunol 2001; 87: 18.

18. Siracusa A, Marabini A, Folletti I, et al. Smoking and occupational asthma. Clin Exp Allergy 2006; 36: 577.

19. Hall W, Solonij N. Adverse effects of cannabis. Lancet 1998; 352: 1611.

20. Contoli M, Canamori G, Mallia P, et al. Mechanisms of respiratory virus-induced asthma exacerbations. Clin Exp Allergy 2005; 35: 137.

21. Wark PA, Johnston SL, Moric I, et al. Neutrophil degranulation and cell lysis in association with severity of virus-induced asthma. Eur Respir J 2002; 19: 68.

22. Cartier A. Occupational asthma: what have we learned? J Allergy Clin Immunol 1998; 102: S90.

23. Malo J-L, Ghezzo H. Recovery of methacholine responsiveness after end of exposure in occupational asthma. Am J Respir Crit Care Med 2004; 169: 1304.

24. Enarson DA, Vedal S, Schulzer M, et al. Asthma, asthma-like symptoms, chronic bronchitis and the degree of bronchial hyperresponsiveness in epidemiological surveys. Am Rev Respir Dis 1987; 136: 612.

25. Akbari O, Fane JL, Hoyte EG, et al. CD$_4^+$ invariant T-cell-receptor$^+$ natural killer T cells in bronchial asthma. N Engl J Med 2006; 354: 1117.

26. Kimber I, Dearman RJ. What makes a chemical a respiratory sensitizer. Curr Opin Allergy Clin Immunol 2005; 5: 119.

27. Gandevia B. Occupational asthma. Med J Aust 1970; 2: 332.

28. Brooks SM, Lockey J. Reactive airways dysfunction syndrome (RADS); a newly defined occupational disease. Am Rev Respir Dis 1981; 123(suppl): A133.

29. Alberts WM, doPico G. Reactive airways dysfunction syndrome. Chest 1996; 104: 1618.

30. Bardana EJ. Reactive airways dysfunction syndrome (RADS): guidelines for diagnosis and treatment and insight into likely prognosis. Ann Allergy Asthma Immunol 1999; 83: 583.

31. Brooks SM, McCluskey JD. When to suspect reactive airways dysfunction syndrome. J Respir Dis 2002; 23: 506.

32. Malo J-L, Ghezzo H, L'Archeveque J, et al. Is the clinical history a satisfactory means of diagnosing occupational asthma? Am Rev Respir Dis 1991; 143: 528.

33. Berkman N, Avital A, Brewer E, et al. Exhaled nitric oxide in the diagnosis of asthma: comparison with bronchial provocation tests. Thorax 2005; 60: 383.

34. Ameille J, Descatha A. Outcome of occupational asthma. Curr Opin Allergy Clin Immunol 2005; 5: 125.

35. Gautrin D, Lemiere C. Persistence of airway responsiveness to occupational agents: what does it matter?. Curr Opin Allergy Clin Immunol 2002; 2: 123.

part 6

SYSTEMIC IMMUNE DISEASES

Mechanisms of autoimmunity

Antony Rosen

50

Human autoimmune diseases occur frequently (affecting in aggregate more than 5% of the population worldwide), and impose a significant burden of morbidity and mortality on the human population.[1] Autoimmune diseases are defined as diseases in which immune responses to specific self-antigens contribute to the ongoing tissue damage that occurs in that disease. Both the specificity of the immune response and its role in tissue damage are central components of the definition. Autoimmune diseases may be either tissue-specific (e.g., thyroid, β-cells of the pancreas), where unique tissue-specific antigens are targeted, or may be more systemic, in which multiple tissues are affected, and a variety of apparently ubiquitously expressed autoantigens are targeted.[2]

Although the definition appears relatively simple in concept, the complexity of this spectrum of disorders is enormous, and has greatly challenged elucidation of simple shared mechanisms. This complexity affects almost every domain, including genetics, phenotypic expression, and kinetics. In the latter case, there is frequently a prolonged period (weeks to months) between initial onset of symptoms and development of the diagnostic phenotype, and disease may vary in expression in the same individual over time. However, in spite of this enormous complexity, there is a striking association of the clinical phenotype with the targets of the autoimmune response. This association is, in fact, so strong that autoantibodies have been used for diagnosis and prognosis in human autoimmune diseases.[2] For example, autoantibodies recognizing thyroid peroxidase are found in patients with autoimmune thyroiditis, autoantibodies to the Sm splicing ribonucleoprotein complex are diagnostic of systemic lupus erythematosus (SLE), and autoantibodies recognizing topoisomerase-1 are found in patients with the diffuse form of scleroderma. The immune response in autoimmune diseases has features of an adaptive immune response (usually directed against exogenous antigens), but its targets are autoantigens. Since the adaptive immune response is initiated when suprathreshold concentrations of molecules with structure not previously tolerized by the host are encountered in a proimmune context, the association of specific autoantibodies with distinct clinical phenotypes provides critical clues to understanding the initiation and propagation of autoimmune diseases.

This chapter highlights some of the mechanistic principles that underlie autoimmune diseases. The extraordinary breadth and complexity of this disease spectrum mean that the areas included cannot nearly encompass everything relevant.

■ THE DISTINCT PHASES IN THE DEVELOPMENT OF AUTOIMMUNITY ■

A major barrier to understanding mechanisms of autoimmunity comes from difficulty in defining early events in these diseases. Since diseases are only recognizable after development of the diagnostic phenotype, there has been the tendency to interpret findings made at diagnosis with findings present at initiation. By studying the development of autoantibodies over time in patients who subsequently manifest an autoimmune disease, significant recent data have demonstrated that this is only partly true, and that autoimmune diseases should be operationally viewed as having two phases—initiation and propagation.[3] In the case of type I diabetes, development of islet cell autoantibodies frequently precedes diabetes, and additional islet cell autoantibodies accrue over time.[4] Similarly, autoantibodies recognizing citrullinated proteins (rheumatoid arthritis (RA)-specific autoantibodies; see below) may precede the development of RA.[5] These findings might indicate that a threshold needs to be exceeded in terms of tissue damage before symptoms manifest, or that there are two distinct phases in disease development, one marked by

---

■ KEY CONCEPTS

BARRIERS TO DEFINING MECHANISMS OF HUMAN AUTOIMMUNE DISEASE

>> Genetic and phenotypic complexity

>> Interval between initiating events and development of diagnostic phenotype

KEY CONCEPTS

AUTOANTIBODIES IN AUTOIMMUNE DISEASES

>> Some autoantibodies precede the development of any symptoms by years (e.g., antinuclear antibodies and anti-phospholipid antibodies in systemic lupus erythematosus (SLE), anti-CCP in rheumatoid arthritis)

>> Some autoantibodies only occur at around the time of onset of disease manifestations (e.g., anti-Sm and anti-RNP in SLE)

>> There is a striking association of specific autoantibodies with distinct clinical phenotypes (e.g., anti-topoisomerase-1 with diffuse scleroderma and interstitial lung disease)

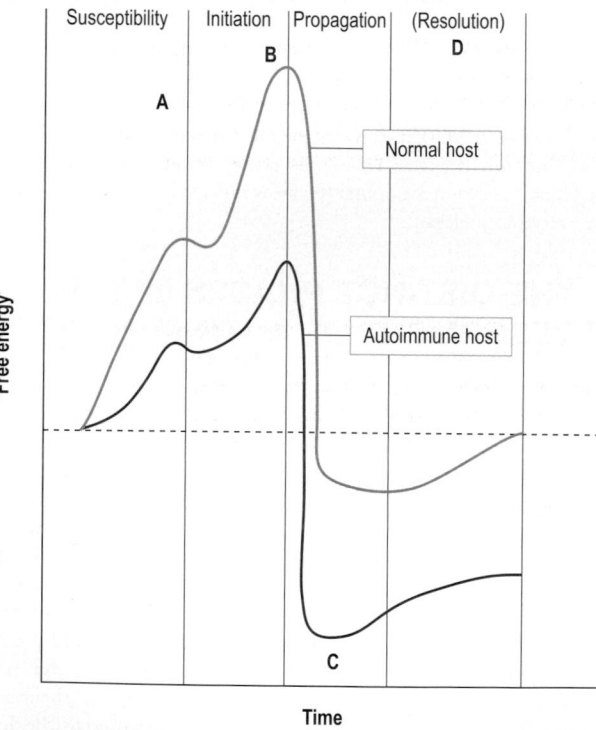

A	Susceptibility
• Impaired tolerance induction • Impaired production of regulatory T cells • Altered immune signaling thresholds	

B	Initiation
• Suprathreshold concentration of autoantigens • Non-tolerized structure • Pro-immune context - infection, malignancy, exposure to adjuvants	

C	Propagation
• Acquisition of adjuvant properties by disease specific autoantigens • Increased autoantigen expression in the target tissue • Immune effector pathways generate/expose autoantigen, which further drives the immune response	

production of a group of autoantibodies, the second by autoamplifying tissue damage. In a landmark study in SLE, Harley and colleagues have provided important insights into this issue.[3] They analyzed sera collected from patients in the US military who subsequently developed SLE. Strikingly, autoantibodies in SLE could be divided into two groups: (1) those that precede the diagnosis of SLE by several years—these included antinuclear antibodies and antiphospholipid antibodies; and (2) those which occurred around the time of onset of symptoms—these included anti-Sm, anti-RNP, and, to a lesser extent, anti-DNA. The observation that one group of autoantibodies precedes symptoms in SLE and that another group appears coincident with the phenotype strongly suggests that the groups mark distinct events in the development of autoimmune disease. Members of the first group are likely markers of disease initiation; members of the second group are likely markers of disease propagation. The antigens targeted by the immune system in this latter phase (i.e., associated with clinical disease) are more likely to have some function in disease propagation, possibly through their possession of proinflammatory or adjuvant functions[6] (see below).

It is therefore useful to examine the development of autoimmune diseases in four phases (Fig. 50.1):

1. Susceptibility phase—before disease, but where one or several preconditions for later initiation are satisfied. This includes impaired tolerance induction, or altered immune signaling thresholds. The susceptibility phase can be either inherited or acquired (and in many diseases, both), permanent or transient.

2. Initiation phase—before onset of clinical disease, but marked by the presence of an autoimmune response (e.g., in the case of SLE—antiphospholipid antibodies).

3. Propagation phase—this corresponds with the onset of clinical disease, marked by propagation-specific immune responses (e.g., in the case of SLE, anti-Sm antibodies).

Fig. 50.1 Autoimmunity: the free-energy model. Autoimmune diseases result from a complex interplay of pathways and events which initially allow autoreactivity to manifest (A), and then, after an initiating event (B), allow development of self-sustaining tissue damage (C). Each of these phases can be viewed as "energy states." Initiation does not occur spontaneously, but requires displacement from equilibrium through exogenous stimuli. The amount of energy input in an autoimmune host required for initiation is lower than that needed in a normal host, where the barriers restraining development of autoimmunity are very stringent. Factors that can decrease the "activation energy" for initiation include abnormalities in tolerance induction, regulatory T-cell (Treg) development, or immune signaling thresholds. Disease initiation is marked by the presence of autoimmunity, but precedes the diagnostic clinical phenotype. The propagation phase—the lowest energy state—is marked by a feed-forward cycle of autoimmunity and tissue damage, in which immune effector pathways cause damage and provide antigen to drive the ongoing immune response. This phase no longer requires significant exogenous energy input to maintain the cycle. In normal hosts, pathways of immunoregulation may dampen this feed-forward loop, and allow resolution to occur (D). Such immunoregulation is likely absent or fails in autoimmune hosts.

4. Regulation/resolution phase—it should also be noted that in many cases during disease propagation, immunoregulatory pathways are also activated, which may result in natural inhibition of clinical disease over time. In rare cases, these inhibitory pathways can lead to permanent resolution. This resolution phase will not be discussed further here but its existence provides important evidence that homeostasis can be re-established even after the amplified phenotype develops.

PHASE I: SUSCEPTIBILITY

Although autoimmune diseases in humans are genetically complex, significant advances in understanding have occurred over the past several years. In some cases, advances have come from the study of autoimmunity with mendelian patterns of inheritance (e.g., APECED, IPEX, C1q deficiency). Advances have also come from genetic association studies of various autoimmune phenotypes (e.g., SLE, type I diabetes mellitus). There have also been important advances in the genetics of autoimmunity in several mouse models. These studies highlight a critical role for pathways of tolerance induction, immunoregulation, and setpoints/thresholds for immune signaling in avoiding emergence of autoimmunity.

Incomplete thymic tolerance induction predisposes to autoimmunity

Significant insights into basic mechanisms can derive from the study of rare human phenotypes. This has been true for autoimmunity, where several monogenic disorders have defined important pathogenic principles. Autoimmune polyendocrine syndrome type I (APS1), also called autoimmune polyendocrinopathy candidiasis ectodermal dystrophy (APECED), is a rare disease in which patients develop multiple autoimmune diseases, often beginning in childhood.[7] While candidiasis and ectodermal dystrophy (including involvement of enamel and nails, as well as keratopathy) are features of the disease, the syndrome is characterized by striking autoimmunity directed against multiple different target tissues. Autoimmune processes include autoimmune hypoparathyroidism, Addison's disease,

autoimmune gastritis with pernicious anemia, type I diabetes, thyroid disease, autoimmune hepatitis, and celiac disease, as well as gonadal failure. Numerous autoantigens have been defined as targets of autoimmunity in APS1, and include enzymes specifically expressed in various endocrine tissues (e.g., steroid 21-hydroxylase, specific for adrenal cortex; steroid 17α-hydroxylase, found in adrenal cortex and gonads; GAD65, found in pancreatic islets, and thyroid peroxidase). The genetic basis of APS1 was mapped to a gene on chromosome 21q22.3, subsequently termed *AIRE* (for autoimmune regulator). *AIRE* expression is highest in the thymus, where it is expressed in medullary thymic epithelial cells. Several predicted structural features of the AIRE protein and its localization in nuclear dots suggested that the protein might be a transcriptional regulator; and significant evidence for this proposal was obtained *in vitro*. Several *AIRE*-deficient mouse models were subsequently generated, which allowed the definition of important pathogenic pathways in APS1 that are likely broadly relevant to the mechanisms of autoimmunity in general. Thus, mice deficient for *AIRE* developed various autoimmune phenotypes, resembling those found in human APS1. These included multiorgan lymphocytic infiltration, autoantibodies, as well as autoimmune eye disease. In an elegant series of experiments, Mathis and colleagues demonstrated that AIRE regulates expression in thymic epithelial cells of various peripheral autoantigens normally expressed exclusively in endocrine target tissues.[8] Thus, AIRE appears to control the ectopic expression in the thymus of tissue-restricted autoantigens, and to provide an antigen source against which to establish central tolerance.[8]

In recent studies, additional strong support for this model has been provided. Anderson and colleagues demonstrated that autoimmune eye disease in AIRE-deficient mice develops as the result of loss of thymic expression of a single eye antigen, interphotoreceptor retinoid-binding protein (IRBP).[9] Interestingly, lack of IRBP expression in the thymus, even in the presence of AIRE expression, is sufficient to induce eye-specific autoimmunity. These data demonstrate that expression of peripheral autoantigens in the thymus constitutes a major barrier to the subsequent development of autoimmunity against these peripheral sites. Although it is likely that similar principles apply to ubiquitously expressed autoantigens targeted in systemic autoimmune diseases, there are currently minimal data directly addressing this issue.

Impaired clearance and tolerance induction by apoptotic cells: susceptibility defect in systemic autoimmunity

Although little is known in humans about the thymic pathways of tolerance induction to ubiquitously expressed autoantigens, there is accumulating evidence to suggest that in the periphery apoptotic cells play an important role in providing a source of autoantigens against which the organism becomes tolerant.[10] Apoptotic cells are generally very efficiently cleared by phagocytic cells; these events are normally associated with the production of anti-inflammatory cytokines and result in tolerance induction.[11] Interestingly, early components of the classical complement pathway (e.g., C1q and C4) and C-reactive protein are required for efficient apoptotic cell clearance, with production of interleukin-10 (IL-10) and transforming growth factor-β (TGF-β). It is of particular note therefore that homozygous C1q deficiency is associated with a striking susceptibility to SLE, suggesting that rapid, efficient, tolerance-inducing clearance of apoptotic cells may play a similar role to AIRE expression in the thymus in preventing subsequent emergence of

---

> ### KEY CONCEPTS
>
> #### MECHANISMS UNDERLYING SUSCEPTIBILITY TO AUTOIMMUNITY
>
> >> Incomplete induction of tolerance in the thymus to peripherally expressed autoantigens (AIRE deficiency causing autoimmune polyendocrinopathy candidiasis ectodermal dystrophy (APECED) syndrome)
>
> >> Impaired clearance and tolerance induction by apoptotic cells (e.g., deficiency of C1q, C4, MFG-E8, Mer)
>
> >> Defective production of regulatory T cells (FOXP3 deficiency causing immune dysregulation, polyendocrinopathy, enteropathy, X-linked (IPEX) syndrome)
>
> >> Altered immune signaling thresholds (e.g., CTLA-4 polymorphisms, PTPN22 polymorphisms)

autoimmunity to ubiquitously expressed autoantigens.[12] Additional support for this model comes from recent studies of milk fat globule-EGF factor 8 (MFG-E8), a glycoprotein secreted from macrophages that is required for the efficient attachment and clearance of apoptotic cells by macrophages and immature dendritic cells. MFG-E8 is also expressed in tingible-body macrophages in the germinal centers of secondary lymphoid tissues. Interestingly, many unengulfed apoptotic cells are present in the germinal centers of the spleen in MFG-E8-deficient mice, which develop a striking lupus-like phenotype.[13] Other examples exist in which defects in clearance of apoptotic cells are associated with development of systemic autoimmunity (e.g., Mer deficiency). Together, the data strongly suggest that efficient, anti-inflammatory clearance of apoptotic cells plays a central role in tolerance induction and prevention of autoimmunity.

Defective production of Treg cells

Although pathways exist that: (1) regulate autoantigen expression at sites of tolerance induction; and (2) guide autoantigens towards tolerance-inducing outcomes, these pathways alone are clearly insufficient to prevent the emergence of autoimmune disease. This fact is highlighted by the emergence of autoimmunity when regulatory T-cell (Treg) differentiation is abnormal in humans with immune dysregulation, polyendocrinopathy, enteropathy, X-linked (IPEX) syndrome, the human equivalent of the *scurfy* mouse. IPEX is a rare, X-linked recessive disorder that is characterized by type I diabetes, thyroiditis, atopic dermatitis, and inflammatory bowel disease, and is caused by mutations in the *FOXP3* gene.[14] *FOXP3* is a member of the forkhead family of transcription factors, and is essential for the development of Tregs, which regulate the activation and differentiation of effector T cells at many different levels. It is therefore likely that induction of tolerance is incomplete under most circumstances, and that self-sustaining autoimmunity is limited by Treg function.

Signaling thresholds and susceptibility to autoimmunity

Several modulators of T-cell signaling have also been defined as important susceptibility determinants in autoimmunity (reviewed in reference 15). For example, CTLA4 polymorphisms are associated with increased risk of a variety of autoimmune diseases, including type I diabetes, Graves disease and rheumatoid arthritis. Similarly, a functional polymorphism in PTPN22 has been identified as a major risk factor for several human autoimmune diseases, including SLE, rheumatoid arthritis and type I diabetes. Although the exact mechanisms underlying susceptibility to autoimmunity remain unclear, in both cases the polymorphisms appear to regulate the balance of stimulatory and inhibitory signaling in effector and regulatory T cells, favoring effector T-cell activation.

There are therefore many barriers to the development of autoimmunity, including effective tolerance induction in the thymus and periphery, tightly regulated immune signaling, and homeostatic pathways of immunoregulation to limit self responses should these occur. It is likely that the genetic susceptibility to autoimmunity in outbred humans represents an integrated threshold involving genes that regulate these various pathways, upon which environmental and stochastic events act to accomplish disease initiation and propagation.

PHASE 2: INITIATION

Initiation of an adaptive immune response requires presentation to T cells of suprathreshold concentrations of molecules with structure not previously tolerized by the host. Such tolerance requires generation of self-determinants in sufficient amounts to be recognized by T cells undergoing deletion in the thymus or anergy in the periphery. One of the more persuasive models proposed to explain the persistence of potentially autoreactive T cells within the repertoire of the host is that of immunodominance of T-cell epitopes. This model provides major insights into the pathogenesis of autoimmunity.[15, 16]

Dominance and crypticity

Studies by Sercarz and colleagues[16] have stressed that, while antigens contain numerous potential determinants that could be presented on major histocompatibility complex (MHC) class II during antigen processing, not all determinants in a particular molecule are equally likely to be efficiently presented. Those determinants that are most efficiently presented are termed 'dominant'; those that are not loaded on to class II to a significant degree are termed 'cryptic.' Since pathways of antigen processing are relatively constant, the outcome in terms of epitope selection for any particular autoantigen–MHC class II combination is predictable and reproducible. For self-antigens, it is likely that a constant set of dominant determinants are generated during antigen processing under most circumstances, with similar outcomes in the thymus and periphery. Antigens processed by the "standard" pathway are therefore fully tolerized, with the T-cell repertoire purged of reactivity to the dominant self. However, since the balance of dominant and cryptic epitopes is significantly influenced by protein structure, post-translational modification, and folding, changes of protein structure may alter the balance of dominant and cryptic determinants that are presented during natural antigen processing. Relevant changes include proteolysis and various post-translational modifications as well as complex formation (including antibodies and other binding partners: see below). Under such conditions, previously cryptic determinants may be revealed, and may stimulate T cells recognizing autoantigens.

KEY CONCEPTS

MECHANISMS THAT CAN ALTER ANTIGEN PROCESSING TO REVEAL CRYPTIC EPITOPES

>> Modification of autoantigen processing through high-affinity binding to ligands or antibodies

>> Distinct proteolytic machinery in the thymus and periphery or differential modification of proteolytic activity

>> Modification of autoantigen structure which modifies its processing by endogenous antigen-presenting cell machinery, generally through post-translational modifications

>> Novel proteolytic events not present in the normal antigen-presenting cell pathways, e.g., novel cleavage during cell death or damage or inflammation

>> Novel forms of autoantigens generated by mutation, truncation, or splicing

It is likely that this paradigm is broadly applicable to autoimmunity, since numerous changes in autoantigen structure occur during various relevant physiological states, and can influence subsequent processing and selection of epitopes presented.[17] Several potential mechanisms that may alter antigen processing to reveal potentially cryptic epitopes are summarized below:

1. Modification of autoantigen processing through high-affinity binding to ligands or antibodies. Several studies have demonstrated that antigen processing can be dramatically altered when the antigen binds with high affinity to a ligand or antibody. Simitsek et al.[18] demonstrated that presentation of T-cell determinants in tetanus toxin can be either enhanced or suppressed as a direct consequence of antibody modulation of antigen processing in human B lymphoblastoid cells. Remarkably, a single bound antibody could simultaneously enhance the presentation of one T-cell determinant by more than 10-fold while strongly suppressing the presentation of a different T-cell determinant. Biochemical analysis showed that both the suppressed and boosted determinants fell within an extended domain of antigen stabilized by this antibody during proteolysis.[18] Thus, ligand-induced changes in processing can destroy dominant determinants or reveal cryptic self-determinants. Similar observations have also been made with numerous other antigen–binding partners, including human immunodeficiency virus (HIV) gp120 and CD4 (with consequent autoimmunity to CD4), and p53-SV40 large T-antigen complexes.[17]

2. Distinct proteolytic machinery in the thymus and periphery or differential modification of proteolytic activity. Watts and colleagues showed that a principal human leukocyte antigen (HLA)-DR2-restricted epitope in myelin basic protein (MBP–MBP[85–99]) contains a processing site for asparagine endopeptidase (AEP), with cleavage by AEP abolishing the epitope. AEP activity is therefore a critical factor in presentation of this epitope.[19] In human antigen-presenting cells (APC), presentation of MBP[85–99] is inversely proportional to the amount of cellular AEP activity, and inhibition of AEP greatly enhances presentation of the MBP[85–99] epitope. Interestingly, both MBP and AEP are expressed in the thymus, AEP at abundant levels. These data suggest that this major epitope in neurological autoimmunity may not be presented under normal circumstances in the thymus due to destruction by AEP, therefore raising the potential for later presentation in the periphery in the setting of decreased AEP activity.

3. Modification of autoantigen structure which modifies its processing by the endogenous APC machinery: various post-translational modifications. It has been known for some time that autoantigens undergo a variety of post-translational modifications, including phosphorylation, proteolytic cleavage, ubiquitination, transglutamination, citrullination, and isoaspartyl modification.[20–22] In several cases, autoantibodies recognize exclusively the modified form of the antigen (e.g., RNA polymerase-II large subunit, SR proteins, citrullinated vimentin and other rheumatoid arthritis autoantigens), indicating that the modified forms of the molecules are important in driving the immune response. Little is known about the circumstances in which such modified antigens are generated in the relevant target tissue *in vivo*, although various pathways of cell injury and death have been proposed to be important in this regard. Doyle and Mamula[20] demonstrated that post-translational modification of autoantigen structure may be much more broadly relevant than can be appreciated by studying autoantibody specificity alone. Their studies centered on the effect of isoaspartyl modifications on antigen processing and presentation. They showed that mouse immunization with a murine cytochrome c peptide (amino acids 90–104) showed no T- or B-cell response. In contrast, immunization with the isoaspartyl form of this peptide resulted in strong T- and B-cell responses. While the autoantibodies that were elicited recognized both the modified and the native form of the antigen, T cells only recognized the isoaspartyl form. Similar observations have also been made for several SLE autoantigens. The difficulty of detecting and quantifying antigen-specific T cells in various autoimmune diseases may reflect their preferential recognition of subtly modified forms of autoantigen. This is an important area for future study–currently there is no systematic way of generating the relevant autoantigen forms.

4. Novel proteolytic events not present in the normal APC pathways, e.g., novel cleavage during cell death or damage or inflammation. Recent studies have provided evidence that single proteolytic events early in the process of antigen processing may play critical roles in defining the epitopes generated. For example, Watts and colleagues conclusively demonstrated that early cleavage by AEP–a protease in the lysosomal pathway that cleaves substrates after asparagines–determines subsequent proteolytic events, and thus which epitopes are selected during natural processing of whole antigens. Modifications of the antigen that affect this early cleavage dramatically change the epitopes loaded on to MHC class II.[23]

This property creates significant potential to load distinct epitopes if unique proteolytic activities are expressed in different tissues or inflammatory microenvironments. Activated inflammatory cells constitute a major source of such proteases, including various cytotoxic lymphocyte granule proteases (granzymes), as well as numerous neutrophil and monocyte granule proteases. It is of interest that numerous autoantigens targeted in systemic autoimmune diseases are substrates for these inflammatory proteases, and that unique autoantigen fragments are generated through the activity of granzyme B and potentially other similar proteases.[24] Such autoantigen forms are not generated during other forms of cell damage or death. Furthermore, similar activity is not observed against nonautoantigens, suggesting that novel proteolytic cleavage of intracellular autoantigens during activity of cytotoxic immune effector pathways may provide a source of cryptic epitopes not generated during homeostatic "tolerance-inducing" tissue turnover. Direct evidence that inflammatory protease-mediated revelation of cryptic epitopes is relevant to initiation of autoimmunity *in vivo* is still needed.

5. Novel forms of autoantigens generated by mutation, truncation, or splicing. Since the final epitopes generated and loaded on to MHC class II can be profoundly influenced by single early cleavage events during antigen processing, relatively minor but critically placed changes in the primary structure of autoantigens may have the capacity to influence peptide selection. A recent study of the melanoma and vitiligo-associated autoantigens (tyrosinase-related proteins 1 and 2) has strikingly demonstrated that this mechanism may play an important role in generating immune responses to self and tumor antigens.[25] In this study, Engelhorn and colleagues studied whether mutated-self gene products are more likely to initiate immunity, and used a systematic approach to define some of the principles that determine this. They used an error-prone polymerase in polymerase chain reactions to generate cDNA libraries encoding large numbers

of random mutations in syngeneic TRP proteins. Individual gene copies had a mean of 15–20 mutations, and each copy was predicted to contain a unique set of mutations. The investigators then used a DNA immunization approach into black mice to test the immunogenicity of pools of mutated cDNAs, by looking for the development of vitiligo or resistance to melanoma challenge. Immunization with nonmutated proteins induced no detectable immune responses, consistent with establishment of tolerance to the full-length molecules. In contrast, the DNA pools elicited both autoimmune depigmentation and the ability to reject tumors. Additional analysis showed that autoimmunity resulted from mutations that altered autoantigen cell biology, particularly as regards degradation rates and pathways. Mutations also created new helper T-cell epitopes, and induced recognition of nonmutated but previously cryptic epitopes. Interestingly, mutations themselves did not form part of CD8 epitopes that drive the anti-self and anti-tumor immune responses. Mutated molecules that were immunogenic were frequently truncated, leading the authors to propose that inappropriately truncated self-proteins may provoke autoimmunity when present in a proinflammatory environment. Although there are not yet good examples where natural autoimmunity arises due to the progressive accumulation of somatic mutations over time, with the expression of mutant, truncated forms of autoantigens, this study does provide an important mechanistic underpinning for the proposal that accumulated mutations have a role in the initiation of autoimmunity.

Indeed, there are substantial data that link autoimmunity and cancer. While many initial reports of a temporal association of malignancy and various autoimmune processes were anecdotal, and thought to be chance observations, evidence demonstrating that this relationship is real and likely of mechanistic significance has been growing. For example, the association of cancer with dermatomyositis is present in ~20% of individuals with dermatomyositis, with a striking temporal clustering of cancer diagnosis around the time of diagnosis of the myositis.[26] Similarly, there is evidence for an association of SLE with cancer, particularly lymphoma, again clustered within the first 2 years of SLE diagnosis.[27] These associations, both with timing of diagnosis as well as preferentially with specific tumor types, are strongly indicative of a nonrandom clustering of potential mechanistic significance. There is also growing evidence that, when associated with 'paraneoplastic' autoimmune syndromes, cancers are frequently smaller at the time of diagnosis and thus may have a better prognosis. Perhaps the most striking evidence for a potential mechanistic association between autoimmunity and effective anti-cancer immunity comes from recent studies showing that development of autoimmunity during immunotherapy for a variety of different cancers is a very striking predictor of a better cancer outcome. This is true for metastatic melanoma, where development of vitiligo is a predictor of an effective anti-tumor response.[28] Perhaps even more striking is the recent observation that this powerful anti-cancer response is observed not only when autoimmunity to melanocytes is induced, but also when immunotherapy (in this case using systemic high-dose adjuvant interferon-α_{2b} therapy) induces evidence of systemic autoimmunity (defined by newly detected autoantibodies).[29]

The likelihood that the significant accumulation of somatic mutation with age in human populations and its association with malignancy play important roles in the genesis of some forms of human autoimmunity is very high. Additional studies to confirm this and elucidate the underly-

ing mechanisms remain a high priority. However, the barriers to such studies in humans are very significant, as effective anti-cancer immunity may be phenotypically silent, and convenient technologies to quantify somatic mutation and specific immune responses in normal individuals will be needed to draw conclusions of causality.

Antigen mimicry

The process of antigen mimicry (see below) has frequently been proposed as a potential initiator of autoimmune diseases.[30, 31] This mechanism, particularly when isolated, is only likely relevant to those autoimmune processes clearly associated with antecedent infections, and particularly those that resolve spontaneously and subsequently recur upon re-exposure to the offending agent. The mechanism may, however, also play a role in initiation of the autoimmune response in self-sustaining autoimmune processes, but in this case, requires that T-cell responses to the cross-reacting self-antigen are initiated.

Foreign antigens, which often differ from their homologous self-antigens in some areas, may nevertheless bear significant structural similarity to self-antigens in other regions. Initiation of an immune response to the foreign antigen may generate a cross-reactive antibody response that also recognizes the self-protein (antigen mimicry). When the antigen is a cell surface molecule, antibody-mediated effector pathways can lead to host tissue damage. Although the antibody response is cross-reactive with self-molecules, the T cells that drive this response are generally directed at the foreign antigen, at least initially (see below). Diseases involving this sort of "antigen mimicry" therefore tend to be self-limited, although they can recur upon re-exposure to the offending antigen. It is important to realize that antigen mimicry alone cannot explain self-sustaining autoimmune diseases, which are driven by self-antigens and autoreactive T cells. In these cases, there is a requirement for overcoming T-cell tolerance to the self protein. The central issues in this regard are: (1) how T-cell tolerance to self-antigens might initially be broken; and (2) once this has occurred, why these antigens continue to drive the immune response to self. The simultaneous liberation of self-antigen in the presence of the cross-reactive antibody response has been proposed to play critical roles in this regard. For example, several studies suggest that when a humoral response to a foreign protein is induced that cross-reacts with the self-antigen, a strong helper T-cell response specific for the self-antigen can occur. The simultaneous liberation of significant amounts of self-antigen in the setting of a cross-reactive antibody response may allow effective presentation of cryptic epitopes in the self-antigen to autoreactive T cells by activated cross-reactive B cells. If continued release of self-antigen occurs, a specific, adaptive immune response to self will be sustained. Antigen release from tissues likely plays a critical role in driving this autoimmune process. Understanding the mechanisms of ongoing antigen release at sites of tissue damage in autoimmune disease (e.g., unique pathways of cell injury and death) is a high priority for future work, as it provides a novel target for therapy (see below).

It is clear from the above discussion that extraordinary complexity is operative in initiation of the human autoimmune diseases. The patient population is genetically heterogeneous, the human immune system is complex and extremely plastic, and it interacts with a plethora of environmental stimuli and stochastic events. The simultaneous confluence of susceptibility factors and initiation forces to set off the self-sustained and autoamplifying process is therefore a rare occurrence. In contrast, once

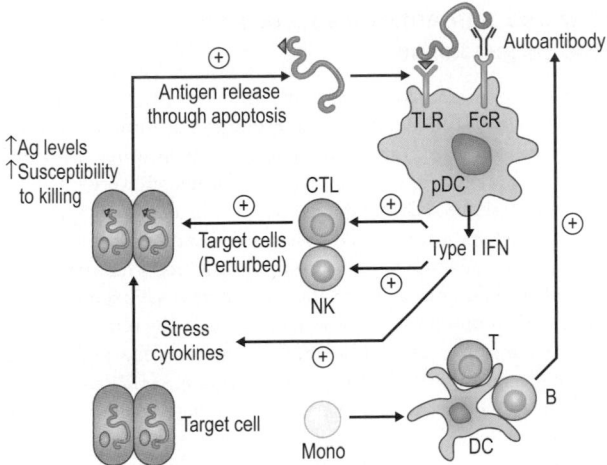

Fig. 50.2 The propagation phase in autoimmune diseases. Target cells in normal tissues express low levels of autoantigens. Under conditions of stress, damage, and exposure to cytokines, antigen levels increase, likely associated with changes in antigen structure (various post-translational modifications). Furthermore, type I interferons sensitize target cells to killing pathways, maximizing antigen release through apoptosis or other forms of cell death. Autoantigens released from this perturbed target cell have adjuvant capacity. In the setting of the immune response generated during the initiation phase, this dual property of autoantigens allows effective stimulation of plasmacytoid DCs (pDC), which secrete type I interferons (IFN) in large amounts. Type I IFNs have multiple effects which conspire to drive additional immune responses to self (including B and T cells), regulate monocyte (mono) differentiation into mature antigen-presenting DCs, increase target cell killing, and enhance autoantigen (Ag) expression. These multiple interacting loops that reinforce each other likely play important roles in generating self-sustaining tissue damage.

activation of autoreactive T cells has occurred, the ability of the immune system to respond vigorously to low concentrations of antigen, to amplify the specific effector response to those antigens, and to spread the response to additional antigens in that tissue, greatly reduces the stringency that must be met to keep the process going.

PHASE III: PROPAGATION (FIG. 50.2)

Principles of amplification

One of the central features of human autoimmunity is the tendency of the process to amplify progressively with the accumulation of significant immune-mediated tissue damage. Furthermore, in the vast majority of cases, once such amplification begins, the process is very unlikely to resolve spontaneously. Properties of autoantigens themselves may be very important in this phase, in terms of both acquisition of adjuvant properties, as well as regulation of expression. The essential features of amplification are a substrate cycle, in which antigen expression and adjuvant properties induce an immune response, which induces increased antigen expression and tissue damage, further driving the immune response. The importance of tissue-specific autoantigen expression in focusing such immune responses is only beginning to be recognized.

Acquisition of adjuvant properties by disease-specific autoantigens

In spite of the fact that tens of thousands of molecules could be targeted by the immune system in autoimmunity, the number of molecules that are frequently targeted in the different phenotypes are markedly restricted – limited perhaps to 100 or so molecules. This has led to the proposal that frequently targeted autoantigens may themselves have properties that make them proimmune. Recent work by Howard et al provided important support for this proposal (reviewed in reference 32). They observed that the autoantigenic histidyl aminoacyl tRNA synthetase (HRS), which is targeted in autoimmune myositis (but not nonautoantigenic lysyl- and aspartyl-aminoacyl tRNA synthetases), is chemoattractant to immature dendritic cells and other leukocytes. In the case of HRS, chemoattraction occurs in a CCR5-dependent way. The authors suggested that the selection of a self-molecule as a target for an autoantibody response may be a consequence of proinflammatory properties of the molecule itself. Plotz further suggested that modification of autoantigen structure during processes of cell damage or death may be critical in recruiting these additional functions of autoantigens.

One of the most likely receptor systems to sense and transduce the proinflammatory properties of autoantigens is the Toll-like receptor (TLR) family, which is the primary innate immune system transducer of pathogen-associated molecular patterns[6, 33] (Chapter 3). Ligands for TLRs include both microbial and endogenous molecules, the latter group being particularly relevant to autoimmunity (see below). Microbial ligands include components of Gram-positive bacteria, Gram-negative bacteria, yeast, and protozoans. For example, lipoteichoic acid and fungal products (e.g., zymosan) signal through TLR-2, lipopolysaccharide activates TLR-4 signaling, dsRNA signals through TLR-3, flagellin through TLR-5, ssRNA through TLR-7 and TLR-8, bacterial or viral DNA through TLR-9, and *Toxoplasma* profilin through TLR-11.[6] Although viral and bacterial nucleic acids are the most likely ligands for TLRs, accumulating data demonstrate that complexes containing endogenous nucleic acids are clearly able to signal through TLRs. Although the exact nature and source of endogenous ligands for TLRs *in vivo* remain unclear, recent studies have demonstrated that components from stressed, injured, and dying cells may play critical roles in this regard.[34]

Working in several models, numerous investigators have now provided evidence that the targeting of frequently targeted nucleoprotein autoantigens (which contain DNA or RNA) results from the ability of these nucleic acid components to ligate TLRs. Early studies demonstrated that anti-chromatin immune complexes could activate dendritic cells through the cooperation of FcγR and TLR-9. Similarly, B cells could be activated by immune complexes that could serve as ligands for both FcγR and TLR-9. Similar results have been demonstrated for TLR-7 and RNA-containing immune complexes. While the *in vitro* data demonstrating that nucleic acid-containing autoantigens have the capacity to signal through TLRs is very clear, it was important to demonstrate that such signaling is of relevance *in vivo* to autoimmunity. Such data have recently been obtained in various *in vivo* studies using mice deficient in TLR-9 and/or TLR-7. For example, when TLR-9 deficiency is bred on to MRL-lpr mice, which are an excellent model of SLE, animals no longer get autoantibody responses to chromatin. Interestingly, these animals nevertheless manifest the SLE phenotype, in some cases, more severely than the TLR-9-sufficient animals.[33] In another model, Ehlers et al. showed that TLR-9 deficiency both inhibits anti-DNA responses and also abrogates the development of renal disease.[35] Similarly, when mice are rendered TLR-7-deficient, the autoantibody response to Sm is markedly inhibited, and severity of the SLE phenotype is improved.[33] Thus, TLR-9 and TLR-7 deficiency appeared to have dramatic and different effects on clinical disease in lupus-prone mice.

These data confirm that autoantigens frequently selected in different autoimmune phenotypes likely have the dual property of being able to activate simultaneously the innate and adaptive immune systems, and that the ability to co-ligate TLRs plays a critical role. Whether other frequently targeted autoantigens in autoimmunity, which do not have nucleic acids as intrinsic components, can similarly ligate TLRs or innate immune receptors remains to be determined. Importantly, these approaches have underscored the significant complexity of the system, and the importance of defining the balance between signaling through different TLRs in integrating the overall outcome of exposure to various combinations of autoantigens.

The source, form, and uptake of nucleic acids appear to pay a large role in determining adjuvant activity. For example, while bacterial and viral DNA, and oligonucleotides with CpG motifs have significant adjuvant activity,[36] mammalian genomic DNA, in which CpG is usually methylated, has very poor adjuvant activity. In contrast, human DNA present within immune complexes in SLE serum activates plasmacytoid dendritic cells effectively, in a DNA-dependent way. Several potential explanations have been advanced to explain these observation.[6] First, that FγR-mediated uptake effectively captures self-DNA bound by anti-DNA antibodies and directs it to the correct endosomal compartment for TLR signaling. Second, that co-ligation of TLR-9 and either B-cell receptor or FγR alters the signaling threshold of immune complexes. Last, that the difference lies in the nucleic acid itself, with additional modifications of DNA and RNA structure occurring in cells under different physiologic circumstances (e.g., cell death) and regulating nucleic acid binding to TLRs.

The TLR–interferon interface has been recognized as critical in the propagation phase of systemic autoimmune diseases, and has been reviewed extensively.[37, 38] Although it is likely that the TLR effects in autoimmunity are expressed in a wide variety of cell types, much attention has been focused on plasmacytoid dendritic cells, a relatively rare class of immature dendritic cell that can secrete large amounts of type I interferons upon TLR ligation, and that express TLR-7 and TLR-9 at high levels. Lovgren and colleagues recently demonstrated that, when added to material from apoptotic or necrotic cells, autoantibodies from SLE and Sjögren's syndrome patients with specificity for DNA or RNA autoantigens induce striking interferon secretion.[34] IFN-α-inducing activity is abrogated by chloroquine or bafilomycin, agents that interfere with endosome acidification and TLR-7 and TLR-9 signaling. Type I interferons have a broad set of functions that likely contribute to the feed-forward, propagation phase of systemic autoimmune diseases.[6, 39] For example, they: (1) promote the differentiation of monocytes into mature dendritic cells, which drive autoreactive T- and B-cell responses; (2) increase target cell sensitivity to killing pathways; (3) upregulate cytotoxic effector pathways; and (4) upregulate expression of autoantigens like Ro52.

This general ability of autoantigens, particularly in the context of immune complexes, to stimulate interferon and other cytokine secretion, is likely a critical principle in the initiation and propagation of autoimmunity.

Enhanced autoantigen expression in the target tissue

The striking association of specific autoantibody responses with distinct phenotypes suggests that autoantigen expression or form in specific target tissues may play an important role in both focusing the immune response and generating tissue damage. Unfortunately, very little is currently known about such parameters *in vivo* in relevant target tissues, both in normal and pathologic circumstances. Recent studies on human autoimmune myopathies have begun to provide important insights into this problem. Thus, myositis-specific autoantigens are expressed at very low levels in control muscle, but at high levels in myositis tissue, where antigen expression is at highest levels in regenerating muscle cells.[40] Interestingly, histidyl tRNA synthetase expression (HRS antibodies are associated with autoimmune myopathies with interstitial lung disease) is also found at high levels in lung. These data suggest that enhanced autoantigen expression in the target tissue may be a feature of disease propagation, and that antigen expression during tissue repair may provide an ongoing antigen source to sustain and amplify tissue damage. Defining whether similar principles are operating in other autoimmune diseases, and elucidating the pathways of antigen expression in relevant target tissues, is an important focus of future studies, as the regulation of antigen expression (rather than exclusively pathways of immune-mediated damage) may have important therapeutic potential.

◼ REFERENCES ◼

1. Davidson A., Diamond B.. General features of autoimmune disease. In: Rose N., Mackay I. (eds) The Autoimmune Diseases. St Louis: Elsevier; 2006: 25–36.

2. von Muhlen CA, Tan EM. Autoantibodies in the diagnosis of systemic rheumatic diseases. Semin Arthritis Rheum 1995; 24: 323–358.

3. Arbuckle MR, McClain MT, Rubertone MV, et al. Development of autoantibodies before the clinical onset of systemic lupus erythematosus. N Engl J Med 2003; 349: 1526–1533.

4. Wasserfall CH, Atkinson MA. Autoantibody markers for the diagnosis and prediction of type 1 diabetes. Autoimmun Rev 2006; 5: 424–428.

5. Nielen MM, van Schaardenburg D, Reesink HW, et al. Specific autoantibodies precede the symptoms of rheumatoid arthritis: a study of serial measurements in blood donors. Arthritis Rheum 2004; 50: 380–386.

6. Marshak-Rothstein A. Toll-like receptors in systemic autoimmune disease. Nat Rev Immunol 2006; 6: 823–835.

7. Peterson P, Nagamine K, Scott H, et al. APECED: a monogenic autoimmune disease providing new clues to self-tolerance. Immunol Today 1998; 19: 384–386.

8. Anderson MS, Venanzi ES, Klein L, et al. Projection of an immunological self shadow within the thymus by the aire protein. Science 2002; 298: 1395–1401.

9. Devoss J, Hou Y, Johannes K, et al. Spontaneous autoimmunity prevented by thymic expression of a single self-antigen. J Exp Med 2006; 203: 2727–2735.

10. Steinman RM, Turley S, Mellman I, et al. The induction of tolerance by dendritic cells that have captured apoptotic cells. J Exp Med 2000; 191: 411–416.

11. Voll RE, Herrmann M, Roth EA, et al. Immunosuppressive effects of apoptotic cells. Nature 1997; 390: 350–351.

12. Manderson AP, Botto M, Walport MJ. The role of complement in the development of systemic lupus erythematosus. Annu Rev Immunol 2004; 22: 431–456.

13. Hanayama R, Tanaka M, Miyasaka K, et al. Autoimmune disease and impaired uptake of apoptotic cells in MFG-E8-deficient mice. Science 2004; 304: 1147–1150.

14. Bennett CL, Christie J, Ramsdell F, et al. The immune dysregulation, polyendocrinopathy, enteropathy X-linked syndrome (IPEX) is caused by mutations of FOXP3. Nat Genet 2001; 27: 20–21.

15. Gregersen PK, Behrens TW. Genetics of autoimmune diseases – disorders of immune homeostasis. Nat Rev Genet 2006; 7: 917–928.

16. Sercarz EE, Lehmann PV, Ametani A, et al. Dominance and crypticity of T cell antigenic determinants. Annu Rev Immunol 1993; 11: 729–766.

17. Lanzavecchia A. How can cryptic epitopes trigger autoimmunity? J Exp Med 1995; 181: 1945–1948.

18. Simitsek PD, Campbell DG, Lanzavecchia A, et al. Modulation of antigen processing by bound antibodies can boost or suppress class II major histocompatibility complex presentation of different T cell determinants. J Exp Med 1995; 181: 1957–1963.

19. Manoury B, Mazzeo D, Fugger L, et al. Destructive processing by asparagine endopeptidase limits presentation of a dominant T cell epitope in MBP. Nat Immunol 2002; 3: 169–174.

20. Doyle HA, Mamula MJ. Posttranslational modifications of self-antigens. Ann NY Acad Sci 2005; 1050: 1–9.

21. Utz PJ, Anderson P. Posttranslational protein modifications, apoptosis, and the bypass of tolerance to autoantigens. Arthritis Rheum 1998; 41: 1152–1160.

22. Rosen A, Casciola-Rosen L. Autoantigens as substrates for apoptotic proteases: implications for the pathogenesis of systemic autoimmune disease. Cell Death Differ 1999; 6: 6–12.

23. Antoniou AN, Blackwood SL, Mazzeo D, et al. Control of antigen presentation by a single protease cleavage site. Immunity 2000; 12: 391–398.

24. Casciola-Rosen L, Andrade F, Ulanet D, et al. Cleavage by granzyme B is strongly predictive of autoantigen status: implications for initiation of autoimmunity. J Exp Med 1999; 190: 815–825.

25. Engelhorn ME, Guevara-Patino JA, Noffz G, et al. Autoimmunity and tumor immunity induced by immune responses to mutations in self. Nat Med 2006; 12: 198–206.

26. Hill CL, Zhang Y, Sigurgeirsson B, et al. Frequency of specific cancer types in dermatomyositis and polymyositis: a population-based study. Lancet 2001; 357: 96–100.

27. Bernatsky S, Boivin JF, Joseph L, et al. An international cohort study of cancer in systemic lupus erythematosus. Arthritis Rheum 2005; 52: 1481–1490.

28. Phan GQ, Yang JC, Sherry RM, et al. Cancer regression and autoimmunity induced by cytotoxic T lymphocyte-associated antigen 4 blockade in patients with metastatic melanoma. Proc Natl Acad Sci USA 2003; 100: 8372–8377.

29. Gogas H, Ioannovich J, Dafni U, et al. Prognostic significance of autoimmunity during treatment of melanoma with interferon. N Engl J Med 2006; 354: 709–718.

30. James JA, Harley JB, Scofield RH. Epstein–Barr virus and systemic lupus erythematosus. Curr Opin Rheumatol 2006; 18: 462–467.

31. Fourneau JM, Bach JM, Van Endert PM, et al. The elusive case for a role of mimicry in autoimmune diseases. Mol Immunol 2004; 40: 1095–1102.

32. Plotz PH. The autoantibody repertoire: searching for order. Nat Rev Immunol 2003; 3: 73–78.

33. Christensen SR, Shupe J, Nickerson K, et al. Toll-like receptor 7 and TLR9 dictate autoantibody specificity and have opposing inflammatory and regulatory roles in a murine model of lupus. Immunity 2006; 25: 417–428.

34. Lovgren T, Eloranta ML, Bave U, et al. Induction of interferon-alpha production in plasmacytoid dendritic cells by immune complexes containing nucleic acid released by necrotic or late apoptotic cells and lupus IgG. Arthritis Rheum 2004; 50: 1861–1872.

35. Ehlers M, Fukuyama H, McGaha TL, et al. TLR9/MyD88 signaling is required for class switching to pathogenic IgG2a and 2b autoantibodies in SLE. J Exp Med 2006; 203: 553–561.

36. Krieg AM. CpG motifs in bacterial DNA and their immune effects. Annu Rev Immunol 2002; 20: 709–760.

37. Ronnblom L, Eloranta ML, Alm GV. The type I interferon system in systemic lupus erythematosus. Arthritis Rheum 2006; 54: 408–420.

38. Banchereau J, Pascual V. Type I interferon in systemic lupus erythematosus and other autoimmune diseases. Immunity 2006; 25: 383–392.

39. Blanco P, Pitard V, Viallard JF, et al. Increase in activated CD8+ T lymphocytes expressing perforin and granzyme B correlates with disease activity in patients with systemic lupus erythematosus. Arthritis Rheum 2005; 52: 201–211.

40. Casciola-Rosen L, Nagaraju K, Plotz P, et al. Enhanced autoantigen expression in regenerating muscle cells in idiopathic inflammatory myopathy. J Exp Med 2005; 201: 591–601.

Systemic lupus erythematosus

Cynthia Aranow, Betty Diamond, Meggan Mackay*

Systemic lupus erythematosus (SLE) is a systemic autoimmune disease characterized by the production of autoantibodies and a diversity of clinical manifestations. It most commonly presents in women during their child-bearing years. Although the etiology of SLE is unknown, both genetic and environmental factors contribute to loss of self-tolerance. Current therapeutic modalities are anti-inflammatory and immunosuppressive.

■ EPIDEMIOLOGY ■

The American College of Rheumatology (ACR) classification[1] (Table 51.1) is the most widely accepted instrument for 'diagnosing' lupus; however, these criteria do not represent the full spectrum of disease. They were created to identify SLE patients for clinical studies. Patients fulfilling four out of the 11 criteria are classified with SLE with approximately 95% certainty, although many individuals who meet only two or three criteria are 'diagnosed' with SLE. During the child-bearing years, the ratio of women to men with lupus is approximately 9:1. This ratio is less in younger and older populations, supporting a role for hormonal factors in disease induction. The majority of lupus presents during adulthood and approximately 20% are diagnosed in the pediatric population.

Lupus occurs throughout the world; susceptibility is linked to ethnicity. Overall incidence rates reported during the last 25 years in North America vary from 2 to 7 per 100 000. Incidence rates in African-Americans, Afro-Caribbeans, Hispanics, and Asians are approximately three times greater. The prevalence in the USA ranges from 50 to 80 per 100 000. Clinical manifestations of disease are also modulated by ethnicity (Table 51.2).

■ IMMUNOPATHOGENESIS ■

The immune system is designed to protect the host against foreign pathogens without damaging self. To accomplish this, a complex system has evolved that treads a delicate balance between self-defense and autoreactivity. Clearly, with the universal production of autoantibodies and characteristic pathological findings of inflammation, vasculitis, vasculopathy,

and immune complex deposition, SLE patients display a failure to down-regulate autoreactivity. The heterogeneity of disease manifestations reflects the multiplicity of genetic, hormonal, and immune abnormalities contributing to clinical disease (Table 51.3). Progression from initial autoreactivity to clinical disease occurs over time (Fig. 51.1).

AUTOANTIBODIES

Most autoantibodies in lupus bind nuclear antigens, although some bind cell membrane antigens, plasma proteins, and extracellular matrix antigens. Antinuclear antibodies (ANA) are present in over 98% of patients diagnosed with SLE. Their presence is not specific to SLE as they are present in patients with other autoimmune diseases (e.g., rheumatoid arthritis, scleroderma, Sjögrens's disease), malignancies, infections including viral (hepatitis) and parasitic (malaria) as well as in response to environmental triggers such as therapeutic agents (see section on drug-induced lupus, below). Furthermore, ANA are found in low titer in 5% of the general population with prevalence increasing with age. In commercial laboratories ANA are typically detected by their binding to Hep-2 cells. Common ANA specificities found in lupus patients include dsDNA, ssDNA, extractable nuclear antigens (such as Sm RNP, Ro and La), histones, and chromatin. Specific ANA are associated with disease subsets such as anti-Ro antibodies with subacute cutaneous and neonatal SLE, and anti ds-DNA antibodies with renal disease. The titers of most autoantibodies do not correlate with disease activity; anti-dsDNA antibodies are a notable exception, fluctuating with disease activity, thereby suggesting a pathogenic role for this autoantibody in disease pathogenesis.

THE PREDISPOSED HOST: GENETIC CONTRIBUTIONS

SLE is a multigenic disease. Most disease-associated alleles are present in healthy individuals in the population. Only when these alleles are present in combination and interact with an appropriate environmental trigger will a lupus-like phenotype arise. The degree of familial disease clustering and the higher disease concordance in monozygotic versus dizygotic twins suggest

---

* Authors contributed equally and are listed in alphabetical order.

Table 51.1 American College of Rheumatology criteria for systemic lupus erythematosus

Criteria	Description
Malar rash	Fixed malar erythema, flat or raised
Discoid rash	Erythematous raised patches with adherent keratotic scaling and follicular plugging; atrophic scarring may occur in older lesions
Photosensitivity	Skin rash as an unusual reaction to sunlight, by patient history or physician observation
Oral ulcers	Oral and nasopharyngeal ulcers, usually painless, observed by physician
Arthritis	Nonerosive arthritis involving two or more peripheral joints, characterized by tenderness, swelling, or effusion
Serositis	Pleuritis (convincing history of pleuritic pain or rub heard by physician or evidence of pleural effusion) *or* Pericarditis (documented by electrocardiogram or rub or evidence of pericardial effusion)
Renal disorder	Persistent proteinuria >0.5 protein:creatinine ratio or >3+ if quantification not performed *or* Cellular casts, may be red cell, hemoglobin, granular, tubular, or mixed
Neurologic disorder	Seizures–in the absence of offending drugs or known metabolic derangements, e.g., uremia, ketoacidosis, or electrolyte imbalance *or* Psychosis–in the absence of offending drugs or known metabolic derangements, e.g., uremia, ketoacidosis, or electrolyte imbalance
Hematologic disorder	Hemolytic anemia–with reticulocytosis *or* Leukopenia (< 4000/mm^3 total on two or more occasions) *or* Lymphopenia (< 1500/mm^3 on two or more occasions) *or* Thrombocytopenia (< 100 000/mm^3 in the absence of offending drugs)
Immunologic disorder	Anti-ds DNA: antibody to native DNA in abnormal titer *or* Anti-Sm: presence of antibody to Sm nuclear antigen *or* Positive finding of antiphospholipid antibodies based on: (1) an abnormal serum level of IgG or IgM anticardiolipin antibodies; (2) a positive test for lupus coagulant using a standard method; or (3) a false-positive serologic test for syphilis known to be positive for at least 6 months and confirmed by *Treponema pallidum* immobilization or fluorescent treponemal antibody absorption test
Antinuclear antibodies	An abnormal titer of antinuclear antibody by immunofluorescence or an equivalent assay at any point in time and in the absence of drugs known to be associated with 'drug-induced lupus' syndrome

Ig, immunoglobulin.

both an underlying genetic susceptibility and the importance of environmental or epigenetic factors. Presumed susceptibility genes identified in humans include those affecting differentiation and survival of B cells, lymphocyte activation, proliferation and apoptosis, cytokine production, antigen presentation, and clearance of apoptotic debris. Many of these genes are also implicated in susceptibility to other autoimmune diseases (e.g., CTLA-4 in Graves disease and type 1 diabetes,[2] PTPN22 polymorphisms in rheumatoid arthritis and type 1 diabetes[3]). Candidate genes are evaluated individually for disease association by looking for different frequencies of specific gene polymorphisms between affected individuals and normal controls. Alternatively, in linkage studies genetic information is assessed statistically, looking for co-inheritance of specific polymorphisms associated with clinical disease in families with multiple affected members.

Genes associated with antigen presentation

Polymorphisms of major histocompatability complex (MHC) genes determine the peptides of self antigens and microbial and foreign antigens presented within the MHC that select the naïve T-cell repertoire. Human leukocyte antigen (HLA) DR2 haplotypes in Afro-American, African, Taiwanese, and Korean populations and HLA DR3 haplotypes in Caucasian populations have been associated with a two- to threefold increased risk for developing SLE.[4] Recent evidence demonstrating close associations between anti-Ro antibodies with HLA-DR3 and anti-La antibodies with HLA-DR25 is consistent with the concept of an antigen-driven process involving T-cell recognition.

Table 51.2 American College of Rheumatology criteria in different ethnic cohorts

	†Hispanic PROFILE cohort[a] (n=78)	†Hispanic Puerto Rican[b] (n=134)	‡Caucasian Spain[c] (n=239)	‡Caucasian USA[d] (n=46)	†Caucasian PROFILE cohort[a] (n=260)	†Caucasian Norwegian[e] (n=346)	†Caucasian Danish[f] (n=513)	†African American PROFILE cohort[a] (n=216)	‡Chinese[d] (n=175)
Malar rash	64.1	71.6	NA	23.9	67.3	40	48	44.7	57.7
Discoid rash	6.4	10.4	27	23.9	11.9	13	14	32.7	5.7
Photosensitivity	59	76.9	29	45.7	72.3	41	43	46.1	30.7
Oral/nasal ulcers	57.7	29.9	18	6.5	57.3	1	11	45.6	14.9
Arthritis	91	67.2	71	54.4	86.9	83	67	88.5	54.3
Seizure/psychosis	11.5	9	5.8	4.4	9.2	8	13	15.7	8.6
Renal	59	29.9	23	54.4	22.7	17	45	54.4	28.6
Serositis	64.1	27.6	33	26.1	41.5	34	39	59.5	10.9
Cytopenias	84.6	76.9	55	82.6	62	36	67	81.6	57.7
Antinuclear antibody	97.4	93.3	100	82.6	96.5	99	98	97.2	95.4
Immunologic	83.3	NA	NA	56.5	65.4	57	98	79.3	80.6

†Cumulative data.
‡Inception data.
a. Alarcon GS, et al. Baseline characteristics of a multiethnic lupus cohort: PROFILE. Lupus 2002; 11: 95–101.
b. Vila LM, et al. Clinical and immunological manifestations in 134 Puerto Rican patients with systemic lupus erythematosus. Lupus 1999; 8: 279–286.
c. Bujan S, et al. Contribution of the initial features of systemic lupus erythematosus to the clinical evolution and survival of a cohort of Mediterranean patients. Ann Rheum Dis 2003; 62: 859–865.
c. Thumboo J, et al. A comparative study of the clinical manifestations of systemic lupus erythematosus in Caucasians in Rochester, Minnesota, and Chinese in Singapore, from 1980 to 1992. Arthritis Rheum 2001; 45: 494–500.
e. Gilboe IM, Husby G. Application of the 1982 revised criteria for the classification of systemic lupus erythematosus on a cohort of 346 Norwegian patients with connective tissue disease. Scand J Rheumatol 1999; 28: 81–87.
f. Jacobsen S, et al. A multicentre study of 513 Danish patients with systemic lupus erythematosus. I. Disease manifestations and analyses of clinical subsets. Clin Rheumatol 1998; 17: 468–477.

Table 51.3 Factors contributing to autoimmunity

Genetic factors
Loss of peripheral tolerance
• B-cell abnormalities
• T-cell abnormalities
• Dendritic cell abnormalities
Cytokine milieu
Hormonal influences
Environmental triggers

Genes associated with impaired clearance of apoptotic debris

Patients with severe deficiencies of C2, C4, and C1q display disease risks of 10%, 75%, and 90% respectively for SLE.[6] Reduced uptake of apoptotic cells has been implicated in disease initiation in murine models of SLE and is seen histopathologically in lymph nodes of lupus patients.[7] Though homozygotes for null alleles of C2, C4, and C1q are at significantly increased risk, these genetic haplotypes are rare. Polymorphisms of mannose-binding lectin (MBL) and C-reactive protein (CRP), acute-phase reactants that facilitate opsonization and phagocytosis of immune complexes, apoptotic debris and microbes, associate with SLE susceptibility; MBL haplotypes appear to be more important in Chinese and Spanish populations than in Caucasians.

Genes associated with lymphocyte activation, proliferation, and function

The Fcγ receptors, FcγR1 (CD 64), FcγRII (CD32), and FcγRIII (CD16), have different binding affinities for immunoglobulin G (IgG) and immune complexes, as well as different cell-specific expression and function. FcγRI, FcγRIIa, and FcγRIIIa and IIIb are all activating receptors. Cross-linking results in degranulation, phagocytosis, antibody-dependent cellular cytotoxicity, cytokine gene transcription, and release of inflammatory mediators. In contrast, FcγRIIb is an inhibitory receptor. Cross-linking of FcγRIIb and the B-cell receptor (BCR) results in decreased intracellular calcium flux and decreased B-cell activation and proliferation. Engagement of FcγRIIb on dendritic cells also delivers an inhibitory signal. Deficiency in FcγRIIb results in a lower threshold for B-cell activation and unopposed activating FcR signaling in dendritic cells and macrophages. Substitutions

of one or more amino acids in the activating FcγR genes–arginine (R) for histidine (H) at position 131 in FcγRIIA and phenylalanine (F) for valine (V) at position 158 in FcγRIIIA–results in functional polymorphisms of these FcγRs with decreased binding affinity for IgG immune complexes. Associations between the FcγRIIA R131H allele and disease susceptibility or nephritis occur in Brazilian, Thai, Korean, German, and African-American populations. The recent finding that the FcγRIIa R131H allele predicts the efficacy of rituximab-induced B-cell depletion in SLE patients suggests that FcR polymorphisms may also predict a therapeutic response.[8] FcγRIIIA F158V and FcγRIIIB NA2/NA2 polymorphisms are reported to associate with disease susceptibility in Dutch, Korean, Thai, and Caucasian populations. The FcγRIIb I232T allele leads to the inability of the receptor to enter lipid rafts and is associated with SLE in Asian populations.[9] The collective results of these studies suggest substantial ethnic variation in these genetic polymorphisms.

CTLA-4 is upregulated on T cells after activation and dampens the inflammatory response. It has a higher affinity than CD28 for binding to B7.1 (CD80) and B7.2 (CD86), thereby competitively inhibiting engagement of CD28, and blocking the co-stimulatory signal required for activation. CTLA-4 ligation of B7 also activates indoleamine 2,3-dioxygenase (IDO) expression, an enzyme involved in tryptophan metabolism, and diminishes T-cell proliferation. Finally, CTLA-4 is critical for activation of regulatory T cells. In its absence, an uncontrolled, lethal inflammatory response occurs in mice. CTLA-4 alleles with decreased production of soluble CTLA4 are implicated in the pathogenesis of several autoimmune diseases, including Sjögren's disease, ulcerative colitis, psoriasis, type 1 diabetes, and multiple sclerosis, as well as SLE.[2]

The PTPN22 gene encodes a tyrosine phosphatase responsible for downregulating T-cell receptor activation. A polymorphism in PTPN22 resulting in diminished ability to control T-cell receptor activation has been reported in SLE. Similar to CTLA-4, the same polymorphism in PTPN22 is associated with other autoimmune diseases (rheumatoid arthritis, type 1 diabetes), suggesting a common mechanism of immune dysregulation in multiple autoimmune diseases.

Genes encoding cytokines and chemokines

Monocyte chemoattractant protein (MCP-1) is a potent chemoattractant for monocytes, memory T cells and natural killer T cells. MCP-1 expression is upregulated in renal tubular cells and glomeruli in lupus nephritis. Urinary levels of MCP-1 are increased in patients with active

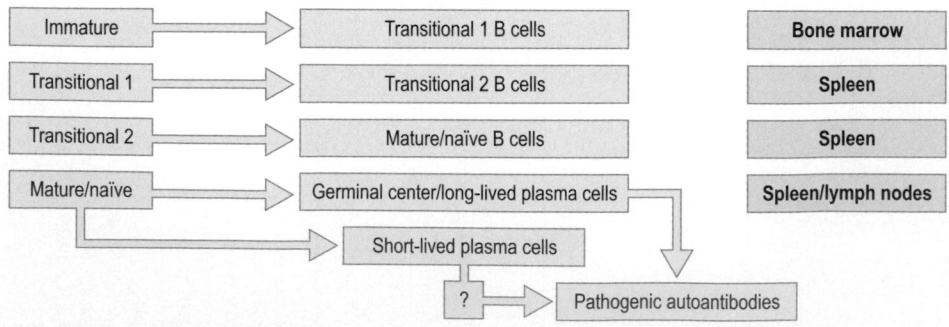

Fig. 51.1 Autoreactive B-cell checkpoints. There are tolerance checkpoints at every stage of B-cell activation and maturation. How many checkpoints need to be breached to achieve a pathogenic state and clinical disease is not known.

lupus nephritis. A functional MCP-1 polymorphism resulting in increased production of MCP-1 has been associated with SLE nephritis.[10] Polymorphisms in the tyrosine kinase-2 (tyk2) gene are associated with increased expression of type I interferons (IFN-α, IFN-β) in SLE. IFN-α-regulated genes are highly expressed in peripheral blood cells from SLE patients compared to healthy controls (the interferon signature).[11] IFN-α mediates maturation of dendritic cells and monocytes, increasing the capacity for T-cell activation, and promotes B-cell differentiation and Ig class switching. However, in two murine models of lupus, decreases in type 1 interferons unexpectedly led to worsening disease, suggesting that the effect of IFN-α on autoimmunity is more complex than currently appreciated.

Multiple polymorphisms in the IL-10 gene have been reported, with conflicting results with respect to SLE susceptibility. A meta-analysis of 15 studies concluded that some IL-10 polymorphisms do associate with SLE but their importance is modulated by ethic background.[12]

In the NZB/W murine model, a tumor necrosis factor (TNF) allele associated with low production is linked with disease, and treatment with TNF decreases autoantibody production. Consistent with this observation, TNF blockade for rheumatoid arthritis or inflammatory bowel disease leads to autoantibody production and infrequently to frank lupus. Several polymorphisms for genes encoding TNF-α and TNF-β (lymphotoxin-α) have been associated with SLE; these associations are also influenced by ethnicity.[13]

Genes associated with cell survival

Fas ligand (expressed on activated T cells) binding to Fas (CD95) stimulates a signaling pathway resulting in apoptotic death of the Fas-expressing cell. Fas-induced apoptosis of activated cells contributes to the elimination of autoreactive B and T lymphocytes. Lymphopenia in SLE has been associated with increased Fas expression on lymphocytes and Fas and Fas ligand alleles have been linked to disease susceptibility.[14]

Bcl-2 family genes encode intracellular proteins that are either pro- or anti-apoptotic. Increased expression of Bcl-2, an anti-apoptotic molecule, leads to a lupus-like serology and nephritis in mice with certain genetic backgrounds. Increased intracellular levels of Bcl-2 are reported in SLE. In Chinese and Mexican populations, Bcl-2 alleles are associated with increased risk of SLE. The combination of a Bcl-2 susceptibility allele and interleukin-10 (IL-10) susceptibility allele confers a 40-fold increased risk of SLE, demonstrating that *infelicitous* combinations potentiate risk.[15]

B CELLS

B-cell selection

Autoreactive B cells *per se* do not confer autoimmunity. The process of immunoglobulin variable region gene rearrangement produces large numbers of self-reactive B cells. To avoid autoimmunity, B cells displaying self-reactive immunoglobulin are deleted centrally in the bone marrow and at subsequent checkpoints in the periphery (Fig. 51.1). Several of these checkpoints appear deficient in SLE. Analysis of antibodies cloned from bone marrow-derived and peripheral blood B cells from healthy donors reveals that up to 75% of antibodies cloned from early immature B cells are autoreactive; 60% of these autoantibodies demonstrate an antinuclear staining pattern. The percent of autoreactive B cells decreases significantly as B cells progress through normal development. The first checkpoint occurs in the marrow at the immature B-cell stage,

where autoreactive B cells may undergo anergy, deletion, or receptor editing. Consequently, the frequency of autoreactive B-cell clones among newly minted B cells in the blood decreases to 40%. The frequency of autoreactive cells decreases further to 20% in the mature naïve B-cell population, although the mechanisms are not fully understood. The IgM cross-reactive autoantibodies made by these remaining autoreactive mature naïve B cells are thought to facilitate clearance of apoptotic cells, decreasing the development of potentially pathogenic T- and B-cell responses to self antigens.

Another important peripheral checkpoint is entry into the T-cell-dependent, long-lived memory compartment. Focusing on a population of B cells (9G4 B cells) that express antibodies encoded by the VH 4.34 gene reactive with *N*-acetyllactosamine (NAL) determinants of glycoproteins on blood group antigens targeted by cold agglutinins, gangliosides, gastrointestinal mucins, glycolipids, and CD45 on B lymphocytes, it is possible to track the fate of autoreactive peripheral B cells.[16]

9G4 B cells are present in 5–10% of the naïve B-cell population in healthy donors as well as in the IgM memory compartment. However, 9G4 B cells are excluded from the T-cell-dependent IgG memory and plasma cell populations, suggesting that these autoreactive cells fail to cross a developmental checkpoint following activation in normal individuals. Evaluation of tonsillar biopsies and spleens from healthy donors shows that the frequency of germinal centers with 9G4+ cells is less than 1%, implying that negative selection of autoreactive cells occurs at the transition of naïve to germinal center cells. In contrast to these findings from healthy donors, tonsillar biopsies from SLE patients demonstrate that 15–20% of germinal centers are positive for autoreactive 9G4 B cells. Autoreactive B cells surviving negative selection in the germinal center join the pool of long-lived antibody-producing plasma cells that home to the marrow. These cells tend to be refractory to treatment with cytotoxic drugs or anti-CD20 antibody.

Pathogenic B-cell autoimmunity

Autoantibodies characteristic of SLE are somatically mutated, IgG autoantibodies reflective of germinal center maturation. While studies demonstrate a failure to tolerize naïve autoreactive B cells, it is possible that some pathogenic autoantibodies are not derived from

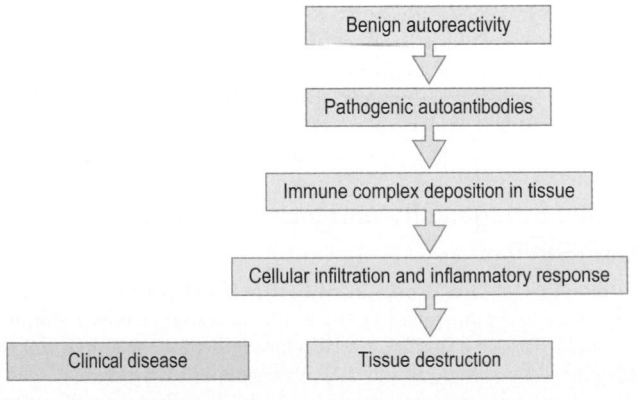

Fig. 51.2 Spectrum of autoimmunity.

natural autoantibodies, but are derived from an antibody with no autoreactive specificity. Support for this hypothesis includes the back mutation of a few anti-DNA antibodies to their germline-encoded precursors which lack autoreactivity. The failure of censoring mechanisms in germinal centers may reflect intrinsic B-cell abnormalities or abnormalities in co-stimulatory molecules, cytokines, dendritic cell, and T-cell interactions.

B-cell signaling

Hyperactive B-cell responses to immunologic stimulation are implicated in the production of pathogenic antibodies. SLE B cells have increased intracellular Ca2+ flux in response to BCR signaling.[17] Increased intracellular Ca2+ flux in SLE B cells is attributed, in part, to FcγRIIb dysfunction, including defective upregulation of FcγRIIb on memory B cells, decreased availability of the FcRIIb-associated intracellular SHIP protein, and an FcγRIIb polymorphism (Ile 232 Thr) that prevents partitioning of the receptor into lipid rafts where it usually associates with the BCR.[9]

The intracellular protein tyrosine kinase Lyn has both positive and negative effects on BCR signaling. Decreased expression of Lyn results in increased intracellular Ca2+ flux; B-cell hyperactivity is present in Lyn-deficient mice. Lyn expression is decreased in one-half to two-thirds of resting and activated B cells in SLE patients, suggesting that Lyn may modulate negative regulation of BCR signaling in human disease. A mutation in mice leading to increased expression of Lyn also results in an autoimmune phenotype with autoantibody production and severe glomerulonephritis.

B-cell rescue

B lymphocyte stimulator (BAFF; also known as BLyS) is a member of the TNF family and participates in B-cell maturation and survival. BAFF enhances survival of B cells through ligation of several receptors—BCMA, BAFF-R, and TACI. There is strong evidence supporting a role for BAFF in autoreactive B-cell rescue and SLE; mice overexpressing BAFF have a lupus-like disease.[18] In humans BAFF is encoded in an SLE susceptibility locus and elevated serum levels of BAFF are reported in patients (although this may be secondary to the lymphopenia seen in SLE).

CD40/CD40 ligand (CD40L) interactions are essential for germinal center formation and differentiation of memory cells into plasma cells. The interaction between T cells expressing CD40L and B cells expressing CD40 results in B-cell proliferation. Immature autoreactive B cells can be rescued from antigen-induced apoptosis by engagement of CD40 or by IL-4.[19] SLE T and B cells have upregulated CD40L, providing a critical molecule to mediate B-cell rescue.

B-cell pathogenicity unrelated to antibody production

An essential role for B cells in SLE that is independent of antibody production is demonstrated by the T-cell activation, kidney inflammation, and increased mortality in MRL/lpr lupus-prone mice that lack the ability to secrete antibody and their absence in mice that lack B cells. B cells are efficient antigen-presenting cells; B cells with self-reactive specificity that have escaped tolerance are likely to present self-peptides

to autoreactive T cells. These animal data are supported by initial observations of SLE patients treated with B-cell-depleting therapy demonstrating improvement in disease activity and normalization of B-cell compartments despite persistent elevation of serum autoantibody levels.

T CELLS

T cells in lupus contribute to the abrogation of self-tolerance by providing help to autoreactive B cells and facilitating the production of somatically mutated, high-affinity, pathogenic autoantibodies. Lupus T cells display increased expression of activation markers. Upon stimulation of the T-cell receptor (TCR), there is an abnormally increased intracellular influx of Ca2+ caused by a substitution of TCR ζ-chain for the γ-chain of the Fc receptor. Although there is a heightened Ca2+ influx after TCR stimulation, activation is impaired and IL-2 production is decreased. Lupus T cells are additionally less susceptible to activation-induced cell death.

Self-tolerance is maintained in part by the suppressive actions of regulatory T cells (Tregs). Studies of Tregs in patients with SLE have demonstrated reduced numbers of peripheral CD4+CD25+ cells in patients with active disease.[20]

■ HORMONAL INFLUENCES ■

The most compelling evidence for the role of sex hormones in SLE is the fact that lupus affects women of child-bearing age. The female-to-male ratio is 2:1 prior to menarche, 8–9:1 in the fourth decade, and 2:1 after menopause. Numerous case reports and studies of disease flares correlating with pregnancy, menstruation, and use of oral contraceptives containing high doses of estrogen suggest a role for estrogen in disease activity. A significant correlation in SLE between plasma levels of estradiol and clinical disease activity and increased α hydroxylation of estrogen in SLE yielding the more active metabolite 16α-hydroxyestrone is also reported.[21] No significant differences in levels of sex hormones (including estrogen, testosterone, prolactin) are noted in male SLE patients, suggesting that the development of SLE in females may be more closely related to sex hormones than in men. Randomized, controlled studies of estrogen in SLE suggest that the use of exogenous estrogen in patients with stable disease may be safe; however, a subset of patients appear to have an estrogen-sensitive disease. Mild to moderate flare rates were significantly increased in postmenopausal women treated with hormone replacement therapy.

Most of what we understand about hormonal modulation of B-cell development comes from mouse studies.[19] Estrogen treatment of NZB/W and MRL/lpr mice or castration of male lupus-prone mice exacerbates disease whereas oophorectomy of females ameliorates disease. Treatment of lupus-prone mice with the selective estrogen receptor modulator tamoxifen also ameliorates disease.

Estrogen and prolactin promote the loss of B-cell tolerance in mice that are not genetically predisposed to spontaneous autoimmunity. In nonautoimmune BALB/c mice that are transgenic for the heavy chain of a nephritogenic anti-DNA antibody, DNA-reactive B cells are regulated by negative selection and serum titers of the transgene-encoded anti-DNA antibody are low. After exposure to estrogen (at doses similar to those present during follicular and luteal phases of the

CLINICAL PEARLS

>> Systemic lupus erythematosus (SLE) is a systemic disease with the potential to affect any organ system

>> The differential diagnosis of a lupus flare mandates consideration of infection, drug toxicities, or other etiologies

>> In the absence of data from randomized trials, use of aggressive treatment must be balanced against associated toxicity

>> SLE patients are at high risk of developing atherosclerotic disease, osteoporosis, malignancy, diabetes mellitus and hypertension (HTN); screening for and reduction of modifiable risk factors are essential

>> Appropriate vaccinations are advisable

estrus cycle), there is a significant increase in serum titers of the transgene-encoded antibody and a selective expansion and maturation of transgene-bearing autoreactive cells into marginal-zone B cells. Several estrogen-responsive genes have been identified in B cells, including cd22 and shp-1; both result in diminished B-cell responsiveness to BCR cross-linking and less stringent negative selection. Bcl-2 is also upregulated by estrogen and known to facilitate escape of autoreactive B cells from tolerance mechanisms. Two intracellular estrogen receptors, ERα and ERβ, mediate the response to estrogen. Polymorphisms of the ERα gene are associated with age of disease onset and disease severity in some human SLE populations.

Elevated prolactin levels are reported in 20% of patients with SLE and increased prolactin exposure in lupus-prone mice exacerbates disease activity. While treatment of patients with bromocriptine yielded equivocal results, treatment of NZB/W lupus mice with bromocriptine results in improved survival. Transmembrane prolactin receptors are present on a variety of cells, including T and B cells. Similar to the findings with estrogen treatment, prolactin treatment of BALB/c mice transgenic for the nephritogenic anti-DNA heavy chain leads to the development of a lupus-like serologic profile. Prolactin treatment, however, results in an expansion of autoreactive B cells with a follicular phenotype. Upregulation of both Bcl-2 and CD40 on B cells and CD40L on T cells occurs in response to prolactin, identifying two pathways that may be involved in the prolactin-mediated rescue of autoreactive B cells.

■ CLINICAL MANIFESTATIONS ■

SYSTEMIC FEATURES

The most common features of lupus are constitutional and include fatigue (which may be severe), malaise, low-grade fever, anorexia, and lymphadenopathy. These symptoms may accompany other, more severe organ system manifestations of active disease or may occur alone. Although frequent, these symptoms are nonspecific and do not aid in making the diagnosis of SLE nor in distinguishing flare in individuals with known disease. Infection must be excluded in a patient who presents with constitutional symptoms. Symptoms of fatigue and malaise may also represent fibromyalgia, which co-occurs with SLE.[22]

MUSCULOSKELETAL INVOLVEMENT

The musculoskeletal system is the most common organ system involved, affecting the joints, muscles, soft tissues, and bones. In approximately 50% of patients, joint pain is the presenting symptom.

Arthritis and arthralgia

The pattern of joint involvement is usually symmetric, affecting the small joints of the hands, wrists, and knees. Pain in the ankles, elbows, shoulders, or hips or monoarticular involvement is less typical. The duration of joint pain and stiffness is variable, with morning stiffness typically lasting only for several minutes. Frequently, the subjective complaints of pain are greater than the objective findings of warmth, swelling, and, occasionally, erythema. Lupus arthritis is characteristically nonerosive and nondeforming. Some lupus patients do develop a hand deformity with hypermobile joints secondary to tendon and ligamentous laxity (Jacoud's arthritis) (Fig. 51.3). Erosions are seen on plain radiographs in fewer than 5% of cases and patients with erosions are said to have 'rhupus,' which is typically associated with deforming arthritis, Sjögren's syndrome, subcutaneous nodules, and serologies that include a positive rheumatoid factor. Utilization of more sensitive imaging techniques such as magnetic resonance imaging (MRI) may show erosions in patients without deforming arthritis. Proliferative tenosynovitis, synovitis, and capsular swelling are other features of soft-tissue involvement that may be seen on MRI.

Joint effusions, when they occur, are usually small. The fluid is clear, yellow with normal viscosity, and able to form a mucin clot. It is typically noninflammatory with a normal glucose level and a white blood cell (WBC) count of less than 2000 cells/ml that is predominantly lymphocytic. Occasionally joint effusions are exudates, with leukocyte counts approaching 15,000 cells/ml and increased protein levels. ANA performed on the synovial fluid may be positive and LE cells may be present. Synovial fluid complement levels may be normal or depressed. Synovial histology in lupus is not specific and shows synovial hyperplasia with fibrin deposition and microvascular changes that include a perivascular infiltrate in the majority of cases.

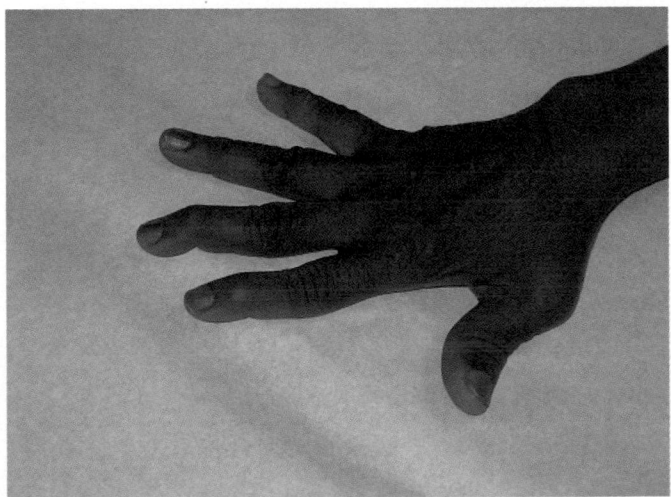

Fig. 51.3 Jacoud's arthritis in systemic lupus erythematosus.

Tendinitis

Tendinitis is not usually attributed to SLE unless associated with tendon rupture. This is an uncommon feature of lupus but, when present, is usually located in the Achilles tendon or the tendons around the knee. Tendon ruptures are more common in males and have been associated with trauma, steroid use, and long disease duration.[22] Biopsy shows a mononuclear infiltrate with tendon degeneration and neovascularization. The diagnosis can be easily demonstrated on MRI.

Myositis/myalgia

Generalized myalgia is extremely common in lupus. It frequently affects the deltoids and quadriceps and occurs during flares of active disease. Muscle disease secondary to treatment with corticosteroids, statins, and anti-malarials or in association with hypothyroidism is also frequent and must be considered in the evaluation of a lupus patient with myalgia. Inflammatory muscle disease with weakness and an elevated creatine phosphokinase is less common and occurs in approximately 10% of lupus patients.[22] Electromyography may be normal or may be characteristic of the myositis observed in polymyositis or dermatomyositis. Muscle biopsy may also be normal or may show changes associated with dermatomyositis such as a perivascular or perifascicular infiltrate and immunoglobulin and complement deposition. Muscle atrophy, fiber necrosis, microtubular inclusions, and/or a mononuclear infiltrate have also been documented. MRI findings are nonspecific.

Avascular necrosis

Avascular necrosis (AVN) has been reported in up to 30% of lupus patients, and is frequently asymptomatic.[23] The most commonly affected site is the femoral head. Groin pain exacerbated with weight-bearing is a common complaint. In addition to the hip, AVN commonly involves the knees, shoulders, and wrists. The majority of AVN is associated with administration of high doses of corticosteroids (> 30 mg/day). Other reported risk factors include Raynaud's phenomenon, hyperlipidemia, and the presence of antiphospholipid antibodies, although these are unconfirmed. Bone biopsy in lupus patients affected by AVN does not reveal unique findings.

MUCOCUTANEOUS MANIFESTATIONS

Skin

The skin is also commonly affected in SLE with numerous types of lesions that are influenced by race and genetic factors as well as environmental exposures and age at onset of disease[24] (Table 51.3). Though rarely life-threatening, cutaneous lesions may be quite disfiguring.

Acute cutaneous SLE

The malar rash typically occurs across the cheeks and nose but may include the forehead and chin, sparing the nasolabial folds (unlike seborrheic dermatitis) (Fig. 51.4). It usually begins as small discrete erythematous macules or papules that coalesce and is frequently associated with sun exposure. Some patients additionally have facial swelling. The

malar rash heals without scarring. The differential diagnosis of a malar rash includes acne rosacea, seborrheic dermatitis, erysipelas, dermatomyositis, and contact dermatitis. Microscopic analysis reveals a sparse inflammatory lymphocytic dermatitis with occasional histiocytes engulfing nuclear debris resembling LE cells found close to the dermoepidermal junction. Immunofluorescent staining for complement components and immunoglobulin at the dermoepidermal junction is positive in 70–80% of patients with a malar rash.

Photosensitivity is common in SLE; many lupus rashes arise in sun-exposed areas and sun exposure can precipitate flares of systemic disease. Typically, a photosensitive rash erupts within hours of sun exposure and consists of tiny pruritic plaques and vesicles lasting several days. Ultraviolet (UV) light induces DNA damage and triggers apoptosis of keratinocytes. SLE patients have increased numbers of apoptotic keratinocytes after exposure to UV light,[25] thus sun exposure may provide a rich source of antigen. UV light and apoptosis have also been implicated in the translocation of nuclear antigens to surface blebs and with increased chemotaxis of plasmacytoid dendritic cells and T cells to skin lesions, with ensuing production of pro-inflammatory cytokines (IL-1, TNF-α, IL-10, IFN-γ). Of note, photosensitivity, along with oral ulcers, alopecia, and Raynaud's phenomenon, has been identified as a predictor of systemic involvement and more severe disease.

Subacute cutaneous lupus (SCLE) is characterized by recurrent, nonscarring, nonindurated skin lesions associated with anti-Ro antibodies. This distinctive rash consists of erythematous papules and plaques, with or without adherent pityriasiform scale, that erupt on the extremities and trunk, usually sparing the head and neck. These lesions may take an annular polycyclic form with a hypopigmented central area and tiny vesicles at the active margins and can be mistaken for erythema multiforme. The differential diagnosis also includes psoriasis, polymorphic light eruption, and tinea corporis. SCLE is exacerbated by UV light and a growing list of medications; common offenders are thiazides and calcium channel blockers (particularly in the elderly). Biopsy reveals a significant lymphocytic dermatitis confined to the superficial and mid dermis, frequently with associated dermal edema, mucinosis, and

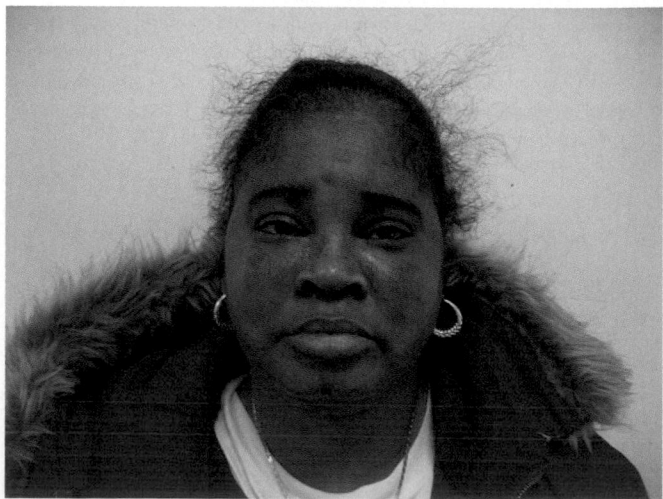

Fig. 51.4 Malar rash in a systemic lupus erythematosus patient.

degenerating keratinocytes. Both TNF-α and IL-6 have been demonstrated in active SCLE lesions. SCLE is most commonly seen in Caucasian populations. Genetic analyses have revealed associations with HLA-A1, B8, and DR3 haplotypes, as well as with deficiencies of C2, C4, and C1q. Sixty to 90% of SCLE patients have anti-Ro antibodies while approximately 50% meet ACR criteria for SLE; only ~10% experience severe, life-threatening internal organ involvement.

Chronic cutaneous SLE

Discoid lesions (DLE) are usually localized to the head and neck in photoexposed areas with a predilection for the ears and periorbital areas (Fig. 51.5). DLE lesions range in diameter from a few millimeters to 10 cm. Early lesions appear as erythematous plaques with or without follicular hyperkeratosis, plugging, and scale and progress to scarring annular lesions with an erythematous, indurated border, adherent scale, and a central area with atrophy and telangectasias. There are no autoantibody associations with DLE and only 5% of patients with DLE develop systemic lupus. High-titer ANA, Raynaud's phenomenon, and the presence of arthralgias may identify patients at risk for systemic evolution. Histopathology characteristically reveals a lymphocytic interface dermatitis with CD4 lymphocytes and plasmacytoid dendritic cells involving follicles and epidermis. There is vacuolar degeneration of the basal layer of epidermal keratinocytes and prominent keratotic follicular plugging. Dermal mucin deposition is also characteristic of DLE lesions and there is usually dense granular deposition of immunoglobulin (predominantly IgG) and C3 at the dermal–epidermal junction. Patients with C2, C4, and C1q deficiencies may be predisposed to DLE and polymorphisms in the promoter regions of genes associated with high IL-10 and low TNF-α are risk factors for DLE.

Lupus profundus typically presents as firm, tender, deep subcutaneous nodules that may atrophy over time. Overlaying epidermal changes include DLE, ulcerations, and dystrophic calcification. Biopsy reveals a lobular panniculitis with patchy lymphoplasmacytic infiltrate in subcutaneous fat lobules. Panniculitis occurs in 10–20% of patients and must be differentiated from a subcutaneous T-cell lymphoma or other variants of panniculitis such as erythema nodosum, pancreatic panniculitis, and morphea.

Nonspecific skin lesions reported in SLE are typically seen during disease flares and are associated with greater disease severity. Theses lesions include, but are not limited to, entities such as cutaneous vasculitis (Fig. 51.6), urticaria, Raynaud's phenomenon, livedo reticularis, alopecia, sclerodactyly, calcinosis cutis, atrophie blanche, bullous lesions, erythema multiforme, and leg ulcers.

The lupus band test (LBT) refers to the deposition of immunoglobulin (IgG, IgM, and/or IgA) and/or C3 along the dermoepidermal junction. Approximately 25% of normal individuals display weak IgM staining at the dermoepidermal junction; 70–80% of SLE patients have a positive LBT in sunexposed, nonlesional skin. Half of SLE patients have a positive LBT in non-sun-exposed, nonlesional skin. It is unclear if the LBT is a consequence of circulating ANA targeting denatured DNA from UV light-damaged keratinocytes, or immune complex deposition or anti-basement membrane antibodies. The test may be useful diagnostically and prognostically as it correlates with increased systemic disease severity.

In summary, the acute cutaneous lesions of malar rash and photosensitivity are strongly associated with systemic disease, whereas 50% of those with SCLE and only 5% of patients with DLE develop systemic disease. Conversely, the incidence of DLE lesions in lupus cohorts is variable (with one report of 73%) and the incidence of SCLE is approximately 5–10%. Nonspecific cutaneous lesions such as cutaneous vasculitis or ulcers are associated with a more aggressive disease course than most of the SLE-specific lesions.

Hair and nail

Hair involvement in SLE includes scarring alopecia resulting in permanent hair loss, induced by DLE. This can be differentiated from other common forms of scarring alopecia by immunofluorescent studies. Patchy or diffuse nonscarring alopecia is frequently associated with disease activity. Histologically, there is a peribulbar lymphocytic infiltrate surrounding shrunken anagen hair bulbs similar to findings in alopecia areata. The diagnosis is made by the presence of other criteria

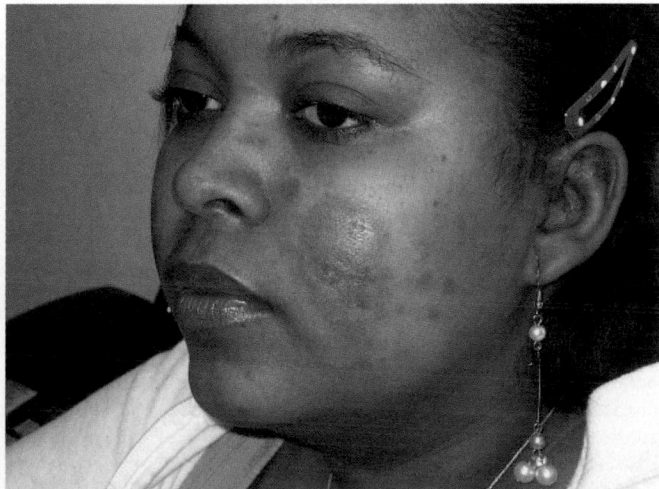

Fig. 51.5 Discoid lesion in systemic lupus erythematosus.

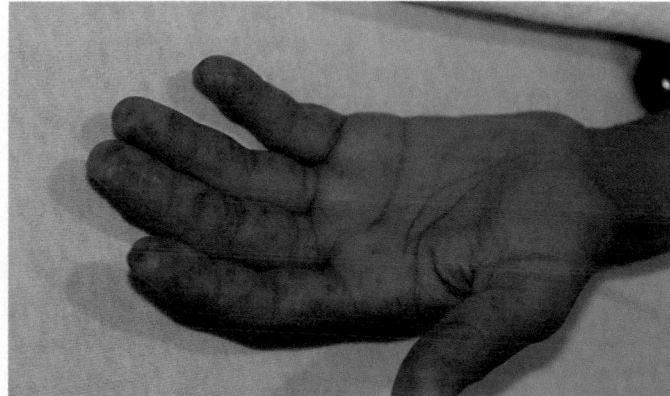

Fig. 51.6 Cutaneous vasculitis affecting the hands in a patient with active systemic lupus erythematosus.

for SLE. Nonscarring alopecia resolves with complete hair regrowth with control of disease activity.

A wide spectrum of nail abnormalities, including pitting, ridging, onycholysis, and dyschromia with blue or black hyperpigmentation, are reported in up to 30% of SLE patients. Nailfold erythema with ragged cuticles and splinter hemorrhages resembling the changes seen in dermatomyositis are common. However, other than rare DLE lesions involving the nailbed, none are lupus-specific.

Oral lesions

The spectrum of oral lesions reported in SLE includes cheilitis, ulcerations, erythematous patches, lichen planus-type plaques on the buccal mucosa and palate, and DLE.[26] Most oral lesions are asymptomatic and must be looked for on exam. Positive immunofluorescent staining on biopsy may be useful to differentiate DLE from lichen planus-like lesions and leukoplakia. Lupus mucosal ulcerations demonstrate an interface mucositis and not leukocytoclastic vasculitis, as previously postulated. The incidence of mucosal lesions is variable depending on ethnicity (Table 51.3).

GASTROINTESTINAL MANIFESTATIONS

Gastrointestinal manifestations of SLE[27] are common; it is often difficult to differentiate between disease activity, side effects of medications, and infectious complications. Most SLE patients require therapy with nonsteroidal anti-inflammatory drugs and/or corticosteroids, increasing the risk of ulcer disease.

Esophagus

The prevalence of esophageal involvement varies. Many of the reviews citing a high incidence of dysphagia and odynophagia predate the advent of proton pump inhibitors and H_2 blockers and the relationship of medication use to symptoms is not clear. Dysphagia and heartburn are reported in 1–50% of patients, although dysmotility documented by decreased esophageal peristalsis and decreased lower esophageal sphincter pressure is observed in up to 72%. An inflammatory process involving esophageal muscle or vasculitic damage to the Auerbach plexus is thought to contribute to the esophageal dysmotility. Ulceration is rarely seen outside the context of infections such as invasive candidiasis, herpes simplex, or cytomegalovirus. SLE patients with a secondary Sjögren's syndrome may have salivary gland dysfunction resulting in decreased saliva contributing to dysphagia.

Abdominal pain/vasculitis

Abdominal pain is commonly seen in SLE with an incidence reported as high as 40%; the clinical challenge is to distinguish active SLE (serositis, pancreatitis, intestinal ischemia/vasculitis) from one of the long list of infectious, metabolic, vascular, mechanical, embolic, and medication-induced causes of abdominal pain.

The most catastrophic gastrointestinal disturbances are related to ischemia of the small and large intestines resulting from medium- and small-vessel vasculitis or thrombotic complications of anti-phospholipid antibodies. The mortality associated with intestinal ischemia is high. In

a review of 51 cases of SLE patients presenting with acute abdominal pain, a significant correlation between SLEDAI scores reflecting disease activity and intestinal ischemia due to vasculitis was found. Alternatively, the presence of a livedoid rash with thrombocytopenia and elevated antiphospholipid antibodies may suggest a thrombosis-related ischemia. Heme-positive stool, an elevated WBC count, and presence of an anion gap acidosis are indicative of perforation. Computed tomography (CT) of the abdomen is the preferred imaging test for evaluation of abdominal pathology. Bowel ischemia is suggested by wall thickening and edema, demonstration of the target sign in the bowel wall, dilatation of intestinal segments, engorgement of mesenteric vessels, and increased attenuation of mesenteric fat. Plain radiographs are useful for detecting free air from a perforated viscus. MR angiography is of limited use due to its decreased sensitivity for small-sized vessels.

Intestinal vasculitis has a reported prevalence of 0.2–53%. Its presentation is not necessarily severe abdominal pain; an insidious, stuttering course, with nausea, vomiting, bloating, diarrhea, post-prandial fullness, anorexia, and weight loss is well recognized. Mesenteric vasculitis preferentially affects the superior mesenteric artery, involving the small intestine more commonly than the large bowel. Vasculitis may occur in the esophagus, stomach, peritoneum, rectum, gallbladder, pancreas, and liver. In cases with an insidious clinical course, endoscopy and colonoscopy may provide evidence of ischemia demonstrating ulcerating or heaped-up lesions and overt vasculitis on biopsy. The lesions are segmental and focal. Histologically, there is a small-vessel arteritis and venulitis with neutrophilic, lymphocytic, and macrophage infiltrates and fibrinoid necrosis of the vessel walls, associated thrombosis, and mononuclear infiltrate in the lamina propria. There may be immunoglobulin, C3, and fibrin deposition in the adventitia and media.

Treatment of acute abdominal pain in SLE is tailored to the underlying cause. Given the potential consequences of undertreating intestinal vasculitis, most patients are treated with high-dose intravenous corticosteroids (1–2 mg/kg per day) and observed closely for progression of disease. Delayed surgical intervention in the event of necrotic bowel is associated with a poorer outcome. Most patients respond after treatment with corticosteroids; the decision to add other immunosuppressive agents is based on anecdotal evidence. There are no randomized trials of immunosuppressive agents to date for the treatment of intestinal vasculitis.

Peritonitis

Inflammation of serosal membranes is well described in SLE; despite evidence of peritoneal inflammation in 63% of autopsy studies, clinical pericarditis and pleuritis occur far more commonly than peritonitis. Acute peritonitis is attributed to peritoneal vasculitis or ischemia and presents with abdominal pain (see above). The finding of ascitic fluid by CT scan or ultrasound mandates an evaluation of the fluid to exclude an infectious etiology. Rarely, ascites may be attributable to hepatic or portal vein thrombosis. Chronic peritonitis characterized by large amounts of painless ascites attributable to SLE and not to heart failure, constrictive pericarditis or severe hypoalbuminemia due to nephrotic syndrome, liver disease, or a protein-losing enteropathy is rare. In lupus peritonitis, the ascitic fluid is generally exudative with a predominance of lymphocytes; LE cells, autoantibodies and low complement levels are frequent. Exclusion of malignancy and indolent infection (tuberculosis, fungal infections) is essential. On biopsy, the peritoneum is usually edematous, and sometimes hemorrhagic with lymphocytic perivascular infiltrates.

Pancreatitis

Pancreatitis attributable to SLE is rare, with an annual reported incidence of 0.4–1/1000. In a recent review of 77 reported cases, most patients with pancreatitis had evidence of other clinical or serological manifestations of disease.[28] Although corticosteroids and azathioprine are medications known to trigger pancreatitis, 34% of reported cases are not on these medications at the onset of pancreatitis and most patients respond to steroid therapy. The clinical presentation of pancreatitis is similar in patients with and without SLE: abdominal pain, nausea/vomiting, fever, and pain radiating to the back. In 97% of cases, the diagnosis is made based on elevated levels of amylase or lipase. CT and ultrasound as well as endoscopic retrograde cholangiopancreatography are useful, but less sensitive, diagnostic tools. Leukopenia, thrombocytopenia, and anemia are commonly observed. Histologic findings show inflammation and necrosis; there is a single report of pancreatic vasculitis. Mortality rates are reported from 18% to 27%; poor outcome is associated with increased systemic SLE activity (particularly low complement and thrombocytopenia) and the development of complications of pancreatitis. Patients receiving steroid therapy tend to have a better outcome.

Liver

Controversy continues over the existence of "lupoid hepatitis."[29] Analysis of SLE livers from 52 autopsies in Japan revealed a variety of findings, including congestion (40/52), fatty liver (38/52), arteritis (11/52), cholestasis (9/52), and a few cases each of chronic persistent hepatitis, nodular regenerative hyperplasia, hemangioma, and cholangiolitis. Cirrhosis is an extremely rare complication of liver involvement in SLE. The distinction between subclinical liver inflammation related to SLE (lupus hepatitis/LH) and autoimmune hepatitis (AIH) is important since therapy and prognosis are different. In contrast to the mild enzyme abnormalities associated with lupus hepatitis, AIH is a progressive disease frequently leading to hepatic failure. Both conditions share a predilection for young women and both demonstrate features of autoimmunity, including hypergammaglobulinemia, arthralgias, and serum autoantibodies. Histologically, biopsies of LH reveal lobular and periportal lymphocytic infiltrates, in contrast to the periportal and piecemeal necrosis with dense lymphocytic infiltrates seen in AIH with progression to panlobular or multilobular necrosis and cirrhosis. Serologically, anti-ribosomal P antibodies are associated with liver disease in LH but not AIH; AIH is associated with antibodies to liver and kidney microsomes. Anti-smooth-muscle antibodies are observed in 60–80% of patients with AIH compared to 30% of patients with LH. Although both have a favorable response to steroids, AIH usually requires additional immunosuppressive agents.

Distinguishing LH from hepatitis C (HCV) can be difficult. Up to 30% of patients chronically infected with HCV have low titers of ANA and other autoantibodies (anti-DNA, anti-cardiolipin antibodies, and rheumatoid factor). They may also have cryoglobulins and associated cryoglobulinemic vasculitis. It is necessary to confirm a positive enzyme-linked immunosorbent assay (ELISA) for HCV with polymerase chain reaction (PCR) in patients presenting with arthritis, cutaneous vasculitis, and a positive ANA as SLE patients may have false-positive serological tests for HCV.

Protein-losing enteropathy

Profound hypoalbuminemia in the absence of severe nephrotic syndrome, liver disease, or constrictive pericarditis should trigger a consideration of protein-losing enteropathy (PLE). The diagnosis is confirmed with an increased α_1-antitrypsin level in a 24-hour stool collection. A review of the 31 cases reported prior to 2002 found that only half the patients experienced diarrhea; endoscopy was either normal or revealed edematous bowel.[30] In biopsies from 22 patients, normal or edematous villi were seen in 12 patients, lymphangiectasia in two, dilated lymphatic vessels in two, inflammation in two, and venulitis in one. These biopsy results implicate a potential role of TNF-α and IFN-γ in the increased vascular and enterocyte permeability in PLE.

PULMONARY INVOLVEMENT

Lupus affects the lungs in diverse ways involving the pleura, lung parenchyma, and blood vessels. The most frequent and important complicating feature is infection, which must be considered before attributing a respiratory symptom to SLE.

Pleuritis

Pleuritis is the most common pulmonary manifestation of SLE, reported in 40–56%.[31] Pleural involvement in up to 93% of lupus patients at autopsy suggests that much pleuritis may be asymptomatic. Clinically, patients note typical pleuritic pain. On physical exam, the most frequent abnormality is tachypnea; a pleural friction rub is present in some cases and pleural effusions occur in more severe cases. Pleural fluid is usually exudative with normal glucose and pH and elevated protein levels. The leukocyte count is variable and may range from several hundred to 20 000 cells/mm3; both a lymphocytic and neutrophilic predominance are reported. Immunologic testing on pleural fluid may show reduced complement levels and the presence of ANA, anti-DNA antibodies, and LE cells. Although these tests are commonly obtained, these results are neither sensitive nor specific to diagnose lupus pleuritis.

Lupus pneumonitis

Lupus pneumonitis is uncommon, occurring in up to 10% of patients. Patients present with dyspnea, cough, mild pleuritic chest pain, and fever. Pulmonary infiltrates are present on plain radiograph or CT. This presentation must be distinguished from an infectious etiology with

KEY CONCEPTS

>> Continued heightened awareness of SLE to shorten the time between onset of symptoms and diagnosis will improve outcomes

>> Lupus is a disease characterized by recurrent flares

>> Attentive monitoring, even during periods of disease remission, leads to early recognition of impending flare, better control, and better prognosis

>> Lupus is a chronic disease; the importance of emotional/social support and patient education cannot be overemphasized

appropriate cultures. Histologic examination of affected lung tissue shows alveolar edema and hemorrhage with hyaline membrane formation; immunofluorescent staining reveals immune complex deposition.

Pulmonary hemorrhage

Pulmonary hemorrhage is a rare but potentially fatal complication of SLE. Typically, symptoms include shortness of breath and hemoptysis or a cough productive of blood-tinged sputum accompanied by a fall in hemoglobin, usually occurring in the context of multiorgan involvement from SLE. Imaging may show patchy infiltrates. Lung function is marked by an increased diffusion capacity of the lung for carbon monoxide (DLCO) (secondary to alveolar blood). Histopathology shows bland intra-alveolar hemorrhage and hemosiderin-laden macrophages, although microangiitis with an inflammatory infiltrate and necrosis of the alveolar septa can occur. As hemorrhage into the lung may be secondary to thrombotic thrombocytopenia, demonstration of an inflammatory process in the pulmonary vessels or tissue is helpful to establish a diagnosis of primary pulmonary hemorrhage.

Chronic diffuse interstitial lung disease

Chronic diffuse interstitial lung disease is a relatively uncommon manifestation of SLE. Patients with anti-Ro antibodies may be at increased risk. It usually has a progressive course with a chronic nonproductive cough with dyspnea and pleuritic chest pains. Physical exam is frequently remarkable for basilar rales with diminished diaphragmatic movement. Pulmonary function tests demonstrate a restrictive pattern with decreased diffusion capacity; oxygen saturation is decreased. Imaging often shows interstitial fibrosis that is more prominent at the lung bases. High-resolution CT (HRCT) is a sensitive technique used for detection of parenchymal abnormalities. A recent study reported that 38% of lupus patients without known pulmonary involvement and normal chest radiographs had abnormal HRCT scans with reduced DLCO on pulmonary function testing. HRCT is also useful to determine the extent of treatable disease, i.e., fibrosis (honeycombing) versus inflammation (ground glass). The most reliable method to assess the extent of pulmonary inflammation in comparison to fibrotic damage is by histologic examination. Evaluation of bronchial alveolar lavage fluid helps to exclude infection.

Pulmonary hypertension

Pulmonary hypertension unrelated to chronic pulmonary emboli or interstitial lung disease occurs in SLE. Severe cases are rare; the recent recognition of milder cases may be partially attributed to the availability of newer effective therapies. Patients note progressive dyspnea commonly occurring in the absence of infiltrates on chest radiographs or significant hypoxemia. Chest pain and a chronic nonproductive cough are also frequently present. Pulmonary function testing reveals a reduced DLCO. Elevated pulmonary artery pressure is documented with cardiac angiogram or echocardiogram. Biopsy or autopsy specimens of the lung reveal 'plexiform' lesions that resemble those seen in primary pulmonary hypertension.

Shrinking-lung syndrome

The shrinking-lung syndrome refers to the rare findings of shortness of breath occurring in the absence of pleuritis or interstitial lung disease plus a chest X-ray showing elevated hemidiaphragms. Pulmonary function testing shows a restrictive pattern with loss of lung volume. It is generally accepted that this syndrome results from diaphragmatic weakness (from a myopathic process) or chest wall restriction. There is no definitive therapy, although immunosuppressive therapy with cytotoxic agents usually results in an improvement of lung function and respiratory symptoms.

CARDIAC INVOLVEMENT

There are a number of ways in which lupus affects the cardiovascular system. The myocardium, valves, pericardium, and vessels can be affected.

Myocardium

Myocardial dysfunction in SLE is likely to be secondary to factors other than lupus, including hypertension, medications, or coronary artery disease (CAD). However, a cardiomyopathy resulting from immune-mediated myocardial inflammation does occur, either in isolation or concomitant with systemic disease, including myositis. Inflammatory myocarditis is often associated with anti-RNP antibodies. Histopathology typically shows a mononuclear, inflammatory cell infiltrate. Perivascular or myocardial wall deposits of immune complexes and complement have been demonstrated. Myocardial biopsy is useful for diagnosis as well as for determination of the extent of active inflammatory disease and fibrosis. Symptoms and signs of myocarditis include unexplained tachycardia, an abnormal electrocardiogram (with ST and T-wave abnormalities), cardiomegaly; and heart failure. Echocardiography may show systolic and diastolic ventricular dysfunction. Myocardial involvement without overt clinical signs occurs commonly and may be documented using Doppler echocardiography. A noninflammatory cardiomyopathy may be seen in association with high-dose cyclophosphamide, usually of the magnitude used to treat malignancy. This potential complication of therapy may become increasingly concerning as patients are exposed to greater cumulative doses of cyclosphophamide over time, or to doses of cyclophosphamide that are used in immunoablation protocols.

Valvular heart disease

Valvular abnormalities, with thickening, regurgitation, or verrucous vegetations, occur commonly in SLE and are documented by transesophageal echocardiography in 50–60% of patients.[32] The characteristic Libman–Sacks lesion, nonbacterial verrucous vegetations, is observed at autopsy in 15–60% of patients. Mitral, aortic, and tricuspid valves are most frequently involved. Clinically these lesions are usually asymptomatic and hemodynamic compromise, rupture of the chordae tendinae, or infection are rare events. On histologic examination, mononuclear cells, hematoxylin bodies, fibrin and platelet thrombi, and immune complexes are present. Anti-phospholipid antibodies may be associated with the development of valvular heart disease, although their pathogenic role is still unproven.

Pericarditis

Serosal inflammation of the pericardium is a frequent manifestation of SLE. While asymptomatic pericarditis is common, occurring in greater than 50% of patients, clinical pericarditis is seen in only 25% of patients. Pericardial fluid and thickening can be detected by echocardiography; cardiac silhouette enlargement on plain films is seen in the presence of large effusions. There are no unique signs and symptoms of pericarditis in lupus patients. Cardiac tamponade and constrictive pericarditis are infrequent. The histologic findings of acute pericarditis in lupus are inflammation with a monuclear cell infiltrate accompanied by immunoglobulin and complement deposition. The pericardial fluid is usually an exudate with elevated protein concentrations, normal or low glucose levels, and an elevated WBC count that is primarily neutrophilic. Complement levels in the fluid are low and autoantibodies (ANA, dsDNA) and LE cells have been reported. Analogous to pleural fluid, results of pericardial fluid analysis are neither sensitive nor specific.

Coronary artery disease

Myocardial infarction, angina, and sudden death resulting from CAD are well described in SLE. Estimates of the prevalence of CAD vary widely; however, the risk of myocardial infarction is 50-fold greater in young women with lupus than in normal age-matched controls.[33] Coronary artery vasculitis is a potential cause of CAD but is exceedingly rare and surgical and postmortem specimens commonly show atherosclerotic plaque. The underlying mechanisms that result in accelerated atherosclerosis are unknown. The prevalence of traditional risk factors for CAD, such as hypertension, diabetes, and hyperlipidemia, is increased in lupus patients. However, lupus *per se* confers an additional increased risk for CAD. Lupus-related factors that have been reported include duration of SLE, duration of corticosteroid use, and absence of use of hydroxychloroquine. The potential contributing influence of antibodies to phospholipids or disease activity continues to be explored. There is a growing body of evidence supporting a risk conferred by inflammation *per se*. Patients with rheumatoid arthritis are recognized to have an increased risk of atherosclerotic events; increased atherosclerosis has also been reported in patients with systemic vasculitis. The pathogenic link between accelerated atherosclerosis and autoimmune inflammatory disease is not known; however, atherosclerosis involves more than the accumulation of lipid in an arterial wall. The atherosclerotic plaque is infiltrated by activated monocytes, macrophages, and T cells and expression of proinflammatory cytokines. If endothelial dysfunction and vascular injury are the events triggering atherosclerosis, there are multiple potentially responsible processes in lupus, including autoantibodies directed to endothelial cells, immune complexes, and enhanced cleavage of membrane endothelial protein C receptor.[34]

RENAL INVOLVEMENT

Lupus nephritis is a common manifestation of disease with significant impact on morbidity and mortality. The prevalence of nephritis ranges from 50% to 75% in reported cohorts. Renal disease is more prevalent and more aggressive in Afro-Americans and Hispanics, who exhibit a greater incidence of proliferative nephritis than Caucasians. Low socioeconomic status, independent of ethnicity, is predictive of poor prognosis. Additionally pediatric lupus and male lupus are both associated with a greater incidence of, and more aggressive, nephritis. Onset of nephritis occurs at any time and monitoring for potential renal activity is an ongoing obligation. Clinically, patients are asymptomatic unless they are nephrotic or have developed end-stage renal disease. Renal disease is usually detected by abnormalities seen on examination of the urine, although a rising

creatinine or hypertension may herald renal involvement. The development of proteinuria on urinalysis or the presence of hematuria (> 5 red blood cells (RBCs)/high-power field) or pyuria (> 5 WBCs/high-power field) in the absence of other etiologies should prompt an evaluation for nephritis. Although not sought routinely in commercial laboratories, dysmorphic RBCs indicate a glomerular or tubulointerstitial source of the RBCs rather than the bladder. A 24-hour urine collection remains the most accurate measurement of urinary protein loss; however the protein/creatinine ratio in a spot urine is useful for following a patient with existing proteinuria. Monitoring serum creatinine as a surrogate for the glomerular filtration rate is a component of standard patient care; however, creatinine is an insensitive marker of lupus renal disease and should be used in conjunction with other assays. Renal activity is usually preceded or accompanied by serologic activity. Antibodies to dsDNA are almost always elevated or rising whereas measurements of serum complement (C3, C4, or CH_{50}) are usually low or dropping.

The World Health Organization (WHO) classification of lupus nephritis was recently modified by the International Society of Nephrology/Renal Pathology Society (ISN/RPS).[35] In general, membranous nephritis (class V) presents with a bland urinary sediment (i.e., no RBCs, WBCs or casts), nephritic-range proteinuria, a normal to mildly elevated creatinine, a normal blood pressure, normal complement components, and without anti-dsDNA. Patients with mesangial disease (class II) present with a bland or minimally active sediment, low-grade proteinuria (less than 500 mg/24 hours) and a normal serologic profile. Class III (focal) and class IV (diffuse) proliferative nephritis are characterized by an active urinary sediment, proteinuria, active serologies, and frequently with hypertension and elevated serum creatinine. Class III is defined as ≤ 50% glomerular involvement and class IV is defined as > 50%. The extent of proteinuria, urinary sediment activity, serologic abnormalities, and creatinine elevation is often less in class III than in class IV renal disease. Most cases of class II nephritis do not require initiation of cytotoxic therapy and the renal prognosis (i.e., lack of progression to end-stage renal disease) is good. The prognosis of class III disease is dependent upon the degree of activity. Patients with greater activity, i.e., 40–50% of glomerular involvement, have a prognosis similar to that of patients with class IV disease. In addition to high-dose corticosteroid therapy, cytotoxic therapy is usually required to induce a clinical response in patients with class III or IV disease. Even with potent immunosuppressant therapy such as cyclophosphamide or mycophenolate mofetil, a partial or complete response is induced in only about 80% of patients. Relapses and flares of renal disease are not infrequent, particularly when tapering corticosteroids or discontinuing immunosuppressive treatment.

HEMATOLOGIC

Hemocytopenias occur frequently in SLE. Severity is influenced by gender and ethnicity (Table 51.4). Though the sensitivity of any cytopenia for diagnosing SLE is low (18–46%), the specificity is high (89–98%).[36] Evaluation for medication effects is essential before attributing a cytopenia to an immune-mediated mechanism.

Anemia

Antibody-mediated peripheral destruction of red blood cells, autoimmune hemolytic anemia (AHA), occurs in 5–14% of SLE patients (Table 51.4). The anti-erythrocyte antibody is usually an opsonizing IgG. The

Table 51.4 Incidence of cytopenias in different ethnic cohorts

	Caucasian/ British[a] (%)	Hispanic/ Texas[b] (%)	Hispanic/ Puerto Rico[b] (%)	Latin American GLADEL[c] (%)	Caucasian/ Danish[d] (%)	African American[e] (%)	Caucasian/ USA[e] (%)
Leukopenia		27	33	42.3	25	20	15
Lymphopenia		62	54	59	42	23	19
Thrombocytopenia	17	21	3.7	19.2	24	10	12
Hemolytic Anemia	5	8.6	3.7	11.8	11	14	7

a. Sultan SM, Begum S, Isenberg DA. Prevalence, patterns of disease and outcome in patients with systemic lupus erythematosus who develop severe haematological problems. Rheumatol (Oxf 2003; 42: 230–234.

b. Vila LM, Alarcon GS, McGwin G Jr, et al. Early clinical manifestations, disease activity and damage of systemic lupus erythematosus among two distinct US Hispanic subpopulations. Rheumatol (Oxf) 2004; 43: 358–363.

c. Pons-Estel BA, Catoggio LJ, Cardiel MH, et al. The GLADEL multinational Latin American prospective inception cohort of 1,214 patients with systemic lupus erythematosus: ethnic and disease heterogeneity among "Hispanics". Medicine (Baltimore) 2004; 83: 1-17.

d. Jacobsen S, Petersen J, Ullman S, et al. A multicentre study of 513 Danish patients with systemic lupus erythematosus. I. Disease manifestations and analyses of clinical subsets. Clin Rheumatol 1998; 17: 468–477.

e. Cooper GS, Parks CG, Treadwell EL, et al. Differences by race, sex and age in the clinical and immunologic features of recently diagnosed systemic lupus erythematosus patients in the southeastern United States. Lupus 2002; 11: 161–167.

specificities of the anti-erythrocyte antibodies in SLE have not been clearly defined; the only nonrhesus-specific antigen reported in SLE is the membrane band 3 anion transporter protein. The presence of AHA is associated with increased disease severity and decreased survival and is readily diagnosed by a positive Coombs test, elevated lactate dehydrogenase and total bilirubin, and the presence of spherocytes on the peripheral smear. There are also reports of an association between AHA and anti-phospholipid antibodies, which may reflect cross-reactivity with erythrocyte membrane antigens.[37]

Anemia of chronic disease is the most common cause of anemia in SLE. The inhibitory effects of pro-inflammatory cytokines on erythrocyte production may be compounded by an inadequate erythropoietin response. Low erythropoietin levels in SLE may be attributable to renal disease as well as anti-erythropoietin antibodies. Although hemophagocytosis of hematopoietic cells is frequently noted on bone marrow biopsies, the hemophagocytic syndrome characterized by spiking fevers, tender hepatosplenomegaly, anemia, leucopenia, and markedly elevated serum ferritin is rare.

Lupus is also associated with a thrombotic microangiopathic hemolytic anemia with schistocytes, helmet cells, and triangular fragments of red blood cells. The clinical constellation of high fever, renal insufficiency, neurologic symptoms, and thrombocytopenia is characteristic of thrombotic thrombocytopenic purpura (TTP). Coexistent TTP and SLE is a rare and frequently fatal phenomenon, with fewer than 50 reported cases; its pathogenesis is unclear. Antibodies to ADAMTS 13 (von Willebrand factor cleaving protease) have been found in some SLE patients;[38] up to 50% of SLE patients with coexistent TTP have anti-phospholipid antibodies.

Leukopenia

Leukopenia, either neutropenia or lymphopenia, occurs in 15–50% of patients (Table 51.4). Both neutropenia and lymphopenia may reflect disease activity and predispose to infection. Anti-neutrophil antibodies directed against membrane components of mature and progenitor cells

are implicated in neutropenia; Western blot analysis of target antigens reveals several bands, including a 60-kDa band that shares sequence with the 60-kDa Ro antigen. Functional consequences of these anti-neutrophil antibodies include decreased phagocytosis and accelerated apoptosis. Antibodies against granulocyte colony-stimulating factor (G-CSF) and hyposensitivity of myeloid cells to G-CSF also contribute to SLE neutropenia. Binding of TNF-related apoptosis-inducing ligand (TRAIL) to TRAIL receptors on neutrophils accelerates neutrophil apoptosis.[39] One of four known TRAIL receptors is unable to transduce the death signal and functions as a decoy receptor; this receptor is reduced in SLE patients with neutropenia and is upregulated by steroid therapy.

Lymphopenia occurs with a reported incidence of 19–62% (Table 51.4). There are reduced numbers of circulating CD4 T cells in SLE and a decreased CD4-to-CD8 ratio. Lymphocytotoxic antibodies, increased apoptosis related to Fas and Fas ligand upregulation, and increased serum IL-10 levels have all been implicated in pathogenesis. It has been suggested that B cells expressing the 9G4 idiotype found on V_H 4.34 heavy chains may be responsible for production of anti-lymphocyte antibodies. In general, in the absence of recurrent infection, leukopenia in SLE rarely warrants treatment. Increased steroids may increase the leukocyte count but also contribute to the risk of infection.

Thrombocytopenia

Low platelet counts are seen in approximately 25% of patients, although severe thrombocytopenia is reported in fewer than 10% of patients (Table 51.4). Immune-mediated consumption is the most frequent cause, but rarely platelet consumption occurs together with a microangiopathic hemolytic anemia, TTP or as part of the hemophagocytic syndrome. A pathogenic role for antibodies against platelet membrane glycoproteins (IIb/IIIa antigen) is well established.[40] Other possible mechanisms include antibodies to thrombopoeitin, and antiphospholipid and anti-CD40-ligand antibodies that bind to platelets, resulting in platelet sequestration.

CENTRAL AND PERIPHERAL NERVOUS SYSTEM

Neurologic and psychiatric manifestations of SLE are diverse and frequently occur irrespective of systemic disease activity. Neuropsychiatric symptoms may be focal or diffuse, peripheral or central; they may occur in an isolated or complex fashion. Little is known about the pathogenesis of most of these syndromes.

In 1999 the ACR developed a nomenclature and case definitions for neuropsychiatric lupus (NPSLE).[41] The consensus committee developed reporting standards, case definitions, and recommendations for laboratory and imaging studies for 19 neurologic, psychiatric, and cognitive syndromes (Table 51.5). Diagnosis of an NPSLE syndrome requires the exclusion of infections, metabolic disturbances, bleeding disorders, malignancy, and medication toxicities. Using this new nomenclature, NPSLE is common, with a prevalence of 57–95%. Headache is the most frequent manifestation, followed by mood disorders, strokes, and transient ischemic attacks, cognitive dysfunction, seizures, and psychosis. Polyneuropathy, demyelinating disease, mononeuritis, myasthenia gravis, chorea, cranial neuropathy, myelopathy, and Guillain–Barré syndrome are uncommon.

Focal presentations attributable to specific central nervous system lesions occur frequently in association with anti-phospholipid antibodies. These presentations include strokes, transient ischemic attacks, seizures, movement disorders, and cranial neuropathies. Global dysfunction without focal impairment presents as intractable headaches, coma, delirium, cognitive dysfunction, and psychiatric syndromes, e.g., psychosis, mania, and depression. Cerebrospinal fluid (CSF) examination is useful for excluding infection or malignant cells. Active NPSLE is characterized by a lymphocytosis and evidence of intrathecal immunoglobulin synthesis with elevated total protein, IgG index, and oligoclonal bands; however, these abnormalities are not consistently present. While numerous autoantibodies (ANA, anti-dsDNA, anticardiolipin, anti-ribosomal P, anti-neuronal) and various cytokines have been identified in the CSF of patients with SLE, none is specific for active NPSLE and routine testing is not recommended. MRI is extremely sensitive for detection of structural lesions and new ischemic lesions; it is not helpful in differentiating between active NPSLE and old changes. Furthermore MRI studies may be normal in patients with psychiatric syndromes and global dysfunction.[42] Positron emission tomography (PET) and single-photon emission computed tomography (SPECT) scans measuring cerebral glucose uptake and blood flow, respectively, correlate to a limited extent with diffuse NPSLE. These scans must be interpreted carefully since atrophy with neuronal cell loss leads to changes in metabolism and blood flow. Atrophy is a common finding on brain imaging in SLE and newer imaging techniques demonstrate that neuronal function may be compromised during flares of NPSLE. The sensitivity and specificity of the newer imaging modalities, magnetic resonance spectroscopy, and functional MRI for detecting active NPSLE are currently under investigation. Cerebral angiograms may be helpful if a diagnosis of cerebral vasculitis is considered; however, central nervous system vasculitis is rare. Autopsy studies have documented the presence of true vasculitis in only 5–8% of cases. More commonly, a bland vasculopathy with degenerative and proliferative changes in small vessels, perivascular infiltrates, microinfarcts, and microhemorrhages is present.

There are no serologic tests specific for NPSLE. Serologic evidence of disease activity (elevated anti-DNA antibodies and low complement) may help to diagnose NPSLE, particularly if combined with other clinical signs of active disease. However, NPSLE may also flare in the absence of serologic and clinical disease activity. Anti-neuronal and anti-ribosomal

Table 51.5 Neuropsychiatric syndromes in systemic lupus erythematosus

Headache
Cerebrovascular disease
Seizures
Acute confusional state
Anxiety disorder
Cognitive dysfunction
Mood disorder
Psychosis
Aseptic meningitis
Autonomic disorder
Demyelinating syndrome
Mononeuropathy
Movement disorder
Myasthenia gravis
Myelopathy
Cranial neuropathy
Plexopathy
Polyneuropathy
Polyradiculopathy

THERAPEUTIC PRINCIPLES

>> Suppression of inflammation
>> Induction of remission
>> Maintenance of remission
>> Preservation of organ function
>> Suppression of immune activation
>> Modulation of the immune response
>> Management/prevention of drug-related toxicities

P antibodies are known to bind neurons; however, no functional consequences of these antibodies binding to tissue have been elucidated and no clear associations with NPSLE have been identified.[43] Antibodies to neuronal NMDA receptors (NMDAR's) have been identified in the sera, CSF, and brain of SLE patients and are associated with cognitive and depressive syndromes in some SLE patients. Animal studies demonstrate that binding of these autoantibodies to the NMDAR results in excitotoxic death of neurons leading to cognitive and emotional disturbances.[44] In summary, the clinical evaluation of a patient with presumed NPSLE involves an exhaustive search for other potential causes, and is guided by the presence of focal or diffuse symptomatology.

Antiphospholipid antibody syndrome is described in detail in Chapter 61.

Drug-induced lupus

Until recently, drug-induced lupus referred to a clinical syndrome that resembled mild lupus and occurred following exposure to a number of drugs (most notably procainamide, hydralazine, chlorpromazine, and methyldopa). Constitutional symptoms, musculoskeletal symptoms (arthritis and arthralgia), and serositis were common and renal and

CLINICAL MANIFESTATIONS

neurologic involvement were rare. Autoantibodies, including a positive ANA and anti-histone antibodies, were characteristically observed while anti-DNA and anti-Sm antibodies were unusual. Symptoms generally began weeks to months following the initiation of the inciting therapeutic agent and resolved within weeks after the drug was discontinued; autoantibodies could persist for up to 12 months. Host factors such as a decreased ability to metabolize the drug (e.g., slow acetylation of procainamide and hydralazine) contributed to the risk of developing drug-induced lupus. Multiple potential mechanisms resulting in the loss of self-tolerance have been suggested for this classic model. One of the most extensively explored is inhibition of DNA methylation, resulting in overexpression of co-stimulatory molecules such as LFA-1 on T cells and enhanced T-cell help.[45]

Since the introduction of anti-TNF agents, a different type of drug-induced lupus has been recognized. Up to 30% of patients receiving TNF blockade develop autoantibodies, including a positive ANA and antibodies to dsDNA. A minority develop a drug-induced clinical syndrome that can include anti-DNA antibodies, nephritis, and vasculitis. The pathogenesis of immunologic dysregulation resulting in the formation of autoantibodies and triggering of clinical disease is not known, although it is similar to observations made in the NZB/W mouse model of lupus.[46]

Treatment

The goals of lupus treatment are to stop and reverse ongoing organ inflammation, prevent or limit irreversible organ damage, and to suppress the immune response driving the inflammation. The efficacy of therapeutic agents must be balanced against their potential toxicity. Thus, treatment must be tailored to the individual patient and individual disease manifestations. In general, milder disease requires treatment with less potent or lower doses of anti-inflammatory and immunosuppressive medications than more active, severe disease affecting major organs such as the kidney or brain (Table 51.6). However, individual patient responses to a given medication will vary and patients must be monitored closely for a clinical response as well as toxicity.

Some genetic factors predicting risk of toxicity or therapeutic benefit for individual agents have been identified. Polymorphisms of a key enzyme in the metabolism of azathioprine, thiopurine methyltransferase (TPMT), are common; 0.3% and 11% of Caucasians are homozygous and heterozygous (respectively) for mutations associated with a lack of expression of TPMT.[47] TPMT-deficient patients are especially susceptible to leukopenia and pancytopenia associated with azathioprine. Cyclophosphamide is metabolized to its active form by cytochrome P450. Individuals heterozygous or homozygous for a specific cytochrome P450 polymorphism (CYP2C19*2) have a lower probability of developing premature ovarian failure, but also show a poorer response to therapy.[48]

Although corticosteroids are the foundation of treatment, exposure must be minimized to the greatest extent given their multiple and frequent side effects, including hypertension, diabetes mellitus, increased susceptibility to infection, bone loss, and weight gain. Currently available agents that are commonly used include antimalarials such as hydroxychloroquine (400 mg/day), anti-metabolites such as azathioprine (1–2.5 mg/kg per day), methotrexate (7.5–25 mg/week), leflunomide (10–20 mg/day), and mycophenolate mofetil (2–3 g/day) and alkylating agents such as cyclophosphamide (monthly pulse 0.5–1.0 g/m2). When more conventional therapies have failed, anecdotal reports, case series, and open-label studies suggest that use of intravenous immunoglobulin (2 g/kg over 2–5 days), thalidomide (50–100 mg/day) or cyclosporine (3–5 mg/kg per day) may be beneficial. Medications such as dapsone, danazol, and chlorambucil may be efficacious in cutaneous disease, hematologic disease, and in severe refractory disease (respectively), but in general these medications are not commonly used due to their toxicity, and the introduction and availability of better-tolerated, efficacious agents.

There are a number of newer agents on the horizon for treatment of SLE. Some are currently available but approved for other indications, whereas others are still in developmental stages. These therapies, in general, have more specific immunologic targets than standard treatments. Although there are multiple agents that have been tested in animal models of disease, we will only focus on therapies that have been given to humans.[49] Some

Table 51.6 Treatments for systemic lupus erythematosus disease manifestations

	NSAIDs	Antimalarials †	Low-dose corticosteroids (< 0.5 mg/ kg per day)	High-dose corticosteroids (> 0.5 mg/ kg per day) ‡	Azathioprine	MMF	CTX
Constitutional	+	+	+		+		
Musculoskeletal	+	+	+		+	+	
Mucocutaneous		+	+				
Serositis	+	+	+		+		
Hematologic		+		+	+		
Renal				+	+	+	+
Central nervous system				+			+
Vasculitis				+	+	+	+

†Antimalarials should be given to all patients to sustain remission and reduce damage
‡High-dose corticosteroids are required for remission induction or an inadequate response to low dose therapy
CTX, cyclophosphamide; MMF, mycophenolate mofetil; NSAIDs, nonsteroidal anti-inflammatory drugs.

agents are antigen-targeted. DNase I cleaves DNA, a target, and perhaps inciter, of the lupus autoimmune response. Abetimus sodium (LJP 394), a tetramer of short double-stranded oligonucleotides binds anti-DNA antibodies and may tolerize DNA-specific B cells. Results of phase II and III studies show that treatment with abetimus sodium results in a decrease in antibodies to dsDNA but clinical efficacy remains unproven. Edratide (TV4710) is a peptide derived from the CDR1 on an anti-DNA antibody. Vaccination with this peptide is currently in clinical trial.

B-cell-directed therapies (and their corresponding targets) include epratuzumab (anti-CD22 antibody) targeting all B cells, rituximab (anti-CD20 antibody) targeting all B cells except plasma cells, belimumab (anti-BAFF antibody) targeting a B-cell growth factor, TACI-Ig which blocks both BAFF and April, and antibody to the receptor for IL-6, another B-cell survival factor. R406, an inhibitor of syk, which is a crucial kinase that is activated after BCR engagement, is designed to block B-cell activation.

Potential therapies aimed at the dendritic cells include vitamin D, which blocks dendritic cell maturation and T-cell activation, abatacept (CTLA4-Ig), now approved for use in rheumatoid arthritis, which blocks the interaction of T cells with B7 molecules on dendritic cells and so blocks T-cell activation, and inhibitory oligodeoxynucleotides, which block TLR9 signaling and dendritic cell maturation. Hydroxychloroquine, a standard agent for lupus, interferes with toll-like receptor (TLR)7 and TLR9 signaling by preventing acidification of the endosomal compartment.

Other potential therapies are directed against IFN-α or IL-12, a dendritic cell cytokine (both a monoclonal antibody and an inhibitor). The monoclonal antibody against IL-12 has demonstrated efficacy in Crohn's disease. Studies of a monoclonal antibody against IFN-α are under way. Novel interventions directed at T cells include therapies interfering with the CD40–CD40L interaction. Initial clinical studies of antibodies against T-cell CD40L were accompanied by an unacceptable increase in thrombosis. Thus, antagonistic antibodies to CD40 are under development.

Eclizumab is an antibody directed against C5 which blocks cleavage of C5 and the subsequent triggering of the complement cascade. C5b is a potent chemotactic factor for both neutrophils and monocytes. Alicaforsen, an antisense oligodeoxynucleotide that inhibits ICAM-1 expression, decreases inflammation in both rheumatoid arthritis and Crohn's disease. Efalizumab, a monoclonal antibody against CD11a (a LFA-1 subunit that interacts with ICAM-1), benefits patients with psoriasis. Although there are no chemokine targeted therapies in clinical trial in lupus, a CCR1 antagonist slowed disease progression in a mouse model of lupus and has been tested in patients with rheumatoid arthritis. FTY720, an agonist for the sphingosine-1 phosphate receptor which prevents egress of lymphocytes from secondary lymphoid organs and inflamed tissues, has beneficial effects in the MRL/lpr mouse model of lupus; it has been given to transplant recipients and to patients with multiple sclerosis. TNF-α is a potent inflammatory cytokine; TNF-α antagonism results in disease reduction in rheumatoid arthritis. However, up to 20% of patients develop autoantibodies and a minority develop lupus. TNF-α is involved in renal inflammation in SLE and monoclonal antibody to TNF-α appears to improve lupus nephritis, showing that agents can abort inflammation and yet exacerbate autoimmunity. The potential efficiency and safety of short-term use of TNF-α blockade in lupus are under study. Another potential therapy in patients with severe unremitting lupus is ablation with high-dose chemotherapy followed by immune reconstitution using

autologous or allogeneic hematopoietic stem cells. Initial efficacy, the associated toxicity and morbidity of these treatments, as well as the durability of both response will be determined in a clinical trial which is now under way.

■ CONCLUSIONS ■

SLE is a heterogeneous disease, with different patterns of immune dysregulation leading to ANA production and target organ inflammation. The goal in therapy must be to eliminate autoreactivity while maintaining immunocompetence. Restoration of normal immune homeostasis and immunocompetence requires treatment during and after remission induction with multiple agents, each modulating a different aspect of immune dysregulation. Among the challenges we now face are the careful phenotyping of patients to identify etiopathologically distinct subpopulations and new clinical trial designs to allow the use of combinations of agents, each of which alone may have a negligible effect on disease course.

■ REFERENCES ■

1. Tan EM, Cohen AS, Fries JF, et al. The 1982 revised criteria for the classification of systemic lupus erythematosus. Arthritis Rheum 1982; 25: 1271–1277.
2. Wong M, Tsao BP. Current topics in human SLE genetics. Springer Semin Imunopathol 2006; 99–102.
3. Ueda H, Howson JM, Esposito L, et al. Association of the T-cell regulatory gene CTLA4 with susceptibility to autoimmune disease. Nature 2003; 423: 506–511.
4. Orozco G, Sanchez E, Gonzalez-Gay MA, et al. Association of a functional single-nucleotide polymorphism of PTPN22, encoding lymphoid protein phosphatase, with rheumatoid arthritis and systemic lupus erythematosus. Arthritis Rheum 2005; 52: 219–224.
5. McHugh NJ, Owen P, Cox B, et al. MHC class II, tumour necrosis factor alpha, and lymphotoxin alpha gene haplotype associations with serological subsets of systemic lupus erythematosus. Ann Rheum Dis 2006; 65: 488–494.
6. Manderson AP, Botto M, Walport MJ. The role of complement in the development of systemic lupus erythematosus. Annu Rev Immunol 2004; 22: 431–456.
7. Baumann I, Kolowos W, Voll RE, et al. Impaired uptake of apoptotic cells into tingible body macrophages in germinal centers of patients with systemic lupus erythematosus. Arthritis Rheum 2002; 46: 191–201.
8. Anolik JH, Barnard J, Cappione A, et al. Rituximab improves peripheral B cell abnormalities in human systemic lupus erythematosus. Arthritis Rheum 2004; 50: 3580–3590.
9. Floto RA, Clatworthy MR, Heilbronn KR, et al. Loss of function of a lupus-associated FcgammaRIIb polymorphism through exclusion from lipid rafts. Nat Med 2005; 11: 1056–1058.
10. Tucci M, Barnes EV, Sobel ES, et al. Strong association of a functional polymorphism in the monocyte chemoattractant protein 1 promoter gene with lupus nephritis. Arthritis Rheum 2004; 50: 1842–1849.

11. Crow MK. Interferon pathway activation in systemic lupus erythematosus. Curr Rheumatol Rep 2005; 7: 463–468.

12. Nath SK, Harley JB, Lee YH. Polymorphisms of complement receptor 1 and interleukin-10 genes and systemic lupus erythematosus: a meta-analysis. Hum Genet 2005; 118: 225–234.

13. Schotte H, Willeke P, Tidow N, et al. Extended haplotype analysis reveals an association of TNF polymorphisms with susceptibility to systemic lupus erythematosus beyond HLA-DR3. Scand J Rheumatol 2005; 34: 114–121.

14. Wu J, Metz C, Xu X, et al. A novel polymorphic CAAT/enhancer-binding protein beta element in the FasL gene promoter alters Fas ligand expression: a candidate background gene in African American systemic lupus erythematosus patients. J Immunol 2003; 170: 132–138.

15. Mehrian R, Quismorio FP Jr, Strassmann G, et al. Synergistic effect between IL-10 and bcl-2 genotypes in determining susceptibility to systemic lupus erythematosus. Arthritis Rheum 1998; 41: 596–602.

16. Milner EC, Anolik J, Cappione A, Sanz I. Human innate B cells: a link between host defense and autoimmunity?. Springer Semin Immunopathol 2005; 26: 433–452.

17. Pugh-Bernard AE, Cambier JC. B cell receptor signaling in human systemic lupus erythematosus. Curr Opin Rheumatol 2006; 18: 451–455.

18. Mackay IR. The hepatitis–lupus connection. Semin Liver Dis 1991; 11: 234–240.

19. Grimaldi CM, Hill L, Xu X, et al. Hormonal modulation of B cell development and repertoire selection. Mol Immunol 2005; 42: 811–820.

20. Miyara M, Amoura Z, Parizot C, et al. Global natural regulatory T cell depletion in active systemic lupus erythematosus. J Immunol 2005; 175: 8392–8400.

21. McMurray RW. Bromocriptine in rheumatic and autoimmune diseases. Semin Arthritis Rheum 2001; 31: 21–32.

22. Zoma A. Musculoskeletal involvement in systemic lupus erythematosus. Lupus 2004; 13: 851–853.

23. Aranow C, Zelicof S, Leslie D, et al. Clinically occult avascular necrosis of the hip in systemic lupus erythematosus. J Rheumatol 1997; 24: 2318–2322.

24. Werth VP. Clinical manifestations of cutaneous lupus erythematosus. Autoimmun Rev 2005; 4: 296–302.

25. Tebbe B. Clinical course and prognosis of cutaneous lupus erythematosus. Clin Dermatol 2004; 22: 121–124.

26. Orteu CH, Buchanan JA, Hutchison I, et al. Systemic lupus erythematosus presenting with oral mucosal lesions: easily missed?. Br J Dermatol 2001; 144: 1219–1223.

27. Hallegua DS, Wallace DJ. Gastrointestinal manifestations of systemic lupus erythematosus. Curr Opin Rheumatol 2000; 12: 379–385.

28. Breuer GS, Baer A, Dahan D, et al. Lupus-associated pancreatitis. Autoimmun Rev 2006; 5: 314–318.

29. Kaw R, Gota C, Bennett A, et al. Lupus-related hepatitis: complication of lupus or autoimmune association? Case report and review of the literature. Dig Dis Sci 2006; 51: 813–818.

30. Yazici Y, Erkan D, Levine DM, et al. Protein-losing enteropathy in systemic lupus erythematosus: report of a severe, persistent case and review of pathophysiology. Lupus 2002; 11: 119–123.

31. Lawrence E. Systemic Lupus Erythematosus and the Lung. New York: John Wiley; 1987.

32. Moder KG, Miller TD, Tazelaar HD. Cardiac involvement in systemic lupus erythematosus. Mayo Clin Proc 1999; 74: 275–284.

33. Manzi S, Meilahn EN, Rairie JE, et al. Age-specific incidence rates of myocardial infarction and angina in women with systemic lupus erythematosus: comparison with the Framingham Study. Am J Epidemiol 1997; 145: 408–415.

34. Sesin CA, Yin X, Esmon CT, et al. Shedding of endothelial protein C receptor contributes to vasculopathy and renal injury in lupus: in vivo and in vitro evidence. Kidney Int 2005; 68: 110–120.

35. Weening JJ, D'Agati VD, Schwartz MM, et al. The classification of glomerulonephritis in systemic lupus erythematosus revisited. J Am Soc Nephrol 2004; 15: 241–250.

36. Kao AH, Manzi S, Ramsey-Goldman R. Review of ACR hematologic criteria in systemic lupus erythematosus. Lupus 2004; 13: 865–868.

37. Sultan SM, Begum S, Isenberg DA. Prevalence, patterns of disease and outcome in patients with systemic lupus erythematosus who develop severe haematological problems. Rheumatol (Oxf) 2003; 42: 230–234.

38. Musio F, Bohen EM, Yuan CM, et al. Review of thrombotic thrombocytopenic purpura in the setting of systemic lupus erythematosus. Semin Arthritis Rheum 1998; 28: 1–19.

39. Matsuyama W, Yamamoto M, Higashimoto I, et al. TNF-related apoptosis-inducing ligand is involved in neutropenia of systemic lupus erythematosus. Blood 2004; 104: 184–191.

40. Michel M, Lee K, Piette JC, et al. Platelet autoantibodies and lupus-associated thrombocytopenia. Br J Haematol 2002; 119: 354–358.

41. American College of Rheumatology. The American College of Rheumatology nomenclature and case definitions for neuropsychiatric lupus syndromes. Arthritis Rheum 1999; 42: 599–608.

42. Govoni M, Castellino G, Padovan M, et al. Recent advances and future perspective in neuroimaging in neuropsychiatric systemic lupus erythematosus. Lupus 2004; 13: 149–158.

43. Karassa FB, Afeltra A, Ambrozic A, et al. Accuracy of anti-ribosomal P protein antibody testing for the diagnosis of neuropsychiatric systemic lupus erythematosus: an international meta-analysis. Arthritis Rheum 2006; 54: 312–324.

44. Girardi G, Redecha P, Salmon JE. Heparin prevents antiphospholipid antibody-induced fetal loss by inhibiting complement activation. Nat Med 2004; 10: 1222–1226.

45. Kaplan MJ, Deng C, Yang J, et al. DNA methylation in the regulation of T cell LFA-1 expression. Immunol Invest 2000; 29: 411–425.

46. Jacob CO, McDevitt HO. Tumour necrosis factor-alpha in murine autoimmune 'lupus' nephritis. Nature 1988; 331: 356–358.

47. Yates CR, Krynetski EY, Loennechen T, et al. Molecular diagnosis of thiopurine S-methyltransferase deficiency: genetic basis for azathioprine and mercaptopurine intolerance. Ann Intern Med 1997; 126: 608–614.

48. Takada K, Arefayene M, Desta Z, et al. Cytochrome P450 pharmacogenetics as a predictor of toxicity and clinical response to pulse cyclophosphamide in lupus nephritis. Arthritis Rheum 2004; 50: 2202–2210.

49. Wiesendanger M, Stanevsky A, Kovsky S, et al. Novel therapeutics for systemic lupus erythematosus. Curr Opin Rheumatol 2006; 18: 227–235.

Rheumatoid arthritis

Andrew P. Cope

52

Rheumatoid arthritis (RA) is one of the most common chronic inflammatory diseases and has become the prototype disease entity for defining the molecular and pathological basis of chronic inflammatory syndromes. The term 'rheumatoid arthritis' was coined by Garrod in 1859. However, this was probably an inappropriate use of the term because it encompassed polyarticular osteoarthritis, as well as inflammatory polyarthritis. For many years there has been considerable debate as to whether RA is in fact a new disease, a hypothesis based more on negative data and inconclusive deductions from archive material, including the visual arts and archaeological artifacts. In spite of references to inflammatory afflictions of joints by the likes of Galen, Sydenham and Heberden, the first convincing case reports of the disease, described in terms that would be recognizable today, were published in 1800 by Landré-Beauvais, who labelled the disease 'la goutte asthénique primitive.'[1] This description was distinct, as all patients were female, an observation that was significant when the most important differential diagnosis at that time was polyarticular gout, a disease predominantly of males.

Today we recognize RA as a chronic inflammatory disorder of joints of unknown etiology in which the major target tissue is the synovial lining of joints, bursae and tendon sheaths.[2] Despite being traditionally considered an autoimmune disease, RA differs from organ-specific autoimmune disease entities in several respects. From the outset of RA, the immunoinflammatory process, driven by cytokines and other inflammatory mediators, promotes the activation and proliferation of stromal joint tissues, in particular the fibroblastic synovial lining layer. In contrast, organ-specific autoimmune diseases such as type I diabetes or autoimmune thyroiditis are characterized by an antigen-driven inflammatory process that leads directly to cellular destruction of pancreatic β-islet or thyroid tissue cells. It is only during the later phase of chronic, severe and progressive disease (representing only a subset of patients) that the invasive synovium, or pannus, invades and erodes underlying cartilage and bone. Unlike some autoimmune diseases that target single organs or tissues, RA is a systemic inflammatory disease that probably encompasses a heterogeneous syndrome. It exhibits marked variations in clinical expression that most clinicians today would acknowledge is more than one disease entity. Indeed, over a period of several decades it has become increasingly apparent that the disease is heterogeneous, not only clinically, but also pathologically, serologically and genetically, presenting major challenges to the immunologist and physician.

■ EPIDEMIOLOGY ■

The incidence of RA (the rate of new cases arising in a given period) is 0.1–0.2 per 1000 of the population for males, and 0.2–0.4 per 1000 for females.[3] These rates plateau between the ages of 45 and 75 years in some series but can increase steadily with age until the seventh decade, declining thereafter. The largest difference in incidence between the sexes occurs in those under 50 years of age. Recent evidence indicates that the incidence may be in decline, suggesting an environmental influence. The disease prevalence (the number of existing cases) should ideally include all past and inactive cases. For RA, large cross-sectional population samples indicate that the figure ranges from 0.5% to 2% for caucasian European and North American populations over the age of 15, with a female to male excess of 2 to 4.[3] Despite similar prevalence estimates for these geographically diverse populations, greater diversity has been documented for rural African populations, where the prevalence has been reported to be as low as 0.1%, and Native Americans (including the Pima, Yakima and Chippewa tribes), where the prevalence may be as high as 5%.

Complex polygenic autoimmune syndromes such as RA are diseases of low penetrance, where thresholds of disease expression may be higher in males. This is based in part on the observation that the increased risk of disease in siblings of probands is rather small. Twin studies provide perhaps the most compelling evidence for genetic effects, given the excess concordance rates for monozygotic (12–15%) compared to dizygotic twins (<5%, and probably nearer to 3.5%).[4] Compared to a background prevalence of 1% in outbred populations, these figures translate to a striking contribution of genetic factors, calculated to be of the order of 53–65%.[5] This leaves a substantial contribution for disease susceptibility from environmental factors, influenced by occupation, socioeconomic status, exposure to infectious pathogens and lifestyle factors.

Two of the more intriguing factors contributing to disease occurrence are age and gender. Age-associated changes in susceptibility to infection, neoplastic disease and autoimmunity suggest that a common mechanism

---

KEY CONCEPTS

IMPORTANT RISK FACTORS FOR DEVELOPING RA

>> Female gender

>> Nulliparity, or during first three months postpartum

>> Low androgen or high estrogen status (in men)

>> Smoking > 25 cigarettes per day for > 20 years. Relative risk increased to 15-fold depending on HLA-DRB1 status

>> Prolonged exposure to unidentified environmental antigens (e.g. infectious pathogens)

>> Urban dwelling

>> Immune senescence

>> Serum autoantibodies to citrullinated protein antigens (anti-CPA)

>> First-degree relative with RA. Relative risk 1.5

>> Inheritance of allelic variants including *HLADRB1* and *PTPN22*

---

could be responsible. Immune senescence is one possibility, where age-related decline in host immunity is characterized at the cellular and molecular level by massive expansions of lymphocyte clones, corresponding contractions of the naïve T- and B-cell repertoires, and telomere erosion of leukocytes, indicative of an extensive proliferative history.[6] When combined with oxidative stress and a range of biochemical derangements of pathways integral to antigen responsiveness and immune regulation, these factors may combine to (1) increase susceptibility to foreign pathogens; (2) augment reactivity to self-tissue antigens (themselves modified post-translationally as a consequence of the ageing process); and (3) generate a repertoire of lymphocytes defective in terms of tumor surveillance. Thus, immune senescence should be considered a risk factor for RA.

The female preponderance implies that hormonal and reproductive factors strongly influence risk. On the one hand, nulliparity is a risk factor for RA. Women entering the first 3 months of the postpartum period are also at increased risk. By contrast, oral contraceptive use, pregnancy and breastfeeding are associated with reduced risk or less severe disease.[7] Several possible immune mechanisms have been proposed. For example, maternofetal mismatch at the MHC locus has been associated with higher disease remission rates during pregnancy. In mice, pregnancy has been shown to be associated with quantitative changes in the numbers of regulatory T cells. An influence of hormonal factors is further suggested in studies of men where disease is associated with lower androgenic testosterone and dehydroepiandrosterone (DHEA) levels and increased estradiol, compared to a cohort of healthy control male subjects.

ETIOLOGY AND PATHOGENESIS

ENVIRONMENTAL AND NONGENETIC FACTORS

Most studies have reported an association between RA and smoking. One of the largest studies comprising over 370 000 women from the Women's Health Cohort Study reported a relative risk of 1.4 for women

who smoked more than 25 cigarettes per day for more than 20 years, compared to nonsmokers.[8] The association appears to be more closely related to duration of smoking rather than the amount of tobacco exposure, and may influence severity, as smokers are more likely to have seropositive, erosive disease with extra-articular manifestations. The effect may be fully reversible in those individuals who stop smoking for 10 years or more. Further evidence of gene–environment interactions with respect to smoking have been documented more recently in a population based case–control study of Swedish RA patients.[9] In this study the relative risk of developing rheumatoid factor-positive (RF+) RA was calculated according to smoking status and HLA-DRB1 genotype. The relative risk of developing RA increased from 2.5 in nonsmokers with disease-associated HLA-DRB1 genes to 7.5 and 15.7 in smokers who carried one or two copies of the susceptibility alleles, respectively. The association between smoking and seropositive disease was explored further in a follow-up study that demonstrated more robust associations with smoking, HLA-DRB1 status, and the presence of autoantibodies to citrullinated protein antigens (anti-CPA).

Being female, a smoker, and carrying specific disease-associated genes may be highly associated (but not sufficient) for the initiation of chronic inflammatory arthritis. Other environmental triggers may be involved. Not least among these are exposure to foreign pathogens.[10] This association has gained much credibility because of the presumed link not only between infection and autoimmunity but also between immunodeficiency and autoimmune disease. Nonetheless, no single pathogen or group of pathogens has been defined. This could imply that aberrant host responses (either exaggerated innate inflammatory responses or failure to terminate such responses) may occur following a wide range of infectious insults. Indeed, bacteria such as *Proteus mirabilis*, or bacterial products including superantigens, *Mycoplasma* species, viruses (including herpes family, parvovirus and retroviruses) and fungi have all been implicated, but data have been insufficient to prove causation. Epstein–Barr virus (EBV) infection has been a particularly attractive candidate as infection is common, antibodies to EBV nuclear antigens have been reported in patients with RA, EBV is a polyclonal activator of B lymphocytes, EBV-specific T cells reactive to EBV gp110 have been identified in RA synovial joints, and EBV RNA has been isolated from the synovium.

Another possible link between infection and autoimmunity comes from the observation that components of the mycobacterium used in Freund's adjuvant to induce arthritis in rodents include heat shock proteins (hsp), especially hsp65, which in turn promotes T cell-specific immunity.[11] One hypothesis suggests that these highly conserved chaperones may cross-react with self proteins, thereby provoking reactivity to host tissues. More recent data suggest that exposure of the immune system to hsp at sites of tissue damage evokes a danger signal that may ultimately result in the expansion of subsets of regulatory T cells that contribute to the resolution of the inflammatory response.[11]

IMMUNOGENETICS

RA is a clinically heterogeneous disease and so it has been very difficult to identify disease susceptibility genes, in spite of heritability estimates of up to 60%. With the exception of the MHC, these genes confer low to moderate risk and have low penetrance. Nevertheless, five genome-wide linkage scans of multiplex families with RA have established an important contribution of the MHC.[12] This lends support to a wealth of epidemiological and genetic data describing associations between RA and specific

HLA-DRB1 alleles, in particular HLA-DR4 subtypes. While this association was first described by Stastny in the 1970s, it was shown more than a decade later that susceptibility to RA across different ethnic populations correlated closely with the expression of a specific consensus amino acid sequence (referred to as the 'shared epitope,' hereafter SE) within the HLA-DRβ chain α helix (Table 52.1).[13] This sequence was subsequently shown by several groups of investigators to be encoded by HLA-DRB1 alleles, including HLA-DR4 (*0401, *0404, *0405 and *0408), but also HLA-DR1 (*0101), DR6 (*1402) and DR10 (*1001) alleles, among others. These shared epitope-carrying alleles have recently been reclassified (Table 52.1). According to this model, RA is associated with the rheumatoid arthritis-associated (RAA) shared epitope sequence (72–74 positions) and the association is modulated by the amino acids at positions 70 and 71, resulting in six genotypes with RA risks varying from 4.4 to 22.2. On the other hand, the finding of DERAA encoding HLA-DRB1 alleles (DRB1*0103, *0402, *1102, *1103, *1302 and *1304) conferring lower disease risk, and more importantly reduced radiographic progression in RA even in the presence of one copy of the SE, raises the possibility that specific subsets of MHC class II genes may confer an independent protective role.[14]

Specific genotypes co-segregate with distinct clinical features.[15] For example, in population-based studies different HLA-DRB1 alleles influence the severity of disease, with DRB1*0401 being found in patients with severe, seropositive, erosive RA (often with extra-articular features such as vasculitis and Felty's syndrome in *0401 homozygous or *0401/*0404 compound homozygote individuals), whereas DRB1*0101 and *1001 are observed at a higher frequency in patients with less severe, seronegative, nonerosive disease. Inheriting two copies of alleles that express the consensus sequence increases disease penetrance, time of onset and severity. Thus, rather than a hierarchy of phenotypes of a single disease, these genetic associations, which are by no means uniform, are reflected clinically as distinct disease entities.

On the basis of early observations, two principal models were proposed to account for the association between RA and the consensus DRβ chain sequence.[16] Both were based on the assumption that the shared epitope is the critical genetic element linked directly to disease. The first model proposed that the shared epitope determines specific peptide binding, and that 'pathogenic' peptides bind only to disease-associated HLA class II molecules (Fig. 52.1). This model predicted that a gradient of affinities of disease-inducing peptide for MHC class II molecules might account for the differences in susceptibility and/or severity conferred by different HLA-DR molecules. Along the same lines, disease-associated alleles may preclude the binding of peptides required for the generation of naturally occurring regulatory T cells specific for self-peptide antigens. The second model proposed that the shared epitope influences T-cell receptor (TCR) recognition by binding and selecting autoreactive T cells during thymic maturation, and expanding these populations in the peripheral compartment; again, perturbations of a repertoire of regulatory T cells could arise through opposing influences of the shared epitope sequence.

Two recent lines of experimental evidence provide further insights into HLA–disease associations. The first is the association between HLA-DR4 subtypes and telomere erosion in RA patients and healthy donors, detectable before the age of 20.[6] Telomeres are reiterative nucleotide sequences found at the end of chromosomes that become eroded with successive rounds of cell division. Their loss has been associated with aging and immunosenescence. Whether this implies a direct contribution

of HLA-DR4 expression to accelerated differentiation of hematopoietic cells in the context of a chronic inflammatory process is intriguing, but certainly warrants further investigation. The second line of evidence pointing to specific functions of SE⁺ alleles has arisen through analysis of autoantibodies in RA patients typed at the HLA-DRB1 locus.[17] These studies, replicated in European and US RA cohorts, demonstrated associations between SE frequencies and antibodies to cyclic citrullinated peptides (anti-CCP). Specifically, compared to healthy controls, the odds ratio for the association between one or two copies of the SE and anti-CCP positivity was 4.4 and 11.8, respectively. These findings point to SE associating not with RA per se, but with a clinical phenotype, in this case autoantibodies to modified proteins.[17]

Linkage studies have generated only nominal evidence of linkage at non-MHC loci. Nevertheless, leading candidates include genomic fragments on chromosomes 1p13, 1q41-43, 6q16, 16p and 18q.[12] This has meant that large cohorts are required to confirm evidence of definite linkage across these intervals. Nonetheless, one allelic variant whose association with RA has now been validated in multiple disease cohorts is found in the gene *PTPN22*, which encodes the hematopoietic protein tyrosine phosphatase Lyp. Combining all studies, the odds ratio is no higher than 1.8. Some studies have revealed an association between the RA-associated variant PTPN22 (R620W) with RF and anti-CCP positivity, which is also independent of SE. The data suggest that PTPN22 may influence autoantibody production and be involved in the initiation of disease, as distinct from regulating severity. *PTPN22* mutations have also been described in type I diabetes, a subset of systemic lupus erythematosus patients, oligoarticular JIA, vitiligo, Addison's disease and autoimmune thyroid disease, but not multiple sclerosis or psoriasis, pointing to a more generic link with pathogenic autoantibodies in a range of syndromes.[12] Recently, the disease-associated Lyp 620W variant was shown to be a gain-of-function mutant, leading to hyporesponsiveness to TCR engagement through attenuated receptor proximal signaling, reduced IL-2 production and proliferative responses. Although the genetic data suggest that the impact of this mutation may be weak relative to MHC genes, this hyporesponsive phenotype could alter thymic selection, or mechanisms of peripheral tolerance that are critically dependent on TCR signaling.

SYNOVIAL PATHOLOGY

RA targets diarthrodial joints, structures characterized by hyaline cartilage lining opposing articulating surfaces and a cavity of viscous synovial fluid lined by synovial membrane lacking a basement membrane but encased by a fibrous joint capsule. Normal synovial tissue comprises a lining layer, no more than a few cells in depth, of stromal fibroblast-like synoviocytes (FLS; also known as type B synoviocytes) and sublining macrophages (type A synoviocytes). The synovium serves to line noncartilaginous surfaces, and although blood vessels are sparse, it functions to provide essential nutrients to avascular structures, including cartilage, tendons and bursae.

INCREASED VASCULARITY AND CELL MIGRATION

The range of pathology observed in patients with RA perhaps most convincingly emphasizes the heterogeneity of the disease. The earliest changes observed relate to increases in vascularity characterized by vascular congestion and thrombosis with obliteration of small vessels in

Table 52.1 Classification of HLA–DRB1 alleles according to the third hypervariable region of the DRβ chain and their association with RA in French caucasian patients (Data adapted from du Montcel et al. New classification of HLA-DRB1 alleles supports the shared epitope hypothesis of rheumatoid arthritis susceptibility. Arthritis Rheum 2005; 52: 1063–1068)

HLA–DRB1 allele¶	DRβ–chain amino acid (shared epitope)								Disease Association#
	67	68	69	70	71	72	73	74	
S_{3P}									**Int risk**
DRB1*0101	L	L	E	Q	R	R	A	A	+
DRB1*0102	–	–	–	–	–	–	–	–	+
DRB1*0404	–	–	–	–	–	–	–	–	+
DRB1*0405	–	–	–	–	–	–	–	–	+
DRB1*0408	–	–	–	–	–	–	–	–	+
DRB1*1001	–	–	–	R	–	–	–	–	+
DRB1*1402	–	–	–	–	–	–	–	–	+
S_{3D}									**Low risk**
DRB1*1101	–	F	–	D	–	–	–	–	–
DRB1*1104	–	F	–	D	–	–	–	–	–
DRB1*12	–	I	–	D	–	–	–	–	–
DRB1*16	–	F	–	D	–	–	–	–	–
S_1									**Low risk**
DRB1*0103	–	I	–	D	E	–	–	–	–
DRB1*0402	–	I	–	D	E	–	–	–	–
DRB1*1102	–	I	–	D	E	–	–	–	–
DRB1*1103	–	F	–	D	E	–	–	–	–
DRB1*1301	–	I	–	D	E	–	–	–	–
DRB1*1302	–	I	–	D	E	–	–	–	–
DRB1*1323	–	I	–	D	E	–	–	–	–
DRB1*15	I	–	–	–	A	–	–	–	–
S_2									**High risk**
DRB1*0401	–	–	–	–	K	–	–	–	+
DRB1*1303	–	I	–	D	K	–	–	–	+
X									**Low risk**
DRB1*03	–	–	–	–	K	–	G	R	+/–
DRB1*0403	–	–	–	–	–	–	–	E	–
DRB1*0407	–	–	–	–	–	–	–	E	–
DRB1*0411	–	–	–	–	–	–	–	E	–
DRB1*07	–	I	–	D	–	–	G	Q	–
DRB1*08	–	F	–	D	–	–	–	L	–
DRB1*09	–	F	–	R	–	–	–	E	–
DRB1*1401	–	–	–	R	–	–	–	–	–
DRB1*1404	–	–	–	R	–	–	–	E	–

¶Allele frequencies were S_1 = 24%; S_2 = 9%; S_{3D} = 10%; S_{3P} = 21%; and X = 36%.
#Based on the RAA sequence at 72–74 modulated by the amino acid at codon 71
*Hierarchy of risk genotypes: $S_2/S_{3P} > S_2/S_2 > S_{3P}/S_{3P} > S_2/X > S_{3P}/X > X/X$.
+Stronger association;– weak, neutral or even protective association with disease.

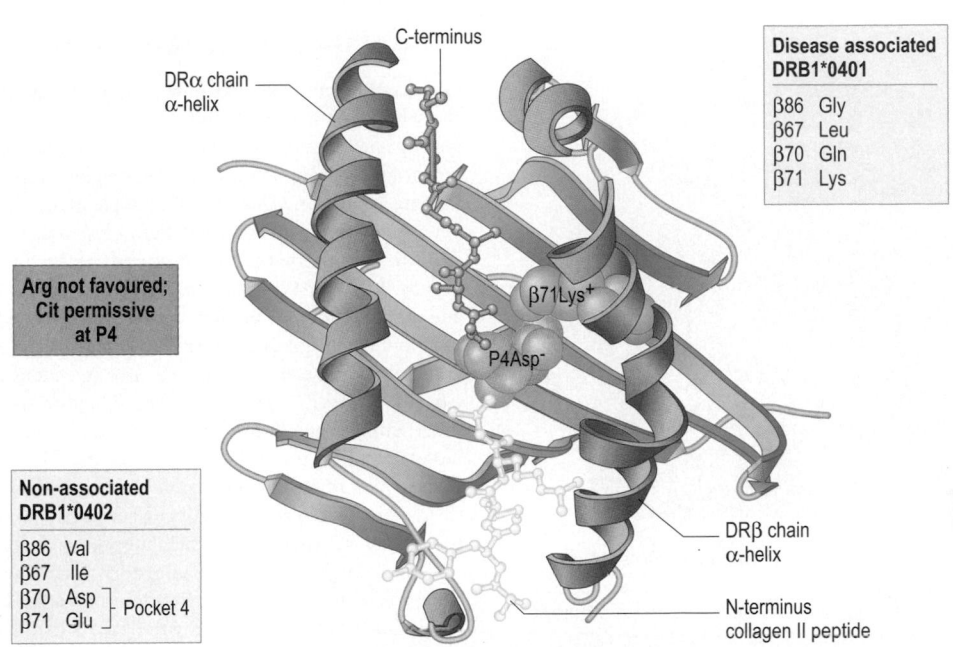

Fig. 52.1 Crystal structure of a collagen II peptide/HLA-DR4 complex ribbon model of an immunodominant collagen II peptide (1168–1180) complexed to HLA-DR4 (DRA*0101/DRB1*0401); a view of the MHC/peptide complex as seen from the T-cell surface. DRα- and DRβ-chain helices are shown in red, whereas the β-pleated sheet comprising the floor of the peptide-binding groove is shown in blue. Residues 67–74 of the DRβ chain, components of the third hypervariable region, derive the 'shared epitope.' The ball-and-stick model of the CII peptide is shown. Interacting residues of the peptide position 4 (Asp – orange) and DRβ-chain residue (β71Lys – green), which make up part of pocket 4, are depicted as van der Waals' spheres. Differences in amino acid sequence between the closely related disease associated DRB1*0401 and nonassociated DRB1*0402 gene products are illustrated. Note that whereas Arg would not be favored at position 4 in the peptide, modification of Arg→Cit by deimination would be permissive. (Figure generated by R. Visse and A. Cope, based on crystal data derived by Wiley and colleagues in Dessen A, Lawrence CM, Cupo S, et al. X-ray crystal structure of HLA-DR4 (DRA*0101, DRB1*0401) complexed with a peptide from human collagen II. Immunity 1997; 7: 473–481.)

association with perivascular inflammatory infiltrates.[18] Hyperplasia of the synovial lining layer is a typical early finding. These changes are rather nonspecific and certainly not diagnostic.

A key checkpoint that defines the switch from acute to chronic persistent inflammation is the sustained activation of microvascular endothelium, phenotypic changes in the high endothelial venules (reminiscent of tissue injury), and the concomitant upregulation of adhesion molecules such as intercellular adhesion molecule (ICAM)-1 and vascular cell adhesion molecule (VCAM)-1.[19] With chemoattractants derived from synovial stromal cells, these changes herald the rolling, adhesion and transmigration of mononuclear cells through endothelial barriers into the synovial membrane, and contribute to the progressive synovial hypertrophy and hyperplasia, sometimes with villous-like projections more typical of chronic, established inflammation. Neovascularization further promotes the influx of inflammatory cells. To what extent this is driven by the hypoxic environment is not clear, but angiogenic growth factors such as vascular endothelial growth factor (VEGF) and hypoxia-inducible factor (HIF) make important contributions.[20] It has been proposed that influx of inflammatory lymphocytes and cells of monocytic lineage far outweighs the egress of cells from synovial tissue, possibly due to chemokine gradients. Once in the synovium egress may be regulated or blocked

through integrin/adhesion molecule interactions, e.g., between antigen-specific T cells and dendritic cells/APC, through TCR-dependent signals that abrogate chemokine responsiveness, or perhaps through highly selective and specific inactivation of chemokines by proteolysis, e.g., stromal-derived factor (SDF)-1 cleavage by cell surface dipeptidyl peptidase CD26. Recent data suggest that generalized cytokine and inflammatory signals rather than antigen drive may trigger the migration of effector memory T-cell subsets such as $CD4^+CD28^{null}CXCR4^+NKG2D^+$ T cells from lymph nodes to synovium.[21] This is an important distinction because it suggests that nonspecific innate inflammatory signals rather than antigen-specific signals might precipitate disease flares in patients with RA.

ORGANIZATION OF LYMPHOID TERTIARY MICROSTRUCTURES

Tissue microstructure dictates and facilitates immune responses in secondary lymphoid organs but also in the gastrointestinal tract. The same concept probably holds for peripheral tissues in chronic inflammatory disease, where the topology of infiltrates appears to be a stable trait over time. Thus, in established disease the rheumatoid synovium

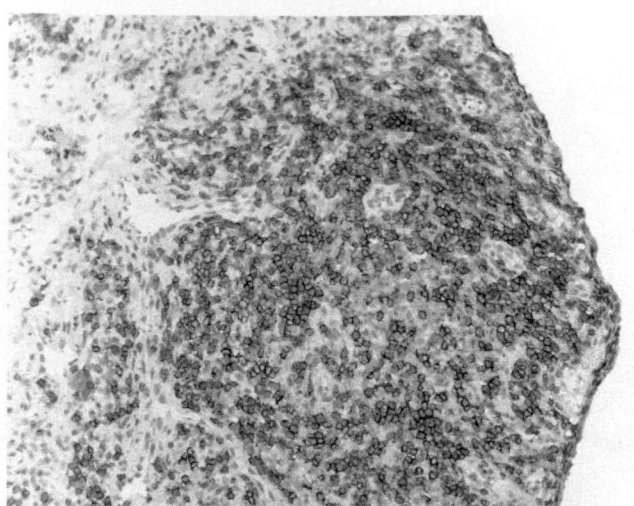

Fig. 52.2 Lymphoid follicular structures in inflamed RA synovial tissue. A characteristic hematoxylin and eosin-stained tissue section from a patient with active RA showing a large follicular-like structure. This section is also stained with monoclonal antibodies to CD3ε, followed by a three-step immunoperoxidase staining protocol (CD3+ T cells stained dark red). (Image provided by and reproduced with kind permission of Professor P.P. Tak.)

appears to be uniquely suited to supporting distinct patterns of cellular infiltrates.[22] These include diffuse, rather disorganized lymphocytic infiltrates, and comprise the most common form of synovitis. In 40–50% of patients more organized follicular structures may exist (Fig. 52.2). Based on immunohistochemical analysis, approximately 25% of these follicular structures include organized germinal centers in which there are zones of proliferating B cells undergoing affinity maturation, in addition to a distinct T-cell zone. In aggregates lacking germinal centers, follicular dendritic cells are also absent. A fourth histological pattern has been described in a much smaller subset of patients characterized by granulomatous reactions. From a clinical standpoint, it has been suggested that these distinct patterns not only reflect the heterogeneity of the disease, but also a spectrum of disease severity, with the presence of germinal centers or granulomatous reactions in tissues that are densely vascularized being associated with more severe, destructive disease. Several molecular determinants of synovial lymphoid structures have been defined. For example, the presence of germinal centers has been associated with tissue production of selected chemokines and the cytokine lymphotoxin.[22]

There is growing evidence from murine models that mononuclear cells invading the synovium can also originate from the bone marrow, passing through enlarged bone canals that connect the marrow to the synovium. This may explain the orientation and localization of invading tissue or 'pannus' (derived from the Greek, meaning 'tongue'). The regulation of this process is not known, but may be a key checkpoint for the initiation and tissue tropism of the inflammatory process. It also has a clinical correlate in early RA in terms of periarticular osteopenia on plain radiographs and bone marrow edema seen by magnetic resonance imaging (MRI).

GENE EXPRESSION SIGNATURES

Gene array technology has now permitted analysis of synovial tissue at the whole genome level, and, like genetic, serological and histological analysis, provides further evidence of disease heterogeneity. This strategy makes the assumption that each disease phenotype should be represented in gene expression signatures of multiple genes. Remarkable variation in gene expression signatures has been observed, although initial analyses seem to suggest that these signatures can be divided broadly into two groups.[23] The first is characterized by upregulation of immune response and inflammatory genes; these tissues are enriched for MHC and immunoglobulin gene products. In some tissues this signature may resemble an antiviral response consistent with prior infectious insult, and, more specifically, a STAT-1-dependent gene signature (promoting protective or proinflammatory effects).[23] This has also been observed in peripheral blood lymphocytes (PBL) from patients. The second group is more indicative of tissue remodeling, more reminiscent of that seen in osteoarthritis. Most interestingly, distinct FLS genotypes and phenotypes match the type of RA tissue from which they derived. For example, FLS signatures from high-intensity inflammatory tissue resemble that of TGF-β/activin A-induced expression profiles in myofibroblasts, whereas growth factors such as insulin-like growth factor 2 and insulin-like growth factor-binding protein 5 characterize FLS from tissues with low-intensity inflammation. These data support the notion of RA heterogeneity being reflected in FLS as a stable, if not a transformed, trait. They would also be consistent with a model of T cell-dependent RA that progresses with time to a relatively T cell-independent process, characterized by autonomous, invasive and aggressive FLS.[24]

■ IMMUNOBIOLOGY OF RA ■

INITIATION OF THE IMMUNE RESPONSE

Synovial fibroblasts are exquisitely sensitive to inflammatory cytokines such as IL-1, TNF-α and IL-6.[24] Accumulating evidence indicates that fibroblast-like synoviocytes (FLS) also express a range of Toll-like receptors (TLRs) that may respond to exogenous, pathogen-derived PAMPS, or indeed a growing range of self-tissue proteins.[25] Endogenous ligands especially relevant to inflammatory arthritis include heat shock proteins, fibrinogen fragments, antibody–DNA complexes, high-mobility group box (HMGB)-1 and hyaluronan oligosaccharides. Indeed, adjuvant arthritis models, as well as the streptococcal cell wall model, are dependent on such ligand receptor pathways. Recent data suggest that synovial FLS, as well as synovial macrophages, express TLR2 *in situ*. Expression is upregulated following stimulation with IL-1 and the TLR2 ligand peptidoglycan. TLR2 engagement induces cytokines such as IL-6, matrix metalloproteinases, adhesion molecules, and an array of chemokines, including granulocyte chemotactic protein (GCP)-2, RANTES, monocyte chemoattractant protein (MCP)-2, IL-8, growth-related oncogene-2, and to a lesser extent, macrophage-inflammatory protein 1α, MCP-1, EXODUS, and CXCL-16. Data suggest that TLR3, TLR4, TLR7 and TLR9 are also expressed at mRNA and possibly protein level,[25] and may augment inflammatory cytokine expression by dendritic cells from patients with RA.

Dendritic cells are likely to be important antigen-presenting cells in RA. Indeed, the proinflammatory environment would certainly favor maturation of DC in regional lymph nodes as well as in inflamed

Table 52.2 Characteristics of resident and infiltrating synovial mononuclear cells

Cellular phenotypes of synovial mononuclear cell subsets	
Cell lineage/marker	Significance or function of marker
T cell/NK cell	
CD45RO$^+$RA–RB^{dim}	Memory subset
CD62L$^-$CCR7$^-$	Homing, effector memory subset
DR$^+$CD69$^+$	Activation marker
LFA-1$^+$CD29^{bright}VLA-1$^+$VLA-4$^+$	Activation, homing and cell adhesion makers
Bcl-2-Bax^{bright}Fas$^+$	Pro-apoptotic markers
CD3^{int}TCRς^{dim}	Markers of prior antigen experience
CD28^{null}NKG2D$^+$perforin$^+$CD40L$^-$	Immune senescent effector T cells
CCR5$^+$CXCR3/4$^+$,CCR4$^+$	Chemokine responsive subsets
TNF/LTβ$^+$CD40L$^+$	Effector cytokines (lymphoid tissue, B-cell help)
IFNγ$^+$IL-10$^+$	Dominant cytokine phenotype (after stimulation)
CD26^{dim}	Impaired chemokine proteolysis
RANKL$^+$	Promote osteoclast differentiation
RANKL$^+$CD40L$^+$	Promote monocyte/DC interactions
CD4$^+$CD25^{bright}Foxp3$^+$	Regulatory T cells
CD3-CD56^{bright}TCRς^{neg}IFNγ$^+$	Effector NK cells
B cell	
CD19$^+$CD20$^+$CD40$^+$CD23$^+$	Differentiating B cells
CD27$^-$CD38$^+$	Memory B cells
CD20$^+$CD38$^-$	Subset of B cells hyporesponsive to proliferation
CD19$^+$CD20$^-$CD38$^+$BCMA$^+$	Autoantibody producing plasma cells
BAFF-R$^+$	Differentiating and mature B cells
Dendritic cell (DC)	
CD33^{dim}CD14^{dim}CD16–	Immature myeloid DC phenotype
DR/DQ^{bright}CD11c$^+$CD33^{bright}	Differentiating myeloid DC phenotype
CD14^{dim}	
plus CD8$^+$RelB$^+$	Functionally mature myeloid DC
DR$^+$CD11c-CD123$^+$RelB$^-$	Plasmacytoid DC
BDCA2$^+$BDCA4$^+$	Subset of plasmacytoid DC
CD33^{bright}CMRF44/56$^+$CD83$^+$	Differentiating DC
Macrophage	
CD68L$^+$	Fully differentiated subset
DR$^+$CD14$^+$FcR$^+$	Activation markers
FLS	
CD45$^-$CD14$^-$CD68$^-$	Key negative markers
CD55$^+$CD44$^+$CD90$^+$cadherin–11$^+$	Surface markers used to characterize FLS
VCAM–1^{high}ICAM–1$^+$CD58$^+$	Cell adhesion
LTβR$^+$	Stromal signal for lymphoid organogenesis
TLR2,3,4,7,9	PRR for PAMPs or endogenous ligands

tissue.[26] Thus, in peripheral blood, dendritic cell precursors express either an immature CD33^{dim}CD14^{dim}CD16$^-$ or a more mature HLA-DR/D Q^{bright}CD11c$^+$CD33^{bright}CD14^{dim} surface phenotype typical of myeloid DC (mDC) (Table 52.2); neither population expresses co-stimulatory molecules. In contrast, synovial fluid and tissue mDC subsets resemble mature peripheral blood cells, but in addition a subset expresses high levels of CD86 and can support allogeneic mixed leukocyte reactions (Table 52.2). More recent data indicate that they may differentiate further *in situ*, as suggested by nuclear translocation of RelB in perivascular DC infiltrates, consistent with prior cytokine receptor or TLR engagement *in vivo*. Perivascular RA synovium also contains populations of HLA-DR$^+$CD11c-CD123$^+$ plasmacytoid DC (pDC); in contrast to the myeloid DC subset, these are RelB$^-$ and comprise ~ 30% of all synovial DC. A subset of pDC express BDCA2 and may be capable of producing

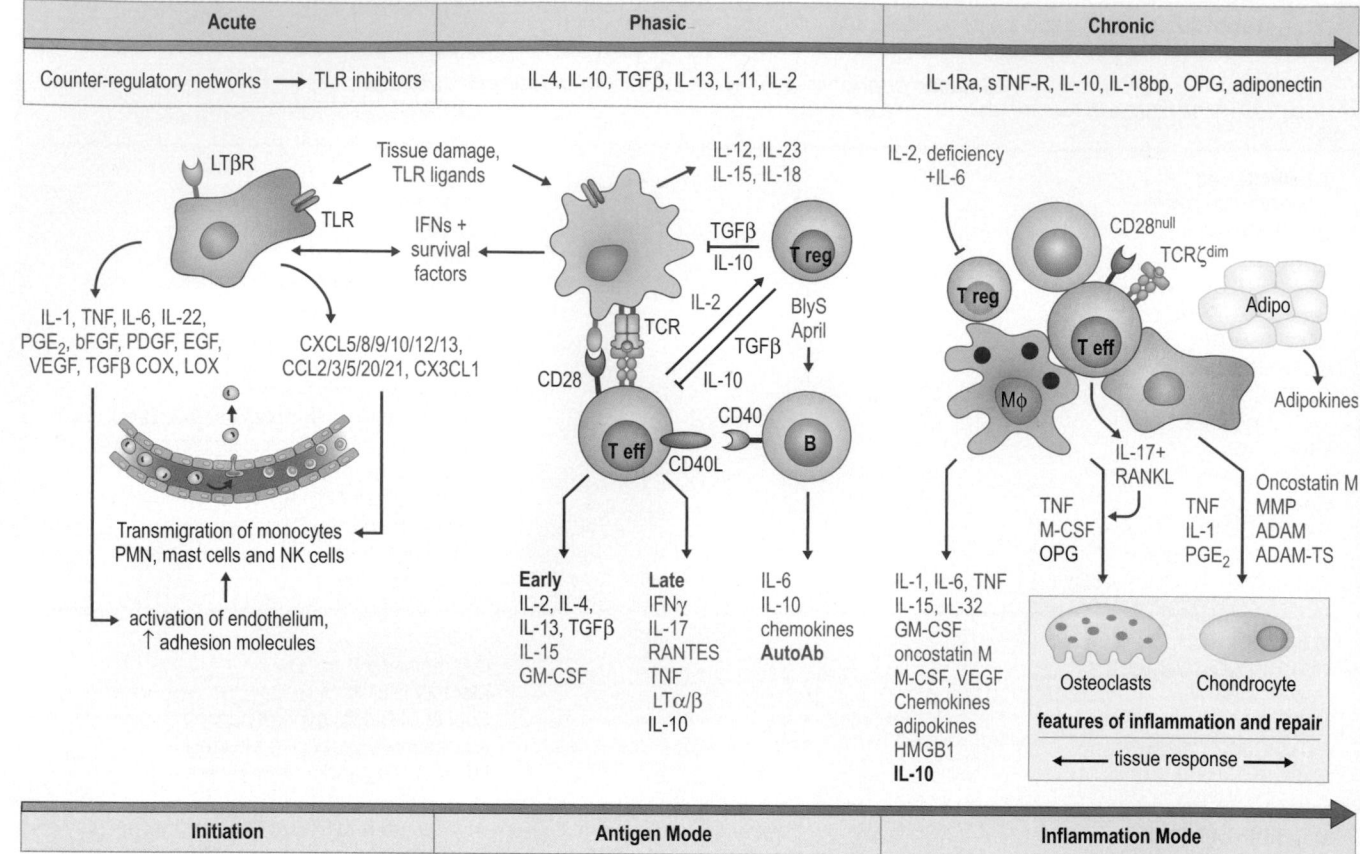

Acute	Phasic	Chronic
Counter-regulatory networks → TLR inhibitors	IL-4, IL-10, TGFβ, IL-13, L-11, IL-2	IL-1Ra, sTNF-R, IL-10, IL-18bp, OPG, adiponectin

| Initiation | Antigen Mode | Inflammation Mode |

Fig. 52.3 Cytokine networks in RA. The pathogenesis of RA can be thought of as a series of complex and closely related pathways regulated both temporally and spatially. These include: (1) an acute insult that may trigger the disease, characterized by stimulation of fibroblast-like synoviocytes (FLS) by inflammatory stimuli and the generation of cytokines and chemokines that promote the migration and infiltration by cells of the innate immune system; (2) repeated episodes of antigen-specific adaptive immune responses (in lymph node, bone marrow as well as in situ). Failure to resolve adaptive immunity is a key checkpoint which may lead to (3), a cytokine-driven chronic inflammatory phase where multiple cellular and molecular components sustain the response. Through multiple pathways acting on many cell types, this process leads to tissue injury. Proinflammatory pathways are shown in blue (text) and red (arrows), and anti-inflammatory, counter-regulatory pathways are shown in black (text and arrows). FLS, fibroblast-like synoviocytes; DC, dendritic cell; T$_{eff}$, effector T-helper cell; TCR, T-cell antigen receptor; Treg, regulatory T cell; B, B cell; AutoAb, autoantibodies; Mφ, macrophage; Adipo, adipocyte.

IFN-α *in situ*. Unlike their peripheral blood counterparts, synovial pDC efficiently activate allogeneic T cells to proliferate, as well as to produce IFN-γ, TNF-α and IL-10. Thus, many cellular and molecular components exist in RA synovium that could both initiate and serve to perpetuate the immune inflammatory response.

This initial wave of inflammation has two major consequences. First, inflammatory cytokines will promote the activation of vascular endothelium, changes that occur very early in disease (see above and Fig. 52.3). Under the influence of locally generated cytokines synovial postcapillary venules undergo morphological changes to an extent that they resemble high endothelial venules similar to those observed in secondary lymphoid organs. The second major consequence is the migration of inflammatory leukocytes, including polymorphonuclear leukocytes and immature or undifferentiated monocytes. This is possible because of chemokines produced on the one hand by resident stromal as well as infiltrating cells (Fig.

52.3), including IL-8/CXCL8, RANTES/CCL5, MIP-1α/CCL3, SDF-1/CXCL12, IP-10/CXCL10, and MCP-1/CCL2,[27] and the upregulation on endothelium of cell surface adhesion molecules, including intracellular adhesion molecule-1 (ICAM-1), vascular cell adhesion molecule-1 (VCAM-1) and E-selectin.[19] C-X-C, C-C, C and C-X₃-C chemokines all play a role, exerting chemotactic activity towards neutrophils, lymphocytes and monocytes, but also influencing the topology of inflammatory infiltrates, as discussed above. They are invariably early activation genes, in response to inflammatory stimuli. In synovial joints, macrophages are probably the dominant source of such factors. Crucially, the expression of chemokine receptors such as CCR4, CCR5, CXCR3 and CX3CR1 on inflammatory cell subsets will contribute to the selectivity of cellular recruitment (Table 52.2).[27] These events characterize the acute phase of an innate immune response, a key checkpoint that precedes the progression to subsequent events that herald the onset of the chronic inflammatory phase.

Table 52.3 Autoantigens in RA

Antigen	Sensitivity (%)	Specificity (%)
Fillagrin	40	92–99
HnRNP-A2	32	90–96
Vimentin	42	98
BiP/grp78	68	97
Collagen I	32	99
eIF4G1	50	97
CCP2	75–80	98–99
Fibronectin	14	nd
α-Enolase	46	nd
IgM RF	73	82
HMG1/2	25–40	nd
p68 (heavy chain BP)	64	90
Glucose-6-phosphate isomerase	64	95
Calpastatin	45	nd
Proteoglycan/aggrecan	nd	nd
Cartilage link protein	nd	nd
HCgp-39	1–8	nd
Osteopontin	<3	45
Hsp60	nd	nd
DNAJ	nd	nd
IR-3 (EBV)	nd	nd
p205	63	nd
Calreticulin	nd	nd
gp130-RAPS	73	97

AUTOANTIGENS IN RA

Although current models of adaptive immune responses would suggest that DC carry antigens derived from damaged or dying synovial tissue, the molecular nature of disease-associated antigens has, until recently, remained an enigma. Many RA-associated autoantigens have been described (Table 52.3). Other candidate autoantigens have been vigorously validated in animal models.[28] The best described are collagen II, HCgp-39, and more recently glucose-6 phosphate isomerase. However, when used as recombinant antigens none of these have been found to elicit reproducible and/or robust T- or B-cell responses in a significant proportion of patients. There are several plausible explanations for this. The most obvious are that antigens that drive autoimmune arthritis are not the same in mice and humans, or that detectable T-cell responses occur very early and are blunted in established disease. Another possibility is that the autoantigens used to test lymphocyte reactivity *in vitro* do not carry the post-translational modifications (i.e., the neo-epitopes) recognized by autoantibody or antigen receptor. Good examples are the carbohydrate moieties of collagen II epitopes that serve as key TCR contacts in collagen II immunity, and the citrullination of key arginine residues in triple helical CII peptides that appear to be the immunodominant autoantibody epitopes.

GENERATION OF NEOEPITOPES BY DEIMINATION

In 1998, van Venrooij and colleagues[29] first reported that patients with RA carried antibodies that recognized deiminated peptides of fillagrin, the substrate that was found to be the antigen recognized in rat keratinized epithelium. This substrate formed the basis of the anti-perinuclear factor (APF) assay. Using new generation anti-cyclic citrullinated peptide (anti-CCP)-based assays, the presence of these antibodies, now collectively termed anti-citrullinated protein antigens, have now been shown by many groups to be both sensitive (up to 80%) and highly specific (> 95%) for the diagnosis of RA.[29] Indeed, serum anti-CCP levels are stable with disease, they have been detected as early as 14 years prior to disease onset, and have been shown to be predictors of radiographic progression. Citrullination is not specific for RA (Fig. 52.4). Indeed, citrullination may be inflammation specific, as it has been documented in inflamed synovium derived from patients with reactive arthritis and psoriatic arthritis as well as RA, but not OA. What appears specific for RA is the immune response to citrulline (Fig. 52.4). A link between anti-CCP and HLA-DRB1 alleles, specifically SE+ alleles, has now been established.[17] Linkage analysis across chromosome 6 has documented a large peak, with LOD scores of >10 for anti-CCP+ patients but not for those who do

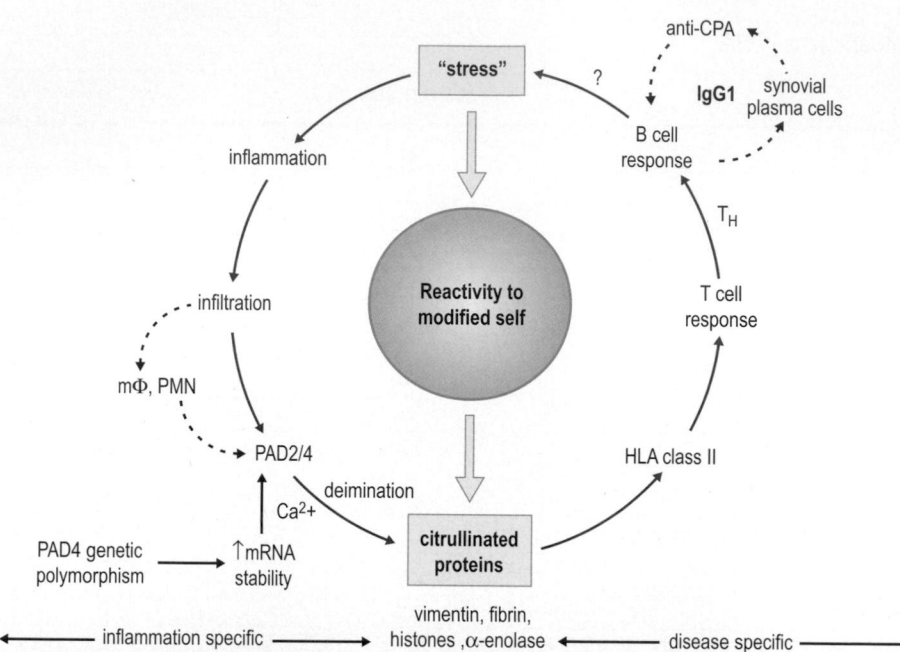

Fig. 52.4 The generation of autoantibodies to citrullinated protein antigens. The stressed and inflamed synovium is characterized by an influx of inflammatory cells, including macrophages and neutrophils that express peptidyl-arginine deiminases (PAD). In the presence of sufficient [Ca^{2+}], PADs deiminate target proteins, including, among others, vimentin, fibrin, histones and α-enolase. This is inflammation, but not disease specific. The combination of environmental stimuli (including inflammation and tobacco smoke) and the inheritance of specific HLA-DRB1 alleles favor T- and B-cell immune responses to the host's derivatized neo-epitope peptide antigens. Th, T-helper effector cell; anti-CPA, autoantibodies to citrullinated protein antigens.

not carry these antibodies. This relationship is independent of RF status, as the SE allele frequencies in anti-CCP+ patients are twice those of anti-CCP- patients, even those who are RF+. Indeed, the risk of carrying SE in RF+anti-CCP- patients is no different from that in the healthy control population. These data would be consistent with a model where T cells from patients with RA can recognize peptide autoantigens modified by citrullination if they carry SE+ DRB1 alleles. Studies in HLA class II transgenic mice suggest that the conversion of positively charged arginine at key residues in antigenic peptides from candidate autoantigens to neutral citrulline is permissive for peptide binding and the induction of antigen-specific immune responses *in vivo*.

Finally, citrullination is widespread in multiple tissues in response to appropriate provocations. Although the molecular basis for these triggers is poorly understood, recent data point to a link between smoking, an environmental exposure known to be linked with RA, citrullination, and individuals carrying SE.[30] Thus, cells derived from bronchoalveolar lavage from smokers express citrulline, but not those from nonsmokers. The association between the development of RA and smoking has now been linked to anti-CCP+ patients, whose relative risk increases to 20 if they smoke and carry two copies of the SE+ DRB1 alleles, compared to patients with anti-CCP-disease showing much weaker or no such relationship. These data may have clinical significance; at the outset of disease, they may provide useful predictors of patients who are more likely to progress to develop severe erosive joint disease.

LYMPHOCYTE BIOLOGY

Flow cytometric analysis of dissociated synovial mononuclear cell cultures indicates that infiltrating T lymphocytes can make up approximately 10–35% of cells in inflamed tissue. The ratio of CD4 to CD8 T cells seen in peripheral blood is skewed in favor of the CD4 subset. Much of the information on phenotype and function is derived from detailed analyses of synovial fluid, and, to a lesser extent, synovial tissue subsets (Table 52.2). Similar enrichment of these subsets is commonly detected in PBL. The majority of synovial T cells express phenotypic markers of antigen-experienced, terminally differentiated T cells with enhanced migratory capacity. Thus synovial T cells would typically be cell surface HLA-DR+, LFA-1+, VLA-1+, CD69+, CD45RO+, CD45RA-, CD45RB^dim, CD29^bright, CD27-, CD25- (Table 52.2).[31] Synovial B cells also express a typical memory/differentiated phenotype. Indeed, analysis of the variable regions of the Ig heavy and light chains confirms that antigen-specific activation and differentiation of B cells into plasma cells takes place in the chronically inflamed synovial tissue of patients with RA. Analysis of synovial T cells reveals that expression of the TCR invariant chain subunits CD3ε and TCRζ are found at lower density than that found in corresponding peripheral blood T cells, consistent with evidence of prior antigen engagement. Although synovial fluid T cells are also FasL+, Bcl2-, Bax^bright, favoring a pro-apoptotic state, it is thought that environmental cues transduced through common γ-chain receptor signaling cytokines such as IL-2, IL-7 and IL-15, as well as type I interferons, prevent apoptosis of T cells *in situ*.[32] Synovial tissue-derived lymphocytes may be different. Consistent with their state of terminal differentiation, synovial T cells comprise populations of T cells with a contracted oligoclonal repertoire, based on assessment of TCR gene rearrangements.[22] A subset of these cells are CD28[null], while at the same time expressing a range of NK-cell surface receptors that are thought to contribute to effector function independently of cognate antigen.[22] Nevertheless, to date there exists no common TCRVB family that might suggest expansion of such clones by a common RA-specific antigen. A subset of IFN-γ-producing CD56[bright]TCRζ[neg] NK cells also appears to accumulate in RA synovial joints.

This state of terminal differentiation or immunosenescence of lymphocytes has several consequences.[6, 33] First, synovial T cells are hyporesponsive to TCR ligation. This may directly reflect a state of proliferative exhaustion, exacerbated by the effects of the inflammatory milieu, including cytokines, reactive oxygen intermediates, and depletion of essential nutrients such as tryptophan or arginine, which target the expression and function of key TCR proximal signaling molecules, including TCRζ, p36 LAT and small GTP-binding molecules, all of which play a specialized role in transmitting signals from the antigen receptor to downstream signaling pathways. Second, these defects may also be detected in the periphery, manifesting themselves as a state of 'anergy,' with impaired DTH skin tests. It is also possible that this state of hyporesponsiveness contributes to the twofold enhanced susceptibility to infection (skin, joint and respiratory tract), especially in patients with more severe disease. Third, the profile of cytokines in SF from patients with very early RA suggests evidence of early Th2 differentiation (arising perhaps from a mast cell-derived IL-4 environment), this profile changes rapidly as the inflammatory process evolves, as synovial T cells from patients with established disease express barely detectable levels of T cell-derived cytokines, including IL-2, IL-4, IL-5 and IL-13, and only small subsets express IFN-γ, some of which also express IL-10. This finding has formed the principle argument against T cells playing a role in established disease. Nevertheless, the finding of reproducible levels of IFN-γ by a subset of synovial T cells has implied a bias toward a Th1 response. The contribution of IL-17 expressing T cells is not clear.

MOLECULAR BASIS OF PERSISTENCE

Understanding the molecular basis of persistence is of major importance in diseases such as RA. Whereas inflammatory infiltrates persist in patients with active disease, the local synovial stromal microenvironment provides a unique niche for the development of follicular lymphoid microstructures in a subset of patients.[34] As mentioned above, these are stable over time and are found in multiple joints from the same patient. For their persistence these structures have been shown to be associated with the expression of LTβ, LTβR and the chemokines CCL19 and CCL21.[35] LTβ is expressed on activated T and B cells, and the rather more restricted expression of LTβR is confined to synovial stromal cells. The importance of LTβ-LTβR signaling, which utilizes both canonical (IKKβ/IKK2) and alternative (IKKα/IKK1) pathways of NF-κB activation, has been firmly established in LTβ- and LTβR-deficient mice, which exhibit severe defects in lymphoid organogenesis. The tumor repressor p53 and PTEN may also contribute to the survival of synovial stroma. It is not surprising, therefore, that these structures (which are associated with more severe, seropositive, erosive disease) also provide a local niche for B-cell differentiation and immunoglobulin production. Indeed, it has been shown that follicular B cells are a source of local autoantibody production, including

RF and anti-CCP. B cells can also contribute to antigen-presenting functions,[36] as well as being a major source of chemokines and inflammatory cytokines, including IL-6. The direct contribution of immune complexes to local inflammation and tissue destruction has long been implied, mediated in part through engagement of activating FcR.[37] Nevertheless, local complement consumption in the synovium has long been recognized, and evidence from the KRN serum transfer arthritis model suggests that local deficiency of naturally occurring inhibitors of complement activation may contribute to the tissue specificity of the inflammatory response.

It is now well established that enhanced expression of inflammatory cytokines is one of the hallmarks of chronic inflammatory diseases such as RA.[38] With few exceptions, most cytokines are expressed in inflamed synovium at mRNA or protein levels. For example, unlike PBL from healthy donors, explants of synovial mononuclear cells constitutively express IL-1, IL-6, IL-8, GM-CSF and a vast array of chemokines, as well as growth factors, including FGF, VEGF and PDGF (Fig. 52.3). Although anti-inflammatory or immunoregulatory cytokines, including IL-4, IL-10, IL-11, TGF-β and specific naturally occurring inhibitors of IL-1α/β (IL-1Ra) and TNF-α (soluble TNF-R) may also be detected, functional bioassays suggest that the overriding response is inflammatory. Indeed, levels of IL-1Ra and sTNF-R are significantly upregulated in synovial fluid compared to serum from patients with RA. Yet IL-1 and TNF bioactivity persists in spite of this, suggesting that attempts to suppress cytokine activity are insufficient. The specific activity of subsets of cytokines, their networks, and how they may contribute to RA is illustrated in Figure 52.3. In many cases, the pathogenic roles of cytokines have been established in rodent models, either by selectively blocking their function (e.g. with specific monoclonal antibodies or soluble receptor fusion proteins) or by gene targeting approaches. Perhaps the best documented include the inflammatory arthritides documented in transgenic mice over-expressing human TNF-α, in IL-6 signaling gp130 mutant mice and ZAP-70 mutant SKG mice.[39] Disruption of immunoregulatory or inhibitory cytokines, including IL-1ra, IL-10 and TGF-β, leads to severe auto-inflammatory syndromes targeting different organs, depending on genotype.

A major challenge has been to identify the pathways that promote chronic cytokine and chemokine expression *in vivo*. One possible mechanism is that of cell contact-dependent stimulation of macrophages and fibroblasts by activated T cells (Fig. 52.3).[40] This is an appealing pathway, given that T cell-derived products such as IFN-γ that prime macrophages to produce TNF, IL-1 and IL-6 are relatively deficient in inflamed synovium. Physical contact of activated but not resting T cells induces abundant TNF-α, IL-1β, IL-8, MCP-1 and MMP production by monocytes (Fig. 52.3). This can be reproduced using T-cell plasma membrane preparations, and prevented by interrupting cell contact. Interestingly, the effector response depends on the nature of the T-cell stimulus. Thus, Th2 T cells produce relatively more monocyte-dependent IL-1Ra than IL-1β and higher ratios of TIMP than MMP. Contact between T cells and synovial fibroblasts has also been shown to induce IL-6, MMPs and PGE$_2$ (Fig. 52.3), each of which may contribute to distinct aspects of downstream effector pathways.

IMMUNE REGULATION

The recent emergence of interest in regulatory cell subsets and their anti-inflammatory properties has perhaps more firmly established the concept that failure of the default mechanisms of immune regulation may underpin autoimmune diseases. Experiments in gene-deficient mice (e.g., Foxp3, IL-2, IL-2R, IL-2R signaling, STAT5, IL-10, TGF-β) lend support to this concept. In RA the data remain less clear.[41] For example, there is *in vitro* evidence for a relative deficiency of constitutive IL-10 expression in synovial cell cultures, and yet clinical trials of IL-10 were rather disappointing; TGF-β is yet to be tested. These results may reflect the complex role of these cytokines in disease pathogenesis. The identification of defective numbers and/or function of CD4+CD25bright regulatory T cells (Tregs) has been suggested by several investigators, but reports are conflicting. Some studies have shown a clear reduction in the numbers of peripheral blood Tregs in patients with RA, but others have shown no difference; interestingly, Tregs appear deficient in numbers in subsets of children with juvenile idiopathic arthritis (JIA) whose disease tends to progress. In synovial joints the data are more consistent, with many reports showing substantial increases in Treg numbers in synovial tissue and fluid compared to paired peripheral blood. However, some studies have reported normal function at a cellular level, whereas others have shown depressed regulatory function.

Two recent reports which both studied Treg phenotype and function in patients receiving anti-TNF therapy have provided some insight into the relationship between inflammation and defective regulatory function. Ehrenstein and colleagues[42] demonstrated that whereas PB Tregs from patients with active RA could suppress the proliferation of CD4+CD25- effector T cells, they failed to suppress IFN-γ and TNF-α production. Treatment with infliximab reversed this defect, but also conferred the capacity of CD4+CD25- precursors to become regulatory cell subsets. A second study demonstrated that TNF at high doses suppresses the expression of Foxp3,[43] a helix–loop–helix transcription factor family member whose deficiency causes Scurfy disease and IPEX in mice and humans, respectively, and is expressed relatively selectively in Tregs (more specific for mouse than human Tregs). In this study, infliximab treatment restored Foxp3 expression in PBL. The data provide a crucial link between inflammation and failure of immune regulation, and may go some way to explain the immunomodulatory properties and sustained clinical benefit of anti-TNF, not only in RA but in a wide range of other chronic inflammatory diseases.

IMPACT OF THE IMMUNE RESPONSE ON CARTILAGE AND BONE

For many years it was thought that the terminal effector phase of chronic inflammation that led to cartilage destruction and bone resorption was driven almost exclusively by inflammatory cytokines and proteinases. IL-1, MMPs (MMP1, 3, 8, 13) and more recently aggrecanases (ADAMTS 4 and 5) were and remain the major culprits. Attempts to establish more directly a link between adaptive immunity and destruction of target tissue failed, not least because of the lack of direct contact between lymphocytes, chondrocytes and bone. A breakthrough came in the late 1990s with the identification of the TNF/TNF-R family member receptor for activation of NF-κB ligand (RANKL)/TRANCE/ODF and its counter-receptor RANK, and the dissection of the molecular and cellular components required for differentiation of osteoclasts from monocyte precursors.[44] According to contemporary paradigms, RANKL is necessary and sufficient for osteoclast differentiation. TNF, M-CSF and IL-17 probably contribute, and RANKL-independent pathways may also play a role. RANKL is expressed on synovial fibroblasts and osteoblasts, but also on activated T cells, its counter-receptor being expressed on myeloid lineage cells including monocytes, osteoclast

precursors and dendritic cells. Its expression is regulated by inflammatory mediators including TNF and PGE₂. RANKL is shed, probably through the action of several membrane-associated proteases, including MT1-MMP (MMP14). Gene targeting of RANKL or RANK in mice leads to inhibition of osteoclastogenesis and a profound osteoporotic bone phenotype. Deletion of OPG, the naturally occurring decoy soluble receptor for RANK, leads to unbridled osteoclast differentiation and bone resorption, and substantially reduced bone mass. A good example of the link between adaptive immunity and bone resorption comes from CTLA4−/− mice, characterized by sustained chronic T-cell activation.[45] T cells from these mice over-express RANKL. Importantly, the bone, but not the inflammatory phenotype, is rescued by inhibition of RANK/RANKL signaling. In RA, several studies have demonstrated perturbations of serum RANKL/OPG ratios, a parameter currently under investigation as a biomarker for bone homeostasis.

■ CLINICAL FEATURES ■

DISEASE ONSET

RA is a heterogeneous disease that does not conform to a single clinical entity.[2] Whereas 10% of patients may have an acute severe onset and 20% a more subacute onset, in up to 70% of patients the onset of signs and symptoms may be insidious. A more episodic or palindromic onset has also been described. A common presentation, more likely during the winter months, is that of a female in the fourth to fifth decades of life who complains of diffuse symmetrical joint pain, swelling and stiffness of small peripheral joints. Patients frequently complain that they can no longer make a fist, especially in the early morning. The targeting of afflicted synovial joints may be symmetrical in most cases, typically affecting the small joints of the hands and feet, as well as the wrists. Less frequent are those with slow-onset monoarticular disease. Patients not fulfilling the diagnostic classification criteria for RA (see below) may, at this point, be ascribed the more appropriate diagnostic label of undifferentiated arthritis, as in a proportion of cases signs and symptoms may resolve spontaneously. At 1 year approximately 30% will progress to develop the syndrome we call RA.

ARTICULAR SIGNS AND SYMPTOMS

Systematic examination of the musculoskeletal system and careful documentation of the pattern of joint involvement (e.g., symmetry, axial versus peripheral joint involvement) are crucial to establishing an unambiguous clinical diagnosis of RA. Patients will often present with swelling, in addition to pain, which affects the whole surface of small joints, in contrast to weightbearing joints. Swelling may arise as a consequence of the disease process affecting intra-articular structures, typically presenting with soft tissue swelling and joint fluid (demonstrated clinically by fluctuation), or periarticular structures including the joint capsule, which is very sensitive to stretching and distension. Tenderness and swelling most closely reflect the intensity of the inflammatory process, but erythema, more characteristic of crystal arthropathies or articular sepsis, is unusual. Surprisingly reliable indicators of the intensity of inflammation include early morning stiffness (as distinct from immobility stiffness), commonly occurring for more than 1 hour per day, poor grip strength, and pain on passive joint movement. In the absence of swelling of specific joints, pain elicited on lateral compression of metacarpophalangeal (MCP) or metatarsophalangeal (MTP) joints (the

MCP or MTP joint 'squeeze') is predictive not only of active disease but of progression to erosive disease. Less frequent are those patients presenting with inflammatory disease of other synovial structures in isolation, such as bursitis. The presence of flexor tenosynovitis at the outset is more common.

HANDS

There is a variety of well-recognized clinical signs that arise as a consequence of more progressive joint inflammation. This is prominent in both upper and lower limb peripheral joints. Symmetrical involvement of PIP joints may lead to fusiform swelling of the joints. Disease of associated structures, including tendons and synovial sheaths, commonly coexists, and together these contribute to impairment in grip strength, whereas distal interphalangeal (DIP) joint involvement is more likely to reflect coincidental osteoarthritis. Specific deficiencies in articular and periarticular structures may arise through variable effects of muscle atrophy, tendon laxity or shortening, tendon rupture, weakening of the joint capsule, and cartilage destruction where an imbalance of forces is transmitted across the joint. Classic joint deformities besides synovitis include joint subluxation, ulnar drift, Boutonnière's and swan-neck deformities; where the thumb is affected, flail, Boutonnière's or duck-bill deformities may develop. Often deformities may occur in combination, such as the subluxation that occurs at MCP joints associated with ulnar drift due to weakening of both dorsal and radial structures and lengthening of collateral ligaments.

WRISTS

Symmetrical involvement of the wrist is common, and loss of wrist extension is an early clinical sign. Typical signs include swelling over the ulnar styloid, whose prominence may be further exacerbated by a predilection for ulnar synovitis, supination–subluxation at the carpus, and disruption of the triangular ligament which promotes volar rotation. Subluxation predisposes to erosion of the floor of the extensor compartments, leading to extensor tendon rupture. Unremitting progressive synovitis at the wrist may ultimately promote fibrosis and then bony ankylosis of the carpus.

ANKLES AND FEET

Hindfoot disease, leading to ankle, subtalar and talonavicular synovitis, is more common than is generally appreciated. Progressive pain, stiffness and peroneal muscle spasm often cause valgus deformity, which increases as cartilage destruction and bone erosion develop. This invariably leaves the patient with a spastic flat foot as flattening of the longitudinal arch progresses. Spontaneous fusion is not uncommon. Disease of the metatarsal heads associated with synovitis of the metatarsophalangeal joints and flexor tenosynovitis is classic, and in very early disease tenderness in response to lateral compression of MTP joints is predictive of progressive, erosive disease.

INVOLVEMENT OF LARGE JOINTS

Although disease of the large joints is well documented they may be spared, especially at the onset and during the early phase of disease. Synovitis of the elbow is a useful sign as it occurs much less frequently in other inflammatory arthritides. The earliest sign is loss of full extension, which may not influence function to any great extent. As disease progresses, the humeroulnar joint is the first to develop erosive changes. With advanced disease this may herald proximal movement of the radial head. Once this affects elbow flexion function is invariably compromised, as supination may also become restricted. RA of the shoulder is observed in more progressive disease and may not become symptomatic or affect day-to-day function until the joint disease is more advanced. Erosive synovitis may target not only the humeral head or glenoid fossa, but also the acromioclavicular joint.

Large joint disease affecting the lower limbs occurs more commonly in the knees than the hips. Whereas the hip may be spared at the outset, hip disease can present with groin discomfort and abnormal gait. Range of movement at this joint may become compromised once synovitis has induced loss of cartilage. As the inflammatory process progresses erosive disease will lead to protrusion of the acetabula. Osteonecrosis is relatively common at the hip, and may arise more often in those patients exposed to long-term corticosteroid therapy. Knee disease is more obvious and can present as small yet obvious effusions (elicited through the 'bulge sign'), and then fixed flexion deformities and popliteal fullness (progressing to Baker's cyst). With active, chronic synovitis progression to erosion and loss of articular cartilage is almost inevitable. At this stage, laxity of collateral or cruciate ligaments further promotes joint instability, detected clinically by lateral or medial movement of the distal limb against the femur, or by the 'draw sign,' respectively. Depending on loading, these deformities may progress to valgus or, less commonly, varus deformities.

DISEASE OF OTHER JOINTS AND TISSUES

Disease of other synovial structures such as the temporomandibular and cricoarytenoid joints is well documented though relatively rare, as is involvement of the ossicles of the ear. Disease of the axial skeleton is restricted to diarthrodial joints of the upper cervical spine (C1–C2). In the early phase this may present with little in the way of pain, but with restriction of movement, especially in lateral flexion, stiffness, and a sensation of 'clunking' at extremes of movement. Synovitis of the articulation between the transverse ligament of the atlas and the posterior aspect of the odontoid peg compromises the transverse ligament allowing forward slip of the atlas (C1) on the axis (C2; atlantoaxial subluxation). The dens may also erode. With severe unremitting synovitis encroachment onto the apophyseal joints may permit basilar invagination of the odontoid into the foramen magnum, threatening both upper cervical cord and the medullary structures. This is potentially life-threatening and poses a significant pre- and perioperative anesthetic risk. Synovitis of the dorsolumbar spine is confined to the apophyseal joints, which, when the synovium is hypertrophied, can lead to compromise of the cord or nerve roots; in the lower lumbar spine this may present with typical signs of lumbar canal stenosis. It should be noted that through different mechanisms, chronic inflammatory diseases such as RA are associated with accelerated loss of bone mass, and bone mineral density may be rapidly compromised further in those patients taking corticosteroids.

■ SYSTEMIC AND EXTRA-ARTICULAR MANIFESTATIONS ■

In addition to generalized polyarthralgia and/or myalgia, common associated signs and symptoms can include systemic features such as anorexia, weight loss or low-grade fever. Fatigue is a particularly good indicator of systemic inflammation but is hard to quantify clinically, being reflected

SYSTEMIC AND EXTRA-ARTICULAR MANIFESTATIONS

Table 52.4 Systemic and extra-articular features of RA

General	Neurological
Fever, sweats	Myelopathy
Lymphadenopathy	Entrapment neuropathy
Weight loss	Peripheral neuropathy
Fatigue, weakness	Mononeuritis multiplex

Dermatological	Haematological
Palmar erythema	Anemia
Subcutaneous nodules	Thrombocytosis
Vasculitis	Lymphocytosis or lymphopenia
Ulceration, neutrophilic	Felty's syndrome
dermatoses	Large granular lymphocytes
	Lymphoproliferative disease

Ophthalmic	Renal
Episcleritis	Interstitial nephritis
Scleritis	Renal tubular acidosis
Choroid and retinal nodules	Amyloidosis
Keratoconjunctivitis sicca	

Pulmonary	Gastrointestinal
Pleuritis	Xerostomia
Nodules	Transaminitis
Interstitial pneumonitis	NSAID enteropathy
Bronchiolitis obliterans	
Arteritis	
Pulmonary hypertension	

Cardiac	Musculoskeletal
Pericarditis	Myositis, muscle weakness
Myocarditis	Osteoporosis
Coronary vasculitis	
Atheromatous disease	
Valvular nodulosis	

CLINICAL PEARLS

PREDICTORS OF POOR OUTCOME IN RA

>> Chronic, unremitting disease onset, especially at advanced age

>> Female gender

>> Poor functional status determined by validated functional disability indices such as the Stanford Health Assessment Questionnaire (HAQ) and the Arthritis Impact Measurement Scale (AIMS)

>> Low socioeconomic status

>> Systemic and extra-articular features

>> Comorbidity, e.g., infection, cardiovascular disease, renal impairment

>> Early erosive disease (in first 6–12 months, often associated with anti-CPA autoantibodies)

>> Persistent acute-phase response (e.g., time integrated CRP levels)

>> Autoantibodies (RF and anti-CPA) and HLA-DRB1 status (SE⁺)

>> Significant delay in early use of DMARD and corticosteroids

CPA, citrullinated protein antigens; CRP, C-reactive protein; RF, rheumatoid factor; SE, shared epitope; DMARD, disease-modifying antirheumatic drug.

more by levels of inactivity or failure to undertake routine daily activities. Other manifestations are more obvious and are listed in Table 52.4.

NATURAL HISTORY, CLINICAL COURSE AND PROGNOSTIC FACTORS ASSOCIATED WITH DISEASE PROGRESSION

Many studies have attempted to identify clinical variables relating to disease onset, or its initial progression, that reproducibly predict patterns of long-term outcome. It is generally agreed that gender, disease activity and functional status at onset, the use of early disease-modifying antirheumatic drugs (DMARDs) and tight control most consistently influence outcome. For those patients with established RA, Wolfe and Cathey[45a] have applied the Stanford Health Assessment Questionnaire

(HAQ) and Functional Disability Index (FDI) in 1274 RA patients followed for 12 years to demonstrate that the progression of disability is most rapid in the first few years after onset. Loss of function was severe over 2–6 years and very severe by 10 years. Progression was found to be more rapid in older women, especially those with longer disease duration, as well as patients with poor grip strength, more pain, and higher global severity scores. Extra-articular and systemic features were also associated with greater functional loss. Simpler composite scores comprising grip strength, button test and walking time produced comparable results. These parameters also predicted longevity, translating to a twofold increase in standardized mortality rates in those patients with severe disease, equivalent to Hodgkin's lymphoma or triple-vessel coronary artery disease. Indeed 5-year survival rates in patients with severe RA have been estimated to be between 40% and 50%. Comorbidity and increased mortality may be related directly to cardiovascular disease associated with chronic inflammation, increased susceptibility to infection, and gastrointestinal adverse events.

DIAGNOSIS

CLASSIFICATION CRITERIA

The American College of Rheumatology criteria for the classification of RA are a set of clinical and laboratory parameters that serve as a guide for the diagnosis of RA, and were established largely for epidemiological purposes. They are relatively straightforward and easy to apply, especially to patients with established disease. However, failure of a patient with early signs and symptoms of an inflammatory arthropathy to fulfill

Table 52.5 1987 revised criteria for the classification of RA

1. Stiffness in and around the joints lasting 1 hour before maximal improvement

2. Soft tissue swelling (arthritis) of 3 or more joint areas, simultaneously, observed by a physician

3. Swelling (arthritis) of the proximal interphalangeal, metacarpophalangeal, or wrist joints

4. Symmetric swelling (arthritis)

5. Rheumatoid nodules

6. The presence of rheumatoid factor

7. Radiographic erosions and/or periarticular osteopenia in hand and/or wrist joints

- four of seven criteria are required to classify a patient as having RA
- criteria 1–4 must be present for at least 6 weeks
- criteria 2–5 must be observed by a physician

them does not mean that she or he does not have RA. The revised 1987 criteria have been further simplified by removing the 'probable,' 'definite' and 'classic' subclassifications (Table 52.5).[46] These new criteria have a sensitivity for RA of 91–94% and a specificity of 89% in the clinical setting. Although these 1987 criteria are used regularly in clinical practice and research, it is likely that as subgroups of patients become defined based on molecular parameters that are clinically meaningful in terms of prognosis and therapy, the criteria may become more sophisticated; stratification of disease according to anti-CCP status is one good example.

LABORATORY FINDINGS

Routine laboratory hematologic and biochemical anomalies, such as normochromic, normocytic anemia, thrombocytosis, and perturbations in the leukocyte count, may inform disease activity but are neither specific nor helpful in diagnosis. The same can be said of the myriad acute-phase proteins, in addition to the ESR, including CRP, fibrinogen, α-macroglobulin, serum amyloid protein and ferritin, although their levels may provide a useful indication of disease activity and longer-term prognosis when measured over time. As with serum biomarkers, analysis of synovial fluid, although undertaken quite frequently in the clinical setting, is rarely, if ever, diagnostic. A typical RA synovial fluid exudate may be turbid due to cellularity ($> 50\,000/mm^3$, although more typically in the 20–40 000/mm^3 range) and contain abundant PMNs, with reduced viscosity. Invariably, the exclusion of sepsis or crystals is most useful with respect to SF analysis.

Until the late 1990s, IgM rheumatoid factors (RF) – autoantibodies that recognize the Fc subunit of IgG – remained one of the few parameters of value in the clinical setting, forming the basis of the seropositive versus seronegative stratification of RA, and identifying those patients more likely to progress to erosive disease with or without extra-articular features.[47] Nevertheless, RF can be detected in up to 5% of the healthy population and between 10% and 20% of the aging population (> 65

years of age), and is found in a range of rheumatic conditions, including Sjögren's syndrome, SLE, and cryoglobulinemia, as well as in acute infectious and neoplastic disease entities, influencing its diagnostic utility. In general RF is not of value for monitoring responses to therapy.

The discovery of antibodies to cyclic citrullinated antigens (anti-CPA) is likely to change diagnostic practice once the assays become more widely available, not least because they are found very early in disease.[29] They also have prognostic value in terms of radiographic progression. The new generation of anti-CCP kits has demonstrated a diagnostic sensitivity of 80% and a specificity of 98%. It is likely that as the range of RA-associated autoantigens expands, and as the repertoire of deiminated target autoantigens is defined, multiplex assay of serum autoantibodies will play an increasingly important role in the diagnosis and prognosis of subsets of inflammatory arthritides. Other biomarkers used in either clinical or investigative settings are listed in Box 52.3.

IMAGING

Plain radiographs of the hands and feet are rarely useful during the first 6–12 months of disease other than to confirm soft tissue swelling, which is invariably present on clinical examination. Nevertheless, they provide an important baseline against which to compare subsequent studies. Beyond this time, abnormalities may include periarticular osteopenia, cortical breaks, loss of articular cartilage (manifest as joint space narrowing) and early bone erosions, especially at the head of metacarpals and metatarsals, or at the base of proximal phalanges (Fig. 52.5). Late changes include subluxation, and eventually bony destruction and ankylosis. High-resolution ultrasound (HRUS) has gained much support, especially as it is cheap and possible to use at the bedside. In combination with power color Doppler imaging modalities, which detect vascularity in addition to inflammation, HRUS has proved to be superior to plain radiographs in detecting early cortical erosions (which require confirmation in longitudinal and transverse planes). It is also useful for detecting subclinical tenosynovitis. Although not all joints are accessible, HRUS has proved especially useful for the monitoring of MCP joints and wrist disease. More expensive, but more sensitive still, is magnetic resonance imaging (MRI), which can detect erosions and bone marrow edema at very early stages of disease, as well as defining periarticular structures, which are more selectively involved in the seronegative arthropathies.

■ TREATMENT ■

Contemporary management of patients with RA requires a multidisciplinary approach, with emphasis on reduction of pain, suppression of inflammation and restoration of function.[2] This is possible only through a coordinated input from a team comprising physician, physiotherapist, occupational therapist, psychologist and surgeon. In current practice, suppression of inflammation is a realistic goal with aggressive and intensive therapy and monitoring. The immunological goal is to halt the underlying disease process by restoring immune homeostatic mechanisms, but this has yet to be achieved routinely in humans.

DISEASE MODIFYING ANTI-RHEUMATIC DRUGS

Over the last two decades there has been a dramatic paradigm shift in the therapy of RA from control of symptoms to the control of the disease process.[48] This has come about through a growing appreciation of the

CLINICAL RELEVANCE

Biomarkers in RA	Clinical association
Autoantibodies	
IgM RF	May antedate disease; associated with more severe ±extra-articular disease; predictor of radiographic progression
IgA RF	Extra-articular disease
Anti-CPA	May antedate disease onset;
(APF, AKA, anti–Sa,	HLA–DRB1 (SE⁺) status; smoking
Anti-vimentin,	Predictor of radiographic progression
Anti-α-enolase)	
Anti-GPI	Felty's syndrome, vasculitis
Acute-phase response	
ESR	Active disease; time integrated levels associated with radiographic progression
CRP	
IL–6	Active disease
Synovial vascularity	
VEGF	Radiographic progression
Cartilage metabolism	
MMP1 and 3	Radiographic damage
COMP	High levels in early RA associated with more severe disease in large and small joints
Aggrecan cleavage fragments	Slow-onset destructive disease in small and large joints
C-terminal/helical	Urinary levels associated with radiographic progression
Cross-linked	
CII peptides	
Bone metabolism	
Pyridinoline cross-links carboxy-terminal	Disease activity
CI telopeptides	Predictor of joint damage in early RA

RF, rheumatoid factor; CPA, citrullinated protein antigen; APF, anti-perinuclear factor; AKA, anti-keratin antibodies; VEGF, vascular endothelial growth factor; MMP, matrix metalloproteinase; COMP, cartilage oligomeric protein; CI/II, collagen type I/II.

relationship between joint inflammation and joint destruction, and the development of imaging technology that has documented evidence of erosive changes within the first 6–12 months of disease. The impact of this paradigm shift in therapeutic terms is striking. Traditional 'go-low, go-slow' regimens of the 1970s and 1980s included the initiation of nonsteroidal anti-inflammatory drugs (NSAIDs), followed by implementation of disease-modifying anti-rheumatic drugs only after destructive disease became evident. Depending on the clinical response, sequential monotherapy was the norm. Although this strategy may still be appropriate for patients with mild disease, current practice now dictates aggressive combination therapy (two or more conventional DMARDs) from the outset for patients with poor prognostic factors, with preference for the faster-acting DMARDs such as methotrexate, leflunomide and sulfasalazine (onset 3–6 weeks) over slower-acting agents, hydroxychloroquine, gold and D-penicillamine (onset 3–6 months), but with the addition of low-dose prednisolone (<10 mg/day). The rationale for combination therapy is far from clear and

has yet to be established in well-designed clinical trials, but could relate to the targeting of distinct pathogenic pathways by different agents, a strategy favored by oncologists for decades. Corticosteroids have a major place in clinical practice when administered as a single intramuscular injection, either as therapy for disease flares, as bridging therapy until DMARDs take effect, or when administered as an intra-articular injection to treat isolated joint synovitis. Some regimens favor high initial dose stepdown corticosteroid protocols. Regardless of the route of administration, evidence points to the value of corticosteroid use early in the disease process. Alternative DMARDs such as cyclosporine A, azathioprine and leflunomide are valuable adjuncts, but used less often as first-line therapy in some countries. Regardless of the specific agent, meta-analyses have demonstrated better response and retention rates when multiple DMARDs are used early. Adverse events are no more frequent with combination therapy. More recent data suggest that the specific choice of therapy may be less important than the strategy. For example, the TICORA and BeST studies[49, 50] both

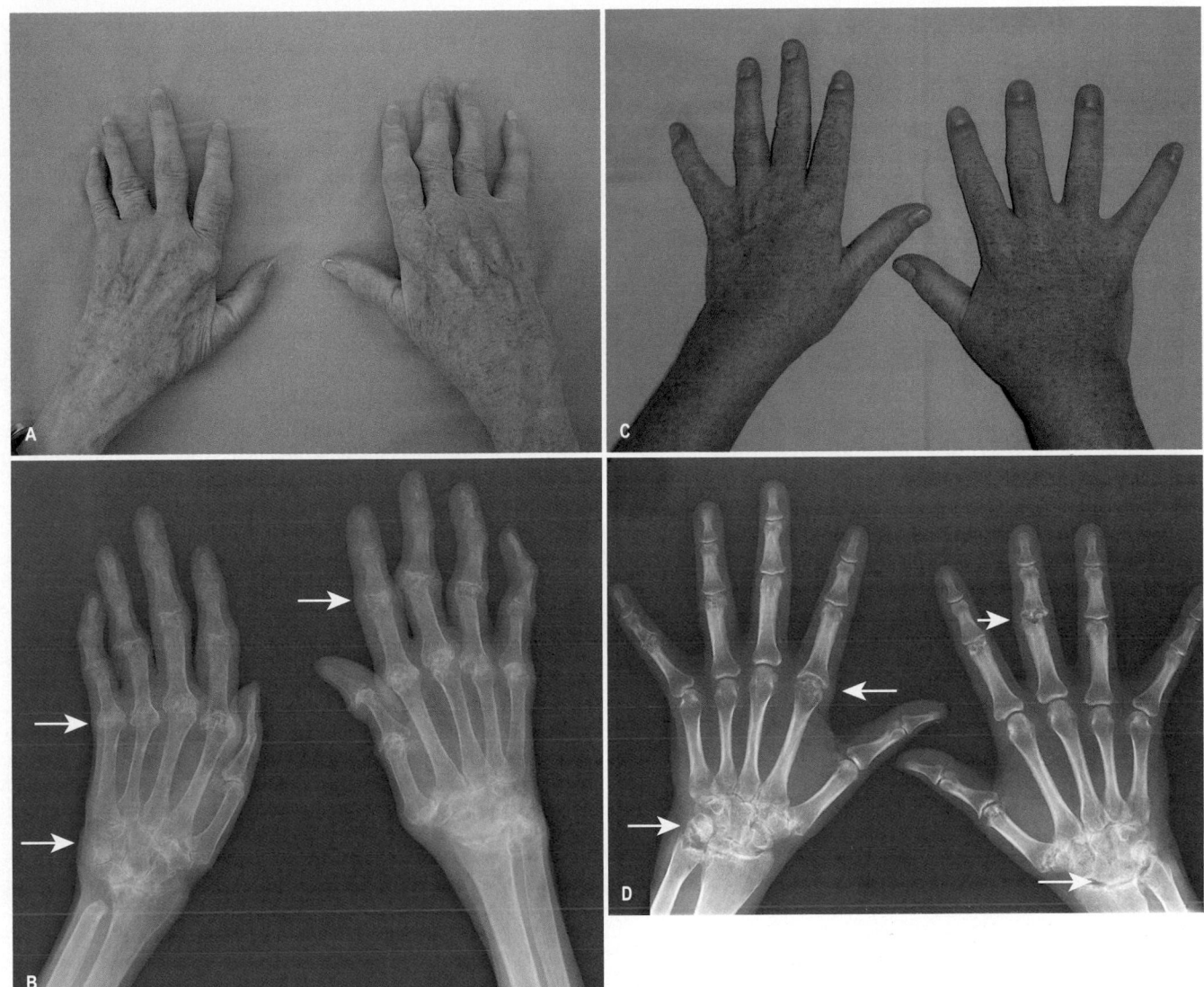

Fig. 52.5 The spectrum of disease severity in RA (**A** and **B**) Chronic, severe and erosive RA showing joint swelling and classic deformities. (**C** and **D**) Milder variant of RA in which bony erosions are detected by X-ray, but disfigurations and functional disabilities are much less pronounced. White arrows indicate major areas of bone and cartilage destruction. (Reproduced with the permission of the patients.)

indicate that intensive treatment combined with intensive control most convincingly influences outcome measures, including clinical response, retention, functional status and radiographic progression.

THE IMMUNOBIOLOGY OF DMARD THERAPY

The traditional paradigm of antigen-driven lymphocyte effector responses in RA promoted the application of a range of immunosuppressive drugs for treatment of the disease.[48] These contrast with more anti-inflammatory DMARDs, such as sulfasalazine (a scavenger of reactive oxygen intermediates with effects on prostanoid synthesis), gold (an inhibitor of AP-1 and NF-κB transcription factor DNA binding and/or transcriptional activity),

D-penicillamine (a modulator of sulfhydryl groups with effects on surface receptor function, intracellular signaling and transcription factor binding), antimalarials (which perturb lysosome acidification and intracellular trafficking), and low-dose corticosteroids (with anti-inflammatory actions related to *trans*-activation and *trans*-repression of inflammatory gene expression as well as effects on inflammatory gene mRNA stability). The best-characterized immunosuppressive agents include methotrexate (a dihydrofolate reductase inhibitor that targets T cells and the production of inflammatory cytokines as well as IL-2), azathioprine (whose active metabolite, 6-mercaptopurine, suppresses lymphocyte proliferative and cytokine responses as well as immunoglobulin synthesis), cyclosporine A (an inhibitor of the phosphatase calcineurin and NFAT transcriptional activity) and

THERAPEUTIC PRINCIPLES

TREATMENT PARADIGMS IN RA

>> Education and counselling through early involvement of multidisciplinary team, including a specialist nurse; appropriate balance of rest and exercise during disease flares

>> Adequate nutrition (especially important with severe, active disease)

>> Comprehensive assessment of disease activity, including imaging

>> Aim for complete suppression of inflammation early in disease, with tight control through regular and frequent reassessments

>> Early relief of pain with judicious use of NSAID or COX2 inhibitors according to safety/risk profile

>> Early use of DMARD/SAARDs

>> Early use of corticosteroids (e.g., low doses ~ 7.5 mg/day), including use of intra-articular injections to suppress inflammation

>> Use of stepup combination therapy in severe disease

>> Appropriate use of biologics, e.g., early use of anti-TNF in severe disease

>> Monitoring for drug toxicity

>> Effective contraception, where appropriate

>> Bone protection

>> Monitoring for risk factors of cardiovascular disease

>> Vaccination (preferably before instituting immunosuppressive agents)

NSAID, nonsteroidal anti-inflammatory drug; COX, cyclo-oxygenase; DMARD, disease-modifying anti-rheumatic drug; SAARD, slow acting antirheumatic drugs.

leflunomide (an inhibitor of dihydro-orotate dehydrogenase that affects a rate-limiting step in de novo pyrimidine synthesis that inhibits lymphocyte proliferative responses, which may favor Th2 differentiation). Somewhat paradoxically, most of these DMARDs may restore the cell-mediated immune response under circumstances where there is robust suppression of inflammation. On the other hand, significant changes in autoantibody titers, especially rheumatoid factor (RF), are less frequently observed.

THE IMMUNOBIOLOGY OF BIOLOGICAL THERAPY

Anti-cytokine therapy

The introduction to the clinic of targeted therapy using biological agents (e.g., chimeric or fully humanized antibodies to ligands or receptors, soluble receptor fusion proteins, or recombinant receptor antagonists) has transformed the treatment of RA. The prototype is TNF-α blockade.[51] The rationale for inhibiting TNF-α bioactivity is based upon its pleiotropic effects on cell activation, cellular adhesion and migration, induction of cytokine and inflammatory gene mRNA and protein, and the regulation

of cartilage catabolic factors such as IL-1 and matrix metalloproteinases (see Fig. 52.3). TNF-α and other inflammatory cytokines such as IL-1, IL-6, IL-15 and IL-17 are expressed constitutively in inflamed synovial tissue at mRNA and protein level. In many cases the expression of their high-affinity cognate receptors is upregulated and the functional activity of the corresponding naturally occurring inhibitors (e.g., soluble TNF-R or IL-1Ra) is reduced (although levels of protein may be increased, reflecting an attempt to restore homeostasis). As proof of principle, inhibition of cytokine activity, including that of TNF-α, IL-1, IL-6, IL-15 and IL-17, has been shown to have benefit in animal models of arthritis. Further, mice over-expressing hTNF-α as a transgene develop a spontaneous inflammatory destructive arthritis with 100% penetrance.

Chimeric anti-TNF monoclonal antibodies (infliximab; Remicade) were first used to treat RA in open-label clinical trials in 1992. Humanized antibodies (adalimumab; Humira) and the soluble p75 TNF-R IgG fusion protein (etanercept; Enbrel) were tested subsequently, with comparable therapeutic effects.[51–54] TNF-α blockade leads to dramatic and rapid reductions in the symptoms (pain, stiffness and fatigue) and signs (joint pain and swelling) of arthritis in a dose-dependent fashion, and in a significant proportion of patients (~ 60–70%) who have failed conventional DMARDs. These biological agents can be used repeatedly, and when used in combination with methotrexate are superior to either drug alone. The mechanism is not clear, but may be related to reductions in immunogenicity of the therapeutic antibody (i.e., the anti-chimeric antibody response), or perhaps the effects of combining anti-cytokine and anti-T-cell agents. Radiographic progression is attenuated over 2–3 years, even in subsets of patients with poor clinical responses, and in some patients radiographic scores improve, suggesting that healing of joint tissues may take place. TNF-α blockers when used early demonstrate superior remission rates. Some studies have shown that a significant proportion of patients remain in remission even after withdrawal of anti-TNF, possible evidence of immune modulation. The immunobiology of TNF-α in vivo, and its contribution to host defence, is further suggested by the increased incidence of upper respiratory tract, cutaneous and articular infections, and the significantly increased risk of reactivation of latent tuberculosis in patients treated with these agents. The risk of malignancy, particularly lymphoma, which is already increased in the RA population as a whole, does not appear to be increased with anti-TNF therapy. The development of antinuclear antibodies in 8–15% patients, as well as rare cases of demyelination, point to effects that may be related to restoration of immune responsiveness following TNF-α inhibition.

The clinical benefit of TNF-α blockade has prompted extensive mechanism of action studies which have been informative.[51] Anti-TNF reduces the acute-phase response, including IL-6 serum levels. Leukocyte trafficking is inhibited, as demonstrated through an early (within hours) and dramatic rise in lymphocyte counts through demargination, a more prolonged and sustained exclusion of leukocytes based on reductions in cellularity of synovial tissue biopsies after treatment and suppression of markers of angiogenesis, including VEGF. The effects of anti-TNF treatment on cell viability and apoptosis remain controversial, however. TNF-α blockade has also been shown to downregulate markers of cartilage and bone destruction, including the collagenases MMP1 and 3, and to reduce the ratio of RANKL and OPG in serum, effects that might partly explain the joint-preserving effects of anti-TNF in vivo. Finally, there is additional evidence of anti-TNF-induced immune homeostasis, based on restoration of cell-mediated immune responses to recall antigens and mitogens, but also an increase in both the numbers and function of $CD4^+CD25^{high}$ regulatory T cells, at least in some studies. This effect could be explained in part by the effect of TNF blockade on restoring the expression of the Treg-associated transcription factor FoxP3. Given that, at least in mice, IL-2 is a critical factor for maintaining Treg metabolic fitness, enhanced IL-2 production by effector T cells may contribute to immune homeostasis.

The IL-1 receptor antagonist (IL-1Ra) is the only IL-1 inhibitor currently licensed for use in RA.[55] It has good effects in animal models of arthritis, with potent joint protection, but has proved less effective in patients with RA compared to anti-TNF. Nevertheless, it has been used effectively to treat patients who have failed TNF-α blockade, and has been shown to slow radiographic progression. Blockade of IL-6 activity should be beneficial in RA because of the effects of IL-6 on the immune response, the acute-phase response, osteoclastogenesis, B-cell activation and immunoglobulin production, angiogenesis and cell adhesion. Indeed, anti-IL-6R has recently been proved in clinical trials to suppress the signs and symptoms of RA, with response rates comparable to those achieved with TNF blockade. However, the onset of disease suppression appears to be slower.

Anti-T-cell therapy

Although methotrexate, cyclosporine A and other immunosuppressive agents have claimed a place in the armamentarium for treating established RA, T cell-targeted therapeutic agents have been relatively disappointing as a group. Depleting anti-CD4 monoclonal antibodies were among the first specific agents to target this cell subset. Clinical efficacy was observed with responder rates consistently less than 30%, perhaps because of ineffective depletion of CD4 T cells in synovial joints, or because the antibody did not distinguish between T-cell effector and regulatory subsets. Theoretically, nondepleting anti-CD4 should be more effective, but this has yet to be confirmed in large phase III studies.

In contrast, the contribution of co-stimulatory signals ('signal 2') transduced through CD28 to priming and activation of naïve cells and amplification of cytokine gene expression and proliferative responses has provided a rationale for testing co-stimulatory blockade in patients. This has been achieved using a nondepleting humanized IgG1–CTLA4 fusion protein, which prevents CD80 and CD86 (B7 family members) from engaging CD28 (but also CTLA4) expressed on T cells. Initial studies confirmed that the agent was safe and well tolerated.[56] When administered as an intravenous infusion on days 1, 15 and 30, and then monthly thereafter, at a dose of 10 mg/kg combined with methotrexate, 60% of patients achieved ACR20 compared to 35.3% of controls; ACR50 responses were 36.5% versus 11.8%, respectively. CTLA4-Ig (licensed as Abatacept) has since been shown to inhibit radiographic progression and structural damage by ~50%, and is also effective in treating those patients who have had an inadequate response to TNF blockade as well as to methotrexate. From an immunological standpoint the data are interesting in several respects. First, the time to peak effect, which may take up to 1 year for some patients, is longer than for anti-TNF or anti-IL-6R therapy. This could reflect the presence of a significant number of co-stimulation-independent T cells (e.g., $CD4^+CD28^{null}$) involved in disease progression, or perhaps the cumulative impact of blocking the activation and differentiation of naïve T-cell precursors over time. Second, inhibition of CD28 signals does not block the development of regulatory T cells, as might have been predicted from mouse studies.

Anti-B-cell therapy

Rituximab is a humanized monoclonal antibody (IDEC-2B8) that recognizes human CD20, a 33–37 kDa membrane-associated phosphoprotein expressed on pre-B, immature and mature B cells but not plasma cells. Although CD20 ligation promotes B-cell activation, differentiation and cell cycle progression, its function is still poorly understood. The therapeutic effects of anti-CD20 are related to profound B-cell depletion due to antibody-dependent cell cytotoxicity, complement-mediated cell lysis, and/or triggering of intracellular pathways for apoptotic cell death.[57]

The initial open-label studies in RA patients combined rituximab with cyclophosphamide and steroids, and so the precise contribution of rituximab to the clinical response was unclear. A pivotal placebo-controlled trial of rituximab therapy randomized 161 patients with rheumatoid factor-positive RA and compared the efficacy and safety of methotrexate alone (standard therapy) versus methotrexate plus rituximab (1000 mg on days 1 and 15), rituximab alone, or rituximab plus cyclophosphamide.[58] All groups received a 17-day course of steroids, which may facilitate B-cell depletion. Up to 43% of patients receiving combination of rituximab with methotrexate achieved a 50% improvement in clinical and laboratory parameters after 24 weeks (based on American College of Rheumatology response criteria – the ACR50), and this was at least as good as the rituximab/cyclophosphamide combination (41% achieving ACR50) and superior to methotrexate (13%) or rituximab alone (33%). The overall incidence of infection was similar across treatment groups, but seven serious infections were reported in rituximab-treated patients.

Detailed analysis of this and subsequent studies in RA patients indicate that the B-cell depletion, which may depend on *FCGR3* allelic variants, is profound (< 2%), with no major differences in infection rates between groups, with the possible exception of lower respiratory tract infections. Repopulation occurs at a mean of 8 months after treatment, comprises immature $IgD^+CD38^+CD27^-CD5^+$ B cells, and is associated with increased serum BLyS levels. Early relapse is associated with reconstitution of $CD27^+$ memory B cells. The effects on serum immunoglobulin levels are modest, with levels remaining in the normal range. Selective and rapid decreases in pathogenic IgM, IgG and IgA rheumatoid factor (~ 60%) and IgG anti-CCP autoantibodies have been documented; these changes are more striking in rituximab responders. Antibody titers to tetanus toxoid or to pneumococcal capsular polysaccharides were only modestly affected (~ 25%). These changes are intriguing, given that terminally differentiated plasma cells do not express CD20. One possibility is that germinal center and marginal zone B cells may be resistant to anti-CD20. These encouraging results pave the way for testing alternative B cell-targeted therapies, of which anti-IL-6R should be included, but also LymphoStat-B (belimumab), TACI-Ig, and monoclonal antibody to BLyS/BAFF.

FUTURE PROSPECTS FOR THERAPY

There remain unmet needs in the treatment of RA. First among these must be the fact that for the majority of patients treatment is invariably lifelong, imposing a greater risk of toxicity and, as the immune system degenerates, an increased risk of infection or lymphoproliferative disease. There is little doubt that early treatment with tight control offers the best outcome. From an immunological perspective, there remains a pressing need to develop immunological tools or immune biomarkers that can redefine disease subsets and measure effector and regulatory cell subsets using technology readily accessible to routine clinical laboratories. Although such tools may provide a better insight into disease pathogenesis, they can also be adapted to monitor the impact of therapeutic intervention, whether this turns out to be cell-based therapy or the application of novel immune modulators.

■ REFERENCES ■

1. Snorrason E. Landré-Beauvais and his goutte asthénique primitive. Acta Med Scand 1952; 142: 115.

2. Harris ED. Rheumatoid arthritis; pathophysiology and implications for therapy. N Engl J Med 1990; 322: 1277.

3. Silman AJ, Hochberg MC. Epidemiology of rheumatic diseases. Oxford: Oxford University Press, 1993.

4. Silman AJ, MacGregor AJ, Thomson W, et al. Twin concordance rates for rheumatoid arthritis: results from a nationwide study. Br J Rheumatol 1993; 32: 903.

5. MacGregor AJ, Snieder H, Rigby AS, et al. Characterizing the quantitative genetic contribution to rheumatoid arthritis using data from twins. Arthritis Rheum 2000; 43: 30.

6. Weyand CM, Goronzy JJ. Stem cell aging and autoimmunity in rheumatoid arthritis. Trends Mol Med 2004; 9: 426.

7. Spector TD, Roman E, Silman AJ. The pill, parity, and rheumatoid arthritis. Arthritis Rheum 1990; 33: 782.

8. Karlson EW, Lee IM, Cook NR, et al. A retrospective cohort study of cigarette smoking and risk of rheumatoid arthritis in female health professionals. Arthritis Rheum 1999; 42: 910.

9. Padyukov L, Silva C, Stolt P, et al. A gene–environment interaction between smoking and shared epitope genes in HLA-DR provides a high risk of seropositive rheumatoid arthritis. Arthritis Rheum 2004; 50: 3085.

10. Carty SM, Snowden N, Silman AJ. Should infection still be considered as the most likely triggering factor for rheumatoid arthritis?. Ann Rheum Dis 2004; 63: 46.

11. van Eden W, van der Zee R, Prakken B. Heat-shock proteins induce T-cell regulation of chronic inflammation. Nature Rev Immunol 2005; 5: 318.

12. Gregersen PK. Pathways to gene identification in rheumatoid arthritis: PTPN22 and beyond. Immunol Rev 2005; 204: 74.

13. Gregersen PK, Silver J, Winchester RJ. The shared epitope hypothesis. An approach to understanding the molecular genetics of susceptibility to rheumatoid arthritis. Arthritis Rheum 1987; 30: 1205.

14. van der Helm-van Mil AH, Huizinga TW, Schreuder GM, et al. An independent role of protective HLA class II alleles in rheumatoid arthritis severity and susceptibility. Arthritis Rheum 2005; 52: 2637.

15. Weyand CM, McCarthy TG, Goronzy JJ. Correlation between disease phenotype and genetic heterogeneity in rheumatoid arthritis. J Clin Invest 1995; 95: 2120.

16. Nepom GT. Major histocompatibility complex-directed susceptibility to rheumatoid arthritis. Adv Immunol 1998; 68: 315.

17. Huizinga TW, Amos CI, van der Helm-van Mil AH, et al. Refining the complex rheumatoid arthritis phenotype based on specificity of the HLA-DRB1 shared epitope for antibodies to citrullinated proteins. Arthritis Rheum 2005; 52: 3433.

18. Bresnihan B, Tak PP. Synovial tissue analysis in rheumatoid arthritis. Baillières Best Pract Res Clin Rheumatol 1999; 13: 645.

19. Haskard DO. Cell adhesion molecules in rheumatoid arthritis. Curr Opin Rheumatol 1995; 7: 229.

20. Taylor PC, Sivakumar B. Hypoxia and angiogenesis in rheumatoid arthritis. Curr Opin Rheumatol 2005; 17: 293.

21. Zhang X, Nakajima T, Goronzy JJ, Weyand CM. Tissue trafficking patterns of effector memory CD4+ T cells in rheumatoid arthritis. Arthritis Rheum 2005; 52: 3839.

22. Goronzy JJ, Weyand CM. Rheumatoid arthritis. Immunol Rev 2005; 204: 55.

23. van der Pouw Kraan TC, van Gaalen FA, Kasperkovitz PV, et al. Rheumatoid arthritis is a heterogeneous disease: evidence for differences in the activation of the STAT-1 pathway between rheumatoid tissues. Arthritis Rheum 2003; 48: 2132.

24. Firestein GS. Evolving concepts of rheumatoid arthritis. Nature 2003; 423: 356.

25. Drexler SK, Sacre S, Foxwell BM. Toll-like receptors: a new target in rheumatoid arthritis?. Expert Rev Clin Immunol 2006; 2: 585–599.

26. Pettit AR, Thomas R. Dendritic cells: the driving force behind autoimmunity in rheumatoid arthritis? Immunol Cell Biol 1999; 77: 420.

27. Szekanecz Z, Kim J, Koch AE. Chemokines and chemokine receptors in rheumatoid arthritis. Semin Immunol 2003; 15: 15.

28. Holmdahl R, Andersson M, Goldschmidt TJ, et al. Type II collagen autoimmunity in animals and provocations leading to arthritis. Immunol Rev 1990; 118: 193.

29. van Venrooij WJ, Vossenaar ER, Zendman AJ. Anti-CCP antibodies: the new rheumatoid factor in the serology of rheumatoid arthritis. Autoimmun Rev 2004; 3: S17–19.

30. Klareskog L, Stolt P, Lundberg K, et al. A new model for an etiology of rheumatoid arthritis: smoking may trigger HLA-DR (shared epitope)-restricted immune reactions to autoantigens modified by citrullination. Arthritis Rheum 2006; 54: 38.

31. Cush JJ, Lipsky PE. Phenotypic analysis of synovial tissue and peripheral blood lymphocytes isolated from patients with rheumatoid arthritis. Arthritis Rheum 1988; 31: 1230.

32. Salmon M, Scheel-Toellner D, Huissoon AP, et al. Inhibition of T cell apoptosis in the rheumatoid synovium. J Clin Invest 1997; 99: 439.

33. Cope AP. Studies of T-cell activation in chronic inflammation. Arthritis Res 2002; 4: S197.

34. Parsonage G, Filer AD, Haworth O, et al. A stromal address code defined by fibroblasts. Trends Immunol 2005; 26: 150.

35. Takemura S, Braun A, Crowson C, et al. Lymphoid neogenesis in rheumatoid synovitis. J Immunol 2001; 167: 1072.

36. Takemura S, Klimiuk PA, Braun A, et al. T cell activation in rheumatoid synovium is B cell dependent. J Immunol 2001; 167: 4710.

37. Winchester RJ. Characterization of IgG complexes in patients with rheumatoid arthritis. Ann NY Acad Sci 1975; 256: 73.

38. Feldmann M, Brennan FM, Maini RN. Role of cytokines in rheumatoid arthritis. Annu Rev Immunol 1996; 14: 397.

39. Sakaguchi S, Sakaguchi N. Animal models of arthritis caused by systemic alteration of the immune system. Curr Opin Immunol 2005; 17: 589.

40. Dayer JM, Burger D. Cell-cell interactions and tissue damage in rheumatoid arthritis. Autoimmun Rev 2004; 3: S14.

41. Leipe J, Skapenko A, Lipsky PE, Schulze-Koops H. Regulatory T cells in rheumatoid arthritis. Arthritis Res Ther 2005; 7: 93.

42. Ehrenstein MR, Evans JG, Singh A, et al. Compromised function of regulatory T cells in rheumatoid arthritis and reversal by anti-TNF-alpha therapy. J Exp Med 2004; 200: 277.

43. Valencia X, Stephens G, Goldbach-Mansky R, et al. TNF downmodulates the function of human CD4+CD25hi T-regulatory cells. Blood 2006; 108: 253.

44. Schett G, Hayer S, Zwerina J, et al. Mechanisms of disease: the link between RANKL and arthritic bone disease. Nature Clin Pract Rheumatol 2005; 1: 47.

45. Theill LE, Boyle WJ, Penninger JM. RANK-L and RANK: T cells, bone loss, and mammalian evolution. Annu Rev Immunol 2002; 20: 795.

45a. Wolfe F, Cathey MA. The assessment and prediction of functional disability in rheumatoid arthritis. J Rheumatol 1991; 18: 1298–1306.

46. Arnett FC, Edworthy SM, Bloch DA, et al. The American Rheumatism Association 1987 revised criteria for the classification of rheumatoid arthritis. Arthritis Rheum 1988; 31: 315.

47. Shmerling RH, Delbanco TL. The rheumatoid factor: an analysis of clinical utility. Am J Med 1991; 91: 528.

48. Lee DM, Weinblatt ME. Rheumatoid arthritis. Lancet 2001; 358: 903.

49. Grigor C, Capell H, Stirling A, et al. Effect of a treatment strategy of tight control for rheumatoid arthritis (the TICORA study): a single-blind randomised controlled trial. Lancet 2004; 364: 263.

50. Goekoop-Ruiterman YP, de Vries-Bouwstra JK, Allaart CF, et al. Clinical and radiographic outcomes of four different treatment strategies in patients with early rheumatoid arthritis (the BeSt study): a randomized, controlled trial. Arthritis Rheum 2005; 52: 3381.

51. Feldmann M, Maini RN. Anti-TNF alpha therapy of rheumatoid arthritis: what have we learned?. Annu Rev Immunol 2001; 19: 163.

52. Lipsky PE, van der Heijde DM, St Clair EW, et al. Anti-Tumor Necrosis Factor Trial in Rheumatoid Arthritis with Concomitant Therapy Study Group. Infliximab and methotrexate in the treatment of rheumatoid arthritis. N Engl J Med 2000; 343: 1594.

53. Bathon JM, Martin RW, Fleischmann RM, et al. A comparison of etanercept and methotrexate in patients with early rheumatoid arthritis. N Engl J Med 2000; 343: 1586.

54. Klareskog L, van der Heijde D, de Jager JP, et al. TEMPO (Trial of Etanercept and Methotrexate with Radiographic Patient Outcomes) Study Investigators. Therapeutic effect of the combination of etanercept and methotrexate compared with each treatment alone in patients with rheumatoid arthritis: double-blind randomised controlled trial. Lancet 2004; 363: 675.

55. Jiang Y, Genant HK, Watt I, et al. A multicenter, double-blind, dose-ranging, randomized, placebo-controlled study of recombinant human interleukin-1 receptor antagonist in patients with rheumatoid arthritis: radiologic progression and correlation of Genant and Larsen scores. Arthritis Rheum 2000; 43: 1001.

56. Kremer JM, Westhovens R, Leon M, et al. Treatment of rheumatoid arthritis by selective inhibition of T-cell activation with fusion protein CTLA4Ig. N Engl J Med 2003; 349: 1907.

57. Edwards JC, Cambridge G. B-cell targeting in rheumatoid arthritis and other autoimmune diseases. Nature Rev Immunol 2006; 6: 394.

58. Edwards JC, Szczepanski L, Szechinski J, et al. Efficacy of B-cell-targeted therapy with rituximab in patients with rheumatoid arthritis. N Engl J Med 2004; 350: 2572.

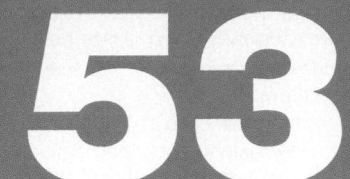

Juvenile idiopathic arthritis

Angelo Ravelli, Alberto Martini

53

The term juvenile idiopathic arthritis (JIA) includes all forms of arthritis which begin before the 16th birthday, persist for more than 6 weeks, and for which no cause is known.[1,2] Therefore, there is no clinical or laboratory feature that is pathognomonic of JIA which represents an exclusion diagnosis that gathers together all forms of childhood chronic arthritis of unknown cause.

Over the years this heterogeneous material has been analyzed using different classification criteria in order to identify discrete clinical subsets that could correspond to different diseases. In the 1970s two classification systems were created: one in the USA (the juvenile rheumatoid arthritis (JRA) criteria) and one in Europe (the juvenile chronic arthritis (JCA) criteria). Although similar, these two classifications had a number of important differences that have prevented interchangeable use and comparative research. To try to overcome these problems, about 10 years ago, the International League of Associations for Rheumatology (ILAR) created a new classification system that could be transatlantically shared.[3] This classification, in which the term JIA has been chosen instead of JRA or JCA, has the great merit of having unified classification criteria and terminology on the basis of current knowledge and represents a useful tool for international research. However, it still requires validation and consensus, has the limits inherent to any classification based on clinical criteria, and will probably be modified as new information on pathogenesis becomes available.[4]

For sake of simplicity, in the present chapter the term JIA will be used, even when studies performed using the JRA or JCA classification systems are quoted.

EPIDEMIOLOGY

Studies in American and northern European populations have reported an incidence and prevalence of JIA varying from 2 to 20 and from 16 to 150 per 100 000 respectively. Marked differences have been noted in the incidence of JIA subtypes according to geographical areas or ethnicity. In western countries the most common subtype is oligoarthritis; this subtype is rare in Costa Rica, India, New Zealand, and South Africa, where polyarthritis predominates.[1,2]

JIA SUBTYPES

In order to be classified as JIA, arthritis must begin before the 16th birthday, persist for more than 6 weeks, and be of unknown origin. In the ILAR classification[3] the various subtypes are identified by a definition and several exclusion items (Table 53.1) on the basis of the features presented in the first 6 months of disease.

SYSTEMIC ARTHRITIS

Systemic arthritis[1,2] is quite distinct from the other JIA subtypes (Table 53.1). Although all subtypes share as a common feature the presence of arthritis and the risk of joint damage, systemic arthritis is also characterized by prominent systemic manifestations. The disease occurs as often in boys as in girls, does not show a preferential age at onset, and represents about 10% of all JIA cases. It can also occur in adults where it is known as 'adult-onset Still's disease.'

The hallmark is a high spiking daily fever greater than 39°C. Another characteristic feature is an evanescent, nonfixed, erythematous rash that typically occurs with fever peaks but may be produced by scratching (Koebner phenomenon); sometimes it can be urticaria-like and quite pruritic (Fig. 53.1). Hepatomegaly, splenomegaly, and generalized

KEY CONCEPTS

>> Juvenile idiopathic arthritis (JIA) is not a single disease but includes a number of different conditions: some of these are not observed in adults whereas others are much more frequent in children than in adults or vice versa. Appropriate therapy and monitoring require a proper subtype diagnosis

>> There are no laboratory or radiological features that are pathognomonic of JIA. The diagnosis is clinical and is based on meeting clinical criteria as well as excluding other diseases that cause chronic arthritis

Table 53.1 The International League of Associations for Rheumatology classification of juvenile idiopathic arthritis (JIA) (second revision)[3]

Systemic arthritis

Arthritis with, or preceded by, daily fever of at least 2 weeks' duration, that is documented to be quotidian for at least 3 days, and accompanied by one or more of the following:

1. Evanescent, nonfixed, erythematous rash
2. Generalized lymph node enlargement
3. Hepatomegaly and/or splenomegaly
4. Serositis

Exclusions: a, b, c, d (see below)

Oligoarthritis

Arthritis affecting 1–4 joints during the first 6 months of disease. Two subcategories are recognized:

1. Persistent oligoarthritis: affects no more than four joints throughout the disease course
2. Extended oligoarthritis: affects a total of more than four joints after the first 6 months of disease

Exclusions: a, b, c, d, e (see below)

Polyarthritis (rheumatoid factor-negative)

Arthritis affecting five or more joints during the first 6 months of disease: tests for rheumatoid factor are negative

Exclusions: a, b, c, d, e (see below)

Polyarthritis (rheumatoid factor-positive)

Arthritis affecting five or more joints during the first 6 months of disease: tests for rheumatoid factor are positive

Exclusions: a, b, c, e (see below)

Psoriatic arthritis

1. Arthritis and psoriasis *or*
2. Arthritis and at least two of the following:
   a. Dactylitis
   b. Nail pitting or onycholysis
   c. Psoriasis in a first-degree relative

Exclusions: b, c, d, e (see below)

Enthesitis-related arthritis

1. Arthritis and enthesitis
2. Arthritis or enthesitis with at least two of the following:
   a. Sacroiliac joint tenderness and/or inflammatory lumbosacral pain
   b. Presence of human leukocyte antigen (HLA) B27
   c. Onset of arthritis in a male after age 6 years
   d. Ankylosing spondylitis, enthesitis-related arthritis, sacroiliitis with inflammatory bowel disease, Reiter's syndrome or acute anterior uveitis in a first-degree relative

Exclusions: a, d, e (see below)

Undifferentiated arthritis

Arthritis that does not fulfill inclusion criteria for any category, or is excluded by fulfilling criteria for more than one category

Exclusion criteria for the classification of JIA

a. Psoriasis in the patient or a first-degree relative
b. Arthritis in an HLA B27-positive male with arthritis onset after 6 years of age
c. Ankylosing spondylitis, enthesitis-related arthritis, sacroiliitis with inflammatory bowel disease, Reiter's syndrome, acute anterior uveitis in a first-degree relative
d. Presence of immunoglobulin M rheumatoid factor on at least two occasions more than 3 months apart
e. Presence of systemic arthritis

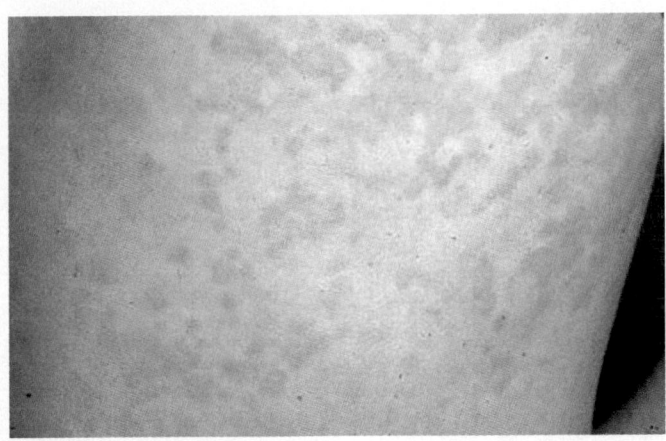

Fig. 53.1 Rash associated with systemic arthritis. This evanescent, nonfixed, salmon-colored rash typically occurs with fever peaks; it may resemble urticaria and be quite pruritic.

lymph node enlargement are found in a sizable number of patients but are usually mild. Pericarditis or pleuritis occurs in a minority of patients and is more often mild and asymptomatic. Cardiorespiratory distress due to myocarditis or cardiac tamponade is very unusual.

Myalgias and abdominal pain may be intense during fever peaks. Arthritis is more often symmetrical and polyarticular. It may be absent at onset in about 30% of cases and develops during disease course.

Laboratory examinations show leukocytosis (with neutrophilia), very high erythrocyte sedimentation rate (ESR) values, and marked thrombocytosis. Anemia, sometimes profound, is common and microcytic. Different from the anemia of chronic disease observed in adult rheumatoid arthritis (RA), it appears mostly related to interleukin-6 (IL-6)-induced iron sequestration in the reticuloendothelial system.[5,6]

About 5–8% of patients with systemic arthritis may develop a life-threatening complication called macrophage activation syndrome (MAS).[1,2] MAS may follows an intercurrent viral illness or a change in medication. The syndrome includes a persistent (instead of spiking) high fever, pancytopenia, hepatosplenomegaly, liver insufficiency, coagulopathy with hemorrhagic manifestations, and neurologic symptoms. Laboratory features include elevated triglycerides and lactic dehydrogenase, low sodium levels, and markedly increased ferritin concentrations. The demonstration of active phagocytosis of hematopoietic cells by macrophage in the bone marrow is common. The syndrome is a life-threatening complication and has to be promptly recognized and treated.

OLIGOARTHRITIS

Oligoarthritis is defined on the presence of arthritis affecting one to four joints during the first 6 months of disease and the exclusion of other JIA subtypes which may present with arthritis in only a small number of joints (Table 53.1).

Although oligoarthritis as a whole is probably heterogeneous, by far the largest group of patients belongs to a quite well-defined form of

JIA.[1,2] This form, which is not observed in adults, is characterized by an asymmetric arthritis, early onset (before 6 years of age), female predilection, high frequency of positive antinuclear antibodies (ANA), and high risk for developing chronic anterior uveitis. In support of the concept that these patients represent a homogeneous entity, a strong association with selected HLA alleles has been found (see section on genetic contribution, below). In Europe and the USA oligoarthritis represents about 50% of all forms of JIA whereas, as mentioned above, it is rare in other countries such as Costa Rica, India, New Zealand, and South Africa.[1,2]

The knee is the most commonly affected joint, followed by the ankle. Other joints are affected less frequently. In about 30–50% of cases a single joint is involved at presentation. Joints are obviously swollen but in general not particularly painful, although joint contractures are frequent.

Acute-phase reactants are usually normal or moderately increased, although in some instances ESR may be quite high. ANA are detected in significant titers in about 70–80% of patients and represent a risk factor for the development of anterior uveitis.

The ILAR classification distinguishes two categories in the oligoarthritis subtype: *persistent oligoarthritis*, in which the disease remains confined to four joints or fewer and *extended oligoarthritis*, in which arthritis extends to more than four joints after the first 6 months of disease. In our opinion most of the patients classified as having either persistent or extended oligoarthritis belong to the same clinical entity.[4] Indeed, the clinical characteristics of ANA-positive patients belonging to these two categories have been found to be homogeneous with respect to age at onset, sex ratio, asymmetry of articular involvement, and frequency of uveitis.[7] This suggests that extended oligoarthritis is the same disease as persistent oligoarthritis but with a more severe outcome. The involvement of an upper limb and higher sedimentation rate at onset have been suggested as predictors for an evolution to the extended phenotype, which occurs in up to 50% of patients.[8]

Uveitis

A chronic, asymptomatic, nongranulomatous, anterior uveitis affecting the iris and the ciliary body (iridocyclitis) that can cause severe visual impairment is a characteristic feature of oligoarthritis and affects about 30% of patients.[1,2] The onset is insidious and often entirely asymptomatic, in contrast with the painful acute uveitis that can be observed in enthesitis-related arthritis. One or both eyes may be involved. In fewer than 10% of patients uveitis is detected before the onset of arthritis and in about half of patients it occurs at the time of JIA diagnosis or shortly thereafter. Most children who develop uveitis do it within 5–7 years from the onset of arthritis. The course of uveitis may be relapsing or chronic and does not parallel the clinical course of arthritis. ANA-positive patients are at higher risk.

Uveitis can occur in other JIA subtypes such as rheumatoid factor (RF)-negative polyarthritis or psoriatic arthritis, especially if ANA-positive. As discussed later, there is evidence suggesting that ANA-positive patients represent a single disease entity, currently classified into different categories. Since uveitis is asymptomatic, children with JIA should be screened periodically by slit-lamp examination. Any patient with oligoarthritis or polyarthritis of early onset or, in general, with ANA-positive, RF-negative JIA should undergo slit-lamp examination at least every 3 months.

CLINICAL PEARLS

>> *Uveitis in Juvenile idiopathic arthritis (Jia)*

>> Chronic anterior uveitis is a complication of JIA and can lead to blindness. It is mainly observed in oligoarthritis; antinuclear antibody positivity represents a risk factor. Since the onset is asymptomatic, patients at risk must undergo frequent ophthalmologic examinations. Early recognition and therapy are essential for prognosis

>> *Macrophage activation syndrome*

>> Macrophage activation syndrome is a life-threatening complication of systemic arthritis and requires prompt recognition. It shares many similarities with the other forms of hemophagocytic lymphohistiocytosis

RHEUMATOID FACTOR-POSITIVE POLYARTHRITIS

RF-positive polyarthritis is defined as an arthritis that affects five or more joints during the first 6 months of disease in patients who test positive for immunoglobulin M (IgM) rheumatoid factor (Table 53.1). It represents a small minority (< 5%) of all cases of JIA. It is the same disease as adult RF-positive RA[1, 2] and is usually observed in adolescent girls. Differences with respect to adults are related to the impact of the disease in a young person or in a child who is still growing.

RHEUMATOID FACTOR-NEGATIVE POLYARTHRITIS

RF-negative polyarthritis is defined as an arthritis that affects five or more joints during the first 6 months of disease in the absence of IgM RF (Table 53.1). It accounts for about 15–20% of all JIA cases and is the least defined and probably the most heterogeneous JIA subtype.[1, 2] At least three distinct subsets can be identified from a clinical point of view.

Early-onset, ANA-positive polyarthritis

This form affects about one-third of patients and is characterized by the following common features: polyarthritis, asymmetric at the onset, affecting both large and small joints, and with onset before 6 years of age; ANA positivity; female predominance; and an elevated risk of developing chronic anterior uveitis. In this group of patients (see genetic contribution, below) a higher prevalence of human leukocyte antigen (HLA)-DRB1*0801 has been observed. All these features, including the HLA association, are identical to those observed in the majority of patients with oligoarthritis.[4] This view has been supported by the demonstration that ANA-positive oligoarthritis shares homogeneous clinical features with ANA-positive RF-negative polyarthritis but not with ANA-negative RF-negative polyarthritis.[7] The hypothesis that ANA-positive RF-negative polyarthritis and ANA-positive oligoarthritis are the same disease is also strongly supported by studies on the frequency of the various JIA subsets in different ethnic populations. Indeed, in those countries in which ANA-positive, early-onset, iridocyclitis-associated oligoarthritis is rare, ANA-positive, early-onset, iridocyclitis-associated RF-negative polyarthritis is also seldomly observed.[4]

Prolific symmetric synovitis

This is the more classic form of RF-negative polyarthritis.[1, 2] Joint involvement is symmetric and affects large joints as well as the small joints of hands and feet. ESR is often elevated and ANA are usually negative. Age at onset is about 7–9 years. The relation between this form of arthritis and the RF-negative form that represent 25% of all forms of adult RA is unknown, since no reliable markers exist for both conditions.

Dry sinovitis

A subgroup of patients with polyarticular RF-negative arthritis show little palpable synovial thickening but gradually contract up in a manner which later leads to marked loss of function.[1, 2] They tend to be about 7 or 8 years of age at presentation. There is usually little pain in the affected joints. The disease often follows a destructive course and is poorly responsive to common treatments. ESR in these patients is often normal or only modestly raised and ANA are negative. This type of RF-negative polyarthritis is uncommon; the peculiarities of its clinical picture suggest that it may include patients affected by some yet unknown genetic disease.

PSORIATIC ARTHRITIS

Psoriatic arthritis is defined by the presence of arthritis plus psoriasis or some psoriatic features (Table 53.1)[1, 2] and represents about 5% of all cases of JIA, although estimates of its prevalence are very variable. It is our opinion that this subtype does not represent a clearly defined entity.[4] Most patients who meet the ILAR criteria for psoriatic arthritis, in which patients with enthesitis are by definition excluded, have an early onset, an asymmetric oligoarthritis, are at risk for the development of iridocyclitis, and are frequently ANA-positive. All these characteristics are very similar to those observed in children with oligoarthritis. The main difference is that patients with psoriatic arthritis have a higher frequency of dactylitis and both small and large joints are involved. In previous studies on children with psoriasis and arthritis in which patients with enthesitis were not excluded, a proportion of patients presented with arthritis and enthesitis or developed sacroiliitis during follow-up, similarly to a sizable proportion of adult patients with psoriatic arthritis who share features with spondyloarthropathies.[1, 2] So it appears that the association of psoriasis with arthritis does not define a unique entity.

ENTHESITIS-RELATED ARTHRITIS

This form of arthritis accounts for about 10% of JIA cases and mainly affects males after the age of 6 years.[1, 2] It is characterized by the association of enthesitis and arthritis. Most patients are HLA-B27-positive. Enthesitis usually occurs around the foot and knees. The most common sites are the calcaneal insertions of the Achilles tendon or plantar fascia and the plantar fascia attachments to the metatarsal heads. Arthritis commonly affects the joints of the lower extremities. At variance with the other JIA subtypes, hip involvement is common at disease presentation. The disease is often remitting and may be mild. About half of patients have four joints or fewer affected during the entire course of the disease. A variable percentage progressively develop involvement of the axial skeleton.

Although characterized by increased extra-axial symptoms compared to adults, enthesitis-related arthritis belongs to the group of spondyloarthropathies. It can be viewed as an umbrella term that encompasses children with juvenile ankylosing spondylitis (who fulfill the criteria for adult ankylosing spondylitis) and with undifferentiated spondyloarthritides, including those with the formerly called seronegative enthesitis and arthritis syndrome.[1, 2] ILAR criteria for the enthesitis-related arthritis category have been criticized because they do not consider psoriatic arthritis and reactive arthritis to be part of the juvenile spondyloarthritides and limit arthritis of inflammatory bowel disease to being only a descriptor of the disease.

UNDIFFERENTIATED ARTHRITIS

Undifferentiated arthritis does not represent a separate subset, but identifies patients who do not fulfill inclusion criteria for any category, or who are excluded by fulfilling criteria for more than one category.

■ ETIOLOGY AND PATHOGENESIS ■

The etiopathogenesis of JIA is still poorly understood. Moreover, the heterogeneity of JIA implies that multiple etiopathogenetic factors are involved.

As previously mentioned, RF-positive polyarticular JIA is considered the childhood equivalent of adult RF-positive RA. Enthesitis-associated arthritis, although characterized by increased extra-axial symptoms and modest sacroiliitis compared to adults, appears to belong pathogenetically to the spondyloarthropathies. Psoriatic arthritis is still a poorly defined condition in children and no reliable specific pathogenic studies have been performed in childhood.

GENETIC CONTRIBUTION

The attempt to define the genetic components of juvenile arthritis has been hampered by disease heterogeneity and classification problems. In addition, small numbers of patients have reduced the power of the studies. Despite these difficulties, it is clear that many diseases classified under the term JIA have a genetic component.[9]

Twin and affected siblings pairs studies

Data on disease concordance in identical twins are scanty. A Finnish study of JIA multicase families identified eight sets of monozygotic twins, two of whom were concordant for arthritis, giving a concordance rate of 25%. In the large US registry for JRA affected sibling pairs (ASPs), of 14 pairs of twins, 13 were concordant for disease onset (10 oligoarticular, 3 polyarticular).[10]

λ_s is calculated as the prevalence of the disease in siblings of affected individuals divided by the prevalence of the disease in the general population. Using the large US registry for JRA ASPs, the λ_s for juvenile arthritis has been estimated to be ~15; the HLA-DR accounted for ~17% of the risk for juvenile arthritis.[9, 10] The most common onset type among 164 nontwin ASPs was oligoarticular (65% overall), supporting the concept that the shared genetic makeup between siblings plays a role in determining this onset type in particular.[11] The systemic-onset subtype did not show a high concordance rate and involved a small number of ASPs, suggesting a weak genetic component for this subtype.

HLA associations

Many associations between JIA subsets and HLA molecules have been described and some of these have been confirmed in several studies.[1, 2, 9, 10]

Oligoarticular JIA has been consistently associated with HLA antigens. Positive associations include HLA-A2, HLA-DRB1*11 (a subtype of HLA-DR5), and HLA-DRB1*08. In contrast, HLA-DRB1*04 and HLA-DRB1*07 have been found to be significantly decreased. These associations are particularly significant in children with oligoarthritis and an early disease onset and have been confirmed with linkage analysis in ASPs.

RF-positive JIA is considered to be the childhood equivalent of adult RF-positive RA and, as in adults, is associated with HLA-DR4.

RF-negative polyarthritis is a heterogeneous condition and indeed HLA associations are not well defined. Interestingly, several groups have reported an increase in HLA-DR8, especially in RF-negative polyarticular patients with early age at onset, ANA positivity, and presence of iridocyclitis, supporting the view that this subset of polyarticular seronegative JIA and early-onset oligoarthritis are the same disease.[4]

Like adult spondyloarthritides, enthesitis-related arthritis has a strong association with HLA-B27. Systemic JIA (sJIA) has shown a poor association with HLA antigens.

Non-HLA associations

The non-HLA association in JIA have been less reproducible.[10, 12] They included T-cell receptor variable genes, the proteasome LMP2 gene (LMP2BB), the transporters associated with antigen-processing genes (TAP1 and TAP2), the major histocompatibility complex (MHC) class I chain-related (MIC) A gene, neuroendocrine genes, the PTPN22 gene, osteopontin, and several cytokine genes (interferon (IFN)-regulatory factor 1, IL-1α, TNF-α, IL-10, IL-6, and macrophage inhibitory factor (MIF)).

A single nucleotide polymorphism (SNP) (-174) in the regulatory region of the IL-6 gene that determines transcriptional response of the IL-6 gene to IL-1 and lipopolysaccharide has been associated with sJIA.[13] A polymorphism in the '5 flanking region (-173) of MIF has been found to be associated with JIA.[14] This polymorphism results in higher endogenous MIF production in the serum of healthy individuals and in higher MIF production in both the serum and synovial fluids of JIA cases. Moreover, in patients with sJIA, the carriage of this MIF polymorphism has been found to be correlated with worse long-term functional outcome.[15] An SNP in the protein tyrosine phosphatase N22 (PTPN22) gene, an apparent negative regulator of T-lymphocyte activation, has been associated with various autoimmune diseases, including JIA.[16] The results of the first genome-wide scan performed in 121 families containing 247 children with juvenile arthritis classified according to the JRA criteria have been published. The data support the hypothesis that multiple genes, including at least one in the HLA region, influence susceptibility to JRA, which is consistent with findings in other autoimmune diseases.[17]

ENVIRONMENTAL FACTORS

The hypothesis that an infection triggers the disease in genetically susceptible individuals, although attractive, remains unproven.[1, 2] It is suggested by similarities with infection-induced arthritides such as Lyme arthritis, reactive arthritis, and parvovirus B19 and rubella virus-induced arthritis. The early age at onset characteristic of oligoarthritis suggests that the disease may be secondary to an altered immunological response to common infectious agents that are encountered very early in life. It has also been suggested that the genetic association of oligoarticular JIA with HLA-DR alleles could be explained by mimicry with peptides from virus antigens such as Epstein–Barr virus.[18]

IMMUNE ABNORMALITIES

A large number of immunological abnormalities have been reported in JIA.[1, 2] Many are similar to those reported in adult RA and will be briefly summarized. Others are related to aspects that are more specific to JIA and will be described in more detail.

Autoantibodies

IgM RF is observed in RF polyarticular JIA, the childhood equivalent of adult RF-positive RA. Similarly, anti-cyclic citrullinated peptide antibodies are found in children with RF polyarticular JIA but not in other JIA subsets.[1, 2] Children with the other JIA subtypes can produce other types of RF, including "hidden RF" which are undetectable by traditional assays because they are bound to autologous IgG[1]; however, the significance of these other antiglobulins is uncertain.

ANA, mainly associated with oligoarthritis, have been found to react against different chromatin constituents and against the DEK nuclear protein, a putative oncoprotein; however, none of these molecular targets is specific for oligoarticular JIA.[1]

Synovitis

The inflammatory synovitis in JIA is similar to that observed in adult RA and does not appear to differ significantly among the different JIA subtypes.[1, 2] The synovium shows marked hyperplasia of the lining layer and an exuberant infiltration of the sub-lining layer with mononuclear cells, including T cells, B cells, macrophages, dendritic cells, and plasma cells. Aggregates of T and B cells can be observed in many patients either in the presence or absence of a germinal center reaction.[19, 20] The T-cell aggregates are composed predominantly of CD4 cells. The inflammatory T cells in the joints are highly Th-1 skewed, predominantly show an activated memory phenotype and express high levels of the chemokine receptors CCR5 and CXCR3.[21, 22] The hypertrophied synovial tissue is rich in microvessels. The pro-angiogenic factor vascular endothelial growth factor (VEGF) is highly expressed in synovial tissue; osteopontin correlates with new vascularization.[1, 2] The inflammatory process leads to pannus formation with cartilage and bone erosions mediated by degradative enzymes such as metalloproteinases.[1, 2]

Cytokines and calgranulins

Several studies have evaluated blood and synovial cytokine levels in children with the various JIA subtypes.[1, 2] However, with the exception of IL-6 in sJIA (see below), the results have often been quite inconsistent. These discrepancies may be due to differences in samples used (i.e., serum or plasma), sample handling, immunoassays, and patient classification criteria. TNF, IL-1, and IL-6 have been variably reported to be elevated in serum and synovial fluids of the various JIA subgroups.[23] As for adult RA, the observed potent therapeutic effect of anti-TNF agents in many

patients (see below) supports an important pathogenic role for this cytokine. Serum MIF levels have been shown to be increased in patients with JIA, with the highest levels observed in patients with systemic-onset JIA.[24] IL-18 has also been found to be increased in patients with sJIA.[25]

The phagocyte-specific calcium-binding proteins known as calgranulins (S100A8, S100A9, and S100A12) have been detected in serum and synovial fluid of patients with JIA. Children with sJIA have serum concentrations of calgranulins up to 20-fold higher than those found in patients with other inflammatory disorders.[26]

Type 2 cytokines

In a study investigating the pattern of expression of type 1 and type 2 cytokines in synovial tissues and fluids, IL-4 mRNA was identified significantly more often in patients with oligoarticular-onset disease than in those with polyarticular disease or adult RA. Similarly, IL-4 mRNA was detected more often in patients with a persistently pauciarticular disease course compared to those with a polyarticular course. Moreover, the combination of IL-4 and IL-10 mRNA was found more frequently in nonerosive compared with erosive disease, suggesting that IL-4, possibly in combination with IL-10, has an anti-inflammatory or disease-restricting role in JIA.[27]

The expression of the chemokine receptor CCR4, associated with a Th2 response and selective accumulation of CCR4+ cells, has not been found in RA. A study has shown the presence in the synovial fluid of JIA patients of CD4+CCR4+ lymphocytes, which produced more IL-4 and less IFN-γ than CD4+CCR4- cells. Increased numbers of CCR4+ cells were observed in samples collected early in the disease process.[28]

Heat shock proteins

Heat shock proteins (hsp) are stress proteins that are increasingly produced when a cell is confronted with an environmental stress. In the adjuvant arthritis model, a T-cell clone specific for a mycobacterial hsp65 was found to induce disease by eliciting a cross-reactive response against cartilage proteoglycan.[29] Subsequently it was found that preimmunization with mycobacterial hsp65 protects rats against subsequent induction not only of adjuvant arthritis but also of most of the other experimental models of arthritis. The subsequent analysis of T-cell epitopes of mycobacterial hsp65 showed that only conserved epitopes with a high degree of homology with the homologous rat peptide and capable of inducing T-cell responses to 'self' rat hsp60 can be protective, suggesting the induction of functional regulatory T cells.[29] Significant T-cell proliferative responses to human hsp60 have been found in patients with oligoarticular JRA early in disease; T-cell reactivity to human hsp60 seemed to be associated with disease remission.[29] Cells responsive to hsp60 express CD30 and produce IL-10.[29] More recently,[30] using computer algorithms for the identification of potential pan-DR-binding epitopes, the reactivity toward eight potential epitopes (from both self and microbial HSP60) binding to many HLA-DR have been studied in patients with oligoarticular and polyarticular JIA. Five of the eight peptides yielded proliferative T-cell responses in 50–70% of JIA patients irrespective of MHC genotype, but not in healthy or disease controls. Only peripheral blood mononuclear cells (PBMC) from patients with the disease produced IL-10, suggesting that in patients with oligoarticular disease the immune response to the identified HSP epitopes could contribute to disease remission.

Regulatory T cells

Regulatory T cells are T lymphocytes that suppress the activity of other T cells. Several different regulatory T-cell types have been described. There is now clear evidence that the population of naturally occurring regulatory T cells which constitutively express CD4 and CD25 plays an essential role in controlling autoimmunity. The development and function of regulatory T cells is critically dependent on the transcriptional repressor FoxP3.

In a recent study[31] the CD4+CD25+ population in synovial fluid of JIA patients (mostly oligoarticular JIA) was shown to comprise both regulatory and effector T cells that could be distinguished by expression of CD27. CD4+CD25+CD27- cells expressed low amounts of FoxP3, produced effector cytokines, and did not suppress T-cell proliferation. In contrast, CD4+CD25+CD27+ cells expressed a high amount of FoxP3, did not produce IL-2, IFN-γ, or TNF, and suppressed T-cell proliferation in vitro. These findings suggest that the combination of CD25 and CD27 allows identification of most regulatory T cells in inflamed tissues. These regulatory cells were, on a per-cell basis, fourfold more potent than the corresponding peripheral blood population, suggesting an activated state in vivo. The ratio of regulatory to activated T cells was found to be higher in patients with oligoarticular course than in those with polyarticular course. IL-7 and IL-15, present in synovial fluid of JIA patients, when added in vitro, were found to abrogate the suppressive activity of regulatory T cells, suggesting that in target tissues the function of regulatory T cells may be substantially limited by these cytokines.

Another study[32] has found that patients with persistent oligoarticular JIA display a significantly higher frequency of CD4+CD25bright T cells with concomitant higher levels of mRNA FoxP3 in the peripheral blood than extended oligoarticular patients. The frequency of CD4+CD25total cells in synovial fluid was higher in patients with persistent than in those with extended oligoarticular JIA. Analysis of FoxP3 mRNA levels revealed a high expression in SF CD4+CD25bright T cells of both patient groups and also a significant expression of FoxP3 mRNA in the CD4+CD25int T-cell population. The CD4+CD25bright T cells of both patient groups and the CD4+CD25int T cells of persistent oligoarticular JIA were able to suppress responses of CD25negative cells in vitro. SF CD4+CD25bright cells showed an increased regulatory capacity in vitro compared to peripheral blood CD4+CD25bright T cells.

IL-6 and IL-1

The cytokines critical to the pathogenesis of systemic JIA appear to be different from those in other JIA subtypes. Anti-TNF agents have indeed shown a rather limited effectiveness in systemic JIA as compared to other JIA subtypes.[33]

Circulating levels of IL-6 are markedly elevated in patients with systemic JIA, increase during the peak of fever, and correlate with the extent and severity of joint involvement and with platelet counts.[34, 35] Both circulating and synovial fluid levels of IL-6 in systemic JIA are significantly higher than in polyarticular and oligoarticular JIA or in adult RA.[36] The overproduction of IL-6 could well explain many of the extra-articular manifestations of systemic JIA, including anemia[5, 6] and growth failure.[37] Together these findings led to the hypothesis that sJIA could be an IL-6-mediated disease.[36] Recently a study on 11 children with sJIA showed that treatment with a monoclonal antibody directed against the IL-6

receptor was associated with marked clinical improvement and normalization of the acute-phase reactants.[38]

A subsequent paper[39] reported that the administration of the recombinant IL-1 receptor antagonist (IL-1Ra) to 9 patients with systemic JIA was also associated with a similar marked improvement and that serum from systemic JIA patients induces the transcription of innate immunity genes, including IL-1, in healthy peripheral blood mononuclear cells. These findings bear striking similarities to those observed in patients with autoinflammatory disorders due to a mutation in the NALP3/cryopirin gene, in which IL-β is involved in disease pathogenesis and in which treatment with IL-Ra resolves the clinical symptoms and normalizes acute-phase reactants. Of note, these diseases are characterized as systemic JIA by elevated serum IL-6 levels that normalize rapidly during IL-1Ra therapy. These observations raise the possibility that at least some forms of systemic JIA could represent autoinflammatory diseases.

Macrophage activation syndrome

As previously mentioned, for unknown reasons MAS occurs much more frequently in systemic arthritis than in other rheumatic diseases. MAS is characterized by a highly stimulated but ineffective immune response and is very similar to the other forms of hemophagocytic lymphohistiocytosis (HLH), the best known of which is familial HLH (FHLH).[40] Several independent genetic loci related to the release of cytolytic granules from natural killer (NK) and CD8 T lymphocytes have been associated with FHLH: perforin mutations have been observed in about 40% of patients. These mutations cause a severe impairment of cytotoxic function which, through mechanisms that have not yet been well elucidated, leads to an excessive expansion and activation of cytotoxic cells with hypersecretion of proinflammatory cytokines. These cytokines are produced by activated T cells and histiocytes that infiltrate all tissues and lead to tissue necrosis and organ failure. In perforin-deficient mice, the animal model of FHLH, although the serum levels of multiple cytokines, including IL-6, IL-18, and IFN-γ, are increased, only antibody to IFN-γ prolongs survival.

The mechanisms leading to cytolytic defects in immune-competent patients with acquired HLH are less clear.[40] Patients with virus-associated HLH also have very low or absent cytolytic NK cell activity. However, in contrast to FHLH, this phenomenon appears to be related to profoundly decreased number of NK cells rather than to impaired perforin expression. Notably, NK function has been found to recover completely in some patients after the resolution of the acute phase.[40]

Depressed NK activity, with or without abnormal perforin expression, may also be involved in the pathogenesis of MAS associated with systemic JIA.[40] NK activity was investigated in 7 patients with systemic arthritis and MAS during the acute stage or after resolution. In some patients, decreased NK activity was associated with very low numbers of NK cells but mildly increased levels of perforin expression in NK cells and cytotoxic CD8 T lymphocytes, a pattern somewhat similar to that in virus-associated HLH. In other patients, very low NK activity was associated with only mildly decreased numbers of NK cells but very low levels of perforin expression in all cytotoxic cell types, a pattern indistinguishable from that seen in FHLH. Remarkably, most of the patients with low perforin expression had a history of multiple episodes of MAS.[40] Hepatic biopsies in patients with various types of HLH, including MAS, revealed extensive infiltration of the liver by IFN-γ-producing CD8 T lymphocytes and hemophagocytic macrophages

> ## KEY CONCEPTS
>
> ### PATHOGENESIS OF JUVENILE IDIOPATHIC ARTHRITIS (JIA)
>
> >> The various JIA subtypes presumably correspond to different multifactorial diseases and likely represent complex genetic traits
>
> >> The pathogenic features of systemic arthritis appear to be different from those of the other JIA subtypes and share similarities with those of autoinflammatory disorders

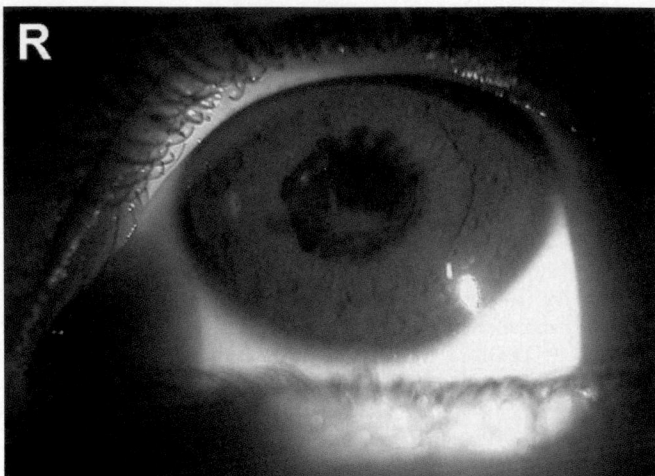

Fig. 53.2 Posterior synechiae, a complication of chronic anterior uveitis associated with juvenile idiopathic arthritis. The irregularities of the margins of the pupil are due to fibrous adhesions between the iris and the lens capsule.

secreting TNF-γ and IL-6.[41] It has been suggested that hyperproduction of IL-18 (which strongly induces Th-1 responses and IFN-γ production and enhances NK cell cytotoxicity) and an imbalance between levels of biologically active free IL-18 and those of its natural inhibitor (the IL-18-binding protein) may also play a role in secondary hemophagocytic syndromes, including MAS.[42] In a child with systemic JIA and MAS, the bone marrow was identified as the origin of the increased serum IL-18.[43]

COURSE AND PROGNOSIS

JIA is not a benign condition; a sizable proportion of patients develop articular damage and enter adult life with still-active disease.[1,2] It would therefore be of great importance to predict early in the disease course the ultimate outcome in order to tailor treatment to the risk of disability. However, although most children can be categorized in one of the various JIA subsets after the first 6 months of disease, this does not allow a reliable prediction of the potential outcome since evolution can differ greatly among patients belonging to the same onset type.

SYSTEMIC ARTHRITIS

Systemic arthritis has a variable course.[1,2] In about half of patients the disease is characterized by a monocyclic or an intermittent course with relapses followed by intervals of remission; in these cases the arthritis accompanies the episodes of fever but remits when systemic features are controlled. The long-term prognosis of these patients is usually good. In the other half of patients the disease follows an unremitting course. In many cases systemic symptoms eventually resolve, leaving chronic arthritis as the major long-term problem. This second group of patients with an unremitting disease course is probably the most severe among all JIA subtypes and can lead to severe joint destruction. Death was once principally related to the development of amyloidosis, that now appears to be a very uncommon complication. Nowadays, MAS remains the most serious and potentially fatal threat and has to be promptly recognized and treated.

OLIGOARTHRITIS

In general patients with oligoarthritis have the best outcome. Moreover, their prognosis has greatly improved in the last decades thanks to the widespread use of intra-articular steroids for the prevention of deformities

secondary to joint contractures. Nevertheless, some series have reported rates of remission after 6–10 years of disease of only 23–47%.[1,2] The percentage of patients who develop extended oligoarthritis has been reported to vary between 20 and 50%.[9,59] As may be expected, joint erosions occur more frequently in patients with a polyarticular course.[8]

The outcome of uveitis depends very much on early diagnosis and treatment. Prior to careful monitoring for uveitis with periodic slit-lamp examinations, a severe outcome was observed in more than one-third of patients. Now only a minority of patients suffer complications which can however be significant and include posterior synechiae (between the iris and the lens), cataract, and band keratopathy (Fig. 53.2). A small minority of patient may experience progressive disease leading to blindness despite adequate monitoring and treatment.[1]

OTHER SUBTYPES

RF-positive polyarthritis has the same poor long-term outcome as RF-positive adult RA. RF-negative polyarthritis has a variable outcome, reflecting the heterogeneity of the subtype. The prognosis of psoriatic arthritis as defined by the current ILAR criteria is not yet defined. In general, patients have a poorer outlook compared with those with oligoarthritis, with more frequent involvement of small joints and an increase in the number of affected joints. A variable percentage of patients with enthesitis-related arthritis progressively develops involvement of the joints of the axial skeleton.

GROWTH ANOMALIES

A characteristic feature of chronic arthritis in children is the effect it may have on bone and joint development.[1,1] Local growth disturbances occur at sites of inflammation resulting in either overgrowth or undergrowth of

mandibular asymmetry, and bilateral involvement may cause marked micrognatia. Similarly, involvement of the cervical spine, which is frequent in patients with JIA, may cause undergrowth of the vertebral bodies, resulting ultimately in a short neck. Anomalies in growth and morphogenesis of skeletal segments also result from anomalous tractions, on growing structures, secondary to muscular spasm and periarticular fibrosis. They are more marked in children with precocious onset of arthritis and very active disease. A characteristic developmental anomaly of the hip is often observed in children with early onset of arthritis. It includes enlargement and flattening of the femoral head, incompletely covered by an underdeveloped acetabulum, and a short, squat, valgus and anteverted femoral neck.

General growth abnormalities may be secondary to treatment with glucocorticoids as well as to the inflammatory process, particularly in patients with severe, persistently active, systemic JIA.

In affected joints periarticular osteoporosis is common. The use of corticosteroids may lead to generalized osteoporosis.

■ DIFFERENTIAL DIAGNOSIS ■

Since JIA is an exclusion diagnosis, by definition any other cause of chronic arthritis has to be ruled out. With the exception of enthesitis-related arthritis in which joint involvement can be quite painful or transient and recurrent, the arthritis of JIA is characterized by persistent joint swelling which is often not particularly painful, especially in the oligoarticular subtype. As in other inflammatory arthritides, joint stiffness is very common.

A wide range of different conditions can cause swelling and limitation of motion in a joint. These include other inflammatory or autoimmune diseases, infectious and post-infectious conditions, hematologic and neoplastic disorders, metabolic diseases, and congenital or acquired disorders of bones. The differential diagnosis is therefore very vast and beyond the scope of this chapter.

The condition that is essential to exclude immediately is septic arthritis, which is usually monoarticular and characterized by extreme joint tenderness and refusal to move the joint. The next most critical conditions to be excluded are neoplastic diseases and in particular leukemia and neuroblastoma. They are often characterized by severe bone pain which may have periods of exacerbation and remission: the pain is out of proportion to physical findings.

Monoarticular swelling can be caused by various conditions, including septic arthritis, hemofilia, osteochondritis dissecans, synovial hemangioma, and tuberculosis. Tuberculosis is characterized by an indolent course that can mimic JIA; therefore a purified protein derivative test has to be performed in any child with monoarthritis, especially of the knee. Hip involvement is very uncommon in JIA at presentation, with the exception of enthesitis-related arthritis. Lyme disease can cause mono- as well as oligoarthritis and has to be considered especially in endemic areas. Gouty arthritis as well as other crystal-induced arthropathies is extremely rare in children and is usually associated with a genetic disease. Chronic uveitis associated with rash and an oligoarthritis with marked periarticular involvement is characteristic of Blau syndrome.

Inflammatory bowel diseases can mimic JIA at presentation. Other inflammatory or autoimmune diseases such as systemic lupus erythematosus, rheumatic fever, Henoch–Schönlein purpura, Kawasaki disease, or other vasculitides can usually be differentiated from JIA on both articular

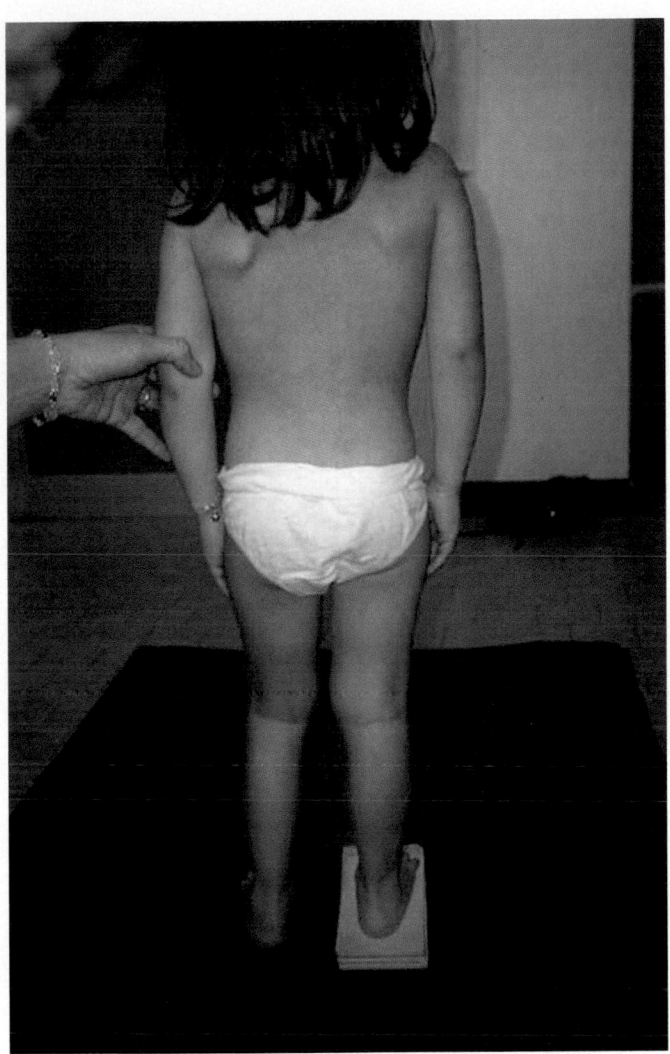

Fig. 53.3 Leg-length inequality secondary to asymmetric knee involvement. The overgrowth of the juxta-articular bone extremities is due to accelerated development of ossification centers, possibly related to inflammation-induced increased vascularization and growth factor release.

the juxta-articular bone extremities. Overgrowth is due to accelerated development of ossification centers, possibly related to inflammation-induced increased vascularization and growth factor release. Asymmetric knee involvement often results in lengthening of the affected leg with leg-length inequality (Fig. 53.3). Many inequalities resolve with growth if arthritis is controlled.

Undergrowth is secondary to growth center damage or premature fusion of epiphyseal plates. When extremities are involved, it may be symmetric, resulting in small hands or feet, or it may be isolated with selective brachydactyly. Arthritis of the wrist may cause growth failure of the ulnar head with shortened ulna and ulnar deviation of the carpus. Unilateral involvement of the temporomandibular joint may result in

THERAPEUTIC PRINCIPLES

>> Children are not small adults and juvenile idiopathic arthritis (JIA) is different from adult rheumatoid arthritis. Therefore, the evaluation of the safety and efficacy of any new drug in JIA needs appropriately designed controlled trials

>> Treatment approaches differ among the various JIA subtypes

>> Growth and developmental abnormalities can be unique complications in young patients

and extra-articular features. Progressive joint contractures are observed in metabolic diseases such as mucopolysaccaridosis and mucolipidosis.

Bacterial infections and malignancy as well as other causes of persistent fever must be ruled out before considering the diagnosis of systemic arthritis. MAS requires a prompt diagnosis and must not be confused with septic shock or other causes of hemophagocytic lymphohistiocytosis.

■ TREATMENT ■

Although we still do not possess drugs that are able to 'cure' the disease, the prognosis of JIA has greatly improved, with respect to even a decade ago, thanks to substantial progresses in disease management. Since JIA is not a single disease, treatment approach also varies among JIA subtypes. Since the course (even within each subtype) is difficult to predict, it is impossible at onset to tell what medications will be needed to control the disease. The goal of treatment is to gain complete control of the disease, to preserve the physical and psychological integrity of the child, and to prevent any long-term consequence related to disease or therapy. Periodic X-ray examination of the affected joints is needed to document progression of erosive disease.[44]

Optimal management of JIA requires a multidisciplinary approach that involves pediatric rheumatologists, nurses, physical and occupational therapists, social workers and, when indicated, psychologists, orthopedic surgeons, and ophthalmologists.

MEDICAL TREATMENT

Oligoarthritis and polyarthritis

Nonsteroidal anti-inflammatory drugs (NSAIDs) have been the mainstay of JIA treatment for decades.[1, 2] Their role remains important and most children with JIA are started on an NSAID. Just a few NSAIDs are approved for use in children; the most commonly used include naproxen, ibuprofen, and indomethacin. They are usually quite well tolerated and side effects are less common than in adults. Acetylsalicylic acid is much less used than in the past because of the less favorable safety profile. Experience with cyclooxygenase-2 inhibitors in children is very limited.

Intra-articular steroid injections with triamcinolone hexacetonide are frequently needed at disease onset or during disease course. In mono- or oligoarticular arthritis they are often used and may be indicated in association of or in substitution for NSAIDs. They are rapidly effective and, most importantly, they break the vicious circle that leads to deformities

(such as valgus knee) secondary to contractures. Although they are not curative, their effect may last for long periods.

In those children in whom the disease is not well controlled by NSAIDs and steroid injections, a second-line agent is often needed. These patients usually have arthritis with a polyarticular onset or course. There is general consensus that in these patients second-line therapy should be introduced quite early in the disease course in order to try to prevent disease progression. The second-line agent of first choice in JIA is methotrexate (MTX). A controlled study has shown its efficacy at a dose of 10 mg/m² per week.[45] A further study has shown that the plateau of efficacy is reached at 15 mg/m² per week and that higher doses are not accompanied by a better effect.[46] MTX is usually well tolerated, especially if associated with the administration of folic or folinic acid. At doses > 10 mg/m² per week, parenteral administration is advisable. Improvement is usually apparent in 6–12 weeks.[47]

In those patients who have an unsatisfactory response to MTX and in whom the disease remains active, treatment with anti-TNF agents is indicated. A controlled study has shown the efficacy of etanercept, at a dose of 0.4 mg/kg subcutaneously twice a week in patients with JIA who were resistant or intolerant to MTX.[48] Subsequently, other studies have confirmed the remarkable and rapid efficacy and the good safety profile of the drug in JIA. Since cases of reactivated tuberculosis have been reported during treatment with TNF inhibitors, all children should have a documented negative tuberculosis test before starting therapy.[1, 2] Etanercept is at present the only anti-TNF agent registered for pediatric use. However, controlled trials with other anti-TNF agents such as infliximab and adalimubab have recently been performed and the results will soon be published. To underline the need for controlled studies specifically performed in children, the infliximab study has shown that, although both the dosages of 3 and 6 mg/kg were effective, children treated with 3 mg/kg developed a much higher percentage of antibodies against infliximab and experienced a higher rate of infusion reactions.[49] Anti-TNF agents have also been reported to be effective in juvenile spondyloarthritides.[50]

As for the other second-line agents, seminal studies performed many years ago have shown that hydroxychloroquine and D-penicillamine are not more effective than placebo in RF-negative JIA.[1] Sulfasalazine[1, 2] may be considered as the second-line agent, especially in enthesitis-related arthritis, although there are no data showing that it is better than MTX for this indication; it has to be avoided in systemic arthritis for the increased risk of toxicity. A recent trial has shown the efficacy of leflonomide in JIA[51] but experience with this drug is still limited.

Systemic steroids (prednisone) are used only as a bridge drug when the disease is very active and time is required before second-line agents (such as MTX) can show their efficacy.

RF-positive polyarthritis is the equivalent of adult RF-positive RA and the therapeutic approach is the same.

Systemic arthritis

Systemic arthritis frequently does not respond to NSAIDs alone. In this case, when the diagnosis is firmly established, prednisone therapy is often indicated. Once disease control is reached, steroid therapy has to be progressively tapered. Indeed, the use of steroids should be limited as much as possible because of their severe side effects which, in children, also include growth retardation. Vitamin D and calcium supplements to try to prevent osteoporosis as well as dietary counseling are indicated. Treatment of MAS relies on prompt recognition of this complication and the use of high-dose steroids and Cyclosporine.[1,2] In children characterized by a polycyclic course, steroids and NSAIDs may be sufficient to control episodes of disease activity. In unremitting disease, steroid tapering is often accompanied by recurrence of systemic symptoms and arthritis. Although systemic symptoms often, but not always, fade during disease course, arthritis persists and often represent the main determinant for disease outcome. MTX is probably less effective in systemic arthritis than in other JIA subtypes.[1,2] Etanercept is also less effective in systemic arthritis than in other JIA subtypes.[33] The use of thalidomide has been proposed for resistant systemic arthritis.[52] In patients with very severe unremitting disease autologous bone marrow transplantation has been performed.[53] In the rare cases that develop amyloidosis, alkylating agents are indicated.[1,2]

As mentioned above, IL-6 has been suggested to play a major role in the pathogenesis of systemic JIA and an uncontrolled trial using a monoclonal antibody against the IL-6 receptor has shown very promising results in 11 patients with systemic JIA.[38] Moreover, recently treatment with IL 1Ra has also been associated with marked clinical improvement in 9 patients with systemic JIA.[39] The efficacy of these potentially very useful treatments requires confirmation in controlled clinical trials. In our experience (manuscript in preparation) some patients with systemic arthritis respond very well to IL-Ra, others have only a partial response, while others are resistant. It is therefore conceivable that treatment with these two cytokine inhibitors could represent not only a very important therapeutic advance but could also help in unraveling the clinical heterogeneity of systemic arthritis.

Uveitis

Early diagnosis is very important for the success of therapy, which has to be managed by an ophthalmologist.[1,2] The initial approach consists of glucocorticoid eye drops with mydriatics to dilate the pupil and prevent the occurrence of posterior synechiae. Concurrent therapy with NSAIDs is often used. In patients with disease resistant to topical therapy systemic steroid administration and/or subtenon injection of corticosteroids are required. In disease not controlled by the above measures several drugs have been claimed to be effective, including MTX, Cyclosporine, and alkylating agents. However no controlled trials exist. The efficacy of etanercept is controversial while infliximab has been anecdotally reported to be of benefit.

■ OTHER THERAPEUTIC ASPECTS ■

Physiotherapy and occupational therapy are important components of the therapeutic approach to any patients with JIA. In general, children limit their activities by themselves and should not be restricted. Swimming and bicycle riding, which do not put significant weight on the joints, should be encouraged. An orthodontic approach is often indicated in case of temporomandibular joint involvement.

Arthroscopic synovectomy may be indicated in a few cases to debulk proliferative synovitis resistant to other treatments. Soft-tissue release may be useful in selected cases but the intervention as well as the following postoperative rehabilitation have to be performed by experienced personnel.

Total arthroplasty, in particular of the hip and knee, represents a successful option in the presence of severe functional impairment and is generally delayed until growth has stopped. It presents special problems and has to be performed by orthopedic surgeons with specific experience.

JIA has a great psychological impact on the child and family. Children should be encouraged to attend school normally as well as take part in all the activities that are appropriate for their age. Parents may tend to protect the child excessively and limit activities; this can affect the proper development of the child's personality and prevent him or her from acquiring adequate self-confidence and self-esteem. When indicated, psychological support can be required. A website with information for families of children with rheumatic diseases is available in 50 languages.[54]

■ REFERENCES ■

1. Cassidy JT, Petty RE, Laxer RM, et al. Textbook of Pediatric Rheumatology, 5th edn. Philadelphia: Elsevier, 2005.
2. Szer Is, Kimura Y, Malleson PN, et al. Arthritis in Children and Adolescents, New York: Oxford University Press, 2006.
3. Petty RE, Southwood TR, Manners P, et al. International League of Associations for Rheumatology classification of juvenile idiopathic arthritis: second revision, Edmonton, 2001. J Rheumatol 2004; 31: 390–392.
4. Martini A. Are the number of joints involved or the presence of psoriasis still useful tools to identify homogeneous disease entities in juvenile idiopathic arthritis?. J Rheumatol 2003; 30: 1900–1903.
5. Martini A, Ravelli A, Di Fuccia G, et al. Intravenous iron therapy for severe anaemia in systemic-onset juvenile chronic arthritis. Lancet 1994; 344: 1052–1054.
6. Cazzola M, Ponchio L, De Benedetti F, et al. Defective iron supply to erythropoiesis and adequate endogenous erythropoietin production in the anemia associated with systemic-onset juvenile chronic arthritis. Blood 1996; 87: 4824–4830.
7. Ravelli A, Felici E, Magni-Manzoni S, et al. Patients with antinuclear antibody-positive juvenile idiopathic arthritis constitute a homogeneous subgroup irrespective of the course of joint disease. Arthritis Rheum 2005; 52: 826–832.
8. Guillaume S, Prieur AM, Coste J, et al. Long-term outcome and prognosis in oligoarticular-onset juvenile idiopathic arthritis. Arthritis Rheum 2000; 43: 1858–1865.
9. Glass DN, Giannini EH. Juvenile rheumatoid arthritis as a complex genetic trait. Arthritis Rheum 1999; 42: 2261–2268.
10. Thomson W, Donn R. Juvenile idiopathic arthritis genetics – what's new? What's next?. Arthritis Res 2002; 4: 302–306.
11. Moroldo MB, Chaudhari M, Shear E, et al. Juvenile rheumatoid arthritis affected sibpairs: extent of clinical phenotype concordance. Arthritis Rheum 2004; 50: 1928–1934.
12. Rosen P, Thompson S, Glass D. Non-HLA gene polymorphisms in juvenile rheumatoid arthritis. Clin Exp Rheumatol 2003; 21: 650–656.
13. Fishman D, Faulds G, Jeffery R, et al. The effect of novel polymorphisms in the interleukin-6 (IL-6) gene on IL-6 transcription and plasma IL-6 levels, and an association with systemic-onset juvenile chronic arthritis. J Clin Invest 1998; 102: 1369–1376.

14. Donn R, Alourfi Z, Zeggini E, et al. A functional promoter haplotype of macrophage migration inhibitory factor is linked and associated with juvenile idiopathic arthritis. Arthritis Rheum 2004; 50: 1604–1610.

15. De Benedetti F, Meazza C, Vivarelli M, et al. Functional and prognostic relevance of the -173 polymorphism of the macrophage migration inhibitory factor gene in systemic-onset juvenile idiopathic arthritis. Arthritis Rheum 2003; 48: 1398–1407.

16. Hinks A, Barton A, John S, et al. Association between the PTPN22 gene and rheumatoid arthritis and juvenile idiopathic arthritis in a UK population: further support that PTPN22 is an autoimmunity gene. Arthritis Rheum 2005; 52: 1694–1699.

17. Thompson SD, Moroldo MB, Guyer L, et al. A genome-wide scan for juvenile rheumatoid arthritis in affected sibpair families provides evidence of linkage. Arthritis Rheum 2004; 50: 2920–2930.

18. Massa M, Mazzoli F, Pignatti P, et al. Proinflammatory responses to self HLA epitopes are triggered by molecular mimicry to Epstein–Barr virus proteins in oligoarticular juvenile idiopathic arthritis. Arthritis Rheum 2002; 46: 2721–2729.

19. Murray KJ, Luyrink L, Grom AA, et al. Immunohistological characteristics of T cell infiltrates in different forms of childhood onset chronic arthritis. J Rheumatol 1996; 23: 2116–2124.

20. Gregorio A, Gambini C, Gerloni V, et al. Lymphoid neogenesis in juvenile idiopathic arthritis. Rheumatology 2007; 46: 308–313.

21. Wedderburn LR, Robinson N, Patel A, et al. Selective recruitment of polarized T cells expressing CCR5 and CXCR3 to the inflamed joints of children with juvenile idiopathic arthritis. Arthritis Rheum 2000; 43: 765–774.

22. Gattorno M, Prigione I, Moranti F, et al. Phenotypic and functional characterization of CCR7+ and CCR7- CD4+ memory T cells homing to the joints in juvenile idiopathic arthritis. Arthritis Res Ther 2005; 7: R256–R267.

23. De Benedetti F, Ravelli A, Martini A. Cytokines in juvenile rheumatoid arthritis. Curr Opin Rheumatol 1997; 9: 428–433.

24. Meazza C, Travaglino P, Pignatti P, et al. Macrophage migration inhibitory factor in patients with juvenile idiopathic arthritis. Arthritis Rheum 2002; 46: 232–237.

25. Maeno N, Takei S, Nomura Y, et al. Highly elevated serum levels of interleukin-18 in systemic juvenile idiopathic arthritis but not in other juvenile idiopathic arthritis subtypes or in Kawasaki disease: comment on the article by Kawashima, et al. Arthritis Rheum 2002; 46: 2539–2541.

26. Foell D, Roth J. Proinflammatory S100 proteins in arthritis and autoimmune disease. Arthritis Rheum 2004; 50: 3762–3771.

27. Murray KJ, Grom AA, Thompson SD, et al. Contrasting cytokine profiles in the synovium of different forms of juvenile rheumatoid arthritis and juvenile spondyloarthropathy: prominence of interleukin 4 in restricted disease. J Rheumatol 1998; 25: 1388–1398.

28. Thompson SD, Luyrink LK, Graham TB, et al. Chemokine receptor CCR4 on CD4+ T cells in juvenile rheumatoid arthritis synovial fluid defines a subset of cells with increased IL-4:IFN-gamma mRNA ratios. J Immunol 2001; 166: 6899–6906.

29. van Eden W, van der Zee R, Prakken B. Heat-shock proteins induce T-cell regulation of chronic inflammation. Nat Rev Immunol 2005; 5: 318–330.

30. Kamphuis S, Kuis W, de Jager W, et al. Tolerogenic immune responses to novel T-cell epitopes from heat-shock protein 60 in juvenile idiopathic arthritis. Lancet 2005; 366: 50–56.

31. Ruprecht CR, Gattorno M, Ferlito F, et al. Coexpression of CD25 and CD27 identifies FoxP3+ regulatory T cells in inflamed synovia. J Exp Med 2005; 201: 1793–1803.

32. de Kleer IM, Wedderburn LR, Taams LS, et al. CD4+CD25 bright regulatory T cells actively regulate inflammation in the joints of patients with the remitting form of juvenile idiopathic arthritis. J Immunol 2004; 172: 6435–6443.

33. Quartier P, Taupin P, Bourdeaut F, et al. Efficacy of etanercept for the treatment of juvenile idiopathic arthritis according to the onset type. Arthritis Rheum 2003; 48: 1093–1101.

34. De Benedetti F, Massa M, Robbioni P, et al. Correlation of serum interleukin-6 levels with joint involvement and thrombocytosis in s ystemic juvenile rheumatoid arthritis. Arthritis Rheum 1991; 34: 1158–1163.

35. De Benedetti F, Massa M, Pignatti P, et al. Serum soluble IL-6 receptor and IL-6/soluble IL-6 receptor complex in systemic juvenile rheumatoid arthritis. J Clin Invest 1994; 93: 2114–2119.

36. De Benedetti F, Martini A. Is systemic juvenile rheumatoid arthritis an interleukin 6 mediated disease?. J Rheumatol 1998; 25: 203–207.

37. De Benedetti F, Alonzi T, Moretta A, et al. IL-6 causes growth impairment in transgenic mice through a decrease in insulin-like growth factor-1: a model for stunted growth in children with chronic inflammation. J Clin Invest 1997; 99: 643–650.

38. Yokota S, Miyamae T, Imagawa T, et al. Therapeutic efficacy of humanized recombinant anti-interleukin-6 receptor antibody in children with systemic onset juvenile idiopathic arthritis. Arthritis Rheum 2005; 52: 818–825.

39. Pascual V, Allantaz F, Arce E, et al. Role of interleukin-1 (IL-1) in the pathogenesis of systemic onset juvenile idiopathic arthritis and clinical response to IL-1 blockade. J Exp Med 2005; 201: 1479–1486.

40. Grom AA. Natural killer cell dysfunction: a common pathway in systemic-onset juvenile rheumatoid arthritis, macrophage activation syndrome, and hemophagocytic lymphohistiocytosis? Arthritis Rheum 2004; 50: 689–698.

41. Billiau AD, Roskams T, Van Damme-Lombaerts R, et al. Macrophage activation syndrome: characteristic findings on liver biopsy illustrating the key role of activated, IFN-gamma-producing lymphocytes and IL-6- and TNF-alpha-producing macrophages. Blood 2005; 105: 1648–1651.

42. Mazodier K, Marin V, Novick D, et al. Severe imbalance of IL-18/IL-18BP in patients with secondary hemophagocytic syndrome. Blood 2005; 106: 3483–3489.

43. Maeno N, Takei S, Imanaka H, et al. Increased interleukin-18 expression in bone marrow of a patient with systemic juvenile idiopathic arthritis and unrecognized macrophage-activation syndrome. Arthritis Rheum 2004; 50: 1935–1938.

44. Magni-Manzoni S, Rossi F, Pistorio A, et al. Prognostic factors for radiographic progression, radiographic damage, and disability in juvenile idiopathic arthritis. Arthritis Rheum 2003; 48: 3509–3517.

45. Giannini EH, Brewer EJ, Kuzmina N, et al. Methotrexate in resistant juvenile rheumatoid arthritis. Results of the U.S.A.–U.S.S.R. double-blind, placebo-controlled trial. The Pediatric Rheumatology Collaborative Study Group and the Cooperative Children's Study Group. N Engl J Med 1992; 326: 1043–1049.

REFERENCES

46. Ruperto N, Murray KJ, Gerloni V, et al. A randomized trial of parenteral methotrexate in intermediate versus higher doses in children with juvenile idiopathic arthritis who failed standard dose. Arthritis Rheum 2004; 50: 2191–2201.

47. Ravelli A, Martini A. Methotrexate in juvenile idiopathic arthritis: answers and questions. J Rheumatol 2000; 27: 1830–1833.

48. Lovell DJ, Giannini EH, Reiff A, et al. Etanercept in children with polyarticular juvenile rheumatoid arthritis. Pediatric Rheumatology Collaborative Study Group. N Engl J Med 2000; 342: 763–769.

49. Ruperto N, Lovell DJ, Cuttica R, et al. Comparison of safety, efficacy and pharmacokinetics for 3 and 6 mg/kg infliximab plus methotrexate therapy in JRA patients. Clin Exp Rheumatol 2005; 23. S-67.

50. Tse SM, Burgos-Vargas R, Laxer RM. Anti-tumor necrosis factor alpha blockade in the treatment of juvenile spondylarthropathy. Arthritis Rheum 2005; 52: 2103–2108.

51. Silverman E, Mouy R, Spiegel L, et al. Leflunomide or methotrexate for juvenile rheumatoid arthritis. N Engl J Med 2005; 352: 1655–1666.

52. Lehman TJ, Schechter SJ, Sundel RP, et al. Thalidomide for severe systemic onset juvenile rheumatoid arthritis: a multicenter study. J Pediatr 2004; 145: 856–857.

53. De Kleer IM, Brinkman DM, Ferster A, et al. Autologous stem cell transplantation for refractory juvenile idiopathic arthritis: analysis of clinical effects, mortality, and transplant related morbidity. Ann Rheum Dis 2004; 63: 1318–1326.

54. Ruperto N, Garcia-Munitis P, Villa L, et al. PRINTO/PRES international website for families of children with rheumatic diseases: www.pediatric-rheumatology.printo.it Ann Rheum Dis 2005; 64: 1101–1106.

REFERENCES

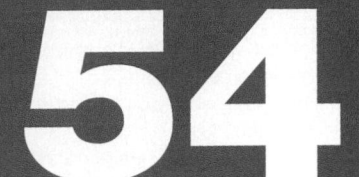
Sjögren's syndrome

54

Stanley R. Pillemer

Sjögren's syndrome (SS) is a debilitating systemic autoimmune disorder in which inflammation of the epithelial tissues, including exocrine glands, is prominent.[1] Salivary and lacrimal gland involvement is very common and associated with decreased production of saliva and tears. Other epithelial components of the body are commonly involved, including the skin, as well as the urogenital, respiratory, and gastrointestinal tracts. In addition, other systemic autoimmune manifestations occur, including synovitis, neuropathy, vasculitis, elevated immunoglobulin levels and autoantibodies, particularly antinuclear antibodies, anti-SSA, anti-SSB, and rheumatoid factor. SS may be associated with malignancies, especially non-Hodgkin's lymphoma.[2]

■ EPIDEMIOLOGY ■

Reported prevalences of primary SS vary from 0.05% to 4.8% of the population,[3, 4] and SS appears to increase in frequency with age.[3] Likely, the prevalence of primary SS is on the order of 0.3–0.6%.[4] The incidence of new cases of primary SS is estimated at ~4 per 100 000 population per year.[3] The diagnosis is most frequently made in mid-life, but can occur at any age. The onset is most often insidious, and diagnosis may be delayed for a number of years.[5] The female-to-male ratio is about 9:1.

Mortality rates in SS may be increased, perhaps more so for secondary SS than primary SS.[6] Approximately 5% of patients with primary SS develop B-cell lymphomas, which may contribute to excess mortality.[2] However, it is not yet clear whether the overall mortality from all causes for primary SS is increased when compared with the general population.[6] Differences in classification criteria may complicate the interpretation of epidemiological data.

■ CLASSIFICATION CRITERIA AND DIAGNOSIS ■

Published classification criteria for SS have included the requirement of keratoconjunctivitis sicca (KCS), xerostomia (XS), and autoantibodies. Preliminary European criteria were revised by the American–European Consensus Group because it was possible for individuals without evidence of autoimmunity (negative labial salivary gland biopsy and negative serology) to meet them.[7] Those criteria, shown in Table 54.1, are currently the most widely used. Rules for applying the criteria and the exclusions for SS are shown in Table 54.2. Patients meeting these current classification criteria may be considered for practical purposes to have a diagnosis of SS. The differential diagnosis for SS includes the disorders listed as exclusions.

SS may be categorized into primary and secondary forms.[8] If SS coexists with other autoimmune diseases, such as rheumatoid arthritis, systemic lupus erythematosus (SLE), scleroderma, polymyositis, and polyarteritis nodosa, it is referred to as secondary SS.[8] Otherwise it is called primary SS. However, this terminology is misleading. For example, as sometimes occurs, a patient with primary SS may subsequently develop SLE. The patient is then said to have secondary SS. There is no evidence that the SS is secondary to SLE in such cases. Such a case could equally be regarded as a case of primary SS with secondary SLE.

■ PATHOGENESIS ■

Although the cause of SS remains unknown, a considerable body of research spanning decades has elucidated many features of the immunopathogenesis of the disorder.[5, 9, 10] Damage to epithelial cells by unknown environmental agents, such as viruses or toxins, might initiate a cascade of events in genetically prone hosts, resulting in the development of SS. A number of viruses have a tropism for salivary glands.[11] Viruses implicated in SS include herpes viruses, such as Epstein–Barr virus, cytomegalovirus, as well as human herpes virus (HHV)-6 and HHV-8; and retroviruses, such as human T-cell lymphotropic virus-1, human retrovirus 5 and human immunodeficiency virus (HIV)-1. However, the salivary involvement in HIV infection affects a higher proportion of males and is associated with CD8 T cells, rather than the increase in CD4 cells occurring in SS, and autoantibodies are less frequent. Hepatitis C virus can also result in salivary gland swelling and may masquerade as SS. Enteroviruses, such as coxsackievirus, have been recently implicated in SS. Coxsackie viral RNA and enteroviral capsid protein VP1 were found in minor salivary gland epithelial cells and lymphocytic infiltrates from SS patients, but not controls.[12] However, of the

Table 54.1 Revised classification criteria for Sjögren's syndrome

I. **Ocular symptoms:** a positive response to at least one of the following questions:
Have you had daily, persistent, troublesome dry eyes for more than 3 months?
Do you have a recurrent sensation of sand or gravel in the eyes?
Do you use tear substitutes more than three times a day?

II. **Oral symptoms:** a positive response to at least one of the following questions:
Have you had a daily feeling of dry mouth for more than 3 months?
Have you had recurrently or persistently swollen salivary glands as an adult?
Do you frequently drink liquids to aid in swallowing dry food?

III. **Ocular signs,** i.e., objective evidence of ocular involvement defined as a positive result for at least one of the following two tests:
Schirmer's I test, performed without anesthesia (≤5 mm in 5 minutes)
Rose Bengal score or other ocular dye score (≥4 according to van Bijsterveld's scoring system).

IV. **Histopathology:** in minor salivary glands (obtained through normal-appearing mucosa) focal lymphocytic sialoadenitis, evaluated by an expert histopathologist, with a focus score≥ 1, defined as a number of lymphocytic foci which are adjacent to normal-appearing mucous acini and contain more than 50 lymphocytes per 4 mm^2 of glandular tissue.

V. **Salivary gland involvement:** objective evidence of salivary gland involvement defined by a positive result for at least one of the following diagnostic tests:
1. Unstimulated whole salivary flow (≤1.5 ml in 15 minutes)
2. Parotid sialography showing the presence of diffuse sialectasias (punctate, cavitary, or destructive pattern), without evidence of obstruction in the major ducts
3. Salivary scintigraphy showing delayed uptake, reduced concentration, and/or delayed excretion of tracer

VI. **Autoantibodies:** presence in the serum of the following autoantibodies:
Antibodies to Ro(SSA) or La(SSB) antigens, or both

Table 54.2 Revised rules for classification

For primary SS
In patients without any potentially associated disease, primary SS can be defined as follows:
1. The presence of *any four out of the six items* is indicative of primary SS, as long as either item IV (histopathology) or VI (serology) is positive
2. The presence of *any three of the four objective criteria items* (i.e., items III, IV, V, VI)
3. *The classification tree procedure* represents a valid alternative method for classification, although it should be more properly used in clinical-epidemiological surveys (Fig. 54.2)

For secondary SS
In patients with a potentially associated disease (for instance, another well-defined connective tissue disease), the presence of *item I or item II plus any two from among items III, IV, and V* may be considered as indicative of secondary SS

Exclusion criteria: past history of head and neck radiation therapy, hepatitis C infection, acquired immunodeficiency disease (AIDS), pre-existing lymphoma, sarcoidosis, graft-versus-host disease, use of anti-cholinergic drugs (within four half-lives of the drug).

---

viral infections implicated in SS in the past, no specific organism has emerged as the cause of SS.[11] Bacteria, such as *Helicobacter pylori* have been considered as potential agents involved in the pathogenesis of SS. However, this organism appears to be no more common in SS patients than healthy controls and not all patients carry *H. pylori*.[13]

Sex and other genetically determined factors have a role in host susceptibility to SS.[9] SS and other autoimmune diseases, such as SLE, are more common in females than males. Females show greater humoral and cellular immune responses than males. Hormonal factors, such as a relative lack of androgens, may have a pathogenic role in SS.[14] In addition, pregnancy is associated with modulation of autoimmune diseases. The severity of a number of autoimmune diseases change during pregnancy and postpartum,

suggesting a role for hormonal fluctuations. Besides the possible role of sex hormones, hypofunction of the hypothalamic–adrenal–pituitary adrenal (HPA) axis occurs in SS and other autoimmune rheumatic diseases.[14] Such HPA axis abnormalities can be congenital or acquired.

Genetic factors other than those above may contribute toward the development of SS.[9] Family members may have an increased prevalence of SS and autoantibodies, mostly anti-Ro/SSA. The HLA-DR3 and HLA-DQ2 alleles are more common in white patients with primary SS. Different alleles predominate in African-Americans and Japanese patients.[15] Identical twins appear to have phenotypically similar disease, including the fine specificities of anti-Ro.[9] In some patients, the transporters associated with antigen processing (TAP) gene alleles, TAP1 (0101) and TAP2 (0101), and microsatellite a2 alleles may be more frequent.[15]

Whether the disease is congenital or acquired, patients with SS appear to have a greater tendency toward apoptosis of the epithelial cells in the salivary glands.[1] An overview of the pathogenesis of SS is shown in key concepts. Apoptotic epithelial cells release material including RNA and RNA-binding proteins, such as Ro/SSA and La/SSB, allowing for the development of autoantibodies directed against Ro/SSA and La/SSB.[10] Immune complexes containing Ro/SSA-anti-Ro/SSA occur in SS, and can bind to Fc receptors on plasmacytoid dendritic cells, become internalized, and activate Toll-like receptors (TLRs).[10] The activation of TLRs results in a cascade of events that increases the production of type I interferons (IFN), such as IFN-α.[10] This is consistent with the type 1 IFN signature seen in salivary gland tissue in SS and represented by increased expression of type 1 IFN response genes. The upregulation of type I IFN response genes can increase expression of IFN-γ and B-lymphocyte stimulator (BLyS; also known as BAFF). BLyS promotes the survival and proliferation of B cells. Expansion of B cells capable of undergoing random mutations may partly account for the relatively high frequency of B-cell lymphomas in SS.

KEY CONCEPTS

PATHOGENESIS OF SJÖGREN'S SYNDROME

>> Sjögren's syndrome is a systemic autoimmune disease that shows characteristic tissue inflammation, which occurs in lacrimal and salivary glands, as well as other exocrine and epithelial tissues; autoantibodies, such as anti-SS-A and anti-SS-B; and increased expression of type 1 interferon response genes

>> Environmental agents and genetic factors likely result in apoptosis of epithelial cells that release RNA, RNA-binding proteins, such as SS-A and SS-B, and other debris

>> Autoantibodies directed against SS-A (60 and 52-kDa proteins) and SS-B (48-kDa proteins) result in SS-A/anti-SS-A and SS-B/anti-SS-B immune complexes

>> Immune complexes can bind to Fc receptors on plasmacytoid dendritic cells in the target tissues. Internalization of immune complexes may occur, resulting in the activation of Toll-like receptors (TLRs), which may result in the increased production of type I interferons, such as interferon-α

>> Interferon-α induces T cells in tissue infiltrates to produce BlyS/BAFF that facilitates the survival and proliferation of B cells. These effects may relate to the increase risk of B-cell lymphomas in Sjögren's syndrome

>> Although B cells have an important role in Sjögren's syndrome, the predominant infiltrating cells in the glands and mucosa-associated lymphoid tissues (MALT) in which lymphomas may arise are CD4 T cells that release Th1-type cytokines.

The distinctive features of SS include focal periductal mononuclear cell infiltration in exocrine tissues.[1] The exocrine infiltrate contains mostly T cells and, to a lesser extent, B cells, macrophages, and mast cells.[1,10] The majority of the T cells are CD4 helper cells of the CD45RO memory cell phenotype. These cells express the α/β T-cell receptor and activated lymphocyte function-associated antigen type 1 (LFA-1), and may have a role in promoting B-cell hyperactivity. Adhesion molecules and LFA-1 facilitate homing in exocrine tissue, which at times results in the formation of follicular structures similar to those seen in lymph nodes. Despite increased expression of Fas, the infiltrating periductal lymphocytes appear to be resistant to apoptosis, favoring persistence of autoreactive cells in the exocrine tissues. Apoptosis may be suppressed by the proto-oncogene Bcl-2.[1]

In SS, both salivary and lacrimal gland epithelial cells express HLA-DR molecules. This enables these epithelial cells to present exogenous antigens and autoantigens to CD4 T cells,[1] promoting the production of cytokines and the stimulation of B-cell proliferation and differentiation. In addition, B-cell activation is typical in SS and may evolve into B-cell lymphoid malignancy.[1] Proinflammatory cytokines, IL-1β, IL-6, and tumor necrosis factor-α (TNF-α) are elaborated by epithelial cells, whereas IL-10 and IFN-γ are mostly made by infiltrating T cells. IL-10 promotes B-cell proliferation and IFN-γ heightens expression of HLA-DR and La/SSB by exocrine glandular epithelial cells.

In SS, activated B cells produce increased amounts of immunoglobulins with autoantibody reactivity for IgG (rheumatoid factor), Ro/SSA, and La/SSB.[13] Evidence suggests that the B cells may produce antibodies targeting the muscarinic M3 receptor.[16] This is reminiscent of myasthenia gravis, an autoimmune disorder in which the target antigen is a postsynaptic receptor for acetylcholine at the neuromuscular junction. In SS, the blockade of the muscarinic (acetylcholine) receptor in exocrine tissue would diminish the production of secretions.

Several other possible explanations exist for the decline in exocrine secretions seen in SS. If tissue destruction is extensive, there may be insufficient tissue to produce secretions. However, total destruction of the salivary tissue is rarely seen in salivary gland biopsies in SS. Significant dryness may occur in individuals that have lost about half of the ducts and acini.[15] Interestingly, patients with little or no tissue destruction may have significant or severe dryness. This suggests that immune-mediated mechanisms may directly or indirectly result in dryness in SS patients. Cytokines may interact directly with epithelial cells. Autoantibodies, other than those directed against muscarinic M3 receptors, could interfere with the nerve supply, resulting in diminished secretions out of proportion to tissue destruction.

Researchers have studied the pathogenesis and genetic factors in SS in a number of animal models, including the nonobese diabetic (NOD) mouse, the NOD.B10, NOD.SCID, and MRL/lpr mouse.[1,9,15] The NOD mouse has an immunological profile and decrease in saliva production similar to that seen in human disease. Also, the transforming growth factor β (TGF-β) knockout mouse develops salivary and lacrimal gland exocrinopathy, suggesting a possible role for this cytokine in SS. TGF-β facilitates certain immune responses and acinar cell differentiation, and could possibly have a role in the early stages of SS.[9] Recently, new mouse models for SS have been explored, including the NOD.H2h4 mouse, the IQI/Jic mouse, and the NFS/sld mouse model. In addition, BALB/c mice immunized with 60-kDa Ro (SS-A) peptides developed a disease similar to SS with lymphocytic infiltration of salivary glands and decreased saliva production.

CLINICAL SPECTRUM OF SS

The classifying manifestations of SS include oral and ocular symptoms and signs of dryness, the presence of autoantibodies, especially anti-Ro/SSA and anti-La/SSB antibodies, and a positive labial salivary gland biopsy. Masaki and Sugai have suggested that primary SS can be divided into three stages according to the extent of organ damage and the course of the disease.[17] In stage I, representing about 45% of the patients, only sicca symptoms are present without systemic involvement. In stage II, affecting about half of the cases, lymphocytic organ damage occurs, which may affect the skin, lungs, kidney, liver, and hematological systems. In stage III, affecting about 5% of patients, malignant lymphomas occur. It is useful to think about the severity of the disease in terms of these stages. However, a caveat is that not all patients progress stepwise through these stages. Patients may be diagnosed in stage I or stage II or could present with lymphoma and features consistent with SS.

CLINICAL CONSIDERATIONS IN THE ASSESSMENT OF PATIENTS WITH SJÖGREN'S SYNDROME

>> Sjögren's syndrome is a systemic autoimmune disease characterized by objective signs of ocular and oral dryness, focal mononuclear cell infiltrates in labial minor salivary gland biopsies, and anti-SS-A or anti-SS-B autoantibodies

>> Salivary gland swelling that occurs in conjunction with meals is more likely to have an obstructive than an inflammatory cause

>> When angular cheilitis is seen, examine the mouth and pharynx carefully for possible candidiasis

>> Unlike rheumatoid arthritis, the arthritis of SS is generally nonerosive. An arthropathy similar to that seen in systemic lupus erythematosus (SLE) may occur

>> Both primary SS and SLE have antinuclear antibodies. SS patients often have, and SLE patients may have, antibodies to SS-A. In primary SS, the double-stranded anti-DNA is negative, in contrast to SLE. Kidney disease in SS is mostly interstitial nephritis and renal tubular acidosis, whereas glomerulonephritis is more common in SLE. The cutaneous manifestations of SS patients are mainly dryness and vasculitic lesions, whereas malar rashes, discoid lupus, and maculopapular eruptions are more common in SLE

>> The vasculitis of SS most often involves the lower limbs in dependent areas, and individual lesions tend to resolve within 48 hours. The vasculitis may occur as leukocytoclastic vasculitis, which tends to be associated with cryoglobulinemia. Vasculitis is often associated with peripheral neuropathy

>> Peripheral neuropathy occurs in about 20% of patients and is easily missed since patients may not be aware of lower-limb sensory loss. Screening by testing sensation, particularly vibration sense, is useful

>> Patients with purpura or cutaneous vasculitis, low serum C3 or C4 complement levels, and low peripheral blood CD4 T-cell counts, and possibly persistent salivary gland swelling, lymphadenopathy, and splenomegaly, are at higher risk for the development of lymphoma, and should be followed closely

OCULAR FEATURES

Precorneal tear fluid represents a complex biochemical mixture that includes water, electrolytes, mucins, antimicrobial proteins (e.g., lactoferrin and lysozyme), immunoglobulins, and growth factors (e.g., TGF-α). Three layers of precorneal tear film starting from the corneal surface are mucus, water, and oil layers.[18] The precorneal mucus, protein, and aqueous components form a hydrated gel. Without the gel, KCS occurs. The barrier to fluorescein dye decreases, contrast sensitivity declines, and irregularity of the corneal surface increases. The outer layer of the precorneal tear film covers the hydrated gel, and is made by the meibomian gland; it consists of a complex mixture of nonpolar and polar lipids.

The relationships between dry eyes and the tear layers are shown in Figure 54.1. In SS, dry eyes result from aqueous tear deficiency (ATD). However, ATD is not pathognomonic of SS, but may occur because of other lacrimal gland diseases, lacrimal duct obstruction, and loss of reflex tearing. Dry eyes resulting from evaporative tear deficiency may be caused by meibomian gland disease, contact lenses, and blink abnormality. SS patients often experience a sensation of sand or grit in the eyes. Dry eyes may be assessed by performing a Schirmer's I test, where abnormal tear production is considered to be present when 5 mm or less of wetting of a standard rectangular strip of filter paper occurs in 5 minutes. In addition, a fluorescein tear film breakup time of less than 10 seconds, observed on slit-lamp examination, is consistent with dry eyes. The extent of staining of the ocular surface by Rose Bengal or other vital dyes can be evaluated using the van Bijsterveld scoring system. In the USA and UK, ophthalmologists commonly use lissamine green, since Rose Bengal staining tends to be more irritating to the eye. Keratinization may also be assessed as a measure of dryness of the ocular surface. Further evaluations of ocular dryness may include surface cytology, lacrimal gland biopsy, and, in a research setting, analysis of tear composition.

ORAL FEATURES

Often, patients with SS experience awareness of decreased saliva, oral dryness that interferes with eating, the need to drink liquids to facilitate the swallowing of dry foods, a chronic burning sensation, intolerance of spicy foods, and altered taste.[19] Oral dryness can result in speech difficulties that may hamper social interactions. Patients with occupations such as teaching, that make demands on speech, may have to retire early. Patients should be asked about their current and past medications, since more than 400 medications have been reported to be associated with dry-mouth symptoms, including a number of commonly prescribed drugs for hypertension, depression, and insomnia.[19] A history of radiation therapy for head and neck tumors should be sought, since this may produce severe oral dryness.[19] Radioactive iodine for thyroid disorders also accumulates in exocrine glands, particularly the salivary glands, potentially resulting in oral dryness. Examination often shows erosions of the teeth and caries, as shown in Figure 54.2, especially at the gingival margins and on the incisal edges of the teeth. Soft-tissue changes are common. The tongue may become furrowed, and the mucosa dry, as shown in Figure 54.3, and sticky. Mucosal erythema and white patches are found in candidiasis, a common complication of dry mouth.[19] When angular cheilitis is present (shown in Figure 54.4), candidiasis should be suspected. Decreased or absent saliva pooling can often be observed on examination. Dysphagia can be investigated by barium swallows or ultrasound studies, which may show esophageal dysmotility.

Major salivary enlargement glands may be observed, as shown in Figure 54.5. The parotid gland may displace the earlobe and the swelling may extend downward over the angle of the jaw. Medial to the angle of the jaw, submandibular salivary gland swelling may be visible or, more frequently, palpated. Tenderness of the glands is variable, and the swelling is often recurrent, thus distinguishing it from mumps. The salivary gland swelling of SS may be transient or chronic. Transient recurrent swelling of rapid onset occurring with eating or drinking suggests salivary duct obstruction. Causes of such obstruction include sialolithiasis and strictures of the duct.

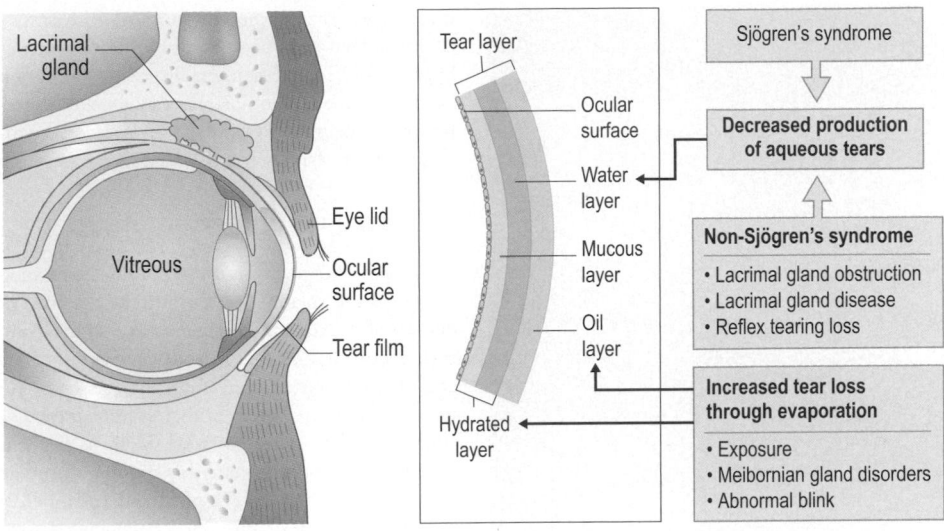

Fig. 54.1 Causes of dry eyes.

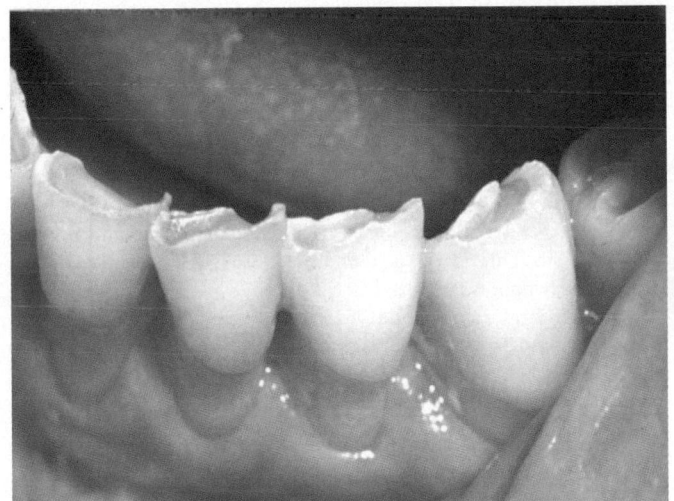

Fig. 54.2 Dental erosions.

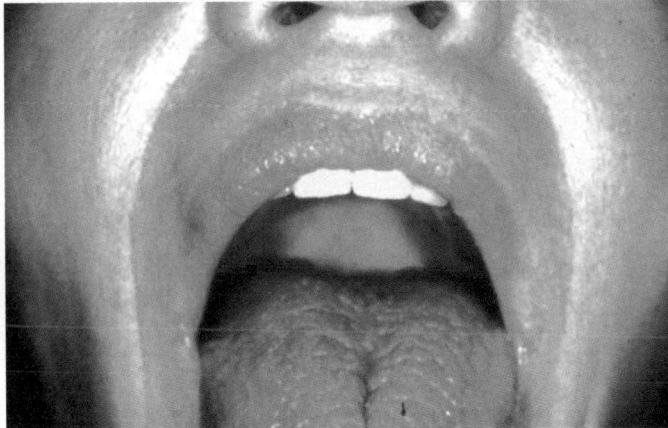

Fig. 54.3 Dry mouth.

MUSCULOSKELETAL FEATURES

Systemic rheumatic symptomatology may include fatigue, myalgias, arthralgias, low-grade fever, and lymphadenopathy.[20] Patients may develop a symmetrical polyarthritis that resembles rheumatoid arthritis. However, as in SLE, it is usually nondeforming. The arthritis of SS tends to respond well to standard treatments used in rheumatoid arthritis. These include nonsteroidal anti-inflammatory drugs, methotrexate, azathioprine, and other agents. The role, though, of TNF-α blockers in more severe cases of arthritis in SS patients is unclear. In so-called secondary SS, rheumatoid arthritis, or SLE, may occur and may begin before or after the onset of SS. Although an increased frequency of sicca symptoms have been described in fibromyalgia, it is unclear whether fibromyalgia occurs more frequently in SS.

CUTANEOUS FEATURES

Dry skin occurs in about half of patients affected with SS.[21] Sweating may be decreased. Pruritus may be associated with dry skin, and in some cases with the dysesthesia of peripheral neuropathy. Repeated scratching may result in hyperpigmentation, excoriations, and lichenification of the skin. In addition, palpable or nonpalpable purpura and petechiae occur in some patients, most frequently on the legs, in showers of lesions lasting up to 4 days. These lesions are histologically consistent with either leukocytoclastic vasculitis, which is typically associated with anti-Ro(SS-A) and La (SS-B), rheumatoid factor, antinuclear antibodies, cryoglobulins, hypocomplementemia, hypergammaglobulinemia, and

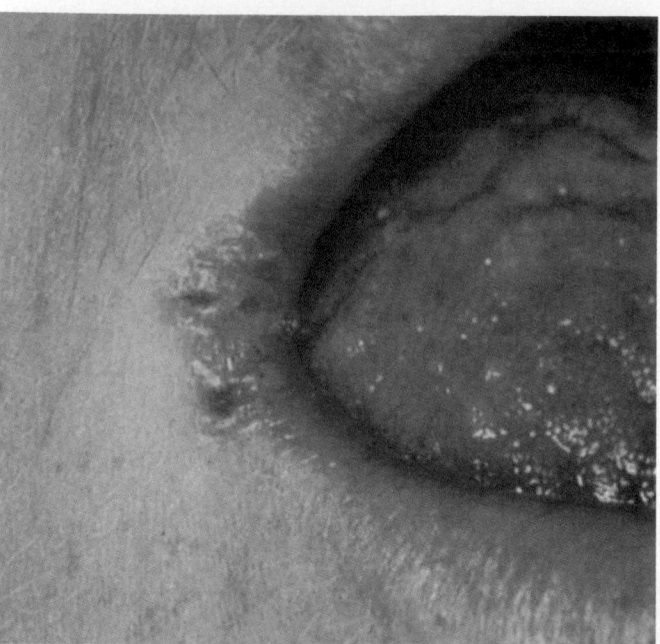

Fig. 54.4 Angular cheilitis.

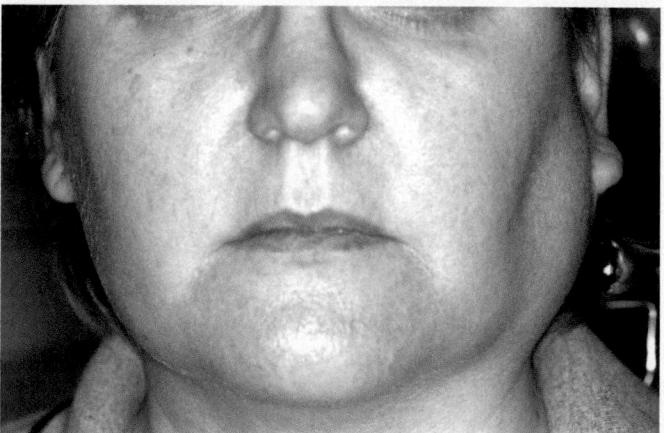

Fig. 54.5 Parotid enlargement.

circulating immune complexes, or mononuclear inflammatory vasculopathy, which is not usually associated with seroreactivity and hypocomplementemia. Vasculitic lesions may also have the appearance of urticaria, erythema multiforme, erythematous macules, patches, or nodules, and digital ulcers. The presence of erythema nodosum should raise the suspicion of sarcoidosis.

NEUROLOGICAL FEATURES

Peripheral neuropathy occurs in about 20% of patients with SS and is most prominent in the lower limbs, and to a lesser extent the upper limbs.[22] It is most often sensory. Trigeminal and other dermatomal involvement may occur. Autonomic neuropathy may occur, and should be considered in patients with symptoms such as unexplained postural hypotension. In addition, involvement of the central nervous system has been described, and lesions have been noted in imaging studies. Peripheral neuropathy tends to be associated with vasculitis, although it may occur in the absence of vasculitis.

HEMATOLOGICAL FEATURES

Lymphoid malignancy is an important hematologic complication of SS. Amongst the rheumatic autoimmune diseases, SS has the highest frequency of B-cell lymphomas.[2, 13] Reported frequencies have varied. The early report of a 44-fold increase in the frequency of B-cell lymphomas among SS patients compared to the general population was not population-based. Subsequent estimates were lower;[3] Theander et al. found about a 16-fold increased risk.[2] While as many as 10% of patients with SS may develop malignant lymphoma, a multicenter European study showed lymphoma in 4.3% of SS patients; these were mostly low-grade B cell lymphoma of the mucosa-associated lymphoid tissue (MALT) type.[2, 13]

What are the risk factors for the development of B-cell lymphomas in SS? A low CD4/CD8 T-lymphocyte ratio was recently reported as a risk factor in a longitudinal population-based study.[2] This increased risk of developing lymphoma in that study was only seen in patients who met the American European classification criteria for SS,[2] requiring either tissue inflammation or autoantibodies (anti-Ro/SSA or La/SSB). This illustrates the importance of case definition and subject selection in the interpretation of epidemiological studies of the risk factors for SS. Purpura or skin vasculitis and low C3 and low C4 were also risk factors in that study.[2] Others have suggested that parotid enlargement, lymphadenopathy, and splenomegaly are risk factors for the development of lymphoma. Although indolent MALT lymphomas are more often reported in SS, Theander et al. found that 58% had high-grade, diffuse, large B-cell lymphomas.[2]

Often cervical lymph nodes and salivary glands are involved. Although nonmalignant glandular swelling with reactive changes occurs more often, malignancy should be ruled out in patients with significantly or prominently swollen salivary glands or nodes in the neck. Diagnostic imaging, such as computed tomographic scans, needle aspirates for cytological and flow cytometric analyses, or biopsy should be considered.

RESPIRATORY FEATURES

Most patients with SS who have pulmonary involvement do not develop progressive disease.[23] Those who do may require more aggressive treatment with immunosuppressive agents such as azathioprine. Dry cough is not uncommon and is probably related to tracheal dryness and diminished mucus production.[24] The cough may also reflect hyperreactive airways in both primary and secondary SS. Smaller airways may be obstructed with minor abnormalities in pulmonary function tests, and lymphocytic infiltrates may be observed in bronchiolar walls. Mucosal biopsies and bronchoalveolar lavage show increased submucosal CD4 T lymphocytes. Interstitial pulmonary disease that is generally mild and rheumatoid-like pulmonary nodules may occur in SS. Metastatic carcinoma, granulomatous lesions, such as sarcoidosis, and other causes should be considered in the differential diagnosis and follow-up of such

THERAPEUTIC PRINCIPLES

TREATMENT OF SJÖGREN'S SYNDROME

>> Sicca symptoms may be ameliorated by decreasing loss of moisture by evaporative loss from body surfaces (such as by using viscous artificial tears), coating dry surfaces with liquid (artificial saliva and tears), and stimulating existing exocrine tissue to increase secretions (muscarinic M3 agonists, such as pilocarpine and cevimeline)

>> Local inflammation of the ocular surface can be treated with anti-inflammatory substances such as topical cyclosporine

>> Systemic inflammation of SS is generally treated in a similar manner to systemic lupus erythematosus. Most commonly hydroxychloroquine and nonsteroidal anti-inflammatory drugs are used. In more severe cases, particularly with arthritis, various disease-modifying antirheumatic drugs, such as methotrexate, azathioprine, and other agents may be used. In the most severe cases brief treatment with glucocorticoids and in some cases cytotoxic agents (such as cyclophosphamide) may be used, such as in cases of life-threatening vasculitis

>> Tumor necrosis factor blockers are best avoided as they do not appear to benefit patients with SS

nodules. Sarcoidosis manifestations include hilar adenopathy, elevated angiotensin-converting enzyme levels, and granulomatous lesions on salivary gland biopsy. Pleural effusions may be noted in primary SS, and may contain antibodies to SS-A, SS-B, and increased lymphocyte counts.

UROGENITAL FEATURES

Irritable bladder symptoms, including urinary frequency, are not uncommon.[25, 26] Urinary frequency may also be caused by drinking excessive fluid to alleviate oral dryness. Renal manifestations include decreased ability to concentrate urine in about half of the cases, distal renal tubular acidosis in about 15%, nephrocalcinosis, renal stones and, less frequently, interstitial nephritis and glomerular disease. Urine pH is generally above 5.5 in renal tubular acidosis and the disorder is associated with systemic acidosis, which results in mobilization of calcium from bone, promoting osteoporosis and resulting in hypercalciuria. In addition, urinary citrate, which normally complexes a substantial proportion of urine calcium, is low. The risk of calcium phosphate stones is increased. Tubular proteinuria occurs in about half the SS cases. Glomerular disease occurs in about 2% of patients, especially in those with longer disease duration, and tends to be associated with cryoglobulins.[26] Patients with glomerulonephritis tend to have mixed cryoglobulinemia and low C4 levels in the serum.

Women with SS often have symptoms of vaginal dryness, which is commonly associated with dyspareunia.[27] Vaginal dryness may be the initial presenting symptom of SS. Obstetric complications in SS, including the risks of prematurity, pre-eclampsia, intrauterine growth retardation, and fetal loss, tend to be related to concomitant autoimmune disease, mostly SLE. However, these problems do not appear to be increased in primary SS.[27] Since anti-SSA (Ro) antibodies occur in SS, there is a risk of congenital heart block, although the frequency is low.

THYROID

Thyroid disease, particularly hypothyroidism, is common in SS patients.[28] This has led to the impression that autoimmune thyroiditis may be a manifestation of SS. However, evidence for a convincing association is lacking. Ramos-Casals and coworkers found no significant differences in the prevalence of thyroid disease in SS patients compared with individuals of similar age and gender.[28]

LABORATORY FEATURES

SS is frequently associated with positive tests for rheumatoid factor (90%), anti-Ro/SSA or anti-La/SSB (50–90%), and hypergammaglobulinemia.[20] Antinuclear antibodies occur in about 80% of cases. The 52-kDa Ro is more often associated with SS, while 60-kDa Ro appears to be more frequent in SLE. Autoantibodies that precipitate Ro/SSA are associated with systemic manifestations of the disease, including anemia, leukopenia, thrombocytopenia, purpura, cryoglobulinemia, hypocomplementemia, lymphadenopathy, and vasculitis.

Other autoantibodies occur in SS, including those directed against carbonic anhydrase, pancreatic antigen, α fodrin, 97-kDa Golgi complex, mitotic spindle apparatus, M3 muscarinic acetylcholine receptors, Fcγ receptors, and centromeres.[20] However, these autoantibody specificities are currently not used in the diagnosis and monitoring of the disease.

■ TREATMENT OF SJÖGREN'S SYNDROME ■

A general approach to SS is to educate patients on the disease and how best to cope with it, and to treat sicca symptoms and inflammatory manifestations. The treatment of sicca symptoms involves minimizing the loss of moisture from body surfaces, covering dry surfaces with liquid, as in the sipping of fluids and use of eye drops, and stimulation of existing secretory tissue with secretogogues, such as pilocarpine or cevimeline. The treatment of inflammation involves the use of drugs such as hydroxychloroquine, corticosteroids, methotrexate, azathioprine, and other immunomodulatory or immunosuppressive drugs.

PATIENT EDUCATION AND SELF-CARE

As in any chronic disease, it is important to help the patient develop strategies for self-management and coping with physical, mental, and social challenges associated with the condition. Patient education on the manifestations, course, prognosis, complications, and treatment of the disease and actions that they make take to minimize complications are extremely important.[20] Since there is often a lag of years before the diagnosis is made, acknowledging the patient's concerns is important.

SICCA SYMPTOMS

Keratoconjunctivitis sicca

Treatment includes tear replacement and conservation, and topical ocular and systemic medications.[29] Artificial tear eye drops are cellulose derivatives and are used frequently for symptoms of dry eyes. Since preservatives can irritate or damage the ocular surface and cause allergies, they are best avoided. Artificial tears in small individual dispensers lessen infections from bacterial contamination. Also, to reduce the risk of infection, patients should avoid rubbing the eyes and rinsing the ocular surface with tap water.

When artificial tears are insufficient to control symptoms, hydroxypropylcellulose pellets can be placed under the lower eyelids. Artificial tears are used to dissolve the pellets, which retain moisture in the eye. Ointments, which decrease evaporative tear loss, are used during the night, as these viscous materials may interfere with vision. Artificial tears can leave crusts on the eyelashes, and ointments may potentially obstruct meibomian glands. By washing eyelashes with baby shampoo, the development of blepharitis can be prevented or treated. Topical steroids, cyclosporine eyedrops, and intraocular androgens may be beneficial in the treatment of KCS. Evidence suggests that intraocular androgens may have a role in treating ocular inflammation and dryness. Systemic pilocarpine appears to improve ocular symptoms, and cevimeline has been approved for this indication. The role of systemic treatment for ocular inflammation of SS remains unclear.

When dry-eye symptoms are unresponsive to the above approaches, punctal plugs can be used. Collagen plugs dissolve over 2 days. Silicon plugs last longer and can be taken out if they result in epiphora. If the use of temporary punctal plugs improves the ocular surface without excessive tears, permanent occlusion can be achieved by punctal cautery.

Xerostomia

Frequent dental care is important.[19] Daily topical fluoride use and antimicrobial mouth rinses may help to prevent caries in patients with reduced salivary flow. Medications that promote oral dryness may be exchanged for more appropriate ones. Artificial saliva and lubricants may ameliorate symptoms in some patients. Sugar-free chewing gum or candies may stimulate residual salivary secretions to ameliorate oral dryness. Patients should be counseled on an appropriate diet and the importance of limiting sugar intake. Humidifiers may decrease sicca symptoms. Problems with swallowing may be treated with oral moisturizers and lubricants, and through dietary modifications.

Secretagogues such as pilocarpine and cevimeline may enhance secretions in patients with sufficient exocrine tissue.[30] Usually, pilocarpine 5 mg orally four times a day is given, and the total daily dose does not generally exceed 30 mg. Adverse effects include increased sweating, feeling hot and flushed, as well as symptoms associated with increased bowel and bladder motility. When bronchspasm is present, caution must be exercised. Patients with adverse effects may benefit from one to three 5 mg doses per day at times to ameliorate symptoms at the most troublesome time of day. Cevimeline can also be used to treat dry mouth in a dosage of 30 mg orally three times daily. It is a muscarinic agonist similar to pilocarpine that enhances production of saliva, and possibly tears and other secretions. Cevimeline is contraindicated for patients with uncontrolled asthma, iritis, and narrow-angle glaucoma.

Oral candidiasis, a common complication of dry mouth in SS, is treated by sucking oral troches or vaginal suppositories of antifungal agents, such as nystatin or clotrimazole. Angular cheilitis may require topical antifungal agents.[19] Bacterial parotitis should be treated with warm compresses, massage of the parotid gland, and, if necessary, antibiotics.

The exocrine or systemic inflammatory manifestations may be treated by various immunomodulatory drugs. Hydroxychloroquine is commonly used for milder systemic manifestations, such as rashes and arthritis. Whether or not hydroxychloroquine is effective for the exocrine manifestations is unclear, although serological measures improve in SS patients on this medication.[31, 32] Drugs such as methotrexate, prednisone, azathioprine, and other immunomodulatory drugs tend to be used in patients with prominent systemic manifestations in an approach similar to that used to treat SLE.[31, 33] However, few randomized, double-blind clinical trials have been performed to demonstrate whether or not these agents are beneficial in SS. Small underpowered, randomized, controlled trials of prednisone and azathioprine showed no benefit.[31, 33] Despite the initial results of an uncontrolled trial of infliximab, subsequent investigations revealed no evidence that TNF-α blockade has any benefit in SS.[34]

ORGAN INVOLVEMENT

Special attention is needed in the treatment of certain organ complications in SS. In patients with renal tubular acidosis, treatment with oral alkaline preparations containing sodium and potassium citrate in a dose of 1–2 mEq/kg per day is used to correct the acidosis and decrease the risk of stones. In addition, the urine calcium should be monitored and patients should receive potassium supplementation. Patients with renal tubular acidosis have increased mobilization of calcium from bone, which requires appropriate monitoring and treatment. Bronchodilators may be useful in patients with chronic cough, since SS is associated with increased airways reactivity. The management of thyroid disorders in SS patients is no different from that for those without the disease.[28] The arthritis of SS tends to respond well to standard treatments for rheumatoid arthritis. Cutaneous dryness is treated with lubricants and decreased frequency of bathing. Pruritus may be treated with mentholated lotions. Superficial vasculitis and dermatitis are managed with steroids. Vaginal dryness and dyspareunia may respond to water-soluble lubricants, and vaginal estrogen preparations may be beneficial in postmenopausal females.

■ FUTURE TREATMENTS ■

While advances continue in our understanding of SS, only symptomatic treatments have been specifically approved for the treatment of this debilitating disorder. Immunomodulatory treatments, replacement of destroyed salivary gland tissue by artificial salivary glands, and the possibilities for gene therapies are under active investigation.

Currently, there is great interest in a number of immunomodulatory treatments for SS.[35] Approaches specifically targeting B cells are the most active area. Candidate therapies include anti-CD20, anti-CD22, and anti BLyS antibodies. Rituximab, an anti-CD20 antibody, has been investigated in autoimmune diseases, including rheumatoid arthritis, SLE, and SS. A number of SS cases treated with rituximab have been reported and studies are currently in progress. Although rituximab has not been approved for the treatment of SS, apparently some clinicians are already treating patients with severe SS with this drug, but the results of sufficiently large double-blinded, randomized, controlled trials are lacking.

Despite the lack of success with TNF-α blockers, antagonism of various cytokines, such as IL-6 and IFNs has the potential to emerge as new therapies for SS within the next decade. Given the observation that patients with SS display a type I IFN signature, it is possible that blockade of type 1 IFN might be explored for the treatment of SS.[10]

It is also possible that IFN-γ antagonists may have a role in the treatment of the disease. Apoptotic epithelial cells may release material containing RNA-binding proteins, such as Ro/SSA.[10] If a way can be found to slow the rate of epithelial apoptosis in SS, this could theoretically be an approach to treatment. There is evidence that immune complexes containing Ro/SSA-anti-Ro/SSA are formed in SS, and can bind to Fc receptors on plasmacytoid dendritic cells, become internalized, and activate TLRs.[10] It is therefore possible that blockade of Fc receptors, or TLR could be an approach toward controlling the disease. In addition, the modulation or destruction of dendritic cells and T cells may be considered as a novel therapeutic strategy. Modulation of cell traffic by targeting integrins and selectins is another possible approach for future treatment. Bone marrow transplantation may be discussed as a means to remove autoreactive cells and reconstitute a normal immune system.

Work continues on the development of adeno-associated virus (AAV) vectors for gene therapy.[35] Experiments have been conducted using cytokine genes in AAV vectors in animal models of SS. Aquaporins, particularly aquaporin 5, which transports water through salivary and lacrimal epithelial cells, may have a role in the pathogenesis of SS. It is possible that viral vectors containing aquaporins may be considered in the future as an intraductal treatment directed toward increasing the capacity for water transport in residual epithelial cells.

Hormonal therapies are also under consideration. Androgens and various estrogens have been investigated as interventions in animal models of SS.

Work studying the differentiation of glandular epithelial cells also continues. Possibly, bone marrow cells may be capable of differentiating into glandular epithelial cells. This may present a future therapeutic opportunity in which precursor cells might be induced to reconstitute damage to epithelial tissue. Finally, research continues in the area of tissue engineering, exploring whether salivary or lacrimal glands can be grown in vitro and implanted to facilitate the production of secretions.

■ REFERENCES ■

1. Tapinos NI, Polihronis M, Tzioufas AG, et al. Sjögren's syndrome. Autoimmune epithelitis. Adv Exp Med Biol 1999; 455: 127–134.

2. Theander E, Henriksson G, Ljungberg O, et al. Lymphoma and other malignancies in primary Sjögren's syndrome: a cohort study on cancer incidence and lymphoma predictors. Ann Rheum Dis 2006; 65: 796–803.

3. Pillemer SR, Matteson EL, Jacobsson LT, et al. Incidence of physician-diagnosed primary Sjögren syndrome in residents of Olmsted County, Minnesota. Mayo Clin Proc 2001; 76: 593–599.

4. Bowman SJ, Ibrahim GH, Holmes G, et al. Estimating the prevalence among Caucasian women of primary Sjögren's syndrome in two general practices in Birmingham UK. Scand J Rheumatol 2004; 33: 39–43.

5. Anaya JM, Talal N. Sjögren's syndrome comes of age [editorial] [see comments]. Semin Arthritis Rheum 1999; 28: 355–359.

6. Martens PB, Pillemer SR, Jacobsson LT, et al. Survivorship in a population based cohort of patients with Sjögren's syndrome, 1976–1992. J Rheumatol 1999; 26: 1296–1300.

7. Vitali C, Bombardieri S, Moutsopoulos HM, et al. Preliminary criteria for the classification of Sjögren's syndrome. Results of a prospective concerted action supported by the European Community. Arthritis Rheum 1993; 36: 340–347.

8. Bloch KJ, Buchanan WW, Wohl MJ, et al. Sjögren's syndrome. A clinical, pathological, and serological study of sixty-two cases.1965.. Medicine (Baltimore) 1992; 71: 386–401.

9. Bolstad AI, Jonsson R. Genetic aspects of Sjögren's syndrome. Arthritis Res 2002; 4: 353–359.

10. Lovgren T, Eloranta ML, Kastner B, et al. Induction of interferon-alpha by immune complexes or liposomes containing systemic lupus erythematosus autoantigen- and Sjögren's syndrome autoantigen-associated RNA. Arthritis Rheum 2006; 54: 1917–1927.

11. Venables PJ, Rigby SP. Viruses in the etiopathogenesis of Sjögren's syndrome. J Rheumatol 1997; 24(Suppl 50): 3–5.

12. Triantafyllopoulou A, Tapinos N, Moutsopoulos HM. Evidence for coxsackievirus infection in primary Sjögren's syndrome. Arthritis Rheum 2004; 50: 2897–2902.

13. Pillemer SR. Lymphoma and other malignancies in primary Sjögren's syndrome. Ann Rheum Dis 2006; 65: 704–706.

14. Johnson EO, Vlachoyiannopoulos PG, Skopouli FN, et al. Hypofunction of the stress axis in Sjögren's syndrome. J Rheumatol 1998; 25: 1508–1514.

15. Fox RI, Tornwall J, Michelson P. Current issues in the diagnosis and treatment of Sjögren's syndrome. Curr Opin Rheumatol 1999; 11: 364–371.

16. Waterman SA, Gordon TP, Rischmueller M. Inhibitory effects of muscarinic receptor autoantibodies on parasympathetic neurotransmission in Sjögren's syndrome. Arthritis Rheum 2000; 43: 1647–1654.

17. Masaki Y, Sugai S. Lymphoproliferative disorders in Sjögren's syndrome. Autoimmun Rev 2004; 3: 175–182.

18. Pflugfelder SC. Advances in the diagnosis and management of keratoconjunctivitis sicca. Curr Opin Ophthalmol 1998; 9: 50–53.

19. Atkinson JC, Wu AJ. Salivary gland dysfunction: causes, symptoms, treatment. J Am Dent Assoc 1994; 125: 409–416.

20. Bell M, Askari A, Bookman A, et al. Sjögren's syndrome: a critical review of clinical management [published erratum appears in J Rheumatol 1999;26: 2718]. J Rheumatol 1999; 26: 2051–2061.

21. Provost TT, Watson R. Cutaneous manifestations of Sjögren's syndrome. Rheum Dis Clin North Am 1992; 18: 609–616.

22. Morgen K, McFarland HF, Pillemer SR. Central nervous system disease in primary Sjögren's syndrome: the role of magnetic resonance imaging. Semin Arthritis Rheum 2004; 34: 623–630.

23. Davidson BK, Kelly CA, Griffiths ID. Ten year follow up of pulmonary function in patients with primary Sjögren's syndrome. Ann Rheum Dis 2000; 59: 709–712.

24. Cain HC, Noble PW, Matthay RA. Pulmonary manifestations of Sjögren's syndrome. Clin Chest Med 1998; 19: 687–699, viii.

25. Viergever PP, Swaak TJ. Renal tubular dysfunction in primary Sjögren's syndrome: clinical studies in 27 patients. Clin Rheumatol 1991; 10: 23–27.

26. Goules A, Masouridi S, Tzioufas AG, et al. Clinically significant and biopsy-documented renal involvement in primary Sjögren syndrome. Medicine (Baltimore) 2000; 79: 241–249.

27. Skopouli FN, Papanikolaou S, Malamou-Mitsi V, et al. Obstetric and gynaecological profile in patients with primary Sjögren's syndrome. Ann Rheum Dis 1994; 53: 569–573.

28. Ramos-Casals M, Garcia-Carrasco M, Cervera R, et al. Thyroid disease in primary Sjögren syndrome. Study in a series of 160 patients. Medicine (Baltimore) 2000; 79: 103–108.

29. Pflugfelder SC, Solomon A, Stern ME. The diagnosis and management of dry eye: a twenty-five-year review. Cornea 2000; 19: 644–649.

30. Vivino FB, Al Hashimi I, Khan Z, et al. Pilocarpine tablets for the treatment of dry mouth and dry eye symptoms in patients with Sjögren syndrome: a randomized, placebo-controlled, fixed-dose, multicenter trial. P92-01 Study Group. Arch Intern Med 1999; 159: 174–181.

31. Oxholm P, Prause JU, Schiodt M. Rational drug therapy recommendations for the treatment of patients with Sjögren's syndrome. Drugs 1998; 56: 345–353.

32. Kruize AA, Hene RJ, Kallenberg CG, et al. Hydroxychloroquine treatment for primary Sjögren's syndrome: a two year double blind crossover trial. Ann Rheum Dis 1993; 52: 360–364.

33. Price EJ, Rigby SP, Clancy U, et al. A double blind placebo controlled trial of azathioprine in the treatment of primary Sjögren's syndrome. J Rheumatol 1998; 25: 896–899.

34. Mariette X, Ravaud P, Steinfeld S, et al. Inefficacy of infliximab in primary Sjögren's syndrome: results of the randomized, controlled Trial of Remicade in Primary Sjögren's Syndrome (TRIPSS). Arthritis Rheum 2004; 50: 1270–1276.

35. Lodde BM, Baum BJ, Tak P, et al. Experience with experimental biological treatment and local gene therapy of Sjögren's syndrome: implications for exocrine pathogenesis and treatment. Ann Rheum Dis. 2006 Jul 31; 65: 1406–1416.

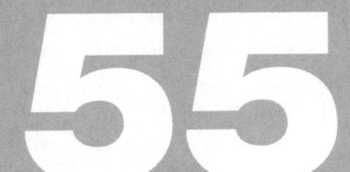

Systemic sclerosis

John Varga, Fredrick M. Wigley

Systemic sclerosis (SSc) is a chronic multisystem connective tissue disease characterized by autoimmunity and inflammation, widespread functional and structural abnormalities in small blood vessels, and progressive fibrosis of the skin and visceral organs. Multiple cell types and their products interact to mediate the pathogenetic processes that underlie the diverse clinical manifestations of SSc.

PREVALENCE AND EPIDEMIOLOGY

Systemic sclerosis is a sporadic disease with worldwide distribution. Incidence estimates in the USA range from nine to 19 cases per million per year, and prevalence rates range from 28 to 253 cases per million. The only community-based survey of SSc yielded a prevalence of 286 cases per million population.[1] Age, gender and ethnicity are important factors determining disease susceptibility.[2] Like other connective tissue diseases, SSc is more prevalent in women, with the most common age of onset in the age range 30–50 years. The incidence of SSc is higher among African-Americans than in whites, and disease onset occurs at an earlier age. Furthermore, African-Americans are more likely to have diffuse skin involvement and pulmonary fibrosis, and to have a worse prognosis.

ETIOLOGY AND PATHOGENESIS

GENETIC FACTORS

Systemic sclerosis is not inherited in a mendelian fashion. Monozygotic and dizygotic twin pairs show a similarly low rate (<5%) of disease concordance.[3] Nonetheless, 1.6% of SSc patients have a first-degree relative with the disease, representing a relative risk of 13, indicating an important role for genetic background in disease susceptibility. In contrast to other connective tissue diseases, HLA linkages with SSc are weak, although specific HLA haplotypes do associate with distinct autoantibody responses. Genetic investigations in SSc have focused primarily on polymorphisms of candidate genes. Weak associations of specific single nucleotide polymorphisms (SNP) have been reported in genes involved in regulation of immunity and inflammation, vascular function, and connective tissue homeostasis.[4]

ENVIRONMENTAL FACTORS

Viruses and exposure to environmental and occupational agents and drugs have been implicated as potential etiologic factors. There are reports that patients with SSc have increased serum antibodies to human cytomegalovirus (hCMV). Furthermore, a study suggests that in a subset of SSc patients autoantibodies to topoisomerase-I recognize antigenic epitopes present on hCMV-derived proteins, providing some evidence that molecular mimicry may be a mechanistic link between hCMV infection and SSc. Evidence of human parvovirus B19 infection has also been presented. These studies need to be confirmed, and the etiologic role of virus in SSc remains conjectural. Although reports of apparent geographic clustering of SSc cases suggest shared environmental exposures, careful investigations have failed to substantiate these clusters. Epidemics of multisystem illnesses with features suggestive of SSc have been linked to contaminated rapeseed cooking oils in Spain (the toxic oil syndrome), and L-tryptophan dietary supplements in the USA (eosinophilia–myalgia syndrome). Although both of these apparently novel syndromes were characterized by chronic scleroderma-like skin induration, they showed clinical and pathological features clearly that distinguished them from SSc. An increased incidence of SSc has been noted among men with occupational exposure to silica, such as miners. Other occupational exposures linked with an increased risk of SSc include polyvinyl chloride, trichloroethylene and organic solvents. Drugs potentially implicated in SSc-like illnesses include bleomycin, pentazocine and cocaine, and appetite suppressants associated with pulmonary hypertension. The occurrence of SSc in women with silicone breast implants raised concern regarding a possible association, but careful subsequent epidemiologic investigations could not substantiate an increased risk.[5]

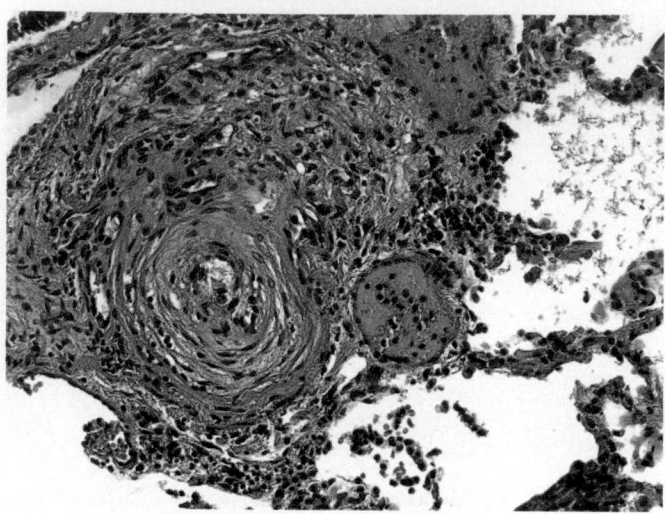

Fig. 55.1 Pulmonary arterial involvement. Significant intimal layer hyperplasia is seen, leading to narrowing of the vascular lumen. (Courtesy of Dr Anjana Yeldandi.)

PATHOLOGY

The characteristic pathological features of SSc are a noninflammatory vasculopathy involving small arteries and arterioles in multiple vascular beds and fibrosis of the skin and internal organs. Although patients with established SSc display pathological changes in the absence of inflammation, in relatively early-stage disease cellular infiltrates may be found in many organs. In the skin, the infiltrates are located predominantly around blood vessels and in the reticular dermis, and are composed primarily of CD4 T lymphocytes.

Vascular injury is likely to be the initial event in the pathogenesis of SSc. In patients with established SSc, widespread vascular lesions are found and are characterized by bland intimal proliferation in the small and medium-sized arteries. The heart, lungs, kidneys and intestinal tract are most prominently affected (Fig. 55.1). Vasculitic lesions are virtually never found. In late stages, perivascular fibrosis may be prominent.

Fibrosis is prominent in the skin, lungs, gastrointestinal tract, heart, tendon sheaths and perifascicular tissue surrounding skeletal muscle. Accumulation of homogeneous connective tissue composed of type I collagen, fibronectin, proteoglycans and other structural macromolecules in these organs leads to progressive disruption of tissue architecture, resulting in functional impairment. In the skin, fibrosis causes massive dermal expansion and obliteration of hair follicles, sweat glands and other skin appendages. Collagen fiber accumulation is prominent in the reticular dermis, and the process invades the subjacent adipose layer with entrapment of fat cells. In the lungs, patchy infiltration of the alveolar walls with lymphocytes, plasma cells, macrophages and eosinophils is seen in early disease. With established disease, fibrosis and vascular damage predominate, often coexisting in the same lesions. However, in patients with limited cutaneous SSc the vascular lesions may predominate. Intimal thickening of the pulmonary arteries, best seen with elastin stain, underlies pulmonary hypertension, and at autopsy is often associated with multiple pulmonary emboli and myocardial fibrosis.

Pulmonary fibrosis is characterized by expansion of the alveolar interstitium, with local accumulation of collagen and other connective tissue

proteins. Progressive thickening of the alveolar septa results in obliteration of the air spaces and honeycombing, and loss of pulmonary blood vessels. This process impairs gas exchange and contributes to worsening of pulmonary hypertension. In the gastrointestinal tract, prominent pathological changes can occur at any level from the mouth to the rectum. The esophagus is frequently involved, with fibrosis of the lamina propria, submucosa and muscular layers, and the development of characteristic vascular lesions. Replacement of the normal intestinal architecture results in disordered peristaltic activity, with gastroesophageal reflux and small bowel dysmotility, obstruction and bacterial overgrowth. Chronic gastroesophageal reflux leads to esophageal inflammation, ulcerations and stricture formation, and premalignant Barrett's metaplasia.

The heart is frequently affected, with prominent myocardial contraction band necrosis reflecting ischemia–reperfusion injury, and patchy areas of myocardial fibrosis. In the kidneys vascular lesions predominate, and glomerulonephritis is rare. Chronic renal ischemia is associated with shrunken glomeruli. Patients with scleroderma renal crisis show dramatic changes in small renal arteries, with reduplication of elastic lamina, marked intimal proliferation and narrowing of the lumen, often with microangiopathic hemolysis.

PATHOGENESIS

An integrated picture of the complex pathogenesis of SSc must account for the vasculopathy, deregulated cellular and humoral immunity, and fibrosis of multiple organs. As illustrated in Figure 55.2, a complex and incompletely understood interplay between these distinct processes initiates, amplifies and sustains tissue damage in SSc.[6]

Vascular involvement

It is currently thought that vascular injury may be the initiating event in the pathogenesis of SSc. Evidence of vascular involvement is an early and widespread feature, with important clinical consequences. Vascular endothelial cell injury is initially associated with functional alterations, with altered blood flow response to vasomotor or cold challenge, and altered production of and responsiveness to factors that mediate vasodilatation (nitric oxide and prostacyclins) and vasoconstriction (endothelins). Microvessels show increased permeability, enhanced transendothelial leukocyte migration, activation of fibrinolytic cascades and platelet aggregation culminating in thrombosis. Endothelial cells show increased expression of surface adhesion molecules and release endothelin-1, which further promotes leukocyte adhesion and smooth muscle cell proliferation. Ensuing intimal and medial hypertrophy and fibrosis of the adventitial layer leads to luminal narrowing. Combined with endothelial cell apoptosis, the process culminates in the characteristic striking absence of blood vessels seen on angiograms of the hands and kidneys of SSc patients with late-stage disease. In addition, the process of revascularization appears to be defective in SSc, possibly due to a defect in bone marrow-derived CD34+ circulating endothelial progenitor cells.[7]

Cellular and humoral immune responses

In the early stages of SSc, activated T cells and macrophages accumulate in skin and lung lesions, where they secrete important mediators, including transforming growth factor-β (TGF-β), cytokines and chemokines. These molecules can activate fibroblasts as well as endothelial

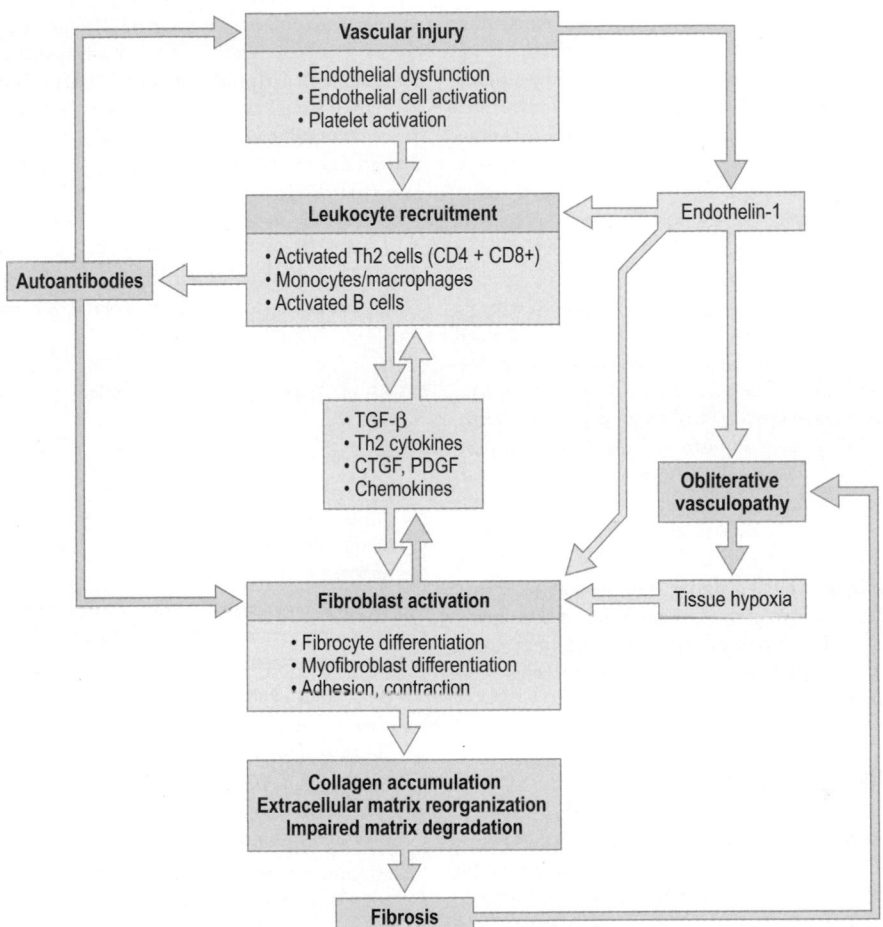

Fig. 55.2 Pathogenesis: fibrosis. Schema illustrating the interactions of cellular and molecular events involved in the pathogenesis of vascular and immune dysfunction resulting in fibrosis associated with systemic sclerosis.

cells, and initiate the fibrotic response. Because TGF-β in particular can induce its own production, as well as that of other growth factors such as connective tissue growth factor (CTGF), initial cytokine secretion associated with inflammation can result in sustained and amplified cytokine production and autocrine and paracrine signaling. The levels of TGF-β are elevated in the skin and lungs of patients with SSc, and receptors for TGF-β are over-expressed on lesional fibroblasts.

Virtually all patients with SSc have serum autoantibodies that are highly specific and mutually exclusive (see below). These SSc-specific autoantibodies show a strong association with individual disease phenotypes, and their titers may fluctuate with disease activity. Multiple mechanism(s) have been proposed to account for autoantibody generation in SSc. B cells from SSc patients are hyperresponsive.[8] Additionally, it has been proposed that in SSc, specific self-antigens undergo post-translational modifications such as proteolytic cleavage, increased expression or altered subcellular localization that result in their recognition as nonself by the immune system. Although SSc-associated autoantibodies have well-established clinical utility as diagnostic markers, their contributions to disease manifestations remain uncertain. Emerging evidence

indicates that antibodies to fibroblasts and endothelial cells, platelet-derived growth factor (PGDF) receptor, and matrix metalloproteinases may potentially play a direct role in the tissue damage of SSc.

Fibrosis: Cellular and molecular components

Interstitial and vascular fibrosis in multiple organs, the hallmark of SSc, is characterized by replacement of normal tissue architecture with dense connective tissue, and is responsible for substantial morbidity and mortality. Fibroblasts and related mesenchymal cells are key effectors of fibrosis. Under the influence of appropriate signals such as TGF-β, CTGF, chemokines, endothelin-1 and hypoxia, these cells proliferate, migrate, elaborate collagens and other matrix macromolecules, adhere to and remodel connective tissue, secrete growth factors and cytokines and express surface receptors for them, and undergo transdifferentiation into contractile myofibroblasts. Together, these biosynthetic, contractile and adhesive functions enable fibroblasts to mediate effective wound healing. Whereas under physiologic conditions the fibroblast repair program is self-limited, in pathological fibrotic responses fibroblast activation is sustained and amplified, resulting in exaggerated matrix accumulation and remodeling. Inappropriate fibroblast activation is the fundamental pathogenetic alteration underlying fibrosis in SSc. In addition to fibroblasts normally residing in tissues, bone marrow-derived mesenchymal progenitor cells also participate in the fibrotic response. For instance, peripheral blood mononuclear cells can differentiate into fibroblasts *in vitro*, and this process is enhanced by TGF-β. The factors that regulate mobilization of mesenchymal progenitor cells from the bone marrow remain largely unknown, including their trafficking to lesional tissue, and their *in situ* differentiation into matrix-producing adhesive and contractile fibroblasts.

Fibroblasts explanted from lesional SSc tissues display an abnormal phenotype indicative of autonomous activation characterized by enhanced synthesis of collagen and other extracellular matrix molecules, expression of α smooth muscle actin and cell surface adhesion molecules, and resistance to apoptosis. The activated scleroderma phenotype persists during the serial passage of lesional fibroblasts *in vitro*, and may be due, in part, to autocrine TGF-β signaling in these cells.[9] Abnormalities in TGF-β pathways have been noted in SSc: lesional fibroblasts secrete TGF-β and exhibit TGF-β hyper-responsiveness due to elevated TGF-β surface receptors and latent TGF-β activation. Furthermore, SSc fibroblasts show evidence of activated intracellular signal transduction pathways that may contribute to the persistence and progression of fibrogenic responses.[10] Targeted therapies that block TGF-β signaling and abrogate other fibrogenic pathways mediated by chemokines, endothelins and CTGF are under development.

CLINICAL FEATURES

Systemic sclerosis is highly variable in its clinical expression and thus represents a broad spectrum of disease. Whereas the disease process targets the skin, blood vessels, lungs, heart, gastrointestinal tract, kidneys and musculoskeletal system, subsets of patients exist with unique clinical features and distinct clinical outcomes. Raynaud's phenomenon is virtually universal in SSc, suggesting that perturbation of the terminal arteries of the circulation is a fundamental process that links the different subsets of the disease. Thickening of the skin distinguishes SSc from other rheumatic diseases (Table 55.1): scleroderma (hard skin) is the most specific and prominent physical finding. Patients vary in the expression of the skin changes, and are classified into two major subsets defined by the degree of clinically involved skin. In the diffuse skin variant called diffuse cutaneous SSc (dcSSc), fibrosis of the skin is widespread and the illness is more violent in expression, with rapid onset and an increased risk of serious and internal organ disease. In contrast, the limited skin variant called limited cutaneous SSc (lcSSc) presents with long-standing Raynaud's phenomenon, skin fibrosis limited to the fingers or distal limbs, and a generally indolent course. Limited SSc is less likely to be associated with organ failure or shortened life expectancy.

Although classification of SSc as diffuse and limited cutaneous is useful, disease expression is far more complex and several distinct phenotypes are recognized within each of the two subsets. For example, 10–15% of patients with lcSSc develop severe pulmonary arterial hypertension without significant lung fibrosis. Other patients develop systemic features of SSc without appreciable skin involvement, a phenotype that is termed systemic sclerosis sine scleroderma. Predictors of elevated mortality rates among SSc patients include diffuse skin disease and internal organ involvement, female gender, African-American race, and later age of disease onset.[11, 12] Unique clinical phenotypes of SSc associate with

specific autoantibodies (Table 55.2). For example, anticentromere antibodies associate with lcSSc, whereas anti-topoisomerase-I antibodies associate with early interstitial lung disease. Some patients with SSc have 'overlap' features, where SSc coexists with clinical and laboratory evidence of another autoimmune disease, such as polymyositis, autoimmune thyroid disease, Sjögren's syndrome, polyarthritis, autoimmune liver disease or systemic lupus erythematosus (Table 55.2).

In contrast to SSc, the term 'scleroderma' is now properly used to describe patients with localized disease, a group of related fibrosing skin disorders that primarily affect children (Table 55.2). Localized scleroderma is infrequently associated with significant systemic

---

Table 55.1 Classification of systemic sclerosis

Diffuse cutaneous scleroderma – skin thickening on the trunk in addition to the face, proximal and distal extremities

Limited cutaneous scleroderma – skin thickening limited distal to the elbow and knee; may also involve the face and neck

CREST syndrome (C, subcutaneous calcinosis; R, Raynaud's phenomenon; E, esophageal dysmotility; S, sclerodactyly; T, telangiectasis)

Sine scleroderma – no apparent skin thickening but characteristic visceral organ involvement, vascular and serologic features

Overlap syndrome – criteria for SSc, coexisting with features of systemic lupus erythematosus, rheumatoid arthritis or inflammatory muscle disease

Mixed connective tissue disease – overlap syndrome with anti-U1RNP antibodies

Early disease – Raynaud's phenomenon with clinical and/or laboratory features of SSc; specific autoantibodies, abnormal nailfold capillaroscopy, finger edema and ischemic injury

---

KEY CONCEPTS

CLINICAL SUBSETS OF SYSTEMIC SCLEROSIS

Limited cutaneous scleroderma

>> Distal skin sclerosis (sclerodactyly); trunk spared

>> Severe Raynaud's phenomenon with digital ischemia

>> Numerous telangiectasia

>> Isolated pulmonary arterial hypertension

Diffuse cutaneous scleroderma

>> Rapidly progressing widespread skin involvement

>> Scleroderma renal crisis

>> Interstitial lung disease

>> Severe gastrointestinal dysmotility

>> Cardiomyopathy

involvement. Morphea, a form of localized scleroderma, can occur as solitary or multiple lesions of expanding circular patches of thickened skin. Linear scleroderma presents as a streak of thickened skin, generally in one or both lower extremities. Linear scleroderma often involves the subcutaneous tissues, with fibrosis and atrophy of supporting structures, muscle and bone, and radiographs may show melorheostosis of the long bones. In children with linear scleroderma, the growth of affected long bones can be retarded. When the lesions cross joints, significant contractures of the affected joint can develop.

SYMPTOMS

Characteristically, the earliest symptoms of SSc are nonspecific and include fatigue, musculoskeletal distress (stiffness or pain) and feeling ill. Cold sensitivity and Raynaud's phenomenon occur early in the course and may be the only clinical clue. Symptoms of esophageal dysfunction with heartburn are common, and along with Raynaud's phenomenon may precede other manifestations of SSc by years. Visible capillary abnormalities at the nailfold (dilatation and loss or dropout of capillaries) are almost a universal finding in SSc, and precede other manifestations of the disease. An individual presenting with Raynaud's phenomenon, abnormal nailfold capillaries and the presence of a SSc-specific autoantibody can be diagnosed with SSc even before other manifestations are noted.[13]

DIFFUSE SSc

In general, patients with dcSSc have a short interval between Raynaud's phenomenon and the onset of other symptoms. Soft tissue swelling, intense pruritus and burning, and nonpitting edema are signs of the early inflammatory or 'edematous' phase of the diffuse cutaneous form of the disease. The skin of the fingers, hands, distal limbs and face are usually affected first, and more severely than other body areas (Fig. 55.3). Carpal

tunnel syndrome can be present as a consequence of soft tissue inflammation around the hands and wrists. Patients may note skin hyperpigmentation (patches or generalized tanning). Other early skin changes include vitiligo-like hypopigmentation ('salt and pepper' appearance), often on the chest or the back (Fig. 55.4). Escalating musculoskeletal symptoms are common, and are associated with muscle weakness and reduced joint mobility. Significant finger and hand/wrist disease limits the patient in performing simple chores or providing self-care.

The early edematous phase of dcSSc has prominent inflammatory features, with significant skin edema and erythema, and is associated with inflammatory cell infiltration in the dermis. After a period of weeks to months, the inflammatory phase evolves into the 'fibrotic' phase as the skin thickens, with thick folds on palpation and decreased skin flexibility. The fibrotic process starts in the dermis and is associated with loss of body hair, reduced production of skin oils, and a decline in sweating capacity as these cutaneous structures atrophy. Gradually the subcutaneous

CLINICAL PEARLS

CLINICAL FEATURES OF EARLY SYSTEMIC SCLEROSIS

>> Definite Raynaud's phenomenon
>> Gastroesophageal reflux with heartburn
>> Swelling of the fingers and hands
>> Musculoskeletal pain and stiffness
>> Dilated nailfold capillaries
>> Hyper- or hypopigmentary changes of the skin

Table 55.2 Autoantibody/phenotype association in SSc (From Harris ML, Rosen A. Autoimmunity in scleroderma: the origin, pathogenetic role, and clinical significance of autoantibodies. Curr Opin Rheumatol 2003; 15: 778–784, with permission)

Antigen	SSc Subtype	Clinical phenotype
Topoisomerase I (Scl-70)	Diffuse	Pulmonary fibrosis, cardiac involvement and cancer
RNA polymerase III	Diffuse	Severe skin involvement, renal crisis
Centromere proteins B, C	Limited (CREST)	Ischemic digital loss, sicca
U3-RNP (fibrillarin, Mpp 10, hU3-55K)	Diffuse or limited	Pulmonary arterial hypertension, cardiac and skeletal muscle involvement
B23	Diffuse or limited	Pulmonary arterial hypertension, Lung disease
Th/To-RNP	Limited	Lung disease, small bowel involvement, renal crisis
PM/Scl	Overlap	Myositis
U1-RNP	Overlap	SLE, myositis, polyarthritis

CREST, calcinosis; Raynaud's phenomenon, esophageal dysfunction, sclerodactyly, telangiectasia syndrome; RNP, ribonucleoprotein; SLE, systemic lupus erythematosus.

SYSTEMIC IMMUNE DISEASES

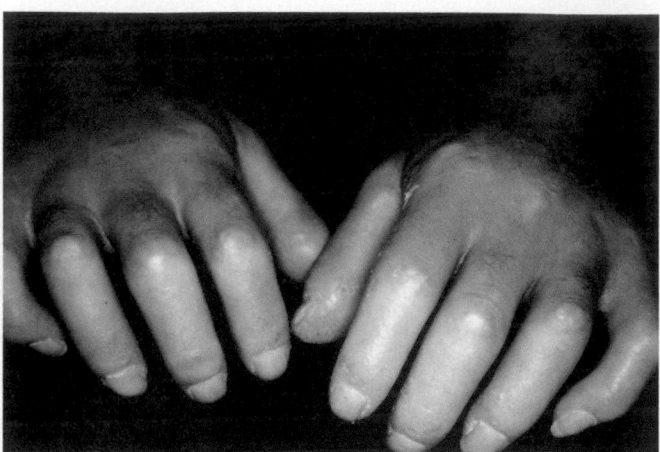

Fig. 55.3 Skin fibrosis in systemic sclerosis. Severe fibrosis of the skin of the hands and forearms causing joint contractures and skin ulcerations in a woman with diffuse cutaneous systemic sclerosis.

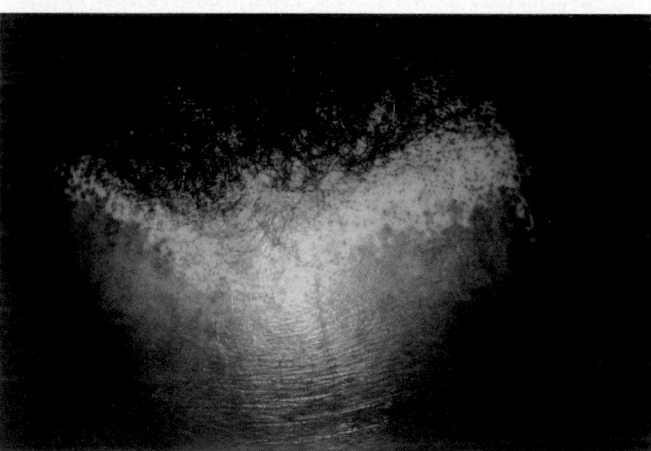

Fig. 55.4 Pigmentation changes in the skin. Vitiligo ('salt and pepper' appearance) of the involved skin in an African-American man with diffuse cutaneous systemic sclerosis.

tissue becomes affected, with atrophy of subcutaneous fat and fibrosis of underlying fascia, muscle and other soft tissue structures. During the fibrotic phase patients note pain, progressive loss of flexibility, distressing disfigurement and profound weight loss. Progressive flexion contractures of the fingers ensue. Other joints, including the wrist, elbow, shoulder, hip girdle, knees, and ankles, are also affected due to fibrosis of the supporting joint structures (Fig. 55.3). Thick ridges at the neck caused by firm adherence of the skin to the underlying platysma muscle interfere with neck extension. Tendon friction rub is a prominent crepitation that can be felt or even heard over tendons of the lower and upper extremity. Tendon friction rubs are due to fibrosis in the tissues surrounding the affected joints, and their presence is a marker of rapidly progressive and aggressive skin disease. Fibrosis of the skin of the face yields a characteristic facial appearance, with a diminished oral aperture, loss of facial expression,

vertical lines around the lips, loss of lip thickness and protrusion of the teeth. In the late stages of dcSSc involved skin may become thin or atrophic and bound down to underlying structures. Skin ulcerations often complicate the fibrotic, atrophic and avascular skin (Fig. 55.3).

The natural history of skin disease in SSc tends to be monophasic, and relapse after the edematous and active fibrotic phase is uncommon (<5%). The period from the first signs of skin involvement to its maximal extent is characteristically less than 3 years; cutaneous inflammation and progressive fibrosis gradually cease after 3 years, and the regression of skin involvement may occur. However, this timeframe is highly variable between patients, with many demonstrating rapid skin regression whereas others show chronically active disease over years. When the skin reaches its maximum involvement the skin disease appears to stop and dramatic recovery can occur, with a return to normal-appearing skin in those areas spared from severe end-stage fibrosis.

Whereas skin involvement is generally the most dramatic and visible manifestation of dcSSc, internal organ involvement occurs during the early active stage of advancing skin disease. Patients with dcSSc have a significant risk for interstitial lung disease, severe gastrointestinal dysfunction, SSc renal crisis, abrupt heart disease and recurrent digital ulcers during the active phases of the skin disease. In practical terms, this means that in dcSSc the initial 4 years is the period during which the systemic process is most active; if organ failure does not occur during this period, the systemic process may stabilize without further progression.

LIMITED CUTANEOUS SSc

The disease course in the limited cutaneous variant of SSc is more indolent and often relatively benign. After the onset of Raynaud's phenomenon, several years may pass before additional symptoms or signs are recognized. The most common non-Raynaud's symptoms in patients with lcSSc are those of upper gastrointestinal disease with dysphagia and gastroesophageal reflux. Dilated capillaries form visible erythematous vascular lesions (telangiectasia), seen most commonly on the fingertips, nailfold areas of the digit, palms, face, lips, and inside the oral cavity (Fig. 55.5). The CREST syndrome (subcutaneous calcinosis, Raynaud's phenomenon, esophageal dysfunction, sclerodactyly and telangiectasia) is a subtype of lcSSc with distinctive features, an overall good prognosis and associated with the presence of anticentromere antibodies. Subcutaneous calcinosis, due to deposition of calcium hydroxyapatite crystals, occurs commonly at sites of tissue ischemia and recurrent trauma, such as the fingertips, forearm or elbow.

Although significant internal organ disease occurs with lower frequency in patients with lcSSc, isolated pulmonary arterial hypertension (PAH) develops in 10–15% of patients and may be life-threatening.[14] Severe Raynaud's phenomenon with macrovascular occlusive involvement occurs more frequently in lcSSc than in dcSSc, and may be associated with critical digital ischemia, ischemic ulcerations, gangrene, and a need for amputation. Overlap with other autoimmune syndromes, including the sicca complex, polyarthritis, cutaneous vasculitis and autoimmune liver disease, such as biliary cirrhosis, is seen primarily in the lcSSc subset of SSc.

RAYNAUD'S PHENOMENON

The skin has a unique vascular architecture designed to help maintain a stable central body temperature. This system has superficial and deep vascular plexuses connected by arteriovenous shunts that allow shunting

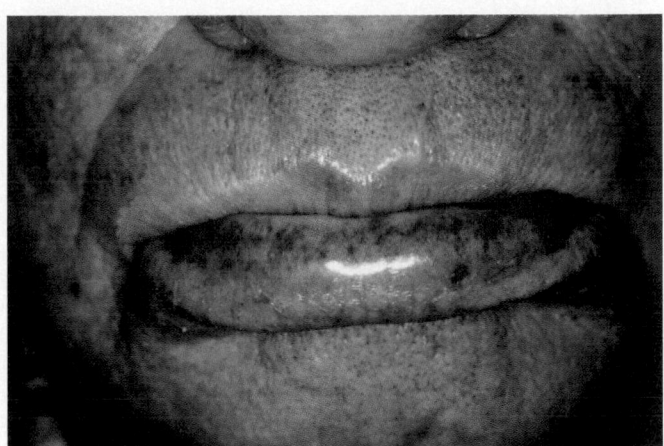

Fig. 55.5 Telangiectasia. Characteristic telangiectasia on the lip in a woman with limited cutaneous systemic sclerosis.

of blood away from the skin surface during exposure to cold. Temperature-activated receptor ion channels on the ends of unmyelinated nerve fibers located in the skin sense the ambient temperature and then send impulses to the dorsal root ganglion and the central nervous system. Following this input, efferent signals via the sympathetic nervous system directly determine vascular reactivity in the skin. Raynaud's phenomenon-associated increase in vascular tone is due in part to a defect in the vascular response to normal sympathetic signals. Recent studies find that α_{2c}-adrenergic receptors on smooth muscle cells of cutaneous vessels are responsive to cold and may be over-expressed in patients with Raynaud's phenomenon.[15]

Raynaud's phenomenon is clinically defined as cold- or emotional stress-induced vascular constriction of arteriovenous shunts, arterioles, and small arteries in the skin and tissues of the digits. Raynaud's phenomenon is manifested as pallor of the digits (the phase of complete loss of blood flow) followed by cyanosis of the skin (low flow with deoxygenated blood) and hyperemia as blood flow rebounds after rewarming the skin. Raynaud's phenomenon affects as much as 3–5% of the general population. In most cases it represents a genetic trait, with cold sensitivity due to abnormal cutaneous vessel reactivity. Raynaud's phenomenon is considered to be primary when there is no other associated disease state. In SSc, the disease targets blood vessels, and is one of many disease states that can alter the normal vascular response to ambient temperature and present with secondary Raynaud's phenomenon. Patients with SSc often have severe Raynaud's phenomenon, with multiple and often prolonged daily episodes associated with critical ischemia, leading to digital infarction or tissue gangrene. There is evidence that abnormal vascular reactivity in SSc is systemic, with recurrent bouts of vasospasm in the pulmonary, renal, gastrointestinal and coronary circulations.

Treatment must be individualized and adjusted according to the severity of the disease. Initial therapy should include avoidance of cold exposure and methods of stress reduction. The best-studied medications to treat Raynaud's phenomenon are the calcium channel blockers (e.g., nifedipine), and they remain the recommended first choice of therapy. Other vasoactive drugs reported to be helpful include the angiotensin II receptor blockers (e.g., losartan); the α_1-adrenergic receptor blocker

prazosin, phosphodiesterase inhibitors including sildenafil, pentoxifylline, and cilostazol; serotonin reuptake inhibitors such as fluoxetine; nitrates including topical nitroglycerine; and intravenous prostaglandins.[16] Bosentan, an endothelin-1 receptor inhibitor, was recently shown to reduce the occurrence of new digital ulcers in patients with SSc, but did not alter the frequency of Raynaud's events.[17]

GASTROINTESTINAL INVOLVEMENT

Gastrointestinal disease is the most frequent initial symptom after Raynaud's phenomenon. Patients with lcSSc and dcSSc are equally at risk. Gastrointestinal involvement is characterized by abnormal motility of the esophagus, stomach, small and large bowel and rectum. Pathological studies show that the smooth muscle (circular greater than longitudinal) of the bowel atrophies, without significant fibrosis, vascular injury or inflammation.[18] Functional and pharmacological studies have shown that a neurogenic process precedes smooth muscle dysfunction. Virtually every patient with SSc demonstrates evidence of distal esophagus dysfunction. Clinically, this may present with dysphagia and dyspepsia typical of gastroesophageal reflux disease. Esophageal manometric evaluation reveals the characteristic triad of low or absent primary and secondary peristaltic activity in the distal esophagus, normal proximal esophageal (striated muscle) motility, and loss of lower esophageal sphincter tone. Complications such as reflux esophagitis, esophageal strictures, mucosal erosions and bleeding, Barrett's metaplasia or, very rarely, adenocarcinoma may develop.

Early satiety, bloating, nausea, periodic vomiting and decreased appetite with weight loss are common, and may be secondary to poor gastric emptying and retention of food and liquids in the stomach. Dilatation of mucosal capillaries is common in the gastrointestinal tract, particularly in the gastric antrum. This lesion, also called watermelon stomach, can be associated with recurrent occult gastrointestinal bleeding and significant anemia. Intestinal dysmotility may involve the small and large bowel. Patients may note a change in bowel habits, or may present with episodes of pseudo-obstruction with severe abdominal pain, bloating, abdominal distension and vomiting. Persistent diarrhea can be a manifestation of malabsorption of fats due to bacterial overgrowth in atonic small bowel, and can be associated with dramatic weight loss and malnutrition. In the late stages the bowel wall thins out and traps air (pneumatosis cystoides intestinalis). Wide-mouthed diverticuli develop in the colon or the bowel, and may rupture.

PULMONARY INVOLVEMENT

Lung disease is now the leading cause of death in patients with SSc and accounts for significant lifetime morbidity. Even in patients without respiratory symptoms, sensitive methods of pulmonary function testing reveal abnormalities, and 40% of SSc patients have clinically significant lung involvement. The most common and serious forms of lung involvement are interstitial lung disease (ILD) and pulmonary vascular disease. Risk factors for severe ILD include African-American race, diffuse skin involvement, and the presence of topoisomerase-I autoantibodies. Additional pulmonary manifestations of SSc include aspiration pneumonitis, pulmonary hemorrhage due to endobronchial telangiectasia, bronchiolitis obliterans with organizing pneumonia, pleural reactions and pneumothorax. The risk of lung cancer is increased in patients with SSc.

Interstitial lung disease

In patients with SSc, interstitial lung disease is most commonly characterized by the histologic pattern of non-specific interstitial pneumonitis (NSIP).[19] Inflammatory alveolitis and subsequent tissue fibrosis cause a restrictive ventilatory defect and abnormal gas exchange. Patients with ILD may experience a rapid initial decline in lung function during the early period of active skin disease. About 20% of patients with ILD continue to progress to severe end-stage disease. In early disease, most patients have no respiratory symptoms. The most sensitive method to detect early lung disease is pulmonary function testing. Imaging by high-resolution computed tomography (HRCT) can be used to demonstrate fibrosis and ground-glass opacities, and can provide an indication of the activity of the process; the degree of fibrosis correlates with decline in forced vital capacity (FVC). Bronchoalveolar lavage (BAL) is sometimes performed to determine the level of activity, to predict outcome, and to rule out occult pulmonary infection. An increase in the total number of cells (mostly macrophages) in the BAL fluid, and an elevated proportion of neutrophils (>3%) and/or eosinophils (>2%), is considered a positive BAL result. In one study, 70% of untreated SSc patients who had positive BAL had a poor outcome, with a clinically significant decline in lung function.[20] Recent multicenter clinical trials comparing cyclophosphamide (oral or intravenous) against placebo demonstrated modest but statistically significant stabilization of lung function (FVC) in the active treatment group, along with improvement in skin score, respiratory symptoms, and a variety of clinical measures. [21,21a] However, the clinical response was not durable after 1 year. The safety and efficacy of prolonged cytotoxic or immunosuppressive therapy remain to be evaluated.

Pulmonary arterial hypertension

Pulmonary arterial hypertension (PAH) is increasingly recognized as a frequent and severe complication of SSc, is detected in 12–15% of patients, it may occur as the sole pulmonary manifestation of the disease, or in association with ILD. The natural history of PAH is highly variable. In many patients with SSc it follows a relentless downhill course with right heart failure and significant mortality. Risk factors for PAH in SSc include limited cutaneous disease, late age at disease onset, history of severe Raynaud's phenomenon, and the presence of U1 RNP, anti-fibrillarin or anti-B23 antibodies. Current therapy for SSc-associated PAH is focused on supportive care, reduction of cardiac workload and vasoactive drugs.[22] Short-acting prostacyclin analogs, including intravenous (epoprostenol or treprostinil) or inhaled (iloprost) prostaglandins, have been in use for several years. More recent interventions include selective and nonselective endothelin-1 receptor inhibitors (bosentan, ambrisentan), and phosphodiesterase type 5 inhibitors (sildenafil). In relatively short-term clinical trials, each of these treatments has been shown to improve exercise tolerance and hemodynamics, with variable benefit on disease progression. Lung transplantation remains an option for selected SSc patients with severe lung disease.

CARDIAC INVOLVEMENT

Heart disease is more prevalent among patients with dcSSc than in patients with lcSSc. Most patients with heart involvement remain asymptomatic until the later stages, when heart failure or serious arrhythmia occur. Clinical evidence of heart disease, such as the presence of a large pericardial effusion, is a poor prognostic indicator. Although generally asymptomatic, pericardial disease can cause typical pericarditis, and rarely significant hemodynamic compromise and tamponade. Myocarditis is less common but can be life-threatening. Severe cardiomyopathy is associated with evidence of polymyositis.[23]

RENAL INVOLVEMENT

The most dreaded complication of SSc is acute renal involvement, called scleroderma renal crisis. It develops in 10–15% of patients, most commonly those with dcSSc, and is generally a relatively early (<3 years) complication of the disease.[24] The presence of tendon friction rubs, pericardial effusion, new unexplained anemia, and RNA polymerase III autoantibodies is associated with elevated risk of renal crisis. Several studies have indicated an association with recent corticosteroid use. Scleroderma renal crisis characteristically presents as malignant hypertension and rapidly progressive oliguric renal failure. Proteinuria, microhematuria, and evidence of a microangiopathic hemolytic process with thrombocytopenia are present. Patients with scleroderma renal crisis who present with a creatinine >3 mg/dL have a poor outcome, with permanent hemodialysis and high mortality. Prompt recognition and aggressive intervention with angiotensin-converting enzyme (ACE) inhibitors to achieve good blood pressure control before evidence of renal dysfunction significantly improves the prognosis.

MUSCULOSKELETAL COMPLICATIONS

Although musculoskeletal complaints are among the earliest symptoms of SSc, inflammatory erosive polyarthritis is uncommon. Joint involvement is usually due to fibrosis of the overlying skin, the supporting joint structures and the joint capsule itself. Flexion contractures associated with 'friction rubs' over tendons are typical of advanced dcSSc, most prominent over the ankles, knees, shoulders and wrists. Muscle weakness is common, and may reflect deconditioning or disuse, malnutrition and weight loss, as well as inflammatory myositis, muscle fibrosis and atrophy.

OTHER DISEASE MANIFESTATIONS

Many patients develop dry eyes and mouth (sicca complex). Unlike Sjögren's syndrome, in SSc these manifestations are due to fibrosis rather than lymphocytic infiltration of the minor salivary and tear glands. Furthermore, in SSc the sicca complex is associated with anticentromere, rather than Ro/SSA or La/SSB autoantibodies, a serological profile that also associates with a subset of patients with primary Sjögren's syndrome. Primary biliary cirrhosis is a rare complication of lcSSc, and is associated with antimitochondrial antibodies. Autoimmune hepatitis may also occur. Up to 20% of SSc patients are hypothyroid, owing to direct thyroid fibrosis or a consequence of autoimmune thyroiditis. The central nervous system is generally spared in SSc, but cases of trigeminal neuralgia have been reported. Erectile dysfunction frequently develops and is due to a combination of microvascular disease and corporeal fibrosis. In some patients with SSc, erectile failure is the initial manifestation of the disease. Because SSc affects every aspect of a patient's life and is disfiguring, it is not surprising that significant depression is common.[25] Chronic pain and the lack of social support are major causes of depression, and therefore vigorous pain control and antidepressant medication are important considerations in the management of SSc.

CLINICAL PEARLS

RECOMMENDED APPROACH TO THE EVALUATION OF A PATIENT WITH SYSTEMIC SCLEROSIS

>> Determine skin score to define clinical subtype.

>> Frequent clinical reassessment to define disease activity.

>> Careful clinical history to evaluate for gastrointestinal dysmotility.

>> Monitor for new onset hypertension: prevent renal crisis.

>> Pulmonary function test: early detection of interstitial lung disease.

>> Doppler echocardiography: screen for pulmonary arterial hypertension.

>> Obtain serology profile to help predict clinical outcome.

THERAPEUTIC PRINCIPLES

TREATMENT OF SYSTEMIC SCLEROSIS

Organ-specific therapy

>> Vasodilator therapy for Raynaud's phenomenon

>> Proton pump inhibitor for gastroesophageal reflux

>> ACE inhibitor for renal crisis

>> Vasodilator therapy for pulmonary arterial hypertension

>> Anti-inflammatory therapy for arthritis

>> Immunosuppressive therapy for interstitial lung disease

Disease-modifying agents

>> No ideal treatment available; immunomodulatory, anti-inflammatory, vasoactive and anti-fibrotic agents are used and/or under study

TREATMENT

Organ specific

The management of patients with SSc must be individualized and treatment decisions based on thorough assessment and careful monitoring. Most successful SSc treatments are directed to the specific organ(s) involved. Therapy is focused on an organ-specific disease process (e.g., ACE inhibitor in SSc renal crisis), or to aid a failing organ (e.g., proton pump inhibitors or metoclopramide for gastroesophageal reflux disease).[26] A recent placebo-controlled clinical trial investigated the efficacy of daily oral cyclophosphamide versus placebo in SSc patients with symptomatic early active alveolitis. The results showed that at 12 months of therapy cyclophosphamide was associated with stabilization of lung function, providing evidence that immunosuppressive therapy may be helpful in selected patients.[21] Potentially safer immunosuppressive (e.g., mycophenolate mofetil), anti-inflammatory (e.g. anti-CCR2) or anti-fibrotic agents (e.g., imatinib) are currently being evaluated for the treatment of lung involvement in SSc.[21]

DISEASE MODIFICATION

To date, no drug or intervention has been shown to be effective and safe for modifying the disease course. Therefore, it is important to characterize the patient's clinical phenotype carefully and define the level of disease activity before deciding on therapy. For example, a patient with lcSSc who has no evidence of visceral organ involvement is likely to have a benign course requiring only symptomatic therapy (e.g., treatment of gastroesophageal reflux disease and Raynaud's phenomenon): disease-modifying drugs would not be indicated. It is also important to distinguish disease activity from severity or advanced cumulative organ damage. For example, a patient with late-stage dcSSc is unlikely to benefit from aggressive immunosuppressive or anti-inflammatory therapy. Intervention with currently available drugs should be initiated early, ideally during the edematous active inflammatory phase of the disease. It is during the early stages that immunosuppression, anti-inflammatory and anti-fibrotic agents have the greatest potential to control disease progression. Clinical experience teaches that once the edematous phase of the disease shifts to the more indolent fibrotic phase, current treatments are largely ineffective to control the progression and tissue damage. Few well-designed controlled studies have been carried out for the treatment of early active disease; most reports are anecdotal uncontrolled experiences complicated by investigator bias and the highly variable natural course of SSc. Medications that have been used in SSc but appear to have little or no benefit include colchicine, DMSO, para-aminobenzoic acid, interferon (IFN)-γ, photopheresis, minocycline, and anti-tumor necrosis factor (TNF)-β agents. Controlled clinical trials have failed to provide evidence for the efficacy of D-penicillamine, a drug long in widespread use for SSc, or for recombinant relaxin.

Immunosuppressive drugs are used to control *early active* dcSSc because of the evidence that this is an autoimmune disease, initiated and/or propagated by an immune process. However, no rigorous trials have evaluated the efficacy of popular approaches to dcSSc. Drugs reported to have benefit include cyclophosphamide and mycophenolate mofetil. Additional reports suggest benefit with Cyclosporine, intravenous γ-globulin, anti-thymocyte globulin, thalidomide and methotrexate. The use of cyclophosphamide is limited by bone marrow suppression and bladder toxicity; mycophenolate mofetil by the issue of long-term immunosuppression; intravenous γ-globulin by its expense; Cyclosporine by frequent renal toxicity; thalidomide by skin rashes and peripheral neuropathy; and methotrexate by its potential to induce or exacerbate liver or lung fibrosis. Treatments targeting B cells with rituximab are under consideration. Multicenter clinical trials of immunoablative therapy with high-dose cyclophosphamide, alone or with radiation, followed by stem cell rescue, are in progress. High-dose cyclophosphamide without stem cell rescue is also under study. The use of novel biologic agents such as anti-cytokines (TGF-β), anti-chemokines (CCR2) or inhibitors of growth factors (CTGF) is being explored. Physicians are encouraged to refer patients with early dcSSc to specialty centers focusing on clinical trials.

OTHER SCLERODERMA-LIKE FIBROSING DISEASES

Several disorders can cause skin fibrosis and mimic SSc or scleroderma.[27] These include localized forms of scleroderma, eosinophilic fasciitis, scleromyxedema (papular mucinosis) and scleredema (Table 55.3).

SYSTEMIC IMMUNE DISEASES

Table 55.3 Differential diagnosis of SSc and scleroderma

Disorders characterized by similar presentations
Systemic lupus erythematosus
Sjögren's syndrome
Rheumatoid arthritis
Polymyositis/dermatomyositis
Primary Raynaud's phenomenon

Disorders characterized by similar visceral features
Primary pulmonary hypertension
Primary biliary cirrhosis
Idiopathic intestinal hypomotility
Idiopathic pulmonary fibrosis
Malignant hypertension

Disorders characterized by skin thickening
Scleromyxedema
Scleredema (of Buschke), diabetic scleredema
Nephrogenic fibrosing dermatopathy
Eosinophilic fasciitis/diffuse fasciitis with eosinophilia
Eosinophilia–myalgia syndrome
Generalized morphea
Chronic graft-versus-host disease
POEMS syndrome
Amyloidosis
Carcinoid syndrome
Pentazocine-induced scleroderma
Diabetic digital sclerosis
Vinyl chloride disease
Toxic oil syndrome
Bleomycin exposure
Werner's syndrome
Phenylketonuria
Porphyria cutanea tarda
Vibration white finger syndrome
Chronic reflex sympathetic dystrophy

A novel syndrome labeled nephrogenic fibrosing dermopathy has been described in patients with end-stage renal disease.[28] Because many patients with this syndrome have evidence of visceral organ fibrosis in addition to skin involvement, 'nephrogenic systemic fibrosis' has been proposed as an alternate name. SSc can be distinguished from these scleroderma-like fibrosing conditions by its characteristic clinical, pathological and laboratory features. These include evidence of widespread vasculopathy with abnormal skin capillaries and Raynaud's phenomenon, the characteristic distribution pattern of skin changes and typical dermatopathological features, the unique pattern of visceral organ involvement, and the presence of SSc-specific serum autoantibodies.

REFERENCES

1. Maricq HR, Weinrich MC, Keil JE, et al. Prevalence of scleroderma spectrum disorders in the general population of South Carolina. Arthritis Rheum 1989; 32: 998–1006.

2. Mayes MD, Lacey JV Jr., Beebe-Dimmer J, et al. Prevalence, incidence, survival, and disease characteristics of systemic sclerosis in a large US population. Arthritis Rheum 2003; 48: 2246–2255.

3. Feghali-Bostwick C, Medsger TA Jr., Wright TM. Analysis of systemic sclerosis in twins reveals low concordance for disease and high concordance for the presence of antinuclear antibodies. Arthritis Rheum 2003; 48: 1956–1963.

4. Feghali-Bostwick CA. Genetics and proteomics in scleroderma. Curr Rheumatol Rep 2005; 7: 129–134.

5. Janowsky EC, Kupper LL, Hulka BS. Meta-analyses of the relation between silicone breast implants and the risk of connective-tissue diseases. N Engl J Med 2000; 342: 781–906.

6. Varga J, Abraham D. Systemic sclerosis: a prototypic multisystem fibrotic disorder. J Clin Invest 2007; 117: 555–567.

7. Kuwana M, Okazaki Y, Yasuoka H, et al. Defective vasculogenesis in systemic sclerosis. Lancet 2004; 364: 603–610.

8. Sato S, Fujimoto M, Hasegawa M, Takehara K. Altered blood B lymphocyte homeostasis in systemic sclerosis: expanded naive B cells and diminished but activated memory B cells. Arthritis Rheum 2004; 50: 1918–1927.

9. Gardner H, Shearstone JR, Bandaru R, et al. Gene profiling of scleroderma skin reveals robust signatures of disease that are imperfectly reflected in the transcript profiles of explanted fibroblasts. Arthritis Rheum 2006; 54: 1961–1973.

10. Mori Y, Chen SJ, Varga J. Expression and regulation of intracellular SMAD signaling in scleroderma skin fibroblasts. Arthritis Rheum 2003; 48: 1964–1978.

11. Krishnan E, Furst DE. Systemic sclerosis mortality in the United States: 1979–1998. Eur J Epidemiol 2005; 20: 855–861.

12. Ioannidis JP, Vlachoyiannopoulos PG, Haidich AB, et al. Mortality in systemic sclerosis: an international meta-analysis of individual patient data. Am J Med 2005; 118: 2–10.

13. LeRoy EC, Medsger TA Jr. J Rheumatol. Criteria for the classification of early systemic sclerosis 2001; 28: 1573–1576.

14. Mukerjee D, St George D, Coleiro B, et al. Prevalence and outcome in systemic sclerosis associated pulmonary arterial hypertension: application of a registry approach. Ann Rheum Dis 2003; 62: 1088–1093.

15. Bailey SR, Eid AH, Mitra S, et al. Rho kinase mediates cold-induced constriction of cutaneous arteries: role of alpha 2C-adrenoceptor translocation. Circ Res 2004; 94: 1367–1374.

16. Boin F, Wigley FM. Understanding, assessing and treating Raynaud's phenomenon. Curr Opin Rheumatol 2005 Nov; 17: 752–760.

17. Korn JH, Mayes M, Matucci Cerinic M, et al. Digital ulcers in systemic sclerosis: prevention by treatment with bosentan, an oral endothelin receptor antagonist. Arthritis Rheum 2004; 50: 3985–3993.

18. Roberts CG, Hummers LK, Ravich WJ, et al. A case-controlled study of the pathology of oesophageal disease in systemic sclerosis (scleroderma). Gut 2006; 55: 1697–1703.

19. Veeraraghavan S, Nicholson AG, Wells AU. Lung fibrosis: new classifications and therapy. Curr Opin Rheumatol Nov; 13: 500–504.

20. White B, Moore WC, Wigley FM, et al. Cyclophosphamide is associated with pulmonary function and survival benefit in patients with scleroderma and alveolitis. Ann Intern Med 2000; 132: 947–954.

21. Tashkin DP, Elashoff R, Clements PJ, et al. Scleroderma Lung Study Research Group. Cyclophosphamide versus placebo in scleroderma lung disease. N Engl J Med 2006; 354: 2655–2666.

21a. Hoyles RK, Ellis RW, Wellsbury J, et al. A multicenter, prospective, randomized, double-blind, placebo-controlled trial of corticosteroids and intravenous cyclophosphamide followed by oral azathioprine for the treatment of pulmonary fibrosis in scleroderma. Arthritis Rheum 2006; 54: 3962–3970.

22. Jain M, Varga J. Bosentan for the treatment of systemic sclerosis-associated pulmonary arterial hypertension, pulmonary fibrosis and digital ulcers. Expert Opin Pharmacother 2006; 7: 1487–1501.

23. Follansbee WP, Zerbe TR, Medsger TA Jr. Cardiac and skeletal muscle disease in systemic sclerosis (scleroderma): a high risk association. Am Heart J 1993; 125: 194–203.

24. Steen VD. Scleroderma renal crisis. Rheum Dis Clin North Am 2003; 29: 315–333.

25. Haythornthwaite JA, Heinberg LJ, McGuire L. Psychologic factors in scleroderma. Rheum Dis Clin North Am 2003; 29: 427–439.

26. Denton CP, Black CM. Targeted therapy comes of age in scleroderma. Trends Immunol 2005; 26: 596–602.

27. Mori Y, Kahari VM, Varga J. Scleroderma-like cutaneous syndromes. Curr Rheumatol Rep 2002; 4: 113–122.

28. Cowper SE, Boyer PJ. Nephrogenic systemic fibrosis: an update. Curr Rheumatol Rep 2006; 8: 151–157

Inflammatory muscle diseases

Lisa Christopher-Stine, Paul H. Plotz

56

The idiopathic inflammatory myopathies (IIM) – dermatomyositis (DM), polymyositis (PM), and inclusion body myositis (IBM) – constitute the largest subgroup of the acquired myopathies. They are a heterogeneous group and are rare among immunologic illnesses. However, the IIM share many clinical features and laboratory abnormalities, including related autoantibodies, and are closely related to major autoimmune diseases. Because their presentation and major clinical manifestations are weakness and/or rash, the differential diagnosis necessarily includes many more common diseases familiar to neurologists and dermatologists.

CLINICAL FEATURES

The clinical hallmark of polymyositis and dermatomyositis is the gradual onset over weeks to months of symmetric proximal muscle weakness. In some cases, myalgia may be the presenting or most bothersome symptom, but more often the patient is evaluated for the physical limitations imposed by weakness: difficulty arising from a low chair or bed, or combing and brushing hair. Rash is the first feature in a considerable proportion of patients who have dermatomyositis, but muscle weakness usually follows within a few months. A subset of patients with dermatomyositis, clinically amyopathic dermatomyositis (C-ADM), may present only with rash in the absence of muscle weakness throughout the course of their illness. These patients are also at risk for pulmonary involvement, as are those with classic DM. The prevalence of interstitial pneumonitis in C-ADM has not yet been determined; however, it may approach 5–10% (compared to 40% of patients with classic DM) based on an estimate made from the current published literature.[1] Arthritis, Raynaud's phenomenon, fever, or lung disease presenting as cough or dyspnea may dominate the clinical picture. Cardiac and gastrointestinal symptoms other than dysphagia in severe cases are rarely early manifestations. Renal and central nervous system (CNS) involvement are almost never a part of the IIM.

Some of the rashes of dermatomyositis are virtually pathognomonic; others are not disease specific (Fig. 56.1). The heliotrope rash, a violaceous discoloration of the eyelids, is sometimes no more than a line along the margin of the upper lid, but may also affect both upper and lower lids completely, and may be associated with edema mimicking thyroid disease.

A reddish, sometimes raised and/or scaly eruption over the metacarpophalangeal joints is known as Gottron's papules. In more advanced cases, the metatarsophalyngeal joints, elbows, knees, and malleoli show a similar rash. Both heliotrope and Gottron's rashes can occur rarely in cases of frank systemic lupus erythematosus (SLE) without muscle involvement. Other common rashes include a flat red blanching eruption of the upper chest (often in a V distribution), the upper back (where a shawl would touch), and sometimes the extensor surfaces of the upper arms and thighs. Another rash that mimics the malar rash of lupus on the face may be present, but, in contrast to lupus, does not spare the nasolabial folds. Although found on sun-exposed parts of the body, these rashes are often not photosensitive in nature. As in other connective tissue diseases, nailfold capillary dilatation and infarcts and cuticular overgrowth occur. A roughening and cracking of the radial sides of the fingers and the palm, resembling a condition found in people who labor with their hands (mechanic's hands), is characteristic of a subset of myositis patients with the 'antisynthetase syndrome'.

CLASSIFICATION

In the past 40 years, several investigators have proposed diagnostic classification criteria for IIM. For clinicians, the criteria proposed by Bohan and Peter[2, 3] three decades ago remain the most familiar and accepted definitions of PM and DM. They combine clinical, laboratory, electrodiagnostic, and pathological features. These criteria currently serve as the gold standard for clinical diagnosis and for inclusion in clinical trials. However, they are limited by their poor specificity in distinguishing PM from other entities, including late-onset muscular dystrophies. The resultant misclassification limits the homogeneity of the patients included in previous observational and interventional studies. Additionally, the Bohan and Peter criteria completely omit the diagnosis of IBM, the most frequent type of IIM in patients over 50 years of age.[4]

Additional classification criteria have been proposed by Tanimoto et al.[5] and by Targoff et al.[6] (Table 56.1), but neither classification has been widely used. The Targoff classification scheme suggests the incorporation of MRI, but the sensitivity and specificity of this scheme have not been

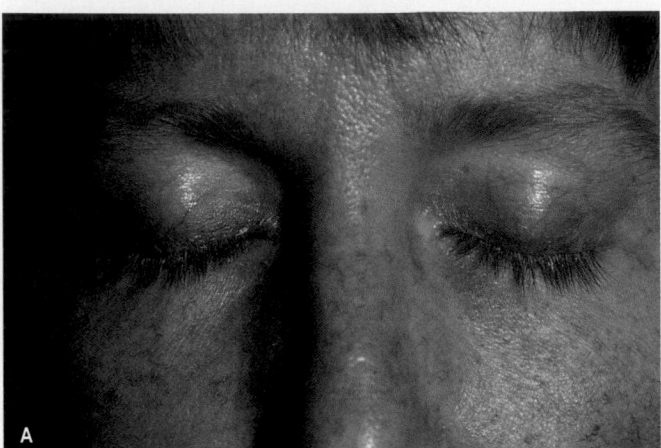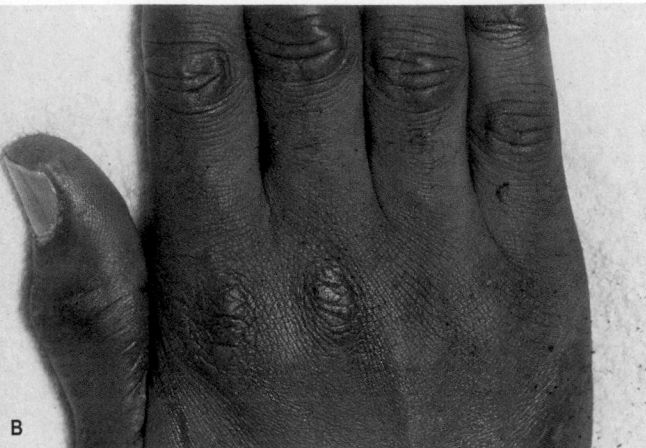

Fig. 56.1 Dermatomyositis rash. (**A**) In addition to the heliotrope rash on the eyelids of this patient with dermatomyositis, there is a flat red rash on the nose and cheeks. (**B**) A raised shiny red rash – Gottron's papules – is apparent on the interphalangeal and the second and third metacarpophalangeal joints of this man with dermatomyositis.

KEY CONCEPTS

DEFINITION AND INCIDENCE OF IDIOPATHIC INFLAMMATORY MYOPATHIES (IIM)

>> Polymyositis, dermatomyositis, and related inflammatory muscle diseases are called IIM.

>> Indistinguishable muscle inflammation may accompany other autoimmune connective tissue diseases or limb girdle muscular dystrophies.

>> The annual incidence in the USA is 5–10 cases per million. DM and PM are more common in women than men in all age groups; IBM is more common in men.

KEY CONCEPTS

CHARACTERISTIC HALLMARKS OF INFLAMMATORY MYOSITIS

>> The clinical hallmark is proximal limb and neck weakness, rarely associated with muscle pain.

>> The laboratory hallmarks are elevated serum levels of creatine kinase (CK), aldolase, lactic dehydrogenase, and the transaminases, and a characteristic pattern ('irritable myopathy') on electromyography (EMG). Elevated serum levels of autoantibodies are common.

>> The pathologic hallmarks are focal muscle necrosis, degeneration, regeneration, and inflammation.

---

validated.[5] The Tanimoto criteria lack quantification or specific requirements for satisfying some criteria, and do not include MRI.[6] Separate classification criteria systems for IBM have been devised (Table 56.2), but characteristic muscle biopsy changes remain the defining feature in IBM.

It has been useful for some purposes to divide cases into groups: polymyositis, dermatomyositis, juvenile myositis, myositis associated with another connective tissue disease (usually systemic sclerosis, SLE, or Sjögren's syndrome), cancer-associated myositis (usually cases in which the diagnoses are made within 6–12 months of one another), inclusion body myositis, and a miscellaneous group that includes such rare entities as eosinophilic myositis (Table 56.3). This classification has allowed recognition of unique clinical and pathogenetic features and response to therapy. In the case of cancer-associated myositis, a more rational approach to workup based on recognition of groups at risk is now possible.

Autoantibodies unique to myositis – the so-called 'myositis-specific autoantibodies' – have allowed a useful alternative classification (Table 56.4). For example, patients with antibodies to one or another of a group of enzymes – the aminoacyl-tRNA (transfer RNA) synthetases, of which Jo-1 is the best known – have a characteristic syndrome that usually includes interstitial lung disease, nondeforming inflammatory arthritis, fevers, mechanic's hands, and Raynaud's phenomenon, in addition to myositis. Those with antibodies to the signal recognition particle (anti-SRP) have severe disease of abrupt onset, often in the autumn, unaccompanied by rash. Recent work has shown that cardiac involvement is less common and survival is better in patients with anti-SRP than has previously been reported.[7] Those with antibodies to the nuclear antigen Mi-2 almost always have the V and shawl rashes and cuticular overgrowth in addition to myositis. Each of the different autoantibody-associated groups also has a predominant histocompatibility type and clinical course (Table 56.4).[2]

Inclusion body myositis (IBM) is becoming increasingly recognized. The diagnosis of IBM is important because, unlike patients with other inflammatory myopathies, those with IBM rarely improve in strength with immunosuppressive therapy. Patients with IBM tend to be older than others with myositis, and in contrast to patients with PM and DM, who are predominantly women, IBM patients are commonly men. They have gradual, painless, progressive weakness and focal atrophy that develop over years, and may complain of frequent falls. The forearms of

Table 56.1 Current idiopathic inflammatory myopathy: diagnostic criteria

Bohan and Peter criteria	Targoff proposed criteria	Tanimoto proposed criteria
1. Symmetrical proximal muscle weakness	1. Symmetrical proximal muscle weakness	1. Symmetrical proximal muscle weakness
2. Skeletal muscle enzyme elevation	2. Skeletal muscle enzyme elevation	2. Skeletal muscle enzyme elevation
3. Abnormal EMG*	3. Abnormal EMG*	3. Abnormal EMG*
4. Muscle biopsy abnormalities	4. Muscle biopsy abnormalities**	4. Muscle biopsy abnormalities**
5. Typical skin rash of DM***	5. Typical skin rash of dermatomyositis***	5. Typical skin rash of dermatomyositis***
	6. One of the myositis specific antibodies (MSAs)	6. Muscle pain
	7. MRI may substitute for criterion 1 or 2	7. Positive Anti-Jo-1 antibody
		8. Nondestructive arthritis/arthralgia
		9. Systemic inflammatory signs†

*Polyphasic, short, small motor- unit potentials; fibrillation, positive sharp waves, increased insertional irritability; bizarre, high-frequency, repetitive discharges.
**Degeneration/regeneration, perifascicular atrophy, necrosis, phagocytosis, fiber size variation, and mononuclear inflammatory infiltrate.
***Gottron's sign, heliotrope rash.
†fever>37° C, elevated CRP, elevated ESR>20 mm by Westergren method.

For the Bohan and Peter criteria
Possible PM = any two of the first four criteria; Possible DM = criterion 5 (rash) + any two criteria
Probable PM = any three of the first four criteria: Probable DM = criterion 5 (rash) + any three criteria
Definite PM = all four of the first four criteria; Definite DM = criterion 5 (rash) + all four other criteria

For the Targoff criteria
Possible IIM = any two criteria
Probable IIM = any three criteria
Definite IIM = any four criteria
MRI results consistent with inflammation may be substituted for criterion 1 or 2

For the Tanimoto criteria
Rash plus at least four of the other eight items = DM
Four of the items excluding rash = PM
(There are no definite/probable/possible categories)

these patients exhibit a scalloped appearance, attributed to muscle atrophy. There are few signs of disease outside the skeletal musculature. Difficulties with swallowing can be a complaint of patients with any inflammatory myopathy, and are frequently a major problem in patients with IBM. The creatine kinase (CK) and other skeletal muscle-associated serum enzymes are normal in about one-quarter of patients with IBM, and only moderately elevated in the remainder. The electromyogram in IBM frequently demonstrates both myogenic and neurogenic features secondary to the effective denervation of some muscle cells by inflammation and necrosis.

Proposed criteria for the diagnosis of IBM rely on both pathologic and clinical features. In the clinical setting of an inflammatory myopathy, the presence on light microscopy (with confirmation by electron microscopy) of the characteristic inclusions or rimmed vacuoles is diagnostic. The origin of the vacuoles in IBM has been the focus of investigation and remains a source of speculation. Among the inflammatory myopathies, IBM is distinguished by substantial numbers of rimmed cytoplasmic vacuoles with tubulofilamentous material within myofibers. A variety of proteins have been found by immunohistochemistry in the muscle cells in IBM, including ubiquitin, β-amyloid precursor protein, phosphorylated t, and the transcription factor NF-κB, but it is not yet possible to tie them to the pathogenesis of the illness.[8] The infiltrates in the muscle of patients with IBM are composed predominantly of CD8 lymphocytes, closely resembling those found in the inflammatory infiltrate in the muscles of patients with polymyositis.[9] There may be increased expression of HLA class I molecules in the muscle of patients with IBM.

IBM must be distinguished from other myopathies because of its chronic nature. These include acquired myopathies, such as those caused by toxins, and genetically determined myopathies, such as some muscular dystrophies and the metabolic myopathies. There are several important differences between IBM and these other myopathies. The separation, however, is not as defined as might be anticipated. Although some of the familial forms of IBM have a distinctive clinical presentation, often early in life, there have been several families with the typical late onset and inflammatory picture of the presumed sporadic cases. Several genetic loci have been identified in familial IBM, so it will be important to assess any identified mutations in familial IBM-associated genes in sporadic cases.[10] A further complexity is that IBM has been described decades after typical dermatomyositis.

necrosis followed by atrophy appear in a perifascicular pattern. Perivascular lymphocytic infiltrates, typical of later disease, have not been described as an early change. Dermatomyositis may thus be the result of an immune complex deposition or a primary attack on endothelial cells. As in SLE, interferon-α/β-inducible gene and protein expression may contribute to the pathogenesis of DM. This innate immune response is characterized by plasmacytoid dendritic cell invasion.[22] Consistent with the importance of immune complexes, histological abnormalities in the skin in dermatomyositis are indistinguishable from the changes in lupus.

In contrast to dermatomyositis, polymyositis and IBM do not demonstrate marked capillary changes, perivascular infiltrates are less pronounced, and T-cell infiltrates in the perimysial and endomysial regions are more pronounced. Nonnecrotic fibers may be surrounded by T lymphocytes and macrophages. The T cells are enriched for the CD8 subset. Attempts to culture these cells and look for lysis of autologous myocytes have met with limited success. There is negligible evidence of NK cell-like activity. Should cytotoxic T cells prove to be the major effector cells, it will be necessary to clone T cells to identify the antigenic targets. Most cytotoxic T cells are of the CD8 phenotype and therefore recognize their antigenic peptide in association with MHC class I molecules. Although resting normal muscle has very low class I expression, it is upregulated in regenerating and degenerating fibers found in both inflammatory and noninflammatory myopathies. Interestingly, in dermatomyositis, class I expression is upregulated predominantly in the perifascicular regions, around sites of atrophy, and near sites of cellular invasion. In contrast, in polymyositis, class I expression may be diffusely upregulated even where there is no cellular infiltrate. IBM shows a more focal class I distribution in regions of T-cell invasion. The presence of focal regions of MHC class I expression in nonnecrotic fibers at the site of activated CD8 T cells is compatible with cytotoxicity as a prime mechanism of myocyte necrosis in IBM and polymyositis. A pivotal study using transgenic mice demonstrated that abnormal accumulation of MHC class I molecules in the endoplasmic reticulum (ER) of muscle may initiate the ER stress response.[23]

Proposed pathogenic mechanisms for the development of both the familial and the sporadic forms of IBM include the concept of increased transcription and accumulation of the β-amyloid precursor protein and its proteolytic fragments; abnormal accumulations of the components of lipid metabolism, including cholesterol; and oxidative stress.[24] These characteristics, in concert with the theory of misfolded or unfolded proteins in the context of a cellular aging milieu, appear to contribute to the pathogenesis of IBM. One of the most intriguing steps forward in the study of IBM in recent years has been the identification of mutations in the UDP-N-acetylglucosamine 2-epimerase/N-acetylmannosamine kinase gene in the recessive familial quadriceps-sparing IBM first described in Iranian Jews, but now more extensively recognized.

The role of MHC class II molecules remains to be clarified. Cultured myoblasts constitutively express high levels of class I and are negative for class II. Class II has been found to be upregulated in the endothelial cells of patients with dermatomyositis, but its expression on T cells, a marker of activation, is more prominent in polymyositis.

Finally, γδ TCR T lymphocytes have been cloned from the muscle biopsy of one patient with polymyositis. Subsequent evaluation of his biopsy demonstrated γδ T cells and a 65 kDa heat shock protein in the endomysial region. The relative importance of γδ T cells in the spectrum of IIM is unknown.

The role of the B cells within affected muscles is not understood. It is not yet known whether they produce any autoantibodies, particularly the myositis-specific antibodies, or whether they play a role in antigen presentation for the T cells.

The pathogenic role of the autoantibodies found in patients with IIM remains uncertain. Myositis-specific antibodies (MSA) are found in 30–40% of patients, appear to delineate specific clinical entities, and each group has a strong but not absolute HLA association. In a patient with myositis and antihistidyl-tRNA synthetase (Jo-1) autoantibodies, sera available from long before the onset of symptoms or biochemical damage to muscle tissue contained the autoantibodies, suggesting that the autoantibodies were not merely a response to release of tissue antigens. The extraordinary specificity of myositis-specific antibodies for IIM and the lack of evidence for strong polyclonal stimulation in these diseases suggest that MSA are related to the fundamental causative process in IIM. Although 80–90% of patients with IIM are found to have antibodies to myosin or myoglobin, these antibodies are also found in patients with noninflammatory myopathies.

The structures bound by MSA are mostly intracellular ribonucleoproteins involved in protein synthesis, such as the aminoacyl-tRNA synthetases and the signal recognition particle (SRP). These autoantigens are found in every nucleated cell. The antibodies in general bind to conformational epitopes and, at least in the case of the antisynthetases, block enzymatic activity. It is possible that a structural property of muscle allows these particular proteins to be presented to the immune system when the cells are damaged, or, alternatively, the capacity of muscle fibers to degenerate alongside intense regeneration within the same fiber may allow these proteins to be efficiently displayed.[25] Recent experiments have suggested that some aminoacyl-tRNA synthetases have a direct proinflammatory role through a subsidiary chemokine-like action.[26]

A landmark study recently determined that cultured myoblasts express high levels of autoantigens, which are strikingly downregulated as cells differentiate into myotubes in vitro. These data strongly associate regenerating rather than mature muscle cells as the source of continuous autoantigen supply in autoimmune myositis.[25]

GENETICS

The IIM do not exhibit a simple mode of inheritance, and the rare familial cases mostly reflect IBM of early onset. As noted above, there are HLA associations for particular myositis-specific autoantibodies. Specifically, HLA-DR52 has a strong association (90%) with antisynthetase-positive myositis in both Caucasians and African-Americans.[27]

KEY CONCEPTS

DIFFERENTIAL FEATURES OF MYOSITIS

>> In dermatomyositis the earliest changes involve vessel walls, and B cells and CD4 T cells predominate in the muscle biopsy.

>> In polymyositis and inclusion-body myositis the dominant pathologic feature is targeting and invasion of muscle cells by CD8 cytotoxic cells.

NATURAL HISTORY

The prognosis for patients with IIM varies greatly with clinical type, autoantibodies, extraskeletal muscle involvement, and the interval between diagnosis and the start of treatment.

Patients with dermatomyositis or myositis accompanying another connective tissue disease are likely to recover most of their strength with prompt and adequate therapy. Although recurrences are common, persistent profound weakness does not usually occur. Most patients with anti-Mi-2 autoantibodies also usually respond well to therapy. Strength usually recovers well in patients whose myositis is cancer related, but overall mortality due to the tumor is high. Indeed, an accompanying tumor remains one of the most frequent causes of death in patients with an IIM. The diagnostic value of serum tumor markers (CEA, CA125, CA19-9 and CA15-3) was investigated in a study that demonstrated that serial CA125 and CA19-9 assessment could be useful markers in predicting which patients will develop cancer, especially in the subset of patients without interstitial lung disease.[28]

Patients with polymyositis fare less well, even when those with IBM are rigorously excluded. A return to normal strength is very unusual, and each recurrence is likely to be followed by greater residual weakness, even if inflammation is fully controlled. IBM has a poorer prognosis, but it is possible that the gradual decline in strength can be halted for long periods by corticosteroid and/or cytotoxic therapy if continuing inflammation is present. Severe muscle weakness and atrophy are prominent features in patients with anti-SRP autoantibodies. They have traditionally had the worst prognosis because there is rampant muscle destruction at the very outset. Those with anti-Jo-1 autoantibodies or antibodies to another synthetase are likely to respond to therapy initially, but to require continuing immunosuppression to treat frequent recurrences. In this group morbidity and mortality are heavily influenced by the progression of lung involvement. Longitudinal studies of outcomes in DM and PM patients are few. Cardiac involvement, respiratory involvement, and cancer were the main causes of death in several cohort analyses.[28–30] Disease course is monocyclic in approximately 20% of patients, polycyclic in 20%, and chronic in the remainder.[30] Relapses have been noted in the initial years of therapy and after prolonged disease-free intervals; therefore, periodic surveillance is warranted for at least 2 years following remission.[31, 32]

PATIENT MANAGEMENT

The treatment of myositis is based on controlling skeletal muscle inflammation and damage. Immunosuppressive therapy is used in the initial stages of the disease to reduce inflammation and muscle damage. To date, there are very few randomized controlled trials of any of the immunosuppressive agents used; thus, therapeutic regimens and responses have remained largely anecdotal. Clinical trials to assess the efficacy of TNF-α inhibitors, tacrolimus, and rituximab are currently under way. After the initial inflammation is controlled, strengthening exercises are useful in improving functional capabilities.

CORTICOSTEROIDS

Corticosteroids are the main immunosuppressive agents used in the treatment of myositis. An initial course of pulses of methylprednisolone may be helpful, particularly in disease of acute onset, and may also be helpful in managing disease flares. If active muscle inflammation persists or the side-effects of corticosteroids are severe, other immunosuppressive treatments are employed.

SECOND-LINE IMMUNOSUPPRESSIVE THERAPIES

The most frequently used second-line agents in the treatment of myositis are azathioprine and methotrexate. Azathioprine has been shown to reduce long-term disability.[33] Methotrexate is useful in patients with little or no response to corticosteroid therapy.[34, 35] Combination therapies, such as methotrexate with azathioprine, are useful even if patients have failed to respond to one of the agents alone.[36] High-dose intravenous immunoglobulin is of proven benefit in dermatomyositis.[37] Its usefulness in polymyositis is less predictable. Apheresis proved ineffective in a controlled blinded study.[38] Both cyclosporine and tacrolimus have been effective in some cases, as have cyclophosphamide and chlorambucil. The most recent therapeutic options include mycophenolate and rituximab.

MONITORING DISEASE ACTIVITY

Improvement in strength and normalization of serum CK activity are the best indirect measures of disease activity. A decrease in serum CK activity may herald clinical improvement, but corticosteroid treatment alone may reduce CK activity without associated clinical improvement. A lack of improvement in strength in a corticosteroid-treated patient may be due to the resistance of the inflammatory process, the presence of a corticosteroid-induced myopathy, and/or misdiagnosis. A diagnostic and therapeutic taper of the corticosteroids may then be warranted. If inflammation is present concurrently, other immunosuppressive agents are useful as the dosage of corticosteroids is lowered. If the CK value begins to rise, even if it is still within the normal range, and the symptoms of myositis are worsening in a patient whose disease has previously been controlled with corticosteroids, an increase in the dose may be warranted.

TREATMENT-RESISTANT MYOSITIS

Some treatment-resistant polymyositis patients have another disease. In such cases IBM or a limb girdle muscular dystrophy should be suspected. Unlike other myositis patients, those with IBM rarely, if ever, improve in strength with immunosuppressive therapy, but stabilization of strength may be achieved in some IBM patients with immunosuppressive agents.[39, 40] Patients with limb-girdle muscular dystrophies may mimic polymyositis clinically. They may have inflammation on muscle biopsy, and occasionally have associated autoantibodies. Thus, patients with a suspected IIM who do not respond to immunosuppressive therapy should undergo further evaluation, including genetic testing, to search for a limb-girdle muscular dystrophy.

NONSKELETAL MUSCLE INVOLVEMENT

Other organs frequently involved in myositis include the skin, lungs, and joints. Such organ involvement and the systemic features of myositis (fever and weight loss) usually improve with immunosuppressive therapy that controls inflammation in the skeletal muscle. Hydroxychloroquine and other antimalarials are useful in controlling the rashes associated with myositis.

DIAGNOSTIC TOOLS, EVALUATION, AND DIFFERENTIAL DIAGNOSIS

Clinical, laboratory, pathologic, and electrodiagnostic findings contribute to the proper diagnosis of IIM. Even in individuals with typical clinical features of IIM, it is essential to exclude other diseases that may have similar symptoms and signs (Table 56.5). Certain clinical features should suggest a different diagnosis. These include a family history of a similar illness; sensory, reflex, or other neurologic changes; fasciculations; a relationship of the weakness to exercise, food intake, or fasting; major muscle cramping, myotonia (difficulty relaxing a contracted muscle), or myasthenia (increasing weakness with repeated contractions); significant early muscle atrophy or hypertrophy; marked asymmetry; weakness in the distribution of the cranial nerves; and dyspnea due to diaphragmatic weakness rather than lung fibrosis.

The single most useful laboratory feature of muscle destruction is elevation of the serum CK, although this is nonspecific, and a small proportion of patients – probably < 5% – have a bona fide inflammatory muscle disease without ever having an elevated CK. Elevations of the serum levels of aldolase, serum glutamic-oxaloacetic transaminase (SGOT), serum glutamate pyruvate transaminase (SGPT), and lactate dehydrogenase (LDH) are as frequent but less specific for muscle disease. Unlike other autoimmune inflammatory diseases, inflammatory markers such as the erythrocyte sedimentation rate and C-reactive protein are often not elevated. Although some studies have shown ESR to be elevated in 50% of patients, most experts find a substantially lower proportion of IIM patients to have an elevated ESR, even with active disease.[41] Likewise, hematologic abnormalities, including anemia, are uncommon and rarely related to the underlying myopathy. If a significant abnormality is found, the physician should be alert to another cause for it.

Electromyographic (EMG) abnormalities are frequently present. Although the test is useful to exclude some neurologic diseases that resemble IIM, it is painful for many patients and not useful for following the course of the illness.

Magnetic resonance imaging (MRI), especially a combination of the T_1 and the fat-suppressed T_2 (STIR) sequences, is remarkably useful in defining the extent of involvement and planning a biopsy (Fig. 56.2). Whole-body MRI was recently shown to facilitate the characterization of inflammatory myopathy, as certain patterns of muscle and subcutaneous tissue inflammation were predictive of the IIM subset (DM, PM, or IBM).[42] Although not specific, the changes of inflammatory myopathy can provide considerable assistance in confusing cases, as well as help in choosing a site to biopsy.

A muscle biopsy should be performed in every suspected case of myositis (Fig. 56.3). Although the patchy involvement means that the biopsy may occasionally miss inflammation, confounding diagnoses, for example amyloidosis, eosinophilic myositis, dystrophy, or some metabolic myopathies as well as the important variant IBM, can only be diagnosed definitively by biopsy. The identification of autoantibodies, particularly the myositis-specific autoantibodies, has distinct clinical and prognostic use. MSAs are highly specific for myositis compared to other neuromuscular diseases, and are not simply associated with muscle inflammation.[43]

At present, of these autoantibodies only anti-Jo-1 is commercially available, but tests for the others are carried out in research centers, and some will eventually become more widely available.

PITFALLS

It is increasingly apparent that the boundary between IIM and some genetically determined myopathies cannot be cleanly drawn. In the last several years, dystrophies with an extraordinary variety of clinical manifestations (with regard to age and distribution of weakness) have also been described.[44] Not only can inflammation be seen on

Table 56.5 Differential diagnosis of IIM

Neuromuscular disorders
Genetic muscular dystrophies
Metabolic myopathies
  Disorders of carbohydrate metabolism: McArdle disease, phosphofructokinase deficiency, adult acid maltase deficiency, and others
  Disorders of lipid metabolism: carnitine deficiency, carnitine palmitoyl transferase deficiency
  Disorders of purine metabolism: myoadenylate deaminase deficiency
Mitochondrial myopathies
Spinal muscular atrophies
Neuropathies: Guillain–Barré and other autoimmune polyneuropathies, diabetes mellitus, porphyria
Myasthenia gravis and Eaton–Lambert syndrome
Amyotrophic lateral sclerosis
Myotonic dystrophy and other myotonias
Familial periodic paralysis

Endocrine and electrolyte disorders
Hypokalemia, hypercalcemia, hypocalcemia, hypomagnesemia
Hypothyroidism, hyperthyroidism
Cushing syndrome, Addison's disease

Toxic myopathies (partial list)
Alcohol
Chloroquine and hydroxychloroquine
Cocaine
Colchicine
Corticosteroids
D-Penicillamine
Ipecac
Statins and other lipid-lowering agents
Zidovudine (AZT)

Infections
Viral: HIV, HTLV-1, influenza
Bacterial: staphylococcus, streptococcus, clostridia
Parasitic: toxoplasmosis, trichinosis, schistosomiasis, cysticercosis

Miscellaneous
Polymyalgia rheumatica
Vasculitis
Eosinophilia myalgia syndrome
Paraneoplastic syndromes

biopsy in some patients, but a partial clinical response to corticosteroids can occur. Furthermore, it is increasingly recognized that mitochondrial abnormalities can be limited to groups of skeletal muscles, leading to confusion with IIM. Toxic myopathies, of course, will continue to occur with the release of new drugs, and will continue to be a possible source of diagnostic confusion.

Thus, not only must the history, physical examination, and biopsy be performed and interpreted with compulsiveness and care, but molecular diagnostic techniques must be employed by clinicians in pursuit of an

CLINICAL PEARLS

CLINICAL FEATURES THAT SUGGEST A NON-IIM DIAGNOSIS

>> Family history of a similar illness

>> Weakness related to exercise, eating, or fasting

>> Sensory, reflex, or other neurologic signs

>> Cranial nerve involvement

>> Fasciculations

>> Muscle cramping (severe)

>> Myasthenia (increasing weakness with repeated contractions)

>> Myotonia (difficulty relaxing a contracted muscle)

>> Significant atrophy or hypertrophy early in the illness

>> Marked asymmetry

>> Dyspnea due to diaphragmatic weakness with normal chest X-ray

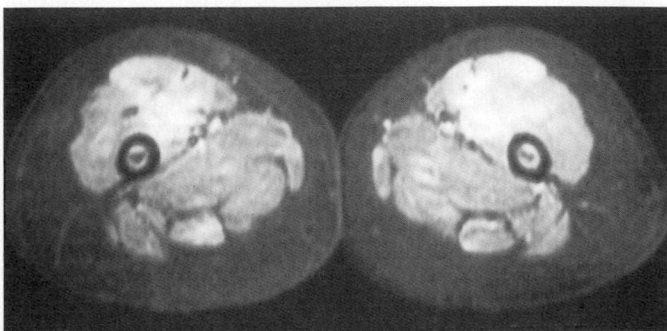
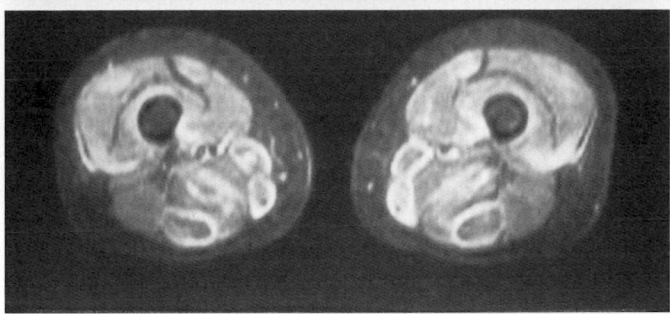

Fig. 56.2 Magnetic resonance images of the upper and lower thighs of a patient with dermatomyositis using the fat-suppressed T$_2$ (STIR) technique. With this technique inflammation appears as a bright signal; normal muscle is gray; and bone, fat, fascia, and normal skin are dark. Blood vessels may appear as bright spots. Note the remarkable symmetry of the inflammation. In this patient most of the involvement is in the quadriceps in the upper thighs and around the periphery of the hamstring muscle group.

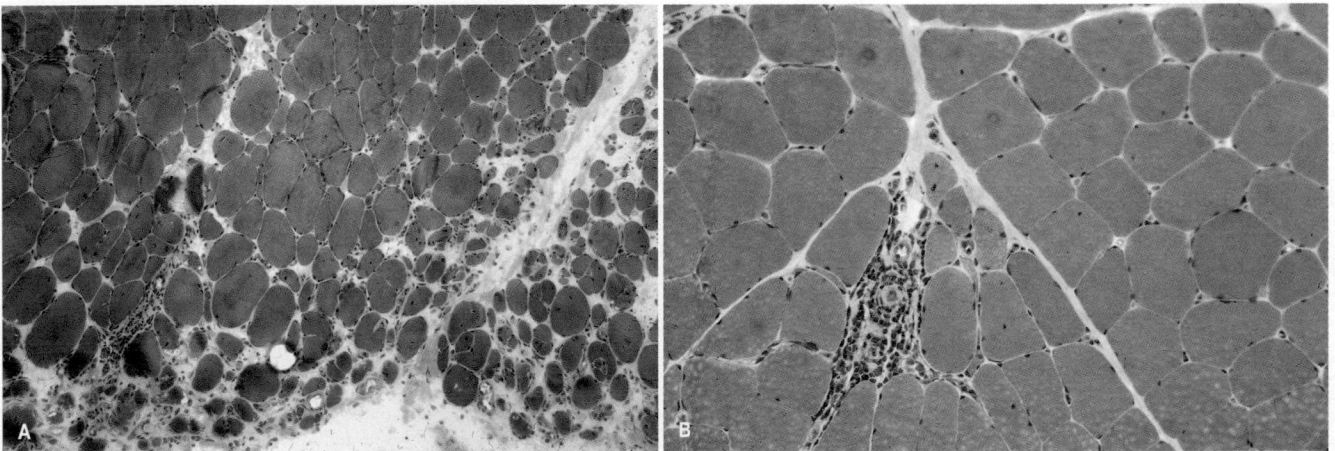

Fig. 56.3 Biopsy in dermatomyositis. (**A**) Low-power (original magnification × 100) view of a muscle biopsy from a patient with dermatomyositis. Note the marked variation in fiber size and the large number of atrophic myocytes, particularly at the periphery of the fascicles. (**B**) High-power (original magnification × 200) view of inflammation around the vessels in the muscle biopsy of a patient with dermatomyositis. There are nearby atrophic cells and cells whose nuclei have moved away from the periphery of the cell (centralized nuclei).

accurate diagnosis and appropriate therapy. The correct response to disease that persists in the face of powerful immunosuppressive therapy is a careful re-thinking of the diagnosis, including, on occasion, re-biopsy and molecular consultation.

◼ REFERENCES ◼

1. Sontheimer RD. Dermatomyositis: an overview of recent progress with emphasis on dermatologic aspects. Dermatol Clin 2002; 20: 387–408.

2. Bohan A, Peter JB. Polymyositis and dermatomyositis (second of two parts). N Engl J Med 1975; 292: 403–407.

3. Bohan A, Peter JB. Polymyositis and dermatomyositis (first of two parts). N Engl J Med 1975; 292: 344–347.

4. Badrising UA, Maat-Schieman M, van Duinen SG, et al. Epidemiology of inclusion body myositis in the Netherlands: a nationwide study. Neurology 2000; 55: 1385–1387.

5. Tanimoto K, Nakano K, Kano S, et al. Classification criteria for polymyositis and dermatomyositis. J Rheumatol 1995; 22: 668–674.

6. Targoff IN, Miller FW, Medsger TA Jr, Oddis CV. Classification criteria for the idiopathic inflammatory myopathies. Curr Opin Rheumatol 1997; 9: 527–535.

7. Kao AH, Lacomis D, Lucas M, et al. Anti-signal recognition particle autoantibody in patients with and patients without idiopathic inflammatory myopathy. Arthritis Rheum 2004; 50: 209–215.

8. Yang CC, Askanas V, Engel WK, Alvarez RB. Immunolocalization of transcription factor NF-kappa B in inclusion-body myositis muscle and at normal human neuromuscular junctions. Neurosci Lett 1998; 254: 77.

9. Engel AG, Arahata K, Emslie-Smith A. Immune effector mechanisms in inflammatory myopathies. Res Publ Assoc Res Nerv Ment Dis 1990; 68: 141.

10. Argov Z, Eisenberg I, Mitrani-Rosenbaum S. Genetics of inclusion body myopathies. Curr Opin Rheumatol 1998; 10: 543.

11. Mathews MB, Bernstein RM. Myositis autoantibody inhibits histidyl-tRNA synthetase: a model for autoimmunity. Nature 1983; 304: 177.

12. Leff RL, Love LA, Miller FW, et al. Viruses in idiopathic inflammatory myopathies: absence of candidate viral genomes in muscle. Lancet 1992; 339: 1192.

13. Smith RD, Konoplev S, DeCourten-Myers G, Brown T. west Nile virus encephalitis with myositis and orchitis. Hum Pathol 2004, 35: 254–258.

14. Petersen LR, Marfin AA. West Nile virus: a primer for the clinician. Ann Intern Med 2002; 137: 173–179.

15. OHanlon T, Koneru B, Bayat E, et al. Environmental Myositis Study Group. Immunogenetic differences between Caucasian women with and those without silicone implants in whom myositis develops. Arthritis Rheum 2004; 50: 3646–3650.

16. Walji S, Rubenstein J, Shannon P, Carette S. Disseminated pyomyositis mimicking idiopathic inflammatory myopathy. J Rheumatol 2005; 32: 184–187.

17. Adams EM, Kirkley J, Eidelman G, et al. The predominance of beta (CC) chemokine transcripts in idiopathic inflammatory muscle diseases. Proc Assoc Am Phys 1997; 109: 275.

18. Lundberg I, Brengman JM, Engel AG. Analysis of cytokine expression in muscle in inflammatory myopathies, Duchenne dystrophy, and non-weak controls. J Neuroimmunol 1995; 63: 9.

19. Lundberg I, Ulfgren AK, Nyberg P, et al. Cytokine production in muscle tissue of patients with idiopathic inflammatory myopathies. Arthritis Rheum 1997; 40: 865.

20. Nagaraju K, Raben N, Villalba ML, et al. Costimulatory markers in muscle of patients with idiopathic inflammatory myopathies and in cultured muscle cells. Clin Immunol 1999; 92: 161.

21. Estruch R, Grau JM, Fernandez-Sola J, et al. Microvascular changes in skeletal muscle in idiopathic inflammatory myopathy. Hum Pathol 1992; 23: 888.

22. Greenberg SA, Pinkus JL, Pinkus GS, et al. Interferonα/βmediated innate immune mechanisms in dermatomyositis. Ann Neurol 2005; 57: 664–678.

23. Nagaraju K, Casciola-Rosen L, Lundberg I. Activation of the endoplasmic reticulum stress response in autoimmune myositis: potential role in muscle fiber damage and dysfunction. Arthritis Rheum 2005; 52: 1824–1835.

24. van der Pas J, Hengstman GJ, ter Laak HJ, et al. Diagnostic value of MHC class I staining in idiopathic inflammatory myopathies. J Neurol Neurosurg Psychiatry 2004; 75: 136–139.

25. Casciola-Rosen L, Nagaraju K, Plotz P, et al. Enhanced autoantigen expression in regenerating muscle cells in idiopathic inflammatory myopathy. J Exp Med 2005; 201: 591–601.

26. Wakasugi K, Schimmel P. Two distinct cytokines released from a human aminoacyl-tRNA synthetase. Science 1999; 284: 147.

27. Goldstein R, Duvic M, Targoff IN, et al. HLA-D region genes associated with autoantibody responses to histidyl-transfer RNA synthetase (Jo-1) and other translation-related factors in myositis. Arthritis Rheum 1990; 33: 1240.

28. Amoura Z, Duhaut P, Huong DTL, et al. Tumor antigen markers for the detection of solid cancers in inflammatory myopathies. Cancer Epidemiol Biomarkers Prev 2005; 14: 1279–1282.

29. Danko K, Ponyi A, Constantin T, et al. Long-term survival of patients with idiopathic inflammatory myopathies according to clinical features. Medicine 2004; 83: 35–42.

30. Bronner IM, van der Muelen M FG, de Visser M, et al. Long-term outcome in polymyositis and dermatomyositis. Ann Rheum Dis 2006; 65: 1456–1461. Epub 2006; Apr 10.

31. Ponyi A, Constantin T, Balogh Z. Disease course, frequency of relapses and survival of 73 patients with juvenile or adult dermatomyositis. Clin Exp Rheumatol 2005; 23: 50–56.

32. Agarwal SK, Monach PA, Docken WP. Characterization of relapses in adult idiopathic inflammatory myopathies. Clin Rheumatol 2005; 25: 1–6.

33. Bunch TW. Prednisone and azathioprine for polymyositis: long-term followup. Arthritis Rheum 1981; 24: 45.

34. Metzger AL, Bohan A, Goldberg LS, et al. Polymyositis and dermatomyositis: combined methotrexate and corticosteroid therapy. Ann Intern Med 1974; 81: 182.

35. Joffe MM, Love LA, Leff RL, et al. Drug therapy of the idiopathic inflammatory myopathies: predictors of response to prednisone, azathioprine, and methotrexate and a comparison of their efficacy. Am J Med 1993; 94: 379.

36. Villalba L, Hicks JE, Adams EM, et al. Treatment of refractory myositis: a randomized crossover study of two new cytotoxic regimens. Arthritis Rheum 1998; 41: 392.

37. Dalakas MC, Illa I, Dambrosia JM, et al. A controlled trial of high-dose intravenous immune globulin infusions as treatment for dermatomyositis. N Engl J Med 1993; 329: 1392–1393.

38. Miller FW, Leitman SF, Cronin ME, et al. Controlled trial of plasma exchange and leukapheresis in polymyositis and dermatomyositis. N Engl J Med 1992; 326: 1380.

39. Leff R, Miller F, Hicks J, et al. The treatment of inclusion body myositis (IBM): A retrospective review and a randomized, prospective trial of immunosuppressive therapy. Medicine (Baltimore) 1993; 72: 225.

40. Sayers ME, Chou SM, Calabrese LH. Inclusion body myositis: analysis of 32 cases. J Rheumatol 1992; 19: 1385.

41. Rider LG, Miller FW. Laboratory evaluation of the inflammatory myopathies. Clin Diagn Lab Immunol 1995; 2: 1–9.

42. Cantwell C, Ryan M, O'Connell M, et al. A comparison of inflammatory myopathies at whole-body turbo STIR MRI. Clin Radiol 2005; 60: 261–267.

43. Hengstman GJ, van Brenk L, Vree Egberts WT, et al. High specificity of myositis specific autoantibodies for myositis compared with other neuromuscular disorders. Neurology 2005; 252: 534–537.

44. Emery AE. The muscular dystrophies. Br Med J: 317–991.

REFERENCES

Table 57.1 Current classification criteria for spondyloarthritis

A. European Spondyloarthropathy Study Group (ESSG) criteria for spondyloarthritis
1. Inflammatory back pain or synovitis (asymmetric, lower extremity) *plus* one of the following:
   (a) Alternating buttock pain
   (b) Sacroiliitis
   (c) Heel pain (enthesitis)
   (d) Positive family history
   (e) Psoriasis
   (f) Crohn's disease, ulcerative colitis
   (g) Urethritis or cervicitis or acute diarrhea in the preceding 4 weeks

B. The modified New York criteria for ankylosing spondylitis[4]
1. Clinical criteria:
   (a) Low-back pain and stiffness for more than 3 months which improves with exercise, but is not relieved by rest
   (b) Limitation of motion of the lumbar spine in both the sagittal and frontal planes
   (c) Limitation of chest expansion relative to normal values correlated for age and sex
2. Radiological criterion:
   Sacroiliitis grade ≥ 2 bilaterally or grade 3–4 unilaterally
   Definite ankylosing sponylitis if the radiological criterion is associated with at least one clinical criterion

C. The classification criteria for psoriatic arthritis (CASPAR) criteria for psoriatic arthritis
1. Inflammatory joint disease plus at least three points from the following features
   (a) Current psoriasis (assigned a score of 2; all others assigned a score of 1)
   (b) History of psoriasis
   (c) Family history of psoriasis
   (d) Dactylitis
   (e) Juxta-articular new bone formation
   (f) Rheumatoid factor seronegativity
   (g) Nail dystrophy

D. Criteria for reactive arthritis (proposed at the International Workshop on Reactive Arthritis, 1996)
1. An acute inflammatory arthritis, inflammatory low-back pain, or enthesitis
2. Evidence of an infection preceding this condition by 4–8 weeks[11]

E. The International League Against Rheumatism (ILAR) Juvenile Idiopathic Arthritis Classification Criteria for Enthesitis-Related Arthritis (ERA)
Arthritis and enthesitis
or
Arthritis or enthesitis with at least two of:
1. Sacroiliac joint tenderness and/or inflammatory spinal pain
2. Presence of human leukocyte antigen (HLA)-B27
3. Family history in at least one first- or second-degree relative of medically confirmed HLA-B27-associated disease
4. Anterior uveitis that is usually associated with pain, redness, or photophobia
5. Onset of arthritis in a boy after 8 years of age

Exclusions
Psoriasis confirmed by a dermatologist in at least one first- or second-degree relative
Presence of systemic arthritis

Table 57.2 The epidemiology of spondyloarthritis

Ethnic group	HLA-B27 frequency (%)	Prevalence of AS	Prevalence of PsA	Prevalence of SpA
Circumpolar groups				
Eskimos (Alaska)	40	0.4	1.5	1.5
Sami (North Norway)	24	1.8	0.23	n.a.
Asia				
China	2-9	0.11–0.26	n.a.	0.5-1.0
Taiwan	5.7	0.19–0.54	n.a.	n.a.
Vietnam	n.a.	0.05	n.a.	0.28
Thailand	4.0	n.a.	n.a.	0.12
Japan	< 1	0.007	n.a.	0.01
Europe and North America				
Norway	16	1.1–1.4	0.195	n.a.
Moravia	16	0.5	n.a.	n.a.
Greece	5.4	0.24	0.17	0.49
France	8	0.2	0.19	0.3
Italy	n.a.	0.37	0.42	n.a.
Germany	9	0.7	1.9	1.9
USA	6-8	0.2–0.5 (estimated)	0.1	0.4–1.2 (estimated)

AS, ankylosing spondylitis; HLA, human leukocyte antigen; n.a., not available; PsA, psoriatic arthritis; SpA, spondyloarthritis

The prevalence of IBD is 100–200 per 100 000 in Caucasians, with equal male-to-female ratio.[8, 11] It is rare in people of African and Asian descent. The risk of spondylitis and peripheral arthritis varies in different reports, perhaps reflecting the subspecialty of the observer. Spondylitis occurs in as many as 15–20% of those with IBD. In general, peripheral arthritis occurs less frequently in those with UC (up to 10%) than in those with Crohn's disease (up to 20%), although its frequency tends to be higher in series where the assessor was a rheumatologist.[8, 10, 11]

■ PATHOGENESIS ■

GENETICS OF SPONDYLOARTHRITIS

Familial aggregation

Susceptibility to AS is clearly attributable to genetic factors, with a sibling recurrence risk ratio as high as 82 and twin-based studies estimating disease heritability to exceed 90%.[12–14] The concordance rate for AS in identical twins has been reported to be as high as 63%, compared to 23% in non-identical twins.[12] The concurrence rate for psoriasis in monozygotic twins is 70% versus 15–30% in dizygotic twins. Recurrence risk for parents and sibs of patients with Crohn's disease is 4.8% and 7%, respectively, and for UC 0.9% and 1.2%, respectively.[13]

HLA-B27 and spondyloarthritis

HLA-B27, which is encoded in the MHC class I region, confers the greatest known risk for AS, and is found in up to 95% of AS patients of European ancestry[12–14] (Table 57.3).

Approximately 70% of patients with ReA have HLA-B27, except in Africa, where no association of HLA-B27 is seen in those with HIV-associated SpA.[13, 14] HLA-B27 does not confer susceptibility to the initial triggering infections in ReA but does correlate with ReA severity.[13]

HLA-B27 is found in 60–70% of patients with psoriatic spondylitis and in 25% of those with peripheral PsA.[13, 14] Up to 70% of those with IBD-associated spondylitis have HLA-B27, although no HLA-B27 association is seen with asymptomatic sacroiliitis. Approximately 50% of patients with AAU alone are HLA-B27-positive.[1]

Over 35 molecular subtypes of HLA-B27 have been described this far (Table 57.4). The most common subtypes (*HLA-B*2705, B*2702, B*2704, B*2707, B*2714*) are clearly associated with SpA. Two subtypes of HLA-B27, *HLA-B*2706* and *B*2709*, found in Southeast Asia and Sardinia, respectively, appear not to be associated with AS,[14] possibly due to amino acid differences in the 'B' pocket of the HLA antigen-binding cleft at positions 114 and 116 that could alter the composition and anchoring of peptides presented by these HLA-B27 subtypes. The other subtypes of HLA-B27 are too rare to have had disease associations established. One subtype, *HLA-B*2722*, was due to a sequencing error and has been withdrawn. These subtypes evolved

Table 57.3 Genetic factors implicated in spondyloarthritis

Factor	Ankylosing spondylitis (%)	Reactive arthritis (%)	Psoriasis/psoriatic arthritis/spondylitis (%)	IBD/enteropathic arthritis/spondylitis (%)
HLA-B27 frequency	90%	70%	24/60/70	7/7/70
Other MHC genes	B60 (B*4001), DRB1*0101	DR4	*C*0602, B*38, B*39, DRB1*04, DRB1*07*	None/*DRB1*0103*/none
Non-MHC genes	*CYP2D6*, interleukin-1 ?ANKH		Interleukin-1 KIR TNF	*Nod2*, IL-23R
Chromosomal regions implicated in genome scans	6p (MHC)-definite 10q, 16q-suggestive 1q, 3q, 5q, 6q, 9q, 17q and 19q-nominal		6p (PSORS1)	

HLA, human leukocyte antigen; MHC, major histocompatibility complex; TNF, tumor necrosis factor.

KEY CONCEPTS

THE GENETIC BASIS OF SPONDYLOARTHRITIS

>> Human leukocyte antigen (HLA)-B27 comprises nearly half of the overall susceptibility to ankylosing spondylitis (AS), and contributes heavily to susceptibility to reactive arthritis, psoriatic and enteropathic spondylitis

>> Additional influences seem to come from other major histocompatibility complex (MHC) genes, including *C*0602* for psoriasis, whose identification has been confounded by linkage to HLA-B27

>> Genetic modeling has suggested up to six additional non-MHC influences

>> Analyses of genomewide scans implicated regions, in addition to the MHC, on chromosomes 10 and 16, and possibly on chromosomes 1, 3, 5, 17, and 19.

>> Non-MHC genes that have been confirmed thus far include the interleukin-1 gene complex on chromosome 2q and the CYP2D6 locus on chromosome 22

>> Genomewide association studies utilizing dense SNP mapping will likely locate many of the remaining genes in AS susceptibility

from the parent allele *HLA-B*2705* along three lines (Fig. 57.1) in three distinct geographic regions.

The exact mechanism underlying the effect of HLA-B27 on disease susceptibility has still not been determined. One theory suggests that SpA results from a unique set of antigenic peptides, either bacterial or self, that are bound and presented by all disease-associated HLA-B27 subtypes (but not by other HLA class I molecules) to CD8 T cells, resulting in an HLA-B27-restricted cytotoxic T-cell response found only in joints and other affected tissues (the so-called *arthritogenic peptide* hypothesis). Recent data suggest that the differential association of HLA-B27 subtypes with SpA is more likely related to differentially bound peptides than to altered antigenicity of shared ligands. The strongest evidence against this theory is that a specific 'arthritogenic peptide' has yet to be demonstrated.

An alternative concept focuses on self-association as a unique property of the HLA-B27 molecule. HLA-B27 heavy chains can form homodimers *in vitro* that are dependent on disulfide binding through their cysteine-67 residues in the extracellular α_1 domain (as well as other cysteine residues in other domains) (Fig. 57.2).[13–15] This occurs as a result of B27 misfolding within the endoplasmic reticulum. The accumulation of misfolded protein results in a proinflammatory intracellular stress response through the stimulation of interferon-β secretion. Also, HLA-B27 homodimers are detectable at the cell surface in patients with SpA, are capable of peptide binding, and are more abundantly expressed when the cell's antigen-presenting function is impaired. They are ligands for a number of natural killer (NK) and related cell surface receptors. Populations of synovial and peripheral blood monocytes, and B and T lymphocytes from patients with SpA and controls, carry receptors for HLA-B27 homodimers, including KIR3DL1 and KIR3DL2, which are receptors for NK cells, and immunoglobulin-like transcript 4 (ILT4).[13–15] It is possible that these homodimers may act as a proinflammatory target or receptor for humoral or cell-mediated autoimmune responses. However, it is not yet known whether HLA-B27 homodimer formation is specific for, or even correlates with, the presence of SpA; in fact, most HLA-B27-positive individuals do not develop disease.

Table 57.4 Amino acid sequence of human leukocyte antigen (HLA)-B27 subtypes in the diversity regions of the first and second domains

Position	60	70	80	90	100	110	120 131	151	160 172
B*270502	EYW	DRETQICKAK	AQTDREDLRT	LLRYYNQSEA	GSHTLQNMYG	CDVGPDGRLL	RGYHQDAYDG	SSWTA	RVAEQLRAYLE-GECVEWLRRYL
B*2701	---	----------	---Y-N---	A--------	----------	----------	----------	-----	------------
B*2702	---	----------	----N-I--	A--------	----------	----------	----------	-----	------------
B*2703	-H-	----------	----------	----------	----------	----------	----------	-----	------------
B*2704	---	----------	---S-----	----------	----------	----------	--D-Y----	-----	---E--------
B*2706	---	----------	---S-----	----------	---S-----	----------	--HN-Y---	R----	--E---------
B*2707	---	----------	---S-N---	--RG-----	----------	----------	----------	-----	------------
B*2708	---	----------	---S-N---	--RG-----	----------	----------	----------	-----	------------
B*2709	---	----------	----------	----------	----------	----------	----H----	-----	---E--------
E*2710	---	----------	----S----	--RG-----	---S-----	----------	--HN-Y---	R----	------------
E*2711	---	----------	----S----	----------	----------	----------	----------	-----	------------
E*2712	---	------TN--	T---S-N--	----------	----------	----------	----------	-----	--E------T--
E*2713	---	----------	----------	----------	----------	----------	----------	-----	---E--------
B*2714	---	----------	----------	----------	--W-T----	------L---	----------	-----	------------
B*2715	---	------TN--	---S-----	----------	----------	----------	----------	-----	------------
B*2716	---	----------	T--------	----------	----------	----------	----------	-----	------------
B*2717	-F-	----------	----------	----------	----------	----------	----------	-----	------------
B*2718	---	----S-TN--	T-Y-S--N-	--RG-----	--II-R---	----------	----------	-----	---E--------
B*2719	---	----------	---S-----	----------	----------	----------	--HN-Y---	-----	---E--------
B*2720	---	----------	---S-----	----------	----R----	----------	--D-Y----	R----	---E--------
B*2721	---	-N--F-TN--	----------	----------	----------	----------	----------	-----	---E--------
B*2723	---	----------	T--Y-S---	----------	----------	----------	--HN-Y---	-----	------------
B*2724	---	----------	---S-----	----------	---S-----	----------	----------	R----	---E--------
B*2725	---	-------Q--	---S-----	--RG-----	----------	----------	--HN-Y---	-----	---E--W---L-
B*2726	---	----------	----------	----------	----------	----------	----------	-----	------------
B*2727	---	----------	----------	----------	--II-R---	----------	----------	-----	------------
B*2728	---	---S-TN--	T-Y------	A--------	----------	----------	----------	-----	----------T---H
3*2729	---	----------	----N-I--	A--------	----------	----------	----------	-----	------------
3*2730	---	-------Q--	---S-----	----------	----------	----------	----------	-----	------------
3*2731	---	----------	---S-----	----------	---S-----	----------	--HN-----	R----	------------
3*2732	---	----------	----------	--RG-----	---S-----	----------	--HD-----	R----	------------
B*2733	---	----------	---S-----	----------	---S-----	----------	----N----	-----	------------
B*2734	---	----------	----------	----------	----------	----------	----------	-----	------------
B*2735	---	----------	----------	----------	----------	----------	----------	-----	------------
B*2736	---	----------	---S-----	----------	----------	----------	----------	-----	------------

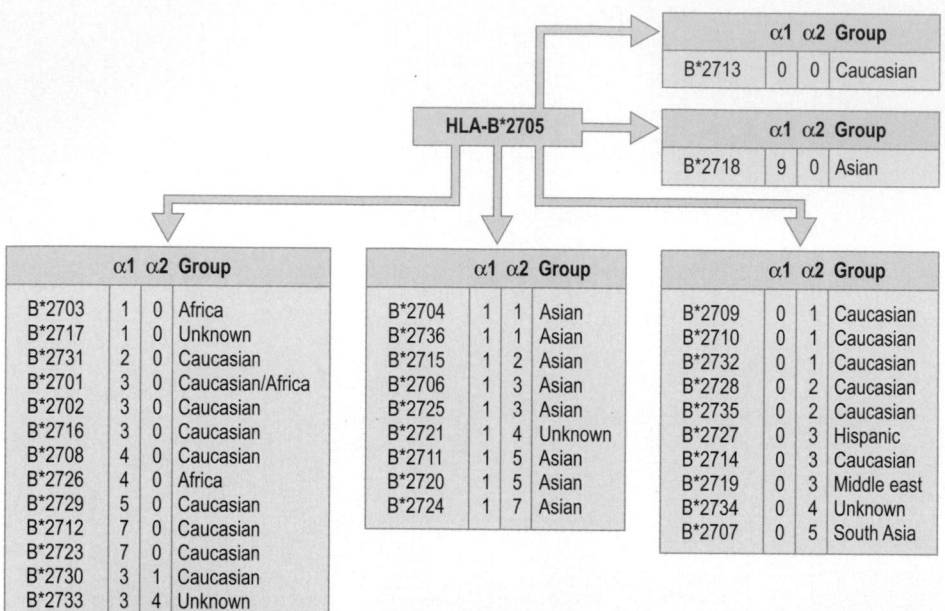

	α1	α2	Group
B*2713	0	0	Caucasian

	α1	α2	Group
B*2718	9	0	Asian

HLA-B*2705

	α1	α2	Group
B*2703	1	0	Africa
B*2717	1	0	Unknown
B*2731	2	0	Caucasian
B*2701	3	0	Caucasian/Africa
B*2702	3	0	Caucasian
B*2716	3	0	Caucasian
B*2708	4	0	Caucasian
B*2726	4	0	Africa
B*2729	5	0	Caucasian
B*2712	7	0	Caucasian
B*2723	7	0	Caucasian
B*2730	3	1	Caucasian
B*2733	3	4	Unknown

	α1	α2	Group
B*2704	1	1	Asian
B*2736	1	1	Asian
B*2715	1	2	Asian
B*2706	1	3	Asian
B*2725	1	3	Asian
B*2721	1	4	Unknown
B*2711	1	5	Asian
B*2720	1	5	Asian
B*2724	1	7	Asian

	α1	α2	Group
B*2709	0	1	Caucasian
B*2710	0	1	Caucasian
B*2732	0	1	Caucasian
B*2728	0	2	Caucasian
B*2735	0	2	Caucasian
B*2727	0	3	Hispanic
B*2714	0	3	Caucasian
B*2719	0	3	Middle east
B*2734	0	4	Unknown
B*2707	0	5	South Asia

Fig. 57.1 The three major families of human leukocyte antigen (HLA)-B27 subtypes (*HLA-B*2713* and *B*2718* are assumed to have evolved separately) are denoted in relationship to the 'parent' subtype *HLA-B*2705*. Most B27 subtypes have evolved through three patterns of evolution along geographic lines. The first group, including *HLA-B*2703-B*2723* (and *B*2730*), appears to have evolved in Africa and Europe, and entails anywhere from one to seven amino acid substitutions in the first (α1) domain, and has the second (α2) domain identical to *B*2705*. The second group, including *HLA-B*2704-B*2724*, evolved in Asia and includes a uniform amino acid substitution in the α1 domain and anywhere from one to seven substitutions in the α2 domain. The third group, including *HLA-B*2709-B*2707*, evolved in southern Asia, the Middle East, and Sardinia and has an α1-domain identical to *B*2705* and an α2 domain with one to seven amino acid substitutions. Notable exceptions include *HLA-B*2713*, which has an amino acid substitution outside α1 and α2, *B*2718*, which appears to have evolved separately in Asia, and *B*2730*, which shares features of the first and third groups.

OTHER MHC GENES AND SPA SUSCEPTIBILITY

HLA-B27 is not the only genetic factor involved in AS and SpA susceptibility (Table 57.3). Fewer than 5% of HLA-B27-positive individuals in the general population become affected,[13, 14] whereas up to 20% of HLA-B27-positive relatives of AS patients will develop SpA. Family studies have suggested that HLA-B27 contributes less than 40% of the overall genetic risk for SpA[12] while the entire effect of the MHC, on the other hand, is about 50%.[12, 16]

HLA-B60, a serologically defined HLA specificity that correlates with *HLA-B*4001* on DNA analysis, has been described as augmenting the risk for AS in both HLA-B27-positive and negative individuals from Europe and Taiwan.[13, 14] Other HLA-B associations that have been reported include PsA-associated alleles HLA-B38 and B39,[14] as well as HLA-B35 and B62 in Caucasian[14] patients lacking HLA-B27.

Other MHC genes have also been implicated in AS in addition to B27, although their identification is complicated by the tight linkage disequilibrium found within the MHC, and many of the associations described thus far might be better explained by linkage to B27. These include MICA, located adjacent to HLA-B27, which encodes a marker of 'stress' in epithelial cells, and acts as a ligand for cells expressing a common activator NK receptor (NKG2D), as well as tumor necrosis factor (TNF), heat shock protein (HSP)-70, LMP-2 and LMP-7, *HLA-DRB1*01*, and *DRB1*04* alleles.[13, 14] In addition, *HLA-DRB1*08* has been implicated both in susceptibility to uveitis in the setting of AS and to juvenile-onset AS.[1, 13, 14] Both *HLA-DRB1*04* and *07* alleles have been implicated in PsA, and *HLA-DRB1*0103* has been associated with enteropathic peripheral arthritis.[13]

LINKAGE STUDIES OF NON-MHC GENES

Recurrence risk modeling suggests that AS is an oligogenic disease (probable up to three to nine genes in total) with predominantly multiplicative interaction between loci.[12–14] A recent meta-analysis of three genome-wide linkage studies in AS or undifferentiated SpA from the UK, North America, and France,[16] including genotype data from 589 affected sibling pairs with AS, showed strongest evidence of linkage of AS to the MHC (Table 57.3), with suggestive linkage on chromosomes 10q and 16q, and areas of nominal linkage on chromosomes 1q, 3q, 5q, 6q, 9q, 17q, and 19q (Table 57.3). Although no genome-wide scans have been conducted in PsA, those in psoriasis itself have mapped a major susceptibility locus to a 60-kb interval telomeric to HLA-C in the MHC known as PSORS1, recently suggested to be HLA-Cw6,[17] as well as other regions on chromosome 17q (PSORS2) and others on other chromosomes 1, 3, 4 and 19 (PSORS3-9) (Fig. 57.3). Since the first genome-wide scan for IBD was published in 1996, numerous other scans have identified seven genomic susceptibility regions, designated IBD1-9,

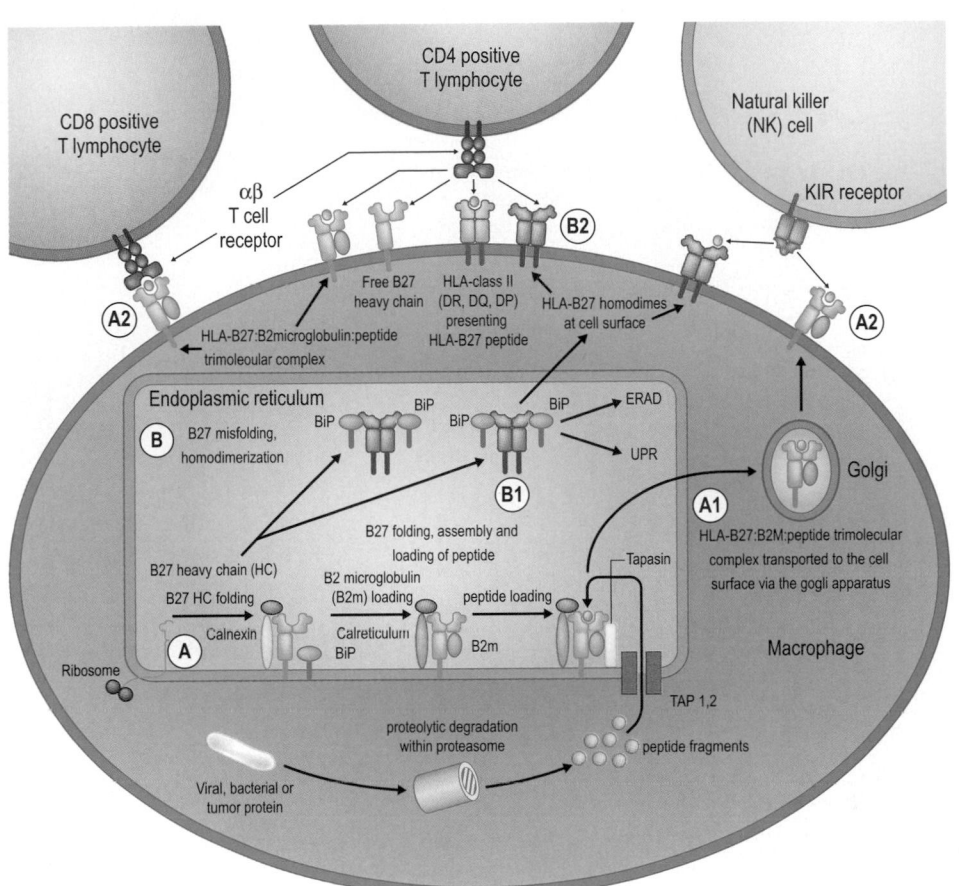

Fig. 57.2 After transcription of the human leukocyte antigen (HLA)-B27 heavy chain on ribosomes in macrophages, it is inserted into the endoplasmic reticulum (ER), glycosylated, and two pathways ensue. (A) The B27 heavy chain is retained through binding with calnexin and ERp57, folded into its tertiary structure and bound to β_2-microglobulin. After that calnexin releases the complex and it is associated with calreticulum, which in turn chaperones the formation of the peptide loading on to the complex of heavy chain, β_2-microglobulin and antigenic peptide, via the TAP proteins and tapasin. Then the trimolecular peptide complex (HLA-B27 heavy chain, β_2-microglobulin and peptide) travels through the Golgi apparatus (A1) to the cell surface, where the antigenic peptide is presented either to the α:β T-cell receptor on CD8-positive T lymphocytes or to the killer immunoglobulin (KIR) receptor on natural killer (NK) cells (A2); or (B) the HLA-B27 heavy chain misfolds in the ER, forming B27 homodimers and other misfoldings which are bound to the ER chaperone BiP. Then, they either (B1) accumulate there, causing either ER-associated degradation (ERAD) or a proinflammatory ER unfolded protein response (UPR); or (B2) the B27 homodimers migrate to the cell surface where they either become antigenic themselves or present peptide to receptors on T cells and natural killer (NK) cells.

located on chromosomes 1, 5, 6, 12, 14, 16, and 19. However, only IBD1, at chromosome 16q12, has been universally replicated (Fig. 57.3).[12, 13]

NON-MHC GENES IN SUSCEPTIBILITY TO SPONDYLOARTHRITIS

The interleukin-1 (IL-1) complex lies on chromosome 2q and includes the genes encoding the proinflammatory cytokines IL-1α, IL-1β, and their naturally occurring inhibitor, IL-1 receptor antagonist (IL-1RA), as well as six other homologous genes of unclear function named *IL-1F5–IL-1F10*. Although numerous studies have suggested a role for genes in this region in AS susceptibility, the actual gene(s) has yet to be identified. Recent studies from the UK, Canada, Taiwan, and the USA[14] have suggested that the IL-1B association may be better explained by linkage disequilibrium with

IL-1A, which may be the primary IL-1 complex gene associated with AS. Nevertheless, it is likely that more than one IL-1 complex gene is involved in AS susceptibility, although the other associated genetic variant(s) remain to be determined. The extensive linkage disequilibrium across this region will make this identification challenging. Two studies have now also reported *IL-1A* associations with PsA.[14]

Approximately 5–10% of Caucasians have deficient function of the cytochrome P450 gene debrisoquine 4-hydroxylase (*CYP2D6*), an autosomal recessive trait leading to poor oxidative drug metabolism (known as the poor metabolizer, or *pm* phenotype). This gene is located at chromosome 22q13.1, and both case-control and family linkage studies support a role in AS susceptibility.[13–15]

The *ank/ank* murine model of AS has mutations in genes influencing PPi transport, leading to low extracellular PPi levels. Different *ANKH*

PATHOGENESIS

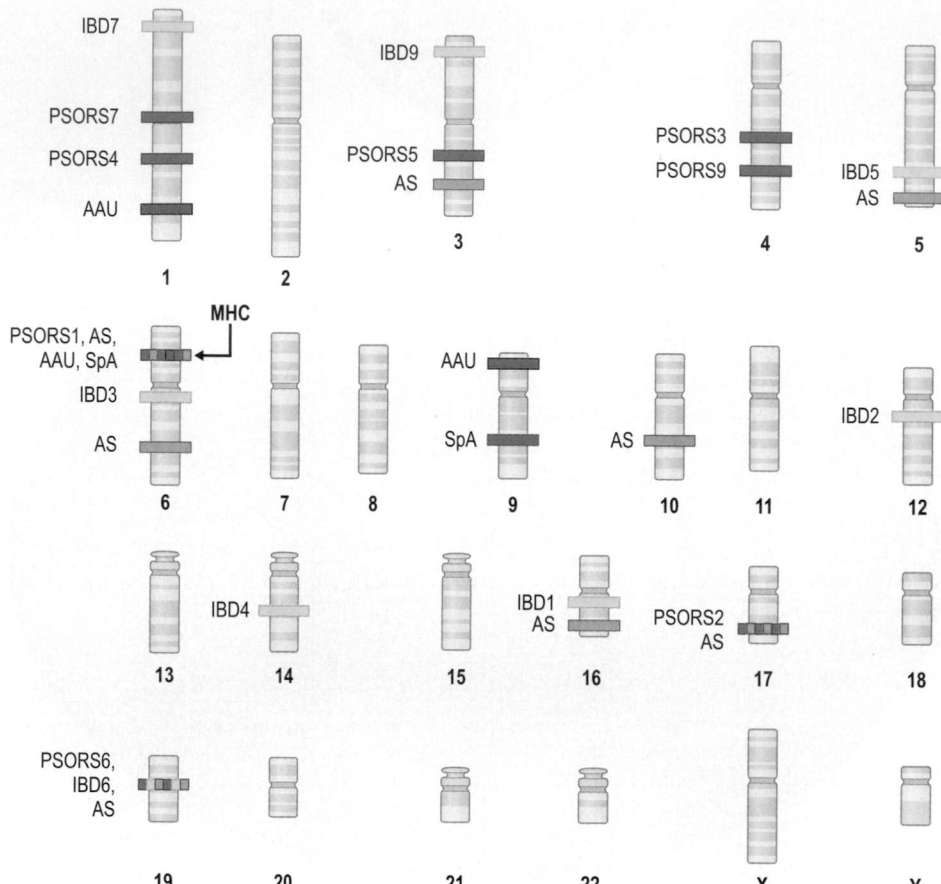

Fig. 57.3 Chromosomal location of susceptibility regions indicated in genome-wide scans of ankylosing spondylitis (AS) (meta-analysis data only shown,[16] psoriasis (PSORS), inflammatory bowel disease (IBD), acute anterior uveitis (AAU), spondyloarthritis (SpA), indicated to the left of the colored bar indicating the designation chromosomal region. Green, AS; red, PSORS; yellow, IBD; blue, SpA; pink, AAU.

variants have been associated with susceptibility to AS[14] in men versus women with AS. However, this was not confirmed in a larger British study.[13–15]

A number of other genes have been examined and not found to play a role in AS susceptibility, including *NOD2/CARD15*, which is a susceptibility factor for Crohn's disease, transforming growth factor-β_1 (TGF-β_1), the α/β T-cell receptor, IL-10, IL-6, *TLR4, CD14, NFKB1, MMP3, PTPN22*, α_1-antitrypsin, androgen receptor genes, secretor status, and immunoglobulin allotypes.[14] However many of these studies included only small to moderate numbers of patients, lacking adequate power to prove (or disprove) a true association for a 'small-impact' gene.

Both susceptibility to and severity of PsA have been associated with a variety of cytokine genes, including *TNF*-α-308 and *TNF*-β +252 polymorphisms,[13, 14] which may explain, at least in part, the reason for the utility of TNF blockers in patients with PsA (see below), as well as IL-1A. In addition, a recent study has also implicated a role for killer immunoglobulin-like receptor (KIR) genes in patients with PsA.

GENES AND SEVERITY OF SpA

Disease severity in AS also has a hereditary component.[13, 14] Defining severity by disease activity, and loss of function, the Oxford group demonstrated that these traits are highly heritable.[13, 14] A region on chromosome 18 was linked to disease activity, age at symptom onset with a region of chromosome 11p, and functional impairment with a region on chromosome 2q (outside the IL-1 region). No evidence was found for an MHC contribution to severity.

INFECTION

A role for triggering infections has been better documented in SpA than in most other rheumatic diseases. The most frequent type of ReA in developed countries follows urogenital infections with *Chlamydia trachomatis* (endemic ReA).[13, 15] Postdysenteric ReA, more commonly encountered in 'less technologically advanced countries,' follows various *Shigella* and *Salmonella* (especially *S. typhimurium* and *S. enteriditis*), *Campylobacter jejuni* and *C. fetus* and, in

CLINICAL FEATURES

Europe, *Yersinia enterocolitica* species. Microorganisms implicated in ReA share common biologic features: (1) they can invade mucosal surfaces and replicate intracellularly; and (2) they contain lipopolysaccharide in their outer membrane. Of particular note, antigens from *Salmonella*, *Yersinia*, and *Chlamydia* have been found in synovial tissues and fluids of patients with ReA,[13, 15] often many years after the initial infection. While only bacterial fragments of the enteric pathogens have been found, evidence for viable *Chlamydia trachomatis* and perhaps *C. pneumoniae* have been demonstrated in several studies.[13, 15] *Chlamydia* and other organisms have also been reported in the joints of healthy individuals, thus questioning the pathogenic significance of these findings.[13] Other data, however, support the likelihood that bacterial persistence plays an important role in ReA, including the finding of specific immunoglobulin A (IgA) antibodies and synovial T-cell proliferation to the initiating infectious agent.[13]

The contribution of infection to other types of SpA is less clear. In older studies *Klebsiella pneumoniae* was implicated in the pathogenesis of AS, although recent data have not borne this out.[13] An analysis of fecal microflora in patients with AS has instead suggested that *Bacteroides* may play a role.[13] It may also be significant that there are high serum IgA levels in AS, although studies seeking significant IgA antibodies to a variety of organisms have been unrewarding. In fact, it has been proposed that there might be no specific infectious trigger in AS, that this may result from gut flora and may thus be 'ubiquitous.'[12]

THE GUT AND SPONDYLOARTHRITIS

In studies from Belgium and from Scandinavia, up to 50% of patients with AS have microscopic ileal inflammation seen on ileocolonoscopy.[18] Moreover, two-thirds of patients with undifferentiated SpA have histologic gut inflammation. Gut inflammation in AS appears to be immunologically related to that seen in Crohn's disease. These observations have raised speculation that the inciting event in the SpA may be a breakdown of the gut–blood barrier to intestinal bacteria, though such has yet to be proven. It has been established that patients with AS and their relatives have increased intestinal permeability compared to healthy controls.[17]

■ PATHOLOGY OF SpA ■

One of the biggest problems with studies of the synovium in SpA and PsA is that most lesions are examined late in the course of disease, i.e., in the hips, and this only at joint replacement. Few data exist from early disease, and the difficulty with tissue access further complicates this.[18–20] Nonetheless, striking advances have occurred. For the most part the synovium in SpA resembles that of rheumatoid arthritis, with some notable differences. The synovium in SpA displays a tortuous vascular morphology compared to rheumatoid synovium, which is linear, and to have dimished lymphoid aggregates. This may be due to vascular endothelial growth factor (VEGF) and the angiogenic growth factor Ang2, whose mRNA have been observed at higher levels in the synovium in PsA compared to rheumatoid arthritis. VEGF is particularly interesting because it can synergize with RANK ligand (RANKL) to induce bone resorption and also synergize with bone morphogenetic proteins to trigger bone formation, both processes typical of the altered bone remodeling seen in PsA and SpA.[19]

Increased production of CD163 in both the lining and sublining layers is seen in SpA compared to rheumatoid arthritis.[18] Local production of soluble CD163 inhibits synovial T-cell activation, and levels of synovial CD163 fall with effective treatment. Increased expressions of Toll-like receptors 2 and 4 (TLR2, 4) have been shown in SpA on CD163+ peripheral blood mononuclear cells in patients with synovitis, which decreases with TNF-α blockade. This leads to the speculation that SpA represents an exaggerated inflammatory response of the innate immune system in genetically susceptible patients.[18, 19]

Osteoclasts also appear to have a role, and have also been observed at the bone–pannus junction in PsA. In addition, CD14+ monocytes that are committed to becoming osteoclasts or osteoclast precursors are increased in the circulation of PsA patients compared to healthy controls, and decline rapidly following treatment with TNF antagonists. The clinical improvement is accompanied by a MRI-defined reduction of bone marrow edema.[19]

Even fewer data exist on enthesitis (the enthesium being the insertion of tendons, ligaments, joint capsules, or fascia into bone). Pathological examination of enthesitis in AS demonstrates local inflammation, fibrosis, erosion, and ossification. Immunohistochemical staining for phosphorylated smad1/5 in entheseal biopsies of patients with SpA reveals active bone morphogenetic protein signaling.[20]

The pathology of psoriasis consists of an inflammatory cell infiltration in the dermis, with localized increased cytokine production and hyperproliferation of keratinocytes. CD4 cells are prominent in the dermis, CD8 in the epidermis; Langerhans cells are suspected to function as antigen-presenting cells. The synovium is infiltrated with CD8 T cells, is less cellular, more vascular than rheumatoid arthritis, and contains numerous B cells and macrophages.

■ CLINICAL FEATURES ■

ANKYLOSING SPONDYLITIS

Musculoskeletal symptoms

The first symptoms of AS usually appear in adolescence or early adulthood and usually start before the age of 40. The hallmark of AS is the presence of inflammatory back pain.[5] This is a dull, persistent ache, usually described by the patient in the buttocks or hips, that is worst in the early-morning hours (between 2 and 5 a.m.), and is associated with morning stiffness lasting more than 30 minutes (and sometimes several hours to all day). The pain is classically worsened by rest or recumbency, and improves with activity. One important component of inflammatory back pain is the striking improvement that results from the use of nonsteroidal anti-inflammatory drugs (NSAIDs: usually in high doses). Although the pain may be unilateral or intermittent at first (in fact, *alternating buttock pain* is a cardinal feature of the disease),[5] within a few months it usually becomes persistent and bilateral, and the lower lumbar area becomes stiff and painful.[4, 5] Occasionally the first symptom of AS may come from extraspinal sources, such as AAU, peripheral arthritis, or enthesitis, especially in patients with disease onset in childhood.

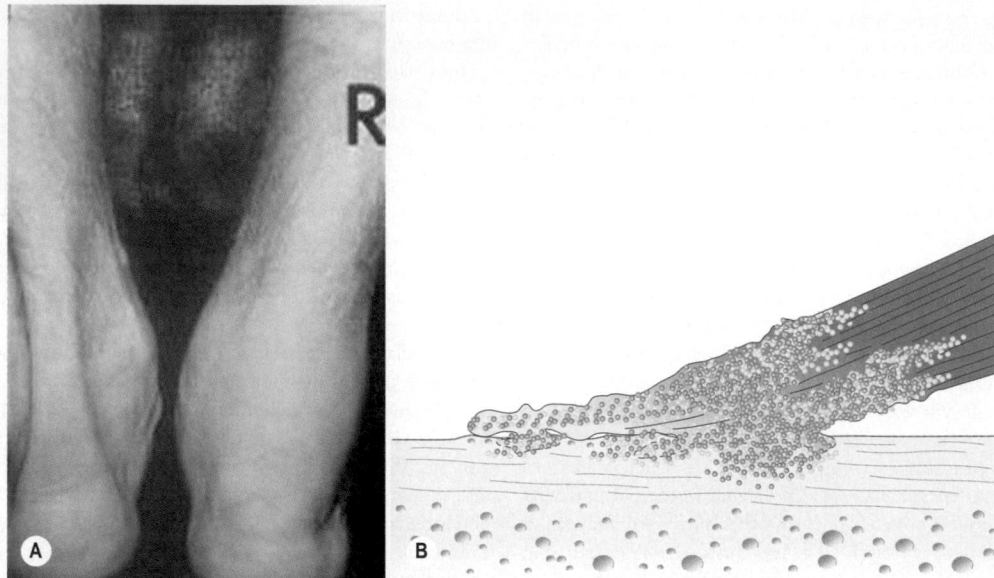

Fig. 57.4 (A) Achilles tendinitis/enthesitis in a patients with reactive arthritis. (B) Schematic drawing of enthesitis, showing periosteal new bone formation, and subchondral bone inflammation and resorption.

KEY CONCEPTS

CLINICAL FEATURES OF INFLAMMATORY BACK PAIN

>> Low-back pain that is present every day for at least 3 months

>> Age of onset at less than 40 years

>> Morning stiffness in the back lasting at least 30 minutes

>> Pain that is relieved by exercise and worsened by rest

>> Alternating-buttock pain

>> Relief with nonsteroidal anti-inflammatory agents

The most commonly affected joints in AS patients outside the spine are in the hips and shoulders (in up to 50% of patients),[21] with rapidly progressive destructive arthritis that necessitates joint arthroplasty at an early age. A characteristic radiographic finding is a fairly characteristic osteophytic collar that forms at the junction of the femoral head and the neck.[22] Peripheral arthritis other than in the hips and shoulders is uncommonly seen in AS patients, but when present is typical of that seen in other types of SpA, with an asymmetric oligoarthritis presenting predominantly in the lower extremities.

Chest pain, often pleuritic, can be seen in patients with AS due to involvement of the costovertebral and manubriosternal joints. This and progressive thoracic spinal involvement can result in fusion of the costovertebral joints, with loss of chest expansion and a mechanical restrictive ventilatory defect.

Enthesitis (inflammation of the origin and insertion of ligaments, tendons, aponeuroses, annulus fibrosis, and joint capsules) is a classic feature of AS and other SpA (Fig. 57.4). The most common (and most disabling) sites for enthesitis are in the foot, at the insertion of the Achilles tendon, and of the plantar fascia on to the calcaneus.[20]

Three physical measurements have been validated and recommended by the Assessment in Ankylosing Spondylitis (ASAS) working group as useful for evaluating patients with AS specifically and with inflammatory back pain in general.[13] The Schober test is measured as the increase with maximal forward spinal flexion with locked knees of a 10-cm segment marked on the patient's back with the inferior mark at the level of the posterior superior iliac spines. The measured distance should increase from 10 cm to at least 15 cm in an adult.[13] Chest wall expansion with inspiration is measured with a tape measure placed circumferentially around the chest wall at the fourth intercostal space.[13] Normal chest expansion in an adult is greater than 5 cm, although this may vary with age and gender. An occiput-to-wall distance of more than 2.5 cm is definitely abnormal. To measure the occiput-to-wall distance, the patient stands with heels and buttocks touching the wall behind and with the knees straight. The patient is asked how far back he/she can get the head, still keeping the chin in the normal position. In the straight position, the distance between the posterior convexity of the occiput and the wall is measured to the nearest 0.1 cm. The better of two attempts is recorded.[13] Anything greater than zero is regarded as abnormal.

Another measure that is increasingly commonly employed is the measurement of lateral bending. Here the patient stands with the heels and back against the wall. There is no flexion of the knees, nor bending forward. The distance between the patient's middle fingertip and the floor is measured. The patient then bends sideways without bending the knees or lifting the heels. A second reading is taken and the difference between the two is recorded. The best of two tries is recorded for left and right. The mean of left and right gives the final result (in centimeters to the nearest 0.1 cm). Normal is greater than 10 cm.

Extra-articular manifestations

Uveitis. The anterior portion of the uvea consists of the iris and ciliary body while the posterior portion is known as the choroid. Inflammation of the anterior uveal tract is known as anterior uveitis or iritis. When the adjacent ciliary body is also inflamed, the process is known as iridocyclitis. AAU represents the typical uveitis found in SpA, occurring in about 40% of patients with AS,[1] of whom approximately 90% are HLA-B27-positive (Table 57.2).[1] Typically, AAU presents unilaterally with sudden onset, is self-limiting, and tends to be recurrent. Symptoms may include redness, pain, blurred vision, increased lacrimation, photophobia, and miosis. The diagnosis is characteristically confirmed by slit-lamp examination, which is also useful in monitoring response to treatment.

Prognosis is favorable in AAU, with resolution of symptoms within a few weeks. However, if treatment is delayed or inadequate, complications can occur; these include anterior synechiae (adherence of the iris to the cornea), posterior synechiae (adherence of the iris to the lens), which can lead to cataracts, and cystoid macular edema.[1] Rarely, increased ocular pressure is seen.[1] Macular edema has been shown to be the main factor that determines visual outcome in cases of uveitis.[1] Although AAU is the most common uveitis associated with AS, posterior uveitis has been reported and tends to be more severe, especially in those with coexistent IBD.[1]

Cardiac manifestations. The characteristic cardiac abnormalities in AS are aortitis, aortic regurgitation and conduction abnormalities that are seen in up to 9% of patients with AS followed over many years. Less commonly associated cardiac conditions include pericarditis, cardiomyopathy, and mitral valve disease. HLA-B27 is an important genetic risk factor for these cardiac conditions. Aortic regurgitation is well characterized and distinguished from aortic valvular dysfunction in other disorders. Three factors contribute to the development of incompetent aortic valves: dilatation of the aortic root, fibrotic thickening and downward retraction of the bases of the cusps, and inward rolling of the edges or margins of the cusps. Aortic regurgitation is present in 2–10% of patients with AS and increases in likelihood with greater disease duration.

Cardiac conduction abnormalities, including atrioventricular and intraventricular blocks, have been regarded as the most common cardiac complication in patients with AS. Complete heart block has been found in 1–9% of patients with AS. Electrophysiologic studies show that the preferential level of block is in the atrioventricular node itself, which is in contrast with most cases of acquired complete heart block, where 80% are within or below the bundle of His. Rare complications include myocardial involvement, mitral regurgitation, and pericarditis.

Pulmonary manifestations. The incidence of pleuropulmonary involvement in AS is estimated to be 1%. The most frequently recognized manifestations are upper-lobe fibrosis, mycetoma formation, and pleural thickening. Fusion of the costovertebral joints caused by inflammation and ankylosis of the thoracic spine can lead to restrictive ventilatory impairment on pulmonary function testing. The upper-lobe fibrosis tends to be progressive. Another common finding is the presence of bilateral symmetric apical pleural thickening. Several recent studies have demonstrated that high-resolution computed tomography is more sensitive than chest radiography in detecting the presence of pulmonary abnormalities in AS, suggesting that pulmonary involvement in AS is more common than once thought. The clinical implications of these observations remain unclear as lung involvement in AS is usually asymptomatic.

Renal manifestations. Renal involvement in AS, although uncommon, may include secondary renal amyloidosis (AA type), NSAID nephropathy, and glomerulonephritis.

Osteoporosis. Measuring bone mineral density in patients with spondylitis is complicated by false increases in spinal density from dense syndesmophyte formation, leading some to recommend quantitative computer tomography over standard dual-energy X-ray absorptiometry (DEXA) for bone mineral density measurements. Nevertheless, up to half of patients with long-standing AS have been reported as having osteopenia or osteoporosis.[23] The etiology of osteoporosis in AS is still not completely understood. Although treatment factors and decreased mobility or physical activity may lead to the development of osteoporosis in AS, histological examinations point to an osteoclast/osteoblast imbalance.[24]

Spondylodiscitis and spinal fractures. An uncommon but well-recognized complication of AS is spondylodiscitis, a destructive discovertebral lesion also called Andersson lesion.[22] Typically, these lesions are confined to the thoracic and lumbar spine, sometimes with multiple-level involvement; however, cervical spondylodiscitis has been reported. Pain and tenderness localized to the affected disk are the most common presenting features of spondylodiscitis, although it can be asymptomatic and only detected on routine radiographic examination many years later. Spondylodiscitis usually occurs at an advanced stage of AS under the form of an erosive condition related to both mechanical factors and osteoporosis. However, early spondylodiscitis can occur as a result of the inflammatory process. Patients may or may not give a history of preceding trauma.

Even trivial falls can be catastrophic for AS patients, who are at risk for spinal fractures due to their spinal rigidity and osteoporosis. The estimated prevalence of vertebral fractures in AS varies from 4% to 18%. Fractures through the disk space, the weakest point in the ankylosed spine, are most common, with the cervical spine being the most frequently affected region, followed by the thoracolumbar junction, and may, or may not, be complicated by injury to the spinal cord ranging from mild sensory loss to quadriplegia. Spontaneous atlantoaxial subluxation is also rarely seen.

Neurological manifestations. Neurological involvement in AS is most often related to spinal fracture, atlantoaxial subluxation, or cauda equina syndrome. The *cauda equina syndrome* in AS is characterized by a slow insidious progression and a high incidence of dural ectasia, although a rapid onset secondary to a traumatic event has been reported. It tends to be a late manifestation of AS, often when the disease is no longer active. The prevalence of neurologic findings in cauda equina syndrome in AS is very high, presenting with a prodrome of sensory, motor, or reflex loss before the progression to sphincter disturbance. About half of patients have pain in the rectum or lower limbs that is presumably neurogenic in origin. Case reports have also been published about the occurrence of AS with a multiple sclerosis-like syndrome and transverse myelitis, although the association is not conclusive.

Fatigue and psychosocial manifestations. Fatigue is a common problem in patients with AS and seems to be associated with more severe disease. Sleep disturbance has also recently been reported to be as high as nearly 81% of female AS patients and 50% of male AS patients. The disturbance is closely related to pain during the night characteristic of active disease. A high level of depressive symptoms has been reported in approximately one-third of patients with AS, with women reporting more depression than men. Pain was found to be a major determinant of depression for women, but was of lesser importance for men.

AS in women. AS in women may not be as severe as it is in men, and may present with isolated neck pain in the absence of typical back pain.[24] There tends to be a greater delay in the diagnosis of AS in women compared to men.[24] Women tend to have less severe involvement of the spine, with peripheral joint involvement. A large review of the impact of AS on reproductive events on women concluded that AS did not adversely affect the ability to conceive, pregnancy outcome, or neonatal health.[24]

REACTIVE ARTHRITIS

The classic triad of *arthritis, urethritis,* and *conjunctivitis,* representing what was formerly known as Reiter's syndrome, is a presenting feature of only a minority of patients with ReA (comprising only a third of the cases in some series). In ReA, the clinical features are today viewed more as a spectrum ranging from the classic triad to undifferentiated SpA. In fact, the manifestations vary among patients, depending on the genetic makeup, the triggering event, and the sequential immunologic reaction.

Typically, the features start 1–4 weeks after a triggering event, frequently identified as an enteric or urogenital infection, but often the event passes unnoticed without any specific symptoms. The syndrome starts with constitutional symptoms such as fatigue, malaise, and fever, and then is typically manifested by *asymmetric, additive lower-extremity oligoarticular inflammatory arthritis* along with an array of different extra-articular features, including a sterile oligoarticular or monoarticular and asymmetric arthritis of the lower extremities, especially the knees, ankles, and, occasionally, hips. Upper-extremity involvement is encountered less commonly. *Dactylitis* occurs in the toes or fingers, resulting in the 'sausage digits' which represent inflammation not only of the interphalangeal joints of the hands and feet, but also of the surrounding soft-tissue structures, including the tendons and subcutaneous tissue.

Sacroiliitis and *spondylitis* are less common than peripheral arthritis, although inflammatory back pain does occur. Unilateral and bilateral sacroiliac involvement and even spondylitis occur, especially in those with chronic or long-standing disease. The most common sites for enthesitis are the Achilles tendon and plantar fascia insertions, although tenderness over the symphysis pubis, iliac crest, ischial tuberosity, greater trochanters, and thoracic cage ribs can also occur.

Mucocutaneous lesion also occur that can be difficult to distinguish from PsA, especially *circinate balanitis* and *keratoderma blenorrhagica.* Circinate balanitis is an ulcerative mucosal lesion over the glans or shaft of the penis that is demarcated by a serpiginous erythematous border. The lesion is usually painless and sterile unless a superimposed

infection occurs. Keratoderma blenorrhagica is a painless desquamative psoriatic-like papulosquamous eruption and is sometimes referred to as pustulosis palmoplantaris and occurs on the palms and soles of the feet. Oral lesions have been described as shallow, painless ulcers or patches on the palate and tongue, or mucositis of the soft palate and uvula. Conjunctivitis and AAU also occur, as described in AS. Conjunctivitis may be unilateral or bilateral and is usually an early feature manifesting with irritation, erythema, and lacrimation. It is usually associated with a sterile discharge unless a superimposed infection occurs due to eye rubbing. It can be severe and occasionally progress to episcleritis, scleritis, or keratitis. Other findings seen in AS, such as cardiac involvement, do rarely occur. Although renal involvement is mainly described in the context of the urogenital triggering infectious process, sterile pyuria in conjunction with proteinuria and microscopic hematuria are sometimes encountered, although documentation of glomerulonephritis is rarely described.

JUVENILE SPONDYLOARTHRITIS

Basically there are two clinical subsets of JSpA. *Undifferentiated* JSpA, which includes peripheral arthritis and enthesitis, primarily affects the lower limbs, may also present with sacroiliac tenderness and/or inflammatory spinal pain, and also includes isolated episodes of arthritis, enthesitis, tendinitis, dactylitis, and seronegative enthesopathy and arthropathy (SEA) syndrome.[25] *Differentiated* JSpA (juvenile AS, PsA, IBD-related arthropathy) includes peripheral arthritis and enthesitis *plus* evidence of structural changes in JAS (radiographic sacroiliitis, spinal disease, or tarsal ankylosis) and/or specific extra-articular symptoms (e.g., psoriasis or IBD). The SEA syndrome was originally referred to the combination of enthesitis and arthritis or arthralgia as an idiopathic disease or as part of a well-defined SpA.[25]

PSORIATIC ARTHRITIS

Skin involvment exhibits four clinical patterns. The most common type is *psoriasis vulgaris.* Nearly as common is *guttate* psoriasis. The most severe type is the *erythrodermic* variety. Finally, *pustular psoriasis* is the type most closely associated with HLA-B27. Usually the disease appears coincident with or after the onset of skin manifestations, although approximately 15–20% of patients will have pre-existent arthritis. The joint disease likewise occurs in different subtypes, as defined by the Moll and Wright classification (Fig. 57.5), including oligoarticular, asymmetric, polyarticular, symmetric, distal interphalangeal (DIP)-predominant, spondylitis (sacroiliitis), arthritis mutilans, inflammation of DIP joints (often with nail involvement (~80%)), dactylitis: 'sausage digits,' and enthesitis.[26] Extra-articular features include nail pitting (which correlates best with DIP involvement) and uveitis (which occurs in some series as high as 33% but in most far less). Radiographically, large eccentric erosions are encountered.

ENTEROPATHIC ARTHRITIS

The arthritis associated with IBD (enteropathic arthritis) is most commonly nondestructive and reversible. Two patterns have been recognized (Table 57.5): type 1 is oligoarticular, involving the knees and ankles more than the upper extremeties. It tends to resolve in < 6 weeks. The second type has a polyarticular presentation, is more likely to involve

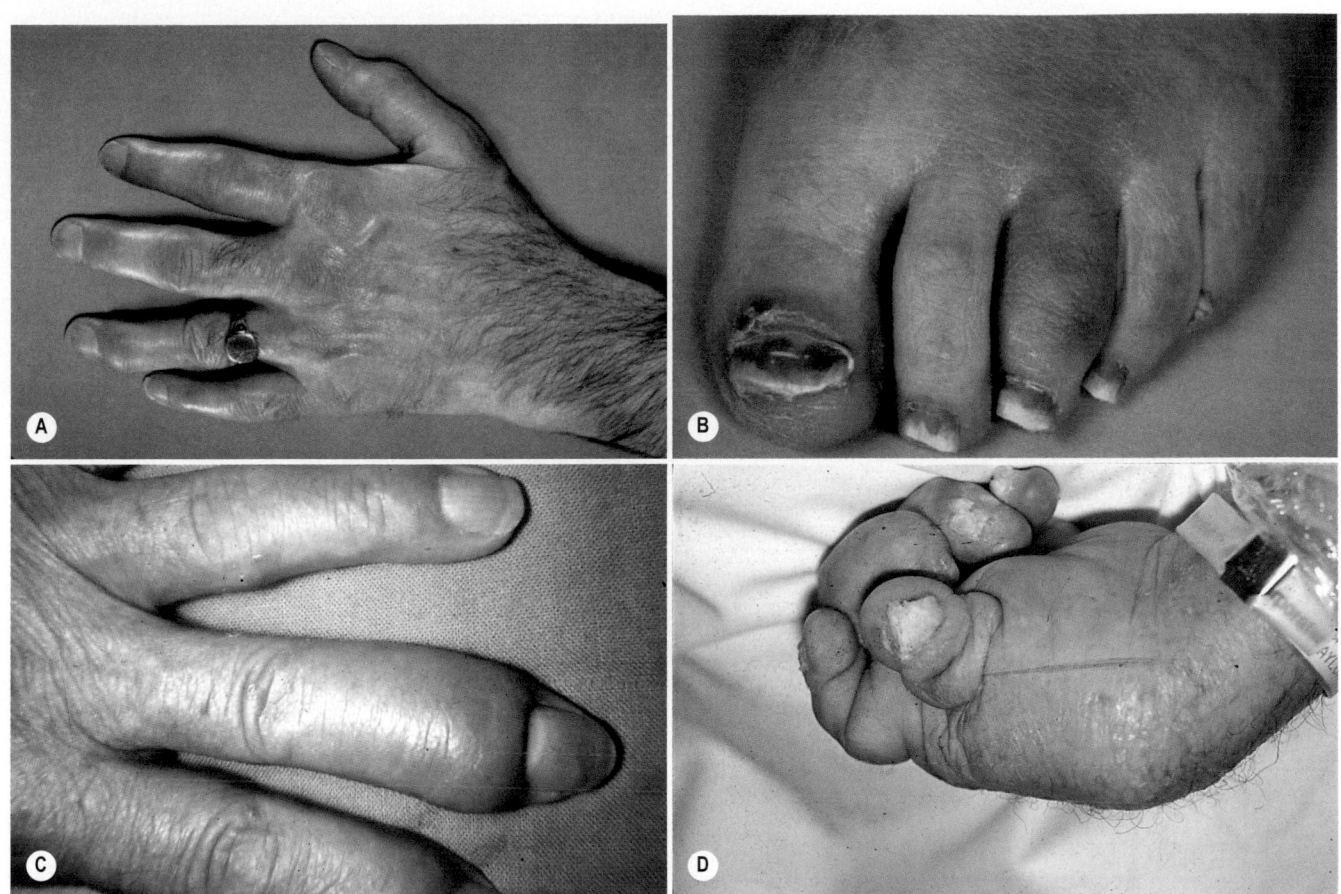

Fig. 57.5 Patterns of psoriatic arthritis, showing **(A)** rheumatoid-like distribution; **(B)** sausage digits; **(C)** distal interphalangeal involvement; and **(D)** psoriatic arthritis mutilans.

the metacarpophalangeal (MCP) and proximal interphalangeal (PIP) joints more than the lower extremities, and is more likely to have a chronic course. The symptoms of peripheral arthritis tend to coincide with activity of the bowel disease in UC but not in Crohn's disease. Total colectomy is associated with remission of arthritis in half of patients. In contrast, axial involvement may precede the development of IBD, has no gender predilection, and resembles the development of AS. The axial symptoms do not parallel activity of bowel disease. In addition to spondylitis, an isolated sacroiliitis occurs that is often asymmetric and not associated with HLA-B27.

Mucocutaneous complications of IBD include erythema nodosum, which occurs in fewer than 10% of those with Crohn's disease and is rare in UC; pyoderma gangrenosus, seen in slightly over 1% of those with Crohn's disease and rarely ocurring in those with UC; and, rarely, erythema multiforme. Painful aphthous ulcers occur in about 8% of those with UC and are rare in Crohn's disease.

The uveitis with IBD that is bilateral, posterior, insidious in onset, and/or chronic in duration contrasts with the uveitis associated with other types of SpA, which is predominantly anterior, unilateral, sudden in onset, and limited in duration. Only 46% of patients with uveitis associated with IBD are HLA-B27-positive, as opposed to 89% of the

Table 57.5 Extraintestinal manifestations of inflammatory bowel disease

Feature	Crohn's disease (%)	Ulcerative colitis (%)
Peripheral arthritis	15	10
Axial arthritis	15–20	10–15
Septic arthritis	Rare	No association
Skin	< 9	< 1
Aphthous ulcers	Rare	8
Nephrolithiasis	< 15	No association
Liver disease	3–5	7
Uveitis	13	4
Vasculitis	Takayasu's arteritis	< 5
Clubbing of fingers	4–13	1–5

Table 57.6 Frequencies of different symptoms and signs in patients with undifferentiated spondyloarthritis

Feature	Percent
Demographic	
Males	62–88
Mean age at onset (years)	16–23
Clinical	
Low-back pain	**52–80**
Peripheral arthritis	**60–100**
Polyarthritis	40
Enthesopathy	56
Heel pain	20–28
Mucocutaneous involvement	16
Conjuctivitis	33
Genitourinary disease	**28**
Inflammatory bowel disease	4
Cardiac abnormalities	8
Laboratory	
Elevated erythrocyte sedimentation rate	19–30
Human leukocyte antigen (HLA)-B27 positive	80–84
Radiographic	
Sacroiliitis	16–30
Spinal radiographic changes	20

Adapted from Chen CH, Lin KC, Yu DT, et al. Serum matrix metalloproteinases and tissue inhibitors of metalloproteinases in ankylosing spondylitis: MMP-3 is a reproducibly sensitive and specific biomarker of disease activity. Rheumatol (Oxf) 2006; 45: 414–420.

patients with SpA. Episcleritis, scleritis, and glaucoma are more common among patients with IBD than in those with SpA.

UNDIFFERENTIATED SPONDYLOARTHRITIS

Patients are regarded as having undifferentiated SpA who do not meet criteria or clinical features of the 'classic' spondyloarthritides. Generally, at presentation, about 40% of patients will be classified as having undifferentiated SpA,[27] and the frequency of HLA-B27 reaches around 80% in Caucasians (Table 57.6). Follow-up studies suggest that over time about one-third will go in to remission and more than half will develop a 'classical' SpA, usually AS.[28]

■ LABORATORY INVESTIGATIONS ■

The most useful investigations in SpA come from musculoskeletal imaging, but some laboratory tests can be informative.

Data on the correlation of erythrocyte sedimentation rate (ESR) and C-reactive protein (CRP) in the assessment of disease activity in SpA show

UTILITY OF HUMAN LEUKOCYTE ANTIGEN (HLA)-B27 TESTING IN THE EVALUATION OF INFLAMMATORY BACK PAIN AND SPONDYLOARTHRITIS

➤➤ Not indicated where the diagnosis is unquestionable, as it has little value in prognosis

➤➤ Although patients with spondyloarthritis of African and Middle Eastern ancestry are more likely to be human leukocyte antigen (HLA)-B27-negative, the finding of HLA-B27 in these patients has higher predictive value

➤➤ Most useful in patients with either inflammatory back pain without radiographic changes or with other features of spondyloarthritis (unexplained lower-extremity arthritis in a young adult, uveitis, etc.)

➤➤ If serologic testing is used to ascertain HLA-B27, insure the blood sample arrives in the laboratory within 24 hours of being drawn (false negatives due to cell death)

ambiguous results, although most studies suggest that CRP performs better. A recent literature review on the validity aspects of ESR and CRP in AS concluded that ESR and CRP do not comprehensively represent the disease process and thus do not have the same validity as in rheumatoid arthritis.[13, 29] Generally, it is felt that patients with peripheral joint involvement or with IBD more often have elevated ESR and CRP than those patients with axial disease.[13] However, a normal ESR and/or CRP does not exclude the presence of clinically active AS. Synovial fluid does not differ in appearance or cytology from that of any inflammatory joint disease.

■ DIAGNOSIS ■

In most cases, SpA is largely diagnosed, or at least initially suspected, on clinical grounds. Current criteria for AS demand that the patient have radiographic sacroiliitis (at least grade II bilaterally or grade III unilaterally) in conjunction with clinical signs of inflammatory back pain and limitation of spinal mobility. However, given that up to 10 years can pass from the onset of inflammatory back pain and the development of radiographic sacroiliitis,[5] many of those with inflammatory back pain might not have radiographic evidence of sacroiliitis.[5] With the development of effective treatments (i.e. anti-TNF blockers), much recent emphasis has come on formulating criteria for earlier diagnosis of axial SpA, which are currently under development.[5] These criteria take into account recent advances in MRI scanning as well as the added benefit provided in HLA-B27 testing.[5]

MEASURES OF SpA ACTIVITY AND SEVERITY

In the past few years, outcome measures have been developed and validated to quantitate disease activity, and disease severity; these are summarized in Table 57.7, including disease activity, functional impairment, metrology, and quality of life. These instruments are extensively validated and easy to administer in clinical practice, and have been shown to perform well in clinical trials.[13]

Table 57.7 Measurements of disease outcome in spondyloarthritis

Ankylosing spondylitis
Disease activity
Bath Ankylosing Spondylitis Disease Activity Index (BASDAI)
Patient and Physician Global Assessments
Function
Bath Ankylosing Spondylitis Functional Index (BASFI)
Dougados Functional Index
Quality of Life
SF-36
Ankylosing Spondylitis Quality of Life Index (ASQOL)
Metrometry
Schober's test (lumbar flexion)
Chest expansion
Occiput-to-wall distance
Bath Ankylosing Spondylitis Metrology Index (BASMI) lateral ending
Imaging
Standard radiographs
Computed tomography scanning
Magnetic resonance imaging
Assessment in Ankylosing Spondylitis (ASAS) 20
An improvement of > 20% and absolute improvement of ≥ 10 units on a 0–100 scale in ≥ three of the following four domains:
1. Patient global assessment (by visual analog scale (VAS) global assessment)
2. Pain assessment (the average of VAS total and nocturnal pain scores)
3. Function (represented by BASFI)
4. Inflammation (the average of the BASDAI's last two VAS concerning morning stiffness, intensity, and duration)
Absence of deterioration in the potential remaining domain (deterioration is defined as 20% worsening)

Psoriatic arthritis
Arthritis
ACR response criteria
Psoriatic Arthritis Response Criteria (PsARC)
Ritchie Articular Index
Skin response
Psoriasis Area and Severity Index (PASI)
Target lesion score
Static global assessment
Quality of life (HAQ, SF-36, DLQI)
Radiographic

RADIOGRAPHIC IMAGING OF SPONDYLOARTHRITIS

Axial spondyloarthritis

The bottom line in the diagnosis of AS is the demonstration of radiographic sacroiliitis (Fig. 57.6).[27] Two outcome instruments have been introduced in the assessment of disease damage and progression in AS: the Bath Ankylosing Spondylitis Radiographic Index (BASRI) and the

CLINICAL PEARLS

OPTIMAL UTILIZATION OF X-RAYS IN THE DIAGNOSIS AND MANAGEMENT OF SPONDYLOARTHRITIS

>> Patient education and physiotherapy should be initiated early in the disease course
>> Nonsteroidal anti-inflammatory drugs (NSAIDs) remain 'first-line' treatment
>> Disease-modifying anti-inflammatory drugs (DMARDs: sulfasalazine, methotrexate) for peripheral arthritis
>> Intra-articular/intralesional corticosteroidal injections
>> Anti-tumor necrosis factor agents for axial disease refractory to nonsteroidal anti-inflammatory drugs (NSAIDs), peripheral arthritis refractory to DMARDs, and entheseal lesions refractory to NSAIDs
>> Don't forget to treat coexistent/complicating conditions (inflammatory bowel disease, psoriasis, osteoporosis)

modified Stokes Ankylosing Spondylitis Scoring System (mSASSS).[30] As a rule, they have a low sensitivity to change (7.5% over 2 years), have been validated in long-duration disease only, and their predictive effect for disease activity is not yet ascertained.

One problem with radiographic imaging is the average decade-long interval from the onset of inflammatory back pain to the appearance of radiographic sacroiliitis.[5] The introduction of MRI imaging of the spine and entheses has allowed not only correct anatomic description of spinal structures, but also differentiation of AS-related and unrelated inflammatory spinal lesions earlier than is possible by standard radiographs.[31] MRI of the sacroiliac joints and spine is currently the only imaging tool to localize and quantify spinal inflammation accurately (Fig. 57.7), and is being developed as a measure of disease activity and treatment response.

Psoriatic arthritis

PsA has some rather characteristic radiographic manifestations, including asymmetric involvement, involvement of the DIP joints, and the classical 'pencil-in-cup' deformities. Also seen are periostitis, bony ankylosis, and bony erosions with new bone formation. Radiographic severity is quantitated by the modified Sharp scoring method used in rheumatoid arthritis.

The measures used in PsA to assess disease severity include the ACR response criteria, the Psoriatic Arthritis Response Criteria (PsARC), which entail improvement in at least two of the following four criteria: (1) physician; and (2) patient global assessments (on 0–5 visual analog scales); (3) tender and swollen joint scores (> 30% improvement), with improvement in at least one of these two joint scales; and (4) no worsening in any criteria. The Ritchie Articular Index is also used. The Psoriasis Area and Severity Index (PASI) is used to assess the extent of skin involvement, as well as general measures such as the target lesion score, and the static global assessment. The PASI is a composite index of skin disease severity, including an overall evaluation and quantitation of the extent of scaling, erythema, and induration weighted: (1) by severity; and (2) by body surface area. A target lesion is a single lesion > 2 cm in diameter evaluated over time by a dermatologist and that is graded for size, elevation, erythema, and scaling.

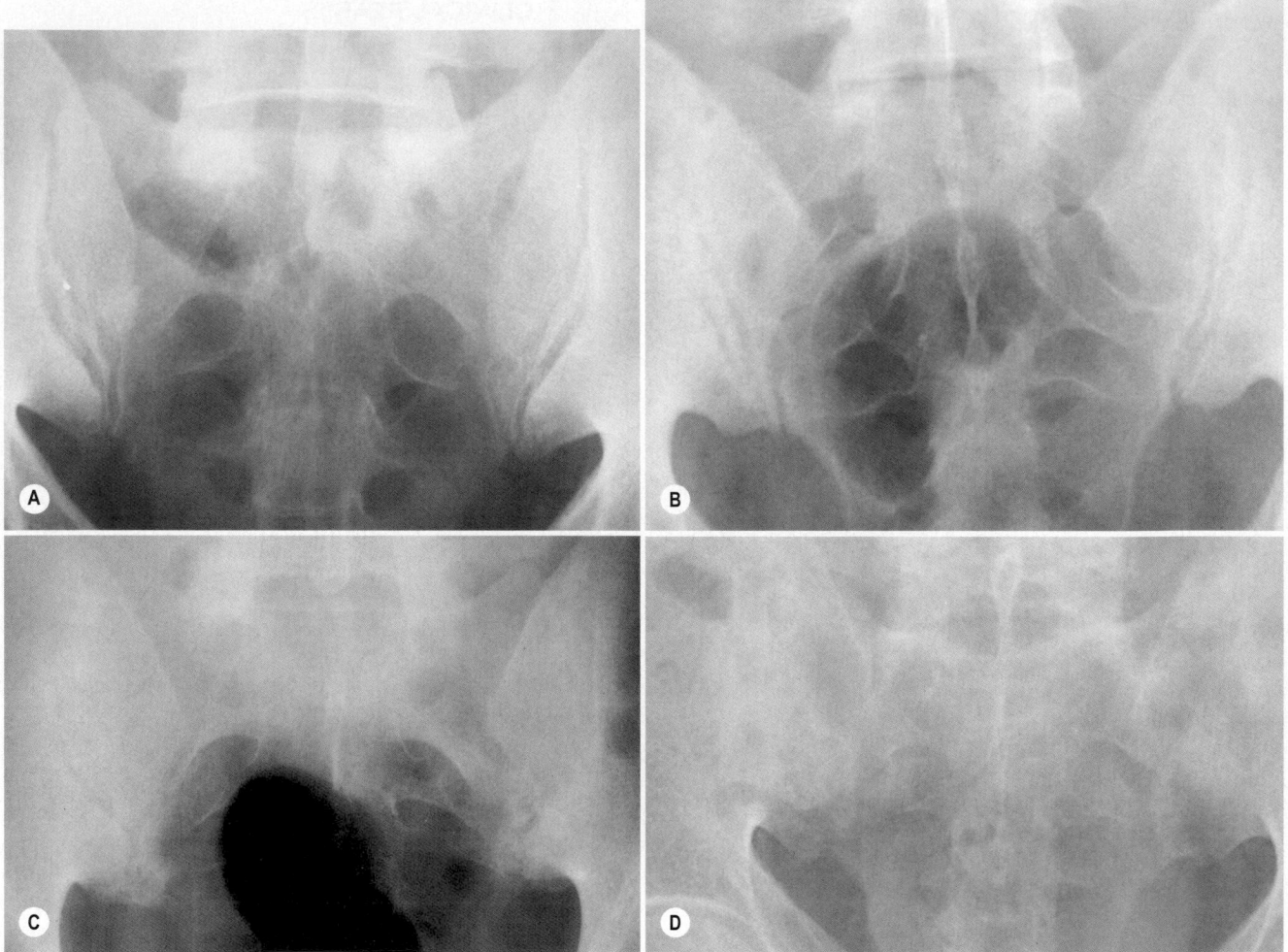

Fig. 57.6 Grading of radiographic sacroiliitis, including: **(A)** grade 0–1 (normal); **(B)** grade 2–3, with sclerosis and small erosions; **(C)** advanced grade 3, with joint space narrowing and large erosions; and **(D)** grade 4 (total sacroiliac fusion).

■ DISEASE COURSE AND PROGNOSIS ■

ANKYLOSING SPONDYLITIS

Although AS is a chronic condition that can frequently have an unpredictable course, some studies suggest that those with higher levels of disease activity early in the course of the disease are more likely to have subsequent active disease in the future[30] (Fig. 57.8). Hip involvement has been shown to be a predictive factor for severe disease.[30] Other factors that may be suggestive of severe disease and severe outcome include: ESR > 30 mm/hour, unresponsiveness to NSAIDs; limitation of lumbar spine; 'sausage' digits; oligoarthritis; or onset at < 16 years.[30] Longitudinal studies in patients with AS revealed that deformities and disability occur within the first 10 years of disease.[30] Most of the loss of function occurred during the first 10 years, and correlated significantly with the occurrence of peripheral arthritis,

radiographic changes of AS in the spine, and the development of 'bamboo' spine.[30]

Significant risk factors for work disability from several studies include older age, longer disease duration, lower level of education, reduced physical functioning, pain, and more physically demanding jobs.[29] Patients with AS have an overall frequency of disability and economic costs similar to that of rheumatoid arthritis.[13, 27] However, the impact of newer agents, such as anti-TNF drugs, on the natural history of this disease remains to be seen.

REACTIVE ARTHRITIS

Early studies of outcome in ReA suggested a relatively poor prognosis. More recent studies, however, have found that, in general, the prognosis of ReA appears to be fairly good.[32] Most cases appear to remit within 6 months of onset. Given the introduction of highly effective biologic agents such as anti-TNF blockers, it is likely that the long-term prognosis in ReA will improve even further.

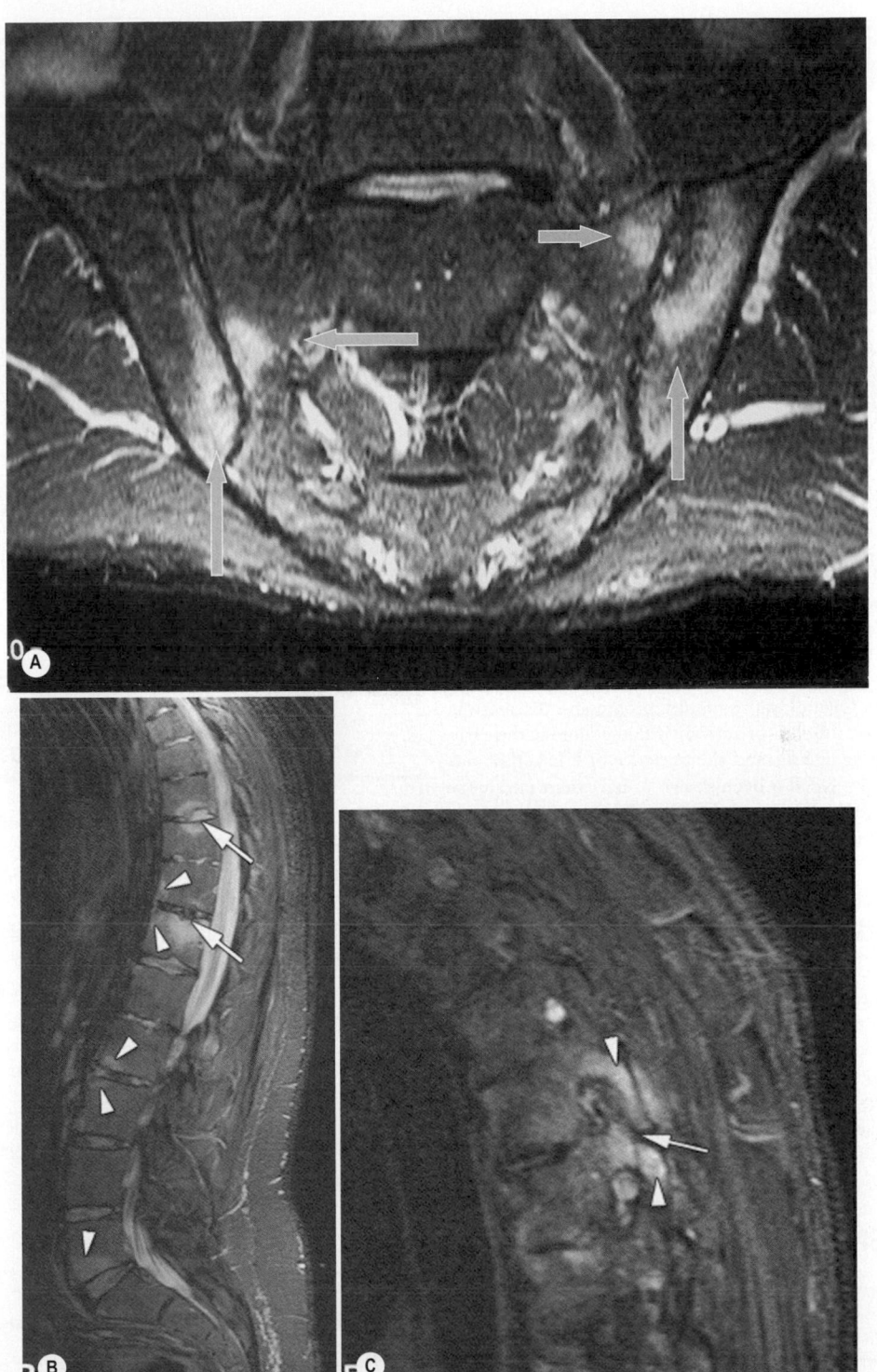

Fig. 57.7 **(A)** Magnetic resonance imaging of the sacroiliac joints, showing areas of marrow edema (indicated by arrows) on STIR sequences. **(B)** Lateral spine, showing enhancement of the insertion of the annulus fibrosis on the disk (arrowheads) and subchondral bone (arrows). **(C)** Involvement of the subchondral bone of the apophyseal joints.

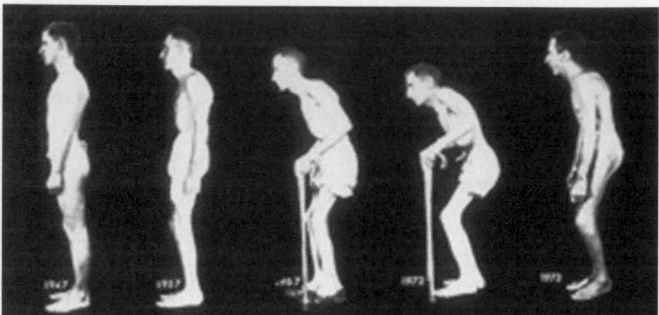

Fig. 57.8 The 'classical' course of ankylosing spondylitis, showing disease progression from shortly after disease onset in 1947 until just before the patient's death in 1973. The slight improvement between 1972 and 1973 was due to his having gotten total hip arthroplasties.

Table 57.8 Treatment of spondyloarthritis
Patient education
Physiotherapy
Medications
Nonsteroidal anti-inflammatory drugs
Disease-modifying antirheumatic drugs
Sulfasalazine (especially for peripheral arthritis)
Methotrexate (especially for psoriatic arthritis, psoriasis)
Leflunomide
Corticosteroids
Systemic
Intra-articular, intralesional
Biologic agents
Tumor necrosis factor blockers
Alefacept (psoriasis)
Treatment of osteoporosis
Surgery
Hip replacement
Corrective spinal surgery

PSORIATIC ARTHRITIS

Recent studies – although before the introduction of biologic treatments – have shown that the prognosis of PsA is worse than previously suggested.[17, 19, 26] In one large cohort, 40–57% of patients had deforming arthritis, 17% had[3] five deformed joints, and up to 19% of patients had disability. Overall, more rapidly progressive disease was associated with a greater number of actively inflamed joints, the early use of disease-modifying agents, and the presence of HLA-B27 and B39. Patients with PsA have also been shown to have increased mortality, which is associated with a high ESR, high 'advanced' medication usage, and early radiographic damage.

JUVENILE SPONDYLOARTHRITIS

Although not extensively studied, the prognosis in JSpA is guarded.[25] Available data suggest that children with disease activity for more than 5 years are more likely to be disabled. In fact, the probability of remission was only 17% after 5 years of disease. Nearly 60% of children with JSpA have moderate to severe limitation after 10 years of disease. What is not clear is the extent to which the outcome in juvenile-onset AS is different from that in adult-onset disease.

■ TREATMENT (TABLE 57.8) ■

PATIENT EDUCATION AND PHYSIOTHERAPY

A great deal of educational information is available for patients (www.spondylitis.org and www.arthritis.org). Unsupervised recreational exercise improves pain and stiffness, and back exercise improves pain and function in patients with AS and other types of SpA, but these effects differ with disease duration. Health status is improved when patients perform recreational exercise at least 30 minutes per day and back exercises at least 5 days per week.[13]

MEDICAL TREATMENT

Nonsteroidal anti-inflammatory drugs

NSAIDs remain the starting point of treatment, and many patients will attain satisfactory symptom control with these agents alone. There are no strong data to suggest the superiority of any specific NSAID in patients with SpA. NSAIDs when taken regularly (not on an as-needed basis) and at full anti-inflammatory doses seem to slow down the radiographic progression of AS.[32] Cyclooxygenase-2 antagonists are recommended mainly for patients with proven peptic ulcer disease. Of concern is the association of the use of NSAIDs with flares of colitis, suggesting they should be used with care in this setting.

Disease-modifying anti-inflammatory drugs (DMARDs)

Sulfasalazine. The efficacy of sulfasalazine in the treatment of peripheral joint involvement in AS and other SpA has been shown in many controlled trials, including two large multicenter studies in the USA and France.[33] Its efficacy in axial disease is unproven; in fact, it has not been shown to be effective in most studies. Coincident with improvement in peripheral arthritis is a fall in acute-phase reactants such as the ESR and CRP.

Other DMARDs. Although less well studied than sulfasalazine, methotrexate has been shown to be effective in the treatment of peripheral arthritis and psoriasis in patients with AS and other SpA. Its efficacy in treating axial arthritis has not been established.

The use of leflunomide in patients with SpA has not been well examined. Limited data suggest it is useful in the treatment of peripheral joint involvement in SpA as well as PsA, although not for axial involvement.

Corticosteroids. Although not well studied in patients with AS, many clinicians add low-dose glucocorticoids to the management of active SpA where NSAIDs or DMARDs fail to achieve a satisfactory response. On occasion pulse steroids have also been utilized. Given the lack of controlled data as to their effectiveness, the side effects of long-term glucocorticoid therapy (including osteoporosis, a major cause of morbidity in AS patients, and possible worsening of psoriasis) and the emergence of more effective treatments, their use is not recommended unless more effective treatments are not available.

Intra-articular/intralesional corticosteroids

Intra-articular and peritendinous injections of depot steroid preparations are frequently employed by clinicians for symptomatic relief of local flares, although they have not been extensively studied in controlled trials. Injecting around the Achilles tendon is generally not recommended because of the risk of tendon rupture.

Antibiotics

Early data suggested that a 3-month course of antibiotics in the acute phase after disease onset may have a beneficial effect on the course of ReA, specifically in those with *Chlamydia trachomatis*-triggered ReA, but not in other patients.[34] Recent long-term follow up data, however, suggest that tetracycline treatment did not change the natural history of the disease.[34] In another recent study, however, a 3-month course of ciprofloxacin in the acute phase was found to have a beneficial effect on the long-term prognosis.[34] It is clear that early antibiotic therapy for chlamydial genital infections can prevent ReA, although the same is not true for enteric pathogens. For patients at risk for enteric infections and ReA, prophylactic antibiotics should be considered. There is no evidence that antibiotics have any place in the management of other SpA.

TNF-α blockers

Infliximab. The use of a chimeric monoclonal antibody to TNF-α (infliximab) at 5 mg/kg of infliximab every 6 weeks has been shown to be beneficial in both the axial and peripheral manifestations of AS in both open-label[35] and in placebo-controlled clinical trials.[36] The onset of action is quite rapid, usually following the first infusion, with over 80% of patients achieving > 20% improvement in measures of disease activity. Improvement was seen not only clinically but also radiographically, with clearing of lesions suggestive of disease activity on MRI.

Etanercept. The soluble TNF-α receptor, etanercept, given 25 mg subcutaneously twice weekly, has been shown to be effective in the treatment of AS in patients in a 4-month randomized double-blind placebo-controlled study of 40 AS patients.[37] Improvement was sustained in an open-label extension of this study for over 10 months. Similar positive results were seen in another longitudinal study of 10 SpA patients studied in the UK, with statistically significant improvement seen not only in all clinical and functional parameters, but also in MRI-detectable entheseal lesions, of which 86% either regressed completely or improved.[38] Similar positive results have been reported in PsA,[35] where substantial improvement was seen in both the joint and entheseal involvement as well as in the extent and severity of the psoriatic skin lesions. The Food and Drug Administration has approved the use of etanercept in the treatment of both AS and PsA.

The use of TNF blockers in the treatment of AAU is less clear, however. Recent data suggest they are useful, at least those comprised of monoclonal antibodies.[1]

Adalimumab. Adalimumab has been approved by the Food and Drug Administration for the treatment of AS and psoriatic arthritis, used at a dose of 40 mg every other week.[38] In patients in whom biweekly dosing does not suffice, weekly administration may be necessary.

ASAS guidelines for the use of TNF blockers. Because of the high cost and potential side-effect profiles of TNF blockers, as well as the finding that many patients with AS are well controlled with NSAIDs or sulfasalazine alone, the ASAS working group formulated and subsequently revised guidelines for the use of TNF blockers. These take into account both the patient's and physician's assessments of disease activity (Table 57.9).[39]

SURGICAL TREATMENT OF AS COMPLICATIONS

Because the hip is the joint most commonly involved in patients with AS, total hip arthroplasty is the most common surgical procedure.[21] Heterotopic new bone formation can be a potential problem.

Limited prevalence data suggest that patients with AS, even those with mild disease, are at increased risk for vertebral fracture, often resulting in neurologic compromise.[24] In general, halo vest immobilization is recommended. Surgical intervention may be necessary when neurological impairment is seen. The fixed kyphotic deformities seen in patients with advanced AS are of considerable distress to patients and can result in substantial functional impairment. A small minority of AS

Table 57.9 International Assessment in Ankylosing Spondylitis (ASAS) consensus statement for the use of antitumor necrosis factor (TNF) agents in patients with ankylosing spondylitis (AS)

1. For the initiation of anti-TNF-α therapy:
   (a) a diagnosis of definitive AS
   (b) presence of active disease for at least 4 weeks as defined by both a sustained Bath AS Disease Activity Index (BASDAI) of at least 4 *and* an expert opinion based on clinical features, acute-phase reactants, and imaging modalities
   (c) presence of refractory disease defined by failure of at least two nonsteroidal anti-inflammatory drugs during a single 3-month period, failure of intra-articular steroids if indicated, and failure of sulfasalazine in patients with peripheral arthritis
   (d) application and implementation of the usual precautions and contraindications for biological therapy

2. For the monitoring of anti-TNF-α therapy: both the BASDAI and the ASAS core set for clinical practice should be followed regularly

3. For the discontinuation of anti-TNF-α therapy: in nonresponders, consideration should be made after 6-12 weeks' treatment. Response is defined as improvement of
   (a) at least 50% or 2 units (on a 0–10 scale) of the BASDAI
   (b) expert opinion that treatment should be continued

patients will seek surgical correction of their spinal deformities. In general, open, polysegmental, and closing wedge osteotomies are employed. Loss of correction is seen least commonly in closing wedge osteotomy. In a meta-analysis of the literature between 1945 and 1998, an average correction of 37–40° degrees was seen, with perioperative mortality of 4% due to pulmonary, cardiac, and intestinal problems.[40]

CONCLUSION

Great progress has been made in the classication and epidemiology of SpA, particularly in the elucidation of the factors involved in the SpA pathogenesis in recent years. It has become clear that HLA-B27, the primary genetic factor identified in the pathogenesis of SpA, functions in a variety of roles, including 'classical' antigen presentation. How these lead to disease remains to be seen. Genome-ide scans have identified a number of regions that may contain other susceptibility genes for SpA, and these are being examined. Non-MHC genes that contribute to SpA susceptibility are currently being elucidated and a number of promising candidates have been identified.

On the other hand, less recent progress has been made in nongenetic factors. Despite what has been learned in ReA, no infectious trigger has been identified in AS (and in fact there might be no specific trigger). The link of gut inflammation to the triggering of AS is strongly suggested by data thus far, but has still not been defined. This is clearly an area of promise for further investigation.

Novel outcome measures have been developed that will help us to care better for ourpatients, especially in the area of imaging. Most exciting has been the advances in treatment, particularly in the development of biologic treatments, which hold promise for a better future for patients with these diseases.

REFERENCES

1. Monnet D, Breban M, Hudry C, et al. Ophthalmic findings and frequency of extraocular manifestations in patients with HLA-B27 uveitis: a study of 175 cases. Ophthalmology 2004; 111: 802–809.

2. Bergtfeldt L. HLA-B27 associated cardiac disease. Ann Intern Med 1997; 127: 621–629.

3. Dougados M, et al. The European Spondylarthropathy Study Group preliminary criteria for the classification of spondylarthropathy. Arthritis Rheum 1991; 34: 1218–1227.

4. van der Linden S, Valkenburg HA, Cats A. Evaluation of diagnostic criteria for ankylosing spondylitis. A proposal for modification of the New York criteria. Arthritis Rheum 1984; 27: 361–368.

5. Rudwaleit M, van der Heijde D, Khan MA, et al. How to diagnose axial spondyloarthritis early. Ann Rheum Dis 2004; 63: 535–543.

6. Taylor W, Gladman D, Helliwell P, et al. Classification criteria for psoriatic arthritis: development of new criteria from a large international study. Arthritis Rheum 2006; 54: 2665–2673.

7. Braun J, Kingsley G, van der Heijde D, et al. On the difficulties of establishing a consensus on the definition of and diagnostic investigations for reactive arthritis. Results and discussion of a questionnaire prepared for the 4th International Workshop on Reactive Arthritis, Berlin, Germany, July 3–6, 1999. J Rheumatol 2000; 27: 2185–2192.

8. Lawrence RC, Helmick CG, Arnett FC, et al. Estimates of the prevalence of arthritis and selected musculoskeletal disorders in the United States. Arthritis Rheum 1998; 41: 778–799.

9. Maurer K. Basic data on arthritis: knee, hip and sacroiliac joints in adults ages 25–74 years, United States, 1971–1975. Vital Health Stat 1979; 11: 213.

10. Sieper J, Rudwaleit M, Khan MA, et al. Concepts and epidemiology of spondyloarthriits. Best Pract Res Clin Rheumatol 2006; 20: 401–417.

11. Loftus EV. Clinical epidemiology of inflammatory bowel disease: incidence, prevalence, and environmental influences. Gastroenterology 2004; 126: 1504–1517.

12. Brown MA, Kennedy LG, MacGregor AJ, et al. Susceptibility to ankylosing spondylitis in twins: the role of genes, HLA, and the environment. Arthritis Rheum 1997; 40: 1823–1828.

13. Reveille JD, Arnett FC. Spondyloarthritis: update on pathogenesis and treatment. Am J Med 2005; 118: 592–603.

14. Reveille JD. The genetic basis of ankylosing spondylitis. Curr Opin Rheumatol 2006; 18: 332–341.

15. Smith JA, Marker-Hermann E, Colbert RA. Pathogenesis of ankylosing spondylitis: current concepts. Best Pract Res Clin Rheumatol 2006; 20: 571–591.

16. Carter KW, Pluzhnikov A, Timms AE, et al. Meta-analysis of three whole genome linkage scans for ankylosing spondylitis. Rheumatol (Oxf), 2006; in press.

17. Elder JT. PSORS1. Linking genetics and epidemiology. J Invest Dermatol 2006; 126: 1205–1206.

18. Mielants H, De Keyser F, Baeten D, et al. Gut inflammation in the spondyloarthropathies. Curr Rheumatol Rep 2005; 7: 188–194.

19. Ritchlin CT, Pathogenesis of psoriatic arthritis. Curr Opin Rheumatol 2005; 17: 406–412.

20. McGonagle D, Gibbon W, Emery P. Classification of inflammatory arthritis by enthesitis. Lancet 1998; 352: 1137–1140.

21. Sweeney S, Gupta R, Taylor G, et al. Total hip arthroplasty in ankylosing spondylitis: outcome in 340 patients. J Rheumatol 2001; 28: 1862–1866.

22. Mitra D, Elvins DM, Speden DJ, et al. The prevalence of vertebral fractures in mild ankylosing spondylitis and their relationship to bone mineral density. Rheumatol (Oxf). 2000; 39: 85–89.

23. Maillefert JF, Aho LS, El Maghraoui A, et al. Changes in bone density in patients with ankylosing spondylitis: a two-year follow-up study. Osteoporos Int 2001; 12: 605–609.

24. Lee W, Reveille JD, Davis JC, et al. Are there gender differences in the severity of ankylosing spondylitis: results from the PSOAS cohort. Ann Rheum Dis 2006 Nov 24. [Epub ahead of print].

25. Burgos Vargas R. Juvenile onset spondyloarthritides. Rheum Dis Clin North Am 2002; 28: 541–560.

26. Mease PJ, Goffe BS, Metz J, et al. Etanercept in the treatment of psoriatic arthritis and psoriasis: a randomised trial. Lancet 2000; 356: 385–390.

27. van der Heijde D, Landewe S, van der Linden S. How should treatment effect on spinal radiographic progression be measurred? Arthriits Rheum 2005; 52: 1979–1985.

28. Zeidler H, Brandt J, Schnarr S. Undifferentiated spondyloarthritis. In: Weisman MH, Reveille JD van der Heijde D, (eds) Ankylosing Spondylitis and the Spondyloarthropathies. Philadelphia, PA: Elsevier; 2006: 75–93.

29. Chen CH, Lin KC, Yu DT, et al. Serum matrix metalloproteinases and tissue inhibitors of metalloproteinases in ankylosing spondylitis: MMP-3 is a reproducibly sensitive and specific biomarker of disease activity. Rheumatol (Oxf) 2006; 45: 414–420.

30. Ward MM, Weisman MH, Davis JC, et al. Risk factors for functional limitations in patients with long-standing ankylosing spondylitis. Arthritis Rheum 2005; 53: 710–717.

31. Maksymowych WP, Inman RD, Salonen D, et al. Spondyloarthritis Research Consortium of Canada magnetic resonance imaging index for assessment of sacroiliac joint inflammation in ankylosing spondylitis. Arthritis Rheum 2005; 53: 703–709.

32. Sairanen E, Paronen I, Mahonen H. Reiter's syndrome: a follow-up study. Acta Med Scand 1969; 185: 57–63.

33. Wanders A, van der Heijde D, Landewe R, et al. Nonsteroidal anti-inflammatory drugs reduce radiographic progression in patients with ankylosing spondylitis: a randomized clinical trial. Arthritis Rheum 2005; 52: 1756–1761.

34. Clegg DO, Reda DJ, Abdellatif M. Comparison of sulfasalazine and placebo for the treatment of axial and peripheral articular manifestations of the seronegative spondylarthropathies: a Department of Veterans Affairs cooperative study. Arthritis Rheum 1999; 42: 2325–2329.

35. Gorman J, Sack KE, Davis JC Jr. Treatment of ankylosing spondylitis by inhibition of tumor necrosis factor α. N Engl J Med 2002; 346: 1349–1356.

36. Laasila K, Laasonen L, Leirisalo-Repo M. Antibiotic treatment and long term prognosis of reactive arthritis. Ann Rheum Dis 2003; 62: 655–658.

37. Braun J, Brandt J, Listing J, et al. Treatment of active ankylosing spondylitis with infliximab: a randomised controlled multicentre trial. Lancet 2002; 359: 1187–1193.

38. Van der Heijde D, Kivitz A, Schiff MH, et al. Efficacy and safety of adalimumab in patients with ankylosing spondylitis: results of a multicenter, randomized, placebo-controlled trial. Arthritis Rheum 2006; 54: 2136–2146.

39. Braun J, Pham T, Sieper J, et al. International ASAS consensus statement for the use of anti-tumour necrosis factor agents in patients with ankylosing spondylitis. Ann Rheum Dis 2003; 62: 817–824.

40. Van Royen BJ, De Gast A. Lumbar osteotomy for correction of thoracolumbar kyphotic deformity in ankylosing spondylitis. A structured review of three methods of treatment. Ann Rheum Dis 1999; 58: 399–406.

Small- and medium-vessel primary vasculitis

58

John H. Stone, David B. Hellmann

Vasculitis is defined as inflammation within blood vessel walls. Inflamed blood vessels are liable to narrow, thrombose, or rupture, and thereby cause tissues served by those vessels to undergo ischemic damage. The many different forms of vasculitis offer several challenges. First, these diseases often begin with nonspecific symptoms and signs, unfolding in an enigmatic fashion. Thus, vasculitis is one of the great diagnostic challenges in medicine. Knowledge of the clinical disguises by which vasculitis can present often permits the physician to suspect or diagnose the condition at the bedside. Second, with therapy, most patients improve, some enter disease remissions, and a substantial portion – variable according to disease type – are cured. Treating patients with vasculitis can therefore be even more rewarding than making the diagnosis. Finally, rapidly expanding knowledge of the pathophysiology of vasculitides promises more specific and more effective therapies for these diseases in the near future.

CLASSIFICATION OF VASCULITIS

More than 20 different forms of vasculitis are recognized; because the causes of most forms are not known, the vasculitides are distinguished by their clinicopathologic differences.[1] Classification schemes have traditionally categorized the different forms of vasculitis according to the size of blood vessels affected (Table 58.1). Beyond vessel size, the vasculitides can also be distinguished by considerations such as the typical host, the organs most commonly affected, and the presence of certain pathologic features. For example, within the small-vessel vasculitides, Henoch–Schönlein purpura (HSP) most commonly occurs in children, typically affects the gut, skin, joints, and kidneys, and produces vasculitis characterized by deposition of immunoglobulin A (IgA). In contrast, Wegener's granulomatosis (WG) usually strikes adults, has a predilection for the upper airways, lungs, and kidneys, and causes granulomatous inflammation. Finally, disorders in which vasculitis is the central cause of the symptoms and signs are designated 'primary.' 'Secondary' forms of vasculitides are those in which vasculitis complicates another type of disease, such as systemic lupus erythematosus (SLE) (Chapter 51) or rheumatoid arthritis (RA) (Chapter 52). This chapter focuses on primary vasculitides.

PATHOGENESIS

With few exceptions among the vasculitides, the etiologies of these diseases are not known, and precise knowledge of how the various effector cells of the immune system, the endothelial cells, cytokines, and other mediators interact to cause vascular inflammation is incomplete. Nevertheless, discussion of what is known about a few forms of vasculitis provides a framework for considering how perturbations of the immune system might play a role. The mechanisms described below are models of disease pathophysiology that have been proposed to explain anti-neutrophil cytoplasmic antibody (ANCA)-associated and immune complex (IC)-mediated vasculitis, respectively.

ANCA MODEL

ANCA are directed against different enzymes contained within primary granules of neutrophils and macrophages. These antibodies are usually detected by adding a patient's serum to a preparation of neutrophils, followed by the addition of an antibody tagged with a fluorescent label. In vasculitis, two main patterns of immunofluorescence (IF) are seen: a cytoplasmic pattern (C-ANCA) (Fig. 58.1) or a perinuclear pattern (P-ANCA). The C-ANCA pattern, usually caused by antibodies to serine proteinase 3 (PR-3), is highly specific for WG.[2] The P-ANCA pattern, typically caused by antibodies to myeloperoxidase (MPO), is much less specific, being found in some patients with WG, microscopic polyangiitis (MPA), the Churg–Strauss syndrome (CSS), and other diagnoses.

Two murine models of ANCA-associated vasculitis (AAV) reveal that adoptive transfer of autoantibody alone is sufficient to induce a necrotizing vasculitis that closely resembles human disease. These models involved two types of genetically altered mice: the MPO knockout mouse and the recombinase-activating gene 2 (RAG-2)-deficient mouse. The latter species lacks both T and B cells. These models provide *in vivo* evidence for the pathogenic potential of ANCA. In the MPO knockout model,[3] mice were initially immunized with mouse MPO, resulting in the formation of anti-MPO T cells and B cells and anti-MPO antibodies. RAG-2-deficient mice were subsequently injected with either anti-MPO

Table 58.1 Major categories of primary vasculitis

Large-vessel vasculitis

Giant-cell arteritis
Takayasu's arteritis

Medium-vessel vasculitis

Polyarteritis nodosa
Kawasaki's disease
Primary central nervous system vasculitis
Buerger's disease

Small-vessel vasculitis

Anti-neutrophil cytoplasmic antibody (ANCA)-associated
small-vessel vasculitis:
- Microscopic polyangiitis
- Wegener's granulomatosis
- Churg–Strauss syndrome
- Drug-induced ANCA-associated vasculitis

Immune-complex small-vessel vasculitis:
- Hypersensitivity vasculitis
- Cryoglobulinemic vasculitis
- Connective tissue disorders
- Urticarial vasculitis
- Behçet's disease
- Goodpasture's syndrome
- Serum sickness
- Infection-induced vasculitis

Paraneoplastic small-vessel vasculitis
Inflammatory bowel disease vasculitis

(Adapted from Jennette J, Falk R. Small vessel vasculitis. *N Engl J Med* 1997; 337: 1512.)

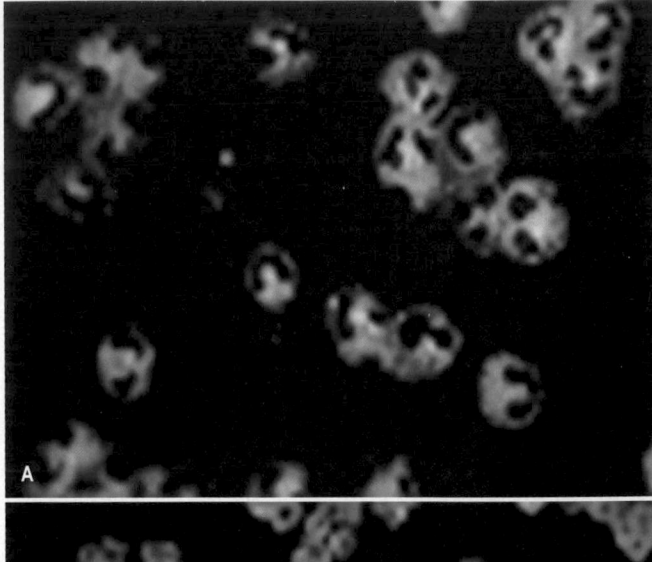
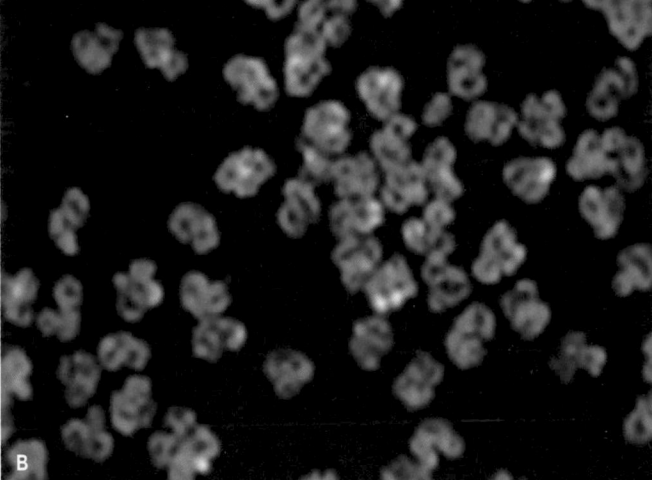

Fig. 58.1 Anti-neutrophil cytoplasmic antibody (ANCA) patterns. **(A)** Immunofluorescence study of serum on the substrate of human neutrophils, demonstrating cytoplasmic immunofluorescence (a positive ANCA assay, C-ANCA pattern). **(B)** Perinuclear immunofluorescence (P-ANCA pattern).

splenocytes or control splenocytes, which did not produce anti-MPO antibodies. RAG-2 mice that received anti-MPO splenocytes developed clinical features of AAV, including crescentic glomerulonephritis and systemic necrotizing vasculitis. By comparison, RAG-2 mice that received non-MPO antibody-producing splenocytes displayed only a relatively mild IC glomerulonephritis. In the RAG-2 model, RAG-2-deficient and wild-type mice were injected with anti-MPO or control immunoglobulins. Only mice receiving anti-MPO antibodies developed a pauci-immune glomerulonephritis.

Potential disease triggers in humans

For AAV in humans, a variety of infectious, genetic, and environmental risk factors (and combinations of all three) have been considered as triggers. Because the symptoms of WG at disease onset overlap substantially with those due to infectious processes, research efforts have focused upon the identification of pathogens that may precipitate WG in individuals of the proper genetic background. However, attempts to identify an infectious cause or causes for WG have not been fruitful. Efforts to define genetic risk factors have also met with limited success.[4–6]

Given the frequency with which the first symptoms of WG occur in the respiratory tract, exposure to noninfectious agents or toxins via the inhalational route is another possible inciting event. One such candidate is silica dust. The odds ratio of exposure to silica dust has been reported to be 4.4 times higher for patients with AAV than in a comparison group of patients with renal disease caused by lupus or other conditions.[7] However, exact relationships between environmental exposures and vasculitis are complicated by difficulties in obtaining reliable measurements of exposures, the likelihood of recall bias among patients who are diagnosed with AAV, and the choice of appropriate control groups.

Because alpha-1 antitrypsin (AAT) is the primary *in vivo* inhibitor of PR-3, the observation that patients with AAT deficiency are at increased risk for WG suggests a potential pathogenic role in this disease for deficient PR-3 clearance from sites of inflammation.[8, 9] Decreased local concentrations of AAT caused by genetic polymorphisms or alterations in the enzyme's functionality induced by inflammation may therefore lead to protease/antiprotease imbalance in the disease microenvironment. Although unproven, these events may be responsible for generating immunogenic forms of PR-3 in these patients.

Mechanisms of ANCA production

Autoantibodies reactive to ANCA are probably generated against newly exposed epitopes (i.e., cryptic sites) of the target autoantigen. Following the production of ANCA, the antibody response may generalize to the rest of the molecule or to other components of a macromolecular protein complex via the process of epitope spreading. With WG, these neoepitopes may arise at the sites of initial tissue injury. Since it is an antigen-driven process, the disease may heavily depend upon help from T cells.

This hypothesis is supported by the finding that lymphocytes have a significant role in AAV:

- Patients with active WG have much higher levels of activated CD4 T cells and monocytes than do patients in remission or healthy controls.[10]
- Very high levels of the Th1 cytokines tumor necrosis factor-α (TNF-α) and interferon (IFN)-γ are observed in patients with active WG. Monocytes from these patients release large quantities of interleukin 12 (IL-12), a major inducer of Th1 cytokines.
- Population-based studies of WG patients reveal a diminished frequency of a major inhibitory CTLA-4 allele.[11] This may contribute to increased T-cell activation in these patients.

These findings suggest that IL-10, a known antagonist of monocyte activation, may inhibit the Th1 pathway in this disease by impairing the production of IL-12. In one study, for example, IL-10 treatment of peripheral blood mononuclear cells from active WG patients impaired the production of IFN-γ in vitro.[10]

The roles of ANCA isotypes and Fc receptors

In theory, the isotype of ANCA in a given individual may have pathophysiological importance. Most patients with AAV, for example, produce isotype-switched IgG ANCA, implying a T-cell-dependent immune response. However, studies regarding the relative importance of IgG subtypes and other types of ANCA (e.g., IgM, IgA) have been inconclusive and contradictory. Presently, there is no clear evidence that particular ANCA isotypes influence the susceptibility to or clinical expression of AAV. The magnitude of enhanced neutrophil activation by ANCA may also be influenced by antibody specificity for different PR-3 epitopes, IgG subclass, and the type of Fcγ-R engaged. The Fcγ-RIIIB allele polymorphism NA1, which allows more efficient neutrophil activation by ANCA, is overrepresented in patients with severe forms of WG.[12]

ANCA and neutrophil activation

The significant role described above for lymphocytes in AAV does not exclude an important role for ANCA themselves. Because Th1 cytokines are effective stimuli of both neutrophils and monocytes, the production of ANCA may further enhance tissue injury by augmenting the damage caused by mononuclear cells. The effects of ANCA are determined by the state of neutrophil activation. PR-3 and MPO, located in the cytosol, can be relatively inaccessible to antibody binding. However, neutrophils primed with TNF as well as those undergoing apoptosis express increased quantities of membrane-associated PR-3,[13, 14] a process known as neutrophil 'priming.' In some individuals, a higher proportion of nonactivated neutrophils may express membrane-associated PR-3, which may be a risk factor for vasculitis, or for more severe manifestations of vasculitis.

Once neutrophils have been activated by priming, ANCA are able to bind relevant membrane-bound antigens, causing abnormal constitutive activation via either the cross-linking of MPO or PR-3 or the binding of Fc receptors. Persistent ANCA binding to neutrophils on the endothelial surface can enhance the degree of vascular injury. The rate at which primed neutrophils degranulate and release chemoattractants and cytotoxic oxygen free-radical species into the local tissue environment is also increased by ANCA. In addition, primed neutrophils can adhere to and damage vascular endothelial cells and attract additional neutrophils to the site of damage, thereby creating an auto-amplifying loop.

Patients with AAV have increased numbers of primed neutrophils in renal biopsy specimens, paralleling the activity of the disease. In addition, persistent membrane expression of PR-3 during periods of disease remission is associated with an increased risk of relapse in WG patients. Enhanced generation of reactive oxygen species by circulating neutrophils in these patients compared to controls may also occur.

ANCA-associated activation can induce neutrophil actin polymerization, resulting in increased neutrophil rigidity.[15] Such activated neutrophils can become sequestered in small-sized vessels since they are unable to adapt morphologically to arterioles; this may help explain the predilection for small blood vessels in ANCA-associated disease.

Role of the endothelial cell

Whether endothelial cells produce PR-3 and display this molecule upon activation is controversial. In the early stages of AAV, however, endothelial cells are known to recruit inflammatory cells and enhance their adhesion to sites of vascular injury. The subsequent release of PR-3 (from infiltrating leukocytes, at a minimum) and other neutrophil proteases may induce endothelial synthesis and secretion of IL-8, a potent neutrophil chemoattractant, thereby attracting additional neutrophils. PR-3 released by neutrophils can also enhance the adhesion of accumulating neutrophils and mononuclear cells to the endothelial surface via the induction of adhesion molecules, such as vascular cell adhesion molecule-1 (VCAM-1). VCAM-1 is known to be expressed *in situ* within the renal lesions of patients with AAV. The soluble endothelial protein C receptor binds activated neutrophils via interactions with PR-3, providing a link between neutrophil priming, vascular inflammation, and the coagulation cascade. This may explain, in part, the increased risk of venous thrombotic events observed in WG.[16] Organ-specific anti-endothelial antibodies have also been reported, albeit the precise antigens and role in disease development are unclear.

The role of B cells

B cells may also play an important role in AAV. The number of activated B cells in circulation correlates with disease activity scores in AAV.[17] Furthermore, B-cell depletion therapy in AAV has shown encouraging results.[18, 19] The rationale for why B-cell depletion may be effective in

AAV is not clear, but possibilities include the complete removal or substantial reduction of ANCA production; diminution of the contribution of B cells to antigen presentation and cytokine production; and the inhibition of B-cell/T-cell cross-talk.

IMMUNE COMPLEX MODEL

Another established mechanism for causing vasculitis is the deposition of circulating ICs. ICs are known to contribute substantially to a number of types of vasculitis in humans. IC deposition is thought to be the prevailing disease mechanism, for example, in HSP, hypersensitivity vasculitis, mixed cryoglobulinemia, and hepatitis B-associated polyarteritis nodosa (PAN). After the formation of soluble ICs, the complexes are deposited in the subendothelium, an event facilitated by the release of vasoactive amines (e.g., histamine) from platelets and basophils. Once trapped in the subendothelial space, ICs fix complement and generate chemotactic factors for the recruitment and activation of neutrophils. Degranulation of these neutrophils leads to the release of oxygen radicals and lysosomal enzymes, which in turn damage the blood vessel walls.

The IC model is compatible with the transient vasculitis known as serum sickness that develops following exposure to some foreign antigens. Antigens as varied as the horse serum formerly used in immunizations, antibiotics (e.g., penicillin), virus-associated antigens (e.g., hepatitis B or C) or self-antigens (e.g., double-stranded DNA) are capable of causing IC-mediated vasculitis in humans. In cases involving a 'one-shot' antigen exposure, the vasculitis resolves as the antigen is cleared. However, when the antigen persists, e.g., in chronic viral hepatitis, SLE, or RA, the vasculitis can be chronic (albeit the precise antigen is not always known).

Formation of ICs is common, even in healthy individuals, but the occurrence of vasculitis is relatively rare. Several factors determine the pathogenicity of ICs. Antigen load is one determinant, as only amounts of antigen large enough to overwhelm the reticuloendothelial system (RES) provoke a pathologic IC response. Another important factor is solubility of the IC, which changes with the ratio of antigen to antibody. When the antigen-to-antibody ratio is very high, for example, complexes of antibody and antigen do not form. Conversely, when antibody is present in large excess compared to the antigen, the RES clears the antigen rapidly. ICs formed in slight antigen excess are most likely to be pathogenic, because they are both soluble and of sufficient size to deposit in blood vessel walls. Finally, physical forces such as pressure within the blood vessel (which can damage vessels), temperature (certain ICs such as cryoglobulin form at colder temperatures), or locations of vascular branch points (where turbulence favors IC deposition) can influence the development of vasculitis.

GENERAL CLUES TO DETECTING VASCULITIS

Inflamed vessels produce clinical symptoms and signs either by being associated with the release of inflammatory cytokines that cause malaise, fever, and weight loss, or by causing direct ischemic damage to specific tissues, such as the induction of digital gangrene. Since the vasculitides demonstrate predilections for certain tissues and organs, their presenting manifestations vary greatly. However, most of the vasculitides share four general features: first, they unfold in a subacute fashion, over weeks or months; second, pain is often a prominent feature of a vasculitis, be it from mononeuritis multiplex, scleritis, migratory oligoarthritis/arthralgias, myalgias, mesenteric ischemia, or another consequence of vascular

---

inflammation; third, signs of inflammation, such as fever, rashes, and weight loss are also prominent; fourth, evidence of multiorgan system dysfunction is common. Although not every case of vasculitis adheres strictly to all four of these guidelines, bearing these clues in mind helps clinicians to identify patients whose symptoms and signs may be caused by vasculitis.

THE ANCA-ASSOCIATED VASCULITIDES

In a landmark 1954 paper, Godman and Churg[20] noted similar pathological features among three clinically distinct disease entities: WG, MPA, and CSS. These diseases, Godman and Churg noted, 'group themselves into a compass, [ranging from] necrotizing and granulomatous processes with angiitis, through mixed forms, to vasculitis without granulomata.' Over the past 15 years WG, MPA, and CSS have become recognized as the cardinal forms of vasculitis associated with ANCA. They are commonly termed ANCA-associated vasculitides or AAV, although not all patients who meet the clinical definitions of these diseases have ANCA. The hallmarks of WG, MPA, and CSS are displayed in Table 58.2.

SEROLOGIC TESTING FOR ANCA

Two types of ANCA tests, IF and enzyme immunoassay (EIA), are now in common use. IF tests are highly operator-dependent, require a high degree of experience for proper interpretation, and are not antigen-specific. They are, however, generally superior to EIA in terms of sensitivity. In contrast to IF assays, EIAs are antigen-specific and demonstrate substantially higher positive predictive values for AAV. A widely adopted strategy for optimizing the utility of ANCA tests, therefore, is to screen patients with potential AAV by IF testing, and then to perform EIAs on patients who test positively.[21] Capture EIAs, available at some centers, do not have clear advantages over these other assays.

WG, MPA, and CSS have variable strengths of association with ANCA (Table 58.2). The strength of association for each disease is affected by several factors, including disease activity, disease extent, and intensity of therapy. Even in WG, the disease for which the association

Table 58.2 Hallmarks of Wegener's granulomatosis (WG), microscopic polyangiitis (MPA), and Churg–Strauss syndrome (CSS)

	WG	MPA	CSS
ANCA positive	80–90%	75%	50%
Typical immunofluorescence/	C-ANCA/PR-3	P-ANCA/MPO	P-ANCA/MPO
Enzyme immunoassay results			
Upper respiratory tract	Nasal septal perforation Saddle-nose deformity Subglottic stenosis	Mild	Nasal polyps Allergic rhinitis
Lung	Nodules Cavitary lesions	Alveolar hemorrhage	Asthma Fleeting infiltrates
Kidney	NCGN, occasional granulomatous features	NCGN	NCGN (severe renal disease unusual)
Distinguishing feature	Destructive upper airway disease	No granulomatous inflammation	Allergy Eosinophilia

(Adapted from Rao JY, Weinberger M, Oddone EZ, et al. The role of antineutrophil cytoplasmic antibody (C-ANCA) testing in the diagnosis of Wegener's granulomatosis. Ann Intern Med 1995; 123: 425.)
ANCA, anti-neutrophil cytoplasmic antibody; C-ANCA, cytoplasmic ANCA; MPO, myeloperoxidase; NCGN, necrotizing crescentic glomerulonephritis; P-ANCA, perinuclear ANCA; PR-3, proteinase 3.

CLINICAL PEARLS

VASCULITIDES ASSOCIATED WITH ANTI-NEUTROPHIL CYTOPLASMIC ANTIBODIES (ANCA)

>> Wegener's granulomatosis (WG), microscopic polyangiitis (MPA), and the Churg–Strauss syndrome (CSS) have become recognized as the types of vasculitis associated with ANCA

>> Shortcomings of reliance upon ANCA to define this group of complex diseases:

>> Not all patients with these diseases have a positive test for ANCA

>> A variety of systemic illnesses, including infections, malignancies, and other conditions, may be associated with a positive ANCA test, particularly when positive immunofluorescence tests are not confirmed by enzyme immunoassay

>> Even when ANCA are present, they are unreliable indicators of disease activity

KEY CONCEPTS

ANTI-NEUTROPHIL CYTOPLASMIC ANTIBODY (ANCA) PATTERNS AND ASSOCIATIONS WITH ANTIGENS AND DISEASES

Pattern	Antigen	Disease association
C-ANCA	Proteinase-3	Wegener's granulomatosis
P-ANCA	Myeloperoxidase	Wegener's granulomatosis
		Microscopic polyangiitis
		Churg–Strauss syndrome

with ANCA is the strongest, most series indicate that 10–20% of patients with active, disseminated, and untreated disease are ANCA-negative. For WG patients with limited WG, defined as the absence of an immediate threat to either the function of a vital organ or the patient's life, 30% or more of patients lack ANCA. In MPA, estimates of ANCA positivity approximate 70%. Finally, although relatively few data exist regarding the prevalence of ANCA in CSS, several studies have indicated that only about 50% of such patients are ANCA-positive.

When carefully employed and properly interpreted, ANCA assays constitute an important, albeit imperfect, adjunct to diagnosis. In rare instances, in the setting of classic clinical presentations and highly consistent ANCA test results (e.g., C-ANCA IF and PR-3 ANCA), the combination of clinical findings and ANCA assays may preclude the need for tissue biopsies to confirm the diagnosis. Despite advances in ANCA testing techniques, however, histopathology remains the cornerstone of diagnosis in AAV. When the diagnosis is unconfirmed, all reasonable attempts to obtain a tissue diagnosis should be pursued.

With regard to predicting disease flares, several studies indicate that elevations in ANCA titers do not predict disease flares; i.e., the temporal relationship between an increase in ANCA and the development of a clinical disease flare is poor.[22, 23] Moreover, disease flares may also occur in the absence of an ANCA titer elevation.

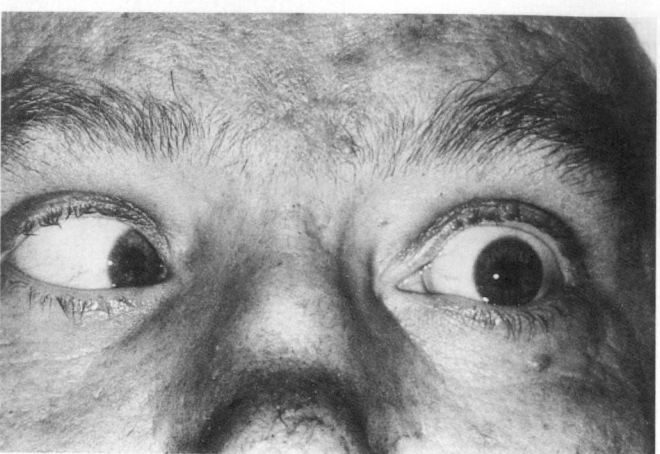

Fig. 58.2 Saddle-nose deformity in Wegener's granulomatosis. Saddle-nose deformity and a left sixth cranial nerve lesion (the latter caused by meningeal inflammation) in a patient with Wegener's granulomatosis. (Reproduced with permission from Jinnah H, Dixon A, Brat D, et al. Chronic meningitis with cranial neuropathies in Wegener's granulomatosis: case report and review of the literature. Arthritis Rheum 1997; 40: 573.)

In the following sections, each of the three major forms of AAV is discussed. Treatment strategies for these disorders are discussed together in the final part of this section.

WEGENER'S GRANULOMATOSIS

In 1936 a German pathologist, Friedrich Wegener, reported 3 patients in their mid-30s whose innocuous presentations were those of a 'common cold.'[24] Within 7 months, all had succumbed to systemic inflammatory illnesses that culminated in uremia. Three years later, Wegener provided a more detailed description of this disease, which he referred to as 'a peculiar rhinogenic granuloma with particular involvement of the arterial system and the kidney.'[25]

Godman and Churg recognized the three pathologic hallmarks of WG[20]: (1) necrotizing granulomas in the upper and/or lower respiratory tract; (2) necrotizing vasculitis affecting arteries or veins; and (3) segmental glomerulonephritis, associated with necrosis and thrombosis of capillary loops, with or without granulomatous lesions. WG is regarded as one of the most common forms of systemic necrotizing vasculitis, with an annual incidence of 8.5 cases/million.[26] Although the disease occurs in all races, there is a strong predilection for individuals of northern European heritage. Classic WG involves the upper respiratory tract, the lungs, and the kidneys, but distinctive features of this disease may also occur in the eye, ear, and other organs. Involvement of tissues as diverse as the prostate gland and meninges has been reported.

The numerous disease manifestations of WG throughout the respiratory tract have long engendered suspicion that the disease results from interactions between an inhaled microbial pathoallergen(s) and a susceptible host. Approximately 90% of patients with WG have nasal involvement.[27] The nasal manifestations of WG include crusting, bleeding, and obstruction. Cartilaginous inflammation may lead to nasal septal perforation and even to collapse of the nasal bridge, a condition known as a saddle-nose deformity (Fig. 58.2). Most patients with nasal (or sinus) disease eventually develop secondary infections of these tissues.

Erosive sinus disease is highly characteristic of WG. Among the AAV, only WG is likely to cause destructive lesions of the bony sinuses. Subglottic stenosis, resulting from a peculiar predilection of WG to cause scarring inflammation in the region of the trachea inferior to the vocal cords, is a potentially disabling disease feature. Subglottic involvement is often asymptomatic and may manifest itself only as a subtle hoarseness. However, some patients present with the subacute onset of respiratory stridor. With time, airway scarring occurs, sometimes accompanied by profound tracheal narrowing. Severe cases require tracheostomy. Subglottic stenosis, particularly when associated with scarring and fibrosis, often responds poorly to immunosuppressive therapy. The most effective therapeutic approach to subglottic stenosis in these cases is usually mechanical, i.e., surgical dilatations to enlarge the airway narrowing, combined with local glucocorticoid injections.

Two principal forms of ear disease, conductive and sensorineural hearing loss, are typical of WG. Mixed hearing loss, the conjoint occurrence of both auditory lesions, is also common. Conductive hearing loss results from granulomatous involvement of the middle-ear cavity, most often leading to serous otitis media. In contrast, the mechanism of inner-ear disease in WG is poorly understood. Granulomatous inflammation in the middle ear may compress the seventh cranial nerve (which courses through the middle-ear cavity), leading to a peripheral facial nerve palsy. Less commonly, vasculitic neuropathy infarcts the nerve at some point during its path through the temporal bone.

WG may be associated with several clinically important ocular lesions (Fig. 58.3). Retrobulbar masses, among the most treatment-refractory WG lesions, may lead to proptosis and visual loss through ischemia of the optic nerve. Scleritis, which causes eye pain and an angry, purplish scleral hue, may lead to scleromalacia perforans and visual loss (Chapter 73). Other ocular manifestations of WG include episcleritis, peripheral ulcerative keratitis, uveitis, conjunctivitis, nasolacrimal duct obstruction (characteristically leading to wet rather than dry eyes), and, occasionally, occlusion of the retinal arteries or veins.

Although the histological features of pulmonary WG are similar to those found in specimens from other tissues, the full pathologic spectrum may be more apparent in lung biopsy specimens (Fig. 58.4). Both vasculitic and necrotizing granulomatous features, which do not invariably coexist, may be confirmed in lung biopsy specimens. In addition to these two processes, pulmonary WG frequently demonstrates an extensive, nonspecific inflammatory background. The leukocytoclastic vasculitis in the lung may involve arteries, veins, and capillaries, with or without granulomatous features. Vascular necrosis begins as clusters of neutrophils within the blood vessel wall (microabscesses) that degenerate and become surrounded by palisading histiocytes. Coalescence of such neutrophilic microabscesses leads to extensive regions of 'geographic' necrosis. The range of granulomatous inflammation found in WG may include palisading granulomas, scattered giant cells, and poorly formed granulomas.

The clinical manifestations of pulmonary WG are equally diverse, ranging from asymptomatic lung nodules to fulminant alveolar hemorrhage. The most common radiographic findings are pulmonary infiltrates and nodules. The infiltrates, which may wax and wane, are often initially misdiagnosed as pneumonia. Nodules are usually multiple and bilateral, and often result in cavitation (Fig. 58.5). Hilar and/or mediastinal adenopathy is rare in WG, but has been reported.

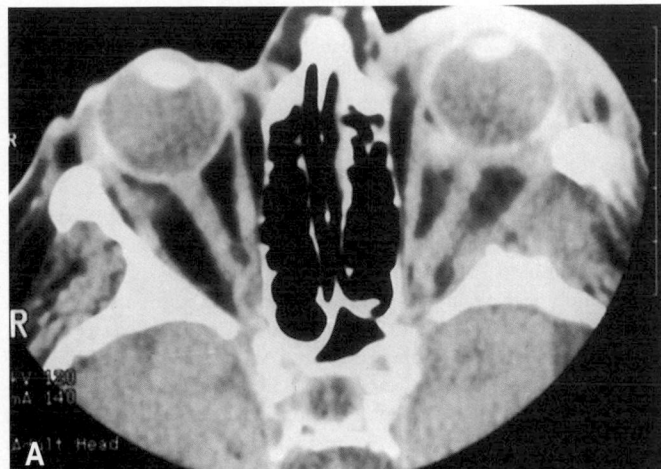

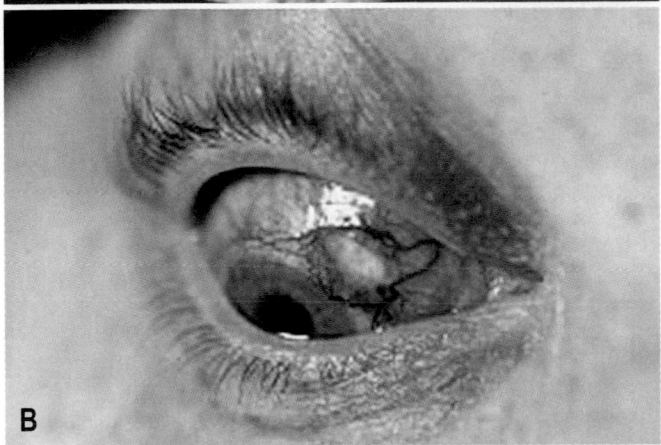

Fig. 58.3 Ocular manifestations of Wegener's granulomatosis.
(A) Bilateral retro-bulbar masses, causing proptosis of the left eye;
(B) necrotizing scleritis.

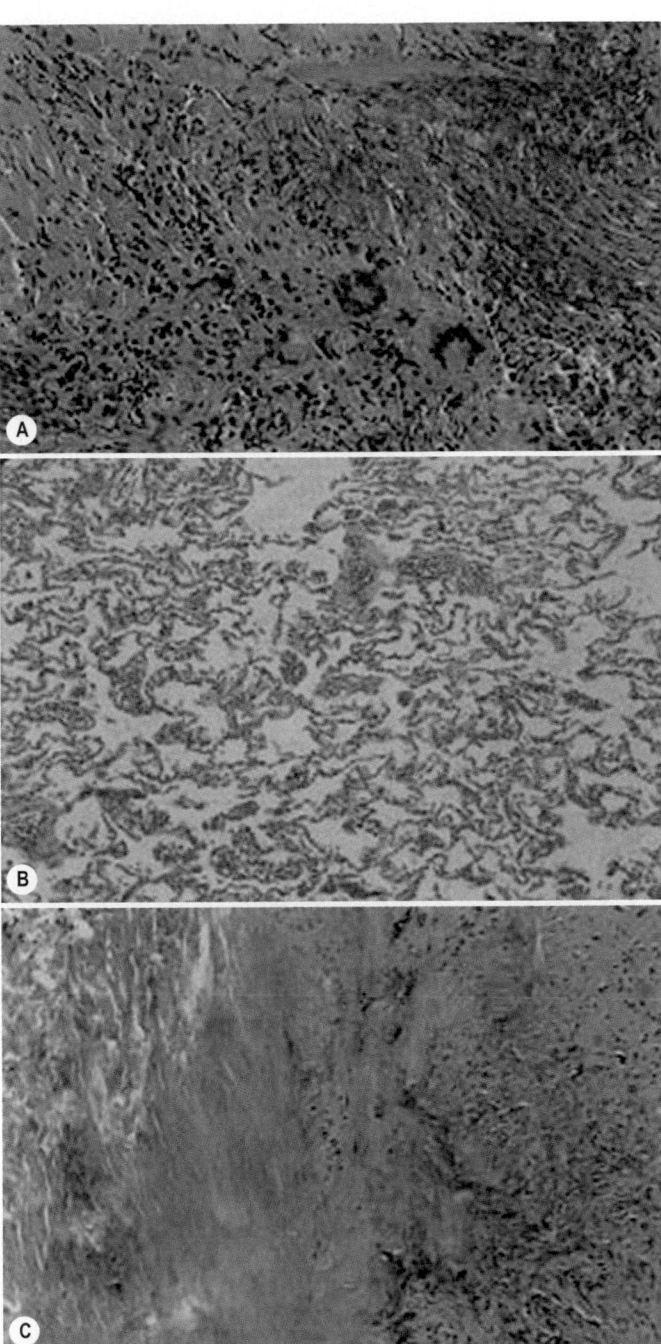

Fig. 58.4 Histopathology of Wegener's granulomatosis. The
pathologic features of Wegener's granulomatosis: **(A)** Langerhans giant
cells and palisading granulomatous inflammation; **(B)** small-vessel
vasculitis and fibrinoid necrosis of the lung; **(C)** 'geographic' necrosis.

Renal involvement is the most ominous clinical manifestation of WG.
The typical lesion of WG (indeed, of all forms of AAV) is segmental
necrotizing glomerulonephritis, usually associated with the formation of
glomerular crescents (Chapter 67). The histopathology of renal disease in
AAV – in contrast to mixed cryoglobulinemia and SLE, for example – is
pauci-immune in nature (i.e., scant immunoglobulin or complement
deposition). Thrombotic changes in the glomerular capillary loops are
among the earliest histologic changes evident in AAV. Granulomatous
changes, although frequently present, are identified only rarely in renal
biopsies. The clinical presentation of renal disease in WG is that of rapidly progressive glomerulonephritis: hematuria, red blood cell casts, proteinuria (usually nonnephrotic), and progressive renal insufficiency.
Without appropriate therapy, end-stage renal disease ensues within days
to weeks. A commonly observed clinical occurrence is acceleration of the
overall disease process once renal involvement is evident.

Less classic but nevertheless common features in WG are involvement
of the musculoskeletal system, skin, and nervous system. Approximately
half of all patients with WG are rheumatoid factor-positive, and RA is

a common misdiagnosis early in the disease course when nonspecific arthralgias and arthritis may occur. Migratory oligoarthralgias and arthritis are a common presentation of disease flares. Unlike RA, the arthritis of WG tends to involve large joints and to spare the small joints of the hands. Splinter hemorrhages, digital ischemia, and digital gangrene resulting from inflammation in large digital arteries are under-appreciated as manifestations of WG. Skin lesions in WG include the full panoply of lesions associated with cutaneous vasculitis (see section on hypersensitivity vasculitis, below). Although involvement of the brain parenchyma with WG has been reported, meningeal inflammation presenting as excruciating headaches and cranial neuropathies is a more common central nervous system manifestation of this disease. Finally, devastating mononeuritis multiplex may accompany WG, but this feature is less characteristic of WG than of the other major forms of AAV – MPA and CSS.

The clinical course of WG is marked by a tendency to recur following tapering or cessation of treatment. In one clinical trial, somewhat less than half of patients achieved disease remissions and maintained them

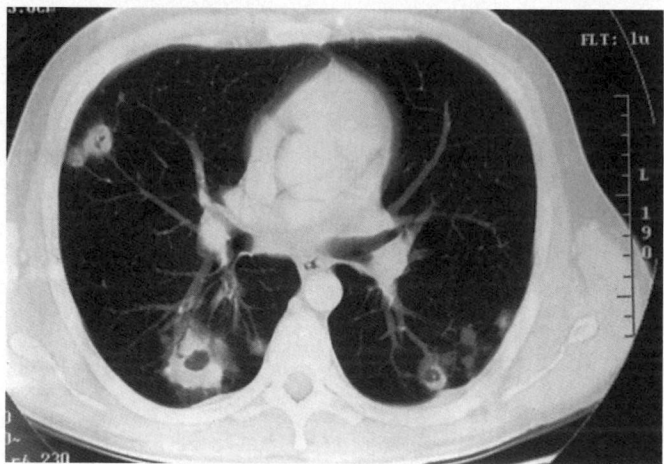

Fig. 58.5 Chest computed tomography abnormalities in Wegener's granulomatosis. Multiple, bilateral pulmonary nodules, several of which have cavitated.

throughout the trial, which had a mean follow-up of approximately 2 years.[28] The requirement for repeated administration of the potentially toxic treatments in WG (discussed below) leads to substantial long-term morbidity.

MICROSCOPIC POLYANGIITIS

In 1948, Davson et al.[29] suggested the division of PAN patients into two groups based on the presence or absence of glomerulonephritis. One group of patients, Davson noted, demonstrated renal vasculitis only in medium-sized vessels of the kidneys (sparing the glomerulus). In contrast, patients in the other group had glomerular inflammation (i.e., small-vessel vasculitis, with or without medium-sized vessel involvement). This subset of patients with small-vessel vasculitis of the kidney was designated as having microscopic PAN. More recently, microscopic PAN has been renamed "microscopic polyangiitis," in recognition of the tendency of MPA to involve not only arteries but also capillaries and veins as well.

The distinction of MPA from PAN was emphasized by the 1994 Chapel Hill Consensus Conference on the nomenclature of vasculitides,[1] which defined MPA as a process: (1) involving necrotizing vasculitis with few or no immune deposits; (2) affecting small blood vessels (capillaries, venules, or arterioles) as well as (perhaps) medium-sized arteries; and (3) demonstrating a tropism for the kidneys (glomerulonephritis) and lungs (pulmonary capillaritis). Microscopic poly*angiitis* (as opposed to poly*arteritis*) is the preferred term for this disorder, because the disease may affect arterioles, capillaries, venules, veins, and arteries in addition to arteries. Table 58.3 compares the principal features of MPA with those of classic PAN.

As with WG, a dominant feature of MPA is necrotizing glomerulonephritis with crescent formation (Fig. 58.6). In one study of 34 MPA patients with glomerulonephritis, the percentage of patients with functioning kidneys was only 55% and the actuarial survival only 65% at 5 years of follow-up, despite aggressive immunosuppressive therapies.[30] Pulmonary capillaritis, most typical of MPA, may rapidly lead to life-threatening hemorrhage from the lungs, requiring prompt, aggressive treatment (Fig. 58.7). In aggregate, the AAV constitute a far more common cause of this pulmonary renal syndrome than does anti-glomerular basement membrane (GBM) disease. In some cases, both ANCA and anti-GBM antibodies occur in the same patient, with disease outcomes generally worse than with either antibody alone.

Table 58.3 Features of microscopic polyangiitis versus classic polyarteritis nodosa

Feature	Microscopic polyangiitis	Classic polyarteritis nodosa
Granulomas	No	No
Vessel size	Small (and medium)	Medium
Renovascular hypertension	No	Yes
Rapidly progressive glomerulonephritis	Yes	No
Lung involvement	Alveolar hemorrhage	No
Mononeuritis multiplex	Yes	Yes
Anti-neutrophil cytoplasmic antibody (ANCA)-positive	P-ANCA (anti-myeloperoxidase)	Rare
Hepatitis B association	No	Sometimes (10%)
Vascular aneurysms	Occasionally	Commonly

In one series of MPA patients,[31] renal manifestations (79%), weight loss (73%), mononeuritis multiplex (58%), and fever (55%) were the most common disease manifestations. Alveolar hemorrhage occurred in 12%. Upper respiratory tract symptoms in MPA are much milder than those associated with WG. MPA is not associated with erosion of the bony sinuses, scarring of the subglottic region, or saddle-nose deformities. The essential difference between MPA and WG, however, is the absence of granulomatous inflammation in MPA.

THE CHURG–STRAUSS SYNDROME

In 1951, Churg and Strauss reported a series of 13 patients with 'peri-arteritis nodosa' who demonstrated severe asthma and an unusual constellation of symptoms: 'fever . . . hypereosinophilia, symptoms of cardiac failure, renal damage, and peripheral neuropathy, resulting from vascular embarrassment in various systems of organs.'[32] The investigators believed the syndrome to represent a new disease entity, which they termed 'allergic angiitis and allergic granulomatosis.' Three histologic criteria for this disorder, subsequently known as CSS, were specified: (1) presence of necrotizing vasculitis; (2) tissue infiltration by eosinophils (Fig. 58.8); and (3) extravascular granulomas. Today the diagnosis is often made on the basis of looser clinical criteria, because finding all three criteria in a single patient is challenging outside the autopsy room.

The 1990 American College of Rheumatology criteria for the classification of CSS[33] are intended to distinguish patients with CSS from those with other vasculitic disorders (Table 58.4). The presence of four or more of the six disease criteria yielded a sensitivity and specificity of 85% and 99.7% for CSS, respectively. The Chapel Hill Consensus Conference defined CSS as the presence of eosinophil-rich, granulomatous inflammation involving the respiratory tract, with necrotizing vasculitis of small to medium-sized vessels, associated with asthma and eosinophilia.[1] In addition to the other vasculitides, CSS must be distinguished from a group of hypereosinophilic disorders: Löffler syndrome, eosinophilic gastroenteritis, chronic eosinophilic pneumonia, the hypereosinophilic syndrome (HES), eosinophilic fasciitis, and eosinophilic leukemia.

Greater than 90% of CSS patients have histories of asthma. Typically the asthma is either of new onset or constitutes a significant exacerbation of long-standing disease. Upon encroachment of the vasculitis phase of CSS, patients' asthma may improve substantially, even before therapy for vasculitis is begun. Following successful treatment of the vasculitic phase, however, glucocorticoid-dependent asthma persists in many patients.

Chest radiographs are normal in the majority of CSS patients. Radiographic abnormalities are usually limited to fleeting pulmonary infiltrates, detected in one-third of patients. Pulmonary hemorrhage is unusual, and cavitary lesions should suggest the alternative diagnosis of WG. The pathological features of lung disease in CSS vary according to the disease phase: in the prodromal phase, there is extensive eosinophilic

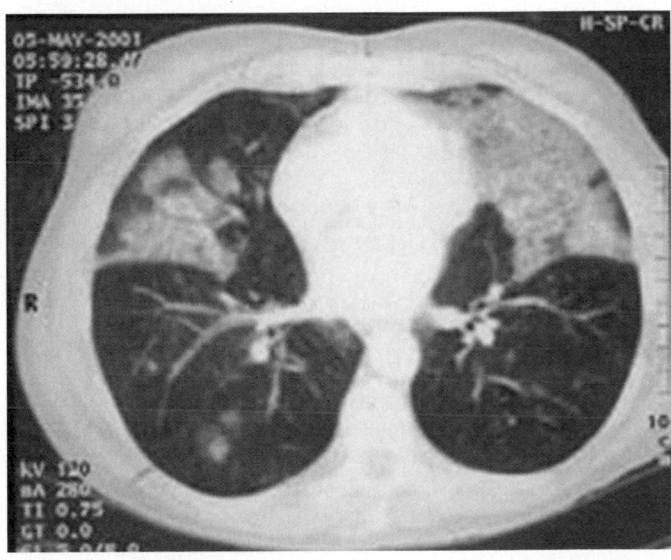

Fig. 58.7 Alveolar hemorrhage in microscopic polyangiitis.

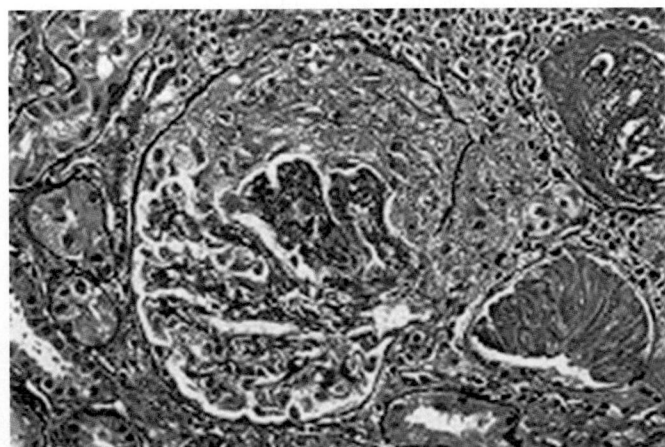

Fig. 58.6 Crescentic glomerulonephritis in microscopic polyangiitis. Glomerular crescent in a patient with rapidly progressive glomerulonephritis secondary to microscopic polyangiitis.

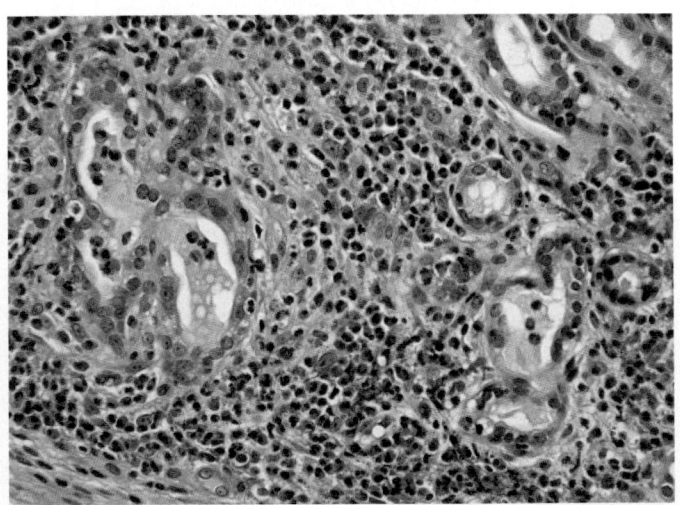

Fig. 58.8 Eosinophilic infiltration of a salivary gland.

infiltration of the alveoli and interstitium; during the vasculitic phase, necrotizing vasculitis and granulomas are evident. Upper-airway disease in CSS usually takes the form of nasal polyps or allergic rhinitis. A high percentage of patients have histories of nasal polypectomies, often long before the diagnosis is considered. Although pansinusitis occurs frequently, destructive upper-airway disease is not characteristic of CSS.

In contrast to WG, mononeuritis multiplex occurs with a remarkable frequency in CSS. This potentially disabling complication was evident in 74 of the 96 patients (77%) in one series.[34] Cardiac involvement (usually congestive heart failure) also occurs with a disproportionate frequency in CSS; cardiac complications are a common mode of death in CSS. Renal disease in CSS has been described as less common and less malignant compared to that associated with other AAV. When it occurs, histopathological findings are often indistinguishable from those of WG, MPA, and other forms of pauci-immune glomerulonephritis, with the possible exception of increased eosinophils in CSS biopsies.

Peripheral blood eosinophilia is a hallmark of CSS, with eosinophils accounting for up to 60% of the white blood cell count (before treatment). Approximately 50% of CSS patients test positive for ANCA, which is usually directed to MPO.

CLINICAL PEARLS

THREE PHASES OF THE CHURG–STRAUSS SYNDROME (CSS)

>> Prodromal phase, characterized by the presence of allergic disease (typically asthma or allergic rhinitis), which may last from months to many years

>> Eosinophilia/tissue infiltration phase, in which remarkably high peripheral eosinophilia may occur and tissue infiltration by eosinophils is observed in the lung, gastrointestinal tract, and other tissues

>> Vasculitic phase, in which systemic necrotizing vasculitis afflicts a wide range of organs, ranging from the heart and lungs to peripheral nerves and skin

---

Although clinical remissions may be obtained in more than 90% of patients with CSS, disease recurrences are common upon cessation of therapy (as with other AAVs). In the largest series reported to date, flares were detected in more than 25% of the patients.[34] In most cases, relapses were heralded by the return of eosinophilia. Many patients develop steroid-dependent asthma after the vasculitic phase of their disease appears to have subsided. Distinguishing simple asthma flares from CSS recurrences can be challenging in such cases.

■ TREATMENT OF THE ANCA-ASSOCIATED VASCULITIDES ■

Patients with WG, MPA, or CSS whose symptoms constitute immediate threats to either the function of vital organs or to the patient's life urgently require treatment with both a cytotoxic agent (usually cyclophosphamide) and high doses of glucocorticoids. The current standard of care for patients with severe disease of this nature is cyclophosphamide for 3–6 months, followed by azathioprine for an additional 18 months.[35, 36] Limited forms of WG may respond to the combination of glucocorticoids and methotrexate, thus sparing patients the potential side effects of cyclophosphamide. Increasing experience with methotrexate and prednisone has demonstrated, however, that durable remissions of WG with this regimen are rare, and smoldering or recurrent disease that reactivates upon taper of the medications is the rule. A substantial number of patients with CSS achieve satisfactory responses with glucocorticoids alone, and monotherapy is a reasonable first approach for many of these patients. However, patients with evidence of rapidly progressive glomerulonephritis or symptoms of mononeuritis multiplex should be treated promptly with both cyclophosphamide and glucocorticoids to halt these devastating disease manifestations.

Practice regarding the use of either daily or intermittent (e.g., monthly intravenous) cyclophosphamide varies from center to center. Remission is induced with either daily or intermittent regimens of cyclophosphamide (combined with glucocorticoids) in high percentages of patients. Regardless of the route by which cyclophosphamide is administered, however, the medication is associated with potential hazards. Careful monitoring, particularly of the white cell count, is essential. Complete blood counts every 2 weeks are advised for patients on cyclophosphamide. The induction of

---

Table 58.4 American College of Rheumatology classification criteria for Churg–Strauss syndrome

Criterion	Definition
Asthma	History of wheezing or diffuse high-pitched rales on expiration
Eosinophilia	Eosinophilia > 10% on white blood cell differential count
Mononeuropathy or polyneuropathy	Development of mononeuropathy, multiple mononeuropathies, or polyneuropathy (i.e., stocking/glove distribution)
Pulmonary infiltrates, nonfixed	Migratory or transitory pulmonary infiltrates on radiographs
Paranasal sinus abnormality	History of acute or chronic paranasal sinus pain or tenderness, or radiographic opacification of the paranasal sinuses
Extravascular eosinophils	Biopsy including artery, arteriole, or venule, showing accumulations of eosinophils in extravascular areas

(From Masi A, Hunder G, Lie J, et al. The American College of Rheumatology 1990 criteria for the classification of Churg–Strauss syndrome (allergic granulomatosis and angiitis). Arthritis Rheum 1990; 33: 1094.)

THERAPEUTIC PRINCIPLES

TREATMENT OF ANTI-NEUTROPHIL CYTOPLASMIC ANTIBODIES (ANCA)-ASSOCIATED VASCULITIDES

>> The presence of symptoms that constitute immediate threats to either function of vital organs or to survival requires urgent treatment with both a cytotoxic agent and high doses of glucocorticoids

>> In patients with severe disease, cyclophosphamide is the cytotoxic drug of choice

>> Limited forms of Wegener's granulomatosis may respond to a combination of glucocorticoids and methotrexate, but durable remissions with this regimen are rare

>> In Churg–Strauss syndrome patients without serious organ involvement, treatment with glucocorticoids is a reasonable first approach. However, the presence of glomerulonephritis or mononeuritis multiplex requires immediate treatment with cyclophosphamide and glucocorticoids

neutropenia is not required to achieve a therapeutic effect in AAV, and avoidance of this side effect is highly desirable as a strategy to prevent opportunistic infections. Cyclophosphamide should be temporarily withheld if the WBC count falls below $4.0 \times 10^6/\mu l$. The multitude of side effects associated with long-term use of cyclophosphamide has inspired the use of shorter courses of induction treatment (e.g., 3–6 months), followed by longer-term maintenance of remission with either azathioprine or methotrexate. A wide array of other therapies, e.g., plasmapheresis or intravenous immunoglobulin, has been employed in small numbers of patients, but insufficient data exist to judge their efficacy. The use of IFN-α in the treatment of CSS appears promising,[37] but larger studies are required.

Results of a recent trial of etanercept (a soluble TNF inhibitor) added to standard therapy for remission maintenance were instructive.[28] Although at least temporary disease control was achieved in a high proportion of patients – 87% in the etanercept group, 91% in the control group – this disease control was due to the conventional therapies that patients in both treatment arms received. Disease flares were common in both groups, with a total of 118 in the etanercept group (23 severe, 95 limited) and 134 in the control group (25 severe, 109 limited). With regard to the trial's primary outcome, sustained remission, the percentages of patients who achieved this measure were not different: 70% in the etanercept group, 75% in the control group. Most strikingly, in the WGET cohort overall, only 49% of patients achieved disease remissions and maintained them throughout the trial. In the two groups combined, 57% of the patients suffered at least one severe or life-threatening adverse event (no difference between groups). Most adverse effects, with the possible exception of solid malignancies,[38] were attributable to conventional therapies rather than to etanercept. There were 6 deaths, but none from overwhelming WG.

Two other randomized trials in ANCA-associated vasculitis[35, 39] confirm the high likelihood of controlling the disease with conventional therapies but also the high likelihood of disease flares once these therapies are tapered. Particularly critical in the maintenance of remission appears to be some dose of maintenance glucocorticoid.[40]

POLYARTERITIS NODOSA

PAN, the grandfather of all the vasculitides, was described in 1866 by Kussmaul and Maier.[41] The patient was a 27-year-old journeyman tailor who died from a multisystem illness characterized by fever, weight loss, polyneuropathy, and abdominal pain. The nodular swellings found along the course of muscular arteries at autopsy prompted Kussmaul and Maier to term the disease 'periarteritis nodosa.' The term was unfortunate because in fact the inflammatory process consists of a panarteritis that involves the entire thickness of the vessel wall. Subsequent authors have adopted the more accurate name 'polyarteritis nodosa.'

PAN can begin in childhood or in the eighth decade of life, but the average age of onset is about 40–45 years. Series vary in the proportion of men and women afflicted. Some 10–30% of patients develop the disease related to infection with hepatitis B, due to the deposition of ICs containing viral antigens.[42] In the remainder of cases, the etiology remains unknown. No genetic susceptibility to PAN has been identified, and familial PAN is exceedingly rare.

CLINICAL FEATURES

The initial symptoms of PAN are usually nonspecific, such as malaise, fatigue, fever, and extremity pain from myalgia or arthralgia (Table 58.5). Typically, it is not until weeks or months later that patients develop signs of vasculitis. The most helpful clinical clues often come from the skin and peripheral nerves because these areas are affected relatively early, and their manifestations of vasculitis are distinctive. Skin lesions of PAN include livedo reticularis, subcutaneous nodules, leg ulcers, palpable purpura, and digital gangrene.[43]

Mononeuritis multiplex, a peripheral neuropathy characterized by the segmental infarction of named nerves, is both one of the most specific clues to vasculitis and a hallmark of PAN. Mononeuritis multiplex most often affects the peroneal, tibial, ulnar, median, and radial nerves, leading to foot or hand symptoms (e.g., foot or wrist drop). Mononeuritis multiplex almost always causes sensory abnormalities, particularly painful dysesthesias. Motor involvement occurs in one-third of patients. Sometimes patients with PAN appear to have a (nonspecific) symmetrical polyneuropathy. In such cases, electrodiagnostic testing may unmask greater asymmetry to the process than is evident clinically, and also confirm that the pattern of nerve injury is one of axonal degeneration.

The gastrointestinal tract is also frequently involved in PAN.[44] The classic manifestation is 'intestinal angina' – periumbilical pain starting 30–60 minutes after eating. The pain results from intestinal ischemia occurring because the increased metabolic demands of the bowel after eating cannot be met by the limited blood flow in inflamed mesenteric vessels. Ischemic bowel can be difficult to recognize, especially in patients receiving glucocorticoids, which blunt the signs of acute abdomens. Vasculitis of individual organs can mimic cholecystitis and appendicitis.

Renal involvement is nearly universal at autopsy in PAN, but tends to produce few clinical symptoms. The new onset of hypertension, hematuria, and rising serum creatinine are the most common signs. Renin-mediated hypertension, a hallmark of PAN, is rare in ANCA-associated vasculitis, which tends to involve smaller vessels and glomeruli rather than medium-sized interlobar renal arteries.

Cardiac involvement, often striking at autopsy, is usually inconspicuous during life. Pericardial effusions, cardiomyopathy, and myocardial infarctions are the most common manifestations. Central nervous system

Table 58.5 Clinical features in patients with polyarteritis nodosa

Clinical feature	Percentage with finding
General	
Fever	71
Weight loss	54
Organ system involvement	
Kidney	70
Musculoskeletal system:	64
• Arthritis/arthralgia	53
• Myalgias	31
Hypertension	54
Peripheral neuropathy	51
Gastrointestinal tract	44
• Abdominal pain	43
• Nausea/vomiting	40
• Cholecystitis	17
• Bleeding	6
• Bowel perforation	5
• Bowel infarction	1
Skin	43
• Rash/purpura	30
• Nodules	15
• Livedo reticularis	4
Cardiac	36
• Congestive heart failure	12
• Myocardial infarction	6
• Pericarditis	4
Central nervous system	23
• Cerebral vascular accident	11
• Altered mental status	10
• Seizure	4

(From Cupps T, Fauci A. Systemic necrotizing vasculitis of the polyarteritis nodosa group. In: Smith LH (ed) The Vasculitides. Major Problems in Internal Medicine, vol. 21. Philadelphia: WB Saunders; 1981:26.)

The pathologic changes in PAN involve small and medium-sized arteries and may be macroscopic and microscopic. Involved arteries may show readily visible aneurysmal bulges of the vessel wall. Infarctions, ruptured aneurysms, and gangrenous tissue may be easily visible. Histological sections show inflammatory cells infiltrating the vessel wall (Fig. 58.9), leading to fibrinoid necrosis. Varying degrees of intimal proliferation and thrombosis occur. Lesions tend to be segmental and to favor branch points. In the acute phase of the illness, the inflammatory infiltrate consists chiefly of neutrophils, whereas mononuclear cells predominate in the chronic phase. Granulomas are absent in PAN, and eosinophils are rarely prominent.

DIAGNOSIS

Criteria for the classification of PAN have been developed by the American College of Rheumatology (ACR) (Table 58.6).[45] Diagnostic certainty requires a positive biopsy or an angiogram demonstrating characteristic microaneurysms (Fig. 58.10). Biopsies of symptomatic sites such as nerve, muscle, or testicle are often useful (sensitivity, 60–70%; specificity ~97%). In the absence of a symptomatic site to biopsy, mesenteric angiography may demonstrate telltale microaneurysms (sensitivity ~60%; specificity, 99%).

TREATMENT AND PROGNOSIS

For patients with idiopathic PAN, treatment usually consists of prednisone and cyclophosphamide. In the precorticosteroid era, only 13% of patients survived 5 years. With high doses of glucocorticoids, it is estimated that approximately half of all patients can achieve remission with prednisone alone. Although there have been few controlled trials (and even case series of PAN are contaminated by patients with other diagnoses, such as MPA or CSS), the only randomized controlled trial comparing prednisone alone with prednisone and cyclophosphamide showed no difference in 10-year survival – approximately 70% in both treatment groups.[46] Patients treated with cyclophosphamide, however, experienced fewer relapses than those treated with prednisone alone (9% versus 38% of patients). Thus, for severe PAN or for cases that are refractory to initial therapy with prednisone, the combination of glucocorticoids and cyclophosphamide is the standard of care. When using cyclophosphamide to treat PAN, achieving leukopenia is neither required nor desirable. Indeed, frequent monitoring of the white blood cell count (e.g., every 2 weeks) is advisable so that leukopenia can be detected early and cyclophosphamide reduced or stopped as needed. The relative efficacy of daily versus intermittent (e.g., monthly) cyclophosphamide is not clear.

Most patients begin to improve within 2–4 weeks of starting treatment. Tapering of prednisone may begin after the first month and is slowly continued until the drug is stopped after 6–12 months. Whenever possible, cyclophosphamide should be discontinued after 6 months and replaced by a less toxic medication (e.g., azathioprine) for the completion of one full year of therapy.

Antiviral agents have revolutionized the treatment of PAN associated with hepatitis B. Before the availability of antiviral agents, all survivors of PAN treated with immunosuppression alone became chronic carriers of hepatitis B and assumed the risks of cirrhosis and hepatoma. The availability of antiviral agents permitted a treatment strategy based on an understanding of disease pathogenesis.[47] Initially patients are treated with prednisone (1 mg/kg per day) to suppress the inflammation. After the first week, prednisone is rapidly tapered and then discontinued over 3–7 days, and antiviral therapy (e.g., lamivudine 100 mg/day or entecavir

disease usually results from hypertension rather than intracranial vasculitis, but involvement of cerebral blood vessels sometimes occurs. Scleritis is the most common ocular manifestation. Testicular infarction can occur early in the course, causing acute pain and swelling that mimics torsion of the testicle. Remarkably, as noted by Kussmaul and Maier, PAN spares the lung parenchyma.

Although PAN typically involves multiple organs, limited forms have been described. Cutaneous PAN is a medium-vessel vasculitis limited to the skin, causing nodules or ulcers. Over time, some of these patients develop systemic disease. Some cases of cutaneous PAN are induced by drugs (especially minocycline and propylthiouracil) and are associated with ANCA.

The laboratory features of PAN, though frequently strikingly abnormal, are nonspecific. Anemia, mild thrombocytosis (except in perforation of the gut, which is associated with thrombocytopenia), elevation of the erythrocyte sedimentation rate (ESR), and microscopic hematuria are common.

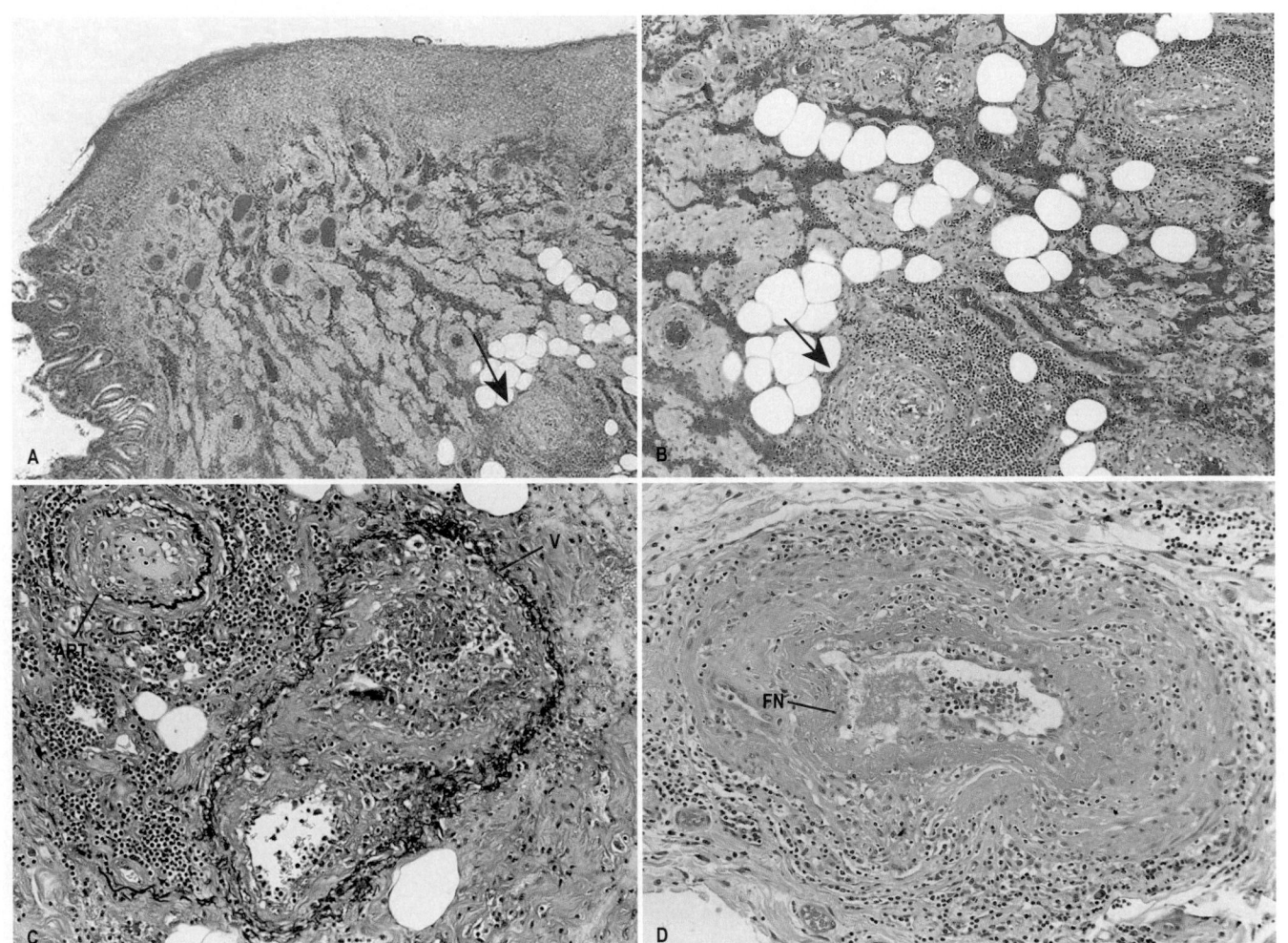

Fig. 58.9 Polyarteritis nodosa histopathology. Photomicrographs of a jejunal specimen obtained at laparotomy from a 74-year-old man who died of complications of mesenteric ischemia related to polyarteritis nodosa. **(A)** Viable-appearing jejunal mucosa with the loss of villi is seen in the lower left corner of the photomicrograph. In the remainder of the visible lumen, the mucosa is replaced by a highly inflamed, ischemia-induced ulcer. In the lower right corner, there is a narrowed, chronically inflamed, medium-sized artery (arrow) surrounded by a lymphocytic infiltrate. **(B)** Higher-powered view of the artery shown in Figure 58.9A (arrow), along with several other inflamed arteries. The extensive lymphocytic infiltrate indicates the chronic nature of the inflammatory process. **(C)** Elastin stain of an artery (ART) and a vein (V) within the wall of the jejunum. The internal elastic lamina of the artery has been disrupted focally by the inflammatory process, and fibrinoid necrosis is present. **(D)** Medium-sized muscular artery from the jejunum, characterized by chronic lymphocytic inflammation, abundant fibrinoid necrosis (FN), and luminal narrowing. (Reproduced with permission from Levine SM, Hellmann DB, Stone JH. Gastrointestinal involvement in polyarteritis nodosa (1986–2000): presentation and outcomes in 24 patients. Am J Med 2002; 112: 386.)

0.5 mg/day) is started. For several weeks throughout this period, plasma exchange is carried out 2–3 times a week for an average of about 20 exchanges per patient, depending on clinical response. With this regimen, 80% of patients survive the vasculitis and 56% no longer demonstrate serologic evidence of hepatitis B replication.

Treatment for PAN associated with hepatitis C

The treatment of hepatitis C-associated PAN is discussed in the section on cryoglobulinemia.

■ MIXED CRYOGLOBULINEMIA ■

Wintrobe discovered cryoglobulins in 1931 when, in the course of evaluating a 56-year-old woman with anemia, Raynaud's phenomenon, and symptoms of hyperviscosity – she ultimately turned out to have myeloma – he refrigerated a tube of the patient's blood and noted the formation of a precipitate in her plasma.[48] To share his discovery with colleagues, he placed the tube in his coat pocket and walked to the wards. Pulling the tube from his warm pocket he was startled to see that his discovery had vanished. This experience helped to define the

Table 58.6 Criteria for classification of polyarteritis nodosa

1. Weight loss ≥ 4 kg
2. Livedo reticularis
3. Testicular pain or tenderness
4. Myalgias, weakness, or leg tenderness
5. Mononeuropathy or polyneuropathy
6. Diastolic blood pressure > 90 mmHg
7. Elevated blood urea nitrogen or creatinine
8. Hepatitis B virus
9. Arteriographic abnormalities
10. Biopsy of small or medium-sized artery containing polymorphonuclear cells in the vessel wall

For classification purposes, a patient shall be said to have polyarteritis nodosa if at least three of these 10 criteria are present (From Lightfoot R, Michel B, Bloch D, et al. The American College of Rheumatology 1990 criteria for the classification of polyarteritis nodosa. Arthritis Rheum 1990; 33: 1088.)

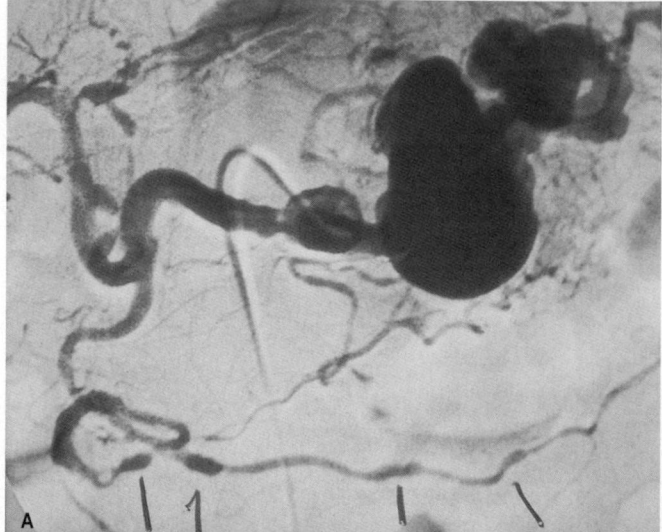

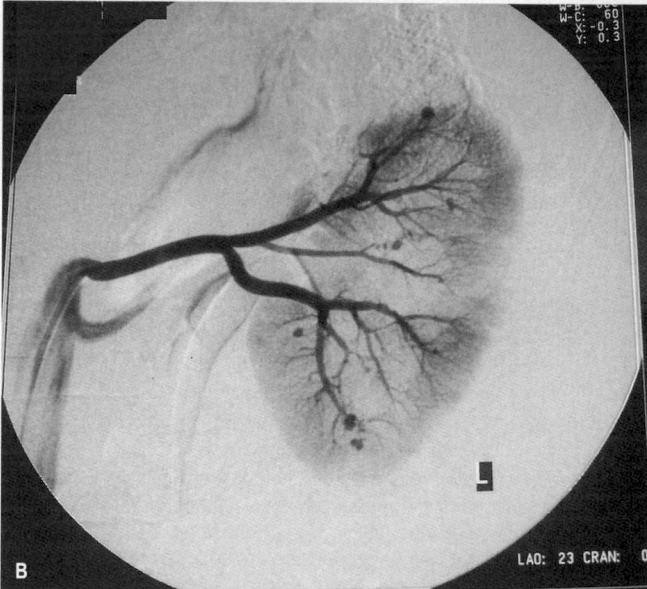

Fig. 58.10 Angiograms in polyarteritis nodosa. **(A)** Large aneurysms in the distribution of the splenic artery in a 60-year-old woman with polyarteritis nodosa. The largest of these aneurysms ruptured, requiring an emergent laparotomy. **(B)** Multiple microaneurysms within the renal parenchyma in a 24-year-old man with polyarteritis nodosa. (Reproduced with permission from Levine SM, Hellmann DB, Stone JH. Gastrointestinal involvement in polyarteritis nodosa (1986–2000): presentation and outcomes in 24 patients. Am J Med 2002; 112: 386.)

hallmark of cryoglobulins – antibodies that precipitate under conditions of cold and solubilize on rewarming (see below).[49]

Cryoglobulins are classified into three types (I, II, or III) (Table 58.7) based on whether or not they are monoclonal, and demonstrate rheumatoid factor activity.[50, 51] Type I cryoglobulins, characteristically found in hematopoietic malignancies, are monoclonal but do not have rheumatoid factor activity. Cryoglobulin types II and III, which typically occur in autoimmune disorders and infections, are designated mixed cryoglobulins, because they consist of both IgG and IgM. The IgM component in type II and type III cryoglobulinemia has rheumatoid factor activity. In type II cryoglobulinemia, the IgM is monoclonal, whereas in type III it is polyclonal. Not all patients with cryoglobulins have symptoms. Indeed, half of all patients with hepatitis C have demonstrable cryoglobulins, yet vasculitis occurs in < 1%. Vasculitis results when ICs containing cryoglobulins and antigenic components deposit in blood vessel walls and activate complement.

The clinical syndrome and underlying disease can be predicted from the type of cryoglobulin present. For example, monoclonal cryoglobulins without rheumatoid factor activity (type I) do not activate complement effectively and are more likely, as in Wintrobe's patient, to cause hyperviscosity than vasculitis. In contrast, the mixed cryoglobulinemias (types II and III) often activate complement efficiently, and are prone to cause vasculitis.

After the discovery of hepatitis C virus (HCV), it quickly became evident that this infection accounted for more than 80% of the cases of 'essential' mixed cryoglobulinemia (EMC). The precise mechanism by which HCV and other infections induce cryoglobulins and the syndrome of EMC is not clear.

Among patients with HCV and mixed cryoglobulinemia, approximately one-third have type II cryoglobulins and two-thirds have type III. Type II mixed cryoglobulinemia developed a mean of 7.6 years after infection, and type III mixed cryoglobulinemia after a mean of 13.7 years following infection.[52] The genetic susceptibility of individual patients to EMC, the duration of HCV infection, and the genotype of particular HCV subspecies may explain why only some patients with HCV develop EMC.

Table 58.7 Classification of cryoglobulins and their immunochemical features and clinical associations

Type	Rheumatoid factor activity	Monoclonal association	Clinical syndrome	Disease present
I	Yes (usually IgG)	No	Hyperviscosity	Malignancy
II	Yes (IgM)	Yes	Vasculitis	Hepatitis C Rheumatic diseases Malignancy Idiopathic
III	No	Yes	Vasculitis	Hepatitis C Rheumatic diseases Idiopathic

Ig, immunoglobulin.

Mixed cryoglobulinemia causes small-vessel vasculitis with a predilection for the skin, peripheral nerves, and kidney. The most common manifestation is recurrent crops of palpable purpura on the legs (Fig. 58.11). Other common manifestations are dysesthesias and mononeuritis multiplex caused by vasculitic neuropathy, glomerulonephritis, arthralgias, malaise, and fatigue. Some patients develop mesenteric vasculitis, Raynaud's phenomenon, livedo reticularis, or secondary Sjögren's syndrome. Lung and heart disease are uncommon. Some patients with mixed cryoglobulinemia develop a severe medium-vessel vasculitis with large, painful ulcerations that are clinically indistinguishable from those of PAN.

Most patients with mixed cryoglobulinemia have anemia, an elevated ESR, and elevated liver transaminases. Those with type II mixed cryoglobulinemia usually show an IgM-γ monoclonal spike. Ninety percent of patients with mixed cryoglobulinemia vasculitis are hypocomplementemic, with C4 levels characteristically more depressed than C3. Biopsies of petechial lesions in the skin or gastrointestinal tract show leukocytoclastic vasculitis, with IF studies revealing IgG and IgM deposition in both medium and small blood vessels. Renal biopsies in patients with type II mixed cryoglobulinemia typically show membranoproliferative glomerulonephritis (Chapter 67). The diagnosis of cryoglobulinemic vasculitis is established by isolating type II or type III cryoglobulins following refrigeration at 4°C for several days and by demonstrating vasculitis pathologically (usually by skin biopsy).

The treatment of mixed cryoglobulinemia is often challenging. For patients with mild symptoms such as infrequent crops of purpura, no therapy is required. For those with HCV-associated mixed cryoglobulinemia, frequent purpura, and a mild vasculitic neuropathy, pegylated IFN (1.5 µg/kg per week) and ribavirin (1000–1200 mg/day) may be effective.[53] Fewer than half of patients with HCV-associated mixed cryoglobulinemia respond to antiviral therapy. Patients younger than 60 who do not have HCV genotype 1 (the most common in Americans) are more likely to respond. This regimen eliminates purpura, reduces the cryocrit, normalizes complement levels, and eliminates HCV-RNA in 30–60% of patients. Unfortunately, up to 90% of patients relapse (clinically or serologically) if the therapy is discontinued. For this reason, antiviral therapy is sometimes continued indefinitely (albeit at lower doses). For those with life-threatening vasculitides, high-dose prednisone, cyclophosphamide (in doses identical to those used in

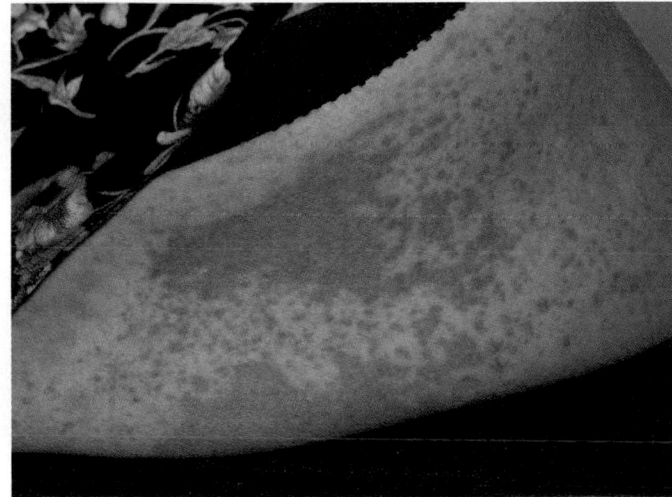

Fig. 58.11 Purpura in vasculitis. Palpable purpura in a patient with cryoglobulinemic vasculitis.

PAN), and plasmapheresis are recommended. If the vasculitis improves and the immunosuppression can be tapered, then antiviral therapy is added.

HYPERSENSITIVITY VASCULITIS

The proliferation of names for cutaneous vasculitis is principally due to the fact that, compared to the relatively limited number of disorders that cause large- or medium-vessel arteritis, a host of disorders can be associated with small-vessel vasculitis of the skin. These disorders include both primary vasculitides and secondary causes of vasculitic inflammation. Whereas some of these conditions cause only cutaneous vasculitis, others can also cause organ- or life-threatening involvement of vital organs, such as the lungs or kidney. This section focuses on types of small-vessel vasculitis confined to the skin. Other prominent causes of cutaneous vasculitis, e.g., cryoglobulinemia, HSP, urticarial vasculitis, the ANCA-associated disorders, and cutaneous PAN, are discussed separately in other sections of this chapter.

In 1952, in the first classification scheme ever devised for the vasculitides, Zeek[54] coined the term 'hypersensitivity vasculitis.' The purpose of this term was to distinguish a form of necrotizing arteritis that involved only small blood vessels from PAN, which has a predilection for larger vessels. The word 'hypersensitivity' stemmed from animal models of vasculitis induced by the administration of horse serum, sulfonamides, and other drugs. These vasculitis models – attempts to develop an animal model of PAN – differed from PAN in their prominent cutaneous involvement, their involvement of the venous as well as the arterial circulation, and their involvement of small blood vessels, i.e., arterioles, venules, and capillaries. Moreover, in contrast to PAN, all of the lesions in hypersensitivity vasculitis tended to occur in "crops," and thus were approximately the same age. Finally, in contrast to the characteristically unrelenting nature of PAN, hypersensitivity vasculitis was self-limited.

Since Zeek's first description of hypersensitivity vasculitis, the term has been narrowed to denote small-vessel vasculitis confined principally to the skin and not associated with any other primary vasculitis (e.g., HSP, WG, or cryoglobulinemia). The identification of an inciting antigen for the vasculitis is not a prerequisite to the diagnosis, because no such provocation is found in many patients who fit the clinical and pathological picture of the disease.

The ACR-formulated criteria for the classification of hypersensitivity vasculitis included: (1) age of onset greater than 16 years; (2) medication at disease onset; (3) palpable purpura; (4) maculopapular rash; and (5) biopsy of arteriole or venule showing granulocytes in a perivascular or extravascular location.[55] The presence of three of five criteria resulted in sensitivity of 71% and specificity of 84%.

The 1994 Chapel Hill Consensus Conference on nomenclature of the vasculitides proposed an alternative term for hypersensitivity vasculitis – cutaneous leukocytoclastic angiitis – because of the frequent failure to identify a precipitant (no manifest cause of hypersensitivity). This designation is also problematic, however, because although most lesional skin biopsies demonstrate a neutrophil predominance, others show a primarily lymphocytic infiltration. Moreover, these two histopathological patterns do not appear to represent different evolutionary stages of the same process, but rather (at a minimum) two distinct processes, underscoring the difficulty of using a single term to define all patients with this clinical phenotype.

Regardless of the name, certain similarities exist among patients who present with symptoms and signs of cutaneous vasculitis. First, the lesions typically occur first in dependent regions, i.e., the lower extremities or buttocks. Second, the lesions may be asymptomatic, but are usually accompanied by a burning or tingling sensation. A wide array of skin lesions may occur, including palpable purpura, papules, urticaria/angioedema, erythema multiforme, vesicles, pustules, ulcers, and necrosis. The simultaneous occurrence of livedo reticularis usually indicates the involvement of medium-sized arteries as well. Most cases with a clearly identified precipitant resolve over a period of 1–4 weeks, often with some residual hyperpigmentation or, in the case of ulcerated lesions, scars. A subset of patients, however, have recurrent disease that remains confined to the skin and requires prolonged therapy.

The pleiomorphic lesions of cutaneous vasculitis and the large number of mimics of vasculitis make confirmation of the diagnosis by skin biopsy essential. Biopsy of an active lesion (<48 hours old, if possible) usually demonstrates leukocytoclastic vasculitis of the postcapillary venules (Fig. 58.12). IF shows variable quantities of immunoglobulin and complement deposition, confirming the importance of ICs to the underlying disease process but not demonstrating a diagnostic pattern. The performance of IF studies, however, is an important (and often neglected) part of the workup, critical for the exclusion of HSP, urticarial vasculitis, and cryoglobulinemia. The workup for a patient with possible HSV includes a number of other laboratory studies to exclude internal organ involvement and to differentiate from other diseases (Table 58.8).

Treatment strategies for hypersensitivity vasculitis are largely empiric. The type, intensity, and duration of therapy are based on the degree of disease severity in an individual patient. For cases in which a precipitant can be identified, removal of the offending agent usually leads to resolution of hypersensitivity vasculitis within days to weeks. Mild cases may be treated simply with leg elevation and the administration of nonsteroidal anti-inflammatory drugs (and/or H_1 antihistamines). Colchicine,

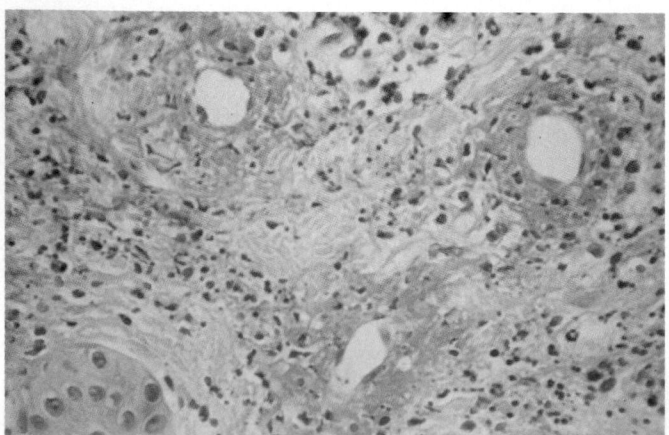

Fig. 58.12 Histopathology of hypersensitivity vasculitis. Necrotizing vasculitis of a small cutaneous vessel, with fibrinoid necrosis.

Table 58.8 Workup for patient with possible cutaneous vasculitis

Skin biopsy with immunofluorescence
Complete blood count
Serum creatinine
Liver transaminases
Serum and urine electrolytes
Urinalysis with microscopy
Chest radiograph
Antinuclear antibody assay
Serum complement levels
Anti-neutrophil cytoplasmic antibodies
Cryoglobulins
Hepatitis C antibody
Erythrocyte sedimentation rate

hydroxychloroquine, or dapsone may be tried for persistent disease that does not lead to cutaneous gangrene. For refractory or more severe disease, immunosuppressive agents may be indicated, generally beginning with glucocorticoids. Failure of the patient to tolerate a steroid taper over some weeks or the requirement for excessive glucocorticoids dictates the use of an additional immunosuppressive agent. Azathioprine is commonly used for this purpose.

■ HENOCH–SCHÖNLEIN PURPURA ■

HSP is a distinct form of small-vessel vasculitis characterized by nonthrombocytopenic purpura, arthritis, abdominal pain, and renal disease.[56, 57] The histopathologic findings are those of a leukocytoclastic vasculitis with IgA deposition. HSP can develop at any age, but occurs most frequently in children. Indeed, HSP is the most common form of vasculitis in children. The mean age of children with HSP is 5.9 years, and 93% of affected children are less than 9 years old. The disease often remits spontaneously but sometimes causes life-threatening or chronic complications, most notably gastrointestinal hemorrhage (especially in children) and nephritis (especially in adults). Although the cause is unknown, an infectious trigger is suggested by the fact that two-thirds of patients experience an acute, virus-like, upper respiratory illness an average of 10 days before the onset of HSP, and by the seasonal variation of the disease (cases are more likely in the fall and winter months). The central role of IgA in the pathogenesis of HSP is emphasized by the demonstration that most patients have increased serum IgA levels, IgA-containing circulating ICs, and IgA deposition in inflamed blood vessels.

Table 58.9 Clinical features in 100 children with Henoch–Schönlein purpura

Feature	Percentage
Purpura	100
Arthritis	82
Abdominal pain	63
Gastrointestinal bleeding	33
• Occult bleeding	23
• Gross bleeding	10
Nephritis	
• Hematuria	40
• Gross hematuria	7
• Proteinuria	25
• Nephrotic syndrome	3
Miscellaneous	
• Orchitis	5 (9% of boys)
• Duodenal obstructions	1
Recurrence of symptoms	33

(From Saulsbury F. Henoch–Schönlein purpura in children. Medicine 1999; 78: 395.)

Typically, patients present with acute onset of fever, palpable purpura on the lower extremities and buttocks, abdominal pain, arthritis, and hematuria (Table 58.9). The purpura tends to be extensive, producing lesions too numerous to count. Although the purpura is most extensive on the legs and buttocks, it can involve the arms and, infrequently, the trunk. In some patients, the cutaneous involvement takes the form of maculopapular lesions, blisters, and ulcers. The abdominal pain is often colicky and may worsen after eating (i.e., intestinal angina). Some patients experience nausea, vomiting, and upper or lower gastrointestinal bleeding. Joint disease manifests as arthralgias or arthritis in large joints, especially the knees and ankles, and to a lesser degree, the wrists and elbows. Migratory patterns can be seen.

The clinical hallmark of nephritis in HSP is hematuria, which is usually microscopic. Proteinuria almost never occurs in the absence of hematuria. Unlike gastrointestinal disease and arthritis, which occasionally precede the onset of purpura, nephritis almost always follows the appearance of skin disease. Other organs are rarely involved, but pulmonary involvement can be manifested by hemoptysis, and central nervous system involvement can result in subarachnoid or intracerebral bleeding. With the exception of renal disease, HSP is self-limited, lasting an average of 4 weeks (range, 3 days–2 years).

The manifestations of HSP vary with age. Among children with HSP, infants have milder disease. Children under the age of 2 are less likely than older children to develop nephritis or abdominal complications. As a group, children differ from adults with HSP in having more frequent gastrointestinal symptoms and less frequent renal disease. Gastrointestinal involvement in children can cause intussusception, which rarely occurs in adults. Renal disease, which affects 50–85% of adult HSP patients, is also more likely to lead to renal insufficiency compared to children.

Routine blood tests show few abnormalities other than a mild leukocytosis. The ESR is elevated in only about a third of patients. Urinalysis reveals hematuria, proteinuria, and red cell casts, but the serum creatinine is usually normal. Approximately 60% of patients have an elevated serum IgA. Although there are two subclasses of IgA, HSP is associated with increases only in IgA_1.[57] Serum complement levels are usually normal.

Leukocytoclastic vasculitis is the dominant finding in most affected organs, including the skin and gut. Deposition of IgA can be demonstrated in most lesional skin biopsies. Renal lesions range from minimal-change disease to focal or diffuse proliferative glomerulonephritis with crescents. IF studies characteristically demonstrate IgA deposition in the mesangium.

Classification criteria for HSP have been established by the ACR to help differentiate this disease from other vasculitides.[58] The differential diagnosis of HSP includes other disorders that cause leukocytoclastic vasculitis. Cryoglobulinemia shares the predilection of HSP for producing purpura, hematuria, and abdominal pain. Cryoglobulinemia is more likely than HSP to recur chronically. Tests for cryoglobulin and HCV help to distinguish the two conditions, and the finding of IgA deposition within lesional biopsies strongly favors HSP. Hypersensitivity vasculitis, unlike HSP, should not be associated with hematuria or gastrointestinal complaints. Unlike AAV, which can also produce purpura, hematuria, and arthritis, HSP seldom affects the lungs. Patients with AAV also differ from those with HSP in that the ANCA associated with those diseases are typically IgG and the glomerulonephritis is pauci-immune, not associated with substantial IgA deposition. Infrequently, bacterial endocarditis and other infections can produce purpura and hematuria that resemble HSP. The purpuric lesions associated with thrombocytopenia are usually extremely fine, very small (albeit diffuse), and not palpable.

Treatment of HSP has not been studied extensively. Most patients, especially children, have a self-limited disease course. Nonsteroidal anti-inflammatory drugs may alleviate arthralgias but can aggravate gastro-intestinal symptoms and should be avoided in any patient with renal disease. Although glucocorticoids have not been evaluated rigorously in HSP, they appear to ameliorate joint and gastrointestinal symptoms. Glucocorticoids do not appear to improve the rash, however, and their effectiveness in renal disease is controversial.[57] Uncontrolled trials suggest that high-dose methylprednisolone followed by oral prednisone or high-dose prednisone combined with azathioprine or cyclophosphamide may help patients with severe nephritis (i.e., nephrotic syndrome and > 50% crescents). Chronic renal failure is rare except in adults with more than 50% crescents on renal biopsy.

■ BEHÇET'S DISEASE ■

The triad of recurrent mouth ulcers, genital ulcers, and eye inflammation was first recognized as a distinct syndrome in 1937 by the Turkish dermatologist, Dr Hulusi Behçet.[59] In addition to these manifestations, Behçet's disease can affect nonmucosal surfaces of skin, the central nervous system, the gastrointestinal tract, and other organs. Most of the tissue damage in Behçet's disease results from vasculitis. Although Behçet's disease most commonly affects small and medium arteries, it can involve larger arteries and has a proclivity – in contrast to PAN, for example – to involve veins as well as arteries. The cause is unknown. Most patients are in their 20s or 30s at disease onset. Behçet's disease is rare in North America, where it affects only 1 out of 500 000 people, but is 100 times more common along the ancient Silk Route, which includes Greece, Turkey, Saudi Arabia, Iran, Korea, China, and Japan. Genetic factors also affect susceptibility to the disease, especially in Asia, where up to 80% of patients have the human leukocyte antigen (HLA)-B51 allele.

The diagnosis of Behçet's disease rests upon a set of established criteria (Table 58.10). No single clinical or laboratory feature is pathognomonic, but the diagnosis is untenable in the absence of recurrent aphthous ulcers of the mouth (Fig. 58.13). The mouth ulcers usually number 2–10 and can affect the tongue, buccal mucosa, gums, and pharynx. The oral ulcers can cause such severe odynophagia that some patients lose weight and become dehydrated. Most patients also experience intermittent painful genital ulcers. Ocular disease, which most commonly presents as anterior or posterior uveitis, can cause substantial disability in Behçet's disease. The anterior uveitis, typically associated with a red, photophobic eye, may be so intense that pus in the anterior chamber produces a white meniscus, called a hypopyon, evident on examination. Scar tissue or synechiae formation between the iris and the lens can lead to distortion of the pupil. With posterior uveitis, essentially a retinal vasculitis, lesions may be

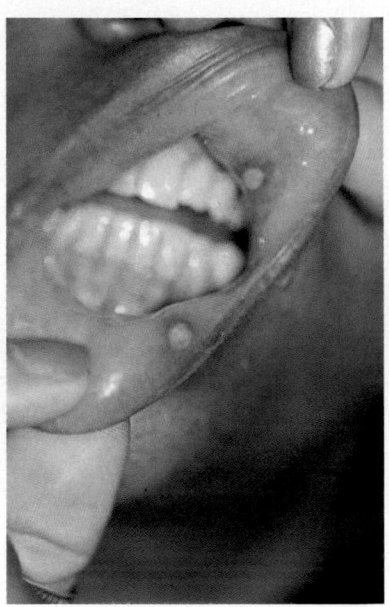

Fig. 58.13 Aphthous oral ulcers in a patient with Behçet's disease.

Table 58.10 Criteria for the diagnosis of Behçet's disease

Finding	Definition
Recurrent oral ulceration	Minor aphthous, major aphthous, or herpetiform ulcers observed by the physician or patient, which have recurred at least three times over a 12-month period
Recurrent genital ulceration	Aphthous ulceration or scarring observed by the physician or patient
Eye lesions	Anterior uveitis, posterior uveitis, or cells in the vitreous on slit-lamp examination; or retinal vasculitis detected by an ophthalmologist
Skin lesions	Erythema nodosum observed by the physician or patient, pseudofolliculitis, or papulopustular lesions, or acneiform nodules observed by the physician in a postadolescent patient who is not receiving corticosteroids
Positive pathergy test	Test interpreted as positive by the physician at 24–48 hours

The criteria were drawn up by the International Study Group for Behçet's disease.[86] For the diagnosis to be made, a patient must have recurrent oral ulceration plus at least two of the other findings in the absence of other clinical explanations.

subclinical until significant portions of the retina have been damaged. Skin lesions (Table 58.10) may include folliculitis and erythema nodosum, which (in contrast to the erythema nodosum of sarcoidosis and inflammatory bowel disease) has a tendency to ulcerate. In most cases, the "erythema nodosum" of Behçet's disease is actually a medium-vessel vasculitis, rather than a septal panniculitis. Finally, the phenomenon of pathergy – the development of pustules at the sites of sterile needle pricks – occurs rarely except in Turks.[60]

Manifestations of Behçet's disease are not limited to those encompassed by the diagnostic criteria. For example, meningoencephalitis, which produces recurrent "sterile meningitis" with fever and encephalopathy, rivals uveitis as the most common cause of permanent disability. Strokes may also complicate Behçet's disease. Additional features seen in some patients include peripheral arthritis (usually nondeforming, oligoarticular, involving large joints in an asymmetrical pattern), sacroiliitis, thrombophlebitis (often migratory), gastrointestinal disease (mimicking Crohn's disease), epididymitis, coronary angiitis, and large-artery vasculitis.

Laboratory tests during active disease usually show mild leukocytosis, thrombocytosis, and an elevated ESR. The cerebrospinal fluid of patients with meningoencephalitis shows a lymphocytosis and elevated protein. Biopsies of the ulcers in the mouth, genital area, or colon show ulcerations and infiltration with mononuclear cells. Granulomas are not seen, a feature that helps to distinguish Behçet's disease of the bowel from Crohn's disease. Biopsies in other affected organs usually reveal vasculitis.

Treatment depends on the type and severity of the disease. Colchicine is sometimes effective for mild oral and genital ulcers. Severe disease in any organ system almost always requires high doses of prednisone (e.g., 1 mg/kg per day). Chlorambucil or cyclophosphamide is useful for the most severe forms of uveitis or meningoencephalitis. Azathioprine, Cyclosporine, methotrexate, IFN-α, and pentoxifylline have been reported to be effective in some patients. Of these latter agents, only azathioprine has been studied in large clinical trials. TNF inhibitors are reputed to be effective in at least some cases, but controlled trials of this approach are lacking. Because disease activity in Behçet's disease tends to remit and relapse, drug therapy is slowly tapered once the patient improves.

■ BUERGER'S DISEASE ■

In 1908, Dr Leo Buerger reported pathological studies on the blood vessels obtained from 11 amputated lower extremities of patients with a disorder he termed 'thrombo-angiitis obliterans.' [61] Buerger wrote that the disorder usually occurred in young adults between the ages of 25 and 40, and was characterized by a thrombotic process in the arteries and veins, followed by organization and recanalization. Portions above and below the diseased segment appear normal.

Buerger proceeded to describe the typical presentation and evolution of this disorder, from the onset of 'indefinite pains in the foot, in the calf of the leg, or in the toes, and particularly of a sense of numbness or coldness whenever the weather is unfavorable.' The initially nonspecific symptoms of Buerger's disease sometimes suggest a primary neuropathic process. Buerger observed that 'Some of these cases give the typical symptoms of intermittent claudication.' Upon the development of critical limb ischemia by the patient, Buerger described the development of a 'blister, hemorrhagic bleb, or ulcer ... near the tip of one of the toes ... and when this condition ensues the local pain becomes intense.' Finally, Buerger reported, the condition resulted in dry gangrene and often in amputation because of unbearable pain.

Except for the remarkably strong association of Buerger's disease with the use of tobacco (see below), relatively little has been learned of this peculiar condition since the time of Buerger's original description. The classic patient with Buerger's disease is a young male who smokes cigarettes heavily. However, in populations where smoking is highly prevalent among females, Buerger's disease may afflict women as well. Although Buerger's disease has a predilection for the distal lower extremities, the distal upper extremities may also be severely involved.

Angiography of the extremities may suggest the diagnosis, but the findings are not pathognomonic (Fig. 58.14). The vessels most commonly involved are the digital arteries of the fingers and toes, as well as the palmar, plantar, tibial peroneal, radial, and ulnar arteries. Obliteration of these vessels leads to the development of collaterals that frequently have a 'corkscrew' appearance. Examination of the proximal vasculature by aortography is essential to exclude embolic sources and to demonstrate normality of the proximal vessels, which is characteristic of Buerger's disease.

Buerger's disease is unusual among the vasculitides in several respects: (1) the disease involves veins as well as arteries (even though the most striking symptoms are secondary to arterial involvement); (2) despite the intense involvement of medium-sized arteries, there is virtually no involvement of internal organs or any tissues besides the extremities; (3) although associated with the formation of a highly inflammatory thrombus, compared to other vasculitides there are fewer inflammatory changes within blood vessel walls, and fibrinoid necrosis is absent; and finally (4) Buerger's disease is not responsive to immunosuppression.

Buerger's disease does not occur in the absence of exposure to tobacco, usually large accounts of cigarette smoking. Once established, the disease may be maintained by even small exposures to tobacco (even smokeless tobacco or second-hand smoke), so cessation of smoking is essential in the treatment of this disease. Failure to stop smoking is associated with a dramatic increase in the risk of limb loss by amputation.[62] Although smoking is necessary, it is clearly not sufficient on its own to cause Buerger's disease. Other factors, including genetic factors and abnormalities of cellular and humoral immunity, are currently under investigation.

In addition to encouraging cessation of smoking in the strongest possible terms, the therapy of Buerger's disease requires meticulous local wound care, avoidance of trauma to the involved areas, and ample use of narcotic analgesia. A variety of empiric therapies may be employed, including calcium channel blockers, pentoxifylline, iloprost, and sympathectomy, but there is currently little evidence to support their efficacy. The impact of anti-coagulation appears to be minimal. Thrombolytic therapies have not been studied in detail.

■ COGAN SYNDROME ■

In 1945, Cogan reported 4 young patients (aged 20–35) who presented with either nonsyphilitic interstitial keratitis (bilateral eye pain, erythema, and photophobia) or symptoms of severe inner-ear dysfunction (disabling vertigo, tinnitus, and progressive bilateral deafness). Regardless of which organ (eye or ear) became involved first, the onset of symptoms in one was followed within days to weeks by the development of symptoms in the other. Interstitial keratitis in the patients reported by Cogan waxed and waned, with only mild long-term ocular morbidity. In contrast, 3 of the 4 patients reported by Cogan suffered inexorable declines in auditory function, leading to deafness.

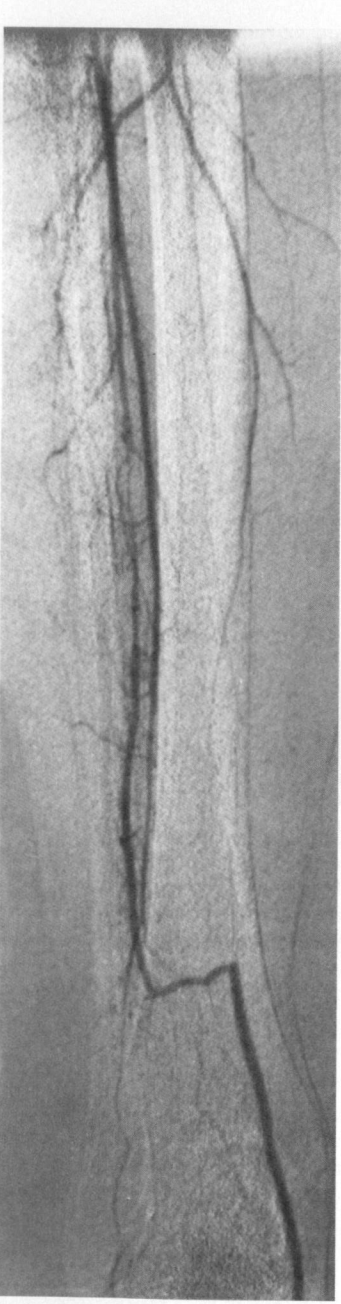

Fig. 58.14 Angiogram in Buerger's disease. Lower-extremity arteriogram in a 20-year-old woman with Buerger's disease. The anterior tibial artery attenuates in the mid-calf. The posterior tibial artery is occluded proximally, but is reconstituted above the ankle by collateral circulation from the peroneal artery. Distal to its reconstitution, the posterior tibial artery appears normal, consistent with the segmental nature of Buerger's disease.

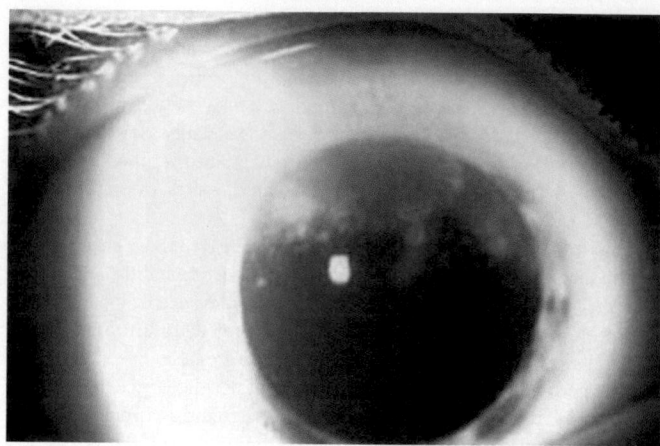

Fig. 58.15 Interstitial keratitis in Cogan syndrome. Nonsyphilitic interstitial keratitis, demonstrated by slit-lamp examination in a patient with Cogan syndrome.

The combination of inflammatory eye disease and vestibulo/auditory dysfunction is the *sine qua non* of Cogan syndrome. The classic presentation is that of interstitial keratitis and sensorineural hearing loss. This disorder afflicts young adults, with no gender predominance. In approximately 10% of cases, eye and ear inflammation is associated with arthritis of medium- and large-sized vessels (including aortitis).[63, 64] The ocular manifestations (and presumably the inner-ear disease) of Cogan syndrome are also vasculitic in nature.

Interstitial keratitis leads to the sensation of ocular irritation, excessive lacrimation, and photophobia, and is accompanied by moderate reductions (generally reversible) in visual acuity. The eye findings may be evanescent, and often require repeated examination for detection. Examination of the cornea by slit lamp (Fig. 58.15) reveals stromal clouding in the anterior and middle cornea. Pathologically, the cornea shows lymphocyte and plasma cell infiltration into the deep layers of the cornea, with varying degrees of neovascularization. Although nonsyphilitic interstitial keratitis is the ophthalmological hallmark of Cogan syndrome, virtually any type of inflammatory eye disease may occur in this disease, including conjunctivitis, uveitis, episcleritis, scleritis, exophthalmos, papilledema, retinal vasculitis, and inflammation of the optic papilla that suggests optic neuritis.

The greater cause of long-term morbidity in Cogan syndrome is the ear manifestations. Failure to recognize the nature of the problem promptly and institute appropriate therapy leads to more than half of the patients with Cogan syndrome suffering some degree of irreversible hearing loss. A substantial percentage become profoundly deaf in at least one, if not both, ears, and become candidates for cochlear implantation. Audiologic testing reveals sensorineural hearing loss. The vestibular manifestations may also be severe, and usually present with the abrupt onset of vertigo, ataxia, tinnitus, and nausea and vomiting. The severity of these symptoms is often sufficiently great to confine patients to bed. Vestibular dysfunction may lead to the disabling visual complaint of oscillopsia, in which patients perceive objects to jiggle back and forth.

Access to tissue at any stage of ear involvement in Cogan syndrome is rare. Consequently, knowledge of the pathology of this disorder stems mostly from temporal bone specimens from patients with long-standing, intensively treated disease. These findings include endolymphatic hydrops, acute labyrinthitis resulting in atrophy of the hair cells and their supporting structures, focal or diffuse proliferation of fibrous tissue and bone (neo-osteogenesis), and neuronal degeneration. Once again, definitive evidence of vasculitis in these tissues is absent.

Medium- and large-vessel arteritis may lead to a host of complications in patients with Cogan syndrome, including aortitis, aortic regurgitation, coronary artery inflammation, mesenteric vasculitis, and limb claudication. The large-vessel disease of Cogan's syndrome must be distinguished from that of Takayasu's arteritis (Chapter 59).

Interstitial keratitis generally responds well to topical steroid therapy, which must often be administered chronically. In contrast, sensorineural hearing loss must be treated early and aggressively, with high doses of systemic glucocorticoids. Failure to institute such therapy within the first 2 weeks of symptoms frequently results in irreversible hearing loss. Most patients who will respond generally do so within 2 weeks. Cytotoxic agents such as cyclophosphamide may also be considered for either the eye or ear manifestations if sufficiently severe. Because of the recurrent nature of Cogan syndrome in many cases, the cumulative morbidity from treatment may be substantial. Once the disease is controlled, a moderate remission maintenance regimen should be considered, particularly in patients who have experienced disease flares before.

■ PRIMARY ANGIITIS OF THE CENTRAL NERVOUS SYSTEM ■

Primary angiitis of the central nervous system (PACNS), a rare disease of unknown etiology, is characterized by small- and medium-sized vessel vasculitis limited to the brain or spinal cord.[65] Some authors prefer the term 'isolated angiitis of the central nervous system.'[66] The once commonly used label 'granulomatous angiitis' has dropped out of favor because not all patients with vasculitis limited to the central nervous system demonstrate granulomatous inflammation, and other forms of vasculitis, including systemic diseases such as sarcoidosis and WG, can cause granulomatous vasculitis in the brain. Vasculitis limited to the central nervous system is the most difficult form of vasculitis to diagnose accurately. The protean manifestations of the disease, the unreliability of noninvasive diagnostic tests, and the difficulty of obtaining adequate brain biopsies all contribute to the diagnostic conundrum of PACNS.

Classically, patients with PACNS manifest the triad of headache, encephalopathy, and multifocal strokes. However, only a minority of patients present with all three features, and many develop a wide range of other neurological manifestations. Most patients present in the fourth or fifth decade of life, but may range in age from 3 to 74. The disease affects women and men equally often. The disease can begin suddenly or develop slowly. The first symptom is usually headache, often severe and sometimes associated with nausea and vomiting. Almost all patients eventually develop encephalopathy with lethargy, confusion, and memory loss. Some develop multifocal strokes, seizures, evidence of increased intracranial pressure, or myelopathy. Constitutional symptoms, a hallmark of most forms of vasculitis, are notably absent in patients with PACNS.

In keeping with the isolated nature of the inflammation of PACNS, routine laboratory tests are usually normal. The majority of patients do not have anemia or an elevated ESR. The lumbar puncture yields abnormal cerebrospinal fluid in approximately 80% of cases: the most common abnormalities are a modest cerebrospinal fluid monocytosis and an increased cerebrospinal fluid protein. Oligoclonal bands and elevated

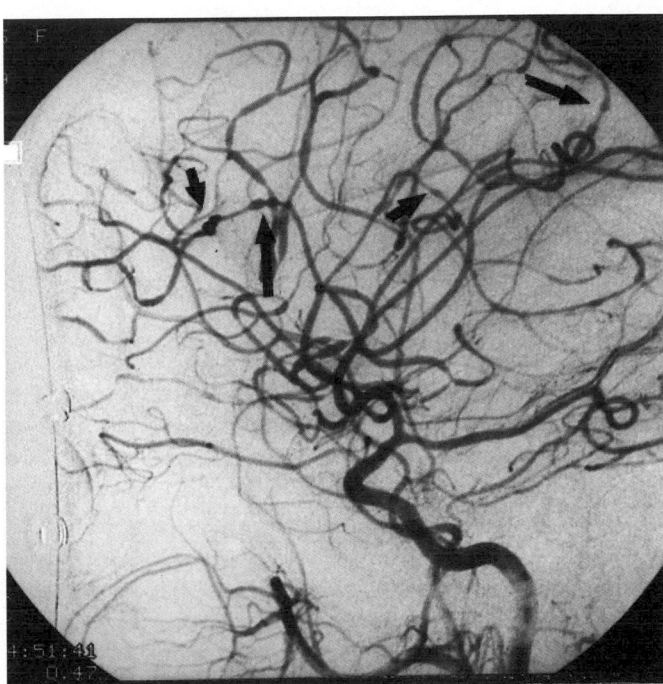

Fig. 58.16 Cerebral angiogram in primary angiitis of the central nervous system. The angiogram illustrates the typical dilatations and narrowing of arteries.

IgG indices in the cerebrospinal fluid do not appear to be either sensitive or specific for PACNS.

The clinical and laboratory features described above apply to patients who are diagnosed by brain biopsy. Over the last 30 years, an increasing number of cases have been reported in which the diagnosis is based on central nervous system angiography alone, without the performance of a brain biopsy.[67] These patients differ from those with biopsy-confirmed cases in that the majority are women, the onset tends to be more abrupt, the neurological signs less severe, and the lumbar puncture normal.

Of the noninvasive imaging tests, magnetic resonance imaging (MRI) is more sensitive than computed tomography (CT).[68, 69] The false-negative rate of MRI appears to be less than 10% in most series. Most commonly the MRI shows multiple, bilateral, bland infarctions, distributed in the subcortical white matter, cortical gray matter, deep gray matter, deep white matter, or cerebellum. Hemorrhagic lesions and mass lesions also occur. No MRI pattern is specific for PACNS. The classic abnormality on angiography is the "string of beads" pattern produced by segmented arterial narrowing alternating with dilatations (Fig. 58.16). Vascular occlusions, collateral formation, and prolonged circulation time may also be seen. Microaneurysms, so frequently seen on visceral angiograms in patients with PAN, rarely occur in PACNS. Unfortunately, no angiographic pattern is pathognomonic, and other disorders, including intravascular lymphoma, systemic infections, and vasospasm can produce similar angiographic abnormalities (see below). Indeed, in one study of 35 patients who had undergone angiography and brain biopsy because of suspected PACNS, no patient with a "classic" angiogram had a positive biopsy. Conversely, none who had a positive brain biopsy for vasculitis had a classic angiogram.[70] Angiograms are falsely negative in about 35% of patients with PACNS.[65]

The diagnosis of PACNS is definite if the patient: (1) presents with multifocal strokes or encephalopathy accompanied by headache; (2) has a cerebral angiogram showing changes consistent with vasculitis; (3) has no evidence of systemic infection, neoplasm, or toxic exposure; and (4) has a biopsy of the leptomeninges or brain cortex demonstrating vasculitis in the absence of other causes. The diagnosis of PACNS should be considered possible when the patient meets all criteria except that of a positive brain biopsy. In patients not having a positive biopsy, systemic vasculitides and other diseases that can mimic vasculitis must be excluded.

Histological specimens in PACNS show vasculitis of small and medium-sized leptomeningeal and cortical arteries. Veins and venules are involved less often. The inflammatory infiltrate varies, but consists predominantly of lymphocytes admixed with histiocytes. Langerhans and foreign-body giant cells occur in about half of the cases. The inflammation usually targets the intima and media and produces variable degrees of necrosis.

The rarity of PACNS has prevented prospective treatment trials. Prednisone and cyclophosphamide are recommended for patients who have severe neurological deficits and a positive brain biopsy. Prednisone alone (beginning at 1 mg/kg per day) appears to be adequate therapy for some patients, especially those who experience a sudden onset of mild to moderate abnormalities that are not progressive, have a normal cerebrospinal fluid, and whose diagnosis is supported by an angiogram in the absence of a brain biopsy. Mortality rates, once as high as 95% in untreated patients, have plummeted to less than 10% for treated patients. Most patients improve with treatment; the degree of recovery correlates inversely with the severity of deficits at diagnosis and the age of the patient.

■ URTICARIAL VASCULITIS ■

In 1973, Mayo Clinic investigators described 4 patients with recurrent attacks of urticarial lesions and combinations of synovitis, abdominal symptoms, and glomerulonephritis.[71] Although transient, urticaria in these patients generally persisted for at least 24 hours (longer than the 6–8 hours typically associated with chronic idiopathic urticaria) and sometimes left traces of hyperpigmentation, indicative of red blood cell extravasation through damaged capillaries. Low complement levels were present in all of the patients during periods of active disease, and skin biopsies demonstrated evidence of an IC-mediated disease process. Investigations excluded SLE and mixed cryoglobulinemia, leading to the report of a previously undescribed disorder now known as the hypocomplementemic urticarial vasculitis syndrome (HUVS).

HUVS is now recognized as one of a group of disorders known as urticarial vasculitis. At least three subtypes of urticarial vasculitis are known[72]: (1) a normocomplementemic form, which is generally idiopathic and benign; (2) a hypocomplementemic form, which is often associated with a systemic inflammatory disease; and (3) HUVS, a potentially severe condition usually associated with autoantibodies to the collagen-like region of C1q. Most patients with urticarial vasculitis have the hypocomplementemic subtype and demonstrate low C3, C4, and CH50. Patients with urticarial vasculitis who show evidence of complement activation are much more likely to manifest signs of a systemic disorder than those with normal complement levels. The majority of urticarial vasculitis patients (80–90%) have an underlying systemic disorder, usually SLE, Sjögren's syndrome, or cryoglobulinemia.

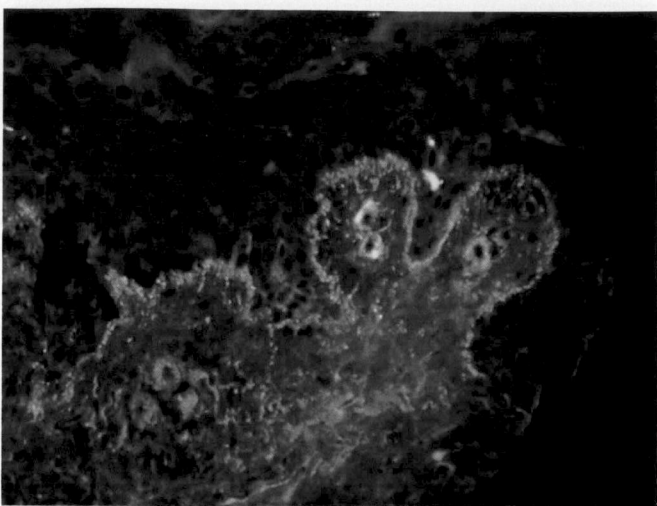

Fig. 58.17 Immunofluorescence study of a skin biopsy from a patient with hypocomplementemic urticarial vasculitis syndrome (HUVS). There is positive staining for immunoglobulin G along the basement membrane and around small arteries in the dermal papillae.

The lesions of urticarial vasculitis must be distinguished from chronic idiopathic urticaria, which is encountered far more commonly in clinical practice. Only about 10% of patients with chronic urticaria have urticarial vasculitis. In contrast to chronic idiopathic urticaria (the principal symptom of which is pruritus), urticarial lesions associated with vasculitis are often accompanied by stinging or burning. Urticarial vasculitis affects the capillaries and postcapillary venules, and the classic features of leukocytoclastic vasculitis may be evident on light microscopy. IF reveals both immunoglobulin and complement deposition in or around blood vessels of the upper dermis and/or the dermal–epidermal junction (Fig. 58.17).

HUVS frequently mimics SLE. As with SLE, HUVS has a striking female predominance, with a female-to-male ratio of 8:1. However, SLE-specific antibodies (e.g., those to dsDNA and the Sm antigen) do not occur in HUVS, and there are several distinguishing clinical features. For example, HUVS may be associated with angioedema, ocular inflammation, and chronic obstructive pulmonary disease (COPD), all of which are highly atypical of SLE. Although exacerbated by tobacco use, COPD may occur in the absence of any history of cigarette smoking, and may be severe. The few cases of lung biopsies in patients with this complication have not demonstrated vasculitis, but rather have shown panacinar emphysema. As in SLE, kidney biopsies in HUVS patients may reveal mesangial inflammation or membranoproliferative glomerulonephritis, but progression to end-stage renal disease in HUVS is unusual. Severe cardiac valve disease and Jaccoud's arthropathy have also been reported in HUVS.

Most patients with HUVS make C1q precipitins, i.e., IgG autoantibodies to the collagen-like region of C1q.[72] Whether or not anti-C1q antibodies contribute to the pathogenesis of HUVS remains unclear. Anti-C1q antibodies are also detected in up to one-third of patients with SLE, and in more than 80% of SLE patients with glomerulonephritis. Despite the prevalence of these antibodies in SLE, few patients who are seropositive for anti-C1q antibodies develop urticarial lesions. Glomeruli from patients with lupus nephritis may contain large quantities of anti-C1q antibodies.

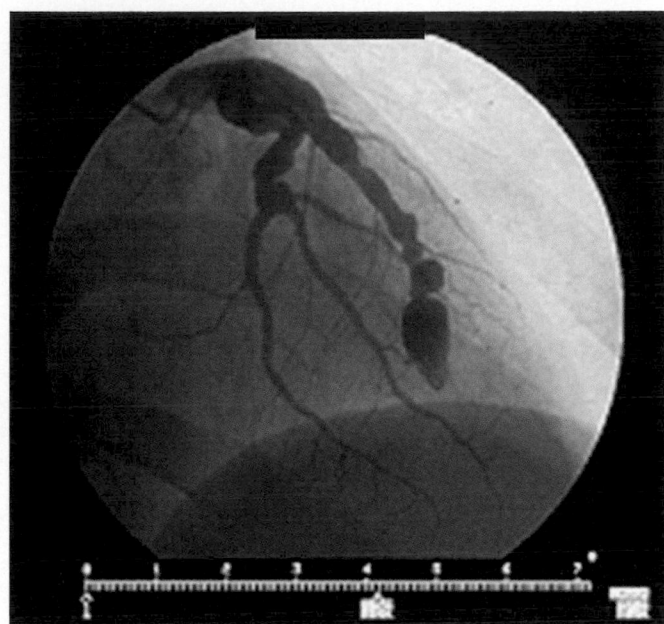

Fig. 58.18 Coronary angiogram in a 38-year-old patient with history of Kawasaki's disease as a child. Febrile illness at the age of 4 led to coronary artery aneurysms, one of which thrombosed at the age of 38, leading to a myocardial infarction.

The natural history of urticarial vasculitis is difficult to predict. Some cases, particularly those with normal complement levels during attacks, are self-limited and require little therapy. Other cases, especially HUVS, may cause life-threatening involvement of the lungs or other organs, and require periods of intensive immunosuppression. The rarity of HUVS means that there exists little consensus regarding the optimal therapeutic strategy, and treatment decisions must be individualized according to each patient's clinical status. For hypocomplementemic urticarial vasculitis limited to the skin, antimalarial agents, dapsone, and low doses of glucocorticoids may be useful.

KAWASAKI'S DISEASE

The first case of the disease now known as Kawasaki's disease was described in 1939[73, 74] and involved a 5-year-old girl who presented with high fever, sore throat, and rash and subsequently died from rupture of a coronary artery aneurysm. In 1961, Tomisaku Kawasaki evaluated a Japanese child with similar disease features, and also noted prominent cervical adenopathy. Over the next 6 years he performed a careful clinical and epidemiological study of the new disorder, and eventually reported the disease in the Japanese literature as 'mucocutaneous lymph node syndrome' in 50 patients.[74, 75] Formal diagnostic criteria for Kawasaki's disease have been developed.[76] The disease has a predilection for Asian children, but occurs in all races. Eighty percent of all cases occur in children younger than 5 years of age. The annual attack rate in Japan is approximately 80–90 cases per 100 000 children under the age of 5, compared to roughly 10 per 100 000 among Caucasian children in the USA.[77]

In all of the patients described initially by Kawasaki, the symptoms resolved without sequelae within 1 month. In subsequent years, however, mortality from cardiac complications (usually coronary artery thrombosis) was reported. Cardiac complications of Kawasaki's disease result from a severe panvasculitis, leading to narrowing of the coronary lumina by the migration of myointimal cells from the media through the fragmented internal elastic lamina. Although catastrophic heart complications occur in only a small minority of patients, evidence suggests that the preponderance of patients with Kawasaki's disease have at least some cardiac involvement. Heart lesions may include myocarditis, pericarditis, aneurysmal dilatation and thrombosis of the coronary arteries, and myocardial infarction (Fig. 58.18). The tropism of the vascular inflammation for coronary arteries and its unusual propensity to cause aneurysm formation remain unexplained. The prompt institution of high-dose intravenous immunoglobulin (IVIG) may prevent this complication (see treatment, below).

Certain clinical features of Kawasaki's disease (fever, conjunctivitis, stomatitis, erythema multiforme-like rash, and the overwhelming predominance of the disease in young children) bear strong resemblance to a number of childhood exanthems. Moreover, the disease epidemiology of Japanese outbreaks is reminiscent of the classic spread of infectious agents. However, the profound disturbances of immunoregulation in Kawasaki's disease, e.g., the unusual degree of T-cell and monocyte activation, far exceed the abnormalities accompanying most other febrile childhood illnesses. Skewing of the T-cell receptor Vβ distribution has been reported by some investigators, but not confirmed by others. The degree of immune activation in Kawasaki's disease and the acute but generally self-limited nature of the illness have implicated superantigens in the disease pathogenesis (Chapter 6). Substantial attention has focused on toxic shock syndrome toxin-1 (TSST-1), an exotoxin produced by *Staphylococcus aureus*, but the true relationship of this and other potential superantigens to the etiology of Kawasaki's disease remains unclear.

Before the availability of effective therapy, at least 20% of patients with Kawasaki's disease developed coronary aneurysms and 2% succumbed to the disease. To confirm earlier reports of efficacy of IVIG in Kawasaki's disease, seven pediatric centers in the USA enrolled 168 children with acute disease into a randomized trial. Half of the patients received IVIG 400 mg/kg per day on four consecutive days plus high-dose aspirin (100 mg/kg per day), and the other half received aspirin alone.[78] IVIG reduced the incidence of coronary aneurysms by 78% and relieved the symptoms of Kawasaki's disease with dramatic swiftness, establishing the combination of IVIG and aspirin as the standard for therapy of Kawasaki's disease. The mechanism of action of IVIG in this disorder remains unknown, but the rapidity of its benefit has implicated an anti-cytokine effect. The optimal dose of IVIG in Kawasaki's disease has not been defined: meta-analyses suggest a lower rate of coronary aneurysms in patients who receive higher IVIG doses.

REFERENCES

1. Jennette J, Falk R, Andrassy K, et al. Nomenclature of systemic vasculitides. Proposal of an international consensus conference. Arthritis Rheum 1994; 37: 187.

2. Hoffman G, Specks U. Antineutrophil cytoplasmic antibodies. Arthritis Rheum 1998; 41: 1521.

3. Xiao H, Heeringa P, Hu P, et al. Antineutrophil cytoplasmic autoantibodies specific for myeloperoxidase cause glomerulonephritis and vasculitis in mice. J Clin Invest 2002; 110: 955.

4. Huang D, Giscombe R, Zhou Y, et al. Polymorphisms in CTLA-4 but not tumor necrosis factor-alpha or interleukin 1beta genes are associated with Wegener's granulomatosis. J Rheumatol 2000; 27: 397.

5. Zhang L, Jayne DRW, Zhao MH, et al. Distribution of MHC class II alleles in primary systemic vasculitis. Kidney Int 1995; 47: 294.

6. Cotch FM, Fauci AS, Hoffman GS. HLA typing in patients with Wegener's granulomatosis. Ann Intern Med 1995; 122: 635.

7. Hogan SL, Satterly KK, Dooley MA, et al. Silica exposure in antineutrophil cytoplasmic autoantibody-associated glomerulonephritis and lupus nephritis. J Am Soc Nephrol 2001; 12: 134.

8. Audrain MA, Sesboue R, Baranger TA, et al. Analysis of anti-neutrophil cytoplasmic antibodies (ANCA): frequency and specificity in a sample of 191 homozygous (PiZZ) alpha1-antitrypsin-deficient subjects. Nephrol Dial Transplant 2001; 16: 39.

9. Elzouki AN, Segelmark M, Wieslander J, et al. Strong link between the alpha 1-antitrypsin PiZ allele and Wegener's granulomatosis. J Intern Med 1994; 236: 541.

10. Ludviksson BR, Sneller MC, Chua KS, et al. Active Wegener's granulomatosis is associated with HLA-DR+ CD4+ T cells exhibiting an unbalanced Th1-type T cell cytokine pattern: reversal with IL-10. J Immunol 1998; 160: 3602.

11. Zhou Y, Huang D, Paris PL, et al. An analysis of CTLA-4 and proinflammatory cytokine genes in Wegener's granulomatosis. Arthritis Rheum 2004; 50: 2645.

12. Tse WY, Abadeh S, Jefferis R, et al. Neutrophil FcgammaRIIIb allelic polymorphism in anti-neutrophil cytoplasmic antibody (ANCA)-positive systemic vasculitis. Clin Exp Immunol 2000; 119: 574.

13. Falk R, Terrell R, Charles L, et al. Anti-neutrophil cytoplasmic autoantibodies induce neutrophils to degranulate and produce oxygen radicals in vitro. Proc Natl Acad Sci USA 1990; 87: 4115.

14. Masutani K, Tokumoto M, Nakashima H, et al. Strong polarization toward Th1 immune response in ANCA-associated glomerulonephritis. Clin Nephrol 2003; 59: 395.

15. Tse WY, Nash GB, Hewins P, et al. ANCA-induced neutrophil F-actin polymerization: implications for microvascular inflammation. Kidney Int 2005; 67: 130.

16. Merkel PA, Lo GH, Holbrook JT, et al. Incidence of venous thrombotic events among patients with Wegener's granulomatosis. Ann Intern Med 2005; 142: 620.

17. Popa ER, Stegeman CA, Bos NA, Differential B-, et al. T-cell activation in Wegener's granulomatosis. J Allergy Clin Immunol 1999; 103: 885–894.

18. Keogh KA, Wylam ME, Stone JH, et al. Induction of remission by B lymphocyte depletion in eleven patients with refractory antineutrophil cytoplasmic antibody-associated vasculitis. Arthritis Rheum 2005; 52: 262–268.

19. Keogh KA, Ytterberg SR, Fervenza FC, et al. Rituximab for refractory Wegener's granulomatosis: report of a prospective, open-label trial. Am J Respir Crit Care Med 2006; 173: 180–187.

20. Godman G, Churg J. Wegener's granulomatosis: pathology and review of the literature. Arch Pathol Lab Med 1954; 58: 533.

21. Hagen E, Daha M, Hermans J, et al. Diagnostic value of standardized assays for anti-neutrophil cytoplasmic antibodies in idiopathic systemic vasculitis. Kidney Int 1998; 53: 743.

22. Boomsma MM, Stegeman CA, van der Leij MJ, et al. Prediction of relapses in Wegener's granulomatosis by measurement of antineutrophil cytoplasmic antibody levels: a prospective study. Arthritis Rheum 2000; 43: 2025.

23. Finkielman, Merkel PA, Schroeder D, et al. Antineutrophil cytoplasmic antibodies against proteinase 3 do not predict disease relapses in Wegener's granulomatosis. Ann Intern Med (In press, November, 2007).

24. Wegener F. Ueber generalisierte, septische Gefasserkrankungen. Verh Dtsch Ges Pathol 1936; 29: 202.

25. Wegener F. Ueber eine eigenartige rhinogene Granulomatose mit besonderer Beteiligung des Arteriensystems und der Nieren. Beitr Pathol Anat Allg Pathol 1939; 36: 36.

26. Watts R, Carruthers D, Scott D. Epidemiology of systemic vasculitis: changing incidence or definition? Semin Arthritis Rheum 1995; 25: 28.

27. Hoffman G, Kerr G, Leavitt R, et al. Wegener's granulomatosis: an analysis of 158 patients. Ann Intern Med 1992; 116: 488.

28. The WGET Research Group. Etanercept in addition to standard therapy in patients with Wegener's granulomatosis. N Engl J Med 2005; 352: 351–361.

29. Davson J, Ball J, Platt R. The kidney in periarteritis nodosa. Q J Med 1948; 17: 175.

30. Savage C, Winearls C, Evans D, et al. Microscopic polyarteritis: presentation, pathology, and prognosis. Q J Med 1985; 56: 467.

31. Guillevin L, Durand-Gasselin B, Cevallos R, et al. Microscopic polyangiitis. Arthritis Rheum 1999; 42: 421.

32. Churg J, Strauss L. Allergic granulomatosis, allergic angiitis, and periarteritis nodosa. Am J Pathol 1951; 27: 277.

33. Masi A, Hunder G, Lie J, et al. The American College of Rheumatology 1990 criteria for the classification of Churg–Strauss syndrome (allergic granulomatosis and angiitis). Arthritis Rheum 1990; 33: 1094.

34. Guillevin L, Cohen P, Gayraud M, et al. Churg–Strauss syndrome: clinical study and long-term follow-up of 96 patients. Medicine 1999; 78: 26.

35. Jayne D, Rasmussen N, Andrassy K, et al. A randomized trial of maintenance therapy for vasculitis associated with antineutrophil cytoplasmic autoantibodies. N Engl J Med 2003; 349: 36.

36. Wung PK, Stone JH. Therapeutics of Wegener's granulomatosis. Nature Clinical Rheum 2006; 2: 192.

37. Tatsis E, Schnabel M, Gross W. Interferon-alpha treatment of four patients with the Churg–Strauss syndrome. Ann Intern Med 1998; 129: 370.

38. Stone JH, Holbrook JT, Marriott MA, et al. Solid malignancies in the Wegener's Granulomatosis Etanercept trial. Arthritis Rheum 2006; 54: 1608–1618.

39. De Groot K, Rasmussen N, Bacon PA. Randomized trial of cyclophosphamide versus methotrexate for induction of remission in early systemic antineutrophil cytoplasmic antibody-associated vasculitis. Arthritis Rheum 2005; 52: 2461.

40. Goek ON, Stone JH. Randomized controlled trials in vasculitis associated with anti-neutrophil cytoplasmic antibodies. Curr Opin Rheumatol 2005; 17: 257.

41. Kussmaul A, Maier R. Ueber eine bisher nicht beschriebene eigenthumliche Arterienerkrankung (periarteritis nodosa), die mit Morbus brightii und rapid fortschreitender allgemeiner Muskellahmung einhergeht. Dtsch Arch Klin Med 1866; 1: 484.

42. Guillevin L, Mahr A, Callard P, et al. Hepatitis B virus-associated polyarteritis nodosa: clinical characteristics, outcome, and impact of treatment in 115 patients. Medicine 2005; 84: 313–322.

43. Stone JH, Nousari HC. Essential cutaneous vasculitis: What every rheumatologist should know about vasculitis of the skin. Curr Opin Rheumatol 2001; 13: 23.

44. Levine SM, Hellmann DB, Stone JH. Gastrointestinal involvement in polyarteritis nodosa (1986–2000): presentation and outcomes in 24 patients. Am J Med 2002; 112: 386.

45. Lightfoot R, Michel B, Bloch D, et al. The American College of Rheumatology 1990 criteria for the classification of polyarteritis nodosa. Arthritis Rheum 1990; 33: 1088.

46. Guillevin L, Jarrousse B, Lok C. Longterm followup after treatment of polyarteritis nodosa and Churg–Strauss angiitis with comparison of steroids, plasma exchange and cyclophosphamide to steroids and plasma exchange. A prospective randomized trial of 71 patients J Rheumatol 1991; 18: 567.

47. Guillevin L, Mahr A, Callard P, et al. Hepatitis B virus-associated polyarteritis nodosa: clinical characteristics, outcome, and impact of treatment in 115 patients. Medicine (Baltimore) 2005; 84: 313.

48. Wintrobe M, Buell M. Hyperproteinemia associated with multiple myeloma. Bull Johns Hopkins Hosp 1933; 52: 156.

49. Lamprecht P, Gause A, Gross W. Cryoglobulinemic vasculitis. Arthritis Rheum 1999; 42: 2507.

50. Meltzer M, Franklin E. Cryoglobulinemia – a study of 29 patients. I. IgG and IgM cryoglobulins and factors affecting cryoprecipitability. Am J Med 1966; 40: 828.

51. Brouet J, Clauvel J, Danon F, et al. Biologic and clinical significance of cryoglobulins. A report of 86 cases. Am J Med 1974; 57: 775.

52. Lunel F, Musset L, Cacoub P, et al. Cryoglobulinemia in chronic liver diseases: role of hepatitis C virus and liver damage. Gastroenterology 1994; 106: 1291.

53. Cacoub P, Saadoun D, Limal N, et al. PEGylated interferon alfa-2b and ribavirin treatment in patients with hepatitis C virus-related systemic vasculitis. Arthritis Rheum 2005; 52: 911.

54. Zeek P. Periarteritis nodosa: a critical review. Am J Clin Pathol 1952; 221: 777.

55. Calabrese L, Michel B, Bloch D, et al. The American College of Rheumatology 1990 criteria for the classification of hypersensitivity vasculitis. Arthritis Rheum 1990; 33: 1108.

56. Gairdner D. The Schönlein–Henoch syndrome (anaphylactoid purpura). Q J Med 1948; 17: 95.

57. Saulsbury F. Henoch–Schönlein purpura in children. Medicine 1999; 78: 395.

58. Mills J, Michel B, Bloch D, et al. The American College of Rheumatology 1990 criteria for classification of Henoch–Schönlein purpura. Arthritis Rheum 1990; 33: 1114.

59. Behçet H. Ueber rezidivierende Aphthose, durch ein Virus verursachte Gerschwure am Mund, am Auge und der Genitalie. Dermatol Wochenschr 1937; 105: 1552.

60. Sakane T, Tekeno M, Suzuki N, et al. Behçet's disease. N Engl J Med 1999; 341: 1284.

61. Buerger L. Thromboangiitis obliterans: a study of the vascular lesions leading to presenile spontaneous gangrene. Am J Med Sci 1908; 136: 567.

62. Olin J, Young J, Graor R, et al. The changing clinical spectrum of thromboangiitis obliterans (Buerger's disease). Circulation 1990; 82(5 Suppl): IV3–8.

63. Haynes B, Kaiser-Kupfer M, Mason P, et al. Cogan syndrome: studies in 13 patients, long-term follow-up, and a review of the literature. Medicine 1980; 59: 426.

64. Vollertsen R, McDonald T, Younge B, et al. Cogan's syndrome: 18 cases and a review of the literature. Mayo Clin Proc 1986; 61: 344.

65. Calabrese L, Duna G, Lie J. Vasculitis in the central nervous system. Arthritis Rheum 1997; 7: 1189.

66. Moore P. Vasculitis of the central nervous system. Semin Neurol 1994; 14: 307.

67. Calabrese L, Gragg L, Furlan A. Benign angiopathy: a distinct subset of angiographically defined primary angiitis of the central nervous system. J Rheumatol 1993; 20: 2046.

68. Stone J, Pomper M, Roubenoff R, et al. Sensitivities of non-invasive tests for CNS vasculitis: a comparison of LP, CT, and MRI. J Rheumatol 1994; 21: 1277.

69. Pomper M, Miller T, Stone J, et al. Central nervous system vasculitis: MR imaging and correlation with angiography. Am J Neuroradiol 1999; 20: 75.

70. Kadkhodayan Y, Abdulrahman A, Moran CJ, et al. Primary angiitis of the central nervous system at conventional angiography. Radiology 2004; 233: 878.

71. McDuffie F, Sams W Jr, Maldonado J, et al. Hypocomplementemia with cutaneous vasculitis and arthritis. Mayo Clin Proc 1973; 48: 430.

72. Wisnieski J, Baer A, Christensen J, et al. Hypocomplementemic urticarial vasculitis syndrome: clinical and serological findings in 18 patients. Medicine 1995; 74: 24.

73. Spector S. Scarlet fever, periarteritis nodosa, aneurysm of the coronary artery with spontaneous rupture, hemopericardium. Arch Pediatr 1939; 25: 319.

74. Kawasaki T. Acute febrile mucocutaneous syndrome with lymphoid involvement with specific desquamation of the fingers and toes in children [in Japanese]. Jpn J Allerg 1967; 3: 178.

75. Kawasaki T, Kosaki F, Okawa S, et al. A new infantile acute febrile mucocutaneous lymph node syndrome (MLNS) prevailing in Japan. Pediatrics 1974; 54: 271.

76. Centers for Disease Control. Kawasaki disease. MMWR 1980; 29: 61.

77. Yanagawa H, Yashiro M, Nakamura Y, et al. Epidemiologic pictures of Kawasaki disease in Japan: from the nationwide incidence survey in 1991 and 1992. Pediatrics 1995; 95: 475.

78. Newburger J, Takahashi M, Burns J, et al. The treatment of Kawasaki syndrome with intravenous gamma globulin. N Engl J Med 1986; 315: 341.

Large-vessel vasculitides

Cornelia M. Weyand, Jörg J. Goronzy

59

Whereas most tissues have compensatory mechanisms that allow them to sustain the damaging effects of acute and chronic inflammation, this is not the case for the body's main blood vessels. Medium and large arteries are organs without redundancy and regenerative capacity; their uncompromised function is required to sustain life. Accordingly, inflammatory damage to such arterial vessels leads to severe clinical consequences, immediately posing a threat for the loss of vital functions. When affected by inflammation, the aorta and its branches have two possible response patterns: inflammatory destruction of the vessel wall leads to dilatation, aneurysm formation, and, infrequently, dissection and hemorrhage; or the inflammation initiates an injury response that results in luminal occlusion, disruption of blood supply, and ischemic damage of dependent organ structures.

In contrast to other vasculopathies, especially those related to atherosclerosis, vasculitides of the larger blood vessels are almost always associated with a syndrome of intense systemic inflammation.[1] Recent evidence has challenged the traditional view that systemic inflammation represents a spill-over of inflammatory mediators from the vasculitic lesions. Instead, systemic activation of the innate immune system may be an early event and initiate the processes leading to vessel wall inflammation. The coincidence of malaise, fever, wasting, and myalgias with signs of ischemia due to vascular failure remains a critical clue for the physician when diagnosing and treating large-vessel vasculitis.

The two major forms of large-vessel vasculitis are giant-cell arteritis (GCA) and Takayasu arteritis (TA). In addition, aortitis can infrequently be seen in other diseases, such as infections, connective tissue diseases, sarcoidosis, and inflammatory bowel disease; and, occasionally, also as an idiopathic syndrome. Polymyalgia rheumatica (PMR) is a condition closely related to GCA, occurs in the same patient population, and often precedes or follows the clinical diagnosis of GCA.[2] Patients with PMR do not have typical vascular lesions, but have a systemic inflammatory syndrome indistinguishable from GCA. About 10% of PMR patients will eventually progress to full-blown vasculitis. Similarities in the vascular lesions of GCA and TA have supported the concept that the immunopathogenesis of these vasculitides is analogous. Whether the systemic inflammatory reactions accompanying GCA, TA, and PMR have disease-specific elements remains unknown. Excellent progress has been made in unraveling the pathogenesis of GCA over the last decade, and this will inevitably lead to improvements in diagnosis, long-term management, and broadening of the therapeutic armamentarium.

■ EPIDEMIOLOGY ■

GCA may be a very old disease, as suggested by historic evidence that more than 1000 years ago removal of the temporal artery was recommended by a physician in Baghdad. In 1932, Horton and colleagues at the Mayo Clinic in Minnesota recognized that GCA was an inflammatory vasculopathy when they found dense inflammation in the temporal arteries of two systemically ill patients with severe headaches. The first reports of TA, or 'pulseles disease,' in young women surfaced in Japan in the 19th century. The syndrome was named after Dr. Takayasu, an ophthalmologist who in 1905 described peculiar optic fundus abnormalities.

The strongest risk factor for GCA, TA, and PMR is age.[3,4] GCA and PMR are essentially absent in individuals younger than 50 years of age, and their incidence climbs continuously during the 7th and 8th decades of life. TA is exclusively diagnosed in individuals younger than 40 years of age, with peak incidence during the 2nd and 3rd decades of life. All three syndromes affect women much more often than men, with a 2:1 ratio in PMR and GCA and a 9:1 ratio in TA.[3,4]

Marked geographic variations in the incidence and prevalence of GCA, TA, and PMR have given rise to speculations about environmental exposures as key factors in disease pathogenesis. GCA is the most frequent vasculitis in the western world, with yearly incidence rates reaching 10–20 cases per 100 000 persons over 50 years of age.[3] In general, PMR is diagnosed three- to fourfold more frequently, with a prevalence of up to 1 case per 133 individuals older than 50.[2] Iceland, Norway, Sweden, and Denmark are high-risk areas; also, higher incidence rates are maintained in Scandinavian immigrant populations in the USA. The risk is significantly lower in Hispanics and African-Americans. Although TA can afflict all races, a predilection exists for individuals of Asian, and Central and South American origins. Japan, Thailand, India, Turkey, and nations in Central and South America are considered high-incidence

CLINICAL PEARLS

CLINICAL AND EPIDEMIOLOGIC CLUES IN GIANT-CELL ARTERITIS

>> Patient older than 50 years of age

>> Female

>> Northern European heritage

>> Laboratory findings of a highly activated acute-phase response

>> Insidious onset of nonspecific symptoms (weight loss, night sweats, malaise, fever)

>> Ischemia of ocular structures, cranial muscles, scalp, or upper extremities

regions. TA is a rare disease with an annual incidence of 1–2 cases/million. The typical patient is a female in her 20s to 30s. In middle-aged men and women, it can be challenging to differentiate TA from rapidly progressing atherosclerotic disease, especially as both disease processes may coexist.[5]

ETIOLOGY AND PATHOGENESIS

Vasculitides affecting medium and large human arteries are caused by dysregulated immune responses.[1, 6, 7] Studies from the last decade have revealed that vasculitis involves a combination of multiple effector mechanisms used by the innate and adaptive immune systems. Inflammation is a critical host defense response protecting against infection and tissue injury, but it invariably contributes collateral damage to the very tissue site in which it intends to destroy microbes and remove the injured self. If initiated in the absence of an instigator or persistent stimulus, despite the successful removal of the inciting infection or injury, inflammation will eventually become the cause of disease as tissue damage accumulates and, in the case of vasculitis, will leave the host with malfunctional arteries.

The similarities in the tissue tropisms and the histologic lesions of GCA and TA suggest overlapping disease pathways, justifying their discussion in the context of either disease. Marked progress has been made in understanding early and late events in GCA from studies focusing on a human artery-severe combined immunodeficiency (SCID) mouse model. The etiopathogenesis of PMR is less well understood, but experimental evidence suggests that it represents a *forme fruste* of GCA in which inflammatory attack to the vessel wall remains below a threshold, and standard histology describes noninflamed arteries.

THE HUMAN ARTERY-SCID MODEL OF VASCULITIS

The unique components of GCA/TA pathogenesis are chronically persistent inflammatory infiltrates settled within the wall of arteries with three distinct layers and well-developed elastic membranes. To overcome limitations encountered in animal models of vasculitis, which cannot mimic the vessel size, vessel wall structure, or aging

component of the host, a novel experimental model for GCA was established by implanting GCA-affected or normal human arteries into immunodeficient mice. Within 1 week, the human arteries are engrafted and supplied with blood through their vasa vasorum trees.[8] Chimeras can then be treated with cell-depleting antibodies, anti-cytokine reagents, or with adoptive transfer of immuno-inflammatory cells. This model has been extremely helpful in deciphering which cells and mediators sustain vasculitis. Equally importantly, the model has allowed for vasculitis induction in normal arteries, thereby illustrating the early pathogenic steps that precede establishment of granulomatous mural lesions.[9]

EARLY STEPS IN VASCULITIS

Normal human arteries of the medium and large categories are not immunologically inert. To the contrary, they possess populations of dendritic cells (DC) distributed amongst wall-residing cells.[10] Among these vascular DCs, a population strategically positioned at the media–adventitia border has been implicated in initiating wall inflammation.[11] In contrast to other DC-containing tissues, normal human arteries do not elicit T-cell stimulation when implanted into SCID mice. This immunologic quiescence, despite being equipped with DC networks, has given rise to the hypothesis that the primary function of vascular DCs lies in maintaining a very high threshold for the induction and persistence of adaptive immune responses. A principal role for vascular DCs in functioning as tolerance inducers would fit well with the host's need to avoid inflammatory damage in such critical and nonregenerative organs as arteries.

The tolerant state of vascular DCs can, however, be broken if the artery is exposed to a microbial environment (Fig. 59.1). Human arteries detect infections through Toll-like receptors (TLR) expressed on vascular DCs.[12] TLRs are a family of pattern recognition receptors employed by nature to detect motifs shared by groups of bacterial and viral microorganisms. By sensing common microbial structures through their TLRs, DCs initiate the first line of defense against infections. Injection of lipopolysaccharide, a moiety conserved across Gram-negative bacteria, into human artery-SCID chimeras, leads to robust activation of wall-residing DCs and is sufficient to initiate adaptive immune responses (Fig. 59.2).[13] Specifically, CD4 T cells are recruited to the vessel, migrate toward the adventitia–media junction, receive activating signals, and undergo *in situ* activation. Arteries harvested from patients with PMR, despite having no sign of inflammation, have mature DCs and do not require exposure to lipopolysaccharide. Spontaneously, they recruit and activate T cells from co-implanted and human leukocyte antigen (HLA)-matched GCA arteries.[9] Thus, DC maturation is a very early step in the initiation of vasculitis, occurring long before the chronic phase of wall inflammation.

The potential of pathogen-derived molecules to start inflammatory responses in arterial tissues has rekindled old discussions on whether vasculitis is elicited by infection. In this context it is important to mention that recurring reports of finding infectious organisms in inflamed temporal arteries from GCA patients have failed to find confirmation in more comprehensive studies.[9] If the role of microbial agents is to stimulate adventitial DCs, the presence of the organism in the affected artery is obviously not necessary, but infections located elsewhere in the patient may still have a facilitating role in disease initiation.

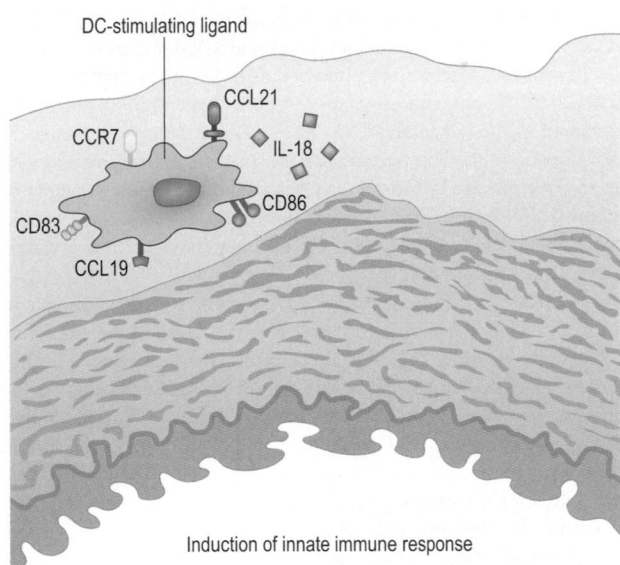

Induction of innate immune response

Fig. 59.1 Pathogenic pathways in giant-cell arteritis (GCA). Under physiologic conditions, dendritic cells (DCs) in the adventitia are immature and resting. In polymyalgia rheumatica and GCA, adventitial DCs undergo activation with the induction of co-stimulatory ligands and chemokines. Under experimental conditions, adventitial DCs can be triggered with Toll-like receptor ligands, e.g., pathogen-derived molecules.

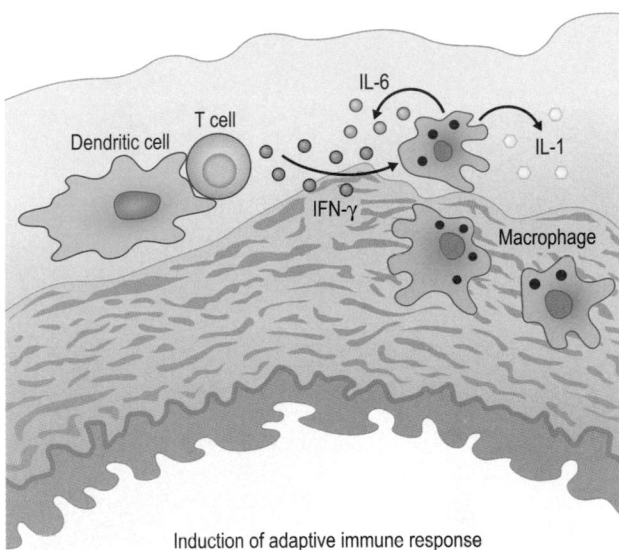

Induction of adaptive immune response

Fig. 59.2 Pathogenic pathways in giant-cell arteritis (GCA). CD4 T cells are recruited to the adventitia of blood vessels by activated dendritic cells and undergo *in situ* stimulation. Interferon-γ is a key cytokine in GCA and regulates activation of macrophages and other proinflammatory pathways.

KEY CONCEPTS

>> Medium and large human arteries have multiple wall layers and a wall structure substantial enough to be the target of transmural inflammation

>> Vasculitis causes the rapid and concentric growth of hyperplastic intima, leading to luminal occlusion and ischemia of dependent tissues. Intramural inflammation of the aorta may occasionally result in wall damage followed by aneurysm formation and rupture

>> Due to the vital function and nonregenerative nature of large human arteries, the threshold for the induction and persistence of innate and adaptive immune responses in the wall structures of such arteries must be explicitly high

>> Inflammatory infiltrates typical for granulomatous vasculitis enter the vessel from the 'back door,' the adventitia, and not from the lumen

>> Besides their critical role in securing blood flow, medium and large blood vessels also possess immunoregulatory functions mediated by dendritic cells indigenous to the vascular wall

ADAPTIVE IMMUNE RESPONSES IN GIANT-CELL ARTERITIS

Chronic inflammatory infiltrates occupying all layers of the affected artery are comprised of CD4 T cells, a few CD8 T cells, and macrophages. Typically, these cells form granulomas. Multinucleated giant cells

are found in about 50% of patients and are often localized close to the intima–media border adjacent to the lamina elastica interna. Fragmentation of that elastic membrane is a hallmark of GCA. Functionally important products of CD4 T cells include interferon-γ (Fig. 59.2), the tissue level of which correlates closely with patterns of clinical manifestations.[14] Maintenance of the complex granulomatous arrangements also requires T cells. Even the process of neoangiogenesis, which is necessary to promote the growth of the lumen occlusive neointima, is closely correlated with interferon-γ levels, thus assigning a key position to this T-cell product in multiple interrelated disease processes.[15] In TA, direct cytotoxic function of CD8 T cells, natural killer cells, and γδ T cells has been implicated in local tissue injury.[16]

CD4 T cells continue to receive instructive signals from DCs even in chronically established disease since DC depletion effectively disrupts granulomatous inflammation.[9] In mature vasculitic lesions, DCs are the sole producers of CCL19 and CCL21, chemokines implicated in T-cell recruitment. Also, they express CD86 and thus provide necessary co-stimulatory signals to maintain T-cell responses.[11] Naturally, the question of whether a unique antigen exists that drives adaptive immune responses in GCA has been raised. Studies with T-cell lines established from inflamed temporal arteries have suggested that the T-cell populations are nonrandom and clonally selected. Identical CD4 T cells dominating the inflammatory infiltrate in the right and left temporal arteries of patients with bilateral biopsies have added weight to these findings.[17] The spectrum of possible antigens includes microbes, products of injured or stressed cells, and altered self. An alternative hypothesis puts emphasis on the uniqueness of the tissue compartment and the dysfunction of T-cell homeostasis and T-cell regulation in the aged host, and considers ordinary self antigens as sufficient to drive these misplaced immune responses.[1, 12]

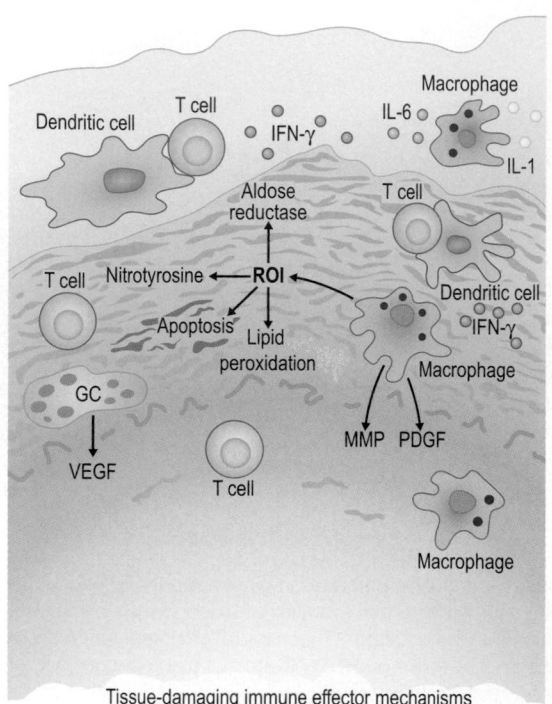

Tissue-damaging immune effector mechanisms

Fig. 59.3 Pathogenic pathways in giant-cell arteritis (GCA). Fully developed GCA is a panarteritis with transmural T-cell and macrophage infiltrates. Macrophages in different wall layers commit to distinct damage pathways involving production of proinflammatory cytokines, reactive oxygen intermediates (ROI), metalloproteinases, or growth factors. Multinucleated giant cells also provide growth and angiogenic factors that promote intimal hyperplasia and luminal occlusion.

IMMUNE-MEDIATED TISSUE INJURY AND THE ARTERY'S CONTRIBUTION TO VASCULAR FAILURE

Accumulated data support the premise that a major part of the tissue injury in the arterial wall is actually mediated by macrophages (Fig. 59.3).[1] Remarkably, wall-invading macrophages commit to selected pathways of maturation according to their placement in the wall structure.[18] Macrophages positioned in the adventitia mainly produce proinflammatory monokines, such as interleukin-6 (IL-6) and IL-1 (Fig. 59.2). Their major function may lie in supporting ongoing T-cell responses. Intimal macrophages have been described to express nitric oxide synthase, and peroxynitrite generation has been associated with endothelial dysfunction.[19] Macrophages captured in the medial smooth-muscle cell layer have a portfolio of tissue-damaging functions (Fig. 59.3).[20, 21] They release metalloproteinases, likely contributing to digestion of the elastic structures. They are potent in secreting reactive oxygen species, facilitating oxidative damage to smooth-muscle cells and endothelial cells. Most importantly, they are the source for platelet-derived growth factor and vascular endothelial growth factor.[15, 22] Through providing these growth and angiogenesis factors, macrophages support wall-resident cells in their injury response pattern. Myofibroblasts migrate towards the intima, proliferate, and produce matrix. The unfortunate consequence is

intimal hyperplasia, the essential mechanism underlying luminal stenosis and vascular failure. Notably, in both GCA and TA, destruction of the arterial wall with subsequent rupture and hemorrhage is the exception. Instead, a fast, concentric, and almost complete intimal hyperproliferation leads to obstruction of the lumen and ischemic damage of dependent organs. Not all GCA patients develop vascular stenosis. In these patients mural inflammation does not lead to intimal hyperplasia and the lumen is maintained. Patients with nonobstructive vasculitis have a distinct clinical presentation; vascular malfunction is not noticeable but they have an intense systemic inflammatory syndrome.

Failure of the inflamed arteries, presenting as lumen obstruction, would not be possible without the active contribution of the arterial wall residents. Proliferating myofibroblasts, rather than immune cells, build the scaffold of the lumen-obstructive neotissue.[22] Also, neoangiogenesis effectively supports the artery's response-to-injury reaction, supplying oxygen and nutrients to the thickening wall.[15] In essence, the immune system emerges as an instructor to a maladaptive response of the vessel itself. The critical participation of vascular components may provide an explanation for the stringent tissue tropism of large-vessel vasculitides, which selectively target certain vascular territories.

■ CLINICAL FEATURES IN GIANT-CELL ARTERITIS ■

Clinical manifestations of GCA reflect the combination of a systemic inflammatory syndrome with vascular insufficiency (Table 59.1).[2, 23] Depending on the preferred target of vascular inflammation, patients fall into the category of either cranial GCA or large-vessel GCA. In addition, there exists another subpopulation of patients in whom the clinical consequences of arterial inflammation are minimal, and they come to clinical attention with a wasting syndrome.

In cranial GCA, symptoms result from vascular stenosis of the neck and head arteries, most prominently in the branches of the external carotid artery. Arteritis of the scalp arteries leads to the typical presentations of headaches and scalp tenderness. Patients report difficulties with wearing glasses or combing their hair. The headaches are often intense and unresponsive to standard analgesics. Headaches are a nonspecific clinical symptom, yet in a patient of the appropriate age with other findings indicating an inflammatory syndrome, physicians need to complete a workup for GCA. Insufficient blood flow to the masseter muscles and the tongue causes jaw claudication, elicited by prolonged chewing and talking. Although this type of claudication is present in less than 30% of patients, it is clinically helpful as it rarely occurs outside GCA. Similarly, painful dysphagia can be a useful clinical clue.

The orbita and the optic nerve are strictly dependent on blood supply from the external carotid system, particularly the ophthalmic artery. GCA in branches of the ophthalmic artery, specifically the posterior ciliary arteries, leads to anterior ischemic optic neuropathy, presenting as sudden and painless vision loss. Typically patients lose vision in the early-morning hours or wake up blind. Involvement of one eye may be followed by visual loss in the partner eye if the disease is not diagnosed and treated promptly. Besides anterior optic neuropathy, GCA can cause a number of ischemic complications in the orbita and along the visual axis, which may present as diplopia or partial vision loss. If recognized and treated immediately, vasculitis-associated sight loss is preventable, thus making GCA an ophthalmologic emergency.

Table 59.1 Clinical features of giant-cell arteritis (GCA), polymyalgia rheumatica (PMR), and Takayasu arteritis (TA)

Organ system	Clinical features	Frequencies GCA	PMR	TA
Vascular	Headaches	***		*
	Limb claudication	*		***
	Scalp tenderness	**		
	Jaw claudication	**		
	Absent or asymmetric pulses	*		***
	Asymmetric blood pressure readings	*		***
	Bruit	*		***
	Tongue claudication	*		
	Tissue gangrene	*		
	Abdominal angina			*
	Cough (dry, nonproductive)	*		*
Constitutional	Malaise	**	**	***
	Wasting syndrome	*	**	*
	Weight loss	**	**	**
	Fever	*	*	*
Nervous system				
Central nervous system	Ocular symptoms	**		*
	Stroke/transient ischemic attack	*		*
	Ischemia of the central nervous system	*		*
Peripheral nervous system	Peripheral neuropathy	*		
Cardiac	Aortic dilatation and regurgitation	*		*
	Myocardial infarction	*		*
	Congestive heart failure			*
Musculoskeletal	Proximal stiffness/muscle pain	**	***	
	Synovitis of peripheral joints		*	
Others	Intense acute-phase response	***	***	***
	Normochromic or hypochromic anemia	**	*	**

Key: *** = high frequency (>70%); ** = moderate frequency (20–70%); * = low frequency (<20%).

Chronic nonproductive cough has been suspected to be related to arteritis in branches of the pulmonary arteries. If the vertebral and basilar arteries develop vasculitic stenosis, ischemia of the central nervous system manifests with transient ischemic attacks or frank stroke.

In patients with large-vessel GCA, cranial symptoms may be minimal, and temporal artery biopsy is often negative.[24] Instead, vascular insufficiency is focused on the upper-extremity vessels and the aorta. In rare cases, lower extremities are affected. Typically, patients have asymmetric blood pressure readings or totally lose upper-extremity blood pressures and pulses. The underlying lesions are occlusions in the distal subclavian arteries, often extending into the axillary sections (Fig. 59.4). Patients with subclavian GCA are on average about 10 years younger at disease onset than are those with dominant cranial manifestations. Diagnosis of large-vessel GCA can be delayed as symptoms are nonspecific, and the systemic inflammatory component is less pronounced. Ischemic pain in the hands when using the arms is often combined with coolness and bluish discoloration. Gangrene of the fingertips is rare. Disability can be significant, as patients have difficulties with activities of daily living. With stenotic lesions of the subclavian arteries, blood pressure readings can be unreliable or totally

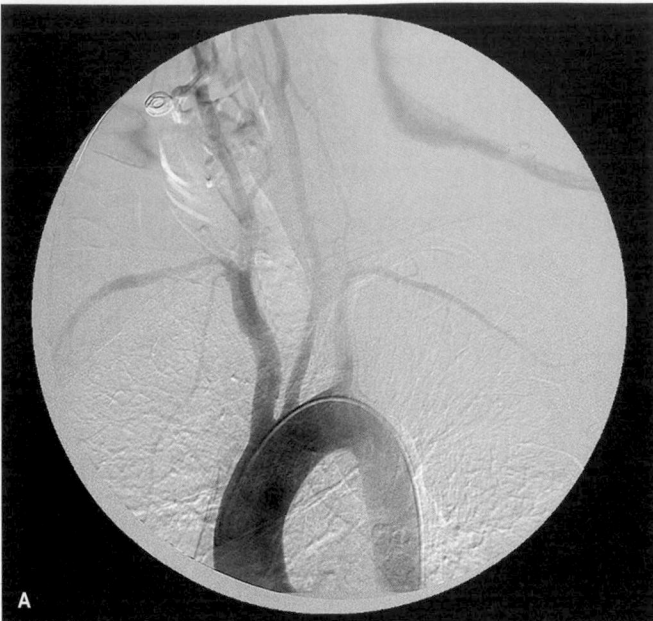

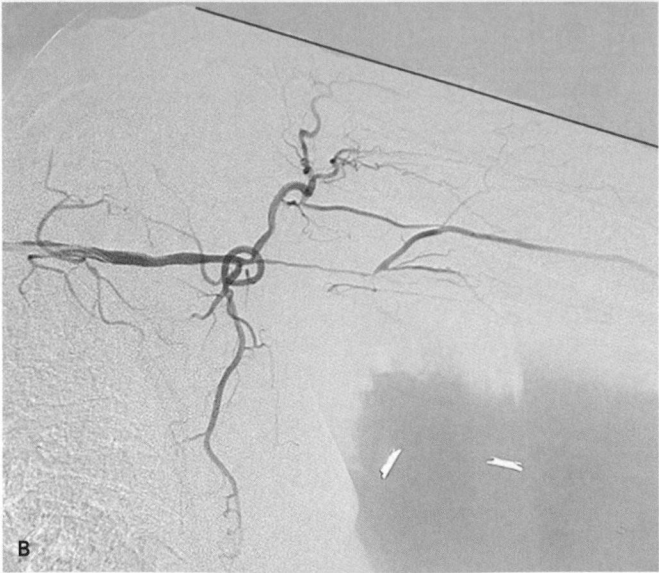

Fig. 59.4 Involvement of the subclavian axillary artery in giant-cell arteritis. Angiography of aortic arch and primary branches shows luminal irregularities in both distal subclavian arteries **(A)**. The digital subtraction angiogram focuses on the left subclavian axillary junction and demonstrates a high-degree, long-segment stenosis that is smooth-walled and tapered **(B)**. Newly formed collateral vessels branching off the distal subclavian supply blood to the arm.

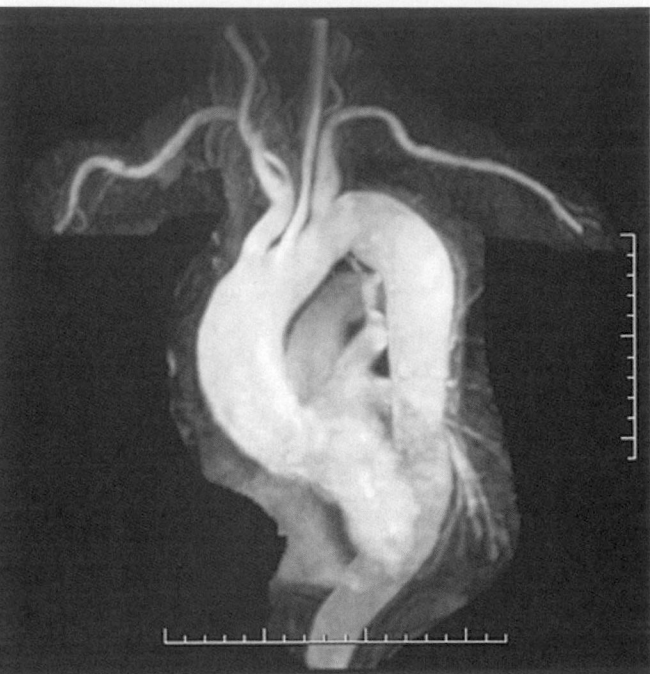

Fig. 59.5 Aortic aneurysm in giant-cell arteritis. A three-dimensional reconstruction of a magnetic resonance angiography demonstrating wall irregularities and ectasia throughout the thoracic aorta of a 63-year-old female with biopsy-proven giant-cell arteritis is shown. The ascending aorta appears most affected. The origins of the subclavian and innominate arteries are dilated, indicating inflammatory damage of the wall. Mild irregularities of the subclavian apex are seen, without evidence for stenosis.

may lead to aortic insufficiency. Aortic aneurysms are often clinically silent. The diagnosis may first be made from tissue obtained surgically during aortic aneurysm repair. In extreme cases, the aortic wall ruptures.

The response pattern of arteries to wall inflammation may not include intimal hyperplasia, thus sparing luminal compromise and vascular failure. In such patients, the systemic inflammatory component dominates the clinical presentation. Fever, fatigue, malaise, weight loss, and depression are intense enough to prompt a workup for a malignancy. GCA needs to be on the list of differential diagnosis in all cases of fever of unknown origin, particularly in elderly individuals. Whereas patients with cranial GCA have abnormally thick and tender temporal arteries exhibiting nodularity and loss of pulses, clinical findings in non-stenosing GCA can be bland and unremarkable. Temporal artery biopsy should be pursued even if clinical examination does not suggest the diagnosis.

■ CLINICAL FEATURES IN POLYMYALGIA RHEUMATICA ■

PMR is diagnosed in patients presenting with pronounced stiffness and pain in the shoulder and pelvic girdle muscles (Table 59.1).[2] Laboratory testing shows a systemic inflammatory syndrome; arterial biopsy is

absent, requiring alternative strategies for blood pressure monitoring. Although carotid involvement is considered infrequent, it can be challenging to distinguish atherosclerotic and vasculitic disease clearly. Patients with carotid GCA are at high risk for cerebral ischemic events. Aortic involvement preferentially targets the thoracic aorta and infrequently the abdominal aorta (Fig. 59.5). Dilation of the aortic root

Table 59.2 Takayasu arteritis: relationship between clinical symptoms and affected vascular territories

Vascular bed involvement	Approximate frequency (%)	Predominant clinical symptoms
Subclavian	90	Arm claudication, pulselessness
Common carotid	60	Visual defects, strokes, transient ischemic attack, syncope
Abdominal aorta	45	Claudication, hypertension, abdominal angina
Renal	35	Hypertension
Aortic arch/root	35	Aortic insufficiency, congestive heart failure
Vertebral	35	Dizziness, visual impairment
Celiac axis	20	Abdominal angina
Superior mesenteric	20	Abdominal angina
Iliac	20	Claudication
Pulmonary	10	Dyspnea, chest pain
Coronary	10	Myocardial infarction, angina

negative for arteritis. It is estimated that about 10% of PMR patients who have no signs of vascular inflammation will eventually develop full-blown vasculitis. Notably, PMR often occurs in patients with GCA and is present in about 40% of GCA patients at disease onset. Tapering of immunosuppressive therapy in GCA is frequently associated with new or remittent PMR symptoms.[24] Complaints are focused on muscle pain and stiffness, classically affecting the neck, the shoulder girdle, and the pelvic girdle. Muscles of the torso may be involved. Peripheral arms and legs are spared. Muscle pain is most intense in the early morning and improves during the day. Inability to get out of bed, stand up from a chair, or get off the toilet seat should alert the physician to consider PMR. Some patients with PMR have synovitis or bursitis in their shoulder and hip joints,[2, 25] making them difficult to distinguish from those with seronegative rheumatoid arthritis. No diagnostic procedure is available that allows for the diagnosis of PMR; the syndrome remains an exclusion diagnosis in cases of myalgia combined with laboratory signs of systemic inflammation. On clinical examination, passive motion of shoulder and hip joints is maintained, but active motion is restricted due to pain. Muscle strength is normal. Careful evaluation of the temporal arteries is warranted to avoid missing fully developed GCA.

CLINICAL FEATURES IN TAKAYASU ARTERITIS

The clinical manifestations of TA are diverse and depend on the vascular territory preferentially affected (Tables 59.1 and 59.2).[26, 27] Initial symptoms are usually nonspecific, such as fever, cough, malaise, weight loss, night sweats, myalgias, and arthralgias. Signs of vascular deficiency develop later in the disease course and are most frequently ischemic in nature. Geographical variations in disease pattern have been reported, likely reflecting the interplay between host risk genes and this inflammatory vasculopathy. In North American, Japanese, and Korean patient populations, the aortic arch and its primary cervical and upper-extremity

branches are preferentially targeted, giving rise to aortic insufficiency, cerebral ischemia, face and neck pain, ocular ischemia, and the typical presentation of 'pulseless disease' (Fig. 59.6). In India, the abdominal aorta and renal arteries are more commonly affected, causing renovascular hypertension and the long-term risk of cardiac failure (Fig. 59.7).[28]

Nonspecific complaints of headaches, syncope, and face and neck pain are often misinterpreted as stress-related problems, particularly in young women. Consequently, the diagnosis may be missed for months. Only few patients come to clinical attention with catastrophic neurological symptoms related to brain ischemia. Helpful clues are differences in blood pressure, loss of pulses, and vascular bruits heard on clinical examination. Retinal neoangiogenesis, induced by hypoperfusion of the eye, is now relatively rare, but fleeting visual abnormalities may indicate transient ischemic attacks. Signs of aortic insufficiency are unlikely to be encountered in early disease, but continuous monitoring for aortic dilation is part of follow-up care. Coronary artery stenosis in a young patient must prompt the physician to rule out TA. In a subset of patients, the origins of mesenteric arteries are involved by stenosing vasculitis. Clinical consequences include weight loss, nausea, vomiting, diarrhea, and abdominal claudication, typically elicited by the increased intestinal blood demand following a meal.

Renal artery stenosis may be clinically silent and is often noticed in routine screening. Correct measurement of blood pressures can represent a pressing clinical problem if the upper-extremity arteries are affected. Involvement of the infrarenal aorta may lead to lower-extremity claudication. Musculoskeletal examinations are usually unrevealing, although joint and muscle pains are common complaints.

DIAGNOSIS

Classification criteria have been developed for GCA and TA in order to differentiate patients with large-vessel vasculitis from those with other vasculitic entities (Tables 59.3–59.5).[29–31] Age at disease onset and the pattern of arteritis are clearly important for establishing the diagnosis and

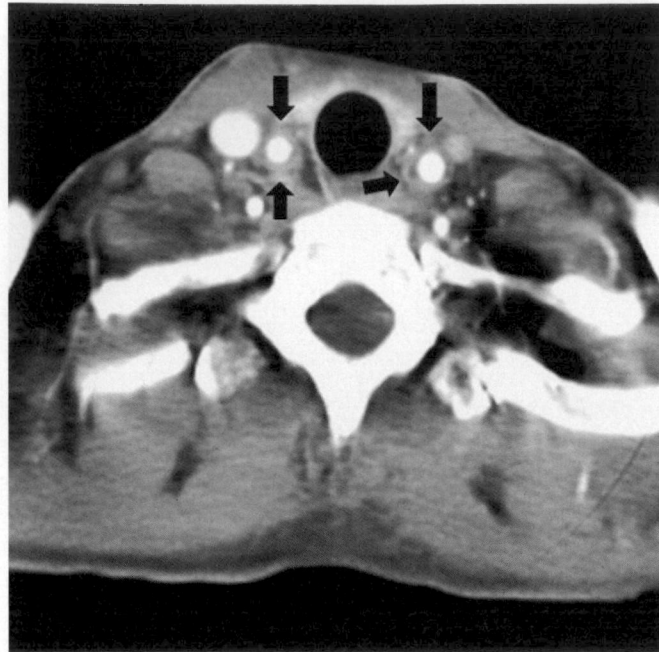

Fig. 59.6 Diagnosis of vascular involvement of Takayasu arteritis by chest computed tomography angiography. Axial images show marked thickening of the circumferential wall of both common carotid arteries (arrows). The vessel lumen is patent without evidence for hemodynamic stenosis. Lumen and wall of the vertebral arteries are normal.

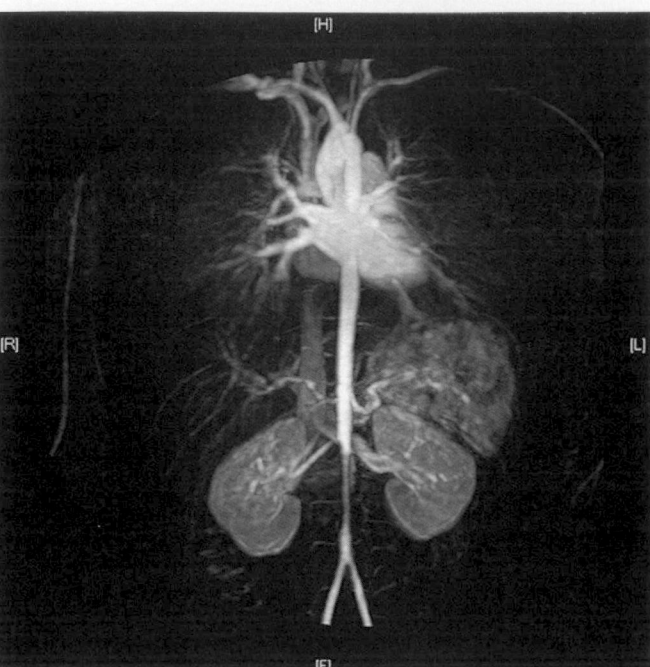

Fig. 59.7 Magnetic resonance angiography of Takayasu arteritis. The three-dimensional reconstruction shows normal caliber of the ascending and descending aorta in a 16-year-old female with Takayasu arteritis. The infrarenal abdominal aorta is narrowed diffusely over a 7-cm segment. Here the lumen measures only 5 mm. Mild narrowing of the common iliac arteries bilaterally, just distal to the aortic bifurcation.

distinguishing between these two related vasculopathies. Diagnostic criteria for PMR remain a challenge (Table 59.3) as they rely on nonspecific symptoms, such as muscle pain and stiffness and elevated erythrocyte sedimentation rate (ESR), all of which occur in many diseases.[2] No pathogenic test is currently available to diagnose PMR. Therapeutic responsiveness of PMR patients to low-dose corticosteroids continues to be clinically helpful but stresses the need for objective diagnostic criteria.

LABORATORY TESTS

In all three conditions, GCA, PMR, and TA, the vast majority of patients have laboratory findings of an intense acute-phase response.[2, 23, 26] Generally, this is captured by measuring ESR or C-reactive protein (CRP). It is important to note, however, that a subset of GCA patients has normal ESR readings, even before initiation of immunosuppressive therapy. A normal ESR or CRP reading is not sufficient to exclude the diagnosis, and further diagnostic workup is required if clinical presentation is suspicious for vasculitis. Other acute-phase proteins, such as fibrinogen and serum amyloid A, have been reported to be elevated as well. The cytokine IL-6 is a potent inducer of acute-phase proteins in the liver and, being located upstream of ESR and CRP, has been found to be a sensitive marker of continuous systemic inflammation.[32] Other laboratory abnormalities, such as elevation of alkaline phosphatase, thrombocytosis, and anemia, are in line with a robust acute-phase response.

Autoantibody measurements are not helpful beyond excluding differential diagnoses, such as rheumatoid arthritis, systemic lupus erythematosus, or anti-neutrophil cytoplasmic antibody (ANCA)-related vasculitides. No disease-specific autoantibodies for GCA and TA have been described, emphasizing that B cells are not involved in the pathogenic events leading to granulomatous inflammation of large vessels.

TISSUE BIOPSY

In patients with TA, tissue biopsies are rarely available unless the patient had to undergo vascular reconstructive surgery. In most patients, the diagnosis is made based on imaging procedures revealing luminal and wall abnormalities in affected blood vessels.

In contrast, arterial biopsy remains a critical diagnostic approach in patients with GCA. Temporal arteries are easily accessible, and a segment of these arteries can be removed in an outpatient setting. Recommendations include harvesting 2–3 cm of the temporal artery, starting at the most symptomatic side. Frozen tissue sections can lead to a quick diagnosis of granulomatous vasculitis. Whether the second side should be biopsied during the same surgical procedure remains a matter of debate. In cohorts including several hundred patients, vasculitis was detected in 2–3% of tissue samples from the second side if the first side was negative. If the clinical suspicion is strong, biopsy confirmation may be sought from a second-side biopsy immediately after the first biopsy or after

Table 59.3 American College of Rheumatology 1990 classification criteria for giant-cell arteritis[a] and polymyalgia rheumatica

Age at disease onset ≥ 50 years

New onset or new type of headache

Temporal artery tenderness or decreased artery pulse

Elevated erythrocyte sedimentation rate (≥ 50 mm/hour)

Histologic incidence of arteritis

(characterized by a predominance of mononuclear cell infiltrates or a granulomatous process with multinucleated giant cells)

(Reprinted from Hunder GG, Bloch DA, Michel BA, et al. The American College of Rheumatology 1990 criteria for the classification of giant cell arteritis. Arthritis Rheum 1990; 33: 1122–1128, with permission of Wiley-Liss, Inc., a subsidiary of John Wiley & Sons, Inc. ©1990.)
[a]A patient is classified as having giant-cell arteritis if at least three of the five criteria are present.

careful monitoring of the patient several weeks later. Negative findings on temporal artery biopsy do not exclude the diagnosis of GCA. In a retrospective cohort study, about half of all patients with subclavian GCA had no evidence of vasculitis in the temporal arteries, emphasizing that the disease may display clear preference for certain vascular territories.[33]

Corticosteroid therapy does not eradicate pathologic findings of vascular wall infiltrates and biopsy can still be valuable in making the diagnosis in patients already on steroids.[34] Nevertheless, it is possible that treatment with steroids leads to a false-negative biopsy result in some patients.

Histomorphologic reports describe mononuclear cell infiltrates penetrating through all layers of the vessel wall (Fig. 59.8).[1] Since the disease process enters the vessel wall through the adventitia, this may be the only site of inflammation. The finding of isolated inflammatory cell clusters in the adventitia, although not diagnostic, should at least be considered as highly suspicious. Multinucleated giant cells may or may not be found. They have a tendency to lie along the internal elastic lamina, at the junction between the media and the intima. Media destruction is not unusual, but findings of fibrinoid necrosis should prompt a search for a different vasculitic entity. The vessel lumen is more or less compromised by hyperplastic intima formed from proliferating fibroblasts, smooth-muscle cells, and deposition of acid mucopolysaccharides.

Histology of TA is similar to that in GCA, making it difficult to dissect both syndromes in tissue samples derived from the aorta or its primary branches.[35] Lymphocytes and plasma cells accumulate around vasa vasorum. Marked wall thickening with inflammatory tissue extending into perivascular structures is typical for TA (Fig. 59.9). Destruction of elastic membranes is often extensive and combined with patchy areas of media necrosis. Weakening of the vessel wall may lead to aneurysm formation. Notably, inflammatory lesions can be arranged in a 'skipped' pattern with normal vessel wall segments alternating with stretches of intense destructive inflammation.

Physicians can be confronted with morphologic findings of granulomatous aortitis in patients undergoing aortic aneurysm repair without any prior diagnosis of vasculitis. Detailed workup of these patients is necessary to identify those with undiagnosed PMR, GCA, or TA. Rare causes of aortitis, including inflammatory bowel disease, sarcoidosis, syphilis, and connective tissue disease, should be ruled out. Isolated granulomatous aortitis is diagnosed as idiopathic aortitis. The pathogenesis and prognosis of this condition are essentially unknown, but relatively good outcomes have been described in patients who did not receive anti-inflammatory therapy.

DIAGNOSTIC IMAGING

Applying modern imaging modalities to the diagnosis and management of large-vessel vasculitis has been a major advance in caring for these patients.[23] Indeed, diagnosing TA mostly depends on identifying vascular lesions in typical distribution by imaging.[36]

Conventional angiography still has its place in presurgical planning and can be combined with intravascular interventions. It provides ideal visualization of the vascular lumen not only for large but also for medium-sized arteries such as the axillary and brachial arteries (Fig. 59.4). Ultrasound (US)-based methods are extremely useful for screening carotid arteries but also emerge as the method of choice for initial assessment of the distal subclavian arteries, vertebral arteries, renal arteries, and femoral arteries. Also, US examination is the optimal method for long term monitoring of vessel bypasses in patients who received surgical reconstruction. With its sensitivity to submillimeter changes and its noninvasiveness, US is gaining a dominant role as a diagnostic tool in the management of vasculitis.

Magnetic resonance (MR) imaging and MR angiography, as well as computed tomography (CT), are now widely used for evaluating the vascular tree. Both methods provide excellent information on abnormalities of the vascular lumen and wall, but are still limited to larger vessels and provide insufficient information about the distal subclavian arteries or the 2nd to 5th branches of the aorta. CT imaging is fast, well tolerated by claustrophobic patients, and allows excellent assessment of the aorta and its wall (Fig. 59.6). However, it has the disadvantages of contrast loading and radiation exposure. With its inherent multiplanar imaging capabilities, MR is used to examine neck vessels, the aorta, and its primary branches (Figs 59.5 and 59.7). Great hope was placed on its potential to measure wall edema and intramural vascularity, which would make MR a useful tool in estimating disease burden and responses to therapy. However, a carefully conducted study comparing imaging results with laboratory parameters of inflammation to results from surgically harvested vessel biopsies has been disappointing, cautioning that edema-weighted MR should not be used as a sole means of measuring disease activity and therapeutic responsiveness.[37]

■ THERAPEUTIC MANAGEMENT ■

With increasing knowledge of the disease process and refinement of diagnosis and long-term treatment, the prognosis for large-vessel vasculitis patients has significantly improved. Life expectancy of patients with GCA is not shorter than of age-matched controls. Follow-up studies of Japanese patients with TA suggest good control of disease activity in about 75% of patients, with only 25% experiencing serious complications and cardiac manifestations that dominate long-term outcome. Recent discussions have focused on the question of whether vasculitis

THERAPEUTIC MANAGEMENT

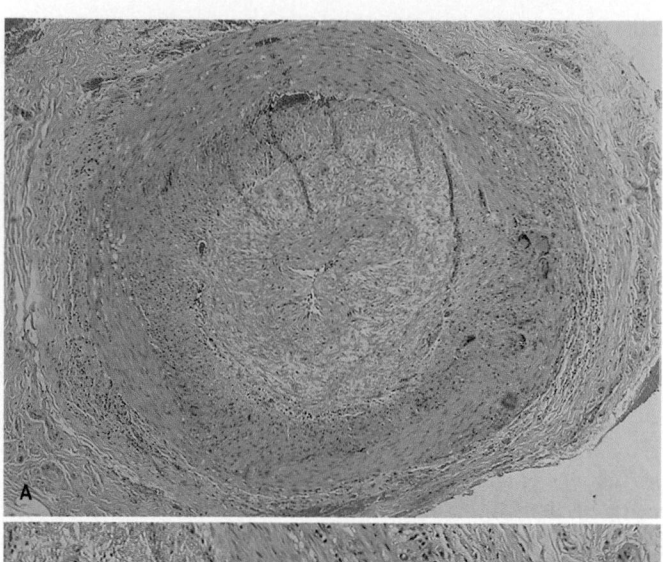

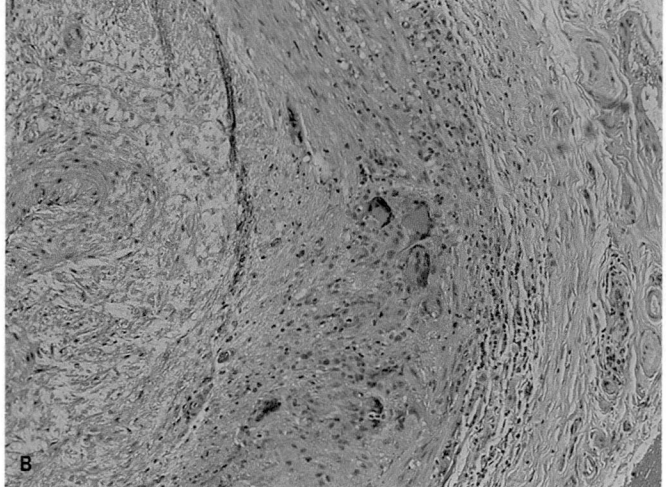

Fig. 59.8 Histomorphology of giant-cell arteritis. **(A)** Temporal artery cross-section with mononuclear infiltrates throughout all wall layers. The adventitia is infiltrated by round cells with cuffing of vasa vasorum by lymphocytes. The vessel lumen is occluded by intimal hyperplasia. **(B)** Higher magnification showing intense granulomatous inflammation with multinucleated giant cells in the proximal media and at the media–intima junction.

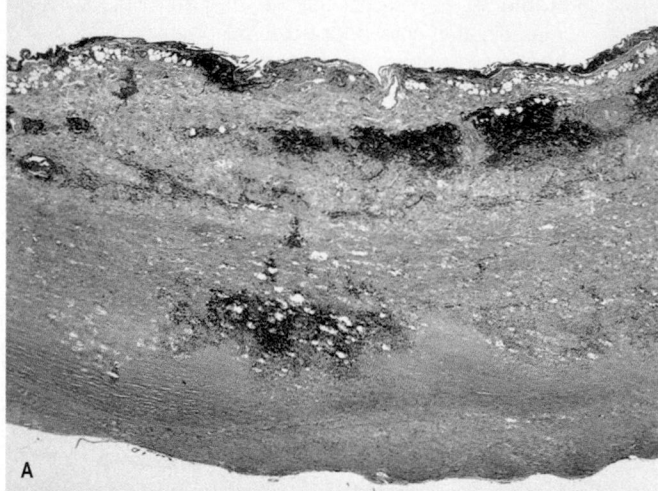

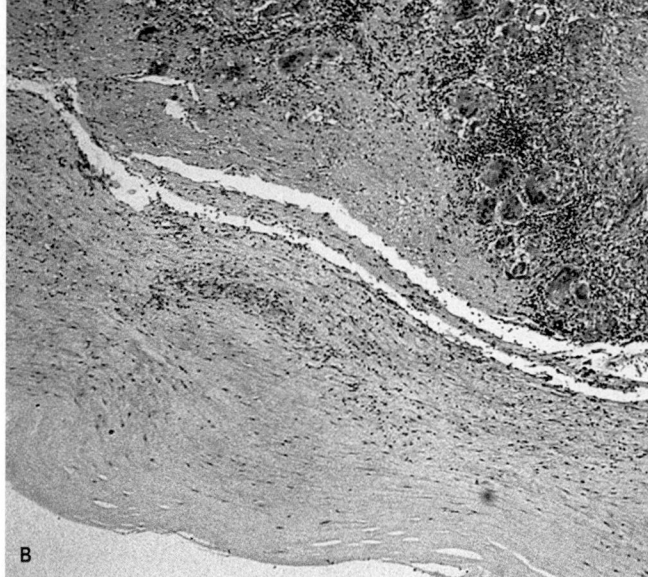

Fig. 59.9 Histopathology of Takayasu arteritis. **(A)** Full-thickness section of the aortic wall shows dense mononuclear infiltrates in the adventitia and media. The intima is thickened and wavy; hematoxylin and eosin (H&E). **(B)** Florid granulomatous inflammation along the media–intima junction with numerous giant cells; H&E.

predisposes patients to accelerated atherosclerotic disease, given the combination of chronic inflammation and injury to vessel wall structures. It is not known whether progression of atherosclerosis and its complications require a different management approach or whether standard vasoprotective measures (such as treating hypertension and hyperlipidemia and advising patients to avoid smoking) are sufficient.[5]

Pathogenic studies have pointed out that the traditional view of GCA as a self-limiting disease is incorrect.[33] To the contrary, granulomatous vasculitis has shown surprising resistance to immunosuppression in models of the disease, such as the temporal artery-SCID chimeras.[38] The paradigm of GCA as a chronic smoldering condition is supported by studies showing that sensitive markers of systemic inflammation remain elevated even in patients who are clinically asymptomatic and are weaned off immunosuppression. It is currently unknown whether this persistent smoldering disease process needs to be treated. Unchanged life expectancy in this population of elderly patients with an average age of 75 years at disease onset suggests that current management is adequate. It could be argued that intensification of immunosuppressive therapy is necessary to prevent long-term complications, such as aortic aneurysm/dissection from GCA aortitis. However, the number of patients developing such complications is low, and no evidence has been provided so far to indicate that therapy can stop progression of aortic wall destruction. The ultimate

Table 59.4 Diagnostic criteria for polymyalgia rheumatica

Age at disease onset ≥50 years

Pain persisting for ≥1 month and involving two of these areas: neck, shoulders, and pelvic girdle

Morning stiffness lasting >1 hour

Elevated erythrocyte sedimentation rate (> 40 mm/hour)

Rapid response to prednisone (≤ 20 mg/day)

Absence of other diseases capable of causing the musculoskeletal symptoms

(Reprinted from Healey LA. Long-term follow-up of polymyalgia rheumatica: evidence for synovitis. Semin Arthritis Rheum 1984; 13: 322–328, with permission of Wiley-Liss, Inc., a subsidiary of John Wiley & Sons, Inc. ©1984.)

THERAPEUTIC PRINCIPLES

>> To prevent vision loss, patients with giant-cell arteritis (GCA) require immediate treatment. Similarly, with the threat of catastrophic cerebral ischemia in Takayasu arteritis (TA), prompt initiation of therapy is imperative

>> Corticosteroids are the immunosuppressive drug of choice for large-vessel vasculitis. Often, they have to be given over a prolonged period of several years but may be clinically effective at very low doses

>> Clinical trials have failed to show steroid-sparing effects for either methotrexate or antitumor necrosis factor-α therapy in patients with GCA

>> Clinical experience (not evidence-based therapeutic trials) suggests that a combination of methotrexate, mycophenolate mofetil, or tumor necrosis factor-α-blocking agents with corticosteroids may be beneficial in disease control in some patients with TA

>> Close monitoring for diabetes, hypertension, and hyperlipidemia combined with bone-saving therapy should be part of the treatment regime in patients with large-vessel vasculitis on long-term corticosteroids

>> It is currently unknown whether the smoldering disease activity persisting beyond the acute phase of disease requires immunosuppressive therapy and whether the benefits of chronic immunosuppressive therapy outweigh the potential risks

decision depends on the cost–benefit analysis comparing the risk from smoldering disease with the risks imposed by long-standing immunosuppression.

The immunosuppressants of choice in GCA, TA, and PMR are corticosteroids. Notably, modern anti-cytokine reagents have failed to show therapeutic efficacy in GCA and PMR; however, they may have a place for a subset of TA patients.[39] Also, methotrexate, an anti-folate widely used in rheumatology to suppress chronic autoimmune inflammation, appears to lack steroid-sparing action in GCA and PMR,[40] but may have a limited effect in TA.[39] The unparalleled response pattern of patients with large-vessel vasculitis to corticosteroids emphasizes disease-specific pathogenic pathways in these syndromes that are distinct from most other autoimmune entities. Equally remarkable is the fact that patients with GCA, PMR, and TA improve within hours after being started on steroid therapy. The response is usually dramatic, with improvements within 24–48 hours. The promptness of clinical improvement is so exceptional that it has been suggested as a diagnostic criterion for PMR. Much of the acute clinical benefit must relate to suppression of the systemic inflammatory syndrome. Signs and symptoms of vascular stenosis are much less responsive. Reduction in wall edema may help to re-establish some blood flow. Over time, formation of collateral blood vessels is an important mechanism for dealing with tissue ischemia.

Patients with GCA are started on a daily prednisone dose of 40–60 mg (about 1 mg/kg body weight). Once stabilized, steroid tapering is guided by close monitoring of the clinical presentation as well as laboratory markers of inflammation. In general, steroids should be reduced 10–20% every 2 weeks. Monthly monitoring of ESR and CRP is mandatory to adjust therapy. Patients frequently return with signs or symptoms of recurrent disease as immunosuppression is lowered. Fortunately, disease exacerbations causing vision loss are infrequent. Disease flares typically present with PMR symptoms or nonspecific manifestations of malaise and failure to thrive. In most patients, disease control can be reinstated by a transient small increase in the steroid dose.

A recent study has suggested that initial treatment of vasculitis may alter the patient's long-term course. Guided by experiments in human artery-SCID chimeras, patients with biopsy-proven GCA were treated with pulse corticosteroids as induction therapy.[41] After receiving pulses of 1000 mg methylprednisolone for three consecutive days, therapy was continued on oral prednisone, and daily doses were swiftly tapered. Compared to patients in the control arm of the study, those who received the three initial steroid pulses had lower likelihoods of disease flares. Particularly, once they reached steroid doses close to 10 mg/day, these patients could tolerate steroid withdrawal significantly better, and the majority were taking 5 mg/day prednisone at 36 weeks.[41] The benefit from initial pulse therapy continued over subsequent months of managing these patients. This study suggests that intense immunosuppression during early disease may be more effective in disrupting underlying immune abnormalities, thereby shortening the overall course of disease duration.

When given to human artery-SCID chimeras, acetylsalicylic acid (aspirin) has marked anti-inflammatory activities with suppression of the key cytokine interferon-γ in vascular lesions.[42] Clinical trials are needed to test whether this immunosuppressive action can translate into corticosteroid sparing. Given that arteries are the primary target of large-vessel vasculitis, the use of aspirin as an anti-platelet agent should be routinely recommended.

There is no evidence that other immunosuppressants such as azathioprine and cyclophosphamide reduce the need for prednisone, prevent vascular complications, or shorten the duration of corticosteroid use.

An integral part of chronic immunosuppression with prednisone is regular monitoring for diabetes and hypertension. Patients should be encouraged to increase physical activity, as steroid-induced myopathy is a frequent finding in this population. A major issue of chronic steroid

Table 59.5 American College of Rheumatology 1990 criteria[a] for the classification of Takayasu arteritis

Disease onset at ≤ 40 years

Claudication of an extremity

Decreased brachial artery pulse

> 10 mmHg difference in systolic blood pressure between arms

Bruit over the subclavian arteries or the aorta

Arteriographic evidence of narrowing or occlusion of the entire aorta, its primary branches, or large arteries in the proximal upper or lower extremities

(Reprinted from Arend WP, Michel BA, Bloch DA, et al. The American College of Rheumatology 1990 criteria for the classification of Takayasu arteritis. Arthritis Rheum 1990; 33: 1129–1134, with permission of Wiley-Liss, Inc., a subsidiary of John Wiley & Sons, Inc. ©1990.)
[a]For purposes of classification, a patient is classified as having Takayasu arteritis if more than three of the six criteria are fulfilled.

treatment, particularly in elderly individuals, is the potential of excessive bone loss, possibly as a result of both increased bone resorption and impaired bone formation. A number of effective and safe therapies for osteoporosis are currently available. Obviously, calcium and vitamin D supplementation should be part of the therapeutic regimen.

Most patients can be discontinued from immunosuppressive treatment 18–24 months after diagnosis. Markers of systemic inflammation may remain elevated, and continuous monitoring for aortic involvement and recurrence of cranial arteritis is recommended.

In patients with PMR who have no evidence for frank vasculitis, much lower doses of steroids are necessary to induce prompt relief of symptoms. Most patients are sufficiently treated with an initial dose of 20 mg of prednisone per day. In some patients, 10 mg of prednisone can induce and sustain a clinical response. Physicians should aim at titrating steroids to minimally needed doses to avoid side effects; tapering usually needs to be slow, over many months.

In TA, initial therapy is similar to that in GCA, but long-term management needs to be tailored to individual patient conditions.[39] It has been discussed that patients should be maintained on a low dose of corticosteroids, such as 5–7 mg prednisone daily, even after successful control of active disease. Given the age at disease onset in TA, preventive measures to counteract accelerated atherosclerosis and optimize blood pressure control are important aspects of management.

It has been suggested that up to 50% of TA patients may require a second immunosuppressive agent.[39] Steroid-sparing effects of methotrexate have been reported for some patients. Similarly, mycophenolate mofetil may have clinical efficiency, although published data are only available on a small patient cohort. Finally, there may be a place for agents blocking tumor necrosis factor-α in patients with persistent disease activity. The dilemma is that well-designed placebo-controlled treatment trials testing the efficiency of such immunosuppressive drugs are lacking, mostly due to the infrequency of TA.

Detecting and treating hypertension is an essential component of caring for patients with TA. Untreated hypertension leads to acceleration of atherosclerosis and cardiac insufficiency. In patients with upper-extremity involvement, obtaining accurate blood pressure measurements is a challenge and requires education of the patient and caregivers.

Besides pharmacologic therapy, revascularization procedures – including both surgical and endovascular interventions – have vastly broadened therapeutic options in patients with TA and large-vessel GCA.[39] To minimize the risk of complications, such as rapid reocclusion, an effort has to be made to suppress vascular wall inflammation optimally before subjecting the patients to revascularization treatment. Conventional bypass grafts are still considered the method of choice. Percutaneous transluminal angioplasty can be useful in managing renal artery stenosis or other short-segment lesions. Bypass surgery is needed in patients with cerebrovascular ischemia in whom catastrophic strokes may be prevented by bypassing critical stenosis of cervical vessels with grafts originating from the aortic arch. Re-establishing flow in upper- and lower-extremity arteries can be complicated by multiple and long-segment stenosis, and arterial reconstructions with prosthetic graft materials or vein may be the only alternative to obtain long-term patency. Placing of conventional stents may be complicated by eliciting rapid restenosis, and it is not known whether outcomes can be improved by drug-eluting stents. Occlusive disease of the coronary arteries usually represents a challenging clinical scenario, and most physicians opt for conventional bypass surgery. Depending on symptoms, patients with aortic regurgitation may require repair of the weakened aortic wall.

■ REFERENCES ■

1. Weyand CM, Goronzy JJ. Medium- and large-vessel vasculitis. N Engl J Med 2003; 349: 160–169.

2. Salvarani C, Cantini F, Boiardi L, et al. Polymyalgia rheumatica and giant-cell arteritis. N Engl J Med 2002; 347: 261–271.

3. Nordborg E, Nordborg C. Giant cell arteritis: epidemiological clues to its pathogenesis and an update on its treatment. Rheumatology (Oxford) 2003; 42: 413–421.

4. Vanoli M, Bacchiani G, Origg L, et al. Takayasu's arteritis: a changing disease. J Nephrol 2001; 14: 497–505.

5. Numano F, Kishi Y, Tanaka A, et al. Inflammation and atherosclerosis. Atherosclerotic lesions in Takayasu arteritis. Ann NY Acad Sci 2000; 902: 65–76.

6. Seko Y. Takayasu arteritis: insights into immunopathology. Jpn Heart J 2000; 41: 15–26.

7. Weyand CM, Ma-Krupa W, Goronzy JJ. Immunopathways in giant cell arteritis and polymyalgia rheumatica. Autoimmun Rev 2004; 3: 46–53.

8. Weyand CM, Goronzy JJ. Arterial wall injury in giant cell arteritis. Arthritis Rheum 1999; 42: 844–853.

9. Ma-Krupa W, Jeon MS, Spoerl S, et al. Activation of arterial wall dendritic cells and breakdown of self-tolerance in giant cell arteritis. J Exp Med 2004; 199: 173–183.

10. Weyand CM, Ma-Krupa W, Pryshchep O, et al. Vascular dendritic cells in giant cell arteritis. Ann NY Acad Sci 2005; 1062: 195–208.

11. Krupa WM, Dewan M, Jeon MS, et al. Trapping of misdirected dendritic cells in the granulomatous lesions of giant cell arteritis. Am J Pathol 2002; 161: 1815–1823.

12. Ma-Krupa W, Kwan M, Goronzy JJ, et al. Toll-like receptors in giant cell arteritis. Clin Immunol 2005; 115: 38–46.

13. Rodriguez-Pla A, Stone JH. Vasculitis and systemic infections. Curr Opin Rheumatol 2006; 18: 39–47.

14. Weyand CM, Tetzlaff N, Bjornsson J, et al. Disease patterns and tissue cytokine profiles in giant cell arteritis. Arthritis Rheum 1997; 40: 19–26.

15. Kaiser M, Younge B, Bjornsson J, et al. Formation of new vasa vasorum in vasculitis. Production of angiogenic cytokines by multinucleated giant cells. Am J Pathol 1999; 155: 765–774.

16. Seko Y, Minota S, Kawasaki A, et al. Perforin-secreting killer cell infiltration and expression of a 65-kD heat-shock protein in aortic tissue of patients with Takayasu's arteritis. J Clin Invest 1994; 93: 750–758.

17. Weyand CM, Schonberger J, Oppitz U, et al. Distinct vascular lesions in giant cell arteritis share identical T cell clonotypes. J Exp Med 1994; 179: 951–960.

18. Wagner AD, Goronzy JJ, Weyand CM. Functional profile of tissue-infiltrating and circulating CD68+ cells in giant cell arteritis. Evidence for two components of the disease. J Clin Invest 1994; 94: 1134–1140.

19. Borkowski A, Younge BR, Szweda L, et al. Reactive nitrogen intermediates in giant cell arteritis: selective nitration of neocapillaries. Am J Pathol 2002; 161: 115–123.

20. Rittner HL, Hafner V, Klimiuk PA, et al. Aldose reductase functions as a detoxification system for lipid peroxidation products in vasculitis. J Clin Invest 1999; 103: 1007–1013.

21. Rittner HL, Kaiser M, Brack A, et al. Tissue-destructive macrophages in giant cell arteritis. Circ Res 1999; 84: 1050–1058.

22. Kaiser M, Weyand CM, Bjornsson J, et al. Platelet-derived growth factor, intimal hyperplasia, and ischemic complications in giant cell arteritis. Arthritis Rheum 1998; 41: 623–633.

23. Weyand CM, Goronzy JJ. Giant-cell arteritis and polymyalgia rheumatica. Ann Intern Med 2003; 139: 505–515.

24. Brack A, Martinez-Taboada V, Stanson A, et al. Disease pattern in cranial and large-vessel giant cell arteritis. Arthritis Rheum 1999; 42: 311–317.

25. Salvarani C, Cantini F, Olivieri I, et al. Proximal bursitis in active polymyalgia rheumatica. Ann Intern Med 1997; 127: 27–31.

26. Kerr GS, Hallahan CW, Giordano J, et al. Takayasu arteritis. Ann Intern Med 1994; 120: 919–929.

27. Numano F, Kobayashi Y. Takayasu arteritis – beyond pulselessness. Intern Med 1999; 38: 226–232.

28. Kobayashi Y, Numano F. 3. Takayasu arteritis. Intern Med 2002; 41: 44–46.

29. Hunder GG, Bloch DA, Michel BA, et al. The American College of Rheumatology 1990 criteria for the classification of giant cell arteritis. Arthritis Rheum 1990; 33: 1122–1128.

30. Healey LA. Long-term follow-up of polymyalgia rheumatica: evidence for synovitis. Semin Arthritis Rheum 1984; 13: 322–328.

31. Arend WP, Michel BA, Bloch DA, et al. The American College of Rheumatology 1990 criteria for the classification of Takayasu arteritis. Arthritis Rheum 1990; 33: 1129–1134.

32. Roche NE, Fulbright JW, Wagner AD, et al. Correlation of interleukin-6 production and disease activity in polymyalgia rheumatica and giant cell arteritis. Arthritis Rheum 1993; 36: 1286–1294.

33. Weyand CM, Fulbright JW, Hunder GG, et al. Treatment of giant cell arteritis: interleukin-6 as a biologic marker of disease activity. Arthritis Rheum 2000; 43: 1041–1048.

34. Achkar AA, Lie JT, Hunder GG, et al. How does previous corticosteroid treatment affect the biopsy findings in giant cell (temporal) arteritis?. Ann Intern Med 1994; 120: 987–992.

35. Johnston SL, Lock RJ, Gompels MM. Takayasu arteritis: a review. J Clin Pathol 2002; 55: 481–486.

36. Steeds RP, Mohiaddin R. Takayasu arteritis: role of cardiovascular magnetic imaging. Int J Cardiol 2006; 109: 1–6.

37. Tso E, Flamm SD, White RD, et al. Takayasu arteritis: utility and limitations of magnetic resonance imaging in diagnosis and treatment. Arthritis Rheum 2002; 46: 1634–1642.

38. Brack A, Rittner HL, Younge BR, et al. Glucocorticoid-mediated repression of cytokine gene transcription in human arteritis-SCID chimeras. J Clin Invest 1997; 99: 2842–2850.

39. Liang P, Hoffman GS. Advances in the medical and surgical treatment of Takayasu arteritis. Curr Opin Rheumatol 2005; 17: 16–24.

40. Hoffman GS, Cid MC, Hellmann DB, et al. A multicenter, randomized, double-blind, placebo-controlled trial of adjuvant methotrexate treatment for giant cell arteritis. Arthritis Rheum 2002; 46: 1309–1318.

41. Mazlumzadeh M, Hunder GG, Easley KA, et al. Treatment of giant cell arteritis using induction therapy with high-dose glucocorticoids: a double-blind, placebo-controlled, randomized prospective clinical trial. Arthritis Rheum 2006; 54: 3310–3318.

42. Weyand CM, Kaiser M, Yang H, et al. Therapeutic effects of acetylsalicylic acid in giant cell arteritis. Arthritis Rheum 2002; 46: 457–466.

Autoinflammatory fever syndromes

Jeroen C. H. van der Hilst, Jos W.M. van der Meer, Joost P.H. Drenth

60

Autoinflammatory syndromes, also known as hereditary periodic fever syndromes, encompass a group of genetic disorders characterized by lifelong recurrent febrile attacks of noninfectious origin. Each syndrome is characterized by a typical mix of symptoms that may include abdominal symptoms, arthralgias, arthritis, lymphadenopathy, and skin manifestations. Attacks of fever are always accompanied by an intense acute-phase response with elevated C-reactive protein (CRP), serum amyloid A (SAA), and leukocytosis.[1]

Autoinflammatory syndromes can be distinguished from autoimmune diseases on several grounds. First, periodic fever is not a typical feature of autoimmune disorders. Moreover, several serological and cellular parameters such as the presence of autoantibodies or antigen-specific T cells do not play a role in the pathogenesis of autoinflammatory syndromes. In recent years, important steps have been made in understanding the pathogenesis of the autoinflammatory syndromes.

Without exception, autoinflammatory syndromes are disorders with a clear mendelian inheritance pattern. The progress in molecular genetics over the last decade has allowed the discovery of the genes implicated in a number of autoinflammatory disorders. The discovery of these genes and the corresponding proteins led to the identification of a new family of inflammatory proteins and their scaffold (named the inflammasome) that have a role in innate immunity. Recent research efforts have broadened the understanding of the mechanism of inflammation. Collectively this group of syndromes can be regarded as gain-of-function disorders in which the causative mutations lead to inappropriate and increased secretion of inflammatory cytokines, such as interleukin (IL)-1β. In turn, this has led to the development of effective treatment strategies for these rare syndromes. This chapter describes the clinical pathology of six autoinflammatory disorders (Table 60.1).

The cornerstone of the diagnosis of the autoinflammatory diseases is clinical assessment. This includes a detailed medical and family history and clinical observation of an attack. Based on age of onset of symptoms, family history, ethnic background, accompanying symptoms, and duration of fever, most autoinflammatory syndromes can be differentiated on clinical grounds (Table 60.2).

Despite the fact that clinical assessment allows the identification of a number of syndromes, we fail to make a classifiable diagnosis in the majority of patients who consult us with periodic fever. It is therefore to be expected that study of the pathogenesis of the various autoinflammatory syndromes will identify new proteins and pathways implicated in hitherto unrecognized syndromes.

◼ EPIDEMIOLOGY ◼

It is important to realize that autoinflammatory diseases are rare and that the incidence of the different autoinflammatory syndromes depends on the background population as the gene distribution depends to some extent on ethnicity. Without doubt, familial Mediterranean fever (FMF) is the most prevalent of these diseases, with more than 10 000 persons affected worldwide. It is found in persons originating from the Mediterranean basin, including Turks, Jews (primarily non-Ashkenazi), Armenians, and Arabs. However, sporadic cases in other ethnic groups have been described. With

Table 60.1 The autoinflammatory syndromes: names and acronyms

Name	Acronym
Familial Mediterranean fever	FMF
Hyperimmunoglobulin D and periodic fever syndrome	HIDS
Tumor necrosis factor receptor-associated periodic syndrome	TRAPS
Familial cold autoinflammatory syndrome	FCAS
Muckle–Wells syndrome	MWS
Neonatal-onset multisystemic inflammatory disease (also known as chronic infantile neurologic cutaneous and articular syndrome)	NOMID/CINCA
Cryopyrin-associated periodic syndrome	CAPS

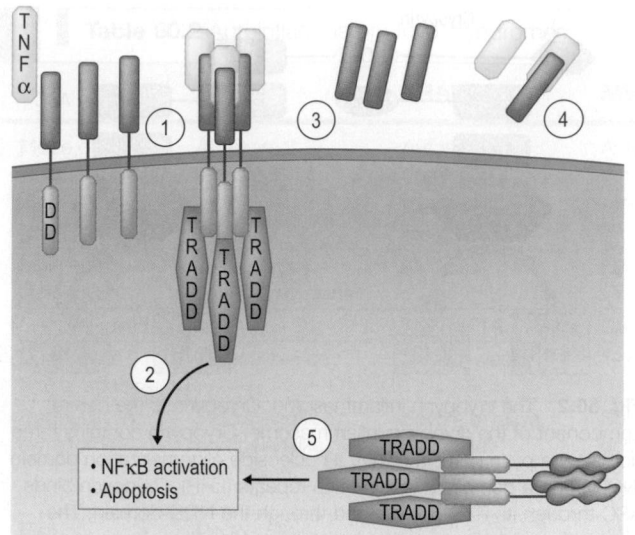

Fig. 60.3 Proposed pathophysiology of tumor necrosis factor receptor-associated periodic syndrome (TRAPS). (1) Tumor necrosis factor (TNF) binds to the TNF receptor on the surface of inflammatory cells (2). After receptor triggering, TRADD is recruited and a signal leads to apoptosis and cytokine production (3). In healthy individuals the receptors are shed from the surface, leading to a pool of receptors that dampen immune response (4). In patients with TRAPS there is diminished shedding, which may lead to a proinflammatory state by ongoing stimulation of retained cell surface receptors. Alternatively, the deficiency of soluble TNF receptors reduces scavenging of excess TNF. (5) Other research has shown that mutated TNF receptors form aggregates and are retained intracellularly. These aggregated receptors are capable of binding TRADD and stimulate ligand-independent cytokine production.

addition to a number of nonsterol isoprenoids. Isoprenoids are essential compounds in diverse cellular function and include ubiquinone, heme A, farnesyl, and geranyl. How a reduced activity of mevalonate kinase leads to an autoinflammatory condition in not known. It can be caused by a lack of isoprenoids or by an excess of the substrate of mevalonate-kinase: mevalonic acid. Proinflammatory cytokine production by mononuclear cells of patients with HIDS is strongly enhanced.[16] Furthermore, a defect in apoptosis of HIDS lymphocytes has been detected.[17] It has been hypothesized that this leads to an inability to curtail an excessive cytokine response after a trivial stimulus.

FAMILIAL MEDITERRANEAN FEVER

Clinical features

FMF is an autosomal recessive disease. Over 90% of patients become symptomatic within the first two decades of life. Typically an attack has an abrupt onset with high fever, reaching a peak soon after onset, lasting from 12 hours to 3 days and then rapidly subsiding.[18] There are no consistent triggers, but in some patients vigorous exercise, emotional stress, or menstruation precedes an attack. The frequency of attacks varies

greatly between patients, from once every week to only once every few years. Even in a given patient the frequency can vary greatly. Signs of painful serositis accompanying the fever are the hallmark of the disease.

Abdominal pain of 1 or 2 days' duration occurs in > 95% of patients. The abdominal pain may originally be focal, and then progresses to become more generalized. It is caused by a sterile peritonitis with a major influx of neutrophils. Many patients have undergone exploratory abdominal surgery because of an acute abdomen, with the resection of an uninflamed appendix. Sometimes adhesions are seen, presumably the result of recurrent peritoneal inflammation. Pelvic adhesions can reduce fertility in female patients.

Other serosal and synovial membranes are often involved. Pleural inflammation presenting as unilateral pleural pain is experienced by ~40% of patients. Synovitis presenting as monoarthritis with effusion of the knee, ankle, or wrist occurs in half to three-quarters of patients. An arthritic attack may have a more protracted course, with fever lasting up to a week. The synovitis usually resolves completely without joint destruction. Pericarditis is rare (< 1%). Erysipelas-like skin lesions are reported in 7–40 % of patients.[19] The lesions mimic acute infectious cellulitis occurring on the lower extremities. Other less frequently encountered symptoms include vasculitis, such as polyarteritis nodosa and Henoch–Schönlein purpura, orchitis, aseptic meningitis, and myalgia. The literature is replete with genotype–phenotype studies, and the most consistent finding is that the M694V/M694V genotype carriers have earlier onset of symptoms and higher frequency of arthritis. The life expectancy of patients depends on receiving appropriate treatment to prevent amyloidosis (see related paragraphs).

Laboratory investigation

There is no specific biological marker for FMF. During attacks patients show a strong acute-phase response with high CRP concentrations and leukocytosis. During remission laboratory analysis shows signs of persistent inflammation despite the fact that patients are clinically well.[20] Proteinuria (more than 0.5 g of protein per 24 hours) in patients with FMF is highly suggestive of amyloidosis.

Diagnosis

FMF is a clinical diagnosis (Table 60.3). A set of validated diagnostic criteria has been designed at the Sheba Medical Center at Tel Hashomer in Tel Aviv, Israel.[21] When applied in a population with high pretest probability, it has a high positive and negative predictive value. It is unknown whether these criteria can be applied to other populations with lower disease frequency. In general, when a patient has a typical medical history and stems from a high-prevalence ethnic group, the diagnosis is not difficult to make. FMF has been described in a wide variety of ethnic groups, so ancestry should no be used to rule out the diagnosis. In atypical cases and in patient from low-prevalence ethnic groups, genetic testing can be useful in the diagnostic process.

CRYOPYRIN-ASSOCIATED PERIODIC SYNDROME

Originally, CAPS was identified as three different syndromes with distinct clinical features. All types of CAPS are autosomal dominantly inherited. With the discovery of the incriminated gene there is increasing awareness that there are many patients with overlapping symptoms.[22] Furthermore, a particular genetic mutation can result in different

Table 60.3 Criteria for the diagnosis of familial Mediterranean fever

Major criteria
Typical attack* with abdominal symptoms
Typical attack with pleural symptoms
Typical attack with monoarthritis
Typical attack with only fever
Incomplete attack[†] with abdominal symptoms

Minor criteria
Favourable response to colchicine
Incomplete attack with monoarthritis
Exertional leg pain

*Typical attacks are defined as at least three attacks with fever > 38ºC.
[†]Incomplete attacks are painful and recurrent attacks not meeting the criteria for typical attack. The diagnosis of familial Mediterranean fever requires one major or two minor criteria. The sensitivity and specificity of these two criteria sets were > 95% and > 97%.[21]

phenotypes, suggesting the role of other disease-modifying genes. Though each of the cryopyrin-associated syndromes has distinctive clinical features, the common genetic basis and the many overlapping clinical manifestations support the notion of a continuous spectrum of diseases with different severities.

FAMILIAL COLD AUTOINFLAMMATORY SYNDROME

Clinical features

Familial cold autoinflammatory syndrome (FCAS) has an almost complete penetrance. The disease becomes clinically manifest in early childhood. In 60% of patients, the first symptoms develop within the first days of life. Symptoms typically occur after a few minutes to a maximum of 3 hours after being exposed to temperatures lower than 22°C. A recurrent characteristic rash is always present. The rash usually starts on the extremities and can extend to other parts of the body. It is described by patients as itchy or burning. Most attacks are accompanied by fever and chills, recurrent arthralgia, and conjunctivitis. Other commonly reported symptoms are profuse sweating, headache, extreme thirst, and nausea.[23] Attacks generally resolve spontaneously after a few hours to a day. Localized exposure to cold does not provoke an attack, which distinguishes it from acquired cold urticaria. Many patients with FCAS also show evidence of chronic inflammation between attacks, particularly a daily pattern of rash developing in the afternoon that can be associated with headaches, myalgia, and fatigue. The symptoms tend to become less severe with advancing age.

Laboratory investigation

The most consistent finding during attacks is a polymorphonuclear leukocytosis, with white blood cell counts up to 36 000/mm³. Erythrocyte sedimentation rate can be moderately elevated, as are other acute-phase reactants. No cold agglutinins or cryoglobulins are present. Skin biopsies from the urticarial rash show neutrophil efflux.

Diagnosis

FCAS is diagnosed based on the typical clinical features in combination with a positive family history.[24] Genetic testing is available.

MUCKLE–WELLS SYNDROME

Clinical features

This autosomal dominant disorder was originally described by Muckle and Wells as a triad of urticaria, deafness, and amyloidosis in a large family. Patients with Muckle–Wells syndrome (MWS) have short bouts of inflammation (12–48 hours); sometimes the attacks are triggered by cold exposure, minor trauma, or emotional stress. The age of onset is variable and ranges from neonatal onset to adolescence. Inflammatory attacks are preceded or accompanied by an urticarial skin rash. The trunk and extremities are most frequently involved, more rarely the face. Arthralgias are a common feature of attacks and can be disabling. Sometimes they are accompanied by large-joint effusion. Arthralgias tend to subside when skeletal growth ceases. Other symptoms may include conjunctivitis, uveitis, severe fatigue, and aphthous ulcers.[25] A distinctive feature of MWS is sensorineural deafness. It has been reported to occur in about 70% of patients. The progressive loss of hearing usually starts in early childhood, but late onset of perceptive deafness is not uncommon.

Laboratory investigation

Leukocytosis and elevated acute-phase reactants are invariably present. Skin biopsies of the lesions show a polymorphonuclear infiltrate.

Diagnosis

Most patients have a positive family history, but isolated cases have been reported. The diagnosis is made on clinical grounds in combination with genetic testing. Genetic testing of rare disorders, such as MWS, is commercially available (www.genedx.com).

NEONATAL-ONSET MULTISYSTEM INFLAMMATORY DISEASE

Clinical features

Neonatal-onset multisystem inflammatory disease (NOMID) is an autosomal dominant inherited condition characterized by a triad of cutaneous, articular, and neurological symptoms. Patients have chronic inflammation with episodic bouts of fever and worsening of symptoms. NOMID has a much more severe clinical course than the other two cryopyrin-associated syndromes. Typically, patients are born prematurely and have a nonpruritic urticarial-like rash. Central nervous system manifestations include chronic aseptic meningitis, increased intracranial pressure, hydrocephalus, seizures, and sensorineural deafness.[11] Chronic papilledema with optic nerve atrophy can result in loss of vision. Headache caused by aseptic meningitis is a prominent

PATHOGENESIS

feature. Magnetic resonance studies from the brain show ventriculomegaly and mild-to-moderate cerebral atrophy. High-resolution images show arachnoid adhesions and cochlear enhancement. The central nervous system involvement often leads to mental retardation. Articular symptoms are a prominent feature of NOMID.[26] A highly characteristic arthropathy, with distinct radiographic findings of premature patellar and epiphyseal long bone ossification and resultant osseous overgrowth, develops early in life. It leads to short stature, severe contractures, and disability. It is unclear whether the bone manifestations are caused by IL-1β-driven inflammation or result from impaired apoptosis of chondrocytes. The prognosis is grave, with a reported mortality rate of 20% before adulthood due to infection, vasculitis, and amyloidosis.

Laboratory investigations

Patients with NOMID have a continuous inflammation, with elevated SAA and CRP and elevated leukocyte counts. There is meningeal inflammation with increased protein concentrations and elevated white-cell counts in the cerebral spinal fluid.

Diagnosis

NOMID can be diagnosed based on characteristic clinical manifestations. Mutational analysis is available (www.genedx.com), but in some patients no mutations are found.

TUMOR NECROSIS FACTOR RECEPTOR-ASSOCIATED PERIODIC SYNDROME

Clinical features

TRAPS is inherited in an autosomal dominant manner. The age of onset varies widely, but most patients become symptomatic within the first few years of life. The median age of onset is 3 years. The usual duration of episodes in TRAPS is considerably longer than in the other autoinflammatory syndromes. An attack persists for a minimum of 3 days, but can last for weeks. The interval between attacks can vary substantially within a single patient. Localized myalgia affecting a limb associated with fever is found in virtually all patients.[27] Patients describe it as a deep cramping muscle pain, often severely disabling. The symptoms are probably due to a monocytic fasciitis. Cutaneous manifestations are present in the large majority of patients during attacks. They consist of localized erythematous macules and patches that tend to migrate to the distal part of the extremities.[28] Abdominal pain, often accompanied by vomiting, constipation, and bowel obstruction, occurs in almost all patients. Arthralgia and monoarticular arthritis involving hips, knees, and ankles are present in a quarter of patients at some point in the natural history of their disease. Chest pain is a frequent feature and may be either pleural in origin or reflect musculoskeletal involvement.

Characteristic ocular symptoms in TRAPS range from conjunctivitis and periorbital pain to severe uveitis and iritis. Periorbital edema with conjunctival injection is another distinctive but infrequent feature of TRAPS. Other less frequently observed symptoms are pericarditis, and inflammation of the tunica vaginalis, leading to scrotal pain. Lymphadenopathy is rare.

Laboratory investigations

During an attack of TRAPS laboratory investigations indicate an acute-phase response, with elevated erythrocyte sedimentation rate, CRP, haptoglobin, fibrinogen, and ferritin. A large proportion of patients also demonstrate an elevated acute-phase response between clinically symptomatic attacks. Complete blood count may demonstrate neutrophilia, thrombocytosis, and anemia of chronic disease. Polyclonal gammopathy as well as small monoclonal gammopathy occur. Autoantibodies, including antinuclear antibodies, anti-cardiolipin antibodies and rheumatoid factor are negative or are found at low titers.

Diagnosis (Table 60.4)

Hull et al. have proposed a set of diagnostic criteria for TRAPS.[27] However, these criteria have not been validated, and information about sensitivity and specificity of this diagnostic test is lacking. Genetic testing is the mainstay in the diagnosis of TRAPS.

HYPERIMMUNOGLOBULIN D AND PERIODIC FEVER SYNDROME

Clinical features

HIDS is an autosomal recessively inherited disease that was first recognized as a separate disease entity in 1984. Patients with HIDS have recurrent fever attacks of 4–6 days' duration that start in early childhood.[16] The inflammatory attacks occur on average every 4–6 weeks, although there is considerable variation within a single patient and between patients. An attack begins with chills followed by a sharp rise in temperature. Factors known to provoke an attack are infection, trauma, vaccination, and both physical and emotional stress, although often a trigger is not obvious. Typically, parents recall the first attack of their child occurring after the first childhood vaccination. The febrile episodes are accompanied by cervical lymphadenopathy and abdominal pain with vomiting and diarrhea. Cutaneous manifestations of HIDS present primarily as erythematous macules and papules, urticaria, and different forms of rash and exanthema (Fig. 60.4). A minority of patients have painful oral and genital aphthus ulcers. Arthralgias and arthritis accompany attacks in nearly 70% of patients, involving the large joints in a polyarticular fashion. Synovial aspirates show a leukocyte-rich fluid

Table 60.4 Diagnostic indicators for tumor necrosis factor receptor-associated periodic syndrome

Recurrent episodes of inflammatory symptoms spanning a period of more than 6 months' duration. Inflammatory symptoms include fever, abdominal pain, myalgia, rash, conjunctivitis/periorbital oedema, chest pain, and arthralgia or monoarticular synovitis
Episodes lasting more than 5 days
Responsiveness to glucocorticosteroids, but not colchicine
Affected family members (not always present)
Any ethnicity may be affected

negative for bacterial growth. Other findings in HIDS are splenomegaly, hepatomegaly, and tendinitis. After 4–6 days there is gradual defervescence, leaving patients completely asymptomatic in between attacks. Patients with HIDS have a normal life expectancy. The frequency and severity of attacks tend to decrease later in life.

It should be noted that the genetic abnormality in HIDS – mevalonate kinase deficiency – is also present in a more severe disease: mevalonatic aciduria. In this inborn error of metabolism there is also periodic fever, but the clinical picture is dominated by psychomotor retardation, ataxia, failure to thrive, cataract, and dysmorphic facies. Most patients die in early childhood.

Laboratory investigation

Laboratory evaluation at the time of attack reveals a vigorous acute-phase response with leukocytosis, raised serum concentrations of CRP, and proinflammatory cytokines such as IL-6, TNF-α, and interferon-γ. Even in between attacks, when patients are asymptomatic, half the patients have laboratory evidence of continuing inflammation. The principal laboratory finding is a persistent elevation of polyclonal immunoglobulin D (IgD). In 80% of patients this is accompanied by an elevation of IgA as well. IgD concentrations do not correlate with disease activity. The mechanism of elevation of IgD is unknown. During attacks traces of mevalonic acid in the plasma can be found, but the increase is only slight.

Diagnosis

The diagnosis of HIDS can be established by characteristic clinical findings in combination with persistent elevated IgD (> 100 IU/ml). Elevation of IgD is not pathognomonic as it also occurs in other inflammatory conditions, including FMF. Furthermore, in the very young, IgD levels can be normal, and in a small number of patients IgD levels remain

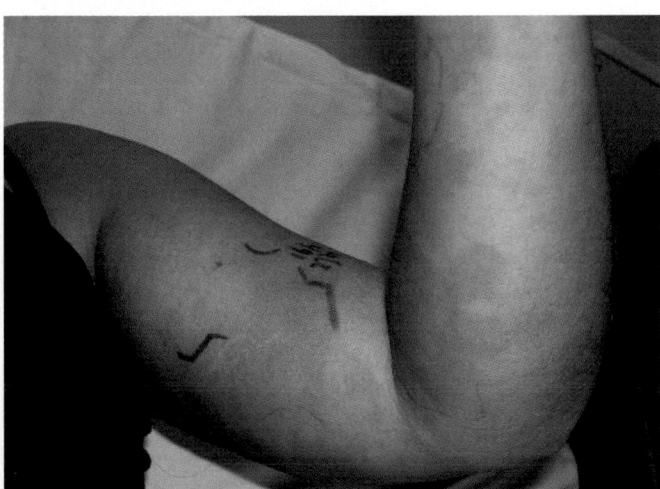

Fig. 60.4 Migrating erythemateous macular rash during an inflammatory attack in a tumor necrosis factor receptor associated periodic syndrome (TRAPS) patient.

low. The diagnosis can be confirmed by DNA analysis; however, in almost half the patients with a periodic fever, elevated acute-phase response, and elevated IgD, no mutations in *MVK* are found. The latter group, which has been described as variant HIDS,[9] suffers from less severe disease, usually with a later onset and IgD concentrations that are not as high as in classic HIDS.

AMYLOIDOSIS

Reactive or type AA amyloidosis is a serious complication of all autoinflammatory syndromes.[29] It is caused by the deposition of insoluble fibrils in the extracellular matrix of organs and tissues, most notable the kidneys, spleen, and liver. The fibrils are composed of a degradation product of SAA. Since SAA is an acute-phase reactant there is a close relationship between the continuous elevation of SAA and the development of amyloidosis. Before the recognition of colchicine as an effective treatment for FMF, amyloidosis occurred in up to 75% of patients. Even before the advent of effective treatment, not all FMF patients developed amyloidosis, suggesting that other factors contribute to the risk of developing amyloidosis.

In FMF there is a strong correlation between ethnicity and risk of amyloidosis, with the highest risk for Sephardic Jews. Another identified risk factor for developing amyloidosis is single nucleotide polymorphisms (SNPs) in the *SAA* gene. Two SNPs define three different SAA proteins: SAA 1.1, 1.3, and 1.5. Patients with the *SAA* 1.1/1.1 genotype have a three- to sevenfold increased risk of developing amyloidosis.[30]

Up to a quarter of TRAPS patients develop amyloidosis. There seems to be a strong family predilection. In some families almost all adults are affected whereas in other families no cases of amyloidosis are found. Hopefully, with the recent progression in treatment, the number of new cases of amyloidosis will decrease in the near future.

Although MWS was originally described as a triad of deafness, urticaria, and amyloidosis, not all patients with MWS develop amyloidosis. Approximately one-third of patients develop amyloidosis, and there is familial clustering. Several cases have been described in FCAS and NOMID, but numbers are too small to make an accurate estimate of the prevalence.

Patients with HIDS have a relatively small risk of developing amyloidosis. In fact, only recently the first cases of amyloidosis were described. Still there is a remarkably lower incidence of amyloidosis in HIDS compared to the other periodic fever syndromes, despite a similar acute-phase response.

A diagnosis of amyloidosis is confirmed by Congo red staining of affected tissues, showing a typical apple-green birefringence under polarized light microscopy (Fig. 60.5). Biopsy of subcutaneous fat or rectal tissue can be used to detect amyloid fibrils. If these are negative and there is a high index of suspicion, a direct biopsy from an affected organ can be considered.

The prognosis of patients with established amyloidosis is grave, with a median survival of 24–53 months. The natural history of amyloidosis is progression to renal failure. If inflammation cannot be controlled, amyloid deposits in a variety of organs (liver, spleen, gastrointestinal tract, heart) occur. As a consequence malabsorption with severe diarrhea may ensue. Cardiac failure and rhythm disturbances are typical manifestations of cardiac involvement. The progression of amyloidosis is strongly dependent on the ability to control the underlying inflammatory process.

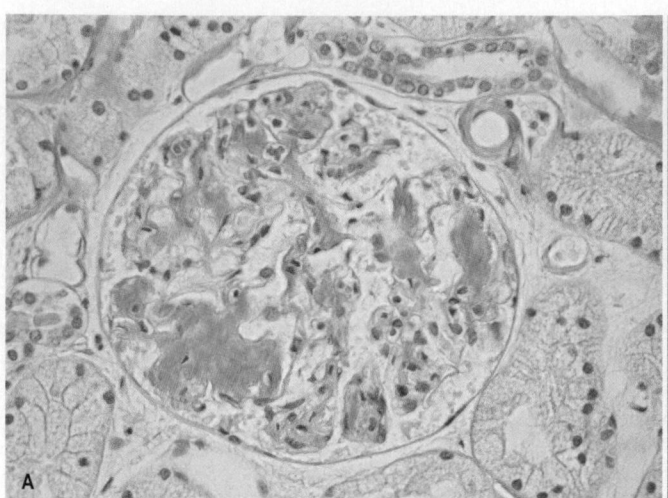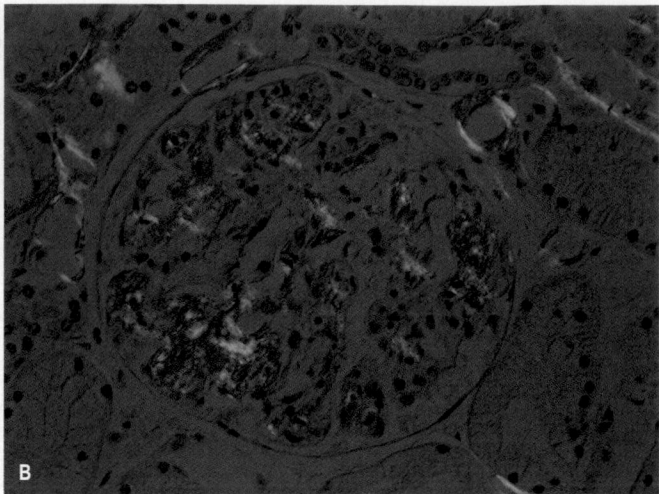

Fig. 60.5 Tissue section of a renal biopsy from a patient with AA amyloidosis. Amyloid deposits are visualized by staining with Congo red **(A)**. Under polarized light microscopy amyloid deposits shows typical apple-green birefringence **(B)**.

If the SAA concentration can be kept under 10 mg/l, progression of amyloidosis can be halted in many cases, and in some the amyloid mass even slowly regresses.[31]

■ TREATMENT ■

COLCHICINE

Colchicine is the treatment of choice in FMF.[32] It is highly effective in preventing attacks. In fact, it is so effective in preventing attacks that response to colchicine has been used as a clinical criterion for diagnosing FMF. The mechanism of action is unknown. Colchicine therapy is also very efficient in preventing amyloidosis. Therefore, all patients with FMF should receive colchicine, regardless of the severity and frequency of attacks. In patients who already have amyloidosis, intensive treatment can sometimes arrest progression or even partially reverse the process.

The average daily dose is 1 mg/day. In cases in which this is not sufficient to prevent attacks the dose can be increased to up to 3 mg. There is a small subset of patients who do not respond to colchicine. The most encountered side effect, gastrointestinal discomfort with diarrhea, usually resolves with dose reduction. Myopathy, neuropathy, and leukopenia are rare, but serious, side effects that primarily occur in patients with renal or liver impairment. In animal studies teratogenic effects are only seen at extremely high dosages. The potential teratogenic role of colchicine arises from its effect on microtubules, and there has been some concern that colchicine could therefore increase inborn errors, especially trisomy 21. However, recent data suggest that colchicine is safe to use during pregnancy. It can also be used while breastfeeding. In therapeutic dosages colchicine does not interfere with sperm quantity or quality. Furthermore, a clinical series of male patients on colchicine did not detect a negative effect on fertility. There is no place for colchicine in the treatment of autoinflammatory syndromes other than FMF.

SOLUBLE TNF RECEPTOR

The initial observation of reduced concentrations of soluble TNF receptors in the serum of TRAPS patients raised the possibility of etanercept as a therapeutic agent. Etanercept is a fusion protein consisting of two chains of the recombinant TNF-α receptor p75 monomere fused with the Fc domain of human IgG1. There are several reports of successful treatment with etanercept, although most patients do not have complete remission of symptoms. In TRAPS patients with established amyloidosis, etanercept can significantly reduce proteinuria. Etanercept has also been tried in HIDS with promising results in a small number of patients. The arthropathy in chronic infantile neurologic cutaneous and articular syndrome (CINCA) may respond to etanercept therapy.

ANAKINRA

Anakinra is a recombinant form of human IL-1Ra that competitively inhibits binding of IL-1α and IL-1β to the IL-1 receptor type 1. With the advances in the understanding of the genetic and molecular basis of the autoinflammatory syndromes, the concept emerged that IL-1β plays a key role in inflammation, and the successful intervention with anakinra in these syndromes provides the best evidence for such a role of IL-1. Recently there has been a focus on the effects of anakinra in CAPS, TRAPS, and HIDS, and although preliminary, the results are very promising. In 2003, Hawkins and Lachman described a patient with MWS who had been unsuccessfully treated with an array of immunosuppressive drugs, but who had a virtual instant and complete response to anakinra.[25] These beneficial effects were confirmed in a larger study of 22 patients. Anakinra is well tolerated and gives a complete resolution of fever, rash, conjunctivitis, and joint symptoms. Furthermore, because of the suppression of acute-phase reactants it can probably prevent amyloidosis.

These favorable results triggered research in other cryopyrin-associated syndromes. In NOMID, a similar dramatic response was found in a clinical study of 18 patients.[11] The skin rash disappears within 24 hours of start of treatment. Also, neurological symptoms resolve and in many patients hearing improves. Further, steroids can be tapered in the majority of patients. The follow-up has been too short to evaluate the effects of anakinra on prevention of bone deformities. FCAS also responds to anakinra treatment. In a well-designed provocation model, Hoffman et al. showed that anakinra effectively prevented attacks when given prior to cold stimulation.[23] In TRAPS no controlled trials are available, but there are reports in the literature indicating a similar improvement in symptoms.

Evidence is accumulating that blocking IL-1β is effective in treatment in HIDS.[33] Anakinra can prevent attacks when given before a trigger, and it has been shown effective in reducing attacks in severe cases. On theoretical grounds, anakinra may be effective in FMF, but since colchicine is so effective, this option has not been studied to a great extent. In a patient with colchicine-resistant FMF we observed a clinical response to anakinra.

An unsettled question is in which way anakinra should be given. One option is chronic suppression of the inflammatory response by daily injections, and this is probably the best regimen in the cryopyrin-associated syndromes, where there is continuous inflammation. In HIDS and TRAPS it is less clear. Here, one may consider patient-initiated treatment at the first sign of an attack. It is unclear as yet how long treatment should be given under these circumstances. With continuous treatment with anakinra in TRAPS we have observed breakthrough attacks, of which the mechanisms are unclear. Under such circumstances we have been able to induce a remission for several weeks with a couple of intravenous injections of 300 mg of anakinra. The latter observation suggests that in patients who do not readily respond to anakinra, a higher dose (intravenously) should be considered.

CORTICOSTEROIDS

A course of steroids (30 mg daily for 1 week) can be used to treat attacks of TRAPS. Severe attacks may respond to high doses of corticosteroids, such as 1 g methylprednisolone infusion. Corticosteroids, however, while reducing the severity of symptoms, do not alter the frequency of attacks, and often escalating dosages are needed over time. In NOMID, corticosteroids can ameliorate skin manifestations and joint symptoms, but remission cannot usually be induced. Corticosteroid treatment is ineffective in FMF and HIDS.

SIMVASTATIN

The possibility that the inflammatory phenotype in HIDS is caused by an excess of mevalonic acid would make an inhibitor of the preceding enzyme, i.e., HMG-coA reductase inhibitors, a therapeutic option. A small controlled trial has demonstrated some advantage of simvastatin over placebo in terms of reduction of the number of days of illness, but the overall efficacy is limited.[34]

OTHER IMMUNOSUPPRESSIVE DRUGS

Testament to the problems in treating the autoinflammatory diseases are the multiple therapeutic agents that have been tried. The often disabling features and the lack of therapeutic agents might lead to a trial-and-error practice exposing these patients to empirical treatment with an array of immunomodulating drugs, such as Cyclosporine, thalidomide, dapsone, azathioprine, mycophenol, and infliximab. Results are disappointing and there is no evidence to support the use of these agents.

CLINICAL PEARL

An 18-year-old woman was seen because of recurrences of fever and skin rash. Her medical history started 2 hours after birth when a maculopapular skin rash appeared, resembling the systemic rash of juvenile chronic arthritis. The rash remained present on a daily basis, but was not triggered or exacerbated by cold exposure. At the age of 2 years, the patient developed fever episodes, approximately 3 days per week. Typically, she had a single fever spike a day, usually in the evening, and body temperature was in the range of 39°C.

The patient is of European ancestry and the family history is negative for autoinflammatory conditions. Articular symptoms were absent, and she had a normal audiometry, while dysmorphic features, meningitis, myalgias, abdominal pain, and lymphadenopathy were absent.

Based on the clinical presentation (daily rash and spiking fever), a cryopyrin-associated periodic syndrome (CAPS) was suspected and targeted gene analysis performed. This showed an R260W mutation of the *CIAS1* gene. This mutation has been found in Muckle–Wells syndrome as well as in patients with familial cold autoinflammatory syndrome. Thus, the patient has a CAPS. However, since she has symptoms consistent with each of the three separate disease entities and lacks other distinguishing symptoms, the patient should not be classified in one of the three distinct syndromes. This illustrates that CAPS is a continuous spectrum of diseases that show great phenotypical overlap. After making the diagnosis the patient was successfully treated with anakinra.

CONCLUSION

The autoinflammatory syndromes are a still expanding group of disorders, characterized by incapacitating attacks of inflammation. In recent years, the genetic background, the molecular pathophysiology, the focus point of the inflammasome, and a key role for IL-1 have surfaced. These insights have provided us with tools for diagnosis and counseling and also for effective treatment. An important challenge is to find other – preferably orally effective – drugs that interfere with IL-1 action.

Although the autoinflammatory syndromes are rare, the study of these diseases has contributed to the insight into important mechanisms of inflammation in general. In the future, with advancing knowledge, we expect new syndromes to be discovered that can contribute to further insight into basic mechanisms of inflammation.

REFERENCES

1. Drenth JPH, van der Meer JWM. Hereditary periodic fever. N Engl J Med 2001; 345: 1748–1757.

2. Touitou I. The spectrum of familial Mediterranean fever (FMF) mutations. Eur J Hum Genet 2001; 9: 473–483.

3. van der Meer JWM, Vossen JM, Radl J, et al. Hyperimmunoglobulinaemia D and periodic fever: a new syndrome. Lancet 1984; 1: 1087–1090.

Table 61.1 Revised Sapporo Classification Criteria for the Antiphospholipid Syndrome.[1]

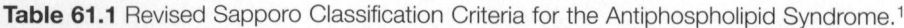

Clinical criteria

1. Vascular thrombosis:[1]
(a) One or more clinical episodes[2] of arterial, venous, or small vessel thrombosis[3], in any tissue or organ
2. Pregnancy morbidity:
(a) One or more unexplained deaths of a morphologically normal fetus at or beyond the 10th week of gestation, *or*
(b) One or more premature births of a morphologically normal neonate before the 34th week of gestation because of eclampsia, severe pre-eclampsia, or recognized features of placental insufficiency[4], *or*
(c) Three or more unexplained consecutive spontaneous abortions before the 10th week of gestation, with maternal anatomic or hormonal abnormalities and paternal and maternal chromosomal causes excluded

Laboratory criteria[5]

1. Lupus anticoagulant present in plasma, on two or more occasions at least 12 weeks apart, detected according to the guidelines of the International Society on Thrombosis and Hemostasis
2. Anticardiolipin antibody of IgG and/or IgM isotype in serum or plasma, present in medium or high titer (i.e. >40 GPL or MPL, or >the 99th percentile), on two or more occasions, at least 12 weeks apart, measured by a standardized enzyme-linked immunosorbent assay (ELISA).
3. Anti-β_2 glycoprotein-I antibody of IgG and/or IgM isotype in serum or plasma, (in titer >the 99th percentile) present on two or more occasions, at least 12 weeks apart, measured by a standardized ELISA

Definite APS is present if at least one of the clinical criteria and one of the laboratory criteria are met. Classification of APS should be avoided if less than 12 weeks or more than 5 years separate the positive aPL test and the clinical manifestation. In studies of populations of patients who have more than one type of pregnancy morbidity, investigators are strongly encouraged to stratify groups of subjects according to a, b, or c above.

[1]Coexisting inherited or acquired factors for thrombosis are not reasons for excluding patients from APS trials. However, two subgroups of APS patients should be recognized, according to: (a) the presence, and (b) the absence of additional risk factors for thrombosis. Indicative (but not exhaustive) such cases include: age (>55 in men, and >65 in women), and the presence of any of the established risk factors for cardiovascular disease (hypertension, diabetes mellitus, elevated LDL or low HDL cholesterol, cigarette smoking, family history of premature cardiovascular disease, body mass index ≥30 kg/m2, microalbuminuria, estimated GFR <60 mL/min), inherited thrombophilias, oral contraceptives, nephritic syndrome, malignancy, immobilization, and surgery. Thus, patients who fulfill criteria should be stratified according to contributing causes of thrombosis.
[2]A thrombotic episode in the past could be considered as a clinical criterion, provided that thrombosis is proved by appropriate diagnostic means and that no alternative diagnosis or cause of thrombosis is found.
[3]Superficial venous thrombosis is not included in the clinical criteria.
[4]Generally accepted features of placental insufficiency include: (i) abnormal or non-reassuring fetal surveillance test(s), e.g. a non-reactive non-stress test, suggestive of fetal hypoxemia, (ii) abnormal Doppler flow velocimetry waveform analysis suggestive of fetal hypoxemia, e.g. absent end-diastolic flow in the umbilical artery, (iii) oligohydramnios, e.g. an amniotic fluid index of 5 cm or less, or (iv) a postnatal birth weight less than the 10th percentile for the gestational age.
[5]Investigators are strongly advised to classify APS patients in studies into one of the following categories: I, more than one laboratory criteria present (any combination); IIa, LA present alone; IIb, aCL antibody present alone; IIc, anti-β_2-glycoprotein-I antibody present alone.

β_2-glycoprotein-I polymorphisms influence the generation of aPL in individuals, but have only a weak relationship to the occurrence of aPL-related clinical events.[15] Persons congenitally lacking β_2GPI?[16] and β_2GPI-knockout mice[17] appear normal.

In humans, although cross-sectional and prospective cohort studies demonstrate that aPL can predict future thrombosis, the pathogenic mechanism is unknown; more than one mechanism may be involved, as outlined in Table 61.2. Because high-titer antibody may persist for years in asymptomatic persons, and because positive aPL tests may precede symptoms for many years, it is likely that vascular injury and/or endothelial cell activation immediately precede thrombosis in those bearing the antibody. Platelet activation followed by binding of aPL to platelet membrane phospholipid-bound annexins may initiate platelet adhesion and thrombosis.[18] Antiphospholipid antibodies may inhibit phospholipid-dependent reactions in the coagulation cascade, for example fibrinolysis, antithrombin III activity, or protein C and protein S activation.[19] Interaction between aPL

KEY CONCEPTS

>> Antiphospholipid antibodies (aPL) exist as a family of autoantibodies directed against phospholipid-binding plasma proteins, most commonly β_2-glycoprotein-I.

>> The origin of aPL is unknown but is hypothesized to be an incidental exposure to environmental agents inducing aPL in susceptible individuals.

>> In humans, although cross-sectional and prospective cohort studies demonstrate that aPL can predict future thrombosis, the pathogenic mechanism is unknown; more than one mechanism may be involved.

>> Concomitant prothrombotic risk factors may promote clotting in an additive manner in aPL-positive patients

Table 61.2 Possible mechanisms of aPL-induced thrombosis

Endothelial cells–aPL interaction

Endothelial cell damage or activation (via increased expression of adhesion molecules)
Coexisting anti-endothelial antibodies
aPL-induced monocyte adhesion to endothelial cells
Increased tissue factor expression

Platelet–aPL interaction

Platelet activation
Stimulation of thromboxane production

Coagulation system–aPL interaction

Inhibition of activation of protein C by the thrombomodulin–thrombin complex
Inhibition of activation of protein C via its cofactor protein S
Interaction between aPL and substrates of activated protein C such as Factors Va and VIIIa
Interaction between aPL and an annexin V anticoagulant shield

Complement activation

Table 61.3 The clinical spectrum of antiphospholipid antibodies (aPL)

Asymptomatic* aPL-positivity

Antiphospholipid syndrome with vascular events

Catastrophic antiphospholipid syndrome

Antiphospholipid syndrome with only pregnancy morbidity

Asymptomatic* aPL-positivity with noncriteria aPL manifestations

*No history of thrombosis or pregnancy morbidity as per the Sapporo Criteria [1]

---

and an annexin V anticoagulant shield is another proposed but less well accepted mechanism.[20] Recent studies also demonstrate that aPL increase tissue factor (a physiologic initiator of coagulation) expression on monocytes.[21] A cluster of 50 upregulated genes may distinguish between aPL-positive patients with and without thrombosis.[22]

In experimental animal models, aPL causes fetal resorption (a proxy for recurrent fetal loss) and increase in size and duration of trauma-induced venous and arterial thrombi. Inhibiting complement activation prevents experimental aPL-induced fetal death, and C5 knockout mice carry pregnancies normally despite the presence of aPL, implying that a complement-mediated effector mechanism is an absolute requirement for fetal death to occur.[23]

In the currently accepted 'second-hit hypothesis,' a second trigger event (such as oral contraceptive use or surgical procedures), which may not otherwise be sufficient to cause thrombosis, may be necessary for an asymptomatic aPL-positive patient to develop thrombosis. Acquired (oral contraceptive use) and heritable thrombotic risk factors (deficiencies of protein C, protein S, or antithrombin III; mutations of factor V [A506G, factor V_{Leiden}], prothrombin [G20210A], or methylene tetrahydrofolate reductase [MTHFR C677T, hyperhomocysteinemia]) may increase the risk of aPL patients (see Table 61.1 footnote).

A proposed pathogenesis for aPL-mediated thrombosis and placental injury begins with the activation or apoptosis (by unknown triggers, possibly infectious or traumatic) of platelets, endothelial cells, or trophoblast. The negatively charged phosphatidylserine migrates from the inner to the normally electrically neutral outer cell membrane. Circulating β_2GPI then binds to phosphatidylserine, followed by the aPL binding to a β_2GPI dimer, activating complement and, through C5a, initiating a signaling cascade that induces cell surface tissue factor (TF) expression and adhesion molecules (e.g., ICAM-1). Other components of the innate immune system can also be activated. Platelets aggregate and initiate

thrombosis. In addition, aPL adversely affect the formation of a trophoblast syncytium, placental apoptosis, and trophoblast invasion, all processes required for normal establishment of placental function. *In vitro*, pathogenic aPL induce adhesion molecules and enhance adherence of leukocytes to cultured endothelial cells.

DIAGNOSIS

CLINICAL MANIFESTATIONS

The clinical manifestations of aPL represent a spectrum from asymptomatic to catastrophic APS (Table 61.3). The principal manifestations of APS are venous or arterial thromboses and pregnancy loss. Except for its severity, the youth of affected patients, and unusual anatomic locations (Budd–Chiari syndrome and sagittal sinus and upper extremity thromboses), thromboses in APS do not clinically differ from thromboses attributable to other causes. Stroke and transient ischemic attack are the most common presentation of arterial thrombosis, whereas deep vein thrombosis, often accompanied by pulmonary embolism, is the most common venous manifestation of APS. Glomerular capillary endothelial cell injury or thrombosis of renal vessels (thrombotic microangiopathy) causes proteinuria without celluria or hypocomplementemia and may lead to severe hypertension and/or renal failure.

Many patients have livedo reticularis (a lattice-like pattern of superficial skin veins) (Fig. 61.1), cardiac valve disease (vegetations, valve thickening and dysfunction), or other nonthrombotic manifestations described in several studies but not included in the revised Sapporo criteria[1] owing to nonspecificity or rarity (Table 61.4). These manifestations do not by themselves classify a patient as having APS for clinical studies, but they add information to the diagnosis of individual patients. The pathogenesis of cardiac valve disease in APS is unknown; valve replacement may be necessary. A putative association of aPL and increased risk of atherosclerosis exists but is controversial; in studies of atherosclerosis in patients with SLE, aPL protected against atherosclerosis.[24] Some patients develop nonfocal neurologic symptoms, such as lack of concentration, forgetfulness, and dizzy spells. Multiple small, hyperintense lesions seen on magnetic resonance imaging (MRI), primarily in the periventricular white matter, do not correlate well with clinical symptoms (Fig. 61.2).

Pregnancy losses in patients with aPL typically occur after 10 weeks' gestation (fetal loss), but early losses also occur (pre-embryonic or embryonic losses).[25] APS patients may develop severe, early pre-eclampsia and HELLP

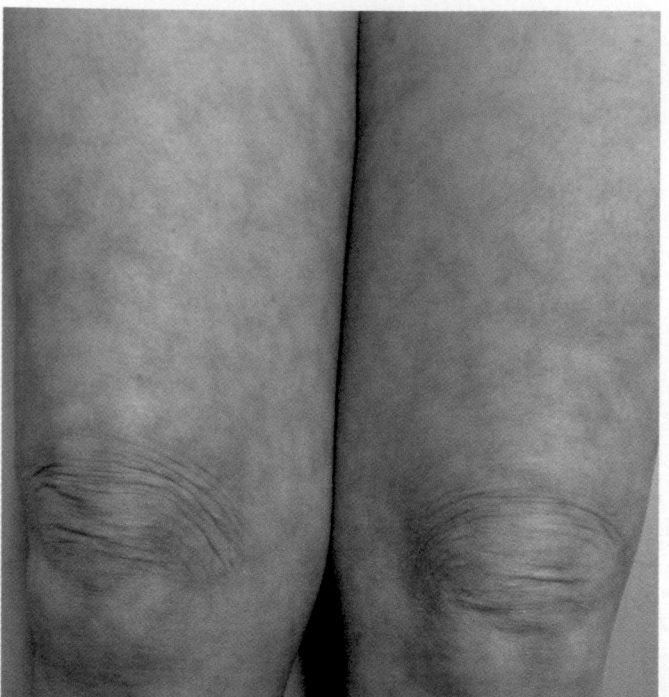

Fig. 61.1 Livedo reticularis in a patient with primary antiphospholipid syndrome.

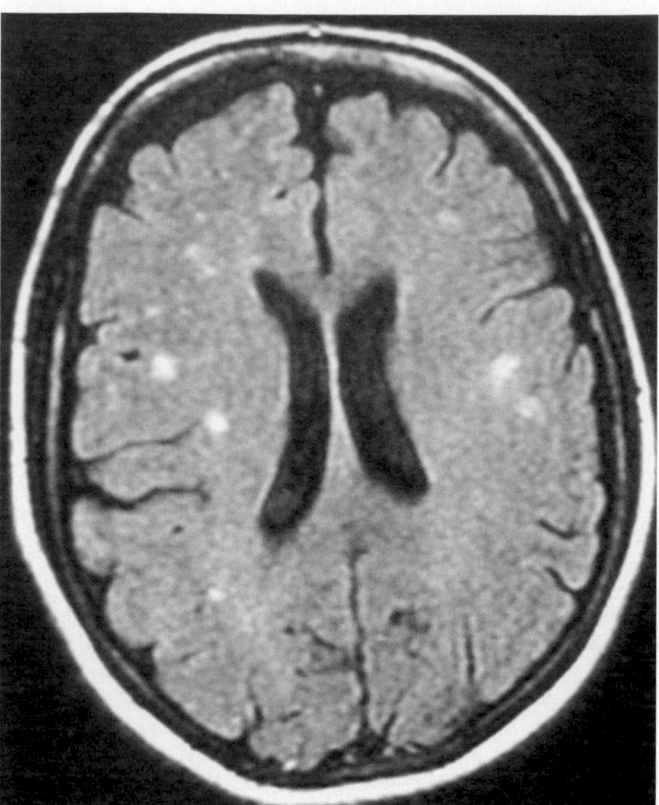

Fig. 61.2 Magnetic resonance imaging demonstrating multiple periventricular white matter hyperintense lesions.

(*h*emolysis, *e*levated *l*iver enzymes, *l*ow *p*latelets) syndrome. Although placental infarction may be a cause of fetal growth restriction or death, nonthrombotic mechanisms of placental dysfunction are probably more important.

Catastrophic APS (CAPS) is a rare, abrupt, life-threatening complication. It consists of multiple thromboses of medium and small arteries occurring (despite apparently adequate anticoagulation) over a period of days, causing stroke, cardiac, hepatic, adrenal, renal, and intestinal infarction and peripheral gangrene. Proposed formal criteria for this syndrome are shown in Table 61.5.[26] Acute adrenal failure may be the initial clinical event, often heralded by unexplained back pain and vascular collapse (e.g., severe hypotension) CAPS patients often have moderate thrombocytopenia; erythrocytes are less fragmented than in the hemolytic–uremic syndrome or thrombotic thrombocytopenic purpura; fibrin split products are not strikingly elevated. Renal failure and pulmonary hemorrhage may occur. Tissue biopsies show noninflammatory vascular occlusion of both very small and medium-sized vessels.

Antibodies to prothrombin (factor II) sometimes accompany aPL[27] and may cause hemorrhage by depleting prothrombin (lupus anticoagulant hypoprothrombinemia syndrome).[28]

LABORATORY TESTS

In the presence of characteristic clinical events, APS is diagnosed when patients have persistent aPL that includes moderate- to high-titer IgG and/or IgM aCL, moderate- to high-titer IgG and/or IgM aβ_2GPI, and/or positive lupus anticoagulant test.[1] Approximately 80% of patients with positive LA tests have aCL, and 20% of patients positive for aCL,

have positive LA tests. IgA aCL can occur rarely as the only aPL in APS patients; some of these patients are aCL negative, but only aβ_2GPI positive. These tests (IgA aCL and aβ_2GPI), when positive, justify a diagnosis of APS in LA and aCL IgG/M test-negative patients with clinically typical disease. Lupus anticoagulant test-positive patients have a higher risk for thrombosis than do LA test-negative patients.[1] Although several studies state that aβ_2GPI-positive patients are also at higher thrombosis risk, these claims are inconsistent.[29]

The lupus anticoagulant test is a functional coagulation assay that measures the ability of aPL to inhibit the conversion of prothrombin to thrombin. Guidelines of the International Society on Thrombosis and Hemostasis[30] for the diagnosis of LA require: (a) demonstration of a prolonged phospholipid-dependent coagulation screening test, such as activated partial thromboplastin time (aPTT) or dilute Russell viper venom time (dRVVT); (b) failure to correct the prolonged screening test by mixing the patient plasma with normal platelet-poor plasma, demonstrating the presence of an inhibitor; (c) shortening or correction of the prolonged screening test by the addition of excess phospholipid, demonstrating phospholipid dependency; and (d) the exclusion of other coagulopathies. A positive screening coagulation test without confirmatory steps is not a positive LA test.

Interpretation of positive tests should take into account the following rules: moderate- to high-titer (> 40 U) aCL is more strongly associated with clinical events than is low-titer aCL;[1] LA is a more specific but less

Table 61.4 Noncriteria features of the antiphospholipid syndrome

Type	Features
Clinical	Livedo reticularis Cardiac valve disease Autoimmune hemolytic anemia Thrombocytopenia (usually 50 000–100 000/mm3) Multiple sclerosis-like syndrome and other myelopathy Nonfocal neurologic symptoms Chorea
Laboratory	IgA anticardiolipin and anti-β_2-glycoprotein-I antibodies Anti-phosphatidylserine, phosphatidylinositol, phosphatidylglycerol, hosphatidylethanolamine antibodies Anti-prothrombin antibodies Anti-phosphatidylserine–prothrombin antibodies

Table 61.5 Preliminary criteria for the classification of catastrophic APS[26]

1. Evidence of involvement of three or more organs, systems, and/or tissues[1]

2. Development of manifestations simultaneously or in less than 1 week

3. Confirmation by histopathology of small vessel occlusion in at least one organ or tissue[2]

4. Laboratory confirmation of the presence of aPL[3]

Definite catastrophic APS:
  All four criteria

Probable catastrophic APS:
  Criteria 2–4 and two organs, systems and/or tissues involved
  Criteria 1–3, except no aPL confirmation 6 weeks apart due to the early death of a patient not tested before catastrophic episode
  Criteria 1, 2, 4; or
  Criteria 1, 3, 4 and development of a third event more than 1 week but less than 1 month after first, despite anticoagulation

[1]Usually, clinical evidence of vessel occlusions, confirmed by imaging techniques when appropriate. Renal involvement is defined by a 50% rise in serum creatinine, severe systemic hypertension and/or proteinuria.
[2]For histopathological confirmation, significant evidence of thrombosis must be present, although vasculitis may occasionally coexist.
[3]If the patient had not been previously diagnosed as having APS, laboratory confirmation requires that presence of aPL must be detected on two or more occasions at least 6 weeks apart (not necessarily at the time of the event), according to the proposed preliminary criteria for the classification of APS.

sensitive predictor of thromboses than is aCL[31]; multiple positive aPL tests impart a worse prognosis than does any single type of test; and positive aPL tests require a repeat test after 12 weeks to exclude transient aPL.[1]

Laboratory variability in these assays is moderately high: stability of assay in individual patients over time is assured about 80% of the time.[32] Based on same-day specimens, the consistency of aCL results among different commercial laboratories ranges from 64% to 88%, with moderate agreement for IgG and IgM, and with marginal agreement for aCL IgA.[32]

Antiphospholipid antibody tests developed based on phosphatidylserine, phosphatidylinositol, phosphatidylethanolamine or prothrombin are not well standardized or widely accepted; their clinical significance is unknown. A false positive test for syphilis is not diagnostic for APS.

Antinuclear and anti-DNA antibodies occur in approximately 45% of APS patients who are not diagnosed as having SLE. Thrombocytopenia in APS is usually modest (>50 000/mm3); proteinuria and renal insufficiency occur in patients with thrombotic microangiopathy. Erythrocyte sedimentation rate (ESR), hemoglobin, and leukocyte count are usually normal in patients with uncomplicated APS, except during acute thrombosis. Complement levels are usually normal or only modestly low.

IMAGING STUDIES

Magnetic resonance imaging (MRI) studies show vascular occlusion and infarction consistent with clinical symptoms, without special characteristics, except that multiple otherwise unexplained cerebral infarctions in a

CLINICAL PEARLS

>> The clinical manifestations of aPL represent a spectrum (from asymptomatic to catastrophic antiphospholipid syndrome [APS]); thus patients should not be evaluated and managed as having a single disease manifestation.

>> Stroke and transient ischemic attack are the most common presentation of arterial thrombosis; deep vein thrombosis, often accompanied by pulmonary embolism, is the most common venous manifestation of APS.

>> Pregnancy losses in patients with aPL typically occur after 10 weeks' gestation (fetal loss), but early losses also occur (pre-embryonic or embryonic losses).

>> Catastrophic APS is a rare, abrupt, life-threatening complication of APS, which consists of multiple thromboses of medium and small arteries occurring over a period of days.

>> Antiphospholipid syndrome diagnosis should be made in the presence of characteristic clinical manifestations and *persistently* (at least 12 weeks apart) positive aPL.

young person suggest the syndrome. Multiple small hyperintense white matter lesions are common and do not unequivocally imply brain infarction (Fig. 61.2). Occlusions usually occur in vessels below the resolution limits of angiography; hence angiography or magnetic resonance angiography is not indicated unless clinical findings suggest medium or large vessel disease. Echocardiography or cardiac MRI may show severe Libman–Sacks endocarditis and intracardiac thrombi.

PATHOLOGIC STUDIES

Skin, renal, and other tissues show noninflammatory occlusion of all caliber arteries and veins, acute and chronic endothelial injury and its sequelae, and recanalization in late lesions. The finding of inflammatory necrotizing vasculitis suggests concomitant SLE or other connective tissue disease. There are no other diagnostic immunofluorescence or electron microscopic findings.

TREATMENT

Treatment recommendations for persistently aPL-positive patients are summarized in Table 61.6. Anticoagulation with unfractionated heparin or low molecular weight heparin (LMWH) followed by warfarin is the treatment for APS patients with vascular events. Heparin inhibits complement, a fact that theoretically makes it a preferred but impractical agent except in the treatment of pregnancies. For those patients with a positive LA test that elevates the aPTT, the heparin dose can be monitored by measuring peak and trough activated Factor Xa levels. For well-anticoagulated patients who continue to have thromboses, antiplatelet drugs, hydroxychloroquine, statins, intravenous immunoglobulin (IVIG), and plasmapheresis have a theoretical basis for efficacy and have all been used. Rituximab is under experimental evaluation. Clinical experience suggests that thrombolytic agents for acute thrombosis are unhelpful,

because re-occlusion rapidly occurs. There are no systematic studies of treatment for catastrophic APS. Detailed reviews conclude that the most effective treatment combines full-dose anticoagulation, high-dose corticosteroid, plasma exchange, and IVIG.[33]

Recent prospective controlled studies conclude that recurrence of thromboses in APS patients can be prevented with moderate-intensity warfarin to an international normalized ratio (INR) of 2.0–3.0.[34, 35] Although these studies provide strong evidence for moderate-intensity anticoagulation following an aPL-related venous event, the intensity of the anticoagulation is still a matter of debate for APS patients with arterial events, because such patients constituted a minority of patients in these controlled studies. Although some APS patients may require high-intensity anticoagulation, in the absence of risk-stratified studies the definition of high-risk is currently based on clinical judgment. No prospective controlled data demonstrate the superiority of high-intensity anticoagulation in APS patients.

Most aPL-positive patients receive warfarin after ischemic strokes; however, the Antiphospholipid Antibody in Stroke Study (APASS) concluded that for selected aPL-positive patients who have neither atrial fibrillation nor high-grade arterial stenosis, aspirin and warfarin therapy (at an INR of 2.2) are equivalent in both efficacy and major bleeding complications.[36] The generalizability of these results is limited, however, as the study group had an average age of 60 years (much higher than the average for APS population), the aPL determination was performed only once at study entry, and the cut-off for assigning a patient to the positive aCL group was very low. However, based on APASS results, aspirin is an option for patients with a single low positive aCL test who present with stroke.

Venous thrombosis in aPL-positive patients has a high recurrence rate if anticoagulation is discontinued, and lifelong anticoagulation is usually recommended. It is unknown whether patients whose event was triggered by an acquired and reversible thrombotic risk factor can discontinue anticoagulation or switch to aspirin when the trigger factor is eliminated. Normalization of the LA or aCL tests is *not* a clear indication to discontinue anticoagulation.

Asymptomatic persons serendipitously found to have aPL need no preventive therapy. Elimination of reversible thrombosis risk factors (smoking, oral contraceptives) and prophylaxis during high-risk periods (such as surgical interventions or prolonged immobilization) are advised for primary thrombosis prophylaxis in persistently aPL-positive individuals. The necessity for and effectiveness of low-dose aspirin in asymptomatic aPL-positive patients remains to be demonstrated. Estrogen and estrogen-containing oral contraceptives are deemed unsafe for APS patients, or even for asymptomatic women serendipitously known to bear high-titer antibody. There is no reliable information regarding the safety of progestin-only contraceptives, 'morning after' contraception, or raloxifene, bromocriptine, or leuprolide in APS patients. However, progestin-only contraception is theoretically safer than estrogen-based contraception. A small retrospective review of women undergoing artificial reproductive technology (IVF) procedures demonstrated no thrombotic events.

Persistence of aPL for decades without clinical events is well documented, although some patients with positive aPL tests have clinical events of ambiguous meaning (dizzy or confusional episodes, nonspecific visual disturbance, very early pregnancy loss). There is no consensus for the treatment of such persons. Because full anticoagulation carries a high risk, many physicians prescribe low-dose (81 mg) aspirin daily and/or hydroxychloroquine. No published data support or repudiate this

Table 61.6 Treatment recommendations in persistently antiphospholipid antibody-positive patients

Clinical circumstance	Recommendation
Asymptomatic	No treatment*
Venous or arterial thrombosis	Warfarin INR 2–3.0 indefinitely
Recurrent thrombosis	Warfarin INR 3–3.5 indefinitely ± low-dose aspirin
First pregnancy	No treatment*
Single pregnancy loss, <10 weeks	No treatment*
Recurrent fetal loss or loss after 10 weeks, history of no thrombosis	Prophylactic dose** heparin with low-dose aspirin throughout the pregnancy, discontinue heparin 6–12 weeks postpartum
Recurrent fetal loss or loss after 10 weeks, history of thrombosis	Therapeutic dose heparin*** with low-dose aspirin throughout pregnancy, warfarin postpartum
Catastrophic APS	Anticoagulation + corticosteroids + intravenous immunoglobulin or plasma exchange
Livedo reticularis	No treatment
Valve nodules or deformity	No known effective treatment; full anticoagulation if emboli or intracardiac thrombi is demonstrated
Thrombocytopenia >50 000/mm^3	No treatment
Thrombocytopenia, <50 000/mm^3	Prednisone and/or intravenous immunoglobulin

*Aspirin 81 mg/day may be given
**Prophylactic dose such as enoxaperin 30–40 mg subcutaneously (SQ) once daily.
***Therapeutic dose such as enoxaperin 1 mg/kg SQ twice daily or 1.5 mg/kg SQ once daily

recommendation. Corticosteroids and/or IVIG are the first-line treatments for platelet counts less than 50 000/mm3.

Pregnancy is a prothrombotic state; management strategies in persistently aPL-positive patients should focus on prevention of both pregnancy morbidity and maternal thrombotic complications.[37] In pregnancy, a combination of heparin and low-dose aspirin increases fetal survival rate from 50% to 80% among women who have had a fetal loss and who have unequivocally positive tests for aPL. If patients fail this regimen, the next step is to add IVIG, an approach not supported by controlled studies. Most experts in the field now use LMWH such as enoxaparin because of the lower risk of thrombocytopenia and osteoporosis: prophylactic doses for women who have had only pregnancy morbidity, or full anticoagulant doses for women who have had prior thromboses (Table 61.5). Treatment begins after confirmation of pregnancy, continues until 48 hours before anticipated delivery (to allow epidural anesthesia), and resumes for 8–12 weeks postpartum. No studies unequivocally justify the treatment of young women with aPL during a first pregnancy, women with only very early losses, or women whose aPL titers are low or transient. Nonetheless, it is common to offer such patients low-dose aspirin.

Serious perioperative complications may occur despite prophylaxis. APS patients are at additional risk for thrombosis when they undergo surgery. Thus, perioperative strategies should be clearly identified before any surgical procedure, pharmacological and physical anti-thrombosis interventions vigorously employed, periods without anticoagulation kept to an absolute minimum, and any deviation from a normal course be considered a potential disease-related event.[38]

THERAPEUTIC PRINCIPLES

>> Secondary thrombosis prevention in persistently aPL-positive individuals lack a risk-stratified approach; although the current recommendation is lifelong warfarin, the *intensity* and *duration* of warfarin treatment are still debated. The effectiveness of high-intensity anticoagulation in APS patients with vascular events is not supported by prospective controlled studies.

>> Primary thrombosis prevention in persistently aPL-positive individuals lacks an evidence-based approach; elimination of reversible thrombosis risk factors and prophylaxis during high-risk periods (such as surgical procedures) are crucial.

>> Catastrophic APS patients usually receive a combination of anticoagulation, corticosteroids, intravenous immunoglobulin (IVIG), and plasma exchange.

>> A common strategy to prevent fetal loss in aPL-positive patients with history of pregnancy morbidities is low-dose aspirin and heparin; if patients fail this regimen, the next step is to add IVIG, although this approach is not supported by controlled studies.

>> Currently, there is no evidence that anticoagulation is effective for nonthrombotic manifestations of aPL, such as livedo reticularis, thrombocytopenia, hemolytic anemia, or heart valve disease.

TREATMENT

part

ORGAN SPECIFIC INFLAMMATORY DISEASE

Immunohematologic disorders

Pierre Noel, Margaret E. Rick, McDonald Horne, Roger Kurlander, Steven J. Lemery

■ IMMUNE-MEDIATED ANEMIA ■

Immune-mediated hemolysis can be autoimmune or alloimmune, idiopathic or secondary to drugs or other diseases, but it consistently involves either immunoglobulin G (IgG) or IgM (rarely IgA) antibodies to antigens on the red cell membrane (Table 62.1).[1,2]

ANTI-ERYTHROCYTE ANTIBODIES AND THEIR ANTIGENS

The antigens for anti-erythrocyte IgG are usually proteins, including the clinically important antigens (D, C, c, E, e) on the Rh-associated glycoprotein (RhAG).[3] In contrast, anti-erythrocyte IgM is directed at polysaccharides, which include the ABO and I-antigens (I, i) found on the anion and glucose transporter proteins in the red cell membrane.[4,5] During the first few months after birth isoantibodies to A and B develop if these antigens are absent on the neonate's red cells. The isoantibodies presumably follow exposure to A and B antigens present on plants and bacteria ubiquitous in the environment.

IgG and IgM antibodies are also distinguished by being 'warm-' and 'cold-' reactive respectively, meaning that they can bind to their antigens at core body temperature (warm) or they bind preferentially at lower temperatures (cold) in the peripheral circulation or *ex vivo*. This distinction results from the different thermodynamics of binding to protein (hydrophobic) and polysaccharide (electrostatic) antigens.[5]

IgG and IgM also differ in their ability to fix complement, and this affects their mechanism of hemolysis. In order to attach the first component of complement, two IgG molecules must bind to the red cell in close proximity. However, because of its pentameric structure, a single IgM molecule can initiate complement activation.

MECHANISMS OF ANTIBODY-MEDIATED HEMOLYSIS

Erythrocyte-bound IgG becomes attached to the Fc receptors of splenic macrophages, which may engulf all or part of the cell or release lysosomal enzymes that digest its membrane (antibody-dependent

cell-mediated cytotoxicity: ADCC).[6] Red cell fragments escaping from this encounter lose more membrane than cytoplasm and become spherical to compensate for this change in their surface-to-volume ratio. If IgG has initiated complement activation on the cell surface, phagocytosis in the spleen will be augmented by binding of C3b to splenic macrophages.[7]

When IgM fixes complement, the process begins in the cooler peripheral circulation where the IgM can bind to the red cells. If the amount of IgM bound is relatively high and if at least some of it remains on the cell at 37°C (e.g., anti-A or anti-B isoantibodies), the cascade of complement reactions goes to completion. Doughnut-shaped holes are formed in the cell membrane that allow the influx of water and sodium, inducing intravascular osmotic rupture of the cell.[6] However, if the IgM elutes from the red cell as it returns to body core temperature, the complement reactions diminish. Under these circumstances the components remain on the cell but do not cause intravascular hemolysis. Instead, they can be cleared by hepatic macrophages with complement-binding sites.[8]

PATHOPHYSIOLOGIC CONSEQUENCES OF HEMOLYSIS

Antibody-mediated hemolysis causes variable degrees of anemia and reticulocytosis. Intravascular hemolysis releases hemoglobin into the circulation. However, the amount of hemoglobin swept away as macrophages are engulfing red cells is generally too small to cause measurable hemoglobinemia, but it will result in consumption of haptoglobin, which quickly becomes depleted. In contrast, when hemolysis results from by complement-mediated lysis, such as follows an ABO-incompatible blood transfusion, hemoglobinemia becomes massive, overcoming the scavaging capacity of plasma hemoglobin binders (haptoglobin, hemopexin, albumin) and resulting in hemoglobinuria. Because hemoglobin is toxic to the renal tubular epithelium, renal function may become impaired. Red cell membrane fragments released by massive intravascular hemolysis are procoagulant and can cause disseminated intravascular coagulation.

The consequences of extravascular hemolysis (i.e., by phagocytosis) are much less severe. In macrophages iron is removed from the hemoglobin

Table 62.1 Classification of immune hemolytic disorders

Autoimmune
  Warm antibody-mediated
  Idiopathic
  Secondary
  Drugs, lymphoid malignancies, infections
  Other autoimmune diseases
  Cold antibody-mediated
  Cold agglutinin disease
  Idiopathic
  Secondary
  Infection, lymphoid malignancies
  Paroxysmal cold hemoglobinuria
  Idiopathic
  Secondary to infections

Alloimmune
  Secondary to red cell transfusions (alloantibodies, isoantibodies)
  Secondary to fetomaternal hemorrhage
  Secondary to transplanted lymphocytes

and recycled to the circulation to support a compensatory reticulocytosis while the heme porphyrin is metabolized to bilirubin.

TESTING FOR RED CELL ANTIBODIES

With few exceptions, if the mechanism is immune-mediated, an anti-red cell antibody can be demonstrated, either on the red cell surface, in the serum or in both circumstances.[1, 2] With autoimmune hemolysis immunoglobulin (IgG or IgM) and/or complement components can be identified by a direct antibody test (DAT), originally known as a direct Coombs test (Fig. 62.1). For this assay a patient's red cells are washed and suspended in buffer. Surface-bound IgG is detected by adding anti-IgG antibody, which, being divalent, can bind to IgG on adjacent red cells and agglutinate them into visible aggregates. Because of its pentameric structure, IgM on the cells can cause agglutination without the addition of a second antibody. Even when IgM has previously eluted from the cell surface, its earlier presence *in vivo* can be detected by telltale remnants of complement that are fixed to the red cell. Detection requires the addition of anti-complement (e.g., anti-C3dg) antibody.

Alloantibodies can also be detected by the DAT if allogenic red cells are still circulating from a previous transfusion. If these have been cleared, however, red cell antibodies can be identified in the patient's serum by adding the serum to a panel of red cells carrying different antigens. Agglutination is detected as described above; this constitutes the indirect antibody test.

AUTOIMMUNE HEMOLYSIS MEDIATED BY WARM ANTIBODY

Although warm-antibody autoimmune hemolytic anemia is rare, it increases in prevalence above the age of 50 and tends to be more common in women than in men. In this condition the DAT is positive

for IgG and may also be positive for complement components. Although the autoantibody is most often against an Rh antigen, a variety of other antigens have also been targeted. The specificity of the antibody, however, does not affect the presentation or management of the disease.

The short-term prognosis of warm-antibody hemolysis depends upon the severity of the anemia, which can develop rapidly and be fatal if not properly treated.[1] The long-term prognosis depends upon the underlying disease when present (Table 62.1) and upon the risks of chronic immunosuppression, which is often required to control the disease. Based upon series of patients treated 40–50 years ago, the overall mortality related to warm-antibody autoimmune hemolysis in adults is 20–40% over 10 years.[2] More recent estimates are not available, but surely must be less. In children the prognosis is better because many cases are related to infections and therefore transient.[9] The estimated mortality is 11%, all due to chronic cases indistinguishable from that in adults.

If the anemia is severe, the patient must be transfused with allogenic red cells, which will be destroyed as rapidly as the patient's own red cells but may be life-saving nevertheless. The challenge for the transfusion service is to avoid giving the patient blood that could cause an additional acute hemolytic reaction due to alloantibodies from previous transfusions or pregnancy. Alloantibodies can be detected using the patient's own cells that have been stripped of autoantibody.[10] Since these are autologous, they can be used to adsorb more autoantibody from the patient's serum, while leaving behind any alloantibodies, which can be detected once the autoantibody has been completely removed.

The mainstay of treatment is immunosuppression with corticosteroids, which usually produce significant benefit within 2 weeks.[1, 11] About 20% of patients achieve a lasting remission with steroids and can stop therapy. The majority, however, require continuous treatment. When long-term steroid treatment is too toxic, splenectomy is usually the next treatment, preferably done laparoscopically. This often produces complete responses. If splenectomy fails, however, a variety of other immunosuppressant medications can be tried (e.g., azathioprine, danazol, rituxamab, cyclosporine).

DRUG-INDUCED IMMUNE HEMOLYSIS

Over 100 drugs have been associated with immune hemolysis.[12] Second- and third-generation cephalosporins currently account for over 80% of cases. The prognosis of this type of immune hemolysis is much better than that of the idiopathic variety because the hemolysis stops once the offending drug has been removed.

Although the biochemical mechanisms leading to drug-related immune hemolysis are not completely clear, several hypotheses are generally accepted. The most common cases appear to be mediated by immune complexes of drug and IgG and/or IgM that adsorb to the red cell surface where they fix complement. The resultant hemolysis is acute and often severe enough to cause renal failure.

A second mechanism is far less common and develops primarily in patients receiving very high doses of penicillin (rarely used any more) for at least a week. High-titer anti-penicillin IgG develops and binds to penicillin that is covalently attached to the red cell membranes. The resultant hemolysis is less acute than that caused by immune complexes but can be life-threatening.

In a third mechanism the drug stimulates the production of an antibody that reacts with the patient's red cells independently of the drug. Serologically this antibody is indistinguishable from an idiopathic autoantibody. These autoantibodies have become rare as the use of the primary

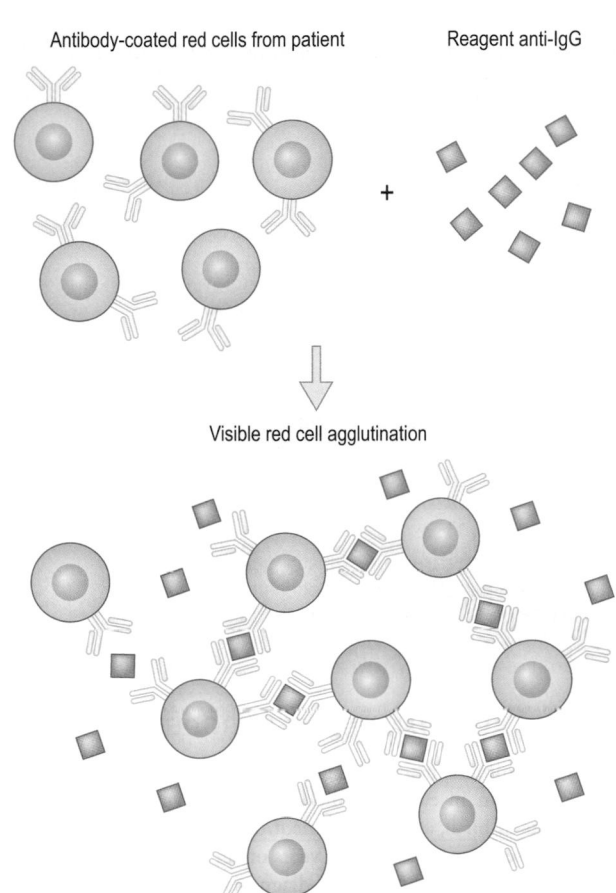

Antibody-coated red cells from patient   Reagent anti-IgG

Visible red cell agglutination

Fig. 62.1 The direct antibody test (DAT). The test is positive when immunoglobulin G (IgG: light blue triangles)-coated red cells are cross-linked by anti-IgG antibody (dark blue triangles) to form visible cell aggregates. Cell-bound complement and/or IgM can be detected by using anti-complement or anti-IgM reagent antibodies.

causal agent, methyldopa, has dwindled. Although these autoantibodies commonly cause positive DATs, they rarely actually cause hemolysis, and when they do, it usually ceases within 2 weeks of discontinuing the drug.

HEMOLYTIC DISEASE OF THE NEWBORN (HDN)

When a fetus inherits red cell antigens unshared by its mother and when the mother becomes immunized against these antigens by fetal–maternal hemorrhage during delivery, there is the possibility that subsequent fetuses will suffer intrauterine and postnatal hemolysis caused by maternal alloantibodies.[13] The majority of anti-A and anti-B isoantibodies are not a problem because they are IgM, and cannot traverse the fetoplacental circulation. Although a variety of antigenic incompatibilities can cause HDN, Rh (specifically D antigen) is the most common. The incidence of HDN has dropped dramatically since 1968 when routine prophylaxis for Rh-negative new mothers began. Since then, mothers at risk receive

intramuscular anti-D after delivery to destroy any fetal cells in their circulation before they can induce a maternal immune response.

The severity of HDN varies from mild jaundice to life-threatening anemia and brain-damaging hyperbilirubinemia (kernicterus) to intrauterine death (fetal hydrops). Treatment varies from irradiation of jaundiced infants with fluorescent lights to postpartum exchange transfusion or intrauterine transfusion.

HEMOLYTIC TRANSFUSION REACTIONS

Because individuals with group O red cells have preformed isoanti-A and -B, they must only be transfused with group O cells. Similarly, individuals with group A red cells and therefore anti-B isoantibodies must only receive group A red cells, and individuals with group B red cells must only receive group B red cells. Because of the absence of either group A or B antigens on the surface of group O red cells, such cells can be used in transfusion of A, B, or AB individuals in emergent situations. Failure to abide by these rules results in acute intravascular hemolysis that can cause renal failure, disseminated intravascular coagulation, and death.

Other hemolytic transfusion reactions are caused by alloantibodies, predominantly IgG. Therefore, a multiply-transfused patient is at risk for hemolysis from alloantibodies if the patient receives incompatible blood. Multiparous women are at similar risk because of exposure to foreign fetal red cell antigens. Fortunately, for unclear reasons, most red cell antigens do not elicit an immune response. The most immunogenic are the Rh, Kell, Kidd, and Duffy. However, exposure particularly to Kidd or Duffy antigens may stimulate alloantibody formation that can rise to sufficient titer to cause hemolysis a week later. Such delayed transfusion reactions may be subtle or cause an abrupt drop in hemoglobin with jaundice and hemoglobinuria.

IMMUNE HEMOLYSIS ASSOCIATED WITH TRANSPLANTATION

Any transplanted tissue may contain 'passenger' lymphocytes that will survive if the recipient is sufficiently immunosuppressed.[14] When the red cells of the recipient carry A- or B-antigen and the donor is ABO-incompatible, the transplanted lymphocytes will respond to the recipient red cells as foreign, and alloanti-A or anti-B antibodies will be produced that can lead to significant hemolysis. If the transplant involves hematopoietic stem cells, this dilemma will resolve once the donor's erythropoiesis prevails and the donor lymphocytes are no longer exposed to recipient red cells.

COLD AGGLUTININ DISEASES

These are mediated predominantly by anti-I or anti-i IgM that agglutinates red cells at temperatures below 37°C.[15] Red cell aggregates formed in the cooler peripheral circulation can obstruct small vessels and lead to acrocyanosis. In addition, complement fixed to red cells induces clearance, primarily by liver macrophages, causing varying degrees of anemia. The severity of the clinical illness depends upon the concentration of the IgM and its "thermal amplitude." Thermal amplitude describes the temperature dependence of its binding to red cells: for example, antibodies that exclusively bind at 4°C are only active *in vitro*, whereas those that bind at > 30°C can bind to red cells in the peripheral circulation and begin the process of complement fixation, which can be continued as the cells return to body core

Using a sophisticated antigen discovery strategy, patients with Felty's syndrome were found to have a high incidence of antibodies against an intracellular antigen eukaryotic elongation factor 1A-1 (eEF1A-1). Although the finding has been confirmed, this antibody probably does not play a crucial role in the pathophysiology of neutropenia since it is also present in nonneutropenic patients with autoimmune disease.

Detection of anti-neutrophil antibodies

Antibodies are assayed clinically using indirect assays, i.e., by measuring the binding of antibodies from patient sera to fixed granulocytes from unrelated individuals. The granulocyte immunofluorescence test (GIFT), which exploits flow cytometry for detection, is most commonly used because of its high sensitivity. The granulocyte agglutination test (GAT) is less sensitive but it is particularly valuable used in conjunction with GIFT to detect antibodies against HNA-3a or HNA-1b. Once the presence of an antibody has been confirmed, monoclonal antibody-specific immobilization of granulocyte antigens (MAIGA) is a valuable technique in identifying the target molecule recognized by the antibody, information which may be very helpful in identifying antibody specificity and in distinguishing granulocyte-specific antibodies from alloantibodies directed against HLA determinants. More precise epitope typing still requires a panel of granulocytes of varied phenotype. Unfortunately, to date, granulocyte panels are both difficult to prepare and impossible to store. Consequently, antibody typing remains a laborious, difficult task. At the second international granulocyte serology workshop, 12 centers independently tested a series of unknown sera. Many laboratories could detect strong HNA-1a antibodies, but the success rate was much lower in defining HNA-1b or HNA-2a antibodies, and individual laboratories varied greatly in their proficiency.[26]

Patterns of antibody specificity

Isoimmune neonatal neutropenia

Maternal IgG iso or autoantibodies can be generated in response to each of the polymorphic alloantigens noted above, particularly polymorphisms affecting FcγRIIIb.

Immune neutropenia in childhood

Antibodies in these patients are IgG and most commonly directed against the autoantigens HNA-1a and/or HNA-1b.[25] Sera from affected patients often also bind (albeit more weakly) to neutrophils expressing the alternative allele, and in some series more than half the patients with this entity produce antibodies capable of binding to nonpolymorphic elements within FcγRIIIb. Using MAIGA to search for antibodies directed against other neutrophil surface molecules, more complex patterns can be recognized. In one study, autoantibodies against CD11b/CDI8 (CR3) were seen in 21%, CD35 (CR1) in 14%, and FcγRII in 2% of patients.[27] Prognostically, patients with antibody responses confined to HNA-1a and/or HNA-1b are more likely to have uncomplicated, self-limited disease; patients with specificity for nonpolymorphic determinants on the FcγRIIIb molecule and other antigens more often have a generalized immune disorder and more persistent neutropenia.[25] Although anti-neutrophil assays are not highly quantitative, a recent retrospective study suggests patients with low levels of anti-neutrophil antibodies may have a more favorable long-term prognosis.[28]

Immune neutropenia in adults

It is often difficult clinically to distinguish immune from nonimmune idiopathic neutropenia in adults. Consequently, the sensitivity and specificity of antibody assays in this setting are uncertain. In general, antibody against HNA-1a or HNA-1b are less common, and antibodies against surface receptors such as CD11b/CD18 (CR3) are more common in older children and adults than in young children.

Felty's syndrome and T-LGL leukemia

Sera from patients with Felty's syndrome[18] and T-LGL leukemia[19] are often positive in anti-neutrophil antibody assays. Interpretation of these results is complicated by the high incidence of immune complexes in these populations, which may bind nonspecifically through Fc and complement receptors to the neutrophil surface. Indeed, because it is difficult to distinguish these two types of binding, the incidence of "true" anti-neutrophil antibodies in these syndromes remains uncertain. Where carefully studied, detectable anti-neutrophil antibodies are low in titer or absent in most patients with either diagnosis.[18, 19]

Impact of antibodies and immune complexes on neutrophil survival

There is sound experimental evidence that both anti-neutrophil antibodies and immune complexes can induce neutropenia in vivo. The relative importance of reversible sequestration and neutrophil destruction in inducing neutropenia varies with the experimental model, the character of the antibody/immune complex, spleen size, and presumably other factors as well.

The detection of anti-neutrophil antibodies in serum, however, does not automatically imply accelerated immune clearance of neutrophils in vivo. Some antibodies bind well to neutrophils under assay conditions, without provoking neutrophil destruction in vivo.[29] In part this reflects the inability of these crude assays to distinguish effective from ineffective binding of immunoproteins. For example, in attempts to correlate levels of allospecific anti-neutrophil antibody in serum from allosensitized individuals with neutrophil survival after transfusion, it was noted that antibodies capable of agglutinating neutrophils in vitro were associated with shorted neutrophil survival, but lymphocytotoxic or granulocytotoxic antibodies capable of promoting complement-mediated cytotoxicity did not. Clinical assays for detecting immune complexes share the same limitation.[22] The impact of immune complexes on neutrophil sequestration varies markedly with the complex size, composition, and complement-fixing activity. Consequently, positive results in an anti-neutrophil antibody or immune complex assays may support, but do not prove, immune destruction is occurring in vivo. Because assay sensitivity is limited, a negative result reduces, but does not eliminate, the possibility of immune-mediated neutrophil clearance. In sum, anti-neutrophil antibodies and immune complexes can alter neutrophil trafficking and survival in the circulation, but our ability to predict this bioactivity prospectively is very limited.

>> The palliative treatment of neutropenia is reserved for patients with a neutrophil count below 500/mm³ or recurrent infection

>> Recombinant granulocyte- and granulocyte–macrophage colony-stimulating factor are the most effective single agents for palliating neutropenia

>> Immunosuppressive agents, steroids, and splenectomy are reserved for patients with persistent or refractory neutropenia or with other detrimental manifestations of systemic autoimmunity

KEY CONCEPTS

>> Immune neutropenia in children is caused by anti-neutrophil antibodies

>> Immune neutropenia in adults has a more complex etiology

>> Immune complex-mediated neutrophils clearance and cell-mediated suppression of myelopoiesis often play a major role

Myelopoiesis in immune neutropenia

In primary immune neutropenia the marrow is typically normocellular or mildly hypercellular with an increased proportion of early myeloid forms (particularly myelocytes and promyelocytes) and decreased mature forms (neutrophils, stabs, and metamyelocytes), a pattern designated maturation arrest. Although maturation arrest can also be seen in a number of other diseases, in this setting it suggests an expansion in immature precursors with early release of mature components into the blood. Rigorous kinetic studies in children with primary neutropenia are not available, but the available data suggest myelopoiesis in this setting is increased.

The findings are more complex in Felty's syndrome and T-LGL leukemia. *In vivo* neutrophil kinetic studies and *in vitro* assays of marrow function often document reduced myelopoiesis in these settings.[18, 19] This has been attributed to T-cell- and cytokine-mediated suppression. T-LGL leukemia cells constitutively express Fas ligand on their surface and also release significant quantities into plasma *in vivo*. Reduced myelopoiesis in T-LGL leukemia and some patients with Felty's syndrome may be linked to apoptosis provoked by the binding of Fas ligand on the abnormal cells to Fas expressed on the surface of myeloid precursors.[19] Whatever the precise mechanism, reductions in myelopoiesis appear to be a common element in patients with these forms of secondary immune neutropenia.

DIAGNOSIS

Clinical presentation

Isoimmune neutropenia presents at birth and may persist for up to 6 months. Self-limited primary autoimmune neutropenia typically presents in early childhood. In older children and adults, neutropenia is more commonly associated with other systemic autoimmune disease, especially rheumatoid arthritis and SLE or T-LGL leukemia. Drug-induced neutropenia must always be considered in patients taking medications.

Since neutrophil destruction *per se* is clinically silent, patients often first seek medical attention because of bacterial infections, particularly involving the skin, upper respiratory tract, or middle ear. More serious systemic infections such as sepsis or meningitis are less common. Splenomegaly, skin lesions, and other manifestations of systemic autoimmunity are common in secondary variants, but not in the primary syndrome.

Laboratory findings

Blood counts typically demonstrate isolated neutropenia, sometimes with monocytosis. More generalized leukopenia, anemia, and/or thrombocytopenia should suggest concurrent SLE or a primary bone marrow disorder, especially aplastic anemia or myelodysplasia.

Examination of the blood film for evidence of abnormalities in other cell lines or increased numbers of LGL is essential. The persistent presence of >2000 LGL/mm³ for 6 months in itself is diagnostic of T-LGL leukemia; however, normal LGL counts in blood do not rule out this diagnosis. Perhaps a quarter of patients with T-LGL leukemia and immune neutropenia have fewer than 500 monoclonal LGL/mm³ in blood.[19] The evaluation of patients with small T-LGL clones detected in blood on flow cytometric or molecular testing without clear tissue infiltration remains problematic. At least some of these patients probably have self-limited "T-cell gammopathies of unknown origin" unassociated with overt lymphoproliferation or autoimmunity.

Bone marrow findings in immune neutropenias (as briefly reviewed above) can vary substantially. Perhaps the most important function of the bone marrow exam is to rule out hypoplasia/aplasia, myelocathexis, marked megaloblastic dysplastic changes, or abnormal infiltration with nonhematopoietic cells, which might suggest an alternative diagnosis. The marrow exam may also be helpful in confirming T-LGL leukemia.[30]

Clinical use of anti-neutrophi antibody studies

In young children with neutropenia, a positive result is very helpful in distinguishing between immune-mediated and congenital causes. Isoimmune and congenital disease may be apparent from birth and the former usually resolves within 2 months. Using GIFT or GAT assays, anti-neutrophil antibodies can be detected in more than 70% of children with primary immune neutropenia. When both are used in tandem the yield increases further. A strong positive result strongly supports the diagnosis of immune neutropenia. On the other hand, a negative study does not exclude the diagnosis.[28]

Primary autoimmune neutropenia in adults is difficult to distinguish from the ill-defined entity chronic idiopathic neutropenia.[1] Since there is no "gold standard" for distinguishing immune from nonimmune disease in this setting, the diagnostic sensitivity and specificity of the anti-neutrophil antibody assays are unclear. Assays are positive in perhaps a third of adults referred with chronic neutropenia, and a positive result in the absence of other systemic autoimmune disease certainly supports a diagnosis of immune neutropenia. Again a negative result does not preclude an immune etiology, but it is more consistent with chronic idiopathic neutropenia.

In patients with systemic autoimmune disease or T-LGL leukemia, hyperglobulinemia and circulating immune complexes greatly complicate laboratory evaluation. Anti-neutrophil assays are frequently positive even in the absence of neutropenia. Since the specificity of a positive result is low, its diagnostic value is very limited, and the clinician must be vigilant for other possible causes, especially drug-induced neutropenia.

Clinical overlap between Felty's syndrome and T-LGL leukemia

At the extremes these syndromes are easily separable. Patients with classical Felty's syndrome have severe rheumatoid arthritis, usually requiring anti-inflammatory therapy, incidentally complicated by late neutropenia. This is quite different from the pattern in patients with isolated T-LGL and neutropenia in the absence of clinical autoimmune disease.

Nonetheless, confusing overlap can occur in two settings:

1. More than half of patients with a clinical Felty's syndrome may have detectable T-LGL clones in their blood when studied with sensitive flow cytometric or molecular techniques.[19] There have been attempts in the past to classify this pattern as pseudo-Felty's syndrome, but the clinical findings and course are often indistinguishable from "classical" Felty's syndrome.

2. About half of patients with clinically apparent T-LGL leukemia have circulating rheumatoid factor and immune complexes in their blood; about a third, usually patients expressing HLA-DR4, develop clinically significant arthritis sometimes requiring anti-inflammatory agents.

Although the reason why clonal T-LGL disorders and autoimmunity often coexist remains unclear, the tendency toward overlap is clear. Since the pathophysiology and therapy of both conditions are similar, these problems in classification usually have little impact on the initial management of neutropenia. When a patient with "Felty's syndrome" develops aggressive T-LGL leukemia, or a patient with T-LGL manifests severe rheumatologic symptoms, the clinician must be prepared to alter therapy as needed to fit the clinical picture.

While some have attempted to develop clinical criteria for distinguishing Felty's syndrome from T-LGL with pseudo-Felty's syndrome, there is now substantial evidence that clonal T-LGL are often present in rheumatology patients and that patients with clonal disorders seldom develop a progressive, neoplastic disorder. Conversely, although T-LGL leukemia patients have a malignancy, it is often extremely indolent. In these cases, the clinical course is often dominated by rheumatologic complication and/or neutropenia and not by progressive neoplastic disease.

THERAPY

Overview

All patients with neutrophil counts below 1000/mm^3 have some increased risk of infection, but some remain asymptomatic even with absolute neutrophil counts of 500/mm^3 or less. Growth factors can usually improve neutropenia and reduce the risk of infection, but given their expense, inconvenience, and possible side effects, they should be reserved for use in patients with a very low count, or a previous pattern of frequent infection. The indications for immunosuppressives, steroids, and splenectomy are more complex.

Colony-stimulating factors (CSF)

Controlled trials are lacking in this disease setting, but granulocyte-CSF (G-CSF) or granulocyte–macrophage-CSF (GM-CSF) usually enhance neutrophil counts in each of the clinical groups discussed. Because of their safety, speed, and efficacy, they have replaced steroids and splenectomy as first-line symptomatic therapy. They should be used at the lowest effective dose, with particular caution in patients with systemic autoimmune disease, who are prone to leukoclastic vasculitis as a complication of therapy.[22]

Immunosuppressive agents

Because disease is usually self-limited and responsive to G-CSF, immunosuppressive agents are seldom used in children with primary immune neutropenia. Chronic low-dose oral therapy with methotrexate is often effective in treating neutropenia (and other autoimmune symptoms) in patients with Felty's syndrome and/or T-LGL. Cyclosporine is the preferred second-line therapy in T-LGL, and cyclophosphamide, cyclosporine, and gold are often considered second-line treatment for Felty's syndrome when total disease control is desired.

Steroids and splenectomy

Each of these treatments can be effective in reversing neutropenia, but their use has diminished considerably in recent years. Intravenous immunoglobulin (IVIG) can temporarily reverse neutropenia, particularly in children, probably by blocking Fc receptors responsible for triggering neutrophil destruction. However, G-CSF, which is more convenient to administer and at least as effective, has largely replaced this agent.

Splenectomy and steroids can each reduce immune destruction by suppressing the body's capacity to clear IgG- and complement-coated cells. Over a longer time frame these treatments may also suppress antibody production, in the first case by removing a major site of production, and in the second by reducing anti-neutrophil antibody production and blocking T-cell-mediated myelosuppression. They can reverse neutropenia in many patients, but their long-term impact on outcome remains unclear. Given their risk and side effects, both modalities are generally reserved for patients resistant to CSFs and low-dose immuno-suppressives.

Prophylactic antibiotics

Where recurrent infection is a problem, oral trimethoprim-sulfamethoxazole is commonly used for prophylaxis, particularly in children. This approach is very reasonabl, given its success in other immunocompromised groups, but it has not been tested in a controlled trial.

■ IMMUNE THROMBOCYTOPENIAS AND COAGULATION INHIBITORS ■

Antibodies can cause destruction or dysfunction of platelets and coagulation factors as the primary manifestation of a disease, or they may be part of an immune disorder that stimulates a spectrum of antibodies causing multiple symptoms in the patient. Antibodies against platelets may cause profound thrombocytopenia as a result of increased platelet clearance or through decreased platelet production when antibodies reduce megakaryocyte production and maturation.[31] They can also alter

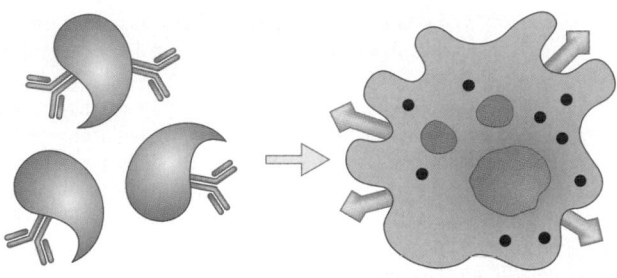

Platelets with bound IgG   Macrophage with FcRγIIA receptor

Fig. 62.3 Platelets with bound antibody are cleared from the circulation by the binding of the antibodies to FcγIIIA receptors on macrophages and other cells. The cross-linking of the macrophage receptors sets off a cascade of internal signaling that leads to increased expression of the inhibitory FcγIIB receptors (not shown).

platelet function by binding to platelet surface proteins necessary for hemostasis. Antibodies directed against coagulation factors or phospholipid coagulation factor complexes can inhibit their function or mediate their clearance from the circulation, causing a bleeding diathesis. One class of antibodies, the lupus anti-coagulants (LAC), predisposes to thrombosis

IMMUNE THROMBOCYTOPENIC PURPURA (ITP)

Pathogenesis

ITP, also called idiopathic or autoimmune thrombocytopenic purpura, is a diagnosis of exclusion and is caused by autoantibodies that promote increased platelet clearance and may decrease platelet production. The stimulus for this autoantibody production is unknown; however, it has been demonstrated that antibody-coated platelets are removed from the circulation through an Fcγ receptor-dependent mechanism,[32] and that T-cell abnormalities are also important in ITP.[33] Antibodies specific for several platelet surface and megakaryocytic proteins have been detected in patients with ITP.[34]

Both activating and inhibiting Fc receptors on cells are important in the platelet destruction of ITP. Murine models have shown that agents that are used therapeutically in humans with ITP, IVIG and anti-D, decrease the removal of antibody-coated platelets either by increasing the expression of the inhibitory FcγIIB receptor (CD32),[35] or by decreasing the expression of a different Fcγ receptor, activating FcγIIIA (CD16).[36] Specific FcγIIIA receptor blockade using a murine antibody has been successful in transiently increasing the platelet count in ITP patients, but this treatment could not be continued because of the formation of human–antimouse antibodies.[37]

Diagnosis and clinical course

The diagnosis of ITP is based on history, physical examination, complete blood count, examination of the peripheral smear, and review of the patient's medications and exposures.[38] The diagnosis is established when a patient has isolated thrombocytopenia without other causes and in whom the bleeding symptoms are consistent with the decrease in platelet numbers. The low sensitivity of current assays for platelet antibodies and

the technical difficulty in performing them limit their clinical use as a diagnostic criterion for ITP; they detect antibodies in 31–88% of patients.[39, 40] ITP in children often occurs after a viral illness and usually follows a course with spontaneous recovery occurring within months; it is generally a less serious illness than adult ITP.[32, 38] ITP in adults most often follows a chronic course with few spontaneous remissions. The diagnosis is strengthened when a patient has a good response to treatment with immunosuppressive medications such as IVIG or prednisone. A bone marrow examination may be appropriate in certain situations, such as in elderly patients where underlying myelodysplasia or lymphoproliferative disease may be suspected, prior to splenectomy, in patients who are unresponsive to immunosuppressive medications, and when other unexplained cytopenias are present.

In children, persistent thrombocytopenia may indicate a congenital disorder, and factors that point to a congenital platelet disorder include abnormalities in platelet size, high-frequency hearing loss, congenital anomalies, and renal function abnormalities. Bleeding out of proportion to the thrombocytopenia may indicate type 2B von Willebrand disease. Human immunodeficiency virus (HIV) testing is important because treatment of HIV may improve an associated immune thrombocytopenia. Review of the patient's medications is also important to exclude drug-induced thrombocytopenia, and in certain populations testing for *Helicobacter pylori* may be indicated. Remissions after treatment of the bacterium have been reported in Italy and Japan, but unfortunately results have been less impressive in the USA.[40]

Treatment

The primary goal in the treatment of patients with ITP is to prevent bleeding. Treatment must be individualized, taking into account the level of activity of the patient's lifestyle, the presenting platelet count, and whether signs of bleeding are present. Usually patients with platelet counts of 30 000/μl or greater do not have significant bleeding, and treatment may be deferred.[32, 38, 40] For a patient with severe thrombocytopenia (<20 000/μl) or bleeding that requires immediate treatment, IVIG and prednisone are usually the treatments of choice.[32, 38, 40] Platelet transfusions and/or plasmapheresis are added to the regimen if the bleeding is life-threatening. For patients with less serious bleeding who require treatment, prednisone (1 mg/kg) is usually given for 2–4 weeks or until a response occurs; it is then slowly tapered, at about 3-week intervals, with monitoring of the platelet counts. For patients who continue to have persistent severe thrombocytopenia (<30 000/μl) or whose platelet counts drop to unacceptable levels during the tapering of steroids, splenectomy is usually the treatment of choice. Complete responses occur in about two-thirds of patients after splenectomy.[41] Patients should receive immunizations with the pneumococcal, *Hemophilus influenzae* b, and the quadrivalent meningococcal vaccines prior to splenectomy.[38] In some patients who are stable with a platelet count of < 30 000/μl, splenectomy is deferred and a more prolonged trial of anti-D or anti-CD20 therapy (rituximab) is given.[40] The latter therapy is not approved by the US Food and Drug Administration for ITP; however rituximab resulted in response rates of greater than 30% in phase II clinical trials.[42]

Therapy for chronic severe ITP that is refractory to splenectomy can be challenging. The primary goal continues to be the prevention of bleeding, and this must be balanced by the potential long-term side effects of different therapies. Anti-CD20 treatment can be used after splenectomy in addition to steroid-sparing agents that include mycophenolate mofetil, danazol, and cyclosporine. If these are not successful, other therapeutic agents utilized are azathioprine, low-dose cyclophosphamide, and vincristine. Adjunctive therapy with antifibrinolytic agents such as ε-aminocaproic acid can help decrease mucosal bleeding. Higher-risk therapy includes combination chemotherapy or high-dose cyclophosphamide with autologous stem cell rescue.[38,40,43] These options should be reserved for patients with severe thrombocytopenia who have bleeding symptoms and have failed more conservative therapy. A new approach showing some efficacy in preliminary clinical trials is the use of thrombopoietic factors[40]; the use of recombinant activated factor VII needs to be studied for efficacy for severe bleeding episodes in ITP patients.

ITP during pregnancy and the neonatal period

Immune thrombocytopenia should be distinguished from other causes of thrombocytopenia during pregnancy such as benign gestational thrombocytopenia, disseminated intravascular coagulation, hemolysis, elevated liver ezymes, and low platelet count (HELLP) syndrome, thrombotic thrombocytopenic purpura, and the acute fatty liver of pregnancy. ITP is more likely when there is a previous diagnosis of ITP, with early presentation during pregnancy, and with profound thrombocytopenia (<50 000/μl). In general, women with a platelet count of greater than 50 000/μl should not be treated because of the potential deleterious effects

---

THERAPEUTIC PRINCIPLES

IMMUNE THROMBOCYTOPENIC PURPURA (ITP)

>> Primary goal – prevent bleeding

>> Treatment not usually necessary if platelets > 30 000/μl

>> Prednisone and/or intravenous immunoglobulin usual first medications

>> Splenectomy for persistent disease

>> >> Immunize patient before surgery

>> >> Anti-D may avert/delay splenectomy

>> Treat refractory ITP with immunosuppressives

>> >> Mycophenolate, cyclosporine, cyclophosphamide, rituximab (not approved by the Food and Drug Administration for this use)

---

of corticosteroids to the mother and the fetus.[38] IVIG is often effective in temporarily increasing platelet counts, and it is useful prior to delivery or epidural anesthesia.

About 4% of infants born to mothers with ITP will have severe thrombocytopenia; fortunately, the danger of intracerebral hemorrhage is low in these infants. Previous neonatal outcomes are the best predictor of the risk during future pregnancies.[40] Platelet counts should be monitored for at least 4 days after birth because platelet count nadirs can be delayed in these neonates.[38] If the infant's platelet count is less than 50 000/μl, brain imaging should be obtained to rule out hemorrhage.[38,40] Treatment with IVIG and prednisone is administered if the platelet count is less than 20 000/μl, or if there is bleeding regardless of the platelet count.

NEONATAL ALLOIMMUNE THROMBOCYTOPENIA AND POSTTRANSFUSION PURPURA

Neonatal alloimmune thrombocytopenia is caused by maternal antibodies against human platelet antigens that the fetus carries, but that the mother lacks (most commonly human platelet antigen-1a (PLA-1)). It is more likely to cause intracerebral hemorrhage (10–20% of cases) compared with children born to mothers with ITP, and it is very likely to recur if it has occurred in a previous pregnancy.[44] IVIG and platelet transfusions using maternal platelets (to insure that the offending antigen is not present in the transfused product) are often necessary.

Antibodies against human platelet antigens are also responsible for posttransfusion purpura, in which the recipient has an acquired antibody directed against a platelet antigen on the donor platelets. For reasons not entirely understood, the antibodies also destroy the patient's own "antigen-negative" platelets. Treatment consists of IVIG and corticosteroids and sometimes plasma exchange.[45]

DRUG-INDUCED THROMBOCYTOPENIA

Drugs can cause thrombocytopenia through multiple mechanisms. They may decrease platelet production, or cause peripheral destruction by stimulating antibody formation:

- A platelet epitope may be altered by the binding of drug to the platelet.
- A neoantigen may be created by the formation of an epitope consisting of the drug–membrane complex (hapten).
- The drug itself may be antigenic, and antibody plus the drug may form an immune complex that binds to platelets by Fc receptors.[46]

If a drug is suspected of causing immune thrombocytopenia, it should be discontinued and the platelet count followed. If the patient has bleeding, platelet transfusions are administered. The platelet count usually recovers in about 5–7 days. Among the common drugs that may cause thrombocytopenia by antibody destruction are penicillin, sulfonamides, gold salts, and anti-seizure medications such as phenytoin.[47]

Heparin-induced thrombocytopenia (HIT), which is caused by antibodies to platelet factor 4 (PF4)–heparin complex, is a special case that can be associated with life-threatening thrombosis. The antibody–PF4–heparin complex activates platelets, resulting in a high risk of both arterial and venous thrombotic events.[48] Thrombocytopenia occurs due to clearance of platelet aggregates caused by the antibody and usually appears 5–7 days after treatment with heparin (or low-molecular-weight heparin) unless a patient has been exposed to heparin in the past 100 days. In this instance, thrombocytopenia can occur within 1 day of heparin administration. Even small doses of heparin given as "flushes" to maintain intravenous catheter patency can be sufficient to cause HIT. In cases of suspected HIT, all heparins should be stopped and an alternative anti-coagulant agent should be used, such as the direct thrombin inhibitors argatroban and lepirudin. Fondaparinux is a pentasaccharide anti-coagulant that may become a third option for treatment of HIT. In cases of confirmed or strongly suspected HIT, anti-coagulation should be continued for 3 months because the risk of thrombosis persists in this group of patients. Coumadin is generally used for long-term anti-coagulation; it should be started by overlapping with one of the agents above because of the increased risk of thrombosis due to the initial depletion of anti-coagulant factors (proteins C and S).

ANTIBODIES TO COAGULATION FACTORS

Antibodies to coagulation factors arise most frequently in patients who have a hereditary deficiency of a factor and receive replacement therapy (alloantibodies); others arise spontaneously as autoantibodies, most commonly to factor VIII (anti-hemophilic factor). Serious bleeding can result in both instances. In contrast, the most common acquired anti-coagulant, the lupus anti-coagulant (LAC), predisposes to thrombosis.

LUPUS ANTI-COAGULANTS

LACs are autoantibodies that target proteins bound to phospholipid, usually β_2-glycoprotein I or prothrombin (Fig. 62.4); they are defined in the laboratory by a prolongation of phospholipid-dependent steps in the coagulation cascade.[49] LACs and/or anti-cardiolipin antibodies (antibodies defined by enzyme-linked immunosorbent assay testing), along with clinical symptoms of venous or arterial thrombosis or recurrent pregnancy morbidity, comprise the anti-phospholipid syndrome (APS). APS is a thrombotic syndrome that is most common in women and often occurs in individuals with autoimmune diseases such as SLE, but also occurs in other inflammatory conditions or infections (Chapters 51 and 61). Besides recurrent venous and/or arterial thrombosis and fetal loss,

the syndrome may include thrombocytopenia, autoimmune hemolytic anemia, livido reticularis, cardiac valve disease (Libman–Sacks), and central nervous system manifestations including headache, seizure, and stroke. The mechanisms by which these antibodies lead to thrombosis are not fully defined, but specific causes include antibody activation of endothelial cells and platelets, inhibition of fibrinolysis, inhibition of activation of the natural anti-coagulant protein C, disruption of annexin V binding to cell surfaces (allowing coagulation factors access to cell surface phospholipid and to possible activation), and inhibition of the natural anti-coagulant action of β_2-glycoprotein I which normally prevents binding of von Willebrand factor to its platelet receptor.

The diagnosis is established when a clotting test that requires phospholipid to create a fibrin clot is prolonged and

- is not "corrected" by a 1:1 mixing study with normal plasma
- but is corrected by the addition of excess phospholipid.[50]

In practice, the partial thromboplastin time is the most commonly performed test that initially detects a LAC, so a LAC may be discovered during routine coagulation screening prior to invasive procedures or during a medical evaluation. Several more specific assays are available to detect LACs, and at least two different assays should be performed if suspicion of a LAC is high, since one test may be negative and others may be positive. The tests indicate a LAC when the abnormal clotting time in the assay is "corrected" during a second assay in which extra phospholipid is added. If correction is not present with the added phospholipid, the test is negative for a LAC. Since these antibodies can be transient, they or anti-cardiolipin antibodies must remain positive for longer than 12 weeks (along with the history of thrombosis and/or pregnancy morbidity) to allow the diagnosis of APS.

Treatment is not indicated for a positive test alone. Treatment for acute thrombosis in patients who have APS consists of routine anti-coagulation starting with heparin and followed by coumadin for at least 6 months. Treatment is prolonged if the thrombosis has occurred in an unusual site such as a mesenteric or hepatic artery or vein or has resulted in a major pulmonary embolus. When patients with LACs have more than one thrombotic episode, lifelong anti-coagulation is usually prescribed unless the patient has a high risk of bleeding. Pregnancy morbidity is treated with heparin (unfractionated, subcutaneously, or low-molecular-weight heparin) and low-dose aspirin.

FACTOR VIII INHIBITORS

Antibodies to factor VIII occur in up to 30% of severe hemophiliacs as a result of exposure to factor VIII replacement therapy.[51] They are IgG antibodies, often of the IgG$_4$ subclass. The antibodies greatly complicate

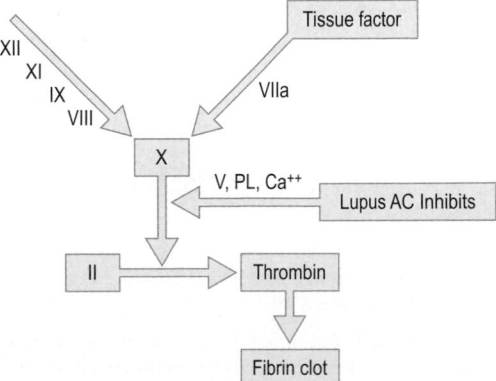

Fig. 62.4 Lupus anti-coagulants inhibit the coagulation cascade assays by interfering with the activation of prothrombin (factor II) to thrombin. This step requires phospholipid (PL) along with the other cofactors, factor V and ionized calcium (Ca^{++}).

> ### KEY CONCEPTS
>
> #### LUPUS ANTICOAGULANTS
>
> » Antibody(ies) versus protein–phospholipid complexes
> » Diagnosis based on phospholipid-dependent clotting tests
> » May cause serious arterial or venous thrombosis
> » Does not cause bleeding; other associated antibodies may cause bleeding

therapy, since they inhibit factor VIII that would normally be given to prevent or stop bleeding. Inhibitors are suspected when a patient does not respond to usual factor VIII replacement therapy. They are confirmed by detecting a shortened factor half-life after replacement and by a factor VIII inhibitor assay. The inhibitor assay uses a mixture of patient plasma (as the source of antibody) and normal pooled plasma (as the source of factor VIII) in 1:1 proportions; after incubation, the mixture is assayed for residual factor VIII activity and the antibody is quantified in Bethesda units. One unit of inhibitor is the quantity of antibody that inhibits 50% of the factor VIII in the normal plasma pool after 2–4 hours' incubation at 37°C. Usually several dilutions of the patient plasma containing the antibody must be incubated with normal plasma to determine the amount of antibody that will inhibit 50% of the factor VIII in the normal plasma; the units of inhibitor are the inverse of the dilution that inhibits 50% of starting factor VIII activity.

Acquired inhibitors to factor VIII are rare, estimated to affect 1 in 2 million individuals; fatal outcomes, however, are reported in up to 20% of patients.[52] Bleeding often occurs in soft-tissue, retroperitoneal, genitourinary, or gastrointestinal sites rather than in joints. These antibodies can be associated with allergic drug reactions, malignancies, autoimmune diseases, and the postpartum state, or they may appear spontaneously. Diagnosis is made in the laboratory with a prolonged activated partial thromboplastin time and a low factor VIII, a positive factor VIII inhibitor assay.

Treatment for bleeding episodes in patients who have inhibitors to factor VIII may include very high doses of factor VIII concentrates (if the inhibitor titer is < 5 Bethesda units), porcine factor VIII, recombinant human factor VIIa, and prothrombin complex concentrates that bypass the step requiring factor VIII during fibrin formation.[52] Plasmapheresis is also used to remove the inhibitor temporarily in serious bleeding situations. To decrease antibody production, prednisone, cyclophosphamide, azathioprine, IVIG, cyclosporine, and, more recently rituximab, are used. Individuals with acquired inhibitors usually respond within 3–8 months. In hemophilic patients who have inhibitors, immune tolerance regimens that include daily or less frequent injections of factor VIII are utilized for long-term treatment; these patients may require over 12 months of therapy.

THERAPEUTIC PRINCIPLES

FACTOR VIII (FVIII) INHIBITORS

>> For acute bleeding episodes for FVIII inhibitors:

>> FVIII concentrates if inhibitor < 5 Bethesda units

>> Recombinant FVIIa or prothrombin complex concentrations for inhibitor titers > 5 Bethesda units

>> For chronic persistent inhibitors in hemophilia A patients with inhibitors:

>> >> Immune tolerance regimens

>> Acquired inhibitor patients:

>> >> Immunosuppressive medications

INHIBITORS TO OTHER COAGULATION FACTORS

Antibodies to von Willebrand factor (VWF) can lead to mucocutaneous bleeding, including gastrointestinal bleeding.[53] Although rare, they occur in conjunction with autoimmune, lymphoproliferative, and myeloproliferative diseases as well as other illnesses. Although VWF and factor VIII levels are decreased in these patients, the antibodies are notoriously difficult to demonstrate *in vitro*, in some cases because they cause immune complexes of antibody-VWF which are cleared from the circulation, thereby lowering the VWF level. The diagnosis is made in a patient who lacks a past personal and family history of bleeding and has decreased VWF and factor VIII levels. These patients often respond to treatment with IVIG or desmopressin (desmopressin releases VWF and factor VIII from body storage sites). Factor VIII/VWF concentrates may be administered if the response is not adequate.

Acquired antibodies to other coagulation factors are also rare.[52] They are usually detected in a patient who presents with a bleeding diathesis and is found to have an abnormal clotting test that does not "correct" to normal in a 1:1 mixing study with pooled normal plasma. Further testing reveals which factor is decreased, and an inhibitor assay shows the presence of an antibody inhibitor. A specific antibody to prothrombin, which causes clearance of the factor, is found in about 5–10% of patients with LACs; this is a separate antibody from the LAC, and it may cause significant bleeding. Patients with acquired inhibitors may respond to replacement therapy using a specific factor concentrate or fresh frozen plasma; they may also require immunosuppressive therapy to abolish the inhibitor.

■ REFERENCES ■

1. Gehrs BC, Friedberg RC. Autoimmune hemolytic anemia. Am J Hematol 2002; 69: 258–271.

2. Petz LD, Garratty G. Classification and clinical characteristics of autoimmune hemolytic anemias. In: Petz LD, Garratty G, (eds) Immune Hemolytic Anemias, 2nd edn. Philadelphia, PA: Churchill Livingstone; 2004): 61.

3. Avent ND, Reid ME. The Rh blood system: a review. Blood 2000; 95: 375–387.

4. Mollison PL, Engelfriet CP, Contreras M. Immunology of red cells. In: Mollison PL, Engelfriet CP, Contreras M, (eds) Blood Transfusion in Clinical Medicine, 10th edn. London: Blackwell Science, 1997: 60.

5. Hughes-Jones NC. Red-cell antigens, antibodies and their interaction. Clin Haematol 1975; 4: 29–43.

6. Petz LD, Garratty G. Mechanisms of immune hemolysis. In: Petz LD, Garratty G, (eds) Immune Hemolytic Anemias, 2nd edn. Philadelphia, PA: Churchill Livingstone 2004: 133.

7. Kurlander RJ, Rosse WF, Logue GL. Quantitative influence of antibody and complement coating of red cells on monocyte-mediated cell lysis. J Clin Invest 1978; 61: 1309–1319.

8. Frank MM, Schreiber AD, Atkinson JP, et al. Pathophysiology of immune hemolytic anemia. Ann Intern Med 1977; 87: 210–222.

9. Habibi B, Homberg J-C, Schaison G, et al. Autoimmune hemolytic anemia in children. A review of 80 cases. Am J Med 1974; 56: 61–69.

10. Petz LD. "Least incompatible" units for transfusion in autoimmune hemolytic anemia": should we eliminate this meaningless term? A commentary for clinicians and transfusion medicine professionals. Transfusion 2003; 43: 1503–1507.

11. King KE, Ness PM. Treatment of autoimmune hemolytic anemia. Semin Hematol 2005; 42: 131–136.

12. Arndt PA, Garratty G. The changing spectrum of drug-induced immune hemolytic anemia. Semin Hematol 2005; 42: 137–144.

13. Moise KJ. Red blood cell alloimmunization in pregnancy. Semin Hematol 2005; 42: 169–178.

14. Petz LD. Immune hemolysis associated with transplantation. Semin Hematol 2005; 42: 145–155.

15. McNicholl FP. Clinical syndromes associated with cold agglutinins. Transfusion Sci 2000; 22: 125–133.

16. Maheshwari A, Christensen RD, Calhoun DA. Immune-mediated neutropenia in the neonate: ActaPaediatv Suppl 2002; 91. 98–103.

17. Capsoni F, Sarzi-Puttini P, Zanella A. Primary and secondary autoimmune neutropenia. Arthritis Res Ther 2005; 7: 208–214.

18. Balint GP, Balint PV. Felty's syndrome. Best Pract Res Clin Rheumatol 2004; 18: 631–645.

19. Burks EJ, Loughran TP Jr. Pathogenesis of neutropenia in large granular lymphocyte leukemia and Felty syndrome. Blood Rev 2006; 29: 1274–1283.

20. Lamy T, Loughran TP Jr. Clinical features of large granular lymphocyte eukemia. Semin Hematol 2003; 40: 185–195.

21. Berliner N, Horwitz M, Loughran TP Jr. Congenital and acquired neutropenia. Hematology (Am Soc Hematol Educ Program) 2004: 63–79.

22. Starkebaum G. Chronic neutropenia associated with autoimmune disease. Semin Hematol 2002; 39: 121–127.

23. Bhatt V, Saleem A. Review: Drug-induced neutropenia – pathophysiology, clinical features, and management. Ann Clin Lab Sci 2004; 34: 131–137.

24. Bux J. Molecular nature of granulocyte antigens. Transfus Clin Biol 2001; 8: 242–247.

25. Bruin MC, von dem Borne AE, Tamminga RY, et al. Neutrophil antibody specificity in different types of childhood autoimmune neutropenia. Blood 1999; 94: 1797–1802.

26. Bux J, Chapman J. Report on the second international granulocyte serology workshop. Transfusion 1997; 37: 977–983.

27. Bux J, Behrens G, Jaeger G, et al. Diagnosis and clinical course of autoimmune neutropenia in infancy: analysis of 240 cases. Blood 1998; 91: 181–186.

28. Kobayashi M, Nakamura K, Kawaguchi H, et al. Significance of the detection of antineutrophil antibodies in children with chronic neutropenia. Blood 2002; 99: 3468–3471.

29. McCullough J, Weibler BJ, Clay M, et al. Effect of leukocyte antibodies on the fate in vivo of indium-111-labelled granulocytes. Blood 1981; 58: 164–170.

30. Morice WG, Kurtin PJ, Tefferi A, et al. Distinct bone marrow findings in T-cell granular lymphocytic leukemia revealed by paraffin section immunoperoxidase stains for CD8. TIA-1, and granzyme B. Blood 2002; 99: 268–274.

31. McMillan R, Wang L, Tomer A, et al. Suppression of in vitro megakaryocyte production by antiplatelet autoantibodies from adult patients with chronic ITP. Blood 2004; 103: 1364–1369.

32. Cines DB, Blanchette VS. Immune thrombocytopenic purpura. N Engl J Med 2002; 346: 995–1008.

33. Semple JW, Freedman J. Abnormal cellular immune mechanisms associated with autoimmune thrombocytopenia. Transfus Med Rev 1995; 9: 327–338.

34. McMillan R, Tani P, Millard F, et al. Platelet-associated and plasma anti-glycoprotein autoantibodies in chronic ITP. Blood 1987; 70: 1040–1045.

35. Samuelsson A, Towers TL, Ravetch JV. Anti-inflammatory activity of IVIG mediated through the inhibitory Fc receptor. Science 2001; 291: 484–486.

36. Song S, Crow AR, Siragam V, et al. Monoclonal antibodies that mimic the action of anti-D in the amelioration of murine ITP act by a mechanism distinct from that of IVIg. Blood 2005; 105: 1546–1548.

37. Soubrane C, Tourani JM, Andrieu JM, et al. Biologic response to anti-CD16 monoclonal antibody therapy in a human immunodeficiency virus-related immune thrombocytopenic purpura patient. Blood 1993; 81: 15–19.

38. George JN, Woolf SH, Raskob GE, et al. Idiopathic thrombocytopenic purpura: a practice guideline developed by explicit methods for the American Society of Hematology. Blood 1996; 88: 3–40.

39. McMillan R. The role of antiplatelet autoantibody assays in the diagnosis of immune thrombocytopenic purpura. Curr Hematol Rep 2005; 4: 160–165.

40. Cines DB, Bussel JB. How I treat idiopathic thrombocytopenic purpura (ITP). Blood 2005; 106: 2244–2251.

41. Kojouri K, Vesely SK, Terrell DR, et al. Splenectomy for adult patients with idiopathic thrombocytopenic purpura: a systematic review to assess long-term platelet count responses, prediction of response, and surgical complications. Blood 2004; 104: 2623–2634.

42. Vesely SK, Perdue JJ, Rizvi MA, et al. Management of adult patients with persistent idiopathic thrombocytopenic purpura following splenectomy: a systematic review. Ann Intern Med 2004; 140: 112–120.

43. Huhn RD, Fogarty PF, Nakamura R, et al. High-dose cyclophosphamide with autologous lymphocyte-depleted peripheral blood stem cell (PBSC) support for treatment of refractory chronic autoimmune thrombocytopenia. Blood 2003; 101: 71–77.

44. Rothenberger S. Neonatal alloimmune thrombocytopenia. Ther Apher 2002; 6: 32–35.

45. Gonzalez CE, Pengetze YM. Post-transfusion purpura. Curr Hematol Rep 2005; 4: 154–159.

46. Aster RH. Drug-induced immune thrombocytopenia: an overview of pathogenesis. Semin Hematol 1999; 36: 2–6.

47. George JN, Raskob GE, Shah SR, et al. Drug-induced thrombocytopenia: a systematic review of published case reports. Ann Intern Med 1998; 129: 886–890.

48. Warkentin TE, Greinacher A. Heparin-induced thrombocytopenia: recognition, treatment, and prevention: the Seventh ACCP Conference on Antithrombotic and Thrombolytic Therapy. Chest 2004; 126: 311S–337S.

49. Levine JS, Branch DW, Rauch J. The antiphospholipid syndrome. N Engl J Med 2002; 346: 752–763.

50. Miyakis S, Lockshin MD, Atsumi T, et al. International consensus statement on an update of the classification criteria for definite antiphospholipid syndrome (APS). J Thromb Haemost 2006; 4: 295–306.

51. Dimichele DM. Management of factor VIII inhibitors. Int J Hematol 2006; 83: 119–125.

52. Boggio LN, Green D. Acquired hemophilia. Rev Clin Exp Hematol 2001; 5: 389–404.

53. Federici AB. Acquired von Willebrand syndrome: an underdiagnosed and misdiagnosed bleeding complication in patients with lymphoproliferative and myeloproliferative disorders. Semin Hematol 2006; 43: S48–S58.

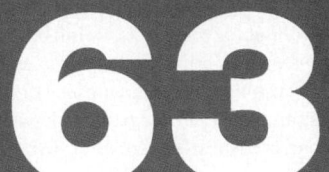
Bullous diseases of the skin and mucous membranes

Khaled M. Hassan, Russell P. Hall III

■ PEMPHIGUS ■

Pemphigus is the term used to describe a group of diseases that have in common superficial blistering of the skin and mucous membranes. Pemphigus can be separated into four distinct groups: pemphigus vulgaris (PV), pemphigus foliaceus (PF), paraneoplastic pemphigus, and intraepidermal immunoglobulin A (IgA) neutrophilic dermatosis.

PEMPHIGUS VULGARIS

PV is the most severe form of pemphigus. PV presents most often in the fourth to sixth decades, but has been reported to occur at any age. Clinically, patients with PV are characterized by the presence of flaccid blisters and erosions of the skin and mucous membranes. Virtually all patients with PV will develop oral erosions at some point during the course of their disease. Most present with oral erosions and many have oral erosions as their only disease manifestation for months to years. These lesions are often persistent, shaggy erosions that can involve all areas of the oral mucosa, extending into the esophagus. In severe cases other mucous membranes, such as the conjunctiva, nasal, anal, cervical, or urethral mucosa, can also be affected.

The blisters seen in patients with PV are flaccid, easily ruptured, and can occur on either inflamed or noninflamed skin. The ease with which these blisters rupture is the origin of the Nikolsky sign, which is elicited

KEY CONCEPTS

PEMPHIGUS VULGARIS

>> Flaccid blisters with denuded epidermis

>> Oral mucous membrane lesions common

>> Suprabasilar blister with 'row of tombstones'

>> Immunoglobulin G deposits on keratinocyte cell surface (antigenic target = desmoglein-3)

when lateral traction on the skin results in desquamation of the superficial layer of the skin. This sign, although helpful, is not unique to PV. Once broken these blisters leave large, nonhealing erosions. Blisters can occur on any area of the skin, most often beginning on the head and neck or trunk. Generalized blistering is not uncommon, especially if diagnosis and/or treatment has been delayed.

Pemphigus vegetans is an unusual variant of PV in which lesions develop that are localized primarily to the axilla, groin, and other flexural areas. The lesions are characterized as hypertrophic granulation tissue with occasional pustules. This presentation can occur *de novo* or after healing of PV lesions. The etiology of this unusual clinical presentation is not known.

Before the advent of systemic glucocorticoid therapy, PV was almost uniformly fatal, with patients developing large areas of denuded skin and dying from overwhelming sepsis. Since the introduction of systemic glucocorticoids the mortality rate has fallen to approximately 10%. The residual mortality is due in large part to side effects of the high doses of systemic glucocorticoids required to treat the disease, particularly in debilitated or elderly patients.

Histologically, PV is characterized by the presence of an intraepithelial blister, with acantholysis or breaking apart of the suprabasilar portion of the epidermis. Biopsy of an early lesion of PV reveals that the basal cells of the epidermis remain attached to the dermis, forming a 'row of tombstones,' with loss of attachment of individual keratinocytes to each other, resulting in the formation of an intraepidermal blister.

A major advance in the understanding of PV occurred in the early 1960s, when Beutner and co-workers described IgG antibodies bound to the epithelial keratinocyte cell surface in the skin of patients with PV.[1] They also demonstrated that the serum of patients with PV had IgG antibodies that bound in an identical pattern to normal human skin *in vitro*.[2] These findings demonstrated that PV is an autoimmune disease directed against a normal component of stratified squamous epithelium.

PEMPHIGUS FOLIACEUS

PF is characterized by blisters within the epidermis, resulting in the development of superficial erosions with scaling and crusting (Fig. 63.1). Unlike patients with PV, those with PF rarely develop mucous membrane lesions. Because of the superficial nature of the blister many patients present with only erythematous, scaling, and crusted plaques on the head, neck, and trunk. The prognosis for patients with PF is markedly better than for those with PV, although patients with severe disease do occasionally die, usually as a result of infectious complications of the disease and/or therapy. The better prognosis is likely secondary to the more superficial nature of the blistering process.

An unusual variant of PF is the endemic form of the disease, fogo selvagem (Portuguese for 'wild fire').[3] This is identical to the sporadic form of PF but is endemic to certain rural areas of South America. The epidemiology suggests an infectious etiology, and preliminary data suggest that an arthropod vector may be involved in spreading the disease.

Pemphigus erythematosus, or Senear–Usher syndrome, is another variant of PF. These patients have typical features of PF with additional characteristics suggestive of systemic lupus erythematosus. The clinical course tends to parallel that of PF, and most patients do not develop systemic lupus erythematosus. The pathogenesis of this form of PF is poorly understood.

PF can also be associated with drugs. The most common agents that induce pemphigus are D-penicillamine and captopril, or other angiotensin-converting enzyme inhibitors.[4] Although these drugs may induce a PV-like picture, the clinical manifestations are most often similar to those of PF. Patients with drug-induced pemphigus have autoantibodies directed against the keratinocyte cell surface but the pathogenetic mechanisms that lead to formation of these antibodies are unknown. It has been postulated that reactive sulfhydryl or amide groups, common to many of the drugs that are associated with drug-induced pemphigus, may be important elements in this reaction.[4]

The histology of a PF blister reveals a superficial, intraepidermal blister with acantholysis of only the most superficial portion of the skin. This blistering occurs in the region of the granular cell layer of the skin, with the result that blisters have a base of epithelium and not the single basal cell layer that is seen in patients with PV.

The immunohistologic features of PF observed are indistinguishable from those seen in PV (Fig. 63.2). Cell surface deposits of IgG are seen in the skin of patients with PF, and circulating IgG, which binds to normal stratified squamous epithelium, is present in the serum of patients with PF.[3] Although the immunofluorescence patterns are virtually identical between PF and PV, the antigenic targets of these autoantibodies are different, as discussed below.

PARANEOPLASTIC PEMPHIGUS

Anhalt described occasional patients who presented with a heterogeneous picture of severe oral erosions and polymorphic skin lesions suggestive of both PV and erythema multiforme.[5] In each case the patients had an associated malignancy, generally lymphoreticular and including lymphoma, chronic lymphocytic leukemia, or thymomas. The histologic features of the skin lesions in these patients resembled those of PV, including suprabasilar blister formation with the additional finding of keratinocyte cell necrosis, as seen in erythema multiforme. The immunopathology of skin biopsies from these patients revealed IgG bound to keratinocyte cell surfaces, and granular-linear deposits of IgG and C3 at the basement membrane. In addition, the serum of these patients contained circulating IgG antibodies, which bound to normal keratinocyte cell surfaces of squamous epithelium. Although initial reports suggested that this antibody bound to both nonstratified and

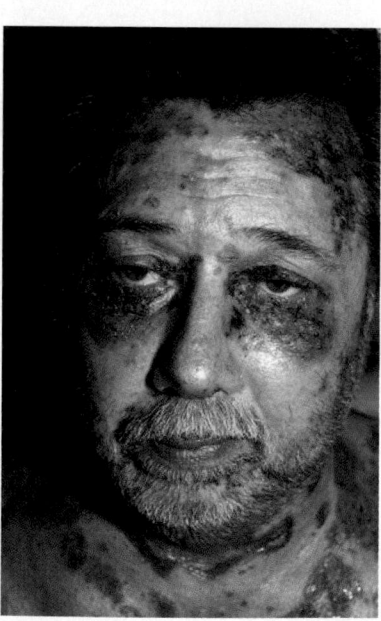

Fig. 63.1 Patient with pemphigus foliaceus showing superficial erosions and crust formation on the head and neck.

KEY CONCEPTS

PEMPHIGUS FOLIACEUS

>> Flaccid blisters with scale and crust

>> Oral mucous membrane lesions rare

>> Intraepidermal blister, granular cell layer

>> Immunoglobulin G deposits on keratinocyte cell surface (antigenic target = desmoglein-1)

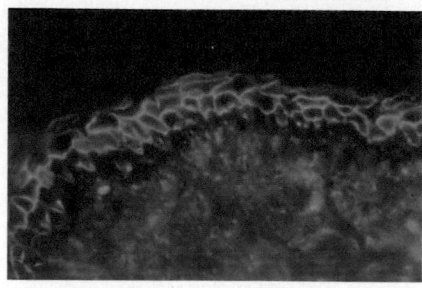

Fig. 63.2 Direct immunofluorescence of perilesional normal-appearing skin from a patient with pemphigus foliaceus using antibodies directed against human immunoglobulin G (IgG). Cell surface IgG deposits are seen on the epidermal keratinocytes. A similar pattern is seen in patients with pemphigus vulgaris.

stratified squamous epithelium, this is not always the case. The antigenic targets of these antibodies are also distinct from both PV and PF, as discussed later.

INTRAEPIDERMAL NEUTROPHILIC IgA DERMATOSIS

In 1985, a patient with an annular, vesiculopustular eruption characterized by intraepidermal blisters with numerous polymorphonuclear leukocytes (PMN) and intercellular deposits of IgA on direct immunofluorescence staining was described by Huff et al., who proposed the name intraepidermal neutrophilic IgA dermatosis.[6] This entity has subsequently been described by other investigators and has been referred to by several different names, including IgA pemphigus, intercellular IgA vesiculopustular dermatosis, and intercellular IgA dermatosis.

Patients with this disorder present with a heterogeneous clinical picture. Some present with tense blisters that enlarge peripherally to form a flower-like grouping, whereas others present with superficial pustules, erosions, and crusts. Sites of involvement include the trunk, abdomen, face, scalp, and extremities, but mucosal involvement has not been reported. Routine histology of lesional skin reveals the presence of either a subcorneal or an intraepidermal blister, with acantholytic cells and a polymorphous infiltrate marked by the predominance of PMN.

Direct immunofluorescence of perilesional skin biopsies from these patients shows IgA deposits on the keratinocyte cell surface. These deposits have been localized to the lower two-thirds of the epidermis in a subset of patients with a subcorneal pustular dermatosis-like disease. Approximately half of these patients have detectable, but low-titer, circulating IgA antibodies specific for epithelium.[6]

PATHOGENESIS

The antigenic targets in pemphigus have been defined as different components of desmosomes, key structures involved in keratinocyte adhesion (Table 63.1). IgG from patients with PF binds to a 160-kDa glycoprotein, desmoglein-1. IgG from patients with PV with only mucosal lesions binds predominantly to a distinct 130-kDa glycoprotein, desmoglein-3, a unique epithelial cadherin with significant homology to desmoglein-1. PV patients with both skin and mucosal disease have IgG antibodies directed against both desmoglein-1 and desmoglein-3.[7]

In paraneoplastic pemphigus, IgG antibodies have been shown to bind to members of the plakin family of desmosomal/hemidesmosomal proteins (desmoplakin I, II, envoplakin, periplakin, plectin, BPAG1) as well as to desmogleins-1 and -3.[5]

Sera from patients with intraepidermal IgA neutrophilic dermatosis have also been used to determine the antigenic targets relevant for this disease. Serum from a patient with the intraepidermal neutrophilic variant recognized a 120-kDa protein from extracts of normal human skin and bovine desmosomes.[8] In contrast, sera from patients with subcorneal pustular dermatosis-like disease recognized proteins in a bovine desmosomal extract that were identified as the desmosomal proteins desmocollin I and II.[8]

In addition to the identification of the specific antigens against which the IgG from patients with pemphigus react, it has been clearly demonstrated that these antibodies are pathogenic. Anhalt and co-workers developed an animal model that demonstrated the pathogenicity of the autoantibodies found in many forms of pemphigus.[9] In this model,

neonatal mice injected with IgG from patients with pemphigus developed cutaneous blisters, histologic changes and immunofluorescence findings consistent with pemphigus. This has been shown with sera from patients with PV, PF, and paraneoplastic pemphigus.[5, 9]

The factors that lead to the development of the autoimmune response are not known. Various investigators have demonstrated an increased frequency of human leukocyte antigen (HLA)-DR4 and HLA-DR6 in patients with PV.[10] Healthy relatives of patients with PV were also shown to have low levels of autoantibodies directed against an epidermal antigen similar to the PV antigen, and the presence of these antibodies was associated with HLA-DR4 or -DR6.[10, 11] Additional studies showed that a specific HLA-DR4 subtype (DRB1*0402) is associated with PV.[12] This DR4 subtype is distinct from those DR4 molecules associated with rheumatoid arthritis (Chapter 52). Studies also showed that T cells from patients with PV secreted high levels of interleukin (IL)-4 and IL-10 in response to specific desmoglein-3 peptides when presented by DRB1*0402.[12] Other workers have further demonstrated that T cells reactive against desmoglein-3 are present in patients with PV, and that T cells from some normal HLA DRB1*0402 subjects also responded to desmoglein-3.[13] It remains unclear what additional factors are required for HLA-susceptible individuals to develop clinical disease, but additional susceptibility genes and/or environmental factors are probably critical for disease development.

Fogo selvagem, a form of PF endemic to certain regions of Brazil, is also associated with particular HLA-DRB1 alleles (DRB1*1042, *1406 and *0404).[14, 15] The prevalence of antibodies against desmoglein-1 is high among normal subjects living in areas where fogo selvagem is endemic, and the onset of disease is preceded by a sustained antibody response.[3] Fogo selvagem has been associated with exposure to the hematophagous black flies found in the endemic areas of Brazil. It has been suggested that the development of fogo selvagem may be related to an immune response to the bite of this fly in the HLA-susceptible individuals who develop cross-reactive antibodies against desmoglein-1.

Despite the clearly demonstrated importance of autoantibodies in disease pathogenesis, the exact mechanism by which they cause acantholysis is not known. Complement components (C3, C1q) are often present in the lesional skin of patients with pemphigus but these autoantibodies can induce acantholysis both in vitro and in the neonatal mouse model without complement activation.[16] In total, these data suggest that, whereas complement may play a role in acantholysis, especially in an additive fashion, pemphigus IgG by itself can attach to the keratinocyte and induce the characteristic loss of cell–cell adhesion. Although early reports suggested that urokinase plasminogen activator was necessary for the development of skin lesions, pemphigus antibodies have been shown to be pathogenic in plasminogen-activator knockout mice.[17] Recent evidence suggests that acantholysis in pemphigus may be related to the intracellular signaling that occurs after the binding of pemphigus antibody to cell surface desmogleins,[18] with inhibition of p38MAPK preventing disease in the mouse model.[19]

THERAPY

Before the advent of systemic glucocorticoids, pemphigus was uniformly fatal. The introduction of high-dose systemic glucocorticoids and improvements in wound care have markedly reduced PV mortality but it remains a serious condition. Most blistering can be controlled with prednisone 1–2 mg/kg per day, usually in divided doses, and the dose can be

Table 63.1 Immunopathology of autoimmune blistering diseases

Disease	Direct IF (patient's skin)	Indirect IF (patient's serum)	Antigen(s)
Pemphigus vulgaris	IgG keratinocyte cell surface	IgG binds keratinocyte cell surface (normal stratified squamous epithelium)	Desmoglein-3 (DSG3) +/- Desmoglein-1 (DSG1)
Pemphigus foliaceus	IgG keratinocyte cell surface	IgG binds keratinocyte cell surface (normal stratified squamous epithelium)	Desmoglein-1 (DSG1)
Paraneoplastic pemphigus	IgG keratinocyte cell surface; C3, granular/linear at epidermal basement membrane (normal stratified and nonstratified squamous epithelium)	IgG binds keratinocyte cell surface	Plakin proteins, DSG1, DSG3
Bullous pemphigoid	Linear IgG, C3 at epidermal basement membrane	IgG binds in linear pattern normal stratified squamous epithelium basement membrane (epithelial side)	180-kDa, BPAg2 230-kDa, BPAg1
Herpes gestationis	Linear C3 at epidermal basement membrane (in 30–50% of patients linear IgG also seen)	IgG binds in linear pattern normal stratified squamous epithelium basement membrane (epithelial side)	180-kDa, BPAg2
Linear IgA bullous dermatosis	Linear IgA at epidermal basement membrane	IgA binds in linear pattern normal stratified squamous epithelium basement membrane (epithelial side)	97-kDa protein (portion of BPAg2)
Epidermolysis bullosa acquisita	Linear IgG epidermal basement membrane (IgA rarely)	IgG binds in linear pattern normal stratified squamous epithelium basement membrane (dermal side)	Type VII collagen (noncollagenous domain)
Dermatitis herpetiformis	Granular IgA dermal papillary tips	Negative	Epidermal transglutaminase (TGase 3)

IF, immunofluorescence; Ig, immunoglobulin.

slowly tapered toward alternate-day therapy. Although many patients are controlled on this regime, disease activity may flare during the corticosteroid taper. These patients require individualized management and often need additional immunosuppresion.

When additional immunosuppressive agents are required, azathioprine, cyclophosphamide, mycophenolate mofetil, methotrexate, or 'Cyclosporine' are most often utilized. However, no prospective controlled trials have demonstrated the superiority of these agents in the treatment of PV compared to corticosteroids alone. The relatively low toxicity of azathioprine (1–3 mg/kg per day) make this drug the first choice as an additional immunosuppressive agent. Other agents, including parenteral gold compounds, plasmapheresis, and extracorporeal photochemotherapy, have also been suggested as adjunctive therapy. Treatment for patients with PF follows many of the principles established for treating PV; however, PF is in general less severe and rarely fatal, and therapy should be designed with this in mind. Dapsone has proved to be the mainstay of therapy for patients with intraepidermal IgA neutrophilic dermatosis, probably owing to its effect on the cutaneous neutrophilic infiltrate.[6] Occasionally systemic glucocorticoid therapy may be needed, either alone or in conjunction with dapsone. Therapy for paraneoplastic pemphigus has been disappointing and in general unsuccessful.

Recently biological agents such as rituximab, infliximab, etanercept, and high-dose intravenous immunoglobulin have been utilized for the treatment of patients with pemphigus with some success, but no controlled studies have been performed to date.

■ BULLOUS PEMPHIGOID ■

CLINICAL FEATURES

Bullous pemphigoid (BP) is characterized clinically by extremely pruritic, tense blisters that can occur on either inflamed or noninflamed skin (Fig. 63.3). These can range in size from small (1–5 mm) vesicles to large bullous lesions several centimeters in diameter. In addition to the characteristic tense blisters, patients with BP can also present with a variety of other skin manifestations, including urticarial lesions, vesicular lesions or, rarely, eczematous dermatitis. Blisters can occur on any part of the skin, but are often found on the extremities, groin, and axilla. Oral and ocular

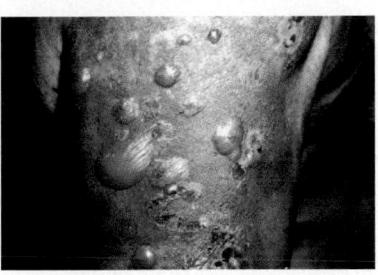

Fig. 63.3 Patient with bullous pemphigoid showing erythematous plaques with tense subepidermal blisters.

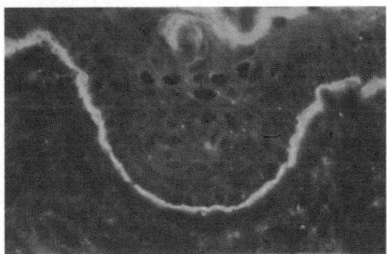

Fig. 63.4 Direct immunofluorescence of perilesional normal-appearing skin from a patient with bullous pemphigoid using antibodies directed against human C3. A linear band of C3 is present at the basement membrane.

KEY CONCEPTS

BULLOUS PEMPHIGOID

>> Tense subepidermal blisters

>> Oral mucous membrane lesions are rare

>> Subepidermal blister, most often with inflammatory infiltrate with eosinophils

>> Linear deposits of immunoglobulin G and C3 at the dermal–epidermal junction (antigenic target 230 and 180-kDa hemidesmosomal proteins)

---

mucosal lesions occur infrequently in patients with BP, in contrast to patients with cicatricial pemphigoid (CP), who have predominantly mucosal lesions.

Although BP is primarily a disease of the elderly, with most patients being over 60, BP can develop at any age. BP has also been reported in association with other diseases, including diabetes mellitus, psoriasis, other autoimmune diseases, and malignancy. The association with malignancy has been noted in case reports and retrospective studies for many years. However, when age- and sex-matched control studies were performed, no statistically increased incidence of malignancy was documented in patients with BP.[20] BP has also been associated with drugs, with furosemide and phenacetin being the most commonly noted. Finally, environmental factors such as ultraviolet light and therapeutic radiation have been reported to precipitate BP. In general, the prognosis for patients with BP is good, with a 1-year survival in the USA reported to be approximately 90%. European studies, however, have reported a significantly higher mortality rate; the reasons behind this difference are not currently understood.

Biopsy of an early lesion of BP can reveal a number of different patterns, consistent with the polymorphic appearance of the eruption. The classic finding is a subepidermal blister with an inflammatory infiltrate in the dermis, comprised predominantly of eosinophils with an admixture of lymphocytes, histiocytes, and neutrophils. The epidermis over this blister is often intact with minimal abnormality, while the blister cavity is filled with inflammatory cells. Variants of this presentation can be seen, including a neutrophil-predominant inflammatory infiltrate, and a cell-poor variant with few inflammatory cells. Occasionally, an early lesion of

BP may not show a subepidermal blister but just edema of the epidermis, with an infiltrate of eosinophils. Because of the polymorphic histology of BP, it is important to realize that the diagnosis is not solely dependent on the histologic and clinical findings.

Patients with BP usually have IgG and/or C3 deposits present in a linear pattern at the dermal–epidermal junction (DEJ) and many have circulating IgG antibodies that bind in a similar linear pattern at the DEJ of normal human skin. Direct immunofluorescence studies of perilesional skin are key to the diagnosis of BP. Some 90–100% of patients with BP have linear deposits of C3 at the DEJ, whereas 70–90% of patients have linear deposits of IgG at the DEJ (Fig. 63.4). C3 may be the only immunoreactant seen in the skin of some patients with BP. By indirect immunofluorescence analysis, 70–90% of patients with BP have circulating IgG that binds in a linear pattern at the DEJ of normal human skin. Although these antibodies are often present at high levels, no consistent relationship has been demonstrated between the presence or level of antibodies directed against the DEJ and clinical disease activity or prognosis.

Although the immunofluorescent findings in patients with BP are characteristic, they are not diagnostic. Other immunologically mediated blistering diseases, such as the bullous eruption of systemic lupus erythematosus, herpes gestationis (HG), and epidermolysis bullosa acquisita (EBA), can have similar patterns of immunoreactivity. Gammon and co-workers reported that the use of normal human skin split with 1 mol/L NaCl can help in distinguishing antibodies directed against BP antigen(s) and the EBA antigen.[21] NaCl treatment splits the skin within the lamina lucida, and IgG from patients with BP binds to the epidermal side only or to the epidermal and dermal sides, whereas antibodies from patients with EBA bind only to the dermal side (Fig. 63.5). Similar studies with NaCl-treated skin of BP patients demonstrated that IgG deposited *in vivo* is also localized to the epidermal side of the split skin.

PATHOGENESIS

Immunoelectron microscopic studies have demonstrated that the *in vivo* deposits of IgG are localized to the lamina lucida of the basement membrane. The target antigens are components of hemidesmosomes, which are the major attachment site of epidermal basal cells and serve as the site of linkage for cytoskeletal proteins through the plasma membrane to the dermis. Characterization of the antigen–antibody interaction in patients with BP has revealed two predominant antigens that are 230-kDa and 180-kDa proteins.

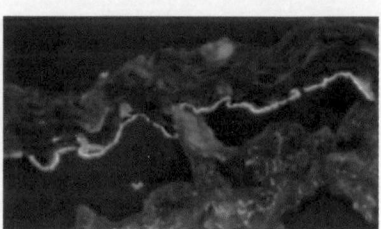

Fig. 63.5 Indirect immunofluorescence using serum from a patient with bullous pemphigoid. Serum was incubated with frozen sections of normal human skin which had been incubated with 1 mol/L NaCl. Immunoglobulin G deposits are present on the epithelial basement membrane associated with the epidermis and not on the dermal side of the split skin.

The 230-kDa and 180-kDa BP antigens have both been cloned and sequenced, confirming that they are distinct proteins, associated as a complex within the hemidesmosome in the native state. The 230-kDa BP antigen (BPAG1) is an intracellular protein with sequence homology to the desmosomal protein, desmoplakin I, a member of an adhesion junction plaque protein family. The 180-kDa BP antigen (BPAG2) contains both intra- and extracellular domains joined by a transmembrane region. The extracellular portion of this protein is remarkable for the presence of alternating collagen and noncollagen domains and has also been termed type XVII collagen. Epitope mapping studies of the 180-kDa protein have identified an immunodominant epitope that maps to an extracellular domain adjacent to the transmembrane region that is also a target for IgG antibodies in the sera of patients with herpes (pemphigoid) gestationis.[22]

Although patients with BP have antibody reactivity against both BPAG1 and BPAG2, the role of these autoantibodies in the pathogenesis of BP has not been clearly established. The 230-kDa BPAG1 is located inside the cell, and it is unclear how the autoantibodies may have access to the antigen. Target disruption of the gene encoding BPAG1 did not result in blister formation or epidermal–dermal adhesion abnormalities. These results suggest that antibodies to BPAG1 may not directly inhibit the function of BPAG1. They may, however, play an important role in maintaining or enhancing the inflammatory response in patients with BP.

Patients with BP and with herpes (pemphigoid) gestationis develop antibodies against a specific noncollagenous, extracellular portion of the BPAG2 molecule.[22] Serum levels of autoantibodies directed against BPAG2 have also been correlated with disease activity in patients with BP.[23] Further evidence for the important role for BPAG2 in BP is provided by the observation that patients with a form of inherited skin blistering and generalized atrophic benign epidermolysis bullosa have a mutation in BPAG2 that results in a dysfunctional or missing protein.[24]

In order to develop an animal model of BP, rabbits were immunized to produce antibodies directed against the region of the mouse BPAG2, which corresponds to the immunodominant region of the human BPAG2. Passive transfer of this rabbit IgG to newborn mice resulted in the development of clinical blisters, an inflammatory infiltrate, and the deposition of immunoreactants. In this model complement activation, mast cell degranulation, and neutrophil infiltration are important in blister formation.[25]

Complement activation and other extracellular mediators also appear to be involved in the pathogenesis of the skin lesions of BP. Complement

and the terminal components of the complement cascade are present in the skin of patients with BP. Early lesions in BP patients contain eosinophil granule proteins, suggesting that eosinophils play an important role in the early development of the lesions. A 92-kDa gelatinase produced by eosinophils present in the skin of patients with BP is capable of cleaving BPAG2.[26] Together, these findings support the hypothesis that the IgG autoantibody binds to the BP antigen, initially most likely BPAG2, and activates the complement cascade and the local production of cytokines, resulting in an accumulation of eosinophils and neutrophils that release enzymes, including gelatinases, leading to blister formation. Recent findings have also demonstrated IgE antibodies directed against BPAG2 in the serum of patients with BP, suggesting that IgE antibodies may play an important role in the early lesions of BP and the development of the eosinophil-dominant inflammatory infiltrate.[27]

The factors that induce the development of autoantibodies in patients with BP are unknown. T cells from patients with BP respond *in vitro* to the extracellular region of the BPAG2,[28] and this reactivity is restricted by HLA-DQB1*0301. Normal HLA-DQB1*0301 subjects showed similar T-cell reactivity, but whereas T cells from the patients with BP produced both Th1- and Th2-type cytokines, normal subjects only produced Th1-type cytokines. These results suggest that the ability to mount a Th2 T-cell response to the BP antigen(s) may play a critical role in the development of the disease.

THERAPY

The mainstay of therapy for patients with BP is systemic glucocorticoids. The majority respond rapidly to 0.5–2.0 mg/kg per day of oral prednisone. Mild or localized disease can sometimes be managed by the use of potent topical corticosteroids; however, this form of BP often progresses to more severe involvement, necessitating systemic therapy. When new blister formation has stopped and healing has begun, a slow taper of the systemic steroids can be commenced. The speed of the taper is often dictated by the severity of the patient's initial disease and the minor flares that may occur during the taper. The majority of patients can be tapered off systemic steroids completely within 6–18 months. Recurrence of active disease is not uncommon. These episodes should be managed with the minimal amount of systemic steroids possible and can occasionally be treated just using topical corticosteroid therapy. In general, BP is a self-limiting process, which usually lasts between 1.5 and 5 years, and responds promptly to treatment with systemic glucocorticoids.

A minority of patients require prolonged high-dose systemic glucocorticoids. In these individuals the addition of immunosuppresive agents such as azathioprine, cyclophosphamide, or methotrexate will often allow tapering or discontinuation of systemic steroid therapy. Few prospective, controlled studies have been done to determine which of these drugs, if any, is superior as a steroid-sparing agent. One controlled study failed to demonstrate any substantial benefit from using either plasmapheresis or azathioprine in addition to systemic glucocorticoids in BP.[29] It is important to note, however, that this study did not address the utility of these agents in patients who had initially been unable to discontinue therapy with systemic glucocorticoids. Other unproven adjunctive therapies that may help in some patients include mycophenolate mofetil, dapsone, cyclosporine and tetracycline with niacinamide. When additional therapy is needed, we favor the use of azathioprine at doses of 1–2 mg/kg per day. A recent analysis of controlled trials published for the treatment of patients with BP concluded

KEY CONCEPTS

EPIDERMOLYSIS BULLOSA ACQUISITA (EBA)

>> Classic EBA with subepidermal blisters, extreme fragility of acral skin

>> Inflammatory EBA with subepidermal blisters similar to bullous pemphigoid

>> Oral, conjunctival, and other mucous membrane lesions frequent

>> Linear deposits of immunoglobulin G at the dermal–epidermal junction, localized to the dermis (antigenic target = type VII collagen)

that very potent topical steroids may be effective and safe and that starting doses of prednisolone above 0.75 mg/kg per day do not offer any greater benefit.[30]

EPIDERMOLYSIS BULLOSA ACQUISITA

EBA is a chronic subepidermal blistering disease that typically presents in the fourth to sixth decades. Patients with the classic form of EBA present with peripherally distributed blisters that heal with scarring and milia formation. The skin of these patients is extremely fragile, often resulting in numerous erosions in areas of mechanical trauma, such as the hands, feet, elbows, and knees. Oral mucous membrane lesions, including esophageal involvement, are often seen. In addition, patients with classic EBA may develop lesions in the ocular, vaginal, urethral, and rectal mucosae. Ocular changes are common and these patients may clinically resemble those with CP. Other cutaneous manifestations include scarring alopecia and variable degrees of nail dystrophy. Patients can also present with a nonclassic or inflammatory type of EBA, the clinical presentation of which is essentially identical to that seen in BP, with widespread tense blisters on an erythematous base, which heal without scarring.

EBA has been associated with a variety of other diseases, particularly inflammatory bowel disease and systemic lupus erythematosus. Part of the explanation for these associations may be the result of the association of EBA with the specific HLA type, DR-2.

Skin biopsies of early lesions from patients with EBA reveal subepidermal blisters with variable degrees of inflammatory response. In patients with classic EBA lesional skin biopsies often have a minimal inflammatory cell infiltrate. In contrast, patients with the inflammatory variant may have substantial collections of inflammatory cells in the superficial dermis, usually consisting of an admixture of mononuclear cells, PMN, and eosinophils.

Direct immunofluorescence shows deposition of immunoreactants, most often IgG, at the DEJ in patients with EBA. Direct immunofluorescence of perilesional skin biopsies from patients with EBA displays a pattern of immunoreactants similar to that seen in patients with BP, with linear deposits of IgG at the DEJ. Linear deposits of C3, IgM, IgA, and

fibrinogen have also been reported in patients with EBA. However, the immunoreactants in the skin of patients with EBA have a different localization from those in the skin of patients with BP. In EBA, the immunoreactants are localized exclusively below the lamina lucida. This distinctive localization of immunoreactants can be visualized by incubating the patient's skin biopsy with 1 mol/L NaCl, which splits the skin at the basement membrane zone. Direct immunofluroesence testing of this "split skin" from patients with EBA will localize the in vivo-deposited IgG to the floor of the in vitro-generated blister, whereas in patients with BP, the IgG localizes to the blister roof.

Indirect immunofluorescence using stratified squamous epithelia such as normal human skin shows circulating anti-basement membrane-zone antibodies in 30–50% of patients with EBA. When NaCl-treated split skin is used as a substrate, however, IgG antibody can be detected in up to 85% of patients, making this a more sensitive and specific substrate for clinical testing. As would be expected based on the in vivo deposition pattern, IgG from patients with EBA localizes to the blister floor. With the improved immunologic characterization of patients with EBA it has become apparent that patients with various other clinical presentations also have antibodies in sera and skin identical to those seen in EBA. One such group includes patients with the bullous eruption of systemic lupus erythematosus, who have a vesiculobullous eruption that is clinically and histologically similar to dermatitis herpetiformis (DH). However, many of these patients have a linear band of IgG at the DEJ that localizes to the floor of 1 mol/L NaCl split skin. Another clinical presentation with EBA-like antibodies against the DEJ of skin is CP. These patients have a limited blistering eruption of the skin with marked mucosal involvement, including oral and ocular inflammation and scarring. These phenotypes are now included in the spectrum of EBA on the basis of the immunologic studies described above, as well as the discovery that antibodies against type VII collagen are demonstrable in each of them.

PATHOGENESIS

Immunoelectron microscopy has shown immunoglobulin deposits in patients with EBA localized to the lamina densa zone of the basement membrane, below the lamina lucida. Standard transmission electron microscopy of lesional skin of patients with EBA shows that the anchoring fibrils are decreased or absent. These findings may be relevant in the development of the clinically evident skin fragility, as anchoring fibrils are postulated to play a role in epidermal–dermal adherence via the linkage of the hemidesmosome through the basement membrane. The lack of an inflammatory infiltrate in many patients with EBA suggests that these autoantibodies may disrupt the interaction between anchoring fibrils and dermal matrix proteins.

The target antigen for the IgG autoantibodies present in the sera of patients with EBA is type VII collagen, a 300-kDa glycoprotein composed of a 145-kDa noncollagenous domain (NC1) at the amino-terminal end, an 18-kDa noncollagenous domain (NC2) at the carboxy-terminus, and a central collagenous domain. IgG antibodies from patients with EBA appear to be specific for epitopes within the NC1 noncollagenous domain of the protein. Type VII collagen is the major structural component of anchoring fibrils and is produced by both epithelial keratinocytes and dermal fibroblasts. Recently, passive transfer experiments using mice, as well as active immune models, have provided additional support for the critical role of antibodies directed against type VII collagen in the pathogenesis of EBA.[31]

TREATMENT

Spontaneous resolution is infrequent in EBA, and management is difficult. The main goals of therapy are to minimize blistering and scar formation, with particular concern for ocular and oral mucosal lesions. Systemic glucocorticoids are the mainstay of therapy, especially for patients with the inflammatory variant of EBA. Unfortunately, even high-dose systemic steroids do not usually affect fragility and trauma-induced blister formation of the skin. Mucosal lesions often respond to systemic steroids in doses of 0.5–1.5 mg/kg per day, but recur with tapering and/or discontinuation of steroids. Several agents have been proposed as adjunctive agents, including azathioprine, cyclophosphamide, dapsone, hydroxychloroquine, and plasmapheresis. However, none has been consistently demonstrated to be effective. Cyclosporine has been used to treat patients with EBA with some success, although toxicity has limited therapy in some cases. Photophoresis and intravenous immunoglobulin have also been reported to be effective in some patients with refractory EBA.[32] Rituximab has also been used succesfully in EBA in a single case report.[33]

Mucous membrane lesions can prove particularly difficult to manage and may necessitate systemic therapy. Ocular lesions should be followed by an ophthalmologist and may require systemic glucocorticoids to prevent conjunctival scarring. Oral mucous membrane lesions can sometimes be managed with frequent application of potent topical steroid ointments or gels (0.05% clobetasol propionate, 0.05% fluocinonide). If this fails and the degree of oral erosions is inhibiting the maintenance of appropriate nutrition, systemic glucocorticoid therapy may be required. In addition, clinicians should always be aware of possible involvement of the esphogeal and/or tracheal mucosa and involve appropriate specialists to monitor and treat these potentially severe complications.

The management of chronic skin wounds is of primary importance in the care of EBA patients. Protection of the skin from trauma and the early use of topical and systemic antibiotics when infections develop are critical to improving the rate of healing. The recent development of new biological dressings for chronic ulcers has also proved helpful in the management of these wounds.

■ HERPES (PEMPHIGOID) GESTATIONIS ■

HG is a rare, itchy blistering disease of pregnancy and the puerperium characterized by linear deposits of IgG and C3 at the DEJ.[34] The descriptor of 'herpes' was initially chosen because of the frequent appearance of groups of vesicular lesions, similar to those seen in primary herpetic infections of the skin. However, HG has no relationship to herpes virus infections. Recently some workers have proposed renaming this eruption pemphigoid gestationis, emphasizing its close association with BP.

HG is rare, occurring in fewer than 1 per 50 000 pregnancies in North America. It usually presents in the third trimester or in the immediate postpartum period. Although it may recur in subsequent pregnancies, this is not absolute. Disease flares in the immediate postpartum period do occur, and patients have been reported to develop blisters when menses return or when oral contraceptives are used.

HG presents as tense blisters, often on an urticarial base, ranging in size from small (3–5 mm) vesicles to large (1–2 cm) bullae. The blisters often begin on the abdomen, although the entire body can be involved. Pruritus is a common feature and can be quite severe.

HG is associated with maternal morbidity and increased fetal morbidity and mortality. The maternal morbidity is mainly related to the skin disease, with extensive itching and blister formation. Fetal morbidity and mortality were previously estimated to range as high as 30%, but several subsequent studies have suggested that this figure is too high.[35] Prematurity and low birth weight may be associated with HG. Infants born to mothers with HG may also develop skin lesions similar to those seen in the mother, due to transplacental passage of maternal autoantibodies. The skin lesions seen in these infants resolve spontaneously with the clearance of maternal immunoglobulin.

The histopathology of HG lesions is not diagnostic. Subepidermal blisters are seen with a perivascular infiltrate containing eosinophils, neutrophils, lymphocytes, and monocytes. Necrotic basal keratinocytes can also be seen. None of these findings is sufficiently distinct, however, to separate HG from other subepidermal blistering diseases on the basis of histologic appearance alone.

Direct immunofluorescence studies of the skin of patients with HG reveal a linear pattern of C3 at the DEJ. In addition, 30–50% of patients have linear deposits of IgG in a similar pattern. Occasionally other immunoreactants, including IgA, IgM, C1q, C4, properidin, factor B and C5, may be present, localized to the lamina lucida region of the DEJ. Indirect immunofluorescence reveals circulating IgG antibodies directed against the epidermal basement membrane in only ~30% of patients. If, however, a complement fixation technique is used, 50–75% of patients will have evidence of IgG antibody directed against epithelial basement membrane. This IgG anti-basement membrane antibody is detected by its ability to fix complement *in vitro*, but cannot be directly detected by routine indirect immunofluorescence due to its low concentration. This autoantibody can cross the placenta, and infants born to mothers with HG will often have C3 deposits at the DEJ, even in the absence of clinical skin disease. The use of 1 mol/L NaCl split skin as the substrate for indirect immunofluorescence has revealed that the IgG antibody present in the serum of patients with HG binds to the epithelial side of the split skin,[36] a pattern identical to that seen in BP.

PATHOGENESIS

Sera from most patients with HG bind to the 180-kDa BPAG2, but do not react with the 230-kDa BPAG1 antigen.[36] In addition, T cells from patients with HG react to peptides from BPAG2.[37] The critical role of pregnancy and other hormonal factors in the development of HG is not understood.

An increased frequency of the HLA-DR3 haplotype has been demonstrated in patients with HG, and the greatest relative risk is associated with the presence of both HLA-DR3 and -DR4. It has also been reported that patients with HG have an increased frequency of anti-HLA antibodies compared to multiparous control subjects. Although some data suggest that the paternal haplotype is important in the pathogenesis of HG, further prospective studies are indicated. Patients with HG are also reported to have an increased frequency of the C4 null allele, although this has been postulated to be secondary to the increased frequency of HLA-DR3 in this patient population.

TREATMENT

Therapy of patients with HG is directed at relieving the significant pruritus and preventing the development of new blisters. If the extent of disease is limited, patients can be managed with topical glucocorticoids and antihistamines.[34] Most patients, however, have more significant disease and require the use of systemic glucocorticoids. Treatment with prednisone 20–60 mg/day is sufficient to control both the pruritus and new blister formation in the vast majority of cases. Every attempt should be made to reduce the corticosteroids to the lowest possible effective dose. Occasionally it may be possible to stop prednisone before delivery. However, the physician should be aware that flares of HG are often seen in the immediate postpartum period. Only rarely will patients require therapy beyond the initial postpartum period. In patients who require prolonged therapy postpartum, immunosuppressive agents such as those used in the other blistering diseases should be considered. Patients being treated with either systemic steroids or immunosuppressive drugs should be counseled with regard to breast-feeding restrictions.

Occasionally infants born to mothers with HG will have skin lesions.[34] These are limited in extent and resolve spontaneously with the disappearance of maternal IgG from the infant's circulation.

■ CICATRICIAL PEMPHIGOID ■

CP is a rare, chronic, scarring blistering disease that predominantly affects the oral and conjunctival mucosae. Involvement of the conjunctiva can range from a mild conjunctivitis to severe conjunctival inflammation leading to symblepharon formation, entropion, trichiasis, corneal scarring and, eventually, blindness in some patients. Oral mucosal lesions include gingivitis, often with erosions and desquamation, as well as erosions and ulcerations on the buccal mucosa and the hard and soft palates. Rarely esophageal and laryngeal involvement is seen with resultant scarring and stenosis. Other mucosal sites that can be involved include the genitalia, rectum, and nasopharynx. Cutaneous involvement occurs in 10–25% of patients, although it is often limited in extent and located predominantly on the scalp, back, or face.[38]

Mucosal biopsies reveal a subepidermal blister with a cellular infiltrate that is usually composed of lymphocytes and plasma cells. Increased numbers of neutrophils or eosinophils have also been reported. Skin biopsies of lesions in patients with CP are essentially indistinguishable from those seen in BP.

Direct immunofluorescence of perilesional skin or mucosal samples reveals a linear deposit of immunoreactants at the basement membrane zone.[39] The majority of patients with CP have IgG and C3 deposits at the basement membrane, although the presence of other immunoreactants, including IgA, IgM, and fibrin, has also been reported. It is important to note that, in patients with ocular or oral mucosal CP who do not have skin lesions, an undirected skin biopsy for immunofluorescence is of little diagnostic use. Similarly, biopsy of the conjunctiva can sometimes yield negative immunofluorescence results in patients with otherwise typical CP. This may be due to the inflammation present in the conjunctiva. In such patients a careful evaluation for mucosal lesions and biopsy of the perilesional mucosa is often diagnostic. On immunoelectron microscopy, immunoreactants have been localized within both the lamina lucida and the lamina densa.

Circulating anti-basement membrane-zone antibodies may be present in low titer, but are usually absent in patients with CP. Attempts to improve the yield of indirect immunofluorescence by using a variety of tissue substrates, including oral and conjunctival mucosa, normal human skin, and normal human split skin, have for the most part been unsuccessful.

PATHOGENESIS

Our understanding of the pathogenesis of CP has been hampered by both the heterogeneous clinical presentation and the lack of high-titer serum antibodies. The identification of different immunoglobulin classes at the basement membrane using immunofluorescence and the different localization of those immunoglobulins in the basement membrane on immunoelectron microscopy support the hypothesis that CP is a heterogeneous disease, with a variety of basement membrane-zone proteins serving as relevant targets. Chan and co-workers have correlated the clinical presentation, immunopathology, and target antigens in a group of patients with immune-mediated subepithelial blistering disorders of the mucous membranes.[39] About 90% of patients with both skin and mucous membrane lesions or mucous membrane lesions alone had immunoreactants present on direct immunofluorescence. In contrast, only 40% of patients with isolated ocular disease had C3 and/or IgG deposits. This finding may reflect the difficulty encountered in biopsies of the inflamed conjunctiva. Of more interest, however, were the results of indirect immunofluorescence: 11 of 14 (81%) patients with skin and mucous membrane disease had circulating IgG anti-basement membrane-zone antibodies, of which 9 identified BPAG1 and BPAG2 by immunoblot and/or immunoprecipitation. In contrast, only 3 of 24 patients with only oral mucosal lesions or ocular lesions had positive indirect immunofluorescence, one of which reacted with the BP antigens.

Other investigators have reported antibody reactivity in patients with CP to a variety of epidermal and dermal proteins. Sera from patients with CP have been shown to react with BPAG2. Sera from ocular CP patients have been reported to react with a 205-kDa protein that has homology with the cytoplasmic domain of β_4-integrin and a 45-kDa protein. Some patients with a clinical phenotype suggestive of CP have autoantibodies directed against epiligrin, a ligand for major keratinocyte integrins ($\alpha_3\beta_1$ and $\alpha_6\beta_4$). Characterization of patients with anti-epiligrin CP is of importance due to the increased risk of malignancy in these individuals.[40] These data suggest that the clinical presentation of CP is associated with a heterogeneous group of autoantibodies that react with multiple antigens of the skin basement membrane zone. The different clinical presentations may therefore result from not only different target antigens, but also perhaps different antibody-binding sites on antigens such as the BP antigen.

The HLA antigen DQB1*0301 has been found to occur with an increased frequency in Caucasian patients with isolated ocular, or with ocular and oral mucosal CP.[41, 42] Chan and co-workers reported that this association was not found in patients with oral mucosal disease without ocular disease, and suggested that the increased frequency of the DQB1*0301 allele may play a role in the development of ocular disease.[42] These results need to be confirmed in larger populations.

THERAPY

Treatment of CP is difficult and directed at minimizing the scarring and resultant complications that can occur in the eye. Dapsone in doses of 100–200 mg/day has been found by many investigators to be effective at controlling the early inflammatory response in patients with CP.[43] Some investigators have also found that tetracyclines, often in combination with nicotinamide, can control the inflammatory process seen in patients with CP. If this therapy is unsuccessful, treatment with systemic glucocorticoids (1–2 mg/kg per day), often with adjunctive immunosuppressive therapy such as azathioprine or cyclophosphamide, may be needed. Intravenous immunoglobulin has been reported to be useful by some authors, but no controlled studies have been performed. Isolated case reports also suggest that therapy with mycophenolate mofetil or plasmapheresis may be of benefit in some patients with CP, but again no control studies or large series using these therapies have been reported. It is important to note that the clinical course of CP is difficult to predict and that the response to treatment in some patients is often suboptimal. Some patients are able to achieve long-lasting remissions, but active disease frequently recurs and patients in remission should be followed closely.

Ocular mucosal lesions may often be severe and can represent significant morbidity in patients with CP. Consultation with an ophthalmologist is important in managing the potentially severe ocular complications seen in patients with CP. Physicians should also be aware of the potential for esophageal and tracheal disease activity and consultation with physicians with expertise in gastroenterology and otolaryngology is often required for patients with severe disease. Oral mucosal lesions can often be managed with potent topical corticosteroids (0.05% clobetasol propionate ointment, 0.05% fluocinonide gel) applied frequently to lesions. In severe cases dapsone or systemic glucocorticoids may be needed. Patients with limited amounts of skin disease can often be managed with topical therapy alone. If this fails, management techniques such as those discussed for patients with BP are usually successful.

■ LINEAR IgA BULLOUS DISEASES ■

Linear IgA bullous disease (LABD) is a clinically heterogeneous blistering disease in which direct immunofluorescence of perilesional skin biopsies reveals the presence of a linear band of IgA at the basement membrane zone.[44] The majority of patients with LABD present with pruritic vesicles and papules, localized primarily to the extensor surfaces, similar to the clinical pattern seen in patients with DH. Patients with LABD do not, however, have an associated gluten-sensitive enteropathy, are not able to control their disease by a gluten-free diet, and do not have the characteristic HLA associations of patients with DH.

Other patients with linear IgA deposits may present with a clinical picture more suggestive of BP, with pruritic tense blisters on an erythematous base. Other clinical presentations have been described with clinical as well as histologic and immunopathologic overlap between patients with LABD and CP or EBA. Finally, children can develop a subepidermal blistering disease with linear IgA deposits; this was previously termed chronic bullous disease of childhood.[44] In these cases the blisters occur mainly in flexural areas, with pruritus that is more variable in degree than in many other blistering diseases.

Routine histopathology of lesional skin of patients with LABD reflects the clinical heterogeneity seen in these patients. Biopsy usually reveals collections of neutrophils in the dermal papillary tips in a pattern virtually identical to that seen in biopsies from patients with dermatitis herpetiformis (DH). However, subepidermal blisters with eosinophils, as observed in patients with BP, may also be seen.

Direct immunofluorescence of perilesional skin in patients with LABD reveals a linear band of IgA at the basement membrane zone,

which has been characterized to be almost exclusively IgA$_1$.[44] Further characterization of these IgA deposits in the skin has revealed that both κ and λ light chains are present, indicating that the antibodies are polyclonal. In addition, J chain has not been detected, suggesting that the IgA is monomeric and may not be of gut origin. Immunoelectron microscopic localization of the immunoreactants has most often revealed IgA deposits in the lamina lucida; however, sublamina densa IgA deposits have also been noted. Circulating IgA antibodies against the basement membrane zone of stratified squamous epithelium have been detected in only 10–30% of patients (children and adults) with linear IgA deposits. Other immunoreactants, especially IgG and C3, have been found in 30–40% of these patients.

PATHOGENESIS

The absence of circulating antibody has made it difficult to determine the antigenic target in LABD. Zone et al. reported that sera from both adults and children with linear IgA deposits within the lamina lucida reacted with a 97-kDa protein that is identical to a portion of the 180-kDa BP antigen BPAG2.[45] In patients with LABD or linear IgA disease of childhood and who have sublaminar densa IgA deposits, investigators have identified reactivity to type VII collagen, and to an unknown 285-kDa dermal protein.[46] These findings support the hypothesis that the target antigens in LABD, including linear IgA disease of childhood, are heterogeneous. Regardless of the location of the IgA deposits or the specific antigenic target, the mechanism of lesion formation in patients with LABD remains unknown.

THERAPY

Dapsone is the mainstay of therapy of patients with all forms of LABD. The exact mechanism of its action is not known, but, as discussed above, this drug seems most useful in diseases with marked neutrophil infiltrates in lesional skin. The dosage needed to control the cutaneous eruption ranges from 25 to 200 mg/day. Most patients can be controlled with 100 mg/day, with minimal side effects. Although dapsone is well tolerated by most patients, it does have significant pharmacologic and idiosyncratic adverse effects and should only be used by physicians experienced in its use. Occasionally patients may not respond to dapsone alone. In these cases the addition of low doses of systemic glucocorticoids (prednisone 10–20 mg/day) may result in significant improvement. If patients cannot tolerate dapsone, systemic glucocorticoids in doses of 40–60 mg/day are usually effective. However, as most adult patients with LABD require long-term therapy, treatment with prednisone should be avoided whenever possible.

■ DERMATITIS HERPETIFORMIS ■

CLINICAL FEATURES

DH is an intensely pruritic blistering disease that classically presents in the second or third decade with erythematous papules and/or vesicles localized over the extensor surfaces (Fig. 63.6). Patients often present with a broad spectrum of lesions. The severe pruritus leads to patients scratching the small papules and vesicles and as a result they often present with multiple erosions. Patients can also present with urticarial

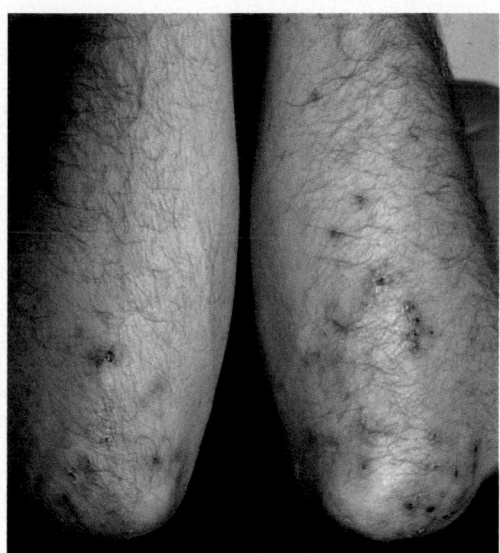

Fig. 63.6 Patient with dermatitis herpetiformis showing erythematous papules with crusts on the elbows. Rare intact vesicles are present.

KEY CONCEPTS

DERMATITIS HERPETIFORMIS

>> Extremely itchy, small blisters on extensor surfaces

>> Associated with asymptomatic/gluten-sensitive enteropathy

>> Increased frequency of human leukocyte antigen (HLA)-B8, -DR3, -DQ2 haplotype

>> Granular deposits of immunoglobulin A at the dermal–epidermal junction (antigenic target unknown)

>> Skin disease controlled by gluten-free diet

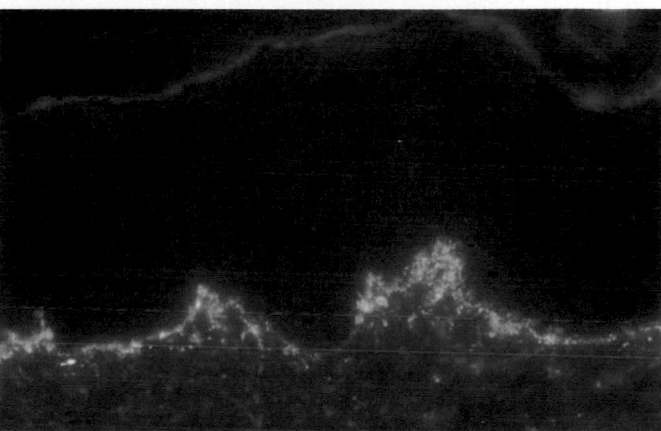

Fig. 63.7 Direct immunofluorescence of normal-appearing perilesional skin of a patient with dermatitis herpetiformis using antibodies against human immunoglobulin A (IgA). Granular deposits of IgA are present at the dermal–epidermal junction.

plaques or, more rarely, frank bullae. Lesions are most often symmetrically distributed over the extensor surfaces, especially the elbows, knees, buttocks, back, and posterior hairline. Symptomatic mucous membrane lesions are rarely present. One clinical hallmark of DH is the extreme pruritus that patients experience. They characteristically report feeling a severe burning or stinging 12–24 hours before the appearance of a lesion, which persists until the vesicle is broken and the crust forms. Although the clinical manifestations of DH may wax and wane, DH is generally a lifelong dermatosis. The wide variety of clinical presentations of DH often suggests a long differential diagnosis, including erythema multiforme, HG, BP, transient acantholytic dermatitis, papular urticaria, scabies, bug bites, and neurotic excoriations.

The frequency of DH varies in different ethnic groups. In Anglo-Saxon and Scandinavian populations it has been estimated to be between 10 and 39 per 100 000 persons, whereas DH occurs much less frequently in other populations, such as African-Americans and Asians. This relates in part to the different frequency of the DH-associated HLA antigens in different populations.

Biopsy of an early lesion of DH reveals a characteristic neutrophilic infiltrate in the dermal papillae with the presence of fibrin, neutrophilic fragments, edema, and variable numbers of eosinophils. This histologic pattern is not specific; it has been reported in patients with BP, linear IgA disease, the bullous eruption of systemic lupus erythematosus, and leukocytoclastic vasculitis. When older bullous lesions are biopsied in patients with DH, the histologic features are often indistinguishable from those seen with other blistering disorders.

IgA is present at the DEJ of the skin of patients with DH (Fig. 63.7). Two patterns of IgA deposition were initially described in patients with identical clinical findings: 85–90% of patients had granular deposits of IgA at the DEJ, and 10–15% had a linear band of IgA at the DEJ. These patterns, consistent within a given individual, have now been shown to distinguish between two different diseases. Patients with linear IgA deposits have LABD (see previous section), whereas patients with

granular deposits of IgA are considered to have true DH. The granular deposits of IgA at the DEJ are specific for patients with DH and have not been found in those with isolated gluten-sensitive enteropathy (GSE) or asymptomatic relatives of patients with DH.[47]

Granular deposits of IgA are found in both involved and uninvolved skin of patients with DH, including the oral mucosa. Consistent regional variations in the amount of IgA in the skin of patients with DH have not been reported. However, Zone and co-workers reported that IgA was either markedly decreased or absent in skin in which the patient reported never having had any lesions.[48] These observations suggest that biopsies taken for direct immunofluorescence studies should be obtained from normal-appearing perilesional skin in order to maximize the diagnostic yield.

IgG, IgM, and IgE are not usually found in the skin of patients with DH. The third component of complement, C3, along with early components of the alternative complement pathway, may be present in skin biopsies of patients with DH. The neoantigens of the C5–C9 membrane attack complex have also been reported to be present in normal-appearing skin of patients with DH. However, the co-localization of vitronectin with the C9 neoantigen suggests that the C5–C9 neoantigen is deposited in DH skin as part of the nonlytic C5–C9 complex, and that the lytic membrane attack complex of complement may not play a primary role in the development of DH skin lesions.[49]

Characterization of IgA in DH skin has shown that it contains both κ and λ light chains, indicating that the IgA is polyclonal. Secretory component, a transport protein bound to secretory IgA, has not been found in these IgA deposits. IgA$_1$ is the predominant subclass found in the skin of patients, with either minimal or no deposits of IgA$_2$ detected.[50] Although this would seem to suggest that the IgA in DH skin may not be mucosal in origin, IgA$_1$ is also the predominant subclass in the gastrointestinal secretions of patients with DH.[51]

In 1966 Marks and co-workers noted a gastrointestinal abnormality in 60–70% of patients with DH, which was histologically similar to that seen in isolated GSE.[52] This abnormality was reversible with the avoidance of dietary gluten, confirming that DH was a gluten-sensitive disease. The histologic changes seen in the small bowel of patients with DH are characterized by flattening of the normal villous architecture of the jejunal epithelium, with elongation of the intestinal crypts and a mononuclear cell infiltrate both within the lamina propria and in an intraepithelial location. This disease is often patchy in character in both DH and isolated GSE, and in general the findings in patients with DH are less severe than those seen in isolated GSE. Essentially all patients with the clinical features of DH and granular IgA deposits have associated GSE.

Despite the morphological similarity of the intestinal abnormality seen in patients with DH and those with isolated GSE, most patients with DH have no gastrointestinal symptoms. Only 10% of patients with DH have the typical symptoms of isolated GSE, such as bloating, diarrhea, and malabsorption, whereas 20–30% may have mild steatorrhea. However, many patients with DH do have abnormal intestinal function, as documented by abnormal absorption of D-xylose, iron, folate, glucose, water, and bicarbonate.

Despite the asymptomatic nature of the GSE associated with DH, it is clear that it plays a critical role in the pathogenesis of DH. The observations that patients with DH who adhere to gluten-free diets can control their skin disease, normalize the morphologic changes of the small intestine, and after years of gluten avoidance lose the cutaneous IgA deposits, are strong evidence that the GSE plays a fundamental role in the pathogenesis of DH. However, the exact relationship between the skin disease, the cutaneous IgA deposits, and the associated GSE remains unknown.

Initial studies of HLA associations in patients with DH and granular deposits of IgA revealed that 70–90% of those with DH express the HLA class I antigen B8, compared to only 20–30% of control subjects. Subsequent studies showed that 90–95% of patients with DH express HLA-DR3, compared to about 23% of controls. In addition, 95–100% of DH patients express HLA-DQ2 (which is in linkage disequilibrium with HLA-B8 and -DR3), compared to 40% of controls. The HLA-DR and HLA-DQ alleles involved in the pathogenesis of DH are DQB1*0201, DQA1*0501, and DRB1*0301 and are essentially identical to those that have been described for patients with isolated GSE.

In addition to the striking association of DH with gluten-sensitive enteropathy, a number of other disease associations have been noted. For example, patients with DH have an increased frequency of gastric atrophy and gastric hypochlorhydria. Thyroid abnormalities, including hypothyroidism, hyperthyroidism, thyroid nodules, and thyroid cancer, also occur more frequently in patients with DH. A number of other autoimmune diseases, including systemic lupus erythematosus, dermatomyositis,

myasthenia gravis, Sjögren's syndrome, and rheumatoid arthritis, have also been reported in patients with DH. It is thought that many of these associations are related to the high frequency of the HLA-B8, -DR3, DQ-2 haplotype in patients with DH. Another important clinical association in patients with DH is an increased frequency of malignancy, specifically lymphomas. An increased standardized incidence ratio of 6.0 for non-Hodgkin's lymphoma has been reported, but no increased mortality was detected.[53]

PATHOGENESIS

The pathogenesis of DH rests on three distinct associations: (1) granular deposits of IgA in the skin at the DEJ; (2) gluten-sensitive enteropathy (albeit most often asymptomatic); and (3) an increased frequency of the HLA-DR3/DQ2 haplotype. Attempts to understand DH must integrate all these factors.

The mechanism by which IgA binds to DH skin is not known. Circulating antibodies that bind to normal human skin *in vitro* have not been detected in patients with DH. The IgA deposits also do not appear to be the result of the presence of IgA-containing circulating immune complexes. These complexes have been found in 25–35% of patients with DH, but have also been detected in the serum of patients with isolated GSE, who do not have cutaneous IgA deposits.[54] Although these data suggest that circulating IgA immune complexes are not responsible for the IgA found in DH skin, it is possible that pathogenic immune complexes may have escaped detection by the available techniques.

A third mechanism by which IgA might bind to DH skin is that IgA produced in the gut, as a response to wheat or other dietary antigens, may reach the circulation where it could either bind to wheat protein deposited in skin or cross-react with normal structures or molecules in the skin. IgA antibodies against endomysium, a connective tissue element surrounding smooth muscle, have been found in the serum of patients with DH and have been determined to be directed against tissue transglutaminase.[55] Recent studies have demonstrated that patients with DH have IgA antibodies against epidermal transglutaminase with a higher avidity than found in patients with isolated GSE. In addition, the IgA deposits in DH skin have been found to co-localize with epidermal transglutaminase, suggesting that the IgA in the skin of DH patients is directed against epidermal transglutaminase.[56] However, the mechanism whereby the IgA deposits remains unknown.

In vitro studies have demonstrated that treatment of gliadin with tissue transglutaminase modifies gliadin peptides to allow recognition by T cells from the gut of patients with isolated GSE.[57] These observations suggest that modification of the wheat protein by tissue transglutaminase may play a role in the development of immunity to wheat seen in patients with isolated GSE and DH. The cytokine profile in the gut of patients with DH differs from that in patients with symptomatic isolated GSE: gut biopsies from patients with isolated GSE expressed significantly more interferon-γ than those with DH, while gut biopsies from DH patients expressed more IL-4.[58] It remains to be determined whether these findings relate to the lack of gut symptoms in patients with DH.

The presence of an ongoing mucosal immune response in patients with DH has been shown to result in systemic signs of inflammation, including elevated serum levels of soluble IL-2 receptor and IL-8, increased neutrophil expression of CD11b, and increased expression of endothelial cell E-selectin in the skin.[59] These findings suggest that the mucosal immune response results in a proinflammatory environment in the skin that, when coupled with cutaneous IgA deposits, may result in the development of the typical skin lesions of DH.

THERAPY

DH can be treated either with dapsone or by adherence to a gluten-free diet, and the choice of therapy should be individualized to each patient. The treatment of choice for most patients with DH is dapsone or sulfapyridine, owing to the lack of gastrointestinal symptoms in most cases, as well as the difficulty of adhering to a strict gluten-free diet. Dapsone 100–200 mg/day is sufficient to control the cutaneous eruption in the majority of cases, with minimal side effects. Dapsone results in an almost immediate cessation of symptoms of the skin disease. It does not, however, affect the gastrointestinal mucosal defect or the gastrointestinal symptoms. Patients with DH on dapsone therefore have an ongoing (albeit low-grade) gluten-sensitive enteropathy. The exact mechanism of action of dapsone remains unknown. Dapsone appears to function at the level of the effector cells in the skin lesions, most likely the PMN, rather than affecting the mucosal immune response to wheat protein. Dapsone is a potentially toxic drug and patients should not increase the dose when disease flares occur without first consulting their physician.

The second mechanism of controlling the cutaneous eruption of DH is by strict adherence to a gluten-free diet. Nearly 80% of patients with DH who follow such a diet are able to stop or substantially reduce the dose of dapsone required to control their skin disease.[60] Patients may require at least 5 months on a gluten-free diet before being able to reduce their dose of dapsone, and 8–48 months of such a diet are necessary before they can discontinue their dapsone. Gluten-reduced diets, in which gluten content is not totally eliminated, appear to be less effective in controlling the cutaneous manifestations of DH, but may provide some relief. Patients on a gluten-reduced diet are able to decrease their dapsone dosage by approximately 50% compared to a 75% or greater reduction in patients on a gluten-free diet. Strict adherence to a gluten-free diet controls the cutaneous manifestations of DH in most patients, reverses the morphological changes in the small intestine, and after many years may result in disappearance of the cutaneous IgA deposits.[60] The cutaneous IgA has been found to return upon rechallenge with dietary gluten in these patients.[60]

Rarely, patients with DH do not respond to a gluten-free diet despite what appears to be total dietary compliance. This has also been reported in patients with isolated GSE, and other dietary factors have been postulated to play a role. In support of this concept is the observation that the skin lesions and gastrointestinal changes of DH may also respond to an elemental diet, often within only 2–3 weeks of starting the diet. Of interest, these patients responded to an elemental diet even in the presence of dietary gluten. These results imply that other proteins besides gluten play a role in the pathogenesis of DH. Although a gluten-free diet is an attractive alternative to medication for many patients, it is difficult to maintain. Gluten is present in most common grains (wheat, rye, barley) but not in rice and maize. Recently it has been established that eating oats appears to be safe for patients with DH, but it is important to remember that oat products may be contaminated with wheat protein. The patient should be informed that the success or failure of the diet cannot generally be assessed until at least a year of therapy has been completed.

■ REFERENCES ■

1. Beutner EH, Lever WF, Witebsky E, et al. Autoantibodies in pemphigus vulgaris: responses to an intracellular substance of epidermis. JAMA 1965; 192: 682–688.

2. Beutner EH, Jordon RE. Demonstration of skin antibodies in the sera of pemphigus vulgaris patients by indirect immunofluorescent staining. Proc Soc Exp Biol Med 1964; 117: 505–510.

3. Warren SJ, Lin MS, Giudice GJ, et al. The prevalence of antibodies against desmoglein 1 in endemic pemphigus foliaceus in Brazil. Cooperative Group on Fogo Selvagem. N Engl J Med 2000; 343: 23–30.

4. Korman NJ, Eyre RW, Zone J, et al. Drug-induced pemphigus: autoantibodies directed against the pemphigus antigen complexes are present in penicillamine and captopril-induced pemphigus. J Invest Dermatol 1991; 96: 273–276.

5. Anhalt GJ. Paraneoplastic pemphigus. J Invest Dermatol Symp Proc 2004; 9: 29–33.

6. Huff JC, Golitz LE, Kunke KS. Intraepidermal neutrophilic IgA dermatosis. N Engl J Med 1985; 313: 1643.

7. Ishii K, Amagai M, Hall RP, et al. Characterization of autoantibodies in pemphigus using antigen-specific enzyme-linked immunosorbent assays with baculovirus-expressed recombinant desmogleins. J Immunol 1997; 159: 2010–2017.

8. Hashimoto T, Kiyokawa C, Mori O, et al. Human desmocollin 1 (Dsc1) is an autoantigen for the subcorneal pustular dermatosis type of IgA pemphigus. J Invest Dermatol 1997; 109: 127–131.

9. Anhalt GJ, Labib RS, Voorhees JJ, et al. Induction of pemphigus in neonatal mice by passive transfer of IgG from patients with the disease. N Engl J Med 1982; 306: 1189–1196.

10. Scharf SJ, Friedman A, Brautbar C, et al. HLA class II allelic variation and susceptibility to pemphigus vulgaris. Proc Natl Acad Sci USA 1988; 85: 3504–3508.

11. Ahmed AR, Mohimen A, Yunis EJ, et al. Linkage of pemphigus vulgaris antibody to the major histocompatibility complex in healthy relatives of patients. J Exp Med 1993; 177: 419–424.

12. Wucherpfennig KW, Yu B, Bhol K, et al. Structural basis for major histocompatibility complex (MHC)-linked susceptibility to autoimmunity: charged residues of a single MHC binding pocket confer selective presentation of self-peptides in pemphigus vulgaris. Proc Natl Acad Sci USA 1995; 92: 11935–11939.

13. Hertl M, Amagai M, Sundaram H, et al. Recognition of desmoglein 3 by autoreactive T cells in pemphigus vulgaris patients and normals. J Invest Dermatol 1998; 110: 62–66.

14. Hans-Filho G, Aoki V, Rivitti E, et al. Endemic pemphigus foliaceus (fogo selvagem) – 1998. The Cooperative Group on Fogo Selvagem Research. Clin Dermatol 1999; 17: 225–235.

15. Moraes JR, Moraes ME, Fernandez-Vina M, et al. HLA antigens and risk for development of pemphigus foliaceus (fogo selvagem) in endemic areas of Brazil. Immunogenetics 1991; 33: 388–391.

16. Rock B, Labib RS, Diaz LA. Monovalent Fab' immunoglobulin fragments from endemic pemphigus foliaceus autoantibodies reproduce the human disease in neonatal Balb/c mice. J Clin Invest 1990; 85: 296–299.

17. Mahoney MG, Wang ZH, Stanley JR. Pemphigus vulgaris and pemphigus foliaceus antibodies are pathogenic in plasminogen activator knockout mice. J Invest Dermatol 1999; 113: 22–25.

18. Berkowitz P, Hu P, Liu Z, et al. Desmosome signaling: inhibition of p38MAPK prevents pemphigus vulgaris IgG-induced cytoskeleton reorganization. J Biol Chem 2005; 280: 23778–23784.

19. Berkowitz P, Hu P, Warren S, et al. p38MAPK inhibition prevents disease in pemphigus vulgaris mice. Proc Natl Acad Sci USA 2006; 103: 12855–12860.

20. Venning VA, Wojnarowska F. The association of bullous pemphigoid and malignant disease: a case control study. Br J Dermatol 1990; 123: 439–445.

21. Gammon WR, Kowalewski C, Chorzelski TP, et al. Direct immunofluorescence studies of sodium chloride-separated skin in the differential diagnosis of bullous pemphigoid and epidermolysis bullosa acquisita. J Am Acad Dermatol 1990; 22: 664–670.

22. Giudice GJ, Emery DJ, Zelickson BD, et al. Bullous pemphigoid and herpes gestationis autoantibodies recognize a common non-collagenous site on the BP180 ectodomain. J Immunol 1993; 151: 5742–5750.

23. Schmidt E, Obe K, Brocker EB, et al. Serum levels of autoantibodies to BP180 correlate with disease activity in patients with bullous pemphigoid. Arch Dermatol 2000; 136: 174–178.

24. McGrath JA, Darling T, Gatalica B, et al. A homozygous deletion mutation in the gene encoding the 180-kDa bullous pemphigoid antigen (BPAG2) in a family with generalized atrophic benign epidermolysis bullosa. J Invest Dermatol 1996; 106: 771–774.

25. Nelson KC, Zhao ML, Schroeder PR, et al. Role of different pathways of the complement cascade in experimental bullous pemphigoid. J Clin Invest 2006; 116: 2892–2900.

26. Stahle-Backdahl M, Inoue M, Guidice GJ, et al. 92-kD gelatinase is produced by eosinophils at the site of blister formation in bullous pemphigoid and cleaves the extracellular domain of recombinant 180-kD bullous pemphigoid autoantigen. J Clin Invest 1994; 93: 2022–2030.

27. Fairley JA, Fu CL, Giudice GJ. Mapping the binding sites of anti-BP180 immunoglobulin E autoantibodies in bullous pemphigoid. J Invest Dermatol 2005; 125: 467–472.

28. Budinger L, Borradori L, Yee C, et al. Identification and characterization of autoreactive T cell responses to bullous pemphigoid antigen 2 in patients and healthy controls. J Clin Invest 1998; 102: 2082–2089.

29. Guillaume JC, Vaillant L, Bernard P. Controlled trial of azathioprine and plasma exchange in addition to prednisolone in the treatment of bullous pemphigoid. Arch Dermatol 1993; 129: 49–53.

30. Khumalo NP, Murrell DF, Wojnarowska F, et al. A systematic review of treatments for bullous pemphigoid. Arch Dermatol 2002; 138: 385–389.

31. Sitaru C, Chiriac MT, Mihai S, et al. Induction of complement-fixing autoantibodies against type VII collagen results in subepidermal blistering in mice. J Immunol 2006; 177: 3461–3468.

32. Mohr C, Sunderkotter C, Hildebrand A, et al. Successful treatment of epidermolysis bullosa acquisita using intravenous immunoglobulins. Br J Dermatol 1995; 132: 824–826.

33. Schmidt E, Benoit S, Brocker EB, et al. Successful adjuvant treatment of recalcitrant epidermolysis bullosa acquisita with anti-CD20 antibody rituximab. Arch Dermatol 2006; 142: 147–150.

34. Lin MS, Arteaga LA, Diaz LA. Herpes gestationis. Clin Dermatol 2001; 19: 697–702.

35. Shornick JK, Black MM. Fetal risks in herpes gestationis. J Am Acad Dermatol 1992; 26: 63–68.

36. Diaz LA, Ratrie H, Saunders WS, et al. Isolation of a human epidermal cDNA corresponding to the 180-kD autoantigen recognized by bullous pemphigoid and herpes gestationis sera. Immunolocalization of this protein to the hemidesmosome. J Clin Invest 1990; 86: 1088–1094.

37. Lin MS, Gharia MA, Swartz SJ, et al. Identification and characterization of epitopes recognized by T lymphocytes and autoantibodies from patients with herpes gestationis. J Immunol 1999; 162: 4991–4997.

38. Chan LS, Ahmed AR, Anhalt GJ, et al. The first international consensus on mucous membrane pemphigoid: definition, diagnostic criteria, pathogenic factors, medical treatment, and prognostic indicators. Arch Dermatol 2002; 138: 370–379.

39. Chan LS, Yancey KB, Hammerberg C, et al. Immune-mediated subepithelial blistering diseases of mucous membranes. Pure ocular cicatricial pemphigoid is a unique clinical and immunopathological entity distinct from bullous pemphigoid and other subsets identified by antigenic specificity of autoantibodies. Arch Dermatol 1993; 129: 448–455.

40. Egan CA, Lazarova Z, Darling TN, et al. Anti-epiligrin cicatricial pemphigoid and relative risk for cancer. Lancet 2001; 357: 1850–1851.

41. Delgado JC, Turbay D, Yunis EJ, et al. A common major histocompatibility complex class II allele HLA-DQB1* 0301 is present in clinical variants of pemphigoid. Proc Natl Acad Sci USA 1996; 93: 8569–8571.

42. Chan LS, Wang T, Wang XS, et al. High frequency of HLA-DQB1*0301 allele in patients with pure ocular cicatricial pemphigoid. Dermatology 1994; 189: Suppl-101.

43. Kirtschig G, Murrell D, Wojnarowska F, et al. Interventions for mucous membrane pemphigoid/cicatricial pemphigoid and epidermolysis bullosa acquisita: a systematic literature review. Arch Dermatol 2002; 138: 380–384.

44. Wojnarowska F, Bhogal BS, Black MM. Chronic bullous disease of childhood and linear IgA disease of adults are IgA1-mediated diseases. Br J Dermatol 1994; 131: 201–204.

45. Zone JJ, Taylor TB, Meyer LJ, et al. The 97 kDa linear IgA bullous disease antigen is identical to a portion of the extracellular domain of the 180 kDa bullous pemphigoid antigen, BPAg2. J Invest Dermatol 1998; 110: 207–210.

46. Wojnarowska F, Whitehead P, Leigh IM, et al. Identification of the target antigen in chronic bullous disease of childhood and linear IgA disease of adults. Br J Dermatol 1991; 124: 157–162.

47. Lawley TJ, Strober W, Yaoita H, et al. Small intestinal biopsies and HLA types in dermatitis herpetiformis patients with granular and linear IgA skin deposits. J Invest Dermatol 1980; 74: 9–12.

48. Zone JJ, Meyer LJ, Petersen MJ. Deposition of granular IgA relative to clinical lesions in dermatitis herpetiformis. Arch Dermatol 1996; 132: 912–918.

49. Dahlback K, Lofberg H, Dahlback B. Vitronectin colocalizes with Ig deposits and C9 neoantigen in discoid lupus erythematosus and dermatitis herpetiformis, but not in bullous pemphigoid. Br J Dermatol 1989; 120: 725–733.

50. Olbricht SM, Flotte TJ, Collins AB, et al. Dermatitis herpetiformis. Cutaneous deposition of polyclonal IgA1. Arch Dermatol 1986; 122: 418–421.

51. Hall RP, McKenzie KD. Comparison of the intestinal and serum antibody response in patients with dermatitis herpetiformis. Clin Immunol Immunopathol 1992; 62: 33–41.

52. Marks J, Shuster S, Watson AJ. Small bowel changes in dermatitis herpetiformis. Lancet 1966; 2: 1280–1282.

53. Viljamaa M, Kaukinen K, Pukkala E, et al. Malignancy and mortality in patients with coeliac disease and dermatitis herpetiformis: 30-year population based study. Dig Liver Dis 2006; 38: 374–380.

54. Hall RP, Lawley TJ, Heck JA, et al. IgA-containing circulating immune complexes in dermatitis herpetiformis, Henoch–Schönlein purpura, systemic lupus erythematosus and other diseases. Clin Exp Immunol 1980; 40: 431–437.

55. Dieterich W, Laag E, Bruckner-Tuderman L, et al. Antibodies to tissue transglutaminase as serologic markers in patients with dermatitis herpetiformis. J Invest Dermatol 1999; 113: 133–136.

56. Sardy M, Karpati S, Merkl B, et al. Epidermal transglutaminase (TGase 3) is the autoantigen of dermatitis herpetiformis. J Exp Med 2002; 195: 747–757.

57. Molberg O, McAdam SN, Korner R, et al. Tissue transglutaminase selectively modifies gliadin peptides that are recognized by gut-derived T cells in celiac disease. Nat Med 1998; 4: 713–717.

58. Smith AD, Bagheri B, Streilein RD, et al. Expression of interleukin-4 and interferon-γ in the small bowel of patients with dermatitis herpetiformis and isolated gluten-sensitive enteropathy. Dig Dis Sci 1999; 44: 2124–2132.

59. Hall RP, Takeuchi F, Benbenisty K, et al. Cutaneous endothelial cell activation in normal skin of patients with dermatitis herpetiformis associated with increased serum levels of IL-8, sE-Selectin and TNF-γ. J Invest Dermatol 2006; 126: 1331–1337.

60. Leonard J, Haffenden G, Tucker W, et al. Gluten challenge in dermatitis herpetiformis. N Engl J Med 1983; 308: 816–819.

REFERENCES

Myasthenia gravis

Arnold I. Levinson

■ INTRODUCTION ■

Myasthenia gravis (MG) is a disease characterized by weakness of striated muscles. The weakness is due to impaired neuromuscular transmission resulting from a reduction in the number of receptors for the neurotransmitter acetylcholine (ACh) at the postsynaptic myoneural junction. This reduction is caused by the action of anti-acetylcholine receptor (anti-AChR) antibodies. The disease occurs with a reported prevalence of 0.5–5/100 000 and an incidence of 0.4/100 000 per year. Although MG can occur at any age, it typically presents in the second and third decades of life, with a later peak occurring after age 50 (late-onset disease). A female preponderance (3:1–4:1) has been reported in the first 40 years of life; thereafter the incidence is comparable between the sexes.

■ CLASSIFICATION ■

MG patients have traditionally been divided into two categories: those with generalized disease and those presenting with disease limited to the ocular muscles.[1] Within these two groups, patients can be further subdivided on the basis of age of onset. Neonatal MG affects 10–20% of offspring born to myasthenic mothers. Disease manifestations are those of generalized MG (see below) but are transient, dissipating with the metabolism of maternal anti-AChR antibodies that had been transferred across the placenta during the third trimester of pregnancy. Several congenital myasthenic syndromes have been described. For the most part, these manifest during the neonatal period, persist into adulthood, and are not considered to have an autoimmune basis. Juvenile MG describes those patients who present with disease between 1 year of age and puberty. Apart from the age of onset, juvenile myasthenics behave like adult patients with MG.

Adults may present with ocular involvement or signs of more generalized disease. The ocular involvement is characterized by impaired ocular muscle motility and lid weakness, manifesting as diplopia and ptosis, respectively. The vast majority of MG patients will experience ocular involvement, with roughly 50% of patients presenting with ocular signs at the time of diagnosis. Those generally at risk of disease progression are: (1) patients with evidence of subclinical disease on electrophysiological testing of limb muscles; and (2) patients who have markedly elevated titers of anti-AChR antibodies. Typically, patients with ocular symptoms for longer than 2 years will not progress to a more generalized form of disease.

In the generalized disease group patients can be classified into mild, moderate, and severe on the basis of clinical activity. Any skeletal muscle group may be affected, but typically the palatal, pharyngeal, and upper esophageal muscles are involved. This results in dysarthria, dysphagia, and difficulty in handling secretions. Involvement of the diaphragm and intercostal muscles produces dyspnea and may lead to respiratory failure. Involvement of the muscles of the extremities and trunk occurs in 20–30% of patients at initial presentation and causes difficulties with activities of daily living. The hallmark of all of muscle involvement in MG is its variability over time, with weakness usually exacerbated by repetitive use.

■ DIAGNOSIS ■

The differential diagnosis is extremely broad, encompassing neuropathies, primary and secondary myopathies, muscular dystrophy, demyelinating disorders, degenerative diseases, cerebrovascular accidents, mass lesions, and infectious diseases. The clinical features that point to a diagnosis of MG include the variable nature of the muscle weakness, normal sensation, and normal deep tendon reflexes. The diagnosis can usually be

> ## CLINICAL PEARLS
>
> ### TELLTALE SIGNS OF MYASTHENIA GRAVIS
>
> >> Variable muscle weakness
> >> Weakness in cranial nerve distribution
> >> Normal reflexes and sensation

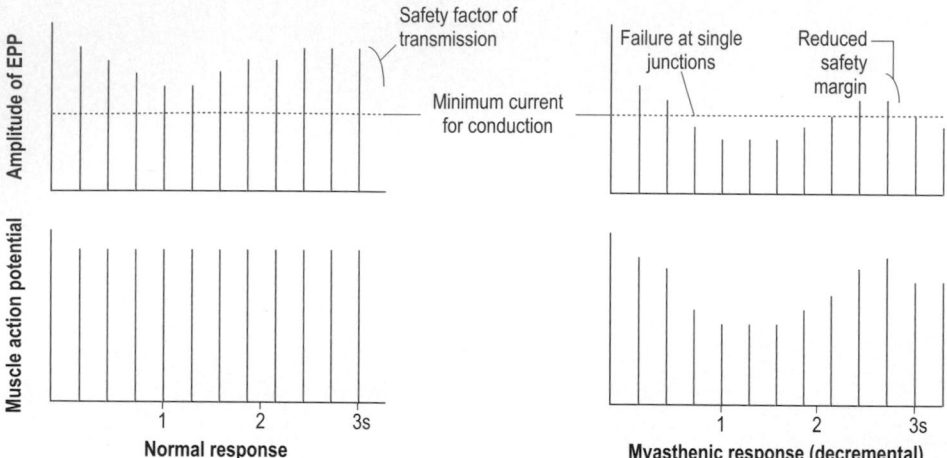

Fig. 64.1 Neuromuscular transmission in normal and myasthenic subjects. With repetitive stimulation there is a reduction in the efficiency of acetylcholine (ACh) release, with a subsequent recovery in efficiency as the train of stimuli continues. Although the endplate potential (EPP) fluctuates at the normal junction, sufficient current is generated to stimulate an action potential of constant magnitude. At the myasthenic junction, however, the amplitude of the EPP in response to a given amount of ACh is reduced. Under conditions of inefficient ACh release, e.g., repetitive stimulation, the minimum current for conduction is not generated, resulting in a profile of action potentials that shows a progressive decline or decrement with subsequent recovery.

confirmed by pharmacologic and electrophysiologic testing. A decremental pattern is characteristically seen following repetitive nerve stimulation (Fig. 64.1) and this pattern is normalized following treatment with the anticholinesterase agent tensilon. Further confirmation rests on detecting anti-AChR antibodies, which are found in 85–90% of patients with generalized disease. In the standard assay, sera are reacted with a nicotinic AChR preparation labeled with ^{125}I-α-bungarotoxin, a snake venom polypeptide that binds irreversibly to the receptor. Bound antibodies are immunoprecipitated by an anti-immunoglobulin reagent or staphylococcal protein A, and the quantity of antibodies detected is expressed in terms of the amount of α-bungarotoxin bound.

■ ACETYLCHOLINE RECEPTOR STRUCTURE ■

The nicotinic AChR (nAChR) is a member of a larger family of ligand-gated ion channels. The muscle-type receptor, which is involved in myasthenia, can be further subclassified into mature junctional receptors, and immature, extrajunctional, or denervated receptors. The nAChR at a mature myoneural junction is composed of four subunits, labeled α, β, δ, and ϵ (Fig. 64.2). In fetal muscle and adult denervated muscle or nonjunctional membrane, a γ-subunit replaces the ϵ-subunit found in mature innervated muscle endplates. This form of the receptor differs from the mature junctional form by its lower density (500 receptors/μm^2) and its distribution over most of the surface of the sarcolemma. The immature receptor also has a lower conductance, a longer open time, a more rapid turnover, and a decreased half-life.

The genes for the α-, δ-, and γ-subunits are located on chromosome 2 in humans, and subunits β and ϵ on chromosome 17. There are two

isoforms of the α-subunit, which are generated by alternative splicing.[2] The larger, which includes an additional sequence of 25 amino acids between exons 3 and 4, is found only in humans and other primates. The subunits of the AChR are homologous to each other and to their counterparts across species, with the greatest conservation of sequence being in the α-subunit. Two α-subunits and one of each of the other subunits are assembled to form an asymmetric hourglass channel spanning the membrane. Each subunit has a large amino-terminus located extracellularly, four transmembrane regions, and a short cytoplasmic tail formed by a loop between the third and fourth transmembrane domains. The receptor appears as a dimer owing to disulfide bonding between the δ-subunits of two receptors. The two α-subunits are not contiguous in each receptor but are separated by another subunit. One ACh-binding site is found on each of the α-subunits around the pair of cysteines at amino acids 192 and 193. The binding of ACh to the α-subunits is believed to engender a conformational change, possibly resulting in rearrangement of charged groups. The binding of ACh to both α-subunits increases the probability of transition of the channel to an open conformation. Binding of curare or α-bungarotoxin to the α-subunits blocks this channel.

In normal innervated neuromuscular junctions there are two forms of the AChR, the predominant form having a long half-life, and a small subset that is rapidly turned over.[3] The rapidly turned-over receptors are the precursors of the stable receptors. It is not clear how these two types differ, or how they are regulated. The receptors are concentrated at the top of the folds in the muscle endplate, adjacent to the nerve terminus, at a density of 10 000/μm^2. This localization reflects the action of agrin, a nerve-derived synaptic organizing molecule.[4] The AChRs are organized into clusters by rapsyn, a 43-kDa cytoplasmic protein.[4] The clustered AChRs are linked to the cytoskeleton by connections between rapsyn and a dystrophin–glycoprotein complex.

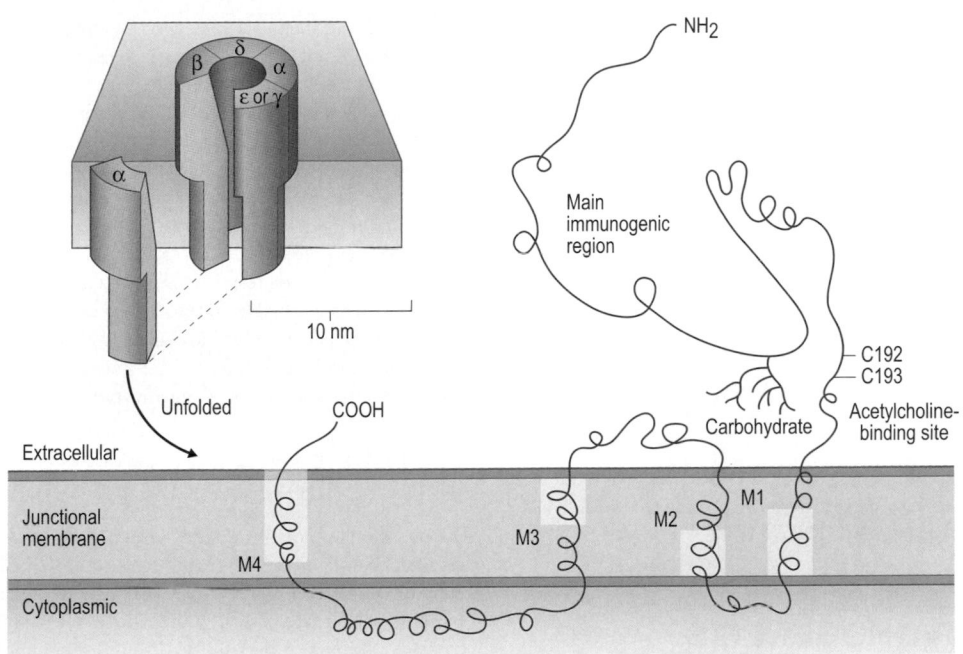

Fig. 64.2 The acetylcholine receptor. The subunits of the acetylcholine receptor – α, β, δ, and γ or ε – are arranged like barrel staves around the central ion pore. Each subunit winds through the junctional membrane four times (sites M1, M2, M3, and M4). In the unfolded view of the α-subunit, the amino-terminal end of the α-subunit is extracellular, where it is accessible to acetylcholine, which binds at the site shown (amino acids 192 and 193). In myasthenia gravis, autoantibodies may bind to various epitopes of all subunits, but a high proportion of antibodies bind to the main immunogenic region of the α-subunit.

■ NEUROMUSCULAR TRANSMISSION ■

When an impulse is transmitted along an axon terminal it results in the release of the neurotransmitter ACh across its presynaptic membrane (Fig. 64.3). ACh diffuses across a 50-nm synaptic cleft, where it interacts with AChRs that are displayed in greatest density at the tops of the junctional folds of the postsynaptic muscle membrane or endplate. This interaction leads to a local depolarization or endplate potential caused by increased membrane permeability to sodium and potassium. The endplate potential is terminated by acetylcholinesterases, which are present in highest concentrations in the synaptic cleft around the junctional folds. If the summation of endplate potentials attains a prescribed threshold it produces an action potential that depolarizes the surrounding sarcolemma and causes muscle contraction. In a healthy individual the arrival of an impulse at the presynaptic membrane of a motor nerve releases considerably more ACh than is required to generate an action potential. This reserve, roughly four times the current needed for propagation of the impulse, is referred to as the safety factor of neuromuscular transmission. Because of the severe reduction in receptor number in MG, the electrical threshold for propagation of an action potential cannot be attained and muscle contraction is prevented. With a less severe reduction in receptor numbers neuromuscular transmission may proceed normally unless the efficiency of presynaptic vesicle release is compromised, as occurs with repetitive use of muscles. The combination of decreasing availability of ACh and the reduced

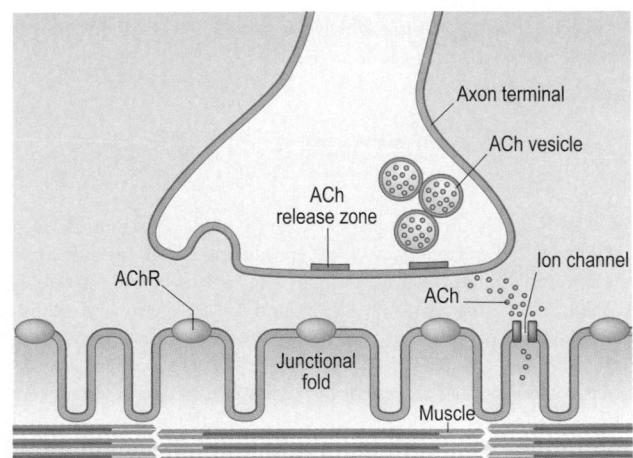

Fig. 64.3 Schematic representation of the myoneural junction. Vesicles of acetylcholine (ACh) release their contents at active zones across from ACh receptors (AChRs) in response to impulses conducted down nerve axons. ACh diffuses across synaptic cleft and binds to AChRs, with opening of the ion channel and the generation of endplate potential. Action potential is propagated to muscle when sufficient amplitude of summated endplate potentials is attained.

number of receptors accounts for the characteristic decremental nerve conduction pattern seen on electromyograms of patients with MG following repetitive nerve stimulation (Fig. 64.1).

IMMUNOPATHOGENESIS OF MYASTHENIA GRAVIS

Anti-AChR antibodies are detected in 85–90% of MG patients and are responsible for the impaired neuromuscular transmission.[5] There are many lines of evidence to support this contention. Immunoglobulin G (IgG), along with C3 and the terminal attack complex (C5–C9), is deposited at AChR-containing areas of the postsynaptic membrane, and anti-AChR–AChR complexes can be extracted from the muscles of patients with MG. Transfer of myasthenic serum from mother to fetus, or from human to mouse, results in symptoms or signs of myasthenia in the recipient. Plasmapharesis, which decreases anti-AChR antibody levels, is associated with clinical improvement.

PROPERTIES OF ANTI-ACHR ANTIBODIES AND CHARACTERIZATION OF B-CELL EPITOPES

Anti-AChR antibodies are produced by a small subset of B cells in affected people. The frequency of IgG-producing AChR-specific peripheral blood mononuclear cells is estimated to be 1 in 15 000–70 000. IgG anti-AChR-secreting cells are also found in the peripheral blood of healthy volunteers, albeit in much lower numbers. The proportion of immunoglobulin-producing AChR-specific B cells or plasma cells is greater in the germinal centers of hyperplastic thymuses, but still only 1 in 1000–10 000 antibodies produced is AChR-specific. Anti-AChR antibodies are predominantly IgG_1 and IgG_3 but IgG_2 and IgG_4 isotypes have also been found. IgA and IgM anti-AChR antibodies are present in some patients, but never in the absence of IgG anti-AChR antibodies. The IgA and IgM anti-AChR antibodies tend to appear in patients whose disease is of longer duration and greater severity, and in association with high IgG titers.

The pathogenic anti-AChR antibodies in MG are thought to be directed to conformationally dependent structures. Immunization of animals with irreversibly denatured AChR leads to the formation of anti-AChR antibodies capable of binding to native AChR, but the antibodies are not capable of causing disease. This observation indicates that conformationally dependent epitopes are important in the induction of disease. Many of the anti-AChR antibodies are directed against the α-subunit, particularly to a small region on the extracellular portion referred to as the main immunogenic region (Fig. 64.2). Approximately 60% of the anti-AChR antibodies are directed against this region, which encompasses a set of overlapping epitopes clustered around amino acids 67–76 of the α-subunit.[6] The reason for the predominant role of the α-chain in the antibody response in myasthenia is not known. Not all disease-producing antibodies in humans or rats appear to be directed to this region. Many patients also have antibodies recognizing the γ-containing embryonic form of AChR. This observation has spawned speculation about a nonmuscle source of sensitization.

ANTI-ACHR ANTIBODY LEVELS AND RELATIONSHIP TO DISEASE ACTIVITY

The relationship of anti-AChR antibody and disease activity in MG is complicated. In general, serum levels of anti-AChR antibody or anti-AChR–AChR complexes correlate poorly with disease severity. Among patients within one clinical grade, anti-AChR antibody levels can vary by several orders of magnitude. In addition, approximately 10–15% of patients with clinical MG have no anti-AChR antibody by standard assays. Anti-AChR antibodies are more likely to be present if the disease is generalized or severe, and there is a tendency for higher levels of anti-AChR antibody to correlate with more severe disease. Also, in an individual patient an increase or decrease in anti-AChR antibody levels often accompanies deterioration or improvement, respectively, in clinical activity.

As the quantity of anti-AChR antibodies produced does not fully explain disease severity, studies have also focused on qualitative differences in these antibodies among different patients. These studies, however, have not been able to distinguish properties of anti-AChR antibodies that lead to greater pathogenicity. Differences in specificity and avidity of binding to AChR have not been associated with particular functional effects or disease severity. Anti-AChR antibodies that bind or compete for the same region of AChR can have different functional effects. Anti-AChR antibodies show extensive heterogeneity by isoelectric focusing, but this characteristic also does not correlate with pathogenic potential.

As noted above, 10–15% of MG patients are persistently antibody-negative. Recently a subset of these patients has been discovered to have serum IgG antibodies specific for muscle-specific tyrosine kinase (MuSK).[7] The prevalence of these antibodies in seronegative patients varies across geographical locales with 60–70%, 40–50%, and 4% reported in patients in the UK (some sera from patients in other European countries), USA, and Taiwan, respectively. Unlike patients with MG and anti-AChR antibodies (see below), most MuSK antibody-positive patients do not have thymic pathology. They tend to be young adult females with bulbar, neck, or respiratory muscle weakness. There is also evidence that some of the so-called antibody-negative patients have anti-AChR antibodies that are not detected by the routine assay systems. For example, plasma from some of these patients can passively transfer a defect in neuromuscular transmission, and disease activity in some seronegative patients improved with plasmapheresis. Anti-AChR antibodies have been demonstrated in some of these patients by rosetting assays using BC3H1 cells (a mouse tumor cell line that expresses AChR on its surface). Anti-AChR-secreting B cells have also been identified in seronegative patients by immunospot assay. Consistent with this finding, human IgG was demonstrated at the neuromuscular synapse when peripheral blood mononuclear cells from seronegative patients were transferred to severe combined immunodeficiency (SCID) mice. These findings are difficult to reconcile with those from mice administered plasma from seronegative patients. Although these mice had impaired neuromuscular transmission on electromyography, immunoglobulin was not detected at the myoneural junction.

Patients with MG associated with thymoma show distinct patterns of antibody production. Almost all patients with thymoma are anti-AChR antibody-positive and most produce antistriational antibodies.[8] These antibodies react with titin, a giant filamentous protein of striated muscle. Titin filaments are involved in muscle assembly and contribute to the muscle's ability to recoil following stimulation. Such antistriational antibodies are also found in approximately 50% of the sera of older, nonthymoma MG patients who have thymic atrophy, but are not frequently detected in patients with early-onset disease and thymic hyperplasia. The finding of antistriational antibodies in an MG patient less than 40 years old strongly suggests the presence of thymoma. There is no evidence that antistriational antibodies are involved in muscle weakness.

MG sera also contain antibodies reacting with the ryanodine receptor.[8] These receptors, which are critically involved in muscle contraction, are Ca^{2+} release channels located in the sarcoplasmic reticulum of striated muscles. Antibodies to ryanodine receptors are found in 50% of MG patients with thymoma, and patients with high levels have a worse prognosis than do antibody-negative MG patients with thymoma. *In vitro* studies have suggested a pathogenic role for these autoantibodies in MG.

Antirapsyn antibodies have been detected in a small subset of MG patients.[9] Seropositive patients with MG are indistinguishable from seronegative patients with regard to clinical and laboratory features of disease. The presence of this autoantibody specificity is not specific for MG, having been detected in the sera of an occasional multiple sclerosis patient and a majority of the lupus patients tested.

PATHOGENIC EFFECTS OF ANTI-ACHR ANTIBODIES

Complement-mediated damage

The critical problem in MG is the anti-AChR antibody-mediated reduction in the number of nAChRs at the myoneural junction. There are several possible mechanisms by which the anti-AChR antibodies could lead to impaired neuromuscular transmission.[10] Ultramicroscopic studies show marked destructive changes in some endplates, particularly at the peaks of the postsynaptic folds, where AChR is usually present in the greatest concentration. The architecture of the muscle endplate is simplified, with loss of junctional folds and widening of the synaptic cleft that contains membrane debris. C3, C9, and the membrane attack complex are deposited at the muscle endplate, suggesting a role for complement in membrane destruction.[11] Indeed, the anti-AChR antibodies in many patients can fix complement *in vitro* when bound to skeletal muscle, and can damage cultured rat myotubes with a resultant decrease in AChR content.

Although antibody-directed complement-mediated destruction is important in the pathophysiology of MG, it is not the entire story. The rapid clinical improvement in MG following certain therapeutic interventions and the lack of destructive changes in many neuromuscular junctions of symptomatic areas despite prominent immunoglobulin deposition suggest that a more readily reversible process is also likely to be involved in the neuromuscular block.

ACCELERATION OF ACHR DEGRADATION

In vitro and *in vivo* studies have shown that anti-AChR antibodies can accelerate the rate of degradation of extrajunctional and junctional receptors, respectively.[12] This reaction is complement-independent and is due to the endocytosis of AChRs via shallow depressions, presumably clathrin-coated pits. Other membrane receptors are not affected. Both stable and rapidly turned-over receptors appear to be affected, thereby explaining the greater than expected antibody-mediated loss of AChRs observed at neuromuscular junctions. The reaction requires cross-linking of adjacent AChRs, as it can be mediated by $F(ab')_2$ fragments, but not Fab fragments, of anti-AChR antibodies. The effect of antibody on the synthesis of new AChR is controversial.

RECEPTOR BLOCKADE

The inhibition of ACh binding has been assessed by studying the effects of MG serum on the binding of the neurotoxin α-bungarotoxin to AChRs. Such blocking antibodies are found in a variable number of MG sera. Blockade has been generally attributed to steric hindrance of the ligand-binding site, rather then direct binding to the ACh-binding site.[13] The importance of these antibodies in the pathophysiology of MG remains unclear. However, in one study the functional ability of an individual serum to accelerate degradation and cause blockade of AChRs paralleled most closely the clinical status of the patient. The *in vivo* significance of such antibodies has also been demonstrated by passive transfer of certain rat monoclonal anti-AChR antibodies into chicks. Complete paralysis was observed within 1 hour of the transfer, presumably before there was time for complement-mediated damage. In MG patients it has been reasoned that such blocking antibodies could further immune response directed at thymic nAChRα is indeed responsible for initiating or perpetuating disease.

IMMUNOLOGIC

From an immunologic standpoint, the MG thymus has unique features that could reflect pathogenic involvement and help explain some of the histologic abnormalities.[22] Although B cells and Ig-secreting cells are rare intramedullary inhabitants of normal thymi, they are increased in cell suspensions of MG thymus, particularly hyperplastic thymus relative to control thymus (obtained from subjects undergoing elective cardiothoracic surgery). When stimulated *in vitro* with the polyclonal B-cell activator pokeweed mitogen, both MG and normal thymus cell suspensions produced surprisingly large amounts of immunoglobulin, with the IgG isotype greatly exceeding IgM.

There has been great interest in determining whether the heightened B-cell activity in MG thymus reflects local immune events. Single-cell suspensions from thymi of MG patients with follicular hyperplasia secrete anti-AChR antibody *in vitro* without addition of B-cell activators.[22] However, the thymic B-cell repertoire also includes anti-influenza specificity and antitetanus toxoid specificity. The latter is only detected when patients are booster-immunized to tetanus toxoid 3–4 weeks prior to thymectomy. Thus, the B-cell repertoire in the MG thymus may reflect systemic as well as local immune events.

AChR-reactive CD4⁺ T cells have been detected and propagated as long-term lines and clones from MG thymus (both thymoma and hyperplasia), but not from normal thymus. These antigen-specific T cells seem to be enriched in the thymus relative to the blood of the same MG patient. Migration of T cells reactive to foreign antigen into the thymus is known to occur.[30] Therefore, it is not clear whether AChR-reactive T cells in MG thymus are sensitized in the periphery with subsequent intrathymic localization, or are sensitized *in situ*.

In addition, hyperplastic MG thymus showed increased numbers of IL-1 and IL-6-producing cells. These cells were found largely in the perifollicular areas and connective tissue adjacent to the septa of disrupted cortex. Cells producing IL-2 were less prominent and largely confined to perifollicular areas. This distribution of cytokine production was not seen in normal thymus or in hyperplastic lymph nodes.

Together, the above studies indicate that MG thymus contains the cellular constituents necessary for an immune response directed against AChR. These include AChR-reactive B cells and helper T cells, cytokines that can facilitate B-cell activation, chemokines that attract immigrant lymphocytes, and a local source of the autoantigen. MG thymus also appears to contain normal numbers of CD4⁺CD25⁺ regulatory T cells.[31] However, these cells are characterized by reduced expression of the transcription factor FOXP3 and decreased suppressive function. Such impaired thymic regulatory T-cell function could impede the development or maintenance of T-cell tolerance to locally expressed AChR. Nevertheless, it is still not known whether autosensitization occurs in the thymus with spillover to the myoneural junction, or whether the thymic pathology is causally related to the pathogenesis of MG. As previously mentioned, thymic pathologic changes are not typically seen in the thymi of rodents with actively or passively induced MG. Thus, the pathologic changes seen in MG thymus are not secondary to the systemic autoimmune response and may be linked to the etiopathogenesis of this disease. The trigger for the putative intrathymic sensitization remains to be determined.

■ ETIOLOGIC FACTORS ■

GENETIC FACTORS

Similar to most autoimmune diseases, the MHC represents an important genetic susceptibility locus for the development of MG. Studies indicate that the MHC haplotype with HLA-B8, DR3, and DQ2 is associated with early-onset MG and hyperplastic thymus in Caucasian individuals. An association with HLA-B7 and DR2, although weaker, has also been described for patients with onset of MG after the age of 40 years associated with atrophic thymic histology. In murine studies the MHC class II molecules I-Aᵇ and I-Eᵏ have been associated with suceptibility to EAMG.[16] In EAMG the permissive MHC class II molecules are capable of binding AChR peptides that are recognized by antigen-specific CD4 T cells.

Studies have also addressed the potential genetic contributions of other immune system-related genes in the pathogenesis of MG. An association has been reported for a particular IL-1β allele and MG[32] and increased serum levels of this cytokine have been reported. This was most pronounced in patients who lacked disease-susceptible HLA genes. Several groups have reported an association between MG and the presence of particular TNF-α polymorphisms.[33, 34] Polymorphisms in the IL-10 promoter region have been reported to be associated with distinct patterns of thymic histology.[35] No correlations have been made between IL-4 alleles and MG. Finally, allotypic markers on IgG and FcγRIIa receptors have been associated with the coexistence of MG and thymoma.

EXOGENOUS FACTORS

Whether or not sensitization to AChR occurs in the thymus or the periphery, the stimulus for this autoimmune response remains a conundrum. Moreover, it remains to be determined whether the stimulus is self-antigen (AChR) or a foreign antigen that mimics the receptor's molecular structure. In this regard, several examples of molecular mimicry between AChRα chain and other molecules have been reported. Studies carried out with certain monoclonal anti-AChR antibodies demonstrated epitope sharing between the receptor and several bacteria, including *Klebsiella pneumoniae*, *Escherichia coli*, *Proteus vulgaris*, and *Yersinia enterocolitica*. However, for the most part no difference was observed in the binding of polypeptides from these organisms by either MG patient or control sera. A computer search of protein banks revealed a sequence homology between AChRα chain and a short peptide in herpes simplex glycoprotein D, although the significance of this finding is unknown. Finally, similarities were reported between idiotypic determinants on anti-AChR antibodies and antibodies reactive with α1,3 dextran. Interestingly, anti-dextran antibodies were detected in approximately 13% of MG patients but rarely in normal controls.[36] α1,3 Dextran is found in the cell walls of several common enteric pathogens and thus represents a potential ubiquitous source of immunogen. This type of idiotypic network connectivity led the investigators to postulate that an unregulated anti-idiotypic response to anti-α1,3 dextran antibodies might lead, in certain individuals, to an anti-AChR antibody response. Unfortunately, there has been no follow-up to these observations.

A striking association has been reported between the development of MG and treatment with the drug penicillamine,[37, 38] particularly in individuals with HLA DR1. MG developed in patients with rheumatoid

TREATMENT OF MYASTHENIA GRAVIS

THERAPEUTIC PRINCIPLES

THERAPEUTIC APPROACHES

>> Anticholinesterase agents

>> Thymectomy

>> Plasmapheresis

>> Corticosteroids

>> Immunosuppressive agents

>> Intravenous γ-globulin

arthritis and patients with Wilson's disease treated with this agent. After discontinuation of penicillamine, resolution of MG symptoms was reported in some patients but not others. Penicillamine treatment was associated with the development of anti-AChR antibodies that appeared to have the same type of specificity profile as found in idiopathic myasthenia. Additional evidence suggests that penicillamine may directly interfere with neuromuscular transmission. Although penicillamine has been shown to have diverse effects on the immune response in the normal host, and has reactive sulfhydryl groups capable of modifying self-antigens, its role in the development of MG remains to be determined.

TREATMENT OF MYASTHENIA GRAVIS

Therapeutic intervention in MG usually proceeds in a stepwise manner, beginning with anticholinesterase agents.[39]

ANTICHOLINESTERASES

Anticholinesterases are the mainstay of treatment. These agents protect ACh from hydrolysis by cholinesterase, thereby increasing the amount of neutrotransmitter and the number of contacts with the reduced number of receptors at the postsynaptic junction. This in turn raises the probability of attaining the necessary threshold for neuromuscular transmission. In addition, some of the anticholinesterase agents have a direct agonist effect at the postsynaptic junction. The three most popular agents in this group are neostigmine bromide (prostigmine), pyridostigmine bromide (mestinon), and ambenonium chloride (mytelase). Although there are only slight differences between these agents, mestinon remains the most commonly used. It has an onset of action of 30–60 minutes, peak action at about 2 hours, and loss of activity occurring after 4 hours. The drug is usually initiated at a dose of 60 mg every 3–4 hours and increased if necessary in 30–60-mg increments. Additional benefit is not usually seen at doses higher than 240 mg every 3–4 hours or 120 mg every 2 hours. It is important to individualize the dosing schedule for each patient according to needs. For example, the patient with bulbar symptoms should be instructed to take anticholinesterase 30 minutes to 1 hour before meals. Adverse effects of these agents are due to excessive stimulation of nicotinic and muscarinic receptors. The nicotinic side effects include fasciculations, muscle cramps, and increased weakness. Muscarinic side effects include

diarrhea, abdominal cramps, palpitations, increased sweating, and nasal and bronchial secretions. Adding atropine or an atropine analog to the regimen can minimize the latter group of reactions. This provides a cushion for increasing the amount of drug, and hence, its effect at the postsynaptic junction. Auxiliary drugs that have been purported to have a salutary effect on neuromuscular transmission are ephedrine and xanthine derivatives (theophylline), which are thought to increase the presynaptic release of ACh. The minimal effect of their added benefit has not warranted their common usage.

THYMECTOMY

Another mainstay in the therapy of the adult with generalized MG is thymectomy.[39] The benefit is greatest in younger patients and those with thymic hyperplasia, although many centers include older patients as well. Although no controlled study has ever been carried out, the accumulated experience indicates that thymectomy is associated with an excellent outcome, measured as either remission or an improvement in clinical symptoms. In one study 90% of patients were asymptomatic or in complete remission within a few years of thymectomy, and 46% were off all medications. With improvements in preoperative care, anesthesia, surgical technique, and postoperative care, thymectomy has become a very safe procedure, but its value and safety in children and older patients are less well established. There is still some controversy over what represents the best surgical procedure, although the transsternal approach is the choice in most centers. Unlike the transcervical approach, it is less likely to be complicated by residual thymic tissue. The mechanism responsible for the salutary effect of thymectomy remains to be elucidated. No obvious effects on immunoregulatory mechanisms have been demonstrated, although anti-AChR titers tend to fall months after the procedure. Thymectomy is also the recommended treatment for patients of all ages suspected of having thymoma.

CORTICOSTEROIDS

Corticosteroids are used in patients with generalized MG who fail to respond to anticholinesterase agents or thymectomy, and in patients needing optimization of their clinical condition in preparation for thymectomy. They are generally not used as a first-line agent to replace thymectomy. They are also used in patients with ocular myasthenia who fail to respond to anticholinesterases. Corticosteroids are initially given on a daily basis, with therapy begun in hospital. This cautious approach is followed because of the fear of clinical deterioration that occurs in some patients during the introduction of corticosteroids. Because of this concern, some groups advocate starting patients on alternate-day therapy, which is not typically associated with clinical deterioration and can be carried out on an outpatient basis. Daily corticosteroids are usually started in patients with generalized MG at a dose > 1 mg/kg prednisone. Patients should be continued on this dose until clinical improvement is maintained for several days, and then gradually weaned on to alternate-day therapy. With improvement sustained over several months, an effort should be made to reduce the dose (usually in 5-mg decrements) administered on the alternate day. Although a recent Cochrane review underscored the dearth of controlled trials, the improvement rate is generally estimated to be 60–90%.[40] Complete remission is rare and most patients will require some dose of steroids indefinitely. The physician should be alert to the possibility that anticholinesterase requirements may decrease as the patient responds to corticosteroids.

PLASMAPHERESIS

Plasmapheresis has enjoyed popularity since its introduction as an auxiliary treatment modality in 1976, particularly as a temporizing measure.[41] It appears to be most beneficial in patients in myasthenic crisis and in those experiencing progressive deterioration despite treatment with anticholinesterases and corticosteroids. Plasmapheresis has also proved to be useful in preparing patients for thymectomy whose course is complicated by involvement of the bulbar and respiratory musculature. Such patients may also require short-term plasmapheresis during the postoperative period. Although there are no hard and fast rules, the average exchange is 1–2 l/day for 7–14 days. Improvement is usually observed within a few days of concluding the treatment course, although patients in crisis often benefit more quickly. The mechanism of action most likely involves the removal of the pathogenic autoantibody, as a reduction in titer of anti-AChR antibody correlates with clinical improvement. However, it is also possible that the removal of other phlogistic humoral factors contributes to clinical efficacy.

IMMUNOSUPPRESSIVE AGENTS

Immunosuppressive drugs have been tried primarily in patients who have failed treatment with anticholinesterases, thymectomy, plasmapheresis, and corticosteroids.[7] Most of the experience has been obtained with azathioprine, which has strong anti-inflammatory effects as well as immunosuppressive activity. The dose of azathioprine has varied between 1 and 3 mg/kg per day, with improvement seen between 5 and 20 weeks. The drug is usually started at a lower dose and escalated weekly to achieve the maintenance dose. Patients should be followed with complete blood counts, particularly during the initiation of therapy, as azathioprine has a suppressive effect on the bone marrow. A white blood cell count below 2500μm³ or a neutrophil count below 1500μm³ should prompt a reduction or termination of the dosage. The results of a randomized double-blind placebo-controlled trial indicated that the addition of azathioprine (2.5 mg/kg) to alternate-day prednisolone was associated with a reduction of the prednisolone dose, fewer treatment failures, longer remissions, and fewer side effects.[42] There is considerably less experience with cyclophosphamide, another powerful immunosuppressive agent. It is associated with more adverse effects and does not appear to offer any significant advantage. Methotrexate has been used in some uncontrolled studies but there is no information to indicate that it is more efficacious or safer than azathioprine and its onset of action may take as long as several months. As is true for corticosteroid therapy, it is the rare patient who enjoys a permanent remission following institution of immunosuppressive therapy, and those who show some improvement often require treatment indefinitely.

Cyclosporine, a potent immunosuppressive agent, has been investigated because it interferes with IL-2-mediated T-cell proliferation and thus would be expected to interfere with the generation of T cells that would "help" the anti-AChR antibody response.[7] A recent retrospective study suggested cyclosporine provided benefit in patients whose disease was refractory to corticosteroids and azathioprine. Serious renal toxicity and treatment withdrawal, which plagued earlier studies, were reduced by careful selection of patients. In a 12-month European trial, cyclosporine

A appeared to be as efficacious as azathioprine in producing clinical improvement. Tacrolimus has a similar mechanism of action to cyclosporine A. When used in low dosage, it has proved as effective as cyclosporine A as a corticosteroid-sparing agent with fewer side effects.

Mycophenolate mofetil is another immunosuppressive agent that affects both T and B cells. This agent has now been used in sufficient numbers of MG patients to conclude that it is effective 70–75% of the time, although probably less so in refractory MG.[7] It has an acceptable saftey profile with adverse effects largely related to gastrointestinal intolerance. Benefit may require many weeks of adminstration.

INTRAVENOUS IMMUNOGLOBULIN

The potential utility of intravenous immunoglobulin (IVIG) was suggested by several uncontrolled trials.[43] Interest in the use of this agent grew out of its demonstrated efficacy in other autoimmune diseases, most notably autoimmune thrombocytopenia. IVIG has generally been administered at a dose of 2 g/kg over 2–4 days, although a recent controlled study suggested that 1 g/kg administered on one day was as beneficial as the standard higher dosing.[44] The results of these trials suggest that IVIG therapy can be associated with rapid clinical improvement in some patients, independent of whether they had undergone thymectomy or were being treated concurrently with corticosteroids or immunosuppressive agents. In some patients improvement was sustained over a period of several weeks. The mechanism(s) of this apparent salutary effect is unknown; improvement was not always accompanied by a consistent reduction in anti-AChR antibody titers.

POSSIBLE FUTURE THERAPEUTIC OPTIONS

There are a number of possible experimental avenues of approach that have been spawned by studies in EAMG. These are aimed at interrupting the sensitization process of helper CD4+ T cells, interrupting their effector function, or interdicting the action of downstream action of proinflammatory molecules. Studies directed at CD4+ T-cell-orchestrated responses include blocking the presentation of immunogenic AChR peptides by antigen presenting cells with nonimmunogenic forms of peptides, impeding activation by inhibitors of the co-stimulatory molecules CD28 and ICOS, the induction of anergy or apoptosis of AChR-reactive T cells, and suppression of AChR-specific Th1 responses by the induction of regulatory T cells or NKT cells, recently shown to be essential for the development of AChR-specific regulatory T cells[45] In addition, inhibition of the cytokines TNF or IL-1 by anti-TNF reagents and an IL-1 receptor antagonist, respectively, have shown efficacy in EAMG.

Two biologics that have begun to receive attention in clinical MG trials are rituxamab and etanercept. The former is a monoclonal antibody specific for CD20, a protein expressed on B lymphocytes. The latter is a fusion protein consisting of the extracellular ligand-binding portion of the human p75 TNF receptor linked to the Fc portion of human IgG₁. Rituxamab, developed as a therapeutic for B-cell malignancies, has shown efficacy in a number of autoimmune disorders, including some in which T cells, rather than B cells, are regarded as the principal effector mechanism. Anecdotal reports of improvement of MG following administration of rituxamab provide a basis for further exploring its utility of this autoimmune disease. Etanercept also appears promising as a type of imunomodulatory agent in MG. However, a recent trial suggested that patients most likely to benefit are those with low plasma IL-6 and IFN-γ.[46]

■ ACKNOWLEDGMENT ■

This work was supported by National Institutes of Health (NIH) grant NS19546.

■ REFERENCES ■

1. Lisak RP, Barchi RL. Myasthenia gravis. In: Walton JN, ed: Major Problems in Neurology, vol. 11. Philadelphia, PA: WB Saunders; 1982: 5.

2. Beeson D, Vincent A, Morris A, et al. cDNA and genomic clones encoding the muscle acetylcholine receptor. Ann NY Acad Sci 1993; 681: 165.

3. Karlin A. Explorations of the nicotinic acetylcholine receptor. Harvey Lect 1991; 85: 71.

4. Sanes JR, Apel ED, Gautam M, et al. Agrin receptors at the skeletal neuromuscular junction. Ann NY Acad Sci 1998; 841: 1.

5. Levinson AI, Zweiman B, Lisak RP. Immunopathogenesis and treatment of myasthenia gravis. J Clin Immunol 1987; 7: 187.

6. Papadouli I, Sakarellos C, Tzartos SJ. High-resolution epitope mapping and fine antigenic characterization of the main immunogenic region of the acetylcholine receptor: Eur J Biochem 1993; 211: 227.

7. Vincent A, Leite MI. Neuromuscular junction autoimmune disease: muscle specific kinase antibodies and treatments for myasthenia gravis. Curr Opin Neurol 2005; 18: 519.

8. Aarli JA, Skeie GO, Mygland A, et al. Muscle striation antibodies in myasthenia gravis. Ann NY Acad Sci 1998; 841: 505.

9. Agius MA, Zhu S, Kirvan CA, et al. Rapsyn antibodies in myasthenia gravis. Ann NY Acad Sci 1998; 841: 516.

10. Drachman DB, Adams RN, Josifek LF, et al. Antibody-mediated mechanisms of ACh receptor loss in myasthenia gravis: clinical relevance. Ann NY Acad Sci 1981; 377: 175.

11. Engel AG, Sahashi K, Fumagalli G. The immunopathology of acquired myasthenia gravis. Ann NY Acad Sci 1981; 377: 158.

12. Drachman DB, Angus CW, Adams RN, et al. Myasthenic antibodies cross-link acetylcholine receptors to accelerate degradation. N Engl J Med 1978; 298: 1116.

13. Richman DP, Wollmann RL, Maselli RA, et al. Effector mechanisms of myasthenic antibodies. Ann NY Acad Sci 1993; 681: 264.

14. Conti-Fine B, Navaneetham D, Karachunski PI, et al. T cell recognition of the acetylcholine receptor in myasthenia gravis. Ann NY Acad Sci 1998; 841: 283.

15. Patrick J, Lindstrom J. Autoimmune response to acetylcholine receptor. Science 1973; 180: 871.

16. Christadoss P, Poussin M, Deng C. Animal models of myasthenia gravis. Clin Immunol 2000; 94: 75.

17. Pachner AR, Kantor FS. The relation of clinical disease to antibody titre, proliferative response and neurophysiology in murine experimental autoimmune myasthenia gravis. Clin Exp Immunol 1983; 51: 543.

18. Bellone M, Ostile N, Lei S, et al. Experimental myasthenia gravis in congenic mice. Sequence mapping and H-2 restriction of T helper epitopes on the α subunits of *Torpedo californica* and murine acetylcholine receptors. Eur J Immunol 1991; 21: 2303.

19. Karachunski PI, Ostlie NS, Okita DK, et al. Interleukin-4 deficiency facilitates development of experimental myasthenia gravis and precludes its prevention by nasal administration of CD4[+] epitope sequences of the acetylcholine receptor. J Neuroimmunol 1999; 95: 73.

20. Poussin MA, Tuzun E, Goluszko E, et al. B7-1 costimulatory molecule is critical for the development of experimental autoimmune myasthenia gravis. J Immunol 2003; 170: 4389.

21. Dong C, Flavell R, Christadoss P. ICOS is essential for the development of experimental autoimmune myasthenia gravis. J Neuroimmunol 2004; 153: 16.

22. Levinson AI, Wheatley LM. The thymus and the pathogenesis of myasthenia gravis. Clin Immunol Immunopathol 1995; 78: 1.

23. Wheatley LM, Urso D, Zheng Y, et al. Molecular analysis of intrathymic nicotinic acetylcholine receptor. Ann NY Acad Sci 1993; 681: 74.

24. Schultz A, Hoffacker V, Wilisch A, et al. Neurofilament is an autoantigenic determinant in myasthenia gravis. Ann Neurol 1999; 46: 167.

25. Zheng Y, Wheatley LM, Liu T, et al. Acetylcholine receptor alpha subnit mRNA expression in human thymus: augmented expression in myasthenia gravis and upregulation by interferon-γ. Clin Immunol 1999; 91: 170.

26. Galy AHM, Spits H. IL-1, IL-4, and IFN-γ differentially regulate cytokine production and cell surface molecule expression in cultured human thymic epithelial cells. J Immunol 1991; 147: 3823.

27. Berrih-Aknin S, Arenzana-Seisdedos F, Cohen S, et al. Interferon-gamma modulates HLA class II antigen expression on cultured human thymic epithelial cells. J Immunol 1985; 35: 1165.

28. Poea-Guyon S, Christados P, Le Panse R, et al. Effects of cytokines on acetylcholine receptor expression: implications for myasthenia gravis. J Immunol 2005; 174: 5941.

29. Wheatley L, Urso D, Tumas K, et al. Molecular characterization of the nicotinic acetylcholine receptor alpha chain in mouse thymus. J Immunol 1992; 148: 3105.

30. Naparstek Y, Ben-Nun A, Holoshitz J, et al. T lymphocyte lines producing or vaccinating against autoimmune encephalomyelitis (EAE). Functional activation induces peanut agglutinin receptors and accumulation in the the brain and thymus of line cells. Eur J Immunol 1983; 13: 418.

31. Balandina A, Lécart S, Dartevelle P, et al. Functional defect of regulatory CD4[+]CD25[+] T cells in the thymus of patients with autoimmune myasthenia gravis. Blood 2005; 105: 735.

32. Huang D, Pirskanen R, Hjelmstrom P, et al. Polymorphisms in IL-1beta and IL-1 receptor antagonist genes are associated with myasthenia gravis. J Neuroimmunol 1998; 81: 76.

33. Skeie GO, Pandey JP, Aarli JA, et al. TNFA and TNFB polymorphisms in myasthenia gravis. Arch Neurol 1999; 56: 457.

34. Huang DR, Pirskanen R, Matell G, et al. Tumour necrosis factor-alpha polymorphism and secretion in myasthenia gravis. J Neuroimmunol 1999; 94: 165.

35. Huang DR, Zhou YH, XiaSQ, et al. Markers in the promoter region of interleukin-10 (IL-10) gene in myasthenia gravis: implications of diverse effects of IL-10 in the pathogenesis of the disease. J Neuroimmunol 1999; 94: 82.

36. Dwyer DS, Vakil M, Bradleg RT, et al. A possible cause of myasthenia gravis: idiotypic networks involving bacterial antigens. Ann NY Acad Sci 1987; 505: 461.

37. Bever CT Jr, Chang HW, Penn AS, et al. Chemical alteration of acetylcholine receptor by penicillamine: a mechanism for induction of myasthenia gravis. Neurology 1982; 32: 1077.

38. Penn A, Jacques JJ. Cells from mice exposed chronically to D-penicillamine show proliferative responses to D-penicillamine-treated self (macrophage/dendritic cells): a graft-versus-host response?. Ann NY Acad Sci 1993; 681: 319.

39. Genkins G, Sivar M, Tartte PI. Treatment strategies in myasthenia gravis. Ann NY Acad Sci 1993; 681: 603.

40. Schneider-Gold C, Gajdos P, Toyka K, et al. Corticosteroids for myasthenia gravis. Cochrane Database Syst Rev 2005; 18: CD002828.

41. Seybold M. Plasmapheresis in myasthenia gravis. Ann NY Acad Sci 1987; 505: 584–594.

42. Palace J, Newsom-Davis J, Lecky B. A randomized double-blind trial of prednisolone alone or with azathioprine in myasthenia gravis. Myasthenia Gravis Study Group. Neurology 1998; 50: 1778.

43. Dalakas MC. The use of intravenous immunoglobulin in the treatment of autoimmune neuromuscular diseases: evidence-based indications and safety profile. Pharmacol Ther 2004; 102: 177.

44. Gajdos P, Tranchant C, Clair B, et al. Myasthenia Gravis Clinical Study Group. Treatment of myasthenia gravis exacerbation with intravenous immunoglobulin: a randomized double-blind clinical trial. Randomized Controlled Trial. Arch Neurol 2005; 62: 1689.

45. Liu R, La Cava A, Bai XF, et al. Cooperation of invariant NKT cells and CD4+CD25+ T regulatory cells in the prevention of autoimmune myasthenia. J Immunol 2005; 175: 7898.

46. Tüzün E, Meriggioli MN, Rowin J, et al. Myasthenia gravis patients with low plasma IL-6 and IFN- benefit from etanercept treatment. J Autoimmun 2005; 24: 261.

Multiple sclerosis

65

Irene Cortese, Henry F. McFarland

Multiple sclerosis (MS) is an inflammatory, demyelinating, relapsing or progressive disorder of the central nervous system (CNS) and is a major cause of disability in young adults. MS usually presents between 20 and 40 years of age and at least 350 000 individuals in the USA alone are affected with MS. Pathologically MS is characterized acutely by multifocal areas of demyelination, loss of oligodendrocytes, and astrogliosis with relative preservation of axons. However, many chronic lesions and some acute lesions are now known to have significant axonal damage. Further, involvement of gray matter is now known to be common, as are diffuse pathological changes throughout the white matter. The etiology of MS remains unclear, but current data suggest that the disease develops in genetically susceptible individuals exposed to environmental triggers. The long-favored hypothesis in MS implicates autoreactive T cells generated in the periphery that access the CNS, where they persist and induce an inflammatory cascade that results in the injury of previously normal neural tissues.

Clinically, MS most often presents as a relapsing remitting disease (relapsing remitting MS) slowly evolving into a course associated with progressive accumulation of disability (secondary progressive MS). In a small number of cases the disease begins with progression independent of acute relapses (primary progressive MS).

KEY CONCEPTS

>> Multiple sclerosis disease course can be relapsing remitting, secondary progressive, primary progressive, or relapsing progressive

>> Typical relapses are characterized by gradual-onset focal neurological deficits with spontaneous improvement over weeks to months

>> Typical symptoms include sensory changes, weakness and loss of dexterity, decrease in visual acuity, double vision, difficulty with coordination or balance

■ CLINICAL PRESENTATION AND CLASSIFICATION ■

MS can cause a wide variety of clinical features. The course of the illness, which is also variable, represents an important consideration in the diagnosis of MS.[1]

Sensory symptoms are the most common presenting symptoms in MS (21–55%) and ultimately develop in nearly all patients. These present as loss of sensation, paresthesias, dysesthesias, and hyperesthesias that can occur in any distribution. A large proportion of MS patients have persistent sensory loss, usually consisting of diminished vibratory and position sensation in the distal extremities.

Motor symptoms are the presenting manifestation of MS in 32–41% of all cases, although their prevalence in long-standing MS is higher than 60%. Pyramidal tract dysfunction causes weakness, spasticity, loss of dexterity, and hyperreflexia.

In 14–23% of patients, the initial symptom of MS is optic neuritis (ON); however more than 50% experience an episode of ON during their lifetime. Clinically the patient presents with visual loss in one eye that evolves over a few days, often accompanied or preceded by periocular pain, especially with eye movement. Most patients begin to recover within 2 weeks, with significant visual recovery being common.

Cerebellar involvement is frequent during the course of MS with manifestations that include dysmetria, dysdiadochokinesia, telekinetic tremor, dysrhythmia, breakdown of complex motor movements, and loss of balance.

Urinary urgency, frequency, and urge incontinence (due to detrusor hyperreflexia or detrusor sphincter dyssynergia) are common in MS patients, with the combined incidence of bowel and bladder dysfunction in MS being higher than 70%. Symptoms of bladder dysfunction may be transient in the setting of a relapse but are often persistent.

Internuclear ophthalmoplegia, caused by a lesion in the medial longitudinal fasciculus, is the most common cause of diplopia in MS patients.

Cognitive disorders are present in 40–70% of MS patients.[2] The signs can be subtle and may therefore be missed on a standard mental status examination. The pattern of cognitive decline is characterized by decrease

Table 65.1 Revised McDonald diagnostic criteria for multiple sclerosis (MS)

Clinical presentation	Additional data needed for multiple sclerosis diagnosis
Two or more attacks[a]; objective clinical evidence of two or more lesions	None[b]
Two or more attacks[a]; objective clinical evidence of one lesion	Dissemination in space, demonstrated by: MRI[c] or Two or more MRI-detected lesions consistent with MS plus positive CSF[d] or
One attack[a]; objective clinical evidence of two or more lesions	Await further clinical attack[a] implicating a different site Dissemination in time, demonstrated by: MRI[e] or Second clinical attack[a]
One attack: objective clinical evidence of one lesion (monosymptomatic presentation; clinically isolated syndrome)	Dissemination in space, demonstrated by: MRI[c] or Two or more MRI-detected lesions consistent with MS plus positive CSF[d] and Dissemination in time, demonstrated by: MRI[e] or Second clinical attack[a]
Insidious neurological progression suggestive of MS	One year of disease progression (retrospectively or prospective determined) and Two or more of the following: Positive brain MRI (nine T2 lesions or four or more T2 lesions with positive VEP) Positive spinal cord MRI (two focal T2 lesions) Positive CSF[d]

CSF, cerebrospinal fluid; MRI, magnetic resonance imaging; VEP, visual evoked potential.

If criteria are fulfilled and there is no better explanation for the clinical presentation, the diagnosis is MS; if suspicious, but the criteria are not completely met, the diagnosis is 'possible MS'; if another diagnosis arises during the evaluation that explains the entire clinical presentation better, then the diagnosis is 'not MS.'

[a]An attack is defined as an episode of neurological disturbance for which causative lesions are likely to be inflammatory and demyelinating in nature. There should be subjective report (backed up by objective findings) or objective observation that the event lasts for at least 24 hours.

[b]No additional tests are required; however, if tests (MRI, CSF) are undertaken and are negative, extreme caution needs to be taken before making a diagnosis of MS. Alternative diagnoses must be considered. There must be no better explanation for the clinical picture and some objective evidence to support a diagnosis of MS.

[c]MRI demonstration of space dissemination must fulfill the criteria detailed in Table 65.2.

[d]Positive CSF determined by oligoclonal bands detected by established methods (isoelectric focusing) different from any such bands in serum, or by an increased immunoglobulin G index.

[e]MRI demonstration of time dissemination must fulfill the criteria in Table 65.1.

Adapted from Polman CH, et al. Diagnostic criteria for multiple sclerosis: 2005 revisions to the 'McDonald criteria.' Ann Neurol 2005; 58: 840–846.

isoelectric focusing of CSF proteins often reveals discrete bands of immunoglobulin, each representing a monoclonal antibody. Unique banding patterns in the CSF, not present in the serum, are known as oligoclonal bands (OCBs) and are indicative of intrathecal humoral immune response. Between 85% and 95% of MS patients have OCBs; however, early in the course of disease they are not as prevalent. Once present, OCBs persist and the pattern does not vary, although new bands occasionally appear. The antigenic specificity of OCBs is unknown.[1]

Evoked potentials are summed cortical electrical responses to peripheral sensory stimulation that can be used to localize sites of pathology and measure conduction velocity along sensory pathways. VEP and somatosensory evoked potentials can detect subclinical sites of demyelination, thus providing evidence of multifocality of MS lesions. Some 85% of patients with MS have abnormalities on VEPs, even when the history of ON is absent.[1]

KEY CONCEPTS

>> Multiple sclerosis is a multifactorial disease most likely due to exposure to environmental triggers in a genetically susceptible individual

>> The inflammatory phase is thought to be driven by autoreactive CD4 T cells specific for myelin epitopes

>> It is not clear if the neurodegenerative phase is a consequence of immune-mediated injury or has an unrelated cause

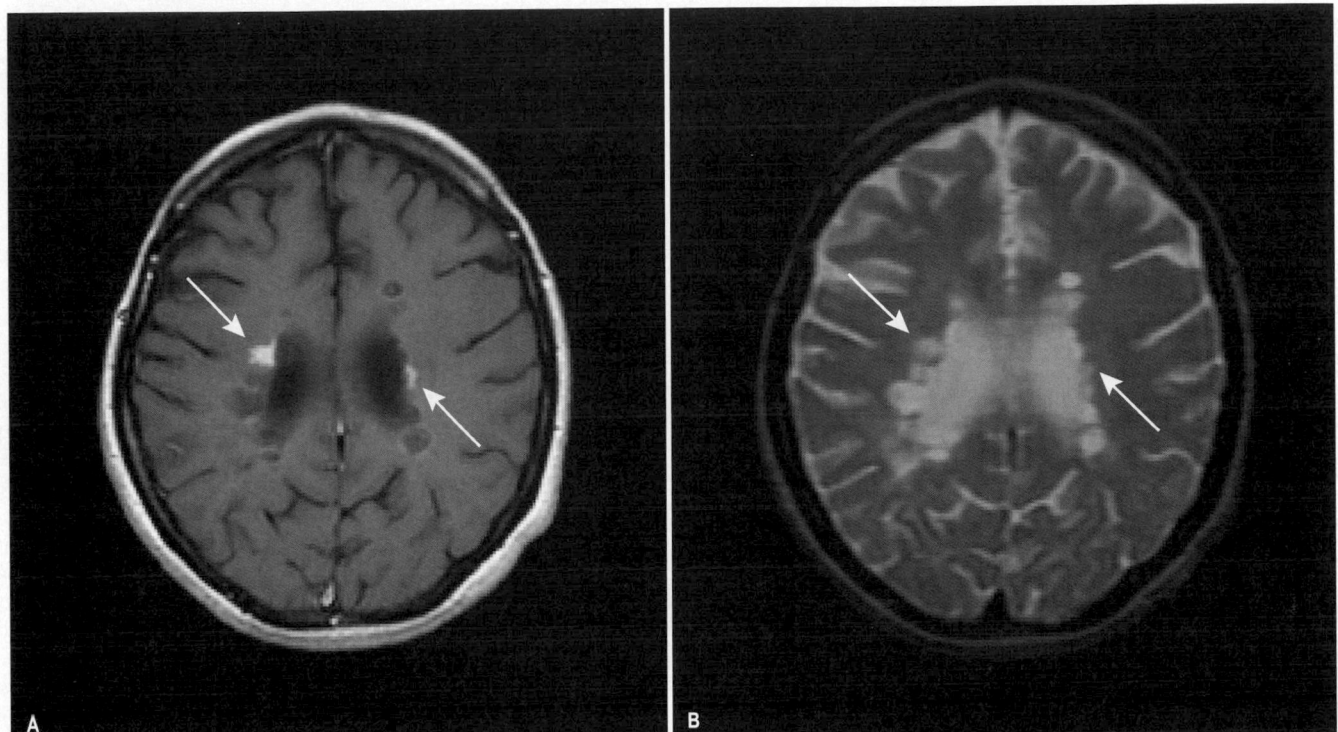

Fig. 65.2 Magnetic resonance imaging (MRI) in multiple sclerosis (MS). **(A)** T1-weighted spin echo (WSE) post contrast MRI obtained in an MS patient after the injection of a single dose (0.1 mmol/kg of body weight) of gadolinium diethylenetriamine pentacid (Gd-DTPA). Two active lesions are visible on the MRI, indicated by the arrows. Several chronic hypointense lesions (T1 'black holes') are seen surrounding the ventricles. **(B)** T2-WSE MRI showing both chronic and acute MS lesions in the same patient.

Table 65.2 Magnetic resonance imaging criteria to demonstrate dissemination of lesions in time

There are two ways to show dissemination in time using imaging:
- Detection of gadolinium enhancement at least 3 months after the onset of the initial clinical event, if not at the site corresponding to the initial event
- Detection of a new T2 lesion if it appears at any time compared with a reference scan done at least 30 days after the onset of the initial clinical event

Adapted from Polman CH, et al. Diagnostic criteria for multiple sclerosis: 2005 revisions to the 'McDonald criteria.' Ann Neurol 2005; 58: 840–846.

Table 65.3 Magnetic resonance imaging criteria to demonstrate brain abnormality and demonstration of dissemination in space

Three of the following:
At least one gadolinium-enhancing lesion or nine T2 hyperintense lesions if there is no gadolinium-enhancing lesion
At least one infratentorial lesion
At least one juxtacortical lesion
At least three periventricular lesions

Note: A spinal cord lesion can be considered equivalent to a brain infratentorial lesion: an enhancing spinal cord lesion is considered to be equivalent to an enhancing brain lesion, and individual spinal cord lesions can contribute together with individual brain lesions to reach the required number of T2 lesions

Adapted from Polman CH, et al. Diagnostic criteria for multiple sclerosis: 2005 revisions to the 'McDonald criteria.' Ann Neurol 2005; 58: 840–846.

A set of criteria have also been established for the diagnosis of primary progressive MS. By definition, all patients with primary progressive MS have a slowly progressive and often monosymptomatic course, frequently consisting of spastic paraparesis without clinical signs of dissemination in the CNS. A proportion of patients may have multiple symptoms at onset.[10] Just as in relapsing remitting MS, in addition to the clinical history, CSF findings, VEPs, and abnormal MRI are often helpful in making a diagnosis. In this case, exclusion of other causes of slowly progressive degenerative disease is essential[11] (Table 65.4).

Table 65.4 Diagnosis of multiple sclerosis in disease with progression from onset

One year of disease progression (retrospectively or prospectively determined) *plus* two of the following:
Positive brain magnetic resonance imaging (MRI) (nine T2 lesions or four or more T2 lesions with positive visual evoked potential)
Positive spinal cord MRI (two focal T2 lesions)
Positive cerebrospinal fluid (isoelectric focusing evidence of oligoclonal immunoglobulin G (IgG) bands or increased IgG index, or both)

Adapted from Polman CH, et al. Diagnostic criteria for multiple sclerosis: 2005 revisions to the 'McDonald criteria.' Ann Neurol 2005; 58: 840–846.

NEUROPATHOLOGY

MS is a CNS disease histopathologically characterized by discrete areas of myelin, oligodendrocyte, and axonal loss, called plaques or MS lesions. These lesions are seen in the cerebral hemispheres, the brainstem, spinal cord, optic nerves and chiasm, and the cerebellum. Although MS has long been regarded as a white-matter disease, MS lesions occur in all CNS parenchymal areas, including cerebral cortex and deep gray matter. Studies have confirmed that the extent of cortical demyelination does not correlate with the extent of focal white-matter demyelination. Extensive cortical demyelination is associated with the progressive phases of disease, while less cortical demyelination has been seen in relapsing remitting MS.

The pathological hallmarks of MS lesions are inflammatory infiltrates with T cells, B cells, and macrophages/microglia; demyelination with oligodendrocyte loss; and a variable degree of remyelination, axonal loss, and gliosis. The mechanisms of tissue damage in MS lesions are not yet fully understood. Besides the inflammatory-demyelinating component, an additional neurodegenerative component appears to be involved, leading to extensive neuroaxonal damage in the chronic MS brain. Regenerative processes such as remyelination are also present in the MS brain and may be extensive, especially early in the course of disease.

The terms active/acute, subacute or chronic active and chronic inactive are used to stage MS lesions. Active/acute lesions have traditionally been defined as showing demyelination with inflammatory infiltrates, while chronic lesions show demyelination with little or no inflammation. The subacute or chronic active lesion is one with a chronic core and active edge, or else one with a low level of inflammatory activity.[12]

The hallmark of the acute lesion is a robust inflammatory response, consisting of lymphocytes, macrophages, occasional plasma cells, or even eosinophils, which may also be scattered in chronic lesions. These form the active rim of expanding chronic active or subacute lesions. The T cells seen in MS lesions consist of both CD4 and CD8 cells.[12]

Investigators examining brain specimens from patients who have diagnostic brain biopsies or from patients with MS who have died have resulted in the description of four pathological patterns.[5] Pattern 1 (macrophage-associated demyelination), representing 15% of lesions, shows inflammatory demyelination marked by macrophage infiltration. The most common is Pattern 2 (antibody-associated demyelination) found in 58% of lesions,

which demonstrates well-demarcated zones of demyelination and striking T-cell inflammation. With the use of specific stains it can be shown that all myelin proteins are lost simultaneously. This lesion is characterized by the striking deposition of complement, especially C9neo component, around blood vessels and on myelin. On MRI, the edges of these lesions show gadolinium enhancement, indicative of BBB breakdown. Oligodendrocytes are relatively well preserved, and remyelination is frequently found.

In Pattern 3, the next most common lesion type at 26%, demyelination and inflammation occur. However the plaque is less sharply delineated. These lesions are characterized by oligodendrocyte apoptosis, marked reduction in oligodendrocytes, and minimal remyelination. In this pattern, there is selective loss of myelin-associated glycoprotein (MAG) compared with the other myelin proteins, which is suggestive of a lesion at the level of the oligodendroglial cell body. For this reason, this pattern has been termed a distal oliogodendrogliopathy. In these cases, Balo-like rings are often found and on MRI there tends to be little gadolinium enhancement.[6, 12]

Pattern 4 (primary oligodendrocyte degeneration) is a rare form that shows nonapoptotic oligodendrocyte death in the normal-appearing adjacent periplaque white matter. The demographic and clinical features of these patients, however, are indistinguishable from those of typical MS patients.[6, 12]

These various patterns of demyelination have suggested the existence of multiple etiologies and pathogenesis between patients and point to the possibility of MS as a heterogeneous disease. Supporting lesion heterogeneity is the observation of differential expression of chemokine receptors on monocytes/macrophages in actively demyelinating lesions.[13] The pathological heterogeneity of the MS lesion remains an area of active research.

Recent pathological studies on a limited number of patients, conducted on tissue just hours after the onset of disease exacerbation, noted the presence of lesions characterized by areas with apoptotic oligodendrocytes and macrophage activity with a paucity of inflammatory cells. These lesions have been termed early apoptotic oligodendrocyte lesions, and it has been postulated that all MS lesions may start this way. An ischemic or metabolic insult to the oligodendrocyte is hypothesized to be the initiating event, and presumably inflammatory changes would be secondary events due to the oligodendrocyte injury.[14, 15] These findings are not, however, substantially different from those found in pattern 3 described above, where a similar anoxic/toxic insult is suggested.

Previously unrecognized diffuse white-matter involvement in the areas that appear grossly normal has been clearly demonstrated by sophisticated forms of MR examination, including reduced magnetization transfer ratios, changes in diffusion coefficient, and decreased N-acetyl aspartic acid (neuronal marker) by MR spectroscopy. Pathological examination of these areas has shown active demyelination, with macrophages filled with myelin components in varying stages of degradation, diffuse, mainly CD8+ T-cell infiltrates, microglial activation, diffuse axonal injury with axonal spheroids, gliosis, and even some remyelination.[6, 12] It is unclear if these represent lesions in their first stages of development or secondary Wallerian degeneration, serial imaging studies have shown subsequent typical plaque formation in the same areas highlighted by these imaging methods.[12]

Significant destruction of axons in MS has been recognized from the time of the earliest pathological descriptions, but the degree of axonal damage and the presence of axonal destruction in the acute MS lesion have only recently been characterized. Axonal degeneration correlates with the presence of permanent black holes on T1-weighted MRI and the extent of atrophy in the spinal cord. Because these imaging parameters correlate with clinical disability, axonal damage is likely responsible for irreversible clinical disability in MS. This is one of the striking pathological features of progressive MS. The extent of axonal transection in early active lesions correlates with inflammation; the magnitude of axonal loss in chronic lesions suggests that mechanisms other than inflammatory demyelination may contribute to axonal damage at later stages. A slow subclinical inflammatory process has been suggested, continuing throughout the disease course and not causing clinical relapses or gadolinium enhancement (the standard markers of acute inflammation). However, other possibilities include loss of trophic factors from oligodendrocytes and myelin, loss of a physical barrier protecting the axon from exposure to destructive factors, or rearrangement of Na^+ and K^+ channels on demyelinated axons that may place an undue metabolic stress on the axons.[12]

The CNS is capable of remyelination, and this occurs commonly in MS. The extent of remyelination in MS varies, with up to 28% of plaques being remyelinated. Efficient remyelination requires the presence of undamaged axons and a sufficient number of residual oligodendrocytes or oligodendrocyte precursors. Areas of extensive remyelination in correspondence with acute and early MS plaques are referred to as 'shadow plaques.'[6]

A unique pathological finding is Balo's concentric sclerosis, which was originally described as a distinct disease entity. Pathologically it consists of ring-shaped lesions composed of alternating bands of demyelination and normally preserved myelin. Similar tigroid lesions are found in MS. The demyelinated bands contain high levels of inducible nitric oxide synthetase, a mediator of inflammatory damage, while preserved myelin contains high levels of proteins involved in hypoxic preconditioning, such as hypoxia-inducing factor (HIF), heat shock protein 70 (HSP-70), and D-110 molecules. These observations suggest that hypoxia may play an important role in mediating tissue injury and contributing to the concentricity typical of this pattern of demyelination. Because of the neuroprotective effects of HIF and HSP-70, it has been hypothesized that the inflammatory process induces hypoxic stress in the periphery of the lesion, the preserved band, rendering this area more resistant to subsequent ischemic assaults. This is consistent with the presence of Balo-like changes in the pattern 3 MS lesions, in which a possible hypoxic etiology has been postulated.[12]

Few pathological studies have focused on patients with primary or secondary progressive MS. The most relevant findings in these reports are the presence of slowly expanding plaques with foamy macrophages containing lipids, especially in periplaque white matter. The description of absent or modest perivascular cuffs in the lesions, but the presence of lymphocytes and plasma cells in the periplaque white matter, is consistent with reduced inflammatory activity. Recently, demyelination in the cerebral cortex, diffuse injury in the form of focal axonal swelling and axonal spheroids, and diffuse rather than focal inflammation (defined as diffuse T-cell infiltration and microglial activation) were shown to be significantly increased in primary progressive and secondary progressive compared to relapsing remitting MS. Results of these studies seem to indicate that inflammation remains an important aspect of pathological changes in secondary progressive MS, albeit with different patterns than in the relapsing remitting MS.[4]

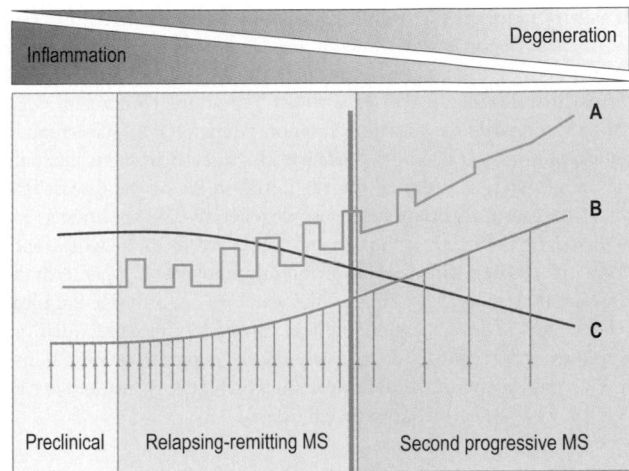

Fig. 65.3 Multiple sclerosis (MS) disease phases. MS disease course over time is characterized by progressive reduction in inflammation and progressive prevalence of neurodegenerative features. This is reflected in the decrease of clinical relapses over time with accumulation of disability (A), the accumulation of T2 lesion load by MRI (B), the decrease of contrast-enhancing lesions (vertical lines), and the irreversible loss of myelin and axons with progressive brain atrophy and decline in brain volume (C).

Most authors now consider MS a biphasic disease, with an early inflammatory period and a subsequent degenerative process, characterized by a progression to brain and spinal cord atrophy in the absence of overt relapses and significant inflammation (Fig. 65.3). Two observational studies of MS natural history found that the progression of disability is not affected by relapses, either those before the onset of the progressive phase or those that occur during this phase. However, the rate of cerebral atrophy is greatest in patients with the highest inflammatory lesion burden before treatment, suggesting these two features are not entirely independent.[16] The answer as to how progression and episodic disease activity are related will be demonstrated by effectiveness of early treatment in eliminating new episodes and accumulation of disability and onset of progression.

■ PATHOGENESIS ■

The long-favored hypothesis in MS implicates autoreactive T cells against myelin components, generated in the periphery, that access the CNS where they persist and induce an inflammatory cascade that results in the injury of previously normal neural tissues. Data in the animal model experimental autoimmune encephalomyelitis (EAE), that is initiated by systemic immunization with neuronal autoantigens, or by transfer of CD4 T cells sensitized with neuronal antigen, have provided support for an autoimmune process in MS.

Considerable evidence now exists for an immunological basis of the acute MS lesion. Various forms of immunosuppression and/or immunomodulation can substantially alter both the frequency of relapses as well as the frequency of contrast-enhancing lesions on MRI. However, most of these therapies have failed to produce a substantial effect on the progression of disability. The discrepancy has led some to argue that MS is primarily a degenerative disease with the immune component occurring as a secondary process. Since immnomodulation does have a modest effect on progression when used early in the disease, it seems likely that immunopathology is essential for the initial stages of the disease. Less clear is the cause of the more diffuse degenerative process that is now recognized. It is not clear if the damage seen in axons in the white matter and gray matter is a direct result of the immunopathology, is secondary to damage occurring at the time of the acute lesion, or has a completely unrelated cause. Most likely the damage caused by the acute, inflammatory process sets the stage for a subsequent degenerative process. Clearly MS is a complex, multifactorial disease in which genetic, nongenetic, and immunological aspects need to be considered.

■ NONGENETIC FACTORS ■

The relatively low concordance rate of identical twins indicates a contribution of nongenetic factors to MS etiology. Both infectious agents and behavioral or lifestyle influences have been proposed to induce or contribute to disease expression.

Different lines of evidence point to the role of environmental contributions. A north–south gradient in disease prevalence on the northern hemisphere and the opposite on the southern hemisphere, which cannot be explained by genetic factors alone, has been repeatedly documented. Migration studies have shown that individuals migrating from areas of high prevalence of MS to areas of low prevalence before the age of 15–16 acquire low risk of MS development, whereas migration after 15–16 does not change the risk. These epidemiological data support exposure to environmental factors in childhood as important in determining risk of disease development. Infections are the favored interpretation of this data; however dietary fatty acids and vitamin D levels have recently received attention. In addition, other factors such as ultraviolet radiation exposure, organic solvent exposure, and cigarette smoking have also been invoked.[17]

Viral and bacterial infections are logical candidates as environmental triggers of MS. Of interest, EAE studies show that almost 100% of transgenic mice expressing a T-cell receptor (TCR) that is specific for an encephalitogenic peptide of myelin basic protein (MBP) develop EAE when they are housed under nonpathogen-free conditions, whereas the same animals housed in a specific-pathogen-free facility remain disease-free. While reports of associations between infections are extensive, no single infectious agent has been detected reproducibly. Current data suggest that MS could be induced or exacerbated by many different microbial infections, and the responsible agents are most likely ubiquitous pathogens that are highly prevalent in the general population.

Viruses that induce persistent infections, such as herpes or retroviruses, have been studied extensively in MS. Herpes viruses are of particular interest due to their neurotropism, ubiquitous nature, and tendency to produce latent, recurrent infections. Among these, human herpes virus 6 (HHV-6) and Epstein–Barr virus (EBV) are leading candidates. The seroprevalence in the general population for both is high. Observations suggest that HHV-6 may play a role in MS, including its detection in oligodendrocytes in MS plaque tissue (but also in normal brain), infection of astrocytes, and the presence of HHV-6 DNA and anti-HHV-6

IgG and IgM antibodies in the serum and CSF of MS patients. DNA and serological data, however, are controversial; the existence of two different HHV-6 variants may account for some of the discrepancies. EBV has also been linked with MS. Anti-EBV antibodies are elevated in patients with MS (seropositivity is 100% versus 90% in the general population) and MS patients reactivate latent EBV infections more often, correlating with relapses.[17, 18]

Molecular mimicry and bystander activation, or a combination of these, are the main mechanisms used to explain how infections could induce MS. The recognition of self-antigens at intermediate levels of affinity by T cells during thymic maturation leads to positive selection and export of these T cells to the periphery. Cross-reactivity of these potentially self-reactive T cells with foreign antigens (molecular mimicry) can lead to activation during infection. Previously immune reactivity was thought to be strictly specific and complete sequence homology was thought to be necessary for molecular mimicry to occur. It is now clear that cross-reactivity can occur with peptides that share no amino acids in their sequence and that each amino acid in a peptide contributes independently and additively to recognition by the TCR.[19] This suggests that molecular mimicry could occur more frequently than previously expected. Despite this, there is little evidence that molecular mimicry occurs in human autoimmune disease.

Bystander activation refers to a mechanism by which autoreactive T cells are activated as a consequence of nonspecific inflammatory events during infections. Cytokines, superantigens, and infectious-derived, proinflammatory agents such as lipopolysaccharide are capable of activating autoreactive T cells.[17]

■ HLA AND GENETICS ■

Familial aggregation has long been noted in MS. First-, second-, and third-degree relatives of people with MS have a greater risk of developing MS than the general population; this risk varies with degree of relatedness, with MS being 20–40 times more common in first-degree relatives, and dropping off rapidly thereafter. Adoption studies have shown that adoptive relatives, although raised from infancy with the MS patient, were no more likely to develop MS than expected for the general population, suggesting that familial aggregation is due to genetic sharing rather than shared family environment. Half-sibling studies support this data. Twin studies have shown there is an excess of monozygotic concordance (25–30%) compared with dizygotic concordance (3–5%).[20]

As in other T-cell-mediated autoimmune diseases, human leukocyte antigen (HLA)-DR and -DQ molecules are by far the strongest genetic risk factors in MS. In Caucasians, the specific genes that confer risk are the HLA-DR15 haplotype (DRB1*1501, DRB5*0101, DQA1*0102, DQB1*0602). A dose effect in DR15 homozygotic MS patients has also been described. Links with other DR molecules in ethnically more distant populations have been described.[17, 18] The association of MS with HLA class I alleles appears to be much lower. However, HLA-A3 and -B7 are overrepresented in MS patients, and HLA-A201 has shown protective effects.[17] Recently, compelling evidence has been reported that polymorphisms in IL7R, which encodes the interleukin 7 receptor alpha chain, contribute to the non-HLA genetic risk in multiple sclerosis. [41,42]

Two other promising candidate genes have emerged. Polymorphisms of the cytokine interferon-γ (IFN-γ) and the haplotypes formed between them are associated with MS susceptibility. This has not, however, been confirmed in all tested populations. Apolipoprotein E (APOe) genotype has been associated with MS disease severity, although consensus here too is lacking. APOe3 and e4 have been associated with neuronal loss, APOe2 is associated with less severe disease in women, and APOe4 has been associated with progressive disease in women and cognitive impairment in men with MS. These associations further suggest the presence of genetic contributions to MS etiology and phenotype.[21]

■ IMMUNOLOGY ■

The activation of autoreactive CD4 T cells in the periphery is considered to be the first important immunological event in MS. This is supported by data obtained from the animal model EAE, which is initiated by systemic immunization with neuronal autoantigens or by transfer of CD4 T cells sensitized with neuronal antigen. Transfer of antibodies alone or of activated monocytes does not result in disease, and myelin-specific CD8 T cells induce EAE only under special circumstances. An increased frequency of CD4 myelin-reactive T cells in the peripheral blood of MS patients compared with healthy donors, seemingly derived from the memory T-cell pool, implicates prior sensitization with disease-relevant antigens.[22] Such clones have been shown to exist in the peripheral blood for long periods of time and may be reactivated during disease exacerbation. Interestingly, it appears that regulation of CD4 T-cell apoptosis is perturbed in MS, with increased expression of anti-apoptotic molecules, that is further heightened during disease exacerbation and downregulation by IFN-β. Myelin-specific T cells in MS are relatively skewed toward a Th1 proinflammatory phenotype. Fluctuations of cytokine secretion have been linked to MRI-documented inflammatory activity: elevated expression of the proinflammatory cytokines IFN-γ and tumor necrosis factor-α (TNF-α) have correlated with disease activity, while IL-10 has shown relatively higher levels during remissions. All these data, as well as the association of MS with distinct HLA class II molecules, support a central role for CD4 T cells in the pathogenesis of MS.[17]

The activation of CD4 T cells is thought to occur following exposure to environmental influences, the favored trigger being infectious agents. This could lead to activation through molecular mimicry, bystander activation, or a combination of these. Alterations in the activation thresholds of autoreactive CD4 T cells due to abnormal requirements for co-stimulation probably play a role. CD4 myelin-specific T cells, as well as T cells with specificity for other antigens, are either less dependent or independent of co-stimulation.[23] In addition, the number and function of CD4+CD25+ immunoregulatory T cells (Tregs) appear reduced in MS patients. CD4 Tregs, characterized by CD25[high] expression and expression of the transcription factor FOX-P3, suppress T-cell proliferation by both cell–cell contact and cytokine-mediated mechanisms.[24] The alteration of this population of regulatory cells could facilitate the activation of autoreactive CD4 T cells in the periphery.

Recent evidence suggests that the innate immune system may also be involved in immune regulation. Natural killer (NK) cells have reduced activity in MS, and their function appears to fluctuate in relation to disease exacerbations.[25] Of interest are the results from a recent phase II clinical trial with daclizumab, a humanized monoclonal antibody against the IL-2 receptor α-chain, in which an expansion of the NK population associated with increased function was seen to correlate strongly with a reduction of inflammatory activity in the brains of treated patients.[17, 26]

Activated autoreactive T cells adhere to the BBB endothelium via adhesion molecules (LFA-1 and VLA-4), and transmigrate into the brain parenchyma through cerebrovascular endothelial cells. Proinflammatory cytokines (IFN-γ and TNF-α) produced by these cells activate adhesion molecules (ICAM-1, VCAM-1, and E-selectin) on the BBB. Activated CD4 T cells also produce proteolytic enzymes (MMP-2 and MMP-9) that facilitate passage through the subendothelial basement membrane.[17, 27] Thus, access to the CNS permits interaction of autoreactive T cells wich the target antigen/s.

MBP is the best-studied myelin protein in MS. It is the second most abundant myelin protein (approximately 30–40%) after proteolipid protein (PLP). The highly basic MBP is positioned at the intracellular surface of myelin membranes, and via interactions with acidic lipid moieties is involved in maintaining the structure of compact myelin. MBP induces EAE in numerous mouse and rat strains, guinea pigs, and non-human primates. In humanized transgenic mouse models carrying MBP-specific TCRs from MS patients, EAE could be readily induced. In one of these models, about 4% of the animals developed spontaneous disease, clearly showing that MS patient-derived MBP-specific T cells have encephalitogenic potential.[28, 29]

PLP is the most abundant CNS myelin protein (about 50%). When comparing PLP and MBP, the former is a stronger and dominant encephalitogen in some EAE models. Upon EAE induction with whole spinal cord homogenate, the dominant T-cell response is directed against PLP.[30] PLP TCR transgenic mice on SJL/J background develop spontaneous EAE with high frequency.[31]

Myelin oligodendrocyte glycoprotein (MOG), a transmembrane glycoprotein of the Ig superfamily, is much less abundant than the major myelin proteins (0.01–0.05%), and it is not located in compact myelin but rather on the outer surface of the oligodendrocyte membrane. Owing to this location, it is directly accessible to antibodies and therefore an easy target for both cellular and humoral immune responses in MS. Of interest, a MOG-TCR transgenic mouse model demonstrates spontaneous EAE in only a small fraction of animals, while 35% develop spontaneous ON.[32]

Other candidate antigens which have been studied include MAG, 2',3'-cyclic nucleotide 3' phosphodiesterase (CNPase), myelin-associated oligodendrocytic basic protein (MOBP), oligodendrocyte-specific glycoprotein (OSP), alpha-b crystalline, S100b protein, transaldolase-H, and lipid components.[17]

Destruction of CNS tissue during autoimmune inflammation leads to release of self-antigens, which can then be processed and presented by antigen-presenting cells, resulting in the *de novo* activation of autoreactive T cells. This cascade of events can also lead to epitope spreading, in which the initial epitope-specific T-cell response broadens to include other epitopes on the same molecule and on different antigens. This process probably plays an important role in the progression and perpetuation of the autoimmune response.

Upon local reactivation, proinflammatory cytokines (IFN-γ, IL-23, TNF-α, lymphotoxin) and chemokines released by the CD4 T cells activate resident cells, such as microglia and astrocytes, recruit other immune cells, including monocytes, CD8 T cells, B cells, and mast cells from the peripheral blood, and contribute to the formation of the inflammatory lesion. A significant number of chemokines and the corresponding receptors have been detected in MS brain lesions, supporting a pathogenic role in MS. These include CCL3 (MIP-1a), CCL4 (MIP-1b), and CCL5 (RANTES), CCL2 (MCP-1), CCL7 (MCP-3), CCL8 (MCP-2), and CXCL10 (IP-10), all of which have also been found in active MS lesions.[17, 27]

Ultimately numerous processes contribute to myelin/oligodendrocyte and axonal damage, including free radicals, cytokines, direct complement deposition, antibody-mediated complement activation and antibody-dependent cellular cytotoxicity via Fc-receptors, myelin phagocytosis, direct lysis of axons by CD8 cytotoxic T lymphocytes, the secretion of proteases, lysis of oligodendrocytes by γδ T cells, and apoptosis of oligodendrocytes.

Only a low level of B cells (< 1%) are able to cross the intact BBB; however, once inflammation disrupts the BBB, B cells, antibodies, and complement can enter the CNS. B cells, plasma cells, and myelin-specific antibodies are detected in MS plaques and in areas of active demyelination in MS patients. The observation of increased immunoglobulins in the CSF in MS patients, but not in the serum, indicates intrathecal production. These CSF Igs are typically oligoclonal, although their specificity is unknown. Within the CNS, B cells can serve as antigen-presenting cells and can provide co-stimulatory signals to autoreactive T cells, thereby contributing to inflammatory process. B cells and tissue-bound Ig can recruit further autoreactive T cells to the CNS. Furthermore, the activation of idiotope-specific T cells by CSF Igs has been described. The production of myelin-specific antibodies and the destruction of myelin within plaques are probably the most significant contributions of B cells to MS pathogenesis.[17, 33]

Different lines of evidence suggest contribution by CD8 T cells in pathogenesis. Except for microglia, none of the resident CNS cells express MHC class II constitutively including oligodendrocytes and neurons, however they can be recognized by CD8 T cells. Clonally expanded CD8 memory T cells have been found in the CSF and in MS brain tissue, and a persistence of CD8 T-cell clones is seen in CSF and blood. In the MS lesion, CD8 T cells predominate. HLA class I-restricted myelin epitopes have been described and the CD8 cytotoxic T-cell response to MBP is increased in MS patients. In addition, histological evidence suggests CD8 T cells may act as effector cells in axonal loss, with an increased frequency of CD8 T cells significantly correlating with the presence of increased amyloid precursor protein (APP), a marker of axonal damage, within neuronal axons.[17, 34]

In addition to these mechanisms of injury, evidence suggests that denuded axons are especially vulnerable to the inflammatory environment of acute lesions. The release of excessive quantities of glutamate by macrophages can cause excitotoxicity and death of neurons and oligodendrocytes. Markers for glutamate production and glutamate receptors are upregulated in MS lesions and appear to correlate with disease severity and axonal damage.[27]

The inflammatory event lasts from a few days to 2 weeks. The natural resolution of the inflammatory process may be explained in part by the function of the subpopulation of regulatory T cells, as well as by activated NK cells that have been shown to have suppressive effects of antigen-specific Th1 responses and to favor Th2 function.[27] The result is characterized by stretches of denuded axons, apoptotic oligodendrocytes and T cells, axon transections, macrophages loaded with phagocytosed myelin lipids, and the activation and proliferation of astrocytes. Besides clearing debris, further lesion resolution includes a relative dominance of Th2/Th3 cytokines, such as IL-10 and transforming growth factor-β, and the secretion of various growth factors (brain-derived neurotrophic factor, platelet-derived growth factor, ciliary neurotropy factor, and fibroblast growth factors) by both resident cells and T cells. Oligodendrocyte precursors that are still present in the adult CNS are also activated, and surviving oligodendrocytes begin to remyelinate denuded internode areas. The original thickness of the compact myelin is not reached again and therefore nerve conduction velocity remains slower in these regions.[17] Myelin debris contains several inhibitory molecules, including Nogo-A, MAG, and OMgp, all of which are physiologically relevant during maturation of the CNS and can impede the repair process.

It appears that the failure of adequate remyelination is the result of an inhospitable environment within the plaque or lack of sufficient signals for extensive myelination rather than a lack of myelin precursor cells.[18] During the months and years following an inflammatory event, the cellular composition of the lesion changes dramatically. Chronic plaques can show smoldering inflammation, but are often devoid of inflammatory cells and characterized by loss of myelin and axons, relative increases in astrocytes and gliosis.

■ TREATMENT ■

During the past decade, the advent of disease-modifying treatments has substantially changed the approach to relapsing remitting MS. Early treatment initiation is now recommended to maximize the efficacy of currently available therapies that are known to act mainly against the inflammatory components of MS. By contrast, the understanding and treatment of the progressive phase of MS, which is characterized by the steady accumulation of fixed disability, are suboptimal.

Treatment of acute exacerbations of disease and disease-modifying therapy are considered below. Most patients with MS are also managed with symptomatic treatment directed at specific issues, such as bladder dysfunction, paresthesias, pain, spasticity, depression, and fatigue. Moreover, many patients benefit from physical therapy and occupational therapy, and the use of assistive devices such as ankle–foot orthotics, canes, or walkers. These strategies are essential for the global care of MS patients.

Corticosteroids are the most commonly used treatment for acute exacerbations of MS, although there have been few studies to address their efficacy. The current recommendation is to treat disabling attacks with 500–1000 mg of intravenous methylprednisolone per day for 3–5 days with or without a short tapering dose of oral corticosteroids. Evidence suggests that intravenous steroids may also have long-term effects on disease progression when given at regular intervals. Up to one-third of patients do not have adequate recovery after relapse despite use of corticosteroids. Plasma exchange was found to be beneficial in a substantial proportion of patients with severe inflammatory demyelinating episodes who had failed treatment with intravenous methylprednisolone.[35]

Several drugs have been approved as disease-modifying agents in the treatment of MS. The treatment of different phases of the disease must be considered separately as the recommendations are different.[36, 37]

For the treatment of clinically definite MS, different options are available. IFN-β are a class of peptides that have antiviral and immunoregulatory functions. IFN-$β_{1b}$ was the first drug approved by the US Food and Drug Administration specifically for the treatment of MS. A large clinical study in relapsing remitting MS demonstrated a reduction in the frequency of relapses by about one-third. The severity of the relapses was also lessened and there was a striking effect on MRI measures of disease activity. No difference was found in disability levels however. IFN-$β_{1a}$ has the same amino acid sequence as natural IFN-β and differs from IFN-$β_{1b}$ by one amino acid and by the presence of carbohydrate moieties. This drug was found to have effects similar to that of IFN-$β_{1b}$ in reducing the frequency of MS relapses and in addition seems to have a favorable effect on disability. IFN-β has been shown to upregulate and increase the shedding of adhesion molecules, induce IL-10, and neurotrophic factors, block the opening of the BBB via inhibition of MMP-2 and -9, and reduce cell adhesion to the BBB.

Glatiramir acetate (GA) is a synthetic mixture of polypeptides produced by the random combination of four amino acids that are frequent in MBP. This drug has demonstrated a 29% reduction in relapse rate. GA reduces new lesion formation, the number of T2-enhancing lesions, lesion volumes, and the percentage of new lesions that will evolve into black holes, although the MRI effect is not apparent until the agent has been used for at least 6 months. The effect of GA that is probably most important is the induction of a relative skewing towards Th2 reactivity. GA has also been shown to displace autoantigenic peptides from HLA class II binding grooves; induce polyclonal T cell activation; act as a partial agonist, induce Th2 activation and cross-reactivity with myelin

peptides; shift the antibody response toward IgG_4; interfere with dendritic cell differentiation; and induce brain-derived neurotrophic factors.

Natalizumab is a humanized monoclonal antibody directed against the $α_4$-subunit of $α_4β_1$-integrin, a cellular adhesion molecule (CAM) that is expressed on the surface of leukocytes and binds to vascular CAM1 (VCAM1) on the surface of endothelial cells of the brain and spinal cord. Such binding allows the leukocytes to cross the BBB into the CNS, and blockage of this interaction prevents this influx. Two trials conducted to date on the use of natalizumab alone or in combination with IFN-$β_{1a}$ showed that this drug is more effective than other available drugs, with a decrease in relapse rate by 60% and disability progression by 40% over a 2-year period. Concerns about safety have been raised because of an increased incidence of progressive multifocal leukoencephalopathy. This risk appears to be increased if patients are on concurrent immunosuppressive treatment.[38]

Mitoxantrone is a cytotoxic anthracededione with potent immunosuppressive activity. This drug has been approved for worsening relapsing remitting MS, secondary progressive MS, and progressive relapsing MS. The major toxicity of mitoxanthrone is cardiac, and a cumulative dose-related cardiotoxicicty limits lifetime exposure.

Several off-label therapies are used in the treatment of MS, including cyclophosphamide, azathioprine, methotrexate, cladribine, cyclosporine, and intravenous immunoglobulin.[1,39]

Some disagreement exists regarding when treatment should be implemented, in part reflected in regional differences in reimbursement for therapy. Evidence supports the use of IFN-β in early treatment in patients presenting with a first attack of presumed MS (CIS), with a

Table 65.5 Multiple sclerosis therapies under investigation

Therapy	Proposed mechanism	Disease phase
HMG-CoA reductase inhibitors (statins)	Immunomodulatory actions. Reduces inflammatory mediators	Active disease
Daclizumab (zenapax)	Enhances immunoregulatory mechanisms	Active disease
FTY720 (sphingosine 1-phosphatase receptor agonist) (fingolimod)	Sequesters T cells in lymphoid organs	Active disease
Rituximab (antiCD20)	Depletes B cells	Uncertain. May be found to be effective in limiting tissue damage
Terifluromide (dihydro-orotate dehydrogenase inhibitor)	Immunomodulatory	Active disease
Alemtuzmab (Campath) (antiCD52)	T-cell-depleting	Active disease
BG00012 (fumaric acid)	Immunomodulatory	Active disease
Minocycline	Anti-inflammatory inhibition of microglial activation	Uncertain. Possible neuroprotective effect
Mycophenolate mofetil (Cellcept)	Immunosuppression	Active disease
Hematopoietic stem cell transplant	Immunosuppression	Active disease
Estrogen derivatives	Immunoregulation	Active disease
Laquinimod	Immunomodulation	Active disease

reduced conversion to clinically definite MS. There is, however, concern for initiating chronic, aggressive treatment of patients who might not have gone on to develop progressive disease. The recently developed diagnostic criteria for MS based on MRI permit a reasonable prediction of disease course over brief time periods (3 months), even when patients have presented only one clinical episode. This allows one to partially reconcile the push toward early treatment with the need for diagnostic certainty.

On the other end of the spectrum, after approximately 15 years from the onset of disease, almost 60% of relapsing remitting MS patients enter the secondary progressive phase of the disease. The treatment of this phase has been less satisfactory. A detailed analysis of two trials of IFN-β_{1b} in secondary progressive MS provided insight into this issue. These trials showed conflicting results of the effect of this drug on disease progression. A comparison revealed baseline differences in the populations studied, with one trial having patients with shorter disease duration and continued relapses and the other having patients with longer disease duration and less relapses, likely accounted for the discrepancy. The results of these trials indicate the mechanisms underlying disease progression probably differ in different stages of the disease. The presence of continued inflammatory activity, as suggested by continued disease relapses and contrast-enhancing lesions by MRI, may characterize a population of patients who could continue to benefit from immunomodulatory therapy, such as IFN. In contrast, IFN appears to be ineffective in modifying the progression of disability related to ongoing destruction independent of, or remote to, the acute inflammatory component of the illness.[40] Similar considerations must be made for other therapies targeting immune mechanisms, such as mitoxantrone. To date, there are no approved therapies for the treatment of primary progressive MS. Currently numerous molecules in various stages of development are being studied in clinical trials. A summary is shown in Table 65.5.

■ SUMMARY ■

Over the past two decades significant progress has been made in understanding the immune mechanisms underlying MS. Several approved therapies are now available, albeit with only moderate impact on disease course. As the understanding of the pathogenesis of MS improves, newer, more targeted therapies will likely emerge. Clarifying the nature of the clinical and pathological heterogeneity, elucidating the neurodegenerative aspects and the dynamic interplay with immune mechanisms are a main focus of current research. This is expected to lead to new treatment strategies in neuroprotection and regeneration that will likely be used in combination with immunomodulatory therapies, and possibly be tailored to individuals, thereby opening a new era in the management of this disease.

■ REFERENCES ■

1. Pirko I, Noseworthy JH. Demyelinating disorders of the central nervous system. In: Goetz CG, ed: Textbook of Clinical Neurology, 2nd edn. Pennsylvania, PA: WB Saunders, 2003. .

2. Achiron A, Polliack M, Rao SM, et al. Cognitive patterns and progression in multiple sclerosis: construction and validation of percentile curves. J Neurol Neurosurg Psychiatry 2005; 76: 744–749.

3. Lublin F, Reingold SC. Defining the clinical course of multiple sclerosis: results of an international survey. Neurology 1996; 46: 907–911.

4. Rovaris M, Confavreux C, Furlan R, et al. Secondary progressive multiple sclerosis: current knowledge and future challenges. Lancet Neurol 2006; 5: 343–354.

5. Lucchinetti CF, Reingold SC; Eden G; Brueck W, Rodriguez M, et al. Multiple sclerosis: lessons from neuropathology. Semin Neurol 1998; 18: 337–349.

6. Luchinetti CF, Parisi J, Bruck W. The pathology of multiple sclerosis. Neurol Clin 2005; 23: 77–105.

7. Polman CH, Reingold SC, Edan G, et al. Diagnostic criteria for multiple sclerosis: 2005 revisions to the "McDonald criteria". Ann Neurol 2005; 58: 840–846.

8. Napoli SQ, Bakshi R. Magnetic resonance imaging in multiple sclerosis. Rev Neurol Dis 2005; 2: 109–116.

9. McDonald IW, Compston A, Edan G, et al. Recommended diagnostic criteria for multiple sclerosis: guidelines from the international panel on the diagnosis of multiple sclerosis. Ann Neurol 2001; 50: 121–127.

10. Montalban X. Primary progressive multiple sclerosis. Curr Opin Neurol 2005; 18: 261–266.

11. Thompson AJ, Montalban X, Barkhof F, et al. Diagnostic criteria for primary progressive multiple sclerosis: a position paper. Ann Neurol 2000; 47: 831–835.

12. Ludwin SK. The pathogenesis of multiple sclerosis: relating human pathology to experimental studies. J Neuropathol Exp Neurol 2006; 65: 305–318.

13. Bruck W, Stadelmann C. The spectrum of multiple sclerosis: new lessons from pathology. Curr Opin Neurol 2005; 18: 221–224.

14. Barnett MH, Prineas JW. Relapsing and remitting multiple sclerosis: pathology of the newly forming lesion. Ann Neurol 2004; 55: 458–468.

15. Barnett MH, Sutton I. The pathology of multiple sclerosis: a paradigm shift. Curr Opin Neurol 2006; 19: 242–247.

16. Compston A. The basis for treatment in multiple sclerosis. Acta Neurol Scand 2006; 113: 41–47.

17. Sospedra M, Martin R. Immunology of multiple sclerosis. Annu Rev Immunol 2005; 23: 683–747.

18. Hauser SL, Oksenberg JR. The neurobiology of multiple sclerosis: genes, inflammation, and neurodegeneration. Neuron 2006; 52: 61–76.

19. Hemmer B, Vergelli M, Gran B, et al. Predictable TCR antigen recognition based on peptide scans leads to the identification of agonist ligands with no sequence homology. J Immunol 1998; 160: 331–363.

20. Dyment DA, Ebers GC, Sadovnick AD. Genetics of multiple sclerosis. Lancet Neurol 2004; 3: 104–110.

21. Kantarci O, Wingerchuk D. Epidemiology an dnatural history of multiple sclerosis: new insights. Curr Opin Neurol 2006; 19: 248–254.

22. Prat A, Antel J. Pathogenesis of multiple sclerosis. Curr Opin Neurol 2005; 18: 225–230.

23. Markovic-Plese S, Cortese I, Wandinger KP, et al. CD4+CD28- costimulation independent T cell sin multiple sclerosis. J Clin Invest 2001; 108: 1185–1194.

24. Viglietta V, Baecher-Allan C, Weiner HL, et al. Loss of functional suppression by CD4+CD25+ regulatory T cells in patients with multiple sclerosis. J Exp Med 2004; 199: 971–979.

25. Kastrukoff LF, et al. A role for natural killer cells in the immunopathogenesis of multiple sclerosis. J Neuroimmunol 1998; 86: 123–133.

26. Bielekova B, Catalfamo M, Reichert-Scrivner S, et al. Regulatory CD56(bright) natural killer cells mediate immunomodulatory effects of IL2Ralpha-targeted therapy (daclizumab) in multiple sclerosis. Proc Natl Acad Sci USA 2006; 103: 5941–5946.

27. McQualter JL, Bernard CCA. Multiple sclerosis: a battle between destruction and repair. J Neurochem 2006; 10: 1471–1474.

28. Madsen LS, Andersson EC, Jansson L, et al. A humanized model for multiple sclerosis using HLA-DR2 and a human T-cell receptor. Nat Genet 1999; 23: 343–347.

29. Quandt J, Baig M, Yao K, et al. Unique clinical and pathological features in HLA-DRB1*0401-restricted MBP 111-129-specific humanized transgenic mice. J Exp Med 2004; 200: 223–234.

30. Kennedy MK, Tan LJ, Dal Canto MC, et al. Inhibition of murine relapsing experimental autoimmune encephalomyelitis by immune tolerance to proteolipid protein and its encephalitogenic peptides. J Immunol 1990; 144: 909–915.

31. Waldner H, Whitters MJ, Sobel RA, et al. Fulminant spontaneous autoimmunity of the central nervous system in mice transgenic for the myelin proteolipid protein-specific T cell receptor. Proc Natl Acad Sci USA 2000; 97: 342–347.

32. Bettelli E, Pagany M, Weiener HL, et al. Myelin oligodendrocyte glycoprotein-specific T cell receptor transgenic mice develop spontaneous optic neuritis. J Exp Med 2003; 197: 1073–1081.

33. Owens GP, Bennett JL, Gilden DH, et al. The B cell response in multiple sclerosis. Neurol Res 2006; 28: 236–244.

34. McDole J, Johnson AJ, Pirko I. The role of CD8+ T-cells in lesion formation and axonal dysfunction in multiple sclerosis. Neurol Res 2006; 28: 256–261.

35. Weinschenker BG, O'Brien PC, Petterson TM, et al. A randomized trial of plasma exchange in acute central nervous system inflammatory demyelinating disease. Ann Neurol 1999; 46: 878–886.

36. Multiple sclerosis therapy consensus group. Escalating immunotherapy of multiple sclerosis: new aspects and practical application. J Neurol 2004; 251: 1329–1339.

37. Stangel M, Gold R, Gass A, et al. Current issues in immunomodulatory treatment of multiple sclerosis: a practical approach. J Neurol 2006; 253(Suppl 1). I/32–I/36.

38. Bennett JL. Natalizumab and progressive multifocal leukencephalopathy: migrating towards safe adhesion molecule therapy in multiple sclerosis. Neurol Res 2006; 28: 291–298.

39. Sorensen PS. Treatment of multiple sclerosis with intravenous immunoglobulin: review of clinical trials. Neurol Sci 2003; 24: S227–S230.

40. Kappos L, Weinshenker B, Pozzilli C, et al. Interferon beta-1b in secondary progressive MS: a combined analysis of the two trials. Neurology 2004; 63: 1779–1787.

41. Gregory SG, Schmidt S, Seth P, et al. Interleukin 7 receptor a chain (IL7R) shows allelic and functional association with multiple sclerosis. Nat Gen 2007; 39: 1083–1091.

42. Lundmark F, Duvelfelt K, Iacobaeus E, et al. Variation in interleukin 7 receptor a chain (IL7R) influences risk of multiple sclerosis. Nat Gen 2007; 39: 1108–1113.

REFERENCES

> **Table 66.1** Common autoimmune neuropathies
>
> Guillain–Barré syndrome(s)
> Chronic inflammatory demyelinating polyneuropathy (CIDP)
>   and its variants
> Polyneuropathy associated with paraproteinemias
>   Polyneuropathies with IgM monoclonal gammopathies
>   IgG and IgA monoclonal gammopathy
>   Polyneuropathy, organomegaly, endocrinopathy, myeloma,
>   and skin changes (POEMS) syndrome
>   Cryoglobulinemic polyneuropathy
> Multifocal motor neuropathy with conduction block
> Paraneoplastic neuropathies associated with anti-Hu antibodies
> Autoimmune autonomic neuropathies
> Vasculitic neuropathies
> Infectious neuropathies (HIV, CMV, EBV, herpes, Lyme,
> leprosy, Chagas' disease, diphtheria, others)

- *Acute motor–sensory axonal neuropathy (AMSAN)*, which is like AMAN but with involvement of the sensory axons. AMSAN is histologically characterized by a large number of macrophages invading the axonal membrane of motor and sensory nerves.

- *C. Miller-Fisher syndrome*, which is characterized by acute onset of ophthalmoplegia, gait ataxia, and areflexia. The ataxia can occur in a setting of normal sensation, although 50% of patients complain of tingling paresthesias.[2] Muscle weakness may be absent at onset in two-thirds of cases, but in approximately a third of all patients weakness leading to paralysis with pharyngeal, facial, trunk, and respiratory muscle involvement can occur.[2] Nerve conduction studies are consistent with proximal demyelination. The C. Miller-Fisher syndrome is a distinct variant, as supported by the presence of a unique IgG antibody against GQ1b ganglioside.

- *Sensory ataxic GBS* due to involvement of roots and ganglionic neurons. In these patients, antibodies against the GD1b ganglioside have been found, suggesting that ataxic GBS and Miller-Fisher variants form a continuum and share autoantibodies with the same fine specificity of sialic groups.

- *Acute pandysautonomic neuropathy.*[4] In these cases, there is no evidence of detectable demyelination, and the target antigen is probably a component of the autoimmune system and ganglionic neurons.

DIAGNOSIS

The classic laboratory abnormalities in GBS patients are elevated cerebrospinal fluid (CSF) protein and abnormal nerve conduction studies consistent with active demyelination.

The CSF protein may be normal in the early phase of the disease, but it can be as high as 1000 mg/dL by the sixth week of illness. The elevation of CSF protein may be due to involvement of the roots related to inflammation, but, as the blood–nerve barrier becomes impaired, serum albumin and IgG may enter freely into the CSF, contributing further to protein elevation. The CSF cell count is normal unless GBS occurs in a setting of HIV infection or in conjunction with other viral infections,

such as CMV or EBV. Mild lymphocytosis is not a sign against the diagnosis of GBS, but rather is suggestive of a coexisting viral illness or a lymphomatous process. When the CSF protein is very high, papilledema may develop because of impaired reabsorption of CSF and raised intracranial pressure. Oligoclonal IgG bands can be also seen.

The differential diagnosis of GBS should include other forms of acute flaccid paralysis, such as: brainstem stroke; brainstem encephalitis; acute paralytic poliomyelitis or West Nile Virus infection; acute myelopathy; other causes of acute neuropathy such as rabies-vaccine neuropathy, diphtheria, heavy metals, acute intermittent porphyria, vasculitis, critical illness neuropathy or lymphomatous neuropathy; disorders of neuromuscular transmissions such as myasthenia gravis, botulism, or other industrial toxins; and disorders of muscles such as hypokalemia, inflammatory myopathy, acute rhabdomyolysis, or periodic paralysis.

ANTECEDENT ILLNESSES OR EVENTS

Two-thirds of patients with GBS give a history of a flu-like illness with upper respiratory signs or acute dysenteric episodes that precede the development of GBS by 1–3 weeks.[1, 2] Among the implicated viruses are cytomegalovirus, Epstein–Barr virus (EBV), herpes viruses, outbreaks of hepatitis A, and HIV. Among bacteria *Mycoplasma pneumoniae* and, most importantly, *Campylobacter jejuni* are serologic markers of infection that may be present in 15–20% of patients. *Campylobacter* is of special interest because it contains glycoconjugates that share epitopes with the peripheral myelin. Cytomegalovirus (CMV) can directly infect the nerve and cross-react with GM2 glycolipid and Po protein of the peripheral nerve. Two vaccines – one against rabies and the other against the swine flu A/New Jersey influenza strain that caused an outbreak of GBS in 1976[1, 2] – have been convincingly connected with the development of GBS. Rabies vaccine that contains brain material is followed by GBS in about one in 1000 cases. Apart from these vaccines, however, there is no convincing evidence that the incidence of GBS is increased in connection with other vaccines, in spite of anecdotal reports of patients who developed GBS 1–3 weeks after vaccination.

Surgery can precede the development of GBS in up to 10% of patients.[2] Surgical stress, the release of nerve autoantigens, and infections have been proposed as possible explanations for this association.

There are only three drugs causally associated with acute demyelinating neuropathy: gold, perhexiline, and suramin.[5] Other drugs cause a chronic or subacute axonal and predominantly sensory neuropathy. In the author's experience, suramin, when used at high doses for the treatment of prostatic carcinoma, caused acute GBS with respiratory involvement. The currently used lower doses of suramin, with concurrent monitoring of the drug levels, do not cause GBS but an axonal, mostly motor, neuropathy with predilection for the proximal muscles (Dalakas, unpublished observations).

GBS has occurred in patients who suffer from neoplasms, especially lymphoma, melanoma and Hodgkin's disease. Interestingly, in spite of the autoimmune nature of GBS, the disease is rarely seen as part of another connective tissue disorder.[1, 2]

IMMUNOPATHOLOGY

GBS is an inflammatory demyelinating polyneuropathy in which the peripheral myelin, the axon or the Schwann cells are the target antigens of an immune attack, possibly triggered by the various antecedent events discussed above. Both the cellular and the humoral components of the immune system have been implicated in the immunopathogenesis of GBS. In spite of newly identified myelin antigens, the exact target antigen is still unknown.

CELLULAR FACTORS

The nerves of GBS patients possess two prominent histologic features: (1) perivascular and endoneurial inflammatory infiltrates consisting of lymphocytes and macrophages, found throughout the cranial nerves, ventral and dorsal roots, plexuses, and peripheral nerves;[1, 2] and (2) segmental demyelination in areas associated with the lymphoid infiltrates. Although among the infiltrates CD4 T cells appear to predominate over CD8 T cells and macrophages, if one takes into account that 70% of tissue macrophages express CD4, the dominant cells are the macrophages. By electron microscopy, macrophages break through the basement membrane of healthy Schwann cells and make direct contact with the outermost myelin lamellae, leading finally to lysis of the superficial myelin sheath. Macrophages may exert their myelinolytic activity via lymphokines, especially interleukin (IL)-1. Interferon (IFN)-γ released by the activated T cells, or complement activation, may also serve as a chemotactic factor, increasing capillary permeability and enhancing recruitment of additional macrophages. When the demyelination is extensive, it is followed by axonal degeneration.[1, 2] At sites of segmental demyelination there is a proliferation of Schwann cells along the denuded axons, whereas in areas of axonal degeneration the Schwann cells proliferate in columns to guide the regenerating axons. The proliferating Schwann cells are responsible for remyelination and axonal regeneration, which may begin even during the phase of active myelin breakdown. The degree and effectiveness of remyelination and axonal regeneration dictate the degree of clinical recovery.

A number of studies indicate that activated T cells play a role in GBS. Peripheral blood lymphocytes from GBS patients exert myelinotoxic activity when applied to cultures of myelinated axons. Further, levels of IL-2 and soluble IL-2 receptors are increased in the serum during the acute phase of GBS and decline during recovery, suggesting ongoing T-cell proliferation.

A more convincing role for a T cell-mediated process in GBS is derived by analogy to the animal model of experimental allergic neuritis (EAN), which resembles GBS in both its pathology and its clinical course. Animals sensitized to whole human nerve or to various myelin proteins such as Po, P2, and the neutral glycolipid galactocerebroside, develop segmental demyelination with mononuclear cell infiltrates consisting of macrophages and T cells. In EAN, the T cells are sensitized against myelin, and T cells from EAN animals or cloned P2-specific T-cell lines can passively transfer the disease to healthy animals.

HUMORAL FACTORS AND ANTI-GANGLIOSIDE ANTIBODIES

There is much stronger evidence that circulating serum factors are responsible for GBS. On clinical grounds, this is supported by the beneficial effect of plasmapheresis, presumably by removing putative antibodies. On laboratory grounds it is supported by the variety of autoantibodies detected in the serum of patients with acute GBS. This conclusion is based on the following observations. Serum from the acute phase of GBS can demyelinate rodent dorsal root ganglionic extracts in a complement-dependent manner. Further, GBS serum injected into rat

sciatic nerves causes demyelination and conduction block. Immunocytochemical studies on the peripheral nerves of GBS patients show deposits of IgG, IgM, and membranolytic attack complex, implying complement-fixing antibody activity of the serum immunoglobulin.[2] This observation is further supported by the report of complement-fixing IgM antibodies against a human neutral glycolipid of peripheral nerve myelin that contains carbohydrate epitopes as well as high-titer antibodies against various sulfated or acidic glycosphingolipids.[6, 7]

Antibodies that react with GM1, GD1a, GalNAc-GD1a and GM1b are found in 80% of cases with motor axonal form of GBS (AMAN and AMSAN). In the common AIDP subtype, however, these antibodies are not frequent. Among the gangliosides, the one that clearly correlates with a specific clinical syndrome is the GQ1b.[8] Anti-GQ1b IgG antibodies appear to be specifically associated with the C. Miller-Fisher variant of GBS because they are present in more than 90% of these patients. Anti-GQ1b IgG antibodies are also found in post-infectious ophthalmoplegias as well as in GBS patients with ophthalmoplegia, but not in GBS patients without ophthalmoplegia or in other autoimmune conditions.[8] Of interest, anti-GQ1b antibody immunostains the paranodal regions of oculomotor nerves III, IV, and VI, suggesting that damage to these regions blocks impulse generation at the nodes of Ranvier, resulting in a conduction block that is characteristic for GBS. Although anti-GQ1b antibodies have been found in patients with IgM paraproteinemic polyneuropathies (discussed later), in ophthalmologic GBS these antibodies are of IgG class and do not recognize other polysialogangliosides. In the author's judgment, anti-GQ1b IgG antibodies should be considered specific for the C. Miller-Fisher variant. Many patients with antibodies to GQ1b also have antibodies to GD1a.

It is important to emphasize that although anti-GM1 antibodies of IgM class are seen in other neuropathies, in GBS patients these antibodies are mostly of the IgG class.

In clinical practice, anti-ganglioside antibodies are identified by ELISA using purified gangliosides, but for more detailed analysis TLC (thin-layer chromatography) overlay is utilized. Gangliosides are present in all tissues but are especially abundant in the nervous system. Their lipid portion lies in the cell membrane, and their signature sugar residues are exposed at the extracellular surface bearing one or more sialic acid molecules, such as one sialic acid ganglioside (GM1), two (GD1a), three (GT1a) or four (GQ1b). Although they do not form a common 'GBS antigen,' different gangliosides are involved in different GBS subtypes. The antibodies against these gangliosides are of pathogenic relevance because immunization of rabbits with GM1 and GD11b induces acute neuropathy with histological features of AMAN.[9] Their pathogenicity was also confirmed by an inadvertent experiment in humans who had received ganglioside injections for various maladies and developed AMAN with GM1 antibodies.[10] Additionally, antibodies to GQ1b or GD1a cause conduction block at the motor nerve terminals in a preparation of mouse phrenic nerve.[9] Similarly, antibodies to GalNAc-Gd1a from a patient with AMAN blocked neuromuscular transmission in a mouse spinal cord muscle co-culture system.

The reasons for different syndromes in connection with specific gangliosides remains unclear, but distribution and accessibility may be critical factors. The gangliosides are distributed differently within the peripheral nervous system, a phenomenon that could explain the different subtypes. For example, there is more GM1 in ventral than in dorsal roots, hence the predominantly motor neuropathy seen with GM1 antibodies; there is also more GQ1b in the ocular motor nerves, which

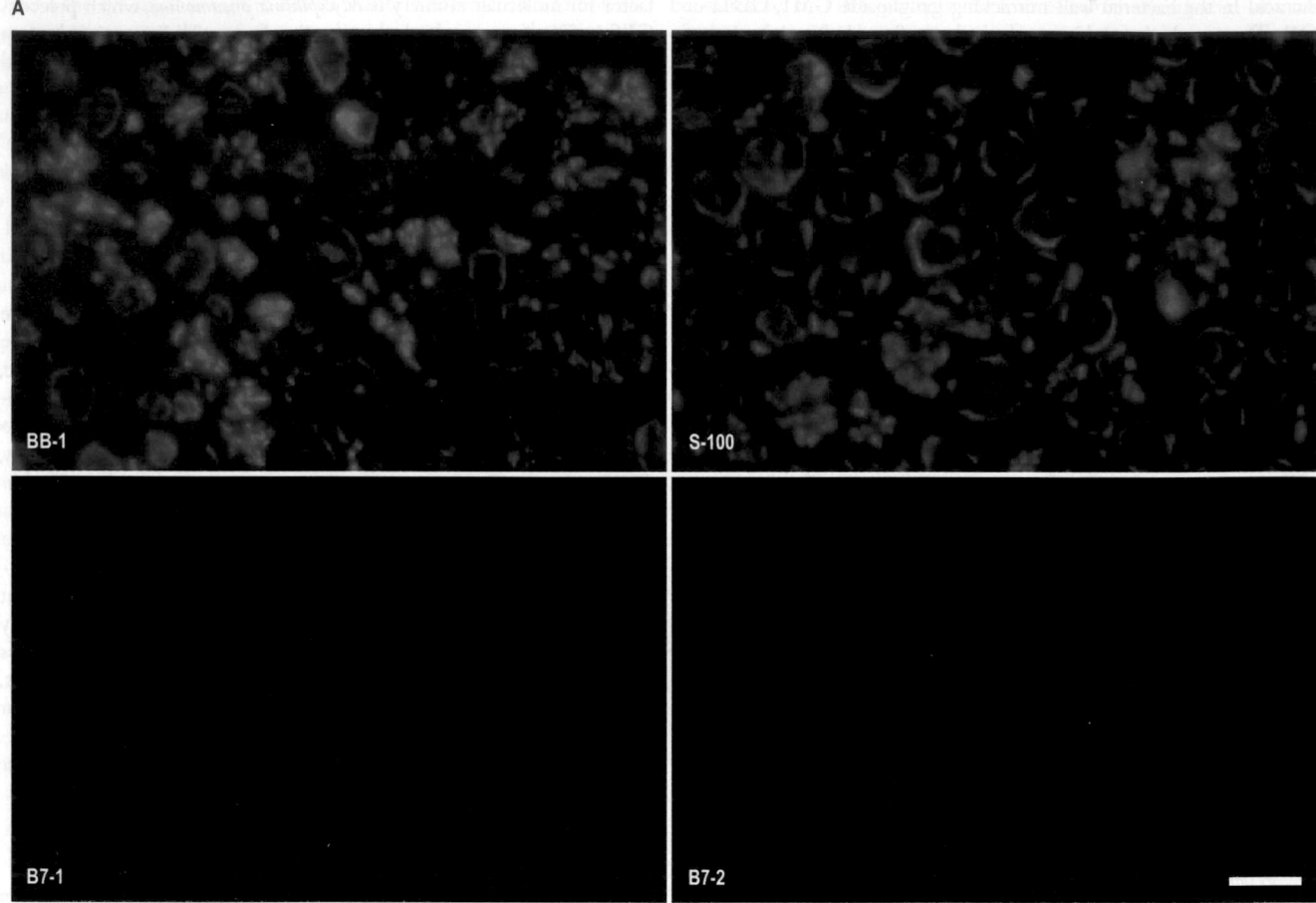

Fig. 66.2 **(A)** The co-stimulatory molecule BB-1, but not B7-1 or B7-2, is expressed on S-100-positive Schwann cells. (From Murata and Dalakas, Brain 2000.)

are prolonged, and an associated conduction block in one or more nerves, with dispersion of the compound muscle action potentials, is noted.[13] An associated axonal loss is not unusual; in the majority of cases needle electromyography (EMG) shows denervation.

As several therapeutic studies have been carried out in CIDP, variations of the diagnostic criteria have been introduced. In all cases, however, it appears to be consensus that CSF examination and nerve biopsy are not mandatory.

CIDP may mimic the following APN: (1) the multifocal motor neuropathy with conduction block,[14] when the sensory findings are not prominent; (2) the demyelinating neuropathies associated with IgA or IgG gammopathies; (3) the intermediate form of GBS when the onset of GBS is not very acute and its maximum deficit is reached between 4 and 8 weeks; and (4) the relapsing form of GBS. Up to 3% of GBS patients relapse,[2] but in some cases the new relapse may not be as acute and typical as the original attack but slower, resembling the intermediate form. Variants of CIDP have been recently recognized.[14] These include a multifocal sensorimotor but asymmetric form, and a multifocal regional form with a predominantly upper or lower limb involvement.

KEY CONCEPTS

AUTOIMMUNITY IN CIDP

>> Activated macrophages are the predominant endoneurial cell, displacing the Schwann cell cytoplasm, disrupting myelin, and lyzing superficial myelin lamellae.

>> Complement-fixing IgG and IgM antibodies are deposited on the myelin sheath.

>> IgG antibodies to acidic glycolipids LM1, GM1, or GD1b and against the 28 kDa Po myelin proteins, are detected in the serum of some patients.

>> There is upregulation of DR and B-7 co-stimulatory molecules in the Schwann cells and macrophages.

>> The serum IgG can induce conduction block when injected into rat nerves.

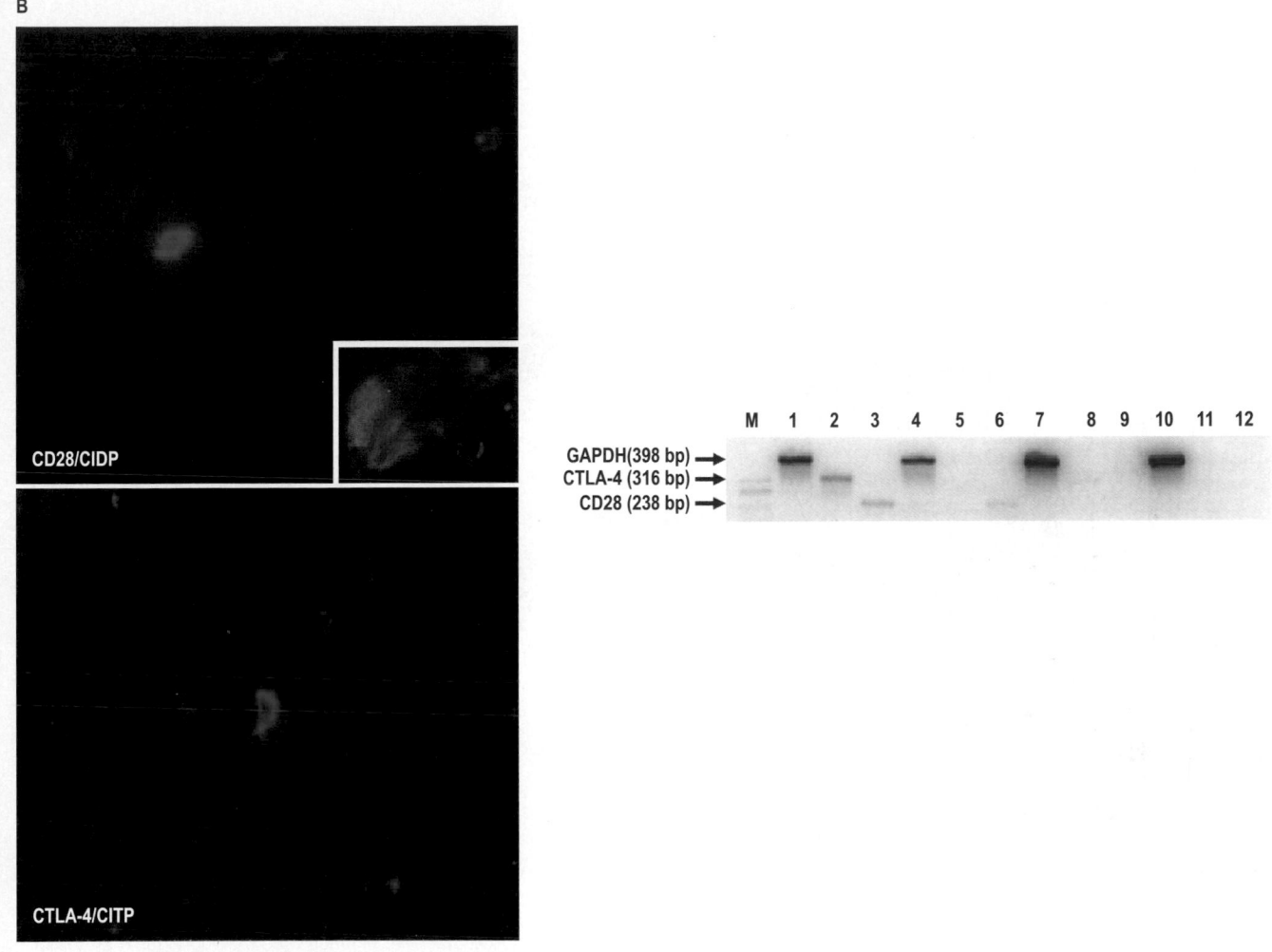

Fig. 66.2 Cont'd (B) The counter-receptors CD28 and CTLA-4 are upregulated on CD4-positive T cells. At the mRNA level, there is upregulation of CD28 and CTLA-4. (Murata K, Dalakas MC Expression of co-stimulatory molecules BB-1, the ligands CTLA-4 and CD28 in patients with chronic inflammatory demyelinating polyneuropathy. Brain 2000; 123: 1660–1666.)

In contrast to GBS, patients with CIDP do not have increased incidence of infections, vaccinations, or traumas preceding the development of the neuropathy. The significance of a few isolated case reports that followed an infectious illness[13] is unclear. CIDP is a chronic disease; although it responds to immunotherapies, a number of patients have incomplete recovery and are left with residual weakness.[14]

IMMUNOPATHOGENESIS

Although CIDP is defined as an inflammatory polyneuropathy, there are only minimal signs of inflammation with hematoxylin and eosin stains in the sural nerve biopsies. The T-cell populations that have been identified are heterogeneous, belonging to both CD4 and CD8 T subsets. Elevated soluble adhesion molecules, chemokines, cytokines and metalloproteinases are detected in the sera and CSF, and this facilitates lymphoid cell transmigration across the blood–nerve barrier. Within the endoneurium cytokines activate the resident macrophages that appear to be the predominant endoneurial mononuclear cell in CIDP nerves.[12] Electron-microscopic studies have demonstrated that the demyelinating process in CIDP is always associated with the presence of macrophages, which sequentially penetrate the basement membrane of the Schwann cell, displace the cytoplasm, and finally disrupt the myelin by focal lysis of the superficial myelin lamellae.[12] Similarities may exist in this regard with GBS and the chronic or relapsing–remitting form of experimental allergic neuritis, in which macrophages, activated T cells, and deposits of membranolytic attack complex C5b-9 are noted on the myelin sheath. In CIDP, macrophages and Schwann cells may serve as antigen-presenting cells. They express HLA-DR and co-stimulatory molecules B7-1, B7-2, whereas their counter-receptors CTLA-4 and CD28 are expressed on rare endoneurial CD4 T cells[15] (Fig. 66.2A and B). The cellular immune response appears to be tightly regulated at the transcriptional level, as

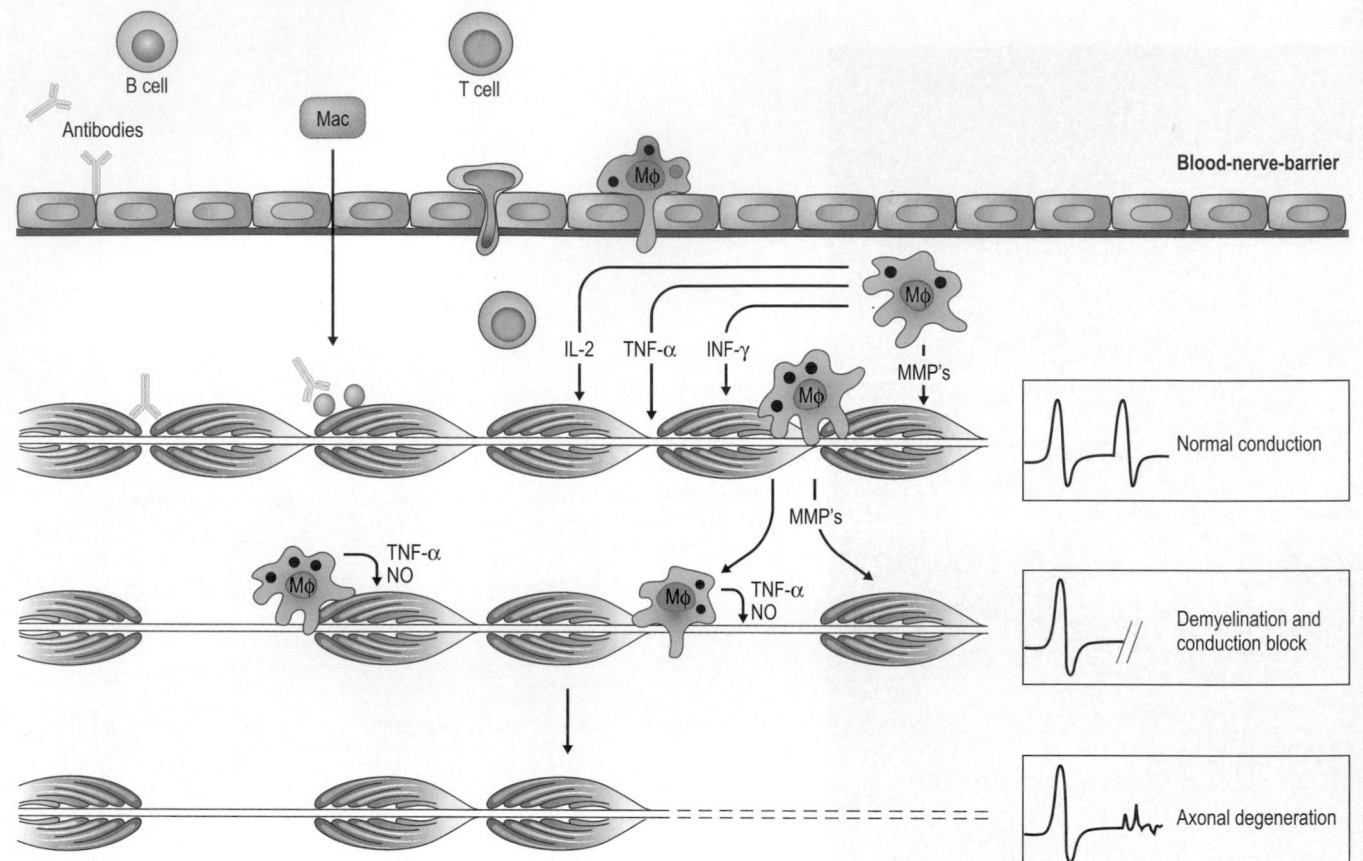

Fig. 66.3 Diagrammatic scheme of the main cellular elements that seem to play a major role in the demyelinating process of CIDP. Activated macrophages (Mφ) and T cells cross the endothelial cell wall of the blood–nerve barrier and reach the myelinated fibers. Activated, TNF-α-positive Mφ invade the myelin sheath, causing Mφ-mediated segmental demyelination. Axonal loss secondary to demyelination, probably enhanced by TNF-α and metalloproteinases, may become prominent in the chronic phases of the disease. Other cytokines, T cells sensitized to unidentified antigens and putative antibodies may participate. IL, interleukin; INF, interferon; MMP, metalloproteinase; Mφ, activated macrophage; TNR, tumor necrosis factor.

supported by the activation of the transcriptional factor NF-κB in the macrophages.

Humoral factors may play a major role in CIDP. Complement-fixing IgG and IgM are deposited on the patient's myelin sheath, indicative of antimyelin antibodies.[16] Antibodies to glycolipids LM1, GM1, or GD1b are also seen in some CIDP patients, but less frequently than in GBS patients and more frequently than in the controls. Serum reactivity against nonmyelin antigens on Schwann cells has been reported in 12 of 45 patients, and passive transfer experiments have demonstrated that serum IgG can induce conduction block in rat nerve. The 28 kDa myelin protein Po was identified as a putative antigen in up to 20% of the patients. Finally, the beneficial effect of plasmapheresis may be indirect evidence that circulatory factors play a pathogenetic role. The immunopathogenetic scheme proposed for GBS (Fig. 66.1) is also appropriately applied to CIDP, with some modification to denote the axonal loss that accompanies the demyelination (Fig. 66.3).

Molecular mimicry can be implicated in CIDP associated with melanoma. Carbohydrate epitopes such as GM3, GM2, GD3 are expressed on melanoma, and antibodies against melanoma cells react with myelin glycoproteins. A molecular mimicry was demonstrated in a patient with CIDP between the GM2-positive melanoma cells and the peripheral myelin because her serum recognized GM2 epitopes present in both the nerve and the tumor.[17]

■ PARAPROTEINEMIC POLYNEUROPATHIES ■

A distinct subset of acquired polyneuropathies has been associated with a circulating monoclonal protein (Chapter 78). Although neuropathy occurs in a setting of myeloma, plasmacytoma, or Waldenström's macroglobulinemia, the majority of paraproteinemic neuropathies occur in patients without an underlying lymphoproliferative disease. The gammopathy in such patients is of undetermined significance, even though most of the time the IgM monoclonal protein recognizes specific antigenic determinants of the human myelin.

Until 1979, the association of neuropathy with benign monoclonal gammopathy was thought to be rare and coincidental because a causal relationship between the neuropathy and the paraproteinemia had not been established. Further, benign gammopathies occur, nonspecifically, in many chronic inflammatory or infectious conditions, and their incidence increases with age, occurring in up to 2% of normal people over 70 years of age. In 1979, in the largest series of 11 such patients,[18] the author stressed that this is a distinct immune-mediated association because the paraprotein binds to peripheral nerve, and in a number of patients the neuropathy responds to immunosuppressive therapy. Two years later, the causal association between the paraprotein and the neuropathy was strengthened when it was shown that the monoclonal IgM of a patient with demyelinating polyneuropathy had a specific anti-myelin activity directed against myelin-associated glycoprotein (MAG).[19] Today, polyneuropathies with monoclonal gammopathy comprise 10% of patients with acquired neuropathy,[20, 21] and paraproteinemic polyneuropathy is a potentially treatable APN.

A monoclonal gammopathy is considered benign when the patients have the following: (1) <3 g/dL of monoclonal protein in their serum and rarely the same monoclonal protein in the urine; (2) <5% plasma cells in the bone marrow aspirate; (3) no systemic signs of renal insufficiency, osteolytic or osteosclerotic lesions in the bone survey, or signs of anemia and hypercalcemia; (4) no suppression of the rest of the uninvolved polyclonal immunoglobulins (background immunoglobulins); (5) no signs of a lymphoproliferative disease; and (6) a stable amount of the monoclonal protein during follow-up examinations. In contrast, ominous signs of malignant plasma cell dyscrasia are lytic bone lesions, Bence Jones proteinuria, a reduction of the uninvolved (background) immunoglobulin level, abnormal bone marrow examinations, and a progressively increased amount of monoclonal protein in serial measurements. Even in the benign gammopathies, however, there is a 1% probability per year that a malignant plasma cell dyscrasia may evolve,[22] hence the need for periodic screening.

A free light chain is more often associated with amyloidosis. If it is present in a patient with gammopathy and neuropathy, deposits of amyloid should be thoroughly sought in the nerve, muscle, skin, abdominal fat or bone marrow.

FREQUENCY OF POLYNEUROPATHIES IN PATIENTS WITH MONOCLONAL GAMMOPATHY

A benign monoclonal gammopathy may occur in up to 1% of normal people over 50 of age.[17] The incidence increases to 1.7% above age 70 and reaches up to 6% above the age of 90.[22] Monoclonal gammopathies, however, are 10 times more frequent in patients with polyneuropathy than in an age-matched control population, and almost 10% of patients with acquired polyneuropathy have an associated monoclonal gammopathy.[20] If one categorizes these gammopathies into subclasses, the incidence of polyneuropathy among patients with IgM monoclonal proteins can be as high as 50%,[21] implying that almost 50% of patients with IgM monoclonal gammopathy may have or will develop polyneuropathy. The association of monoclonal gammopathy with peripheral neuropathy is not therefore fortuitous.

Some patients with paraprotein may have an associated amyloidosis derived from the variable region of the immunoglobulin light chain.

When amyloidosis is present, the neuropathy is often painful and has a strong autonomic component. In addition to painful paresthesias in the hands and feet, these patients have mild to moderate distal weakness, often with pedal edema, and autonomic symptoms consisting of orthostatic hypotension, dizziness, impotence, impaired gastric motility, or frequent diarrhea. The disease is difficult to treat, and, apart from symptomatic therapy (mostly opiates), immunosuppressive therapies have been largely unsuccessful. The diagnosis is made via a muscle or nerve or fat biopsy that demonstrates amyloid deposits in the connective tissue or around blood vessels. In the author's hands, the muscle and skin biopsy has a higher yield than nerve biopsy for finding amyloid deposits.

POLYNEUROPATHIES ASSOCIATED WITH IgG OR IgA MONOCLONAL GAMMOPATHIES

Patients with polyneuropathy and benign IgG or IgA monoclonal gammopathy usually have an axonal neuropathy, and their IgG or IgA does recognize specific neuronal or myelin antigens. Sometimes, when the neuropathy is demyelinating, it behaves like CIDP and responds to immunotherapy. The causal association between the monoclonal protein and neuropathy in these patients has not been established. The monoclonal spike may represent a nonspecific response to a chronic inflammatory process, or it may be due to an underlying lymphoproliferative disease that is slow and restrained.

POLYNEUROPATHY, ORGANOMEGALY, ENDOCRINOPATHY, MYELOMA, AND SKIN CHANGES (POEMS)

A subset of patients with malignant IgG or IgA gammopathy have polyneuropathy with osteosclerotic myeloma. Most of them comprise the POEMS syndrome (*p*olyneuropathy, *o*rganomegaly, *e*ndocrinopathy, *M* protein, and *s*kin changes).[23] Not included in the acronym are several features such as sclerotic bone lesions, Castleman's disease, papilledema, pleural effusion, edema, ascites and thrombocytosis.[23] More than 50% of patients with osteosclerotic myeloma of IgA or IgG type have a sensorimotor, symmetric polyneuropathy with mixed demyelinating and axonal features and high (usually 200 mg/dL) CSF protein.[23] Pure axonal neuropathies can be also seen. In POEMS the neuropathy tends to be associated with edema in the legs, with hyperpigmentation, sclerodermatous thickening or papular angiomas of the skin, and hypertrichosis with dark hair.[23] Endocrinopathy most often includes gonadal failure, amenorrhea, impotence, gynecomastia, hypothyroidism, diabetes, or elevated prolactin levels. The IgG class is slightly more common than the IgA class, but the λ light chain is present in the majority (up to 95%) of the patients.[23] Computed tomography (CT) of the abdomen may reveal an enlarged spleen and calcifications. The bone lesions can be sclerotic, solitary, or multiple, sparing the skull and the extremities. Pathologic changes in the lymph nodes, which can also be enlarged, may at times resemble those of Castleman's disease, which can also be associated with polyneuropathy.[23] Not all patients with POEMS, however, have all these features. When sclerotic lesions are absent, patients are said to have Crow–Fukase syndrome.[24] POEMS appears to be mediated by an imbalance of proinflammatory cytokines. IL-1b, IL6 and TNF-α are increased. Vascular endothelial growth factor (VEGF) may play a major role because it induces a rapid increase in vascular permeability and is a growth factor important in angiogenesis and endothelial cells.[23, 24]

The neuropathy in some patients responds to steroids, tamoxifen, or alkylating agents. In others, it may respond to the removal or irradiation of the solitary sclerotic lesion, suggesting that the tumor may secrete neurotoxic factors, perhaps neurotoxic light chains. IVIG and plasmapheresis are ineffective. The role of autologous stem cell transplantation or cytokine modulation remains untested. The median survival is 165 months.[23]

POLYNEUROPATHIES ASSOCIATED WITH IgM MONOCLONAL GAMMOPATHIES

This entity is composed of an immunochemically and clinically heterogeneous group of neuropathies in which the immunoglobulin appears to be an antibody to various glycoproteins or glycolipids of the peripheral nerve. These neuropathies can be best divided into the following subsets.

- *Demyelinating polyneuropathy with IgM anti-MAG or ganglioside antibodies.* Sera from approximately 50% of patients with IgM monoclonal gammopathy and neuropathy react with myelin-associated glycoprotein (MAG), a 100-kDa glycoprotein of the central and peripheral nerve myelin, as well as other glycoproteins or glycolipids that share antigenic determinants with MAG.[21] Most patients with anti-MAG antibodies present with a sensory, large-fiber, demyelinating polyneuropathy that manifests as sensory ataxia.[25] Other patients have a sensorimotor polyneuropathy with mixed features of demyelination and axonal loss. The CSF protein is elevated, up to 250 mg/dL (normal is ≤50 mg/dL). The monoclonal IgM may also enter the CSF compartment, in spite of its high molecular weight, via dorsal root ganglia that lack a blood–CSF barrier or from a disrupted root–CSF barrier. Nerve conduction studies demonstrate slow conduction velocity and a rather characteristic prolonged distal motor and sensory latency. Sural nerve biopsy demonstrates a diminished number of myelinated axons (Fig. 66.3). Lymphocytic infiltrates are rarely seen within the endoneurial parenchyma. On electron microscopy there is splitting of the outer myelin lamellae, linked to the presence of IgM deposits in the same area of the split myelin sheath.[26]

- *Anti-MAG and SGPG antibodies.* MAG is the most extensively studied antigen recognized by the IgM paraproteins. The antigenic determinant for the anti-MAG IgM paraprotein resides in the carbohydrate component of the MAG molecule, as demonstrated by the loss of reactivity following deglycosylation of purified human MAG[27] (Fig. 66.4). An important finding was the observation that the anti-MAG IgM paraproteins co-react with an acidic glycolipid in the ganglioside fraction of the human peripheral nerve, which is separated from the whole ganglioside fraction by ion-exchange chromatography.[28] This antigenic glycolipid, chromatographed between GM1 and GD1a, has been identified as a sulfoglucuronyl glycosphingolipid, SGPG (Fig. 66.5). In contrast to MAG, which is mostly present in the CNS, SGPG is found only in peripheral nerves.

- *Anti-ganglioside antibodies.* The sera of some patients with IgM monoclonal gammopathy and demyelinating polyneuropathy may not react with MAG, in spite of clinical similarities to the anti-MAG-reacting paraproteins, but with various gangliosides. Most common gangliosides reacting with IgM, especially in patients with

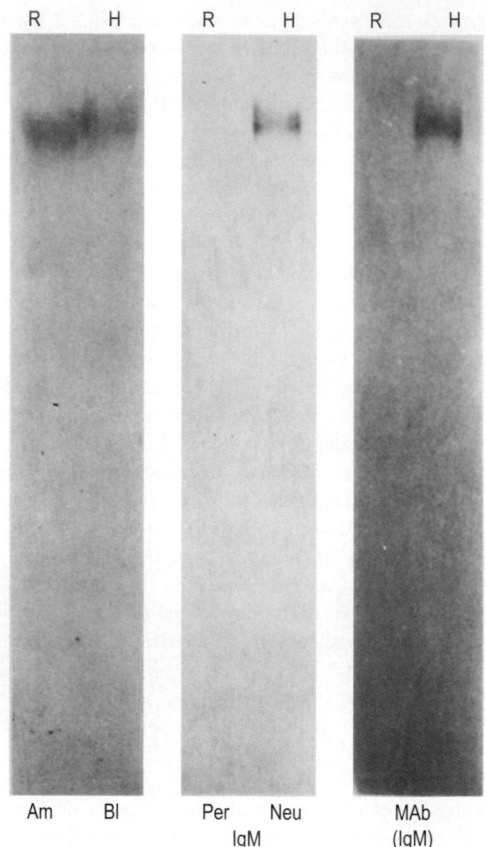

Fig. 66.4 Immunoblots showing binding of IgM to purified human MAG. Immunoblots of sodium dodecyl sulfate gels with purified rat MAG in lane 1 (R) and purified human MAG in lane 2 (H). (**A**) Purified MAG 10 μg in each lane are stained for protein with amido black; (**B**) 500 ng of purified MAG in each lane immunostained with a 1:50 dilution of serum from a patient with IgM monoclonal gammopathy, followed by peroxidase-labeled goat antihuman IgM; (C) the same blots, loaded as in (B) but stained with the mouse IgM monoclonal antibody produced against human MAG, are visualized by peroxidase-labeled goat anti-mouse IgG and IgM.

pure sensory neuropathies, are those that contain either a disialosyl moiety, such as GD1b, GQ1b, GT1b, the GalNac-GM1b and Gal-NAc-GD1a, or two gangliosides that share epitopes with GM2, or a combination of GM2 and GM1, GM1 and GD1b.[29, 30]

- *Motor, axonal neuropathies or neuronopathies with monoclonal IgM anti-GM1-antibodies.* A small number of patients with IgM paraprotein have a predominantly motor neuropathy that resembles a lower motor neuron syndrome. The IgM in some of these patients shows strong immunoreactivity to GM1 and asialoGM1 and, to a lesser degree, to GD1b. Because GM1 is present on the surface of motor neurons and the nodes of Ranvier, these findings led to a search for polyclonal GM1 antibodies in patients with a variety of conditions, including motor neuron diseases, multifocal motor neuropathy with conduction block, and Guillain–Barré syndrome and CIDP.

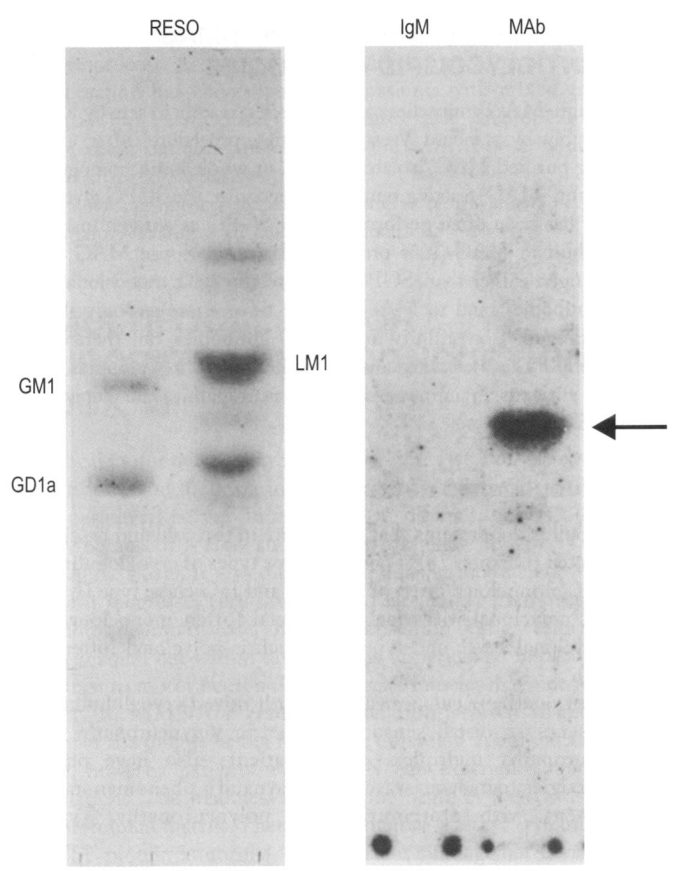

Fig. 66.5 Thin-layer chromatography overlay experiments demonstrating the reactivity of an anti-MAG monoclonal antibody from a neuropathy patient with glycolipid antigens of human sciatic nerve. The panel on the left shows the resorcinol-stained ganglioside fractions (10 µg sialic acid) isolated from human brain (CNS left lane) and human sciatic nerve (PNS right lane). The prominent chromatography GM1 and GD1a gangliosides of brain and LM1 ganglioside of nerve are labeled for reference. The panel on the right is an autoradiograph obtained after overlaying the same TLC plate with the patient's serum followed by radioiodinated antihuman IgM. The major glycolipid antigen in the PNS is indicated by the arrow, and two minor glycolipid antigens are seen migrating just above and below the major antigen.

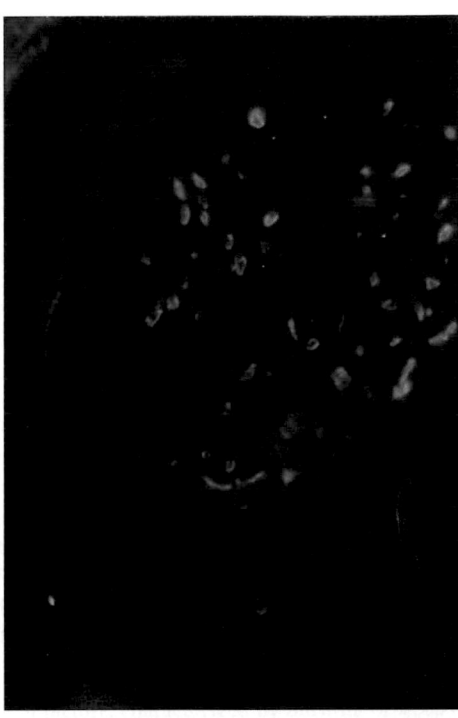

Fig. 66.6 Cross-section of a sural nerve from a patient with IgM paraproteinemia and demyelinating polyneuropathy. Fresh-frozen nerve specimen stained with FITC-conjugated antibodies to human IgM reveals IgM deposits in many myelinated fibers.

CAUSAL RELATIONSHIP BETWEEN ANTI-MAG ANTIBODIES AND NEUROPATHY

Because MAG is present in small amounts in the peripheral nervous system (PNS) but abundant in the CNS, which is spared in these patients, it was suggested that the reactivity of IgM to MAG may represent nonspecific binding to carbohydrate antigens. However, the discovery of the PNS-specific glycolipid SGPG, with which all the anti-MAG-reacting monoclonal IgMs react immunologically, has led to the proposal that the glycolipids, rather than the glycoproteins, may serve as primary antigenic targets. More than half of the IgM paraproteins recognize MAG and SGPG, and 75% of the rest recog-

nize ganglioside antigens, indicating that acidic glycolipids are the most common antigenic epitopes. Although the role of these antibodies in the pathogenesis of the neuropathy remains still unclear, the following factors suggest that they are related to the cause of the neuropathy:

- IgM and complement are deposited on the homologous myelinated nerve fibers on the patient's sural nerve biopsy,[18, 31] which suggests that activated complement may be needed in the induction of demyelination (Fig. 66.6).

- The IgM recognizes neural cell adhesion molecules and co-localizes with MAG on the areas of the split myelin lamellae,[26] suggesting involvement in myelin disadhesion. Skin biopsies from these patients have also confirmed the presence of IgM, complement C3d, and MAG deposition on the dermal myelinated fibers and the concurrent loss of nerve fibers.[32]

- Injection of serum from patients with IgM anti-MAG/SGPG paraprotein supplemented with fresh complement into feline peripheral nerve causes complement-dependent demyelination and conduction block within 2–9 days of the injection.[33] The IgM injected intraneurally also localizes to the outer layer of the myelin sheath. Moreover, systemic transfusion of anti-MAG IgM paraproteins produces segmental demyelination in chickens,[34] with deposition of IgM on to the outer lamellae of the myelin along with splitting of the myelin lamellae, similar to that observed in the human neuropathy.

■ AUTOIMMUNE AUTONOMIC NEUROPATHIES ■

Autoimmune autonomic neuropathy (AAN) is a recently recognized entity highlighted by circulating antibodies against the ganglionic nicotinic acetylcholine receptors (AChR).[37] These patients present with a subacute (within 4 weeks) or chronic (within months) onset of neurogenic orthostatic hypotension, defined as a systolic blood pressure reduction of at least 30 mmHg or mean blood pressure reduction of at least 20 mmHg that occurs within 3 minutes of head tilting. The subacute onset is often preceded by a viral infection. In addition, patients demonstrate three or four parasympathetic/enteric symptoms: sicca (dry eyes and dry mouth); abnormal pupillary response to light; upper gastrointestinal symptoms (early satiety, postprandial nausea and vomiting that lead to severe weight loss); and neurogenic bladder. Plasma norepinephrine values are reduced. Patients with more severe cholinergic impairment have higher-titer antibodies against ganglionic AChR, suggesting that these antibodies may be pathogenic.

The pathogenic role of these antibodies was further supported by the observation that some symptoms can be passively transferred to mice injected with the patient's IgG. Further, rabbits immunized with a fragment of ganglionic AChR protein exhibit autonomic failure, similar to that noted in patients with subacute and chronic AAN.[38] Because ganglionic AChR have also been found in small-cell lung carcinoma cell lines, cancer may be a potential initiator of ganglionic AChR autoimmunity. AChR antibodies may therefore be implicated in the pathogenesis of diverse neurological disorders, especially paraneoplastic syndromes.[38]

■ LOCALIZED, ISOLATED VASCULITIS OF THE PERIPHERAL NERVES ■

Polyneuropathy is a common manifestation of systemic vasculitis.[39] It occurs in patients with polyarteritis nodosa; vasculitis associated with connective tissue diseases, such as rheumatoid arthritis, Sjögren's syndrome, or systemic lupus erythematosus; hypersensitivity vasculitis; or temporal arteritis, in which it may occur up to 14% of cases. There is, however, a distinct vasculitic entity localized only to the peripheral nerve,[39] known as isolated peripheral nerve vasculitis (PNV).

PNV involves the small and medium-sized arteries of the epineurium and perineurium and causes ischemic changes within the peripheral nerve. The presentation is similar to that of the vasculitic neuropathy seen in patients with systemic vasculitis – the only difference is the lack of systemic organ involvement. The diagnosis is confirmed with nerve biopsy either of the sural, the superficial peroneal, or the superficial radial nerve. When nerve biopsy is combined with a muscle biopsy, the diagnostic yield is higher. PNV has a better prognosis than the systemic vasculitides and is a treatable form of neuropathy.

An evaluation for PNV should include all the tests needed to exclude systemic vasculitis and cryoglobulinemia, including hepatitis B and C infection, which is often associated with vasculitis of the peripheral nerve.

■ NEUROPATHY WITH VIRUSES AND HIV ■

Neuropathy can be seen in a setting of infectious, viral, or bacterial processes. In patients with Lyme disease, various neuropathies, including Guillain–Barré syndrome and mononeuritis (Bell's palsy), have been noted. Other infections, such as CMV, hepatitis, herpes, leprosy, Chagas' disease and diphtheria, can affect peripheral nerves, triggering an autoimmune peripheral neuropathy.

HIV-RELATED PERIPHERAL NEUROPATHIES

The most common neuropathies seen today in a setting of a viral infection are those associated with HIV.

Peripheral neuropathies usually develop in a stage-specific fashion in HIV-infected adults.[40] Two immune neuropathies, GBS and CIDP, may occur early in the infection, or they may be the presenting manifestation of unsuspected HIV infection. The only difference between HIV-negative GBS or CIDP and the HIV-associated condition is that in the latter there is often pleocytosis in the spinal fluid. Sural nerve biopsy shows segmental demyelination associated with a large number of macrophages within the endoneurial parenchyma. Perivascular inflammation can be also seen. Less common peripheral neuropathies that may develop in early-stage HIV infection include acute ganglioneuronitis coincident with seroconversion, and mononeuritis multiplex.

The most common neuropathy in AIDS patients occurs in the later stage of the infection. This is a painful sensory axonal neuropathy that may affect up to 70% of adults with AIDS. Pathologic studies at autopsy indicate that peripheral nerve pathology is ubiquitous in AIDS patients, whether or not they had clinical evidence of peripheral neuropathy. Painful axonal neuropathy can also complicate therapy with the nucleoside analogues ddI or ddC, and may represent the cumulative effect on the peripheral nerves of various endogenous or exogenous neurotoxins related to a multisystem disease and dysfunction of many organs and toxicity to mitochondria. Despite the relative lack of motor involvement, severe neuropathic pain in such patients can be disabling. Pain may be so severe that even contact with light stimuli (e.g., bed sheets) is intolerable. Clinical findings include distal pansensory loss or hypesthesia, areflexia, and, in advanced cases, distal weakness.

Another neuropathy seen in later-stage HIV infection is a lumbosacral polyradiculoneuropathy that affects roots and sensory ganglia, often related to CMV infection. CMV polyradiculoneuropathy presents with lower-extremity muscle weakness, sacral and distal paresthesias, areflexia, and atrophy, mostly of the legs, associated with sphincteric dysfunction resembling a cauda equina syndrome. The spinal fluid may show pleocytosis or harbor CMV detected by culture or cytologic examination. CMV inclusions are often found within Schwann cells or endothelial cells (Fig. 66.8). The disease is thought to represent reactivated CMV infection of the nerve root rather than primary infection. Recognition is important because anti-CMV therapy with ganciclovir or foscarnet is helpful.

Although zidovudine (AZT) is myotoxic, the two other antiretroviral drugs, ddC and ddI, are neurotoxic, causing a dose-dependent and reversible axonal painful sensory neuropathy.[41] The major feature that distinguishes a ddI- or ddC-related painful neuropathy from the painful sensory axonal neuropathy of AIDS is that the latter tends to be progressive, whereas the nucleoside-related peripheral

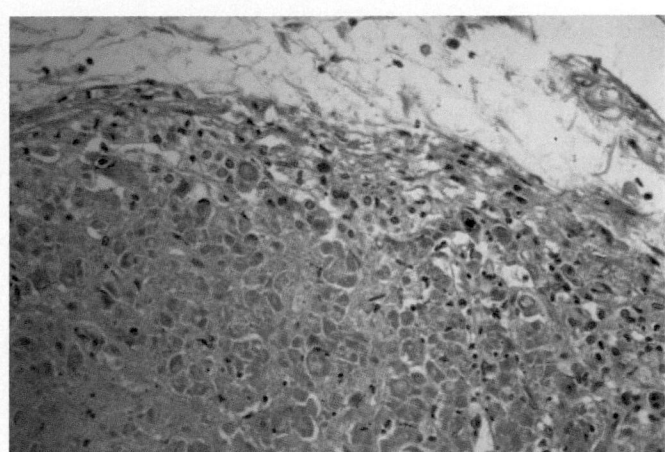

Fig. 66.8 Cross-section of a root from a patient with HIV-associated Guillain–Barré syndrome shows cytomegalovirus inclusions within the Schwann cell.

neuropathies tend to improve when the drugs are discontinued. Another clinical feature of nucleoside neuropathy is 'coasting,' or worsening of symptoms for a period after the drug is discontinued, followed by clinical improvement. The cause of ddC neuropathy is dysfunction of the nerve's mitochondria, which leads to depletion of mitochondrial DNA.[41]

PATHOGENESIS OF PERIPHERAL NEUROPATHIES IN HIV INFECTION

The possible mechanisms include direct viral infection, immune alterations triggered by the viral illness, complications of antiretroviral therapy, sequelae of chronic illness, and a combination of all these.

HIV has been cultured from peripheral nerves, and the author has amplified HIV viral RNA from sural nerve biopsy sections in two patients. However, there is no convincing evidence that the neuropathy results from direct infection of peripheral nerves with the virus. The author's own immunocytochemical studies using double-binding techniques on sural nerve biopsies have shown that HIV is present only in rare endoneurial macrophages, but not within the Schwann cells or the axons. With immunocytochemistry, the endoneurial infiltrates in sural nerve biopsies from such patients consist mostly of macrophages; CD8 and CD4 T cells are sparse. There is also strong expression of HLA class I and class II molecules on Schwann cells, endothelial cells, and/or macrophages, as shown in serial sections (Fig. 66.9). The macrophages express co-stimulatory molecules and may behave as antigen-presenting cells.[16] It is possible that systemic viral infection or rare HIV-infected endoneurial lymphoid cells may release lymphokines and cytokines that expose new nerve antigens against which there is no self-tolerance, generating a tissue-specific autoimmune attack. Proliferating macrophages may play a major role as immune effector cells or as sensitized cytotoxic cells responsible for a macrophage-mediated demyelination, similar to that described previously for the Guillain–Barré syndrome in HIV-negative patients. The frequency of anti-myelin or GM1-specific autoantibodies in the

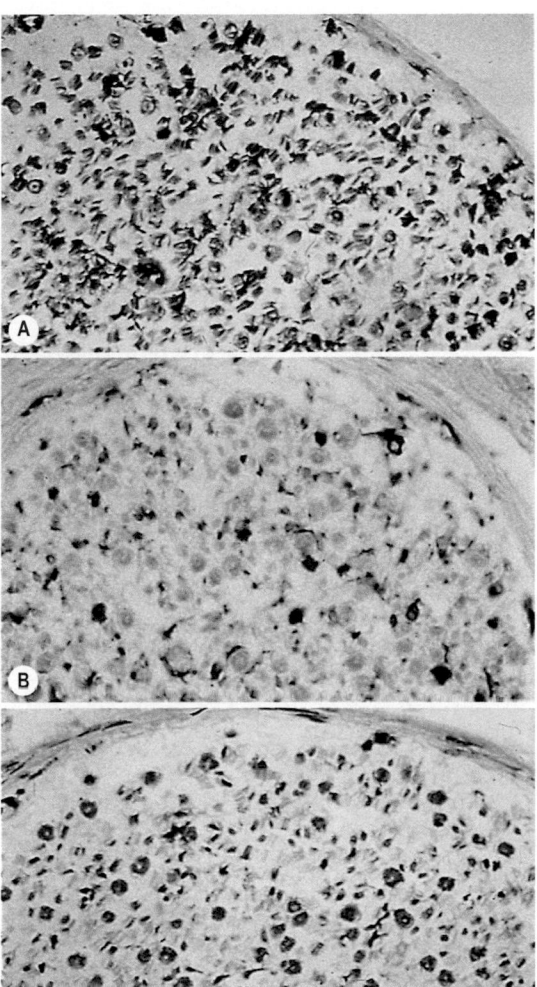

HLA-DR, Macrophages, CD8(+)T cells

Fig. 66.9 Serial sections of a new biopsy from a patient with HIV-chronic inflammatory demyelinating polyneuropathy stained for (**A**) HLA-DR, (**B**) macrophages, and (**C**) CD8 T shows that the majority of the endoneurial cells are macrophages. Only rare CD8+ cells are noted.

serum of these patients is also similar to that in HIV-negative patients with demyelinating polyneuropathies.

■ TREATMENT ■

APN are clinically important because they comprise potentially treatable disorders amenable to various immunosuppressive, immunomodulating, or chemotherapeutic agents. The selection of an effective protocol is based on the results of experimental therapeutic trials, clinical experience, and the risk–benefit ratio of available therapies. The author's approach to the treatment of these disorders is described below.

GUILLAIN–BARRÉ SYNDROME

Supportive care

The dramatic reduction in the mortality of GBS is mainly due to the availability of ICUs, improvement of respiratory support, antibiotic therapy, and control of autonomic cardiac dysregulation. A GBS patient is best monitored in ICU, even if respiratory compromise is not evident at the time of admission. When forced vital capacity (FVC) drops or bulbar weakness is severe, intubation is in order. A team approach provides the best results.

Plasmapheresis

In several double-blind studies[42] plasmapheresis has been shown to be effective if performed early in the course of the illness. A continuous-flow machine is preferable and a central venous catheter may be required for some patients. Based on two controlled studies, plasma exchange should begin within the first week from onset to be effective. A series of five or six exchanges, with one exchange every other day, is sufficient. Early relapses can occur in up to 20% of patients, who may require a second series of plasma exchanges to abort the relapse. Plasmapheresis has been shown to be effective even in mild cases of GBS; two exchanges are sufficient for mild GBS and four are optimal for moderate cases, but there is no difference between those who receive four plasma exchanges and those who receive six.

High-dose intravenous immunoglobulin

On the basis of two controlled studies using intravenous immunoglobulin (IVIG) versus plasmapheresis,[43] IVIG, given at 2 g/kg over 2–5 days, has been shown to be equally effective as plasmapheresis, with no added benefit when the two procedures are combined. The decision as to which treatment to use first, plasmapheresis or IVIG, is governed by circumstances, availability of the treatment modality, experience, age of the patient, and other associated conditions. Early relapses can also occur with IVIG, as often as with plasmapheresis. Because IVIG is easy to administer and more readily available, and because time to initiate treatment is of the essence, IVIG has become the therapeutic choice worldwide.

Steroids are ineffective in GBS and may even increase the incidence of future relapses. A new study combining IVIG with IV methylprednisolone showed a marginal added benefit, but this was not statistically significant.[44]

CIDP

Prednisone

CIDP is a classically steroid-responsive polyneuropathy. The efficacy of steroids was proven in a controlled study. A high-dose regimen of 80–100 mg prednisone daily is begun, and then tapered to every other day.[13] The starting dose can be a little lower and the tapering faster in patients with coexisting cardiac disease or severe osteoporosis, or the elderly. The goal is to increase strength, and strength is the single parameter to follow. Azathioprine, cyclosporine, or mycophenolate can be used as steroid-sparing agents.

IVIG

In several controlled studies[45] IVIG has been effective in the majority of patients with CIDP. The more chronic the disease and the more severe the axonal degeneration that has taken place, the fewer the chances that the recovery will be complete or significant. IVIG can be used effectively as a first-line therapy to avoid steroid-related side effects.

Plasmapheresis

Plasmapheresis has been also effective in controlled studies.[46] After a series of six plasma exchanges, maintenance therapy, with one exchange at least every 8 weeks, may be required if this therapy is beneficial. IVIG has now replaced plasmapheresis, although in the author's experience some patients may benefit more from steroids, others more from IVIG, and still others more after plasmapheresis.

POLYNEUROPATHY WITH PARAPROTEINEMIAS

Patients with benign IgG or IgA demyelinating polyneuropathies respond like CIDP patients. Patients with malignant paraproteinemias should be treated with chemotherapy as needed for the underlying disease. Often the neuropathy responds to chemotherapy. When the neuropathy is axonal, treatments are generally disappointing.

For the IgM anti-MAG demyelinating polyneuropathies, the treatments that have been used are prednisone plus chlorambucil, plasmapheresis, and IVIG,[47] but the benefit from these therapies has been marginal. Recent studies using rituximab, a monoclonal antibody against CD20, appear promising.[48] A double-blind study conducted by the author involving 27 patients has now been completed and the results are analyzed.

■ MULTIFOCAL MOTOR NEUROPATHY ■

This neuropathy responds very well to IVIG, which is the treatment of choice based on controlled trials. In difficult cases, aggressive treatment with cyclophosphamide followed by plasmapheresis and then IVIG has also been shown to be of benefit in the author's experience. Rituximab is also promising in difficult cases, but no controlled study has been carried out.[5]

PARANEOPLASTIC NEUROPATHY

Anecdotally, some of these patients have responded to plasma exchange or IVIG, but overall this neuropathy is not easily responding to available therapies.

VASCULITIC NEUROPATHIES

Patients with isolated peripheral nerve vasculitis are treated less aggressively than those with systemic vasculitis. A combination of prednisone 1.5 mg/kg/day, and oral cyclophosphamide 2 mg/kg/day, is the treatment of choice. Although treatment may vary between patients, the administration of cyclophosphamide may not be necessary for more than 12 months as in systemic vasculitis. Often 6–12 months of treatment may suffice. Plasmapheresis has been tried in cryoglobulinemic neuropathies, with variable results.

HIV NEUROPATHIES

The demyelinating neuropathies GBS and CIDP are treated with the same immunomodulatory therapies as used in HIV-negative patients. In uncontrolled studies, plasmapheresis and IVIG have each been effective. The author's preference is IVIG, because it augments rather than suppresses immune function, and it is easily administered.

Ganciclovir appears to be effective in CMV-related polyradiculoneuropathy. Painful sensory neuropathy can be quite disabling because of intractable pain, even though muscle weakness may be minimal. Tricyclic antidepressants, nonsteroidal anti-inflammatory drugs, anticonvulsants (carbamazepine, gabapentin), narcotic analgesics and topical capsaicin in various combinations provide some relief from neuropathic pain, although symptomatic management of this condition is a notoriously difficult clinical problem.

■ ACKNOWLEDGMENTS ■

The author thanks the various Neurology Fellows in the Neuromuscular Diseases Section who provided excellent care to his patients; and Drs Amjad Ilyas and Richard Quarles for help with immunochemistry.

■ REFERENCES ■

1. Asbury AK, Arnason BG, Adams RD. The inflammatory lesion in idiopathic polyneuritis: its role in pathogenesis. Medicine (Baltimore) 1969; 48: 173–215.

2. Hughes RA, Cornblath DR. Guillain–Barré syndrome. Lancet 2005; 366: 1653–1666.

3. Feasby TE, Hahn AF, Brown WF, et al. Severe axonal degeneration in acute Guillain–Barré syndrome: evidence of two different mechanisms? J Neurol Sci 1993; 116: 185–192.

4. Feldman EL, Bromberg MB, Blaivas M, Junck L. Acute pandysautonomic neuropathy. Neurology 1991; 41: 746–748.

5. LaRocca RV, Meer J, Gilliatt R et al. Suramin-induced polyneuropathy. Neurology 1990; 40: 954–960.

6. Ilyas AA, Mithen FA, Chen ZW, Cook SD. Search for antibodies to neutral glycolipids in sera of patients with Guillain–Barré syndrome. J Neurol Sci 1991; 102: 67–75.

7. Willison HJ, Yuki N. Peripheral neuropathies and anti-glycolipid antibodies. Brain 2002; 125: 2591–2625.

8. Chiba A, Kusunoki S, Obata H. Serum anti GQ1b IgG antibody is associated with ophthalmoplegia in Miller-Fisher syndrome and Guillain–Barré syndrome. Neurology 1993; 43: 1911–1917.

9. Yuki N, Susuki K, Koga M, et al. Carbohydrate mimicry between human ganglioside GM1 and *Campylobacter jejuni* lipooligosaccharide causes Guillain–Barré syndrome. Proc Natl Acad Sci USA 2004; 101: 11404–11409.

10. Illa I, Ortiz N, Gallard E, et al. Acute axonal Guillain–Barré syndrome with IgG antibodies against motor axons following parenteral gangliosides. Ann Neurol 1995; 38: 218–224.

11. Ang CW, Jacobs BC, Laman JD. The Guillain–Barré syndrome: a true case of molecular mimicry. Trends Immunol 2004; 25: 61–66.

12. Koller H, Kieseier BC, Jander S, Hartung HP. Chronic inflammatory demyelinating polyneuropathy. N Engl J Med 2005; 352: 1343–1356.

13. Dalakas MC, Engel WK. Chronic relapsing (dysimmune) polyneuropathy: pathogenesis and treatment, Ann Neurol 1981; 10: 134–145.

14. Dalakas MC. Advances in chronic inflammatory demyelinating polyneuropathy: disease variants and inflammatory response mediators and modifiers. Curr Opin Neurol 1999; 12: 403–409.

15. Murata K, Dalakas MC. Expression of the co-stimulatory molecule BB-1, the ligands CTLA-4 and CD28 and their mRNAs in chronic inflammatory demyelinating polyneuropathy. Brain 2000; 123: 1660–1666.

16. Dalakas M, Engel WK. Immunoglobulin deposits in chronic relapsing polyneuropathies. Arch Neurol 1980; 37: 637–640.

17. Weiss MD, Luciano CA, Semino-Mora C, et al. Molecular mimicry in chronic inflammatory demyelinating polyneuropathy and melanoma. Neurology 1998; 51: 1738–1741.

18. Dalakas MC, Engel WK. Polyneuropathy and monoclonal gammopathy: studies of 11 patients. Ann Neurol 1981; 10: 45–52.

19. Latov N, Braun PE, Gross RB et al. Plasma cell dyscrasia and peripheral neuropathy: identification of the myelin antigens that react with human paraproteins. Proc Natl Acad Sci USA 1981; 78: 7139.

20. Kelly JJ, Kyle RA, O'Brien PC, Dyck PJ. The prevalence of monoclonal gammopathy in peripheral neuropathy. Neurology 1981; 31: 1480–1483.

21. Latov N, Hays A, Sherman WH. Peripheral neuropathy and anti-MAG antibodies. Crit Rev Neurobiol 1988; 3: 301–332.

22. Kyle RA, Therneau TM, Rajkumar SV, et al. Prevalence of monoclonal gammopathy of undetermined significance. N Engl J Med 2006; 354: 1362–1369.

23. Dispenzieri A, Kyle RA, Lacy MQ, et al. POEMS syndrome: definitions and long-term outcome. Blood 2003; 101: 2496–2506.

24. Nakanishi T, Sobue I, Toyokura Y et al. The Crow–Fukase syndrome: a study of 102 cases in Japan. Neurology 1984; 34: 712–720.

25. Dalakas MC. Chronic idiopathic ataxic neuropathy. Ann Neurol 1986; 19: 545–554.

26. Mendell JR, Sahenk Z, Whitaker JN et al. Polyneuropathy and monoclonal gammopathy: studies on the pathogenetic role of anti-myelin-associated glycoprotein antibody. Ann Neurol 1985; 17: 243–254.

27. Ilyas AA, Quarles RH, McIntosh TD et al. IgM in a human neuropathy related to paraproteinemia binds to a carbohydrate determinant in the myelin-associated glycoprotein and to a ganglioside. Proc Natl Acad Sci USA 1984; 81: 1225–1229.

28. Ilyas AA, Quarles RH, Dalakas MC, Brady RO. Polyneuropathy with monoclonal gammopathy: glycolipids are frequently antigens for IgM paraproteins. Proc Natl Acad Sci USA 1985; 82: 6697–6700.

29. Ilyas AA, Li SC, Chou DKH et al. Gangliosides GM$_2$, IV^{4}Gal NaC GM$_{1B}$, and IV^{4}Gal NaC GD1a as antigens for monoclonal immunoglobulin M neuropathy associated with gammopathy. J Biol Chem 1988; 263: 4369–4373.

30. Duane GC, Farrer RG, Dalakas MC, Quarles RH. Sensory neuropathy associated with monoclonal IgM to GD1b ganglioside. Ann Neurol 1992; 31: 683–685.

31. Monaco S, Bonetti B, Ferrari S et al. Complement dependent demyelination in patients with IgM monoclonal gammopathy and polyneuropathy. N Engl J Med 1990; 322: 844–852.

32. Lombardi R, Erne B, Lauria G, et al. IgM deposits on skin nerves in antimyelin-associated glycoprotein neuropathy. Ann Neurol 2005; 57: 180–187.

33. Willison HJ, Trapp BD, Bacher JD et al. Demyelination induced by intraneural injection of human antimyelin associated glycoprotein antibodies. Muscle Nerve 1988; 11: 1169–1176.

34. Tatum AH. Experimental paraprotein neuropathy; demyelination by passive transfer of human IgM anti-MAG. Ann Neurol 1993; 33: 502–506.

35. Van Asseldonk JT, Franssen H, Van den Berg-Vos RM, et al. Multifocal motor neuropathy. Lancet Neurol 2005; 4: 309–319.

36. Darnell RB, Posner JB. Paraneoplastic syndromes affecting the nervous system. Oncology 2006; 33: 270–298.

37. Vernino S, Low PA, Fealey RD, et al. Autoantibodies to ganglionic acetylcholine receptors in autoimmune autonomic neuropathies. N Engl J Med 2000; 343: 847–855.

38. Lennon VA, Ermilov LG, Szurszewski JH, Vernino S. Immunization with neuronal nicotinic acetylcholine receptor induces neurological autoimmune disease. J Clin Invest 2003; 111: 907–913.

39. Chalk CH, Dyck PJ, Conn DL. Vasculitic neuropathy. In: Dyck PJ, Thomas PK, Griffin JW, et al., eds: Peripheral neuropathy, Philadelphia: WB Saunders, 1993; 1424–1436.

40. Dalakas MC, Pezeshkpour GH. Neuromuscular diseases associated with human immunodeficiency virus infection. Ann Neurol 1988; 23: 38–48.

41. Dalakas MC. Peripheral neuropathy and antiretroviral drugs. J Periph Nerv Syst 2001; 6: 14–20.

42. McKhann GM, Griffin JW, Cornblath DR. The Guillain–Barré Syndrome Study Group. Plasmapheresis and Guillain–Barré syndrome: analysis of prognostic factors and the effect of plasmapheresis. Ann Neurol 1988; 23: 347–353.

43. Van der Meche FGA, Schmitz PIM. The Dutch Guillain–Barré syndrome. N Engl J Med 1992; 326: 1123–1129.

44. Van Koningsveld R, Schmitz PIM, van der Meché FGA, et al. Effect of methylprednisolone when added to standard treatment with intravenous immunoglobulin for Guillain–Barré syndrome: randomised trial. Lancet 2004; 363: 192–196.

45. Hahn AF, Bolton CF, Zochodne D, Feasby TE. Intravenous immunoglobulin treatment in chronic inflammatory demyelinating polyneuropathy. A double-blind, placebo-controlled, cross-over study. Brain 1996; 119: 1067–1077.

46. Hahn AF, Bolton CF, Pillay N, et al. Plasma-exchange therapy in chronic inflammatory demyelinating polyneuropathy. A double-blind, sham-controlled, cross-over study. Brain 1996; 119: 1055–1066.

47. Dalakas MC, Quarles RH, Farrer RG, et al. A controlled study of intravenous immunoglobulin in demyelinating neuropathy with IgM gammopathy. Ann Neurol 1996; 40: 792–795.

48. Pestronk A, Florence J, Miller T, et al. Treatment of IgM antibody associated polyneuropathies using rituximab. J Neurol Neurosurg Psychiatry 2003; 74: 485–489.

Immunologic renal diseases

James E. Balow, Monique E. Cho, Howard A. Austin III

67

Immunologic renal diseases encompass a broad range of clinicopathologic entities, some of which are limited to kidney disease (primary) whereas in others the kidney involvement is one component of a systemic disease (secondary). The immune mechanisms underlying these diverse conditions are equally complex and diverse.[1] This chapter considers the more common immune-mediated diseases of native kidneys, but not those involving immune mediated diseases of renal allografts.

Collectively, immune-mediated kidney diseases represent the third most common cause of end-stage renal failure (after diabetic and hypertensive nephropathies). Disappointingly large numbers of patients first present for medical attention in advanced renal insufficiency. Several factors contribute to the late diagnosis and treatment of immune-mediated kidney disease. Patients with primary glomerular diseases tend to experience few symptoms that prompt them to seek medical evaluation. Shortcomings in the medical system also contribute to late diagnosis and treatment: subtle abnormalities in urinary screening tests are too commonly overlooked or misattributed to inconsequential intercurrent conditions. It is clear from both experimental and clinical studies that early detection is one of the most important determinants of the success of treatment in both primary and secondary forms of immune-mediated renal disorders.

Appropriate evaluation of patients with immune-mediated kidney diseases requires particular attention to the findings of urinalysis, tests of renal functions, and renal biopsy.[2] Urinalysis plays a pivotal role in the assessment of urinary disorders. The physician should be mindful of the many 'false negative' urinalyses reported by practice-oriented clinical pathology laboratories with high throughput. As a general rule, reports of positive findings are much more likely to be accurate than are negative reports. The thorough clinician should personally review microscopic urinalysis in any case in which there is a reasonable index of suspicion of immune-mediated renal disease.

HEMATURIA

Evaluation of hematuria should begin with determination of whether the bleeding is due to upper urinary tract (glomerular and/or tubulointerstitial) pathology or to lower urinary tract abnormalities. Urinary erythrocyte morphology helps to determine the cause of hematuria. Red blood cells that emanate from lesions of the calices, ureters, bladder or urethra tend to maintain their normal morphology; when nondysmorphic red blood cells are present, it is usually appropriate to refer the patient to urology for further evaluation. Red blood cells that result from glomerular or tubulointerstitial pathology are more likely to appear dysmorphic (abnormal shapes and sizes, fragmented); when dysmorphic red blood cells are present, it is usually appropriate to refer the patient to nephrology for further evaluation. Erythrocyte and/or leukocyte casts are indicative of glomerulonephritis (or interstitial nephritis). Cellular casts can be formed from erythrocytes and/or leukocytes that enter the tubular lumen because of glomerular or tubular inflammation (Fig. 67.1).

PROTEINURIA

Proteinuria is a cardinal feature of renal parenchymal disease and may indicate glomerular or tubular pathology. Glomerular proteinuria results from a loss of the size-selective and/or charge-selective properties of the glomerular capillary wall and disruptions of the glomerular epithelial cells (podocytes), allowing plasma proteins (especially albumin) to leak into the filtrate. Tubulointerstitial nephropathy often leads to impaired tubular absorption of other normally filtered low molecular weight proteins; this so-called 'tubular proteinuria' exhibits a characteristic pattern on urine protein electrophoresis (low fraction of albumin), rarely exceeds 2 g/day, and is often associated with other manifestations of tubular dysfunction.

The validity of 24-hour urine collections for determination of quantitative proteinuria is often an issue; under- and over-collections are common and must be countered with explicit instructions to patients regarding urine collection. Owing to the high prevalence of collection errors, many clinicians have turned to estimates of proteinuria based on the protein-to-creatinine concentration ratio in random urine samples. Normally, the urine protein-to-creatinine ratio is less than 0.1. This random urine sample method has continued to gain favor as an efficient, cost-effective method to monitor proteinuria in both children and adults.

Filtration of abnormal plasma proteins may be responsible for proteinuria (e.g., multiple myeloma or immunoglobulin light-chain disease). This type of proteinuria (paraproteinuria) may be undetected or underestimated by the dipstick method of evaluation. Abnormal immunoglobulin

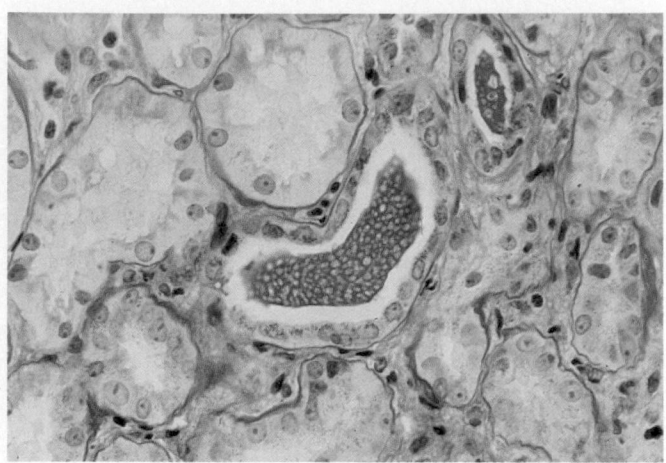

Fig. 67.1 Red blood cell cast. Cast present in situ within the lumen of a distal renal tubule. (PAS stain.)

Table 67.1 Indications for renal biopsy

1. Active 'nephritic' urine sediment
   Dysmorphic erythrocytes: > 10 per high-power field
   Cellular casts: erythrocyte or leukocyte

2. Proteinuria >2 g/day

3. Abnormal renal function
   Associated with the above features of active nephritis
   Particularly important if the duration of renal disease and/or rate of change are unknown

4. Document indications for use of high risk therapeutic interventions

---

light-chain excretion may be detected by urine protein electrophoresis, but immunofixation electrophoresis is particularly important for detection and definitive diagnosis of paraproteinuria.

NEPHROTIC SYNDROME

The nephrotic syndrome is characterized by substantial degrees of proteinuria (> 3.5 g/day) resulting in hypoalbuminemia, edema, hyperlipidemia and lipiduria. The degree of proteinuria may offer a helpful diagnostic clue because some immune-mediated conditions with typically diffuse glomerular disease (e.g., membranous nephropathy, systemic lupus, amyloidosis) are more likely than others with typically focal disease (e.g., IgA nephropathy, microscopic polyangiitis, Wegener's granulomatosis) to be associated with the nephrotic syndrome.

ACUTE NEPHRITIC SYNDROME

The acute nephritic syndrome is characterized by hematuria (dysmorphic cells), erythrocyte casts, abnormal proteinuria, fluid retention, azotemia and hypertension. Histologically, this constellation of clinical findings is due to proliferative glomerulonephritis. A variant of this syndrome, called rapidly progressive glomerulonephritis, is defined by 50% or greater loss of glomerular filtration rate over 3 months, along with cellular crescents on renal biopsy. It is important to recognize that rapidly progressive glomerulonephritis may present subtly as hematuria and/or proteinuria without oliguria, edema, hypertension or azotemia, yet become an explosive manifestation of several immunologic renal diseases, particularly Wegener's granulomatosis, microscopic polyangiitis, Henoch–Schönlein nephritis, and proliferative lupus nephritis.

CHRONIC GLOMERULONEPHRITIS

Chronic glomerulonephritis is not a diagnosis, but rather is a stage in the evolution of immune-mediated renal disease. The urinalysis often provides valuable clues regarding the duration of glomerular disease. Broad and waxy casts are features of chronic renal disease that are not likely to be seen in recent-onset acute glomerulonephritis.

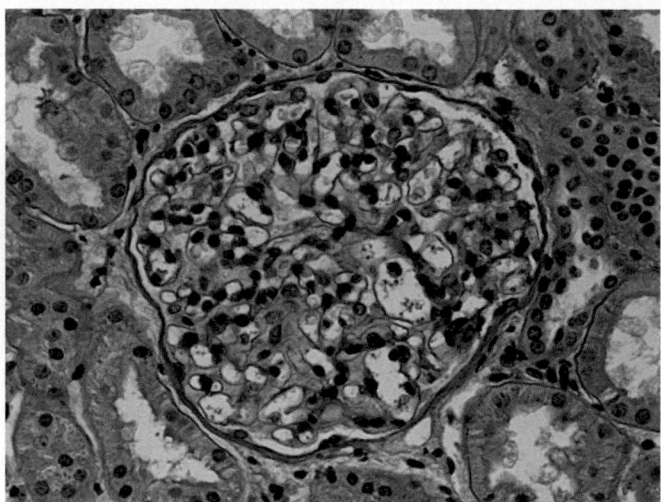

Fig. 67.2 Normal glomerular architecture. Note the thin, delicate capillary walls. Neither cells nor matrix encroach upon the patency of the capillary lumina. (PAS stain.)

RENAL BIOPSY

After extensive clinical and laboratory evaluations, a renal biopsy may be indicated to establish or confirm a tissue diagnosis, to clarify the precise type of renal involvement, to formulate a prognosis, and to direct therapy. Some of the more important indications for renal biopsy are listed in Table 67.1. To assist the reader in recognizing patterns of glomerular diseases addressed in subsequent discussions, a normal glomerulus is illustrated in Figure 67.2. An excellent color atlas of glomerular diseases is available.[3]

■ MINIMAL CHANGE NEPHROPATHY (LIPOID NEPHROSIS) ■

Nephrotic syndrome of childhood is mainly due to minimal change nephropathy.[4] Minimal change nephropathy is an uncommon cause of nephrotic syndrome in neonates and infants, where genetic conditions should receive first consideration. The frequency of minimal change nephropathy in adults with nephrotic syndrome is low compared to other entities discussed below, but this disease has been seen even into the ninth decade of life.

CLINICAL FEATURES

Minimal change nephropathy characteristically presents with a rather precipitous onset of severe nephrotic syndrome in the absence of signs of a systemic disease. Massive generalized edema and ascites can be very debilitating; these features may be difficult to control with diuretics because of the typically extreme hypoalbuminemia. There are no specific tests short of kidney biopsy to establish a diagnosis of minimal change nephropathy; standard immunologic screening tests are usually normal.

ETIOLOGY AND PATHOGENESIS

The cause of minimal change nephropathy is largely unknown, but this entity is inferentially considered an immune-mediated kidney disease because of its association with some allergic reactions and its characteristic response to immunosuppressive drugs. Reactions to nonsteroidal anti-inflammatory drugs have been invoked in some cases of minimal change nephropathy. Rare cases have been associated with systemic interferon (IFN) treatment, but interestingly not with interleukin (IL)-2. Lymphatic malignancies, particularly Hodgkin's lymphoma, have occasionally been associated with minimal change nephropathy.

The basic lesion of minimal change nephropathy is loss or neutralization of the normal high density of anionic proteoglycans in the glomerular capillary loops. Dissipation of the negative charge barrier allows anionically charged albumin to pass freely. The pathogenic factors that are responsible for massive proteinuria remain elusive. Interdigitating foot processes normally joined by intercellular bridges, called slit diaphragms, form a second barrier to the passage of protein into the urinary space. Characteristically, the podocyte foot processes and slit diaphragms are also disrupted in minimal change nephropathy, although there is uncertainty as to whether these changes are the cause or effect of proteinuria. Recently, mutations of one or more components of the proteins constituting the slit pore complex have been recognized. Recognition of several genetic forms of nephrotic syndrome has led some clinicians to challenge the traditional practice of administering an empiric trial of steroid therapy based on a presumptive diagnosis of classic minimal change nephropathy prior to establishing a specific pathologic diagnosis by renal biopsy and potentially obviating the risk of empiric immunosuppressive therapy.

PATHOLOGY

On light microscopy the renal biopsy is essentially normal, including glomerular tuft cellularity and capillary wall thickness. The characteristic pathologic lesion is seen by electron microscopy where there is fusion of the foot processes of the epithelial cells (podocytes) diffusely around glomerular capillaries. No deposits of antibody or complement components are typically seen.

TREATMENT

Minimal change nephropathy is characteristically exquisitely sensitive to glucocorticoids (remitting within the first few weeks of therapy in over 90% of children). The response rate to glucocorticoids in adults is

---

> ## KEY CONCEPTS
>
> ### MINIMAL CHANGE NEPHROPATHY
>
> >> Most common cause of nephrotic syndrome in children
>
> >> High rate of response to glucocorticoids
>
> >> Cyclophosphamide is useful for frequent relapsers
>
> >> Renal prognosis is excellent
>
> >> Subset may evolve to focal segmental glomerulosclerosis

somewhat lower and more delayed than in children. A substantial portion of patients with minimal change nephropathy face long-term difficulties with the disease and its therapy: some are steroid-resistant from the start; others are steroid-dependent for control of nephrotic syndrome; still others become frequent relapsers and suffer substantial steroid toxicity with repeated treatments. Controlled trials have shown that alkylating agents (cyclophosphamide or chlorambucil) increase response rates, but in particular reduce rates of relapse. Cyclosporine and mycophenolate mofetil have also been shown to be promising alternatives to prolonged and repeated courses of steroid therapy.

The risk of progression to end-stage renal failure is extremely low in true minimal change nephropathy. However, there is a relationship between minimal change nephropathy and focal segmental glomerulosclerosis, the latter being typically more refractory to therapy and having a much more adverse renal prognosis. Renal biopsy sampling errors account for a mistaken diagnosis of minimal change disease in a proportion of cases that are in fact focal segmental glomerulosclerosis. It is also debated whether a subset of minimal change nephropathy can progress to focal segmental glomerulosclerosis.

■ FOCAL SEGMENTAL GLOMERULOSCLEROSIS ■

Few clinical features distinguish patients with new-onset idiopathic nephrotic syndrome due to minimal change nephropathy and focal segmental glomerulosclerosis (FSGS). Patients with FSGS have a higher frequency of microscopic hematuria, higher frequency of persistent nephrotic syndrome, a poorer response to immunosuppressive drug therapies, and a higher risk of progression to end-stage renal failure.[5] The incidence of FSGS is clearly increasing as a cause of nephrotic syndrome, particularly among black patients, in whom the search for genetic factors is ongoing.

ETIOLOGY AND PATHOGENESIS

The etiology and pathogenesis of FSGS are largely unknown. Evidence that there are multiple forms of FSGS further complicates our understanding of this entity. Studies of alterations in podocyte structures and functions are the central focus of research attempting to elucidate the pathogenesis of various subsets of FSGS. The characteristic renal pathology includes segmental areas of podocyte damage and detachment, irregular foot process fusion, and collapse of glomerular capillaries

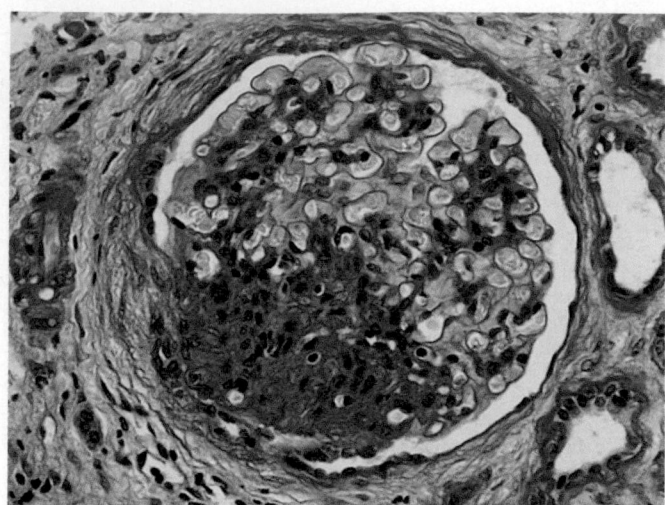

Fig. 67.3 Focal segmental glomerulosclerosis. Glomerular capillary loops at the lower left are collapsed and obliterated by excessive matrix and connective tissue. (PAS stain.)

KEY CONCEPTS

FOCAL SEGMENTAL GLOMERULOSCLEROSIS

>> Nephrotic syndrome with progressive renal insufficiency

>> Glomerular permeability factor in plasma of some cases

>> Unpredictable responses to glucocorticoids or cyclophosphamide

>> Cyclosporine effective but relapses common

>> Moderately high relapse rate in renal allografts

associated with marked local increase in matrix and collagen accumulation (Fig. 67.3). Segmental sclerotic areas typically stain with antisera to IgM and C3 (but not IgG or IgA), particularly areas of glomerular tuft hyalinosis (representing trapped plasma constituents), but none of these collections should be considered to represent classic immune complexes.

Although there is consensus that there are several forms of FSGS, classification schemes for the FSGS variants are somewhat arcane and have not been widely adopted in routine clinical practice.[6] The collapsing variant of FSGS has been associated with viral infections, notably HIV, and follows a particularly aggressive course. Some forms of FSGS, such as those associated with morbid obesity, appear to result from nonimmunologic glomerular hyperfiltration injury. Potential new insights into the pathogenesis of FSGS emanate from the discovery of plasma factors that, *in vitro*, increase the permeability of normal glomerular capillaries to albumin.[7] Clinical support for the theory of soluble mediator pathogenesis derives from cases of mother–child transfer of FSGS in utero, and from cases in which fulminant recurrence of FSGS occurs shortly after renal transplantation. Albeit controversially, some investigators have found permeability factors in a subset of cases of FSGS; levels of these factors correlate with remissions and exacerbations of nephrotic syndrome in some cases. Finally, recent evidence indicates that some cases of FSGS are familial and result from mutations in constitutive components of the slit diaphragm filtration barrier.[8]

TREATMENT

It is important to consider the possibility of genetic forms of FSGS before beginning immunosuppressive drug therapy. Treatment of genetic and hyperfiltration-induced forms of FSGS is focused mostly on renoprotection with angiotensin antagonists and lipid-lowering agents. The treatment of other forms of primary FSGS is basically similar to that of minimal change nephropathy and includes prednisone, cyclophosphamide, cyclosporine and mycophenolate. Recent controlled trials have shown that cyclosporine is much more effective than prednisone alone in inducing remission of nephrotic syndrome and in preserving renal

function in patients with steroid-resistant FSGS.[9] Preliminary studies have suggested some potential benefit of plasma exchange therapy with or without cyclophosphamide in patients with high plasma levels of permeability factors, and in those relapsing after renal transplant. Complete remission of proteinuria is less commonly achieved than in minimal change nephropathy; however, achievement of even partial remission of proteinuria is associated with improved prognosis and is a laudable goal of treatment.

MEMBRANOUS NEPHROPATHY

Membranous nephropathy is identified in approximately 20% of adults who undergo renal biopsy for the nephrotic syndrome. It is a less frequent cause of nephrotic syndrome in children. Primary membranous nephropathy is a diagnosis of exclusion after considering secondary causes such as medication reactions, infections, neoplasms and systemic illnesses.

ETIOLOGY AND PATHOGENESIS

Membranous nephropathy is characterized by subepithelial (epimembranous) immune deposits containing IgG and complement components. The leading hypothesis based on experimental models is that immune complexes are formed in situ by the interaction of a pathogenic antibody with an endogenous glomerular antigen or with an antigen that had been ectopically planted in the glomerulus. Detailed reviews of the immunopathogenesis of membranous nephropathy have recently been published.[10, 11]

CLINICOPATHOLOGIC FEATURES

The majority of patients with membranous nephropathy present with the nephrotic syndrome. Some are discovered by detection of asymptomatic proteinuria on routine urinalysis. Renal biopsy is usually required to establish the diagnosis of membranous nephropathy. In the early stages of the disease, glomeruli may appear normal by light microscopy. In most cases, light microscopy shows uniform thickening of the glomerular capillary walls without endocapillary cell proliferation (Fig. 67.4). Characteristic subepithelial (epimembranous) and/or intramembranous deposits are seen on electron microscopy (Fig. 67.5). Diagnosis of secondary membranous nephropathy depends on concurrent abnormalities in clinical and laboratory data.

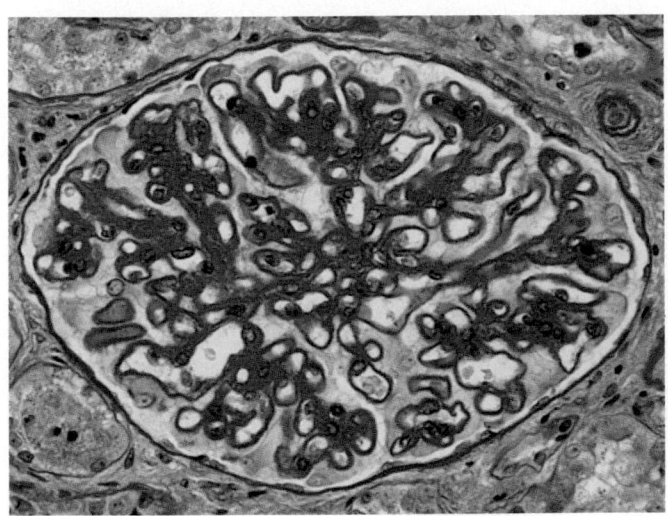

Fig. 67.4 Membranous nephropathy. Capillary walls are nearly uniformly thickened but remain widely patent. Cellularity of the glomerulus is normal. (PAS stain.)

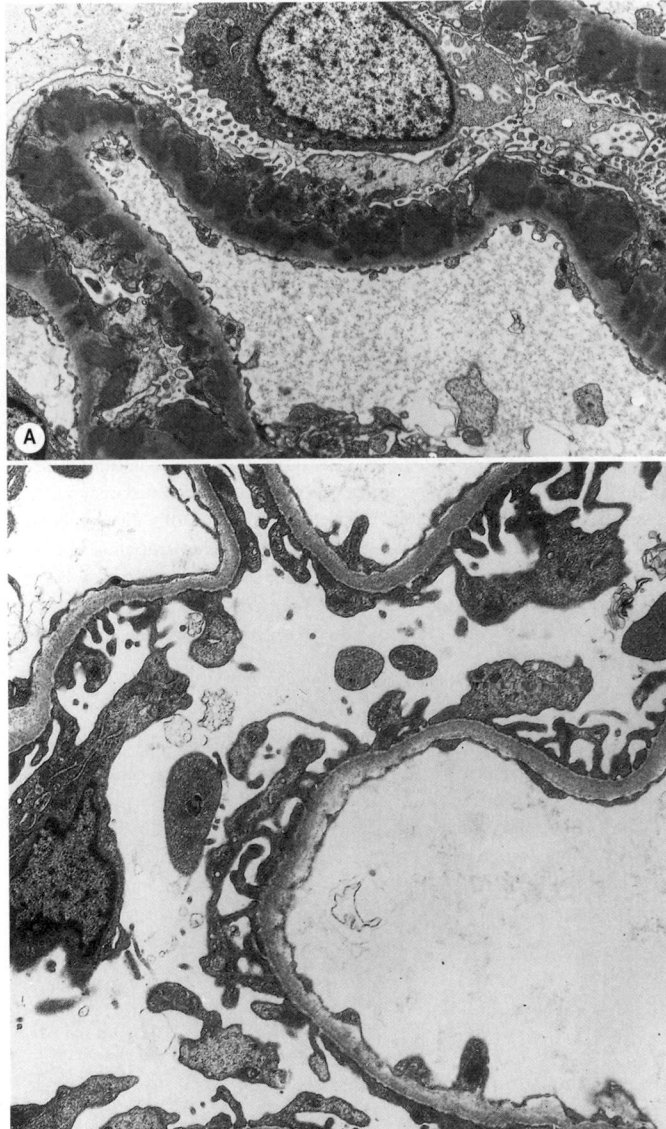

Fig. 67.5 Membranous nephropathy (ultrastructure). (**A**) Electron micrograph demonstrates heavy, dark-staining immune complex deposits along the outer surface of the glomerular basement membrane and beneath the epithelial foot processes (hence the terms subepithelial or epimembranous deposits). Note the thickening and projections of the gray-staining basement membrane between the electron-dense deposits. (**B**) Ultrastructure of a normal glomerular capillary wall for comparison. (Electron micrographs courtesy of Dr S. Sabnis, Armed Forces Institute of Pathology; Washington, DC.)

NATURAL HISTORY

The clinical course of idiopathic membranous nephropathy is highly variable. On average, about one-quarter of adult patients progress to end-stage renal failure within 10 years. Another quarter experience a spontaneous remission of proteinuria. The majority are likely to have persistent proteinuria and moderately impaired renal function over an extended period of observation. Patients with sustained hyperlipidemia are at risk for premature cardiovascular disease. Reduction of cardiovascular risk may be as important an element in the rationale for treatment as is preserving kidney function.

It is difficult to predict the clinical course of individual patients with membranous nephropathy. Patients with severe nephrotic syndrome, hypertension and azotemia on presentation have been associated with a poor prognosis in several studies. Protracted high-grade nephrotic-range proteinuria is a relatively strong predictor of an adverse renal outcome. On the other hand, complete or partial remission of proteinuria is associated with excellent long-term prognosis.

TREATMENT

Management of patients with membranous nephropathy usually includes diuretics to reduce edema, lipid-lowering drugs (for severe hyperlipidemia), anticoagulant therapy for thromboembolic complications, and antihypertensive agents. Angiotensin antagonists have been shown to have a substantial anti-proteinuric effect. Whereas patients with severe nephrotic syndrome due to membranous nephropathy are often treated with high-dose alternate-day prednisone, it is generally considered that prednisone does not significantly reduce the risk of progression to renal failure. There is evidence that a combination of prednisone and cytotoxic drug therapy is more effective than prednisone alone. Azathioprine has not been widely used for the treatment of membranous nephropathy. Several small, nonrandomized

studies of the related drug, mycophenolate mofetil, in patients resistant to other immunosuppressive therapies showed encouraging evidence of benefit. The most compelling results from controlled trials have shown that patients with membranous nephropathy treated with alternating monthly courses of pulse methylprednisolone and chlorambucil or cyclophosphamide were more likely than controls to experience a remission of the nephrotic syndrome and achieve stable renal function.[12]

Several anecdotal series and controlled trials of cyclosporine in membranous nephropathy have suggested a moderate benefit on proteinuria and renal function.[13] Relapses of proteinuria are common, particularly after a short course of cyclosporine therapy. Preliminary studies suggest that rituximab (which depletes CD20 B lymphocytes) may be a useful alternative for treatment of membranous nephropathy.[14]

MEMBRANOPROLIFERATIVE GLOMERULONEPHRITIS ■

Membranoproliferative glomerulonephritis (MPGN) is a rare condition that is sometimes referred to as mesangiocapillary glomerulonephritis (Fig. 67.6). Besides the presence of pathologic immunoreactants in glomerular sites, the immune-mediated nature of this disease is suggested by the high frequency of persistent hypocomplementemia. It is of interest that both congenital complement deficiencies (e.g., C3 deficiency) and sustained hypocomplementemia induced by nephritic factor autoantibodies or circulating immune complexes have all been associated with MPGN.

PATHOLOGIC VARIANTS

The nomenclature of MPGN includes two main pathological subsets: type I, MPGN with subendothelial deposits (Fig. 67.7A), and type II, MPGN with dense intramembranous deposits (Fig. 67.7B).[15] Although most cases of MPGN are of unknown etiology, studies over the past decade have shown that chronic hepatitis C infection, particularly when accompanied by cryoglobulinemia, accounts for a substantial portion of cases of type I MPGN.

Types I and II idiopathic MPGN are clinically indistinguishable. Typically, asymptomatic hematuria and proteinuria are discovered incidentally. Judging from the chronicity found on initial renal biopsies, MPGN probably goes undetected for long periods in most patients. Although it is characteristically a chronic low-grade nephropathy, some patients experience complicated nephrotic syndrome and even rapidly progressive and crescentic disease phases.

NEPHRITIC FACTORS

Patients with type II MPGN, and to a lesser extent type I, exhibit a complement-activating antibody called nephritic factor.[16] The typical nephritic factor is an IgG autoantibody that binds to the alternative pathway convertase called C3b,Bb. Nephritic factor stabilizes and prolongs the activity of the enzyme by interfering with normal factors controlling the convertase activity. This leads to sustained activation and

▌ KEY CONCEPTS

MEMBRANOUS NEPHROPATHY

>> Common cause of idiopathic nephrotic syndrome in adults

>> Several secondary causes: systemic lupus, drugs, chronic hepatitis, certain malignancies

>> One-quarter of patients have spontaneous remission

>> One-quarter of patients develop ESRD within a decade

>> Protracted nephrotic syndrome confers risks of cardiovascular and thromboembolic events

>> Therapy: steroids, alkylating agents, lipid-lowering drugs, angiotensin antagonists

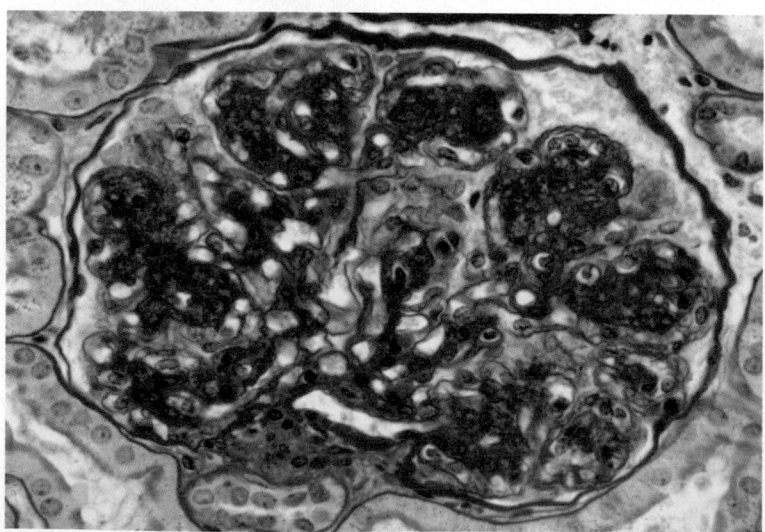

Fig. 67.6 Membranoproliferative glomerulonephritis (MPGN). Glomerulus exhibits the typical lobulated appearance of this disease. Markedly increased mesangial cells and matrix in all of the lobules. Mesangium extends outward into the capillary loops and forms double contours with the glomerular basement membrane. (PAS stain.)

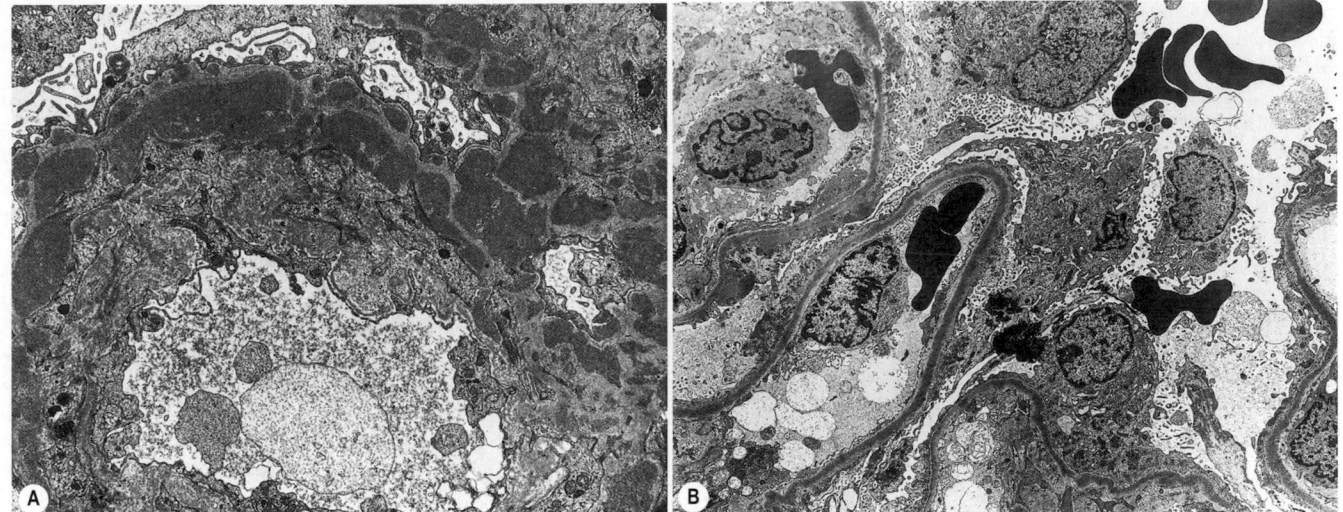

Fig. 67.7 Membranoproliferative glomerulonephritis (MPGN) ultrastructure. (**A**) Type I MPGN: capillary wall is markedly thickened and contains heavy, dark-staining electron dense immune complexes in the subendothelial space. Mesangium (lighter material) extends into the capillary loop, where it is interposed between the basement membrane and the endothelium; the process gives the appearance of a massively thickened capillary loop on hematoxylin and eosin staining, and the split appearance by PAS and silver stains. (**B**) Type II MPGN (dense intramembranous deposit disease): capillary loops contain smooth, continuous linear dense material within the basement membrane. (Electron micrographs courtesy of Dr S. Sabnis, Armed Forces Institute of Pathology; Washington, DC.)

severe depletion of serum C3 levels, which is a hallmark of MPGN. Whether or how C3 nephritic factor plays a role in the pathogenesis of either form of MPGN is unknown. Interestingly, in type II MPGN there are no immunoglobulin components in the dense intramembranous deposits, although there are heavy linear deposits of C3 complement, possibly indicating an effect of the prolonged C3 activation.

TREATMENT

There is no consensus about the treatment of MPGN. The overwhelming opinion is that no therapy is effective in inducing remission or in protecting against progressive renal failure. Overall, renal survival is approximately 50% at 10 years from diagnosis, although a subset of patients have a rapidly progressive course if they develop superimposed crescentic glomerulonephritis. Alternate-day prednisone is commonly tried in children with MPGN, but no controlled trials are available and the long-term prognosis remains unfavorable. The efficacy of cytotoxic drug therapy, anticoagulants, and anti-platelet drugs are similarly unproven. Both forms of MPGN tend to recur in renal allografts; recurrences of both types of MPGN have a detrimental effect on graft survival.

POSTINFECTIOUS NEPHROPATHIES

An ever-expanding list of infectious agents has been implicated in the pathogenesis of immune-mediated nephropathies.[17] Some are acute and self-limited, but many of the nephritogenic infections are protracted and are associated with circulating immune complexes, cryoglobulins, high-titer rheumatoid factor, and hypocomplementemia.

KEY CONCEPTS

MEMBRANOPROLIFERATIVE GLOMERULONEPHRITIS (MPGN)

>> Rare form of chronic nephritis mostly discovered as asymptomatic hematuria, variable proteinuria and/or insidious chronic renal insufficiency

>> Type I MPGN: subendothelial immune complex deposits

>> Type II MPGN: dense intramembranous deposits (containing C3 complement)

>> Hypocomplementemia associated with C3 nephritic factor, an autoantibody to C3 convertase of the alternative complement pathway

>> Response to immunosuppressive drug treatment generally poor

>> Both types MPGN tend to recur in renal allografts

VIRAL INFECTIONS

HEPATITIS B

Chronic hepatitis B virus (HBV) has been associated with membranous nephropathy, membranoproliferative glomerulonephritis, and polyarteritis nodosa.[18] The available evidence suggests that HBV-associated nephropathy is immune-complex mediated. Nearly all patients with chronic HBV have HBsAg, anti-HBc antibodies and elevated serum aminotransferase levels. Serum C3 and C4 are reduced in some patients.

Hepatitis B-associated nephropathy most frequently presents as nephrotic syndrome accompanied by microscopic hematuria; only rarely is there evidence of renal functional impairment or progressive liver disease on presentation. Renal biopsy most commonly shows membranous nephropathy; membranoproliferative glomerulonephritis is less common in HBV-associated renal disease. Immunofluorescence studies usually show immunoglobulin, C3 and viral antigens, particularly HBsAg and HBeAg. Electron microscopy shows subepithelial and intramembranous deposits, but unlike in idiopathic membranous nephropathy there may also be mesangial and even some subendothelial deposits.

Therapy for hepatitis B renal disease has focused on antiviral drugs, as glucocorticoids and cytotoxic agents may promote viral replication. Currently, the three drugs approved for hepatitis B infection in adults are recombinant human IFN-α, lamivudine and adefovir. IFN-α has been shown to produce remission of both liver and kidney disease. Lamivudine should be used for at least 1 year, and continued for at least 6 months after HBeAg seroconversion. Adefovir has been evaluated as monotherapy for adults with chronic hepatitis B infection and those resistant to lamivudine.

HEPATITIS C

Hepatitis C virus (HCV) is a major cause of both transfusion-associated and sporadic chronic hepatitis. Persistent infection occurs in approximately 50% of patients and may result in chronic active hepatitis, cirrhosis, cryoglobulinemia, and MPGN. The pathogenesis of the renal disease is unknown, but may relate to deposition within glomeruli of immune complexes containing HCV, anti-HCV antibody and virus-related (or unrelated) cryoglobulins.

Treatment of hepatitis C focuses on antiviral drugs.[19] Combination therapy with IFN-α and ribavirin can be effective in reducing viral replication and improving renal and liver disease. Rituximab and plasma exchange are currently under investigation for the treatment of patients with severe refractory cryoglobulin-related renal disease or vasculitis.

HUMAN IMMUNODEFICIENCY VIRUS (HIV)

Patients with the acquired immunodeficiency syndrome (AIDS) develop a wide variety of renal abnormalities, including focal segmental glomerulosclerosis and drug-induced interstitial nephritis.[20] Black patients and intravenous drug abusers are more likely to develop an aggressive form of glomerular disease, currently designated HIV-associated nephropathy (HIVAN). HIVAN is characterized by focal segmental glomerulosclerosis (collapsing type) with extensive tubular ectasia and interstitial fibrosis. Treatment with highly active antiretroviral therapies has somewhat ameliorated the otherwise poor renal prognosis of HIVAN, although complications of the drug therapy itself have been observed. The use of standard immunosuppressive drug therapies for HIVAN is controversial.

■ BACTERIAL INFECTIONS ■

POST-STREPTOCOCCAL GLOMERULONEPHRITIS

Post-streptococcal glomerulonephritis is the result of skin or throat infection with nephritogenic strains of group A streptococci. Nephritic syndrome characteristically appears around 2 weeks after the infection. Whereas the role of streptococcal infection in causing the disease is widely accepted, the demonstration of streptococcal antigens and antibodies in glomeruli has been controversial.

Post-streptococcal glomerulonephritis is characterized by a nephritic syndrome consisting of smoky or rust-colored urine, generalized edema, hypertension, and nephritic urine sediment. Proteinuria is typically mild. Patients have rising titers of anti-streptolysin and depressed C3 levels early in nephritis but normal or minimally depressed C4 levels, indicating activation of the alternative complement pathway.

Complete clinical resolution of nephritis is the rule, and therefore renal biopsy is not usually indicated in children. In adults, biopsy is often necessary for diagnosis. Proliferative glomerulonephritis with polymorphonuclear leukocyte and monocyte infiltration, granular immune deposits of IgG and C3, and dome-shaped electron-dense subepithelial deposits (humps) are characteristic. The prognosis is excellent: almost all children will recover with supportive care. Progressive renal failure accompanied by severe hypertension appears to be more common in adults.

GLOMERULONEPHRITIS ASSOCIATED WITH FOCAL INFECTIONS

Renal disease has been associated with infective endocarditis, infection of artificial vascular devices, and localized chronic abscesses. A variety of organisms have been implicated in the pathogenesis of renal disease, which seems to be immune-complex mediated. Overlap with renal vasculitic diseases is common. Renal biopsy findings in fulminant infections resemble those of acute post-streptococcal glomerulonephritis. In subacute forms (e.g., endocarditis), focal segmental proliferative glomerulonephritis is more common. The course and prognosis are variable. Antibiotic therapy in most cases is associated with improvement in the renal lesions.

SYPHILIS

Nephropathy may occur in both congenital and acquired syphilis. In acquired syphilis the nephropathy usually becomes apparent during the secondary phase of the infection. Most patients present with nephrotic syndrome and have secondary membranous nephropathy on renal biopsy. Patients with concurrently positive syphilis serologies and antinuclear antibodies may have lupus-related rather than syphilis-associated membranous nephropathy. Following the institution of antimicrobial therapy most, but not all, patients with syphilis-associated nephropathy recover.

■ PARASITIC DISEASES ■

SCHISTOSOMIASIS

Schistosomal infections affect millions of patients in tropical countries. Nephropathy usually occurs after the development of the chronic hepatosplenic infection with *Schistosoma mansoni* and is characterized by proteinuria, hypertension and chronic renal failure. Renal biopsy usually demonstrates focal segmental glomerulosclerosis or membranoproliferative glomerulonephritis. Long-standing schistosomiasis rarely produces secondary renal amyloidosis. Treatment of the underlying schistosomiasis or the nephropathy with corticosteroids and immunosuppressive therapy do not seem to affect the progression of the schistosomiasis-associated nephropathy.

IgA NEPHROPATHY

Idiopathic IgA nephropathy (also known as Berger's disease) is among the most common forms of glomerular disease in many parts of the world, especially southern Europe, Australia and Asia.[21] The high frequency of IgA nephropathy in these countries appears partly to reflect widespread routine screening of healthy schoolchildren and military recruits for urinary abnormalities, and frequent use of renal biopsy to evaluate asymptomatic, isolated hematuria. Renal histologic features and aspects of immunopathogenesis are comparable to those of Henoch–Schönlein nephritis.[22]

CLINICAL FEATURES

IgA nephropathy may affect patients of all ages, especially children and young adults, with a male preponderance. Unexplained is the fact that IgA nephropathy is rare in black patients. This observation and examples of familial clustering of IgA nephropathy favor an important element of genetic susceptibility. IgA nephropathy may be discovered as asymptomatic microscopic hematuria. Alternatively, patients (especially children) may present with recurrent episodes of macroscopic hematuria that occur within 24–48 hours after an intercurrent infection, usually an upper respiratory or gastrointestinal tract infection. A transient elevation in serum creatinine has been associated with macroscopic hematuria in about one-third of cases. This has been attributed to tubular injury and obstruction caused by intraluminal red blood cell casts. An episode of macroscopic hematuria is occasionally associated with extensive cellular crescent formation, rapidly deteriorating renal function, hypertension and nephrotic syndrome.

NATURAL HISTORY

IgA nephropathy typically has a benign renal prognosis. However, it is recognized that at least one-third of patients with IgA nephropathy eventually progress to end-stage kidney failure. Twenty years after apparent disease onset the probability of renal failure is 25%, and the probability of some renal dysfunction is 50%. Hypertension occurs frequently as the disease progresses and forebodes a poor prognosis.

Other clinical features that have been associated with a poor prognosis include older age at apparent disease onset, persistent proteinuria (>1 g/day), and persistent azotemia. On renal biopsy evaluation extensive cellular crescents, endocapillary proliferation, and extension of immune deposits to the peripheral glomerular capillary walls are indicative of severe immune-mediated glomerulonephritis and a poor prognosis. Evidence of irreversible renal parenchymal injury (glomerular sclerosis, interstitial fibrosis and tubular atrophy) also identifies high-risk patients.

TREATMENT

The treatment of progressive IgA nephropathy remains undefined.[23, 24] Angiotensin antagonists are recommended to achieve blood pressure control, to reduce proteinuria, and to slow the rate of deterioration of renal function. There are conflicting data about the value of fish oil dietary supplements (eicosanoids) in preventing renal progression in patients with IgA nephropathy. The risk–benefit of corticosteroids is unclear, but these agents are generally used in patients with persistent proteinuria >1 g/day despite maximally tolerated angiotensin antagonist therapies. Cytotoxic drugs are indicated in a small subset of patients with crescentic rapidly progressive IgA glomerulonephritis.

HENOCH–SCHÖNLEIN NEPHRITIS

Henoch–Schönlein purpura (HSP) is a generalized vasculitis that usually affects children and typically involves the skin, joints, kidneys and gastrointestinal tract. Classic Henoch–Schönlein disease, manifested as

---

KEY CONCEPTS
INFECTIOUS-RELATED NEPHROPATHIES

>> *Viral:* Hepatitis B – membranous nephropathy; hepatitis *C* – cryoglobulinemic membranoproliferative glomerulonephritis; HIV – focal segmental glomerulosclerosis (HIV nephropathy)

>> *Bacterial (mainly gram-positive):* Nephritogenic streptococcal infections, prosthetic device (shunt) infections, subacute bacterial endocarditis, chronic deep tissue abscesses – mainly diffuse or focal proliferative glomerulonephritis; secondary syphilis – membranous nephropathy

>> *Parasitic:* Schistosomiasis mansoni (chronic hepatosplenic form) – focal segmental glomerulosclerosis and membranoproliferative glomerulonephritis

>> Effective control of renal disease in most conditions (except perhaps schistosomiasis) depends on eradication of the organism; immunosuppressive or anti-inflammatory drug therapies are rarely indicated

---

KEY CONCEPTS
IgA NEPHRITIS

>> Common cause of asymptomatic microscopic hematuria, recurrent macroscopic hematuria, and/or low-grade proteinuria

>> Spectrum of disease, including idiopathic IgA nephritis and Henoch–Schönlein purpura nephritis; IgA in skin and renal biopsies

>> Mostly benign prognosis, especially in children

>> Patients with progressive renal insufficiency and/or crescentic glomerulonephritis warrant trial of glucocorticoids and/or cytotoxic drug therapy

purpuric rash with features of joint, kidney and/or gastrointestinal involvement, is readily recognized. Characteristic skin and renal biopsy findings may support the diagnosis. Skin biopsies reveal leukocytoclastic vasculitis with granular deposits of IgA along dermal vessels of purpuric and uninvolved skin.

Whereas in most patients the disease remits spontaneously, some patients develop serious renal and/or gastrointestinal complications. Evidence of immune complex causation has prompted recommendations for immunosuppressive treatment of severe Henoch–Schönlein nephritis, but the data are uncontrolled and controversial.

CLINICAL FEATURES

Urinary abnormalities were seen in about one-third of a largely unselected sample of children with Henoch–Schönlein purpura. Microscopic hematuria is detected in nearly all cases of Henoch–Schönlein nephritis, and is accompanied by variable proteinuria in more than 90% of cases. Approximately 40% of patients reported from referral centers had nephrotic-range proteinuria, and in two-thirds of those there were complicating features, including various combinations of hypertension, azotemia, and hypoproteinemia. Renal biopsy findings range from mild mesangial proliferation to crescentic glomerulonephritis. Immune deposits are predominantly mesangial and characteristically contain IgA.

NATURAL HISTORY

Most patients with Henoch–Schönlein nephritis follow a relatively benign clinical course. The probability of maintaining life-supporting renal function is nearly 90% at 10 years. It is debated whether adults are at greater risk for renal failure than children. Patients who present with microscopic hematuria without proteinuria rarely progress to renal failure. Approximately 80% of patients who initially manifest hematuria and proteinuria have normal renal function with little or no urinary abnormality after extended observation; another 10% are likely to progress to renal failure. Patients who present with proteinuria >1 g/day, impaired renal function and hypertension are at considerable risk for end-stage kidney failure. The renal biopsy also provides useful prognostic information. Widespread cellular crescents, interstitial fibrosis and tubular atrophy portend an increased risk of renal failure.[25]

THERAPY

Decisions regarding the treatment of Henoch–Schönlein nephritis are made difficult by a lack of compelling data from prospective randomized therapeutic trials and by the highly unpredictable nature of this disease. Corticosteroids and cytotoxic drugs should be reserved for the high-risk patients described above. Pulse intravenous methylprednisolone seems to offer additional benefit. Uncontrolled observations also suggest that azathioprine, cyclosporine, plasma exchange, anticoagulants, dipyridamole and urokinase may be useful, but additional studies are needed. Renal transplantation is a reasonable option for patients who progress to terminal renal failure, provided the disease has been in remission for several months preoperatively.

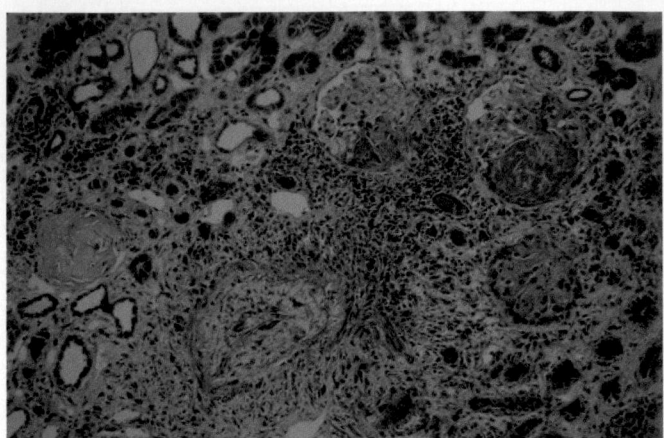

Fig. 67.8 Renal vasculitis showing both glomerular and arteriolar lesions. Small renal vessel shows healing arteritis with proliferation, edema, and fibrosis which severely compromise the lumen. Lesions in the four glomeruli include segmental fibrinoid necrosis (upper right), cellular crescent (lower right) and hyalinized glomerulus (middle left). Tubular atrophy and interstitial fibrosis are prominent. (Masson stain. Micrograph courtesy of Dr S. Sabnis, Armed Forces Institute of Pathology; Washington, DC.)

■ NEPHROPATHIES ASSOCIATED WITH ANTI-NEUTROPHIL CYTOPLASMIC ANTIBODIES (CLASSIC POLYARTERITIS, MICROSCOPIC POLYANGIITIS, WEGENER'S GRANULOMATOSIS, AND IDIOPATHIC NECROTIZING CRESCENTIC GLOMERULONEPHRITIS) ■

Systemic vasculitis is covered in detail in Chapters 58 and 59. This discussion is limited to the renal components of the major vasculitic syndromes.

CLINICAL AND PATHOLOGIC FEATURES

Renal involvement is common in the systemic vasculitides but varies in type and severity. In classic polyarteritis nodosa the vasculitis affects mainly arteries outside the glomerulus, producing ischemia, hypertension, segmental infarctions, and renal failure. In microscopic polyangiitis, Wegener's granulomatosis and renal-limited necrotizing and crescentic glomerulonephritis, the vasculitis occurs mainly within the glomerulus. The glomerular abnormalities are similar among these groups (Fig. 67.8). The lesions are characteristically focal and segmental in distribution, with fibrinoid necrosis and crescent formation but few, if any, immune deposits (some use the term pauci-immune glomerulonephritis). Clinically, rapidly progressive glomerulonephritis is a common manifestation of these renal vasculitides, making early detection of glomerulonephritis critically important in management.

Table 67.2 Prevalence of ANCA in renal vasculitis

Type of renal vasculitis	ANCA test positivity (%)	
	P-ANCA or Anti-MPO	C-ANCA or Anti-PR3
Polyarteritis nodosa	10-20	10-20
Microscopic polyangiitis	50-80	10-20
Wegener's granulomatosis	10-20	80-90
Necrotizing and crescentic GN	50-80	10-20

MPO = myeloperoxidase; PR3 = proteinase 3

KEY CONCEPTS

RENAL VASCULITIS

>> Renal vasculitis with glomerular involvement includes microscopic polyangiitis, Wegener's granulomatosis, and necrotizing crescentic glomerulonephritis (renal-limited vasculitis)

>> Associated with anti-neutrophil cytoplasmic antibodies (ANCA)

>> Rapidly progressive glomerulonephritis is common; early treatment includes pulse methylprednisolone, cyclophosphamide (possibly adjunctive plasma exchange)

>> Maintenance therapy: azathioprine, mycophenolate, methotrexate

Another common feature of the renal vasculitides is the presence of autoantibodies to neutrophil cytoplasmic antigens. As shown in Table 67.2, microscopic polyangiitis, Wegener's granulomatosis and idiopathic necrotizing crescentic glomerulonephritis all express anti-neutrophil cytoplasmic antibodies (ANCA), but in somewhat different patterns. There is a strong correlation between the presence of ANCA and glomerular involvement in systemic vasculitis. Recent murine models with anti-myeloperoxidase antibodies have demonstrated the role of ANCA in the pathogenesis of the vasculitic diseases.[26]

TREATMENT AND PROGNOSIS

Renal vasculitis tends to be severe and fulminant. Even with early diagnosis, approximately one-third of patients will progress to renal failure within 5 years. Relapsing courses are common in patients with microscopic polyangiitis, and particularly Wegener's granulomatosis. Glucocorticoids are important in the early treatment of renal vasculitis, but their efficacy is limited and maintenance should include alternate-day therapy whenever possible.

In patients with severe pulmonary hemorrhage or rapidly progressive glomerulonephritis due to renal vasculitis, pulse methylprednisolone followed by prednisone and daily cyclophosphamide are clearly indicated. Adjunctive plasma exchange is commonly used in cases of aggressive pulmonary–renal syndrome.

Although controversial, some recent experience indicates that intermittent pulse cyclophosphamide may be substituted for daily cyclophosphamide in order to reduce the toxicity of extended therapy in ANCA-associated glomerulonephritis. Wegener's granulomatosis is generally considered an exception, in which case most investigators advocate daily cyclophosphamide for remission induction therapy with conversion to azathioprine, mycophenolate, or methotrexate for maintenance. Cyclosporine has not proved to be an effective alternative to conventional cytotoxic drug therapy, either as primary therapy or in preventing renal relapse following kidney transplantation. Pilot studies of anti-TNF-α therapy have not shown promising results in the treatment of patients with systemic vasculitis.[27]

ANTI-GBM ANTIBODY-MEDIATED NEPHRITIS: GOODPASTURE'S DISEASE

Goodpasture's disease is a rare but classic immune-mediated cause of severe pulmonary–renal syndrome.[28] Its essential components include pulmonary hemorrhage and rapidly progressive glomerulonephritis, both of which are characteristically (but not universally) fulminant. The cardinal pathogenic factor is autoantibody to a component of type IV collagen present in the capillary basement membranes of the lung and kidney; this IgG factor is called anti-glomerular basement membrane (anti-GBM) antibody because glomerular antigens are normally used for its detection in immunoassays.

The genesis of anti-GBM antibodies in sporadic cases is unknown. Iatrogenic cases have occurred when normal kidneys have been transplanted into patients with hereditary Alport's nephropathy (who lack normal Goodpasture antigen and tolerance thereto); thus, recipients mount an anti-GBM antibody response to the new donor Goodpasture antigen. It appears that anti-GBM antibodies are expressed for a limited duration (weeks to months) in sporadic cases of Goodpasture's disease. This is of little consolation because of the devastating nature of the disease during the height of the pulmonary–renal syndrome. Hence, aggressive treatments with pulse methylprednisolone, cyclophosphamide and plasma exchange are indicated early in the course of Goodpasture's disease. Reversibility of renal disease is unlikely if renal function is substantially impaired or oliguria ensues before treatment is begun. Immunosuppressive treatment is normally continued until the

KEY CONCEPTS

GOODPASTURE'S DISEASE

>> Circulating anti-GBM antibody

>> Pulmonary hemorrhage: treated mostly with pulse methylprednisolone

>> Rapidly progressive glomerulonephritis with cellular crescents and linear deposits of IgG: treated with high-dose steroids, cyclophosphamide, plasma exchange

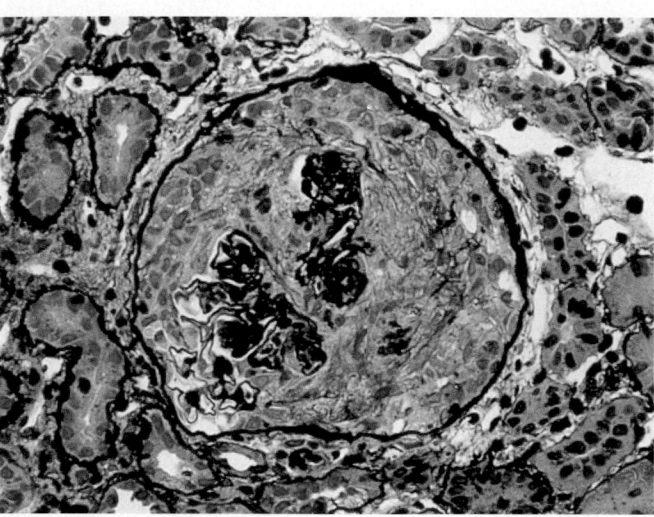

Fig. 67.9 Goodpasture's disease. Circumferential cellular crescent fills Bowman's capsule and compresses the glomerular tuft. (Silver stain.)

patient has been in sustained clinical remission and anti-GBM titers are minimal or absent for at least 3 months.

◼ LUPUS NEPHRITIS (CHAPTER 51) ◼

Glomerular disease affects the majority of patients with SLE, but lupus nephritis has a wide spectrum of disease expression and outcomes among different patient populations; in particular, lupus nephritis generally exhibits a substantially more ominous prognosis and a poorer response to treatment in black patients than in white patients. Nephritis is a major cause of morbidity and mortality, and accounts for a large portion of all hospital admissions in lupus patients. The majority experience chronic renal disease with remissions and exacerbations. Patients rarely enter permanent remission or achieve complete cure of SLE.

PATHOGENESIS

Several different mechanisms appear to be involved in the pathogenesis of lupus nephritis, resulting in a wide spectrum of renal lesions. Deposition of immune complexes from the circulation into the kidney appears to be the initiating event in proliferative lupus nephritis; however, only a subset of immune complexes appears to be nephritogenic. DNA and anti-DNA antibodies are known to be concentrated in glomerular deposits in the subendothelial location and are likely to play a central role in the pathogenesis of proliferative lupus nephritis. Unfortunately, there are fewer insights into the pathogenesis of lupus membranous nephropathy with its characteristic epimembranous immune deposits. Although T cells are almost certainly involved in autoantibody production, it is unknown whether they have a direct role in the pathogenesis of lupus nephritis.

CLINICAL FEATURES

Asymptomatic hematuria or proteinuria may be the presenting features, but they often progress to nephritic and/or nephrotic syndromes.[29] Nephrotic syndrome is seen in both severe proliferative and membranous forms of lupus nephritis. Hypertension, azotemia, nephritic urine sediment (with hematuria and cellular casts), hypocomplementemia and high anti-dsDNA titers are more commonly found in patients with proliferative lupus nephritis. Rapidly progressive glomerulonephritis is usually associated with the appearance of cellular crescents and may be superimposed on severe proliferative or membranous forms of lupus nephritis.

DIAGNOSIS

Proper evaluation of the urinary sediment is very helpful in assessing and monitoring renal disease activity. Active glomerulonephritis is indicated by hematuria (with dysmorphic erythrocytes) as well as cellular casts. Broad and/or waxy casts indicate long-standing or advanced glomerulonephritis. Serum complement levels (especially C3 and C4) have been found to correlate with activity of glomerular disease on renal biopsy. Falling levels of complement components may indicate a flare of lupus nephritis; other tests (including anti-dsDNA antibodies) are less reliable. Therapeutic decisions should not be based on serologic tests alone, because none of these tests have adequate sensitivity or specificity to justify treatment decisions. Renal biopsy is indicated only if the patient has laboratory evidence of urinary abnormalities.

The former World Health Organization (WHO) classification of renal biopsy in lupus nephritis has recently been revised by an international committee (Figs 67.9–67.12).[30] A summary of the histologic features in each class of lupus nephritis can be found in Table 67.3.

TREATMENT

Treatment of mesangial lupus nephritis is usually not indicated unless protein excretion exceeds 2 g/day. However, the distinction between early mesangial lesions that are in transition to more ominous classes from those that reflect mild and stable nephropathy is difficult. Patients with focal or diffuse proliferative glomerulonephritis and a relative paucity of activity and/or chronicity features on renal biopsy may benefit from oral glucocorticoids or monthly pulses of intravenous methylprednisolone. A prolonged course of intravenous cyclophosphamide pulses is more efficacious than pulses of methylprednisolone in patients with severe focal or diffuse proliferative nephritis.[31] Plasmapheresis does not offer any significant advantage over cytotoxic therapy. Controlled studies have shown that intermittent pulse cyclophosphamide is more efficacious than either high-dose conventional prednisone or extended courses of pulse methylprednisolone.[32, 33] In general, treatment should continue for at least 1 year after remission of renal disease to prevent exacerbations. Recent short-term studies have shown that mycophenolate is equivalent to cyclophosphamide for both induction and maintenance therapy in lupus nephritis.[34–36]

Neither pulse cyclophosphamide nor mycophenolate is universally effective in the management of lupus nephritis, hence the search for more efficacious alternative treatment regimens, including rituximab, immunoablation without or with stem cell reconstitution, and immunological co-stimulation inhibitors (e.g., CTLA4-Ig), continues.

No definitive therapeutic guidelines have been established for lupus membranous nephropathy. High-dose alternate-day glucocorticoids,

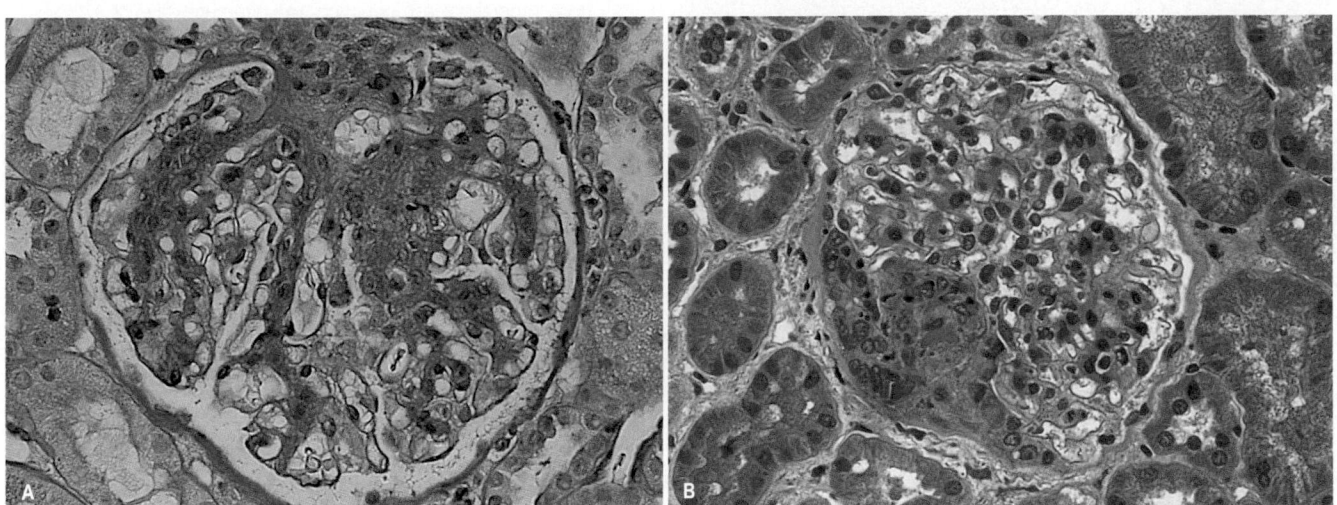

Fig. 67.10 Classes of the pathology of lupus nephritis (1). (**A**) Class II, mesangial proliferative lupus nephritis. Mesangial areas are expanded by cells and matrix but the peripheral capillary loops remain widely patent. PAS stain. (**B**) Class III, focal lupus nephritis. Solid lesion at the lower right portion of this glomerulus demonstrates segmental fibrinoid necrosis. Note the nuclear fragments (karyorrhexis) in the fibrinous exudate. (Hematoxylin and eosin stain.)

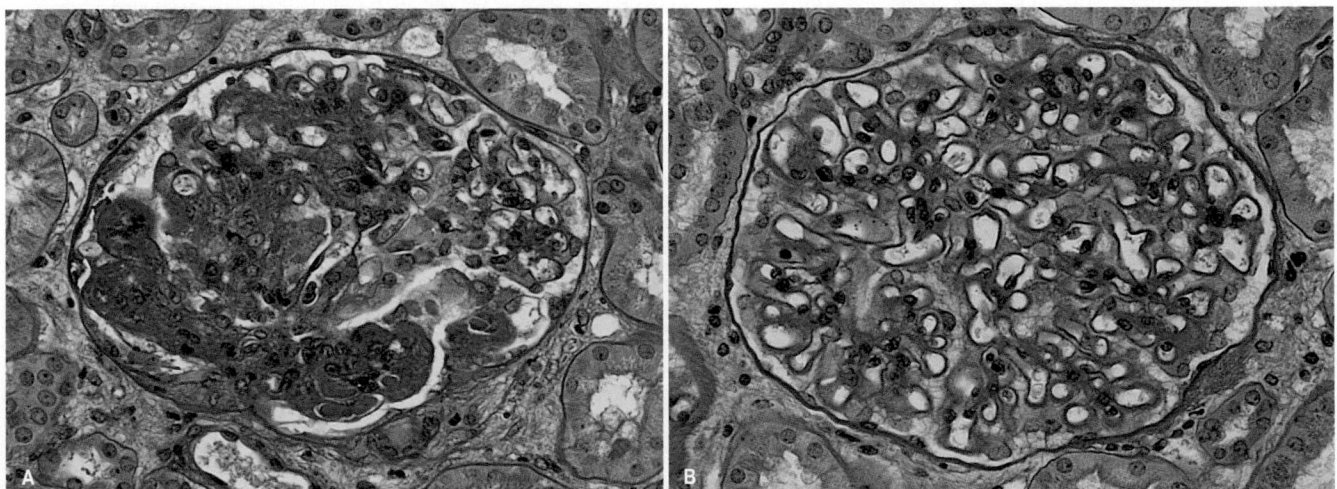

Fig. 67.11 Classes of the pathology of lupus nephritis (2). (**A**) Class IV, diffuse lupus nephritis. Glomerulus with irregular but nearly global changes including obliteration of many capillary loops due to endocapillary hypercellularity, 'wire loop' thickening and hyaline thrombi. (PAS stain.) (**B**) Class V, membranous lupus nephritis. Glomerulus shows minimally increase mesangial cellularity with thickened but widely patent capillary loops. (PAS stain.)

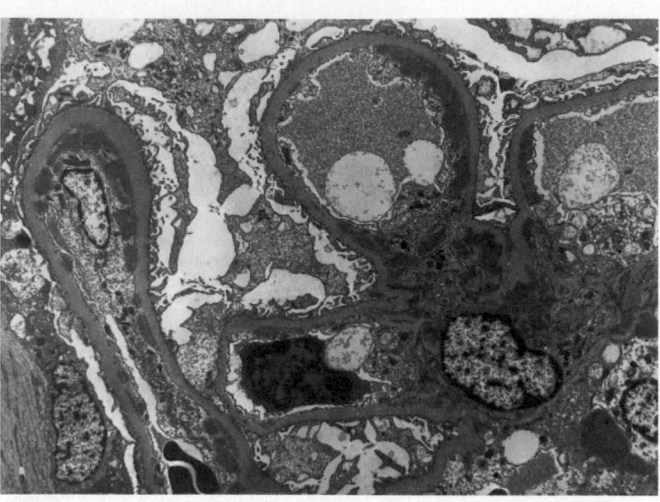

Fig. 67.12 Ultrastructure of proliferative lupus nephritis. Electron micrograph demonstrates the characteristic mesangial deposits (dark materials interspersed within the centrally located amorphous, gray mesangial matrix) and subendothelial deposits (dark materials extending along the peripheral capillary loops).

KEY CONCEPTS

LUPUS NEPHRITIS

>> Class II, mesangial: no treatment indicated unless transforms to class III or IV disease

>> Class III, focal nephritis and class IV, diffuse nephritis: high-dose prednisone for induction with alternate-day maintenance with adjunctive immunosuppressive therapy options of: (a) pulse cyclophosphamide or (b) mycophenolate mofetil; azathioprine may be used as more cost effective maintenance therapy

>> Membranous nephropathy: alternate-day prednisone with bimonthly pulse cyclophosphamide or low-dose daily cyclosporine

Table 67.3 International Society of Nephrology/Renal Pathology Society 2004 Classification of Lupus Nephritis

Class	Histologic features/comments
I. Minimal mesangial	Normal light microscopy (LM); mesangial deposits by immunofluorescence (IF) and electron microscopy (EM)
II. Mesangial proliferative	Pure mesangial hypercellularity and matrix expansion; *IF and EM:* mesangial immune deposits
III. Focal	Glomerular capillary obliteration in < 50% of nephrons owing to proliferation or sclerosis; *LM:* Increased numbers of mesangial, endothelial and/or hematogenous cells. Active inflammatory lesions (karyorrhexis, fibrinoid necrosis, adhesion to Bowman's capsule, cellular crescents, interstitial inflammatory infiltrates). Wire loop lesions. Hyaline thrombi; *IF and EM:* Mesangial and peripheral capillary loop (subendothelial) immune complex deposits
IV. Diffuse	Qualitatively similar histologic lesions as in class III. Glomerular capillary obliteration involving > 50% of nephrons. Subsets defined as primarily global (class IV-G) or primarily segmental (class IV-S) involvement
V. Membranous	*LM:* Regular thickening of the peripheral capillary loops of the glomerulus. Mesangial expansion; *EM:* Subepithelial, intramembranous, mesangial (but no or very rare subendothelial) immune complex deposits
VI. Advanced sclerosis	More than 90% global sclerosis without residual active lesions

cyclophosphamide, and cyclosporine have been used, with mixed results. Preliminary results of a prospective controlled trial indicate that both cyclophosphamide and cyclosporine are more effective than steroids alone in inducing complete remission of proteinuria in lupus membranous nephropathy.[37]

SCLERODERMA (SYSTEMIC SCLEROSIS) (CHAPTER 55)

Renal disease occurs in the diffuse form of systemic sclerosis and is a major cause of morbidity and mortality in these patients.[38] Patients with early (within the first year of disease onset) renal disease may experience rapidly progressive disease and early death. Acute scleroderma renal crisis

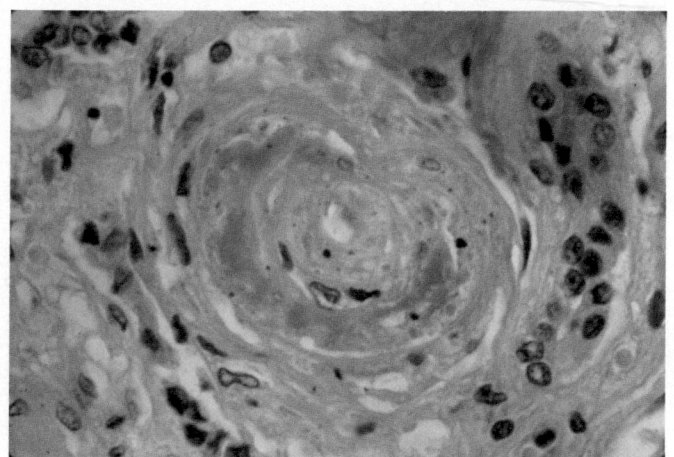

Fig. 67.13 Scleroderma renal crisis. Renal arteriole demonstrates extensive fibrin deposition (dark material) within multiple layers of its wall. The lumen is further compromised by severe swelling and intimal hyperplasia. (Masson trichrome stain.)

is particularly ominous. Proteinuria, urine sediment abnormalities (hematuria or pyuria), hypertension and renal insufficiency are clinical markers of renal disease. Renal disease is more common in the first 5 years of the disease, especially if there is rapid progression of skin disease. A significant decrease in renal function, proteinuria in excess of 500 mg/day, or urinary sediment abnormalities should alert the physician. Plasma renin activity increases with the onset of renal injury, but there is no convincing evidence that the rise precedes the onset of scleroderma renal crisis.

Scleroderma renal crisis is characterized by renin-mediated malignant hypertension, rapid deterioration of renal function, and proteinuria (usually nonnephrotic). The primary pathogenic process appears to be a renal vasculopathy involving predominantly the interlobular arteries and arterioles. Marked intimal thickening with an attendant 'mucoid' appearance, and fibrinoid necrosis in the absence of vasculitis, are common and characteristic of the disease (Fig. 67.13). Immune deposits are rarely observed by fluorescence or electron microscopy studies.

Although a variety of treatments have been proposed for patients with scleroderma, none has been proved to be consistently efficacious. The most significant therapeutic advance in the treatment of renal involvement is the use of angiotensin antagonists, which have dramatically increased the 1-year survival of patients with scleroderma renal crisis. Despite this initial improvement, approximately half will subsequently progress to death or renal failure. Survival of patients undergoing any form of treatment for end-stage renal disease due to scleroderma (hemodialysis, peritoneal dialysis or transplantation) has been poor.

SJÖGREN'S SYNDROME (CHAPTER 54)

A variety of renal manifestations occur in approximately one-third of patients with primary Sjögren's syndrome, including tubular dysfunction (distal or proximal tubular acidosis, nephrogenic diabetes insipidus), nephrocalcinosis, interstitial nephritis, pseudolymphoma, necrotizing vasculitis and glomerulopathy. Mild, nonspecific glomerular changes are common in patients with Sjögren's syndrome. However, overt primary glomerular disease is rare. Membranous nephropathy and proliferative glomerulonephritis (focal or diffuse, and membranoproliferative) have been reported in primary Sjögren's syndrome. In such cases the possibility of overlap with systemic lupus should be considered.

RHEUMATOID ARTHRITIS (CHAPTER 52)

Although early studies described a condition called 'rheumatoid glomerulonephritis,' several investigators have questioned whether a specific rheumatoid nephritis does in fact exist. From a clinical standpoint, renal disease due to drugs used for its therapy, or secondary amyloidosis developing as a result of chronic debilitating disease, are more common.

Membranous nephropathy, formerly seen as a complication of gold or D-penicillamine therapy, is rarely seen during the course of the more commonly used contemporary therapies for rheumatoid arthritis. Mesangial glomerulonephritis has been described in several patients with rheumatoid arthritis who had renal biopsy because of hematuria and/or proteinuria. No consistent type of glomerular disease has been seen, suggesting the possible coincident diseases. However, an association between high titers of rheumatoid factor and the occurrence of mesangial nephritis has been described, leading to the hypothesis that the renal lesion represents a functional response of the mesangium to remove IgM rheumatoid factor–IgG complexes. Proliferative glomerulonephritis is extremely rare and may be found in patients with rheumatoid vasculitis.

RENAL DISEASES IN DYSPROTEINEMIAS AND PARA-PROTEINEMIAS (SEE CHAPTER 78)

MULTIPLE MYELOMA

Multiple myeloma results from a neoplastic proliferation of plasma cells that produce one or more abnormal monoclonal proteins (M-proteins). Abnormal bands of light or heavy chains of immunoglobulin are present

AMYLOIDOSIS

in the urine of 50–70% of patients with myeloma. These paraproteins have a predilection to precipitate in the tubular lumina to produce the so-called cast nephropathy or myeloma kidney. Acute renal failure (precipitated by dehydration or contrast dyes) and chronic renal failure may result from the cast tubulopathy. Distal renal tubular acidosis is also a common manifestation of myeloma protein deposition in renal tubules. Myeloma paraproteins are not detected by urine protein dipstick methods. Urinary protein electrophoresis and immunofixation electrophoresis are critically important for diagnosis.

LIGHT-CHAIN DEPOSITION DISEASE

In this systemic disease, monoclonal immunoglobulin light chains, usually κ type, are commonly deposited in the vessel walls of multiple organs, especially the renal glomeruli. Proteinuria (accompanied by nephrotic syndrome in about 30% of cases), microscopic hematuria, hypertension and progressive renal failure are common. Renal biopsy shows nodular sclerosing glomerulonephritis (Fig. 67.14) similar in light-microscopic appearance to diabetic glomerulosclerosis and amyloidosis. Diagnosis depends on finding monoclonal light chains by immunofluorescence studies of renal biopsy tissue. Treatment with prednisone and alkylating agents may halt or reverse the progression of renal failure. Stem cell transplantation has been successful in advanced cases.[39]

AMYLOIDOSIS

The glomerular and renal vasculature is a common locus for deposition of amyloid fibrils in patients with systemic amyloidosis. Both immunoglobulin-associated (primary, AL) and protein A-associated (secondary, AA) amyloid have been associated with renal involvement.

Proteinuria (often within the nephrotic range) is the most frequent indicator of renal involvement. Hematuria and hypertension are uncommon. Long-standing amyloidosis is regularly accompanied by autonomic neuropathy and postural hypotension. Glomerular involvement is found in all cases of AA amyloidosis, whereas in AL amyloidosis glomerular disease is present in only half of patients.

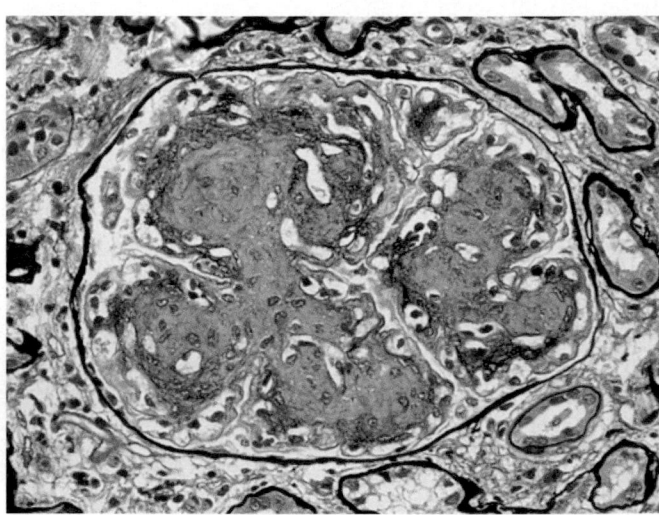

Fig. 67.14 Light-chain nephropathy. Glomerulus has the characteristic appearance of an extrinsic deposition disease. The mesangial areas are filled with pale-staining material which produces a lobular pattern and severely compromises the capillary loops. Immunofluorescence studies are needed to distinguish the light-chain deposits from amyloid infiltration. (Silver stain.)

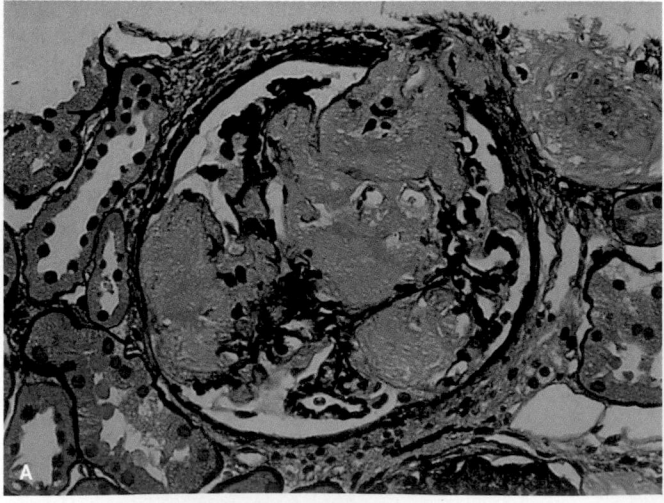

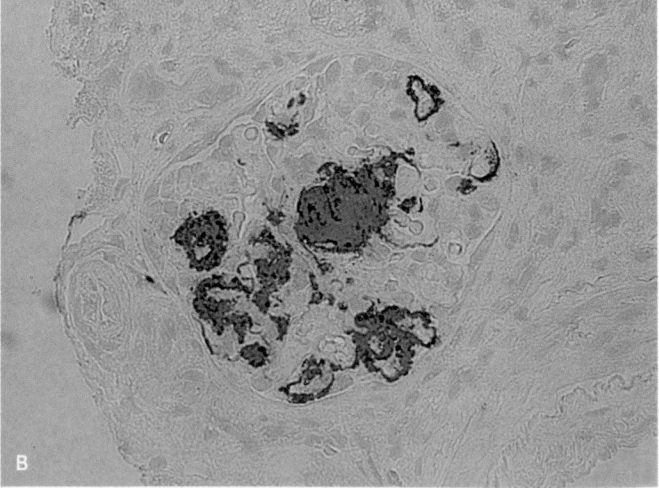

Fig. 67.15 Amyloidosis of the kidney. (**A**) Glomerulus contains nodules of pale-staining amorphous material distorting and compromising the capillary loops. (Silver stain.) (**B**) Immunohistochemistry of glomerular amyloid deposits demonstrated by peroxidase-labeled antibody specific for AA proteins. (Immunoperoxidase technique.)

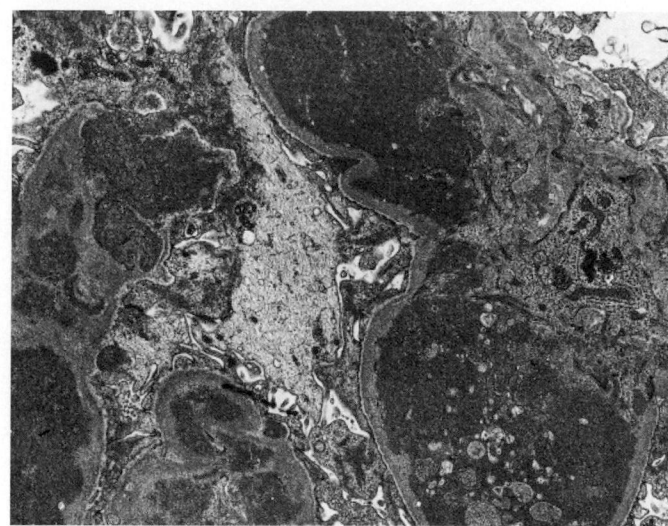

Fig. 67.16 Cryoglobulinemic nephropathy. Electron micrograph demonstrates dense material completely filling the glomerular capillary lumina. On light microscopy these capillary 'plugs' have the appearance of microvascular thrombi, but ultrastructural studies show the crystalline structure of immune aggregates, not fibrin tactoids. (Electron micrographs courtesy of Dr S. Sabnis, Armed Forces Institute of Pathology; Washington, DC.)

Deposition of amyloid protein is recognized by the characteristic staining with metachromatic dyes such as Congo red, which exhibits birefringence on polarized light microscopy. Involvement is typically generalized and diffuse in distribution, and not associated with any significant cellular proliferation or glomerular inflammation (Fig. 67.15)A. Immunohistochemical staining may be used to define the type of amyloid deposit (Fig. 67.15)B. Amyloid deposits initially involve the mesangium, but with disease progression they extend on to the glomerular capillary surfaces (which become markedly and irregularly thickened); this ultimately results in capillary luminal occlusion, glomerular obliteration, and end-stage renal disease. Amyloid deposits are also found in the intrarenal vasculature, resembling hyaline arteriosclerosis on hematoxylin and eosin-stained sections. Electron microscopic findings of fibrillar material of characteristic morphology confirm the diagnosis.

Treatment of primary AL amyloidosis with cytotoxic agents has generally not resulted in a favorable long-term outcome. However, there are some recent very encouraging reports of salutary effects of aggressive cytotoxic drug therapy followed by stem cell reconstitution.[40] For patients with secondary amyloidosis control of the underlying diseases may prevent, stabilize or even reverse this process.[41] Colchicine and anti-tumor necrosis factor therapies can prevent deposition of amyloid if started early in familial Mediterranean fever.

CRYOGLOBULINEMIA

Cryoglobulins (immunoglobulins which reversibly precipitate on cooling) are present in the serum of patients with a wide variety of autoimmune, lymphoproliferative and infectious diseases. Cryoglobulinemia with MPGN is commonly associated with chronic hepatitis C.[42] Essential mixed cryoglobulinemia (ECM) refers to an idiopathic clinical syndrome consisting of recurrent episodes of palpable purpura involving the lower extremities, constitutional symptoms, arthralgias, vasculitis, hepatosplenomegaly, lymphadenopathy, and neuropathy.

Renal complications are common with mixed cryoglobulinemia. A waxing and waning course is characteristic of this disease. Glomerular involvement may develop acutely, particularly after dehydration or exposure to cold, and may be associated with oliguric acute renal failure. Other clinical syndromes may also occur, including nephrotic syndrome, hematuria, renal insufficiency, and chronic or rapidly progressive glomerulonephritis. Deposition of cryoglobulins usually occurs in the glomerular subendothelial space, and these deposits exhibit a unique fibrillar appearance on electron microscopy (Fig. 67.16). The glomerulonephritis is typically membranoproliferative and/or crescentic in nature. Large eosinophilic, PAS-positive intraluminal deposits ('thrombi') are found in more than one-third of patients.

Treatments with combinations of glucocorticoids, cytotoxic drugs, rituximab and plasma exchange have been successful in controlling cryoglobulinemic nephritis. IFN-α has been shown in small, nonrandomized studies to be efficacious even in patients refractory to conventional therapy.[43]

REFERENCES

1. Nangaku M, Couser WG. Mechanisms of immune-deposit formation and the mediation of immune renal injury. Clin Exp Nephrol 2005; 9: 183–191.

2. Rosner MH, Bolton WK. Renal function testing. Am J Kidney Dis 2006; 47: 174–183.

3. Churg J, Bernstein J, Glassock RJ. Renal disease: classification and atlas of glomerular diseases, 2nd edn. New York: Igaku-Shoin, 1995; 1–541.

4. Eddy AA, Symons JM. Nephrotic syndrome in childhood. Lancet 2003; 362: 629–639.

5. Meyrier A. Mechanisms of disease: focal segmental glomerulosclerosis. Nature Clin Pract Nephrol 2005; 1: 44–54.

6. Thomas DB, Franceschini N, Hogan SL et al. Clinical and pathologic characteristics of focal segmental glomerulosclerosis pathologic variants. Kidney Int 2006; 69: 920–926.

7. McCarthy ET, Sharma M, Sharma R, et al. Sera from patients with collapsing focal segmental glomerulosclerosis increase albumin permeability of isolated glomeruli. J Lab Clin Med 2004; 143: 225–229.

8. Johnstone DB, Holzman LB. Clinical impact of research on the podocyte slit diaphragm. Nature Clin Pract Nephrol 2006; 2: 271–282.

9. Cattran DC, Appel GB, Hebert LA, et al. A randomized trial of cyclosporine in patients with steroid-resistant focal segmental glomerulosclerosis: North America Nephrotic Syndrome Study Group. Kidney Int 1999; 56: 2220–2226.

10. Nangaku M, Shankland SJ, Couser WG. Cellular response to injury in membranous nephropathy. J Am Soc Nephrol 2005; 16: 1195–1204.

11. Ronco P, Debiec H. Molecular pathomechanisms of membranous nephropathy: from Heymann nephritis to alloimmunization. J Am Soc Nephrol 2005; 16: 1205–1213.

12. Ponticelli C, Altieri P, Scolari F, et al. A randomized study comparing methylprednisolone plus chlorambucil versus methylprednisolone plus cyclophosphamide in idiopathic membranous nephropathy. J Am Soc Nephrol 1998; 9: 444–450.

13. Cattran DC. Management of membranous nephropathy: when and what for treatment. J Am Soc Nephrol 2005; 16: 1188–1194.

14. Salama AD, Pusey CD. Drug insight: rituximab in renal disease and transplantation. Nature Clin Pract 2006; 2: 221–230.

15. Appel GB, Cook HT, Hageman G, et al. Membranoproliferative glomerulonephritis type II (dense deposit disease): an update. J Am Soc Nephrol 2005; 16: 1392–1403.

16. Walport MJ. Complement. N Engl J Med 2001; 344: 1058–1066.

17. Montseny JJ, Meyrier A, Kleinknecht D, et al. The current spectrum of infectious glomerulonephritis: experience with 76 patients and review of the literature. Medicine (Baltimore) 1995; 74: 63–73.

18. Lai AS, Lai KN. Viral nephropathy. Nature Clin Pract Nephrol 2006; 2: 254–262.

19. Kamar N, Rostaing L, Alric L. Treatment of hepatitis C-virus-related glomerulonephritis. Kidney Int 2006; 69: 436–439.

20. Cho ME, Kopp JB. HIV and the kidney: a status report after 20 years. Curr HIV/AIDS Rep 2004; 1: 109–115.

21. Barratt J, Feehally J. IgA nephropathy. J Am Soc Nephrol 16: 2088–2097.

22. Davin JC, Ten Berge IJ, Weening JJ. What is the difference between IgA nephropathy and Henoch–Schönlein purpura nephritis?. Kidney Int 2001; 59: 823–834.

23. Appel GB, Waldman M. The IgA nephropathy treatment dilemma. Kidney Int 2006; 69: 1939–1944.

24. Locatelli F, Del Vecchio L, Pozzi C. IgA glomerulonephritis: beyond angiotensin-converting enzyme inhibitors. Nature Clin Pract Nephrol 2005; 2: 24–31.

25. Coppo R, Andrulli S, Amore A, et al. Predictors of outcome in Henoch–Schönlein nephritis in children and adults. Am J Kidney Dis 2006; 47: 993–1003.

26. Jennette JC, Xiao H, Falk RJ. Pathogenesis of vascular inflammation by anti-neutrophil cytoplasmic antibodies. J Am Soc Nephrol 2006; 17: 1235–1242.

27. Morgan MD, Harper L, Williams J, et al. Anti-neutrophil cytoplasm-associated glomerulonephritis. J Am Soc Nephrol 2006; 17: 1224–1234.

28. Bolton WK. Goodpasture's syndrome. Kidney Int 1996; 50: 1753–1761.

29. Balow JE. Clinical presentation and monitoring of lupus nephritis. Lupus 2005; 14: 25–30.

30. Weening JJ, D'Agati VD, Schwartz MM, et al. The classification of glomerulonephritis in systemic lupus erythematosus revisited. J Am Soc Nephrol 2004; 15: 241–250.

31. Boumpas DT, Austin HA, Vaughan EM, et al. Controlled trial of pulse methylprednisolone versus two regimens of pulse cyclophosphamide in severe lupus nephritis. Lancet 1992; 340: 741–755.

32. Austin HA, Klippel JH, Balow JE, et al. Therapy of lupus nephritis: controlled trial of prednisone and cytotoxic drugs. N Engl J Med 1986; 314: 614–619.

33. Illei GG, Austin HA, Crane M, et al. Combination therapy with pulse cyclophosphamide plus pulse methylprednisolone improves long-term renal outcome without adding toxicity in lupus nephritis. Ann Intern Med 2001; 135: 248–257.

34. Contreras G, Pardo V, Lecleercq B, et al. Sequential therapies for proliferative lupus nephritis. N Engl J Med 2004; 350: 971–980.

35. Ginzler EM, Dooley MA, Aranow C, et al. Mycophenolate mofetil or intravenous cyclophosphamide for lupus nephritis. N Engl J Med 2005; 353: 2219–2228.

36. Chan TM, Tse KC, Tang CS, et al. Long-term study of mycophenolate mofetil as continuous induction and maintenance treatment for diffuse proliferative lupus nephritis. J Am Soc Nephrol 2005; 16: 1076–1084.

37. Austin HA, Illei GG. Membranous lupus nephritis. Lupus 2005; 14: 65–71.

38. Donohoe JF. Scleroderma and the kidney. Kidney Int 1992; 41: 562–577.

39. Weichman K, Dember LM, Prokaeva T, et al. Clinical and molecular characteristics of patients with nonamyloid light chain deposition disorders, and outcome following treatment with high-dose melphalan and autologous stem cell transplantation. Bone Marrow Transplant 2006; 38: 339–343.

40. Gertz A. Leung N, Lacy MQ, et al. Myeloablative chemotherapy and stem cell transplantation in myeloma or primary amyloidosis with renal involvement. Kidney Int 2005; 68: 1464–1471.

41. Gillmore JD, Hawkins PN. Drug insight: emerging therapies for amyloidosis. Nature Clin Pract 2006; 2: 263–270.

42. D'Amico G. Renal involvement in hepatitis C infection: cryoglobulinemic glomerulonephritis. Kidney Int 1998; 54: 650–671.

43. Pagnoux C, Cohen P, Guillevin L. Vasculitides secondary to infections. Clin Exp Rheumatol 2006; 24: S71–S81.

Inflammation and atherothrombosis

Prediman K. Shah

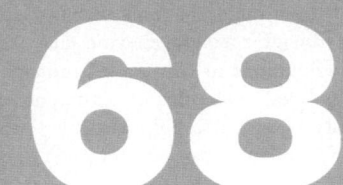

Arterial occlusive disorders include atherosclerosis of native arteries, accelerated atherosclerosis involving vein grafts and arteries of transplanted organs, and restenosis following angioplasty and stenting. Atherosclerotic vascular disease is a leading cause of death and disability throughout the USA and other industrialized nations and consumes enormous fiscal resources. An improved understanding of the pathophysiology of atherosclerosis and thrombosis is likely to lead to improved prevention, diagnosis, and treatment of this common disorder.

Atherosclerosis involves the development of a plaque composed of variable amounts of lipoproteins, extracellular matrix (collagen, proteoglycans, glycosaminoglycans), calcium, vascular smooth-muscle cells, inflammatory cells (chiefly monocyte-derived macrophages, T lymphocytes, mast cells, dendritic cells), and new blood vessels (angiogenesis). A body of evidence now suggests that atherosclerosis represents a chronic inflammatory response to vascular injury caused by a variety of agents that activate or injure endothelium and promote lipoprotein infiltration, retention, and modification, combined with leukocyte retention and activation.[1]

KEY CONCEPTS

PATHOPHYSIOLOGY OF ATHEROSCLEROSIS

>> Atherosclerosis is a chronic immunoinflammatory disease

>> Immune activation and inflammation are involved in the initiation, progression, and destabilization of atherosclerosis

>> Most lethal consequences of atherosclerosis result from thrombosis superimposed on a ruptured or eroded atherosclerotic plaque

>> Plaque composition rather than the luminal stenosis severity is the major determinant of vulnerability to plaque rupture

>> Plaques that are rupture-prone have a large acellular lipid core, intimal and adventitial inflammation, enhanced plaque neovascularity and hemorrhage, and outward adventitial remodeling

■ SHEAR STRESS AND ENDOTHELIAL INFLAMMATORY GENE ACTIVATION AT SITES OF PREDILECTION ■

The sites of predilection for atherosclerosis are characterized by low shear stress, evidence of endothelial activation with expression of proinflammatory genes such as leukocyte adhesion molecules, and increased influx and/or prolonged retention of lipoproteins[2] (Table 68.1 and Fig. 68.1). Specific arterial sites, such as branches, bifurcations, and curvatures, cause characteristic alterations in the flow of blood, including decreased shear stress and increased turbulence. Changes in flow alter the expression of genes that have elements in their promoter regions that respond to shear stress. For example, the genes for intracellular adhesion molecule-1, platelet-derived growth factor B chain, and tissue factor in endothelial cells have these elements, and their expression is increased by reduced shear stress.[3-6] Rolling and adherence of inflammatory cells (monocytes and T cells) occur at these sites as a result of the upregulation of adhesion molecules on both the endothelium and the leukocytes. At these sites, specific molecules form on the endothelium that are responsible for the adherence, migration, and accumulation of monocytes and T cells. Such adhesion molecules, which act as receptors for glycoconjugates and integrins present on monocytes and T cells, include several selectins, intercellular adhesion molecules (ICAM), and vascular cell adhesion molecules (VCAM).[3-6]

Molecules associated with the migration of leukocytes across the endothelium, such as platelet endothelial cell adhesion molecules, act in conjunction with chemoattractant molecules generated by the endothelium, smooth muscle, and monocytes – such as monocyte chemotactic protein-1 (MCP-1), osteopontin, and modified low-density lipoprotein (LDL) – to attract monocytes and T cells into the artery.[2-6] Chemokines may be involved in the chemotaxis and accumulation of macrophages in fatty streaks.[7] Activation of monocytes and T cells leads to upregulation of receptors on their surfaces, such as the mucin-like molecules that bind selectins, integrins that bind adhesion molecules of the immunoglobulin superfamily, and receptors that bind chemoattractant molecules.

These ligand–receptor interactions further activate mononuclear cells, induce cell proliferation, and help define and localize the inflammatory response at the site of lesions.

In genetically modified mice that are deficient in apolipoprotein E (and have hypercholesterolemia), ICAM-1 is constitutively increased at lesion-prone sites long before the lesions develop.[5] In contrast, VCAM-1 is absent in normal mice but is present at the same sites as ICAM-1 in mice with apolipoprotein E deficiency.[5] Mice that are completely deficient in ICAM-1, P-selectin, CD18, or combinations of these molecules have reduced atherosclerosis in response to lipid feeding. Proteolytic enzymes may cleave adhesion molecules such that in situations of chronic inflammation it may be possible to measure the 'shed' molecules in plasma as markers of a sustained inflammatory response to help identify patients at risk for atherosclerosis or other inflammatory diseases.[8, 9]

KEY ROLE OF ENDOTHELIAL ACTIVATION/DYSFUNCTION AND INFLAMMATION IN ATHEROGENESIS

Several studies have suggested that one of the earliest steps in atherogenesis is endothelial activation or injury/dysfunction with infiltration and retention and modification of atherogenic lipoproteins (predominantly the apo B-containing lipoproteins) in the subendothelial space of the vessel wall (Table 68.2).

Various factors that can contribute to endothelial activation or the development of endothelial injury/dysfunction predisposing to atherosclerosis include risk factors such as elevated and modified LDL/very-low-density lipoprotein (VLDL) cholesterol; reduced high-density lipoprotein (HDL) cholesterol; oxidant stress caused by cigarette smoking, hypertension, and diabetic mellitus; genetic alterations; elevated plasma homocysteine concentrations; infectious microorganisms such as herpes viruses or *Chlamydia pneumoniae*; estrogen deficiency; and advancing age.[10] Endothelial activation and injury/dysfunction may manifest in: (1) increased adhesiveness of the endothelium to inflammatory cells (leukocytes) or platelets; (2) increased vascular permeability; (3) change from an anti-coagulant to a procoagulant phenotype; (4) change from a vasodilator to a vasoconstrictor phenotype; or (5) change from a growth-inhibiting to a growth-promoting phenotype through elaboration of cytokines.

Abnormal vasomotor function has been one of the best-studied manifestations of endothelial dysfunction in subjects with either established atherosclerosis or in those with risk factors for atherosclerosis. Normal healthy endothelium produces nitric oxide from arginine through the action of a family of enzymes known as nitric oxide synthases.[10] Nitric oxide acts as a local vasodilator by increasing smooth-muscle cell cyclic guanosine monophosphate (GMP) levels while at the same time inhibiting platelet aggregation and smooth-muscle cell proliferation.[10] In the presence of risk factors, a reduced vasodilator response to endothelium-dependent vasodilator stimuli or even paradoxical vasoconstrictor response to such stimuli has been observed in large vessels as well as in the microcirculation, even in the absence of structural abnormalities in the vessel wall.[10] These abnormal vasomotor responses have been attributed to reduced bioavailability of endothelium-derived relaxing factor(s), specifically nitric oxide, due to rapid inactivation of nitric oxide by oxidant stress or excess generation of asymmetric dimethylarginine and/or increased production of vasoconstrictors such as endothelin.[10]

One of the major contributors to endothelial injury is LDL cholesterol modified by processes such as oxidation, glycation (in diabetes), aggregation, association with proteoglycans, or incorporation into immune complexes.[10–12] Oxidized LDL has been shown to be present in the atherosclerotic lesions of both experimental animals as well as in humans. Subendothelial retention of LDL particles results in progressive

---

Table 68.1 Key steps in atherogenesis highlighting role of inflammation at various steps

1. Endothelial activation with increased infiltration of atherogenic lipoproteins at sites of low or oscillating shear stress (branch points and flow dividers)
2. Subendothelial retention and modification of atherogenic lipoproteins (low-density lipoprotein/very-low-density lipoprotein)
3. Endothelial activation with increased mononuclear leukocyte (inflammatory cell) adhesion, chemotaxis, and subendothelial recruitment
4. Subendothelial inflammatory cell activation with lipid ingestion through monocyte scavenger receptor expression resulting in foam cell formation
5. Intimal migration and proliferation of medial/adventitial smooth-muscle cells/myofibroblasts in response to growth factors released by activated monocytes with matrix production and formation of fibrous cap and fibrous plaque
6. Abluminal plaque growth with positive (outward) arterial adventitial remodeling preserving lumen size in early stages; later, plaque growth or negative remodeling results in luminal narrowing
7. Neoangiogenesis due to angiogenic stimuli produced by inflammatory cells (macrophages) and other arterial wall cells (vascular endothelial growth factor, interleukin-8)
8. Death of foam cells by necrosis/apoptosis leading to necrotic lipid core formation
9. Plaque disruption (rupture of fibrous cap or endothelial erosion) due to inflammatory cell-mediated matrix degradation and death of matrix-synthesizing smooth-muscle cells
10. Exposure of thrombogenic substrate (lipid core-containing tissue factor derived from inflammatory cells) following plaque disruption with arterial thrombosis

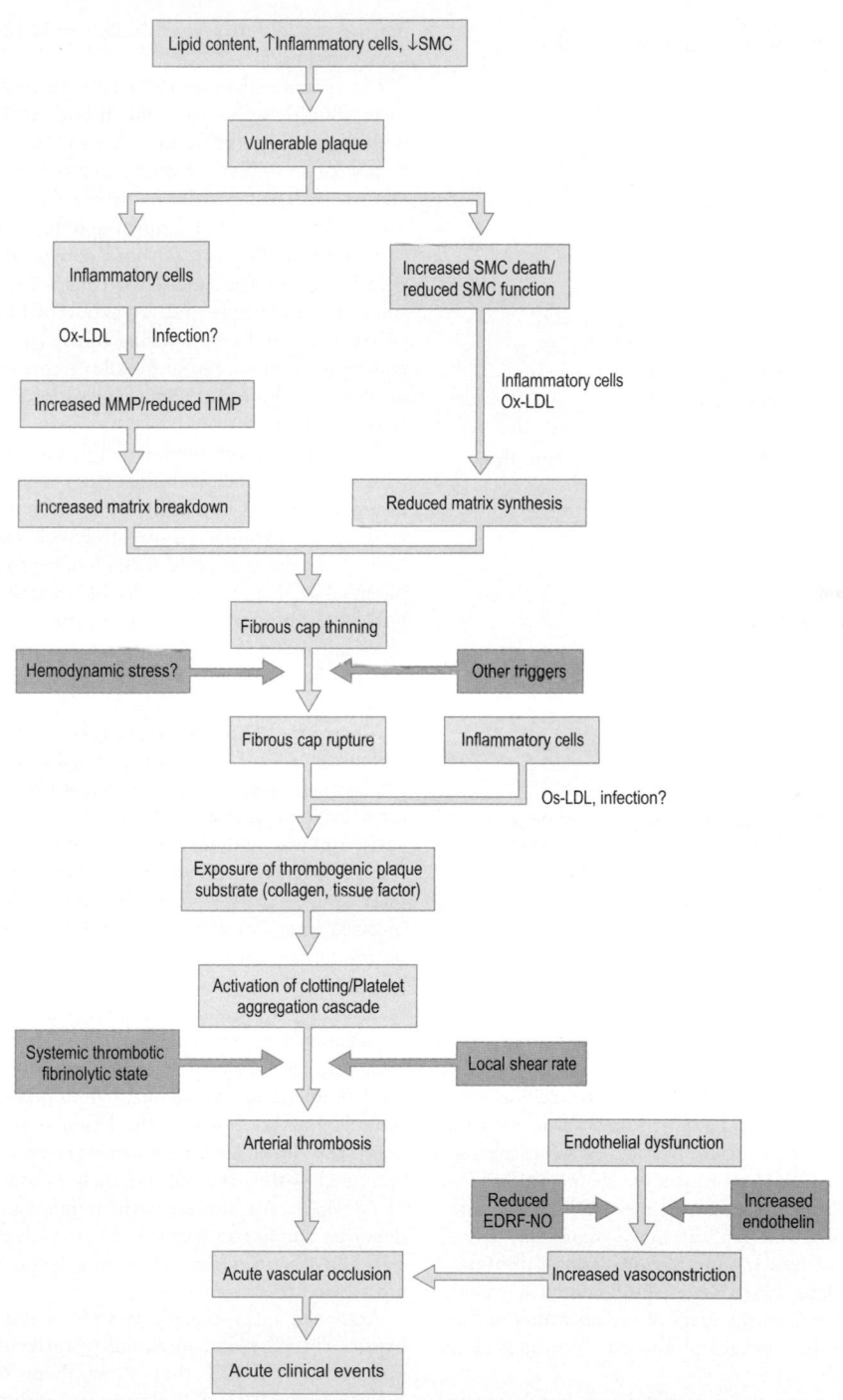

Fig. 68.1 Different shear stress patterns, resulting from different flow patterns in the athero-prone segment versus athero-resistant segment of a human carotid artery, as measured by ultrasound technique, are shown. Note that the low shear stress flow pattern in athero-prone segments is able to induce inflammatory genes in endothelial cells in culture; this may contribute to propensity for lesion localization at athero-prone sites. (Adapted from Dai G, Kaazempur-Mofrad MR, Natarajan S, et al. Distinct endothelial phenotypes evoked by arterial waveforms derived from atherosclerosis-susceptible and -resistant regions of human vasculature. Proc Natl Acad Sci USA 2004; 101: 14871–14876.)

Table 68.2 Endothelial activation/dysfunction in atherosclerosis

Phenotypic features

Reduced vasodilator and increased vasoconstrictor capacity
   Enhanced oxidant stress with increased inactivation of nitric oxide
   Increased expression of endothelin
Enhanced leukocyte (inflammatory cell) adhesion and recruitment
   Increased adhesion molecule expression (ICAM, VCAM)
   Increased chemotactic molecule expression (MCP-1, IL-8)
Increased prothrombotic and reduced fibrinolytic phenotype
Increased growth-promoting phenotype

Factors contributing to endothelial activation/dysfunction

Dyslipidemia and atherogenic lipoprotein modification
   Elevated LDL, VLDL, LP(a)
   LDL modification (oxidation, glycation)
   Reduced HDL
Increased angiotensin II and hypertension
Insulin resistance and diabetes
Estrogen deficiency
Smoking
Hyperhomocysteinemia
Advancing age
Infection?

HDL, high-density lipoprotein; ICAM, intercellular adhesion molecules; IL-8, interleukin-8; LDL, low-density lipoprotein; LP, lipoprotein; MCP-1, monocyte chemotactic protein-1; VCAM, vascular cell adhesion molecules; VLDL, very-low-density lipoprotein.

oxidation and its subsequent internalization by macrophages through the scavenger receptors. The internalization leads to the formation of lipid peroxides and facilitates the accumulation of cholesterol esters, even finally resulting in the formation of foam cells. Once modified and taken up by macrophages, LDL activates the foam cells. In addition to its ability to injure these cells, modified LDL is chemotactic for other monocytes and can upregulate the expression of genes for macrophage colony-stimulating factor (M-CSF) and monocyte chemotactic protein derived from endothelial cells.[13] Thus, it may help expand the inflammatory response by stimulating the replication of monocyte-derived macrophages and the entry of new monocytes into lesions. Continued inflammatory response stimulates migration and proliferation of smooth-muscle cells that accumulate within the areas of inflammation to form an intermediate fibroproliferative lesion resulting in thickening of the artery wall.

The inflammatory and immune response in atherosclerosis consists of accumulation of monocyte-derived macrophages and specific subtypes of T lymphocytes at every stage of the disease.[14, 15] The fatty streak, the earliest type lesion, common in infants and young children, consists of monocyte-derived macrophages, macrophage-derived foam cells, and T lymphocytes. The critical role of the macrophage in atherogenesis is supported by the virtual absence (or drastic reduction) of atherosclerosis when M-CSF null genotype is introduced in murine models of severe dyslipidemia induced by diet or genetic manipulation.[16]

Continued inflammation results in increased numbers of macrophages and lymphocytes, which both emigrate from the blood and multiply within the lesion. Activation of these cells leads to the release of proteolytic enzymes, cytokines, chemokines, and growth factors, which can induce further damage and eventually lead to focal necrosis. Necrosis and/or apoptosis of foam cells results in the formation of the necrotic lipid core in the plaque. Thus, cycles of accumulation of mononuclear cells, migration and proliferation of smooth-muscle cells, and formation of fibrous tissue lead to further enlargement and restructuring of the lesion, so that it becomes covered by a fibrous cap that overlies a core of lipid and necrotic tissue, resulting in the formation of an advanced and complicated atherosclerotic plaque.

The inflammatory response itself can influence lipoprotein transfer within the vessel wall. Proinflammatory cytokines, such as tumor necrosis factor-α (TNF-α), interleukin-1 (IL-1), and M-CSF increase binding of LDL to endothelium and smooth muscle and increase the transcription of the LDL receptor gene.[1] After binding to scavenger receptors *in vitro*, modified LDL initiates a series of intracellular events that include the induction of proteases and inflammatory cytokines.[1] Thus, a vicious circle of inflammation, modification of lipoproteins, and further inflammation can be maintained in the artery by the presence of these modified lipoproteins.

Monocyte-derived macrophages are present in various stages of atherosclerosis and act as scavenging and antigen-presenting cells. They produce cytokines, chemokines, growth-regulating molecules, tissue factor, metalloproteinases, and other hydrolytic enzymes. The continuing entry, survival, and replication of monocytes/macrophages in lesions depend in part on growth factors, such as M-CSF and granulocyte–macrophage colony-stimulating factor (GM-CSF), whereas IL-2 is involved in a similar manner for T lymphocytes. Recent experimental observations suggest that in and out trafficking of macrophages within the atherosclerotic vascular wall may be regulated by the microenvironment within the lesion with ingress and retention being promoted by a proinflammatory milieu related to oxidized lipids, whereas egress via the lumen or via transformation into migratory dendritic cells and subsequent immigration to regional lymph nodes is associated with reduced proinflammatory lipids in the lesion – an environment promoted by high HDL levels favoring lesion regression.[17] Dendritic cells have been identified within the subendothelium and the adventitia of normal blood vessels. An increase in the number and activity of subendothelial dendritic cells has been observed in the atherosclerotic lesion, raising the possibility that dendritic cells may be involved in the pathophysiology of atherosclerosis.[18]

Activated macrophages as well as lesional smooth-muscle cells express class II histocompatibility antigens such as human leukocyte antigen (HLA)-DR that allow them to present antigens to T lymphocytes.[1, 14, 15] Atherosclerotic lesions contain both CD4 and CD8 T cells, implicating the immune system in atherogenesis.[14, 15] T-cell activation, following antigen processing, results in production of various cytokines, such as interferon-γ (INF-γ) and TNF-α and β, which can further enhance the inflammatory response.[1] Antigens presented include oxidized LDL and heat shock protein 60 (HSP60), which may participate in the immune response in atherosclerosis.[2, 14, 15]

Macrophages, T cells, endothelial and smooth-muscle cells in the atherosclerotic lesions express CD40 ligand and its receptor, which may play a role in atherogenesis by regulating the function of inflammatory cells.[19] The anti-atherogenic effects of CD40-blocking antibodies in the murine model of atherosclerosis suggest that CD40-mediated signaling may play an important role in atherogenesis.[20]

Platelet adhesion and mural thrombosis are ubiquitous in the initiation and generation of the lesions of atherosclerosis in animals and humans.[1] Platelets can adhere to dysfunctional endothelium, exposed collagen, and macrophages. When activated, platelets release their granules, which contain cytokines and growth factors that, together with thrombin, may contribute to the migration and proliferation of smooth-muscle cells and monocytes. Activation of platelets leads to the formation of free arachidonic acid, which can be transformed into prostaglandins such as thromboxane A_2, one of the most potent vasoconstricting and platelet-aggregating substances known, or into leukotrienes, which can amplify the inflammatory response.

Angiotensin II, a potent vasoconstrictor, may also contribute to atherogenesis by stimulating the growth of smooth muscle, increasing oxidant stress, inducing LDL oxidation, and promoting an inflammatory response.[1, 20–22]

Elevated plasma homocysteine concentrations, resulting from enzymatic defects or vitamin deficiency, may facilitate atherothrombosis by inducing endothelial dysfunction with reduction in vasodilator capacity and enhanced prothrombotic phenotype and smooth-muscle replication.[23–25] Hyperhomocysteinemia is associated with an increased risk of atherosclerosis of the coronary, peripheral, and cerebral arteries.[23–25] Recently completed clinical trials have failed to demonstrate clinical cardiovascular benefits from reduction of plasma homocysteine levels by vitamins.[25]

POTENTIAL ROLE OF INFECTION IN ATHEROTHROMBOSIS

It is likely that a number of stimuli are responsible for provoking and sustaining a chronic inflammatory response in the vessel wall in atherosclerosis. Among the key potential culprits are the modified lipoproteins and infectious agents. Oxidatively modified lipoproteins can induce a variety of proinflammatory genes in the vessel wall that are responsible for recruiting and activating inflammatory cells such as ICAM- and VCAM-type adhesion molecules, chemotactic cytokines such as MCP-1 and IL-8, and colony-stimulating factors such as M-CSF. In addition to modified lipoproteins, there is now a body of evidence suggesting that arterial wall infections with organisms such as *Chlamydia pneumonia*, cytomegalovirus/herpes virus, as well as remote infections such as chronic bronchitis, gingivitis, and *Helicobacter pylori* infection, may affect inflammation, thereby contributing to atherogenesis and/or plaque disruption and thrombosis in the presence of pre-existing atherosclerosis[23–31] (Table 68.3). Increased titers of antibodies to these organisms have been used as a predictor of further adverse events in patients who have had a myocardial infarction.

Organisms, particularly *Chlamydia pneumoniae*, have been identified in atheromatous lesions in coronary arteries and in other organs obtained at autopsy. The case for *C. pneumoniae* is of

Table 68.3 Potential role of infection in atherosclerosis and thrombosis

Infectious organisms implicated
Viruses
Herpes virus
Cytomegalovirus
Bacteria
Chlamydia pneumoniae
Helicobacter pylori
Porphyromonas gingivalis?

Mechanism(s) by which infections may contribute to atherothrombosis
Direct infection of the vascular wall with endothelial injury, inflammatory cell recruitment, and activation (*Chlamydia pneumoniae*, herpes virus, cytomegalovirus)
Immune-mediated vascular injury through molecular mimicry (*Chlamydia pneumoniae*)
Remote infections with systemic activation of the inflammatory response (*Helicobacter pylori*, *Porphyromonas gingivalis*)

particular interest since both in the hypercholesterolemic rabbit as well as in genetically hyperlipidemic mice, acceleration of atherosclerosis with *C. pneumoniae* infection has been demonstrated.[30] In addition, pilot clinical trials of anti-chlamydial macrolide antibiotics have raised the possibility that such therapy may reduce the risk of recurrent coronary events.[31, 32] *In vitro* studies have suggested that *C. pneumoniae* can trigger proatherogenic events, such as foam cell formation, procoagulant activity, and metalloproteinase activity in monocytes, probably mediated by its HSP60. Molecular antigenic mimicry between certain *Chlamydia* antigens and myosin has also raised the additional possibility that such antigenic mimicry could be involved in an immune-mediated vascular and myocardial injury. However, recent large-scale clinical trials have failed to demonstrate any clinical benefit of using antibiotics targeting *C. pneumoniae*, raising questions about the link between infection and atherothrombosis.[33–36]

TOLL-LIKE RECEPTORS, INNATE IMMUNITY AND ATHEROSCLEROSIS

Toll-like receptors (TLR) are a family of transmembrane receptors that serve as signaling receptors in the innate immune system; their ligation by exogenous and possibly endogenous ligands triggers a proinflammatory signaling cascade in various cells linking innate immunity to inflammation[37] (Chapter 3). Recent studies have shown that TLRs are expressed in murine and human atherosclerotic lesions and that hyperlipidemia induces proinflammatory signaling, in part through these receptors and their downstream adaptor molecules such as MyD88 (myeloid differentiation factor) contributing to vascular inflammation, neointimal hyperplasia, and atherosclerosis in murine models.[38, 39]

ANGIOGENESIS IN ATHEROSCLEROSIS

Angiogenesis or neovascularization is an essential process that supports chronic inflammation and fibroproliferation, processes that are involved in atherogenesis. Several studies have demonstrated increased neoangiogenesis in atherosclerotic lesions and hypercholesterolemia has been shown to increase adventitial neovascularity in porcine arteries before the development of an atherosclerotic lesion.[40] Proinflammatory chemokines such as IL-8 and other angiogenic growth factors such as vascular endothelial growth factor (VEGF) have been demonstrated in atherosclerotic lesions where they could contribute to angiogenesis. Angiogenesis may contribute to plaque progression by providing a source of intraplaque hemorrhage that in turn may provide red cell membrane-derived cholesterol, contributing to the expansion of the necrotic lipid core. In addition neovascular channels may also provide a source of inflammatory cells into the vessel wall; thus angiogenesis and inflammation appear to be linked pathophysiologic processes.[41] The ability of macrophages to undergo transdifferentiation into functional endothelial cells has been demonstrated, suggesting a more direct link between inflammation and angiogenesis.[42] Preliminary data demonstrating an inhibitory effect of angiostatin in murine models of atherosclerosis suggest the potential proatherogenic role for angiogenesis.[43]

ROLE OF INFLAMMATION IN PLAQUE RUPTURE, PLAQUE EROSION, AND THROMBOSIS

Thrombosis complicating atherosclerosis is the mechanism by which atherosclerosis leads to acute ischemic syndromes of unstable angina, non-Q- and Q-wave myocardial infarction and many cases of sudden cardiac death.[44–46] In most cases, coronary thrombosis occurs as a result of uneven thinning and rupture of the fibrous cap, often at the shoulders of a lipid-rich lesion where macrophages and T cells enter, accumulate, and are activated, and where apoptosis may occur[44–46] (Figs 68.2–68.4)). Thinning of the fibrous cap may result from elaboration of matrix-degrading metalloproteinases (MMPs) such as collagenases (MMP-1, MMP-13), gelatinases (MMP-2, MMP-9), elastases (MMP-12), and stromelysins (MMP-3), and/or other proteases such as cathepsins, by inflammatory cells, chiefly macrophages.[44–48] These proteases may be induced or activated by oxidized LDL, cell-to-cell interaction between macrophages and activated T cells, CD40 ligation, mast cell-derived proteases, oxidant radicals, matrix proteins such as tenascin-C, and infectious agents.[44–48] Thinning can also result from increased smooth-muscle cell death by apoptosis/necrosis and consequent reduced matrix production; increased smooth-muscle cell death may result from oxidized LDL, cleavage products of tenascin-c or by direct contact with plaque-infiltrating CD4 T cells expressing TNF-related apoptosis-inducing ligand (TRAIL).[49–51]

Inflammatory cells, specifically the macrophages, are also the main source of tissue factor in the atherosclerotic plaque.[52] Tissue factor, when exposed to circulating blood, interacts with activated factor VII to generate activated factor X; activated factor X in turn cleaves thrombin from prothrombin. Thrombin is involved in recruiting and activating platelets as well as the clotting cascade, thereby initiating thrombus formation. Tissue factor

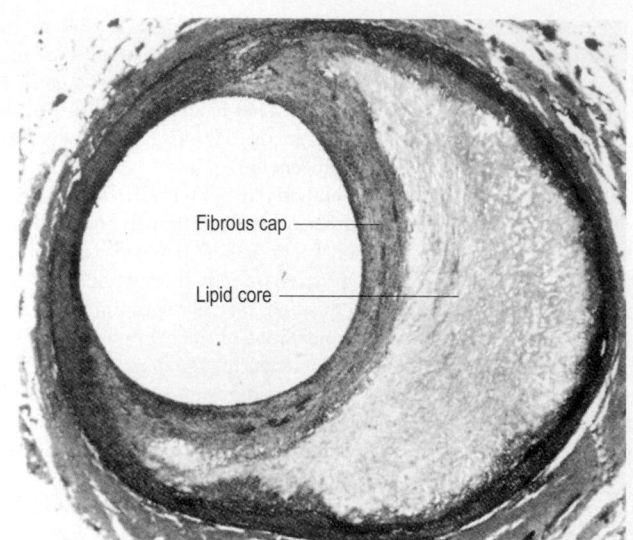

Fig. 68.2 An atherosclerotic plaque in a human coronary artery depicting various components of the lesion.

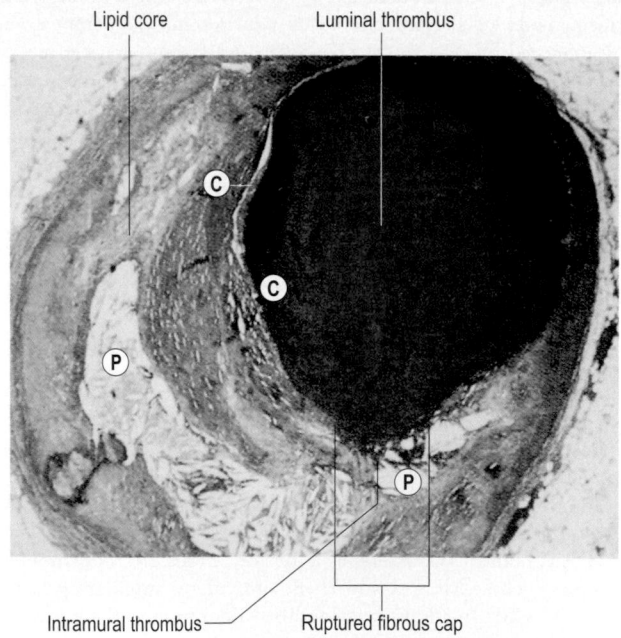

Fig. 68.3 Coronary thrombosis resulting from rupture of the fibrous cap of a lipid-rich coronary artery plaque (plaque rupture). P, plaque; C, cap.

expression is increased in atherosclerotic plaques, particularly in unstable coronary syndromes.[52] The lipid core of the atheromatous lesion is heavily impregnated with tissue factor derived from dead (possibly apoptotic) macrophages and foam cells, accounting for its high thrombogenicity. Macrophage tissue factor expression may be induced by a variety of signals in the atherosclerotic plaque, including various cytokines, infectious agents, and oxidized

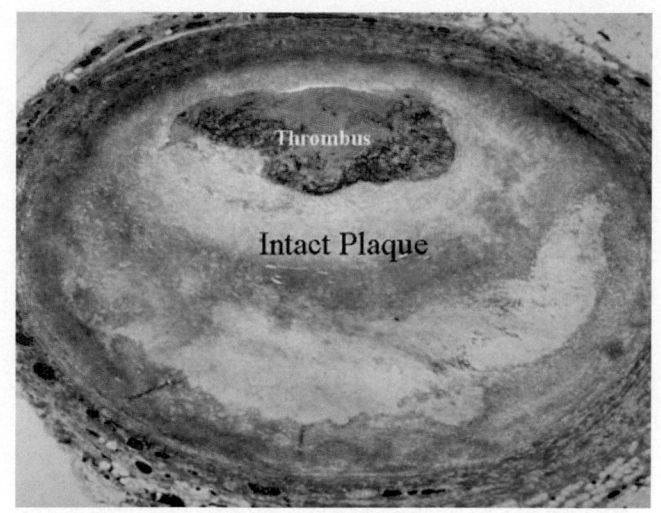

Fig. 68.4 Coronary thrombosis resulting from superficial endothelial erosion without rupture of the plaque (plaque erosion).

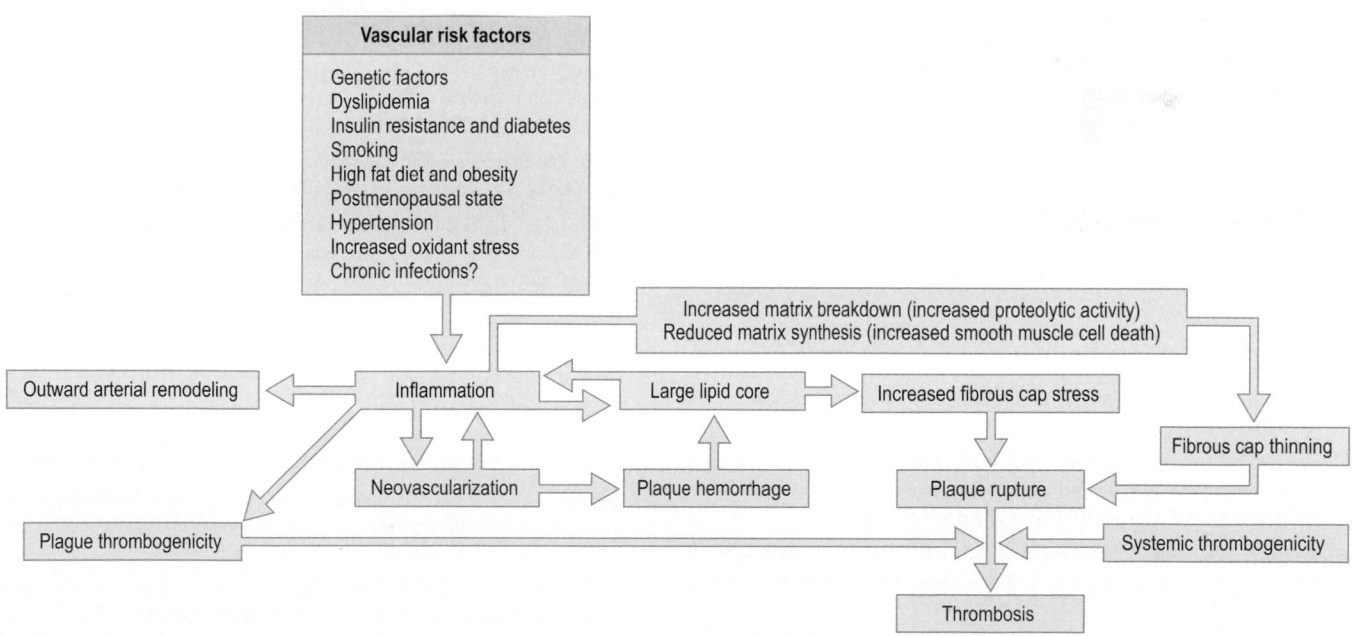

Fig. 68.5 Scheme showing the pathophysiology of plaque rupture and thrombosis.

lipoproteins. Thrombosis may also occur on a proteoglycan-rich matrix without a large lipid core, and in such cases, evidence of superficial endothelial erosion is found.[53] This plaque erosion may account for thrombosis in a relatively higher proportion of young victims of sudden death, particularly in women and smokers.[54] The precise molecular basis for these plaque erosions is not clear, although endothelial desquamation through activation of basement membrane-degrading MMP may be involved.[48]

Plaques with a large core, active inflammatory infiltration, and a thinned fibrous cap are therefore considered vulnerable or unstable plaques. Their identification can be particularly difficult because they may not produce symptoms due to lack of flow-limiting stenoses and may thus escape detection by stress testing and even angiography. Inflammation in atherosclerosis may be accompanied by elevation of circulating proinflammatory markers such as C-reactive protein (CRP), IL-6, serum amyloid A, and a variety of soluble leukocyte adhesion molecules.[54-56] Elevated CRP levels predict an increased risk of adverse cardiac events in patients with symptomatic vascular disease as well as in asymptomatic subjects at risk for vascular disease.[54]

CONCLUSIONS

Atherosclerosis is a complex disease process that involves lipoprotein influx, lipoprotein modification, increased pro-oxidant stress, and inflammatory, angiogenic, and fibroproliferative responses intermingled with extracellular matrix and lipid accumulation, resulting in the formation of an atherosclerotic plaque. Endothelial activation/dysfunction is common in atherosclerosis and often manifests as a reduced vasodilator or enhanced vasoconstrictor phenotype that contributes to luminal compromise. Thrombosis resulting from plaque rupture or superficial erosion complicates atherosclerosis, often resulting in abrupt luminal occlusion with resultant acute ischemic syndromes (Fig. 68.5). Infectious agents may contribute to the inflammatory response and thus to destabilization of lesions. An improved understanding of the pathophysiology of atherosclerosis is providing novel directions for its prevention and treatment. In particular, the recognition of the important role of inflammation could lead to novel therapeutic interventions directed at selective inhibition of inflammatory cascade in the vessel wall. Targeting inflammatory triggers such as lipoproteins, angiotensin II, possible infectious agents, and others is likely to lead to improved outcomes in patients with atherosclerosis.

REFERENCES

1. Ross R. Atherosclerosis: an inflammatory disease. N Engl J Med 1999; 340: 115–126.
2. Dai G, Kaazempur-Mofrad MR, Natarajan S, et al. Distinct endothelial phenotypes evoked by arterial waveforms derived from atherosclerosis-susceptible and -resistant regions of human vasculature. Proc Natl Acad Sci USA 2004; 101: 14871–14876.
3. Nagel T, Resnick N, Atkinson WJ, et al. Shear stress selectively upregulates intercellular adhesion molecule-1 expression in cultured human vascular endothelial cells. J Clin Invest 1994; 94: 885–891.
4. Resnick N, Collins T, Atkinson W, et al. Platelet-derived growth factor B chain promoter contains a cis-acting fluid shear-stress-responsive element. Proc Natl Acad Sci USA 1993; 90: 4591–4595.
5. Nakashima Y, Raines EW, Plump AS, et al. Upregulation of VCAM-1 and ICAM-1 at atherosclerosis-prone sites on the endothelium in the ApoE-deficient mouse. Arterioscler Thromb Vasc Biol 1998; 18: 842–851.
6. Giachelli CM, Lombardi D, Johnson RJ, et al. Evidence for a role of osteopontin in macrophage infiltration in response to pathological stimuli in vivo. Am J Pathol 1998; 152: 353–358.
7. Boisvert WA, Santiago R, Curtiss LK, et al. A leukocyte homologue of the IL-8 receptor CXCR-2 mediates the accumulation of macrophages in atherosclerotic lesions of LDL receptor-deficient mice. J Clin Invest 1998; 101: 353–363.
8. Herren B, Raines EW, Ross R. Expression of a disintegrin-like protein in cultured human vascular cells and in vivo. Faseb J 1997; 11: 173–180.
9. Hwang S-J, Ballantyne CM, Sharrett AR, et al. Circulating adhesion molecules VCAM-1, ICAM-1, and E-selectin in carotid atherosclerosis and incident coronary heart disease cases: the Atherosclerosis Risk in Communities (ARIC) study. Circulation 1997; 96: 4219–4225.
10. Kinlay S, Ganz P. Role of endothelial dysfunction in coronary artery disease and implications for therapy. Am J Cardiol 1997; 80: 111–161.
11. Steinberg D. Low density lipoprotein oxidation and its pathobiological significance. J Biol Chem 1997; 272: 20963–20966.
12. Khoo JC, Miller E, McLoughlin P, et al. Enhanced macrophage uptake of low density lipoprotein after self-aggregation. Arteriosclerosis 1988; 8: 348–358.
13. Han J, Hajjar DP, Febbraio M, et al. Native and modified low density lipoproteins increase functional expression of the macrophage class B scavenger receptor, CD36. J Biol Chem 1997; 272: 1654–1659.
14. Hansson GK, Jonasson L, Siefert PS, et al. Immune mechanisms in atherosclerosis. Arteriosclerosis 1989; 9: 567–578.
15. Stemme S, Faber B, Holm J, et al. T lymphocytes from human atherosclerotic plaques recognize oxidized low density lipoprotein. Proc Natl Acad Sci USA 1995; 92: 3893–3897.
16. Qiao J-H, Tripathi J, Mishra NK, et al. Role of macrophage colony-stimulating factor in atherosclerosis: studies of osteopetrotic mice. Am J Pathol 1997; 150: 1687–1699.
17. Llodra J, Angeli V, Liu J, et al. Emigration of monocyte-derived cells from atherosclerotic lesions characterizes regressive, but not progressive, plaques. Proc Natl Acad Sci USA 2004; 101: 11779–11784.
18. Lord RS, Bobryshev YV. Clustering of dendritic cells in athero-prone areas of the aorta. Atherosclerosis 1999; 146: 197–198.
19. Schonbeck U, Mach F, Sukhova GK, et al. Regulation of matrix metalloproteinase expression in human vascular smooth muscle cells by T lymphocytes: a role for CD40 signaling in plaque rupture?. Circ Res 1997; 81: 448–454.
20. Mach F, Schonbeck U, Sukhova GK, et al. Reduction of atherosclerosis in mice by inhibition of CD40 signaling. Nature 1998; 394: 200–203.
21. Gibbons GH, Pratt RE, Dzau VJ. Vascular smooth muscle cell hypertrophy vs. hyperplasia: autocrine transforming growth factor-beta 1 expression determines growth response to angiotensin II. J Clin Invest 1992; 90: 456–461.
22. Lacy F, O'Connor DT, Schmid-Schonbein GW. Plasma hydrogen peroxide production in hypertensive and normotensive subjects as genetic risk of hypertension. J Hypertens 1998; 16: 291–303.
23. Nehler MR, Taylor LM Jr, Porter JM. Homocysteinemia as a risk factor for atherosclerosis: a review. Cardiovasc Surg 1997; 6: 559–567.
24. Nygard O, Nordrehaug JE, Refsum H, et al. Plasma homocysteine levels and mortality in patients with coronary artery disease. N Engl J Med 1997; 337: 230–236.
25. Kaul S, Zadeh AA, Shah PK. Homocysteine hypothesis for atherothrombotic cardiovascular disease not validated. Preventing coronary heart disease: B vitamins and homocysteine. J Am Coll Cardiol 2006; 48: 914–923.
26. Jackson LA, Campbell LA, Schmidt RA, et al. Specificity of detection of Chlamydia pneumoniae in cardiovascular atheroma: evaluation of the innocent bystander hypothesis. Am J Pathol 1997; 150: 1785–1790.

27. Melnick JL, Adam E, Debakey ME. Cytomegalovirus and atherosclerosis. Eur Heart J 1993; 14(suppl. K): 30–38.

28. Nicholson AC, Hajjar DP. Herpesviruses in atherosclerosis and thrombosis: etiologic agents or ubiquitous bystanders? Arterioscler Thromb Vasc Biol 1998; 18: 339–348.

29. Shah PK. Plaque disruption and coronary thrombosis: new insight into pathogenesis and prevention. Clin Cardiol 1997; 20: 38–44.

30. Muhlestein JB, Anderson JL, Hammond EH, et al. Infection with *Chlamydia pneumoniae* accelerates the development of atherosclerosis and treatment with azithromycin prevents it in a rabbit model. Circulation 1998; 97: 633–636.

31. Gurfinkel E, Bozovich G. Daroca A, et al. Randomized trial of roxithromycin in non-Q-wave coronary syndromes: ROXIS Pilot Study. ROXIS Study Group [see comments]. Lancet 1997; 350: 404–407.

32. Gupta S, Leatham EW, Carrington D, et al. Elevated *Chlamydia pneumoniae* antibodies, cardiovascular events, and azithromycin in male survivors of myocardial infarction. Circulation 1997; 96: 404–407.

33. Cercek B, Shah PK, Noc M, et al. Effect of short-term treatment with azithromycin on recurrent ischemic events in patients with acute coronary syndrome in the Azithromycin in Acute Coronary Syndrome (AZACS) trial: a randomised controlled trial. Lancet 2003; 361: 809–813.

34. O'Connor CM, Dunne MW, Pfeffer MA, et al. Azithromycin for the secondary prevention of coronary heart disease events. the WIZARD study: a randomized controlled trial. JAMA 2003; 290: 1459–1466.

35. Cannon CP, Braunwald E, McCabe CH, et al. Antibiotic treatment of *Chlamydia pneumoniae* after acute coronary syndrome. N Engl J Med 2005; 352: 1646–1654.

36. Grayston JT, Kronmal RA, Jackson LA, et al. Azithromycin for the secondary prevention of coronary events. N Engl J Med 2005; 352: 1637–1645.

37. Xu XH, Shah PK, Faure E, et al. Toll-like receptor-4 is expressed by macrophages in murine and human lipid-rich atherosclerotic plaques and upregulated by oxidized LDL. Circulation 2001; 104: 3103–3108.

38. Michelsen KS, Wong MH, Shah PK, et al. Lack of Toll-like receptor 4 or myeloid differentiation factor 88 reduces atherosclerosis and alters plaque phenotype in mice deficient in apolipoprotein E. Proc Natl Acad Sci USA 2004; 101: 10679–10684.

39. Bjorkbacka H, Kunjathoor VV, Moore KJ, et al. Reduced atherosclerosis in MyD88-null mice links elevated serum cholesterol levels to activation of innate immunity signaling pathways. Nat Med 2004; 10: 416–421.

40. O'Brien ER, Garvin MR, Dev R, et al. Angiogenesis in human atherosclerotic plaques. Am J Pathol 1994; 145: 883–894.

41. Virmani R, Kolodgie FD, Burke AP, et al. Atherosclerotic plaque progression and vulnerability to rupture: angiogenesis as a source of intraplaque hemorrhage. Arterioscler Thromb Vasc Biol 2005; 25: 2054.

42. Sharifi BG, Zeng Z, Wang L, et al. Pleiotrophin induces transdifferentiation of monocytes into functional endothelial cells. Arterioscler Thromb Vasc Biol 2006; 26: 1273–1280.

43. Moulton KS, Heller E, Konerding MA, et al. Angiogenesis inhibitor endostatin or TNP-470 reduces intimal neovascularization and plaque growth in apolipoprotein E deficient mice. Circulation 1999; 99: 1726–1732.

44. Falk E, Shah PK, Fuster V. Pathogenesis of plaque distribution. In: Fuster V, Ross R, Topol EJ (eds) Atherosclerosis and coronary artery disease, vol. 2. Philadelphia: Lippincott-Raven, 1996: 492–510.

45. Shah PK. Role of inflammation and metalloproteinases in plaque disruption and thrombosis. Vasc Med 1998; 3: 199–206.

46. Shah PK. Plaque disruption and thrombosis. Potential role of inflammation and infection. Cardiol Clin 1999; 17: 271–281.

47. Xu XP, Meisel SR, Ong JM, et al. Oxidized low-density lipoprotein regulates matrix metalloproteinase-9 and its tissue inhibitor in human monocyte-derived macrophages. Circulation 1999; 99: 993–998.

48. Rajavashisth TB, Xu XP, Jovinge S, et al. Membrane type 1 matrix metalloproteinase expression in human atherosclerosis plaques: evidence for activation by proinflammatory mediators. Circulation 1999; 99: 3103–3109.

49. Wallner K, Chen Li, Shah PK, et al. The EGF-L domain of tenascin-C is pro-apoptotic for cultured smooth muscle cells. Arterioscler Thromb Vasc Biol 2004; 24: 1416–1421.

50. Sato K, Niessner A, Kopecky SL, et al. Trail expressing T cells induce apoptosis of vascular smooth muscle cells in atherosclerotic plaque. J Exp Med 2006; 203: 239–250.

51. Pryschep S, Sato K, Goronzy JJ, et al. T cell recognition and killing of vascular smooth muscle cells in acute coronary syndromes. Circ Res 2006; 98: 1168–1176.

52. Moreno PR, Bernardi VH, López-Cuéllar J, et al. Macrophages, smooth muscle cells, and tissue factor in unstable angina. Implications for cell-mediated thrombogenicity in acute coronary syndromes. Circulation 1996; 94: 3090–3097.

53. Burke AP, Farb A, Malcom GT, et al. Effect of risk factors on the mechanism of acute thrombosis and sudden coronary death in women. Circulation 1998; 97: 2110–2116.

54. Ridker PM, Cushman M, Stampfer MJ, et al. Inflammation, aspirin, and the risk of cardiovascular disease in apparently healthy men. N Engl J Med 1997; 336: 973–979.

55. Haverkate F, Thompson SG, Pyke SD, et al. Production of C-reactive protein and risk of coronary events in stable and unstable angina: European Concerted Action on Thrombosis and Disabilities Angina Pectoris Study Group. Lancet 1997; 349: 462–466.

56. Levenson J, Giral P, Razavian M, et al. Fibrinogen and silent atherosclerosis in subjects with cardiovascular risk factors. Arterioscler Thromb Vasc Biol 1995; 15: 1263–1268.

REFERENCES

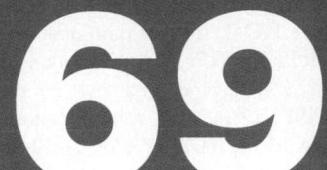

Autoimmune thyroid diseases

69

Su He Wang, James R. Baker Jr.

Autoimmune thyroid disease (AITD) is the most common organ specific autoimmune disorder. AITD includes a group of thyroid diseases that share the common finding of altered thyroid function, with susceptibility determined by a combination of genetic and environmental factors. The pathogenesis of AITD is associated with autoimmune responses against specific components of thyroid tissues, including cell membrane proteins, receptors, and enzymes. AITD affects 1–2% of the population, and is 5–10-fold more common in women. AITD is generally divided into two entities: autoimmune hyperthyroidism and autoimmune thyroiditis. The details of these disorders are listed in Table 69.1.

The concept of autoimmune responses to thyroid antigens originated more than 50 years ago when antithyroid antibodies were found in the serum of patients with Hashimoto's thyroiditis (HT), followed by the induction of experimental autoimmune thyroiditis in animals.[1] Subsequently, the long-acting thyroid stimulator (LATS) was discovered to be an immunoglobulin that caused Graves' disease (GD).[2] We continue to progress in our ability to understand the pathogenesis of AITD, and especially of GD and HT, the two most common thyroid disorders.

■ GRAVES' DISEASE ■

GD accounts for most cases of hyperthyroidism. It is named after the Irish physician Robert J. Graves, who first gave a clinical description of the disease in 1835, although the symptoms of hyperthyroidism were noted in the early 1800s. It was 51 years after Graves' description, however, that excessive production of thyroid hormones was proposed as the cause of the disease. After several decades' active study of hyperthyroid-related hormones, in 1956 Adams and Purves discovered an abnormal thyroid stimulator protein named LATS in the serum of patients with GD.[2] The nature of LATS was later identified as an autoantibody against thyroid follicular cell thyrotropin receptors, and since that time GD has been classified as an autoimmune disease.

GENETIC AND ENVIRONMENTAL FACTORS

GD is a common disorder in the general population, with an incidence of 1–1.5 cases/1000 population. The etiology is largely unknown; however, development of the disease appears predominantly in genetically susceptible individuals. Family members of a patient with GD are more likely than would be expected by chance to have AITD or other organ-specific autoimmune diseases. Studies on monozygotic twins have indicated that the disease has a concordance rate of only 30–60%.[3] Another study of 8966 pairs of twins showed that 35% of monozygotic twins (versus 3% of dizygotic twins) were concordant for GD.[4] The result provides a measure of the relative contribution of genetic as opposed to environmental factors to disease susceptibility. It is estimated that up to 79% of the predisposition to GD is the result of genetic factors.[4] However, the expression of GD in genetically susceptible individuals is certainly regulated by environmental agents and endogenous factors in either permissive or protective ways.

One of the most significant pathological features seen in GD is an infiltrate of activated lymphocytes in the thyroid gland, which exhibit increased expression of major histocompatibility complex (MHC) class II molecules. MHC genes and their products play a crucial role in determining immune responses, particularly through antigen presentation (Chapter 5). There is overwhelming evidence that loci in the human leukocyte antigen (HLA) region (chromosome 6p21) are important, providing a relative risk of 1.9–4.0 for GD.[5] An association between GD and HLA-DR3 in Caucasian populations has been noted, although this might not be the case in other races.[6] Other studies indicate that HLA-DR3 is in strong linkage disequilibrium with DQB1*0201 and DQA1*0501, both of which are strongly associated with GD.[7] HLA-DQB1*0303 has been suggested to be a race-specific susceptible allele for GD in Hong Kong Chinese.[6] Two HLA-DRB1 alleles might contribute independently to GD susceptibility.[8] Within the crystal structure of HLA-DRB1, residues characteristic of alleles that are positively and negatively associated with GD have been identified. There are also reports indicating no significant linkage between MHC genes and GD.[9] The HLA locus did not co-segregate with disease in DR3-positive

GRAVES' DISEASE

1023

families,[10] suggesting that HLA genes may not be the major genes for AITD expression, even within DR3-positive families. However, considering that HLA-DR3 was associated with GD in the probands,[7] it is most likely that the DR3 gene is a modulating gene that contributes to the effect of other susceptibility genes. Nevertheless, the above data suggest that controversy exists on the actual role of HLA in the development of GD.

Several non-MHC genes may also be linked to the pathogenesis of GD (Table 69.2). These genes include the cytotoxic T lymphocyte antigen-4 (CTLA-4) gene, the thyroid-stimulating hormone receptor (TSHR) gene, GD-1, an X-chromosome gene, vitamin D receptor (VDR), CD40, interferon (IFN)-γ, interleukin-4 (IL-4), IL-1 receptor antagonist (IL-1RA) gene, and the lymphoid protein tyrosine phosphatase (PTPN22). CTLA-4, located on chromosome 2q33, plays an important role in the regulation of T-cell activation (Chapter 13). The linkage between the CTLA-4 gene and GD has been found in different races and geographical locations.[22] Primary susceptibility has now been mapped to CTLA-4 itself, with an odds ratio of 1.5 (confidence interval (CI), 1.31–1.75; $P = 2.72 \times 10^{-8}$) for GD.[22] CTLA-4 gene polymorphisms are also thought to be linked to thyroid autoantibody production,[12] suggesting a broad role of CTLA-4 in immune modulation, as opposed to being specific for GD. In some GD pedigrees, CTLA-4 polymorphisms synergistically enhanced the risk conferred by MHC alleles. CTLA-4 splice variants may regulate immunoregulatory pathways that

Table 69.1 The classification of autoimmune thyroid disease

Autoimmune hyperthyroidism
Graves' disease
Autoimmune thyroiditis
Hashimoto's (lymphocytic) thyroiditis
Postpartum thyroiditis

Table 69.2 Genes associated with Graves' disease

Gene or locus	Reference
CD40	11
Cytotoxic T-lymphocyte antigen-4 (CTLA-4)	12
Graves' disease-1 (GD-1, 14q31)	13
Human leukocyte antigen (HLA)-DR,DQ	6, 7
Interferon (IFN)-gamma	14
Interleukin-1 receptor antagonist (IL-1RA)	15
Interleukin-4	16
Thyroid-stimulating hormone receptor	17
Tyrosine phosphatase (PTPN22)	18, 19
Vitamin D receptor	20
X-chromosome at Xq21.33-22	21

are essential (but not sufficient) for autoimmunity in both mice and humans.[22]

Many cytokine gene polymorphisms have been examined among patients with GD. A significant reduction in the frequency of the variant T allele of the IL-4 promoter (C/T single nucleotide polymorphism (SNP); position -590) was found in GD.[16] However, other studies have failed to support this finding.[23] One case-control study reported that the frequency of an allele for the IL-1RA gene was significantly increased in patients with GD.[15] However, similar to IL-4, the result has been difficult to replicate.[24] In addition to IL-4 and IL-1RA, there is an important association between IFN-γ microsatellite polymorphisms and GD.[14] However, it is likely that these microsatellite polymorphisms play only a minor role in the susceptibility to GD. A genome-wide screen in GD has suggested the presence of a major GD susceptibility gene on chromosome 20q11.2,[25] designated GD-2. Subsequently, the gene encoding CD40, which stimulates lymphocyte proliferation and differentiation, was mapped to this region, and a C/T polymorphism in the 5′ untranslated region of the CD40 was associated with the susceptibility to and the phenotype of GD.[11] Several reports have indicated that VDR polymorphisms are associated with GD.[20] However, VDR polymorphism analysis needs to be stratified according to the population background.[20] The gene encoding lymphoid PTPN22 may be a general susceptibility locus for several autoimmune diseases, including GD.[18] It is proposed that autoimmune-associated lymphoid tyrosine phosphatase is a gain-of-function variant.[19]

Several studies have failed to show any significant role of the TSHR gene locus in the genetics of GD.[26] GD-1, a locus located on chromosome 14q31, has been suggested as being a major GD-susceptible gene,[27] and this location is close to the multinodular goiter-1 locus. An unknown gene(s) located on the X-chromosome at Xq21.33-22 has also been linked to GD.[21] Considering that GD is a female-predominant disease, this preliminary result is very interesting.

In summary, GD appears to be a polygenic disorder in which each gene contributes a certain amount to an individual's susceptibility. Although a number of susceptible genes have been associated with GD, their relative contributions to pathogenesis have yet to be clearly defined. Moreover, additional nongenetic factors significantly contribute to the etiology of this disorder.

Both human and animal studies have indicated that chronic excess iodine supplementation may modulate the expression of AITD in genetically susceptible individuals. Iodine can stimulate B lymphocytes to increase immunoglobulin production, enhance T-lymphocyte activity, and influence the expression of MHC antigens. Although excess iodine is unlikely to cause GD *de novo* in normal subjects, recurrence is almost certainly affected by iodine intake. Patients given iodine supplementation after discontinuing treatment with antithyroid drugs are more likely to relapse than those who do not receive iodine. GD is more likely to recur in areas of high iodine intake than in areas of normal iodine intake following thyroidectomy.[28] Comparable doses of antithyroid drugs are more likely to cause hypothyroidism in patients with GD who reside in an area of iodine deficiency than in those residing in an area of iodine sufficiency.[29]

Studies have implicated stress in changing thyroid function by increasing uptake of iodine and stimulating secretion of TSH and thyroid hormones.[30] The incidence of GD is significantly increased in populations exposed to major wars.[30] While there is strong evidence that stress is related to the development of GD, it is unlikely that, in and of itself, it can induce the disease.

CLINICAL PEARLS

SUSPECTED ENVIRONMENTAL RISK FACTORS IN GRAVES' DISEASE

Clinical/epidemical phenomenon observed	Pathogenic factors suggested
Increased incidence or recurrent rate in high iodine intake areas	Excess iodine
Increased incidence in populations exposed to war	Stress
Female predominance	Female hormones
Occurrence after viral or bacterial infections	Infections

KEY CONCEPTS

IMMUNOLOGIC FEATURES IN GRAVES' DISEASE

>> Presence of autoantibodies, particularly thyroid-stimulating hormone-stimulating antibodies (TSAb)

>> Infiltration of T cells into the thyroid parenchyma, mostly CD4 T cells

>> Thyroid expression of major histocompatibility complex (MHC) class II antigens, especially human leukocyte antigen (HLA)-DR antigen

>> Recognition of thyroid antigens by T cells

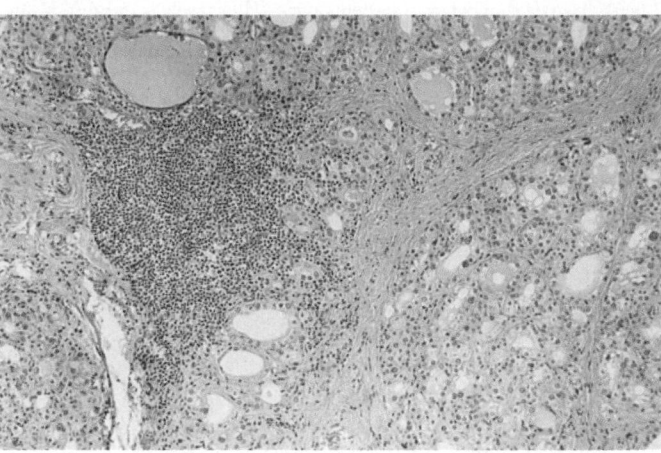

Fig. 69.1 Graves' disease, showing epithelial hyperplasia, lymphocytic infiltration and fibrous bands. (Courtesy of Dr. Thomas Giordano, Department of Pathology, University of Michigan.)

There is increasing evidence showing a connection between infectious agents and GD. Many studies suggest that GD often occurs after infection. The frequency of antibodies to *Yersinia enterocolitica*, a Gram-negative bacillus, is significantly increased in patients with GD. Furthermore, *Y. enterocolitica* appears to have saturable TSH-binding sites[31]; this bacillus may contain antigenic determinants that cross-react with human thyroid autoantigens. Other microorganisms may also be predisposing agents in GD by breaking tolerance to autoantigens, stimulating cytokine production, changing host cell components, and through molecular mimicry (Chapter 50).

PATHOGENESIS

An immune response is initiated when T-cell receptors recognize foreign peptides or self-peptide fragments bound to HLA molecules. HLA class II molecules are usually only expressed on antigen-presenting cells, such as B cells, dendritic cells, and macrophages, and not on epithelial cells such as thyrocytes. As mentioned above, several HLA molecules encoded by the class II gene region have been reported to be associated with GD. Abnormal or aberrant expression of these antigens on thyrocytes and lymphocytes may play a key role in the development of GD.

GD is characterized by lymphocytic infiltration of the thyroid gland. It is believed that T cells and B cells accumulate in the thyroid gland (Fig. 69.1), as a result of various factors such as viral/bacterial infection, stress, sex hormones, and genetic abnormality. Cytokines and other molecules released during initial steps of the disease may upregulate the expression of MHC class I and class II molecules on the surface of thyroid cells, which may become adequate antigen-presenting cells and present TSHR peptides.

Alternatively, infection might produce mimic peptides or alter host cell components such that they could be attacked by the immune system.

Analysis of the phenotypic profile of intrathyroidal T lymphocytes in GD reveals CD4 T-cell dominance; only a few infiltrating T cells are CD8. CD4 T cells are capable of helping locally abundant B cells to produce antibodies. Mechanisms leading to the selection of relevant CD4 T cells in the thyroid tissue remain unclear. The number of intrathyroidal CD4 T cells decreased, whereas CD8 T cells increased in patients treated with antithyroid medicines.

TSHR is the dominating force in regulating thyroid gland growth and differentiation. TSHR can undergo different intramolecular cleavage and/or conformational changes into three functional epitopes or subunits, A, B, and C.[32] These three epitopes can function as autoantigens to initiate different pathological reactions. Autoantibodies that bind to epitope A can mimic TSH, causing thyroid stimulation, and thus they are named TSHR-stimulating antibodies (TSAb). By binding to the epitope A on thyroid follicular cells, TSAb stimulate excessive cyclic adenosine monophosphate (cAMP) synthesis and induce excess production of thyroid hormones, leading to hyperthyroidism or GD. Shed epitope A can act as a systemic antigenic stimulus and may contribute to the breakdown of TSHR tolerance in susceptible individuals.[32] In healthy individuals, thyroid hormone release is normally regulated by feedback inhibition from TSH, but the presence of TSAb disrupts this system because the generation of TSAb is independent of thyroid hormones. As a result, the TSHR is under continuing stimulation by TSAb.

Epitope B comprises a small part of the ectodomain and the transmembrane region. Autoantibodies against epitope B can block the thyrotropic action of TSH, causing hypothyroidism.[32] Therefore, these autoantibodies are termed TSHR-blocking antibodies (TBAb). Some patients with GD may eventually develop hypothyroidism, not because the thyroid gland itself is destroyed by autoreactive cells, but because the nature of the TSAb generated switches from agonist to antagonist.

Epitope C is a region located in the N-terminus of the TSHR ectodomain cleaved from the holoreceptor. Autoantibodies bind to epitope C but result in no signal transduction. Therefore, these autoantibodies are designed as TSHR-neutral autoantibodies (TNAb). The presence of TNAb has been reported in patients with GD as well as in normal subjects.[32] The physiological or pathophysiological relevance of TNAb remains unclear. However, TNAb may inhibit TSHR cleavage and, as a consequence, prolong the half-life of the TSHR.

In addition to autoantibodies against TSHR, other nonspecific autoantibodies against various components of the thyroid gland, including thyroid peroxidase (TPO), thyroid Na/iodine transporter and thyroglobulin, can also be present in GD.

▪ PREVENTION AND PATIENT MANAGEMENT ▪

There is no effective way of preventing the occurrence of GD. Prior to a confirmatory diagnosis, an effective means of controlling symptoms is the use of inhibitors of β-adrenergic receptors, such as propranolol. These β-adrenergic blocking agents can also be used after diagnosis with other therapies.

Treatment of GD focuses on decreasing the overproduction of thyroid hormones and returning the patient to an euthyroid state. There are three standard methods available for treatment: antithyroid medication, radioactive ablation, and surgical thyroidectomy. Table 69.3 shows the various medications available for the treatment of GD and the sites of their actions. Propylthiouracil and methimazole are the two antithyroid drugs that are most frequently used. They not only inhibit the production of thyroid hormones, relieving hyperthyroidism, but also decrease the size and vascularity of the goiter, making it more amenable to a definitive therapy with surgery or radioactive iodine if necessary. Both radioactive iodine and surgical subtotal thyroidectomy are final, ablative therapies. The destructive therapy with ^{131}I is beneficial because patients do not relapse, but it may increase the risk of posttreatment orbitopathy or worsening of existing orbitopathy. Corticosteroids, lithium, ipodate, and amiodarone have also been used in the treatment of GD.

One study has reported that combining antithyroid drugs with thyroxine (T_4) initially and then suppressive doses of T_4 alone maintains a continually low level of TSAb and thus prevents the recurrence of hyperthyroidism.[33] However, other groups have been unable to obtain the same result.[34]

In order to determine the efficiency of therapy, dose of use, and length of maintenance, some pathological markers need to be monitored during the treatment. Among many markers, thyroid hormone and TSH concentrations are perhaps the most useful. The measurement of TSAb levels has also been used to assess the response to treatment and to predict relapse or remission.[32]

▪ PATIENT EVALUATION AND DIFFERENTIAL DIAGNOSIS ▪

GD typically presents with a diffuse goiter and thyrotoxicosis. The classic signs of hyperthyroidism are heat intolerance; hand tremors; nervousness; irritability; warm, moist skin; weight loss; muscle reflex changes; hyperdynamic cardiovascular status with tachycardia; hyperdefecation; and changes in mental status.

Approximately 20–25% of patients who present with clinical thyroid-associated ophthalmopathy are characterized by proptosis. However, subclinical thyroid-associated ophthalmopathy can be found in a majority of patients with GD when more sensitive imaging techniques (computed tomography scan or magnetic resonance imaging) are used. Surprisingly, some patients with clinical thyroid-associated ophthalmopathy can present without any evidence of Graves' hyperthyroidism, though autoantibodies against the thyroid may exist. TSH receptors are known to be expressed in the orbital connective tissues, but the potential role of the TSH receptor has yet to be established. Thyroid-associated dermopathy usually presents as a swelling in the pretibial area (myxedema) and in the feet, face, or hands, and rarely in other parts of the body. Furthermore, dermopathy typically coexists with and sometimes precedes thyroid-associated ophthalmopathy.

Laboratory findings in patients with hyperthyroidism include elevated levels of total and free triiodothyronine (T_3) and T_4. Because T_4 and T_3 are usually bound to proteins, testing for free T_4 is more accurate because it is the only thyroid hormone that is free to enter tissues.[35] TSH levels are low or undetectable because the stimulation of the thyroid gland is exogenous, rather than from the pituitary axis, and the elevated levels of the thyroid hormones cause a feedback inhibition of the pituitary TSH secretion. The appearance of TSAb is regarded as a specific and pathogenic marker for GD. This autoantibody can be demonstrated in about 90% of GD patients. A detectable rate less than 100% is probably due to the insensitive methodology that is currently available, rather than to the absolute absence of TSAb because thyroid glands of GD patients always show an increased uptake of radioactive iodine. Finally, a diffuse homogeneous uptake on a radioisotopic scan of the thyroid is almost pathognomonic of GD.

A differential diagnosis of GD involves exclusion of other thyroid disorders with hyperthyroidism, such as HT, pituitary tumors, or thyroid adenomas. Most of these can be ruled out by determining that the thyroid gland has a diffused increase in iodine uptake. The presence of ophthalmopathy is good diagnostic evidence of GD. Sometimes it is difficult to differentiate between GD and HT. Fine-needle biopsy helps the diagnosis. In HT, the lymphocytic infiltrate is usually diffuse and is considerably more intense than in GD. Oxyphilic cells, typical of HT, are usually absent in GD.

The hypermetabolic state of pregnancy can be confused with GD. Systemic symptoms such as fatigue, heat intolerance, emotional liability, and hyperhidrosis are often part of normal pregnancy. A normal pregnancy may also be associated with a slight increase in the size of the thyroid gland and warm and moist skin. Therefore, these nonspecific symptoms cannot be used in making a diagnosis of hyperthyroidism. However, a failure to gain weight adequately may serve as a useful sign. Laboratory confirmation of the clinical suspicion is essential. Radioisotope tests should be avoided because of the risk to the fetus.

Table 69.3 Therapies available for the treatment of Graves' disease

Beta-blockers	Inhibition of peripheral thyroxine (T_4) conversion to the active hormone triiodothyronine (T_3) Block of sympathetic action
Iodine	Inhibition of thyroid hormone release Inhibition of thyroid-stimulating hormone action on thyroid
Ipodate	Inhibition of thyroid hormone synthesis Decrease of serum T_3 and increase of serum rT_3
Lithium	Inhibition of T_4 release
Steroids	Immunosuppressive actions Inhibition of peripheral monodeiodination, causing a decrease in serum T_3 and an increase in serum rT_3
Thionamides	Inhibition of thyroglobin synthesis Correction of abnormal immune responses

■ HASHIMOTO'S THYROIDITIS ■

HT was first described by H. Hashimoto in 1912 as struma lymphomatosa. The autoantibodies present in this disorder were identified in 1956 by Roitt et al. [36, 41] HT is characterized by lymphocytic infiltration of the parenchyma (Fig. 69.2) (causing a dense accumulation of lymphocytes, plasma cells, and macrophages sometimes with germinal center formation) and by the presence of thyroid autoantibodies to thyroglobulin and to TPO. HT is the most common underlying cause for hypothyroidism. It has been estimated that about 3–4% of the population suffers from HT. This disorder is most commonly found in middle-aged and elderly females, but it also occurs in other age groups. HT is distributed throughout the world without racial and ethnic restriction. It occurs more commonly in families where another member has an AITD or another organ-specific autoimmune disease, such as systemic lupus erythematosus.

GENETIC AND ENVIRONMENTAL FACTORS

The etiology of HT is not known, but, similar to GD, it is believed to be an interplay between genetic and environmental factors. The relative contribution of each is not clearly defined and may vary from patient to patient. Thyroid antibodies are found with high frequency among first-degree relatives, and there is a high degree of concordance among twins and triplets. Siblings of adult patients with HT have about a 50% chance of developing thyroid autoantibodies[36]; however, the mode of inheritance has not been defined. Most of the genetic studies look at the HLA region (Table 69.4). There is increasing evidence to support the association between HT and HLA-DR3.[40]

Studies on both human and animal models have indicated that the autoimmune process in HT is a multistep process (Fig. 69.3). Initially it is believed that the immune system in susceptible individuals is altered by environmental factors. Such alterations in the immune system may result in defective immunoregulatory pathways, such as reduced function of the coinhibitory molecule or in CTLA-4, CD4+CD25+ T regulatory cells (CD4+CD25+ Treg cells).[46] Genetic elements are apparent from the fact that 95% of patients who acquire the disease are women,[47] strongly suggesting a role for sex hormones in

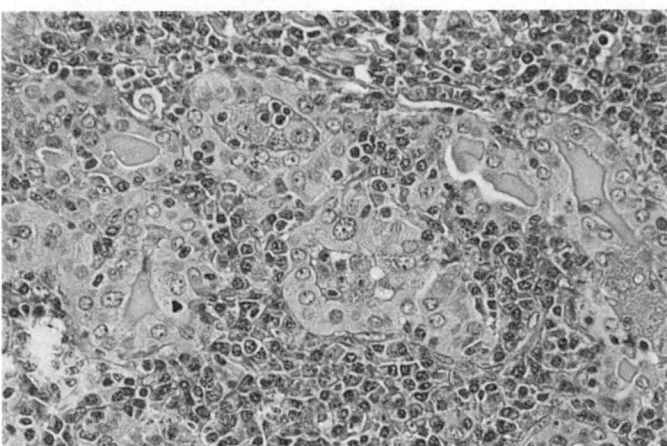

Fig. 69.2 Hashimoto's thyroiditis, with prominent infiltration by lymphocytes, plasma cells, and oncocytic metaplasia of residual follicular epithelium. (Courtesy of Dr. Thomas Giordano, Department of Pathology, University of Michigan.)

disease. Testosterone suppresses and estrogen exacerbates experimental autoimmune thyroiditis induced by immunization of mice or by thymectomy; castration of male animal increases the severity of experimental autoimmune thyroiditis.[48] Furthermore, the expression of a functional estrogen receptor in thyroid cells suggests that thyrocytes may be sex-hormone-responsive.[49] Infection, iodine, and irradiation might also increase the risk of developing HT.

There is increasing evidence that CD4+CD25 Treg cells represent an important mechanism for the maintenance of self-tolerance (Chapter 16). Removal of CD4+CD25+ Treg cells from mice that do not develop autoimmune disease can result in autoimmune thyroiditis. Furthermore, CD4+CD25+ Treg cells are able to prevent experimental autoimmune thyroiditis.[46] CD4+CD25+ Treg cells produce a number of molecules that are known to have immunosuppressive effects, including CD25, IL-2,

CTLA-4, IL-10, GITR, LAG-3, Foxp3, and transforming factor-β (TGF-β). It is currently believed that immunosuppressive mechanisms of Treg cells in patients with HT are defective due to intrinsic factors in the thyroid microenvironment. Reduction of several of these molecules may enhance the activity of B cells, which produce autoantibodies against TPO, and thyroglobulin. Depending upon the method of detection, 55–90% of patients with HT exhibit anti-thyroglobulin antibodies, while 82–91% exhibit anti-TPO antibodies.[50, 51]

On the other hand, a defect in CD4+CD25+ Treg cells may promote the production of Th1 cytokines and thus increase the levels of IL-1β, IFN-γ and tumor necrosis factor-α (TNF-α), all of which are known to play an important role in triggering apoptosis in thyroid cells.[52, 53] Thyroid follicles are either destroyed or damaged, and therefore their

Table 69.4 Association of human leukocyte antigen (HLA) types with Hashimoto's thyroiditis

Population studied	HLA associated	Reference
Caucasian (Canada)	DR4, DR5	37
Caucasian (Canada + UK)	DR4, DR5	38
Caucasian (Denmark)	Dw5	39
Caucasian (Hungary)	DR3	40, 41
Caucasian (UK)	DR3	40, 41
Oriental (China)	DR9, Bw46	42
Oriental (Japan)	DRB4*0101, A2	43
Oriental (Japan)	DR53	44
Oriental (Korea)	DR8, DQB1*0302	45

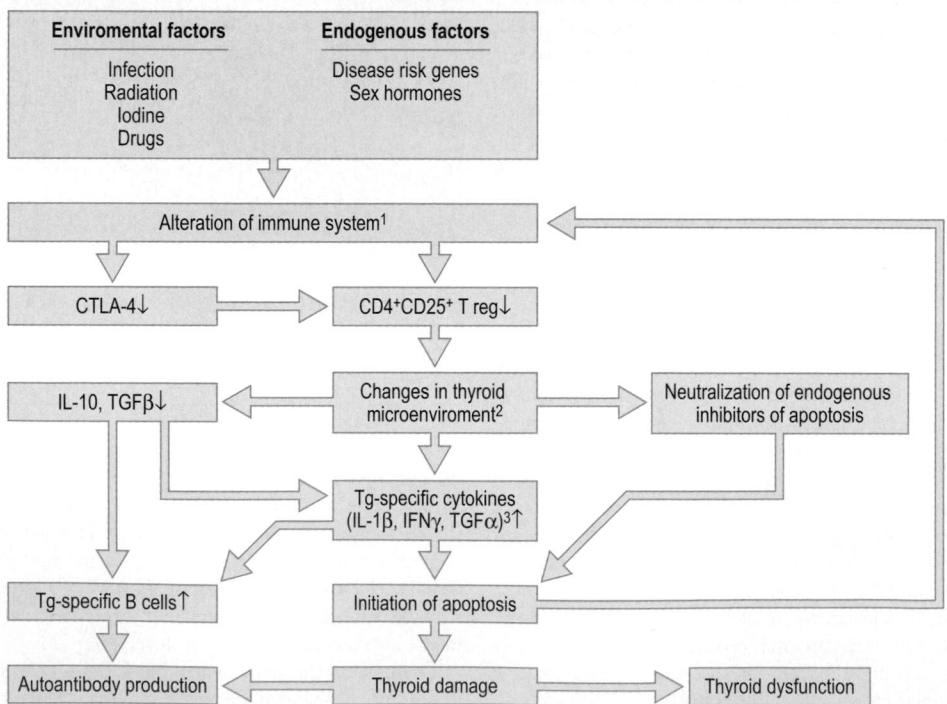

Fig. 69.3 Hashimoto's thyroiditis: pathways of thyroid cell damage. With the influence of environmental factors, the immune system in genetically susceptible individuals loses its surveillance function. A defect in CD4+CD25+ regulatory T cells occurs, which leads to changes in the thyroid microenvironment. Subsequently, the production of Th1 cytokines is increased and apoptosis inhibition is removed. The thyroid is damaged by apoptosis.

numbers are reduced. Traditionally it has been thought that thyroid follicles are injured by cytotoxicity, but now there is increasing evidence that apoptosis plays a key role in the loss of thyroid cells.[52-54] Figure 69.4 shows that apoptosis occurs in follicular thyroid cells. Thyroid cells are known to express apoptotic molecules, such as TNF, Fas, and TNF-related apoptosis-inducing ligand (TRAIL)[55] (Chapter 14). The Fas apoptosis pathway is implicated in CD8-T-cell-mediated cytotoxicity. Under physiologic conditions, these apoptotic molecules may remain inactivated. The process of lymphocytic infiltration into an inflamed thyroid can be inhibited by direct injection of a FasL-expression vector,[56] suggesting that FasL can induce apoptosis of the infiltrating lymphocytes. Although Fas is known to be expressed constitutively on thyrocytes (Fig. 69.5), normally it does not cause apoptosis even in the presence of excess anti-Fas antibodies. The Fas–FasL pathway may therefore be regulated in thyrocytes, and certain combinations of inflammatory cytokines may reverse the inhibition.[52, 53]

PATHOGENESIS

Basement membranes on thyroid follicular cells from HT are shown to stain positive for immune complexes and terminal complement components.[41] In an inflammatory or immunologic response, thyroid cells may express the intercellular adhesion molecules ICAM-1, VCAM-1, and LFA-3. Adhesion molecules have been implicated not only in cell adhesion but also in signal transduction, leading to cellular activation and proliferation. The presence of these adhesion molecules may induce thyroid follicular cells to bind T cells and thus significantly increase thyroid cell damage mediated by cytotoxic T cells. One of the important characteristics of HT is the formation of germinal centers within the thyroid gland. Germinal centers constitute a specialized microenvironment essential for the induction of antibody synthesis, affinity maturation of B cells, memory B-cell formation, and maintenance of T-cell memory. The interactions among thyroid follicular cells, dendritic-like cells, infiltrating B cells, and T cells in germinal centers may have a key role in the generation of thyroid

autoantibodies, the production of cytokines, and the formation of memory B and T cells.

PREVENTION AND PATIENT MANAGEMENT

The cause of HT is largely unknown, and no preventive approaches are available. The treatment usually consists of thyroid hormone replacement for hypothyroidism, which is generally required lifelong. In response to thyroid hormone therapy, levels of antithyroid antibodies often decrease. In patients with symptomatic goiter, thyroid hormones at doses that suppress TSH secretion may decrease the size of the gland. Although immunosuppressive (corticosteroid) therapy may regress thyroid enlargement, it is not recommended because corticosteroids have serious side effects. Patients with coexisting thyrotoxicosis should be treated with antithyroid drugs and should be carefully monitored for levels of thyroid hormones. An appropriate therapy is not available for patients who are euthyroid but have enlarged glands. Thyroid hormone therapy may decrease the size of the gland in some cases and increase it in others.

Occasionally, HT coexists with GD, often presenting with hyperthyroidism. Antithyroid treatment should be handled with extreme caution because patients with both diseases are more likely to become hypothyroid after surgical or radioactive iodine therapy than patients with GD alone.

With recent advances in understanding of how the thyroid is damaged, several experimental therapies have emerged for the treatment of autoimmune thyroiditis. One such new approach is enhancement of the activity of CD4+CD25+ Treg cells, which has successfully resulted in the suppression of mTg-specific effector T cells and the inhibition of damage in the thyroid.[46] Interestingly, it has been shown that exogenous TRAIL can suppress the development of autoimmune thyroiditis via altering the function of immune response cells.[57] This finding may lead to the design of a novel therapeutic strategy for treatment of autoimmune thyroiditis.

PATIENT EVALUATION AND DIFFERENTIAL DIAGNOSIS

HT primarily presents with symptoms of altered thyroid function. Early in the course of the disease, the patient is usually euthyroid but can experience clinical thyrotoxicosis because of the breakdown of thyroid

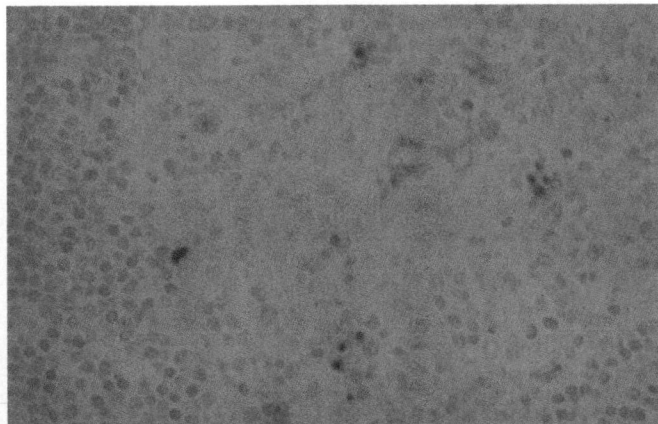

Fig. 69.4 Apoptosis occurs in thyrocytes from Hashimoto's thyroiditis. The apoptotic cells were detected with ApopTag staining Kit, where the nuclear fragmented DNA is detected by the brown color.

KEY CONCEPTS

IMMUNOLOGIC FEATURES IN HASHIMOTO'S THYROIDITIS

>> Expression of major histocompatibility complex (MHC) class II antigens, especially human leukocyte antigen (HLA)-DR antigen on thyrocytes

>> Possible defects in CD4+CD25+ regulatory T cells

>> Changes in the thyroid microenvironment

>> Cytokine-induced apoptosis in thyrocytes

>> Recognition of thyroid antigens by T cells

>> Production of antithyroid peroxidase (TPO) antibody and antithyroglobulin antibody

>> Production of immune complexes

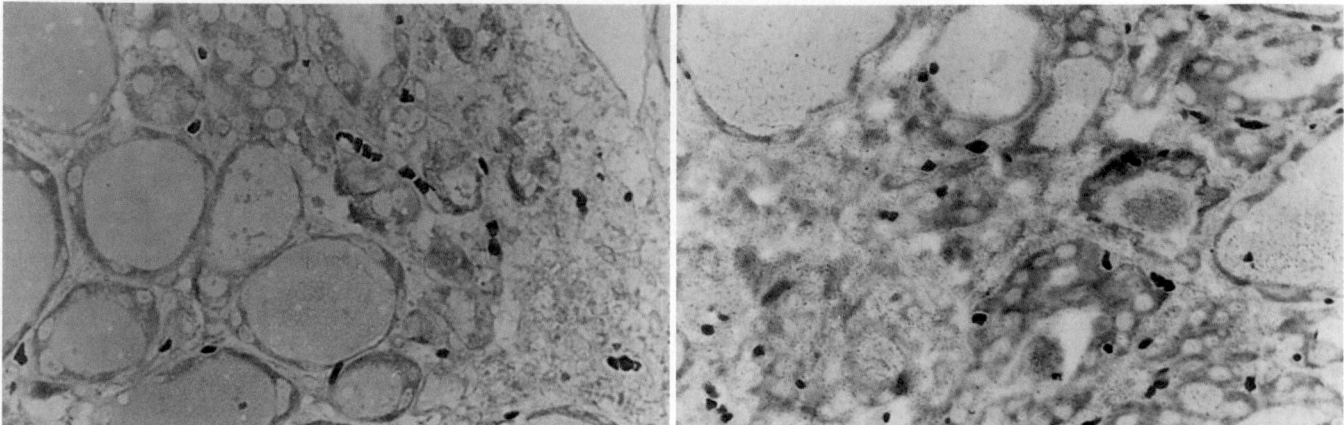

Fig. 69.5 Expression of Fas in Hashimoto's thyroiditis. Fas is constitutively expressed in thyrocytes from Hashimoto's thyroiditis. Left panel: control antibody; right panel: anti-Fas antibody.

follicles with the release of thyroid hormones. In contrast, late in the disease, the patient is often hypothyroid due to progressive destruction of the thyroid gland. The most common outcome of HT is hypothyroidism. HT is not usually life-threatening, but its natural history is quite long in evolution and may confound clinicians.

A consistent physical sign seen in HT is an enlarged thyroid gland. The goiter is often symmetrically large and feels very firm, with fine nodularity present. The size of an enlarged thyroid gland and the number of nodules are variable, depending on the amount of lymphocytic infiltration, the formation of fibrosis, and the degree of compensatory hyperplasia. Lymph nodes surrounding the gland often become enlarged, and lymphoma must be excluded. Sometimes patients show symptoms of other autoimmune diseases, such as generalized vasculitis with urticaria and nephritis, and these are believed to be caused by the cross-reaction of antithyroid autoantibodies with other tissues or the presence of circulating immune complexes containing thyroid antigens, predominantly thyroglobulin.

General laboratory findings are not very useful in making a diagnosis of HT other than conducting tests of the thyroid status. However, screening tests for specific autoantibodies against thyroid (antithyroglobulin and antithyroid TPO) may be helpful. In the early phase of the disease, thyroid hormone levels may be normal, high, or low. An increased TSH in the presence of normal thyroid hormones (T_4 and T_3) may presage clinical hypothyroidism. HT patients with hyperthyroidism are differentiated from those with GD by the demonstration of patchy or decreased uptake on a radioiodine scan of the thyroid.

Sometimes it may be difficult to differentiate HT from GD and other types of thyroiditis (focal lymphocytic thyroiditis, subacute thyroiditis, Riedel's thyroiditis). On occasion, the rapid enlargement of one lobe of the thyroid gland in HT also needs to be differentiated from malignant lymphoma or thyroid carcinoma. The fibrous variant of HT may also mimic carcinoma. In subacute thyroiditis, the involvement of the gland is focal, whereas in HT the gland is diffusely nodular and only rare nodules may be spared from the process. Often, fine-needle biopsy will be necessary to provide pathologic diagnosis. Cytologically, HT is characterized by the presence of lymphoid infiltration of follicules, follicular cells with oxyphilic changes of varying degrees, polymorphous lymphocyte populations, and histiocytes.

■ POSTPARTUM THYROIDITIS ■

Postpartum thyroiditis is characterized by the development of transient thyrotoxicosis and/or hypothyroidism during the first 6 months of the postpartum period. A significant percentage of patients (25–30%) will suffer from chronic hypothyroidism. The symptoms of postpartum thyroiditis were first described by H.E.W. Robert in 1948, but the nature of the disease was not fully established until 1976. The incidence of postpartum thyroiditis has been reported to range from 2% to 21% in different races and geographical locations. However, a much narrower range of 5–8% is generally accepted.

GENETIC AND ENVIRONMENTAL FACTORS

The development of postpartum thyroiditis, like other AITDs, is thought to involve genetic and environmental factors. A familial form of postpartum thyroiditis has been reported.[58] HLA haplotypes (DR3, DR4, DR5, DR7) are positively or negatively associated with disease risk, emphasizing the role of genetic predisposition.

Iodine consumption may affect the incidence or severity of postpartum thyroiditis and this concept is in agreement with the fact that the administration of iodine exacerbates AITD.[28, 29, 59] One study performed by Kampe *et al.* showed that the administration of 150 µg of iodine daily increased the severity of hypothyroidism in women with postpartum thyroiditis.[59] A history of smoking may also be a risk factor in the development of postpartum thyroiditis.[60]

PATHOGENESIS

Complement-fixing TPO antibodies are present in a majority of patients with postpartum thyroiditis, and the titer of this autoantibody is closely associated with the severity of the disease.[61] Although the TPO antibody response is significant and dramatic, the role it plays in the pathogenesis of postpartum thyroiditis remains unknown. As the histomorphologic changes seen in postpartum thyroiditis are the same as in HT, it is possible that the antibody only reflects the degree of damage to the thyroid gland and that the damage is executed by lymphocyte-, complement-, and apoptosis-mediated mechanisms similar to HT. However, it should be noted that the pathways leading to the final presentation of the disease appear somewhat different between these two types of thyroiditis.

It has been well known that pregnancy can induce dramatic suppression of both humoral and cell-mediated immunity, for example, a decrease in helper T-cell number and an increase in suppressor T-cell number.[62] In the postpartum state, reversal of this phenomenon may induce rebound activation of autoimmune diseases. Obviously, rebound of suppressive immunity itself is not the sole factor in inducing postpartum thyroiditis. A number of studies have indicated that HLA antigens, particularly DR antigens, are associated with the disease. There is a positive correlation of the syndrome with DR5. Negative correlation between the disorder and DR2 has been observed,[63] suggesting that DR2 might confer a protective effect. Frequencies of DR3, DR4, and DR7 have been found to be increased in postpartum thyroiditis.[64]

Lymphocyte subsets and functions are significantly altered in postpartum thyroiditis. The ratio of B cells to T cells within thyroid glands is increased, as is the ratio of helper T cells to suppressor T cells.[65] Functionally, T-cell activation is significantly increased.[62] All these changes may present a picture very similar to the one seen in HT. Involvement of an apoptotic process in postpartum thyroiditis is possible. 2-Methoxyestradiol, an endogenous estrogen metabolite, is able to induce thyroid cell apoptosis,[66] suggesting that there may be a link between thyrocyte apoptosis and female hormones or their metabolites.

PATIENT MANAGEMENT

Treatment is not usually recommended for the thyrotoxic phase unless symptoms are severe. As thyrotoxicosis in postpartum thyroiditis is caused by hormone release from the damaged gland and is not secondary to increased synthesis and secretion of thyroid hormones, antithyroid medicines are not useful.

In the hypothyroid phase of postpartum thyroiditis, the management of this disorder is somewhat similar to that of hypothyroidism caused by other diseases. Therefore, thyroid hormone therapy is not required unless the hypothyroidism is clinically and biochemically significant. Administration of T_4 prevents hypothyroid symptoms, but it does not alter the course of the disease.

PATIENT EVALUATION AND DIFFERENTIAL DIAGNOSIS

The classic clinical course of postpartum thyroiditis consists of a sequence of two phases, hyperthyroidism and hypothyroidism. The hyperthyroid phase is followed by the hypothyroid phase and the recovery. The hyperthyroidism is often too mild to be recognized or even does not occur at all. During this phase, irritability and lack of energy are prominent, even in autoantibody-positive women who do not develop thyroid dysfunction. In contrast, the symptoms of the hypothyroid phase may be profound. Because psychomotor retardation is a prominent feature of both diseases, thyroid function studies are recommended in the evaluation of women with clinically significant symptoms of postpartum depression.

About 80% of the patients are euthyroid within 12 months after delivery. However, many of them will have a recurrence of postpartum thyroiditis with subsequent pregnancies, and they are also at a greater risk of becoming permanently hypothyroid. In addition, patients are more likely to become persistently hypothyroid when they have relatively high autoantibody titers or lack a hyperthyroid phase of the disease.

Results from laboratory tests need to be analyzed with consideration given to the two phases in the course of the disease. The levels of TSH are usually a little lower or at the lower limit of detection in the hyperthyroid phase, whereas its levels are increased during the hypothyroid phase. Thyroid hormones are also consistent with the two-phase changes. Antithyroid autoantibodies, especially the anti-TPO antibodies, are present in most patients. TRAb is usually not found unless there is coexisting GD.

The first phase (hyperthyroidism) of postpartum thyroiditis is sometimes difficult to distinguish from GD, although the latter commonly ameliorates during pregnancy. If necessary, the thyroid radioactive iodine uptake (RAIU) test can be performed to differentiate between these two diseases. In postpartum patients, I-123 should be used rather than I-131, and appropriate preventions should be taken to avoid exposure to the child. A low RAIU uptake is consistent with postpartum thyroiditis, while a high one is consistent with GD.

The relation between women with postpartum thyroiditis and the outcome of their babies has received much attention. Infants born to women who suffer from the disease show a decrease in their growth during the first 30 days, though Apgar scores, birth weight and length, and levels of thyroid hormones are not significantly different from those of infants born to unaffected women.[67] Low IQ is also associated with postpartum thyroiditis of the mother.[68]

■ REFERENCES ■

1. Rose NR, Witebsky E. Studies on organ-specificity. V. Changes in the thyroid gland of rabbits following active immunization with rabbit thyroid extract. J Immunol 1956; 76: 417–427.

2. Adams DD, Purves HD. Abnormal responses in the assay of thyrotropin. Proc Univ Otago Med Sch 1956; 34: 11–12.

3. Tomer Y, Davies TF. The genetic susceptibility to Graves' disease. Baillieres Clin Endocrinol metab 1997; 11: 431–450.

4. Brix TH, Kyvik KO, Christensen K, et al. Evidence for a major role of heredity in Graves' disease: a population-based study of two Danish twin cohorts. J Clin Endocrinol Metab 2001; 86: 930–934.

5. Hunt PJ, Marshall SE, Weetman AP, et al. Histocompatibility leucocyte antigens and closely linked immunomodulatory genes in autoimmune thyroid disease. Clin Endocrinol (Oxf) 2001; 55: 491–499.

6. Wong GWK, Cheng SH, Dorman JS. The HLA-DQ associations with Graves' disease in Chinese children. Clin Endocrinol 1999; 50: 493–495.

7. Chuang LM, Wu HP, Chang CC, et al. HLA DRB1/DQA1/DQB1 haplotype determines thyroid autoimmunity in patients with insulin dependent diabetes mellitus. Clin Endocrinol 1996; 45: 631–636.

8. Larizza D, Calcaterra V, Martinetti M, et al. Helicobacter pylori infection and autoimmune thyroid disease in young patients: the disadvantage of carrying the human leukocyte antigen-DRB1*0301 allele. J Clin Endocrinol Metab 2006; 91: 176–179.

9. Roman SH, Greenberg D, Rubinstein P, et al. Genetics of autoimmune thyroid disease: lack of evidence for linkage to HLA within families. J Clin Endocrinol Metab 1992; 74: 496–503.

10. Ban Y, Davies TF, Greenberg DA, et al. The influence of human leucocyte antigen (HLA) genes on autoimmune thyroid disease (AITD): results of studies in HLA-DR3 positive AITD families. Clin Endocrinol 2002; 57: 81–88.

11. Kurylowicz A, Kula D, Ploski R, et al. Association of CD40 gene polymorphism (C-1T) with susceptibility and phenotype of Graves' disease. Thyroid 2005; 15: 1119–1124.

12. Tomer Y, Greenberg DA, Barbesino G, et al. CTLA-4 and not CD28 is a susceptibility gene for thyroid autoantibody production. J Clin Endocrinol Metab 2001; 86: 1687–1693.

13. Tomer Y, Barbesina G, Greenberg DA, et al. Linkage analysis of candidate genes in autoimmune thyroid disease. III. Detailed analysis of chromosome 14 localizes Grave's disease-1 close to multinodular goiter (MNG-1). J Clin Endocrinol Metab 1998; 83: 4321–4327.

14. Siegmund T, Usadel KH, Donner H, et al. Interferon-gamma gene microsatellite polymorphisms in patients with Graves' disease. Thyroid 1998; 8: 1013–1017.

15. Blakemore AIF, Waston PF, Weetman AP, et al. Association of Graves' disease with an allele of the interleukin-1 receptor antagonist gene. J Clin Endocrinol Metab 1995; 80: 111–115.

16. Hunt PJ, Marshall SE, Weetman AP, et al. Cytokine gene polymorphisms in autoimmune thyroid disease. J Clin Endocrinol Metab 2000; 85: 1984–1988.

17. De Roux N, Shields DC, Misrahi M, et al. Analysis of the thyrotropin receptor as a candidate gene in familial Graves' disease. J Clin Endocrinol Metab 1996; 81: 3483–3486.

18. Skorka A, Bednarczuk T, Bar-Andziak E, et al. Lymphoid tyrosine phosphatase (PTPN22/LYP) variant and Graves' disease in a Polish population: association and gene dose-dependent correlation with age of onset. Clin Endocrinol 2005; 62: 679–682.

19. Vang T, Congia M, Macis MD, et al. Autoimmune-associated lymphoid tyrosine phosphatase is a gain-of-function variant. Nature Genetics 2005; 37: 1317–1319.

20. Ramos-Lopez E, Kurylowicz A, Bednarczuk T, et al. Vitamin D receptor polymorphisms are associated with Graves' disease in German and Polish but not in Serbian patients. Thyroid 2005; 15: 1125–1130.

21. Barbesina G, Tomer Y, Concepcion E, et al. Linkage analysis of candidate genes in antoimmune thyroid disease. II. Selected gender-related genes and the X-chromosome. J Clin Endocrinol Metab 1998; 83: 3290–3295.

22. Ueda H, Howson JM, Esposito L, et al. Association of the T-cell regulatory gene CTLA4 with susceptibility to autoimmune disease. Nature 2003; 423: 506–511.

23. Tait KF, Nithiyananthan R, Heward JM, et al. Polymorphisms of interleukin 4 receptor gene and interleukin 10 gene are not associated with Graves' disease in the UK. Autoimmunity 2004; 37: 189–194.

24. Muhlberg T, Kirchberger M, Spitzweg C, et al. Lack of association of Graves' disease with the A2 allele of the interleukin-1 receptor antagonist gene in a white European population. Eur J Endocrinol 1998; 138: 686–690.

25. Tomer Y, Barbesino G, Greenberg DA, et al. A new Graves disease-susceptibility locus maps to chromosome 20q11.2. International Consortium for the Genetics of Autoimmune Thyroid Disease. Am J Human Genet 1998; 63: 1749–1756.

26. Ban Y, Greenberg DA, Concepcion ES, et al. A germline single nucleotide polymorphism at the intracellular domain of the human thyrotropin receptor does not have a major effect on the development of Graves' disease. Thyroid 2002; 12: 1079–1083.

27. Chistiakov DA, Savost'anov KV, Turakulov RI. Screening of SNPs at 18 positional candidate genes, located within the GD-1 locus on chromosome 14q23-q32, for susceptibility to Graves' disease: a TDT study. Mol Genet Metab 2004; 83: 264–270.

28. Thjodleifsson B, Hedley AJ, Donald D, et al. Outcome of sub-total thyroidectomy for thyrotoxicosis in Iceland and Northeast Scotland. Clin Endocrinol (Oxf) 1975; 7: 367–376.

29. Azizi F. Environmental iodine intake affects the response to methimazole in patients with diffuse toxic goiter. J Clin Endocrinol Metab 1985; 61: 374–377.

30. Winsa B, Adami HO, Bergstrom R, et al. Stressful life events and Graves' disease. Lancet 1991; 338: 1475–1479.

31. Weiss M, Inghar SH, Winbald S, et al. Demonstration of a saturable binding site for thyrotropin in Yersinia enterocolitica. Science 1983; 219: 1331.

32. Davies TF, Ando T, Lin RY, et al. Thyrotropin receptor-associated diseases: from adenomata to Graves disease. J Clin Invest 2005; 115: 1972–1983.

33. Hashizume K, Ichikawa K, Sakurai A, et al. Administration of thyroxine in treated Graves' disease: effects on the level of antibodies to thyroid-stimulating hormone receptors and on the risk of recurrence of hyperthyroidism. N Engl J Med 1991; 324: 947–953.

34. McIver B, Rae P, Beckett G, et al. Lack of effect of thyroxine in patients with Graves' hyperthyroidism who are treated with an antithyroid drug. N Engl J Med 1996; 334: 220–224.

35. Mastorakos G, Doufas AG, Mantzos E, et al. T_4 but not T_3 administration is associated with increased recurrence of Graves' disease after successful medical therapy. J Endocrinol Invest 2003; 26: 979–984.

36. Hall R, Owen SG, Smart GS. Evidence for genetic predisposition to formation of thyroid autoantibodies. Lancet 1964; 2: 187–188.

37. Vargas MT, Bropnes-Urbina R, Gladman D, et al. Antithyroid microsomal autoantibodies and HLA-DR5 are associated with postpartum thyroid dysfunction: evidence supporting an endocrine pathogenesis. J Clin Endocrinol Metab 1988; 67: 327–333.

38. Badenhoop K, Schwarz G, Walfish PG, et al. Susceptibility to thyroid autoimmune disease: molecular analysis of HLA-D region genes identifies new markers for goitrous Hashimoto's thyroiditis. J Clin Endocrinol Metab 1990; 71: 1131–1137.

39. Thomsen M, Ryder LP, Bech K, et al. HLA-D in Hashimoto's thyroiditis. Tissue Antigens 1983; 21: 173–175.

40. Levin L, Ban Y, Concepcion E, et al. Analysis of HLA genes in families with autoimmune diabetes and thyroiditis. Hum Immunol 2004; 65: 640–647.

41. Weetman AP. Autoimmune thyroiditis: predisposition and pathogenesis. Clin Endocrinol 1992; 36: 307–323.

42. Hawkins BR, Lam KSL, Ma JTC, et al. Strong association between HLA-DRw9 and Hashimoto's thyroiditis in southern Chinese. Acta Endocrinol 1987; 114: 543–546.

43. Wan XL, Kimura A, Dong RP, et al. HLA-A and DRB4 genes in controlling the susceptibility to Hashimoto's thyroiditis. Hum Immunol 1995; 42: 131–136.

44. Onuma H, Ota M, Sugenoya A, et al. Association between HLA and Hashimoto thyroiditis in Japanese. In: Nagataki S, Mori T, Torizuka K (eds) Eighty Years of Hashimoto Disease, Amsterdam: Elsevier Science; 1993 : 65–68.

45. Cho BY, Chung JH, Lee HK, et al. Immunogenetic heterogeneity of atrophic antoimmune thyroiditis according to thyrotropin receptor blocking antibody. In: Nagataki S, Mori T, Torizuka K (eds) Eighty Years of Hashimoto Disease, Amsterdam: Elsevier Science; 1993 :45–50.

46. Verginis P, Li HS, Carayanniotis G. Tolerogenic semimature dendritic cells suppress experimental autoimmune thyroiditis by activation of thyroglobulin-specific CD4+CD25+ T cells. J Immunol 2005; 174: 7433–7439.

47. Levine SN. Current concepts of thyroiditis. Arch Intern Med 1983; 143: 1952–1956.

48. Ansar Ahmed S, Young PR, Penhale WJ. The effects of female sex steroids on the development of autoimmune thyroiditis in thymectomized and irradiated rats. Clin Exp Immunol 1983; 54: 351.

49. Clark OH, Gerend PL, Davis M, et al. Estrogen and thyroid-stimulating hormone (TSH) receptors in neoplastic and nonneoplastic human thyroid tissue. J Surg Res 1985; 38: 89–96.

50. Baker Jr JR. Immunologic aspects of endocrine diseases. Ann Intern Med 1988; 108: 26–30.

51. Bonger U, Finke R, Hegedus L, et al. Cytotoxicity and antithyroid peroxidase antibodies in patients with autoimmune thyroiditis. In: Nagataki S, Mori T, Torizuka K, eds: Eighty Years of Hashimoto Disease, Amsterdam: Elsevier Science, 1993 :383–388.

52. Wang SH, Mezosi E, Wolf JM, et al. IFNgamma sensitization to TRAIL-induced apoptosis in human thyroid carcinoma cells by upregulating Bak expression. Oncogene 2004; 23: 928–935.

53. Mezosi E, Wang SH, Utsugi S, et al. Interleukin-1beta and tumor necrosis factor (TNF)-alpha sensitize human thyroid epithelial cells to TNF-related apoptosis-inducing ligand-induced apoptosis through increases in procaspase-7 and bid, and the down-regulation of p44/42 mitogen-activated protein kinase activity. J Clin Endocrinol Metab 2004; 89: 250–257.

54. Baker JR Jr. Dying (apoptosing?) for a consensus on the Fas death pathway in the thyroid. J Clin Endocrinol Metab 1999; 84: 2593–2595.

55. Arscott PL, Baker JR Jr. Apoptosis and thyroiditis. Clin Immunol Immunopathol 1998; 87: 207–217.

56. Batteux F, Tourneur L, Trebeden H, et al. Gene therapy of experimental autoimmune thyroiditis by in vivo administration of plasmid DNA coding Fas ligand. J Immunol 1999; 162: 603–608.

57. Wang SH, Cao Z, Wolf JM, et al. Death ligand tumor necrosis factor-related apoptosis-inducing ligand inhibits experimental autoimmune thyroiditis. Endocrinology 2005; 146: 4721–4726.

58. Singer PA, Gorsky JE. Familial postpartum transient hypothyroidism. Arch Intern Med 1985; 145: 240–242.

59. Kampe O, Jansson R, Karlsson FA. Effects of L-thyroxine and iodide on the development of autoimmune postpartum thyroiditis. J Clin Endocrinol Metab 1990; 70: 1014–1018.

60. Jansson R, Dahlberg PA, Karlsson FA. Postpartum thyroiditis. Baillieres Clin Endocrinol Metab 1988; 2: 619–635.

61. Jansson R, Bernander S, Karlsson A, et al. Autoimmune thyroid dysfunction in the postpartum period. J Clin Endocrinol Metab 1984; 58: 681–687.

62. Stagnaro-Green A, Roman SH, Cobin RH, et al. A prospective study of lymphocyte-initiated immunosuppression in normal pregnancy: evidence of a T-cell etiology for postpartum thyroid dysfunction. J Clin Endocrinol Metab 1992; 74: 645–653.

63. Kologlu M, Fung H, Darke C, et al. Postpartum thyroid dysfunction and HLA status. Eur J Clin Invest 1990; 20: 56–60.

64. Parkes AB, Darke C, Othman S, et al. Major histocompatibility complex class II and complement polymorphisms in postpartum thyroiditis. Eur J Endocrinol 1996; 134: 449–453.

65. Mizukami Y, Michigishi T, Nonomura A, et al. Postpartum thyroiditis. A clinical, histologic, and immunopathologic study of 15 cases. Am J Clin Pathol 1993; 100: 200–205.

66. Wang SH, Phelps E, Utsugi S, et al. Susceptibility of thyroid cancer cells to 7-hydroxystaurosporine-induced apoptosis correlates with Bcl-2 protein level. Thyroid 2001; 11: 725–731.

67. Bech K, Hertel J, Rasmussen NG, et al. Effect of maternal thyroid autoantibodies and post-partum thyroiditis on the fetus and neonate. Acta Endocrinol 1991; 125: 146–149.

68. Pop VJ, de Vries E, van Baar AL, et al. Maternal thyroid proxidase antibodies during pregnancy: a marker of impaired child development. J Clin Endocrinol Metab 1995; 80: 3561–3566.

Diabetes and related autoimmune diseases

George S. Eisenbarth

70

DIAGNOSIS

Diabetes mellitus is a heterogeneous group of disorders characterized by glucose intolerance and hyperglycemia. The clinical manifestations of this disease are the result of either an absolute or a relative deficiency of insulin secretion. An expert committee of the American Diabetes Association proposed four categories of diabetes, based on etiology rather than the age of disease onset (e.g. juvenile-onset versus adult-onset) or the requirement for insulin therapy (insulin-dependent versus noninsulin-dependent).[1] The categories are type 1 (formerly termed insulin-dependent diabetes – IDDM); type 2 (with a major component of insulin resistance); diabetes with known genetic mutations (e.g. the maturity-onset diabetes of youth syndromes with mutations in glucokinase, hepatic nuclear factor genes etc.); and gestational diabetes (Table 70.1). Type 1 diabetes is divided into types 1A (immune mediated) and 1B (idiopathic loss of insulin secretion), depending primarily on the presence or absence respectively of anti-islet autoantibodies.

The subject of this chapter is type 1A or immune-mediated diabetes, and there is now convincing evidence that this form results from immune-mediated destruction of the cells that produce insulin. Despite older designations for this category, approximately the same number of adults develop type 1A diabetes as do children, and many individuals early in the course of type 1A diabetes are not 'insulin dependent' but can transiently be treated with oral hypoglycemic agents. The incidence of type 2 diabetes increases dramatically with age, whereas that of type 1A changes relatively little with age (less than threefold).[2] Thus, when a child develops diabetes they usually (>90% for non-Hispanic white children) have type 1A diabetes mellitus. There is, however, heterogeneity of diabetes even among children with the disorder. For example, almost half of African-American and Hispanic-American children who develop diabetes do not have type 1A, but rather primarily type 2.[3] Given such heterogeneity, it is likely that the diagnostic classification of diabetes will in the future depend upon the immunologic parameters to be discussed and the identification of specific genetic mutations associated with specific disorders of glucose metabolism.

The information indicating that type 1A diabetes is an immune-mediated autoimmune illness has greatly increased during the past two decades. The recognition that there might be a form of 'juvenile' or

insulin-dependent diabetes of autoimmune origin came from the observation that diabetes was often associated with disorders thought to be of autoimmune origin, such as Addison's disease, Graves' disease and thyroiditis. Nevertheless, considerable confusion existed because of the failure to separate diabetes into distinct disease categories (type 1 versus type 2). Although insulitis had been observed in a few children who had come to autopsy shortly after the development of diabetes, this was an extremely rare event for diabetes as a whole.[4]

Studies of monozygotic twins with diabetes revealed very different patterns of inheritance for insulin-dependent and noninsulin-dependent diabetes mellitus, and two major forms of the disease were proposed. Specific HLA alleles were found to be associated with the insulin-dependent form,[5] and in 1974 cytoplasmic islet cell autoantibodies were found for diabetic patients with polyendocrine autoimmunity (e.g. Addison's disease).[6] Islet cell autoantibodies were then found to be

KEY CONCEPTS

TYPE 1A DIABETES IS AN AUTOIMMUNE DISEASE

>> Genetic and familial clustering of diabetes and additional autoimmune disorders

>> Presence of high-affinity autoantibodies and T cells reactive to islet cell autoantigens

>> Strong HLA association (DR3/DR4)

>> Ability to transfer the disease in animal models through adoptive transfer of islet cell-reactive T-cell clones

>> Recurrence of disease in pancreas transplanted between identical twins

>> Regulatory T cells important; their loss in IPEX syndrome leads to neonatal diabetes

1035

Table 70.1 Classification of diabetes mellitus (DM)

Diabetes mellitus	Previous designations	Etiologic distinctions	Clinical distinctions
Type 1 A. Immune-mediated B. Idiopathic	Juvenile onset/IDDM Type 1.5/Flatbush DM	β-cell destruction Immune Unknown	Both result in insulin dependence, with loss of β-cells
Type 2	NIDDM	Insulin resistance and relative insulin deficiency	Oral hypoglycemic agents are effective early in the disease
Other specific types	MODY Secondary diabetes	Specific genetic defects Pancreatic disease Endocrinopathies Chemical induced Infection related Immune-mediated forms Genetic syndromes	Specific mutations identified and defined clinical syndromes
Gestational	Unchanged		Onset during pregnancy

IDDM, insulin-dependent diabetes; MODY, maturity-onset diabetes of youth; NIDDM, non-insulin dependent diabetes.

present prior to the development of diabetes, and studies of monozygotic twins of patients with type 1 diabetes led to the observation that this was a chronically progressive autoimmune disorder.[7] In identical twins developing diabetes, islet cell autoantibodies and loss of insulin secretion preceded the development of diabetes by years. As discussed below, the measurement of anti-islet autoantibodies has improved dramatically during the past two decades, and for many individuals the development of type 1A diabetes can now be predicted.

Despite the emphasis on anti-islet autoantibodies, most investigators believe that T cells, and not autoantibodies, mediate the immune destruction of insulin-producing cells.[8] Studies of T cells have benefited from the discovery of two animal models of type 1A diabetes, the NOD mouse and the BB rat.[8] In animal models diabetes can be transferred to nondiabetic animals by T-cell clones. In addition, a clinical observation by Sutherland and co-workers[9] was particularly informative in terms of demonstrating the importance of T cells in this disease. They transplanted the tail of the pancreas from monozygotic twins who had not developed diabetes into their respective twin pairs with more than a decade of diabetes. The transplanted islets were invaded by lymphocytes, and islet β cells (the cells that produce insulin) were specifically and rapidly destroyed.

Despite considerable progress in studies of type 1A diabetes, a series of basic and clinical questions remain unanswered or have only partial answers (Table 70.2). This chapter reviews current knowledge concerning many of these questions.

■ DIAGNOSIS ■

The demonstration of elevated plasma glucose is the sine qua non for diagnosis of diabetes mellitus. Recent recommendations by the American Diabetes Association have lowered the diagnostic level of fasting glucose from 140 mg/dl (7.8 mmol/L) to 126 mg/dL (7.0 mmol/L). Other

Table 70.2 Key questions in type 1A diabetes

Basic science questions
What genes determine type 1A diabetes susceptibility?
What triggers or suppresses the activation of autoimmunity?
What are the major target molecules and is there a primary autoantigen?
What are the effector mechanisms for islet destruction?

Clinical questions
Is type 1A diabetes predictable?
Is the rate of progression to overt diabetes predictable?
Is type 1A diabetes preventable?

diagnostic criteria include a random plasma glucose level >200 mg/dL (11.1 mmol/L) or a plasma glucose level >200 mg/dL (11.1 mmol/L) 2 hours after ingestion of 75 g oral glucose (the oral glucose tolerance test – OGTT).

The clinical signs and symptoms associated with hyperglycemia and osmotic diuresis (e.g. polyuria and polydipsia) are recognized by clinicians and lay people alike, making the diagnosis relatively straightforward. Insulin deficiency, if untreated, leads to the utilization of fats for fuel, with subsequent metabolism of fatty acids and the production of ketoacids. Thus, the presentation of ketonuria, ketonemia and ketoacidosis, often associated with nausea or hyperventilation, is an important clinical feature. Unexplained weight loss, along with the classic signs and symptoms mentioned above, is highly suggestive of the diagnosis of diabetes. Despite the classic signs and symptoms, approximately 1 in 200 children die at the onset of type 1 diabetes. If the first healthcare provider to see the child fails to make a diagnosis of diabetes, the child may subsequently present with severe ketoacidosis and may develop cerebral edema, which is usually fatal.

Although not specifically recommended as a diagnostic criterion, an elevated glycosylated hemoglobin concentration (HbA1c) may also be useful for diagnosis. The HbA1c level correlates with mean glucose levels over several months and eventually with the development of diabetic complications, including diabetic retinopathy.

The diagnosis of specific diabetic syndromes, including type 1A diabetes, requires further information. Several clinical criteria increase or reduce the probability that an individual has type 1A diabetes (e.g. increase: onset at age <35, nonobese, presence of ketoacidosis, immediate therapy with insulin required, family or personal history of organ-specific autoimmunity; decrease: age of onset >35, effective therapy with oral hypoglycemic agents, African-American or Hispanic-American child, obesity). These clinical criteria are, however, imprecise guidelines at best. For example, as many as 10% of obese white adults presenting with diabetes have type 1A. The hallmark of type 1 versus type 2 diabetes is the early (several years after diagnosis) development of severe insulin deficiency. The connecting peptide (C-peptide) of the proinsulin molecule is secreted in equimolar quantity to insulin by pancreatic β cells. Within 3 years of the onset of type 1A diabetes, most children have a severe impairment of insulin secretion with low C-peptide. The range of C-peptide secretion, however, is large at the onset in both type 1 and type 2 diabetes. Secretion is influenced by metabolic control, such that determination of C-peptide at onset has limited diagnostic utility in distinguishing type 1 from type 2 diabetes. The maintenance of C-peptide secretion can also be used as a measure of effective immunotherapy in clinical trials.

It should be recognized that both type 1A and type 2 diabetes are relatively common disorders, and thus individuals might have both diseases. Type 2 diabetes would be manifested by resistance to insulin, such that overt hyperglycemia will present earlier in the course of the islet β-cell destruction associated with type 1A diabetes. It has been proposed ('accelerator hypothesis') that type 1A and type 2 diabetes both result from metabolic changes associated with insulin resistance, and that type 1A represents a more severe form of diabetes with anti-islet autoimmunity. Data leading to this hypothesis are slightly faster growth and higher body mass index (BMI) in children who develop type 1A diabetes.[10]

Given the improved genetic prediction of type 1A diabetes with genes influencing immune function, it is unlikely that insulin resistance is a major factor in the initiation of islet autoimmunity,[11] although insulin resistance is likely to reveal overt hyperglycemia earlier in the course of immune-mediated β-cell destruction

The best immunologic markers for distinguishing type 1A from other forms of diabetes is the presence of islet cell autoantibodies. Diagnostic accuracy depends on the sensitivity and specificity of the autoantibody assays employed. Assays for autoantibodies reacting with insulin, glutamic acid decarboxylase (GAD65) and ICA512 (IA-2), when performed with fluid-phase assays (not ELISA), can be set such that fewer than 1 in 100 nondiabetic individuals are positive. One or another of these three autoantibodies is present in approximately 95% of children with recent-onset type 1A diabetes. However, approximately half of Hispanic-American children presenting with diabetes do not express any of the three anti-islet antibodies (compared to approximately 10% of non-Hispanic white children). We believe that the majority of the antibody-negative population represent a type 2 diabetes variant, although there are important genetic variants, including half of neonatal diabetes determined by mutations of the sulfonylurea receptor Kir6.2 gene[12] and multiple MODY genes.[13]

EPIDEMIOLOGY/INCIDENCE

Type 1A diabetes is one of the most common chronic diseases of childhood and is the most common type of diabetes in persons under 40. Diabetes is the leading cause of blindness, amputations and end-stage renal disease, and is a major factor contributing to cardiovascular disease and premature death. It typically presents in children (with a peak onset at 12–13 years of age), but it may occur at any age and in all racial groups, with approximately similar prevalence in both females and males.

CLINICAL PEARLS

>> Type 1A diabetes can occur at any age. Testing of islet cell autoantibodies identifies 10% of adults (thought to have type 2 diabetes) as having type 1A diabetes.

>> Half of African-American and Hispanic-American children are negative for anti-islet autoantibodies and have type 2 or type 1B diabetes.

>> Organ-specific autoimmunity (in particular celiac disease, thyroid disease, Addison's disease and pernicious anemia) is greatly increased in patients with type 1A diabetes.

>> The more common the organ-specific autoimmune disease in the general population the more common the disease in patients with type 1A diabetes. For example, thyroid autoimmunity is common and routine TSH testing is advised.

>> In diabetic patients with decreasing insulin need or severe hypoglycemia, rule out Addison's disease.

KEY CONCEPTS

EPIDEMIOLOGY AND INCIDENCE OF TYPE 1A DIABETES

>> One of the most common chronic diseases of childhood and the most common type of diabetes in persons under 40 years of age.

>> The leading cause of blindness, amputations, and end-stage renal disease, and contributes to premature death.

>> Peak age of onset is 12–13 years, but may occur at any age, in all racial groups, with equal prevalence between males and females.

>> More children are diagnosed in the fall and winter months, but it is likely that this reflects factors that bring children to medical attention.

>> The incidence of type 1A diabetes has been increasing in many countries.

>> No conclusive evidence exists for an association between vaccination and incidence of type 1A diabetes.

The annual incidence of type 1A diabetes varies dramatically. In children the incidence is approximately 15/100 000 in the United States, 35/100 000 in Finland, and fewer than 1/100 000 in Japan. The prevalence in the USA is approximately 1/300, and 90% of children developing diabetes do not have a first-degree relative with the disorder. Approximately 1/20 first-degree relatives of patients develop the disease. The risk to offspring of a father with type 1A diabetes is approximately twice that of offspring of an affected mother. In the US, non-Hispanic white Americans are approximately 1.5 times more likely to develop type 1A diabetes than are other groups.

The prevalence of type 1A diabetes is greatest in countries where the predominant population is Caucasian. For example, it is most prevalent in Finland and Sardinia and rare in Japan, Korea and China. A child in Finland has a 35 times greater risk of developing diabetes than a child in Japan. In Japan, for example, monozygotic twins of patients with type 1A diabetes and their first-degree relatives have a risk of diabetes similar to that of twins and relatives in the USA.[14] This suggests that the bulk of differences between countries relates to genetic differences and not environmental factors. Studies of migrant populations from developed countries have failed to reveal major differences in the incidence of diabetes based on migration from a high-incidence to a lower-incidence country.[15] Nevertheless, there are less well characterized populations where the incidence may have changed dramatically with migration, e.g., Yemenite Jews migrating to Israel.[16]

Seasonal variations in the incidence of type 1A diabetes have been well documented, with more children presenting with the disease in the fall and winter months. This seasonal variation has been ascribed to potential viral infections that destroy β cells; however, with increased knowledge of the natural history of type 1A diabetes it is more likely that such seasonal variation may simply reflect factors (such as viral infections) that either bring children to medical attention or produce insulin resistance when limited islet β-cell mass remains.

■ NATURAL HISTORY ■

Studies over the past decade in humans are defining details of the chronology of development of type 1A diabetes. In addition, studies in animal models have contributed to a greater understanding of the pathogenesis of the disease. At present, there are three major hypotheses (described below) concerning the natural history of type 1A diabetes, with a fourth having almost no supporters. The fourth hypothesis, which was prominent two decades ago, was that type 1A diabetes was an acute disorder induced by viral infection. If the development of diabetes is acute it is likely to be extremely rare, given studies of both relatives and the general population. Anti-islet autoantibodies almost always precede diabetes by years, as does the loss of first-phase insulin secretion.[17,18]

● *Hypothesis 1* Type 1A diabetes is a chronic and progressive disorder resulting from immune-mediated destruction of islet β cells.[7,19] A corollary of this hypothesis is that as immunologic and immunogenetic assays are refined, one should be able to predict both the risk of diabetes and the approximate time of progression to diabetes, with different individuals progressing at different rates. This hypothesis is encapsulated in the division of type 1A diabetes into a series of stages (I, genetic susceptibility; II, triggering of autoimmunity; III, active immunity; IV, loss of insulin secretion; and V, overt diabetes) (Fig. 70.1).[7,19]

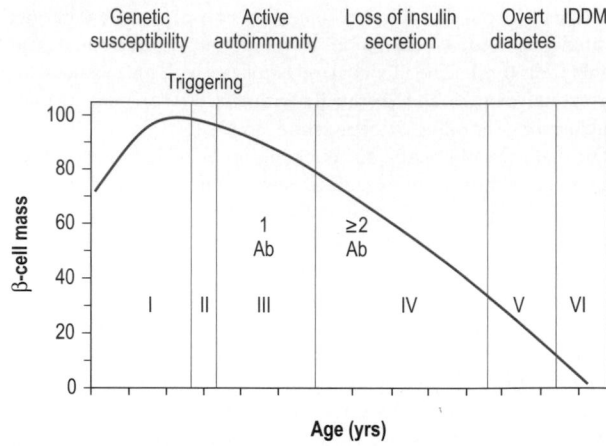

Fig. 70.1 Stages in the development of type 1A diabetes. (From Eisenbarth GS. Type I diabetes mellitus. A chronic autoimmune disease. N Engl J Med 1986; 314: 1360.)

● *Hypothesis 2* Type 1A diabetes is preceded by a long prodromal phase of autoimmunity, but actual islet β-cell destruction is acute and occurs at the end of the process.

● *Hypothesis 3* Type 1A diabetes results from 'multiple' hits, perhaps viral, and thus develops slowly, but would be difficult to predict as the 'hits' are not predictable.[20]

It is possible that a combination of all three hypotheses will eventually be found to apply to different individuals developing diabetes. For example, an identical twin with diabetes who receives half of the pancreas from their nondiabetic twin rapidly develops recurrent diabetes within several weeks.[9] Thus, the immune system has the potential to rapidly destroy human β cells. Nevertheless, there is considerable evidence that the first hypothesis is generally applicable. It reflects the progressive loss of first-phase insulin secretion that precedes diabetes, and the chronic loss of C-peptide secretion (over years) after the diagnosis of diabetes. This hypothesis is also consistent with recent analysis of β-cell loss and regeneration in NOD mice prior to diabetes.[21]

Despite evidence for progressive loss of β cells in the NOD mouse,[21] there is evidence for important changes in the immune system at the onset of diabetes. In the NOD mouse, splenocytes from recently diabetic – but not nondiabetic – mice transfer diabetes. Close to the time of diabetes, but not at early ages, NOD mice destroy islet transplants.[22] Finally, anti-CD3 therapy produces long-term improvement in blood sugar levels if given at the onset of disease, but not with early treatment.[23]

■ STAGE I: GENETIC SUSCEPTIBILITY ■

TWIN STUDIES

Monozygotic twins of patients with type 1A diabetes have approximately a 50% concordance rate for type 1A diabetes. This concordance is markedly different from that of dizygotic twins (5%), who have a risk similar to a sibling of a patient with type 1A diabetes. This difference reflects a significant role for genetic factors, but suggests that environmental and possibly somatic mutations or other stochastic events may also play a significant role in the pathogenesis. Although the risk of a discordant twin progressing to type 1A diabetes decreases proportionally with the duration of discordance, twins can become concordant after many years. In a prospective study involving 187 monozygotic twins from the UK and the USA who were discordant at the time of enrolment, 47 became concordant, with a range of time of onset of 0.4–39 years. The median discordance time of the twin pairs was 4.2 years, and 25% became concordant after 14 years of discordance.[24]

HLA GENES

A major determinant of genetic susceptibility resides in the MHC class II region (*IDDM1*). HLA class II molecules, particularly DR and DQ, account for approximately 50% of the genetic risk for type 1A diabetes.[25] As the MHC region displays a significant degree of linkage disequilibrium (e.g. specific DQ and DR alleles are nonrandomly associated with each other) associations of HLA with disease must be thought of as haplotype specific and not allele specific. Class I HLA alleles can also influence disease, and it is possible that unknown genes linked to the HLA region are important. Nevertheless, the identification of HLA class II alleles associated with high, moderate, low risk and even 'protection' is useful in disease prediction (Table 70.3).

Individuals with the highest risk for type 1A diabetes in the USA express both DQA1*0501-DQB1*0201 (DQ2), which is almost always

inherited with DRB1*0301, and DQA1*0301-DQB1*0302 (DQ8), inherited with DRB1*0401 or *0402. These individuals have been referred to as DR3/DR4 or DQ2/DQ8 heterozygotes. The genotype, DQ2/DQ8 (DR3/DR4), is commonly observed in type 1A diabetics. Although only 2% of children in the USA have this genotype, they constitute approximately 40% of those developing diabetes.[26] Observations of transmission frequencies of particular haplotypes have helped illustrate the importance of certain haplotypes in contributing to diabetes susceptibility. For example, analysis of the Human Biological Data Interchange (HBDI) family collection has revealed that DQA1*0501-DQB*0201 and DQA1*0301-DQB1*0302 are transmitted to more than 80% of diabetic children. DQB1 alleles without an aspartic acid at position 57 of the β chain have been proposed to determine diabetes risk. However, no simple amino acid rule adequately describes the risk associated with DQ alleles.

HLA DQ alleles have also been associated with dominant protection from type 1A diabetes.[27] Approximately 20% of the general population have DQA1*0102-DQB1*0602, the HLA haplotype that provides dominant protection from type 1A diabetes. Interestingly, autoantibody-positive relatives of affected individuals who express the HLA haplotype DQA1 0102, DQB1*0602 are protected from progression to diabetes, albeit not completely.[28]

HLA class I and DP alleles are also associated with diabetes risk. For example, the A24 allele is associated with early age of onset of type 1A diabetes.[29] There are probably additional loci linked to HLA, such as loci near microsatellite D6S2223, also conferring risk.

NON-HLA GENES

Genome-wide screens for loci linked with diabetes (using microsatellite markers from all of the chromosomes) have led to the identification of 18 genetic loci contributing to diabetes susceptibility in the NOD mouse, and over 15 in humans, with variable statistical significance (Table 70.4). However, for the great majority of these putative loci no actual genes have been identified.

Because the autoimmune response against the β cell-specific molecule insulin is a major component of type 1A diabetes, the insulin gene would be an ideal candidate locus. In fact, polymorphisms in the 5′ flanking sequence (promoter region) of the insulin gene have been associated with diabetes risk, and account for about 10% of the familial aggregation of type 1A diabetes.[30] The insulin gene is located on the short arm of chromosome 11 and has been termed *IDDM2*. Polymorphisms in the 5′ sequence leading to alterations in insulin gene expression could be envisaged as potentially modulating the development of tolerance in the thymus or yolk sac. A low level of insulin gene expression in the thymus may allow insulin-reactive T cells to escape negative selection. The insulin gene polymorphism (larger repeat region), which results in greater thymic expression of proinsulin, is associated with protection.[31,32] The mutated gene underlying the autoimmune polyendocrine syndrome type I (APS-I), namely AIRE (autoimmune regulator gene) appears also to control insulin expression in the thymus and hence diabetes risk[33]

Some of the loci identified through genome-wide screens for linkage have not been replicated by different groups, although a few, such as PTPN22, have been confirmed in multiple studies.[34] The reasons for this lack of reproducibility may include the following: genetic heterogeneity in different populations; heterogeneity of disease phenotypes; ethnic differences; statistical 'artifacts'; and differences in the markers used. It is possible

Table 70.3 High-risk and protective HLA haplotypes

High risk			
DR3	DRB1*0301	DQA1*0501	DQB1*0201
DR4	DRB1*0401	DQA1*0301	DQB1*0302
	DRB1*0402	DQA1*0301	DQB1*0302
	DRB1*0405	DQA1*0301	DQB1*0302
Moderate risk			
DR1	DRB1*01	DQA1*0101	DQB1*0501
DR8	DRB1*0801	DQA1*0401	DQB1*0402
DR9	DRB1*0901	DQA1*0301	DQB1*0303
Protective			
Strong protection			
DR2	DRB1*1501	DQA1*0102	DQB1*0602
DR6	DRB1*1401	DQA1*0101	DQB1*0503
DR7	DRB1*0701	DQA1*0201	DQB1*0303
Moderate protection			
DR5	DRB1*1101	DQA1*0501	DQB1*0301
Weak protection			
DR4	DRB1*0401	DQA1*0301	DQB1*0301
	DRB1*0403	DQA1*0301	DQB1*0302
DR7	DRB1*0701	DQA1*0201	DQB1*0201

that genetic heterogeneity between different families having different non-MHC genes may underlie the inability of sibling-pair studies to identify loci accounting for a major proportion of the familial aggregation of type 1A diabetes. Three potential patterns of inheritance for diabetes will be addressed: monogenic, polygenic and oligogenic (Table 70.5).

In 1989, Pnini Vardi identified a unique family with a high frequency of type 1A diabetes[86]. This Bedouin Arab family consisted of over 250 members, of whom 18 were affected (Fig. 70.2). A genome-wide scan for linkage in this family revealed that the risk for diabetes was associated with a

susceptibility locus on chromosome 10 which is termed *IDDM17*. In family members expressing the DR3 or DR4 haplotypes, the risk for diabetes was 30%, as opposed to <2% for those members who did not have a DR3 or DR4 haplotype. Linkage analysis and association studies revealed that in this family a pattern of oligogenic inheritance may underlie disease susceptibility.

■ RODENT MODELS ■

Studies in animal models have contributed greatly to our understanding of the pathogenesis of type 1A diabetes. Numerous models exist, both induced (e.g. with alloxan, streptozotocin treatment) and spontaneous (e.g. NOD mouse, BB rat) (Table 70.6). Some important advantages of an autoimmune model include access to the pancreas at various stages in the immunopathology; ability to breed and genetically manipulate the animals; and intervention strategies that can be employed at various disease stages (e.g. preinsulitis, insulitis/presymptomatic stage etc.).

NOD MOUSE

The best-studied animal model for type 1A diabetes is the nonobese diabetic (NOD) mouse, which develops diabetes spontaneously. In the NOD mouse, cellular and humoral immune responses specific for β cells are present, anti-insulin autoantibodies precede overt diabetes, and disease is associated with specific MHC alleles. Pancreatic insulitis in the NOD mouse can be detected as early as 2 weeks with electron microscopy, and becomes detectable by light microscopy at 4–5 weeks of age. Approximately 80% of female mice and 20% of male mice progress to diabetes by 30 weeks of age. The reason for the excess of female cases is unknown, but may be related to the effects of sex hormones.

Multiple genetic loci in this mouse determine disease susceptibility, with the MHC (termed *Idd1*) being necessary but not sufficient for disease. The class II region in NOD mice encodes the I-A^{g7} molecule, the ortholog of the human class II DQ8 and DQ2. I-A^{g7} is unique among the known I-A molecules in that it has a serine instead of an aspartic acid at position 57 of the β chain. Like a number of normal strains, NOD mice do not express I-E (the murine ortholog of HLA-DR) because of a mutation in the Eα promoter. The introduction of a normal I-Eα gene inhibits

Table 70.4 IDDM loci in humans

Locus	Chromosome	Comment
– *IDDM1*	6p21.31	Major histocompatibility locus
– *IDDM2*	11p15.5	Insulin gene 5′ VNTR
	1p13	PTPN22
IDDM3?	15q26	
IDDM4?	11q13	
– *IDDM5*	6q25	
IDDM6?	18q21	
IDDM7	2q31-33	
IDDM8	6q27	
IDDM9	3q21	
IDDM10?	10p11-q11	
IDDM11?	14q24.3-14q31	
IDDM12	2q33	CTLA4
IDDM13	2q34	
– *IDDM15*	6q21	Confirmed multiple studies
IDDM17	10q25.1	Single Bedouin Arab family

?, negative evidence for linkage in two or more large linkage studies.
–, evidence for linkage found in more than one major study.
Underlined, definitive evidence for linkage or association.

Table 70.5 Three genetic models of type 1A diabetes inheritance

Monogenic model
Susceptibility to type 1A diabetes and other endocrine and nonendocrine autoimmune diseases can be determined by a mutation in a single gene. An example is the autoimmune polyendocrine syndrome type I (APS-I) with a mutation in the autoimmune regulator (AIRE) gene.[48]

Polygenic model
A major role for class II molecules (DQ, DR) in determining susceptibility for type 1A diabetes is well recognized. In the NOD mouse model more than 15 non-MHC loci have been found to contribute to diabetes risk. The idea that multiple genetic polymorphisms, each contributing a small component to disease susceptibility, is a popular model.

Oligogenic model
Diabetes risk may be determined by HLA alleles in conjunction with one or two non-MHC disease genes in each family. For different families the specific major 'diabetogenes' would differ. This model is supported by studies of a large Bedouin Arab family[49] and the finding of a risk of 40% for DQ2/DQ8 siblings of patients with type 1A diabetes.[39]

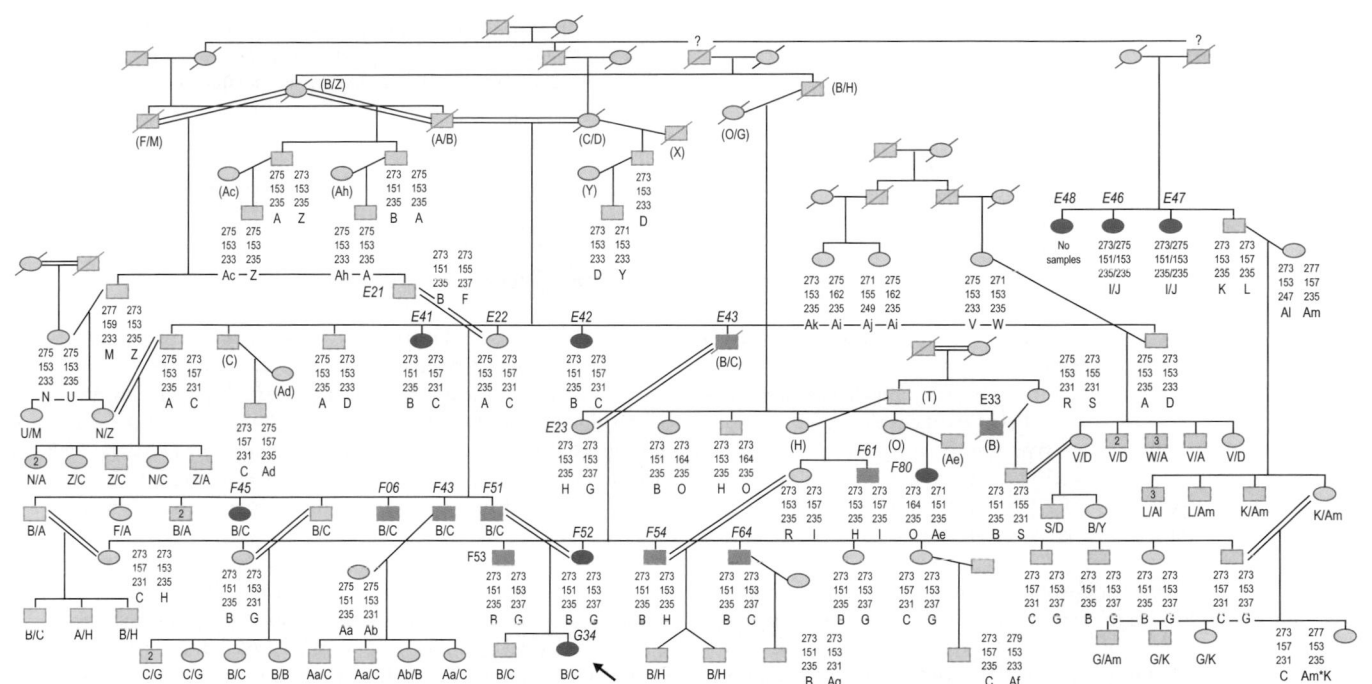

Fig. 70.2 Type 1A diabetes inheritance. Family tree in which 18 members have developed type 1 diabetes and diabetes appears to be inherited as an autosomal recessive mutation at a locus on chromosome 10 plus typical type 1 HLA alleles. The B haplotype on chromosome 10 occurs in the majority of patients with diabetes (numbers refer to chromosome 10q25.1 microsatellite alleles) and diabetics have homologous B like 10q25.1 regions for other diabetic haplotypes (e.g. haplotypes, Ae, O, I, J, C, G, and H).

Table 70.6 Spontaneous animal models of type 1A diabetes

BB rat (oligogenic inheritance)
Homozygosity lymphopenia gene (Ian gene)
RT1-U MHC class II alleles
Additional loci

NOD mouse (polygenic inheritance of diabetes)
I-A^{g7}; I-Eα deletion; class I allele
IL-2 polymorphism
More than 15 additional IDDM loci

Tokushima rat (oligogenic inheritance)
RT1-U MHC alleles
Homozygosity chromosome 11 (Cblb gene)

the development of diabetes in the NOD mouse, implying that its absence is important.[35] Transgenic NOD mice expressing a 'normal' I-A, or with amino acid substitutions at positions 56 and 57 of the NOD I-A^{g7}, are protected from disease. Recent studies suggest that insulin may be a primary autoantigen for the disorder, and mutation of a single amino acid of insulin prevents the development of diabetes.[36]

BB RAT

The BB rat also develops diabetes spontaneously, with equal frequency among males and females.[8] Ninety percent of both sexes developing insulitis progress to overt diabetes between 50 and 90 days of age. Selective breeding of BB rats resulted in the production of a diabetes-prone (DP) and a diabetes-resistant (DR) strain.

Genetic susceptibility for type 1A diabetes in the BB rat is also determined in part by the MHC genes. In the BB rat, diabetes is independent of class I alleles but requires the MHC class II haplotype RT-1U (*Iddm2*), in which at least one allele must be present for diabetes to develop. A second locus (*Iddm1*) is inherited in an autosomal recessive manner and is responsible for T-cell lymphopenia in these animals, determined by a frameshift mutation of an Ian (immune associated nucleotide) gene.[37] The DP-BB rat is deficient in T cells expressing the surface antigen RT6. RT6 is a surface marker that appears to distinguish a subset of T cells capable of immunoregulation, as adoptive transfer of these cells into a DP-BB rat abrogates diabetes. In addition, monoclonal antibodies targeting RT6 can induce β-cell destruction in nonlymphopenic, diabetes-resistant (DR) BB rats.

The DR-BB rats are nonlymphopenic and diabetes can be induced either by the administration of RT6 monoclonal antibodies or by infection with the Kilham rat virus. The Kilham rat virus does not infect β cells but is believed to alter immune regulation.[38] Table 70.6 lists several animal models of type 1A diabetes.

■ TRANSGENIC MODELS ■

The use of transgenic and knockout technology has allowed investigators to begin to determine the role of various immune factors in the etiology and pathology of type 1A diabetes. In these models, the breakdown of organ-specific tolerance can be examined by creating DNA constructs that allow tissue-specific expression of the transgene under the control of tissue-specific promoters (e.g. insulin promoter). Most of the transgenic models of type 1A diabetes involve the NOD mouse, and a brief summary of some of these studies is provided (Table 70.7).

NOD mice that have been crossed with mice having a target mutation of the μ chain in the IgM heavy chain do not develop diabetes,[39] suggesting that B lymphocytes play an important role in the disease process. As autoantibodies do not appear to be directly pathogenic to β cells, the role of B cells in the pathogenesis of type 1A diabetes appears to be that of antigen presentation. When B cell-deficient (MT$^{-/-}$) mice were crossed with NOD mice expressing a B7.1 transgene in the pancreatic β cells, progression to diabetes was accelerated, suggesting that B-cell presentation can be bypassed.

The perhaps overly simplistic hypothesis that Th1 cells are destructive and Th2 protective is the basis for efforts to skew the cytokine environment towards Th2 cytokines. In support of this idea, the administration of IL-4 or IL-10 has been associated with disease protection in NOD mice, whereas systemic administration of Th1-type cytokines, IL-12 and TNF-α[40] can precipitate disease. However, studies of transgenic and knockout NOD models involving cytokines have suggested that the Th1/Th2 paradigm is an oversimplification. For example, NOD mice expressing an IL-4 transgene specifically in the islet β cells show protection from diabetes, whereas IL-4 knockout NOD mice do not show accelerated diabetes. In addition, anti-IFN-γ treatment prevents diabetes developing in the NOD mouse, but IFN-γ-deficient NOD mice continue to develop diabetes, albeit at a reduced rate.[41] Furthermore, whereas NOD mice administered IL-10 are protected from diabetes,[33] mice expressing an IL-10 transgene specifically in the islet β cells develop accelerated diabetes.[42] Although the reasons for these differences remain to be clarified, it suggests that the ability to dissect out the role of individual cytokines may be complicated by a variety of factors that can all muddy the waters of cytokine regulation of the disease process. Such factors may include functional redundancy in cytokine action; the fact that individual cytokines may modulate the expression of other cytokines and/or chemokines; cytokine influence may vary at different periods during disease development; and the microenvironment of cytokine production. Though the Th1/Th2 paradigm can relate to aspects of pathogenesis, it is clear that regulatory T cells can prevent type 1A diabetes in animal models and are implicated in humans.[43,44] The key importance of such regulatory T cells is revealed by children with the IPEX syndrome (immune dysfunction, polyendocrinopathy, enteritis, X-linked) with a mutation of the gene FoxP3, a transcription factor that drives the development of regulatory T cells.[45]

Several caveats should be considered when evaluating animal models. First, no single model exactly replicates the disease process in humans, and genus-specific differences can contribute to this variance. In addition, the highly inbred nature of these models (owing to multiple brother–sister matings) and the controlled housing environment of these animals implies that the model is not directly analogous to humans, in that inbred mice are monoallelic at all loci. Despite these disadvantages, animal models remain an invaluable tool to research immunopathology.

■ STAGE II: TRIGGERING OF AUTOIMMUNITY (POTENTIAL ENVIRONMENTAL FACTORS) ■

Environmental factors suggested to influence the development of type 1A diabetes include viral infections, bacterial and/or viral superantigens, dietary components and environmental toxins. Many investigators support a viral etiology for type 1A diabetes. However, so far there has been no formal demonstration that viral infections directly cause type 1A diabetes in humans. Congenital rubella (and only congenital infection) is associated with diabetes risk, but such infection increases the risk of a series of autoimmune disorders.

The mechanism by which microbial infections might influence the autoimmune process of type 1A diabetes is poorly defined. Hypotheses include: (1) microbial-specific T and B cells may cross-react with self-antigens (molecular mimicry); (2) virally infected β cells may be directly destroyed by cytotoxic T lymphocytes reacting to viral epitopes displayed on MHC class I; (3) indirect or 'bystander' activation of autoreactive lymphocytes may occur owing to a local increase in inflammatory cytokines associated with viral infection; and (4) the effects of congenital infection (e.g., rubella) on the developing immune system may contribute to disease susceptibility. Without convincing epidemiological evidence for relevant environmental factors, it is difficult to test these hypotheses.

RUBELLA VIRUS

Congenital rubella infection is a well-defined environmental factor contributing to the development of type 1A diabetes in humans. Approximately 12–20% of individuals infected with rubella in utero develop diabetes in 5–20 years, in what appears to be an autoimmune process. One hypothesis to explain this association involves a molecular mimicry mechanism, supported by the fact that there is a shared epitope between a rubella viral noncapsid protein and a 52 kDa islet autoantigen. Alternatively, the rubella virus may alter β-cell antigens as it buds from the membrane, resulting in the formation of a novel antigenic determinant. A separate hypothesis would be that rubella infection might modulate T-cell development and result in abnormal immunologic tolerance to islet and thyroid tissues.[46]

COXSACKIE B VIRUSES

Coxsackie viruses are RNA-containing picornaviruses that have been implicated in the etiology of type 1A diabetes. The Coxsackie viruses are members of the enterovirus class and have six B serotypes (B1–B6). The specific role these viruses play in the etiology of type 1A diabetes has yet to be defined.

Sequence similarity exists between the Coxsackie viral protein 2C (P2-C) and the glutamic acid decarboxylase (GAD65) autoantigen that is expressed in the pancreas. This amino acid sequence homology is highly conserved in Coxsackie B4 isolates, and the relevant peptide has

Table 70.7 Summary of transgenic and knockout studies on the NOD background

Transgene	Observation	Conclusion
I-Eα	Diabetes prevented	I-E prevents diabetes
I-Aβ proline 56, Asp57	Diabetes prevented	I-A sequence is important
Proinsulin with Class II promoter	Diabetes prevented	Insulin 'key' autoantigen
GAD65 with Class II promoter	No decrease in diabetes	Heat-shock protein with Class II promoterSmall decrease in diabetes
GAD65/67 antisense transgene	Two strains with decreased diabetes	Potential importance of HSP
IL-2 B6 variant	Diabetes decreased	GAD65 not essential
		Controversial manuscript
		IL-2 polymorphisms contribute to diabetes
Expression in β cells	Accelerated diabetes	Neutrophil infiltration induced
TNF-α	Accelerated diabetes	B7.1 Costimulation is important
IL-10	Accelerated diabetes	TGF-β may induce suppression of islet-reactive
FasL	Accelerated diabetes	CD4 T cells and/or induce regulatory T-cell
B7.1	Decreased incidence of diabetes	subsets
TGF-β	Abrogates insulitis and development of diabetes	IL-4 may induce a 'protective' Th2 response
IL-4		
Expression in T cells	Protection with limited diabetes	
IL-10		
Expression in α cells (paracrine effect)	Protected against spontaneous and cyclophosphamide-induced diabetes	Paracrine TGF-β is important for suppressing autoimmunity, perhaps through induction of regulatory T cells
TGF-β		
In vitro	Protected from IL-1β, TNF-α, IFN-γ-induced destruction	Bcl-2 antiapoptotic factor blocks Cytokine-induced apoptosis
Bcl-2 transgenic islet cells		
Knockout/inactivating mutation	Diabetes prevented	T-cell receptors or Igs are essential
Rag, SCID	Diabetes prevented	B cells important
Mu chain of immunoglobulin	Diabetes prevented	B-cell expression of class II important
Class II deficient B lymphocytes	Diabetes prevented	Class I and CD8 T cells are important
β2-microglobulin ('class I knockout')	Pancreatic infiltration/seldom insultls/diabetes prevented	CD4 T cells needed for progression to insulitis and diabetes
CIITA 'Class II transactivator' (deficient in MHC II and peripheral CD4 T cells)	Insulitis severity unchanged	Perforin-dependent cytotoxicity is important in the late effector phase of disease
Perforin	Incidence/onset of diabetes is reduced and delayed	Fas is important for autoimmune β-cell destruction
Fas	Fas−/− prevents diabetes	GAD65 is not required
Knockout insulin 1 and 2 gene Diabetes prevented Altered insulin sequence	Diabetes rate/incidence unchanged	GAD67 not tested
IA-2 and IA-2β	Not required NOD diabetes	TNFR1 signaling is important for progression to diabetes
GAD65	Diabetes rate/incidence unchanged	Other cytokines may substitute
GAD67	Normal islet development but perinatal death unrelated to diabetes (respiratory distress)	Other cytokines may substitute
IFN-γ	Develop diabetes at a slower rate	
TNF Receptor 1	Insulitis but no diabetes	
IL-12	Diabetes unchanged	
IL-4	Diabetes unchanged	

finding is observed when NOD mice are treated with a monoclonal antibody against CD8. Recently, Wong and colleagues[62] identified insulin as the autoantigen recognized by a NOD-derived pathogenic CD8 T cell. Interestingly, the region recognized by the CD8 T cells overlapped with the portion of the insulin B chain recognized by the majority of the insulin-reactive CD4 T cells.

Despite the importance of T lymphocytes for the development of type 1A diabetes, both in humans and in animal models, T-cell assays useful for the prediction or follow-up of the diabetes process are essentially nonexistent. It is hoped that with improved knowledge of T-cell autoimmunity better assays will be developed and, for instance, there is evidence that ELISPOT or Tetramer assays can detect autoreactive T lymphocytes,[63] but a major limitation is likely to be the frequency of autoreactive T cells outside the islets that are available for study.

HISTOPATHOLOGY

Studies in the NOD model have provided the opportunity to examine the islets at various stages of the natural history of the disease. Through these studies it has become clear that intra-islet infiltration evolves from a stage of peri-insulitis and MHC class I hyperexpression in the NOD islet β cells. The perivascular and periductal T-cell infiltration, termed peri-insulitis, is usually observed at 4–6 weeks of age. Animals at this stage have been described by some authors as being in a state of 'benign autoimmunity', in which case the peri-insulitis is thought to be nondestructive. The conversion to invasive insulitis and β-cell destruction ('malignant autoimmunity') in these mice was reported to occur abruptly and in an unpredictable fashion as the mice aged. However, O'Brien[85] and colleagues reported that apoptosis in the NOD islets was detectable throughout the period of peri-insulitis. Apoptotic death of the islets preceded lymphocytic infiltration and then declined when progression to overt diabetes occurred. In another study, NOD mice were observed to have an early increased 'compensatory' β-cell proliferation. This was unable to keep pace with the progressive β-cell destruction and resulted in a reduction in β-cell mass that became worse with time and correlated with a decrease in the insulin secretory response.[21]

Histological analyses of the islets in humans have been limited for several reasons, which include the relative inaccessibility of the pancreas for biopsy; the fact that the islets make up only 2–3% of the pancreatic tissue; and the fact that histologic examination of the islets at the time of disease onset (which precedes clinical presentation) has not been possible. Histological evaluation of pancreases from children who have died at disease onset also suggests a slowly evolving autoimmune process in type 1A diabetes.[4] Foulis and colleagues[64] have described three histologically distinguishable types of islet in patients with new-onset diabetes: insulin-deficient islets, which make up the largest fraction (approximately 70%); insulin-containing islets with a chronic inflammatory cell infiltrate; and insulin-containing islets that appear normal. T cells make up most of the infiltrate, with CD8 T cells comprising a larger fraction than CD4 in some studies. Butler and colleagues[65] have described greatly decreased numbers of β cells in pancreases from long-term patients, but nevertheless evidence of β-cell apoptosis.

In contrast to the characteristic peri-insulitis associated with the early stages of immunopathology in the NOD mouse, peri-insulitis does not appear to be a common feature in humans. Another distinction is that insulitis in the NOD mouse is associated with massive mononuclear cell infiltrates not typically seen in humans. The mechanisms that underlie these differences remain unclear. It is, however, a good reminder that the NOD mouse, albeit an excellent model, is clearly not identical to humans.

◼ TYPE 1A DIABETES PREDICTION ◼

By the time a diagnosis of type 1A diabetes is made, approximately 80–90% of the β cells may have been destroyed. Therefore, the ability to predict who will develop type 1A diabetes among high-risk individuals (siblings of type 1A diabetics) has become an important goal. Using HLA haplotype analysis and 'combinatorial' autoantibody analyses, clinicians should be able to identify high-risk individuals. Because the autoimmune process in type 1A diabetes begins years before the progression to overt symptoms, the chance of early intervention is feasible. Furthermore, if a definable environmental trigger exists for type 1A diabetes, as it does for celiac disease (wheat gliadin), preventing exposure may be important.

The most important risk factor for disease development is the expression of multiple anti-islet autoantibodies,[65] particularly two or more of GAD65, ICA512 (IA-2) or insulin autoantibodies (Fig. 70.3). However, there is a subset of relatives who express a single autoantibody, and an even smaller subset expressing multiple autoantibodies, who have the 'protective' HLA alleles DQA1*0102, DQB1*0602. In individuals with DQB1*0602 the risk of progressing to diabetes is low, but still present. Approximately 1% (versus 20% of the general population) of patients with type 1A diabetes have this allele.

◼ THERAPEUTIC PRINCIPLES

>> Autoantibody testing in combination with HLA testing can be used to predict type 1A diabetes.

>> Insulin therapy is mandatory in type 1A patients who are ketosis prone. Testing of islet cell autoantibodies identifies 10% of adults (thought to have type 2 diabetes) as having type 1A diabetes.

>> Prevention of diabetic complications is feasible; it requires routine screening for retinal lesions and microalbuminuria.

◼ PREVENTION ◼

IMMUNOSUPPRESSION

The first major trial of general immunosuppressive therapy for newly diagnosed subjects involved the administration of cyclosporine A (CyA).[66] CyA was effective in prolonging insulin secretion when treatment lasted 1 year and was initiated during the first 6 weeks of insulin therapy. Long-term benefit was limited, however, with relapse of hyperglycemia

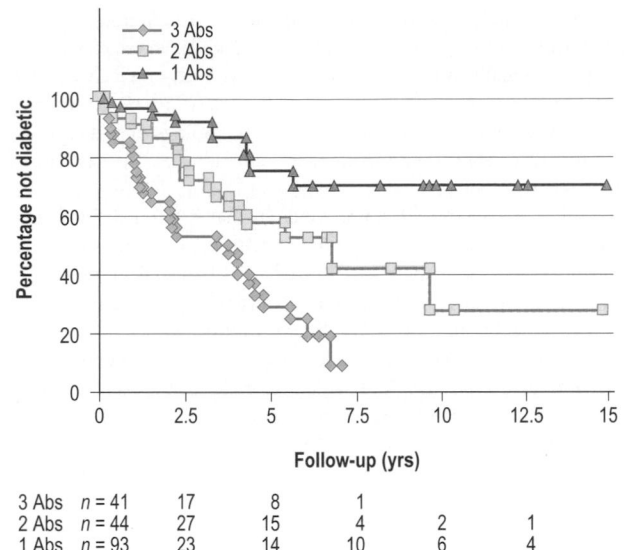

3 Abs	*n* = 41	17	8	1	
2 Abs	*n* = 44	27	15	4	2	1
1 Abs	*n* = 93	23	14	10	6	4

Fig. 70.3 Life table analysis of progression to type 1A diabetes in relatives of affected patients subdivided by the number of autoantibodies (GAD65, insulin, ICA512) expressed.

occurring within 3 years despite continued CyA therapy, and despite continued maintenance of improved insulin secretion as measured with C-peptide. When CyA was discontinued, insulin secretion was rapidly lost. Because of the potential for nephrotoxicity and the risk of malignancy associated with long-term treatment, CyA therapy has not been adopted. Other immunosuppressive agents have been studied, including prednisone, anti-CD5, anti-CD25, anti-thymocyte globulin andanti-T12, but so far they have had little success in providing long-term protection. Recent studies of anti-T cell antibodies (in particular modified anti-CD3 antibodies) have shown promise.[67, 68]

AUTOANTIGEN ADMINISTRATION

The administration of certain islet cell autoantigens, such as insulin and GAD, and derivatives of these autoantigens can prevent diabetes in animal models. For example, in the NOD mouse long-term (up to 1 year) oral ingestion of these autoantigens has been reported to delay the onset and/or reduce the incidence of disease.[69] Subcutaneous and intranasal administration of the insulin B chain B9-23 can prevent diabetes in the NOD mouse.[70] Although the precise mechanism by which subcutaneous administration of the insulin peptide mediates immunoprotection is unknown, the isolation of B9-23-reactive CD4 T-cell clones[71] expressing TGF-β suggests that protection may be mediated by regulatory T cells. Much evidence exists that in type 1A diabetes a Th1-dominant response enhances β-cell destruction, whereas a Th2 response is protective. Autoantigen administration appears to dampen the autoimmune response via bystander suppression through the generation of regulatory T cells secreting a Th2 cytokine profile.[72] In the USA individuals at moderate risk for type 1A diabetes are being randomized to receive either oral insulin or placebo in the Diabetes Prevention Trial-1 (DPT-1). In this same study, individuals at high risk are being randomized to parenteral insulin therapy. Insulin therapy did not overall decrease progression to diabetes, but there was evidence in a subgroup (those with high levels of insulin autoantibodies) of a significant delay in progression.[73]

ADJUVANTS

In the NOD mouse a single injection of complete Freund's adjuvant prevents the development of diabetes[74] but not insulitis. A single injection of incomplete Freund's adjuvant (IFA) was unable to induce this effect. However, when combined with an injection of B chain of insulin or the B9-23 peptide, IFA was able to prevent diabetes in the NOD mouse.[70] Vaccination with the bacillus Calmette–Guérin (BCG) strain of *Mycobacterium bovis* has also been found to prevent diabetes in the NOD mouse.[75] In several randomized double-blinded placebo-controlled trials intradermal BCG vaccination did not alter remission rate or protect β cells.

NICOTINAMIDE

In the NOD mouse large doses of the vitamin nicotinamide delayed the development of diabetes, and preliminary uncontrolled trials suggested that such therapy might also be successful in humans. In light of this, two randomized controlled trials of nicotinamide, the small German DENIS (Deutsche Nicotinamide Trial) trial and the larger ENDIT (European Nicotinamide Trial) trial in Europe, were initiated and no protection was found.[76]

■ TREATMENT WITH INSULIN ■

Insulin is administered subcutaneously to millions of individuals with diabetes. Over the past three decades, not only has the purity of the insulin preparations improved, but in developed countries human insulin has essentially replaced the use of porcine or bovine insulin. Porcine insulin differs from human insulin by only one amino acid, whereas bovine insulin differs by three amino acids. Multiple recombinant forms of human insulin and an additional route of administration have been introduced into clinical practice. For fast-acting insulins the change in the insulin molecule disrupts the natural ability of insulin to form hexamers and greatly speeds subcutaneous absorption. Although the insulin is modified, modifications have not been associated with an increase in insulin antibodies or greater immunologic reactions to insulin.

Essentially, all patients treated with insulin, even human insulin, develop a low level of antibodies that cross-react with native insulin. These antibodies are of relatively low affinity compared to the insulin autoantibodies of pre-diabetic patients, and do not usually interfere with insulin action. Insulin resistance due to induced insulin antibodies (defined as patients requiring more than 200 U of insulin per day, and insulin antibodies with a capacity that usually exceeds 50 U of insulin per liter of serum) was always rare and appears to be nearly disappearing as human insulin replaces animal insulins. Allergic or hypersensitivity reactions to insulin and (in the past) lipoatrophy or lipohypertrophy at the site of insulin injection, are also very rare at present. Such allergic reactions can be treated by changing the formulation of insulin used (e.g. NPH insulin to Lente insulin) or, for delayed hypersensitivity, adding small amounts of glucocorticoids to the insulin preparation.

ASSOCIATED AUTOIMMUNE DISORDERS ■

Type 1A diabetes is associated with several autoimmune diseases, including Addison's disease, thyroiditis, Graves' disease, pernicious anemia, celiac disease, myasthenia gravis and vitiligo.[77] The association with other organ-specific autoimmune diseases points to the importance of screening for these diseases in type 1A patients. Several commonly associated diseases or unique syndromes are discussed in this section.

AUTOIMMUNE POLYENDOCRINE SYNDROMES

Polyendocrine syndromes are characterized by multiple autoimmune disorders. Two distinct forms have been described: autoimmune polyendocrine syndrome I (APS-I) and II (APS-II).

Autoimmune polyendocrine syndrome type I (APS-I)

APS-I consists of a triad of chronic mucocutaneous candidiasis, hypoparathyroidism and Addison's disease, which often present in that order. Other endocrine and nonendocrine disorders can also be present or develop later in patients with this syndrome (Table 70.9). Eighteen percent of patients develop type 1A diabetes. APS-I is also known as autoimmune polyendocrinopathy candidiasis ectodermal dystrophy (APECED), and is an autosomal recessive disorder in which males and females are equally affected. In contrast to APS-II, in which the manifestations of disease usually occur in middle age, APS-I usually manifests in infancy or early childhood. In both syndromes the detection of autoantibodies against endocrine and nonendocrine tissues precedes overt disease.

APS-I is of considerable importance in that it has a defined monogenic etiology. In addition, no association with HLA alleles is found. The gene underlying the pathogenesis of APS-I is localized to the long arm of chromosome 21 (21q22.3) and is termed autoimmune regulator (AIRE).[78] AIRE has two zinc-finger motifs and a DNA-binding domain, and is localized to the nucleus, suggestive of a role in modulating transcription. Studies by Anderson and colleagues[79] have led to the hypothesis that the AIRE gene is important for induction of tolerance to 'peripheral' antigens such as insulin, expressed at low levels in the thymus.

Autoimmune polyendocrine syndrome type 2 (APS-II)

APS-II, or Schmidt's syndrome, is the most common of the polyendocrine syndromes and, in contrast to APS-I, the incidence is two to three times higher in females than in males, with onset typically in adulthood. The classic triad of APS-II involves Addison's disease, autoimmune

Table 70.9 Autoimmune polyendocrine syndrome types I and II

	APS-I[a]	APS-II[b]
Inheritance	Autosomal recessive AIRE gene 21q22.3	Autosomal dominant polygenic/oligogenic
HLA association	None	HLA DR3 and DR4
Immunodeficiency	Mucocutaneous candidiasis, asplenism	Not well defined
Age of onset	Infancy or early childhood	Adulthood (peak 20–60)
Sexual prevalence	Equal among males and females	Greater in females (by 2–3-fold)
[a]Mucocutaneous candidiasis	73–100%	Not associated
[a]Hypoparathyroidism	80–89%	Not associated
[a,b]Addison's disease	60–72%	70%
[b]Type 1 diabetes	4–15%	52%
[b]Autoimmune thyroid disease	10–40%	70%
Gonadal failure	38–60% of females	3.5–10% of females
	7–14% of males	5–50% of males
Vitiligo	4–9%	4.5%
Hepatitis	10–15%	Rare
Pernicious anemia	12–15%	<1%
Malabsorption	18%	With celiac disease

[a]Classic triad for APS-I.
[b]Classic triad for APS-II.

thyroid disease and type 1A diabetes, but other endocrine and nonendocrine disorders can be seen in affected patients. Unlike APS-I, APS-II is strongly associated with HLA alleles and susceptibility is probably determined by an interaction between multiple genetic loci and environmental factors. The class II HLA alleles associated with most of the component disorders of APS-II are DR3 (DQB*0201) and DR4 (DQB1*0302).

ADDISON'S DISEASE

Addison's disease, or primary adrenocortical insufficiency, is an autoimmune disease characterized by the presence (in 70% of patients) of autoantibodies directed predominantly against 21-hydroxylase, a key regulator of mineralocorticoid and glucocorticoid synthesis. The myriad clinical manifestations of Addison's disease, including muscle weakness and fatigue, hypotension and hyponatremia, and loss of axillary and pubic hair in women, are the result of cortisol, aldosterone and sex hormone deficiencies, respectively. Addison's disease is the principal component disorder of APS-II.

In 'DR4' patients with Addison's disease DRB1*0404 is the DR4 allele most often carried. Individuals with type 1A diabetes have a 100 times greater risk of developing Addison's disease. This significant increase justifies anti-21-hydroxylase autoantibody screening in type 1A diabetics. The MICA-5.1 allele is an additional major independent determinant of Addison's disease. This nontraditional class I allele has an extra nucleotide that disrupts the transmembrane portion of the molecule.

CELIAC DISEASE

Celiac disease is a common autoimmune disease (incidence of 1 in 250 in the USA) characterized by immune-cell-induced intestinal lesions which may lead to malabsorption and growth failure. The highest incidence occurs in type 1A diabetics and their relatives, with most of these patients expressing DQA1*0501; DQB1*0201 (DR3, DR3/3 or DR5/7).[80] Of the autoimmune diseases, celiac disease is unique in that intestinal pathology is entirely dependent on the ingestion of cereal proteins, namely wheat, rye and barley. Remarkably, the removal of wheat gliadin from the diet resolves the intestinal lesions and also leads to the disappearance of autoantibodies associated with the disease.

Tissue transglutaminase (tTG), an enzyme that catalyzes the cross-linking of proteins via glutamyl–lysine bonds, has been shown to be the primary autoantigen of the autoantibodies directed to the intestinal tissues (anti-endomysial antibodies).[81] Glutamine residues make up over 40% of the amino acid residues of the gliadin protein, making it a good substrate for transglutaminase. It is postulated that gliadin may become cross-linked to transglutaminase, creating a novel antigenic determinant that is then recognized by T cells.

Tissue transglutaminase IgA antibodies have been assessed using both an enzyme-linked immunoabsorbent assay (ELISA)[81] and a radioisotope-binding assay.[82] Ten percent of all type 1A diabetics are positive for tTG autoantibodies. Using the radioisotope-binding assay, 22 of 68 (32%) of type 1A diabetics homozygous for HLA-DQ2 express tTG autoantibodies, as opposed to <2% of those lacking DQ2 or DQ8.[82] Approximately 70% of anti-glutaminase-positive patients have celiac disease on biopsy, and the finding of high serum levels of these antibodies revealed a 100% positive predictive value for biopsy evidence of intestinal lesions.

PITFALLS/CONTROVERSIES

GENERAL POPULATION SCREENING

Current trials that target individuals at increased risk for the development of type 1A diabetes, such as the large multicenter randomized trial headed by the National Institutes of Health (Diabetes Prevention Trial), are aimed at intervening in the pre-diabetic stage with the hope of either delaying or preventing disease onset. The success of such trials relies partly on our ability to reliably detect at-risk individuals (e.g., siblings of affected patients). However, 90% of patients with type 1A diabetes do not have an affected first-degree relative, making prediction in the general population an important goal.

General population screening depends on the development of effective interventions that can be instituted prior to the development of diabetes, and potentially prior to autoimmunity. Given the natural history of type 1A diabetes (for many individuals), this will mean that treatment would need to be initiated in infancy. Further complicating this strategy is that only a subset of genetically susceptible individuals progress to diabetes. This subset is highest (40–50%) for DQ8/DQ2 heterozygous first-degree relatives of patients with type 1A diabetes. Trials can be designed that will determine whether autoantibodies, and subsequently disease, are preventable. Because only 10% of first-degree relatives of patients with type 1A diabetes are DQ8/DQ2 heterozygous, such trials will require the screening of more than 1000 neonates. This is obviously a logistical hindrance to such trials, but the major impediment is likely to be the consideration that antigen-based trials have some probability of activating disease. Thus, it is likely that therapies will initially be evaluated in patients with recent-onset type 1A diabetes, and in individuals expressing autoantibodies and progressing to diabetes, before instituting trials involving individuals with genetic susceptibility alone. Increased knowledge of the basic mechanisms of disease and mechanisms of immunotherapies and new assays that predict efficacy are a high priority, so that safe and effective preventive trials can be carried out.

DISTINGUISHING VARIOUS FORMS OF DIABETES

Not all children presenting with diabetes mellitus have type 1A diabetes. Whereas only 10% of non-Hispanic white children do not express GAD65, ICA512 or insulin autoantibodies, as many as 50% of Hispanic and African-American children do not express these antibodies. For patients with type 2 diabetes oral hypoglycemic agents may be the more appropriate therapy. In such cases, clinicians need to carefully monitor these patients for possible decompensation requiring insulin treatment.

In a fraction of adults presenting with what appears to be type 2 diabetes, anti-islet autoantibodies can be detected.[83] When these patients are followed, most eventually require exogenous insulin for control of glycemia. It is likely that such patients, who represent approximately 5–10% of adults presenting with diabetes mellitus, actually have type 1A diabetes. One goal for clinicians is to identify both of the groups described above to ensure that they receive the appropriate therapy in a timely fashion.

Large quantities of antibodies to insulin can occur separately from treatment with insulin as part of the insulin autoimmune syndrome (also termed Hirata syndrome). The two forms of this syndrome, both very rare, are characterized by high-titer anti-insulin antibodies. In the rarest form, monoclonal insulin autoantibodies are produced. The form of the syndrome with polyclonal anti-insulin autoantibodies is frequently associated with ingestion of sulfhydryl-containing drugs such as methimizole (treatment for Graves' disease) in East Asian patients. In both syndromes hypoglycemia and not insulin resistance is the usual presenting abnormality. The polyclonal syndrome is strongly associated with a specific DRB1 allele (DRB1*0406) and usually resolves with discontinuation of the inciting drug. Ninety-six percent of Japanese patients (48/50) were found to have DR4, and 42 of these had DRB1*0406.[84]

Autoantibodies to the insulin receptor are present in a rare syndrome characterized by both hypoglycemia and hyperglycemia in the same patient at different times. It is thought that the anti-insulin receptor antibodies can act as agonists or antagonists. Patients with this syndrome frequently have systemic autoimmune disorders such as lupus erythematosus, rheumatoid arthritis and Sjögren's syndrome. There are case reports of a favorable response to immunosuppression (e.g., with cyclosporine).

■ REFERENCES ■

1. Gavin JR, Alberti G, Davidson MB, et al. Report of the Expert Committee on the Diagnosis and Classification of Diabetes Mellitus. Diabetes Care 1997; 20: 1183.

2. Rewers M, Norris JM, Kretowksi A Epidemiology of type I diabetes. In: Eisenbarth GS, ed. Type I diabetes: molecular, cellular, and clinical immunology. web book at www.barbaradaviscenter.org 7/14/06 publisher Barbara Davis Center, Denver, CO.

3. Pinhas-Hamiel O, Dolan LM, Daniels SR, et al. Increased incidence of noninsulin dependent diabetes mellitus among adolescents. J Pediatr 1996; 128: 608.

4. Foulis AK, Liddle CN, Farquharson MA, et al. The histopathology of the pancreas in type I diabetes (insulin dependent) mellitus: a 25-year review of deaths in patients under 20 years of age in the United Kingdom. Diabetologia 1986; 29: 267.

5. Johnston C, Pyke DA, Cudworth AG, Wolf E. HLA-DR typing in identical twins with insulin-dependent diabetes: difference between concordant and discordant pairs. Br Med J 1983; 286: 253.

6. Bottazzo GF, Florin-Christensen A, Doniach D. Islet-cell antibodies in diabetes mellitus with autoimmune polyendocrine deficiencies. Lancet 1974; 2: 1279.

7. Eisenbarth GS. Type I diabetes mellitus. A chronic autoimmune disease. N Engl J Med 1986; 314: 1360.

8. Mordes JP, Bortell R, Doukas J, et al. The BB/Wor rat and the balance hypothesis of autoimmunity. Diabetes Metab Rev 1996; 12: 103.

9. Sutherland DE, Sibley R, Xu XA, et al. Twin-to-twin pancreas transplantation: reversal and reenactment of the pathogenesis of type I diabetes. Trans Assoc Am Phys 1984; 97: 80.

10. Betts P, Mulligan J, Ward P, et al. Increasing body weight predicts the earlier onset of insulin-dependant diabetes in childhood: testing the 'accelerator hypothesis' (2). Diabet Med 2005; 22: 144–151.

11. Ladner MB, Bottini N, Valdes AM, Noble JA. Association of the single nucleotide polymorphism C1858T of the PTPN22 gene with type 1 diabetes. Hum Immunol 2005; 66: 60–64.

12. Ashcroft FM. K(ATP) channels and insulin secretion: a key role in health and disease. Biochem Soc Trans 2006; 34: 243–246.

13. Porter JR, Barrett TG. Monogenic syndromes of abnormal glucose homeostasis: clinical review and relevance to the understanding of the pathology of insulin resistance and beta cell failure. J Med Genet 2005; 42: 893–902.

14. Ikegami H, Ogihara T. Genetics of insulin-dependent diabetes mellitus. Endocrinol J 1996; 43: 605.

15. Muntoni S, Fonte MT, Stoduto S, et al. Incidence of insulin-dependent diabetes mellitus among Sardinian-heritage children born in Lazio region, Italy. Lancet 1997; 349: 160.

16. Weintrob N, Sprecher E, Israel S, et al. Type 1 diabetes environmental factors and correspondence analysis of HLA class II genes in the Yemenite Jewish community in Israel. Diabetes Care 2001; 24: 650–653.

17. Bingley PJ, Bonifacio E, Williams AJK, et al. Prediction of IDDM in the general population: strategies based on combinations of autoantibody markers. Diabetes 1997; 46: 1701.

18. Rewers M, Norris JM, Eisenbarth GS, et al. Beta-cell autoantibodies in infants and toddlers without IDDM relatives: Diabetes Autoimmunity Study in the Young (Daisy). J Autoimmun 1996; 9: 405.

19. Eisenbarth GS. Prediction of type I diabetes: the natural history of the pre-diabetic period. In: Eisenbarth GS. Type I diabetes: molecular, cellular, and clinical immunology. web book at www.barbaradaviscenter.org 7/14/06 publisher Barbara Davis Center, Denver.

20. Greenbaum CJ, Sears KL, Kahn SE, Palmer JP. Relationship of B-cell function and autoantibodies to progression and nonprogression of subclinical type 1 diabetes. Diabetes 1999; 48: 170.

21. Sreenan S, Pick AJ, Levisetti M, et al. Increased β-cell proliferation and reduced mass before diabetes onset in the nonobese diabetic mouse. Diabetes 1999; 48: 989.

22. Gazda LS, Charlton B, Lafferty KJ. Diabetes results from a late change in the autoimmune response of NOD mice. J Autoimmun 1997; 10: 261.

23. Chatenoud L, Thervet E, Primo J, Bach JF. Anti-CD3 antibody induces long-term remission of overt autoimmunity in nonobese diabetic mice. Proc Natl Acad Sci USA 1994; 91: 123.

24. Redondo MJ, Yu L, Hawa M, et al. Heterogeneity of type 1 diabetes: analysis of monozygotic twins in Great Britain and the United States. Diabetologia 2001; 44: 354–362.

25. Pugliese A, Eisenbarth GS. Type I diabetes mellitus of man: genetic susceptibility and resistance. In: Eisenbarth GS (ed) Type I diabetes: molecular, cellular, and clinical immunology.web book at www.barbaradaviscenter.org 7/14/06 publisher Barbara Davis Center, Denver.

26. Rewers M, Bugawan TL, Norris JM, et al. Newborn screening for HLA markers associated with IDDM: diabetes autoimmunity study in the young (DAISY). Diabetologia 1996; 39: 807.

27. Redondo MJ, Babu S, Zeidler A, et al. Specific HLA DQ influence on expression of anti-islet autoantibodies and progression to type 1 diabetes. J Clin Endocrinol Metab 2006; 91: 1705–1713.

28. Pugliese A, Gianani R, Moromisato R, et al. HLA-DQB1*0602 is associated with dominant protection from diabetes even among islet cell antibody-positive first-degree relatives of patients with IDDM. Diabetes 1995; 44: 608.

29. Nakanishi K, Kobayashi T, Murase T, et al. Human leukocyte antigen-A24 and -DQA1*0301 in Japanese insulin-dependent diabetes mellitus: independent contributions to susceptibility to the disease and additive contributions to acceleration of beta-cell destruction. J Clin Endocrinol Metab 1999; 84: 3721.

30. Bennett ST, Lucassen AM, Gough SCL, et al. Susceptibility to human type I diabetes at IDDM2 is determined by tandem repeat variation at the insulin gene minisatellite locus. Nature Genet 1995; 9: 284.

31. Pugliese A, Zeller M, Fernandez A, et al. The insulin gene is transcribed in the human thymus and transcription levels correlate with allelic variation at the INS VNTR-IDDM2 susceptibility locus for type I diabetes. Nature Genet 1997; 15: 293.

32. Vafiadis P, Bennett ST, Todd JA, et al. Insulin expression in human thymus is modulated by INS VNTR alleles at the IDDM2 locus. Nature Genet 1997; 15: 289.

33. Su MA, Anderson MS. A IRE: an update. Curr Opin Immunol 2004; 16: 746–752.

34. Smyth D, Cooper JD, Collins JE, et al. Replication of an association between the lymphoid tyrosine phosphatase locus (LYP/PTPN22) with type 1 diabetes, and evidence for its role as a general autoimmunity locus. Diabetes 2004; 53: 3020–3023.

35. Nishimoto H, Kikutani H, Yamamura K, Kishimoto T. Prevention of autoimmune insulitis by expression of I-E molecules in NOD mice. Nature 1987; 328: 432.

36. Nakayama M, Abiru N, Moriyama H, et al. Prime role for an insulin epitope in the development of type 1 diabetes in NOD mice. Nature 2005; 435: 220–223.

37. Moralejo DH, Park HA, Speros SJ, et al. Genetic dissection of lymphopenia from autoimmunity by introgression of mutated Ian5 gene onto the F344 rat. J Autoimmun 2003; 21: 315–324.

38. Zipris D, Lien E, Xie JX, et al. TLR activation synergizes with Kilham rat virus infection to induce diabetes in BBDR rats. J Immunol 2005; 174: 131–142.

39. Akashi T, Nagafuchi S, Anzai K, et al. Direct evidence for the contribution of B cells to the progression of insulitis and the development of diabetes in nonobese diabetic mice. Int Immunol 1997; 9: 1159.

40. Yang XD, Tisch R, Singer SM, et al. Effect of tumour necrosis factor alpha on insulin-dependent diabetes mellitus in NOD mice. I., The early development of autoimmunity and the diabetogenic process. J Exp Med 1994; 180: 995.

41. Hultgren B, Huang X, Dybdal N, Stewart TA. Genetic absence of γ-interferon delays but does not prevent diabetes in NOD mice. Diabetes 1996; 45: 812.

42. Wogensen L, Lee M-S, Sarvetnick N. Production of interleukin 10 by islet cells accelerates immune-mediated destruction of β cells in nonobese diabetic mice. J Exp Med 1994; 179: 1379.

43. Masteller EL, Warner MR, Tang Q, et al. Expansion of functional endogenous antigen-specific CD4+CD25+ regulatory T cells from nonobese diabetic mice. J Immunol 2005; 175: 3053–3059.

44. Bisikirska B, Colgan J, Luban J, et al. TCR stimulation with modified anti-CD3 mAb expands CD8 T cell population and induces CD8CD25 Tregs. J Clin Invest 2005; 115: 2904–2913.

45. Wildin RS. Freitas A. IPEX and FOXP3: Clinical and research perspectives. J Autoimmun 2005; 25: 56–62.

46. Rabinowe SL, George KL, Loughlin R, et al. Congenital rubella. Monoclonal antibody-defined T cell abnormalities in young adults. Am J Med 1986; 81: 779.

47. Hyöty H, Hiltunen M, Knip M, et al. A prospective study of the role of Coxsackie B and other enterovirus infections in the pathogenesis of IDDM. Diabetes 1995; 44: 652.

48. Salminen KK, Vuorinen T, Oikarinen S, et al. Isolation of enterovirus strains from children with preclinical Type 1 diabetes. Diabet Med 2004; 21: 156–164.

49. Graves PM, Rewers M. The role of enteroviral infections in the development of IDDM: limitations of current approaches. Diabetes 1997; 46: 161.

50. Akerblom HK, Virtanen SM, Ilonen J, et al. Dietary manipulation of beta cell autoimmunity in infants at increased risk of type 1 diabetes: a pilot study. Diabetology 2005; 48: 829–837.

51. Martin JM, Trink B, Daneman D, et al. Milk proteins in the etiology of insulin-dependent diabetes mellitus (IDDM). Ann Med 1991; 23: 447.

52. Pietropaolo M, Castano L, Babu S, et al. Islet cell autoantigen 69kDa (ICA69): molecular cloning and characterization of a novel diabetes associated autoantigen. J Clin Invest 1993; 92: 359.

53. Couper JJ, Steele C, Beresford S, et al. Lack of association between duration of breast-feeding or introduction of cow's milk and development of islet autoimmunity. Diabetes 1999; 48: 2145.

54. Jun HS, Yoon CS, Zbytnuik L, et al. The role of macrophages in T cell-mediated autoimmune diabetes in nonobese diabetic mice. J Exp Med 1999; 189: 347.

55. Palmer JP, Asplin CM, Clemons P, et al. Insulin antibodies in insulin-dependent diabetics before insulin treatment. Science 1983; 222: 1337.

56. Achenbach P, Bonifacio E, Koczwara K, Ziegler AG. Natural history of type 1 diabetes. Diabetes 2005; 54: S25–S31.

57. Koczwara K, Bonifacio E, Ziegler AG. Transmission of maternal islet antibodies and risk of autoimmune diabetes in offspring of mothers with type 1 diabetes. Diabetes 2004; 53: 1–4.

58. Ujihara N, Daw K, Gianani R, et al. Identification of glutamic acid decarboxylase autoantibody heterogeneity and epitope regions in type I diabetes. Diabetes 1994; 43: 968.

59. Gianani R, Rabin DU, Verge CF, et al. ICA512 autoantibody radioassay. Diabetes 1995; 44: 1340.

60. Barker JM, Barriga K, Yu L, et al. Prediction of autoantibody positivity and progression to type 1 diabetes: Diabetes Autoimmunity Study in the Young (DAISY). JCEM 2004; 89: 3896–3902.

61. Simone E, Daniel D, Schloot N, et al. T cell receptor restriction of diabetogenic autoimmune NOD T cells. Proc Natl Acad Sci USA 1997; 94: 2518.

62. Wong FS, Karttunen J, Dumont C, et al. Identification of an MHC class I-restricted autoantigen in type 1 diabetes by screening an organ-specific cDNA library. Nature Med 1999; 5: 1026.

63. Mallone R, Nepom GT. Targeting T lymphocytes for immune monitoring and intervention in autoimmune diabetes. Am J Ther 2005; 12: 534–550.

64. Itoh N, Hanafusa T, Miyazaki A, et al. Mononuclear cell infiltration and its relation to the expression of major histocompatibility complex antigens and adhesion molecules in pancreas biopsy specimens from newly diagnosed insulin-dependent diabetes mellitus patients. J Clin Invest 1993; 92: 2313.

Clinical manifestations

The incidence and prevalence of IPF remain unknown, although recent studies have reported prevalence rates for men and women as 20.2 per 100 000 and 13.2 per 100 000, respectively.[4] Both the incidence and prevalence of IPF increase with age, with most patients presenting between 40 and 70 years of age. Although the clinical features of IPF are variable, most patients present with the insidious onset of exertional dyspnea and a dry, nonproductive cough. Physical examination typically reveals dry, end-inspiratory crackles; clubbing may be present in 25–50% of patients.

The chest radiograph typically shows diffuse reticular opacities, predominantly in the lower zone and lung periphery. Ground-glass opacities, small cysts (honeycombing), and reduced lung volumes may also be seen (Fig. 71.1A). These radiographic changes often precede the onset of symptoms, and serial chest radiographs usually reveal progression with associated volume loss. High-resolution computed tomography (HRCT) findings include bibasal peripheral reticular opacities (Fig. 71.1B).[5] Honeycombing, traction bronchiectasis, and subpleural fibrosis may also be present. The finding of ground-glass opacities on the initial HRCT suggests alveolar inflammation and may identify patients with IPF who are more likely to respond to glucocorticoid therapy.

The typical physiologic abnormalities in IPF are those of a restrictive lung disease with a low diffusing capacity for carbon monoxide and severe gas exchange abnormalities exacerbated by exercise.

Histopathology

The gross appearance of the lungs in IPF shows a nodular pleural surface while histopathologic examination reveals UIP. UIP is characterized by nonuniform and variable distribution of the interstitial changes. At low magnification, alternating zones of interstitial fibrosis, inflammation, honeycombing, and normal lung may be seen (Fig. 71.2A). At higher magnification, findings include derangement of alveolar walls with edema, fibrinous exudate, fibroblast proliferation, and fibrosis. Honeycomb

▌ CLINICAL PEARLS

IDIOPATHIC PULMONARY FIBROSIS (IPF)

›› IPF is one of the most common causes of diffuse parenchymal lung disease of unknown etiology and is characterized by insidious onset of cough and dyspnea

›› The histopathologic pattern of IPF is usual interstitial pneumonitis

›› A confident diagnosis of IPF based on high-resolution computed tomography can only be made in two-thirds of cases

›› IPF is generally a fatal disorder, characterized by relentless progression and a 5-year survival of 30–50%

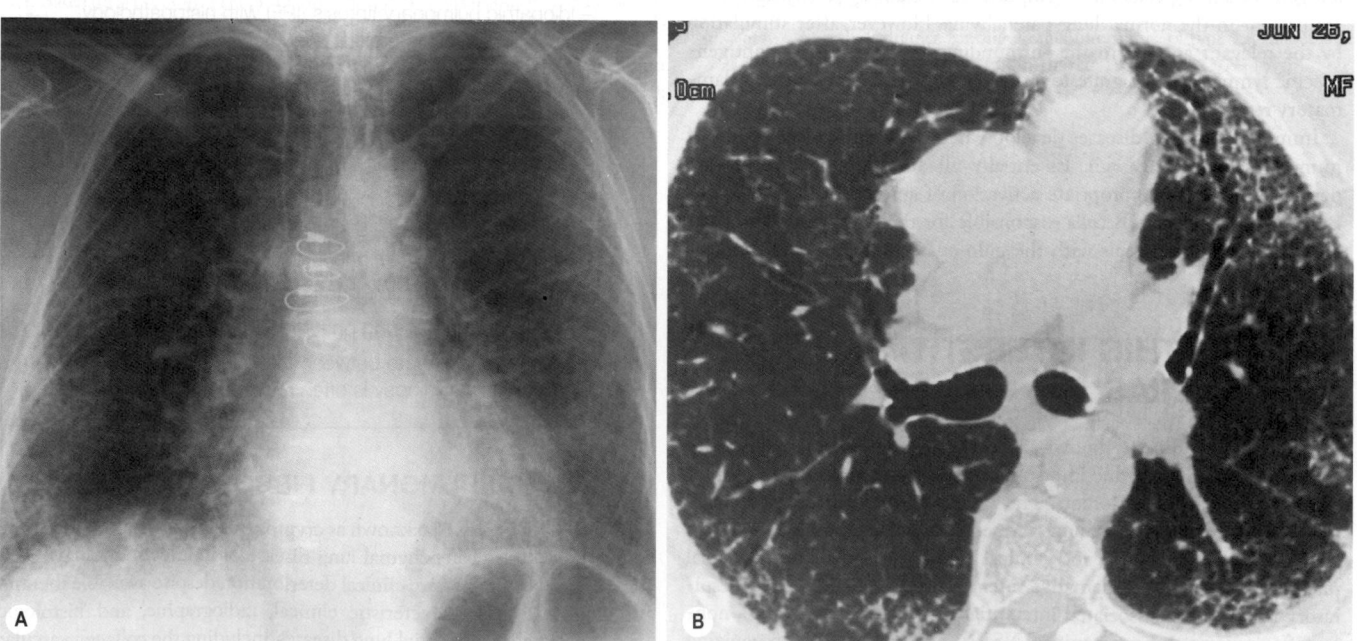

Fig. 71.1 Radiographic manifestations of idiopathic pulmonary fibrosis. **(A)** Chest radiograph in a patient with idiopathic pulmonary fibrosis showing diffuse, coarse reticular opacities with a lower-lung zone predominance. Cystic radiolucencies, consistent with honeycombing, are evident. **(B)** High-resolution computed tomography shows peripheral reticular opacities, honeycombing, and traction bronchiectasis.

change refers to enlarged airspaces lined by metaplastic bronchial epithelium and surrounded by walls thickened with collagen (Fig. 71.2B). The earliest finding in UIP is thought to be the "fibroblast focus," a lesion consisting of distinct clusters of fibroblasts and myofibroblasts in a loose connective tissue matrix within the alveolar wall, with minimal interstitial inflammation or intra-alveolar macrophage accumulation (Fig. 71.2C).[6] Tables 71.1 and 71.2 compare the clinical and pathologic features of UIP, DIP, RB-ILD, and NSIP.

Pathogenesis

The etiologic agent(s) responsible for the initiation of IPF remains unknown. Evidence suggests that an interaction between genetic, environmental, and viral factors may be involved (Fig. 71.3). Some cases of IPF are familial, inherited as an autosomal dominant trait with variable penetrance.[7] A recent study suggested that a functionally uncharacterized gene, ELMOD2, may be a candidate gene for susceptibility in familial IPF.[8]

At present, the mechanisms involved in the induction of the inflammatory events that lead to the development of lung fibrosis remain poorly understood. However, little doubt exists regarding the immunologic nature of this disease. For example, an identical pathologic process can be seen in several immune-mediated diseases such as CVD, inflammatory bowel disease, and primary biliary cirrhosis. In addition, no single stimulus is responsible for all causes of pulmonary fibrosis. More likely, the fibrotic response represents a final common pathway following certain immune and inflammatory events.

In the normal lung, the interstitium is thin and delicate with few lymphoid cells and fibroblasts. Following the initiation of the inflammatory process, damage to the alveolar epithelium occurs, followed by infiltration of the interstitium with activated immune cells. In addition, immune complexes have been identified in the serum and lungs of IPF patients. Activated alveolar macrophages secrete interleukin-1 (IL-1), IL-8, tumor necrosis factor-α (TNF-α), platelet-derived growth factor (PDGF), and insulin-like growth factor-1 (IGF-1). This cytokine milieu promotes the activation and recruitment of neutrophils and lymphocytes to the area of alveolitis.

T lymphocytes, which accumulate in the alveolar space and interstitium, express an activated phenotype, including the expression of human leukocyte antigen (HLA)-DR and IL-2 receptor. Following activation, CD4 T cells evolve into two major subsets distinguished by the cytokines produced (Chapters 10 and 17).[9] In IPF, T cells expressing a Th2-type phenotype predominate, producing IL-4, IL-5, IL-10, and IL-13. Th2 cells are mainly involved in the development of humoral immunity by helping B cells through the promotion of class switching and enhancement of the production of certain IgG isotypes and production of IgE. Evidence suggests that a switch to Th2-type cells may be important in the development of fibrosis through the deposition of matrix components. Thus, a switch to Th2-type cells may occur in IPF followed by the release of Th2-type cytokines stimulating production of extracellular matrix as well as attracting the influx of fibroblasts.

In addition to their role as scavengers, alveolar macrophages are vital in the repair phase of inflammation. However, the distinguishing feature between a self-resolving inflammatory process and a fibrotic response, as seen in IPF, is the accumulation of collagen. Current evidence suggests that the fibrotic process in IPF is a consequence of dysregulation of both collagen synthesis and degradation. Macrophage-derived growth factors, including transforming growth factor-β (TGF-β), PDGF, and IGF-1,

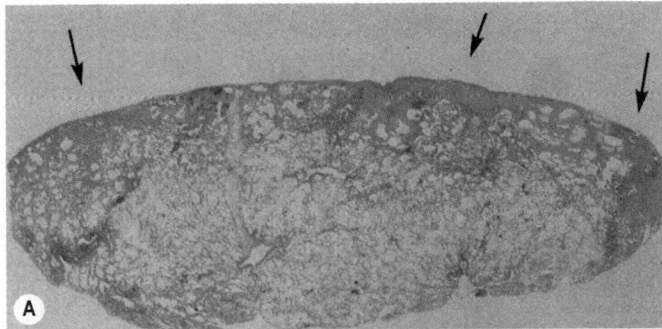

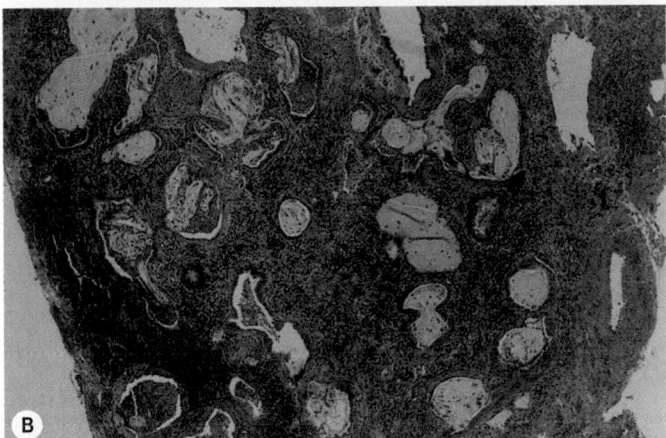

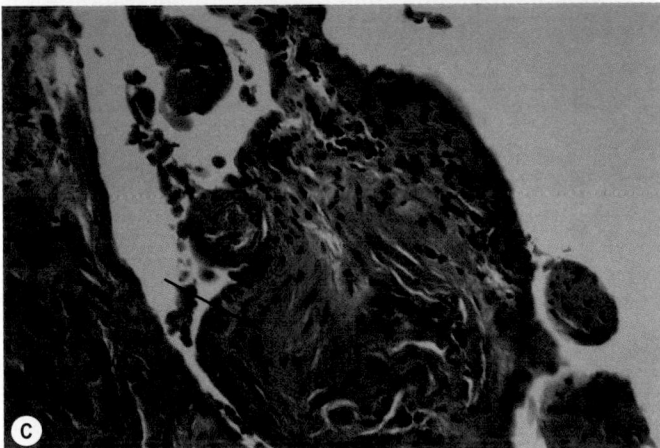

Fig. 71.2 Histopathology of usual interstitial pneumonitis (UIP). **(A)** Low-magnification photomicrograph of UIP showing the variegated appearance from one field of view to the next with areas of dense subpleural fibrosis (arrows) separated from other areas of normal lung. **(B)** High-magnification photomicrograph of UIP showing honeycomb change characterized by enlarged airspaces filled with mucin and separated by fibrosis. **(C)** Fibroblast focus in UIP is characterized by clusters of spindle-shaped fibroblasts (arrow) in a loose connective tissue matrix within the alveolar wall.

Table 71.1 Clinical features of the idiopathic interstitial pneumonias

	UIP	DIP	RB-ILD	AIP	NSIP
Mean age (years)	57	42	36	49	49
Childhood	No	Rare	No	Rare	Occasionally
Onset	Insidious	Insidious	Insidious	Acute	Subacute, insidious
Mortality (mean survival)	68% (5–6 years)	27% (12 years)	0%	62% (1–2 months)	11% (17 months)
Response to steroids	Poor	Good	Good	Poor	Good
Recovery possible	No	Yes	Yes	Yes	Yes

AID, acute interstitial pneumonitis; DIP, desquamative interstitial pneumonitis; NSIP, nonspecific interstitial pneumonitis; RB-ILD, respiratory bronchiolitis-associated interstitial lung disease; UIP, usual interstitial pneumonitis.
Adapted from Katzenstein AL, Myers JL. Idiopathic pulmonary fibrosis: clinical relevance of pathologic classification. Am J Respir Crit Care Med 1998; 157: 1301.

Table 71.2 Histopathologic features of the idiopathic interstitial pneumonias

	UIP	DIP/RB-ILD	AIP	NSIP
Temporal appearance	Variegated	Uniform	Uniform	Uniform
Interstitial inflammation	Scant	Scant	No	Prominent
Collagen/fibrosis	Patchy	Diffuse (DIP) Focal (RB-ILD)	No	Diffuse
Fibroblast proliferation	Fibroblast foci prominent	No	Diffuse	Rare
BOOP	No	No	No	Focal
Honeycomb change	Yes	No	No	Rare
Intra-alveolar macrophages	Focal	Diffuse (DIP) Focal (RB-ILD)	No	Patchy
Hyaline membranes	No	No	Focal	No

AIP, acute interstitial pneumonitis; BOOP, bronchiolitis obliterans organizing pneumonia; DIP, desquamative interstitial pneumonitis; NSIP, nonspecific interstitial pneumonitis; RB-ILD, respiratory bronchiolitis-associated interstitial lung disease; UIP, usual interstitial pneumonitis.
Adapted from Katzenstein AL, Myers JL. Idiopathic pulmonary fibrosis: clinical relevance of pathologic classification. Am J Respir Crit Care Med 1998; 157: 1301.

stimulate fibroblast proliferation and collagen deposition.[10] Adequate resolution of an inflammatory process requires matrix degradation. Metalloproteases produced by macrophages and fibroblasts are involved in matrix degradation, and control of metalloprotease production involves substances known as tissue inhibitors of metalloproteases (TIMPs). TIMPs are elevated in the lungs of patients with IPF. In addition, TGF-β can markedly augment TIMP production. Thus, there appears to be a loss of balance between the events mediating resolution and those mediating perpetuation of the inflammatory response, setting the stage for lung injury, tissue remodeling, and the development of irreversible pulmonary fibrosis.[11]

Diagnosis

The diagnostic evaluation of a patient with diffuse parenchymal lung disease includes a thorough history and physical examination with particular attention to symptoms and signs that could indicate CVD, occupational and environmental exposures, or medication and drug usage. A careful family history is also important.

The history and physical findings in IPF are nonspecific. However, extrapulmonary involvement does not occur: the presence of fever, arthralgias, myalgias, or pleuritis should suggest a collagen vascular disorder. Antinuclear antibodies and rheumatoid factor are present in

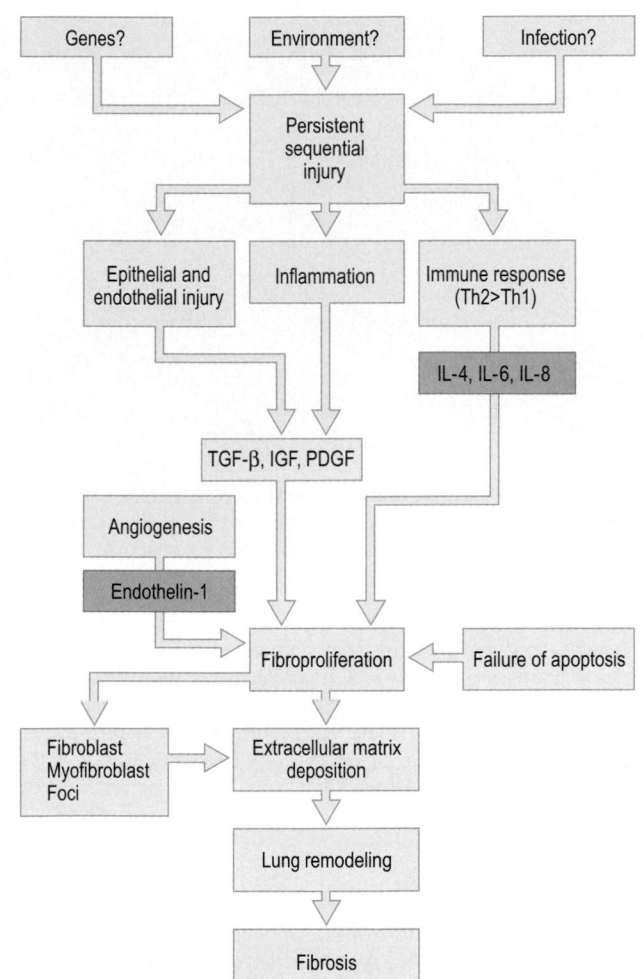

Fig. 71.3 Events hypothesized to be involved in the pathogenesis of idiopathic pulmonary fibrosis. The initiating event(s) leading to persistent lung injury remains poorly understood. The interaction between genetic factors, environmental exposures, and infectious agents leads to epithelial and endothelial injury, resulting in the secretion of macrophage-derived growth factors, including transforming growth factor-β (TGF-β), insulin-like growth factor-1 (IGF-1), and platelet-derived growth factor (PDGF). This cytokine milieu stimulates fibroblast proliferation and collagen deposition. In addition, the resulting Th2 immune response stimulates extracellular matrix production and fibroblast proliferation, resulting in lung remodeling and, eventually, lung fibrosis.

KEY CONCEPTS

PATHOGENESIS OF THE IDIOPATHIC INTERSTITIAL PNEUMONIAS

>> Although the inciting event(s) is unknown in the different diseases, a common result is a dysregulated fibroproliferative response (similar to wound healing), which leads to excessive extracellular matrix production and lung remodeling

>> A genetically determined inability to repair and re-epithelialize the denuded basement membranes adequately may be a contributing factor and may relate to the familial occurrence of some cases of idiopathic pulmonary fibrosis

>> The presence of a chronic stimulus (autoantigen), as is seen in the pneumoconioses, may result in a persistent inflammatory and immune response and lead to a failure in the normal healing process

>> The release of transforming growth factor-β following epithelial injury stimulates collagen synthesis and the prevention of apoptosis of proliferating fibroblasts in the lung and may impair collagen degradation by inhibiting the production of metalloproteases

>> A predominant Th2 response in the lung and the absence of interferon-γ favor the development of a fibrotic response

hypersensitivity pneumonitis, bronchiolitis obliterans organizing pneumonia (BOOP), or NSIP.

A surgical lung biopsy is recommended in suspected IPF patients without a definitive HRCT appearance and who do not have contraindications to the procedure. This is especially important in patients with atypical clinical or radiographic findings, which could suggest the possibility of one of the other histologic patterns of the idiopathic interstitial pneumonias and an improved prognosis. Biopsy may be omitted in elderly patients with cardiovascular disease, or those with evidence of extensive honeycomb change. Video-assisted thoracoscopic (VATS) biopsy is the preferred surgical technique and has been associated with less morbidity and a decreased hospital stay compared with open lung biopsy.

Treatment and outcome

The usual course of IPF is relentless progression without spontaneous remission, commonly with a fatal outcome. Recent studies in patients with biopsy-proven IPF indicate a shorter survival than previously thought (30–50% 5-year survival). Currently available treatment options include glucocorticoids or immunosuppressant drugs, either alone or in combination. However, despite the fact that the glucocorticoids are considered the mainstay of therapy for IPF, no prospective, randomized, double-blind, placebo-controlled trial has demonstrated their efficacy in the treatment of IPF. Moreover, a recent study showed that the combination of prednisone and cyclophosamide did not alter survival of IPF patients.[13] Thus, there is no good evidence to support the use of any specific therapy in the management of IPF. Large controlled trials are under way to confirm the potential usefulness of newer agents such as IFN-γ$_{1b}$,[14] pirfenidone, and

10–20% of IPF patients, but titers greater than 1:160 should suggest the possibility of an alternative diagnosis.

The majority of patients with IPF have an abnormal chest radiograph at the time of presentation. Basal peripheral reticular opacities are the characteristic radiographic findings of IPF. A confident diagnosis of IPF from HRCT of the lung requires the presence of patchy, peripheral bibasal reticular abnormalities.[12] The presence of extensive ground-glass opacities on HRCT should suggest an alternative diagnosis, such as DIP,

THERAPEUTIC PRINCIPLES

TREATMENT OF PATIENTS WITH IDIOPATHIC PULMONARY FIBROSIS (IPF)

>> No data exist to show that any currently available therapy alters survival and improves quality of life

>> Therapy is not recommended in all IPF patients (e.g., age >70 years, end-stage honeycomb lung, and significant comorbid diseases such as cardiac disease or diabetes mellitus)

>> Until studies define the best therapeutic regimen in IPF, combined therapy should include prednisone 0.5 mg/kg per day for 4 weeks followed by a taper to 0.125 mg/kg per day plus azathioprine or cyclophosphamide 2mg/kg per day

>> At least 3 months are needed to determine an objective response to any intervention

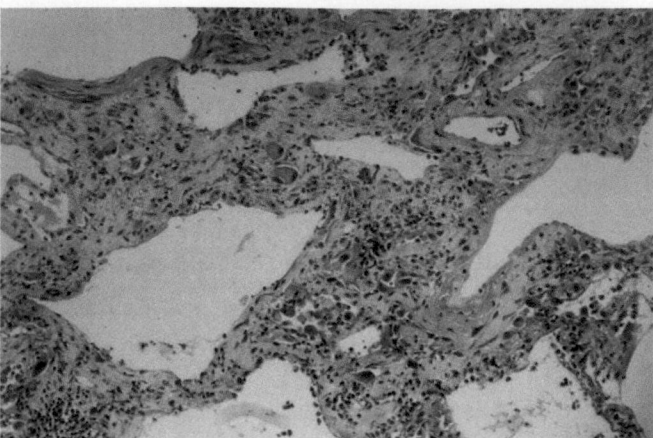

Fig. 71.4 Histopathology of acute interstitial pneumonitis. Diffuse thickening of the alveolar septum with an infiltration of mononuclear cells is the characteristic abnormality. The temporal uniformity of this process is also apparent.

bosentan. Lung transplantation should be considered in patients with progressive clinical and physiologic deterioration who meet established criteria. Early listing is crucial since the waiting time may exceed 2 years.

The most common cause of death in patients with IPF is progression of the underlying disease.[15] In one study, 39% of IPF patients died of respiratory failure, with cardiovascular complications (ischemic heart disease, heart failure, stroke) accounting for 27% of the deaths. Other causes of death in IPF include bronchogenic carcinoma (10%), infection (7%), and pulmonary embolism (3%).

ACUTE INTERSTITIAL PNEUMONIA

Acute interstitial pneumonia (AIP) is a fulminant form of idiopathic interstitial pneumonia. Although it was previously thought to represent an acute phase of UIP, recent studies indicate that it may be a distinct entity. However, in patients with documented UIP/IPF, acute exacerbations may demonstrate the pathology of AIP superimposed on the features of UIP.

Clinical manifestations

AIP usually presents with acute onset of dyspnea followed by rapid progression to respiratory failure. The clinical, radiographic, physiologic, and histologic features are identical to those of the adult respiratory distress syndrome but without any identifiable cause. Most patients are previously healthy individuals over 40 years of age. Men and women are equally affected. A viral prodrome is common, with symptoms including fever, nonproductive cough, and dyspnea. Laboratory studies are nonspecific. Chest radiographs show diffuse, bilateral airspace opacities, and on HRCT there is ground-glass attenuation. A similar presentation may complicate or represent the initial manifestation of a CVD.

Histopathology

AIP is characterized by diffuse interstitial fibrosis that is temporally uniform (Fig. 71.4).[16] The changes are identical to the organizing phases of diffuse alveolar damage, as seen in ARDS. Within the thickened interstitial space, there is active, diffuse fibroblast proliferation similar to the focal fibroblast foci seen in UIP. If this is progressive, honeycomb change occurs. However, these airspaces are lined with alveolar epithelium as opposed to the bronchiolar epithelium lining honeycomb spaces. Other features of acute lung injury, which are frequently seen in AIP, are intra-alveolar hyaline membranes.

Diagnosis

The diagnosis of AIP requires a clinical syndrome of idiopathic ARDS and the presence of organizing diffuse alveolar damage on lung biopsy. Thus, an openlung biopsy or VATS lung biopsy is suggested to secure the diagnosis and exclude other causes of acute interstitial lung disease.

Treatment and outcome

No effective therapy exists for patients with AIP. Glucocorticoids are utilized in most cases, but no survival benefit has been shown. One study shows that the additional use of anticoagulation improves survival. Overall, the prognosis of patients with AIP is poor, with mortality rates ranging from 50% to 88%. Half of patients die within 6 months of disease onset. However, those individuals who survive may have complete recovery of lung function. Once recovered, AIP rarely recurs.

DESQUAMATIVE INTERSTITIAL PNEUMONITIS

DIP represents fewer than 3% of all cases of interestitial lung disease.[17] However, it is a distinct clinicopathological entity that differs substantially from UIP.

Clinical manifestations

DIP affects individuals in their fourth to fifth decades of life; a male predominance is noted in most studies. This disease occurs predominantly in cigarette smokers. Clinically, most individuals present with

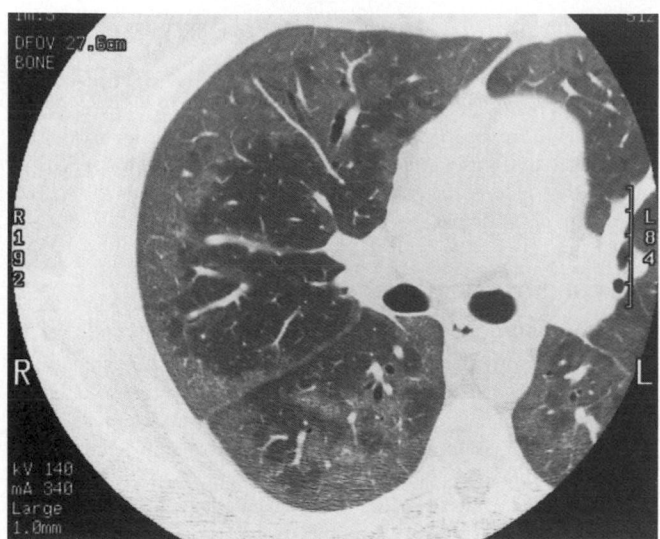

Fig. 71.5 Radiographic manifestations in desquamative interstitial pneumonitis. High-resolution computed tomography in a patient with desquamative interstitial pneumonitis shows ground-glass attenuation in the periphery of the upper and lower lung fields.

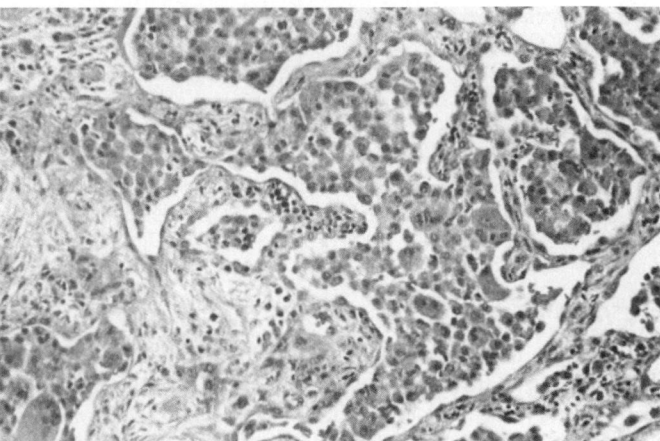

Fig. 71.6 Histopathology of desquamative interstitial pneumonitis. A high-magnification photomicrograph of desquamative interstitial pneumonitis shows the uniform, diffuse accumulation of macrophages within the alveolar space with associated thickening of the alveolar septum. These aggregates of macrophages almost completely fill the alveolar spaces.

subacute onset of a dry, nonproductive cough and dyspnea. Clubbing is present in approximately 50% of DIP patients. Laboratory evaluation is usually nonspecific.

The chest radiograph typically reveals bibasal ground-glass opacities that are not disease-specific. Reticulonodular interstitial infiltrates have also been reported. In addition, a normal chest radiograph may be seen in up to 20% of symptomatic individuals. HRCT confirms the chest radiograph findings, showing ground-glass attenuation in the periphery of the lower lung zones (Fig. 71.5). Pulmonary function testing shows a restrictive defect with an associated decreased diffusing capacity and hypoxemia.

Histopathology

DIP is a misnomer. It was initially thought that the intra-alveolar cells represented sloughed or desquamated alveolar epithelial cells. However, DIP is pathologically characterized by uniform, diffuse accumulation of macrophages in the alveolar space (Fig. 71.6).[16] At low magnification, the overall appearance is one of uniformity from one field of view to the next as opposed to the variegated appearance of UIP. In addition, scant interstitial inflammation with varying degrees of fibrosis of the alveolar septum is present.

Diagnosis

The diagnosis of DIP requires tissue confirmation of the pathologic lesion. This is important since this process has a better prognosis and response to therapeutic intervention compared to IPF. A DIP-like lesion is frequently seen in the other idiopathic interstitial pneumonias as well as in eosinophilic granuloma, drug reactions, and other unrelated conditions. Thus, the diagnosis of DIP requires careful correlation of pathologic findings with clinical and radiologic findings.

Treatment and outcome

The primary intervention in DIP is smoking cessation. Since there are a limited number of cases, it is unclear whether glucocorticoids alter the natural history of this disease. A mortality rate of 28% with a mean survival of 12 years was initially reported, compared to a 66% mortality and a mean survival of 5.6 years in UIP. Of note, 22% patients improved spontaneously and 60% responded to glucocorticoid therapy. This improvement is dramatically different from IPF, in which spontaneous improvement rarely, if ever, occurs and a response to glucocorticoids is seen in only 10–15% of patients. There are, however, a number of patients with DIP who fail to respond to treatment and progress to respiratory failure, secondary to advanced fibrosis.

RESPIRATORY BRONCHIOLITIS-ASSOCIATED INTERSTITIAL LUNG DISEASE

RB-ILD is a distinct clinical entity that occurs in current or former cigarette smokers. However, it remains unclear whether RB-ILD and DIP represent different diseases or different ends of the spectrum of the same disease process.[17] DIP occurs predominantly and RB-ILD occurs exclusively in cigarette smokers, suggesting a common pathogenesis related to cigarette smoke.

Clinical manifestations

In the two studies to date evaluating RB-ILD, the mean age at presentation was 36 years. A male predominance was noted, and all individuals with RB-ILD were cigarette smokers. The most common symptoms were a dry, nonproductive cough and dyspnea. Clubbing is absent in RB-ILD, in contrast to its frequent presence in patients with DIP.[18] Laboratory evaluation is nonspecific.

The chest radiograph typically shows diffuse, fine reticular or nodular interstitial opacities with normal lung volumes. Additional findings include bronchial wall thickening and a prominent peribronchovascular interstitium. HRCT may reveal ground-glass opacification as well as emphysema.

Pulmonary function tests most commonly reveal a mixed restrictive–obstructive pattern with a reduced diffusing capacity and mild hypoxemia. An isolated elevation of the residual volume may also be observed.

Histopathology

The pathology of RB-ILD has similarities to DIP. However, in RB-ILD, the intra-alveolar macrophages accumulate primarily within the peribronchiolar airspaces and are associated with thickening of the alveolar septum in these areas (Fig. 71.7). The differentiation of this lesion from DIP requires sparing of distal airspaces with the lesion confined to the peribronchiolar airspaces in RB-ILD.

Diagnosis

RB-ILD should be suspected in young individuals with a history of cigarette use who complain of cough and dyspnea with a chest radiograph or HRCT showing nodular and/or reticular interstitial opacities. The diagnosis requires tissue confirmation of the pathologic findings noted above.

Treatment and outcome

The key therapeutic intervention in RB-ILD is cessation of smoking. The use of glucocorticoids has been associated with favorable results. At present, the clinical course and prognosis of patients with RB-ILD are unknown. In most clinical series, patients either improved or stabilized with no deaths reported.

NONSPECIFIC INTERSTITIAL PNEUMONITIS

The term NSIP was first used to describe cases of interstitial pneumonia that did not demonstrate a pattern of UIP, AIP, or DIP.[19] Currently, the term NSIP is applied to an idiopathic interstitial pneumonia or to a similar histologic pattern that occurs in CVD, hypersensitivity pneumonitis, or drug-induced lung disease. In fact, 16% of patients in the original description of NSIP had one of the CVD.[19]

Clinical manifestations

Idiopathic NSIP is most often seen in middle-aged individuals, and a slight female predominance has been noted.[20] A dry, nonproductive cough and exertional dyspnea are the most common symptoms, although fever is present in 25% of patients. Symptoms are usually present for 6–10 months prior to diagnosis. As in other interstitial pneumonias, the laboratory evaluation is nonspecific.

The chest radiograph usually shows bilateral interstitial infiltrates and sometimes can be normal in a symptomatic patient. The HRCT characteristically shows bilateral, patchy ground-glass attenuation indistinguishable from DIP or RB-ILD.[5]

Histopathology

NSIP is characterized by varying but temporally uniform degrees of fibrosis and inflammation of the alveolar septum, without histopathologic features indicative of UIP, AIP, or DIP (Fig. 71.8). Katzenstein and Fiorelli[19] divided NSIP cases into three groups depending on the presence or absence of interstitial fibrosis: interstitial lymphoplasmacytic inflammation (48% of cases); inflammation and fibrosis (38%); and fibrosis (14%). Although the changes are temporally uniform, they may be patchy with intervening areas of normal lung.

This temporal uniformity is in contrast to the variegated pattern seen in UIP. Fibroblast foci, the earliest lesion seen in UIP, are found in 20%

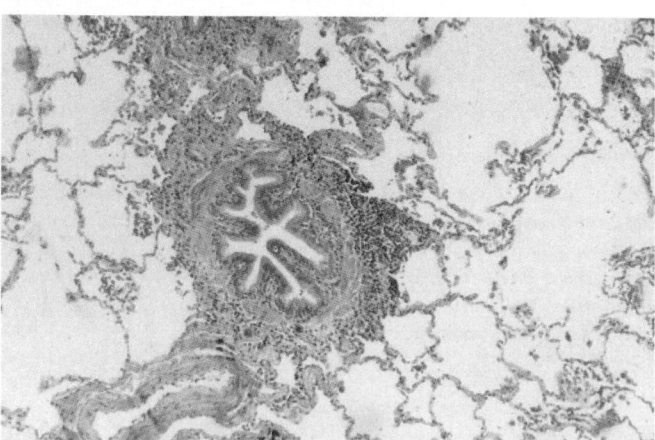

Fig. 71.7 Histopathology of respiratory bronchiolitis – interstitial lung disease. An ectatic bronchiole with a thickened wall is shown, with a mononuclear infiltrate extending into the immediately surrounding alveoli.

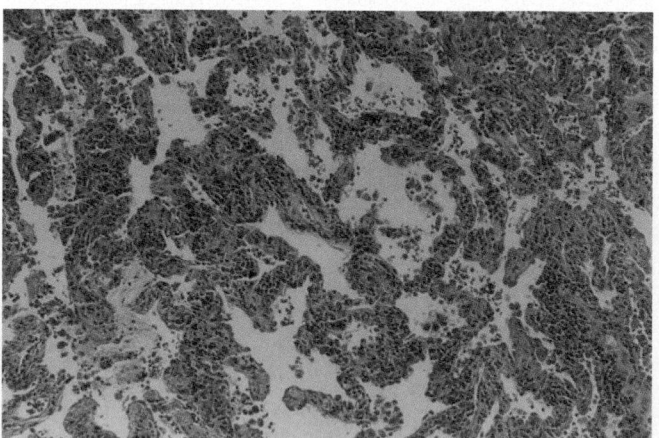

Fig. 71.8 Histopathology of nonspecific interstitial pneumonitis. Low-magnification photomicrograph of cellular nonspecific interstitial pneumonitis shows diffuse uniform thickening of the alveolar septum due to the presence of a lymphoplasmacytic infiltrate.

of patients with NSIP, making the differentiation of fibrotic NSIP from UIP difficult. The key feature in this circumstance is the temporal uniformity of the lesion in NSIP.

Treatment and outcome

Unlike patients with UIP, individuals with NSIP have a favorable prognosis. In the original description of the disease, 45% of subjects completely recovered while another 42% remained stable or improved.[19] Only 11% of patients died, with a mean survival of 16 months. All of the individuals with an aggressive course were in the fibrotic group. Ten-year survival in the cellular group was 90%, compared to 35% in patients with the fibrotic pattern. Despite the worse prognosis of NSIP with a fibrosing pattern, this is still significantly better than the 10-year survival rate of UIP patients (15%).[21]

CRYPTOGENIC ORGANIZING PNEUMONIA

COP or idiopathic BOOP is a specific clinicopathologic disorder of unknown etiology characterized by excessive proliferation of granulation tissue within the lumen of the distal airspaces.[22] The term COP is reserved for cases demonstrating BOOP without an obvious cause, since this histologic appearance also occurs in a variety of inflammatory lung disorders, including CVD, malignancy, infections, and those caused by medications.

Clinical manifestations

The onset of disease is usually in the fifth to sixth decades of life; men and women are affected equally. Most individuals have symptoms for less than 2 months prior to diagnosis. The initial presentation is characterized by a dry, nonproductive cough with flu-like symptoms, including fever, sore throat, and malaise. This is followed by progressive dyspnea and cough. Routine laboratory evaluation is nonspecific.

The chest radiograph is characterized by diffuse, often patchy alveolar opacities in the setting of normal lung volumes (Fig. 71.9A). These opacities can be migratory and can have a peripheral distribution similar to those seen in chronic eosinophilic pneumonia. Other rare radiographic manifestations include linear or nodular interstitial opacities and honeycombing. The presence of a pleural effusion or pleural thickening should suggest an associated CVD.

HRCT of the chest shows patchy airspace consolidation more commonly located in the lung periphery with a lower-lung zone predominance (Fig. 71.9B). Other findings include ground-glass attenuation, small nodular opacities, and bronchial wall thickening.

As in other interstitial lung diseases, a restrictive ventilatory defect is the most common pulmonary function abnormality. Gas exchange abnormalities are common and are accompanied by decreased diffusing capacity, widening of the alveolar–arterial gradient, and exercise-induced hypoxemia.

Histopathology

The histopathology of COP is characterized by excessive proliferation of granulation tissue in the small airways and alveolar ducts with associated chronic inflammation in the alveolar walls (Fig. 71.10).[23] The intraluminal fibrotic buds (Masson bodies) consist of loose collagen-embedding fibroblasts and myofibroblasts and have a tendency to extend from one alveolus to the next, giving a characteristic "butterfly" pattern. The lesions are patchy in nature and have a uniform temporal appearance at low magnification with preservation of the underlying lung parenchyma. COP has been described as the prototypical healing response of the lung to a variety of insults.

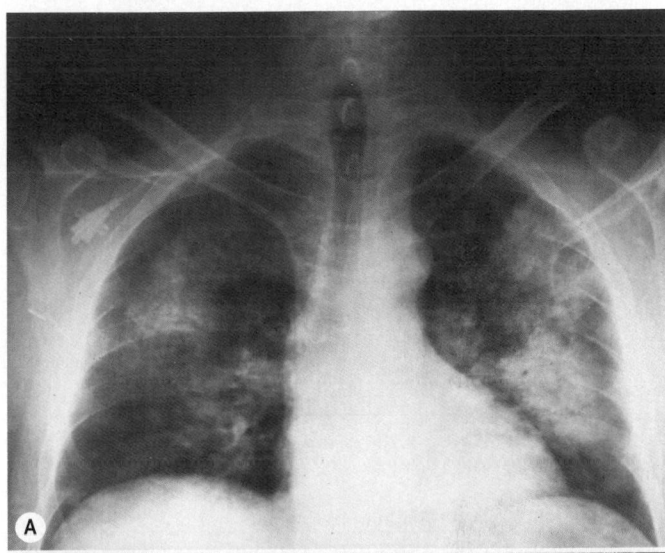

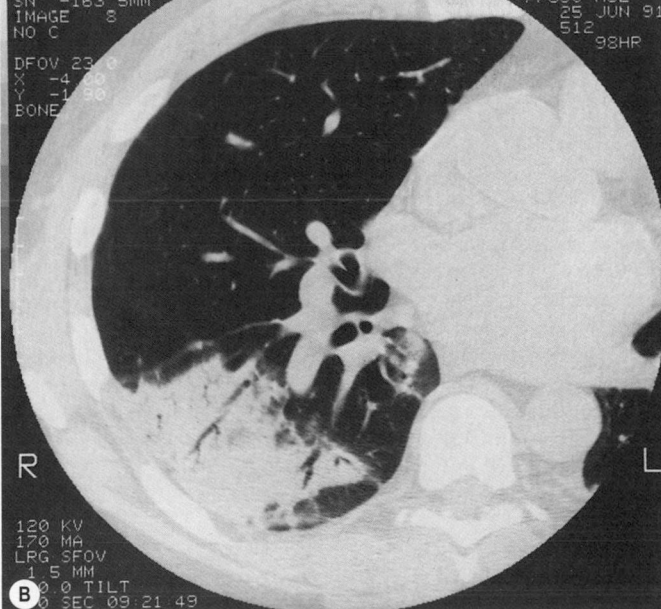

Fig. 71.9 Radiographic findings in cryptogenic organizing pneumonia. **(A)** Chest radiograph in a patient with cryptogenic organizing pneumonia shows bilateral patchy alveolar opacities with a peripheral distribution in the setting of normal lung volumes. **(B)** Chest computed tomography shows a dense right lower lung consolidation with the presence of air bronchograms.

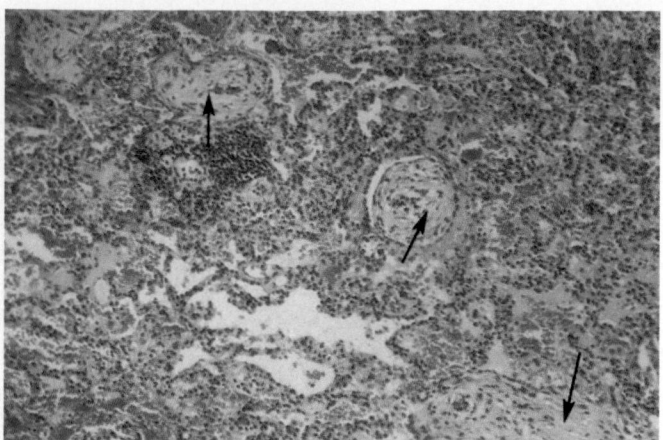

Fig. 71.10 Histopathology of cryptogenic organizing pneumonia. A photomicrograph of cryptogenic organizing pneumonia shows intra-alveolar fibroblast proliferation (arrows) and early collagen production. In addition, thickening of the alveolar septa with a lymphoplasmacytic infiltrate consistent with cellular nonspecific interstitial pneumonitis is present.

Diagnosis

The presence of BOOP in a lung biopsy does not necessarily represent COP since this is a diagnosis of exclusion. Organizing pneumonia is a nonspecific response to many lung injuries and may occur in conjunction with another pathologic process or as a component of other primary pulmonary disorders such as infections, irradiation, CVD, hypersensitivity pneumonitis, Wegener's granulomatosis (WG), or chronic eosinophilic pneumonia (Table 71.3).

Treatment and outcome

Treatment with glucocorticoids usually offers dramatic clinical and radiographic improvement within days to weeks.[23] Complete clinical, physiologic, and radiographic recovery occurs in two-thirds of cases. However, in the remainder, persistent disease with progression to fibrosis can be expected. It is common for relapses to occur with glucocorticoid tapering, followed by improvement with reintroduction of treatment; consequently at least 6 months of therapy is recommended. The 5-year survival in COP is 73%, compared to 5-year survival rates of 44% in patients with BOOP due to other causes (e.g., CVD) or 30% for IPF.

■ VASCULITIS ■

The primary systemic vasculitides are a heterogeneous group of disorders of unknown etiology with a wide spectrum of clinical manifestations (Chapter 58). The complexity of the clinical and histopathologic features, as well as the potential for overlap, can make specific diagnosis difficult. The 1992 Chapel Hill International Consensus Conference was convened to reconcile definition and classification schemata.[24] This nomenclature is based on histopathologic criteria including size of vessels

Table 71.3 Disorders associated with a bronchiolitis obliterans organizing pneumonia (BOOP) pattern

Idiopathic BOOP (cryptogenic organizing pneumonia)
Collagen vascular diseases
- Systemic lupus erythematosus
- Rheumatoid arthritis
- Polymyositis/dermatomyositis
- Sjögren syndrome

Hypersensitivity pneumonitis
Chronic eosinophilic pneumonia
Drug-induced
- Gold
- Penicillamine
- Amiodarone
- Bleomycin
- Sulfa drugs

Wegener's granulomatosis
Bone marrow transplantation
Lung transplantation/rejection
Inhalational injury
Neoplasms
Lung irradiation
Virus-associated
- Human immunodeficiency virus (HIV)
- Influenza
- Adenovirus

involved and the presence or absence of serum anti-neutrophil cytoplasmic antibody (ANCA).

Most of the pulmonary vasculitides are systemic in nature. Consequently, the lung is one of many organ systems involved in the disease process. The systemic vasculitides, which typically involve the small vessels of the lung, include WG, Churg–Strauss syndrome (CSS), and microscopic polyangiitis. Involvement of alveolar capillaries (pulmonary capillaritis) in the inflammatory process results in intra-alveolar bleeding and the clinical syndrome known as diffuse alveolar hemorrhage (DAH).

WEGENER'S GRANULOMATOSIS

WG (Chapter 58) is a systemic vasculitis of small arteries and veins involving the upper and lower respiratory tract, often with associated glomerulonephritis. A limited form of WG involving only the upper and lower respiratory tract has been observed in 28% of patients.[25] Classically, the inflammatory lesions include necrosis, granulomatous inflammation, and vasculitis.

Clinical manifestations

The incidence of WG is unknown. Men and women are affected equally; the mean age at presentation is 40 years, with approximately 15% of patients presenting prior to the age of 19 years. The clinical presentation is characterized by upper respiratory tract signs and symptoms, including recurrent epistaxis, mucosal ulcerations, and septal perforation. At initial presentation, 90% of patients have evidence of upper

Treatment and outcome

The recommended therapy for WG consists of cyclophosphamide (2 mg/kg per day) and prednisone (1 mg/kg per day). The prednisone dosage is tapered once remission is achieved; cyclophosphamide is continued for 6–12 months after the disappearance of symptoms and gradually tapered over the next several months.

With this regimen, a partial remission can be achieved in 90% of patients and a complete remission occurs in 75% patients.[28] Approximately 50% of patients who experience a complete remission suffer one or more relapses. Although this regimen has converted a previously fatal disease into a treatable disorder with prolonged survival and often a cure, it is associated with significant toxicity. Treatment-related side effects include infections, hemorrhagic cystitis, bladder cancer, and myelodysplasia. The increased incidence of *Pneumocystis jiroveci* pneumonia in patients with WG has led to the recommendation that all WG patients who are receiving daily glucocorticoids should be given chemoprophylaxis against *P. jiroveci*.[28] The elimination of B cells via treatment with anti-CD20 monoclonal antibody has been attempted with success, warranting the performance of clinical trials.[29]

CHURG–STRAUSS SYNDROME

CSS, previously referred to as allergic angiitis and granulomatosis, is a rare disorder characterized by allergic rhinitis, asthma, eosinophilia, and a granulomatous vasculitis.[30] The lung is the most common organ affected. The diagnosis is sometimes unclear due to similarities with other vasculitides, such as WG.

Clinical manifestations

The incidence and prevalence of CSS are unknown. The mean age at diagnosis is 38 years; men and women are affected equally. In most cases there are three phases of the disease. The prodromal phase is characterized by atopy (rhinitis and asthma) and occurs during the second and third decades of life. This is followed by the eosinophilic phase with peripheral blood eosinophilia and eosinophilic tissue infiltration, including chronic eosinophilic pneumonia. Finally, the vasculitic phase is heralded by the onset of life-threatening vasculitis affecting medium and small vessels. This classic presentation is not universal, and, in 20% of cases, asthma, eosinophilia, and vasculitis develop simultaneously.

Asthma and allergic rhinitis are the most consistent nonvasculitic findings in CSS. Complications related to vasculitis include skin changes in two-thirds of patients, manifesting as subcutaneous nodules and palpable purpura. The most common neurologic complication is a peripheral neuropathy due to mononeuritis multiplex. Cardiovascular involvement includes pericarditis, coronary arteritis, and eosinophilic myocarditis, and accounts for approximately 50% of the deaths due to CSS. Renal involvement is more common than previously reported, with one study showing some degree of renal involvement in approximately 90% of patients.

Laboratory tests are nonspecific, but abnormalities include peripheral blood eosinophilia (5–10 × 10^9/l), anemia, leukocytosis, and an elevated erythrocyte sedimentation rate. Approximately 50% of CSS patients are p-ANCA-positive, usually with autoantibodies to myeloperoxidase. BAL shows eosinophilia, but this is nonspecific.

---

and lower respiratory tract involvement. The most frequent lower respiratory symptoms are cough, dyspnea, and hemoptysis. DAH is an uncommon presenting manifestation of WG, occurring in 5% of patients. Only 18% of patients have renal involvement at initial presentation, but 75% will go on to develop glomerulonephritis within 2 years of presentation. Other nonspecific findings include fever, malaise, and weight loss.

Laboratory findings in WG include elevated erythrocyte sedimentation rate, mild anemia, leukocytosis, and thrombocytosis. c-ANCA, an autoantibody directed against a neutrophil cytoplasmic serine protease, proteinase 3, is highly specific (> 95%) for WG. The sensitivity of c-ANCA parallels disease activity and may be as low as 65–70% in patients with inactive disease. In limited WG, the sensitivity of the c-ANCA is only 65%. Thus, a negative c-ANCA in the setting of limited WG does not exclude the diagnosis.

The most common radiographic findings in WG are single or multiple pulmonary nodules with or without cavitation.[26] Less common findings include pleural effusions, bilateral alveolar opacities representing DAH, hilar adenopathy, and the presence of an aspergilloma in a pre-existing cavity. Occasionally, endobronchial involvement can cause lobar atelectasis.

Histopathology

The pulmonary histopathology of WG is characterized by vasculitis, parenchymal necrosis, and granulomatous inflammation, accompanied by a mixed infiltrate of neutrophils, lymphocytes, histiocytes, and eosinophils.[27] The necrotizing granulomas vary from punctate microabscesses to large geographic zones of necrosis, while the vasculitis typically involves pulmonary arteries, veins, and capillaries.

The histopathologic correlate of DAH in WG is pulmonary capillaritis. Even though the frequency of this manifestation of WG is low, capillaritis was observed in 35% of granulomatous lesions, usually adjacent to the granulomatous process.

The renal histopathology in WG shows a focal, segmental necrotizing glomerulonephritis with or without crescent formation (Chapters 58 and 67). This lesion is not specific for WG as it also occurs in other small-vessel vasculitides and Goodpasture syndrome.

The chest radiograph is abnormal in about 70% of cases, with the most common abnormality being transient, patchy alveolar opacities. Pleural effusions are present in over 15% of cases, and eosinophils usually comprise more than 60% of pleural fluid cells.

Histopathology

The major histologic findings of CSS include eosinophil infiltration of vascular media and perivascular tissues accompanied by lymphocytes, plasma cells, and histiocytes. There is a necrotizing vasculitis of small arteries and veins and necrotizing extravascular granulomatosis.

Diagnosis

Using the American College of Rheumatology criteria,[31] a sensitivity of 85% and a specificity of 99.7% are obtained if four or more of the following criteria are met: (1) asthma; (2) greater than 10% peripheral blood eosinophilia; (3) mononeuritis or polyneuropathy; (4) paranasal sinus abnormality; (5) transient alveolar opacities on chest radiograph; and (6) extravascular eosinophils on a vessel biopsy. The finding of a positive p-ANCA further strengthens the diagnosis.

Treatment and outcome

Glucocorticoids are the mainstay of therapy. Most patients respond favorably to prednisone administered at a dose of 0.5–1.5 mg/kg per day. Persistent ANCA positivity does not appear to correlate with underlying disease activity. Without treatment, CSS is characterized by a 50% mortality at 3 months. In contrast, with treatment a 5-year survival rate of 70% has been reported. Cardiac involvement, gastrointestinal disease, renal insufficiency, proteinuria, or central nervous system involvement are poor prognostic factors.

GOODPASTURE SYNDROME

Goodpasture syndrome is a rare disorder characterized by DAH and rapidly progressive glomerulonephritis, related to the production of autoantibodies reactive with glomerular and alveolar basement membranes. This syndrome is part of a spectrum of diseases known as anti-basement membrane antibody (ABMA) diseases (also referred to as anti-glomerular basement membrane (AGBM) diseases). In the majority of cases, lung and renal involvement occurs simultaneously (Goodpasture syndrome). However, in approximately one-third of cases, glomerulonephritis is the sole manifestation of disease and, in fewer than 5% of patients, DAH occurs without clinical evidence of renal involvement.

Clinical manifestations

The disease occurs two to three times more commonly in men than in women, with a peak incidence in the second and third decades of life. A genetic basis for ABMA production is suggested by its association in Caucasians with certain HLA alleles, including DRB1*1501 and DRB1*1502.[32] Patients with Goodpasture syndrome who express these histocompatibility molecules experience severe renal disease with an associated poor prognosis.[32]

Goodpasture syndrome commonly presents with cough, dyspnea, and hemoptysis. Fatigue, due to a combination of iron-deficiency anemia and

renal failure, may be the presenting symptom in patients without DAH. Gross hematuria and hypertension are uncommon, but microscopic hematuria, proteinuria, and red blood cell casts are common, as well as an increased serum creatinine. The chest radiograph shows patchy or diffuse alveolar infiltrates, and pulmonary physiology reveals increased diffusion capacity during periods of active bleeding (because of increased availability of hemoglobin to bind carbon monoxide).

The presence of serum or tissue ABMA in a patient with DAH and/or glomerulonephritis establishes the diagnosis of ABMA disease. These antibodies are almost always IgG, and most commonly of the subclass IgG_1. The level of the ABMA in the serum correlates with the severity of the renal disease but not with that of the lung disease.

Histopathology

The DAH in Goodpasture syndrome represents either bland pulmonary hemorrhage or pulmonary capillaritis. In those with capillaritis, alveolar wall necrosis is not seen. Similar to renal involvement in the systemic vasculitides (Chapters 58 and 67), the renal histology shows focal segmental necrotizing glomerulonephritis with crescent formation. Immunofluorescent staining of alveolar and glomerular basement membranes shows an uninterrupted linear deposition of immunoglobulin (Fig. 71.11).

Pathogenesis

The pathologic damage in Goodpasture syndrome is related to the binding of autoantibodies directed against the noncollagenous domain (α_3-chain) of type IV collagen in the basement membrane.[33] Two dominant epitopes (E_A and E_B) have been identified in the α_3-chain of type IV collagen. Despite the widespread distribution of type IV collagen in the body, disease expression is limited to the lungs and kidneys. This limited disease expression suggests the possibility that other factors allow exposure of this autoantigen selectively in alveolar or glomerular basement membranes. Since the epitopes in the α_3-chain of type IV collagen are typically hidden, it is likely that some additional injury is necessary in order to reveal the hidden epitopes to the immnue system.[33] For example, the clinical onset of alveolar hemorrhage has been associated with influenza A2 infection, hydrocarbon exposure, and cigarette smoking. On the other hand, the glomerular basement membrane is directly exposed to the vascular compartment through endothelial fenestrations, which probably explains the positive association between the level of ABMA and the severity of the glomerulonephritis.

Molecular mimicry has been linked to the pathogenesis of several autoimmune disorders, including multiple sclerosis and type I diabetes mellitus (Chapter 50). This concept proposes that a susceptible host is exposed to an infectious agent that has antigens that are immunologically similar to the host but sufficiently different to induce an immune response. Subsequently, tolerance to the autoantigen breaks down, and the pathogen-specific immune response is generated that cross-reacts with host structures, resulting in tissue damage. The possibility of molecular mimicry between basement membrane antigens and antigens from infectious agents is suggested by the finding of sequence homology between the α_3-chain of type IV collagen in the basement membrane and a segment of influenza A hemagglutinin.[33]

Autoreactive CD4 T cells are also required for the pathologic autoimmune response.[34] These autoreactive CD4 T cells require CD28 co-stimulation since blockade of CD28 reduces anti-basement membrane

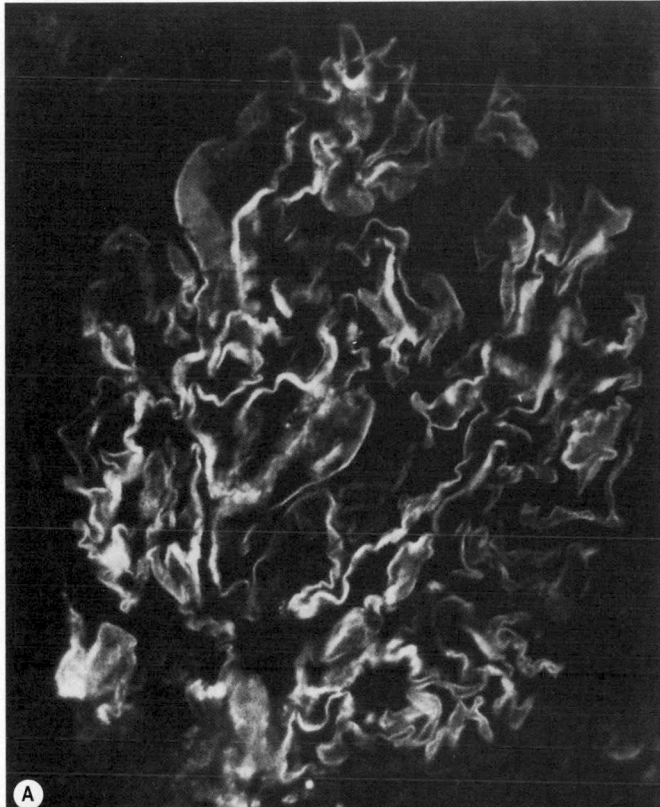

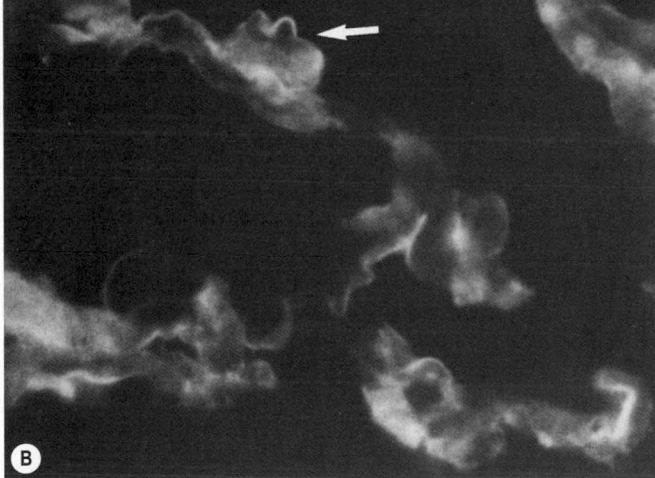

Fig. 71.11 Immunofluorescence staining patterns of Goodpasture syndrome with immunoglobulin G deposits on the basement membrane. The characteristic linear deposit of antibody reacting with the continuously distributed basement membrane antigen(s) of **(A)** glomerular basement membrane (GBM) in the kidney and **(B)** alveolar basement membrane in the lung can be appreciated; this pattern easily distinguishes this condition from the more common granular or interrupted patterns of staining seen with immune complex forms of immune renal injury.

antibody production and prevents the development of experimental autoimmune glomerulonephritis.[35]

Treatment and outcome

The establishment of a rapid diagnosis is essential since the severity of the renal lesion at the time of presentation correlates with the potential recovery of renal function. Prior to the introduction of plasmapheresis, the mortality of Goodpasture syndrome was between 75% and 90%. In patients with DAH alone, glucocorticoids are effective, but if glomerulonephritis is present (with or without alveolar hemorrhage) monotherapy is usually unsuccessful. Cytotoxic therapy, usually azathioprine or cyclophosphamide, may reverse the renal dysfunction, but the main role of these medications is to control alveolar hemorrhage. However, the combination of plasmapheresis, glucocorticoids, and cytotoxic therapy may be the most efficacious regimen, particularly for patients with oliguria who do not require hemodialysis. Plasmapheresis (3–6 l/day) is generally continued for 2 weeks.

The 2-year survival of patients with Goodpasture syndrome is approximately 50%, with the majority dying from alveolar hemorrhage, often precipitated by a concomitant infection. Severe renal failure reduces survival to 50% at 6 months. Renal biopsy provides both a diagnosis and prognostic information. Involvement of less than 30% of the glomeruli with crescent formation is associated with preserved renal function, significant response to therapy, and prolonged survival. However, when greater than 70% of the glomeruli are involved with crescent formation, progressive renal dysfunction is expected, requiring hemodialysis and consideration of renal transplantation.

■ LUNG INVOLVEMENT IN COLLAGEN VASCULAR DISEASES ■

CVD are a heterogeneous group of systemic autoimmune diseases, that frequently involve the lungs. The pleuropulmonary manifestations of these diseases are diverse, affecting all parts of the respiratory tract (i.e., airways, alveoli, blood vessels, and pleura) (Table 71.4). Although pulmonary complications generally occur in patients with well-established disease, occasionally the lung involvement is the first manifestation of the autoimmune disorder. This section discusses the pleuropulmonary manifestations of systemic lupus erythematosus (SLE), rheumatoid arthritis (RA), systemic sclerosis (SS), and polymyositis/dermatomyositis (PM/DM) (for a discussion of other manifestations in these diseases, see Chapters 51–56).

SYSTEMIC LUPUS ERYTHEMATOSUS

SLE is a disease of unknown etiology characterized by the presence of autoantibodies directed against various nuclear antigens. These autoantibodies and the resultant immune complexes mediate many of the manifestations of SLE (Chapter 51). This disease primarily affects young women (female-to-male ratio > 8:1) and may involve and derange the function of virtually every organ system. Pleuropulmonary involvement occurs at some point in the disease course in 38–89% of cases.[36] Thus, the respiratory system is affected more commonly in SLE than in any other CVD. That said, infectious pneumonia remains the commonest cause of pulmonary disease in this patient population, and infection is a common cause of death. Thus, in SLE patients presenting with a febrile illness and pulmonary infiltrates, a community-acquired or opportunistic infection must be promptly excluded.

Table 71.4 Pleuropulmonary manifestations of collagen vascular diseases

	SLE	RA	SS	PM/OM
Pulmonary hypertension	+	+	+++	±
Vasculitis	+	±	±	–
Pleural disease	+++	+++	+	–
Bronchiolitis obliterans	±	++	+	+
Aspiration pneumonia	–	–	++	++
Diaphragmatic dysfunction	++	–	–	±
Lung nodules	–	++	–	–
Diffuse alveolar damage	+	±	±	+
BOOP	±	+	±	+
UIP	+	++	+++	++
Capillaritis	++	+	±	±
LIP	+	+	+	±
NSIP	+	++	+	++

BOOP, bronchiolitis obliterans organizing pneumonia; LIP, lymphocytic interstitial pneumonitis; NSIP, nonspecific interstitial pneumonitis; PM/DM, polymyositis/dermatomyositis; RA, rheumatoid arthritis; SLE, systemic lupus erythematosus; SS, systemic sclerosis; UIP, usual interstitial pneumonitis.

Acute lupus pneumonitis

Acute lupus pneumonitis is an uncommon pulmonary manifestation of SLE, occurring in fewer than 5% of cases.[37] The clinical presentation mimics that of an infectious pneumonia with the abrupt onset of fever, cough, and dyspnea. Serum complement levels are often low and the chest radiograph typically shows diffuse alveolar opacities. It may be accompanied by pericarditis and often pleuritis and pleural effusion.

It can be difficult to distinguish acute lupus pneumonitis from an infectious pneumonia: BAL followed by thoracoscopic lung biopsy is often recommended prior to instituting corticosteroid therapy. The histopathology varies and includes diffuse alveolar damage, BOOP, NSIP, or a combination of these.

There are no controlled trials of therapy for acute lupus pneumonitis. Treatment includes high-dose glucocorticoids (1–2 mg/kg per day) with or without accompanying cytotoxic drugs, such as cyclophosphamide. Mortality rates as high as 50% have been reported. In those patients who fail to respond to treatment, respiratory failure is the usual cause of death.

Diffuse alveolar hemorrhage

DAH occurs in fewer than 5% of patients with SLE, and it represents the initial manifestation of disease in 11–20% of those cases.[38] However, most cases develop in individuals with well-established diagnoses of SLE, usually with pre-existing lupus nephritis.

The symptoms of DAH mimic those of infectious pneumonia and acute lupus pneumonitis.[39] Hemoptysis is present in 42–66% of patients at presentation. Therefore, the absence of hemoptysis does not exclude the diagnosis, particularly in the setting of a falling hematocrit, diffuse pulmonary infiltrates, and blood-stained BAL fluid. When it is possible to test diffusing capacity (often not possible due to respiratory failure), this will be elevated because of the increased availability of hemoglobin to bind carbon monoxide. DAH in SLE is most often due to pulmonary capillaritis, but it can also be caused by diffuse alveolar damage. Immunofluorescence studies show granular deposits of IgG and C3 along alveolar walls, interstitium, and capillary endothelial cells.

There are no controlled trials for the treatment of alveolar hemorrhage in SLE. Glucocorticoids, cytotoxic drugs, and plasmapheresis have all been used in various combinations. The mortality rate associated with DAH is approximately 50%. Poor prognostic factors include the need for mechanical ventilation, presence of infection, and prior treatment with cyclophosphamide.

Lupus pleuritis

The pleura is the most common site of respiratory involvement in SLE, with pleurisy and pleural effusions occurring in 50–80% of patients. Lupus pleuritis may be the presenting manifestation of disease, but, more commonly develops in patients with established SLE. It is often recurrent. The clinical manifestations include chest pain, fever, and dyspnea, and the chest radiograph typically shows bilateral pleural effusions. The pleural fluid is serous or serosanguineous and exudative in nature. Compared to effusions in RA, the glucose is higher and the lactate dehydrogenase level is lower. The most helpful measurement is a pleural fluid antinuclear antibody titer greater than 1:160. Examination of the pleura reveals infiltration with plasma cells and lymphocytes accompanied by pleural thickening and fibrosis. Treatment with nonsteroidal anti-inflammatory drugs and/or glucocorticoids is usually effective for relief of pleural discomfort.

Interstitial lung disease

The presence of ILD in SLE was once thought to be uncommon, especially when compared to SS or RA.[37] However, minor interstitial abnormalities can be found on HRCT in approximately one-third of SLE patients who have a normal chest radiograph and physiological testing. The significance and natural history of these subclinical findings are uncertain. The presence of anti-SSA (Ro) has been noted in approximately 80% of lupus patients with interstitial changes. In addition, the prevalence of ILD is increased in a subset of SLE patients with sclerodermatous skin changes.

The diagnosis of SLE is usually well established in the subgroup of patients who develop the insidious form of ILD. The disease course is characterized by progressive dyspnea and cough; the chest radiograph shows reduced lung volumes and reticular interstitial infiltrates. A restrictive lung function pattern with reduced diffusing capacity and exercise-induced hypoxemia are typical. The histopathology of chronic interstitial disease in SLE resembles UIP, although cases of BOOP, lymphocytic interstitial pneumonitis (LIP), and NSIP have been described. Response to therapy depends on the underlying histopathology with the UIP like form being least responsive (see above).

Pulmonary vascular disease

In acutely ill SLE patients, a syndrome of acute reversible hypoxemia has been described. These patients have hypoxemia and a widened alveolar–arterial oxygen gradient with a normal chest radiograph and ventilation–perfusion scan. The etiology of this syndrome is unknown, but complement-mediated intravascular neutrophil aggregation has been suggested. The hypoxemia usually resolves with glucocorticoid treatment.

Although previously thought to be unusual, the development of pulmonary hypertension secondary to plexogenic arteriopathy has been increasingly noted in SLE, with an incidence ranging from 5% to 14%. Pulmonary hypertension in SLE has been associated with the presence of Raynaud syndrome, serositis, digital vasculitis, and antiphospholipid antibodies.[40] Dyspnea and fatigue, despite a normal chest radiograph, is the most common presentation. As the pulmonary hypertension advances, the central pulmonary arteries enlarge. Pulmonary function testing shows an isolated decrease in the diffusing capacity for carbon monoxide. Ventilation–perfusion scanning and pulmonary angiography may be indicated in order to exclude thromboembolic disease. Treatment consists of oxygen and calcium-channel blockers. It remains unknown whether the use of continuous intravenous epoprostenol can alter exercise capacity and cardiopulmonary hemodynamics in patients with secondary pulmonary hypertension due to SLE.

Respiratory muscle dysfunction

The *shrinking or vanishing-lung syndrome* is due to diaphragmatic weakness as well as weakness of other respiratory muscles.[41] This entity accounts for the findings of dyspnea without evidence of interstitial infiltrates or pulmonary vascular disease. It is estimated to occur in 25% of patients with SLE. The chest radiograph typically shows elevated diaphragms and basilar atelectasis. The pathogenesis of respiratory muscle weakness is unknown, but it is not associated with generalized muscle weakness. Glucocorticoids are frequently ineffective in the treatment of this syndrome. Improvement has been noted with inhaled β-agonist and theophylline therapy. Despite a variable response to therapy, it is unusual for this manifestation of SLE to be progressive.

RHEUMATOID ARTHRITIS

RA is characterized by the presence of a symmetric, inflammatory polyarthritis occurring more frequently in women, with a 2:1 female-to-male ratio (Chapter 52). Disease onset is most commonly in the fourth to fifth decades of life. The pleuropulmonary complications of RA occur more commonly in individuals with subcutaneous nodules, high titers of rheumatoid factor, and more severe chronic articular involvement. Although RA itself is more common in women, the pleuropulmonary manifestations have a higher incidence in men. The pleuropulmonary complications of RA are numerous, but it is important to remember that treatment-related lung toxicity and pulmonary infections are sometimes difficult to differentiate from the primary pleuropulmonary manifestations of the disease.

Pleuritis and pleural effusions

As in SLE, pleural abnormalities are one of the most common pulmonary complications of RA.[42] Pleural effusions are clinically evident in approximately 5% of patients, and these may occur prior to the development

---

CLINICAL PEARLS

LUNG INVOLVEMENT IN RHEUMATOID ARTHRITIS (RA)

>> RA is more common in women, but pleuropulmonary complications occur more frequently in men

>> Factors associated with pleuropulmonary complications of RA include more severe articular involvement, subcutaneous nodules, and high levels of rheumatoid factor

>> Pleural effusions are the most common complication, characterized by an exudate and a low glucose and low pH

>> The differentiation of rheumatoid nodules from malignant lesions can be difficult

>> The rapid growth of a nodule should prompt aggressive investigation for a malignant cause

---

of arthritis. Pleural disease is often discovered as an incidental finding on routine chest radiographs, but nonspecific chest pain, dyspnea, and fever are not unusual. The effusion may be unilateral or bilateral and may coexist with interstitial lung disease.

Typically, the effusion is an exudate, with a glucose level less than 30 mg/ml in 70–80% of cases. The mechanism underlying the low pleural fluid glucose is impaired membrane transport of glucose. A low pleural fluid pH is thought to occur secondary to impaired carbon dioxide exit from the pleural space. If the effusion is chronic, the cholesterol concentration can be increased, and the pleural fluid may have a milky appearance (pseudochylothorax). Cytologic examination typically reveals multinucleated giant cells, spindle-shaped macrophages, and necrotic debris.

Most rheumatoid effusions are small and asymptomatic, and therefore require no treatment. They resolve over several months without complications. Occasionally, fibrothorax can occur. The use of glucocorticoids for active articular disease hastens the resolution of the pleural process.

Rheumatoid nodules

Rheumatoid or necrobiotic nodules are the only pleuropulmonary manifestation specific for RA. These nodules are most commonly seen in men with active articular disease, high rheumatoid factor titers, and subcutaneous nodules. Most individuals are asymptomatic and are diagnosed on routine chest radiograph. Radiographically, these nodules may be singular or multiple with an upper to mid-lung zone predominance. Cavitation occurs in approximately 50% of cases. HRCT of the lung indicates a higher frequency of nodules than previously thought. Rarely, subpleural necrobiotic nodules can erode into the pleural space, resulting in a pneumothorax with a complicating bronchopleural fistula. It can be difficult to differentiate these nodules from malignant lesions, and frequently open-lung biopsy is necessary. Evidence on chest radiograph of rapid growth should prompt an aggressive diagnostic evaluation. Usually, no treatment is necessary.

Caplan syndrome refers to the rapid development of pulmonary nodules with an upper-lung-zone predominance, originally described in Welsh coalminers with RA. Histologically, these nodules are identical to necrobiotic nodules. Other occupational dust exposures have also been associated with this syndrome.

Pulmonary vascular disease

Although systemic vasculitis with nailfold infarcts, cutaneous ulcers, mononeuritis multiplex, and digital ischemia can develop in RA, pulmonary vascular disease is the least common pleuropulmonary complication of RA. Rarely, pulmonary capillaritis can result in DAH.[43] In contrast to SLE and SS, primary pulmonary vascular disease resulting in pulmonary hypertension is rare.

Airway disease

Airflow limitation is a common finding in patients with RA, being present in approximately one-third of patients. The mechanism(s) responsible for airway disease is poorly understood. The interplay of cigarette smoking and RA may play a role.

A life-threatening complication of RA is upper-airway obstruction, resulting from synovitis of the cricoarytenoid joint. Common presenting complaints include a sore throat, hoarseness, and fullness in the throat. It can progress to inspiratory stridor and upper-airway obstruction. This complication occurs more commonly in women, particularly in those with advanced RA. Seventy-five percent of patients were found to have cricoarytenoid abnormalities when screening with direct or indirect laryngoscopy and computed tomography was utilized. The treatment of cricoarytenoid arthritis includes anti-inflammatory medications.

Bronchiolitis obliterans is a progressive form of obstructive lung disease that is being increasingly recognized as a complication of RA.[44] This entity was thought to develop secondary to the use of penicillamine for the treatment of RA, but most cases occur in the absence of this therapy. The histopathologic lesion of bronchiolitis obliterans is constrictive bronchiolitis, which is characterized by concentric submucosal and peribronchiolar fibrosis resulting in extrinsic compression and obliteration of the bronchiolar lumen. The typical clinical presentation is with insidious onset of cough and dyspnea, with a normal or hyperinflated chest radiograph. This complication occurs more commonly in women than in men. Pulmonary function studies show airflow limitation with hyperinflation and a reduced diffusing capacity. Expiratory HRCT shows multiple areas of air trapping (mosaic pattern). Some individuals respond to high-dose glucocorticoids and cytotoxic drugs, but most patients with bronchiolitis obliterans progress to respiratory failure.

Bronchiectasis occurs at an increased frequency in RA, usually in individuals with long-standing articular disease. Productive cough and dyspnea are the most common respiratory symptoms. In most patients, bronchiectasis is not clinically significant. Recurrent pneumonia and respiratory failure are potentially fatal complications of this problem.

Interstitial lung disease

Although ILD is a common complication of RA, the incidence is difficult to determine, since different methods of detection have been employed and dissimilar populations of patients have been studied. However, clinically significant ILD occurs in approximately 14% of patients.[45] The development of ILD in relation to the onset of arthritis is variable. Most often, the ILD develops subsequent to arthritis, but, in approximately 20% of patients, the lung disease precedes the onset of arthritis.

The most common histopathologies identified in this patient population are UIP, LIP, NSIP, and BOOP (see above). The clinical manifestations of ILD in RA resemble those seen in idiopathic disease and include a dry, nonproductive cough and dyspnea on exertion. The chest radiograph and HRCT show increased reticular markings with a predilection for the periphery and lower-lung zones. Often, pleural abnormalities accompany the interstitial changes. With advanced disease, progression to honeycomb lung occurs. LIP usually occurs in cases of RA complicated by Sjögren syndrome: the presence of keratoconjunctivitis sicca and xerostomia in a patient with RA and ILD should suggest this histologic type.

In general, ILD in RA appears more indolent than in idiopathic interstitial pneumonitis. Thus, due to uncertain treatment benefits and possible adverse effects, the decision to institute therapy should be based on clinical, radiographic, and physiologic deterioration.

Drug-induced lung disease

Methotrexate and gold are the two main anti-RA drugs capable of causing lung injury. Methotrexate administered weekly (10–20 mg/week) is associated with the development of interstitial changes in 1–5% of patients with RA.[46] No correlation with age, sex, disease duration, or cumulative dose has been identified. The clinical presentation is subacute in nature, with fever, cough, and dyspnea occurring 1–5 months after the initiation of the drug. The chest radiograph shows mixed interstitial–alveolar infiltrates. Nonspecific laboratory abnormalities include leukocytosis, sometimes with mild eosinophilia, and an elevated erythrocyte sedimentation rate. In most cases, BAL reveals a lymphocytosis. Histologically, cellular NSIP is seen with areas of organizing pneumonia. Noncaseating, granulomatous inflammation similar to that seen in hypersensitivity pneumonitis may also be present. The primary treatment of methotrexate-induced pneumonitis is withdrawal of methotrexate, plus appropriate supportive care.

Gold-induced pneumonitis occurs in fewer than 1% of RA patients treated with gold. Dyspnea and cough usually begin after 4–6 weeks of therapy; eosinophilia occurs in a minority of patients. The chest radiograph typically reveals mixed alveolar–interstitial opacities with an upper-lung zone predilection. The histology is similar to that seen in RA patients with ILD. Thus, the differentiation of gold-induced pneumonitis from RA-associated interstitial lung disease can only be established when discontinuation of the medication results in remission.

SYSTEMIC SCLEROSIS (SCLERODERMA)

SS is characterized by excessive deposition of extracellular matrix in the skin and internal organs, and vascular involvement (Chapter 55). The degree of visceral organ involvement determines morbidity and mortality. Pulmonary involvement occurs in 70–100% of patients with SS. There is no correlation with the degree of extrapulmonary disease. Interstitial lung disease is the most common pulmonary manifestation of SS. Of note, with the improved mortality associated with renal involvement in SS, lung disease has become the most important cause of morbidity and mortality.[47]

Interstitial lung disease

The incidence of ILD in SS depends on the method of detection. Autopsy studies have reported an ILD incidence of 60–100% of cases, whereas studies based on chest radiographs have noted interstitial changes in only 14–66% of cases.

Similar to other ILD, cough and dyspnea on exertion are the most common symptoms. Physical examination reveals bibasal rales. Clubbing is unusual, due perhaps to capillary destruction in the nail beds. Radiographic findings include basal reticulonodular infiltrates, enlargement of pulmonary arteries, and progressive volume loss with associated honeycomb change. Pulmonary function testing reveals restrictive lung disease, preservation of flow rates, and decreased diffusing capacity. A disproportionate decrease in diffusing capacity compared to lung volume changes should suggest pulmonary hypertension, especially in individuals with limited scleroderma (calcinosis, Raynaud's phenomenon, esophageal dysmotility, sclerodactyly, telangectasia [CREST] syndrome). The predominant histopathologic abnormality is UIP with honeycomb changes and is identical to that seen in IPF. Rarely, LIP may complicate cases of SS associated with Sjögren syndrome. Although the 5-year survival for SS patients with ILD is 38–45%, it is better than that of patients with IPF.[48]

Pulmonary vascular disease

Pulmonary hypertension is a frequent complication of SS, occurring in approximately 30% of patients with diffuse scleroderma and in 10–50% of those with limited scleroderma (Chapter 55). The pulmonary hypertension may either be associated with interstitial fibrosis or result from involvement of small and medium-sized arteries and arterioles with smooth-muscle hyperplasia, medial hypertrophy, and intimal proliferation (plexogenic). Direct involvement of the pulmonary circulation is more common with limited scleroderma while pulmonary hypertension in patients with diffuse scleroderma is more likely associated with ILD.

The clinical presentation is characterized by the insidious onset of fatigue and dyspnea on exertion. Physical examination and chest radiographs show signs typical of pulmonary hypertension, while decreased diffusing capacity is seen on pulmonary function testing.

The prognosis of isolated pulmonary hypertension, with a 2-year survival rate of 40%, is worse than that for pulmonary hypertension associated with interstitial fibrosis.[49] A recent study using continuous intravenous epoprostenol in patients with hypertension associated with scleroderma showed improvement in exercise capacity and cardiopulmonary hemodynamics as compared to control subjects treated with conventional therapy alone.[50]

Pleural disease

Clinically significant pleural disease is uncommon in SS, although pleural fibrosis and adhesions are frequent findings in postmortem studies.

Aspiration pneumonia

Patients with SS have an increased incidence of esophageal dilatation and decreased peristalsis: this esophageal dysmotility predisposes to aspiration pneumonia. However, it is unclear if there is any relationship between gastroesophageal reflux and the development of lung disease. One study showed that gastroesophageal reflux did not correlate with physiologic impairment of the lung in these patients.[51]

POLYMYOSITIS/DERMATOMYOSITIS

Polymyositis and dermatomyositis are idiopathic inflammatory myopathies characterized by proximal muscle weakness and, in the case of DM, a characteristic skin rash (Chapter 56). Pulmonary complications in PM/DM are important causes of morbidity and mortality and may overshadow the muscle involvement. Approximately 40% of patients with PM/DM have pulmonary involvement. As compared to the other collagen vascular diseases, lung involvement in PM/DM does not primarily affect the airways or the pleura.

Aspiration pneumonia

Aspiration pneumonia is the most common pulmonary complication in patients with PM/DM. Upper-airway protection is impaired, secondary to a reduced cough reflex resulting from weakness of striated muscles of the soft palate, pharynx, and upper esophagus. This weakness results in dysphagia, and, as a consequence, aspiration pneumonia occurs in 15–20% of PM/DM patients. A history of aspiration pneumonia carries a poor prognosis since it tends to occur in patients with more extensive muscle involvement.

Respiratory muscle dysfunction

Hypercapnic respiratory failure secondary to generalized respiratory muscle dysfunction occurs infrequently in patients with PM/DM. Mucus plugging with resultant atelectasis occurs secondary to the inadequate cough reflex. Chest radiograph may reveal reduced lung volumes with associated bibasal atelectasis. The respiratory muscle weakness results in both inspiratory and expiratory dysfunction, and measurement of maximal inspiratory and expiratory pressures is useful in the determination of respiratory muscle dysfunction as the cause of restrictive lung disease in patients with PM/DM. Sequential measurements are useful to monitor the clinical course and response to therapy.

Interstitial lung disease

Depending on the method of screening, 5–30% of patients with PM/DM have interstitial lung disease.[48] UIP is the commonest histopathologic lesion, but NSIP, DAH secondary to capillaritis, diffuse alveolar damage, and BOOP may also occur. There is no relationship between the interstitial changes and the degree of skin and/or muscle involvement.

Depending on the underlying lung pathology, several clinical syndromes may occur. The most common presentation is insidious onset of cough and dyspnea due to UIP or NSIP. Laboratory findings include elevated creatine phosphokinase and anti-Jo-1 antibodies, which are directed against histidyl-tRNA-synthetase. This autoantibody specificity serves as a marker for the subset of PM/DM patients who have interstitial fibrosis, being present in 50% of these individuals (Chapter 56). The chest X-ray appearance of ILD in PM/DM is similar to that seen in IPF. Physiologic testing shows a restrictive pattern with reduced diffusing capacity. The natural history and optimal treatment of interstitial lung disease in PM/DM are unknown.

Some PM/DM patients present with acute onset of diffuse alveolar infiltrates and associated respiratory failure. The underlying histopathologic lesion may be diffuse alveolar damage, capillaritis, or BOOP. The differentiation of diffuse alveolar damage from capillaritis and BOOP is critical since the response to treatment and survival are dramatically different. In diffuse alveolar damage, recovery is unusual despite aggressive anti-inflammatory and immunosuppressive treatment. On the other hand, both BOOP and capillaritis are responsive to standard therapeutic options.

■ REFERENCES ■

1. Martinez FJ. Idiopathic interstitial pneumonias: usual interstitial pneumonia versus nonspecific interstitial pneumonia. Proc Am Thorac Soc 2006; 3: 81–95.

2. Noble PW, Homer RJ. Idiopathic pulmonary fibrosis: new insights into pathogenesis. Clin Chest Med 2004; 25: 749–758.

3. Selman M, Thannickal VJ, Pardo A, et al. Idiopathic pulmonary fibrosis: pathogenesis and therapeutic approaches. Drugs 2004; 64: 405–430.

4. Coultas DB, Zumwalt RE, Black WC, et al. The epidemiology of interstitial lung diseases. Am J Respir Crit Care Med 1994; 150: 967–972.

5. Lynch DA, Travis WD, Muller NL, et al. Idiopathic interstitial pneumonias: CT features. Radiology 2005; 236: 10–21.

6. Cool CD, Groshong SD, Rai PR, et al. Fibroblast foci are not discrete sites of lung injury/repair: the fibroblast reticulum. Am J Respir Crit Care Med 2006; 174: 654–658.

7. Lee HL, Ryu JH, Wittmer MH, et al. Familial idiopathic pulmonary fibrosis: clinical features and outcome. Chest 2005; 127: 2034–2041.

8. Hodgson U, Pulkkinen V, Dixon M, et al. ELMOD2 is a candidate gene for familial idiopathic pulmonary fibrosis. Am J Hum Genet 2006; 79: 149–154.

9. O'Garra A. Cytokines induce the development of functionally heterogeneous T helper cell subsets. Immunity 1998; 8: 275–283.

10. Lee CG, Homer RJ, Zhu Z, et al. Interleukin-13 induces tissue fibrosis by selectively stimulating and activating transforming growth factor beta(1). J Exp Med 2001; 194: 809–821.

11. Strieter RM. Pathogenesis and natural history of usual interstitial pneumonia: the whole story or the last chapter of a long novel. Chest 2005; 128: 526S–532S.

12. Lynch DA, David Godwin J, Safrin S, et al. High-resolution computed tomography in idiopathic pulmonary fibrosis: diagnosis and prognosis. Am J Respir Crit Care Med 2005; 172: 488–493.

13. Collard HR, Ryu JH, Douglas WW, et al. Combined corticosteroid and cyclophosphamide therapy does not alter survival in idiopathic pulmonary fibrosis. Chest 2004; 125: 2169–2174.

14. Raghu G, Brown KK, Bradford WZ, et al. A placebo-controlled trial of interferon gamma-1b in patients with idiopathic pulmonary fibrosis. N Engl J Med 2004; 350: 125–133.

15. Martinez FJ, Safrin S, Weycker D, et al. The clinical course of patients with idiopathic pulmonary fibrosis. Ann Intern Med 2005; 142: 963–967.

16. Katzenstein AL, Myers JL. Idiopathic pulmonary fibrosis: clinical relevance of pathologic classification. Am J Respir Crit Care Med 1998; 157: 1301–1315.

17. Ryu JH, Myers JL, Capizzi SA, et al. Desquamative interstitial pneumonia and respiratory bronchiolitis-associated interstitial lung disease. Chest 2005; 127: 178–184.

18. Yousem SA, Colby TV, Gaensler EA. Respiratory bronchiolitis-associated interstitial lung disease and its relationship to desquamative interstitial pneumonia. Mayo Clin Proc 1989; 64: 1373–1380.

19. Katzenstein AL, Fiorelli RF. Nonspecific interstitial pneumonia/fibrosis. Histologic features and clinical significance. Am J Surg Pathol 1994; 18: 136–147.

20. Flaherty KR, Martinez FJ, Travis W, et al. Nonspecific interstitial pneumonia (NSIP). Semin Respir Crit Care Med 2001; 22: 423–434.

21. Travis WD, Matsui K, Moss J, et al. Idiopathic nonspecific interstitial pneumonia: prognostic significance of cellular and fibrosing patterns: survival comparison with usual interstitial pneumonia and desquamative interstitial pneumonia. Am J Surg Pathol 2000; 24: 19–33.

22. Cordier JF. Cryptogenic organizing pneumonia. Clin Chest Med 2004; 25: 727–738.

23. Epler GR. Bronchiolitis obliterans organizing pneumonia. Arch Intern Med 2001; 161: 158–164.

24. Jennette JC, Falk RJ, Andrassy K, et al. Nomenclature of systemic vasculitides. Proposal of an international consensus conference. Arthritis Rheum 1994; 37: 187–192.

25. Fauci AS, Haynes BF, Katz P, et al. Wegener's granulomatosis: prospective clinical and therapeutic experience with 85 patients for 21 years. Ann Intern Med 1983; 98: 76–85.

26. Lohrmann C, Uhl M, Kotter E, et al. Pulmonary manifestations of Wegener granulomatosis: CT findings in 57 patients and a review of the literature. Eur J Radiol 2005; 53: 471–477.

27. Travis WD, Hoffman GS, Leavitt RY, et al. Surgical pathology of the lung in Wegener's granulomatosis: review of 87 open lung biopsies from 67 patients. Am J Surg Path 1991; 15: 315–333.

28. Hoffman GS, Kerr GS, Leavitt RY, et al. Wegener's granulomatosis: an analysis of 158 patients. Ann Intern Med 1992; 116: 488–498.

29. Specks U, Fervenza FC, McDonald TJ, et al. Response of Wegener's granulomatosis to anti-CD20 chimeric monoclonal antibody therapy. Arthritis Rheum 2001; 44: 2836–2840.

30. Gross WL. Churg–Strauss syndrome: update on recent developments. Curr Opin Rheumatol 2002; 14: 11–14.

31. Masi AT, Hunder GG, Lie JT, et al. The American College of Rheumatology 1990 criteria for the classification of Churg–Strauss syndrome (allergic granulomatosis and angiitis). Arthritis Rheum 1990; 33: 1094–1100.

32. Phelps RG, Rees AJ. The HLA complex in Goodpasture's disease: a model for analyzing susceptibility to autoimmunity. Kidney Int 1999; 56: 1638–1653.

33. Hudson BG, Tryggvason K, Sundaramoorthy M, et al. Alport's syndrome, Goodpasture's syndrome, and type IV collagen. N Engl J Med 2003; 348: 2543–2556.

34. Cairns LS, Phelps RG, Bowie L, et al. The fine specificity and cytokine profile of T-helper cells responsive to the alpha3 chain of type IV collagen in Goodpasture's disease. J Am Soc Nephrol 2003; 14: 2801–2812.

35. Reynolds J, Tam FW, Chandraker A, et al. CD28-B7 blockade prevents the development of experimental autoimmune glomerulonephritis. J Clin Invest 2000; 105: 643–651.

36. Orens JB, Martinez FJ, Lynch JP 3rd. Pleuropulmonary manifestations of systemic lupus erythematosus. Rheum Dis Clin North Am 1994; 20: 159–193.

37. Cheema GS, Quismorio FP Jr. Interstitial lung disease in systemic lupus erythematosus. Curr Opin Pulm Med 2000; 6: 424–429.

38. Santos-Ocampo AS, Mandell BF, Fessler BJ. Alveolar hemorrhage in systemic lupus erythematosus: presentation and management. Chest 2000; 118: 1083–1090.

39. Badsha H, Teh CL, Kong KO, et al. Pulmonary hemorrhage in systemic lupus erythematosus. Semin Arthritis Rheum 2004; 33: 414–421.

40. Fagan KA, Badesch DB. Pulmonary hypertension associated with connective tissue disease. Prog Cardiovasc Dis 2002; 45: 225–234.

41. Oud KT, Bresser P, ten Berge RJ, et al. The shrinking lung syndrome in systemic lupus erythematosus: improvement with corticosteroid therapy. Lupus 2005; 14: 959–963.

42. Balbir-Gurman A, Yigla M, Nahir AM, et al. Rheumatoid pleural effusion. Semin Arthritis Rheum 2006; 35: 368–378.

43. Torralbo A, Herrero JA, Portoles J, et al. Alveolar hemorrhage associated with antineutrophil cytoplasmic antibodies in rheumatoid arthritis. Chest 1994; 105: 1590–1592.

44. Schwarz MI, Lynch DA, Tuder R. Bronchiolitis obliterans: the lone manifestation of rheumatoid arthritis?. Eur Respir J 1994; 7: 817–820.

45. Gabbay E, Tarala R, Will R, et al. Interstitial lung disease in recent onset rheumatoid arthritis. Am J Respir Crit Care Med 1997; 156: 528–535.

46. Barrera P, Laan RF, van Riel PL, et al. Methotrexate-related pulmonary complications in rheumatoid arthritis. Ann Rheum Dis: 53434–53439.

47. Arroliga AC, Podell DN, Matthay RA. Pulmonary manifestations of scleroderma. J Thorac Imaging 1992; 7: 30–45.

48. Kocheril SV, Appleton BE, Somers EC, et al. Comparison of disease progression and mortality of connective tissue disease-related interstitial lung disease and idiopathic interstitial pneumonia. Arthritis Rheum 2005; 53: 549–557.

49. Trad S, Amoura Z, Beigelman C, et al. Pulmonary arterial hypertension is a major mortality factor in diffuse systemic sclerosis, independent of interstitial lung disease. Arthritis Rheum 2006; 54: 184–191.

50. Badesch DB, Tapson VF, McGoon MD, et al. Continuous intravenous epoprostenol for pulmonary hypertension due to scleroderma spectrum of disease: A randomized controlled trial. Ann Intern Med 2000; 132: 425.

51. Troshinsky MB, Kane GC, Varga J, et al. Pulmonary function and gastroesophageal reflux in systemic sclerosis. Ann Intern Med 1994; 121: 6–10.

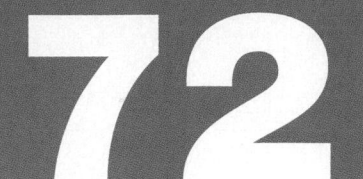
Sarcoidosis

David R. Moller

72

Sarcoidosis is a multisystem disorder of unknown etiology characterized by noncaseating epithelioid granulomas in affected organs.[1][3] The disease most commonly affects the lungs and intrathoracic lymph nodes, although granulomatous inflammation may be present in any organ system. The clinical manifestations and course of sarcoidosis vary greatly.[4] An estimated 30–60% of patients with sarcoidosis are asymptomatic, usually with isolated bilateral hilar adenopathy. Symptomatic manifestations most frequently involve the respiratory system, with symptoms of cough, dyspnea, and chest discomfort. Löfgren syndrome is a form of acute sarcoidosis characterized by erythema nodosum, bilateral hilar adenopathy, polyarthritis, and often uveitis. Other clinical manifestations depend on the range and extent of extrapulmonary involvement (Table 72.1).

EPIDEMIOLOGY

Sarcoidosis is found worldwide, though there are striking differences in the prevalence of the disease in different geographic areas and racial groups.[5] In Europe and North America the prevalence is estimated to range from 10 to 64 cases per 100 000, with higher rates in African-American populations. In countries where tuberculosis is common and health care uncertain, no reliable epidemiologic data are available because of the difficulty in distinguishing between sarcoidosis and tuberculosis. Worldwide there is a slight female preponderance. Although all ages can be affected, more than 80% of cases are diagnosed between the ages of 20 and 50 years.

The frequency of different clinical manifestations and disease severity varies among different groups.[4, 5] Löfgren syndrome has a particularly high frequency in Scandinavian countries and Ireland, but occurs in fewer than 5% of African-American patients with sarcoidosis. Lupus pernio, a disfiguring nodular facial condition associated with chronic sarcoidosis, is more frequent in patients of African descent. Cardiac sarcoidosis affects up to 50% of Japanese patients with sarcoidosis, but fewer than 10–25% of European and North American patients. In a study of mortality data from hospitals in the USA from 1979 to 1991, age-adjusted mortality was consistently higher among blacks than whites, and among women compared with men. Retrospective studies suggest that sarcoidosis is the direct cause of death in < 1–6% of cases, usually from pulmonary, cardiac, or neurologic involvement.

GENETICS

There is substantial evidence for a genetic predisposition to sarcoidosis. This was initially suggested from the familial clustering that occurs in approximately 5–16% of patients. A recent US-based multicenter study of sarcoidosis called ACCESS compared 706 newly diagnosed, biopsy-proven sarcoidosis cases to age-, sex-, and race-matched controls.[6] This

KEY CONCEPTS

>> Sarcoidosis is characterized by noncaseating epithelioid granulomas and mononuclear cell inflammation, usually in multiple organ systems

>> Genetic susceptibility to sarcoidosis and its various clinical presentations is suggested by family studies and associations with major histocompatibility complex (MHC) haplotypes

>> Granulomatous inflammation in sarcoidosis is characterized by oligoclonal expansions of Th1 cells and activated mononuclear phagocytes producing tumor necrosis factor (TNF)-α, interleukin-12 (IL-12), and IL-18

>> Pulmonary involvement with bilateral hilar adenopathy, restrictive or obstructive interstitial lung occurs in over 90% of patients

>> Symptomatic, extrapulmonary sarcoidosis is often chronic, requiring treatment to prevent serious permanent organ damage

>> Standard treatment for progressive, symptomatic sarcoidosis involves corticosteroid therapy, although the long-term benefits remain unproven

Table 72.1 Major clinical features of systemic sarcoidosis

Organ system (approx. % involvement)	Major clinical features
Pulmonary (90)	Bilateral hilar adenopathy, restrictive and obstructive disease, fibrocystic disease, bronchiectasis, mycetomas
Upper airway (5–10)	Hoarseness, laryngeal or tracheal obstruction, nasal congestion, sinusitis, saddle-nose deformity
Ocular (25)	Anterior and posterior uveitis, chorioretinitis, conjunctivitis, optic neuritis, glaucoma, lacrimal gland enlargement
Skin (20)	Erythema nodosum, chronic nodules and plaques, lupus pernio, alopecia
Hepatic (10)	Hepatomegaly, pruritus, jaundice, cirrhosis
Cardiac (5–10)	Arrhythmias, heart block, cardiomyopathy, sudden death
Central nervous system (5–10)	Cranial neuropathy, e.g., Bell's palsy, aseptic meningitis, brain mass, seizures, obstructing hydrocephalus, myelopathy, polyneuropathy, mononeuritis multiplex
Salivary and parotid gland (10)	Salivary and parotid gland enlargement, sicca syndrome
Hematologic (30–50)	Lymphadenopathy, splenomegaly, hypersplenism, anemia, lymphopenia, thrombocytopenia
Joints/musculoskeletal (10–20%)	Polyarthritis, bone cysts, Achilles tendinitis, heel pain, myopathy
Endocrine (< 10)	Hypercalciuria (more common), hypercalcemia, hypopituitarism, diabetes insipidus
Renal (< 5)	Renal calculi, nephrocalcinosis, renal failure, epididymitis, testicular mass

study found a higher relative risk in siblings of sarcoidosis cases (odds ratio (OR) ~ 5.8) than in parents (OR ~ 3.8). Both the ACCESS study and a UK study found higher adjusted familial relative risk estimates for Caucasians than blacks, suggesting that genetic factors have a greater influence in susceptibility to sarcoidosis in Caucasians.

Genetic association studies support a consensus view that major histocompatibility complex (MHC) class II alleles are the major contributor to disease susceptibility across different ethnic populations in sarcoidosis. Human leukocyte antigen (HLA)-DR3 is associated with increased sarcoidosis risk in Scandinavian and European populations whereas HLA-DR1 and -DR4 alleles are associated with disease protection. The ACCESS study found a significant association between HLA-DRB1*1101 in both African-Americans and Caucasians, whereas HLA-DRB1*1501 was associated with sarcoidosis risk only in Caucasians.[7]

HLA class II alleles have also been associated with clinical course. DR3 haplotypes and specifically HLA DRB1*0301 or the closely linked DQB1*0201 alleles are associated with favorable outcomes (Löfgren syndrome, acute arthritis, stage I chest radiograph, or remission within 2 years) whereas DR14 and DR15 are associated with severe, chronic disease, in European and Japanese populations.[8] The ACCESS study found DRB1*1501 or the closely linked DQB1*0602 alleles were associated with more severe or chronic disease.

Studies of non-HLA polymorphisms have yielded few clues to the genetic basis of sarcoidosis. Polymorphisms of the angiotensin-converting enzyme (ACE) gene have been associated with sarcoidosis risk in Japan, but not elsewhere. In one study, specific tumor necrosis factor-α (TNF-α) gene polymorphisms were associated with patients with Löfgren syndrome, although the overall disease frequency of the

sarcoidosis cohort did not differ from that of a control group. Two studies report associations with sarcoidosis and the CC chemokine receptors CCR2 and CCR5.

Family linkage studies confirm the importance of genes from the MHC locus in determining susceptibility to sarcoidosis. A German study employing genome-wide microsatellite analysis found strongest linkage to the MHC class II locus on chromosome 6p with minor linkage peaks on chromosomes 1, 3, 9, and X.[9] A US-based study of African-Americans called SAGA found the highest linkage peak on chromosome 5q and minor peaks on chromosome 1, 2, 9, 11, and 20.[10] No significant linkage to the MHC region on chromosome 6 was found in the SAGA study, possibly due to the influence of Caucasian gene admixture among African-Americans in the USA. Recently, German and US investigators report that the butyrophilin-like 2 (BTNL2) gene within the MHC locus is associated with sarcoidosis risk in Caucasians and, to a lesser extent, African-American populations.[11] BTLN2 is a member of the B7 receptor family that functions in T-cell co-stimulation, leading to the hypothesis that this gene plays a role in the polarized Th1 granulomatous response in sarcoidosis.

ENVIRONMENTAL FACTORS

Environmental factors have been implicated in the etiology of sarcoidosis with reports of time–space clustering and a higher incidence of disease in spring months. Health care workers, military personnel and firefighters may have a higher incidence of sarcoidosis.

The largest reported study of sarcoidosis etiology (ACCESS) failed to detect any environmental or occupational risk factor that carried an

OR > 2.0 and an exposure prevalence of > 5% (pre-study goal).[12] Weak positive associations (OR ~ 1.5) were found for insecticide use at work, mold/mildew exposures at work, and musty odors, suggesting possible links to microbial-rich environments. Sarcoidosis was not found to be associated with exposure to heavy metals, including beryllium, wood dusts, or rural residence. The ACCESS study found a robust negative association of smoking and sarcoidosis risk, confirming earlier studies. The lack of a single dominant exposure associated with sarcoidosis risk is consistent with the concept that gene–environment interactions are important in causing disease.

Since the initial descriptions of sarcoidosis, investigators have postulated an infectious cause of the disease based on its clinical similarities to other infectious diseases, most notably tuberculosis. Reports of acid-fast organisms and cultivatable mycobacterial or cell wall-deficient organisms have not been confirmed in other centers. Studies using polymerase chain reaction (PCR) methods find mycobacterial DNA or RNA in 0–80% of tissues from patients with sarcoidosis; the variability of results from different centers precludes a consensus on a role for mycobacterial organisms in sarcoidosis.[13] Japanese investigators report the presence of *Propionibacterium acnes* or *granulosum* genomes in 80–98% of sarcoidosis tissues from Japan and Europe but also in 0–60% of control tissues.[14] Given that these organisms are part of the normal skin and upper-airway flora, a pathogenic role for these organisms remains uncertain. The presence of high titers of antibodies against many viral agents (Epstein–Barr virus, human herpes virus-8, cytomegalovirus, parainfluenzae, adenovirus) and bacterial antigens (*Chlamydia* spp., *Borrelia burgdorferi*) in sarcoidosis sera are thought to reflect generalized B-cell activation and not a direct causal relationship. An infectious etiology of sarcoidosis is supported by observations of apparent transmissibility of systemic granulomas by allogeneic bone marrow or cardiac transplantation derived from individuals with sarcoidosis.

One clue to sarcoidosis etiology is the observation made in the 1940s by A. Kveim that the intradermal inoculation of a suspension of sarcoidosis tissue results in a nodular skin reaction with sarcoid-like granulomas in patients with suspected sarcoidosis. In this reaction, well-formed granulomas take 2–4 weeks to develop. The active component appears to be a poorly soluble microparticulate with relative resistance to neutral detergents, nucleases, proteases, heat, and acidity.[15]

A recent study used a limited proteomic approach to identify potential pathogenic antigens in sarcoidosis tissues based on the biochemical properties of the Kveim reagent and not on *a priori* hypotheses regarding specific infectious or autoimmune causes. This approach detected the mycobacterial catalase-peroxidase protein (mKatG) in over 50% of sarcoidosis tissues.[16] Immunoglobulin G (IgG) responses to mKatG were detected in ~50% of sarcoidosis patients, supporting the premise that mKatG is a pathogenic antigen and that mycobacterial organisms trigger a subset of sarcoidosis.

Although direct demonstration of an infectious etiology remains unproven, many investigators favor the hypothesis that certain classes of microbial organisms trigger sarcoidosis in those with genetic susceptibility. Whether autoimmunity plays a role in sarcoidosis is unknown, since there are no disease-specific autoantibodies.

■ IMMUNOLOGY/PATHOGENESIS ■

The histologic hallmark of sarcoidosis is the presence of discrete, compact noncaseating granulomas (Fig. 72.1). The dominant cell in the central core is the epithelioid cell, thought to be a differentiated form of mononuclear phagocyte. CD4 lymphocytes and mature macrophages are interspersed throughout the epithelioid core, whereas both CD4 and CD8 lymphocytes are seen around the periphery of the granuloma. Multinucleated giant cells, often containing cytoplasmic inclusions such as Schaumann bodies or asteroid bodies, are scattered throughout the inflammatory locus. In the lung, granulomas tend to form along areas that are rich in lymphatic vessels, such as bronchovascular, bronchial

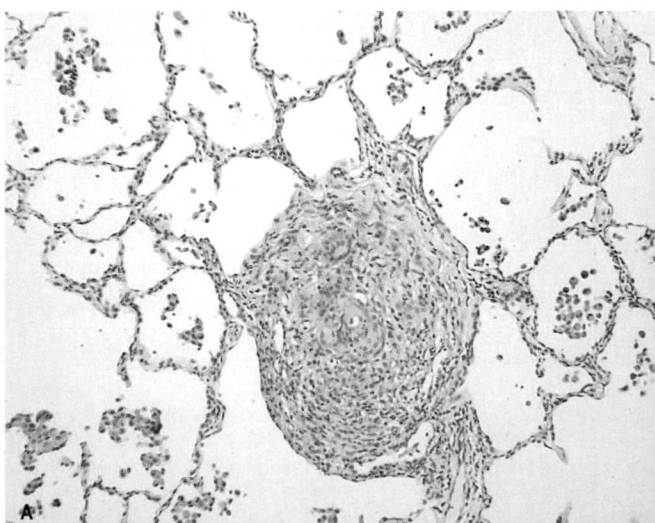
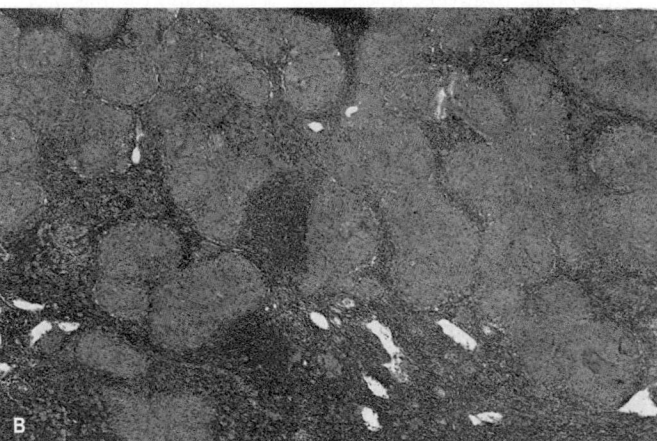

Fig. 72.1 **(A)** Open-lung biopsy showing typical noncaseating epithelioid granuloma, giant cells, and lymphocytic infiltrates in lung parenchyma in sarcoidosis. **(B)** Lymph node biopsy showing extensive replacement with well-defined epithelioid granulomas in a patient with sarcoidosis.

submucosal, subpleural, and interlobular septal regions, as well as alveolar and bronchial walls. Granulomas in sarcoidosis tend to vary from cellular forms to acellular, hyalinized ghosts of granulomas that probably reflect an evolution to an inactive or fibrotic form.

The concept of sarcoidosis as a disorder of enhanced cell-mediated immune processes at sites of granulomatous inflammation was based on landmark studies in the 1980s using bronchoalveolar lavage (BAL). These studies demonstrated increased proportions and numbers of activated CD4 BAL lymphocytes in pulmonary sarcoidosis. Prior to these findings, sarcoidosis had been thought of as a disease of immune depression exemplified by circulating lymphopenia and cutaneous anergy. In sarcoidosis, most BAL T cells are CD4 with a CD45RO "memory" phenotype expressing high levels of activation molecules DR and very late activation antigen-1 (VLA-1, CD49a) and reduced surface density of the CD3:T-cell receptor (TCR) complex.

Direct evidence that sarcoidosis is an antigen-driven disorder is provided by studies analyzing TCR gene expression. These studies document the expansion of oligoclonal populations of lung (BAL), blood or skin (Kveim biopsy) T cells expressing specific $V\alpha$ or $V\beta$ TCR genes. The most compelling data derive from DR17(3)/DQ2 Swedish patients who have greatly expanded numbers of $V\alpha2.3(AV2S3)$ T cells in the lung.[17] Sequence analyses demonstrate that expanded oligoclonal $\alpha\beta+$ T-cell subsets in sarcoidosis often contain shared amino acid motifs in the CDR3 region of their $V\beta$ or $V\alpha/J\alpha$ genes, consistent with a conventional antigen-driven T-cell response. Despite intense efforts, the specificities of these expanded T-cell clones have yet to be identified.

As many as 30% of sarcoidosis patients have greater proportions of $\gamma\delta+$ T cells in their blood, predominantly of the $V\gamma_9V\delta_2$ subset. As $\gamma\delta+$ T cells are rarely found around granulomas in lymph nodes or skin, their role in the pathogenesis of sarcoidosis remains uncertain.

Alveolar macrophages are thought to play a central role in the development of granulomatous inflammation in sarcoidosis by presenting disease-specific antigens and producing cytokines that regulate granuloma formation.[18] Alveolar macrophages from patients with sarcoidosis express higher levels of surface class II MHC molecules, leukocyte function associated–antigen-1 (LFA-1), intracellular adhesion molecule-1 (ICAM-1), and the accessory molecules CD86 (B7.2), CD80 (B7.1), and CD40 than do alveolar macrophages from healthy controls. These characteristics probably contribute to the enhanced ability of sarcoidosis alveolar macrophages to present antigen to autologous T cells compared to normal alveolar macrophages. Importantly, sarcoidosis alveolar macrophages spontaneously produce the proinflammatory cytokines TNF-α, interleukin (IL)-6, IL-1α, and IL15. These lung cells also produce increased amounts of lysozyme, ACE, reactive oxygen species, fibronectin, and insulin-like growth factor-1 (IGF-1) and lower than normal amounts of the counterinflammatory prostaglandin E$_2$.

Several chemotactic cytokines (chemokines) are expressed by BAL cells in sarcoidosis, including monocyte chemotactic protein (MCP)-1, RANTES, macrophage inflammatory protein (MIP)-1, monokine-induced by interferon (IFN)-γ (MIG), IL-8, and osteopontin (early T-lymphocyte activation protein). These chemokines probably assist in the recruitment of T cells, blood monocytes, and granulocytes to inflammatory loci in sarcoidosis. Natural killer (NK) cells, B cells, and mast cells are also occasionally seen around granulomas; their contributions to the inflammatory response are uncertain.

The granulomatous inflammation in sarcoidosis is dominated by a polarized Th1 cytokine profile at time of diagnosis (Fig. 72.2).[19] DAL

studies demonstrate increased mRNA and protein levels of IFN-γ and IL-2, with low or undetectable levels of IL-4 and IL-5 in pulmonary sarcoidosis. Consistent with a polarized Th1 process, IL-12 and IL18 are upregulated in BAL fluid and in cells from the lungs and lymph nodes of patients with sarcoidosis,[19] while most sarcoidosis BAL T cells express a functional, high-affinity IL-12 receptor with β_2-chains and the chemokine receptors CXCR3 and CCR5. It is not known whether this Th1

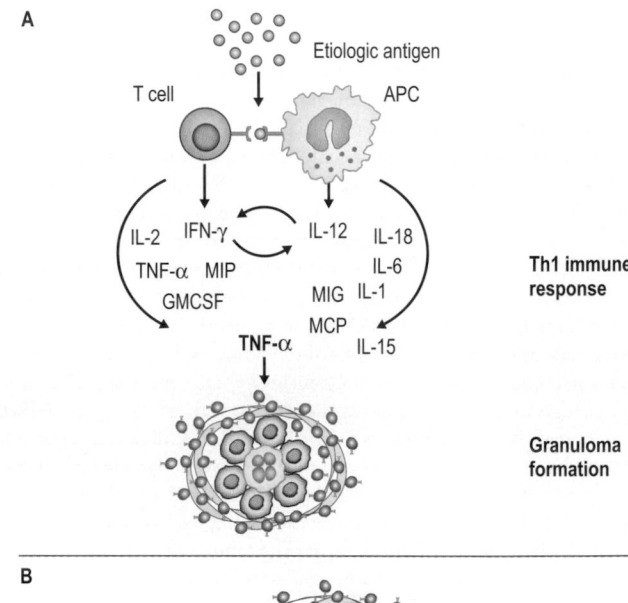

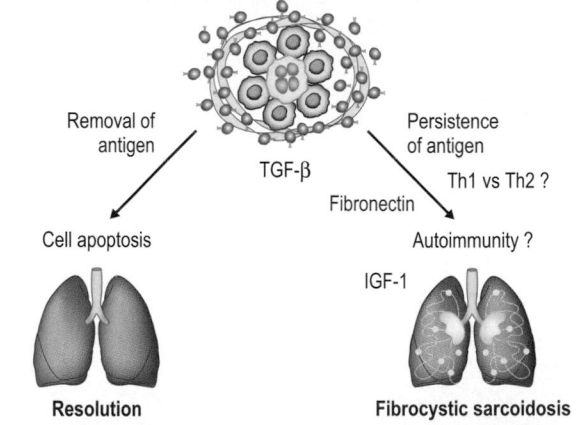

Fig. 72.2 Hypothetical model of the immunopathogenesis of sarcoidosis. **(A)** Granuloma formation in sarcoidosis results from stimulation by an insoluble antigen that evokes an adaptive T-cell immune response and stimulates the production of tumor necrosis factor (TNF) and interleukin-12 (IL-12) along with other cytokines from mononuclear phagocytes and dendritic cells. **(B)** Remission versus chronic fibrotic sarcoidosis. After the removal of stimulating antigen(s), suppression of Th1-driven granuloma formation is mediated in part by transforming growth factor-β (TGF-β), followed by granuloma resorption with cell apoptosis. Progressive fibrosis results from persistent, possibly autoimmune, antigenic stimulation in the presence of either Th1 or Th2 cytokines and TGF-β, insulin-like growth factor-1 (IGF-1), and other profibrotic mediators.

polarization persists in chronic, fibrotic sarcoidosis or there is a transition to a more profibrotic Th2 cytokine profile. Recent reports of increased IL-13 expression in some sarcoidosis patients are consistent with this latter possibility.

Over 50% of all patients with sarcoidosis have remission of their disease. The determinants of this outcome are unknown. One study found that patients with active sarcoidosis who underwent spontaneous remission within 6 months had significantly greater production of transforming growth factor-β (TGF-β) from cultured BAL cells at the time of initial evaluation than did patients who later required therapy or who demonstrated progressive disease.[18] Because TGF-β is a potent endogenous inhibitor of IL-12 and CD4 Th1 development, these observations suggest that TGF-β may downregulate Th1-driven granulomatous responses in sarcoidosis in the absence of persistent antigenic stimulation. Two studies have found reduced numbers of immunoregulatory CD1d-restricted Vα24 NKT cells in the blood of patients with nonremitting sarcoidosis, suggesting a deficiency of these cells may play a role in chronic sarcoidosis. Another study reports that immunoregulatory CD4+CD25(bright)FoxP3+ T cells accumulate at the periphery of sarcoidosis granulomas, in BAL fluid, and in peripheral blood of patients with active disease.[20] These T regulatory (Treg) cells exhibited powerful antiproliferative activity *in vitro*, yet did not completely inhibit TNF-α production, suggesting that an expanded Treg population was insufficient to control local inflammation but could account for the cutaneous anergy that is typical in sarcoidosis.

■ PATIENT EVALUATION AND DIFFERENTIAL DIAGNOSIS ■

PULMONARY SARCOIDOSIS

The most common symptoms of pulmonary sarcoidosis are progressive shortness of breath, nonproductive cough and ill-defined, variably severe chest discomfort (Table 72.1). Chronic sputum production and hemoptysis are more frequent in advanced fibrocystic disease. Typically, there are few physical findings in pulmonary sarcoidosis. Lung crackles are heard in fewer than 20% of patients and clubbing is rare. Findings of pulmonary hypertension or cor pulmonale are seen in 1–4% of patients, usually those with severe fibrocystic sarcoidosis or, rarely, a granulomatous vasculitis of the pulmonary vessels.

Chest radiographs are abnormal in more than 90% of patients with sarcoidosis. By international convention, the chest radiograph is divided into the following stages or types:

Stage 0: normal chest radiograph

Stage I: bilateral hilar adenopathy

Stage II: bilateral hilar adenopathy + interstitial infiltrates

Stage III: interstitial infiltrates only (nonfibrotic)

Stage IV: fibrocystic interstitial lung disease

A normal chest X-ray is found in 5–10% of patients with sarcoidosis. Stage I changes are seen in 40–50% of cases at presentation. Typically, the hilar adenopathy is discrete, symmetric, and often accompanied by right paratracheal adenopathy. A stage II chest radiograph, often with mid- or

upper-zone infiltrates, is initially seen in 20–30% of cases (Fig. 72.3). A stage III radiograph is initially seen in 10–20% of cases. Chest radiographs with fibrocystic changes and scarring are rare at presentation and carry a poor outcome (Fig. 72.4). Mycetomas are mobile fungus balls that colonize pre-existing cystic spaces in fibrocystic sarcoidosis. More unusual patterns of pulmonary sarcoidosis include large, well-defined nodular infiltrates, miliary disease, or a pattern of patchy airspace consolidation with air bronchograms, termed "alveolar sarcoidosis." Pleural effusions and pneumothorax are rare.

Computed tomography (CT) of the chest is more sensitive than plain radiography in demonstrating enlarged lymph nodes and pulmonary infiltrates. Chest CT typically demonstrates nodular infiltrates that follow central bronchovascular structures (Fig. 72.5).

Pulmonary function tests do not correlate well with chest radiographs. In patients with stage I chest radiographs pulmonary function tests are normal in about 80% of cases, or have only an isolated reduction in diffusing capacity for carbon monoxide (DLco). When pulmonary infiltrates are present on chest radiography, restrictive impairment with reduction in lung volumes, forced vital capacity and forced expiratory volume in 1 second, or a reduction in DLco is found in 40–70% of cases. Obstructive impairment is found in < 30–50% of patients, most often in advanced fibrocystic sarcoidosis. Bronchial hyperreactivity is present in 10–30% of patients. Gas exchange is usually preserved unless extensive fibrotic changes are evident.

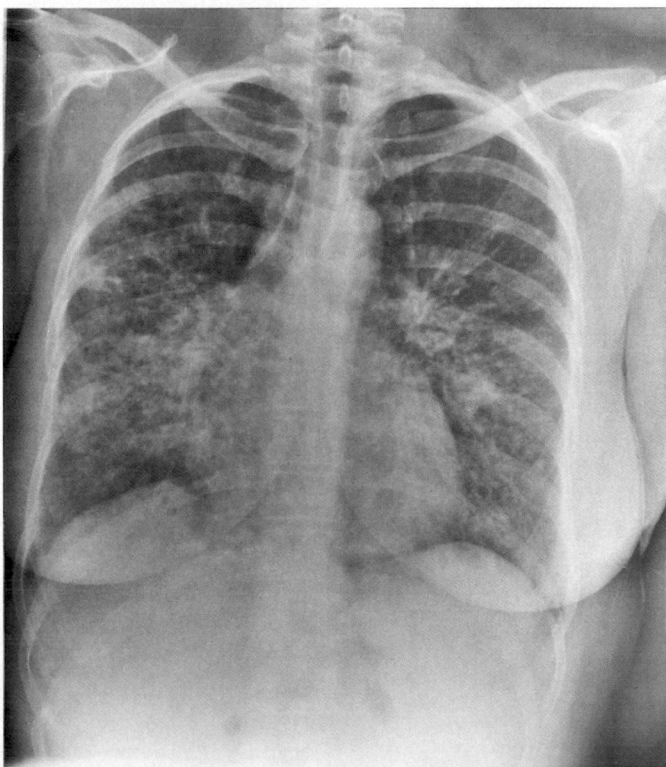

Fig. 72.3 Chest radiograph demonstrating a stage II pattern with bilateral hilar adenopathy and reticulonodular infiltrates.

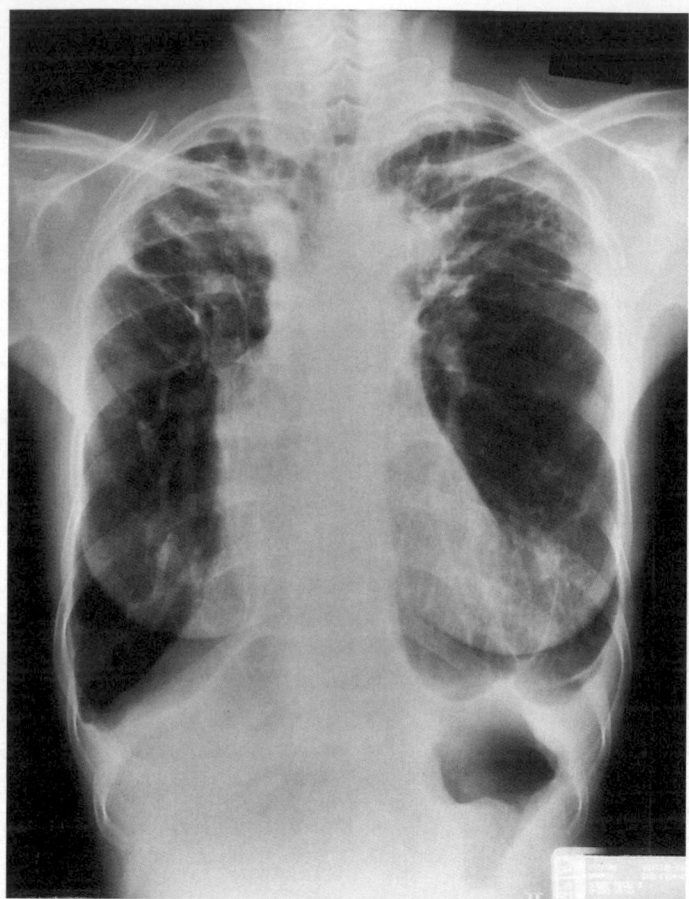

Fig. 72.4 Fibrocystic (stage IV) pulmonary sarcoidosis with typical upward hilar retraction and multiple cystic and bullous changes.

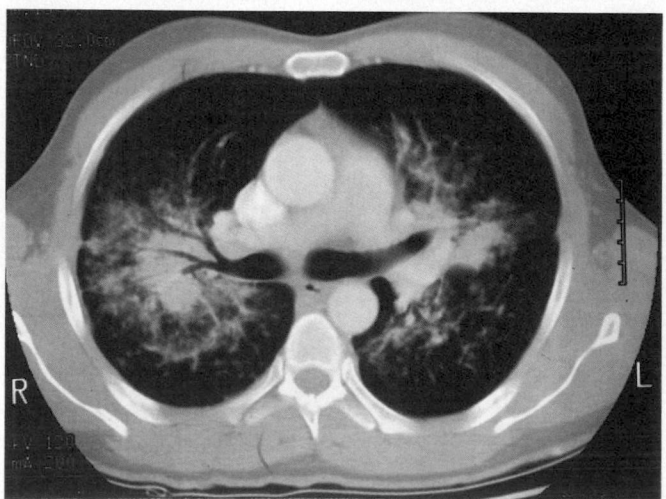

Fig. 72.5 Computed tomography scan of the chest in a patient with biopsy-proven pulmonary sarcoidosis, demonstrating bilateral hilar, paratracheal, and para-aortic lymphadenopathy with interstitial infiltrates in a dominantly central bronchovascular distribution.

EXTRAPULMONARY SARCOIDOSIS

Most patients have clinically important involvement of more than one organ, either with or without pulmonary sarcoidosis (Table 72.1).[21] Rare manifestations are usually the result of either an uncommon pattern of systemic involvement or granulomatous inflammation developing in an unusual location for sarcoidosis.[22]

SARCOIDOSIS OF THE UPPER RESPIRATORY TRACT

Sarcoidosis of the upper respiratory tract occurs in approximately 5–10% of patients, usually those with long-standing disease. Involvement of the mucosa of the nasal septum, inferior turbinates, and nasopharynx may lead to nasal congestion, dizziness, crusting, epistaxis, anosmia, or rhinorrhea. Nasal septal perforation, a 'saddle-nose' deformity, or palatal perforation or bone erosion may occur, particularly in patients with previous submucous resections. Sarcoidosis may affect the maxillary, ethmoid, and sphenoid sinuses, leading to obstruction and sinusitis. Laryngeal sarcoidosis is an uncommon feature, occurring in < 1–5% of patients. Patients may manifest with hoarseness, dysphonia, dysphagia, dyspnea or, rarely, stridor and acute respiratory failure.

OCULAR SARCOIDOSIS

Unilateral or bilateral anterior uveitis is the most common ocular manifestation of sarcoidosis and is often associated with bilateral hilar adenopathy. Chronic uveitis occurs in as many as 20% of patients with chronic sarcoidosis, more frequently in black populations. Other manifestations include posterior uveitis, granulomatous conjunctivitis or severe chorioretinitis, or optic neuritis; these latter conditions may present acutely with blindness.

CUTANEOUS SARCOIDOSIS

Erythema nodosum is a component of Löfgren syndrome, and may recur. Chronic skin sarcoidosis usually manifests as nontender, nonpruritic plaques and subcutaneous nodules around the hairline, eyelids, ears, nose, mouth, and the extensor surfaces of the arms and legs. Lupus pernio is a particularly disfiguring form of cutaneous sarcoidosis of the face, with violaceous plaques and nodules covering the nose, nasal alae, malar areas, and around the eyes.

CARDIAC SARCOIDOSIS

Cardiac sarcoidosis is clinically apparent in < 5–10% of patients with sarcoidosis in North America and Europe, though autopsy studies suggest up to 25% may be affected. In Japan, cardiac involvement may be present in > 50% of patients. Complete heart block is the most common manifestation; other less common patterns include ventricular arrhythmias, bundle-branch blocks, sudden death, cardiomyopathy, supraventricular arrhythmias, and valvular dysfunction. Most deaths due to cardiac sarcoidosis are caused by arrhythmias, heart block, or congestive heart failure.[23]

HEPATIC SARCOIDOSIS

Symptomatic hepatic sarcoidosis manifests with fever, tender hepatomegaly, or intense pruritus. Characteristically, the serum alkaline phosphatase and γ-glutamyltransferase are elevated proportionally higher than the aspartate aminotransferase (AST) and alanine aminotransferase (ALT) and bilirubin, though all patterns can be seen. Hepatic sarcoidosis may mimic primary biliary cirrhosis, except that antimitochondrial antibodies are absent. The term 'abdominal sarcoidosis' is often used for patients manifesting with liver, spleen, and abdominal lymph node involvement, often with hypercalcemia; pulmonary involvement may not be evident.

JOINTS AND BONES

Arthralgias are common in active multisystem sarcoidosis, although joint radiographs are usually negative. Acute, often incapacitating, migratory polyarthritis involving the ankles, feet, knees, and wrists may be seen in Löfgren syndrome. Persistent joint disease is found in fewer than 5% of patients with chronic sarcoidosis. Pain, swelling, and tenderness of the phalanges of the hands and feet are the commonest symptoms. Joint radiographs may demonstrate 'punched-out' lesions with cystic changes and marked loss of trabeculae but without evidence of erosive chondritis. Cystic lesions of the long bones, pelvis, sternum, skull, and vertebrae rarely occur.

NEUROSARCOIDOSIS

Neurosarcoidosis occurs in approximately 5% of sarcoidosis patients.[24] The most common manifestation is cranial neuropathy, with bilateral or unilateral seventh-nerve (Bell's) palsy or, less commonly, glossopharyngeal, auditory, oculomotor, or trigeminal palsies. The palsy may resolve spontaneously or with corticosteroids, but sometimes recurs years later. Optic neuritis can result in blurred vision, field defects, and blindness. Manifestations of central nervous system (CNS) involvement include mass lesions, aseptic meningitis, obstructive hydrocephalus, and hypothalamic/pituitary dysfunction. Seizures, headache, change in mental status, confusion, and diabetes insipidus may be presenting symptoms. Spinal cord compression syndromes are rare, but paraparesis, hemiparesis, and back and leg pain have been described. Peripheral neuropathies account for about 15% of cases of neurosarcoidosis, often presenting as mononeuritis multiplex or a primary sensory neuropathy. Small-fiber neuropathy occurs frequently in sarcoidosis, particularly in chronic disease. A subset of patients meets diagnostic criteria for fibromyalgia. Both conditions may be associated with pain that is resistant to anti-inflammatory drugs.

SALIVARY, PAROTID, AND LACRIMAL GLAND SARCOIDOSIS

Parotid or lacrimal gland enlargement or sicca syndrome can occasionally be the dominant clinical manifestations of sarcoidosis. Herefordt syndrome, also known as uveoparotid fever, manifests as fever, parotid and lacrimal gland enlargement, uveitis, and bilateral hilar adenopathy. This uncommon presentation of acute sarcoidosis can be associated with cranial neuropathies, usually facial palsy.

HEMATOLOGIC SARCOIDOSIS

Peripheral lymph node enlargement occurs in 20–30% of patients as an early manifestation of sarcoidosis, but then typically undergoes spontaneous remission. Persistent, bulky lymphadenopathy occurs less than 10% of the time. Splenomegaly, occasionally massive, occurs in fewer than 5% of cases and is often associated with hepatomegaly or hypercalcemia. Nonclonal hypergammaglobulinemia is present in 25% or more of patients.

SARCOIDOSIS MYOPATHY

Although muscle granulomas can be found at autopsy in most sarcoidosis patients, symptomatic myopathy with weakness and tenderness is uncommon. Rarely, sarcoidosis presents as a polymyositis with profound weakness and elevated serum creatine kinase and aldolase.

HYPERCALCEMIA, HYPERCALCIURIA, AND RENAL DISEASE

Hypercalcemia is present in 2–5% of patients; hypercalciuria is more common. Abnormal calcium regulation is thought to be due to an increased conversion of 1-hydroxy (OH) vitamin D_3 to active 1,25-$(OH)_2$ vitamin D_3 by macrophages and epithelioid cells from granulomas. Chronic hypercalcemia or hypercalciuria most commonly manifests as kidney stones. Renal failure from chronic clinically silent nephrocalcinosis can occur. Granulomatous involvement of the kidneys is uncommon and usually not a cause of renal failure.

PSYCHOSOCIAL MANIFESTATIONS

Depression has been found in 30–60% of symptomatic patients with sarcoidosis. In the ACCESS study, depression was associated with female sex, lower socioeconomic status, poor access to care, and increased disease severity, but not race.

ASSOCIATED CONDITIONS

Sarcoidosis and pregnancy

Usually pregnancy has little effect on the course of sarcoidosis, although some patients experience spontaneous improvement. In those who improve, exacerbation frequently follows several months after delivery. The reasons for the temporary clinical improvement are not known but might be related to suppressed Th1 immunity during pregnancy.

Th1-promoting therapeutics

The administration of Th1-promoting therapeutics such as IFN-α, IFN-γ, IL-2, and IFN-β may be associated with initiation or recrudescence of sarcoidosis.

Common variable immunodeficiency

Sarcoidosis is associated with common variable immunodeficiency (CVID) in both adult and pediatric sarcoidosis. A high index of suspicion must be maintained for CVID in sarcoidosis patients who have recurrent infections or in any child with sarcoidosis, given the low frequency of sarcoidosis in this age group.

Human immunodeficiency virus (HIV)

Sarcoidosis may develop in HIV-infected patients with immune reconstitution following initiation of highly active antiretroviral therapy, perhaps from reconstituted Th1 immunity. Granulomatous inflammation of the lungs or skin is the commonest presentation.

Autoimmune disorders

Sarcoidosis has been described in association with autoimmune diseases such as Crohn disease, ulcerative colitis, primary biliary cirrhosis, scleroderma, Sjögren syndrome, autoimmune hemolytic anemia, and autoimmune endocrinopathies. These associations could be the result of a common, predisposing altered Th1 immunity.

Cancer

Epithelioid granulomas are reported in ~3–10% of tumors and in ~4% of regional draining lymph nodes. Much less commonly, multisystem sarcoidosis can develop in patients with a recent or past diagnosis of cancer or following chemotherapy treatment. Several cases of sarcoidosis have developed in patients with 5q-myelodysplasia that results in deletion of several Th2 genes (IL-4, IL-13, colony-stimulating factor-2) that probably lead to dysregulated Th1/Th2 immunity.

DIAGNOSIS

A diagnosis of sarcoidosis is based on a compatible clinical picture, histologic evidence of noncaseating granulomas, and the absence of other known causes of this pathologic response.[2] Tuberculosis, fungal disease, and lymphoma are the most important diseases to be excluded in patients with chest disease. Chronic beryllium disease and hypersensitivity pneumonitis must be excluded when there is a compatible history and clinical findings are confined to the lung. In the absence of defined multisystem disease a diagnosis of sarcoidosis should be presumed, as local 'sarcoid' reactions may occur in response to infection, tumor, or foreign material. Biopsy confirmation of sarcoidosis is not usually necessary in Löfgren syndrome, except in regions where histoplasmosis is endemic.

In general, biopsy of the easiest, most accessible abnormal tissue site is used to confirm the diagnosis. Biopsy of a skin nodule, superficial lymph node, lacrimal gland, nasal mucosae, conjunctivae, or salivary gland (lip biopsy) may establish a diagnosis. Biopsy of the liver or bone marrow is nonspecific and should be used to support a diagnosis of sarcoidosis only after malignancy, infectious granulomatous diseases, or other organ-specific diagnoses have been excluded. Imaging techniques such ^{18}F-fluorodeoxyglucose (FDG)-positron emission tomography (PET) scanning or gallium-67 scanning are occasionally helpful in defining appropriate sites for biopsy.

Biopsy by fiberoptic bronchoscopy is frequently used to diagnose pulmonary sarcoidosis because of its relative safety and high yield. The yield of transbronchial biopsy is operator-dependent, but approaches 80–90% when pulmonary infiltrates are seen radiographically (Figs 72.3–72.5). Bronchial or transbronchial needle aspiration biopsies may increase the yield further. Mediastinoscopy or thoracoscopic or surgical lung biopsy should be considered when lymphoma or other intrathoracic malignancy cannot be reasonably excluded.

The initial diagnostic evaluation of a patient with possible sarcoidosis should include tests to evaluate the presence and extent of pulmonary involvement and screen for extrathoracic disease.[2] In the presence of cardiac symptoms, two-dimensional echocardiography and 24-hour electrocardiograph recording are indicated. Radionuclide imaging with gated 201-thallium or technetium-99m sestamibi has greater sensitivity in detecting segmental areas of decreased uptake that correspond to areas involved with granulomatous inflammation or fibrosis. When uncertainty persists, cardiac magnetic resonance or cardiac PET have even greater theoretical resolution, but are nonspecific and there is limited experience in sarcoidosis. A diagnosis of cardiac sarcoidosis is usually made clinically, with biopsy confirmation of a noncardiac site. Endomyocardial biopsy is positive in < 10–25% of cases of cardiac sarcoidosis, owing to the patchiness of the granulomatous inflammation; thus, a negative biopsy never excludes the diagnosis.

When CNS sarcoidosis is considered, magnetic resonance imaging (MRI) with gadolinium enhancement is now considered the optimal test to detect the characteristic inflammatory lesions that have a propensity for periventricular and leptomeningeal areas.[24] A normal scan does not exclude neurosarcoidosis, particularly for cranial neuropathies or while taking corticosteroids. Cerebrospinal fluid characteristically demonstrates lymphocytic pleocytosis and/or elevated protein levels. A diagnosis of neurosarcoidosis is usually confirmed by biopsy of a non-CNS site, generally by bronchoscopic or lymph node biopsy. Rarely, brain biopsy is

CLINICAL PEARLS

TESTS RECOMMENDED FOR AN INITIAL EVALUATION OF A PATIENT WITH SARCOIDOSIS

>> Chest radiograph

>> Pulmonary function tests
  - Spirometry
  - Diffusing capacity
  - Lung volumes
  - Flow–volume loop (if suspected upper-airway obstruction)

>> Slit-lamp examination (to exclude subclinical uveitis)

>> Liver and renal function tests

>> Calcium level

>> Complete blood count

>> Electrocardiogram

>> Purified protein derivative skin test

>> Organ specific testing for symptomatic involvement

needed to exclude infectious or malignant disease. In suspected cases of peripheral neuropathy or myopathy, electromyogram or nerve conduction studies should be considered.

OTHER DIAGNOSTIC STUDIES

There are no noninvasive tests that have been shown to be useful in assisting the clinician in making a diagnosis of sarcoidosis. Serum ACE (SACE) levels are elevated in 40–90% of patients with clinically active disease, but may be found in other granulomatous diseases and in some nongranulomatous conditions, such as hyperthyroidism, hepatic cirrhosis, diabetes mellitus, and Hodgkin disease. This lack of specificity limits the use of SACE in confirming a diagnosis of sarcoidosis.[2,3] Although > 90% of nonsmoking patients with pulmonary sarcoidosis have increased proportions of CD4 BAL T cells, typically with a CD4:CD8 ratio of 3–10:1 compared to 2:1 in healthy individuals, these findings are not sufficiently specific to establish a diagnosis of sarcoidosis.[2,3]

PREVENTION AND PATIENT MANAGEMENT

The clinical course of sarcoidosis is highly variable.[2,4] Overall, 50–65% of patients undergo spontaneous remission, usually (> 85%) within the first 2 years. The prognosis is best for those with Löfgren syndrome, 70–80% of whom have a spontaneous remission. Peripheral adenopathy, salivary and parotid gland enlargement, and Bell palsy generally subside spontaneously or with treatment, and do not recur. Elevated serum liver function tests can also revert to normal without treatment. The rate of spontaneous remission in pulmonary sarcoidosis differs according to the initial chest X-ray pattern. Approximately 50–80% of patients with a stage I chest radiograph have remission, whereas 30–60% with a stage II radiograph and 20–30% with a stage III radiograph undergo remission.

Patients with a stage IV chest radiograph with fibrocystic changes rarely (< 5%) undergo remission. Extrapulmonary disease that is symptomatic and severe on presentation tends to persist and require treatment. Patients with lupus pernio, bony involvement, nephrocalcinosis, and splenomegaly rarely undergo spontaneous remission.

The intensity of surveillance of sarcoidosis depends on the severity of clinical presentation, but should include serial tests of organ-specific function. When sarcoidosis undergoes remission, the disease rarely recurs; exceptions often involve neurologic or ocular manifestations. Noninvasive tests such as BAL, SACE, and other biochemical measurements have not been shown to be useful in management decisions.[2,3]

TREATMENT

Corticosteroids remain the mainstay of therapy for serious or progressive pulmonary or extrapulmonary sarcoidosis.[2,3] Corticosteroids provide symptomatic relief acutely and reverse organ dysfunction in > 90% of patients with symptomatic disease. Although there is controversy regarding their overall effectiveness in altering the long-term course of the disease, there is widespread agreement that early treatment is indicated for serious pulmonary or extrapulmonary disease. When the condition is not serious or organ-threatening, a period of observation is often indicated to evaluate whether the patient will undergo spontaneous remission.

The optimal doses and duration of corticosteroid treatment have not been established by rigorous clinical studies. Initial treatment with corticosteroids usually employs no more than 20–40 mg/day of prednisone for 2–4 weeks, followed by a slow tapering regimen over several months to a maintenance dose of 5–15 mg/day.[25] Alternate-day therapy is suggested by some investigators, although such a regimen may not be effective in a subgroup of patients who then respond to daily dosing. Treatment is ordinarily continued for a minimum of 8–12 months, as premature tapering is likely to result in relapse. Recurrent, progressive pulmonary disease occurs in 16–74% of patients as corticosteroid therapy is tapered; those patients with repetitive relapses usually benefit from indefinite suppressive therapy to minimize loss of lung function.[26] Inhaled corticosteroids may be helpful in reducing symptoms of endobronchial sarcoidosis, such as cough or airway irritability, but have not been proven useful as sole agents in pulmonary sarcoidosis, except possibly in mild disease.

Low-dose corticosteroid therapy is often well tolerated, although weight gain, hypertension, hyperglycemia, glaucoma, and osteoporosis are serious complications. Because of the risk of hypercalcemia and hypercalciuria, supplemental calcium and vitamin D are not routinely given. Bisphosphonate therapy is often recommended for documented osteoporosis, but clinical studies of their efficacy in sarcoidosis are lacking.

SPECIFIC SITUATIONS

LÖFGREN SYNDROME

Nonsteroidal anti-inflammatory drugs are recommended for the relief of constitutional symptoms and joint pains. For disabling arthritis or severe constitutional symptoms, corticosteroids are almost immediately effective. Generally, the steroids can be tapered over a few weeks to months without recrudescence of symptoms.

THERAPEUTIC PRINCIPLES

INDICATIONS FOR CORTICOSTEROID THERAPY IN PATIENTS WITH SARCOIDOSIS

>> Pulmonary involvement
- Moderate or severe, symptomatic pulmonary disease
- Progressive, symptomatic pulmonary disease
- Persistent pulmonary infiltrates or abnormal lung function for 1–2 years with mild symptoms to assess reversibility
- Advanced fibrocystic disease

>> Extrapulmonary involvement
- Threatened organ failure: severe ocular, cardiac, or central nervous system disease
- Posterior uveitis or anterior uveitis not responding to local steroids
- Persistent hypercalcemia
- Persistent renal or hepatic dysfunction
- Pituitary disease
- Myopathy
- Palpable splenomegaly or evidence of hypersplenism such as thrombocytopenia
- Severe fatigue and weight loss
- Painful lymphadenopathy
- Disfiguring skin disease

OCULAR SARCOIDOSIS

Anterior uveitis can often be treated effectively with topical corticosteroids alone. Oral corticosteroids are usually necessary for posterior uveitis, chorioretinitis, and optic neuritis. The latter two may present as ocular emergencies requiring high doses of intravenous corticosteroids initially.

CARDIAC SARCOIDOSIS

Treatment consists of antiarrhythmic therapy, diuretics, and afterload-reducing agents for heart failure, in addition to anti-inflammatory drugs. Corticosteroids are recommended in moderate doses since such treatment is associated with improved cardiac function and outcomes and may reverse heart block or reduce arrhythmias.[27] Initial therapy often begins with prednisone 40–60 mg/day, followed by a slow taper to a maintenance dose of 10–20 mg/day. Automatic implantable defibrillators or pacemakers are indicated in patients at risk for sudden death from serious arrhythmias or heart block, though indications for their prophylactic placement have not been established.

NEUROSARCOIDOSIS

High doses of oral corticosteroids (60–80 mg/day) or high-dose pulse intravenous therapy are often employed for serious CNS involvement.[24] Tapering should be performed over several months after evidence of suppression of inflammation by objective criteria (e.g., serial MRI scans). With the exception of cranial neuropathies, neurosarcoidosis tends to be chronic and requires long-term therapy.

■ ALTERNATIVE THERAPIES ■

Alternative therapies are frequently employed for chronic, progressive sarcoidosis when corticosteroid adverse effects significantly degrade quality of life.[28] None of these therapies has been proven effective by rigorous clinical trials. Large case series suggest these therapies are effective in only subsets of patients, and may require concomitant corticosteroid therapy.

ANTI-INFLAMMATORY THERAPIES

Hydroxychloroquine is often tried as a first-line treatment for mucocutaneous disease, including lupus pernio, other disfiguring skin disease, and nasal, sinus, and laryngeal sarcoidosis when corticosteroids are not immediately needed. The beneficial effects may not be evident for 2–3 months, with an overall 40–50% response rate. Hydroxychloroquine is often tried as a potential steroid-sparing drug for pulmonary or systemic disease, though with lower effectiveness. Chloroquine may be effective in some patients unresponsive to hydroxychloroquine, but has a greater potential for ocular toxicity and requires periodic drug-free intervals.

Pentoxifylline, a phosphodiesterase inhibitor, was found to be beneficial in one study of mild pulmonary sarcoidosis, though wider experience suggests only a small minority of patients respond. Gastrointestinal side effects often limit the dose that is tolerated.

Small case series suggest that thalidomide may be beneficial in severe cutaneous sarcoidosis, including lupus pernio. However, the drug does not appear to be effective for pulmonary disease. Peripheral neurotoxicity and the well-known teratogenicity of the drug mandate careful patient selection.

The tetracyclines, minocycline and doxycycline, have been reported to be effective in a small number of patients with cutaneous sarcoidosis and even less frequently as a steroid-sparing drug in pulmonary sarcoidosis. These antibiotics have anti-inflammatory effects that likely explain their mechanism of action as other antibiotics have not been found effective in sarcoidosis.

IMMUNOSUPPRESSIVE THERAPIES

Methotrexate in low weekly doses (10–20 mg/day) is often used as an alternative therapy in corticosteroid-recalcitrant pulmonary, cardiac, ocular, cutaneous, and neurologic sarcoidosis.[28] Success rates range from 50% to 70% as a corticosteroid-sparing drug, but it may take 6 months or longer to show effectiveness. Potential serious complications include hepatotoxicity, opportunistic infections, bone marrow suppression, and pulmonary toxicity.

Limited clinical studies suggest that azathioprine in a dose of 100–200 mg/day may be useful in corticosteroid-recalcitrant sarcoidosis, often combined with low doses of corticosteroids. More recently, mycophenolate mofetil has been used with anecdotal benefit and, possibly, an improved safety profile over azathioprine. Beneficial effects are usually apparent by 2–4 months. Potential drug toxicities include bone marrow suppression, gastrointestinal symptoms, skin rashes, arthralgias, and possibly a slightly increased risk of malignancy. There are some anecdotal reports of using cyclophosphamide in steroid-recalcitrant sarcoidosis, particularly refractory neurosarcoidosis, though its use is severely limited because of its oncogenic potential.

Cyclosporine, a drug known to inhibit T-cell activation, appears to be ineffective, except possibly in a few cases of severe neurosarcoidosis.

ANTI-TNF INHIBITORS

The use of TNF inhibitors in sarcoidosis is based on the established role of TNF in experimental models of granuloma formation. One recent multicenter study found infliximab to have a modest effect on one of several primary endpoints (improved forced vital capacity after 24 weeks of therapy).[29] Anecdotal cases suggest adalimumab may also be effective, but etanercept was ineffective in a small clinical trial. Risks of these therapies include allergic reactions and infectious complications, including sepsis and reactivation tuberculosis. Given these risks, further clinical trials are needed before these therapies could be routinely recommended in sarcoidosis.

ROLE OF TRANSPLANTATION IN SARCOIDOSIS

Lung, heart, kidney, and liver transplantations have been performed successfully in small numbers of patients with sarcoidosis. Recurrent granulomas are found in the transplanted organs of some patients but are generally transient, self-limited, and responsive to an increase in immunosuppression. Pulmonary hypertension is an independent predictor of reduced survival in patients with advanced pulmonary sarcoidosis awaiting lung transplantation.[30] Overall, the survival rate for lung transplantation for end-stage pulmonary sarcoidosis appears to be similar to that of other organ-specific diseases.

INFORMATION FOR PATIENTS

An updated primer on sarcoidosis sponsored by the US National Heart, Lung and Blood Institute is available on the internet for interested patients and physicians.[31]

■ REFERENCES ■

1. Mitchell DN, Scadding JG. Sarcoidosis. Am Rev Respir Dis 1974; 110: 774.

2. Joint Statement of the American Thoracic Society (ATS), the European Respiratory Society (ERS) and the World Association of Sarcoidosis and Other Granulomatous Disorders (WASOG) adopted by the ATS Board of Directors and by the ERS Executive Committee, February 1999. Statement on sarcoidosis. Am J Respir Crit Care Med 1999; 160: 736.

3. Drent M, Costabel U, (eds) Sarcoidosis, vol. 10, Monograph 32 of the European Respiratory Society. Wakefield, UK: Charlesworth Group, 2005.

4. Siltzbach LE, James DG, Neville E. Course and prognosis of sarcoidosis around the world. Am J Med 1974; 57: 847.

5. Hosoda Y, Yamaguchi M, Hiraga Y. Global epidemiology of sarcoidosis. What story do prevalence and incidence tell us? Clin Chest Med 1997; 18: 681.

6. Rybicki BA, Iannuzzi MC, Frederick MM, et al. Familial aggregation of sarcoidosis: a case control etiologic study of sarcoidosis (ACCESS). Am J Respir Crit Care Med 2001; 164: 2085.

7. Rossman MD, Thompson B, Frederick M, et al. HLA-DRB1*1101: a significant risk factor for sarcoidosis in blacks and whites. Am J Hum Genet 2003; 73: 720.

8. Berlin M, Fogdel-Hahn A, Olerup O, et al. HLA-DR predicts the prognosis in Scandinavian patients with pulmonary sarcoidosis. Am J Respir Crit Care Med 1997; 156: 1601.

9. Schurmann M, Lympany PA, Reichel P, et al. Familial sarcoidosis is linked to the major histocompatibility complex region. Am J Respir Crit Care Med 2000; 162: 861.

10. Iannuzzi MC, Iyengar SK, Gray-McGuire C, et al. Genome wide search for sarcoidosis susceptibility genes in African Americans. Genes Immun 2005; 6: 509.

11. Valentonyte R, Hampe J, Huse K, et al. Sarcoidosis is associated with a truncating splice site mutation in BTNL2. Nat Genet 2005; 37: 357.

12. Newman LS, Rose CS, Bresnitz EA, et al. A case control etiologic study of sarcoidosis: environmental and occupational risk factors. Am J Respir Crit Care Med 2004; 170: 1324.

13. Hance AJ. The role of mycobacteria in the pathogenesis of sarcoidosis. Semin Respir Infect 1998; 13: 197.

14. Eishi Y, Suga M, Ishige I, et al. Quantitative analysis of mycobacterial and propionibacterial DNA in lymph nodes of Japanese and European patients with sarcoidosis. J Clin Microbiol 2002; 40: 198.

15. Munro CS, Mitchell DN. The Kveim response: still useful, still a puzzle. Thorax 1987; 42: 321.

16. Song Z, Marzilli L, Greenlee BM, et al. Mycobacterial catalase-peroxidase is a tissue antigen and target of the adaptive immune response in systemic sarcoidosis. J Exp Med 2005; 201: 755.

17. Katchar K, Wahlstrom J, Eklund A, et al. Highly activated T-cell receptor AV2S3(+) CD4(+) lung T-cell expansions in pulmonary sarcoidosis. Am J Respir Crit Care Med 2001; 163: 1540.

18. Muller-Quernheim J. Sarcoidosis: immunopathogenetic concepts and their clinical application. Eur Respir J 1998; 12: 716.

19. Moller DR, Forman JD, Liu MC, et al. Enhanced expression of IL-12 associated with Th1 cytokine profiles in active pulmonary sarcoidosis. J Immunol 1996; 145: 4952.

20. Miyara M, Amoura Z, Parizot C, et al. The immune paradox of sarcoidosis and regulatory T cells. J Exp Med 2006; 203: 359.

21. Baughman RP, Tierstein AS, Judson MA, et al. Clinical characteristics of patients in a case control study of sarcoidosis. Am J Respir Crit Care Med 1885; 2001: 164.

22. Moller DR. Rare manifestations of sarcoidosis. In: Drent M, Costabel U, eds: Sarcoidosis, vol. 10. Monograph 32 of the European Respiratory Society, Wakefield, UK: Charlesworth Group, 2005: 233–250.

23. Chapelon-Abric C, de Zuttere D, Duhaut P, et al. Cardiac sarcoidosis: a retrospective study of 41 cases. Medicine (Baltimore) 2004; 83: 315.

24. Stern BJ. Neurological complications of sarcoidosis. Curr Opin Neurol 2004; 17: 311.

25. Johns CJ, Michele TM. The clinical management of sarcoidosis – a 50-year experience at the Johns Hopkins Hospital. Medicine 1999; 78: 65.

26. Gibson GJ, Prescott RJ, Muers MF. British Thoracic Society Sarcoidosis Study: effects of long-term corticosteroid treatment. Thorax 1996; 51: 238.

27. Yazaki Y, Isobe M, Hiroe M, et al. Prognostic determinants of long-term survival in Japanese patients with cardiac sarcoidosis treated with prednisone. Am J Cardiol 2001; 88: 1006.

28. Baughman RP, Lynch JP. Difficult treatment issues in sarcoidosis. J Intern Med 2003; 253: 41.

29. Baughman RP, Drent M, Kavuru M, et al. Infliximab therapy in patients with chronic sarcoidosis and pulmonary involvement. Am J Respir Crit Care Med 2006; 174: 795–802.

30. Arcasoy SM, Christie JD, Pochettino A, et al. Characteristics and outcomes of patients with sarcoidosis listed for lung transplantation. Chest 2001; 120: 873.

31. National Heart, Lung, and Blood Institute (NHLBI): Sarcoidosis. Available online at: http://www.nhlbi.nih.gov/health/dci/Diseases/sarc/sar_whatis.html.

REFERENCES

Immunologic ocular disease

73

James T. Rosenbaum, Matthias D. Becker,
Justine R. Smith

The immune system can induce disease in virtually any portion of the eye. Examples include conjunctivitis, keratitis, keratoconjunctivitis, uveitis, scleritis, optic neuritis, and orbital inflammation. The anatomy of the eye is depicted schematically in Figure 73.1. Two relatively common immunologically mediated ocular diseases discussed elsewhere in this volume are sicca syndrome secondary to Sjögren's syndrome (Chapter 54) and anterior ischemic optic neuropathy secondary to giant cell arteritis (Chapter 59). Before considering those additional ocular disorders that are the most common and visually significant, it is critical to review some unique considerations related to ocular immunology.

OCULAR IMMUNE PRIVILEGE

Many of the mechanisms that drive inflammation in the eye are identical to those operating at other tissue sites. The major difference between the immunopathology of intraocular inflammation and that of systemic inflammatory disease relates to the fact that the eye, like the brain and the testis, is an immunologically privileged site. During uveitis, keratitis, and scleritis, as well as following corneal transplantation, a variety of local immunosuppressive mechanisms act to limit the damage caused by infiltrating leukocytes, and, consequently, to influence the patient's clinical course. One of the most important factors is the constitutive expression of Fas ligand (FasL) within the eye. In addition, normal ocular tissues produce relatively high levels of immunomodulatory cytokines and immunosuppressive neuropeptides, as well as complement regulatory proteins. Other factors include the blood–aqueous and blood–retinal anatomical barriers, limited MHC expression, a paucity of lymphatic drainage channels within the eye, and, in the case of the cornea, the complete absence of blood vessels. Anterior chamber-associated immune deviation (ACAID) describes the suppression of a cell-mediated immune response when soluble antigen is directly injected into the aqueous humor. ACAID presumably results from some or all of the above factors.

FAS LIGAND

Many immune cells, including neutrophils, monocytes, macrophages and lymphocytes, express Fas (CD95) on their surface. The interaction between Fas and its receptor FasL (CD95L) triggers apoptosis of the Fas-bearing cell. FasL is constitutively expressed within the eye, being detected in normal cornea, anterior uvea and retina. The importance of FasL to ocular immune privilege has been demonstrated primarily in experimental models of ocular inflammation. Corneal allografts from FasL-negative mice into recipients of normal phenotype are rejected in all cases, whereas approximately half of FasL-positive grafts survive.[1] When injected into the eyes of FasL-deficient mice, herpes simplex virus causes a severe invasive infection. A similar procedure in normal phenotype control animals results in relatively minor inflammation. Levels of FasL in aqueous humor during human acute anterior uveitis are capable of inducing apoptosis in Fas-positive lymphoid cells. In this self-limiting condition, as well as in relevant rodent models, apoptosis of infiltrating T cells is observed early in the course of the inflammation. In addition to FasL, the local expression of TRAIL (TNF-related apoptosis-inducing ligand) by corneal endothelium also contributes to enhanced apoptosis and immune privilege within the eye.[2]

CYTOKINE NETWORK, NEUROPEPTIDES AND COMPLEMENT

Tissues in both the anterior and the posterior segments of the human eye constitutively express the immunomodulatory cytokine transforming growth factor-β (TGF-β).[3] The concentration of TGF-β in the aqueous humor is sufficient to inhibit T-cell activation and proliferation in a variety of assays.[4] As might be anticipated, significantly lower levels of this activated cytokine are measured in the aqueous of patients with a variety

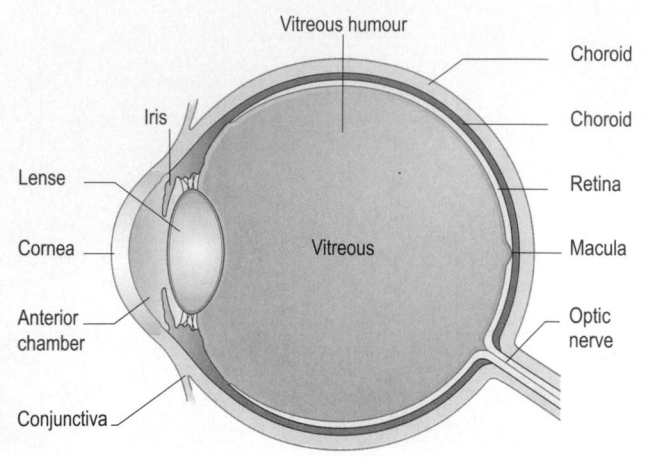

Fig. 73.1 Schematic representation of the eye.

of uveitis syndromes compared to levels present in normal eyes. The inflammatory cytokine interleukin (IL)-1 has been implicated in the pathogenesis of various ocular inflammatory diseases. There is expression of IL-1 receptor antagonist (IL-1Ra) in normal cornea[5] and retinal pigment epithelium, implying that this tissue contains a control mechanism for responses mediated by IL-1. Interestingly, topical application of IL-1Ra has a significantly positive effect in promoting experimental corneal allograft survival. The aqueous humor contains neuropeptides, including α-melanocyte stimulating hormone, vasoactive intestinal peptide and calcitonin gene-related peptide, that inhibit the activities of T cells and macrophages. Complement is active at low levels in the healthy eye, regulated by complement regulatory proteins that are expressed both on intraocular cell membranes and within the intraocular fluid; this system may participate in the destruction of pathogens invading the eye.[6] However, interestingly, iC3b, generated because of this activation, appears to inhibit antigen-specific delayed type hypersensitivity.

■ ANTERIOR CHAMBER-ASSOCIATED IMMUNE DEVIATION ■

Anterior chamber-associated immune deviation is 'a stereotypic, systemic immune response to antigens placed in the anterior chamber (of the eye) in which delayed hypersensitivity is avoided and suppressed.' The molecular events that are responsible for this phenomenon include the following:[7] Entry of an antigen into the eye stimulates production of tumor necrosis factor-α, and hence the upregulation of cell adhesion molecules; secretion of IL-10 by the infiltrating T cells; and sensitization of these cells for FasL-mediated killing. TGF-β also induces ocular antigen-presenting cells to secrete IL-10 during antigen processing.[8] Apoptotic T cells pass in the bloodstream to the spleen, where they are phagocytosed and induce activation of Th2-type CD4 T cells. The Th2-type cells control Th1 function by secreting various immunomodulatory cytokines. T-cell receptor α-chain fragments from apoptotic cells are presented in the class I pathway. This event generates CD8 killer cells, which are capable of deleting the CD4 T cells that would otherwise mediate a delayed-type hypersensitivity response. CD8 T cells that

secrete immunomodulatory cytokines, including IL-10 and TGF-β, are also generated. ACAID is also dependent on the presence of invariant natural killer T cells.

■ IMMOBILITY OF DENDRITIC CELLS WITHIN THE ANTERIOR CHAMBER ■

A recently appreciated phenomenon within the iris is that the vast majority of cells that phagocytose foreign antigen fail to migrate after antigen uptake. This is clearly demonstrable by intravital microscopy and correlates with the failure of these antigen-bearing cells to migrate to the local lymph nodes.[9] The inability to migrate is consistent with the known lack of lymphatics within the eye, and must mean that soluble antigen injected into the anterior chamber is not presented in the regional lymph node in a manner that is comparable to what follows antigen exposure in an organ such as the skin.

■ UVEITIS ■

UVEITIS AS A DIAGNOSTIC ENTITY

The uveal tract is the middle layer of the eye, divided into the anterior uvea (iris, ciliary body) and posterior uvea (choroid). The uvea is sandwiched between an outer layer (sclera) and an inner layer (retina). The anterior segment is separated from the posterior segment by the lens. Uveitis is an extremely variable spectrum of different diseases that includes a variety of infections and immune-mediated diseases (Table 73.1). It is the third leading cause of preventable blindness worldwide. Inflammatory disorders of the retina (retinitis) and sclera (scleritis) frequently involve the adjacent uveal tract. Many different immune mechanisms could result in uveitis, as evidenced in animal models. These mechanisms include an immune response to a sequestered self-antigen, molecular mimicry, immune complex deposition, and the response to a toxin.

The differential diagnosis of uveitis is facilitated by identifying characteristic clinical features. Uveitis can be classified by location: anterior (iritis, iridocyclitis), intermediate (pars planitis, vitritis) or posterior (retinitis, choroiditis, retinochoroiditis, chorioretinitis, retinal vasculitis). Some forms of uveitis involve all portions of the uveal tract (panuveitis). Uveitis can be classified by course (self-limited, chronic, or recurrent); by onset (sudden, insidious); by symmetry (unilateral, bilateral); by associated complications such as glaucoma, cystoid macular edema (Figs. 73.2–73.4), synechiae (for example, adhesion of the iris to the lens) (Fig. 73.5), retinal detachment, or band keratopathy (the deposition of calcium in the epithelium of the cornea) (Fig. 73.6); and by the appearance of inflammatory keratic precipitates on the endothelium of the cornea within the eye (granulomatous, nongranulomatous) (Fig. 73.7). Granulomatous diseases with large cellular concretions on the cornea or nodules within the iris include tuberculosis, syphilis, sarcoidosis, Vogt-Koyanagi–Harada disease and sympathetic ophthalmia. The group of nongranulomatous diseases includes ankylosing spondylitis, reactive arthritis, and juvenile idiopathic arthritis. Table 73.2 shows how these parameters contribute to the differential diagnosis. Additionally, ethnic and geographic considerations factor into the differential diagnosis. For example sarcoidosis, Behçet' syndrome, and Vogt Koyanagi Harada

Table 73.1 Diagnostic categories of uveitis

Diagnostic group		Diagnosis
Infectious Causes	Viral	Herpes simplex
		Herpes zoster
		Cytomegalovirus
		HTLV-1
		Mumps
		West Nile
	Bacterial or spirochetal	Atypical Mycobacterium
		Bacterial endocarditis
		Bartonella
		Brucellosis
		Leprosy
		Leptospirosis
		Lyme disease
		Propionibacterium
		Tuberculosis
		Leprosy
		Syphilis
		Whipple's disease
	Parasitic (protozoan or helminthic)	Acanthameba
		Cysticercosis
		Onchocerciasis
		Pneumocystis carinii
		Toxoplasmosis
		Toxocariasis
	Fungal	Histoplasmosis
		Coccidioidomycosis
		Candidiasis
		Aspergillosis
		Sporotrichosis
		Blastomycosis
		Cryptococcosis
Immune Mediated		Ankylosing spondylitis
		Behçet's disease
		Crohn's disease
		Drug or hypersensitivity reaction (such as rifabutin or cidofovir)
		Familial granulomatous synovitis with uveitis
		Interstitial nephritis
		Juvenile idiopathic arthritis
		Kawasaki disease
		Multiple sclerosis
		Psoriatic arthritis
		Reactive arthritis
		Relapsing polychondritis
		Rheumatic fever
		Sarcoidosis
		Scleritis
		Sjogren's syndrome
		Sweet's syndrome
		Systemic lupus erythematosus

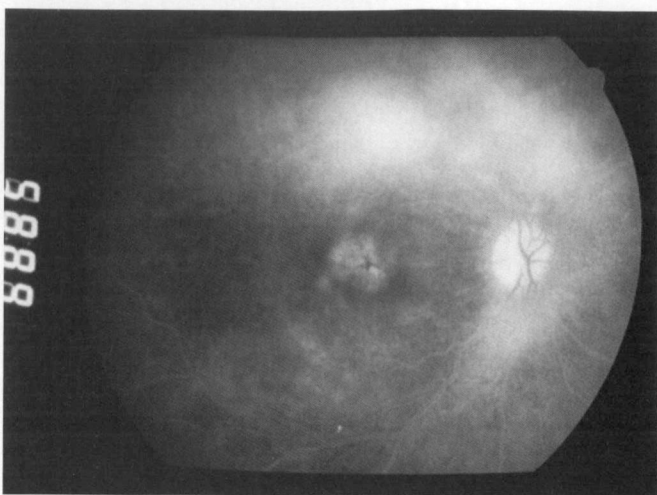

Fig. 73.2 Fundus fluorescein angiogram showing cystoid macular edema. Fluorescein, which appears as a white stain, should be absent from the center of this photograph because the macular area is avascular.

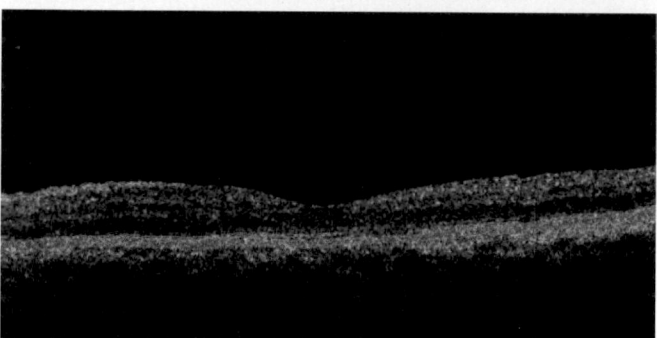

Fig. 73.3 Ocular coherence tomogram (OCT). This is an image of a normal eye. An OCT allows precise quantification of macular thickening. In this image, the macula shows a normal dimple or indentation.

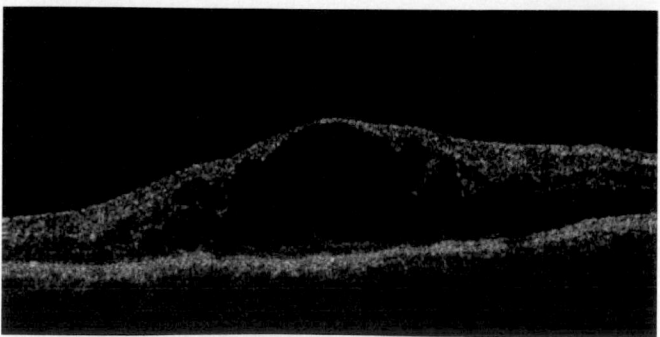

Fig. 73.4 OCT image showing marked macular edema. The macula is markedly elevated.

disease have strong ethnic predispositions, whereas certain infections such as cytomegalovirus in association with AIDS, leprosy, or onchocerciasis vary in prevalence based on geographic area. Together with a medical history, gender, and age, these findings help to narrow the differential diagnosis of uveitis.

The following case vignettes illustrate how important a precise and critical history and examination are. A 22-year-old man with low back pain and a red painful eye due to episodic, unilateral, sudden onset anterior uveitis is highly likely to have a spondyloarthropathy (Chapter 57). A 6-year-old girl with no ocular complaints but biomicroscopic findings of bilateral band keratopathy and leukocytes in the anterior chamber is likely to suffer from the pauciarticular subset of juvenile idiopathic arthritis (Chapter 53).

The most obvious sign of uveal inflammation is the presence of biomicroscopically visible leukocytes in the anterior or the posterior chamber of the eye. Most patients with anterior uveitis will experience pain, redness, photophobia, miosis and a variable degree of visual loss. In contrast, many forms of uveitis that affect the posterior segment will cause no redness, no pain, no change in pupil size (no macroscopically apparent signs of an inflamed eye). Instead, disturbances in visual acuity may vary from normal vision to seeing floaters, to blurred vision to blindness.

EPIDEMIOLOGY

The incidence and prevalence of the different types of uveitis varies among regions of the world, depending on numerous factors: level of development, HLA distribution, prevalence of different infectious diseases in each region, and also the methodology employed by each physician to evaluate and classify uveitis (Table 73.3).[10] Using a northern California database for enrollees in a health maintenance study, Gritz and Wong[10a] recently reported an incidence of 52.4 per 100 000 per year and a prevalence of 115.3/100 000. Anterior uveitis is much more common than intermediate or posterior uveitis.

PREVENTION AND PATIENT MANAGEMENT

Uveitis can be the first sign of occult, potentially severe, systemic disease (for example sarcoidosis, syphilis, or central nervous system lymphoma). Despite the difficulty of successful systemic anti-inflammatory/ immunosuppressive treatment, there are some diagnoses that can be treated to complete recovery, such as syphilis. Therefore it is essential to identify as accurately as possible the cause of uveitis. A targeted approach is preferable, with a limited work-up guided by the type and severity of uveitis and the presence of systemic findings. The history assumes greater importance than in any other ophthalmic entity. The minimal work-up for uveitis of unknown etiology requires an extensive and careful review of systems, a syphilis serology, and a chest X-ray.[11]

Most practitioners use a stepladder approach to the treatment of uveitis. The first step is treatment with corticosteroids for all patients with noninfectious uveitis (topical, especially for anterior uveitis, local peribulbar injection, intravitreal injection, or systemic administration). A surgically implantable intravitreal device to release fluocinolone continuously for approximately 2.5 years is an additional option that is limited by cost and complications, which can include cataract, glaucoma, and scleral thinning.[12] Systemic immunosuppressive therapy should be used in cases of inadequate benefit from corticosteroids or unacceptable steroid side

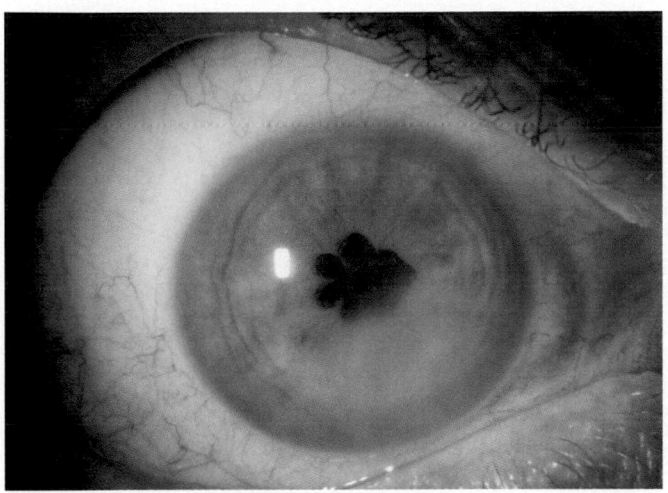

Fig. 73.5 Posterior synechiae. The cloverleaf appearance of the pupil is due to the iris adhering to the lens.

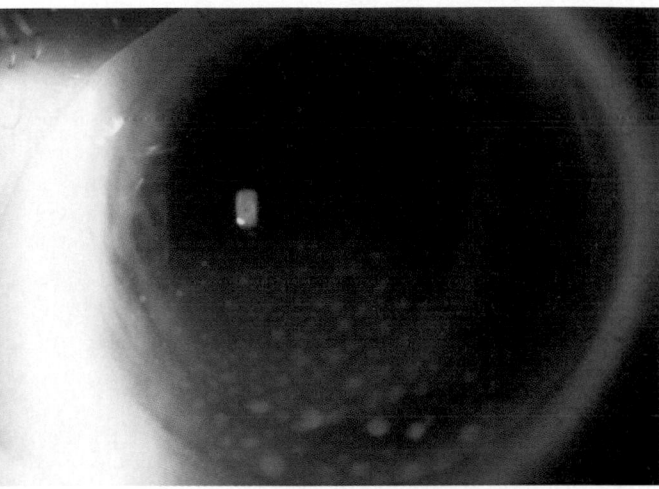

Fig. 73.7 Granulomatous keratic precipitates. Round white dots are scattered in a triangular shape. The dots represent concretions of leukocytes adherent to the corneal endothelium.

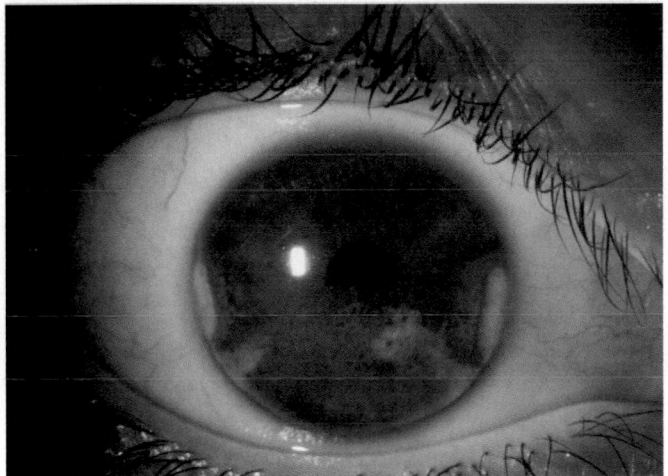

Fig. 73.6 Band keratopathy. Calcium deposition in the corneal endothelium complicates the iridocyclitis in a patient with juvenile idiopathic arthritis.

effects. Immunosuppression is usually reserved for bilateral forms of uveitis with a severity sufficient to alter activities of daily living, and is frequently chosen for eye involvement with Behçet's disease. Immunosuppression may be contraindicated by active infection in the eye or elsewhere.

OVERVIEW OF THE MOST COMMON UVEITIS DIAGNOSES

Ankylosing spondylitis (AS) is the most common systemic diagnosis associated with uveitis in western nations. A genetic predisposition with the HLA-B27 marker is found in 88–96% of patients with AS. About 40% of AS patients develop anterior uveitis transiently during their

lifetime; conversely 30% of anterior uveitis patients have AS. Approximately 50% of patients with a sudden onset anterior uveitis are HLA-B27 positive. In some studies, 80–90% of individuals with HLA B27-associated iritis have a systemic disease, either ankylosing spondylitis or reactive arthritis. Ankylosing spondylitis should be considered in any patient with sudden onset, primarily anterior, unilateral uveitis associated with redness and pain. Recurrent disease, fibrin in the anterior chamber, posterior synechiae, relatively brief inflammation that resolves in less than 2 months, and lowered intraocular pressure are additional hallmarks that sometimes help to distinguish HLA-B27-associated iritis from other categories of intraocular inflammation.[13] Cells can be seen in the anterior chamber by slit lamp examination. Inflammation is sometimes so severe that a hypopyon (Fig. 73.8) develops. The posterior segment of the eye is not commonly involved in this disease except for the development of a vision-reducing cystoid macular edema (see Figs 73.2, 73.4), which is a more frequent complication than with other forms of anterior uveitis. The disease usually shows a good response to topical corticosteroids. In frequently recurrent cases, therapy with sulfasalazine or TNF inhibitors has been shown to be effective in reducing the frequency and severity of the attacks.

Ocular manifestations of inflammatory bowel disease (IBD) (Crohn's disease and ulcerative colitis; Chapter 74) include iritis, episcleritis, and scleritis (1–9% of all cases). Twenty percent of patients with IBD may have sacroiliitis; 60% of these are HLA-B27 positive. The anterior uveitis in patients with IBD is often similar to that seen with the HLA-B27 spectrum of joint diseases (ankylosing spondylitis): sudden in onset, unilateral, and self-limited. But Crohn's disease is a granulomatous process: like sarcoidosis, it may result in intraocular inflammation that is insidious in onset, bilateral, posterior to the lens, chronic, or associated with a retinal vasculitis.[14]

Crohn's disease is a complex genetic disease, meaning that multiple genes undoubtedly contribute to susceptibility to this inflammation. One of the best-characterized of these genes is NOD-2, which is also known as CARD-15. This gene seems to function as an intracellular Toll

ORGAN-SPECIFIC INFLAMMATORY DISEASE

Table 73.2 Characteristic features of common forms of uveitis

Parameter	
Location	**Anterior:** Ankylosing spondylitis, reactive arthritis, juvenile idiopathic arthritis **Intermediate:** Pars planitis **Posterior:** Vogt–Koyanagi–Harada syndrome
Onset	**Sudden:** Ankylosing spondylitis, reactive arthritis **Insidious:** Pars planitis, juvenile idiopathic arthritis
Symmetry	**Unilateral:** Ankylosing spondylitis, toxoplasmosis **Bilateral:** Pars planitis, lymphoma, juvenile idiopathic arthritis
Course	**Self-limited:** Toxoplasmosis **Recurrent:** Behçet's disease, ankylosing spondylitis **Chronic:** Pars planitis

Table 73.3 Likelihood of developing uveitis in association with a specific disease

Diagnosis	Likelihood (%)
Ankylosing spondylitis	30
Sarcoidosis	25–50
Behçet's disease	80
Inflammatory bowel disease	1–9
Psoriatic arthritis	7
Juvenile idiopathic arthritis	<2–53
Multiple sclerosis	<1–2

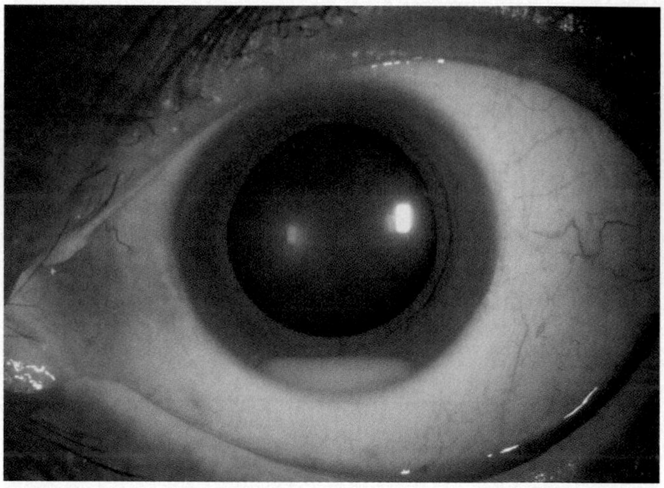

Fig. 73.8 Hypopyon. Intense inflammation has resulted in a creamy exudate (pus), seen as whitening over the inferior portion of the anterior chamber. In this example, hypopyon was secondary to rifabutin, not ankylosing spondylitis.

receptor that recognizes muramyl dipeptide from both Gram-negative and Gram-positive bacteria. The NOD-2 gene has homology to genes implicated in autoinflammatory diseases such as familial cold urticaria. A mutation in the portion of the NOD-2 gene known as the nucleotide-binding domain results in a rare autosomal dominant form of uveitis known as Blau syndrome.

One percent of the population has psoriasis; 7% of psoriasis patients have arthritis; and 7% of patients with psoriasis and arthritis have uveitis. The diagnosis is made clinically with the typical findings of cutaneous changes (erythematous, hyperkeratotic rash) and joint disease. Patients with sacroiliac disease and psoriatic arthritis are especially likely to develop uveitis.

Ocular disease is the initial manifestation of sarcoidosis (Chapter 72) in 20% of patients. The systemic illness begins as ocular inflammation almost as often as it initially presents as pulmonary disease. Between 25% and 50% of patients with systemic sarcoidosis exhibit ocular inflammatory disease. In most case series sarcoidosis accounts for 3–10% of all patients with uveitis, and it therefore follows spondyloarthropathy as the second most common systemic illness associated with uveitis in North America and Europe. The diagnosis of sarcoidosis should always be considered in any patient presenting with a uveitis of unknown etiology.

Sarcoidosis has a strong ethnic association: it occurs in the USA 10 times more frequently among African-Americans than among whites. Because it can affect almost every part of the eye, symptoms of ocular sarcoidosis vary widely depending on the distribution of pathology. Most commonly, patients will have a bilateral chronic granulomatous iridocyclitis.[15] The disease often regresses clinically, with two-thirds of patients symptom-free after 10 years. Typical findings include 'mutton-fat' keratic precipitates of the cornea (Fig. 73.7), Koeppe and Busacca iris nodules, posterior synechiae (Fig. 73.5), and white clumps of cells ('snowballs') in the inferior anterior vitreous. A chest X-ray (or CT scan of the chest[16]) should be included in every basic work-up of patients with uveitis of unknown cause. The diagnosis is most reliably established by a biopsy that demonstrates the noncaseating granuloma in the absence of an infection or beryllium exposure. Possible biopsy sites include lymph nodes, lung, skin, oral mucosa, and conjunctiva. Serological abnormalities

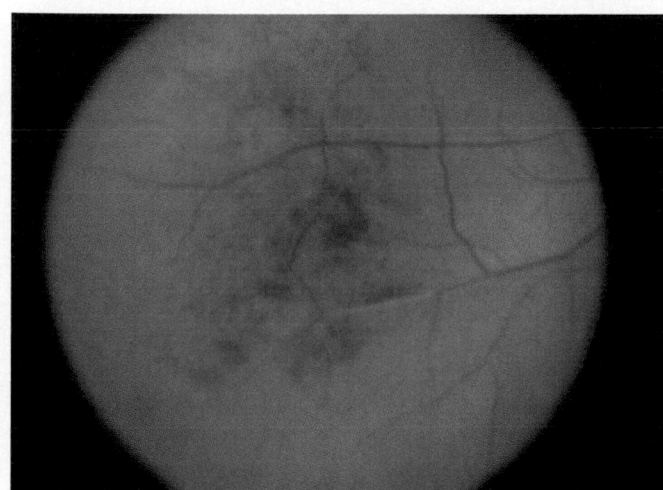

Fig. 73.9 Fundus photograph showing retinal vasculitis. The scattered hemorrhages are secondary to the vasculitis. The patient has Behçet's syndrome.

are not sufficiently unique to establish a diagnosis. They include elevated serum angiotensin-converting enzyme and lysozyme levels. In general, the combination of uveitis and symmetrical hilar adenopathy is specific for sarcoidosis. It is therefore not necessary to obtain tissue confirmation when this presentation occurs. Topical, periocular, and systemic corticosteroids are the mainstay of therapy.

Behçet's syndrome is a generalized occlusive vasculitis of unknown cause (Chapter 58). It accounts for about 2.5% of patients at a North American referral uveitis clinic, and has a strong ethnic relationship. It is most common in Japan (20% of uveitis patients) and prevalent in Middle Eastern countries along the silk road.

The classic complex includes aphthous stomatitis, genital ulceration and iritis, sometimes with hypopyon (30% of patients), and skin lesions. The posterior segment is more commonly involved than the anterior and includes an occlusive retinal vasculitis (Fig. 73.9).[17] Extraocular manifestations most commonly include arthritis, erythema nodosum, diarrhea (mimicking inflammatory bowel disease), and sterile meningitis. There is a strong tendency for the symptoms to remit and exacerbate spontaneously. HLA-B5 or its subset, B51, is more commonly found among Behçet's patients. Behçet's syndrome may lead to blindness if ischemic optic neuropathy and retinopathy are not adequately treated. Patients are often inadequately managed by corticosteroids alone: a regimen with immunosuppressive drugs (cyclosporine A) or azathioprine has been proved useful. Some investigators advocate the use of α-interferon.[18] Infliximab has demonstrated dramatic benefit in studies reported from Europe and Japan.[19]

Although retrobulbar optic neuritis is the ocular inflammation most clearly associated with multiple sclerosis, both intermediate uveitis (pars planitis) and a bilateral granulomatous anterior uveitis are well described in association with this demyelinating central nervous system disease[20] (Chapter 65). The granulomatous inflammation is typically bilateral and may indicate a worse prognosis for the neurologic disease. The HLA-DR2 antigen, strongly associated with MS, is also associated with uveitis.

Patients with juvenile idiopathic arthritis (JIA; Chapter 53) need special consideration as the disease often does not present with a 'red eye:' the uveitis is often a smoldering, silent inflammation with a quiet, white eye. These young patients need to be screened on a routine basis to avoid structural damage to the eye from even low-grade inflammation with resulting blindness. In 20% of all JIA cases the joint involvement is pauciarticular (five or fewer joints affected). Uveitis occurs far more commonly in this pauciarticular subset, and these patients require ophthalmic screening every 3–4 months. Girls are affected four times more often than boys, although boys may be more likely to develop complications.[21] Eighty percent of uveitis cases are positive for anti-nuclear antibodies (ANA) and negative for rheumatoid factor. The onset of ocular disease is usually within 5 years of arthritis. Biomicroscopically, bilateral fine keratic precipitates, band keratopathy (Fig. 73.4), flare and cells in the anterior chamber, posterior synechiae, glaucoma and cataract formation can be found. Topical and periocular corticosteroid treatment with a slow taper is the mainstay of therapy. Systemic therapy with methotrexate can be used as a substitute for corticosteroids in selected cases. Cataract surgery is a special challenge and may require intense perioperative immunosuppression.

KEY CONCEPT

Immune-mediated diseases can affect virtually any portion of the eye. Uveitis, scleritis, keratoconjunctivitis sicca, conjunctivitis, optic neuritis, keratitis, and orbital pseudotumor are examples of eye diseases that are frequently immune mediated.

CLINICAL PEARL

The immune privilege of the eye does not prevent immune-mediated eye disease.

SCLERITIS

DESCRIPTION/NATURAL HISTORY

Scleritis is a relatively uncommon inflammation that affects the sclera, the white tunic that encases the posterior eye. Scleritis is usually presumed to represent a vasculitis of scleral vessels. Approximately 50% of patients with scleritis will have clinical evidence for a systemic vasculitis elsewhere in the body. The most common systemic disease is rheumatoid arthritis (RA; Chapter 52), especially the subset of patients with rheumatoid nodules, high-titer rheumatoid factor, and pleuropericarditis as well as small vessel vasculitis of the lower extremities. Other systemic diseases commonly associated with scleritis are listed in Table 73.4. The epidemiology of scleritis has not been adequately reported. However, rheumatoid arthritis accounts for about one-third of all cases of scleritis. Because only 1% of patients with rheumatoid arthritis develop scleritis and about 1% of the population has RA one can estimate that the prevalence of scleritis is $0.01 \times 0.01 \times 3$, or 3/10 000.

Scleritis is frequently divided into five subsets based on the clinical presentation: diffuse anterior (Fig. 73.10); nodular anterior; necrotizing; scleromalacia perforans (Fig. 73.11); and posterior. Scleromalacia perforans is also known as necrotizing without inflammation. The clinical presentation will vary according to the type, but scleritis is usually a very painful and persistent condition. Even with treatment, a median duration reaches 7 years.

Table 73.4 Systemic immune-mediated diseases associated with scleritis

Rheumatoid arthritis
Wegener's granulomatosis
Inflammatory bowel disease
Polyarteritis nodosa
Temporal arteritis/giant cell arteritis
Systemic lupus erythematosus
Ankylosing spondylitis
Relapsing polychondritis
Rheumatic fever
IgA nephropathy

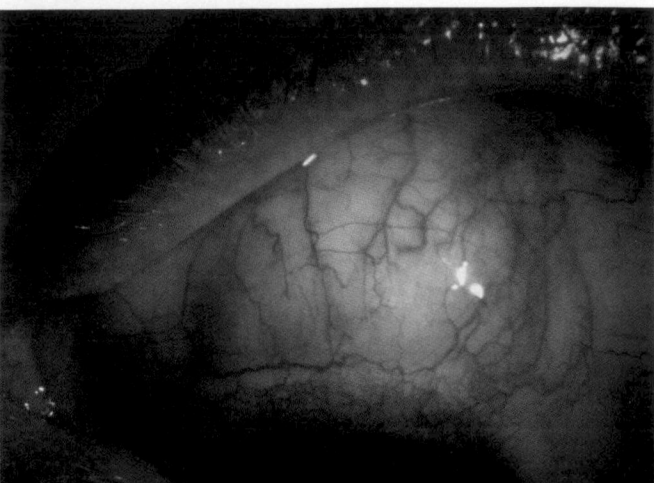

Fig. 73.11 Scleromalacia perforans. Blue sclera is visible secondary to inflammation, resembling a rheumatoid nodule in the eye.

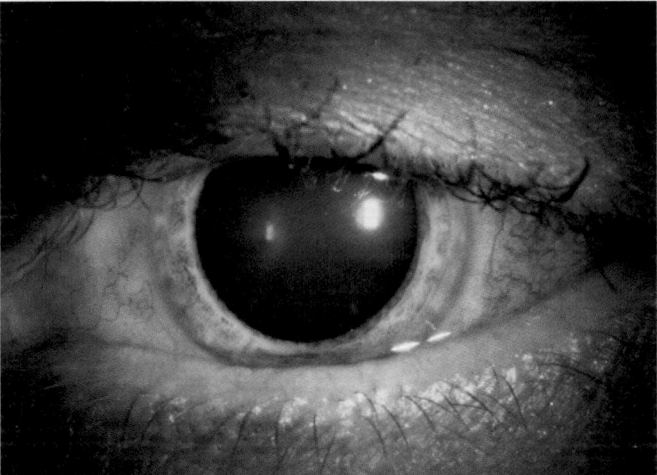

Fig. 73.10 Diffuse anterior scleritis. The red patch of vessels temporally is secondary to scleritis.

GENETIC/ENVIRONMENTAL FACTORS

Genetic factors affecting scleritis have not been adequately studied. Genes that affect the associated systemic diseases, such as RA, Wegener's granulomatosis, and polyarteritis, presumably also influence susceptibility to scleritis. Environmental triggers for scleritis have not been defined, except that some cases of scleritis can be a manifestation of infection, such as herpes zoster ophthalmicus, syphilis, or Lyme disease, as well as other bacterial and fungal infections.

IMMUNOLOGY/PATHOLOGY

Biopsy of the sclera entails some risk. Accordingly, many of the published histological observations are based on end-stage or extremely severe disease. In one pathology study of 55 examples of necrotizing scleritis the histology was divided into four types: zonal necrotizing granulomatous; nonzonal diffuse; necrotizing with microabscess; and sarcoidal granulomatous.[22] Eighty-five percent of patients with zonal necrotizing granulomatous pathology had a systemic disease, usually rheumatoid arthritis.

The pathology associated with RA was not distinct from other systemic diseases such as Wegener's granulomatosis. None of 19 patients with nonzonal diffuse scleral inflammation had a systemic disease. Just over half of the patients with microabscesses had an identifiable infection as the cause of scleritis. Only one patient had 'sarcoidal granulomatous inflammation,' and that patient had sarcoidosis.

PREVENTION/MANAGEMENT

Topical medications are only slightly beneficial for most patients with scleritis. Topical nonsteroidal anti-inflammatory drugs (NSAIDs), such as ketorolac, have not been proved efficacious in a controlled study. A topical corticosteroid can sometimes help in symptomatic control but also has risk, especially the promotion of cataract formation and elevation of intraocular pressure. The role for topical cyclosporine has not been adequately evaluated, but the authors' clinical experience has not been favorable.

Although most forms of scleritis represent a vasculitis, oral NSAIDs can be immensely beneficial. Although not all patients derive adequate control from NSAIDs, a subset will benefit sufficiently such that no other medication is required. Indomethacin has most frequently been reported to be effective,[23] but other NSAIDs have simply not been tested in a sufficiently large sample population. A recent report demonstrates that celecoxib is an effective option.

Many patients with scleritis will not benefit adequately from a nonsteroidal agent and will require immunosuppression. In general, for those with an associated systemic disease the control of that disease will lead to control of the scleritis. For those without a systemic illness, oral corticosteroids are an accepted initial approach to treatment. For example, therapy might begin with a dose of prednisone of 1 mg/kg bodyweight per day. The use of calcium and vitamin D, and other measures to preserve bone mineral density, should be considered for any patient who will be receiving corticosteroid on a chronic basis. If prednisone is not adequate for disease control, or if the medication is toxic, poorly tolerated, and cannot be safely tapered to a modest dosage, it is reasonable to add a steroid-sparing medication such as methotrexate, azathioprine, cyclosporine, mycophenolate, or even an alkylating agent such as cyclophosphamide.

Periocular corticosteroids are very effective for uveitis, but they are relatively contraindicated for patients with necrotizing scleritis. The steroid probably promotes reduced wound healing and thus enhances the likelihood that the sclera might perforate as a result of the inflammation. Scleral inflammation limited to the posterior sclera can probably be safely treated with a periocular steroid injection. Anterior scleritis that is nonnecrotizing also responds to the cautious use of periocular corticosteroid injection.

In choosing to treat with oral corticosteroid or an immunosuppressive, the clinician will, of course, weigh the risk/benefit ratio. The rationale for aggressive therapy is much stronger if the disease is bilateral and is affecting activities of daily living, because of either pain or a reduction in visual acuity.

CLINICAL PEARLS

> Uveitis and scleritis are frequently associated with a systemic illness. These illnesses can usually be diagnosed by history without resorting to extensive laboratory testing.

EVALUATION/DIFFERENTIAL DIAGNOSIS

Patients with scleritis generally have characteristic findings that allow an accurate diagnosis; scleritis can usually be readily distinguished from other causes of a red, painful eye. The most difficult distinction is between scleritis and episcleritis. The episclera overlies the sclera. In general patients with episcleritis do not experience pain, do not have an associated systemic disease, do not have complications such as iritis or glaucoma, and have an excellent prognosis, with complete resolution usually within weeks. The differences between scleritis and episcleritis are highlighted in Table 73.5.

The scleritis associated with a systemic vasculitis is often more severe than scleritis not associated with a systemic illness.[24] The scleritis associated with Wegener's granulomatosis may be particularly destructive and refractory to therapy.[25] Scleritis in association with rheumatoid arthritis is often a poor prognostic sign for the joint disease. For example, the small subset of patients with scleritis in association with rheumatoid arthritis have a shortened life expectancy compared to other patients with RA and no evidence for scleritis.

Posterior scleritis can be an extremely difficult disease to diagnose. If the anterior sclera is uninvolved, no redness is present. Pain with posterior scleritis is much more variable. The examination may show elevation of the adjacent retina and choroid. The diagnosis can be confirmed with an ultrasound examination or, less commonly, with a CT scan of the orbit demonstrating thickening of the sclera. Posterior scleritis is treated similarly to anterior scleritis, except that topical corticosteroids are not useful and a periocular corticosteroid injection can be given safely.

PITFALLS/CONTROVERSY

Some experts believe that scleritis is often a forme fruste of Wegener's granulomatosis. It clearly occurs in association with Wegener's granulomatosis, and patients with scleritis, a positive ANCA test, and no other evidence for Wegener's granulomatosis have been well described.[26]

With the exception of the ANCA, laboratory studies are generally selected according to the history and general physical examination. For example, although rheumatoid arthritis is associated with scleritis, the patients almost always have long-standing severe RA. A rheumatoid factor would not be an appropriate test if no joint disease were present clinically. Similarly, systemic lupus can be associated with scleritis, but one would not diagnose lupus on the basis of a positive ANA, scleritis, and the absence of other findings to suggest lupus. An erythrocyte sedimentation rate can sometimes be helpful in reassuring that a systemic process is not present. Other laboratory tests are largely dictated by the medication that is chosen and how that medication is monitored.

KERATITIS

The cornea is the anteriorly situated window to the eye. Normally it should be clear. It can become opacified due to trauma, exposure to toxins, infection, dryness, calcium deposition, or genetic diseases such as corneal dystrophies. The three main immune-mediated diseases that affect the cornea are corneal melt, Mooren's ulcer, and Cogan's syndrome.

Corneal melt is also known as marginal keratolysis (Fig. 73.12). The majority of patients have an associated systemic form of vasculitis and usually scleritis. The medical therapy is basically the same as that described for scleritis, with emphasis on controlling the underlying systemic illness and the use of immunosuppression. Corneal melt often leads to perforation of the eye. This is usually treated surgically with tissue adhesives, conjunctival flaps, or corneal transplantation, in addition to aggressive systemic

Table 73.5 Contrasting features of scleritis and episcleritis

	Scleritis	Episcleritis
Pain	Prominent	Minimal
Duration	Years	Days to several months
Association with systemic disease	Frequent	Rare
Vessels blanch with topical vasoconstrictor	No	Yes
Associated ocular complications including visual loss	Sometimes present	Never
Vessel color	Deep pink to violaceous	Light pink

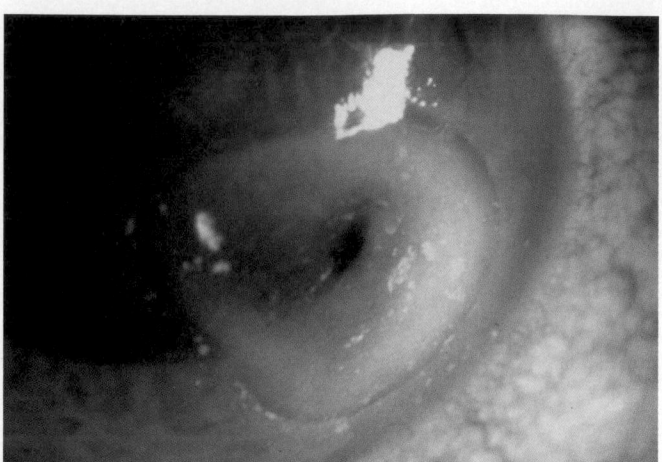

Fig. 73.12 Corneal melt. A pie-shaped wedge of the cornea is thinned. The eye is red secondary to an associated scleritis.

immunosuppression. Corneal melt is fortunately a very rare disease. A melt must also be distinguished from some other causes of corneal thinning, such as Terrien's marginal degeneration or a senile marginal furrow, both of which are generally more benign and rarely lead to perforation.

Mooren's ulcer is clinically very similar to a melt, except that there is no accompanying scleritis and no evidence for a systemic illness. The superior cornea is especially likely to be involved. Mooren's ulcer is too rare for therapeutic options to be studied with randomized clinical trials. It may respond to oral immunosuppression, which is warranted if the severity threatens visual acuity because of impending perforation of the eye. A small study not confirmed by subsequent investigation suggested that Mooren's ulcer is frequently associated with evidence of previous infection with hepatitis C.[27] Some patients with Mooren's ulcer have an autoantibody to calgranulin C. This antigen is expressed in cornea, in neutrophils, and by filarial nematodes.

The cornea is divided into three layers: the epithelium facing the atmosphere, the stroma, and the endothelium abutting the aqueous humor. Opacification of the stroma is known as interstitial keratitis. Congenital syphilis and other infections such as herpes simplex are important causes of this. Cogan's syndrome is defined as an autoimmune disease of the eighth nerve combined with interstitial keratitis, presumably also on an autoimmune basis.[28] Some ophthalmologists also recognize autoimmune eighth-nerve disease associated with other forms of ocular inflammation, such as uveitis, as examples of Cogan's disease.[29] The pathogenesis of Cogan's syndrome is presumed to be a vasculitis, and many patients will have evidence for vasculitis elsewhere in the body. The treatment usually requires aggressive use of systemic immunosuppressive medications.

CORNEAL TRANSPLANTATION AND TRANSPLANT REJECTION

Corneal transplantation involves the replacement of a diseased cornea with healthy cadaver tissue. Since the 1970s, advances in microsurgical techniques and eye banking procedures have lead to widespread acceptance of

this procedure. Currently corneal transplantation is performed 40 000 times annually in the USA alone. The usual indication for a corneal graft is poor vision, although the operation may also be undertaken to relieve ocular pain. Keratoconus, a condition in which myopic astigmatism develops as the cornea becomes progressively more conical in shape, corneal edema following intraocular surgery, and a failed previous corneal graft are the commonest medical conditions leading to corneal transplantation.[30]

Although the eye is an immune privileged site, and corneal transplants enjoy a 91% 1-year survival as shown by Kaplan–Meier survival analyses, only 62% of grafts are functional at 10 years.[30] The commonest cause of transplant failure is immunological rejection.[30] Corneal allograft rejection rarely occurs within 2 weeks, and may occur as late as 20 years following surgery. Animal studies using monoclonal antibodies directed against different T-cell subsets indicate that CD4 T cells play a critical role in the rejection response. However, the exact mechanisms responsible for this process are yet to be elucidated.

Early recognition of a rejection episode is the most important factor in achieving survival of the corneal transplant. In its most florid form, the anterior eye is obviously inflamed, with intense conjunctival injection, a cellular anterior chamber reaction and a Khodadoust line. This line, which is visible with the slit-lamp biomicroscope, is a classic sign of corneal graft rejection. It appears as a linear formation of inflammatory precipitates stretching across the corneal endothelium and represents a wave of lymphocytes marching across the cornea and destroying the endothelium in their path.[31] As endothelial pump function is lost, the cornea becomes waterlogged and opaque. At an early stage of rejection the patient may be asymptomatic, but later, ocular redness, photophobia, halos and blurred vision are frequent complaints.

An intensive and extended course of topical corticosteroids is the mainstay of treatment for a rejecting corneal graft, and in severe cases intravenous and/or oral corticosteroids may also be administered. Patients considered to be at high risk of transplant rejection, such as those with corneal neovascularization or a history of other anterior segment inflammation, are often given perioperative systemic immunosuppression. The ideal prophylactic regimen has not been defined, although various combinations of prednisone, cyclosporine and azathioprine may be used. Despite the critical influence of donor–recipient histocompatibility matching for solid organ transplant survival, the chance of corneal graft survival is not significantly improved by HLA matching.

CANCER-ASSOCIATED RETINOPATHY

Cancer-associated retinopathy (CAR) is a rare paraneoplastic syndrome that is most commonly induced by small cell carcinoma of the lung.[32] In addition, the disease has been documented in association with various tumors of the female reproductive tract, carcinoma of the breast and neuroendocrine bronchial carcinoma. For 50% of patients CAR is the presenting feature of their malignancy. Interestingly, there are now reports of retinopathy mimicking CAR, but occurring in an apparently healthy individual. Melanoma-associated retinopathy is a related syndrome, occurring in patients with metastatic cutaneous melanoma.

Histopathological examinations of postmortem specimens taken from patients with CAR consistently demonstrate loss of inner and outer segments of the retinal photoreceptors. This destruction was initially attributed to the release of a hormone-like substance by the malignant cells, but evidence has now accumulated in support of an autoimmune etiology. Affected individuals produce antibodies against one or more retinal photoreceptor antigens.[33] These antibodies induce experimental CAR when injected into laboratory animals. Although over 15 antigens have been described in relation to CAR, the commonest is the so-called CAR antigen.[33] This 23-kDa protein has been identified as recoverin, a photoreceptor protein that participates in visual adaptation. Experimental work supports the hypothesis that a single mutational event simultaneously activates the recoverin gene and eliminates functional p53, a tumor suppressor protein.[34] Consequently, there is development of a tumor that encodes for CAR antigen and stimulates formation of anti-recoverin antibody. Anti-recoverin antibodies are capable of inducing photoreceptor apoptosis, leading to the characteristic loss of both rods and cones.

Cancer-associated retinopathy generally occurs after the age of 60. Patients usually complain of decreased vision, although other symptoms may include transient visual obscurations, various positive visual phenomena, night blindness, scotomata, glare and photosensitivity. Although visual acuity may be dramatically reduced, other clinical signs are often subtle. Color vision can be impaired. An afferent pupillary defect can be present if the retinopathy is asymmetric. There may be mild iridocyclitis and/or vitritis, narrowing of retinal arterioles, mottling of retinal pigment epithelium and optic disc pallor. Visual field abnormalities occur, the most common being several midperipheral scotomata that later join up as a ring scotoma or central defect. Electroretinography shows either reduced or completely flattened amplitudes. The disease must be differentiated from optic neuritis which, unlike CAR, typically occurs in younger persons, some of whom suffer from multiple sclerosis, and is painful. In contrast to CAR, optic neuritis typically has an abrupt onset. In patients with malignancy, direct tumor spread and the effects of drugs, including chemotherapy agents, must be excluded before CAR is diagnosed.

The natural history of CAR is one of progressive visual loss, although this occurs over a variable period. Treatment directed towards curing or palliating the malignancy does not appear to prevent this loss. A series of case reports have documented improvement of vision in response to systemic corticosteroid therapy. High doses (60–80 mg) of prednisone have been used, but the minimum dose for preservation of vision is uncertain. Corticosteroid-sparing systemic immunosuppression has also been used to treat this disease. It is suggested that monitoring serum antibody levels can be used to guide therapy. However, in some cases advanced photoreceptor damage may be irreversible despite therapy.

■ IMMUNOLOGIC ETIOLOGICAL FACTORS IN 'NONIMMUNOLOGIC' OCULAR DISEASE ■

The eye contains many unique proteins that are sequestered from the immune system in early development, and which, if released systemically during adulthood, could act as autoantigens. Autoantibodies directed against certain ocular proteins have been detected in the serum of patients with a variety of ocular diseases traditionally regarded as nonimmunologic. Examples of such conditions include cataract, glaucoma, age-related macular degeneration (AMD), and retinal degenerative diseases such as retinitis pigmentosa (RP). The unanswered question is whether these antibodies contribute to the pathogenesis of the disease or merely coexist as an epiphenomenon.

Cataract is an opacification of the crystalline lens of the eye. It is the most frequent cause of blindness worldwide, most commonly occurring as an age-related phenomenon. The prevalence of cataract is approximately 70% in those over 75 years of age. The pathogenesis is poorly understood, and many varied mechanisms, including autoimmunity, have been hypothesized. Autoantibodies to sequestered lens proteins termed crystallins are present in some normal individuals, but occur significantly more frequently in patients with cataract. Immune complexes have been demonstrated in human cataractous lenses. Immunization of rabbits with human lens protein can induce cataract formation which is suppressed by systemic corticosteroid therapy. Human sera containing autoantibodies against lens proteins are cytotoxic for lens epithelial cells in culture.[35] On the other hand, it has not been possible to demonstrate T cell-mediated immune responses to lens proteins experimentally, suggesting that a process of active tolerance might prevent these autoantigens from inducing significant inflammation.

In glaucoma, a relative elevation of intraocular pressure is associated with optic nerve damage and visual field loss. More than 3 million people in the world are irreversibly blind owing to this disease, the basic mechanisms of which continue to puzzle clinicians and scientists despite very extensive research. There is recent evidence that autoimmunity may play a role in glaucoma, at least for a subgroup of affected individuals with so-called normal-tension glaucoma, in which there is no apparent elevation in intraocular pressure above population normal levels. Increased titers of various autoantibodies, including antibodies directed against extractable nuclear antigens, retinal heat shock proteins, and the retinal photoreceptor protein rhodopsin, have been measured in patients with normal-tension glaucoma. In addition, autoantibodies to optic nerve head glycosaminoglycans have been detected in the serum and optic nerve of patients with glaucoma, including the normal-tension form. It is postulated that these anti-glycosaminoglycan antibodies may increase the susceptibility of the optic nerve head to glaucomatous disease by altering physical characteristics of the tissue.

Age-related macular degeneration is the leading cause of irreversible visual loss for elderly persons in western nations. A spectrum of pathologies may occur at the macula, ranging from relatively benign focal hypo- and hyperpigmentation of the retinal pigment epithelium to sinister subretinal neovascularizations which may leak serous fluid and blood. The pathogenic stimulus for these aging changes is unknown. Genetic polymorphism of the complement regulatory protein, complement factor H, influences the susceptibility to AMD, suggesting that this disease is related to chronic inflammation.[36] Subretinal scar tissue removed from patients with advanced disease may contain immunoglobulins and complement components. The histopathology of AMD includes a few inflammatory cells, including lymphocyte subsets, and local cell populations may express class II MHC antigens. A mouse model of retinal changes that resemble macular degeneration is associated with the deletion of a receptor for a chemotactic factor for macrophages.[37] Macular drusen, seen early in the course of AMD, may also contain immunoglobulin.

Retinitis pigmentosa is a hereditary pigmentary degeneration of the retina. Just under half of patients have no family history. Various anti-retinal antibodies have been detected in approximately half of patients with this disease, including antibodies directed against the enzymes carbonic anhydrase II and enolase.[38] Interestingly, there is a significant association between the occurrence of cystoid edema at the macula, a dreaded vision-threatening complication of RP, and the presence of the circulating anti-retinal antibodies. The complication has been reported in 90% of affected individuals with antibodies, compared to only 13% of patients who are antibody negative. A less convincing association is that between an accelerated rate of visual field loss and the presence of anti-retinal antibodies.[38]

REFERENCES

1. Stuart P.M., Griffith T.S., Usui N., et al. CD95 ligand (FasL)-induced apoptosis is necessary for corneal allograft survival. J Clin Invest 1997; 99: 396–402.

2. Wang S., Boonman Z.F., Li H.C., et al. Role of TRAIL and IFN-gamma in CD4+ cell-dependent tumor rejection in the anterior chamber of the eye. J Immunol 2003; 171: 2789–2796.

3. Pasquale L.R., Dorman-Pease M.E., Lutty G.A., et al. Immunolocalization of TGF-beta1, TGF-beta2, and TGF-beta3 in the anterior segment of the human eye. Invest Ophthalmol Vis Sci 1993; 34: 23–30.

4. Cousins S.W., McCabe M.M., Danielpour D., Streilein J.W.. Identification of transforming growth factor-beta as an immunosuppressive factor in aqueous humor. Invest Ophthalmol Vis Sci 1991; 32: 2201–2211.

5. Kennedy M.C., Rosenbaum J.T., Brown J., et al. Novel production of interleukin-1 receptor antagonist peptides in normal human cornea. J Clin Invest 1995; 95: 82–88.

6. Sohn J.H., Kaplan H.J., Suk H.J., et al. Chronic low level complement activation within the eye is controlled by intraocular complement regulatory proteins. Invest Ophthalmol Vis Sci 2000; 41: 3492–3502.

7. Ferguson T.A.. The molecular basis of anterior associated immune deviation (ACAID). Ocul Immunol Inflamm 1997; 5: 213–215.

8. D'Orazio T.J., Niederkorn J.Y.. A novel role for TGF-beta and IL-10 in the induction of immune privilege. J Immunol 1998; 160: 2089–2098.

9. Dullforce P.A., Garman K.L., Seitz G.W., et al. APCs in the anterior uveal tract do not migrate to draining lymph nodes. J Immunol 2004; 172: 6701–6708.

10. Vadot E., Barth E., Billet P.. Epidemiology of uveitis – preliminary results of a prospective study in Savoy. In: Saari K.M., ed. Uveitis update New York: Excerpta Medica, 1984; 13–16.

10a. Gritz DC, Wong I.G.. Incidence and prevalence of uveitis in Northern California; the Northern California Epidemiology of Uveitis Study. Ophthalmology 2004; 111: 491–500.

11. Rosenbaum J.T.. An algorithm for the systemic evaluation of patients with uveitis: guidelines for the consultant. Semin Arthritis Rheum 1990; 19: 248–257.

12. Lim L.L., Smith J.R., Rosenbaum J.T.. Retisert (Bausch & Lomb/Control Delivery Systems). Curr Opin Investig Drugs 2005; 6: 1159–1167.

13. Rosenbaum J.T.. Acute anterior uveitis and spondyloarthropathies. Rheum Dis Clin North Am 1992; 18: 143–151.

14. Lyons J.L., Rosenbaum J.T.. Uveitis associated with inflammatory bowel disease compared with uveitis associated with spondyloarthropathy. Arch Ophthalmol 1997; 115: 61–64.

15. James D.G.. Ocular sarcoidosis. Ann NY Acad Sci 1986; 465: 551–563.

16. Kosmorsky G.S., Meisler D.M., Rice T.W., et al. Chest computed tomography and mediastinoscopy in the diagnosis of sarcoidosis-associated uveitis. Am J Ophthalmol 1998; 126: 132–134.

17. Michelson J.B., Chisari F.V.. Behçet's disease. Surv Ophthalmol 1982; 26: 190–203.

18. Kotter I., Zierhut M., Eckstein A.K., et al. Human recombinant interferon alfa-2a for the treatment of Behçet's disease with sight threatening posterior or panuveitis. Br J Ophthalmol 2003; 87: 423–431.

19. Ohno S., Nakamura S., Hori S., et al. Efficacy, safety, and pharmacokinetics of multiple administration of infliximab in Behçet's disease with refractory uveoretinitis. J.Rheumatol 2004; 31: 1362–1368.

20. Lim J.I., Tessler H.H., Goodwin J.A.. Anterior granulomatous uveitis in patients with multiple sclerosis. Ophthalmology 1991; 98: 142–145.

21. Edelsten C., Lee V., Bentley C.R., et al. An evaluation of baseline risk factors predicting severity in juvenile idiopathic arthritis associated uveitis and other chronic anterior uveitis in early childnood. Br J Ophthalmol 2002; 86: 51–56.

22. Riono W.P., Hidayat A.A., Rao N.A.. Scleritis: a clinicopathologic study of 55 cases. Ophthalmology 1999; 106: 1328–1333.

23. Rosenbaum J.T., Robertson J.E,. Jr. Recognition of posterior scleritis and its treatment with indomethacin. Retina 1993; 13: 17–21.

24. Sainz de la Maza M., Foster C.S., Jabbur N.S.. Scleritis associated with rheumatoid arthritis and other systemic immune-mediated diseases. Ophthalmology 1994; 101: 1281–1288.

25. Sainz de la Maza M., Foster C.S., Jabbur N.S.. Scleritis associated with systemic vasculitic diseases. Ophthalmology 1995; 102: 687–692.

26. Soukiasian S.H., Foster S., Niles J.L., Raizman M.B.. Diagnostic value of anti-neutrophil cytoplasmic antibodies in scleritis associated with Wegener's granulomatosis. Ophthalmology 1992; 99: 125–132.

27. Zegans M.E.S., McHugh T., Whitcher J.P., et al. Mooren ulcer in South India: serology and clinical risk factors. Am J Ophthalmol 1999; 128: 205–210.

28. Cogan D.G.. Syndrome of nonsyphilitic interstitial keratitis and vestibuloauditory symptoms. Arch Ophthalmol 1945; 33: 144–149.

29. Allen N.B., Cox C.C., Cobo M., et al. Use of immunosuppressive agents in the treatment of severe ocular and vascular manifestations of Cogan's syndrome. Am J Med 1990; 88: 296–301.

30. Williams K.A., Muehlberg S.M., Lewis R.F., Coster D.J.. Long-term outcome in corneal allotransplantation. Australian Corneal Graft Registry 1997; 29: 983.

31. Khodadoust AA, Silverstein AM. Transplantation and rejection of individual cell layers of the cornea. Invest Ophthalmol Invest Ophthalmol; 8: 180–195.

32. Weleber R.G., Watzke R.C., Shults W.T., et al. Clinical and electrophysiologic characterization of paraneoplastic and autoimmune retinopathies associates with antienolase antibodies. Am J Ophthalmol 2005; 139: 780–794.

33. Thirkill C.E., Keltner J.L., Tyler N.K., Roth A.M.. Antibody reactions with retina and cancer-associated antigens in 10 patients with cancer-associated retinopathy. Arch Ophthalmol 1993; 111: 931–937.

34. McGinnis J.F., Austin B., Klisak I., et al. Chromosomal assignment of the human gene for the cancer-associated retinopathy protein (recoverin) to chromosome 17p13.1. J Neurosci Res 1995; 40: 165–168.

35. Ibaraki N., Lin L.R., Dang L., et al. Anti-beta-crystallin antibodies (mouse) or sera from humans with age-related cataract are cytotoxic for lens epithelial cells in culture. Exp Eye Res 1997; 64: 229–238.

36. Edwards A.O., Ritter R.I., Abel K.J., et al. Complement factor H polymorphism and age-related macular degeneration. Science 2005; 308: 421–424.

37. Ambati J., Anand A., Fernandez S., et al. An animal model of age-related macular degeneration in senescent Ccl-2 or Ccr-2-deficient mice. Nature Med 2003; 9: 1390–1397.

38. Heckenlively J.R., Aptsiauri N., Nusinowitz S., et al. Investigations of antiretinal antibodies in pigmentary retinopathy and other retinal degenerations. Trans Am Ophthalmol Soc 1996; 94: 179–200.

REFERENCES

Immunologic disease of the gastrointestinal tract

Charles O. Elson III, Phillip D. Smith

74

The gastrointestinal tract mucosa is a major immune system organ, contains the majority of lymphocytes and produces the majority of immunoglobulins synthesized in the body. The host immune system interacts with the microbiota and with foreign antigens in food most directly and intimately in the intestine. It is therefore not surprising that the intestine is affected by a variety of immunodeficiencies, by chronic infections of the mucosa, and by autoimmune and idiopathic chronic inflammatory diseases. This chapter describes the spectrum of different immune disorders involving the gastrointestinal tract.

■ GASTROINTESTINAL DISORDERS ASSOCIATED WITH PRIMARY IMMUNODEFICIENCY ■

Primary immunodeficiency diseases are uncommon disorders caused by congenital defects in B, T, or phagocytic cells. These diseases are frequently associated with an array of gastrointestinal illnesses that vary in severity, depending on the type of underlying immunodeficiency, the level of immune dysfunction, and the presence of enteric pathogens.[1] Importantly, the association between gastrointestinal illnesses and immunodeficiency disease emphasizes the fundamental role of systemic and mucosal immunity in maintaining gastrointestinal health. Here we describe the major immunodeficiency diseases and their associated gastrointestinal manifestations.

COMMON VARIABLE IMMUNODEFICIENCY DISEASE

Diagnosis

Common variable immunodeficiency (CVID) is an uncommon disorder (1 in 50 000 Caucasians) characterized by reduced concentrations of most or all immunoglobulin (Ig) isotypes (IgG, IgA, IgE and IgM) with defective specific-antibody production; frequent sinopulmonary and gastrointestinal infections; and less frequent immunologic abnormalities, including autoimmune and lymphoproliferative disorders (Chapter 34).[2] CVID occurs equally in men and women and typically presents in the third decade of life, with a small subset presenting in early childhood. The late presentation of CVID suggests an acquired disease, but a familial association of individuals with CVID is consistent with an inherited disorder.

Individuals with CVID usually have normal numbers of surface Ig-bearing B-cell precursors, but the cells are unable to differentiate into Ig-secreting cells. This defect is accompanied by variable reductions in the secretion of IgA and IgG in most patients, as well as IgM and IgE in many, resulting in corresponding reductions in serum Ig levels and defective antigen-specific antibody responses. Cell-mediated immunity is usually normal in CVID, although a subset of patients display T-cell abnormalities, including impaired T-cell receptor and CD28 signaling, reduced expression of activation molecules, reduced Th2 cytokine secretion, enhanced apoptosis, and deficient inducible co-stimulator molecule expression.[3] These abnormalities lead to a reduction in T-cell activation and proliferation. The role of T cells in regulating B-cell function was demonstrated indirectly by the normalization of reduced Ig levels and impaired antibody responses in a patient with CVID after he acquired HIV-1 infection and depleted his T cells, allowing restoration of B-cell function.[4] Defective myeloid dendritic cell function has also been reported in some patients with CVID.[5]

Clinical manifestations

As a consequence of the above immune defects, patients with CVID have a high incidence of sinopulmonary infections and gastrointestinal manifestations. Recurrent pulmonary infection can lead to irreversible chronic lung disease with bronchiectasis. The most common pathogens include the encapsulated bacteria *Streptococcus pneumoniae* and *Hemophilus influenzae*. In normal persons, IgG antibodies, particularly of the IgG_2 subclass, are directed against encapsulated bacteria and are the major opsinin in mucosal fluids; among patients with CVID, those with IgG_2 deficiency have the highest frequency of infections with encapsulated bacteria.

■ GASTROINTESTINAL DISEASES THAT CAUSE IMMUNODEFICIENCY ■

Protein-losing enteropathy due to gastrointestinal and extra-intestinal disease can lead to excessive loss of proteins, including serum Igs. Causes of protein-losing enteropathy include increased interstitial pressure (intestinal lymphangiectasia, mesenteric lymphatic obstruction, tuberculosis, sarcoidosis, lymphoma, retroperitoneal fibrosis or constrictive pericarditis and congestive heart failure), ulcerative gastric or intestinal/colonic disease (Crohn's disease, pseudomembranous colitis or graft-versus-host disease) and nonulcerative diseases (Ménétrièr's disease, infectious enteropathies, Whipple's disease, eosinophilic gastroenteritis and sprue). Here we discuss intestinal lymphangiectasia and Whipple's disease, two prototype intestinal diseases that can lead to immunodeficiency.

INTESTINAL LYMPHANGIECTASIA

Diagnosis

Intestinal lymphangiectasia (IL) is a rare disease that occurs as a primary congenital disorder (Milroy's disease) or as a secondary disorder due to the causes of increased interstitial pressure listed above. Increased intestinal lymphatic pressure leads to intestinal leakage of lymph, impaired absorption of chylomicrons, and reduced re-entry of intestinal lymphocytes into the circulation. In addition to the leakage of lymph due to increased pressure, lymphatic fistulae may form, allowing intestinal lymph containing serum proteins, Igs, chylomicrons and lymphocytes to drain directly into the intestinal lumen. The normal daily loss of serum protein into the gastrointestinal tract is <2%, but in the presence of intestinal lymphangiectasia may increase to 5–50%.[9] Loss of serum proteins and lymphocytes leads to varying levels of hypogammaglobulinemia, lymphocytopenia and impaired cell-mediated immunity.

Clinical manifestations

Patients with primary IL usually present in the second or third decade of life with prominent edema due to lymphatic obstruction and/or protein-losing enteropathy-induced hypoalbuminemia and gastrointestinal complications. The edema is usually symmetric in the setting of major lymphatic obstruction, and asymmetric when peripheral lymphatic obstruction is present. The gastrointestinal manifestations include diarrhea, abdominal pain, distension, nausea, vomiting, malabsorption, and steatorrhea. Chylous ascites may be present as a result of blockage of serosal and mesenteric lymphatics; chylous pleural effusions may accompany blockage of the thoracic duct. The diagnosis is confirmed by the presence of hypoalbuminemia (<2.0–2.5 g/dL), lymphocytopenia (<1000–1500 cells/mm$_2$) and a jejunal biopsy showing dilated lymphatics. Multiple biopsies may be necessary, because the changes may be patchy.

Clinical management

Treatment of primary IL focuses on therapy of the clinical manifestations, whereas treatment of secondary IL is directed to correcting the underlying cause. Peripheral edema is treated by postural drainage and

stockings. A low-fat diet reduces chylomicrons in obstructed lymphatics, thereby reducing intestinal lymphatic pressure, intestinal leakage of lymph, and the excretion of fat and protein. Replacing long-chain triglycerides with medium-chain triglycerides may reduce the steatorrhea and diarrhea, as medium-chain triglycerides are more water soluble and may be more readily absorbed into the portal venous system. Consistent with intact antigen-specific antibody responses,[9] intestinal infections are not more common in IL.

WHIPPLE'S DISEASE

Diagnosis

Whipple's disease is a systemic infection caused by the Gram-negative actinomycete *Tropheryma whippelii*. Organisms may infect any region of the gastrointestinal tract mucosa, but most commonly the proximal small intestine. Bacilli are identified microscopically in the lamina propria as either free PAS-positive bacilli or as PAS-positive particles within macrophages. The particles represent intact or partially degraded bacilli, causing the macrophages to appear 'foamy.' *T. whippelii* have not so far been cultivated, therefore the diagnosis is based on the presence of clinical features of Whipple's disease and an intestinal biopsy containing PAS-positive, diastase-resistant, acid fast-negative macrophages. The biopsy also often shows dilated lacteals, probably due to compression of the lymphatics by the numerous large macrophages and neutral fat deposits and/or to compression of the mesenteric lymphatics by fibrosis. Other tissues also may contain PAS-positive macrophages, including lymph nodes, liver and spleen. When extra-intestinal PAS-positive macrophages are identified, histoplasmosis, nontuberculous mycobacterial infection and macroglobulinemia should be excluded, as PAS-positive macrophages may accompany these diseases as well.

Clinical manifestations

The classic presentation of Whipple's disease is that of a man (85% of cases) in his fourth or fifth decade with weight loss, diarrhea, abdominal pain and arthralgias. Complications of the gastrointestinal tract and the intestinal lymphatic system dominate the clinical presentation. Diarrhea with fat and carbohydrate malabsorption is present in the majority of patients, although the etiology of the diarrhea is unclear. Intestinal erosions and ulcerations, leading to significant bleeding, are also common. Extra-intestinal disease involves the central nervous system in approximately 10% of patients, most commonly manifesting as dementia, ophthalmoplegia and myoclonus. Migratory arthralgias usually predate the other symptoms, involve large joints, and do not demonstrate inflammation. Cardiac manifestations include pericarditis and endocarditis. Uveitis, retinitis, vitritis and optic neuritis are important ocular manifestations of Whipple's disease. Pleuritis, hyperpigmentation and lymphadenopathy also may be present in a substantial proportion of patients.

Treatment

Without antimicrobial therapy Whipple's disease is fatal. The recommended antibiotic regimen includes procaine penicillin G and streptomycin for 14 days, followed by trimethoprim-sulfamethoxazole for 1 year. Dietary folic acid should also be given.

HUMAN IMMUNODEFICIENCY VIRUS TYPE-1 INFECTION ■

The first cases of the acquired immunodeficiency syndrome (AIDS) were recognized in the USA in 1981, and human immunodeficiency virus type-1 (HIV-1) was identified as the causative agent in 1984. Since then, AIDS has emerged as the greatest pandemic in human history (Chapter 37). Although first recognized in the USA, the epicenter of the epidemic is sub-Saharan Africa, home to 10% of the world's population and by mid-2006 home to 64% of all persons with HIV-1 infection. All African countries (except Angola) have an estimated adult prevalence rate >10%, and in some countries (South Africa, Botswana, Lesotho, Swaziland and Zimbabwe) the rate approaches or exceeds 20%.[10] Next to Africa, the Caribbean has the highest adult prevalence rate in the world. Countries with alarming and increasing rates of HIV-1 infection include India, Brazil and China.

Mucosal surfaces play a fundamental role in HIV-1 transmission, pathogenesis, natural history and vaccine strategy. Heterosexual transmission occurs through the genital mucosa, homosexual transmission through the lower and upper gastrointestinal tract mucosa, and vertical transmission via the upper gastrointestinal tract mucosa. Worldwide, approximately 85% of all HIV-1 infections are transmitted across the genital mucosa. Following inoculation onto a mucosal surface, translocation of virus from the apical surface into the lamina propria probably occurs through dendritic cell trapping, possibly via C-type lectins such as DC-SIGN, which bind HIV-1 gp120, and/or through epithelial cell transcytosis.[11] In the subepithelial lamina propria the virus encounters mononuclear target cells. However, in contrast to monocytes and macrophages in other tissues, resident intestinal macrophages lack the co-receptors necessary for HIV-1 infection.[12, 13] Thus, lymphocytes are the initial mononuclear target cell in mucosal infection. The majority of these cells are activated memory T cells that express chemokine receptor 5 (CCR5), the co-receptor for the entry of CCR5-tropic HIV-1. Studies of simian immunodeficiency SIV (SIV) in macaques, a model for HIV-1 infection, as well as some studies of HIV-1 infection in humans, show rapid and massive depletion of intestinal CD4+ memory T cells within days to weeks of inoculation, regardless of the route of transmission. This depletion localizes to the effector region (lamina propria), persists in untreated subjects, is incompletely restored during antiretroviral therapy, and results in profound immunodeficiency. Viremia during early infection leads to rapid dissemination of virus to lymphoid organs, where persistent infection is established. T-cell activation via virus-induced cytokines and aberrant signaling predispose and enhance virus replication, which in the setting of rapid T-cell turnover promotes destruction of the immune system, perpetuating the immune deficiency and ineffective viral clearance. Rapid virus mutation and evolving glycosylation of the V1-V4 binding region of gp120 contribute to evasion of neutralizing antibodies and cytotoxic T cells. Blood monocytes express CD4, the primary receptor for HIV-1, and CXCR4, the co-receptor for CXCR4-tropic viruses, as well as CCR5, and probably participate in dissemination of the virus and serve as a reservoir in late-stage disease. These virus-induced cellular events predispose to the clinical manifestation of HIV-1 infection, particularly in the gastrointestinal tract.

Diagnosis

The diagnosis of HIV-1 infection is based on the detection of antibodies to viral antigens and/or the detection of viral components. Antibodies to HIV-1 are detected by enzyme immunoassay, which has a sensitivity of >99.5%. A positive or indeterminate test is confirmed by Western blotting. For an indeterminate Western blot, or to monitor the effect of therapy on viral load, a polymerase chain reaction (PCR)-based assay is used to detect viral RNA or proviral DNA. AIDS is diagnosed in a person with either HIV-1 infection plus a T-cell count <200 cells/μL, or HIV-1 infection plus an AIDS-defining opportunistic infection or a pathological process such as encephalopathy.

Clinical manifestations

The first clinical manifestation of HIV-1 infection is a mononucleosis-like syndrome that occurs 2–6 weeks after virus inoculation in 50–70% of acutely infected people. Infrequently, patients will progress rapidly (within months) to late-stage disease, with a prompt decline in CD4+ T cells and the appearance of opportunistic infections, particularly *Candida* infections of the oral cavity and esophagus.[14] After seroconversion and the resultant decline in viremia in response to the anti-HIV-1 antibodies, symptoms of the acute syndrome subside and a prolonged period (median 10 years) of clinical latency follows,[15] despite active virus replication and gradual destruction of the immune system. During this period, the number of CD4 T cells steadily declines and the patient becomes progressively more susceptible to an array of fungal, viral, parasitic and bacterial organisms. When CD4 T-cell numbers reach <200/μL, patients are particularly susceptible to *Pneumocystis jiroveci*, and when the number declines to <50 cells/μL they are at high risk for cytomegalovirus and *Mycobacterium avium* complex infections.[16] The opportunistic organisms that cause gastrointestinal disease, particularly diarrheal illness, in immunosuppressed HIV-1-infected patients are listed in Table 74.1. In addition to infections, gastrointestinal lymphoma is more common in HIV-1-infected than uninfected persons. Kaposi's sarcoma was the most common neoplasm of the gastrointestinal tract at the outset of the epidemic, but is now rare in HIV-1-infected persons.

Treatment

Highly active antiretroviral therapy (HAART) combines reverse transcriptase inhibitor and protease inhibitor drugs into a powerful and highly effective antiviral therapy. HAART has revolutionized the

Table 74.1 Gastrointestinal pathogens associated with immunosuppression in HIV-1 infection

Organ process	Pathogens
Esophagitis, esophageal ulcer	*Candida albicans*; herpes simplex virus; cytomegalovirus
Gastritis, gastric ulcer	Cytomegalovirus; *Mycobacterium avium* complex
Cholecystitis	*Cryptosporidium*; cytomegalovirus; *Microsporidium*; *Isospora belli*
Enteritis, intestinal inflammatory mass	*Cryptosporidium*; *Microsporidium*; *Isospora belli*; *Mycobacterium avium* complex; *Salmonella* sp.; *Campylobacter jejuni*
Colitis, colonic inflammatory mass	Cytomegalovirus; *Cryptosporidium*; *Mycobacterium avium* complex; *M. intracellulare*; *Shigella flexneri*; *Campylobacter jejuni*; *Histoplasma capsulatum*; adenovirus; herpes simplex virus (rectum)

treatment of HIV-1 disease, dramatically reducing the rate of death and the incidence of opportunistic infections as well as increasing the resolution of ongoing opportunistic infections. An additional benefit of HAART is a reduction in the use of antimicrobial agents, resulting in fewer *C. difficile* infections.

Standard antibiotic therapy remains an integral component of the management of HIV-1-associated opportunistic and nonopportunistic pathogens of the gastrointestinal tract. In this regard, the side effects, expense and availability of HAART, as well as HIV-1 resistance to HAART, require that many infections be treated with antibiotics. The management and antibiotic regimens for infectious diarrhea in HIV-1-infected persons have been described in detail elsewhere.[14, 16]

GASTRITIS

Chronic gastritis is common in the general population, particularly in the aged. On clinical grounds chronic gastritis has been categorized as either type A, involving mainly the body of the stomach, or type B, mainly involving the antrum. In most individuals chronic gastritis is silent, although a variety of complaints, such as dyspepsia, fullness, nausea, vomiting, and abdominal pain, are sometimes attributed to it, and in some instances it may well be responsible for symptoms. Inflammation of these two areas of the stomach has different effects on normal physiology. Gastric acid is produced by parietal or oxyntic cells located in the body of the stomach. The antrum does not have parietal cells, but is enriched for endocrine cells that produce gastrin. Gastrin stimulates gastric acid secretion, and acid in turn inhibits gastrin.

Autoimmune gastritis falls into the type A category, and most instances of type B gastritis are due to *Helicobacter pylori* infection, but as noted below the two may be linked.

AUTOIMMUNE GASTRITIS/PERNICIOUS ANEMIA

Autoimmune gastritis occurs with increased frequency in individuals with other organ-specific autoimmune disorders, such as Hashimoto's thyroiditis, hypothyroidism, Graves' disease, insulin-dependent diabetes mellitus, Addison's disease, hyperparathyroidism, and vitiligo.[17]

A number of serologic tests are available if the diagnosis is suspected (Table 74.2), including serum anti-parietal cell antibodies, anti-intrinsic factor antibodies, serum gastrin, and serum pepsinogen I.[18] Individuals with a positive anti-parietal cell antibody and a high gastrin have a high likelihood of having autoimmune gastritis.

The diagnosis is made by endoscopy and gastric biopsy. The histopathologic lesion consists of a mononuclear infiltrate in the gastric mucosa with variable atrophy of the gastric glands. Intestinal metaplasia is commonly associated and can be a precursor of gastric carcinoma. Gastric carcinoids can occur as well. Radiologic tests are not useful in either suspecting or making a diagnosis.

The major clinical manifestation of autoimmune gastritis is that of vitamin B_{12} (cobalamin) deficiency, which results in a megaloblastic anemia (pernicious anemia) and a variety of neuropsychiatric manifestations. Dietary cobalamin is normally released by the acid proteolysis in the stomach. The released cobalamin then binds to a salivary B_{12}-binding protein called haptocorrin. Haptocorrin–cobalamin complexes are degraded by proteases in the intestine, and cobalamin then binds to gastric intrinsic factor; intrinsic factor–cobalamin complexes transit through the small intestine and bind to specific receptors on enterocytes in the distal ileum, triggering endocytosis and absorption. Autoimmune gastritis results in both achlorhydria and an absence of intrinsic factor, both of which contribute to the malabsorption of cobalamin. Cobalamin deficiency manifests as anemia, glossitis, neuropathy, depression, and memory impairment. Such individuals generally have a low vitamin B_{12} level and an elevated serum gastrin. Diagnosis of vitamin B_{12} malabsorption can be confirmed with a Schilling test with and without intrinsic factor. There are many other causes of cobalamin deficiency.

Pathophysiology

Autoimmune gastritis is one of the classic organ-specific autoimmune diseases. The major autoantigens recognized by T and B cells are the α and β subunits of H^+-K^+-ATPase, which is the acid pump that is localized on the canalicular or luminal surface of parietal cells.[19] Parietal cells also produce intrinsic factor. Approximately 90% of patients with autoimmune gastritis have antibodies to parietal cells, and 50–60% have antibodies to intrinsic factor. Experimental models of autoimmune gastritis in the mouse seem to mimic the disorder closely, e.g., the same autoantibodies develop in mice with autoimmune gastritis as are seen in

Table 74.2 Biomarkers useful in the diagnosis of gastritis and gastric atrophy

	Autoimmune Gastritis	H. pylori Gastritis*	Comment
Serum gastrin	↑	↓	Increased in gastric atrophy
Serum pepsinogen I	↓	↓	Decreased in gastric atrophy
IgG antipareital cell antibody	↑	-	Indicates autoimmune gastritis
IgG Anti-H. pylori	-	+	Indicates H. pylori infection

*When H. pylori affects the body of the stomach the pattern becomes more like that of autoimmune gastritis.

humans.[20] The autoantibodies are most likely not directly pathogenic but rather a reflection of T-cell autoreactivity, because in experimental models CD4 T cells are the effector cells that mediate tissue injury.[21] The T-cell epitopes in the α and β chains of H+-K+-ATPase have been defined, and interestingly some murine T-cell epitopes overlap with those recognized by human T cells.[22] These experimental models have also been crucial in the identification of the CD25+ (natural) T regulatory (Treg) cell. Autoimmune gastritis, as well as other organ-specific autoimmune diseases, arises in mice thymectomized at 3 days of life. In a series of classic studies this was found to be due to ablation of the development of CD25+ Treg cells.[23, 24]

A subset of patients with *H. pylori* gastritis can develop gastric atrophy.[25] CD4 T cells that respond to both H+-K+-ATPase and to *H. pylori* antigens have been identified in such patients,[26] suggesting that in some individuals autoreactive CD4 T cells can be activated by cross-cross-reactive epitopes on *H. pylori* via molecular mimicry. In some environments, a high rate of *H. pylori* infection has been found in individuals with autoimmune gastritis, particularly in the younger age groups.[27] Because acid releases iron from food, individuals with gastric atrophy can present with iron deficiency anemia (as well as a megaloblastic anemia), and such iron-deficient individuals may be refractory to oral iron replacement.[28]

Treatment

There is no treatment for autoimmune gastritis. The treatment of vitamin B12 deficiency consists of injections of vitamin B12 100 μg IM monthly, or daily administration of cobalamin 1 mg orally.

HELICOBACTER PYLORI GASTRITIS

Type B chronic gastritis is mainly due to chronic *H. pylori* infection. *H. pylori* is a Gram-negative bacterium that persistently colonizes the mucous layer of the stomach, particularly in the antrum. The bacterium is usually acquired via oral ingestion in childhood and is transmitted within families, particularly in the setting of poor hygiene associated with lower socioeconomic conditions. Consequently, in most developing countries 60–80% of children less than 10 years of age are infected, whereas in industrialized countries less than 10% of similarly aged children are infected.[29] Although most *H. pylori* reside in the mucus, approximately 20% attach to the epithelium, probably facilitated by an adhesin, BabA, that binds to fucosylated Lewis B blood-group antigens

on gastric epithelial cells. Most *H. pylori* that cause disease contain a 29-gene 37 000-bp region called the *cag* pathogenicity island (*cag*PAI). The *cag* genes encode components of the type IV secretory system that is responsible for injecting the CagA protein into gastric epithelial cells, leading to the *cag*PAI-dependent induction of inflammatory responses through the activation of NF-κB.[30]

Diagnosis

H. pylori is identified in the gastric mucosa using noninvasive and invasive tests. These include the urea breath test (sensitivity 90%; specificity 92%), serologic assay for IgG anti-*H. pylori* antibodies (sensitivity 91%; specificity 92%), Warthin–Starry staining (sensitivity 93%; specificity 99%), CLO test for bacterial urease (sensitivity 90%; specificity 100%), and histology for chronic inflammation (sensitivity 100%; specificity 66%).[31] Overall, the serologic assay for *H. pylori* infection is the most convenient test for the detection of the bacterium and for monitoring therapeutic effectiveness, as the antibody titer will decline approximately 50% by 6 months after successful eradication.[32]

Clinical manifestations

Colonization of the stomach by *H. pylori* is the major risk factor for gastritis, peptic ulceration, gastric adenocarcinoma, and gastric lymphoma. Virtually all infected persons develop gastritis, but the course of infection is influenced by *H. pylori*- and host-specific factors. Patients with antral-dominant gastritis have higher gastric acid output and are predisposed to duodenal ulcers but not gastric cancer. In contrast, those with gastritis involving the body of the stomach are predisposed to gastric ulceration and the loss of parietal cells, achlorhydria, gastric atrophy, intestinal metaplasia, dysplasia and gastric cancer.[33] Carcinogenesis is influenced by host genetic diversity, including polymorphisms in the *IL-1β* and *TNF-α* cytokine genes, which are associated with increased corpus cancer, possibly through the acid inhibitory activity of IL-1β and TNF-α.[34] Among *H. pylori*-infected persons the cumulative long-term risk for ulcer disease varies between 2% and 10%, depending on the study population. In developed countries, the overall risk for developing gastric cancer is estimated to be increased sixfold among *H. pylori*-infected persons. Importantly, *H. pylori* loses its ecological niche in the setting of achlorhydria and gastric atrophy; consequently, it is difficult to detect in persons with gastric cancer.

KEY CONCEPTS

CLINICAL MANIFESTATIONS OF *H. PYLORI* INFECTION (INCIDENCE)

>> Chronic gastritis (100%)

>> Gastric and duodenal ulcer (2–10%)

>> Gastric adenocarcinoma (23%)

>> Gastric mucosa-associated lymphoid tissue (MALT) lymphoma (<3%)

>> Iron-deficiency anemia (not known)

The incidence of *H. pylori*-associated gastric lymphoma is probably less than that of gastric adenocarcinoma, but unlike gastric adenocarcinoma, in many *H. pylori*-infected patients gastric lymphoma can be eradicated with antibiotic therapy.

Treatment

In countries with a high prevalence of *H. pylori* infection, the cost and risks associated with antimicrobial treatment do not justify mass eradication programs. However, therapy is indicated in patients with *H. pylori*-related symptoms, or complications such as peptic ulcer, mucosa-associated lymphoid tissue (MALT) lymphoma, or a first-degree relative with *H. pylori* infection. A triple-drug regimen for 2 weeks is usually necessary for successful eradication. The combination of bismuth, tetracycline and metronidazole is highly effective. However, the widespread use of antibiotics has resulted in the development of resistant strains, which may require follow-up evaluation for the persistence or recurrence of symptoms.

■ CELIAC DISEASE ■

Celiac disease is a chronic inflammatory disease of the small intestine induced in genetically susceptible individuals by ingestion of the cereal grains of wheat, barley, and rye that collectively are known as 'glutens.' The inflammation is accompanied by a variable degree of villous atrophy and malabsorption of nutrients, but has many manifestations in other organ systems. It has been called a variety of names, including celiac sprue, gluten-sensitive enteropathy, and nontropical sprue. Celiac disease occurs worldwide and the prevalence seems to range between 1 in 100 and 1 in 300 individuals in various parts of the world.[35] In the USA the prevalence is estimated to be 0.5–1% of the population (http://consensus.nih.gov/cons/118/118cdc_intro.htm). As in many other immune-mediated inflammatory diseases, there are environmental, genetic, and immune components in its pathogenesis. Celiac disease is widely considered an autoimmune disease due to serologic reactivity to tissue matrix autoantigens.

Clinical presentations

The classic gastrointestinal presentation of celiac disease is chronic diarrhea, weight loss or failure to grow, malabsorption, and abdominal distension, particularly in children. This presentation is now recognized to be uncommon.[35, 37] Celiac disease manifestations are quite variable, can start at any age, and can affect organ systems other than the gastrointestinal tract. Other gastrointestinal presentations that can occur include chronic constipation, abdominal pain, bloating, and anorexia. Nongastrointestinal manifestations are shown in Table 74.3 and clearly can affect multiple organ systems. Patients with these manifestations have few or no GI symptoms, and so considering the diagnosis can be quite challenging. In addition to the entities shown in Table 74.3, a number of neuropsychiatric conditions have been associated with celiac disease, including fatigue, depression, anxiety, peripheral neuropathy, cerebellar ataxia, other neurologic syndromes, and migraine headaches.

Dermatitis herpetiformis is now considered a dermatologic manifestation of celiac disease.[38] This condition consists of a pruritic, vesicular, symmetrical rash, particularly on extensor surfaces of the limbs. The diagnosis is made by biopsy, which demonstrates acute inflammatory infiltrates below the dermis and granulated deposits of IgA and complement at the basement membrane by immunohistochemistry. Gliadin peptides have not been formally proven in these immune complexes, but are inferred by the loss of IgA deposits with a gluten-free diet. Most patients with dermatitis herpetiformis have no GI symptoms. The response to a gluten-free diet is slow and takes many months. Anti-inflammatory agents such as dapsone are frequently used for rapid symptom relief. If a biopsy diagnosis of dermatitis herpetiformis is made, there is no need for small bowel biopsy to confirm celiac disease because the two diagnoses are considered equivalent.

Serologic tests

Serologic tests are available to help in the diagnosis of celiac disease. These tests can be used to identify symptomatic individuals who should have a small-intestinal biopsy. Although anti-gliadin antibodies have for many years been measured for this purpose, these antibodies are not sufficiently sensitive or specific and have been largely replaced by the newer tests discussed below.

Endomysial antibodies (EMA) are detected by immunohistochemical tests that detect IgA binding to a connective tissue component surrounding smooth muscle fibers. This test is a more refined version of the older reticulin antibody test. It is operator dependent and thus somewhat subjective, but has high sensitivity and specificity (Table 74.4). The specific antigen detected by these IgA antibodies has been identified as tissue transglutaminase, which has allowed an ELISA to be developed

Table 74.3 Multisystemic presentations of celiac disease

Dermatitis herpetiformis	Elevated transaminase test
Dental enamel hypoplasia of permanent teeth	Infertility
Osteopenia/osteoporosis	Autoimmune endocrine disorders
Delayed puberty	Epilepsy with occipital calcifications
Short stature	Neuropsychiatric symptoms
Iron deficiency anemia	Aphthous stomatitis Depression

Table 74.4 Serologic tests for celiac disease (From Farrell RJ, Kelly CP. Celiac sprue. N Engl J Med 2002;346:180–188)

	Sensitivity (%)	Specificity (%)
IgA anti-gliadin antibody	75–90	82–95
IgG anti-gliadin antibody	69–85	73–90
IgA anti-endomesium (EMA)	85–98	97–100
IgA anti-tissue transglutaminase (TTG)	90–98	94–97

for its measurement. The initial versions of this ELISA used a guinea pig protein, but the second generation of the test now utilizes human recombinant tissue transglutaminase, which is preferred. IgA anti-tissue transglutaminase (TTG) has as high a sensitivity and specificity as the EMA. Either is suitable as a screening assay. Because both of these assays detect IgA antibodies, IgA deficiency is a possible confounder. In symptomatic individuals concomitant measurement of serum IgA can be helpful to interpret a negative result. Both assays can be falsely negative in young children. These serologic tests become negative when celiac patients follow a gluten-free diet. Thus, some clinicians monitor compliance with the diet by periodically re-testing the IgA EMA or IgA TTG.

The application of these newer serologic tests to blood donor populations has identified many positives,[35] and this is the basis of the estimates that 0.5–1% of the population in the USA might have celiac disease. Only a small percentage of the total estimated cases are diagnosed, which has led to the analogy of celiac disease as an iceberg, with diagnosed cases representing only the tip. Such screening of healthy populations and of those at risk has detected individuals with positive serologic tests but no symptoms. Some of these individuals have an abnormal small bowel biopsy compatible with celiac disease, and this group has been termed 'silent' celiac disease. Other individuals have a normal small bowel biopsy despite positive serologies and are thought to have latent celiac disease. Some of the latter individuals will develop typical small intestinal lesions over time, but others do not (Fig. 74.1). The natural history of these two groups is unclear, and whether the 'silent' group should follow a gluten-free diet is at present unknown (http://www.worldgastroenterology.org/globalguidelines/guide13/g_data13_en.htm#sec08).

Because this is the age of the Internet, it is not uncommon that individuals with various symptoms diagnose themselves as having celiac disease. They often then put themselves on a gluten-free diet and later appear in the physician's office wanting to know whether they do indeed have celiac disease. This represents a clinical conundrum, in that both the serologic tests and the biopsy return to negative or normal on a gluten-free diet. One approach is to test such individuals for HLA DQ2 and DQ8, which if negative virtually excludes the diagnosis of celiac disease. Another approach is to put them back on a gluten-containing diet and follow their serologic reactivity. Individuals with positive serology could undergo a small bowel biopsy to establish the diagnosis. There are individuals who do not have celiac disease but have gluten intolerance, i.e., are symptomatic when eating gluten-containing foods. Such individuals can safely remain on a gluten-free diet for life and may be able to tolerate small amounts of gluten without symptoms.

Diagnosis/histology

A small bowel biopsy is obligatory to confirm a diagnosis of celiac disease. The histologic features include increased numbers of intraepithelial lymphocytes, villous shortening or flattening, crypt hyperplasia, and infiltration of the lamina propria with lymphoid cells. These changes form a spectrum from mild to severe, and this spectrum can be quantified using a numerical grading scale called the Marsh criteria. These histopathologic changes are maximal in the proximal small intestine and in severe cases may extend down into the ileum. However, the lesions can transition back to normal, even in the upper jejunum. This variation in the extent of small bowel affected probably accounts for the variability in symptoms seen in patients. Endoscopic biopsies sample only the second and third portions of the duodenum, and thus at present there is no way to measure the length of small bowel affected.

Biopsy is part of the gold standard for diagnosing celiac disease, but other diseases can share similar histopathologic features, including tropical sprue, HIV enteropathy, immunodeficiency states, radiation damage, graft-versus-host disease, chronic ischemia, Crohn's disease, Zollinger–Ellison syndrome, and eosinophilic gastroenteritis, to name but a few. Many of these alternative diagnoses can be eliminated by the clinical situation. Thus, in addition to a compatible small intestinal biopsy, a clinical response to a gluten-free diet is required for a definitive diagnosis to be made. This response should include both symptomatic improvement and conversion of the serologic tests to negative.

Genetics

It has long been recognized that there is a strong genetic component in celiac disease. For example, the prevalence among first-degree relatives is 10%, and the disease concordance in identical twins is up to 70%. There is a strong link to the HLA locus, and within that locus the disease is linked specifically to the DQ2 and DQ8 class 2 alleles (Chapter 5).[39, 40] DQ2 is formed by an α chain encoded by DQA1*05 and a β chain encoded by DQB1*02 and is present in 90–95% of patients with celiac disease. The DQ8 α chain is encoded by DQA1*03 and the β by DQB1*0302 and is present in the 5–10% of celiac patients not bearing DQ2. These alleles form an antigen-binding MHC class II molecule on the surface of antigen-presenting cells that has high affinity for the gluten peptides that trigger disease. Based on the crystal structure of a DQ2–gluten peptide complex, this binding is enhanced by deamidation of selected glutamines to negatively charged glutamic acid residues, which in turn is accomplished by tissue transglutaminase.[41] Populations with a low frequency of DQ2 and DQ8, for example in Japan and China, have low

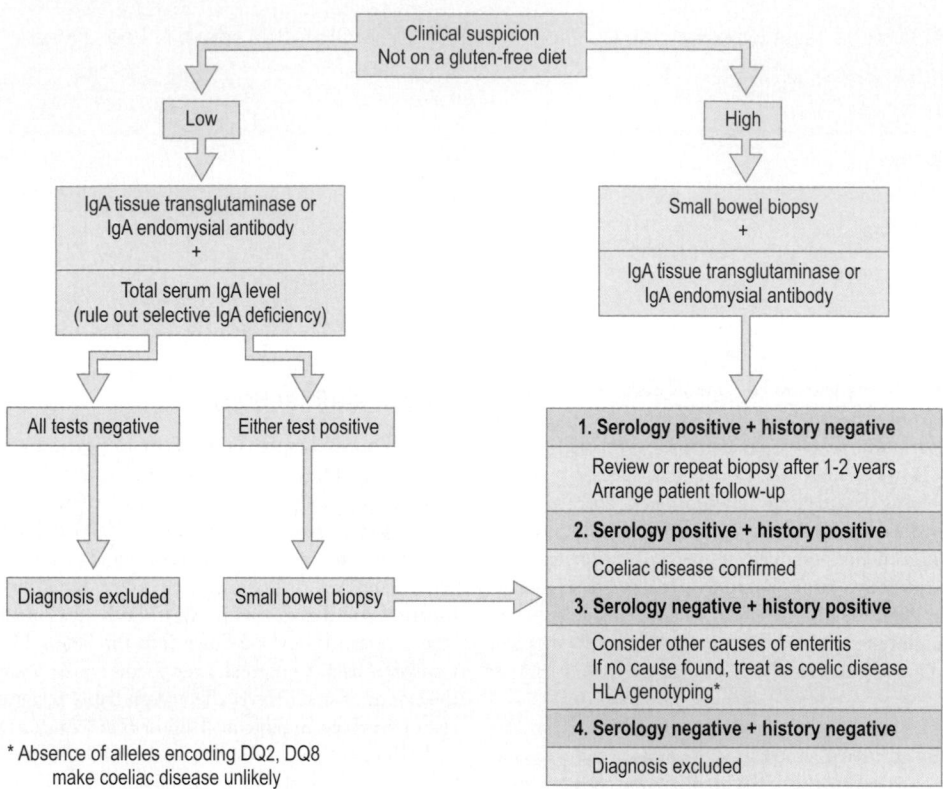

Fig. 74.1 Diagnostic algorithm for celiac disease.

frequency of celiac disease. However, these HLA genes are necessary albeit not sufficient for celiac disease to occur, because in North America and Europe some 30–40% of the population is DQ2 positive. These two alleles account for an estimated 30% of the risk for celiac disease, and thus other genetic loci are probably involved. There are limited data on what these other genes are, but quantitative gene locus mapping has identified at least one locus on chromosome 5q31-33.[42] Interestingly, this same locus is implicated in other chronic inflammatory diseases.

Environmental/dietary factors

Exposure to cereal grains from wheat, barley, and rye is obligatory for celiac disease to manifest, even in genetically susceptible individuals. This is proven by the absence of lesions and symptoms in individuals with celiac disease on a gluten-free diet. Wheat, barley, and rye share a common ancestry in the grass family. Oats are more distantly related and are tolerated in the diet of most celiac disease patients. By definition, gluten refers only to the cereal grain proteins of wheat; the analogous proteins in rye are the hordeins, and in barley are the secalins. However, all three have been collectively and loosely referred to as glutens or gluten peptides. These proteins are responsible for the elasticity and other favorable cooking properties of these grains.

Gluten proteins from all three sources share a high proline and glutamine content, which renders them relatively resistant to degradation by mammalian digestive enzymes. This resistance allows gluten peptides

to remain of a size able to bind to DQ2 or DQ8 and stimulate CD4 T cells. Indeed, T cells have been isolated from the mucosa of patients with celiac disease that react to gluten peptides in the context of HLADQ2 or DQ8.[43] T cells isolated from nonceliac mucosa, even of individuals that are DQ2 positive, do not contain gluten reactive T cells.

Pathogenesis

There is strong evidence that lamina propria CD4 T cells play an important role in the pathogenesis of the celiac lesion.[44] Because these T cells are separated from the gluten peptides by the epithelial layer, such peptides must cross the mucosa in some fashion, but the mechanism of such translocation is unclear. In the lamina propria tissue transglutaminases act on the gluten peptides to deamidate them, converting selected glutamines to negatively charged glutamic acids.[45] The deamidated gliadin peptides have been shown to have a much greater ability to bind to DQ2 and DQ8 antigen-binding grooves that have positively charged binding pockets. In fact, CD4 T cells in the lamina propria of celiac disease patients recognize mainly deamidated gliadin peptides. Although there is great variation in the specific peptide sequences activating T cells obtained from different individuals, a 33-mer peptide has been identified that can activate a large proportion of T-cell clones isolated from celiac mucosa.[47] This motif can be related back to the DQ2 binding groove, whose crystal structure is known.[46] The number of wheat, barley, and rye proteins with the correct binding motifs for DQ2 or

DQ8 have been estimated to be a small fraction of the total sequences potentially present in these grains.[48] The gliadin-reactive CD4 T cells in the lamina propria of celiac disease patients produce interferon (IFN)-γ, suggesting that they are polarized to a Th1 effector phenotype.[43] Such cells are known to activate a variety of downstream inflammatory cytokines and upregulate tissue metalloproteinases, which presumably results in the actual lesion. However, very little information is available about these downstream effects. IFN-γ is also known to increase gut permeability and hence might increase the translocation of more peptides, resulting in a vicious circle. The event that triggers this whole cascade is as yet unclear, but gastrointestinal infections with enteric viruses, for example, have long been suspected as a crucial trigger. The lamina propria is known to contain CD4 Treg cells, but little is known about the role they play in celiac disease.

Less is known about what role the intraepithelial lymphocyte (IEL) plays in disease pathogenesis. Increased numbers of IEL are a consistent feature of the histopathology of celiac disease. Intraepithelial lymphocytes are mainly CD8 T cells that bear either a γδ or an αβ TCR. The numbers of IEL return to normal on a gluten-free diet, and increases in IEL can occur within hours of a gluten challenge. However, there is no evidence that the T-cell receptors on these CD8 T cells are responding directly to gliadin peptides. Rather, this response may be secondary to the lamina propria CD4 T-cell response. IL-15 has been shown to expand certain IEL subsets, including those that bear natural killer (NK) receptors such as NKG2d and CD94.[49] These NK receptors are known to interact with nonclassic MHC class I molecules whose expression is induced by cellular stress or by IFN-γ. The epithelial cells of patients with celiac disease produce high amounts of IL-15; this has been postulated to result in the expansion of IEL expressing these NK cell receptors, which then are cytotoxic for epithelial cells expressing the relevant ligands.[50] Expansion of such NK-like IEL has been identified in individuals with celiac disease that is refractory to a gluten-free diet.[51]

Treatment

The treatment of celiac disease is a gluten-free diet for life, i.e., total avoidance of wheat, barley, and rye in the diet. Oats are allowed, at least in moderate amounts, although there are concerns that oats may be contaminated with these other grains, making them deleterious to some patients. Because gluten is present in a wide variety of foods, education of the patient is required. The ideal way to accomplish this is a consultation with a dietitian who is extremely knowledgeable about gluten-free diets. Not all dietitians have such expertise, and thus a patient can be referred to a variety of local and national support groups who can provide the required information. Patients starting such a diet should be followed with repeated visits to the physician for guidance, encouragement, and to enhance compliance. Many clinicians follow the IgA antitissue transglutaminase as a measure of the adequacy of a gluten-free diet: this test should return to normal if the diet is strict. Alternate forms of therapy that might allow continued ingestion of gluten are under study. These include the production of genetically modified wheat that lacks the relevant peptides, bacterial endopeptidases that degrade the gliadin peptides, drugs that might block intestinal tissue transglutaminase, competitive peptides that might block HLA-DQ2 or -DQ8, and anti-IL-15.

REFRACTORY CELIAC DISEASE

A small subset of patients with confirmed celiac disease fail to respond to a gluten-free diet. The most common cause is continued ingestion of gluten, either deliberately or inadvertently. However, some other conditions that need to be considered include autoimmune enteropathy,[52] lymphoma, ulcerative jejunoileitis, collagenous sprue, or refractory sprue. Patients with refractory sprue can demonstrate abnormal oligoclonal expansions of intraepithelial T cells, a condition that has been called 'cryptic intestinal T-cell lymphoma' and which has a poor prognosis. These oligoclonal expansions can progress into enteropathy-associated T-cell lymphoma (EATL), in which there are monoclonal expansions of these IEL.[53] Patients with refractory sprue may benefit from treatment with corticosteroids, an immune modulator such as azathioprine, cyclosporine, or infliximab.[54] Fortunately, this entity is uncommon.

■ INFLAMMATORY BOWEL DISEASE ■

Crohn's disease and ulcerative colitis are two related but distinct chronic inflammatory diseases of the intestine. Because they have overlapping features, the two are grouped together under the term 'inflammatory bowel disease' (IBD). Crohn's disease is a transmural inflammation that can affect any part of the intestine from the mouth to the anus, but most commonly the distal ileum and colon. The inflammation tends to be focal and discontinuous, with areas of involvement alternating with normal intestine ('skip lesions'). Granulomas in the lesions are a hallmark, but are not needed for diagnosis because they occur in less than half of patients. Mucosal ulcerations are fissuring, i.e., penetrate deep into the intestinal tissue, and can erode through the gut wall to form fistulas or abscesses. Ulcerative colitis is restricted to the rectum and colon and the inflammation and ulceration affect only the surface mucosa. Ulcerative colitis starts in the rectum and extends proximally and contiguously into the colon to a variable extent. The inflammation typically does not affect the deeper layers of the colon, except when the disease becomes very severe.

Clinical presentations

Both diseases affect children and adults, with a peak incidence in the second to third decades, but both can occur at any age. Crohn's disease presents with abdominal pain, watery diarrhea, weight loss, and fever. Ulcerative colitis usually presents as rectal bleeding and diarrhea, but can present with either of these alone. A subset of patients develop extra-intestinal manifestations such as arthralgias, arthritis, uveitis, or skin lesions, and sometimes these are the dominant presenting feature. The prevalence of each disease is approximately 150 per 100 000 population in the USA. It is likely that several subtypes of each disease exist that are currently placed together under these two diagnoses, in that data from experimental models of IBD indicate that multiple genetic deficiencies and different immunologic mechanisms can result in IBD.[55] Research is ongoing to define such disease subgroups using genotype and immunophenotype stratifications.[56]

Diagnosis

The diagnosis of these disorders is based on the clinical symptoms, radiologic imaging, endoscopy, and biopsies. The radiologic tests include barium contrast studies of the colon, stomach, and small intestine, as well as various CT scans of the abdomen and pelvis. A recent addition for the diagnosis of Crohn's disease has been wireless capsule endoscopy, which can image the mucosa of the entire small intestine. Endoscopy is a mainstay of diagnosis and management. However, tissue biopsies or histopathology of intestinal resections are optimal for diagnosis. Serologic tests are available, but their utility for diagnosis has not been established.

Serology

A number of autoantibodies have been found in patients with ulcerative colitis, e.g., multiple autoantibodies to colon epithelial cells have been identified, the best-characterized of these being an antibody to tropomyosin.[57] However, the only antibody in clinical use is serum IgG pANCA (perinuclear anti-nuclear cytoplasmic antibody). This antibody is detected by reactivity to methanol-fixed neutrophils and has a characteristic staining of the perinuclear membrane rather than the cytoplasm, as seen with other ANCAs. pANCA is produced by lamina propria B cells from the lesions of ulcerative colitis, and probably represents cross-reactivity to an antigen of the microbiota.[58] pANCA has no known role in disease pathogenesis. pANCA sensitivity and specificity are not high enough to use alone as a diagnostic test. Serum pANCA may have some prognostic value, in that patients with high-titer pANCA tend to have more severe ulcerative colitis, and a higher proportion of pANCA-positive patients develop chronic pouchitis after colectomy.

Autoantigens have also been found in subsets of patients with Crohn's disease, but again there is no convincing evidence that these play a role in the pathogenesis. Antibodies to multiple microbial antigens have been detected in the serum of patients, and these may have some clinical utility.[59] The best-defined of these is IgG and IgA anti-*Saccharomyces cerevisiae* (ASCA). In addition, patients with Crohn's disease have also been found to selectively express IgA anti-*E. coli* outer membrane protein C, IgA anti-*Pseudomonas fluorescens* I2, and IgG anti-CBir1 flagellin to a greater extent than do patients with ulcerative colitis or disease controls (Table 74.5). It remains to be proved that these tests can be used for diagnosis, for example to distinguish IBD as Crohn's disease. However, these antimicrobial antibodies appear to have some prognostic value, in that patients with high titers have a higher rate of complications as well as a higher frequency of surgery than do patients without these antibody

reactivities.[60] Serum IgG anti-flagellin reactivity, which has only been recently discovered,[61] is independently associated with a poor prognosis.[62] Combining these antibody reactivities considerably improves their sensitivity and specificity for diagnosing Crohn's disease and ulcerative colitis, and such a panel is commercially available.

Histopathology

Because both diseases are within reach of the endoscope, endoscopy with biopsy of affected tissue is the mainstay of histopathologic analysis. Endoscopic biopsies are small and sample only the superficial mucosa, hence it can be difficult to distinguish ulcerative colitis from Crohn's disease by biopsy alone. However, some histopathologic features can be identified in such small biopsies that are characteristic of IBD, including distortion of the crypts, infiltration of lamina propria by mononuclear cells and neutrophils, increased numbers of plasma cells, the location of plasma cells below the base of the crypts, and Paneth cell metaplasia. The hallmark of the lesions of ulcerative colitis is that the inflammation remains confined to the mucosa and immediate adjacent submucosal area, whereas in Crohn's disease the inflammatory infiltrates penetrate through the entire wall. However, these features are only evident in surgical resections. Analysis of such resections has revealed that the lymphoid infiltrates involves all the major leukocyte cell types including B cells, T cells, plasma cells, macrophages, neutrophils, and eosinophils. Among the plasma cells, those producing IgG and IgM are increased more than those producing IgA. Analysis of the TCR repertoire of such resections shows that it is a diverse polyclonal repertoire and is not significantly different in diseased as opposed to unaffected mucosa.

Genetics

It has long been recognized that these diseases have a genetic component. For example, Crohn's disease has a high concordance between monozygotic twins, and both Crohn's disease and ulcerative colitis occur with a higher frequency in family members of patients and in certain ethnic groups, such as Jews.[63] Interestingly, certain of the serologic markers of IBD discussed above appear with a higher frequency in unaffected family members of seropositive patients.[64] A variety of candidate genes have been linked to IBD, including some MHC genes, but the associations have generally been weak and inconsistent among different populations.

A major breakthrough in the genetic basis of IBD came with the advent of genome scanning using microsatellite markers (Chapter 101). In this technique a trait such as the presence of a disease can be linked to

Table 74.5 Serologic tests in inflammatory bowel disease

Antibody to	Isotype	% positive		
		UC	Crohn's	Control
pANCA	IgG	30–70	25	<5
ASCA	IgG, IgA	6–14	40–70	–
I2	IgA	–	50	–
OmpC	IgA	–	55	–
CBir1 flagellin	IgG	6	50	8

a specific location along the chromosomes where one or more genes reside that affect the expression of that trait. An advantage of this approach is that one does not need to know the identify of the gene to find an association; a disadvantage is that the approach does not identify the specific gene involved, but only a chromosomal region, which usually encompasses many genes. Despite these difficulties, a major triumph of this approach has been the identification of NOD2/CARD15 as a major susceptibility gene for Crohn's disease but not ulcerative colitis.[65,66] The gene encodes an intracellular pattern recognition receptor for the muramyl dipeptide component of bacterial peptidoglycan. There are three dominant mutations in the carboxy end of the molecule that are associated with the development of Crohn's disease, one of which is a truncation mutation. The exact mechanism of disease susceptibility caused by the CARD15 gene is as yet unknown but under intense study. However, the identification of a pattern recognition receptor as a susceptibility gene for Crohn's disease is coherent with the abundant data from preclinical experimental models, which is discussed in the next section. Genome scanning has identified many other loci linked to either Crohn's disease, ulcerative colitis, or both, and other candidate genes are being identified.[67]

Environmental factors

In addition to genetic susceptibility, it has long been recognized that there is a major environmental influence on the expression of these diseases. One of the major environmental influences is geographic location. IBD is a disease of westernized, urbanized populations and is rare in the Third World. For example, until recently these diseases had been rare in India and China, but as these countries industrialize IBD is now emerging in both. Interestingly, immigrants into the industrialized countries from less developed areas do not develop IBD; rather, it is their children who are born and raised in the western environment who develop these disorders. The environmental factors that lead to increased susceptibility to these diseases in western countries is unknown, but one interesting hypothesis is that there is a relative lack of appropriate stimulation of the immune system by the flora or by enteric pathogens – the hygiene hypothesis. Only two factors have been identified that can strongly influence the development of either Crohn's disease or ulcerative colitis. Smoking increases susceptibility to Crohn's disease and, conversely, nonsmoking has been associated with a higher frequency of ulcerative colitis. Smoking also affects disease course, in that individuals with Crohn's disease who continue to smoke require immune suppression more frequently.[68] The second factor is appendectomy performed for appendicitis, which reduces the frequency of ulcerative colitis development but has no effect on Crohn's disease incidence.

Pathophysiology

An infectious etiology for both Crohn's disease and ulcerative colitis has long been postulated, but no agent has been consistently identified. One cannot exclude infection with an unknown organism, and certainly the experience with *Helicobacter pylori*-induced gastritis shows that such an organism can elude detection for decades. However, the bulk of the data favors that the inflammatory bowel diseases are disorders of host–microbe interactions in the intestine.[69] This concept is still evolving and has been strongly influenced by results from many experimental models

of IBD. These models have provided important hypotheses that need to be confirmed in human studies. The microbiota itself is poorly understood and largely undefined. Current estimates are of 500–1000 species and ~8000 strains.[70] With regard to host immune interactions with the microbiota, innate, adaptive, and regulatory cells all are involved in the response.

Experimental models demonstrate that gene defects in each of the innate, adaptive, and regulatory compartments can result in IBD.[71] In many models there are abnormalities of more than one component, e.g., IL-10-deficient mice have abnormalities in both innate and regulatory components. Multiple genes are known to be involved in susceptibility to IBD in humans as well. Because humans are unlikely to have the absolute genetic defects that have been induced in experimental models, human disease is more likely to represent partial (10–20%) defects in multiple genes, rather than a major defect in one or a few genes. In combination, such partial defects can result in the phenotype of Crohn's disease or ulcerative colitis, but the individual contribution of each gene will be difficult to detect because each is a small contributor.

With regard to the adaptive immune system, a consistent observation in experimental models has been that the CD4 T cell is the major effector cell leading to chronic intestinal inflammation. Crohn's disease is considered an example of a CD4 Th1-mediated disease. Supporting this idea are increased levels of IL-12 p40, IFN-γ, and STAT4 in active lesions. The recently described IL-23-dependent, CD4 Th17 effector cell lineage may also play a role, in that both IL-23 and IL-17 are increased in the lesions of Crohn's disease, and the CD4 Th17 subset has been shown to play an important role in disease progression in experimental models of colitis. In experimental models the immune reaction is directed at antigens of the microbiota, and the same appears to be the case in patients with Crohn's disease, as demonstrated by the multiple antimicrobial antibodies mentioned above.

Ulcerative colitis does not fit well into the Th1/Th2 paradigm but some have suggested it to be a Th2-like disease. Although IL-4, the hallmark Th2 cytokine, is not increased in the lesions of ulcerative colitis, IL-5 and possibly IL-13 are increased. In one experimental model, an ulcerative colitis-like disease was determined to be due to an IL-13-dependent, CD1d-restricted NK T-cell effector mechanism. A similar mechanism has been postulated for human ulcerative colitis.[72]

Inflammatory cytokines are increased in the active lesions of both UC and CD, including IL-1, IL-6, TNF-α, and many others. These are produced by macrophages and other innate cells. This assortment is no different from those produced in any inflamed tissue. Macrophages present in the normal intestine do not produce cytokines and have down-regulated many surface molecules, such as CD14, a state that has been called 'inflammatory anergy.'[73] In contrast, the macrophages producing inflammatory cytokines in the lesions of IBD are CD14+ and appear to be recent immigrants into the gut from the monocyte pool in the blood. Thus, inhibition of leukocyte trafficking into the intestine is an attractive target for therapy. The inflammatory cytokines have many detrimental effects on tissues, such as recruitment of granulocytes, induction of metalloproteinases that can destroy tissue stroma, etc. TNF seems to play an important central role in this inflammatory cytokine cascade, in that monoclonal neutralization of TNF in patients with both CD and UC can result in rapid inhibition of the inflammatory response. Although these cellular contributors to tissue injury are known, the exact molecular mechanisms underlying tissue injury in these two diseases are yet to be defined.

Medical treatment

The mainstays of medical therapy are nonspecific anti-inflammatory drugs (NSAIDs) to inhibit the inflammatory cascade. These include 5-aminosalicylic acid agents and topical steroids such as budesonide. Patients not responding to this first line of therapy are usually placed on oral or parenteral steroids. Because a significant fraction of patients do not respond to steroids or cannot be weaned off of them, immune modulators are often used, including 6-mercaptopurine or its imidazole derivative azathioprine. These agents act slowly but can allow patients to come off steroids, or at least minimize the dose required in 50–70% of steroid-refractory or steroid-dependent cases. Methotrexate has shown some efficacy as a maintenance agent in Crohn's disease, but does not appear effective in ulcerative colitis. Cyclosporine has shown some efficacy in fulminant ulcerative colitis but is too toxic for prolonged use, and is used as a bridge to one of the traditional immune modulators. Cyclosporine has shown no efficacy in Crohn's disease. Monoclonal antibodies to TNF have shown efficacy in both Crohn's disease and more recently in ulcerative colitis, and are used for patients who are not responding to the standard therapies listed above. The indications for anti-TNF and other biologics are continuing to evolve, and their use earlier in the disease course is being explored. Many other strategies are being developed for the medical management of inflammatory bowel disease, as well as for other immune-mediated diseases, such as inhibitors of leukocyte migration by blockade of adhesion molecules.

Surgical treatment

Surgery is generally reserved for the complications of inflammatory bowel disease rather than as a primary therapeutic modality. A common indication for surgery is disease that does not respond to any of the medical therapies or, in the case of ulcerative colitis, becomes fulminant. For ulcerative colitis, a complete colectomy is required. The operation of choice is a complete proctocolectomy with construction of a neorectum or 'pouch' from the distal ileum, which is attached to the anal canal. Unfortunately, inflammation of this ileal pouch can occur in up to 50% of patients receiving this operation for ulcerative colitis, although pouchitis does not occur in patients having a colectomy for hereditary polyposis. Most patients with pouchitis respond to a short course of antibiotics, but others require many of the same medications used for treatment of the primary disease.

In individuals with Crohn's disease, surgery is reserved for complications of the disease, such as stricture with obstruction, hemorrhage, fistula, abscess, or lack of response to medical therapy. The affected segments are resected and the unaffected bowel reconnected. There is a high rate of recurrence after surgery, which is dependent on the presence of the fecal stream. Such disease often recurs at the anastomosis, e.g., in the neoterminal ileum after an ileocecal resection. At present there is no medication that will prevent the recurrence of Crohn's disease.

■ CONCLUSION ■

The broad spectrum of immune disorders affecting the gastrointestinal tract reflects its unique role as the major interface between the host immune system and the microbial world. The mucosal immune system also has to deal with the large quantities of foreign antigens present in food. Progress has been made in understanding how the mucosal immune system is able to deal with this complex environment while maintaining intestinal homeostasis. These various disorders represent instances in which the normal mucosal immune mechanisms have failed in one way or another. The study of these disorders is important because they are human diseases, but they also provide a window into how the gut immune system accomplishes its amazing ability to balance nonresponsiveness to the microbiota and to food while retaining the ability to actively respond to intestinal pathogens.

■ REFERENCES ■

1. Janoff EN, Smith PD. Approach to gastrointestinal problems in the immunocompromised patient. In : Yamada T, Alpers DH, Laine L,. eds: Textbook of gastroenterology, 4th edn. Philadelphia: Lippincott-Raven. 2003, p 1017–1032.

2. Sneller MC, Strober W, Eisenstein E, et al. New insights into common variable immunodeficiency. Ann Intern Med 1993; 118: 720–730.

3. Bayry J, Hermine O, Webster DA, et al. Common variable immunodeficiency: the immune system in chaos. Trends Mol Med 2005; 11: 370–376.

4. Wright JJ, Birx DL, Wagner DK, et al. Normalization of antibody responsiveness in a patient with common variable hypogammaglobulinemia and HIV infection. N Engl J Med 1987; 317: 1516–1520.

5. Bayry J, Lacroix-Desmazes S, Kazatchkine MD, et al. Common variable immunodeficiency is associated with defective functions of dendritic cells. Blood 2004; 104: 2441–2443.

6. Janoff EN, Smith PD. The role of immunity in *Giardia* infections. In: Meyer EA, ed: Giardiasis, Edinburgh: Elsevier Science; 1990, 215–233.

7. Sperber KE, Mayer LM. Gastrointestinal manifestations of common variable immunodeficiency. Immunol Allergy Clin North Am 1988; 8: 423–434.

8. Teahon K, Webster AD, Price AB, et al. Studies on the enteropathy associated with primary hypogammaglobulinaemia. Gut 1994; 35: 1244–1249.

9. Strober W, Wochner RD, Carbone PO, Waldmann TA. Intestinal lymphangiectasia: a protein-losing enteropathy with hypogammaglobulinemia, lymphocytopenia and impaired homograft rejection. J Clin Invest 1967; 46: 1643–1656.

10. CDC. The Global HIV/AIDS pandemic, 2006. MMWR Morb Mortal Wkly Rep. 2006; 11: 841–844.

11. Meng G, Wei X, Wu X, et al. Primary intestinal epithelial cells selectively transfer R5 HIV-1 to CCR5+ cells. Nature Med 2002; 8: 150–156.

12. Li L, Meng G, Graham MF, Shaw GM, Smith PD. Intestinal macrophages display reduced permissiveness to human immunodeficiency virus 1 and decreased surface CCR5. Gastroenterology 1999; 116: 1043–1053.

13. Meng G, Sellers MT, Mosteller-Barnum M, et al. Lamina propria lymphocytes, not macrophages, express CCR5 and CXCR4 and are the likely target cell for human immunodeficiency virus type 1 in the intestinal mucosa. J Infect Dis 2000; 182: 785–791.

14. Janoff EN, Smith PD. Emerging concepts in gastrointestinal aspects of HIV-pathogenesis and management. Gastroenterology 2001; 120: 607–621.

15. Schrager LK, Young JM, Fowler MG, et al. Long-term survivors of HIV-1 infection: definitions and research challenges. AIDS 1994; 8:s95–s108.

16. Smith PD, Janoff EN. Gastrointestinal infections in HIV-1 disease. In Blaser MJ, Smith PD, Ravdin JI et al., eds: Infections of the gastrointestinal tract, Philadelphia: Lippincott-Raven; 2002, 415–443.

17. Lam-Tse WK, Batstra MR, Koeleman BP, et al. The association between autoimmune thyroiditis, autoimmune gastritis and type 1 diabetes. Pediatr Endocrinol Rev 2003; 1: 22–37.

18. Germana B, Di Mario F, Cavallaro LG, et al. Clinical usefulness of serum pepsinogens I and II, gastrin-17 and anti-*Helicobacter pylori* antibodies in the management of dyspeptic patients in primary care. Dig Liver Dis 2005; 37: 501–508.

19. van Driel IR, Read S, Zwar TD, Gleeson PA. Shaping the T cell repertoire to a bona fide autoantigen: lessons from autoimmune gastritis. Curr Opin Immunol 2005; 17: 570–576.

20. Field J, Biondo MA, Murphy K, et al. Experimental autoimmune gastritis: mouse models of human organ-specific autoimmune disease. Int Rev Immunol 2005; 24: 93–110.

21. Laurie KL, La Gruta NL, Koch N, et al. Thymic expression of a gastritogenic epitope results in positive selection of self-reactive pathogenic T cells. J Immunol 2004; 172: 5994–6002.

22. Bergman MP, Amedei A, D'Elios MM, et al. Characterization of H+,K+- ATPase T cell epitopes in human autoimmune gastritis. Eur J Immunol 2003; 33: 539–545.

23. Sakaguchi S, Sakaguchi N, Shimizu J, et al. Immunologic tolerance maintained by CD25+ CD4+ regulatory T cells: their common role in controlling autoimmunity, tumor immunity, and transplantation tolerance. Immunol Rev 2001; 182: 18–32.

24. McHugh RS. Autoimmune gastritis is a well-defined autoimmune disease model for the study of CD4+CD25+ T cell-mediated suppression. Curr Topics Microbiol Immunol 2005; 293: 153–177.

25. Bergman MP, Vandenbroucke-Grauls CM, Appelmelk BJ, et al. The story so far: *Helicobacter pylori* and gastric autoimmunity. Int Rev Immunol 2005; 24: 63–91.

26. Amedei A, Bergman MP, Appelmelk BJ, et al. Molecular mimicry between *Helicobacter pylori* antigens and H+, K+ -adenosine triphosphatase in human gastric autoimmunity. J Exp Med 2003; 198: 1147–1156.

27. Hershko C, Ronson A, Souroujon M, et al. Variable hematologic presentation of autoimmune gastritis: age-related progression from iron deficiency to cobalamin depletion. Blood 2006; 107: 1673–1679.

28. Hershko C, Hoffbrand AV, Keret D, et al. Role of autoimmune gastritis, *Helicobacter pylori* and celiac disease in refractory or unexplained iron deficiency anemia. Haematologica 2005; 90: 585–595.

29. Torres J, Pérez-Pérez G, Goodman KJ, et al. A comprehensive review of the natural history of *Helicobacter pylori* infection in children. Arch Med Res 2000; 31: 431–469.

30. Brandt S, Kwok T, Hartig R, et al. NFκB activation and potentiation of proinflammatory responses by the *Helicobacter pylori* CagA protein. Proc Natl Acad Science USA 2005; 102: 9300–9305.

31. Cutler AF, Havstad S, Ma CK, et al. Accuracy of invasive and noninvasive tests to diagnose *Helicobacter pylori* infection. Gastroenterology 1995; 109: 136–141.

32. Perez-Perez GI, Cutler AF, Blaser MJ. Value of serology as a noninvasive method for evaluating the efficacy of treatment of *Helicobacter pylori* infection. Clin Infect Dis 1997; 25: 1038–1043.

33. Suerbaum S, Michetti P. *Helicobacter pylori* infection. N Engl J Med 2002; 347: 1175–1186.

34. Peek RMJ, Crabtree JE. *Helicobacter* infection and gastric neoplasia. J Pathol 2006; 208: 233–248.

35. Fasano A, Berti I, Gerarduzzi T. et al. Prevalence of celiac disease in at-risk and not-at-risk groups in the United States: a large multicenter study. Arch Intern Med 2003; 163: 286–292.

36. Green PH, Jabri B. Coeliac disease. Lancet 2003; 362: 383–391.

37. Farrell RJ, Kelly CP. Celiac sprue. N Engl J Med 2002; 346: 180–188.

38. Karpati S. Dermatitis herpetiformis: close to unravelling a disease. J Dermatol Sci 2004; 34: 83–90.

39. Louka AS, Sollid LM. HLA in coeliac disease: unravelling the complex genetics of a complex disorder. Tissue Antigens 2003; 61: 105–117.

40. Margaritte-Jeannin P, Babron MC, Bourgey M, et al. HLA-DQ relative risks for coeliac disease in European populations: a study of the European Genetics Cluster on Coeliac Disease. Tissue Antigens 2004; 63: 562–567.

41. Kim CY, Quarsten H, Bergseng E, et al. Structural basis for HLA-DQ2- mediated presentation of gluten epitopes in celiac disease. Proc Natl Acad Sci USA 2004; 101: 4175–4179.

42. Percopo S, Babron MC, Whalen M, et al. Saturation of the 5q31-q33 candidate region for coeliac disease. Ann Hum Genet 2003; 67: 265–268.

43. Nilsen EM, Lundin KE, Krajci P, et al. Gluten specific, HLA-DQ restricted T cells from coeliac mucosa produce cytokines with Th1 or Th0 profile dominated by interferon gamma. Gut 1995; 37: 766–776.

44. Kagnoff MF. Overview and pathogenesis of celiac disease. Gastroenterology 2005; 128: S10–18.

45. Fleckenstein B, Qiao SW, Larsen MR, et al. Molecular characterization of covalent complexes between tissue transglutaminase and gliadin peptides. J Biol Chem 2004; 279: 17607–17616.

46. Shan L, Molberg O, Parrot I, et al. Structural basis for gluten intolerance in celiac sprue. Science 2002; 297: 2275–2279.

47. Qiao SW, Bergseng E, Molberg O, et al. Antigen presentation to celiac lesion-derived T cells of a 33-mer gliadin peptide naturally formed by gastrointestinal digestion. J Immunol 2004; 173: 1757–1762.

48. Vader LW, Stepniak DT, Bunnik EM, et al. Characterization of cereal toxicity for celiac disease patients based on protein homology in grains. Gastroenterology 2003; 125: 1105–1113.

49. Jabri B, de Serre NP, Cellier C, et al. Selective expansion of intraepithelial lymphocytes expressing the HLA-E-specific natural killer receptor CD94 in celiac disease. Gastroenterology 2000; 118: 867–879.

50. Meresse B, Chen Z, Ciszewski C, et al. Coordinated induction by IL15 of a TCR-independent NKG2D signaling pathway converts CTL into lymphokine-activated killer cells in celiac disease. Immunity 2004; 21: 357–366.

51. Cellier C, Delabesse E, Helmer C, et al. Refractory sprue, coeliac disease, and enteropathy-associated T-cell lymphoma. French Coeliac Disease Study Group. Lancet 2000; 356: 203–208.

REFERENCES

52. Leon F, Olivencia P, Rodriguez-Pena R, et al. Clinical and immunological features of adult-onset generalized autoimmune gut disorder. Am J Gastroenterol 2004; 99: 1563–1571.

53. Meijer JW, Mulder CJ, Goerres MG, et al. Coeliac disease and (extra)intestinal T-cell lymphomas: definition, diagnosis and treatment. Scand J Gastroenterol (suppl) 2004; 241: 78–84.

54. Goerres MS, Meijer JW, Wahab PJ, et al. Azathioprine and prednisone combination therapy in refractory coeliac disease. Aliment Pharmacol Ther 2003; 18: 487–494.

55. Elson CO, Weaver CT. Experimental mouse models of inflammatory bowel disease: new insights into pathogenic mechanisms. In : Targan SR, Shanahan F, Karp LC, eds. Inflammatory bowel disease: From bench to bedside, . 2nd edn, Dordrecht: Kluwer Academic, 2003, p 67–99.

56. Silverberg MS, Satsangi J, Ahmad T, et al. Toward an integrated clinical, molecular and serological classification of inflammatory bowel disease: Report of a Working Party of the 2005 Montreal World Congress of Gastroenterology. Can J Gastroenterol 2005: 19: 5–36.

57. Onuma EK, Amenta PS, Ramaswamy K, et al. Autoimmunity in ulcerative colitis (UC): a predominant colonic mucosal B cell response against human tropomyosin isoform 5. Clin Exp Immunol 2000; 121: 466–471.

58. Seibold F, Brandwein S, Simpson S, et al. pANCA represents a cross-reactivity to enteric bacterial antigens. J Clin Immunol 1998; 18: 153–160.

59. Vasiliauskas EA, Kam LY, Karp LC, et al. Marker antibody expression stratifies Crohn's disease into immunologically homogeneous subgroups with distinct clinical characteristics. Gut 2000; 47: 487–496.

60. Mow WS, Vasiliauskas EA, Lin YC, et al. Association of antibody responses to microbial antigens and complications of small bowel Crohn's disease. Gastroenterology 2004; 126: 414–424.

61. Lodes MJ, Cong Y, Elson CO, et al. Bacterial flagellin is a dominant antigen in Crohn disease. J Clin Invest 2004; 113: 1296–1306.

62. Targan SR, Landers CJ, Yang H, et al. Antibodies to CBir1 flagellin define a unique response that is associated independently with complicated Crohn's disease. Gastroenterology 2005; 128: 2020–2028.

63. Yang H, McElree C, Roth M-P, et al. Familial empirical risks for inflammatory bowel disease: differences between Jews and nonJews. Gut 1993; 34: 517–524.

64. Mei L, Targan SR, Landers CJ, et al. Familial expression of anti-*Escherichia coli* outer membrane porin C in relatives of patients with Crohn's disease. Gastroenterology 2006; 130: 1078–1085.

65. Hugot JP, Chamaillard M, Zouali H, et al. Association of NOD2 leucine-rich repeat variants with susceptibility to Crohn's disease. Nature 2001; 411: 599–603.

66. Ogura Y, Bonen DK, Inohara N, et al. A frameshift mutation in NOD2 associated with susceptibility to Crohn's disease. Nature 2001; 411: 603–606.

67. Ahmad T, Tamboli CP, Jewell D, Colombel JF. Clinical relevance of advances in genetics and pharmacogenetics of IBD. Gastroenterology 2004; 126: 1533–1549.

68. Cosnes J, Carbonnel F, Beaugerie L, et al. Effects of cigarette smoking on the long-term course of Crohn's disease. Gastroenterology 1996; 110: 424–431.

69. Lorenz RG, McCracken VJ, Elson CO. Animal models of intestinal inflammation: ineffective communication between coalition members. Springer Semin Immunopathol 2005; 27: 233–247.

70. Ley RE, Peterson DA, Gordon JI. Ecological and evolutionary forces shaping microbial diversity in the human intestine. Cell 2006; 124: 837–848.

71. Elson CO, Cong Y, McCracken VJ, et al. Experimental models of inflammatory bowel disease reveal innate, adaptive, and regulatory mechanisms of host dialogue with the microbiota. Immunol Rev 2005; 206: 260–276.

72. Fuss IJ, Heller F, Boirivant M, et al. Nonclassical CD1d-restricted NK T cells that produce IL-13 characterize an atypical Th2 response in ulcerative colitis. J Clin Invest 2004; 113: 1490–1497.

73. Smythies LE, Sellers M, Clements RH, et al. Human intestinal macrophages display profound inflammatory anergy despite avid phagocytic and bacteriocidal activity. J Clin Invest 2005; 115: 66–75.

Inflammatory hepatobiliary cirrhosis

75

Carlo Selmi, Michael P. Manns, M. Eric Gershwin

Inflammatory hepatobiliary disease is a generic term that comprises conditions presenting a complex noninfectious etiopathogenesis characterized by chronic inflammatory infiltrate and autoimmune features.[1] Among these, the main distinction is based on the target tissue, whether this is the hepatocyte (as in the case of autoimmune hepatitis (AIH)) or the bile duct cell (as in the case of primary biliary cirrhosis (PBC) or primary sclerosing cholangitis (PSC)). In between, there is a series of conditions sharing characteristics of both groups coined overlap syndromes with peculiar features as to clinical management. Regardless of the subgroup, all conditions eventually lead to liver cirrhosis and ultimately liver failure; however, progression rates vary widely and are likely determined by unknown genetic factors.

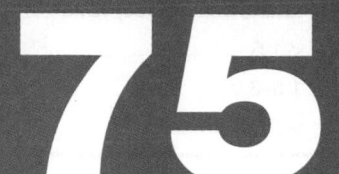

KEY CONCEPTS

INFLAMMATORY HEPATOBILIARY DISEASES

>> An autoimmune pathogenesis is recognized for autoimmune hepatitis, implied for primary biliary cirrhosis, and suggested for primary sclerosing cholangitis

>> In all cases, the etiology remains enigmatic, although the roles of genetic susceptibility and environmental factors are well established

>> The diagnosis of autoimmune hepatitis, primary sclerosing cholangitis, and primary biliary cirrhosis is based on criteria comprising clinical, imaging, and histological factors

>> Overlap syndromes can ensue between the diseases, possibly modifying the natural history and the therapy approach

■ AUTOIMMUNE HEPATITIS ■

CLINICAL FEATURES AND DIAGNOSTIC CHALLENGE

AIH is a chronic disease of unknown etiology resulting from the immune-mediated destruction of hepatocytes secondary to a loss of immune tolerance against liver tissues. AIH major features[1] include striking female predominance, presence of hypergammablubulinemia, significant association with the human leukocyte antigen (HLA) alleles DR3 and DR4, good clinical response to steroids and other immunosuppressive treatments, and detection of serum autoantibodies. In some cases, the diagnosis can be challenging due to the presence of confounding factors or features mimicking other conditions. For these reasons, a scoring system has been developed over the past years to account for all criteria that influence the likelihood of AIH diagnosis. The system, first introduced in 1992 and then modified in 1999, is a practical tool for clinical management and allows a high sensitivity and specificity in the diagnosis (Table 75.1). Factors taken into account in this system include sex, plasma biochemical variables, serum autoantibodies, liver histology, possible co-factors (drugs, alcohol, viruses), and response to medical treatment. The sum of all factors produces a score to be used for determining the likelihood of the AIH diagnosis either

prior to or after medical treatment; in particular, a score > 15 prior to therapy or > 17 after treatment is associated with a definite diagnosis of AIH while scores in the 10–15 (pre-treatment) or 12–17 (post-treatment) ranges characterize a probable case. The 1992 version of the scoring system allowed high sensitivity (89%) with a relatively low specificity, particularly in cases of chronic hepatitis C with autoimmune features (80%) or chronic cholestatic liver diseases (61%). The revised 1999 criteria appear to give a better distinction between PSC and AIH.

AIH is a rare disease estimated to have a prevalence of 170/million persons in Europe. As mentioned above, it affects women of any age more commonly than men, but the female-to-male ratio in AIH is lower compared to PBC. The onset is typically indolent and asymptomatic subjects diagnosed with AIH following a screening examination currently represent the majority of cases. On the other hand, if symptoms are present at diagnosis, these are nonspecific or secondary to end-stage liver disease (jaundice, pruritus, ascites, upper digestive bleeding).

present in the heterogeneous antigenic "cocktail" derived from the aqueous extract of rabbit thymus that is currently used to detect antibodies to extractable nuclear antigens.

Autoantibodies to liver–kidney microsomal antigens

Autoantibodies against microsomal proteins form a heterogeneous group and are associated with several immune-mediated diseases, including AIH and drug-induced hepatitis. Serum autoantibodies against LKM-1 are the main serological markers of type 2 AIH and recognize the proximal renal tubule and hepatocellular cytoplasm. The 50-kDa autoantigen was identified as the cytochrome P450 2D6 (CYP2D6). Interestingly, the sequence between amino acids 316 and 327, which is most likely exposed on the surface of the molecule, appears to be a region capable of differentiating LKM-1 activity in AIH and hepatitis C virus and may represent a key target for autoimmunity. The mechanisms of onset remain enigmatic and solid evidence of a causative role of hepatitis C virus cross-reactivity is still awaited. Similarly, the pathogenic role of anti-LKM-1 and their prognostic significance are debated, despite the development of type 2 AIH animal models following immunization with human CYP2D6 or with adenoviruses in mice transgenic for human CYP2D6. Finally, two other types of serum anti-LKM have been described in patients with ticrynafen-associated hepatitis (anti-LKM-2, directed against CYP2C9) and in 10% of patients with type 2 AIH (anti-LKM-3, directed against UGT1A), either alone or in combination with LKM-1 antibodies.

Autoantibodies to soluble liver antigen/liver pancreas antigen

Anti-SLA/LP antibodies are detectable by radioimmunoassay and enzyme-linked immunosorbent assay but not by immunofluorescence and are directed against different epitopes of a UGA tRNA suppressor. Serum anti-SLA/LP antibodies are occasionally found in patients with AIH who are negative for ANA, SMA, or anti-LKM and are cumulatively detected in 10–30% of cases of type 1 and type 2 AIH. Recent data indicate that anti-SLA/LP antibodies are also detectable in subgroups of pediatric patients with autoimmune cholangitis or adult patients with hepatitis C virus infection when tested with sensitive methods.

Antibodies to liver-cytosol type 1

Anti-LC1 antibodies are detected by indirect immunofluorescence in sera from up to 50% of patients with type 2 AIH and less frequently in type 1 AIH or chronic hepatitis C. Importantly, however, anti-LC1 are the only detectable markers in 10% of AIH cases.

The LC1 autoantigen is the liver formiminotransferase cyclodeaminase, an enzyme involved in folate metabolism. Interestingly, serum anti-LC1 antibodies correlate with AIH severity and progression.

Other autoantibodies

Antibodies to the asialoglycoprotein receptor are observed in up to 90% of all patients with AIH and often coexist with other autoantibodies while lacking specificity for the disease. Similar to anti-LC1, however, anti-asialoglycoprotein titers are associated with a more florid inflammatory disease activity and may monitor treatment response.

Antibodies to neutrophil cytoplasmic antigens (pANCA) can be detected by indirect immunofluorescence in sera from patients with type 1 AIH but also in a subgroup of patients with PSC or chronic viral hepatitis.

PATHOGENESIS

Similar to most autoimmune diseases, the current hypothesis states that environmental factors trigger autoimmunity onset in genetically susceptible individuals. Several microorganisms, particulary viruses, have been suggested as triggers but sound evidence is still awaited. The proposed mechanism is based on molecular mimicry between infectious agent epitopes and human liver antigens. There has been evidence implicating measles virus, cytomegalovirus, and Epstein–Barr virus as initiators of the disease while the most solid data were obtained with hepatitis C virus.[3]

From a genetic standpoint, AIH is considered a complex disease not following a strictly hereditary pattern.[4] In fact, conclusive data of a single genetic locus causing AIH onset have not been obtained and multiple genes are likely to contribute to disease susceptibility. Recently developed technologies such as the genome-wide scan appear promising in unraveling the genetic mysteries of AIH.

Most evidence in AIH genetics comes from the study of major histocompatibility complex (MHC) alleles, critical molecules in the T-cell recognition process (Chapter 7). Data from Caucasian patients in northern Europe and the USA reported an association with HLA DRB1*0301 and DRB*0401 although most reported associations appear to be limited to specific geographical areas or ethnicities. Nevertheless, the association of AIH with DR3 and DR4 alleles is solid to the point of being included in the diagnostic scoring system currently in use. The scenario is further complicated by the possibility that different environmental factors trigger AIH in different areas. HLA alleles associated with AIH not only confer susceptibility towards AIH but also appear to influence the course of the disease. Most strikingly, patients with DRB1*0301 are younger at disease onset and have a lower frequency of response to treatment. HLA DR3 is further associated with a lower probability of remission, manifesting more frequent relapses and need for liver transplantation. Furthermore, associations have also been reported between AIH and tumor necrosis factor-α and carbonic anhydrase gene polymorphisms, although these genes might not represent primary susceptibility genes but rather markers of MHC associations. Outside the MHC cluster, polymorphisms of genes involved in the regulation of immune responses have been investigated, leading to inconclusive data. These include the cytotoxic T-lymphocyte antigen 4 (CTLA-4), cytokines, vitamin D receptor, CD45, and Fas receptor.

NATURAL HISTORY

Data on the natural course of AIH are limited, particularly due to the paucity of clinical trials during the past decades[5] when hepatitis C became manifest as a common confounding factor significantly influencing the disease progression. Accordingly, older studies reported that AIH had a very poor prognosis and 5- and 10-year survival rates of 50% and 10% without treatment while immunosuppressants could significantly improve survival to 10-year rates as high as 90%. At the time of diagnosis, approximately 30% of adult patients have histological evidence of cirrhosis; when appropriately treated, however, only a small number of patients develop cirrhosis during follow-up if an anti-inflammatory response is achieved.

Nevertheless, having cirrhosis at presentation significantly increases the risk of liver-related death or the need for liver transplantation.

The scenarios are different when pediatric or elderly cases are studied. In fact, almost 50% of children with AIH already manifest cirrhosis at diagnosis and the majority of patients require long-term immunosuppressive treatment until adulthood. In elderly patients a more severe initial histology grade should be expected, alongside a similar response rate to immunosuppression. It is still debated if these patients should be treated with higher or lower doses of steroids. Beside age at presentation, race also modifies disease progression data. In fact, cirrhosis is more frequent at younger age in African-American patients with AIH compared to Caucasian subjects from the same areas.

The occurrence of hepatocellular carcinoma in patients with AIH is a rare event and only develops in long-standing cirrhosis. In the absence of solid data on large numbers of cases, primary liver neoplasia incidence should be regarded as similar to other nonviral cases of cirrhosis.

THERAPY

Different from the other autoimmune liver diseases described herein, immunosuppressants are the treatments of choice for AIH, based on the good response in terms of biochemistry, histology, and survival.[6] Corticosteroids (prednisone), as monotherapy or in combination with azathioprine, are the first line of treatment and should be started in patients with aminotransferase levels > 5 times the upper normal limit or histological evidence of bridging or multilobular necrosis. Prednisone and azathioprine appear equally effective. Treatment follows guidelines (Table 75.3) but tailored schedules are encouraged in selected cases. In asymptomatic patients with milder presentation, the opportunity to treat is still a matter of debate since the survival of these patients without treatment is similar to the overall AIH population.[7] Nevertheless, a close follow-up is required in these patients since symptoms develop in 25% of cases. The goal of a biochemical and histological resolution of inflammation as well as the clinical remission of symptoms is observed in up to 80% of patients treated with steroids within the first 3 years, most commonly during the first few months. It should be noted, however, that subgroups of patients manifest disease progression (approximately 10%) or are intolerant to standard therapy (13%). Relapses following therapy discontinuation are common since only 20% of patients remain in sustained remission. Second-choice therapies include cyclosporine A, tacrolimus, cyclophosphamide, mercaptopurine, mycophenolate mofetil, or deflazacort, thus far tested in small populations of patients. Ursodeoxycholic acid (UDCA) is a well-tolerated drug; its efficacy in AIH therapy or in combination with immunosuppressive therapy is still not established, particularly in terms of survival or histological improvement. Finally, patients with end-stage liver disease or fulminant presentation who do not respond to immunosuppressive therapy should be promptly considered for liver transplantation. Patients with AIH undergoing liver transplant have overall 5- and 10-year survival rates of 90% and 75%, respectively, although disease recurrence is common.

■ PRIMARY BILIARY CIRRHOSIS ■

PBC is a chronic cholestatic liver disease of unknown etiology characterized by high-titer serum anti-mitochondrial autoantibodies (AMA) and an autoimmune-mediated destruction of the small and medium-sized intrahepatic bile ducts. It affects women more frequently than men, with a female-to-male ratio of 9:1, the average age at diagnosis is within the 5th and 6th decades of life, and it presents a geographical pattern of prevalence. Table 75.4 illustrates the epidemiological data currently available for PBC. Sporadic cases of PBC onset in pediatric ages have recently been reported. The diagnosis of PBC is based on the presence of two out of three internationally accepted criteria, i.e., detectable serum AMA (titer > 1:40), increased enzymes indicating cholestasis (i.e., alkaline phosphatase) for longer than 6 months, and a compatible or diagnostic liver histology. The classification proposed to indicate a definite diagnosis only when all criteria are met may

Table 75.3 Treatment guidelines for autoimmune hepatitis

Therapeutic stages	Single-drug regimen	Combination regimen
Induction therapy		
Week 1	40–60 mg prednisone/day[a]	40–60 mg prednisone/day + 1–2 mg azathioprine/kg body weight
Week 2	40 mg prednisone/day	
Week 3	30 mg prednisone/day	15 mg prednisone/day + 1–2 mg azathioprine/kg body weight
Week 4	Taper down 5 mg every week, until maintenance therapy	15 mg prednisone/day + 1–2 mg azathioprine/kg body weight
Maintenance therapy	5–15 mg prednisone/day are common	10 mg prednisone/day + 1–2 mg azathioprine/kg body weight dosages *Alternative option:* 2 mg/kg azathioprine as monotherapy
Upon relapse	Like induction therapy	Like induction therapy

[a]Prednisolone may be taken instead of prednisone.

> ## CLINICAL PEARLS
>
> ### PRIMARY BILIARY CIRRHOSIS
>
> >> Primary biliary cirrhosis is a rare disease, affecting middle-aged women more commonly than men
>
> >> Genetic factors are critical, yet not well defined, in the pathogenesis of the disease; environmental factors are important, possibly infectious or chemical
>
> >> The serum hallmark is serum anti-mitochondrial antibodies (AMA), found in >90% of cases
>
> >> At presentation, patients most commonly manifest early stages and have nonspecific symptoms, such as fatigue or pruritus

be too narrow as, for example, patients lacking serum AMA appear to follow a similar natural history when compared to their AMA-positive counterparts.[8] Although it remains critical for the assessment of the histological stage, the issue of whether a liver biopsy is needed for the diagnosis of PBC is still highly debated. Currently, performing a liver biopsy seems not to be indicated when the other two diagnostic criteria are met. In a large number of cases (20–60%) the diagnosis of PBC is established in the absence of symptoms indicating a liver condition or cholestasis, and the proportion of asymptomatic cases at diagnosis has been increasing since the first series were reported.

CLINICAL FEATURES

Symptoms most commonly accompanying PBC at presentation are classically defined as fatigue and pruritus while physical findings may include skin hyperpigmentation, hepatosplenomegaly, and (rarely) xanthelasmas. End-stage symptoms are those of all types of liver cirrhosis, including ascites, jaundice, hepatic encephalopathy, and upper digestive bleeding. *Fatigue* is an incompletely defined, nonspecific symptom that affects up to 70% of patients with PBC and that is often overlooked, particularly in middle-aged women. Importantly, the severity of fatigue is independent of the stage of PBC or its other features (pruritus or severe cholestasis), nor does it depend on psychiatric factors. No medical treatment has been shown to be effective in alleviating this symptom, although fatigue has never been included as an endpoint in any of the large controlled clinical trials.

As many as 70% of patients with PBC and jaundice suffer from *pruritus*. Longitudinal data show that the vast majority of patients will eventually experience this symptom during their lifetime; pruritus might long precede jaundice onset. Typically, pruritus worsens at night, following contact with wool, or in warm climates. The bases of PBC-associated pruritus are not clear and two hypotheses have been proposed: serum bile acid retention secondary to chronic cholestasis or amplified release of endogenous opioids. Treatment of pruritus can be challenging for the clinician. The use of cholestyramine (4 g two or three times a day) ameliorates pruritus. In cases poorly responsive to resins, rifampicin has been used to achieve rapid symptom relief; its prolonged use, however, should be avoided. Based on the opioid theory of pruritus, treatment with opiate antagonists such as naltrexone (50 mg/day) is currently being used, with limited adverse effects. The recently

proposed use of sertraline is encouraged by promising preliminary data but warrants further evaluation.

Portal hypertension is frequently found in patients with PBC and, importantly, does not imply the presence of liver cirrhosis. Over half of untreated patients eventually develop portal hypertension over a 4-year period. The prevention and treatment of PBC-associated portal hypertension are not different from other chronic liver diseases.

Although there are conflicting data, it appears that accelerated bone loss accompanies long-standing cholestasis in PBC compared to sex- and age-matched healthy individuals. It has been coined *metabolic bone disease* secondary to reduced bone deposition. Current treatment of bone loss includes oral calcium supplementation, weight-bearing activity, and oral vitamin D replacement, if deficiency is found. Postmenopausal hormone replacement therapy should be considered but jaundice and other signs of liver failure should be evaluated during the first months of treatment. Efficacy and safety of other treatments are being evaluated.

Hyperlipidemia is common in up to 85% of patients with PBC and both serum cholesterol and triglyceride high levels can be observed. Interestingly, however, such alterations are not accompanied by a proportionally increased incidence of cardiovascular events or atherosclerosis and do not correlate with disease stage. Treatment with bile acid helps reduce blood lipids levels via unknown mechanisms.

Comorbidity is an important feature of PBC. Various disorders, particularly other autoimmune syndromes, are associated with PBC at various degrees. Our epidemiological study of 1032 patients with PBC has demonstrated that one-third of cases are also affected by another autoimmune disease, most commonly Sjögren's syndrome, Raynaud's phenomenon, autoimmune thyroid disease, scleroderma, and systemic lupus erythematosus, while the prevalence of rheumatoid arthritis did not differ from controls.[9] Interestingly, recent data demonstrated that patients affected by both PBC and scleroderma manifest a less aggressive liver disease, thus suggesting an active interaction between the two conditions. Similarly to other types of cirrhosis, end-stage PBC can be complicated by the occurrence of *hepatocellular carcinoma* and patients with intense nodular liver structure at ultrasound should be monitored by computed tomography. Importantly, PBC does not associate with cholangiocarcinoma (CCA) or breast cancer.

BLOOD TESTS

At presentation, PBC is suspected if a biochemical cholestatic pattern represented by increased plasma alkaline phosphatase or γ-glutamyltransferase is present. Such increase is typically not accompanied by an increase of similar magnitude in plasma aminotransferase levels. Serum immunoglobulin M levels are typically elevated in PBC cases without being correlated with AMA titers or levels of other Ig subtypes. Data suggest that this phenomenon might be secondary to an aberrant response of patients' memory B cells to bacterial stimuli[10] but its clinical significance remains enigmatic. Once cirrhosis has developed, biochemical alterations are similar to other types of cirrhosis.

LIVER HISTOLOGY

According to the classification of Ludwig et al.,[11] histology identifies four PBC stages. Stage I manifests with portal tract inflammation with predominantly lymphoplasmacytic infiltrates, resulting in vanishing

Table 75.4 Epidemiological data on primary biliary cirrhosis prevalence, incidence, and sex ratios

Year	Location	No. of cases	Case finding	Diagnosis criteria	Annual incidence (per million)	Prevalence (per million)	Gender ratio (M/F)
1980	Sheffield, UK	34	PS, lab reports	AMA+ and LFTs or liver histology	5.8	54	1:16
1980	Dundee, UK	21	Liver histology	AMA+ and liver histology	10.6	40.2	1:9.5
1983	Newcastle, UK	117	Hospital registers, lab reports, death certificates	AMA+, LFTs, and liver histology	10	37–144	1:14
1984	Malmö, Sweden	33	PS, lab reports, death certificates	AMA+, LFTs, and liver histology	4–24	28–92	1:3
1984	Western Europe	569	PS	Nonuniform	4	23 (5–75)	1:10
1985	Orebro, Sweden	18	Lab reports	AMA+, LFTs, and liver histology	14	128	1:3.5
1987	Glasgow, UK	373	Lab reports	AMA+, liver histology	11–15	70–93	–
1990	Umea, Sweden	111	PS, hospital registers, lab reports	Liver histology	13.3	151	1:6
1990	Ontario, Canada	225	PS	AMA+, liver histology	3.26	22.4	1:13
1990	Northern England	347	PS, hospital admission data, lab reports	AMA+ and LFTs or liver histology	19	129–154	1:9
1995	Victoria, Australia	84	PS, hospital records	AMA+, LFTs, and liver histology	–	19.1	1:11
1995	Estonia	69	PS, hospital admission data, lab reports	AMA+ and LFTs and liver histology	2.27	26.9	1:22
1997	Newcastle, UK	160	PS, hospital admission data, lab reports, death certificates	AMA+, LFTs, and liver histology	14–32	240	1:10
2000	Olmsted county, MN (USA)	46	Hospital records	LFTs, and AMA+ or liver histology	27	402	1:8
2005	Japan	5805	Ministry of Health database	Diagnosis in hospital records	–	–	1:8
2005	US	1032	Tertiary referrals, web-based	LFTs, and AMA+ or liver histology			1:9

AMA, anti-mitochondrial antibodies; LFTs, liver function tests; PS, physician survey.

PRIMARY BILIARY CIRRHOSIS

septal and interlobular bile ducts (diameter < 100 μm). At this stage, bile duct obliteration and granulomas (possibly found at all stages) are strongly suggestive of PBC. In stage II a periportal inflammatory infiltrate is observed and signs of cholangitis, granulomas, and florid proliferation of ductules are typical. Stage III demonstrates septal or bridging fibrosis, with ductopenia (over half of the visible interlobular bile ducts having vanished) and copper deposition in periportal and paraseptal hepatocytes can be seen. Stage IV corresponds to frank cirrhosis. The observation of eosinophils in the portal tract is a specific finding in PBC histology. Finally, the possibility of a sampling error should be considered when evaluating histology in PBC and, in case of variable staging within one biopsy, the highest stage should be accepted. Figure 75.1 illustrates the histological findings in representative cases of early PBC.

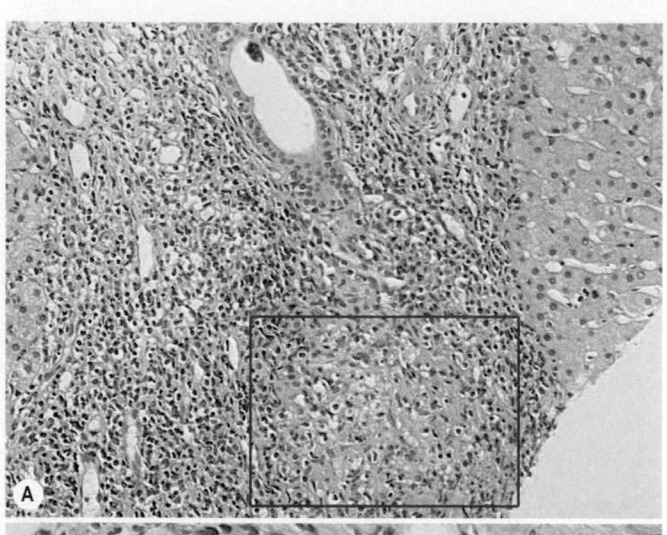
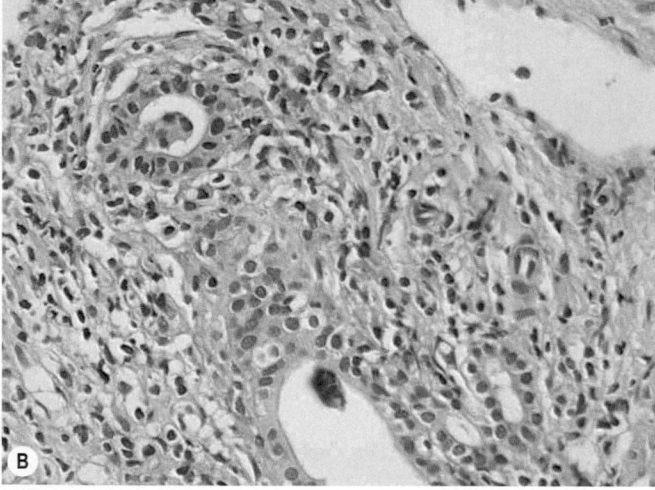

Fig. 75.1 Histological findings in early stages of primary biliary cirrhosis, i.e., nonsuppurative destructive cholangitis, following hematoxilin and eosin staining. **(A)** Mixed lymphocytic and plasma cell periductular inflammation with bile duct infiltration and granulomatous reaction (square). Magnification 200×. **(B)** Detail of bile duct disruption with lymphocytic and plasmacellular periductular and intraepithelial infiltration. Magnification 400×. (Courtesy of Dr. Marco Maggioni, Human Pathology Service, San Paolo Hospital, Milan, Italy.)

SERUM AUTOANTIBODIES

Anti-mitochondrial antibodies

AMA are highly specific for PBC and can be detected in nearly 100% of patients when sensitive diagnostic methodologies based on recombinant antigens are used.[12] In most clinical settings, however, indirect immunofluorescence techniques are used for initial screening of cases and might provide falsely positive or negative results. AMA are directed against components of the 2-oxoacid dehydrogenase (2-OADC) family of enzymes within the mitochondrial respiratory chain,[13] most frequently the E2 and E3-binding protein (E3BP) components of the pyruvate dehydrogenase complex and the E2 components of the 2-oxo glutarate dehydrogenase and branched-chain 2-oxo acid dehydrogenase complexes. In all three antigens epitopes contain the motif DKA, with lipoic acid covalently bound to the lysine (K) residue. The role of lipoic acid in epitope recognition by AMA is unclear. The pathogenic role of AMA is debatable, since no clinical correlation can be found and animal models developing serum AMA do not develop PBC-like liver lesions.

Antinuclear antibodies

As many as 50% of patients with PBC have detectable serum ANA, most commonly producing 'nuclear rim' or 'multiple nuclear dots' patterns. The pattern is based on the recognition by the autoantibodies of gp210 and nucleoporin 62 (within the nuclear pore complex) and Sp100 and promyelocytic leukemia protein (PML) (possibly also cross-reacting with small ubiquitin-like modifiers, SUMO), respectively.[14] ANA-positive patients are more frequently AMA-negative, possibly because of the lack of a masking effect of these latter antibodies in such sera. The pathogenic role of ANA in PBC remains enigmatic, although cross-sectional and longitudinal data demonstrate an association between ANA positivity and a worse prognosis. Finally, patients with PBC and limited systemic sclerosis have detectable serum anti-centromere antibodies in 10–15% of cases.

PATHOGENESIS

Several clinical and experimental findings strongly imply an autoimmune pathogenesis for PBC while two components are necessary for disease onset: a permissive genetic background and an environmental trigger.

Genetics

PBC is more frequent in relatives of affected individuals and the term 'familial PBC' has been coined to indicate families that have more than one case. Our data indicate 6% of cases have a first-degree relative that is also affected.[9] More importantly, the concordance rate observed among monozygotic twins for PBC is 63%, amongst the highest reported in autoimmunity, reinforcing the idea of an important role of genetics in disease susceptibility.[15] Several association studies have attempted to identify genes associated with PBC although no family study of genetic linkage has been performed. Associations are often not applicable to all populations but suggest that a multi-hit genetic model seems to apply to PBC, with different genetic variants conferring susceptibility (first hit) and others influencing disease progression (second hit). The study of the variants of MHC (including type I, II, and III loci) have produced associations that are often weak or limited to specific geographical areas.[14] Similar findings were also reported from the study of the genetic variants of immunomodulatory molecules (such as chemokines and their receptors), enzymes producing vasoactive compounds, and bile acid transporters that have recently been extensively reviewed elsewhere.[16] Recently, Invernizzi and colleagues reported an age-dependent enhanced monosomy X in peripheral white blood cells of women with PBC,[17] thus suggesting that PBC might ensue from a polygenic model with an X-linked major locus of susceptibility in which genes escaping inactivation are the major candidates. On the other hand, it can also be hypothesized that susceptibility to PBC is the result of a multigenic complex inheritance model where Y-linked genes might exert a protective role.

Table 75.5 Risk/protective factors (expressed as odd ratios, OR) for primary biliary cirrhosis. Results of multiple logistic regression models obtained from 1032 patients and 1041 controls are represented[9]

	OR	95% CI
Medical/family history		
Family history of PBC	10.736	4.227–27.268
Family history of SLE	2.234	1.261–3.957
Family history of Sjögren's	5.814	1.279–26.435
History of urinary tract infections	1.511	1.192–1.915
Lifestyle factors		
Ever smoked > 100 cigarettes/day	1.569	1.292–1.905
No passive smoke at work	0.820	0.582–1.155
Don't have a job	1.369	1.095–1.712
Uses of nail polish/year	1.002[a]	1.000–1.003
Number of cigarettes smoked	0.999	0.998–1.000
Each additional smoker in household	0.5078	0.3167–0.8143
Reproductive history[b]		
Ever used hormonal replacement	1.548	1.273–1.882
Never pregnant	0.6118	0.4489–0.8338
Age of first pregnancy	0.9541	0.9331–0.9755

[a]Calculated for each additional use of nail polish/year.
[b]For female cases and controls only.
CI, confidence interval; PBC, primary biliary cirrhosis; SLE, systemic lupus erythematosus

Environmental factors

Although genetics should be regarded as the major determinant in susceptibility to PBC, several other factors have been proposed. Our epidemiological study has demonstrated that a high risk of developing PBC is associated with a positive family history for PBC, a history of urinary or vaginal infections, comorbidity with other autoimmune diseases, lifestyle factors, such as smoking, and previous pregnancies (Table 75.5). Furthermore, we observed that the frequent use of nail polish also slightly increased the risk of having PBC. Experimental studies have focused on two main classes of agents possibly triggering PBC: infectious (bacteria and viruses) and chemical (xenobiotics). Most evidence has been reported for *Escherichia coli*, while contrasting data have been obtained on the role of *Chlamydia pneumoniae*. Finally, we have provided experimental evidence suggesting that *Novosphingobium aromaticivorans*, a ubiquitous xenobiotic-metabolizing Gram-negative bacterium, is the best candidate yet for the induction of PBC.[18] Figure 75.2 illustrates our bacterial theory. A retroviral hypothesis has also been proposed for PBC but direct proof is still awaited after data were not reproduced. Xenobiotics are foreign compounds that may either alter or complex to defined self or nonself proteins, inducing a change in the molecular structure of the native protein sufficient to induce an immune response. Such immune responses may then result in the cross-recognition of the self form, which could in turn perpetuate the immune response, thus leading to chronic autoimmunity. Interestingly, most xenobiotics are metabolized in the liver, thereby increasing the potential for liver-specific alteration of proteins. Data from our laboratory at UC Davis demonstrate that certain chemical compounds can induce AMA or are in fact recognized by patients' sera with higher affinity compared to self proteins[19, 20] and that specific ones are found in common-use products.[21]

NATURAL HISTORY

The progression of PBC varies widely, as represented by patients remaining asymptomatic and others reaching liver failure at young ages. The factors influencing the severity and progression of the disease are largely unknown, although data seem to indicate that genetic factors other than those inducing the disease ('second hit') might play a role. In general terms, the natural history of the disease is into three time periods preceding liver failure, i.e., asymptomatic, symptomatic, and pre liver failure. The duration of these periods can vary significantly but we note that the first step might last for decades, while the third is usually very rapid. The diagnosis of PBC is most commonly made within the first stage; patients presenting with symptoms or advanced disease are currently less frequent compared to older reports.

Having symptoms at presentation is considered the major factor determining survival rates of patients with PBC. In fact, symptomless PBC is accompanied by 10-year survival rates similar to the general population. On the other hand, 67% of precirrhotic patients will develop liver cirrhosis over a 7-year observation period while 70% of asymptomatic patients will develop symptoms. Accordingly, more recent regression models indicate that asymptomatic patients with PBC have significantly lower survival than the general population. Based on the conflicting data, it has been hypothesized that survival rates of asymptomatic patients with PBC are shorter than the general population if symptoms develop during follow-up.[22] An additional confounding factor is provided by the rate of non-liver-related deaths that appears to cause the reduced survival of asymptomatic patients.[23] Further studies on large populations and longer follow-up periods are clearly warranted.

Patients with symptomatic PBC show a more rapid progression to late-stage disease and a worse prognosis than their asymptomatic counterparts with survival time among symptomatic subjects within 6–10 years.[24] Older age at diagnosis and signs of advanced disease (clinical, histological, or biochemical) are associated with a worse prognosis. The establishment of accurate prognostic models to predict survival in patients with PBC is of obvious importance in the clinical practice. The model based on the Mayo score is the only validated and most widely utilized[25]; it is calculated based on clinical (age, presence of ascites) and biochemical variables as represented by cholestasis (bilirubin levels) and liver function (prothrombin time, albumin). We submit that this model is a static representation of a dynamic entity and has a lower accuracy for patients with early disease. Most recently, Invernizzi and colleagues reported that PBC-specific serum ANA, albeit found in a minority of patients, can predict a more aggressive disease, as suggested by longitudinal data collected during long follow-up periods.[14]

THERAPY

The only approved treatment for PBC is the hydrophilic bile acid UDCA. The mechanism of action of UDCA in PBC is incompletely understood but it has been hypothesized that it is based on

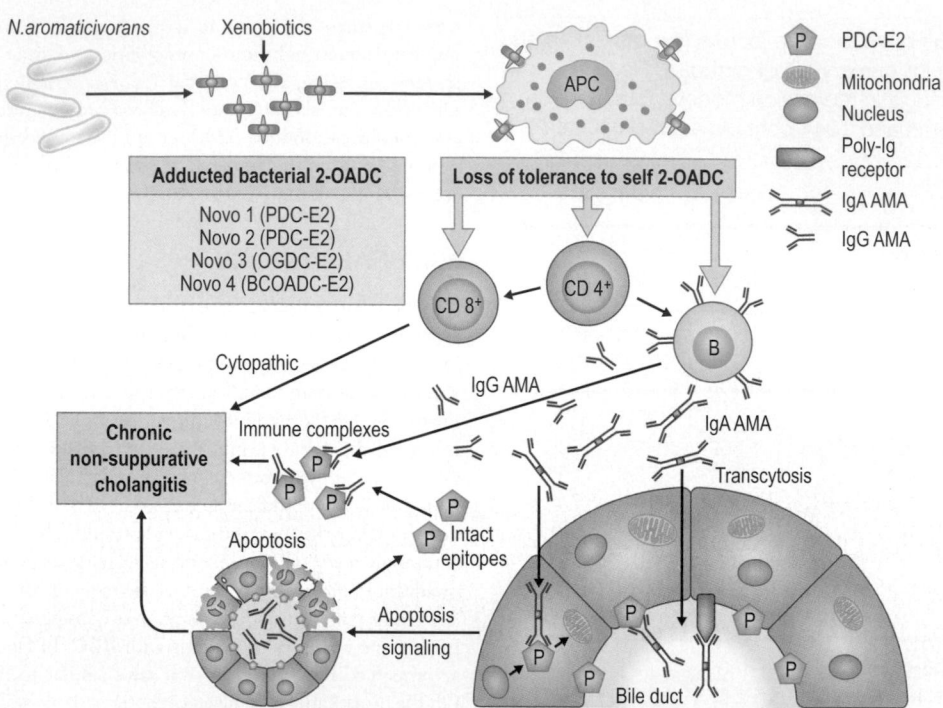

Fig. 75.2 Representation of the proposed theory on the etiopathogenesis of primary biliary cirrhosis based on the suggested role of *Novosphingobium aromaticivorans* in combination with individual susceptibility and environmental factors. The bacterium enters the mucosal system and its lipoylated proteins (Novo) are modified by xenobiotics, thus creating immunoreactive molecules. Modified proteins are then processed by antigen-presenting cells (APC) in the mucosa, thus activating autoreactive T and B cells. While T cells exert a cytopathic effect directly and/or recruit additional lymphocytes, B cells secrete anti-mitochondrial autoantibodies (AMA) of the immunoglobulin G (IgG) and IgA isotype. IgA enter the lumen of biliary epithelial cells (BECs) by transcytosis and then react with molecules mimicking pyruvate dehydrogenase ED (PDC-E2), thus initiating apoptosis. The intact PDC-E2 liberated from apoptotic cells forms immune complexes with circulating AMA IgG. Such immune complexes, the enhanced apoptosis, the direct cytopathic effect of T cells, and possibly AMA eventually lead to the appearance of the histological signs of primary biliary cirrhosis, i.e., chronic nonsuppurative cholangitis.

different factors, including modification of the bile acid pool, reduction in proinflammatory cytokines, effects on apoptosis and on vasoactive mediators.[26] Doses ranging from 13 to 15 mg/kg of UDCA are currently used and lead to optimum bile enrichment. Accordingly, a meta-analysis demonstrated that an increased survival is only obtained when a dose > 13 mg/kg is prescribed,[27] despite the fact that a complete biochemical response to UDCA is achieved in approximately 40% of treated patients. Immunosuppressive drugs have also been used in PBC with poor efficacy, including corticosteroids, azathioprine, cyclosporine, methotrexate, penicillamine, and colchicine. Their use is currently encouraged only in combination with UDCA in selected cases (i.e., when features of AIH are found). Definitive data are still awaited on the efficacy of UDCA plus bezafibrate, mycophenolate mofetil, budesonide, and tamoxifen. Liver transplantation is the ultimate treatment for end-stage PBC, with survival rates of 92% and 85% at 1 and 5 years after transplant, respectively. Recurrence is common and its rates seem to be influenced by certain immunosuppressive regimens, while the use of UDCA for recurrence is safe and recommended.

PRIMARY SCLEROSING CHOLANGITIS ■

PSC is a progressive cholestatic liver disease of unknown etiology presenting with autoimmune features and associated with significant morbidity and mortality. Different from PBC, PSC can affect all tracts of the biliary tree, including the extrahepatic bile ducts. Epidemiological data indicate that annual incidence rates are not increasing over time despite earlier ages at diagnosis and, possibly, longer survival, similar to what was observed in PBC. Recent data from the northern USA (Olmstead County, MN) reported a disease prevalence of 20.9 per 100 000 men and 6.3 per 100 000 women.[28] In fact, different from the vast majority of autoimmune diseases, PSC is more commonly diagnosed in men, with a female-to-male ratio estimated as 1:2.

CLINICAL FEATURES

PSC is currently diagnosed most commonly in the absence of symptoms and during routine blood tests in healthy individuals or patients with inflammatory bowel disease (IBD). In fact, PSC is strongly associated with

IBD, particularly ulcerative colitis (UC) with prevalence rates as high as 4%. Conversely, patients with PSC are affected by IBD in > 75% of cases (more commonly UC). The other important association is with CCA, which is found in 7–13% of patients with PSC. At early stages, PSC symptoms are generally nonspecific and include abdominal pain, jaundice, and fever in the case of bacterial cholangitis. The management of symptoms, which also include pruritus, bone density reduction, and fatigue, is similar to that described for PBC. At more advanced stages, symptoms include those of all types of decompensated cirrhosis or neoplasia. Commonly, PSC is further complicated by episodic bacterial cholangitis favored by biliary strictures. Lastly, subgroups of patients manifest the "small-duct" variant or overlap syndrome.

DIAGNOSIS

PSC is characteristically accompanied by a biochemical cholestatic pattern, as represented by elevated serum alkaline phosphatase and γ-glutamyltransferase, while tests of liver function are normal until late stages. Autoantibodies are of limited use in the diagnosis of PSC due to low sensitivity and specificity. A variable percentage of patients (as low as 33%) have detectable serum atypical p-ANCA, which can also be found in patients with AIH or IBD without PSC. More useful in the diagnosis of PSC are the imaging techniques that demonstrate strictured and dilated tracts within the intrahepatic or extrahepatic bile ducts. Among the imaging approaches in use, endoscopic retrograde cholangiopancreatography (ERCP) and magnetic resonance cholangiopancreatography (MRCP) are currently considered equal for sensitivity but their results are influenced by the operator's skills and experience. Liver histology is crucial in establishing the diagnosis in the case of small-duct PSC (typically characterized by the absence of ERCP or MRCP alterations) or PSC-AIH overlap syndrome.

LIVER HISTOLOGY

Although not necessary for establishing the diagnosis, liver histology is essential for the staging of PSC or when the small-duct variant, an overlap syndrome, or CCA is suspected. The histological picture varies widely, from minimal alterations to cirrhosis with portal inflammation, concentric 'onion-skin' periductal fibrosis, and periportal fibrosis developing into septal and bridging necrosis. Similar to PBC, sampling errors should be considered in the liver sample collection. Histological findings are only diagnostic in one-third of patients. Figure 75.3 illustrates the histological findings in two representative cases of early and advanced PSC.

INFLAMMATORY BOWEL DISEASE

As mentioned above, the majority of patients with PSC are also affected by IBD, often at asymptomatic stages.[29] Alongside the varying genetic background for IBD in different areas, the prevalence of IBD in patients with PSC changes in various part of the world. Accordingly, asymptomatic patients with PSC should undergo endoscopic evaluation with appropriate histological sampling. When IBD is found in this setting, IBD symptoms can ensue several years after diagnosis. Importantly, UC in patients with PSC is clinically different from UC without PSC in that it is often quiescent and rectum-sparing. Furthermore, PSC comorbidity in UC increases the risk of colon dysplasia or carcinoma compared to UC alone.

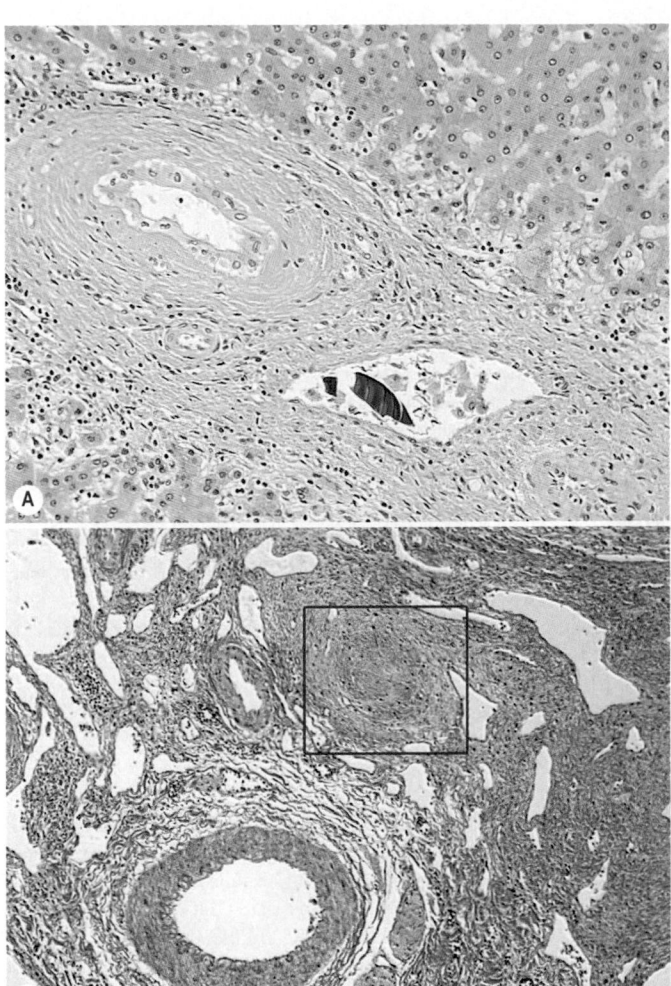

Fig. 75.3 Histological findings in primary sclerosing cholangitis. **(A)** Early disease and periductular fibrosis. Magnification 200×, hematoxylin and eosin staining. **(B)** Advanced disease with cirrhosis and bile duct substitution by fibrous scar (square). Magnification 200×, Masson staining. (Courtesy of Dr. Marco Maggioni, Human Pathology Service, San Paolo Hospital, Milan, Italy.)

PATHOGENESIS

The etiopathogenesis of PSC is unknown, despite growing evidence that (auto)immune-mediated mechanisms play a role.[30] This is indicated by the association with IBD in the majority of patients, the presence of serum autoantibodies, and the reported HLA susceptibility associations. It has been hypothesized that PSC is either an atypical autoimmune disease or an immune-mediated inflammatory disease. From a genetic standpoint, PSC occurs in susceptible individuals, as indicated by several association studies, particularly with HLA haplotypes. Family and twin studies are not available for PSC. Experimental insights into the disease pathogenesis have demonstrated a multistep pathway where innate immunity and microorganisms (possibly derived from an IBD-affected gut) play a role. In particular, cholangiocytes are first activated by bacterial stimuli in the presence of gut-specific chemokines and endothelial cell adhesion molecules in the environment. Further, gut-primed T cells migrate into the portal tracts and peribiliary spaces where focal lesions subsequently appear. Finally, chronic inflammation and progressive fibrosis of the biliary epithelium lead to chronic cholestasis secondary to vanishing bile ducts and ultimately to biliary cirrhosis.

NATURAL HISTORY

Cumulatively, data on the natural history of PSC indicate that the median timespan from diagnosis to liver-related death or liver transplantation can be estimated at 18 years.[31] It is still debated whether medical treatment with UDCA in fact produces a longer survival. The prognosis is clearly influenced by the possible onset of CCA. In most cases, an early diagnosis of CCA is problematic since its clinical presentation is not distinguishable from benign dominant biliary strictures and cytology is not 100% sensitive in the diagnosis of the neoplasia.[32] Similar to forms not associated with PSC, the prognosis of PSC-related CCA at 1 year is extremely poor, with the exception of selected patients undergoing liver transplantation.

Another important distinction in predicting the natural history is small-duct PSC. In fact, the clinical course of this subgroup of patients is relatively benign and only a minority (12%) of patients progresses to develop classical PSC.[33] Importantly, no CCA occurrence was reported in these cases, although IBD comorbidity was equally common (with possibly a higher representation of Crohn's disease), compared to classical PSC.

THERAPY

The treatment of PSC includes medical and endoscopic measures, as well as liver transplantation.[34] Most clinical trials in PSC have investigated the effects of UDCA, with conflicting results (Table 75.6). Taken together, the available evidence suggests that UDCA is not proven to produce a substantial change in the course of PSC, despite remaining the most prescribed drug. However, it appears that high-dose UDCA might reduce the rate of progression[35] and might prevent the development of colon cancer in patients with PSC and UC. Endoscopic measures are indicated to treat complicated PSC through the opening of short- and long-segment stenoses of the common bile duct and short-segment stenoses of the hepatic ducts near to the bifurcation.[36] The treatment can be repeated over time once restenoses ensue and resulting survival rates are higher compared to patients not treated endoscopically. Finally, PSC represents an important indication for liver transplantation since patients are commonly younger compared to other autoimmune liver diseases.[37] Indication is made in the absence of biliary neoplasias (ruled out by bile duct brushing) and timing is challenging due to the variable disease course. Survival rates at 1 year are approximately 90% and are only slightly lower in patients in whom CCA is diagnosed on the explanted liver. Recurrence of disease is common and affects 20–40% of transplanted patients during prolonged follow-up.

■ AUTOIMMUNE CHOLANGITIS ■

The term 'autoimmune cholangitis' was first introduced to indicate AMA-negative PBC, possibly with serum ANA.[38] However, more recently a broader significance has been suggested to include: (1) serum ANA and/or SMA positivity and/or hypergammaglobulinemia; (2) serum

KEY CONCEPTS

PRIMARY SCLEROSING CHOLANGITIS

>> Primary sclerosing cholangitis is a cholestatic liver disease of unknown etiology that is more common in men

>> It might affect any section of the biliary tree, usually producing strictures and dilation

>> Primary sclerosing cholangitis is significantly associated with inflammatory bowel diseases, particularly ulcerative colitis in an often indolent form

>> An increased risk of cholangiocarcinoma is present and the diagnosis is often challenging

THERAPEUTIC PRINCIPLES

INFLAMMATORY HEPATOBILIARY DISEASES

>> Despite common putative pathological mechanisms (i.e., autoimmunity), the treatment of early stages of autoimmune hepatitis (AIH), primary biliary cirrhosis (PBC), and primary sclerosing cholangitis (PSC) differs significantly

>> Immunosuppressants (steroids, azathioprine) are the only effective treatments for AIH

>> Ursodeoxycholic acid (13–15 mg/kg per day) is the only effective treatment for PBC

>> Ursodeoxycholic acid at high doses (> 20 mg/kg per day) for PSC might influence disease progression while endoscopic treatments may ameliorate cholestasis

>> Once liver cirrhosis ensues, treatment of complications (ascites, digestive bleeding) does not differ from other types of cirrhosis

>> Liver transplantation is the only effective treatment for all three conditions, with good survival rates; relapses are common

AMA negativity by immunofluorescence; (3) biochemical and/or histological features of cholestatic and hepatocellular injury; and (4) exclusion of chronic viral, metabolic, or toxic liver disease.[39] This definition possibly includes PBC with atypical presentation, small-duct PSC, idiopathic adulthood ductopenia, and transitional stages of the classic diseases. Consensus is still awaited on this issue.

■ OVERLAP SYNDROMES ■

It is currently estimated that as many as 18% of patients with autoimmune liver disease also manifest features on a second autoimmune liver disease. These patients are considered to have overlap syndromes.[40] Patients with overlap syndromes usually present with both hepatocellular and cholangiocellular injury with biochemical and histological features of AIH and PBC or PSC. When not treated, these patients show a progressive course toward liver cirrhosis and failure. More specifically, AIH–PBC overlap syndrome is found in 10% of adults with AIH or PBC and AIH–PSC

Table 75.6 Available data on ursodeoxycholic acid (UDCA) efficacy for primary sclerosing cholangitis (PSC)[34]

Author	Year	No. of patients	Daily UDCA dose	Duration (months)	Biochemical improvement	Symptom improvement	Histology improvement
O'Brien et al.	1991	12	10 mg/kg	30	Y	Y	–
Beuers et al.	1992	6	13–15 mg/kg	12	Y	N	Y
Lo et al.	1992	23	10 mg/kg	24	Y	N	N
Stiehl et al.	1994	20	750 mg	12–48	Y	N	Y
De Maria et al.	1996	59	600 mg	24	N	–	–
Lindor et al.	1997	105	13–15 mg/kg	34	Y	N	N
Van Hoogastraten et al.	1998	48	10 mg/kg	24	Y	N	–
Mitchell et al.	2001	26	20–25 mg/kg	24	Y	N	Y
Harnois et al.	2001	30	25–30 mg/kg	12	Y	–	–
Okolicsanyi et al.	2003	86	8–13 mg/kg	–	Y	Y	N
Olsson et al.	2004	110	17–23 mg/kg	60	Y	N	–

overlap syndromes in 6–8% of children, adolescents, and young adults with AIH or PSC. Besides overlaps, transitions are also possible in rare cases from PBC to AIH, AIH to PBC, or AIH to PSC. The pathogenesis of overlap syndromes is poorly understood, and few data are available regarding the clinical characteristics and outcome of these syndromes. Thus, the clinical management of overlap syndromes is based on single diseases while medical treatment is empiric. Therefore, UDCA is used for chronic cholestasis and immunosuppressants (steroids and azathioprine) for AIH, while liver transplantation is indicated for end-stage disease.

■ CONCLUDING REMARKS ■

As indicated by the discussed evidence, several aspects of inflammatory hepatobiliary diseases remain enigmatic. Moreover, it appears that PBC, PSC, and AIH share limited features and should be considered as single diseases in clinical practice as well as in bench research. Specifically, medical treatment of those diseases has substantial differences in response and outcomes. Finally, while it appears straightforward in many cases, the diagnosis of these conditions is often challenging. Overlap syndromes and antibody-negative forms are commonly difficult to define and can only be resolved through a collaborative effort by radiologists, pathologists, and hepatologists.

■ REFERENCES ■

1. Batts KP, Ludwig J. Histopathology of autoimmune hepatitis, primary biliary cirrhosis, and primary sclerosing cholangitis. In: Krawitt EL, Wiesner RH, Nishioka M (eds) Autoimmune Liver Diseases, 2nd edn. Amsterdam: Elsevier; 1998. : 115–140.

2. Vergani D, Alvarez F, Bianchi FB, et al. Liver autoimmune serology: a consensus statement from the committee for autoimmune serology of the International Autoimmune Hepatitis Group. J Hepatol 2004; 41: 677–683.

3. Vento S, Cainelli F, Renzini C, et al. Autoimmune hepatitis type 2 induced by HCV and persisting after viral clearance. Lancet 1997; 350: 1298–1299.

4. Donaldson PT. Genetics in autoimmune hepatitis. Semin Liver Dis 2002; 22: 353–364.

5. Czaja AJ. Natural history, clinical features, and treatment of autoimmune hepatitis. Semin Liver Dis 1984; 4: 1–12.

6. Czaja AJ, Bianchi FB, Carpenter HA, et al. Treatment challenges and investigational opportunities in autoimmune hepatitis. Hepatology 2005; 41: 207–215.

7. Feld JJ, Dinh H, Arenovich T, et al. Autoimmune hepatitis: effect of symptoms and cirrhosis on natural history and outcome. Hepatology 2005; 42: 53–62.

8. Invernizzi P, Crosignani A, Battezzati PM, et al. Comparison of the clinical features and clinical course of anti-mitochondrial antibody-positive and -negative primary biliary cirrhosis. Hepatology 1997; 25: 1090–1095.

9. Gershwin ME, Selmi C, Worman HJ, et al. Risk factors and comorbidities in primary biliary cirrhosis: a controlled interview-based study of 1032 patients. Hepatology 2005; 42: 1194–1202.

10. Kikuchi K, Lian ZX, Yang GX, et al. Bacterial CpG induces hyper-IgM production in CD27(+) memory B cells in primary biliary cirrhosis. Gastroenterology 2005; 128: 304–312.

11. Ludwig J, Dickson ER, McDonald GS. Staging of chronic nonsuppurative destructive cholangitis (syndrome of primary biliary cirrhosis). Virchows Arch A Pathol Anat Histol 1978; 379: 103–112.

12. Miyakawa H, Tanaka A, Kikuchi K, et al. Detection of anti-mitochondrial autoantibodies in immunofluorescent AMA-negative patients with primary biliary cirrhosis using recombinant autoantigens. Hepatology 2001; 34: 243–248.

13. Gershwin ME, Ansari AA, Mackay IR, et al. Primary biliary cirrhosis: an orchestrated immune response against epithelial cells. Immunol Rev 2000; 174: 210–225.

14. Invernizzi P, Selmi C, Ranftler C, et al. Antinuclear antibodies in primary biliary cirrhosis. Semin Liver Dis 2005; 25: 298–310.

15. Selmi C, Mayo MJ, Bach N, et al. Primary biliary cirrhosis in monozygotic and dizygotic twins: genetics, epigenetics, and environment. Gastroenterology 2004; 127: 485–492.

16. Selmi C, Invernizzi P, Zuin M, et al. Genetics and geoepidemiology of primary biliary cirrhosis: following the footprints to disease etiology. Semin Liver Dis 2005; 25: 265–280.

17. Invernizzi P, Miozzo M, Battezzati PM, et al. Frequency of monosomy X in women with primary biliary cirrhosis. Lancet 2004; 363: 533–535.

18. Selmi C, Balkwill DL, Invernizzi P, et al. Patients with primary biliary cirrhosis react against a ubiquitous xenobiotic-metabolizing bacterium. Hepatology 2003; 38: 1250–1257.

19. Long SA, Quan C, Van de Water J, et al. Immunoreactivity of organic mimeotopes of the E2 component of pyruvate dehydrogenase: connecting xenobiotics with primary biliary cirrhosis. J Immunol 2001; 167: 2956–2963.

20. Leung PS, Quan C, Park O, et al. Immunization with a xenobiotic 6-bromohexanoate bovine serum albumin conjugate induces anti-mitochondrial antibodies. J Immunol 2003; 170: 5326–5332.

21. Amano K, Leung PS, Rieger R, et al. Chemical xenobiotics and mitochondrial autoantigens in primary biliary cirrhosis: identification of antibodies against a common environmental, cosmetic, and food additive, 2-octynoic acid. J Immunol 2005; 174: 5874–5883.

22. Springer J, Cauch-Dudek K, O'Rourke K, et al. Asymptomatic primary biliary cirrhosis: a study of its natural history and prognosis. Am J Gastroenterol 1999; 94: 47–53.

23. Prince MI, Chetwynd A, Craig WL, et al. Asymptomatic primary biliary cirrhosis: clinical features, prognosis, and symptom progression in a large population based cohort. Gut 2004; 53: 865–870.

24. Pares A, Rodes J. Natural history of primary biliary cirrhosis. Clin Liver Dis 2003; 7: 779–794.

25. Grambsch PM, Dickson ER, Kaplan M, et al. Extramural cross-validation of the Mayo primary biliary cirrhosis survival model establishes its generalizability. Hepatology 1989; 10: 846–850.

26. Lazaridis KN, Gores GJ, Lindor KD. Ursodeoxycholic acid 'mechanisms of action and clinical use in hepatobiliary disorders'. J Hepatol 2001; 35: 134–146.

27. Gluud C, Christensen E. Ursodeoxycholic acid for primary biliary cirrhosis. Cochrane Database Syst Rev2002: CD000551.

28. Bambha K, Kim WR, Talwalkar J, et al. Incidence, clinical spectrum, and outcomes of primary sclerosing cholangitis in a United States community. Gastroenterology 2003; 125: 1364–1369.

29. Broome U, Bergquist A. Primary sclerosing cholangitis, inflammatory bowel disease, and colon cancer. Semin Liver Dis 2006; 26: 31–41.

30. Aoki CA, Bowlus CL, Gershwin ME. The immunobiology of primary sclerosing cholangitis. Autoimmun Rev 2005; 4: 137–143.

31. Levy C, Lindor KD. Primary sclerosing cholangitis: epidemiology, natural history, and prognosis. Semin Liver Dis 2006; 26: 22–30.

32. Jones BA, Gores GJ. Hepatobiliary malignancy. Clin Liver Dis 1998; 2: 437–449. xi–xii.

33. Bjornsson E, Boberg KM, Cullen S, et al. Patients with small duct primary sclerosing cholangitis have a favourable long term prognosis. Gut 2002; 51: 731–735.

34. Cullen SN, Chapman RW. Review article: current management of primary sclerosing cholangitis. Aliment Pharmacol Ther 2005; 21: 933–948.

35. Mitchell SA, Bansi DS, Hunt N, et al. A preliminary trial of high-dose ursodeoxycholic acid in primary sclerosing cholangitis. Gastroenterology 2001; 121: 900–907.

36. Stiehl A. Primary sclerosing cholangitis: the role of endoscopic therapy. Semin Liver Dis 2006; 26: 62–68.

37. Bjoro K, Brandsaeter B, Foss A, et al. Liver transplantation in primary sclerosing cholangitis. Semin Liver Dis 2006; 26: 69–79.

38. Heathcote J. Autoimmune cholangitis. Gut 1997; 40: 440–442.

39. Czaja AJ, Carpenter HA, Santrach PJ, et al. Autoimmune cholangitis within the spectrum of autoimmune liver disease. Hepatology 2000; 31: 1231–1238.

40. Beuers U, Rust C. Overlap syndromes. Semin Liver Dis 2005; 25: 311–320.

part 8

NEOPLASIA AND THE IMMUNE SYSTEM

Lymphoid leukemias

Moshe E. Gatt, Dina Ben-Yehuda, Shai Izraeli

76

The leukemias are a group of malignant clonal diseases arising in the bone marrow, each of which is characterized by a specific set of clinical and laboratory features. This chapter focuses on the two most common lymphoid leukemias, acute lymphoblastic leukemia (ALL) and chronic lymphocytic leukemia (CLL). ALL is the most common leukemia of lymphoid precursors. CLL consists of a clonal accumulation of mature lymphoid cells and is the most common type of leukemia in adults. Special emphasis is given to immunological aspects of both diseases.

◼ ACUTE LYMPHOBLASTIC LEUKEMIA ◼

ALL is characterized by the clonal proliferation and accumulation of malignant lymphoid progenitors. ALL is typically viewed as a developmental disease of the lymphoid system. Indeed, it is believed that most of childhood ALL arise as a 'developmental accident' during normal fetal lymphopoiesis.[1] Studies of chromosomal translocations in ALL cells have identified key genes involved in normal lympho- and hematopoiesis. Conversely, basic studies of the development of the immune system and the immune receptors have provided important tools for the diagnosis and management of ALL. These achievements in basic and clinical research have led to the remarkable transformation of ALL from what was a uniformly fatal disease several decades ago to a disease that is curable in more than 80% of children. Unfortunately, at present adults do not fare as well.[2–4]

EPIDEMIOLOGY AND ETIOLOGY

ALL is the most common malignancy of childhood. One in every 2000 children will develop leukemia by 15 years of age. In contrast ALL accounts for fewer than 20% of leukemias in adults. In developed countries, incidence peaks at 2–5 years of age (to about 55 per million), remains low during later childhood, adolescence, and young adulthood (fewer than 10 per million), and then rises again in individuals older than 65 years of age. In all age groups, males tend to be affected more often than females. The low age peak is characteristic of affluent societies, and

the higher rate of childhood ALL in whites than blacks and in northern America and Europe compared with Asia and Africa has been attributed to socioeconomic factors.[5]

Most ALLs are sporadic. Fewer than 5% are associated with hereditary or constitutional syndromes. Children with Down syndrome have about 20-fold increased risk of ALL. This higher risk may reflect the leukemogenic role of chromosome 21, as extra copies of chromosome 21 are frequently observed in leukemic blasts of sporadic ALL.[6] Other diseases associated with increased risk are inherited genomic instability syndromes such as ataxia-telangiectasia, Bloom syndrome and Li–Fraumeni syndrome. ALL is also more common in patients with other congenital immunodeficiencies, such as X-linked agammaglobulinemia, immunoglobulin A deficiency, and common variable immunodeficiency (Chapter 34).

Studies of leukemia in identical twins have shed light on the etiology of childhood ALL. Although ALL is not hereditary, there is markedly increased risk of leukemias in identical twins. If leukemia occurs in one identical twin, the other twin generally has a 10–20% chance of developing the disease by the age of 10 years. This phenomenon has promoted the hypothesis that at least two genetic hits are required for the development of ALL[5] (Fig. 76.1). The first occurs during fetal lymphopoiesis and results in clonal proliferation of a preleukemic clone. Molecular studies have demonstrated that intrauterine metastasis of such a preleukemic clone from one twin to the other via their shared placental circulation is responsible for the concordant leukemia. These studies have also demonstrated that additional genetic hits in the preleukemic cells occur after birth and are required for the development of full-blown leukemia, which explains the less than 100% concordance. The initial findings in identical twins with leukemia have been extended to sporadic ALL; in at least 70% of patients the preleukemic clone can be detected molecularly in the neonatal blood samples collected after birth (known as Guthrie cards). More recently, molecular analysis of cord blood of normal infants has demonstrated that the occurrence of a preleukemic clone carrying a leukemia-defining chromosomal translocation is very common (up to one of every 20 newborns). Only 1% of children born with such a preleukemic clone will develop leukemia, making a molecular screen for early diagnosis of childhood ALL impractical.

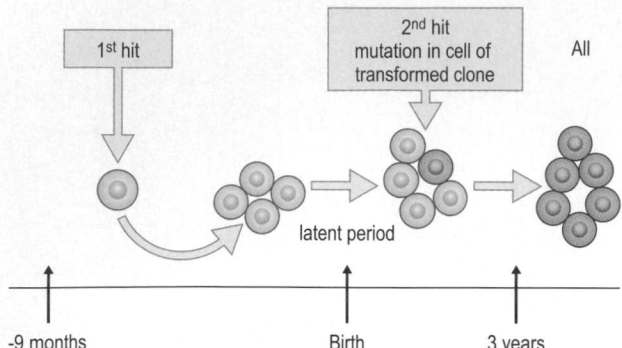

Fig. 76.1 A model for the development of childhood acute lymphoblastic leukemia (ALL). The first acquired genomic hit (e.g., chromosomal translocation or change in chromosomal copy number) occurs during fetal hematopoiesis and results in clonal proliferation of a preleukemic clone. This event is common, occurring in up to 1 in every 20 children. Additional genetic aberrations occurring after birth are required for the development of ALL. These events are rare and are estimated to occur in about 1% of children born with a preleukemic clone.[5]

The causes of the relatively rare postnatal leukemogenic genetic hits are unknown. Although environmental agents such as ionizing radiation and chemical mutagens have been implicated in the induction of ALL, almost all cases lack discernible etiologic factors. As the risk of B-cell precursor ALL during early childhood is markedly increased by higher socioeconomic status and suburban style of living, in which the exposure of children to infectious pathogens is typically delayed beyond the neonatal period, Greaves hypothesized that many childhood cases are the consequence of an abnormally late immunologic response to common infections. One proposed mechanism is that growth-inhibitory factors, such as interferon or transforming growth factor-β (TGF-β), secreted during this immune response, provide a survival advantage to a preleukemic clone, setting the stage for additional leukemogenic mutations.[5] Recently, increased expression of interferon inducible genes has been observed in many cases of hyperdiploid ALL, possibly providing the first direct biological evidence for the potential involvement of the immune system in the pathogenesis of childhood ALL.[7]

IMMUNOLOGIC AND MOLECULAR CLASSIFICATION OF ALL

Immunologic classification

The subtypes of ALL are usually identified by their immunophenotype, which often resembles the lymphoid developmental stage in which the leukemic cell was arrested[8, 9] (Table 76.1).

B-cell precursor leukemias. These are the most common childhood leukemias. Pro-B ALL is characterized by expression of CD19 and CD34 without CD10. This is the most common leukemia of infants that usually contains rearrangements of the MLL gene on chromosome 11q23 and is associated with poor outcome. Leukemic blast cells of early pre-B ALL resemble normal B-lymphoid cell precursors. They express CD19, CD22, and CD79a. CD10 and terminal deoxynucleotidyl

transferase (TdT) are detectable in 90% of cases, and CD34 in more than 75% of cases. This is the most common type of ALL, often called 'common ALL.' In pre-B ALL cases lymphoblasts accumulate cytoplasmic immunoglobulin heavy chains but have no detectable surface immunoglobulins. This subtype also expresses CD19, CD22, and CD79a. This type of leukemia often contains a translocation that fuses the E2A gene on chromosome 19 with the PBX1 gene on chromosome 1.[10] Leukemic cells that express both cytoplasmic and surface immunoglobulin heavy chains have been designated transitional pre-B ALL. The surface μ-chains on these leukemic cells are linked to pseudo-light chains (Chapter 4) as well as to CD79a and CD79b.

Mature B-cell ALL is the leukemic form of Burkitt's lymphoma (Chapter 77). As treatment for mature B-cell ALL is dramatically different from that for B-cell precursor ALL, it must be specifically ruled out before initiating therapy. Mature B-cell ALL cells express surface immunoglobulin μ heavy chains plus either κ or λ light chains. In most cases cells have an L3 morphology and express CD19, CD22, and CD20. They frequently express CD10 and CD23 as well. CD34 is absent.

T-cell ALL. In affluent countries, T-ALL occurs in 10–15% of children with ALL. Its prevalence is higher in nonaffluent countries, probably as a reflection of a lower incidence of the common B-lineage early-childhood peak. T-ALL is also more common in adults. T-ALL has a less favorable prognosis than B-cell precursor ALL.

T-cell ALL cells express surface CD7 and cytoplasmic CD3 (cCD3). More than 90% of T lymphoblasts also express CD2, CD5, and TdT. Three stages of immunophenotypic differentiation can be determined: early (CD7+, cCD3+, surface CD3-, CD4-, and CD8-), intermediate (cCD3+, surface CD3-, CD4+, CD8+, and CD1+) and late (surface CD3+, CD1-, and either CD4+ or CD8+). However, up to one-quarter of T-lineage ALL cases do not conform to one of these maturation stages.[11]

T-cell receptor (TCR) proteins are heterogeneously expressed in T-lineage ALL. In approximately two-thirds of cases membrane CD3 and TCR proteins are absent. However, in half of these cases TCR proteins (TCR-β, TCR-α, or both) are present in the cytoplasm. When membrane CD3 and TCR chains are expressed, the αβ form of the TCR predominates. Only a minority of cases expresses TCR γδ proteins.

The expression of myeloid-associated antigens, such as CD13, CD15, CD33, or CD65, in leukemic lymphoblasts can complicate leukemia classification in early studies. The diagnosis of B-lineage ALL should be made when leukemic cells express cytoplasmic immunoglobulin, CD79a, or CD19 plus CD22, regardless of myeloid-associated antigen expression. Likewise, the diagnosis of T-lineage ALL should be made when leukemic cells express CD7 plus either surface or cytoplasmic CD3. Myeloid-associated antigen expression in ALL has no independent prognostic significance. These ALLs should be distinguished from true biphenotypic leukemias that usually express cytoplasmic myeloperoxidase. Biphenotypic leukemias are associated with poorer outcome and are often treated with acute myeloid leukemia protocols.

Genetic and molecular classification

Virtually every leukemic cell has acquired alterations in more than one oncogene. These alterations are manifest as gross numerical or structural aberrations that can be used to define a specific clinical subtype of ALL. The common and/or clinically significant genetic aberrations that are

Table 76.1 Immunophenotypic classification of acute lymphoblastic leukemia

Subtype	Leukocyte antigen expression (% of cases positive)										Frequency (%)	
	CD19	cCD22	CD79a	CD10	CD7	CD2	cCD3	clg μ	slg μ	slg κ or γ	Children	Adults
Pre-pre-B	100	>95[a]	>95	0	0	0	0	0	0	0	5	10
Early pre-B	100	>95[a]	>95	95	5	<5	0	0	0	0	60–65	50–55
Pre-B	100	100[a]	100	>95	0	0	0	100	0	0	20–25	10
Transitional pre-B	100	100[a]	100	50	0	0	0	100	100	0	1–3	?
B	100	100[a]	100	50	0	0	0	>95	>95	>95	2–3	4
Pre-T	<5	0	0–20	45	100	0	100	0	0	0	1	5
T	<5	0	0–20	45	100	95	100[a]	0	0	0	10–15	15–20

c, cytoplasmic; clg μ, cytoplasmic immunoglobulin μ-chain; slg μ, surface immunoglobulin μ-chain; slg κ or λ, surface immunoglobulin κ- or λ-chains.
[a]Detectable on the cell surface membrane in some cases.

typically found in ALL are reviewed in references 2 and 12 and summarized in Table 76.2.[2, 12]

Numerical chromosomal aberrations. Deviation from the normal chromosomal modal number is called aneuploidy and is the most common chromosomal aberration in cancer. High Hyperdiploid ALL (Fig. 76.2)A, containing between 50 and 60 chromosomes, is the most common type of B-lineage ALL in children and is associated with about 90% cure rate. Typically there is excess of specific chromosomes, most commonly chromosomes 6, 10, 14, 17, 18, 21 and X. Hypodiploid ALL (Fig. 76.2)B, containing less than 45 chromosomes is much rarer and is associated with a very poor prognosis.

Chromosomal translocations can be divided into two general subtypes;[13, 14] The first is the translocation of a proto-oncogene into the proximity of a strong regulatory region, resulting in its marked overexpression. Often these translocations are mediated by the V(D)J recombination machinery (Chapter 4) and can be therefore viewed as unfortunate developmental "accidents" caused by the physiologic lymphocyte specific genomic instability. Such instability is necessary for the creation of the diversity required for the recognition of novel foreign antigens. Examples of these translocations are the activation of *MYC* oncogene by the t(8;14) translocation in Burkitt's lymphoma and, the activation of the *SCL (TAL1)* gene by the t(1;14) translocation near the *SIL* gene on chromosome 1p32 in T-ALL. Most of the chromosomal translocations observed in T-ALL are of the latter type. The second is the creation of novel fusion proteins consisting of parts of the genes that participate in the chromosomal translocation. The mechanisms of these translocations are unclear. Most of the translocations characteristic of B precursor ALL are of this type, for example the t(12;21) fusion of the *TEL (ETV6)* gene on chromosome 12 with the *AML1 (RUNX1)* gene on chromosome 21.

Amplifications and deletions of small chromosomal regions represent a second set of common structural aberrations. For example, deletion of the INK4A locus located on the short arm of chromosome 9, which codes for the tumor suppressor genes *P16* and *P14*, is often observed in T-ALL. Amplification of the AML1 locus on the long arm of chromosome 21,

Table 76.2 Frequencies of major clinically important genetic aberrations in childhood and adult acute lymphoblastic leukemia

Genetic abberation	Children (%)	Adults (%)
B-cell lineage		
Hyperdiploidy (> 50 chromosomes)	30	9
Hypodiploid (< 45 chromosomes)	1	2
Amplified 21q	2	?
TEL-AML1 (t12;21)	25	3
MLL rearrangements	9	13
BCR-ABL	4	33
E2A-PBX1	5	4
MYC rearrangements	2	5
T-cell lineage		
Notch1 mutations	60	70
TAL1 (SCL) cluster	58	33
HOX11 (TLX1) cluster	3	33
HOX11L2 (TLX3) cluster	20	5
LYL1 cluster	12	37
MLL-ENL	2	2
NUP214-ABL	6 (?)	6 (?)

Modified from Armstrong SA, Look AT. Molecular genetics of acute lymphoblastic leukemia. J Clin Oncol 2005; 23: 6306–6315; and Pui CH, Relling MV, Downing JR. Acute lymphoblastic leukemia. N Engl J Med 2004; 350: 1535–1548.

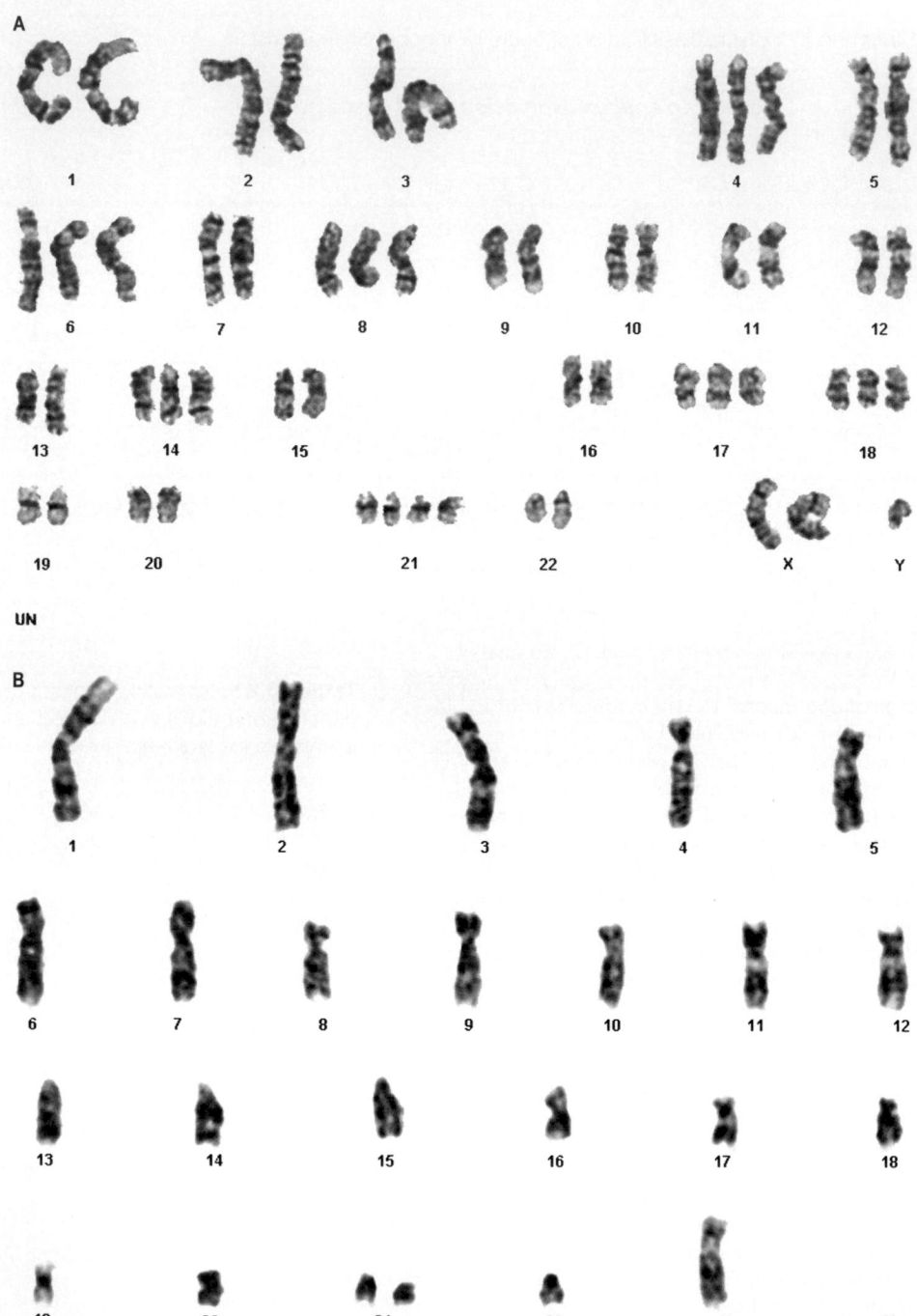

Fig. 76.2 Chromosomal aneupoloidy in acute lymphoblastic leukemia (ALL). A typical karyotype of (**A**) hyperdiploid and (**B**) hypodiploid ALL. (Courtesy of B. Stark and D. Betts.)

found in about 2% of B cell precursor ALL, has been associated with an extremely poor prognosis.

Oncogenic activating mutations in ALL are reported with an increasing frequency. The Notch pathway, which is normally involved in T cell development, has been recently reported to be activated by acquired mutations in more than 60% of T-ALL.[15] This finding is of potential therapeutic significance since novel β-secretase inhibitors, originally developed for treatment of Alzheimer's disease, block the Notch pathway. Another example is mutational activation of the FLT3 growth pathway, which is often observed in hyperdiploid and t(4;11) leukemias.

Table 76.3 Example of hematopoietic genes involved in the pathogenesis of leukemia

Gene(s) names	Normal hematopoietic development	Leukemic involvement
SCL (TAL1)	Hemangioblast specification. Erythro- and megakaryopoiesis	T-ALL
LMO1/2	Similar to SCL	T-ALL
NOTCH	T lymphocytes	T-ALL
HOX11	Spleen	T-ALL
E2A	T and B lymphocytes	BCP-ALL
PAX5	B lymphocytes	BCP-ALL, B-NHL
SLP-65	B lymphocytes	BCP-ALL
TEL	Bone-Marrow Hematopoietic Stem Cells	BCP-ALL, rarely myeloid malignancies
RUNX1 (AML1, CBFA2)	Definite hematopoiesis. Megakaryopoiesis and T lymphocytes	BCP ALL, AML (M0-M1) Hereditary FPD/AML
CBFB	Same as RUNX1	AML (M4e)
C/EBP 1-3	Myeloid cells	AML (M1, M2)
PU.1	Myeloid and Lymphoid stem cells	AML
GATA1	Erythropoiesis, Megakaryopoiesis and Mast cells	AML (M7) associated with trisomy 21
FLT3	Hematopoiesis and lymphopoiesis	AML and ALL
MLL	Hematopoiesis stem cells	AML and ALL

AML, acute myeloid leukemia; BCP-ALL, B cell precursor acute lymphoblastic leukemia; B-NHL, B cell Non Hodgkin Lymphoma; FPD, familial platelet disorder; T-ALL, T-cell acute lymphoblastic leukemia.

Many of the genes modified by chromosomal translocations, amplification, deletions or point mutations play important roles in normal lymphoid or hematopoietic development (Table 76.3). The acquired aberrations of these genes may promote malignant transformation by overexpression or aberrant expression (wrong cell or wrong developmental stage). The activation of Notch in T-ALL is a prime example. Conversely, the acquired genetic aberration may block the normal developmental function of the involved gene(s). For example, the *TEL-AML1 (ETV6-RUNX1)* translocation occurs in about 25% of childhood B-precursor ALLs; *AML1* is required for embryonic hematopoietic development and for differentiation of the lymphoid and the megakaryocytic compartments. It is involved in multiple translocations, resulting in fusion proteins that are thought to block its normal function dominantly. TEL is required for maintenance of the hematopoietic stem cells. The normal TEL allele is lost in the majority of TEL-AML1 leukemia, which implies that inhibition of the normal function of TEL further facilitates the development of this subtype of leukemia.

MAJOR CLINICALLY RELEVANT MOLECULAR SUBTYPES OF ALL (TABLE 76.2)

B-lineage ALL

Hyperdiploid and TEL-AML1 ALL comprise the majority of 'common ALL' leukemias typical of young children, but are rare in adults with ALL. Both are associated with an extremely good prognosis. In contrast, hypodiploidy (fewer than 45 chromosomes) and the internal amplification of chromosome 21q (iAMP 21q) are both associated with a poor prognosis.[16, 17] Another poor-prognosis aberration is the *BCR-ABL* fusion created by the t(9;22) 'Philadelphia chromosome.' Its frequency is low in children (3–5%) but high in adults (at least 30%). These differences may

explain the poorer outcome of ALL in adults compared with children. The *MLL* gene located on chromosome 11q23 is involved in fusion translocations, with more than 80 different partner genes. The most common translocation in ALL fuses the *MLL* with the *AF*4 gene on chromosome 4. This t(4;11) translocation is characteristic of infant leukemia and is associated with poor prognosis. Interestingly, translocations involving the *MLL* gene are commonly seen in secondary leukemias (mostly AMLs) that occur in patients treated with topoisomerase inhibitors for a variety of cancers (e.g., etoposide or doxorubicin). This association raises the possibility that infant leukemias with *MLL* rearrangements are caused by intrauterine exposure to an environmental topoisomerase inhibitor. This has prompted large ongoing epidemiological studies.

The clinical significance of the *E2A-PBX1* fusion caused by the t(1;19) translocation, which occurs in fewer than 5% of childhood ALL, remains unclear. It was associated with a worse prognosis for patients on treatment protocols that were mainly based on antimetabolite chemotherapy. However, with newer protocols that incorporate anthracyclines, this prognostic significance has been lost. Indeed, this type of ALL may be associated with a better outcome. The change in the prognostic significance of this particular translocation with improved therapy exemplifies the general principle that the prognostic impact of a clinical or biological parameter is highly dependent on the specific treatment protocol.[2, 3] The *E2A* gene is rarely fused with the *HLF* gene in the t(17;19) translocation. This is an extremely rare translocation that is associated with a clinical presentation of diffuse intravascular coagulation and hypercalcemia and an extremely poor prognosis.

T-lineage ALL

Although multiple genetic and molecular subtypes of T-ALL have been recently described, their clinical significance is presently unclear.[12, 18] Most of the genetic aberrations in T-ALL result in the abnormal expression of transcription factors. Aberrant overexpression of the bHLH transcription factor SCL (TAL1) is found in at least 60% of T-ALL in children and in about a third in adults. The mechanism of its overexpression is unknown in about half of these patients. The LMO1 or LMO2 proteins are often co-expressed with SCL. Together with SCL, these two proteins regulate very early T-cell development. Their aberrant continued expression is believed to cause the differentiation arrest characteristic of T-ALL. The importance of this gene in leukemogenesis has perhaps been best demonstrated by the development of T-ALL in several patients with severe combined immunodeficiency where there was retroviral insertion into the *LMO2* gene with gene therapy (Chapters 35 and 101). Another set of common abnormalities in childhood T-ALL is the activation of either *HOX11L2 (TLX3)* or, less commonly, *HOX11 (TLX1)* by chromosomal translocations with the TCR loci. Other chromosomal rearrangements in T-ALL involve the bHLH transcription factor LYL1, the *MLL-ENL* fusion, and amplification of the *ABL* oncogene. Activating mutations in Notch1 have been reported in over 60% of patients with all karyotypic subtypes of T-ALL. This finding suggests that activation of the Notch pathway may contribute to enhanced proliferation of T-cell precursors, thereby 'setting the stage' for the occurrence of other leukemogenic translocations. One recent study reported that children with T-ALL carrying *NOTCH* mutations had better survival when treated using Berlin–Frankfort–Munster protocols.[19] This association requires independent verification from other clinical studies.

CLINICAL FEATURES

The clinical signs and symptoms of leukemia reflect the replacement of bone marrow cells by leukemic blasts and the infiltration of extramedullary sites by the leukemic cells. Anemia, thrombocytopenia, and neutropenia that result from bone marrow involvement may manifest as pallor, fatigue, petechiae, bleeding, or fever. Bone pain and arthralgias, the development of a limp, the refusal of the young child to walk, and even frank arthritis are not uncommon. The musculoskeletal symptoms may be confused with osteomyelitis or juvenile idiopathic arthritis, which may delay the diagnosis. Uncommonly, central nervous system (CNS) involvement may present with signs and symptoms of increased intracranial pressure, such as headaches and papilledema, or by cranial nerve palsies, nuchal rigidity and, rarely, as hyperphagia and obesity caused by infiltration of the hypothalamus. Overt testicular leukemia at diagnosis is rare and manifests by painless testicular enlargement. Mediastinal involvement, common in T-ALL, may lead to dyspnea, superior vena cava syndrome, and even frank respiratory failure.

CLINICAL PEARLS

ACUTE LYMPHOBLASTIC LEUKEMIA (ALL) AND RHEUMATOID DISORDERS

>> ALL can mimic juvenile idiopathic arthritis (JIA) and other musculoskeletal disorders

>> Leukemic blasts may be absent from the peripheral blood, hence bone marrow examination should be considered in any child with JIA, especially prior to commencement of steroid therapy.

Clinical laboratory findings often reveal anemia and thrombocytopenia. However, leukocyte counts may vary. Only 20% of children present with leukocyte counts greater than 50 000/μl, whereas up to 40% demonstrate leukocyte counts less than 10 000/μl. Leukemic blasts may or may not be seen on peripheral smears. Therefore the diagnosis of leukemia may occasionally be missed in routine automated blood count. Elevated serum lactate dehydrogenase activity, hyeruricemia, or hyperphosphatemia are commonly observed in patients with a large leukemic cell burden.

The diagnosis of ALL is established by bone marrow examination. The normal bone marrow contains less than 5% blasts. A minimum of 25% lymphoblasts on differential examination of the bone marrow aspirate is necessary for the diagnosis of ALL. Most children with ALL have a hypercellular marrow with blasts constituting 60–100% of the nucleated cells.

Traditionally, CNS leukemia is defined by the presence of at least 5 leukocytes/μl of CSF and the detection of leukemic blast cells, or by the presence of cranial nerve palsy or by retinal involvement, as detected by ophthalmoscopy. While overt CNS leukemia is relatively rare, submicroscopic CNS involvement is present at diagnosis in at least half of the patients, even in the absence of any neurological symptoms. Therefore CNS-directed therapy is routinely included in ALL therapy (see below).

The differential diagnosis of ALL includes neoplastic and nonneoplastic diseases. Because children with ALL present with a variety of nonspecific symptoms, several pediatric nonmalignant conditions may be confused with leukemia. Since treatment with steroids can mask the presence of ALL, *serious consideration of the diagnosis of ALL must be given before starting treatment with steroids to any pediatric nonmalignant disorder*. Bone marrow examination is recommended in case of uncertainty.

Idiopathic thrombocytopenic purpura (ITP) is a common cause of bruising and petechiae in children. ITP is characterized by the absence of any other hematological abnormalities. Bone marrow should be examined if anemia or hepatosplenomegaly is present. Infectious mononucleosis can present with fever, malaise, adenopathy, splenomegaly, rash, and lymphocytosis. Lymphocytosis accompanied by thrombocytopenia and immunohemolytic anemia may further confuse the diagnosis. The atypical lymphocytes may morphologically resemble leukemic lymphoblasts, although an experienced hematologist can usually easily distinguish between the two conditions. Rarely, flow cytometry may be necessary to distinguish between activated atypical lymphocytes and immature leukemic lymphoblasts. Occasionally bone marrow examination is needed. Leukemoid reactions, observed in sepsis, acute hemolysis, and other disorders are usually easy to distinguish from ALL by morphological examination of peripheral blood smear. Since ALL occasionally presents with pancytopenia, aplastic anemia must also be considered.

Between 5% and 10% of children with ALL are first evaluated at pediatric rheumatology clinics. Fever, arthralgias, arthritis, or a limp accompanied by anemia, mild splenomegaly, and lymphadenopathey may frequently be confused with juvenile idiopathic arthritis (JIA) (Chapter 53) or osteomyelitis. Several of these patients receive antibiotics and anti-inflammatory agents for several weeks to months before the diagnosis of ALL. Bone marrow examination should be seriously considered in such patients.

As leukemic lymphoblasts are small round blue cells when stained with hematoxylin and eosin, they may be rarely be confused with metastatic small round-cell pediatric tumors, including neuroblastoma, rhabdomyosarcoma, and retinoblastoma.

SPECIAL DIAGNOSTIC TESTS

The classification and risk stratification for treatment protocols of ALL are based on detailed immunophenotyping and genotyping analysis.[20] Immunophenotyping by flow cytometry is required for confirmation of the diagnosis of ALL and for determination of the specific immunophenotype. Flow cytometry of propidium iodide-stained lymphoblasts can be used to determine the DNA index for the diagnosis of numerical chromosomal aberrations. A high DNA index (> 1.16) is typical for good-prognosis high hyperdiploid ALL, whereas a low DNA index reflects hypodiploidy, which is associated with a poor outcome. Cytogenetic analysis is required for the determination of the major genetic subtypes. In most centers karyotype by classical cytogenetics (Fig. 76.2) is performed. However, because of lack of metaphases, the yield of karyotypic analysis of ALL in multicenter protocols is often less than 70%. Furthermore, the observed karyotype may be derived from normal bone marrow cells and not from leukemia blasts. This drawback can be overcome by interphase fluorescent *in-situ* hybridization (FISH), a technique that does not require metaphases, or by direct examination of the genes or their products (Chapter 101). All clinically relevant structural and numerical chromosomal aberrations can be detected by the use of commercially available FISH probes (Fig. 76.3). Fusion translocations, such as *BCR-ABL, TEL-AML1,* and *MLL-AF4,* can be detected by reverse transcriptase polymerase chain reaction (RT-PCR).

The elucidation of the human genome and the invention of microarray technologies are anticipated to revolutionize the diagnostics of leukemias. Several pioneering studies from St. Jude Children's Research Hospital, Memphis, TN, USA, have demonstrated the diagnostic power of microarray-based gene expression analysis of childhood ALL.[21, 22] Currently several prospective studies are comparing microarray technology with more conventional methods for identification of clinically relevant genetic subtypes of leukemia. It is highly likely that within the next 5 years microarray technology will be incorporated into the clinical diagnostics of leukemia.

PRINCIPLES OF THERAPY[3]

Supportive therapy is given before the initiation of leukemia-specific therapy and this includes hydration, treatment, and preventive therapy of hyperuricemia, blood and platelet transfusion, and treatment of emergencies such as respiratory insufficiency associated with mediastinal leukemia.

It is highly recommended that children and adults with ALL be treated in specialized centers as part of a clinical prospective study. Such clinical trials are the basis for the dramatic improvement in the ALL patient outcome that has been achieved over the last several decades.

Treatment of ALL is initiated with an intensive remission induction regimen. This is usually followed by risk stratification into several treatment arms based on molecular studies and response to initial therapy. An intensification course may be followed by another phase of reinduction. All protocols include a prolonged maintenance phase, which consists of low-dose oral chemotherapy continued for 2–3 years after remission. Continuous chemotherapy for at least 2 years is unique to ALL. This approach differs significantly from chemotherapy regimens involving several very intensive courses for a relatively short time that are typically used for mature B-cell or acute myeloid leukemias. This empiric evolution of vastly different treatment protocols for B-cell precursor ALL versus mature B-cell leukemias likely reflects fundamental differences in the biology of the relevant leukemic stem cell.

Typical remission induction regimens include a glucocorticoid (prednisone, prednisolone, or dexamethasone), vincristine, and L-asparaginase. Several protocols also add anthracycline. The rate of complete remission now ranges between 97% and 99% for children versus 75% and 90% for adults. Intensification therapy incorporates either high doses of multiple agents not used during the induction phase or repeats the induction regimen. Regimens used for children include high-dose methotrexate with or without 6-mercaptopurine; high-dose L-asparaginase given for an extended period; an epipodophyllotoxin plus cytarabine; or a combination of dexamethasone, vincristine, L-asparaginase, doxorubicin, and thioguanine,

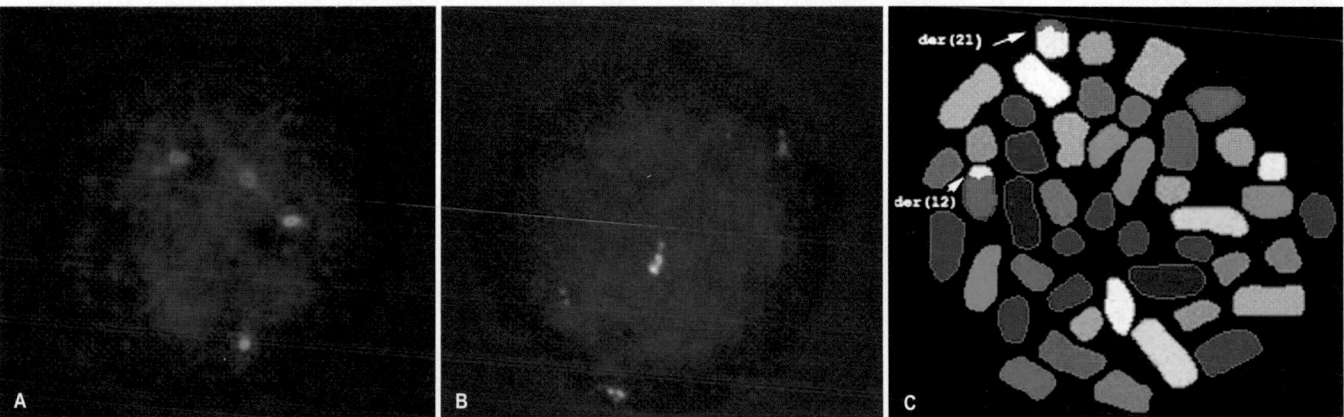

Fig. 76.3 Molecular cytogenetic techniques for the diagnosis of chromosomal translocations in acute lymphoblastic leukemia (ALL). Panels A and B display interphase fluorescent *in-situ* hybridization (FISH) with probes to the *AML1* (RUNX1) gene on chromosome 21 (red) and to the *TEL* (ETV6) gene on chromosome 12 (green). Panel A displays a normal cell, and panel B displays a leukemic cell that has undergone a fusion *TEL-AML1* translocation (arrow). Panel C displays the same translocation as depicted in B, but on metaphase chromosomes. It uses a molecular cytogenetic technique called *spectral karyotyping* (arrows). Classical cytogenetic analysis often misses this translocation. (Courtesy of Dr. L. Trakhtenbrot.)

with or without cyclophosphamide. Another integral component of many protocols is reinduction therapy. This treatment employs drugs similar to those used during the initial phase of induction therapy and has improved the outcomes of both children and adults with ALL. Maintenance therapy consists of a combination of methotrexate administered weekly and mercaptopurine administered daily. Some protocols add intermittent pulses of vincristine and dexamethasone.

CNS prophylactic therapy consisting of cranial irradiation plus intrathecal chemotherapy that is introduced after the induction of complete remission became one of the cornerstones of ALL therapy in the 1970s. More recently, because of concerns about neurotoxicity and the occurrence of brain tumors, the regimen of choice tends to include both intensive intrathecal and systemic chemotherapy.

Allogeneic stem-cell transplantation is reserved for patients who have relapsed or who suffer from refractory leukemia, as well as for patients with very-high-risk leukemia, such as BCR-ABL leukemia with slow response to therapy. With improvements in the prevention of transplant-related toxicities, suitable marrow donors now include matched unrelated donors and, in some situations, two- and three-antigen-mismatched family members, as well as classic human leukocyte antigen (HLA)-identical siblings or single-antigen-mismatched family members. Umbilical cord blood and peripheral blood stem cells have also been used successfully.

PROGNOSTIC FACTORS (TABLE 76.4)

Therapy for ALL is based on adjustment of the intensity of therapy to the risk assessment of the relapse hazard.[3,23] The two major clinical parameters of prognostic significance are age at diagnosis and leukocyte count. Favorable prognostic factors include presentation of the disease when the child is between 1 and 9 years of age and a leukocyte count less than 50×10^9/l. For adults, the outcome of therapy worsens with increasing age and leukocyte count; patients older than 60 years and/or leukocyte count $>100 \times 10^9$/l have a particularly poor treatment response. Girls fare somewhat better than boys and in some protocols boys are treated for 3 instead of 2 years. Hyperdiploidy (> 50 chromosomes) and *TEL-AML1* are favorable prognostic factors that correlate strongly with age and white cell count.

MLL gene rearrangements lead to a less favorable prognosis, especially the *MLL-AF4* fusion. This fusion translocation is mostly detected in infant leukemia. The presence of the Philadelphia chromosome encoding the BCR-ABL fusion also confers a poor prognosis. Patients with either of these abnormalities are stratified into a high-risk treatment arm in all current protocols. Also associated with bad prognosis is hypodiploidy and amplification of the AML1 region on chromosome 21. Traditionally patients with T-ALL tended to fare worse than those with B-lineage ALL. However, these differences appear to have been eliminated with the introduction of many modern protocols.

The most significant prognostic factor is the initial response to therapy. A rapid clearance of leukemic cells from the blood or bone marrow confers a favorable prognosis. A child with BCR-ABL positive ALL who presents with a low leukocyte count and in whom all blasts have disappeared from the peripheral blood after 1 week of steroid therapy is likely to do better than a similar child with hyperdiploid leukemia who has not significantly reduced the blast count after 2 weeks of therapy. The level of minimal residual disease (MRD) after the induction of clinical remission has also emerged as a powerful tool for gauging treatment response and predicting outcome.

WHERE IMMUNOLOGY MEETS ONCOLOGY – MINIMAL RESIDUAL DISEASE

Modern treatment protocols lead to morphological complete remission, defined as less than 5% blasts in the bone marrow examination, in the majority of patients. If treatment is discontinued at that stage, most patients will eventually relapse. Indeed, all prospective clinical studies have shown that ALL should be treated for at least 2 years. These facts indicate that viable clonigenic malignant lymphoblasts continue to persist even after the completion of remission induction, even though the patient may be in clinical and morphological remission. Indeed, by this criterion patients may have as many as 10^{10} undetectable neoplastic cells when in remission. Since leukemic cells have to constitute at least 1–5% of the nucleated cells in the bone marrow in order to be detected by microscopic examination, morphological examination is clearly inadequate for evaluation of the quality of remission. Therefore more sensitive

Table 76.4 Major prognostic factors in acute lymphoblastic leukemia[a]

Prognostic factor	Good prognosis	Worse prognosis
Age at diagnosis	1 < age < 10 (6) years	< 1 year; > 10 years (children) > 60 years (adult)
Peripheral blood WBC	< 50 000/µl	
Response to therapy	Early response to therapy; negative MRD at the end of induction	Slow response to therapy High MRD
Genetic abnormalities	Hyperdiploidy (> 50 chromosomes); TEL/AML1 (ETV6/RUNX1)	BCR/ABL MLL/AF4 Hypodiploidy < 45 chromosomes

MRD, minimal residual disease; WBC, white blood cells.
[a]The most important prognostic factor is the *treatment protocol*. Thus the prognostic significance of various clinical and laboratory variables may differ between protocols. Here, the significant parameters common to most studies are listed.

techniques for detection of rare leukemic cells are required. This is the rationale behind the recent incorporation of modern techniques of detection of MRD into treatment protocols of childhood ALL.

RT-PCR is an extremely sensitive technique for evaluation of residual leukemic cells that carry fusion translocations (such as *BCR-ABL* and *TEL-AML*). However, the majority of the leukemias lack these translocations. During the last decade, two general methologies for sensitive detection of submicroscopic residual leukemic cells have been developed. These methodologies could not be developed without an understanding of the scientific basis of the developmental phenotype of immune cells (Chapters 8 and 9) and of the elaborate process of immunoglobulin gene rearrangements (Chapter 4).

The most widely studied DNA-based MRD methodology is based on the identification of clonospecific rearrangements of immunoglobulin genes or T-cell receptors (IgTCR-PCR).[24] This approach exploits the physiologic process of somatic rearrangement of Ig and TCR gene loci that occurs during early differentiation of any lymphocyte. Thus, any single lymphocyte carries a unique rearrangement that is not shared by any other lymphoid cell. This process ensures the level of diversity of the immune response against an unlimited number of antigens. Since leukemia is clonal, that is, it originates from one lymphoid cell, all the leukemic cells of a particular person carry the same Ig and/or TCR rearrangements. Because leukemic cells are genetically unstable, they often

(> 90% of the cases) carry multiple rearrangements, a fact that facilitates the usefulness of using these rearrangements as a clonal marker for MRD detection. The major advantages of this technique are the exquisite sensitivity (at least 10^{-5}), reliability, reproducibility, and its applicability to more than 90% of children with ALL. Its biggest disadvantages are the costs and complexity.

Current strategies for flow cytometric detection of MRD rely on combinations of leukocyte markers that do not normally occur in cells of the peripheral blood and bone marrow. Such leukemia-associated phenotypes can be identified by two-, three-, or four-color staining techniques (Fig. 76.4).[25] Flow cytometric analysis allows the detection of one leukemic cell among 10^4 or more normal cells. The advantages of flow cytometry for MRD detection are adequate sensitivity and the presence of immunophenotyping facilities in most major centers that facilitates the timely performance of the analysis on fresh cells at a reasonable cost. There are a few disadvantages, however. It requires a flow cytometry operator with a high level of expertise and it is more difficult to standardize compared to PCR. Moreover, it may be difficult to distinguish between regenerating B-cell progenitors and leukemic blasts. Thus flow MRD is most reliable and sensitive at very early stages (up to 4 weeks) of therapy.

Many clinical studies on a relatively small number of patients (which include a total of several hundred patients) enrolled on ALL treatment protocols revealed strikingly similar results. Fast clearance of leukemic

ACUTE LYMPHOBLASTIC LEUKEMIA

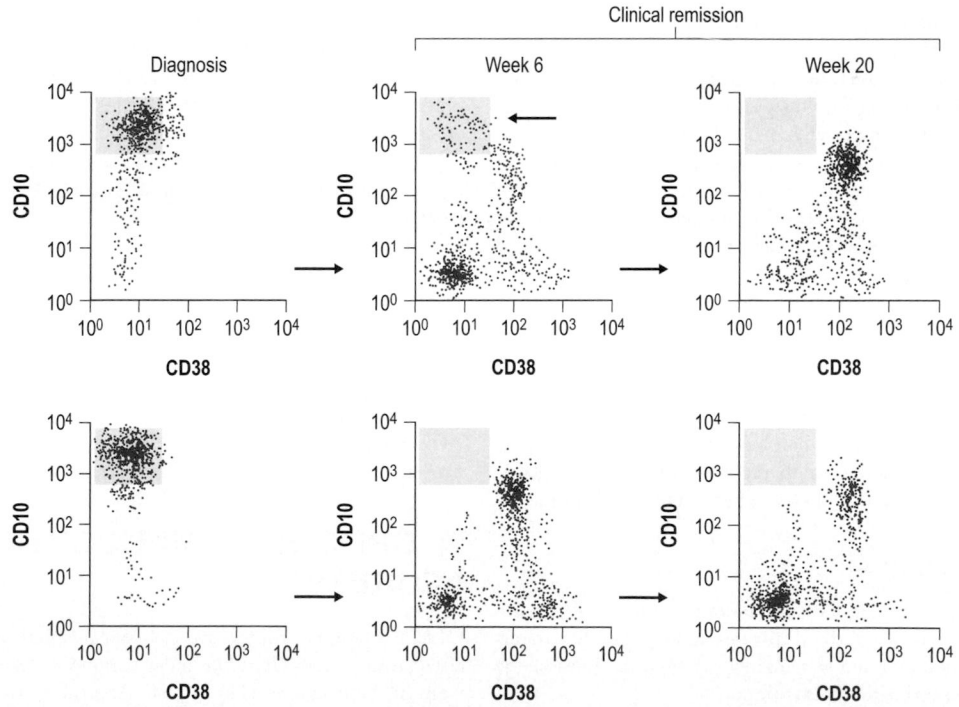

Fig. 76.4 Different kinetics of leukemia cytoreduction revealed by minimal residual disease (MRD) studies with flow cytometry.[51] The left panels illustrate the leukemia-specific immunophenotype (CD10+,CD38−) determined at diagnosis in two children with ALL. This phenotype is not found in normal bone marrow. Bone marrow samples were collected during clinical remission from both patients. In one patient (top panels), 0.04% of mononuclear cells expressed the leukemia-specific phenotype at week 6. MRD was undectable by week 20. In the other patient (bottom panels), a profound remission (MRD < 0.01%) was achieved by week 6 and maintained at week 20.

blasts to below 10^{-4} cells within the first 2–4 weeks of therapy is detected in about 40% of children with ALL and is associated with an extremely good prognosis. Conversely, the presence of more than 0.1% blasts after 2 or 3 months of therapy defines a very high-risk group.[9, 26–29] These initial findings have led the BFM-AEIOP study group to initiate a prospective study on children with ALL that utilize the MRD level determined by IgTCR-PCR for risk classification. Initial, as-yet unpublished analysis of more than 2500 patients (presented in the iBFM Study Group meeting 2006), confirms the strength of PCR MRD over genetic classification as a prognostic marker.

At present MRD studies have been incorporated into most treatment protocols. Patients with high MRD are stratified into a high-risk arm and receive more intensive chemotherapy. A few protocols are also testing whether therapy can be reduced for patients with no detectable MRD after 2–4 weeks of therapy, irrespective of their clinical presentation. While the robustness of MRD as the most sensitive and reliable prognostic indicator in ALL has been confirmed, at present it is unclear if adjustment of therapy to the MRD level will improve survival for these higher-risk patients.

COURSE AND PROGNOSIS

With current protocols, the cure rate of children with ALL is about 80%.[3, 4] More than 90% of children with low-risk leukemia and about 70% of children with high-risk leukemia are cured. The cure rates of adult is significantly lower – around 35–40%[30, 31] – probably because these adults tend to suffer with ALL genetic subtypes that have an inherently unfavorable prognosis.

Most relapses occur during treatment or within the first 2 years after completion of therapy. However, late relapses (even 10 years after diagnosis) are increasingly seen, especially in ALL containing the *TEL-AML1* genotype. In about 5% of cases, the clinical relapse occurs in an extramedullary site, most often the CNS or, in males, the testes. Leukemic relapse occasionally occurs at other sites, including the eye, ear, ovary, uterus, bone, muscle, tonsil, kidney, mediastinum, pleura, and paranasal sinuses. The prognosis of relapse depends on the time from diagnosis (earlier is worse), leukocyte count, immunophenotype, and genotype (similar to the prognostic factors at diagnosis). Isolated extramedullary relapse carries a better prognosis. Although some relapses can be treated by chemotherapy alone, most are being treated by stem-cell transplantation. At present, the most important prognostic factor is the MRD level before transplant. More than half of the late relapses (more than half a year since completion of therapy) in patients with "good-prognosis" ALL are curable. The prognosis of early relapsers is grim.

TREATMENT SEQUELAE

Improvements in supportive care reduced the rate of early death to less than 2% in the 1990s. However, the death rate among elderly patients during remission induction therapy remained as high as 30% due to hematological, hepatic, and cardiac toxicities.

Long-term toxicity is also of major concern for children cured from ALL. Aseptic necrosis of various bones has emerged as a common late toxicity of glucocorticoids, especially in adolescent girls treated with dexamethasone.[32, 33] The rate of long-term neurotoxicity has been reduced due to replacement of cranial irradiation with high-dose and intrathecal methotrexate. However, it remains unclear whether intensive methotrexate therapy may lead to very

late neurodegeneration effects. The dose of anthracyclines used in most ALL protocols is unlikely to produce severe cardiomyopathy. However, secondary cancers are a major concern. The development of therapy-related acute myeloid leukemia has been linked to the use of topoisomerase II inhibitors (teniposide and etoposide), and the risk is apparently dependent on the treatment schedule and the concomitant use of other agents (e.g., L-asparaginase, alkylating agents, and perhaps antimetabolities). Children who received cranial irradiation at 6 years of age or younger are most susceptible to the development of brain tumors. This risk is increased by the intensive use of antimetabolite drugs before and during cranial irradiation.[34]

Recent long-term follow-up studies reported from Scandinavia of children cured of ALL confirm excellent long-term outcome, judged by their socioeducational achievements and by reproductive success resulting in healthy children.[35]

CURRENT CONTROVERSIES AND FUTURE PERSPECTIVE

The high cure rates in patients with ALL (nearly 80% of children and 40% of adults) attest to the steady progress that has been made in treating this disease. A further increase in cure rates will require efforts to maximize the efficacy and minimize the toxicity of current therapy. A major challenge is to improve risk classification to optimize therapy for individual patients. Progress in pharmacogenomics may allow personal tailoring of dosage of specific drugs. The role of microarray gene expression analysis is still unclear, as well as the best technical approach to MRD. Currently MRD measurement can reliably identify the extremely good and poor-risk patients. However, about half of the patients belong to an "intermediate-risk" group in which most of the relapses occur. Optimization of diagnosis and treatment of this group of patients are among the current major challenges.

The development of new treatments for ALL is a major challenge, especially for the high-risk group of patients. Given the rarity of ALL, compared with epithelial cancers, the development of specific new drugs is unlikely. Imatinib, the prototype of targeted therapy against BCR-ABL chronic myeloid leukemia, has only modest activity against BCR-ABL ALL. New ABL and dual kinase inhibitors may prove more promising. Genetic modifications of allogeneic and autologous cells may be another future approach for targeted therapy of ALL. The reliable identification of extremely high-risk ALL patients by MRD measurement permits the examination of new therapies early in the course of therapy, as a phase I/II window. Such studies within the context of large cooperative trials may further improve the survival of patients with high-risk ALL.

■ CHRONIC LYMPHOCYTIC LEUKEMIA ■

CLL is a lymphoproliferative indolent neoplasm of mature peripheral circulating B cells. It is the most common leukemia in adults of the western hemisphere (Fig. 76.5). According to the World Health Organization classification, CLL and small lymphocytic lymphoma (SLL) are considered to be one disease at different stages.[36] CLL originates from a clonal lymphoid-evolved mature stem cell which can be identified by its distinct B-cell immunoglobulin gene rearrangement. Both clinically and at the molecular level, CLL is a heterogeneous disease. Some patients have an indolent course with distinct

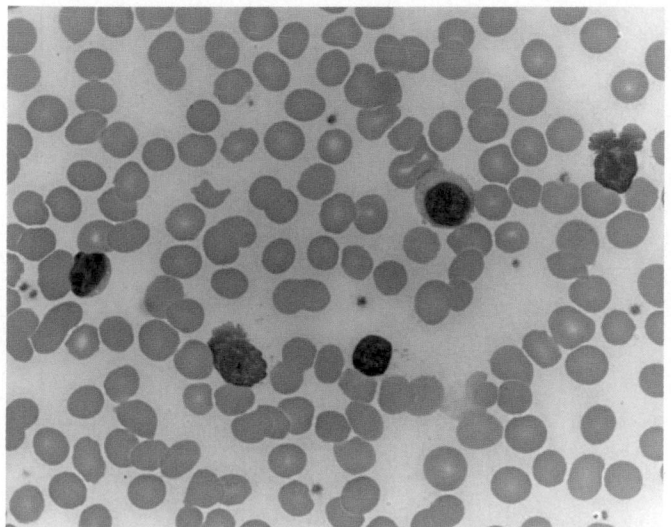

Fig. 76.5 A Giemsa-stained peripheral blood smear displaying chronic lymphocytic leukemia cells.

genetic markers, whereas other suffer with a more rapid and aggressive disease characterized by a separate molecular signature. During its progression, CLL may be associated with significant immune deficiencies and autoimmune phenomena that can complicate its course and treatment. These abnormalities may be so profound that they alter the nature of the disease. They are attributed to the clonal nature of its B-cell origin. More than 95% of patients have a B-CLL phenotype; the remainder express T-CLL.

EPIDEMIOLOGY

The clinical diagnosis of CLL requires absolute lymphocytosis of more than 5000/μl mature lymphocytes in the peripheral blood. The extensive use of automated peripheral blood lymphocyte counts has led to an increase in the rate of diagnosis of asymptomatic patients with CLL. The incidence rate of CLL increases logarithmically from age 35, with a median age at the time of diagnosis of 65 years. There is a male predominance, and the disease exhibits geographic and ethnic variation. In the USA, CLL is reported to occur with equal incidence among residents of sub-Saharan African and European descent, but it is uncommon among those of East Asian descent. The reported incidence is 4.3/100 000 per year. Because many of these patients may never require tissue diagnosis or inpatient treatment, they are not likely to be recorded by a tumor registry. Thus the true annual incidence of the disease is likely to be higher than previously appreciated (6.8/100 000 population).[37] It is important to note that, when techniques of higher sensitivity are used, monoclonal populations of B lymphocytes that are indistinguishable from CLL cells can be found in the blood of 3.5% of persons older than 40 years of age.[38]

The etiology of CLL is largely unknown; however, as with other forms of malignancy, there is increasing evidence for the role of inherited factors in its development. Family surveys show a genetic predisposition in first-degree relatives. Anticipation, the phenomenon of earlier onset and more severe phenotype in successive generations, has been reported in CLL families.[39]

PATHOGENESIS AND THE BIOLOGY OF LEUKEMIC LYMPHOCYTES

CLL was initially considered to be a single homogeneous disease of accumulating immature, immune-competent, minimally self-renewing B cells. It is now viewed as two related entities, both of which originate from B lymphocytes while differing in their state of activation and maturation.[40]

Normal B-lineage cells mature in the bone marrow, where they undergo rearrangement of immunoglobulin variable (V), diversity (D), and joining (J) gene segments to create the rearranged variable domains that encode the antigen-binding portion of their antigen receptor, immunoglobulin (Chapters 4 and 8). When an antigen of adequate affinity engages their B-cell receptor, the cell enters a germinal center located in a lymphoid follicle, where, as a centroblast with appropriate T-cell help, it rapidly divides and its V genes undergo somatic hypermutation. This process introduces mutations in the rearranged gene segments that code for the binding site of the receptor. Through these mutations, the receptors of the descendent B cells, called centrocytes, acquire new properties. Cells with receptors that have enhanced antigen-binding affinity proliferate in the presence of the antigen, whereas centrocytes with receptors that no longer bind the antigen (or bind autoantigens) are normally eliminated. Once the centrocytes are selected, they become plasma or memory B cells (Fig. 76.6). Thus, the CLL cell population may originate from a clone with few or no V-domain mutations, or from a more mature clone whose V domains have undergone the hypermutation process. This creates two separate pools of B cells, both of which originate from antigen-stimulated mature B lymphocytes. In CLL with mutated Ig genes, the proliferating B cell is likely to have traversed a germinal center, whereas in CLL with unmutated Ig genes the malignant B cell is more likely to derive from a pregerminal center naïve B cell.

Mutations of V genes are detected by comparing DNA sequences of the genes in B cells with corresponding genes in the germline. A sequence that differs from its germline counterpart by 2% or more is defined as mutated. This mutational status strongly correlates with prognosis, in that patients with an unmutated clone have a much worse prognosis than patients with mutated clones.[41] These patients may differ also in their association with specific genetic aberrations. 11q22-23 (the ataxia-telangiectasia mutated gene) or 17p13 (the p53 gene) deletions are associated with a poorer outcome and with an unmutated VH profile. These genes regulate apoptosis and resistance to chemotherapy. 13q14 deletion or a normal karyotype are associated with a mutated profile of V genes, and are considered to carry better prognosis. There is controversy as to whether trisomy 12 is associated with an unmutated status.[42] These chromosomal aberrations appear to have separate and independent (unrelated to the mutational status) effects on the patient's prognosis.[43]

Antigens typically found on the surface of the membrane of B-CLL cells include CD19, CD21, and CD23, with reduced levels of membrane IgM, IgD, and CD79b. This is a phenotype most consistent with that observed among mature activated B cells. The pathological features of biopsied lymph node are those of an SLL.[40] The coexpression of CD5, a T-cell-associated antigen, is a phenotypic characteristic and part of the disease-defining criteria. CD5+ B cells can be found in the peripheral blood of normal adults, suggesting that specific subsets of CD5+ B cells from the mantle zone may be the normal counterparts of B-CLL.[40, 44] The low expression of the BCR is the hallmark of CLL cells, and appears to contribute impaired responses to BCR stimulation. Studies analyzing

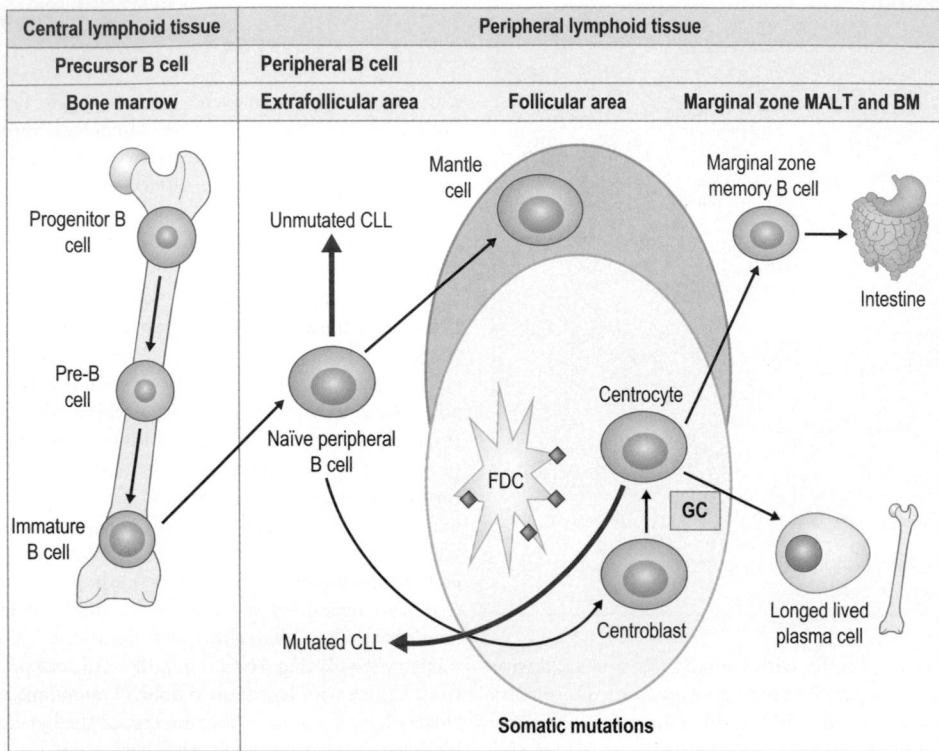

Central lymphoid tissue	Peripheral lymphoid tissue		
Precursor B cell	Peripheral B cell		
Bone marrow	Extrafollicular area	Follicular area	Marginal zone MALT and BM

Fig. 76.6 Chronic lymphocytic leukemia (CLL) and B-cell development. The phenotype displayed by a B-cell lymphoproliferative disorder reflects the stage of normal B-cell development it achieved prior to its final transformation. Development begins in the fetal liver and in fetal and adult bone marrow. Maturing B cells exit to the peripheral blood, but typically require entry into the germinal center (GC) in order to undergo somatic hypermutation. The CLL cells that express unmutated immunoglobulin variable domains thus likely underwent final transformation prior to entry into the GC, whereas those that express mutated variable domains likely transited the GC and then underwent final transformation. Transformation in pro- and pre-B cells typically gives rise to acute lymphoblastic leukemia. Transformation of intermediate stages can give rise to mantle-zone lymphomas. Transformation at later stages can give rise to marginal-zone lymphomas and plasma cell-derived multiple myeloma.

signal competence have shown that unmutated CLLs tended to express higher amounts of the BCR and to respond better to stimulation when compared with mutated CLLs. These results suggest that unmutated CLLs may be more likely to preserve their ability to respond to BCR stimulation, whereas mutated ones most closely resemble the phenotype observed in anergic B cells.[43]

The CD38 surface molecule supports B-cell interactions and differentiation, and under certain circumstances augments signaling of BCR, delivering signals that regulate the apoptosis of B cells.[43] It also correlates with the mutational status of the BCR and confers bad prognosis. Another molecule that influences the BCR is zeta-associated protein 70 (ZAP-70). High levels of this receptor-associated protein tyrosine kinase (usually found in T and natural killer (NK) cells, but not in normal B cells) are detected in the majority of unmutated CLLs. These levels may be measured by routine flow cytometry studies and correlate not only with the an unmutated V domain state, but also independently with prognosis.[45]

The role of the antigenic stimulus for promotion of proliferation has also been studied. The BCRs from various patients are similar, suggesting a common pathogenetic antigen. The source of this putative common antigen – bacteria, virus, or rather an environmental factor – has yet to be identified.[40] The possibility that an autoantigen provokes clonal expansion is supported by the finding of some mutated immunoglobulin V genes that encode poly-reactive receptors.

The microenvironment may also play a role in the pathogenesis of CLL.[40, 46] Interactions with stromal cells rescue CLL cells from apoptosis *in vitro*, activated T cells support the growth of CLL cells, and cytokines such as interleukin-4 (IL-4) and vascular endothelial growth factor and chemokines such as SDF-1 support the expansion of CLL clones.

CLL is classically characterized by the accumulation of mature B cells that evade apoptosis, with high levels of the BCL2 anti-apoptotic protein.[46] Contradicting this dogma is the measurement of CLL kinetics, which has shown CLL cells to proliferate at a high dynamic rate of up to 1% of the clone per day.[47] This finding suggests that CLL may not only be an accumulative disease, but also has a proliferative element.

CLINICAL FEATURES OF CLL

The clinical diagnosis of CLL requires an absolute lymphocytosis of greater than $5000 \times 10^9/l$ mature-appearing lymphocytes in the blood smear and that persists for a period of at least 4 weeks. By immunophenotype, the

CLINICAL PEARLS

CLINICAL MANIFESTATIONS OF CHRONIC LYMPHOCYTIC LEUKEMIA

>> Absolute blood lymphocytosis > 5000/mm³ sustained over a period of 4 weeks (to exclude transient lymphocytosis-related conditions as viral infections)

>> At least 30% lymphocytes in a normo- or hypercellular marrow

>> Lymphocytes are phenotypically monoclonal, i.e., express both B-cell markers (CD19, CD23, CD20) and the pan-T-cell marker (CD5)

>> Lymphocytes are morphologically mature-appearing

>> Most patients will have some degree of lymphadenopathy on physical examination

>> Progression and the need for treatment are according to lymphocyte doubling time, bulky symptomatic disease, anemia, thrombocytopenia, and autoimmune phenomena

cells predominantly display the mature B-cell markers (CD19, CD20, and CD23) as well as the pan-T-cell CD5 antigen in the absence of all other T-cell markers. As many as one-quarter of patients are asymptomatic at the time of diagnosis.[48, 49] For those who are symptomatic, clinical characteristics at presentation include lymphadenopathy (87%), splenomegaly (54%), hepatomegaly (14%), leukocytosis, anemia, and thrombocytopenia (20%). Very high blood cell counts are rare at the time of initial diagnosis, but may develop over time. Hyperleukocytosis causing leukostasis and needing emergency treatment is extremely rare, but has been reported in isolated cases.[50] In addition to the lymphoid tissues, solid organs and the skin may occasionally be affected. A full diagnostic evaluation typically requires a bone marrow aspirate and biopsy. An interstitial or nodular infiltration pattern correlates with a better prognosis than the diffuse type.[49, 51]

A prognostic evaluation, especially in young patients or early stages of CLL, should include evaluation of the CD38 and ZAP-70 immune phenotype, cytogenetic analysis for chromosomal abnormalities, and an assessment of the extent of somatic hypermutation in the CLL immunoglobulin H-chain variable domain. Lymph node biopsy is not necessary, but if performed may lead to the diagnosis of SLL, which is currently considered a separate manifestation of the same disease. A wide spectrum of immune deficiency and autoimmune phenomena is characteristic of CLL, and is discussed in greater detail in the following section on immunologic aspects of the disease. The differential diagnosis includes other low-grade lymphoproliferative disorders such as the leukemic phase of lymphoma and mantle-cell lymphoma (usually negative for CD23), hairy-cell leukemia (CD5 and 21-negative and CD103 and 25-positive), T-cell leukemia (expressing the CD3, CD4, and CD7 T-cell markers) and prolymphocytic leukemia (PLL), which is distinguished by morphologically immature-appearing cells and the presence of FMC7 and CD79b on the cell surface. T-cell CLL is rare (< 5%).

The oldest system of CLL risk stratification relies on measurement of disease bulk. Rai et al.[52] reported a staging classification ranging from stage 0 to 4 that uses lymphadenopathy, splenomegaly, anemia, and thrombocytopenia as markers of progressive disease bulk. Subsequently,

Binet et al.[53] reported a staging system ranging from stages A to C that relies on the number of enlarged lymph node regions and the presence of anemia or thrombocytopenia (Table 76.5).[51] Both staging systems place patients into one of three prognostic groups: good, intermediate, and poor prognosis. Placement into the last group makes the patient a candidate for treatment. These staging systems have been very useful for defining whom to treat at the time of diagnosis, but not at predicting who will subsequently need treatment.[38]

One-third of patients never require treatment and have a long survival. In another third, an initial indolent phase is followed by disease progression. The remaining third tends to exhibit aggressive disease at the onset and needs immediate treatment. However, even in the low-risk group (stage A Binet or stage 0 Rai), over 25% of these indolent cases die of causes related to CLL, 40% progress to advanced stages, and 50% ultimately require treatment. These results demonstrate that neither the Rai nor the Binet staging system is able to predict accurately which patients among the good-prognosis group will eventually develop progressive disease.

The most powerful predictors for rapid and aggressive progression are the mutational status and chromosomal abnormalities, as described above (Fig. 76.7 and Table 76.5).[40] The mutational profile has the advantage of remaining constant during disease evolution, in contrast to genomic aberrations and surface markers such as CD38. Since the ability to sequence immunoglobulin genes is not available in most laboratories, a surrogate assay such as the ZAP-70 molecule, as identified by flow cytometry, may become the laboratory test of choice. This test is still not widely used due to the technically difficult nature of the flow cytometric assay.[51] Another marker, β_2-microglobulin, was reported in retrospective series to correlate with disease burden and prognosis. However, this was not reproduced in a prospective study.[48, 51]

Clonal evolution with the transformation to a more aggressive lymphoid malignancy, termed Richter's transformation, includes other lymphoid malignancies that develop in patients with CLL. Classically defined as high-grade large B-cell lymphoma, its definition has been extended to include PLL, Hodgkin disease (the so-called Hodgkin variant of Richter's transformation), lymphoblastic lymphoma, and hairy-cell leukemia. In rare cases, patients with B-cell CLL may develop high-grade, T-cell non-Hodgkin lymphoma (NHL).[53] These transformations are relatively uncommon (2–14%) and are characterized by progressive lymphadenopathy and constitutional symptoms. The prognosis is generally ominous.

TREATMENT

As CLL remains an incurable tumor, treatment may be delayed and the patient monitored until becoming symptomatic.[48, 49, 51, 55] Guidelines include the development of symptoms, worsening anemia and/or thrombocytopenia, autoimmune cytopenias, progressive splenomegaly, progressive lymphadenopathy, or lymphocyte doubling time of 6 months. No prospective data exist yet to support the early treatment of patients with adverse prognostic features. On the other hand, many patients will be treated with supportive care only because of advanced age and comorbidities.

Chlorambucil, alone or combined with corticosteroids, is the most commonly used drug. It is advantageous in relieving symptoms, even in advanced disease. However, several randomized trials have failed to demonstrate improved survival, and hardly any patient achieves complete

Table 76.5 Major factors associated with prognosis[38, 40–43, 45, 51–52]

	Definition	Median survival (years)	Used in clinical practice
Rai stage			
0	Leukocytosis	12.5	Yes
1	Leukocytosis and lymphadenopathy	8.4	
2	Lymphocytosis plus hepatosplenomegaly	6.9	
3	Lymphocytosis plus anemia (< 11 g/dl)	1.5	
4	Lymphocytosis plus thrombocytopenia (< 100 000 × 10^9/l)	1.5	
Binet stage			
A	Leukocytosis and lymphadenopathy	Age-matched	Yes
B	Lymphadenopathy of more than two involved areas	7	
C	Anemia or thrombocytopenia	2	
β_2-microglobulin	Normal	9.7	Yes
	Elevated	4.5	
CD38			
Early-stage CLL	> 30%	2.9–<10 years	Yes
	< 30%	9–> 26 years	
Chromosomal aberrations (FISH analysis)	17p-	2.7	Sometimes
	11q-	6.5	
	Trisomy 12	9.5	
	Normal karyotype	9.3	
	13q-	11.1	
ZAP70			
Early-stage CLL	> 20%	7.5	Not available
	< 20%	Not reached	
Mutational status	Unmutated	5.7–< 9.9 years	If available
	Mutated	10.2–> 24 years	

CLL, chronic lymphocytic leukemia; FISH, fluorescent in-situ hybridization; ZAP70, zeta-associated protein 70.

remission. Purine analogues with or without cyclophosphamide were demonstrated to induce higher response rates when compared to chlorambucil, with some patients achieving complete remission.

The CD52 antigen is present on lymphocytes (B, T, and NK cells), monocytes, and some granulocytes. The humanized monoclonal anti-CD52 antibody (CAMPATH-1, alemtuzumab) has been shown to have an effect against B-CLL cells. Studies demonstrated high activity of this drug in previously treated and even refractory CLL patients, as well as in eliminating MRD, especially in the bone marrow.[56] Nevertheless, the resulting depletion of B cells and T cells places patients at higher risk for severe infectious complications, particularly CMV reactivation.[45] Anti-CD20 (rituximab, MabThera) as single agent shows limited efficacy in CLL, possibly because of the weak receptor expression on CLL cells. However, in combination with chemotherapy and particularly fludarabine it appears to act synergistically and to achieve high rates of response, including molecular complete remission.[48, 49] The combination of alemtuzumab with rituximab had a good but limited overall response.[56] Other immune-based therapies include lumiliximab (anti-CD23), apolizumab (anti-HLA-DR), and anti-CD40. These are being tested with or without the addition of chemotherapy.

Some immunologic novel futuristic approaches involving expanded autoreactive activated T cells have shown a safe profile and modest clinical improvements in phase I trials, as have vaccination strategies utilizing autologous leukemic cells transduced with different proapoptotic receptors (i.e., CD40 and CD95).[56]

Allogeneic hematopoietic stem cell transplantation (HSCT) is the only curative CLL treatment. Allogeneic HSCT relies on myeloablative doses of chemoradiotherapy, making this treatment unacceptably risky for the majority of CLL patients. In nonmyeloablative or reduced-intensity approaches, rates of engraftment are similar to fully ablative conditioning regimens with lower rates of early toxicity. Early evidence suggests that the graft-versus-leukemia effect is present against the disease. Studies involving autologous transplantation and high-dose chemotherapy for CLL have a limited survival advantage. Relapses are frequent and there is a high incidence of secondary myelodysplastic syndrome and acute myeloid leukemia.

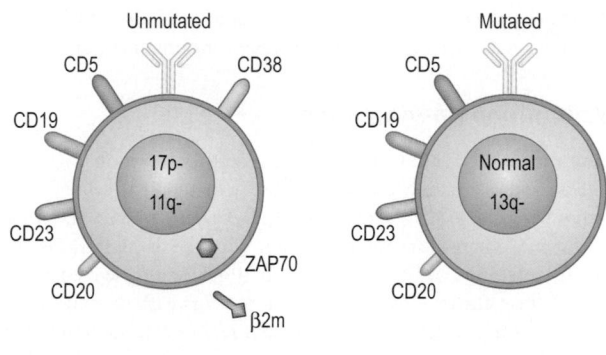

Fig. 76.7 Risk markers and stratification in chronic lymphocytic leukemia (CLL). B-cell CLL can be divided into two different entities. Both express the B-cell surface antigens CD19, CD23, and CD20, the last at low levels. They also express the pan-T-cell antigen CD5. The unmutated form yields a worse prognosis, and features CD38 on its cell surface, intracellular zeta-associated protein 70 (ZAP-70), chromosomal aberrations as 17p- and 11q-, and high levels of soluble β_2-microglobulin (β2m). In contrast, the mutated form has a better prognosis, tends to lack CD38 and ZAP-70, and has a normal karyotype or is 13q-.

The present treatment criteria do not identify patients in early stages with adverse prognostic high-risk features. Nevertheless, the overall survival of CLL patients has globally improved from 5 to 8 years for Binet stage B patients and from 2 to 5 years for stage C patients. This consistent improvement could be due to subsequent treatment advances provided to patients failing to respond initial treatment.[49] Thus, pending ongoing clinical trials, it may become feasible to treat patients with good performance and early-stage status who also demonstrate unfavorable prognostic features.[30]

IMMUNOLOGIC ASPECTS OF CLL

CLL is characterized by multiple immune deficiencies and autoimmune phenomena. It is reasonable to hypothesize that immune incompetence and autoimmunity are two sides of the same coin.[57]

The pathophysiologic rationale

CLL cells secrete TGF-β, which is a potent inhibitor of B-cell proliferation, and release high levels of circulating IL-2 receptor, which downregulates T-helper function. B-CLL cells also fail to present soluble antigen and alloantigens, as do anergic normal B cells. Conversely, normal activated B cells are very effective antigen-presenting cells.[57]

There is increasing evidence of T-cell dysfunction in CLL, which may contribute to the etiology and progress of the disease. An absolute CD8 lymphocytosis correlates with disease progression. Also, as found in autoimmune diseases, low expression of CD4 and CD8 is seen with abnormal expression of other surface molecules. In addition, the T cells in CLL patients were found to have profound abnormalities of their antigen receptor (TCR) repertoire[57] and appear dysfunctional in terms of cytokine secretion. Aberrant levels of interferon-γ, IL-2, IL-4, and

THERAPEUTIC PRINCIPLES

GOAL: TO AMELIORATE SYMPTOMS

>> Chronic lymphocytic leukemia is incurable but the likelihood of complete remission is good and survival appears to be improving for high-risk patients

>> Intervention in asymptomatic early stages should be limited to watchful waiting

>> Supportive care (gammaglobulin replacement, blood supplements and erythropoietin, treatment of infections) should be provided as needed

>> Conventional therapy includes steroids and/or chemotherapy (alkylating agents such as chlorambucil and cyclophosphamide, purine analogues such as fludarabine and cladribine, other lymphoma regimens)

>> Chlorambucil is the most commonly used drug and works well to relieve symptoms

>> Steroids can be very helpful for treating autoimmune phenomenon

>> More recent approaches use targeted monoclonal antibody therapy with or without chemotherapy (i.e., rituximab and alemtuzumab)

>> Autologous and allogeneic stem-cell transplantation are the only curative treatments, but require myeloablative chemoradiotherapy

CLINICAL PEARLS

IMMUNOLOGIC MANIFESTATIONS OF CHRONIC LYMPHOCYTIC LEUKEMIA

>> Pan-hypogammaglobulinemia

>> A monoclonal immunoglobulin peak, usually of the immunoglobulin M type

>> Downregulation of T-cell function and aberrant cytokine production

>> Defects in the complement system

>> High risk of recurrent infections – encapsulated bacteria and opportunistic infections

>> >> Autoimmune-associated phenomena:

>> >> Autoimmune hemolytic anemia

>> >> Autoimmune thrombocytopenia

>> >> Pure red-cell aplasia and autoimmune neutropenia

>> >> Other autoimmune disorders (myositis, vasculitis, pemphigus vulgaris, acquired angioedema, and glomerulonephritis)

CHRONIC LYMPHOCYTIC LEUKEMIA

IL-6 production have been described[58] and are dependent on the number of leukemic B cells and disease stage. It is possible that progression of the disease leads to a decline in T-cell function, greater negative feedback by B cells on the T cells, enhanced cytokine production by the B cells, or a combination of these factors. An imbalance of cytokine production could contribute to the upregulation of BCL-2 anti-apoptotic activity.[59] T-cell dysfunction could also explain the higher incidence of autoimmune complications, such as autoimmune hemolytic anemia (AIHA), among patients treated with purine analogues, which induce T-cell depletion. Assuming that certain T-cell subsets prevent the development of autoreactive B cells, purine analogue-induced depletion of T-cell numbers may permit autoreactive B-cell clones to emerge and expand.[57] However, this last complication is mainly observed among heavily pretreated patients who have received purine analogues as salvage therapy.[49]

Immunologic deficiencies

Patients with CLL are extremely sensitive to various infectious agents. A monoclonal immunoglobulin peak, usually of the IgM type, is found in 5% of CLL, and a small amount of a monoclonal component can be identified in the serum or urine of 60% of patients. Hypogammaglobulinemia occurs in at least 60% of B-CLL cases, and may include all three classes (IgG, IgA, IgM). The pathogenesis of hypogammaglobulinemia in B-CLL is poorly understood, as this phenomenon is rare in other B-cell malignancies except for multiple myeloma. Regulatory abnormalities in T cells may play a role in the induction of hypogammaglobulinemia, but may also result as a consequence of dysfunction of nonclonal normal B cells.[49] Low Ig levels correlate with recurrent infections of encapsulated organisms. Patients who receive intravenous immunoglobulin (Chapter 85) experience a decrease in the incidence of major bacterial infections.[60] Although it is costly, patients who have demonstrated a pattern of repeated serious infections should be treated with prophylactic IgIV.

Infections are a major cause of morbidity and mortality in CLL patients. Impaired humoral and cellular immunity, defects in the complement systems, and variable neutropenia, depending on marrow infiltrates, all contribute to the high rate of infections.[61] It is estimated that up to 50% of patients have recurrent infections, some severe. Bacterial infections are the principal risk in patients treated with conventional therapies. Due to the relative preservation of cellular immunity early in the disease, opportunistic infections are initially uncommon. *Pneumocystis jiroveci* pneumonia and other fungal infections, listeriosis, mycobacterial infections, and respiratory syncytial and herpes virus infections occur in heavily pretreated patients receiving combination chemotherapy and as the consequence of cumulative effects of numerous therapies. Infection risk is increased following purine analogue therapy because of the side effects of myelosuppression and marked lymphopenia with T-cell depletion. The combination of purine analogues with steroids increases this infectious risk substantially. Patients with fludarabine-resistant or partially responsive disease are at highest risk of infection. The addition of rituximab, the anti-B-cell marker CD20 antibody (Chapter 94), to nucleoside analogue-based therapy does not appear to increase the risk of early or late infections, but may increase the rate of neutropenia. The addition of the anti-B- and T-cell marker CD52 antibody alemtuzumab in pretreated patients and as first-line therapy resulted in high levels of infections, particularly in nonresponders.

Active immunization with vaccines is hampered by the patient's inability to generate or retain a long and significant immune response.

Autoimmune phenomenon

Autoimmune-associated features are frequently observed in CLL. These manifestations are mainly directed against hematopoietic cells. The most common known cause of AIHA is CLL.[62] A positive direct antiglobulin test (direct Coombs test) has been reported to be as high as 7–35% of CLL patients, and AIHA itself occurs in 10–25% of patients during the course of their disease – twice as often in patients with unmutated genes as in those with mutated ones. Tumor cells secrete small amounts of idiotypic IgM that may react with autoantigens as the Fc region of IgG, single- and double-stranded DNA, histones, cardiolipin, and other proteins. Nevertheless, in most cases autoantibodies against red blood cells are warm reactive polyclonal IgG and are not secreted by the malignant clone, but rather from normal B cells.[49, 62] Cold agglutinins are rare. AIHA is thought to arise from the imbalance among lymphocyte subsets, contributed by therapy, which results in the emergence of the autoimmune clone. Men, aged patients, and patients with a higher lymphocyte count demonstrate a significantly higher rate of AIHA. It is usually observed in advanced stages of the disease, correlates with a poor prognosis, and has a close relationship with the activity of CLL. After therapy, 70% of patients may achieve the disappearance of the autoimmune antibodies.[63]

ITP is observed in about 2–3% of cases, with increased megakaryocytes in the bone marrow. It should be distinguished from ITP induced by marrow infiltration, which is seen in up to 50% of patients at presentation.[62] Two-thirds of patients with CLL-associated ITP also have AIHA (Evan's syndrome). Pure red-cell aplasia and autoantibodies against neutrophils are only rarely observed, but are part of the CLL-related autoimmunity repertoire. The appearance of autoantibodies may be due to a defect of T-cell subsets controlling the autoantibody-producing B cells. This approach is supported by the observation that autoimmunity is much more common in patients treated with fludarabine, a drug known to induce profound suppression of circulating CD4 T cells.[57] Autoimmune phenomena in patients treated with purine analogues (mostly fludarabine-related) are of a more severe nature and generally trigger AIHA. However, ITP, possibly pure red-cell aplasia, and neutropenia are also seen.

Other rare entities are reported, such as paraneoplastic autoimmune disorders with connective tissue disease manifestations, including polymyositis, dermatopolymyositis, focal myositis,[64] vasculitis,[65] pemphigus vulgaris,[66] and acquired angioedema. These autoimmune disorders are related to T-cell dysfunction and may be associated with purine analogue treatment. Thirty percent of paraneoplastic pemphigus cases are reported to occur in CLL patients, as compared with other lymphoid neoplasms, and may be triggered by chemotherapy and radiotherapy.[62] Glomerulonephritis and nephrotic syndrome are also seldom reported. These are related to different mechanisms and are marked by the presence of cryoglobulins and anti-neutrophil cytoplasmic antibodies.

Therapy of autoimmune phenomenon includes high-dose steroids and disease control.[63] For patients refractory to, or relapsing after, the administration of steroids, further treatment is warranted. High-dose immunoglobulins offer amelioration in some patients, but with only a transient response. Splenectomy may induce some remission, especially in patients with AIHA due to IgG alone and no complement component. Splenic irradiation may substitute for splenectomy in older and debilitated patients.[62] Cytotoxic agents or cyclosporine may represent valid rescue approaches. In patients where the AIHA has been triggered by fludarabine, further exposure is hazardous, although courses combining cyclophosphamide with fludarabine are much less prone to develop AIHA. Withholding treatment to patients with a positive direct antiglobulin (Coombs) test is controversial. Rituximab may be an alternative agent for the treatment of CLL-associated autoimmune diseases,[67] as well as in rare autoimmune phenomena such as pemphigus and pure red-cell aplasia.

CONCLUSION

CLL is a common indolent lymphoid neoplasm that demonstrates a wide clinical heterogeneity. It is suspected and diagnosed more commonly as an incidental finding after performance of routine blood tests. Diagnosis is made with simple immunophenotyping, but an evaluation of prognosis will likely require more extensive laboratory evaluation, including cytogenetics and molecular diagnostic techniques. The origin of CLL is yet to be elucidated, but as data accumulate, two related entities emerge, both originating from antigen-stimulated mature B lymphocytes with different clinical behavior. The complications of CLL appear to be unique to this neoplasm and are part of a failing immune system with T-cell and B-cell dysregulation. A combined immune deficiency may result, predisposing patients to recurrent infections and autoimmune diseases. New molecular and protein markers that identify patients who are at a high risk for progressive disease may provide clues for effective targeted therapies.

■ ACKNOWLEDGMENTS ■

We are grateful to Professor Debora Rund and Dr. Neta Goldschmidt for their aid in writing this chapter.

■ REFERENCES ■

1. Izraeli S. Leukaemia – a developmental perspective. Br J Haematol 2004; 126: 3–10.

2. Pui CH, Relling MV, Downing JR. Acute lymphoblastic leukemia. N Engl J Med 2004; 350: 1535–1548.

3. Pui CH, Evans WE. Treatment of acute lymphoblastic leukemia. N Engl J Med 2006; 354: 166–178.

4. Schrappe M, Camitta B, Pui CH, et al. Long-term results of large prospective trials in childhood acute lymphoblastic leukemia. Leukemia 2000; 14: 2193–2194.

5. Greaves M. Infection, immune responses and the aetiology of childhood leukaemia. Nat Rev Cancer 2006; 6: 193–203.

6. Izraeli S. Perspective: chromosomal aneuploidy in leukemia – lessons from Down syndrome. Hematol Oncol 2006; 24: 3–6.

7. Einav U, Tabach Y, Getz G, et al. Gene expression analysis reveals a strong signature of an interferon-induced pathway in childhood lymphoblastic leukemia as well as in breast and ovarian cancer. Oncogene 2005; 24: 6367–6375.

8. Basso G, Buldini B, De Zen L, et al. New methodologic approaches for immunophenotyping acute leukemias. Haematologica 2001; 86: 675–692.

9. Campana D, Coustan-Smith E. Advances in the immunological monitoring of childhood acute lymphoblastic leukaemia. Best Pract Res Clin Haematol 2002; 15: 1–19.

10. Izraeli S, Henn T, Strobl H, et al. Expression of identical E2A/PBX1 fusion transcripts occurs in both pre- B and early pre-B immunological subtypes of childhood acute lymphoblastic leukemia. Leukemia 1993; 7: 2054–2056.

11. Pui CH, Behm FG, Singh B, et al. Heterogeneity of presenting features and their relation to treatment outcome in 120 children with T-cell acute lymphoblastic leukemia. Blood 1990; 75: 174–179.

12. Armstrong SA, Look AT. Molecular genetics of acute lymphoblastic leukemia. J Clin Oncol 2005; 23: 6306–6315.

13. Look AT. Oncogenic transcription factors in the human acute leukemias. Science 1997; 278: 1059–1064.

14. Aplan PD. Causes of oncogenic chromosomal translocation. Trends Genet 2006; 22: 46–55.

15. Weng AP, Ferrando AA, Lee W, et al. Activating mutations of NOTCH1 in human T cell acute lymphoblastic leukemia. Science 2004; 306: 269–271.

16. Strefford JC, van Delft FW, Robinson HM, et al. Complex genomic alterations and gene expression in acute lymphoblastic leukemia with intrachromosomal amplification of chromosome 21. Proc Natl Acad Sci USA 2006; 103: 8167–8172.

17. Heerema NA, Nachman JB, Sather HN, et al. Hypodiploidy with less than 45 chromosomes confers adverse risk in childhood acute lymphoblastic leukemia: a report from the children's cancer group. Blood 1999; 94: 4036–4045.

18. Ferrando AA, Neuberg DS, Staunton J, et al. Gene expression signatures define novel oncogenic pathways in T cell acute lymphoblastic leukemia. Cancer Cell 2002; 1: 75–87.

19. Breit S, Stanulla M, Flohr T, et al. Activating NOTCH1 mutations predict favorable early treatment response and long term outcome in child-hood precursor T-cell lymphoblastic leukemia. Blood 2006; 108: 1151–1157.

20. van der Does-van den Berg A, Bartram CR, Basso G, et al. Minimal requirements for the diagnosis, classification, and evaluation of the treatment of childhood acute lymphoblastic leukemia (ALL) in the "BFM Family" Cooperative Group. Med Pediatr Oncol 1992; 20: 497–505.

21. Yeoh EJ, Ross ME, Shurtleff SA, et al. Classification, subtype discovery, and prediction of outcome in pediatric acute lymphoblastic leukemia by gene expression profiling. Cancer Cell 2002; 1: 133–143.

22. Ross ME, Zhou X, Song G, et al. Classification of pediatric acute lymphoblastic leukemia by gene expression profiling. Blood 2003; 102: 2951–2959.

23. Schrappe M, Reiter A, Zimmermann M, et al. Long-term results of four consecutive trials in childhood ALL performed by the ALL-BFM study group from 1981 to 1995. Berlin–Frankfurt–Munster. Leukemia 2000; 14: 2205–2222.

24. Szczepanski T, Orfao A, van der Velden VH, et al. Minimal residual disease in leukemia patients. Lancet Oncol 2001; 2: 409–417.

Lymphomas including Hodgkin lymphoma

77

Stefania Pittaluga, Martina Rudelius,
Elaine S. Jaffe

The classification of the malignant lymphomas has undergone significant reappraisal over the past 40 years. These changes have resulted from insights gained through the application of immunological and molecular techniques, as well as a better understanding of the clinical aspects of lymphoma through advances in diagnosis, staging, and treatment. Recently, genomic-scale gene expression profiling has been applied to lymphomas to define their molecular signatures further with the aim of improved understanding of oncogenic pathways and their clinical implications.[1] These studies have led to new prognostic and diagnostic tools and ultimately may lead to more targeted approaches to therapy.

Early classifications were based on architectural and cytological characteristics of the neoplastic elements; however, with increasing knowledge of the complexity of the immune system a more functional approach was sought. This attempt was only partially successful, owing to the limited array of tools available to the pathologist in the 1970s and 1980s. Ideally, lymphomas, like most other tumors, should be classified according to their presumed normal counterpart. This approach should provide the best information about disease biology, natural history, and response to treatment. However, there are difficulties in defining the full extent of the neoplastic clone in individual cases of lymphoma, and some well-defined lymphoma types lack obvious normal counterparts. Differentiation schemes provide useful conceptual frameworks for understanding lymphomas (Fig. 77.1), and current understanding of both the immune system and the lymphomas has been enhanced by the genomic-scale approach offered by high-throughput technologies to move towards a biologically "correct" lymphoma classification.

A more practical approach to lymphoma categorization was adopted by the International Lymphoma Study group in 1994 to define the diseases that could be recognized with the currently available morphologic, immunologic, and genetic techniques.[2] The resulting Revised European–American Lymphoma (REAL) classification departed from previous traditional schemes and represented a new paradigm for the classification of lymphomas. Each variant could be distinguished by a combination of morphologic, immunophenotypic, and genotypic analyses, and each was associated with a characteristic clinical behavior,

KEY CONCEPTS

LYMPHOMA

>> Classification consists of a list of individual disease entities defined by morphologic, immunophenotypic, genetic, and clinical features

>> Neoplastic cells are related to the postulated normal counterpart, when possible

>> Histologic grade should be applied within individual diseases

>> Clinical factors for individual patients, as measured by the International Prognostic Index (IPI) and gene expression profiling, are useful in predicting clinical outcome

pattern of spread, and response to therapy. In addition it stressed the distinction between histologic grade and clinical aggressiveness, and emphasized that histologic grade should be applied within individual diseases and not across the entire spectrum of lymphoid neoplasms. This classification further noted that the site of involvement (e.g., nodal versus extranodal) was often an indicator of important biologic distinctions. It stressed that many disease entities are associated with distinctive clinical presentations and natural histories, even though treatment options may still be limited.

The validity of this approach was confirmed by an international study[3] concluding that the REAL classification enhanced diagnostic accuracy and reduced subjectivity. Immunophenotyping improved reproducibility and was essential in some specific entities, including most peripheral T-cell lymphomas (PTCL). This study also stressed the importance of clinical factors, such as the International Prognostic Index (IPI) for predicting prognosis and providing a guide to clinical management.[4] Applying the IPI, a wide survival range was observed across most disease entities, suggesting that it can be misleading to stratify different diseases into risk groups based only on histologic criteria. It became evident that there was a need to approach each disease individually, considering the

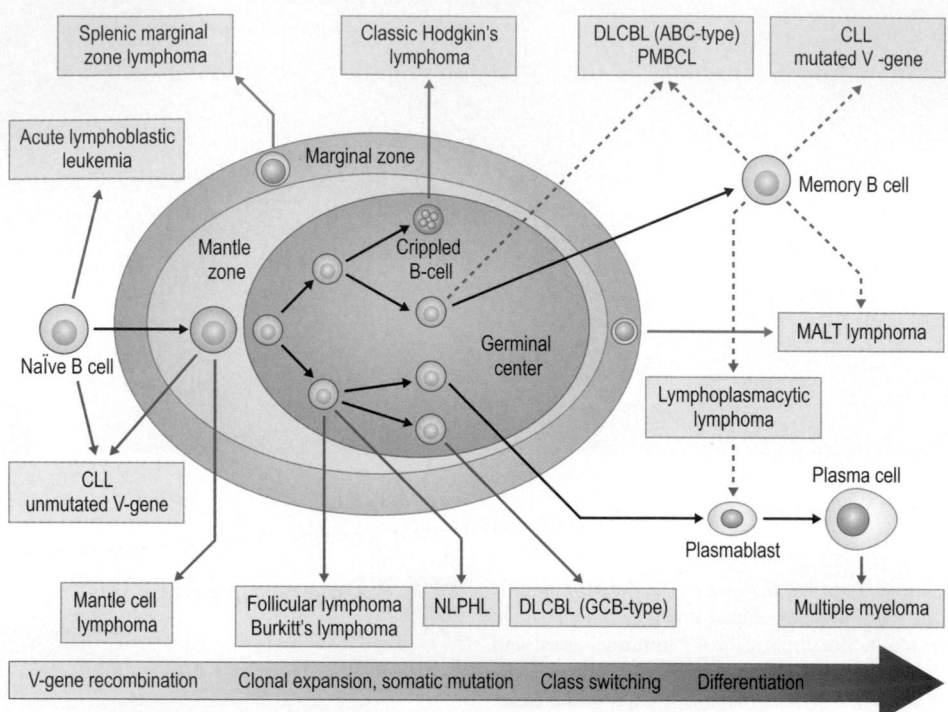

Fig. 77.1 Normal B-cell differentiation in relation to a secondary B follicle, mutational stages of the immunoglobulin genes, and cellular counterparts for B-cell lymphomas. Simplified version of B-cell development indicates points at which V-gene recombination, clonal expansion, and somatic mutations occur in relation to a secondary B follicle. B-cell lymphomas are related to different stages of B-cell differentiation and function. ABC-type, activated B-cell-like type; CLL, chronic lymphocytic leukemia/lymphoma; DLBCL, diffuse large B-cell lymphoma; GCB-type, germinal center B-cell-like type; MALT lymphoma, marginal-zone B-cell lymphoma of mucosa-associated lymphoid tissue (MALT) type; NLPHL, nodular lymphocyte-predominant Hodgkin lymphoma; PMBCL, primary mediastinal B-cell lymphoma.

KEY CONCEPTS

SOMATIC MUTATION IN RELATION TO NORMAL B-CELL DEVELOPMENT

>> Premutational stage: circulating naïve B cells (immunoglobulin (Ig)M+/D+) prior to antigen exposure

>> Stage of somatic mutation, clonal expansion, and isotype switch: at the germinal center

>> Postmutational stage: selected B cells move to the periphery (postgerminal center) or to the recirculating pool (memory B cells), or undergo terminal differentiation (plasma cells)

diagnosis, the patient's risk factors, and the known idiosyncrasies of each disease with regard to treatment.

Utilizing the principles of the REAL classification, a new World Health Organization (WHO) classification for hematological malignancies was developed (Table 77.1).[5] There are strong similarities between the WHO and REAL classification schemes. However, since

the publication of the REAL classification, new data have been generated for some categories. These studies allowed the resolution of entities that were previously listed as provisional; some were retained, whereas others were eliminated from the classification scheme. The recent application of gene expression profiling in lymphomas has generated distinct molecular "signatures" for a variety of disease entities, in some cases corresponding more closely to different stages of lymphoid differentiation, and in other instances offering insights into mechanisms of neoplastic transformation with delineation of derangements in specific pathways. This chapter focuses on the classification of neoplasms derived from mature B cells, T cells, and natural killer (NK) cells, with emphasis on malignant lymphomas.

■ MATURE B-CELL NEOPLASMS ■

LYMPHOPLASMACYTIC LYMPHOMA (LPL)

The definition of LPL is still controversial as specific genetic and immunophenotypic markers have not yet been identified. The previously used terms (lymphoplasmacytoid lymphoma, plasmacytoid lymphocytic lymphoma, or immunocytoma) do not appear to define a single

Table 77.1 Proposed World Health Organization classification for neoplastic diseases of the lymphoid tissue

B-cell neoplasms
Precursor B-cell lymphoblastic leukemia/lymphoma

Mature B-cell neoplasms
Chronic lymphocytic leukemia/small lymphocytic lymphoma
B-cell prolymphocytic leukemia
Lymphoplasmacytic lymphoma
Mantle-cell lymphoma
Follicular lymphoma
Marginal-zone B-cell lymphoma of mucosa-associated lymphoid tissue (MALT) type
Nodal marginal-zone B-cell lymphoma with or without monocytoid B cells
Splenic marginal-zone B-cell lymphoma
Hairy-cell leukemia
Diffuse large B-cell lymphoma
Subtypes: mediastinal (thymic), Intravascular, primary effusion lymphoma
Burkitt's lymphoma
Plasmacytoma
Plasma-cell myeloma

T-cell neoplasms
Precursor T-cell lymphoblastic leukemia/lymphoma
Mature T-cell and natural killer (NK)-cell neoplasms
T-cell prolymphocytic leukemia
T-cell large granular lymphocytic leukemia
NK-cell leukemia
Extranodal NK/T-cell lymphoma, nasal type
Mycosis fungoides
Sézary syndrome
Angioimmunoblastic T-cell lymphoma
Peripheral T-cell lymphoma (unspecified)
Adult T-cell leukemia/lymphoma
Systemic anaplastic large-cell lymphoma (T- and null cell types)
Primary cutaneous anaplastic large-cell lymphoma
Subcutaneous panniculitis-like T-cell lymphoma
Enteropathy-type intestinal T-cell lymphoma
Hepatosplenic T-cell lymphoma

Hodgkin lymphoma (Hodgkin's disease)
Nodular lymphocyte-predominant Hodgkin lymphoma
Classic Hodgkin lymphoma
Hodgkin's lymphoma nodular sclerosis (grades I and II)
Classic Hodgkin lymphoma, lymphocyte-rich
Hodgkin lymphoma, mixed cellularity
Hodgkin lymphoma, lymphocytic depletion

More common entities are in italics.
Morphologic and clinical variants are not listed.
In this chapter we will discuss disease entities that do not appear in other chapters.

CLINICAL PEARLS

INDOLENT LYMPHOMAS

>> Natural history: survival measured in years

>> Least sensitive to therapy

>> Good response to low-dose oral alkylating agents, radiotherapy, and steroids, but no curability

>> Higher response rate and complete remission with combination of standard chemotherapy and anti-CD20 monoclonal antibody

>> Gene expression profiling can help to identify patients who might benefit from high-dose chemotherapy and autologous stem-cell transplantation, which is a potentially curative modality

entity, as used in the literature. Many B-cell neoplasms occasionally show maturation to plasmacytoid or plasma cells containing cytoplasmic immunoglobulin (cIg), including chronic lymphocytic leukemia (CLL), and mantle-cell, follicle center, and marginal-zone cell lymphomas. We suggest that these cases be classified according to their major features, and not as LPLs. There does appear to be a distinct disorder of small lymphoid cells that show maturation to plasma cells without features of other lymphoma types, which corresponds to most cases of Waldenström's macroglobulinemia (WM). The term LPL should be restricted to these cases.

This is a disease of adult life (median age 61) that usually presents with generalized lymphadenopathy, vague constitutional symptoms, anemia, and splenomegaly. Autoimmune hemolytic anemia is a common complication. Peripheral blood involvement with an absolute lymphocytosis is less common in LPL than in B-cell CLL/small lymphocytic lymphoma. IgM monoclonal gammopathy may be associated with increased serum viscosity, leading to neurologic and vascular complications. However, this phenomenon can also be observed in other lymphomas. The course is chronic and indolent, and the disease is not generally curable with the available treatments; median survival is 78 months. Similar to other indolent lymphomas, the survival curve does not show any plateau. The treatment options, which depend on the clinical presentation, include plasmapheresis, the use of nucleoside analogues and alkylator agents, monoclonal antibody anti-CD20, either as single agents or in combination with chemotherapy[6]

The tumor consists of a diffuse proliferation of small lymphocytes, plasmacytoid lymphocytes (cells with abundant basophilic cytoplasm but lymphocyte-like nuclei), and plasma cells, with or without Dutcher bodies. The growth pattern is often interfollicular, with sparing of the sinuses.

The cells have surface and cytoplasmic Ig, usually of IgM type, usually lack IgD, and express B-cell-associated antigens (CD19, 20, 22, 79a). They are negative for CD5, CD10, and CD43; CD25 or CD11c may be faintly positive in some cases. A lack of CD5 and the presence of strong cytoplasmic Ig are useful in distinction from CLL. The postulated normal counterpart is thought to be a postfollicular medullary cord B cell based in part on the presence of somatic mutations in the Ig heavy- and light-chain variable region genes.

MANTLE-CELL LYMPHOMA (MCL)

MCL is a distinct clinicopathologic entity that has been more precisely defined in recent years through the integration of immunophenotypic, molecular genetic, and clinicopathologic studies. This tumor was recognized in the Kiel classification as centrocytic lymphoma and in the modified Rappaport scheme as lymphocytic lymphoma of intermediate differentiation. It tended to surround residual naked germinal centers, and a derivation from the follicular lymphoid cuff was postulated. Tumors with a very conspicuous mantle-zone pattern of growth were also termed 'mantle-zone lymphoma.'

MCL occurs in adults (median age 62), with a high male-to-female ratio. Most patients present with advanced-stage disease at diagnosis. Common sites of involvement include the lymph nodes, spleen, bone marrow, and lymphoid tissue of Waldeyer's ring. Gastrointestinal tract involvement is common and is associated with the picture of lymphomatous polyposis. This tumor appears to be incurable with the available treatments. In data collated from several retrospective studies the prognosis is poor, with a median survival ranging from 20 months to over 52 months. The relapse rate is high, with a median disease-free survival between 10.2 and 25.5 months.[7, 8] The clinical course and survival can be better predicted by gene expression profiling.[9] Genes whose expression is associated with short survival belong to the proliferation signature and are involved in cell cycle progression and DNA synthesis. The proliferation signature provides a quantitative measurement of tumor proliferation rate and can be used to get valuable prognostic information. The central role of proliferation was also stressed in the past by several studies based on scoring of Ki67-positive cells[10, 11]; however, the larger set of genes analyzed by expression profiling offers a more accurate survival stratification compared with a single marker.

It is important to identify at diagnosis those patients who may benefit from a more aggressive therapy versus those with a more indolent clinical disease who may be observed on a watchful waiting protocol. The treatment approach to newly diagnosed patients with MCL depends on the patient's eligibility for stem-cell transplantation (STC). However, because of the frequent bone marrow involvement, purging of the neoplastic cells is difficult to achieve.[12] With the addition of rituximab to standard chemotherapy regimens, an overall response rate of 94% and high rate of clinical remission can be achieved, but this does not yet translate in a prolonged progression-free survival. Therefore new therapeutic strategies, including molecular targeting agents like proteosome inhibitors such as bortezomib, are under investigation.[13]

The hallmark of MCL is a monotonous cytologic composition. In the typical case the cells are slightly larger than a normal lymphocyte, with finely clumped chromatin, scant cytoplasm, inconspicuous nucleoli, and irregular nuclear contour. Cytological (blastoid or blastic) and architectural variants (mantle zone, nodular, and diffuse) have been described and associated with a more aggressive clinical course (blastoid variant) or with a longer median survival (mantle-zone pattern). However, because of the overall poor prognosis and the lack of statistical significance of these architectural/cytological changes, the WHO classification considers MCL and its variants to be one group.[5]

Immunophenotypic and genotypic studies have been helpful in precisely defining MCL. The immunophenotype is distinctive (IgM/IgD$^+$; CD5$^+$, CD10$^-$, and CD23$^-$). In addition, the chromosomal translocation t(11;14) involving *CYCLIN D1* located at the *BCL-1/PRAD1* locus is associated with MCL, but is absent in most other low- and high-grade B-cell malignancies. By Northern analysis virtually 100% of cases of MCL have shown overexpression of cyclin D1, which has not been identified to the same degree in other B-cell malignancies. Cyclin D1 overexpression is believed to be essential in the pathogenesis of MCL; however, a few cases with similar clinical course and gene expression signature that did not overexpress Cyclin D1 have recently been identified.[14] Interestingly, they expressed either Cyclin D2 or Cyclin D3, which may substitute for Cyclin D1 in the pathogenesis of MCL. Additional alterations involving other cell cycle regulatory molecules (RB, p53, CDK inhibitors) have been described in the more aggressive forms of MCL. The INK4a/ARF deletions occur in approximately 20% of cases. The INK4a/ARF locus encodes two key suppressor genes, p16^{INK4a} and p14^{ARF}, which are important negative cell cycle regulators.

The postulated normal counterpart is the CD5$^+$ "virgin" B cell, sIgM$^+$ and sIgD$^+$, that can be found in the peripheral blood and in the mantle of reactive germinal centers.

FOLLICULAR LYMPHOMA (FL)

FL is the most common subtype of non-Hodgkin lymphoma in the USA and accounts for approximately 45% of all newly diagnosed cases. It has a peak incidence in the fifth and sixth decades, and is rare under the age of 20. Men and women are equally affected: FL is found less commonly in African-American and Asian populations. Most patients have stage 3 or 4 disease at diagnosis, with generalized lymphadenopathy and staging evaluation that usually reveals bone marrow involvement. Approximately 10% of patients have circulating malignant cells. However, careful immunophenotypic or molecular analyses may disclose peripheral blood involvement in a higher proportion of patients.

FL is indolent, but currently incurable with available therapeutic modalities. The natural history of the disease, with frequent relapses and relatively long survival, has led to different therapeutic approaches (watchful waiting versus chemotherapy).[15] Several attempts have been made to design predictive models to identify patients for whom aggressive, experimental therapies are warranted. Clinical parameters have been successfully used to develop prognostic indexes (for example, the FLIPI, adjusted from the IPI for aggressive B-cell lymphoma)[16]; however, the prognostic assessment of patients with FL could be improved by including other biological variables, like gene expression signatures or immunohistochemistry, taking into account the environment and infiltrating inflammatory cells.[17, 18]

More recently, new therapeutic avenues have been explored as, following relapses, patients become resistant to chemotherapy. A more aggressive approach with intent to eradicate the disease at the first or second relapse has been tested in clinical trials.[19] The use of monoclonal antibody therapies (especially anti-CD20), either as carriers of toxins or radioisotopes or as direct cytotoxic agents, has opened a new era in the treatment of B-cell lymphomas. The addition of anti-CD20 to conventional chemotherapy (cyclophosphamide, doxorubicin, vincristine and predinisone [CHOP] versus CHOP-rituximab [R]) has improved both remission and duration rates.[20]

The natural history of the disease is associated with histologic progression in both pattern and cell type (Fig. 77.2). A heterogeneous cytologic composition is one of the hallmarks of FL. Usually, all of the follicle center cells are represented, but in varying proportions.

This variation in cytologic composition is the basis for the subclassification of FL. It should be stressed that the variation in cytologic grade is a continuum, and therefore precise morphologic criteria for subclassification are difficult to establish. Most studies have shown that the subclassification of FL is difficult to reproduce among groups of pathologists. According to the WHO clinical advisory committee, FL should be graded and for most clinical purposes the distinction into two grades is sufficient (grade 1, predominantly small cleaved cell together with grade 2, mixed small cleaved and large cell; as distinct from grade 3, predominantly large cell). However, the distinction into three grades continues, with a recommendation for the use of the Berard counting method.[5]

The vast majority of FL (approximately 90%) are associated with a t(14;18) involving rearrangement of the BCL2 gene. This translocation appears to result in constitutive expression of BCL-2 protein, which is capable of inhibiting apoptosis in lymphoid cells. The cells of FL accumulate and are at risk for secondary mutations, which may be associated with

histologic progression. It is interesting that the small subset of grade 3 FL (large cell) is less commonly associated with the BCL2 translocation. Thus, some forms of FL may have a different pathogenesis. It is thought that the BCL2 translocation occurs at a very early stage of B-cell development, during immunoglobulin gene rearrangement. This fact may contribute to the difficulty of eradicating the neoplastic clone with chemotherapy.

Most FL present in lymph nodes while a subset of cases with the morphologic features of FL present in extranodal sites. When these tumors are localized (without lymph node involvement) they usually have a good prognosis. Complete remissions may be obtained with either surgical excision or local radiation therapy. In particular cutaneous follicle center lymphoma, which frequently lacks the BCL2 translocation and BCL2 expression, is considered by the European Organization for the Research and Treatment of Cancer (EORTC)-WHO classification as a separate entity.[21] However, when BCL2 expression is detected, the possibility that this may represent a secondary site of involvement should be considered. FL in children is also often extranodal at presentation[22] and usually of large-cell type (grade 3), suggesting an alternate molecular pathogenesis.[23]

The cells have a mature B-cell phenotype with expression of the B-cell antigens CD19, CD20, and CD22. Surface Ig is positive, most commonly with IgM expression, but IgG or IgA can be seen in many cases. CD10, BCL-6 stains are positive, but CD5 is negative.

FL represents the neoplastic counterpart of the reactive germinal center cells. Consistent with their normal counterparts, intraclonal heterogeneity with high numbers of somatic mutations and ongoing mutations of the Ig genes was detected in the neoplastic cells.[24]

MARGINAL-ZONE B-CELL LYMPHOMA OF MUCOSA-ASSOCIATED LYMPHOID TISSUE (MALT) TYPE

Most lymphomas of marginal-zone derivation present in extranodal sites and have histopathologic and clinical features that are part of the spectrum of MALT lymphomas. MALT lymphomas are characterized by a heterogeneous cellular composition that includes marginal-zone or centrocyte-like cells, monocytoid B cells, small lymphocytes, and plasma cells. In most cases large transformed cells are uncommon, but reactive germinal centers are nearly always present. Therefore, it is not surprising that, based on the heterogeneous cellular composition and the presence of reactive follicles, most MALT lymphomas were in the past diagnosed as pseudolymphomas or atypical hyperplasias. However, recent studies have shown the majority to be composed of monoclonal B cells. When follicular colonization by the neoplastic cells occurs the process can simulate FL.

MALT lymphomas have been described in nearly every anatomic site, but are most frequent in the stomach, lung, thyroid, salivary gland, and lacrimal gland. Other less common sites of involvement include the orbit, breast, conjunctiva, bladder, kidney, and thymus. Most patients present with localized disease, although regional lymph node involvement is common in gastric and salivary gland MALT lymphoma. Widespread nodal involvement is infrequent, as is bone marrow involvement. The clinical course is usually quite indolent and many patients are asymptomatic. MALT lymphomas tend to relapse in other MALT-associated sites.

MALT lymphomas of the salivary gland and thyroid are usually associated with a history of autoimmune diseases. There is a strong association between chronic infection with *Helicobacter pylori* and

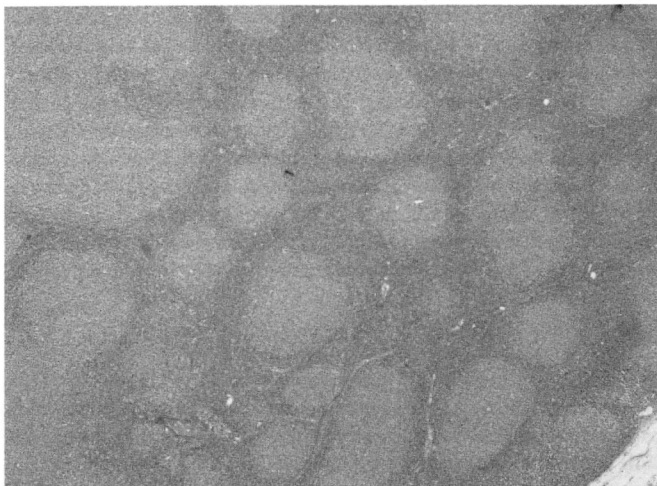

Fig. 77.2 Follicular lymphoma. The neoplastic follicles are similar in size and are partially surrounded by lymphoid cuffs. In contrast to reactive germinal centers, they lack polarization and tingible body macrophages ('starry-sky pattern').

PMLBCL and classic HL.[34,35] TRAF1 expression and c-REL amplification are seen in both types of neoplasms and can be detected with suitable immunohistochemical studies.[46]

BURKITT LYMPHOMA (BL)

BL is most common in children and accounts for up to one-third of all pediatric lymphomas in the USA.[47] It is the most rapidly growing of all lymphomas, with 100% of the cells in cell cycle at any time. It usually presents in extranodal sites. In nonendemic regions, such as the USA, common sites of presentation are the ileocecal region, ovaries, kidneys, or breasts. Jaw presentations, as well as the involvement of other facial bones, are common in African or endemic cases and are occasionally seen in nonendemic regions. Bone marrow involvement is a poor prognostic sign.

BL is one of the more common tumors associated with the human immunodeficiency virus (HIV).[48] It can present at any time during the clinical course. In some patients with HIV infection BL is the initial acquired immunodeficiency syndrome (AIDS)-defining illness.

The pathogenesis of BL is undoubtedly related to the translocations involving the c-MYC oncogene, which are seen in virtually 100% of cases. Most of the translocations involve the Ig heavy-chain gene on chromosome 14. Less commonly the light-chain genes on chromosomes 2 and 22 are involved. African BL occurs in regions endemic for malaria, and it has been postulated that immunosuppression associated with malarial infection puts patients at increased risk. In this regard, the pathogenesis appears similar to that seen with HIV infection.

Epstein–Barr virus (EBV) is closely linked to BL in endemic regions but is less frequently seen (15–20%) in Europe and North America.[47] In other regions, characterized by low socioeconomic status and EBV infection at an early age, BL is often EBV-positive, in the range of 50–70%. These data support the concept the EBV is a cofactor for the development of BL. Differences in the proportion of cases associated with the two EBV strains (types 1 and 2) have also been shown in sporadic and endemic EBV-positive BL.

Cytologically, BL is monomorphic with cells of medium size, round nuclei, and multiple (2–5) basophilic nucleoli. The cytoplasm is deeply basophilic and moderately abundant. These cells contain cytoplasmic lipid vacuoles, which are probably a manifestation of the high rates of proliferation and spontaneous cell death. The starry-sky pattern characteristic of BL is a manifestation of the numerous benign macrophages that have ingested karyorrhectic or apoptotic tumor cells.

BL has a mature B-cell phenotype. The cells express CD19, CD20, CD22, CD79a, and monoclonal surface Ig, nearly always IgM. CD10 is positive in nearly all cases, and CD5, CD23, and BCL-2 are consistently negative.

■ T-CELL AND PUTATIVE NK-CELL NEOPLASMS ■

OVERVIEW OF THE CLASSIFICATION OF T-CELL NEOPLASMS

Whereas the definition of precursor T-cell or lymphoblastic neoplasms is straightforward, the classification of PTCL has been controversial. These are uncommon, representing fewer than 15% of all non-Hodgkin lymphomas. Most previously published classification schemes for the malignant lymphomas in the USA or Europe have been based on the far more common B-cell malignancies. In addition, the molecular pathogenesis of most peripheral T-cell neoplasms has not been defined, and immunophenotypic markers are less specific for apparently distinct disease entities. For these reasons, the WHO classification relies to a considerable extent on clinical presentation to subdivide these tumors.[5]

EXTRANODAL NK/T-CELL LYMPHOMA, NASAL-TYPE

Extranodal NK/T-cell lymphoma, nasal type, is a distinct clinicopathologic entity highly associated with EBV. It is much more common in Asians than in those of European background. Clusters of the disease have also been reported in Central and South America in individuals of Native American heritage, suggesting that ethnic background may play a role in the pathogenesis of these lymphomas. It affects adults (median age 50) and the most common clinical presentation is a destructive nasal or midline facial lesion. Palatal destruction, orbital swelling, and edema can be prominent. NK/T-cell lymphomas have been reported in other extranodal sites, including the skin, soft tissue, testis, upper respiratory tract, and gastrointestinal tract. A leukemic form of the disease has also been reported, with similar morphologic, immunophenotypic, and genotypic features. The clinical course is usually aggressive, with a slightly improved median survival in patients with localized disease. However, with current chemotherapy the outcome remains poor. Radiation therapy may be effective in localized disease.[49]

Extranodal NK/T-cell lymphoma, nasal type, is characterized by a broad cytologic spectrum. The atypical cells can be small or medium in size. Large atypical and hyperchromatic cells can be admixed, or may predominate. If the small cells are in the majority the disease can be difficult to distinguish from an inflammatory or infectious process. In early stages there can also be a prominent admixture of inflammatory cells, causing further difficulty in diagnosis.

Although the cells express some T-cell-associated antigens, most commonly CD2, other T-cell markers, such as surface CD3, are usually absent. Cytoplasmic CD3 can be found in paraffin-embedded sections, but cytoplasmic CD3 can be found in NK cells and is not specific for a T-cell lineage tumor. In addition, molecular studies have not shown a clonal T-cell gene rearrangement, despite clonality being shown by other methods.[50] In favor of an NK-cell origin, the cells are nearly always CD56+, although CD16 and CD57 are usually negative. EBV is invariably positive by in situ hybridization.

A hemophagocytic syndrome is a common clinical complication, and adversely affects survival in extranodal NK/T-cell lymphoma, nasal type. It is likely that EBV plays a role in the pathogenesis of the hemophagocytic syndrome.

ANGIOIMMUNOBLASTIC T-CELL LYMPHOMA (AILT)

AILT was initially proposed as an abnormal immune reaction or form of atypical lymphoid hyperplasia with a high risk of progression to malignant lymphoma. Because the majority of cases show clonal rearrangements of T-cell receptor genes, it is now regarded as a variant of T-cell lymphoma. The median survival is usually less than 5 years, so that the designation as lymphoma is also warranted on clinical grounds.

The nodal architecture is generally effaced, but peripheral sinuses are often open and even dilated. Often regressed follicles containing a proliferation of dendritic cells and blood vessels (so-called 'burned-out') are present and only rarely hyperplastic follicles are noted. At low power there is usually a striking proliferation of postcapillary venules with prominent arborization. Clusters of atypical lymphoid cells with clear cytoplasm may be seen and they are admixed with an inflammatory cellular background containing small lymphocytes, immunoblasts, plasma cells, and histiocytes, with or without eosinophils. The abnormal cells are T cells usually positive for CD4 and CD10; this phenotype has been described in a particular subtype of T-helper cells associated with the germinal centers. More recently CXCL-13, a chemokine involved in B-cell trafficking into the germinal centers, has been described in AILT.[51, 52] These markers provide support for T-helper cell derivation of this lymphoma and also offer powerful diagnostic tools. Another helpful diagnostic feature is the presence of numerous CD21⁺ dendritic reticulum cells, which are especially prominent around postcapillary venules. Polyclonal plasma cells may be numerous.

AILT presents in adults; most patients have generalized lymphadenopathy with prominent systemic symptoms, including fever, weight loss, and skin rash. There is usually a polyclonal hypergammaglobulinemia. Patients may initially respond to steroids or mild cytotoxic chemotherapy, but progression usually occurs. More aggressive combination chemotherapeutic regimens have led to a higher remission rate but patients are prone to secondary infectious complications. Progression to a more monomorphic T-cell immunoblastic lymphoma occurs in some cases, and the proportion of large immunoblastic cells appears to correlate with the clinical course. Rarely, B-cell immunoblastic lymphomas positive for EBV occur in patients with AILT; these latter malignancies appear secondary to the underlying immunodeficiency.

PERIPHERAL T-CELL LYMPHOMAS, UNSPECIFIED

PTCL is a diagnosis of exclusion and is admittedly a heterogeneous category with most cases being nodal in origin. PTCL are characterized by a heterogeneous cellular composition. There is usually a mixture of small and large atypical lymphoid cells. An inflammatory background is common, consisting of eosinophils, plasma cells, and histiocytes. If the epithelioid histiocytes are numerous and clustered, the neoplasm fulfills the criteria for lymphoepithelioid cell lymphoma or Lennert's lymphoma, which is considered in the WHO to be a morphologic variant of PTCL and not a distinctive clinicopathologic entity.

Clinically, PTCL most often present in adults. Most patients exhibit generalized lymphadenopathy, hepatosplenomegaly, and frequent bone marrow involvement. Constitutional symptoms, including fever and night sweats, are common, as is pruritus. The clinical course is aggressive, although complete remissions may be obtained with combination chemotherapy.[53] However, the relapse rate is higher in PTCL than in B-cell lymphomas of comparable histologic grade.[53]

PTCL, as defined in the WHO classification, remains heterogeneous. It is likely that individual clinicopathologic entities will be delineated in the future from this broad group of malignancies. Thus far,

immunophenotypic criteria have not been helpful in delineating subtypes. Most cases have a mature T-cell phenotype and express one of the major subset antigens, with CD4 expression seen more frequently than CD8. These are not clonal markers, and antigen expression can change over time. Loss of one of the pan-T-cell antigens (CD3, CD5, CD2, or CD7) is seen in 75% of cases, with CD7 most frequently being absent.

SYSTEMIC, ANAPLASTIC LARGE-CELL LYMPHOMA (ALCL)

ALCL is characterized by pleomorphic or monomorphic cells that have a propensity to invade lymphoid sinuses. Because of the sinusoidal location of the tumor cells and their lobulated nuclear appearance, this disease was previously interpreted as a variant of malignant histiocytosis. Misdiagnosis as metastatic carcinoma or melanoma was also common.

A consistent feature is the expression of the CD30 antigen, which is a hallmark of this disease. It has been referred to as Ki-1-positive lymphoma. However, CD30 expression is not specific for ALCL and may also be seen in other forms of malignant lymphoma, including HD. Systemic ALCL is associated with a characteristic chromosomal translocation, t(2;5)(p23;q35), involving *ALK/NPM* genes, respectively.[54] A variety of other partners of ALK has been identified and monoclonal antibodies to the cytoplasmic portion of ALK protein have been made, and are able to identify tumor cells regardless of the underlying translocation.[55]

The cells of classic ALCL have large, often lobulated nuclei with small basophilic nucleoli. In some cases the nuclei may be round. The cytoplasm is usually abundant and amphophilic, with distinct cytoplasmic borders. A prominent Golgi region is generally visible. Immunohistochemistry is very valuable in the correct diagnosis of ALCL. The prominent Golgi region usually shows intense staining for CD30 and epithelial membrane antigen (EMA). In the majority of cases the neoplastic cells show nuclear and cytoplasmic staining with antibodies to the ALK protein. In about 15–20% of cases the presence of only cytoplasmic staining for ALK suggests that a variant translocation has occurred.[56]

The cells exhibit an aberrant phenotype with loss of many of the T-cell-associated antigens. Both CD3 and CD45RO, the most widely used pan-T-cell markers, are negative in more than 50% of cases. CD2 and CD4 are positive in the majority of cases, whereas CD8 is usually negative. ALCL cells, despite the CD4⁺/CD8⁻ phenotype, do express the cytotoxic-associated antigens TIA-1, granzyme B, and perforin.[57] In addition clusterin is generally present in ALCL and represents another useful diagnostic marker.[58] Molecular studies in most cases demonstrate T-cell receptor rearrangement, confirming a T-cell origin.

ALCL is most common in children and young adults. However, in elderly patients the t(2;5) or ALK expression is lacking, suggesting that these cases may be part of a different clinicopathologic entity. A marked male predominance, usually presenting with nodal disease, has been noted. However, a high incidence of extranodal site involvement has also been reported (involving skin, bone and soft tissue). About 75% of cases present with advanced stage and systemic symptoms.[59] Although these lymphomas have an aggressive natural clinical history they respond well to chemotherapy; overall survival and disease-free

different forms of treatment should be attempted to determine the optimal approach to this disorder.

CLASSIC HODGKIN LYMPHOMA, NODULAR SCLEROSIS (NSHL)

This variant is most common in adolescents and young adults, but can occur at any age; female cases equal or exceed those in males. The mediastinum is commonly involved; stage and bulk of disease have prognostic importance. NSHL is often curable; however, in long-term survivors the risk of secondary malignancies is increased, especially in those receiving both radiation and chemotherapy.

The tumor has at least a partially nodular pattern, with fibrous bands separating the nodules in most cases. Diffuse areas may be present, as is necrosis. The characteristic cell is the lacunar-type RS cell, which may be very numerous. Diagnostic RS cells are usually also present. The background contains lymphocytes, histiocytes, plasma cells, eosinophils, and neutrophils. Subclassification according to the number of atypical cells may be clinically relevant; several grading schemes exist (NSI/II, syncytial variant, lymphocyte-depleted, cellular phase). However, clinical trials have shown conflicting results. For routine clinical purposes grading is not required according to the WHO clinical advisory report. However, grading may be useful for clinical trials. The grading scheme of the British National Lymphoma Investigation (BNLI) (NSI/II) is recommended. The immunophenotype and genotype are characteristic of classic HD.

CLASSIC HODGKIN LYMPHOMA, MIXED CELLULARITY (HLMC)

Patients are usually adults; males outnumber females and the stage may be more advanced than in nodular sclerosis or lymphoplasmacytic types, involving lymph nodes, spleen, liver, or marrow. The course is moderately aggressive but is often curable.

The infiltrate is diffuse, without band-forming sclerosis, although fine interstitial fibrosis may be present (Fig. 77.4). RS cells are of the classic type, although some lacunar cells may be seen. The inflammatory background is similar to that of other subtypes of classic HL and the immunophenotype and genotype are also similar. The diagnosis is made on routine sections, and immunophenotyping studies are at best an adjunct to the diagnosis.

CLASSIC HODGKIN LYMPHOMA, LYMPHOCYTE DEPLETION (HLLD)

This is the least common variant of HL and is most common in older people, in HIV-positive individuals, and in nonindustrialized countries. It frequently presents with abdominal lymphadenopathy, spleen, liver, and bone marrow involvement, without peripheral adenopathy. The stage is usually advanced at diagnosis; however, response to treatment is reported not to differ from other subtypes.

The infiltrate is diffuse and often appears hypocellular, owing to the presence of diffuse fibrosis and necrosis. Relative to the number of normal lymphocytes there are large numbers of RS cells and occasional bizarre 'sarcomatous' variants, with a paucity of other inflammatory cells. Confluent sheets of RS cells and variants may occur and rarely predominate ('reticular' variant, or 'Hodgkin sarcoma').

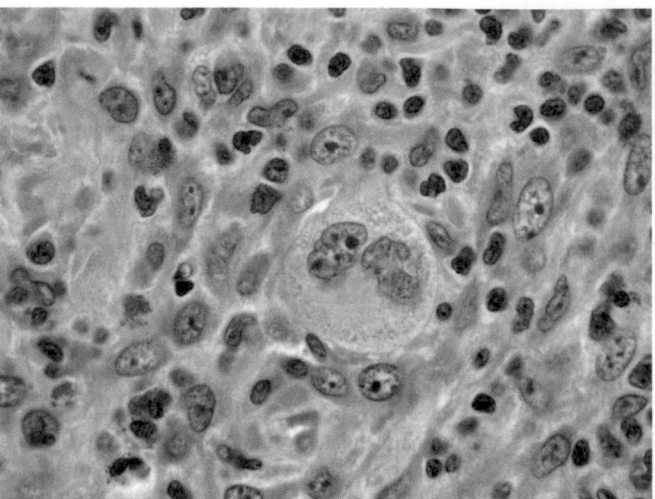

Fig. 77.4 Classic Hodgkin lymphoma, mixed cellularity subtype. A classic Reed–Sternberg cell is shown in a mixed inflammatory background with eosinophils, plasma cells, histiocytes, and small lymphocytes.

The immunophenotype is characteristic of classic HL. Since the histologic differential diagnosis often includes B- or T-large-cell lymphoma or ALCL, immunohistochemistry should be performed in most cases. EBV is positive in the majority of cases.

CLASSIC HODGKIN LYMPHOMA, LYMPHOCYTE-RICH (HLLR)

This type of classic HL may be nodular or diffuse and contains relatively infrequent RS cells, which are of the classic type, rather than the variants seen in NLPHL. Some lacunar cells may be present, in a background of lymphocytes, with infrequent eosinophils or plasma cells. In the past many cases of HLLR were misdiagnosed as nodular or diffuse lymphocyte-predominant HL. In contrast to NLPHL, the RS cells have the morphology and immunophenotype of classic RS cells. The immunophenotype and genetic features are similar to those of the other variants of classic HL. Patients usually present with localized disease.[71] This variant of HL was a provisional form of HD in the REAL classification and has been retained in the WHO classification. The nodular form has been recognized more recently.[72]

■ REFERENCES ■

1. Staudt LM, Dave S. The biology of human lymphoid malignancies revealed by gene expression profiling. Adv Immunol 2005; 87: 163–208.

2. Harris NL, Jaffe ES, Stein H, et al. A revised European–American classification of lymphoid neoplasms: a proposal from the International Lymphoma Study Group. Blood 1994; 84: 1361–1392.

3. The Non-Hodgkin's Lymphoma Classification Project. A clinical evaluation of the International Lymphoma Study Group classification of non-Hodgkin's lymphoma. Blood 1997; 89: 3909–3918.

4. Shipp MA. Prognostic factors in aggressive non-Hodgkin's lymphoma: who has "high risk" disease? Blood 1994; 83: 1165–1173.

5. Jaffe ES, Harris NL, Stein H, et al. Pathology and Genetics of Tumours of Haematopoietic and Lymphoid Tissues. Lyon, France: IARC Press, 2001.

6. Treon SP, Gertz MA, Dimopoulos M, et al. Update on treatment recommendations from the Third International Workshop on Waldenström's macroglobulinemia. Blood 2006; 107: 3442–3446.

7. Fisher RI, Dahlberg S, Nathwani BN, et al. A clinical analysis of two indolent lymphoma entities: mantle cell lymphoma and marginal zone lymphoma (including the mucosa-associated lymphoid tissue and monocytoid B-cell subcategories): a Southwest Oncology Group study. Blood 1995; 85: 1075–1082.

8. Teodorovic I, Pittaluga S, Kluin-Nelemans JC, et al. Efficacy of four different regimens in 64 mantle-cell lymphoma cases: clinicopathologic comparison with 498 other non-Hodgkin's lymphoma subtypes. European Organization for the Research and Treatment of Cancer Lymphoma Cooperative Group. J Clin Oncol 1995; 13: 2819–2826.

9. Rosenwald A, Wright G, Wiestner A, et al. The proliferation gene expression signature is a quantitative integrator of oncogenic events that predicts survival in mantle cell lymphoma. Cancer Cell 2003; 3: 185–197.

10. Lardelli P, Bookman MA, Sundeen J, et al. Lymphocytic lymphoma of intermediate differentiation. Morphologic and immunophenotypic spectrum and clinical correlations. Am J Surg Pathol 1990; 14: 752–763.

11. Katzenberger T, Petzoldt C, Holler S, et al. The Ki67 proliferation index is a quantitative indicator of clinical risk in mantle cell lymphoma. Blood 2006; 107: 3407.

12. Freedman AS, Neuberg D, Gribben JG, et al. High-dose chemoradiotherapy and anti-B-cell monoclonal antibody-purged autologous bone marrow transplantation in mantle-cell lymphoma: no evidence for long-term remission. J Clin Oncol 1998; 16: 13–18.

13. O'Connor O. Targeting histones and proteasomes: new strategies for the treatment of lymphoma. J Clin Oncol 2005; 23: 6429–6436.

14. Fu K, Weisenburger DD, Greiner TC, et al. Cyclin D1-negative mantle cell lymphoma: a clinicopathologic study based on gene expression profiling. Blood 2005; 106: 4315–4321.

15. Horning SJ. Natural history of and therapy for the indolent non-Hodgkin's lymphomas. Semin Oncol 1993; 20: 75–88.

16. Solal-Celigny P, Roy P, Colombat P, et al. Follicular lymphoma international prognostic index. Blood 2004; 104: 1258–1265.

17. Dave SS, Wright G, Tan B, et al. Prediction of survival in follicular lymphoma based on molecular features of tumor-infiltrating immune cells. N Engl J Med 2004; 351: 2159–2169.

18. Farinha P, Masoudi H, Skinnider BF, et al. Analysis of multiple biomarkers shows that lymphoma-associated macrophage (LAM) content is an independent predictor of survival in follicular lymphoma (FL). Blood 2005; 106: 2169–2174.

19. Rohatiner A. Follicle centre cell lymphoma: optimal use of therapeutic options. Ann Oncol 2000; 11: 111–115.

20. Hiddemann W, Kneba M, Dreyling M, et al. Frontline therapy with rituximab added to the combination of cyclophosphamide, doxorubicin, vincristine, and prednisone (CHOP) significantly improves the outcome for patients with advanced-stage follicular lymphoma compared with therapy with CHOP alone: results of a prospective randomized study of the German Low-Grade Lymphoma Study Group. Blood 2005; 106: 3725–3732.

21. Burg G, Kempf W, Cozzio A, et al. WHO/EORTC classification of cutaneous lymphomas 2005: histological and molecular aspects. J Cutan Pathol 2005; 32: 647–674.

22. Heller KN, Teruya-Feldstein J, La Quaglia MP, et al. Primary follicular lymphoma of the testis – excellent outcome following surgical resection without adjuvant chemotherapy. J Pediatr Hematol Oncol 2004; 26: 104–107.

23. Lorsbach RB, Shay-Seymore D, Moore J, et al. Clinicopathologic analysis of follicular lymphoma occurring in children. Blood 2002; 99: 1959–1964.

24. Kuppers R, Zhao M, Hansmann ML, et al. Tracing B cell development in human germinal centres by molecular analysis of single cells picked from histological sections. Embo J 1993; 12: 4955–4967.

25. Farinha P, Gascoyne RD. *Helicobacter pylori* and MALT lymphoma. Gastroenterology 2005; 128: 1579–1605.

26. Wotherspoon A, Doglioni C, Diss T, et al. Regression of primary low-grade B-cell gastric lymphoma of mucosa-associated lymphoid tissue type after eradication of *Helicobacter pylori*. Lancet 1993; 342: 575–577.

27. Farinha P, Gascoyne RD. Molecular pathogenesis of mucosa-associated lymphoid tissue lymphoma. J Clin Oncol 2005; 23: 6370–6378.

28. Campo E, Miquel R, Krenacs L, et al. Primary nodal marginal zone lymphomas of splenic and MALT type. Am J Surg Pathol 1999; 23: 59–68.

29. Isaacson PG, Matutes E, Burke M, et al. The histopathology of splenic lymphoma with villous lymphocytes. Blood 1994; 84: 3828–3834.

30. Algara P, Mateo MS, Sanchez-Beato M, et al. Analysis of the IgV(H) somatic mutations in splenic marginal zone lymphoma defines a group of unmutated cases with frequent 7q deletion and adverse clinical course. Blood 2002; 99: 1299–1304.

31. Fisher RI, Shah P. Current trends in large cell lymphoma. Leukemia 2003; 17: 1948–1960.

32. Rosenwald A, Wright G, Chan WC, et al. The use of molecular profiling to predict survival after chemotherapy for diffuse large-B-cell lymphoma. N Engl J Med 2002; 346: 1937–1947.

33. Shipp MA, Ross KN, Tamayo P, et al. Diffuse large B-cell lymphoma outcome prediction by gene-expression profiling and supervised machine learning. Nat Med 2002; 8: 68–74.

34. Rosenwald A, Wright G, Leroy K, et al. Molecular diagnosis of primary mediastinal B cell lymphoma identifies a clinically favorable subgroup of diffuse large B cell lymphoma related to Hodgkin lymphoma. J Exp Med 2003; 198: 851–862.

35. Savage KJ, Monti S, Kutok JL, et al. The molecular signature of mediastinal large B-cell lymphoma differs from that of other diffuse large B-cell lymphomas and shares features with classical Hodgkin lymphoma. Blood 2003; 102: 3871–3879.

REFERENCES

Monoclonal gammopathies

Robert A. Kyle, Angela Dispenzieri

78

The monoclonal gammopathies (paraproteinemias, dysproteinemias) are a group of disorders characterized by the proliferation of a single clone of plasma cells that produce an immunologically homogeneous (monoclonal) protein (M protein, paraprotein). Each M protein consists of two heavy polypeptide chains of the same class, designated as γ in IgG, α in IgA, μ in IgM, δ in IgD, and ε in IgE, and two associated light chains of the same type (κ or λ).

The monoclonal gammopathies include monoclonal gammopathy of undetermined significance (MGUS), multiple myeloma (MM), smoldering multiple myeloma (SMM), plasma cell leukemia, nonsecretory myeloma, solitary plasmacytoma (bone or extramedullary), POEMS (osteosclerotic myeloma), Waldenström's macroglobulinemia (WM), heavy-chain diseases (HCD), and primary systemic amyloidosis (AL).

The distribution of serum M proteins at Mayo Clinic from 1960 to 2005 is shown in Figure 78.1A and the diseases associated with them are shown in Figure 78.1B.

▌ KEY CONCEPTS

CLASSIFICATION OF MONOCLONAL GAMMOPATHIES

>> Monoclonal gammopathy of undetermined significance (MGUS) (benign monoclonal gammopathy)

>> Multiple myeloma

>> Multiple myeloma variants: smoldering multiple myeloma (SMM), plasma cell leukemia, nonsecretory myeloma, osteosclerotic myeloma (POEMS syndrome)

>> Plasmacytoma: solitary plasmacytoma of bone, extramedullary plasmacytoma

>> Waldenström's macroglobulinemia

>> Heavy-chain diseases (α, γ, and μ)

>> Primary amyloidosis (AL)

▌ RECOGNITION OF M PROTEINS IN SERUM AND URINE ▌

High-resolution agarose gel electrophoresis is preferred for the detection of an M protein. Immunofixation should be used to confirm the presence of an M protein and to identify the heavy-chain type and the light-chain class.[1] Serum protein electrophoresis should be performed whenever MM, WM, or AL is suspected, and if clinical suspicion is high, immunofixation studies should be done despite a normal serum electrophoretic pattern. These studies are also indicated in the presence of unexplained back pain, weakness or fatigue, recurrent infections, anemia, hypercalcemia, renal insufficiency, osteoporosis, or lytic lesions. It should also be performed in all patients with sensorimotor peripheral neuropathy, nephrotic syndrome, orthostatic hypotension, refractory congestive heart failure, carpal tunnel syndrome, or malabsorption of unknown cause because the presence of an M protein in one of these syndromes strongly suggests AL.

An M protein appears as a narrow peak or spike in the densitometer tracing or as a discrete band on agarose gel. In contrast, an excess of polyclonal immunoglobulins (having one or more heavy-chain types and both κ and λ light chains) produces a broad-based peak or band. It is important to differentiate an M protein from a polyclonal increase because the former is associated with a neoplastic process or a potentially malignant condition, whereas a polyclonal increase in immunoglobulins is associated with a reactive or inflammatory process. An M protein may exist even when the total protein level, beta (β)- and gamma (γ)-globulin concentrations, and quantitative immunoglobulin values are all within the normal limits. A monoclonal light chain in the serum (Bence Jones proteinemia) is rarely recognized with agarose gel electrophoresis. Immunofixation is recommended for identification of an M protein.

Rate nephelometry is the preferred method for quantitation of immunoglobulins because it is not affected by molecular size. The nephelometry value for immunoglobulin M (IgM), and occasionally IgG or IgA, is higher than that obtained with the densitometer tracing of serum protein electrophoresis. One must use either electrophoresis or nephelometric quanitation of immunoglobulins throughout the course of a patient's illness instead of alternating the techniques because of the differences in results.

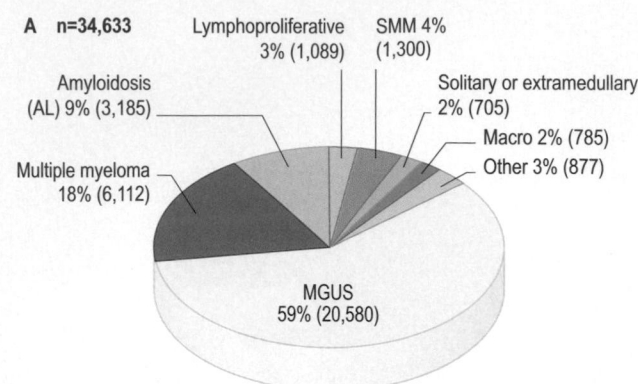

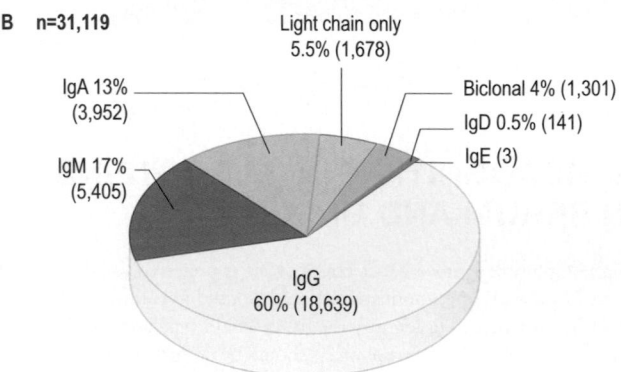

Fig. 78.1 **(A)** Monoclonal gammopathies Mayo Clinic 1960–2005. **(B)** Monoclonal serum proteins Mayo Clinic 1960–2005.

Immunofixation is the preferred technique for identifying a monoclonal light chain in urine. A 24-hour urine specimen should be collected and the amount of M protein calculated on the base of the densitometer tracing and the 24-hour urine protein content. The amount of M protein is a direct reflection of the size of the tumor mass. The heat test for Bence Jones (monoclonal light-chain) proteinuria is unsatisfactory.

Measurement of free light-chain (FLC) has been introduced into clinical practice. This automated nephelometric assay measures the level of free κ and λ light chains in the serum. The normal ratio for FLC κ/λ is 0.26–1.65. In a series of 1020 patients at Mayo Clinic in whom an FLC assay was ordered, 88% had a monoclonal plasma cell disorder. The 121 patients who did not have a monoclonal protein had a normal FLC κ/λ ratio. Among 110 untreated patients with AL, the combination of serum–urine immunofixation and serum FLC detected an abnormal result in 99% of patients.[2]

■ MONOCLONAL GAMMOPATHY OF UNDETERMINED SIGNIFICANCE ■

MGUS is characterized by an M-protein concentration < 3 g/dl; fewer than 10% plasma cells in the bone marrow; no or only small amounts of M protein in the urine; absence of lytic bone lesions, anemia, hypercalcemia,

and renal insufficiency related to the plasma cell proliferative process. Although this disorder has been considered benign, it is known that symptomatic MM or related disorders can develop in many patients and for this reason the term MGUS is more appropriate.

MGUS has been reported in 3% of patients over 70 years and 1% of persons older than 50. In order to determine the prevalence, serum samples were obtained from 21 463 (77%) of the 28 038 enumerated residents of Olmsted County, Minnesota, who were 50 years of age or older.[3] MGUS was identified in 694 (3.2%) of these persons. Age-adjusted rates were higher in men than in women (4% versus 2.7%, P = 0.001). The prevalence of MGUS was 5.3% among persons 70 years of age or older and 7.5% among those 85 years of age or older. In both sexes the prevalence increased with advancing age and was almost four times as high among persons 80 years of age or older than among those 50–59 years of age (Table 78.1). The isotype of the monoclonal protein was IgG in 69% of the 694 with MGUS, IgM in 17%, IgA in 11%, and biclonal in 3%. The concentration of immunoglobulins was less than 1.0 g/dl in 63.5% and at least 2.0 g/dl in only 4.5% of the 694 persons. The median value was 0.5 g/dl. The level of uninvolved (normal, polyclonal) immunoglobulins was reduced in 28% of the 447 patients in whom quantitative immunoglobulins were measured. Urine from 70 persons with MGUS showed a monoclonal kappa protein in 16.5% or lambda in 5%.[3] The incidence of MGUS is higher in African Americans than in Caucasians.[4]

Because of its frequency, it is of great importance to know whether the M protein will remain stable or will progress to MM, WM, AL, or other related disorders. At Mayo Clinic, 241 patients with an apparently benign monoclonal gammopathy have been followed for 3579 person-years (median, 13.7 years; range 0–39 years).[5] The bone marrow contained 1–10% plasma cells (median, 3%).

The actuarial risk of malignant transformation was 17% at 10 years, 34% at 20 years, and 39% at 25 years. The interval from recognition of M protein to the diagnosis of serious disease ranged from 1 to 32 years (median, 10.4 years). In 10 patients, MM was diagnosed more than 20 years after detection of the M protein. The mode of development of MM was variable, in that some patients remained stable for many years and MM developed gradually or suddenly, whereas in others there was a steady increase in the M-protein level until they became symptomatic. The median duration of survival after the diagnosis of MM was 33 months, which is not different from those who develop myeloma *de novo*.

In order to confirm the findings of the 241 Mayo Clinic patients from the USA and other countries, which may be subject to referral bias, we conducted a population-based study of a group of 1384 patients with MGUS from the 11 counties of southeastern Minnesota evaluated at the Mayo Clinic from 1960 to 1994.[6] The median age at diagnosis of MGUS was 72 years compared to 64 years in the 241-patient cohort. Fifty-four percent of patients were men and only 2% were < 40 years of age at diagnosis.[6] The size of the M protein at diagnosis ranged from unmeasurable to 3.0 g/dl (median 1.3 g/dl). The M protein was IgG in 70%, IgM in 15%, IgA in 12%, and biclonal in 3%. The uninvolved (normal or background) immunoglobulins were reduced in 38% of 840 patients who were evaluated. Of the 418 patients who had immunofixation of urine, 31% had a monoclonal light chain. In each case anemia or renal insufficiency, when present, was not attributable to the monoclonal plasma cell process.

The 1384 patients were followed for a total of 11 009 person-years (median, 15.4 years; range, 0–35 years), during which time 963 (70%) died. During follow-up, MM, AL, WM, chronic lymphocytic leukemia, or plasmacytoma developed in 115 patients (8%) (Table 78.2). The

Table 78.1 Prevalence of monoclonal gammopathy of undetermined significance (MGUS) according to age group and sex among residents of Olmsted County, Minnesota

Age (years)	Women	Men	Total
	Number/total number (percent)[a]		
50–59	59/4335 (1.4)	82/4038 (2.0)	141/8373 (1.7)
60–69	73/3155 (2.3)	105/2864 (3.7)	178/6019 (3.0)
70–79	101/2650 (3.8)	104/1858 (5.6)	205/4508 (4.6)
≥ 80	111/1854 (6.0)	59/709 (8.3)	170/2563 (6.6)
Total	344/11,994 (2.9)[b]	350/9469 (3.7)[b]	694/21463 (3.2)[b, c]

From Kyle RA, Therneau TM, Rajkumar SV, et al. Prevalence of monoclonal gammopathy of undetermined significance. N Engl J Med 2006; 354: 1362–1369, with permission from the Massachusetts Medical Society.
[a]The percentage was calculated as the number of patients with MGUS divided by the number who were tested.
[b]Prevalence was age-adjusted to the 2000 US population as follows: men, 4.0% (95% confidence interval, 3.5–4.4); women, 2.7% (95% confidence interval, 2.4–3.0) and total, 3.2% (95% confidence interval, 3.0–3.5).
[c]Prevalence was age- and sex-adjusted to the 2000 US total population.

Table 78.2 Risk of progression among 1384 residents of southeastern Minnesota in whom monoclonal gammopathy of undetermined significance was diagnosed in 1960 through 1994[a]

Type of progression	Observed No. of patients	Expected No. of patients	Relative risk (95% CI)
Multiple myeloma	75	3.0	25.0 (20-32)
Lymphoma	19[b]	7.8	2.4 (2-4)
Primary amyloidosis	10	1.2	8.4 (4-16)
Macroglobulinemia	7	0.2	46.0 (19-95)
Chronic lymphocytic leukemia	3[c]	3.5	0.9 (0.2-3)
Plasmacytoma	1	0.1	8.5 (0.2-47)
Total	115	15.8	7.3 (6-9)

CI, confidence interval.
[a]Expected numbers of cases were derived from the age- and sex-matched white population of the Surveillance, Epidemiology, and End Results program in Iowa,[7] except for primary amyloidosis, for which data are from Kyle et al.[8]
[b]All 19 patients had serum immunoglobulin M (IgM) monoclonal protein. If the 30 patients with IgM, IgA, or IgG monoclonal protein and lymphoma were included, the relative risk would be 3–9 (95% confidence interval, 2.6–5.5).
[c]All 3 patients had serum IgM monoclonal protein. If all 6 patients with IgM, IgA, or IgG monoclonal protein and chronic lymphocytic leukemia were included, the relative risk would be 1.7 (95% confidence interval, 0.6–3.7).
From Kyle RA, Therneau TM, Rajkumar SV, et al. A long-term study of prognosis in monoclonal gammopathy of undetermined significance [see comment]. N Engl J Med 2002; 346: 564–569, with permission from the Massachusetts Medical Society.

cumulative probability of progression to one of these disorders was 10% at 10 years, 21% at 20 years, and 26% at 25 years (Fig.78.2). The overall risk of progression was about 1% per year but it must be emphasized that patients were at risk for progression even after 25 years or more of stable MGUS. In addition, there were 32 patients in whom the monoclonal protein value increased to more than 3 g/dl or the percentage of plasma cells increased to more than 10% but in whom symptomatic MM did not develop. At 20 years, the risk of death for patients with MGUS was 10% from plasma cell disorders and 72% from non-plasma cell disorders.

The number of patients with progression to a plasma cell neoplasm or a related disorder (115 patients) was more than seven times expected on the basis of incidence rates for those conditions in the general population (Table 78.2). The risk of developing MM, WM, or AL was increased 25-fold, 46-fold, and 8.4-fold respectively.

MM was diagnosed more than 10 years after the detection of the monoclonal protein in 24 (32%) of the 75 patients, and after 20 years of follow-up in 5 (7%) patients. Characteristics of these 75 patients were comparable with those of the 1027 patients with newly diagnosed MM

CLINICAL PEARLS

MONOCLONAL GAMMOPATHIES

>> Monoclonal gammopathy of undetermined significance (MGUS) (benign monoclonal gammopathy) occurs in nearly 60% of all patients with a monoclonal gammopathy

>> MGUS occurred in 3.2% of persons older than 50 years and in 5.3% of those older than 70 years in a population-based study of 21 463 residents of Olmsted County, Minnesota

>> The risk of MGUS developing multiple myeloma, primary systemic amyloidosis, macroglobulinemia, or related disorders is 1% per year during long-term follow-up

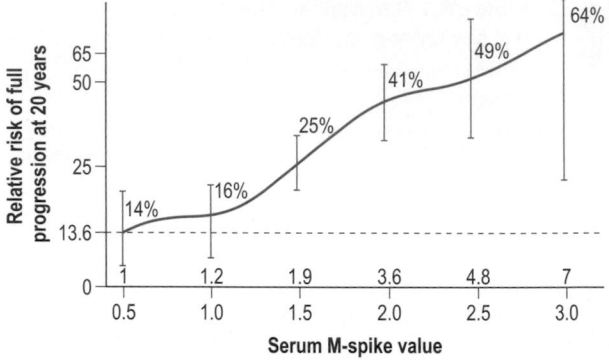

Fig. 78.2 Actuarial risk of full progression by serum monoclonal protein (M protein) value at diagnosis of monoclonal gammopathy of undetermined significance (MGUS) in persons from southeastern Minnesota. (From Kyle et al. Immunological Reviews, 2003; 194: 112–139, with permission of Blackwell Publishing.)

who were referred to the Mayo Clinic from 1985 to 1998, except that the southeastern Minnesota patient population was older (median 72 versus 66 years) and had a smaller percentage of men (46% versus 60%).[9]

Similar findings have been reported in other series: the actuarial risk was 8.5% and 19.2% at 5 and 10 years respectively in one series of 128 patients with MGUS. In a report of 335 patients with MGUS, the frequency of progression after a median follow-up of 70 months was 6.8%.

PROGRESSION OF MGUS

The sequence of events responsible for progression of MGUS to myeloma or a related disorder is poorly understood. This has recently been reviewed.[10] Almost one-half of patients with MGUS have immunoglobulin heavy-chain translocations consisting of t(11;14), t(4;14), and t(14;16). These translocations lead to dysregulation of putative oncogenes. Deletions of chromosome 13 have also been found in MGUS.

Risk factors for progression consist of size of the M-protein at diagnosis, type of M protein, presence of abnormal serum FLC ratio, and bone marrow plasma cell involvement. In a series of 1384 patients with MGUS from southeastern Minnesota, the size of the M-protein at diagnosis was the most important predictor of progression. The risk of progression to MM or a related disorder 20 years after the diagnosis of MGUS was 14% for patients with an initial M protein value of 0.5 g/dl and 49% for those presenting with an M spike of 2.5 g/dl (Fig. 78.2). The risk of progression of a serum M protein of 1.5 g/dl was almost twice the risk of progression with a value of 0.5 g/dl and the risk of progression with 2.5 g/dl was 4.6 times that of a value of 0.5 g/dl. Patients with IgM or IgA protein had an increased risk of progression compared with those with IgG monoclonal protein ($P = 0.001$).

An abnormal FLC ratio was detected in 379 (33%) of 1148 patients from the 1384 patients with MGUS from southeastern Minnesota. The risk of progression with an abnormal FLC ratio was significantly higher than that in patients with a normal ratio (hazard ratio 3.5; $P < 0.001$) and was independent of the size and type of serum M protein. A new stratification model for determining the risk of progression of MGUS was developed in that study.[11] The number of plasma cells in the bone marrow may help predict progression.[12]

In our experience, age; gender; levels of hemoglobin, serum creatinine, and serum albumin; presence, type, and amount of monoclonal urinary light-chain; and reduction of uninvolved immunoglobulins have not helped to determine the risk of progression.

MANAGEMENT OF MGUS

Despite the results of sophisticated laboratory tests, MM is differentiated from MGUS on the basis of clinical factors such as symptoms, anemia, hypercalcemia, renal insufficiency, and lytic bone lesions. The serum and urine M proteins must be measured periodically and a clinical evaluation conducted to determine whether MM, AL, WM, or a lymphoproliferative disorder has developed.

If a patient has no features of MM or AL, the serum protein value (IgG type) is less than 1.5 g/dl and FLC ratio is normal, the serum protein electrophoresis should be repeated in 6–12 months and, if the results are stable, annually.

If the patient has an M-protein value of > 1.5 g/dl, a 24-hour urine specimen should be collected for electrophoresis and immunofixation. A metastatic bone survey and bone marrow aspiration and biopsy should also be done. Determination of the plasma cell labeling index (PCLI), search for circulating plasma cells in the blood, and cytogenetic studies should be performed if available. Levels of β_2-microglobulin and C-reactive protein should also be determined. Serum protein electrophoresis should be performed in 3–6 months and if the results are stable it should be repeated in 6 months and then annually or sooner if symptoms develop. Patients should be instructed to contact their physician if there is any change in clinical condition.

ASSOCIATION OF MONOCLONAL GAMMOPATHIES WITH OTHER DISEASES

Although MGUS frequently exists without any other abnormalities, certain diseases are associated with it, as would be expected in an older population. There may be an apparent association because of differences in the referral practices or in other selected patient groups. Appropriate control populations are essential for determining whether the association is merely a coincidence.

M proteins have been noted in lymphoproliferative disorders, leukemia, other hematologic diseases, connective tissue disorders, and neurologic conditions such as peripheral neuropathy. Dermatologic diseases, including lichen myxedematosus, pyoderma gangrenosum, necrobiotic xanthogranuloma, and plane xanthomatosis, have been associated with an M protein. M proteins have also been found after renal, bone marrow, or liver transplantation as a result of immunosuppressive therapy. More detailed reviews of the association of monoclonal gammopathy with nonplasma cell disorders have been published.[10]

VARIANTS OF MGUS

IgM MGUS

IgM MGUS comprises 20% of all patients with MGUS. IgM MGUS was diagnosed in 213 Mayo Clinic patients who resided in the 11 counties of southeastern Minnesota.[13] Non-Hodgkin's lymphoma (*n*=17), WM (*n*=6), chronic lymphocytic leukemia (*n*=3), or AL (*n*=3) developed in 29 (14%) of the 213 IgM patients with a relative risk of 15, 262, 6, and 16 respectively. The risk of progression was 14%, 26%, 34%, and 41% for concentrations of ≤ 0.5, 1.5, 2.0, and ≥ 2.5 g/dl respectively. Progression occurred at a rate of approximately 1.5%/year.

Biclonal gammopathies

Biclonal gammopathies occur in approximately 4–6% of patients with monoclonal gammopathies and have similar clinical features. Two-thirds of cases of biclonal gammopathy are of undetermined significance.[14] The remainder have MM, AL, WM, or other lymphoproliferative disorders. More than 25 cases of triclonal gammopathy have been reported.

Idiopathic Bence Jones proteinuria

In most patients, the presence of Bence Jones proteinuria indicates MM, AL, WM, or other lymphoproliferative disorders. However, it may follow a benign course for many years. Patients with 'idiopathic' Bence Jones proteinuria must be observed indefinitely, because MM or AL will eventually develop in most of those with > 1 g of Bence Jones proteinuria/24 hours.[15]

■ MULTIPLE MYELOMA ■

MM (myelomatosis, Kahler's disease) is characterized by the neoplastic proliferation of a single clone of plasma cells producing an M protein. This proliferation often results in skeletal destruction, with osteolytic lesions or pathologic fractures producing pain, hypercalcemia, and anemia. An excess of M protein can contribute to renal failure, the hyperviscosity syndrome, or recurrent bacterial infections.

EPIDEMIOLOGY

The annual incidence of MM is 4.3 per 100 000.[16] The apparent increased incidence during the past few decades is probably related more to the increased availability and use of medical facilities in the elderly and to improved diagnostic techniques rather than an actual increased incidence. MM represents 1% of all malignant disease and slightly more than 10% of hematologic malignancies. Its incidence in African Americans is twice that in Caucasians, and it is slightly more frequent in men than in women. MM occurs in all races and all geographic regions, but rates are lower in Asian populations. Only 10% are younger than 50 years and 2% are younger than 40 years. The median age is 66 years.[9]

BIOLOGIC ASPECTS

Plasma cells are cytoplasm Ig (cIg+) and express surface CD38. A small subset of myeloma cells express CD10 and 15–20% express CD20. CD56 (N-CAM) is expressed on the majority of malignant plasma cells, but CD34 is not. The clonogenic cell in MM has not been demonstrated with certainty. There is evidence that plasma cell precursors of myeloma circulate in the peripheral blood. The current hypothesis is that, by means of adhesion molecules, circulating clonogenic myeloma cells home to the bone marrow, where they find an appropriate microenvironment to differentiate and expand further.

Approximately 50% of patients have translocations that involve the immunoglobulin heavy-chain locus on chromosome 14q32 and 1 of 5 partner chromosomes: 11q13(CCND-1), the most common, 4p16.3(FGFR-3 and MMSET), 6p21(CDND-3), 16q23(C-mAF), and 20q11 (mAF-β).[17] Other cytogenetic changes include M-RAS, K-RAS, and P16 methylation.

Conventional cytogenetic studies show abnormal karyotypes in only 30–40% of patients. Newer techniques using interphase fluorescence *in-situ* hybridization (FISH) have detected a higher frequency of abnormalities.

CLINICAL MANIFESTATIONS

Bone pain, usually in the back or chest, is present at the time of diagnosis in about 60% of patients and is usually aggravated by movement.[9] Weakness and fatigue are common and usually associated with anemia. The major symptoms may result from an acute infection, renal failure, hypercalcemia, or amyloidosis. Pallor is the most frequent physical finding.

RENAL INVOLVEMENT

The serum creatinine level is 2 mg/dl or more in one-fifth of patients at diagnosis. Two major causes of renal failure are "myeloma kidney" and hypercalcemia. Myeloma kidney is characterized by the presence of large, dense, waxy, laminated casts in the distal and collecting tubules. Hypercalcemia, which is present in 15% of patients initially, is a major and treatable cause of renal insufficiency. Dehydration, infections, or nonsteroidal antiinflammatory agents may all contribute to renal failure.

SKELETAL INVOLVEMENT

Almost 80% of patients have lytic lesions, osteoporosis, or fractures with conventional radiographs at diagnosis. Magnetic resonance imaging (MRI) or computed tomography (CT) is most helpful in the detection of extramedullary plasmacytomas compressing the spinal cord in patients with severe back pain but no abnormalities on routine radiographs.

NEUROLOGIC INVOLVEMENT

Radiculopathy from nerve compression by an extradural plasmacytoma or by the collapsed bone itself is the most frequent neurologic complication. Compression of the spinal cord occurs in about 5% of patients and must be recognized and treated without delay. Peripheral neuropathy is rare in MM, and, when present, is usually due to amyloidosis. Leptomeningeal myelomatosis is uncommon but is being recognized more frequently. Intracranial plasmacytomas are rare.

THERAPEUTIC PRINCIPLES

TREATMENT OF MULTIPLE MYELOMA

>> Consider an autologous peripheral blood stem-cell transplant in newly diagnosed patients

>> Autologous peripheral blood stem-cell transplantation is not curative

>> Oral melphalan and prednisone for patients ineligible for a peripheral stem cell transplant. The addition of thalidomide is promising

>> Combinations of alkylating agents produce a higher response rate without improved survival compared to melphalan and prednisone

>> Allogenic bone marrow transplant has a significant early mortality and is not recommended

>> Novel agents for multiple myeloma include thalidomide, bortezomib, and lenalidomide

response in 50–60% of patients. Leukocyte and platelet counts should be determined at 3-week intervals after beginning therapy, because the melphalan dosage must be altered until midcycle neutropenia or thrombocytopenia occurs. Chemotherapy should be continued for at least 1 year or until the patient is in a plateau state with stable serum and urine M-protein levels and no progression of disease. Patients should be followed closely during the plateau state and the same chemotherapy should be reinstituted if relapse occurs after 6 months.

Because of the obvious shortcomings of melphalan and prednisone, various combinations of therapeutic agents have been used. In an overview of individual data of 4930 persons from 20 randomized trials comparing melphalan and prednisone with various combinations of therapeutic agents, response rates were significantly higher with combination chemotherapy (60%) than melphalan/prednisone (53%) ($P < 0.00001$). However, there was no significant difference in response duration or overall survival.[26]

Two recent randomized trials have compared melphalan and prednisone to melphalan and prednisone plus thalidomide (MPT).[27, 28] These trials show superior response rates and event-free survival with the latter regimen. Consequently, MPT is an additional standard option for patients with newly diagnosed myeloma who are not candidates for transplantation. MPT is associated with significant greater toxicity, including thrombosis; therefore, care must be exercised in patient selection as well as during therapy.[27]

Maintenance Therapy

Maintenance therapy with interferon-α_2 is of limited value and is seldom used. Recent results from a large intergroup study showed no benefit with interferon as maintenance therapy.[29] Prednisone 50 mg q.o.d. may be useful for maintenance therapy. In a randomized study of 50 mg versus 10 mg of prednisone taken every 48 hours, the progression-free survival (14 versus 5 months) and overall survival (37 versus 26 months) were

significantly longer in the 50-mg regimen.[30] Preliminary results from a French randomized trial showed improvement in event-free overall survival with maintenance thalidomide plus pamidronate.[31]

Allogeneic bone marrow transplantation

Bone marrow transplantation from an identical-twin donor (syngeneic) is the treatment of choice if a donor is available. Results are superior to allogeneic transplantation.

Allogeneic bone marrow transplantation is advantageous because the graft contains no tumor cells and there may be a graft-versus-tumor effect. However, there is a mortality rate of at least 25%. Furthermore, 90–95% of patients with MM are ineligible because of their age, lack of a human leukocyte antigen (HLA)-matched sibling donor, or inadequate renal, pulmonary, or cardiac function. Currently, conventional allogeneic transplantation is associated with too-high a mortality and cannot be recommended. However, efforts are under way to reduce allogeneic transplant-related mortality using T-cell depletion or nonmyeloablative regimens. Nonmyeloablative (mini-allo) allogeneic protocols following ASCT are being pursued. The mortality is 10–15% and graft-versus-host disease occurs in about one-half of patients. Efforts are being made to reduce the toxicity of this approach. Currently, nonmyeloablative approaches should be limited to protocol studies.

REFRACTORY MULTIPLE MYELOMA

Cure rarely occurs, so that almost all patients who respond to chemotherapy or transplantation will eventually have a relapse if they do not die of another disease. Furthermore, at least one-third of patients treated initially do not obtain an objective response. Patients who are initially refractory or who become refractory to alkylating agent therapy generally have a low response to subsequent chemotherapy and a short survival. Until recently the highest response rates in such patients had been with VAD given intravenously for 96 hours or as a bolus injection. Many physicians choose single-agent dexamethasone instead because it accounts for 80% of the effect of VAD.

In the past decade, novel agents for the treatment of MM include thalidomide and its analogue, lenalidomide, and the proteosome inhibitor, bortezomib. Thalidomide is usually given in a dosage of 50–200 mg/daily. Objective responses occur in approximately one-third of patients with a median duration of response of approximately 12 months. The addition of dexamethasone increases the response rate. Side effects from thalidomide include weakness, fatigue, constipation, and somnolence. Thrombotic events, sensory motor peripheral neuropathy, and skin rashes are more troublesome side effects. Lenalidomide, an immunomodulatory derivative, has shown activity in previously treated patients. Phase II studies produce response in 30% of patients and constipation, somnolence, and neuropathy have not been troublesome. The lenalidomide dosage for myeloma is 25 mg orally on days 1–21 every 28 days. Higher response rates are seen when used in combination with dexamethasone. Bortezomib produced objective response in 35% of patients with relapsed, refractory myeloma who had received at least two prior therapeutic regimens. The median duration of response is approximately 12 months. Fatigue, anorexia, nausea and vomiting, fever, diarrhea, constipation, anemia, asthenia, peripheral neuropathy, neutropenia, and thrombocytopenia are adverse side effects.[32]

■ TREATMENT OF COMPLICATIONS OF MULTIPLE MYELOMA ■

LOCAL THERAPY

Palliative radiation in a dosage of 20–30 Gy should be limited to patients with disabling pain who have a well-defined focal process that has not responded to chemotherapy or in the case of symptomatic spinal cord compression. Analgesics in combination with chemotherapy can usually control the pain. This approach is preferred to local radiation because pain frequently occurs in another site and local radiation does not benefit the patient with systemic disease.

HYPERCALCEMIA

Hypercalcemia (7 mg/dl) is present in almost 15% of patients at diagnosis. It should be suspected in the presence of anorexia, nausea, vomiting, polyuria, polydipsia, constipation, confusion, or stupor. Hypercalcemia also contributes to the development of renal insufficiency. Hydration and prednisone, 25 mg q.i.d., are effective in most cases. If not, a bisphosphonate such as zoledronic acid or pamidronate should be given. Patients with MM should be encouraged to be as active as possible because prolonged bedrest contributes to osteopenia and hypercalcemia.

SKELETAL LESIONS

Complications related to lytic skeletal lesions are common in MM. Patients should be encouraged to be as active as possible but to avoid trauma. Fixation of fractures or impending fractures of long bones with an intramedullary rod and methylmethacrylate has produced good results.

In a prospective placebo-controlled study, pamidronate showed a significant reduction in skeletal events (pathologic fractures, need for radiation or surgery to treat or prevent pathologic fractures, or spinal cord compression associated with compression fractures).[28]

Intravenous bisphosphonates should be given to all patients who have lytic lesions, pathologic fractures, or severe osteopenia. Zoledronic acid (Zometa) 4 mg intravenously over 15–30 minutes every 4 weeks and pamidronate (Aredia) 90 mg intravenously over 2–3 hours every 4 weeks are equally efficacious. The dosage of bisphosphonates should be reduced in renal insufficiency. Because renal insufficiency or nephrotic-range proteinuria may occur, serum creatinine and 24-hour urine protein monitoring are necessary. One may consider reducing the intravenous bisphosphonate to every 3 months after 2 years unless there is evidence of progressive skeletal disease. Osteonecrosis of the jaw has been reported in patients receiving bisphosphonates. Although the relationship is unclear, it is essential to obtain a complete dental evaluation and perform preventive dental treatment prior to beginning bisphosphonates. Good oral hygiene should be practiced during therapy. Dental extractions or other invasive procedures should be avoided during bisphosphonate therapy. Management of osteonecrosis of the jaw should be conservative. Clodronate and ibandronate are alternatives and can be given orally.

Both vertebroplasty (injection of methylmethacrylate into a collapsed vertebral body) and kyphoplasty (introduction of an inflatable bone tamp into the vertebral body and, after inflation, the injection of methyl methacrylate into the cavity) have been used successfully to decrease pain and help restore height. Pain relief is generally rapid and can be long-lasting.

RENAL INSUFFICIENCY

Patients should be treated with dexamethasone alone or thalidomide plus dexamethasone or VAD to reduce the tumor mass as quickly as possible in patients with acute or subacute renal failure. A trial of plasmapheresis is reasonable in an attempt to prevent chronic dialysis but this has not been proven. Hemodialysis and peritoneal dialysis are equally effective and are necessary for patients with symptomatic azotemia. Renal transplantation for myeloma kidney may also be helpful. Maintenance of a high (3 l/day) urine output is important for preventing renal failure in patients with Bence Jones proteinuria.

ANEMIA

Anemia occurs in almost all patients during the course of MM. Symptomatic anemia during the plateau phase is benefited by the administration of erythropoietin in at least one-half of patients. Those with low serum erythropoietin values are more likely to respond, but most physicians proceed with a trial of erythropoietin, 150 U/kg three times weekly, or 40 000 U once a week. Darbepoetin (Aranesp), a long-lasting erythropoietin, may be given weekly or biweekly. There are no side effects and the major disadvantage is its cost. Red-cell transfusions may also be needed for anemia.

INFECTIONS

Prompt and appropriate therapy for bacterial infection is essential. Pneumococcal and influenza vaccines should be given to all patients despite their suboptimal antibody response. Intravenous immunoglobulin may be helpful for patients with recurrent infections but is very expensive.

SPINAL CORD COMPRESSION

Spinal cord compression should be suspected in patients with back pain, weakness, or paresthesias of the lower extremities, or bowel dysfunction. MRI or CT must be done immediately. Radiation therapy and dexamethasone are usually helpful and surgical compression is rarely necessary.

EMOTIONAL SUPPORT

All patients with MM need substantial and continuing emotional support. Quality-of-life issues must be in the forefront. The physician's approach must be positive in emphasizing the potential benefits of therapy. It is reassuring for patients to know that some survive for 10 years or more. It is vital that the physician caring for patients with MM has the interest and capacity for dealing with incurable disease over the span of years with assurance, sympathy, and resourcefulness.

■ VARIANTS OF MULTIPLE MYELOMA ■

SMOLDERING MULTIPLE MYELOMA

SMM is characterized by the presence of an M protein > 3 g/dl and/or more than 10% plasma cells in the bone marrow but no evidence of anemia, hypercalcemia, skeletal lesions, or renal insufficiency.[33] SMM accounts for 10–15% of all cases with newly diagnosed MM. The risk of progression to MM is approximately 10% per year for the first 5 years compared to 1% per year for MGUS. Treatment should not be given unless progression occurs.

PLASMA CELL LEUKEMIA

Plasma cell leukemia is defined as the presence of more than 20% plasma cells in the peripheral blood and an absolute plasma cell count > 2×10^9/l. When it presents *de novo* (60% of cases) it is classified as primary, and when it presents as a leukemic transformation of a previously recognized MM it is secondary (40%). Patients with primary plasma cell leukemia are younger and have a greater incidence of hepatosplenomegaly and lymphadenopathy, fewer bone lesions, a smaller serum M component and a longer survival than patients with secondary plasma cell leukemia. Cytogenetic abnormalities are more common than in patients with MM.[34] ASCT after response to high-dose chemotherapy has been beneficial for some patients. Those with secondary plasma cell leukemia rarely respond to chemotherapy because they have already received treatment for MM and are refractory.

NONSECRETORY MYELOMA

Patients with nonsecretory myeloma have no M component in either the serum or the urine and account for only 3% of patients with MM. The FLC assay is abnormal in more than 60% of patients and is useful for monitoring response to therapy. The diagnosis is established by identification of an M protein in the plasma cells by immunofluorescence or immunoperoxidase. The behavior of nonsecretory myeloma is similar to MM, except there is less renal involvement.

SOLITARY PLASMACYTOMA OF BONE

The diagnosis of solitary plasmacytoma of bone is based on the presence of a skeletal plasma cell tumor without evidence of MM. The hemoglobin, calcium, and creatinine values are normal, there are no other bone lesions, and the bone marrow contains no increase in monoclonal plasma cells. Small amounts of M protein may be present in the serum or urine, but they usually disappear after tumoricidal radiation (40–50 Gy). MRI is useful because of the high incidence of MM if additional lesions are seen, in contrast to patients with no additional lesions on MRI.[35] Overt MM develops in approximately 55% of patients during long-term follow-up. New bone lesions or local recurrences develop in about 10%. There is no convincing evidence that chemotherapy affects the incidence of conversion to MM. Progression, when it occurs, is usually evident within 3–4 years.

EXTRAMEDULLARY PLASMACYTOMA

The diagnosis is based on the finding of a plasma cell tumor in an extramedullary location and the absence of MM on bone marrow examination, radiography, and appropriate studies of serum and urine. Approximately 80% of cases involve the upper respiratory tract, producing epistaxis, nasal discharge, or nasal obstruction.[36]

Treatment consists of tumoricidal radiation. Adjuvant chemotherapy does not appear to lower the relapse rate or increase disease-free survival. Local recurrence is approximately 5% or less if tumoricidal radiation is given. A review of 400 publications between 1905 and 1997 found 800 cases. Patients who had combined surgery and radiation had better results than those who had only surgery or only radiation. There was local recurrence in 22% of patients whereas MM developed in 15%.[36]

■ POEMS SYNDROME (OSTEOSCLEROTIC MYELOMA) ■

The major clinical findings in POEMS syndrome are characterized by *p*olyneuropathy, *o*rganomegaly, *e*ndocrinopathy, *M* protein, and *s*kin changes (POEMS).[37] Castleman's disease may also be present. The major clinical findings are chronic inflammatory demyelinating polyneuropathy with predominantly motor disability and sclerotic skeletal lesions. Papilledema may occur. Hepatosplenomegaly and lymphadenopathy may be present. Skin hyperpigmentation and hypertrichosis may be prominent. Gynecomastia, testicular atrophy, and clubbing of the fingers and toes may occur. Pulmonary hypertension has been recognized in several instances. Ascites, pleural effusion, and peripheral edema may be present. The hemoglobin level is usually normal or elevated and thrombocytosis is common. Hypercalcemia and renal insufficiency rarely occur, and the bone marrow usually contains less than 5% plasma cells. Most patients have a λ protein, and IgA is common. The diagnosis is confirmed by the presence of monoclonal plasma cells in an osteosclerotic lesion. Radiation to the localized osteosclerotic lesion usually produces improvement of the neuropathy, but if the lesions are widespread, ASCT should be seriously considered.[38]

■ WALDENSTRÖM'S MACROGLOBULINEMIA ■

WM is a consequence of a malignant proliferation of plasma cells and B-cell lymphocytes producing a monoclonal IgM protein. In a study from the USA, the incidence of WM was 0.3/100 000 in white men and 0.17/100 000 in white women, with approximately 1400 new cases occurring each year. The median age at diagnosis is 63 years; fewer than 1% of our patients are younger than 40 years and approximately 60% are males.[39]

CLINICAL MANIFESTATIONS

The onset is usually insidious and characterized by weakness and fatigue. There may be oozing from the oronasal area or blurring of vision. Weight loss, fever, and night sweats resembling lymphoma may occur. Peripheral neuropathy, pulmonary infiltration with cough, and dyspnea or skin lesions may be evident. Dyspnea and congestive heart failure may be an initial finding. In contrast to MM, renal failure, osteolytic lesions, and AL are rare.

Pallor is a frequent finding on physical examination. Hepatomegaly, splenomegaly, or lymphadenopathy occurs in about a third of patients. Hyperviscosity is often present in WM and can produce oronasal bleeding, blurred vision, headache, vertigo, dizziness, sudden deafness, diplopia, or ataxia. Confusion, dementia, and disturbances of consciousness may occur. Clinical manifestations are rarely due to hyperviscosity if the serum viscosity is less than 4 centipoises (normal = 1.8). The correlation between the serum viscosity and clinical manifestations is not precise. Clinical symptoms and retinal lesions, including hemorrhages, exudates, and venous congestion, are more important in making a therapeutic decision.

LABORATORY FINDINGS

A normocytic, normochromic anemia occurs in almost all cases during the course of the disease. The hemoglobin and hematocrit values are often spuriously reduced because of the increased plasma volume. The serum cholesterol value is often low. Serum protein electrophoresis reveals a sharp narrow spike or dense localized band consisting of monoclonal IgM. A bone marrow aspirate is often hypocellular, but the biopsy specimen is hypercellular and extensively infiltrated by lymphocytes, plasma cells, and lymphoplasmacytoid cells and mast cells. In contrast to MM, lytic lesions and fractures are found in fewer than 5% of patients.

DIFFERENTIAL DIAGNOSIS

Diagnosis depends on the presence of typical symptoms, physical findings, IgM protein in the serum, and a lymphoplasma cell proliferation of more than 10% in the bone marrow. It must be differentiated from MGUS of the IgM type, smoldering WM, lymphoma, other lymphoproliferative diseases, MM, and chronic lymphocytic leukemia.

PROGNOSIS

The median survival is approximately 5 years. Morel and colleagues have constructed a risk stratification model based on age ($\geq$ 65 years), serum albumin (< 4.0 g/dl), and cytopenias. Patients in the low-risk, intermediate-risk, and high-risk groups had 5-year survival rates of 87%, 62%, and 25% respectively.[40] Ghobrial et al.[41] developed a prognostic model based on age more than 65 years and the presence of organomegaly as well as β_2-microglobulin.

TREATMENT

Therapy should be withheld until the patient has constitutional symptoms such as weakness, fatigue, night sweats, weight loss, features of hyperviscosity, anemia, significant hepatosplenomegaly, or lymphadenopathy. Plasmapheresis should be performed based on the patient's symptoms and physical findings, rather than on the magnitude of the viscosity measurement. Therapeutic options include rituximab, the nucleoside analogues, fludarabine, and cladribine (2-chlorodeoxyadenosine), akylating agents such has chlorambucil or cyclophosphamide, corticosteroids, and ASCT. Thalidomide has been disappointing but trials are ongoing with bortezomib and sildenafil. A detailed review of management of WM has recently been published.[42]

■ HEAVY-CHAIN DISEASES ■

The HCD are lymphoplasma cell-proliferative disorders characterized by the production of an M protein consisting of an incomplete heavy chain devoid of light chains. There are three major types: α, γ, and μ.[43]

α-HEAVY-CHAIN DISEASE

α-HCD is the most common type and is characterized by the presence of a monoclonal α-chain with extensive internal deletions encompassing the V_H region and the entire first constant domain.[44] It usually occurs in the second or third decade of life, and about 60% of patients are male. Most have been from the Mediterranean region and Middle East. Gastrointestinal tract involvement is most common and is manifested by malabsorption, with weight loss, diarrhea, and steatorrhea. It is similar to immunoproliferative small intestinal disease (IPSID), but patients with IPSID do not synthesize α heavy chains. Poor hygiene and low socioeconomic status are important risk factors. Rarely, the respiratory tract is involved.

The serum protein electrophoretic pattern shows a broad band in the α_2 or β regions in half of patients and is normal in the remainder. There is no visible spike. The diagnosis depends on the recognition of a monoclonal α heavy chain in the serum, jejunal fluid, or the lymphocytes and plasma cells. The amount of α-chain in the urine is small and Bence Jones proteinuria is absent. The bone marrow is normal. The course of α-HCD is variable but generally progressive. Surprisingly, antibiotics may produce remission. In patients who do not respond to antibiotics and in those with extensive intestinal or mesenteric involvement, chemotherapy with cyclophosphamide, doxorubicin (Adriamycin), vincristine, and prednisone should be given.

γ-HEAVY-CHAIN DISEASE

In γ-HCD, the γ-chain is incomplete, with large deletions of amino acids, including the C_H1 domain and a portion of the V_H1 of the constant region. The median age at diagnosis is over 60 years but several patients younger than 20 years have been recognized. Its clinical picture has been described as a lymphoma-like illness, but its features are variable, ranging from an aggressive lymphoproliferative process to an asymptomatic state.[45] The most frequent presenting symptoms are weakness, fatigue, and fever. Autoimmune disorders such as rheumatoid arthritis, Sjögren's syndrome, systemic lupus erythematosus, Hashimoto's thyroiditis and myasthenia gravis have been noted.

Normocytic, normochromic anemia is found in 80% of cases. The amount of γ heavy-chain protein in the urine ranges from nondetectable to 20 g/24 hours; more than half of patients excrete less than 1 g of protein. Bence Jones proteinuria is not found. The bone marrow and lymph nodes contain an increased number of plasma cells, lymphocytes, and lymphoplasmacytoid cells. The diagnosis depends on demonstration of a monoclonal γ heavy chain in the serum or urine.

The median duration of survival in a series of 23 patients from a single institution was 7.4 years (range 1 month to more than 21 years).[45] Therapy with cyclophosphamide, vincristine, and prednisone is a reasonable choice, but if there is no response, doxorubicin should be added.

Table 78.4 Risk stratification model to predict progression of primary amyloidosis

Risk group	Median survival	
	Patients undergoing stem-cell transplantation (months)	Patients not undergoing stem-cell transplantation (months)
Low risk (cardiac troponin level < 0.035 μg/l and NT-proBNP level < 332 ng/l)	Not reached at 40 months	26.4
Intermediate risk (any one factor abnormal)	Not reached at 40 months	10.5
High risk (cardiac troponin level ≥ 0.035 μg/l and NT-proBNP level ≥ 332 ng/l)	8.4	3.5

NT-proBNP, N-terminal pro-brain natriuretic peptide.
From Rajkumar SV, Dispenzieri A, Kyle RA. Monoclonal gammopathy of undetermined significance, Waldenström macroglobulinemia, AL amyloidosis, and related plasma cell disorders: diagnosis and treatment. Mayo Clin Proc 2006; 81:653–703, with permission.

μ HEAVY-CHAIN DISEASE

μ-HCD is characterized by a monoclonal μ heavy chain in which the V_H domain is absent. Other deletions may also occur. Most patients have a chronic lymphoproliferative process resembling chronic lymphocytic leukemia or lymphoma. A monoclonal peak is found in the serum of 40% of patients. Two-thirds have Bence Jones proteinuria. Increases in lymphocytes, plasma cells, and lymphoplasmacytoid cells in the bone marrow are common. Vacuolization of the plasma cells is an important clue for the diagnosis of μ-HCD, which depends on the demonstration of a μ heavy chain in the serum. The course of the disease is variable; the duration of survival ranges from less than 1 month to 11 years (median, 24 months). Treatment with corticosteroids and alkylating agents has shown benefit.

PRIMARY SYSTEMIC AMYLOIDOSIS

Amyloid consists of rigid, linear, nonbranching fibrils segregated in a beta-pleated sheet confirmation which stains with Congo red and shows apple-green birefringence under polarized light. It is composed of the variable portion of a monoclonal light chain, or rarely, an intact monoclonal light chain, and is the result of a clonal plasma cell proliferative disorder.[46]

DIAGNOSIS

The diagnosis requires the demonstration of amyloid deposits which are composed of monoclonal light chains. It should be suspected in patients with nephrotic syndrome, cardiomyopathy with congestive heart failure, axonal peripheral neuropathy, or orthostatic hypotension, and the presence of a monoclonal light chain in the serum or urine. The source of tissue for diagnosis includes subcutaneous fat aspirate (75% positive), bone marrow biopsy (55% positive), or rectum (75% positive). Biopsy of the liver, kidney, heart, or sural nerve is almost 100% positive. The median age is 65 years. Macroglossia, carpal tunnel syndrome, and purpura involving the periorbital area, face, and neck may occur.

Immunofixation of the serum and urine reveals a positive result in almost 90% of patients at diagnosis. The FLC ratio is abnormal in almost all patients with a negative immunofixation.

PROGNOSIS

The median survival was 13 months in 474 patients seen at the Mayo Clinic within 1 month of diagnosis.[47] On the other hand, the estimated median survival was 40 months for amyloid patients eligible for peripheral stem-cell transplantation.[48] Median survival of patients with detectable cardiac troponin T (≥ 1 μg/L) was significantly shorter than those with undetectable levels (6 versus 22 months, respectively) (Table 78.4).

TREATMENT

Melphalan and prednisone have been the mainstay of treatment, but the results are not satisfactory. Patients who are not eligible for a stem-cell transplant (three or more organs involved, advanced cardiac amyloidosis, major comorbidities, or poor performance) are offered therapy with melphalan plus high-dose dexamethasone. The conditioning regimen for transplantation consists of intravenous melphalan (100–200 mg/m²).

Organ improvement can be achieved in 50% of patients treated with an ASCT. The mortality is approximately 10% compared to 1% for patients with MM. Patients with end-stage cardiomyopathy may be treated with a heart transplant followed by a stem-cell transplant. Thalidomide plus high-dose dexamethasone is another option,[49] but thalidomide is not well tolerated in AL.

REFERENCES

1. Kyle RA, Katzmann JA, Lust JA, et al. Immunochemical characterization of immunoglobulins. In: Rose NR, Hamilton RJ, Detrick B (eds) Manual of Clinical Laboratory Immunology, 6th edn. Washington, DC: ASM Press; 2002: 71–91.

2. Katzmann JA, Abraham RS, Dispenzieri A, et al. Diagnostic performance of quantitative κ and λ free light chain assays in clinical practice. Clin Chem 2005; 51: 878–881.

3. Kyle RA, Therneau TM, Rajkumar SV, et al. Prevalence of monoclonal gammopathy of undetermined significance. N Engl J Med 2006; 354: 1362–1369.

4. Landgren O, Gridley G, Turesson I, et al. Risk of monoclonal gammopathy of undetermined significance (MGUS) and subsequent multiple myeloma among African American and white veterans in the United States. Blood 2006; 107: 904–906.

5. Kyle RA, Therneau TM, Rajkumar SV, et al. Long-term follow-up of 241 patients with monoclonal gammopathy of undetermined significance: the original Mayo Clinic series 25 years later [see comment]. Mayo Clinic Proc 2004; 79: 859–866.

6. Kyle RA, Therneau TM, Rajkumar SV, et al. A long-term study of prognosis in monoclonal gammopathy of undetermined significance [see comment]. N Engl J Med 2002; 346: 564–569.

7. Surveillance, Epidemiology, and End Results (SEER) Program public-use data (1973–1998). Bethesda Md, National Cancer Institute, Cancer Statistics Branch, April 2001.

8. Kyle RA, Linos A, Beard CM, et al. Incidence and natural history of primary systemic amyloidosis in Olmsted County, Minnesota, 1950 through 1989. Blood 1992; 79: 1817–1822.

9. Kyle RA, Gertz MA, Witzig TE, et al. Review of 1027 patients with newly diagnosed multiple myeloma [see comment]. Mayo Clin Proc 2003; 78: 21–33.

10. Kyle RA, Rajkumar SV. Monoclonal gammopathy of undetermined significance. Clin Lymphoma Myeloma 2005; 6: 102–114.

11. Rajkumar SV, Kyle RA, Therneau TM, et al. Serum free light chain ratio is an independent risk factor for progression in monoclonal gammopathy of undetermined significance. Blood 2005; 106: 812–817.

12. Cesana C, Klersy C, Barbarano L, et al. Prognostic factors for malignant transformation in monoclonal gammopathy of undetermined significance and smoldering multiple myeloma. J Clin Oncol 2002; 20: 1625–1634.

13. Kyle RA, Therneau TM, Rajkumar SV, et al. Long-term follow-up of IgM monoclonal gammopathy of undetermined significance. Blood 2003; 102: 3759–3764.

14. Kyle RA, Robinson RA, Katzmann JA. The clinical aspects of biclonal gammopathies. Review of 57 cases. Am J Med 1981; 71: 999–1008.

15. Kyle RA, Greipp PR. "Idiopathic" Bence Jones proteinuria: long-term follow-up in seven patients. N Engl J Med 1982; 306: 564–567.

16. Kyle RA, Therneau TM, Rajkumar SV, et al. Incidence of multiple myeloma in Olmsted County, Minnesota – trend over 6 decades. Cancer 2004; 101: 2667–2674.

17. Kuehl WM, Bergsagel PL. Multiple myeloma: evolving genetic events and host interactions. Nat Rev Cancer 2002; 2: 175–187.

18. Greipp PR, San Miguel J, Durie BG, et al. International staging system for multiple myeloma. J Clin Oncol 2005; 23: 3412–3420.

19. Kyle RA, Rajkumar SV. Multiple myeloma: drug therapy. N Engl J Med 2004; 351: 1860–1873.

20. Rajkumar SV, Kyle RA. Multiple myeloma: diagnosis and treatment. Mayo Clin Proc 2005; 80: 1371–1382.

21. Rajkumar SV, Blood E, Vesole D, et al. Phase III clinical trial of thalidomide plus dexamethasone compared with dexamethasone alone in newly diagnosed multiple myeloma: a clinical trial coordinated by the Eastern Cooperative Oncology Group. J Clin Oncol 2006; 24: 431–436.

22. Cavo M, Zamagni E, Tosi P, et al. Superiority of thalidomide and dexamethasone over vincristine-doxorubicindexamethasone (VAD) as primary therapy in preparation for autologous transplantation for multiple myeloma. Blood 2005; 106: 35–39.

23. Child JA, Morgan GJ, Davies FE, et al. High-dose chemotherapy with hematopoietic stem-cell rescue for multiple myeloma [see comment]. N Engl J Med 2003; 348: 1875–1883.

24. Harousseau JL, Moreau P, Attal M, et al. Stem-cell transplantation in multiple myeloma. Bailliere's Best Pract Clin Hematol 2005; 18: 603–618.

25. Attal M, Harousseau JL, Facon T, et al. Single versus double autologous stem-cell transplantation for multiple myeloma [see comment] [erratum appears in N Engl J Med 2004; 350: 2628]. N Engl J Med 2003; 349: 2495–2502.

26. Group MTC. Combination chemotherapy versus melphalan plus prednisone as treatment for multiple myeloma: an overview of 6633 patients from 27 randomized trials. Myeloma Trialists' Collaborative Group. J Clin Oncol 1998; 16: 3832–3842.

27. Palumbo A, Bringhen S, Caravita T, et al. Oral melphalan and prednisone chemotherapy plus thalidomide compared with melphalan and prednisone alone in elderly patients with multiple myeloma: randomised controlled trial. Lancet 2006; 367: 825–831.

28. Facon T, Mary J, Hulin C, et al. Major superiority of melphalan and prednisone (MP) plus thalidomide (THAL) over MP and autologous stem cell transplantation in the treatment of newly diagnosed elderly patients with multiple myeloma. Blood 2005; 106: A780(abst).

29. Barlogie B, Kyle RA, Anderson KC, et al. Standard chemotherapy compared with high-dose chemoradiotherapy for multiple myeloma: final results of phase III US Intergroup Trial S9321. J Clin Oncol 2006; 24: 929–936.

30. Berenson JR, Lichtenstein A, Porter L, et al. Long-term pamidronate treatment of advanced multiple myeloma patients reduces skeletal events. Myeloma Aredia Study Group. J Clin Oncol 1998; 16: 593–602.

31. Attal M, Harousseau J-L, Leyvraz S, et al. Maintenence therapy with thalidomide improves survival in patients with multiple myeloma. Blood 2006; 108: 3289–3294.

32. Richardson PG, Sonneveld P, Schuster MW, et al. Bortezomib or high-dose dexamethasone for relapsed multiple myeloma. N Engl J Med 2005; 352: 2487–2498.

33. Kyle RA, Greipp PR. Smoldering multiple myeloma. N Engl J Med 1980; 302: 1347–1349.

34. Garcia-Sanz R, Orfao A, Gonzalez M, et al. Primary plasma cell leukemia: clinical, immunophenotypic, DNA ploidy, and cytogenetic characteristics. Blood 1999; 93: 1032–1037.

35. Liebross RH, Ha CS, Cox JD, et al. Solitary bone plasmacytoma: outcome and prognostic factors following radiotherapy. Int J Radiat Oncol Biol Phys 1998; 41: 1063–1067.

36. Alexiou C, Kau RJ, Dietzfelbinger H, et al. Extramedullary plasmacytoma: tumor occurrence and therapeutic concepts. Cancer 1999; 85: 2305–2314.

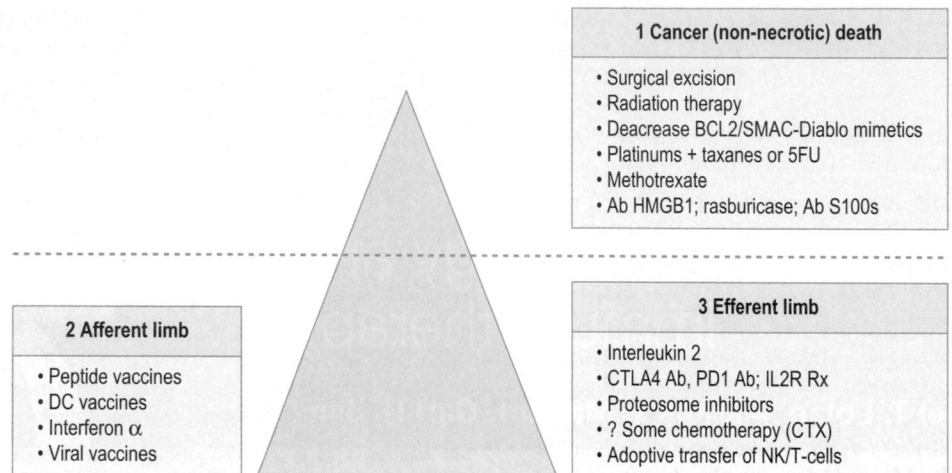

1 Cancer (non-necrotic) death

- Surgical excision
- Radiation therapy
- Deacrease BCL2/SMAC-Diablo mimetics
- Platinums + taxanes or 5FU
- Methotrexate
- Ab HMGB1; rasburicase; Ab S100s

2 Afferent limb

- Peptide vaccines
- DC vaccines
- Interferon α
- Viral vaccines

3 Efferent limb

- Interleukin 2
- CTLA4 Ab, PD1 Ab; IL2R Rx
- Proteosome inhibitors
- ? Some chemotherapy (CTX)
- Adoptive transfer of NK/T-cells

Fig. 79.1 Immunotherapeutic triangle. Traditional therapies for cancer (shown above the dotted line) have involved those designed primarily to (1) kill the tumor cell, largely by mediating necrotic cell death, taking the tumor out or treating with chemotherapy. More recently, it has become apparent that how the tumor cell dies, normally with apoptosis or autophagic death versus necrotic death, is of likely importance. More modern strategies have included use of platinums, which sequester high-mobility group box 1 (HMGB1) in the cytosol, typically in conjunction with taxanes or fluoropyrimidines such as 5 fluorouracil (5FU); radiation therapy, which induces oxidative strand breaks in DNA, limiting necrosis; use of agents such as methotrexate that promote metabolic/autophagic death; or use of means to block anti-apoptotic factors such as BCL2. Antibodies to HMGB1 or S100 proteins or blockade of purine metabolites such as uric acid with enzyme therapies such as rasburicase recognize the critical role of cell death. Below the dotted line are the postulated role of emergent immunotherapies for cancer, which typically focus on enhancing (2) the afferent limb of the immune response through vaccination strategies or application of immune stimulants such as interferon-α or (3) the efferent limb of the immune response with interleukin-2-promoting delivery of immune effectors into the tumor microenvironment, potentiating their cytolytic activity, or use of agents that directly (CTLA4 antibody, or antibodies to other inhibitory pathways) or indirectly (some chemotherapy) limit means of escape from immune detection.

the tumor after heating the skin of the tumor. This was the first clinical experiment in which a purposeful bacterial infection was intended to cure cancer. Subsequently, a New York surgeon, William B. Coley, used a bacterial vaccine to treat inoperable sarcoma, with a reported cure rate of better than 10%.

- Passive immunotherapy. Gilliland et al.[18] and Croce et al.[19] demonstrated that monoclonal antibodies could be used therapeutically, ushering in the application for infectious diseases and cancer. Anti-CD20 monoclonal antibodies (rituximab) were approved by the Food and Drug Administration (FDA) in 1997 for the treatment of B-cell non-Hodgkin lymphoma . Addition of rituximab to standard cyclophosphamide, adriamycin (hydroxydoxorubicin, vincristine, concovin), prednisone (CHOP) chemotherapy provided the first improvement in survival in 2002.[20–22] Transfer of IL-2 activated NK cells to patients with melanoma and other tumors was initially promising but found ineffective in randomized trials; it has had a renaissance in the setting of the treatment of leukemias.[23] More recently, pioneering studies with the adoptive transfer of genetically modified T cells have had demonstrable success with the elimination of large, progressively growing tumors when coupled with lymphodepletion.[24,25] DC therapies have been associated with anecdotal responses in patients with lymphoma and melanoma.[26,27]

- Limiting inhibitory factors. The notion that immunosuppression and regulatory cells (Table 79.1) played a critical role in cancer has been recognized for many years. That this was derived from tumor

factors, now molecularly defined as transforming growth factor-β and damage-associated molecular pattern molecules (DAMPs, see below) was presaged by Revescz (Fig. 79.2), in pioneering studies performed over half a century ago.[28,29] He demonstrated that tumors failed to grow in murine recipients unless irradiated tumors were added to limiting numbers of tumor cells. He suggested that the growth-promoting effect was due to: (1) specific stimulation by homologous cell products; (2) provision of a 'feeder effect' in which the dead cells release essential nutrients; or (3) stimulation provoking an inflammatory response and/or vascularization from the host. This notion has relevance today with novel therapies converting necrotic to apoptotic cell death, which paradoxically both recruits immune cells and also drives reparative epithelial proliferation, angiogenesis, and stromagenesis. More recent strategies include the use of antibodies to CTLA-4, thus enabling clonal expansion of T-cell effectors.

Transferable tumor immunity is dependent on T cells, and less dependent on humoral factors. Thus a generation of immunotherapies ensued, predicated on active immunization with antigens and various adjuvants, with little to show for the effort to date. Passive immunotherapies with the application of monoclonal antibodies targeting cell surface molecules and the role of innate immune cells, although thought to be of less importance in previous studies, are now re-emerging, with TLRs, NLRs, and RLRs signaling cell death pathways.[30,31] Recently the application of histone deacetylase (HDAC) inhibitors to alter gene expression heat shock protein 90 (HSP90, a critical chaperone protein necessary for the function of many

Table 79.1 Darwinian selection and coevolution of cancer in its host: means of escape from immune control

Host	Tumor	Stroma
Immunosuppressive cytokines/factors (TGF-β, IL-10, PGE$_2$), VEGF	Immunosuppressive cytokines/factors (TGF-β, IL-10, PGE$_2$), VEGF	Vascular endothelium in tumor limiting recruitment of host effectors; lack of responsiveness to TNF
Suppressor macrophages	Downregulation of receptors (e.g., TGF-βR)	Nonsenescent fibroblasts
Plasmacytoid dendritic cells producing IDO	Specific downregulation of antigens	Reducing tumor microenvironment
Granulocytes promoting acute inflammatory response	Individual allelic class I MHC molecule expression	Wound repair response to DAMPs (S100 family of molecules, purine metabolites including uric acid and ATP, hyaluronan, heat shock proteins (HSPs), heparin sulfate, and syndecan)
Basophils promoting immunosuppression and angiogenesis	B$_2$-microglobulin loss	
Regulatory T cells limiting immune effectors	Shedding stress receptors such as MICA/MICB	
Blocking antibodies	Tumor antigen loss variants	
Th2–Th4-biased response		

ATP, adenosine triphosphate; DAMPs, damage-associated molecular pattern molecules; IDO, indoleamine 2,3 dioxygene; IL, interleukin; MHC, major histocompatibility complex; MICA, MHC Class I associated A; MICB, MHC Class I associated B; PGE, prostaglandin E; TGF, transforming growth factor; TNF, tumor necrosis factor; VEGF, vascular endothelial growth factor.

proteins) inhibitors as well as small molecules inhibiting the mammalian target of rapamycin (mTOR, a critical pathway regulating growth, differentiation, and survival in many cancers) in clinical trials suggests that modern small-molecule therapies with defined targets could join biologic agents driving important immune-mediated antitumor effects.

ROLE OF PATHOGEN-ASSOCIATED MOLECULAR PATTERN MOLECULES (PAMPs)

Many tumors arise in the setting of chronic microbial infection. Examples include human papillomavirus and cervical cancer, hepatitis B and C and hepatoma, *Helicobacter pylori*, and gastric cancer. Perhaps the most effective strategies to prevent cancer are those designed to limit infections and resultant chronic inflammation. Indeed, immunization to hepatitis B has been shown to limit hepatoma[32] in hepatitis B-carrier children. In those born after initiation of a vaccination program, a lower risk of developing human cervical cancer was identified than those born before the program (risk ratio, 2.3–4.5). Similarly, vaccination to human papillomavirus has led to substantial decreases in cervical carcinoma precursor lesions.[33]

ROLE OF DAMAGE-ASSOCIATED MOLECULAR PATTERN MOLECULES

DAMPs are typically released following necrotic and late apoptotic tumor death (Fig. 79.3). DAMPS include the small calcium-binding S100 family of molecules, purine metabolites including uric acid and

KEY CONCEPTS

DAMAGE-ASSOCIATED MOLECULAR PATTERN MOLECULES (DAMPS) AND PATHOGEN-ASSOCIATED MOLECULAR PATTERN MOLECULES IN TUMOR BIOLOGY

>> Substantial linkage of chronic inflammation with initiation and progression of tumors is found in adults, not in children

>> Immune cells are found throughout epithelial neoplasms and correlate positively with clinical outcome parameters

>> Increased high-mobility group box 1 (HMGB1), a prototypic DAMP, is associated with cancer as well as its receptor, receptor for advanced glycation end products (RAGE)

>> Cancer is associated with release of DAMPs, promoting tumor progression

>> Decreased incidence of hepatoma is noted in endemic areas where children are vaccinated against hepatitis B

>> Decreased incidence of cervical intraepithelial neoplasia is noted in women vaccinated against human papillomavirus

>> Strategies to limit DAMPs in murine models are now in process and could presage novel therapies for patients

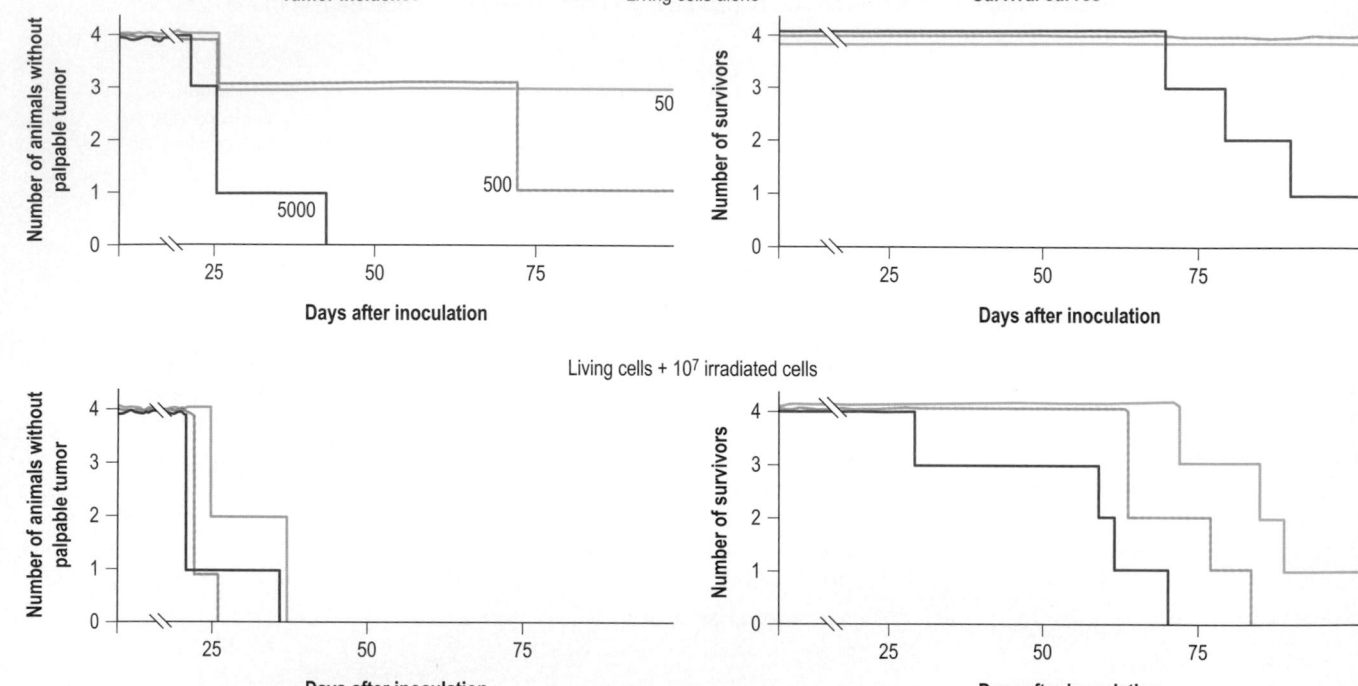

Fig. 79.2 Tumor cell death promotes tumor cell growth. Over 50 years ago, it was recognized that limiting numbers of tumor cells failed to grow in murine hosts unless additional irradiated cells were added. The role of these added cells was considered at the time to mediate its effects by: (1) specific stimulation by homologous cell products; (2) a 'feeder effect' in which the dead cells release essential nutrients; or (3) stimulation through provoking an inflammatory response and/or vascularization from the side of the host. Thus the role of inflammation and immune mechanisms was suggested early as an important part of tumor biology, promoting resultant growth of both primary and metastatic tumors. The factors mediating these effects are recognized today as damage-associated molecular pattern molecules. (Data from Revesz L. Effect of tumor cells killed by x-rays upon the growth of admixed viable cells. Nature 1956; 178: 1391–1392.)

adenosine triphosphate, hyaluronan, HSPs, heparin sulfate, and syndecan.[16] An interesting member of the DAMP family which has cytokine-like properties is the evolutionarily conserved nuclear protein, high-mobility group box 1 (HMGB1).[34] HMGB1 is present in the nuclei and cytoplasm of nearly all cell types.[15, 35] It is released upon necrotic but not apoptotic death (Fig. 79.4), and cytolytic effectors promote release from tumor cells.[14, 35]

ROLE OF INNATE IMMUNE CELLS IN CANCER

Neutrophils and macrophages, particularly M2 macrophages, those promoting wound healing, are associated with poor prognosis. Eosinophils have been found at increased numbers both within tumor tissues and within the bloodstream in cancer patients.[36] Eosinophilic granulocytes belong to a class of inflammatory cells that are often found naturally within tumor tissues.[37] Eosinophilia is also found following effective immunotherapy and the antitumor effects of successful cytokine therapy of cancer with IL-2 have been associated with the identification of degranulating eosinophils within the tumor.[38] In trials of IL-4, Sosman and colleagues[39] found induction of systemic eosinophil degranulation with increases in serum and urine major basic protein. Eradication of melanoma metastases[40] in a mouse model by CD4 Th2 cells is associated with a substantial influx

KEY CONCEPTS

TUMOR BIOLOGY AND THE ROLE OF INFLAMMATION

>> Cancer arises in the setting of genomic instability

>> Genomic instability arises from primary critical genetic alterations arising during meiosis and early rapid expansion of the embryo, in a mendelian fashion from the parents, but most frequently in adults as a consequence of chronic inflammation

>> Pediatric tumors have a paucity of cells associated with adaptive immunity (T cells and myeloid dendritic cells)

>> Adult tumors are frequently associated with both T-cell and dendritic cell infiltrate

>> Adoptive immune responses driven by interleukin-2, interferon-α, or dendritic cell therapy can mediate important antitumor effects

>> Regulatory cells limit immune effector function (M2 macrophages, regulatory T cells, plasmacytoid dendritic cells (PDCs), etc.)

>> The application of approved immunotherapy for cancer, including the cytokines interleukin-2 and interferon-α, likely promotes adaptive immunity

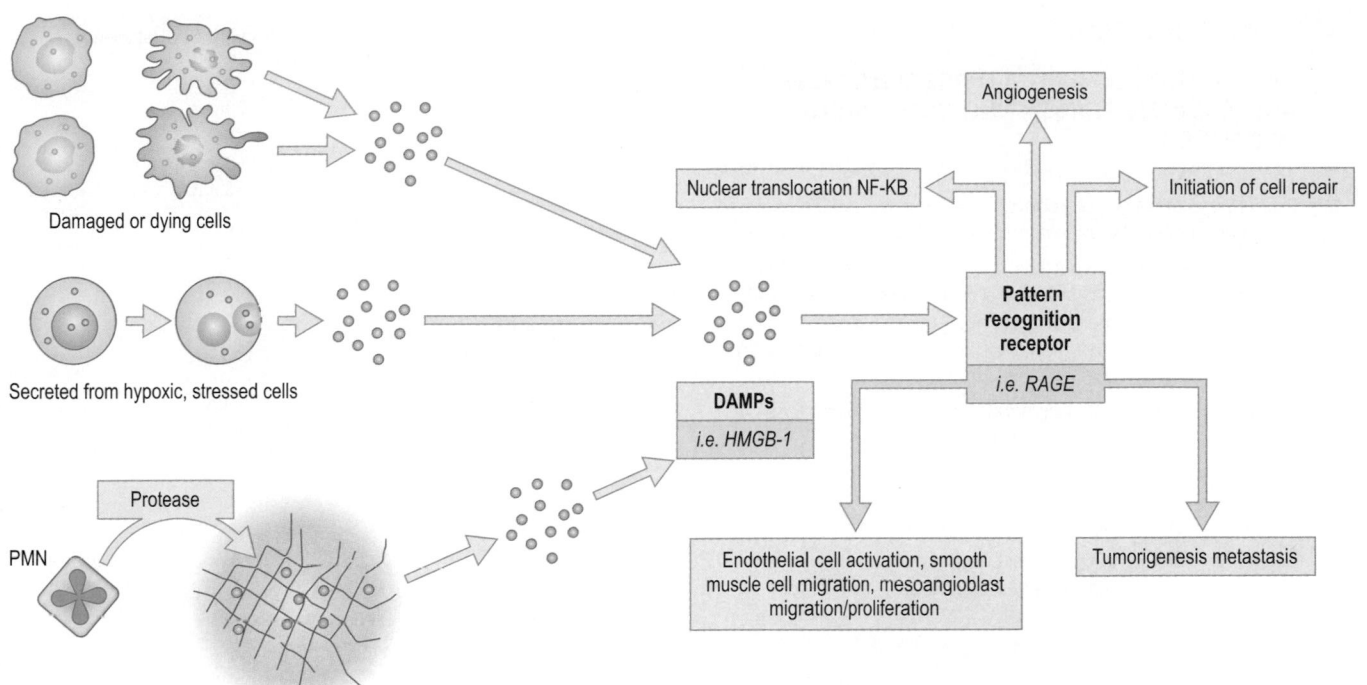

Fig. 79.3 Tumor sources of endogenous damage-associated molecular pattern molecules (DAMPs). In the setting of tumor growth and death, release of DAMPs by damaged or dying cells, actively secreted by hypoxic or stressed cells, or as degradation products derived from proteolytically cleaved tissue matrix, prompted by neutrophils (polymorphonuclear leukocytes, PMNs) collectively leads to recruitment and recognition by innate immune effectors of these products. Together, these changes lead to enhanced survival in viable epithelial cells through upregulation of NF-κB, angiogenesis and stromagenesis, intiation of a wound repair phenotype, and associated with enhanced tumorigenesis, migration, and metastasis.

of eosinophils into the tumor, supporting a role for eosinophil-mediated tumor cytotoxicity. Although incubation of eosinophils with B16 melanoma cells has no direct effects, eosinophil lysates are themselves cytotoxic for tumor.[40] Understanding the relationship between tumor-derived factors such as HMGB1 and eosinophils is important to discern their role in the tumor microenvironment. Recently, mast cells have been shown to promote survival of allogeneic skin grafts[41] and their perceived role in tumor thus also needs to be immunologically reconsidered.

ROLE OF CANCER STEM CELLS AND MESANGIOBLASTS

Most tissues in humans contain a small subset of cells that self-renew, including solid tumors and hematopoietic neoplasms. During tumor expansion, both inflammatory cells and hemangioblasts are recruited to the tumor microenvironment. Whether tumors arise because of changes in nominal tumor stem cells or whether more differentiated cells acquire stem-cell-like properties is as yet unclear. The goals of developing effective immunotherapies for cancer are similar to those using chemotherapy or radiation therapy. It is unknown whether immune effectors target the nominal daughter cells or the functional stem cells.[42]

ANTIGEN PROCESSING AND PRESENTATION IN CANCER; RECRUITMENT AND ROLE OF ADAPTIVE IMMUNE EFFECTORS

The notion of cancer immune surveillance suggests that immune cells take an active role in destroying cancers, thereby leading to darwinian selection and emergence of tumors capable of evading immune detection. Indeed, single allelic loss of MHC class I molecules, antigen-processing machinery losses, and even global loss of MHC class I molecules have been noted in cancer (Table 79.1). Presumably antigen-specific T-cell responses to cancer and concurrent alterations in the ability to be recognized by NK cells through stress receptors enable persistence and expansion of malignant lesions. The means to reverse and overcome tumor cell immune evasion is an area of active research.[43]

WOUND HEALING AND CANCER[44]

The relationship between altered wound healing ('the wound that does not heal') and cancer has been noted for some time. The mechanisms involved and the role of inflammatory and immune cells, however, have been obscure. Fibroblasts can activate an aging process called replicative senescence, possibly providing a barrier against transformation of tissues. The p53 inducible gene plasminogen activator inhibitor-1 is important in replicative senescence, upregulated in stressed fibroblasts,

KEY CONCEPTS

IMPORTANCE OF ANTIGEN PRESENTATION AND ANTIGEN-PRESENTING CELLS (APC) IN CANCER

>> Tumors are infiltrated with conventional dendritic cells and there is a direct relationship between number of cells and prognosis

>> Evidence for immune interaction with tumor cells includes loss of single allelic major histocompatibility complex (MHC) class I molecule expression, global β_2-microglobulin expression loss, or loss of individual elements of the antigen-processing machinery

>> Tumor cell-derived antigens can be processed and cross-presented by antigen-presenting cells

>> In murine models, tumors can be immunologically recognized and eliminated by CD8+ effectors, even in the absence of class I expression on the tumor cells

>> Means to increase antigen presentation include application of agents such as interferon-γ or interferon-α to promote protein processing

>> Means to increase antigen-presenting cells in the tumor include application of agents such as interleukin-2, which increases vascular leak and promotes recruitment of immune cells

>> Antigen-presenting cells can be increased in number by promoting their production with administration of FLT3 ligand, granulocyte–macrophage colony-stimulating factor, or interleukin-3

THERAPEUTIC PRINCIPLES

IMPORTANT FOR THE IMMUNOTHERAPY OF CANCER

>> Assess immune reactivity, and the presence of infiltrating immune cells in the peripheral blood and tumor when available; assess presence of necrosis in the tumor

>> General immune status, delayed-type hypersensitivity (DTH) reactivity to recall antigens

>> Baseline serum and peripheral blood to assess pretreatment immunity to nominal target antigens

>> Determine evidence of damage-associated molecular patterns (DAMPs) in the peripheral blood (high-mobility group box 1 (HMGB1), uric acid, lactate dehydrogenase) and DAMP-Rs/induced (soluble RAGE (sRAGE), interleukin-1 receptor antagonist (RA), neopterin)

and inhibiting the urokinase-type plasminogen activator. Senescence, wound healing, and metastasis are thus linked.[44] The major and crucial roles of epithelia (the origins of most lethal tumors in humans) are: (1) to provide a barrier; and (2) to provide selective transport across that barrier. These are mutually exclusive functions that require guardians, immune effectors that can mediate both tolerance and host defense at this interface. Regulation of the epithelial cell barriers is central to development of immunity and chronic inflammation, and plays a postulated

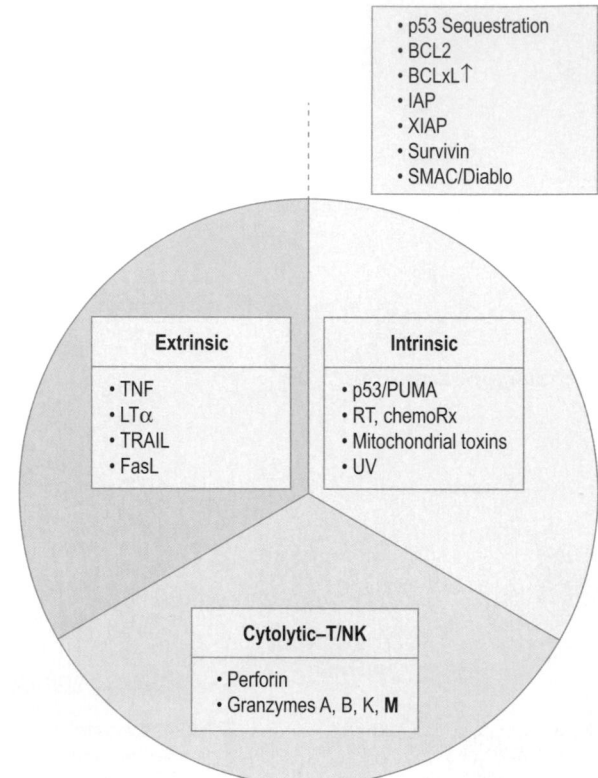

Fig. 79.4 Apoptosis and necrosis in tumor immunobiology. The chevron diagram of apoptotic death involves: (1) intrinsic pathways induced by p53-sensitive induction of cell cycle arrest, and in the absence of genomic repair, upregulation of the BH3 domain containing proteins PUMA and NOXA that promote mitochondrial-mediated cell death and release of SMAC/Diablo and cytochrome C. These are typically induced by radiation therapy, some chemotherapeutic agents, toxins and ultraviolet (UV) irradiation; (2) extrinsic pathways mediated by members of the tumor necrosis factor (TNF) family, including lymphotoxin a (LTa), TNF-related apoptosis-inducing ligand (TRAIL), or Fas ligand (FAS L); or by (3) cytolytic effectors, specifically natural killer (NK) and T cells. Delivery of perforin-mediated pores/membrane disruption and granule exocytosis of the serine proteases, Granzymes A, B, K, and M lead to apoptotic death in normal cells. Paradoxically, in the setting of p53 sequestration in the cytosol, often mediated by mutation, upregulation of the anti-apoptotic proteins, BCL2, BCLxL, IAP, XIAP, and survivin, tumor cells fail to undergo apoptosis or autophagy, but rather, under conditions of genomic, nutrient, or endoplasmic reticulum stress, undergo necrotic cell death. The consequences are release of DAMPs (Fig. 79.3) and resultant recruitment of inflammatory cells. (Data from Zeh HJ 3rd, Lotze MT. Addicted to death: invasive cancer and the immune response to unscheduled cell death. J Immunother 2005; 28: 1–9.)

Table 79.2 Examples of tumor antigens applied in cancer immunotherapy

Altered self	Viral antigens	Oncofetal antigens	Autoantigens
K-ras, p53 mutants	EBV-EBNA	Carcinoembryonic antigen (CEA)	Overexpression – c-myc in lymphomas, leukemias
Products of normally unexpressed genes (MAGE, BAGE, GAGE)	HPV E-6,-7	Alpha-fetoprotein (AFP)	HER-2/neu epidermal growth factor receptor- breast cancer (Herceptin)
Proteins of alternative reading frame, of posttranslational modification	SV40 T Ag	Prostate-specific membrane antigen (PSMA) and PSA	
Melanosomal antigens (MART1/Melan A,gp100, tyrosinase)		Pancreatic oncofetal antigen	
hTERT			
Proteins with altered glycosylation, (mucin-CA125, MUC1)			

EBNA, Epstein Barr nuclear antigen; EBV, Epstein–Barr virus; HPV, human papillomavirus; PSA, prostate-specific antigen

central role in cancer development. Several cytokines and other immune modulators that control tight junctions between epithelial cells play important roles during development, wound healing, infection, chronic inflammation, and cancer.

IMMUNOTHERAPHY OF CANCER

ACTIVE IMMUNOTHERAPY WITH VACCINATION

Long-term survival in patients with cancer has changed little in the last 30 years and introducing effective vaccination to cancer patients remains a major therapeutic challenge. Although cancer vaccines have been practiced in animal models for over 50 years, such immunotherapy in patients remains a novel, unapproved approach, which remains experimental. Active specific immunotherapy in patients with various solid tumors has been carried out for the last 10 years with only modest anecdotal response to nominal common tumor antigens (Table 79.2). In part, this may be because each tumor has its own immunodominant antigens, distinct from histologically similar tumors arising in other individuals. Similarly, overall survival obtained by systemic chemotherapy in patients with advanced cancer has been poor, comparable to the low improvement observed with cancer vaccines.[45] In such trials in 440 patients conducted at the National Institutes of Health Surgery Branch,[45a] the objective response rate was low (2.6%), comparable to poor results obtained by others. Perhaps the greatest experience has been in patients with melanoma as a consequence of the identification of many melanoma antigens recognized by T cells. Clinical trials performed with various vaccination strategies, including whole tumor cells, antigen peptides, antigen-pulsed DCs, recombinant viruses, plasmids or naked DNA, and HSPs, failed to demonstrate efficacy in the few large phase III randomized clinical trials performed to date.

ACTIVE IMMUNOTHERAPY WITH CYTOKINE TREATMENT

Cytokine therapies are designed to alter immune homeostasis with the tumor and provoke or disinhibit immune effectors. Although both IFN-α (Fig. 79.5) and IL-2 (Fig. 79.6) have been approved for the treatment of patients with metastatic renal cell carcinoma and melanoma, no randomized studies have demonstrated substantial (> 10%) efficacy and the high doses necessary to mediate antitumor effects have substantial toxicities, and thus have precluded widespread acceptance. IL-2 is produced by activated T cells and serves as a growth factor for T and NK cells but also induces sensitivity to apoptosis in these same cells. It induces IFN-γ production and cytolysis by T (αβ and γδ) as well as NK cells. Like IL-2 deficiency, IL-2 administration is associated with enteropathy, whereas the hematopoietin IL-15 that shares two receptors with IL-2 is observed to have gut-protective activity. There have been many clinical trials performed and IL-2 is now FDA-approved for the treatment of patients with metastatic melanoma and renal cell carcinoma. We first showed that IL-2 treatment was associated with substantial gastrointestinal toxicity and rare perforation almost 20 years ago. The pathogenic mechanisms have not been studied in detail. Since therapy with high doses are required to mediate important antitumor effects, toxicity becomes a critical issue, leading to reduction in dose and duration of therapy. However, since the initial report over 20 years ago there have essentially been no improvements in the therapy! IL-2 is associated with major hemodynamic changes, including hypotension, profound oliguria, and renal dysfunction, as well as enteropathy, including:

- Anorexia, nausea, vomiting, diarrhea
- Glossitis, xerostomia, stomatitis

In the second approach, polyclonal *ex vivo* activation of the input T cells is done, based on the assumptions that antigen-specific T cells are present in the patient and have been primed *in vivo*.[47] The first approach will guarantee antigen specificity but is costly and labor-intensive. The second approach is technically more facile. Both approaches have been strengthened by the realization that homeostatic expansion of transferred lymphocytes can improve engraftment and effector functions *in vivo*.[48] The rationale for the polyclonal approach has been substantially strengthened by the realization that most patients are already primed to their tumor, and that the major issue is improving the quality and quantity of the natural immune response.

Studies conducted during the past several decades have uncovered a number of principles of adoptive immunotherapy. These principles are to: (1) avoid the induction of immunogenicity of the infused cells; (2) prevent or delay cellular immunosenescence; (3) maximize help; and (4) choose lymphopenic rather than lymphoreplete hosts. Given that the immune system is probably the most efficient biosensor system ever developed, it is not surprising that seemingly trivial modifications to cell culture technologies can have large differences in the immunogenicity and subsequent engraftment of the adoptively transferred cells. Human T cells have finite clonal lifespans *in vitro*, a phenomenon also manifested with other somatic tissue cells and commonly known as the Hayflick limit. Lymphocytes and stem cells belong to a select class of cells that have the capacity for induction of telomerase activity. It is possible that many previous clinical adoptive immunotherapy trials have been unsuccessful because the prolonged *ex vivo* culture process resulted in a population of cells that had reached, or were near, replicative senescence. Recent studies show that the *in vivo* persistence and engraftment of tumor-infiltrating lymphocytes (TIL) correlate with telomere length and tumor regression in patients with melanoma.[49]

Many studies show that the generation and/or maintenance of CD8 memory requires CD4 cell help, and clinical adoptive transfer studies show that the persistence of CD8 effector T cells is enhanced with the concomitant administration of IL-2 or CD4 cells. Host lymphodepletion may also enhance the effectiveness of adoptively transferred T cells.[48] Lymphodepletion eliminates Tregs and other competing elements of the immune system that act as 'cytokine sinks,' enhancing the availability of cytokines such as IL-7 and IL-15. This hypothesis has been tested clinically in patients with metastatic melanoma and myeloma, and initial results suggest that the efficacy of adoptive transfer is improved in patients rendered immunodeficient by cytotoxic chemotherapy.[50, 51]

■ ADOPTIVE TRANSFER OF EFFECTOR T CELLS ■

VIRAL SPECIFIC T CELLS

Virally induced lymphomas that retain some expression of the inciting viral genome are likely to present a good target for adoptive cellular therapy. Unlike most spontaneous tumors, the repertoire of T-cell receptors contains T cells with high-affinity receptors for the viral protein, as a consequence of a lack of deletion of these T cells in the thymus. In patients recovering from allogeneic bone marrow transplantation, a severe defect in the cellular immune system exists, and this often results in the death of the patients from reactivation of systemic cytomegalovirus (CMV) or Epstein–Barr virus (EBV) infection. Donor-derived,

CMV antigen-specific CD8 cytotoxic T lymphocytes (CTL) have been administered to the patients, and represents a promising means of restoring immune function.[46] Even relatively modest doses of T cells (1×10^6 cells/kg) have been shown to be an effective treatment or prophylaxis for patients with EBV-associated lymphoma, with complete remissions recorded in most patients.[52] Pneumonitis and tumor swelling with respiratory obstruction have been reported as adverse events following CTL infusion for lymphoma. Recent studies indicate that EBV-specific CTLs are safe and have significant antitumor activity in Hodgkin's disease and nasopharyngeal carcinoma associated with EBV infection.

TUMOR SPECIFIC CYTOTOXIC T CELLS

Due to recent technical advances that permit the generation of tumor-specific CTLs, their clinical utility has not yet been extensively evaluated. Tumor-specific CTLs generated *ex vivo* with the rapid expansion method appear to have substantial activity in melanoma, as 8 of 10 patients with refractory, metastatic melanoma had minor, mixed, or stable responses.[53] However, studies at the National Cancer Institute suggested that host conditioning can increase the response to adoptive immunotherapy with TIL.[50] Adverse effects included opportunistic infections, and the frequent induction of vitiligo and uveitis, presumably due to autoreactivity by TIL. If confirmed, these results indicate that prior host immunosuppression is useful to improve antitumor efficacy of adoptive immunotherapy.

T REGULATORY CELLS (TREGS)

Suppressor or Tregs were recently rediscovered based on their ability to prevent a number of autoimmune disorders in mice. A congenital deficiency of FoxP3 in humans leads to a deficiency of Tregs and is associated with a variety of autoimmune immunopathologies.[54] Tregs were initially thought to be hypoproliferative; however, recent studies show that they can be expanded *in vitro* sufficiently for potential adoptive therapy approaches.[55] Tregs have not yet been tested in humans; however, based on preclinical studies, graft-versus-host disease (GvHD) following allogeneic hematopoietic stem cell transplantation in adults is likely to be the initial setting for the first human trials with *ex vivo* expanded and adoptively transferred Tregs.

NATURAL KILLER CELLS

Unlike T cells, NK cells are cytolytic for targets, even in the absence of MHC class I expression (Chapter 18). Another hallmark of NK cells is that they use a variety of nonrearranging receptors to initiate cytolytic activity and cytokine production. The ability of NK cells to kill tumors that have diminished MHC class I expression predicts that immunotherapies based on adoptive NK cell transfer should be synergistic with T-cell-based therapies, in that MHC loss variants that emerge as a result of tumor immunoediting by T cells could be 'cleaned up' by NK cell-based approaches.

The availability of recombinant IL-2 enabled the first clinical trials of adoptively transferred autologous NK cells. Due to poor efficacy, adoptive therapy with NK cells was largely abandoned until recently. However, given the recent appreciation that NK cells express both activating and inhibitory (KIR) receptors, a resurgence of interest has occurred.

KEY CONCEPTS

ADOPTIVE IMMUNOTHERAPY WITH GENETICALLY MODIFIED LYMPHOCYTES

>> Antigen specificity can be assured by transduction of chimeric artificial receptors or natural antigen receptors

>> T-cell lifespan can be regulated by incorporation of conditional suicide genes or genes to delay senescence

>> T cells are efficiently transduced with retroviruses and lentiviruses

>> Genetically modified T cells can be used to study engraftment and trafficking of adoptively transferred T cells

>> Genetically modified T cells have been shown to persist for years in patients after adoptive transfer

Infusions of 'alloreactive' NK cells have been shown to mediate antileukemic effects against acute myelogenous leukemia in the setting of mismatched transplantation when KIR ligand incompatibility existed in the direction of GvHD, i.e., MHC class I KIR ligand that is absent in the recipient but present in the donor.[56] Studies indicating that alloreactive NK cells are cytotoxic for melanoma and renal cell cancer cells *in vitro*[57] suggest that HLA-mismatched hematopoietic stem cell transplantation may be an attractive setting to exploit NK-cell adoptive therapies for patients with solid tumors. Once the complexity of the NK system is better understood, it is likely that clinical trials using combinations of tumor-specific T cells and NK cells will be done.

GENETICALLY MODIFIED LYMPHOCYTES

Genetic modification of T cells *ex vivo* to engineer an improved antitumor effect is an attractive strategy for many settings.[58] The advent of lentiviral vectors has greatly increased the efficiency of T-cell engineering, and adoptive therapies with HIV-based lentiviral engineered T cells has shown promise in pilot clinical trials.[59]

A number of issues can be addressed with genetically modified T cells to overcome limitations of natural lymphocytes. The first use of genetically modified T cells was to demonstrate that adoptively transferred cells could persist in the host and traffic to tumor. A second use has been to address the principal limitation of cancer immunotherapy, which is tumor-induced tolerance that results in few natural T cells that have high avidity for tumor-specific antigens. To address this problem, some clinical trials now in progress attempt to endow T cells with novel receptor constructs by introduction of 'T bodies': chimeric receptors that have antibody-based external receptor structures and cytosolic domains that encode signal transduction modules of the T-cell receptor.[58] These constructs can function to retarget T cells *in vitro* in an MHC-unrestricted manner.

Lamers and colleagues recently reported interim results of a pilot trial testing T bodies in 3 patients with metastatic renal cell carcinoma.[60] The T bodies, expressed in autologous T cells using retroviral transduction, were retargeted with a single-chain Fv fragment specific for carboxy-anhydrase-IX (the G250 antigen) that is overexpressed on clear-cell kidney cancers. The subjects were treated with a dose escalation scheme of G250-modified T cells and recombinant IL-2. Infusions of these G250 T bodies were initially well tolerated; however, significant liver toxicity developed that appeared to reflect expression of the G250 antigen in the biliary tract. This finding points to the promise of genetically retargeted T cells and provides a reminder that expression of the targeted antigen on tissues other than the tumor can result in significant toxicity.

Infusions of genetically modified T cells have also been tested in patients with HIV infection. CD4ζ is a genetically engineered, MHC-unrestricted chimeric receptor composed of the γ subunit of the CD3 T-cell receptor, the cytoplasmic domain involved in signal transduction, fused to the transmembrane and extracellular domains of human CD4, which targets HIV env expressed on the surface of infected cells. Upon binding to HIV envelope, CD8 T cells engineered to express the CD4ζ fusion protein proliferate and initiate effector functions such as cytokine secretion and HIV-specific cytolytic activity. In phase I and II trials, CD4ζ-modified T cells were detected in the peripheral blood of all patients following infusion, and sustained mean levels of 1–3% of T cells were detected for about 1 year after infusion. In a randomized phase II trial, adoptive transfer resulted in modest antiviral effects.[61]

GvHD is associated with a potent antitumor effect. The ability to terminate GvHD at will without the use of pharmacologic immunosuppressants following allogeneic T-cell infusions would be useful. Genetically modified T cells that have an inducible 'suicide switch' have been tested in patients after allogeneic hematopoietic stem-cell transplantation. Using this strategy, Bonini and colleagues found that some cases of severe GvHD could be aborted after infusions of allogeneic T cells that had been modified to incorporate this novel conditional suicide switch.[62] Together these clinical results indicate that genetically modified T cells have promise in early-stage clinical trials in patients with cancer and HIV infection. The principal limitation of most strategies that use genetically modified T cells is that the cell transduction process can render the cells immunogenic, resulting in host-mediated elimination of the adoptively transferred cells.

PASSIVE IMMUNOTHERAPY WITH BONE MARROW TRANSPLANTATION

Harnessing the immune system for induction of antitumor responses has been a long-standing dream and goal of generations of immunologists. In fact the successful introduction of monoclonal antibody therapy for the treatment of lymphomas, as demonstrated by anti-CD20 therapy, has proven that immunotherapy of tumors has become a reality. However, in contrast to monoclonal antibody-mediated immunotherapy, induction of autochthonous T-cell-mediated tumor immunity has been less successful and remains a formidable challenge similar to the situation in infectious diseases where induction of neutralizing humoral immunity has been more successful when compared to induction of T-cell immunity. The major reasons for this failure to induce or maintain T-cell-dependent antitumor responses involve different mechanisms of immune escape, including but not limited to downregulation of MHC molecules, direct tolerization of effector cells or induction of Tregs. Conversely, the concept of immunoediting has been suggested to contribute to the selection of more aggressive, immune-resistant tumor variants.

The power of cellular immunotherapy for the treatment of malignancies has been demonstrated clinically by the success of allogeneic hematopoietic stem-cell transplantation and its associated graft-versus-leukemia (GvL) effects (Chapter 82).[1,63] In particular this has been proven by the success of the administration of donor lymphocyte infusions (DLI) for the

25. Muranski P, Boni A, Wrzesinski C, et al. Increased intensity lymphodepletion and adoptive immunotherapy – how far can we go? Nat Clin Pract Oncol 2006; 3: 668–681.

26. Grover A, Kim GJ, Lizee G, et al. Intralymphatic dendritic cell vaccination induces tumor antigen-specific, skin-homing T lymphocytes. Clin Cancer Res 2006; 12: 5801–5808.

27. Palucka AK, Ueno H, Connolly J, et al. Dendritic cells loaded with killed allogeneic melanoma cells can induce objective clinical responses and MART-1 specific CD8+ T-cell immunity. J Immunother 2006; 29: 545–557.

28. Revesz L, Klein G. Quantitative studies on the multiplication of neoplastic cells in vivo. II. Growth curves of three ascites lymphomas. J Natl Cancer Inst 1954; 15: 253–273.

29. Revesz L. Effect of lethally damaged tumor cells upon the development of admixed viable cells. J Natl Cancer Inst 1958; 20: 1157–1186.

30. Martinon F, Tschopp J. Inflammatory caspases and inflammasomes: master switches of inflammation. Cell Death Differ 2007; 14: 10–22.

31. Meylan E, Tschopp J, Karin M. Intracellular pattern recognition receptors in the host response. Nature 2006; 442: 39–44.

32. Chang MH, Chen TH, Hsu HM, et al. Prevention of hepatocellular carcinoma by universal vaccination against hepatitis B virus: the effect and problems. Clin Cancer Res 2005; 11: 7953–7957.

33. Harper DM, Franco EL, Wheeler CM, et al. Sustained efficacy up to 4.5 years of a bivalent L1 virus-like particle vaccine against human papillomavirus types 16 and 18: follow-up from a randomized control trial. Lancet 2006; 367: 1247–1255.

34. Mitola S, Belleri M, Urbinati C, et al. Cutting edge: extracellular high mobility group box-1 protein is a proangiogenic cytokine. J Immunol 2006; 176: 12–15.

35. Dong XD, Ito N, Lotze MT, et al. High mobility group box 1 (HMGB1) release from tumor cells following treatment: implications for development of targeted chemo-immunotherapy. J Immunother 2007; 30:596–606.

36. Lotti R, Lee JJ, Lotze MT. Eosinophilic granulocytes and damage associated molecular pattern molecules (DAMPs). J Immunother 2006; 2007; 30:16–28.

37. Samoszuk M. Eosinophils and human cancer. Histol Histopathol 1997; 12: 807–812.

38. Simon HU, Plotz S, Simon D, et al. Interleukin-2 primes eosinophil degranulation in hypereosinophilia and Wells' syndrome. Eur J Immunol 2003; 33: 834–839.

39. Sosman JA, Bartemes K, Offord KP, et al. Evidence for eosinophil activation in cancer patients receiving recombinant interleukin-4: effects of interleukin-4 alone and following interleukin-2 administration. Clin Cancer Res 1995; 1: 805–812.

40. Mattes J, Hulett M, Xie W, et al. Immunotherapy of cytotoxic T cell-resistant tumors by T helper 2 cells: an eotaxin and STAT6-dependent process. J Exp Med 2003; 197: 387–393.

41. Lu LF, Lind EF, Gondek DC, et al. Mast cells are essential intermediaries in regulatory T-cell tolerance. Nature 2006; 442: 997–1002.

42. Weissman L. Stem cell research: paths to cancer therapies and regenerative medicine. JAMA 2005; 294: 1359–1366.

43. Chang CC, Ferrone S. Immune selective pressure and HLA class I antigen defects in malignant lesions. Cancer Immunol Immunother 2007; 56: 227–236.

44. Kortlever RM, Bernards R. Senescence, wound healing and cancer: the PAI-1 connection. Cell Cycle 2006; 5: 2697–2703.

45. Gattinoni L, Powell DJ Jr, Rosenberg SA, et al. Adoptive immunotherapy for cancer: building on success. Nat Rev Immunol 2006; 6: 383–393.

45a. Rosenberg SA, Yang JC, Restifo NP. Cancer immunotherapy: moving beyond current vaccines. Nature Medicine 2004; 10: 909–915.

45b. Billingham RE, Brent L, Medawar PB. Quantitative studies on tissue transplantation immunity. II. The origin, strength and duration of actively and adoptively acquired immunity. Proc R Soc Lond Biol Sci 1954; 143: 58–80.

46. Riddell SR, Watanabe KS, Goodrich JM, et al. Restoration of viral immunity in immunodeficient humans by the adoptive transfer of T cell clones. Science 1992; 257: 238–241.

47. Milone MC, June CH. Adoptive immunotherapy: new ways to skin the cat?. Clin Immunol 2005; 117: 101–103.

48. Dummer W, Niethanmer AG, Baccala R, et al. T cell homeostatic proliferation elicits effective antitumor autoimmunity. J Clin Invest 2002; 110: 185–192.

49. Zhou J, Shen X, Huang J, et al. Telomere length of transferred lymphocytes correlates with in vivo persistence and tumor regression in melanoma patients receiving cell transfer therapy. J Immunol 2005; 175: 7046–7052.

50. Dudley ME, Wunderlich JR, Robbins PF, et al. Cancer regression and autoimmunity in patients after clonal repopulation with antitumor lymphocytes. Science 2002; 298: 850–854.

51. Rapoport AP, Stadtmauer EA, Aqui N, et al. Restoration of immunity in lymphopenic individuals with cancer by vaccination and adoptive T-cell transfer. Nat Med 2005; 11: 1230–1237.

52. Heslop HE, Ng CY, Li C, et al. Long-term restoration of immunity of Epstein–Barr virus infection by adoptive transfer of gene-modified virus-specific T lymphocytes. Nature Med 1996; 2: 551–5.

53. Yee C, Thompson JA, Byrd D, et al. Adoptive T cell therapy using antigen-specific CD8+ T cell clones for the treatment of patients with metastatic melanoma: in vivo persistence, migration, and antitumor effect of transferred T cells. Proc Natl Acad Sci USA 2002; 99: 16168–16173.

54. Gambineri E, Torgerson TR, Ochs HD. Immune dysregulation, polyendocrinopathy, enteropathy, and X-linked inheritance (IPEX), a syndrome of systemic autoimmunity caused by mutations of FOXP3, a critical regulator of T-cell homeostasis. Curr Opin Rheumatol 2003; 15: 430–435.

55. June CH, Blazar BR. Clinical application of expanded CD4+25+ cells. Semin Immunol 2006; 18: 77–88.

56. Ruggeri L, Capanni M, Urbani E, et al. Effectiveness of donor natural killer cell alloreactivity in mismatched hematopoietic transplants. Science 2002; 295: 2097–2100.

57. Igarashi T, Wynberg J, Srinivasan R, et al. Enhanced cytotoxicity of allogeneic NK cells with killer immunoglobulin-like receptor ligand incompatibility against melanoma and renal cell carcinoma cells. Blood 2004; 104: 170–177.

58. Sadelain M, Riviere I, Brentjens R. Targeting tumours with genetically enhanced T lymphocytes. Nat Rev Cancer 2003; 3: 35–45.

59. Levine BL, Humeau LM, Boyer J, et al. Gene transfer in humans using a conditionally replicating lentiviral vector. Proc Natl Acad Sci USA 2006; 103: 17372–17377.

60. Lamers CH, Sleijfer S, Vulto AG, et al. Treatment of metastatic renal cell carcinoma with autologous T-lymphocytes genetically retargeted against carbonic anhydrase IX: first clinical experience. J Clin Oncol 2006; 24: e20–e22.

61. Deeks SG, Wagner B, Anton PA, et al. A phase II randomized study of HIV-specific T-cell gene therapy in subjects with undetectable plasma viremia on combination anti-retroviral therapy. Mol Ther 2002; 5: 788–797.

62. Bonini C, Ferrari G, Verzeletti S, et al. HSV-TK gene transfer into donor lymphocytes for control of allogeneic graft-versus-leukemia. Science 1997; 276: 1719–1724.

63. Horowitz MM, Gale RP, Sondel PM, et al. Graft-versus-leukemia reactions after bone marrow transplantation. Blood 1990; 75: 555–562.

64. Suchin EJ, Langmuir PB, Palmer E, et al. Quantifying the frequency of alloreactive T cells in vivo: new answers to an old question. J Immunol 2001; 166: 973–981.

65. Aversa F, Tabilio A, Terenzi A, et al. Successful engraftment of T-cell-depleted haploidentical "three-loci" incompatible transplants in leukemia patients by addition of recombinant human granulocyte colony-stimulating factor-mobilized peripheral blood progenitor cells to bone marrow inoculum. Blood 1994; 84: 3948–3955.

66. Aversa F, Tabilio A, Velardi A, et al. Treatment of high risk leukemia with T cell depleted stem cells in patients from related donors with one fully matched haplotype. N Engl J Med 1998; 339: 1186–1193.

67. Shlomchik WD. Antigen presentation in graft-vs-host disease. Exp Hematol 2003; 31: 1187–1197.

68. Reddy P, Maeda Y, Liu C, Krijanovski OI, et al. A crucial role for antigen-presenting cells and alloantigen expression in graft-versus-leukemia responses. Nat Med 2005; 11: 1244–1249.

69. Ferrara JL, Reddy P. Pathophysiology of graft-versus-host disease. Semin Hematol 2006; 43: 3–10.

70. Lowsky R, Takahashi T, Liu YP, et al. Protective conditioning for acute graft-versus-host disease. N Engl J Med 2005; 353: 1321–1331.

71. Wysocki CA, Panoskaltsis-Mortari A, Blazar BR, et al. Leukocyte migration and graft-versus-host disease. Blood 2005; 105: 4191–4199.

72. Kim YM, Sachs T, Asavaroengchai W, et al. Graft-versus-host disease can be separated from graft-versus-lymphoma effects by control of lymphocyte trafficking with FTY720. J Clin Invest 2003; 111: 659–669.

73. Edinger M, Hoffmann P, Ermann J, et al. CD4+CD25+ regulatory T cells preserve graft-versus-tumor activity while inhibiting graft-versus-host disease after bone marrow transplantation. Nat Med 2003; 9: 1144–1150.

74. Hoffmann P, Eder R, Kunz-Schughart LA, et al. Large-scale in vitro expansion of polyclonal human CD4(+)CD25high regulatory T cells. Blood 2004; 104: 895–903.

75. Vodanovic-Jankovic S, Hari P, Jacobs P, et al. NF-kappaB as a target for the prevention of graft-versus-host disease: comparative efficacy of bortezomib and PS-1145. Blood 2006; 107: 827–834.

76. Leng C, Gries M, Ziegler J, et al. Reduction of graft-versus-host disease by histone deacetylase inhibitor suberonylanilide hydroxamic acid is associated with modulation of inflammatory cytokine milieu and involves inhibition of STAT1. Exp Hematol 2006; 34: 776–787.

77. Sun K, Wilkins DE, Anver MR, et al. Differential effects of proteasome inhibition by bortezomib on murine acute graft versus-host disease (GVHD): delayed administration of bortezomib results in increased GVHD-dependent gastrointestinal toxicity. Blood 2005; 106: 3293–3299.

TRANSPLANTATION

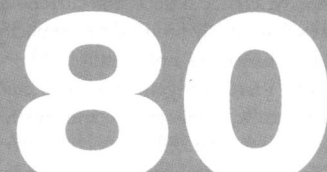
Concepts and challenges in transplantation: rejection, immunosuppression and tolerance

Barry D. Kahan

80

Although transplantation as a cure for disease is richly described in mythic literature, its clinical practice spans only six decades. The legendary exchange of hearts by the Chinese practitioner Pien Ch'iao restored the proper balance of Yin and Yang elements in each recipient; the xenotransplantation of the elephant's head onto the boy, creating the god Ganesha, corrected the mistaken decapitation by the Hindu deity Shiva; and the limb transplant from the cadaveric Ethiopian gladiator to their devout sacristan by the Saints Cosmas and Damien replaced a gangrenous appendage.[1] The powerful symbolism of the chimeric patient in whom diseased organs are replaced by normal ones represents not only the pantheistic ideal of renewal and 'rebirth' of the recipient, but also the immortality of at least remnants of a frequently unexpectedly and catastrophically terminated donor life.

The barrier to transplant success remained a mystery until this century, when the local resistance 'athrepsia' theory of Ehrlich, which had been reinforced by Loeb's concept of incompatible protein templates, was superseded by the observations of Jensen, Schoene, Holman, and, most elegantly, by Medawar, that rejection was due to acquired immunity:[1] foreign grafts confer a state of donor-specific systemic resistance transferable by lymphocytes and abrogated by neonatal exposure. Our current failures to ensure graft success and to achieve full host rehabilitation are due both to gaps in our knowledge of the immunological events, and to a lack of understanding of the pathophysiology of transplanted organs.

■ ALLOGRAFT REJECTION ■

IMMUNE MECHANISMS

Antigenic signals

The transplant presents a mosaic of antigens foreign to the host. Incompatibility for major blood group ABH antigens triggers rapid rejection, due in most cases to the onslaught of natural antibodies. However, if it survives the first month the ABH-incompatible allograft can enjoy survival similar to that of an ABH-compatible transplant. The incompatibility is not absolute: blood group O recipients display far less violent reactions toward grafts from donors of the ABO-A2 than from the -A1 erythrocyte subgroup.

A second system determining transplant outcome is encoded by the 'classic loci' within the major histocompatibility complex (MHC), which encode surface glycoprotein products (Chapter 5). The human class I MHC genes HLA-A and -B heavy chains complexed with β_2-microglobulin are assembled with endogenously generated peptide fragments into heterotrimers. Expression on donor-type antigen-presenting cells (APCs) in the graft interstitium – dendritic cells – powerfully triggers CD8 T cells. In contrast, each class II MHC gene (HLA-DP, -DQ, -DR) encodes two polypeptide chains that, upon cytoplasmic assembly, bind exogenous, endocytosed and endosomally processed antigenic peptides for indirect presentation primarily to CD4 T cells (Chapters 6, 7). Determination of the patient's phenotype for the three MHC loci of greatest import to transplant outcomes – HLA-A, -B, and –DR – has evolved from the use of serologic microcytotoxicity reactions to DNA amplification reactions using selective primers. A six-antigen ('full') match ensures that most living related transplant recipients of a postoperative course are free of serious rejection episodes, provided the patient has not been pre-sensitized. Evidence of pre-sensitization would be provided by the presence of cytotoxic antibodies toward donor-type non-MHC antigens encoded by endothelial, tissue or Lewis erythrocyte markers. The undeniable benefit of HLA identity for living related donor transplants may be explained by the fact that not only the HLA-A, -B, and -DR, but also other, as yet incompletely defined, classic and nonclassic MHC genes encoded on the short arm of human chromosome 6 are shared between donor and recipient. However, even these patients require immunosuppression to counter the modest immunogenicity of non-MHC – so-called 'minor'–histocompatibility loci which, in aggregate, can trigger prompt allograft rejection. Only a graft from an identical twin donor fails to evoke alloimmunity, and thus does not require immunosuppression (unless the recipient's original disease was autoimmune in nature).

In contrast, the impact of HLA matching on the survival of cadaveric donor grafts is controversial. Although it is generally believed that there is a hierarchical relation between the number of HLA matches and the rate of graft survival, data from the large US Renal Data System

80 | **TRANSPLANTATION**

Table 80.1 Rejection characteristics of renal allografts

Type	Timing	Symptoms	Time frame of onset	Vector	Histopathology	Treatment	Success Rate of R_x
Hyperacute	<24 h	Fever, anuria	Hours	C-Ab	Polymorph deposition and thrombosis	None	0%
Accelerated	3–5 days	Fever, graft swelling, oliguria, tenderness	1 day	non C-Ab	Vascular disruption with hemorrhage	Anti-lymphocyte reagents	60%
Acute	6–90 days	Decreased urine output, salt retention, graft swelling/tenderness, infrequently fever	Days to weeks	T cells	'Tubulitis'	Steroids	80%
						Anti-lymphocyte reagents	90%
				Ab	Endovasculitis	Anti-lymphocyte reagents	60%
Chronic	>60 days	Peripheral edema, hypertension, proteinuria, occasional hematuria	Months to years	Ab	Vascular onion-skinning	None	0%

prognosticate the outcome of rejection episodes based on the number of peripheral blood – or even graft-infiltrating – CD8 cells.

B LYMPHOCYTES

Class I antigen-bearing donor cells may serve as APCs to trigger antibody synthesis. Host antidonor pre-sensitization, as a result of prior blood transfusions, pregnancy, or exposure to cross-reactive infectious agents, may presage a poor prognosis. Although donor-directed IgM antibodies produce target cell lysis *in vitro*, they rarely cause graft loss. In contrast, the presence in recipient serum of complement-fixing host antidonor IgG antibodies, particularly directed toward class I antigens – a 'positive cross-match' – represents an absolute contraindication to renal transplantation, owing to its propensity to produce hyperacute rejection. However, liver and heart grafts may be less vulnerable to this outcome.

Clinical rejection responses

The four major forms of allograft rejection are discerned according to time of onset, pathophysiology, and vulnerability to therapeutic reversal[4] (Table 80.1). Renal allograft rejection is described here as the paradigm, as similar types of immune responses can occur in all organ transplants.

Hyperacute rejection occurs within the first 48 hours of transplantation. The binding of cytotoxic antibodies to vascular endothelial cells produces thrombosis following local complement activation and aggregation of FcR-positive leukocytes (PMN) and platelets onto the antibody-coated endothelial cells. These events are frequently heralded by fever as well as by severe allograft dysfunction and markedly reduced graft perfusion. Because this response is not amenable to treatment, the condition demands emergency removal of the transplant. Histopathologic examination showing polymorphonuclear leukocyte infiltration, particularly in the glomeruli of renal allografts, confirms an immunologic vector, as opposed to a 'bland' thrombosis resulting from a technical misadventure during the vascular anastomoses.

Accelerated rejection occurs between 3 and 5 days postoperatively and results from deposition of noncomplement-fixing antibodies that act via FcR-positive K cells and monocytes to produce vascular disruption and interstitial hemorrhage. These events tend to evolve rapidly (within a day), resulting in a clinical picture of fever, graft swelling and tenderness, as well as swiftly deteriorating function. Because of the involvement of a cellular vector and the rapid pace of events, anti-lymphocyte antibodies represent the therapeutic cornerstone. In cases where a positive *post*-transplant cross-match is observed, plasmapheresis combined with administration of an anti-CD20 monoclonal antibody (mAb; rituximab) is useful. Frequently, the condition is only partially reversed, with recurrences of increasing severity, until transplant removal becomes the most appropriate option. Hyperacute and accelerated rejections are anamnestic responses, wherein the antibody vector was either in the circulation at the time of, or its production was immediately triggered after, transplantation. In contrast, acute and chronic rejections result from primary immune responses.

Acute rejection generally occurs between 6 and 90 days post transplant, but may begin later in the transplant course, particularly when triggered by patient or physician noncompliance with the immunosuppressive regimen. Mild and moderate acute rejection episodes produce clinical syndromes of progressive graft dysfunction, swelling and tenderness, infrequently accompanied by fever. The characteristic histopathologic appearance includes a cellular infiltrate containing CD8 cytolytic T cells, and a polymorphic inflammatory response elicited by the release of lymphokines by CD4 T cells. Although perivenous lymphocyte collections characteristic of delayed-type hypersensitivity reactions are frequently present, the typical histopathologic lesion results from direct

KEY CONCEPTS

REJECTION VECTOR/TREATMENT/PROGNOSIS (% 5-YEAR GRAFT SURVIVAL)

Anamnestic responses
>> Hyperacute/none/irreversible (0%)
>> Accelerated/intense anti-lymphocyte antibody ± plasmapheresis/poor (40%)

Primary immune responses
>> Acute cellular/steroids ± anti-lymphocyte antibody/fair (60%)
>> Chronic/none/irreversible (50%)

THERAPEUTIC PRINCIPLES

LIMITATIONS OF IMMUNOSUPPRESSIVE THERAPY

>> Paresis of nonspecific host resistance
>> Excessive T-cell depression
>> Collateral toxicities

lymphocyte contact with parenchymal elements, often accompanied by interstitial edema. For example, in the kidney, lymphocyte penetration of peritubular basement membranes produces 'tubulitis,' a lesion that is almost always reversed by administration of large doses of steroids. Severe bouts of acute rejection frequently include a component that produces endovasculitis, with the infiltration of lymphocytes into the vessel wall below swollen, ischemic endothelial cells. Although administration of anti-lymphocyte antibodies may reverse steroid-refractory cell-mediated lesions, some cases show only transient benefit, followed by recurrent acute episodes and evolution to chronic rejection.

Chronic rejection usually appears at least 60 days post transplant. This insidious condition, which is generally believed to be antibody mediated, includes histopathologic features of smooth muscle cell invasion and proliferation in the intima, disruption of the internal elastic lamina, and vascular immuno-obliteration. Interstitial cicatricial changes are also observed, either associated with or independent of the vascular events. Although the molecular mechanisms by which antibodies trigger these changes are uncertain, cytokines, eicosanoids, and growth factors have been documented to participate in the process. In renal transplantation the clinical picture includes vasculopathic hypertension and glomerulopathy with accelerating proteinuria, followed by microscopic and then gross hematuria. The presence of complement component C4d in peritubular capillaries of the kidney seems to represent a footprint of the humoral immune response. When this histopathologic finding is accompanied by the presence of donor-specific antibody in the serum, a combination of plasmapheresis and anti-CD20 mAb therapy may forestall the inevitable loss of the graft. Liver allografts undergo the 'vanishing bile duct' syndrome; heart transplants, a pernicious form of coronary artery disease; and lung transplants, bronchiolitis obliterans. The chronic rejection lesion shows a treatment-resistant, indolent but progressive course of stepwise deterioration of allograft function over a period of months to years.

IMMUNOSUPPRESSION

Immunosuppressive strategies have evolved slowly during the past century, from the cytotoxic agents benzene and toluene to the anti-proliferative modalities of radiation or anti-metabolites, to the present era of disrupting the production, reception and transduction of cytokine

signals. However, despite this progress, the pharmacologic and antibody reagents currently available are merely nonspecific bludgeons that can engender serious side effects. First, most agents display at least some degree of inhibition of nonspecific host resistance by macrophages, monocytes and polymorphonuclear leukocytes. Second, excessive immunodepression of T and B cells may lead to the emergence of occult viral infections in, or neoplastic diseases of, lymphoid cells. Third, adverse effects on nonimmune organs not infrequently result from the high drug doses that must be administered to achieve adequate immunosuppression. The anti-proliferative and steroid combination used in the original pharmacologic strategies exemplified the first problem; the mAb OKT3, the second problem; and cyclosporine (CsA), tacrolimus (TRL), and sirolimus (SRL), the third. Indeed, in some cases the 'diseases' produced by immunosuppression are of greater consequence than that of allograft rejection: to wit, post-transplant diabetes mellitus engendered by steroids or by TRL. Avoidance of adverse outcomes is currently difficult owing to the lack of assays to quantify the effects of individual immunosuppressive agents; of intermediate immunologic endpoints for early rejection diagnosis prior to tissue damage, and of monitoring reversal to avoid excessive treatment; as well as quantitative, scientifically based individualized algorithms to tailor induction, maintenance and anti-rejection therapies to patient needs. Thus, current clinical practice uses an array of nonspecific therapies of low immunosuppressive or low therapeutic index, rather than strategies that induce donor-specific unresponsiveness.

AGENTS THAT INTERFERE WITH ALLORECOGNITION

Interruption of ischemia/adhesion/migration

Although no agents are currently approved to interdict the initial events in the injury response – leukocyte adhesion and emigration into the graft interstitium – this area represents a major focus for new therapeutic strategies. In experimental animal models some modalities seem to dampen these injuries: endothelin-A receptor antagonists; or molecular antagonists or mAbs blocking selectins, LFA-1, or ICAM-1. However, clinical trials using murine mAb directed against ICAM-1 or LFA-1 failed to show beneficial effects in human renal transplantation. An ongoing trial of a recombinant p-selectin glycoprotein ligand-immunoglobulin conjugate proffers an exciting approach to the problem.[5] Many of these agents may be delivered initially *ex vivo* to saturate the graft, and then administered continuously in the recipient (Fig. 80.3A).

One new class of agent is the synthetic compounds that bind to type 1 sphingosine-1-phosphate receptors. Patients treated with the archetypal sphingosine analog FTY720 displayed depletion from the

THERAPEUTIC PRINCIPLES

THE CYTOKINE PARADIGM OF MODERN IMMUNOSUPPRESSIVE THERAPY

>> Calcineurin antagonists
    Cyclosporine
    Tacrolimus

>> Anti-IL-2 monoclonal antibodies
    Basiliximab (chimeric)
    Daclizumab (humanized)

>> Cytokine signal transduction inhibitors
    Sirolimus
    SDZ-RAD

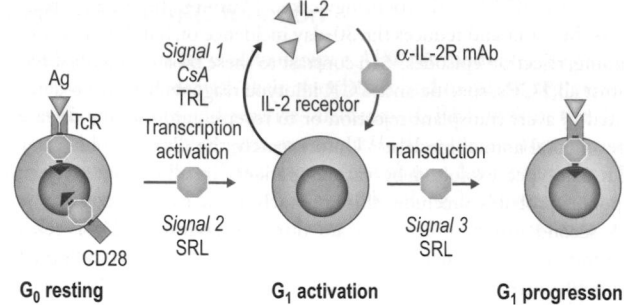

Fig. 80.4 Cytokine paradigm. Complementary sites of action of immunosuppressive drugs during lymphocyte activation. Cyclosporine (CsA) and tacrolimus (TRL) inhibit transcription of T-cell growth-promoting genes (e.g., IL-2). Anti-IL-2 mAbs block binding of IL-2 to its receptor. SRL blocks growth-factor-initiated signal transduction.

Nutley, NJ) to a regimen of CsA, Aza and steroids significantly reduced the incidence of biopsy-proven acute rejection within the first 6 months to 28%, compared to 43% for the placebo-treated group in the USA trial (with Aza-Pred) and with 47% in the European cohort (without Aza; $P = 0.03$).[23] However, at 12 months patients treated with CsA-Aza-Pred failed to display a benefit of adjunctive daclizumab treatment on either rejection episodes or renal function (Daclizumab Product Insert). The immunosuppressive activity of both reagents is limited by two shortcomings. First, the antibodies do not compete effectively with the IL-2 ligand for binding to the IL-2R. Thus, they must be used in circumstances where IL-2 production is low and cannot reverse acute rejection episodes. Second, the specificity of the antibodies for CD25 (IL-2Rα), despite ensuring their reactivity with only activated T cells, does not prevent immune activation generated via other cytokines, such as IL-7 and IL-15, which do not share the α chain and which can be independently recruited to mediate allorejection in IL-2 knockout animals.

Agents disrupting cytokine-stimulated G$_1$ activation

Two agents act on the calcium-independent cytokine transduction events during the G$_1$ phase. Sirolimus (SRL; rapamycin; Rapamune; Wyeth-Ayerst, Princeton, NJ; molecular weight 95 kDa),[25] a macrocyclic lactone produced by an actinomycete, forms complexes with the immunophilin FKBP12, thereby inhibiting a multifunctional kinase – mammalian target of rapamycin (mTOR). This inhibition disables transduction of growth and of cytokine signals in the G$_1$ phase (Fig. 80.3G), both at the relatively early stage of activation of p70^{S6} kinase, and later at the generation of the elongation factor for ribosomal protein synthesis, as well as at steps necessary for cyclin activation. SRL thus inhibits the transduction of a variety of cytokine signals that may promote the vasculo-occlusive phenomena of chronic rejection, namely, the hematologic–vascular stem cell growth factor, vascular endothelial growth factor, and fibroblast derived growth factor, in addition to those of the IL-2 family. However, the broad tissue distribution of mTOR and its participation in a variety of signal transduction processes may explain the dyslipidemic, myelosuppressive and catabolic effects of SRL.

SRL acts in synergistic fashion with CsA, owing to its effects on both G$_1$ progression, and, as recently discovered, the co-stimulatory Signal 2 cascade, namely, blockade of the kinase necessary for generation of c-Rel transcription factors. Thus, we formulated the matrix of CsA, anti-IL-2R mAbs and SRL as the three components of the cytokine paradigm (Fig. 80.4).

Clinical trials have documented the immunosuppressive activity of SRL.[26] The pivotal phase III US and global trials showed that the rates of efficacy failure (a composite of the occurrences of acute rejection episodes, graft loss and/or death) were significantly reduced ($P<0.0001$) among patients treated with either SRL 2 mg/day ($n=511$), or SRL 5 mg/day ($n=493$), versus either placebo ($n=130$), or azathioprine (Aza; $n=161$). Furthermore, fewer patients treated with SRL displayed acute rejection episodes that were graded as moderate or severe by the Banff system, or required antibody therapy for rejection reversal. Because of the 90–96% overall patient and graft survival rates, it was not possible to discern a difference in these outcomes among the groups. As is the case for other immunosuppressive agents, higher (5 mg/day) doses of SRL were necessary to show a therapeutic effect in African-American patients.[27] The trials confirmed preclinical observations that SRL and CsA are metabolized by the same cytochrome P450 isoforms and extruded from cells via p-glycoprotein, leading to intense pharmacokinetic interactions that exacerbate each other's toxicities. The major clinical concern is the potentiation of calcineurin antagonist-induced nephrotoxicity, which is being addressed by marked reductions in the exposure to CsA by as much as 80% to minimize synergistic pharmacodynamic interactions leading to adverse reactions.

Everolimus (EVL, Certican, Novartis, Basel, Switerland), a 25-hydroxy-ethyl derivative of SRL, is slightly more hydrophilic than the parent compound and displays a more rapid clearance rate. Like SRL, the analog drug is rapidly absorbed, reaching a maximum concentration (C$_{max}$) within 2 hours, but, in contrast, EVL displays a half-life of 16–19 hours, which is significantly shorter than that of SRL (30 hours) and thus necessitates twice-daily dosing. EVL concentrations reach steady state by 4 days, in contrast to 7 days for SRL. The pharmacokinetic parameters of both drugs show dose proportionality, with a good correlation between trough and area-under-the-curve (AUC) concentrations. Future studies must gauge whether the EVL analog confers any benefits beyond those achieved with SRL. In a phase I study in stable renal transplant patients[28]

EVL displayed a similar spectrum of side effects to that observed with SRL, and in a preliminary phase II dose-finding trial, the 2 mg/day EVL cohort showed a similar incidence of acute rejection episodes to the SRL 2 mg/day group.[29] However, a phase III multicenter randomized blinded clinical trial showed no benefit of EVL compared to MMF.[30] Another ongoing phase III trial is assessing the role of CsA dose minimization to increase the benefits of EVL therapy.

Recently, attention has focused on disrupting membrane-proximal signal transduction events that are relatively specific for the IL-2 family of lymphokine receptors – IL-2, -4, -7, -9, -13, and -15. A nonspecific inhibitor of Lck and Fyn tyrosine kinases of the Src family, the isoxazol derivative leflunamide (Hoechst, Basle, SZ), has been shown to prolong rodent as well as canine renal allograft survival times.[31] However, its toxic effects in animal models have necessitated caution in de novo administration to human transplant recipients. A recently completed trial has confirmed this concern, and so the drug is unlikely to be utilized in future regimens. An alternate target is Janus kinase 3 (Jak3), an enzyme that transduces membrane receptor IL-2R γ-chain activation to signal transduction and transcription (STAT) factors. An ATP analog with modest selectivity for Jak3 versus Jak2 evoked prolonged survival of renal allografts in subhuman primates and is currently in clinical trials.[32]

Another target is the protein translation process. The selective class of agents – DNA oligonucleotides (oligos) – bind homologous regions of mRNA, thereby disrupting ribosomal synthesis of a specific protein. Oligos that selectively disrupt TNF-α-driven upregulation of ICAM-1 synthesis have been shown to inhibit in vitro proliferation, block expression of this tethering molecule upon perfusion ex vivo, and prolong the survival of vascularized heterotopic cardiac or renal allografts in experimental animals. Although the stability of oligos has been enhanced by substitution of sulfuryl for phosphoryl groups, the clinical application of these agents has been limited by their high negative charge, leading to poor cytoplasmic penetration,[33] an obstacle that is being addressed by methoxyethoxy substitutions on the terminal nucleotides.

De novo nucleoside synthesis inhibitors

The slightly reduced activity of purine salvage enzymes in lymphocytes compared to other rapidly dividing cell types suggests that these immune elements are more dependent on *de novo* nucleoside synthesis of DNA and RNA building blocks (Fig. 80.3H). However, the inhibition of *de novo* nucleoside synthesis produces a low immunosuppressive index, because this effect also inhibits a variety of cell types. Azathioprine (Aza; Burroughs-Wellcome, Research Triangle, NC), mizorbine (MZB; Bredinin, Toyo Jozo, Tokyo, JP) and mycophenolic acid (MPA) all inhibit generation of guanosine monophosphate (GMP), thus mimicking the Lesch–Nyhan syndrome. Aza, a competitive inhibitor of a variety of synthetic pathways, including inosine monophosphate dehydrogenase (IMPDH), the target of MPA and MZB, was developed following the pioneering animal work of Schwartz and Dameshek[34] using 6-mercaptopurine, as well as the clinical trials of its imidazole analog by Calne et al.[35] After 20 years of clinical use Aza was displaced by CsA as the cornerstone of pharmacologic therapy; however, some physicians combine Aza with CsA to enhance the immunosuppressive effect. Although MZB is widely used in Japan, the morpholinylethyl analog of MPA, mycophenolate mofetil (MMF; Roche, Basle, Switzerland) is used throughout the rest of the world, where it is approved for prophylaxis of acute rejection episodes in combination with CsA. Although nonnephrotoxic, MMF is associated with diarrhea and a spectrum of other gastrointestinal complaints, as well as neutropenia, an increased incidence of cytomegalovirus (CMV) and BK virus infections, and possibly posttransplant lymphoproliferative disease.

Randomized, double-blind, multicenter clinical trials conducted in the USA, Canada, Europe and Australia showed that the addition to CsA and Pred of either 2 g or 3 g daily doses of MMF, compared with Aza or placebo, significantly reduced the incidence and severity of acute renal allograft rejection episodes during the first 6 months.[36] However, the addition of MMF showed less effect on African-American than on Caucasian recipients.[37] Furthermore, nonblinded studies have reported that MMF provides better prophylaxis of acute rejection episodes than does Aza in the settings of liver, simultaneous pancreas–kidney, heart and lung transplantations. However, MMF treatment failed to improve patient or graft survivals at 1 or 3 years following cadaveric kidney transplantation, suggesting that the drug did not impede the occurrence or the progression of chronic rejection, a clinical observation that does *not* support the preliminary findings claiming benefits in animal models.[38]

The frequent adverse reactions displayed by patients toward MMF may be overcome with a new enteric-coated formulation of the sodium salt of mycophenolic acid (MPA; Myfortic, Novartis, Basle, Switzerland), which has less tendency to cause adverse gastrointestinal effects, particularly in subjects intolerant to MMF. A 720 mg dose of MPA resulted in drug exposure bioequivalent to that of 1000 mg of MMF. In clinical trials the efficacy and side-effect profile of MPA was similar to that of MMF.[39]

A second class of nucleoside synthesis inhibitors blocks dihydroorotate dehydrogenase, the third enzyme in the de novo synthesis pathway of pyrimidine. Because of the critical role of UDP sugars in the synthesis of glycoproteins, these agents may possess additional immunosuppressive properties beyond anti-proliferative effects. The original drug of this type was brequinar (BQR; DuPont-Merck, Wilmington, DE); it has been claimed that leflunomide also displays this activity. The occurrence of the principal toxicity of BQR, thrombocytopenia, which correlated with high peak plasma concentrations, proved to be so dose-limiting as to obviate any benefit when added to a CsA/steroid-based immunosuppressive regimen. Owing to their lack of lymphocyte specificity and to their failure to display synergistic interactions that would permit dose reduction of calcineurin antagonists, the nucleoside synthesis inhibitors are unlikely to become permanent members of a T cell-selective immunosuppressive armamentarium.

Lymphocyte depletion agents

Polyclonal anti-lymphocyte xenoantibodies have been the primary reagents to achieve lymphocyte depletion. These agents opsonize lymphocytes, granulocytes and platelets by binding to a variety of human-specific surface markers. The opsonized targets are then eliminated by the reticuloendothelial system. The hallmark of this effect is a decreased number of CD2+ lymphocytes. Therapy is generally targeted to reduce the number of CD2+ lymphocytes to 15–50 mm^3 in peripheral blood. However, dose reductions from the starting amounts of 10–15 mg/kg are frequently necessary because of thrombocytopenia and neutropenia. Whereas equine hosts were initially used to raise antibodies, more potent reagents have been prepared in rabbits (thymoglobulin).

Although the starting doses of the rabbit products are more modest (1.5 mg/kg), their side-effect profile is similar to that of the equine reagents. These reagents have been associated with serum sickness reactions, which have not been consistently anticipated using skin test with dilute antibody. Owing to its lack of initial side effects on administration, a humanized monoclonal anti-CD52 antibody has increasingly been substituted, revealing little evidence of early adverse reactions. However, lymphocyte depletion, particularly prolonged and intense, has been associated with this reagent.

THE CLINICAL IMMUNOSUPPRESSIVE MATRIX

Unfortunately, the current therapeutic matrix is based on empiric rather than scientific foundations. Indeed, despite the widely disparate intrinsic immunogenicity of various organs, the various degrees of donor versus host incompatibility, and the well-recognized inter-individual variations in recipient immunoresponsiveness, transplant centers have tended to employ relatively uniform schedules for initial induction and early maintenance immunosuppressive regimens.

Induction of immunosuppression

The first 2 post-transplant weeks pose the greatest therapeutic challenge, owing to the need to establish adequate immunosuppression promptly and thus avert an acute allograft rejection episode. Although calcineurin inhibitors exert maximal benefit when delivered at the time of antigen presentation, the propensity of the drug to produce renal and/or hepatic dysfunction suggests the need for delayed administration, particularly in cases of poor initial graft function. The brief window provided by antilymphocyte antibodies, either monoclonal (anti-IL-2R, anti-CD25, or anti-CD3) or polyclonal, has now been widened by simultaneous treatment with SRL, or to a lesser extent with MMF, both of which tend to be nonnephrotoxic.

We stratify recipients based on putative immunoreactivity, preferring to use anti-IL-2Rα mAbs for induction therapy in weak responders, as they do not carry the potentially severe penalties of depletion agents, namely, excessive global immunodepression enhancing the propensity to viral infection and/or post-transplant lymphoproliferative disease (PTLD). Whereas induction immunosuppression with daclizumab and MMF was attended by an almost 50% incidence of acute rejection episodes,[40] the combination of basiliximab with SRL has permitted extended periods (mean 33 days) of freedom from concomitant CsA treatment, a particularly useful period for recovery of grafts displaying poor initial function (Fig. 80.5). Only 18% of patients experienced acute rejection episodes, which occurred almost exclusively in re-transplant or African-American patients.[41] For these strong responder patients we prefer thymoglobulin induction.[42] Other workers have advocated induction treatment with the anti-CD52 reagent.[43]

In the future the induction period will be the stage for selective immunoregulation. Indeed, a recent preliminary report claimed that one injection of anti-CD52 mAb provided a 'window of opportunity' for donor–host interactions, facilitating the induction of 'almost tolerance,' namely, a state of graft acceptance despite only low doses of immunosuppressive agents.[44] Unfortunately, a recent report of the 5-year follow-up of this cohort failed to document a benefit over conventionally treated patients.[45]

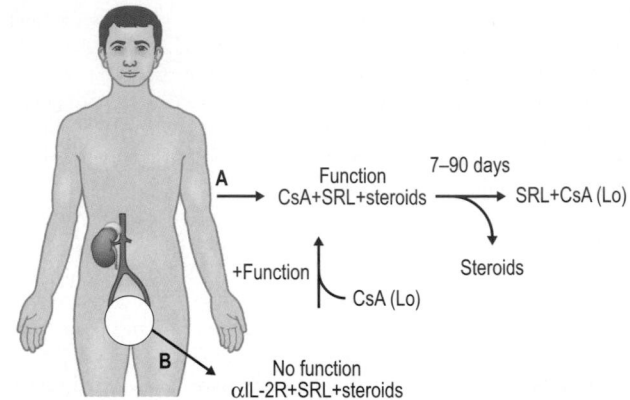

Fig. 80.5 Induction immunosuppression strategies for renal transplantation. (**A**) Regimen for immediate function includes CsA in low doses, SRL, and steroids, with steroid withdrawal. (**B**) Regimen for delayed graft function: αIL-2R mAbs + SRL + steroids, with delayed introduction of low-dose CsA.

Acute rejection prophylaxis

The early immunosuppressive regimen from 2 to 12 weeks seeks to avert allograft rejection episodes, as their mere occurrence, particularly if not totally reversed, presages a greatly increased rate of eventual graft loss. During the past decade, whence CsA and TRL were the therapeutic linchpins, successful rejection prophylaxis at least partly reflected the clinician's expertise to deliver adequate doses of the calcineurin inhibitors tailored to achieve target drug concentrations. For example, the initial 8–10 mg/kg CsA oral dose divided as a twice-daily (b.i.d.) regimen, was adjusted thereafter based on measured trough levels. Although a variety of measurement methods/matrices are available, most workers strive for whole blood CsA concentration targets of 175–350 ng/mL, measured with specific mAbs either in an automated fluorescence device (TDx, Abbott, IL) or in radioimmunoassays with ^{3}H or ^{131}I tracers. The major challenge posed by this dose-finding strategy is the 54-fold inter-individual variation in CsA (and probably TRL) pharmacokinetic parameters and the limited correlation between CsA trough levels and the AUC, a measure of drug exposure during the dosing interval. As pharmacokinetic studies are beyond the expertise of most centers, an abbreviated strategy utilizing a single 2-hour concentration (target ≥1600 ng/mL)

CLINICAL PEARLS

CYCLOSPORINE

>> Mechanism of action to inhibit proinflammatory cytokine m-RNA synthesis.

>> Assure adequate levels of drug: use 2-hour or absorptive phase (0–4)/full area under the curve concentrations.

>> Avoid use in damaged kidney/liver; prefer induction therapy.

>> Synergistic immunosuppressive effect with sirolimus.

CLINICAL PEARLS

SIROLIMUS

>> Mechanism of action to block transduction of virtually every cytokine signal

>> Nonnephrotoxic: use for induction therapy

>> Hyperlipidemia, particularly in diabetics, a major side-effect

>> Pharmacokinetic interaction with CsA (cytochrome P450 3A4; p-glycoprotein)

has been advocated as a method to assure adequate exposure using a CsA-based regimen during the critical drug absorption phase.

Some clinicians seek to compensate for the pharmacokinetic variability by adding 1 g b.i.d. doses of MMF (1.5 g b.i.d. in African-Americans) to augment the immunosuppressive effect of full doses of the calcineurin antagonist. However, this strategy may result in over-immunosuppression. Because SRL acts in synergistic fashion with CsA, combination therapy permits substantial reductions in exposure to each drug, namely, dose ratios of 5–10 mg four times daily (q.i.d.) SRL with 50 mg CsA b.i.d. (C_2 = 200–400 ng/mL). When TRL is used as base therapy, initial oral doses of 10 mg b.i.d. are followed by adjustments targeting an initial trough concentration of 10–15 ng/mL. The addition of SRL to the TRL regimen permits the use of 1–4 mg doses of TRL b.i.d. However, the renal experience has revealed potent pharmacokinetic interactions between SRL and the calcineurin antagonists, which can impair graft function,[27] and the early experience in liver transplant patients suggested an increased incidence of hepatic artery thrombosis. These observations combined with the adverse effects of SRL on wound healing and platelet production have limited the drug's use *de novo*.

The strategy of combining steroids with a calcineurin inhibitor is based on both clinical and experimental data. Steroids inhibit generation of the cytokine IL-1, and of inhibitor κ-kinase (IκK)- α, which would be otherwise activated by co-stimulation, thereby generating NF-κB, a critical transcription factor. Almost all steroid regimens include a massive (250–1000 mg) intraoperative dose of methylprednisolone to dampen graft tissue injury, to drive lymphocytes out of the circulation and away from the allograft, and to blunt T-cell activation. During the immediate postoperative phase, steroid doses are rapidly tapered from 200 mg to 20–30mg/day, followed by a more gradual taper to 15 mg by 30 days, 10 mg

by 60 days, and 5 mg by 90 days. The use of combination therapy with an array of drugs can facilitate early steroid withdrawal or even avoidance, particularly in patients who show weak immunoresponsiveness.

Immunosuppression to reverse acute rejection episodes

The principles of treatment for rejection episodes are relatively uniform across organs and among transplant centers. Whereas some physicians empirically initiate treatment with increased doses of steroids, most centers demand histopathologic confirmation of an immune injury, owing to the substantial penalties of excessive treatment of an adequately immunosuppressed patient. Steroid regimens combining large IV doses of methylprednisolone with an oral prednisone taper are useful for patients with type I pure cellular rejection. The delivery of IV steroids achieves high plasma concentrations and rapid reversal of symptoms, particularly fever, graft swelling and graft tenderness. The acute risks of steroid therapy include exacerbating or inducing diabetes mellitus, producing gastrointestinal irritation/perforation, and triggering psychoses. Administration of more than 7 g of methylprednisolone within the first 30 days post transplant constitutes a risk factor for patient survival, owing to the pronounced depression of nonspecific host resistance. Recycling of oral steroids tends to follow a twofold slower version of the taper used during the first post-transplant week. It is important to reduce the level of steroids to the pre-therapy dose within 1 month, as long-term administration of high doses predisposes to gastrointestinal bleeding, myopathy, osteoporosis, bacterial/fungal infections and hypertension. The advantages of steroid treatment are the low medication costs and the 90% efficacy of rejection reversal. A growing community of transplantologists advocates 'presumptive therapy' based on the presence of subclinical acute rejection processes detected by surveillance renal biopsies. This treatment has been reported to improve graft outcomes.

Acute rejection episodes that include humoral and cellular components are generally resistant to steroid therapy. They may be treated with OKT3. However, administration of doses >75 mg OKT3 has been associated with the development of PTLD among cardiac transplant recipients.[46] Furthermore, as discussed above, the production of neutralizing HAMA occurs in nearly 50% of patients following the initial course of OKT3, which may render a patient resistant to a second course of treatment. Thus, before initiating repeat treatment with OKT3, it is useful to rule out the presence of HAMA. The laboratory at the University of Texas at Houston currently uses OKT3 covalently bound to tosylated dynabeads (M-280) to test for the presence of HAMA. The binding of patient serum to the coated beads is evaluated by flow cytometry after incubation with a fluorescein-conjugated goat anti-human antibody (Jackson ImmunoResearch Laboratories, West Grove, PA). For even more potent treatment, a 10–14-day course of thymoglobulin has been advocated by many physicians.

Refractory rejection therapy

There are considerable differences in the timing at which various transplant centers deem a rejection episode to be actually or potentially steroid resistant. For example, acute rejection episodes that display evidence of vascular injury on histopathologic examination are unlikely to respond to steroids. Some workers define a rejection episode as 'refractory' if it does not reverse after steroid treatment, and suggest a benefit of TRL or

MMF in this setting. A few centers believe that the benefits of steroids, even in the setting of mild rejection episodes, are modest, and favor initial treatment with anti-lymphocyte preparations. After 2–5 days of steroid treatment, most centers assess treatment success based on the remission of symptoms or the onset of improved graft function, or histopathologic evidence of remission. In the clinical setting this assessment may be difficult to make. On the one hand, blood chemistry values reflect tissue damage endpoints, which only slowly reverse even after control of the immune process; on the other hand, delay in the delivery of adequate immunosuppression may condemn the graft to failure or severe permanent impairment.

If the response to steroids is deemed inadequate, the physician proceeds to administer an anti-lymphocyte preparation; the two options are anti-CD3 or polyclonal sera. To minimize OKT3 toxicity, the physician strives to obtain modest and graded cytokine release. Our regimen employs a split-dose approach, delivering 1, 2 and 2 mg IV every 8 hours for the first day, followed by 2.5 mg every 12 hours on the second day, and 5 mg/day thereafter. Each dose is administered with an anti-inflammatory pretreatment cocktail of 100 mg hydrocortisone, 50 mg diphenhydramine and 120 mg acetaminophen. Enumeration of the CD3+ T cells in the peripheral circulation provides an intermediate endpoint for the efficacy of OKT3 therapy: values of <10% are deemed to represent a good therapeutic effect. In addition to the acute complications of cytokine release, excessive OKT3 therapy predisposes to CMV infections and PTLD despite routine antiviral prophylaxis. Unfortunately, there are no secure algorithms to guide the duration of OKT3 treatment, as the therapeutic effect may be delayed by 7–10 days and the long-term toxic effects by 14–30 days. On balance, OKT3 therapy plays an established role to reverse 80% of steroid-resistant acute rejection episodes.

Deterioration in transplant function during OKT3 therapy may be due to the emergence of host HAMA that neutralize the therapeutic agent. However, in most instances OKT3 failures reflect pharmacodynamic resistance caused by the emergence of immune mechanisms not susceptible to the modulation of T-cell function. In these cases some physicians advocate a switch to treatment with polyclonal xenogeneic antibodies in an attempt to obtain lymphocyte depletion; however, because of the limited possibility of success, and the morbidity associated with an additional course of treatment, this strategy is rarely justified. 'Refractory' rejection episodes that fail to respond to a 14- (or preferably 21-) day course of an anti-lymphocyte antibody place the patient at high risk for graft loss. Thus, a rigorous definition of a refractory rejection episode is one that is both steroid and anti-lymphocyte antibody resistant, as documented by the presence of a positive transplant biopsy at the end of these treatments. In this setting addition of SRL to a CsA-Pred[47] regimen may ameliorate renal function. An alternative therapy is high dose anti-CD52 mAb.[48]

Acute humoral rejection

Increasingly, humoral antibody, particularly of the IgG class, is being recognized as an important, pernicious component of acute rejection in humans. Hallmarks of the process include the presence of endothelialitis and of the complement component C4d, which is a footprint in the peritubular capillaries of the kidney transplant. The diagnosis is robustly confirmed by the detection of circulating donor-specific antibody, although the graft may be a site of deposition, depleting peripheral blood of this reactant. Humoral vectors are rarely dampened by steroid therapy and only occasionally abrogated by anti-lymphocyte antibodies. Whereas plasmapheresis can temporarily reduce the antibody content in serum, B cells rebound with the generation of more of this vector. In the past, cyclophosphamide treatment engendered severe myelotoxicity. More recently, intravenous immunoglobulin has been administered with variable outcomes.[49] Recently, a chimeric murine human anti-CD20 mAb (Rituximab) has been used off-label without or with plasmapheresis, showing benefit in 24 of 27 patients.[50]

LONG-TERM MAINTENANCE IMMUNOSUPPRESSION

Although calcineurin inhibitors without or with concomitant MMF administration have reduced the incidence and severity of acute rejection episodes, they have not improved the 5% annual rate of graft attrition previously observed with Aza-Pred therapy. Although it is possible that this failure reflects chronically inadequate or variable CsA exposure owing to reductions in the calcineurin antagonist doses in response to impaired renal function, it is more likely that the host B-cell responses that mediate chronic rejection are less sensitive to these agents than T-cell responses.

Owing to a lack of knowledge concerning the pathophysiologic mechanisms of chronic rejection, long-term immunosuppressive regimens, including CsA, TRL, steroids, MMF, Aza and SRL, show greater inter-center variations than do the short-term strategies. In the chronic rejection setting, long-term SRL administration may confer novel advantages based on the capacity of this agent to block the effects of hematologic–vascular cytokines that stimulate endothelial and smooth muscle cell proliferation, resulting in immuno-obliterative lesions. Although there are currently no data to support this hypothesis, four observations suggest that SRL may prevent the occurrence or slow the progression of chronic rejection.[51] First, SRL inhibits growth factor-driven proliferation of endothelial and smooth muscle cells in vitro, presumably by blocking the action of cytokines critical to producing the immuno-obliterative vascular and bronchial lesions – the histologic hallmarks of chronic rejection. Second, SRL exerts a beneficial effect on the smooth muscle and endothelial cell responses to vascular injury provoked in vivo by balloon catheter injury or observed in aortic allografts. Third, SRL mitigates chronic rejection in rat renal allografts. Fourth, used in combination with CsA in humans, SRL reduces the incidence of acute rejection episodes, which are widely believed to predict an increased risk of chronic rejection. Further, the administration of SRL permits either minimization or elimination of CsA, thereby promoting renal recovery during the early postoperative period and possibly mitigating chronic CsA-induced renal dysfunction, which may exacerbate other processes that contribute to graft attrition.

Although the usual strategy is to attempt steroid withdrawal at the patient's request, where there is good HLA matching or evidence of drug-induced morbidities, the clinician's decision must be based on a perception of the safety of steroid withdrawal. Evidence of host anti-donor hyporesponsiveness in mixed lymphocyte cultures, cell-mediated cytotoxic effector and precursor assays,[52] and suppressor 'three cell' reactions have provided indices to withdraw steroids from or otherwise modulate CsA- or TRL-based regimens. A delay in withdrawal may compromise some of the potential benefits to be gained from a steroid-free regimen, specifically the prevention of cataract formation, amelioration of diabetes mellitus, and mitigation of bone destruction. There is a general impression that drug doses can be reduced over time owing to 'adaptation' of the graft to the host; this phenomenon has been attributed to repopulation of the donor vasculature with host elements. However, transplantation of long-term accepted grafts in experimental animals back into syngeneic donor-strain animal hosts fails to elicit rejection responses, a finding that suggests that the host rather than the donor 'adapts' to this artificial situation. However, virtually every patient who discontinues all immunosuppressive medications rejects the graft; there is currently no clinically applicable strategy to induce tolerance.

■ TRANSPLANTATION TOLERANCE ■

IMMUNO-UNRESPONSIVENESS

The ultimate goal of transplantation research is to achieve selective tolerance toward donor – but not third-party – foreign allografts. Tolerance is the 'cure' for transplant success, whereas immunosuppression is only palliative therapy. One must distinguish tolerance from immuno-unresponsiveness, a state that demands at least some concomitant immunosuppression. Although treatment of experimental animals with relatively abbreviated courses of immunosuppressants produces a propensity towards tolerance, such an evolution occurs only rarely in humans. The presence of donor-type putatively dendritic elements in numerous tissues of organ transplant recipients has been attributed to the presence of an unresponsive state,[53] indicating a 'truce' between host-versus-graft and graft-versus-host reactions. These findings led to the suggestion that the facile acceptance of liver grafts reflects their rich passenger cell component. This hypothesis has not yet been supported by clinical trials: infusion of supplemental donor bone marrow elements concomitant with transplantation of passenger cell-poor cardiac or renal allografts, or even rich orthotopic liver transplants, has neither improved graft survival nor rendered patients tolerant of their grafts.[54] Indeed, the significance of chimerism as a marker for unresponsiveness is controversial; some patients displaying donor cell chimerism have been reported to undergo rejection episodes. Calne and colleagues[55] offer a more conservative proposal: after T-cell depletion with an anti-CD52 mAb, a 1-day interval is allowed to elapse before treatment is started with low-dose CsA in the absence of steroids. These workers suggested that the modest (18%) incidence of rejection observed within 1 year reflected 'prope' (almost) tolerance; however, as noted above, the 5-year data did not show unique benefits in this patient cohort.

Immunological tolerance

The concept of immunologic tolerance evolved from observations that hosts exposed to foreign cells during fetal/neonatal stages subsequently accepted donor-type tissue transplants.[1] In 1914, John Murphy reported that duck or pigeon embryos permit the unrestricted growth of Rous chicken sarcoma cells, unless the embryo had been previously inoculated with adult chicken lymphoid cells. Owen in 1945 demonstrated that nonidentical freemartin calf twins showed erythrocyte chimerism, which he attributed to the exchange of placental blood. Tissue transplant tolerance was demonstrated in fetal or newborn mice by Billingham, in chicken egg embryos by Hasek, and in the first 2 weeks of life of rats by Woodruff.

These phenomena have been explained as an alteration of the 'central' thymic process, which naturally eliminates putatively self-reactive T-cell clones present in the thymus[55] (Chapter 9). A similar cellular 'macro' chimerism has been produced in adult animals following 'debulking' of the immune system by total-body or total-lymphoid[56] irradiation to recreate the 'pristine' fetal state and allow 'space' for reconstitution with donor or F_1 bone marrow cells. Adult allogeneic T cells are 'purged' from the donor bone marrow inoculum with anti-T cell sera, with anti-CTLA-4Ig receptor conjugates,[57] or with anti-CD40 ligand (-CD154) mAbs[58] to prevent graft-versus-host disease. Hosts displaying this 'macro-chimeric' type of tolerance show either an absent or an altered T-cell repertoire, presumably owing to the effects of the newly seeded donor-type dendritic cells in the host thymus. Clinical induction of macro-chimerism is limited by the hazards and logistical demands of pre-transplant radiotherapy, as well as by the mature state of the primate thymus, such that donor-specific tolerance is not readily produced by intra-thymic injection of donor materials combined with peripheral lymphoid depletion using polyclonal antisera.[59]

The primary potential mechanism of central tolerance is clonal deletion or elimination. Tolerance toward kidney grafts has been observed in patients who have previously received donor-type bone marrow infusions after myeloablative therapy as the reconstituted immune system is putatively of donor type. Administration of a nonmyeloablative conditioning regimen, including cyclophosphamide, thymic irradiation and anti-thymocyte globulin combined with a short course of CsA, has reportedly induced functional tolerance and sustained anti-tumor responses following combined bone marrow and kidney transplantation from the same donor.[60] However, this approach has not been successful when the marrow and kidney donors are not HLA identical. Alternative T-cell depletion strategies employing immunotoxin[61] or anti-CD52 mAb[62] have produced equivocal results even when combined with pharmacologic immunosuppressants.

A critical question for the clinical enterprise is whether tolerance can be produced peripherally without 'debulking' or elimination of the host's immune system. The 'horror autotoxicus' concept of Ehrlich postulated that tolerance is a natural immune process that lymphocytes undergo after leaving the thymus. This 'peripheral' form of tolerance occurs despite the persistence of alloantigen-reactive host T cells, an observation elegantly confirmed in transgenic models. The expression of foreign I-E class II molecules restricted to the acinar pancreas and kidney,[63] or to pancreatic islet β cells, failed to elicit rejection responses, although adoptive transfer of naïve T lymphocytes killed the transgenic cells.[64] Durable tolerance in clinically relevant settings probably requires a combination of strategies that affect central and peripheral mechanisms. In humans, several vectors block the emergence of tolerance toward transplants: nonspecific immune responses triggered by tissue injury, the high frequency of alloreactive cells in the repertoire, and cross-reactivity due to recognition of heterologous antigens that generate memory cells which are resistant to depletion or inactivation.

Several mechanisms may explain post-thymic 'peripheral' unresponsiveness: anergy,[65] ignorance,[66] deletion by apoptosis[67] or regulatory (suppressor) cell activity.[68] Anergy represents an unresponsive state of antigen-reactive lymphocytes. Bretscher and Cohn[69] proposed that unresponsiveness was due to the absence of an appropriate second humoral activation signal. Th cells recognize alloantigen, but neither proliferate nor secrete IL-2, the addition of which reverses the anergy. Although in animal models anergy emerges after abrogation of helper–inducer

41. Hong JC, Kahan BD. Use of anti-CD25 monoclonal antibody in combination with rapamycin to eliminate cyclosporine treatment during the induction phase of immunosuppression. Transplantation 1999; 68: 701.

42. Knight RJ, Kerman RH, Schoenberg L, et al. The selective use of basiliximab versus thymoglobulin in combination with sirolimus for cadaveric renal transplant recipients at low risk versus high risk for delayed graft function. Transplantation 2004; 78: 904.

43. Kaufman DB, Leventhal JR, Axelrod D, et al. Alemtuzumab induction and prednisone-free maintenance immunotherapy in kidney transplantation: comparison with basiliximab induction – long-term results. Am J Transplant 2005; 5: 2539.

44. Calne R, Moffatt SD, Friend PJ, et al. Campath IH allows low-dose cyclosporine monotherapy in 31 cadaveric renal allograft recipients. Transplantation 1999; 68: 1613.

45. Watson CJ, Bradley JA, Friend PJ, et al. Alemtuzumab (CAMPATH 1H) induction therapy in cadaveric kidney transplantation – efficacy and safety at five years. Am J Transplant 2005; 5: 1347.

46. Swinnen LJ, Costanzo-Nordin MR, Fisher SG, et al. Increased incidence of lymphoproliferative disorder after immunosuppression with the monoclonal antibody OKT3 in cardiac-transplant recipients. N Engl J Med 1990; 323: 1723.

47. Hong JC, Kahan BD. Sirolimus rescue therapy for refractory rejection in renal transplantation. Transplantation 2001; 71: 1579.

48. Csapo Z, Benavides-Viveros C, Podder H, et al. Campath-1H as rescue therapy for the treatment of acute rejection in kidney transplant patients. Transplant Proc 2005; 37: 2032.

49. Montgomery RA, Zachary AA, Racusen LC, et al. Plasmapheresis and intravenous immune globulin provides effective rescue therapy for refractory humoral rejection and allows kidneys to be successfully transplanted into cross-match-positive recipients. Transplantation 2000; 70: 887.

50. Becker YT, Becker BN, Pirsch JD, Sollinger HW. Rituximab as treatment for refractory kidney transplant rejection. Am J Transplant 2004; 4: 996.

51. Kahan BD. The role of rapamycin in chronic rejection prophylaxis: a theoretical consideration. Graft 1998; 1: 93.

52. Herzog WR, Zanker B, Irschick E, et al. Selective reduction of donor-specific cytotoxic T lymphocyte precursors in patients with a well-functioning kidney allograft. Transplantation 1987; 43: 384.

53. Starzl TE, Demetris AJ, Murase N, et al. Cell migration, chimerism, and graft acceptance. Lancet 1992; 339: 1579.

54. Rolles K, Burroughs AK, Davidson BR, et al. Donor-specific bone marrow infusion after orthotopic liver transplantation. Lancet 1994; 343: 263.

55. Kappler JW, Roehm N, Marrack P. T cell tolerance by clonal elimination in the thymus. Cell 1987; 49: 273.

56. Slavin S, Strober S, Fuks Z, Kaplan HS. Induction of specific tissue transplantation tolerance using fractionated total lymphoid irradiation in adult mice: long-term survival of allogeneic bone marrow and skin grafts. J Exp Med 1977; 146: 34.

57. Blazar BR, Taylor PA, Panoskaltsis-Mortari A, et al. Opposing roles of CD28: B7 and CTLA-4: B7 pathways in regulating *in vivo* alloresponses in murine recipients of MHC disparate T cells. J Immunol 1999; 162: 6368.

58. Buhlmann JE, Gonzalez M, Ginther B, et al. Cutting edge: sustained expansion of CD8+ T cells requires CD154 expression by Th cells in acute graft versus host disease. J Immunol 1999; 162: 4373.

59. Odorico JS, Barker CF, Posselt AM, Naji A. Induction of donor-specific tolerance to rat cardiac allografts by intrathymic inoculation of bone marrow. Surgery 1992; 112: 370. discussion 376–377.

60. Buhler LH, Spitzer TR, Sykes M, et al. Induction of kidney allograft tolerance after transient lymphohematopoietic chimerism in patients with multiple myeloma and end-stage renal disease. Transplantation 2002; 74: 1405.

61. Contreras JL, Wang PX, Eckhoff DE, et al. Peritransplant tolerance induction with anti-CD3-immunotoxin: a matter of proinflammatory cytokine control. Transplantation 1998; 65: 1159.

62. Knechtle SJ, Pirsch JD, H Fechne J Jr., et al. Campath-1H induction plus rapamycin monotherapy for renal transplantation: results of a pilot study. Am J Transplant 2003; 3: 722.

63. Lo D, Burkly LC, Flavell RA, et al. Tolerance in transgenic mice expressing class II major histocompatibility complex on pancreatic acinar cells. J Exp Med 1989; 170: 87.

64. Jones-Youngblood SL, Wieties K, Forman J, Hammer RE. Effect of the expression of a hepatocyte-specific MHC molecule in transgenic mice on T cell tolerance. J Immunol 1990; 144: 1187.

65. Jones LA, Chin LT, Merriam GR, et al. Failure of clonal deletion in neonatally thymectomized mice: tolerance is preserved through clonal anergy. J Exp Med 1990; 172: 1277.

66. Lakkis FG, Arakelov A, Konieczny BT, Inoue Y. Immunologic 'ignorance' of vascularized organ transplants in the absence of secondary lymphoid tissue. Nature Med 2000; 6: 686.

67. Li Y, Li XC, Zheng XX, et al. Blocking both signal 1 and signal 2 of T-cell activation prevents apoptosis of alloreactive T cells and induction of peripheral allograft tolerance. Nature Med 1999; 5: 1298.

68. Jiang S, Lechler RI. Regulatory T cells in the control of transplantation tolerance and autoimmunity. Am J Transplant 2003; 3: 516.

69. Bretscher P, Cohn M. A theory of self-nonself discrimination. Science 1970; 169: 1042.

70. Kingsley CI, Karim M, Bushell AR, Wood KJ. CD25+CD4+ regulatory T cells prevent graft rejection: CTLA-4- and IL-10-dependent immunoregulation of alloresponses. J Immunol 2002; 168: 1080.

71. Walsh PT, Strom TB, Turka LA. Routes to transplant tolerance versus rejection; the role of cytokines. Immunity 2004; 20: 121.

72. Vendetti S, Chai JG, Dyson J, et al. Anergic T cells inhibit the antigen-presenting function of dendritic cells. J Immunol 2000; 165: 1175.

Challenges and potentials of xenotransplantation

Marilia Cascalho, Jeffrey L. Platt

81

Xenotransplantation refers to the transplantation of living cells, tissues, or organs from individuals of species into another species. Among the various fields of transplantation, none has sparked greater excitement and none greater controversy than xenotransplantation. This chapter will consider the various applications that have been proposed for xenotransplantation, as it is these from which the excitement derives. The chapter addresses the hurdles that prevent the application of xenotransplantation for the treatment of disease today, particularly those hurdles stemming from the immune response of the recipient to the graft. It is from these hurdles and the possibility that xenografts might serve as a vehicle for transfer of infectious organisms between species that the controversy derives.

■ APPLICATIONS FOR XENOTRANSPLANTATION ■

Although various types of xenografts were contemplated and even tried during all of history, xenotransplantation was first undertaken in the early years of the 20th century for the treatment of renal failure. Experimental surgeons had recently devised the vascular anastomosis as a way of connecting the cut end of blood vessels, and that advance created the field of vascular surgery. The vascular anastomosis would allow the repair of traumatic wounds and the penetration of surgery deeper into body cavities. However, those who developed the procedure realized the vascular anastomosis might also prove to be the critical technical advance needed to replace a sick organ with a healthy one, i.e., for organ transplantation.[1] As exciting as the prospect of organ replacement seemed to be, it was not clear then how one could obtain an organ from a human for transplantation. It was reasoned then that since some cellular components of the kidney and other organs often remain alive long after a person is deceased, harvesting a kidney from a cadaver would be unethical. Because of this concern, the first application of the vascular anastomosis to replacement of organ function was conducted using animals – swine and sheep – as a source of organs instead of humans.

The most important reason for interest in xenotransplantation today is to provide a plentiful source of organs, in lieu of human organs, for transplantation. By some estimates, the number of human organs available for transplantation equals as little as 5% of the number needed.[2] In the case of the kidney and liver, this shortage may be blunted by the use of living donors. However, for reasons discussed below, the demand for organ transplantation may soon increase further, and dramatically so.

Today, organ transplantation is mainly undertaken to treat severe failure of the kidneys, liver, heart, and lungs. As advances in public health and medicine allow many to live to an advanced age, the prevalence of type 2 diabetes and cardiovascular disease will increase, as will the demand for transplantation. The demand for transplantation could increase further as advances in molecular diagnostics, genomics, and proteomics make it possible to detect tumors and other lethal diseases before they are clinically apparent. The diagnosis of such disease will spark interest in using transplantation to pre-empt these conditions or to spare the patient from the risk of waiting until the tumor can be localized.

Xenotransplantation may even be preferred in some circumstances over human-to-human transplantation. When a virus causes organ failure, xenotransplantation might be preferred to avoid infection of the transplanted organ. This approach has already been attempted for treatment of cirrhosis caused by hepatitis virus and loss of immune competence caused by human immunodeficiency virus (HIV). A xenograft (or at least a xenogeneic organ) might be used as a temporary measure to preserve life or health until healing occurs (or until a human organ becomes available). Thus, the blood of subjects with fulminant hepatic failure has been through swine livers as a way of improving the subject's condition so that the patient could undergo allotransplantation. Xenografts might be used to deliver genes or gene products for complex metabolic pathways, exploiting the ability to express heterologous genes at high levels in genetically engineered animals. Xenografts (human-to-animal) have even been advanced as systems that might coax the differentiation of stem cells into functional tissues and organs.[3]

Unfortunately, despite the many potential uses and the long history of interest in xenotransplantation, daunting biological barriers presently prevent widespread application of xenotransplantation. These barriers include the graft injury caused by the immune response of the recipient against the graft, physiological incompatibilities between the transplant

Perhaps because of uncertainties about the importance of NK cells in the barrier to xenotransplantation, therapeutic strategies for inhibiting these cells have been discussed but so far have not been advanced. Among the considerations are transgenic expression of human leukocyte antigen (HLA)-E or other stimulators of inhibitory receptors.

Inflammation and coagulation as innate barriers to xenotransplantation

Besides those components generally viewed as elements of the innate immune system, phagocytes (neutrophils and macrophages), platelets, and the coagulation system can recognize and react directly with xenografts. Of course, these elements can also be recruited by innate and adaptive immune responses. Whether these cells and pathways cause greater harm by direct action on xenografts or as effectors recruited by immune reactions has not been tested. However, since inhibition of innate and elicited immunity largely prevents acute destruction of xenografts, one suspects that these elements mainly serve an accessory capacity.

ELICITED IMMUNE RESPONSES

T cells

T cells clearly recognize and destroy xenografts since cellular xenografts can survive in nude mice, but not in wild-type mice. To which extent and by what mechanism T cells recognize xenogeneic cells, however, have been matters of controversy. T-cell responses to xenogeneic cells appear to be defective when evaluated *in vitro* because cytokines and co-stimulatory molecules produced by xenogeneic antigen-presenting cells (APCs) act poorly on responding T cells. However, xenogenic APCs can present foreign MHC antigen to T cells, presumably through the use of alternative co-stimulatory pathways and cross-reactive properties of T-cell receptors. T cells may also respond *in vitro* to foreign peptides presented by self-APC. Although the nature and intensity of T-cell responses to xenotransplantation are still not completely known, the response is likely to be at least as intense as the response to allotransplantation, owing to the diverse set of antigenic peptides, an amplifying effect of humoral immunity and inflammation on cellular immune responses, and defective immune regulation.[14]

Elicited antibodies

Xenogeneic cells and tissues elicit powerful and diverse antibody responses. These responses, like other T-cell-dependent responses, are controlled to some extent by immunosuppressive therapy. The elicited immune response has been seen as the critical barrier to transplantation of xenogeneic organs, yet little is known about the specificity. Xenotransplantation does lead to the production of a large amount of anti-Galα1-3Gal antibodies, consisting of a greater fraction of IgG and exhibiting higher affinity than natural anti-Galα1-3Gal antibodies. However, whether these antibodies result from class switch recombination and affinity maturation in B cells producing natural Ig or the activation of novel clones is uncertain. Because production of anti-Galα1-3Gal antibodies or their impact on the graft might be controlled as described above, the elicited antibodies of greater importance are probably T-cell-dependent antibodies specific for other antigens.[15] Unfortunately, little is

known about the specificity of the antibodies; however, these antibodies are now seen as another important barrier to successful transplantation of xenogeneic organs.

IMPACT OF IMMUNE RESPONSES ON THE XENOGRAFTS

If xenotransplantation excites nearly every facet of innate and adaptive immunity, the impact of an immune response is determined not so much by the intensity or diversity of the response as by the type of graft implanted: cell, tissue, or organ. The type of graft determines the impact of the immune response because it determines the means by which the graft receives its supply of blood, and it is the vasculature of grafts that is most vulnerable to immune-mediated injury. Figure 81.1 depicts the various responses observed following xenotransplantation of organs, tissues, and cells. Notice that organs are susceptible to various types of rejection that are not observed in cell and tissue grafts. These types of rejection focus predominantly on the vasculature of the graft.

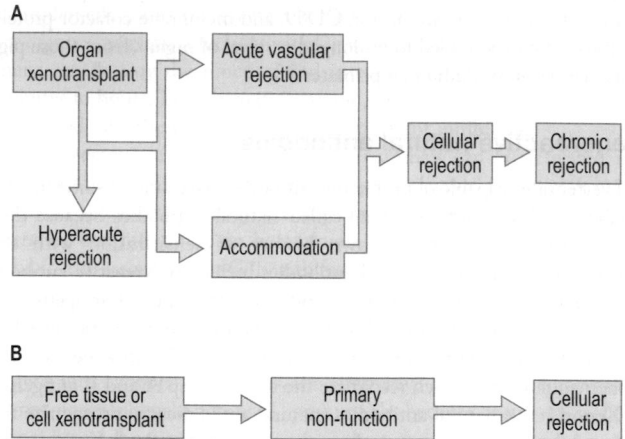

Fig. 81.1 Biological outcome of xenografts. (**A**) The outcome of organ xenotransplants. Organ xenografts are subject to vascular types of rejection, including hyperacute, acute vascular, and chronic rejection. Vascular rejection, particularly hyperacute and acute vascular rejection, are caused by the binding of antibodies and activation of complement of the recipient on xenogeneic blood vessels. Having blood vessels originating with the recipient, cell and tissue xenografts are not subject to this type of problem. Accommodation refers to acquired resistance to injury. Organ xenografts are also susceptible to cellular rejection. (**B**) The outcome of free tissue and cell xenotransplants. Cell and tissue xenografts derive their blood supply through the in-growth of blood vessels of the recipient. Since the blood vessels of these grafts are constructed from cells of the recipient, antibodies of the recipient do not generally bind to the blood vessels, and hence vascular diseases of organ grafts such as hyperacute and acute vascular rejection are not observed. Free tissue and cell xenografts are mainly subject to injury by T cells that have the ability to migrate effectively through blood vessels walls, causing primary nonfunction and cellular rejection.

HYPERACUTE REJECTION

Hyperacute rejection refers to the rejection of an organ graft within 24 hours of reperfusion; it is arguably the most severe and violent immunological reaction as it reflects the loss of graft function and destruction of the organ within a period of hours. Hyperacute rejection begins within minutes of the perfusion of a newly transplanted organ and is characterized by formation of platelet thrombi and bleeding into the graft. Organs transplanted between disparate species are especially susceptible to hyperacute rejection.

The development of hyperacute rejection depends absolutely on activation of complement in an organ graft. In some combinations of organ and recipient species, complement activation is initiated directly through the alternative pathway, owing presumably to species-specific function of factor H. This type of hyperacute rejection is especially severe and resistant to therapy, perhaps because C3b attaches simultaneously to many available sites on blood vessel walls. In clinically relevant combinations of organ and recipient (e.g., swine organs transplanted in higher primates), complement activation is mainly initiated by the classical pathway, owing the binding of xenoreactive antibodies and involvement of the alternative pathway is secondary. In this setting, the kinetics and extent of complement activation are functions of mainly antibody–antigen interaction.

Hyperacute rejection appears to reflect a loss of endothelial cell function. This loss is triggered by terminal complement complexes inserted into endothelial cell membranes. The rate of complement activation appears particularly important, as measures that slow the formation of terminal complexes, such as expression of very low levels of decay-accelerating factor and/or CD59 from the recipient species in blood vessels of the graft may prevent the disease.[5]

Hyperacute rejection can be prevented by any means that hinders activation of complement in the transplant. In pig-to-primate xenografts, such means include the depletion of xenoreactive antibodies from the circulation of the recipient, elimination by gene targeting or other means of the antigen they recognize, and the inhibition of complement reactions, such as through expression as the product of transgenes of complement regulatory proteins of the recipient species.

ACUTE VASCULAR REJECTION

If hyperacute rejection does not occur or if it is prevented, a xenografted organ is susceptible to acute vascular rejection. Acute vascular rejection emerges over a period of days to weeks and is characterized by endothelial swelling, focal ischemia, and intravascular coagulation. Acute vascular rejection, sometimes called delayed xenograft rejection or acute humoral rejection, causes destruction of a xenograft over a period of days to weeks and is now widely seen as a third major hurdle to the clinical application of organ xenotransplantation.[14]

Acute vascular rejection appears to be caused mainly by the action over hours to days of antibodies of the recipient directed against the graft. Besides antibodies, other factors, including macrophages, platelets, and NK cells, have been implicated in this disease. However, most transplant physicians are so persuaded about the importance of antibodies that when this type of rejection occurs in an allograft it is often referred to as 'antibody-mediated' rejection.

Binding of antibodies to blood vessels in a graft is thought to cause acute vascular rejection (if it does not cause hyperacute rejection) by activating endothelium. In some cases at least, activation of endothelium depends on activation of complement and particularly the insertion of sublytic amounts of terminal complement complexes in endothelial cells. Terminal complement complexes activate the interleukin (IL)-1α gene, leading to production of that cytokine; under some conditions, it is that cytokine that determines the subsequent fate (activation versus nonactivation) of endothelium and hence of the graft. Endothelial cell activation changes the posture of blood vessels from anti-coagulant to procoagulant and from anti-inflammatory to proinflammatory.

Several approaches have been pursued in efforts to prevent or treat acute vascular rejection. To the extent that anti-Galα1-3Gal antibodies trigger acute vascular rejection, the induction of immunological tolerance to Galα1-3Gal or the elimination of that saccharide from transplants might prevent the initiation of that process. However, neither tolerance induced by presently available means nor the elimination of Galα1-3Gal can prevent acute vascular rejection of xenografts.[12, 13] In these cases, antibodies elicited against antigens other than Galα1-3Gal appear to incite rejection. Perhaps tolerance might be induced to a broader spectrum of antigens by transplantation of hematopoietic stem cells of the donor species into the recipient. Still another approach to preventing acute vascular rejection of xenotransplants, however, may involve the induction of accommodation.

ACCOMMODATION

Accommodation is an acquired resistance to humoral injury and acute vascular rejection of an organ graft.[6, 16] Accommodation was first observed in the transplantation of kidneys across blood group A and B barriers when transient removal of anti-blood group antibodies from the recipients of the transplants was followed by prolonged function of the transplants after the return of the antibodies to the circulation. Accommodation has been observed in rodent models of xenotransplantation and in porcine organs transplanted into baboons where the organs express human complement regulatory proteins and the xenoreactive antibodies are temporarily depleted from the circulation of the xenograft recipient. Accommodation may exemplify a broader response in which cells exhibit reversal of noxious pathways.[16] The development of accommodation may be important for the successful engraftment of xenogeneic organs because these organs contain numerous antigens that could evoke humoral immune responses.

We originally postulated that accommodation may reflect one or more of three changes following organ transplantation: (1) a change in the nature of xenoreactive antibodies; (2) a change in the antigen-impairing antibody binding; and (3) induction of cellular resistance to humoral injury.[6] Most evidence would presently point to acquired resistance to injury as being central to accommodation. Accommodation in both rodents and pig-to-primate xenografts appears to be associated with expression of various anti-apoptotic proteins and heme oxygenase-1. In other biological systems, accommodation may require the AKT and PI3 kinase system. Which gene(s) and signaling pathways actually bring about accommodation and which are simply needed for cell survival, but not accommodation *per se,* is still uncertain.

CHRONIC REJECTION

Whether or not, and to what frequency, chronic rejection would occur in a vascularized xenograft is uncertain because of the difficulties in overcoming acute vascular rejection. Clearly, ongoing production

8. Landsteiner K. The Specificity of Serological Reactions. New York, NY: Dover Publications; 1962.

9. Cosimi AB, Sachs DH. Mixed chimerism and transplantation tolerance. Transplantation 2004; 77: 943–946.

10. Phelps CJ, Koike C, Vaught TD, et al. Production of alpha 1,3-galactosyl-transferase-deficient pigs. Science 2003; 299: 411–414.

11. Kuwaki K, Tseng YL, Dor FJ, et al. Heart transplantation in baboons using alpha1,3-galactosyltransferase gene-knockout pigs as donors: initial experience. Nat Med 2005; 11: 29–31.

12. Yamada K, Yazawa K, Shimizu A, et al. Marked prolongation of porcine renal xenograft survival in baboons through the use of alpha1,3-galactosyltransferase gene-knockout donors and the cotransplantation of vascularized thymic tissue. Nat Med 2005; 11: 32–34.

13. Chen G, Qian H, Starzl T, et al. Acute rejection is associated with antibodies to non-Gal antigens in baboons using Gal-knockout pig kidneys. Nat Med 2005; 11: 1295–1298.

14. Platt JL. New directions for organ transplantation. Nature 1998; 392: 11–17.

15. McCurry KR, Parker W, Cotterell AH, et al. Humoral responses in pig-to-baboon cardiac transplantation: implications for the pathogenesis and treatment of acute vascular rejection and for accommodation. Hum Immunol 1997; 58: 91–105.

16. Koch CA, Khalpey ZI, Platt JL. Accommodation: preventing injury in transplantation and disease. J Immunol 2004; 172: 5143–5148.

17. Paradis K, Langford G, Long Z, et al. Search for cross-species transmission of porcine endogenous retrovirus in patients treated with living pig tissue. Science 1999; 285: 1236–1241.

18. Ogle BM, Cascalho M, Platt JL. Biological implications of cell fusion. Nat Rev Mol Cell Biol 2005; 6: 567–575.

19. Cascalho M, Platt J. New technologies for organ replacement and augmentation. Mayo Clin Proc 2005; 80: 370–378.

Hematopoietic stem cell transplantation for malignant diseases

Scott Rowley, Thea M. Friedman, Robert Korngold

82

Hematopoietic stem cell transplantation (HSCT) is currently the therapy of choice for most hematological malignancies, including all forms of leukemia, lymphoma, and multiple myeloma that are nonresponsive to first-line chemotherapeutics, as well as the clonal but nonmalignant myelodysplastic and myeloproliferative disorders. Autologous HSCT is commonly used as salvage therapy for patients with malignancies sensitive to chemo-/radiotherapy in a dose-responsive manner. These patients receive very dose-intensive cytoreductive regimens designed to eliminate all tumor cells, but in so doing also destroy the stem cell elements needed to populate the hematopoietic compartment. Infusion of previously collected HSC will rescue the patient from the marrow-ablative effects of this treatment. On the other hand, allogeneic HSCT, which will also reconstitute bone marrow function after dose-intensive chemo-/radiotherapy, is now also used to provide an immunotherapeutic approach with the intention of allowing donor T cells to attack residual tumor cells that remain after the conditioning regimen, reducing the risk of later disease relapse. Thus, allogeneic HSCT does not require the administration of dose-intensive regimens to achieve complete tumor cell kill, and lower-intensity nonmyeloablative regimens may be used to 'condition' the host for transplantation.

Autologous (including syngeneic [identical twin]) HSCT is justified by the dose sensitivity of most hematological malignancies. Although there is some evidence that faster immunological recovery after autologous HSCT predicts a lower risk of relapse, possibly opening an area of research in graft modification to enhance such recovery, treatment of the disease is a result of the chemotherapy administered, with infusion of cells only required to hasten hematological recovery. The primary complications of autologous HSCT result from the administration of the dose-intense pre-transplant regimen and include a period of marrow hypoplasia, possibly requiring blood transfusions and antibiotics. Nonhematological toxicities, including mucositis resulting in inanition, and diarrhea, and damage to other organs such as lung, liver, and kidney, limit the amount of chemotherapy that can be administered. Relapse of disease, however, is the primary cause of death after autologous HSCT, and improvements in the outcome will probably require new strategies to induce effective immune responsiveness to the residual disease.

THERAPEUTIC PRINCIPLES

AUTOLOGOUS VERSUS ALLOGENEIC HSCT

Autologous transplantation

>> Based on chemo-/radiotherapy dose-sensitivity of primary disease
>> Requires collection and storage of adequate HSC, preferably before extensive alkylating agent or purine analog therapy
>> Lower risk of graft failure (no immunologic rejection)
>> No routine post-transplant immunosuppression
>> Minimal or no risk of GvHD
>> Quicker post-transplant immune reconstitution
>> Mimal or no GvL effect
>> Variable risk of tumor cell contamination in donor infusate
>> Not useful for diseases in which normal HSC cannot be collected (e.g., chronic myelogenous leukemia, myelodysplasia)

Allogeneic transplantation

>> Rescues bone marrow function after dose-intense therapy
>> Effective with reduced-intensity conditioning regimens
>> Achieves a GvL effect in many malignancies
>> Risk of GvHD that may be uncontrollable
>> Higher risk of transplant-related complications that may offset the benefit of the GvL effect
>> Risk of immunological graft rejection
>> Slow post-transplant immune reconstitution
>> No risk of tumor cell contamination
>> Risk of disease transmission (viral infections, cancer) from donor

Table 82.1 Clinical grading of acute GvHD (Adapted from Glucksberg H, Storb R, Fefer A, et al. Clinical manifestations of graft-versus-host disease in human recipients of marrow from HLA-matched sibling donors. Transplantation 1974; 18: 295–304)

Overall grade	Skin stage	Liver stage	Gut stage	Functional impairment stage
0 (none)	0	0	0	0
1 (mild)	1–2	0	0	0
2 (moderate)	1–3	1	1	1
3 (severe)	2–3	2–3	2–3	2
4 (life-threatening)	1–4	1–4	1–4	3

Table 82.2 Clinical staging of acute GvHD (Adapted from Glucksberg H, Storb R, Fefer A, et al. Clinical manifestations of graft-versus-host disease in human recipients of marrow from HLA-matched sibling donors. Transplantation 1974; 18: 295–304)

Stage	Skin	Liver	Gut
1	Maculopapular rash <25% BSA	Bilirubin 2–3 mg/dL	Diarrhea 500–1000 ml/day, or Persistant nausea
2	Maculopapular rash 25–50% BSA	Bilirubin 3–6 mg/dL	Diarrhea 1000–1500 ml/day
3	Generalized erythroderma	Bilirubin 6–15 mg/dL	Diarrhea >1500 ml/day
4	Desquamation and bullae formation	Bilirubin >15 mg/dL	Pain ± ileus

CLINICAL ASPECTS OF cGvHD

cGvHD is the leading cause of late TRM among recipients of allogeneic HSCT, and resembles autoimmune disorders such as scleroderma, Sjögren's syndrome, and primary biliary cirrhosis. As with aGvHD, diagnosis is based on clinical observations with secondary laboratory confirmation (Table 82.3).[14] A falling performance status, progressive weight loss, or recurrent infections are usually signs of clinical extensive cGvHD. About 50% of long-term survivors will develop cGvHD at a median of 9 months, and patients must be monitored closely for at least 2 years after transplantation so that appropriate treatment can be started before extensive target end-organ damage ensues.

Factors predictive for the development of cGvHD again include the degree of HLA disparity, but also include the source of HSC in that peripheral blood stem cell (PBSC) transplantation conveys a higher risk than marrow or cord blood transplantation. Patients who develop cGvHD have a higher risk of TRM but a lower risk of relapse as a result of the immunological GvL effect.[15] T-cell depletion may decrease the risk of cGvHD, although this has not been demonstrated in all studies.[16] Most patients require at least two drugs for treatment of cGvHD, the standard initial treatment again being glucocorticoids and a calcineurin

inhibitor. About half of patients with cGvHD do not achieve complete remission (CR) with first-line therapy, although the manifold signs and symptoms of cGvHD complicate the definition of response to treatment.[17] There are no clear recommendations regarding second-line treatments, and a variety of pharmacologic and immunologic techniques have been used. Re-transplantation is ineffective, but a single-center report of low-dose thoracoabdominal irradiation described an 82% response rate, with the best responses observed in patients with fasciitis or oral involvement.[18] Photopheresis has an overall response rate of 50–60%, with many cGvHD patients achieving complete control of this complication.[19]

GvL RESPONSES

An inverse correlation has been observed in allogeneic HSCT patients between the incidence and severity of GvHD and the relapse rate of chronic myeloid leukemia (CML), and to a lesser extent acute myeloid leukemia (AML).[20] This relationship has not been so clear in other forms of hematological malignancy, such as acute lymphocytic leukemia (ALL) or multiple myeloma. Relapses after HSCT are thought to occur because of the survival of a few leukemia lineage stem cells in the bone

Table 82.3 Staging of chronic GvHD[14]

Target organ	Score 0	Score 1	Score 2	Score 3
Performance score	KPS 100%	KPS 80–90%	KPS 60–70%	KPS <60%
Skin	No symptoms	<18% BSA	19–50% or sclerotic, still able to pinch	>50% or 'Hidebound'
Mouth	No symptoms	Mild symptoms, no limitations	Moderate symptoms, decreased oral intake	Severe symptoms with major decrease in intake
Eyes	No symptoms	Mild dry eyes	Moderate dry eyes, drops >3x/day	Severe dry eyes affecting daily activities
GI tract	No symptoms	Symptoms without weight loss	Symptoms with moderate weight loss (5–15%)	Symptoms with weight loss >15%
Liver	Normal LFTs	LFTs elevated <2 × upper limits of normal	LFTs elevated 2–5 × upper limits of normal	LFTs elevated >5 × upper limits of normal
Lungs	No symptoms	Mild symptoms FEV 60–79%	Moderate symptoms FEV 40–59%	Severe symptoms FEV <40%
Joints and fascia	No symptoms	Mild tightness not affecting daily activities	Tightness affecting daily activities	Contractures with significant loss of range of motion
Female genital tract	No symptoms	Symptomatic with middle signs on examination	Symptomatic with dispareunia	Symptomatic with strictures

National Institutes of Health consensus development project on criteria for clinical trials in chronic graft-versus-host disease: I. Diagnosis and staging working group report. Biol Blood Marrow Transplant 2005; 11: 945–956. Mild cGvHD involves only 1 or 2 organs (except lung). Moderate involves at least one organ with clinically significant but not major disability (maximum score of 2, lung score of 1 or 2). Severe cGvHD indicates major disability (a score of 3 for any organ).

marrow after administration of the pre-transplant conditioning regimen, and their outgrowth several months after HSCT. The ability to mediate an effective GvL response probably depends on several factors, including the presentation of appropriate antigens by MHC class I and/or class II molecules on the tumor cells themselves, that can be recognized by effector CD4 or CD8 T cells; the lack of strong regulatory T-cell (Treg) activity that may be induced by cytokines from the tumor cells; tumor cell susceptibility to lysis by effector T cells (e.g., the level of Bcl-2 expression and the ability to resist apoptosis induction); ability of T cells to home to sites of tumor growth; and the direct effect of immunosuppressive cytokines, such as TGF-β, produced by the tumor cells. Many types of tumor cell downregulate expression of MHC on their surface, and perhaps CML and AML are most susceptible to GvL responses because the myeloid lineage is adapted for antigen presentation and high MHC expression.

A number of novel immunotherapeutic approaches are being developed to overcome many of these obstacles and enhance GvLresponses, keeping in mind that GvHD must also be avoided or minimized to improve outcomes (Fig. 82.2). One example is the use of delayed donor lymphocyte infusions (DLI), which are administered months after HSCT, at a time when the recipient cytokine environment is less conducive to GvHD induction.

PBMC components, collected from donors with or without granulocyte colony-stimulating factor (G-CSF) treatment, are also effective as

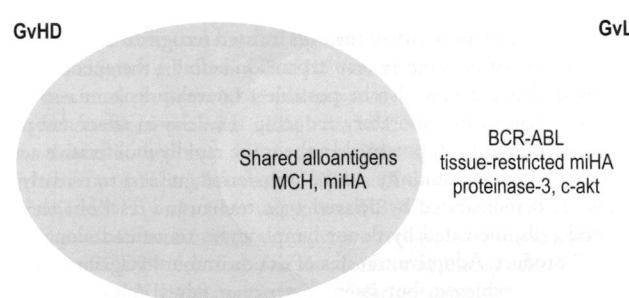

Fig. 82.2 GvHD and GvL responses. Donor T-cell responses to recipient antigens can cause GvHD, but can also target residual leukemia cells. T cells causing GvHD may recognize ubiquitous or tissue-restricted antigens (either MHC or miHA). Many of these recipient antigens may also be expressed by the leukemia cells and allows for a GvL response. Additional leukemia-specific (e.g., bcr-abl, proteinase 3, or c-akt) or tissue-restricted antigens (some miHA, as those expressed only by certain lineages of hematological cells) may be dominantly expressed by the tumor cells and can be targeted by donor T cells without causing GvHD.

donor HSC product by various methods has proved an effective means of reducing the incidence of aGvHD and cGvHD, but this approach increases the risk of graft failure, opportunistic infections, and post-transplant relapse, effectively nullifying the advantage achieved by the lower incidence of GvHD.[4] Higher doses of HSC, which can be achieved by the use of large quantities of PBSC or by combining marrow and PBSC components, will reduce the risk of graft failure. Fixed doses of lymphocytes, as opposed to maximal T-cell depletion may also reduce the risk of graft failure. Some centers are exploring partial T-cell depletion or post-transplant T-cell infusion in an effort to maintain the GvL effect while still reducing the morbidity and mortality of GvHD.

EXPANSION OF HSC PRODUCTS

Ex vivo expansion of HSC contained in UCB products is one potential mechanism to offset the low cell dose and delayed hematological recovery after transplantation.[32] However, no expansion technique has yet achieved this goal, and such endeavors are complicated by the difficulty in identifying pluripotent HSC as opposed to lineage-committed progenitor cells. Furthermore, it is likely that expansion techniques effective for HSC expansion will result in T-cell depletion, resulting in other complications described above.

HEMATOLOGICAL RECOVERY

HSC engraftment encompasses two concepts: recovery of hematopoietic and immunological function of the bone marrow, and the rate at which this occurs. Delay in or failure of sustained engraftment after administration of a myeloablative-conditioning regimen greatly increases the morbidity and cost of the treatment and can result in the death of the patient.[35] Engraftment failure can occur as a result of inadequate quantities of HSC from poor collection or loss in post-collection processing, inadequate host support of the infused cells, post-transplant events or medications, or the immunologically mediated rejection of the allogeneic donor's cells (Fig. 82.3). Failure of engraftment is a very rare complication of autologous HSCT, and is likely only with poor preservation of HSC after collection. For allogeneic transplants, the risk of engraftment failure is proportional to the disparity between donor HLA and miHA, which occurs more commonly in unrelated-donor than in sibling-donor transplantation, and for mismatched rather than HLA-matched transplants. The risk of engraftment failure is also increased by the removal of T cells from the marrow inoculum because of the loss of the GvH effect, mediated by donor alloreactive cells against residual host immune cells.

Assessment of chimerism is important in evaluating poor marrow function after allogeneic HSCT. A fall in peripheral blood counts could indicate HvG-mediated rejection of the graft or early relapse after transplantation, or could be a result of post-transplant events, such as GvHD or viral infection. Documentation of stable persistence of donor cells will help discriminate between these possibilities. It is also important that sustained chimerism be demonstrated if DLI is to be used in the treatment of disease relapse after transplantation. The level of donor–host chimerism after allogeneic HSCT is currently demonstrated through the detection of sex chromosomes using fluorescent in situ hybridization (FISH) techniques, or for same-gender donor–patient pairs, through evaluation of single nucleotide tandem repeats (STR) using molecular analysis techniques (Chapter 101). Obviously, these studies are of no value in assessing engraftment after autologous HSCT.

Much of the emphasis in transplantation has been on myeloid engraftment, because initial patient survival depends on recovery of phagocytes and, to a lesser extent, platelets. Immune reconstitution, and in particular donor T-cell reconstitution, in HSCT patients is often hampered by the age of the recipient, the functional status of the thymus, the cytokine milieu at the time of transplant, and post-transplant immunosuppressive treatments. The thymus involutes rapidly during childhood, and in a normal adult is only able to contribute a very small portion to the mature T-cell compartment. Making matters worse, the thymic tissue may be damaged as a result of a myeloablative conditioning regimen, or it can also be a target of alloreactive donor T cells mediating GvHD. As a result, restoration of the T-cell compartment in patients is often slow, particularly for CD4 T cells, and may be suboptimal for many months to over a year. This situation, of course, endangers the ability of the patient to stave off opportunistic infections, and common complications arise from cytomegalovirus, herpes viruses, and fungal pathogens. If donor T cells are provided in the HSC inoculum, some reconstitution of the T-cell repertoire, mostly CD8 T cells, is provided by the mechanism of nonthymic homeostatic expansion, although the level of diversity may be limited. Experimentally, the administration of cytokines, such as IL-7, after HSCT can enhance thymic function and help donor T-cell reconstitution. Clinical trials are in progress to test this and other novel approaches with the same goal in mind. B-cell reconstitution, on the other hand, is less problematic in terms of the regeneration of the repertoire, although the ability to respond effectively to an infection with antibody production can still depend on the availability of antigen-specific CD4 T cells. Administration of immunoglobulin supplementation to patients with low IgG levels can prevent some of the infectious complications.[39] It should also be mentioned that HSCT patients who are conditioned with myeloablative regimens often attain high levels of donor chimerism in their lymphoid compartment within a few months of transplant. This often correlates with the ability of alloreactive donor T cells, capable of mediating GvHD, to target residual recipient HSC elements so that the primary source of de novo lymphoid reconstitution will be of donor origin. By the same token, high donor chimerism is also associated with a lower incidence of malignant relapse.

▍CONDITIONING REGIMENS ▍

DOSE-INTENSIVE CHEMOTHERAPY

Many cancers treatable by HSCT exhibit chemotherapy sensitivity, and contemporary regimens produce initial tumor regression in most patients. However, for many patients regression may be partial or temporary, and survival is increased by only a few months or years. Chemotherapy-resistant tumor cells that will lead to subsequent relapse of disease may be present before initial treatment, or may develop by mutation during the period of treatment. However, for many cancers, including the hematological malignancies and certain solid tumors, resistance might be relative rather than absolute, justifying the administration of a dose-intense cycle of chemotherapy with HSC support. In this simplified explanation, the infused HSC are intended only to rescue the patient from the marrow toxicity of the intensive regimen. The usual strategy that has evolved in the treatment of patients is 'debulking' with one or more cycles of conventional chemotherapy, followed by high-dose therapy as a late-intensification regimen. This strategy determines the sensitivity of the disease to chemotherapy;

also, patients who come to transplantation with lower burdens of disease generally achieve a better outcome. Randomized and nonrandomized studies in a number of malignancies such as lymphoma, leukemia, and myeloma demonstrate improved survival of patients who undergo autologous HSCT compared to salvage therapy with lower doses of drugs.

Total body irradiation (TBI) became the primary component of myeloablative conditioning regimens because of its efficacy in the treatment of hematological malignancies, its ability to treat sanctuary sites of disease such as the CNS, and for its immunosuppressive effects that can temper HvG rejection of the donor HSC. TBI is usually combined in sequence with chemotherapy agents such as cyclophosphamide or etoposide. The nonhematopoietic toxicities of TBI are reduced by fractioning the dose over several days, allowing higher total doses. Increasing the total dose of TBI decreases the risk of relapse, but increases the risk of transplant-related complications.[40] Often, these effects are offsetting and event-free survival remains the same. The primary dose-limiting toxicities of TBI include pneumonitis, veno-occlusive disease of the liver, renal impairment, and mucositis.

Busulfan-based regimens were developed as alternatives to TBI for the treatment of patients who had received prior dose-limiting radiotherapy, to avoid the effects of TBI on growth and development in children, and to eliminate the difficulty in scheduling patients to the limited availability of appropriate radiotherapy equipment. Initially, one of the limitations to the use of busulfan was the lack of an intravenous preparation, and wide variation in plasma levels with consequent effects on regimen-related toxicities, such as hepatic veno-occlusive disease, failure of engraftment, and relapse of disease.[41–44] Close monitoring of plasma busulfan levels with dose adjustment reduces the risk of treatment failure, as does the recent availability of an intravenous formulation of this drug. A review of several studies to compare the use of busulfan and TBI found no statistically significant difference in overall or disease-free survival for patients with CML or AML.[45]

The myeloablative conditioning regimens currently used have been tested in dose-escalation studies to achieve the maximal tolerated doses in otherwise healthy patients. Further incremental increases in drug or radiation doses, although reducing the risk of relapse, increase the risk of TRM offsetting any gain. New approaches include the addition of targeted therapies to the conditioning regimen, such as tumor-directed monoclonal antibodies or radioimmunoconjugates that will not increase the toxicity to other organs. Tandem transplantation with the combination of a dose-intense regimen with autologous HSCT followed, after recovery from the immediate regimen-related toxicities, by allogeneic HSCT using a reduced-intensity regimen is a novel approach to combine the benefits of each transplant modality.

Nonmyeloablative regimens have been developed for allograft patients ineligible for myeloablative conditioning because of age or comorbid conditions, based on the concept that GvL responses, rather than high-dose cytoreductive therapy alone, are the key to preventing disease relapse. The primary requirement in developing a reduced-intensity regimen is the need to achieve adequate immunosuppression to permit the development of hematopoietic chimerism, which became feasible with the development of the purine analog family of drugs. A variety of regimens are available, including combinations of fludarabine with melphalan, and fludarabine with busulfan. These regimens can pose less immediate risk of regimen-related toxicities, and open the option of combining them with more aggressive immunotherapy in the form of delayed DLI to mediate a GvL effect. Among the least toxic are regimens that involve a single fraction of TBI. Storb et al.[46] proposed that the

HvG reaction leading to HSC rejection and the GvH reaction could both be modified by an appropriate immunosuppressive regimen administered after transplantation, allowing a reduction in the intensity of the pre-transplant conditioning regimen. This group demonstrated in both canine models and human trials the ability to achieve durable donor cell engraftment with low levels of TBI (2 Gy), if high-concentrations of cyclosporine and MMF were maintained after transplantation. Engraftment success in clinical transplantation was subsequently improved with the addition of the purine analog fludarabine.[47]

■ HSCT FOR INDIVIDUAL DISEASES ■

ACUTE MYELOGENOUS LEUKEMIA (AML)

Most patients with AML will achieve a remission with an initial course of chemotherapy, but almost all will rapidly relapse if post-induction consolidation therapy is not administered. Even with appropriate therapy, the majority of patients (~65%) will relapse within 1–2 years, with the presence of cytogenetic abnormalities and the ability to achieve a CR with the initial course of therapy as predictors for long-term disease control. Numerous studies compared standard consolidation therapy to dose intensification with autologous or allogeneic HSCT. In general, autologous HSCT has not proved more effective than nontransplant intensive consolidation chemotherapy. Allogeneic HSCT had the lowest risk of relapse and, despite the higher transplant-related complications, in at least two major studies patients assigned to allogeneic transplantation achieved a significantly better disease-free survival (DFS) than those assigned to either chemotherapy or autologous HSCT. Allogeneic HSCT using related donors achieves about a 60–70% event-free survival, regardless of cytogenetic changes, and is the treatment of choice for patients with adverse risk cytogenetic findings or leukemia arising from prior chemotherapy or other marrow diseases.[48] In addition, a number of phase II studies of autologous HSCT for AML patients in second or later remission reported survival probabilities of ~35%, which is higher than what would be expected with standard chemotherapy regimens.[49]

MYELODYSPLASTIC SYNDROMES (MDS)

MDS comprise a closely related but heterogeneous group of nonmalignant hematological disorders characterized by a clonal HSC abnormality that engenders variable degrees of cytopenia and frequent evolution to AML. Currently, allogeneic HSCT is the only treatment modality that can achieve long-term control of disease; autologous HSCT is not feasible because of the inability to collect normal HSC from these patients. The best results are seen in patients with earlier-stage disease,[50] complicating the decision to undertake this therapy rather than a watchful waiting approach with transplantation performed at the time of disease progression.

CHRONIC MYELOGENOUS LEUKEMIA (CML)

Allogeneic HSCT is an appropriate treatment for CML with long-term survival rates >80% for younger patients undergoing related donor transplantation within the first year after diagnosis. However, newly developed

HODGKIN'S DISEASE

Many patients with Hodgkin's disease will achieve a durable remission with nontransplant chemotherapy and/or radiation therapy, and algorithms for staging and treatment of this disease are well defined. Dose-intense therapy with autologous HSCT is available to those patients who do not achieve a remission or who relapse after initial therapy, and who will succumb without aggressive therapy. For patients who suffer a relapse after achieving a CR, the prognosis with conventional salvage therapy is directly related to the duration of the initial CR. The outcome for patients whose remission lasted less than 1 year is dismal with standard dose second-line treatments, and these patients are best treated with dose-intense chemotherapy and stem cell rescue. Approximately 40–50% of patients with Hodgkin's disease who suffer a relapse within 1 year will achieve a durable remission after autologous HSCT.

Patients with refractory Hodgkin's disease may achieve durable CR with dose-intense chemotherapy and autologous HSCT. Several studies have demonstrated that this approach can overcome drug resistance in Hodgkin's disease and lead to an overall survival rate of 34–50%.

Allogeneic HSCT is not a first choice for the treatment of relapsed Hodgkin's disease because of the higher transplant-related complications, despite the evidence of an effective GvL effect. With the regimen-related mortality of conventional myeloablative allogeneic HSCT approaching 60% in some reports of dose-intense regimens used to salvage patients after a failed prior autologous transplant, nonmyeloablative approaches are being actively studied as an alternative.[62]

SOLID TUMORS

The skin and colonic mucosa are primary targets of both acute and cGvHD, and this suggests that allogeneic HSCT would be effective in the treatment of cancers of these organs. Yet allogeneic HSCT has not been shown to be effective in the control of these cancers, illustrating the discrimination between target antigens of normal tissues, such as the colonic crypt cells, and antigens expressed by tumors derived from these tissues. With the exception of allogeneic HSCT in the treatment of renal cell cancer, in which a graft-versus-tumor effect is clinically evident in some studies,[63, 64] transplantation in the treatment of solid tumors such as neuroblastoma, Wilms' tumor, and germ cell tumors is limited to autologous HSCT after one or more cycles of dose-intense chemotherapy.

■ FUTURE DIRECTIONS ■

Advances in HLA typing, chemotherapy conditioning regimens and supportive care have greatly reduced the toxicity of both autologous and allogeneic HSCT, allowing older patients (those more likely to suffer from malignant hematological disorders) to receive this potentially curative therapy. Although the diseases treatable by HSCT are characterized by dose sensitivity, currently available dose-intense conditioning regimens have been pushed to maximal tolerable doses. New approaches to the treatment of these malignancies include the addition of therapies that are targeted to the malignancy, such as radioimmunoconjugates that will add minimal toxicity to other organs. The availability of reduced-intensity regimens permits tandem transplantation, using dose-intense therapy with autologous HSCT to achieve maximal tumor cell debulking, followed after recovery from transplant-related toxicities by allogeneic HSCT, using a reduced-intensity regimen to achieve an immunological GvL effect. This approach may be especially effective in the treatment of diseases most sensitive to this immunological benefit of allogeneic HSCT. Finally, the ability to use HSCT as a platform for protein or cellular-based vaccination strategies is conceivable, and is the subject of considerable interest.

■ REFERENCES ■

1. Petersdorf EW, Malkki M. Human leukocyte antigen matching in unrelated donor hematopoietic cell transplantation. Semin Hematol 2005; 42: 76–84.

2. Farag SS, Bacigalupo A, Eapen M, et al. The effect of KIR ligand incompatibility on the outcome of unrelated donor transplantation: a report from the Center for International Blood and Marrow Transplant Research, the European Blood and Marrow Transplant Registry, and the Dutch Registry. Biol Blood Marrow Transplant 2006; 12: 876–884.

3. Petersdorf EW, Malkki M. Genetics of risk factors for graft-versus-host disease. Semin Hematol 2006; 43: 11–23.

4. Wagner JE, Thompson JS, Carter SL, Kernan NA; Unrelated Donor Marrow Transplantation Trial. Effect of graft-versus-host disease prophylaxis on 3-year disease-free survival in recipients of unrelated donor bone marrow (T-cell Depletion Trial): a multi-centre, randomised phase II–III trial. Lancet 2005; 366: 733–741.

5. Glucksberg H, Storb R, Fefer A, et al. Clinical manifestations of graft-versus-host disease in human recipients of marrow from HLA-matched sibling donors. Transplantation 1974; 18: 295–304.

6. Beelen DW, Elmaagacli A, Muller KD, et al. Influence of intestinal bacterial decontamination using metronidazole and ciprofloxacin or ciprofloxacin alone on the development of acute graft-versus-host disease after marrow transplantation in patients with hematologic malignancies: final results and long-term follow-up of an open-label prospective randomized trial. Blood 1999; 93: 3267–3275.

7. Bacigalupo A, Lamparelli T, Bruzzi P, et al. Antithymocyte globulin for graft-versus-host disease prophylaxis in transplants from unrelated donors: 2 randomized studies from Gruppo Italiano Trapianti Midollo Osseo (GITMO). Blood 2001; 98: 2942–2947.

8. Van Lint MT, Uderzo C, Locasciulli A, et al. Early treatment of acute graft-versus-host disease with high- or low-dose 6-methylprednisolone: a multicenter randomized trial from the Italian Group for Bone Marrow Transplantation. Blood 1998; 92: 2288–2293.

9. Cragg L, Blazar BR, Defor T, et al. A randomized trial comparing prednisone with antithymocyte globulin/prednisone as an initial systemic therapy for moderately severe acute graft-versus-host disease. Biol Blood Marrow Transplant 2000; 6: 441–447.

10. Ringden O, Uzunel M, Rasmusson I, et al. Mesenchymal stem cells for treatment of therapy-resistant graft-versus-host disease. Transplantation 2006; 81: 1390–1397.

11. Chao NJ, Chen BJ. Prophylaxis and treatment of acute graft-versus-host disease. Semin Hematol 2006; 43: 32–41.

12. Greinix HT, Volc-Platzer B, Kalhs P, et al. Extracorporeal photochemotherapy in the treatment of severe steroid-refractory acute graft-versus-host disease: a pilot study. Blood 2000; 96: 2426–2431.

13. Holmberg L, Kikuchi K, Gooley TA, et al. Gastrointestinal graft-versus-host disease in recipients of autologous hematopoietic stem cells: incidence, risk factors, and outcome. Biol Blood Marrow Transplant 2006; 12: 226–234.

14. Filipovich AH, Weisdorf D, Pavletic S, et al. National Institutes of Health Consensus Development Project on Criteria for Clinical Trials in Chronic Graft-Versus-Host Disease: I. Diagnosis and staging working group report. Biol Blood Marrow Transplant 2005; 11: 945–956.

15. Lee SJ, Klein JP, Barrett AJ, et al. Severity of chronic graft-versus-host disease: association with treatment-related mortality and relapse. Blood 2002; 100: 406–414.

16. Pavletic SZ, Carter SL, Kernan NA, et al. Influence of T-cell depletion on chronic graft-versus-host disease: results of a multicenter randomized trial in unrelated marrow donor transplantation. Blood 2005; 106: 3308–3313.

17. Pavletic SZ, Martin P, Lee SJ, et al. Measuring therapeutic response in chronic graft-versus-host disease: National Institutes of Health Consensus Development Project on Criteria for Clinical Trials in Chronic Graft-versus-Host Disease: IV. Response Criteria Working Group report. Biol Blood Marrow Transplant 2006; 12: 252–266.

18. Robin M, Guardiola P, Girinsky T, et al. Low-dose thoracoabdominal irradiation for the treatment of refractory chronic graft-versus-host disease. Transplantation 2005; 80: 634–642.

19. Couriel D, Hosing C, Saliba R, et al. Extracorporeal photopheresis for acute and chronic graft-versus-host disease: does it work?. Biol Blood Marrow Transplant 2006; 12: 37–40.

20. Kolb H-J, Schmid C, Barrett AJ, Schendel DJ. Graft-versus-leukemia in allogeneic chimeras. Blood 2004; 103: 767–776.

21. Collins RH Jr, Shpilberg O, Drobyski WR, et al. Donor leukocyte infusions in 140 patients with relapsed malignancy after allogeneic bone marrow transplantation. J Clin Oncol 1997; 15: 433–444.

22. Mackinnon S, Papadopoulos EB, Carabasi MH, et al. Adoptive immunotherapy evaluating escalating doses of donor leukocytes for relapse of chronic myeloid leukemia after bone marrow transplantation: separation of graft-versus-leukemia responses from graft-versus-host disease. Blood 1995; 86: 1261–1268.

23. Patterson AE, Korngold R. Infusion of select leukemia-reactive TCR Vβ+ T cells provides graft-versus-leukemia responses with minimization of graft-versus-host disease following murine hematopoietic stem cell transplantation. Biol Blood Marrow Transplant 2001; 7: 187–196.

24. Choudhury A, Gajewski JL, Liang JC, et al. Use of leukemic dendritic cells for the generation of antileukemic cellular cytotoxicity against Philadelphia chromosome-positive chronic myelogenous leukemia. Blood 1997; 89: 1133–1142.

25. Morisaki T, Matsumoto K, Onishi H, et al. Dendritic cell-based combined immunotherapy with autologous tumor-pulsed dendritic cell vaccine and activated T cells for cancer patients: rationale, current progress, and perspectives. Hum Cell 2003; 16: 175–182.

26. Leitch HA, Connors JM. Vaccine therapy for nonHodgkin's lymphoma and other B-cell malignancies. Curr Opin Invest Drugs 2005; 6: 597–604.

27. Stem Cell Trialists Collaborative Group. Allogeneic peripheral blood stem-cell compared with bone marrow transplantation in the management of hematologic malignancies: an individual patient data meta-analysis of nine randomized trials. J Clin Oncol 2005; 23: 5074–5087.

28. Endo T, Sato N, Koizumi K, et al. A preliminary analysis of the balance between Th1 and Th2 cells after CD34+ cell-selected autologous PBSC transplantation. Cytotherapy 2004; 6: 337–343.

29. Vasconcelos ZF, Santos BM, Costa ES, et al. T-lymphocyte function from peripheral blood stem-cell donors is inhibited by activated granulocytes. Cytotherapy 2003; 5: 336–345.

30. Rocha V, Gluckman E; Eurocord and European Blood and Marrow Transplant Group. Clinical use of umbilical cord blood hematopoietic stem cells. Biol Blood Marrow Transplant 2006; 12: 34–41.

31. Barker JN, Weisdorf DJ, DeFor TE, et al. Transplantation of 2 partially HLA-matched umbilical cord blood units to enhance engraftment in adults with hematologic malignancy. Blood 2005; 105: 1343–1347.

32. Shpall EJ, Quinones R, Giller R, et al. Transplantation of ex vivo expanded cord blood. Biol Blood Marrow Transplant 2002; 8: 368–376.

33. Rowley SD, Zuehlsdorf M, Braine HG, et al. CFU-GM content of bone marrow graft correlates with time to hematologic reconstitution following autologous bone marrow transplantation with 4-hydroperoxycyclophosphamide purged bone marrow. Blood 1987; 70: 271–275.

34. Weaver CH, Hazelton B, Birch R, et al. An analysis of engraftment kinetics as a function of the CD34 content of peripheral blood progenitor cell collections in 692 patients after the administration of myeloablative chemotherapy. Blood 1995; 86: 3961–3969.

35. Offner F, Schoch G, Fisher LD, et al. Mortality hazard functions as related to neutropenia at different times after marrow transplantation. Blood 1996; 88: 4058–4062.

36. Dominietto A, Lamparelli T, Raiola AM, et al. Transplant-related mortality and long-term graft function are significantly influenced by cell dose in patients undergoing allogeneic marrow transplantation. Blood 2002; 100: 3930–3934.

37. Ringden O, Barrett AJ, Zhang MJ, et al. Decreased treatment failure in recipients of HLA-identical bone marrow or peripheral blood stem cell transplants with high CD34 cell doses. Br J Haematol 2003; 121: 874–885.

38. Lonial S, Hicks M, Rosenthal H, et al. A randomized trial comparing the combination of granulocyte-macrophage colony-stimulating factor plus granulocyte colony-stimulating factor versus granulocyte colony-stimulating factor for mobilization of dendritic cell subsets in hematopoietic progenitor cell products. Biol Blood Marrow Transplant 2004; 10: 848–857.

39. Sullivan KM, Kopecky KJ, Jocom J, et al. Immunomodulatory and antimicrobial efficacy of intravenous immunoglobulin in bone marrow transplantation. N Engl J Med 1990; 323: 705–712.

40. Demirer T, Petersen FB, Appelbaum FR, et al. Allogeneic marrow transplantation following cyclophosphamide and escalating doses of hyperfractionated total body irradiation in patients with advanced lymphoid malignancies: a Phase I/II trial. Int J Radiat Oncol Biol Phys 1995; 32: 1103–1109.

41. Groshow LB. Busulfan disposition. The role of therapeutic monitoring in bone marrow transplantation induction regimens. Semin Oncol 1993; 20: 18–25.

42. Slattery JT, Sanders JE, Buckner CD, et al. Graft-rejection and toxicity following bone marrow transplantation in relation to busulfan pharmacokinetics. Bone Marrow Transplant 1995; 16: 31–42.

Table 83.1 Hematopoietic stem cell transplantation for primary immune deficiencies in Europe 1968–2004 (Data from the European SCETIDE Registry, courtesy of Paul Landais and Alain Fischer)

Type of Immunodeficiency	Patients with genotypically identical related donor	Patients with phenotypically identical related donor	Patients with mismatched related donor	Patients with matched unrelated donor	Total number of patients
SCID	126	61	367	58	612
Omenn's syndrome	14	9	29	10	62
MHC class II deficiency	20	10	26	5	61
PNP deficiency	2	1	1	1	5
CD40L deficiency	9	0	1	21	31
Other forms of CID	35	7	44	29	115
Di George syndrome	1	0	0	1	2
Other T-cell deficiencies	5	1	5	4	15
WAS	45	8	47	50	150
FHL	26	6	37	19	88
XLP	3	0	1	7	11
Chediak–Higashi syndrome	10	5	3	4	22
Griscelli syndrome	6	2	1	1	10
Agranulocytosis	3	0	2	3	3
CGD	25	0	0	5	30
LAD	13	2	16	1	32
IFN-γ receptor deficiency	2	1	1	0	4
Other phagocytic disorders	2	0	0	1	3
All defects	347	113	581	220	1261

SCID, severe combined immunodeficiency; MHC, major histocompatibility complex; PNP, purine nucleoside phosphorylase; CID, combined immune deficiency; WAS, Wiskott–Aldrich syndrome; FHL, familial hemophagocytic lymphohistiocytosis; XLP, X-linked lymphoproliferative disease; CGD, chronic granulomatous disease; LAD, leukocyte adhesion deficiency.

HSCT from a haploidentical donor

Unfortunately, the option of related HLA-identical HSCT is limited to only a minority of patients. When no such donor is available, stem cell transplantation from a haploidentical parent should be considered, particularly in infants with SCID. The rationale of haploidentical HSCT is based on the ability of donor-derived stem cells to repopulate the recipient's vestigial thymus and give rise to fully mature T lymphocytes. Indeed, this is a life-saving procedure which has been successfully applied to several hundreds of infants with SCID.[2, 3] However, it requires careful removal of T lymphocytes from the graft, as these would otherwise cause severe GvHD. Several methods are now available to attain T-cell depletion.[3]

Soybean lectin allows agglutination of the majority of mature marrow cells that can be removed by sedimentation. This step is followed by further depletion of T lymphocytes by rosetting with sheep erythrocytes (E-rosetting technique) and density gradient centrifugation. Importantly, T-cell depletion by soybean lectin agglutination and E-rosetting maintains all immature marrow cells in the final preparation. In general, the procedure requires a relatively large collection (approximately 1 L) of bone marrow from the donor.

T-cell depletion can also be achieved by incubation of the marrow with monoclonal antibodies to T lymphocytes plus complement. Campath-1G, Leu 1 and other monoclonal antibodies have been used for this purpose, but the degree of T-cell depletion that is achieved is often less effective than with soybean lectin and E-rosetting, possibly because of modulation of antigen expression on the surface of T lymphocytes. Consequently, there is a higher probability that GvHD may develop.

Positive selection of CD34+ cells using monoclonal antibody affinity columns or immunomagnetic beads has been widely used in recent years. However, this approach removes immature CD34− cells and other cells (especially stromal marrow cells) that may facilitate stem cell engraftment. Following the recognition that CD133 is expressed on primitive

KEY CONCEPTS

SOURCES OF STEM CELLS AND SELECTION OF DONORS FOR HEMATOPOIETIC STEM CELL TRANSPLANTATION IN PRIMARY IMMUNODEFICIENCIES

>> Sources of hematopoietic stem cells for transplantation include bone marrow, peripheral blood, and cord blood.

>> If the donor is a genotypically HLA-identical sibling, unmanipulated bone marrow is used as source of stem cells.

>> Whenever the donor is HLA-mismatched to the recipient, T-cell depletion must be performed to eliminate mature T lymphocytes from the graft. Methods for T-cell depletion of the bone marrow include:

  Use of soybean lectin agglutination (± E-rosetting)

  Depletion with monoclonal antibodies plus complement

  Positive selection of stem cells.

>> Cord blood is a rich source of stem cells. However, the volume of cord blood is limited, so that its use is mainly restricted to young patients.

>> The number of volunteers included in Bone Marrow Donor Registries is expanding. Consequently, there is a continuous increase in the number of matched unrelated donor (MUD) transplantations performed for patients with primary immunodeficiencies.

>> Whenever unrelated cord blood or MUD stem cells are used, conditioning regimen is usually given to the recipient prior to transplantation, in order to facilitate engraftment of donor stem cells.

>> Therapeutic options for patients with SCID include transplantation from HLA-genotypically identical donor, or from mismatched related donors. Recently, transplant from MUD has also been successfully used in SCID infants under stable conditions.

>> For other forms of primary immunodeficiencies, whenever no related HLA-identical donor is available, search for a MUD or an unrelated cord blood should be started, as the results of such transplants are better than from related mismatched donors.

Table 83.2 Sources of hematopoietic stem cells for transplantation

HSCT from a related donor
Bone marrow from an HLA-genotypically identical sibling
Bone marrow from an HLA-phenotypically identical family member
Bone marrow from a haploidentical parent
  T cell-depleted by negative selection with soybean lectin agglutination/SRBC
  T cell-depleted by negative selection with monoclonal antibodies
  Positive selection of CD34+ cells (± CD133+ cells)

HSCT from a matched unrelated donor
Unmanipulated bone marrow
T cell-depleted bone marrow by means of positive selection of CD34+/CD133+ cells
Positively selected peripheral blood CD34+ cells

HSCT from unmanipulated related or unrelated cord blood

In utero haploidentical HSCT

The identification of a growing number of immunodeficiency-causing genes has resulted in continuous improvement in prenatal diagnosis, which can now be accomplished on chorionic villi DNA at 10–11 weeks of gestation in most cases of severe immunodeficiency. This has prompted a prenatal transplantation of parental positively-selected CD34+ stem cells in fetuses affected with SCID. This novel strategy has overcome previous largely unsatisfactory experience with fetal liver and other stem cells.

The technique used for in utero HSCT includes injection of purified CD34+ cells into the fetal peritoneum under ultrasound guidance.

The rationale underlying in utero HSCT includes a lower risk of graft rejection due to decreased fetal immunocompetence (although this consideration is not relevant in the case of fetuses with SCID); a presumed induction of tolerance to paternal antigens (which might favor successful engraftment after postnatal transplantation from the same donor); the predicted competition between donor and autologous stem cells at a time when several empty niches should be available for stem cell engraftment; the potential ability to provide pre-emptive treatment (thus reducing the risk of postnatal infection); and the lower cost of the procedure, which does not require prolonged hospitalization. On the other hand, in utero HSCT exposes to the potential risks of fetal loss and of GvHD. Finally, if maternal T cells had engrafted into the fetus with SCID, transplantation of paternal CD34+ cells might cause graft-versus-graft reaction.

In utero HSCT has been attempted in several infants with severe immunodeficiencies, most notably SCID.[5] Five of these transplants have been performed at the authors' institution. All three cases with B+ SCID (two of which were due to γc deficiency and one to IL7Rα deficiency) have survived with evidence of T-cell reconstitution; of the two cases with B− SCID, one has failed to achieve immune reconstitution, in spite of two additional boosting transplants from the same donor (the father) after birth. This patient eventually died of B-cell lymphoproliferative disease (BLPD) after a MUD HSCT. In the fifth patient (with B− SCID due to RAG2 mutation), thymopoiesis has rapidly declined and the patient remains profoundly lymphopenic. Although the overall results of the procedure appear to be

hematopoietic progenitors, positive selection of CD133+ cells with immunomagnetic beads has also been proposed.

Selection of the best donor is another important aspect of T cell-depleted haploidentical HSCT for SCID. In general, the donor is represented by one of the parents, as the volume of bone marrow that can be collected is much higher than it would be in case a haploidentical sibling served as donor. It is also important to recognize that maternal T-cell engraftment is a common finding in infants with SCID. In a survey of 121 SCID patients, Müller et al.[4] identified 48 cases (39.7%) with maternally derived T lymphocytes. In such cases, T cell-depleted HSCT should be performed using the mother as donor if possible, as transplantation from the father might cause graft-versus-graft reaction.

influenced by the nature of the underlying disease, the use of in utero HSCT for SCID is now largely unjustified, in consideration of the fact that early postnatal HSCT for SCID leads to long-term survival in 97% of cases.[3, 6] Furthermore, the observation that engraftment is restricted only to cell lineages that were missing in the affected fetus is a strong argument against the use of in utero HSCT for treatment of PID other than SCID.

HSCT from matched unrelated donors

Since the first successful experience with this technique, performed in 1977 in an infant with SCID,[7] HSCT from MUD has been increasingly used to treat severe primary immunodeficiencies. In particular, use of MUD HSCT has been shown to be more effective than T cell-depleted HSCT in patients with immunodeficiencies other than SCID.[2] More recently, it has been successfully used also in infants with SCID.[8, 9]

Transplantation from MUD has been facilitated by the increasing number of volunteer donors included in registries worldwide. In addition, advances in the quality of the techniques used for HLA typing permits optimization of the identification of a MUD, and a reduction in the risk of GvHD. As of April 2006, more than 10 million donors were included in the Bone Marrow Donors Worldwide (BMDW) registry. At present, it takes 3–4 months on average to identify a MUD. However, the probability of finding a suitable donor is lower for selected ethnic or racial groups that are poorly represented among volunteer donors.

Importantly, MUD HSCT requires the use of a preparative chemotherapy regimen in the recipient (even in the case of SCID) and graft-versus-host prophylaxis (because of more likely disparity between donor and recipient at minor histocompatibility loci), whereas neither one is necessary for related HLA-identical HSCT in SCID infants.

HSCT using unmanipulated cord blood

As opposed to MUD, stored cord blood is readily available as a source of stem cells for transplantation. In addition, it appears that the risk of GvHD is lower when using cord blood than with MUD, so that some HLA disparity with the recipient can be tolerated. On the other hand, a major limitation of cord blood remains the number of cells contained in any defined unit. However, this is not usually a problem for transplants performed in infants with SCID or other severe forms of immunodeficiency, owing to the low weight of the recipient. Indeed, unrelated umbilical cord stem cell transplantation has been successfully used in several patients with severe primary immune deficiencies.[2, 3, 9, 10] In practice, an unrelated hematopoietic stem cell donor should be simultaneously searched for in cord blood banks and in bone marrow donor registries for patients lacking an HLA-identical sibling hematopoietic stem cell donor. The option of performing cord blood transplants should be based on the urgency of the transplant, the cell dose required, and the number of HLA disparities. Like HSCT from MUD, transplantation using unrelated cord blood usually requires pre-transplant conditioning and GvHD prophylaxis, irrespective of the underlying disease.

COMPLICATIONS OF HEMATOPOIETIC STEM CELL TRANSPLANTATION

A variety of complications may compromise the success of HSCT. Among these, incompatibility between donor and recipient may lead to graft rejection by the host immune system or, alternatively, to GvHD,

caused by alloreactivity of donor-derived lymphocytes to the recipient's cells. Furthermore, the use of a conditioning regimen is often responsible for toxicity that may affect several organs. In addition, myeloablative regimens cause anemia, thrombocytopenia, and leukopenia. Consequently, supportive treatment with red blood cell and platelet transfusions is necessary during the aplastic phase. Finally, the leukopenia may expose to an increased risk of infections. The frequency and severity of these complications depend on the type of transplant, the possible use of a conditioning regimen, and specific considerations related to the underlying disorder and to the clinical status of the recipient prior to transplantation.

Graft rejection

Graft rejection reflects the presence of immunocompetent cells in the host that specifically recognize and react to donor-derived stem cells. Several factors influence the likelihood of graft rejection, in particular (a) the degree of immunocompetence of the host; (b) the degree of HLA disparity between donor and recipient; (c) the number of stem cells infused; (d) the type of conditioning regimen used; and (e) the possible pre-sensitization of the host to donor histocompatibility antigens.

In the case of infants with SCID, graft rejection is unlikely because of the profound immunodeficiency that characterizes these conditions. Conversely, in other forms of primary immunodeficiency there is sufficient immune function in the host to allow for rejection of donor-derived stem cells, unless an appropriate conditioning regimen is used prior to HSCT.

In children, the most commonly used preparative regimen consists of busulfan and cyclophosphamide, with or without the addition of anti-thymocyte globulin (ATG). In some forms of congenital immunodeficiencies, such as phagocytic or hemophagocytic cell disorders, a more aggressive conditioning regimen is often used that includes additional drugs.

On the other hand, infants with pre-existing organ damage are highly exposed to the toxic effects of drugs conventionally used in the conditioning regimen. In these cases, nonmyeloablative regimens (e.g., the association of fludarabine and melphalan) have often been preferred.[11] A more vigorous GvHD prophylaxis is often necessary if nonmyeloablative conditioning is used, because of the higher risk of GvHD.

Acute graft-versus-host disease

Acute GvHD (aGvHD) is the result of alloreactivity of donor-derived T lymphocytes to the recipient's antigens, and is one of the most severe complications of HSCT. It may occur as early as 1 week after HSCT and is potentially fatal. Clinical manifestations of aGvHD include high-grade fever, maculopapular skin rash (that tends to be confluent), diarrhea, and liver abnormalities (hepatomegaly, elevated liver enzymes, increased levels of conjugated bilirubin).[12] The disease may progress to severe skin manifestations, with exfoliative dermatitis, and significant liver and gut damage (with intractable watery diarrhea, protein-losing enteropathy, and abdominal pain). In the most severe cases, leakage of intravascular fluids into the interstitium (so-called 'third space filling'), leads to generalized edema. Bone marrow aplasia, and a high susceptibility to infections (including reactivation of herpes virus infections) are also often observed in severe aGvHD. The severity of aGvHD is evaluated according to grading (Table 83.3). The major risk factors for aGvHD include HLA mismatch between donor and recipient; older age of the recipient at HSCT; gender mismatch; or a prior herpes virus infection.[12] However, aGvHD may also be observed following related HLA-identical HSCT, particularly when conditioning regimen is used. Finally, transfusion-associated aGvHD is a very severe complication after HSCT that can be effectively preventing by using irradiated (150–300 Gy) and filtered blood derivatives.

Chronic graft-versus-host disease

GvHD is defined as chronic (cGvHD) if symptoms persist or appear after 100 days since the time of transplantation. The clinical manifestations of cGvHD include skin changes (scleroderma-like lesions, hyperpigmentation, hyperkeratosis, skin atrophy, ulcerations), tissue fibrosis and limitation of joint motility, fibrosis of exocrine glands ('sicca syndrome'), fibrosis of lungs and liver, increased susceptibility to infections, immune dysregulation and autoimmunity. Consequently, cGvHD poses a major burden on the patient's quality of life, and may even be fatal.

Although the incidence of cGvHD is lower in children than in adults treated by allogeneic HSCT, the risk factors and the spectrum of clinical manifestations are similar.[13]

Acute GvHD represents a major risk factor for cGvHD, yet cGvHD may be observed even without a preceding aGvHD, and it does not represent merely the continuation of aGvHD, when present. Older age of the recipient at HSCT, transplantation from a multiparous female

Table 83.3 Grading of acute GvHD

Grade 1: 1+ to 2+ skin rash, without involvement of the gut, and with absent or minimal (no more than 1+) liver involvement
Grade 2: 1+ to 3+ skin rash, with either 1+ to 2+ gut involvement and/or 1+ to 2+ liver involvement. Fever is often observed
Grade 3: 2+ to 4+ skin rash, with 2+ to 4+ gut involvement with or without 2+ to 4+ liver involvement. High-grade fever and deterioration of general conditions are also observed
Grade 4: as in grade 3, but with severe deterioration of the general conditions

donor into a male recipient (with reactivity to Y chromosome-associated antigens), and incompatibility at minor histocompatibility loci represent additional risk factors for cGvHD.[13] Furthermore, it appears that use of peripheral blood stem cells carries an increased risk of cGvHD compared to the use of bone marrow stem cells.

Prevention of GvHD

Prevention is the most effective approach to GvHD, and the use of a fully matched donor represents the best method of prevention. Alternatively, if a related HLA-mismatched donor is used for transplantation, it is essential that the graft is vigorously T-cell depleted.

Whenever a conditioning regimen is used in the transplantation protocol, pharmacological prophylaxis of GvHD must also be included, even in the case of HSCT from a related HLA-identical donor. The most commonly used approaches to prevent GvHD include cyclosporine A daily for 6 months, or methotrexate (15 mg/m^2 on the first day after HSCT, and then 10 mg/m^2 at days 3, 6, and 11 after transplant), or a combination of the two. ATG is also commonly used to prevent GvHD.

Attempts to prevent cGvHD have been less satisfactory. In particular, the use of prolonged immunosuppression after transplant does not reduce the incidence of cGvHD.

Treatment of GvHD

Once GvHD has developed, treatment is based mainly on the use of immunosuppressive drugs, including steroids, ATG, mycophenolate mofetil, cyclosporine A, and a variety of monoclonal antibodies directed to human T-lymphocyte antigens (e.g., anti-CD3) or to Th1-type cytokines (e.g., anti-TNF-α) and cytokine receptors (anti-CD25, daclizumab). These drugs are usually effective for mild and moderate forms of aGvHD, but their efficacy in severe aGvHD is limited.

Treatment of cGvHD is also based on immunosuppression, but with limited efficacy.[13] Topical steroids and calcineurin inhibitors may alleviate mucosal and skin symptoms. Systemic steroids have been shown to improve survival, but at the risk of significant adverse effects. Ursodeoxycholic acid may be useful in cGvHD with significant liver involvement. Extracorporeal photopheresis can be used, with the aim of inducing tolerance; typically, its benefits, if present, are delayed until 2–3 months after the start of treatment. The use of hydroxichloroquine, mycophenolate mofetil, anti-TNF-α monoclonal antibody, and etanercept (a recombinant form of soluble TNF receptor) remains at present investigational.

An interesting approach under consideration is based on the adoptive transfer of regulatory T cells (Treg), which may improve tolerance and prevent autoimmune responses.

Infections

Infections are one of the major complications following HSCT. Patients with severe primary immunodeficiency are intrinsically highly susceptible to infection. For infants with SCID and other forms of combined immunodeficiency, viral and opportunistic infections may develop prior to transplantation and are one of the factors that adversely affect the outcome of HSCT itself.[2] Similarly, treatment-refractory bacterial – and especially fungal – infections may compromise survival after HSCT in children with phagocytic disorders.[14] Regardless of the type of underlying primary immunodeficiency, T cell-depleted HSCT carries a high risk of infections because of the longer time needed to achieve immune reconstitution. Furthermore, the use of a pre-transplant conditioning regimen resulting in myeloablation and immunosuppression, and GvHD prophylaxis, contributes to the increased susceptibility to infections after HSCT.

Strict isolation of the patient during and after HSCT, and prophylactic administration of antibiotics, have been associated with a better survival rate, particularly after related HLA-mismatched transplantation for SCID.[2] In spite of this, infections remain the major cause of death. Challenging viruses in infants with SCID include adenovirus, cytomegalovirus (CMV), parainfluenzae III virus, and Epstein–Barr virus (EBV), although several drugs (e.g., acyclovir, ganciclovir, foscarnet, cidofovir) are now available that give good results especially against CMV.[15] Filtering of blood derivatives removes leukocytes and thus reduces the risk of transfusion-associated infections, such as CMV. Viral infection after HSCT may cause interstitial pneumonia, enteritis, and also encephalitis. EBV may also cause B-cell lymphoproliferative disease (BLPD), especially after T cell-depleted HLA-mismatched transplantation, in particular in patients with Wiskott–Aldrich syndrome (WAS). This complication is now often treated successfully with *in vivo* administration of anti-CD20 monoclonal antibody (rituximab).

Pneumocystis jiroveci is a common cause of pneumonia in severely immunocompromised patients. Treatment is based on intravenous co-trimoxazole (20 mg/kg/day).

Aspergillus infection is a severe complication in patients with chronic granulomatous disease (CGD) and in profoundly neutropenic patients.[14] Voriconazole offers some advantage over liposomal amphotericin B for the treatment of invasive aspergillosis, whereas prophylactic itraconazole reduces the incidence of fungal infections in patients with CGD prior to transplantation.

Bacterial infections are usually amenable to successful treatment, if the pathogen is identified and appropriate and aggressive use of antibiotics is initiated. Prophylactic administration of immunoglobulins following HSCT contributes to reduce the frequency and severity of infections.

Finally, the clinical manifestations of the infection tend to be more severe when initial signs of immune reconstitution appear, as the latter facilitates the development of inflammatory reactions both at the site of infection and systemically.

Toxicity related to conditioning regimen

Chemotherapeutic agents that are used in the conditioning regimen of HSCT are often a cause of significant toxicity. In particular, radiomimetic drugs such as busulfan may cause lung damage, which is often difficult to distinguish from pulmonary infection.

Chemotherapeutic drugs that damage the liver vascular endothelium may cause veno-occlusive disease (VOD), which is marked clinically by painful hepatomegaly, jaundice, ascites, fluid retention, and weight gain, and may ultimately result in fatal multiorgan failure (MOF). Defibrotide and recombinant tissue plasminogen activator (rTPA) are effective in the treatment of VOD.[16, 17]

Pre-transplant conditioning may also lead to hormonal disturbances. Early complications include inappropriate secretion of anti-diuretic hormone, especially when cyclophosphamide is included in the conditioning regimen. Long-term hormonal complications are more common when total body irradiation (TBI) is used. However, cyclophosphamide may cause delayed puberty or sterility, and thyroid dysfunction is frequently observed, even in patients who have not received TBI. In contrast, effects on final height are not significant when regimens other than TBI are used.

■ HSCT FOR THE TREATMENT OF PRIMARY IMMUNODEFICIENCY DISORDERS ■

In 1968, the first successful experience with HLA-identical HSCT in SCID was reported.[1] Shortly thereafter, partial success was achieved also with HSCT in a child with WAS.[18] Since then, over 1300 transplants have been performed in patients with primary immunodeficiencies, most of whom were children with SCID.[2, 3] The increasing number of transplants over the years reflects the improved outcome of the procedure as a result of advances in supportive and critical care before and after HSCT, as well as of increasingly improved strategies for T-cell depletion applied for related HLA-mismatched HSCT, and of the greater availability of MUD and cord blood for transplantation.

HSCT FOR SCID

General considerations

SCID is a medical emergency and is uniformly fatal unless diagnosed promptly and treated successfully. With few exceptions, in which alternative strategies (gene therapy, enzyme replacement therapy) can be used, allogeneic HSCT represents the only and most effective form of treatment (i.e., cure) for these disorders.

SCIDs are also a unique situation in which the virtual lack of T lymphocytes strongly impairs the ability of the recipient to reject the graft. Consequently, immune suppression is not required in these patients. Furthermore, no conditioning regimen is necessary for infants with SCID who have a related HLA-identical donor. Some transplant centers in the USA adopt the same policy also for T cell-depleted mismatched HSCT, whereas such transplants in Europe are usually performed with use of a preparative regimen, unless the patient's conditions are so severe as not to allow the use of chemotherapeutic drugs. Avoiding the use of

CLINICAL PEARLS

CONSIDERATIONS OF STEM CELL TRANSPLANTATION UNIQUE TO SCID

>> Patients with SCID are strongly impaired in their ability to reject allogenic cells, including stem cells. Therefore, no chemotherapy is required in these patients in order to achieve T-cell reconstitution following stem cell transplantation.

>> The quality and the kinetics of T-cell reconstitution following stem cell transplantation depend on the type of transplant. If unmanipulated bone marrow from genotypically HLA-identical related donor is used, mature T cells contained in the graft expand as early as 2 weeks after transplantation and provide a rapid source of immune competence. Following unmanipulated MUD transplantation, however, drugs used in conditioning regimen decrease the degree of early expansion of donor-derived T cells.

>> Appearance of naïve T cells occurs only at 3 months or more after transplantation, regardless of the degree of HLA-matching between donor and recipient. Consequently, following haploidentical transplantation there is a prolonged period during which the recipient remains lymphopenic and at high risk of infections.

>> In the absence of pre-transplant conditioning, following haploidentical transplantation for SCID, engraftment is usually restricted to T (and sometimes NK) lymphocytes. This may cause persistent B-cell dysfunction.

>> Patients with NK+ SCID may show some ability to reject stem cells from HLA-mismatched donors. For these reasons, many centers (particularly in Europe) include pre-transplant conditioning for haploidentical, MUD, or unrelated cord blood transplantation for SCID

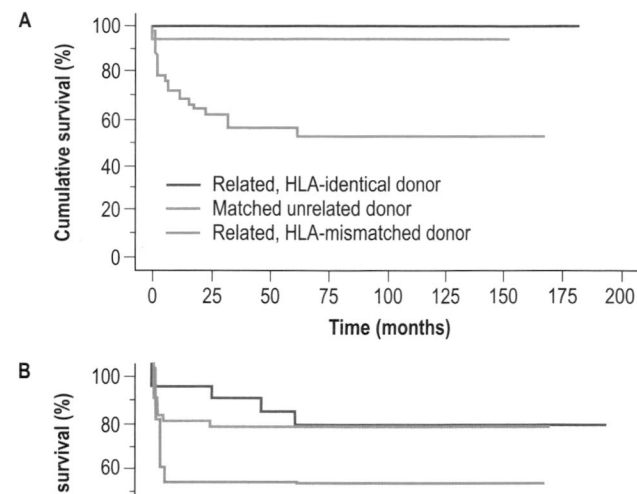

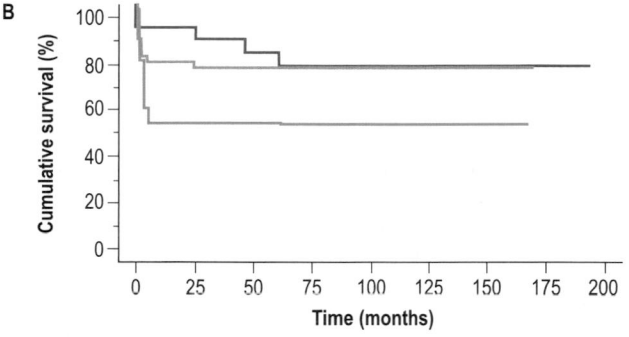

Fig. 83.1 Kaplan–Meyer survival curve for 148 consecutive children with primary immunodeficiency who have received hematopoietic stem cell transplantation (HSCT) at the authors' institution. (**A**) survival after HSCT in 69 infants with SCID, 12 of whom have received related HLA-identical HSCT, 41 a mismatched related transplant, and 16 a MUD HSCT. (**B**) Survival after HSCT in 79 children with immunodeficiency other than SCID. Of these patients, 23 have received related HLA-identical HSCT, 13 a mismatched related HSCT, and 43 a MUD HSCT

conditioning regimens eliminates the risk of drug-related toxicity, and reduces the chance of developing GvHD. On the other hand, the reason why European centers tend to use conditioning regimens prior to mismatched or MUD HSCT for SCID is the resistance to engraftment that may be observed, particularly in SCID with residual autologous NK lymphocytes. Furthermore, unconditioned mismatched related HSCT has been shown to lead to split chimerism, which may affect the quality of immune reconstitution.

Survival following HSCT for SCID

The two largest series of SCID patients treated by HSCT in Europe and at a single center in the USA include 475 and 138 cases, respectively.[2, 3] In the European study, which includes transplants performed from 1968 to 1999, 153 patients had received HSCT from a genotypically ($n = 104$) or phenotypically ($n = 49$) identical related donor, with an overall survival rate of 77%. This figure is clearly superior to the 54% survival rate observed among 294 patients who had received related HLA-mismatched HSCT. Finally, in this report only 28 patients had received HSCT from a MUD, and 63% were alive.[2] At the authors' institution, among 69 infants with SCID treated by HSCT, overall survival rates following related HLA-identical, MUD, and T cell-depleted haploidentical HSCT

were 100%, 94%, and 52%, respectively (Fig. 83.1A). In the most recent report from Buckley and collaborators,[3] the overall survival rate after HSCT for SCID was 78%. In particular, all 16 recipients of related HLA-identical HSCT were reported to be alive, as were 91 of 122 (75%) recipients of T cell-depleted related HLA-mismatched HSCT.

Survival after HSCT for SCID has improved over the years,[2] reflecting more effective treatment and prevention of disease-related and transplantation-associated complications, such as infections and GvHD. In particular, current survival rate after HSCT from HLA-identical related donors is over 90%, whereas survival after HSCT from related HLA-mismatched donors has improved from 35% in transplants performed up to 1985 to 75% in those performed between 1996 and 1999.[2]

Several factors influence survival after HSCT for SCID. In particular, younger age at transplantation leads to superior survival. Among 38 infants who were treated by Buckley and collaborators before 3.5 months of age, 37 (97%) have survived.[3, 6, 19] Importantly, the vast majority of these infants received T cell-depleted HLA-mismatched HSCT from a parent, without any conditioning or GvHD prophylaxis. In Europe, among infants with SCID who received HLA-identical transplantation, survival was clearly better when HSCT was performed at less than 6 months of age (85% survival rate) than at 12 months or more (survival rate 53%).[2]

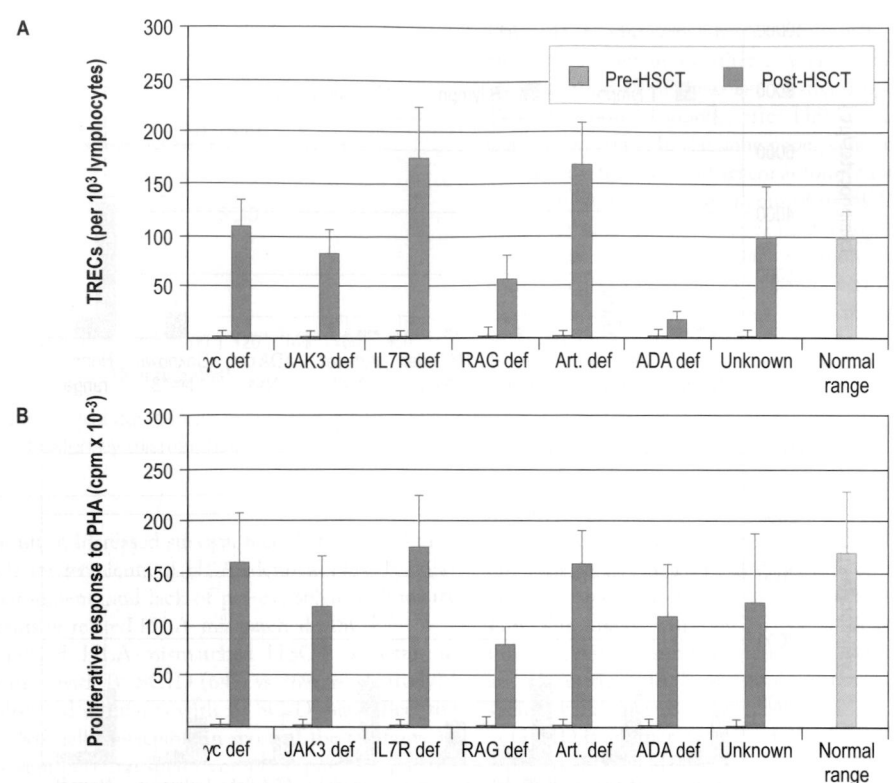

Fig. 83.4 Number of TRECs (**A**) and *in vitro* proliferative response to phytohemagglutinin (PHA) (**B**) before transplantation and at the last follow-up after transplantation in a series of 42 SCID infants treated at the authors' institution, according to the type of SCID.

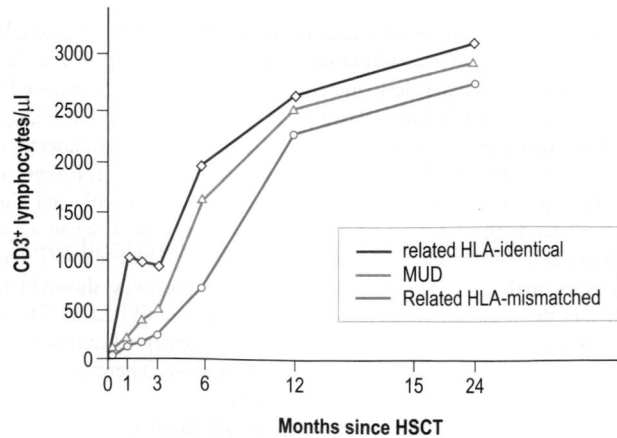

Fig. 83.5 Kinetics of CD3+ T lymphocytes reconstitution in 48 SCID infants following HLA-identical (*n* = 12), MUD (*n* = 15) or haploidentical (*n* = 21) HSCT, performed at the authors' institution. Geometric mean CD3+ T-cell counts are shown.

Quantification of TRECs sequentially after HSCT is a solid approach to assess engraftment of bona fide stem cells and to monitor the persistence of immunity. It has been shown that levels of TRECs tend to decline by 10 years after unconditioned HSCT,[24] when oligoclonal representation of the T-cell repertoire appears, particularly within CD8 T lymphocytes.[23] This decline of thymic function in SCID recipients of HSCT is more rapid than what is observed in normal children. The reasons for this difference are not clear. It is possible that the SCID thymus is not able to sustain active thymopoiesis for as long as a normal thymus. Alternatively, a low dose of infused stem cells, HLA incompatibility between donor and recipient, and GvHD may also contribute to the observed accelerated thymic involution after HSCT. Even if it is not necessary to provide T-cell reconstitution in SCID, the prior use of chemotherapy might facilitate engraftment of stem cells and thus sustain long-term immune reconstitution. However, no studies have compared long-term thymopoiesis in myeloablated MUD HSCT versus unconditioned related HLA-identical HSCT.

In any case, this late decline of T cell-mediated immunity after HSCT is not negligible. Data from the European registry indicate that at the time of last follow-up as many as 16% of recipients of HLA-identical HSCT and 18% of recipients of haploidentical HSCT had a T-cell immunodeficiency (defined as fewer than 1000 T lymphocytes/μL).[2]

Reconstitution of B- and NK-cell immunity

In contrast to what was observed for T lymphocytes, the engraftment of B cells after HSCT for SCID is often problematic and may require 2 years or more to develop.[3] In their series, Buckley and colleagues[19] report that only six of 12 recipients of HLA-identical bone marrow, and 21 of 76 patients treated by unconditioned T cell-depleted haploidentical transplant had evidence of donor-derived B lymphocytes; overall, 62 of 102 survivors were requiring intravenous immunoglobulins. Booster transplants have been used to overcome these problems; 21 of 33 patients who received such boosters at Buckley's institution were reported to be alive, and most of them normalized or improved their immune function.[3] In Europe, the use of pre-transplant conditioning regimens has been advocated in haploidentical HSCT with the goal of facilitating engraftment of stem cells and hence also of B lymphocytes. Among 28 infants with B⁺ SCID treated by HSCT at the authors' institution, all those ($n=11$) who did not receive conditioning failed to achieve engraftment of donor B cells; on the other hand, 12 of 17 of those who received pre-transplant chemotherapy had evidence of B-cell engraftment.

The use of a conditioning regimen is particularly important to achieve B-cell function in patients with B⁻ SCID treated by haploidentical HSCT. In a report from the European series, none of the patients with B⁻ SCID who received unconditioned haploidentical HSCT developed normal B-cell function.[20] In patients with B⁺ SCID, the difficulty of achieving B-cell engraftment after unconditioned HLA-identical HSCT may reflect competition between host and donor early B-cell precursors.[25]

Finally, attainment of a normal B-cell function may also depend on the nature of the genetic defect, as shown by the fact that among infants with B⁺ SCID, those who have an *IL7RA* gene defect usually develop normal B-cell immunity after HSCT even if no donor-derived B cells are present, whereas patients with γc or JAK3 deficiency (both of which compromise B-cell function) often remain dependent on immunoglobulin substitution therapy if engraftment of donor-derived B cells is not achieved.[22]

More limited data are available about reconstitution of NK cell function. In patients with NK⁻ SCID, NK are often the first cells to appear after haploidentical HSCT.[3] Lower NK cell counts have been reported at long-term follow-up after HSCT in patients who originally had an NK⁻ form of SCID (such as γc or JAK3 defects).[19, 22] Whether this may contribute to the occurrence of papillomavirus infection in patients transplanted because of γc or JAK3 defects remains unknown.

HSCT FOR IMMUNODEFICIENCIES OTHER THAN SCID

Immunodeficiencies other than SCID are characterized by residual T cell-mediated immunity that may prove an obstacle to engraftment of donor-derived stem cells. For this reason, a pre-transplant conditioning regimen is required to treat these disorders, even when an HLA-identical donor is available. Furthermore, results of T cell-depleted haploidentical transplant are not particularly good in these diseases. This has prompted the use of HSCT from alternative donors (MUDs and cord blood).

Although these disorders may be severe, they rarely represent a medical emergency and often permit longer survival. Consequently, the decision whether to attempt HSCT for immunodeficiencies other than SCID must be based on a careful evaluation of the patient's clinical history and quality of life, the effectiveness of alternative and more conservative approaches, as well as on current knowledge of the clinical course for that specific disorder and of genotype–phenotype correlation, if known. In many cases, this remains a difficult decision, which must be shared between the physician and the family (and the child, when possible). On the other hand, advances in critical and supportive care, and improved availability of alternative donors, have resulted in more effective application of HSCT even for this difficult set of patients.[2, 3] At the authors' institution, 79 patients with immunodeficiency other than SCID have received HSCT. Of these, 23 were treated by related HLA-identical transplant, 13 by T cell-depleted haploidentical HSCT, and 43 by MUD HSCT. The overall survival rates were 78.5%, 53.8%, and 78.1%, respectively (Fig. 83.1B).

Combined immunodeficiencies other than SCID

Omenn's syndrome is a fatal disorder unless treated with HSCT. In the past, satisfactory results had been obtained with transplantation from related HLA-identical donors (with a survival rate of 75%), whereas other types transplantation had led to poorer outcome (41% survival after haploidentical transplant, and 50% after MUD HSCT).[3] More recent data, however, indicate a lower mortality. Nine of 11 patients with Omenn's syndrome transplanted at the authors' institution are alive; importantly, of these, only one had a matched sibling, whereas two infants had a phenotypically identical related donor, three were treated by MUD HSCT, and five received a haploidentical HSCT.[26]

HSCT has been attempted also in other predominant T-cell immunodeficiencies, such as purine nucleoside phosphorylase deficiency, cartilage–hair hypoplasia, and other forms of T-cell activation deficiency, with an overall survival rate of approximately 50%.[3]

Major histocompatibility complex (MHC) class II deficiency remains a very difficult disease to transplant, with 54% survival rate after HLA-identical HSCT,[3] and only 32% 1-year survival after haploidentical transplant.[2] Possibly, the persistent lack of expression of HLA class II molecules on thymic epithelium may cause failure to attain a normal CD4 T-cell count after transplant.

HSCT for DiGeorge syndrome may be attempted only when an HLA-identical donor is available; in such cases, immune reconstitution is provided by T lymphocytes contained in the graft.[27]

Patients with CD40 ligand (CD40L) deficiency suffer from recurrent bacterial and opportunistic (*Pneumocystis jiroveci, Cryptosporidium parvum*) infections, resulting in a survival rate of only 46% at 25 years of age according to the European Registry (Notarangelo, unpublished). Consequently, HSCT has been advocated as the treatment of choice for this disease. In a series of 38 patients transplanted in Europe, 26 (68.4%) survived.[28] Early age at transplantation and lack of pre-existing pulmonary disease were associated with a more favorable outcome.

Finally, we have recently obtained the first evidence of successful HSCT in a child with CD40 deficiency who has received bone marrow from her HLA-identical sibling.[49]

Pre-existing viral infections and/or organ damage (possibly related to the conditioning regimen) are responsible for most deaths in patients with combined immunodeficiency other than SCID. As an attempt to reduce drug-related toxicity, several groups have used reduced-intensity conditioning. Nineteen of 21 patients with various immunodeficiencies treated by HSCT with a nonmyeloablative regimen were reported to be alive at a median follow-up of 13 months.[29] However, nonmyeloablative conditioning does not always allow for sustained engraftment of donor stem cells, so that repeated transplants are often necessary.

Wiskott–Aldrich syndrome

Bone marrow transplantation for correction of WAS was attempted as early as 1968, with partial success.[18] Full correction following HSCT was first reported in 1978, when a more robust conditioning regimen was used.[30] Since then, results of related HLA-identical HSCT in WAS have been consistently good; in contrast, poorer results have been achieved with T cell-depleted haploidentical transplants. In a survey of the International Bone Marrow Transplant Registry of 170 WAS patients treated with HSCT, the survival rate was 87%, 52%, and 71% for HLA-identical, haploidentical, and MUD transplants, respectively.[31] In this study, MUD HSCT was effective especially in children less than 5 years of age. In Europe, out of 75 patients treated by HLA-identical or haploidentical transplantation, survival rates were 81% and 43%, respectively.[2] Overall, these studies indicate that indications for haploidentical HSCT should be carefully reviewed, and possibly restricted to severely affected patients for whom no alternative donors have been identified.

Recent data support the efficacy of MUD HSCT for WAS. At the authors' institution, 23 WAS patients were transplanted, 16 of whom received MUD HSCT. Overall survival was 78.2%; specifically, survival among recipients of MUD HSCT was 81.2%.

Finally, cord blood transplantation has been increasingly reported as an effective form of treatment for WAS.[32]

Effective prevention and treatment of EBV-related BLPD (a common complication of HSCT in WAS) has been essential to the improved outcome of HSCT for WAS.

Cytotoxicity defects

Familial hemophagocytic lymphohistiocytosis (FHL) comprises a genetically heterogeneous group of disorders of T- and NK cell-mediated cytotoxicity. Although chemotherapy may induce remission, patients with FHL tend to relapse and ultimately die, mostly due to MOF observed in the accelerated phase of the disease. At present, HSCT is the only curative approach to FHL.[33] In an international study on 86 children with FHL who received chemotherapy followed by HSCT, the overall 3-year survival after HSCT was 64%. Survival was similar for related HLA-identical (71%) and MUD (70%) transplantation, but was less good (survival rate 50%) with a mismatched related donor.[33] Also in the European experience, 3-year survival was better for HSCT from genotypically identical than from HLA-mismatched related donors (68% vs 49%, respectively).[2] A single-center report of 48 patients transplanted at Hôpital Necker, France, gave an overall survival of 58.5%, and transplants from related HLA-identical or MUD gave a better outcome than from mismatched related donors.[34] Importantly, a stable donor chimerism ≥20% is sufficient to provide long-term remission. Accelerated disease is the major risk factor for failure of HSCT and death.[33, 34] Furthermore, VOD and pulmonary hypertension have frequently been observed after HSCT for FHL.

The selection of optimal family donors is an important issue for HSCT in FHL. Because of the lack of reliable assays (other than genetic analysis, when possible) to identify affected individuals at a presymptomatic stage, transplant from siblings carries the risk of using an affected individual as a donor. For this reason, whenever the molecular defect in the family is known, genetic testing is strongly recommended before HSCT from a sibling is attempted.

Chediak–Higashi syndrome (CHS) can be cured by bone marrow transplantation;[35] also for this disease, better results have been obtained with HSCT from HLA-identical siblings or MUDs. At the authors' institution, three patients with CHS have been treated and all are alive and in full remission. On the other hand, the long-term outcome of CHS patients treated with HSCT remains unclear, especially as neurological deterioration has been consistently observed several years after transplant.[36]

HSCT has been also shown to be curative for X-linked lymphoproliferative disease (XLP).[3, 10] Ideally, the transplant should be performed before EBV infection.

Phagocytic cell disorders

Although regular administration of prophylactic antibiotics and antifungals (with or without interferon-γ) has clearly improved the outcome in patients with CGD, this remains a severe disorder, with a rather high risk of complications and death. Therefore, there has been a renewed interest in HSCT for CGD. In a survey of the European experience from 1985 to 2000, 27 patients with CGD were treated by HSCT; most of them received unmodified bone marrow from an HLA-identical sibling after myeloablative conditioning. Overall, 23 of 27 patients were reported to be alive, and the disease had been cured in 22 of them.[14] In this study, all 18 patients who were infection free at the time of transplantation survived. Based on these data, HSCT early in life appears to be a safe and effective form of treatment for CGD patients who have a matched sibling.

HSCT is a successful and life-saving procedure also in patients with the complete form of leukocyte adhesion deficiency type 1 (LAD1), even when performed from MUD or related mismatched donors.[35] Recently, HSCT with reduced-intensity conditioning, allowing stable mixed chimerism, has been successfully used in such patients.[37]

Administration of recombinant G-CSF is the treatment of choice for patients with severe congenital neutropenia (SCN). However, a subgroup of these patients fail to respond to G-CSF, and some of these are at high risk for the development of myelogenous leukemia. Data from the SCN International Registry reported that from 1976 to 1998 11 SCN patients were treated with HSCT for reasons other than malignant transformation.[38] Of these, seven of eight who had a matched sibling survived with engraftment, and one rejected and had autologous reconstitution. Of the three patients treated by mismatched transplantation, two died and one developed very severe GvHD. Data from the French SCN Registry indicate that nine patients were transplanted (seven from a MUD and two from a matched sibling). Engraftment occurred in all but one of the patients. Three died, and six are alive in complete remission.[39] Two patients with SCN refractory to treatment with G-CSF have been successfully transplanted from a MUD at the authors' institution.

Other primary immunodeficiencies

Interferon-γ receptor 1 deficiency leads to severe mycobacterial infections, with a high mortality rate early in life. Although HSCT should theoretically correct the disease, with few exceptions the results have been very disappointing. In particular, an international survey on eight patients transplanted showed that only two were in full remission 5 years later.[40] These are the only two who had received HSCT from an HLA-identical sibling after full myeloablative conditioning. The reasons for the unsatisfactory application of HSCT in this disease remain unclear.

Immunodysregulation, polyendocrinopathy, enteropathy, X-linked (IPEX) syndrome often leads to early death. In spite of the fact that partial engraftment after stem cell transplantation in the murine model of the disease is able to induce sustained remission, the experience with HSCT in IPEX patients has not been very successful.[41] We have been able to achieve sustained remission with stable mixed chimerism following HSCT from a matched sibling in one case of IPEX.[42]

Autoimmune lymphoproliferative syndrome (ALPS) is usually treated by immune suppression, and possibly by splenectomy. However, a successful outcome of HSCT has been reported in a few patients with severe ALPS.[43, 44]

■ PERSPECTIVES FOR HSCT IN THE TREATMENT OF PRIMARY IMMUNODEFICIENCIES ■

Although HSCT has clearly shown its efficacy in patients with severe forms of primary immunodeficiency, several goals remain to be met. In particular, the main areas of interest for future development include methods to improve and sustain engraftment of stem cells; strategies to facilitate engraftment and to reduce the incidence of GvHD in recipients of mismatched or matched unrelated transplants; attempts to improve thymopoiesis, with the aim of accelerating immune reconstitution and avoiding or postponing long-term decline of immunity; and amelioration of strategies aiming at reducing the burden of infections after HSCT.

Strategies aimed at improving thymic function after HSCT (reviewed in [45]) may include protection of thymic stroma that supports thymopoiesis; and direct stimulation of early T-cell progenitors. Keratinocyte growth factor (KGF) is potentially attractive because it protects the thymic stroma. Administration of KGF before HSCT has been shown to enhance thymopoiesis and peripheral T-cell numbers, and to reduce the incidence and severity of GvHD in murine models of HSCT.[45] However, more must be learned on the long-term outcome of this treatment before clinical trials can be started.

Recently, a common thymic epithelial precursor for all thymic epithelial cells has been identified in mice.[46] This precursor cell may give rise to a functional thymus *in vivo*. Should a similar element be identified in humans, it might prompt novel strategies aimed at accelerating T-cell recovery after HSCT.

Attempts to accelerate immune reconstitution might be based on the use of cytokines that promote T-cell development and maturation in the thymus, such as IL-7. However, experience in severely immunodeficient mice has shown that infusion of IL-7 provides limited benefit in the MHC-compatible or partially compatible setting, whereas in a fully mismatched setting it has facilitated T-cell development.[47]

Infusion of donor T cells that have anti-infective activity but no GvHD activity might help reduce infection-related mortality after HSCT. Such strategy could be based on removal of alloreactive cells by negative selection using anti-CD25 or anti-CD69 antibodies.

Recognition that B-cell engraftment after HSCT is hampered by competition between host and donor early B-cell precursors[25] may

OUTCOME OF STEM CELL TRANSPLANTATION FOR PRIMARY IMMUNODEFICIENCIES

» For SCID, the overall survival rate of patients transplanted since 1968 is over 70%, and is higher for patients treated by HLA-identical transplantation.

» There has been a continuous improvement in the outcome of the procedure.

» Survival rates are over 90% for HLA-identical transplantation, and 75% for haploidentical transplantation for SCID.

» Improvement in clinical care (both in critical care and in prevention/treatment of infections) has recently led to exploit efficacy of MUD transplantation also for SCID, with excellent results.

» The decision to attempt a MUD transplantation for SCID must be weighed against the risks associated with the time interval required to identify such a donor.

» Factors influencing survival after transplantation for SCID include younger age at transplant, prevention of GvHD, and control of infections. For the latter, isolation in a protected environment, and prophylactic use of antibiotics are effective measures.

» The decline of T-cell function that is observed at 10 years or more after unconditioned transplantation remains a concern, and may cause clinical problems. Therefore, there is a need for improvements in the procedures used to facilitate and sustain stem cell engraftment, and/or to boost donor-derived immunity.

» For primary immunodeficiencies other than SCID, there has been a progressive improvement in the outcome following stem cell transplantation.

» Results are good both for HLA-identical transplants (with a survival rate of 70% or more, depending on the disease), and for MUD or cord blood transplantations.

» Reduced-intensity conditioning regimens have been often used in these patients, in the attempt to reduce the risks of drug-related toxicity.

prompt novel forms of conditioning regimen targeted to host pro-B lymphocytes, with the aim of facilitating the development of donor-derived B cells, even in the HLA-identical setting.

Finally, it has recently been demonstrated in a murine model that endogenous stem cells obstruct the engraftment of donor-derived stem cells, and that the recipient's CD4 T lymphocytes inhibit productive engraftment, possibly by recognizing subtle histocompatibility differences.[48] Novel strategies aimed at interfering more specifically with the mechanisms involved in graft rejection, without requiring full myeloablation, could therefore be envisaged, at least for some severe T-cell immunodeficiency disorders.

■ REFERENCES ■

1. Gatti RA, Meuwissen HJ, Allen HD, et al. Immunological reconstitution of sex-linked lymphopenic immunological deficiency. Lancet 1968; 2: 1366–1369.

2. Antoine C, Muller S, Cant A, et al. Long-term survival and transplantation of hemopoietic stem cells fro immunodeficiencies: report of the European experience 1968–1999. Lancet 2003; 361: 553–560.

3. Buckley RH, Fischer A. Bone marrow transplantation for primary immunodeficiency diseases. In: Ochs HD, Smitch CIE, Puck JM, eds. Primary immunodeficiency diseases: a molecular and genetic approach, 2nd edn. New York: Oxford University Press, 2006.

4. Müller SM, Ege M, Pottharst A, et al. Transplacentally acquired maternal T lymphocytes in severe combined immunodeficiency: a study of 121 patients. Blood 2001; 98: 1847–1851.

5. Muench MO. In utero transplantation: baby steps towards an effective therapy. Bone Marrow Transplant 2005; 35: 537–547.

6. Myers LA, Patel DD, Puck JM, Buckley RH. Hematopoietic stem cell transplantation for severe combined immunodeficiency in the neonatal period leads to superior thymic output and improved survival. Blood 2002; 99: 872–878.

7. O'Reilly RJ, Dupont B, Pahwa S, et al. Reconstitution in severe combined immunodeficiency by transplantation of marrow from an unrelated donor. N Engl J Med 1977; 297: 1311.

8. Grunebaum E, Mazzolari E, Porta F, et al. Bone marrow transplantation for severe combined immunodeficiency. JAMA 2006; 295: 508–518.

9. Tsuji Y, Imai K, Kajiwara M, et al. Hematopoietic stem cell transplantation for 30 patients with primary immunodeficiency diseases: 20 years experience of a single team. Bone Marrow Transplant 2006; 37: 469–477.

10. Ziegner UHM, Ochs HD, Schanen C, et al. Unrelated umbilical cord stem transplantation for X-linked immunodeficiencies. J Pediatr 2001; 138: 570–573.

11. Veys P, Rao K, Amrolia P. Stem cell transplantation for congenital immunodeficiencies using reduced-intensity conditioning. Bone Marrow Transplant 2005; 35: S45–S47.

12. Ferrara JL, Deeg HJ. Graft-versus-host disease. N Engl J Med 1991; 324: 667–674.

13. Lee SJ. New approaches for preventing and treating chronic graft-versus-host disease. Blood 2005; 105: 4200–4206.

14. Seger RA, Gungor T, Belohradsky BH, et al. Treatment of chronic granulomatous disease with myeloablative conditioning and an unmodified allograft: a survey of the European experience, 1985–2000. Blood 2002; 100: 4344–50.

15. Ljungman P. Prevention and treatment of viral infections in stem cell transplant recipients. Br J Haematol 2002; 118: 44–57.

16. Richardson PG, Murakami C, Jin Z, et al. Multi-institutional use of defibrotide in 88 patients after stem cell transplantation with severe veno-occlusive disease and multisystem organ failure: response without significant toxicity in a high-risk population and factors predictive of outcome. Blood 2002; 100: 4337–4343.

17. Bajwa RP, Cant AJ, Abinun M, et al. Recombinant tissue plasminogen activator for treatment of hepatic veno-occlusive disease following bone marrow transplantation in children: effectiveness and a scoring system for initiating treatment. Bone Marrow Transplant 2003; 31: 591–597.

18. Bach FH, Albertini RJ, Joo P, et al. Bone marrow transplantation in a patient with the Wiskott–Aldrich syndrome. Lancet 1968; 2: 1364–1366.

19. Buckley RH. Molecular defects in human severe combined immunodeficiency and approaches to immune reconstitution. Annu Rev Immunol 2004; 22: 625–655.

20. Haddad E, Landais P, Friedrich W, et al. Long-term immune reconstitution and outcome after HLA-nonidentical T-cell-depleted bone marrow transplantation for severe combined immunodeficiency: a European retrospective study of 116 patients. Blood 1998; 91: 3636–3653.

21. Laffort C, Le Deist F, Favre M, et al. Severe cutaneous papillomavirus disease after haemopoietic stem-cell transplantation in patients with severe combined immunodeficiency caused by gamma c cytokine receptor subunit or JAK-3 deficiency. Lancet 2004; 363: 2051–2054.

22. Fischer A, Le Deist F, Hacein-Bey S, et al. Severe combined immunodeficiency. A model disease for molecular immunology and therapy. Immunol Rev 2005; 203: 98–109.

23. Sarzotti M, Patel DD, Li X, et al. T cell repertoire development in humans with SCID after nonablative allogeneic marrow transplantation. J Immunol 2003; 170: 2711–2718.

24. Patel DD, Gooding ME, Parrott RE, et al. Thymic function after hematopoietic stem-cell transplantation for the treatment of severe combined immunodeficiency. N Engl J Med 2000; 342: 1325–1332.

25. Liu A, Vosshenrich CA, Lagresle-Peyrou C, et al. Competition within the early B cell compartment conditions B cell reconstitution after hematopoietic stem cell transplantation in non-irradiatedrecipients. Blood. Apr 13 [Epub ahead of print].

26. Mazzolari E, Moshous D, Forino C, et al. Hematopoietic stem cell transplantation in Omenn syndrome: a single-center experience. Bone Marrow Transplant 2005; 36: 107–114.

27. Goldsobel AB, Haas A, Stiehm ER. Bone marrow transplantation in DiGeorge syndrome. J Pediatr 1987; 111: 40–44.

28. Gennery AR, Khawaja K, Veys P, et al. Treatment of CD40 ligand deficiency by hematopoietic stem cell transplantation: a survey of the European experience, 1993–2002. Blood 2004; 103: 1152–1557.

29. Gaspar HB, Amrolia P, Hassan A, et al. Non-myeloablative stem cell transplantation for congenital immunodeficiencies. Recent Results Cancer Res 2002; 159: 134–142.

30. Parkman R, Rappeport J, Geha R, et al. Complete correction of the Wiskott–Aldrich syndrome by allogenic bone marrow transplantation. N Engl J Med 1978; 342: 1325–1332.

31. Filipovich AH, Stone JV, Tomany SC, et al. Impact of donor type on outcome of bone marrow transplantation for Wiskott–Aldrich syndrome: collaborative study of the International Bone Marrow Transplant Registry and the National Bone Marrow Donor Program. Blood 2001; 97: 1598–1603.

32. Knutsen AP, Steffen M, Wassmer K, Wall DA. Umbilical cord blood transplantation in Wiskott–Aldrich syndrome. J Pediatr 2003; 142: 519–523.

33. Horne A, Janka G, Maarten Egeler R, et al. Haematopoietic stem cell transplantation in haemophagocytic lymphohistiocytosis. Br J Haematol 2005; 129: 622–630.

34. Ouachéè-Chardin M, Elie C, de Saint Basile G, et al. Hematopoietic stem cell transplantation in hemophagocytic lymphohistiocytosis: a single-center report of 48 patients. Pediatrics 2006; 117: 743–750.

35. Fischer A, Landais P, Friedrich W, et al. Bone marrow transplantation (BMT) in Europe for primary immunodeficiencies other than severe combined immunodeficiency: a report from the European Group for BMT and the European Group for Immunodeficiency. Blood 1994; 83: 1149–1154.

36. Tardieu M, Lacroix C, Neven B, et al. Progressive neurologic dysfunctions 20 years after allogeneic bone marrow transplantation for Chediak–Higashi syndrome. Blood 2005; 106: 40–42.

37. Engel ME, Hickstein DD, Bauer TR, et al. Matched unrelated bone marrow transplantation with reduced-intensity conditioning for leukocyte adhesion deficiency. Bone Marrow Transplant 2006; 37: 717–718.

38. Zeidler C, Welte K, Barak Y, et al. Stem cell transplantation in patients with severe congenital neutropenia without evidence of leukemic transformation. Blood 2000; 95: 1195–1198.

39. Ferry C, Ouachéè M, Leblanc T, et al. Hematopoietic stem cell transplantation in severe congenital neutropenia: experience of the French SCN Registry. Bone Marrow Transplant 2005; 35: 45–50.

40. Roesler J, Horwitz ME, Picard C, et al. Hematopoietic stem cell transplantation for complete IFN-gamma receptor 1 deficiency: a multi-institutional survey. J Pediatr 2005; 145: 806–812.

41. Wildin RS, Smyk-Pearson S, Filipovich AH. Clinical and molecular features of the immunodysregulation, polyendocrinopathy, enteropathy, X-linked (IPEX) syndrome. J Med Genet 2002; 39: 537–545.

42. Mazzolari E. Forino C, Fontana M. A new case of IPEX receiving bone marrow transplantation. Bone Marrow Transplant 2005; 35: 1033–1034.

43. Benkerrou M, Le Deist F, De Villartay JP, et al. Correction of Fas (CD95) deficiency by haploidentical bone marrow transplantation. Eur J Immunol 1997; 27: 2043–2047.

44. Sleight BJ, Prasad VS, DeLaat C, et al. Correction of autoimmune lymphoproliferative syndrome by bone marrow transplantation. Bone Marrow Transplant 1998; 22: 375–380.

45. Wils E-J, Cornelissen JJ. Thymopoiesis following allogenic stem cell transplantation: new possibilities for improvement. Blood Rev 2005; 19: 89–98.

46. Gill J, Malin M, Hollander GA, Boyd R. Generation of a complete thymic microenvironment by MTS24+ thymic epithelial cells. Nature Immunol 2002; 3: 635–642.

47. Andre-Schmutz I, Bonhomme D, Yates F, et al. IL-7 effect on immunological reconstitution after HSCT depends on MHC incompatibility. Br J Haematol 2004; 126: 844–851.

48. Bhattacharya D, Rossi DJ, Bryder D, Weissman IL. Purified hematopoietic stem cell engraftment of rare niches corrects severe lymphoid deficiencies without host conditioning. J Exp Med 2006; 203: 73–85.

49. Mattolari E, Lanzi G, Forino C, et al. First report of successful stem cell transplantation in a child with CD40 deficiency. Bone Marrow Transplant 2007; 40: 279–281.

REFERENCES

Thymic reconstitution

84

M. Louise Markert, Blythe H. Devlin

■ INTRODUCTION ■

Thymus transplantation is a promising experimental procedure for reconstitution of thymic function in patients with congenital athymia. Thymus transplantation was initiated in the 1960s and 1970s as a means of reconstituting the T-cell population and function in infants who presented with infections and low T-cell numbers. Although there were some reports of success, most patients died.[1] The poor results at that time may have been secondary to the difficulty in distinguishing athymic patients from those with a genetic defect in bone marrow stem cells. In addition, at the time, reagents such as monoclonal antibodies reactive with thymic epithelium were not available to evaluate the quality of thymus tissue. In the 1990s, with the ability to identify appropriate patients for treatment and with better reagents for assessing graft quality, the feasibility of using thymus transplantation was readdressed.

A summary of results of thymus transplantation by the authors is presented. The clinical trials involve patients with complete DiGeorge anomaly. With follow-up times of up to 12 years, the safety profile and resulting T-cell function are excellent.[2, 3] The transplant recipients continue to be followed to assess the persistence of T-cell numbers and function and to monitor for potential autoimmune disorders. These studies are performed under an Investigational New Drug (IND) application with the Food and Drug Administration.

■ PATIENT POPULATIONS ■

Patients who may benefit from thymus transplantation include infants with congenital athymia from complete DiGeorge anomaly. This is a heterogeneous congenital anomaly in which infants present with variable defects in the heart, parathyroid gland and thymus.[4-7] Of these, fewer than 1 in 200 have athymia and thus are categorized as having 'complete' DiGeorge anomaly.[8] Based on 48 infants with complete DiGeorge anomaly enrolled in transplantation protocols, 39 of whom received thymic transplants, the main genetic and syndromic risk factors for complete DiGeorge anomaly include 22q11 hemizygosity, CHARGE (coloboma, heart anomaly, choanal atresia, retardation, and genital and ear

anomalies) association and diabetic embryopathy (Table 84.1).[9-11] It is notable that less than half of infants with complete DiGeorge anomaly are hemizygous at chromosome 22q11. All athymic patients present at birth with very low T-cell counts (<50/mm^3). They are consequently profoundly immunodeficient and susceptible to infections.

Athymic infants with complete DiGeorge anomaly can develop oligoclonal T-cell populations at varying times after birth, usually within the first 12 months of life. The oligoclonal T cells can infiltrate the skin and other organs. Figure 84.1 panel A shows a typical rash associated with circulating oligoclonal T cells. The rash is similar to severe atopic dermatitis or graft-versus-host disease. On biopsy, the rash appears to be spongiotic dermatitis with T-cell infiltration.[12] Lymphadenopathy develops subsequent to the rash. Upon biopsy, the lymph nodes are typically given the diagnosis of dermatopathic lymphadenopathy. The term atypical complete DiGeorge anomaly is used to characterize these patients. Athymic infants who develop circulating oligoclonal T cells remain susceptible to infections.

DIAGNOSIS OF ATHYMIA

Infants that may benefit from thymic transplantation require prompt diagnosis of athymia for effective treatment. The absence of a typical thymic shadow on chest X-ray, CT scan, or magnetic resonance imaging (MRI) cannot be used to diagnose athymia. The thymus may be embedded in the thyroid, for instance (unpublished findings). A small mass in the location where one anticipates finding the thymus may be a lymph node instead. Therefore, one must rely on blood tests to assess thymic function.

In normal infants, thymic function is revealed by the presence in blood of recent thymic emigrants, also called 'naive T cells.' All T cells express the CD3 proteins, but naive T cells also express the cell surface proteins CD45RA and CD62L.[13] The co-expression of these molecules can be assessed by flow cytometry. Over 50% of a normal infant's T cells are naïve, reflecting active thymic function. Another characteristic of good thymic function is the presence of a broad T-cell receptor repertoire in the blood. The assays to assess these characteristics and the interpretation of the data in the differential diagnosis of athymia in infants with DiGeorge syndrome are described below in greater detail.

In typical complete DiGeorge anomaly, the total number of T cells (and hence the number of naive T cells) is usually $< 50/mm^3$ and thus thymic function is considered to be absent. These T-cell numbers are profoundly depressed compared to a normal infant's T-cell count of $>2000/mm^3$, with over 50% being naive. The evaluation of thymic function is more difficult in patients with atypical complete DiGeorge anomaly because proliferation of the oligoclonal T cells may lead to significantly elevated T-cell numbers.[3, 12] The lack of thymic function in these infants is demonstrated when less than 5% of total T cells are found to be naive by flow cytometry. Figure 84.2 presents an example of an infant with fewer than 5% naive T cells prior to transplantation when the T-cell count was $2113/mm^3$. The very low percentage (<5%) of T cells co-expressing the markers CD45RA and CD62L confirms the diagnosis of athymia. It should be noted that the oligoclonal T cells present in athymic patients may proliferate in response to the mitogen phytohemagglutinin (PHA). Thus, a T-cell proliferative response to mitogens such as PHA cannot be used to confirm the presence of a thymus.[3, 12] The oligoclonal T cells that respond to PHA in patients with atypical complete DiGeorge anomaly do not protect against pathogens, and the patient remains susceptible to infections.

Table 84.1 Syndromic associations in complete DiGeorge anomaly

Genetic or syndromic associations	Percentage*
22q11 hemizygosity	46
CHARGE	25
Infant of diabetic mother	21
Ectodermal dysplasia	2
None	6

*Data based on 48 patients enrolled in protocols.

CLINICAL PEARLS

Perform a T-cell count to diagnosis complete DiGeorge anomaly in all infants with the following:

>> 22q11 hemizygosity
>> CHARGE
>> Primary hypoparathyroidism
>> Truncus arteriosis
>> Interrupted aortic arch type B

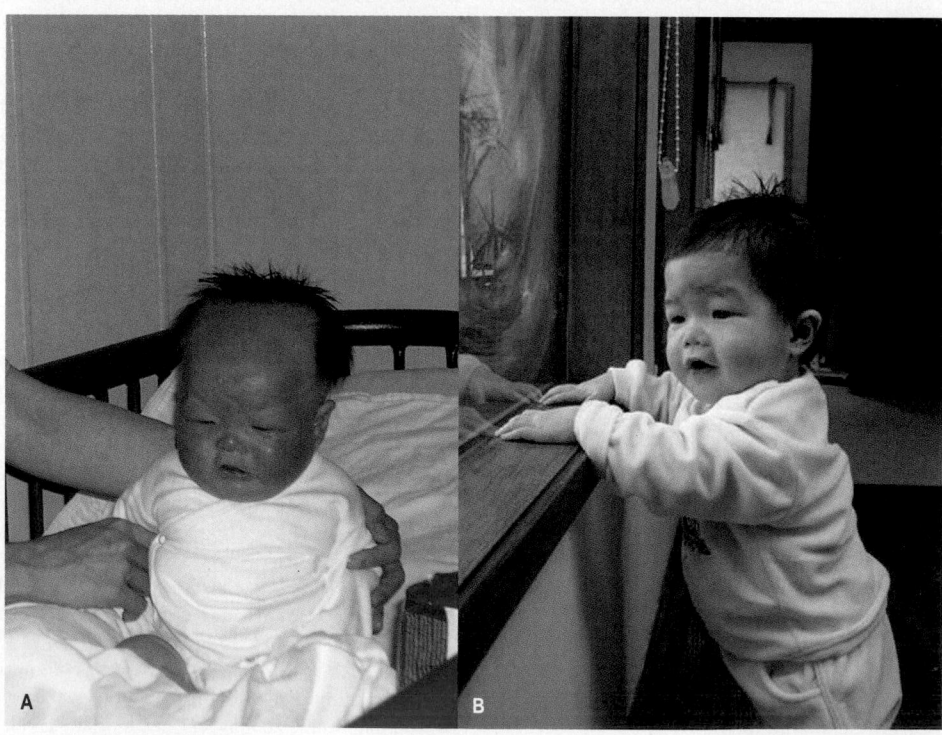

Fig. 84.1 Dermatologic findings in patient with atypical complete DiGeorge anomaly. (**A**) Rash before and (**B**) skin after thymus transplantation. Note hair loss with rash and regrowth after thymus transplantation.

A broad T-cell receptor (TCR) repertoire is found in infants with normal thymic function. Circulating T cells in athymic infants are usually oligoclonal. To support the diagnosis of athymia in patients who have circulating T cells, diversity of the TCR repertoire is evaluated by spectratyping. Spectratyping assesses the repertoire of the TCR β chain variable segment (TCRBV) usage.[2, 3] Most T cells express the TCRαβ receptor. Spectratyping uses PCR to amplify the TCRBV-containing mRNAs for different TCRBV families. In a normal individual with a diverse TCRBV repertoire, a quasi-gaussian distribution of lengths of the mRNAs utilizing each TCRBV segment is present because of the variability of recombination joints between the variable (V), diversity (D), and joining (J) gene segments in the chromosome. Different forward primers specific for the various TCRBV-variable regions are used to amplify cDNA in separate reactions with a single reverse primer that hybridizes with either of the two TCRBV constant regions. The PCR products are end-labeled and size-separated by electrophoresis or capillary gels. Figure 84.3 panel A presents a spectratype from a patient with atypical complete DiGeorge anomaly who has an oligoclonal repertoire. Panel B illustrates a normal quasi-gaussian spectratype from a patient with typical complete DiGeorge anomaly 4.5 years after thymus transplantation. When a patient with DiGeorge anomaly has normal numbers of T cells and very few naïve T cells, as in Figure 84.2, the TCRBV repertoire will be oligoclonal as in Figure 84.3 panel A. This association of oligoclonality with low naive T-cell numbers is related to the loss of CD45RA and the acquisition of CD45RO as T cells proliferate. All patients with atypical complete DiGeorge anomaly who have a very low percentage of naive T cells have had an oligoclonal TCRBV repertoire.

CLINICAL PEARLS

Although the chest X-ray, CT scan or MRI scan can be used to detect the lack of a thymus gland in an infant suspected of the DiGeorge anomaly, immune tests of the blood cells are necessary to confirm the diagnosis. These tests include measurements of total (CD3) T cells and naïve (CD45RA+CD62+) T cells by flow cytometry and assessment of the T-cell receptor β chain variable segment (TCRVβ) repertoire by spectratyping.

KEY CONCEPTS

CHARACTERISTICS OF NAIVE T CELLS

>> Co-expression of CD45RA and CD62L
>> Broad T-cell receptor repertoire

■ THYMUS TRANSPLANTATION ■

PREPARATION OF THYMUS TISSUE FOR TRANSPLANTATION

Thymus tissue is often removed by pediatric cardiac surgeons in order to access the surgical field necessary to repair the heart. For thymus transplantation, informed consent is obtained from the parents of the infant undergoing heart surgery in order to collect discarded tissue. The thymus is collected aseptically and processed in the laboratory. Based on the procedures initially described by Hong,[14] the thymus is sectioned and the slices are maintained in tissue culture for 2–3 weeks. Donor screening includes testing and screening for risk factors as recommended for all cell and tissue products (Code of Federal Regulations Title 21; Part 1270). HLA matching is not required, but the HLA types of the donor and recipient are evaluated.

USE OF IMMUNOSUPPRESSION

Table 84.2 shows the number of patients who were transplanted without immunosuppression and the number given immunosuppression. No immunosuppression was used in 21 patients with typical complete DiGeorge anomaly who had very low T-cell numbers and very depressed T-cell proliferative responses to the mitogen PHA, as these patients cannot reject transplants.[2] Another 18 patients were immunosuppressed with deoxycoformycin (one patient) or pre-transplant rabbit anti-thymocyte globulin (17 patients).[3, 12] Of the group of 17 treated with anti-thymocyte globulin, peri-transplantation cyclosporine was used in six. Peri-transplantation steroids were used in five of these plus one other, who did not receive cyclosporine. Infections and deaths did not increase in the infants who received immunosuppression compared to those who did not.

Immunosuppression is given if an infant has atypical complete DiGeorge anomaly, or if there is an elevation in the T-cell responses to mitogens in patients with typical complete DiGeorge anomaly. The

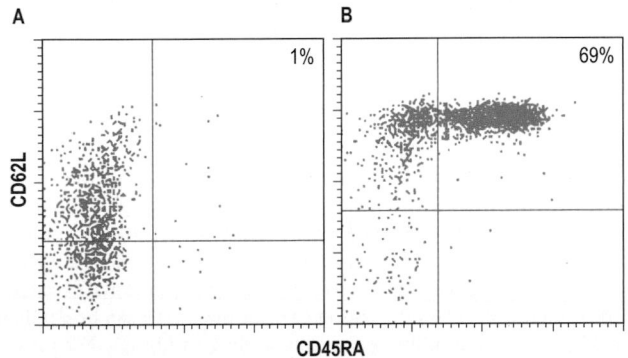

Fig. 84.2 Naïve CD45RA+CD62L+ T cells pre and post thymus transplantation. (**A**) Naive CD3 T cells (1%) on day −8 pre thymus transplantation and (**B**) naïve CD4 T cells (69%) on day 550 (year 1.5) post transplantation in a patient with atypical complete DiGeorge anomaly. This is the same patient whose data are illustrated in Figure 84.6, panels D–F. On day −8 pre transplantation, the patient had 7684/mm³ total T cells with 585/mm³ CD4 T cells, 4594/mm³ CD8 T cells and 2506/mm³ double-negative T cells. On day 550 post transplantation the patient had 1013/mm³ T cells with 674/mm³ CD4 T cells, 251/mm³ CD8 T cells, and 82/mm³ double-negative T cells.

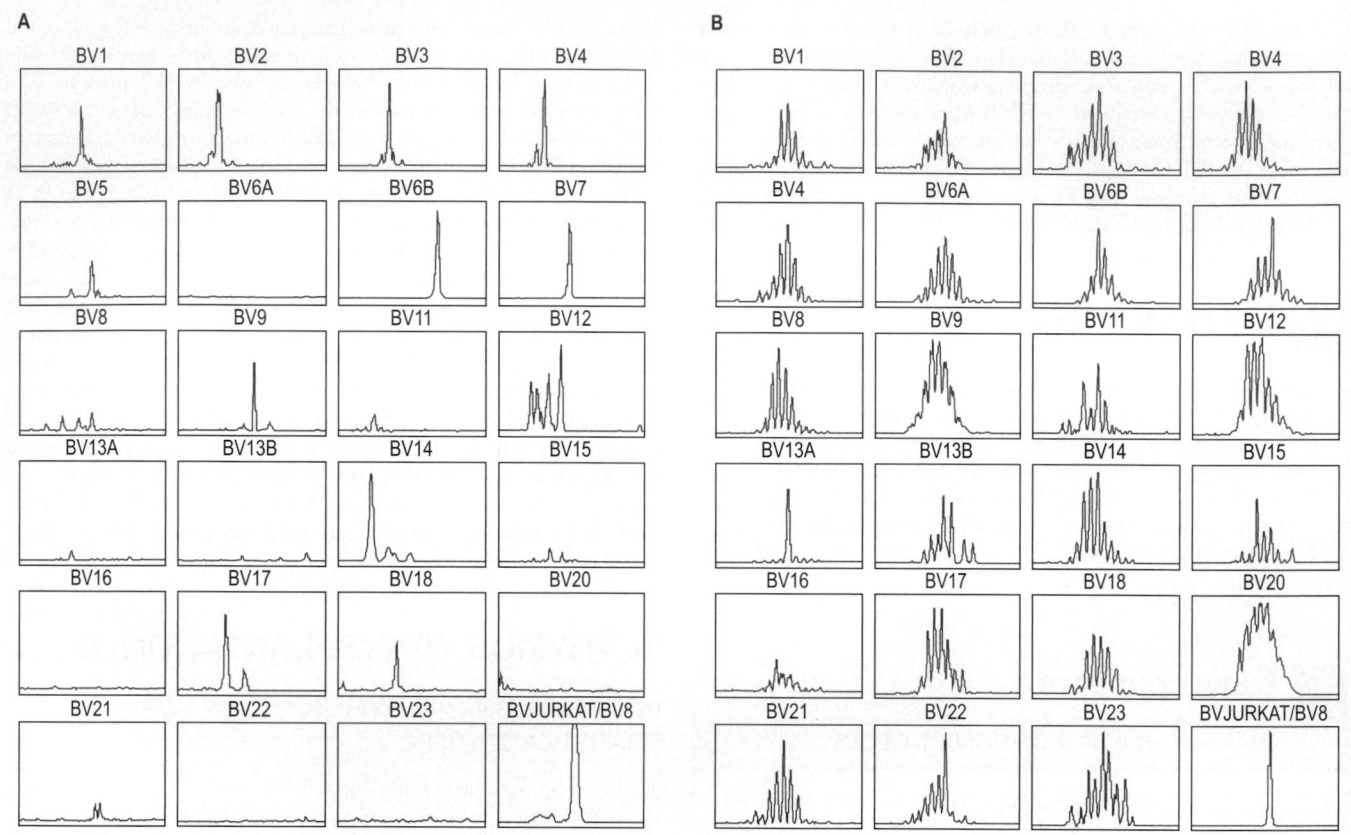

Fig. 84.3 Spectratype evaluation of TCRBV repertoire. (**A**) An oligoclonal CD4 spectratype from an infant with atypical complete DiGeorge anomaly who had 5897/mm^3 circulating T cells with 2726/mm^3 CD4 T cells. (**B**) Post transplantation CD4 T cell immunoscope in a patient with typical complete DiGeorge anomaly 4.5 years after transplantation, when the T-cell count was 998/mm^3 with 729/mm^3 CD4 T cells. The TCRBV family designation is above each panel. The Jurkat/TCRBV 8 control is in the bottom right panel of each spectratype. These spectratypes contrast the oligoclonal extrathymically derived T cells in a patient with athypical complete DiGoerge anomaly with the polyclonal T cells found post thymus transplantation.

Table 84.2 Use of immunosuppression for thymus transplantation

Diagnosis	Treatment*	
	No suppression # surviving/total	Suppression # surviving/total
Typical complete DiGeorge anomaly	16/21 (76%)	6/6 (100%)
Atypical complete DiGeorge anomaly	0/0	8/12 (67%)
Total	16/21 (76%)	14/18 (78%)

*Data based on 39 transplanted patients.

T cells of these infants can reject allografts, even though they do not protect against infection. If an infant has atypical complete DiGeorge syndrome, the authors begin cyclosporine treatment prior to transplantation. Cyclosporine is usually started when the diagnosis of atypical complete DiGeorge anomaly is made because the oligoclonal T cells can be very aggressive. The rash associated with these cells can be debilitating. The T cells can infiltrate the liver, leading to fibrosis. For patients with activated T cells (those expressing high levels of CD25 and HLA-DR), cyclosporine is started at least 1 week prior to the rabbit anti-thymocyte globulin therapy. Rabbit anti-thymocyte globulin is currently used in all subjects who receive immunosuppression. Both infants with typical complete DiGeorge syndrome and elevated PHA responses and all those with atypical complete DiGeorge syndrome are treated prior to thymus transplantation using three doses of the anti-thymocyte globulin at 2 mg/kg over 3 days. The rabbit anti-thymocyte globulin is generally well tolerated. The cyclosporine is usually continued in patients with atypical complete DiGeorge anomaly after transplantation until naive T cells emerge in the blood.

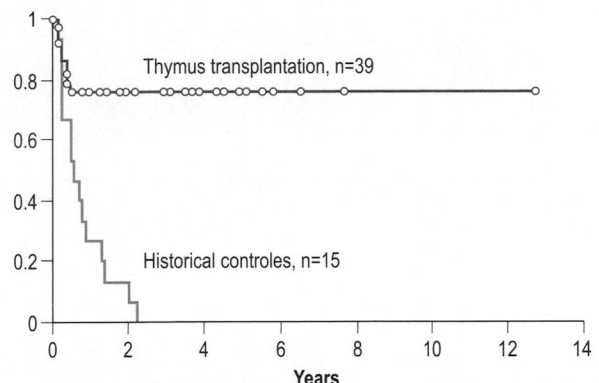

Fig. 84.4 Survival after thymus transplantation. Thirty of 39 (77%) patients treated with thymus transplantation survive.

OPERATIVE PROCEDURE

Thymus transplantation is an open procedure under general anesthesia. The surgeon creates furrows in the quadriceps muscle and places the slices of cultured thymus tissue individually into pockets in the muscle. The quadriceps serves as a good site because it is a relatively large, highly vascularized muscle. To allow the thymus to become vascularized in the first weeks after transplantation, steroids are limited to doses of methylprednisolone ≤2 mg/kg/day. Other surgeries are postponed if possible. As has been described, preparation for thymus transplantation requires careful coordination between immunologist, surgeon, and anesthesiologist.[15]

■ RESULTS OF THYMUS TRANSPLANTATION ■

SURVIVAL

Survival rate after thymus transplantation is 77% (30 of 39) (Fig. 84.4). Seventeen of the 30 surviving transplanted patients are 3 or more years from transplantation. No patient has died later than 6 months post transplantation. Early deaths were not related to the transplantation but were predominantly secondary to infection.

■ IMMUNE OUTCOMES ■

THYMUS GRAFT BIOPSY

Biopsies of the thymus graft 2–3 months post transplantation confirm thymopoiesis (Fig. 84.5). The biopsy illustrated was taken from a patient who was treated with immunosuppression, showing that these treatments do not prevent thymopoiesis. Specifically, the patient whose biopsy is shown had been diagnosed with atypical complete DiGeorge anomaly. This patient had 5151/mm³ T cells 8 days prior to transplantation; he had severe rash and lymphadenopathy. The patient was treated with cyclosporine, rabbit anti-thymocyte globulin, and steroids before transplantation, and with cyclosporine and steroids afterwards. The

biopsy, done 66 days after transplantation while the patient was still on cyclosporine, shows tissue that appears to be normal thymus with cortex and medulla (Fig. 84.5). Thus, pre-transplantation anti-thymocyte globulin and peri-transplantation cyclosporine does not prevent the development of T cells in transplanted thymus tissue.

T-CELL NUMBERS

Typical complete DiGeorge syndrome

Immune findings in the first year after transplantation vary depending on whether the infant has typical or atypical complete DiGeorge anomaly. In patients with typical complete DiGeorge anomaly, who initially have very few T cells and no rash, T cells are first observed in the peripheral blood about 3–4 months post transplantation. Naive T cells appear by 5–6 months. CD4 T cells predominate initially; CD8 T cells develop more slowly. By 2 years post transplantation, a stable total T-cell count reaches the 10th percentile in some patients, but is usually lower. CD8 numbers remain below the 10th percentile in all patients. The CD4:CD8 ratio remains >1 in all patients. A typical pattern of T-cell development is shown in Figure 84.6, panels A-C. By 9 months after thymus transplantation, T-cell proliferative responses to mitogens are normal. At that time patients are immunized with tetanus toxoid. Antigen-specific proliferative responses have developed by 2 years in all except two patients. The repertoire of TCRBV chain usage normalizes by 6–9 months. Although T-cell numbers are low for age, their function and the Vβ chain repertoire are normal. Composite data from these patients have been published elsewhere.[2]

Atypical complete DiGeorge syndrome

The time course of development of T cells in infants with atypical complete DiGeorge anomaly is similar to that in typical patients, except that such infants may have predominantly CD4 single-positive, CD8 single-positive or double-negative (CD3⁺CD4⁻CD8⁻) cells prior to transplantation. An example of a patient with a prominent CD8 single-positive population (greater than the CD4 single-positive or double-negative population) in the peri-transplant period is shown in Figure 84.6 panel D. As observed in other patients, by 4 months post transplantation the number of CD4 T cells equaled the numbers of CD8 and double-negative cells, and by 5 months CD4 T cells outnumbered the sum of CD8 single-positive and double-negative T cells. As in other atypical and typical patients 6 months post transplantation, the presence of naive CD4 T cells indicated thymic function (Fig. 84.6). In all patients treated with immunosuppression, normal proliferative responses and a normal TCRBV repertoire developed over a time course similar to that of typical patients. Composite data have been published on these patients elsewhere.[3]

SPECTRATYPING

Spectratyping of the TCRBV repertoire provides supportive evidence for thymic function, as polyclonal repertoires are seen in the presence of thymic function. As a polyclonal repertoire develops, naive T cells are detected in the peripheral blood by flow cytometry (Fig. 84.2 panel B). Almost all patients develop a polyclonal TCRBV repertoire within 9 months of transplantation.[2, 3] The TCRBV repertoire remains polyclonal in patients for many years, as illustrated in Figure 84.3 panel B.

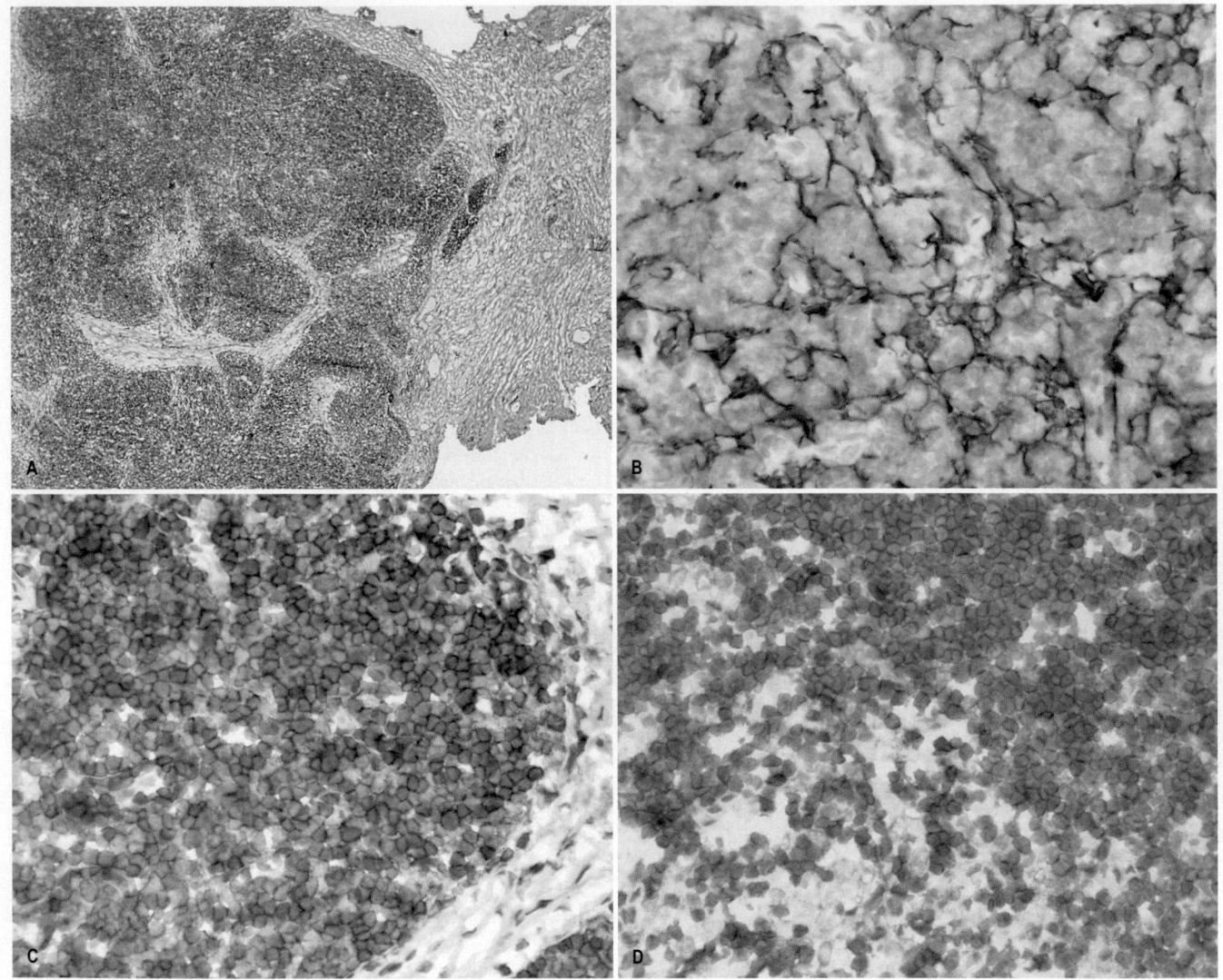

Fig. 84.5 Biopsy of thymus graft. (**A**) Hematoxylin and eosin staining showing cortex and medulla. Fibrous tissue and striated muscle can be seen on the right. (**B**) Cytokeratin staining reveals lacy patterns of cytokeratin. Hassall bodies were identified on other sections. (**C**) CD1 staining shows expression of this marker of normal cortical thymocytes. (**D**) CD3 staining shows many T cells. This biopsy was obtained 66 days after thymus transplantation. As expected, there were no circulating naive T cells at this early time point. Cyclosporine had been started 14 days prior to thymus transplantation and was still being used at the time of this biopsy.

B-CELL FUNCTION

Two years post transplantation, intravenous immunoglobulin is stopped and patients are tested for specific antibody function in response to immunizations with tetanus toxoid and a pneumococcal polysaccharide vaccine (Pneumovax). All patients tested have been shown to make antigen-specific antibodies, demonstrating B-cell function. They remain off replacement immunoglobulin. Patients are then given the normal childhood vaccines, but no live vaccines are used. Future studies include plans to evaluate memory B-cell function by measuring antibody titers to secondary immunizations and the persistence of titers after immunization.

(Note: the one patient who has not developed T-cell proliferative responses against tetanus toxoid has not been tested for specific antibody function.)

■ SAFETY ■

No serious adverse events have been associated with the transplantation or biopsy procedures. In the first 3 months post transplantation three patients had mild wheezing or hypoxemia, controlled by steroids. The respiratory symptoms were associated with development of oligoclonal

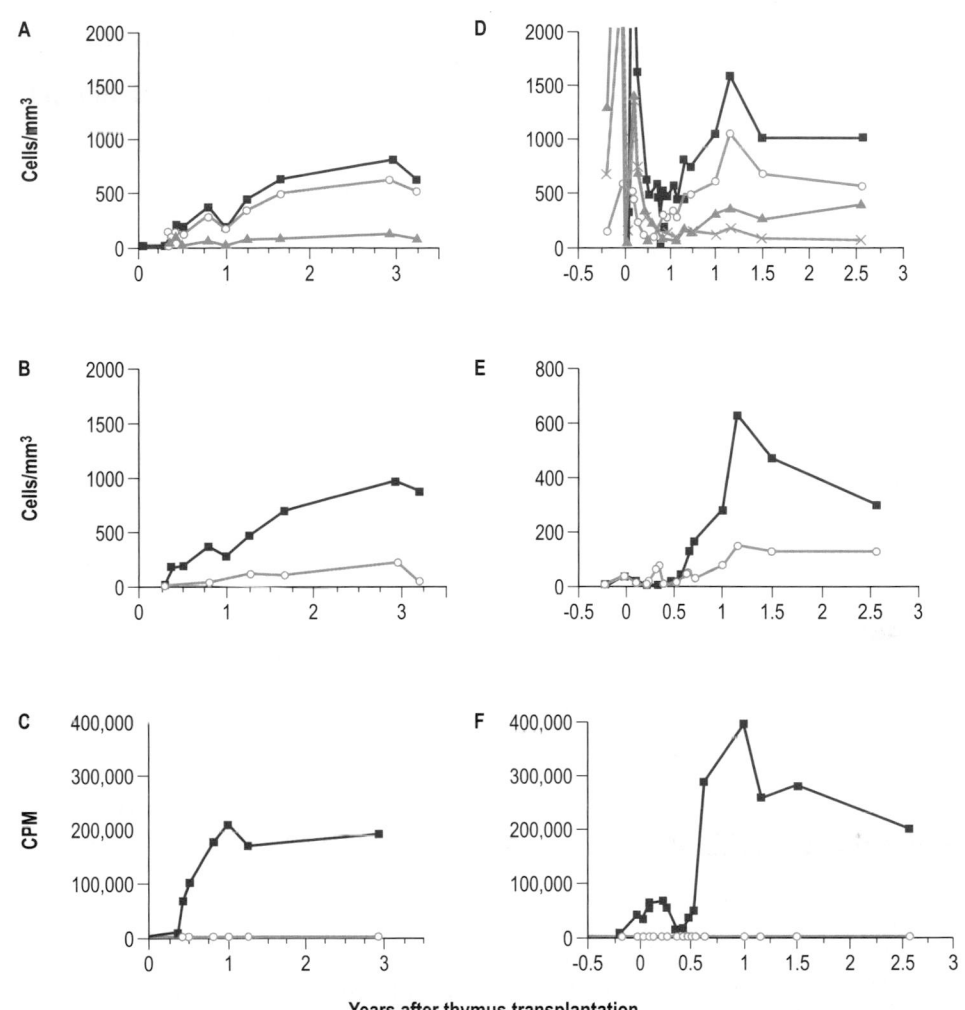

Fig. 84.6 T-cell phenotype and function after thymus transplantation. A patient with typical complete DiGeorge anomaly who was not given immunosuppression is shown in panels A–C. A patient with atypical complete DiGeorge anomaly who was given immunosuppression is shown in panels D–F. Panels A and D show absolute numbers of T-cell subsets in cells per cubic millimeter (mm³), (■) CD3, (o) CD4, (▲) CD8, (x) double negative, CD4⁻CD8⁻, T cells. Panels B and E show (■) naive CD4 and (o) naive CD8 T cell development. Panels C and F present proliferative responses in counts per minute (cpm) to the mitogen phytohemagglutinin (■) and the background of cells without mitogen (o). In panel D, the number of pre-transplantation oligoclonal T cells was 7684/mm³ prior to administration of rabbit anti-thymocyte globulin. Composite graphs for patients receiving transplants with and without immunosuppression have been published.[2,3]

T cells after transplantation prior to the appearance of naive T cells. In one of the patients, low numbers (<500/mm³) of oligoclonal T cells had developed prior to transplantation. The respiratory symptoms only appeared after transplantation, when the T cells increased to over 1500/mm³. Many patients developed post-transplantation rashes, easily managed with topical steroids. No thymus recipient developed graft-versus-host disease. Three patients developed autoimmune-mediated thyroid disease that requires hormone replacement. These patients are discussed in detail in the next section. An additional patient developed nephrotic syndrome, which resolved after a brief course of steroids. Most patients on cyclosporine developed hypertension that required therapy until the cyclosporine was discontinued.

■ CLINICAL ISSUES AFTER TRANSPLANTATION ■

RASHES

Rashes can develop after transplantation prior to the development of naive T cells in the blood. Like the rashes seen with the development of oligoclonal T cells prior to transplantation, biopsies have been diagnosed as spongiotic dermatitis with T cells identified infiltrating the skin. The rashes are usually managed with topical steroid creams. The circulating T cells have been of recipient origin in all patients tested, although one

INFECTIONS

AUTOIMMUNE DISEASE

LONG-TERM OUTCOME

CONCLUSION

REFERENCES

CLINICAL RELEVANCE

part **10**

PREVENTION AND THERAPY OF IMMUNOLOGIC DISEASES

Immunoglobulin therapy: replacement and immunomodulation

Mark Ballow

85

■ INTRODUCTION ■

Plasma and subsequently a cold ethanol fraction of plasma that contained an enriched fraction of gammaglobulin were used over 40–50 years ago as passive immunotherapy for the treatment and protection of infectious pathogens. Drs. Robert Good in Minnesota and Charles Janeway and Fred Rosen in Boston started using this Cohn ethanol fractionation product intramuscularly (IM) as antibody replacement therapy for patients with primary immune deficiency. The goal of immunoglobulin replacement in patients with primary immunodeficiency was to provide adequate antibodies to prevent infections and long-term complications, especially pulmonary disease. This intramuscular immune serum globulin remained the principal form of therapy until 1981, when an intravenous form, i.e., immune globulin, intravenous, or IgIV, became available. Subsequently, Imbach[1] observed that thrombocytopenia resolved when immune-deficient patients were treated with IgIV. This observation led to the use of IgIV in patients with autoimmune idiopathic thrombocytopenia purpura, and an explosion on the use of IgIV as immunomodulatory therapy in a number of autoimmune disorders.

IgIV products are modified to prevent the formation of IgG aggregates to make IgIV suitable for the intravenous route. Other additions, such as sugars, amino acids, or albumin, stabilize the IgG molecules from reaggregation and also protect it during lyophilization. Treatment with solvent and detergent, pasteurization, or nanofiltration is also used as a final step for viral inactivation or removal. IgIV contains a broad spectrum of antibodies with biological activity for a number of infectious pathogens, and maintains biologic activity for Fc-mediated function. Practically, all commercial IgIV preparations are derived from ~10 000 (range 10 000–60 000) donors. Although there is no standardization for the titer of antibodies against common organisms such as *Streptococcus pneumoniae* and *Haemophilus influenzae*, each lot must contain adequate levels of antibody to potential pathogens. These products may vary slightly from each manufacturer and from lot to lot but they are generally comparable for clinical efficacy, although perhaps not tolerability. The characteristics of IgIV preparations available in the USA are reviewed in Table 85.1.

In this chapter the application of IgIV as replacement therapy in patients with primary immune deficiency and in the treatment of autoimmune and inflammatory diseases will be reviewed. The mechanism(s) by which IgIV modulates the immune or inflammatory process in certain disease will be discussed. For a comprehensive review of all disorders treated with IgIV the reader is referred to a recent evidence-based medicine review of the topic elsewhere.[1]

■ REPLACEMENT THERAPY WITH IMMUNE GLOBULIN, INTRAVENOUS ■

Several early trials in the 1980s were conducted to examine the efficacy of IgIV with IM gammaglobulin, and a comparison of low-dose with high-dose IgIV therapy. In a randomized cross-over study of either

KEY CONCEPTS

PROPERTIES OF IMMUNOGLOBULIN, INTRAVENOUS (IGIV)

- ≫ Plasma fractionation (first step) by cold ethanol/Cohn–Oncley modification (fraction II)
  - \> 98% immunoglobulin G (IgG); >90% monomeric IgG
- ≫ Traces of other immunoglobulins, e.g., IgA and IgM, and serum proteins
- ≫ Addition of sugar, amino acids, or albumin stabilizes IgG from aggregation
- ≫ Intact Fc receptor important for biological function
  - – Opsonization and phagocytosis
  - – Complement activation
  - – Antibody-dependent cytotoxicity
- ≫ Normal half-life comparable to serum IgG
- ≫ Normal proportion of IgG subclasses
- ≫ Broad spectrum of antibodies to bacterial and viral agents

Table 85.1 Adverse events associated with intravenous immunoglobuin therapy

Rate-related
Chills
Headache
Back pain
Myalgia
Malaise, fatigue
Fever
Pruritus
Rash
Nausea, vomiting
Tachycardia
Chest pain or tightness
Dyspnea
Hypotension/hypertension

Central nervous system
Severe headaches
Aseptic meningitis[*]

Renal
Azotemia
Renal failure

Thromboembolic events[a]
Thrombosis/cerebral infarction
Myocardial infarction
Pulmonary embolism
Posterior leukoencephalopathy syndrome

Anaphylaxis from anti-immunoglobulin E (IgE) antibodies to IgA

Rare (isolated reports)
Cardiac rhythm abnormalities
Coagulopathy
Hemolysis – alloantibodies to blood type A/B
Cryoglobulinemia
Neutropenia
Alopecia
Uveitis
Noninfectious hepatitis

[a]See text for predisposing risk factors.

KEY CONCEPTS

PROPERTIES OF IMMUNOGLOBULIN, INTRAVENOUS IMMUNOGLOBULIN – VIRAL SAFETY

>> Donor selection

>> Donor screening

>> Donor plasma testing

 – Viral antibody screen

 – Nucleic acid testing (NAT)

>> Donor deferral[a]

>> Mini-pool testing by NAT

>> Viral inactivation[b]

 – Depth filtration
 – Column chromatography
 – Caprylate precipitation
 – Low pH incubation
 – Solvent/detergent treatment
 – Nanofiltration
 – Pasteurization
 – PEG precipitation

[a] Plasma from donor is held for 6 months until donor returns for second plasmapheresis donation.
[b] Not all products use the same virus inactivation/removal steps. Each product uses 2–5 steps.

IgIV therapy between 1982 and 1997. IgIV was given at doses of > 250 mg/kg every 3 weeks with a mean serum trough level of 500–1140 mg/dl (median, 700 mg/dl). The incidence of bacterial infections requiring hospitalizations fell from 0.4 to 0.06 per patient per year. However, enteroviral meningoencephalitis still developed in 3 patients. Of 23 patients evaluated by pulmonary function tests and chest computed tomography, 3 had obstructive disease, 6 had bronchiectasis, and 20 had chronic sinusitis. The authors concluded that, although early treatment with IgIV that achieved a trough serum IgG level of > 500 mg/dl was effective in preventing severe acute bacterial infections, these levels did not prevent pulmonary disease and sinusitis. The authors suggested that more intensive therapy to maintain a higher serum IgG level (e.g., > 800 mg/dl) may improve pulmonary outcome. Most studies show that doses of IgIV of 400 mg/kg or greater have improved efficacy over lower doses in reducing the incidence of infection.[2]

The overall consensus among clinical immunologists is that a dose of IgIV of 400–600 mg/kg per month or a dose that maintains trough serum IgG levels > 500 mg/dl is a good starting point. Immunologists may have to rethink these levels in light of the several studies cited above.[2,3] Generally, 400–600 mg/kg per month should raise the trough serum IgG level near the low normal range 4–8 months after initiating the infusions. On average, peak serum IgG levels increase approximately 250 mg/dl, and trough levels increase 100 mg/dl for each 100 mg/kg of IgIV infused. A rough goal to shoot for is a trough serum IgG level equal to pretreatment levels plus 300 mg/dl. Studies have demonstrated a variation in individual catabolism of infused immunoglobulin.

600 mg/kg or 200 mg/kg of IgIV in 12 patients with antibody deficiency and chronic lung disease, pulmonary function improved on the higher doses of IgIV therapy. Despite adequate serum IgG trough levels (> 500 mg/dl), patients with primary hypogammaglobulinemia and pulmonary abnormalities treated with IgIV can still progress with silent and asymptomatic pulmonary changes. Quartier and associates[2] performed a retrospective study of the clinical features and outcomes of 31 patients with X-linked agammaglobulinemia receiving replacement

Measurement of preinfusion (trough) serum IgG levels at 3-month intervals until a steady state is achieved, and then every 6–12 months if the patients is stable, may be helpful in adjusting the dose of IgIV to achieve adequate serum levels. For persons who have a high catabolism rate of infused IgG, or more frequent infections, infusions every 2–3 weeks of smaller doses may maintain the serum level in the normal range. The rate of elimination of IgG may be higher during a period of active infection; measuring serum IgG levels and adjusting to higher dosages or shorter treatment intervals may be required.

For replacement therapy of patients with primary immune deficiency, all brands of IgIV are probably equivalent, although there are differences in viral inactivation processes (Table 85.1). The choice of products may be dependent on the hospital or home care formulary, and the distributor availability and cost. The dose, manufacturer, and lot number should be recorded for each infusion in order to perform look-back procedures for adverse events or other consequences. It is crucial to record all side effects that occur during the infusion. It is also recommended to monitor liver and renal function tests periodically, approximately once or twice yearly.

To avoid adverse reactions in patients with active infection, especially patients with common variable immunodeficiency, the initial (first) dose should be halved (i.e., 150–200 mg/kg), and the dose repeated 2 weeks later to achieve a full dose.

To minimize cost and inconvenience, self-administration and home treatment have been used successfully. For home therapy, patients need to be selected carefully. Infusions should be done only in the presence of a responsible adult who is ready to provide assistance. Home treatment has been reported to be as effective as hospital treatment in terms of the frequency of infections, days missed from school or work, antibiotics used, and immunoglobulin level achieved. Patients receiving home treatment should be seen as regularly as patients on hospital-based treatment to monitor clinical status, liver function, and serum IgG level.

Berger and colleagues were the first to describe the use of the subcutaneous route for immunoglobulin replacement therapy in 1980.[5] It was reported to be safe, well tolerated, and effective in achieving adequate serum IgG levels. In a multicenter study of 165 patients with primary hypogammaglobulinemia or IgG subclass deficiency those patients receiving subcutaneous infusions (27 030 at home) showed significant reductions in adverse systemic reactions compared with intramuscular or intravenous administration. Anaphylactoid reactions did not occur. Patients achieved significant increases in serum IgG after 6 months of initiating immunoglobulin therapy. The use of subcutaneous infusions instead of intravenous infusions resulted in yearly cost reductions of approximately $10 000. Local tissue reactions to subcutaneous infusions included swelling, soreness, redness, induration, local heat, itching, and bruising. Each subcutaneous infusion requires a small portable syringe driver-type pump together with a 10–20-ml syringe and an infusion set with specialized 25–27-gauge needles. The length of the needle may have to be adjusted for the thickness of the subcutaneous tissue of each patient. Before infusion, the infusion catheter needs to be checked to ensure that there is no blood return. Infusions need to be given weekly at multiple sites or more often if needed to maintain adequate serum IgG levels. Infusion sites are usually on the abdominal wall and lateral thigh. In adults 20–40 ml can be infused into a single subcutaneous site. Before beginning home treatment, patients need to be instructed on the correct technique under close supervision and on how to recognize possible side effects. Recently, a new 16% IgIV for subcutaneous administration was approved by the Food and Drug Administration

(FDA), although any commercial IgIV preparation is suitable. Subcutaneous immunoglobulin infusion is safer, and may be less expensive, better tolerated, and preferred by some patients. It should be considered as an alternative in selected patients, especially those with adverse reactions to Ig IV with the intravenous route. More details on the subcutaneous route can be found in the review by Berger.[5]

■ ADVERSE EVENTS ASSOCIATED WITH IGIV THERAPY ■

RATE-RELATED

Typical rate-related adverse reactions with IgIV include tachycardia, dyspnea, chest tightness, back pain, arthralgia, myalgia, hypertension or hypotension, headache, pruritus, rash, and low-grade fever (Table 85.1). It seems that patients with more profound immunodeficiency or patients with active infections tend to have more severe reactions. The cause of the reactions is thought to be related to the anticomplementary activity of IgG aggregates in the IgIV in which immune complexes form between infused antibodies and antigens of infectious agents in the patient. The other possible mechanism is the formation of oligomeric or polymeric IgG complexes that interact with cell-bound Fc receptors and trigger the release of inflammatory mediators. These rate-related reactions appear to occur less frequently with the newer IgIV products. However, headaches still remain as the most frequent adverse event associated with IgIV infusions. Slowing the infusion rate or discontinuing therapy until symptoms subside may diminish the reaction. Pretreatment with aspirin (15 mg/kg per dose), acetaminophen (15 mg/kg per dose), diphenhydramine (1 mg/kg per dose) and/or hydrocortisone (6 mg/kg per dose, maximum 100 mg) 1 hour before the infusion may prevent adverse reactions.

CENTRAL NERVOUS SYSTEM-RELATED ADVERSE EVENTS

Aseptic meningitis has been reported as one of the complications of IgIV, especially with large doses, rapid infusions, and in the treatment of patients with autoimmune disease.[6] Interestingly, this infrequently occurs in immunodeficient subjects and may be related to a lower dose of IgIV given more slowly. Symptoms, including headache, stiff neck, and photophobia, usually develop within 24 hours after completion of the infusion and may last 3–5 days. Spinal fluid pleocytosis occurs in most patients.[6] Long-term complications are minimal. The etiology of aseptic meningitis is unclear but migraine headaches have been reported as a risk factor and may be associated with recurrence despite the use of different IgIV preparations and slower rates of infusion.

RENAL ADVERSE EVENTS

Acute renal failure is a rare but significant complication of IgIV treatment. Histopathologic findings of acute tubular necrosis, vacuolar degeneration, and osmotic nephrosis were suggestive of osmotic injury to the proximal renal tubules. Most patients (95%) had received large doses for the treatment of autoimmune disease. The majority of the cases were treated successfully with conservative treatment, but deaths were reported in 17 patients who had serious underlying conditions.

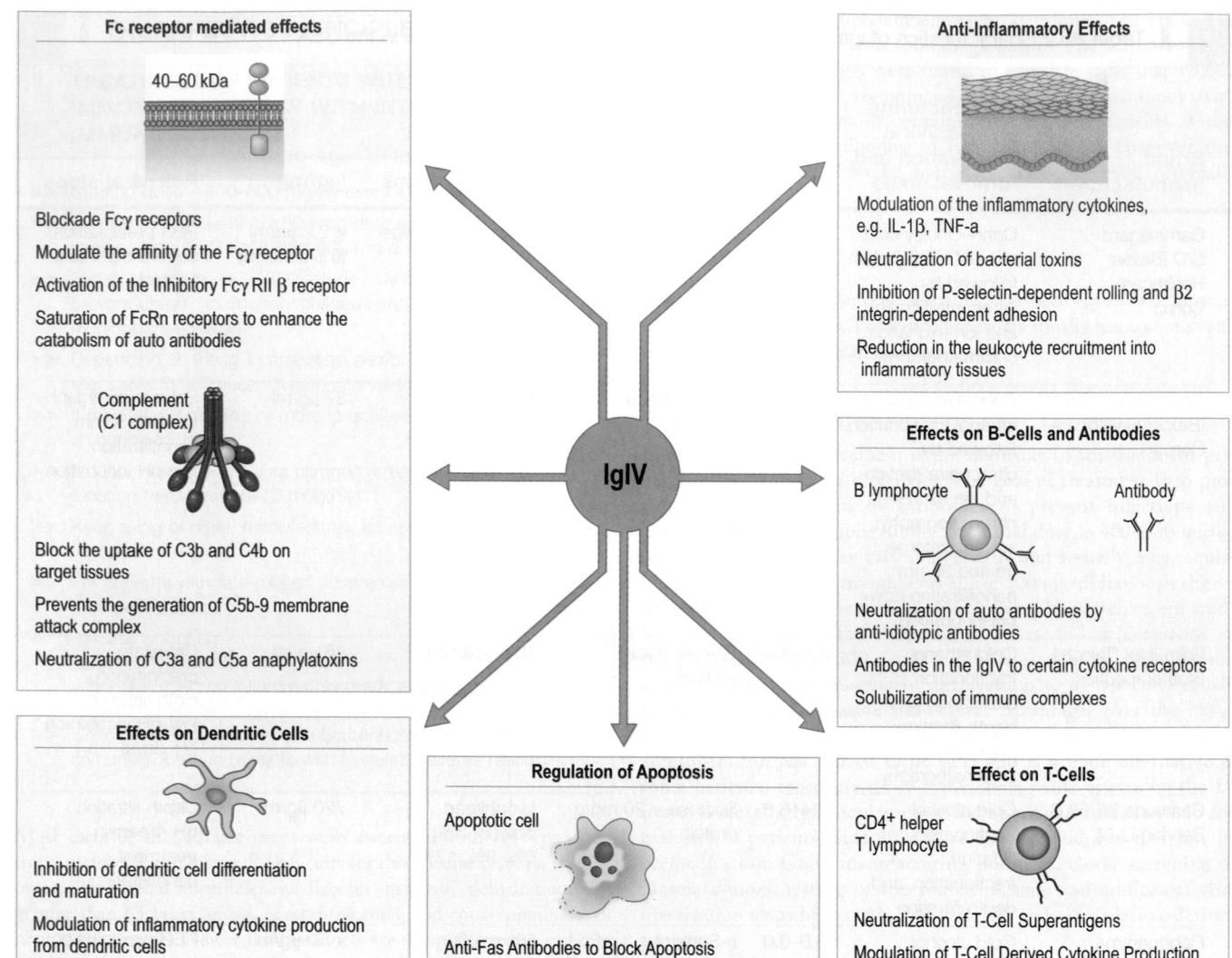

Fc receptor mediated effects

40–60 kDa

Blockade Fcγ receptors

Modulate the affinity of the Fcγ receptor

Activation of the Inhibitory Fcγ RII β receptor

Saturation of FcRn receptors to enhance the catabolism of auto antibodies

Complement (C1 complex)

Block the uptake of C3b and C4b on target tissues

Prevents the generation of C5b-9 membrane attack complex

Neutralization of C3a and C5a anaphylatoxins

Anti-Inflammatory Effects

Modulation of the inflammatory cytokines, e.g. IL-1β, TNF-a

Neutralization of bacterial toxins

Inhibition of P-selectin-dependent rolling and β2 integrin-dependent adhesion

Reduction in the leukocyte recruitment into inflammatory tissues

Effects on B-Cells and Antibodies

B lymphocyte   Antibody

Neutralization of auto antibodies by anti-idiotypic antibodies

Antibodies in the IgIV to certain cytokine receptors

Solubilization of immune complexes

Effects on Dendritic Cells

Inhibition of dendritic cell differentiation and maturation

Modulation of inflammatory cytokine production from dendritic cells

Regulation of Apoptosis

Apoptotic cell

Anti-Fas Antibodies to Block Apoptosis

Effect on T-Cells

CD4+ helper T lymphocyte

Neutralization of T-Cell Superantigens

Modulation of T-Cell Derived Cytokine Production

IgIV

Fig. 85.1 Possible immunomodulatory effects of immunoglobulin, intravenous (IgIV).

AUTOIMMUNE CYTOPENIAS

Idiopathic thrombocytopenic purpura

Idiopathic thrombocytopenic purpura (ITP) results from accelerated platelet destruction attributable to an immunologic process that could result in bleeding, which is sometimes life-threatening (Chapter 62). A number of studies in childhood ITP have shown that IgIV leads to the reversal of the thrombocytopenia. The number of days required to achieve a platelet count of $50 \times 10^9/L$ was significantly fewer in the children given IgIV than in those receiving prednisone or no therapy. IgIV as a single dose at 0.8 g/kg was similar to 1 g/kg on 2 consecutive days, but was more rapid in restoring platelet levels than intravenous anti-D or oral corticosteroids. Studies have shown that intravenous anti-D immunoglobulin is as effective as IgIV in acute childhood ITP.[9] Anti-D IGIV therapy is

FDA-approved for the treatment of ITP in Rho(D)-positive, nonsplenectomized children, children and adults with chronic ITP, and ITP secondary to human immunodeficiency virus (HIV) infection. The main side effect from anti-D IgIV therapy is anemia due to immune hemolysis. Rarely, patients may experience acute hemoglobinemia, hemoglobinuria, acute renal failure, or disseminated intravascular coagulation.[10] Anti-D IgIV therapy has the advantage of ease of administration and lower costs, and most hematologists prefer this form of therapy over IgIV.

Autoimmune hemolytic anemia

Autoimmune hemolytic anemia (AIHA) occurs when autoantibodies bind to determinants on the surface of red blood cell membranes and cause the premature clearance and destruction of erythrocytes (Chapter 62). Conflicting reports have been published regarding the efficacy of IgIV therapy in

THERAPEUTIC PRINCIPLES

TREATMENT OF IDIOPATHIC THROMBOCYTOPENIA PURPURA

>> Corticosteroids, oral – 1-4 mg/kg or 60 mg/m^2 per day until platelet recovery plus 2–3 weeks

  – For severe thrombocytopenia and impending bleed – intravenous methylprednisolone (30 mg/kg per day for 3 days)

>> Intravenous immunoglobulin – 1 g/kg on 2 consecutive days

>> Intravenous anti-D immunoglobulin (Rho (D)-positive individuals) – 50–75 µg/kg

>> Anti-CD20 chimeric monoclonal antibody (rituximab)

>> Splenectomy

KEY CONCEPTS

MECHANISMS OF ACTION OF INTRAVENOUS IMMUNOGLOBULIN IN AUTOIMMUNE CYTOPENIAS

>> Blockade of reticuloendothelial system

>> Fcγ receptor downregulation

>> Idiotype–anti-idiotype interaction between anti-platelet GPIIb/IIIa autoantibodies and the anti-idiotypic antibodies in intravenous immunoglobulin

>> Activation of inhibitory receptor FcγRIIB

>> Saturation of FcRn receptor to accelerate the catabolism of anti-platelet autoantibodies

patients with AIHA. Responses have been limited to patients with warm (IgG) hemolytic anemia. Patients with AIHA respond less frequently than patients with either ITP or autoimmune neutropenia. In addition, the dose of IgIV necessary to obtain a response is higher (up to 5 g/kg).

Autoimmune neutropenia

The largest experience with IgIV therapy in neutropenic states has been reported in autoimmune neutropenia of infancy. This acquired condition typically occurs in the first year of life and is characterized by an absolute neutrophil count of less than 500/mm^3 (Chapter 21). In general, children with this disorder suffer from symptoms of recurrent fever and nonlife-threatening infections (gingivitis, otitis media, gastroenteritis), with recovery occurring by 4 years of age. Treatment is usually limited to antibiotic therapy. However, in children with serious infections, IgIV therapy should be considered. Therapy should be reserved for those patients with severe infections who are responding poorly or not at all to appropriate intravenous broad-spectrum antibiotic therapy.

Mechanisms of action of IgIV in ITP and autoimmune cytopenias

IgIV treatment responses in ITP are due to a blockade of the reticuloendothelial system. Sequential clearance studies of autologous radiolabeled anti-Rh(D)-sensitized erythrocytes in adults with ITP treated with IgIV showed that the increase in platelet count was accompanied by a prolonged immune clearance rate. In a different approach, children with acute ITP treated with intravenous Fcγ fragments showed a rapid increase in platelet counts. The efficacy of Fcγ fragment therapy strengthens the hypothesis that Fcγ receptor blockade is the main mechanism of action of IgIV in ITP. Other studies have suggested that Fcγ receptor downregulation or change in receptor affinity may also be involved. In addition, idiotype–anti-idiotype interactions between anti-platelet GPIIb/IIIa autoantibodies and IgIV could affect autoantibody production in ITP.

Using a murine model of immune thrombocytopenia, Samuelsson et al.[11] showed that the administration of IgIV prevented platelet destruction induced by a pathogenic monoclonal autoantibody. Protection was associated with the induction of the expression of FcγRIIB receptors on splenic macrophages. This inhibitory FcγRIIB receptor was required for the protection of the animals against the pathogenic monoclonal autoantibody since disruption of the receptor by either genetic deletion or a blocking monoclonal antibody reversed the therapeutic effects of IgIV. These studies are consistent with the observation that infusion of Fc IgG fragments are effective therapy for ITP, whereas modified IgG lacking the Fc domain is less effective than intact IgG. In addition, activation of the inhibitory FcγRIIB receptor on macrophages could inhibit macrophage-mediated phagocytosis of autoantibody-coated target cells.

Recently, another mechanism has been proposed for the decrease in serum levels of autoimmune antibodies in patients treated with IgIV. The FcRn (neonatal Fc receptor) was identified as the receptor responsible for protecting IgG from catabolism in the endocytotic vesicles of the endosome, and perhaps explains the relatively long half-life of this plasma protein. IgIV may accelerate the catabolism of IgG autoantibodies by saturating these protective receptors in direct proportion to the relative concentration of exogenous plasma levels of IgG from the IgIV.[12] In a rat model of immune thrombocytopenia, Hansen and Balthasar[13] showed that IgIV enhanced the clearance of anti-platelet antibodies in a dose-dependent manner by saturation of the FcRn receptor.

Autoimmune coagulopathies

Autoantibodies against factor VIII coagulant protein can cause an acquired hemophilia, resulting in a spectrum of bleeding complications.[14] These acquired antibodies can be idiopathic, but are often found in patients with autoimmune disorders, inflammatory bowel disease, pemphigus, malignancy, and in the postpartum state. High-dose IgIV in patients with anti-factor VIII autoantibodies produces rapid and prolonged, although incomplete, suppression of inhibitor.[14] Other studies showed that an F(ab')$_2$ fragment prepared from IgIV inhibited autoantibody activity to factor VIIIc, suggesting an idiotypic–anti-idiotypic interaction between the IgIV and the autoantibodies.

KAWASAKI SYNDROME

Kawasaki syndrome (KS) is an acute multisystem disease of unknown etiology that primarily affects infants and young children (Chapter 58). Although KS occurs worldwide in children of all racial groups, it is most

CLINICAL PEARLS

CLINICAL FEATURES OF ACUTE KAWASAKI SYNDROME[a]

1. Fever of at least 5 days' duration
2. Presence of at least four of the five following conditions:
   >> Bilateral nonexudative conjunctival injection
   >> One of the following changes in the oropharynx: injected or fissured lips, injected pharynx, or 'strawberry tongue'
   >> One of the following extremity changes: erythema of the palms or soles, edema of the hands or feet, or periungal desquamation
   >> Polymorphous rash
   >> Acute nonsuppurative cervical lymphadenopathy
3. Cardiovascular abnormalities:
   >> Myocarditis, arterial aneurysms, pericarditis, aortic or mitral regurgitation, ventricular arrythmias
4. Other:
   >> Arthralgia and arthritis, urethritis with sterile pyuria, hydrops of the gallbladder, diarrhea, vomiting, or abdominal pain, sensorineural hearing loss

[a] Points 1 and 2 constitute the primary diagnostic criteria for Kawasaki syndrome

prevalent in Japan and in children of Japanese ancestry. Although the acute illness is generally self-limited, coronary artery abnormalities related to a generalized inflammation and immune activation of small and medium-sized blood vessels develop in up to 25% of untreated patients. Although the etiology remains unknown, the clinical features and laboratory findings suggest an infectious or postinfectious process.

In a multicenter randomized trial in the USA, the effects of IgIV 400 mg/kg per day for 4 consecutive days plus aspirin were compared to aspirin alone. The results showed that 2 weeks after onset of therapy, coronary artery abnormalities were present in 23% (18 of 78) of children in the aspirin group, as compared with only 8% (6 of 75) in the IgIV plus aspirin group. Seven weeks after enrollment, coronary abnormalities were present in 18% (14 of 79) of children in the aspirin group and in 4% (3 of 79) of the IgIV plus aspirin group. In a follow-up study, the efficacy of a single infusion of IgIV 2 g/kg was compared with 400 mg/kg for 4 consecutive days.[15] The relative prevalence of coronary artery lesions, adjusted for age and sex, among patients treated with the 4-day regimen was almost twice as high as those patients treated with the single-infusion regimen. Laboratory assessments of acute inflammation in the single-infusion group showed a more rapid trend toward normal. Lower serum IgG levels on day 4 were associated with a greater degree of systemic inflammation and with a higher prevalence of coronary abnormalities. A meta-analysis of published studies on the treatment of KS showed a dose response for IgIV with a threshold for decreased incidence of coronary artery aneurysm with IgIV dosages of > 1 g/kg, and that low-dose aspirin (80 mg/kg) was comparable to high-dose aspirin (> 80 mg/kg) when combined with high-dose IgIV.[16] More recently, a retrospective

analysis of retreatment of patients who remained febrile after IgIV (1 g/kg) suggested improved outcome with a higher dose of IgIV (2 g/kg), although these findings need to be confirmed prospectively.

KS is associated with marked activation of T cells and monocytes–macrophages.[17] Based on the immunologic and clinical features overlapping with a bacterial toxic shock-like syndrome, studies were carried out to determine if KS is associated with exposure to a superantigen such as a bacterial toxin.[18] The mechanism by which a superantigen can lead to the clinical manifestations of KS remains to be elucidated. However, acute KS is associated with marked immune activation and increased circulating cytokine levels, including interleukin-1 (IL-1), IL-6, IL-8, IL-4, IL-10, and tumor necrosis factor-α (TNF-α).[18] Some of these cytokines elicit proinflammatory and prothrombotic responses by inducing the expression of leukocyte adhesion molecules, which attach inflammatory cells to vascular endothelial cells. The expression of endothelial leukocyte adhesion molecules has been demonstrated in acute KS and its downregulation correlates with favorable response to IgIV treatment.[17] In contrast, patients treated with aspirin alone show prolonged T- and B-cell activation. The magnitude and persistence of proinflammatory cytokine synthesis have been reported to constitute a risk for the development of coronary artery abnormalities.

IgIV has been shown to contain high titers of specific antibodies that inhibit the activation of T cells by staphylococcal and streptococcal superantigens. These findings may account for the observation that treatment of acute KS with IgIV results in a marked reduction of macrophage and T-cell activation.[18] In this regard, the efficacy of IgIV in suppressing the immune activation associated with KS, and more importantly, its ability to prevent the development of coronary artery abnormalities in this illness may relate to the neutralizing antibody activity of IgIV against these bacterial toxins.[17] The finding that a threshold dose of IgIV is needed to decrease signs of acute inflammation in KS and that some patients require retreatment suggests that IgIV contains variable anti-toxin titers. In addition, toxin neutralization is not likely the only beneficial effect of IgIV in KS. A recent report of the use of different brands of IgIV in patients with KS showed differences in response rate and the development of coronary artery aneurysms.[19] The authors attributed these differences in efficacy to differences in manufacturing processes between the different products that may affect the Fc portion of the IgG molecule. As noted for ITP, the Fc portion may activate the immune-modulating FcγRIIB receptor. Other potential mechanisms of IgIV include immunomodulation of cytokine production or cytokine effects, resulting in the inhibition of endothelial cell activation. Gill and coworkers[20] reported that IgIV inhibits leukocyte recruitment into inflammatory tissues by inhibiting selectin and integrin function. New insights into the pathogenesis of KS will likely help elucidate the mechanisms by which IgIV reduces coronary artery vasculitis.

AUTOIMMUNE NEUROMUSCULAR DISEASES

The autoimmune neuropathies represent the largest group of autoimmune diseases that are treated with IgIV (Chapters 64-66). In fact, autoimmune neurological diseases account for approximately 30–40% of all IgIV use for 'recommended off-label' indications. The autoimmune neuropathies fall into four categories: (1) the *inflammatory demyelinating polyneuropathies*, which include the Guillain–Barré syndrome (GBS); chronic progressive or relapsing remitting inflammatory demyelinating polyneuropathy (CIDP), and multifocal motor neuropathy; (2) the *autoimmune neuromuscular junction defects* such as myasthenia gravis (MG) and Lambert–Eaton syndrome; (3) the *inflammatory myopathies*, which include dermatomyositis (DM), polymyositis, and inclusion-body myositis; and (4) the *central nervous system diseases* such as multiple sclerosis, stiff-person syndrome, and Alzheimer's disease. More information about the use of IgIV in the autoimmune neuromuscular diseases can be found in reviews on this topic elsewhere.[21, 22]

THE INFLAMMATORY DEMYELINATING POLYNEUROPATHIES

Although the etiology of GBS is not known, the pathogenesis of GBS is thought to be an autoimmune process with destruction of peripheral nerve myelin. Patients present with a rapid ascending paralysis, often with autonomic and sensory involvement. Most cases are preceded by an upper respiratory or diarrheal illness. *Campylobacter jejuni* is the most common bacterial pathogen isolated from the gastrointestinal tract. About 80% of GBS patients recover satisfactorily from their disease. The principal approach to the treatment of these patients has been supportive therapy. As summarized by Delakas,[21] a Dutch group reported on a randomized trial comparing plasma exchange and IgIV (0.4 g/kg per day for 5 days). Muscle strength improved by one grade in 34% of those treated with plasma exchange compared to 53% receiving IgIV; median time to improvement was 41 and 27 days, respectively. Also in a large European, multicenter randomized trial of 379 adult patients with GBS, the efficacy of inflammatory demyelinating polyneuropathy (50 ml/kg for 5 exchanges) was compared with IgIV (0.4 g/kg for 5 days), and with a combination regimen of plasma exchange followed by IgIV. There were no differences between any of the treatment groups for the major and secondary outcome measures. Both the French and North American studies concluded that plasma exchange in GBS is most effective when carried out early in the course of the disease. Early recognition and treatment may thus be important for the long-term prognosis of patients who have severe disease and rapid progression.[23] Because IgIV treatment is more readily available, easier, and has fewer side effects than plasma exchange, this modality of treatment might be more useful in GBS patients at the early stage of disease, especially in patients who have evidence of rapid progression, older age, or a history of diarrhea.[23] Several studies looked at optimal dosing that showed that IgIV was most beneficial when given in a full dose of 2 g/kg, especially in patients who needed ventilatory assistance. In children with GBS IgIV therapy was equally as effective as plasmapheresis, and associated with fewer complications.[24]

CIDP is an inflammatory neurologic disease resembling GBS, which may cause prolonged disability.[22] As with GBS, an immune-mediated mechanism for myelin destruction has been postulated in CIDP. In a double-blind placebo-controlled cross-over study of IgIV (0.4 g IgIV per kg per day for 5 consecutive days), all IgIV-treated patients improved on day 8 after therapy; in contrast, none of the patients receiving placebo improved. In other studies comparing IgIV with steroids or plasma exchange, improvements in neurological disability were similar, although the administration of IgIV was less complex than plasma exchange, and IgIV had fewer adverse effects compared to steroids. However, not all patients respond to IgIV and certainly not all patients respond to the same extent. Improvement is usually noticed within the first week of treatment and may last for 6–8 weeks. Many patients can be maintained on IgIV pulse therapy of 1 g/kg body weight prior to the expected relapse. A beneficial response to IgIV was found to be more likely in

patients with acute relapse or with disease of 1 year or less. Patients with sensory signs responded less well. Children with CIDP also respond well to IgIV. Patients with an IgM monoclonal paraprotein associated with a demyelinating peripheral neuropathy may also have a modest response to IgIV treatment. In contrast, patients with a paraneoplastic neurological syndrome and antineuronal autoantibodies (anti-Hu and anti-Yo) did not respond to IgIV therapy.

Multifocal motor neuropathy shares some similarities with GBS and CIDP.[21] This disorder is characterized by progressive distal, asymmetric limb weakness with a conduction block of motor but not sensory nerves. However, several open-label studies and a controlled trial showed that multifocal motor neuropathy responds to IgIV therapy. Of note, the beneficial effects of IgIV are often not long-lasting.

These autoimmune demyelinating polyneuropathies are considered to be immunologically mediated disorders of the peripheral nervous system.[25] An initial lymphocytic infiltration, and later on, an influx of macrophages, leads to demyelination. A variety of cellular and humoral immune perturbations have been described in patients with GBS. Elevated serum levels of several proinflammatory cytokines, including TNF and interferon-γ, have been reported. Other cytokines have been reported to be elevated in the spinal fluids of GBS patients, including IL-1β and IL-6. Antibodies reactive against myelin components, e.g., ganglioside-specific antibodies such as GM_1, GD_{1b}, and GQ_{1b}, are found in the sera of many patients with GBS. Anti-GM_1 antibodies are also found in patients with motor neuropathies and motor neuron disease. Anti-GM_1 antibodies are more prominent in GBS patients lacking sensory symptoms and in those patients who have a prodromal diarrheal disease.

The association of certain viruses and bacteria, and their serologies with GBS, suggests that these microbial agents are involved in the pathogenesis of GBS. Van der Meché and colleagues[26] reported that the sera of GBS patients have antibodies to the ganglioside GM1 which shares epitopes on *Campylobacter* bacteria. Interestingly, the lipopolysaccharides in the capsule of *C. jejuni*, a frequent cause of diarrheal disease preceding GBS, has epitopes related to the ganglioside GM_1 and GQ_{1b}. This has led to the hypothesis of molecular mimicry in which immune responses against *C. jejuni* lipopolysaccharide produce cross-reactive antibodies to myelin with subsequent demyelination.[26] Another possible mechanism leading to demyelination is complement deposition on the surface of Schwann cells and the myelin sheath, which leads to the recruitment of macrophages and complement-mediated damage.

THE AUTOIMMUNE NEUROMUSCULAR JUNCTION DEFECTS

MG is an antibody-mediated autoimmune disease directed against the acetylcholine nicotinic receptor (AChR) which results in abnormalities of neuromuscular transmission leading to fluctuating weakness and fatigability (Chapter 64). A number of case reports and small, uncontrolled clinical trials have been reported, with over 100 patients undergoing treatment with IgIV.[24] A number of different preparations and dosage regimens have been employed. The overall response rate is about 74%, with improvement occurring within 3 weeks from the start of therapy. The duration of the response is variable and seems to be longer if patients are receiving steroids. AChR antibody titers declined in four trials but remained unchanged in three others. Overall, the clinical response did not appear to correlate with AChR antibody levels. Repeated courses of IgIV may be needed to maintain improvement. A recent controlled trial

THERAPEUTIC PRINCIPLES

TREATMENT EFFICACY IN PATIENTS WITH AUTOIMMUNE NEUROMUSCULAR DISEASES

Proven efficacy

Guillain–Barré syndrome
Chronic demyelinating polyneuropathy
Mutifocal motor neuropathy
Dermatomyositis (adults)

Probable treatment efficacy

Myasthenia gravis
Stiff-person syndrome
Multiple sclerosis, relapsing remitting disease

Possible treatment efficacy

Childhood epilepsies

>> West syndrome

>> Lennox–Gastaut syndrome

Obsessive-compulsive disorder (Tourette syndrome)

KEY CONCEPTS

THE IMMUNE PATHOGENESIS OF GUILLAIN–BARRÉ SYNDROME AND CHRONIC INFLAMMATORY DEMYELINATING POLYNEUROPATHY

>> Molecular mimicry between epitopes on capsule of *Campylobacter jejuni* and myelin

    Preceding history of diarrhea
    Positive stool culture for *C. jejuni*

>> Autoantibodies to myelin components, i.e., ganglioside-specific antibodies (GM1, GD$_{1b}$, GQ$_{1b}$)

>> Macrophage influx into lesions

>> Complement deposition on Schwann cell and myelin sheath

comparing the efficacy and side effects of IgIV to plasma exchange in MG patients undergoing exacerbation, using two IgIV dosages, showed similar efficacy, but fewer side effects in the IgIV group.[27]

THE INFLAMMATORY MYOPATHIES

Polymyositis, DM, and inclusion-body myositis are inflammatory muscle disorders characterized by muscle weakness and cellular infiltrates within the skeletal muscles (Chapter 56). Although the pathogenesis of these diseases is thought to be similar, each inflammatory myopathy group has characteristic clinical and immunopathologic features that sets each apart. DM affects the proximal muscles and is associated with a violaceous rash on the face and extremities.

Dalakas and coworkers[28] conducted a double-blind, placebo-controlled study of 15 patients (age 18–55 years) with treatment-resistant DM. Patients were randomly assigned to receive IgIV therapy (2 g/kg) or placebo every month for 3 months. The patients receiving IgIV had significant improvements in muscle strength, neuromuscular symptoms related to daily living, and skin rash. Clinical improvement became noticeable about 15 days after the first IgIV infusion. Serum creatine kinase fell by 50% after the first infusion, with further decreases toward normalization in subsequent infusions. Unfortunately, continued improvement of these patients was variable. Some patients continued to get IgIV less frequently and were able to maintain improvement along with low-dose steroids. Some patients who were unresponsive to steroids during their initial treatment regimen became steroid-responsive following IgIV infusion.

Muscle biopsy studies showed marked improvement in muscle histology after IgIV treatment.[29] The mean muscle fiber diameter and the mean number of capillaries increased. Immunological activation markers, such as major histocompatibility complex class I determinants and ICAM-1 expression, became diminished after IgIV therapy. Transforming growth factor-β (TGF-β), which is upregulated in the muscle tissues of patients with DM, was markedly downregulated. Finally, in muscle biopsies after therapy, the complement-mediated damage was diminished after IgIV therapy.[29]

Inclusion-body myositis is the most common inflammatory muscle disorder in individuals above the age of 50 and is characterized by a slowly progressive muscle weakness and atrophy affecting the proximal and distal muscle groups. Dysphagia is also frequent, occurring in 60% of patients. Initial open-label small trials suggested that IgIV was helpful in some patients with inclusion-body myositis, particularly with activities related to daily living. Other uncontrolled studies showed no benefit of IgIV. A double-blind, placebo-controlled cross-over study in 19 patients with inclusion-body myositis using monthly IgIV infusions of 2 g/kg or placebo for 3 months showed a mild statistical improvement in the IgIV group (6 of 19 patients); the study did not establish efficacy for IgIV treatment. In a follow-up study, combining IgIV therapy with prednisone, there appeared to be no clear benefit. However, some patients may have some transient benefit from IgIV therapy, especially those with severe dysphagia.[21, 29]

THE CENTRAL NERVOUS SYSTEM DISEASES

Multiple sclerosis is the most common demyelinating disorder of the central nervous system, and studies have suggested that the pathogenesis of multiple sclerosis is related to an autoimmune process (Chapter 65). Several uncontrolled and open-label studies have shown a beneficial effect of long-term IgIV therapy in the treatment of acute exacerbations in patients with multiple sclerosis.[30] In a randomized placebo-controlled trial of monthly infusions of IgIV (0.15–0.2 g/kg) therapy in patients with relapsing remitting multiple sclerosis, the number of patients who improved in the IgIV group was 31%, while in the placebo group only 14% of patients improved. Side effects were minimal. Other studies correlated changes in disease activity with changes in multiple sclerosis lesions, as measured by magnetic resonance imaging. A meta-analysis of four controlled trials in patients with relapsing remitting MS showed that IgIV significantly reduced the annual relapse rate, increased the proportion of relapse-free patients, and reduced disease progression, as measured by the change in Kurtzke expanded disability status scale.[30]

Stiff-person syndrome is characterized by fluctuating muscle rigidity, episodic muscle spasms, and high titers of antibodies against glutamic acid decarboxylase. In a placebo-controlled cross-over trial by Dalakas[21, 29] of 16 patients treated with 2 g/kg of IgIV or placebo for 3 months, stiffness scores decreased, heightened sensitivity scores declined, and patients were able to walk and perform work-related or household tasks.

Ten to 20% of childhood epilepsies are intractable, i.e., not controlled adequately with first-line conventional anti-epileptic drug therapy. Children with epilepsy, who were treated with IgIV for recurrent respiratory tract infections, had a decrease in the frequency and severity of their seizures. A number of investigators have suggested that immune mechanisms are important in the pathogenesis of epilepsy, particularly those that are associated with infections or vaccination. A number of reports have appeared on the responsiveness of certain patients with childhood epilepsy to IgIV therapy. The favorable effects of IgIV treatment were especially seen in children with variant forms of epilepsy, such as West syndrome and Lennox–Gastaut syndrome. Placebo-controlled studies showed significant reductions in seizure episodes with IgIV treatment. Additional multicenter placebo-controlled trials are needed to define further the subpopulation of children with intractable seizures who would benefit from IgIV treatment, although the best candidates appear to be those patients with West syndrome and Lennox–Gastaut syndrome and those patients who have postinfectious epileptic encephalopathies. Perlmutter and coworkers[31] reported a placebo-controlled study with plasma exchange and IgIV in patients with obsessive-compulsive disorder and tic disorders (Tourette syndrome). At 1 month the plasma exchange and IgIV groups showed striking improvements on several neuropsychiatric functioning scales. Tic symptoms also significantly improved. Improvement was maintained at 1 year by 82% of the children in both the plasma exchange and IgIV groups.

MECHANISMS OF ACTION OF IgIV IN NEUROMUSCULAR DISEASES

The autoimmune neurologic diseases and inflammatory myopathies provide a broad group of immunologically mediated diseases in which many inflammatory and immune-mediated effector pathways lead to tissue destruction. These neurological and myopathic diseases provide models for the study of the mechanisms of action by which IgIV modulates these autoimmune and inflammatory processes. Several mechanisms have been proposed for the immune-modulating effects of IgIV. IgIV may modulate the inflammatory response by the suppression of cytokine production. Proinflammatory cytokines, e.g., TNF-α and IL-1β, in GBS patients decrease with IgIV therapy. Dalakas[29] documented reduction in muscle levels of ICAM-1, TGF-β, and TGF-β mRNA in patients with inflammatory myopathies after IgIV treatment. Although IgIV may contain antibodies to certain cytokines, other studies suggested that IgIV was downregulating cytokine production by inhibiting gene expression. Of interest, plasma exchange was not associated with a decrease in these proinflammatory cytokines, suggesting that the mechanisms of action of plasma exchange and IgIV in GBS may be quite different.

A number of studies have shown that IgIV contains antibodies with idiotypic specificities that can bind and neutralize potentially pathogeneic autoantibodies such as anti-GM1 antibodies in GBS and CIDP and anti-AchR in MG.[29] Malik and coworkers[32] showed that anti-idiotypic antibodies in the IgIV directed against idiotopes located on the anti-GM$_1$ immunoglobulin molecule blocked the binding of the

anti-GM$_1$ antibodies to its target antigen. Van Doorn et al.,[33] using an immunofluorescence assay, showed that the sera of patients with GBS and CIDP contained antibodies to a cell membrane constituent of a neuroblastoma cell line. Intact IgIV or F(ab')$_2$ fragments blocked these antibodies from binding to the cell membrane of this neuroblastoma cell line. These studies again suggest an idiotype–anti-idiotype interaction as a possible mechanism by which IgIV could modulate the immune-mediated disease process and contribute to remyelination in patients with GBS and CIDP. Support for a similar mechanism in MG comes from the fact that IgG or F(ab')$_2$ fragments in the IgIV preparations are capable of binding to AChR antibodies in vitro.[34] Using in vitro nerve muscle preparations, Buchwald et al.[35] showed that the F(ab')$_2$ portion of IgIV neutralized the 'blocking' effect of serum from patients with acute GBS.

As discussed above for ITP, the administration of large amounts of IgG could saturate the FcRn receptor and accelerate the degradation of the IgG autoantibodies found in many of the autoimmune neuropathies. This mechanism may be applicable to antibody-mediated neuromuscular diseases such as MG, Lambert–Eaton myasthenia syndrome, GBS, stiff-person syndrome, CIDP, and multifocal motor neuropathy.

The principal inflammatory mechanism in DM is complement (C)-dependent microangiopathy with activation of C3 and deposition of the complement C5b-9 membranolytic attack complex (MAC) on the endomysial capillaries.[29] Basta[36] has shown that IgIV can inhibit the uptake of C components on target tissues. In DM patients treated with IgIV, C3 deposition was reduced, with corresponding decreases in MAC expression on endomysial capillaries.[29, 36] IgIV prevents the uptake of complement components and formation of the MAC on the endomysial capillaries in the muscle tissues of patients with DM. Consequently, IgIV allowed neovascularization to occur and reversal of the ischemic process, resulting in muscle tissue healing. This effect of IgIV on complement deposition may be relevant to other autoimmune neurological diseases, such as MG, in which complement may be playing a role in the tissue damage at the postsynaptic junctional membrane.[29, 36]

CONNECTIVE TISSUE DISORDERS

SYSTEMIC VASCULITIS

IgIV has been shown to be useful as adjunct therapy in patients with anti-neutrophil cytoplasmic antibody (ANCA)-positive systemic vasculitis (Chapter 59). High-dose IgIV (e.g., 400 mg/kg per dose given over 5 consecutive days) may benefit the disease activity and circulating ANCA levels. ANCA levels decreased by 51% of pretreatment values, and improvement started 2 days to 3 weeks after IgIV therapy; 5 patients went into full remission. Other investigators also reported beneficial clinical responses following high-dose IgIV treatment. Response rates vary between 60% and 100%, and may be related in some patients to a chronic paravovirus B19 infection. Further placebo-controlled studies are needed.

RHEUMATIC DISEASES

The clinical studies of IgIV therapy in patients with rheumatoid arthritis (Chapter 52) and systemic lupus erythematosus (SLE) (Chapter 51) have been case reports and open-labeled studies.[2] Most have shown little

FOOD AND DRUG ADMINISTRATION-APPROVED INDICATIONS FOR INTRAVENOUS IMMUNOGLOBULIN

>> Patients with primary immunodeficiency disease – replacement therapy

>> Idiopathic thrombocytopenia – prevent severe bleeding

>> Children with human immunodeficiency virus (HIV)/acquired immunodeficiency syndrome (AIDS) and recurrent infections – prevent serious bacterial infections

>> B-cell chronic lymphocytic leukemia with recurrent infections and humoral immune deficiency – prevent bacterial infection

>> Kawasaki disease – to prevent coronary artery aneurysms

>> Bone marrow transplantation – decrease risk of infection, interstitial pneumonia, and graft-versus-host disease in the first 100 days after transplantation

the placebo (albumin 2 g/kg per month) and the two IgIV treatment groups for forced expiratory volume in 1 second, emergency room visits, or days missed from work or school. Adverse events were common in the IgIV groups, especially in the high-dose treatment group. In another double-blind placebo-controlled randomized trial of IgIV in children with severe asthma, there was a significant reduction in oral steroid requirement in both the IgIV and placebo treatment groups.[52] In a subgroup of patients requiring extremely high doses of oral steroids (> 2000 mg in the year before the study), there was a significant steroid-sparing effect by the IgIV. These authors concluded that IgIV was useful in a subgroup of severe asthmatic patients who required high doses of oral steroids. A larger placebo-controlled trial is needed to determine the efficacy of IgIV therapy in oral steroid-dependent asthmatics.

A number of mechanisms have been proposed for the effects of IgIV in asthma. Several studies have shown that IgIV can modulate the synthesis of cytokines. Related to cytokine inhibition, Spahn et al.[53] showed that the addition of IgIV to phytohemagglutinin (PHA)-stimulated lymphocytes shifted the dexamethasone dose–response curve, rendering the cells more sensitive to the suppressive effects of steroids in patients with glucocorticoid-insensitive asthma. In addition, IgIV significantly improved glucocorticoid receptor-binding affinity that may be responsible for the steroid-sparing effects of IgIV.

The mechanism(s) by which IgIV suppresses immunoglobulin synthesis by B cells has been postulated to occur by inhibiting cytokine production and by directly suppressing B-cell function through its low-affinity $Fc\gamma$ receptor. The $Fc\gamma RIIB$ receptor on B cells can provide a negative signal through protein tyrosine phosphatases (SHP-1) to inhibit B-cell proliferation and decrease antibody synthesis. The mechanism for this negative signaling in B cells is thought to occur by the immunoreceptor tyrosine-based inhibition motif (ITIM) that is known to be associated with the intracytoplasmic domain of the $Fc\gamma RIIB$ receptor. Co-ligation of the B-cell receptor and the $Fc\gamma RIIB$ receptor could occur by the binding of IgG in IgIV through its Fc moiety to the $Fc\gamma RIIB$ receptor and the $F(ab')_2$ moiety with anti-idiotypic antibody specificity to the B-cell

antigen receptor. Thus, through pathways that modulate cytokine production and decrease B-cell Ig synthesis, i.e., diminished serum levels of IgE antibodies, IgIV may have both anti-inflammatory and immunomodulating effects in the immunopathogenesis of asthma.

Chronic urticaria

A subset of patients with chronic urticaria (Chapter 42) have IgG autoantibodies directed against the α-chain of the high-affinity receptor for IgE, suggesting an autoimmune etiology. In 10 patients with chronic severe urticaria poorly responsive to conventional therapy, treatment with IgIV (0.4 g/kg per day for 5 days) showed clinical benefit in 9 patients, including 3 who had prolonged remission over a 3-year follow-up period. The majority of responders had a decreased wheal-and-flare response to intradermal autologous serum compared with their pre-IgIV response. Placebo-controlled studies are needed.

CONCLUSIONS

IgIV has been found to be an effective treatment for a wide spectrum of autoimmune and inflammatory diseases. At present, IgIV is FDA-approved for only a few autoimmune and inflammatory diseases, e.g., ITP and KS. However, even in ITP and KS, the mechanism of action of IgIV remains to be fully elucidated. Although no single mechanism can explain the beneficial effects of IgIV, it is likely that several mechanisms of action working together are responsible for the effects of IgIV in the many clinical disorders for which it has been used. It is important to recognize that IgIV contains not only a broad spectrum of IgG antibodies, but also small amounts of other immunoglobulin isotypes, as well as soluble cell membrane products and HLA determinants. These "contaminants" may in fact play an important immunomodulatory role in autoimmune and inflammatory diseases. A better understanding of the pathogenic mechanisms involved in these diseases will undoubtedly lead to more effective therapy with IgIV or more specific, modified forms of this product.

REFERENCES

1. Imbach P, d'Apuzzo V, Hirt A, et al. High-dose intravenous gammaglobulin for idiopathic thrombocytopenic purpura in childhood. Lancet; 1: 1228–1231.

2. Orange JS, Hossny EM, Weiler CR, et al. Use of intravenous immunoglobulin in human disease: a review of evidence by members of the primary immunodeficiency committee of the American Academy of Allergy, Asthma and Immunology. J Allergy Clin Immunol 2006; 117(Suppl): S525–S553.

3. Quartier P, Debre M, DeBlie J, et al. Early and prolonged intravenous immunoglobulin replacement therapy in childhood agammaglobulinemia: a retrospective survey of 31 patients. J Pediatr 1999; 134: 589–596.

4. Busse PJ, Razvi S, Cunningham-Rundles C. Efficacy of intravenous immunoglobulin in the prevention of pneumonia in patients with common variable immunodeficiency. J Allergy Clin Immunol 2002; 109: 1001–1004.

5. Berger M, Cupps TR, Fauci AS. Immunoglobulin replacement therapy by slow subcutaneous infusion. Ann Intern Med 1980; 93: 55–56.

6. Brannagan TH, Nagle KJ, Lange DJ, et al. Complications of intravenous immune globulin treatment in neurologic disease. Neurology 1996; 47: 674–677.

7. Burks A, Sampson H, Buckley R. Anaphylactic reactions after gamma-globulin administration in patients with hypogammaglobulinemia. Detection of IgE antibodies to IgA. N Engl J Med 1986; 314: 560.

8. Thampakkul S, Ballow M. Replacement intravenous immune serum globulin therapy in patients with antibody immune deficiency. Allergy Immunol Clin North Am 2001; 21: 165–184.

9. Tarantino MD, Madden RM, Fennewald DL, et al. Treatment of childhood acute immune thrombocytopenic purpura with anti-D immune globulin or pooled immune globulin. J Pediatr 1999; 134: 21–26.

10. Gaines AR. Disseminated intravascular coagulation associated with acute hemoglobinemia or hemoglobinuria following $Rh_o(D)$ immune globulin intravenous administration for immune thrombocytopenic purpura. Blood 2005; 106: 1532–1537.

11. Samuelsson A, Towers TL, Ravetch JV. Anti-inflammatory activity of IVIG mediated through the inhibitory Fc receptor. Science 2001; 291: 484–486.

12. Yu Z, Lennon VA. Mechanism of intravenous immune globulin therapy in antibody-mediated autoimmune diseases. N Engl J Med 1999; 340: 227–228.

13. Hansen RJ, Balthasar JP. Effects of intravenous immunoglobulin on platelet count and anti-platelet antibody disposition in a rat model of immune thrombcytopenia. Blood 2002; 100: 2087–2093.

14. Schwartz RS, Gabriel DA, Aledort LM, et al. A prospective study of treatment of acquired (autoimmune) factor VIII inhibitors with high-dose intravenous gammaglobulin. Blood 1995; 86: 797–804.

15. Newburger JW, Takahashi M, Beiser AS, et al. A single intravenous infusion of gamma globulin as compared with four infusions in the treatment of acute Kawasaki syndrome. N Engl J Med 1991; 324: 1633–1639.

16. Durongpisitkul K, Gururaj VJ, Park JM, et al. The prevention of coronary artery aneurysm in Kawasaki disease: a meta-analysis on the efficacy of aspirin and immunoglobulin treatment. Pediatrics 1995; 96: 1057–1061.

17. Leung DYM. Immunologic aspects of Kawasaki syndrome. J Rheumatol 1990; (Suppl)24: 15–18.

18. Leung DY. Kawasaki syndrome: immunomodulatory benefit and potential toxin neutralization by intravenous immune globulin. Clin Exp Immunol 1996; (Suppl 1)104: 49–54.

19. Tsai M-H, Huang Y-C, Yen M-H, et al. Clinical responses of patients with Kawasadi disease to different brands of intravenous immunoglobulin. J Pediatr 2006; 148: 38–43.

20. Gill V, Doig C, Knight D, et al. Targeting adhesion molecules as a potential mechanism of action for intravenous immunoglobulin. Circulation 2005; 112: 2031–2039.

21. Dalakas MC. Intravenous immunoglobulin in autoimmune neuromuscular diseases. JAMA 2004; 291: 2367–2375.

22. Fergusson D, Hutton B, Sharma M, et al. Use of intravenous immunoglobulin for treatment of neurologic conditions: a systematic review. Transfusion 2005; 45: 1640–1657.

23. Hughes RA, Raphael JC, Swan AV, et al. Intravenous immunoglobulin for Guillain–Barré syndrome [update of Cochrane Database Syst Rev 2001;(2):CD002063; PMID: 11406030]. Cochrane Database Syst Rev 2004.

24. Bril V, Allenby K, Midroni G, et al. IGIV in neurology – evidence and recommendations. Can J Neurol Sci 1999; 26: 139–152.

25. Sater RA, Rostami A. Treatment of Guillain–Barré syndrome with intravenous immunoglobulin. Neurology 1998; 51(Suppl 5): S9–S15.

26. van der Meché FGA, Visser LH, Jacobs BC, et al. Guillain–Barré syndrome: multifactorial mechanisms versus defined subgroups. J Infect Dis 1997; 176(Suppl 2): S99–S102.

27. Gajdos P, Chevret S, Clair B, et al. Plasma exchange and intravenous immunoglobulin in autoimmune myasthenia gravis. Ann NY Acad Sci 1998; 841: 720–726.

28. Dalakas MC, Illa I, Dambrosia JM, et al. A controlled trial of high-dose intravenous immunoglobulin infusions as treatment for dermatomyositis. N Engl J Med 1993; 329: 1993–2000.

29. Dalakas MC. Mechanism of action of intravenous immunoglobulin and therapeutic considerations in the treatment of autoimmune neurologic diseases. Neurology 1998; 51(Suppl 5): S2–S8.

30. Sorensen PS, Fazekas F, Lee M. Intravenous immunoglobulin G for the treatment of relapsing-remitting multiple sclerosis: a meta-analysis. Eur J Neurol 2002; 9: 557–563.

31. Perlmutter SJ, Leitman SF, Garvey MA, et al. Therapeutic plasma exchange and intravenous immunoglobulin for obsessive-compulsive disorder and tic disorders in childhood. Lancet 1999; 354: 1153–1158.

32. Malik U, Oleksowicz L, Latov N, et al. Intravenous γ-globulin inhibits binding of anti-GM1 to its target antigen. Ann Neurol 1996; 39: 136–139.

33. van Doorn PA, Brand A, Vermeulen M. Anti-neuroblastoma cell line antibodies in inflammatory demyelinating polyneuropathuy: inhibition in vitro and in vivo by IV immunoglobulin. Neurology 1988; 38: 1592–1595.

34. Liblau R, Gajdos PH, Bustarret A, et al. Intravenous γ-globulin in myasthenia gravis: interaction with anti-acetylcholine receptor autoantibodies. J Clin Immunol 1991; 11: 128–131.

35. Buchwald B, Ahangari R, Weishaupt A, et al. Intravenous immunoglobulins neutralize blocking antibodies in Guillain–Barré syndrome. Ann Neurol 2002; 51: 673–680.

36. Basta M. Modulation of complement-mediated immune damage by intravenous immune globulin. Clin Exp Immunol 1996; 104(Suppl 1): 21–25.

37. Mouthon L, Kaveri SV, Spalter SH, et al. Mechanisms of action of intravenous immune globuline in immune-mediated diseases. Clin Exp Immunol 1996; 104: 3–9.

38. Gergely J, Sarmay G. Fc gamma RII-mediated regulation of human B cells. Scand J Immunol 1996; 44: 1–10.

39. Daya S, Gunby J, Clark DA. Intravenous immunoglobulin therapy for recurrent spontaneous abortion: a meta-analysis. Am J Reprod Immunol 1998; 39: 69–76.

40. Scott JR. Immunotherapy for recurrent miscarriage. Cochrane Database Syst Rev2003; CD000112.

41. Jordan SC, Vo AA, Tyan D, et al. Current approaches to treatment of antibody-mediated rejection. Pediatr Transplant 2005; 9: 408–415.

42. Kaul R, McGeer A, Norrby-Teglund A, et al. Intravenous immunoglobulin therapy for streptococcal toxic shock syndrome – a comparative observational study. Clin Infect Dis 1999; 28: 800–807.

43. Ohlsson A, Lacy JB. Intravenous immunoglobulin for suspected or subsequently proven infection in neonates. Cochrane Database Syst Rev 2001; CD001239.

44. Letko E, Papaliodis DN, Papaliodis GN, et al. Stevens–Johnson syndrome and toxic epidermal necrolysis: a review of the literature. Ann Allergy Asthma Immunol 2005; 94: 419–436.

45. Viard I, Wehrli P, Bullanim R, et al. Inhibition of toxic epidermal necrolysis by blockade of CD95 with human intravenous immunoglobulin. Science 1998; 282: 490–493.

46. Faye O, Roujeau JC. Treatment of epidermal necrolysis with high-dose intravenous immunoglobulins (IVIg). Drugs 2005; 65: 2085–2090.

47. Jolles S. High-dose intravenous immunoglobulin (hdIVIg) in the treatment of autoimmune blistering disorders. Clin Exp Immunol 2002; 129: 385–389.

48. Li N, Zhao M, Hilario-Vargas J, et al. Complete FcRn dependence for intravenous Ig therapy in autoimmune skin blistering diseases. J Clin Invest 2005; 115: 3440–3450.

49. Jolles S, Hughes J, Whittaker S. Dermatological uses of high-dose intravenous immunoglobulin. Arch Dermatol 1998; 134: 80–86.

50. Ahmed AR, Dahl M, for the Consensus Development Group. Consensus statement on the use of intravenous immunoglobulin therapy in the treatment of autoimmune bucocutaneous blistering. Arch Dermatol 2003; 139: 1051–1059.

51. Kishiyama JL, Valacer D, Cunningham-Rundles C, et al. A multicenter, randomized, double-blind, placebo-controlled trial of high-dose intravenous immunoglobulin for oral corticosteroid-dependent asthma. Clin Immunol 1999; 91: 126–133.

52. Salmun LM, Barlan I, Wolf HM, et al. Effect of intravenous immunoglobulin on steroid consumption in patients with severe asthma: double-blind, placebo-controlled, randomized trial. J Allergy Clin Immunol 1999; 103: 810–815.

53. Spahn JD, Leung DYM, Chan MTS, et al. Mechanisms of glucocorticoid reduction in asthmatic subjects treated with intravenous immunoglobulin. J Allergy Clin Immunol 1999; 103: 421–426.

Gene transfer therapy of immunologic diseases

Javier Chinen, Fabio Candotti

86

Immunodeficiency diseases comprise a group of clinical conditions characterized by an impairment of one or more components of the immune system, resulting in increased susceptibility to infections and, in some particular diseases, to an increased incidence of neoplastic and autoimmune disorders. According to their etiology, immunodeficiencies can be classified into two major categories: primary and secondary. Primary immunodeficiencies result from inherited or 'de novo' defects in genes encoding proteins that are involved in the development and function of the cells of the immune system. Secondary immunodeficiencies are acquired disorders caused by environmental agents (e.g., infectious agents, radiation, immunosuppressive drugs), or by processes that indirectly affect the immune system, such as malnutrition. Currently, infection by the human immunodeficiency virus (HIV) is the most common form of immunodeficiency found in clinical practice in developed countries. HIV infects and causes the death of CD4 T cells, progressively reducing the ability of the infected individual to activate and develop immune responses. Both primary and secondary immunodeficiencies represent a management challenge for the clinician, who has a limited number of treatment options for these diseases: reversal of most severe primary immunodeficiencies today requires hematopoietic stem cell transplantation (HSCT), and most HIV-infected individuals will require anti-retroviral therapy. However, HSCT has significant mortality and side effects. Also, anti-HIV therapy halts disease progression but seldom eradicates the virus, necessitating lifelong treatment that can be associated with severe adverse effects and the development of anti-retroviral drug resistance.

In the mid 1980s, gene therapy was proposed as an alternative treatment to genetic diseases, including inherited immunodeficiencies with known genetic defects (Table 86.1). Applications of gene therapy strategies were suggested for a wide variety of conditions, including treatment of cancer and HIV infection. In 2006 there were 119 active gene therapy clinical protocols in the USA, 72 of which were directed to the treatment of cancer using genes expected to stimulate the immune response and therefore help to eliminate cancer cells.[1] Five of the studies were proposed for genetic intervention in HIV infection, and five other protocols were directed to gene correction of monogenic diseases. Two of these were designed for primary immunodeficiencies: X-linked severe combined immunodeficiency (XSCID) and adenosine deaminase (ADA) deficiency. The remaining studies tested the safety and efficacy of approaches for the genetic modification of bone marrow cells using nontherapeutic genes.

In this chapter, we review in chronological order the progress achieved in the development of gene therapy for primary immunodeficiencies and for the control of HIV infection, with a focus on its application to the clinical management of affected patients.

GENE THERAPY AS TREATMENT MODALITY

Gene therapy can be described as a therapeutic strategy that involves the genetic modification of a target cell in order to produce biological effects that halt or reverse a disease process. Investigators need to carefully consider at least four aspects of any gene therapy approach: the pathogenesis of the disease; the target cell intended to modify; the therapeutic gene to be used; and the vector to transfer the therapeutic gene into the target gene (Fig. 86.1).

Several viral and nonviral methods have been reported for gene therapy (Table 86.2). Retroviral vectors derived from murine leukemia virus have been the preferred gene vectors for immunodeficiencies, because of their ability to integrate permanently into the genome of the target cells, which is a prerequisite for long-term correction of genetic diseases. The integrated provirus behaves as a gene transcription unit, with the therapeutic gene copied into daughter cells during cell replication. The gene therapy field has accumulated extensive experience with gene transfer of hematopoietic stem cell (HSC) using these vectors (Fig. 86.2) Significant limitations of murine retroviral vectors are the need for cell division for efficient gene transfer, and recent reports of retroviral insertional oncogenesis in animal

Table 86.1 Primary immunodeficiency candidates for gene therapy

	Gene	Gene regulation required	Correction of animal model	*In vitro* human cell correction	Clinical trial
ADA deficiency	*ADA*	No	Yes	Yes	Successful
CGD (X-linked)	*gp91phox*	No	Yes	Yes	Successful
CGD (autosomal)	*p47phox*	No	Yes	Yes	Unsuccessful
LAD type I	*CD18*	No	Yes	Yes	Unsuccessful (two patients treated)
XSCID	*IL2RG*	No	Yes	Yes	Successful
JAK3-SCID	*JAK3*	No	Yes	Yes	Unsuccessful (one patient treated)
Hyper IgM type 1	*CD40L*	Yes	Yes, induced lymphoma	Yes	None
Wiskott–Aldrich syndrome	*WASP*	No	Yes	Yes	None
X-linked agammaglobulinemia	*BTK*	Yes	Yes	Not reported	None
RAG1/2 deficiency	*RAG 1/2*	Yes	Yes, induced lymphoma	Not reported	None
IL7RA deficiency	*IL7RA*	Yes	Yes	Yes	None
Artemis-SCID	*DCLREC1*	Yes	Yes	No	None

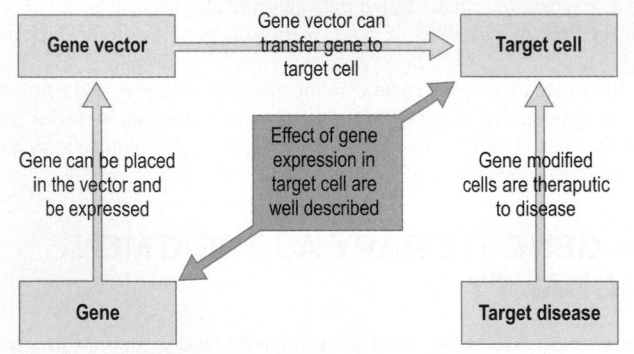

Fig. 86.1 Elements of gene therapy. The diagram shows four elements of gene therapy that need to be identified and carefully studied for all potential applications.

Table 86.2 Viral and non-viral delivery methods used for gene therapy

Viral based	Nonviral based
Retroviruses	Naked DNA
Murine oncoretrovirus	Liposomes
Mammalian lentivirus	Gold-coated DNA
Foamy virus	Molecular conjugates
Feline oncoretrovirus	
Avian sarcoma–leukosis virus	
Adenoviruses	
Adeno-associated viruses	
Herpes simplex virus	
Epstein–Barr virus	

models and humans. However, there is an active development of alternative vectors, for example based on mammalian lentiviruses and foamy viruses. Other efforts are aimed at developing retroviral vectors using viral envelopes with increased efficiency to transduce HSCs.[2]

GENE THERAPY FOR PRIMARY IMMUNODEFICIENCIES

More than 120 genetic defects are known to cause primary immunodeficiency (PI) disorders. The most common PIs are characterized by defective antibody responses, albeit with relatively intact cellular immunity. Patients with these conditions are usually treated with immunoglobulin replacement and achieve an acceptable reduction of the frequency of infections. In contrast, immunodeficiencies associated with defective T-cell function, e.g., SCID, are almost always fatal unless treatment to restore immune function is provided. Currently, the standard curative therapy for many types of SCID and other severe PIs is hematopoietic stem cell transplantation (HSCT).[3] In addition, enzyme replacement is available for patients with genetic defects of ADA.[4] Weekly intramuscular injections of bovine ADA enzyme conjugated to polyethylene glycol (PEG-ADA) improve immune function in most of these patients, but requires continuous administration. HSCT treatment performed in an experienced medical center can rescue up to 75–90% of infants diagnosed with SCID, obtaining the best results if performed in the first 3 months of life, before devastating infections occur.[3] If HSCT is performed using an

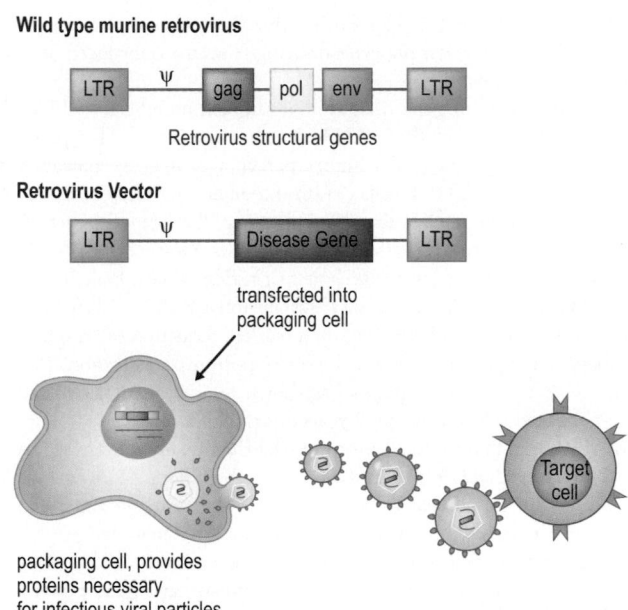

Wild type murine retrovirus

Retrovirus structural genes

Retrovirus Vector

transfected into
packaging cell

packaging cell, provides
proteins necessary
for infectious viral particles

Target
cell

Fig. 86.2 Structure of a typical retroviral vector. Structural retroviral genes are removed from the wild-type retrovirus, which leaves space to insert the gene of interest. Long terminal repeats (LTRs) and packaging signal (ψ) are elements necessary for viral replication. Packaging cells provide the viral capsid and envelope proteins that are necessary to form a complete viral particle able to infect target cells and integrate its genome into the genomic DNA.

Table 86.3 Milestones of gene therapy for primary immunodeficiencies

Year	Milestone
1986	Functional correction of ADA-deficient human T cells by gene transfer Expression of human ADA in murine hematopoietic stem cells by gene transfer
1990	T cell-directed gene therapy for ADA deficiency: First two patients treated showed feasibility of *in vivo* correction of human lymphocytes
1996	Retroviral gene transfer correction of XSCID in a mouse model
1998	Gene transfer to CD34+ cells from ADA deficient patients results in gene-corrected T cells with survival advantage
2000	Gene therapy clinical trial in two XSCID infants demonstrated satisfactory immune reconstitution for the first time
2002	Successful gene therapy trial for ADA-deficient patients, using nonmyeloablative conditioning
2003	Adverse event reported in XSCID gene therapy trial: two patients developed leukemia
2004	Additional gene therapy trials for XSCID and ADA-SCID confirms the efficacy of this experimental treatment
2006	Gene therapy for two CGD patients restored microbicidal capacity of neutrophils and helped clear chronic infections

ADA, adenosine deaminase; XSCID, X-linked severe combined immunodeficiency; CGD, chronic granulomatous disease.

HLA-matched sibling as a donor, the rate of immune reconstitution reaches over 90%. Because of the infrequent availability of a HLA-matched related donor; however, HSCT is usually performed from a haploidentical HLA (parental) donor, which results in a lower probability of success and an increased risk for morbidity and mortality over time. A significant number of patients treated with haploidentical HSCT may achieve only partial or unstable immune reconstitution. Others suffer acute or chronic graft-versus-host disease (GvHD) and, if a myeloablative conditioning regimen is used, side effects due to chemotherapy.

Because of the severity of the clinical phenotype, the infrequent availability of HLA-identical sibling donors and the imperfect results of HSCT, gene therapy has been investigated as an alternative treatment for primary immunodeficiencies, aiming at the correction of gene defects in hematopoietic stem cells (HSC). PIs have played a major role in the development of gene therapy since the inception of this novel area of medicine. (Table 86.3) In the mid 1980s ADA deficiency was identified as one ideal candidate disease, and soon thereafter became the first disease to be treated in an NIH-approved clinical gene therapy trial.[3] Thereafter, preclinical and clinical trials of corrective gene transfer for PIs have advanced the gene therapy field and have reported clear therapeutic successes, as well as the serious adverse events that occurred in a clinical trial for XSCID, described below.

GENE THERAPY FOR ADA-SCID

Genetic mutations affecting ADA function result in a heterogeneous presentation of immunodeficiency characterized, in severe cases, by profoundly reduced numbers of T and B cells and a consequent lack of both cellular and humoral responses (Chapter 35). ADA is an enzyme present in every cell in the body, but its deficiency primarily affects lymphocytes because the purine intermediates that build up in the absence of ADA are particularly toxic to B and T cells. Allogeneic HSCT and enzyme replacement therapy have proved life-saving for affected patients.[3,4] Gene therapy approaches have been developed to improve on the toxicity and limited efficacy that complicate these existing forms of treatment. Recent milestones in the treatment of ADA deficiency are described below.

As mentioned above, ADA deficiency was the first genetic disorder in which the 'proof of concept' of gene therapy was demonstrated. In 1990, two ADA-deficient girls were enrolled in the first single-gene disease clinical trial at the National Institutes of Health.[5] Peripheral blood T cells were obtained by apheresis, expanded *ex vivo* in IL-2-containing media, transduced with a retroviral vector carrying the ADA cDNA, and infused back into the patients. Over a 2-year period the two patients received a series of 11–12 infusions of *in vitro* expanded gene-corrected cells. Clinical follow-up showed a prolonged increase in T-cell numbers, the development of antigen-induced cutaneous delayed-type hypersensitivity, and normalization of isohemoagglutinins

KEY CONCEPTS

GENE THERAPY FOR ADA DEFICIENCY

>> The 'proof of concept' of gene therapy was first demonstrated in a clinical trial involving two patients with ADA deficiency who received autologous gene-modified T cells.

>> The routine use of replacement enzyme, PEG-ADA, might reduce survival advantage for ADA gene-corrected lymphocytes.

>> Successful immunologic reconstitution has been obtained with ADA gene therapy to bone marrow HSCs, with nonmyeloablative conditioning and in the absence of PEG-ADA.

>> Reported side effects in this trial were secondary to cytoreductive therapy, including transient myelosuppression.

titers and antibody responses to vaccines. In patient 1, more than 50% of circulating peripheral blood lymphocytes carried the corrected ADA gene, resulting in measurable ADA activity of nearly 25% of normal levels. Patient 2 showed very low numbers of transduced cells (0.1–1%) and barely detectable ADA enzyme expression. One possible explanation for the different outcomes in the two patients is the development of an immune response in patient 2 against the fetal calf serum used during the *in vitro* gene transfer procedure. T cell-directed gene therapy was also used in the treatment of an ADA-deficient patient in Japan, starting in 1995. Improvements in T-cell numbers and function were observed in this patient, with gene correction of over 15% of circulating lymphocytes and good levels of ADA enzyme activity.[6]

The results of T-cell gene therapy for ADA deficiency were encouraging, with the observation of a series of immune responses that were absent or barely detectable before the genetic treatment. However, all ADA-deficient patients were still receiving PEG-ADA treatment during the trials, which complicates the assessment of clinical benefits that can be exclusively attributed to gene therapy. The T-cell gene therapy studies, however, demonstrated that gene-modified T cells could have very long-term survival *in vivo*, as they have persisted for more than 14 years in the first treated patient. However, the lifespan of these mature lymphocytes cannot be assumed to be unlimited, and this approach intrinsically requires patients to receive periodic treatment to replace dying gene-corrected lymphocytes. The successful genetic correction of the patients' HSCs would theoretically avoid the need for repeated treatments and has been pursued by a series of independent clinical trials.[7]

In 1992, a gene therapy trial targeting bone marrow progenitors and peripheral lymphocytes in two ADA-deficient patients resulted in the improvement of their immune function, with normalization of lymphocytes counts and T-cell proliferation responses to antigens and mitogens.[7] There was also evidence of successful transduction of hematopoietic progenitor cells, demonstrated by the detection of the ADA gene vector in DNA extracted from blood cell colony-forming units (CFUs) in both patients, with frequencies ranging from 0.8% to 8.5%. Molecular analysis suggested that gene transfer into peripheral lymphocytes led to the persistence of gene-corrected cells in the patients'

circulation for the first 6–12 months after the infusion, and thereafter they were replaced by lymphocytes deriving from the transduced hematopoietic progenitors.[7]

A second stem cell gene therapy trial targeted umbilical cord blood-derived CD34+ cells in three ADA-deficient neonates.[7] This protocol resulted in the presence of a higher percentage of gene transduction among peripheral CD3+ T cells (1–10%) than among monocytes and B lymphocytes (0.01–0.1%), thereby indicating that genetic correction provided selective survival advantage to T cells. However, the levels of genetic correction were not sufficient to provide clinical benefit, which was evident when the temporary suspension of PEG-ADA in one patient was unsuccessful, resulting in a marked reduction of lymphocyte numbers and function, followed by an opportunistic infection. Long-term follow-up of these patients has shown the presence of circulating gene-corrected cells for over 5–7 years after treatment.

In 1993, in a multicenter European trial three patients were reported to have received ADA gene transfer into their bone marrow HSCs. Unfortunately, no clinical improvement or long-term presence of the transferred gene could be demonstrated by the investigators.[7]

Altogether, the first series of HSC gene therapy trials for ADA deficiency showed that the efficiency of gene transfer and gene expression was low, and substantiated the need for improvement of gene transfer vectors and transduction procedures. Several research groups in Europe, the USA and Japan have since then proposed various modifications to the gene therapy protocols to increase its efficiency. (Fig. 86.3)

In 2002, Aiuti et al.[8] reported on a gene therapy study in two ADA-deficient SCID patients, which included the administration of nonmyeloablative conditioning (4 mg/kg busulfan) prior to the infusion of gene-corrected autologous bone marrow CD34+ cells, and the absence of PEG-ADA treatment. The authors showed that this protocol resulted in significant immunologic and metabolic improvement. Transient myelosuppression developed, with neutrophil counts returning to minimal normal levels at 21 days. Increases in T, B and NK cells were observed, with an increase in CD4+CD45RA+ naïve T cells and T-cell receptor excision circles (TREC), also suggesting normal thymic function. T-cell proliferation to mitogens and antigens and T-cell receptor repertoire were restored. Serum IgG, IgA and IgM increased to normal levels, which correlated with positive responses to routine immunizations. No adverse effects were observed, and the two patients (and six additional unpublished patients) were apparently well without receiving PEG-ADA treatment or immunoglobulin replacement. The study demonstrated that this form of gene therapy could cure ADA deficiency and yield better results than those obtained in two previous trials performed in the absence of myeloablative chemotherapy.

In 2001, four ADA-deficient patients received gene therapy in the U.S., while continuing PEG-ADA treatment.[9] Retroviral gene transfer into bone marrow CD34+ cells from these patients has resulted in low levels (0.01–0.1%) of retroviral marking and no clinical benefit, suggesting that the presence of PEG-ADA might have interfered with the selective advantage of gene-corrected cells.

Based on this hypothesis, two patients were treated in a Japanese trial after withdrawal of PEG-ADA treatment and in the absence of myeloablation.[10] These patients showed a slow but definite increase in peripheral blood lymphocyte numbers. At the last reported follow-up, 2 years after treatment, the patients were apparently well in the absence of PEG-ADA.

An additional recent trial in London of retroviral ADA gene transfer into bone marrow CD34+ cells by Gaspar and colleagues showed

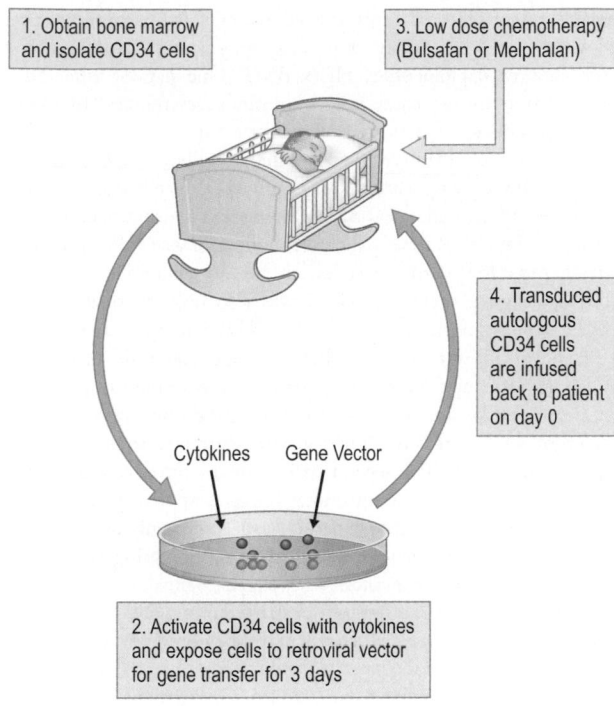

1. Obtain bone marrow and isolate CD34 cells

3. Low dose chemotherapy (Bulsafan or Melphalan)

4. Transduced autologous CD34 cells are infused back to patient on day 0

Cytokines   Gene Vector

2. Activate CD34 cells with cytokines and expose cells to retroviral vector for gene transfer for 3 days

Fig. 86.3   ADA deficiency gene therapy.

successful immune reconstitution after myeloablation and in the absence of PEG-ADA.[11] The future form of gene therapy for ADA deficiency is likely to depend upon the use of cytoreduction, which appears to favor prompt immune reconstitution.

GENE THERAPY FOR CHRONIC GRANULOMATOUS DISEASE

Patients with chronic granulomatous disease (CGD) have increased susceptibility to pyogenic and fungal infections as a result of poor or absent neutrophil oxidase activity (Chapter 21). A defect in any of four proteins of the NADPH oxidase complex can be responsible for this disease, with about two-thirds of the patients with CGD having a deficiency in the X-linked gene encoding one of these proteins, gp91phox. CGD can be cured with an HLA-identical allogeneic bone marrow transplant (BMT); however, haploidentical T cell-depleted BMT is not similarly successful owing to toxicity from myeloablation regimens or to GvHD, resulting in high mortality. Gene therapy experiments have been performed in mice with targeted disruptions of either *p47phox*, the most common gene causing the autosomal recessive form of CGD, or *gp91phox*, demonstrating correction of oxidase activity, protection from bacterial infections, and reduction of excessive inflammatory disease.[12] In addition, studies of CGD female carriers have shown that clinical benefit in humans may require as little as 5% of neutrophils with normal oxidase activity.[12]

After the demonstration of successful *in vitro* correction of human cells, phase I clinical trials were carried out for CGD due to *p47 phox* deficiency and for CGD caused by mutations in *gp91phox*. Mobilized

KEY CONCEPTS

GENE THERAPY FOR CGD

>> Oxidase activity correction of 5% of neutrophils may be sufficient to provide protection against infections and granuloma formation.

>> Sustained clinical and laboratory improvement was reported in two CGD patients who received gene-corrected autologous HSCs, after non myeloablative chemotherapy.

>> Adverse effects, including transient myelosuppression, were secondary to chemotherapy.

>> Corrected cells had retroviral insertions in three genes, *MDS1-EVI1, PRDM16* and *SETBP1*, which caused their activation and non-malignant clonal cell expansion.

peripheral CD34+ cells from CGD patients were collected and transduced with retroviral vectors. Oxidase-positive neutrophils, used as a measure of transduction efficiency, were observed at low frequencies (0.004–0.2%) up to 6 months after infusion. Overall, the modest results of the initial gene therapy trials for CGD were probably the consequence of reduced transduction of early hematopoietic progenitors.[13] Ott and colleagues[14] recently reported significant progress, with clinical improvement in two adults with X-linked CGD following a gene therapy protocol that used a nonmyeloablative chemotherapy regimen consisting of busulfan at 8 mg/kg. CD34+ cells were isolated from peripheral blood after mobilization with G-CSF and transduced with a retroviral vector carrying the *gp91phox* gene. Transient myelosuppression occurred after chemotherapy, and blood cell counts recovered gradually to normal levels around day 30. Gene-modified cells increased from 10–20% of peripheral blood leukocytes soon after infusion to 40–60% after 7 months. The levels of gene-marked T cells were 2–7% in one patient and 0.4–5% in the other. For B cells, the marking was 17% and 11%, respectively. Significantly, both patients had resolution of chronic infections (pneumonia due to *Aspergillus fumigatus* and pulmonary abscesses due to *Staphylococcus aureus*, respectively) within 2 months of gene therapy. Analysis of DNA from leukocytes of these patients showed a nonrandom distribution of retroviral insertions, with clustering in the *MDS1-EVI1*, *PRDM16* and *SETBP1* loci. Clones carrying these integration sites were found to have undergone *in vivo* expansion starting from 3 months after therapy, and stabilization after 10 months. This particular cell expansion probably contributed to the therapeutic efficacy of the procedure. However, whether or not these clones are at increased risk for future malignant transformation remains unclear. One of these two patients died 24 months after the gene therapy from a bacterial infection with colon perforation and sepsis, and it was reported that there had been a decrease in the NADPH oxidase activity of his granulocytes. Investigations are still preliminary.[13]

Compared to the earlier trials, the results of this study suggest that gene therapy protocols for CGD, and other PIs in which there is no physiologic survival advantage for corrected cells, may benefit from myeloablation. In addition, more efficient gene transduction, to generate a large proportion of corrected cells, will improve the clinical benefits. Towards this goal, recent work has focused on the generation of gene transfer vectors based in lentiviruses pseudotyped with the RD114 envelope (derived from a feline retrovirus) and has shown high levels of oxidase correction and increased human cell engraftment in the NOD/SCID mouse model.[2]

■ GENE THERAPY FOR LEUKOCYTE ADHESION DEFICIENCY TYPE I ■

Leukocyte adhesion deficiency (LAD) type I is an autosomal recessive disease caused by deficient expression of CD18, a cell membrane adhesion protein that is essential for migration of neutrophils from blood vessels to sites of inflammation (Chapters 12 and 21). LAD patients have recurrent and severe bacterial infections that shorten their life expectancy. The only curative treatment for LAD has been BMT. A human clinical gene therapy trial was conducted for LAD type 1, using G-CSF-mobilized peripheral CD34[+] HSC transduced with a retroviral vector carrying the CD18 cDNA.[16] One month after infusion of transduced cells, two patients demonstrated that 0.03–0.04% of circulating myeloid cells contained the retrovirally transduced gene. However, these cells had no intrinsic survival advantage and were not detectable at the 2-month post-treatment evaluation. Considering that, as with CGD, LAD neutrophils may not have a survival advantage in their development, future clinical trials may consider including myeloablation to increase the chances of engraftment and differentiation of gene-corrected cells. Experimental results in a canine model using nonmyeloablative conditioning prior to gene therapy support this concept. In 6 of 11 treated dogs with a severe LAD deficiency, up to 8.4% of CD18 leukocytes retained the gene construct one-year later, with reversal or moderation of the phenotype, and marked improvement of neutrophil migration to extravascular spaces.[15]

■ GENE THERAPY FOR X-LINKED SCID ■

X-linked SCID (XSCID) is the most common genetic form of SCID and is caused by deleterious mutations in the *IL2RG* gene that encodes for the IL-2 receptor common γ (γc) chain, a transmembrane protein in the cytokine receptor gene superfamily (Chapter 35). Patients with XSCID do not produce T and NK cells, and their B cells are functionally impaired. *In vitro* experiments with human XSCID cells and *in vivo* mouse models have shown that correction of γc expression and function, as well as the restoration of XSCID immune defects, was possible by using retroviral vector gene transfer.

Two gene therapy trials for XSCID have been conducted in Europe, one at the Necker Hospital in Paris, and the second at Great Ormond Street Hospital in London.[18, 19] These studies have shown that infants with XSCID who received an infusion of autologous bone marrow cells corrected by *IL2RG* gene transfer can experience significant immune reconstitution. In both protocols CD34[+] cells were isolated from bone marrow, activated with cytokines, and exposed to a supernatant containing retroviral vectors carrying *IL2RG* cDNA at high titers. Transduced cells were infused back to patients at a dose of 1.1–22 million cells/kg. Eleven of 14 infants for whom published data are available (10 treated in France and four in England) developed normal T-cell counts, and showed normal proliferative responses to mitogens and antigens.[19, 20] Gene-corrected NK cells were detected, and about 1% of B cells contained the corrected gene. Antibody responses to vaccines were tested and found to be adequate, which allowed most treated patients to discontinue immunoglobulin supplementation, thus suggesting some advantage of the procedure over haploidentical HLA BMT. One patient who did not experience immune reconstitution had previous disseminated BCG infection and an enlarged spleen that might have trapped the gene-corrected cells. The one patient who received less than 3 million transduced CD34[+] cells/kg did not develop a satisfactory number of T cells and later underwent successful haploidentical BMT. Expression and function of γc have persisted to date in all other patients, as long as 6 years after the therapy, suggesting that long-term correction has been obtained.[20]

The same gene therapy protocol was also used to treat two older XSCID patients, aged 20 and 16 years. This attempt was reported to have failed, and it was suggested that older age may limit the efficacy of XSCID gene therapy.[21] One of the patients was followed up to 2 years after treatment: he did not show immunological improvement, and the presence of gene-corrected cell lineages was estimated to be less than 1% by quantitative PCR. The second patient died from severe pre-existing and recurrent skin and lung infections 1.5 years after treatment. He had evidence of gene-corrected peripheral blood T cells only up to 4 months of follow-up. The transient presence of cells containing the retroviral vector in this patient is consistent with engraftment of transduced committed progenitors with a limited lifespan. Among the reasons for the lack of success in these two patients is that the dose of transduced CD34[+] cells may have been inadequate to achieve significant number of corrected T cells and immune reconstitution. One patient received a low dose of 0.7×10^6 transduced CD34[+] cell/kg. The other received 4.5×10^6 CD34[+] cell/kg; however, transduction efficiency was only 13%.

At the National Institutes of Health, a gene therapy clinical trial is being conducted as a salvage treatment for patients who have received BMT and have failed to develop lasting T-cell function.[22] Three patients (10, 13 and 14 years of age, respectively) have been treated using *ex vivo* transduction of CD34[+] cells obtained from peripheral blood by apheresis, after mobilization with granulocyte colony-stimulating factor (G-CSF). Although the presence of peripheral T cells carrying the correct copy of the *IL2RG* gene has been demonstrated in all three patients, only one has shown a high retroviral vector copy number in his T cells (average of 1.11–1.35 vector copies/cell), and progressive replacement of the residual T cells from his previous bone marrow donor with autologous T cells. Up to 18 months post gene therapy, T-cell proliferative responses to mitogen and *Candida* antigen are

■ KEY CONCEPTS

GENE THERAPY FOR XSCID

>> Infants with XSCID were the first individuals to be effectively treated by gene therapy, achieving sustained immunological restoration.

>> Cellular and humoral immune functions of the infants with XSCID are restored by autologous gene-modified bone marrow CD34[+] cells.

>> Development of T-cell lymphoproliferative disease is a risk factor for gene therapy of XSCID.

>> Gene therapy for XSCID is an alternative treatment for patients who do not have an HLA-matched sibling donor for bone marrow transplantation and over 3.5 months of age.

normal in this patient, although antibody response remains poor. The other two patients have not developed significant immunological changes. However, the clinical status of both patients has improved.

The excitement from the gene therapy success in XSCID infants was partially set back by the occurrence of T-cell leukemia-like disease in three patients in the French study, which will be discussed in the next section. Because of this complication, the gene therapy trial in France was stopped voluntarily by the investigators, and in England new enrollees have been considered on a case-by-case basis. In the USA, XSCID gene therapy trials are allowed to recruit patients who have failed a previous HSCT, or who carry clinical complications (e.g., viral infections) that increase the mortality risk of BMT.

LEUKEMIA IN THE XSCID TRIAL GENE THERAPY PROTOCOL

The two youngest infants (respectively 1 and 3 months of age at treatment) in the French XSCID gene therapy trial developed T-cell leukemia respectively 30 and 34 months after the infusion of corrected cells.[23] A third patient, who received gene therapy treatment at 8 months of age, developed T-cell lymphoma 35 months after treatment.[24] For the treatment of their neoplastic diseases all patients received anti-leukemic chemotherapy, and one received an allogeneic BMT when his response to chemotherapy did not eliminate the leukemic clone. This patient later experienced recurrence of his leukemia and died. The other two patients are currently in remission and apparently well, with no antibiotic prophylaxis or immunoglobulin supplementation. The fourth case of leukemia in this trial was recently reported to have occurred 68 months after gene transfer.

The first two patients presented with lymphocytosis, anemia, low platelet counts and splenomegaly. Flow cytometry studies showed that the first patient had a single T-cell clone with a γδ T-cell receptor; the second had three different T-cell clones with αβ T-cell receptors. Inappropriate expression of the LIM-domain-only-2 (LMO-2) transcription factor, due to insertion of the retroviral vector close to the 5′ end of the *LMO2* gene locus, was found in both cases (Fig. 86.4). LMO2 is expressed in early hematopoietic progenitors, and around 10% of T-cell leukemias have chromosomal translocations involving this locus. The third patient had a presentation more like that of lymphoma than leukemia, with enlarged mediastinum and lymph nodes, and with good response to corticosteroids. His T-cell clone was a double-negative CD3⁺CD4⁻CD8⁻ T cell with at least three different retroviral insertions, including LMO2, although the role of this gene in the development of this neoplasia is less clear than in the previous two cases. Before the first case of leukemia in gene therapy patients occurred in 2002, retroviral insertional mutagenesis in hematopoietic cells was assumed to be an event that occurred at random and with a very low probability of adverse consequences. In 2003, a committee of experts appointed by the American Society of Gene Therapy reviewed all published and unpublished studies of HSC transduced with replication-incompetent retroviral vectors.[25] Both animal models and more than 40 clinical trials did not show adverse effects attributable to the integration of the gene vector, with the exception of one study describing myeloid leukemia in a mouse that received mouse bone marrow transduced with a truncated nerve growth factor receptor gene.[26] Clinical trials have used retroviral vectors to transfer marker genes, anti-HIV genes, genes conferring resistance to cancer chemotherapy, and genes to correct inherited disorders,

with follow-up for more than 10 years in some cases, with no evidence of mutagenesis induced by retroviral gene transfer. However, most of these studies achieved only very low levels of retroviral transduction.

In addition to increased transduction efficiency, compared to previous clinical trials of retroviral gene therapy into HSCs, genetic and environmental

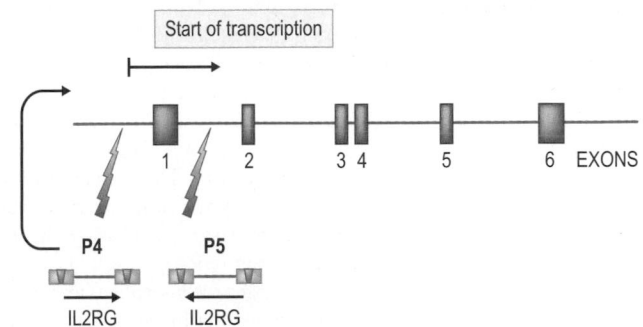

P4 /P5 Patients who presented with retroviral insertions in LO2

▽ Gene transcription enhancer in retroviral vector

Fig. 86.4 Retroviral insertion sites in the LMO2 gene identified in leukemic cells from two patients who received gene therapy for X-linked severe combined immunodeficiency and presented with T-cell proliferative diseases at 30 and 34 months follow-up, respectively. Abnormal constitutive expression is driven by the enhancer element present in the retroviral vector.

CLINICAL RELEVANCE

LEUKEMOGENESIS IN GENE THERAPY

>> Four of 11 XSCID patients in a gene therapy trial conducted in France developed T-cell leukemia between 30 and 68 months after gene therapy. After anti-leukemic treatment, two of the patients are in remission, but one child had a relapse and died.

>> The first two patients were the youngest to be treated with gene therapy (1 and 3 months of age, respectively).

>> T-cell clones from these patients had abnormal expression of the *LMO2* gene, a known oncogene, driven by gene vector insertions. These clones also contained chromosomal abnormalities, such as translocation and trisomy 10.

>> The third patient was 8 months old at the time of treatment, and had T-cell clones with at least three retroviral insertion sites, including *LMO2*.

>> Studies on retroviral integration sites suggest that these occur preferentially near the 5′ end of gene transcription units.

>> The estimated risk and the risk factors for leukemogenesis in gene therapy are unknown. Other XSCID patients treated with gene therapy and followed for a similar period have not presented with similar adverse events.

influences might have contributed to the development of leukemia in the three XSCID patients. The first of these had experienced a varicella infection just before the amplified clone was detected, and had a family history of childhood cancer. Leukemic cells from both patients had cytogenetic abnormalities often found in malignant cells: a chromosome 6;13 translocation in the first patient; trisomy 10 plus a SIL-TAL1 fusion transcript in the second case. An additional potential risk factor in both children was their young age at treatment. Both had been diagnosed with XSCID at birth based on family history, and were treated at 1 and 3 months of age, respectively. The small size of the infants not only resulted in their receiving large doses of gene-corrected cells (18 and 20 million CD34+ cells/kg body weight), but their cells were noted to proliferate more vigorously in the transduction culture than those of the older subjects. HSC obtained from very young patients may, like those from cord blood, have an intrinsically high capacity for replication, possibly increasing their risk of having a harmful gene insertion during retroviral transduction.

The fact that the *LMO2* locus was a target for insertional mutagenesis in both XSCID leukemia cases suggests that inappropriate *LMO2* activation in developing T cells combined with the restored γc chain can lead to excess cell proliferation, accumulation of oncogenic changes, and ultimately leukemia. Dave et al.[27] have provided interesting data that support this hypothesis. In their database of 3000 hematopoietic tumors induced in mice by replication-competent retroviral viruses, they found one case of mouse leukemia with integrations in both *LMO2* and *IL2RG*. The probability for these two integrations to occur by chance in the same tumor is extremely low and suggests synergism between these two genes. However, the molecular mechanisms of how the co-expression of *LMO2* and γc lead to leukemia in pre- or post-thymic cells and many other aspects of the oncogenesis in these patients are not clear.[28] Further clinical and basic research is needed to identify risk factors for the development of neoplasias by insertional mutagenesis. In addition, *in vitro* and *in vivo* models are needed to test safer gene therapy approaches. For example, comprehensive identification of retroviral integration sites has become possible with the availability of the complete human genome sequence.[29] Analysis of the identified integration sites of retrovirus and lentivirus-based vectors in HeLa cells, human peripheral blood cells and CD34+ cells have revealed a tendency of these vectors to integrate in actively transcribed genes.

GENE THERAPY FOR JAK3-SCID

JAK3 is a lymphoid tissue-specific tyrosine kinase that binds to γc and is therefore involved in the signal transduction of IL-2, IL-4, IL-7, IL-9, IL-15, and IL-21. Mutations of *JAK3* can result in an autosomal recessive form of SCID, with clinical characteristics virtually identical to those of XSCID, except for the fact that JAK3 deficiency can also be found in female patients (Chapter 35). Retrovirally mediated gene correction has been effective for reconstitution of IL-2 and IL-4 responses in JAK3-deficient cell lines, and preclinical *in vivo* studies have demonstrated the efficacy of retrovirally mediated gene correction of JAK3 deficiency in JAK3 knockout mice.[30]

Based on these results, a clinical trial was designed at the St Jude Children's Research Hospital in Memphis to attempt genetic correction of bone marrow CD34+ cells of a JAK3-deficient patient who had failed BMT.[31] An infusion of retrovirally transduced cells was carried out twice in this patient, resulting in low levels of marking without significant changes in immunological status. The reasons for these unsatisfactory results remain unclear.

GENE THERAPY FOR WISKOTT–ALDRICH SYNDROME

The Wiskott–Aldrich syndrome (WAS) is an X-linked hematological disorder characterized by eczema, thrombocytopenia, and impaired cellular and humoral immunity. WAS is caused by defects in the WAS protein (WASP), which links the cytoskeleton to intracellular signal transduction pathways (Chapter 35). Severe hemorrhage, disseminated viral or other opportunistic infections, autoimmune disease or lymphoma can cause recurrent and chronic illness and premature death in WAS patients. HSCT from an HLA-identical sibling is the treatment of choice and can be curative, but only a minority of patients have such a donor available. The risks of mortality and adverse effects are much higher when alternative donors are used, such as a haploidentical HLA parent. Gene therapy has therefore been proposed as an alternative, supported by the observation that spontaneous somatic mutations restoring WASP function are associated with a survival advantage of gene-corrected cells over *WASP*-deficient populations; clinical trials of gene therapy for WAS are under development in Europe.

Preclinical studies in *WASP* knockout mice and in human cell lines have shown that retroviral transduction corrects (although mostly only partially) the biological and immunological defects seen in these models (e.g., increased actin polymerization and functional correction of T cells following transduction). Strom et al.[32] reported increased specific T-cell responses to influenza as a result of the transplantation of retrovirally transduced HSC in lethally irradiated mice. They also demonstrated restoration of proliferative and IL-2 responses to TCR stimulation. Most recently, Dupre et al.[33] and Charrier et al.[34] showed efficacy of WAS gene transfer into mice and human HSC using a lentiviral vector containing the WASP gene, driven either by its own promoter or by the PGK promoter.

GENE THERAPY FOR OTHER PRIMARY IMMUNODEFICIENCY DISEASES

There are a number of other PIs being investigated for potential treatment with gene therapy (Table 86.1). In several cases, the proof of principle has been obtained in patient-derived primary cells or cell lines. We briefly discuss some examples in which preclinical studies have progressed to the stage of *in vivo* experimentation in mouse models.

X-linked hyper-IgM syndrome type-1 (XHIM1) is caused by defects in the gene for CD40 ligand (CD40L) and is characterized by lack of immunoglobulin switching and defects in cellular immunity owing to the impaired interaction between CD40L (expressed by normal CD4 T cells) and CD40 on B cells (Chapter 35). Studies in mice exploring the possibility of gene therapy for this disease demonstrated that tightly controlled regulation of the expression of CD40L is important in order to avoid uncontrolled lymphoproliferation. CD40L knockout mice that received bone marrow progenitors transduced with the *CD40L* cDNA developed normal humoral and cellular immunity. However, 12 of 19 mice developed lymphoproliferative disorders.[35] These results emphasize the complexity and danger of gene therapy when it is aimed at correcting highly regulated genes. Efforts to develop human gene therapy for XHIM1 now include effective regulatory elements for CD40L expression.

Deficiency of ZAP-70, another signal transduction protein, results in an absence of mature circulating CD8 T lymphocytes and TCR signal transduction defects in peripheral CD4 T cells (Chapter 35). Preliminary experiments in patient-derived T-cell lines and primary T cells have indicated the feasibility of the gene correction approach for this disease. *In vivo* experiments of retrovirally mediated gene transfer into bone marrow cells of *ZAP-70* knockout animals resulted in the development of mature, polyclonal and functional T lymphocytes in treated animals.[36] Potential deleterious effects of the 'ectopic' expression of *ZAP-70* in cell types other than T cells is a reasonable concern, because of the characteristic restricted expression of the ZAP-70 protein in specific lymphoid lineages. An alternative solution to this problem was recently explored by Adjali et al.,[37] who injected a ZAP-70 lentiviral vector into the thymus of ZAP-70 knockout mice. These experiments resulted in differentiation of mature thymocytes and peripheral ZAP-70-expressing T cells that were responsive to alloantigens both *in vitro* and *in vivo*. Altogether, these data indicate that retrovirally mediated gene transfer of the ZAP-70 gene may prove to have a therapeutic benefit for patients with ZAP-70 deficiency.

Defects in Bruton tyrosine kinase (BTK) cause X-linked agammaglobulinemia (XLA), which presents with an absence of B cells, low immunoglobulin levels and frequent bacterial infections (Chapter 34). Currently, XLA patients receive supportive therapy with prophylactic antibiotics and IVIG; these treatments offer considerable protection, which is, however, expensive and incomplete. Mouse models of XLA have successfully been corrected with retroviral vectors carrying the BTK gene, restoring B-cell numbers and T cell-independent response.[38] A survival advantage of normal B cells over cells with BTK mutations has been demonstrated. The application of gene therapy to this disease would include risks that need to be balanced with the relatively safe administration of IVIG.

Interleukin-7 receptor α-chain (IL7RA)-deficient SCID, and recombinase activating gene 1 (RAG1)/RAG2-deficient SCID are other forms of PI for which murine models of gene therapy have shown functional correction of immune function. In all cases, retroviral transduction of bone marrow cells with therapeutic retroviral vectors was performed, followed by transplantation into the respective knockout mouse model.[18] Successful immune reconstitution of both *RAG1* and *RAG2* knockout mice was achieved by transducing their HSCs with a retroviral vector carrying the RAG1 cDNA or the RAG2 cDNA, respectively.[39, 40] The RAG1 and RAG2 vectors were detected in lymphoid cells, but not in myeloid cells, suggesting the strong survival advantage conferred by these genes similar to other SCID genes. Of note, in the case of RAG1, one of the treated mice developed lymphoproliferative disease, warning investigators of the need for regulated expression of this gene. Splenomegaly secondary to neutrophil infiltration was observed in the *IL7RA* knockout mouse model, suggesting that IL-7 activation signals are not limited to lymphocytes and suggesting potential toxic effects for clinical applications.[18] The correction of a mouse model of a radiosensitive form of SCID, due to mutations in the *Artemis* gene, was achieved by transduction of mouse HSC from the Artemis knockout mice with lentiviral vectors expressing human Artemis and transplant of the gene-modified HSC back to the mice, after they received submyeloablative dose of Busulfan. No side effects were reported.[41]

GENE THERAPY FOR HUMAN IMMUNODEFICIENCY VIRUS (HIV) INFECTION

HIV infection leads to the development of the acquired immunodeficiency syndrome (AIDS), the most common secondary immunodeficiency due to infection in developed countries. Several gene therapy initiatives were developed in the early 1990s, but were unsuccessful owing to the low efficiency of the technology available to transduce HSC. Progression of HIV infection to AIDS is currently being prevented by early detection and the use of a cocktail of antiviral drugs collectively called highly active antiretroviral therapy (HAART). Ten years after the introduction of HAART, experience with these drug regimens is satisfactory but accompanied by significant side effects, poor patient compliance and the development of resistance, secondary to the need for lifelong treatment. No HAART regimen has shown to be able to consistently eradicate viral infection (Chapter 37).

Gene therapy strategies to control HIV infection may have at least an adjuvant role in the current clinical management of the disease. Genetic intervention has been suggested in order either to induce anti-HIV immunity or to introduce anti-HIV protective genes into T cells or into hematopoietic cells. The major HIV genes involved in its replication and pathogenesis have been well characterized, and clever interventions to neutralize these genes have been proposed. These include transdominant negative proteins, intracellular antibodies, antisense sequences, ribozymes and molecular decoys that inhibit or sequester HIV proteins (Table 86.4). In addition, combinations of these mechanisms have also been proposed, such as a triple combination of a ribozyme targeting Tat and Rev, a TAR RNA decoy and an anti-CCR5 ribozyme.[42] Most anti-HIV gene therapy approaches have in common the use of a retroviral vector and being efficient at inhibiting HIV replication in T cells or hematopoietic CD34+ cells *in vitro*. However, only few clinical trials have been reported.[43] In one of the earliest it was shown that transduced CD4 T cells expressing RevM10, a genetically engineered dominant negative mutant protein of HIV Rev, had a survival advantage over cells that were not expressing this gene. This study showed that survival advantage that had been shown *in vitro* could also be demonstrated in HIV-infected patients.[44] Similar results were obtained using ribozyme targeting the HIV promoter and the HIV *tat* RNA message. In addition, more recent studies have focused on the transduction of anti-HIV genes into CD34+ hematopoietic stem cells, to take advantage of their self-renewal capacity and to allow thymic T-cell differentiation. However, the low transduction efficiency of CD34+ cells has resulted in very low levels of engraftment of gene-modified CD34+ cells, although these vector-containing cells persisted for over 3 years in most patients.[43, 44]

Current studies are focused on increasing the effective rate of transduction working with lentivirus-derived vectors, which have the advantage of being more efficient in the transfer of genes to nondividing cells. Perez et al.[45] demonstrated a significant reduction of cytopathic effects and the production of soluble HIV protein p24 when CD4 T cells transduced with an HIV-based gene vector carrying the membrane-bound gp41 fusion inhibitor were challenged with a T-cell tropic HIV strain. Large animal models continue to be fundamental for the development of anti-HIV therapeutic genes, such as the work of Braun et al.[46] in monkeys using a HIV-1 based vector carrying an antisense

Table 86.4 Examples of anti-HIV gene therapy strategies

Inhibitory interventions	Strategies in clinical trials
Transdominant negative proteins	M10Rev (Rev transdominant protein)
Ribozymes	Rrz2 (Tat targeted ribozyme)
Sense avd antisense sequences	VRX496 (antisense for Env gene)

molecule targeting the envelope sequence. Rhesus monkey bone marrow CD34+ cells were transduced and cultured in thymus stroma to induce T-cell development. These gene-modified T cells were resistant to simian HIV replication. Clinical trials using different anti-HIV genes and lentivirus-derived gene vectors are being developed. No definite results have so far been reported.[47]

CONCLUSIONS AND FUTURE DIRECTIONS

Current treatment for many PIs and for HIV infection is not optimal and justifies the search for alternative treatments. For example, in the case of SCID, in many patients enzyme replacement or BMT often remains inadequate, with increased susceptibility to infections, autoimmunity, and/or GvHD. Gene therapy is a promising alternative treatment for primary immunodeficiencies, provided that restoration of an appropriate level of gene expression can be achieved in multipotent, self-renewing stem cells. PIs are the first group of diseases in which gene therapy has been successful in human trials, with complete restoration of immune competence in infants with XSCID and ADA-deficient SCID. Unfortunately, at the same time, the application of gene therapy in XSCID has also made evident for the first time the risk of insertional mutagenesis. Several hypotheses are being investigated concerning the roles of specific gene expression, gene vector dose and patient age. Because of the overall limited clinical experience, it appears that the risk of oncogenesis in gene therapy trials will be realistically estimated only after treating more patients and following them closely over the long term, with careful assessment of insertion sites and clonality. Future directions to improve the safety of gene therapy in this regard include the development of vectors with reduced ability to activate nearby genes, using strategies such as 3′ LTR deletion.

New approaches are being suggested, such as the direct intra-femoral injection of retroviral vectors, as an alternative to avoid deleterious effects of *ex vivo* manipulation. McCauslin et al.[48] used this technique to correct JAK3 knockout mice with a JAK3 cDNA vector. Five of 12 injected mice had increased naïve T-cell counts. Specific antibody titers and mitogen proliferative responses were also improved in two of five treated mice studied. Although a minority of the treated mice were reconstituted, this study demonstrated the feasibility of direct vector injection. Another proposal is the intravenous injection of retroviral vectors, tested in a canine model of XSCID, and a mouse model of ADA-SCID.[50] *In vivo* approaches are appealing to surpass loss of HSC engraftment potential during *in vitro* cultures required for gene transduction; however, the safety issues relating to retroviral insertion in these new approaches may need to be completely addressed before *in vivo* gene therapy is used in clinical trials.

Other methods for gene delivery are being developed to achieve gene transfer targeted to specific genome sites, which would ideally avoid integrations in undesirable regions of the genome, including the vicinity of known oncogenes. These methods include the PhiC31 integrase system,[51] and specific site-directed recombination using modified zinc finger molecules.[52] The PhiC31 uses a rare 34-bp recognition sequence that allows integration in unique specific sites of the genome. Ishikawa et al.[47] demonstrated the feasibility of this approach using a human T-cell line deficient in the γc chain and characterized the insertion of the gene vector, which appeared to reproducibly involve intergenic regions in chromosomes 13 and 18, and lead to stable expression with correction of the IL-2 signaling response. In developing the nuclease/zinc finger approach, Urnov and colleagues[52] demonstrated that gene repair strategies may work by showing modification of an *IL2RG* point mutation in 5% of T cells *in vitro* and the reversion to wild-type sequence in about 10% of K562 cells engineered to carry a point mutation in *IL2RG*. Although these results are encouraging, both approaches require additional vectors to deliver these recombination enzymes into target cells. In addition, more experiments are needed to assess the intrinsic risk of nonspecific recombination events that may be associated with these strategies.

The successes of XSCID, ADA SCID and CGD gene therapy clinical trials, as well as the unexpected adverse events in a small proportion of treated patients, demonstrate that gene therapy for immunodeficiencies is past its infancy, and has the clear potential to become a viable alternative for the treatment of these otherwise fatal disorders.

REFERENCES

1. National Institutes of Health. Genetic Modification Clinical Research Information System Version 4.0 (http://www.gemcris.od.nih.gov, accessed 5/18/06).

2. Brenner S, Malech HL. Current developments in the design of onco-retrovirus and lentivirus vector systems for hematopoietic cell gene therapy. Biochim Biophys Acta 2003; 1640: 1–24.

3. Buckley RH. Molecular defects in human severe combined immunodeficiency and approaches to immune reconstitution. Annu Rev Immunol 2004; 22: 625–655.

4. Hirschhorn R. Immunodeficiency disease due to deficiency of adenosine deaminase. In: Ochs H, Smith CIE, Puck JM, eds. Primary Immunodeficiency Diseases, a Molecular and Genetic Approach, New York, NY: Oxford University Press, 1999: 121–139.

5. Blaese RM, Culver KW, Miller AD, et al. T lymphocyte-directed gene therapy for ADA- SCID: initial trial results after 4 years. Science 1995; 270: 475–480.

6. Onodera M, Ariga T, Kawamura N, et al. Successful peripheral T-lymphocyte-directed gene transfer for a patient with severe combined immune deficiency caused by adenosine deaminase deficiency. Blood 1998; 91: 30–36.

7. Aiuti C, Cattaneo F, Ficara F, et al. Gene therapy for adenosine deaminase deficiency. Curr Opin Allergy Clin Immunol 2003; 3: 461–466.

8. Aiuti A, Slavin S, Aker M, et al. Correction of ADA-SCID by stem cell gene therapy combined with nonmyeloablative conditioning. Science 2002; 296: 2410–2413.

9. Candotti F, Podsakoff G, Schurman SH, et al. Corrective gene transfer into bone marrow CD34+cells for adenosine deaminase (ADA) deficiency: Results in four patients after one year of follow-up. Mol Ther 2003; 7: 1163.

10. Otsu M, Ariga T, Maeyama Y, et al. Clinical trial in Japan of retroviral-mediated gene transfer to bone marrow CD34(+) cells as a treatment of adenosine deaminase (ADA)-deficiency. Mol Ther 2004; 9: 175.

11. Gaspar HB, Bjorkegren E, Parsley K, et al. Successful reconstitution of immunity in ADA-SCID by stem cell gene therapy following cessation of PEG-ADA and use of mild preconditioning. Mol Ther 2006; 14: 505–513.

12. Goebel WS, Dinauer MC. Gene therapy for chronic granulomatous disease. Acta Haematol 2003; 110: 86–92.

13. Malech HL, Maples PB, Whiting-Theobald N, et al. Prolonged production of NADPH oxidase-corrected granulocytes after gene therapy of chronic granulomatous disease. Proc Natl Acad Sci USA 1997; 94: 12133–12138.

14. Ott MG, Schmidt M, Schwarzwaelder K, et al. Correction of X-linked chronic granulomatous disease by gene therapy, augmented by insertional activation of MDS1-EVI1, PRDM16 or SETBP1. Nature Med 2006; 12: 401–409.

15. European Society of Gene Therapy (ESGT). One of three successfully treated CGD patients in a Swiss-German gene therapy trial died due to his underlying disease: A position statement from the European Society of Gene Therapy (ESGT). J Gene Med 2006; 8: 1435.

16. Bauer TR Jr, Hickstein DD. Gene therapy for leukocyte adhesion deficiency. Curr Opin Mol Ther 2000; 2: 383–388.

17. Bauer TR Jr, Hai M, Tuschong LM, et al. Correction of the disease phenotype in canine leukocyte adhesion deficiency using ex vivo hematopoietic stem cell gene therapy. Blood 2006; 108: 3313–3320.

18. Cavazzana-Calvo M, Lagresle C, Hacein-Bey-Abina S, Fischer A. Gene therapy for severe combined immunodeficiency. Annu Rev Med 2005; 56: 585–602.

19. Gaspar HB, Parsley KL, Howe S, et al. Gene therapy of X-linked severe combined immunodeficiency by use of a pseudotyped gammaretroviral vector. Lancet 2004; 364: 2181–2187.

20. Cavazzana-Calvo M, Hacein-Bey S, de Saint Basile G, et al. Gene therapy of human severe combined immunodeficiency (SCID)-X1 disease. Science 2000; 288: 669–672.

21. Thrasher AJ, Hacein-Bey-Abina S, Gaspar HB, et al. Failure of SCID-X1 gene therapy in older patients. Blood 2005; 105: 4255–4257.

22. Chinen J, Davis J, De Ravin SS, et al. Gene therapy improves immune function in preadolescents with X-linked severe combined immunodeficiency. Blood 2007; 110: 67–73.

23. Hacein-Bey-Abina S, Von Kalle C, Schmidt M, et al. LMO2-associated clonal T cell proliferation in two patients after gene therapy for SCID-X1. Science 2003; 302: 415–419.

24. Kaiser J. Panel urges hints on XSCID trial. Science 2005; 307: 1544–1545.

25. Kohn DB, Sadelain M, Dunbar C, et al. American Society of Gene Therapy (ASGT) ad hoc subcommittee on retroviral-mediated gene transfer to hematopoietic stem cells. Mol Ther 2003; 8: 180–187.

26. Li Z, Dullmann J, Schiedlmeier B, et al. Murine leukemia induced by retroviral gene marking. Science 2002; 296: 497.

27. Dave UP, Jenkins NA, Copeland NG. Gene therapy insertional mutagenesis insights. Science 2004; 303: 333.

28. Fischer A, Thrasher A, von Kalle C, Cavazzana-Calvo M. LMO2 and gene therapy for severe combined immunodeficiency. N Engl J Med 2004; 350: 2526.

29. Wu X, Li Y, Crise B, Burgess SM. Transcription start regions in the human genome are favored targets for MLV integration. Science 2003; 300: 1749–1751.

30. Bunting KD, Lu T, Kelly PF, Sorrentino BP. Self-selection by genetically modified committed lymphocyte precursors reverses the phenotype of JAK3-deficient mice without myeloablation. Hum Gene Ther 2000; 11: 2353–2304.

31. Sorrentino BP, Lu T, Ihle J, et al. A clinical attempt to treat JAK3-deficient SCID using retroviral mediated gene transfer to bone marrow CD34+ cells. Mol Ther 2003; 7: S449.

32. Strom TS, Turner SJ, Andreansky S, et al. Defects in T-cell mediated immunity by influenza virus in murine Wiskott–Aldrich syndrome are corrected by oncoretroviral vector-mediated gene transfer into repopulating hematopoietic cells. Blood 2003; 102: 3108–3116.

33. Dupré L, Marangoni F, Scaramuzza S, et al. Efficacy of gene therapy for Wiskott–Aldrich syndrome using a WAS promoter/cDNA-containing lentiviral vector and nonlethal irradiation. Hum Gene Ther 2006; 17: 303–313.

34. Charrier S, Dupre L, Scaramuzza S, et al. Lentiviral vectors targeting WASp expression to hematopoietic cells, efficiently transduce and correct cells from WAS patients. Gene Ther 2007; 14: 415–428.

35. Brown MP, Topham DJ, Sangster MY, et al. Thymic lymphoproliferative disease after successful correction of CD40 ligand deficiency by gene transfer in mice. Nature Med 1998; 4: 1253–1260.

36. Otsu M, Steinberg M, Ferrand C, et al. Reconstitution of lymphoid development and function in ZAP-70-deficient mice following gene transfer into bone marrow cells. Blood 2002; 100: 1248–1256.

37. Adjali O, Vicente RR, Ferrand C, et al. Intrathymic administration of hematopoietic progenitor cells enhances T cell reconstitution in ZAP-70 severe combined immunodeficiency. Proc Natl Acad Sci USA 2005; 102: 13586–13591.

38. Yu PW, Tabuchi RS, Kato RM, et al. Sustained correction of B-cell development and function in a murine model of X-linked agammaglobulinemia (XLA) using retroviral-mediated gene transfer. Blood 2004; 104: 1281–1290.

39. Yates F, Malassis-Seris M, Stockholm D, et al. Gene therapy of RAG-2-/- mice: sustained correction of the immunodeficiency. Blood 2002; 100: 3942–3949.

40. Lagresle-Peyrou C, Yates F, Malassis-Seris M, et al. Long-term immune reconstitution in RAG-1-deficient mice treated by retroviral gene therapy: a balance between efficiency and toxicity. Blood 2006; 107: 63–72.

41. Mostoslavsky G, Fabian AJ, Rooney S, et al. Complete correction of murine Artemis immunodeficiency by lentiviral vector-mediated gene transfer. Proc Natl Acad Sci USA 2006; 103: 16406–16411.

42. Li MJ, Kim J, Li S, et al. Long-term inhibition of HIV-1 infection in primary hematopoietic cells by lentiviral vector delivery of a triple combination of anti-HIV shRNA, anti-CCR5 ribozyme, and a nucleolar-localizing TAR decoy. Mol Ther 2005; 12: 900–909.

43. Strayer DS, Akkina R, Bunnell BA, et al. Current status of gene therapy strategies to treat HIV/AIDS. Mol Ther 2005; 11: 823–842.

44. Podsakoff GM, Engel BC, Carbonaro DA, et al. Selective survival of peripheral blood lymphocytes in children with HIV-1 following delivery of an anti-HIV gene to bone marrow CD34(+) cells. Mol Ther 2005; 12: 77–86.

45. Perez EE, Riley JL, Carroll RG, et al. Suppression of HIV-1 infection in primary CD4 T cells transduced with a self-inactivating lentiviral vector encoding a membrane expressed gp41-derived fusion inhibitor. Clin Immunol 2005; 115: 26–32.

46. Braun SE, Johnson RP. Setting the stage for bench-to-bedside movement of anti-HIV RNA inhibitors – gene therapy for AIDS in macaques. Front Biosci 2006; 11: 838–851.

47. Dropulic B, June CH. Gene-based immunotherapy for human immunodeficiency virus infection and acquired immunodeficiency syndrome. Hum Gene Ther 2006; 17: 577–588.

48. McCauslin CS, Wine J, Cheng L, et al. In vivo retroviral gene transfer by direct intrafemoral injection results in correction of the SCID phenotype in JAK3 knock-out animals. Blood 2003; 102: 843–848.

49. Ting-De Ravin SS, Kennedy DR, Naumann N, et al. Correction of canine X-linked severe combined immunodeficiency by in vivo retroviral gene therapy. Blood 2006; 107: 3091–3097.

50. Carbonaro DA, Jin X, Petersen D, et al. In vivo transduction by intravenous injection of a lentiviral vector expressing human ADA into neonatal ADA gene knockout mice: a novel form of enzyme replacement therapy for ADA deficiency. Mol Ther 2006; 13: 1110–1120.

51. Ishikawa Y, Tanaka N, Murakami K, et al. Phage phiC31 integrase-mediated genomic integration of the common cytokine receptor gamma chain in human T-cell lines. J Gene Med 2006; 8: 646–653.

52. Urnov FD, Miller JC, Lee YL, et al. Highly efficient endogenous human gene correction using designed zinc-finger nucleases. Nature 2005; 435: 646–651.

Glucocorticoids

Frank Buttgereit, Markus J.H. Seibel, Johannes W.J. Bijlsma

87

Glucocorticoids exceed many other drugs in terms of numbers of patients treated, variety of applications and pharmacological experience in humans.[1] Almost 60 years after their introduction into clinical practice, they still represent the most important and most frequently employed class of anti-inflammatory drug, with a steady rise in therapeutic use in recent years.[2] About 10 million new prescriptions for oral glucocorticoids are issued each year in the USA.[2] Community survey data estimate the frequency of oral glucocorticoid use as 0.5% of the general population and 1.75% of women aged over 55 years.[3, 4] Between 56% and 68% of patients with rheumatoid arthritis are treated more or less continuously with glucocorticoids.[1] Glucocorticoids are relatively inexpensive, but owing to the sheer volume prescribed the total market size is about US$10 billion per year.[2]

The major reason for their widespread use is simple: glucocorticoids are the most effective (and cost-effective) anti-inflammatory and immunomodulatory drugs available. At the same time, glucocorticoids are prone to cause frequent and serious side effects, especially when used incorrectly.

■ MECHANISMS OF ACTION ■

The basis for the use of different dosages of glucocorticoids in different clinical conditions is essentially empirical, as evidence to support preferences in specific clinical settings is scarce.[1] It is clear, however, that glucocorticoid dosages increase with clinical activity and the severity of the disease under treatment. The rationale for this (mostly successful) clinical approach is that higher dosages increase glucocorticoid receptor saturation in a dose-dependent manner (Table 87.1), which intensifies the therapeutically relevant, *genomic* glucocorticoid actions; and it is assumed that with increasing dosages, additional and qualitatively different, *nonspecific, nongenomic* actions of glucocorticoids come into play (Table 87.1).

GENOMIC ACTIONS OF GLUCOCORTICOIDS

The anti-inflammatory and immunomodulatory effects of glucocorticoids (GC) are mediated predominantly by genomic mechanisms (Figs 87.1 and 87.2). Binding to cytosolic glucocorticoid receptors (cGCR) ultimately induces ('*transactivation*') or inhibits ('*transrepression*') the synthesis of regulator proteins.[5] Between 10 and 100 genes per cell are directly regulated by glucocorticoids, but many genes are regulated indirectly through interaction with transcription factors and co-activators (see below).[6] It is estimated that glucocorticoids influence the transcription of approximately 1% of the entire genome. In the past few years, our in-depth knowledge of the genomic actions of GCs has greatly increased. Their lipophilic structure and low molecular mass allow GCs to pass easily through the cell membrane and bind to the inactive cGCR (α-form = cGCRα).

CHARACTERISTICS APPLYING TO GENOMIC ACTIONS

>> Physiologically relevant

>> Therapeutically effective at all dosages, even very small ones (low dose therapy).

>> Slow; significant changes in the regulator protein concentrations are not seen within less than 30 minutes because of the time required for cGCR activation/ translocation, transcription and translation effects.

>> The GC-induced synthesis of regulator proteins can be prevented by inhibitors of transcription (e.g. actinomycin D) or translation (e.g. cycloheximide).

Table 87.1 Current knowledge on the relationship between clinical glucocorticoid dosing and cellular glucocorticoid actions (From Buttgereit F, Straub RH, Wehling M, Burmester GR. Glucocorticoids in the treatment of rheumatic diseases. An update on mechanisms of action. Arthritis Rheum 2004; 50: 3408–3417, with permission)

Terminology (mg prednisone equivalent per day)	Clinical application	Genomic actions (receptor saturation)	Unspecific nongenomic actions	cGCR-mediated nongenomic actions
Low dose (≤ 7.5)	Maintenance therapy for many rheumatic diseases	+ (< 50%)	–	?
Medium dose (>7.5–≤30)	Initially given in primary chronic rheumatic diseases	++ (> 50 -<100%)	(+)	(+)
High dose (>30-≤100)	Initially given in subacute rheumatic diseases	++(+) (almost 100%)	+	+
Very high dose (> 100 mg)	Initially given in acute and/or potentially life-threatening exacerbations of rheumatic diseases	+++ ((almost) 100%)	++	+(+?)
Pulse therapy (≥ 250 mg for 1 or a few days)	Particularly severe and/or potentially life-threatening forms of rheumatic diseases	+++ (100%)	+++	+(++?)

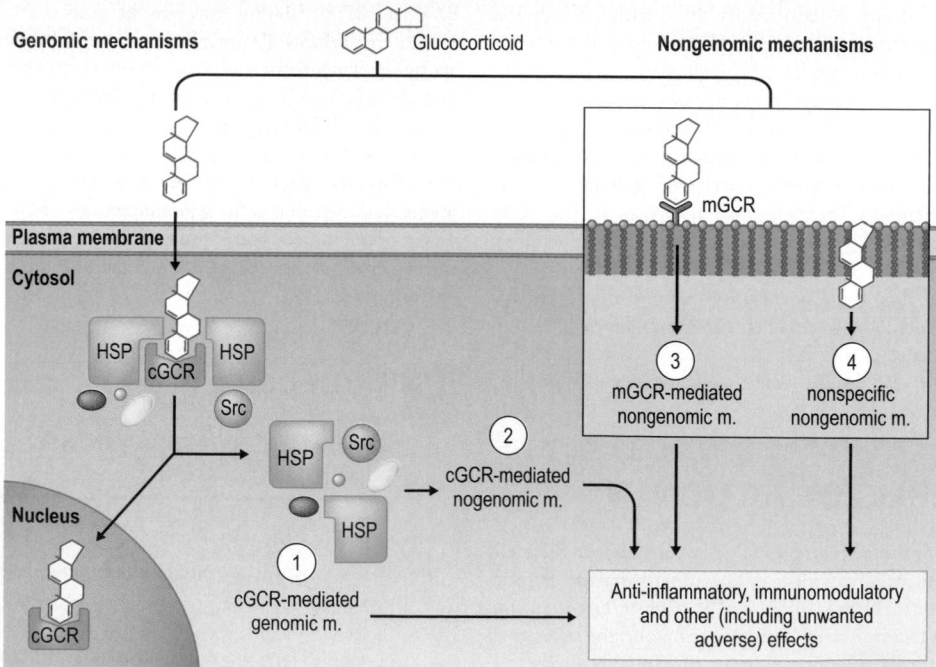

Fig. 87.1 Mechanisms of the cellular action of glucocorticoids. As lipophilic substances, glucocorticoids pass very easily through the cell membrane into the cell, where they bind to ubiquitously expressed cytosolic glucocorticoid receptors (cGCR). This is followed by either the classic cGCR-mediated genomic effects (I) or by cGCR-mediated nongenomic effects (II). Moreover, the glucocorticoid is very likely to interact with cell membranes, either specifically via membrane-bound glucocorticoid receptors (mGCR) (III) or via nonspecific interactions with cell membranes (IV). (From Buttgereit F, Straub RH, Wehling M, Burmester GR, 2004. Glucocorticoids in the treatment of rheumatic diseases. An update on mechanisms of action. Arthritis and Rheumatism 50: 3408–3417.)

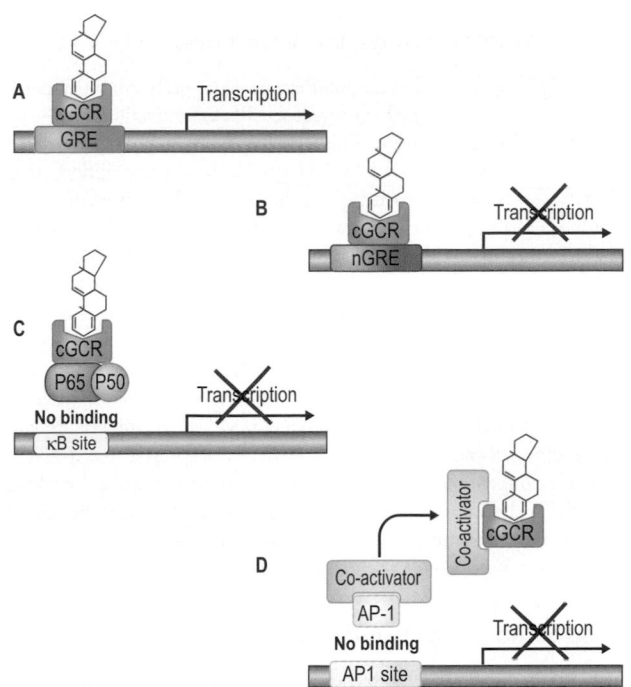

Fig. 87.2 (A–D) Genomic mechanisms of glucocorticoids. This figure illustrates the different mechanisms by which the activated glucocorticoid receptor complex leads to the induction or to the inhibition of transcription and finally translation/synthesis of specific regulator proteins. Details are given in the text. (From Buttgereit F, Straub RH, Wehling M, Burmester GR, 2004. Glucocorticoids in the treatment of rheumatic diseases. An update on mechanisms of action. Arthritis and Rheumatism 50: 3408–3417.)

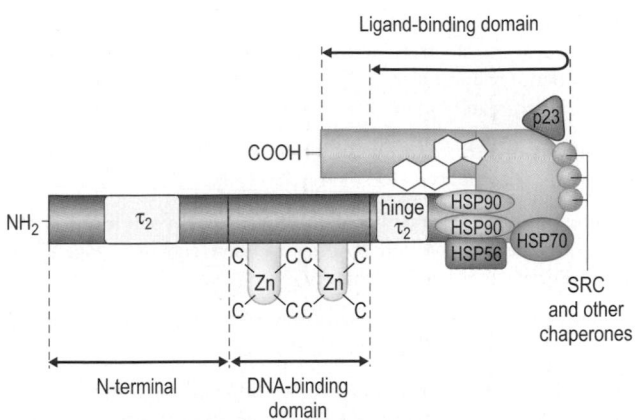

Fig. 87.3 Structure of the cytosolic glucocorticoid receptor. The unactivated (unligated) cGCR is a 94 kDa protein retained in the cytoplasm as a multi-protein complex consisting of several heat shock proteins (hsp), including hsp90, hsp70, hsp56 and hsp40 (chaperones). Furthermore, the cGCR interacts with immunophilins, p23 and several kinases of the mitogen-activated protein kinase (MAPK) signaling system, including Src, which also act as molecular (co-)chaperones. An important function of molecular (co-)chaperones is to stabilize a specific conformational state of the GC which binds ligand with high affinity (see text). The receptor protein itself consists of different domains: an N terminal, a DNA-binding domain (DBD) and a ligand-binding domain (LBD). The N terminal harbors transactivation functions, especially within the so-called τ1 region. Another major transactivation region is τ2, which can interact with the above-mentioned cofactors.(From Buttgereit F, Straub RH, Wehling M, Burmester GR, 2004. Glucocorticoids in the treatment of rheumatic diseases. An update on mechanisms of action. Arthritis and Rheumatism 50: 3408–3417.)

Structure of the cGCR

The unactivated cGCR is a 94 kDa protein held in the cytoplasm as a multi-protein complex consisting of several heat shock proteins (hsp), including hsp90, hsp70, hsp56 and hsp40 (chaperones) (Fig. 87.3). The cGCR interacts with immunophilins, p23 and several kinases of the mitogen-activated protein kinase (MAPK) signaling system, including Src, which also act as molecular (co)chaperones (Figs 87.1 and 87.3).[1,7,8] The general function of molecular (co)chaperones is to bind and stabilize proteins at intermediate stages of folding, assembly, translocation and degradation. With regard to cGCR, they also regulate cellular signaling, which includes (i) stabilizing a specific conformational state of cGCR that binds ligand with high affinity; (ii) simultaneously opening the glucocorticoid binding cleft to access by glucocorticoids; and (iii) stabilizing the binding of GR to the promoter.[1]

The first step in assembling the multi-protein cytosolic complex is ATP- and hsp40(YDJ-1)-dependent formation of a cGCR-hsp70 complex that primes the receptor for subsequent ATP-dependent activation by hsp90, Hop, and p23.[9] The glucocorticoid receptor consists of different domains with distinct functions: an N terminal, a DNA-binding domain (DBD) and a ligand-binding domain (LBD) (Fig. 87.3). The N terminal harbors transactivation functions, especially within the 'τ1' region. A motif common to DNA-interacting proteins, the zinc finger

motif, is found twice within the DBD. The LBD consists of 12 α helices, several of which help form a hydrophobic ligand-binding pocket.[8] The cGCR contains another major transactivation region ('τ2') that can interact with the above-mentioned cofactors (Fig. 87.3). Following glucocorticoid/receptor binding, hsp90 molecules and other chaperones are rapidly shed. This allows translocation into the cell nucleus, where the GC/cGCR complex binds as a homodimer to consensus palindromic DNA sites (GC-responsive elements – GREs).[5]

Translocation into the nucleus

Nuclear translocation of the GC/cGCR complex occurs within 20 minutes. Hormone-directed recruitment of FKBP52 and dynein to the GCR may causes its transport to the nucleus.[10] Depending on the target gene, transcription is then either activated (*transactivation* via positive GRE) or inhibited (*transrepression* via negative GRE) (Fig. 87.2A and B).

Interactions with transcription factors

Besides the interactions of GC/cGCR complexes with GREs, a further important genomic mechanism of GC action is interaction of activated cGCR monomers with transcription factors. Accordingly, although the GC/cGCR complex does not inhibit their synthesis, it modulates the activity of AP-1 (activator protein-1), NF-κB (nuclear factor-κB) and

NF-AT (nuclear factor for activated T cells).[11–15] This leads to inhibition of nuclear translocation and/or function of these transcription factors, and hence to inhibition of the expression of many immunoregulatory and inflammatory cytokines. Possible mechanisms include: [5]

- Synthesis of IκB (a specific inhibitor of NF-κB) induced through GC/cGCR complex–GRE interaction (Fig. 87.2A).

- Protein–protein interaction of the GC/cGCR complex with transcription factors through binding to their subunits (Fig. 87.2C), which prevents their DNA binding.

- Competition for nuclear co-activators between the GC/cGCR complex and transcription factors (Fig. 87.2D).

Inhibition of transcription factor function and the resultant inhibition of protein expression are referred to as *transrepression*. Numerous genes are regulated by this mechanism. It appears that many adverse effects of GC are caused by *transactivation* (i.e., induced synthesis of regulator proteins), whereas many anti-inflammatory effects are mediated by transrepression (i.e., inhibited synthesis of regulator proteins). This differential molecular regulation underlies current drug-discovery programs aimed at developing dissociated cGCR-ligands.[2]

The cGCRβ isoform

An alternative splice variant of the cGCRα exists: the cGCRβ isoform, which does not bind ligand and has been proposed to inhibit classic cGCRα-mediated transactivation. Recent structural research has shown a possible physical explanation for the lack of hormone binding and the dominant negative actions of cGCRβ.[16]

Post-transcriptional and post-translational mechanisms

Glucocorticoids also act through post-transcriptional and post-translational mechanisms, e.g., reduction of cytokine mRNA half-life and downregulation of GCR (via reduced mRNA levels and reduced stability of the GCR protein).[17]

Glucocorticoid receptor resistance

GCR resistance is an interesting field of research. Several different mechanisms may mediate this phenomenon, among them alterations in number, binding affinity or phosphorylation status of the GCR. Other mechanisms being investigated are polymorphic changes and/or over-expression of (co-)chaperones, increased expression of inflammatory transcription factors, over-expression of the GCRβ isoform, the multi-drug resistance pump, and altered mGCR expression.

NONGENOMIC ACTIONS OF GLUCOCORTICOIDS

Some regulatory effects of glucocorticoids arise within seconds or minutes. These are too rapid to be explained as genomic actions, and are attributed to *nongenomic* mechanisms of action. Three different rapid nongenomic actions of glucocorticoids have recently been described.[1, 18–21]

cGCR-mediated nongenomic actions

Croxtall et al.[19] reported that dexamethasone can rapidly inhibit epidermal growth factor-stimulated cPLA$_2$ (cytosolic PLA$_2$) activation with subsequent arachidonic acid release. This effect is thought to be mediated by occupation of cGCR, but not by changes in gene transcription, as the observed effect is RU486 sensitive (i.e., glucocorticoid receptor dependent), but actinomycin insensitive (i.e., transcription independent). It is suggested that chaperones or co-chaperones of the multi-protein complex may act as signaling components to mediate this effect. Following glucocorticoid binding, the cGCR is released from this complex to mediate classic genomic actions. However, there is also a rapid release of Src and other (co-)chaperones of the multi-protein complex, which may cause rapid inhibition of arachidonic acid release. Similarly, cardiovascular protective effects of dexamethasone have been reported which are not genomic (because they occurred too quickly and were actinomycin insensitive) or nonspecific nongenomic effects (because they occurred at a very low dosage (100 nM).[21] These may involve binding of glucocorticoids to the cGCR, leading to nontranscriptional activation of phosphatidylinositol 3-kinase, protein kinase Akt and endothelial nitric oxide synthase.

Nonspecific nongenomic actions

Under certain circumstances glucocorticoids are administered at very high concentrations (e.g., intra-articular injection or IV pulse therapy). Systemically administered daily dosages >100 mg prednisone equivalent are regarded as 'very high dose.' In contrast, 'pulse therapy' is the daily administration of ≥250 mg prednisone equivalent for one or a few consecutive days[22] (Table 87.1). Saturation of all cGCR is almost complete with a daily dose of 100 mg prednisone equivalent, so that specificity, i.e., the exclusivity of receptor-mediated effects, is lost at these high – but clinically relevant – glucocorticoid concentrations.[18] Nonspecific nongenomic actions occur in the form of physicochemical interactions with biological membranes, which probably contribute to the therapeutic effect.[1] A nonspecific intercalation of glucocorticoid molecules into cell membranes is thought to alter cell function by influencing cation transport and increasing mitochondrial proton leak. The resulting inhibition of calcium and sodium cycling across the plasma membrane of immune cells is thought to contribute to rapid immunosuppression and to reduced inflammation.[1, 18]

The use of such high glucocorticoid doses is confined to certain clinical specialties and has been criticized by endocrinologists and pharmacologists. Unfortunately, scientific evidence on this issue is lacking, as there are no randomized controlled trials. However, high-dose glucocorticoid therapy is often used with clinical success in acute exacerbations of life-threatening diseases and various clinical conditions resistant to other therapies. For example, pulsed IV methylprednisolone is effective in the treatment of systemic lupus erythematosus (SLE). However, these studies were mainly uncontrolled and retrospective in nature. A recent review concluded that intravenous pulses of methylprednisolone rapidly immunosuppresses patients with organ- and/or life-threatening manifestations of SLE. However, the gold standard – 1 g/day for 3 consecutive days – is associated with significant infectious complications, and lower doses may be just as useful.[23]

Another example is immune thrombocytopenia associated with SLE where high-dose glucocorticoids are normally (and mostly successfully) used, although comparative studies are lacking.[24] It has been calculated that in situations like these, concentrations are achieved *in vivo* that are high enough (around 10^{-5} mol/L) to cause immediate nonspecific nongenomic effects on immune cells.[1] Intra-articular injections also bring high concentrations of glucocorticoids into contact with inflammatory cells, although it is difficult to assess locally achieved concentrations because crystal suspensions are most often used.

Specific nongenomic actions

Glucocorticoids can also induce specific nongenomic actions mediated through membrane-bound glucocorticoid receptors (mGCR). The existence and function of membrane-bound receptors have recently been demonstrated for various steroids (including mineralocorticoids, gonadal hormones, vitamin D and thyroid hormones).[1, 18, 25] Using immunofluorescence, small numbers of mGCR can be demonstrated on human peripheral blood mononuclear cells (monocytes and B lymphocytes) from healthy controls.[25] The monoclonal antibody used to detect mGCR also recognized cGCR, suggesting that mGCR are probably variants of cGCR produced by differential splicing or promoter switching. It has also been found that immunostimulation with lipopolysaccharide increases the percentage of mGCR+ monocytes; this can be prevented by inhibiting the secretory pathway with brefeldin A. This suggests that mGCR are actively upregulated and transported through the cell following immunostimulation. These *in vitro* findings are consistent with observations that the frequency of mGCR+ monocytes is increased in patients with rheumatic disorders, and is positively correlated with disease activity in rheumatoid arthritis.[25] The function(s) of mGCR remain unclear, but this observation means that mGCR may be implicated in pathogenesis. Alternatively, and perhaps more likely, they may cause negative feedback regulation.

■ GLUCOCORTICOID EFFECTS ON IMMUNE CELLS ■

Through the above mechanisms, glucocorticoids mediate a fascinating range of anti-inflammatory and immunomodulatory effects when used therapeutically, with virtually all primary and secondary immune cells affected to some extent (Table 87.2).[26]

■ THERAPEUTIC USE ■

A wide range of GC molecules are available for clinical use: these share a common basic structure and have been modified to improve their usefulness in various clinical applications (Fig 87.4). Despite their widespread use, the designation of GC treatment regimens is often imprecise. Recommendations for a standardized nomenclature for GC therapy are summarized below.[22]

TERMINOLOGY

What term should be used to describe this class of drugs?

The term 'steroids' (although very often used) is too broad, as it simply describes chemical compounds characterized by a common multiple-ring structure (including, for example, cholesterol, vitamin D and sex hormones); also, the terms 'corticosteroids' or 'corticoids' are not

Table 87.2 Important effects of glucocorticoids on primary and secondary immune cells (From Buttgereit F, Saag K, Cutolo M, et al. The molecular basis for the effectiveness, toxicity, and resistance to glucocorticoids: focus on the treatment of rheumatoid arthritis. Scand J Rheumatol 2005; 34: 14–21, with permission)

Monocytes/macrophages
  ↓ number of circulating cells (↓ myelopoiesis, ↓ release)
  ↓ expression of MHC class II molecules and Fc receptors
  ↓ synthesis of proinflammatory cytokines (e.g., IL-2, IL-6, TNF-α) and prostaglandins
T cells
  ↓ number of circulating cells (redistribution effects)
  ↓ production and action of IL-2 (most important)
Granulocytes
  ↓ number of eosinophil and basophil granulocytes
  ↑ number of circulating neutrophils
Endothelial cells
  ↓ vessel permeability
  ↓ expression of adhesion molecules
  ↓ production of IL-1 and prostaglandins
Fibroblasts
  ↓ proliferation
  ↓ production of fibronectin and prostaglandins

KEY CONCEPTS

GLUCOCORTICOID EFFECTS ON IMMUNE CELLS

>> Inhibit leukocyte traffic and access of leukocytes to the site of inflammation.

>> Interfere with functions of leukocytes, fibroblasts and endothelial cells.

>> Suppress the production and actions of humoral factors involved in the inflammatory process.

sufficiently precise, as the adrenal cortex, from which these designations are derived, synthesizes not only glucocorticoids, but also mineralocorticoids and androgens. For these reasons, the terms 'glucocorticoid' or 'glucocorticosteroid' are scientifically correct, but 'glucocorticoid' is the more widely used.

How can glucocorticoid therapy schedules be described as precisely as possible?

A description has been suggested that is precise regarding the drug, the dosage, the route of administration, and the timing of administration (timing, frequency, duration, sometimes cumulative dosage where appropriate).

Of note is that different glucocorticoid drugs have different potencies. Moreover, glucocorticoids differ in their ability to produce the distinct

exogenous GCs. Glucocorticoid-induced hypertension is dose related and might be less likely with medium- or low-dose therapy. Individual variation in susceptibility and other factors, such as the level of starting blood pressure, dietary salt intake, functional renal mass, associated diseases and drug therapy may also play a role. Patients with essential hypertension require closer surveillance of blood pressure and may need their anti-hypertensive regimen modified while on moderate- to high-dose GC therapy. In patients receiving <10 mg/day, age and elevated pre-treatment blood pressure may better explain significant hypertension than the use of GCs.

Another troublesome but very difficult-to-study potential toxicity of low-dose GCs is the development of premature atherosclerotic vascular disease. Increasing attention to the importance of accelerated atherosclerotic disease in RA and other inflammatory conditions has raised interesting questions about the role of chronic inflammation on the vascular endothelium. A threefold increase in atherosclerosis has been reported in RA patients treated with GCs compared to nonGC-treated patients, although the GC dose and other confounding factors were not reported. Studies evaluating the effects of GCs on lipids and atherosclerosis in RA patients have yielded mixed results. Observational studies of patients on long-term treatment with moderate to high doses of glucocorticoids for renal or cardiac allografts and asthma generally demonstrate elevations in total plasma cholesterol, low-density lipoprotein cholesterol (LDL-C), high-density lipoprotein cholesterol (HDL-C) and triglycerides. The effects of GCs on lipids seem to be dose dependent. In two studies in SLE patients, significant changes in lipid levels were seen only at prednisone doses >10 mg/day. In one report, moderate- to low-dose glucocorticoids (20 mg tapered to 5 mg over 3 months) had no significant adverse effect on lipoprotein levels if other risk factors were controlled. Other studies have even suggested that GCs may reverse unfavorable lipid changes. At present, the existing evidence does not show a strong association between low-dose glucocorticoids and cardiovascular disease in RA, even though atherosclerotic vascular disease is known to be accelerated in patients with Cushing's disease.

Dermatologic adverse effects

Even at low doses, skin thinning and ecchymoses are common adverse events with glucocorticoids. Cutaneous atrophy results from catabolic GC effects on keratinocytes and fibroblasts. Purpura and easy bruising in GC-treated patients is probably due to decreased vascular structural integrity. A cushingoid appearance is very troubling to patients, but is uncommon at doses below the physiologic range. One study reported facial fullness ('moon facies') in 13% of patients receiving 4–12 mg triamcinolone for up to 60 days. All these side effects are observed in over 5% of patients exposed to ≥5 mg prednisone equivalent for ≥1 year. The incidence of iatrogenic Cushing's syndrome is dose dependent and generally becomes evident after >1 month of GC therapy. Alternate-day therapy may reduce the incidence, although data supporting this concept are few. Glucocorticoid acne, hirsutism and striae are other undesirable dermatologic effects that occur even with lower doses.

Gastrointestinal adverse effects

Glucocorticoids are considerably less toxic to the upper gastrointestinal (GI) tract than NSAIDs. If GCs independently increase GI events (e.g., gastritis, ulceration, bleeding), the effect is slight, with estimated relative risks varying from 1.1 (not significant) to 1.5 (marginally significant). There are also anecdotal reports of intestinal rupture, diverticular perforation, and pancreatitis attributed to low-dose GCs. Glucocorticoids are frequently used concurrently with NSAIDs in RA, and meta-analyses confirm that the combination of the two synergistically increases the risk of GI adverse events. In a large-scale study based on the UK General Practice Research Database, the risk of upper GI complications was 1.8 (95% CI, 1.3–2.4) times higher for GC users than for nonusers. The risk tended to be greater for higher GC doses, but the dose gradient was not statistically significant. The risk was >12 times higher for those taking both glucocorticoids and NSAIDs than for those not using either. No studies have yet looked at the GI effects of combining GCs with COX-2-selective NSAIDs.

Infectious diseases

Medium- to high-dose GC therapy, particularly when administered for prolonged periods, may increase the risk of serious infections requiring hospitalization or surgery. However, to our knowledge, no studies have explored the risk of infection in patients on lower doses. The risk of infection appears to be lessened with alternate-day therapy. A meta-analysis showed that infection rates were not significantly increased in patients on <10 mg/day prednisone or a cumulative dose of <700 mg.

In GC-treated patients, physicians should anticipate the risk of infections with both typical and atypical organisms, realizing that GCs may blunt the classic clinical features and delay diagnosis. *Pneumocystis jiroveci* infections can occur with doses as low as 16 mg/day of prednisone for 8 weeks and have been associated with increased risk in one series.[34] Herpes zoster is also more common in RA patients treated with immunosuppressive agents. In one analysis,[35] eight such patients developed zoster compared with only one control (P<0.04). However, it is difficult to separate the independent effects of GC use from those of other commonly used anti-rheumatic agents, such as methotrexate and anti-TNF-α agents. At present, the independent role of GCs in facilitating herpes zoster infection in RA patients remains uncertain.

Adverse effects on glucose metabolism

It is uncommon for frank diabetes mellitus to develop *de novo* as a result of GC therapy. However, patients with pre-existing diabetes will commonly have higher blood glucose levels while taking glucocorticoids. At doses of 1–7.9 mg/day prednisone, the odds ratio for hyperglycaemia is 1.8; this rises progressively to 7 when the dose of prednisone is ≥25 mg/day. The odds ratio of requiring therapy for hyperglycaemia is 1.7 during the first 45 days of GC use, falling to 1.3 between 46–90 days and to 1.1 thereafter. Ketoacidosis is very rare in GC-associated diabetes, as the gluconeogenic and glycogenic effects of GCs protect against this complication.

Adverse effects on the hypothalamopituitary axis

The prevalence of HPA insufficiency appears to depend on both the dose and the duration of GC treatment. High-dose therapy can result in marked and prolonged suppression of ACTH release and adrenal hyporesponsiveness after only 5 days. Spontaneous recovery of the HPA axis is the rule in patients on ≤5 mg/day prednisone; however, low doses (<7.5 mg/day) given for longer periods (e.g., 4–6 weeks) will also blunt

HPA responsiveness. Suppression of the HPA tends to be more pronounced if GCs are given twice daily instead of once daily. Glucocorticoid withdrawal syndrome is not clearly associated with HPA insufficiency, but presents as weakness and arthralgias. Indeed, difficulty in withdrawing patients from GCs is sometimes cited as a compelling reason for not initiating them. Despite these widely held sentiments, the issue of lower dose withdrawal has not been addressed in randomized controlled trials.

Neuropsychiatric adverse effects

Many patients suffering from RA report a slight increase in their overall sense of wellbeing when starting on low-dose GC therapy; this appears to be independent of improvements in disease activity. Symptoms of akathisia, insomnia, and depression are also occasionally observed during low-dose GC therapy. Memory impairment, particularly in older patients, can occur even at low doses and could relate to hippocampus-dependent functions. Daily split-dose therapy tends to be particularly troublesome, because the evening dose disrupts normal diurnal variations in endogenous GC levels and promotes sleep disturbances. True GC psychosis is distinctly uncommon at doses <20 mg/day prednisone.

Ophthalmologic adverse effects

Posterior subcapsular cataracts after prolonged GC use are well described. Some clinicians believe there is no minimal safe dose for this complication. Others note that cataracts rarely occur in patients taking <10 mg/day for <1 year. Cortical cataracts have also been associated with GC use. In addition to cataracts, GC-treated patients may develop increased intra-ocular pressure, which can cause minor visual disturbances. The development of frank glaucoma is rare, particularly with low-dose therapy, and tends only to affect patients already predisposed to the condition. GC-associated glaucoma tends to occur in families, suggesting a genetic basis. Highlighting a potential risk of even low-dose therapy, glaucoma may also occur with inhaled GCs.

■ NEW GLUCOCORTICOID RECEPTOR LIGANDS ON THE HORIZON ■

The various mechanisms of GC action provide interesting opportunities for developing optimized GCs and GC-receptor ligands, which are reviewed below. More detailed information is available elsewhere.[1, 31, 36]

SELECTIVE GLUCOCORTICOID RECEPTOR AGONISTS (SEGRAS)

The existence of the genomic component mechanisms of transactivation and transrepression provides a foundation for developmental research into GC-receptor ligands that cause predominantly transrepression but not transactivation. This research is based on the assumption that the anti-inflammatory properties of GCs are mostly due to repression of AP-1- and NF-κB-stimulated synthesis of inflammatory mediators, whereas most of their adverse effects are associated with transactivation of genes involved in metabolic processes. Investigators have therefore sought novel GCR ligands with high repression but low transactivation

activity. One such compound, A276575, exhibits a high affinity for the GCR and potently represses IL-1α-induced IL-6 production, similarly to dexamethasone. However, unlike dexamethasone, A276575 induces little aromatase activity. Other novel nonsteroidal GCR ligands are being developed which possess high repression activities against inflammatory mediator production, but have lower transactivation activities than traditional GCs. Substances that cause a receptor conformation preferring a GCR/protein interaction and not a GCR/DNA-binding-dependent mechanism are now being called 'dissociated glucocorticoids' or selective glucocorticoid receptor agonists (SEGRAs). At present it cannot be reliably predicted whether SEGRAs will prove clinically useful, as 'improved glucocorticoids'. However, these novel developments are very interesting: further *in vivo* investigations and preliminary clinical trials are needed to define the safety/efficacy profile of SEGRAs.

NITRO-STEROIDS

Recent experimental observations prompt assessment of the clinical impact of another new class of glucocorticoid drugs, nitro-steroids, on RA and inflammatory bowel disease. Nitro-steroids are able to release low levels of nitric oxide (NO) and are endowed with enhanced anti-inflammatory properties and fewer unwanted effects. The prototype of these new steroids, 21-NO-prednisolone (NCX-1015), is much more potent than prednisolone in models of acute and chronic inflammation, including collagen II-induced arthritis. In contrast, in an *in vitro* assay of bone resorption NCX-1015 did not activate primary osteoclast activity, whereas prednisolone did. This lack of effect of NCX-1015 was chiefly due to NO. It has been suggested that post-translational modification of GCR (tyrosine nitration) by NCX-1015 may explain its enhanced anti-inflammatory activity. Moreover, NCX-1015 potently stimulates IL-10 production, suggesting that nitro-steroids induce regulatory T cells that negatively modulate inflammation. However, more studies are needed to confirm that nitro-steroids will be effective as anti-inflammatory agents in clinical practice.

LONG-CIRCULATING LIPOSOMAL GLUCOCORTICOIDS

As previously discussed, the anti-inflammatory efficacy of GCs can be improved by the additional benefits of nongenomic actions at high GC concentrations. This has led to the successful use of long-circulating liposomal GCs. In rats with experimental autoimmune encephalitis, GC-containing liposomes accumulate at sites of inflammation, reaching ultra-high concentrations (> 10^{-5} mol/L for ≥18 hours). These liposomes may thus be therapeutically superior to conventional intravenous high-dose GC therapy, as evidenced by their successful use in rats with adjuvant-induced arthritis. A single injection of 10 mg/kg liposomal prednisolone phosphate resulted in complete remission of the inflammatory response for almost a week. In contrast, the same dose of unencapsulated prednisolone phosphate did not reduce inflammation, and only a slight effect was observed after repeated daily injections. One may conclude that preferential delivery of GC to the site of inflammation leads to very high GC concentrations at the inflamed joint, but lower plasma concentrations with perhaps a lower rate of side effects. These are very promising developments which exploit the broad spectrum of therapeutically relevant genomic and nongenomic GC actions preferentially at the site of inflammation.

In conclusion, recent research has greatly increased our knowledge of conventional GCs as the best anti-inflammatory agents currently available. In particular, new findings on the effects of occupation of cytosolic GCRs on intracellular signaling, transcription processes and gene expression, and on the existence of membrane-bound glucocorticoid receptors as well as the information on dose–effect relationships, have stimulated intensive research activity aimed at bringing this increased knowledge from scientific research into clinical practice as quickly as possible. The new GCR ligands and liposome encapsulation are very promising approaches that will hopefully soon be available in clinical practice to improve the risk–benefit ratio of GC therapy and the wellbeing of patients.

■ REFERENCES ■

1. Buttgereit F, Straub RH, Wehling M, Burmester GR. Glucocorticoids in the treatment of rheumatic diseases. An update on mechanisms of action. Arthritis Rheum 2004; 50: 3408–3417.

2. Schäcke H, Döcke WD, Asadullah K. Mechanisms involved in the side effects of glucocorticoids. Pharmacol Ther 2002; 96: 23–43.

3. Ramsey-Goldman R. Missed opportunities in physician management of glucocorticoid-induced osteoporosis? Arthritis Rheum 2002; 46: 3115–3120.

4. Walsh LJ, Wong CA, Pringle M, Tattersfield AE. Use of oral corticosteroids in the community and the prevention of secondary osteoporosis: a cross section study. Br Med J 1996; 313: 344–346.

5. Almawi WY. Molecular mechanisms of glucocorticoid effects. Mod Aspects Immunobiol 2001; 2: 78–82.

6. Adcock IM, Lane SJ. Mechanisms of steroid action and resistance in inflammation. Corticosteroid-insensitive asthma: molecular mechanisms. J Endocrinol 2003; 178: 347–355.

7. Pratt WB. The hsp90-based chaperone system: involvement in signal transduction from a variety of hormone and growth factor receptors. Proc Soc Exp Biol Med 1998; 217: 420–434.

8. Wikström AC. Mechanisms of steroid action and resistance in inflammation. Glucocorticoid action and novel mechanisms of steroid resistance: role of glucocorticoid receptor-interacting proteins for glucocorticoid responsiveness. J Endocrinol 2003; 178: 331–337.

9. Murphy PJ, Morishima Y, Chen H, et al. Visualization and mechanism of assembly of a glucocorticoid receptor-Hsp70 complex that is primed for subsequent Hsp90-dependent opening of the steroid binding cleft. J Biol Chem 2003; 278: 34764–34773.

10. Davies TH, Ning YM, Sánchez ER. A new first step in activation of steroid receptors. J Biol Chem 2002; 277: 4597–4600.

11. Chen R, Burke TF, Cumberland JE, et al. Glucocorticoids inhibit calcium- and calcineurin-dependent activation of the human IL-4 promoter. J Immunol 2000; 164: 825–832.

12. De Bosscher K, Vanden Berghe W, Vermeulen L, et al. Glucocorticoids repress NF-κB-driven genes by disturbing the interaction of p65 with the basal transcription machinery, irrespective of coactivator levels in the cell. Proc Natl Acad Sci USA 2000; 97: 3919–3924.

13. Heck S, Bender K, Kullmann M, et al. I kappaB alpha-independent downregulation of NF-kappaB activity by glucocorticoid receptor. EMBO J 1997; 16: 4698–4707.

14. Mori A, Kaminuma O, Suko M, et al. Two distinct pathways of interleukin-5 synthesis in allergen-specific human T-cell clones are suppressed by glucocorticoids. Blood 1997; 89: 2891–2900.

15. Vacca A, Felli MP, Farina AR, et al. Glucocorticoid receptor-mediated suppression of the interleukin 2 gene expression through impairment of the cooperativity between nuclear factor of activated T cells and AP-1 enhancer elements. J Exp Med 1992; 175: 637–646.

16. Yudt MR, Jewell CM, Bienstock RJ, Cidlowski JA. Molecular origins for the dominant negative function of human glucocorticoid receptor beta. Mol Cell Biol 2003; 23: 4319–4330.

17. Sanden S, Tripmacher R, Weltrich R, et al. Glucocorticoid dose dependent downregulation of glucocorticoid receptors in patients with rheumatic diseases. J Rheumatol 2000; 27: 1265–1270.

18. Buttgereit F, Scheffold A. Rapid glucocorticoid effects on immune cells. Steroids 2002; 67: 529–534.

19. Croxtall JD, Choudhury Q, Flower RJ. Glucocorticoids act within minutes to inhibit recruitment of signaling factors to activated EGF receptors through a receptor-dependent, transcription-independent mechanism. Br J Pharmacol 2000; 130: 289–298.

20. Falkenstein E, Norman AW, Wehling M. Mannheim classification of nongenomically initiated (rapid) steroid actions(s). J Clin Endocrinol Metab 2000; 85: 2072–2075.

21. Hafezi-Moghadam A, Simoncini T, Yang E, et al. Acute cardiovascular protective effects of corticosteroids are mediated by nontranscriptional activation of endothelial nitric oxide synthase. Nature Med 2002; 8: 473–479.

22. Buttgereit F, da Silva JA, Boers M, et al. Standardised nomenclature for glucocorticoid dosages and glucocorticoid treatment regimens: current questions and tentative answers in rheumatology. Ann Rheum Dis 2002; 61: 718–722.

23. Badsha H, Edwards CJ. Intravenous pulses of methylprednisolone for systemic lupus erythematosus. Semin Arthritis Rheum 2003; 32: 370–377.

24. Vasoo S, Thumboo J, Fong KY. Refractory immune thrombocytopenia in systemic lupus erythematosus: response to mycophenolate mofetil. Lupus 2003; 12: 630–632.

25. Bartholome B, Spies CM, Gaber T, et al. Membrane glucocorticoid receptors (mGCR) are expressed in normal peripheral blood mononuclear cells and upregulated following in vitro stimulation and in patients with rheumatoid arthritis. FASEB J 2004; 18: 70–80.

26. Buttgereit F, Saag K, Cutolo M, et al. The molecular basis for the effectiveness, toxicity, and resistance to glucocorticoids: focus on the treatment of rheumatoid arthritis. Scand J Rheumatol 2005; 34, 14–21.

27. da Silva JAP, Jacobs JWG, Kirwan JR, et al. Long-term glucocorticoid therapy in rheumatoid arthritis: An evidence-based review of potential adverse effects. Ann Rheum Dis 2006; 65: 285–293.

28. Shane E, Rivas M, McMahon JD, et al. Bone loss and turnover after cardiac transplantation. J Clin Endocrinol Metab 1997; 82: 1497–1506.

29. Khanna D, Paulus HE. Corticosteroids. In: St Clair EW, Pisetsky DS, Haynes BF, eds. Rheumatoid arthritis. Baltimore: Lippincott Williams and Wilkins, 2004; 283–302.

30. Gaffney K, Ledingham J, Perry JD. Intra-articular triamcinolone hexacetonide in knee osteoarthritis: factors influencing the clinical response. Ann Rheum Dis 1995; 54: 379–381.

31. Bijlsma JW, Saag KG, Buttgereit F, da Silva JA. Developments in glucocorticoid therapy. Rheum Dis Clin North Am 2005; 31: 1–17.

32. O'Brien C, Jia D, Plotkin L, et al. Glucocorticoids act directly on osteoblasts and osteocytes to induce their apoptosis and reduce bone formation and strength. Endocrinology 2004; 145: 1835–1841.

33. Seibel MJ. Markers of bone turnover in transplantation osteopathy. Clin Lab 1996; 42: 927–937.

34. Yale SH, Limper AH. *Pneumocystis carinii* pneumonia in patients without acquired immunodeficiency syndrome: associated illnesses and prior corticosteroid therapy. Mayo Clin Proc 1996; 71: 5–13.

35. Saag KG, Koehnke R, et al. Low dose long-term corticosteroid therapy in rheumatoid arthritis: an analysis of serious adverse events. Am J Med 1994; 96: 115–123.

36. Song IH, Gold R, Straub RH, et al. New glucocorticoids on the horizon. J Rheumatol 2005; 32: 1199–1207.

Nonsteroidal anti-inflammatory drugs

Maryam Shahbaz-Samavi, Frank McKenna

88

The earliest evidence of the use of willow bark as a medicinal agent is documented in Chinese records from over 7000 years ago. Hippocrates (460–377 BC) described the use of powder made from the bark and leaves of the willow tree to help heal headaches, pains, and fevers. In 1826 Brugnatelli and Fontana obtained a highly impure form of bitter-tasting yellow crystals from willow bark, but working separately 2 years later, Johann Buchner, professor of pharmacy at the University of Munich, Germany, isolated a tiny amount of crystalline material and called it salicin. By 1829, Henri Leroux had improved the extraction procedure to obtain about 30 g from 1.5 kg of bark. In 1838 Raffaele Piria, working at the Sorbonne in Paris, split salicin into a sugar and salicylaldehyde and converted the latter, by hydrolysis and oxidation, to an acid of crystallized colorless needles, which he named salicylic acid. However, salicylic acid was poorly tolerated. In 1853 Charles Frederic Gerhardt created acetylsalicylic acid by buffering salicylic acid with sodium (sodium salicylate) and acetyl chloride, but it was not developed. The method was rediscovered and modified in 1897 by Felix Hoffmann and his colleagues, working for Bayer. Hoffmann's father had arthritis and was intolerant of salicylates but found acetylsalicylic acid to be more effective and well tolerated. Bayer decided to market the compound which they named aspirin from the 'a' in acetyl chloride, the 'spir' in *Spiraea ulmaria* (the plant from which they derived the salicylic acid), and 'in' was a familiar ending for medicines. Aspirin was patented on March 6th, 1889 and in 1915 became the first mass-produced tablet in medicine. Over the last century there have been over 20 other similar anti-inflammatory analgesics developed and licenced, the class being named nonsteroidal anti-inflammatory drugs (NSAIDs).

■ BIOCHEMISTRY AND PHARMACOLOGY ■

All NSAIDs are completely absorbed, have negligible first-pass hepatic metabolism, are tightly bound to albumin, and have small volumes of distribution. Half-lives of the NSAIDs vary from about 2 hours to more than 24 hours, although the duration of biological effect may be significantly longer than the plasma half-life. Patients with hypoalbuminemia may have a higher free serum concentration of the drug. There is a clear individual variation in response to NSAIDs and their toxic effects. These differences have been ascribed to differences in absorption, distribution, and metabolism. In addition, numerous mechanisms of action have been ascribed to the NSAIDs.

Vane established in the 1970s that a major effect of NSAIDs is to inhibit cyclooxygenase (COX or prostaglandin synthase: PGHS), thereby impairing the ultimate transformation of the unsaturated fatty acid arachidonic acid, derived from cellular phospholipids, to prostaglandins, prostacyclin, and thromboxanes (Fig. 88.1).[1] The extent of enzyme inhibition varies among the different NSAIDs, although there are no studies relating the degree of COX inhibition with anti-inflammatory efficacy in individual patients. Two related isoforms of the COX enzyme were discovered in the 1980s: COX-1 (PGHS-1) and COX-2 (PGHS-2).[2] The most important differences between the two isoforms are the regulation and expression of the enzymes in different tissues.

COX-1 is variably expressed in most tissues. It has been described as a 'housekeeping' enzyme, regulating normal cellular processes such as gastric cytoprotection, vascular homeostasis, platelet aggregation, and renal function; its production is stimulated by hormones or growth factors.

COX-2 is constitutively expressed in the brain, kidney, bone, and probably in the female reproductive system, but it is not expressed in normal gastrointestinal mucosa. It is also expressed at other sites during inflammation or in mitotic tissue, and experimentally in response to mitogenic stimuli. Both COX isoforms are regulated by physiological stimuli. In the human kidney COX-2 mRNA is found in normal kidney and increased in certain pathological conditions, including diabetic nephropathy, hypertension, and heart failure.[3] COX-2 is also expressed in malignant cells and a number of studies have found a beneficial therapeutic effect from COX-2 inhibition, most notably in reducing malignant change in adenomatous colonic polyps. There are important differences in the regulation and expression of these enzymes in various tissues. One distinguishing characteristic of COX-2 is that its expression is inhibited by glucocorticoids, which may contribute to the anti-inflammatory effects of glucocorticoids.

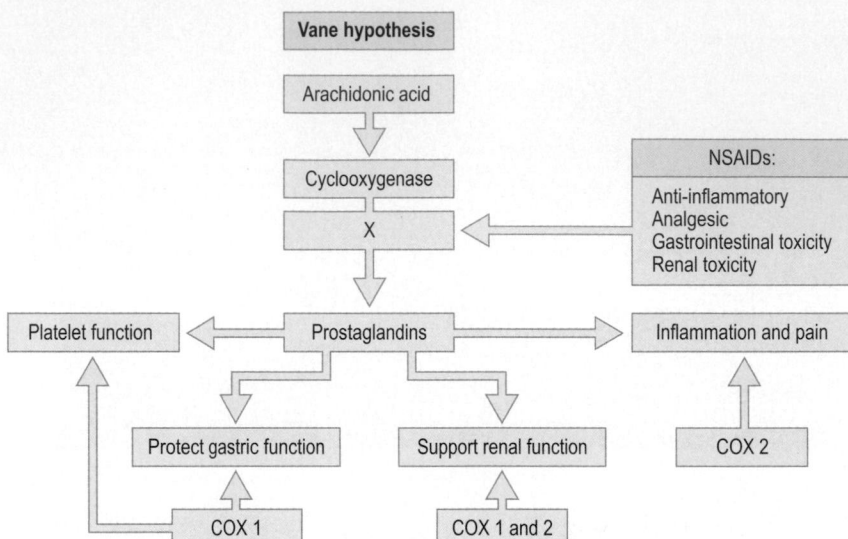

Fig. 88.1 The Vane hypothesis of the mode of action of nonsteroidal anti-inflammatory drugs (NSAIDs). COX, cyclooxygenase.

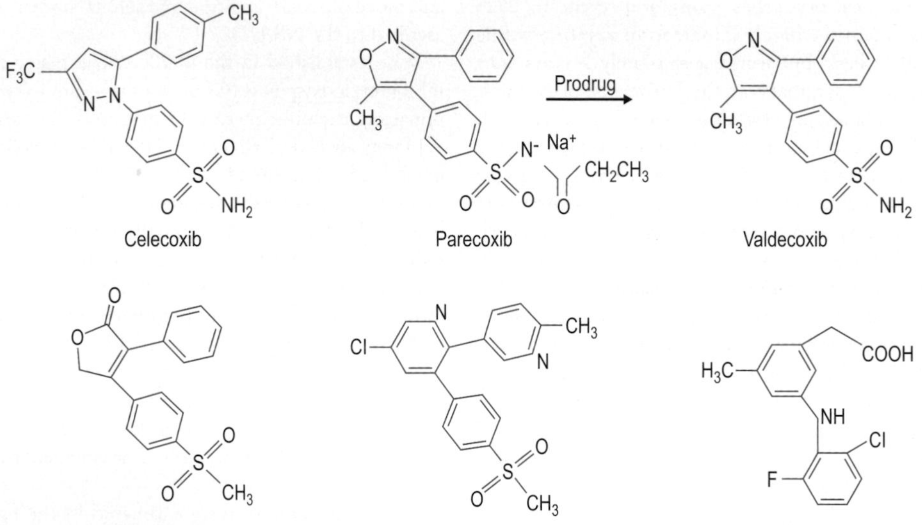

Fig. 88.2 The chemical structure of licenced cyclooxygenase-2 (COX-2) inhibitors.

It is unclear whether there are other biologically active COX enzymes. COX-3 has been described[4, 5]; this is a splice variant derived from the COX-1 gene with an additional peptide sequence derived from intron I. COX-3 appears to be expressed at a high level in the central nervous system, with transcripts for this splice variant accounting for 5% of COX mRNA, although at present it is uncertain whether this enzyme is expressed in humans.

Differences in the extent to which a particular NSAID inhibits an isoform of COX can affect both its activity and toxicity. Most traditional NSAIDs are nonselective inhibitors of both COX-1 and COX-2. Because the toxicity of NSAIDs on the gastrointestinal tract is largely related to the inhibition of COX-1, highly selective COX-2 inhibitors have been developed that do not inhibit COX-1 at therapeutic doses (Fig. 88.2). Celecoxib (Celebrex) and rofecoxib (Vioxx) were initially approved for use in rheumatoid arthritis, osteoarthritis, and acute pain. Etoricoxib (Arcoxia), valdecoxib (Bextra), and lumiracoxib (Prexige) have subsequently been licenced. Rofecoxib was withdrawn worldwide by the manufacturer due to an increased risk of adverse cardiovascular events. Valdecoxib was also withdrawn from the US and European Union markets in April 2005 because of a small but increased risk of Stevens–Johnson syndrome,

KEY CONCEPTS

Two distinct cyclooxygenase (COX) enzymes exist:

>> COX-1 is constitutively expressed in most tissues, and is involved in homeostasis and 'housekeeping' functions

>> COX-2 is constitutively expressed in brain, bone, and kidney, but not in normal gastrointestinal tract. It is induced by cytokines, endotoxin, tumor promoters, growth factors, and gonadotropins

KEY CONCEPTS

The efficacy of both nonsteroidal anti-inflammatory drugs (NSAIDs) and cyclooxygenase-2 (COX-2) inhibitors is mediated by the reduction of inflammatory prostaglandins produced following the action of COX-2 on arachidonic acid

Nonselective NSAIDs inhibit both COX-1 and COX-2, but at therapeutic concentration COX-2 inhibitors do not inhibit COX-1

NSAIDs and COX-2 inhibitors are analgesics with anti-pyretic and weak anti-inflammatory effects

Gastrointestinal toxicity is predominantly a consequence of the inhibition of COX-1, whereas renal toxicity results from inhibition of both COX-1 and COX-2

although parecoxib, a prodrug of valdecoxib, remains available for clinical use. These compounds have been shown to provide comparable analgesia to the nonselective NSAIDs in patients with pain and arthritis, with a reduced risk of gastroduodenal toxicity. Although some older NSAIDs are also relatively selective for COX-2 at low doses (e.g., etodolac inhibits the COX-2 isoform 10 times more than COX-1), it is unclear whether this avoids inhibition of COX-1 at therapeutic doses. Endoscopic studies with COX-2 inhibitors have found an incidence of ulceration comparable to placebo. However, although selective COX-2 inhibition may produce less gastric toxicity, there has been concern that COX-2 inhibition may enhance injury in inflamed tissue and delay healing of gastric erosions or ulcers,[6] an observation that may explain why COX-2 inhibitors have been associated with peptic ulceration.

NONPROSTAGLANDIN-MEDIATED EFFECTS

Although aspirin (the only acetylated NSAID) is not thought to have effects other than those related to inhibition of prostaglandin synthesis, several nonprostaglandin-mediated mechanisms of action have been postulated to explain the actions of the nonacetylated salicylates; these mechanisms may also apply, to a varying degree, to the nonsalicylate NSAIDs. Some of these effects appear to be related to the physicochemical property of NSAIDs that enables them to insert into biological membranes and disrupt important interactions necessary for cell function (e.g., transmembrane anion transport, oxidative phosphorylation, and uptake of arachidonate). Neutrophil function is inhibited by nonacetylated salicylates and other nonsalicylate NSAIDs *in vitro*. As an example, NSAIDs interfere with the neutrophil–endothelial cell adherence that is critical for the ability to respond to inflammation. NSAIDs decrease the expression of L-selectin, which removes a crucial step in the migration of granulocytes to sites of inflammation. The role of these nonprostaglandin-mediated processes in clinical inflammation remains unclear.

NSAIDs have also been shown to inhibit NF-κB-dependent transcription *in vitro*, leading to inhibition of inducible nitric oxide synthetase (iNOS). Nitric oxide synthetase, once induced by cytokines and other proinflammatory mediators, produces nitric oxide in large amounts, thereby leading to increased inflammation (including vasocongestion, cytotoxicity, and vascular permeability). Therapeutic levels of aspirin inhibit expression of iNOS and the subsequent production of nitrite *in vitro*, whereas sodium salicylate, indomethacin, and acetaminophen (paracetamol) have no such effects at pharmacological concentrations.

EFFICACY

ANTI-PYRETIC EFFECT

The synthesis of prostaglandin E_2 (PGE_2) depends on the constitutively expressed COX enzyme, and inhibitors of either COX-1 or COX-2 are potent anti-pyretics. There is a direct correlation of the anti-pyretic potency of various drugs with the inhibition of brain COX. Acetaminophen is a poor inhibitor of COX in peripheral tissue and has no significant anti-inflammatory activity; however, acetaminophen is oxidized in the brain by the cytochrome p450 system, and the oxidized form inhibits COX, which may explain why there is no difference between oral aspirin and acetaminophen in reducing fever in humans. NSAIDs such as naproxen or ibuprofen are also excellent anti-pyretics. However, there appears to be no role for PGE_2 in normal thermoregulation, as chronic use of aspirin or NSAIDs in arthritis does not reduce normal core body temperature.

OSTEOARTHRITIS

NSAIDs are effective in the symptomatic relief of osteoarthritis but there is considerable individual variation in response, with some patients experiencing little or no response to treatment. A meta-analysis of 10 randomized control trials demonstrated that acetaminophen was an effective treatment for osteoarthritis but was inferior to NSAIDs.[7] In cross-over studies between acetaminophen and NSAIDs (Fig. 88.3) or coxibs, the majority of patients with osteoarthritis preferred the anti-inflammatory drugs.[8–10] A minority of patients prefer acetaminophen but unfortunately there are no clinical features that predict which treatment is likely to be most effective. Studies with COX-2 inhibitors have found similar efficacy to nonselective NSAIDs but with better tolerability.[11,12] The American College of Rheumatology treatment guidelines for osteoarthritis support the use of NSAIDs in conjunction with nonpharmacological measures for some acetaminophen-naïve patients, particularly those with more severe pain.[13] EULAR (European League against Rheumatism) guidelines recommend NSAIDs for patients with osteoarthritis of the knee whose pain is inadequately relieved with acetaminophen.[14]

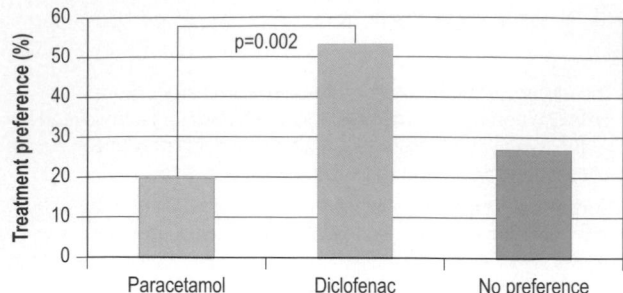

Fig. 88.3 Preference of diclofenac versus acetaminophen (paracetamol) in a cross-over study in patients with osteoarthritis (OA). (Data from Pickavance L, Griffiths G, McKenna F. Br J Rheumatol 1995; 34: (suppl 1): 137.

RHEUMATOID ARTHRITIS

NSAIDs are effective symptomatic therapy for rheumatoid arthritis. However, although they have both analgesic and anti-inflammatory properties, they do not affect objective measures of the inflammatory response and do not alter disease outcomes. Appropriate initial therapy of patients with mild disease consists of an NSAID at full therapeutic dose. Most physicians and patients prefer initiating therapy with an NSAID or COX-2 inhibitor rather than a salicylate, as they are usually better tolerated and have a longer duration of action.

The dose of NSAIDs is titrated to the optimum tolerated level and continued for at least 2 weeks. Therapeutic trials of individual NSAIDs continue until the patient appears to have achieved adequate control of symptoms with minimal side effects. If NSAIDs are combined, there is an increased risk of gastrointestinal toxicity, without any additional therapeutic benefit. NSAIDs will only partially improve symptoms in those with active disease and do not prevent the development of erosive disease. Thus, when there are signs of persistent synovitis (e.g., swollen joints, tender joints, or elevated acute-phase response (erythrocyte sedimentation rate or C-reactive protein)), it is recommended that disease be controlled with intra-articular or intramuscular corticosteroids and one or more disease-modifying anti-rheumatoid drugs (DMARDs) be added.

SYSTEMIC LUPUS ERYTHEMATOSUS

NSAIDs are generally effective for musculoskeletal complaints and mild serositis. COX-2-selective inhibitors may also be effective in such patients. Although celecoxib contains a benzenesulfonamide moiety and should be used with caution in those with a known sulfonamide allergy, celecoxib has been used in systemic lupus erythematosus patients, even those with "sulfa" allergy, without precipitating any allergic response. The potential for allergic responses to NSAIDs is discussed below.

SPONDYLOARTHRITIS

Symptoms of acute arthritis or enthesopathy from reactive arthritis, including Reiter's disease, usually respond to NSAIDs but high doses may be needed. NSAIDs are often very effective in relieving the pain and stiffness from ankylosing spondylitis. Although

indometacin was thought to be the most effective NSAID for ankylosing spondylitis, there is little evidence that any single compound is superior in efficacy. The selection of a particular NSAID to treat ankylosing spondylitis should therefore reflect the presence or absence of risk factors for adverse effects with specific NSAIDs.

CARDIOVASCULAR PROPHYLAXIS

Aspirin has proven efficacy for secondary prevention of cardiovascular disease, and, in selected patients, for primary prevention. With respect to primary prevention, it has been suggested that low-dose aspirin prophylaxis is warranted in patients with an estimated 10-year risk of cardiovascular disease of 6–10%. Aspirin differs from other NSAIDs in binding permanently in circulating platelets. Since other NSAIDs only inhibit platelet function temporarily and they compete with aspirin for the binding site, they should not be ingested with aspirin.[15] This is not a concern with COX-2 inhibitors as they do not bind to platelets. However, following the withdrawal of rofecoxib because of potential cardiac toxicity, there has been concern that other NSAIDs and COX-2 inhibitors may actually increase the risk of cardiac disease (see below).

CEREBROVASCULAR ACCIDENT

The effectiveness of aspirin for preventing ischemic stroke and cardiovascular events is supported by a meta-analysis of 195 randomized clinical trials comparing anti-platelet therapy, primarily aspirin, with placebo in the prevention of stroke, myocardial infarction (MI), and vascular death among high-risk patients with some vascular disease or other condition, implying an increased risk of occlusive vascular disease.[16] Patients treated with anti-platelet therapy (primarily aspirin) had a 25% relative risk reduction in nonfatal stroke compared with placebo. Among the subset of patients with prior cerebrovascular disease (transient ischemic attack or stroke), anti-platelet therapy reduced the risk of secondary stroke, MI, or vascular death by 22%; the absolute benefit was 36 events prevented per 1000 patients treated for 29 months. The benefit of anti-platelet therapy was independent of sex, age, diabetes, or hypertension.

Stopping anti-platelet therapy in high-risk patients may itself increase the risk of stroke. Given the apparent equivalent benefit of different doses of aspirin for ischemic stroke prevention, and the increased risk of bleeding complications with higher-dose aspirin, a dose of 50–81 mg/day when using aspirin for the secondary prevention of ischemic stroke seems reasonable.

NSAIDs AND CANCER

Most epidemiological studies suggest that aspirin use reduces the risk of colorectal cancer by approximately 40–50%.[17] A similar reduction in colorectal adenoma risk is also observed, suggesting that the benefit may occur at early stages of carcinogenesis. Consistent with this pattern, some, but not all, data indicate that up to 10 years of use may be required for a significant effect on colorectal cancer incidence. Nonaspirin NSAIDs, including COX-2-selective inhibitors, appear to have a similar anti-cancer benefit. Nonetheless, the clinical implications of these findings remain unclear because of increased toxicity related to chronic aspirin and NSAID use and the proven efficacy of alternative prevention strategies, particularly colonoscopic screening.[18] The overall risks and benefits of prolonged NSAID use, as well as the risk profile of the individual patient, should be considered before making individual recommendations.

NSAIDs IN ALZHEIMER'S DISEASE

Some epidemiological studies have suggested that NSAIDs protect against the development of Alzheimer's disease.[19] However the results have been conflicting and may be due in part to the timing and duration of NSAID use, and to differences in tracking NSAID use. In addition, all of the studies of this issue are observational studies, which are subject to various forms of bias. Apart from an effect on risk of Alzheimer's disease, long-term use of NSAIDs has also been associated with preservation of cognitive function and prevention of early cognitive decline, although this effect has not been uniform. Use of NSAIDs has also been associated with a decreased incidence of Parkinson's disease, another important cause of dementia. However, at present there are insufficient data to recommend this treatment for prevention of dementia.

◼ TOXICITY ◼

INTOXICATION

NSAIDs are among the most common classes of medications prescribed in the USA. Despite the high rates of acute ingestion, few patients experience poor outcomes, and most require no medical intervention or supportive care alone. Symptoms and signs in NSAID intoxication are generally nonspecific. The most common symptoms are nausea, vomiting, drowsiness, blurred vision, and dizziness. NSAID ingestion of less than 100 mg/kg is unlikely to cause significant symptoms; ingestions greater than 400 mg/kg can cause severe symptoms. Renal failure and renal papillary necrosis are rare but do occur, most commonly in patients with decreased effective arterial volume, age-related underlying renal dysfunction, or massive overdose. Acute central nervous system toxicity related to NSAID use shows a variety of clinical manifestations, ranging from mild drowsiness to seizure or coma.

GASTROINTESTINAL TRACT (FIG. 88.4)

The pathogenesis of symptomatic peptic ulcer disease caused by exposure to NSAIDs is mainly a consequence of systemic inhibition of gastrointestinal mucosal COX activity. Even intravenous or intramuscular administration of aspirin or NSAIDs can cause gastric or duodenal ulcers in animals and humans. Many mucosal functions are altered by endogenous or exogenously administered PGs: this may explain the mucosal protective effects of PGs. Combined mucus and bicarbonate secretion forms an alkaline layer on the surface of the gastric mucosa, which retards diffusion of acid pepsin from the lumen into the mucus. Gastric and duodenal injury by acid and pepsin occurs when these protective functions are compromised and may lead to gastric and/or duodenal ulcer formation with associated risks of bleeding, perforation, or obstruction. Some of the cytoprotective mechanisms of PGs include stimulation of glycoprotein (mucin) secretion, stimulation of bicarbonate secretion, stimulation of phospholipid secretion, increased epithelial cell migration towards the luminal surface (restitution), enhanced epithelial cell proliferation, and enhancement of mucosal blood flow. This last effect may control a number of the other mechanisms.

Generation of nitric oxide may be a key intermediate in cytoprotection.[20] Similar to the role of COX-1, constitutive nitric oxide synthase (NOS) is important in the maintenance of an intact mucosal lining. Two enzymes contribute to the basal, constitutive NOS activity: neuronal NOS (nNOS, type I) and endothelial NOS (eNOS, type III). The cytoprotective mechanisms of nitric oxide parallel PG effects and include mediation of the release of gastric mucus, stimulation of fluid secretion, maintenance of epithelial barrier function, and enhancement of mucosal blood flow.

While inhibition of COX-1 is the major mechanism by which NSAIDs produce gastric injury, mediators besides PGs (and nitric oxide) may also be involved. For example, interference with factors that mediate restitution or adaptive protection may contribute to mucosal injury. Adaptive protection refers to the observation that mild gastric irritants induce enhanced cytoprotection. COX-1, COX-2, and nitric oxide as well as various growth factors, including epidermal growth factor and transforming growth factor (TGF)-β and TGF-α, appear to participate in these adaptive processes.[21] NSAIDs probably interfere with growth factors and other mediators responsible for restitution and adaptive protection, further contributing to their toxicity.

The role of *Helicobacter pylori* (HP) infection in NSAID-induced gastritis or ulcer formation is complex.[22] Although the incidence of ulceration in some studies appears to be similar in HP-positive and -negative patients, other studies have found a reduction in NSAID ulceration after HP eradication. There are also some data indicating that the risk of ulcer hemorrhage may be increased in HP-positive patients.

The risk of developing significant NSAID-induced gastrointestinal bleeding or perforation due to a peptic ulcer has been evaluated in multiple studies.[23] The duration of therapy is important. Administration of NSAIDs for short periods (less than 1 week) in healthy people is unlikely to result in any significant gastroduodenal toxicity. In contrast, longer duration of therapy is associated with an increased risk of complications. Gastroduodenal toxicity may develop even in patients taking low doses of NSAIDs (such as for cardiovascular prophylaxis), which, despite the low dose, can be associated with a significant decrease in gastric mucosal prostaglandin concentrations. Gastric ulceration from NSAIDs is often silent (Fig. 88.5). Several other factors are associated with increased risk of gastroduodenal toxicity and complications such as bleeding from NSAIDs. The most important risk factor is age (Fig. 88.6). The risk increases above the age of 60 with an approximately 10-fold risk in those aged over 75 years.[24] A past history of peptic ulceration or NSAID toxicity, the presence of comorbid diseases, a higher dose of NSAID, or concurrent use of glucocorticoids or anticoagulants all increase the risk of ulceration. Overall the annual risk of admission from regular NSAID therapy is approximately 1% per annum. Among those admitted, mortality is approximately

NSAID GI toxicity
GI ulceration
Oesophageal Gastric Duodenal Small bowel Colon
Small bowel diaphragm formation
Colitis

Fig. 88.4 The spectrum of nonsteroidal anti-inflammatory drug (NSAID)-induced gastrointestinal (GI) damage.

10%, largely in the elderly and frail. The risk is reduced but not eliminated by prescribing COX-2 inhibitors.

The CLASS (celecoxib), VIGOR (rofecoxib) and TARGET (lumiracoxib) studies demonstrated an approximate threefold reduction in the incidence of gastrointestinal complications compared with nonselective NSAIDs, although in both the CLASS and TARGET studies this difference was largely eliminated with co-prescription of low-dose aspirin. (Patients taking low-dose aspirin were excluded from the VIGOR study.) However, none of these studies included a placebo comparator. A retrospective observational study in elderly patients in Ontario[25] found the incidence of gastrointestinal complications related to celecoxib was similar to an age- and gender-matched control group; there was a small but significantly increased incidence from rofecoxib but this was less than the rate seen with either diclofenac/misoprostol combination (Arthrotec) or other nonselective NSAIDs (Fig. 88.7).

The distal small bowel and colon are also susceptible to the deleterious effects of NSAIDs.[26, 27] The ileocecal region is a potential site for a variety of NSAID-induced injuries, including erosions, ulcers, strictures, perforation, and the formation of diaphragms, which can lead to bowel obstruction. NSAIDs can also lead to colitis resembling inflammatory bowel disease, exacerbate pre-existing inflammatory bowel disease, or complicate diverticular disease (i.e., perforation or bleeding). Elderly people and those on long-term NSAID therapy appeared to be at highest risk. Emerging data from video endoscopic studies indicate that there is a significantly greater risk of small-bowel lesions from NSAIDs than COX-2 inhibitors[28] and the risk is not reduced by co-prescription of proton pump inhibitors.

The potential gastroduodenal sparing effect of selective COX-2 inhibitors may be reduced or eliminated by concurrent low-dose aspirin therapy for primary or secondary prevention of cardiovascular or cerebrovascular disease. This may be directly related to the effect of aspirin, which blocks COX-1 in the gastrointestinal tract. In the CLASS and TARGET studies similar rates of ulcers and ulcer complications were noted among those receiving the COX-2 inhibitors plus low-dose aspirin as among patients receiving a nonselective NSAID plus aspirin. Thus, patients receiving both aspirin and a selective COX-2 inhibitor may also require prophylactic anti-ulcer therapy if they are at risk for gastroduodenal toxicity.

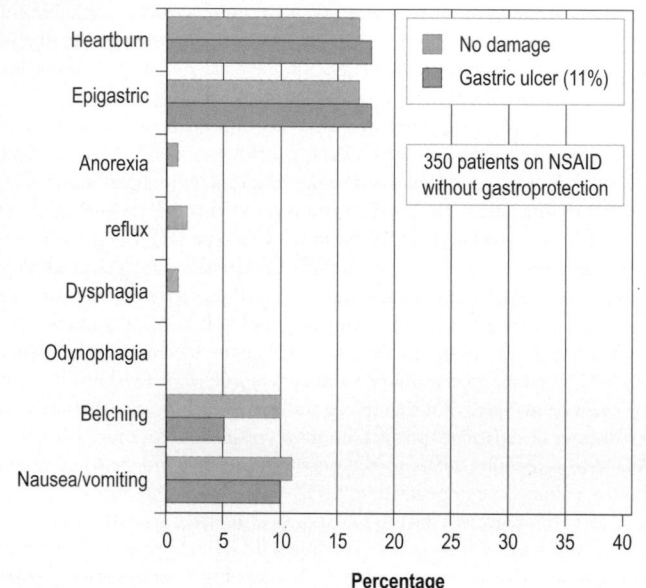

Fig. 88.5 Incidence of dyspeptic symptoms in patients with either a normal upper gastrointestinal endoscopy or a gastric ulcer whilst taking regular nonsteroidal anti-inflammatory drugs (NSAIDs). (Data from Mason J, McKenna F. Ann Rheum Dis 2002; Suppl. 2: 257.)

RENAL

NSAIDs can induce two different forms of acute renal failure: hemodynamically mediated and acute interstitial nephritis (which is often accompanied by the nephrotic syndrome). The former and perhaps the

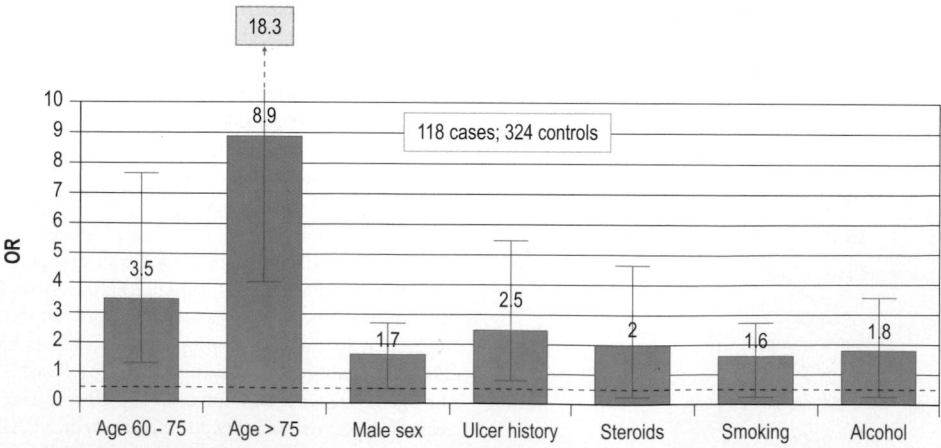

Fig. 88.6 Risk factors for nonsteroidal anti-inflammatory drug (NSAID) ulcer complications. OR, odds ratio. (Data from Hansen JM, Hallas J, Lauritsen JM, et al. Non-steroidal anti-inflammatory drugs and ulcer complications: a risk factor analysis for clinical decision-making. Scand J Gastroenterol 1996; 31: 126–130.)

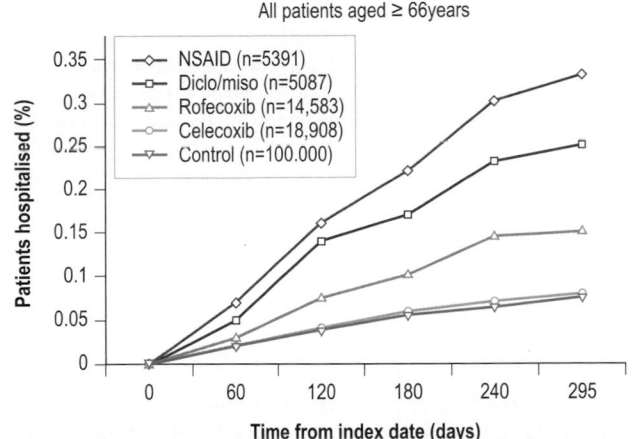

All patients aged ≥ 66years

Fig. 88.7 The rate of upper gastrointestinal (GI) complications in Ontario in elderly patients prescribed nonsteroidal anti-inflammatory drugs (NSAIDs) or cyclooxygenase-2 (COX-2) inhibitors. (Data from Mamdani et al. Br Med J 2002; 325: 624–629.[25])

CLINICAL PEARLS

Gastric ulceration from nonsteroidal anti-inflammatory drugs (NSAIDS) is common and often silent

Complications from NSAID ulceration are more common in the elderly and frail

Cyclooxygenase-2 inhibitors are associated with a significant reduction in gastrointestinal complications

A life-threatening gastrointestinal complication from NSAIDs may occur after as little as 7 days' treatment

---

latter are directly related to the reduction in prostaglandin synthesis induced by NSAIDs.[29]

Although renal prostaglandins are primarily vasodilators, they do not play a major role in the regulation of renal hemodynamics in normal subjects, since the basal rate of prostaglandin synthesis is relatively low. In contrast, the release of these hormones (particularly prostacyclin and PGE_2) is increased by underlying glomerular disease, renal insufficiency, hypercalcemia, and the vasoconstrictors angiotensin II and norepinephrine. The secretion of these latter hormones is increased in states of effective volume depletion, such as heart failure or cirrhosis, and in true volume depletion due to gastrointestinal or renal salt and water losses. Vasodilator prostaglandins act to preserve renal blood flow and glomerular filtration rate by relaxing preglomerular resistance. This is particularly important with effective volume depletion, in which the prostaglandins antagonize the vasoconstrictor effects of angiotensin II and norepinephrine. In glomerular disease, however, the increase in prostaglandin production seems to maintain the glomerular filtration rate even in the presence of a reduction in glomerular capillary permeability.

In some patients inhibition of prostaglandin synthesis with an NSAID may therefore lead to reversible renal ischemia, a decline in glomerular hydraulic pressure, and acute renal failure. The rise in the plasma creatinine

concentration is often seen within the first 3–7 days of therapy, the time required to achieve steady-state drug levels and maximum inhibition of prostaglandin synthesis. The selective COX-2 inhibitors may also precipitate acute renal failure in some patients.[30] How frequently this occurs compared to the nonselective NSAIDs is unclear but it is advisable to consider COX-2 inhibitors to have a similar risk of nephrotoxicity to nonselective NSAIDs.

Acute interstitial nephritis may occur with any nonselective NSAID. There have also been case reports of selective COX-2 inhibitors being associated with this pattern of injury. The mechanism is uncertain but it is possible that COX inhibition results in the preferential conversion of arachidonic acid to leukotrienes, which can then activate helper T cells. Patients usually present with hematuria, pyuria, white cell casts, proteinuria, and an acute rise in plasma creatinine concentration. Fever, rash, and eosinophilia are uncommon. Spontaneous recovery generally occurs within weeks to a few months after therapy is discontinued. Corticosteroids are sometimes used empirically if the renal failure persists for 1–2 weeks after NSAID withdrawal, although the benefit of such treatment is not established. After recovery patients should avoid subsequent administration of NSAIDs as relapse may occur with rechallenge.

CARDIAC FAILURE

NSAIDs may cause an exacerbation of heart failure. The probable cause is an increase in afterload resulting from reduction in vasodilatory prostaglandins such as prostacyclin, plus the renal effect of salt and water retention. In addition, NSAIDs may partially or totally reverse the beneficial effect of angiotensin-converting enzyme inhibition, reversing the improvements in cardiac output, and may also blunt the renal effects of diuretics, causing a further exacerbation of symptoms. There may be differences between drugs. The combined risk of death and recurrent congestive heart failure was higher in patients prescribed NSAIDs or rofecoxib than in those prescribed celecoxib in a population-based retrospective cohort study of 2256 patients aged 66 or more, who were prescribed celecoxib, rofecoxib, or an NSAID after an index admission for congestive heart failure.[31] However, the risks of death and recurrent congestive heart failure, combined and separate, were similar between patients prescribed NSAIDs and rofecoxib.

MYOCARDIAL INFARCTION

The benefit of platelet inhibition by aspirin for the secondary and, in selected patients, primary prevention of cardiovascular disease has been clearly demonstrated. However, concerns were raised that anti-inflammatory drugs may increase the risk of cardiac events following the results of the VIGOR trial, with the observation of a significant increase in cardiac events in those taking rofecoxib compared with naproxen. Although analysis of the CLASS and TARGET studies did not find any significant difference in cardiac events between either celecoxib or lumiracoxib and the comparator nonselective NSAIDs, the results of the VIGOR study raised the question whether selective COX-2 inhibition may increase the risk of MI or whether the anti-platelet effect of naproxen reduced the risk of cardiac events. However, most studies have not found a cardioprotective effect from naproxen.[32] In addition, in placebo-controlled studies evaluating the benefit of COX-2 inhibitors in patients with colonic polyps, there was an increased incidence of events with rofecoxib in standard-dose,[33] and also in one study with high-dose celecoxib.[34] These studies did

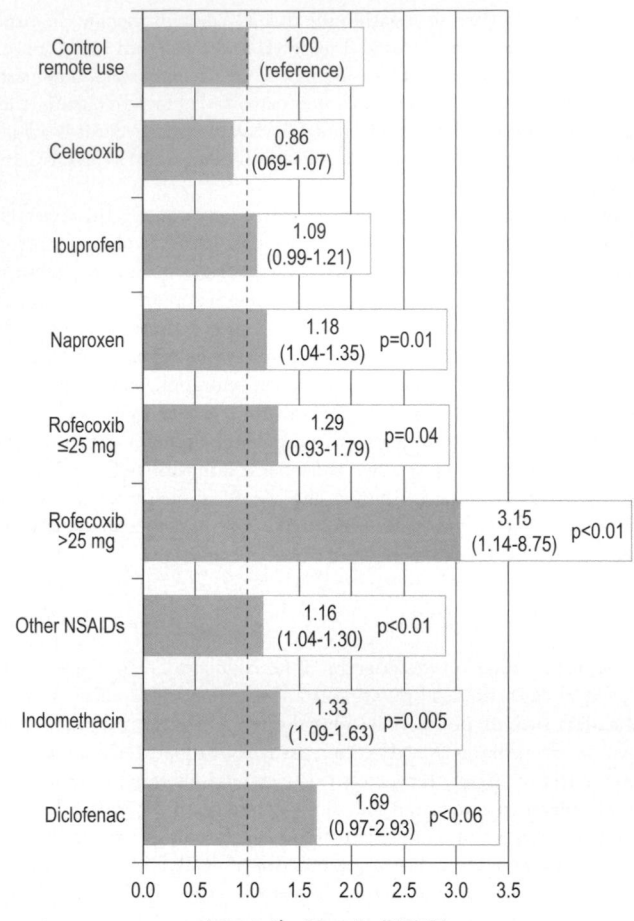

Fig. 88.8 The incidence of myocardial infarction in a prospective study in California in patients taking nonsteroidal anti-inflammatory drugs (NSAIDs) or cyclooxygenase-2 (COX-2) inhibitors. FDA, Food and Drug Administration. Data from Graham DJ et al, Lancet 2005;365:475-81.

not have an NSAID comparator and the number of events were small but indicated the need for further studies.

A number of observational studies have now been undertaken with similar findings. The results from a large prospective observational study conducted by the Food and Drug Administration (FDA) in California are typical (Fig. 88.8). They found a threefold risk of MI with high-dose rofecoxib, and a small but significant increased risk with a number of other NSAIDs but not from celecoxib.[35] Although the risk from celecoxib may have been underestimated, these data do not support the hypothesis that COX-2 inhibition increases the risk of MI any more than other NSAIDs. The risk from rofecoxib, particularly in high dose, appears to be specific to that compound. The mechanism may be related to a greater effect on salt and water retention and blood pressure, but there may be other mechanisms. As a result of these and other data, the FDA placed a black box warning on all NSAIDs and COX-2 inhibitors related to the small but significant risk of cardiac disease with these compounds.

HEMATOLOGICAL

The anti-platelet effects of NSAIDs are due to inhibition of COX-1 and decreased production of thromboxane A_2, which is released by platelets in response to a number of agonists, amplifying the platelet response and leading to aggregation. COX-2 is not expressed in platelets and COX-2 inhibitors do not have any effect on platelet function. NSAIDs should be avoided in patients with pre-existing platelet defects, in patients with thrombocytopenia, and perioperatively.

HEPATIC

Mild elevation of serum aminotransferases (transaminases) is commonly associated with NSAID use, particularly with diclofenac, but liver failure is quite rare. Diclofenac has been reported to cause clinical hepatitis with features including antinuclear antigen positivity and histologic evidence of chronic active hepatitis that can lead to misdiagnosis and inappropriate treatment. Introduction of another class of NSAID in many of these patients appeared to be safe. In a retrospective study of 625 000 patients who received more than 2 million prescriptions for NSAIDs and who were evaluated for newly diagnosed acute liver injury, there were 23 cases of acute liver injury over the 4-year study period.[36]

ALLERGIC AND CUTANEOUS REACTIONS

Various skin reactions may develop in association with the use of NSAIDs. Mostly these are morbilliform rashes and urticaria; severe, potentially life-threatening reactions such as toxic epidermal necrolysis and the Stevens–Johnson syndrome are uncommon.[37] These reactions are characterized by blistering skin lesions that may begin as erythematous macules and by target-like areas anywhere on the body. They may also lead to mucosal blistering or ulceration.

There has been concern that the sulfa-containing COX-2 inhibitors may cause hypersensitivity reactions in those with a known sulfa sensitivity.[38] Celecoxib and valdecoxib have a sulfonamide moiety whereas rofecoxib and etoricoxib have a methylsulfone side chain. Adverse reactions to sulfonamide antimicrobials include type I, or immunoglobulin E-mediated reactions, hypersensitivity syndrome reactions, and severe skin reactions, including toxic epidermal necrolysis and Stevens–Johnson syndrome. The aromatic amine portion of the sulfonamide antimicrobial is considered to be critical in the development of latter two reactions. In susceptible individuals, the hydroxylamine metabolite cannot be detoxified, leading to a cascade of cytotoxic and immunological events that eventually result in the adverse reaction. However, the major difference between sulfonamide antimicrobials and other sulfonamide-containing medications such as furosemide, thiazide diuretics, and celecoxib or valdecoxib, is that sulfonamide antimicrobials contain an aromatic amine group at the N4 position.

This allows for division of the sulfonamides into two groups: aromatic amines (i.e., sulfonamide antimicrobials) and nonaromatic amines. In addition, sulfonamide antimicrobials contain a substituted ring at the N1 position; this group is not found with nonaromatic amine-containing sulfonamides. Since celecoxib and valdecoxib do not contain the aromatic amine, adverse reactions such as hypersensitivity syndrome reactions and toxic epidermal necrolysis would not be expected to occur at the same frequency as they do with sulfonamide antimicrobials. Similarly, for IgE-mediated reactions, the N1 substituent and not the sulfonamide

THERAPEUTIC PRINCIPLES

There is no difference in efficacy between any nonsteroidal anti-inflammatory drug (NSAID) or cyclooxygenase-2 (COX-2) inhibitor when used in maximum doses

NSAIDs and COX-2 inhibitors should be prescribed as a therapeutic trial

They do not have disease-modifying effect and should only be continued if there is significant symptomatic benefit

The lowest effective dose should be used for the shortest time

NSAIDs should be avoided in the elderly and in those who are anti-coagulated, have significant concomitant disease, or with a history of previous gastrointestinal toxicity

Both NSAIDs and COX-2 inhibitors should be avoided in those with significant renal or cardiac disease and in very elderly and frail patients

moiety is important in determining specificity to antibodies. However, postmarketing surveillance studies found that reporting rates for Stevens–Johnson syndrome/toxic epidermal necrolysis with the sulfonamide coxibs were substantially higher than the background rate of 1.9 cases per million population per year, with the valdecoxib rate being 8–9 times that of celecoxib and approximately 25 times that of the background rate.

In the first 2 years of marketing, the reporting rate with valdecoxib was 49 cases per million person-years of use, 6 cases per million person-years for celecoxib and 3 cases per million person-years for rofecoxib.[39] On the basis of these data, the manufacturer withdrew valdecoxib from the market.

RESPIRATORY

The NSAIDs rarely induce pulmonary problems, although the actual incidence of adverse events is unknown. The principal pulmonary reactions that can occur include bronchospasm (which can be quite severe) and pulmonary infiltrates with eosinophilia. Precipitation or exacerbation of airway obstruction may occur in aspirin-sensitive individuals.[40] The syndrome of pulmonary infiltrates with eosinophilia can occur in patients receiving NSAIDs. It is not known whether this syndrome is associated with specific NSAIDs, or a general class effect. In one review, the typical presentation consisted of fever, cough, dyspnea, infiltrates on chest X-ray, and an absolute peripheral eosinophilia. Pathological examination revealed poorly defined granulomas with infiltrating eosinophils. Glucocorticoids were required, along with discontinuation of the drug, in order to reverse the process.

CENTRAL NERVOUS SYSTEM

The reported central nervous system side effects of NSAIDs include aseptic meningitis, psychosis, and cognitive dysfunction.[41] Psychosis and cognitive impairment are more prevalent in elderly patients, particularly those taking indometacin. Aseptic meningitis seems to be more prevalent in patients with systemic lupus erythematosus who are treated with NSAIDs of the phenylproprionic acid class, such as naproxen or ibuprofen, but the diagnosis should be considered in any patient with aseptic meningitis who has been using NSAIDs.

Tinnitus is a common problem, particularly in patients prescribed high doses of salicylates, although it can occur with all the NSAIDs. Tinnitus is typically reversible upon cessation of drug therapy, and should be regarded as a warning sign that patients are developing high blood levels of the drug. However, this may not be as evident in patients at the extremes of age.

PREGNANCY AND LACTATION

Aspirin has a role in prevention of pre-eclampsia and the treatment of the anti-phospholipid syndrome (Chapter 61), and it is not associated with an increased risk of miscarriage when used later in pregnancy. However, the inhibition of prostaglandin synthesis by NSAIDs, particularly by aspirin, can result in premature closure of the ductus arteriosus, and other effects have been suggested, including smaller babies and neonatal bruising. However, the safety of these drugs has not been fully evaluated in pregnant women. If possible, NSAIDs and aspirin should be avoided by women who are trying to conceive and in early pregnancy but may be used during pregnancy in women who have significant rheumatic symptoms unrelieved with other treatment. The drugs should be stopped in the last 2 months of pregnancy to avoid potential bleeding complications and premature closure of the ductus arteriosus.

■ REFERENCES ■

1. Vane JR. Inhibition of prostaglandin synthesis as a mechanism of action for the aspirin-like drugs. Nat New Biol 1971; 231: 232.

2. McKenna F. Cox-2: Separating myth from reality. Scand J Rheumatol 1999; 28(suppl 109): 19–29.

3. Khan KN, Stanfield KM, Harris RK, et al. Expression of cyclooxygenase-2 in the macula densa of human kidney in hypertension, congestive heart failure, and diabetic nephropathy. Ren Fail 2001; 23: 321.

4. Chandrasekharan NV, Dai H, Roos KL, et al. COX-3, a cyclooxygenase-1 variant inhibited by acetaminophen and other analgesic/anti-pyretic drugs: cloning, structure, and expression. Proc Natl Acad Sci USA 2002; 99: 13926.

5. Schwab JM, Schluesener HJ, Laufer S. COX-3: just another COX or the solitary elusive target of paracetamol? Lancet 2003; 361: 981.

6. Perini RF, Ma L, Wallace JL Mucosal repair and COX-2 inhibition. Curr Pharm Des 2003; 9: 2207–2211.

7. Zhang W, Jones A, Doherty M. Does paracetamol (acetaminophen) reduce the pain of osteoarthritis? A meta-analysis of randomised controlled trials. Ann Rheum Dis 2004; 63: 901–907.

8. Pickavance L, Griffiths G, McKenna F. Diclofenac is a better analgesic than paracetamol in patients with osteoarthritis of the hip, knee and lumbar spine. Br J Rheumatol 1995; 34(suppl 1): 3.

9. Pincus T, Koch GG, Sokka T, et al. A randomized, double-blind, crossover clinical trial of diclofenac plus misoprostol versus acetaminophen in patients with osteoarthritis of the hip or knee. Arthritis Rheum 2000; 44: 1477–1480.

10. Pincus T, Koch G, Lei H, et al. Patient Preference for Placebo, Acetaminophen (paracetamol) or Celecoxib Efficacy Studies (PACES): two randomised, double blind, placebo controlled, crossover clinical trials in patients with knee or hip osteoarthritis. Ann Rheum Dis 2004; 63: 931–939.

11. McKenna F, Weaver A, Jfiechtner J, et al. COX-2 specific inhibitors in the management of osteoarthritis of the knee: a placebo-controlled randomized, double-blind study. J Clin Rheumatol 2001; 7: 151–159.

12. McKenna F, Arguelles L, Burke T, et al. Upper GI tolerability of celecoxib compared with diclofenac in the treatment of OA and RA. Clin Exp Rheumatol 2002; 20: 35–43.

13. American College of Rheumatology Subcommittee. Recommendations for the medical management of osteoarthritis of the hip and knee: 2000 update. American College of Rheumatology Subcommittee on Osteoarthritis Guidelines. Arthritis Rheum 2000; 43: 1905.

14. Jordan KM, Arden NK, Doherty M, et al. EULAR recommendations 2003. An evidence based approach to the management of knee osteoarthritis: report of a Task Force of the Standing Committee for International Clinical Studies Including Therapeutic Trials (ESCISIT). Ann Rheum Dis 2003; 62: 1145–1155.

15. Kimmel SE, Berlin JA, Reilly M, et al. The effects of nonselective non-aspirin nonsteroidal anti-inflammatory medications on the risk of nonfatal myocardial infarction and their interaction with aspirin. J Am Coll Cardiol 2004; 43: 985–990.

16. Antithrombotic Trialists' Collaboration. Collaborative meta-analysis of randomised trials of antiplatelet therapy for prevention of death, myocardial infarction, and stroke in high risk patients. Br Med J 2002; 324: 71–86.

17. Chan AT. Aspirin, non-steroidal anti-inflammatory drugs and colorectal neoplasia: future challenges in chemoprevention. Cancer Causes Control 2003; 14: 413.

18. Hawk ET, Levin B. Colorectal cancer prevention. J Clin Oncol 2005; 23: 378.

19. de Craen AJ, Gussekloo J, Vrijsen B, et al. Meta-analysis of nonsteroidal antiinflammatory drug use and risk of dementia. Am J Epidemiol 2005; 161: 114.

20. Whittle BJ. Gastrointestinal effects of nonsteroidal anti-inflammatory drugs. Fundam Clin Pharmacol 2003; 17: 301–313.

21. Tarnawski AS, Jones MK. The role of epidermal growth factor (EGF) and its receptor in mucosal protection, adaptation to injury, and ulcer healing: involvement of EGF-R signal transduction pathways. J Clin Gastroenterol 1998; 27(Suppl 1): S12–S20.

22. Papatheodoridis GV, Sougioultzis S, Archimandritis AJ. Effects of *Helicobacter pylori* and nonsteroidal anti-inflammatory drugs on peptic ulcer disease: a systematic review. Clin Gastroenterol Hepatol 2006; 4: 130–142.

23. Singh G. Gastrointestinal complications of prescription and over-the-counter nonsteroidal anti-inflammatory drugs: a view from the ARAMIS database. Arthritis, Rheumatism, and Aging Medical Information System. Am J Ther 2000; 7: 115–121.

24. Hansen JM, Hallas J, Lauritsen JM, et al. Nonsteroidal anti-inflammatory drugs and ulcer complications: a risk factor analysis for clinical decision-making. Scand J Gastroenterol 1996; 31: 126–130.

25. Mamdani M, Rochon PA, Juurlink DN, et al. Observational study of upper gastrointestinal haemorrhage in elderly patients given selective cyclo-oxygenase-2 inhibitors or conventional nonsteroidal anti-inflammatory drugs. Br Med J 2002; 325: 624.

26. Allison MC, Howatson AG, Torrance CJ, et al. Gastrointestinal damage associated with the use of nonsteroidal anti-inflammatory drugs. N Engl J Med 1992; 327: 749–754.

27. Graham DY, Opekun AR, Willingham FF, et al. Visible small-intestinal mucosal injury in chronic NSAID users. Clin Gastroenterol Hepatol 2005; 3: 55–59.

28. Goldstein JL, Eisen GM, Lewis B, et al. Video capsule endoscopy to prospectively assess small bowel injury with celecoxib, naproxen plus omeprazole, and placebo. Clin Gastroenterol Hepatol 2005; 3: 133–141.

29. Huerta C, Castellsague J, Varas-Lorenzo C, et al. Nonsteroidal anti-inflammatory drugs and risk of ARF in the general population. Am J Kidney Dis 2005; 45: 531–539.

30. Harris RC. COX-2 and the kidney. J Cardiovasc Pharmacol 2006; 47(Suppl 1): S37–S42.

31. Hudson M, Richard H, Pilote L. Differences in outcomes of patients with congestive heart failure prescribed celecoxib, rofecoxib, or nonsteroidal anti-inflammatory drugs: population-based study. Br Med J 2005; 330: 1370.

32. Salpeter SR, Gregor P, Ormiston TM, et al. Meta-analysis: cardiovascular events associated with nonsteroidal anti-inflammatory drugs. Am J Med 2006; 119: 552–559.

33. Bresalier RS, Sandler RS, Quan H, et al. Adenomatous Polyp Prevention on Vioxx (APPROVe) trial investigators. Cardiovascular events associated with rofecoxib in a colorectal adenoma chemoprevention trial. N Engl J Med 2005; 352: 1092–1102.

34. Solomon SD, Pfeffer MA, McMurray JJ, et al. Effect of celecoxib on cardiovascular events and blood pressure in two trials for the prevention of colorectal adenomas. Circulation 2006; 114: 1028–1035.

35. Graham DJ, Campen D, Hui R, et al. Risk of acute myocardial infarction and sudden cardiac death in patients treated with cyclo-oxygenase 2 selective and non-selective non-steroidal anti-inflammatory drugs: nested case-control study. Lancet 2005; 365: 475–481.

36. Garcia Rodriguez LA, Williams R, Derby LE, et al. Acute liver injury associated with nonsteroidal anti-inflammatory drugs and the role of risk factors. Arch Intern Med 1994; 154: 311.

37. Mockenhaupt M, Kelly JP, Kaufman D, et al. The risk of Stevens–Johnson syndrome and toxic epidermal necrolysis associated with nonsteroidal antiinflammatory drugs: a multinational perspective. J Rheumatol 2003; 30: 2234.

38. Knowles S, Shapiro L, Shear NH. Should celecoxib be contraindicated in patients who are allergic to sulfonamides? Revisiting the meaning of 'sulfa' allergy. Drug Safe 2001; 24: 239–247.

39. La Grenade L, Lee L, Weaver J, et al. Comparison of reporting of Stevens-Johnson syndrome and toxic epidermal necrolysis in association with selective COX-2 inhibitors. Drug Safe 2005; 28: 917–924.

40. Jenkins C, Costello J, Hodge L. Systematic review of prevalence of aspirin induced asthma and its implications for clinical practice. Br Med J 2004; 328: 434.

41. Hoppmann RA, Peden JG, Ober SK. Central nervous system side effects of nonsteroidal anti-inflammatory drugs. Aseptic meningitis, psychosis, and cognitive dysfunction. Arch Intern Med 1991; 151: 1309–1313.

Antihistamines

Phil Lieberman, Vivian Hernandez-Trujillo, Jay Lieberman, Anthony J. Frew

89

Histamine is found widely distributed through the body, with highest concentrations in lung, skin, and gastrointestinal tract. The majority is found in mast cells and basophils. Histamine also exists in the central nervous system, epidermal cells, gastric mucosa, and rapidly growing tissue.

■ HISTAMINE RECEPTORS ■

The actions of histamine are mediated by at least four receptor types (H_1, H_2, H_3, H_4). All of these are G protein-coupled receptors.[1] The activities of histamine are summarized in Table 89.1.

In general H_1 receptors exert activity by producing changes in free cytosolic calcium, and H_2 receptors mediate responses by producing elevations in cyclic adenosine monophosphate (cAMP). H_3 and H_4 receptors utilize both mechanisms and can also decrease cyclic AMP.[1]

The histamine-binding site on the H_1 receptor consists of five amino acids. H_1 receptors are probably the most important in relation to the production of symptoms of immediate hypersensitivity reactions. The major effects produced by stimulation of H_1 receptors include bronchial smooth-muscle contraction that can cause wheezing, stimulation of peripheral nerve endings causing pruritus, stimulation of the vagus inducing reflex bronchoconstriction and cough, and an increase in vascular permeability with peripheral vasodilatation resulting in a fall in blood pressure.[2]

The H_2 receptor is a member of the heptahelical receptor family. It is linked to a G protein that activates adenylyl cyclase and thus increases cAMP formation. This increase in cAMP produces a rise in intracellular calcium that mediates calcium-calmodulin actions in the gastric mucosa, vascular smooth muscle, brain, adipocytes, basophils, neutrophils, and other tissues.

The H_3 receptor has been found principally in the central nervous system. H_3 receptors are located in the hippocampus, the thalamus, the amygdala, and the hypothalamus. Most H_3 receptors are on presynaptic sites on histaminergic nerve terminals. They tend to be "inhibitory receptors." H_3 receptors are also found on peripheral nerve afferent neurons and reduce nerve repolarization when stimulated. H_3 receptors have also been detected in vascular beds.

H_4 receptors are found principally on peripheral blood cells. Their distribution suggests that they might be active in regulation of immune responses. They are also located in the bone marrow, colon, small intestine, and lung.

■ ACTIVITY OF HISTAMINE ON TARGET ORGANS ■

VASCULAR BED

The overall effect of histamine on the vascular bed is dilatation, which results in flushing, lowering of peripheral resistance, and a fall in systolic blood pressure.[2] In addition there is an increase in capillary permeability, mainly caused by a separation of the endothelial cells of the postcapillary venules, exposing the permeable basement membrane. Vasodilatation is mediated by both H_1 and H_2 receptors, with maximal vasodilatation achieved when both are stimulated. H_1 receptors have higher affinity for histamine, are stimulated by a lower concentration of histamine, and mediate a rapid-onset and short-lived vasodilatation. The vasodilatation produced by H_2 receptors is slower in onset but longer-lasting. Therefore, H_1 antagonists are more effective in blunting vasodilator responses at low concentrations of histamine and less effective at higher concentrations, which activate the H_2 receptor.[2]

H_2 receptors exert their effect via a direct action on the vascular smooth muscle, whereas H_1 receptors exert their effect not only directly on smooth muscle but also indirectly by stimulation of endothelial cells. Endothelial cell stimulation results in the production of nitric oxide and possibly prostaglandin I_2 (PGI_2). This indirect vasodilatory action plays an important role in the cumulative vasodilatory response mediated by H_1 receptors and is a function solely of the H_1 receptor.

H_3 receptors also play a role in vascular responses, as evidenced by animal models of anaphylaxis[3] and nasal challenge studies involving the application of histamine to the human nasal airway.[4] H_3-receptor stimulation of presynaptic terminals of sympathetic effector nerves innervating the heart and systemic vasculature as well as the nasal vasculature inhibits endogenous norepinephrine release. Since norepinephrine is involved

Table 89.1 Histamine and its activities

Receptor	H$_1$	H$_2$	H$_3$	H$_4$
Signal conduction through	G$_{q/11}$ and others	G$_s$	G$_{i/o}$	G$_{i/o}$ and G$_{15/16}$
Location of receptors	Multiple sites throughout the body, including: smooth-muscle bronchi and gastrointestinal tract, cardiac tissue, blood vessels, sensory nerves, endothelium, central nervous system	Widely expressed, including: mucosa of stomach, cardiac tissue, uterus, smooth-muscle vascular bed, epithelium of mucosa of nose, submucosal glands in nose, central nervous system, immune cells	Mainly expressed on presynaptic nerves in the peripheral sympathetic adrenergic system and histaminergic nerves in the central nervous system. Receptors can be found in airways and gastrointestinal tract	Eosinophils, neutrophils, basophils, mast cells, spleen, liver, lung, colon, epicanthus, and bone marrow
Chromosome location	3p25, 3p14-21	5q35.3	20q13.33	18q11.2
Signal conduction induces	Increased cyclic guanosine monophosphate, increased intracellular cytosolic calcium, activation of phospholipase C, activation of guanyl cyclase, nitric oxide production	Increase in cyclic adenosine monophosphate (AMP), activation adenyl cyclase	Decreased cyclic AMP, induction of mitogen-activated protein (MAP) kinase	Decreased cyclic AMP, MAP kinase induction, phospholipase C activation, formation of diacylglycerol, calcium mobilization
Antagonists (reverse agonists)	Over 40 exist. Examples of 'second generation' include cetirizine, desloratadine, fexofenadine, loratadine, azelastine	Burimamide, cimetidine, dimaprit, famotidine, nizatidine, ranitidine, and others	None available clinically: thioperamide, alobenpropit, and others	None available clinically: has homology with H$_3$ receptor and is also antagonized by same drugs
Activities	Increases vascular permeability, producing a fall in blood pressure, flush, headache, and reflex tachycardia; itch; smooth-muscle contraction in bronchi and gastrointestinal tract; stimulation of vagal nerve receptors producing reflex smooth-muscle contraction in airways; cough via stimulation of sensory nerves in airways; eosinophil chemotaxis; decreased atrioventricular node conduction time; enhancement of release of histamine and arachidonic acid derivatives; nitric oxide formation	Increased gastric acid secretion; increases vascular permeability, producing a fall in blood pressure, flush, headache, and reflex tachycardia; stimulate mucus production in the lungs; direct chronotropic effect on atrium and inotropic action on ventricle; relaxation of esophageal sphincter; stimulation of suppressor T cells; decrease neutrophil and basophil chemotaxis and activation; proliferation of lymphocytes; activity of natural killer cells	Opposes bronchoconstriction and gastric acid; suppression of norepinephrine release at presynaptic nerve endings	Chemotaxis and chemokinesis of mast cells and eosinophils; enhancement of the activity of other chemoattractants (e.g., chemokines) on eosinophils; upregulation of adhesion molecules

in correction of hypotension in shock and in the homeostasis of normal airway patency, such stimulation can prevent compensatory sympathetic response to shock and result in increased nasal airway resistance due to intranasal vascular dilatation. Thus, H$_3$-receptor blockade in animal models of allergic shock improves cardiovascular responses,[3] and H$_3$ antagonists will reverse the intranasal congestion occurring as a result of histamine-induced nasal blockage.[4]

It stands to reason, therefore, that antagonism of all three receptors (H$_1$, H$_2$, and H$_3$) would be beneficial in the context of shock due to anaphylaxis as well as congestion occurring during rhinitis. It has been demonstrated that a combination of H_1 and H_2 antagonism is more effective than either alone in correcting symptoms of flush, headache, and blood pressure changes occurring during intravenous infusion of histamine in human volunteers.[2]

HEART

The effect of histamine on the heart is mainly mediated through the H_2 receptor. However the H_1 receptor also plays a significant role. The vasodilatory response to histamine results in a reflex tachycardia. In addition histamine exerts a direct effect on the heart that is both chronotropic and inotropic. H_2-receptor stimulation increases the rate and force of both atrial and ventricular contraction, probably by enhancing calcium influx. H_1-receptor activation speeds the heart rate by hastening diastolic depolarization of the sinoatrial node. Contraction of the coronary arteries is mediated through the activity of the H_1 receptor.

EXTRAVASCULAR SMOOTH MUSCLE

Histamine produces varying effects on extravascular smooth muscle, including smooth-muscle contraction in the bronchial tree, mediated via the H_1 receptor. The H_1 receptor also produces modest contraction of the smooth muscle of the human uterus, whereas the H_2 receptor can produce uterine relaxation. The gastrointestinal smooth-muscle response varies from species to species, but the predominant effect is contraction, which is mediated through the H_1 receptor.

GLANDULAR SECRETION

An important biologic effect of histamine in hypersensitivity reactions is the excess production of mucus, which appears to be mediated through both H_1 and H_2 receptors. The H_2 receptor increases the amount of mucus glycoprotein secretion from goblet cells and bronchial glands, whereas the H_1 receptor increases the viscosity of the mucus.

IMMUNE REGULATION

Histamine regulation of immune and inflammatory responses is mediated through the H_2 receptor and appears to be directly related to an increase in intracellular cAMP. This results in a negative feedback on basophil (but not mast cell) histamine release. It also produces several effects on lymphocytes *in vitro*, including inhibition of T-cell-mediated cytotoxicity, activation of suppressor T cells, decrease in immunoglobulin production, and suppression of lymphocyte proliferation and lymphokine production. In addition, H_2-receptor stimulation can decrease monocyte secretion of complement components, inhibit neutrophil superoxide production, and modulate neutrophil chemotaxis.

It is reasonable to assume that, since H_4 receptors are found on leukocytes, including eosinophils, histamine might play a role in the immunologic inflammatory response. Stimulation of eosinophils by histamine can induce chemokinesis as well as chemotaxis. Those activities are inhibited by an H_4 antagonist. H_4 antagonists also reduce histamine-induced upregulation of adhesion molecules. H_4 stimulation can also cause chemotaxis of mast cells and thus it can be postulated that the H_4 receptor is active in recruiting mast cells to areas of

> ### KEY CONCEPTS
>
> >> Histamine exerts its activities via four well-characterized G protein-coupled receptors
>
> Major effects via H_1 receptor
> >> Smooth-muscle contraction
> >> Pruritus
> >> Vascular dilatation and permeability
>
> Major effects via H_2 receptor
> >> Gastric acid secretion
> >> Inotropic and chronotropic cardiac stimulation
>
> Major effect via H_3 receptor
> >> Reduced postsynaptic release of norepinephrine
>
> Major effect via H_4 receptor
> Downregulation of activity of eosinophils, basophils, T cells
> Antagonism of the activity of histamine at H_1, H_2, and H_3 receptors could be of benefit in the management of allergic disease.

> ### KEY CONCEPTS
>
> **ANTI-ALLERGIC, ANTI-INFLAMMATORY ACTIVITIES OF SECOND-GENERATION ANTIHISTAMINES**
>
> >> Prevent mast-cell degranulation
> >> Downregulate expression of adhesion molecules
> >> Diminished chemotaxis of eosinophils
> >> Reduction in inflammatory cytokine expression
> >> Enhanced programmed cell death of eosinophils

allergen challenge, thereby amplifying histamine-mediated allergic reactions.

ANTI-ALLERGIC, ANTI-INFLAMMATORY EFFECTS OF ANTIHISTAMINES

Over the last 20 years, there has been increasing interest in the potentially beneficial effects of second-generation antihistamines that are unrelated to their antihistaminic activity. This 'anti-allergic-anti-inflammatory' activity has been demonstrated in numerous spheres with most second-generation antihistamines, in studies mainly targeted at examining the drugs' roles in prevention of mast cell and basophil degranulation, downregulation of adhesion molecules, regulation of eosinophil chemotaxis and apoptosis, and modulation of cytokine production.

EFFECT ON MAST CELL AND BASOPHIL DEGRANULATION

Perhaps the most-researched anti-inflammatory activity of antihistamines relates to their ability to inhibit mediator release from mast cells and basophils. This effect has been demonstrated both *in vitro* and *in vivo*.[5] Suppression of mast cell and basophil degranulation, as measured by either release of preformed proinflammatory mediators (e.g., histamine) and/or newly synthesized molecules (e.g., arachidonic acid metabolites) has been demonstrated for both immunologic and nonimmunologic stimuli including allergen, anti-IgE, N-formyl-methionyl-leucyl-phenylalanine (fMLP), compound 48/80, substance P, concanavalin A, and calcium ionophore A23187.

In general, all second-generation antihistamines show inhibition of inflammatory mediator release from mast cells and basophils *in vitro*, but there is a great degree of heterogeneity between drugs depending on the different stimuli and different experimental conditions. In addition, at higher doses these drugs can induce release (see below). For example, when Okayama et al.[6] studied the effects of terfenadine, ketotifen, and cetirizine on human lung, tonsil, and skin mast cells stimulated immunologically with anti-immunoglobulin E (IgE), they found varying results both between drugs and within the same drug. Terfenadine inhibited mediator release from all tissue mast cells in the 5–10 μM range, while it enhanced release above 10 μM from the lung and skin mast cells, but not from the tonsillar mast cells. Ketotifen, on the other hand, was a weak inhibitor of histamine release, and only induced release from skin mast cells, whereas cetirizine caused inhibition of both histamine and PGD_2 release from all tissues, yet did not induce release from any tissue at higher concentrations.[6] The absence of a comprehensive comparison makes interpretation of the observed differences difficult, but nonetheless most evidence supports the idea of inhibition of mediator release from mast cells and basophils by antihistamines *in vitro*.

In addition to the heterogeneity observed from *in vitro* studies, the clinical studies looking at the effect of antihistamines on release of inflammatory mediators have also been varied. Most of these studies have measured inflammatory mediators in the nose or skin, and have found evidence, once again, to be supportive of the anti-inflammatory role of these drugs. However, there is still inconclusive evidence for a definitive effect *in vivo*.

EFFECTS ON EXPRESSION OF ADHESION MOLECULES

Downregulation of expression of cellular adhesion molecules, specifically intracellular adhesion molecule (ICAM-1), has been shown for levocabastine, fexofenadine, terfenadine, and desloratadine *in vitro*.[7]

Even more persuasive are the clinical trial data over the last decade demonstrating the effects of various antihistamines on ICAM-1 expression and inflammatory infiltration in the nose and eyes. Azelastine, levocabastine, cetirizine, oxatomide, terfenadine, fexofenadine, mizolastine, and loratadine decrease ICAM-1 expression on either nasal and/or conjunctival epithelial cells and reduce inflammatory infiltrate in mucosal tissues *in vivo*, effects observed both after allergen challenge and during natural antigen exposure.[7] In most studies, clinical symptom scores decreased concurrently with ICAM-1 expression.

EFFECTS ON CHEMOTAXIS AND APOPTOSIS

A third anti-inflammatory effect of antihistamines is their ability to regulate eosinophil and neutrophil chemotaxis and to increase eosinophil apoptosis. Fexofenadine, ketotifen, cetirizine, terfenadine, loratadine, and desloratadine decrease eosinophil chemotaxis *in vitro* while ketotifen, terfenadine, azelastine, and cetirizine decrease neutrophil chemotaxis *in vitro*.[5] This inhibition of eosinophil accumulation may be mediated by downregulation of adhesion molecule expression or by a direct antichemotactic effect.[8] In addition to hampering eosinophil migration, two antihistamines, ketotifen and cetirizine, also increase programmed cell death of eosinophils in the presence of interleukin-5 (IL-5).

EFFECTS ON CYTOKINE EXPRESSION

In vitro, desloratadine inhibits IL-4 and IL-13 release from anti-IgE-stimulated human modulate cytokine patterns *in vivo* by diminishing production of TH2-related cytokines and IL-8.[8, 9]

MECHANISMS OF ACTION RELATIVE TO ANTI-ALLERGIC, ANTI-INFLAMMATORY ACTIVITIES

Effects on mast cell and basophil degranulation

The exact mechanism by which antihistamines prevent mast cell and basophil degranulation is unknown. It appears that these effects are not related to H_1-receptor binding affinity, and it is very unlikely that they result from H_1-receptor blockade.

Two hypotheses have been proposed to explain the effects of antihistamines on mast cell and basophil degranulation. Some work suggests that the polar nature of these drugs, which contain both lipophilic and cationic regions, is a factor in their ability to inhibit mast cell mediator release. It is thought that the lipophilic portion, by dissolving into the cell membrane, could, at low concentrations, physically stabilize the membrane and/or interact with proteins involved in signal transduction, decreasing downstream activity. Also, at higher concentrations, the insertion of the lipophilic portion of these drugs into the cell membrane could destabilize it, causing membrane disruption and release of the preformed inflammatory mediators.

The second hypothesis suggests that antihistamines could modify degranulation by modulating calcium flux, either by interfering with calcium channels, thereby competitively inhibiting the binding of calcium to the cell membrane, or by effecting intracellular calcium release.

Effects on expression of adhesion molecules and cytokines

The effects of antihistamines on ICAM and cytokine expression may be mediated by antihistamines regulating expression of proteins, by decreasing activity of transcription factor NF-κB. This has been shown *in vitro* for desloratadine, pyrilamine, cetirizine, loratadine, and fexofenadine. In contrast to the mechanisms proposed to explain inhibition of mast cell degranulation, this downregulation of protein synthesis appears to be directly related to the H_1 receptor, as antihistamines had no effect on NF-κB activity in the absence of the H_1 receptor.[9, 10]

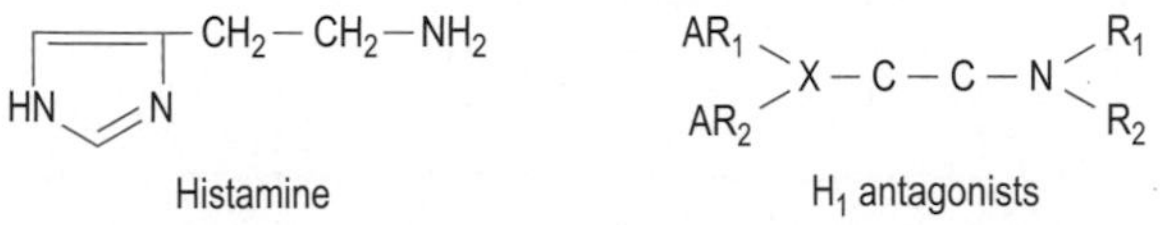

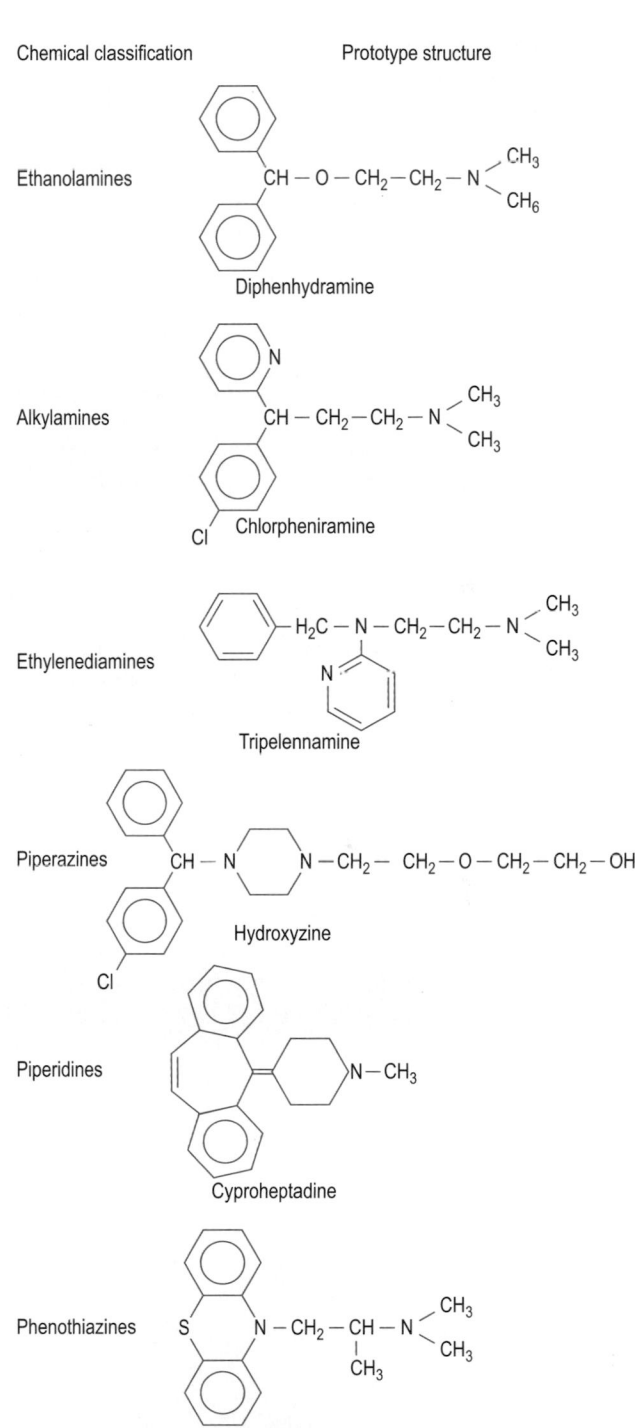

Fig. 89.1 Structure of histamine and the basic formula of classic H_1 antagonist.

CLASSIC, FIRST-GENERATION H_1 ANTAGONISTS

Structure–function relationships and chemical classification

Although it is clear that classification schemes dependent on chemical structure are imperfect, such classification still has merit since it provides insight into mechanisms of action. This traditional classification scheme is outlined in Figures 89.1 and 89.2 and Table 89.2.

Most, but not all, first-generation H_1 antagonists have a structural resemblance to histamine in that they contain a substituted ethylamine moiety. With the development of newer agents that do not have an ethylamine moiety, it has become evident that antihistaminic activity does not require this shared structure. It is now known that most, if not all, available antihistamines are not competitive antagonists, but inverse agonists.[10] This concept is based on the state in which a histamine receptor exists. At equilibrium, the histamine receptor exists in both active and inactive states. Whereas agonists such as histamine preferentially bind the active state, inverse agonists such as antihistamines bind the inactive state. Therefore, when antihistamines bind the histamine receptor, this results in the receptors being held in the inactive state, in which histamine is unable to exert its effects (Fig. 89.3).

The prototype basic structure of the ethylamine-containing first-generation H_1 antagonists (which represent the majority of drugs) is compared to histamine in Figure 89.1. These drugs contain the ethylamine moiety attached to aromatic substituents (AR_1, AR_2) by a nitrogen, carbon, or oxygen linkage (X). The two aromatic rings may be bridged, as in tricyclic antihistamines, or the ethylamine may actually be part of a ring structure. The classification of first-generation H_1 antagonists has traditionally been based on the atom linking the ethylamine grouping to the aromatic substituents (Fig. 89.2). If the link is via oxygen, the drugs are ethanolamines; if via carbon, they are termed alkylamines; and if via nitrogen, they are ethylenediamines. This structural classification does not apply to piperazines, piperidines, and phenothiazines. The aromatic substituents in these compounds make them lipid soluble, so they pass through the blood–brain barrier.

Pharmacokinetics

All first-generation H_1 receptor antagonists are rapidly absorbed after oral administration and reach peak serum concentrations in 2–3 hours when given in liquid form. Most have a duration of action of 4–6 hours, but some have longer durations of action. Studies of diphenhydramine suggest that H_1 antagonists are disseminated throughout the body, including the central nervous system. Antihistamines are secreted in breast milk, and the concentration is dependent upon serum concentration.

Fig. 89.2 Structural classification of classic H_1 antagonists.

Table 89.2 Characteristics of representative first-generation H$_1$ antagonists based upon chemical classification

Chemical class	Examples	Comments
Ethanolamines	Diphenhydramine Clemastine Carbinoxamine	Significant antimuscarinic effects. Can be potent sedatives, but sedative potential varies, with clemastine producing the least amount. Low incidence of gastrointestinal side effects. Can have some anti-motion sickness activity. Diphenhydramine and clemastine both available over the counter
Alkylamines	Chlorpheniramine Brompheniramine Dexchlorpheniramine Triprolidine	Relatively moderate incidence of drowsiness. Moderate anticholinergic effect. No anti-emetic or anti-motion sickness activity. Few gastrointestinal side effects. All available over the counter. Occasional paradoxical central nervous system stimulation, especially in children
Ethylenediamines	Tripelennamine Pyrilamine Antazoline	Mild to moderate sedation. Slight anticholinergic effect. Some local anesthetic effect. Pyrilamine is sold over the counter and is the oldest antihistamine preparation available today. As a group, may have more frequent gastrointestinal side effects
Piperazines	Hydroxyzine Meclizine Cyclizine	Hydroxyzine has highest sedative activity in group. Meclizine and cyclizine relatively low sedative activity, with main use being for vertigo, anti-motion sickness, and anti-emetic activity. Hydroxyzine has significant anticholinergic activity
Piperidines	Cyproheptadine Phenindamine Azatadine	Mild to moderate sedation. Little anticholinergic activity, anti-emetic activity, and anti-motion sickness activity. Cyproheptadine has potent anti-serotonin effect. As a class has relatively high incidence of paradoxical central nervous system stimulatory activity
Phenothiazines	Promethazine Methdilazine Trimeprazine	Usually highly sedating. Strong anti-emetic, anticholinergic activity. Main clinical use is as anti-emetic

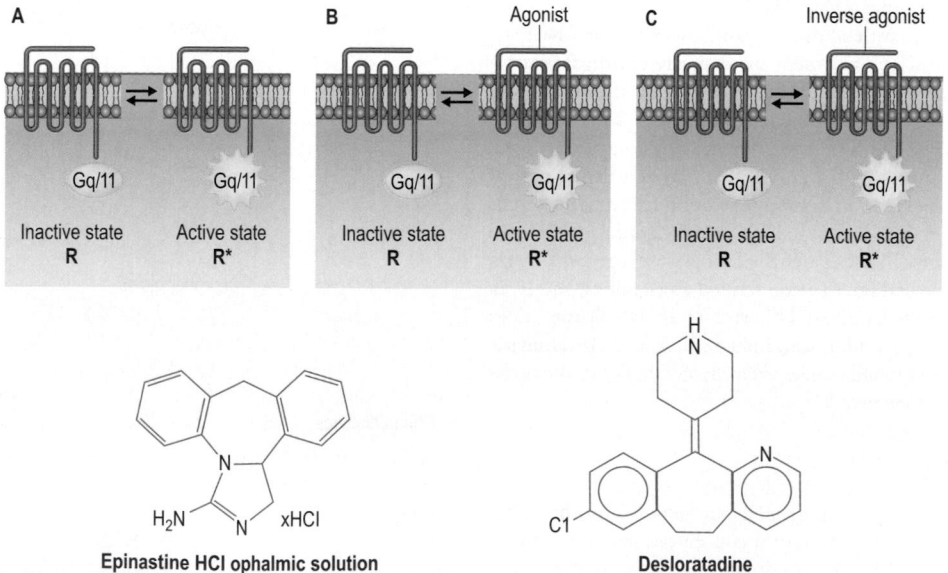

Fig. 89.3 The conformational states of the H$_1$ receptor. (A) Equilibrium exists at rest between active and inactive states. (B) Agonists (such as histamine) bind the active state preferentially, thereby shifting the equilibrium towards the active state. (C) Inverse agonists (such as antihistamines) bind the inactive state preferentially, thereby shifting the equilibrium towards the inactive state. (From Simons FER. Antihistamines. In: Adkins NF, et al. (eds) Allergy Principles and Practice, 6th edn, vol. 1. Philadelphia: Mosby; 2003:834–869 with permission.)

CLINICAL PEARLS

SIDE EFFECTS OF FIRST-GENERATION H₁ ANTAGONISTS

>> Drowsiness

>> Central nervous system impairment that may occur without subjective drowsiness

>> Potentiation of effects of alcohol, tranquilizers

>> Impaired motor skills – driving, flying

>> Paradoxical hyperactivity in some children

>> Dryness of mouth

>> Urinary retention, constipation

CLINICAL PEARLS

KEY CLINICAL FEATURES OF SECOND-GENERATION ANTIHISTAMINES

>> Fexofenadine and desloratadine are nonsedating

>> Loratadine is nonsedating in recommended doses, but may sedate in higher doses

>> Cetirizine and azelastine can produce sedation, but are probably less sedating than first-generation drugs

>> Cetirizine and loratadine are US Food and Drug Administration class B drugs in pregnancy

All first-generation H₁ antagonists are extensively metabolized in the liver, and little, if any, of these drugs is excreted unchanged in the urine. All of these agents are metabolized by the hepatic cytochrome P450 system. Clearance rates are variable and half-lives differ according to the metabolic potential of the patient, such that children have shorter and the elderly have longer elimination half-lives. Severe hepatic dysfunction can prolong the half-life, and dosage regimens must be altered accordingly.

Pharmacodynamics

An important principle of the pharmacodynamic activity of these drugs is that their tissue effect is somewhat delayed compared to serum levels and can extend far beyond the life of the drug in the serum.[11] For example, a single dose of hydroxyzine significantly suppresses histamine-induced wheal and flare for 36 hours, reducing the mean flare size for as long as 60 hours despite a negligible serum concentration. Also, the maximal suppression of wheal and flare does not occur until 7 hours after mean peak serum concentrations have been reached.[11] Thus it is best to administer H₁ antagonists before allergen exposure.

Side effects

By far the most common and significant side effect of first-generation antihistamines is drowsiness. Their soporific activity can clearly be attributed to the fact that these drugs pass through the blood–brain barrier and exert their effect on the central nervous system. The exact mechanism(s) by which these drugs produce drowsiness is unknown but may include antihistaminic, anti-cholinergic, anti-α-adrenergic, anti-serotonergic, and/or calcium channel blocking activities. It should be noted that antihistaminic activity does not necessarily correlate with sedative potential, suggesting that this is not the sole mechanism producing this side effect.

It is crucial to appreciate that the subjective degree of drowsiness does not necessarily correlate with the objective assessment of central nervous system impairment.[12] Since these drugs can produce impairment without apparent sedation and inhibit performance on tests of psychomotor reflexes and driving skills, civilian and military aircraft pilots are prohibited from taking these drugs while flying.

Paradoxical central nervous system stimulation can be encountered in some patients, especially children. Other less common central nervous system side effects include dizziness, tinnitus, blurred vision, and tremor.

The next most frequent group of side effects is due to the anti-muscarinic activity and includes dryness of the mouth, urinary retention and dysuria, blurring of vision, and constipation.

Other side effects are uncommon and include loss of appetite, nausea, abdominal pain, and diarrhea. Drug allergy to antihistamines has been reported. Leukopenia, agranulocytosis, and hemolytic anemia are extremely rare. Although teratogenic effects have been noted in animals, these have not been documented in humans.

Acute toxicity resulting from overdose can produce central nervous system effects, including hallucinations, central nervous system excitement, profound sedation, ataxia, incoordination, and convulsions. Other findings are fixed and dilated pupils, as well as sinus tachycardia, which is frequent, and ventricular arrhythmias, which are less common. The anti-cholinergic effects of dry mouth and urinary retention are usually observed and fever may be present. Fatal overdose reactions have occurred, with profound coma and respiratory collapse.

NONSEDATING, SECOND-GENERATION ANTIHISTAMINES

A variety of second-generation antihistamines are available in different countries. Loratadine, desloratadine, cetirizine, and fexofenadine are administered orally, azelastine is administered orally or by nasal spray, while others (levocabastine, olopatadine, ketotifen, and epinastine) are available for ocular administration.

These drugs are not as easily classified by structure as are the first-generation antihistamines because they do not always contain an ethylamine side chain. Nonsedating antihistamines are of diverse chemical structure, and many can be considered drugs with multiple pharmacologic effects in addition to their antihistaminic activity. The term "non sedating" is actually somewhat of a misnomer since some of these drugs (cetirizine and azelastine) are mildly sedating at standard dosage, and others can be sedating when given in amounts exceeding the recommended dose.

Numerous studies have demonstrated that all second-generation drugs cause less in the way of significant subjective sedation or objectively assessed impairment of function.[13] Many factors may account for the reduced sedative potential of these agents, but the most important seems to be that they do not pass through the blood–brain barrier.

Another postulated mechanism for their lack of sedation is their relative specificity for the H₁ receptor. In general, compared to first-generation antihistamines, they are highly specific for the H₁ receptor

Table 89.3 Single-dose pharmacokinetics of selected second-generation antihistamines in healthy adults

Drug	Major metabolite	Activity of metabolite	Dose (mg)	T_{max} (h)
Loratadine	Descarboethoxy	4 × parent	10 q.d.	1.2 ± 0.3
Desloratadine	3-hydroxydesloratadine	Relative potency unknown	5 q.d.	4
Cetirizine	None	NA	10 q.d.	1.0 ± 0.5
Fexofenadine	None	NA	60 b.i.d.	1.3–2.6
Azelastine	Desmethyl	Relative potency unknown	0.55 b.i.d.	2–3

Table 89.4 Clinical profiles of selected second-generation antihistamines

Drug	Preparations available	Available with decongestant	US FDA approved non sedating	Pregnancy category	Food effect on bioavailability	Dosing frequency
Loratadine	Tablet, syrup, dissolvable wafer	Yes	Yes	B	Increase	q.d.
Cetirizine	Tablets, syrup	No	No	B	None	q.d.
Fexofenadine	Capsule	Yes	Yes	C	Decrease	b.i.d.[a]
Azelastine	Nasal spray	No	No	C	None	b.i.d.

FDA, Food and Drug Administration.
[a]Adjustment only suggested for moderate to severe liver or renal impairment.

Table 89.5 Pharmacodynamics of selected second-generation antihistamines based on suppression of histamine-induced wheal and flare

	Onset (hours)	Duration of action (h)	Persistence of tissue activity after cessation of regular administration (days)
Loratadine	3	24	7
Desloratadine	1	24	NA
Cetirizine	0.7	>24	3
Fexofenadine	2	24	2
Azelastine	1	12	2

NA, not available

Effect of food on absorbtion	$T_{1/2}$ (h)	Plasma protein bound%	Excretion % feces	Excretion % urine	Hepatic metabolism
Increase	7.8 ± 4.2	97–99	40	40	CYP3A4 (P450)CYP2D6 (P450)
None	27	82–87	43.5	43.5	CYP3A4
None	7–10	93	10	70	Not significant
Decrease	14.4	60–70	80	11	Not significant
Not applicable	22	78–88(54)	75	24	P450 (isoform

Pediatric use approved by FDA	Effects as single agent in nonallergic rhinitis	Effects on nasal congestion	Need to alter dose[a] elderly	Need to alter dose[a] liver disease	Need to dose[a] renal disease	Drug interaction
Yes	No	Little to none	–	Possible decrease	Possibly decrease	–
Yes	No	Little to none	–	Possible decrease	Possibly decrease	–
Pending	No	Little to none	–	–	Possibly decrease	Coadministation of erythromycin or ketoconazole increases plasma level of fexofenadine (see text)
Pending	Effective	Most studies indicate beneficial effect	–	–	–	–

Some suppression of histamine-induced skin wheal and flare has been seen after the intranasal administration of azelastine but this effect is probably of little clinical significance and disappears within 48 hours of cessation of the drug.

Azelastine is also somewhat unusual in terms of its clinical effects: it reduces nasal obstruction and decreases postnasal drip. It appears to be effective as monotherapy in chronic nonallergic rhinitis.[23, 24]

The incidence of sedation in clinical trials appears to be low (approximately 2–3%).[24]

■ ANTIHISTAMINES AVAILABLE ONLY FOR OCULAR USE ■

Several antihistamines are available as topical preparations for the treatment of allergic conjunctivitis. These include ketotifen, levocabastine, olopatadine, and epinastine.

KETOTIFEN

Ketotifen, like azelastine, has potent nonantihistamine anti-inflammatory activity. It inhibits mediator release from mast cells and basophils, degranulation of eosinophils and neutrophils, chemotaxis of eosinophils, leukotriene generation, and the generation of platelet-activating factor.[25]

After oral administration, ketotifen is completely absorbed, with peak concentrations occurring at about 3 hours. The absorption half-life is about 1 hour. The absorbed drug is distributed extensively to circulating cells and 16–18% is bound to plasma proteins. Some 69–70% of the dose is excreted as metabolites. Both ketotifen and its metabolites appear to be largely excreted in the urine, with fecal elimination found only after the first 24 hours. Based on the above pharmacokinetic data, it is assumed that any ketotifen that is systemically absorbed after ophthalmic application would be extensively metabolized and eliminated via the urine. The recommended dosage is one drop every 8–12 hours.

REFERENCES

LEVOCABASTINE

Levocabastine absorption from the eye occurs within 1–2 hours. Bioavailability from topical ocular administration ranges from 30% to 60%. Steady-state plasma levels after the application of a 0.05% ophthalmic suspension one drop three times a day are 1.6 µg/l. The drug has a plasma protein binding of approximately 65%.

The half-life of levocabastine is fairly long: between 35 and 40 hours regardless of the route of administration. There is very little hepatic metabolism, with about 75% of the drug excreted unchanged in the urine and 10–20% unchanged in the feces. The recommended dosage is one drop in each eye b.i.d. to q.i.d. Eye drops administered regularly do not suppress histamine-induced skin wheal and flare.[26]

OLOPATADINE

Olopatadine also appears to have significant anti-inflammatory activity, and inhibits histamine release from mast cells. It is a selective H_1 antagonist that is devoid of effects on α-adrenergic, dopaminergic, and muscarinic receptors. The recommended dose is 1–2 drops in each affected eye b.i.d. at an interval of 6–8 hours. Peak serum concentrations are usually reached within 2 hours of dosing. The half-life in plasma is approximately 3 hours and elimination is primarily through renal excretion, with 60–70% of the dose recovered in the urine as the parent drug. Two metabolites are found in low concentrations in the urine: the mono-desmethyl and *N*-oxide moieties.

EPINASTINE

Like ketotifen, olopatadine, and azelastine, epinastine inhibits histamine release from mast cells. Although it is selective for H_1 receptors, it has affinity for H_2, α-adrenergic, and serotonin receptors as well. The peak plasma concentrations are usually reached within 2 hours of dosing. The plasma protein binding of epinastine is 64%, with a terminal plasma elimination half-life of 12 hours. It is excreted unchanged for the most part, with less than 10% of the drug metabolized. Epinastine has 55% excretion in the urine and 30% fecal elimination. The recommended dosage is one drop b.i.d.

SIDE EFFECTS OF SECOND-GENERATION ANTIHISTAMINES

As a class, the second-generation antihistamines have relatively few side effects. Some sedation can occur with azelastine and cetirizine, but its incidence is lower than with first-generation antihistamines.

None of the presently available drugs is known to prolong the Q-T interval, on their own, and none of them therefore carries any warning regarding the production of ventricular arrhythmias.

There is no evidence to date that any of the second-generation antihistamines cause fetal abnormalities in humans. They do, however, cross the placenta. In high doses, loratadine and hydroxyzine cause embryotoxicity in animals, and despite the lack of hard evidence from human studies, regulators and manufacturers advise against using all second-generation antihistamines in pregnancy. It is likely that all second-generation antihistamines are excreted in breast milk,[27] but there is no evidence that they exert any clinically significant side effects in nursing infants. However nursing mothers are warned against their use.

Although astemizole was associated with increase in body weight and appetite, none of the newer antihistamines has been known to affect appetite or weight gain, when administered in standard doses by approved routes of administration.

REFERENCES

1. Parsons M, Ganellin CR. Histamine and its receptors. Br J Pharmacol 2006; 147: S127–S135.
2. Lieberman P. Anaphylaxis and anaphylactoid reactions. In: Middleton Adkinson, Yunginger, et al. (eds) Allergy: Principles and Practice, 6th edn. St Louis, Missouri: Mosby Year Book; 2003: 1497–1522.
3. Chrusch C, Sharma S, Unruh H, et al. Histamine H_3 receptor blockade improves cardiac function in canine anaphylaxis. Am J Respir Crit Care Med 1999; 160: 1142–1149.
4. Taylor-Clark T, Sodha R, Warner B, et al. Histamine receptors that influence blockage of the normal human nasal airway. Br J Pharmacol 2005; 144: 867–874.
5. Gelfand EW, Appajosyula S, Meeves S. Anti-inflammatory activity of H_1-receptor antagonists: review of recent experimental research. Curr Med Res Opin 2004; 20: 73–81.
6. Okayama Y, Benyon RC, Lowman MA, et al. In vitro effects of H_1-antihistamines on histamine and PGD2 release from mast cells of human lung, tonsil, and skin. Allergy 1994; 48: 246–253.
7. Ciprandi G, Tosca MA, Cosentino C, et al. Effects of fexofenadine and other antihistamines on components of the allergic response: adhesion molecules. J Allergy Clin Immunol 2003; 112: S78–S82.
8. Ciprandi G, Cirillo I, Vizzaccaro A, et al. Levocetirizine improves nasal obstruction and modulates cytokine pattern in patients with seasonal allergic rhinitis: a pilot study. Clin Exp Allergy 2004; 32: 958–964.
9. Wu RL, Antes JC, Kreutner W, et al. Desloratadine inhibits constitutive and histamine-stimulated nuclear factor κB activity consistent with inverse agonism at the histamine H_1 receptor. Int Arch Allergy Immunol 2004; 135: 313–318.
10. Simons FER. Antihistamines. In: Adkinson NF, et al. (ed) Allergy Principles and Practice, 6th edn, vol. 1. Philadelphia, PA: Mosby; 2003: 834–869.
11. Simons FER, Simons KJ. H_1 receptor antagonists: clinical pharmacology and use in allergic disease. Pediatr Clin North Am 1983; 30: 899.
12. Meltzer EO. Performance effects of antihistamines. J Allergy Clin Immunol 1990; 8: 613.
13. Slater JW, Zechnich AD, Haxby DG. Second-generation antihistamines. Drugs 1999; 57: 31.
14. Du Buske LM. Clinical comparison of histamine H_1-receptor antagonist drugs. J Allergy Clin Immunol 1996; 98: S307.
15. Timmerman H. Why are nonsedating antihistamines nonsedating?. Clin Exp Allergy 1999; 29: 13.
16. Simons FER, Bergman JN, Watson WTA, et al. The clinical pharmacology of fexofenadine in children. J Allergy Clin Immunol 1996; 98: 1062.

17. Bousquet J, Chanal I, Skassa-Brociek W, et al. Lack of subsensitivity to loratadine during long-term dosing during 12 weeks. J Allergy Clin Immunol 1990; 86: 248.

18. Golightly LK, Greis LS. Second-generation antihistamines: actions and efficacy in the management of allergic disorders. Drugs 2005; 65: 341–384.

19. Bryce PJ, Geha R, Oettgen HC. Desloratadine inhibits allergen-induced airway inflammation and bronchial hyperresponsiveness and alters T-cell responses in murine models of asthma. J Allergy Clin Immunol 2003; 112: 149–158.

20. Murdoch D, Goa KL, Keam SJ. Desloratadine: an update of its efficacy in the management of allergic disorders. Drugs 2003; 63: 2051–2077.

21. Pierson WE. Cetirizine: a unique second-generation antihistamine for treatment of rhinitis and chronic urticaria. Clin Ther 1991; 13: 92.

22. Kontow FTK, Maniatokov G, Pateologis G, et al. Cetirizine inhibits delayed pressure urticaria. Ann Allergy 1990; 65: 520.

23. Berger WE, Fineman SM, Lieberman P, et al. Double-blind trials of azelastine nasal spray monotherapy versus combination therapy with loratadine tablets and beclomethasone nasal spray in patients with seasonal allergic rhinitis. Ann Allergy Asthma Immunol 1999; 82: 535.

24. Lieberman PL, Settipane RA. Azelastine nasal spray: a review of pharmacology and clinical efficacy in allergic and nonallergic rhinitis. Allergy Asthma Proc 2003; 24: 95–105.

25. Nabe M, Miyagawa H, Agrawai DK, et al. The effect of ketotifen on eosinophils as measured at LTC4 release and by chemotaxis. Allergy Proc 1991; 12: 267.

26. Heykants J, Van Peer A, Van de Velde V, et al. The pharmacokinetic properties of topical levocabastine: a review. Clin Pharmacokinet 1995; 29: 221.

27. Horak F, Stubner UP. Comparative tolerability of second generation antihistamines. Drug Safe 1999; 20: 385.

REFERENCES

Immunomodulating pharmaceuticals

90

Edwin S.L. Chan, Stephen N. Oliver, Bruce N. Cronstein

Recent excitement over biologic agents and their ability to regulate immunologic reactions and significantly affect such immunologically mediated diseases as rheumatoid arthritis and Crohn's disease has overshadowed previous emphasis on small molecules for the treatment of immunological diseases. Nonetheless, some small molecules (most notably methotrexate) have proved to be nearly as effective as biological agents when tested head-to-head in patients with immunological diseases, and combining these small molecule therapies with biological agents generally leads to significantly better outcomes than the use of either single agent. Thus, it is likely that many small molecule immunomodulatory drugs will continue to be widely used for many years to come. The most well-accepted and commonly used immunomodulators in current clinical use are reviewed here.

■ METHOTREXATE ■

Now regarded as a landmark agent among immunomodulatory pharmaceuticals, the history of this drug dates back to the 1940s, when Farber et al.[1] first reported temporary remissions achieved in children with acute lymphocytic leukemia. The treatment, aminopterin, a derivative of folic acid, was later to find a new disguise whereby a methyl group substitution resulted in methotrexate (Fig. 90.1). Methotrexate has been employed in the treatment of rheumatoid arthritis (RA) since as early as 1951, but its popularity as an immunomodulatory drug in RA did not come until the 1980s. Over the years, extensive experience with its use in inflammatory diseases as diverse as RA, psoriasis and inflammatory bowel disease has taught us a great deal about its safety, efficacy, and toxicities, as well as its anti-inflammatory mechanisms of action. In this respect, methotrexate, much like corticosteroids, can be justly regarded as a cornerstone of immunomodulatory therapy.

PHARMACOKINETICS OF METHOTREXATE

When used as an anti-inflammatory agent, methotrexate is administered at low doses (usually 10–25 mg/week) once weekly, usually orally, but may also be given via the subcutaneous or intramuscular routes. At these low doses oral bioavailability is high (60–70%), and although transporters are responsible for its absorption from the gastrointestinal tract, no saturation effect occurs with these low doses. A small proportion of methotrexate is metabolized by hydroxylation into 7-hydroxymethotrexate, and both of these compounds are short-lived with a serum half-life of no more than 8 hours. The much longer anti-inflammatory action, which allows for once-weekly dosing, must therefore be attributable to other, longer-lasting metabolites, the polyglutamates. Excretion occurs principally via the urinary tract, but also via the biliary tract. Therefore renal function is an important consideration in methotrexate dosing, and any medication that impairs glomerular filtration may also potentiate both the effect and the toxicity of methotrexate.[1]

MECHANISMS OF ACTION

Methotrexate is an analog of folic acid, which inhibits purine and pyrimidine synthesis and thereby suppresses the cellular proliferation important for the growth of malignant tumors (Table 90.1). These actions are highly dependent on its ability to inhibit dihydrofolate reductase, and hence the toxicity arising from high-dose methotrexate therapy can similarly be treated with folic acid derivatives, such as leucovorin, which is used as an antidote for methotrexate given as a chemotherapeutic agent. However, it may come as a surprise that folic or folinic acid is often given in conjunction with methotrexate in inflammatory diseases to reduce the incidence of side effects such as mucositis and bone marrow suppression, without hampering its anti-inflammatory efficacy. Reductions in the levels of purines and pyrimidines in the serum have indeed been observed following a single dose of methotrexate, along with decreased proliferation of antigen stimulated lymphocytes. However, these changes are transient and insufficient to explain the anti-inflammatory effectiveness of once-weekly dosing. This, and the fact that methotrexate is anti-inflammatory at only one-thousandth of the anti-malignant dose, must mean that the anti-inflammatory actions are mediated mostly through different mechanisms from those responsible for suppression of tumor growth.

Methotrexate is also known to block transmethylation reactions within the cell and to inhibit the production of S-adenosylmethionine.

avoided in patients with known allergy to sulfa drugs, and screening for G6PD deficiency should be carried out where appropriate.

■ AZATHIOPRINE ■

Azathioprine (Fig. 90.3) is an imidazolyl derivative of 6-mercaptopurine that has been widely used in the treatment of rheumatic diseases such as RA and inflammatory bowel disease, as well as to prevent the rejection of solid organ transplants. Cleavage into 6-mercaptopurine and the imidazole moiety occurs rapidly within erythrocytes, both enzymatically by glutathione transferase, and nonenzymatically. Several enzymes (Table 90.3) participate in the metabolism of 6-mercaptopurine into active and inactive compounds. One of these, thiopurine methyltransferase is known to be associated with genetic polymorphisms in the population, and inherited changes in thiopurine methyltransferase activity may have a strong impact on patient response to azathioprine treatment. Xanthine oxidase is another important enzyme that inactivates 6-mercaptopurine by converting it to 6-thiouric acid. As this occurs mainly in the liver, the importance of first-pass metabolism is best observed in enzyme deficiency states, whether due to disease or to drugs such as allopurinol, where toxicity arising from azathioprine therapy is a major threat.

PROPOSED MECHANISMS OF ACTION

The molecular mechanisms by which azathioprine exerts its immunomodulatory effects are still unclear. As purine analogs, the active metabolites interfere with the de novo synthesis of purines and with purine synthesis through the salvage pathway, and are incorporated into RNA and DNA. The proliferation of both T and B lymphocytes is inhibited, and the function of natural killer (NK) cells is also suppressed, without any change in cell numbers. Antibody production is also suppressed, although it is not known which of these effects predominate *in vivo*. Cellular responses to chemoattractants are altered and the production of cytokines such as IL-6 is also affected.

ADVERSE EFFECTS

Azathioprine therapy is generally well tolerated. The most common side effects are gastrointestinal and are generally mild. Pancreatitis may occasionally occur as an idiosyncratic reaction. Hepatotoxicity and cholestasis

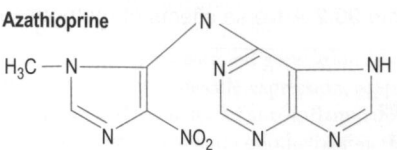

Fig. 90.3 Azathioprine – chemical structure.

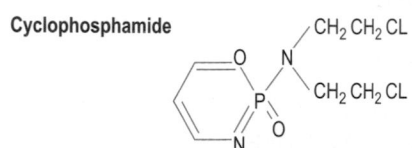

Fig. 90.4 Cyclophosphamide – chemical structure.

Table 90.3 Principal enzymes involved in the metabolism of azathioprine

Enzyme	Action
Glutathione transferase	Cleaves azathioprine into 6-mercaptopurine and imidazole moieties
Thiopurine methyltransferase	Metabolism of 6-mercaptopurine
Xanthine oxidase	Conversion of 6-mercaptopurine to 6-thiouric acid

are not uncommon, but peliosis hepatis and nodular regenerative hyperplasia occur rarely. The possibility of malignant potential has been raised and there have been reports of a possible heightened risk for non-Hodgkin lymphoma, but these events are rare and no definite link between azathioprine administration and the development of malignancies has been established. Bone marrow suppression and opportunistic infections do occur and pose far greater threats.

■ CYCLOPHOSPHAMIDE ■

Alkylating agents were first used in the treatment of inflammatory diseases after promising reports of the application of the first of its kind, nitrogen mustard, in RA. Cyclophosphamide (Fig. 90.4) is a prodrug that is extensively metabolized to produce phosphorymide mustard, an active component responsible for the alkylating actions of cyclophosphamide, as well as acrolein, which is inactive but causes the hemorrhagic cystitis associated with cyclophosphamide therapy. Although it can be given intravenously, bioavailability following oral administration is high (>75%). Its use in inflammatory diseases has been severely limited by toxicity, although it has a useful place in the management of lupus nephritis.

KEY CONCEPTS

MECHANISMS OF ACTION OF SULFASALAZINE

>> Suppresses the proliferation of lymphocytes

>> Suppresses proinflammatory cytokine production

>> Inhibits activation of NF-κB

>> Promotes adenosine accumulation

MECHANISMS OF ACTION

Cyclophosphamide alkylates guanine residues, principally on DNA, but also on RNA, with the result that strands are rendered cross-linkable and hence the processes of transcription and translation are disrupted. This alkylating process is thought to affect resting as well as actively dividing cells. The number of circulating CD4 T lymphocytes is reduced, and to a lesser extent the number of CD8 T cells is reduced as well, thereby reducing the CD4/CD8 ratio. Despite observations of an increase in immunoglobulin-secreting cells, B-cell function is suppressed and overall immunoglobulin synthesis reduced.

ADVERSE EFFECTS

Perhaps the best-known side effect is hemorrhagic cystitis. As this is known to occur more frequently after oral dosing, this route of administration has fallen out of favor. This may relate to continuous exposure of the bladder to the inactive byproduct acrolein, and the acrolein-neutralizing agent Mesna (2-mercaptoethane sulfonate) has been recommended as a prophylactic measure along with a copious amount of hydration. Hemorrhagic myocarditis may also occur, leading to myocardial necrosis, hemopericardium and congestive cardiac failure. Survivors of acute cardiac toxicity do not, however, appear to show any residual EKG or echocardiographic abnormalities.

Apart from bone marrow suppression, reduction of fertility and a heightened risk of infection as a result of immunosuppression, cyclophosphamide therapy has also been associated with secondary malignancies, which may occur years after cessation of the drug. Malignancies of the bladder, often of a transitional cell type, tend to occur only in those with a previous history of treatment-related hemorrhagic cystitis. Myeloproliferative and lymphoproliferative disorders have also been associated with the use of cyclophosphamide.

■ LEFLUNOMIDE ■

A derivative of isoxazole, leflunomide is an inhibitor of de novo pyrimidine synthesis. Leflunomide (Fig. 90.5) is an inactive prodrug which is converted into the long-acting active compound A77 1726 (2-cyano-3-hydroxy-*N*-[4-trifluoromethyl]-butenamide) (Fig. 90.6), which is a reversible inhibitor of dihydro-orotate dehydrogenase, an enzyme involved in pyrimidine synthesis. Because of its long half-life, therapy with leflunomide is usually started with a loading dose so that therapeutic levels can be achieved more quickly. A77 1726 is highly bound to plasma protein and undergoes enterohepatic recirculation.

MECHANISMS OF ACTION

When the synthesis of pyrimidines is inhibited, the availability of pyrimidine nucleotides becomes insufficient to support the growing demands of proliferating immune response cells such as activated T lymphocytes. This deficiency is not adequately replenished by the involvement of salvage pathways, rendering cell proliferation inefficient and thus limiting the clonal expansion of T cells. Proliferation of B cells is similarly suppressed with reduction of Cdk2, a cyclin-dependent

Table 90.4 Adverse effects of thalidomide

Severe	Common	Uncommon or disease specific*
Teratogenicity	Sedation	Thromboembolism*
• Phocomelia	Constipation	Peripheral neuropathy*
• Deafness	Paresthesias	Neutropenia*
• Facial/ocular	Dizziness	Amenorrhea
paralysis	Skin rash	Peripheral edema
Stevens–Johnson	Dry skin	Bradycardia
syndrome	Pruritus	Impotence
Toxic epidermolysis		Hypo- or hyperglycemia
		Hypothyroidism

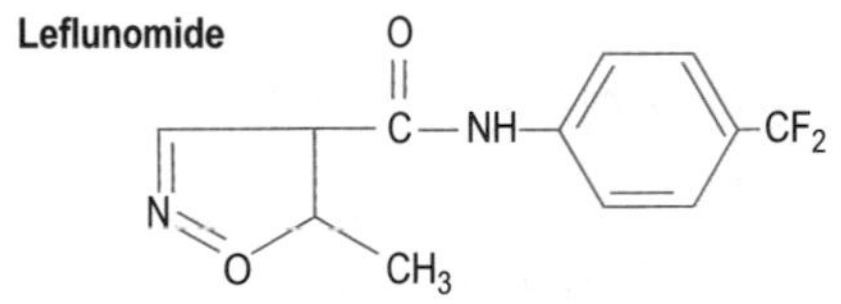

Fig. 90.5 Leflunomide – chemical structure.

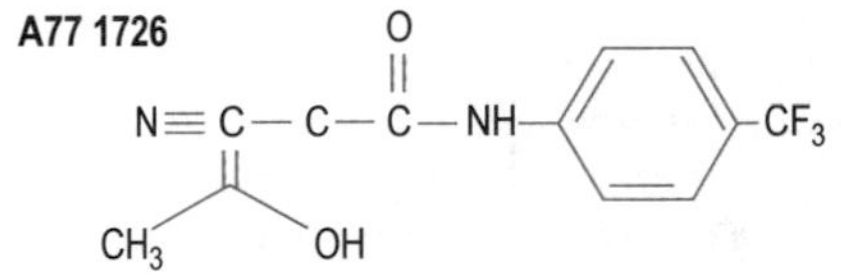

Fig. 90.6 A77 1726 – chemical structure.

kinase. Leflunomide also inhibits activation of the transcription factor NF-κB. Whereas the anti-proliferative actions of moderate concentrations of leflunomide can be reversed *in vitro* by the addition of uridine, this reversal does not occur at higher concentrations, suggesting that at higher concentrations other mechanisms may be important for its immunomodulatory effects. At these higher concentrations, leflunomide inhibits tyrosine kinase activity, although the relevance of this effect *in vivo* remains questionable.

ADVERSE EFFECTS

Liver toxicity is the most important side-effect of leflunomide therapy, although gastrointestinal symptoms appear to be most common. Thus there is some similarity to methotrexate with regard to toxicity profile, and concerns have been raised regarding the co-administration of these two medications. However, clinical trials have shown that these agents can be safely and effectively given together in patients with RA, although transaminasemia occurs more frequently than with methotrexate alone.[6,7] Occasional episodes of fatal fulminant hepatic failure have been reported. Skin reactions are mostly minor rashes, but occasionally more serious manifestations such as Stevens–Johnson syndrome and toxic epidermal necrolysis occur.

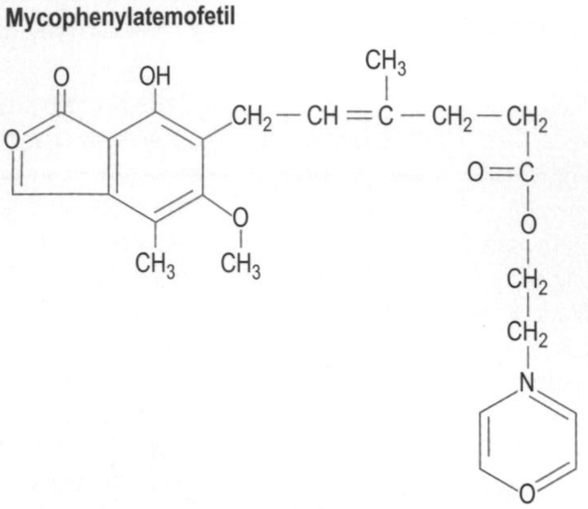

Mycophenylatemofetil

Fig. 90.7   Mycophenolate mofetil – chemical structure.

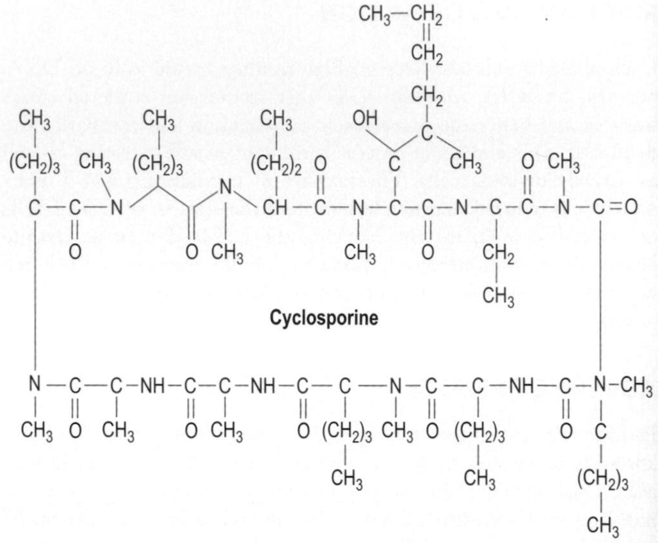

Fig. 90.8   Cyclosporine – chemical structure.

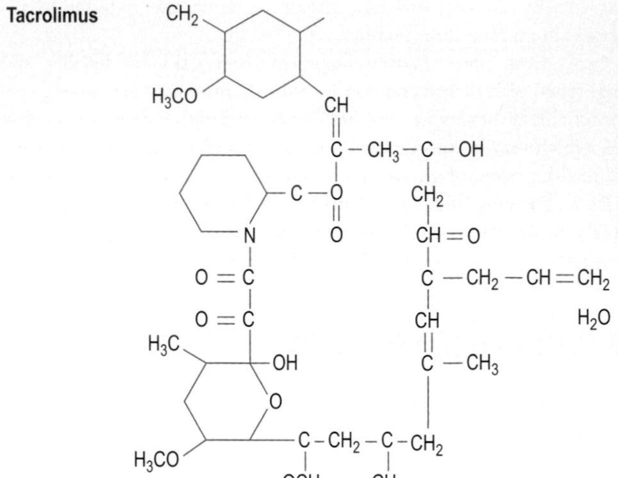

Tacrolimus

Fig. 90.9   Tacrolimus – chemical structure.

MYCOPHENOLATE MOFETIL

Mycophenolate mofetil (Fig. 90.7) has been widely used to prevent rejection in solid organ transplantation, but has also been successfully employed in the treatment of autoimmune diseases such as RA, systemic lupus erythematosus and psoriasis. It is rapidly absorbed and hydrolyzed into the active compound mycophenolic acid, which is a reversible inhibitor of inosine monophosphate dehydrogenase. Because the latter is a key enzyme in the de novo synthesis of guanine nucleotides, its inhibition is most keenly felt in lymphocytes, which are more reliant upon the de novo synthetic pathway rather than on the hypoxanthine–guanine phosphoribosyl transferase salvage pathway of purine synthesis. The reduction in guanine synthesis has many effects on the immune system. Lymphocyte proliferation is suppressed; antibody production and NK cell activity are also reduced; and in vitro cytokine production by activated human mononuclear cells is affected.[8]

ADVERSE EFFECTS

Mycophenolate mofetil is generally well tolerated when used in autoimmune diseases such as RA. The most common side effects are gastrointestinal, such as nausea, vomiting, abdominal discomfort, and diarrhea. Nongastrointestinal side effects include fever, headache, skin rashes, back pain or tremor, but rarely require discontinuation of therapy. Rarer reported side effects include leukopenia and other cytopenias, cutaneous and noncutaneous malignancies, and pancreatitis.

CYCLOSPORINE AND TACROLIMUS (FK506)

Cyclosporine (Fig. 90.8) and tacrolimus (Fig. 90.9) are structurally similar drugs that have been widely used in solid organ transplantation as well as in immunological diseases. Cyclosporine has potent inhibitory effects in damping down the production of proinflammatory mediators such as IL-2 by immunocompetent cells, most importantly T cells. Cyclosporine acts through an association with a binding protein, cyclophilin, which produces a cyclosporine–cyclophilin complex. This complex is a binder of the serine/threonine

KEY CONCEPTS

MECHANISMS OF ACTION OF CYCLOSPORINE

>> Association with cyclophilin
>> Formation of Cyclosporine–cyclophilin complex
>> Binds calcineurin
>> Inactivates calcineurin
>> Regulatory proteins unable to translocate into nucleus
>> Transcription of proinflammatory genes affected

phosphatase known as calcineurin.[9] The binding and inactivation of calcineurin disrupts phosphorylation of regulatory proteins, for which NF-AT (nucleated factor of activated T cells) is a critical component. The result is the inability of these proteins to translocate into the nucleus, and the process of transcription of genes important for the promotion of the inflammatory process such as IL-2, which induces mitogenesis in activated T cells, cannot be effectively activated. Several other cytokines are affected, including interleukin-3, interleukin-6, transforming growth factor-β and interferon-γ. Tacrolimus works in a similar way, binding to another T cell-specific immunophilin, FK506-binding protein (FKBP) a tacrolimus–FKBP complex with resultant calcineurin inhibition.[10]

ADVERSE EFFECTS

Most patients taking long-term oral cyclosporine will experience a decrease in their glomerular filtration rate,[11] and this may lead to a rise in serum creatinine. Some of these may indeed progress to histologically proven nephropathy.[12] Nephrotoxicity has also been a concern during therapy with tacrolimus. Other adverse effects include infections, hepatotoxicity, gastrointestinal upset, rash, tremor, headache and insomnia.

◼ THALIDOMIDE ◼

Historically known primarily for its teratogenic effects, the drug thalidomide (α-[N-phthalimido] glutarimide) has more recently been recognized as a powerful immune modulator and anti-cancer drug. First synthesized in 1954, thalidomide became the drug of choice for pregnant women throughout much of the world for the treatment of morning sickness and nausea. Although initially thought to be completely safe, it soon became apparent that chronic use could cause peripheral neuropathy. More tragically, the drug was also later linked to an epidemic of limb and bowel malformations affecting thousands of children in over 46 nations, resulting in its removal from the world market by 1962.[13]

The serendipitous discovery of thalidomide as an effective anti-inflammatory therapy for erythema nodosum leprosum (ENL) in patients with lepromatous leprosy kept the drug from disappearing completely from the world's formularies. Over the years there were anecdotal reports attesting to thalidomide's efficacy in treating various inflammatory diseases, including Behçet disease, sarcoidosis, Crohn disease and other inflammatory disorders involving the skin and mucosal membranes.[14] In the early 1990s, the discovery that thalidomide was a modulator of cytokine production and blood vessel formation led to a upsurge of interest in its application in immune-mediated diseases, HIV-related conditions and cancer. Approval of thalidomide in the USA was given for the treatment of ENL in 1998 and multiple myeloma in 2005, thus making the drug also available for a multitude of off-label uses by physicians.[15]

PHARMACOKINETICS

Thalidomide is a synthetic derivative of glutamic acid, consisting of a glutarimide ring and a phthaloyl ring (Fig. 90.10).[16] Limited in water solubility, thalidomide is administered orally, with variable peak plasma concentrations from a single dose ranging from 3 to 6 hours, and plasma

Thalidomide

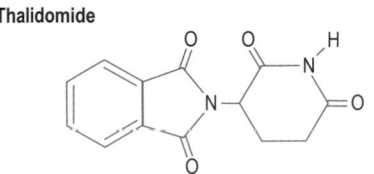

Fig. 90.10 Thalidomide – chemical structure.

◼ **KEY CONCEPTS**

PROPOSED MECHANISMS OF ACTION OF THALIDOMIDE

>> Tumor necrosis factor-α inhibition

>> T-lymphocyte co-stimulation

>> Angiogenesis inhibition

>> Activation of NK cell responses

>> Inhibition of cytokine-induced NF-κB activation

>> Inhibition of neutrophil and monocyte chemotaxis

>> Modulation of cell adhesion molecule expression

>> Inhibition of nitric oxide synthase

half-life between 5 and 14 hours, depending on formulation. Once exposed to an aqueous environment, thalidomide spontaneously and rapidly hydrolyzes into at least 12 hydrolysis products. Having no significant binding to plasma proteins, thalidomide has a large distribution volume and can be found in all bodily fluids, including milk and semen. Most of the absorbed dose is eliminated in the urine, with similar pharmacokinetics observed in renally impaired patients.

PROPOSED MECHANISMS OF ACTION

Despite continued interest in thalidomide over the past half century as a teratogen and immune modulator, its exact mechanism of action remains unclear. The marked species difference in biological effects has suggested that thalidomide may act as a prodrug for one of its hydrolysis products or metabolites. Indeed, although the drug itself is neither a mutagen nor directly toxic to cells, incubation of thalidomide together with liver homogenates or microsomes of rabbit origin produced toxic metabolites that were not found when rodent tissues were used, thereby providing one possible explanation for the species differences in susceptibility to thalidomide's teratogenic effects.

Potential mechanisms to explain thalidomide's biological effects are numerous, suggesting either an as yet undiscovered upstream molecular drug target or a multifaceted mechanism of action. For example, the drug has differential effects on cytokine production, depending on the cell type and stimulus studied.[17] Thalidomide is a broad inhibitor of proinflammatory molecules produced by endotoxin-stimulated monocytes that has been shown to occur by both enhanced mRNA degradation and suppression of NF-κB activation. However, when a T cell-specific stimulus is used, thalidomide acts through the CD28 pathway to exert a co-stimulatory or adjuvant effect on T-cell response and downstream Th1 immunity.[18] In addition, thalidomide has been shown to modulate NK cell numbers and activity, cell surface adhesion molecule expression, and nitric oxide synthesis.[19]

The identification of thalidomide as an *in vivo* inhibitor of fibroblast growth factor-induced angiogenesis (in the cornea micropocket rabbit model) led to a surge of interest in its use against cancer. In particular, thalidomide has been found effective in treating relapsed and refractory multiple myeloma.[20] Proposed mechanisms of action for thalidomide in this disease have included inhibitory effects on bone marrow stromal cell production of IL-6 and TNF-α, important cytokines driving the biology of multiple myeloma.[15] In addition, thalidomide has been shown *in vitro* to activate NK cells to lyse multiple myeloma cells. Potential mechanisms for its effects in solid tumors are less clear.

ADVERSE EFFECTS

Doses of thalidomide reported to be effective clinically range from as low as 25–50 mg/day in cutaneous lupus to 800 mg/day or more in oncology, with the average dosing range for most clinical uses between 100 and 400 mg/day. Adverse effects vary, partly according to dosing levels, but may also be disease specific (Table 90.4). Teratogenicity is the most serious complication, with the period of fetal development sensitive to thalidomide-induced teratogenicity occurring between gestational days 21 and 36. Fetal malformations have been reported with maternal exposure to a single 50 mg dose of the drug. The association of thalidomide with peripheral neuropathies that can be long lasting is another serious side effect that appears unrelated to dose or duration of drug exposure. Sedation, rash, dizziness and constipation are common, but usually self-limiting or clinically manageable. Less common complications include thromboembolism, dry mouth and skin, amenorrhea, neutropenia, bradycardia, weight gain and edema.[19]

THALIDOMIDE ANALOGS

The unique biological effects of thalidomide, coupled with its deleterious effects on fetal development and the nervous system, have driven investigators to develop safer thalidomide analogs with logs-fold more potency as immune modulators.[15, 17] Chemical manipulation of the structure of thalidomide has produced analogs that fall within one of two distinct categories, based on their immune-modulating effects. One group of analogs was noted to be effective inhibitors of endotoxin-induced production of IL-12 and TNF-α by monocytes, but had little effect on other endotoxin-stimulated cytokines. Later investigations revealed that this group achieved its immune-modulating effects through inhibition of phosphodiesterase IV (PDE-4), a well-described anti-inflammatory mechanism by which intracellular cAMP levels are increased. The second group was found, like the parent drug thalidomide, to be broad inhibitors of endotoxin-stimulated production of proinflammatory cytokines as well as having T-cell co-stimulatory effects, albeit having little effect on PDE-4. Currently, clinical trials of the PDE-4 inhibitors have been hampered by dose-limiting side effects, such as nausea and vomiting, common to other drugs of this class. Development of the thalidomide-like analogs has been more successful, resulting to date in the recent approval of lenalidomide (Fig. 90.11) in the USA for the treatment of myelodysplastic syndrome. Lenalidomide has been reported to have reduced sedation and neurotoxicity compared to thalidomide.[15] In addition, this analog has

Lenalidomide

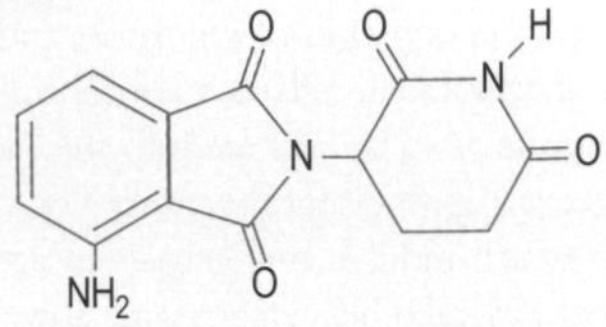

Fig. 90.11 Lenalidomide – chemical structure.

Imiquimod

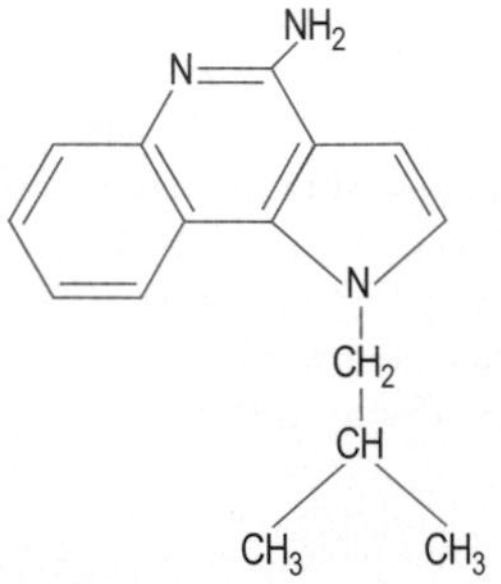

Fig. 90.12 Imiquimod – chemical structure.

been reported to lack teratogenicity in the New Zealand White rabbit, a model that is susceptible to thalidomide.

■ IMIQUIMOD ■

Imiquimod (Fig. 90.12) is an imidazoquinoline drug that is formulated as a dermal cream. It exerts its immune effects by activation of Toll-like receptor-7 and possesses both antiviral and anti-tumor activities.[21] The antiviral properties have been successfully exploited in the treatment of external genital warts, which are caused by infection with the human papillomavirus. Immune amplification responses are induced through stimulation of inflammatory cytokines, as reviewed extensively elsewhere.[22, 23] The production of interferon-α is stimulated, which suppresses the replication of viruses in infected keratinocytes. NK cell activity is also increased, partly through the induction of oligoadenylate synthase. The increase of dermal interferon-α transcript levels is both rapid and dramatic.[24] Other cytokines modulated by imiquimod include tumor necrosis factor-α and IL-12, peripheral blood monocytes being the principal cell type affected.[25, 26] The overall effect appears to be a shift from a Th2-cytokine towards a Th1-cytokine predominant profile. Other dermatological conditions where imiquimod has been found useful include actinic keratosis, herpes simplex, basal cell carcinoma and molluscum contagiosum.

ADVERSE EFFECTS

As this is a topical medication, local reactions at the site of application are the most commonly encountered adverse reaction. However, non-dermatological side effects such as fever, fatigue, myalgia and headache have also been described.

■ REFERENCES ■

1. Farber S, Diamond LK, Mercer RD, et al. Temporary remissions in acute leukemia in children produced by the folic acid antagonist, 4-aminopteroylglutamic acid (aminopterin). N Engl J Med 1948; 238: 787–793.

1a. Chan ES, Cronstein BN. Molecular action of methotrexate in inflammatory diseases. Arthritis Res 2002; 4: 266.

2. Cronstein BN, Naime D, Ostad E. The antiinflammatory mechanism of methotrexate. Increased adenosine release at inflamed sites diminishes leukocyte accumulation in an in vivo model of inflammation. J Clin Invest 1993; 92: 2675.

3. Baggott JE, Morgan SL, Sams WM, Linden J. Urinary adenosine and aminoimidazolecarboxamide excretion in methotrexate-treated patients with psoriasis. Arch Dermatol 1999; 135: 813.

4. Chan ES, Montesinos MC, Fernandez P, et al. Adenosine A(2A) receptors play a role in the pathogenesis of hepatic cirrhosis. Br J Pharmacol 2006; 148: 1144.

5. Amos RS, Pullar T, Bax DE, et al. Sulphasalazine for rheumatoid arthritis: toxicity in 774 patients monitored for one to 11 years. Br Med J (Clin Res Ed) 1986; 293: 420.

6. Kremer JM, Genovese MC, Cannon GW, et al. Concomitant leflunomide therapy in patients with active rheumatoid arthritis despite stable doses of methotrexate. A randomized, double-blind, placebo-controlled trial. Ann Intern Med 2002; 137: 726.

7. Weinblatt ME, Kremer JM, Coblyn JS, et al. Pharmacokinetics, safety, and efficacy of combination treatment with methotrexate and leflunomide in patients with active rheumatoid arthritis. Arthritis Rheum 1999; 42: 1322.

8. Nagy SE, Andersson JP, Andersson UG. Effect of mycophenolate mofetil (RS-61443) on cytokine production: inhibition of superantigen-induced cytokines. Immunopharmacology 1993; 26: 11.

9. Liu J, Farmer JD Jr, Lane WS, et al. Calcineurin is a common target of cyclophilin-Cyclosporine A and FKBP-FK506 complexes. Cell 1991; 66: 807.

10. Baughman G, Wiederrecht GJ, Campbell NF, et al. FKBP51, a novel T-cell-specific immunophilin capable of calcineurin inhibition. Mol Cell Biol 1995; 15: 4395.

11. Wilkinson A, Ross EA, Hawkins R, Danovitch G. Measurement of true glomerular filtration rate in renal transplant patients receiving Cyclosporine. Transplant Proc 1987; 19: 1739.

12. Mihatsch MJ, Antonovych T, Bohman SO, et al. Cyclosporine A nephropathy: standardization of the evaluation of kidney biopsies. Clin Nephrol 1994; 41: 23.

13. Stephens T, Brynner R. Dark remedy: the impact of thalidomide and its revival as a vital medicine. Cambridge: Perseus Publishing, 2001.

14. Koch HP. Thalidomide and congeners as anti-inflammatory agents. Prog Med Chem 1985; 22: 165.

15. Teo SK. Properties of thalidomide and its analogues: implications for anticancer therapy. Am Assoc Pharm Sci J 2005; 7: E14.

16. Teo SK, Colburn WA, Tracewell WG, et al. Clinical pharmacokinetics of thalidomide. Clin Pharmacokinet 2004; 43: 311.

17. Corral LG, Haslett PA, Muller GW, et al. Differential cytokine modulation and T cell activation by two distinct classes of thalidomide analogues that are potent inhibitors of TNF-alpha. J Immunol 1999; 163: 380.

18. LeBlanc R, Hideshima T, Catley LP, et al. Immunomodulatory drug costimulates T cells via the B7-CD28 pathway. Blood 2004; 103: 1787.

19. Wu JJ, Huang DB, Pang KR, et al. Thalidomide: dermatological indications, mechanisms of action and side-effects. Br J Dermatol 2005; 153: 254.

20. Kumar S, Rajkumar SV. Thalidomide and lenalidomide in the treatment of multiple myeloma. Eur J Cancer 2006; 42: 1612.

21. Hemmi H, Kaisho T, Takeuchi O, et al. Small anti-viral compounds activate immune cells via the TLR7 MyD88-dependent signaling pathway. Nature Immunol 2002; 3: 196.

22. Dahl MV. Imiquimod: an immune response modifier. J Am Acad Dermatol 2000; 43: S1.

23. Skinner RB Jr. Imiquimod. Dermatol Clin 2003; 21: 291.

24. Imbertson LM, Beaurline JM, Couture AM, et al. Cytokine induction in hairless mouse and rat skin after topical application of the immune response modifiers imiquimod and S-28463. J Invest Dermatol 1998; 110: 734.

25. Gibson SJ, Imbertson LM, Wagner TL, et al. Cellular requirements for cytokine production in response to the immunomodulators imiquimod and S-27609. J Interferon Cytokine Res 1995; 15: 537.

26. Tyring S. Imiquimod applied topically: A novel immune response modifier. Skin Ther Lett 2001; 6: 1.

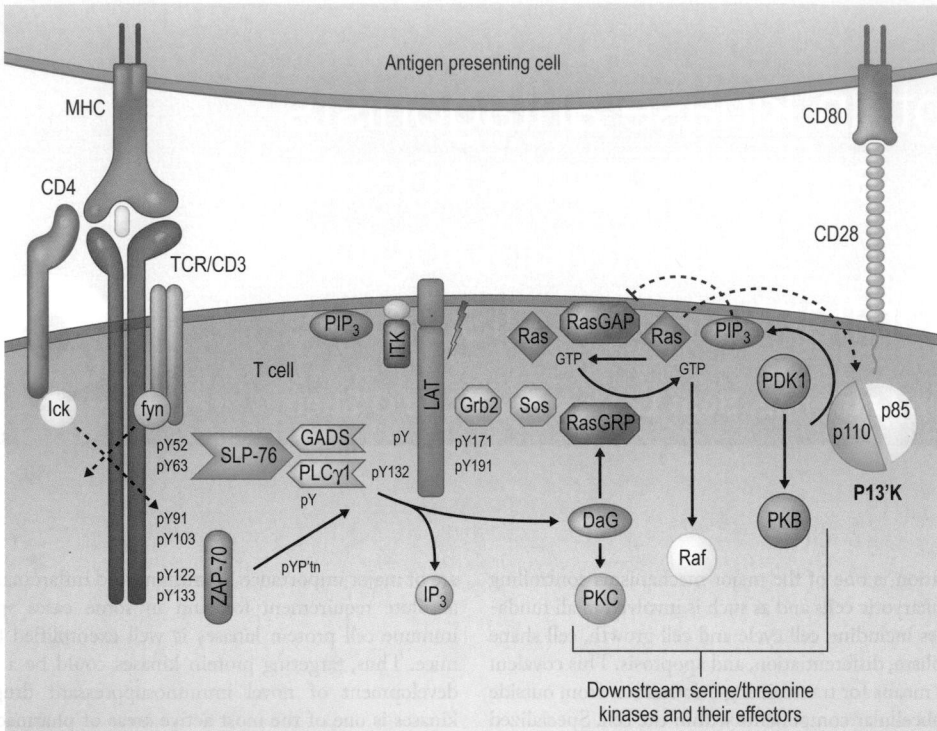

Fig. 91.1 Proximal signaling events in response to T-cell receptor activation by an antigen-presenting cell. Tyrosine and lipid kinases are indicated in red, serine/threonine kinases indicated in blue.

substrate; and (3) the transfer of the γ-phosphate from ATP or GTP to the protein substrate. Despite the huge number of serine/threonine and tyrosine kinases, there is evidence of a common ancestor and this is reflected in structural similarities, particularly in the active (ATP-bound) confirmation. The major kinase domains of all typical protein kinases consist of two lobes (N-lobe and C-lobe) that surround the nucleotide binding site[1] (Fig. 91.2). The smaller N-lobe consists of a cluster of β-pleated sheets with a single α-helix. The larger C-lobe is made up of α-helices. Within the C-lobe lies the substrate-binding site, typically a groove on the surface. A hinge region connects the two lobes. The hinge, together with two loops emerging from each lobe, forms the ATP binding pocket: the primary target for most kinase inhibitors. In many protein kinases a loop emerging from the C-lobe must be phosphorylated in order for the kinase to be fully active (Fig. 91.2). This is known as the activation loop. Substrates of PTKs often include the activation loop of downstream kinases, creating signaling cascades of proteins that in turn phosphorylate each other; examples include the MAPKs (Fig. 91.3).

■ A SHORT HISTORY OF THE FIRST-GENERATION KINASE INHIBITORS ■

Given that protein kinases bind ATP, the notion that therapeutically useful kinase inhibitors could be generated initially met with some skepticism. First, as there are more than 500 human kinases, many of which serve critical cellular functions, would it really be possible to attain the

PROTEIN KINASE SUPERFAMILIES (1.6% OF THE GENOME)

>> Protein tyrosine kinases (90 members, e.g., Jak3)

>> Protein serine/threonine kinases (400 members)

>> AGC kinase family (e.g., protein kinase B/Akt)

>> CAMK kinase family (e.g., calmodulin-dependent kinase)

>> CMGC kinase family (e.g., MAP kinases: ERK, JNK, p38)

>> STE kinase family (e.g., MAPKK kinases, MAPK kinases)

>> TKL kinase family (e.g., IRAK)

>> Others: casein kinase family, GYC kinase family, IKK family

specificity needed? Second, protein kinases are not the only kinases – there are lipid kinases and nucleotide kinases, in addition to numerous other types of ATP-binding proteins. Third, despite the many potential ways of designing a small-molecule kinase inhibitor, in practice the existing successful inhibitors all work by sitting within the ATP-binding pocket.[2] *A priori*, then, one might conclude that it would be impossible to generate an antagonist that did not target some other essential ATP-dependent process. Fortunately, though, this dismal view does not reflect reality.

Table 91.1 The common γ chain receptor family of cytokine receptors

Cytokine receptor	IL-2R	IL-4R	IL-7R	IL-9R	IL-15R	IL-21R
Functions	Control of peripheral self tolerance (mice)	Regulation of B-cell function (in concert with IL-21 and IL-25)	Thymocyte survival and development factor	Goblet-cell hyperplasia	CD8+ memory T-cell survival and proliferation factor	T- and B-cell proliferation factor
	Development and maintenance of T-regulatory cells	Immunoglobulin class switching	Peripheral T-cell survival factor. Mediates homeostatic reconstitution of lymphopenic animals	Mucus production	Peripheral T-cell survival factor. Mediates homeostatic reconstitution of lymphopenic animals	Regulates immunoglobulin production (with IL-4)
	Differentiation of helper and cytotoxic T cells	Differentiation of helper T cells (Th2 lineage)	B-cell progenitor survival factor (mice)		NK cell development, differentiation, and survival factor	NK cell proliferation and activation factor
	In vitro expansion and differentiation of antigen-selected T and NK cells	Co-stimulant for growth in T, B, and mast cells				Differentiation of helper T cells (Th17 lineage)
		Inhibition of Th1 differentiation and macrophage activation				
Downstream signaling pathways	PI3K, Ras, MAPK, STAT1, 3, 5	PI3K, Ras MAPK, STAT 5, 6	PI3K, STAT(1), (3), 5	PI3K, Ras MAPK, STAT1, 3, (5)	PI3K, Ras MAPK, STAT1, 3, 5	PI3K, Ras MAPK, STAT1, 3,(5)

IL, interleukin; MAPK, mitogen activated protein kinases; NK, natural killer.

Table 91.2 The Jak family of tyrosine kinases

Gene	Phenotype associated with gene deletion or mutation	Associated receptor
Jak1	Perinatal lethality, block in thymocyte development	Many, including IL-7R and IFN receptors
Jak2	Embryonic lethality due to anemia	Many, including the Epo receptor
Jak3	T, B, NK-cell lymphopenia, SCID phenotype	Common γ-chain receptor
Tyk2	Failure to clear *Toxoplasma*, reduced arthritis	Many, including the IL-12/23 receptor and the IFN α receptor

IFN, interferon; IL, interleukin; Jak, Janus kinase; NK, natural killer; SCID, severe combined immunodeficiency.

Table 91.3 Selected kinase inhibitors and related drugs

Mechanism	Compound	Kinase inhibited	Comments
Direct binding to the kinase	Imatinib	KIT, PDGFR, and Bcr-Abl	Licensed for the treatment of CML, eosinophilic leukemia and gastric stromal tumors. Under evaluation in multiple types of cancer and in combination with other cancer drugs
	Erlotonib	VEGFR-2 and EGFR tyrosine kinases	In phase III trials for treatment of advanced nonsmall-cell lung cancer.10/05: Granted orphan drug designation by the FDA for treatment of certain rare forms of thyroid cancer. Erlotonib is in phase II development for treatment of medullary thyroid cancer. Also in clinical development for treatment of additional cancers
	Sorafenib	Dual specific inhibitor blocking both tyrosine and serine / threonine kinases including: RAF kinase, VEGFR-2, VEGFR-3, PDGFR-B, KIT, and FLT-3	FDA-approved for treatment of advanced renal cell carcinoma.Also being developed for treatment of additional cancers. Phase III trial in nonsmall-cell lung cancer planned
	Dasatinib	Multiple Src family tyrosine kinases, including BCR-Abl	Filed for approval for treatment of adult CML and Philadelphia chromosome-positive ALL
	Lestaurtinib	FLT3 and Trk	In phase II clinical trials for treatment of AML patients who have an FLT3-activating mutation at first relapse from standard induction chemotherapy
	Lapatinib	ErbB-2 and EGFR kinases	For treatment of breast cancer. Also in development for treatment of renal, gastric, and head and neck cancers
	Sunitinib	Inhibits multiple RTKs including PDGFR3-α, PDGFR-β, VEGFR1 VEGFR2, VEGFR3, Kit, FLT3, CSF-1R, and RET	For treatment of gastrointestinal stromal tumor after disease progression on or intolerance of imatinib mesylate, and for treatment of advanced renal cell carcinoma
	CP-690 550	Jak3	Efficacy shown in animal models of solid-organ transplantation and chronic graft-versus-host disease Phase II trials starting in the treatment of rheumatoid arthritis
	SCIO 469	p38 MAPK	Phase II trials ongoing in rheumatoid arthritis and myeloma
	VX-702		Phase II trials ongoing in rheumatoid arthritis
Indirect binding to kinase	Sirolimus (Rapamycin)	mTOR	Licensed for use in solid-organ and bone marrow transplantation
	Temsirolimus		Phase II clinical trials in the management of mantle-cell lymphoma. A 38% response rate has been reported Small benefit in advanced renal cell carcinoma – currently being fast-tracked by FDA Phase II clinical trials ongoing in multiple sclerosis and rheumatoid arthritis
	Everolimus		Licensed for use with cyclosporine in cardiac and renal transplantation. Clinical trials are assessing its use in rheumatoid arthritis
Monoclonal antibodies binding to receptor tyrosine kinases	Trastuzumab	EGFR-2	Licensed for use in HER2/neu-positive breast carcinoma
	Pertuzumab		Prevents dimerization of the receptor – undergoing phase I/II studies in solid tumors
	Cetuximab	EGFR	Licensed for use in relapsed colorectal cancer in combination with traditional chemotherapy
	Bevacizumab	VEGF – prevents binding to its receptor (FLT-1)	
Other indirect inhibitors of kinase signaling pathways	Tipifarnib	Farnesyl transferase (Ras – MAPK)	Fasnylation inhibitor: inhibits formation of farnesylated signaling proteins (Ras). Phase II clinical trials for MDS/AML

The stem '-inib' denotes a tyrosine kinase inhibitor; '-rolimus' denotes a macrolide immunosupressant. ALL, acute lymphoblastic leukemia; AML, acute myeloid leukemia; CML, chronic myeloid leukemia; EGFR, epidermal growth factor receptor; FDA, Food and Drug Administration; MDS, myelodysplatic syndrome; PDGFR, platelet-derived growth factor receptor; VEGFR,

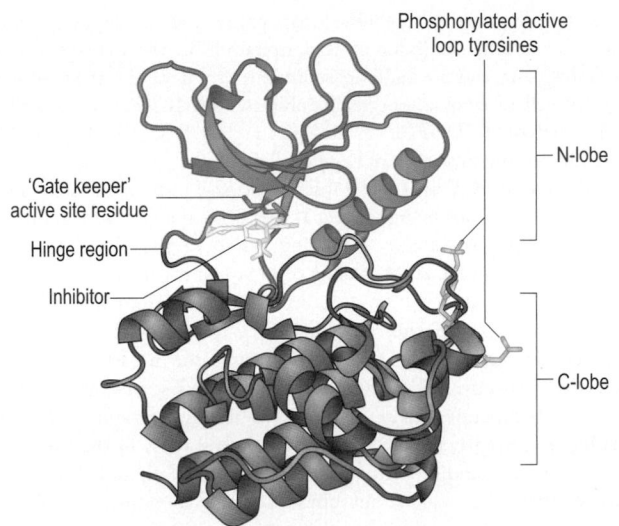

Fig. 91.2 Crystal structure of the Jak3 kinase domain complexed with staurosporine (pdb accession code 1YVJ). This structure captures the active conformation of Jak3 with both active-loop tyrosine residues phosphorylated (green). The molecule can be described in two halves, with the N-terminal lobe presented in blue and the C terminal domain in red. These are linked by a hinge region that forms part of the active site. Highlighted in magenta within the active site is the gatekeeper residue. Bound within this site is an analogue of the inhibitor staurosporine, and its proximity to the gatekeeper residue highlights why this residue and this region are critical for the specificity of inhibitors for individual protein kinases.

IMATINIB AND OTHER FIRST-GENERATION PROTEIN TYROSINE KINASES INHIBITORS

The first Food and Drug Administration (FDA)-approved protein kinase inhibitor is imatinib (Table 91.3). The mutated form of the Abl tyrosine kinase, BCR-Abl, represents a fusion protein that is the result of a chromosomal translocation (Philadelphia chromosome) observed in patients with chronic myeloid leukemia (CML).[3] The pathognomonic presence of BCR-Abl in CML has led to it becoming one of the most intensively studied PTKs. The fusion protein consists of an oligomerization domain, a plecstrin homology (PH) domain and a Dbl/cdc24 guanine nucleotide exchange factor homology domain that contains the N-terminal breakpoint cluster region (BCR) of the protein. The Abl half of the fusion protein contains a tyrosine kinase domain, a Src homology 2 (SH2) domain, and a DNA-binding domain together with nuclear localization and nuclear export motifs. The Abl kinase is constitutively active within the fusion protein and has been implicated in initiating numerous signaling pathways that mediate cell survival and proliferation. In view of this and the essential requirement for BCR-Abl kinase activity in CML, it was thought to be an ideal target for the generation of a selective kinase inhibitor despite the aforementioned caveats with targeting protein kinases. As predicted, imatinib has revolutionized the treatment of CML. This inhibitor has been remarkably successful in arresting the progression of the disease, but is also well tolerated with minimal side effects.

The epidermal growth factor receptor (EGFR) is another intensively studied PTK which is highly expressed and/or frequently mutated in cancers. It too has been considered a good therapeutic target and gefitonib was the first selective EGFR inhibitor. Gefitonib was not efficacious in a nonsmall-cell lung cancer trial; however, erolotinib, another EGFR inhibitor, has been approved by the FDA for the treatment of pancreatic and nonsmall-cell lung cancer.

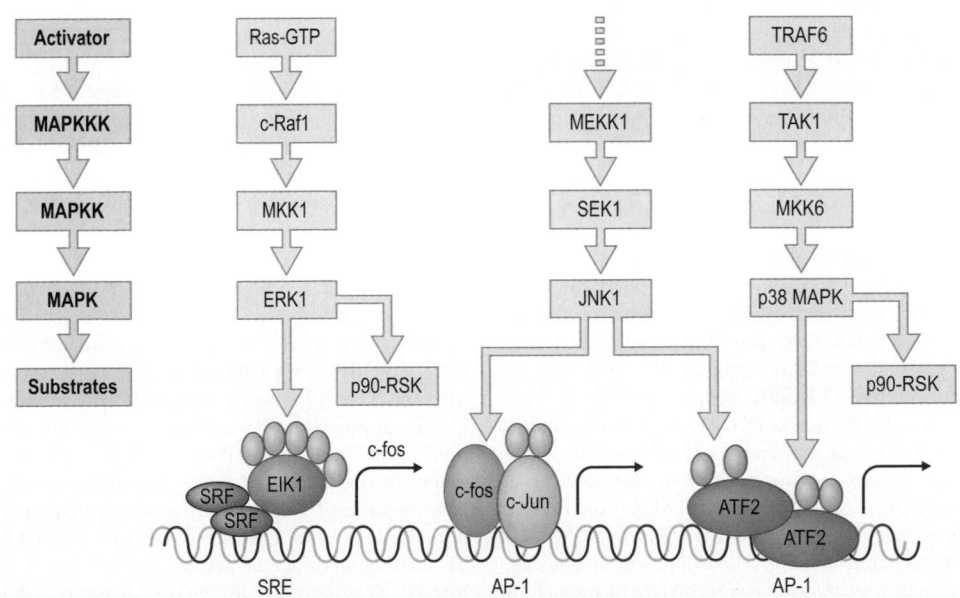

Fig. 91.3 A summary of the mitogen activated protein kinases (MAPK) signal transduction pathways. Examples of receptors that activate Ras include the interleukin-2 (IL-2) receptor and T-cell receptor; examples of receptors that activate TRAF6 include the IL-1 receptor.

While conservation of the kinase ATP-binding pocket has posed a potential problem for designing kinase inhibitors, in practice this has not happened for a number of reasons. Although different kinases are structurally similar in an active ATP-bound confirmation, this is not so in the inactive confirmation – a form that is exploited by many selective inhibitors.[4] The ATP-binding region is made up of six polar amino acid residues that are invariant across whole families of kinases; similarly, there are a number of lipophilic residues that are highly conserved, but within this critical region lies an amino acid with an amide carbonyl that binds to N-6 of adenine in the active confirmation. The side chain of this amino acid sticks into the reaction pocket in the inactive state and for this reason is referred to as the 'gatekeeper' residue. As the side chain is not involved in direct ATP binding, it varies across kinases, and variation of this gatekeeper residue is exploited by a number of inhibitors that are able to bind the inactive confirmation of specific kinases. In the case of Abl kinase the gatekeeper residue is threonine, which binds directly to a methyl group of the phenyl ring of the Abl kinase inhibitor imatinib.[4] Across the collective kinase superfamily almost any amino acid can appear as the gatekeeper, although in practice it is typically a bulky nonpolar residue (methionine, tyrosine, phenylalanine, lysine). Clearly, as more detailed structural information emerges from the many protein kinases, capitalizing upon subtle differences in structure, in principle, would be expected to improve potency and specificity. For instance, cyclin-dependent kinase 2 (CDK2) contains an additional pocket on its C-lobe next to the ATP-binding pocket.[5] A number of CDK2-specific inhibitors exploit this by binding to both pockets.

Of further structural significance is the emergence of tumor drug resistance in response to the chronic use of protein kinase inhibitors. Mutant forms of BCR-Abl, Kit, and EGFR have been associated with loss of drug activity and disease relapse. Interestingly, one of the most common sites of mutation is the otherwise conserved gatekeeper residue. Although a major problem in the treatment of malignancy, this is less likely to be an issue in the treatment of autoimmune disease.

One of the surprises that has emerged regarding imatinib is that, although it was originally thought to be a highly specific inhibitor for Abl kinase, in reality it does have activity against other PTKs.[6] Consequently, it has been found to be useful in the treatment of other tumors and this has led to its successful use in the treatment of gastrointestinal stromal tumor, and hypereosinophilic syndrome through its effects on Kit[7] and platelet-derived growth factor receptor (PDGFR)-FIPIL1[8] kinases respectively. In spite of efforts to develop highly specific kinase inhibitors, there is increasing evidence that a partial inhibition of multiple kinases is efficacious and is potentially less toxic than originally feared. One such broad-spectrum kinase inhibitor is the recently FDA-approved inhibitor sorafenib for use in advanced renal cancer. Sorafenib inhibits the serine/threonine kinase Raf, as well as RTKs, including PDGFR, vascular endothelial growth factor receptor (VEGFR), Kit, and FLT-3.

Many receptors, including RTK, such as EGFR and PDGFR, activate the MAPK signaling pathway via the small p21 GTPase Ras. The MAPK family consists of numerous serine/threonine kinases that can be crudely divided into three groups: (1) the MAPKs themselves; (2) kinases that phosphorylate the MAPKs, the MAPK kinases (MKKs); and (3) the MKK kinases (MKKKs) (Fig. 91.3). Not only is Ras activated by a number of growth factors, but it is also frequently mutated in cancers. Ras activation leads to the activation of the MKKK, Raf. This is turn phosphorylates the MKK, MEK which subsequently phosphorylates and activates the MAPKs ERK1 and 2. Two small-molecule inhibitors of this serine/threonine kinase pathway are undergoing clinical trials: the farsenyl inhibitor of Ras, tipifarnib, in the management of myelodysplasia, and the multikinase inhibitor sorafenib for the treatment of renal cell carcinoma. Sorafenib inhibits the MKKK Raf, as well as RTKs, including PDGFR, VEGFR, Kit, and FLT-3, and is approved by the FDA for the treatment of hepatocellular and renal carcinoma.

Although only four small-molecule kinase inhibitors are FDA-approved for various malignancies at this time, many other candidates against a range of kinases are being tested in the clinic presently. Additionally, though, another class of kinase antagonists exists. These are antibodies that are directed against extracellular domains of RTKs. These include cetuximab, panitumumab, trastuzumab ranibizumab and bevacizumab, which are directed against the EGFR, Her2/Neu, VEGFR, respectively. Pertuzumab, one of the first in a new class of targeted therapeutic agents known as heterodimerization inhibitors (HDIs), is currently being evaluated in clinical trials in the treatment of lung, ovarian, and prostate cancer. It has passed phase I studies that have confirmed its safety but phase II trials in nonsmall-cell lung cancer have to date been disappointing.[9]

In summary, oncology studies have demonstrated unequivocally the safety and efficacy of inhibiting kinases either through small molecules or, in the case of RTKs, with antibodies.

■ TARGETING IMMUNE CELL KINASES ■

The development of therapeutically useful kinase inhibitors for the treatment of immune and inflammatory disease is also an area of intensive research. Although at present there is only one class of kinase inhibitors approved by the FDA for the treatment of immune-mediated disease, the expectation is that many more will follow.

mTOR INHIBITORS

As its name suggests, mammalian target of rapamycin (mTOR) can be inhibited by the macrolide, rapamycin, now licensed for use against graft rejection as the drug sirolimus[10] (Fig. 91.4). mTOR is a critical link in coupling cell growth stimuli with cell cycle progression. It is activated by a number of growth factor receptors, including the interleukin-2 (IL-2) receptor in T cells. Many signaling pathways link growth factor receptors with activation of mTOR, including the AMP-dependant kinase (AMPK), phosphatidyl inositol 3' kinase (PI3'K)[11], and MAPK pathways (discussed below) (Fig. 91.4). mTOR promotes cell growth by activation of p70 S6K1 and inactivation of 4EBP-1.[12] Critical to cell growth is the translation of new protein. This process is initiated by the multi-subunit complex eIF4F; unphosphorylated 4EBP-1 represses the eIF4F complex by binding to one of the subunits, eIF4E. mTOR phosphorylates and inactivates 4EBP-1, allowing the initiation of protein translation. Maintenance of protein translation is further regulated by the phosphorylation of the 40S ribosomal subunit S6. Once phosphorylated, S6 can be recruited to actively translating polysomes; this is performed by the serine/threonine kinase p70 S6K1, which is itself phosphorylated and activated by mTOR.

Sirolimus does not inhibit mTOR by direct binding to the ATP-binding pocket but acts indirectly, associating with FK506-binding

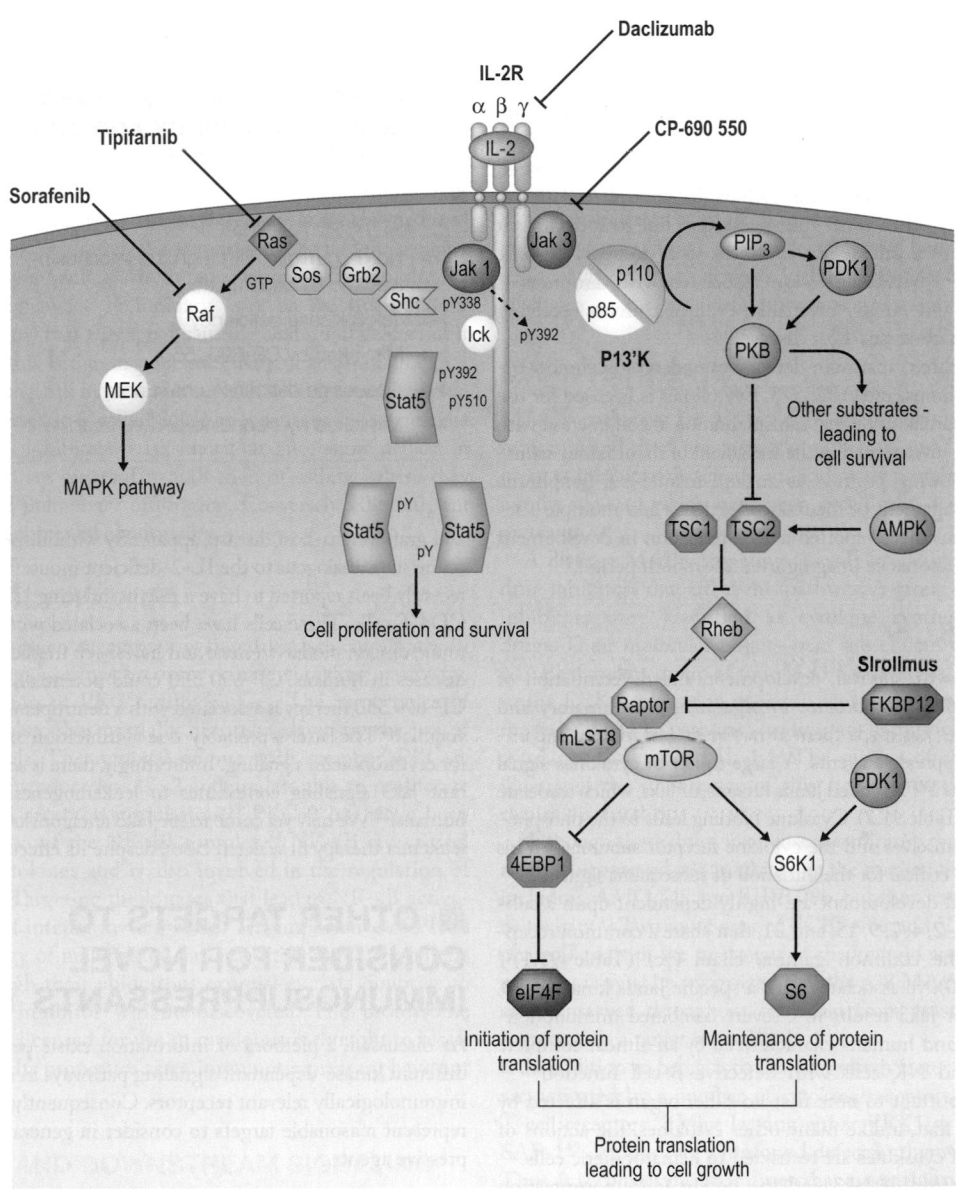

Fig. 91.4 Signal transduction pathways stemming from the interleukin-2 receptor in T cells culminating in the activation of the mTOR serine/threonine kinase. Tyrosine kinases are indicated in red and serine/threonine kinases are indicated in blue.

protein 12 (FKBP12). This in turn inhibits the kinase complex made up of mTOR, mLST8, and raptor (mTORC1).[13] Sirolimus was hoped to be a potent anticancer drug but has met with limited success in this regard. In contrast it has been successfully used as an immunosuppressant typically as part of a combination regimen for allograft rejection prophylaxis.

In a US phase III study sirolimus was compared with azathioprine in patients receiving prednisolone and cyclosporine for renal graft rejection prophylaxis.[14] After 6 months there was a 17% incidence of graft failure in the sirolimus group and a 32% incidence in the azathioprine group, although after 12 months there was no significant difference between the two groups.[14] Further studies have compared sirolimus with cyclosporine in conjunction with mycophenolate and prednisolone in renal transplantation and generally found equivalence.[15] There is more limited experience with sirolimus in transplantation of other solid organs, although it is being used in heart, lung, liver, and pediatric intestinal transplantation. Finally, sirolimus is being used as a second-line agent in the treatment of graft-versus-host disease in bone marrow transplantation.[16]

In view of the ubiquitous expression of mTOR and its role in protein translation, it is not surprising that sirolimus would be associated with varied side effects; these include hyperlipidemia, hypertriglyceridemia, myelosuppression, and delayed wound healing.[17] There is some evidence

THERAPEUTIC CONCEPTS

MECHANISMS OF KINASE INHIBITOR SPECIFICITY

➤➤ Gatekeeper residue within the kinase reaction pocket
  e.g., Imatinib binding to Abl kinase

➤➤ Unique subsidiary binding pockets near the kinase reaction pocket
  e.g., Cyclin-dependent kinase 2

➤➤ Specific protein-binding partners that can be blocked
  e.g., Sirolimus/FKBP12 inhibition of the mTOR–mLST8–Raptor complex

➤➤ Inhibition of kinase activation by upstream signaling
  e.g., Inhibition of Ras-dependent kinases by tipifarnib

disease. Clinical trials are assessing its efficacy in the treatment of multiple sclerosis and Crohn's disease.

CONCLUSION

The success of the anti-cancer BCR-Abl inhibitor imatinib and the immunosuppressive mTOR inhibitor sirolimus has placed the protein kinases center stage as targets of future drug discovery. A primary focus of efforts by drug companies is the development of novel anti-cancer drugs, but as we have seen with sirolimus, many of the kinases central to tumor cell proliferation are also important in T-cell activation. Conversely, inhibition of Jak3 could potentially be used in the treatment of leukemia. Either way, we are likely to see a number of novel immunosuppressants appear both serendipitously and intentionally as new protein kinase inhibitors are developed for a wide range of debilitating illnesses.

REFERENCES

1. Hanks SK, Quinn AM, Hunter T. The protein kinase family: conserved features and deduced phylogeny of the catalytic domains. Science 1988; 241: 42–52.

2. Noble ME, Endicott JA, Johnson LN. Protein kinase inhibitors: insights into drug design from structure. Science 2004; 303: 1800–1805.

3. Sawyers CL. Chronic myeloid leukemia. N Engl J Med 1999; 340: 1330–1340.

4. Schindler T, Bornmann W, Pellicena P, et al. Structural mechanism for STI-571 inhibition of abelson tyrosine kinase. Science 2000; 289: 1938–1942.

5. Davies TG, Pratt DJ, Endicott JA, et al. Structure-based design of cyclin-dependent kinase inhibitors. Pharmacol Ther 2002; 93: 125–133.

6. Buchdunger E, Cioffi CL, Law N, et al. Abl protein-tyrosine kinase inhibitor STI571 inhibits in vitro signal transduction mediated by c-kit and platelet-derived growth factor receptors. J Pharmacol Exp Ther 2000; 295: 139–145.

7. Demetri GD, von MM, Blanke CD, et al. Efficacy and safety of imatinib mesylate in advanced gastrointestinal stromal tumors. N Engl J Med 2002; 347: 472–480.

8. Cools J, DeAngelo DJ, Gotlib J, et al. A tyrosine kinase created by fusion of the PDGFRA and FIP1L1 genes as a therapeutic target of imatinib in idiopathic hypereosinophilic syndrome. N Engl J Med 2003; 348: 1201–1214.

9. Johnson BE, Janne PA. Rationale for a phase II trial of pertuzumab, a HER-2 dimerization inhibitor, in patients with non-small cell lung cancer. Clin Cancer Res 2006; 12: 4436s–4440s.

10. Camardo J. The Rapamune era of immunosuppression 2003 the journey from the laboratory to clinical transplantation. Transplant Proc 2003; 35: 18S–24S.

11. Tee AR, Fingar DC, Manning BD, et al. Tuberous sclerosis complex-1 and -2 gene products function together to inhibit mammalian target of rapamycin (mTOR)-mediated downstream signaling. Proc Natl Acad Sci USA 2002; 99: 13571–13576.

12. Easton JB, Kurmasheva RT, Houghton PJ. IRS-1: auditing the effectiveness of mTOR inhibitors. Cancer Cell 2006; 9: 153–155.

13. Harris TE, Lawrence JC Jr. TOR signaling. Sci STKE 2003: 15.

14. Kahan BD. Efficacy of sirolimus compared with azathioprine for reduction of acute renal allograft rejection: a randomised multicentre study. The Rapamune US Study Group. Lancet 2000; 356: 194–202.

15. Kreis H, Cisterne JM, Land W, et al. Sirolimus in association with mycophenolate mofetil induction for the prevention of acute graft rejection in renal allograft recipients. Transplantation 2000; 69: 1252–1260.

16. Perez-Simon JA, Sanchez-Abarca I, ez-Campelo M, et al. Chronic graft-versus-host disease: pathogenesis and clinical management. Drugs 2006; 66: 1041–1057.

17. Murgia MG, Jordan S, Kahan BD. The side effect profile of sirolimus: a phase I study in quiescent cyclosporine-prednisone-treated renal transplant patients. Kidney Int 1996; 49: 209–216.

18. Kobashigawa JA, Miller LW, Russell SD, et al. Tacrolimus with mycophenolate mofetil (MMF) or sirolimus vs. cyclosporine with MMF in cardiac transplant patients: 1-year report. Am J Transplant 2006; 6: 1377–1386.

19. Sennesael JJ, Bosmans JL, Bogers JP, et al. Conversion from cyclosporine to sirolimus in stable renal transplant recipients. Transplantation 2005; 80: 1578–1585.

20. Witzig TE. Current treatment approaches for mantle-cell lymphoma. J Clin Oncol 2005; 23: 6409–6414.

21. Kappos L, Barkhof F, Desmet A, et al. The effect of oral temsirolimus on new magnetic resonance imaging scan lesions, brain atropy, and the number of relapses in multiple sclerosis: results from a randomized, controlled clinical trial. J Neurol 2005; 252: S46 (abstract).

22. Pesu M, Candotti F, Husa M, et al. Jak3, severe combined immunodeficiency, and a new class of immunosuppressive drugs. Immunol Rev 2005; 203: 127–142.

23. Yamaoka K, Saharinen P, Pesu M, et al. The Janus kinases (Jaks). Genome Biol 2004; 5: 253.

24. Vosshenrich CA, Di Santo JP. Interleukin signaling. Curr Biol 2002; 12: R760–R763.

25. Buckley RH, Schiff RI, Schiff SE, et al. Human severe combined immunodeficiency: genetic, phenotypic, and functional diversity in one hundred eight infants. J Pediatr 1997; 130: 378–387.

26. Borie DC, Changelian PS, Larson MJ, et al. Immunosuppression by the JAK3 inhibitor CP-690,550 delays rejection and significantly prolongs kidney allograft survival in nonhuman primates. Transplantation 2005; 79: 791–801.

27. Paniagua R, Si MS, Flores MG, et al. Effects of JAK3 inhibition with CP-690,550 on immune cell populations and their functions in nonhuman primate recipients of kidney allografts. Transplantation 2005; 80: 1283–1292.

28. Wolff D, Roessler V, Steiner B, et al. Treatment of steroid-resistant acute graft-versus-host disease with daclizumab and etanercept. Bone Marrow Transplant 2005; 35: 1003–1010.

29. Walters DK, Mercher T, Gu TL, et al. Activating alleles of JAK3 in acute megakaryoblastic leukemia. Cancer Cell 2006; 10: 65–75.

30. Orchard J, Ibbotson R, Best G, et al. ZAP-70 in B cell malignancies. Leuk Lymphoma 2005; 46: 1689–1698.

31. Gilbert C, Levasseur S, Desaulniers P, et al. Chemotactic factor-induced recruitment and activation of Tec family kinases in human neutrophils. II. Effects of LFM-A13, a specific Btk inhibitor. J Immunol 2003; 170: 5235–5243.

32. Schwartzberg PL, Finkelstein LD, Readinger JA. TEC-family kinases: regulators of T-helper-cell differentiation. Nat Rev Immunol 2005; 5: 284–295.

33. Pfeifhofer C, Kofler K, Gruber T, et al. Protein kinase C theta affects Ca²⁺ mobilization and NFAT cell activation in primary mouse T cells. J Exp Med 2003; 197: 1525–1535.

34. Manicassamy S, Gupta S, Sun ZM. Selective function of PKC-theta in T cells. Cell Mol Immunol 2006; 3: 263–270.

35. Okkenhaug K, Vanhaesebroeck B. PI3K in lymphocyte development, differentiation and activation. Nat Rev Immunol 2003; 3: 317–330.

36. Walker EH, Pacold ME, Perisic O, et al. Structural determinants of phosphoinositide 3-kinase inhibition by wortmannin, LY294002, quercetin, myricetin, and staurosporine. Mol Cell 2000; 6: 909–919.

37. Vanhaesebroeck B, Leevers SJ, Ahmadi K, et al. Synthesis and function of 3-phosphorylated inositol lipids. Annu Rev Biochem 2001; 70: 535–602.

38. Hirsch E, Katanaev VL, Garlanda C, et al. Central role for G protein-coupled phosphoinositide 3-kinase gamma in inflammation. Science 2000; 287: 1049–1053.

39. Camps M, Ruckle T, Ji H, et al. Blockade of PI3Kgamma suppresses joint inflammation and damage in mouse models of rheumatoid arthritis. Nat Med 2005; 11: 936–943.

40. Mora A, Komander D, van Aalten DM, et al. PDK1, the master regulator of AGC kinase signal transduction. Semin Cell Dev Biol 2004; 15: 161–170.

41. Hinton HJ, Alessi DR, Cantrell DA. The serine kinase phosphoinositide-dependent kinase 1 (PDK1) regulates T cell development. Nat Immunol 2004; 5: 539–545.

42. Braddock M, Quinn A. Targeting IL-1 in inflammatory disease: new opportunities for therapeutic intervention. Nat Rev Drug Discov 2004; 3: 330–339.

43. Lee MR. Dominguez C. MAP kinase p38 inhibitors: clinical results and an intimate look at their interactions with p38alpha protein. Curr Med Chem 2005; 12: 2979–2994.

44. Genot E, Cantrell DA. Ras regulation and function in lymphocytes. Curr Opin Immunol 2000; 12: 289–294.

45. Costello PS, Nicolas RH, Watanabe Y, et al. Ternary complex factor SAP-1 is required for Erk-mediated thymocyte positive selection. Nat Immunol 2004; 5: 289–298.

humans, as well as the strong discovery stimulus provided by ongoing efforts to develop new vaccines for major infectious diseases for which vaccines are not currently available.

Vaccine development today faces a number of significant challenges. There exist tremendous public health needs to address major well-known pandemic diseases, including acquired immunodeficiency syndrome (AIDS), tuberculosis, and malaria, for which no vaccines currently exist and for which natural immunity does not provide a helpful guide for vaccine development. Furthermore, there exists a need to confront effectively newly emerging and re-emerging diseases, ranging from the well-known, but constantly changing, threats from influenza pandemics to the appearance of previously unknown zoonotic infections such as the coronavirus that causes severe acute respiratory syndrome (SARS). With changes in population density, mobility, and social constructs, along with alterations in the global climate, ecological circumstances, and the proximity of humans to animal reservoirs for previously confined infectious agents, the concept of new infectious agents entering human populations and spreading rapidly around the world is no longer novel. In confronting prevalent or newly emerging diseases, vaccines are looked to as the most promising line of defense. However, the speed at which new infectious disease threats have been shown to emerge and spread, and the fact that the pathogens that now need to be confronted may display tremendous genetic variability (e.g., human immunodeficiency virus (HIV)) or an identity that cannot be predicted in advance (e.g., avian influenza or agents like SARS) places unprecedented demands on the vaccine development process.

In addition to these new challenges, there remain unmet needs in the derivation of vaccines that can achieve the greatest public health benefit. These needs include the development of new ways to achieve more effective vaccine-elicited immune responses in neonates whose immune systems are immature (or are impacted by maternal antibodies) (Chapter 32) and in the elderly whose immune system function may be waning as a result of immune senescence (Chapter 33). Fortunately, the scientific foundation provided by basic and applied immunology and the use of new methods for pathogen identification, antigen discovery, vaccine production, adjuvant development, and novel vector derivation afford important opportunities for vaccine development and additionally present the possibility of improving on natural immunity.

Success in vaccine development will be predicated on continuing the historical synergy between advances in vaccine technology and basic immunologic discovery. Toward that end, this chapter focuses on preventive vaccines for infectious diseases and how they are developed. Although current routine vaccine recommendations are reviewed, given the active state of new vaccine introduction and evolving vaccine recommendations, as well as differences in recommendations in different countries, readers are encouraged to refer to up-to-date national resources for the most current information. While vaccine approaches are being actively explored to modify beneficially malignant and immunologic diseases (autoimmunity and allergy), these are beyond the scope of the current discussion.

■ IMPACT OF VACCINATION PROGRAMS ■

Unlike other medical interventions, vaccines confer benefits to both individuals and populations.[4,5] While individuals may be protected from infection or disease by vaccine-induced immune responses, decreasing the number of susceptible hosts in a population also helps break the chain of transmission that pathogens require to spread and persist in human populations by induction of 'herd immunity.' The benefits of herd immunity depend on achieving sufficiently high immunization rates in a population to impact pathogen transmission dynamics (including the potential for extinction of ongoing interhost transmission). The requisite level of vaccination coverage of a population needed to compromise pathogen spread significantly varies between pathogens, and is influenced both by vaccine efficacy (and its duration) and by the reproductive characteristics and infectiousness of the pathogen.

Analysis of the impact of vaccination programs in the USA provides an example of the beneficial impact of vaccines when used routinely and when high coverage levels are achieved.[6] As shown in Tables 92.1 and 92.2, vaccination programs in the USA dramatically decreased the annual morbidity of many vaccine-preventable diseases. In many instances, the disease burden from several vaccine-preventable diseases of childhood has been reduced by over 99% since vaccine introduction (e.g., diphtheria, tetanus, measles, mumps, rubella, and polio). The somewhat lower rate of decline of pertussis (the annual morbidity of which has been reduced by a nonetheless impressive 83%) relates to the limited duration of vaccine-induced immunity, which is estimated to wane within 5–10 years after childhood vaccination. It is anticipated that recent availability of pertussis booster vaccines for use in adolescents and adults will lead to significant further declines in pertussis morbidity. Even for diseases targeted by vaccines that have been in widespread use for less time (< 10 years), impressive decreases in disease morbidity have been seen (e.g., varicella, hepatitis A, and pneumococcal disease). In a notable recent demonstration of the population benefits of vaccines, introduction of the 7-valent pneumococcal conjugate vaccine resulted in a decrease of 73% in disease morbidity in children under 5 years of age within the first 5 years of its introduction. Interestingly, the rate of meningitis and bloodstream infections caused by antibiotic-resistant *Streptococcus pneumoniae* also fell by 81% in this age group. In a striking related finding illustrating how vaccines can impact pathogen transmission dynamics, rates of antibiotic-resistant pneumococcal infections also declined by 49% in individuals over the age of 65 who had not received the vaccine. Thus, direct protection by vaccination of children who represent a reservoir of infection provided, via herd immunity, significant indirect benefits to those who did not themselves receive the vaccine.

In addition to their benefits in preventing disease morbidity and mortality, routine vaccination programs are also impressively cost-effective. Evaluation in the USA of the impact of ten vaccines routinely given as part of the childhood immunization schedule (diphtheria, tetanus, pertussis, *Haemophilus influenzae* b (Hib), polio; measles, mumps, rubella, hepatitis B and varicella) found that more than 14 million cases of disease and more than 33 500 deaths were averted over the lifetime of the immunized birth cohort of children.[7] When the cost of the vaccination program was compared to the economic impact of diseases prevented, these vaccines alone are estimated to save nearly $10 billion each year. When including indirect economic benefits (such as the time parents take off from work to care for sick children), the annual savings to society exceed $40 billion. When 30 preventive services were ranked based on clinically preventable disease burden and cost-effectiveness, childhood immunization received the highest score.[8]

Progress in the development of new vaccines accelerated significantly towards the end of the 20th century, with the development of vaccines against diseases that were not previously preventable by vaccination, but also with the development of improved versions of existing vaccines.

Table 92.1 Comparison of 20th-century peak annual morbidity versus current annual morbidity: United States vaccine-preventable diseases

Disease	20th-century annual morbidity[1]	2005[2]	Decrease (%)
Smallpox	48 164	0	100
Diphtheria	175 885	0	100
Measles	503 282	66	> 99
Mumps	152 209	314	> 99
Pertussis	147 271	25 616	83
Polio (paralytic)	16 316	1[3]	> 99
Rubella	47 745	11	> 99
Congenital rubella syndrome	823	1	> 99
Tetanus	1314	27	98
Haemophilus influenzae	20 000	226[4]	99

[1]Source: Centers for Disease Control. MMWR 1999; 48: 242–264.
[2]Source: Centers for Disease Control. MMWR 2006; 55: 880–893.
[3]Imported vaccine-associated paralytic polio (VAPP).
[4]Type b and unknown (< 5 years of age).
Numbers indicate at- or near- record lows in 2005 (except pertussis).

Table 92.2 Comparison of pre-vaccine-era estimated annual morbidity versus current estimated morbidity: vaccine-preventable diseases, United States

Disease	Pre-vaccine-era estimated annual morbidity[1]	2005 Estimated morbidity[1]	Decrease (%)
Hepatitis A	117 333	19 183	84
Hepatitis B (acute)	66 232	15 352	77
Pneumococcus (invasive)			
All ages	63 067	40 325	36
< 5 years of age	16 069	4 400	73
Varicella	4 085 120	817 024	80

[1]Unpublished Centers for Disease Control data, reported November 2006.

Thus, the number of diseases that can be prevented by vaccines included in the US Centers for Disease Control and Prevention's (CDC) routine childhood and adolescent immunization schedules grew from seven in 1985 to 16 in 2007 (Table 92.3 and Fig. 92.1). Moreover, in the past several years, new vaccines have been introduced for adolescents and young adults (e.g., pertussis booster (Tdap), meningococcal conjugate, and human papillomavirus (HPV) vaccines), and older adults (e.g., Tdap and zoster vaccines) have shown that the value of vaccines extends across the human lifespan (Figs 92.1 and 92.2). New combination vaccines have been developed to increase the simplicity and acceptability of vaccination regimens, as well as to improve overall compliance with the recommended series of vaccines. Such combinations include either those that contain multiple inactivated or recombinant antigens (such as a combination diphtheria, pertussis, tetanus, Hib, and hepatitis B vaccine) or multiple live attenuated viruses (such as a combination measles, mumps, rubella, and varicella vaccine (MMRV)). The development of a combination vaccine is often more complicated than simply combining individual antigens, for when antigens are administered in combination, immunologic interference is sometimes seen. This necessitates titration of antigen combinations (and in the case of combinations of inactivated and/or

DEPARTMENT OF HEALTH AND HUMAN SERVICES • CENTERS FOR DISEASE CONTROL AND PREVENTION

Recommended Immunization Schedule for Persons Aged 7–18 Years—UNITED STATES • 2007

Vaccine ▼ / Age ▶	7–10 years	11–12 YEARS	13–14 years	15 years	16–18 years
Tetanus, Diphtheria, Pertussis[1]	see footnote 1	Tdap	Tdap		
Human Papillomavirus[2]	see footnote 2	HPV (3 doses)	HPV Series		
Meningococcal[3]	MPSV4	MCV4		MCV4[3] / MCV4	
Pneumococcal[4]		PPV			
Influenza[5]		Influenza (Yearly)			
Hepatitis A[6]		HepA Series			
Hepatitis B[7]		HepB Series			
Inactivated Poliovirus[8]		IPV Series			
Measles, Mumps, Rubella[9]		MMR Series			
Varicella[10]		Varicella Series			

Range of recommended ages

Catch-up immunization

Certain high-risk groups

Fig. 92.1 continued.

Age group (yrs) ▶ Vaccine ▼	19–49 years	50–64 years	≥65 years
Tetanus, diphtheria, pertussis (Td/Tdap)[1]*	1-dose Td booster every 10 yrs		
		Substitute 1 dose of Tdap for Td	
Human papillomavirus (HPV)[2]*	3 doses (females)		
Measles, mumps, rubella (MMR)[3]*	1 or 2 doses	1 dose	
Varicella[4]*	2 doses (0, 4–8 wks)	2 doses (0, 4–8 wks)	
Influenza[5]*	1 dose annually	1 dose annually	
Pneumococcal (polysaccharide)[6,7]	1–2 doses		1 dose
Hepatitis A[8]*	2 doses (0, 6–12 mos, or 0, 6–18 mos)		
Hepatitis B[9]*	3 doses (0, 1–2, 4–6 mos)		
Meningococcal[10]	1 or more doses		

Fig. 92.2 Recommended immunization schedule for adults – USA, 2007. This schedule indicates the recommended age groups (A) and medical indications (B) for routine administration of currently licensed vaccines for persons aged 19 years or older, as of October 1, 2006 (published in MMWR 2006; October 13). For detailed recommendations on all vaccines, including those primarily for travelers or that are issued or updated over time, consult the manufacturers' package inserts and the complete statements of the Advisory Committee on Immunization Practices (ACIP) (http://www.cdc.gov/nip/publications/acip-list.htm). Recently issued, provisional ACIP recommendations can be found at www.cdc.gov/nip/recs/provisional_recs/default.htm. See url for footnotes to the figure.

Continued

PRINCIPLES OF IMMUNIZATION

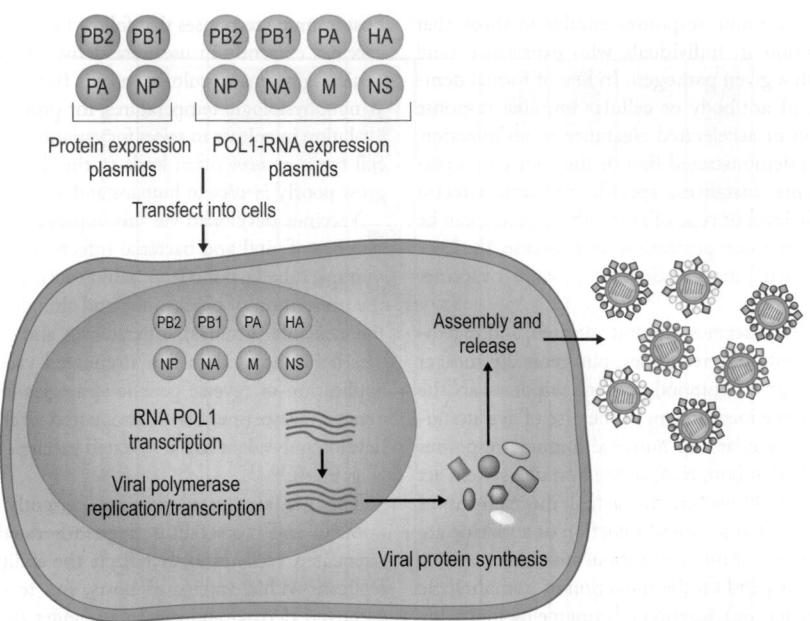

Fig. 92.3 New vaccine strategies: reverse genetic approaches. The term 'reverse genetics' refers to the use of recombinant DNA methods to generate infectious viruses possessing genomes derived from cloned cDNAs. Such cDNAs can be modified to study the impact of specific genetic modifications to viral phenotype, providing a new approach for the generation of live attenuated vaccines via either introduction of targeted mutations or, in the case of segmented viruses, the preparation of vaccines via genetic reassortment (see Fig. 92.4). Reverse genetic methods provide promising tools for the study and defined manipulation of both nonsegmented and segmented negative-strand RNA viruses (such as the respiratory syncytial virus (RSV) and influenza viruses, respectively). The use of reverse genetic strategies to generate infectious viral progeny from cloned cDNAs is shown above. Influenza virus genomes are comprised of eight single-stranded (negative-sense) RNA segments. Initiation of influenza virus RNA (vRNA) transcription from negative-sense genomic RNAs, and the replication of the virus genome, depends on the viral ribonucleoprotein (RNP) complex (which includes viral RNA, the nucleoprotein (NP) and three polymerase proteins (PB1, PB2, and PA)). To generate infectious influenza virus from cDNAs of the vRNA genome segments, cells are cotransfected with all eight segments of vRNA under the control of RNA polymerase promoters. Cellular polymerase I (pol 1) synthesizes vRNAs that are then replicated and transcribed by the viral polymerase and NP proteins that comprise the RNP complex. Reverse genetics strategies are expected to facilitate the generation of novel flu vaccines by enabling preparation of well-defined vaccine preparations comprised of donor 'backbone' viral segments (see Fig. 92.4) that harbor specific attenuating mutations with vRNA segments encoding the hemagglutinin (HA) and neuraminidase (NA) proteins obtained via reverse transcription of vRNA genes from circulating viruses (including those prepared from pandemic strains that may be difficult and/or unsafe to propagate in large manufacturing scale). (Adapted from Marsh GA, Tannock GA. The role of reverse genetics in the development of vaccines against respiratory diseases. Exp Opin Biol Ther 2005; 5: 369–380, with permission from Expert Opinion.)

infectivity. While this approach has the benefit of presenting most of a pathogen's antigenic repertoire to the immune system of the immunized host, it can only be used in instances where the inactivated pathogen does not possess constituents that would confer significant toxicity. Vaccines based on killed pathogens are believed to exert their protective effects via elicitation of pathogen-neutralizing antibodies and the induction of memory B-cell responses (likely in concert with CD4 T-cell memory). However, because inactivated pathogens cannot accomplish *de novo* synthesis of pathogen-derived gene products in antigen-presenting cells (APCs), they do not typically induce CD8 T-cell responses (Chapter 6). In addition, killed vaccines are generally less immunogenic than live attenuated vaccines. As a result, they are commonly administered with an adjuvant (most often alum: see section on Adjuvants, below) to augment their immunogenicity. A number of viral and bacterial vaccines currently in use are killed/inactivated vaccines, including whole-cell *Bordetella pertussis* vaccine and the influenza virus, rabies virus, and hepatitis A virus vaccines.

PURIFIED SUBUNIT VACCINES

A number of bacteria produce toxins that represent the major pathogenic components responsible for disease in infected humans. Examples include *Corynebacterium diphtheriae* and *Clostridium tetani*. Detoxified versions of these toxins are referred to as 'toxoids,' and represent the purified components of vaccines preventing diphtheria and tetanus, respectively. Toxoids have historically been produced by chemical inactivation of toxins, but more recently, genetic inactivation via targeted mutagenesis has been employed. The acellular pertussis vaccine is also a purified subunit vaccine composed of a defined set of protein constituents prepared from cultured *Bordetella pertussis*. The mechanism of immune protection conferred by purified subunit vaccines is the antibody response elicited by vaccination.

Antibodies directed against the capsular polysaccharides present on encapsulated bacteria also confer protective immunity in a number of important instances by inducing antibodies that exert opsonophagocytic

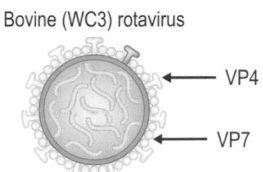

Bovine (WC3) rotavirus

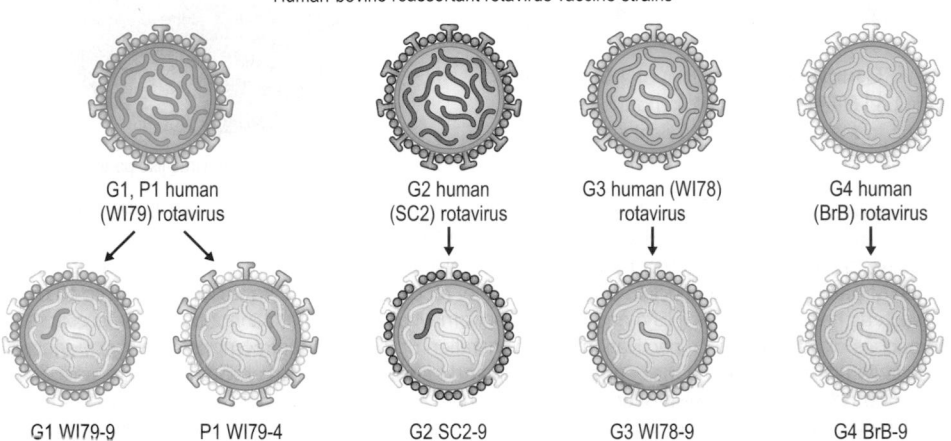

Human-bovine reassortant rotavirus vaccine strains

G1, P1 human (WI79) rotavirus

G2 human (SC2) rotavirus

G3 human (WI78) rotavirus

G4 human (BrB) rotavirus

G1 WI79-9   P1 WI79-4   G2 SC2-9   G3 WI78-9   G4 BrB-9

Fig. 92.4 New vaccine strategies: genetic reassortment approaches. Viruses with segmented genomes provide a now approach for the generation of attenuated vaccines via Mendelian genetic reassortment. If two such segmented viruses with different genetic characteristics are used to infect one cell, the progeny viruses from this mixed infection will carry a range of mixtures of the genes of the two parent viruses. Using either genetic or immunologic screening methods, reassorted viruses carrying the precise gene composition of interest can be selected. This approach has recently been employed to generate live attenuated vaccines against rotavirus and influenza virus. The strategy for generation of the pentavalent bovine–human reassortment rotavirus vaccine is shown above. Rotaviruses have a segmented double-stranded RNA genome comprising 11 independent RNA elements. The outer shell of the virus comprises two proteins VP4 and VP7 that are involved in cell binding and entry and that specify the viral serotype (P type for VP4 and G type for VP7). VP4 and VP7 also represent the targets of virus-neutralizing antibodies. The pentavalent bovine–human rotavirus vaccine was generated by a 'modified Jennerian' approach in which the bovine rotavirus WC3 (which is attenuated in humans as a result of host range restriction) serves as the gene donor for the backbone on to which gene segments encoding four common human rotavirus G types (G1–4) as well as one very common P type (P8) (derived from individual rotavirus isolates) were reassorted via a process of cell co-infection and subsequent selection of the recombinant viruses with the desired composition of bovine and human gene segments. An analogous genetic reassortment approach has also been used to generate live attenuated influenza vaccines. In this instance, three attenuated 'cold-adapted' viral strains (two A types and one type B) are used in co-infections in tissue culture with recent circulating wild-type influenza strains to derive vaccine strains that include the two relevant hemagglutinin (HA) and neuraminidase (NA)-encoding gene segments admixed with the six 'backbone' genes from the attenuated master donor virus for use in annual influenza vaccines.

effects (promoting phagocytosis of antibody-coated bacteria) and, in some instances, bactericidal effects.[17] Initial successful vaccine efforts against *Streptococcus pneumoniae* and *Neisseria meningitidis* utilized purified preparations of capsular polysaccharides. Although such purified polysaccharides can induce protective levels of antibody responses in adults, they are poorly immunogenic in children under 2 years of age (as a function of the relative immaturity of their immune systems). In addition, T-Independent antibody responses elicited by purified capsular polysaccharides are less durable than those that are produced in the presence of CD4 T-cell help. As a means of both augmenting antibody responses against polysaccharide antigens in young children and facilitating their persistence, the development of conjugate vaccines represented an important advance.[18] In this approach, purified polysaccharides are chemically conjugated to a carrier protein (such as diphtheria toxoid or an outer-membrane protein complex (OMPC) derived from *N. meningitidis*). The carrier protein augments CD4 T-cell

helper responses to the polysaccharide antigens, and enables elicitation of durable protective antibody responses even in young children. Polysaccharide-conjugate vaccines have been produced that protect against *Haemophilus influenzae* b, *Streptococcus pneumoniae*, and *N. meningitidis* infections.

RECOMBINANT PROTEIN SUBUNIT VACCINES

The advent of recombinant DNA technologies provided a transformational event in the history of vaccine development. In addition to facilitating the identification and expression of pathogen-derived protective antigens, techniques were developed that enabled their large-scale manufacture as vaccines. Recombinant DNA technologies provided a new path to develop vaccines against pathogens, such as hepatitis B virus (HBV) or HPV, that could not be grown in culture. In addition, recombinant methods provided the potential to derive even safer versions of available vaccines.

Phase II studies also present the first opportunity to identify a potential laboratory immunological correlate of protection from disease – if nature and prior experience have not already done so. In order to do so, the placebo recipients in the phase II trial must experience a sufficient number of cases of disease while vaccine recipients need to exhibit significant evidence of decreased risk of infection or disease. In addition, immunological measurements in the vaccinees need to capture the relevant protective immune responses (e.g., the type and level of antibody and/or cellular immune response that predict protection) and measure them with sufficient precision and reliability. If laboratory measurements of immunity correlate with vaccine protection, subsequent refinements of the vaccine, its adjuvant, its manufacturing process, or its regimen may be assessed by simple immunogenicity studies, rather than repeating efficacy studies. Once efficacy is established for a vaccine, it is very difficult to carry out a double-blinded, placebo-controlled efficacy study.

Vaccines that have been shown to be immunogenic and well tolerated in phase II studies can then advance to pivotal phase III studies required for vaccine licensure by regulatory authorities. Phase III studies are intended to expand further the safety database in a larger number of individuals (who are representative of the specific populations for which the vaccine will ultimately be used), establish definitive evidence of protective efficacy, and to establish clinical consistency of the vaccine made by the process run in the facility intended for licensure and commercialization (www.fda.gov/cber/genetherapy/isct092506jcr.htm). Typically, phase III studies include 10 000 or more subjects in a blinded, placebo-controlled design. This size trial allows the identification of less frequent safety events. It also provides an opportunity to capture data on health care utilization, cost, and impact of the vaccine on these parameters. As a new vaccine will ultimately be included in a vaccine program where multiple vaccines may be administered at the same time, it is also necessary to conduct concomitant-use studies. The developer of the new vaccine must show that the new vaccine does not impact on the immunogenicity of the existing vaccines, and that the existing vaccines do not impact on the immunogenicity of the new vaccine.

LICENSURE AND RECOMMENDATION OF VACCINES

In contrast to drugs, where licensure by the FDA is the primary determinant of how a new product is implemented in medical practice, vaccine use in the USA includes an additional process that evaluates how best to employ a new vaccine to optimize its implementation and public health impact. The US CDC has responsibility for making recommendations about the use of licensed vaccines, and it relies on its Advisory Committee on Immunization Practices (ACIP) for guidance. The ACIP considers several aspects in addition to a vaccine's safety and efficacy, including the anticipated cost-effectiveness and practical feasibility of potential alternative vaccine deployment strategies and consideration of how a new vaccine may be successfully implemented in clinical practice to achieve the greatest public health impact. Once the CDC has received, reviewed, and accepted the recommendation of the ACIP, the recommendation is published in its final official form in *Morbidity and Mortality Weekly Report* (MMWR; www.cdc.gov/nip/publications/acip-list.htm).

VACCINES FOR ROUTINE USE AND IN SPECIAL POPULATIONS

The recommended immunization schedule for children and adolescents (Fig. 92.1) is updated on an annual basis and can be accessed at www.cdc.gov/nip/recs/child-schedule.htm. The recommended adult immunization schedule (Fig. 92.2) is also updated on an annual basis and can be accessed at www.cdc.gov/nip/recs/adult-schedule.htm. The recommended adult immunization schedule includes information concerning use in special populations (such as health care workers and pregnant women) and individuals with specific conditions associated with altered or impaired immune function (such as individuals with congenital and acquired immunodeficiency syndromes, recipients of immunosuppressive therapies, malignancies, asplenia, liver disease, and renal disease). Readers are encouraged to check to ensure that they are following current recommendations.

Pregnancy registries currently exist for four vaccines in the USA. Health care professionals are encouraged to report exposures of pregnant women to the appropriate registry: HBV vaccine (800-670-6126), HPV vaccine (800-986-8999), meningococcal vaccine (800-822-2463), and varicella vaccine (800-986-8999).

VACCINE SAFETY

Unlike drugs that are utilized to treat individuals suffering from a given disease state, vaccines are administered to normal, healthy infants, adolescents, and adults. Consequently, standards for the safety and tolerability of vaccines are set at a very high level. When developing a new vaccine, a graded process of clinical studies is employed that involves increasingly larger numbers of volunteers and that typically progresses from individuals who are selected to be free of any identifiable health problems to those who are selected to be representative of the overall population for whom the vaccine is being developed. If phase I studies reveal no evidence of safety concerns and the desired evidence of immunogenicity, a major focus of the series of larger randomized double-blind, phase II placebo-controlled studies that are then conducted is to explore the safety and tolerability of a vaccine in increasingly vulnerable populations (such as those who may have identified pre-existing health problems or asymptomatic abnormalities detected on screening laboratory studies).

Reflecting the importance of documenting the safety of a new vaccine, phase III studies to assess the safety and efficacy of a new vaccine now typically involve large numbers of volunteers. Indeed, as a result of needing to provide evidence for safety, it is now common to have the size of the phase III trial be significantly larger than would be necessary to document vaccine efficacy. The ability of a study to identify an increased risk of any given adverse event with sufficient statistical power is directly related to the size of the population in the study. As a general rule, a study of 300–400 subjects is needed to measure the risk of an event that happens in one out of 100 individuals. For one in 1000, 3000–4000 subjects are needed. Even in studies of this size, very rare events may not be identified, and if a specific safety concern exists substantially larger trials may be needed.

The recent experience with the development of rotavirus vaccines provides an illustrative example of the importance placed on documenting vaccine safety.[24] Rotavirus is an important cause of serious gastroenteritis in infants and young children, and the associated diarrhea and vomiting can lead to life-threatening dehydration. In developing countries where health care resources and effective rehydration options are limited, over 600 000 infants die of rotavirus gastroenteritis each year.[25] Given the global importance of rotavirus gastroenteritis, the first licensure of an orally administered rotavirus vaccine in 1998 was a very welcome advance. However, as the vaccine entered routine pediatric practice, it was recognized that a low, but increased incidence of intestinal intussusception was seen after the first and second doses (with about one case of intussusception seen per 10 000 vaccinees.)[26] Upon recognition of this association, the vaccine was withdrawn from the market.[27]

With the evident public health need for a safe and effective rotavirus vaccine, it was hoped that alternative rotavirus vaccines then in development (both oral vaccines based either on a combination of bovine–human reassortant viruses (Fig. 92.4) or an attenuated human rotavirus strain) might differ from the first licensed rotavirus vaccine and not result in an increased rate of intussusception. However, to demonstrate that these alternative rotavirus vaccines were safe, and that an increased risk of intussusception was not inherent to rotavirus vaccines as a class, very large-scale safety studies were required. Toward this end, the safety of each of these vaccines was evaluated in studies involving about 70 000 infants – just to evaluate whether the rate of intussusception in vaccinees was discernibly increased compared to the normal background rates seen in the placebo recipients.[10,11] Fortunately, both vaccines were found to be well tolerated and no increase in intussusception was observed in vaccine as compared to placebo recipients. In light of the documented efficacy of these vaccines determined in earlier and significantly smaller phase III trials, both have now been licensed in a number of countries. However, even with the large phase III studies conducted for these newer rotavirus vaccines, they will still be studied in large postlicensure active surveillance safety studies and closely monitored in active and passive vaccine safety surveillance systems (see below).

Following vaccine licensure, safety is tracked via a number of means, including both active and passive surveillance studies of adverse events. Active surveillance includes phase IV postmarketing studies of vaccine safety in larger populations in real-world use. Formal postmarketing studies can include tens of thousands of individuals or more.

An alternative type of postmarketing safety study is carried out by the US FDA and the CDC within the context of the Vaccine Adverse Event Reporting System (VAERS) database (www.vaers.hhs.gov or by telephone: 800-822-7967). The VAERS database accepts spontaneous reports of adverse experiences from health care providers, patients, parents, vaccine manufacturers, and other sources.[28] The best use of the VAERS database is to identify signals in a population that may appear following the introduction of a new vaccine.

A newer vaccine safety surveillance system, known as the Vaccine Safety Database (VSD), has been developed by the CDC in cooperation with seven large health maintenance organizations (HMOs) around the USA.[29] The VSD contains the complete medical records of all the members from the participating HMOs, and the information used to populate the database is entered by health care professionals using relatively consistent terminology, improving the quality, uniformity, and usefulness of the data. Particularly important is that the VSD construct allows comprehensive epidemiological analyses to determine if the incidence rate of a specific adverse event is higher among vaccinees than nonvaccinees. In addition to VAERS and the VSD, the CDC has also created a Clinical

Immunization Safety Assessment Network that reviews patterns of clinical syndromes that may follow vaccination.

While the safety profile of a vaccine can be relatively well defined through the efforts described above, confidence in vaccination programs has often been challenged by public perceptions, either real or unsubstantiated, about vaccine safety. In some instances, specific vaccines have been associated with increased incidence of a specific adverse experience, such as the association between the first-generation rotavirus vaccine and an increased risk of intussusception following vaccination. However, a number of other safety concerns that have emerged are not supported by scientific evidence. An example of this can be found in the case of concerns about the association of whole-cell pertussis vaccines with permanent brain damage – concerns that were later shown to be unfounded. Nevertheless, public concerns about the safety of the whole-cell pertussis vaccine resulted in decreased levels of pertussis vaccination coverage that were soon followed by epidemics of whooping cough in the UK and Japan.[30] Another example is the allegation that certain vaccines, such as the combination measles, mumps, rubella (MMR) vaccine, are associated with autism. Highlighting how perceptions of temporal association can give rise to public concerns, MMR vaccines are generally given around 1 year of age, and autism is generally diagnosed in the second year of life. Although the alleged causal association between MMR and autism has been refuted by thorough scientific analyses, reports in the popular media in the UK resulted in a dramatic drop in vaccination rates, followed by an increased rate of new infections.[31,32]

VACCINES NOT YET AVAILABLE

Although an impressive armamentarium of vaccines is now available, safe and effective vaccines have yet to be developed for a number of very important infectious diseases. The reasons underlying the lack of effective vaccines for an array of important pathogens include biological considerations, safety concerns, and practical constraints. Of these, the biological considerations are often the most important barrier. As discussed above, vaccines have been successfully developed for pathogens whose natural infections give rise to natural immunity wherein the infected host (at least those who survive initial infection) is no longer susceptible to re-infection (such as measles, yellow fever virus, or smallpox) or who experiences significantly less severe clinical sequelae upon re-infection (such as rotavirus). In instances where natural immunity follows natural infection, not only is a precedent for immune protection established, but the nature of protective host responses can be studied, providing a correlate of protection to guide vaccine development efforts. However, for many of the pathogens for which vaccines remain elusive, natural immunity does not follow natural infection. In the absence of natural immunity, not only is a precedent for successful immune containment lacking, but no potential correlates of protection are available to inform vaccine development. In some instances where natural immunity does not follow natural infection, persistent infections are established and maintained by active virus replication that cannot be controlled or cleared by host immune responses (such as HIV and hepatitis C).

Alternatively, other pathogens are able to persist in the host through establishment, via diverse mechanisms, of latent infections that are resistant to host immune clearance (such as tuberculosis or herpes viruses (such as herpes simplex virus (HSV) or Epstein–Barr virus (EBV))). In other instances, even when the host is cleared of an infection via drug

trials. An alternative strategy is based on improving the performance of the BCG vaccine by insertion of genes encoding specific potential protective antigens that it normally lacks. In addition, the development of auxotrophic mutants of *M. tuberculosis* is being explored as a potential immunogenic and specifically attenuated live vaccine. The determination of the sequence of the *M. tuberculosis* genome nearly a decade ago helped identify numerous previously unknown gene products, and increased the repertoire of antigens to be evaluated for their ability to induce protective immune responses.[52] The pathogen sequence is also being used to elucidate virulence determinants and thereby help guide efforts to attenuate *M. tuberculosis* rationally.

RESPIRATORY SYNCYTIAL VIRUS AND PARAINFLUENZA VIRUS (PIV)

Together with influenza virus, RSV and PIV account for a substantial majority of pediatric upper respiratory illness and consequent acute otitis media. A variety of influenza vaccines are licensed for pediatric use, but vaccines to prevent infection with the paromyxoviruses RSV and PIV remain elusive. A significant impediment to vaccine development for RSV and PIV traces back to unanticipated untoward results obtained in clinical studies of inactivated RSV vaccines in the early 1960s.[53] These early-generation RSV vaccines – based on cultured virus that had been inactivated with formalin – raised a potent antibody response in immunized children. However, on subsequent natural exposure to RSV, vaccine recipients exhibited more frequent and significantly more severe lower respiratory tract RSV infections than did unimmunized children. As a similar phenomenon was also seen with a formalin-inactivated measles vaccine in the same era, a common immunopathologic mechanism may be operative.[54] While the mechanism of exacerbation of RSV disease by the early inactivated vaccines is incompletely understood, it has been suggested that chemical inactivation of RSV and measles resulted in modification of a critical neutralizing structure on the surfaces of these viruses, thereby limiting the induction of the most potent neutralizing antibodies and favoring nonneutralizing and potentially immunopathologic antibody responses. (Passive protection against RSV is available for premature infants in the form of monoclonal antibodies that target the RSV F protein (one of the viral envelope glycoproteins); certain anti-RSV antibody responses can clearly mediate protective as opposed to deleterious effects.[46]) Alternatively, or in addition, it has been proposed that inactivated RSV vaccines may have preferentially induced a Th2-type immune response when a Th1-type response may be needed to effect protection of the lower respiratory tract from RSV infection and damage.

While excellent live attenuated measles vaccines have been developed, RSV and PIV have so far resisted the approach used for measles and mumps (these are all members of the Paramyxoviridae family of viruses). Based on the successful precedent provided by the live attenuated measles vaccine, an attenuated or reverse genetics-engineered RSV is considered the most promising approach. However, stable attenuation of RSV has been difficult to achieve and vaccine safety concerns result in their cautious advancement through clinical evaluation.[55]

NEISSERIA MENINGITIDIS GROUP B

Effective vaccines for meningococcus types A, C, Y, and W135 are available as straight capsular polysaccharides and as conjugated polysaccharides.[56] The group B polysaccharide shares chemical similarity with a shorter sugar found on the surface of neuronal tissue.[57] While it is possible to make highly immunogenic conjugates with the group B polysaccharide, theoretical concerns about cross-reactivity with self antigens has impeded the development of this type of vaccine. Current work centers on a handful of relatively well-conserved surface proteins of meningococcus.

GROUP B STREPTOCOCCUS

GBS is a common component of the flora of the female genital tract, and transfer to the neonate is the cause of severe infections that are fatal or have serious sequelae.[58] Short-course intrapartum antibiotics are recommended for culture-positive women, and this approach has cut the incidence of neonatal infections by about two-thirds, thus reducing somewhat the urgency of vaccine development. However, short-course antibiotics could ultimately drive the emergence of antibiotic-resistant GBS. Candidate vaccines have been shown to elicit a protective response.[34] However, aside from a reduced market, the main impediment to development of a GBS vaccine is concern over vaccination of pregnant women or women of childbearing age. Any birth defect might be attributed to the vaccine, and in a litigious society, this would be problematic for a vaccine producer.

HEPATITIS C VIRUS (HCV)

Prior to the advent of effective polymerase chain reaction methods for screening blood donations, HCV was a significant cause of transfusion-related hepatitis. Currently, transmission of HCV among the normal population is quite low; transmission among injection drug users remains high. HCV is another pathogen where infection does not typically result in an immune response that clears the infection. However, a minority of HCV patients do spontaneously clear their infection, suggesting that an appropriate immune response could do the job. Current vaccine work is concentrated on vectored gene delivery vaccines, primarily adenoviruses, intended to raise antiviral cytotoxic T-cell responses.[59]

HERPES SIMPLEX VIRUS

With the exception of the live attenuated varicella-zoster virus (VZV) vaccine used for the primary prevention of chickenpox and reactivation of latent VZV infections (the cause of shingles and postherpetic neuralgia in older individuals), there are no other vaccines available for use in humans to prevent infection with members of the herpes virus family.[60] HSV types 1 and 2 cause recurrent vesicular eruptions "above or below the belt," respectively. Like other herpes viruses, HSV infections are not cleared by the immune system and the virus can persist, remaining in a latent state that is functionally inaccessible to immune recognition and clearance. In addition, like other herpes viruses, HSV encodes a number of gene products that promote evasion of host immune responses. Recent attempts to make HSV2 vaccines have used virus glycoproteins produced by recombinant DNA methods. A recent clinical efficacy trial of this vaccine approach showed partial protection of women, but not men, who were seronegative for HSV1.[61] The reasons for this curious result are not clear, but efforts to develop this type of vaccine continue. In addition, a number of preclinical studies are exploring the ability of cell-mediated immune responses to HSV antigens induced by recombinant vaccine vectors (e.g., adenoviruses: see Novel vaccine vectors, below) to prevent or ameliorate HSV infections. Genetically engineered attenuated HSV variants have also been studied in experimental animal models. It is not clear when these new strategies may advance to clinical evaluation in humans.

KEY CONCEPTS

CONTEMPORARY OPPORTUNITIES AND CHALLENGES IN VACCINE DEVELOPMENT

The processes of vaccine development have changed significantly in recent years – a process facilitated by substantial improvements in understanding of human immune system function, as well as the advent of powerful new technologies for vaccine development. As a result of these advances, vaccine development is now commonly pursued in a hypothesis-driven manner and is a far less empiric pursuit than in the past. However, at the same time, the infectious diseases for which no effective vaccines currently exist represent more challenging targets than those diseases that have yielded to vaccine development efforts in the past. Furthermore, global changes that influence the emergence and rate of spread of infectious diseases place unprecedented challenges on the productivity and pace of new vaccine development efforts.

Current opportunities

>> Improved understanding of human immunology (including the biology of innate immune system function, antigen presentation, and the generation and maintenance of T- and B-cell memory)

>> Improved technologies to measure human cellular and humoral immune responses

>> The advent of genomic and proteomic technologies for new antigen discovery

>> The wealth of recombinant DNA methodologies that enable the isolation and characterization of protective antigens from diverse pathogens (including those that may not be successfully propagated in culture)

>> The development of recombinant and synthetic approaches for the large-scale production of precisely defined vaccine antigens (including the ability to produce immunogens that accurately recapitulate the conformational structure of native antigens, or that, alternatively, alter them so that they serve as more effective immunogens in eliciting desired immune responses)

>> The emergence of new mechanism-based vaccine adjuvants to enhance the immunogenicity of vaccine antigens

Current challenges

>> The need to develop vaccines for infections where natural immunity does not often or ever develop following natural infection (e.g., human immunodeficiency virus (HIV), malaria, hepatitis C)

>> The need to develop vaccines that protect against genetically diverse pathogen variants with a limited number of vaccine immunogens (e.g., HIV, malaria, and influenza)

>> The need to develop vaccines for infections where concerns exist about vaccine elicitation of potentially autoimmune (*Neisseria meningiditis* group B) or immunopathologic (e.g., respiratory syncytial virus) responses by vaccination

>> The challenge of responding rapidly and effectively, with powerful new technologies, to newly emerging infections – including those that haven't been seen in humans before (e.g., severe acute respiratory syndrome (SARs)) or for which novel antigenic variants are anticipated but cannot be predicted (e.g., pandemic influenza)

>> Maximizing the value of innovative new approaches while ensuring the safety of new vaccines so derived

CYTOMEGALOVIRUS (CMV)

Another herpes virus, CMV is a very common infection in humans, with 50–80% of individuals being infected by adulthood. CMV is a cause of severe infections in neonates, causing debilitating neurological sequelae. Following initial infection, CMV persists in infected humans, despite the fact that anti-CMV antibodies are present and that a very sizeable proportion of the overall host CD4 and CD8 immune responses are specific for CMV antigens. Ongoing virus persistence and replication in the face of active host immune responses are likely explained by CMV's sophisticated repertoire of host immune evasion functions (including those that inhibit antigen presentation mechanisms and immune effector responses). For these reasons, to be successful, vaccine development efforts will need to elicit immune responses that are significantly more effective than the quantitatively impressive, but functionally limited, immune responses that are generated in the course of natural CMV infections. Live attenuated vaccines have been investigated sporadically since the 1970s.[62] An attenuated strain, the Towne strain, showed some effect, but was judged to be insufficiently immunogenic. Hybrids of the attenuated Towne strain and the virulent Toledo strain remain in development. Recent work has included recombinant DNA (rDNA)-derived proteins (via either DNA vaccine approaches or recombinant viral vectors, such as attenuated poxviral vectors).[63, 64]

EPSTEIN–BARR VIRUS

EBV is a herpes virus that represents the causative agent of infectious mononucleosis and is widespread among the human population. In concert with incompletely understood environmental (and perhaps additional host) factors, EBV is also etiologically associated with Burkitt's lymphoma. The ability of EBV to establish persistent infections in humans (along with latent infections at the cellular level) despite readily detectable antiviral immune responses suggests that, like other herpes viruses, the development of effective EBV vaccine will likely be challenging. EBV vaccines have been in development since the 1980s with the coat protein, gp220/350, as the most common vaccine antigen studied.[65]

DENGUE FEVER VIRUS

Dengue fever virus is a mosquito-borne flavivirus (the virus family that includes Japanese encephalitis virus and yellow fever virus – for which successful vaccines exist). Dengue virus is endemic in a substantial portion of tropical and subtropical areas and causes febrile disease as well as hemorrhagic fever. There are four distinct serotypes of dengue fever virus. Prior infection with one serotype has been implicated in predisposing for more severe disease following infection with a second dengue fever virus serotype, although the evidence supporting this concept has been questioned and the underlying pathogenic mechanisms are incompletely understood.[66]

VACCINES NOT YET AVAILABLE

PREVENTION AND THERAPY OF IMMUNOLOGIC DISEASES

the benchmark for laboratory studies of adjuvants. CFA is a mixed emulsion of mineral oil, mannide monooleate, and killed mycobacteria. However, it is far too reactogenic for use in humans, causing significant pain and abcesses at the site of injection – reactions that would be exacerbated if CFA were to be used repeatedly. An alternative preparation termed incomplete Freund's adjuvant (IFA) lacks the mycobacterial component, but it too is associated with injection site reactions that are severe enough to limit its use to experimental therapeutic cancer vaccines. Although CFA's toxicity precludes its use as a vaccine adjuvant in humans, many of its constituents (including liposaccharides, DNA, and specific bacterial cell wall components) are now understood to exert their adjuvant effects on vaccine-induced immune responses via engagement of specific TLRs. Similarly, the live attenuated *Mycobacterium bovis* strain, BCG, long widely employed as a vaccine for the prevention of

tuberculosis, includes cell wall, peptidoglycan, and DNA components that activate specific TLRs. Interestingly, the highly effective yellow fever vaccine 17D has been shown to activate multiple TLRs as part of its induction of antiviral immune responses.[87] It is quite likely that other live attenuated viruses that transiently replicate in immunized hosts also activate innate immune responses via engagement of TLRs. In yet another example involving a nonreplicating vaccine immunogen, one version of the Hib polysaccharide conjugate vaccines now licensed for use in children for the prevention of invasive Hib disease includes the meningococcal outer-membrane protein complex (OMPC) as its protein carrier. OMPC conjugates have favorable immunogenic properties that correlate with the ability of OMPC to activate DCs via TLR2.[88]

Hundreds of different adjuvant formulations have been tested in animal models, and a few have been advanced into human studies. With a few

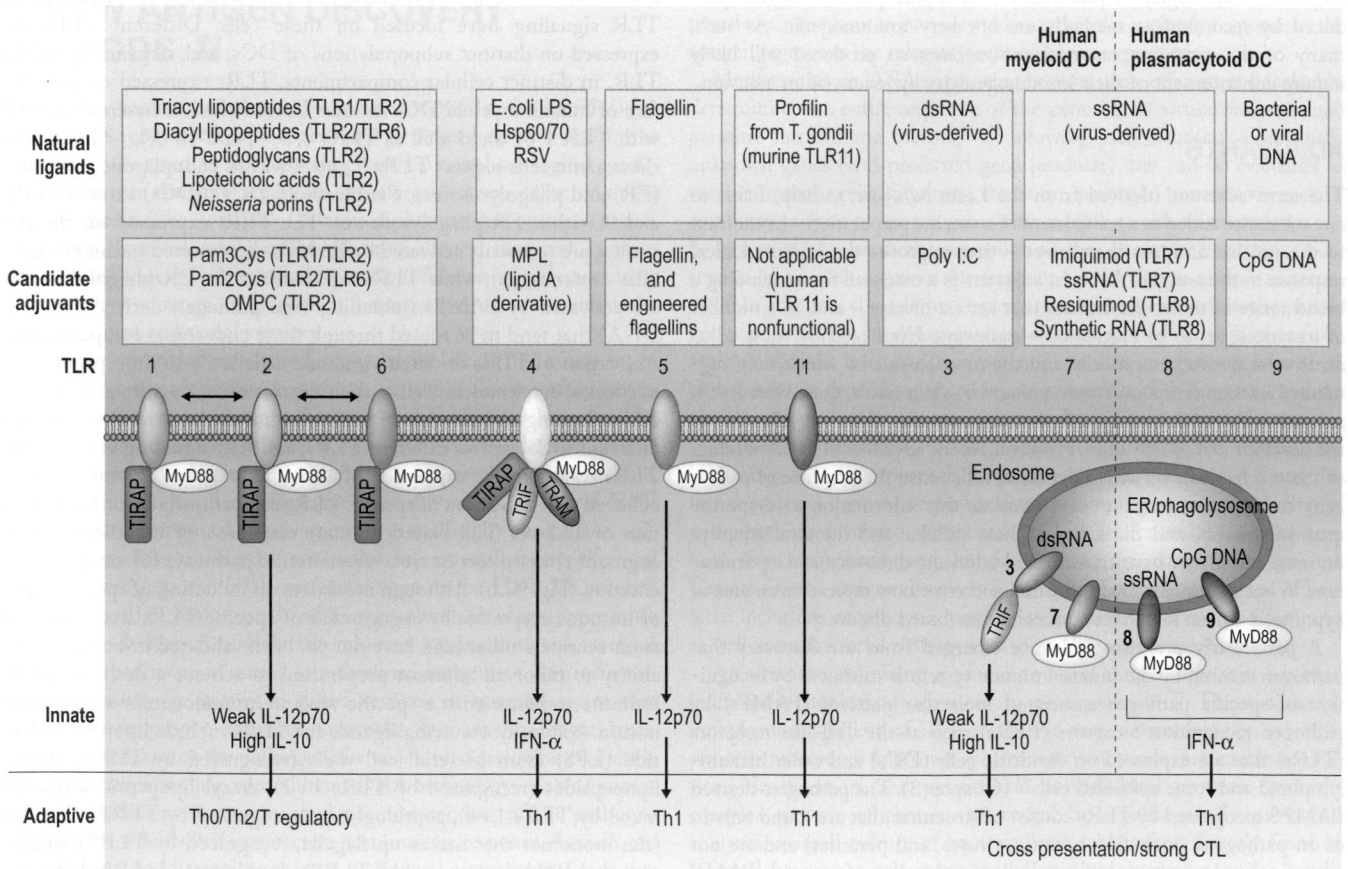

Fig. 92.6 Toll-like receptor (TLR) signaling pathways and mechanism-based adjuvants. The targeted activation of specific dendritic cell (DC) populations via engagement of specific TLRs to initiate innate and adaptive immune responses represents a very promising approach for the development of novel adjuvants based on natural or synthetic versions of the pathogen-associated molecular patterns (PAMPs) that trigger specific TLRs. Specific TLRs and their natural activating ligands are shown above. Different TLRs are associated with different adaptor proteins that propagate intracellular signaling along distinct pathways which favor specific immune responses (e.g., Th1, Th2, cross-presentation or CTL priming). The character of responses from specific TLR engagement illustrated is based on animal and *ex vivo* studies. In humans, TLRs 7 and 9 are expressed in the endoplasmic reticulum (ER)/phagolysosomes of plasmacytoid DCs (pDCs) that represent the major sources of type I interferon production (e.g., IFN-α). Human myeloid DCs (mDCs) express TLR3 (in the ER/phagolysosomes); and TLR2 (heterodimerized with TLRs 1 or 6), and TLRs 4, 5, 8, and 11 on the cell surface. (Adapted from Pulendran B, Ahmed R. Translating innate immunity into immunologic memory: implications for vaccine development. Cell 2006; 124: 849–863, with permission from Elsevier.

notable exceptions, these formulations have not yet been licensed as a vaccine. Major classes of adjuvants now available and in development include: (1) alum; (2) liposomes; (3) immune-stimulating complexes (ISCOMs); (4) virosomes; (5) emulsions; (6) cytokines; and (7) Toll-receptor agonists.

Alum

Alum, the classical adjuvant most often used in vaccines in humans, includes a range of salts of aluminum precipitated under basic conditions, usually aluminum sulfate mixed with sodium or potassium hydroxide plus a variable amount of phosphate.[89] The relative proportions will determine the size, charge, and solubility of alum. The composition of alum used as an adjuvant varies in currently available vaccines and may influence vaccine immunogenicity. Alum is utilized as an adjuvant in many of the currently available vaccines composed of inactivated toxins or recombinant proteins (live attenuated vaccines do not include alum or other adjuvants).

Alum serves two main purposes as an adjuvant. First, it acts as an antigen depot. Vaccine antigens adsorb to alum and elute from it following injection into the host. Second, alum acts a mild irritant, causing the recruitment of leukocytes necessary for generation of an immune response to the site of injection. Adsorption of antigens on to alum routinely improves immunogenicity, particularly the antibody response. Alum does not typically enhance CD8 T-cell responses. Alum has been a component of many vaccines for decades and has an excellent safety record. As new adjuvants are developed, alum may remain as a component of combination adjuvant mixtures (as is the case with some newer adjuvants now approaching clinical use), or it may eventually be supplanted by other agents that more effectively provide favorable depot and local inflammatory responses to accentuate host immune responses.

Liposomes

Using lipids with polar head groups (e.g., triglycerides) and differing types of hydrophobic tails, one can form either micelles (spheres) or multilamellar sheets in aqueous environments.[90] Under the right conditions, antigens can be incorporated into the spheres or between layers of the sheets, providing a potential slow-release depot system. Immunopotentiators such as QS21 or detoxified LPS derivatives (such as monophosphoryl lipid A (MPL)) may be added to the lipid mix.[45]

Immune-stimulating complexes

ISCOMs are a proprietary form of liposomes made of cholesterol, saponins from Quillaia bark (various members of the QS-X family of triterpene glycosides), and phospholipids that form cage-like structures into which antigens can be entrapped or intercalated.[86] ISCOM complexes may provide a depot function, as well as facilitate the delivery, uptake, and processing of vaccine immunogens by APCs.

Virosomes

Purified influenza virus hemagglutinin (HA) and neuraminidase mixed with phosphatidyl choline and phosphatidyl ethanolamine (polar lipids) will form empty particles that have the surface properties of influenza virus. Adding an antigen in solution before mixing the lipids results in the incorporation of the antigen inside the particle. This provides a vehicle for delivering antigens to the interior of a cell, via the influenza HA membrane

fusion process, thereby enabling antigen processing and presentation via both major histocompatibility complex (MHC) class 1 and 2 pathways.[91]

Emulsions

Numerous oil-in-water and water-in-oil emulsions have been tested as adjuvants. One such emulsion, MF59, is used in a licensed influenza vaccine. MF59 consists of squalane, a metabolizable shark oil and two surfactants, polyoxyethylene sorbitan monooleate and sorbitan trioleate, in an oil-in-water emulsion.[92]

Cytokines

Cytokines are host-produced immunomodulators that regulate immune cell action (Chapter 10). Several cytokines are being tested as potential vaccine adjuvants, including granulocyte–macrophage colony-stimulating factor (GM-CSF), interleukin-2 (IL-2), and IL-12.

Toll-receptor agonists

Of the defined TLR agonists being explored as vaccine adjuvants, LPS and its partially detoxified form, MPL, which activate TLR 4, have been most thoroughly explored in clinical trials. With evidence of enhanced ability to increase the percentage of individuals responding with protective antibody levels to hepatitis B as compared to a standard hepatitis B vaccine, one hepatitis B vaccine that employs an adjuvant formulation (termed AS04) consisting of a combination of alum and MPL[93] has been licensed for use in high-risk individuals. In addition, a vaccine against HPV that uses the same adjuvant formulation may be licensed soon, and candidate HSV-1 and malaria vaccines currently being studied in late-stage clinical trials also include this alum–MPL combination adjuvant.

A wide variety of TLR9-specific agonists consisting of oligodeoxynucleotides containing unmethylated CpG motifs (CpG-ODN) are being evaluated in preclinical studies. These CpG-ODNs resemble bacterial DNA, modified to include a phosphorothioate backbone to increase their stability. Two CpG-ODN adjuvants have been evaluated in recent phase I and II trials and shown to increase the timing and magnitude of induction of protective antibody levels, as well as the proportion of responding individuals, to recombinant HBSAg vaccine as compared with the current commercially available version of the vaccine.[94] One of these CpG-ODN adjuvants also elicits protective antibody responses in immunized HIV-infected individuals who had previously failed to respond to the hepatitis B vaccine. This approach is now being studied as a way of inducing protective immune responses to hepatitis B earlier after initiation of the vaccination regimen or with fewer doses of the vaccine.

In addition to the CpG-ODN-based TLR9 adjuvants described above, small chemical compounds with structures that resemble nucleic acid bases have been identified that activate TLR7 (e.g., imiquimod) or both TLR7 and 8 (e.g., resiquimod). These compounds are being evaluated as vaccine adjuvants in preclinical studies. Flagellin, a TLR5 agonist, is also being explored as an adjuvant.

Recently, attention has also been focused on coupling, rather than mixing, TLR agonists to antigens. CpG oligonucleotides conjugated to antigens have been tested in preclinical studies of hepatitis B vaccines[95] and in human clinical trials for treatment of allergy.[96] Ligands for TLR7/8 have been coupled to HIV antigens,[97] and the ligand for TLR5 (flagellin) has been fused to a variety of antigens.[98, 99] In some instances, coupling a TLR ligand to an antigen resulted in a substantial improvement of the immune response compared to mixtures – potentially the result of enabling the antigen and the TLR ligand to co-locate in the same DC compartments.

Numerous preclinical studies have confirmed that many natural and synthetic TLR agonists possess adjuvant activity. Importantly, early human clinical trials of TLR-predicated adjuvants have supported the promise of this approach to mechanism-based strategies to augment vaccine immunogenicity. An important challenge is to define the most potent and best-tolerated variants, and to define rules by which activation of specific TLR pathways might translate into predictable augmentation of desired types of immune responses. It is hoped that general rules will emerge to suggest which of an increasing number of novel adjuvants in development performs best with which type of vaccine immunogen, and if results obtained with a specific type of immunogen–adjuvant combination can be extrapolated to predict the likelihood of enhanced immunogenicity with other vaccines. Although beyond the reach of available experimental results, the ability to tailor, titrate, and otherwise optimize immune responses to vaccines by manipulation of specific TLR pathways appears a realistic future possibility. However, important challenges remain. In particular, a primary challenge for next-generation adjuvant development is finding a combination that retains immunopotentiating action while minimizing vaccine-associated adverse experiences. Short-term adverse experiences, such as local injection site reactions, represent undesirable side effects that may disqualify candidate adjuvants early in clinical development. However, given that vaccines are administered to healthy people to prevent potential future infectious diseases, the potential for rarer adverse experiences (such as autoimmunity) that may only be manifest with much longer latency from the time of vaccine adjuvant administration will undoubtedly be important considerations for use in prophylactic vaccines.

NOVEL VACCINE VECTORS

As induction of cell-mediated immune responses is considered an important component of vaccine strategies for many diseases for which no vaccines are currently available (many of which are caused by intracellular pathogens), there is a need to develop safe and readily scalable approaches to elicit durable CD8 T-cell responses in immunized humans. Further, given the critical role that CD4 T cells play in induction, differentiation, and maintenance of CD8 T-cell responses, any such novel vaccine strategy will likely also require appropriate CD4 T-cell responses. As elicitation of CD8 T-cell responses against a foreign antigen usually depends on the *de novo* expression of the antigen within a host cell and its subsequent processing and presentation via class I MHC pathways (Chapter 6), most novel vaccine strategies are predicated on the need to achieve synthesis of pathogen-derived antigens within APCs of immunized human hosts. With an increasing appreciation of the role that cross-presentation pathways can play in elicitation of class I-restricted CD8 T-cell responses, such *de novo* antigen synthesis may not need to occur within APCs themselves (which may be an advantage for potential vaccine delivery strategies that do not directly target APCs).

One of the many attractive attributes of effective live attenuated vaccines is their ability to recapitulate (to various degrees) many of the processes that lead to the generation of potent immune responses following natural infection. These processes include the fact that replication of

all viruses depends on gaining access to host cells for genome replication and for the synthesis of essential components of virus particles that permit further propagation of the infection within and between hosts. One immunologic benefit of this requirement is that *de novo* synthesis of viral gene products within infected cells provides a key opportunity for viral antigen presentation (via MHC class I pathways) and elicitation of antiviral cellular immune responses. Along with the processing and presentation of intact virus proteins via MHC class II pathways leading to production of antiviral antibody responses, live attenuated viral vaccines have a strong track record for induction of broad cellular and humoral immune responses that likely both contribute to conferring protective immunity. However, despite their track record of success, it is likely that few, if any, new live attenuated viral vaccines will be derived in a manner that resembles previous successful efforts (e.g., the empiric derivation of live attenuated polio, yellow fever, or varicella-zoster vaccines). Important reasons for this change include the desire for safe and well-characterized vaccines whose mechanisms of attenuation are defined and that can be monitored in the course of vaccine production and use. Indeed, most of the recently developed live attenuated vaccines were derived using new approaches for genetic reassortment (Fig. 92.4) wherein genome segments encoding pathogen-derived antigens of interest are recombined with a common set of genome segments that carry attenuating mutations (derived either by use of attenuating viral passage under specific conditions in cell culture (e.g., the cold-adapted influenza vaccine or use of a virus obtained from a nonhuman host that is itself inherently unable to replicate to high levels in humans, e.g., the reassortant rotavirus vaccine prepared via genetic reassortment between human and bovine rotavirus strains (Fig. 92.4)[100]). Although such approaches have proven successful, they are limited in that they can only be applied to homologous viruses (e.g., those derived from the same virus type) whose genomes are segmented and capable of ready genetic reassortment in culture, or to viruses that can be manipulated by reverse genetics.

In response to the desire to produce vaccines that can safely and reliably elicit desired immune responses, especially T-cell responses, several approaches are being explored to develop novel vector systems that permit the expression of pathogen-derived antigens. As many of these approaches are based on viruses distinct from the viral pathogen targeted for induction of host immune responses, the inserted pathogen-derived gene products are expressed via recombinant methods as heterologous antigens. Alternatively, in nonviral expression systems, such as DNA vaccines, the pathogen-derived antigen is expressed in isolation and does not depend on virus-mediated antigen delivery to APCs following host inoculation.

Collectively, such recombinant heterologous expression systems are commonly referred to as 'vaccine vectors.' In some instances, such recombinant vectors express only a specific antigen (in the case of DNA vaccines or certain viral vectors, e.g., adenovirus), while in others both the inserted pathogen-derived antigens and antigens encoded by the viral vector 'backbone' are expressed (e.g., poxvirus vectors). Most new approaches employ expression systems that are inherently nonreplicating (e.g., DNA vaccines) or that employ viral vectors that can replicate at high levels in tissue culture but not *in vivo* (e.g., complemented adenovirus deletion variants or host range-restricted poxviruses). While numerous approaches are being pursued to develop novel vaccine vectors, they will all need to meet certain common criteria to emerge as vaccine approaches applicable for widespread use. In particular, any successful approach must be safe in healthy and immunodeficient humans (given their increased representation in the population as a result of HIV infection and therapeutic immunosuppression), desirably immunogenic (including in individuals who may have been previously exposed to the virus from which the vector was derived, e.g., vaccinia or adenovirus), and able to be produced in large quantities and in a stable manner. A limited number of vaccine vector approaches now being pursued are likely to meet these criteria.

Should successful approaches emerge, there will likely be interest in applying them for use in vaccines targeting diverse pathogens. Thus, while definition of promising, broadly applicable, vaccine vector approaches may help simplify certain aspects of vaccine regulatory review and manufacture, they may also present challenges to prioritize use for specific applications should administration of a given vaccine vector on one occasion compromise or preclude successful administration at a later time. Nevertheless, the development of novel vaccine vectors is laying essential groundwork for the development of next-generation vaccines.

Several novel vaccine vectors currently being studied in preclinical studies and human clinical trials are described below, all of which depend on the delivery and expression of a candidate pathogen-derived gene sequence. In a number of ways, DNA vaccines represent the simplest approach to deliver pathogen-derived genes. Viral vectors similarly serve to deliver pathogen gene sequences to host APCs, either directly or indirectly, but do so in a manner that depends on and takes advantage of the lifecycle and tropism of the virus that is being adapted to express the exogenous pathogen gene products.

DNA vaccines

The ability of purified plasmid DNA containing heterologous antigens expressed under the control of eukaryotic transcriptional regulatory and RNA processing signals to elicit immune responses when injected into experimental animals was discovered serendipitously.[101] However, since the initial, quite surprising, description, the development of so-called DNA vaccines has become an active area of preclinical and clinical vaccine development.[102] Reasons for this enthusiasm include the attractive simplicity and facile preparation of vectors that encode only the defined antigen of interest (which can itself be manipulated via recombinant methods to assume a desired configuration), a reasonably straightforward method for vaccine production, and the inherent stability to temperature (which is much greater than most currently live or subunit vaccines). Although the DNA vector is most commonly injected intramuscularly, the generation of specific immune responses depends on the uptake of the vector DNA by APCs followed by the expression, processing, and presentation of vector-encoded antigens. As tissue and tissue fluids present a hostile environment for purified DNA, and the process of DNA uptake by APCs appears to be relatively inefficient, much of the dose of injected DNA is degraded before it can be reached by an APC that can initiate the desired immune response.

Most DNA vaccine research has been pursued in mice, although studies have now been performed in numerous animal species. Studies have usually utilized intramuscular injection of vaccine vector DNA, but various intradermal and transdermal approaches have also been explored. Murine studies have shown that administration of antigen-encoding plasmid DNA can elicit appreciable cellular and humoral immune responses that may confer protection against experimental challenge. However, translation of these promising results in animal models to humans has proven frustrating. While DNA vaccines have been generally well tolerated in immunized volunteers, in most human studies of DNA vaccines, administration of even substantial quantities of DNA vaccine vectors has elicited relatively low-level immune responses. It is not yet known whether these disappointing results reflects fundamental differences in the immunogenic behavior of DNA vaccines in humans and mice, or the fact that the DNA doses administered to humans do not match those administered to mice (DNA per weight of the immunized host). Given the substantial size differences between humans and mice, it would likely be impractical (for reasons of both vaccine supply and the actual process of administration of sufficiently high doses of DNA) to administer the relative murine dose to humans. As such, a variety of approaches are being explored to prolong DNA survival in tissue, promote more efficient targeting of DNA to APCs, or to develop novel adjuvants that might specifically amplify immune responses to DNA vaccines.[103, 104]

DNA vaccines are currently being used as candidate preventive vaccines for a wide variety of infectious diseases, including HIV, tuberculosis, malaria, and CMV.

Poxviruses

Poxviruses represent the family of viruses that are physically the largest viruses and that possess the largest genomes. Much of the poxvirus genome encodes gene products that serve to evade host immune responses, and that are not required for virus replication in tissue culture. Further, facile techniques for the insertion and deletion of specific viral genes have been developed. The ability to accommodate sizeable foreign gene inserts is, in part, a function of the large size of the poxvirus genome (and the large packaging capacity of poxvirus virions). As a result of these favorable attributes, poxviruses have been utilized extensively in laboratory studies of virus biology, recombinant protein production, and host immune responses.[105] Although poxviruses encode multiple gene products that help the virus evade host immune responses, they are, nevertheless, potent immunogens. Studies of individuals immunized decades ago with vaccinia virus (in the course of smallpox eradication efforts) have shown that this virus induces long-lasting memory T- and B-cell immune responses.

In contrast to most of the other viral vectors currently being developed, poxviruses can replicate readily in culture and do not require an engineered host cell to support propagation *ex vivo*. One important limitation of all poxvirus vectors developed to date is that, given the large size of the poxvirus genomes and the multitude of gene products they naturally express, even large inserts derived from foreign pathogens of interest will present only a minority of the vaccine vector antigens delivered to and recognized by the host immune system. To be effective, approaches to focus immune responses on the antigen of interest will need to be developed. Toward this end, a variety of so-called 'prime–boost'[106] approaches are being explored where the host immune response is primed with one type of recombinant vaccine vector (such as a DNA vaccine or adenovirus vector) and then boosted with subsequent delivery of poxvirus vectors encoding the same antigen. In this manner, immune responses to antigens of interest have been significantly augmented in a number of preclinical studies.

Vaccinia virus represents the prototypic vaccine vector. This virus is the same one that was employed in the successful smallpox eradication campaign, and has been used as a laboratory tool for decades. However, given current high expectations for vaccine safety, and the increased number of immunodeficient individuals present in the population (as a result of the emergence of the HIV pandemic and the increased use of immunosuppressive therapies in clinical medicine) at high risk of serious adverse events, and potentially fatal consequences, from vaccinia immunization, the original vaccinia strains used in smallpox eradication efforts are not considered safe for general use. However, studies of vaccinia-based vaccine vectors have provided a strong basic foundation for research on other more highly attenuated poxvirus variants.

Modified vaccinia Ankara (MVA) is an attenuated vaccinia virus that was originally derived by prolonged passage of a vaccinia virus isolate on chicken embryo fibroblasts in culture. In the course of extensive passage in culture, a viral variant emerged that had fortuitously deleted large sections of the viral genome, including those that encode important poxvirus immune evasion genes and those that determine the ability of the virus to replicate on cells obtained from different animal species. Specifically, while MVA grows well on chicken cells, it cannot replicate in human cells in culture or *in vivo,* conferring an inherent safety feature.

MVA was safely administered to over 100 000 individuals at high risk of adverse consequence for vaccinia immunization toward the end of the smallpox eradication effort. More recently, it has garnered renewed interest as a potential safer smallpox vaccine in the wake of concerns about bioterrorism threats. Even though MVA cannot replicate in mammalian cells, the virus demonstrates favorable immunogenic properties. MVA has been used as a vector expressing genes for a wide variety of genes, including HIV and malaria antigens either alone or, as described above, in 'prime–boost' regimens, where MVA has been administered following initial priming immunizations with other vaccine vectors. A concerted effort is under way to improve further the performance of MVA by manipulating a series of poxvirus genes that dampen the human immune response to the virus (and to any antigens inserted in it).[107]

Avipox is a family of poxviruses that infect birds and cause respiratory diseases in poultry. Canarypox, a member of the avipox group, has been adapted as a vaccine vector. Canarypox replicates well on avian cells in culture but cannot replicate on human cells in culture or in humans *in vivo.* As a result, canarypox, like MVA, provides an interesting vector system with inherent safety features.[108] Canarypox vectors carrying HIV genes have been tested in several clinical studies, either alone, or in 'prime–boost' regimens following priming with adenovirus vectors and recombinant protein antigens. In a large ongoing phase III HIV vaccine trial, a recombinant canarypox vector is being used as a priming vector, followed by boosting with a recombinant version of the HIV gp120 surface Env protein. To date, the results from human clinical trials of canarypox vectors have been disappointing, with only low-level specific immune responses generated in human volunteers.[109]

Adenoviruses

Adenoviruses, one of the common causes of upper respiratory and gastrointestinal infections, have seen extensive use in clinical trials and were one of the first gene therapy vectors.[110] Most adenovirus vectors currently being studied in preclinical and clinical settings are disabled by deletion of the early E1 genes that are necessary for replication in an immunized host. Most adenovirus vaccine vectors developed have used the well-characterized and readily produced adenovirus serotype 5 (Ad5) as the vector 'backbone.' Disabled adenovirus vectors are grown in cells that express the E1 genes artificially inserted into the cell's genome.[111] Once these disabled vectors, encoding a heterologous pathogen-derived antigen of interest, enter a cell, the pathogen gene product is expressed,

processed, and presented by host APCs. As adenoviruses can directly infect dendritic cells, they promise to provide efficient vaccine vectors. Robust antibody and CD8 T-cell responses to heterologous antigen genes expressed by adenovirus vectors have been observed in preclinical animal models. Furthermore, in early-phase human clinical trials, adenovirus vectors have been generally well tolerated, and proven to be the most effective of any recombinant vector system studied to date in eliciting high-level CD8 T-cell responses.

The main potential drawback to widespread use of adenovirus vectors in humans is that, depending on the adenovirus type and the geographic location, variable levels of pre-existing immunity are found in humans as a result of prior naturally acquired adenovirus infections. High levels of antibody against the adenovirus vector might blunt the immunogenicity and efficacy of an adenovirus vector-based vaccine, but it remains to be seen if this will be a significant limitation.[112] Should pre-existing immunity to adenovirus vectors derived from epidemiologically prevalent serotypes (e.g., Ad5) limit vaccine immunogenicity, current efforts to develop vaccine vectors based on serotypes that are rare in human populations or novel adenovirus vectors specifically designed to avoid pre-existing antibody responses may yield effective alternative approaches.

Adenovirus vectors are currently used in clinical trials for vaccines against HIV,[113] malaria, influenza, and a range of other pathogens.

Alphaviruses

Alphaviruses are RNA viruses that cause zoonotic diseases, such as Venezuelan equine encephalitis. These viruses do not normally circulate in humans, so immunity to these viruses is quite rare in humans. Alphaviruses have a strategy for overexpressing the proteins that make up the virion by making a separate subgenomic RNA specifically encoding these gene products. Current recombinant alphavirus vaccine vector strategies take advantage of this subgenomic transcript, replacing the viral genes with selected genes for other antigens, but maintaining the signals for translation and protein production. In addition, through use of genetic complementation, it is possible to generate virus particles that only contain this heterologous antigen-encoding expression cassette. Such virus particles can efficiently mediate infection of host cells, but because they lack other alphavirus genes needed for virus replication cannot spread beyond the initial target cell infected.[114, 115] Alphavirus vectors rival the adenoviruses in efficiency of protein production in tissue culture and have induced robust antibody and T-cell responses in preclinical studies.[116] One current limitation of the alphavirus vector system is the difficulty of scaling the production system; however, this is a technical matter that should be addressable. In addition, ample safety data will be needed before widespread use of alphavirus vaccines achieves endorsement by regulatory authorities for use in healthy populations.

Adeno-associated virus

Adeno-associated viruses (AAV) belong to a family of single-stranded DNA viruses (parvoviruses) that include the B19 parvovirus that causes a rash in children known as 'fifth disease' (measles, mumps, rubella, and varicella make up the first four). AAV is transmitted in conjunction with adenovirus infection, and is not known to cause any significant disease. It is poorly immunogenic in the course of natural infections.[117] AAV can integrate into the genome of the infected cell, usually in a particular place on chromosome 19, although integration

product for a long time without the immune system killing the infected cell. Recently, efforts have been made to adapt replication-defective AAV as a vaccine vector. Although encouraging results have been reported in preclinical studies, phase I studies in humans have demonstrated disappointing immunogenicity.

■ SUMMARY ■

The challenges to optimizing the full public health potential of existing vaccines largely relate to programmatic considerations. In contrast, the terrible impact of infectious diseases that cannot now be prevented by vaccines (such as the 'big three' killers of HIV, tuberculosis, and malaria) pose direct challenges to the scientific community to develop new generations of vaccines that overcome the largely biological obstacles to control and elimination of these diseases. The nature of the challenges posed by such pathogens necessitates that future vaccine efforts will not simply recapitulate the immune responses engendered by natural infection (as has been the premise of traditional vaccine development efforts), but rather, substantially improve upon them.

As the development of vaccines to prevent infections with the so-far refractory pathogens is pursued, improved understanding of the immune response to natural infection, as well as delineation of the reasons why host immune responses fail either to clear incipient infections or prevent future new ones, will be essential. Fortunately, early empiric approaches have now been replaced with hypothesis-driven strategies enabled by improved insight into the functioning of the human immune system, as well as new technologies, including higher-resolution tools to describe and quantitate pathogen-specific immune responses; novel methods for antigen discovery and targeted optimization of immunogenicity; the development of new, mechanism-based adjuvants; and the advent of innovative methods for vaccine vector-mediated antigen delivery. Thus, although the challenges may be vexing, the scientific and technical foundations on which vaccine development efforts rest have never been stronger.

■ REFERENCES ■

1. Ten great public health achievements – United States, 1900–1999. MMWR Morb Mortal Wkly Rep 1999; 48: 241–243.

2. Henderson DA. Principles and lessons from the smallpox eradication programme. Bull World Health Organ 1987; 65: 535–546.

3. Berndt ER, Glennerster R, Kremer MR, et al. Advance market commitments for vaccines against neglected diseases: estimating costs and effectiveness. Health Econ 2007; 16: 491–511.

4. Heymann DL, Aylward RB. Mass vaccination: when and why. Curr Top Microbiol Immunol 2006; 304: 1–16.

5. Anderson RM, May RM. Immunisation and herd immunity. Lancet 1990; 335: 641–645.

6. Peter G, Gardner P. Standards for immunization practice for vaccines in children and adults. Infect Dis Clin North Am 2001; 15: 9–19.

7. Zhou F, Santoli J, Messonnier ML, et al. Economic evaluation of the 7-vaccine routine childhood immunization schedule in the United States, 2001. Arch Pediatr Adolesc Med 2005; 159: 1136–1144.

KEY CONCEPTS

VACCINE APPROACHES BEING EXPLORED TO IMPROVE ON NATURAL IMMUNITY

For many important infectious diseases for which no vaccines are currently available, successful derivation of effective vaccines will depend on improving upon natural immunity, especially in those instances where natural immunity does not follow natural infection (such as human immunodeficiency virus (HIV) and malaria) or where safety concerns limit the development of specific protective antigens (*Neisseria meningitidis* group B). In addition, for other pathogens that typically manifest significant genetic (and antigenic) diversity (such as influenza, HIV, and bacteria such as *Streptococcus pneumoniae*), a need exists to develop novel vaccines that can protect against a wide range of variants with a limited number of vaccine immunogens. Towards these ends, a number of new approaches, enabled by new vaccine technologies, are being pursued, including:

>> Targeted alteration of protective antigens to increase their ability to elicit protective immune responses (e.g., efforts to alter the structure of the HIV Env glycoproteins gp120 and gp41 so that they elicit higher-level, more potent, neutralizing antibody responses than their native counterparts)

>> The development of synthetic consensus antigens able to elicit broader immune responses than would sequences obtained from individual pathogen isolates (e.g., efforts to develop consensus immunogens able to elicit cytotoxic T-lymphocyte (CTL) responses against genetically diverse HIV-1 variants)

>> Techniques for new antigen discovery to identify novel conserved antigens within otherwise genetically diverse pathogens (e.g., *Streptococcus pneumoniae*) or those for which currently known protective antigens cannot be developed as vaccines (e.g., *Neisseria meningitidis* group B)

>> The use of novel adjuvants or vaccine vectors to enable generation of higher-level and/or more functional immune responses to pathogen antigens by vaccination than are seen following natural infection, and to enable high-level, fully functional memory immune responses to be activated at the time of initial infection (e.g., efforts to elicit high-level HIV-specific or hepatitis C virus-specific CTLs by recombinant viral vectors)

>> Use of novel methods to shift relative immunodominance of specific pathogen gene products to increase the immunogenicity of conserved antigens from otherwise diverse pathogen genomes that are typically poorly immunogenic in the course of natural infections (e.g., efforts to augment the antibody response to the influenza A virus M2 protein via the use of potent adjuvants or conjugation to immunogenic carrier proteins)

does not appear to be efficient or site-specific when replication-defective adenoviruses of the type being developed as vaccine vectors are used. The propensity for chromosomal integration and poor immune response to the virus made AAV a good candidate for gene therapy; cells with an integrated viral genome could deliver a gene

8. Coffield AB, Maciosek MV, McGinnis JM, et al. Priorities among recommended clinical preventive services. Am J Prev Med 2001; 21: 1–9.

9. Cross AS, Opal S, Cook P, et al. Development of an anti-core lipopolysaccharide vaccine for the prevention and treatment of sepsis. Vaccine 2004; 22: 812–817.

10. Ruiz-Palacios GM, Perez-Schael I, Velazquez FR, et al. Safety and efficacy of an attenuated vaccine against severe rotavirus gastroenteritis. N Engl J Med 2006; 354: 11–22.

11. Vesikari T, Matson DO, Dennehy P, et al. Safety and efficacy of a pentavalent human-bovine (WC3) reassortant rotavirus vaccine. N Engl J Med 2006; 354: 23–33.

12. Stewart AJ, Devlin PM. The history of the smallpox vaccine. J Infect 2006; 52: 329–334.

13. Tizard I. Grease, anthraxgate, and kennel cough: a revisionist history of early veterinary vaccines. Adv Vet Med 1999; 41: 7–24.

14. Dowdle WR, De Gourville E, Kew OM, et al. Polio eradication: the OPV paradox. Rev Med Virol 2003; 13: 277–291.

15. Falk LA, Chandler DK, Richman P. Review of current preclinical testing strategies for bacterial vaccines. Dev Biol Stand 1998; 95: 25–29.

16. Kreeftenberg JG. Standardization of acellular pertussis vaccines. Biologicals 1999; 27: 115–117.

17. Lesinski GB, Westerink MA. Vaccines against polysaccharide antigens. Curr Drug Targets Infect Disord 2001; 1: 325–334.

18. Lockhart S. Conjugate vaccines. Exp Rev Vaccines 2003; 2: 633–648.

19. Hilleman MR. Newer directions in vaccine development and utilization. J Infect Dis 1985; 151: 407–419.

20. Zuckerman AJ. The development of novel hepatitis B vaccines. Biochem Soc Symp 1987; 53: 39–49.

21. Kirnbauer R, Booy F, Cheng N, et al. Papillomavirus L1 major capsid protein self-assembles into virus-like particles that are highly immunogenic. Proc Natl Acad Sci USA 1992; 89: 12180–12184.

22. Garland SM, Hernandez-Avila M, Wheeler CM, et al. Quadrivalent vaccine against human papillomavirus to prevent anogenital diseases. N Engl J Med 2007; 356: 1928–1943.

23. Villa LL, Ault KA, Giuliano AR, et al. Immunologic responses following administration of a vaccine targeting human papillomavirus types 6, 11, 16, and 18. Vaccine 2006; 24: 5571–5583.

24. Shaw AR. The rotavirus vaccine saga. Annu Rev Med 2006; 57: 167–180.

25. Parashar UD, Hummelman EG, Bresee JS, et al. Global illness and deaths caused by rotavirus disease in children. Emerg Infect Dis 2003; 9: 565–572.

26. Simonsen L, Morens D, Elixhauser A, et al. Effect of rotavirus vaccination programme on trends in admission of infants to hospital for intussusception. Lancet 2001; 358: 1224–1229.

27. Matson DO. RotaShield: the ill-fated rhesus-human reassortant rotavirus vaccine. Pediatr Ann 2006; 35: 44–50.

28. Geier DA, Geier MR. A review of the Vaccine Adverse Event Reporting System database. Exp Opin Pharmacother 2004; 5: 691–698.

29. Verstraeten T, DeStefano F, Chen RT, et al. Vaccine safety surveillance using large linked databases: opportunities, hazards and proposed guidelines. Exp Rev Vaccines 2003; 2: 21–29.

30. Griffith AH. Permanent brain damage and pertussis vaccination: is the end of the saga in sight? Vaccine 1989; 7: 199–210.

31. Afzal MA, Ozoemena LC, O'Hare A, et al. Absence of detectable measles virus genome sequence in blood of autistic children who have had their MMR vaccination during the routine childhood immunization schedule of UK. J Med Virol 2006; 78: 623–630.

32. Burgess DC, Burgess MA, Leask J. The MMR vaccination and autism controversy in United Kingdom 1998–2005: inevitable community outrage or a failure of risk communication? Vaccine 2006; 24: 3921–3928.

33. Tsai CM. Molecular mimicry of host structures by lipooligosaccharides of *Neisseria meningitidis*: characterization of sialylated and nonsialylated lacto-*N*-neotetraose (Galbeta1-4GlcNAcbeta1-3Galbeta1-4Glc) structures in lipooligosaccharides using monoclonal antibodies and specific lectins. Adv Exp Med Biol 2001; 491: 525–542.

34. Healy CM, Baker CJ. Prospects for prevention of childhood infections by maternal immunization. Curr Opin Infect Dis 2006; 19: 271–276.

35. Johnston MI, Fauci AS. An HIV vaccine – evolving concepts. N Engl J Med 2007; 356: 2073–2081.

36. Garber DA, Silvestri G, Feinberg MB. Prospects for an AIDS vaccine: three big questions, no easy answers. Lancet Infect Dis 2004; 4: 397–413.

37. Johnson VA, Brun-Vezinet F, Clotet B, et al. Update of the drug resistance mutations in HIV-1: 2004. Top HIV Med 2004; 12: 119–124.

38. HIV gp120 vaccine – VaxGen: AIDSVAX, AIDSVAX B/B, AIDSVAX B/E, HIV gp120 vaccine – Genentech, HIV gp120 vaccine AIDSVAX – VaxGen, HIV vaccine AIDSVAX – VaxGen. Drugs R D 2003; 4: 249–253.

39. Shiver JW, Emini EA. Recent advances in the development of HIV-1 vaccines using replication-incompetent adenovirus vectors. Annu Rev Med 2004; 55: 355–372.

39a. Steinbrook R. One step forward, two steps back — will there ever be an AIDS vaccine? N Engl J Med 2007; 357: 2653–2655.

40. Smith TA, Leuenberger R, Lengeler C. Child mortality and malaria transmission intensity in Africa. Trends Parasitol 2001; 17: 145–149.

41. Snow RW, Trape JF, Marsh K. The past, present and future of childhood malaria mortality in Africa. Trends Parasitol 2001; 17: 593–597.

42. Malaguarnera L, Musumeci S. The immune response to *Plasmodium falciparum* malaria. Lancet Infect Dis 2002; 2: 472–478.

43. Achtman AH, Bull PC, Stephens R, et al. Longevity of the immune response and memory to blood-stage malaria infection. Curr Top Microbiol Immunol 2005; 297: 71–102.

44. Ballou WR. Malaria vaccines in development. Exp Opin Emerg Drugs 2005; 10: 489–503.

45. Bojang KA. RTS,S/AS02A for malaria. Exp Rev Vaccines 2006; 5: 611–615.

46. Wizel B, Houghten RA, Parker KC, et al. Irradiated sporozoite vaccine induces HLA-B8-restricted cytotoxic T lymphocyte responses against two overlapping epitopes of the *Plasmodium falciparum* sporozoite surface protein 2. J Exp Med 1995; 182: 1435–1445.

47. Maher D, Raviglione M. Global epidemiology of tuberculosis. Clin Chest Med 2005; 26: 167–182. v.

48. Skeiky YA, Sadoff JC. Advances in tuberculosis vaccine strategies. Nat Rev Microbiol 2006; 4: 469–476.

49. Fine PE, Rodrigues LC. Modern vaccines. Mycobacterial diseases. Lancet 1990; 335: 1016–1020.

50. Orme IM. Tuberculosis vaccines: current progress. Drugs 2005; 65: 2437–2444.

51. Orme IM. Preclinical testing of new vaccines for tuberculosis: a comprehensive review. Vaccine 2006; 24: 2–19.

52. de Jonge MI, Brosch R, Brodin P, et al. Tuberculosis: from genome to vaccine. Exp Rev Vaccines 2005; 4: 541–551.

53. Fulginiti VA, Eller JJ, Sieber OF, et al. Respiratory virus immunization. I. A field trial of two inactivated respiratory virus vaccines; an aqueous trivalent parainfluenza virus vaccine and an alum-precipitated respiratory syncytial virus vaccine. Am J Epidemiol 1969; 89: 435–448.

54. Wilson S, Aprile MA. Sensitizing versus immunizing properties of inactivated measles vaccine. Prog Immunobiol Stand 1970; 4: 657–660.

55. Schmidt AC, McAuliffe JM, Murphy BR, et al. Recombinant bovine/human parainfluenza virus type 3 (B/HPIV3) expressing the respiratory syncytial virus (RSV) G and F proteins can be used to achieve simultaneous mucosal immunization against RSV and HPIV3. J Virol 2001; 75: 4594–4603.

56. Pichichero ME. The new meningococcal conjugate vaccine. A profile of its safety, efficacy, and indications for use. Postgrad Med 2006; 119: 47–54, 64.

57. Finne J, Leinonen M, Makela PH. Antigenic similarities between brain components and bacteria causing meningitis. Implications for vaccine development and pathogenesis. Lancet 1983; 2: 355–357.

58. Schrag S, Gorwitz R, Fultz-Butts K, et al. Prevention of perinatal group B streptococcal disease. Revised guidelines from CDC. MMWR Recomm Rep 2002; 51: 1–22.

59. Mikkelsen M, Bukh J. Current status of a hepatitis C vaccine: encouraging results but significant challenges ahead. Curr Infect Dis Rep 2007; 9: 94–101.

60. Ferenczy MW. Prophylactic vaccine strategies and the potential of therapeutic vaccines against herpes simplex virus. Curr Pharm Des 2007; 13: 1975–1988.

61. Stanberry LR. Clinical trials of prophylactic and therapeutic herpes simplex virus vaccines. Herpes 2004; 11(Suppl. 3): 161A–169A.

62. Plotkin SA, Huygelen C. Cytomegalovirus vaccine prepared in WI-38. Dev Biol Stand 1976; 37: 301–305.

63. Adler SP, Plotkin SA, Gonczol E, et al. A canarypox vector expressing cytomegalovirus (CMV) glycoprotein B primes for antibody responses to a live attenuated CMV vaccine (Towne). J Infect Dis 1999; 180: 843–846.

64. Zhong J, Khanna R. Vaccine strategies against human cytomegalovirus infection. Exp Rev Anti Infect Ther 2007; 5: 449–459.

65. Moutschen M, Leonard P, Sokal EM, et al. Phase I/II studies to evaluate safety and immunogenicity of a recombinant gp350 Epstein–Barr virus vaccine in healthy adults. Vaccine 2007; 25: 4697–4705.

66. Stephenson JR. Understanding dengue pathogenesis: implications for vaccine design. Bull World Health Organ 2005; 83: 308–314.

67. Whitehead SS, Blaney JE, Durbin AP, et al. Prospects for a dengue virus vaccine. Nat Rev Microbiol 2007; 5: 518–528.

68. Ramos BV. A method for the screening of fusion protein expression by lambda-GT11 recombinant clones without the preparation of lysogens. Nucleic Acids Res 1989; 17: 6421.

69. Jones P. Antibody screening of bacteriophage lambda gt-11 DNA expression libraries. Methods Mol Biol 1998; 80: 439–447.

70. Wack A, Rappuoli R. Vaccinology at the beginning of the 21st century. Curr Opin Immunol 2005; 17: 411–418.

71. Rappuoli R. Reverse vaccinology, a genome-based approach to vaccine development. Vaccine 2001; 19: 2688–2691.

72. Muzzi A, Masignani V, Rappuoli R. The pan-genome: towards a knowledge-based discovery of novel targets for vaccines and antibacterials. Drug Discov Today 2007; 12: 429–439.

73. Grandi G. Genomics and proteomics in reverse vaccines. Methods Biochem Anal 2006; 49: 379–393.

74. Tang CM, Hood DW, Moxon ER. Haemophilus influence: the impact of whole genome sequencing on microbiology. Trends Genet 1997; 13: 399–404.

75. Gardner MJ, Hall N, Fung E, et al. Genome sequence of the human malaria parasite Plasmodium falciparum. Nature 2002; 419: 498–511.

76. Nilsson CL. Bacterial proteomics and vaccine development. Am J Pharmacogenomics 2002; 2: 59–65.

77. Klade CS. Proteomics approaches towards antigen discovery and vaccine development. Curr Opin Mol Ther 2002; 4: 216–223.

78. Hillen N, Stevanovic S. Contribution of mass spectrometry-based proteomics to immunology. Exp Rev Proteomics 2006; 3: 653–664.

79. Strong M, Goulding CW. Structural proteomics and computational analysis of a deadly pathogen: combating Mycobacterium tuberculosis from multiple fronts. Methods Biochem Anal 2006; 49: 245–269.

80. Chitlaru T, Gat O, Grosfeld H, et al. Identification of in vivo-expressed immunogenic proteins by serological proteome analysis of the Bacillus anthracis secretome. Infect Immun 2007; 75: 2841–2852.

81. Klade CS, Voss T, Krystek E, et al. Identification of tumor antigens in renal cell carcinoma by serological proteome analysis. Proteomics 2001; 1: 890–898.

82. Janeway CA Jr, Medzhitov R. Innate immune recognition. Annu Rev Immunol 2002; 20: 197–216.

83. Blander JM, Medzhitov R. On regulation of phagosome maturation and antigen presentation. Nat Immunol 2006; 7: 1029–1035.

84. Pulendran B, Ahmed R. Translating innate immunity into immunological memory: implications for vaccine development. Cell 2006; 124: 849–863.

85. Medzhitov R, Janeway CA Jr. Innate immune induction of the adaptive immune response. Cold Spring Harb Symp Quant Biol 1999; 64: 429–435.

86. Kersten GF, Crommelin DJ. Liposomes and ISCOMs. Vaccine 2003; 21: 915–920.

87. Querec TD, Pulendran B. Understanding the role of innate immunity in the mechanism of action of the live attenuated yellow fever vaccine 17D. Adv Exp Med Biol 2007; 590: 43–53.

88. Latz E, Franko J, Golenbock DT, et al. Haemophilus influenzae type b outer membrane protein complex glycoconjugate vaccine induces cytokine production by engaging human Toll-like receptor 2 (TLR2) and requires the presence of TLR2 for optimal immunogenicity. J Immunol 2004; 172: 2431–2438.

89. Hem SL, White JL. Structure and properties of aluminum-containing adjuvants. Pharm Biotechnol 1995; 6: 249–276.

90. Desjardins R, Krzystyniak K, Therien HM, et al. Immunoactivating potential of multilamellar liposome vesicles (MLV) in murine popliteal lymph node (PLN) test. Int J Immunopharmacol 1995; 17: 367–374.

91. Gluck R, Burri KG, Metcalfe I. Adjuvant and antigen delivery properties of virosomes. Curr Drug Deliv 2005; 2: 395–400.

92. Atmar RL, Keitel WA, Patel SM, et al. Safety and immunogenicity of nonadjuvanted and MF59-adjuvanted influenza A/H9N2 vaccine preparations. Clin Infect Dis 2006; 43: 1135–1142.

93. Kundi M. New hepatitis B vaccine formulated with an improved adjuvant system. Exp Rev Vaccines 2007; 6: 133–140.

94. Cooper CL, Davis HL, Angel JB, et al. CPG 7909 adjuvant improves hepatitis B virus vaccine seroprotection in antiretroviral-treated HIV-infected adults. Aids 2005; 19: 1473–1479.

95. Payette PJ, Ma X, Weeratna RD, et al. Testing of CpG-optimized protein and DNA vaccines against the hepatitis B virus in chimpanzees for immunogenicity and protection from challenge. Intervirology 2006; 49: 144–151.

96. Broide DH. Immunostimulatory sequences of DNA and conjugates in the treatment of allergic rhinitis. Curr Allergy Asthma Rep 2005; 5: 182–185.

97. Wille-Reece U, Flynn BJ, Lore K, et al. HIV Gag protein conjugated to a Toll-like receptor 7/8 agonist improves the magnitude and quality of Th1 and CD8+ T cell responses in nonhuman primates. Proc Natl Acad Sci USA 2005; 102: 15190–15194.

98. Huleatt JW, Jacobs AR, Tang J, et al. Vaccination with recombinant fusion proteins incorporating Toll-like receptor ligands induces rapid cellular and humoral immunity. Vaccine 2007; 25: 763–775.

99. McDonald WF, Huleatt JW, Foellmer HG, et al. A west nile virus recombinant protein vaccine that coactivates innate and adaptive immunity. J Infect Dis 2007; 195: 1607–1617.

100. Clark HF, Offit PA, Ellis RW, et al. The development of multivalent bovine rotavirus (strain WC3) reassortant vaccine for infants. J Infect Dis 1996; 174(Suppl 1): S73–S80.

101. Wells DJ. Intramuscular injection of plasmid DNA. Mol Cell Biol Hum Dis Ser 1995; 5: 83–103.

102. Ulmer JB, Donnelly JJ, Parker SE, et al. Heterologous protection against influenza by injection of DNA encoding a viral protein. Science 1993; 259: 1745–1749.

103. Liu MA, Wahren B, Karlsson Hedestam GB. DNA vaccines: recent developments and future possibilities. Hum Gene Ther 2006; 17: 1051–1061.

104. Laddy DJ, Weiner DB. From plasmids to protection: a review of DNA vaccines against infectious diseases. Int Rev Immunol 2006; 25: 99–123.

105. Franchini G, Gurunathan S, Baglyos L, et al. Poxvirus-based vaccine candidates for HIV: two decades of experience with special emphasis on canarypox vectors. Exp Rev Vaccines 2004; 3(Suppl): S75–S88.

106. Kent S, De Rose R, Rollman E. Drug evaluation: DNA/MVA prime-boost HIV vaccine. Curr Opin Invest Drugs 2007; 8: 159–167.

107. Abaitua F, Rodriguez JR, Garzon A, et al. Improving recombinant MVA immune responses: potentiation of the immune responses to HIV-1 with MVA and DNA vectors expressing Env and the cytokines IL-12 and IFN-gamma. Virus Res 2006; 116: 11–20.

108. Taylor J, Tartaglia J, Riviere M, et al. Applications of canarypox (ALVAC) vectors in human and veterinary vaccination. Dev Biol Stand 1994; 82: 131–135.

109. Goepfert PA, Horton H, McElrath MJ, et al. High-dose recombinant Canarypox vaccine expressing HIV-1 protein, in seronegative human subjects. J Infect Dis 2005; 192: 1249–1259.

110. McConnell MJ, Imperiale MJ. Biology of adenovirus and its use as a vector for gene therapy. Hum Gene Ther 2004; 15: 1022–1033.

111. Graham FL, Prevec L. Adenovirus-based expression vectors and recombinant vaccines. Biotechnology 1992; 20: 363–390.

112. Schulick AH, Vassalli G, Dunn PF, et al. Established immunity precludes adenovirus-mediated gene transfer in rat carotid arteries. Potential for immunosuppression and vector engineering to overcome barriers of immunity. J Clin Invest 1997; 99: 209–219.

113. Casimiro DR, Wang F, Schleif WA, et al. Attenuation of simian immunodeficiency virus SIVmac239 infection by prophylactic immunization with DNA and recombinant adenoviral vaccine vectors expressing Gag. J Virol 2005; 79: 15547–15555.

114. Caley IJ, Betts MR, Davis NL, et al. Venezuelan equine encephalitis virus vectors expressing HIV-1 proteins: vector design strategies for improved vaccine efficacy. Vaccine 1999; 17: 3124–3135.

115. Perri S, Greer CE, Thudium K, et al. An alphavirus replicon particle chimera derived from Venezuelan equine encephalitis and sindbis viruses is a potent gene-based vaccine delivery vector. J Virol 2003; 77: 10394–10403.

116. Riezebos-Brilman A, de Mare A, Bungener L, et al. Recombinant alphaviruses as vectors for anti-tumour and anti-microbial immunotherapy. J Clin Virol 2006; 35: 233–243.

117. Sun JY, Anand-Jawa V, Chatterjee S, et al. Immune responses to adeno-associated virus and its recombinant vectors. Gene Ther 2003; 10: 964–976.

Immunotherapy of allergic disease

Anthony J. Frew

93

Specific allergen immunotherapy (SIT) involves the administration of allergen extracts to modify or abolish symptoms associated with atopic allergy. The general principles of managing allergic conditions are to make an accurate diagnosis, to identify relevant trigger factors, to institute appropriate interventions in order to reduce the impact of those triggers, and to control symptoms and disease progression. Allergen avoidance measures may be helpful, but may be difficult to implement, and are rarely sufficient to allow patients to do without other therapy. Drug treatments can be very effective, but only work as long as they are taken, so there is clearly a need for additional and long-lasting therapy. SIT is the only current therapy that modifies the immune response to allergens. The process is specific, in that the treatment is targeted at those allergens recognized by the patient and physician as responsible for symptoms. While claims for bystander benefits have been made, there is little convincing evidence that treating for one allergen will alleviate symptoms caused by a different allergen. Before deciding to use SIT it is therefore essential to assess the patient's condition carefully, with particular emphasis on the role of allergic triggers.

SIT was pioneered at the end of the 19th century and then reported formally in 1911 by Noon and Freeman at St. Mary's Hospital, London.[1] Immunotherapy then became popular in North America and in Europe, but some differences in practice have gradually developed either side of the Atlantic. In particular, American allergists tend to treat for all sensitivities identified on skin testing, using mixtures of extracts prepared from bulk vials, whereas in Europe patients are normally only treated with a single allergen, which is supplied direct from the manufacturer. Mixed allergen extracts are available and used in some parts of Europe, but only as custom mixes from manufacturers. Another difference in clinical practice is that allergen extracts used in Europe are usually dialyzed to remove low-molecular-weight components, and are standardized according to their ability to elicit a wheal, whereas in the USA, extracts may not be dialyzed and standardization is based on ability to elicit erythema rather than wheal.

Whichever form of extract is chosen, patients are started on a very low dose of allergen, and the dose is then increased, usually at weekly intervals until a plateau or maintenance dose is achieved. The maintenance dose is then given at 4–6-weekly intervals for 3–5 years. Alternative induction regimes may give several doses on each day (semi-rush protocol), or may give the whole series of incremental injections in a single day (rush protocol). The main drawback to rush and semi-rush protocols is the risk of adverse reactions, which are much commoner than in conventional protocols. On the other hand, full protection can be attained in a few days as compared to the 3 months required in the conventional regime. Normally the doses are given by subcutaneous injection, but in recent years there has been an upsurge of interest in alternative routes of administration, especially the sublingual route, which is popular in Italy, France, and Germany and is gaining ground elsewhere in Europe, but not yet in the USA.

■ MECHANISMS ■

Several mechanisms have been proposed to explain the beneficial effects of immunotherapy (Table 93.1). Following subcutaneous injection of allergen extracts, a small proportion of the allergenic material is taken up by phagocytic cells and carried to the regional lymph nodes. The process is fairly inefficient and less than 1% of a radiolabeled dose actually reaches the lymph nodes. Almost all studies have shown that SIT induces allergen-specific immunoglobulin G (IgG) antibodies that increase progressively over the course of treatment. This has led to suggestions that SIT might work by inducing antibodies that intercept the allergen and "block" the allergic response. In patients treated for venom anaphylaxis, the development of allergen-specific IgG antibody correlates with clinical efficacy but, for other allergens, the magnitude of the IgG response is not closely related to the degree of efficacy. Moreover, the rise in IgG follows the onset of clinical benefit, rather than preceding it. Initially there is an increase in allergen-specific IgE antibodies, but the usual rise in IgE seen during natural seasonal exposure is blunted.[2] Over the course of several years, the amount of allergen-specific IgE declines, but it does not disappear. In keeping with this there is little effect on immediate skin test responses to allergen. In contrast, the late-phase skin test response is virtually abolished after successful SIT. Similar patterns are observed for late-phase nasal and airway responses.[3]

SIT also has clear effects on allergen-specific T cells (Fig. 93.1). Both in the skin and in the nose, successful SIT is accompanied by a reduction in

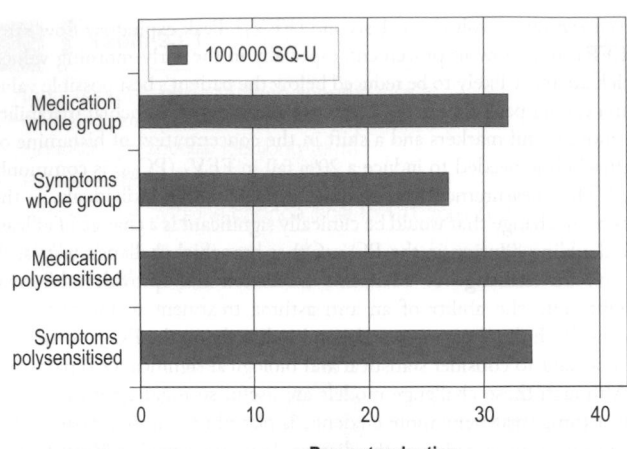

Fig. 93.2 Effect of grass-pollen specific allergen immunotherapy on symptom scores and medication use in a clinical trial of 410 subjects. Polysensitized subjects responded at least as well as those who were monosensitized to grass pollen. (Data adapted from Frew AJ, Powell RM, Corrigan CJ, et al. Efficacy and safety of specific immunotherapy with SQ allergen extract in treatment-resistant seasonal allergic rhinoconjunctivitis. J Allergy Clin Immunol 2006; 117: 319–325.)

perennial symptoms. Allergy to housedust mite is common and does not always cause symptoms. Conversely, there are other causes of perennial rhinitis, including vasomotor instability, infection, and aspirin sensitivity. Nevertheless, clinical trials have shown a definite benefit provided the subjects are appropriately selected.[10] Clearer evidence of efficacy has been obtained in rhinitis due to pet allergy. Several studies have shown a marked improvement in tolerance of cat exposure after SIT, confirmed both on challenge tests (Fig. 93.3) and in simulated natural exposure.[11]

As with any therapy, the risks and cost-effectiveness of SIT need to be assessed on a case-by-case basis. Current drug therapy for rhinitis can be very effective, but about 60% of patients with seasonal allergic rhinitis report inadequate symptom control, even when taking maximal doses of antihistamines and intranasal glucocorticoids. Others experience nose bleeds from intranasal steroids and drowsiness from antihistamines. Moreover, we are now more aware of the adverse effects of rhinitis on quality of life. SIT offers a useful option for these patients as well as a logical approach to dealing with the underlying problem.

SIT FOR ASTHMA

Immunotherapy was widely used to treat allergic asthma in the UK prior to 1986 but evidence of severe adverse reactions, including a small number of fatalities, led to SIT being abandoned for asthma treatment in the UK, although asthma remains a common indication for SIT in North America and continental Europe.[11, 12] There is no doubt that SIT is effective on asthma symptoms and protects against specific and nonspecific triggers. However, the role of allergic sensitization in ongoing asthma is less clear than for rhinitis, and the risks of therapy are undoubtedly greater in asthma. Current drug therapies for asthma aim to suppress the airways inflammation and smooth-muscle contraction that are characteristic features of asthma. None of these treatments are curative

and asthma rapidly recurs on ceasing treatment. Moreover, none of the current drug therapies is directed against agents that might cause asthma. Allergen avoidance has been proposed as a potentially useful maneuver in those with allergic asthma, but although asthma control can be improved by extreme forms of allergen avoidance (e.g., admission to hospital, sending children to holiday homes at altitude), there is little evidence that similar benefits can be achieved using the type of allergen avoidance that can be achieved in suburban homes. There is thus scope for improving asthma care and for identifying allergen-specific therapies. SIT offers the possibility of deviating the immune response away from the allergic pattern and towards a more protective or less damaging response.

The efficacy of SIT in adult asthma has been assessed in many trials over the last 50 years. The results of these studies have often been difficult to interpret, either because poor-quality allergen extracts were used or because of poor study design. Many trials were not placebo-controlled; they were either open or single-blind, and in most cases only small numbers of patients were treated. A recently updated meta-analysis identified 75 papers published between 1954 and 2001.[13] Thirty-six of these were for mite allergy, 20 for pollen allergy, 10 for animal dander allergy, two for mold allergy, one for latex allergy, and six used combinations of allergens. Concealment of allocation was clearly adequate in only 15 trials. A wide variety of different measurements were made, which makes it difficult to reach a firm view on the overall effectiveness of SIT. Symptom scores improved in the treated groups – it was necessary to treat four patients to prevent one from exacerbating, and to treat five to prevent one from needing an increase in medication. SIT reduced the airways response to inhalation of specific allergen and also improved nonspecific bronchial reactivity.

The economics of using SIT to treat asthma are that some reduction can be achieved in anti-asthma drug costs, but these do not offset the costs of SIT. This means that the cost–benefit analysis depends greatly on the value placed on symptom reduction and perhaps the prevention of progression.

SIT reduces the early asthmatic response to inhaled allergen in cat-allergic asthmatics and attenuates responses to cat room exposure. Interestingly, these studies showed a clear delay in onset of symptoms and an overall reduction in symptoms and peak flow recordings after exposure to cats, but there was no protection against allergen-induced increases in nonspecific bronchial hyperresponsiveness. In contrast, SIT with a dog dander extract has not been shown to be effective in clinical trials.

Several double-blind placebo-controlled studies have examined the effects of SIT in asthmatic patients sensitive to housedust mite. Early studies showed conflicting results, but recent studies using more modern extracts have found beneficial effects on symptoms, anti-asthma drug use, and bronchial hyperresponsiveness.

COMPARISON OF SIT WITH OTHER THERAPIES

The majority of clinical trials of SIT for asthma have compared SIT either with untreated historical controls or with a matched placebo-treated group. To date, the effectiveness of SIT in asthma has rarely been compared with conventional management (avoidance measures and inhaled or oral anti-asthma drugs). One study assessed SIT in asthmatic children receiving conventional drug therapy and found no additional benefit in patients who were already receiving optimal drug therapy.[14]

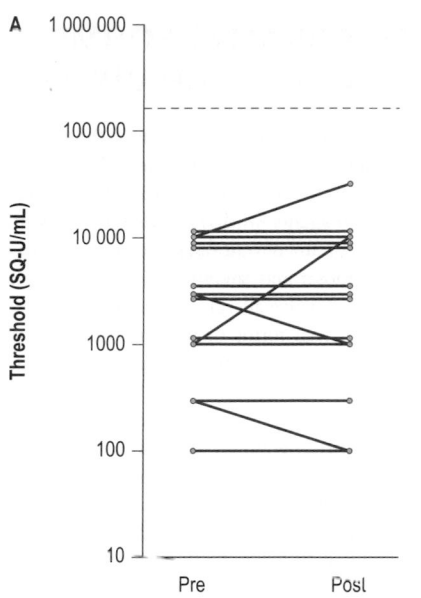 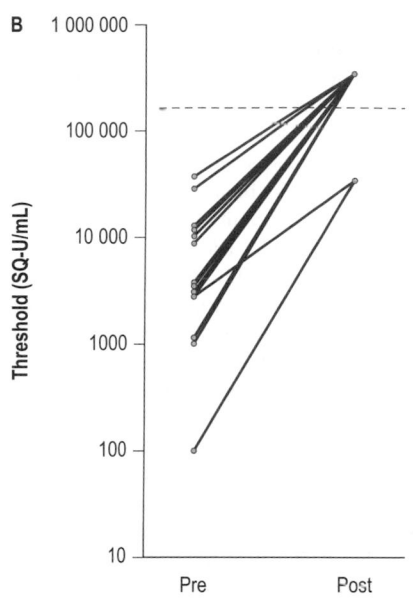

Fig. 93.3 Effect of specific allergen immunotherapy with cat dander extract on conjunctival provocation test threshold. (From Varney VA, Edwards J, Tabbah K, et al. Clinical efficacy of specific immunotherapy to cat dander: a double blind placebo controlled trial. Clin Exp Allergy 1997; 27: 860–867.)

There are some flaws in the design of this study and further work of this type is urgently needed.

EFFECTS OF SIT ON THE NATURAL HISTORY OF ALLERGIC DISEASE

A proportion of patients with allergic rhinitis go on to develop asthma each year. This annual rate of progression has been estimated at 5% in college students,[15] but this is perhaps surprisingly an area of considerable ignorance. A number of long-term epidemiological studies are now in progress under the auspices of the International Study of Asthma and Allergies in Childhood (ISAAC) and these should eventually shed light on the rate of progression at different ages and the extent of regional and international variation. It has been suggested that SIT may modify the natural history of asthma in children who have allergic rhinitis but have not yet developed asthma. Only limited data are available to support this proposition. In the key study, a group of 205 children aged 6–14, without previously diagnosed asthma, were treated with SIT for birch or grass-pollen allergy in an open randomized design. Three years after completing treatment 45% of the untreated group had developed asthma whereas only 26% of the treated group had asthma. These results have been sustained to 7 years after completing therapy. Thus four children had to be treated to prevent one case of asthma, which makes this an extremely effective therapy.[16] SIT may also modify the progression of established asthma. An early open study using uncharacterized mixed allergen extracts supported this view, with about 70% of treated children losing their asthma after 4 years' therapy, compared to about 19% of untreated controls, a result that was sustained up to the age of 16 years. The proportion of children whose asthma was severe at age 16 was also much lower in the treated group.[12] By modern standards, this study was not well designed, and it needs repeating with modern SIT extracts in an up-to-date trial design.

CLINICAL PEARLS

FACTORS ASSOCIATED WITH ADVERSE REACTIONS TO SPECIFIC ALLERGEN IMMUNOTHERAPY

Dosage errors

Asthma, especially uncontrolled/severe

Highly sensitive patients

Concurrent treatment with β-adrenergic blockers

Accelerated regimens (rush, ultra-rush)

Injections from new vials (especially with nonstandardized extracts)

Injections during periods of exacerbation of symptoms

Injections given during active viral or bacterial respiratory tract infections

SIT can also prevent the development of new sensitizations.[10] In both open and double-blind studies, monosensitized children were much less likely to acquire new sensitivities, as shown by skin tests, than comparable control groups. It seems probable that this effect is indirect. In other words it is unlikely that SIT with housedust mite directly affects B cells that recognize cat or grass pollen, but by treating the housedust mite allergy, SIT may reduce inflammation in the nose, and hence modify the likelihood of exposure to other allergens proceeding to sensitization. There is as yet no evidence to support claims that SIT is different from drug therapy in terms of influencing the evolution of established asthma. In part this reflects the reluctance of physicians to

The recent introduction of monoclonal antibodies directed against IgE offers another alternative. Treatment with anti-IgE reduces immediate and late-phase responses to inhaled allergen[32] and should also reduce the risk of adverse effects from SIT injections. Moreover, when anti-IgE is combined with conventional SIT, the effects are additive against seasonal allergic rhinitis.[33] However, the high cost of anti-IgE and the need for regular infusions are likely to limit its use to patients with severe allergic disease that cannot be managed by other means.

■ CONCLUSIONS ■

SIT is established as a treatment for allergic rhinitis and for venom hypersensitivity, but is more controversial when used to treat allergic asthma. When used in appropriately selected patients, SIT is effective and acceptably safe, but care is needed to recognize and treat adverse reactions. Appropriate training of allergists and SIT clinic support staff is essential. Despite a century of use, the precise mechanisms of action of SIT remain uncertain. Current emphasis on the role of T-regulatory cells is leading to renewed attempts to simplify SIT regimes and reduce its risks. Future directions in SIT include the development of vaccines that are better standardized, and the use of recombinant allergens, both of which should improve the safety profile of SIT. In parallel, and perhaps in the longer term, we should look for the development of general immunomodulatory therapies, which would be particularly advantageous for those patients sensitized to multiple allergens.

■ REFERENCES ■

1. Freeman J. Vaccination against hay fever: report of results during the first three years. Lancet 1914; 1: 1178.

2. Creticos P, van Metre TA, Mardiney MR, et al. Dose–response of IgE and IgG antibodies during ragweed immunotherapy. J. Allergy Clin Immunol 1984; 73: 94–104.

3. Iliopoulos O, Proud D, Adkinson NF, et al. Effects of immunotherapy on the early, late and rechallenge nasal reaction to provocation with allergen: changes in inflammatory mediators and cells. J Allergy Clin Immunol 1991; 87: 855–866.

4. Durham SR, Ying S, Varney VA, et al. Grass pollen immunotherapy inhibits allergen-induced infiltration of CD4+ T-lymphocytes and eosinophils in the nasal mucosa and increases the number of cells expressing mRNA for interferon-gamma. J Allergy Clin Immunol 1996; 97: 1356–1365.

5. Ebner C, Siemann U, Bohle B, et al. Immunological changes during specific immunotherapy of grass pollen allergy: reduced lymphoproliferative responses to allergen and shift from Th2 to Th1 in T-cell clones specific for Phl p1, a major grass pollen allergen. Clin Exp Allergy 1997; 27: 1007–1015.

6. Jutel M, Akdis M, Blaser K, et al. Mechanisms of allergen specific immunotherapy – T-cell tolerance and more. Allergy 2006; 61: 796–807.

7. Golden DB, Kagey-Sobotka A, Norman PS, et al. Outcomes of allergy to insect stings in children, with and without venom immunotherapy. N Engl J Med 2004; 351: 668–674.

8. Frew AJ, Powell RM, Corrigan CJ, et al. Efficacy and safety of specific immunotherapy with SQ allergen extract in treatment-resistant seasonal allergic rhinoconjunctivitis. J Allergy Clin Immunol 2006; 117: 319–325.

9. Durham SR, Walker SM, Varga EM, et al. Long-term clinical efficacy of grass pollen immunotherapy. N Engl J Med 1999; 341: 468–475.

10. Bousquet J, Lockey RF, Malling H-J. Allergen immunotherapy: therapeutic vaccines for allergic diseases. J Allergy Clin Immunol 1998; 102: 558–562.

11. Varney VA, Edwards J, Tabbah K, et al. Clinical efficacy of specific immunotherapy to cat dander: a double blind placebo controlled trial. Clin Exp Allergy 1997; 27: 860–867.

12. Johnstone DE, Dutton A. The value of hyposensitization therapy for bronchial asthma in children. A 14 year study. Pediatrics 1968; 42: 793.

13. Abramson MJ, Puy RM, Weiner JM. Allergen immunotherapy for asthma. Cochrane Database Syst Rev 2003; (4): CD003093.

14. Adkinson NF, Eggleston PA, Eney D, et al. A controlled trial of immunotherapy in allergic children. N Engl J Med 1997; 336: 324–331.

15. Horak F. Manifestation of allergic rhinitis in latent sensitised patients. A prospective study. Arch Otorhinolaryngol 1985; 242: 242–249.

16. Niggemann B, Jacobsen L, Dreborg S, et al. Five-year follow-up on the PAT study: specific immunotherapy and long-term prevention of asthma in children. Allergy 2006; 61: 855–859.

17. Bernstein DI, Wanner M, Borish L, et al. Twelve-year survey of fatal reactions to allergen injections and skin testing: 1990–2001. J Allergy Clin Immunol 2004; 113: 1129–1136.

18. Wilson DR, Lima MT, Durham SR. Sublingual immunotherapy for allergic rhinitis: systematic review and meta-analysis. Allergy 2005; 60: 4–12.

19. Radcliffe MJ, Lewith GT, Turner RG, et al. Enzyme-potentiated desensitisation in treatment of seasonal allergic rhinitis: double-blind randomised controlled study. Br Med J 2003; 327: 251–254.

20. Reilly DT, Taylor MA, McSharry C, et al. Is homeopathy a placebo response? Controlled trial of homeopathic potency with pollen in hay fever as a model. Lancet 1986; ii: 881–886.

21. Jutel M, Akdis M, Blaser K, et al. Allergen-specific immunotherapy with recombinant grass pollen allergens. Allergy 2006; 61: 796–807.

23. Corrigan CJ, Kettner J, Doemer C, et al. Efficacy and safety of preseasonal-specific immunotherapy with an aluminium-adsorbed six-grass pollen allergoid. Allergy 2005; 60: 801–807.

24. Larche M. Peptide immunotherapy. Immunol Allergy Clin North Am 2006; 26: 321–332.

25. O'Hehir RE, Yssel H, Verma S, et al. Clonal analysis of differential lymphokine production in peptide and superantigen-induced T-cell anergy. Int Immunol 1991; 3: 819–826.

26. Norman PS, Ohman JL, Long AA, et al. Treatment of cat allergy with T-cell reactive peptides. Am J Respir Crit Care Med 1996; 154: 1623–1628.

27. Jain VV, Kitagaki K, Kline JN. CpG DNA and immunotherapy of allergic airway diseases. Clin Exp Allergy 2003; 33: 1330–1335.

28. Tighe H, Takabayashi K, Schwartz D, et al. Conjugation of immunostimulatory DNA to the short ragweed allergen Amb a1 enhances its immunogenicity and reduces its allergenicity. J Allergy Clin Immunol 2000; 106: 124–134.

29. Creticos PS, Eiden JJ, Broide D, et al. Immunotherapy with immunostimulatory oligonucleotides linked to purified ragweed Amb a 1 allergen: effects on antibody production, nasal allergen provocation and ragweed seasonal rhinitis. JACI 2002; 109: 743–744.

30. Hsu CH, Chua KY, Tao MH, et al. Immunoprophylaxis of allergen-induced IgE synthesis and airway hyperresponsiveness in vivo by genetic immunisation. Nat Med 1996; 2: 540–544.

31. Hartl A, Hochreiter R, Stepanoska T, et al. Characterisation of the protective and therapeutic efficiency of a DNA vaccine encoding the major birch pollen allergen Bet v1a. Allergy 2004; 59: 65–73.

32. Fahy J, Fleming HE, Wong HH, et al. The effect of an anti-IgE monoclonal antibody on the early and late-phase responses to allergen inhalation in asthmatic subjects. Am J Respir Crit Care Med 1997; 155: 1828–1834.

33. Rolinck-Werninghaus C, Hamelmann E, Kcil T, et al. The co-seasonal application of anti-IgE after preseasonal specific immunotherapy decreases ocular and nasal symptom scores and rescue medication use in grass pollen allergic children. Allergy 2004; 59: 973–979.

REFERENCES

Following a series of case reports, two controlled trials evaluated IFN-α in Behçet's disease (BD). In a placebo-controlled randomized double-blind study 15/23 IFN-α-treated patients responded compared to 3/21 placebo recipients. In another open-label nonrandomized study, 92% of the 50 patients with BD and posterior uveitis and/or retinal vasculitis responded to IFN-α.[6]

SJÖGREN'S SYNDROME

In several phase II studies low-dose natural human IFN-α administered by the oral mucosal route improved salivary output and decreased complaints of xerostomia in patients with primary Sjögren syndrome. In a phase III study, IFN-α increased unstimulated whole saliva flow significantly more than placebo, the co-primary endpoints of stimulated whole saliva flow and oral dryness were not significantly improved in the IFN-α group relative to placebo.[7] Further studies are needed to establish the efficacy of IFN-α in Sjögren's syndrome.

FIBROSING DISEASES

IFN-γ, a potent inhibitor of collagen synthesis, was tested as a treatment for pulmonary fibrosis and systemic sclerosis. In a large randomized controlled trial IFN-γ did not improve lung function but there was a trend toward improved survival in the treated group.[8] A follow-up trial is under way, with death as the primary endpoint. A randomized controlled trial of 44 patients with systemic sclerosis showed no significant benefit in improving skin thickness in the 27 treated patients compared to placebo.[9] In spite of its significant antifibrotic effects, thus far the data suggest that IFN-γ alone is not likely to have a major impact on fibrosing autoimmune diseases.

INFLAMMATORY BOWEL DISEASE

Many autoimmune diseases, such as inflammatory bowel diseases and inflammatory arthritides, are characterized by local inflammation and a relative paucity of anti-inflammatory cytokines, such as interleukin-10 (IL-10) and IL-11, suggesting their possible therapeutic potential.

The encouraging results seen in early pilot studies of recombinant human IL-10 in Crohn's disease (Chapter 74) were not confirmed by three large placebo-controlled trials.[10] Similarly, the effect of IL-10 in rheumatoid and psoriatic arthritis was marginal at best and IL-10 is currently not being pursued as a therapeutic option.

In addition to its thrombocytopoietic effects, IL-11 has been shown to have anti-inflammatory effects. In a phase II study in patients with active Crohn's disease, IL-11 led to a 37% remission rate compared to 16% in the placebo group. In another study the long-term remission rate was similar (21%) in patients treated with recombinant human IL-11 or prednisolone.[10]

SUMMARY OF CYTOKINE THERAPY IN AUTOIMMUNE DISEASES

The success of interferon treatment in various diseases established the viability of cytokine therapy in autoimmune diseases. Further studies are needed to improve the modest clinical responses seen with other cytokines. Targeted delivery of cytokines to the site of inflammation or immune activation or the combination of various cytokines will enhance the specificity and efficacy of cytokine therapy.

■ CYTOKINE THERAPY IN ALLERGIC DISEASE ■

Cytokines and chemokines are important in the initiation and long-term maintenance of allergic disorders.[11] It has been suggested that the development of allergen-specific T cells with a Th2 cytokine profile (IL-4, -5, -9, and -13) plays a critical role in allergic rhinitis, asthma, atopic dermatitis, and hypereosinophilic disorders. Studies have focused on the effects of the Th2-derived cytokines and demonstrated that these cytokines mediate many of the pathological changes associated with these diseases. However, it has also been shown that proinflammatory cytokines (including tumor necrosis factor-α (TNF-α) and IFN-γ) are present in these diseases and can also mediate detrimental effects. While it is not as simple as tipping the balance from Th2 to Th1 cytokine expression, it is believed that by altering the levels of these proteins through antibody or cytokine treatment, the severity of disease can be alleviated.

ASTHMA

Asthma is not a single disease, but rather a complex disorder sharing the characteristics of reversible bronchial constriction, pulmonary inflammation and airway remodeling (Chapter 39). Current therapies include corticosteroids, leukotriene modifiers, and β-agonists that provide symptomatic control. None of these agents are able to provide long-term immunomodulation of the disease and reverse the observed pathological changes.

Given the understanding that asthma is characterized as a Th2-mediated disease, IL-4 was an obvious cytokine choice to target therapeutically (Fig. 94.1 and Table 94.1). To date, every anti-IL-4 therapy has failed during clinical evaluation, with the exception of human anti-IL-4 receptor antibody, which is still under preclinical development. All drugs were safe with no adverse reactions during treatment and there was no evidence of autoantibody production. The question is: why did the trials with these agents fail to show a significant improvement in asthma? Anti-IL-4 therapy is believed to involve immune deviation, resulting in a decrease in the number and activity of Th2 cells, so one concern is the

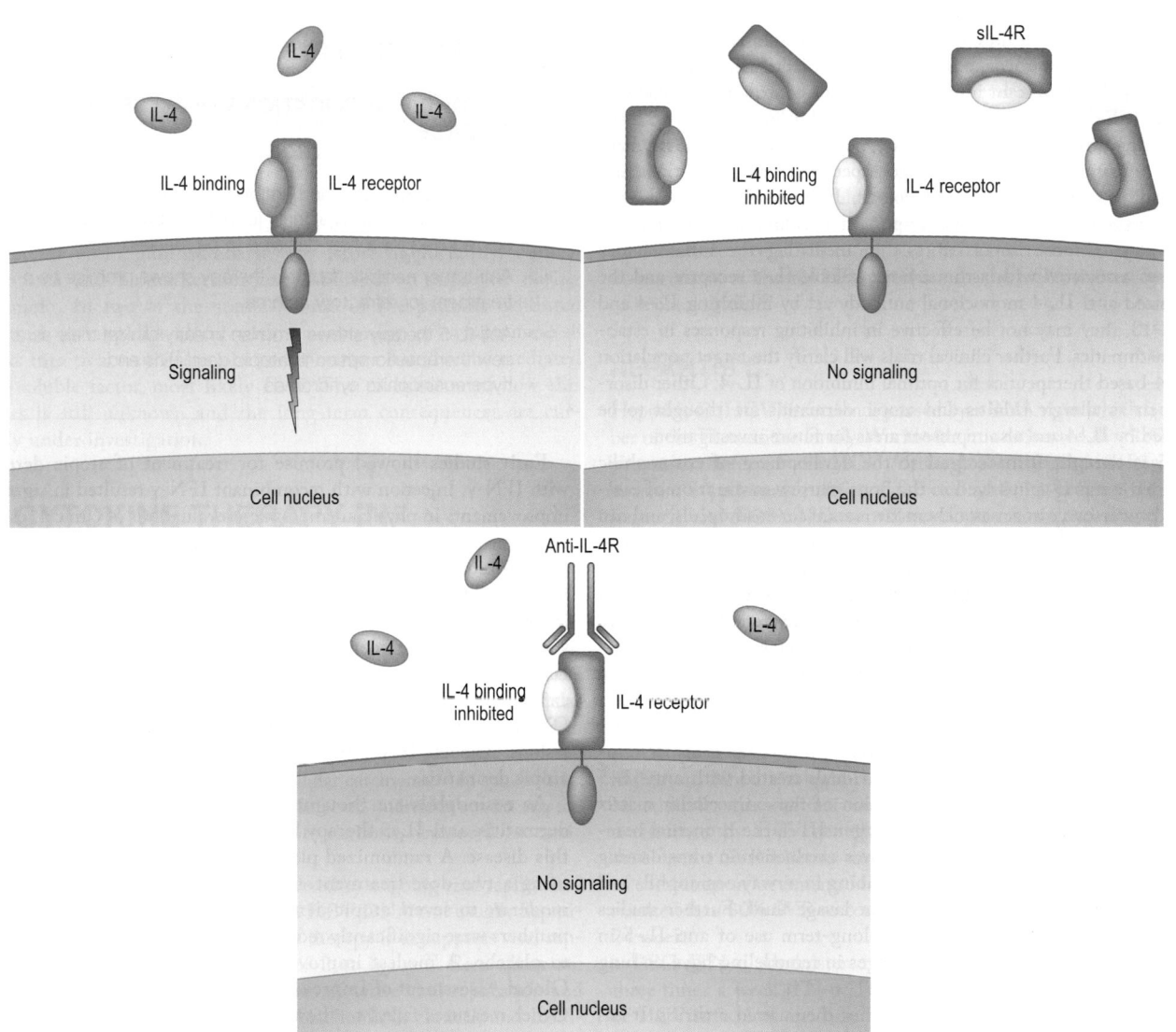

Fig. 94.1 Approaches to interleukin-4 (IL-4) signaling blockade. (A) IL-4 signaling. (B) IL-4 blockade utilizing soluble IL-4 receptor (sIL-4R). (C) IL-4 blockade utilizing anti-IL-4 receptor (IL-4R) antibody.

Table 94.1 Therapeutic agents with interleukin-4-inhibitory activity

Agent	Soluble human IL-4 receptor	IL-4 double mutein	IL-4/IL-13 trap	Humanized anti-IL-4 antibody	Human anti-IL-4 receptor antibody
Inhibition of IL-4	Yes	Yes	Yes	Yes	Yes
Inhibition of IL-13	No	Yes	Yes	Yes	Yes
Half-life	5 days	4–6 hours	5 days	18–21 days	18–21 days
Route of administration	Inhaled	Systemic	Systemic	Systemic	Systemic
Active in immune synapse	No	Yes	No	No	Yes

IL4 mutein – IL4 protein with two point mutations that has no agonist activity; IL4/IL13 trap-protein based drug candidate that binds IL4 and IL13 to prevent cell surface interaction.

CONDYLOMATA ACUMINATA AND RECURRENT RESPIRATORY PAPILLOMATOSIS

Studies of IFN effectiveness in the treatment of diseases caused by papillomaviruses date back to 1974, when leukocyte IFN was injected into a patient's plantar warts, causing the warts to disappear and reappear upon discontinuation of the IFN injections.[39] Numerous studies have followed, demonstrating effectiveness of local injections of IFN-β in treating common warts,[40] subcutaneous injections of IFN-γ, or systemic IFN-α for treating condylomata acuminata and local injections of IFN-α for treating condylomata acuminata.[41] However studies comparing IFN to other forms of local therapy, for example, cryotherapy or imiquimod, have not been done.[42] IFN-α is FDA-approved for the treatment of condylomata acuminata.

Recurrent respiratory papillomatosis (RRP) is a disease that occurs primarily in children and is caused by human papillomaviruses. It is characterized by recurrent growth of benign papillomas throughout the respiratory tract. Treatment includes endoscopic laser excisions and surgery; however, papillomas often regrow, requiring further therapy. For those patients with aggressive RRP, IFN-α has been successfully used. In 1988, Leventhal et al. reported the results of a randomized, cross-over trial of IFN-α in 66 patients with juvenile-onset RRP.[43] During periods of drug administration there was a statistically significant improvement observed. Nine of 57 patients with assessable airway disease achieved complete remission while no patients achieved complete remission during 6 months of observation alone. However, as was seen in prior reports, the patients who discontinued drug therapy showed a significant regrowth of papillomas within 4 months.

A long-term follow-up of this study was published in 1991, revealing approximately a 40% complete remission and a 40% partial remission rate over a 5-year period.[44] Based on the results of this study it has been recommended that patients with RRP who require surgery every 2–3 months be given a 6-month trial of IFN-α. To date a clinical trial establishing the optimal dose and duration of treatment with IFN-α for RRP has not been published.

HUMAN IMMUNODEFICIENCY VIRUS

HIV infection results in a severe cellular immunodeficiency disease characterized by decreased CD4 T cells that results in the development of opportunistic infections and other complications (Chapter 38). Treatment of HIV-infected patients consists of anti-microbial prophylaxis and combination anti-retroviral therapy to suppress HIV replication. Although much success has been achieved with these therapies, complete suppression of viral replication is not possible with current anti-retroviral medications. One complementary treatment approach is the use of IL-2.

IL-2 is a T-cell-derived cytokine with many effects on the immune system, including activation, proliferation, and differentiation of T, B, and natural killer (NK) cells (Chapter 10). Early in vitro studies culturing peripheral blood mononuclear cells from patients with acquired immunodeficiency syndrome (AIDS) in IL-2 demonstrated improvement in immune function, including T-cell proliferative responses to antigen and mitogen, NK-cell activity, antigen-specific cytotoxic lymphocyte activity, and IFN-γ production.[45]

In 1996, Kovacs et al. published a randomized controlled study of IL-2 therapy in HIV-infected patients in which 60 patients with CD4 cell counts above 200 cells/mm^3 were randomized to receive either nucleoside analogue anti-retrovirals alone or in combination with six cycles of intravenous IL-2 administered every 2 months, for 5 days, starting at a dose of 18 million IU/day.[46] At the end of 12 months, the mean CD4 count increased from 428 ± 25 cells/mm^3 at baseline to 916 ± 128 cells/mm^3 in the IL-2 group, compared to a decrease in the mean CD4 count from 404 ± 29 cells/mm^3 to 349 ± 41 cells/mm^3 in the control group ($P < 0.001$) (Fig. 94.2). Numerous studies have since corroborated these findings, including studies using IL-2 administered subcutaneously, IL-2 therapy in individuals with CD4 counts of less 350 cells/mm^3, and IL-2 administration to individuals not receiving anti-retroviral drugs with CD4 counts of greater than 350 cells/mm^3.[47, 48]

Recent publications have provided insights into possible reasons for the increase in CD4 cells following IL-2 administration. In vivo labeling studies have demonstrated a preferential increase in survival of both naïve and central memory CD4 cells (with half-lives that can exceed 3 years) following IL-2 administration that is critical to the sustained expansion of the CD4 cells.[49] In addition, a unique subset of naïve CD4 cells, CD4/CD45RO/CD25 cells, has been described that is distinct from antigen-triggered cells and regulatory T cells, and may play a role in the maintenance of a state of low T-cell turnover and sustained expansion of the CD4 T-cell pool.[50]

Whether these findings will translate into improved clinical outcomes in HIV-infected patients is still not known. Three international, multicenter, phase III clinical end-point trials, SILCAAT, ESPRIT, and STALWART, are currently under way to address this question. IL-2 is not an FDA-approved therapy for HIV-1 infection and should only be administered to individuals as part of clinical trials designed to elucidate further the role of IL-2 in the management of individuals who are infected with HIV.

Other cytokines, including IL-7 and IL-15, are important in the regulation of T-cell homeostasis. IL-7 is a cytokine that increases the proliferation and survival of T cells. A multicenter, randomized single-blind study of subcutaneous IL-7 versus placebo in HIV-1-infected patients is currently under way.

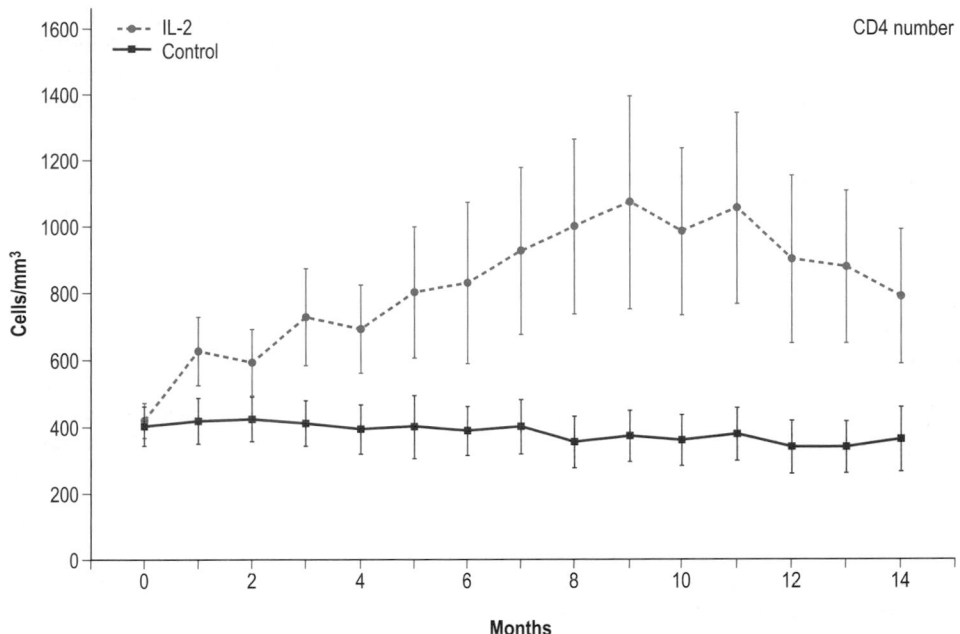

Fig. 94.2 CD4 count changes with rIL-2. Change in CD4 lymphocyte counts during a randomized trial of intravenously administered IL-2 and anti-retroviral drugs or antiretroviral drugs alone. (Modified from Kovacs JA, Vogel S, Albert JM, et al. Controlled trial of interleukin-2 infusions in patients infected with the human immunodeficiency virus. N Engl J Med 1996; 335: 1350.)

IFN-α, known to inhibit HIV-1 replication in cell culture, has been studied since the 1980s for the treatment of patients infected with HIV-1. Results of these studies have yielded variable results; however some did reveal significantly lower plasma HIV RNA levels in the groups randomized to receive IFN-α.[45] The decreases in HIV-1 RNA levels were modest at best and these studies were conducted prior to the availability of potent anti-retroviral therapy.

AIDS-ASSOCIATED KAPOSI'S SARCOMA

Kaposi sarcoma (KS) is a tumor of vascular origin, with four clinical variants including classic KS, endemic KS, immunosuppression-associated or transplantation-associated KS, and AIDS-associated KS. These variants have identical histologic features, but differ in the specific populations of patients affected, the sites involved, and the clinical course. In 1994, herpes virus-like DNA sequences were identified in tissues from patients with AIDS-associated KS.[51] KS-associated herpesvirus (KSHV) or herpesvirus-8 (HHV-8) have since been identified in all variants of KS.

The AIDS-associated variant was one the first recognized manifestations of AIDS. In 1983, in an open-label study, IFN-α was found to be effective in the treatment of patients with KS.[52] High doses of IFN-α ere used and yielded dramatic tumor regression of lesions in the skin, lymph nodes, oral cavity, and gastrointestinal tract, with up to a 40% response rate seen. Numerous studies since have corroborated these findings, leading to the FDA approval of IFN-α for the treatment of AIDS-associated KS.

With the use of highly active anti-retroviral therapy (HAART) in the mid-1990s for HIV, it became clear that HAART was also an important component of AIDS-associated KS treatment.[53] Lower doses of IFN-α (1 MU/day) in combination with nucleoside analogue anti-retroviral

medications was shown to induce tumor regression. Currently trials of PEG IFN-α in combination with HAART are under way.

LEPROMATOUS LEPROSY

Nathan et al. first used IFN-γ in the treatment of lepromatous leprosy at a dose of 1–10 μg/day injected directly into the cutaneous lesion daily for 3 days in addition to anti-microbials.[54] IFN-γ was shown to enhance granuloma formation and markers of local inflammation and to decrease cutaneous bacterial burden. Other small studies confirmed these findings and in long-term studies of IFN-γ, erythema nodosum leprosum (ENL), a toxic immune response leading to nerve damage, was a complicating phenomenon, but was readily suppressible with thalidomide. Sixty percent of patients treated with the combination of IFN-γ and anti-mycobacterial drugs developed ENL compared to 17% of those treated with anti-mycobacterial drugs alone.[55] It is not clear if this effect is related to long-term IFN-γ therapy; but if this is the case, it may limit the use of IFN-γ in this disease.

Low-dose IL-2, given intradermally, has been shown to reduce numbers of *Mycobacterium leprae* both at the injection site and at remote skin sites.[56] In addition, cutaneous infiltration of CD4 lymphocytes, monocytes, and Langerhans cells and increased levels of circulating antibody to *M. leprae* antigens were observed.[57]

LEISHMANIAL INFECTIONS

Leishmaniasis is a protozoal infection caused by intracellular parasites of the *Leishmania* species. It has various clinical presentations, including localized cutaneous, mucocutaneous, and visceral forms (kala-azar), of

■ REFERENCES ■

1. Goodin DS. Treatment of multiple sclerosis with human beta interferon. Int MS J 2005; 12: 96–108.

2. Rio J, Montalban X. Interferon-beta 1b in the treatment of multiple sclerosis. Exp Opin Pharmacother 2005; 6: 2877–2886.

3. Samuels J, Spiera R. Newer therapeutic approaches to the vasculitides: biologic agents. Rheum Dis Clin North Am 2006; 32: 187–200, xi.

4. Mazzaro C, Zorat F, Caizzi M, et al. Treatment with peg-interferon alfa-2b and ribavirin of hepatitis C virus-associated mixed cryoglobulinemia: a pilot study. J Hepatol 2005; 42: 632–638.

5. Cacoub P, Saadoun D, Limal N, et al. PEGylated interferon alfa-2b and ribavirin treatment in patients with hepatitis C virus-related systemic vasculitis. Arthritis Rheum 2005; 52: 911–915.

6. Kotter I, Gunaydin I, Zierhut M, et al. The use of interferon alpha in Behçet disease: review of the literature. Semin Arthritis Rheum 2004; 33: 320–335.

7. Cummins MJ, Papas A, Kammer GM, et al. Treatment of primary Sjogren's syndrome with low-dose human interferon alfa administered by the oromucosal route: combined phase III results. Arthritis Rheum 2003; 49: 585–593.

8. Raghu G, Brown KK, Bradford WZ, et al. A placebo-controlled trial of interferon gamma-1b in patients with idiopathic pulmonary fibrosis. N Engl J Med 2004; 350: 125–133.

9. Charles C, Clements P, Furst DE. Systemic sclerosis: hypothesis-driven treatment strategies. Lancet 2006; 367: 1683–1691.

10. Ardizzone S, Bianchi Porro G. Biologic therapy for inflammatory bowel disease. Drugs 2005; 65: 2253–2286.

11. Steinke JW, Borish L. Cytokines and chemokines. J Allergy Clin Immunol 2003; 111: S460–S475.

12. Borish LC, Nelson HS, Lanz MJ, et al. Interleukin-4 receptor in moderate atopic asthma. A phase I/II randomized, placebo-controlled trial. Am J Respir Crit Care Med 1999; 160: 1816–1823.

13. Leckie MJ, ten Brinke A, Khan J, et al. Effects of an interleukin-5 blocking monoclonal antibody on eosinophils, airway hyper-responsiveness, and the late asthmatic response. Lancet 2000; 356: 2144–2148.

14. Flood-Page P, Menzies-Gow A, Phipps S, et al. Anti-IL-5 treatment reduces deposition of ECM proteins in the bronchial subepithelial basement membrane of mild atopic asthmatics. J Clin Invest 2003; 112: 1029–1036.

15. Howarth PH, Babu KS, Arshad HS, et al. Tumor necrosis factor (TNF-α) as a novel therapeutic target in symptomatic corticosteroid dependent asthma. Thorax 2005; 60: 1012–1018.

16. Berry MA, Hargadon B, Shelley M, et al. Evidence of a role of tumor necrosis factor α in refractory asthma. N Engl J Med 2006; 354: 697–708.

17. Grassegger A, Hopfl R. Significance of the cytokine interferon gamma in clinical dermatology. Clin Exp Dermatol 2004; 29: 584–588.

18. Oldhoff JM, Darsow U, Werfel T, et al. Anti-IL-5 recombinant humanized monoclonal antibody (mepolizumab) for the treatment of atopic dermatitis. Allergy 2005; 60: 693–696.

19. Butterfield JH. Interferon treatment for hypereosinophilic syndromes and systemic mastocytosis. Acta Haematol 2005; 114: 26–40.

20. Klion AD, Law MA, Noel P, et al. Safety and efficacy of the monoclonal anti-interleukin-5 antibody SCH55700 in the treatment of patients with hypereosinophilic syndrome. Blood 2004; 103: 2939–2941.

21. Plotz SG, Simon HU, Darsow U, et al. Use of an anti-interleukin-5 antibody in the hypereosinophilic syndrome with eosinophilic dermatitis. N Engl J Med 2003; 349: 2334–2339.

22. Malik AH, Lee WM. Chronic hepatitis B virus infection: treatment strategies for the next millennium. Ann Intern Med 2000; 132: 723–731.

23. Wong DK, Cheung AM, O'Rourke K, et al. Effect of alpha-interferon treatment in patients with hepatitis B e antigen-positive chronic hepatitis B. A meta-analysis. Ann Intern Med 1993; 119: 312–323.

24. Niederau C, Heintges T, Lange S, et al. Long-term follow-up of HBeAg-positive patients treated with interferon alfa for chronic hepatitis B. N Engl J Med 1996; 334: 1422–1427.

25. Lau GK, Piratvisuth T, Luo KX, et al. Peginterferon alfa-2a, lamivudine, and the combination for HBeAg-positive chronic hepatitis B. N Engl J Med 2005; 352: 2682–2695.

26. Marcellin P, Lau GK, Bonino F, et al. Peginterferon Alfa-2a HBeAg-Negative Chronic Hepatitis B Study Group. Peginterferon alfa-2a alone, lamivudine alone, and the two in combination in patients with HBeAg-negative chronic hepatitis B. N Engl J Med 2004; 351: 1206–1217.

27. Keeffe EB, Dieterich DT, Han SH, et al. A treatment algorithm for the management of chronic hepatitis b virus infection in the United States: an update. Clin Gastroenterol Hepatol 2006; 4: 936–962.

28. NIH Consensus Statement on Management of Hepatitis C: 2002. NIH Consens State Sci Statements 2002; 19: 1–46.

29. Poynard T, Yuen MF, Ratziu V, et al. Viral hepatitis C. Lancet 2003; 362: 2095–2100.

30. Strader DB, Wright T, Thomas DL, et al. AASLD Practice Guideline Diagnosis, management, and treatment of hepatitis C. Hepatology 2004; 4: 1147–1171.

31. Davis GL, Balart LA, Schiff ER, et al. Treatment of chronic hepatitis C with recombinant interferon alfa. A multicenter randomized, controlled trial. Hepatitis Interventional Therapy Group. N Engl J Med 1989; 321: 1501–1506.

32. Di Bisceglie AM, Martin P, Kassianides C, et al. Recombinant interferon alfa therapy for chronic hepatitis C. A randomized, double-blind, placebo-controlled trial. N Engl J Med 1989; 321: 1506–1510.

33. McHutchison JG, Gordon SC, Schiff ER, et al. Interferon alfa-2b alone or in combination with ribavirin as initial treatment for chronic hepatitis C. Hepatitis Interventional Therapy Group. N Engl J Med 1998; 339: 1485–1492.

34. Poynard T, Marcellin P, Lee SS, et al. Randomized trial of interferon alpha2b plus ribavirin for 48 weeks or for 24 weeks versus interferon alpha2b plus placebo for 48 weeks for treatment of chronic infection with hepatitis C virus. International Hepatitis Interventional Therapy Group. Lancet 1998; 352: 1426–1432.

35. Manns MP, McHutchison JG, Gordon SC, et al. Peginterferon alfa-2b plus ribavirin compared with interferon alfa-2b plus ribavirin for initial treatment of chronic hepatitis C: a randomised trial. Lancet 2001; 358: 958–965.

36. Fried MW, Shiffman ML, Reddy KR, et al. Peginterferon alfa-2a plus ribavirin for chronic hepatitis C virus infection. N Engl J Med 2002; 347: 975–982.

37. Hadziyannis SJ, Sette H Jr, Morgan TR, et al. Peginterferon-alpha2a and ribavirin combination therapy in chronic hepatitis C: a randomized study of treatment duration and ribavirin dose. Ann Intern Med 2004; 140: 346–355.

38. Marcellin P, Boyer N, Gervais A, et al. Long-term histologic improvement and loss of detectable intrahepatic HCV RNA in patients with chronic hepatitis C and sustained response to interferon-alpha therapy. Ann Intern Med 1997; 127: 875–881.

39. Strander HA. Interferon in the treatment of human papilloma virus. Med Clin North Am(Suppl.): 19–23.

40. Niimura M. Intralesional human fibroblast interferon in common warts. J Dermatol 1983; 10: 217–220.

41. Reichel RP, Fitz R, Neumann R, et al. Clinical study with recombinant interferon gamma versus interferon alpha-2c in patients with condylomata acuminata. Int J STD AIDS 1992; 3: 350–354.

42. Gibbs S, Harvey I, Sterling J, et al. Local treatments for cutaneous warts: systematic review. Br Med J 2002; 325: 461–469.

43. Leventhal BG, Kashima HK, Weck PW, et al. Randomized surgical adjuvant trial of interferon alfa-n1 in recurrent papillomatosis. Arch Otolaryngol Head Neck Surg 1988; 114: 1163–1169.

44. Leventhal BG, Kashima HK, Mounts P, et al. Long-term response of recurrent respiratory papillomatosis to treatment with lymphoblastoid interferon alfa-N1. Papilloma Study Group. N Engl J Med 1991; 325: 613–617.

45. Smith KL, Jacobson EL, Giordano M, et al. Restoration of immunity with interleukin-2 therapy. AIDS Reader 1999; 9: 56–72.

46. Kovacs JA, Vogel S, Albert JM, et al. Controlled trial of interleukin-2 infusions in patients infected with the human immunodeficiency virus. N Engl J Med 1996; 335: 1350–1356.

47. Allende MC, Lane HC. Cytokine-based therapies for HIV infection. AIDS 2001; 15(Suppl. 5): S183–S191.

48. Youle M, Emery S, Fisher M, et al. A randomised trial of subcutaneous intermittent interleukin-2 without antiretroviral therapy in HIV-infected patients: the UK-Vanguard study. PLoS Clin Trials 2006; 1: e3. Epub 2006 May 19.

49. Kovacs JA, Lempicki RA, Sidorov IA, et al. Induction of prolonged survival of CD4+ T lymphocytes by intermittent IL-2 therapy in HIV-infected patients. J Clin Invest 2005; 115: 2139–2148.

50. Sereti I, Imamichi H, Natarajan V, et al. In vivo expansion of CD4CD45RO-CD25 T cells expressing foxP3 in IL-2-treated HIV-infected patients. J Clin Invest 2005; 115: 1839–1847.

51. Chang Y, Cesarman E, Pessin MS, et al. Identification of herpesvirus-like DNA sequences in AIDS-associated Kaposi's sarcoma. Science 1994; 266: 1865–1869.

52. Krown SE, Real FX, Cunningham-Rundles S, et al. Preliminary observations on the effect of recombinant leukocyte A interferon in homosexual men with Kaposi's sarcoma. N Engl J Med 1983; 308: 1071–1076.

53. Vanni T, Sprinz E, Machado MW, et al. Systemic treatment of AIDS-related Kaposi sarcoma: current status and perspectives. Cancer Treat Rev. 2006; 32: 445–455.

54. Nathan CF, Kaplan G, Levis WR, et al. Local and systemic effects of intradermal recombinant interferon-gamma in patients with lepromatous leprosy. N Engl J Med 1986; 315: 6–15.

55. Sampaio EP, Moreira AL, Sarno EN, et al. Prolonged treatment with recombinant interferon gamma induces erythema nodosum leprosum in lepromatous leprosy patients. J Exp Med 1992; 175: 1729–1737.

56. Kurkcuoglu N, Tandogdu R. Interferon gamma therapy for cutaneous leishmaniasis [letter]. Arch Dermatol 1990; 126: 831–832.

57. Villahermosa LG, Abalos RM, Walsh DS, et al. Recombinant interleukin-2 in lepromatous leprosy lesions: immunological and microbiological consequences. Clin Exp Dermatol 1997; 22: 134–140.

58. Reed SG, Scott P. T-cell and cytokine responses in leishmaniasis. Curr Opin Immunol 1993; 5: 524–531.

59. Akuffo H, Kaplan G, Kiessling R, et al. Administration of recombinant interleukin-2 reduces the local parasite load of patients with disseminated cutaneous leishmaniasis. J Infect Dis 1990; 161: 775–780.

60. Holland SM, Eisenstein EM, Kuhns DB, et al. Treatment of refractory disseminated nontuberculous mycobacterial infection with interferon gamma. A preliminary report. N Engl J Med 1994; 330: 1348–1355.

61. Altare F, Jouanguy E, Lamhamedi S, et al. Mendelian susceptibility to mycobacterial infection in man. Curr Opin Immunol 1998; 10: 413–417.

62. Levin M, Newport M. Understanding the genetic basis of susceptibility to mycobacterial infection. Proc Assoc Am Phys 1999; 111: 308–312.

63. Boehm U, Klamp T, Groot M, et al. Cellular responses to interferon-gamma. Annu Rev Immunol 1997; 15: 749–795.

64. Appelberg R, Orme IM. Effector mechanisms involved in cytokine-mediated bacteriostasis of *Mycobacterium avium* infections in murine macrophages. Immunology 1993; 80: 352–359.

65. Feng CG, Jankovic D, Kullberg M, et al. Maintenance of pulmonary Th1 effector function in chronic tuberculosis requires persistent IL-12 production. J Immunol 2005; 174: 4185–4192.

66. Gallin JI, Farber JM, Holland SM, et al. Interferon-gamma in the management of infectious diseases. Ann Intern Med 1995; 123: 216–224.

67. Jouanguy E, Doffinger R, Dupuis S, et al. IL-12 and IFN-gamma in host defense against mycobacteria and salmonella in mice and men. Curr Opin Immunol 1999; 11: 346–351.

68. Kampmann B, Hemingway C, Stephens A, et al. Acquired predisposition to mycobacterial disease due to autoantibodies to IFN-gamma. J Clin Invest 2005; 115: 2480–2488.

69. Condos R, Raju B, Canova A, et al. Recombinant gamma interferon stimulates signal transduction and gene expression in alveolar macrophages in vitro and in tuberculosis patients. Infect Immun 2003; 71: 2058–2064.

70. Squires KE, Brown ST, Armstrong D, et al. Interferon-gamma treatment for *Mycobacterium avium*-intracellular complex bacillemia in patients with AIDS. J Infect Dis 1992; 166: 686–687.

71. The International Chronic Granulomatous Disease Cooperative Study Group. A controlled trial of interferon gamma to prevent infection in chronic granulomatous disease. N Engl J Med 1991; 324: 509–516.

72. Marciano BE, Wesley R, De Carlo ES, et al. Long-term interferon-gamma therapy for patients with chronic granulomatous disease. Clin Infect Dis 2004; 39: 692–699.

73. Cunningham-Rundles C, Kazbay K, Hassett J, et al. Brief report: enhanced humoral immunity in common variable immunodeficiency after long-term treatment with polyethylene glycol-conjugated interleukin-2. N Engl J Med 1994; 331: 918–921.

74. Rump JA, Jahreis A, Schlesier M, et al. A double-blind, placebo-controlled, crossover therapy study with natural human IL-2 (nhuIL-2) in combination with regular intravenous gammaglobulin (IVIG) infusions in 10 patients with common variable immunodeficiency (CVID). Clin Exp Immunol 1997; 110: 167–173.

75. Cunningham-Rundles C, Bodian C, Ochs HD, et al. Long-term low-dose IL-2 enhances immune function in common variable immunodeficiency. Clin Immunol 2001; 100: 181–190.

76. Key LL Jr, Ries WL, Rodriguiz RM, et al. Recombinant human interferon gamma therapy for osteopetrosis. J Pediatr 1992; 121: 119–124.

77. Key LL Jr, Rodriguiz RM, Willi SM, et al. Long-term treatment of osteopetrosis with recombinant human interferon gamma. N Engl J Med 1995; 332: 1594–1599.

Monoclonal antibodies and fusion proteins

Susan J. Lee, Arthur F. Kavanaugh

95

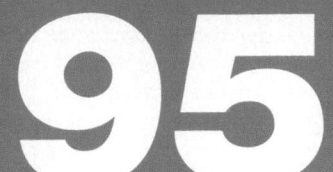

The immune system is composed of a complex array of diverse immunocompetent cells and pro- and anti-inflammatory mediators that exist in complex networks. These components interact through cascades and positive- and negative-feedback circuits to maintain normal inflammation and immunity. In various autoimmune and allergic diseases, a foreign or autoantigen may upset this fine balance, leading to dysregulated inflammation and ultimately pathologic findings characteristic of a disease. In recent years, there has been tremendous progress delineating the specific components of the immune system that contribute to various aspects of normal immunity and to specific disease states. With progress in biotechnology, these components have become targets for more specific immunomodulatory therapies.

Traditionally, the treatment for most autoimmune diseases consisted largely of potent immunosuppressive agents. Although effective, treatment of autoimmune diseases with immunosuppressive agents rarely achieved the full extent of clinical response desired. This generated a substantial unmet therapeutic need. Moreover, because such drugs nonspecifically inhibited numerous parts of the immune response, treatment had the untoward effect of predisposing patients to generalized immunosuppression and significant toxicities such as infections. These considerations, in conjunction with the progress in biotechnology, provided the thrust for the development of a new class of therapeutic agents commonly called 'biologic agents.' Development in this area has been brisk, and in recent years more than two dozen therapeutic biologic agents have been approved by regulatory agents for use in the clinic. The two most common classes of biologic agents approved to date are monoclonal antibodies (mAb) and fusion proteins. The notable potential for these agents derives from their ability to inhibit targets, for example particular components of the immune system, with exquisite specificity. This has the potential both to optimize outcomes by more thorough modulation of specific parts of the dysregulated immune response as well as to minimize potential adverse events related to more broad methods of immunosuppression.

The mechanisms of action of mAb and fusion proteins are diverse. The simplest mechanism of action would be inhibition of the function of a target molecule, either soluble or cell surface, by binding to it, and thereby preventing ligation with its counter-receptor. The potential targets are myriad, and include specific molecules on B cells, T cells, and other immunocompetent cells. Such targets would be those with effector functions key to the cells' role in the disease being treated. In addition, various soluble inflammatory mediators, such as cytokines, chemokines, complement proteins, enzymes, immunoglobulin molecules, or their surface receptors, can also be targeted. The effects of such inhibition derive most directly from the removal of a particular interaction, for example the blocking of an inflammatory cytokine from binding its cell surface receptor and thereby transducing a signal. Such inhibition may interfere with the normal function of the target molecule, such as binding of a cell surface adhesion molecule. Simple competitive inhibition of a key ligand/receptor pair could induce diverse downstream effects, as has been seen for the inhibitors of tumor necrosis factor-α (TNF). Alternatively, biologic agents may alter cell populations by binding a target on a specific cell, and then engaging effector functions such as activation of the complement cascade or antibody-dependent cellular cytotoxicity (ADCC). All mAbs and many fusion proteins have immunoglobulin G (IgG) Fc pieces as part of their construct. If such Fc pieces remain functional, then these effector mechanisms can be utilized if the binding characteristics of the target are appropriate. Because the regions of the Fc piece mediating the processes are distinct, biologic agents affecting either complement ligation or ADCC can be constucted. Cell depletion could also be induced by apoptosis related to ligation of an appropriate cell surface target. Relevant targets for cell-depleting therapy would include lineage-specific molecules or activation molecules.

■ MONOCLONAL ANTIBODIES ■

MAbs to human targets are generated most readily in other species, for example in mice. Although murine mAbs can be effective, and several have been brought to the clinic as therapeutic agents, they are suboptimal for most indications. Being foreign, these relatively large protein molecules are immunogenic. The development of antibodies to the treating agent can potentially result in several undesirable consequences, such as a decrease in half-life due to more rapid elimination, and interference with the intended therapeutic function. Moreover, the development of antibodies to the treating agent can directly cause severe allergic reactions, such as anaphylaxis. For these reasons, there has been great interest in developing mAbs that are composed of less foreign material (Fig. 95.1). With chimeric mAb, the variable region of a murine-derived mAb is fused through genetic engineering with the Fc piece of a human IgG molecule. The resulting construct is approximately one-quarter murine and three-quarters human origin. For humanized mAb, only the complementarity-determining regions (CDR) from the original murine mAb are retained, resulting in a construct that is approximately 95% human. There are a number of theoretical approaches towards creating human mAb to human targets, including immunizing human/severe combined immunodeficient (SCID) mouse chimeras, or using Epstein–Barr virus-transformed human B cells. One of the most commonly employed has been repertoire cloning. In this procedure, target antigen is used to capture human CDR generated from vast human cDNA libraries, with the mAb then constructed to incorporate the generated CDR.

The standard nomenclature for mAbs makes note of their source as the last four or five letters of the mAb name: -omab, murine; -ximab, chimeric; -zumab, humanized; -umab, fully human. The middle part of the name refers to the disease indication for which the mAb is intended: thus, '-lim-' for immune and inflammatory diseases, '-cir-' for cardiovascular disorders, and '-tu-' for tumors or neoplastic conditions. The first three or four letters are chosen by the sponsor/developer. In general, the more human the construct, the less immunogenic the mAb. Therefore, human mAb are less immunogenic than humanized mAb, which in turn are less immunogenic than chimeric mAb. As the consequences of antibodies developing to the treating mAb include not only decreased efficacy but also potentially adverse reactions, less immunogenicity is desirable. However, there are several caveats that should be noted. Even small molecules whose amino acid sequence is identical to human, such as recombinant insulin, can be immunogenic. In the case of mAb, even fully human mAb have certain potential differences from native Ig, such as patterns of glycosylation. In addition, although mAb with greater murine components are more immunogenic, much of the reactivity appears to be idiotypic. Thus, patients who develop antibodies after treatment with one chimeric mAb might not be expected to demonstrate reactivity to another chimeric mAb. Also, other key factors that are relevant to the immunogenicity of a compound include those factors long known to affect the outcome of an immune challenge, including: route of administration (intravenous versus subcutaneous), treatment paradigm (continuous versus intermittent), and concurrent immunosuppressive therapy. In clinical practice, these factors have proven to be relevant considerations for the therapeutic use of mAb. While numerous mAbs have been approved by the US Food and Drug Administration (FDA) and other regulatory agencies, this chapter will focus on several key mAbs used in the treatment of allergic and autoimmune conditions: omalizumab, natalizumab, infliximab, adalimumab, rituximab, and efalizumab (Table 95.1).

FUSION RECEPTORS

Fusion proteins are typically composed of the extracellular domains of native transmembrane proteins, such as cell surface receptors, linked to another molecule. In most cases, the linker that has been used has been the Fc portion of human Ig, which achieves the desired effect of enhancing the pharmacokinetic properties of the construct. The Fc portion of the fusion receptor can be maintained to be functional and bind to complement and to cell surface Fc receptors. This allows effector function, and has been used for the compounds etanercept and alefacept. Alternatively, the construct can be engineered such that the Fc piece is unable to execute effector functions, as in the case of abatacept, which does not activate complement. As their primary mechanism of action, fusion receptors competitively inhibit the binding of a ligand to its specific receptor and thereby prevent downstream effects, such as activation of inflammatory cascade. However, ligation of certain molecules by fusion receptors may induce other functions as well. In this chapter, the focus will be on several important fusion receptors that have been brought to the clinic for autoimmune diseases: etanercept, abatacept, and alefacept (Table 95.1).

■ AGENTS THAT INHIBIT PROINFLAMMATORY CYTOKINES ■

Cytokines are small proteins that regulate diverse aspects of the function of the immune system and the inflammatory response. Individual cytokines often exhibit multiple effects and their activities are often synergistic with, or antagonistic to, the actions of other cytokines. Cytokines and inflammatory cells exist in a complex network where they interact through cascades of stimulation and inhibition. In a susceptible patient, an imbalance in the cytokine cascade can help the initiation and propagation of the immune-driven inflammation characteristic of autoimmune diseases. For example, in inflammatory arthritides such as rheumatoid arthritis (RA), psoriatic arthritis (PsA), and ankylosing spondylitis (AS), the important proinflammatory cytokines TNF-α and interleukin-1 (IL-1) have been shown to play a central role in disease pathogenesis and sustenance. TNF in particular appears to play a central role in inflammatory reactions, and has proven to be an especially attractive target for biologic agents. Among its sundry proinflammatory and immune-regulating activities, TNF activates various cell types, promotes accumulation of immunocompetent cells at sites of inflammation by activation of the vascular endothelium and upregulation of adhesion molecules, stimulates synthesis of other proinflammatory cytokines (e.g., IL-1, IL-6, granulocyte–macrophage

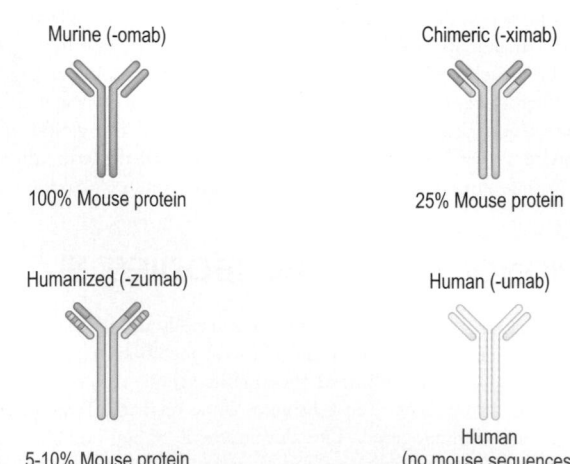

Monoclonal antibodies

Murine (-omab)

100% Mouse protein

Chimeric (-ximab)

25% Mouse protein

Humanized (-zumab)

5-10% Mouse protein

Human (-umab)

Human
(no mouse sequences)

Fig. 95.1 Monoclonal antibodies.

Table 95.1 Food and Drug Administration-approved therapeutic biologics[a]

Drugs	Description	Indications
Abciximab	Chimeric monoclonal Fab fragment to platelet IIb/IIIa	Acute MI; post-PTCA
Adalimumab	Human mAb to TNF-α	RA, PsA
Agalsidase beta	Recombinant human α-galactosidase A enzyme	Fabry disease
Aldesleukin	Recombinant IL-2	Metastatic renal cell cancer
Alefacept	Recombinant LFA-3/IgG Fc construct	Psoriasis
Alemtuzumab	Humanized mAb to CD52	Chronic lymphocytic leukemia
Alteplase	Recombinant tPA	Acute MI, massive PE
Anakinra	Recombinant IL-1R antagonist	RA
Anti-thymocyte globulin (ATG)	Horse anti-human T-cell Ig	Acute renal transplant rejection, aplastic anemia
Basiliximab	Chimeric mAb to IL-2R	Acute renal transplant rejection
Becaplermin	Recombinant human PDGF gel	Diabetic ulcer
Bevacizumab	Humanized mAb to VEGF	Metastatic colorectal cancer
Cetuximab	Chimeric mAb to EGFR	Metastatic cancer
Daclizumab	Humanized mAb to IL-2R	Acute renal transplant rejection
Darbepoetin alpha	Recombinant erythropoietin	Anemia related to chemotherapy
Denileukin diftitox	Recombinant diphtheria toxin/IL-2 construct	Cutaneous T-cell lymphoma
Digoxin immune Fab	Fab against digoxin	Digoxin toxicity
Drotrecogin alfa	Recombinant activated protein C	Severe sepsis
Efalizumab	Humanized mAb to LFA-1 (CD11a)	Psoriasis
Etanercept	Recombinant soluble TNF-R/IgG Fc construct	RA, JIA, PsA, AS, psoriasis
Filgrastim	Recombinant G-CSF	Neutropenia
Galsulfase (rhASB)	Recombinant N-acetylgalactosamine 4-sulfatase	Mucopolysaccharidosis VI
Gemtuzumab ozogamicin	Humanized mAb to CD33	Acute myelocytic leukemia
Ibritumomab	Murine mAb to CD20	NHL
Infliximab	Chimeric mAb to TNF-α	RA, Crohn's, UC, PsA, AS
IFN-α (2a, 2b, etc)	Recombinant IFN-α	Hepatitis C, hairy cell leukemia, Kaposi sarcoma, hepatitis B, condyloma, melanoma, NHL
IFN-β (1a,1b)	Recombinant IFN-β	Multiple sclerosis
IFN-γ	Recombinant IFN-γ	Chronic granulomatous disease, osteopetrosis
Laronidase	Recombinant human α₁-iduronidase	Mucopolysaccharidosis I
Natalizumab	Humanized mAb to α₄β₁ integrin	Multiple sclerosis
Omalizumab	Humanized mAb to IgE	Severe allergic asthma

[a]Accessed 4/06: modified from www.fda.gov/cder/biologics and www.drugs.com.
AS, ankylosing spondylitis; EGFR, epidermal growth factor receptor; Fab, fragment, antigen-binding; Fc, fragment, crystallizable; G-CSF, granulocyte colony-stimulating factor; HER, human epidermal growth factor receptor 2; IFN, interferon; IgE, G, immunoglobulin E, G; IL-2, interleukin-2; JIA, juvenile idiopathic arthritis; LFA, leukocyte function antigen; mAb, monoclonal antibody; MI, myocardial infarction; NHL, non-Hodgkin's lymphoma; PDGF, platelet-derived growth factor; PE, pulmonary embolism; PsA, psoriatic arthritis; PTCA, percutaneous transluminal coronary angiogram; RA, rheumatoid arthritis; RSV, respiratory syncytial virus; TNF, tumor necrosis factor; tPA, tissue plasminogen activator; UC, ulcerative colitis; VEGF, vascular endothelial growth factor

AGENTS THAT INHIBIT PROINFLAMMATORY CYTOKINES

Continued

Table 95.1 Food and Drug Administration approved therapeutic biologics[a]—cont'd

Drugs	Description	Indications
Oprelvekin	Recombinant IL-11	Thrombocytopenia
Palivizumab	Humanized mAb to RSV	Severe RSV
Rasburicase	Recombinant uricase	Post-chemotherapy hyperuricemia
Reteplase	Recombinant tPA	Acute MI
Rituximab	Chimeric mAb to CD20	NHL, RA
Tenecteplase	Recombinant tPA	Acute MI
Tositumomab	Murine mAb to CD20	NHL refractory to rituximab
Trastuzumab	Humanized mAb to HER-2	Metastatic breast cancer

KEY CONCEPTS

THE ROLE OF TUMOR NECROSIS FACTOR (TNF) INHIBITORS IN CROHN'S DISEASE

>> Treatment with monoclonal antibodies has been effective both as single therapy and as maintenance therapy

>> Combination therapy with immunomodulators appears to enhance efficacy and minimize immunogenicity

>> At doses studied to date, etanercept has not been effective in Crohn's disease, whereas anti-TNF monoclonal antibodies available have been effective

>> Treatment with TNF inhibitor monoclonal antibodies also appears to be effective in ulcerative colitis

colony-stimulating factor), chemokines (e.g., IL-8), and other inflammatory mediators. IL-1, another inflammatory cytokine, also stimulates production of other proinflammatory cytokines, angiogenic factors, and endothelial adhesion molecules. Both TNF and IL-1 activate macrophages to release mediators destructive to bone and cartilage, including matrix metalloproteinases such as collagenase and prostaglandins.

■ TNF INHIBITORS ■

As of 2006, more than 1 million people worldwide have received one of the three currently available TNF inhibitors: (1) infliximab, a chimeric monoclonal anti-TNF-α antibody initially approved in 1998 for Crohn's disease; (2) etanercept, a recombinant soluble p75 TNF-receptor (CD120b)-IgG Fc fusion protein initially approved in 1998 for RA; and (3) adalimumab, a human monoclonal anti-TNF-α antibody initially approved in 2002 for RA (Table 95.2).

The conditions for which patients have most commonly received TNF inhibitors are RA and Crohn's disease. In Crohn's disease, there has been an evolution in the manner in which TNF inhibitors have been utilized.

Initially, treatment was for the most severe, refractory disease, and treatment was given as a single course. Following upon the successes achieved in this group of patients, repeated treatments and more chronic dosing regimens have been assessed. Also, the efficacy of TNF inhibitor therapy in another form of inflammatory bowel disease, ulcerative colitis (UC), has also been explored. To date, although the mAb TNF inhibitors have been effective in inflammatory bowel disease, the fusion protein construct has not been.

In RA, the effects of TNF inhibitor therapy have been dramatic. Initially, these agents were tested in patients with the most severe and active disease that had been refractory to all other available treatments. In this population, the TNF inhibitors not only substantially improved the signs and symptoms of disease, but also resulted in significantly improved functional status and enhanced quality of life. Most notably, treatment with TNF inhibitors was capable of attenuating the progression of joint damage as assessed radiographically, a characteristic of RA previously considered to be inexorable despite any form of therapy. Following upon the experience in refractory RA, the TNF inhibitors have also been tested in patients with earlier onset of disease. In early RA, the same breadth of positive responses that had been noted for more established RA was seen; however, the extent of clinical responses was even greater in these patients. The clinical success achieved by the TNF inhibitors in RA has been so dramatic that the introduction of this therapeutic approach has resulted in an alteration in the treatment paradigm for RA, with the goals of therapy being set higher than they had been prior to their introduction.

In addition to RA, other types of arthritis have also responded to treatment with TNF inhibitors. PsA, a form of inflammatory arthritis associated with skin psoriasis, often has clinical resemblance to RA. It is sometimes classified as one of the spondyloarthropathies, as a subset of patients has spinal involvement. As was observed in RA, treatment of PsA patients with the TNF inhibitors improved not only the signs and symptoms of arthritis, but also functional status and quality of life as well. In addition, prevention of the progression of radiographic joint damage was also demonstrated. Moreover, dramatic improvements in skin psoriasis were achieved, as were improvements in extra-articular involvement characteristic of PsA, such as dactylitis and enthesitis. Improvement in skin psoriasis with TNF inhibitor therapy has likewise been noted in patients without arthritis. In AS, although previously available therapies had the potential for some clinical improvement

Table 95.2 Characteristics of biologics: dosing, half-life, and indications

Agent	Dosing	Mode of delivery	Half-life
Cytokine inhibitors			
Etanercept	RA: 25 mg biweekly or 50 mg weekly JIA: 0.4 mg/kg biweekly	SQ	4–5 days
Infliximab	3–10 mg/kg every 4–8 weeks	IV	8–9.5 days
Adalimumab	40 mg every week–every other week	SQ	12–14 days
Anakinra	100 mg qd	SQ	4–6 hours
B-cell modulators			
Rituximab	NHL: 375 mg/m² weekly × 4 doses RA: 500–1000 mg every 2 weeks × 2 doses	IV	60–170 hours
T-cell modulators			
Abatacept	RA: 10 mg/kg then every 4 weeks	IV	14.7 days
Alefacept	15 mg IM weekly × 12 weeks (can be repeated after 12-week observation period)	IM	270 hours
Adhesion-cell modulators			
Efalizumab	1–2 mg/kg weekly × 12 weeks	SQ	3–5 days
Natalizumab	300 mg every 4 weeks	IV	11 days
Immunoglobulin inhibitor			
Omalizumab	0.016 mg/kg IgE (IU/ml)/month divided every 2–4 weeks	SQ	26 days

IM, intramuscular; IgE, immunoglobulin E; JIA, juvenile arthritis; NHL, non-Hodgkin's lymphoma; RA, rheumatoid arthritis.

in peripheral arthritis, no therapy was effective at alleviating spinal inflammation. Therefore, the ability of the TNF inhibitors to improve spinal inflammation, both in terms of signs and symptoms as well as with imaging, such as magnetic resonance imaging (MRI), is all the more notable. While the success of TNF inhibitors in these autoimmune conditions has been remarkable, it is worth noting that, almost uniformly, treatment failed to induce long-term treatment-free remission or immunological tolerance. Thus, maintenance of clinical response requires continuous therapy.

TNF inhibitors have not proven effective in several other conditions, including several wherein there was pathophysiologic evidence for a role for this cytokine in the disease process. Among autoimmune conditions, TNF inhibitor therapy has been notably ineffective to date in several forms of vasculitis, including Wegener's granulomatosis and polymyalgia rheumatica/temporal arteritis. This is perhaps surprising, given the role of TNF in granuloma formation and maintenance. Also, in Sjögren's syndrome, therapy was not effective. In congestive heart failure (CHF), data from animal models implicated TNF as a key

mediator of deteriorating cardiac function, and hence an attractive target. However, TNF inhibitors have failed to improve patients with CHF in clinical trials, and sometimes resulted in worsened clinical outcome. Although they were limited, studies of TNF inhibitors that had negative results in multiple sclerosis, along with anecdotal reports of the development or worsening of demyelinating symptoms among RA patients treated with these agents, would seem to preclude further development of these agents in that condition. TNF inhibitors are still being actively investigated in a variety of other diseases, including Behçet's disease, uveitis, asthma, dermatomyositis/polymyositis, and others.

As regards safety, in general, TNF inhibitors have been well tolerated in clinical trials. *In vitro* evidence from studies assessing various aspects of immune function among patients receiving treatment with TNF inhibitors has suggested that TNF inhibitors do not cause broad immune system suppression. It appears that these agents selectively decrease proinflammatory cytokines while preserving both the humoral and cell-mediated arms of the immune response. In longer-term follow-up

KEY CONCEPTS

THE ROLE OF TUMOR NECROSIS FACTOR (TNF) INHIBITORS IN RHEUMATOID ARTHRITIS

>> Inhibition of a single cytokine can be highly effective

>> Substantial improvement seen in signs and symptoms of disease, functional status, and quality of life

>> Treatment can inhibit progression of joint damage, as assessed radiographically

>> Most patients require continuous treatment for efficacy

>> Long-term treatment-free remission is rare

>> Switching from one TNF inhibitor to another TNF inhibitor can be effective

>> Treatment with a TNF inhibitor plus methotrexate appears to have additive or synergistic efficacy, particularly as regards joint damage

>> Combination therapy of a TNF inhibitor and methotrexate represents the current 'gold standard' for the treatment of rheumatoid arthritis

KEY CONCEPTS

THE ROLE OF TUMOR NECROSIS FACTOR (TNF) INHIBITORS IN ANKYLOSING SPONDYLITIS (AS), PSORIASIS, AND PSORIATIC ARTHRITIS (PsA)

>> In AS, treatment improves signs and symptoms of axial arthritis, peripheral arthritis, and extra-articular involvement, such as uveitis

>> In AS, treatment appears to attenuate spinal inflammation, as assessed with magnetic resonance imaging

>> In psoriasis and PsA, treatment improves signs and symptoms of disease, functional status, and quality of life

>> In PsA, improvement has been noted in peripheral arthritis, dactylitis, enthesitis, and skin psoriasis

>> In PsA, treatment can result in attenuation in the progression of joint damage, as assessed radiographically

CLINICAL PEARLS

LENGTH OF TREATMENT WITH TUMOR NECROSIS FACTOR (TNF) INHIBITORS

>> Almost uniformly, treatment with TNF inhibitors fails to induce long-term treatment-free remission or immunological tolerance. Thus, maintenance of clinical response requires continuous therapy

CLINICAL PEARLS

LACK OF EFFECT OF TUMOR NECROSIS FACTOR (TNF) INHIBITORS

>> TNF inhibitors have been shown to be ineffective in patients with congestive heart failure, multiple sclerosis, Wegener's granulomatosis, Sjögren's syndrome, temporal arteritis, and polymyalgia rheumatica

trials. As will be discussed below, the risk of infection with TNF inhibitor therapy has been shown to be substantially increased when combined with other biologic agents. For example, combination therapy with the TNF inhibitor etanercept and the IL-1 receptor antagonist anakinra resulted in a higher rate of serious infections in RA patients, despite the failure to achieve any additive clinical benefit. Data, particularly from pharmacovigilance, have noted a number of opportunistic infections (e.g., *Pneumocystis jiroveci* pneumonia listeriosis, coccidioidomycosis) among those patients treated with TNF inhibitors. Interpretation of the excess risk of infections attributable to therapeutic intervention in RA needs to take into account the increased baseline risk of infections among RA patients. Thus, without a control group, it is sometimes difficult to ascertain the excess infection risk specifically attributable to TNF inhibitors in RA.

Another potential sequela of immunosuppression is malignancy. With a few notable exceptions, the bulk of the data to date do not support an increased risk of solid tumors related to TNF inhibitor therapy. However, greater numbers of hematological malignancies, particularly non-Hodgkin's lymphoma, have been observed. Like the problem with infections, complicating the assessment of the risk attributable to therapy is the increased baseline risk of lymphoma among RA patients. This risk, which seems to vary directly with disease activity and severity, would be expected then to introduce bias towards observing cases among patients treated with TNF inhibitors as the most severe and active RA patients are often the most common type of patients treated. However, if the observed increase related entirely to the subset of patients treated, one might anticipate that in years to come the incidence of lymphoma should decrease, as disease activity is diminished in such patients. Obviously this is an area of great interest and further long-term data are needed. In conditions being treated with TNF inhibitors, the relative impact of dose and duration of therapy and host factors such as comorbidities, relevant genetic polymorphisms, and concomitant medications on the risk of infections and malignancy remain incompletely defined. For example, patients with early RA, AS, or PsA tend to

studies of patients from clinical trials, and, more importantly, in postmarketing pharmacovigilance assessments, a number of relevant safety issues regarding the use of TNF inhibitors have emerged.[1] Adverse events associated with TNF inhibitors may be broadly classified as target/class-related or agent-related (Table 95.3).

Target-related adverse effects include those potentially attributable to the immunosuppression inherent in blocking a key component of the immune system such as an inflammatory cytokine. This would include the sequelae of impaired immunosurveillance, such as an increased susceptibility to infections and malignancies. Safety data from clinical trials have shown a small but consistent increase in infections among treated patients, although generally the risk of serious infections was not substantially greater, perhaps related to the close follow-up patients receive in clinical

Table 95.3 Safety issues with tumor necrosis factor inhibitors

	Target-related	Agent-related
Definite		Injection site reactions, infusion reactions, immunogenicity (e.g., serum sickness, anaphylaxis)
Probable	Infections, serious infections opportunistic infections (e.g. coccidioidomycosis), tuberculosis autoantibodies, lupus-like syndromes, hepatotoxicity	
Possible	Malignancies (lymphoma), demyelinating disorders (multiple sclerosis), hematologic abnormalities, congestive heart failure	

be younger and have fewer comorbidities than patients with long-standing RA, and would therefore be expected to have a lower incidence of certain adverse effects such as infection. The extent to which this may be true is still being investigated.

In addition to those adverse effects noted above, which might be associated with various immunomodulatory approaches, inhibition of TNF may predispose patients to a variety of untoward effects that seem to be specific to inhibition of the TNF molecule. These include an increased susceptibility to tuberculosis (TB), autoantibody production, hepatotoxicity, the development of demyelinating disease such as multiple sclerosis, and clinical worsening of CHF. Regarding TB, there is a fair amount of animal and *ex vivo* data supporting the important role played by TNF in controlling this infectious agent. Although few cases of TB were seen in early clinical trials, a number of cases were noted, including fatalities, soon after the more widespread use of TNF inhibitors, particularly in geographic locations where TB was endemic. Many cases were initially missed due to atypical presentations. In contrast to typical presentation of acute TB as pneumonia, about half of the cases of TB related to TNF inhibitors presented as extrapulmonary or disseminated TB. The majority of these TB cases appear to be reactivation of latent TB, with infection occurring within the first few months of therapy; however, newly acquired cases have been well described. The incidence of cases may be greater with the mAb TNF inhibitors than with the fusion protein inhibitor. Fortunately, screening for latent TB before initiating TNF inhibitor therapy has been an effective strategy, with a reduction in incidence of new TB cases by approximately 85%.

Treatment with TNF inhibitors has also been associated with development of autoantibodies. Although the mechanism of this is unknown, it does not appear to result from general immunosuppression, but rather to an aspect of TNF itself, perhaps induction of apoptosis. The autoantibodies typically generated include the generic antinuclear antibody (ANA, which develops in about half of RA patients treated with TNF inhibitors), antibodies to double-stranded DNA (anti-dsDNA, which develops in approximately 10–15% of patients treated with TNF inhibitors), and anticardiolipin antibodies. The clinical implications of these autoantibodies remain to be defined, as progression to a lupus-like illness appears to be uncommon.

THERAPEUTIC PRINCIPLES

ADVERSE EFFECTS OF BIOLOGIC AGENTS

>> Adverse effects can be globally considered to be agent-related or target-related

>> Target-related effects derive from inhibition of the target; for immunomodulatory therapies, this often includes immunosuppression and its potential sequelae (e.g., infection)

>> Agent-related adverse effects relate to the specific agent; they may be mechanistic (e.g., cell lysis) or idiosyncratic (e.g., immunogenicity)

Agent-related adverse effects such as allergic reactions and antigenicity are idiosyncratic reactions that relate to the particular agent used. Antibodies to TNF inhibitor construct have been noted, with the highest rates being noted for the chimeric antibody infliximab. However, antibodies to adalimumab and etanercept have also been observed. As noted above, intermittent use and use without concomitant immunosuppressants have been associated with a greater propensity for the development of antibodies to TNF inhibitor. The extent to which these antibodies influence response rates or the duration of response to treatment remains to be fully defined.

Despite their shared ability to inhibit TNF, there are some notable differences between the three currently approved TNF inhibitors. Infliximab and adalimumab are IgG_1 mAb that are specific for TNF-α; etanercept is a fusion protein of the type II TNF receptor, that therefore binds both TNF-α and lymphotoxin-α (previously known as TNF-β). The clinical relevance of this distinction is unknown. In addition, the binding characteristics of the mAb and the fusion protein differ slightly. While all agents bind soluble TNF with high affinity, the mAb have slightly higher affinity for membrane-bound TNF than the soluble TNF receptor, presumably related to the physical constraints of the binding domains of the soluble TNF receptor. Whether these differences may account for variability in efficacy (e.g., in Crohn's disease) or as regards any particular adverse effects remains to be seen.

INFLIXIMAB

Infliximab, a chimeric IgG_1 mAb specific for TNF-α, has been proven effective in RA.[2–4] Initially in patients with well-established severe yet active disease, infliximab was shown to improve the signs and symptoms of RA, functional status, and quality of life. In early studies, it was demonstrated that the combination therapy with infliximab and methotrexate (MTX), a traditional disease-modifying anti-rheumatic drug (DMARD) used for RA, was synergistic. Part of this may relate to pharmacokinetic effects; concomitant treatment with MTX increases the area under the curve for infliximab concentrations by about 25%. Since these earlier studies, almost all studies of infliximab in RA patients have used it in conjunction with MTX. In addition to its use in established RA, infliximab was also tested in patients with early RA, defined as less than 3 years of disease. In early RA, even higher levels of response were noted with the combination of infliximab and MTX. In addition to the beneficial effect on signs and symptoms, the most notable result from the studies of infliximab in RA has been its ability to arrest in radiographic progression. This is quite distinct from, and superior to, results among patients receiving traditional DMARDs. In the trial of patients with early RA, while most patients on MTX monotherapy had a progression of radiographic damage, approximately 90% of patients on the combination therapy had no radiographic progression.[4] Interestingly, inhibition of radiographic progression of disease seemed to be dissociated from clinical efficacy as measured by the typically utilized composite scoring measures, such as the American College of Rheumatology 20% improvement criteria (ACR 20). Thus, some patients who did not achieve an ACR 20 response still experienced inhibition of damage on X-ray.[3] Although some of this dissociation probably relates to the inexactness of the ACR 20 in capturing the entire spectrum of clinical benefit, it does raise the possibility that distinct outcomes in RA may relate to different immunological process.

Infliximab has been shown to improve signs and symptoms of disease in patients with AS.[5, 6] Because MTX is not a standard therapy for spinal involvement in AS, infliximab monotherapy has been used in this condition. While the majority of outcome measures utilized in clinical trials focus on spinal inflammation, improvement with infliximab therapy has also been observed in peripheral arthritis, as well as in some extra-articular manifestations of disease such as uveitis. Interestingly, those with elevated acute-phase reactants at study entry, as well as those with evidence for spinal inflammation on MRI, tended to respond more favorably to TNF inhibitors. Paralleling data from RA, infliximab provided rapid clinical improvement, often as early as 2 weeks. Also, continued treatment was necessary to sustain the response, and all patients flared within a few months of discontinuing therapy. The ultimate goal in treating AS would be to stop the progression of spinal ankylosis. However, structural effects of TNF inhibitors or any drug on axial disease are difficult to assess due to the slow rate of skeletal progression in AS. In fact, such studies could probably not currently be done, as the amount of time necessary to see a meaningful difference in radiographic change between treatment and control would far exceed the time span considered ethical given the dramatic effect of TNF inhibitor therapy on the signs and symptoms of disease. Therefore, it is quite encouraging that TNF inhibitors have been shown to attenuate spinal inflammation on a sensitive imaging modality such as MRI.[7]

The treatment of patients with PsA requires consideration of the various potential areas of disease involvement, including peripheral arthritis, axial arthritis, skin and nail involvement, dactylitis, and enthesitis. Similar to RA, the level of TNF-α is notably increased in biopsy samples of skin and synovial tissues from patients with PsA, providing rationale for TNF inhibitors in the treatment of PsA and psoriasis. All three currently approved TNF inhibitors have been associated with improvements in signs and symptoms of peripheral arthritis, dactylitis, and enthesitis associated with PsA as well as functional status and quality of life.[8–11] For all three agents, studies have allowed, but not required, patients to be on concomitant MTX. In all studies, the use of concomitant MTX has not seemed to affect any outcomes; however, given the study design, this does not address the important issue of whether there is synergy between the agents in PsA or psoriasis. In addition to improving the signs and symptoms of peripheral arthritis, treatment of PsA patients with TNF inhibitors also attenuated the progression of radiographic damage. As regards skin manifestations, all three TNF inhibitors induced clinical improvement. Interestingly, while the extent of improvement in peripheral arthritis was comparable among TNF inhibitors, the extent of improvement in skin psoriasis appears to be greater with the mAbs than with the soluble receptor construct. Whether this difference relates to differential mechanisms, dosages used, or some other factor remains to be defined. Preliminary analysis of individual patient responses shows that there may be a discordance between dermatologic and articular outcomes in individual patients, suggesting potential heterogeneity to pathophysiologic mechanisms underlying different clinical manifestations.

The levels of TNF-α are increased in the mucosa of inflamed intestine and thought to exert deleterious effects relevant to the pathophysiology of inflammatory bowel disease (Crohn's disease and UC). Infliximab has been shown to improve both clinical and endoscopic luminal fistulas and bowel mucosal inflammation associated with Crohn's disease.[12–14] In Crohn's disease, the use of infliximab in combination with immunosuppressives (e.g., MTX, azathioprine), enhances efficacy and decreases immunogenicity. More recently, infliximab has been approved for the treatment of UC after promising results from two large phase III studies. Approximately 65% of patients receiving infliximab in addition to conventional therapy had a clinical response, with less rectal bleeding, compared to 31–35% in the placebo group.[15]

ETANERCEPT

Etanercept has been shown to improve signs and symptoms of arthritis rapidly and retard radiographic progression in both early and established RA.[16–19] In long-term extension studies, many patients on etanercept were also able to decrease the doses of their concomitant MTX and/or corticosteroids. Although etanercept has been proven to be effective as monotherapy, and although there is no pharmacokinetic interaction, combination therapy with MTX appears to provide additional benefits. Thus, patients on combination therapy had the greatest radiographic protection compared to those on either etanercept or MTX alone.[19]

Etanercept is the only TNF inhibitor currently approved for the treatment of juvenile idiopathic arthritis (JIA). In a long-term follow-up study of more than 60 children with MTX-resistant polyarticular juvenile RA, etanercept provided sustained clinical improvement without an increase in the incidence of adverse effects.[20] Studies are ongoing to assess the efficacy and safety of infliximab and adalimumab in JIA.

Etanercept has been shown to improve signs and symptoms of arthritis and quality of life in patients with AS.[21] In AS, the characteristics and the degree of clinical and radiographic response appeared comparable among all three TNF inhibitors. As noted above, because MTX is not an effective therapy for spinal inflammation in AS, it has not been utilized in studies of the TNF inhibitors. Whether there may be any synergistic effect of the combination of TNF inhibitor and MTX on radiographic progression in AS remains to be seen. Etanercept has also been shown effective in improving the signs and symptoms of arthritis and quality of life in patients with PsA.[9]

ADALIMUMAB

Adalimumab has also been shown to improve signs and symptoms of arthritis and quality of life, and to retard radiographic progression in both early and established RA.[22–24] Similar to etanercept, adalimumab can be given as monotherapy or in combination with MTX. However, the combination therapy has been associated with greater clinical response and radiographic inhibition than either adalimumab or MTX alone.[22–24] Similar to infliximab and etanercept, adalimumab has also been effective in improving signs and symptoms of arthritis and functional status in AS patients, and in psoriasis and PsA. Adalimumab has also shown promising results in decreasing fistulas and bowel inflammation associated with Crohn's disease.[25]

INTERLEUKIN-1 RECEPTOR ANTAGONIST

IL-1 is synthesized as an inactive precursor. Upon cleavage by IL-1β-converting enzyme, it activates a variety of cells that can then release mediators destructive to bone and cartilage. In the RA synovium, although there is an increase in the naturally occurring IL-1 receptor antagonist (IL-1Ra) that prevents the binding of IL-1 to its receptor, IL-1R, the levels are apparently insufficient to counteract the effects of IL-1. Anakinra, approved in 2001 for the treatment of RA, is a recombinant competitive IL-1Ra that differs from the endogenous antagonists by a single amino acid addition at the amino-terminus. Compared to the TNF inhibitors, the clinical responses achieved by anakinra are modest; combined with cost and the need for daily injections, this has led to its relatively infrequent use in the treatment of RA. However, it has been gaining renewed interest in the treatment of treatment of familial cold autoinflammatory syndrome and Muckle–Wells syndrome, with promising results. These autosomal dominant disorders are characterized by mutated cryopyrin genes resulting in increased IL-1 activity. Similar to TNF inhibitors, anakinra can also modulate normal immune responses and potentially lead to adverse effects such as infections. In clinical studies, the overall rate of serious infections and malignancies has been comparable between the treated and the control groups. The most commonly reported infections were pneumonias, occurring more frequently in patients with underlying asthma, and cellulitis. However, as noted above, the combination of TNF inhibitor and IL-1Ra did lead to a higher incidence of serious infections. Because there was also no clinical benefit achieved with such an approach, this combination is not recommended for clinical use.[1]

■ AGENTS THAT INHIBIT T CELLS ■

There is a large body of evidence suggesting autoreactive T cells, especially CD4 Th1 T cells, serve a key role orchestrating the immune-driven inflammatory responses in autoimmune diseases such as RA,

Crohn's disease, PsA, and psoriasis. Early attempts at eliminating CD4 cells with anti-CD4 mAb achieved a biologic effect, with reduction in circulating cells, but did not achieve a beneficial clinical effect. This may have been related to several factors, including insufficient effect at the tissue level, preferential targeting of naïve rather than memory T cells, deleterious effects on regulatory T cells, or others. Further attempts at manipulating T-cell function have utilized different approaches.

Productive CD4 T-cell responses require two signals (Chapter 13). The first signal comes from the binding of specific antigen appropriately presented in the context of major histocompatibility complex class II molecule to the T-cell receptor complex. The second signal comes from co-stimulatory molecules. If T cells fail to receive the second signal, then tolerance or ignorance of the antigen ensues, and a productive immune response is not generated. Co-stimulation can occur through several pairs of cell surface molecules on antigen-presenting cells (APCs) and T cells. Among the most important molecules is CD28, which binds CD80 and CD86. CD28 and its natural inhibitor, cytotoxic T-lymphocyte–associated antigen 4 (CTLA-4; CD152) are present on T cells and bind to CD80 and CD86 on APCs. CD28 ligation results in stimulation of T cells while CTLA-4 serves an inhibitory role. CTLA-4, which binds CD80 and CD86 with substantially higher affinity than CD28, inhibits the stimulatory effects of CD28 by competitively binding to CD80 and CD86.[26]

ABATACEPT

Abatacept (CTLA-4 Ig) is a soluble chimeric human protein consisting of the extracellular domain of CTLA-4 (CD152) and the Fc portion of a human IgG$_1$ (Table 95.2). Abatacept has been developed in an attempt to downregulate T-cell responses and induce T-cell anergy by preventing CD28-mediated T-cell co-stimulation. Abatacept was approved for the treatment of refractory RA in 2005. It has been shown to be effective both in RA patients who had active disease despite concomitant MTX, and also in patients who had failed therapy with one or more TNF inhibitors.[26, 27] Because of the larger clinical experience to date with TNF inhibitors, it is likely that it may be used initially in the clinic in patients who have previously tried TNF inhibitor therapy. Abatacept therapy has also been shown to attenuate the progression of radiographic damage in RA patients, and to improve functional status and quality of life. Treatment, which is given as a 30-minute intravenous infusion monthly, is generally very well tolerated.

Recently, a safety study assessed the combination of abatacept and TNF inhibitor therapy. In that study, a higher incidence of serious adverse effects, including infections, was seen at 1-year follow-up in the patients receiving combination therapy compared to those on monotherapy.[28] Although clinical efficacy was not rigorously tested in that study, at present the combination of these agents is not recommended in routine clinical use.

■ ALEFACEPT ■

The interaction of LFA-3 on APCs and CD2 on T cells is thought to be important in T-cell activation and in the development of cells into memory T cells. Alefacept is a fusion protein of a soluble form of the extracellular domain of LFA-3 attached to the Fc portion of an IgG$_1$ molecule. Alefacept was approved in 2003 for the treatment of chronic plaque psoriasis. It binds and depletes CD2$^+$ T cells, utilizing cell-based effector mechanisms via its Fc portion. Other cells also bear CD2 receptors, including natural killer cells and some bone marrow B cells, although the effects on these cells are less pronounced than on circulating memory T cells. Although the exact mechanism of action of alefacept is unknown, it is thought to improve psoriasis by inducing memory T-cell apoptosis, inhibiting inflammatory gene expression, and preventing T-cell migration into psoriatic plaques.[29] Alefacept, either as monotherapy or in combination with MTX, has been shown to be effective for skin psoriasis. T-cell depletion related to therapy did not correlate nor predict the response rate during treatment or follow-up. Despite its ability to produce a long-lasting depletion of memory T cells and lymphopenia, alefacept has been well tolerated without an increase in adverse effects, including infections and malignancies. Furthermore, both primary and secondary antibody response to neoantigen and memory response to recall antigen appeared to be intact.[29] Studies are ongoing to assess the long-term safety of repeated and/or combination therapy as well as its use in other autoimmune diseases.

IL-2 RECEPTOR INHIBITORS

Daclizumab is a humanized IgG_1 mAb, and basiliximab is a chimeric IgG_1 mAb. Both are directed against the IL-2 receptor on the surface of activated T lymphocytes. Both mAb bind to IL-2 receptors and prevent IL-2-mediated activation of lymphocyte in response to antigenic challenges. They are approved for the prevention of acute kidney transplant rejection and are used in combination with other immunosuppressive agents, such as cyclosporine and corticosteroids. Despite their potential to induce severe immunosuppression, IL-2 receptor inhibitors have overall been well tolerated.[30]

AGENTS THAT INHIBIT B CELLS

Recent data suggest that B cells may contribute significantly to the initiation and perpetuation of the immune response in various autoimmune diseases. Not only can B cells produce potentially pathologic autoantibodies (e.g., rheumatoid factor, ANA) and proinflammatory cytokines, but they can also present antigens to T cells and provide co-stimulatory signals essential for T-cell activation, clonal expansion, and effector function.

Rituximab is a chimeric monoclonal IgG_1 antibody directed against B-lymphocyte surface antigen, CD20. It is thought to induce B-cell lysis by several mechanisms, including complement activation, ADCC, and induction of apoptosis. CD20 is restricted to the surface of pre-B and activated mature B cells. Within 24–48 hours of infusion, rituximab markedly depletes peripheral B cells ($CD19^+$, $CD20^+$). This effect can last up to 9 months after a single course of therapy. Despite its actions on B cells, the overall levels of serum Ig generally remain stable during treatment.[31] However, some patients may exhibit an impaired humoral immune response with less robust B-cell proliferation to simple haptens and recall antigen challenge, presumably related to depletion of memory B cells with rituximab.

Rituximab was initially approved in 1997 for the treatment of relapsed or refractory low-grade or follicular CD20-positive B-cell non-Hodgkin's lymphoma. In 2006 its indication was expanded to include RA that had been refractory to TNF inhibitor therapy. In early studies, it was shown that rituximab combined with MTX or with cyclophosphamide was more effective than as monotherapy.[32] Later studies used this combination in patients who were naïve to or refractory to TNF inhibitor therapy.[32–34] Rituximab has also been suggested to be effective in other autoimmune diseases such as systemic lupus erythematosus, primary Sjögren's syndrome, idiopathic thrombocytopenic purpura, chronic inflammatory demyelinating polyneuropathy, and vasculitis. Additional trials are under way that should answer questions regarding dosing, treatment intervals, safety, and tolerability in these conditions. Despite the potential for immunodeficiency related to depletion of mature B cells, no significant increases in infections, either serious or opportunistic, were reported in both RA and non-Hodgkin's lymphoma patients treated with rituximab.[35] This could be related to preserved function of plasma cells, which lack CD20 and are, therefore, not depleted by rituximab given as a single course. However, if rituximab is used as a recurrent or maintenance therapy for autoimmune conditions, this may become more of a safety concern as plasma cells are not replenished by memory B cells. While treatment has overall been well tolerated, infusions have been associated with hypersensitivity reactions, Stevens–Johnson syndrome, and type III serum sickness-like illness, and cytokine release syndrome.[29] The infusion reactions are more common during the first infusion, and may occur more in lymphoma than in RA. Other notable adverse effects include rare neutropenia and reactivation of hepatitis B infection.

AGENTS THAT INHIBIT CELL ADHESION AND/OR MIGRATION

Activated T lymphocytes must migrate to sites of inflammation and lymph tissue to exert their diverse effects. The entry of lymphocytes into specific sites occurs through several specific interactions between the adhesion molecules on lymphocytes, including the integrins, and their ligands on endothelial cells. Two ligand pairs that are particularly important for lymphocyte migration and homing are LFA-1 and its counter-receptors intercellular adhesion molecule-1 (ICAM-1) and ICAM-2 and very late antigen-4 (VLA-4) and its counter-receptor vascular cell adhesion molecule-1 (VCAM-1).

NATALIZUMAB

Natalizumab, approved in 2004 for the treatment of multiple sclerosis, is a recombinant humanized IgG_4 mAb directed against the α_4-subunit of $\alpha_4\beta_1$ integrin; it also binds to and inhibits the function of the $\alpha_4\beta_7$ integrins, whose ligand is mucosal addressin-cell adhesion molecule-1 (MadCAM-1). In addition to blocking the migration of lymphocytes into the central nervous system and intestinal parenchyma, natalizumab induces T-cell apoptosis and anergy and prevents T-cell binding to osteopontin and fibronectin, thereby attenuating T-cell-mediated inflammation.[36] In two large clinical trials, natalizumab, either alone or in combination with interferon-β_{1a}, was associated with significantly lower relapse rates, disability, and fewer new multiple sclerosis lesions on MRI. However, only months after FDA approval, natalizumab was withdrawn from the market after three cases of progressive multifocal leukoencephalopathy (PML) were reported.[36, 37] Natalizumab may be brought back to the market with appropriate care and assessment of its long-term safety. The exact role of natalizumab in the development of PML remains unknown but it highlights the importance of pharmacovigilance and potential unforeseen long-term adverse effects related to biological agents.

EFALIZUMAB

Efalizumab, approved in 2003 for the treatment of psoriasis, is a humanized IgG_1 mAb directed against the cell adhesion molecule CD11a. CD11a is a subunit of the LFA-1 molecule on T cells that binds to ICAM-1 on APCs and endothelial cells. In addition to inhibiting activation of T cells, efalizumab also blocks trafficking of lymphocytes into skin by blocking LFA-1/ICAM-1 interaction.[38] Efalizumab has been shown to provide greater improvement in skin psoriasis after 3 months of therapy with continued increase in response if therapy was continued for another 3-month cycle. Also, efalizumab therapy significantly improved health-related quality of life and other patient-reported outcomes (e.g., psoriasis symptom assessment and patient global psoriasis assessment) in patients with moderate to severe psoriasis.[38] Overall, efalizumab was well tolerated, with most adverse events being mild and occurring most frequently during the first two doses. Due to its ability to modulate adhesion molecules, efalizumab is also being evaluated for the treatment of other autoimmune conditions.

■ AGENTS THAT INHIBIT IMMUNOGLOBULINS ■

Immunoglobulins play a significant role in inflammation and have been a target of novel therapeutic agents, especially in the treatment of allergic asthma. For example, immediate hypersensitivity reactions associated with allergic asthma are mediated by complex interaction between IgE, precipitating antigen, and inflammatory cells (e.g., mast cells, basophils). Upon cross-linking of the Fab of IgE to multivalent antigen, IgE activates inflammatory cells through its Fc receptors to release effector mediators (e.g., histamine).

OMALIZUMAB

Omalizumab, approved in 2003 for the treatment of asthma, is a humanized IgG_1 mAb directed against free circulating IgE.[39] It binds to IgE in the region of its C3 domain, thereby blocking its interaction with Fcε receptor on mast cells and basophils. This specific binding region is important in two ways: first, it prevents the drug from binding to and cross-linking IgE that is already cell-bound, and therefore does not trigger mast cell activation and degranulation. Second, by not binding the variable region of IgE, it forms complexes with IgE of any specificity. The complex formed is biologically inert and cleared by the reticuloendothelial system without activating complement. Omalizumab has been shown to be effective in reducing the number of asthma exacerbations (by 50%) and decreasing the dose of inhaled corticosteroid.[39] Omalizumab was well tolerated with only mild adverse effects such as injection site reaction and respiratory tract infections.

■ FUTURE DIRECTIONS ■

The factors that drove the initial introduction of the biologic agents – a clinical need for better outcomes, greater delineation of pathophysiology allowing definition of various targets, and progress in biotechnology allowing development of agents – will no doubt continue to fuel progress in this area. It can be expected that additional mAbs and fusion receptors, both directed at existing targets as well as against novel targets, will continue to be developed and brought to the clinic. Regarding TNF inhibitors, several molecules are already in late-stage development, including golimumab (a human IgG_1 anti-TNF-α mAb), and certolizumab pegol (a polyethylene glycol-treated humanized anti-TNF-α mAb Fab fragment), and others are in earlier phases of development. Along with the number of agents, it is anticipated that the conditions for which these agents are utilized will also expand. For existing biologic agents, a number of questions remain as to the optimum treatment paradigms and most appropriate patient populations for their use; this will be germane for newer agents as well.

Great progress is being made in developing and fusion receptors that have additional mechanisms of action. Largely in oncology, bispecific mAb, as well as mAb conjugated with various compounds including toxins, chemotherapeutic drugs, or cytokines, are in development.[40] Such constructs might also find use in nonneoplastic conditions.

As always, the balance between achieving higher levels of efficacy, with disease remission being the ultimate goal, needs to be balanced against safety considerations. For macromolecules, such as mAbs and soluble receptors, there is the potential for optimizing their characteristics, including ease of use, immunogenicity, and cost. For certain targets, it is possible that small-molecule inhibitors may be developed that can address some of these issues. However, as these molecules can be anticipated to have pharmacokinetic, mechanistic, and other important differences from their macromolecular counterparts, this may translate into variable safety and efficacy. Therefore, newer agents of a different class, even those whose putative target is the same as existing therapies, need to be assessed with the same rigor as the currently available agents.

■ REFERENCES ■

1. Lee SJ, Kavanaugh A. Adverse events related to biologic agents. J Allergy Clin Immunol 2005; 116: 900–905.

2. Maini R, St Clair EW, Breedveld F, et al. Infliximab (chimeric anti-tumour necrosis factor α monoclonal antibody) versus placebo in rheumatoid arthritis patients receiving concomitant methotrexate: a randomized phase III trial. ATTRACT Study Group. Lancet 1999; 354: 1932–1939.

3. Lipsky PE, van der Heijde DM, St Claire EW, et al. Infliximab and methotrexate in the treatment of rheumatoid arthritis. N Engl J Med 2000; 343: 1594–1602.

4. St Clair EW, van der Heijde DM, Smolen JS, et al. Combination of infliximab and methotrexate therapy for early rheumatoid arthritis: a randomized, controlled trial. Arthritis Rheum 2004; 50: 3432–3443.

5. Braun J, Brandt J, Listing J, et al. Treatment of active ankylosing spondylitis with infliximab: a randomised controlled multicentre trial. Lancet 2002; 359: 1187–1193.

6. van der Heijde D, Dijkmans B, Geusens P, et al. Efficacy and safety of infliximab in patients with ankylosing spondylitis. Arthritis Rheum 2005; 52: 582–591.

7. Sieper J, Baraliakos X, Listing J, et al. Persistent reduction of spinal inflammation as assessed by magnetic resonance imaging in patients with ankylosing spondylitis after 2 years of treatment with the anti-tumor necrosis factor agent infliximab. Rheumatol 2005; 44: 1525–1530.

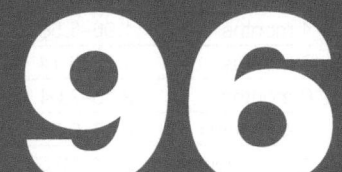

Assessment of proteins of the immune system

Henry A. Homburger, Ravinder Jit Singh

96

Clinical and research laboratories use a variety of analytical methods to detect and measure immunoglobulins and antibodies – the most numerous proteins of the immune system. These methods have been developed over decades and vary considerably in analytical sensitivity and specificity, ease of use, reliability, scope of application in large and small laboratories, and usefulness in clinical medicine and research applications. This chapter provides a broad overview of analytical methods for the detection, qualitative assessment and measurement of immunoglobulins and antibodies. Discussion of this subject is complicated by the fact that methods developed years ago are still in widespread use alongside much newer methods. It is important to provide at least some discussion of older analytical methods in order to understand the basic principles of measurement of immunoglobulins and antibodies. Several of the measurement methods mentioned in this chapter are more appropriate for research applications than for clinical use, and these distinctions are mentioned where they apply.

Measurements of immunoglobulins and antibodies must also be considered from the perspective of their usefulness in different clinical situations. Comprehensive consideration of this subject is beyond the scope of this chapter, but references are made to common clinical applications of measurements of immunoglobulins and antibodies in other chapters devoted to individual immunologic diseases. It is also important to consider immunoglobulins and antibodies from the perspective of their use as reagents in analytical systems of various types, referred to collectively as immunoassays. Reagent antibodies are key ingredients in all the analytical methods discussed in this chapter, irrespective of whether the analyte being measured is an immunoglobulin molecule, a specific antibody, or an unrelated molecule such as a microbial antigen or endogenous antigen.

The chapter is divided into sections devoted to consideration of the qualitative and quantitative assessment of immunoglobulin proteins, the measurement of antibodies by qualitative, semi-quantitative and quantitative methods, advanced analytical methods for the identification and qualitative analysis of proteins and antibodies (proteomic techniques), and proficiency testing programs designed to determine the performance of laboratories that perform clinical tests for immunoglobulins and antibodies. Throughout the chapter, the discussion of older analytical

methods is approached from the perspective of principles of immunochemistry illustrated by these methods. In some instances several different analytical methods are in widespread use for the same clinical applications, e.g., detection of monoclonal immunoglobulin paraproteins (M-proteins) or measurement of autoantibodies, and the advantages and limitations of each method are mentioned.

It is important at the outset to recognize an essential difference between immunoglobulins and antibodies as analytes in immunoassays. When measuring an immunoglobulin, the analytical method relies upon the fact that all molecules of immunoglobulin protein that react in the assay possess a common chemical structure, i.e., an epitope defined by several amino acids associated with the constant region of the immunoglobulin heavy or light chain.[1] Immunoglobulin molecules that possess the epitope all react in the immunoassay regardless of differences in the molecular structure or amino acid sequence of other domains of the heavy or light chains. By contrast, immunoassays that measure antibodies rely on the fact that all the antibodies of interest react with an antigen of defined structure. The antibodies that are detected often vary extensively in the strength with which they bind to the target antigen, a property referred to by the terms affinity and avidity, and thus are not chemically identical even in the portion of the molecules that react with antigen.[2] For this reason, it is more difficult to measure antibodies quantitatively, and it is often difficult to compare the results of antibody measurements performed by different analytical methods. Examples of this phenomenon are presented in the sections devoted to the measurement of antibodies.

■ IMMUNOGLOBULINS: QUALITATIVE ASSESSMENT AND CHARACTERIZATION ■

The common structural elements of immunoglobulins are the heavy and light polypeptide chains. There are five different polypeptide heavy chains, γ, α, μ, δ and ε, and two different polypeptide light chains, κ and λ. Each heavy chain and light chain is composed of several domains that contain common structural elements (constant regions) and a variable

KEY CONCEPTS

QUALITATIVE AND SEMI-QUANTITATIVE IMMUNOGLOBULIN TESTING

Protein electrophoresis:

>> Useful to evaluate body fluids for the presence of monoclonal immunoglobulins (M-proteins).

>> Useful to estimate changes in the concentrations of M-proteins.

Immunofixation electrophoresis, capillary zone electrophoresis with immunosubtraction, and immunoelectrophoresis:

>> Useful to characterize the heavy and light chains of M-proteins.

>> Capable of identifying small M-proteins present in low concentrations that may not be apparent on protein electrophoresis.

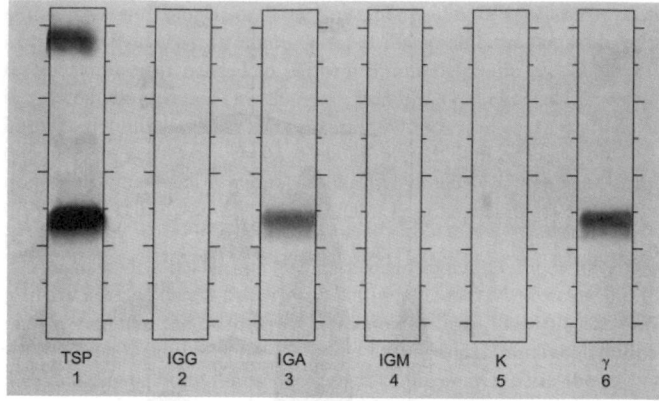

Fig. 96.3 Immunofixation of serum from a patient with an IgA-λ M-protein. Lane 1 shows a serum protein electrophoresis. Lanes 2–6 represent serum samples from the same patient reacted with monospecific antisera to IgG, IgA, IgM, κ and λ.

further evaluated by other methods and hypogammaglobulinemia should be confirmed by quantifying the levels of IgG, IgM and IgA. Densitometric analysis of stained proteins after SPEP is an acceptable method for following the response to therapy of diseases characterized by M-proteins once the specific diagnosis has been established.

IMMUNOFIXATION ELECTROPHORESIS

Immunofixation electrophoresis (IFE) has largely replaced immunoelectrophoresis (IEP) (see below) for establishing the presence and isotype of a monoclonal immunoglobulin M-protein[8, 9] (Fig. 96.3). IFE is easier to perform, is somewhat more sensitive, and is easier to interpret than IEP. IFE combines the resolution of zone electrophoresis and the specificity of an antigen–antibody precipitin reaction. The initial step in the IFE procedure involves creating replicate lanes of high-resolution protein electrophoresis. After the proteins are separated, but before staining, the replicate electrophoretic strips are each incubated with a different specific antiserum, either in solution or with an antiserum-soaked membrane. Laboratories usually include antisera to the heavy chains of IgG, IgA and IgM, and κ and λ light chains, but leave one lane blank to observe the appearance of an untreated (standard) SPEP. The quality of antisera used to stain the separated immunoglobulins is critical in that they must be specific for the intended targets and of high titer. The protein band and its antiserum form a precipitate on the gel at the region of antibody–antigen equivalence (see below), which is then washed to remove unreacted proteins. Following staining with amido black or Coomassie blue, the gel is reviewed manually. The location of the immunoprecipitate depends on the electrophoretic mobility of the specific M-protein.

Most laboratories use IFE after screening samples with the SPEP test and/or quantitative immunoglobulin measurements.[9] Although serum is the most common sample source, urine or cerebrospinal fluid can also be examined to detect and/or characterize M-proteins or their fragments. IFE has several advantages over IEP, including rapid turnaround time (2 hours, versus overnight incubation); increased sensitivity; better resolution; and ease of interpretation compared to IEPs. IFE is particularly useful for characterizing small M-proteins and nonIgG M-proteins.

CLINICAL PEARLS

ASSESSMENT OF IMMUNOGLOBULINS

>> Initial assessment is performed by protein electrophoresis and by quantification of immunoglobulins and free light chains by nephelometry.

>> Useful in the diagnosis of a monoclonal immunoglobulin (M-protein, multiple myeloma or Waldenström's macroglobulinemia).

>> Useful to estimate the quantity of M-protein or response to therapy:

Electrophoresis is often more useful than nephelometry for following the level of a monoclonal M-protein.

>> Second order testing is performed by immunofixation analysis or immunoglobulin analysis by capillary zone electrophoresis with immunosubtraction to identify and characterize the heavy and light chains of monoclonal M-proteins.

The disadvantages of IFE include the increased quality, quantity and cost of antisera required. Optimal resolution requires that the amounts of antisera be determined for each patient sample to avoid either excess dilution or excess antibody. In addition, because of the increased sensitivity of IFE, smaller bands are more frequently identified. These may be of uncertain clinical significance, leading to some difficulties in interpretation.

CAPILLARY ZONE ELECTROPHORESIS (CZE)

This is a more recent electrophoretic technique that provides increased sensitivity, speed, and the potential for automation.[10] Commercial instruments aimed at detecting M-proteins are available and are an attractive alternative to IFE for those laboratories that process large numbers of samples.

In a typical CZE analysis, samples are aspirated into narrow-bore, negatively charged capillary tubes. An electrical current is applied and proteins migrate toward the cathode. The fractions are optically quantified at a wave length of 215 nm to produce a virtual electropherogram similar to those seen with traditional SPEP. There is no staining of the proteins and up to 40 samples per hour can be processed. CZE has been used to characterize M-proteins by a process called immunosubtraction.[10, 11] The patient's specimen is absorbed with beads to which individual specific antisera, including anti-μ, anti-γ, anti-α, anti-κ, and anti-λ, are bound. An M-protein present before immunosubtraction is diminished or absent following incubation with appropriate class-specific antiserum. Recent comparisons of CZE and agarose electrophoresis with IFE indicate similar analytical sensitivity for detecting and characterizing M-proteins.[11] CZE and immunosubtraction are relatively new techniques. Larger laboratories will be drawn to the possibility of automation, speed, and potential cost savings. Clinicians will be drawn to the speed and potential improvement in sensitivity of this technology compared to older analytical methods.

IMMUNOELECTROPHORESIS

Immunoelectrophoresis (IEP) is an older method for qualitative analysis of M-proteins in serum and urine. IEP is a two-step procedure that combines the principles of zone electrophoresis and immunodiffusion. The method is mentioned here as it is still used by some clinical laboratories. In a typical IEP analysis, serum proteins are first separated by electrophoresis in a supporting medium such as agarose bound to a glass slide or plastic sheet. The separated proteins are reacted for up to 72 hours with specific antisera placed in troughs parallel to the electrophoretic migration. Antigen and antibody diffuse toward each other, forming elliptical precipitin arcs. The shape, position, and size of each arc demonstrate the specific characteristics of each protein. γ-Globulin from a healthy individual will form a balanced, evenly distributed smooth arc when reacted with antisera specific for the more prevalent heavy chains or light chains. Excess monoclonal production of any one isotype of immunoglobulin leads to distortion by thickening or bowing of the uniformity of the precipitation arc. In this way, M-proteins are visualized qualitatively. The quality and quantity of antisera used are not as critical as in IFE.

IEP has been largely supplanted for evaluating immunoglobulins in serum and other body fluids. Nevertheless, many small laboratories throughout the world still use IEP to detect and/or characterize M-proteins in the serum or urine. IEP is slower, less sensitive, and more difficult to interpret than IFE. IEP fails to detect some small monoclonal M-proteins because the most rapidly migrating immunoglobulins present in the highest concentrations may obscure the presence of small M-proteins.

■ QUANTITATIVE METHODS FOR MEASURING IMMUNOGLOBULINS: PRECIPITIN METHODS ■

The levels of immunoglobulins in a healthy population vary markedly with age, and to a lesser extent with gender, racial background, environmental factors and genetic makeup.[12] Each laboratory must verify the reference values for immunoglobulins by age, often by assessing a group of healthy individuals and comparing those results with data in the literature and/or data supplied by the reagent manufacturer. Although there are international standards for immunoglobulin measurements, variations in methods and techniques have been associated with differences between laboratories in reference ranges for immunoglobulins.[12]

Immunoglobulin levels outside the reference range include low levels seen in hypogammaglobulinemia and increased levels associated with polyclonal hypergammaglobulinemia. Polyclonal hypergammaglobulinemia is often associated with chronic inflammatory diseases, including infectious diseases, autoimmune diseases and chronic liver diseases. Monoclonal hypergammaglobulinemia is a hallmark of multiple myeloma and Waldenström's macroglobulinemia. Immunoglobulins are commonly quantified to evaluate suspected deficiency, to monitor immunoglobulin replacement therapy, and to monitor levels in patients with monoclonal immunoglobulins. Adequate monitoring of a monoclonal M-protein often requires the use of other qualitative techniques, as described above.[9]

RADIAL IMMUNODIFFUSION (RID)

RID is an older method based on the classic precipitin reaction in which antigen and antibodies react to form precipitates in liquid or semi-fluid media.[13] Under conditions of antibody excess, the quantity of the precipitate is directly related to the quantity of antigen in the test sample. Ouchterlony[26] demonstrated that precipitins form in agar or agarose media in a manner related to the relative quantities of each. In a typical RID analysis, the amount of precipitin, as measured in distance migrated from the antigen well, is mathematically related to the concentration of antigen added to the well.

RID uses a predetermined dilution of specific antiserum mixed with agar or agarose in a Petri dish or on a glass slide. A series of small wells are cut in the agar and filled with samples containing antigen. As the antigen diffuses into the agar it forms a precipitate with the antibodies contained in the gel. Once antigen–antibody equivalence is reached, an opaque precipitin ring develops around the antigen well. The diameter of the precipitin ring is proportional to the concentration of antigen in the test solution or standard added to the center well. The diameter may be measured either at the endpoint, when the antigen has completely reacted with antibody (typically 48–72 hours), or after a fixed diffusion time, usually 24 hours. The concentration of the unknown sample is estimated by measuring the diameter of the ring produced by the sample and plotting this on a concentration–diameter curve, established using standards containing known amounts of the antigen. The lower limit of sensitivity of RID is approximately 0.5 mg/L. Within limitations, the ring diameter for a given antigen concentration can be increased by reducing the antiserum concentration in the gel.

RID is used in many smaller laboratories to measure the concentrations of common proteins, including serum immunoglobulins and IgG subclasses. The method is simple to perform and requires very little equipment. The major limitations include the amount of time required, the relative imprecision of the assay, with coefficients of variation often greater than 10%, relative insensitivity, and dependence on antigen quantity and configuration. In rare situations RID can lead to large errors in estimates of immunoglobulin concentrations, including

> ## KEY CONCEPTS

> ### QUANTITATIVE IMMUNOGLOBULIN TESTING
>
> Nephelometry:
> >> Most commonly used method for measuring immunoglobulin levels.
> >> Can be used to measure immunoglobulins, immunoglobulin subclasses and free light chains.
> >> Less variable and more sensitive than radial immunodiffusion.
> Radial immunodiffusion:
> >> Used by some small laboratories to quantify immunoglobulins and other serum proteins.
> >> More variable and slower to perform than nephelometry.

estimations of IgM levels in patients with 7S IgM M-proteins, patients with high levels of rheumatoid factor, and some patients with IgA deficiency who may have antibodies that react with antisera used to prepare the RID plate.

ELECTROIMMUNODIFFUSION (EID)

Electroimmunodiffusion is a modification of RID used in occasional cases and in some research settings to measure specific proteins.[14] The technique differs from radial immunodiffusion in its use of an electric field to induce migration of the protein antigen into an antibody-containing gel. Antigen–antibody complexes form a visible precipitate in the form of a cone or 'rocket.' The height of the cone is proportional to the amount of antigen in the sample. A standard curve is constructed and the concentration of the protein unknown is extrapolated from the curve. The sensitivity of the EID method is of the order of 0.01–0.05 mg/L.

NEPHELOMETRY

Nephelometry has largely replaced RID in most clinical laboratories as the preferred method for measuring intact immunoglobulins, immunoglobulin light chains and many other proteins in body fluids.[12, 15] Nephelometry is a modification of the basic precipitin reaction that relies on light-scattering by soluble immune complexes in solution (Figs 96.4 and 96.5). The amount of scatter produced by soluble immune complexes is measured in a photoelectric cell as optical density. As the concentration of antigen increases, scattered light increases. In contrast to the standard precipitin reaction, which requires that the concentrations of antigen and antibody be at equivalence, nephelometry often performs best with excess antibody.

In a typical nephelometric assay for immunoglobulin, a standard curve is developed by reacting increasing concentrations of the antigen of interest with a constant, large quantity of specific antiserum. Increasing amounts of immune complexes scatter more light, and the intensity of scattered light is directly related to the concentration of antigen. Antigen can be measured accurately in the antibody excess portion of the precipitin curve, and to maintain this relationship, increased antigen concentration requires additional dilutions of the sample.

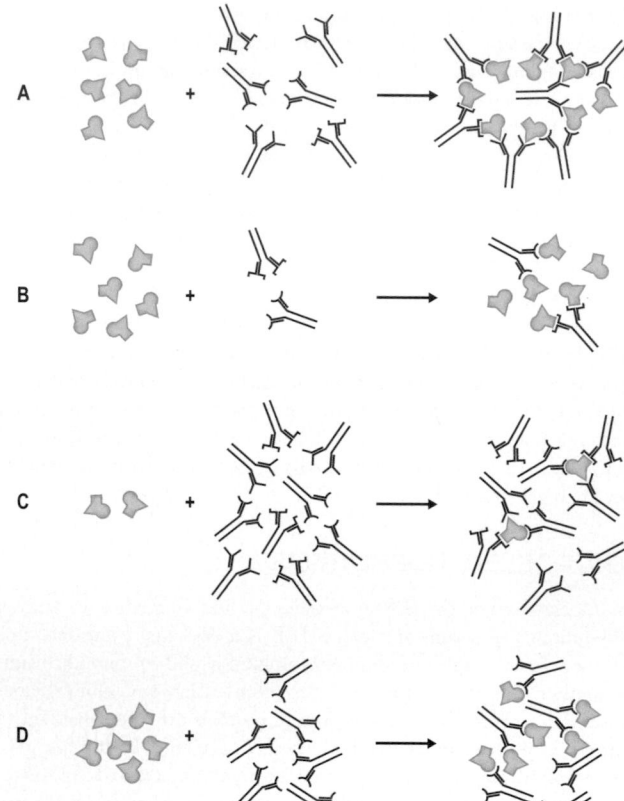

Fig. 96.4 Precipitin reaction. Antigen molecules are represented as having three different antigenic sites (epitopes) on their surface. Three different types of antibodies are illustrated, each having binding regions for one of the three types of antigenic sites. (A) Near the equivalence point, lattice formation occurs and a precipitate forms. (B) In the presence of excess antigen the concentration of antibody is insufficient for cross-linking. Lattice formation does not occur and complexes are soluble. (C) In the presence of excess antibody, lattice formation does not occur and complexes are soluble. (D) In the presence of a monoclonal antibody each antigen molecule is bound at a single site. No cross-linking can occur and complexes remain soluble.

Endpoint (or fixed-time) nephelometry measures the maximum scattered light after an antigen–antibody reaction has reached equilibrium, or after a fixed reaction time. The antigen concentration in the unknown sample is calculated from a response curve produced with reference standards containing known amounts of the antigen tested under identical conditions.

Rate or kinetic nephelometry is an alternative method in which the peak rate of immune complex formation is measured.[15, 16] As soluble immune complexes are formed during an antigen–antibody reaction, the quantity of light scattered over time can be plotted as a sigmoid curve. The upper inflection point in the curve represents the peak rate of immune complex formation and is directly proportional to the antigen concentration. The antigen concentration of an unknown sample is calculated by comparing the sample's peak rate of light scatter to an established reference curve. Rate nephelometry has been automated by

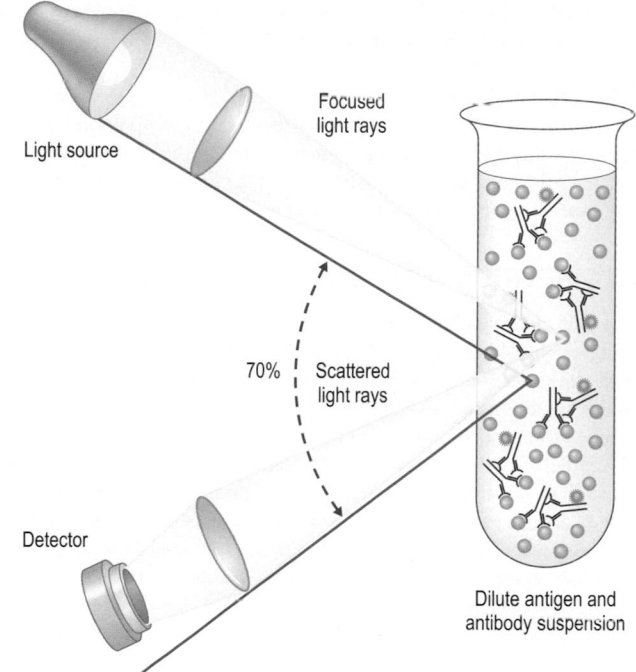

Fig. 96.5 Nephelometry. Light scatter by soluble immune complexes is measured at an acute angle to the incident light source.

> **KEY CONCEPTS**
>
> **IMMUNOASSAYS**
>
> Precipitin assays:
>
> ➤➤ Useful for measuring both immunoglobulins and antibodies.
>
> ➤➤ Except for nephelometry and certain agglutination methods, less sensitive than immunometric assays and immunofluorescent microscopy.
>
> ➤➤ Tend to be used in smaller laboratories and for infrequent analyses.
>
> Immunometric assays:
>
> ➤➤ Useful for measuring immunoglobulins and antibodies.
>
> ➤➤ Measurements based on competitive displacement or two-site (sandwich) techniques.
>
> ➤➤ Antigen or antibody is labelled with an enzyme, fluorophore or chemiluminescent molecule.
>
> ➤➤ Sensitive to nanogram or picogram quantities of analyte.

several commercial manufacturers. Available instruments provide an automated platform of reagents, with barcoding of test specimens and rapid analysis with high throughout. The coefficients of variation for measurements of intact immunoglobulins and free immunoglobulin light chains are typically in the range of 5%.

According to recent inter-laboratory proficiency surveys from the College of American Pathologists, the vast majority of clinical laboratories use nephelometric methods to measure immunoglobulins.[17] Fewer than 2% use RID. Some disadvantages of nephelometry include increased costs for instruments and reagents, although these are compensated for by savings in personnel costs. Other potential problems include reagent antisera, i.e., poor reactivity of certain commercial antisera with unusual M-proteins; poor linearity of measurement of some M-proteins leading to inaccurate quantification; and temperature maintenance problems with the measurement of cryoglobulins. In general, from a clinical perspective it is preferable to monitor the quantity of an M-protein during therapy of a plasma cell proliferative disease by electrophoresis with densometric quantification.[9] Nephelometric methods can also be subject to interferences caused by particles or pigments in serum that increase background light scatter and make interpretation difficult or impossible.

IMMUNOMETRIC METHODS

The first widely adopted immunometric assays were competitive displacement radioimmunoassays used to measure hormones in human plasma.[18] More recently, radiolabeled antigens have been largely supplanted by enzyme or chemiluminescent labels in most displacement

assays.[19, 20] In a typical competitive displacement assay, labeled and unlabeled antigen are incubated with limited quantities of first-stage antibody. The two species of antigen compete for binding to the first-stage antibody. A standard curve is developed by adding standards that contain increasing quantities of unlabeled antigen. The degree of inhibition of the trace amount of labeled antigen by unlabeled antigen provides an indirect measure of the concentration of the unlabeled species. After incubation, the antigen–antibody complexes are separated from unbound labeled and unlabeled antigen, and 'bound' or 'free' labeled antigen is measured to construct a standard curve.

Noncompetitive immunometric assays are now more popular than displacement assays.[20] In a noncompetitive (sandwich) assay, specific antibody bound to a solid phase, e.g., a polystyrene particle or microtiter plate, is used to 'capture' the antigen of interest. An aliquot of test specimen is incubated with antibody bound to the solid phase, allowing the antigen to react with the first-stage antibody. The excess specimen is washed away and a second labeled antibody, also reactive with the antigen, is added. Excess second-stage labeled antibody is washed away after a second incubation, and the binding of standards and unknowns is measured. Unknowns are compared to a standard curve generated with calibrator materials having known concentrations of antigen. Noncompetitive immunometric methods are approximately as sensitive as displacement methods. Sensitivity is determined by the affinities of reagent antibodies, and by the amplified signal obtained from the chemical label.[21]

In general, immunometric assays of either type have excellent sensitivity, reasonable precision with coefficients of variation in the range of 10% for measurements of proteins, and may be used to measure antigens of all types in human body fluids. Immunoglobulins present in serum in very low concentrations, especially IgE, are effectively measured by these techniques.

Enzyme-linked immunosorbent assay (ELISA) is the most popular technical version of immunometric assay in current use. There are many variations of the basic ELISA method, including both competitive and

> ### KEY CONCEPTS
>
> #### SPECIFIC ANTIBODY TESTING
>
> ▶▶ Can be performed by a variety of methods, including precipitin-based immunoassays, fluorescence microscopy, and immunometric assays (ELISA).
>
> ▶▶ Most measurements are semi-quantitative and quite variable.
>
> ▶▶ Tests performed with crude antigens are often used for screening.

noncompetitive assays. As noted above, ELISA is a sensitive method capable of measuring proteins in nanogram or picogram quantities, without the use of radionuclides. ELISA assays are so named because reagent enzymes are used to label either the antigen standard or the second-stage antibody in competitive displacement and noncompetitive (sandwich) assays, respectively (see below).

■ DETECTION AND MEASUREMENT OF SPECIFIC ANTIBODIES ■

Laboratory testing for specific antibodies and autoantibodies is useful clinically to screen for disease, to establish specific diagnoses, and to monitor the clinical courses of certain diseases. This is particularly true for diseases in which the antibody response is involved in the pathogenesis, e.g., immediate hypersensitivity diseases, or where antibodies serve empirically as disease-specific markers or independent prognostic indicators.

Antibodies are routinely detected and measured by a variety of immunoassay methods. In virtually all cases, the methods rely on the use of antigens as analytical reagents. Reagent antigens can be complex mixtures of molecules, e.g., an allergen mixture in a test for IgE antibodies or highly purified 'native' or recombinant molecules, e.g., small nuclear ribonucleoproteins in a test for IgG antibodies to extractable nuclear antigens. Many reagent antigens of clinical interest are large molecules with several antigenic sites (epitopes) that react with antibodies of clinical interest in patients' specimens.[22, 23]

Clinical applications of tests for specific antibodies are directly related to the nature of the reagent antigens. For example, tests that employ crude or complex antigen preparations, such as the tissue substrates used in the test for antinuclear antibodies, are useful primarily as screening tests, whereas tests that employ highly purified or recombinant antigens, such as tests for antibodies to some microbial antigens or extractable nuclear antigens, detect antibodies that are disease-specific markers.[24]

Tests performed with purified or recombinant antigens are often used to detect disease-specific antibodies. The nature of the reagent antigen also influences the precision and accuracy of antibody measurements. Measurements performed using a crude antigen as reagent tend to be semi-quantitative and imprecise, with the result often expressed as a titer (i.e., the reciprocal of the dilution of test specimen used in the assay). In contrast, a highly purified antigen may be used to prepare a pure preparation of specific antibodies by affinity chromatography,

which enables calibration of the assay system either in mass units (e.g., micrograms of antibody protein per liter) or in arbitrary quantitative units.

The antigens of interest in clinical immunology belong to several different chemical classes, including proteins and glycoproteins, lipids, nucleic acids, carbohydrates and haptens. Many of the analytic methods discussed below are adaptable for use with each of these classes of antigen. Exceptions are noted where they apply.

PRECIPITATION METHODS

Analytical methods that rely on the principles of immunoprecipitation are among the oldest methods in clinical immunology. They are applicable to the detection of both specific antibodies and immunoglobulin proteins (as discussed above). Precipitation methods are based on the antigen–antibody precipitin reaction originally described by Heidelberger and Kendall.[25] In this reaction, a multivalent antigen reacts with antibodies in a fluid or semi-solid matrix such as agar gel to form an insoluble lattice of antigen–antibody complexes. The presence of a precipitin indicates the presence of specific antibodies to one or more of the antigens in the antigen reagent. Precipitation occurs over a range of concentrations of antigens and antibodies referred to as the zone of equivalence (Fig. 96.4). If the concentration of either reactant is too great, precipitation does not occur and only soluble complexes are formed.

A modification of the basic immunoprecipitation technique, called double immunodiffusion, is commonly used in both research and clinical laboratories to detect specific antibodies.[26, 27] In this adaptation of the precipitin method, an aqueous solution of reagent antigen is placed in the center well of an agar slide and positive control sera and specimens to be tested for the presence of specific antibodies are pipetted into surrounding wells. After 24–48 hours of incubation, which permits diffusion of antigens and antibodies throughout the gel, precipitin lines form that can be detected visually. The specificity of antibodies in the test specimen is evaluated by examining the pattern of convergence between the unknown precipitins and a control that contains antibodies of known specificities. The possible reactions include identity (fusion), partial identity (one spur) and nonidentity (two spurs), (Fig. 96.6).

The double immunodiffusion method is simple to perform and requires no special equipment. However, the technique is qualitative and is sensitive only to concentrations of antibodies greater than approximately 0.1 µg/mL. The relative lack of sensitivity of this method limits its application in the clinical laboratory to situations in which patients' sera contain relatively high concentrations of specific antibodies. The results of double immunodiffusion tests are also subject to errors of interpretation. False negative results may occur if the concentration of antigen is not carefully adjusted to produce a zone of equivalence with the concentration of antibodies usually encountered in patients' specimens. In addition, multiple precipitin lines of unknown specificity can be seen with clinical specimens, and these precipitins can obscure identification of specific antibodies of clinical interest. The double immunodiffusion method cannot be used to detect antibodies to haptens and monovalent antigens, which fail to form an insoluble lattice. Despite these limitations, the method is still in widespread use in clinical laboratories for the detection of autoantibodies, including antibodies to small nuclear ribonucleoproteins (SSA/Ro, SSB/La, Sm, and SmRNP) and enzymes (topoisomerase 1 and RNA synthetases) in patients with systemic rheumatic diseases.

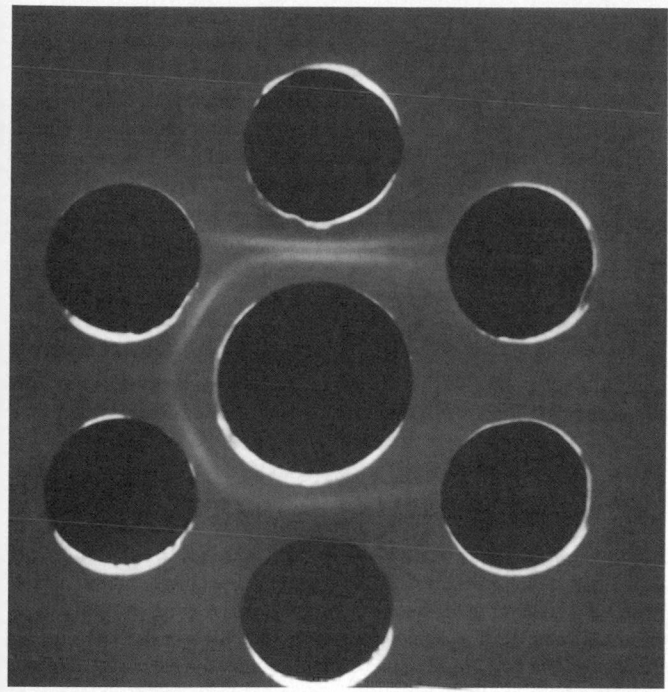

Fig. 96.6 Double immunodiffusion for autoantibodies to extractable nuclear antigens U_1RNP and Sm. The center well was loaded with U_1RNP/Sm antigen. Outside wells were loaded with control sera or patients' sera as follows (counterclockwise from top well): anti-U_1RNP and anti-Sm control, patient 1 in duplicate; anti-U_1RNP control, patient 2 in duplicate. Precipitin formed with serum from patient 1 shows line of identity (fusion of precipitins) with anti-U_1RNP control sera.

Counterimmunoelectrophoresis (CIEP) is another modification of the basic immunoprecipitation technique that utilizes electrophoresis to enhance the rate of migration of antigen and antibodies in a gel matrix. By adjusting the pH of the electrophoresis buffer, antigens and specific antibodies are made to migrate in opposite directions toward the center of the slide, where immunoprecipitation can occur. CIEP is a somewhat more sensitive technique than conventional double immunodiffusion, but it is technically demanding and has limited application in the clinical laboratory for detecting most specific antibodies.[28]

AGGLUTINATION METHODS

Agglutination is the aggregation or clumping of visible, discrete particles in an antigen–antibody reaction to form a larger mass.[13, 29] The fundamental immunologic principle of agglutination reactions is the same as previously described for precipitin reactions. Initially, antigen–antibody recognition occurs, followed by binding, and visible aggregation of antigen particles. Occasionally agglutination is incomplete because the necessary antibody bridging of adjacent antigen particles fails to occur.

Agglutination assays for specific antibodies can be performed using insoluble native antigens such as bacterial cells, antigen-coated particles such as latex beads, or red blood cells to which antigens have been attached by chemical coupling. Agglutination assays require a stable particle on which antigen is accessible for binding, and a reaction solution of proper ionic strength and viscosity to prevent incomplete agglutination. Most commercially available agglutination tests that are designed to detect antibodies specify the use of serum (not plasma) or cerebrospinal fluid. The sensitivity and specificity of these tests are determined by the purity of the antigens coupled to the insoluble indicator particles.

In general, the advantages of agglutination methods are their ease of performance; speed of performance, usually requiring less than 10 minutes; their high degree of analytic sensitivity (often comparable to immunometric methods); and the enormous variety of antibodies that can be detected. In addition, with the exception of cold agglutinins (typically IgM antibodies), the tests are usually not affected by temperature. One of the major disadvantages of agglutination methods is that the reactions are at best semi-quantitative. For example, although qualitative test results are highly reproducible, for most test systems the results are only accurate to a fourfold difference in antibody titer. The other important disadvantage of agglutination methods is their susceptibility to false negative reactions caused by the prozone phenomenon. Prozone refers to the absence of agglutination in conditions of extreme antibody excess, which results in poor lattice formation.

Agglutination techniques are routinely used in the diagnosis of infectious diseases, in transfusion medicine for typing of blood cells, and in commercial assays for the detection of autoantibodies in patients with autoimmune diseases. Numerous agglutination-based diagnostic tests are available because of the ease with which test reagents can be developed. For example, some red blood cells, bacteria, and fungi can be agglutinated directly by serum antibodies. Indirect agglutination tests are also available in which a vast repertoire of soluble antigens can be passively adsorbed or chemically coupled to red blood cells or inert particles.

Direct agglutination

Direct agglutination is the aggregation of particles brought about by the interaction of specific antibodies with particulate antigens. To agglutinate an antigen, all that is required is a reaction solution of the proper ionic strength and an antibody with two or more receptors that cross-link adjacent antigen particles (Fig. 96.7). IgM antibodies are more efficient than IgG antibodies in agglutination reactions. IgM antibodies usually aggregate particulate antigens based on the size of the antibody molecule, whereas IgG antibodies may require the addition of substances such as bovine serum albumin or dextran to alter the viscosity and charge of the reaction solution before agglutination can occur.[29] In some direct agglutination tests, red blood cells or bacteria are treated with enzymes such as papain or DNase to increase the exposure of surface antigens, remove allosteric interferences, or alter the configuration of external membrane components to enhance the agglutination reaction. For direct agglutination tests, if the techniques are highly standardized the only reagents necessary for a functional assay are positive and negative controls for qualitative tests, a serum that can be diluted for quantitative tests, some measurement of antigen concentration (such as a McFarland standard for opacity), and a control for nonspecific agglutination.

The most common clinical use of the direct agglutination test procedure is in transfusion medicine, i.e., ABO typing of erythrocytes.[30] Direct agglutination tests are also widely used for serotyping of bacteria, e.g., *Campylobacter* and other enteric pathogens involved in outbreaks of

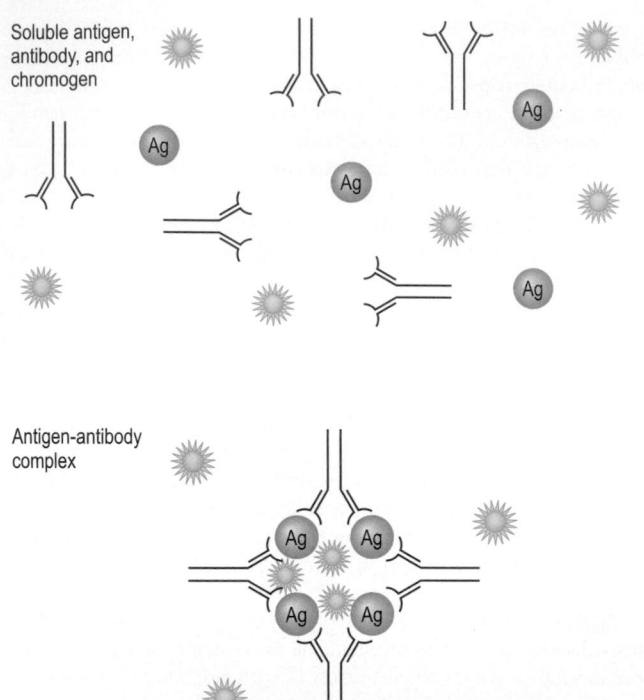

Soluble antigen, antibody, and chromogen

Antigen-antibody complex

Fig. 96.7 Direct agglutination reaction. Particulate antigen reacts with specific antibodies to form an insoluble matte. Chromagen particles are trapped in the matte, indicating that the reaction has taken place.

foodborne human gastroenteritis, and in the diagnosis of certain infectious diseases.[31, 32]

Indirect agglutination

The most widely used agglutination methods are so-called indirect assays in which antigen is attached to a carrier particle, either covalently or by adsorption. The two most common indirect agglutination methods use red blood cells and polystyrene beads as carriers. A number of bacterial antigens, viruses and microbial toxins adsorb directly to red blood cells, but for many applications of the indirect hemagglutination method it is necessary to treat the carrier cells with coupling reagents such as tannic acid, bisdiazobenzidine or glutaraldehyde to couple the antigen to the carrier cells.[29] Covalent coupling of antigens to polystyrene beads is often performed using carbiodimides or other chemical coupling reactions. Indirect agglutination assays that use polystyrene carrier beads are used to detect antibodies to bacteria, fungi, rickettsial and parasitic antigens, as well as certain viruses, including rubella, HIV, rotaviruses and Epstein–Barr virus. Indirect agglutination assays are also available to detect autoantibodies, including antibodies to various nuclear antigens and dsDNA.

A third form of agglutination test is the antibody-mediated incomplete agglutination reaction. The direct antiglobulin test used in the diagnosis of autoimmune and drug-induced immune hemolytic anemia and to determine antibody to Rh antigens on erythrocytes is an example. In this technique, antiglobulin antibodies produced in a heterologous species are added to detect subagglutinating or nonagglutinating

amounts of anti-erythrocyte antibodies. The direct antiglobulin test detects specific antibodies or other serum proteins that bind to a patient's erythrocytes. The indirect antiglobulin test is a two-stage reaction in which the patient's serum is first incubated with commercially available red blood cells, after which an antiglobulin antiserum is added. Still another variation of the indirect antiglobulin test uses enzyme-treated erythrocytes to increase assay sensitivity.

Finally, flocculation, a term used mainly in syphilis serology, describes the reaction of a microscopically visible particulate antigen with an invisible substance (antibody) to form aggregates that either can be seen microscopically, as in the Venereal Disease Research Laboratory (VDRL) slide test, or visualized by the addition of an inert particle such as charcoal, which becomes entrapped in the antigen–antibody lattice, as in the rapid plasma reagin (RPR) card test for syphilis. In these tests the antigen–antibody reaction particles stay suspended rather than settling in a clump or forming a matte pattern.[33]

IMMUNOFLUORESCENCE METHODS

Indirect immunofluorescence (IF) is the technique most commonly used in clinical laboratories to screen for specific antibodies that react with cellular antigens. IF is more sensitive than immunodiffusion methods and faster to perform. Its increased sensitivity enables the detection of human antibodies in concentrations less than 0.1 µg/mL. The technique is semi-quantitative, with results expressed in titers, and is readily adaptable to the detection and measurement of many clinically important antibodies.[34]

IF tests are performed by incubating diluted patients' sera with thin sections of animal or human tissues or cultured cells that have been fixed chemically to allow intracellular penetration of specific antibodies. After incubation, unbound antibodies and serum proteins are washed off the slide and a second-stage, fluorochrome-conjugated anti-human immunoglobulin of desired specificity, is pipetted onto the substrate. Reagent antibody binds to any specific antibodies that have been captured by antigens in the substrate. Depending upon the specific test application, a fluorochrome-labeled anti-human immunoglobulin reagent can be chosen that reacts with any or all of the prevalent isotypes of human immunoglobulin, including IgG, IgM, and IgA. Bound anti-human immunoglobulin antibody is visualized by use of a fluorescent microscope. Incident light at a wavelength optimal to excite the fluorochrome is directed at the substrate slide, and light emitted by the fluorochrome is isolated by appropriate filters and transmitted to the microscope objective, where it can be visualized.[35] The presence of specific antibodies is indicated by fluorescence of the tissue or cells on the substrate slide.

The accurate performance of IF testing for specific antibodies requires careful attention to quality control of the test specimen, substrate slides, and fluorochrome-conjugated anti-human immunoglobulin antiserum. Sera from fasting patients are optimal for testing, as lipemic or hemolyzed sera may produce increased background fluorescence. In addition, each assay must include known negative- and positive-control sera. Long-term quality control requires comparison testing of successive lots of substrate slides with known negative- and positive-control sera to insure that there is minimal nonspecific binding of human immunoglobulins in the negative sera and comparable binding of specific antibodies, defined by similar endpoint titers (plus or minus one dilution), for the positive-control sera. Successive lots of

CLINICAL PEARLS

ASSESSMENT OF SPECIFIC ANTIBODIES #2

>> Tests for the detection of specific antibodies are useful for diagnosis in patients with autoimmune diseases, immune mediated inflammatory diseases, immediate hypersensitivity diseases and infectious diseases.

>> Most tests for specific antibodies are semi-quantitative.

>> Repeated tests for specific antibodies are not recommended for following the clinical course of most allergic diseases and many autoimmune diseases.

>> Clinicians must use caution in interpreting the results of antibody tests, as differences in analytical methods can be associated with significant differences in the diagnostic reference values for particular tests.

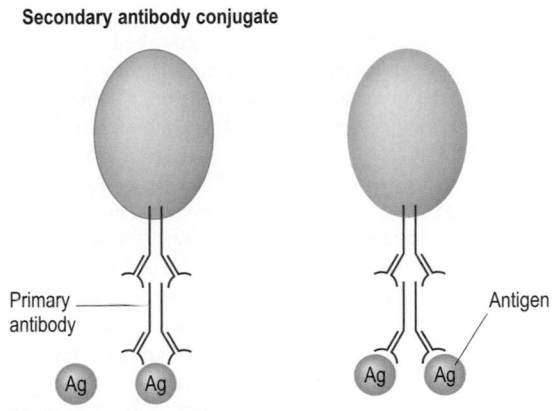

Fig. 96.8 Enzyme linked immunosorbent assay (see text for explanation).

anti-human immunoglobulin antisera are also compared to ensure reproducibility and analytical sensitivity. Anti-immunoglobulin reagents are characterized in terms of their antibody to total protein content, fluorochrome to protein ratio (typically in the range of 3 molecules of fluorochrome per mole of protein), and the dilution of reagent antiserum that yields maximal specific to nonspecific fluorescence, as demonstrated with well-characterized positive- and negative-control sera.[36] In most IF assays it is also desirable periodically to test a weakly reactive, positive-control serum to ensure that there has been no loss of analytic sensitivity from storage of the substrate slides or fluorochrome-conjugated antiserum. IF is routinely used in clinical laboratories to detect and measure antibodies associated with immune-mediated inflammatory diseases and antibodies to some bacteria and spirochetes in infectious diseases.

It is useful here to point out the relative advantages and disadvantages of this technique compared to ELISA methods as discussed below. IF has a long history of use in clinical laboratories and an established base of clinician users. Most physicians are familiar with IF test reports, which include reference ranges expressed as titers accompanied by comments about the pattern or morphologic appearance of fluorescence observed microscopically.[37] In addition, IF is suitable for use in both small and large laboratories, provided there are trained personnel available to perform the test and interpret the appearance of slides. For certain applications, one substrate slide can be used to detect several different antibodies simultaneously, e.g., tests for antinuclear antibodies and mitochondrial antibodies can be performed on the same substrate. Disadvantages of the IF method include the time required to perform endpoint titrations of positive sera, subjectivity in the interpretation of fluorescence morphology, and the need for highly trained technologists to perform the test. Nevertheless, it is worth noting that fluorescence microscopy remains useful for the discovery of autoantibodies, e.g., the recently described autoantibodies in patients with neuromyelitis optica.[38] IF can also be adapted to create novel test substrates for the clinical laboratory by transfecting cell lines with genetic material that codes for autoantigens of clinical interest e.g., a recently developed test for autoantibodies to proteinase 3 uses transfected human basophilic leukemia cells.[39]

IMMUNOMETRIC ASSAY METHODS

Immunometric methods, including ELISA, are widely used, versatile analytical systems for the detection and measurement of specific antibodies. These methods make use of reagent antigens immobilized on solid phases (immunosorbents) to capture specific antibodies from patients' specimens. Specific antibodies bound to the immunosorbent in the first stage of the assay are detected in the second stage by incubating with a polyclonal or monoclonal anti-human immunoglobulin antibody labeled with an enzyme or fluorophore. In the final stage of the assay, the amount of labeled second-stage antibody that has been bound to the immunosorbent is determined by measuring a colored or fluorescent product generated by the enzyme label or fluorophore (Fig. 96.8).

Immunometric methods offer several advantages that account for their popularity. A variety of methods have been developed to couple antigens covalently or noncovalently to solid-phase immunosorbents; and each of the principal chemical classes of antigen mentioned previously, including some haptens, has been used as an immunosorbent. Antigen immunosorbents can be prepared from crude antigen mixtures for use in screening tests e.g., the microtiter plate ELISA for antinuclear antibodies, or from highly purified antigens for use in the measurement of marker autoantibodies.[36] Immunometric methods are more sensitive than precipitin or agglutination techniques and are similar in sensitivity to IF. Analytical sensitivity is in the range of 1–10 ng of antibody protein/mL, which is adequate for measurement of specific antibodies of all human isotypes and subclasses, including IgE and IgG subclasses. The enhanced analytical sensitivity of immunometric assays is largely a result of amplification of the signal produced by the binding of labeled, second-stage anti-immunoglobulin antibody. As noted above, the second-stage antibody is typically labeled with an enzyme or fluorophore. Commonly used enzyme labels, such as alkaline phosphatase, generate many moles of measurable product for each mole of second-stage antibody bound to the immunosorbent, and reagent fluorophores emit light that can be counted to a predetermined endpoint. The analytic sensitivity of immunometric methods is limited primarily by the ratio of specific to nonspecific binding of immunoglobulin in the first stage of the assay.[13, 37] Immunosorbents with low levels of nonspecific binding afford maximum analytical sensitivity.

The most common immunometric assay for specific antibodies is the ELISA. In a typical ELISA, antigen is adsorbed noncovalently to the wells of a polystyrene microtiter plate. Different types of plates have been developed to maximize the adsorption of different chemical classes of antigen, including proteins and glycoproteins, phospholipids and nucleic acids, and to minimize nonspecific binding of immunoglobulins. ELISA methods can be used to detect specific antibodies qualitatively, or to make semi-quantitative measurements of specific antibodies by use of a standard curve calibrated in arbitrary units. For qualitative applications, the absorbance in wells incubated with an unknown (e.g., diluted patient serum) is compared to a calibrator that contains a low concentration of antibody. The absorbance of the calibrator is typically at least four times the background level. Positive results are indicated by absorbances significantly greater than the negative control and at least as great as the calibrator. In semi-quantitative applications, the absorbance in wells that contain an unknown specimen is compared to a standard curve prepared by plotting the absorbances of several calibrators. In either application, positive and negative control sera must be run with each assay to ensure that all steps in the procedures have been performed properly. There are limitations on the accuracy and precision of semi-quantitative tests performed by ELISA. Microtiter ELISA methods are inherently quite variable, and inter-assay coefficients of variation for positive sera may exceed 15%. In addition, the standard curve of absorbance versus antibody level is usually nonlinear. Consequently, even though results are reported on a continuous numerical scale in units, the results must be considered semi-quantitative. Results are often interpreted as falling within ranges, e.g., negative, borderline, weakly positive and strongly positive, with each category defined by a range of values expressed in units. Truly quantitative applications of the basic ELISA method are less common. These methods require calibration based on reference preparations that contain known concentrations of the antibody of interest, e.g., WHO Wo/80 for dsDNA antibodies.[40]

As noted above, the most common ELISA method is performed in polystyrene microtiter plates in which an antigen is adsorbed noncovalently to the plate. In other applications, antigen may be coupled covalently to a solid phase. This is particularly common with allergen immunosorbents used to test for specific IgE antibodies (Chapter 100).[41] The principal advantages of covalent coupling are that the antigen immunosorbents are stable indefinitely, and successive lots can be characterized in terms of the amount of antigen coupled per gram of solid phase, and by the capacity to bind antibodies from well-characterized positive control pools.

Given the large number of commercially available, US FDA-approved ELISA assays for antibodies, it is useful to point out the responsibilities of the manufacturer and end-user for validating the performance of these assays in the clinical environment.[36] It is generally accepted that the manufacturer is responsible for providing accurate information about the following parameters: expected values of test results in various populations, e.g., blood donor normals and certain relevant clinical groups; analytical assay performance, e.g., accuracy, precision, analytical specificity and reportable range of results; stability of the reagents; and quality control parameters to assess the validity of each test run. The end-user is responsible for validating the analytical performance characteristics mentioned above, and for establishing reference ranges appropriate to the clinical situations in which testing is likely to be performed. This latter point may be difficult to achieve, and clinical reference ranges may be based on peer-reviewed published clinical studies when it is not possible to conduct studies with clinical specimens obtained locally.

■ EMERGING ANALYTICAL CONCEPTS: PROTEOMICS, AND MICROARRAY AND MULTIPLEX TESTING FOR ANTIBODIES ■

PROTEOMIC METHODS

Analytical methods now applied to the qualitative analysis and measurement of proteins include liquid chromatography (LC) techniques and mass spectrometry (MS).[42, 43] Test methods that employ these techniques are regarded as the methods of choice for several analytes routinely measured in clinical laboratories, including drugs, drug metabolites, and steroid and peptide hormones.[44–46] However, for routine measurement of most proteins, including immunoglobulins, immunoassay techniques such as nephelometry and immunometric methods are preferred. The matrix of blood plasma is very complex and may cause artifacts in the measurement of proteins by chromatographic methods. A common problem is suppression of the analytical signal in chromatographic assays which results in low signal-to-noise ratios. Improved analytical sensitivity and specificity for clinically relevant protein analytes has been accomplished by immunoaffinity chromatography and by immunosubtraction techniques.[43]

An application of advanced proteomic techniques that has gained acceptance in recent years is the analysis of therapeutic antibodies. Monoclonal antibodies are now widely used as therapeutic agents to treat several immune-mediated and autoimmune diseases. For example, antibodies to tumor necrosis factor (TNF) are used to treat rheumatoid arthritis and inflammatory bowel diseases (Chapters 52 and 74).

The pharmaceutical industry standard for therapeutic monoclonal antibodies is to have the purest immunoglobulin with no contamination with other variants. C-terminal modification of the heavy chains with variable numbers of lysines in these drugs is a common structural variation during the manufacturing process and demands careful analysis.[47] Using capillary isoelectric focusing chromatography, these variants can be readily separated and analyzed, as shown in Figure 96.9A.

Carbohydrate modifications are also known to influence the function and thermodynamic stability of immunoglobulins. Carbohydrate moieties on immunoglobulins can be analyzed using a variety of techniques, such as capillary electrophoresis chromatography and MS spectrometry.[48] An example of such an analysis is shown in Figure 96.9B.

Chromatography and mass spectrometry methods have been reported to have good precision, linearity, and accuracy. We anticipate that these methodologies will gain acceptance for the analysis of intact immunoglobulins. The methods are rapid, can be automated, and require minimal sample preparation. It is predicted that multidimensional liquid chromatography, e.g., LC-LC-LC-MS, will become a routine analytical tool in the manufacture and quality assessment of reagents. It is likely that improvements in separation technologies will make it possible to lower the manufacturing costs of antibody production and significantly improve the quality of the clinical assays in routine laboratories.

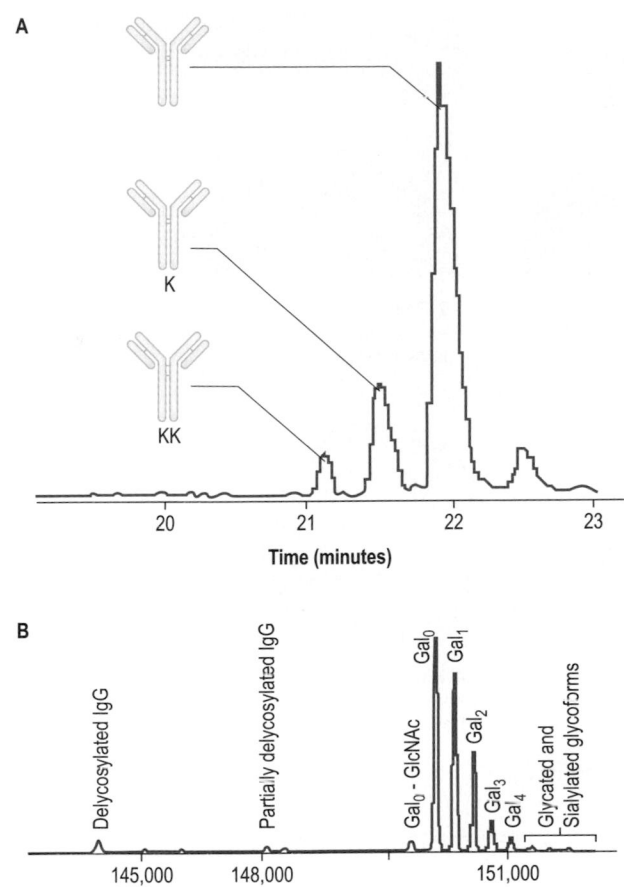

A

K

KK

Time (minutes)

B

Delycosylated IgG

Partially delycosylated IgG

Gal$_0$ - GlcNAc

Gal$_0$

Gal$_1$

Gal$_2$

Gal$_3$

Gal$_4$

Glycated and Sialylated glycoforms

Molecular Wt

Fig. 96.9 Identification of the C-terminal lysine (lys) variants of an antibody (A) and analysis of carbohydrate modified antibodies (B). (A) Capillary isoelectric focusing separates 0-Lys and -Lys fractions of an IgG antibody. MS. (B) Glycated immunoglobulins have been analyzed using MS. Deconvoluted mass spectra of intact immunoglobulin containing low levels of completely deglycosylated, as well as partially deglycosylated species (with one deglycosylated and one glycated heavy chain), and typical IgG glycoforms are shown.

SIMULTANEOUS DETECTION AND MEASUREMENT OF MULTIPLE ANTIBODIES

New technologies for the simultaneous detection and measurement of multiple antibodies include microarray methods and multiplex immunoassay.[49, 50] Both require that large amounts of data be acquired and analyzed rapidly, which is now possible using digital signal processing technology. Microarray methods consist of multiple simultaneous, qualitative or semi-quantitative immunoassays using activated silica microchips or nitrocellulose paper coated in individual microdots with antigens of interest. This technique has been used in research applications to detect IgE antibodies to both crude and recombinant allergens, and to identify IgG antibodies that react with nuclear antigens or tumor-associated peptides. Binding of antibodies is detected as in a conventional immunometric assay by the use of anti-immunoglobulin antibodies conjugated with an enzyme or fluorophore. Bound anti-immunoglobulin antibody is visualized by scanning the microarray in a fluorescent microscope or by densitometric scanning of antigen immunodots. Preliminary data indicate that microarrays display good sensitivity; nanogram quantities of Ig can be detected reliably; and they require very small (nanoliter) volumes of test specimen. Microarray systems also can be automated, thus making it possible to test large numbers of samples. Disadvantages of current microarray methods include relatively high analytical variability compared to conventional immunometric techniques and possible interference in detecting antibodies of one isotype due to competition from another isotype. Enhanced susceptibility to interference results from the use of very small quantities of antigen in immunometric microarray systems compared to conventional immunometric assay systems.

Multiplex immunoassay analysis offers another approach to the simultaneous detection of multiple antibodies. Several US FDA-approved multiplex immunoassays are currently available for semi-quantitative measurement of autoantibodies associated with systemic rheumatic diseases, celiac disease and antibody-mediated vasculitides; and quantitative multiplex immunoassays have been described to measure IgG antibodies to bacterial antigens, including up to 23 different *Streptococcus pneumoniae* serotypes. The principle of one multiplex immunoassay is illustrated in Figure 96.10. Polystyrene microspheres are impregnated with varying proportions of two different fluorescent dyes to create a family of microspheres, each with a unique fluorescent signature. Individual microspheres are then coupled covalently with reagent antigens. Different coupling reactions can be used to synthesize protein, nucleic acid or polysaccharide-coupled microspheres. Individual microspheres coupled with different antigens, e.g., individual extractable nuclear antigens in the test for ENA antibodies, can be mixed in a single tube to create an immunosorbent cocktail capable of binding several different antibodies simultaneously. After incubating with a test specimen, standard or calibrator, the microspheres are washed to remove unbound immunoglobulin and an anti-immunoglobulin antibody labeled with another fluorophore is added. The microspheres are then aspirated and separated in a flow cell, where they are illuminated with lasers that simultaneously identify each microsphere by its fluorescent signature and detect antibody bound to the surface by measuring the second fluorescent signal. The ability to measure multiple antibodies simultaneously allows the user to identify an antibody 'phenotype' for each specimen based on the presence of several different antibodies. With this methodology it is also possible to sample specimens in a random access mode rather than creating batches of specimens, and all tests are performed using the same data reduction. It is likely that multiplex immunoassay testing will gain wide acceptance in laboratories that process large numbers of specimens and offer a large repertoire of tests.

ASSESSMENT OF LABORATORY PERFORMANCE ■

Given the wide variety of analytic methods available to perform laboratory tests for immunoglobulin proteins and antibodies, clinicians and laboratories need a source of information with which to judge the performance (sensitivity and specificity, and market penetrance or acceptability) of the methods they have access to. Much information can be

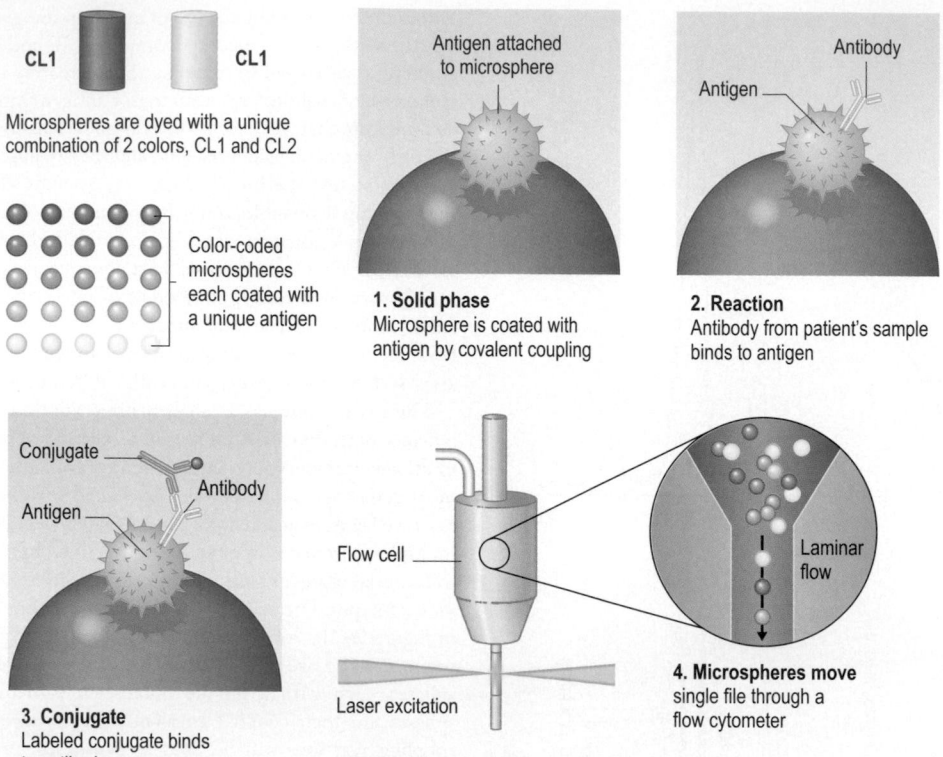

Fig. 96.10 Multiplex cytometric analysis for antibodies. See text for explanation.

found from the results of federally mandated laboratory proficiency testing programs. The US Clinical Laboratory Improvement Amendment of 1988 (CLIA88) established a single set of federal standards that apply to laboratories testing human specimens.[51] Periodic proficiency testing is a mandatory part of this program. Data from large inter-laboratory proficiency testing programs often include results from hundreds of different laboratories. These data are useful to indicate the performance of each individual laboratory compared to the entire group of laboratories, or of peer laboratories that use the same analytic methods. Proficiency surveys often reveal significant differences for clinically important analytes that may exist among otherwise similar analytical methods.

■ REFERENCES ■

1. Virella G, Wang AC. Immunoglobulin structure. Immunology 1993; 58: 75–90.

2. Tonegawa S. The Nobel lectures in immunology. The Nobel Prize for physiology or medicine. Somatic generation of immune diversity 1987; 38: 303–319.

3. Kipps TJ. Immunoglobulin genes. In: Detrick B, Hamilton RG, Folds JD, (eds) Manual of molecular and clinical laboratory immunology, 7th edn. Washington, DC: ASM Press, 2006; 56–68.

4. Keren DF. Protein electrophoresis in clinical diagnosis. London: Arnold, 2003.

5. Keren DF, Warren JS, Lowe JB. Strategy to diagnose monoclonal gammopathies in serum: high-resolution electrophoresis, immunofixation, and kappa/lambda quantification. Clin Chem 1998; 34: 2196–2201.

6. Keren DF, Humphrey RL. Clinical indications and applications of serum and urine protein electrophoresis. In: Detrick B, Hamilton RG, Folds JD, eds: Manual of molecular and clinical laboratory immunology, 7th edn. Washington, DC: ASM Press, 2006; 75–87.

7. Kunkel HG, Tiselius A. Electrophoresis of proteins on filter paper. J Gen Physiol 1951; 35: 39–118.

8. Katzmann JA, Kyle RA. Immunochemical characterization of immunoglobulins in serum, urine, and cerebrospinal fluid. In: Detrick B, Hamilton RG, Folds JD, eds: Manual of molecular and clinical laboratory immunology, 7th edn. Washington, DC: ASM Press, 2006. : 88–100.

9. Keren DF, Alexanian R, Goeken JA, et al. Guidelines for clinical and laboratory evaluation of patients with monoclonal gammopathies. Arch Pathol Lab Med 1999; 123: 106–107.

10. Henskens Y, de Winter J, Pekelharing M, et al. Detection and identification of monoclonal gammopathies by capillary electrophoresis. Clin Chem 1998; 44: 1184–1190.

11. Katzmann JA, Clark R, Sanders E, et al. Prospective study of serum protein capillary zone electrophoresis and immunotyping of monoclonal proteins by immunosubtraction. Am J Clin Pathol 1998; 110: 503–509.

12. Warren JS. Immunoglobulin quantification and viscosity measurement. In: Detrick B, Hamilton RG, Folds JD, eds. Manual of molecular and clinical

laboratory immunology, 7th edn. Washington, DC: ASM Press, 2006; 69–74.

13. Remaley AT, Hortin GL. Protein analysis for diagnostic applications. In: Detrick B, Hamilton RG, Folds JD, eds: Manual of molecular and clinical laboratory immunology, 7th edn. Washington, DC: ASM Press, 2006; 7–21.

14. Laurel C. The use of electroimmunoassay for determining specific proteins as a supplement to agarose gel electrophoresis. J Clin Pathol 1975; 6: 22–26.

15. Finely PR. Nephelometry; principles and clinical laboratory applications. Lab Manage 1982; 20: 34.

16. Tiffany TO. Fluorometry, nephelometry, and turbidimetry. In: Burtis CA, Ashwood ER, eds. Tietz textbook of clinical chemistry. Philadelphia: WB Saunders, 1999; 94–112.

17. College of American Pathologists Diagnostic Immunology Participant Summary. Surveys 2005. CAP, 325 Waukegan Rd, Northfield, IL 60093–62750.

18. Yalow RS, Berson SA. Assay of plasma insulin in human subjects by immunological methods. Nature 1959; 184: 1648–1649.

19. Wu JT. Quantitative immunoassays: a practical guide for assay establishment, troubleshooting, and clinical application. Washington, DC: AACC Press, 2000.

20. Gosling JP. Immunoassays: a practical approach. Oxford: Oxford University Press, 2000.

21. Diamandis EP, Christopoulos TK. The biotin (strept) avidin system; principles and applications in biotechnology. Clin Chem 1991; 37: 625–636.

22. Benjamin DC, Berzofsky JA, East IJ, et al. The antigenic structure of proteins: a reprisal. Annu Rev Immunol 1984; 2: 67.

23. Sela M. Antigenicity: some molecular aspects. Science 1969; 166: 1365.

24. Tan EM. Antinuclear antibodies: diagnostic markers for autoimmune diseases and probes for cell biology. Adv Immunol 1989; 44: 93.

25. Heidelberger M, Kendall FE. A quantitative study of the precipitin reaction between type III pneumococcus polysaccharide and purified homologous antibody. J Exp Med 1929; 50: 809.

26. Ouchterlony O, Nilsson LA. Immunodiffusion and immunoelectrophoresis. In: Wier DN, ed. Handbook of experimental immunology, Vol 32. St Louis: Blackwell, 1986. 655–707.

27. Reeves WH, Satoh M, Lyons R, et al. Detection of autoantibodies against proteins and ribonucleoproteins by double immunodiffusion and immunoprecipitation. In: Detrick B, Hamilton RG, Folds JD, eds. Manual of molecular and clinical laboratory immunology, 7th edn. Washington, DC: ASM Press, 2006; 1007–1018.

28. Dee TH. Detection of aspergillus fumigatus serum precipitins by counterimmunoelectrophoresis. J Clin Microbiol 1975; 2: 482–485.

29. Kassahara Y. Agglutination immunoassays. In: Rose NR, de Marcario EC, Folds JD, et al., eds. Manual of clinical laboratory immunology, 5th edn. Washington, DC: ASM Press, 1997; 7.

30. Johnson CL. Blood group antigens and antibodies. In: Tilton RC, Balows A, Hohnadel DC, et al., eds. Clinical laboratory medicine, St Louis: Mosby-Yearbook, 1992; 1064–1084.

31. Lepow ML, Hughes PA. *Corynebacterium diphtheriae* and *Clostridium tetani*: immune response and diagnostic methods. In: Detrick B, Hamilton RG, Folds JD, eds. Manual of molecular and clinical laboratory immunology, 7th edn. Washington, DC: ASM Press, 2006; 444–447.

32. Pasetti MF, Nataro JP, Levine MM. Immunologic methods for diagnosis of infections caused by diarrheagenic enterobacteriaceae and Vibrionaceae. In: Detrick B, Hamilton RG, Folds JD, eds. Manual of molecular and clinical laboratory immunology, 7th edn. Washington, DC: ASM Press, 2006; 448–461.

33. Pope V, Ari MD, Schriefer ME, et al. Immunologic methods for diagnosis of spirochetal diseases. In: Detrick B, Hamilton RG, Folds JD, eds: Manual of molecular and clinical laboratory immunology, 7th edn. Washington, DC: ASM Press, 2006; 477–492.

34. Collins AB, Colvin RB, Nousari CH. Immunofluorescence methods in the diagnosis of renal and skin diseases. In: Detrick B, Hamilton RG, Folds JD, eds. Manual of molecular and clinical laboratory immunology, 7th edn. Washington, DC: ASM Press, 2006; 414–423.

35. Ploem J. The use of a vertical illuminator with interchangeable dichroic mirrors for fluorescent microscopy with incidental light. Z Wiss Mikrosk 1967; 68: 129–142.

36. Lightfoote MM, Chirmule N, Homburger HA. Quality assurance of laboratory tests for autoantibodies to nuclear antigens: (1) indirect fluorescence assay for microscopy and (2) microtiter enzyme immunoassay methods; approved guideline. Clinical and Laboratory Standards Institute, 2006.

37. Tan EM. international cooperative activities in standardization of antinuclear antibodies. In: van Venrooij WJ, Maini RN, eds: Manual of biological markers of diseases. Norwell, MA: Kluwer Academic, 1993; AI: 1–5.

38. Wingerchuk DM, Pittock SJ, Lennon VA, et al. Neuromyelitis optica diagnosis criteria revisited: validation and incorporation of the NMO-IgG serum autoantibody. Neurology 2005; 64: A38.

39. Specks U, Wiegert EM, Homburger HA. Human mast cells expressing recombinant proteinase 3 (PR3) as substrate for clinical testing for antineutrophil cytoplasmic antibodies (ANCA). Clin Exp Immunol 1997; 109: 286–295.

40. Feltkamp TEW, Kirkwood TBL, Maini RN, et al. The first international standard for antibodies to doublestranded DNA. Ann Rheum Dis. 1988; 47: 740–746.

41. Hamilton RG, Adkinson NF Jr. In vitro assays for IgE mediated sensitivities. J Allergy Clin Immunol 2004; 114: 213–225.

42. Shen Y, Kim J, Strittmatter EF, et al. Characterization of the human blood plasma proteome. Proteomics 2005; 5: 4034–4045.

43. Pieper R, Gatlin CL, Huang ST, et al. Multi-component immunoaffinity subtraction chromatography: an innovative step towards a comprehensive survey of the human plasma proteome. Proteomics 2003; 3: 422–432.

44. Nelson RE, Grebe SK, O'Kane DJ, et al. Liquid chromatography-tandem mass spectrometry assay for simultaneous measurement of estradiol and estrone in human plasma. Clin Chem 2004; 50: 373–384.

45. Shou WZ, Pelzer M, Addison T, et al. An automatic 96-well solid phase extraction and liquid chromatography-tandem mass spectrometry method for the analysis of morphine-3-glucuronide in human plasma. J Pharm Biomed Anal 2002; 27: 143–152.

46. Rogatsky E, Tomuta V, Cruikshank G, et al. Direct sensitive quantitative LC/MS analysis of C-peptide from human urine by tow dimensional reverse phase/reverse high-performance liquid chromatography. J Separation Sci 2006; 29: 529–537.

47. Santora LC, Krull IS, Grant K. Characterization of recombinant human monoclonal tissue necrosis factor-alpha antibody using cation-exchange HPLC and capillary isoelectric focusing. Anal Biochem 1999; 275: 98–108.

REFERENCES

48. Siemiatkoski J, Lyubarskaya Y, Houde D, et al. A comparison of three techniques for quantitative carbohydrate analysis used in characterization of therapeutic antibodies. Carbohydrate Res 2006; 341: 410–419.

49. Podzorski RP. Introduction to molecular methodology. In: Detrick B, Hamilton RG, Folds JD, eds. Manual of molecular and clinical laboratory immunology, 7th edn. Washington, DC: ASM Press, 2006. : 26–51.

50. Meheus L, van Venrooij WJ, Wiik A, et al. Multicenter validation of recombinant, natural and synthetic antigens used in a single muliparameter assay for the detection of specific anti-nuclear autoantibodies in connective tissue disorders. Clin Exp Rheumatol 1999; 17: 205–214.

51. Federal Register 1992; 57(40) Washington, DC, United States Government Printing Office, pp 7139, 7245

Flow cytometry

Thomas A. Fleisher, João Bosco de Oliveira

Flow cytometry has become a standard laboratory tool in the evaluation of hematopoietic cells, including the identification of lymphocyte populations and subpopulations, a method referred to as immunophenotyping. The clinical application of this technology has been facilitated by the development of instruments and data analysis systems suitable for routine use in diagnostic laboratories. In addition, the expanded range of monoclonal antibodies specific for lymphocyte (and other hematopoietic cell) surface antigens directly conjugated to a number of different fluorescent indicators (fluorochromes) provide an extensive panel of reagents that facilitate multicolor studies.

The clinical needs that drove this technology relate to the emergence of absolute CD4 T-cell counts as a critical measure for disease assessment and follow-up in patients infected with the human immunodeficiency virus (HIV). Flow cytometry applied in the monitoring of HIV infection was followed by the routine application of cell characterization by flow cytometry in the evaluation of lymphoproliferative disorders, and more recently in the study of immunodeficiency disorders as well as other immune-mediated diseases.

The assessment of cell surface characteristics is now often coupled with the evaluation of intracellular parameters, including the detection of specific intracellular proteins including cytokines, and the identification of changes linked to cellular activation and apoptosis. Intracellular flow cytometry also can be applied to evaluate cell cycle status (i.e., G_0–G_1, S, G_2–M) based on DNA staining useful in evaluating tumor cells and assessing the *in vitro* lymphocyte response to various stimuli. Functional testing of lymphocytes can also be performed with cell tracking dyes that allow quantification of the rounds of cell division. Finally, characterization of antigen-specific T cells associated with normal and/or abnormal immune responses in association with disease states or following immunization can be accomplished using multimer technology and intracellular cytokine detection following antigen exposure.

This chapter focuses on the basic concepts of flow cytometry, including instrument characteristics, data management, lymphocyte gating and directed use of test reagents. In addition, a brief overview of intracellular probes, cell activation studies, cell cycle analysis, apoptosis detection and multimer technology is provided, focusing on the appropriate application of these approaches as well as their limitations.

■ INSTRUMENTATION ■

The basic components of a flow cytometer, as shown in Figure 97.1, include the illumination source, optical bench, fluidic system, electronics and computer.[1] Illumination in standard clinical instruments is generated by two air-cooled lasers, each of which provides a specific monochromatic light source (e.g., an argon laser generates a 488 nm wavelength [blue] beam and a helium neon [HeNe] laser generates a 633 nm wavelength [red] beam). The point where the light illuminates the cell in analytical instruments occurs within a flow cell, whereas in cell sorters the beam intersects cells flowing as a stream in air. The optical bench contains lenses that shape and focus the illumination beam to ensure consistent excitation energy at the point of analysis. The illumination of a cell generates both nonfluorescent and fluorescent signals that are collected and measured by optically coupling the signal to a detection system consisting of filters linked to a photodetector. The filters are chosen to allow the nonfluorescent signals to be measured at the same wavelength as the excitation signal (e.g., 488 nm), whereas those for the fluorescence channels are linked to the emission signals of specific fluorochromes (e.g., green, orange or red; see Fluorochromes).

The fluidic system lies at the heart of a flow cytometer and consists of isotonic sheath fluid that moves the sample stream containing the cells. This is accomplished by injecting the cell sample into the moving sheath fluid, establishing a hydrodynamically focused single-file flow of cells that move through the analysis point while maintaining the cell stream in a constant, central location.[2] The centrally focused cell stream ensures that the illumination of all cells is virtually equivalent. Thus, the difference in magnitude of the emission signal generated from each cell reflects biologic differences between the cells (not the result of variation in the illumination energy). The use of hydrodynamic focusing has the additional advantage of producing little or no change in cell shape, although it may have an effect on cell orientation. The consistency in maintaining cell shape makes it easier to distinguish 'architectural' differences between specific leukocyte types (see Gating).[3] The choice and arrangement of the filters allows for the simultaneous evaluation of multiple colors (parameters) for each cell, and a recent report described a modified clinical instrument that was capable of evaluating 17 colors simultaneously from each cell contained in the sample.[4] Thus,

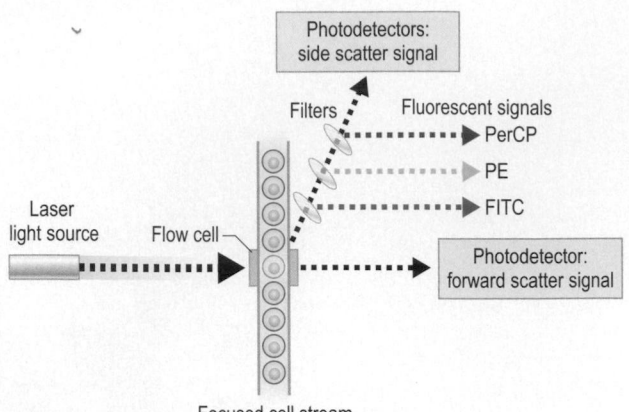

Fig. 97.1 Simplified design of a flow cytometer with one illumination source (laser) set up to collect five parameters. These include the two nonfluorescent parameters (blue light) forward and side scatter, as well as three fluorescent parameters, green (FITC), orange (PE) and red (PerCP) light.

a flow cytometer provides a platform with the capacity to assess multiple pieces of discrete information (parameters) generated from each individual cell contained within a large number of cells present in the test sample, and these are typically accrued at rates of 1000–2000 (or more) cells per second.

The internal electronics in the flow cytometer provide the system for converting analog light signals (photoelectrons) received at the photodetectors into digital signals for acquisition and storage in a computer. The intensity of these converted signals is measured on a relative scale that is generally set in either 256 or 1024 equal increments (referred to as channels) for display and analysis. A number of specialized analysis programs are available and results are depicted graphically as a single-parameter histogram displaying specific light (fluorescence) intensity (x-axis) versus cell number (y-axis) (Fig. 97.2). Two-color (parameter) studies can be evaluated with a pair of histograms (one for each color) or with a single (dot or contour) plot displaying both parameters (Fig. 97.3).

Specialized computer software enables data analysis, which in immunophenotyping studies is typically directed at defining cell subpopulations based on the presence or absence of specific antibody binding. Cell cycle analysis evaluates fluorescence intensity as a measure of cellular DNA content. Most programs enable the operator to evaluate the number of events, percentage of events, mean and/or median channel fluorescence, and selected statistical measures for each identified cell, and these are aggregated into specific populations and/or subpopulations of cells. The mean or median channel fluorescence is a measure of fluorescence intensity and can be used to determine the mean or median number of antigen molecules per cell compared to fluorescence calibration standards.[5]

The evaluation of clinical immunophenotyping data usually involves establishing criteria for the boundaries between negative or nonstained cells and positive (stained) cells. This is a very common technique used in clinical laboratories that provides relatively consistent criteria for negative versus positive cell discrimination. When dealing with DNA staining, a consistent cellular source of DNA (e.g. chicken erythrocytes) should be used as an internal reference for evaluating DNA content and cell cycle distribution.

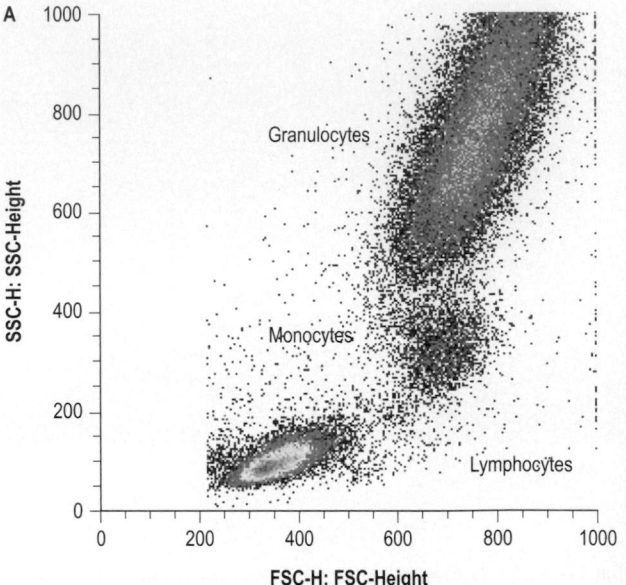

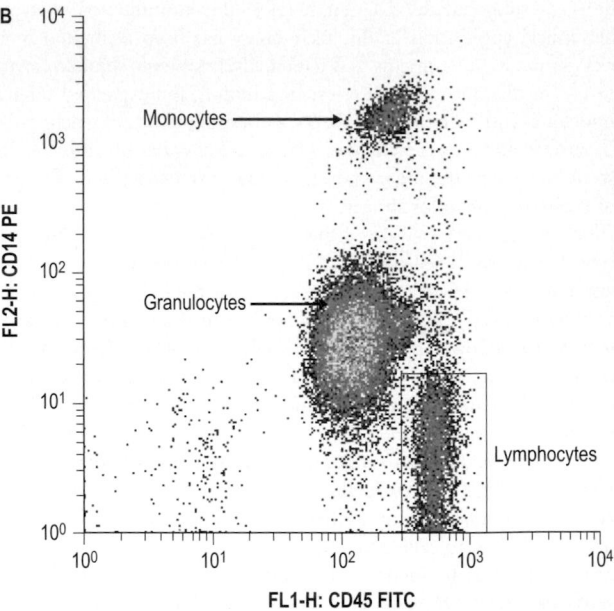

Fig. 97.2 (**A**) Forward- and side-scatter dot plots on a lysed whole blood sample, demonstrating the basic three-part leukocyte differential with lymphocytes, monocytes and granulocytes. (**B**) Dot plot with CD45/CD14 gating reagents showing the fluorescence distribution of all the three leukocyte types identified to include lymphocytes, monocytes and granulocytes, as well as a small number of nonlysed red blood cells and/or debris.

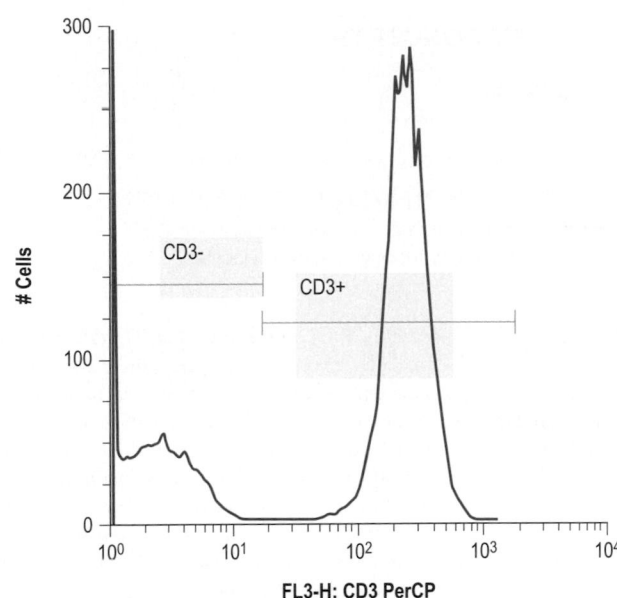

Fig. 97.3 Single-parameter histogram for CD3 expression on lymphocytes demonstrating the negative non-T-cell population (autofluorescence and nonspecific antibody binding) and a positive T-cell population. Integrating the area under each curve would provide the numbers and percentage of cells present in each respective subpopulation.

FLUORESCENCE REAGENTS

Standard monoclonal antibody reagents for clinical use are typically directly conjugated to a fluorochrome, a dye that absorbs and emits light of different wavelengths resulting from the energy lost during the return of excited electrons to their ground state.[6] Thus, the emitted light has a longer wavelength (lower energy) than that of the excitation beam. Direct staining involves the use of directly conjugated reagents, whereas indirect staining involves an unlabeled primary monoclonal antibody followed by a wash step and the addition of a fluorochrome-conjugated antibody reactive with the first antibody (e.g., goat anti-murine immunoglobulin when using a murine monoclonal antibody as the primary reagent). The direct method is technically easier and more readily adaptable to multicolor studies, but the indirect method may be more sensitive (although it often has higher background 'noise'). The three most commonly used fluorochromes in immunophenotyping when using an instrument with a single argon laser (488 nm excitation beam) are fluorescein isothiocyanate (FITC), phycoerythrin (PE), and peridin chlorophyll protein (PerCP), which emit green, orange and red light, respectively. In addition, an alternative third color (red) has been developed based on energy transfer using one fluorochrome (e.g., PE) to provide the excitation energy (light) for a second fluorochrome (e.g., a cyanine dye such as Cy5) that is the source of emitted light. There are now a number of additional standard fluorochromes and energy transfer based fluorochrome conjugates available to extend the number of colors per study. Most of the current clinical instruments have moved to two (or more) air-cooled lasers and collect at least four fluorescence signals; an eight-color, three-laser

clinical instrument has recently been marketed. The fluorescent signals are usually complemented by collecting two nonfluorescence signals (forward and side scatter). The number of events (cells) analyzed typically ranges from 10 000 to 20 000 in routine clinical studies, but must be increased when evaluating very small subpopulations of cells in order to produce statistically relevant data such as would be necessary in rare event analysis.

Studies of intracellular parameters require the reagents to traverse the cell membrane and gain entry to the cell. This is typically accomplished by cell fixation and permeabilization. Depending on the target area within the cell, an additional step may be required to enable entry to the cell nucleus. Activation-induced changes involve probes including calcium-sensitive dyes (e.g., fluo-3), glutathione-sensitive dyes (e.g., monochlor-bimane) and H_2O_2-responsive dyes (e.g., dihydrorhodamine 123).[7, 8] DNA content can be assessed with dyes that intercalate double-stranded DNA and RNA, including propidium iodide and ethidium bromide.[9] In addition, there are ultraviolet-excited dyes that are highly specific for DNA, including Hoechst 33258 and 4,6-diamidino-2-phenylindole (DAPI); acridine orange is used for simultaneous staining of DNA/RNA.

One recent exciting advance in the field of fluorescent labeling of molecules was the development of fluorescent semiconductor nanocrystals, named quantum dots.[10] Quantum dots are usually composed of a CdSe core coated with a layer of ZnS. Quantum dots have a broad absorption spectrum and a sharp, discrete emission spectrum, which varies according to their core size. This means that quantum dots of different sizes (and consequently of different emission spectra, or 'colors') can be excited with a single light source, such as UV light, allowing simpler multiplexing. In addition, quantum dots have high quantum yield, high molar extinction coefficients, high photobleaching resistance, and extraordinary resistance to photo- and chemical degradation. These qualities make them perfectly suitable for use in biological studies, including intracellular *in vivo* imaging, fluorescence resonance energy transfer (FRET) analysis, and dynamic imaging of single proteins for longer periods.

IMMUNOPHENOTYPING

GATING

The proper assessment of specific cell types within a mixture requires initial identification of lineage-specific cells, an approach referred to as gating. In practical terms, immunophenotyping focused on lymphocytes requires minimization of the nonlymphocytes included in the evaluation, and this is accomplished by lymphocyte gating. The standard sample for clinical studies is anticoagulated whole blood, and directing the study to lymphocytes requires elimination of the great majority of nonlymphocytes from the collected data, such that the percentage of a specific cell subpopulation is an accurate measurement. Without gating the data can also be negatively affected by co-expression of surface antigens on different cell lineages (e.g., CD4 is found at differing densities on lymphocytes and monocytes). In addition, nonspecific binding of monoclonal reagents through Fcγ receptors and the level of cytophilic human immunoglobulin varies between cell types, making appropriate gating crucial to generate valid data. These techniques are also used to focus the evaluation on other hematopoietic cells, including monocytes, granulocytes, eosinophils, erythrocytes and platelets.

Initial gating to focus on a specific leukocyte population typically involves using the two nonfluorescent parameters, forward angle

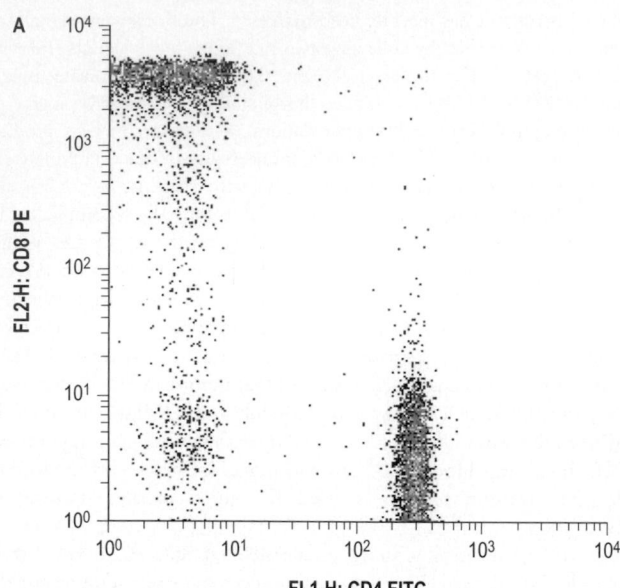

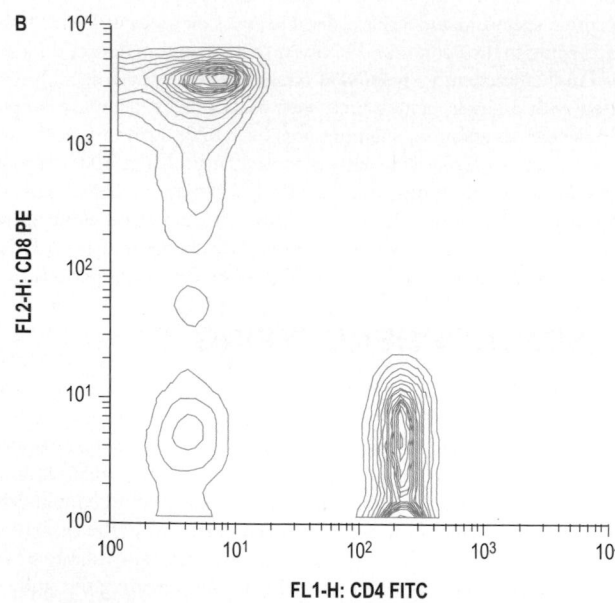

Fig. 97.4 Examples of (**A**) dot and (**B**) contour displays based on the same two-color data. Both techniques enable simultaneous evaluation of both parameters in this case evaluating the expression of CD4 and/or CD8 on CD3+ T cells. These plots identify four populations of cells: those expressing only CD 4 or CD8, those expressing both CD4 and CD8 (virtually absent) and those expressing neither CD4 nor CD8 (double-negative T cells).

KEY CONCEPTS

GATING

>> Method to define cell population of interest

>> Typically performed using forward and side scatter

>> Should be confirmed with gating reagents (CD45 and CD14 for lymphocytes and monocytes)

(low angle, FSC) and side (90°, SSC) light scatter (Fig. 97.4A).[3] Forward scatter is a reflection of cellular cross-sectional area (direct relationship to cell size) and refractile index, whereas side scatter is an indication of cellular granularity and surface irregularity. The combination of these two nonfluorescent parameters provides a three-part differential that distinguishes between normal lymphocytes, monocytes and granulocytes (in the absence of contaminating red blood cells and platelets). As can be seen in Figure 97.4A, lymphocytes have the lowest forward and side scatter, monocytes have higher forward and side scatter, and granulocytes have the greatest side scatter. In most circumstances this method is effective in distinguishing a relatively pure population of lymphocytes. However, the presence of nucleated red cells, large platelets or other particulate debris can produce contaminating events (cells) within this 'lymphocyte gate.' Furthermore, malignant lymphoid cells may not fit into the previously outlined standard light scatter patterns.

A method to confirm the integrity of the light scatter-based lymphocyte gate uses the directly conjugated monoclonal reagents CD45 and CD14.[11] These 'gating reagents' more accurately identify the three-part differential. Lymphocytes have the highest level of CD45 binding but are negative for CD14; granulocytes have a lower level of CD45 binding and an intermediate level of CD14 expression; and monocytes have high levels of both CD45 and CD14 expression (Fig. 97.4B). Importantly, nonleukocytes, including erythrocytes and platelets, are negative with both reagents. In addition, malignant leukocytes that have characteristics of early precursor cells often have altered CD45 and/or CD14 expression. Gating reagents provide a reliable means of checking the light scatter-based lymphocyte gate for the frequency of nonlymphocytes within the gate and the extent of lymphocyte exclusion from the gate. Guidelines for an acceptable degree of contamination within the lymphocyte gate, as well as the level of lymphocyte exclusion, are contained within the US Clinical and Laboratory Standards Institute (formerly the National Committee for Clinical Laboratory Standards) guideline for lymphocyte immunophenotyping.[12] In some situations, CD45 has to be included in every analysis tube to refine the gate and prevent cell contamination that cannot be excluded using the standard nonfluorescent parameters (forward and side scatter) for gating.

DATA PRESENTATION

The simplest method for demonstrating flow cytometry data is the single-parameter histogram (see Fig. 97.2), a graphic presentation of cell number on the *y*-axis versus fluorescence (light) intensity from a single fluorochrome on the *x*-axis. Integration of curve areas provides the number of cells, and often there are two distinct distributions: one referred to as negative identifies cells that are not bound specifically by the monoclonal reagent, and the second represents cells bound by the antibody. Negative actually reflects low-level fluorescence resulting from cellular autofluorescence together with any nonspecific binding of the monoclonal reagent(s); the magnitude of the latter varies between different cell types. The interpretation of the data is simplified when there are distinct two cell populations (i.e. negative and positive), whereas evaluation of two overlapping distributions is more difficult.

Multicolor data can be evaluated using a series of single-parameter histograms that consider each fluorochrome independently. However, it is more informative to present two parameters simultaneously using a correlated display (Fig. 97.3), and two-color displays are recommended for clinical flow cytometry.[13] This approach enables the characterization of four different phenotypes: CD4+/CD8-, CD4-/CD8+, CD4+/CD8+ and CD4-/CD8- (using the two reagents anti-CD4 and anti-CD8). When three reagents are used simultaneously, eight different subsets can be identified that would typically be interpreted by first dividing the cells into positive or negative with one reagent, and then evaluating these two defined populations for the remaining two reagents using a two-color approach. The simultaneous use of n monoclonal reagents could identify a total of 2^n subpopulations. The multicolor approach can provide a means to further resolve subpopulations, and has been particularly useful in the evaluation of cellular differentiation, activation and functional correlates, as well as clarifying overlapping cell subpopulations.

A commonly used convention to differentiate between negative and positive cells in a control sample is to establish a marker (discriminator) at the fluorescence histogram channel number such that it includes 98–99% of the negative cells. As previously noted, negative refers to the aggregate of baseline cellular autofluorescence plus nonspecific reagent binding. The latter is generally established by using directly conjugated control monoclonal antibodies of the appropriate class or subclass (e.g., IgG$_1$, IgG$_{2a}$, IgG$_{2b}$ or IgM) that are not specifically reactive with human lymphocyte surface antigens. The negative cell discrimination can be relatively simple to apply unless there is significant overlap between two populations, in which case this approach underestimates the frequency of positive cells.

The level of fluorescence produced by different fluorochromes varies: the brightest of the three standard immunophenotyping dyes is phycoerythrin (PE). This observation has been used to demonstrate that varying the fluorochrome can alter the resolution of antigens expressed at low concentrations. As a general rule, phycoerythrin is particularly suited for evaluating 'dim' positive markers.

It should also be noted that the fluorescence signals emitted by different fluorochromes are not completely separated by the filters. This can lead to signal overlap that is corrected by electronic subtraction of the overlapping signal, a process referred to as compensation. The overlap is particularly significant when using FITC and PE in combination, as FITC produces orange light in addition to the primary green signal emitted by this fluorochrome. The compensation process involves subtraction of the orange signal produced by FITC from the orange signal produced by PE. The availability of tandem conjugates adds another level of complexity, as does four-color flow cytometry, particularly when performed with a single light source. Overlap between fluorochrome combinations must be compensated, and a general approach to successfully accomplish this has been published.[13]

The fluorescence intensity of histogram patterns can be compared between different samples when the same reagent and experimental set-up are used. This enables semi-quantitative comparison of antigen densities between the various cells studied. However, fluorescence data obtained using different reagents generally should not be compared

KEY CONCEPTS

DATA PRESENTATION

>> Fluorescence intensity is plotted versus cell number.

>> Can present cummulative data on more than one parameter for each cell.

>> Multicolor data presentation may increase cell subpopulation resolution.

because of the variability that results from differences in antibody affinity and fluorochrome-to-protein ratio for the two reagents.

Quality control is a critical component of clinical flow cytometry to ensure optimal results.[13] This includes monitoring instrument set-up and performance, as well as optimizing sample preparation and reagents and standardizing controls and data interpretation. Quantitative flow cytometry based on a fluorescence standard curve provides quantitative data in units referred to as molecular equivalents of soluble fluorochrome (MESF). When properly constructed standard curves are used, quantitative data for different reagents can be generated and compared.[5, 14] Finally, participation in inter-laboratory proficiency testing surveys, such as the triannual samples provided by the College of American Pathologists (CAP), is an important additional measure to monitor laboratory performance and is mandated in US clinical laboratories by the Clinical Laboratory Improvement Amendment of 1988 (CLIA 88).

METHODS

Whole-blood lysis is the most common technique used for sample preparation and consists of mixing a fixed volume of anticoagulated whole blood (or bone marrow) with one or more directly conjugated monoclonal antibodies, followed by incubation at a designated temperature and time.[11, 15, 16] Next the red blood cells are lysed, the sample is washed and then run into the flow cytometer, usually following fixation in paraformaldehyde to reduce the risk of infection. The nonlysed cells remaining include all peripheral blood leukocytes, as well as any nonlysed red cells, platelets and debris. The heterogeneity of the sample necessitates careful lymphocyte gating in order to generate accurate immunophenotyping data. The advantages of the whole-blood lysis method include fewer preparation steps, less sample handling, and a lower likelihood of differential lymphocyte loss. This last point can occur when density gradient techniques are used to prepare mononuclear cells for analysis. Alternative sources of cells (e.g., bronchial alveolar lavage fluid, fine-needle aspirates) can also be evaluated with flow cytometry.[17] Patient studies must be determined with the same methods and reagents as used in the determination of the control ranges to ensure comparability.

The application of control ranges must take into account the fact that significant changes take place in lymphocyte distribution during childhood, as well as in the very elderly.[18, 19] There are also immunophenotypic differences induced by drugs, including tobacco products, such that information on current medications should be obtained whenever possible.[20] Other factors can also have an impact on lymphocyte distribution, including race, gender, diurnal variation, and recent or intercurrent infection.[21]

Table 97.1 Selected lymphocyte surface antigens for immunophenotyping

T cells
Pan-T cell: CD3, CD2, CD7, CD5
Major T-cell subset: CD4, CD8
Surface antigens associated with function: CD28, CD38, CD45RA, CD45RO, CD62L
Activation antigens: CD25, CD40L, CD69, CD71, HLA-DR

B cells
Pan-B cell: CD19, CD20, surface immunoglobulin
Major B-cell subset: CD5, CD21
Surface antigens associated with function: CD27, CD40
Activation antigens: CD23, CD25

NK cells
Pan-NK cell: CD16, CD56
NK subset: CD2, CD8, CD57

The choice of immunophenotyping reagents depends on the cells being studied and the question being asked. However, regardless of the specific set-up, the inclusion of a tube with gating reagents (CD45 and CD14) to confirm the integrity of the standard lymphocyte gate is recommended.[11] In addition, control reagents should be included to establish the fluorescence intensity of negative cells. Additional important controls include a pan-T cell, B-cell, and NK-cell marker for every sample (Table 97.1) as this provides an internal control, based on the principle that the whole is the sum of its parts. Thus, the total percentage of lymphocytes in the gate determined by the gating reagents should approximately equal the sum of the percentages for T cells, B cells, and NK cells. A technical or biological explanation must be identified when this relationship does not hold. Biological explanations for a significant difference would include the presence of immature or malignant cells that were not identified by standard pan-T cell, B-cell and NK-cell reagents. In addition, if the gating reagents (CD45/CD14) had not been included, contaminating cells (e.g., myeloid precursors, nucleated red blood cells, large platelets) with forward- and side-scatter characteristics similar to those of lymphocytes could not be ruled out. Potential technical problems include reagent or fluorochrome degradation, failure to add a reagent, and a host of others. Evidence of a major technical error should result in repeating the study.

Additional data that can be used for controls depend on the set-up. For example, the availability of multiple antibodies that identify a similar cell (sub)population can serve as a useful check (e.g., total T cells by comparing CD3 and CD5 or CD2; total B cells by comparing CD19 and CD20). In addition, the use of specific reagents in more than one tube enables comparison between the repeat values as a measure of consistency. The application of internal checks should be performed by the flow operator as a simple means of confirming the validity of the data. Insights regarding unusual biological findings may also be uncovered through this type of evaluation (e.g. the presence of an increased population of CD4$^-$/CD8$^-$ double-negative T cells).[22]

The challenge in performing immunophenotyping is to accurately identify cells with specific surface characteristics (antigens). As previously noted, the capacity to discriminate cell subpopulations is often enhanced through the directed use of antibody combinations. The typical data generated consist of the percentage of negative versus positive cells when using one reagent, and multiple subpopulations when using more than one reagent. Regardless of the experimental design, it is important to consider not only the percentage of cells within each subpopulation, but also the absolute number of cells. This is most commonly obtained by multiplying the relevant percentage from the flow cytometer by the absolute lymphocyte count obtained using a white blood count and differential. For example, when assaying for CD4 T-cell counts, the percentage of CD4$^+$ cells is multiplied by the peripheral lymphocyte count to yield the absolute CD4 count. A potential problem with this approach is the requirement for two separate procedures (i.e., dual platforms) to generate the final result. This introduces the possibility of additive error, based on the inherent errors of the two different methods. It has also fueled a search for approaches that facilitate the performance of both tasks by flow cytometry (i.e., a single platform). One alternative involves the inclusion of a fixed number of fluorescent beads (in a defined volume) in each tube as a reference standard to generate absolute numbers without requiring the use of the complete blood count and differential to generate a lymphocyte count. Regardless of the approach, it is necessary to report both percentages and absolute numbers when immunophenotyping peripheral lymphocytes.

The object of evaluating malignant cells is often to characterize the lineage and differentiation level of the abnormal cells, rather than to quantify subpopulations.[23] The pattern of reactivity combined with fluorescence intensity is often useful in identifying leukemic patterns, whereas the absolute number of cells may not be required. However, flow cytometric detection and quantification of rare abnormal cells can be useful in evaluating for minimal residual disease in lymphoproliferative disorders.

IMMUNOPHENOTYPING STUDIES

The majority of immunophenotyping studies are directed at quantifying specific cell subpopulations, evaluating for the presence or absence of particular surface antigens, identifying the differentiation level of specific cells, determining cell lineage, evaluating for functional correlates based on specific antigen expression, examining for evidence of cell activation, and/or establishing monoclonality.

CLINICAL RELEVANCE

IMMUNOPHENOTYPING STUDIES

>> Can be used to identify cell subsets, lineage, stage of cell differentiation, state of cell activation, and clonality.

>> Lymphocyte results should be checked with T cells + B cells + NK cells = 100%.

>> Immunophenotyping studies are not the equivalent of lymphocyte function studies.

A particular cell subpopulation can be readily quantified with flow cytometry. The evaluation of absolute CD4 T-cell counts has formed the basis for monitoring patients infected with HIV.[24] Quantification of CD34+ hematopoietic stem cells in donor peripheral blood or bone marrow is used in many cellular reconstitution protocols.[25] Subpopulation characterization can also be useful in the evaluation of patients with clinical history and laboratory findings suggestive of immunodeficiency. These studies identify the presence or absence of cells and surface proteins associated with specific functional attributes, but do not assess the actual functional status of the cells. This point is clearly illustrated by the finding of normal B-cell numbers in most patients with common variable immunodeficiency, despite the fact that these patients fail to produce immunoglobulins normally.[26] However, changes in the characteristics of the cells present may provide insight into the basis of a disorder, an observation that has been made in some patients with CVID, and provides additional support for heterogeneity of patients with this disorder.[27] Because of the limitations of immunophenotyping, it is common practice when evaluating the status of the immune system to test cell function in parallel.

Flow cytometry can be used to test for the presence or absence of a specific cell surface antigen. An example of this type of application is in the evaluation of a patient with a history of recurrent skin infections, delayed wound healing and persistent granulocytosis that suggests a diagnosis of type 1 leukocyte adhesion deficiency.[28] This disorder results from a defect in the gene encoding CD18, preventing the expression of three different heterodimeric adhesion molecules each containing CD18 (Chapter 21). This disorder can usually be diagnosed by studying granulocytes (and lymphocytes) for the expression of CD18 (as well as the three isoforms of CD11). Patients often have reduced rather than absent CD18 expression, and the diagnosis can be further confirmed by demonstrating a failure of CD18 (and CD11a, 11b, 11c) upregulation following cell activation.

The directed use of a panel of monoclonal reagents can help address questions regarding the level of cell differentiation. Antibodies that are specific to proteins expressed by early (precursor) cells represent one approach, which would include evaluating for the thymocyte marker CD1, or the pre-B-cell marker CD10 (CALLA). However, many surface antigens are expressed throughout differentiation. Examples of these include CD2 and CD7 found on thymocytes and circulating T cells, or CD19 and HLA-DR found on pre-B cells as well as B cells. Thus the pattern of surface antigen expression can also help distinguish the level of differentiation. Defining the developmental level of a particular cell population or subpopulation is best accomplished using a panel of reagents that span the natural history of the cell lineage. This approach represents the standard for testing leukemias and lymphomas, enabling improved classification of the malignant cells relative to prognosis and therapy. Focusing on the presence or absence of specific antigens also involves evaluating the level of expression. Malignant cells may express antigens associated with different lineages, such that lineage-directed studies can provide insight into shared expression of specific antigens. Additionally, malignant cells may have altered forward- and side-scatter characteristics, as well as diminished or absent CD45 expression.[23] Thus, the approach to gating may have to be modified when studying hematopoietic malignancies.

Issues of monoclonality can be dealt with using flow cytometry when analyzing B cells, and in some circumstances when studying T cells. Normally B cells are a heterogeneous mixture of mutually exclusive κ or λ light chain-positive cells. The distribution of light-chain expression can be evaluated for clonal excess using a method called the Kolgomorov–Smirnov D value comparison.[29, 30] Light-chain clonal excess will usually be accompanied by an excess in B cells expressing one particular heavy chain (α,γ, μ or ε). The capacity to evaluate T-cell monoclonality by flow cytometry is less definitive and consists of using T-cell antigen receptor β-variable chain-specific reagents looking for evidence of significant over-representation of one β-chain family.

The state of lymphoid activation can be addressed by evaluating for the presence of surface antigens that are either found only on activated cells or are upregulated following activation. These include receptors for specific growth factors (e.g., IL-2 receptor α chain, CD25), receptors for critical elements required for cell growth (e.g., transferrin receptor [CD71]), ligands that are critical for cell–cell communication following activation (CD40 ligand [CD152] on CD4 T cells), and surface antigens that are upregulated as a result of activation (e.g., adhesion molecules, HLA-DR, CD69). In addition, the memory status of both T and B cells can be assessed based on differential surface molecule expression associated with prior antigen encounter. This enables a distinction to be made between naïve T cells that express CD45RA, CD62L and CXCR7 from memory T cells that express the alternative CD45 isoform CD45RO (and varied CD62L or CXCR7, depending on whether the cells are central or effector memory cells).[31, 32] In addition, memory B cells can be detected by the expression of CD27 and be further divided into isotype switched or nonswitched, based on their pattern of surface immunoglobulin expression.[27, 33]

INTRACELLULAR EVALUATION

CELLULAR ACTIVATION

Ligand binding and transmembrane signal transduction resulting in cellular activation can be evaluated using flow cytometry. Changes in intracellular ionic calcium concentration (Ca^{2+}) are frequently used to monitor cell activation after ligand binding. These changes are associated with the activation of phospholipase C and protein kinase C. In general, three reagents have been used to measure Ca^{2+}: quin 2, indo-1, and fluo-3. Quin 2 has a low excitation coefficient and is not useful for

---

CLINICAL RELEVANCE

INTRACELLULAR FLOW CYTOMETRY

>> Activation-directed studies:
>> Calcium flux
>> Intracellular protein phosphorylation
>> Oxidative burst: neutrophils
>> Intracellular cytokine studies:
>> Clarify the Th1/Th2 status of an immune response
>> Can be assessed in an in vitro antigen specific response
>> Can be combined with evaluation of cell surface studies

flow cytometry; indo-1 requires ultraviolet excitation; fluo-3 can be excited by 488 nm but does not permit ratiometric analysis. Nevertheless, because of its ease of use, fluo-3 is currently the most widely used probe for intracytoplasmic Ca^{2+} evaluation by flow cytometry. Strict attention must be paid to loading conditions, the presence or absence of free Ca^{2+} in the media, experimental temperature, baseline measurements and calibration. This approach can be combined with cell surface marker or cell cycle evaluation.[7]

Intracellular pH changes related to cellular activation also can be evaluated. The most useful probe for pH is SNARF-1.[7] This probe can be excited at 488 nm and allows for ratiometric analysis with detection wavelengths set for 575 and 640 nm. Glutathione (glutamylcysteinylglycine, GSH) is an important antioxidant generated during cell activation that can be measured by flow cytometry.[7] The fluorescent probe monochlorobimane is most commonly used for this measurement, but is complicated by the need to determine GSH by an independent method such as HPLC.

Additional approaches to evaluate cellular activation include assessment of intranuclear markers (Ki-67, PCNA) as well as surface proteins that are upregulated following cellular activation (e.g., CD69, CD25, CD71).[34] Actual cell division can be evaluated using lipophilic membrane dyes (e.g., PKH26), also referred to as cell tracking dyes, which lose 50% of their fluorescence with each round of cell division.[35] This approach has become more common in the clinical assessment of lymphocyte function because of its capacity to evaluate specific lymphocyte subpopulations responding to mitogenic and antigenic stimuli. Lipophilic membrane dyes also can be used to label target cells in cell-based cytotoxicity assays.[36]

Functional evaluation of cell activation can be accomplished with flow cytometry-directed detection of the generation of phosphorylated intracellular proteins associated with specific activation signals. An example of this is the detection of phosphorylated STAT-1 following interferon-γ stimulation of monocytes, which has been found to be more sensitive than immunoblotting.[37] This type of assay requires fixation and permeabilization to allow the entry of the specific reagent, and has now been extended to a number of additional intracellular proteins that are phosphorylated after specific exposure of the cell to specific stimuli. Currently, a number of intracellular signaling proteins that undergo phosphorylation following a specific activation signal can be assessed with flow cytometry using commercially available reagents in kit form.

The assessment of oxidative burst following cell stimulation plays a central role in neutrophil function testing using the hydrogen peroxide-sensitive dye dihydrorhodamine 123. This procedure involves loading the granulocytes with the dye, stimulating with phorbol myristate acetate (PMA), and evaluating for fluorescence by flow cytometry.[8] This test has proved to be extremely accurate in diagnosing patients with chronic granulomatous disease (CGD) and carriers of X-linked CGD.[38] A major advantage is its sensitivity, which allows the detection of one normal cell in a population of 1000 abnormal cells. This makes assessment of oxidative burst a useful tool in following allogeneic granulocyte survival after transfusion into patients with CGD, as well as in evaluating the effectiveness of allogeneic stem cell transplantation and gene therapy in CGD.

INTRACELLULAR CYTOKINE DETECTION

Flow cytometry provides a platform to evaluate cytokine production at the single-cell level using cytokine-specific directly conjugated monoclonal antibodies following fixation and permeabilization of cells.[39, 40]

This approach allows for the simultaneous detection of two or more intracellular cytokines combined with cell surface markers or other intracellular markers. Important aspects of intracellular cytokine detection include the use of a protein transport inhibitor during activation, the use of proper controls, and the choice of antibodies. As there is little or no spontaneous cytokine production in circulating human lymphocytes, intracellular cytokine detection requires *ex vivo* activation. Initial experience was based on supraphysiological stimulation using PMA and ionomycin, but antigen-specific activation systems have also proved feasible. It should be emphasized that, regardless of the activation method, the duration of activation is an important variable, as individual cells reach maximum cytokine production at different times. In addition, different cytokines have different optimal periods of activation. It is recommended that a proper kinetic profile be established for the biological system or clinical condition being studied.[39]

To increase the amount of intracellular cytokines, inhibitors of intracellular protein transport, such as monensin or brefeldin, are commonly used and lead to the accumulation of proteins within the cell. Nonspecific binding of the antibody reagents is an issue, as permeabilization allows access not only to the cytokine of interest, but also to other proteins present in much greater quantities than on the cell surface. In addition, fixation further increases nonspecific binding and the use of both a negative control sample, which contains an excess of unlabeled or 'cold' anticytokine antibody, and a subclass-matched control sample provide the optimal control. When the conjugated anti-cytokine is added to the negative control sample it can only bind to other proteins in a nonspecific manner, thereby providing a measure to discriminate between specific and nonspecific binding.[39] The use of directly conjugated anti-cytokine antibodies not only simplifies the staining procedure, but also provides the best distinction between specific and nonspecific binding. Because the fixation agent may change the native state of certain epitopes, it is also important when combining cell surface characterization with intracellular cytokine evaluation to use antibodies that recognize antigens after fixation.

One of the main applications of intracellular cytokine detection by flow cytometry has been the study and refinement of the Th1/Th2 paradigm.[40] It has recently become clear that the regulated secretion of cytokines can be used to study the response of individual T cells to both polyclonal stimuli and specific antigens. Measuring antigen-specific T-cell cytokine expression in response to specific antigen offers a useful alternative to the tetramer-based approach (discussed later) to quantify the frequency of antigen-specific T cells (Fig. 97.5).[41]

CELL CYCLE ANALYSIS

In addition to surface immunophenotyping and cytoplasmic characterization, flow cytometry is also used in cell cycle analysis. Propidium iodide (PI) is the most commonly used fluorochrome owing to its optimal linear DNA-binding capacity in a variety of different cell types. Thus, a single-parameter histogram of DNA content using PI readily permits the determination of cell cycle compartments, expressed as the percentage of cells in G_0–G_1, S and G_2–M (Fig. 97.6A). In addition to these conventional parameters, the presence or absence of aneuploidy can be determined by inspection of the G_0–G_1 peak and/or use of a DNA index (ratio of abnormal DNA content to a diploid DNA standard). Also, elevation in the S and/or G_2–M phases can be detected. The optimal display

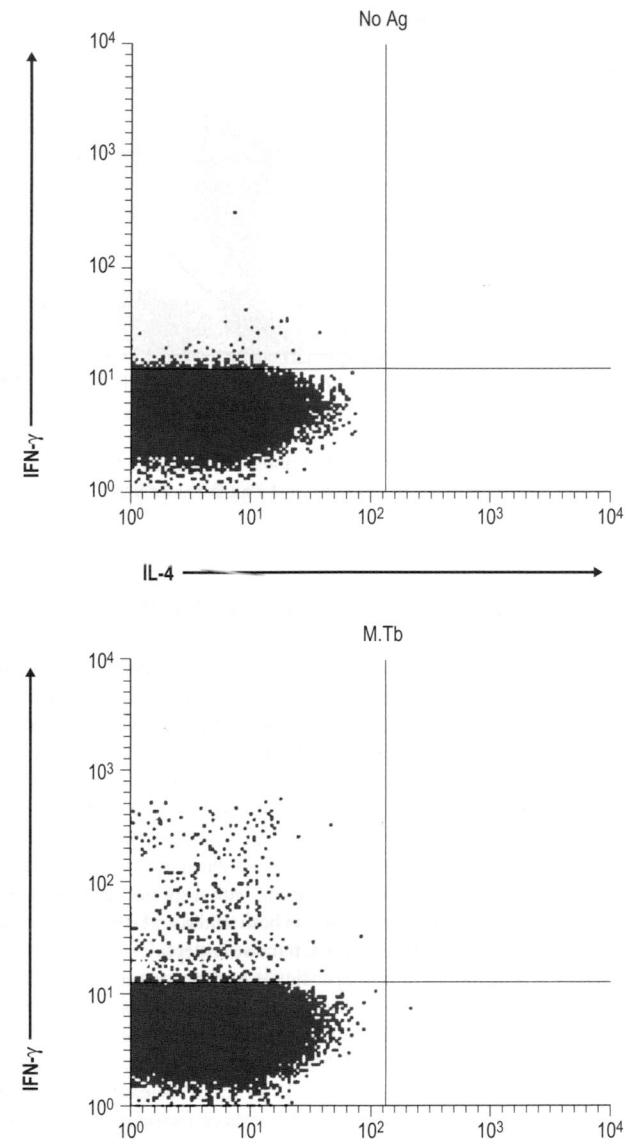

No Ag

M.Tb

Fig. 97.5 Two-color dot plots of CD3+ T cells evaluated for intracytoplasmic interferon-γ and IL-4 expression. The donor had a positive skin test to PPD and demonstated a Th1 pattern of cytokine expression (interferon-γ) in response to *Mycobacterium tuberculosis* antigen, with an absence of a Th2 cytokine pattern (IL-4). (Courtesy of Dr Calman Prussin.)

of these data uses a combination of side scatter versus DNA content. Cells observed on the histogram in the area below the level of G_0–G_1 may be undergoing apoptosis.[42]

It should be noted that several different computer algorithms have been developed to determine the relative proportion of each cell cycle compartment, and the selection of a software program is not a trivial

CELL CYCLE ANALYSIS

>> Useful to screen percentage of S phase and aneuploidy.
>> Can be combined with cell surface studies.
>> Can be combined with markers of apoptosis.

process. The major instrument manufacturers supply cell cycle analysis programs, and there are also third-party programs available. Generally the optimal program should be capable of modeling two or more aneuploid populations, subtracting debris (particularly if formalin-fixed paraffin-embedded archival material is used) and accurately estimating S-phase cells.[9, 43] The combination of a surface marker and cell cycle has been very useful in differentiating normal cell populations from tumor cell populations.[44] One example is the use of either anti-κ, anti-λ or B-cell reagents to separate the aneuploid B-cell clone from the remaining normal, reactive B cells in a lymphoid cell mixture. Another uses cytokeratin as a marker to distinguish between the tumor cells and the inflammatory cells that are present.

The other major event that has occurred in cell cycle analysis has been the development of technology using the incorporation of bromodeoxyuridine.[44] This thymidine analog is used to directly determine the percentage of S-phase cells. Also, when used in kinetic studies it permits a determination of the individual times for the components of the cell cycle and a determination of the growth fraction. Finally, recent developments have resulted in the availability of two anticyclin reagents to evaluate cell cycle transition points in malignant cells.[45]

■ APOPTOSIS DETECTION ■

Flow cytometry has become the method of choice for the detection and quantification of cellular apoptosis.[46] This is due partly to its capacity for rapid assessment of a large number of cells and samples. Many distinct features of an apoptotic cell can be evaluated by flow cytometry based on light scatter, plasma membrane changes, mitochondrial transmembrane potential, DNA content and DNA integrity.

The light-scattering properties of a cell undergoing programmed cell death are the simplest attributes that can be assessed by flow cytometry. Dying cells typically shrink, producing a loss in forward light scatter (FSC) and, despite an initial transient increase in side scatter (SSC), also ultimately demonstrate a decrease in SSC (Fig. 97.6B). The use of light scatter can be combined with cell surface staining to help characterize the dying cells. However, scatter changes alone are not specific to apoptosis, and should be accompanied by an additional characteristic associated with cell death. Live cells have phospholipids asymmetrically distributed in the inner and outer plasma membrane, with phosphatidylcholine and sphingomyelin on the outer surface and phosphatidylserine (PS) on the inner. Early during apoptosis cells lose asymmetry, exposing PS on the outside. Annexin V is a protein that binds preferentially to negatively charged phospholipids such as PS, and directly conjugated annexin V is a useful reagent for the specific detection of apoptotic cells.[47]

23. Knowles DM, Chadburn A, Inghirami G, et al. Immunophenotypic markers useful in diagnosing and classification of hematopoietic neoplasms. In: Knowles DM, ed. Neoplastic hematopathology. Baltimore: Williams & Wilkins, 1992, 73–167.

24. Yarchoan R, Venzon DJ, Pluda JM, et al. CD4 count and the risk for death in patients infected with HIV receiving antiretroviral therapy. Ann Intern Med 1991; 115: 184.

25. Sekhsaria S, Fleisher TA, Vowells SJ, et al. G-CSF recruitment of CD34+ progenitors: impaired mobilization in chronic granulomatous disease and ADA deficient patients. Blood 1996; 88: 1104.

26. Wright JJ, Wagner DK, Blaese RM, et al. Characterization of common variable immunodeficiency: characterization of patients with distinctive immunophenotypic and clinical features. Blood 1990; 76: 2046.

27. Warnatz K, Denz A, Drager R, et al. Severe deficiency of switched memory B cells (CD27(+)IgM(-) IgD(-)) in subgroups of patients with common variable immunodeficiency: a new approach to classify a heterogeneous disease. Blood 2002, 99: 1544.

28. Rosenzweig SD, Holland SM. Phagocyte immunodeficiencies and their infections J Allergy Clin Immunol 2004; 1113: 620.

29. Berliner N, Ault KA, Martin P, Weinberg DS. Detection of clonal excess in lymphoproliferative disease by κ/λ analysis: correlation with immunoglobulin gene rearrangement. Blood 1986; 67: 80.

30. Young IT. Proof without prejudice. Use of the Kolgomorov–Smirnov test for the analysis of histograms from flow systems and other sources. J Histochem Cytochem 1977; 25: 935.

31. Stockinger B, Kassiotis G, Bourgeois C. CD4 T-cell memory. Semin Immunol 2004; 16: 295.

32. Klebanov CA, Gattinoni K, Restifo NP. CD8+ T-cell memory in tumor immunology and immunotherapy. Immunol Rev 2006; 211: 214.

33. Avery DR, Ellyard JT, Mackay F, et al. Increased expression of CD27 on activated human memory B cells correlates with their commitment to the plasma cell lineage. J Immunol 2005; 174: 4034.

34. Mardiney MM III, Brown MR, Fleisher TA. Measurement of CD69 expression: a rapid and efficient means to assess mitogen or antigen induced proliferative capacity in normals. Cytometry 1996; 26: 305.

35. Allsopp CE, Nicholls SJ, Langhorne J. A flow cytometric method to assess antigen-specific proliferative response of different subpopulations of fresh and cryopreserved human peripheral blood mononuclear cells. J Immunol Meth 1998; 214: 175.

36. Slezak SE, Horan PK. Cell-mediated cytotoxicity. A highly sensitive and informative flow cytometric assay. J Immunol Meth 1989; 117: 205.

37. Fleisher TA, Dorman SE, Anderson JA, et al. Detection of intracellular phosphorylated STAT-1 by flow cytometry. Clin Immunol 1999; 90: 425.

38. Vowells SJ, Fleisher TA, Sekhsaria S, et al. Genotype dependent variability in flow cytometric evaluation of reduced nicotinamide adenine dinucleotide phosphate oxidase function in patients with chronic granulomatous disease. J Pediatr 1996; 128: 104.

39. Prussin C. Cytokine flow cytometry: understanding cytokine biology at the single-cell level. J Clin Immunol 1997; 17: 195.

40. Rostaing LM, Tkaczuk J, Durand M, et al. Kinetics of intracytoplasmic Th1 and Th2 cytokine production assessed by flow cytometry following in vitro activation of peripheral blood mononuclear cells. Cytometry 1999; 35: 318.

41. Suni MA, Picker LJ, Maino VC. Detection of antigen-specific T cell cytokine expression in whole blood by flow cytometry. J Immunol Meth 1998; 212: 89.

42. Wheeless LL, Coon JS, Cox C, et al. Precision of DNA flow cytometry in inter-institutional analyses. Cytometry 1991; 12: 405.

43. Shankey TV, Rabinovitch PS, Bagwell B, et al. Guidelines for implementation of clinical DNA cytometry. Cytometry 1993; 14: 472.

44. Gray JW, Dolbeare F, Pallavicinic M, et al. Flow cytokinetics. In: Gray JW, Darzynkiewicz Z, eds: Techniques in cell cycle analysis, Clifton NJ: Humana Press, 1987; 93–137.

45. Gong J, Tragonos F, Darzynkiewicz Z. Expression of cyclins B and E in individual MOLT-4 cells and in stimulated human lymphocytes during their progression through the cell cycle. Int Oncol 1993; 3: 1037.

46. Hotz MA, Gong J, Tragonos F, et al. Flow cytometric detection of apoptosis: comparison of assays of in situ DNA degradation and chromatin changes. Cytometry 1994; 15: 232.

47. Shounan Y, Feng X, O'Connell PJ. Apoptosis detection by annexin V binding: a novel method for quantitation of cell-mediated cytotoxicity. J Immunol Meth 1998; 217: 61.

48. Altman JD, Moss PAH, Goulder PJR, et al. Phenotypic analysis of antigen-specific T lymphocytes. Science 1996; 274: 94.

49. M Ruan GP, Ma L, Meng MJ, et al. Improved preparation of class I HLA tetramers and their use in detecting CMV-specific CTL. J Immunol Meth 2006; 312: 148.

50. Mallone R, Nepom GT. MHC class II tetramers and the pursuit of the antigen-specific T cells: define deviate and delete. Clin Immunol 2004; 110: 232.

51. Kern F, LiPira G, Gratama JW, et al. Measuring Ag-specific immune responses: understanding immunopathogenesis and improving diagnostics in infectious disease, autoimmunity and cancer. Trends Immunol 2005; 6: 477.

Assessment of functional immune responses

Jack J. H. Bleesing, Kimberly A. Risma

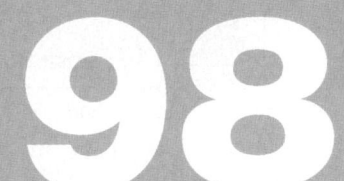

A comprehensive clinical evaluation of the immune system, whether to diagnose immunodeficiency or other immune-mediated disorders, ideally includes both quantitative and qualitative aspects. According to the principle: 'form follows function,' important clues to the functional status of the immune system are provided by the assessment of form (quantity), as determined by the cellular phenotype of lymphocytes and other cell populations and by the measurement of secreted/produced factors (complement factors, antibodies, cytokines, etc.).[1] For example, lack of memory B cells, as determined by flow cytometric measurement of CD27 expression on B cells (Fig. 98.1C), can guide appropriate functional testing of the B-cell compartment. This theme of interconnected determination of form and function will be a central thread throughout this chapter. Rather than describing in great detail the technical aspects of individual assays, the emphasis of this chapter will be on providing a general overview in the context of indication and interpretation. For more in-depth discussions on the assays themselves, the reader is referred to other sources, such as *Current Protocols in Immunology*[1a] and the *Manual of Molecular and Clinical Laboratory Immunology*,[1b] among others. Most of the assays described in this chapter are performed in highly specialized laboratories that often have a dual clinical/research mission. This dual role has been artificially separated into clinical and research sections in this chapter.

Despite enormous advances in technology, not much has changed in the day-to-day practical assessment of lymphocyte function, as routinely performed in clinical laboratories. In addition, it has been well recognized that certain immunologic conditions defy commonly used tools of laboratory investigation. This may be due to the fact that the "wrong" populations of cells are studied; the method of *in vitro* testing does not appropriately mimic the *in vivo* situation, and other factors. Thus new assays need to make their way into the clinical laboratory to capture these "emerging" disorders. Some of these assays are almost ready for clinical "prime time," whereas others are still in the early phases of development.

■ CLINICAL IMMUNOLOGY ■

GENERAL CONSIDERATIONS

Since the immune system operates in a profoundly intricate matter that is difficult to define by straightforward *modi operandi*, it is generally necessary to assess immunologic function according to pragmatic models

KEY CONCEPTS

BASIC CONCEPTS OF FUNCTIONAL TESTING

>> Immunologic form follows immunologic function

>> The right assay(s) for the right clinical scenario

>> An abnormal result invites several essential considerations:

   Does it reflect a biologically accurate and reproducible finding (confirmation)?

   What is its relevance (interpretation; pattern recognition)?

   What is its significance (further studies, patient care issues)?

   Is it reflective of disease and/or age (age-appropriate controls)?

>> With the exception of completely normal and abnormal test results, speculation is invariably involved in data/result interpretation (the gray zone)

>> *In vitro* assays that provide increasingly detailed information are also increasingly more demanding and prone to variation and artifacts, requiring rigorous quality control measures

or schemes. This approach divides the immune system into compartments, such that essentially every aspect of immune function can be studied through *in vivo*, *ex vivo*, or *in vitro* measurements. Focusing on the lymphoid system, functional assessment of T-, B-, and natural killer (NK)-cell compartments can be separated in phases of activation, and by functional output (Table 98.1). Another approach to dissect the complexities of lymphocyte function is to assay lymphocyte function following various methods of activation to reveal its normal (or abnormal) function (Table 98.2). Finally, functional assays can be distinguished based on whether they test function *in vivo* (measured *ex vivo*), or *in vitro*.

As with all laboratory studies, interpretation of abnormal immunologic studies leads to three basic questions. First, does the abnormality reflect a biologically accurate and reproducible finding? It is important to confirm test results, also paying attention to correct procurement and processing – including labeling – of specimens. Second, what is the relevance of the finding? In other words, what is the underlying basis for

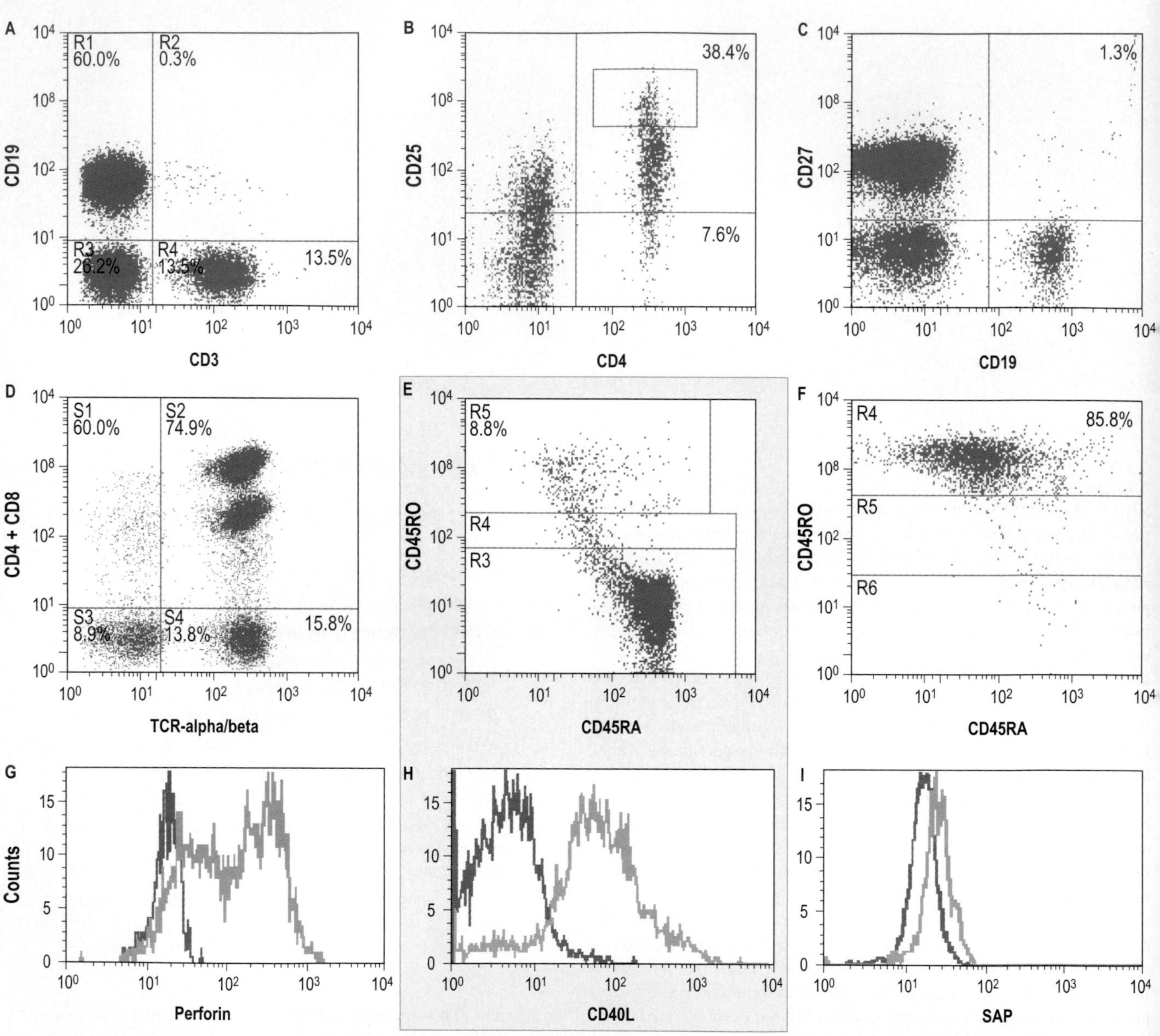

Fig. 98.1 Immunologic form follows immunologic function. Examples of abnormal immunologic form, detected by flow cytometry (dual-parameter dotplots A–F; single-parameter histograms G–I, showing patients in purple and controls in green). **(A)** Reduced T-cell compartment in patient with DiGeorge syndrome (gated on total lymphocytes, 13.5% versus 60–70% of lymphocytes in controls). **(B)** Activated CD25-expressing (CD4+) T cells in patient with chronic rejection of orthotopic liver transplantation (gated on total T cells). **(C)** Lack of memory B cells in patient with common variable immunodeficiency (CVID), as determined by CD27expression (gated on total lymphocytes; 1.3% versus >15% of B cells in controls). **(D)** Presence of T cells expressing the T-cell receptor (TCR)-alpha/beta but lacking CD4 and CD8 in a patient with autoimmune lymphoproliferative syndrome (ALPS, gated on total T cells; 15.8% versus <2% of lymphocytes in controls). **(E)** Lack of CD45RO-positive T cells in young adult with X-linked hyper-IgM syndrome (gated on total T cells, see H for associated functional assay). **(F)** Lack of CD45RA-positive T cells in patient 12 months post bone marrow transplantation (gated on total T cells). **(G)** Lack of intracellular perforin in natural killer (NK) cells (and associated defective NK-cell function) in patient with familial form of hemophagocytic lymphohistiocytosis on the basis of mutations in the perforin gene (FHLH, gated on total NK cells). **(H)** Lack of CD40L upregulation on (CD4+) T cells following 4-hour T-cell stimulation (gated on CD8-negative T cells). **(I)** Lack of intracellular Signaling Lymphocyte Activation Molecule (SLAM)-Associated Protein (SAP) expression in (CD8+) T cells in patient with X-linked lymphoproliferative disease (XLP, gated on CD8-positive T cells; cytolytic functions were abnormal in the presence of Epstein–Barr virus infection).

Table 98.1 Lymphocyte function as reflected by phases or events of activation

Phases/events of/in activation
Expression of cell surface proteins required to respond to antigenic stimuli (TCR, BCR, CD3, CD19)
Calcium influx
Expression and/or up- or downregulation of cell surface receptors, important in early activation (CD69, CD25, CD40L)
Blastogenesis (mitogenesis) and cell division (measured by a wide range of 'read-out' systems)
Up- or downregulation of markers indicating chronic activation, antigen priming (CD71, CD45RO, CCR7, CD62L)
Apoptosis (cell death)

Outcome
Production of cytokines in response to polyclonal or antigen-specific stimulation (Th1/Tr1 versus Th2/Tr2)
Production of polyclonal or antigen-specific immunoglobulins
Specific and non-specific cytolytic activity (see Table 98.3)
Measuring suppressive effects (T-regulatory activity, suppression of immunoglobulin secretion)

BCR, B-cell receptor; TCR, T-cell receptor.

the abnormal value(s); does it fit with an immunologic condition? Third, what are the consequences (significance) for the patient? Are immediate interventions indicated, such as intravenous immunoglobulin (IVIG), antibiotics, and patient isolation? When dealing with pediatric patients, a fourth question should be asked: how do the patient's laboratory results compare to age-appropriate normal values/reference ranges?

Controls (i.e., presumed healthy individuals) play important roles in all immunologic assays. Broadly categorized, there are assay controls and interpretation controls. Assay controls are needed to ensure that the assay is performing adequately (including shipping controls if the blood has to travel to the laboratory). In addition to a healthy control, the patient or subject constitutes an internal assay control (i.e., intra-assay control) to distinguish between 'noise' and 'signal' (e.g., cells cultured in the presence (signal) and in the absence (noise) of mitogens). Controls are also needed in the interpretation of the results, providing a framework for comparison. This includes the results of the healthy control, analyzed in parallel with the patient, and results from other control subjects, captured in a reference (normal) range. As mentioned in the introduction, the use of demographics-matched controls (age – both young and old – gender, ethnicity) is important for many assays.

The patient should be the starting point and the endpoint of the immunologic investigation. To guide the appropriate choice of functional assays for immune competence, it is imperative to have an initial assessment of immunologic phenotype (that could follow from function or lack thereof), linked to a specific question that is posed by the patient's clinical scenario. In many or most cases, clues to the nature of the functional defect are provided by abnormal phenotype (examples in Fig. 98.1). It is recommended to develop concepts as to the likely explanation of abnormal phenotype and the associated clinical scenario, anticipating how the data/results of functional assays will fit in these concepts. This approach should, however, be balanced by keeping an open mind, especially if few clues are available, or if clues seem contradictory. *An important aspect of functional testing is in fact obtaining the right assay(s) for the right scenario.* For example, obtaining a proliferation assay to

CLINICAL PEARLS

AVOIDING PITFALLS OF *IN VITRO* ASSAYS

What do we need to know about the patient?

Demographic data (age, sex, ethnicity, smoking)

Exposure history (natural infections, vaccinations)

Medications (immunosuppression)

Relevant (current) medical scenario (viral infection, trauma, cancer)

Interfering factors *in vivo* (rheumatoid factor, heterophile antibodies)

What do we need to know about the assay?

Cell source and viability (fresh, shipped, cryopreserved)

Cell manipulation, requirement for other cells (antigen-presenting cells, interfering suppressor T cells)

Controls (assay controls, including intra-assay, interpretation controls)

Data scoring (ELISPOT), calculation, and representation (e.g., counts per minute, lytic units)

measure T-cell responses to recall antigens would be of no value if the antigen has not been experienced and thus cannot "recall." Many other such examples can be envisioned.

FUNCTIONAL ASSAYS OF T-CELL IMMUNE COMPETENCE

Functional assays of T cells are generally intended to determine: (1) global immune competence; (2) specific (selective) immune competence; (3) *in vivo* state of immune activation; (4) recovery of *in vivo*

Table 98.2 Methods of lymphocyte activation *in vitro*

Frequency[a]	Stimulator	Target	Remarks
	Phorbol esters		
	PMA	Protein kinase C	Stimulates both T and B cells (similar for ionophores)
~80–90%	**Ionophores**		
	Ionomycin	Ion channels	PMA+ionomycin: bypasses cell surface receptors and early signaling molecules
~60–70%	**Mitogens**		
	PHA	Multiple receptors	T-cell stimulator (carbohydrate-recognizing lectin) (mitogen stimulation assay)
	ConA	Multiple receptors	T-cell stimulator (carbohydrate-recognizing lectin) (mitogen stimulation assay)
	PWM	Multiple receptors	T-cell stimulator and T-cell-dependent B-cell stimulator (mitogen stimulation assay)
~40–50%	**Antibodies/ligands**		
	Anti-TCR	TCR–CD3 complex	
	Anti-CD3	TCR–CD3 complex	Mild mitogen in soluble form; potent if immobilized on membranes or beads
	Anti-CD28	CD28 on T cells	Not mitogenic unless used in combination with TCR/CD3 stimulation
	Anti-IgM	BCR	Potent if immobilized; ±T cells or T-cell supernatant to test regulatory T-cell effects
	Anti-CD40 or sCD40L	CD40	Polyclonal immunoglobulin secretion; isotype determined by cytokine addition
~20–30%	**Microbial antigens**		
	SEB	TCR (noncognate)	Superantigen, stimulates ~20% of T cells through an invariant domain of the TCR
	SAC	BCR	SAC+IL-2: polyclonal immunoglobulin secretion in the absence of T cells
~5–10%	**Allogeneic cells**	TCR + others	One-way, two-way mixed lymphocyte culture (MLC)
< 1%	**Recall antigens**		
	Tetanus	TCR (cognate)	Dependent on prior *in vivo* exposure to tetanus (vaccination) (antigen proliferation assay)
	Candida	TCR (cognate)	Dependent on prior *in vivo* exposure to *Candida* spp. (antigen proliferation assay)

[a]Estimates of frequencies of responding T cells.
BCR, B-cell receptor; ConA, concanavalin-A; IgM, immunoglobulin M; IL-2, interleukin-2; PHA, phytohemagglutinin; PMA, Phorbol myristate acetate; SAC, *Staphylococcus aureus* Cowan strain; SEB, Staphylococcal enterotoxin B; TCR, T-cell receptor.

immune activation following immunosuppression; (5) appropriate downregulation of immune activation, and induction of cell death; (6) determination of prior exposures to foreign antigens (through infection or immunization); and (7) major histocompatibility complex (MHC) transplantation compatibility and evidence of prior exposure to alloantigens.

It should be possible to obtain a fairly detailed assessment of the T-cell compartment with a combination of immunophenotyping (Chapter 97) and functional assays (Table 98.2). This should allow hypotheses, regarding the immunologic nature of the clinical scenario, to be accepted or rejected. Depending on the complexity of the clinical circumstance, immunophenotyping can vary from a screening assessment of basic lymphocyte subsets to an advanced-flow cytometric analysis of subset, activation, effector, adhesion and many other cell surface and intracellular markers (beyond the scope of this chapter). The choice of functional assays is also determined by the complexity of the clinical situation (and pretest determination of form). For patients with immunodeficiency states that are predominantly characterized by issues with host defense (infections), performing a mitogen stimulation assay, employing combinations of phytohemagglutinin (PHA), concanavalin-A (Con-A), and pokeweed mitogen (PWM), immobilized anti-CD3, and/or an antigen stimulation assay are sufficient for the assessment of T-cell immune competence.[2–5]

In patients with suspected complex cellular immunodeficiency states, combinations of functional assays that have different cellular requirements and/or divergent pathways and modes of activation may be helpful to develop an understanding of the underlying defect(s), especially if these assays impose an incremental stringency on the T-cell compartment (e.g., the estimated percentage of T cells that can respond to the stimulus). For example, PMA and ionomycin can bypass relevant cell surface receptors, such as the T-cell receptor (TCR)–CD3 complex and upstream signaling components, connected to these receptors, allowing the vast majority of T cells to show a response. On the other end of the spectrum is the response to recall antigens, which typically involves less than 1% of the entire T-cell compartment (see Table 98.2 for a global overview). Adding growth factors (e.g., interleukin-2 (IL-2)) may provide additional information regarding the functional status of the cell population. Two examples of this principle are demonstrated in Figure 98.2, showing differential responses to phorbol esters, ionophores, mitogens, and the effect of exogenous cytokines (IL-2) in 2 patients with relatively similar clinical scenarios, characterized by infections and T-cell immunodeficiency.[6] Similar studies are helpful in other scenarios (e.g. ZAP70 defects that show abnormal TCR/CD3 stimulation but normal responses to stimuli that bypass the ZAP70 adaptor protein, such as achieved with PMA and ionomycin).[7]

As with most functional assays, the clinical utility of the assays described above depends on the ability of the clinician to translate raw data into an appropriate interpretation of the results. It seems self-evident that completely normal and completely abnormal results are relatively easy to explain; everything in between (the gray zone) is, more or less, a matter of an educated interpretation. Detailed functional analysis, as shown in Figure 98.2, can help in making the gray zone easier to navigate. This of course is balanced by the added technical challenges (and potential pitfalls) of these labor-intensive assays. In the event that the results of the functional assay do not fit with the observed form, an attempt should be made to explain whether this discrepancy has a biological basis or is due to assay-related artifacts (technical issues). Thus, it is crucial that adequate quality control programs are in place to ensure that data interpretation and its consequence on clinical management are valid. Essentially every aspect of functional assays is subject to variation that can influence its performance. An evaluation of T-cell immune competence can be achieved without obtaining a blood sample. Delayed-type hypersensitivity skin testing constitutes an *in vivo* method for determining (screening) cellular immunity based on prior exposure to certain pathogens. Its major advantages are convenience, availability, and quick turnaround time (~48–72 hours). In addition, DTH skin tests measure both the afferent (e.g., antigen presentation) and efferent loops of the immune response (e.g., T cell infiltration, mediator release). An obvious limitation is that exposures to the agents used in DTH must

have taken place. Clinical relevance and use of DTH tests to detect incompetent T-cell function are limited by the facts that the response cannot be adequately quantified and that there are many causes of false-negative results (anergy). Among the latter are young and advanced age, concurrent infections, use of immunosuppressive medications, malnutrition, atopic dermatitis, and others. Thus, DTH tests ideally include at least a combination of several recall antigens (e.g., tetanus toxoid, *Candida*, mumps) placed by intradermal injection to increase the probability of a positive response (i.e., erythema and induration at 48 and 72 hours after application). This testing should not performed on children under the age of 1–2 years and negative results should be interpreted with great caution (positive results can be used to plan subsequent *in vitro* studies, if necessary).[8, 9]

ASSESSMENT OF CYTOLYTIC FUNCTION

Assays which measure proliferation to mitogens, antigens, and cytokines reveal the ability of T cells to divide appropriately and produce soluble products in response to stimulation. However, the effector function of cytotoxic lymphocytes requires both proliferation and the ability to kill target cells. Cytolytic function pertains to subsets of T and NK cells. There are several types of cytolytic activity that differ in respect to effector cell population, specificity (e.g., MHC restriction), requirement for prior sensitization to the target, and other features (Table 98.3).[10–12] While both T-cell subsets and NK cells can function as non-MHC-restricted cytolytic cells, only T cells have the ability to kill target cells via cognate (MHC/peptide) recognition, a process that requires prior exposure to the target or antigens derived from the target.[13, 14] Antibody-dependent cellular cytotoxicity (ADCC) is a cytolytic process that is dependent on the cooperative interaction of several different cellular and humoral constituents of the immune system. In ADCC, effector cells with receptors for the Fc portion of antibodies (e.g., CD16) infer target cell lysis by using these Fc receptors to attach to antibody-coated target cells.[15, 16] Lymphokine activated killer (LAK) cells are cytotoxic cells, mostly, but not exclusively, derived from NK cells that, through activation by IL-2, acquire more potent cytolytic function to "traditional" targets, as well as broaden the repertoire of potential targets (e.g., fresh tumor cells).[17, 18]

Cytolytic activity can be divided into three phases that can be assessed *in vitro*. The process starts with conjugate formation between target and effector cells, mediated by many receptor/ligand pairs. Following cellular contact, the cytolytic cells are triggered, i.e., prepared for imminent killing. This process can be measured on the basis of calcium flux or by intracellular phosphorylation events. The process is completed (and can be repeated with other targets) by lysis of target cells through membranolytic/secretory (perforin and granzymes) and by nonsecretory receptor-mediated (Fas/Fas ligand) mechanisms.[19–22]

Reasons for obtaining cytolytic assays broadly follow the same considerations as for assays measuring T-cell immune competence. It has long been recognized that abnormal cytolytic function is found in patients with a variety of disorders that include primary and acquired immunodeficiency disorders, viral infections, cancer, trauma/burns, and other conditions, some of which are better characterized than others (e.g., chronic fatigue syndrome).[12, 23] From a practical standpoint, however, it is often difficult to translate the results of these assays into meaningful interpretations that are actually helpful in the diagnosis and management of these conditions. Development of new therapeutic options for some

focused on studying patients with dysregulated lymphoproliferation, autoimmunity, allergy, or malignancy. Here again, the diagnosis is not readily discovered in the clinical immunology laboratory.

In Figure 98.1D, an example is shown with normal function, as measured by standard clinical assays of T-, NK- (and B-) cell function. Nonetheless, the presence of abnormal T cells, that lack expression of CD4 and CD8 and express TCR-α/β (double-negative T cells), is a direct consequence of defective function, namely abnormal Fas-mediated apoptosis (cell death). Apoptosis assays are becoming relevant in the comprehensive evaluation of the immune system as our appreciation for the importance of downregulation and termination of immunologic function has evolved.[46] Determination of apoptosis in vitro is part of the evaluation of autoimmune lymphoproliferative syndrome (ALPS), linking a defined clinical scenario and abnormal immunologic function due to a fundamental defect in Fas-mediated cellular suicide (apoptosis).[47] Again, an important consideration in the design and execution of apoptosis assays is the right assay for the right setting. For ALPS, the in vitro assay must approximate the in vivo relevance of Fas-mediated apoptosis. Resting (circulating) T cells are typically not sensitive to undergo Fas-mediated apoptosis in vivo. Thus, PBMC (or isolated T cells) are placed in a primary culture system, similar to mitogen or antigen proliferation assays (for example, 2–3 days with PHA, followed by several days of additional culture with exogenous IL-2). This induces the T cells to become sensitive to Fas-mediated apoptosis. At this stage, cells are incubated with anti-Fas antibodies for a 24–48-hour period, after which apoptosis of T cells is measured, using any of a multitude of flow cytometric read-out systems. As has been the theme of this chapter, intra-assay (the patient/subject) and interassay (healthy subject) controls should be included. In addition, it is recommended to test non-Fas-mediated apoptosis pathways, for example using chemotherapeutic drugs (staurosporine) and gamma irradiation, to determine specificity of the apoptotic defect. Further development and refinement of apoptosis assays appear to indicate the existence of other defects in specific modes and pathways of apoptosis, some with their own clinical scenarios and observed altered form.[46]

Expression of CD25 on (CD4+) T cells (Fig. 98.1B) does not only, or always, reflect a state of T-cell activation. Within this population, recent advances in basis science have identified unique T cells, often designated CD25^{bright} (see box in Fig. 98.1B), that function as regulatory T cells (i.e., T-regulatory cells (Tregs); Chapter 16). Further characterization has shown these cells to be positive for intracellular expression of cytotoxic T-lymphocyte-associated protein 4 (CTLA4) and forkhead box P3 (FOXP3). Tregs are found in peripheral blood, thymus, lymph nodes, and a variety of other tissues, including gut and endocrine organs.[48] The importance of Tregs is illustrated by a primary immunodeficiency disorder, designated immune dysregulation, polyendocrinopathy, enteropathy, X-linked syndrome (IPEX) (Chapter 35). This disorder occurs in boys who are deficient in the X-linked gene encoding FOXP3.[49] Patients present with diarrhea or failure to thrive, rash, insulin-dependent diabetes, and other autoimmune endocrinopathies, as well as immune-mediated cytopenias. The underlying genetic defect in IPEX is a direct result of defective generation and function of these regulatory cells. Their unique function is to suppress the proliferation of activated (other) T cells, thereby limiting the immune response to self antigens, and perhaps nonself antigens as well. Functional assays for Tregs have been established in research laboratories. They are based on isolating CD4/CD25^{bright} T cells from PBMC and incubating them in a pre-established concentration with the nonisolated, remaining

(CD25$^-$), T cells, antigen-presenting cells, and other cells. Standard proliferation assays are set up using mitogens, anti-CD3, or specific antigens (Table 98.2). In the presence of Tregs, proliferation, as measured by [^{3}H]-thymidine incorporation in dividing T cells, is reduced, while in the absence of these cells, normal proliferation is detected.

Although IPEX is a rare disorder, Tregs have fast become a popular cell population because of their impact on immune-mediated disorders and, consequently, their potential application in counteracting these disorders. It can be envisioned that clinical scenarios, resulting from abnormal regulatory T-cell function (Tregs and other cell populations) will become part of contemporary clinical immunology, following the same principle that abnormal immunologic form reflects abnormal immunologic function.[48, 49]

Together these groups of disorders, including defects in host defense and in immune regulation, will provide ample opportunity for the development and refinement of novel assays of immunologic function. In addition, as has been the case for many other functional assays that seem to have been part of the clinical laboratory since inception, new discoveries will be made that will increase our understanding of the human immune system and how it functions.

REFERENCES

1. Bleesing JJ, Fleisher TA. Immunophenotyping. Semin Hematol 2001; 38: 100–110.

1a. Coligan JE, Bierer BE, Marguiles DH, Shevach EM, Strober W (eds). Current Protocols in Immunology. John Wiley & Sons, New Yoark, 2007.

1b. Detrick B, Hamilton RG, Folds JD (eds). Manual of Molecular and Clinical Laboratory Immunology. American Society for Microbiology (ASM) Press, 7th edition. Washington DC, 2006.

2. Stobo JD. Phytohemagglutin and concanavalin A: probes for murine 'T' cell activation and differentiation. Transplant Rev 1972; 11: 60–86.

3. Greaves M, Janossy G, Doenhoff M. Selective triggering of human T and B lymphocytes in vitro by polyclonal mitogens. J Exp Med 1974; 140: 1–18.

4. Vine JB, Geppert TD, Lipsky PE. T4 cell activation by immobilized phytohemagglutinin: differential capacity to induce IL-2 responsiveness and IL-2 production. J Immunol 1988; 141: 2593–2600.

5. Geppert TD, Lipsky PE. Activation of T lymphocytes by immobilized monoclonal antibodies to CD3. Regulatory influences of monoclonal antibodies to additional T cell surface determinants. J Clin Invest 1988; 81: 1497–1505.

6. Flomenberg N, Welte K, Mertelsmann R, et al. Immunologic effects of interleukin 2 in primary immunodeficiency diseases. J Immunol 1983; 130: 2644–2650.

7. Chan AC, Kadlecek TA, Elder ME, et al. ZAP-70 deficiency in an autosomal recessive form of severe combined immunodeficiency. Science 1994; 264: 1599–1601.

8. Gordon EH, Krouse HA, Kinney JL, et al. Delayed cuteneous hypersensitivity in normals: choice of antigens and comparison to in vitro assays of cell-mediated immunity. J Allergy Clin Immunol 1983; 72: 487.

9. Palmer DL, Reed WP. Delayed hypersensitivity skin testing. II. J Infect Dis 1974; 130: 138.

10. Roberts K, Lotze MT, Rosenberg SA. Separation and functional studies of the human lymphokine-activated killer cell. Cancer Res 1987; 15: 4366–4371.

11. Whiteside TL, Vujanovic NL, Herberman RB. Natural killer cells and tumor therapy. Curr Top Microbiol Immunol 1998; 230: 221–244.

12. Sanderson CJ. The mechanism of lymphocyte-mediated cytoxicity. Biol Rev 1981; 56: 153–197.

13. Rees RC. MHC-restricted and nonrestricted killer lymphocytes. Blood 1990; 4: 204–210.

14. Greenberg AH, Shen LA. Class of specific cytotoxic cells demonstrated in vitro by arming with antigen-antibody complexes. Nat New Biol 1973; 245: 282–285.

15. Johnson WJ, Steplewski Z, Matthews TJ, et al. Cytolytic interactions between murine macrophages, tumor cells, and monoclonal antibodies: characterization of lytic conditions and requirements for effector activation. J Immunol 1986; 136: 4707–4713.

16. Melder RJ, Walker ER, Herberman RB, et al. Surface characteristics, morphology, and ultrastructure of human adherent lymphokine-activated killer cells. J Leukoc Biol 1990; 48: 163–173.

17. Melder RJ, Walker E, Herberman RB, et al. Adhesion characteristics of human interleukin 2-activated natural killer cells. Cell Immunol 1991; 132: 177–192.

18. Berke G. The binding and lysis of target cells by cytotoxic lymphocytes: molecular and cellular aspects. Annu Rev Immunol 1994; 12: 735–773.

19. Russell JH, Ley TJ. Lymphocyte-mediated cytotoxicity. Annu Rev Immunol 2002; 20: 323–370.

20. Podack ER, Hengarner H, Lichtenheld MG. A central role of perforin in cytolysis? Annu Rev Immunol 1991; 9: 129–157.

21. Brunner T, Wasem C, Torgler R, et al. Fas (CD95/Apo-1) ligand regulation in T cell homeostasis, cell-mediated cytotoxicity and immune pathology. Semin Immunol 2003; 15: 167–176.

22. Whiteside TL, Bryant J, Day R, et al. Natural killer cytotoxicity in the diagnosis of immune dysfunction: criteria for a reproducible assay. J Clin Lab Anal 1990; 4: 102–114.

23. Whiteside TL, Herberman RB. Role of human natural killer cells in health and disease. Clin Diag Lab Immunol 1994; 1: 125–133.

24. Sullivan KE, Delaat CA, Douglas SD, et al. Defective natural killer cell function in patients with hemophagocytic lymphohistiocytosis and in first degree relatives. Pediatr Res 1998; 44: 465–468.

25. Villanueva J, Lee S, Giannini EH, et al. Natural killer cell dysfunction is a distinguishing feature of systemic onset juvenile rheumatoid arthritis and macrophage activation syndrome. Arthritis Res Ther 2005; 7: R30–R37.

26. Grom AA, Villanueva J, Lee S, et al. Natural killer cell dysfunction in patients with systemic-onset juvenile rheumatoid arthritis and macrophage activation syndrome. J Pediatr 2003; 142: 292–296.

27. Bryant J, Day R, Whiteside TL, et al. Calculation of lytic units for the expression of cell-mediated cytotoxicity. J Immunol Methods 1992; 146: 91–103.

28. Junghans RP, Waldmann TA, Landolfi NF, et al. Anti-Tac-H, a humanized antibody to the interleukin 2 receptor with new features for immunotherapy in malignant and immune disorders. Cancer Res 1990; 50: 1495–1502.

29. Sorensen RU, Moore C. Antibody deficiency syndromes. Pediatr Clin North Am 2000; 47: 1225.

30. Bleesing JJ, Fleisher TA. Human B cells express a CD45 isoform that is similar to murine B220 and is downregulated with acquisition of the memory B-cell marker CD27. Cytometry B Clin Cytom 2003; 51: 1–8.

31. Avanzini MA, Locatelli F, Dos Santos C, et al. B lymphocyte reconstitution after hematopoietic stem cell transplantation: functional immaturity and slow recovery of memory CD27+ B cells. Exp Hematol 2005; 33: 480–486.

32. Stiehm ER, Ochs HD, Winkelsein JA. Immunodeficiency disorders: general considerations. In: Stiehm ER, Ochs HD, Winkelsein JA (eds): Immunologic Disorders in Infants and Children, 5th edn. Philadelphia, PA: Elsevier Saunders, 2004. .

33. Pyuan KH, Ochs HD, Wedgwood RJ, et al. Human antibody responses to bacteriophage phiX174: sequential induction of IgM and IgG subclass antibody. Clin Imunol Immunopathol 1989; 51: 252–263.

34. Curtis JE, Hersh EM, Harris JE, et al. The human primary immune response to keyholder limpet haemocyanin: interrelationships of delayed hypersensitivity. Clin Exp Immunol 1970; 6: 473.

35. Brinkman DM, Jol-van der Zijde CM, ten Dam MM, et al. Vaccination with rabies to study the humoral and cellular immune response to a T-cell dependent neoantigen in man. J Clin Immunol 2003; 23: 528–538.

36. Dunbar PR, Ogg GS. Oligomeric MHC molecules and their homologues: state of the art. J Immunol Methods 2002; 268: 3–7.

37. Mallone R, Nepom GT. MHC class II tetramers and the pursuit of antigen-specific T cells: define, deviate, delete. Clin Immunol 2004; 110: 232–242.

38. Whiteside TL. Monitoring of antigen-specific cytolytic T lymphocytes in cancer patients receiving immunotherapy. Clin Diagn Lab Immunol 2000; 7: 327–332.

39. Hickling JK. Measuring human T-lymphocyte function. Expert Review Molecular Medicine, 1998. Available online at: www.-ermm.cbcu.cam.ac.uk (link verified 4/27/06)

40. Zeng C, MaWhinneya S, Baróna AE, McFarland EJ. Evaluating ELISPOT summary measures with criteria for obtaining reliable estimates. J Immunol Methods 2005; 297: 97–108.

41. Orange JS, Levy O, Geha RS. Human disease resulting from gene mutations that interfere with appropriate nuclear factor-kappaB activation. Immunol Rev 2005; 203: 21–37.

42. Ku CL, Yang K, Bustamante J, et al. Inherited disorders of human Toll-like receptor signaling: immunological implications. Immunol Rev 2005; 203: 10–20.

43. Cardenes M, von Bernuth H, Garcia-Saavedra A, et al. Autosomal recessive interleukin-1 receptor-associated kinase 4 deficiency in fourth-degree relatives. J Pediatr 2006; 148: 549–551.

44. Rosenzweig SD, Holland SM. Defects in the interferon-gamma and interleukin-12 pathways. Immunol Rev 2005; 203: 38–47.

45. Haverkamp MH, van Dissel JT, Holland SM. Human host genetic factors in nontuberculous mycobacterial infection: lessons from single gene disorders affecting innate and adaptive immunity and lessons from molecular defects in interferon-gamma-dependent signaling. Microbes Infect 2006; 8: 1157–1166.

REFERENCES

maturation stages of neutrophil development.[10] Granules are classified into four distinct populations: azurophilic, specific, gelatinase, and secretory granules. Azurophilic granules contain myeloperoxidase, lysozyme, antimicrobial peptides, defensins, proteases, and the lysosomal acid hydrolases. The specific granules contain lactoferrin, lysozyme, and vitamin B_{12}-binding protein, and also serve as storage pools for CD11b/CD18 and cytochrome b_{558} of the O_2^- generating enzyme, NADPH oxidase. The gelatinase granules are a subset of the specific granules that have a high content of gelatinase. The secretory granules are highly mobilizable intracellular vesicles that contain alkaline phosphatase and other surface antigens.

As the phagosome forms, the azurophilic granules fuse with the phagosomal membrane, forming the phagolysosome and releasing their complement of acid hydrolases, defensins, and myeloperoxidase. These enzymes can potentiate the digestive and microbicidal activities of the neutrophil. The secretion of specific and secretory granules is thought to release mediators of inflammation (such as lactoferrin) and mediate the translocation of additional receptors (CD11b/CD18, fMLF receptor, and laminin receptors, as well as cytochrome b_{558} of the NADPH oxidase) to the plasma membrane. Translocation of these receptors modulates neutrophil adhesion, movement, phagocytosis, and respiratory burst activity. Factors that can affect signal transduction, metabolic activity, microfilament rearrangement, and microtubule assembly can regulate the degranulation process.

Accompanying the fusion of the granule to the phagolysosome is the assembly of the multicomponent O_2^--generating enzyme, NADPH oxidase or phagocyte oxidase (*phox*), an enzyme complex consisting of at least two cytosolic components,[11] p47*phox* and p67*phox*, and two membrane components, p22*phox* and, gp91*phox*, that constitute cytochrome b_{558}.[12, 13] This enzyme reduces molecular O_2 to O_2^- using NADPH generated by the oxidation of glucose through the pentose phosphate pathway. O_2^- either spontaneously or enzymatically converts to H_2O_2. In the presence of a metal such as Fe^{2+}, H_2O_2 and O_2^- can react to form the highly reactive hydroxyl radical, OH•. Alternatively, the azurophilic granule constituent, myeloperoxidase, catalyzes the formation of hypochlorous acid from H_2O_2 and Cl^-. The combined activities of reactive O_2 species, antimicrobial peptides, and lysosomal hydrolases result in the ultimate destruction of the microorganism. Excess production of reactive O_2 species and release of lysosomal hydrolases into the extracellular milieu can lead to tissue damage and inflammation.

Neutrophils display a diverse array of cellular functions. Abnormalities in these functions can severely compromise host defense, leading to recurrent bacterial and fungal infections. To localize specific deficiencies of neutrophil function, assays have been developed that mimic these functions both *in vivo* and *in vitro*. Often, a preliminary screening of several neutrophil functions is performed to localize deficits and then more vigorous testing of specific function is performed. Assays to assess neutrophil function should address several limitations – the number of cells required for the assay, the type of cell preparation needed (isolated neutrophils versus whole blood), the overall incubation time for the assay, the complexity of the assay, and the rapidity of data collection. These issues become more critical if multiple functional assays are planned concurrently. Since neutrophils cannot be stored or frozen and maintain viability, control neutrophils from a normal volunteer are generally assayed in parallel to validate the results. Generally, this doubles the number of assays to be performed. Additionally, isolation of neutrophils can take 1–2 hours, limiting the time available for functional assays. Fluorescent probes have increased the sensitivity of many of the assays and eliminated the need for radioactive probes. The use of multi-well plates and multi-well microplate readers has reduced the number of cells required and has facilitated the collection of data.

■ ISOLATION OF NEUTROPHILS ■

CLINICAL INDICATIONS AND IMPLICATIONS

Assays that avoid neutrophil isolation are preferred because of the artifactual priming of neutrophils during isolation.[14] However, most assays require isolated neutrophils to eliminate any possible contributions of other leukocytes and blood components. In general, blood should be drawn using either citrate or heparin (10 units/ml) as anticoagulant and maintained at 20–25°C in polypropylene containers. Most isolation protocols require 1–2 hours to obtain purified neutrophils.

PRINCIPLE AND INTERPRETATION OF LABORATORY ASSESSMENT

Most neutrophil isolation protocols use differences in the cell density as the basis for the separation. The relative densities of blood cells are as follows: erythrocytes > neutrophils and eosinophils > monocytes, lymphocytes, and basophils > platelets. Ficoll-Hypaque is a solution of sodium diatrizoate (a dense, iodine-containing molecule) and Ficoll (a polysaccharide) with a density (1.083 g/cc) that falls between that of neutrophils and that of the mononuclear cells. To isolate neutrophils,[15] whole blood is diluted with saline and underlayed with Ficoll-Hypaque. After centrifugation for 30 minutes at 500 g, the less dense monocytes,

---

■ KEY CONCEPTS

>> The stepwise reduction of O_2 leads to reactive oxygen intermediates and finally to H_2O

$$2H^+$$

$$O_2 \xrightarrow{e^-} O_2^- \xrightarrow[2H^+]{e^-} H_2O_2 \xrightarrow{e^-} OH^• + OH^- \xrightarrow{e^-} H_2O + \tfrac{1}{2}O_2$$

Oxygen	Superoxide anion	Hydrogen peroxide	Hydroxyl radical	Water

---

■ KEY CONCEPTS

>> Because of: (1) the short lifespan of neutrophils and (2) the time required to isolate neutrophils, assays of neutrophil function should have minimal complexity and rapid data collection

lymphocytes, basophils, and platelets remain at the upper interface of the Ficoll-Hypaque while the denser erythrocytes and neutrophils pass through the Ficoll-Hypaque and pellet at the bottom. The mononuclear cells are carefully harvested and the remaining Ficoll-Hypaque aspirated. The erythrocyte/neutrophil pellet is resuspended with saline and mixed with 3% dextran. Dextran promotes the formation of rouleaux by the erythrocytes, causing them to sediment rapidly at 1 g. The neutrophil-enriched supernatant fluid is harvested from the bulk of the erythrocytes. Contaminating erythrocytes are removed by a brief (30-second) hypotonic lysis with 0.2% saline. The isotonicity is quickly restored with an equal volume of 1.6% saline. A second hypotonic lysis removes many of the red cell ghosts. In general, $1–2 \times 10^6$ neutrophils can be isolated per milliliter of whole blood from a normal subject with a normal white blood cell count. A second neutrophil isolation protocol that uses a discontinuous gradient of plasma/Percoll has often been used to minimize exposure of neutrophils to trace contamination by bacterial LPS and reduce neutrophil priming.[16]

In our laboratory, isolated neutrophils are routinely frozen in aliquots of 5×10^6 cells/vial. For Western blot studies, neutrophils (1×10^6 cells/ml of buffer) are pretreated for 20 minutes with the cell permeant, irreversible serine protease inhibitor, diisopropylfluorophosphate (DFP, 5mM). The cells are then centrifuged and the supernatant fluid removed prior to freezing. In addition, these frozen neutrophils, though not viable, provide an excellent source of material for isolation of DNA for subsequent genetic analysis.

■ NEUTROPHIL ADHERENCE ■

CLINICAL INDICATIONS AND IMPLICATIONS

Adherence of neutrophils to the endothelium is a prerequisite step to the migration of neutrophils into the tissues. Neutrophils isolated from patients with leukocyte adhesion deficiency type 1 (LAD-1) who lack the common β_2 integrin subunit CD18 exhibit abnormal adherence to endothelium,[17] and therefore are not able to migrate efficiently into the surrounding tissues, often resulting in marked granulocytosis[18] (Chapter 21). LAD-2 is a milder form of the disease in which patients exhibit a defect in fucose metabolism and glycoprotein biosynthesis.[19] Neutrophils from patients with LAD-2 exhibit abnormal expression of the glycoprotein, L-selectin, and fail to roll along the endothelium. However, they do exhibit normal β_2-integrin mediated adherence.

PRINCIPLE AND INTERPRETATION OF LABORATORY ASSESSMENT

The adhesive function of phagocytes is commonly assessed by passage of 1 ml of whole blood through a column filled with nylon wool. Adherence is measured as the difference in the absolute neutrophil count of the pre-column sample and of the sample after passage through the nylon wool column.

Alternatively, isolated neutrophils can be induced to bind to plastic using a 96-well plate either uncoated, or coated with fetal bovine serum or a specific extracellular matrix protein such as fibrinogen or fibronectin. Endothelial cell monolayers harvested from human umbilical veins may serve as a more physiological substrate for the measurement of cell adhesion. Isolated neutrophils are pre-loaded with the cell permeant, acetoxymethyl ester derivative of the fluorescent dye, calcein (calcein-AM). Nonspecific esterases in the cytosol cleave the ester linkage, trapping the fluorescent probe in the cytosol. The labeled neutrophils are added to each well and incubated in the absence or presence of phorbol myristate acetate (PMA) to promote adherence through activation of the integrins. At the end of the incubation, the wells are washed three times to remove nonadherent cells. The fluorescence of each well is determined with a fluorescent microplate reader and compared to the fluorescence of a control well with a fixed number of fluorescent cells. As shown in the left panel of Figure 99.1, under control conditions, fewer than 10% of the neutrophils adhere to plastic or to plastic coated with fetal bovine serum. Slightly more neutrophil adherence is observed on wells coated with fibrinogen. Treatment of normal neutrophils with PMA for 30 minutes results in the adherence of > 90% of the neutrophils under all conditions. This adherence assay is valuable in the diagnosis of patients with leukocyte adhesion deficiency. As shown in the right panel of Figure 99.1, neutrophils isolated from patients with LAD-1 generally exhibit < 5% adherence under control conditions and do not increase adherence after treatment with PMA.

■ NEUTROPHIL CHEMOTAXIS ■

CLINICAL INDICATIONS AND IMPLICATIONS

Neutrophil migration is a prerequisite for neutrophil accumulation at sites of inflammation. Patients with leukocyte chemotactic defects usually show recurrent skin abscesses and occasional life-threatening invasive infections.

PRINCIPLE AND INTERPRETATION OF LABORATORY ASSESSMENT

Assessment of neutrophil chemotaxis *in vivo* can be evaluated using skin windows. Skin blisters are gently raised on the volar surface of the forearm using a vacuum pump and an 8-well blister device, with little hemorrhage and vascular damage. The roof of the blister is removed and the exposed skin lesion is bathed with autologous serum using a skin window chamber. In 24 hours, exudative neutrophils accumulate in the autologous serum bathing the skin lesion. The skin chamber provides a mechanism for characterizing the immune cells, as well as soluble immune mediators, that accumulate in the autologous serum during the evolution of the inflammatory response.[20]

Chemotaxis *in vitro* is generally measured using a Boyden chamber. The Boyden chamber includes three components: a lower (chemoattractant) chamber, a nitrocellulose or polycarbonate filter layer, and an upper cell chamber. The lower compartments of the Boyden chamber are filled with a chemoattractant such as fMLF (10^{-8} M) or IL-8 (10 ng/ml). Recently, a rapid fluorescence-based measurement of neutrophil chemotaxis has been

---

| KEY CONCEPTS

>> In general, $1–2 \times 10^6$ neutrophils can be isolated per milliliter of whole blood from a normal subject with a normal white blood cell count

PRINCIPLE AND INTERPRETATION OF LABORATORY ASSESSMENT

Stimulation of neutrophils with various secretagogues can result in the release of granular enzymes into the extracellular fluid. Treatment of the neutrophils with cytochalasin b (5 μg/ml) disrupts microfilament assembly and facilitates the release of both specific and azurophilic enzymes. Since stimulation of neutrophil degranulation is often accompanied by O_2^- generation and oxidative inactivation of enzymes, both the cell supernatant fluid and the cell pellet should be analyzed to determine the percentage of enzyme released. To differentiate degranulation from cell lysis, release of the cytosolic enzyme lactate dehydrogenase should be monitored simultaneously.

The release of azurophilic granules can be assessed by determination of β-glucuronidase activity. Supernatant fluids or cell extracts obtained from stimulated neutrophils are incubated with 4-methylumbelliferyl-β-D-glucuronide. The reaction is stopped with the addition of ammonium hydroxide/glycine buffer and the fluorescence compared to a standard curve of 4-methylumbelliferone. Alternatively, myeloperoxidase can be determined using commercially available enzyme-linked immunoassays. CD63 is also found in the membrane of azurophilic granules and migrates to the neutrophil surface after stimulation with fMLF in the presence of cytochalasin b.

The release of specific granules can be assessed by determination of lactoferrin levels using an enzyme-linked immunoassay. The carcinoembryonic antigen CD66b (formerly CD67) is found on the neutrophil surface and the specific granules, and its expression on the surface of the neutrophils is increased after stimulation with fMLF or LPS. The secretory granules usually contain proteins that are translocated into the membrane from cytosol during degranulation. Detection of the constituents of secretory granules can be assessed by flow cytometric analysis of the change in expression of surface proteins such as adhesion molecules, and cytochrome b_{558} of the NADPH oxidase.

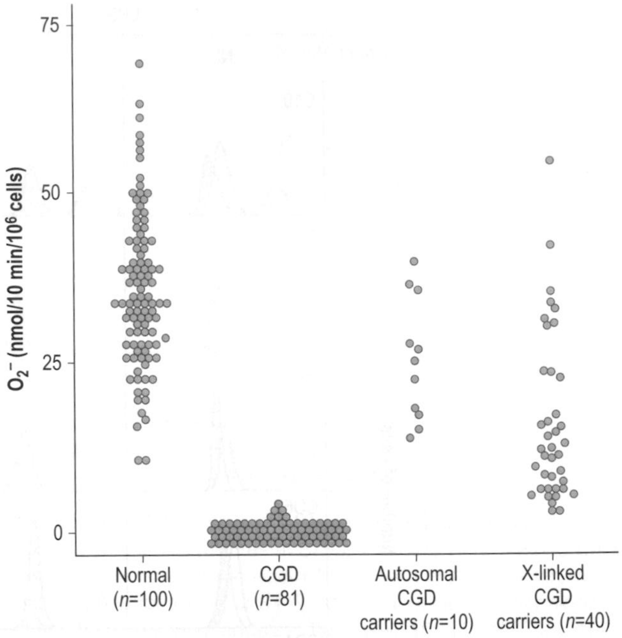

Fig. 99.3 O_2^- generation from normal subjects, chronic granulomatous disease (CGD) patients, and CGD carriers. Neutrophils (1×10^6/ml HBSS) were incubated in the presence of 100 μM cytochrome c with phorbol myristate acetate (PMA: 100 ng/ml) for 10 minutes at 37°C. The reaction was terminated by centrifugation at 4°C. Reduction of cytochrome c was monitored at an analytical wavelength of 549.5 nm and a micromolar extinction coefficient of 0.0211. An identical tube containing superoxide dismutase (100 μg/ml) served as a blank.

◼ GENERATION OF REACTIVE OXYGEN INTERMEDIATES ◼

CLINICAL INDICATIONS AND IMPLICATIONS

The release of reactive oxygen intermediates (ROI) such as O_2^- and H_2O_2 is an important component of neutrophils' bactericidal machinery. Neutrophils isolated from patients with chronic granulomatous disease (CGD) have a defect in the NADPH oxidase and are unable to generate ROI, resulting in an oxygen-dependent bactericidal defect (Chapter 21). Microorganisms causing infections in patients with CGD are usually catalase-positive, such as *Staphylococcus aureus* and *Escherichia coli*, but not catalase-negative bacteria, because neutrophils isolated from CGD patients can utilize the H_2O_2 generated by the catalase-negative bacterium to enhance the bactericidal activity. NADPH, the source of reducing potential utilized by the oxidase, is provided by metabolism of glucose through the pentose phosphate pathway.

PRINCIPLES AND INTERPRETATION OF LABORATORY ASSESSMENTS

The production of superoxide (O_2^-) can be detected using the reduction of cytochrome c. Because O_2^- causes a one-to-one stoichiometric reduction of ferricytochrome c to ferrocytochrome c, the resultant increase in the absorption spectrum at 550 nM can be used to quantitate the production of O_2^-. Superoxide dismutase is added to an identical tube to control for the nonspecific reduction of cytochrome c. However, since cytochrome is not permeable to the cells, the detection of O_2^- is limited to that released into the extracellular milieu. Neutrophils isolated from normal volunteers produce 0.42 ± 0.67 nmol/10^6 neutrophils per 10 minutes under resting conditions. As shown in Figure 99.3, treatment of normal neutrophils with PMA results in 35.92 ± 11.92 nmol/10^6 neutrophils per 10 minutes. An estimate of normal O_2^- production over 60 minutes can be obtained by reducing the number of neutrophils in the assay to 2×10^5. Neutrophils isolated from patients with CGD fail to produce O_2^- in response to PMA in 10 minutes. However, some patients with autosomal forms of CGD have low, but detectable O_2^- production in 60 minutes. Neutrophils isolated from X-linked heterozygous carriers of CGD can yield a full spectrum of O_2^- production, while neutrophils from autosomal recessive carriers of CGD generally yield a normal response. Although the detection of O_2^- by reduction of cytochrome c is useful in the diagnosis of patients with CGD, it cannot be used in the diagnosis of carriers because of the wide spectrum of responses that result from the degree of X chromosome lyonization. Recent studies have shown that O_2^- determinations sufficiently reliable to diagnose CGD can be obtained from neutrophils isolated from heparinized whole blood that has been stored overnight. Hence, analyses can be performed on blood samples shipped by overnight express. A normal control blood sample should accompany the sample to ensure adequate shipment handling. By 48 hours of storage, however, there are marked reductions in the PMA response and the data are no longer valid.

The extracellular release of H_2O_2 can be measured using horseradish peroxidase-induced oxidation of either phenol red or Amplex red. Polymorphonuclear neutrophil suspensions in the presence of horseradish peroxidase and one of the chromophores are exposed to either PMA or buffer alone. Changes in optical density of phenol red at 600 nm can be determined with a standard microplate reader. Amplex red is a much more sensitive fluorescent chromophore and H_2O_2-dependent changes in fluorescence can be determined with a fluorescence microplate reader.

The nitroblue tetrazolium (NBT) test is a qualitative assay of O_2^- production. Either whole blood or isolated neutrophils are mixed with NBT in a chamber slide and stimulated with PMA for 15–30 minutes at 37°C. The neutrophils are allowed to settle on the slide. The slide is air-dried, counterstained with 0.1% safranin, and examined under a microscope. The NBT test yields a visual record of the reduction of the NBT dye to the insoluble, blue-black deposits of formazan. Normal neutrophils, but not neutrophils from CGD patients, reduce the yellow dye to black-brown blue aggregates in the cells (Fig. 99.4). Because of the random inactivation of the X chromosome, X-linked carriers of CGD exhibit both NBT (+) and NBT (−) neutrophils. The percentage of NBT (+) neutrophils in X-linked carriers of CGD ranges from 5% to 95%. The drawback of the NBT test is the manual counting necessary to obtain an accurate reflection of the percentage of positive cells. The NBT can be used to diagnose X-linked carriers of CGD but cannot differentiate autosomal carriers from normal subjects.

An alternative to the NBT test is a flow cytometric assay using the dye, dihydrorhodamine-1,2,3.[24] Neutrophils are loaded with the nonfluorescent dye, and then stimulated with PMA for 15 minutes at 37°C. The H_2O_2 produced oxidizes the dye and results in increased fluorescence, detectable with a flow cytometer. Catalase is added to prevent cell-to-cell diffusion of H_2O_2. Since dye is localized to the cytoplasm, and catalase is present in the extracellular fluid, the dihydrorhodamine-1,2,3 assay detects the intracellular production of reactive oxygen metabolites. As shown in Figure 99.5, stimulation of normal neutrophils (A) with PMA results in a two-log shift in the fluorescence intensity. Neutrophils from an X-linked carrier of CGD (B) exhibit mosaicism with a negatively stained (abnormal) population and a brightly stained positive population. Neutrophils from a patient with X-linked CGD that lack gp91phox (C) express little increase in fluorescence while neutrophils from a patient with a deficiency in p47phox exhibit a slight increase in fluorescence. The major advantages of the dihydrorhodamine-1,2,3 assay are the sensitivity, the signal-to-noise ratio, and the ease of counting a large number of cells. Moreover, it has been shown that the dihydrorhodamine-1,2,3 assay yields reliable results on ethylenediaminetetraacetic acid (EDTA) or heparin-treated blood samples that have been stored overnight. In general, more than 90% of the neutrophils from the control blood samples will exhibit increased dihydrorhodamine-1,2,3 fluorescence. For this same reason, however, overnight samples should not be used

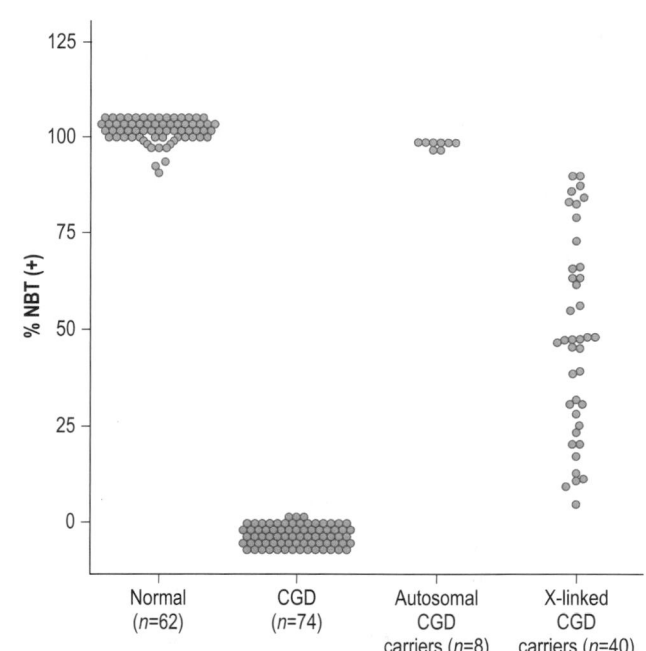

Fig. 99.4 Nitroblue tetrazolium tests from normal subjects, chronic granulomatous disease (CGD) patients, and CGD carriers. Neutrophils (1×10^6/ml HBSS) were incubated in the presence of nitroblue tetrazolium (1 mg/ml) and phorbol myristate acetate (PMA: 100 ng/ml) for 30 minutes at 37°C in a slide chamber. The slide was washed twice with HBSS and counterstained with safranin O. Two hundred cells were manually counted using a microscope and scored as the percent nitroblue tetrazolium (+).

to rule out X-linked heterozygosity since a highly lyonized CGD carrier (> 90%) could yield similar results.

■ BACTERICIDAL ACTIVITY ■

CLINICAL INDICATIONS AND IMPLICATIONS

Assessment of bactericidal activity is a general test that encompasses a broad spectrum of neutrophil function. To show normal bactericidal activity, the neutrophil must be able to recognize and ingest bacteria, and then activate a potent microbicidal response that may include both oxidative and nonoxidative mechanisms.

PRINCIPLES AND INTERPRETATION OF LABORATORY ASSESSMENT

Challenging neutrophils with viable bacteria at a fixed bacteria:neutrophil ratio is a useful assay to assess the ability of neutrophils to recognize, ingest, and kill bacteria. In our laboratory, we typically use *Staphylococcus aureus*, substrain 502A. The bacteria are suspended in trypticase soy broth and grown in a shaker water bath at 37°C, monitoring growth until the bacteria are in log phase. In order to add a known number of bacteria, preliminary studies should be performed to determine the number of viable bacteria (i.e., colonies) versus the $OD_{650 \text{ nm}}$. In our laboratory, an $OD_{650 \text{ nm}}$ of 0.250 yields $0.8–1 \times 10^8$ bacteria/ml.

■ REFERENCES ■

1. Bainton DF. The cells of inflammation: a general view. In: Weissman G, (ed) The Cell Biology of Inflammation, 2nd edn. New York: Elsevier/North-Holland, 1980.

2. Athens JW, Raabs SO, Haab OP, et al. Leukokinetic studies. IV. The total blood, circulating and marginal pool and the granulocyte turnover rate in normal subjects. J Clin Invest 1961; 40: 989.

3. Bainton DF. Developmental biology of neutrophils and eosinophils. In: Gallin JI, Snyderman R, (eds) Inflammation: Basic Principles and Correlates, 3rd edn. Philadelphia, PA: Lippincott Williams & Wilkins, 1999.

4. Hallett MB. The significance of stimulus-response coupling in the neutrophil for physiology and pathology. In: Hallett MB, (ed) The Neutrophil: Cellular Biochemistry and Physiology, Boca Raton, FL: CRC Press, 1989.

5. Springer TA. Adhesion receptors of the immune system. Nature 1990; 346: 425.

6. Kishimoto TK, Baldwin ET, Anderson DC. The role of β2 integrins in inflammation. In: Gallin JI, Snyderman R, (eds) Inflammation: Basic Principles and Correlates, 3rd edn. Philadelphia, PA: Lippincott Williams & Wilkins; 1999.

7. Gallin JI, Rosenthal AS. The regulatory role of divalent cations in human granulocyte chemotaxis. Evidence for an association between calcium exchanges and microtubule assembly. J Cell Biol 1974; 62: 594.

8. Vaporciyan AA, Delisser HM, Yan H-C, et al. Involvement of platelet-endothelial cell adhesion molecule-1 in neutrophils recruitment in vivo. Science 1993; 262: 1580.

9. Shaw DR, Griffin FM Jr. Phagocytosis requires repeated triggering of macrophage phagocytic receptors during particle ingestion. Nature 1981; 289: 409.

10. Borregaard N, Cowland BJ. Granules of the human neutrophilic polymorphonuclear leukocyte. Blood 1997; 89: 3503.

11. Volpp BD, Nauseef WM, Clark RA. Two cytosolic neutrophil oxidase absent in autosomal recessive chronic granulomatous disease. Science 1988; 242: 1295.

12. Parkos CA, Dinauer MC, Walker LE, et al. Primary structure and unique expression of the 22-kilodalton light chain of human neutrophil cytochrome b. Proc Natl Acad Sci USA 1988; 85: 3319.

13. Segal AW, Cross AF, Garcia RC. Absence of cytochrome b-245 in chronic granulomatous disease: a multicenter European evaluation of its incidence and relevance. N Engl J Med 1983; 308: 245.

14. Kuijpers TW, Tool ATJ, van der Schoot CE, et al. Membrane surface antigen expression on neutrophils: a reappraisal of the use of surface markers for neutrophil activation. Blood 1991; 78: 1105.

15. Boyum A. Isolation of mononuclear cells and granulocytes from human peripheral blood. Scand J Clin Lab Invest 1968; 21: 77.

16. Haslett C, Guthrie LA, Kopaniak MM, et al. Modulation of multiple neutrophil functions by preparative methods or trace concentrations of bacterial lipopolysaccharide. Am J Pathol 1985; 119: 101.

17. Buescher EB, Gaither T, Nath J, et al. Abnormal adherence-related functions of neutrophils, monocytes, and Epstein–Barr virus-transformed B cells in a patient with C3bi receptor deficiency. Blood 1985; 65: 1382.

18. Anderson DC, Schmalsteig FC, Finegold MJ, et al. The severe and moderate phenotypes of inheritable Mac-1, LFA-1 deficiency: their quantitative definition and relation to leukocyte dysfunction and clinical features. J Infect Dis 1985; 152: 668.

19. Etzioni A, Frydmann M, Pollack S, et al. Recurrent severe infections caused by a novel leukocyte adhesion deficiency. N Engl J Med 1992; 327: 1789.

20. Kuhns DB, DeCarlo E, Hawk DM, et al. Dynamics of the cellular and humoral components of the inflammatory response in skin blisters in humans. J Clin Invest 1992; 89: 1734.

21. Frevert CW, Wong VA, Goodman RB, et al. Rapid fluorescence-based measurement of neutrophil migration in vitro. J Immunol Methods 1998; 213: 41.

22. Anderson DC, Springer TA. Leukocyte adhesion deficiency: and inherited defect in the Mac-1, LFA-1, and p150, 95 glycoproteins. Annu Rev Med 1987; 38: 175.

23. Kuhns DB, Long Priel DA, Gallin JI. Endotoxin and IL-1 hyporesponsiveness in a patient with recurrent bacterial infections. J Immunol 1997; 158: 3959.

24. Emmendörfer A, Hecht M, Lohmann-Matthes ML, et al. A fast and easy method to determine the production of reactive oxygen intermediates by human and murine phagocytes using dihydrorhodamine-1,2,3. J Immunol Methods 1990; 131: 269.

25. Decleva E, Menegazzi R, Busetto S, et al. Common methodology is indadequate for studies on the microbicidal activity of neutrophils. J Leuk Biol 2006; 79: 87.

Assessment of human allergic diseases

Robert G. Hamilton

100

Human allergic disease comprises a spectrum of IgE-mediated immediate-type hypersensitivity reactions that manifest as reactions in the skin (urticaria, dermatitis), respiratory tract (asthma or rhinitis), gastrointestinal tract and, in their most extreme condition, systemic anaphylaxis. These reactions are precipitated by exposure of a genetically predisposed and sensitized individual to a variety of environmental substances that are ubiquitous and usually well tolerated by most healthy individuals. This chapter reviews the principles and performance characteristics of analytical methods used in the diagnosis and management of individuals with allergic disease. It examines *in vivo* and *in vitro* methods for the quantification of total and allergen-specific IgE. Other analytes used in the diagnostic work-up and management of the allergic patient are discussed including total 'free' IgE, mast cell tryptase, eosinophil cationic protein, precipitating IgG antibodies, and the environmental assessment of aeroallergens in indoor environments.

■ BIOLOGICAL PROPERTIES OF IGE ■

In 1921, Prausnitz and Kustner (PK)[1] reported that an intradermal injection of serum from an allergic individual into the skin of an unsensitized (nonallergic) individual, followed 24 hours later by injection of specific antigen into the same skin site, induced local itching and swelling surrounded by a zone of erythema. This passively transferred allergic or *PK reaction* reached a maximum within 10 minutes, persisted for about 20 minutes, and gradually disappeared. The antibody mediating this reaction was shown to be thermolabile, losing its sensitizing activity after heating serum at 56°C for several hours. In 1967, this antibody was identified as a fifth human immunoglobulin isotype and designated IgE[2–4] (see also Chapter 4).

Serum IgE concentrations are the lowest of the five human immunoglobulin isotypes (0–0.0001 g/L, 0.004% of the total adult serum immunoglobulin).[5] Approximately 50% of IgE is localized in the extravascular space. Its short biological half-life in peripheral blood of 1–5 days is due primarily to a relatively high fractional catabolic rate (71% intravascular pool catabolized/day). IgE does not pass the placenta or activate the classic complement pathway. Its reaginic (mast-cell

sensitizing) activity is dependent upon its ability to bind to the α chain of the high-affinity IgE Fc-ε receptor (α-FcεRI) that resides on the membrane surface of basophils and mast cells. The interaction between IgE Fc and the α-FcεRI is blocked by the therapeutic subcutaneous administration of omalizumab (a humanized IgG_1-κ anti-IgE Fc), as discussed below.

■ TOTAL SERUM IGE ■

The concentration of IgE in the serum is highly age dependent.[5] Cord serum IgE concentrations are low, usually <2 kU/l (<4.88 μg/L), because IgE does not readily cross the placenta. Serum IgE levels progressively increase in healthy children up to the age of 10–15 years. The rate of this rise towards adult levels is slower than that of IgG but comparable to the observed rise in IgA. Atopic infants have an earlier and steeper rise in serum IgE levels during their early years compared to age-matched nonatopic controls.[6] Total serum IgE gradually declines in an age-dependent manner from the second to the eighth decades of life.

Clinically, a patient's serum IgE level should be compared to reference intervals established with sera from an age-stratified, healthy skin test-negative (nonatopic) population such as the one reported by Barbee et al.[6] After age 14, serum IgE levels >333 kU/l (>800 μg/L) are considered abnormally elevated and strongly associated with atopic disorders, such as allergic rhinitis, extrinsic asthma and atopic dermatitis. Extreme elevations in serum IgE are commonly observed in parasite infections and are necessary for the diagnosis of the hyper-IgE (Jobs) syndrome. Normal or low total IgE levels in some individuals with asthma suggest that IgE-mediated mechanisms play only a minor or insignificant role in the pathogenesis of their condition. Low total serum IgE levels can thus support the diagnosis of nonallergic (intrinsic) asthma and help to exclude bronchopulmonary aspergillosis. The reported overlap between IgE levels in atopic and nonatopic populations, however, is considerable.[6–8] Thus although an elevated serum IgE can be useful in confirming the clinical diagnosis of allergic respiratory or skin diseases, a low or normal value does not eliminate the possibility of an IgE antibody-mediated mechanism. This is illustrated by the observation that a group of adults with allergic asthma had a mean serum IgE level of 1589 ng/mL (range 55–12750 ng/mL), with only about half of them having IgE concentrations >800 ng/mL. In contrast, approximately 90% of patients with atopic dermatitis had elevated total serum IgE levels (mean 978 kU/L, range 1.3–65208 kU/L, where 1 IU = 2.44 ng). Parasitic infections, selected immunodeficiency states, cancer (Hodgkin's disease, bronchial carcinoma), rheumatoid arthritis, liver disease and atopic dermatitis (eczema) are other disease states that have been associated with a dysregulation of total serum IgE levels. The total serum IgE must therefore be interpreted carefully within the relevant clinical context for each patient.

Owing to the wide overlap between atopic and nonatopic individuals, total serum IgE measurements had largely been surplanted in the diagnosis of allergic disease by the quantification of allergen-specific IgE antibody. However, this changed when IgE became the focus of a novel therapeutic intervention that involved the subcutaneous administration of anti-IgE antibodies specific for the region on the heavy chain of IgE that interacts with α-FcεR1.[9] A recombinant, humanized IgG_{1}-κ monoclonal anti-human IgE Fc (omalizumab) was licensed in 2003 for the treatment of moderate to severe persistent allergic asthma based on the strategy of blocking IgE binding to the α-FcεR1. The binding of omalizumab to IgE *in vivo* reduces both the number of free IgE molecules able to interact with the α-FcεR1 and the number of FcεR1 receptors on the surface of effector cells. The consequence is a reduction in mediator release and allergy symptoms following allergen exposure.[10] Because dosing of omalizumab is dependent on the pre-treatment level of total serum IgE to achieve the desirable molar ratios of omalizumab to IgE of between 10:1 and 50:1, the measurement of total serum IgE has reclaimed a level of importance in the management of allergic disease using omalizumab.

ALLERGEN-SPECIFIC IGE

In contrast to total serum IgE, the presence of allergen-specific IgE antibody on basophils or skin mast cells or in the serum is highly predictive of an individual's propensity to exhibit an allergic response upon re-exposure to that allergen. Before its identification as a novel immunoglobulin in 1967, IgE was only detectable with *in vivo* bioassays (skin test, bronchial or nasal provocation tests). Purification of IgE myeloma protein and the subsequent production of antisera specific for IgE led to the development of the first *in vitro* assay (radioallergosorbent test or RAST) for the detection of allergen-specific IgE antibody in serum.[4, 11] Since then, many commercial variants based on the original noncompetitive cellulose paper disc solid-phase radioallergosorbent test design have been developed.

A number of historical studies have compared the diagnostic sensitivity and specificity of *in vivo* and the early *in vitro* assays in the diagnosis of human allergic disease. Such inter-method comparisons, albeit limited in their scope, have shown that the presence of IgE antibody as measured by serologic immunoassay methods usually agreed well with the presence of IgE detected in leukocyte and mast-cell histamine release assays, and provocation tests such as the skin test, food challenge and inhalation provocation test.[12] However, these early studies emphasized the important issue that detection of IgE antibody either *in vivo* or *in vitro* should be considered at best a confirmatory measurement of sensitization that

supports the diagnosis of allergic disease once a patient's medical, family and environmental histories identify a temporal association between allergic symptoms and allergen exposure. The clinical importance of differences in diagnostic sensitivity between skin test and serologic detection of IgE antibody may be less important for patients with allergies to inhaled (pollen, dust mite and epidermal) allergens than in those facing life-threatening anaphylactic reactions caused by Hymenoptera stings, drug administration or occupational exposure to natural rubber latex allergen. In these latter cases, skin tests are preferable to *in vitro* immunoassay analyses for the detection of allergen-specific IgE antibodies.[13] Immunoassay analyses of IgE antibody in serum may, however, be helpful in certain cases where the patient has taken antihistamines, β-receptor stimulants or high-dose steroids, which can reduce the provocation test's measured response in children, pregnant women and elderly patients, in whom skin testing may not be well tolerated; and when dealing with allergens (e.g., foods, molds) where commercial extracts can be highly variable or labile.[14]

DIAGNOSTIC METHODS

A combination of *in vivo* provocation and *in vitro* laboratory tests may be useful as confirmatory tests to support the clinical diagnosis of allergic disease. The actual tests selected will ultimately depend on the nature of the disease process under investigation (e.g., extrinsic asthma, urticaria/angioedema, rhinitis/sinusitis or anaphylaxis).

INITIAL CLINICAL LABORATORY TESTS

Following a medical history and physical examination, the patient who is suspected of having allergic disease may undergo several preliminary blood tests. A complete blood count and/or a total blood eosinophil count, if performed, should be obtained before any systemic corticosteroids or epinephrine are administered. Normal whole blood eosinophil levels range from 0 to 500 cells/mm^3. Children generally have higher normal levels (mean 240 cells/mm^3, 95% confidence limit = 0–740 cells/mm^3), with peak levels occurring at 4–8 years of age. Most laboratories consider a differential white blood cell count with an eosinophil level >5–10% of the total white cell count to be abnormal. Blood, sputum and nasal secretion eosinophilia is characteristic of asthma, whether or not allergy is present. In a bronchitic sputum specimen, neutrophils predominate. A neutrophilic nasal discharge is characteristic of sinusitis. Other laboratory tests that may be ordered include pulmonary function tests and a chest X-ray or sinus CT, as indicated.

IN VIVO PROVOCATION TESTING

Both the skin test and nasal/bronchial/gastrointestinal provocation tests are useful diagnostic tools for the confirmation of immediate-type hypersensitivity reactions associated with allergic disease, and in the identification of the offending allergens in the work-up for avoidance, or management with pharmacotherapy, immunotherapy or anti-IgE therapy.

SKIN TESTS

Guerin and Watson[15] described a three-phase response that occurs in the skin during an immediate-type skin test reaction following the administration of a stimulus (allergen or histamine-positive control). First, a bluish-white area appears that involves the constriction of capillaries and which typically disappears within minutes. Second, an erythemic peripheral halo or flare appears as a result of arteriole dilatation. Finally, a circular urticarial papule or wheal is observed, as a result of extravasation of plasma into the skin, which is generally maximal by 15–20 minutes. The immediate wheal and flare reaction can be followed by a late-phase reaction 5–6 hours later that appears as a poorly defined edema-like reaction which usually disappears by 24 hours. An allergen extract can be administered either by a prick/puncture or by intradermal injection.[16]

Puncture skin testing involves placing a drop of allergen extract on the skin of the forearm or back and the introduction of allergen into the epidermis by a needle puncture. A variety of single-point, multipoint and bifurcated needles have been used.[17] After the prick or puncture, the excess allergen is removed by blotting with tissue paper or gauze. An immediate reaction (wheal and erythema) is read at 15–20 minutes as it reaches its maximum size. Care is taken to space individual tests sufficiently far from each other as not to produce overlapping erythema. Because of the direct skin irritation, with some crude allergen extracts bleeding can produce false positive results.

The intradermal skin (ID) test is 1000–10 000 times more sensitive by concentration than is the puncture test. A 0.01–0.05 mL volume (optimally 0.02 mL) of diluted allergen extract in a 0.5–1.0 mL syringe is injected intracutaneously through a 26–27 gauge needle. An 0.02 mL injection will initially produce a superficial 2–3 mm diameter bleb. Like the puncture test, the ID skin test is read at 15–20 minutes, when the reaction is maximal. Dilutions of extract >1:1000 w/v are commonly used to minimize false positive irritation and the potential for systemic reactions. Subcutaneous administration of the allergen may lead to a false negative result. The volume of allergen extract that is injected only slightly influences the size of the wheal and flare reaction, whereas its concentration is the most important determinant of final ID skin test results. Intradermal testing allows an investigator to perform a skin test titration to determine quantitatively the patient's skin sensitivity. For serial titration, the same volume (e.g., 0.02 mL) of 3–10-fold serial dilutions of allergen extract is injected into different sites in the skin and the concentration of allergen required to produce a wheal or erythema of a defined mean diameter (e.g., 8 mm wheal) is interpolated. The higher the concentration of allergen required to induce the defined size of wheal or erythema, the less sensitive the patient is to that allergen preparation.

Figure 100.1 shows the relationship between the ng/mL level of *Dermatophagoides pteronyssinus* (*Dpt*, dust mite) specific IgE antibody in sera from 30 dust mite-allergic subjects, as measured in serum by an *in vitro* assay, and the ID skin test midpoint *Dpt* allergen extract titer required to produce an 8 mm wheal in the same individual. Using the same *Dpt* extract in both tests, a higher degree of skin sensitivity (i.e., lower titer of antigen required to induce an 8 mm wheal) was strongly correlated ($r2 = 0.77$, $P < 0.001$) with higher serum IgE antibody levels in those with the higher levels of skin sensitivity (<10 ng/mL midpoint). Figure 100.2 shows the strong correlation in wheal size that is observed in the same *Dpt*-allergic patients receiving the same dust mite extract in a single puncture skin test and a midpoint intradermal skin test titration.

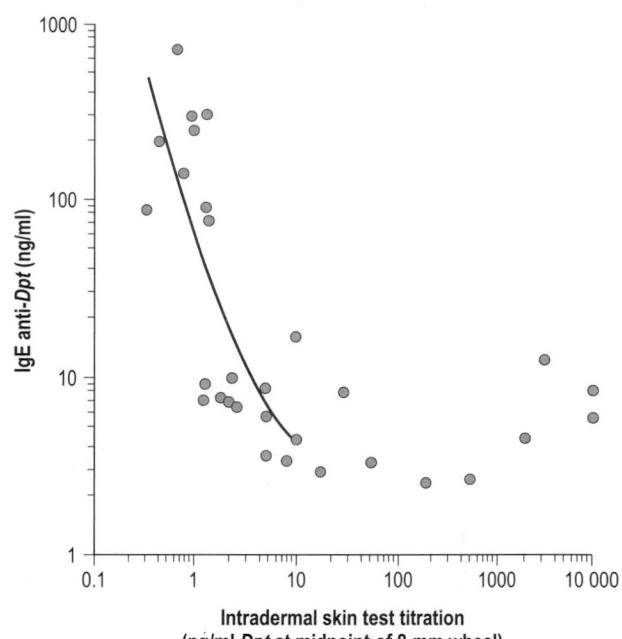

Fig. 100.1 Relationship between IgE anti-*D. pteronyssinus* (*Dpt*) in the skin (x-axis, intradermal skin test titration; ng/mL of *Dpt* required to produce an 8mm wheal) and in the serum serum (y axis, ng/ml of IgF anti-*Dpt* as measured by RAST; sensitivity = 2 ng/mL). These results were obtained by testing the skin and serum of 30 dust mite-allergic individuals with varying degrees of clinical sensitivity using the same *Dpt* extract in both the RAST and the ID skin test titration study. A lower 'titer' of antigen required to induce an 8 mm wheal (e.g., higher degree of skin sensitivity) was strongly correlated ($r = 0.77$; $P < 0.001$) with a higher serum IgE antibody level in individuals with the higher level of skin sensitivity (<10 ng/mL midpoint). Less sensitive patients (titers >10 ng/mL *Dpt*) had lower levels of serum antibody (2–15 ng/mL) that did not relate well with skin sensitivity.

Both the puncture and the ID skin test procedures produce a maximal wheal and flare size by 15–20 minutes, which is measured with a millimeter ruler or caliper. The maximal diameter and the midpoint perpendicular diameter are averaged to generate an index. A permanent record of the skin reaction can be made by applying adhesive cellulose tape over the wheal and flare skin area, which has previously been outlined with a felt-tip or ballpoint pen. Using a single concentration of allergen, the ID skin test can be graded according to one of several reported systems[16, 17] (Table 100.1). Alternatively, a midpoint titer may be interpolated from a skin test titration including serial three or 10-fold dilutions of the allergen extract. Some investigators prefer to use the erythema (flare) size rather than the wheal size obtained during titration studies because the slope of the flare's regression line with dose is steeper.[18] The strong relationship between the size of the intradermal erythema and wheal observed with the mean of 304 duplicate skin tests is shown in Figure 100.3. This relationship is useful to know, because in many dark-skinned subjects the erythema is difficult or impossible to assess.

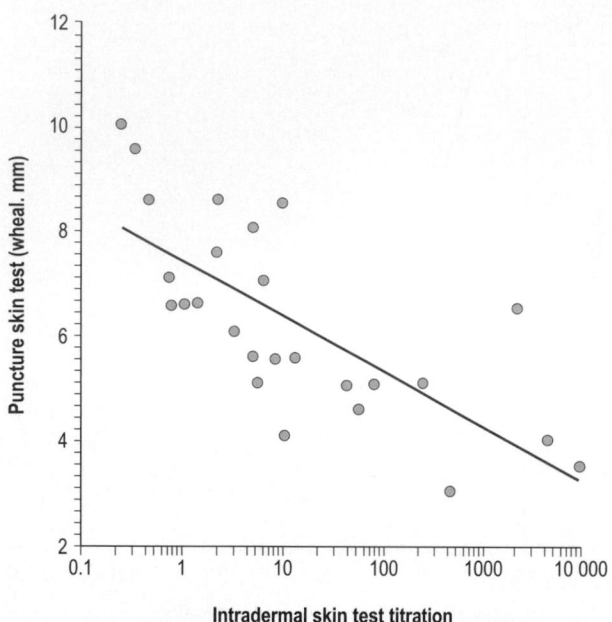

Fig. 100.2 The wheal size in millimeters at a single dose of *Dpt* allergen administered in a puncture skin test compared to the titer or ng/mL of the same *Dpt* allergen obtained in an ID skin test titration on the same 26 dust mite-allergic patients to produce an 8 mm wheal. These data indicate that the wheal size obtained with a single dose of allergen by the less labor-intensive puncture skin test is as predictive ($r2 = 0.72$, $P < 0.001$) of relative patient sensitivity as the more technically complex intradermal skin test titration study, which involves the administration of seven increasing concentrations of the same allergen into different skin sites.

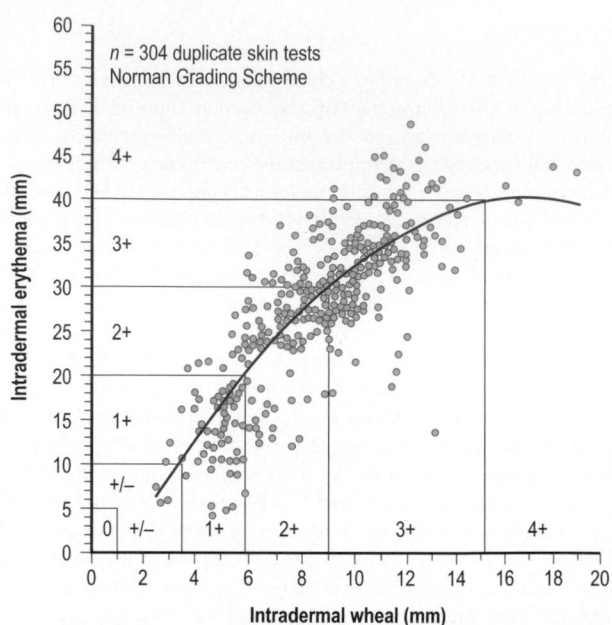

Fig. 100.3 Correlation plot of the mean wheal (*x*-axis) and erythema (*y* axis) in millimeters for the mean of 304 duplicate intradermal skin tests to dust mite (*D. pteronyssinus*) obtained in a population of dust mite-sensitive individuals. The relationship is highly correlated ($r = 0.82$, $P < 0.001$) in grades 0–3+, indicating that either can be used to judge the degree of intradermal skin sensitivity. In highly allergic individuals (>35 mm erythema), however, the slope declines dramatically, indicating that wheal size may be more discriminating than erythema.

BRONCHIAL AND NASAL PROVOCATION TESTS

Bronchial and nasal provocation challenges are performed primarily as research procedures to identify a relationship between an inhaled substance and a change in the patient's bronchial or nasal physiology. Bronchoprovocation studies with methacholine can also be useful in the diagnosis of difficult cases of asthma. The bronchoprovocation procedure involves the administration of either methacholine or histamine via a calibrated nebulizer, starting at doses of 0.05–0.1 mg/mL and doubling the concentration up to 10–25 mg/mL. Alternatively, allergen extracts can be administered in increasing doses. Pulmonary function is monitored after each dose. A positive response is usually defined as the concentration of agonist that results in a drop in the forced expiratory volume per second (FEV_1) of 20% or more from the baseline (which must be >70% of that predicted for valid interpretation). More extensive details regarding the methods and interpretation of bronchial challenges are presented elsewhere.[19]

Nasal provocation in its simplest form involves the controlled administration of buffer (human serum albumin–saline) or increasing concentrations of allergen into a washed nasal passage. The symptoms (e.g., number of sneezes) induced and/or mast cell mediators released into nasal lavage fluids (e.g., TAME esterase and histamine) after each concentration of allergen indicates the relative level of sensitivity to that allergen. Nasal airway resistance is a less satisfactory end-point because of high intrinsic variations. Details of the procedure and applications can be found elsewhere.[20]

A hooded exposure chamber has been described for simultaneous nasal and bronchial challenges as a diagnostic procedure for assessing occupationally induced latex allergy.[21] The challenge involves bathing the subject's conjunctiva and upper and lower airways with air alone, placebo (untreated) cornstarch, and then graded concentrations of latex cornstarch, each for 3-minute intervals separated by 15 minutes. Following each challenge the peak expiratory flow rates (PEFR) and chest and rhinoconjunctival symptoms scores are monitored.[22] This procedure has been particularly useful in problematic diagnostic cases involving a discordant clinical history and IgE anti-latex skin test and/or serological test result.

DOUBLE-BLIND PLACEBO-CONTROLLED FOOD CHALLENGE

Food-induced gastrointestinal reactions (e.g., nausea, colic, vomiting and diarrhea) may occur minutes to hours after the consumption of food allergens by a sensitized individual.[23] Commonly eaten foods

Table 100.1 Grading system for puncture and intradermal skin testing using histamine as a reference[a], [b] (Modified from Norman PS. Skin testing. In: Middleton E, Ellis EF, Reed CE, eds. Allergy: principles and practice, 2nd edn. St Louis: CV Mosby, 1982, with permission from Elsevier.)

Skin testing grading system

Grade or Class	Wheal size (mm)	Erythema size (mm)
0	No discernible wheal	
1+	$\leq \frac{1}{2} \times$ histamine wheal	
2+	$> \frac{1}{2} \times$ histamine and $< 1 \times$ histamine wheal	
3+	= size of histamine wheal ± 1mm	
4+	$> 1 \times$ histamine wheal and $< 2 \times$ histamine wheal	
5+	$> 2 \times$ histamine wheal	

Alternative skin test grading system for intradermal skin testing only involving interpretation of wheal and erythema responses[b]

0	<5	<5
+/−	5–10	5–10
1+	5–10	11–20
2+	5–10	21–30
3+	10–15	31–40
4+	> 15 with pseudopods	41–50

[a]Prick/puncture histamine (3–10 mg/mL), ID histamine (100 mg/mL). Modified from Norman PS. In: Middleton E, Ellis EF, Reed CE (eds). Allergy: principles and practice, 2nd edn. St. Louis, CV Mosby, 1982.

that are known to contain potent allergens include cow milk (caseins, β-lactoglobulin, α-lactalbumin), chicken egg white (ovalbumin, ovomucoid, ovotransferrin), cereal grains (wheat, rye, barley, oats), legumes (peanut, soybean, white bean), fish and seafood (shrimp, crabs, lobsters, oysters). Diagnosis of a food allergy begins with a medical history, which includes an assessment of diet diaries and elimination diets as necessary. Skin tests and serological tests for IgE antibody to extracted food allergens and open food challenges with fresh and cooked foods may also be used to confirm sensitization to suspected foods. No evidence is available to indicate that food-specific IgG or IgG$_4$ antibody levels have any diagnostic value. The double-blind placebo-controlled food challenge (DBPCFC) is considered the definitive diagnostic test for food allergy.[23, 24] An extensive discussion of the DBPCFC and variables influencing its outcome is presented elsewhere.[23–25]

In 2001, prospectively collected sera from 100 children and adolescents who had been previously evaluated by a skin test and DBPCFC were analyzed in the Phadia ImmunoCAP system for food-specific IgE antibody.[25] The investigators were able to identify a diagnostic level of IgE antibody for egg (7 kIUa/L), milk (17 kIUa/L), peanut (14 kIUa/L) and fish (20 kUa/L), above which they could predict clinical reactivity in this group with more than 95% certainty. They concluded that by measuring the concentration of food-specific IgE antibody with the ImmunoCAP system, it was possible to identify a subset of children who were highly likely (>95%) to experience a clinical reaction to egg, milk, peanut or fish. Quantitative serological measurements for food-specific IgE antibody may therefore be able to eliminate the need for time-consuming DBPCFCs in a significant number of children who are suspected of having food allergy.

CLINICAL LABORATORY (*IN VITRO*) TESTING

Most diagnostic allergy laboratories offer a variety of serological tests that can be useful in the diagnosis and management of human allergic disease. Analytes commonly measured in these laboratories include the total serum IgE, allergen-specific IgE, Hymenoptera venom-specific IgG, the venom-RAST inhibition test, and mast cell α and β tryptase. IgG antibody measurements to allergens other then Hymenoptera venom have not been shown to be clinically useful. Basophil histamine release (BHR), although rarely offered as a clinical test because of the requirement for fresh blood, is a useful investigational method that will also be reviewed in this section.

TOTAL SERUM IgE

Of the diagnostic allergy tests that are performed in the clinical immunology laboratory, total serum IgE is currently the only analyte regulated under the US Clinical Laboratory Improvement Amendment of 1988 (CLIA88). Currently five FDA-cleared commercial assays are used by clinical laboratories in the USA to measure the total level of IgE in serum (see College of American Pathologists [CAP] proficiency survey).[26] At present, free total IgE measurements for patients receiving omalizumab are only available with research enzyme immunoassays,[27] and the clinical utility of free IgE levels in assessing the efficacy of Xolair (anti-IgE) treatment still needs to be confirmed by prospective clinical studies.

Radioisotopes such as ^{125}I have been largely replaced by nonisotopic labels such as enzymes (horseradish peroxidase, alkaline phosphatase, β-galactosidase) or fluorophors. The minimum detectable concentration

KEY CONCEPTS

IgE (REAGINIC) ANTIBODY DETECTION

>> Allergen-specific IgE can be detected in skin test by a puncture or intradermal administration of allergen or in the serum by laboratory-based immunoassays.

>> In general, the intradermal skin test is more sensitive than a puncture skin test, which is roughly comparable to the best *in vitro* methods for IgE antibody detection in serum.

>> Because the results of *in vitro* tests for IgE antibody vary considerably between methods, proficiency testing surveys are essential to evaluate performance.

>> Double-blind placebo-controlled food challenge is the gold standard for definitive diagnosis of food allergies.

of most commercial assays is between 0.5 and 1 μg/L. The inter-method agreement of the different commercial IgE assays is excellent (e.g. inter-method coefficents of variation [CVs] typically <10% for serum IgE levels = 30 kIU/L).[28] Nonatopic age-adjusted reference intervals for total serum IgE must be used for normative interpretation.[5]

ALLERGEN-SPECIFIC IgE

Laboratories performing clinical diagnostic allergy testing need to use an FDA-cleared procedure and perform successfully in an external diagnostic allergy proficiency survey (e.g., CAP SE Survey [26]). Of the 11 earlier versions commercial IgE antibody assays, only three have remained in active use in the USA. The two most widely used (Phadia ImmunoCAP System and Siemens Immulite 2000) are assays that use automated platforms with high-quality control reagents and calibrators. These assays have achieved unsurpassed intra-assay precision and inter-assay reproducibility and a high degree of quantification. Their basic assay design can be traced back to the first IgE antibody assay, the radioallergosorbent test or RAST, reported by Wide et al. in 1967.[11]

The most highly variable component of the IgE antibody assay is the allergen-containing reagent. The US Clinical and Laboratory Standards Institute (CLSI) (formally the National Committee on Clinical Laboratory Standards [NCCLS]) has an established 1997 guideline that is currently being revised.[29] It defines the performance characteristics of immunologic assays for human IgE antibodies to specific allergens and provides a glossary of ~400 allergens of clinical interest. Some of these share structurally similar or cross-reactive epitopes, and others possess entirely unique IgE antibody-binding determinants. Allergens as a whole have been conveniently grouped into extracts of weed pollen, grass pollen, tree pollen, animal epidermals, molds, house dust mites, parasites/insects, occupational allergens, drugs, venoms and foods. Among different species of a genus, such as ragweed (e.g., Canyon, Desert, Giant, Short, Silver, Southern, Western), there is extensive allergenic cross-reactivity. Extensive allergenic cross-reactivity has also been documented within particular pollen groups, such as the grasses (June, Brome, Timothy, Perennial Rye, Fescue, Orchard, Red Top, Salt, Sweet Vernal, Velvet). In contrast, certain grass pollens, such as those produced by Bermuda Grass, Johnson Grass and cultivated corn, oat and wheat, are minimally cross-reactive (allergenically distinct). Variations in the allergenic content of

source materials, the extraction process from the raw source material, allergen-reagent manufacturing methods, differential binding to various allergosorbent supports, instability during storage, heterogeneity of internal reference allergen standards, and differences in characterization procedures (antisera, assays) make the production of reproducible allergens for *in vitro* use a challenge. Table 100.2 lists the most commonly requested allergen specificities that are available as diagnostic products.

The second attribute that varies widely among commercially available IgE antibody assays is the unitage that provides an estimate of IgE antibody content in a serum. The CLSI guideline[29] has been instrumental in establishing expectations for the units reported from IgE antibody assays. Because clinically used allergen-specific IgE antibody immunoassays are now calibrated using a heterologous total IgE calibration curve[30] traceable to the WHO 75/502 IgE international reference preparation, quantitative interpolated results should be reported in kIUa/L. At least for one IgE antibody assay (the ImmunoCAP system), there is evidence that absolute quantification has been achieved. Using IgE chimeric antibodies with adsorption and depletion analysis, 1 kIUa/L of allergen-specific IgE antibody has been shown in this assay to be equivalent to 1 kIU/L of total serum IgE.[31]

Some investigators have proposed that IgE antibody to 10–15 aeroallergen specificities may account for much aeroallergen-related disease. Although the particular 10–15 allergen specificities may vary for children and adults, or for individuals in Europe, Asia and the USA, it has been possible to develop a single 'multiallergen' IgE antibody screening test that is highly predictive of the results obtained by a panel of skin tests or *in vitro* IgE antibody tests. In these assays, a panel (e.g., 10–15) of common complex allergen mixtures crossing the aeroallergen groups are insolubilized on a single solid phase (e.g., Phadiatop) or comparable purified native or recombinant allergens are adsorbed onto triplicate dots of a single solid support (silicone chip).[14, 32] These screening assays are useful in confirming the absence of significant atopic disease in individuals suspected of having an intrinsic or nonIgE-mediated disease process. Their negative predictive value as a single test is higher than total serum IgE in identifying nonatopic individuals. Such a test can minimize the need for multiple *in vivo* or *in vitro* allergen-specific IgE measurements in patients with a low clinical probability of atopic disease. The use of such screening tests in unselected populations sometimes generates positive results of questionable clinical significance, however, as IgE antibody responses are more frequent than is symptomatic disease. Most recently, multiple allergens have been adsorbed in single or multiple bands on one nitrocellulose strip and configured in a lateral flow assay cassette analogous to over-the-counter pregnancy type assays.[33] This semi-quantitative 'point of care' test is designed for use with a drop of whole blood from a finger stick. It is unclear what impact these lateral flow assays will have on the diagnosis of allergic disease when used by patients or primary care physicians.

The quality of allergen-specific IgE antibody results reported from clinical diagnostic allergy laboratories is not uniformly equivalent.[34] For this reason, physicians requesting IgE antibody testing bear some responsibility for determining the quality of the results they receive. In the USA, testing should be performed in a clinical laboratory that is federally licensed for highly complex immunology clinical testing under CLIA-88 (verified by requesting a copy of the federal laboratory license). The requesting physician should inquire about the assay method used, the source of its reagents and how assays are quality controlled by the laboratory.

Table 100.2 Selected allergen specificities

Weeds

Common ragweed (short)
Western ragweed
Giant ragweed (tall)
False ragweed
Wormwood (sagebrush)
Mugwort (sagebrush)
Oxeye daisy
Dandelion
English plantain
Lamb's quarters
Russian thistle
Goldenrod
Cocklebur
Rough pigweed
Scale
Rough marsh elder
Firebrush (Kochia)
Sheep sorrel

Grasses

Sweet vernal
Bermuda
Orchard
Meadow fescue
Timothy
Common reed grass
June Grass–Kentucky
Red top (Bent)
Johnson grass
Brome
Cultivated rye
Velvet
Wheat pollen
Meadow foxtail
Canary (Reed)

Trees

Maple (Box elder)
Alder
BirchParsley
Hazel nut
Beech
Mountain cedar
Oak
Malt
Elm
Olive
Walnut
Sycamore

Willow
White pine
Eucalyptus
Acacla
Mesquite
Melaleuca
Pecan
Italian cypress
Cottonwood
White ash

Epidermals

Cat dander
Dog epithelium
Horse dander
Cow dander
Dog dander
Guineapig epithelium
Pigeon droppings
Goose feathers
Mouse epithelium
Mouse urine proteins
Rat epithelium
Rat urine proteins
Rat serum proteins
Mouse serum proteins
Budgerigar droppings
Budgerigar feathers
Budgerigar serum
Duck feathers

Molds

Penicillium notatum
Cladosporium herbarum
Aspergillus fumigatus
Candida albicans
Alternaria tenuis
Botrytis cinerea blue
Helminthosporium halodes
Fusarium moniliforme
Stemphylium botryosum
Rhizopus nigricans
Aureobasidium pullulans
Phoma betae
Epicoccum purpurascens
Trichoderma viride

House dust mites

Dermatophagoides pteronyssinus
Dermatophagoides farinae

House dust

House dust – Greer
House dust – Hollister Stier

Insects

Cockroach
Mosquito

Occupational

Wild silk
Silk
Isocyanate TDI
Isocyanate MDI
Isocyanate HDI
Ethylene oxide
Phtallic anhydride
Formaldehyde
Natural rubber latex
Cotton seed
Sunflower seed
Trimellitic anhydride
Natural rubber latex

Foods

Egg white
Milk
Codfish
Barley
Oat
Corn
Rice
Sesame seed
Pea
Peanut
Soybean
White bean
Hazel nut
Brazil nut
Almond
Crab
Shrimp
Tomato
Pork
Orange
Potato
Coconut
Tuna
Salmon
Strawberry
Baker's yeast

Continued

Table 100.2 Selected allergen specificities—Cont'd

Garlic	Celery	Human insulin
Apple	Parsley	Protamine
Egg yolk	Melons	Vancomycin
Chicken meat	Lamb	**Venoms**
α-Lactalbumin	Mustard	
β-Lactoglobulin	Malt	White-faced hornet
Casein	Mango	Yellowjacket
Gluten	Cacao	*Polistes* paper wasp
Lobster		Yellow hornet
Cheese (Cheddar)	**Drugs**	Honey bee
Cheese, mold type	Penicilloyl G/V	Bumble bee
Kiwi fruit	Beef/pork insulin	Imported fire ant

COMPETITIVE IGE ANTIBODY INHIBITION ASSAY

The soluble allergen, competitive inhibition format of the IgE antibody assay (e.g., ImmunoCAP, Immulite 2000), or its isotopic counterpart (the RAST inhibition assay), has been widely used by researchers, allergen manufacturers and regulators to determine the relative potency of allergen extracts. One practical research application of the IgE antibody inhibition assay has been as a tool for monitoring the concentration of allergens released into environments (e.g., air sampling of airplanes for aerosolized peanut allergen). Latex allergen, for instance, that is released into the air from powdered latex gloves or onto mucosal surfaces from condoms, or the dental use of latex gloves, has been monitored using this assay as manufacturers change their production methods in an effort to reduce leachable allergen content. In the diagnostic allergy laboratory, the competitive IgE antibody inhibition assay has been used analytically to confirm an IgE antibody assay's minimum detectable dose (sensitivity) and nonspecific binding, and to document the allergen specificity of IgE antibody binding as a part of a quality control program.

The one clinical application of the IgE antibody inhibition assay has been as an adjunct to define the appropriate therapeutic composition of venoms for insect sting-allergic patients who have multiple potentially cross-reactive sensitivities and have elected to receive immunotherapy[35] (Chapter 93). The primary indication for this test is a strong skin reactivity or a high level of serum IgE antibody to Yellow jacket venom (YJV) and a weak skin reactivity or low level of serum IgE antibody specific for *Polistes* wasp venom (PWV). The structural similarity between vespid and *Polistes* wasp phospholipase A1/B (*Ves g* I; *Pol a* I) and hyaluronidase (*Ves g* II; *Pol a* II) frequently produces IgE antibody cross-reactivity. Sera from 305 Hymenoptera venom-allergic patients with >2 ng/mL of IgE antibody to YJV and PWV were evaluated in the IgE antibody inhibition assay to document its utility. The clinical question for these patients was whether PWV should be included in their venom immunotherapy together with Yellow jacket or mixed vespid venom. Using this procedure, the venom RAST inhibition assay identified one-third (36.4%) of subjects with a primary YJV sensitivity who were candidates for exclusion of PWV from their immunotherapy regimen because their IgE anti-PWV was >95% cross-inhibitable with soluble YJV.[35]

CLINICAL PEARLS

CLINICAL UTILITY OF HYMENOPTERA VENOM RAST INHIBITION TEST

>> Useful in identifying venom cross-reactive IgE antibodies and selecting appropriate venoms for immunotherapy.

>> One-third of venom-allergic patients with concomitant Yellowjacket venom (YJV) and *Polistes* wasp venom (PWV) sensitivity can be treated with YJV alone or mixed vespid venoms, owing to >95% cross-reactive IgE anti-PWV with soluble YJV.

ALLERGEN-SPECIFIC IgG

Allergen injections during immunotherapy are known to enhance the production of specific IgG 'blocking' antibodies. Quantitative measurements of total IgG antibodies or IgG subclass antibodies in studies of allergic rhinitis have not generally correlated with the control of clinical symptoms in individual patients. However, clinically successful immunotherapy is almost always accompanied by high serum levels of allergen-specific IgG.[36] In contrast, the presence or levels of IgG antibodies specific for food antigens have shown no correlation with the results of positive double-blind placebo-controlled food challenges.

Allergen-specific IgG antibody measurements may be helpful in determining optimal therapy in patients with Hymenoptera venom sensitivity. In a prospective study, Hymenoptera venom-specific IgG antibodies were monitored in the serum of 109 venom-allergic patients to examine whether IgG antibody levels could predict the risk of a systemic reaction after a sting challenge in patients receiving venom immunotherapy.[37] The highest rate of allergic reactions (26%) occurred in patients who had both a venom-specific IgG antibody level <3 μg/mL and fewer than 4 years of venom immunotherapy.[3] Therefore, quantitative venom-specific IgG antibody levels appear to be of value in individualizing the dose and frequency of injections while maximizing the protective effects. The clinical utility of the IgG antibody measurement may be restricted to the first 4 years of venom immunotherapy

CLINICAL PEARLS

IGG ANTIBODY MEASUREMENTS

>> Clinically successful aeroallergen immunotherapy is almost always accompanied by high serum levels of allergen-specific IgG.

>> Quantitative venom-specific IgG antibody levels can be of value in individualizing venom doses and frequencies for patients on immunotherapy for up to 4 years.

>> Food-specific IgG and IgG4 assay results do not correlate with the results of double-blind placebo-controlled food challenges.

MAST-CELL TRYPTASE

Two types of mast cells have been identified in skin, respiratory and digestive tract connective tissues based on the types of neutral proteases present in their secretory granules. One group contains only tryptase, whereas the other contains both tryptase and chymase[38] (Chapter 22). Upon activation of mast cells, these proteases are released in parallel with pre-stored histamine and newly generated vasoactive mediators. Mast-cell tryptase (MW 134 kDa) is a serine esterase with four subunits, each having an enzymatically active site. A resting mast cell contains 10–35 pg of tryptase that is stored attached to heparin. When dissociated from heparin, it rapidly degrades into its monomers and loses enzymatic activity. As basophils are a rather insignificant source of tryptase release, tryptase in serum has been proposed as a marker of mast-cell activation. The concentration of α-tryptase in blood is considered a measure of mast cell numbers. It is estimated by subtracting the measured β-tryptase level from the total serum tryptase concentration. The level of β-tryptase is considered a measure of mast cell activation.

A noncompetitive two-site fluorescent enzyme immunoassay (Phadia, ImmunoCAP) is available to measure total tryptase in serum.[39] Total tryptase levels in the serum of healthy (nondiseased) adults average 5 μg/L (range 1–10 μg/L). Elevated levels of tryptase (>10 μg/L) can be detected in serum from 1 to 4 hours after the onset of systemic anaphylaxis with hypotension.[40] Baseline levels >20 μg/L suggest systemic mastocytosis. β-tryptase levels <1 μg/L are observed in nondiseased individuals and >1 μg/L indicates mast cell activation. Recommended serum collection times for tryptase quantification range from 30 minutes to 4 hours after the onset of an acute event. Although postmortem specimens are often difficult to analyze for tryptase because of high viscosity related to gross hemolysis, tryptase levels >10 μg/L suggest systemic anaphylaxis as one probable cause of death. Elevated β-tryptase resulting from an insect sting-induced anaphylaxis can peak at more than 5 μg/L by 30–60 minutes after the sting, and then decline with an approximate half-life of 2 hours.[41] This contrasts with histamine, which peaks within 5–10 minutes after an event, and may return to baseline levels in less than 1 hour. Tryptase has also been detected in bronchoalveolar lavage fluid, nasal lavage fluid, tears and skin chamber fluid, but there are currently no clinical indications for such measurements. The diagnostic value of tryptase as a marker of anaphylaxis and mastocytosis is extensively reviewed elsewhere.[42]

BASOPHIL MEDIATOR RELEASE ASSAYS

Histamine release assay

The potent vasoactive mediator histamine is stored in cytoplasmic granules of basophilic leukocytes and mast cells and released along with other mediators of inflammation in response to both immunologic and nonimmunologic stimuli.[37, 43] The basophil histamine release (BHR) assay has been particularly useful as a quantitative assay of allergen potency, and as an *in vitro* model for the study of triggering mechanisms of mediator release from basophils. In its most basic form, peripheral blood leukocytes are isolated from a donor and incubated with varying concentrations (e.g., 3–10-fold dilutions) of allergen extract or anti-human IgE as a positive control. Histamine release is complete within 30 minutes, and then histamine in the supernatant is measured by enzymatic, radiometric or spectrophotofluorometric techniques.[44] Details of the BHR assay are given elsewhere.[44]

Patient sensitivity for a given allergen can be determined with a positive BHR test. The results are highly correlated with those determined by skin testing[44] and bronchoprovocation.[45] Although the BHR test has been most widely used in research laboratories owing to its expense, time-consuming nature and the need for fresh blood (<24 hours old), it can be successfully applied to the clinical diagnosis of allergy in selected cases, as the results obtained parallel those of other IgE antibody tests. BHR has also been a useful tool for clarifying discrepancies between skin test and serological IgE antibody test results.

Leukotriene C4 (LTC4) release assay

An assay method for measuring LTC4 released from allergen-activated basophils has been reported as the cellular antigen stimulation test (CAST)–ELISA.[46] The LTC4 assay is designed for use with either whole blood preparations or washed leukocytes. A number of clinical studies have compared the predictive value of the CAST to skin testing using dust mite, food, Hymenoptera venoms and drugs as challenges. The observed diagnostic sensitivity of the CAST compared to the combination of a clinical history and skin test ranged from 18% with aspirin to 85% for selected food allergens. The reported diagnostic specificity of the CAST in the same studies ranged from 67% to 100%. These data indicate that the CAST assay is not sufficiently sensitive for effective clinical use in the diagnosis of IgE-mediated sensitivities to β-lactam or nonsteroidal anti-inflammatory drugs. Its utility in the diagnosis of sensitization to other allergen specificities appears more promising, but further documentation involving clinical studies is required.[47]

Utility of mediator release assays as diagnostic tests

Despite their unquestioned value as research methods, the basophil histamine and LTC4 release assays are rarely used clinically in the routine diagnosis of human allergic disease. Moreover, it is unlikely that this trend will change in the foreseeable future.

FLOW CYTOMETRY BASOPHIL ACTIVATION ASSAYS

In the late 1990s, basophils were shown to upregulate the expression of a number of surface proteins (e.g., CD45, CD63, CD69 and CD203c) when activated by allergen.[48–50] CD63 is a member of the transmembrane-4

<table>
<tr><td>

CLINICAL PEARLS

INDOOR AEROALLERGEN ANALYSES

>> Predominant indoor aeroallergens include dust mites, cockroaches, epidermal allergens (cat, dog, mouse, rat) and a limited number of molds.

>> Quantitative analysis of house dust samples enables allergic subjects to assess the individual risk for symptoms and/or sensitization in a particular home and to monitor the effects of environmental control.

</td></tr>
</table>

between the means of allergen levels across participating laboratories. The data provided confirmation that aeroallergen results from CLIA-88-licensed reference laboratories that use enzyme immunoassay procedures display a level of accuracy and precision that is acceptable for distinguishing environments with high aeroallergen levels (e.g. expected to trigger asthma in predisposed individuals) from those with lower levels considered to be safe.

Allergens that are measured in reservoir dust can be considered 'indicator' molecules because they allow the clinician and the patient to track the relative levels of associated allergen source(s) by room throughout a house, school or workplace. Figure 100.4 shows a representative distribution of *D. farinae* (*Der f* 1) and *D. pteronyssinus* (*Der p* 1) group 1 allergen levels as measured by enzyme immunoassay in respectively 647 and 741 fine dust specimens from across the USA. Levels of *Der p* 1 and/or *Der f* 1 allergen >2000 ng/g of fine dust have been associated with an increased risk of allergic symptoms in sensitized individuals, whereas levels >10 000 ng/g of fine dust have been associated with an increased risk of sensitization.[60] For cat, *Fel d* 1 levels >8000 ng/g of fine dust have been proposed as a threshold for sensitization. Any cockroach allergen, mouse and rat allergen detected in an environment identifies an indoor area that places individuals allergic to cockroach, mouse or rat at risk for symptoms and sensitization. Finally, viable mold spore levels above 25 000 colonies/g of fine dust place the mold content in the environment above the 75th percentile for homes monitored across the USA. Where these proposed threshold levels are exceeded, the allergic individual is encouraged to take action to reduce the levels. A detailed discussion of strategies for doing this can be found elsewhere.[60] Repeat household dust allergen measurements following an intervention allows monitoring and documentation of allergen reduction.

OUTDOOR ENVIRONMENTS

In most major cities across the USA, aerobiology stations have been established to perform a daily evaluation of the outdoor air for pollen and mold spore levels. Daily information is often transmitted to local weather stations and newspapers for public use, or posted in allergists' offices for their patients to review. An aerobiology network has been established by the American Academy of Allergy, Asthma and Immunology to certify participating laboratories and monitor their performance. This network also collates and disseminates pollen and mold data across the nation throughout the allergy season.

REFERENCES

1. Prausnitz C, Kustner H. Studine uber die Ueberempfindlichkeil. Zentrabl Bakteriol Mikrobiol Hyg 1921; 86: 160.

2. Ishizaka K, Ishizaka T. Physiochemical properties of reaginic antibody. I. Association of reaginic activity with an immunoglobulin other than gamma A or gamma G globulin. J Allergy 1967; 37: 169.

3. Johansson SGO. Raised levels of a new immunoglobulin class (IgND) in asthma. Lancet 1967; 2: 951.

4. Hamilton RG. The science behind the discovery of IgE. J Allergy Clin Immunol 2005; 115: 648.

5. Hamilton RG. Human immunoglobulins. In: Leffell MS, Rose N, eds: Handbook of human immunology, Boca Raton: CRC Press, 1998; 65–109.

6. Barbee RA, Halomen M, Lebowitz M, et al. Distribution of IgE in a community population sample: correlations with age, sex and allergen skin test reactivity. J Allergy Clin Immunol 1981; 68: 106.

7. Wittig HJ, Belloit J, DeFillippi I, et al. Age-related serum IgE levels in healthy subjects and in patients with allergic disease. J Allergy Clin Immunol 1980; 66: 305.

8. Dati F, Ringel KP. Reference values for serum IgE in healthy nonatopic children and adults. Clin Chem 1982; 28: 1556.

9. Cameron L, Vercelli D. Synthesis and regulation of immunoglobulin E. In: Adkinson NF Jr., Yunginger JW, Busse WW, et al. eds: Allergy: principles and practice, 6th edn. Philadelphia: Mosby, 2003; 87.

10. Lin H, Boesel KM, Griffith DT, et al. Omalizumab rapidly decreases nasal allergic response and FcεR1 on basophils. J Alllergy Clin Immunol 2004; 113: 297.

11. Wide L, Bennich H, Johansson SGO. Diagnosis by an in vitro test for allergen specific antibodies. Lancet 1967; 2: 1105.

12. Yunginger JW, Ahlstedt S, Eggleston PA, et al. Quantitative IgE antibody assays in allergic diseases. J Allergy Clin Immunol 2000; 105: 1077.

13. Hamilton RG. Diagnostic methods for insect sting allergy. [Review]. Curr Opin Allergy Clin Immunol 2004; 4: 297.

14. Hamilton RG, Adkinson NF Jr.. In vitro assays for IgE mediated sensitivities. [Review] J Allergy Clin Immunol 2004; 114: 213–225.

15. Guerin B, Watson RD. Skin tests. Clin Rev Allergy 1988; 6: 211.

16. DemolyPiette PV, Bousquet J. In vivo methods for study of allergy: Skin tests, techniques and interpretation. In: Adkinson NF Jr., Yunginger JW, Busse WW, et al. eds: Allergy: principles and practice, 6th edn. Philadelphia: Mosby, 2003; 631.

17. Nelson HS. In vivo testing for immunoglobulin E mediated sensitivity. In: Leung DYM, Sampson HA, Geha RS, Szefler SJ, eds: Pediatric allergy: principles and practice, Philadelphia: Mosby, 2003; 243.

18. Turkeltaub PC, Rastogi SC, Baer H, et al. A standardized quantitative skin test assay of allergen potency and stability. Studies on the allergen dose-response curve and effect of wheal, erythema and patient selection on assay results. J Allergy Clin Immunol 1982; 70: 343.

19. Fish JE, Peters SP. Bronchial challenge testing. In: Adkinson NF Jr., Yunginger JW, Busse WW, et al. eds: Allergy: principles and practice, 6th edn. Philadelphia: Mosby, 2003; 657.

20. Rajakulasingam K. Nasal provocation testing. In: Adkinson NF Jr., Yunginger JW, Busse WW, et al. eds: Allergy: principles and practice, 6th edn. Philadelphia: Mosby, 2003; 644.

21. Kurtz KM, Hamilton RG, Adkinson NF Jr. Role and application of provocation in the diagnosis of occupational latex allergy. Ann Allergy Asthma Immunol 1999; 83: 634.

22. Pipkorn U, Granerus G, Proud D. The effect of a histamine synthesis inhibitor on the immediate nasal allergic reaction. Allergy 1987; 42: 496.

23. Sampson HA. Adverse reactions to foods. In: Adkinson NF Jr., Yunginger JW, Busse WW, et al. eds: Allergy: principles and practice, 6th edn. Philadelphia: Mosby, 2003; 1619.

24. Bock SA, Sampson HA, Atkins FM, et al. Double-blind placebo controlled food challenge as an office procedure: a manual. J Allergy Clin Immunol 1988; 82: 986.

25. Sampson HA. Utility of food specific IgE concentrations in predicting symptomatic food allergy. J Allergy Clin Immunol 2001; 107: 891.

26. Diagnostic Allergy [SE-A-2006] Proficiency Survey Participant Summary, College of American Pathologists (CAP). 325 Waukegan Road, Northfield, IL 60093–2750: p 1–21.

27. Hamilton RG, Marcotte GV, Saini SS. Immunological methods for quantifying free and total serum IgE in asthma patients receiving Omalizumab (Xolair) therapy. J Immunol Meth 2005; 303: 81–91.

28. Hamilton RG. Accuracy of Food and Drug Administration-cleared IgE antibody assays in the presence of anti-IgE (Omalizumab). J Allergy Clin Immunol 2006; 117: 759–766.

29. National Committee on Clinical Laboratory Standards [currently Clinical and Laboratory Standards Institute] (Matsson P, Hamilton RG, eds) Evaluation methods and analytical performance characteristics of immunological assays for human IgE antibody of defined allergen specificities: approved guideline 1/LA20-A, 1997.

30. Hamilton RG, Butler JE. Quantitation of specific antibodies: methods of expression, standards solid phase considerations and specific applications. In: Butler JE, ed: Immunochemistry of solid phase immunoassays. Boca Raton: CRC Press, 1991; Chapter 9.

31. Kober A, Perborn H. Quantitation of mouse-human chimeric Allergen-specific IgE antibodies with ImmunoCAP technology. J Allergy Clin Immunol 2006; 117: S219. [Abstract 845].

32. Jahn-Schmid B, Harwanegg C, Hiller R, et al. Allergen microarray: comparison to microarray using recombinant allergens with conventional diagnostic methods to detect allergen-specific serum immunoglobulin E. Clin Exp Allergy 2003; 33: 1443–1449.

33. Nystrand M, Kober A, Stderstrom L. A semi-quantitative point of care (POC) test for rapid detection of specific IgE antibodies. J Allergy Clin Immunol 2006; 117: S219. [Abstract 844].

34. Wood RA, Segall N, Ahlstedt S, Williams PB, Accuracy of IgE antibody laboratory results. Ann Allergy Asthma Immunol 2007; 99: 34–41.

35. Hamilton RG, Wisenauer JA, Golden DB, et al. Selection of Hymenoptera venoms for immunotherapy based on patient's IgE antibody crossreactivity. J Allergy Clin Immunol 1993; 92: 651.

36. Lichtenstein LM, Norman PS, Winkenwerder WL. A single year of immunotherapy of ragweed hay fever: immunologic and clinical studies. Ann Intern Med 1971; 75: 663.

37. Golden DBK, Lawrence ID, Hamilton RG, et al. Clinical correlation of the venom-specific IgG antibody level during maintenance venom immunotherapy. J Allergy Clin Immunol 1992; 90: 386.

38. Craig CS, Schwartz LB. Tryptase and chymase: markers of distinct types of human mast cells. Immunol Res 1989; 8: 130.

39. Enander I, Matsson P, Anderson AS, et al. A radioimmunoassay for human serum tryptase released during mast cell activation. J Allergy Clin Immunol 1990; 85: 154–159.

40. Van der Linden PW, Hack CE, Poortman J, et al. Insect sting challenge in 138 patients: relation between clinical severity of anaphylaxis and mast cell activation. J Allergy Clin Immunol 1992; 90: 110–118.

41. Miller JS, Schwartz LB. Tryptase levels as an indication of mast cell activation in a patient with Hymenoptera anaphylaxis and mastocytosis. N Engl J Med 1987; 316: 1622.

42. Schwartz LB. Diagnostic value of tryptase in anaphylaxis and mastocytosis. Immunol Allergy Clin North Am. 2006; 26: 451–463.

43. Lichtenstein LM, Osler AG. Studies on the mechanisms of hypersensitivity phenomenon. IX. Histamine release from human leukocytes by ragweed pollen. J Exp Med 1964; 120: 507.

44. Siraganian RP. Automated histamine analysis for in vitro allergy testing. II. Correlation of skin test results with in vitro whole blood histamine release in 82 patients. J Allergy Clin Immunol 1977; 59: 214.

45. Wegner F, Hockamp R, Rutschke A, et al. Superiority of the histamine release test above case history, prick test and radioallergosorbent test in predicting bronchial reactivity to the house dust mite in asthmatic children. Klin Wochenschr 1983; 61: 43.

46. de Weck AL. Cellular allergen stimulation test (CAST): a new dimension in allergy diagnostics. ACI News 1993; 1/5: 9–14.

47. Maly FE, Marti-Wyss S, Blumber S, et al. Mononuclear blood cell sulpholeukotriene generation in the presence of interleukin 3 and whole blood histamine release in honeybee and yellow jacket venom allergy. J Invest Allergy Clin Immunol 1997; 7: 217–224.

48. Moneret-Vautrin DA, Sainte-Laudy J, Kanny G, Fremont S. Human basophil activation as measured by CD63 expression and LTC4 release in IgE mediated food allergy. Ann Allergy Asthma Immunol 1999; 82: 33.

49. Bochner BS, Sterbinsky SA, Saini SA, et al. Studies of cell adhesion and flow cytometric analyses of degranulation, surface phenotype and viability using human eosinophils, basophils and mast cells. Methods 1997; 13: 61–68.

50. Sanz ML, Gamboa PM, Antepara I. Flow cytometric basophil activation test by detection of CD63 expression in patients with immediate type reactions to beta lactam antibiotics. Clin Exp Allergy 2002; 32: 277–286.

51. Buhring HJ, Sieffert M, Giesert C. The basophil activation marker defined by antigen 97A6 is identical to ectonucleotide pyrophosphate/phosphodiesterase 3. Blood 2001; 97: 3303–3305.

52. Platz I, Binder M, Marxer A, et al. Hymenoptera venom induced up regulation of basophil activation marker ecto-nucleotide pyrophosphatase/phosphoesterase 3 (E-NNP3, CD203c) in sensitized individuals. Int Arch Allergy Immunol 2001; 126: 335–342.

53. Ebo DG, Hagendorens MM, Bridts CH, et al. In vitro allergy diagnosis: should we follow the flow?. [Review] Clin Exp Allergy 2004; 34: 332–339.

KEY CONCEPTS

HUMAN GENOMICS

>> The human genome encompasses approximately 25 000 protein-coding genes, but each cell expresses only a subset of those genes.

>> Genetic and physical maps of the genome are essential to molecular diagnosis of immune system diseases.

>> Genetic maps depend on the co-inheritance of DNA segments – linkage – to derive gene order on individual chromosomes.

>> Physical maps of the genome describe the exact gene locations on a chromosome. The genome DNA sequence is the finest-scale physical map of the genome.

allele frequency with the age of polymorphism, i.e., the older the polymorphism the greater the allele frequency and the greater the likelihood that it will be observed in all ethnic groups. Indeed, the more common allele is most often ancestral within the whole human population, in the sense that it is generally the base observed at the homologous position in chimpanzee and other primates. Polymorphisms are the key to tracking the inheritance of whole segments of adjacent DNA and are thus used to follow disease genes in families.

During the formation of the haploid germ cells – ova and sperm – one member (homolog) of each parental chromosome pair is segregated to one of two daughter nuclei (first meiotic division; Fig. 101.1). Because each chromosome is essentially independent of the others, genes on different chromosomes are independently segregated and unlinked. If any position along a pair of chromosomes differs between the two, then the variants are called *alleles*. The arrangement of alleles along a chromosome is called the *haplotype*. For each autosome there are literally two chromosome-length haplotypes per individual. During meiosis, *recombination* between homologous chromosomes leads to intermixing of the two parental genomes. Each chromosome may cross over an average of two to three segments per meiosis. When loci are close together on the same chromosome there is less chance for recombination between them and the *phase* in which they start is more likely to be unaltered through meiosis (Fig. 101.2). If the loci are far apart on a chromosome then it is likely that at least one crossover will come between them during meiosis. Because the physical distance between two loci determines whether they will be inherited as a block during meiosis, a statistical relationship can be developed that indicates how likely two segments are to be co-inherited. *Linkage* between two loci can be quantified as the recombination fraction $-\theta$. Linkage is present if the fraction of recombination is <0.5 (i.e., a 50:50 chance of co-inheritance). θ is often expressed in centimorgans (cM), so that if two loci are 1 cM apart then there is a 1% chance of recombination at meiosis. 1 cM is on average equivalent to approximately 1 million base pairs (bp) of DNA. However, the recombination rate between two loci can be affected by factors other than physical distance, e.g., the presence of repeat sequences that may favor recombination or proximity to the centromere that may suppress recombination. The same processes of haplotype formation and shuffling of haplotype segments by recombination along chromosomes shapes the correlations between markers in the population as whole.

Genes can be mapped in relation to one another by a linkage map. Genes that are physically close can be shown to be predominantly co-inherited. The usual way to express this relationship within a family linkage study is with the LOD score – log of the odds of linkage – which compares the chance of two gene segments being co-inherited with the situation in which they are unlinked. Conventionally, if the LOD is >3.0 (or 1000:1 in favor of the genes being linked) the results are considered significant. One major achievement of the human genome project has been to develop linkage maps for humans. The use of marker loci that show a high degree of polymorphism is particularly useful for this. Whereas linkage in this sense is best observed in families, the same phenomenon persists at a very fine scale in the population. The correlation of alleles among markers that are very close to each other in the genome is called *linkage disequilibrium* (LD). LD occurs because the mutation that creates a polymorphism occurs on a single chromosome. Then various demographic factors (drift, migration, and selection) cause the variant to become more frequent over time. The arrangement of alleles, however, is broken up by recombination over time as well. Hence, only markers that are relatively close to each other continue to have significant LD. A large international project (HapMap) has recently created a dense map of SNP markers allowing a view of LD in several reference populations.

Linkage mapping played a large role in the identification of the X-linked immunodeficiency genes (Chapters 21, 34–36). Linkage has been much less useful for the identification of autosomal recessive genes responsible for rare immunodeficiencies because average families are not large enough to be used by themselves. Another difficulty is that similar diseases can be caused by mutation in more than one gene locus (locus heterogeneity). Extremely dense LD maps have recently become available,[2] and these are expected to facilitate the identification of many more disease genes using powerful new study designs in large populations.

PHYSICAL MAPS AND MOLECULAR CYTOGENETICS

Genetic or linkage maps can be contrasted with the physical gene map. Physical maps are different from the genetic map in that they describe how genes are arranged in the DNA on a scale as large as a whole chromosome and as fine as a single nucleotide. At the coarsest level of the physical map, genes are placed in chromosome segments corresponding to the Giemsa stain banding pattern of metaphase chromosomes. This physical map is encompassed in a set of bacterial artificial chromosome (BAC) clones that have DNA inserts of approximately 90 000–250 000 nucleotides that provided the scaffold for the public genome sequencing project. BAC clones now provide extremely useful reagents for both research and clinical purposes.

A very important way to localize genes after they have been cloned is to hybridize them directly to a chromosome spread. The technique, called fluorescence in situ hybridization (FISH), allows the detection of signals from the chromosome spread to directly localize genes.[3] FISH is used for cytogenetic examination of tumors, leukemias, and lymphomas. In the DiGeorge syndrome, characteristic deletions of chromosomes 22q11 or 10p13 cannot be detected by chromosome analysis only (Chapter 35). FISH is now gradually being replaced by microarray comparative genome hybridization (CGH), which examines many hundreds of chromosomal positions simultaneously on a printed array of BAC clones.[4] Newer high-density oligonucleotide arrays promise whole genome resolution of <100 Kb. These methods are detailed below.

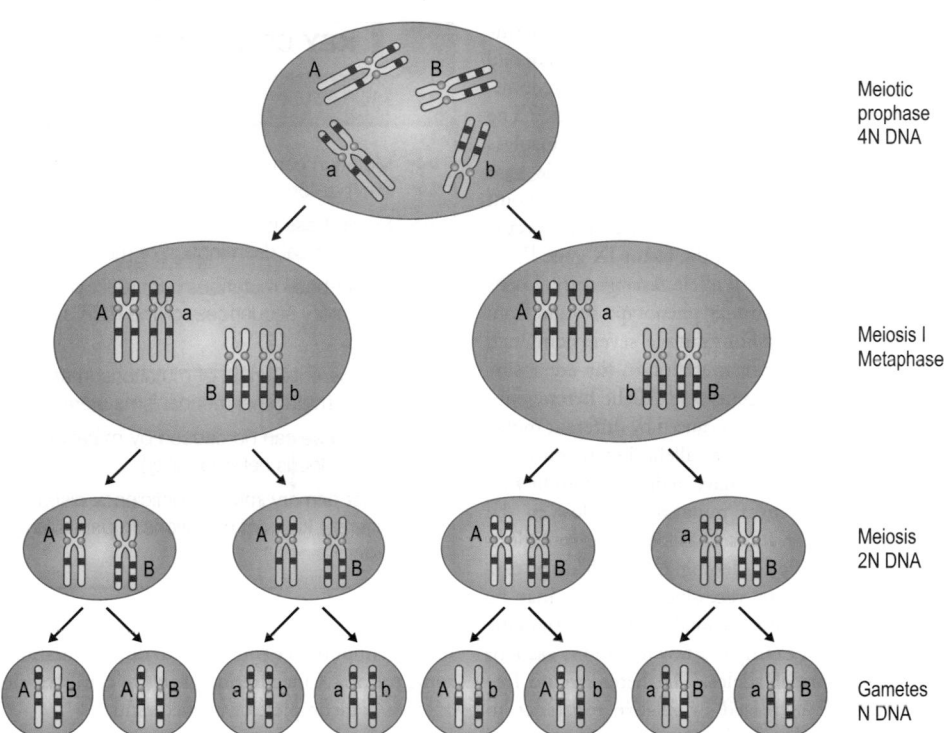

Fig. 101.1 Independent segregation of chromosomes during meiosis. The diploid adult cells give rise to all combinations of parental chromosomes. Genes on different chromosomes are unlinked. Detection of this phenomenon depends on distinguishing allelic polymorphisms, i.e., A or a, B or b.

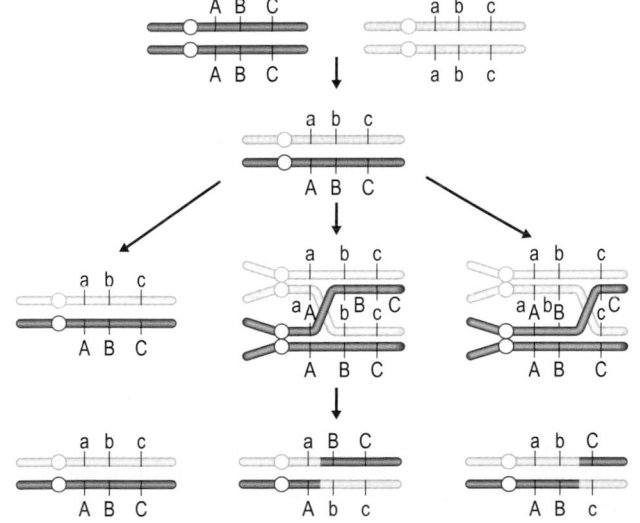

Fig. 101.2 Recombination.

MUTATION

Mutations may involve small or large deletions, insertions, inversions, or duplications. Some mutations may have no measurable or functionally significant phenotypic effect. They become one of the huge pool of neutral polymorphisms in the genome. Single base substitutions in a triplet amino acid codon often disturb the normal function of proteins. These are described as missense (i.e. causing an amino acid substitution) or nonsense (i.e. terminating translation). Mutations affecting regulatory or splice signal sequences in RNA can also be deleterious. Primary mechanisms of mutation are misincorporation of nucleotides and faulty repair of chemically damaged nucleotides (e.g., 8-oxodG) during DNA replication by DNA polymerases.[5, 6] Another important mechanism underlying single base or 'point' mutations occurs at CpG dinucleotides.[7] The cytosine is often methylated, and chemical deamination of the methylated cytosine gives the base thymidine. At the next round of replication the CG may be changed to TG or CA, depending on which DNA strand was altered. CG is found in the amino acid codons of Arg, Ser, Pro, Thr, and Ala. These amino acids are frequently involved in coding sequence mutations. Small insertion and deletion (indel) mutations are also very common. Indels occurring in protein coding sequence are frequently deleterious as they may cause frameshifts (changing the reading frame, usually leading to translation termination within a few codons). They result from strand slippage in repetitive sequence and misaligned intermediates during DNA synthesis.[8] Finally, an entirely different and novel mechanism for mutation is expansion of unstable triplet repeat segments.[9] So far, no disorder that affects the immune system has been associated with this mechanism. As outlined below, mutation screening will have a continuing and expanding role in clinical molecular testing.

PCR AND OTHER NUCLEIC ACIDS AMPLIFICATION TECHNIQUES

DNA amplification using the polymerase chain reaction (PCR) was a watershed advance in the detection of specific nucleic acid sequences.[26] PCR depends on the ability of two short synthetic oligonucleotides to find the DNA that closely matches each one (Fig. 101.4). A thermostable enzyme is added that can synthesize new DNA using each oligonucleotide as a primer, resulting in a doubling of the segment between the primers. The presence of the complementary oligonucleotide allows a second strand of complementary DNA to be synthesized. This constitutes one cycle of PCR. When this cycle is repeated, the segment of DNA in between the oligonucleotides is geometrically increased. RNA can also be amplified by first synthesizing complementary DNA (cDNA) using viral reverse transcriptase (RT-PCR). The amount of product then becomes great enough to detect, either by hybridization or by direct visualization on an ethidium bromide-stained gel. PCR can theoretically detect a single molecule of DNA or RNA. Thus, small cell or tissue samples can be analyzed very rapidly. One variation is to label one of the oligonucleotides, either with a radioactive molecule such as ^{32}P or with a fluorescent tag. PCR provides the starting point for linkage assays, mutation analysis, and DNA sequencing. RT-PCR is finding use in the quantification of mRNA from blood cells, e.g. in measuring cytokine transcription from activated T and B cells. Using specially designed instrumentation it has become possible to monitor and quantify the synthesis of DNA at each cycle of amplification in a PCR. These methods are called 'real-time' PCR and they provide sensitive assays for quantification of DNA and RNA, e.g., in assessment of HIV load.[27] The real-time PCR instrument detects fluorescent reporters such as SYBR Green (fluoresces when bound to double-stranded DNA). TaqMan and molecular beacons are related techniques in which oligonucleotide probes are dual-labeled with a fluorescent reporter and a

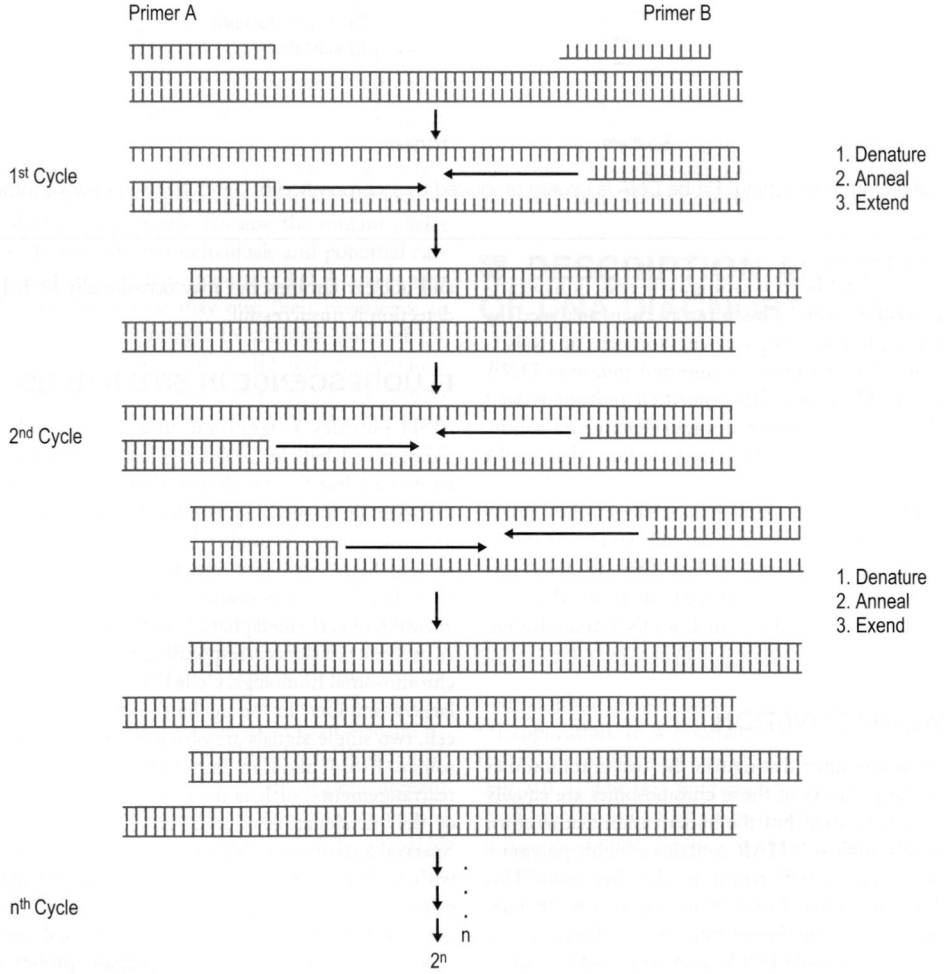

Fig. 101.4 Polymerase chain reaction. (**A**) Primers that hybridize to the target sequence are used to initiate multiple cycles of synthesis, melting, annealing, and synthesis. In practice, the potential geometric increase in DNA tapers off as reaction components become limiting. (**B**) Primers. PCR flanking a triplet (AAT)$_n$ repeat segment at DXS101 allows the detection of allelic differences. This polymorphism is tightly linked to the XLA locus and can be used to track inheritance of the disease in a family.

quencher moiety. Molecular beacons are oligonucleotides that can form stem-loops in which the loop can hybridize to a specific target DNA sequence. A fluorescent dye is covalently linked to one end of the stem and the quencher is attached to other end. The probe anneals to PCR products, causing the arm sequences to separate such that the amount of fluorescence is proportional to the increasing amount of target DNA in the reaction at each cycle. The TaqMan reaction is described in the section on detection of known mutations, but the same technique is also useful for quantification of specific nucleic acids.

There are a variety of other amplification techniques with application in clinical diagnostic laboratories. PCR uses cycles of denaturation and annealing of double-stranded DNA to achieve amplification, but there are also isothermal (processes occur at a single temperature) methods for nucleic acid amplification. Nucleic acid sequence-based amplification (NASBA) utilizes reverse transcriptase, RNAse H and T7 polymerase in an isothermal process that produces single-stranded RNA as the amplification product.[28] Transcription-mediated amplification (TMA) amplifies RNA using reverse transcriptase (RT) and RNA polymerase.[29] The RT makes double-stranded DNA copies that are used by the RNA polymerase to synthesize multiple copies of the single-stranded RNA. The branched-DNA assay uses the accumulation of branched enzyme-conjugated DNA probes on target DNA trapped on a solid phase.[30] Pre-amplifier and amplifier molecules are then hybridized to the captured target. Labeled oligonucleotides hybridize to the branched DNA complex and are then detected using a chemiluminescent enzyme substrate.

Segments of DNA that are variable in length between individuals can be readily detected by PCR. A class of polymorphism that is easily distinguished by PCR is called a microsatellite. These short tandem repeat polymorphisms (STRP) are principally dinucleotide, trinucleotide, and tetranucleotide elements that vary in the number of repeat subunits between individuals.[31] STRs have much higher mutation rates than

single nucleotide positions (~1000 times greater).[32] This instability creates extensive families of alleles. In general, the longer the uninterrupted repeat segments, the greater the chance that the element will be polymorphic. At many of these loci the heterozygosity is 70–90%. Polymorphic short tandem repeats are distributed in the genome approximately every 40 000 bases. It has been possible to identify them either close to or within most genes of medical interest. Their high degree of heterozygosity and the ease of the assay have made microsatellites an important tool for disease gene mapping and positional cloning. Improved technology for SNP detection has largely displaced STRPs for research.[33]

DNA SEQUENCING

The direct determination of a DNA sequence is fundamental to mutation identification (Fig. 101.5). The most commonly used method (called Sanger sequencing) depends on termination of DNA synthesis by chemically modified nucleotides (dideoxy-NTPs). A single-stranded DNA template is hybridized to a primer that can recognize a short known segment of DNA. The single-stranded DNA is obtained from bacterial plasmid/phage vectors, or may be produced by DNA amplification. The primer acts as a starting point for DNA synthesis by a DNA polymerase that is added to the reaction. Four separate reactions are set up, each 'spiked' with one of the four possible dideoxynucleotides (ddATP, ddTTP, ddCTP, or ddGTP). As synthesis proceeds, some of the strands incorporate a dideoxynucleotide and no further extension can take place. In each reaction a family of molecules is synthesized whose unit lengths are determined by whether the reaction had been terminated by incorporation of a specific dideoxynucleotide at a given position. Either the primer or the nucleotides may be labeled. Automated instrumentation for DNA sequencing using laser scanning of fluorophore-labeled reactions has largely replaced other labeling schemes. By using four different fluorescent labels the reaction products

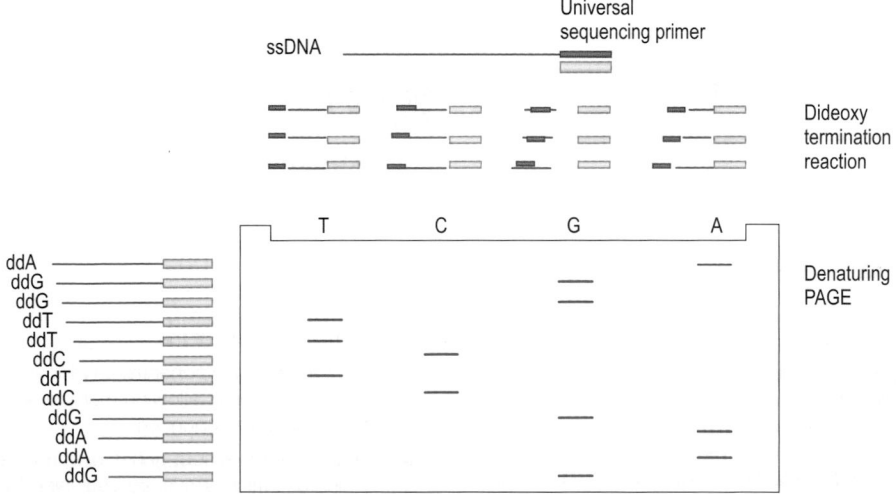

Fig. 101.5 DNA sequencing by dideoxy-NTP chain termination. Copying of the DNA by the polymerase is terminated at specific positions when a ddNTP is incorporated. The ddNTP is added mixed with dNTPs so that, in each reaction, only some new strands terminate whereas others continue through to the next complementary nucleotide. The sequencing products can be visualized by autoradiography or by laser scanning in an automated sequencer.

DHPLC system. An individual bearing a homozygous mutation at an autosomal locus or a hemizygous mutation at an X-linked locus will produce only homoduplexes. Depending on the nature of the mutation, the mutant homoduplexes may not be reliably distinguished from wild-type sequence based only on their elution profile on the column. Intentional introduction of wild-type DNA or PCR products as a secondary procedure can then be employed.

DETECTION OF A KNOWN MUTATION

Once a mutation has been identified in a patient, the entire family can be tested. One of the simplest methods is called oligonucleotide ligation assay (OLA).[50] In this procedure, pairs of specific oligonucleotides are designed to match exactly the wild-type and variant sequences. After a denaturing step, the temperature is reduced to one at which the oligos can hybridize with the single-strand template. Thermal-stable ligase is used to ligate the two oligos and the cycle is repeated. One popular method is to capture the ligated oligos in an ELISA so that the ligated products can be detected by conventional antibody and enzyme processes and quantified in a standard 96-well format plate reader. Amplification refractory mutation system (ARMS, Fig. 101.8A) and allele-specific primer extension (ASPE) are related techniques in which specific primer oligonucleotides are designed for each allele or mutation to be detected.[51] Oligos with a perfect match will not allow either PCR or primer extension reactions. ASPE has been developed into an FDA-approved clinical test that achieves multiplexing by incorporating a tag address system with detection of fluorescent beads (Luminex; Fig. 101.8B). 'Molecular beacons' are specialized oligonucleotides that contain a fluorophore and a fluorescence-quencher group at opposite ends of the molecule[52] (Fig. 101.9A). The probe oligos are designed to form a stem structure with an intervening loop that is complementary to the target sequence. In solution, the molecular beacon assumes a hairpin structure in which the fluorescence emission is quenched. In the presence of a perfectly matched target, the molecular beacon unfolds, placing the fluorophore and quencher far enough apart so that the fluorophore is no longer quenched. Fluorescence emission increases during PCR amplification. To determine whether a known mutation is present, specific probe oligos are designed to be exact matches for the wild-type and mutant DNA sequences. Different fluorophores with minimally overlapping emission spectra are used for each probe oligo, and their differential hybridization is monitored at each cycle of amplification. Specialized instrumentation is used to monitor single reactions or reactions in a 96-well format during the PCR amplification process. Another technique, the TaqMan reaction[53] (Fig. 101.9B), uses the same kind of instrumentation to monitor the PCR reaction in real time, but employs a slightly different approach to allele recognition. In the TaqMan method, the fluorophore is attached to the 5' end of the probe and a quencher to the 3' end. The 3' end is modified so that it cannot be used as a primer for polymerase extension. In its native state this oligo is quenched. The TaqMan probe hybridizes to the target sequence as it is produced in the PCR reaction. As the Taq polymerase extends on the template, the probe oligo is displaced and the 5' end becomes a substrate for the exonuclease activity of the polymerase. Cleavage of the 5' base from the oligo releases the fluorophore and the quenching is relieved. The increase in fluorescence emission as the PCR reaction proceeds is monitored in the instrument. Allele-specific genotyping for mutant or wild-type forms is again accomplished by designing specific probe oligos for each sequence.

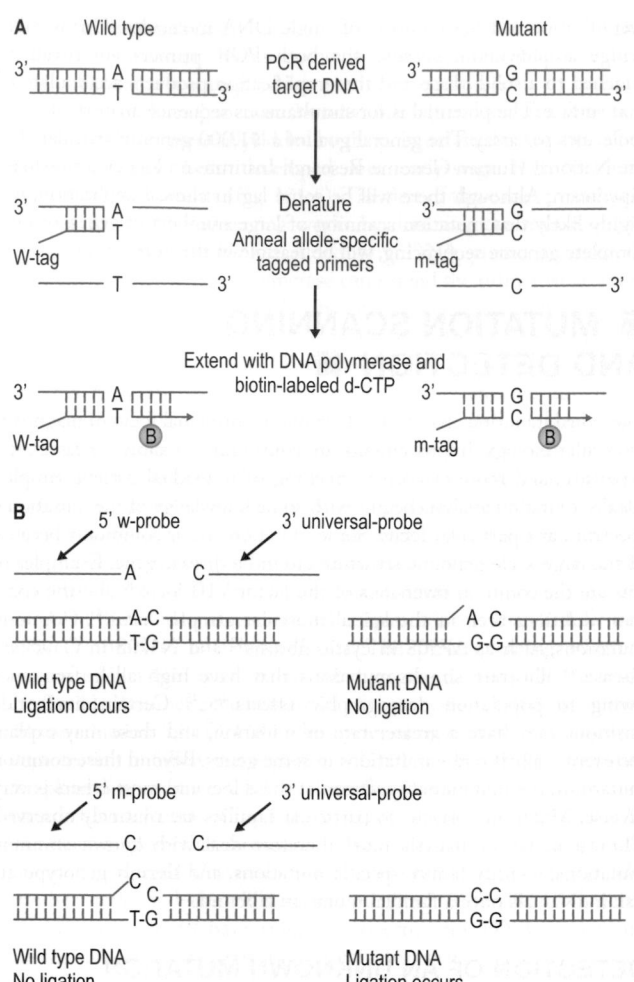

Fig. 101.8 Detecting known mutations. (**A**) Amplification refractory mutation system (ARMS). In this assay primers specific for the normal and mutant allele are synthesized. In its simplest form the presence or absence of amplification products can be detected on an agarose gel. The scheme depicted in the diagram shows tagged primers that allow capture of the amplification products on a solid phase and then detection by immunoenzyme recognition of the biotin label. (**B**) Oligonucleotide ligation assay (OLA). In this assay there are again specific oligonucleotides corresponding to exact matches with either the wild-type or mutant allele together with a 3' universal probe that exactly matches the adjacent sequence. After annealing the probes that match the target sequence may be ligated. The ligated products can be detected in various ways not shown in this diagram.

These will compete with one another, and the fluorescence emission will correspond to the oligo that exactly matches the target sequence. Both molecular beacons and TaqMan reactions are robust and, because they occur in solution without need for electrophoretic fragment separation, they lend themselves to scale-up automation. Limitations include the need for very precise probe design (which may require several rounds of optimization), the cost of custom fluorophore-tagged oligos, and the requirement for at least four oligos for each reaction.

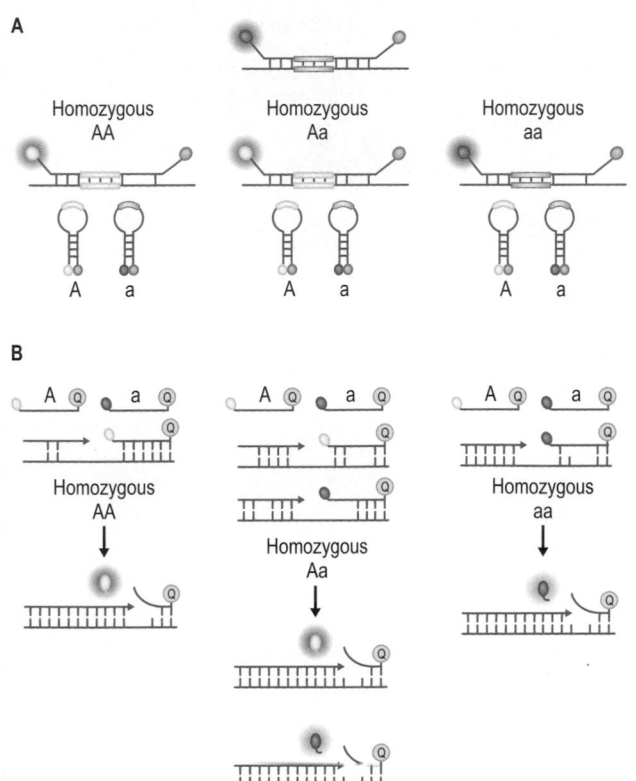

DNAs or oligonucleotides to be spotted on activated glass surfaces.[55–57] Distribution of oligos onto beads has also been used.[58, 59] An alternative approach is direct synthesis of oligonucleotides on a silicon surface using photoactive chemistry and masking templates.[60] This process is very similar in principle to the fabrication of microelectronics devices, and so has given these arrays the nickname of 'gene chips'. For expression analysis, cDNA 'target' derived from the tissue or cell source is labeled with fluorophores and used to determine complementary binding by massively parallel hybridization to the probes fixed on the array. Such arrays are extraordinarily useful for monitoring gene expression at thousands of loci in a single assay. Diagnostic and prognostic information about lymphomas,[61, 62] leukemias,[63, 64] and autoimmunity derived from expression arrays has already had a large impact on research and is likely to enter clinical diagnostic practice shortly.[65]

Microarrays have been used both to assay for known mutations and polymorphisms and for the primary screening process – a kind of sequencing by hybridization. There are several limitations to this approach relating to the specificity of the hybridization, i.e., it is difficult to obtain conditions of specific and sensitive hybridization across many thousands of unique sites. Robust chemistries that can analyze standard sets of >500 000 SNPs in a single assay are now routine (Fig. 101.10). Nonamplified genomic DNA is too complex (i.e. the concentration of any particular sequence is too low) to be analyzed directly. High-throughput genotyping assays require an array-based readout and scalable, multiplex assay chemistry. This is extremely challenging because of the complexity of the human genome, i.e., any particular unique sequence in the mixture has a low molar concentration and because of the need for exquisite specificity at the single base level. An important general principle for achieving single base specificity is the detection of physically coincidental events.[66] This is exactly the route taken by PCR, in which specific annealing of both primers is required for the reaction to take place.

The molecular inversion probe (MIP) assay[67, 68] and the GoldenGate assay[69] are examples that exploit a combination of linked specificity steps with a universal PCR. In both MIP and GoldenGate, specificity requires two-step recognition through annealing of 5′ and 3′ oligos flanking the SNP site. In MIP both the upstream and downstream locus-specific probes are physically linked in a single long oligonucleotide. The resulting enhanced binding kinetics allow lower concentrations of each probe and thus aids the multiplexing. MIP obtains allele discrimination by separating the reaction into nucleotide-specific reactions in which successful single base fill-in enables a subsequent ligation step. GoldenGate uses allele-specific primer extension in which the upstream and downstream probes are separate. But GoldenGate achieves high specificity by binding the target genomic DNA onto a bead, which can then be washed very stringently. Both MIP and GoldenGate use universal PCR to amplify the diverse locus-specific assays, a process that allows multiplexing at a level in which thousands of genomic loci are interrogated in parallel in the same reaction. The amplicons in this PCR reaction all contain short unique 'address tags' that are used as indicators for the individual assays. Both MIP and GoldenGate are read out through hybridization of the multiplex PCR products to a standardized array of oligonucleotides complementary to the address sequences. A severe problem in multiplex PCR is the potential formation of hybridization products, called primer dimers, between the various primers. The key to the universal PCR is the use of primers that include locus-specific 3′ and 5′ connected to universal primer sequences common to all assays in the

Fig. 101.9 Detecting known mutations and SNPs. (**A**) Molecular beacons. Fluorophore-tagged oligonucleotides specific for the wild-type and mutant allele are hybridized during a PCR reaction to the DNA amplimers. The opening of the oligo hairpin allows the fluorophore to emit light at its characteristic wavelength, and the result is quantitatively detected as the PCR reaction progresses. (**B**) TaqMan reaction. Allele-specific fluorophore-tagged oligonucleotides are hybridized to single-strand DNA produced during a PCR reaction. Strand displacement leads to cleavage of the fluorophore and release from quenching. The intensity and wavelength of the emitted light is monitored during the course of the PCR.

Given that an increasing number of common mutations have been identified that may be screened in many unrelated patients, multiplex genotyping assays have begun to find wide application. One of the methods that has proved itself in both research and diagnostic applications is matrix-assisted laser desorption ionization time of flight (MALDI-TOF) mass spectroscopy.[54] In MALDI-TOF short amplification products are analyzed and the subtle differences in molecular weight are used to infer the base sequence. The method is highly sensitive, and by careful amplimer design can be used to analyze three to five amplimers per sample. By combining this analytical system with a single-base extension approach, multiplexing of up to 24-plex can be achieved.

MICROARRAYS

BAC and oligonucleotide arrays are having a revolutionary impact on RNA expression analysis, SNP genotyping and comparative genome hybridization. Array printing allows hundreds to thousands of BAC

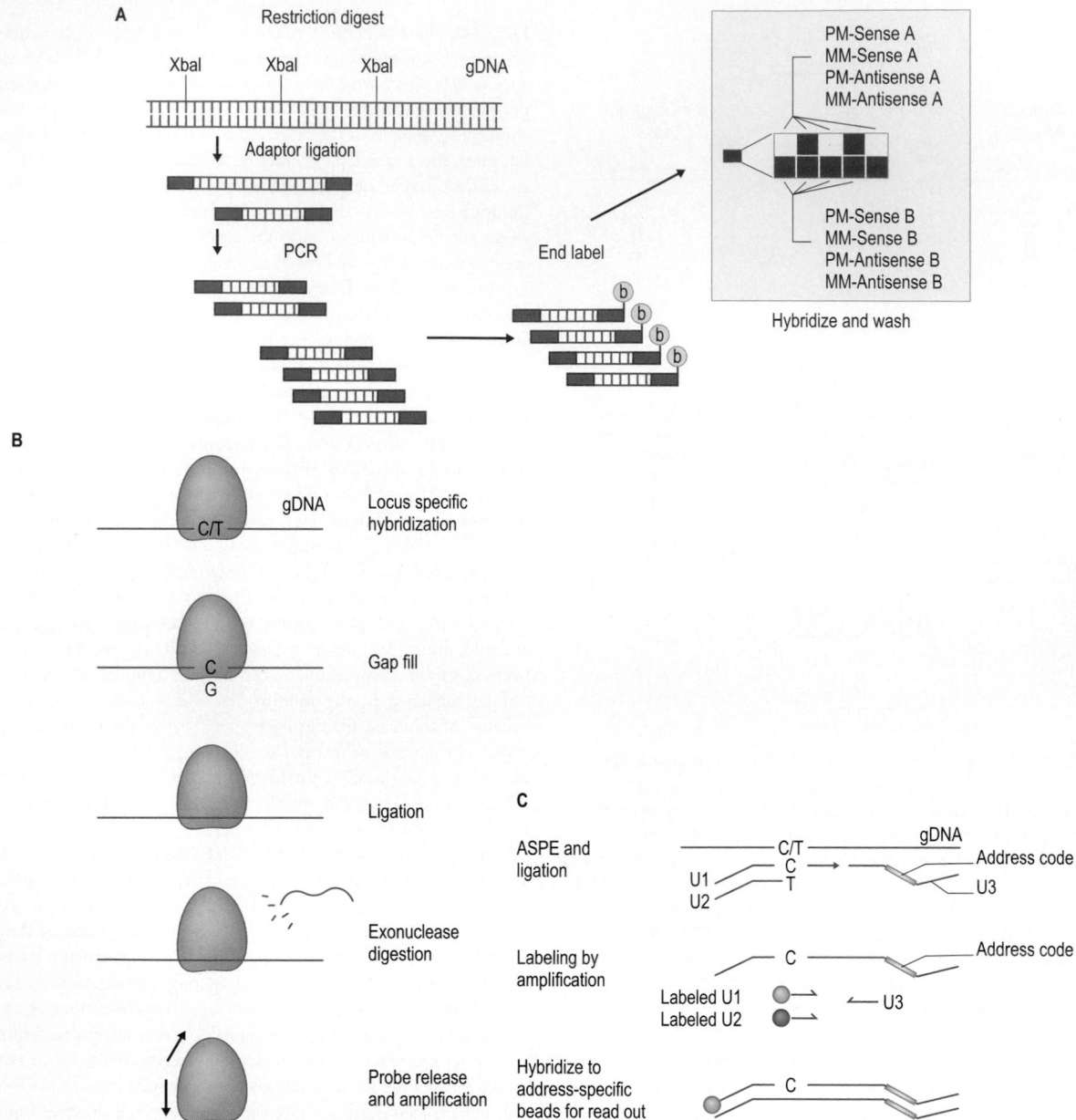

Fig. 101.10 Microarray genotyping. Oligonucleotides are printed or synthesized on a glass surface. Arrays based on oligonucleotide attachment to microbeads are also widely employed. Allele-specific hybridization is detected by the position in the array either employing locus-specifc hybridization or address tags. Four methods are depicted that either detect standard sets of SNPs (**A, D**) or allow for custom assay design by the end-user (**B, C**). Each method is described in the text. (**A**) Whole genome sampling and amplification (WGSA). End-labeled PCR products which constitute a sample from the genome are hybridized to oligo sets on standard chips. The oligos are organized into 'probe quartets' consisting of perfect matches (PM) and single-base mismatches (MM) for each allele, A and B. Separate quartets for the sense and antisense strand of DNA help to ensure specifity and in the actual assay these quartets are repeated three to five times on the chip. (**B**) This type of assay has been developed to test a standard panel of >1 M SNPs per sample. Molecular inversion probe (MIP). This assay is employed when genotyping several thousand SNPs that require custom design. The probe pools consist of very long oligonucleotides that allow the formation of a 'padlock' after allele-specific fill-in and ligation. The detection system involves a set of address oligos built into the original probes. After labeling these addresses are used to detect which allele is present in the target DNA by hybridization to a standard chip (not shown). (**C**) GoldenGate. This assay combines an allele-specific primer extension (ASPE) recognition with an address code system. Labeled universal primers (U1 and U2) assigned to each allele along with a fixed universal 3' primer (U3) are used to amplify a highly multiplexed reaction (up to ~1500-plex). Each SNP assay is identified with an address code sequence and the resulting amplification products are read out on a dense bead array (not shown).

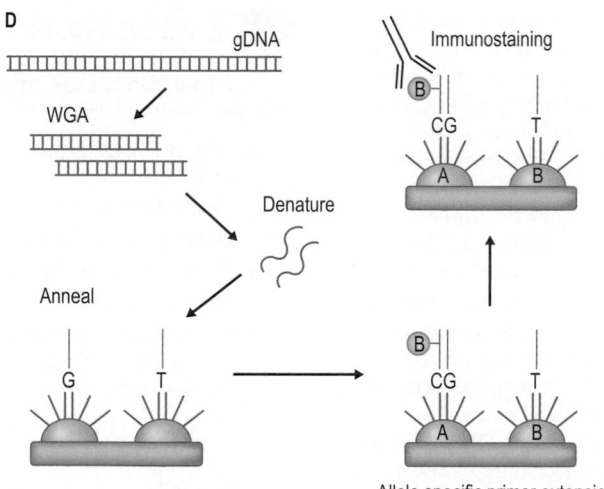

Fig. 101.10—Cont'd (**D**) Infinium. This assay uses whole genome amplification (WGA) to increase the molar concentration of target DNA. ASPE on arrays of tagged microbeads allows allele discrimination and the resulting products are detected by immunostaining (signal amplification). This assay has been used for assays of >600 000 SNPs per sample.

primer pool. One approach, called homo-tag nondimer system (HANDS), uses reaction temperature variation to first allow locus-specific recognition and a subsequent switch to a higher annealing temperature that favors the universal primer reaction.

Whole genome sampling and amplification (WGSA) allows parallel amplification of short DNA segments (200–1100 bp) that are then labeled and hybridized to oligonucleotide probe arrays.[70] The oligonucleotides are specific for each allele of SNPs and the resulting hybridization intensities can be used to derive the genotypes. These assays are fixed in the sense that the investigator uses the information from a standardized array but cannot add SNPs for particular purposes. An alternative approach, incorporated in the Infinium assays (Illumina), involves the detection of allele-specific primer extension or single base extension products on a self-assembling high-density microbead array.[71] In the Infinium assays genomic DNA is first subjected to whole genome amplification (WGA) and those products are hybridized to an array of locus-specific 50-mer capture probes. Either primer extension or ligation reactions on the array surface are used to accomplish allele discrimination. Signal amplification with methods familiar to users of ELISA assays are used to enhance the sensitivity. A distinct advantage of this class of assays is that the 'assay conversion' (percent SNPs that actually allow inference of the genotype in the final assay mixture) is very high. This allows great latitude in the selection of SNPs, and thus might prove highly useful in assays of human mutations.

■ BIOINFORMATICS ■

Bioinformatics has emerged as a fundamental discipline in molecular biology as enormous DNA and protein sequence databases, linkage maps, physical maps, and other integrated data sets have been generated by individual laboratories and the human genome project. The growing number of genetic loci that are already known to be important in immunological disease renders it critical that both research and diagnostic laboratories make maximal use of automated processes in sample archiving, data acquisition, data analysis, and reporting.

INTERNAL DATABASES AND DATA ACQUISITION

Laboratory information management (LIM) systems are widespread and each laboratory must deal with the generic operational problems of sample accession, tracking, and reporting. DNA diagnostic laboratories have several unique problems and requirements that deserve comment. Relational databases (usually implemented on Oracle or SQL servers) should integrate sample accession, physical archive, quality control, and genotype information. Automated data acquisition is an important component of DNA sequencing and genotyping. Instrument-specific and secondary base-calling programs are necessary for data interpretation. More sophisticated statistical models of sequencing and genotyping data are greatly improving the ability to handle datasets per individual that would be far too large for manual analysis.[72] Automated procedures for exporting data files to analytical software and data archiving on indelible media are also important issues. The number of patient-specific data records and the complexity of relationships in family-based testing make it difficult for manual processes to achieve the required reliability.

DATA INTERPRETATION AND PUBLIC SEQUENCE DATABASES

Computer-based methods for genotype and DNA sequence data interpretation are necessary for efficiency and cost-effectiveness. Estimation of genetic risks based on genotype data requires a knowledge of specialized statistical procedures whose description is beyond the scope of this chapter. The development of specialized training programs in molecular genetics and molecular genetic pathology by the American Boards of Medical Genetics and Pathology[73] highlights the recognition by professional groups that this area of clinical testing is exceptionally complex. Although inferences made about disease diagnosis and carrier status based on direct detection of mutations are inherently categorical, data interpretation should incorporate known genotype–phenotype correlations, variable disease expression/severity, incomplete penetrance, gender-specific risk, and other available data. In the future, as DNA testing is employed in the assessment of more complex traits such as autoimmune and neoplastic diseases, genotype data will perhaps be expressed as 'relative risk' and incorporate gene–gene and gene–environment interactions. The reliability of these estimates will require standard data acquisition algorithms and constant updating of population-based data.

The reference human genome sequence is complete (http://genome. ucsc.edu/) and has fueled the rapid expansion of clinical sequencing and genotyping. Diagnostic laboratories must actively use information contained in the public sequence databases to interpret the biological consequences of mutations and polymorphisms. There are at least several broad databases that are likely to have an important role over the next decade: (1) GenBank, which contains the nonredundant cDNA and protein sequences, finished human genomic sequences (http://www.ncbi.nlm. nih.gov/entrez); (2) dbSNP, which contains more than 10 000 000 common single-nucleotide polymorphisms; and (3) the Human Mutation Database, which assembles mutation information on known disease loci (http://www.hgmd.cf.ac.uk/ac/index.php). Public tools are available for DNA sequence comparisons of patient-specific data with the reference sequences (http://www.ncbi.nlm.nih.gov/BLAST/). The Smith–Waterman algorithm estimates local sequence similarity. The most common implementations employ variations on the basic alignment search tool (BLAST) which quantifies local similarity using the maximal segment pair (MSP) score. A very large database of SNPs genotyped in four reference population samples (northern Europeans from Utah; Yoruba from Ibadan, Nigeria; Han Chinese from Beijing; and Japanese from Tokyo) was produced by the International Haplotype Map Project (www. hapmap.org). This database is expected to enable mapping of genes that underlie complex traits such as human autoimmune diseases. The reference genotypes and their associated haplotypes give important information about the short-range correlations between markers (called linkage disequilibrium) and allow the selection of marker sets that efficiently capture most of the genetic information in a population sample.[74, 75]

Interpretation of sequence and genotype information is the final output of a molecular diagnostic test. If a mutation has been observed in the proband and other family members are tested, then the expectation is that the mutation will exactly segregate with the disease. An example would be testing for a mutation in X-linked SCID in two brothers. The causal mutation will be present in both. When the proband is the only affected individual, then one may look to the research literature and locus-specific public databases (http://bioinf.uta.fi/base_root/mutationdatabases.php) to determine whether the specific mutation has previously been observed in another affected person. However, it is not uncommon to find a mutation that has not previously been observed, and as mutation analysis by DNA sequencing becomes more common this will be a frequent occurrence. Assessment of the functional consequence of a newly observed sequence variant is problematic as there is no guarantee that the variant is anything more than a rare, but neutral, polymorphism. Nonsense and frameshift mutations are relatively clear. Mutations in sites flanking coding exons known to be required for splicing are easily categorized. Missense substitutions are more difficult. Several methods based on sequence conservation and the chemical properties of amino acids have been developed. These are available in software called SIFT (*Sorting Intolerant From Tolerant*, http://blocks.fhcrc.org/sift/SIFT.html)

KEY CONCEPTS

PRINCIPLES OF MOLECULAR DIAGNOSTICS

>> DNA diagnostics can play an important role in the diagnosis of specific diseases in affected patients and in genetic risk assessment for their family members.

>> Genotyping can be used to conduct prenatal diagnoses.

>> Prenatal diagnosis may be used not only for elective termination of pregnancy but also for treatment planning.

>> Provision of genetic testing results to patients and their families carries responsibilities for sensitivity and confidentiality.

and PolyPhen (http://coot.embl.de/PolyPhen/). As the growing database of protein crystal structures (http://www.ncbi.nlm.nih.gov/Structure/) is extended, alignment methods, called 'threading,' will permit evaluation of the effect of an amino acid substitution on catalytic and interaction sites.

■ RECOMMENDATIONS FOR USE ■

Molecular diagnostic techniques have a wide range of potential applications in clinical immunology. DNA diagnostic procedures are used to (a) perform HLA genotyping; (b) analyze neoplastic disease; (c) provide identification or DNA 'fingerprinting'; (d) monitor bone marrow engraftment; (e) establish a genetic diagnosis in a symptomatic individual; (f) determine the risk of occurrence of a disease in offspring; and (g) to establish a prenatal diagnosis. The use of DNA analysis for HLA typing is described in Chapter 5. DNA techniques are used in leukemias and lymphomas, primarily for investigation of cell lineage, proliferative clonality, and measurement of residual abnormal cells after therapy. Molecular analysis, and especially molecular cytogenetic analysis, is important in guiding initial and follow-up therapy (see Chapters 76 and 77).

GENETIC COUNSELING

There is a role for molecular testing in genetic risk assessment in primary immune deficiencies.[76] Testing is usually applied to families whose risk of recurrence has been signaled by the birth of an affected child. Almost every case has to be treated as a problem requiring initial mutation identification. The rarity of the individual disorders and the frequent occurrence of new mutations in the X-linked diseases preclude population-wide heterozygote screening.

In the recessive immune deficiencies, carrier status is assumed in the parents once an affected child has been diagnosed. A much lower risk of having an affected child is attached to other carriers in a family, as their mates are unlikely to bear a mutant disease gene allele unless they are themselves lineal relatives of the index case. In the X-linked immune deficiencies the situation is strikingly different. In those cases the origin of mutation should be investigated to ascertain the carrier status of all the at-risk women. In a family with a single affected child carrying the diagnosis of an X-linked immune deficiency, there is a substantial risk that the mother is a carrier. The risk of carrier status in such women is 67–80%, depending on the locus. After the birth of a second affected child, and if the mutation has not been directly identified, the mother would be considered an obligate carrier (although somatic mosaicism is also a less likely possibility[77–79]). Women sharing a common lineage between two affected individuals in an extended pedigree, e.g., affected first cousins, would also be considered obligate carriers.

Genetic information, like any medical information, may be unsettling to patients and families. However, there are some special considerations that attach themselves to genetic testing, and practitioners need to be aware of this and appropriately cautious (http://www.ornl.gov/sci/techresources/Human_Genome/elsi/elsi.shtml). A fundamental principle of genetic testing for clinical or research purposes should be informed consent. The testing itself, as well as the plan for sample preservation or disposal, should be described in detail to the patient and family and, where appropriate, written consent obtained. An unintended consequence of genotyping may be to reveal nonpaternity of the stated father. The possibility that this might emerge from genetic testing should be sensitively conveyed to the prospective clients and may be a reason for avoiding further laboratory testing. In addition, pedigree analysis may uncover unsuspected risk in other family members who may not be seeking genetic information. Some have argued for a 'duty to inform' at-risk family members. Prospective testing, particularly carrier testing, in children before the age of individual consent raises troubling issues that have not been resolved. The latent possibility of employment or insurance discrimination with the incorporation of genotype information into the medical record is another area receiving a great deal of attention. It is important to emphasize in the presentation of the information that the occurrence of new mutation is a natural accident. Where possible, it is strongly preferred that genetic risk information be provided by professionals with experience and training in clinical genetics. There is currently a great deal of concern for the preservation of confidentiality relating to all genetic information.

PRENATAL DIAGNOSIS

Prenatal diagnosis is accomplished either by direct measurement of the defective function, e.g., enzyme activity in ADA deficiency, or by genetic methods. Because many immune disorders affect cells of the blood system exclusively, the former would mean fetal blood sampling. This is accompanied by a higher risk of fetal loss than either amniocentesis or chorion villus sampling (CVS). DNA-based methods may be equally applied to CVS samples or amniocytes. An important technical consideration in the use of CVS is examination for maternal cell contamination, as this could lead to an erroneous diagnosis. DNA diagnosis may employ linkage analysis, in which an inference is made using neighboring DNA markers about whether the developing fetus has inherited the same mutated chromosomal segment(s) as the index case. However, direct mutation identification in the index case and then use of a direct mutation detection procedure in the developing fetus is always preferred. There is now much more experience with pre-implantation genetic diagnosis (PGD), but this remains a highly specialized and expensive procedure.[80] PGD involves the removal of a single blastomere at the eight-cell stage. PCR methods are used to carry out genetic analysis. Recent publications have illustrated the use of PGD to select offspring with compatible HLA types for siblings requiring hematopoietic stem cell transplantation.[81, 82]

Prenatal diagnosis is used for either pregnancy management or treatment planning. In the case of a positive diagnosis of a primary immune deficiency, the couple should then have access to detailed information from an experienced clinical immunologist regarding the current treatment options and prognosis. The perception of the burden of disease may be colored by a previous bad therapeutic outcome caused by late diagnosis and its consequent complications. Prenatal diagnosis allows appropriate treatment planning to be carried out for isolation, prospective intravenous immunoglobulin therapy, prophylactic antibiotic therapy, and planning for bone marrow stem cell transplantation (Chapter 83).

Despite current successes in clinical management of immune deficiency, clinicians involved in providing prenatal genetic services should be prepared to be supportive toward the couple regarding decisions made to terminate an affected pregnancy. Although the ideal of genetic medicine is nondirective counseling, it has been pointed out that by offering to conduct prenatal testing, physicians are communicating a value judgment about the severity, treatability, and burden of a disease. Physicians involved in prenatal diagnosis for genetic immune deficiency should be aware of the particular couple's balance in decision making, opinions or pressures from extended family, and religious outlook.

LABORATORY STANDARDS AND REPORTING

All US laboratories providing any clinical data are subject to the regulatory requirements embodied in the Clinical Laboratory Improvement Amendments of 1988 (CLIA88).[83] Research laboratories that do not report patient-specific information are specifically exempt, but CLIA88 is clearly intended to preclude an arrangement where research laboratories perform diagnostic tests and prenatal diagnoses. CLIA88 mandates biannual laboratory inspections, quality control, quality assurance, proficiency testing, and personnel training standards. The American College of Medical Genetics has also produced guidelines for diagnostic laboratories conducting molecular genetics testing (http://www.faseb.org/genetics/acmg/stds/stdsmenu.htm). A clear argument can be made for the cost-effectiveness of prenatal diagnosis for such diseases, but it is unknown whether family analysis and carrier detection are ultimately effective in either reducing the number of affected individuals or improving their clinical outcome.

FUTURE DIRECTIONS

The next decade will bring further improvements in our ability to identify family-specific mutations for all the known disease genes. Sequencing technology will move increasingly to microscale formats, perhaps even employing 'nanotechnology' devices that integrate both chemical reactions and analytical devices. Highly parallel sequence analysis should increase production rates and reduce the cost per sample. DNA arrays for genotyping and mutation screening should ultimately replace current single-assay formats. As our understanding of the role of polymorphisms in disease risk increases the importance of low-cost, high-throughput genotyping of standard variant panels will also increase. The importance of bioinformatics in data analysis will become increasingly apparent as large amounts of individual genotype data are produced. International mutation databases will play an important role in both diagnosis and

81. Fiorentino F, Kahraman S, Karadayi H, et al. Short tandem repeats haplotyping of the HLA region in preimplantation HLA matching. Eur J Hum Genet 2005; 13: 953–958.

82. Kuliev A, Rechitsky S, Tur-Kaspa I, Verlinsky Y. Preimplantation genetics: Improving access to stem cell therapy. Ann NY Acad Sci 2005; 1054: 223–227.

83. Rivers PA, Dobalian A, Germinario FA. A review and analysis of the clinical laboratory improvement amendment of 1988: compliance plans and enforcement policy. Health Care Manage Rev 2005; 30: 93–102.

APPENDICES

Appendix:

Selected CD molecules and their characteristics

1

Selected CD molecules and their characteristics

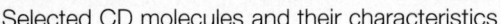

CD molecule	Predominant distribution	Identity/function
CD1a–e	Thymocytes, subset of lymphocytes, antigen-presenting cells	MHC class I-like molecules; presentation of non-peptide antigens to T cells; thymic T-cell development
CD2	T cells	Binds to LFA-3; receptor for CD48; T-cell activation; adhesion
CD3	T cells	T-cell signaling complex; associated with T-cell receptor (TCR)
CD4	T-cell subset	TCR co-receptor; interacts with MHC class II molecules on antigen presenting cells; identifies T cells with helper function; signal transduction
CD5	Most T cells, thymocytes, B-cell subset	Binds to CD72; regulation of cell proliferation/activation; identifies B-1 B-cell subset
CD6	Thymocytes, T cells, B-cell subset	Binds CD166 (ALCAM); adhesion; mediates binding of developing thymocytes with thymic epithelial cells; thymic development; T-cell activation
CD7	Pluripotent hematopoietic cells, thymocytes, T cells	T-cell and NK-cell development
CD8	T-cell subset	TCR co-receptor; interacts with MHC class I molecules on antigen-presenting cells; identifies T cells with cytotoxic function
CD10	B cells	Neutral endopeptidase; enkephalinase; B-cell development; common acute lymphoblastic leukemia antigen (CALLA)
CD11a	Leukocytes	α chain of LFA-1; pairs with CD18; interacts with ICAM; adhesion and cellular migration
CD11b	Monocytes, granulocytes, NK cells	α chain of complement receptor 3 (CR3); pairs with CD18; adhesion molecule
CD11c	Monocytes, granulocytes, NK cells	α chain of complement receptor 4 (CR4); pairs with CD18; adhesion molecule

Continued

Selected CD molecules and their characteristics—cont'd

CD molecule	Predominant distribution	Identity/function
CD14	Granulocytes, monocytes/macrophages	Receptor for LPS/LPB complex; myeloid differentiation antigen; cell activation
CD16a,b	NK cells, monocytes/macrophages, neutrophils	FcγRIIIA and FcγRIIIB (low- affinity IgG receptors-type III); phagocytosis; ADCC
CD18	Leukocytes	β chain of $β_2$-integrin molecules, including LFA-1, CR3, and CR4; pairs with CD11a, b, and c
CD19	B cells	BCR co-receptor; signal transduction; complexes with CD21
CD20	B cells	Role in B-cell activation/differentiation
CD21	B cells; follicular dendritic cells	Complement receptor type 2 (CR2): C3d receptor; B-cell co-receptor subunit; EBV receptor
CD22	B cells	Associates with BCR; signaling; regulation of B-cell activation; adhesion
CD23	B cells, macrophages, eosinophils, platelets, follicular dendritic cells	FcεRII; (Low-affinity IgE receptor)
CD24	Leukocytes	Heat-stable antigen; co-stimulation; adhesion
CD25	Activated T cells and B cells	α chain of IL-2 receptor, low-affinity IL-2 binding; signaling for cell proliferation/ differentiation
CD26	Activated T cells and B cells; macrophages	Dipeptidyl peptidase; role in extracellular adhesion; cell activation
CD27	T cells; B cell subset	Co-stimulation; T-cell proliferation, memory B cells
CD28	T cells	Binds B7-1 (CD80) and B7-2 (CD86); T-cell co-stimulation; signal transduction
CD29	Leukocytes	Integrin $β_1$ chain; pairs with CD49a-CD49f to form VLA-1-VLA-6 integrins, respectively; adhesion; signal transduction; development
CD30	Activated B cells and T cells	Binds to CD153; T cell activation/ regulation/differentiation
CD31	Monocytes, granulocytes, platelets, endothelial cells, B cells	PECAM-1; Binds to CD38; adhesion; signal transduction
CD32	B cells, monocytes/macrophages, granulocytes, eosinophils	FcgRII (low-affinity IgG receptor-type II) phagocytosis; ADCC; B cell regulation
CD33	Myeloid progenitors, granulocytes	Binds sialic acid
CD34	Hematopoietic progenitor cells; capillary endothelium	Mucosialin; binds to CD62L; adhesion
CD35	Leukocytes; erythrocytes	Complement receptor 1 (CR1); C3b and C4b receptor; phagocytosis
CD36	Monocytes/macrophages; endothelium; platelets	Binds oxidized LDL; scavenger receptor; binds apoptic cells; adhesion and endocytic receptor; GPIIIb; platelet adhesion and aggregation
CD38	NK cells; T- and B-cell subsets; monocytes	Binds CD31; cyclase; hydrolase; cell activation

Selected CD molecules and their characteristics—cont'd

CD molecule	Predominant distribution	Identity/function
CD40	B cells; antigen-presenting cells	Binds CD154 (CD40 ligand); B-cell proliferation differentiation, and survival; T-cell co-stimulation
CD41	Megakaryocytes/platelets	Glycoprotein IIb; a IIb integrin chain; binds fibronectin, fibrinogen, von-Willebrand factor, thrombospondin; extracellular adhesion; platelet aggregation
CD43	Leukocytes (except resting B cells)	Leukocyte sialoglycoprotein; may bind CD54; signal transduction; adhesion; anti-adhesion
CD44	Leukocytes; memory T cells; erythrocytes	Binds hyaluronan (H-CAM), collagen, fibronectin, laminin, osteopontin; extra- and intercellular adhesion; T-cell co-stimulation; leukocyte homing
CD45	Leukocytes (pan-leukocyte marker)	Protein tyrosine phosphatase; cell differentiation; lymphocyte signal transduction and activation
CD45RA	Naive T-cell marker (in conjunction with CD62L); B cells, monocytes	CD45 isoform
CD45RB	B- and T-cell subsets, monocytes/macrophages, granulocytes	CD45 isoform
CD45RO	Memory and activated T cells; B cells, B cells, monocytes/macrophages	CD45 isoform
CD46	Hematopoietic cells	Membrane cofactor protein (MCP); binds to C3b and C4b and regulates complement pathway
CD47R	Leukocytes; endothelium	Integrin-associated protein (IAP); leukocyte migration, extravasation and activation
CD48	Leukocytes (not neutrophils)	Binds CD2; adhesion; co-stimulation
CD49a-f	Various distributions	Integrin a1-6 chain; binds to CD29 to form VLA-1 to VLA-6; binds extracellular matrix components such as fibronectin, laminin, collagen (CD49D binds VCAM-1, fibronectin, MadCAM-1, invasin); lymphocyte homing; extracellular adhesion; embryonic development
CD50	Thymocytes, B cells, T cells, monocytes, granulocytes	ICAM-3; adhesion
CD51	Platelets/megakaryocytes, granulocytes, monocytes, T cells	Integrin α chain; associates with CD61; binds vitronectin, fibronectin, fibrinogen; extracellular adhesion; T-cell co-stimulation; epithelial inflammatory response
CD52	Leukocyes	GPI linked, signaling, defined by CAMPATH-1
CD54	Broad distribution; increased on activated leukocytes	ICAM-1; binds LFA-1; adhesion; leukocyte transendothelial migration, rhinovirus receptor
CD55	Hematopoietic cells and some nonhematopoietic cells	Decay accelerating factor (DAF); binds complement fragment C3b; regulation of complement activation
CD56	NK cells	NKH-1; adhesion

Continued

Selected CD molecules and their characteristics—cont'd

CD molecule	Predominant distribution	Identity/function
CD57	NK cells, T-cell subset, B cells, monocytes	Oligosaccharide expressed on cell surface glycoproteins
CD58	Hematopoietic cells and nonhematopoietic cells	LFA-3; binds CD2; adhesion; lymphocyte co-activation
CD59	Hematopoietic cells and non-hematopoietic cells	Binds complement components C8 and C9 and regulates assembly of complement membrane attack complex
CD61	Platelets/megakaryocytes, macrophages	Integrin β_3 subunit; associates with CD41 or CD51
CD62E	Endothelium	ELAM-1 or E-selection; binds sialyl-Lewis X; adhesion; mediates rolling interaction of neutrophils on endothelium and neutrophil extravasation
CD62L	B cells, T cells, monocytes, NK cells	LECAM-1, LAM-1 (or L-selectin); binds CD34 and GlyCAM; adhesion; mediates rolling interactions with endothelium and call extravasation
CD62P	Platelets/megakaryocytes, endothelium	P-selectin; binds sialyl-Lewis X; mediates interaction of platelets with neutrophils and monocytes; mediates rolling interaction of neutrophils with endothelium
CD64	Monocytes/macrophages	FcγR1 (High affinity IgG receptor)
CD68	Monocytes/macrophages	Macrosialin; early activation antigen; role in phagocytic activity
CD69	Activated T cells, B cells, macrophages, NK cells	Early activation antigen; co-stimulation
CD70	Activated B and T cells; macrophages	Binds to CD27; co-stimulation
CD71	Activated leukocytes	Transferrin receptor; cell activation
CD72	B cells	Ligand for CD5; B-cell activation and differentiation; co-stimulation
CD73	B- and T-cell subsets	Ecto-5′ nucleotidase; allows nucleoside uptake
CD74	MHC class II-expressing cells	MHC class II-associated invariant chain; involved in antigen processing and peptide presentation in antigen-presenting cells
CD77	Germinal center B cells	
CD79a,b	B cells	Iga, Igb; components of BCR complex that mediate signal transduction
CD80	Monocytes/macrophages, dendritic cells, activated B cells	B7-1; ligand for CD28 and CTLA-4; T-cell interaction with antigen-presenting cells; co-stimulation
CD81	Lymphocytes	Associates with CD19 and CD21 to form B-cell co-receptor complex; co-stimulation; adhesion
CD86	Monocytes, activated B cells	B7-2; ligand for CD28 and CTLA-4; T cell interaction with antigen-presenting cells; co-stimulation
CD87	Granulocytes; monocytes/macrophages, activated T cells	Urokinase plasminogen activator receptor
CD88	Granulocytes, macrophages, mast cells	Complement component fragment C5a receptor
CD89	Monocytes/macrophages, granulocytes, B and T cell subsets	FcαR (IgA receptor)

Selected CD molecules and their characteristics—cont'd

CD molecule	Predominant distribution	Identity/function
CD91	Monocytes	α_2-macroglobulin receptor
CD94	NK cells, T-cell subset	Inhibits killing
CD95	Broad distribution	Fas or Apo-1; induces apoptosis after being bound by Fas ligand
CD97	Activated B and T cells, monocytes, PMN	Activation antigen
CD102	Resting lymphocytes, monocytes, endothelial cells	ICAM-2; binds LFA-1 (CD11a/CD18); adhesion; T-cell co-stimulation
CD103	Intraepithelial lymphocytes, T-cell subset	aE integrin; T-cell development and co-stimulation
CD104	Epithelial cells, Schwann cells	β_4-integrin; epidermal adhesion to basement membrane
CD105	Endothelial cells, bone marrow cell subset, activated macrophages	Endoglin; adhesion
CD106	Endothelial cells	VCAM-1; ligand for VLA-4; lymphocyte adhesion; embryonic development
CD107a,b	Epithelial cells, subsets of monocytes, granulocytes, and lymphocytes	LAMP-1 and LAMP-2; adhesion
CD110	Hematopoietic stem cells, megakaryocytes, platelets	Thrombopoietin receptor; megakaryocyte proliferation and differentiation
CD114	Granulocytes	G-CSF receptor; regulates granulopoiesis
CD115	Monocytes/macrophages	M-CSF receptor; cell differentiation
CD116	Monocytes, neutrophils, eosinophils	GM-CSF a chain receptor; cell differentiation
CD117	Hematopoietic progenitors	c-kit; stem cell factor (SCF) receptor; hematopoietic cell differentiation
CD118	Broad distribution	Type 1 interferon (interferon-α/β) receptor
CD119	Broad distribution	Interferon-γ receptor
CD120a	Hematopoietic cells, nonhematopoietic cells, myeloid cells	TNF receptor-type 1; signal transduction; apoptosis
CD120b	Hematopoietic cells, nonhematopoietic cells, myeloid cells	TNF receptor-type II; signal transduction, apoptosis
CD121a	Thymocytes, T-cell subset, fibroblasts, epithelial cells, and brain cells	IL-1 receptor-type I; signal transduction
CD121b	T-cell subset, mycloid cell subsets	IL-1 receptor-type II
CD122	NK cells, T-cell and B-cell subset	IL-2 and IL-15 receptor β chain; signal transduction; regulation of lymphocyte development, differentiation, activation and proliferation
CD123	Bone marrow stem cells, granulocytes, monocytes, megakaryocytes	IL-3 receptor α chain; cell development and differentation
CD124	Mature B and T cells, hematopoietic precursor cells	IL-4 receptor; signal transduction; lymphocyte development, activation, differentiation and proliferation
CD125	Eosinophils, basophils, B cell subset	IL-5 receptor; eosinophil and B-cell growth and differentiation
CD126	Activated B cells, plasma cells, T cells, granulocytes, monocytes/macrophages; also expressed on epithelial cells, fibroblasts, hepatocytes, and neural cells	IL-6 receptor α chain; regulation of B- and T-cell differentiation and function; hematopoiesis
CD127	Bone marrow lymphoid precursors, pro-B cells, T cell precursors, T-cell subset, monocytes	IL-7 receptor α chain; signal transduction; B- and T-cell proliferation and differentiation

Continued

Selected CD molecules and their characteristics—cont'd

CD molecule	Predominant distribution	Identity/function
CD128	Neutrophils, basophils, T-cell subset	IL-8 receptor; neutrophil activation and migration
CD129	T cells	IL-9 receptor α chain; T-cell proliferation
CD130	Broad distribution	IL-6 receptor β chain (with CD126); signal transduction
CD131	Lymphocytes, granulocytes, monocytes	IL-3, IL-5 and GM-CSF receptor; common β chain; signal transduction; see CD123 and CD125
CD132	Lymphocytes	Common γ chain of high-affinity receptor for IL-2 (with CD25 and CD122), IL-4 (with CD124), IL-7 (with CD127), IL-9 (with CD129), and IL15 (with CD122) receptors; signal transduction
CD134	Activated T cells	OX-40 antigen of TNFR superfamily (binds OX-40 ligand); T-cell–B-cell interaction and T-cell co-stimulation
CD135	Lymphoid and myeloid cell progenitor subsets	Flt3 ligand receptor; development of mycloid and lymphoid progenitors
CD137	Activated T cells	4-1BB; binds 4-1BB ligand and extracellular matrix components; T-cell–B-cell interaction and T-cell co-stimulation; extracellular adhesion; signal transduction
CD138	B cell subset, plasma cells	Syndecan-1; binds interstitial matrix proteins; B-cell–matrix interactions
CD140a,b	Endothelial cells	PDGF receptor α and β chain; embryonic development; signal transduction; chemotaxis
CD141	Endothelium	Thrombomodulin (binds thrombin); regulates coagulation
CD142	Endothelium	Tissue factor; binds plasma factors VII/VIIa; hemostasis, coagulation, and angiogenesis
CD143	Endothelium	Angiotensin-converting enzyme (ACE); binds angiotensin 1; regulates blood pressure
CD144	Endothelium	VE-cadherin; cell–cell adhesion; maintenance of endothelium integrity
CD146	Activated T-cell subset	Mel-CAM, adhesion molecule during development
CD150	T- and B-cell subsets	Surface lymphocyte activation marker (SLAM); B-cell–T-cell interaction; co-stimulation
CD151	Not defined	PETA-3; regulates platelet aggregation and mediator release
CD152	Activated T cells	CTLA-4; binds B7-1 (CD80) and B7-2 (CD86); T-cell co-stimulation-negative signal
CD153	T cells	CD30 ligand; T-cell activation, differentiation, and regulation
CD154	Activated T cells	CD40 ligand; T-cell co-stimulation
CD156a	Leukocytes, B cells	Transmembrane glycoprotein; disintegrin and metalloproteinase domain (ADAM) family member; leukocyte adhesion and protease function; infiltration of myelomonocytic cells

Selected CD molecules and their characteristics—cont'd

CD molecule	Predominant distribution	Identity/function
CD156b	Broad distribution	TNF-α-converting enzyme (TACE); disintegrin and metalloproteinase domain (ADAM) family member; cleaves TNF and transforming growth factor-α from cell surface, thereby releasing soluble form
CD158	NK cells	Killer cell immunoglobulin (Ig)-like receptors (KIR); family of molecules that inhibit NK cytotoxic activity
CD159a	NK cells	NKG2A (killer cell lectin-like receptor)
CD161	NK cells	Natural killer cell receptor-P1; target cell recognition; NK cell activation
CD162	Granulocyte and T cell subsets	P-selectin glycoprotein ligand-1 (PSGL-1); adhesion
CD166	Activated T cells, B cells	ALCAM; binds CD6; T-cell activation; thymocyte development
CD167a	Epithelial cells	Discoidin domain receptor 1 (DDD1); tyrosine kinase receptor; binds to collagen; cell–cell contact and adhesion
CD178	Activated T cells; various tissue cells	Fas ligand (ligand for CD95); binding to Fas triggers apoptosis
CD179a	Pro-B and pre-B cells	VpreB; forms surrogate light chain with CD179b; early B-cell differentiation
CD179b	Pro-B and pre-B cells	λ5; forms surrogate light chain with CD179a; early B-cell differentiation
CD180	B cells	RP105; toll-like receptor family; regulates B-cell recognition and signaling of LPS
CD183	Effector/memory T cells, NK cells, eos	CXCR3 receptor for interferon-inducible chemokines IP10, Mig, and I-TAC; chemotactic migration of effector T cells into areas of inflammation
CD184	Leukocytes; hematopoietic progenitors	CXCR4 receptor for chemokines such as stromal cell-derived factor-1 (SDF-1) (fusin); chemotaxis; HIV-1 co-receptor
CD195	Broad distribution; myeloid cells, lymphocytes, T lymphocytes, neurons, epithelium, endothelium	CCR5 receptor for chemokines such as macrophage inflammatory proteins, MIP-1a and MIP-1b, and RANTES; chemotaxis; HIV-1 co-receptor
CDw197	Lymphoid tissues, B cells, T-cell subset	CCR7 chemokine receptor; chemotaxis; T-cell homing and migration
CD201	Endothelial cells	Protein C receptor; coagulation
CD204	Myeloid cells, monocytes/macrophages	Macrophage scavenger receptor-1 (MSR1); mediates binding, internalization and processing of various negatively charged macromolecules
CD206	Dendritic cells, macrophages, myeloid cells, endothelial cells	Mannose receptor, C-type 1; binds microorganisms; phagocytosis
CD207	Dendritic cells, Langerhans' cells	Langerin; mannose receptor; phagocytosis and internalization of antigen for processing
CD208	Dendritic cells	DC-LAMP
CD209	Dendriic cells	DC-SIGN
CDw210	Broad distribution	I1-10 receptor α and β chain;

Continued

Selected CD molecules and their characteristics—cont'd

CD molecule	Predominant distribution	Identity/function
CD212	T cells, NK cells	IL-12 receptor β_1 chain;
CD213a1,a2	Lymphocytes, bronchial epithelial and smooth muscle cells	IL-13 receptor α_1 and α_2 chains
CDw217	Activated T-cell subset	IL-17; cytotoxic T-lymphocyte-associated serine esterase 8; stimulates cell activation; induces osteoclast differentiation factor (ODF)
CD220	Broad distribution	Insulin receptor; stimulates glucose uptake
CD molecule	Predominant distribution	Identity/function
CD221	Broad distribution	Insulin-like growth factor 1 receptor; cell signaling; activation, and differentiation
CD222	Broad distribution	Mannose-6-phosphate receptor; insulin-like growth factor-2 receptor
CD226	NK cells, platelets, monocytes, T-cell subset	Platelet and T-cell activation antigen 1 (PTA1); adhesion
CD233–241	Erythrocytes	Various erythrocyte membrane antigens, including blood group-associated glycoproteins
CD242	Erythrocytes	ICAM-4
CD246	T cells	TCR or CD3 ζ chain; associated with TCR and CD3; couples TCR recognition with T-cell signaling
CD247	T cells	T cells ζ chain of the TcR
CD252	Activated B cells	OX40 ligand
CD253	Activated T cells	TRAIL, death receptor
CD254	Activated T cells, LN and BM stroma	RANK ligand
CD256	Monocytes, macrophages	APRIL, binds TACI and BCMA
CD261	Activated T cells, peripheral leukocytes	TRAIL-R2, DR5, death receptor
CD262	Peripheral lymphocytes	TRAIL-R1, DR4, death receptor
CD263	Peripheral lymphocytes	TRAIL-R3, DcR1, death receptor
CD264	Peripheral lymphocytes	TRAIL-R4, DcR2, death receptor
CD265	Broad distribution	RANK
CD267	B cells, activated T cells	TACI
CD268	B cells	BAFFR, binds BLys, mature B-cell survival
CD269	Mature B cells	BCMA, binds APRIL and BAFF, B-cell survival and proliferation
CD275	B cells, dendritic cells, monocytes	ICOSL, costimulation, cytokine production
CD278	Activated T cells	ICOS, T-cell co-stimulation
CD257	Activated monocytes	BLyS, BAFF, binds TACI, BCMA, BAFFR, induces B-cell proliferation

ADCC, antibody dependent cellular cytotoxicity; ALCAM, activated leukocyte cell adhesion molecule; BCR, B cell receptor for antigen; EBV, Epstein–Barr virus; ELAM, endothelial leukocyte adhesion molecule; G-CSF, granulocyte colony-stimulating factor; GM-CSF, granulocyte macrophage colony-stimulating factor; ICAM, intercellular adhesion molecule; LAM, leukocyte adhesion molecule;
LAMP, latent membrane protein; LDL, low density lipoproteins; LECAM, lymphocyte endothelial cell adhesion molecule; LFA, lymphocyte function antigen; LPB, lipopolysaccharide binding protein;
LPS, lipopolysaccharide; M-CSF, macrophage colony-stimulating factor; MHC, major histocompatibility complex; NK cells, natural killer cells; PDGF, platelet-derived growth factor; PECAM, platelet endothelial cell adhesion molecule; PETA, platelet-endothelial cell tetraspan antigen; TCR, T-cell receptor for antigen; TNF, tumor necrosis factor; TNFR, tumor necrosis factor receptor; VCAM, vascular cellular adhesion molecule; VLA, very late antigen.
This list was adapted from the results of the Eighth International Workshop on Human Leukocyte Differentiation Antigens (HLDA8) held in Adelaide, Australia, in December 2004 (Cell Immunol 2005; 236: 1–187).

Appendix:
Laboratory reference values

2

Immunoglobulin levels (age-related reference ranges; see Chapter 96)

	Immunoglobulin levels (mg/mL)		
	IgG	IgM	IgA
Cord blood	6.36–16.06	0.06–0.25	0.01–0.03
1 month	2.51–9.06	0.20–0.87	0.01–0.53
2 months	2.06–6.01	0.17–1.05	0.02–0.46
3 months	1.76–5.81	0.24–0.89	0.04–0.46
4 months	1.96–5.58	0.27–1.01	0.04–0.73
5 months	1.72–8.14	0.33–1.09	0.08–0.68
6 months	2.15–7.04	0.35–1.02	0.08–0.68
7–9 months	2.17–9.04	0.34–1.26	0.11–0.90
10–12 months	2.94–10.69	0.41–1.49	0.16–0.84
1 year	3.45–12.13	0.43–1.73	0.14–1.06
2 years	4.24–10.51	0.48–1.68	0.14–1.23
3 years	4.41–11.35	0.47–2.00	0.22–1.59
4–5 years	4.63–12.36	0.43–1.96	0.25–1.54
6–8 years	6.33–12.80	0.48–2.07	0.33–2.02
9–10 years	6.08–15.72	0.52–2.42	0.45–2.36
Adult	6.39–13.49	0.56–3.52	0.70–3.12

Total serum IgE (IU/mL)

Age	Gender	Geometric mean	Upper 95% confidence limit
6–14 years	M	42.7	527
	F	43.3	344
15–24 years	M	33.6	447
	F	18.6	262
25–34 years	M	16.8	275
	F	16.6	216
35–44 years	M	21.7	242
	F	19.3	206
45–54 years	M	19.2	254
	F	13.3	177
55–64 years	M	21.3	354
	F	11.7	148
65–74 years	M	21.2	248
	F	11.5	122
>75 years	M	18.4	219
	F	9.2	124
6–75 years	all M	22.9	317
	all F	14.7	189

Data generated using skin-prick test-negative (i.e. house dust mite, Bermuda grass, tree mix, weed mix, mold mix) individuals (From Barbee RA, et al. J Allergy Clin Immunol 1981; 68: 106, with permission.)

Lymphocyte immunophenotype: adult reference range (95% confidence interval)

Surface antigens	Percent positive	Cells/mm^3
T cells		
CD3	57–86	650–2108
CD5	56–84	638–2099
CD2	76–93	876–2258
CD3/CD4	29–57	358–1259
CD3/CD8	13–47	194–836
CD4/CD45RO	12–34	203–976
CD4/CD45RA	2.5–25	31–533
CD8/CD45RO	3–14	34–309
CD8/CD45RA	7–28	101–636
CD3/CD8/CD28	9.5–23	155–441
CD3/CD8/CD57	≤16	≤239
CD3/HLA–DR	≤ 15.1	≤ 291
CD3/CD25	≤ 37.4	≤ 756
B cells		
CD19	3.5–15.5	49–424
CD20	3.5–17	47–409
CD20/CD5	1.5–8.5	13–145
CD20/CD23	1.6–13.2	38–360
CD20/CD27	0.7–6.3	16–118
NK cells		
CD3$^-$/CD16$^+$CD56$^+$	4.5–30	87–505
Lymphocytes	17–41	1173–2640

Data gererated in the Flow Cytometry Section, Immunology Service, DLM, CC, NIH, Bethesda, MD. The 95% confidence interval for the WBC is 4300–9200/mm^3.

Age-dependent lymphocyte immunophenotype reference range (80% confidence interval)

T cells

Age	CD3		CD4		CD8	
	Percent positive	Cells/mm³	Percent positive	Cells/mm³	Percent positive	Cells/mm³
0–3 mo	53–84	2500–5500	35–64	1600–4000	12–28	560–1700
3–6 mo	51–77	2500–5600	35–56	1800–4000	12–23	590–1600
6–12 mo	49–76	1900–5900	31–56	1400–4300	12–24	500–1700
1–2 yr	53–75	2100–6200	32–51	1300–4300	14–30	620–2000
2–6 yr	56–75	1400–3700	28–47	700–2200	16–30	490–1300
6–12 yr	60–76	1200–2600	31–47	650–1500	18–35	370–1100
12–18 yr	56–84	1000–2200	31–52	530–1300	18–35	330–920

CD4 T-cell subpopulations

Age	CD4/CD45RA		CD3/CD4/CD45RO		CD4/HLA–DR	
	Percent CD4 positive	Cells/mm³	Percent CD3/CD4 positive	Cells/mm³	Percent CD4 positive	Cells/mm³
0–3 mo	64–95	1200–3700	2–22	60–900	2–6	40–180
3–6 mo	77–94	1300–3700	3–16	120–630	2–10	60–280
6–12 mo	64–93	1100–3700	5–18	160–800	2–11	50–260
1–2 yr	63–91	1000–2900	7–20	210–850	2–11	70–280
2–6 yr	53–86	430–1500	9–26	220–660	3–12	50–180
6–12 yr	46–77	320–1000	13–30	230–630	3–13	40–120
12–18 yr	33–66	230–770	18–38	240–700	4–11	30–100

CD8 T-cell subpopulations

Age	CD8/CD45RA		CD3/CD4–/CD45RO		CD8/HLA–DR	
	Percent CD8 positive	Cells/mm³	Percent CD3/CD4- positive	Cells/mm³	Percent CD8 positive	Cells/mm³
0–3 mo	80–99	450–1500	1–9	30–330	2–20	20–160
3–6 mo	85–98	550–1400	1–7	30–290	3–17	30–170
6–12 mo	75–97	480–1500	1–8	40–330	4–27	40–290
1–2 yr	71–98	490–1700	2–12	60–570	6–33	60–600
2–6 yr	69–97	380–1100	4–16	90–440	7–37	70–420
6–12 yr	63–92	310–900	4–21	70–390	6–29	40–270
12–18 yr	61–91	240–710	4–23	60–310	5–25	30–180

Continued

Age-dependent lymphocyte immunophenotype reference range (90% confidence interval)—cont'd

	B cells and NK cells				
	CD19			CD3–/CD16–56+	
Age	Percent positive	Cells/mm^3		Percent positive	Cells/mm^3
0–3 mo	6–32	300–2000		4–18	170–1100
3–6 mo	11–41	430–3000		3–14	170–830
6–12 mo	14–37	610–2600		3–15	160–950
1–2 yr	16–35	720–2600		3–15	180–920
2–6 yr	14–33	390–1400		4–17	130–720
6–12 yr	13–27	270–860		4–17	100–480
12–18 yr	6–23	110–570		3–22	70–480

Data generated by Shearer WT, et al. J Allergy Clin Immunol 2003; 112: 973–980.

Lymphocyte proliferation – counts per minute

Mitogens

Unstimulated	252–2425
PHA 10 µg/ml	165,549–307,659
Con A 50 µg/ml	93,548–245,877
PWM 100 µg/ml	42,095–138,816

Antigens

Unstimulated	273–3808
Tetanus toxoid (0.08 LF µ/ml)	206–17,279
Candida (1:100 wt/vol)	634–26,130

Data generated by the Allergy Immunology Department, Texas Children's Hospital, Baylor College of Medicine, Houston, TX.

Appendix:
Chemokines

Chemokines

Class	Systemic name	Chemokine		Receptor(s)	Receptor(s) expressed on	Receptor class
CXC (α)	CXCL1	GRO-α, MGSA	Growth-related oncogene-α	CXCR2 / Duffy	NK, M, N, Ba / Erythrocytes	CXC / XC
	CXCL2	GRO-β	Growth-related oncogene-β	CXCR2	NK, M, N, Ba	CXC
	CXCL3	GRO-γ	Growth-related oncogene-γ	CXCR2	NK, M, N, Ba	CXC
	CXCL4	PF4	Platelet factor 4			
	CXCL5	ENA-78	Epithelial cell derived neutrophil attractant-78	CXCR1, CXCR2	NK, DC, M, N, Ba, Plt	CXC
	CXCL6	GCP-2	Granulocyte chemoattractant protein-2	CXCR1, CXCR2	NK, DC, M, N, Ba, Plt	CXC
	CXCL7	NAP-2	Neutrophil activating peptide-2	CXCR2 / Duffy	N, M, T, NK / Erythrocytes	CXC / XC
	CXCL8	IL-8	Interleukin-8	CXCR1, CXCR2 / Duffy	NK, DC, M, N, Ba, Plt / Erythrocytes	CXC / XC
	CXCL9	MIG	Monokine-induced by interferon γ	CXCR3 / CCR3 (Antag)	B, T, NK, M, Eo	CXC / CC
	CXCL10	IP-10	Interferon γ-inducible protein-10	CXCR3 / CCR3 (Antag)	B, T, NK, M, Eo	CXC
	CXCL11	I-TAC	Interferon inducible T cell α chemoattractant	CXCR3 / CCR3 (Antag)	B, T, NK, M, Eo	CXC / CC
	CXCL12	SDF-1 / PBSF	Stromal cell-derived factor 1 / Pre-B-cell growth-stimulating factor	CXCR4	SC, B, P, Thy, T, NK, NKT, DC, M, N, Ba, Eo, Plt	CXC
	CXCL13	BCA-1	B cell-attracting chemokine-1	CXCR3, CXCR5	B, T, NK, M, Eo	CXC
	CXCL14	BRAK	Chemokine isolated from breast and kidney tissue			
	CXCL16	Sexckine		CXCR6	P, T, NKT	CXC
CC (β)	CCL1	I-309	Inducible 309	CCR8	T, M	CC
	CCL2	MCP-1	Monocyte chemoattractant protein-1	CCR1, CCR2, D6 / Duffy	B, T, NKT, DC, M, N, Ba, Eo, Plt / Erythrocytes	CC / XC

Continued

Chemokines—cont'd

Class	Systemic name	Chemokine		Receptor(s)	Receptor(s) expressed on	Receptor class
	CCL3	MIP-1α	Macrophage inflammatory protein 1α	CCR1, CCR5, CCR9	B, P, Thy, T, NKT,NK,	CC
		LD78α			NKT, NK	
		MIP-1αS	Macrophage inflammatory protein 1αS		DC, M, Ba, Eo	
	CCL4	MIP-1β	Macrophage inflammatory protein 1β	CCR5, CCR8, D6	B, P, Thy, T, NKT,NK,	CC
		LD78β		CCR1 (Antag)	NKT, NK	
					DC, M, Ba, Eo	
	CCL5	RANTES	Regulated on activation of normal Tβ cells expressed & secreted	CCR1, CCR3, CCR5, D6	B, P, Thy, T,	CC
					NKT, NK	
					DC, M, Ba, Eo	
				Duffy	Erythrocytes	XC
	CCL7	MCP-3	Monocyte chemoattractant protein-3	CCR1, CCR2, CCR3, D6, CCR5 (Antag)	B, P, Thy, T, NKT, NK, DC, M, Ba, Eo	CC
	CCL8	MCP-2	Monocyte chemoattractant protein-2	CCR1, CCR2, CCR3, CCR5, D6	B, P, Thy, T, NKT,NK, NKT, NK, DC, M, Ba, Eo	CC
	CCL11	Eotaxin-1		CCR3, CCR5, D6, CCR2 (Antag)	B, P, Thy, T, NKT, NK, DC, M,	CC
				CXCR3 (Antag)	N, Ba, Eo, Plt	CXC
	CCL13	MCP-4	Monocyte chemoattractant protein-4	CCR1, CCR2, CCR3, D6	B, P, Thy, T, NKT, DC, M, N,	CC
	CCL14a	HCC-1	Hemofiltrate CC chemokine-1	CCR1, CCR5, D6	B, T, NKT, NK, DC, M, N, Ba, Eo, Plt	CC
	CCL14b	HCC-3	Hemofiltrate CC chemokine-3			
	CCL15	HCC-2	Hemofiltrate CC chemokine-2	CCR1, CCR3	B, P, Thy, T, NKT, DC, M, N, Ba, Eo, Plt	CC
		LKN-1	Leukotactin			
	CCL16	HCC-4	Hemofiltrate CC chemokine-4	CCR1, CCR2, CCR5, CCR8	B, T, NKT, NK, DC, M, N, Ba, Eo, Plt	
		LEC	Liver-expressed chemokine			
	CCL17	TARC	Thymus and activation-regulated chemokine	CCR4, CCR8	Thy, T, NKT, DC, M, Plt	CC
	CCL18	DC-CK1	Dendritic cells chemokine-1	CCR7	B, Thy, T,	CC
		PARC	Pulmonary and activation-regulated chemokine		NK, DC	
	CCL19	ELC	EBV-Induced gene 1 -ligand chemokine	CCR7	B, Thy, T,	CC
		MIP-3β	Macrophage inflammatory protein-3β	CCX-CKR	NK, DC, M	
	CCL20	LARC	Liver & activation-regulated chemokine	CCR6	B, T. NKT, DC	CC
		MIP-3α	Macrophage inflammatory protein-3α			
	CCL2l	SLC	Secondary lymphoid tissue chemokine	CXCR3	B, Thy, T,	CXC
		6Ckine		CCR7	NK, DC,	CC
				CCX-CKR	M, Eo	
	CCL22	MDC	Macrophage derived chemokine	CCR4	Thy, T, NKT, DC, Plt	CC

Continued

Chemokines—cont'd

Class	Systemic name	Chemokine		Receptor(s)	Receptor(s) expressed on	Receptor class
	CCL23	MPIF-1	Myeloid progenitor inhibitory factor-1	CCR1	B, T, NKT, DC, M, N, BA, Eo, Plt	CC
	CCL24	Eotaxin-2		CCR3	P, Thy, T, Ba, Eo, Plt	CC
	CCL25	TECK	Thymus-expressed chemokine	CCR9 CCX-CKR	P, Thy, T, DC	CC
	CCL26	Eotaxin-3		CCR3	P, Thy, T, Ba, Eo, Plt	CC
	CCL27	CTACK Eskine	Cutaneous T cell-attracting chemokine	CCR10	P, T	CC
	CCL28	MEC		CCR3, CCR10	P, Thy, T, Ba, Eo, Plt	CC
CX_3C (γ)	CX3CL1	Fractalkine		CX_3CR1	T, NK, M	CX_3C
XC (δ)	XCL1	Lymphotactin-α		XCR1	NK	XC
	XCL2	Lymphotactin-β		XCR1	NK	XC

Abbreviations for cells: B, B cells; Ba, Basophils; DC, Dendritic cells; Eo, Eosinophils;M, Macrophages/Monocytes; N, Neutrophils; NK, Natural Killer cells ; NKT, NK T cells; P, plasma cells; Plt, platelets; SC, hematopoietic stem cells; T, T cells.
Other abbreviations: Antag (Antagonist)

Appendix:
Cytokines

Cytokines

Cytokine	Abbreviation	Receptor	Receptor family	Signaling	Source
Cardiotrophin 1	CT1		Type I (hematopoietin) gp130-utilizing	Jak1, Stat3	myocardial cells
Ciliary neutrotrophic factor	CNTF	CNTFR, LIFR	Type I gp130-utilizing	Jak1, Stat3	Schwann cells, astrocytes
Colony stimulating factor 1	CSF1 (M-CSF)	FMS (CSF1R)	receptor tyrosine kinases	Ras/Raf/MAPK	macrophages, endothelium, fibroblasts, other
Colony stimulating factor 2	CSF2 (GM-CSF)	CSF2R	Type I βc utilizing	Jak2, Stat5	T cell, macrophages, endothelium, fibroblasts
Colony stimulating factor 3	CSF3 (G-CSF)	CSF3R	Type I homodimeric	Jak2, Stat3	macrophages, endothelium, fibroblasts, other
Erythropoietin	EPO	EPOR	Type I homodimeric	Jak2, Stat5	kidney, liver
FMS-related tyrosine kinase 3 ligand	FLT3 ligand	FLT3	receptor tyrosine kinases	Ras/Raf/MAPK	diverse tissues
Growth hormone	GH	GHR	Type I homodimeric	Jak2, Stat5b	two GH genes, pituitary, placental
Interferon-α/β	IFNα/β	IFNAR	Type II (interferons) heterodimeric	Jak1, Tyk2, Stat1, Stat2	macrophages, fibroblasts, other
Interferon-γ	IFNγ	IFNGR	Type II heterodimeric	Jak1, Jak2, Stat1	Th1 T cells, NK cells
Interleukin-1α/β	IL1α/β	IL1R	IL-1/TLR	IRAK, MyD88, TRAF6, NF-κB	many cells, especially macrophages
Interleukin-2	IL2	IL2R (TAC,CD25)	Type I γc-utilizing	Jak1, Jak3, Stat5	T cells
Interleukin-3	IL3	IL3R	Type I βc utilizing	Jak2, Stat5	T cells
Interleukin-4#	IL4#	IL4R	Type I γc-utilizing	Jak1, Jak3, Stat6	Th2 T cells, mast cells
Interleukin-5	IL5	IL5R	Type I βc utilizing	Jak2, Stat5	Th2 T cells
Interleukin-6	IL6	IL6R	Type I gp130-utilizing	Jak1, Stat3	macrophage, fibroblasts, endothelium, epithelium, T cells, other
Interleukin-7	IL7	IL7R	Type I γc-utilizing	Jak1, Jak3, Stat5	bone marrow, thymic stromal cells, spleen
Interleukin-9	IL9	IL9R	Type I γc-utilizing	Jak1, Jak3, Stat5	Th2 T cells
Interleukin-10	IL10	IL10R	Type II heterodimeric	Jak1, Tyk2, Stat3	Th2 T cells, other cells
Interleukin-11	IL11	IL11R	Type I gp130-utilizing	Jak1, Stat3	stromal cells
Interleukin-12	IL12	IL12R	Type I heterodimeric	Jak2, Tyk2, Stat4	macrophages, B cells
Interleukin-13	IL13	IL13R	Type I heterodimeric	Jak1, Tyk2, Stat6	activated T cells
Interleukin-15#	IL15#	IL15R	Type I γc-utilizing	Jak1, Jak3, Stat5	many cells

Target	Action	Knockout phenotype
myocardium	growth	
neuronal cells	survival	progressive atrophy and loss of motor neurons
committed myelomonocytic progenitors	differentiation, proliferation, survival	monocytopenia, osteopetrosis, female infertility
immature and committed myelo-monocytic progenitors, mature macrophages, granulocytes, DC	growth, differentiation, survival, activation	pulmonary alveolar proteinosis
committed progenitors	differentiation, activates mature granulocytes	neutropenia
erythroid precursors	erythroid differentiation	embryonic lethal, severe anemia
Myeloid cells, especially DC	proliferation, differentiation	reduced repopulating hematopoietic stem cells; reduced B cell precursors
diverse tissues	growth, adipocyte differentiation, induces IGF-1	dwarfism*
all NK cells	antiviral, antiproliferative, increased MHC class I activation	susceptibility to viral infections
macrophages, endothelium, NK cells	activation, increased MHC Class II expression, increased antigen presentation	susceptibility to bacterial infections*
CNS, endothelial cells, liver, thymocytes, macrophages	fever, anorexia, activation, acute phase reactants, costimulation, activation, cytokine secretion	
T cells, B cells, NK cells, macrophages	proliferation, cytotoxicity, IFNγ secretion, antibody production	lymphoproliferation*
immature hematopoietic progenitors of multiple lineages	growth, differentiation, survival	no defects in basal hematopoiesis
T cells, B cells, macrophages	proliferation, Th2 differentiation, IgG1 and IgE production, Inhibition of cell-mediated immunity	defective Th2 differentiation and IgE production, Decreased allergic responses
eosinophils, B cells	proliferation, activation	decreased eosinophilia, defective CD5+, B1 cell development
liver, B cells, T cells, thymocytes, myeloid cells, osteoclasts	acute phase reactants, proliferation, differentiation, costimulation	reduced Ig, esp IgA, T lymphopenia, impaired acute phase response
Thymocytes, T cells, B cells	growth, differentiation, survival	SCID*
T cells, mast cell precursors	proliferation	
macrophages	decreased MHC class II expression, decreased antigen presentation	exaggerated inflammatory response and autoimmune disease
hematopoietic stem cells	proliferation	
T cells, NK cells	Th1 differentiation, proliferation, cytotoxicity	defective Th1 differentiation, susceptibility to bacterial infections*
B cells, macrophages	costimulator of proliferation, IgE, increased CD23 and MHC class II, inhibits cytokine secretion and cell-mediated immunity	defective Th2 responses and IgE production, decreased allergic responses
T cells, especially memory cells, NK cells	proliferation, survival	absence of NK and memory cells

Continued

Cytokines—cont'd

Cytokine	Abbreviation	Receptor	Receptor family	Signaling	Source
Interleukin-17	IL17	IL17R			Th17 helper cells, cytotoxic T cells
Interleukin-17B	IL17B	IL17R			spinal cord, testis, small intestine
Interleukin-17F	IL17F, ML1				activated CD4 T cells, monocytes, other cells
Interleukin-18	IL18	IL18R	IL-1/TLR	IRAK, MyD88, TRAF6, NF-κB	
Interleukin-19	IL19		Type I γc-utilizing	Jak1, Jak3, Stat5	Th2 T cells
Interleukin-20	IL20	IL20R	Type II heterodimeric	Jak1, Tyk2, Stat3	Th2 T cells, other cells
Interleukin-21	IL21	IL21R	Type I gp130-utilizing	Jak1, Stat3	stromal cells
Interleukin-22	IL22	IL22R	Type I heterodimeric	Jak2, Tyk2, Stat4	macrophages, B cells
Interleukin-23	IL23	IL23R	Type I heterodimeric	Jak1, Tyk2, Stat6	activated T cells
Interleukin-24	IL24		Type I γc-utilizing	Jak1, Jak3, Stat5	many cells
Interleukin-25	IL-25 (IL-17E)	IL17RH1	Type I		various tissues
Interleukin-26	IL26	IL26R	Type II heterodimeric	Stat3	T cells
Interleukin-27	IL27 (IL30/EBI3)	IL27R	Type I gp130-utilizing	Jak1, Stat3	CD4 T cells, NK T cells
Interleukin-28	IL28	IL28R	Type II heterodimeric	Jak1, Stat1	
Interleukin-29	IL29	IL28R	Type II heterodimeric	Jak1, Stat1	
Interleukin-31	IL31	IL31R (GLMR)	Type I gp130-utilizing	Jak1, Stat3, Stat5	
Interleukin-32	IL32				activated T cells, NK cells
Leptin	LEP	LEPR	Type I homodimeric	Jak2, Stat3	adipoctyes
Leukemia inhibitory factor	LIF	LIFR	Type I gp130-utilizing	Jak1, Stat3	uterus, macrophage, fibroblasts, endothelium, epithelium, T cells
Lymphotoxin-α	LTA	TNFR	TNF		activated T cells and B cells
Oncostatin M*	OSM	OSMR	Type I gp130-utilizing	Jak1, Stat3	macrophage, fibroblasts, endothelium, epithelium, T cells, others
Prolactin	PRL	PRLR	Type I homodimeric	Jak2, Stat5a	two Prl genes pituitary, uterus
Stem cell factor	SCF, c-kit ligand	c-kit	receptor tyrosine kinases	Ras/Raf/MAPK	bone marrow stromal cells
Thrombopoietin	THPO	THPOR	Type I homodimeric	Jak2, Stat5	liver, kidney
Tissue necrosis factor	TNF	TNFR	TNFR	TRAFs, TRADD, FADD, Caspases, NF-kB	macrophages, T cell
Transforming growth factor β 1, 2, 3	TGFB 1, 2, 3	TGFBR	TGF-β receptor serine kinase family	SMADs, SARA, FAST-1, TAK1	T cells, macrophages, other

*Asterisks denote human disease
#note that two forms of the IL-4 and IL 15 receptor exist

Target	Action	Knockout phenotype
fibroblasts, osteoclasts	T cell activation, osteoclastogenesis	
	induces expression of TGFB, inhibits angiogenesis	
T cells, mast cell precursors	proliferation	
macrophages	decreased MHC class II expression, decreased antigen presentation	exaggerated inflammatory response and autoimmune disease
hematopoietic stem cells	proliferation	
T cells, NK cells	Th1 differentiation, proliferation, cytotoxicity	defective Th1 differentiation, susceptibility to bacterial infections*
B cells, macrophages	costimulator of proliferation, IgE, increased CD23 and MHC class II, inhibits cytokine secretion and cell-mediated immunity	defective Th2 responses and IgE production, decreased allergic responses
T cells, especially memory cells, NK cells	proliferation, survival	absence of NK and memory cells
MHC class II expressing non-T, non-B accessory cells	induction of proinflammatory cytokines	increased susceptibility to experimental autoimmune encephalomyelitis
triggers expansion of naïve CD4 T cells, promotes polarization to Th1	augments INFG secretion by CD4 T cells to help initiate Th1 differentiation	weak IFNG primary responses, susceptibility to parasitemia
	stimulates production of TNF	
hypothalamus, thyroid	satiety, controls metabolic rate	obesity
embryonic stem cells, neurons, hematopoietic cells	survival	decreased hematopoietic progenitors, defective blastocyst implantation
many cells	cytolysis, lymph node architecture, activation	aberrant lymph node structure
myeloid cells, liver, embryonic stem cells	differentiation, acute phase induction	
mammary epithelium	growth, differentiation	infertility, lactation defects
pluripotent stem cells	activation, growth	defective hematopoietic stem cell proliferation, melanocyte production and germ cell development
committed stem cells, megakaryocytes	platelet	severe thrombocytopenia
neutrophils, macrophages, endothelium, CNS, muscle, fat, many cells	adhesion, activation, adhesion, cytokines, coagulation, fever, cachexia, cytolysis	fever deregulation *
T cells, macrophages, other	inhibits growth and activation	

Index

Note: page numbers in *italics* refer to figures and tables

A

Abatacept, 1406, *1407, 1409,* 1413
Abl kinase inhibitor, 1346
ABO blood group system, 93
Abortion, recurrent spontaneous, 1276
Accommodation by organ grafts, 1219–1220
Acetaminophen in osteoarthritis, 1309, *1310*
Acetylcholine, 953–954
Acetylcholine (ACh) receptors
  autoimmune autonomic neuropathy, 990
  blockade, 955–956
  degradation acceleration, 955
  intrathymic, 957
  myasthenia gravis, 951, 952, 955–956, 1273
  structure, 952, *953*
Acid phosphatase, 662
Acquired immunity, 3–4
  atopic dermatitis, 671
  basis 5
  Cryptosporidium parvum, 435, 443–444
  Entamoeba histolytica infection, *435,* 442
  Giardia lamblia infection, *435,* 443
  helminth parasites, 452
  intracellular bacteria, 400–406
  Leishmania infection, *435,* 437–438
  mucosal surfaces, 378
  Plasmodium infection, *435,* 436–437
  protozoal infections, 433, *435*
  Toxoplasma gondii infection, *435,* 441
  Trichomonas vaginalis, 435, 444
  Trypanosoma cruzi infection, *435,* 439
Acrodermatitis
  chronica atrophica, 412
  enteropathica, 465
ActA, 400
Actin, polymerization, 400
Activated factor X, 1020

Activation-induced cell death (AICD), 135, 266
  CTL help process, 276
  Fas/FasL pathway, 272
  IL-2 signal loss, 268
Activation-induced cytidine deaminase (AID), 122–123
  hyper IgM syndrome, 520, 521
Acute disseminated encephalomyelitis (ADEM), 965
Acute hemorrhagic leukoencephalitis (AHLE), 965
Acute inflammatory demyelinating polyneuropathy (AIDP), 977
Acute interstitial pneumonia, 1058
Acute lymphoblastic leukemia (ALL), 1131–1140
  B-lineage, 1135
  chromosomal aberrations, 1133–1135
  clinical features, 1136
  course, 1140
  cure rates, 1140
  diagnosis, 1136
  diagnostic tests, 1137
  epidemiology/etiology, 1131–1132
  genetic classification, 1132–1135
  hematopoietic stem cell transplantation, 1232
  immunologic classification, 1132, *1133*
  minimal residual disease, 1138–1140
  molecular classification, 1132–1135
  molecular subtypes, 1135–1136
  oncogenic activating mutations, 1134
  prognosis, 1138, 1140
  prophylaxis, 1138
  reinduction therapy, 1138
  stem cell transplantation, 1138
  T-cell, 1132
  treatment, 1137–1138
    sequelae, 1140
Acute motor axonal neuropathy (AMAN), 977, 979–980
  Campylobacter jejuni, 980–981
Acute motor–sensory axonal neuropathy (AMSAN), 978

Acute myeloid/myelogenous leukemia (AML)
  hematopoietic stem cell transplantation, 1231
  severe congenital neutropenia, 329
Acute pandysautonomic neuropathy, 978
ADA gene, 537–538
Adalimumab, *1409,* 1411, 1413
  ankylosing spondylitis, 1413
  rheumatoid arthritis, 1413
  spondyloarthritis, 855
ADAM33, 603
Adaptive immune effectors, cancer, 1185
Adaptive immune response, 79–80
  Borrelia burgdorferi, 417
  dendritic cells in transition, 189
  protozoal infections, 433
Adaptive immunity, 39, *40*
  aging, 504–505, *507*
  APCs, 424
  chemokines, 189–191
  complement, 314–315
  giant-cell arteritis, 887
  immunological memory, 426
  TLR-mediated response, *43*
  viral infections, 423–426
Adaptor proteins, 216–219, 220–221
Addison's disease, 1048–1049
Addressins, 201
  lymphocyte homing, 291
Adeno-associated virus vectors, 1378–1379
Adenosine, release by methotrexate, 1332
Adenosine deaminase deficiency, *464,* 465, *473*
  case study, 471–472
  gene therapy, 1282, 1283–1285
  late-onset, 538
  polyethylene glycol treatment, 1284, 1285
  SCID, 537–538
Adenosine triphosphate (ATP), 1341–1342
Adenovirus vectors, 1378
Adhesion cascade, 200
Adhesion molecules, 27
  atherosclerosis, 1013, 1014
  diagnostic targets, 207
  inflammation, 199

Index